KU-069-405

VASCULAR SURGERY

VASCULAR SURGERY

FIFTH EDITION

ROBERT B. RUTHERFORD, M.D., F.A.C.S., F.R.C.S. (Glasg.)

Emeritus Professor of Surgery

University of Colorado School of Medicine

Denver, Colorado

W.B. SAUNDERS COMPANY
A Division of Harcourt Brace & Company
Philadelphia London Sydney Toronto

W.B. SAUNDERS COMPANY
A Division of Harcourt Brace & Company

The Curtis Center
Independence Square West
Philadelphia, Pennsylvania 19106

Library of Congress Cataloging-in-Publication Data

Vascular surgery [edited by] Robert B. Rutherford. —5th ed.

p. cm.

Includes bibliographical references and index.

ISBN 0-7216-8078-X (set)

1. Blood-vessels—Surgery. I. Rutherford, Robert B.

[DNLM: 1. Vascular Surgical Procedures. WG 170 V3311 2000]
RD598.5.V37 2000

617.4′13—dc21

DNLM/DLC 98-52324

ISBN 0-7216-8078-X
Vol. 1 ISBN 0-7216-8100-X
Vol. 2 ISBN 0-7216-8101-8

VASCULAR SURGERY

Printed in the United States of America.

Last digit is the print number: 9 8 7 6 5 4 3 2 1

To my wife Kay, who has sacrificed more than anyone, in lost time and patience strained, as I happily labored through all these editions.

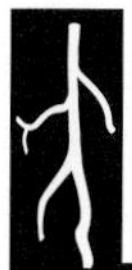

EDITORS

ASSOCIATE EDITORS

JACK L. CRONENWETT, M.D.
Professor of Surgery and Chief, Section of Vascular Surgery, Dartmouth Medical School, Hanover, New Hampshire, and Dartmouth-Hitchcock Medical Center, Lebanon, New Hampshire.

PETER GLOVICZKI, M.D.
Professor of Surgery, Mayo Medical School. Vice Chair, Division of Vascular Surgery, Mayo Clinic and Foundation. Staff Surgeon, Saint Mary's Hospital of Rochester and Rochester Methodist Hospital, Rochester, Minnesota.

K. WAYNE JOHNSTON, M.D., F.R.C.S.(C.)
Professor of Surgery and Chair, Division of Vascular Surgery, University of Toronto, Toronto, Ontario, Canada.

RICHARD F. KEMPCZINSKI, M.D.
Emeritus Professor of Surgery, University of Cincinnati College of Medicine, Cincinnati, Ohio.

WILLIAM C. KRUPSKI, M.D.
Professor of Surgery, University of Colorado School of Medicine. Chief, Vascular Surgery, University of Colorado Health Sciences Center, Denver, Colorado.

ASSISTANT EDITORS

JULIE A. FREISCHLAG, M.D.
Professor of Surgery, University of California at Los Angeles, UCLA School of Medicine. Chief of Vascular Surgery, The Gondo Vascular Center, Los Angeles, California.

KIMBERLEY J. HANSEN, M.D.
Professor of Surgery, Division of Surgical Sciences, Department of General Surgery, Wake Forest University School of Medicine. Winston-Salem, North Carolina.

KAJ H. JOHANSEN, M.D., PhD.
Professor of Surgery, University of Washington School of Medicine. Director, Surgical Education, Providence Medical Center, Seattle, Washington.

KENNETH OURIEL, M.D.
Professor of Surgery, Ohio State University College of Medicine. Chairman, Department of Vascular Surgery, Cleveland Clinic Foundation, Cleveland, Ohio.

THOMAS S. RILES, M.D.
Professor of Surgery and Director, Division of Vascular Surgery, New York University School of Medicine. Attending Physician, Tisch Hospital and Bellevue Hospital, New York, New York.

ANTON N. SIDAWY, M.D.
Professor of Surgery, George Washington University School of Medicine and Health Sciences and Georgetown University School of Medicine. Chief, Veterans Affairs Medical Center, Washington, DC.

LLOYD M. TAYLOR, JR., M.D.
Professor of Surgery, Oregon Health Sciences University School of Medicine, Portland, Oregon.

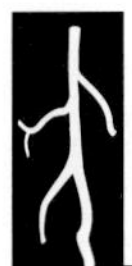

CONTRIBUTORS

ALI F. AbuRahma, M.D.
Professor, Department of Surgery, West Virginia University School of Medicine and Robert C. Byrd Health Sciences Center. Chief, Vascular Section, and Medical Director, Vascular Laboratory, Charleston Area Medical Center, Charleston, West Virginia.
Causalgia and Post-traumatic Pain Syndromes

C. ALAN ANDERSON, M.D.
Assistant Professor of Neurology and Emergency Medicine, University of Colorado School of Medicine, Denver, Colorado.
Diagnosis, Evaluation, and Medical Management of Patients with Ischemic Cerebrovascular Disease

ENRICO ASCHER, M.D.
Professor of Surgery, State University of New York Health Science Center at Brooklyn. Director, Division of Vascular Surgery, Maimonides Medical Center, Brooklyn, New York.
Secondary Arterial Reconstructions in the Lower Extremity

J. DENNIS BAKER, M.D.
Professor of Surgery, University of California, UCLA School of Medicine. Chief, Vascular Surgery Section, West Los Angeles Veterans Affairs Medical Center, Los Angeles, California.
The Vascular Laboratory

WILLIAM H. BAKER, M.D., F.A.C.S.
Professor of Surgery, Loyola University Stritch School of Medicine. Chief, Division of Vascular Surgery, Loyola University Medical Center, Maywood, Illinois.
Arteriovenous Fistulae of the Aorta and Its Major Branches

JEFFREY L. BALLARD, M.D., F.A.C.S.
Associate Professor of Surgery, Loma Linda University School of Medicine. Program Director, Vascular Surgery Residency, and Medical Director, Noninvasive Vascular Laboratory, Loma Linda University Medical Center, Loma Linda, California.
Cervicothoracic Vascular Injuries

DENNIS F. BANDYK, M.D.
Professor of Surgery and Director, Division of Vascular Surgery, University of South Florida College of Medicine, Tampa, Florida.
Infection in Prosthetic Vascular Grafts

RICHARD A. BAUM, M.D.
Assistant Professor of Radiology, University of Pennsylvania School of Medicine, Philadelphia, Pennsylvania.
Magnetic Resonance Imaging and Angiography

B. TIMOTHY BAXTER, M.D.
Professor of Surgery, University of Nebraska College of Medicine. Chief of Vascular Surgery, Omaha Veterans Affairs Hospital, Omaha, Nebraska.
Arterial Aneurysms: Etiologic Considerations

MICHAEL BELKIN, M.D.
Associate Professor of Surgery, Harvard Medical School. Program Director in General Surgery, Brigham and Women's Hospital, Boston, Massachusetts.
Infrainguinal Bypass

MARSHALL E. BENJAMIN, M.D.
Vascular Fellow, Division of Surgical Sciences, Department of General Surgery, Wake Forest University School of Medicine, Winston-Salem, North Carolina.
Techniques of Operative Management

THOMAS M. BERGAMINI, M.D.
Associate Professor of Surgery, University of Louisville School of Medicine. Chief, Section of Vascular Surgery, Veterans Administration Medical Center, Louisville, Kentucky.
Long-Term Venous Access

JOHN J. BERGAN, M.D., F.A.C.S.
Professor of Surgery, University of California, San Diego, School of Medicine, San Diego; Loma Linda University School of Medicine, Loma Linda, California; and U.S. United Health Service, Bethesda, Maryland. Attending Surgeon, Scripps Memorial Hospital, La Jolla, California.
Adventitial Cystic Disease of the Popliteal Artery; Varicose Veins: Treatment by Surgery and Sclerotherapy

RAMON BERGUER, M.D., Ph.D.
Professor of Surgery, Wayne State University School of Medicine. Chief, Section of Vascular Surgery, Harper Hospital, Detroit, Michigan.
Vertebrobasilar Ischemia: Indications, Techniques, and Results of Surgical Repair

SCOTT S. BERMAN
Associate Professor of Biomedical Engineering and Associate Professor of Clinical Surgery, University of Arizona College of Medicine. Section Head, Vascular Surgery, Carondelet St. Mary's Hospital. Medical Director, Vascular Program, Tucson Heart Hospital, Tucson, Arizona.
Patient Evaluation and Preparation for Amputation

VICTOR M. BERNHARD, M.D.
Visiting Scholar, Department of Surgery, Section of Vascular Surgery, University of Chicago, Chicago, Illinois.
Profundaplasty

MICHAEL J. BLOCH, M.D.
Instructor, Department of Medicine, Division of Hypertension, Cornell University Medical College. Assistant Attending Physician, Department of Medicine, New York Presbyterian Hospital, New York, New York.
Renal Artery Imaging: Alternatives to Angiography

FRED BONGARD, M.D.
Professor of Surgery, University of California, Los Angeles, UCLA School of Medicine, Los Angeles. Chief, Division of Trauma and Critical Care, Department of Surgery, Harbor–UCLA Medical Center, Torrance, California.
Thoracic and Abdominal Vascular Trauma

THOMAS C. BOWER, M.D.
Associate Professor of Surgery, Mayo Graduate School of Medicine. Program Director, Vascular Surgery Fellowship Program, Mayo Clinic and Mayo Foundation, Rochester, Minnesota.
Diagnosis and Management of Tumors of the Inferior Vena Cava

DAVID C. BREWSTER, M.D.
Clinical Professor of Surgery, Harvard Medical School. Attending Surgeon, Division of Vascular Surgery, Massachusetts General Hospital, Boston, Massachusetts.
Prosthetic Grafts; Direct Reconstruction for Aortoiliac Occlusive Disease

JOHN G. CALAITGES, M.D.
Clinical Instructor in Surgery, University of Missouri–Columbia School of Medicine. Vascular Resident, University of Missouri–Columbia Hospitals and Clinics, Columbia, Missouri.
Principles of Hemostasis; Antithrombotic Therapy

KEITH D. CALLIGARO, M.D.
Associate Clinical Professor of Surgery, University of Pennsylvania School of Medicine. Chief, Section of Vascular Surgery, Pennsylvania Hospital, Philadelphia, Pennsylvania.
Renal Artery Aneurysms and Arteriovenous Fistulae

RICHARD P. CAMBRIA, M.D.
Associate Professor of Surgery Harvard Medical School. Visiting Surgeon, Massachusetts General Hospital, Boston, Massachusetts.
Thoracoabdominal Aortic Aneurysms

ROBERT A. CAMBRIA, M.D., F.A.C.S.
Associate Professor of Surgery, Medical College of Wisconsin, Milwaukee, Wisconsin.
Iatrogenic Complications of Arterial and Venous Catheterizations

MICHAEL T. CAPS, M.D., M.P.H.
Assistant Professor of Surgery, University of Washington School of Medicine, Seattle, Washington.
The Epidemiology of Vascular Trauma

JEFFREY P. CARPENTER, M.D.
Associate Professor of Surgery, University of Pennsylvania School of Medicine, Philadelphia, Pennsylvania.
Magnetic Resonance Imaging and Angiography

KENNETH J. CHERRY, JR., M.D.
Professor of Surgery, Mayo Medical School. Chair, Division of Vascular Surgery, Mayo Clinic, Rochester, Minnesota.
Arteriosclerotic Occlusive Disease of Brachiocephalic Arteries

JAE-SUNG CHO, M.D.
Senior Staff Surgeon, Henry Ford Hospital, Division of Vascular Surgery, Detroit, Michigan.
Surgical Treatment of Chronic Deep Venous Obstruction

G. PATRICK CLAGETT, M.D.
Jan and Bob Pickens Professor of Medical Science; Chairman, Division of Vascular Surgery, and Director, Center for Vascular Disease, University of Texas Southwestern Medical Center at Dallas. Chief of Vascular Surgery and Attending Staff, Zale Lipshy University Hospital and Parkland Memorial Hospital. Attending Staff, Vascular General Surgery, and Consulting Member, Department of Surgery, Children's Medical Center, Dallas, Texas.
Upper Extremity Aneurysms

ELIZABETH T. CLARK, M.D.
Chief, Section of Vascular Surgery, Catholic Health Partners, Chicago, Illinois.
Anastomotic and Other Pseudoaneurysms

ALEXANDER W. CLOWES, M.D.
Professor of Surgery, University of Washington School of Medicine. Attending Surgeon, University of Washington Medical Center, Seattle, Washington.
Pathologic Intimal Hyperplasia as a Response to Vascular Injury and Reconstruction

JON R. COHEN, M.D.
Professor of Surgery, Albert Einstein College of Medicine of Yeshiva University, Bronx, New York. Chairman, Department of Surgery, and Chief of Vascular Surgery, Long Island Jewish Medical Center, New Hyde Park, New York.
Ruptured Abdominal Aortic Aneurysms

ANTHONY J. COMEROTA, M.D., F.A.C.S.
Professor of Surgery, Department of Surgery, Temple University School of Medicine. Chief of Vascular Surgery, Temple University Hospital, Philadelphia, Pennsylvania.
Clinical and Diagnostic Evaluation of Deep Venous Thrombosis

DANIEL P. CONNELLY, M.D.
Assistant Professor of Surgery, Uniformed Services University of the Health Sciences, Bethesda, Maryland. Chairman, Department of Surgery, Overland Park Regional Medical Center, Overland Park, Kansas.
The Arterial Autograft

JOHN P. COOKE, M.D., Ph.D.
Associate Professor, Division of Cardiovascular Medicine, Stanford University School of Medicine, Stanford, California.
Atherogenesis and the Medical Management of Atherosclerosis

MICHAEL A. COOPER, M.D.
Assistant Clinical Professor, University of Colorado School of Medicine. Attending Physician, Rose Medical Center, Denver, Colorado.
Neurogenic Thoracic Outlet Syndrome

ENRIQUE CRIADO, M.D., F.A.C.S.
Associate Professor of Surgery, University of North Carolina at Chapel Hill, Chapel Hill, North Carolina. Head, Vascular Surgery Unit, Fundación Hospital de Alcorców, Madrid, Spain.
Physiologic Assessment of the Venous System

JACK L. CRONENWETT, M.D.
Professor of Surgery and Chief, Section of Vascular Surgery, Dartmouth Medical School, Hanover, New Hampshire, and Dartmouth-Hitchcock Medical Center, Lebanon, New Hampshire.
Overview, Section XII; Abdominal Aortic and Iliac Aneurysms

MICHAEL D. DAKE, M.D.
Associate Professor of Radiology and Medicine (Pulmonary), Stanford University School of Medicine. Chief, Cardiovascular and Interventional Radiology, Stanford University Hospital and UC San Francisco–Stanford Health Care, Stanford, California.
Radiographic Evaluation and Treatment of Renovascular Disease; Endovascular Treatment of Chronic Occlusions of Large Veins

HERBERT DARDIK, M.D.
Clinical Professor of Surgery, Mount Sinai School of Medicine of the City University of New York. Chief of Vascular Surgery, Englewood Hospital and Medical Center, Englewood, New Jersey.
Biologic Grafts for Lower Limb Revascularization

RICHARD H. DEAN, M.D.
Interim Vice-President for Health Affairs, Wake Forest University School of Medicine, Winston-Salem, North Carolina.
Atherosclerotic Renovascular Disease: Evaluation and Management of Ischemic Nephropathy; Techniques of Operative Management

JONATHAN S. DEITCH, M.D.
Vascular Fellow, Wake Forest University School of Medicine, Winston-Salem, North Carolina.
Renal Complications

RALPH G. DePALMA, M.D., F.A.C.S.
Professor of Surgery, Vice Chair Department of Surgery, and Associate Dean, University of Nevada School of Medicine. Chief of Surgery, Veterans Affairs Medical Center, Reno, Nevada.
Vasculogenic Impotence; Superficial Thrombophlebitis: Diagnosis and Management

LARRY-STUART DEUTSCH, M.D., C.M. F.R.C.P.(C.)
Professor and Chief-of-Service, University of California, Irvine, College of Medicine, Irvine. Chief-of-Service, Vascular and Interventional Radiology, UC Irvine Medical Center, Orange, California.
Anatomy and Angiographic Diagnosis of Extracranial and Intracranial Vascular Disease

JOHN A. DORMANDY, D.Sc., F.R.C.S.
Professor of Vascular Sciences, St. Georges Hospital Medical School. Consultant Vascular Surgeon, Department of Vascular Surgery, St. George's Hospital, London, England.
Circulation-Enhancing Drugs

MATTHEW J. DOUGHERTY, M.D.
Assistant Clinical Professor of Surgery, University of Pennsylvania School of Medicine; Section of Vascular Surgery, Pennsylvania Hospital, Philadelphia, Pennsylvania.
Renal Artery Aneurysms and Arteriovenous Fistulae

JOSEPH R. DURHAM, M.D., R.V.T.
Chairman, Department of Surgery, Oak Forest Hospital of Cook County, Oak Forest, Illinois.
Lower Extremity Amputation Levels: Indications, Determining the Appropriate Level, Technique, and Prognosis

JAMES M. EDWARDS, M.D.
Associate Professor of Surgery, Oregon Health Sciences University School of Medicine, Portland, Oregon.
Upper Extremity Ischemia: Approach to Diagnosis; Occlusive and Vasospastic Diseases Involving Distal Upper Extremity Arteries—Raynaud's Syndrome

BO EKLOF, M.D., Ph.D.
Clinical Professor of Surgery, John A. Burns School of Medicine, University of Hawaii. Vascular Surgeon, Straub Clinic and Hospital, Honolulu, Hawaii.
Interventional Treatments for Iliofemoral Venous Thrombosis

ERROL E. ERLANDSON, M.D.
Clinical Associate Professor of Surgery, University of Michigan Medical School. Director, Noninvasive Vascular Laboratory, St. Joseph Mercy Hospital, Ann Arbor, Michigan.
Upper Extremity Revascularization

CALVIN B. ERNST, M.D.
Professor of Surgery, MCP Hahnemann University School of Medicine. Chief, Division of Vascular Surgery, MCP Hahnemann University Hospital, Philadelphia, Pennsylvania.
Aortoenteric Fistulae; Infected Aneurysms; Colon Ischemia Following Aortic Reconstruction

MICHAEL M. FAROOQ, M.D.
Assistant Professor of Surgery, University of California, Los Angeles, UCLA School of Medicine. Attending Vascular Surgeon, UCLA Medical Center, UCLA Olive View Medical Center, West Los Angeles Veterans Affairs Medical Center, Los Angeles.
Peritoneal Dialysis

RISHAD M. FARUQI, M.B.B.S., F.R.C.S.(Eng.), F.R.C.S.(Ed.)
Clinical Instructor of Surgery, Division of Vascular Surgery, University of California, San Francisco School of Medicine, San Francisco, California.
The Arterial Autograft

CARLOS M. FERRARIO, M.D.
Professor, Wake Forest University School of Medicine. Director, Hypertension and Vascular Disease Center, North Carolina Baptist Hospitals, Inc., Winston-Salem, North Carolina.
Pathophysiology, Functional Studies, and Medical Therapy of Renovascular Hypertension

MARK F. FILLINGER, M.D.
Assistant Professor of Surgery, Dartmouth Medical School, Hanover, New Hampshire, and Dartmouth-Hitchcock Medical Center, Lebanon, New Hampshire.
Computed Tomography and Three-Dimensional Reconstruction in Evaluation of Vascular Disease

DANIEL F. FISHER, JR., M.D., F.A.C.S.
Associate Professor, Department of Surgery, University of Tennessee, Chattanooga, College of Medicine. Chief of Surgery, Erlanger Medical Center, Chattanooga, Tennessee.
Complications of Amputation

D. PRESTON FLANIGAN, M.D.
Clinical Professor of Surgery, University of California, Irvine, College of Medicine, and UC Irvine Medical Center, Orange, California.
Postoperative Sexual Dysfunction After Aortoiliac Revascularization

RICHARD J. FOWL, M.D.
Associate Professor of Surgery, Mayo Medical School. Vascular Surgeon, Mayo Clinic, Scottsdale, Arizona.
Popliteal Artery Entrapment

JULIE A. FREISCHLAG, M.D.
Professor of Surgery, University of California at Los Angeles, UCLA School of Medicine. Chief of Vascular Surgery, The Gondo Vascular Center, Los Angeles, California.
Hemodialysis Access; Peritoneal Dialysis

GAIL L. GAMBLE, M.D.
Assistant Professor, Mayo Medical School. Co-Director, Lymphedema Center, and Consultant, Department of Physical Medicine and Rehabilitation, Mayo Clinic, Rochester, Minnesota.
Nonoperative Management of Chronic Lymphedema

HUGH A. GELABERT, M.D.
Associate Professor, Division of Vascular Surgery, University of California, UCLA School of Medicine, Los Angeles, California.
Hemodialysis Access

BRUCE L. GEWERTZ, M.D., F.A.C.S.
Dallas B. Phemister Professor and Chairman, Department of Surgery, The University of Chicago Pritzker School of Medicine, Chicago, Illinois.
Anastomotic and Other Pseudoaneurysms; Acute Occlusive Events Involving the Renal Vessels

JOSEPH M. GIORDANO, M.D.
Professor of Surgery, George Washington University School of Medicine. Chairman, Department of Surgery, George Washington University Medical Center, Washington, DC.
Embryology of the Vascular System; Takayasu's Disease: Nonspecific Aortoarteritis

SEYMOUR GLAGOV, M.D.
Professor of Pathology, Medicine, and Surgery, University of Chicago Pritzker School of Medicine, Chicago, Illinois.
Artery Wall Pathology in Atherosclerosis

BOBBY S. GLICKMAN, M.D.
Resident in General Surgery, University of Nebraska Medical Center, Omaha, Nebraska.
Arterial Aneurysms: Etiologic Considerations

PETER GLOVICZKI, M.D.
Professor of Surgery, Mayo Medical School. Vice Chair, Division Vascular Surgery, Mayo Clinic and Foundation, Rochester, Minnesota. Staff Surgeon, Saint Mary's Hospital of Rochester and Rochester Methodist Hospital, Rochester, Minnesota.
Principles of Venography; Lymphatic Complications of Vascular Surgery; Venous Disease: An Overview; Management of Perforator Vein Incompetence; Surgical Treatment of Chronic Deep Venous Obstruction; Surgical Treatment of Superior Vena Cava Syndrome; Lymphedema: An Overview; Clinical Diagnosis and Evaluation of Lymphedema; Nonoperative Management of Chronic Lymphedema; Lymphatic Reconstructions

JERRY GOLDSTONE, M.D.
Professor of Surgery, University of California, San Francisco, School of Medicine. Chief, Vascular Surgery, San Francisco General Hospital, San Francisco, California.
Aneurysms of the Extracranial Carotid Artery

MICHAEL J. V. GORDON, M.D., F.A.C.S.
Associate Professor and Director, Hand Surgery, University of Colorado School of Medicine; University Hospital, Veterans Administration Medical Center, The Children's Hospital, Denver Health Medical Center, Denver, Colorado.
Upper Extremity Amputation

FRANK A. GOTTSCHALK, M.D., F.R.C.S.Ed., F.C.S.(S.A.)Orth.
Professor, Orthopaedic Surgery, University of Texas Southwestern Medical Center at Dallas Southwestern Medical School. Orthopaedic Consultant, Zale Lipshy University Hospital, Parkland Memorial Hospital, and University of Texas Southwestern Medical Center, Dallas, Texas.
Complications of Amputation

LINDA M. GRAHAM, M.D.
Professor of Surgery, University of Michigan Medical Center. Chief of Vascular Surgery at Department of Veterans Affairs Medical Center, Ann Arbor, Michigan.
Femoral and Popliteal Aneurysms

ROY K. GREENBERG, M.D.
Instructor in Surgery, The University of Rochester School of Medicine and Dentistry, Rochester, New York.
Arterial Thromboembolism

LAZAR J. GREENFIELD, M.D.
Frederick A. Coller Distinguished Professor and Chairman, Department of Surgery, The University of Michigan Medical School. Surgeon-in-Chief, University of Michigan Hospitals, Ann Arbor, Michigan.
Caval Interruption Procedures

NAVYASH GUPTA, M.D.
Fellow, Vascular Surgery, The University of Chicago Hospitals, Chicago, Illinois.
Acute Occlusive Events Involving the Renal Vessels

JOHN W. HALLETT, JR., M.D., F.A.C.S.
Professor of Surgery, Associate Dean for Faculty Affairs, Mayo Medical School. Attending Physician, Mayo Clinic, Rochester, Minnesota.
Iatrogenic Complications of Arterial and Venous Catheterizations

SHARON L. HAMMOND, M.D.
Vascular Surgeon, Rose Medical Center, and Chairman, President Health Center, Denver, Colorado.
Neurogenic Thoracic Outlet Syndrome

KIMBERLEY J. HANSEN, M.D.
Professor of Surgery, Division of Surgical Sciences, Department of General Surgery, Wake Forest University School of Medicine.
Renal Complications; Renovascular Disease: An Overview; Atherosclerotic Renovascular Disease: Evaluation and Management of Ischemic Nephropathy; Techniques of Operative Management

JOHN P. HARRIS, M.S., F.R.A.C.S., F.R.C.S., F.A.C.S., D.D.U.
Professor of Vascular Surgery, University of Sydney. Chairman, Division of Surgery, Royal Prince Alfred Hospital, Sydney, Australia.
Upper Extremity Sympathectomy

DOMINIC F. HEFFEL, M.D.
Resident, Division of General Surgery, University of California, Los Angeles, UCLA School of Medicine, Los Angeles, California.
Excisional Operations for Chronic Lymphedema

W. SCOTT HELTON, M.D.
Professor of Surgery, University of Illinois College of Medicine, Chicago, Illinois.
Operative Therapy for Portal Hypertension

NORMAN R. HERTZER, M.D.
Staff Vascular Surgeon, Department of Vascular Surgery, The Cleveland Clinic Foundation, Cleveland, Ohio.
Postoperative Management and Complications Following Carotid Endarterectomy

WILLIAM R. HIATT, M.D.
Professor of Medicine, University of Colorado School of Medicine and University of Colorado Health Sciences Center. Executive Director, Colorado Prevention Center, Denver, Colorado.
Atherogenesis and the Medical Management of Atherosclerosis

JOHN R. HOCH, M.D.
Assistant Professor of Surgery, University of Wisconsin Medical School. Chief, Section of Vascular Surgery, William S. Middleton Veteran Affairs Medical Center, Madison, Wisconsin.
Long-Term Venous Access

KIM J. HODGSON, M.D.
Professor and Chief of Peripheral Vascular Surgery, Southern Illinois University School of Medicine. Attending Surgeon, Memorial Medical Center and St. John's Hospital, Springfield, Illinois.
Principles of Arteriography; Fundamental Techniques in Endovascular Surgery

GARY S. HOFFMAN, M.D.
Chairman, Department of Rheumatic and Immunologic Diseases, Cleveland Clinic Foundation, Cleveland, Ohio.
Takayasu's Disease: Nonspecific Aortoarteritis

DOUGLAS B. HOOD, M.D.
Assistant Professor of Surgery, University of Southern California School of Medicine; USC University Hospital, Los Angeles, California.
Vascular Injuries of the Extremities

RICHARD L. HUGHES, M.D.
Associate Professor of Neurology, University of Colorado School of Medicine. Chief, Neurology, Denver Health Medical Center, Denver, Colorado.
Diagnosis, Evaluation, and Medical Management of Patients with Ischemic Cerebrovascular Disease

RUSSELL D. HULL, M.B.B.S., M.Sc.
Professor of Medicine, University of Calgary Faculty of Medicine. Foothills Hospital, Calgary, Alberta, Canada.
Prevention and Medical Treatment of Acute Deep Venous Thrombosis

SCOTT N. HURLBERT, M.D.
Clinical Vascular Fellow, Southern Illinois University School of Medicine, Springfield, Illinois.
Subclavian-Axillary Vein Thrombosis

KARL A. ILLIG, M.D.
Assistant Professor of Surgery, University of Rochester School of Medicine and Dentistry. Associate Attending Physician, Strong Memorial Hospital and Rochester General Hospital, Rochester, New York.
Perioperative Hemorrhage

GLENN R. JACOBOWITZ, M.D.
Assistant Professor of Clinical Surgery, Division of Vascular Surgery, New York University School of Medicine, New York, New York.
Peripheral Arteriovenous Fistulae

DENNIS M. JENSEN, M.D.
Professor of Medicine, University of California, Los Angeles, UCLA School of Medicine. Staff Physician, Division of Digestive Diseases, UCLA Center for the Health Sciences, West Los Angeles Veterans Affairs Medical Center, and CURE: Digestive Disease Research Center, Los Angeles, California.
Initial Management of Upper Gastrointestinal Hemorrhage in Patients with Portal Hypertension

KAJ H. JOHANSEN, M.D., Ph.D.
Professor of Surgery, University of Washington School of Medicine. Director, Surgical Education, Providence Medical Center, Seattle, Washington.
Compartment Syndrome: Pathophysiology, Recognition, and Management; Portal Hypertension: An Overview; Operative Therapy for Portal Hypertension

GEORGE JOHNSON, JR., M.D.
Emeritus Professor of Surgery, University of North Carolina at Chapel Hill, Chapel Hill, North Carolina.
Superficial Thrombophlebitis: Diagnosis and Management

K. WAYNE JOHNSTON, M.D., F.R.C.S.(C.)
Professor of Surgery and Chair, Division of Vascular Surgery, University of Toronto Faculty of Medicine, Toronto, Ontario, Canada.
Overview, Section VII; Ischemic Neuropathy; Upper Extremity Ischemia: Overview

DARRELL N. JONES, Ph.D.
Research Associate in Vascular Surgery, University of Colorado Health Sciences Center. Associate Director, Vascular Diagnostic Laboratory, University Hospital, Denver, Colorado.
Integrated Assessment of Results: Standardized Reporting of Outcomes and the Computerized Vascular Registry

JOHN W. JOYCE, M.D.
Professor of Medicine, Emeritus, Mayo Medical School, Rochester, Minnesota.
Uncommon Arteriopathies

VIKRAM S. KASHYAP, M.D.
Fellow in Vascular Surgery, University of California, Los Angeles, UCLA School of Medicine, Los Angeles, California.
Principles of Thrombolytic Therapy

JEFFREY L. KAUFMAN, M.D.
Associate Professor of Surgery, Tufts University School of Medicine. Vascular Surgeon, Department of Surgery, Baystate Medical Center, Springfield, Massachusetts.
Atheroembolism and Microthromboembolic Syndromes (Blue Toe Syndrome and Disseminated Atheroembolism)

ANDRIS KAZMERS, M.D., M.S.P.H.
Associate Professor of Surgery, Wayne State University School of Medicine. Medical Director, Vascular Surgery Laboratory, Harper Hospital, Detroit, Michigan.
Intestinal Ischemia Caused by Venous Thrombosis

RICHARD F. KEMPCZINSKI, M.D.
Emeritus Professor of Surgery, University of Cincinnati College of Medicine, Cincinnati, Ohio.
Vascular Conduits: An Overview; The Chronically Ischemic Leg: An Overview; Popliteal Artery Entrapment; Vasculogenic Impotence

K. CRAIG KENT, M.D.
Professor, Department of Surgery, Division of Vascular Surgery, Cornell University Medical College. Attending Physician, Department of Surgery, New York Presbyterian Hospital, New York, New York.
Renal Artery Imaging: Alternatives to Angiography

ROBERT K. KERLAN, JR., M.D.
Clinical Professor of Radiology, University of California, San Francisco, School of Medicine. Interventional Radiologist, Chief, Interventional Radiology, Mount Zion Medical Center of UC–San Francisco, San Francisco, California.
Percutaneous Interventions in Portal Hypertension

LAWRENCE L. KETCH, M.D., F.A.C.S., F.A.A.P.
Associate Professor and Chief, Plastic and Reconstructive Surgery, University of Colorado School of Medicine. Chief, Pediatric Plastic Surgery, The Children's Hospital, Denver, Colorado.
Upper Extremity Amputation

EDOUARD KIEFFER, M.D.
Professor of Vascular Surgery, Pitre-Salpetriere University. Chief, Department of Vascular Surgery, Pitre-Salpetriere University Hospital, Paris, France.
Arterial Complications of Thoracic Outlet Compression; Dissection of the Descending Thoracic Aorta

ROBERT L. KISTNER, M.D.
Clinical Professor of Surgery, University of Hawaii, John A. Burns School of Medicine. Department of Vascular Surgery, Straub Clinic and Hospital, Honolulu, Hawaii.
A Practical Approach to the Diagnosis and Classification of Chronic Venous Disease

STEVEN J. KNIGHT, R.V.T.
Instructor in Surgery, University of Vermont College of Medicine. Technical Director, Vascular Diagnostic Laboratory, Fletcher Allen Health Care, Inc., Burlington, Vermont.
The Role of Noninvasive Studies in the Diagnosis and Management of Cerebrovascular Disease

THOMAS O. G. KOVACS, M.D.
Associate Professor of Medicine, Division of Digestive Diseases, University of California, Los Angeles, UCLA School of Medicine. Director, Cure Clinical Trials Unit, West Los Angeles Veterans Affairs Medical Center, Los Angeles, California.
Initial Management of Upper Gastrointestinal Hemorrhage in Patients with Portal Hypertension

WILLIAM C. KRUPSKI, M.D.
Professor of Surgery, University of Colorado School of Medicine. Chief, Vascular Surgery, University of Colorado Health Sciences Center, Denver, Colorado.
Cardiac Complications and Screening; Thromboendarterectomy for Lower Extremity Arterial Occlusive Disease; Overview, Section XII; Abdominal Aortic and Iliac Aneurysms; Indications, Surgical Technique, and Results for Repair of Extracranial Occlusive Lesions; Uncommon Disorders Affecting the Carotid Arteries; Overview of Extremity Amputations, Section XXI

JEANNE M. LaBERGE, M.D.
Associate Professor of Radiology, University of California, San Francisco, School of Medicine. Interventional Radiologist, The Medical Center at UC San Francisco, San Francisco, California.
Percutaneous Interventions in Portal Hypertension

LEWIS J. LEVIEN, M.B., B.Ch., Ph.D., F.C.S.(S.A.)
Honorary Lecturer, Department of Surgery, University of the Witwatersrand. Vascular Surgeon, Milpark Hospital, Johannesburg, South Africa.
Advential Cystic Disease of the Popliteal Artery

PAVEL J. LEVY, M.D.
Assistant Professor, Wake Forest University School of Medicine. Attending Physician, North Carolina Baptist Hospitals, Inc., Winston-Salem, North Carolina.
Pathophysiology, Functional Studies, and Medical Therapy of Renovascular Hypertension

ROBERT P. LIDDELL, M.S.
Royal College of Surgeons and Beaumont Hospital, Dublin, Ireland.
Endovascular Treatment of Chronic Occlusions of Large Veins

ROBERT C. LOWELL, M.D., F.A.C.S., R.V.T.
Vascular Surgeon, The Longstreet Clinic, Gainesville, Georgia.
Lymphatic Complications of Vascular Surgery

JAMES M. MALONE, M.D., F.A.C.S.
Clinical Professor of Surgery, University of Arizona College of Medicine, Tucson, Arizona, and Mayo Graduate School of Medicine, Rochester, Minnesota.
Revascularization Versus Amputation

M. ASHRAF MANSOUR, M.D., F.A.C.S.
Assistant Professor of Surgery, Loyola University Stritch School of Medicine. Attending Vascular Surgeon, Director of Residency Training and Education, Loyola University Medical Center, Maywood, Illinois.
Arteriovenous Fistulae of the Aorta and Its Major Branches

ELNA M. MASUDA, M.D.
Assistant Professor of Surgery, University of Hawaii John A. Burns School of Medicine. Vascular Surgeon and Director of Vascular Laboratory, Straub Clinic and Hospital, Honolulu, Hawaii.
A Practical Approach to the Diagnosis and Classification of Chronic Venous Disease

JAMES MAY, M.D., M.S., F.R.A.C.S., F.A.C.S.
Bosch Professor of Surgery, University of Sydney. Vascular Surgeon, Royal Prince Alfred Hospital, Sydney, Australia.
Endovascular Grafts; Upper Extremity Sympathectomy; Endovascular Treatment of Aortic Aneurysms

KENNETH E. McINTYRE, JR., M.D.
Professor of Surgery, Division of Vascular Surgery, University of Texas Southwestern Medical Center at Dallas Southwestern Medical School. Chief, Vascular Surgery, St. Paul Medical Center, Dallas, Texas.
Patient Evaluation and Preparation for Amputation

W. BURLEY McINTYRE, M.D.
Vascular Surgeon, Everett Clinic, Everett, Washington.
Cervicothoracic Vascular Injuries

MICHAEL A. McKUSICK, M.D.
Assistant Professor of Radiology, Mayo Graduate School of Medicine. Vascular and Interventional Radiologist, Mayo Clinic, Rochester, Minnesota.
Principles of Venography

ROBERT H. MEIER, III, M.D.
Director, Amputee Services of Colorado, Sunspectrum Outpatient Rehabilitation, Thornton, Colorado.
Rehabilitation of the Person with an Amputation

MARK H. MEISSNER, M.D.
Assistant Professor, Department of Surgery, University of Washington School of Medicine; Department of Vascular Surgery, Harborview Medical Center, Seattle, Washington.
Venous Duplex Scanning; Pathophysiology and Natural History of Acute Deep Venous Thrombosis

LOUIS M. MESSINA, M.D.
Professor of Surgery and Chief, Division of Vascular Surgery, University of California, San Francisco, School of Medicine. Attending Surgeon, UC San Francisco–Stanford Hospital, San Francisco, California.
Endarterectomy; Renal Artery Fibrodysplasia and Renovascular Hypertension

MARK MEWISSEN, M.D.
Clinical Associate Professor of Radiology, Medical College of Wisconsin. Interventional Radiologist, Wisconsin Heart and Vascular Clinics, Milwaukee, Wisconsin.
Interventional Treatments for Iliofemoral Venous Thrombosis

TIMOTHY A. MILLER, M.D., F.A.C.S.
Professor of Plastic and Reconstructive Surgery, University of California, Los Angeles, UCLA School of Medicine. Chief, Plastic and Reconstructive Surgery, West Los Angeles Veterans Administration Hospital, Los Angeles, California.
Excisional Operations for Chronic Lymphedema

MARC E. MITCHELL, M.D.
Assistant Professor of Surgery, Division of Vascular Surgery, University of Pennsylvania School of Medicine, Philadelphia, Pennsylvania.
Basic Considerations of the Arterial Wall in Health and Disease

GREGORY L. MONETA, M.D.
Professor of Surgery, Oregon Health Sciences University School of Medicine, Staff Surgeon, Veterans Affairs Medical Center, Portland, Oregon.
Natural History and Nonoperative Treatment of Chronic Lower Extremity Ischemia; Diagnosis of Intestinal Ischemia; Treatment of Acute Intestinal Ischemia Caused by Arterial Occlusions; Treatment of Chronic Visceral Ischemia; Pathophysiology of Chronic Venous Insufficiency; Nonoperative Treatment of Chronic Venous Insufficiency

WESLEY S. MOORE, M.D.
Professor of Surgery, University of California, Los Angeles, UCLA School of Medicine. Vascular Surgeon, UCLA Center for the Health Sciences, Los Angeles, California.
Fundamental Considerations in Cerebrovascular Disease; Indications, Surgical Technique, and Results for Repair of Extracranial Occlusive Lesions

MARK R. NEHLER, M.D.
Assistant Professor of Surgery, University of Colorado School of Medicine and University of Colorado Health Sciences Center, Denver, Colorado.
Cardiac Complications and Screening; Pathophysiology of Chronic Venous Insufficiency

AUDRA A. NOEL, M.D.
Division of Vascular Surgery, Mayo Clinic and Foundation, Rochester, Minnesota.
Lymphatic Reconstructions

SEAN P. O'BRIEN, M.D.
Vascular Surgery Fellow, MCP Hahnemann University Hospitals, Philadelphia, Pennsylvania.
Aortoenteric Fistulae

JEFFREY W. OLIN, D.O.
Chairman, Department of Vascular Medicine, Cleveland Clinic Foundation, Cleveland, Ohio.
Thromboangiitis Obliterans (Buerger's Disease)

KENNETH OURIEL, M.D.
Professor of Surgery, Ohio State University College of Medicine, Columbus. Chairman, Department of Vascular Surgery, The Cleveland Clinic Foundation, Cleveland, Ohio.
Perioperative Hemorrhage; Acute Limb Ischemia; Arterial Thromboembolism

MARC A. PASSMAN, M.D.
Fellow, Division of Vascular Surgery, Department of Surgery, University of North Carolina at Chapel Hill School of Medicine, Chapel Hill, North Carolina.
Physiologic Assessment of the Venous System

GRAHAM F. PINEO, M.D.
Professor of Medicine, University of Calgary Faculty of Medicine; Foothills Hospital, Calgary, Alberta, Canada.
Prevention and Medical Treatment of Acute Deep Venous Thrombosis

JOHN M. PORTER, M.D.
Professor of Surgery (Head), Oregon Health Sciences University School of Medicine, Portland, Oregon.
Natural History and Nonoperative Treatment of Chronic Lower Extremity Ischemia; Upper Extremity Ischemia: Approach to Diagnosis; Occlusive and Vasospastic Diseases Involving Distal Upper Extremity Arteries—Raynaud's Syndrome; Treatment of Acute Intestinal Ischemia Caused by Arterial Occlusions; Treatment of Chronic Visceral Ischemia; Pathophysiology of Chronic Venous Insufficiency; Nonoperative Treatment of Chronic Venous Insufficiency

WILLIAM J. QUIÑONES-BALDRICH, M.D.
Professor of Surgery, University of California, Los Angeles, UCLA School of Medicine. Vascular Surgeon, UCLA Center for the Health Sciences, Los Angeles, California.
Principles of Thrombolytic Therapy; Indications, Surgical Technique, and Results for Repair of Extracranial Occlusive Lesions

RICARDO T. QUINTOS II, M.D.
Clinical Research Fellow, Montefiore Medical Center, New York, New York.
Techniques for Thromboembolectomy of Native Arteries and Bypass Grafts; Secondary Arterial Reconstructions in the Lower Extremity

SESHADRI RAJU, M.D.
Emeritus Professor of Surgery, University of Mississippi School of Medicine. Honorary Surgeon, University Hospital, Jackson, Mississippi.
Surgical Treatment of Deep Venous Valvular Incompetence

DANIEL J. REDDY, M.D.
Head, Division of Vascular Surgery, Program Director, Vascular Fellowship, Henry Ford Hospital, Detroit, Michigan.
Infected Aneurysms

JASON P. REHM, M.D.
Resident in General Surgery, University of Nebraska Medical Center, Omaha, Nebraska.
Arterial Aneurysms: Etiologic Considerations

JEFFREY M. RHODES, M.D.
Clinical Fellow, Division of Vascular Surgery, Mayo Clinic, Rochester, Minnesota.
Management of Perforator Vein Incompetence

MICHAEL A. RICCI, M.D.
Associate Professor of Surgery, University of Vermont College of Medicine. Director, Vascular Diagnostic Laboratory, Fletcher Allen Health Care, Inc., Burlington, Vermont.
The Role of Noninvasive Studies in the Diagnosis and Management of Cerebrovascular Disease

LAYTON F. RIKKERS, M.D.
A.R. Curreri Professor and Chairman, University of Wisconsin Medical School, Madison, Wisconsin.
Operative Therapy for Portal Hypertension

THOMAS S. RILES, M.D.
Professor of Surgery and Director, Division of Vascular Surgery, New York University School of Medicine. Attending Physician, Tisch Hospital and Bellevue Hospital, New York, New York.
Overview, Section XIII; Peripheral Arteriovenous Fistulae; Congenital Vascular Malformations

STEVEN P. RIVERS, M.D.
Associate Professor of Surgery, Albert Einstein College of Medicine of Yeshiva University, Bronx, New York. Division of Vascular Surgery, Montefiore Medical Center, New York, New York.
Nonocclusive Mesenteric Ischemia

THOM W. ROOKE, M.D.
Associate Professor, Mayo Graduate School of Medicine. Head, Section of Vascular Medicine, Mayo Clinic, Rochester, Minnesota.
Uncommon Arteriopathies; Nonoperative Management of Chronic Lymphedema

ROBERT J. ROSEN, M.D.
Associate Professor of Radiology, New York University School of Medicine. Director of Vascular and Interventional Radiology, New York University Medical Center, New York, New York.
Peripheral Arteriovenous Fistulae; Congenital Vascular Malformations

CARLO RUOTOLO, M.D.
Assistant Professor of Surgery, Pitre-Salpetriere University. Staff Surgeon, Department of Vascular Surgery, Pitre-Salpetriere Hospital, Paris, France.
Arterial Complications of Thoracic Outlet Compression

ROBERT B. RUTHERFORD, M.D., F.A.C.S., F.R.C.S.(Glasg.)
Emeritus Professor of Surgery, University of Colorado School of Medicine, Denver, Colorado.
Initial Patient Evaluation: The Vascular Consultation; Evaluation and Selection of Patients for Vascular Interventions; Integrated Assessment of Results: Standardized Reporting of Outcomes and the Computerized Vascular Registry; Basic Vascular Surgical Techniques; Causalgia and Post-traumatic Pain Syndromes; Extra-anatomic Bypass; Endovascular Interventions in the Management of Chronic Lower Extremity Ischemia; Lumbar Sympathectomy: Indications and Technique; Subclavian-Axillary Vein Thrombosis; Abdominal Aortic and Iliac Aneurysms; Diagnostic Evaluation of Arteriovenous Fistulae; Extracranial Fibromuscular Arterial Dysplasia; Interventional Treatments for Iliofemoral Venous Thrombosis

DAVID SACKS, M.D.
Head, Interventional Radiology, The Reading Hospital and Medical Center, West Reading, Pennsylvania.
Angiography and Percutaneous Vascular Interventions: Complications and Quality Improvement

LUIS A. SANCHEZ, M.D.
Associate Professor of Surgery, Albert Einstein College of Medicine of Yeshiva University, Bronx, New York. Chief of Vascular Surgery, Jack D. Weiler Hospital, New York, New York.
Secondary Arterial Reconstructions in the Lower Extremity

RICHARD J. SANDERS, M.D.
Clinical Professor of Surgery, University of Colorado School of Medicine and Health Sciences Center. Attending Surgeon, Rose Medical Center, Denver, Colorado.
Neurogenic Thoracic Outlet Syndrome

ALVIN H. SCHMAIER, M.D.
Professor, Hematology and Oncology Division, Department of Internal Medicine and Pathology, University of Michigan Medical School. Director, Coagulation Laboratory, University of Michigan Medical Center, Ann Arbor, Michigan.
Vascular Thrombosis Due to Hypercoagulable States

PETER A. SCHNEIDER, M.D.
Clinical Assistant Professor of Surgery, University of Hawaii John A. Burns School of Medicine. Vascular and Endovascular Surgeon, Hawaii Permanente Medical Group, Honolulu, Hawaii.
Endovascular Interventions in the Management of Chronic Lower Extremity Ischemia; Extracranial Fibromuscular Arterial Dysplasia

LEWIS B. SCHWARTZ, M.D.
Assistant Professor of Surgery, University of Chicago Pritzker School of Medicine, Chicago, Illinois.
Anastomotic and Other Pseudoaneurysms

GARY R. SEABROOK, M.D.
Associate Professor, Division of Vascular Surgery, Medical College of Wisconsin, Milwaukee, Wisconsin.
Management of Foot Lesions in the Diabetic Patient

CHARLES J. SHANLEY, M.D.
Assistant Professor of Surgery, University of Michigan Medical School, Ann Arbor, Michigan.
Pulmonary Complications in Vascular Surgery

CYNTHIA K. SHORTELL, M.D.
Assistant Professor of Surgery, University of Rochester School of Medicine and Dentistry. Attending Surgeon, Strong Memorial Hospital and Rochester General Hospital, Rochester, New York.
Perioperative Hemorrhage

ANTON N. SIDAWY, M.D.
Professor of Surgery, George Washington University School of Medicine and Health Sciences and Georgetown University School of Medicine. Chief, Surgical Services, Veterans Affairs Medical Center, Washington, DC.
Basic Considerations of the Arterial Wall in Health and Disease

DONALD SILVER, M.D.
Emeritus Professor of Surgery, University of Missouri–Columbia School of Medicine, Columbia, Missouri.
Principles of Hemostasis; Antithrombotic Therapy; Diagnosis of Intestinal Ischemia

SUZANNE M. SLONIM, M.D.
Assistant Professor of Radiology, Stanford University School of Medicine, Stanford, California. Chief, Cardiovascular and Interventional Radiology, Palo Alto Veterans Administration Medical Center, Palo Alto, California.
Radiographic Evaluation and Treatment of Renovascular Disease

RICHARD K. SPENCE, M.D., F.A.C.S.
Director of Surgical Education, Baptist Health System, Birmingham, Alabama.
Blood Loss and Transfusion in Vascular Surgery

JAMES C. STANLEY, M.D.
Professor of Surgery, University of Michigan Medical School. Head, Section of Vascular Surgery, University Hospital, Ann Arbor, Michigan.
Splanchnic Artery Aneurysms; Arterial Fibrodysplasia; Renal Artery Fibrodysplasia and Renovascular Hypertension

ANTHONY STANSON, M.D.
Associate Professor of Radiology, Mayo Medical School. Consultant, Department of Diagnostic Radiology, Mayo Clinic and Mayo Foundation, Rochester, Minnesota.
Diagnosis and Management of Tumors of the Inferior Vena Cava

RONALD J. STONEY, M.D.
Professor of Surgery, Division of Vascular Surgery, University of California, San Francisco, School of Medicine, San Francisco, California.
Endarterectomy; The Arterial Autograft

D. EUGENE STRANDNESS, JR., M.D.
Professor, Department of Surgery, University of Washington School of Medicine, Seattle, Washington.
Pathophysiology and Natural History of Acute Deep Venous Thrombosis

DAVID S. SUMNER, M.D.
Distinguished Professor of Surgery Emeritus, Southern Illinois University School of Medicine, Springfield, Illinois.
Essential Hemodynamic Principles; Physiologic Assessment of Peripheral Arterial Occlusive Disease; Evaluation of Acute and Chronic Ischemia of the Upper Extremity; Hemodynamics and Pathophysiology of Arteriovenous Fistulae; Diagnostic Evaluation of Arteriovenous Fistulae

GENE Y. SUNG, M.D.
Assistant Professor, Neurology, University of Colorado School of Medicine. Director, Neurocritical Care and Stroke, University of Colorado Health Sciences Center, Denver, Colorado.
Diagnosis, Evaluation, and Medical Management of Patients with Ischemic Cerebrovascular Disease

SCOTT W. TABER, M.D.
Assistant Professor of Surgery, University of Louisville School of Medicine, Department of Surgery, Louisville, Kentucky.
Long-Term Venous Access

LLOYD M. TAYLOR, JR., M.D.
Professor of Surgery, Oregon Health Sciences University School of Medicine, Portland, Oregon.
Natural History and Nonoperative Treatment of Chronic Lower Extremity Ischemia; Upper Extremity Ischemia: Approach to Diagnosis; Treatment of Acute Intestinal Ischemia Caused by Arterial Occlusions; Treatment of Chronic Visceral Ischemia

JONATHAN B. TOWNE, M.D.
Professor and Chairman, Division of Vascular Surgery, Medical College of Wisconsin, Milwaukee, Wisconsin.
The Autogenous Vein; Profundaplasty; Management of Foot Lesions in the Diabetic Patient

J. JEAN E. TURLEY, M.D., F.R.C.S.(P.)
Associate Professor, Department of Medicine, University of Toronto Faculty of Medicine. Attending Physician, St. Michael's Hospital, Toronto, Ontario, Canada.
Ischemic Neuropathy

WILLIAM W. TURNER, JR., M.D.
James D. Hardy Professor and Chairman, Department of Surgery, The University of Mississippi School of Medicine, Jackson, Mississippi.
Acute Vascular Insufficiency Due to Drug Injection

R. JAMES VALENTINE, M.D.
Associate Professor, University of Texas Southwestern Medical Center at Dallas Southwestern Medical School. Attending Surgeon, Parkland Memorial Hospital, Zale Lipshy University Hospital, Veterans Affairs Medical Center, Dallas, Texas.
Anatomy of Commonly Exposed Arteries; Acute Vascular Insufficiency Due to Drug Injection

FRANK J. VEITH, M.D.
Professor of Surgery, Albert Einstein College of Medicine of Yeshiva University, Bronx, New York. Chief, Vascular Surgical Services, Montefiore Medical Center, New York, New York.
Techniques for Thromboembolectomy of Native Arteries and Bypass Grafts; Secondary Arterial Reconstructions in the Lower Extremity; Nonocclusive Mesenteric Ischemia

OMAIDA C. VELÁZQUEZ, M.D.
Instructor in Surgery, University of Pennsylvania School of Medicine, Philadelphia, Pennsylvania.
Magnetic Resonance Imaging and Angiography

TERRI J. VRTISKA, M.D.
Department of Diagnostic Radiology, Mayo Clinic and Foundation, Rochester, Minnesota.
Surgical Treatment of Superior Vena Cava Syndrome

HEINZ W. WAHNER, M.D., F.A.C.P.
Professor Emeritus of Radiology, Mayo Clinic, Rochester, Minnesota.
Clinical Diagnosis and Evaluation of Lymphedema

THOMAS W. WAKEFIELD, M.D.
Professor, Section of Vascular Surgery Department of Surgery, University of Michigan Medical School. Director, Noninvasive Diagnostic Vascular Unit, University of Michigan Medical Center. Staff Surgeon, Ann Arbor Veterans Administration Medical Center, Ann Arbor, Michigan.
Arterial Fibrodysplasia; Vascular Thrombosis Due to Hypercoagulable States

DANIEL B. WALSH, M.D.
Professor of Surgery, Dartmouth Medical School, Hanover, New Hampshire. Vice Chair, Department of Surgery, Dartmouth-Hitchcock Medical Center, Lebanon, New Hampshire.
Technical Adequacy and Graft Thrombosis

JAMES C. WATSON, JR., M.S., M.D.
Clinical Instructor, University of Washington School of Medicine; Advanced Surgical Associates, PLLC; Northwest Hospital and Providence Medical Center, Seattle, Washington.
Compartment Syndrome: Pathophysiology, Recognition, and Management

FRED A. WEAVER, M.D., F.A.C.S.
Associate Professor of Surgery, University of Southern California School of Medicine. Chief, Division of Vascular Surgery, USC University Hospital, Los Angeles, California.
Vascular Injuries of the Extremities

ERIC S. WEINSTEIN, M.D.
Assistant Clinical Professor, University of Colorado School of Medicine, Denver. Attending Physician, Swedish Medical Center, Englewood, Colorado; and Rose Medical Center and Porter Medical Center, Denver, Colorado.
Thromboendoarterectomy for Lower Extremity Arterial Occlusive Disease; Neurogenic Thoracic Outlet Syndrome

KURT WENGERTER, M.D.
Director of the Vascular Laboratory, Englewood Hospital and Medical Center, Englewood, New Jersey.
Biologic Grafts for Lower Limb Revascularization

GEOFFREY H. WHITE, M.D., F.R.A.C.S.
Clinical Associate Professor, University of Sydney. Vascular Surgeon, Department of Vascular Surgery, Royal Prince Alfred Hospital, Sydney, Australia.
Endovascular Grafts; Endovascular Treatment of Aortic Aneurysms

JOHN V. WHITE, M.D.
Chairman, Department of Surgery, Lutheran General Hospital, Park Ridge, Illinois.
Integrated Assessment of Results: Standardized Reporting of Outcomes and the Computerized Vascular Registry

THOMAS A. WHITEHILL, M.D.
Associate Professor of Surgery, University of Colorado School of Medicine. Chief of Vascular Surgery, Veterans Administration Medical Center, Denver, Colorado.
Uncommon Disorders Affecting the Carotid Arteries

WALTER M. WHITEHOUSE, JR., M.D.
Clinical Associate Professor of Surgery, University of Michigan Medical School. Chairman, Department of Surgery, St. Joseph Mercy Hospital, Ann Arbor, Michigan.
Upper Extremity Revascularization

ANTHONY D. WHITTEMORE, M.D.
Professor of Surgery, Harvard Medical School. Chief of Vascular Surgery, Brigham and Women's Hospital, Boston, Massachusetts.
Infrainguinal Bypass

KENT WILLIAMSON, M.D.
Surgery Resident, Oregon Health Sciences University School of Medicine, Portland, Oregon.
Upper Extremity Ischemia: Approach to Diagnosis

GARY G. WIND, M.D.
Professor of Surgery, Uniformed Services University of the Health Sciences. Staff Surgeon, National Naval Medical Center, Bethesda, Maryland.
Anatomy of Commonly Exposed Arteries

CHARLES L. WITTE, M.D.
Professor of Surgery, University of Arizona College of Medicine, Tucson, Arizona.
Circulatory Dynamics and Physiology of the Lymphatic System

MARLYS H. WITTE, M.D.
Professor of Surgery and Director, Medical Student Research Program, University of Arizona College of Medicine, Tucson, Arizona.
Circulatory Dynamics and Pathophysiology of the Lymphatic System

JAMES S. T. YAO, M.D., Ph.D.
Magerstadt Professor of Surgery, Northwestern University Medical School. Acting Chair, Department of Surgery, Northwestern Memorial Hospital, Chicago, Illinois.
Occupational Vascular Problems

ALBERT E. YELLIN, M.D., F.A.C.S.
Professor of Surgery, University of Southern California School of Medicine. Associate Chief of Staff, Medical Director of Surgical Services, Los Angeles County–University of Southern California Medical Center, Los Angeles, California.
Vascular Injuries of the Extremities

CHRISTOPHER K. ZARINS, M.D.
Chidester Professor of Surgery, Stanford University School of Medicine. Chief of Vascular Surgery, Stanford University Medical Center, Stanford, California.
Artery Wall Pathology in Atherosclerosis

GERALD B. ZELENOCK, M.D.
Professor of Surgery, Section of Vascular Surgery, University of Michigan Medical School; Attending Staff, Section of Vascular Surgery, University Hospital, and Vascular Surgery Service, Veterans Administration Hospital, Ann Arbor, Michigan.
Pulmonary Complications in Vascular Surgery; Splanchnic Artery Aneurysms

R. EUGENE ZIERLER, M.D.
Professor of Surgery, Department of Surgery, Division of Vascular Surgery, University of Washington School of Medicine. Attending Staff, University of Washington Medical Center, Seattle, Washington.
Physiologic Assessment of Peripheral Arterial Occlusive Disease

ROBERT M. ZWOLAK, M.D., Ph.D.
Associate Professor, Dartmouth Medical School, Hanover, New Hampshire. Director, Noninvasive Vascular Laboratory, Mary Hitchcock Memorial Hospital, Lebanon, New Hampshire.
Arterial Duplex Scanning

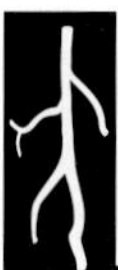

PREFACE

The fifth edition of *Vascular Surgery* comes at the millennium, a time when everyone tends to reflect on changes occurring over the past century, the past 25 years, or at least the past decade. I will spare the reader this and will focus primarily on the changes that have occurred in the practice of vascular surgery since the fourth edition and their impact on the current edition.

The inevitable trend of more vascular surgery being done by fewer but better-trained surgeons, who are more committed to this field as their primary or sole activity, has continued. This is just as well, for it offsets other negative trends. The pressure from superimposed cost-containment measures has resulted not only in more conservative indications for intervention, which is mostly appropriate, but also in far less compensation per procedure, which is not. Vascular surgery, dealing as it does primarily with an elderly population (e.g., Medicare participants) has never been compensated on the same scale as some other surgical specialties with which it has been targeted. Endovascular procedures, on the other hand, have not suffered the same fate, even though their relative costs have climbed because of the new technology involved (e.g., better imaging equipment, special devices, catheters and introducers, and other improvements). While the overall number of traditional (i.e., open) vascular surgical procedures might have declined, from the inroads made by managed care and endovascular procedures, this has been offset, for the most part, in the majority of vascular surgery practices by the dwindling numbers of part-time or "occasional" vascular surgeons, the aging of the population, and the increasing degree to which vascular surgeons in North America and Europe have acquired the necessary skills with which to perform endovascular interventions themselves or in collaboration with interventional radiologists. This latter trend was given a boost by the advent of endografts that, at the outset at least, *required* involvement by vascular surgeons but that also honed their skills at manipulations under fluoroscopic monitoring to the point where balloon dilations and stenting and other simpler procedures were reasonably within reach.

This change is reflected in this new edition in an expanded coverage of *endovascular procedures* and *alternative imaging options* in addition to angiography, topics written principally by surgeons. New chapters are devoted to the various types of endovascular grafts, to the endovascular treatment of abdominal aortic aneurysms (AAAs), to the complications of angiography and of endovascular interventions, and to endovascular interventions for lower extremity occlusive disease. Endovascular treatments are also presented in other chapters dealing with the management of variceal hemorrhage, renovascular disease, acute deep venous thrombosis, and chronic large vein obstruction.

Despite the inroads made by imaging-based radiologists into the field of noninvasive vascular diagnosis, vascular surgeons have managed to keep a firm control on duplex scanning by showing the way in extending and standardizing its clinical applications (e.g., as the sole preoperative imaging method for most cases of carotid endarterectomy and in selected cases of lower extremity revascularization). Vascular surgeons have also demonstrated the continued value of certain of the indirect physiologic tests, which are less expensive than duplex scans but foreign to most radiologists. Nevertheless, in this edition separate chapters describe peripheral arterial and venous duplex scanning, and the application in the diagnosis of mesenteric and renal disease has been given expanded coverage.

Other trends that had just surfaced during the writing of the last edition have continued. Thrombolytic therapy has continued to flourish and has become an integral part of the management of acute arterial thromboses, even though several randomized trials have had difficulty in showing advantages, in overall results, over surgery. These disappointing trial results are partly due to a higher than expected (but "real life?") failure to gain access and achieve lysis (i.e., initial technical failure) and to flaws in protocol design, particularly the linking of thrombolysis with the ultimate treatment of the underlying lesion by percutaneous transluminal angioplasty (PTA), even when surgery would have been more effective. Post hoc analysis has helped to identify the settings in which catheter-directed thrombolysis is likely to be of benefit and demonstrated the clear need for careful case selection. Two chapters address these issues, and another one fully discusses the use of catheter-directed thrombolysis in deep venous thrombosis.

Angioaccess, particularly for hemodialysis, continues to play a major role in the practice of many vascular surgeons, and new techniques that improve the opportunity to create autogenous fistulae and enhance the patency of prosthetic shunts have been introduced. Periodic surveillance of surgical and endovascular revascularizations has become a standard of care, even though appropriate reimbursement for these efforts has lagged shamefully behind. The criteria for identifying critical restenoses and the most cost-effective monitoring intervals need to be better defined, but reasonable options have been identified. The advantages and limitations of PTA and stenting for renal artery stenosis have become better recognized, and its relative role vis à vis surgical revascularization has been better delineated. However, the preferred techniques for renal revascularization have clearly shifted away from a clear dominance by aortorenal vein bypass to relatively more endarterectomies, prosthetic grafts, and extra-anatomic bypasses, each used selectively in certain settings.

Carotid endarterectomy has survived its challenge from

randomized prospective trials versus the best medical therapy and, despite the incurable negativity of some neurologists, has come out stronger than ever. Rather than stand pat, however, we have seen a sweeping trend toward the use of duplex scanning instead of arteriography as the preoperative imaging method in the majority of patients, same-day admission for surgery, selective avoidance of monitoring in intensive care units, and discharging a sizable portion of patients from the hospital on the day after surgery. Although these measures have been instigated by competitive pressures related to increased managed care, they have not reduced the safety of carotid endarterectomy—which, if anything, has continued to improve while becoming less costly. This is just as well, for carotid endarterectomy must meet the new challenge of carotid stenting. Critical appraisal of the initial and current results of stenting, particularly in regard to some deceiving reporting practices, suggests that it should not constitute a major threat to modern-day carotid endarterectomy, but the pressures of continued open use by enthusiasts, industry-driven uncontrolled "trials," and its potential attractiveness to patients, have finally prompted proper randomized trials, even though the matter of clinical equipoise is still being debated. The recent announcement that the CAVITAS trial has shown "no significant difference" ensures that its details will be hotly debated and puts more pressure on the CREST trial. I predict that, in the absence of unforeseen major technologic innovations, carotid stenting will still end up having limited applications (e.g., in technical or operative high-risk patients, such as postendarterectomy restenoses and in the patient with a hostile neck from previous cancer surgery or irradiation).

Although not a major part of the practice of most vascular surgeons, operations for the complications of portal hypertension and for congenital vascular malformations have continued to decline. Operations for mesenteric insufficiency and for upper and lower extremity occlusive disease have not declined, except for aortoiliac occlusive disease. Even there, however, when long-term, lesion-specific stratified data become available, particularly for the more extensive lesions that are being treated percutaneously since the advent of stents, and the impact of reintervention is included in outcome assessment, the pendulum can be expected to swing back.

The management of venous disease has made great strides, the major exception being in direct reconstructive surgery for chronic venous *valvular* insufficiency (as opposed to obstructive disease); even here, however, the selective use and results have been more clearly defined, suggesting that it would be better limited to primary cases rather than postphlebitic cases.

The advances in the management of venous disease are reflected in this book in an expanded section, "Management of Venous Diseases." A new section, "Basic Principles in Vascular Disease," includes chapters on embryology of the vascular system, anatomy of commonly exposed arteries, and vascular biology of the arterial wall in health and disease. The acutely ischemic limb and vascular trauma are now covered in separate sections, the latter with two new chapters.

Considering these and many other changes not detailed here, the fifth edition of *Vascular Surgery* has again undergone major revision. The number of chapters totals 166 instead of 153, but there are more new chapters than the numerical difference would suggest. Some chapters have actually been consolidated, so that almost 20 chapters are topically new. In addition, 87 chapters have been written by new authors or a new primary author. Many other primary authors have enlisted new coauthors in bringing about major revisions. Thus, more than two thirds of the chapters are new or have been extensively revised, and the remainder have been appropriately updated. Even those chapters dealing with slowly changing subjects (e.g., lymphedema and amputation, hemodynamic principles, basic vascular surgery techniques, endarterectomy technique, ischemic neuropathy, and the hemodynamics and pathophysiology of arteriovenous fistulae) have not remained the same.

I owe my deep appreciation to the associate and assistant editors who have shared the hard work of putting together yet another comprehensive and thoroughly updated edition. With each new edition, we resist the temptation to cut back or at least to hold it to the same size, for knowledge in this field is increasing and we believe that there should be one text in this field that endeavors to be almost encyclopedic, one in which the reader can expect almost every aspect to be covered. As this textbook is not meant to be read from cover to cover, there is deliberate repetition in addition to thorough cross-referencing.

The associate and assistant editors join me in thanking each and every author and coauthor of the many chapters. Writing chapters is usually a thankless job, with no reward other than being recognized for one's expertise and the satisfaction of contributing to updating and perpetuating a textbook that has become, by these efforts and the efforts of past contributors, a valuable resource in one's chosen field.

Needless to say, I have benefited the most from all these efforts, being given undue credit for the work of so many others. It is my hope that they all will share my pride in a job well done and that their unselfish efforts will continue to sustain *Vascular Surgery* in the role into which it has grown—that of vascular surgery's main textbook—and that they will see it as a legacy worth perpetuating with future editions, long after I cease to wheedle yet one more chapter from them and then cajole them to produce it on time.

ROBERT B. RUTHERFORD

NOTICE

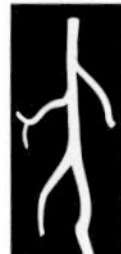

CONTENTS

SECTION XI

SECTION XII

SECTION XIII

SECTION XIV

SECTION XV

SECTION XVI

SECTION XVII

SECTION XVIII

SECTION XIX

Plate I

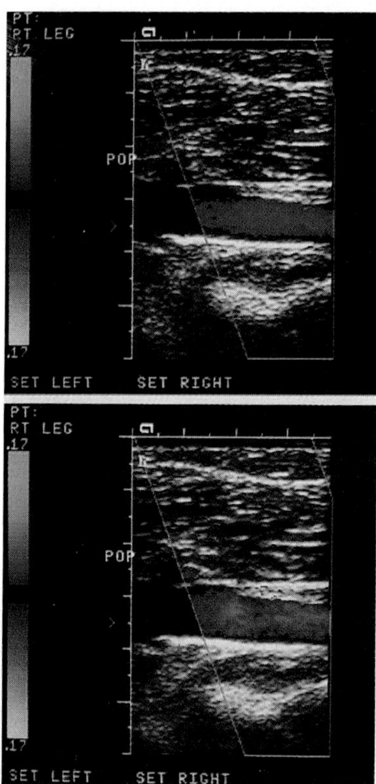

FIGURE 11–14. Real-time imaging with color flow duplex scanning allows quick assessment of venous incompetence by identifying bidirectional flow. In color flow images of an incompetent popliteal (POP) vein, blue hue *(top)* represents flow away from the transducer and red hue *(bottom)* represents flow toward the transducer (reversed flow).

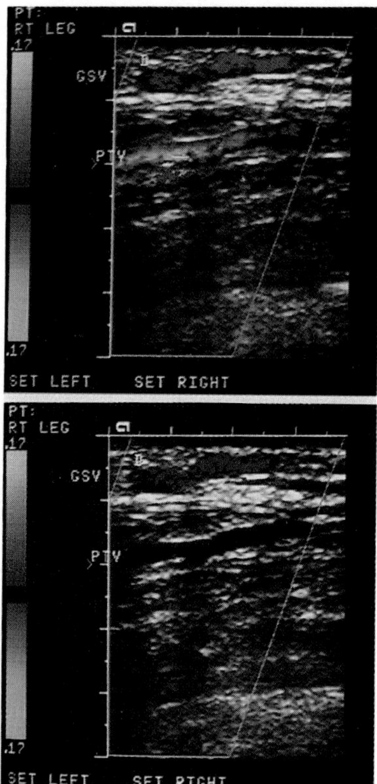

FIGURE 11–15. Simultaneous color flow real-time images of the posterior tibial vein (PTV) and the greater saphenous vein (GSV). *Top,* Both veins show flow toward the transducer (blue hue). *Bottom,* Greater saphenous vein shows no color because flow has ceased, which implies valvular competence in the posterior tibial vein.

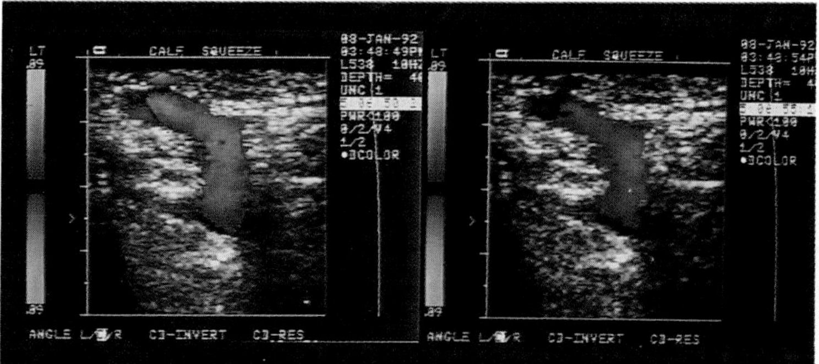

FIGURE 11–21. Color flow images of an incompetent calf perforating vein. *Right,* Transverse calf insonation demonstrating flow from the greater saphenous vein to the deep calf vein. *Left,* Flow reversal (red hue) after the release of distal calf compression.

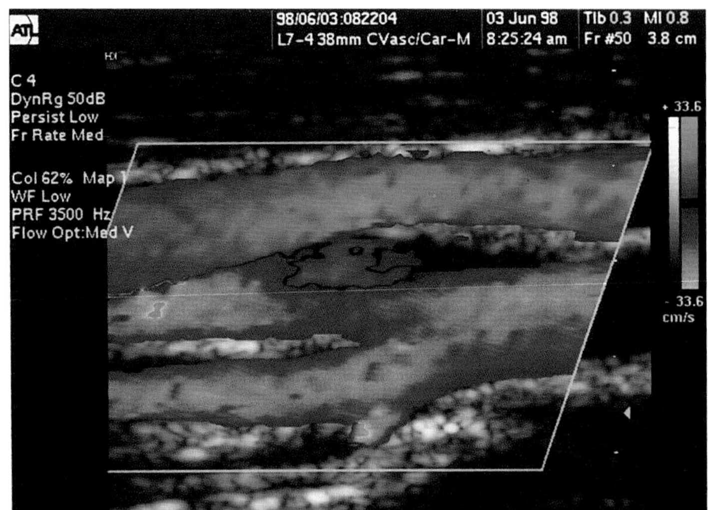

FIGURE 12–1. Color flow duplex image of normal carotid bifurcation. The superior thyroid branch is visible, originating from the external carotid. Small region of color flow reversal in the carotid bulb is a normal finding in patients entirely free of carotid atherosclerosis.

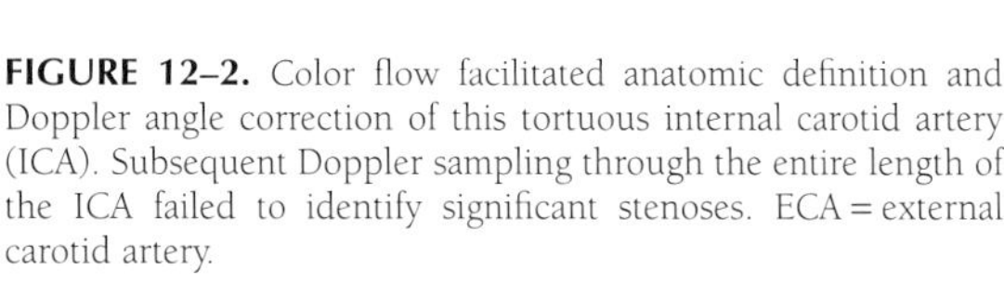

FIGURE 12–2. Color flow facilitated anatomic definition and Doppler angle correction of this tortuous internal carotid artery (ICA). Subsequent Doppler sampling through the entire length of the ICA failed to identify significant stenoses. ECA = external carotid artery.

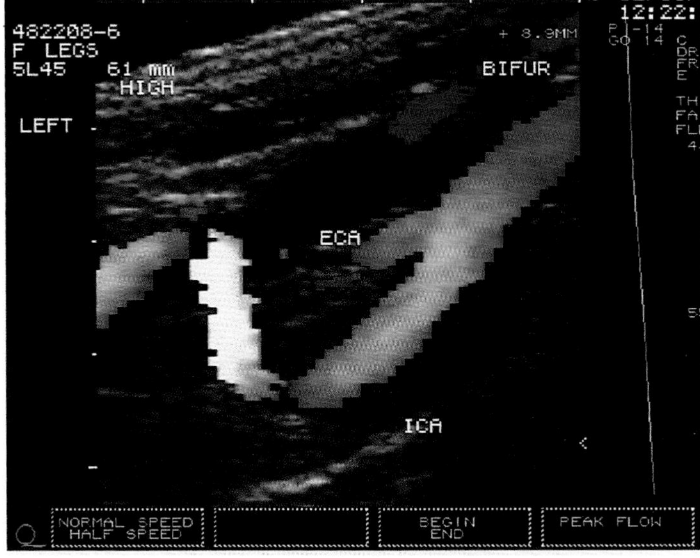

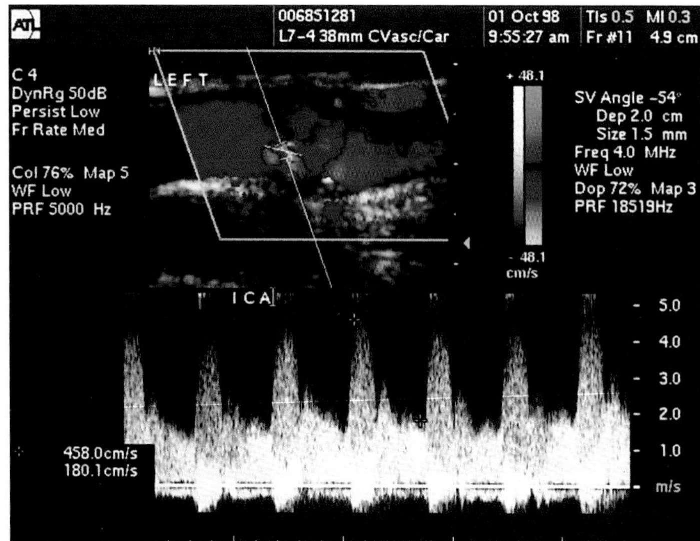

FIGURE 12–3. Identification of carotid stenosis is best performed using angle-corrected Doppler velocity and spectral analysis. In this study, the sample volume is placed in a region of disordered blood flow, indicated by the focal color variation in the color flow inset. Recorded peak systolic velocity (PSV) of 458 cm/sec and end-diastolic volume of 180 cm/sec fall well above thresholds for 70% stenosis on all published grading scales. Common carotid artery (CCA) PSV of 65 cm/sec (not shown) produced calculated ICA:CCA ratio of 7.0, also indicating greater than 70% stenosis by all published grading scales. ICA = internal carotid artery.

Plate III

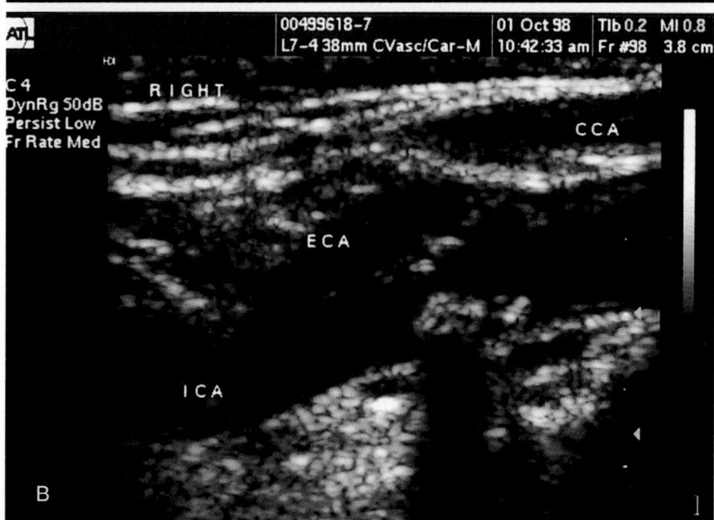

FIGURE 12–4. Examination of the carotid bifurcation with gray scale B-mode imaging is the best method for evaluating atherosclerotic plaque characteristics. *A,* The Doppler spectral window is clear, and velocities are minimally elevated. Color flow gain is well adjusted, and by visual interpretation the far wall plaque is unremarkable. *B,* The same carotid bifurcation is examined using magnified B-mode without color flow. A focal, bulky plaque is apparent. Even in the absence of severe stenosis, a plaque of this magnitude may occasionally be the source of atheroembolic symptoms. CCA = common carotid artery; ECA = external carotid artery; ICA = internal carotid artery.

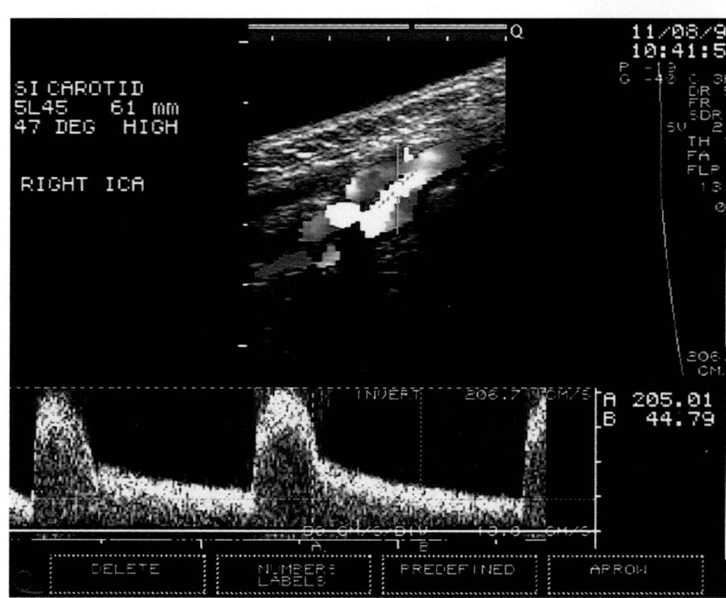

FIGURE 12–5. The Doppler spectrum in this image was obtained at the region of highest internal carotid artery velocity. With an angle-corrected peak systolic velocity (PSV) of 205 cm/sec and end-diastolic volume of 45 cm/sec, this lesion would be interpreted as greater than 60% stenotic by at least one published scale, but less than 60% by several others. The example reinforces the need for local validation of whichever scale is chosen for interpretation. ICA = internal carotid artery.

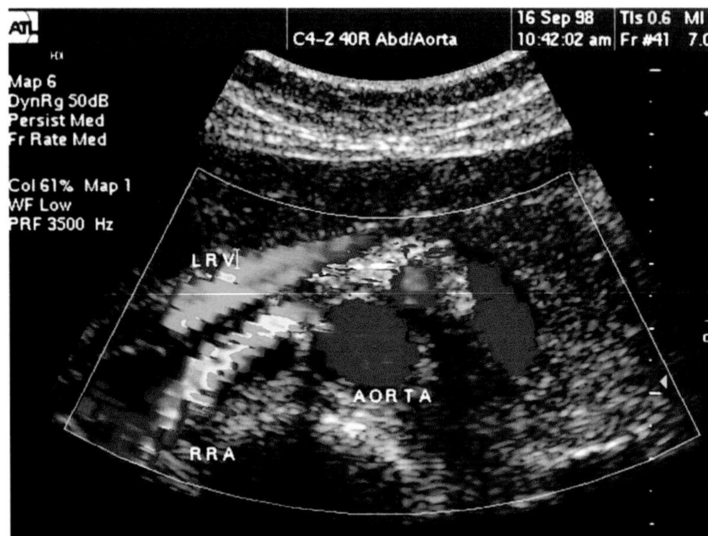

FIGURE 12–6. Transverse view of aorta, right renal artery (RRA), left renal vein (LRV), and origin of left renal artery (unlabeled). This is a typical color flow landmark enabling the examiner to begin Doppler spectral data collection in the renal arteries.

FIGURE 12–7. Color flow image of left renal artery from aorta to renal pelvis. After the artery is located, its entire length is sampled for Doppler velocities and spectra.

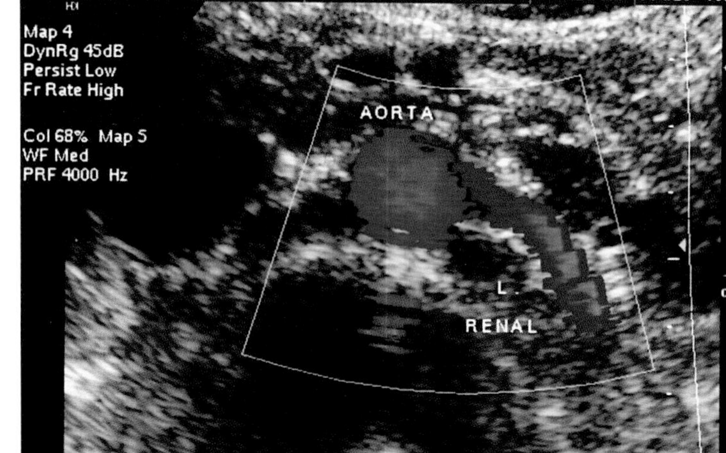

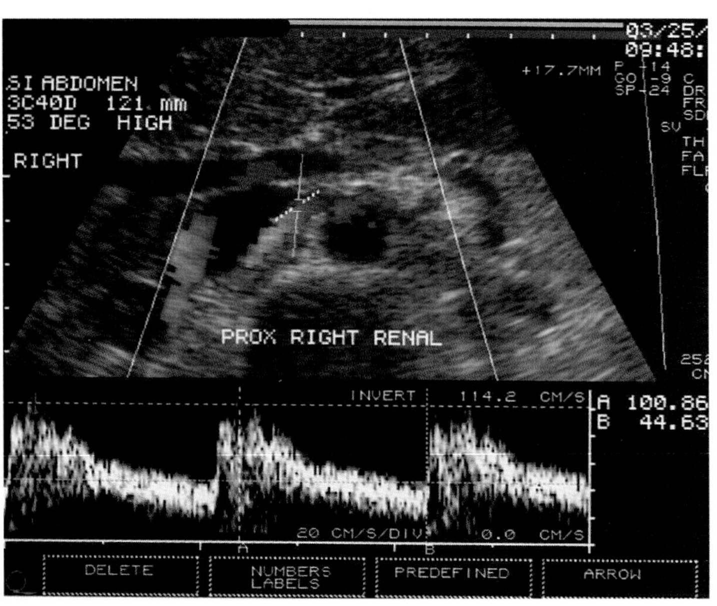

FIGURE 12–8. Normal Doppler spectrum sampled from proximal right renal artery. Waveform has rapid upstroke and high flow throughout diastole. This low resistance morphology indicates normal low resistance of the renal parenchyma.

Plate V

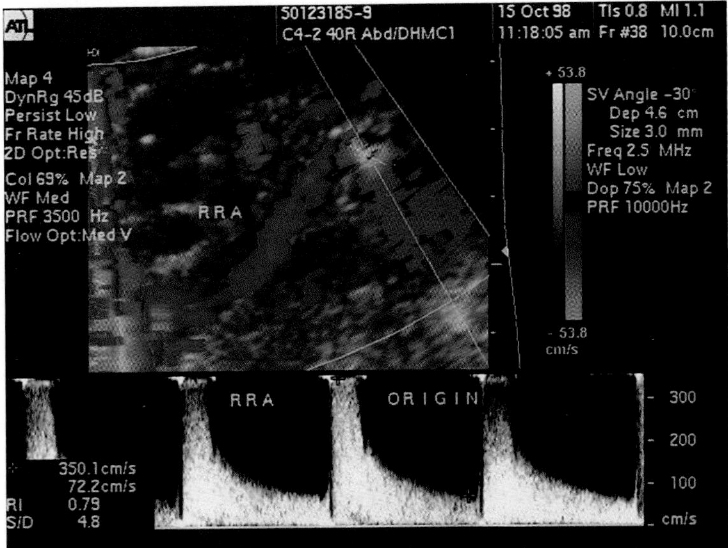

FIGURE 12–9. Abnormal right renal artery (RRA) with a peak systolic velocity (PSV) of 350 cm/sec. Aortic PSV was 70 cm/sec, resulting in a renal-aortic ratio of 5.0. Stenosis was subsequently confirmed by angiography. The image demonstrates the importance of accurate angle correction in tortuous renals.

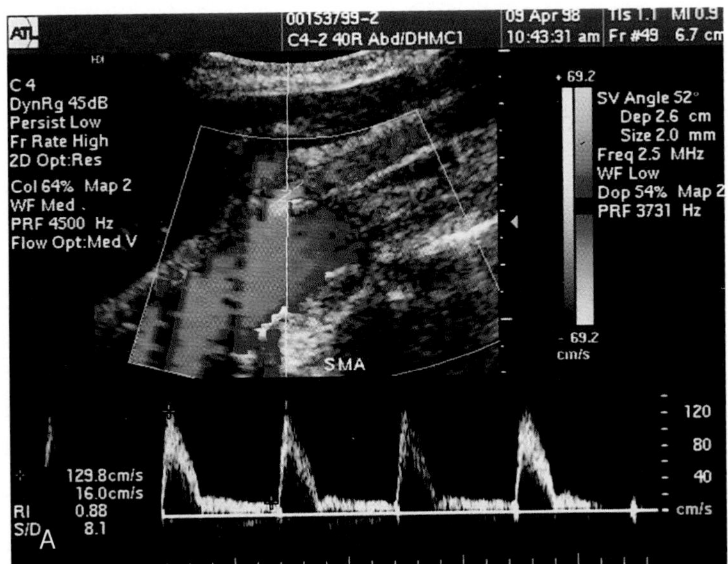

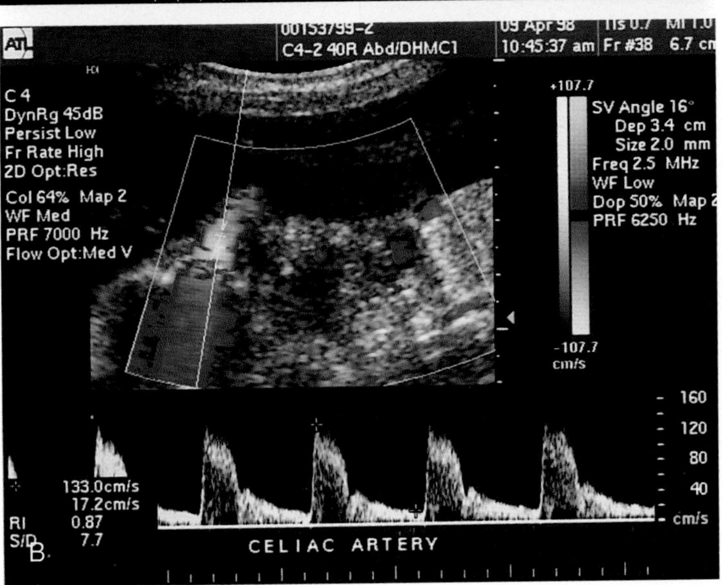

FIGURE 12–10. *A*, Normal, fasting, high-resistance waveform in the superior mesenteric artery (SMA). Angle correction is crucial as the SMA curves sharply beyond its origin from the aorta. *B*, The celiac origin has a low-resistance Doppler waveform.

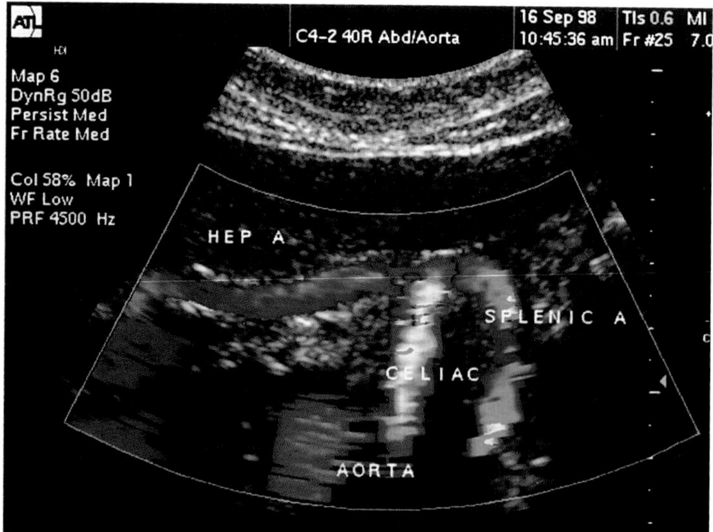

FIGURE 12–11. Color flow appearance of the celiac axis and bifurcation into the splenic and common hepatic arteries. Common hepatic artery flow direction may be retrograde if the celiac artery is severely stenotic or occluded. Visual impression of flow direction based on color flow must be confirmed by Doppler sampling.

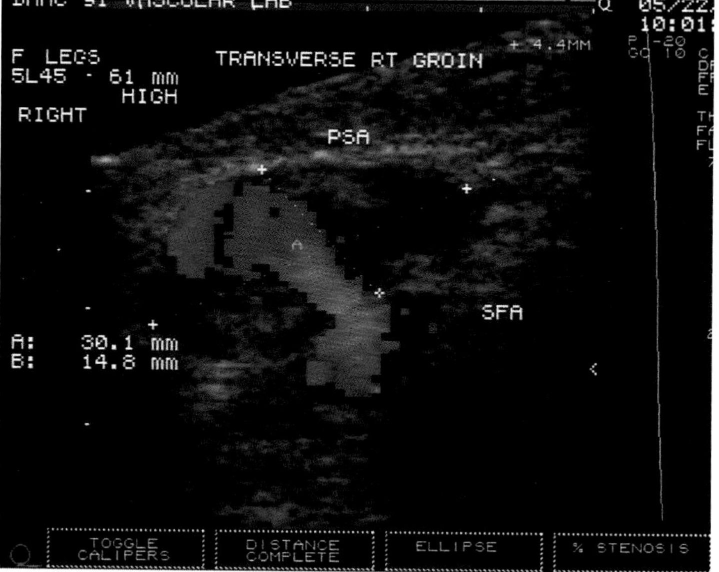

FIGURE 12–12. Pseudoaneurysm arising from the superficial femoral artery (SFA) just beyond the femoral bifurcation. Pseudoaneurysm (PSA) is partially thrombosed. Swirling blood is seen in the remainder. Compression over the PSA neck is frequently successful in achieving complete thrombosis. (See also Figure 48–6.)

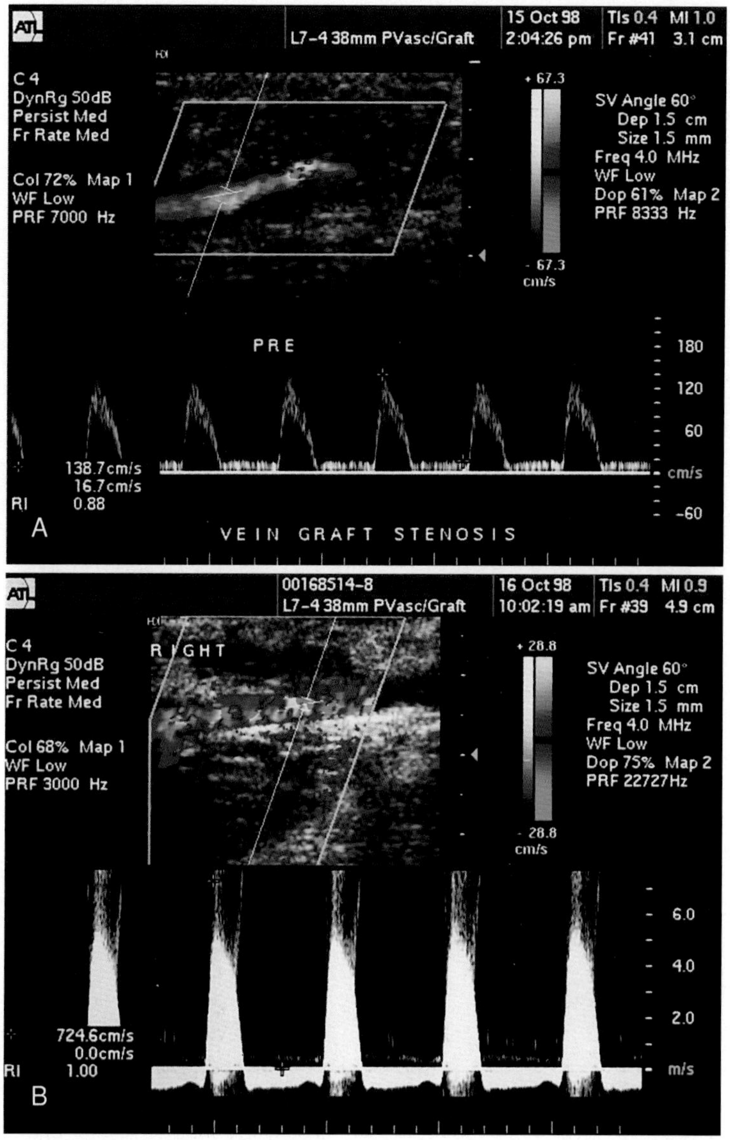

Plate VII

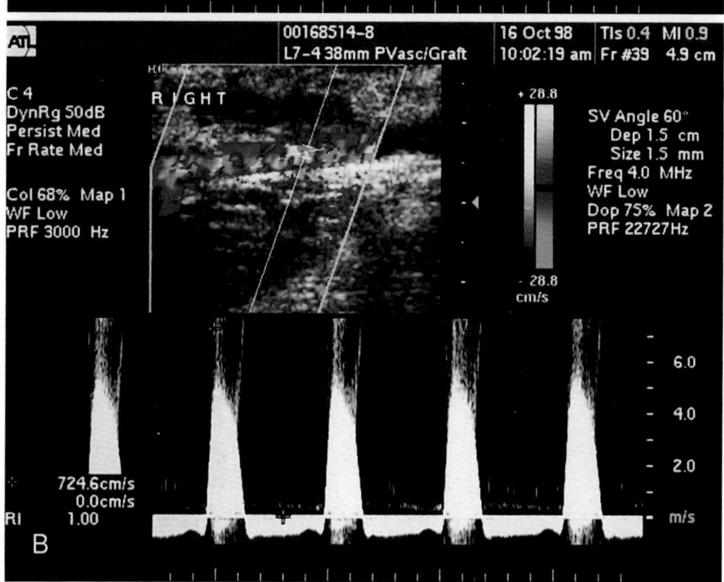

FIGURE 12–13. *A,* Bypass graft Doppler spectrum proximal to a vein graft stenosis reveals a peak systolic velocity (PSV) of 139 cm/sec with a clear systolic window. *B,* Region of bypass stenosis with markedly elevated PSV (725 cm/sec), spectral broadening, and tissue vibration causing color pixels outside the flow channel.

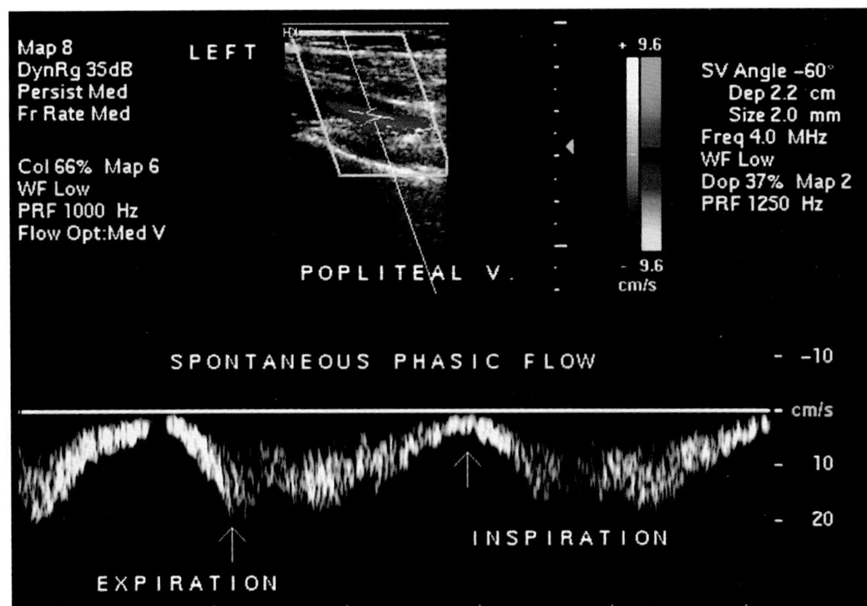

FIGURE 13–2. Doppler spectrum common femoral vein. Antegrade flow in the common femoral vein is displayed below the baseline. Unobstructed venous flow in the proximal veins is spontaneous with respiratory variation. Flow velocity increases with a reduction in intra-abdominal pressure during expiration and is damped or ceases during inspiration.

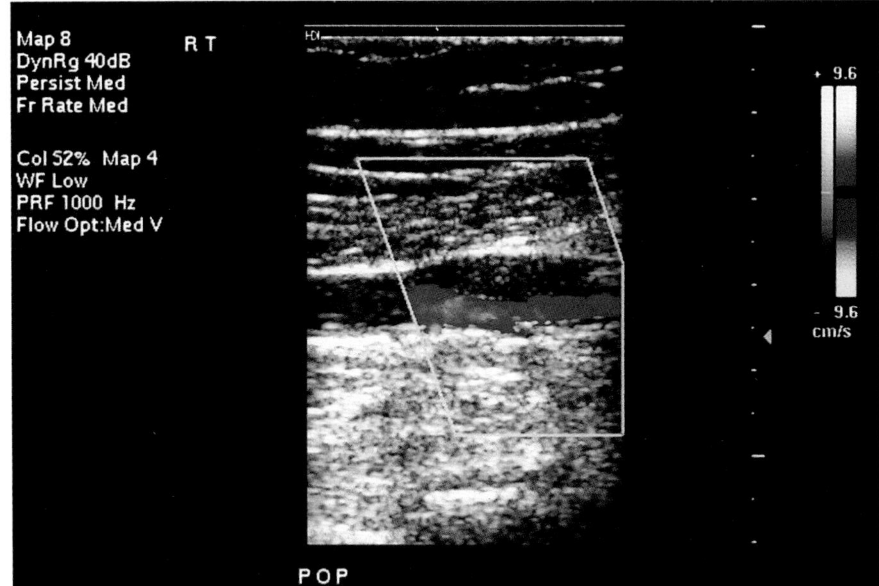

FIGURE 13–3. Partially occlusive popliteal vein thrombosis. Echogenic thrombus encroaches on the color flow Doppler image.

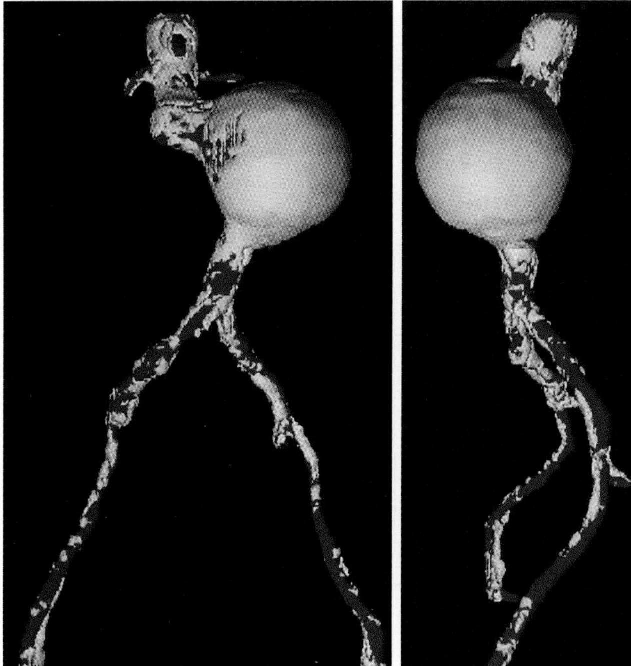

FIGURE 14–10. Multiple-object surface-shaded display (SSD), anteroposterior *(left)* and left lateral *(right)* views of the same abdominal aortic aneurysm seen in Figures 14–8 and 14–9. Contrast-enhanced blood flow is displayed in red, thrombus and noncalcified plaque are displayed in yellow, and calcified plaque is white. In this type of three-dimensional reconstruction, all of the components of the aneurysm are seen. Multiple views are helpful, and it is preferable if the display can be rotated and viewed at will on a computer screen. This type of display is most helpful in determining the true extent of an aneurysm, since thrombus is clearly visible.

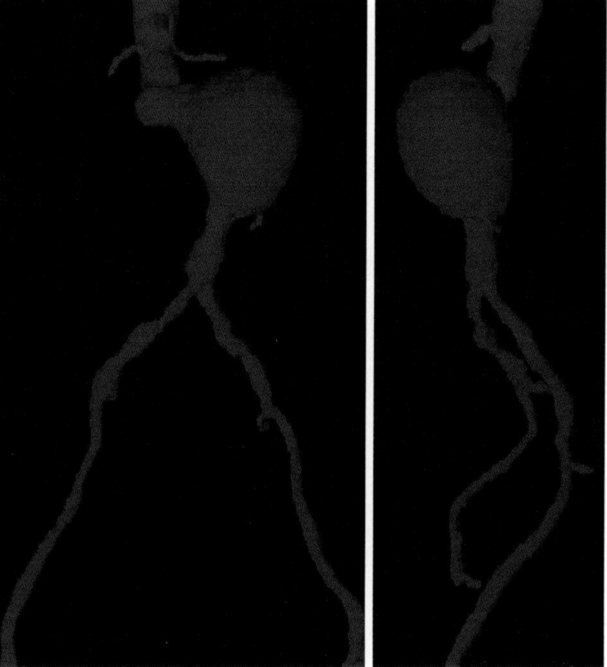

FIGURE 14–11. Multiple-object, surface-shaded display (SSD) from Figure 14–10 with all structures made invisible except blood flow, using the same anteroposterior *(left)* and left lateral *(right)* views. With calcified plaque made invisible, the degree of occlusive disease becomes apparent in the iliac arteries. A key point is that calcified plaque was modeled separately and has been made invisible; thus, this three-dimensional reconstruction does *not* have the same appearance as the typical one-object SSD shown in Figure 14–8. For surgical planning, it is preferable if the objects can be made visible or invisible at will on a computer screen. An alternative is to print hard copy images in multiple views with the various components sequentially highlighted, transparent, or invisible.

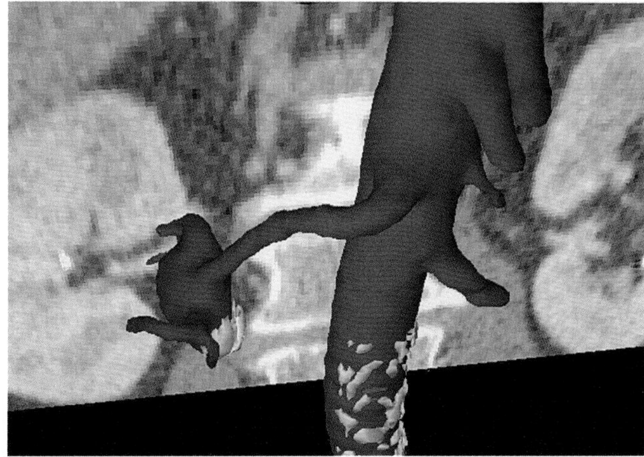

FIGURE 14–12. Multiple-object, surface-shaded display with a CT slice displayed in the context of the model in three-dimensional space. Thus, the right renal artery aneurysm is displayed with its branches heading toward the CT display of the right kidney. The central branch exiting the aneurysm is cut off as it disappears into the CT slice.

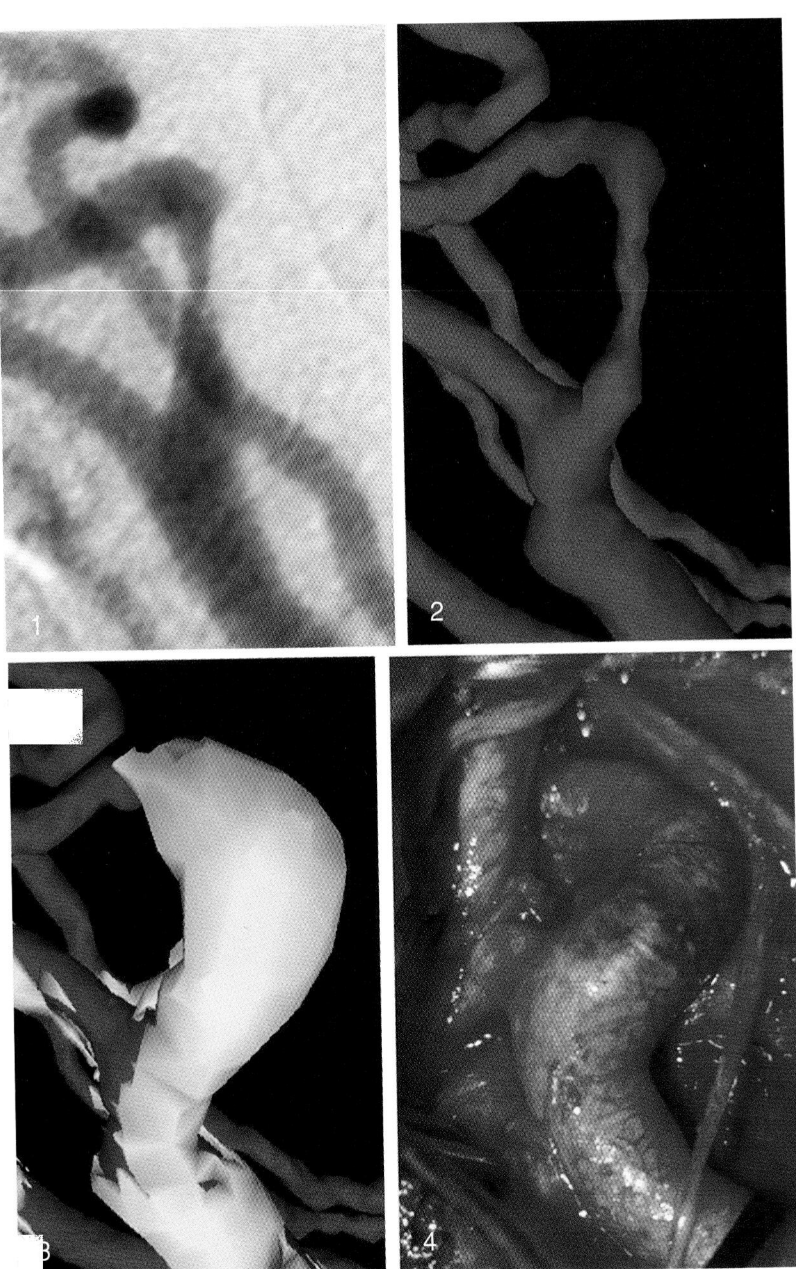

FIGURE 14–19. Demonstration of carotid artery disease. From *left* to *right:* *1,* Angiogram of an internal carotid artery stenosis; *2,* three-dimensional (3-D) reconstruction of blood flow (red) in the same location; *3,* 3-D reconstruction of blood flow and plaque or thrombus (yellow); and *4,* intraoperative photograph of the same location. There is obviously a striking similarity despite rotation of the head and neck in the operative photograph.

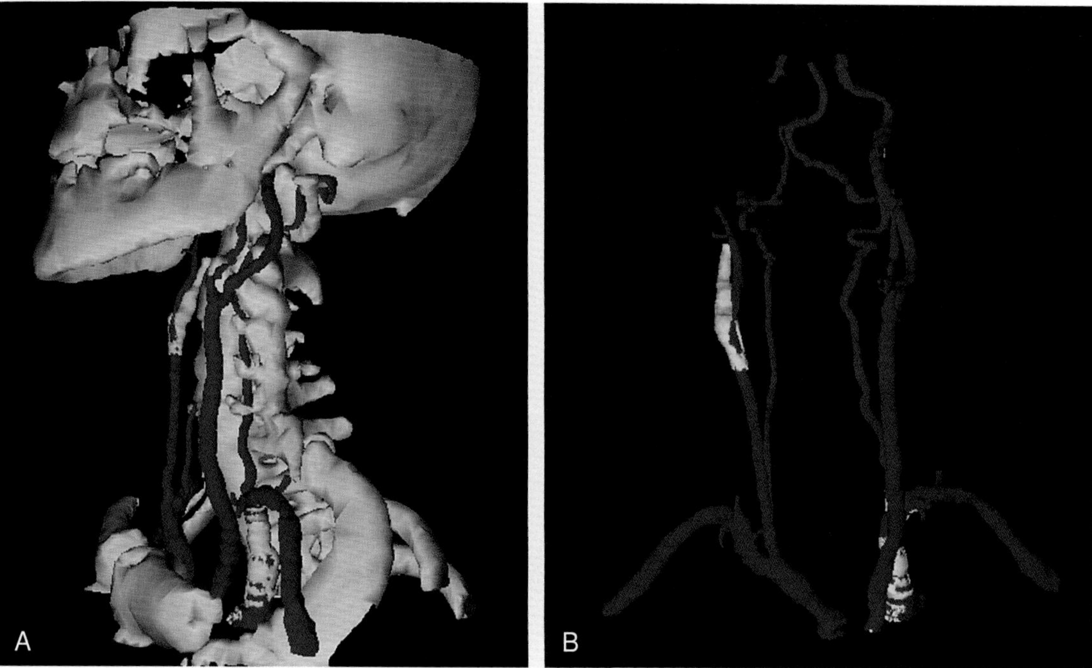

FIGURE 14–20. Multiple-object, three-dimensional reconstruction can demonstrate the relationship of the extracranial vessels and the bony structures as an aid to surgical planning. A *with* and B *without* bony structures.

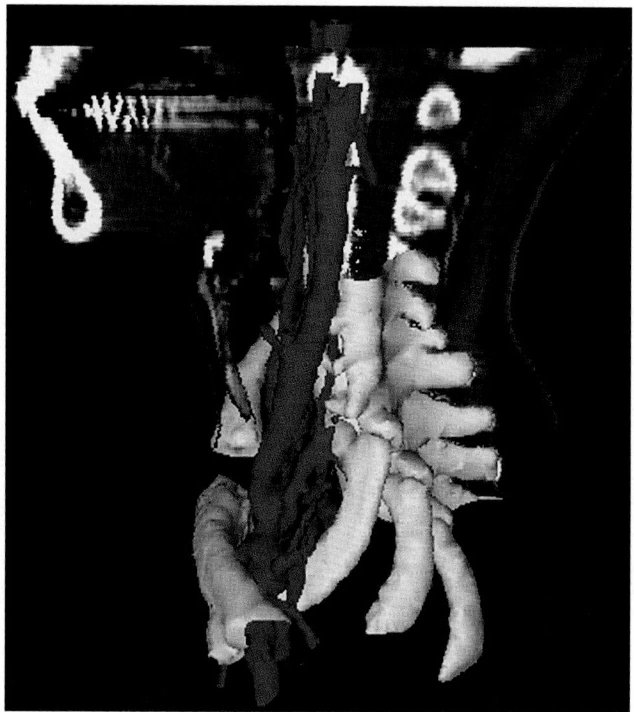

FIGURE 14–22. Three-dimensional reconstruction of the bony and vascular structures of the thoracic outlet.

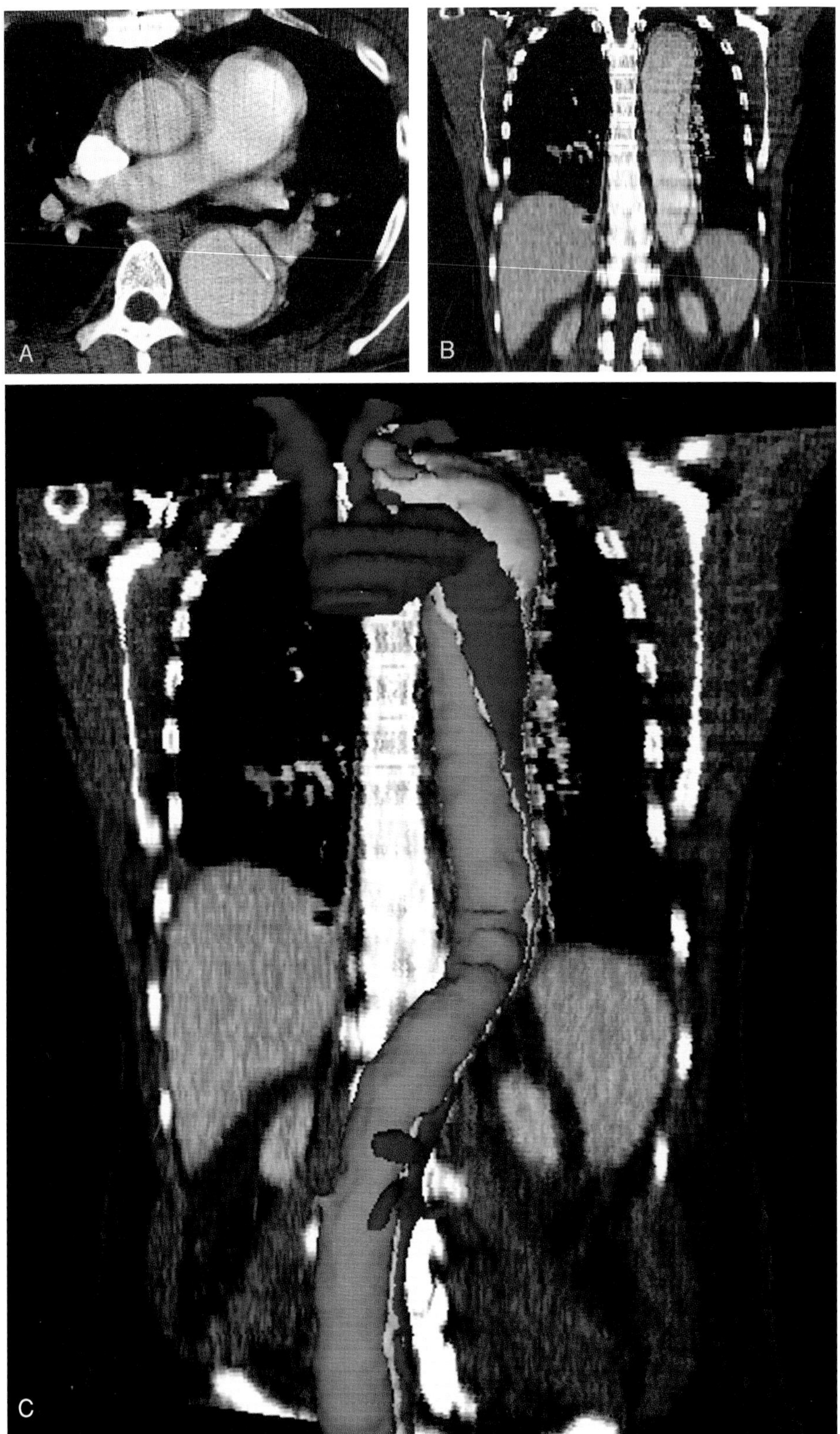

FIGURE 14–23. Dissection of the thoracic aorta. *A*, Axial CT demonstrates dissection within the descending thoracic aorta. Compare this picture with the artefacts in Figure 14–17. CT artefacts can create the impression of a dissection, but these can usually be distinguished from genuine pathology. *B*, Coronal reformat demonstrates the dissection in a consistent manner over a long segment of aorta. *C*, Three-dimensional (3-D) reconstruction depicts (1) the blood from the true lumen supplying the celiac, superior mesenteric artery, and left renal artery (red); (2) blood from the false lumen involving the left subclavian artery and supplying the right renal artery (magenta); and (3) thrombus (yellow). This illustration demonstrates how a 3-D reconstruction can rapidly convey a large amount of information. A coronal CT slice has been placed within the model at the appropriate location to lend context.

Plate XIII

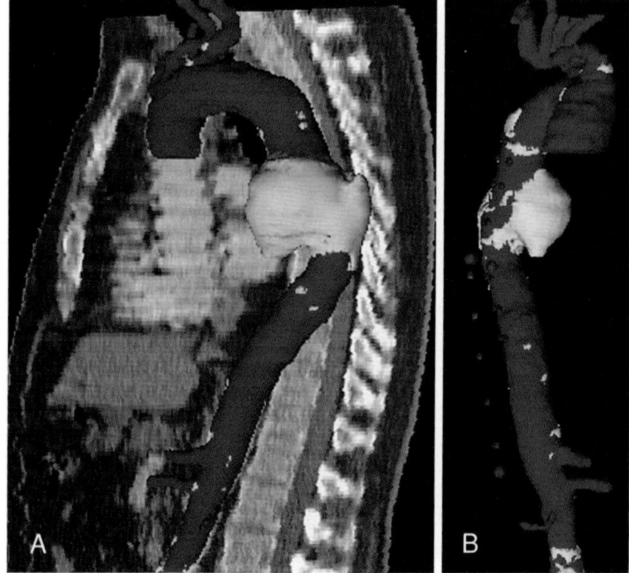

FIGURE 14–25. *A*, Aneurysm of the thoracic aorta demonstrated using three-dimensional (3-D) reconstruction with simultaneous display of a sagittal CT slice to lend context. Motion artefact is much greater around the heart and proximal ascending aorta. The focal blebs displayed in the model were verified at the time of surgery. *B*, Intercostal arteries are marked on the CT slices and are displayed on the 3-D model using interactive software (blue marks). The red marks were placed to denote the top of the eighth thoracic vertebra (T8) and the bottom of the 12th thoracic vertebra. The large intercostal artery near the top of T8 was identified and preserved at the time of operation.

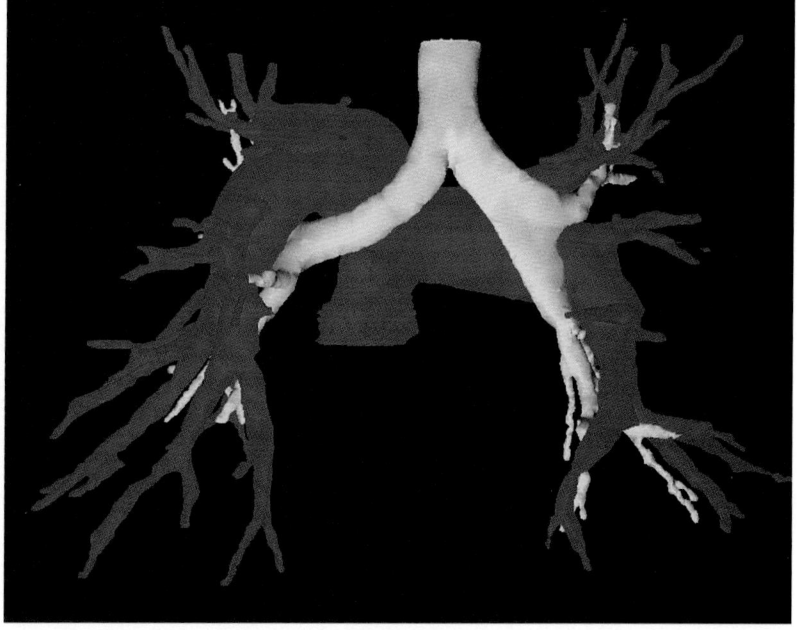

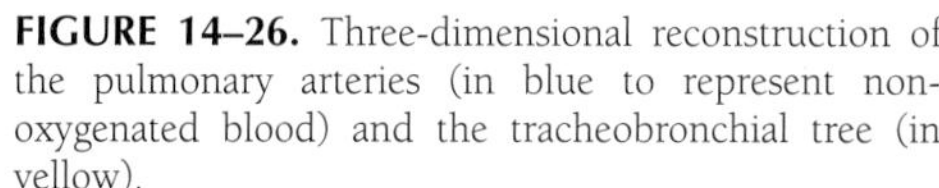

FIGURE 14–26. Three-dimensional reconstruction of the pulmonary arteries (in blue to represent non-oxygenated blood) and the tracheobronchial tree (in yellow).

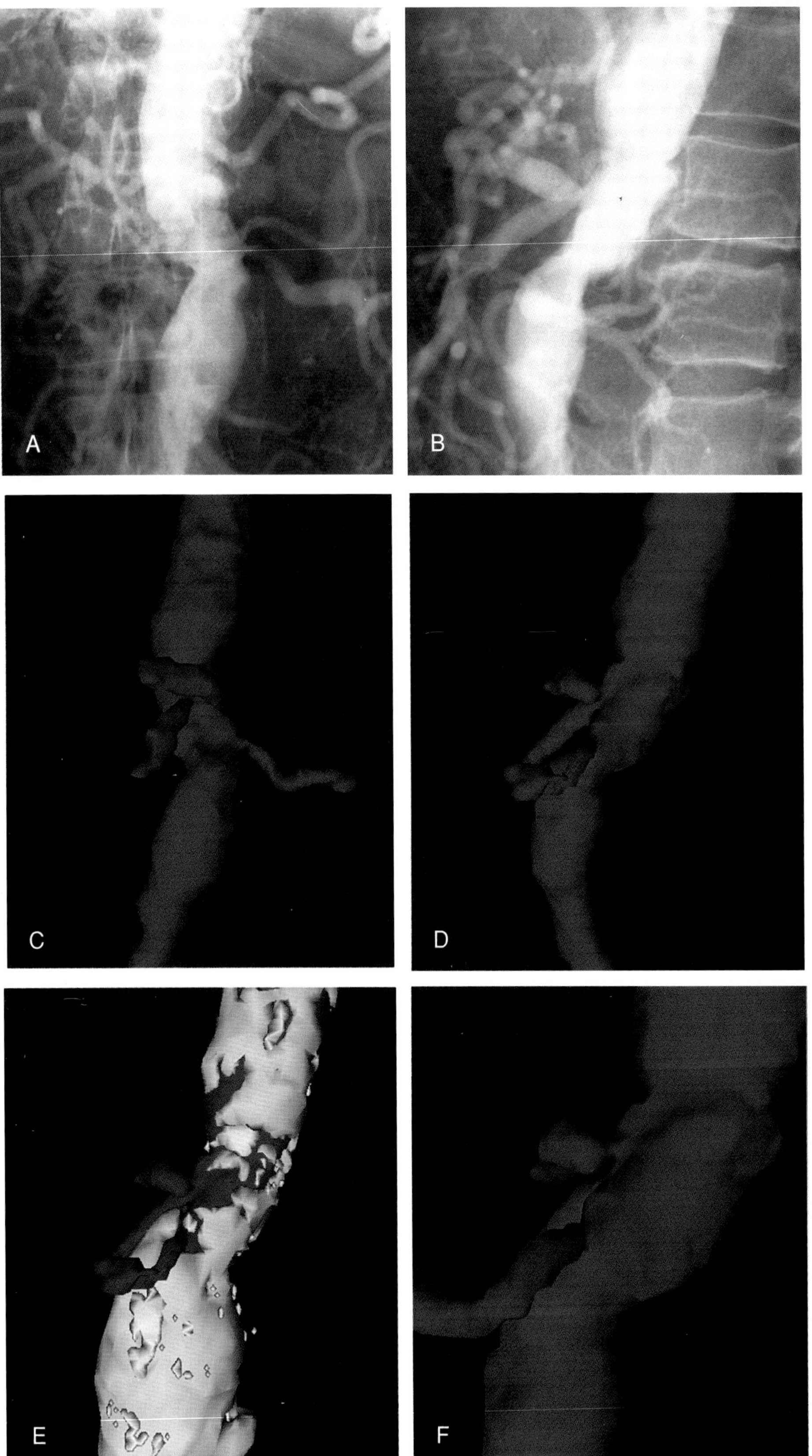

FIGURE 14–27. Anteroposterior (AP) *(A)* and lateral aortographic views *(B)* of what appears to be an infrarenal abdominal aortic aneurysm (AAA). The right renal artery is occluded and the left renal artery has a mild stenosis. *C* and *D,* AP and lateral three-dimensional (3-D) reconstruction images of only the contrast-enhanced blood flow demonstrate the same findings. *E,* Multiple-object 3-D reconstruction with calcified plaque (white) and thrombus (yellow) made visible demonstrates that the AAA actually involves the suprarenal aorta, including the origin of the superior mesenteric artery. This was confirmed at operation. This view of the reconstruction was very useful for determining a good location for the aortic cross-clamp (proximal to the celiac artery) and for determining that beveled anastomosis could be performed along the relatively normal aorta. The left renal artery was reimplanted on an aortic patch following endarterectomy of the plaque at the renal artery origin. *F,* Celiac artery stenosis is demonstrated on a magnified and rotated 3-D reconstruction image with only blood flow made visible. The lesion was confirmed at operation. The celiac stenosis was missed by angiography because it overlapped the superior mesenteric artery on the lateral view.

Plate XV

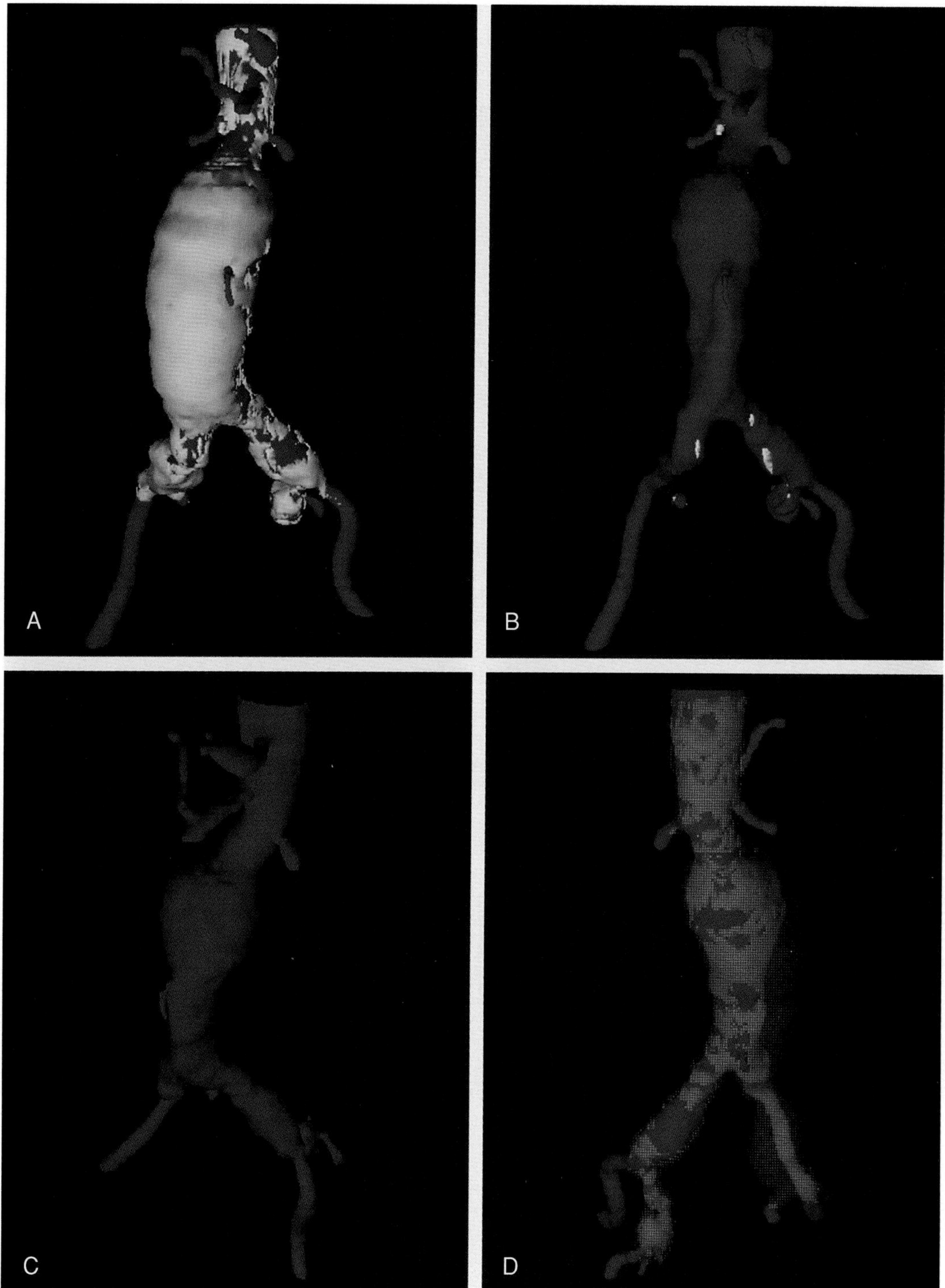

FIGURE 14–33. Demonstration of several abnormalities on one 3-D reconstruction, highlighting the utility of multiple views and a multiple-object display. This study was obtained to evaluate a possible infrarenal abdominal aortic aneurysm (AAA) and also revealed a celiac artery aneurysm, a replaced right hepatic artery arising from the superior mesenteric artery, multiple iliac artery aneurysms, and a right internal iliac artery occlusion. We can best understand the various abnormalities by rotating the model and changing the visibility of thrombus, which can be done in real time on a workstation or a personal computer with specialized software. *A,* Anteroposterior (AP) view of a multiple-object 3-D reconstruction with blood flow (red), thrombus or noncalcified plaque (yellow), and calcified plaque (white) all included in the model. *B,* A 3-D reconstruction with thrombus made invisible demonstrates the right internal iliac artery occlusion. *C,* Oblique view of the 3-D reconstruction demonstrates the celiac artery aneurysm and the replaced right hepatic artery better than other views. *D,* The outflow branches of the left internal iliac artery aneurysm are best seen on a posterior view with thrombus made transparent.

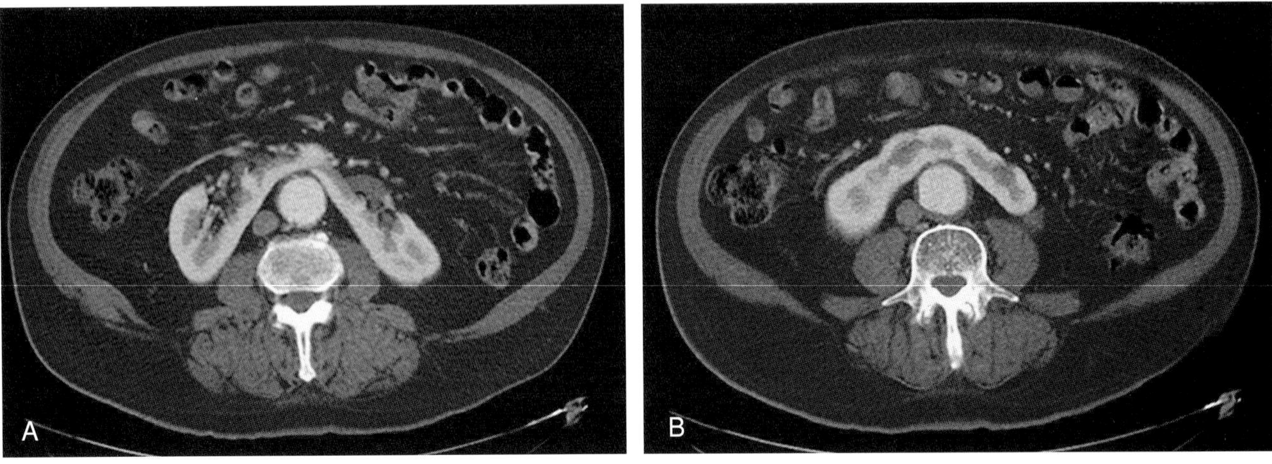

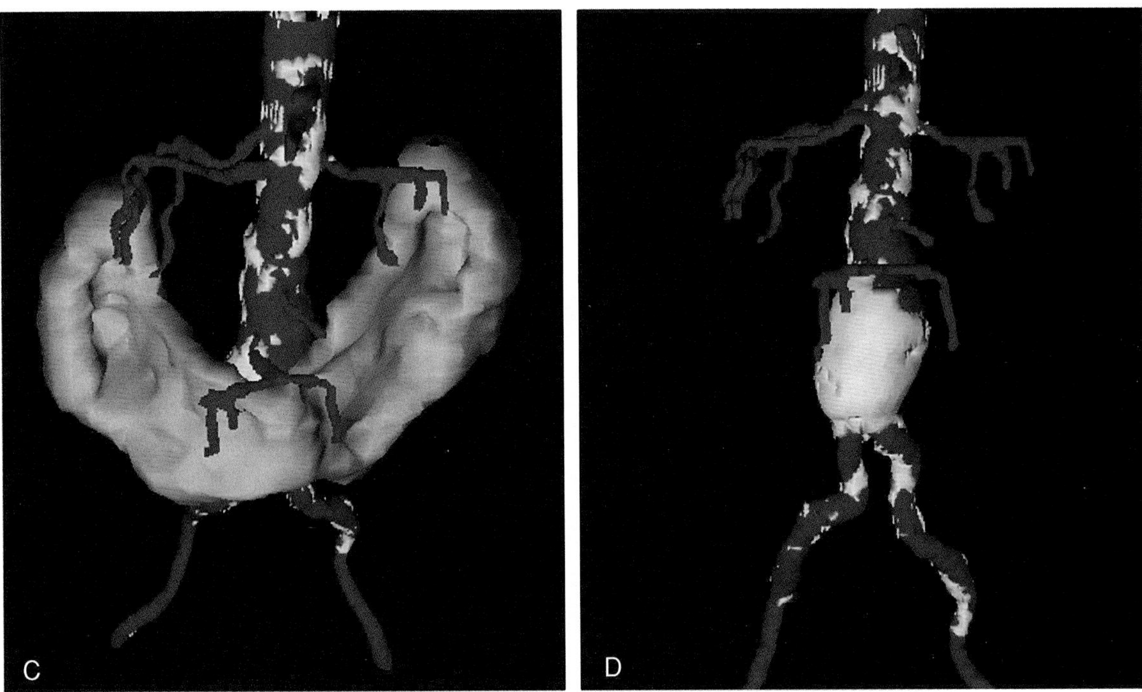

FIGURE 14–34. *A,* Horseshoe kidney on axial CT scan. *B,* The portion of the horseshoe kidney that crosses the midline is often relatively thin, but in this case the parenchyma does not appear to be attenuated. *C,* A 3-D reconstruction with the horseshoe kidney and associated complex blood supply clearly visible. The reconstruction is rotated slightly to demonstrate a stenosis in the lowest midline renal artery near its origins. A very large amount of information is gained rapidly using this technology, as it would be extremely difficult to trace the renal arteries through their course on CT slices. Angiography does not provide a 3-D prospective of the renal parenchyma. *D,* Anteroposterior view of the 3-D reconstruction with the kidney made invisible, demonstrating a small abdominal aortic aneurysm arising just distal to the lowest renal artery (which is in the midline).

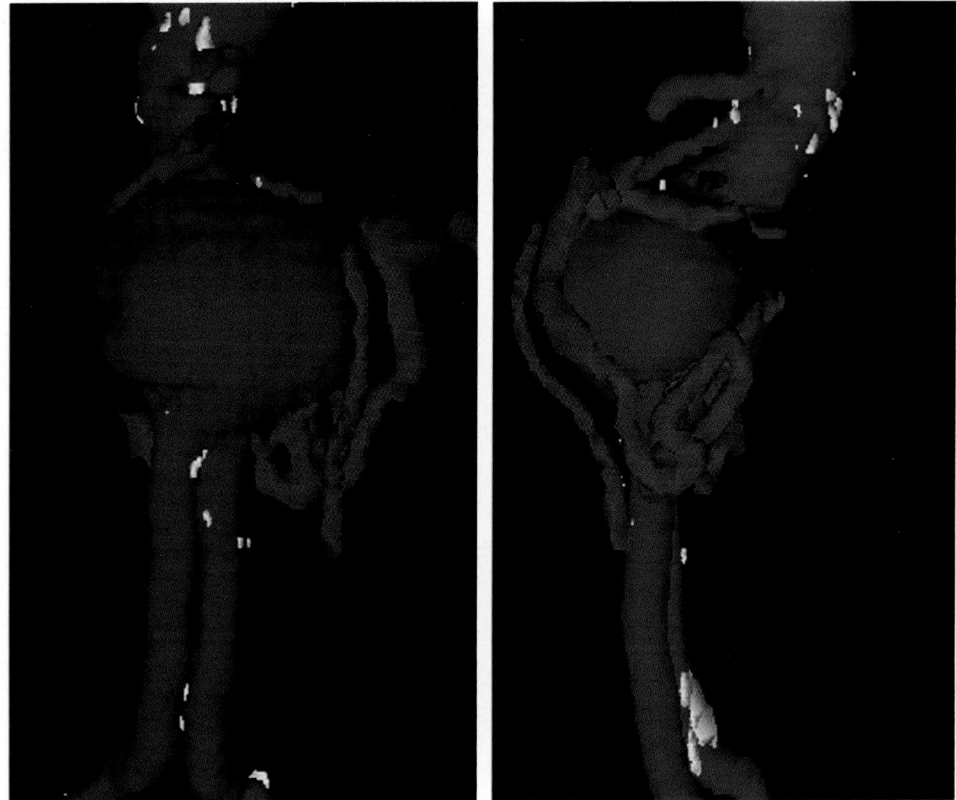

FIGURE 14–36. Three-dimensional (3-D) reconstruction image of a patient with occlusion of the left renal vein by an 8-cm aneurysm, which developed proximal to an infrarenal abdominal aortic aneurysm (AAA) repair many years earlier. Huge left-sided venous collaterals and their 3-D relationship to the AAA are easily seen. In this case, 3-D reconstruction changed the operative approach from retroperitoneal to transabdominal.

Plate XVIII

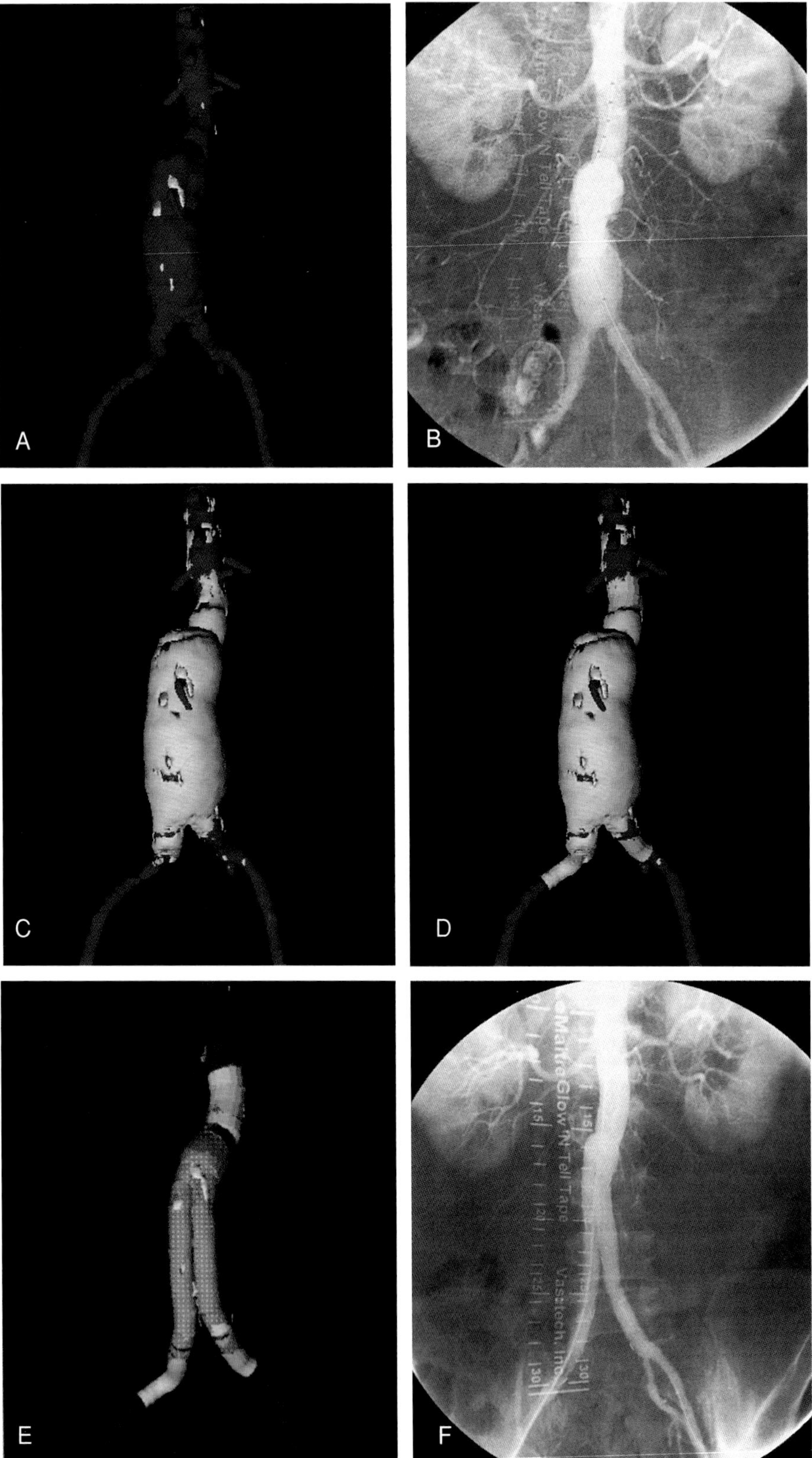

FIGURE 14–39. Use of CT with three-dimensional (3-D) reconstruction and specialized software in endovascular abdominal aortic aneurysmal repair.

A, Preoperative 3-D reconstruction showing contrast-enhanced blood flow (red) and calcified plaque (white). Owing to the accuracy of this technique, preoperative angiograms are not necessary.

B, Angiogram performed on the operating table at the time of the procedure, which is necessary to deliver the device even if a preoperative angiogram had been performed. Note the similarity to the 3-D reconstruction.

C, Preoperative 3-D reconstruction including thrombus, demonstrating the need for CT prior to endovascular repair. The iliac arteries are aneurysmal proximally, especially on the left. The endograft cannot be implanted into thrombus and must be long enough to achieve a seal in the normal common iliac artery.

D, Preoperative planning with a "virtual graft," which is displayed in bright yellow. The brighter yellow of the simulated endograft protrudes beyond the red blood flow and the lighter yellow of the thrombus for sufficient lengths proximally and distally; thus, this 3-D reconstruction demonstrates that the proposed graft is appropriately oversized to achieve a seal at the neck of the infrarenal aorta and in the iliac arteries. This view rapidly provides a check to be sure that the proposed endograft is not too small or excessively oversized. It also graphically demonstrates the quality and length of the "seal zone."

E, Preoperative stimulation using the virtual endograft, in this case with thrombus invisible and blood flow made transparent to better demonstrate the anticipated course of the proposed endograft. The prediction here is that the endograft will dilate as it exits the aortic neck (consistent with the degree of oversizing) and deviate slightly at the same location because it must follow the aortic lumen. It is anticipated that some deviation and constriction of the limbs will occur at the aortic bifurcation, but this does not appear to be excessive. This same technology and display is used to evaluate graft length along the center line of the lumen or along a user-defined path. In this case, the length and diameter of the endograft were simulated to coincide with an available graft size. An endograft of this length is anticipated to end just above the left internal iliac artery origin and extend beyond the right iliac artery stenosis if it is deployed appropriately (with the proximal endograft just below the renal arteries).

F, Completion angiogram at the time of the procedure verifies the accuracy of the preoperative computer simulation. The endograft was deployed just below the renal arteries and ends just above the left internal iliac artery origin. The endograft also extends beyond the right iliac stenosis, which is no longer apparent.

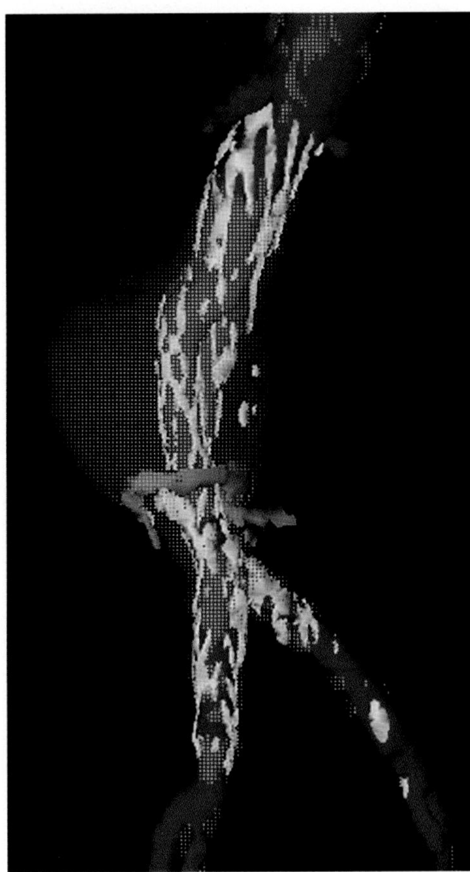

FIGURE 14–40. Perigraft flow (endoleak) following endovascular abdominal aortic aneurysmal repair, as displayed on three-dimensional (3-D) reconstruction image. 3-D reconstruction (created from the CT data) is rotated to a posterolateral view. Multiple-object 3-D display includes the densities consistent with contrast-enhanced lumen (red); thrombus and noncalcified plaque (yellow, made transparent to display the endoleak); calcified plaque and metallic stent (white); and contrast-enhanced endoleak (magenta). The 3-D display demonstrates that the endoleak is associated with a patent lumbar artery and a patent inferior mesenteric artery (IMA).

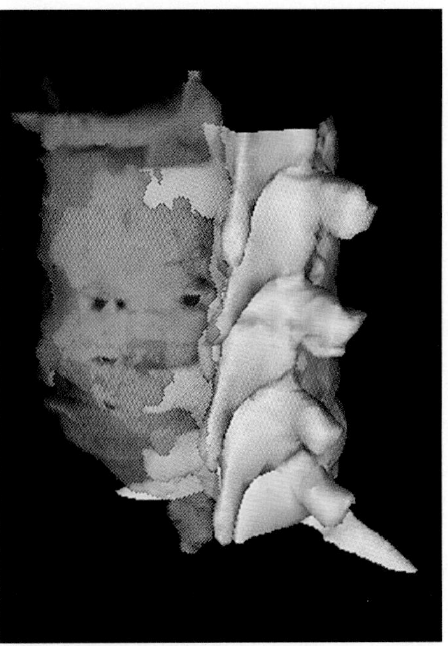

FIGURE 14–43. Arteriovenous malformation adjacent to the spine on three-dimensional (3-D) reconstruction derived from the CT data. On the 3-D reconstruction, the spine is white, the contrast-enhanced vessels are red and the surrounding structures are yellow (made transparent to reveal the vasculature).

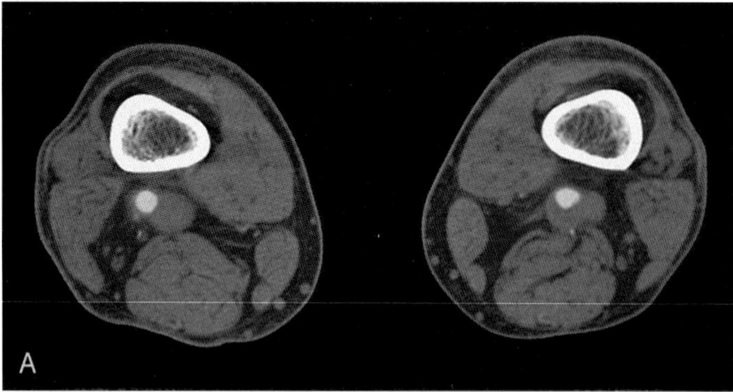

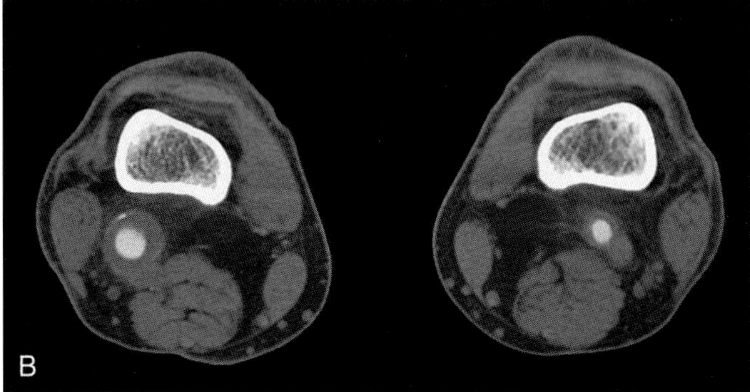

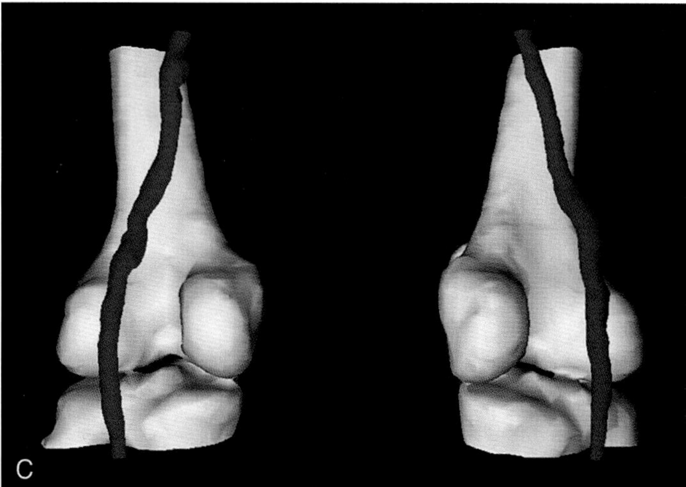

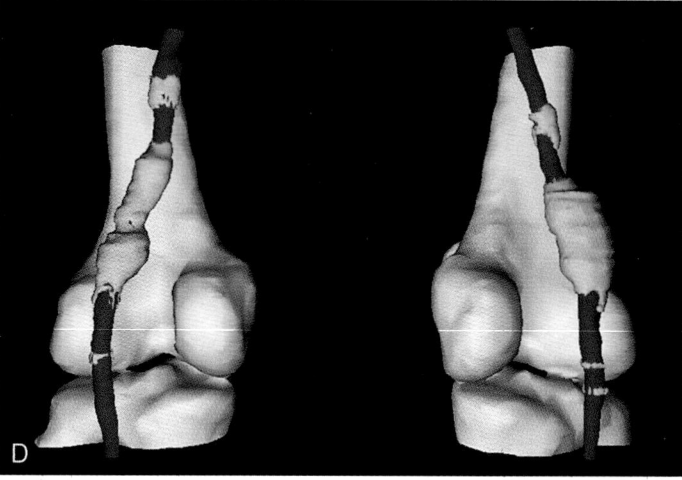

FIGURE 14–41. Bilateral popliteal aneurysms. *A,* The lumen can have a variable appearance, as demonstrated by the eccentric cross section on the patient's left *(right)*. *B,* This axial CT cross section demonstrates a more characteristic circular lumen with circumferential thrombus on the patient's right *(left)*. As with other aneurysms, the diameter of the contrast-enhanced lumen does not correlate with the outer diameter of the vessel, thus making angiography a poor diagnostic modality. *C,* Posterior view of the 3-D reconstruction with only the contrast-enhanced blood flow (red) and bones (white) made visible. This view is similar to an angiogram and would not depict the full extent of the aneurysms. The patient had no occlusive disease on ultrasound examination or ankle-brachial indices. *D,* This posterior view of the 3-D reconstruction with thrombus and plaque added nicely depicts the full extent of the aneurysms. In this case, bypass of the lesions could be performed without angiography.

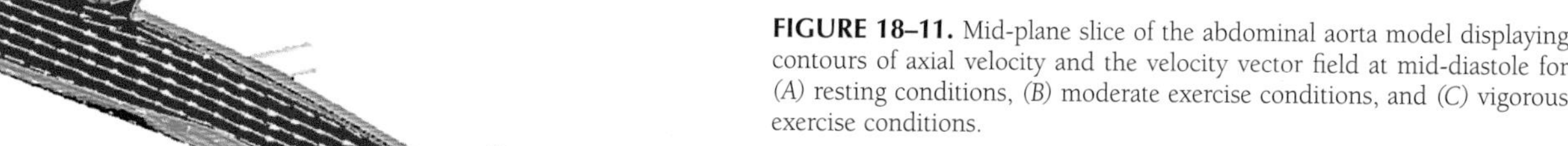

FIGURE 18–11. Mid-plane slice of the abdominal aorta model displaying contours of axial velocity and the velocity vector field at mid-diastole for *(A)* resting conditions, *(B)* moderate exercise conditions, and *(C)* vigorous exercise conditions.

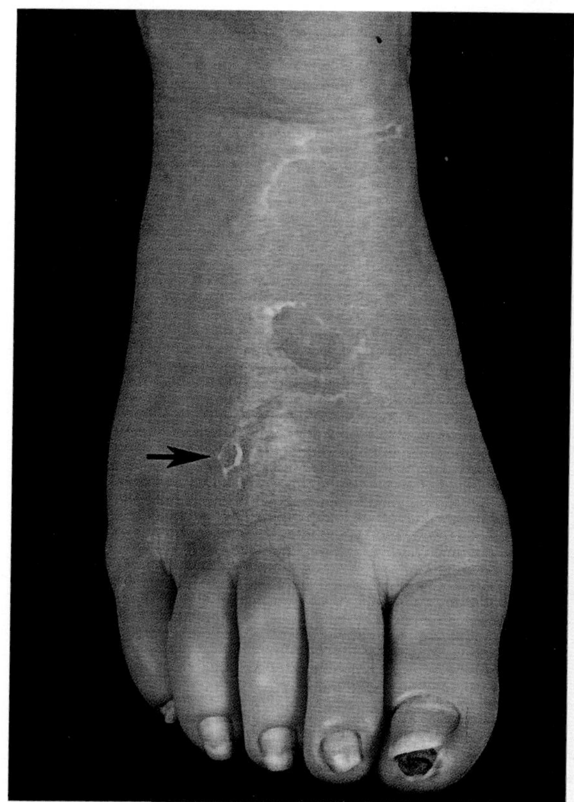

FIGURE 20–4. Ischemic ulcer on the distal portion of the right great toe in a young man with acute Buerger's disease. Note the superficial thrombophlebitis on the dorsum of the foot *(arrow)* with marked erythema around the phlebitis. (From Olin JW, Lie JT: Thromboangiitis obliterans. *In* Cooke JP, Frohlich ED [eds]: Current Management of Hypertension and Vascular Disease. Philadelphia, BC Decker, 1992, pp 265–271.)

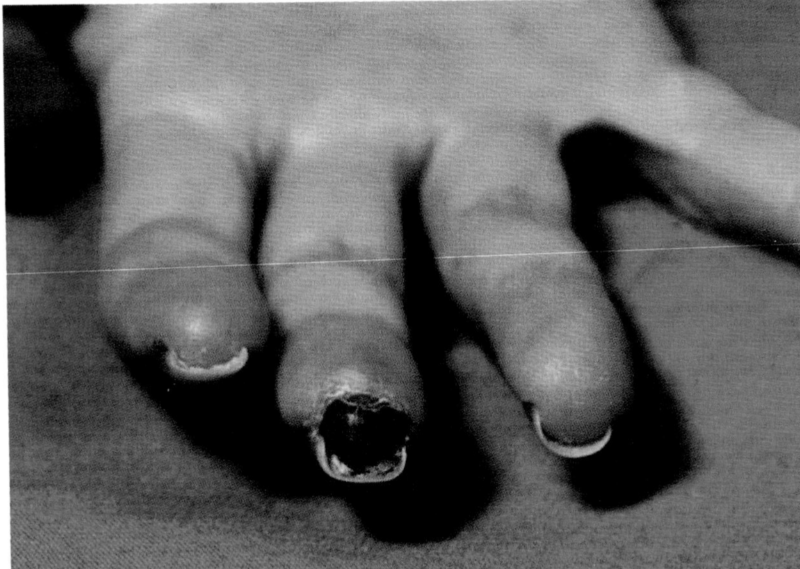

FIGURE 20–5. Ischemic ulcers on the index and middle fingers of a patient with Buerger's disease. Base of little finger is on left.

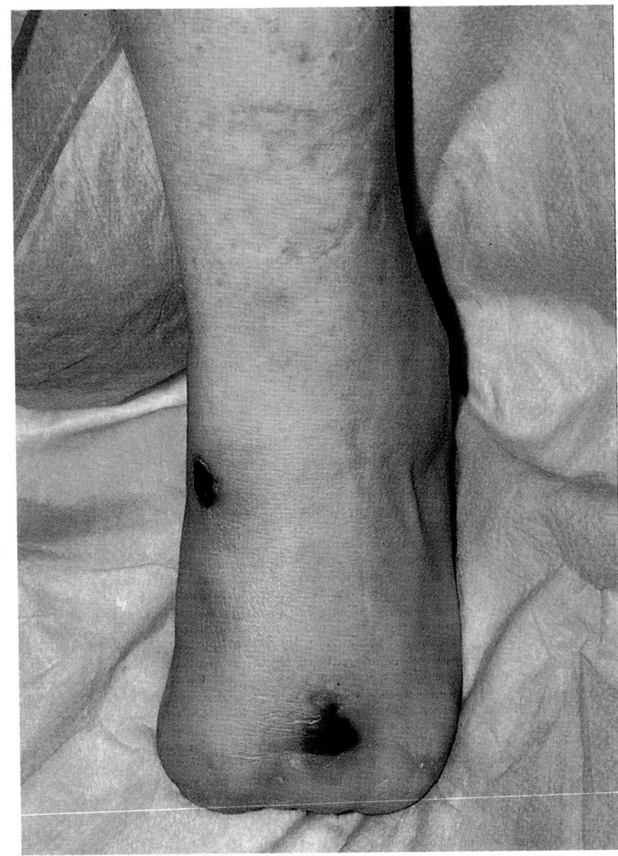

FIGURE 20–12. This patient underwent a transmetatarsal amputation in the past. He continued to smoke and has developed several areas of ischemic ulceration on the foot, two of which are visible.

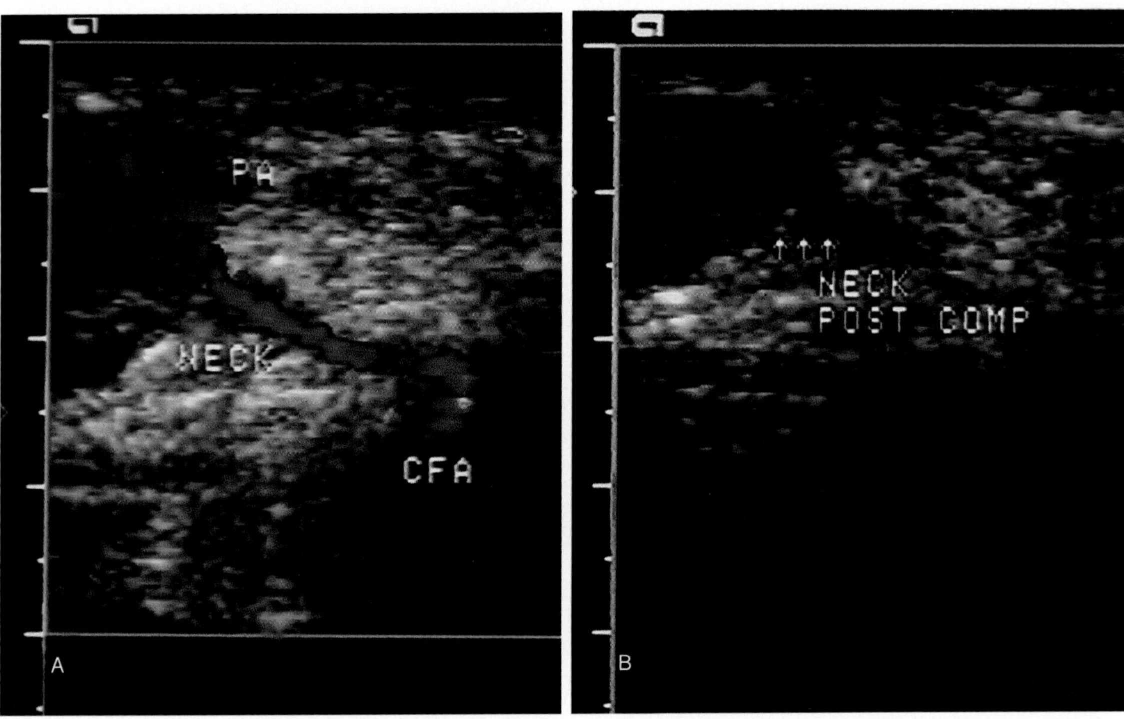

FIGURE 48–6. Common femoral artery (CFA) iatrogenic pseudoaneurysm in a 42-year-old woman 1 day after cardiac catheterization. *A,* Duplex image with color flow mapping showing the CFA, pseudoaneurysm neck (NECK), and pseudoaneurysm cavity (PA). *B,* Duplex image at same location after successful ultrasound-guided compression. Note the obliteration of the neck following compression *(arrows).*

SECTION I

BASIC APPROACHES TO VASCULAR PROBLEMS

ROBERT B. RUTHERFORD, M.D.

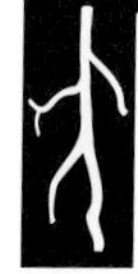

CHAPTER 1

Initial Patient Evaluation: The Vascular Consultation

Robert B. Rutherford, M.D.

BASIC CONSIDERATIONS

The vascular surgeon is usually consulted in order to establish a diagnosis and to recommend or carry out appropriate treatment. This process involves (1) reaching a presumptive diagnosis on clinical grounds; (2) using noninvasive diagnostic measures to either confirm the diagnosis or grade the functional severity of the condition; (3) weighing the degree of disability and natural course of the underlying disease, with best medical treatment, against the risk and success rate of various interventional options; and (4) when necessitated by a likely need to intervene, confirming the diagnosis and the extent and degree of involvement by angiography (Fig. 1–1). When percutaneous, catheter-directed interventions are likely options, tentative arrangements should be made to proceed with an appropriate procedure at the time of angiography to avoid duplication of risk, time, and effort.

One can make the final decision only by combining the sociologic, pathologic, anatomic, and physiologic findings in the individual patient. All but the precise anatomy of the responsible lesion should be known after the initial consultation, the assessment of risk factors, and hemodynamic studies in the vascular laboratory. At this point or at the time of angiography, the surgeon should be prepared to make a definitive recommendation regarding best therapy. With the increasing introduction of percutaneous treatments, it is even more important that a basic strategy be worked out before angiography so that a definitive recommendation can be made at that time. A superficial evaluation sufficient to recommend angiography with subsequent review before final recommendation (a common practice in earlier times) will often result in decision making by others.

Experience and judgment make this important process of patient evaluation and selection of appropriate therapy relatively straightforward in most cases, but there will always be some patients in whom the disease process or its management is neither obvious nor definitive. There are few areas in medicine in which the conditions encountered lend themselves so readily to diagnosis solely on the basis of thoughtful history and careful physical examination as do vascular diseases. Specialists in this field are often surprised at their colleagues' difficulties in assessing peripheral vascular problems and, conversely, surprise them with their clinical acumen.

The majority of vascular problems are caused, in the Western world at least, by one of two basic disease processes: arteriosclerosis or thrombophlebitis. These processes predominantly affect the circulation of the lower extremity rather than of the upper extremity or the viscera; the presenting manifestation is either pain, some form of tissue loss (ulceration or gangrene), or a change in appearance or sensation (swelling, discoloration, or temperature change). By applying a systematic, problem-oriented approach to these complaints, clinicians soon find that they can often predict the likely status of the arterial circulation even before examination, recognize the postphlebitic leg at a glance, determine the cause of leg or foot ulcerations by their location and appearance, and predict the cause of leg swelling by its distribution and associated skin changes.

Unfortunately, there is a tendency—as the clinician becomes adept at this, is able to turn the anticipated 1-hour consultation with a new patient into a 15-minute interview and spot diagnosis, and can handle a clinic full of patients with chronic but familiar vascular problems in an hour or two—to bypass the systematic approach with increasing frequency and to abbreviate consultation notes and clinical records. Eventually, the ability to transmit this knowledge to others (colleagues, students, house staff) in an organized fashion becomes lost or stinted. It may be useful, therefore, for experienced as well as inexperienced clinicians, to have and maintain some formal framework on which these diagnostic skills can be superimposed. This need can be filled by a diagnostic checklist or evaluation form, such as the one presented in Figure 1–2. This approach not only avoids embarrassing oversights but also preserves the details of

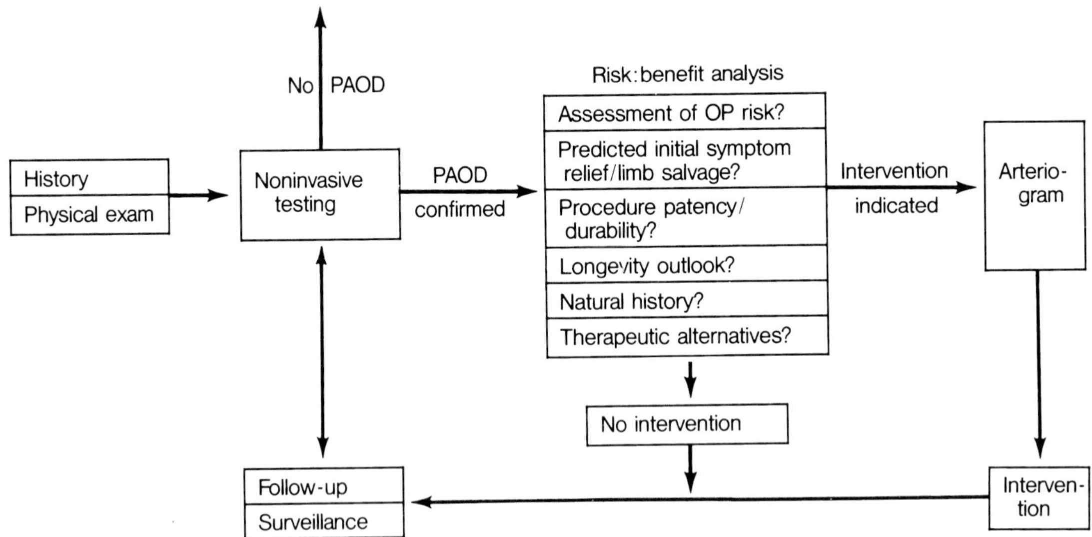

FIGURE 1–1. This algorithm shows the stepwise evaluation and management of patients presenting with peripheral arterial occlusive disease (PAOD). Note the central role played by noninvasive testing and the relegation of arteriography to therapeutic, *not diagnostic*, indications. OP, operative.

the initial evaluation for later dictation and can function as a temporary record until the transcribed note reaches the files.

Understandably, it is difficult for the experienced clinician to adhere to such a comprehensive approach. He or she will automatically proceed in algorithmic fashion, following the branches of a decision tree out to the area of appropriate focus. Nevertheless, organized evaluation forms like this can still serve as a guideline for students, house staff, and fellows as they first begin evaluating vascular problems. Auxiliary personnel may fill in parts, and in larger clinic practices (such as tabular checklists, particularly if modified for each of the major disease entities or operations encountered) can provide the basis for clinical investigation and computer-based records and a vascular registry.

The form shown here is intended only as an example. It is more elaborate than most will need, and physicians should develop their own versions. For most purposes, only the major historical subheadings need to be listed on the form (e.g., location, duration, frequency, course, influencing factors). Further, instead of using tabular forms for pulses, the location of edema, discoloration, or ulceration, one can use and mark an anatomic silhouette, with or without an outline of the arterial tree, to note the pertinent physical findings.

Finally, work forms destined to feed information into a vascular registry must be simpler still, because only essential and unambiguous categorical information should be stored in computers (see Chapter 3).

HISTORY AND PHYSICAL EXAMINATION

Patients with vascular diseases usually present with key complaints that often can be developed by pointed questioning into a reasonable presumptive diagnosis even before physical examination is performed. The major diagnostic considerations for the various forms of vascular disease are covered later in appropriate sections of this book. The intention at this point is to demonstrate, mainly with the lower extremity as an example, the value of knowing which questions to ask and which physical signs to seek. This problem-oriented approach is preferred to simply describing an uncorrelated list of vascular signs and symptoms.

The Painful Extremity

The most common presenting symptom in lower extremity vascular disease is pain. Knowing the pain's character, severity, location, frequency and duration, and temporal pattern and determining what precipitates or aggravates the pain or makes it subside can allow one to diagnose or rule out arterial and venous diseases with more than 90% certainty *before* the physical examination begins.

Acute arterial occlusion does not always produce the well-known "five Ps":

- Pain
- Pallor
- Pulselessness
- Paresthesias
- Paralysis

Pain may be evanescent, cyanosis often replaces pallor, pulses may be difficult to evaluate in those with preexisting arterial occlusive disease, and early changes in sensation and muscle strength may be easily missed. Early sensory deficits may be subtle. Light touch, two-point discrimination, vibratory perception, and proprioception are usually lost well before appreciation of deep pain and pressure. Similarly, most foot movements are produced by more proximal muscles (e.g., dorsiflexion or plantar flexion of toes is produced by muscles originating just below the knee), where ischemia may be far less profound than distally. Therefore, to detect early motor weakness, the physician should also test the function of intrinsic muscles of the foot, remembering that in some patients these muscles are not well developed. Capillary filling is usually impaired, the limb segments below the obstruction are noticeably cool, and venous filling may be diminished. These findings and the palpation of pulses should always be compared with the contralateral extremity.

The pain of *acute limb ischemia* is variable. In lesser degrees of ischemia, the pain may be absent or evanescent. If the pain is not severe and sustained and if the patients do not experience motor or sensory loss, they may not even seek immediate medical help and the absence of pulses may not be detected until later, when patients present with claudication or are examined for other reasons. Nevertheless, the initial pain of acute arterial occlusion usually is fairly characteristic. It is not identical to the ischemic rest pain of chronic severe ischemia (see later). It is not as well localized to the distal forefoot, nor is it clearly affected by gravity. It may share the same compelling intensity but tends to be more diffuse, often extending above the ankle in severer cases. It begins suddenly and reaches a peak rapidly in the case of arterial embolism, and patients may describe a sensation of the leg's being "struck" by a severe, shocking pain that renders it weak. If standing at the time, they may be forced to sit down immediately or may even crumple to the ground as the extremity gives way.

With *arterial thrombosis*, the clinical presentation is not usually as dramatic as with embolism, but the patient is usually aware of some sudden change in status; when the severity of ischemia is truly limb-threatening, pain quickly supervenes. The pain may subside in intensity, and depending on the severity of the ischemia that remains after the initial wave of vasospasm has passed and collateral channels are recruited, it may either resolve completely or settle into one of the typical pain patterns of chronic ischemia. The persistence of pain, particularly if followed by numbness, weakness, or both, indicates that one is dealing with severe, limb-threatening ischemia.

Chronic arterial insufficiency of the lower extremity causes two very characteristic types of pain:

- Intermittent claudication
- Ischemic rest pain

Claudication, although derived from the Latin word for limp *(claudicatio)*, has by usage come to mean a discomfort or disability associated with exercise. Depending on the level and extent of the arterial occlusive disease, the patient may present with buttock and thigh claudication, calf claudication, or foot claudication, either singly or in contiguous combination. The most common presentation—*calf claudication*—is easily recognized as a "cramping" pain in the calf that can be consistently reproduced by the same degree of exercise and that is completely relieved by a minute or so of rest. These calf cramps are not to be confused with those that occur at night in older patients, some of whom may even have pulse deficits or other signs of arterial occlusive disease. Nocturnal muscle cramps have no known vascular basis; rather, they are thought to result from an exaggerated neuromuscular response to stretch. Experienced clinicians can quickly differentiate between these two unrelated causes of leg cramps. They also realize that it is not unusual for older patients to experience no symptoms from superficial femoral artery occlusion because their sedentary existence protects them from claudication, and the occlusive process is gradual enough to allow concomitant development of collateral circulation, so that there is no ischemia at rest.

Pain or discomfort associated with tightness in the calf and precipitated by exercise may result from a *chronic compartment compression syndrome* (see Chapter 62). The patient is often an athlete or a runner with large calf muscles. Muscle swelling, increased compartment pressure, and impaired venous outflow constitute a vicious circle. However, this pain usually comes on after considerable exercise and does not quickly subside with rest.

Patients with arterial occlusive disease of more proximal (aortoiliac) distribution usually suffer from buttock and thigh claudication, although a significant number also complain of calf claudication. Buttock and thigh claudication does not usually produce the severe cramping muscular pain experienced in the calf. The sensation is more of an "aching" discomfort associated with *weakness*. These patients may even deny the existence of pain per se, complaining only that their hip or thigh "gives out" or "tires" after they have walked a certain distance. Patients with *osteoarthritis* of the hip or knee may complain of similar extremity discomfort that is also brought on by exercise; however, important differentiating factors are as follows:

1. The amount of exercise causing their symptoms is variable.
2. The pain does not disappear as promptly with rest.
3. The pain varies in severity from day to day, frequently in association with changes in weather conditions or physical activity.

Neurospinal compression, caused by osteophytic narrowing of the lower (lumbar) neurospinal canal, may simulate claudication secondary to aortoiliac occlusive disease. Usually, however, it is more of a numbing weakness that is also produced by standing (or anything increasing lumbar lordosis) rather than just ambulation, and it is not relieved by stopping unless the patient sits down or leans against a lamp post or tree with the upper body bent forward, and straightens out the lumbar spine. Further questioning often reveals that this weakness is associated with either numbness or paresthesias, sometimes involving the perineum. Because older patients not infrequently have diminished femoral pulses and proximal bruits, reflecting some degree of aortoiliac occlusive disease, it is not unusual for these other painful conditions to be wrongly ascribed to vascular disease. This is a classic example of the importance of matching symptoms and signs in terms of severity and distribution. It is unusual to have significant hip or buttock pain from iliac artery stenosis without associated thigh claudication. Furthermore, aortic or complete iliac artery occlusion with absence of femoral pulses on at least one side is usually necessary for such proximally distributed symptoms.

Finally, bilateral aortoiliac occlusive disease severe enough to produce disabling claudication is nearly always associated with impotence in men. The absence of impotence in a man with bilateral hip or thigh pain suggests that the pain may not be due to aortoiliac occlusive disease unless the occlusive lesions are limited to the external iliac arteries. Although true claudication is attributable to arterial occlusive disease, thigh claudication can also be experi-

PERIPHERAL VASCULAR WORKSHEET

Name ______ **Date** ______

Past History

Allergies ______ Operations ______
Injuries ______ Major illnesses ______
Pregnancies ______ Phlebitis ______
Pulmonary embolism ______ Serious infections ______
Cardiac: angina ______ CHF ______ MI ______
arrhythmia ______ DOE ______ orthopnea ______
Respiratory ______
Diabetes ______
Hypertension ______
Renal ______
Neurological: cerebrovascular ______
peripheral ______
Venereal disease ______
Arthritis, collagen vascular ______
Other ______

Family History

Same condition ______ Other vascular ______
Diabetes ______ Hypertension ______ CVA ______ Cardiac ______
Clotting abnormalities ______

Personal and Social

Alcohol ______ Tobacco ______
Education ______ Psychological ______
Occupations ______
Travel ______
Drug use: past ______
present ______

PERIPHERAL VASCULAR WORKSHEET

Name ______ **Date** ______

I. Complaints:	**Rank**	**Severity**	**Descriptive Comments**
Pain			
Weakness			
Hot/cold			
Numb/sensitive			
Discoloration			
Swelling			
Ulceration			
Varicose veins			

II. Location: R/L, medial/lateral, dorsal/ventral
Toes ______ Foot ______ Ankle ______ Leg ______ Knee ______
Fingers Hand Wrist Forearm Elbow
Thigh ______ Hip ______ Back ______ Other ______
Arm Shoulder Neck ______

III. Onset: sudden/gradual
IV. Duration: ______ days/weeks/months/years
V. Frequency: ______ times/day/week/month/year
VI. Temporal Pattern: continuous/intermittent/day/night/none
VII. Course: static/better/worse/fluctuates
VIII. Interferes With: sleep/work/exercise/other
IX. Influencing Factors (A-aggravates, R-relieves, O-no effect):
Elevation ______ Dependency ______ Exercise ______ Rest ______ Heat ______
Cold ______ Weather change ______ Menses ______ Emotions ______ Vibration ______
Pressure ______ Position ______
Activity ______
Other (including Rx) ______

FIGURE 1–2. Diagnostic checklist for vascular evaluation.

PERIPHERAL VASCULAR WORKSHEET

Physical Examination

Name ______ **Date** ______
Ht.______ Wt. ______ Pulse______ Temperature______ B.P.______
General ______ Head and neck ______
Heart______
Lungs______ Abdomen ______

Extremities		**Upper** right	left	**Lower** right	left
Skin	Warm/cool				
	Atrophied/thickened				
	Cyanosis/mottling				
	Pallor/rubor				
	Capillary filling				
	Hair growth				
	Nails				
Edema	Brawny/pitting/spongy				
	Degree				
	Extent				
	Subcutaneous atrophy fibrosis				
	Ulceration/tissue loss				
	Discoloration/pigmentation				
	Erythema/cellulitis				
	Lymphangitis				
Musculoskeletal	Symmetry/atrophy				
	Hypertrophy				
	Joint enlargement/swelling				
	Range of motion				
	Reflexes				
	Sensory				
	Motor				

PERIPHERAL VASCULAR WORKSHEET

Arterial Survey	**Right** pulse	bruit	aneurysm	**Left** pulse	bruit	aneurysm
Carotid						
Subclavian						
Brachial						
Radial						
Ulnar						
Abdominal aorta						
Iliac						
Femoral						
Popliteal						
Dorsalis pedis						
Posterior tibial						

Venous Survey **Code:** N = normal; P = prominent, tense; V = varicose; T = thrombosed

	Right	**Left**
Greater saphenous		
Lesser saphenous		
Anterolateral thigh		
Posteromedial thigh		
Anterior tibial		
Posterior arch		
Perforators		
Intracutaneous venules		
Tourniquet test		

Demographic Data
Name______ Date ______ History no. ______
Address______ Occupation ______
Age______ Sex ______ Nationality/race______
Referring physician ______ Telephone no. ______
Address______

FIGURE 1–2 *Continued*

enced because of venous occlusion. This venous "claudication" usually results because recanalization has not occurred after iliofemoral venous thrombosis. At rest, collateral vessels allow venous outflow to match arterial inflow without the development of high venous pressures but cannot handle the severalfold increases in arterial inflow associated with exercise. The venous channels in the thigh or leg become engorged and tense, and it is this high venous pressure—not ischemia—that is the source of the pain, which is often appropriately described as a "bursting" pain or a tight, heavy sensation. Because this venous engorgement is slow to subside, the pain does not abate as quickly as that of claudication due to arterial occlusive disease.

Foot claudication occurring on an ischemic basis is very rare. It may exist independently of calf claudication if the occlusive lesions are diffuse and involve all the infrapopliteal arteries distally, but it is just as commonly associated with more proximal occlusions and calf pain. It has a greater relative frequency in thromboangiitis obliterans than in arteriosclerosis obliterans because of the typically more distal distribution of occlusive lesions in the former condition. The patient usually complains of a painful ache, a "drawing" pain or cramp in the forefoot, associated only with walking. Patients usually also complain of a "wooden" sensation or numbness in the same distribution and of a persistently cold foot at night. Frequently, they have visited several podiatrists or have tried a variety of arch supports or "orthopedic" shoes. This rarest form of lower extremity claudication usually occurs only with advanced degrees of arterial insufficiency and, therefore, is commonly associated with ischemic rest pain of the foot. This form of claudication can be confused with arthritic or inflammatory processes involving the foot (e.g., rheumatoid arthritis, plantar fasciitis, or metatarsalgia, with the latter two often seen in joggers). With these other conditions, however, the relationship with exercise and rest is variable and not as precisely precipitated and relieved. Table 1–1 outlines the differential diagnosis of claudication at these three levels with the conditions that mimic them.

One may encounter cases in which either the clinical diagnosis of arterial claudication is not clear-cut or the symptoms and findings, although compatible with the diagnosis, do not match it in severity. In such cases, noninvasive testing can be extremely helpful (see Chapter 10). For example, the ankle pressure after exercise sufficient to reproduce the pain should fall to the vicinity of 50 mmHg or below. If not, the patient may have two causes of leg pain, the lesser of which is related to arterial insufficiency.

Ischemic rest pain, as seen in *chronic critical ischemia*, is typically a nocturnal pain of disturbing severity that diffusely involves the foot distal to the tarsal bones, although pain may be sharply localized to the vicinity of an ischemic ulcer or gangrenous toe. The pain may be so severe that it is not relieved even by substantial doses of narcotics. Patients who sleep in a *horizontal* position are typically awakened by this pain and forced to get up and do something about it. They may sit up and rub or hold the painful foot, get up and pace the floor, or walk to the medicine cabinet to take an analgesic. Any of these responses may relieve the pain fairly promptly, but only by the unwitting recruiting of the help of gravity in improving the perfusion pressure to the distal tissues. Although patients may at first wrongly attribute the relief to rubbing the foot, walking, or even an amazingly fast-acting analgesic, eventually they learn to sleep with the foot *dependent*, either dangling it over the side of the bed and resting it on a chair, or sleeping out the night in a lounge chair. This pain pattern is too characteristic to be missed by the careful interrogator, but the unwary may be thrown off by the rubor and apparent prompt capillary filling of the toes, observed when seated patients remove their shoes. This "dependent pallor" is matched by "cadaveric pallor" if the leg is elevated (Buerger's signs; see later), but many physicians do not go beyond the erroneous initial impression.

Occasionally, patients with arthritic changes in the small bones of the feet (metatarsals, usually) can experience "metatarsalgia" that occurs primarily at night and is relieved by standing. This can be seen with either degenerative osteoarthritis or rheumatoid arthritis. Its occurrence is irregular (i.e., it may be present or absent for several days to weeks), thus distinguishing it from ischemic rest pain, which occurs whenever the patient lies down for any length of time.

Pain associated with *venous disease* of the lower extremity is not as characteristic as the arterial pain syndromes. Fortunately, venous conditions usually are easily recognized by their associated physical findings. The example of pain associated with activity seen in proximal venous obstruction has already been mentioned, but most pain from chronic venous insufficiency is a consequence of valve reflux in patent veins. Severe pain is not a common complaint of patients with *primary varicose veins*. In fact, one must be suspicious when older patients with varicose veins present with pain, particularly if the varicosities are of long standing and have not previously been painful. Such patients may be suffering from extremity pain of another, more obscure etiology, although blaming it on the visible varicosities and leading the physician into the same trap. Occasionally, varicose veins produce a "pulling," "pricking," "burning," or "tingling" discomfort that is well localized to the varicose veins themselves, unlike the diffuse sensation of fatigue or heaviness that is commonly associated with pain and ache in patients with deep venous insufficiency. Although these symptoms, as with all venous discomfort, are relieved by elevation, the tingling and burning sensation often worsens during the initial period of elevation before it subsides.

Venous thrombosis in the lower extremity may cause little or no *acute* pain unless the associated inflammatory reaction is significant, in which case there may also be localized tenderness along the course of the involved vein. Swelling, either early or later in the postphlebitic period, is not uncommonly associated with a moderate aching discomfort and a tight or heavy sensation; severe, "bursting" pain, however, is rare unless the patient is spending too much time in the upright position or still has significant residual obstruction to venous outflow *(venous claudication)*. Although the symptoms associated with venous valvular insufficiency or obstruction (in the absence of associated inflammation) are extremely variable, their aggravation by standing and relief by elevation are consistent, and this relationship should always be explored. The presence of significant discomfort after standing for long periods or walking with chronic venous valvular insufficiency or ob-

TABLE 1–1. DIFFERENTIAL DIAGNOSIS OF CLAUDICATION

CONDITION	LOCATION OF PAIN OR DISCOMFORT	CHARACTERISTIC DISCOMFORT	ONSET RELATIVE TO EXERCISE	EFFECT OF REST	EFFECT OF BODY POSITION	OTHER CHARACTERISTICS
Intermittent Claudication (Calf)						
Venous compartment syndrome	Calf muscles	Cramping pain	After *same* degree of exercise	Quickly relieved	None	Reproducible
	Calf muscles	Tight, bursting pain	After *much* exercise (e.g., jogging)	Subsides very slowly	Relief speeded by elevation	Typically heavy muscled athletes
Venous claudication	Entire leg, but usually worse in thigh and groin	Tight, bursting pain	After walking	Subsides slowly	Relief speeded by elevation	History of iliofemoral deep venous thrombosis, signs of venous congestion, edema
Nerve root compression (e.g., herniated disc)	Radiates down leg, usually posteriorly	Sharp lancinating pain	Soon, if not immediately after onset	Not quickly relieved (also often present at rest)	Relief may be aided by adjusting back position	History of back problems
Intermittent Claudication (Hip, Thigh, Buttock)						
Hip arthritis	Hip, thigh, buttocks	Aching discomfort, weakness	After *same* degree of exercise	Quickly relieved	None	Reproducible
	Hip, thigh, buttocks	Aching discomfort	After *variable* degree of exercise	*Not* quickly relieved (and may be present at rest)	More comfortable sitting, weight taken off legs	*Variable,* may relate to activity level, weather changes
Neurospinal root compression	Hip, thigh, buttocks (follows dermatome)	Weakness more than pain	After walking or standing for same length of time	Relieved by stopping only if position changed	Relief by lumbar spine flexion (sitting or stooping forward)	Frequent history of back problems; provoked by increased intra-abdominal pressure
Intermittent Claudication (Foot)						
Arthritic, inflammatory processes	Foot, arch	Severe deep pain and numbness	After *same* degree of exercise	Quickly relieved	None	Reproducible
	Foot, arch	Aching pain	After *variable* degree of exercise	*Not* quickly relieved (and may be present at rest)	May be relieved by not bearing weight	*Variable,* may relate to activity level

struction (respectively) stands in marked contrast to the lack of discomfort associated with lymphedema (see later).

Patients with other forms of extremity pain are often referred to the vascular surgeon under the false presumption that the pain is circulatory in origin, and therefore the surgeon must be able to recognize the nonvascular extremity pain syndromes or at least the common ones associated with nerve or musculoskeletal derangements. As previously pointed out, the pain of *arthritis* or *sciatica* usually is fairly characteristic and easily distinguishable from that caused by vascular disease. However, two other conditions cause extremity pain that can masquerade as vascular disease because of the associated vascular signs. One is a painful *peripheral neuritis* commonly seen in diabetics and, because their peripheral pulses may be diminished and they may have rubor and trophic skin changes, the examiner may mistake the problem for arterial insufficiency rather than the early stage of diabetic neuropathy. Later stages of diabetic neuropathy are characteristically painless, and the associated neurologic signs are obvious, but in the early "neuritic" stages, the neurologic signs may be subtle, often no more than a patchy loss of light touch, vibratory sense, and two-point discrimination.

The other misleading type of extremity pain is *reflex sympathetic dystrophy*, or *minor causalgia*. Like the neuritis, the pain it produces is usually burning in character. *Major causalgia*, associated with incomplete nerve injury, usually is easily recognized; the minor variety, which may follow relatively minimal trauma or acute circulatory problems such as venous or arterial thrombosis, must always be kept in mind by the vascular surgeon. Similarly, there is the patient with residual discomfort following back surgery (disc operations, lumbar fusions), which is often labeled "arachnoiditis." However, this is actually a form of causalgic pain resulting from the "trauma" of long-standing nerve compression.

Typically, there are the signs of autonomic imbalance, the "vascular" signs that originally attracted the attention of the referring physician. The causalgic extremity may be warm and dry initially, but later becomes cool, mottled, or cyanotic. Eventually, trophic changes develop that are not unlike those of arterial insufficiency. The pain is not always classically superficial, burning, and localized to the distribution of a somatic nerve as originally described. If there are reasonable grounds for suspicion after initial evaluation, relief of the pain by a proximal arterial injection of 10 to 15 mg of tolazoline, confirmed later by a paravertebral sympathetic block, establishes the diagnosis (see Chapter 63).

Physical examination of the painful extremity is usually carried out by a "prejudiced" examiner if a careful history has been taken, for the reasons already given, and it is difficult to be systematic when physical findings confirming one's suspicions immediately catch the eye. A complete and thorough initial examination, however, should be carried out. Discovery of a previously undetected diastolic hypertension, carotid bruit, fibrillating heart, or abdominal aortic aneurysm may be the dividend of such thoroughness. Furthermore, documentation of the state of the peripheral pulses may well have future value.

Examination of the abdomen should consist of more than a brief palpation for an occult aneurysm. For example, lower abdominal bruits may provide the only physical clue of aortoiliac occlusive disease in a patient with buttock and thigh claudication, since there may be no signs of chronic ischemia and a femoral pulse may be readily palpated because a hemodynamically significant iliac artery stenosis may produce a pressure gradient of as little as 10 mmHg at rest.

If such patients (with "critical" stenoses) exercise to the point of claudication, they usually temporarily "lose" the previously palpable pedal pulses because of the marked decrease in vascular resistance that occurs in exercising muscle distal to an obstruction and the increased distribution of flow to muscle beds proximal to the obstruction. This is the basis for the practice of monitoring ankle pressure following a standard treadmill exercise (see Chapter 10).

Another example of claudication with palpable pulses should be kept in mind. If one elicits a good history of claudication in a *young* patient with palpable pedal pulses, one should suspect popliteal entrapment (see Chapter 75) and recheck the pulses during active plantar flexion or passive dorsiflexion.

Palpating Pulses

Femoral pulses may be difficult to palpate in muscular or obese patients unless the hips are externally rotated and the vessels are palpated over the pubic ramus of the ilium, where they lie 1½ to 2 fingerbreadths lateral to the pubic tubercle and are covered by less fat. Even for the experienced examiner, the *popliteal pulses* are often difficult to palpate—so difficult, in fact, that the knowledgeable vascular surgeon who feels them too easily usually suspects at once the possibility of a fusiform popliteal aneurysm. Holding the supine patient's knee partially flexed plus allowing it to fall gently back into the examiner's hand, which is positioned so that the proximal interphalangeal joints hook the tendons while the fingertips sink gently into the middle of the popliteal space, is just as effective a means of palpating popliteal pulses as having the patient turn into the prone position with the knee flexed.

The location of the *posterior tibial pulse* in the hollow behind the medial malleolus and that of the *dorsalis pedis pulse* along the dorsum of the foot between the first and the second metatarsal bones are well known. It is less well appreciated that one or the other of these pedal pulses is not palpable in almost 10% of normal persons. In such cases, the lateral tibial artery, the terminal branch of the peroneal artery, should be sought higher in the foot, just below the ankle and medial to the bony prominence of the fibula. A warm room and a light touch are the best combination for the most accurate detection of pedal pulses. Otherwise, it must be hoped that the examiner's and the patient's pulses are distinctly different in rate.

Finally, it is important to listen for bruits over the course of these major arteries, especially at or above the most proximal pulse that feels weaker than normal. It is surprising how often the telltale bruit of an iliac stenosis is not even auscultated.

Signs of Advanced Ischemia

Severe claudication may be associated with atrophy of the calf muscles; unless this is unilateral and produces asymmetry, however, it may escape detection. Loss of hair growth over the dorsum of the toes and foot is another relatively common sign of arterial insufficiency, and this may be accompanied by thickening of the toenails secondary to slowness of nail growth. More advanced ischemic changes, however, such as atrophy of the skin and its appendages and the subcutaneous tissue, so that the foot becomes shiny, scaly, and "skeletonized," usually do not appear in the absence of ischemic rest pain. Delayed return of the capillary blush after pressure on the pulp of the digit and slow venous filling after dropping the elevated extremity back into the dependent position are also signs of advanced ischemia.

Buerger's sign (i.e., cadaveric pallor on elevation and rubor on dependency) occurs with very restricted arterial inflow and chronic dilatation of the peripheral vascular bed beyond, particularly the postcapillary venules. The dependent toes may appear so red and may refill so rapidly after pressure application that the uninitiated may mistakenly consider this to be evidence of hyperemia rather than an expression of severe ischemia. Localized pallor or cyanosis associated with poor capillary filling is usually a prelude to ischemic gangrene or ulceration. At this advanced stage of chronic critical ischemia, the foot may be edematous from being continually kept in the dependent position in an attempt to relieve the ischemic pain.

Signs of Venous Insufficiency

As previously stated, lower extremity pain secondary to venous disease is inconstant. In addition, the discomfort caused by venous distention from whatever cause is similar in character, as is its relief by elevation. Therefore, the physical findings associated with these venous problems may be extremely helpful in differentiating between them. For example, *varicose veins* may be the result of primary saphenofemoral incompetence or may be secondary to deep venous and perforator incompetence. In the untreated state, the latter produces brawny edema, stasis dermatitis, and ulceration. By contrast, the edema associated with primary uncomplicated varicose veins is mild and rarely appears early in the day, dermatitis with pigmentation is restricted to the skin immediately overlying prominent varicosities, and ulceration does *not* occur in early cases. Furthermore, primary varicose veins typically involve the main saphenous vein and its major branches rather than scattered tributaries, and they do not refill quickly on standing after a tourniquet has been applied to the upper thigh (positive tourniquet test).

An acutely thrombosed superficial vein feels like a cord; it is tender and may be surrounded by erythema, skin pigmentation, warmth, swelling, induration, and other localized signs of inflammation. Even acute thrombosis of a deep vein, if associated with a sufficient inflammatory reaction, may result in tenderness along its course. Usually, however, it produces a more generalized edema distally. If the deep calf veins are thrombosed, there may be pain on dorsiflexion *(Homans' sign)*, tenderness on anteroposterior but not lateral compression of the calf *(Bancroft's sign)*, and prompt pain in the calf caused by inflating a sphygmomanometer cuff around it to a pressure of 80 mmHg *(Löwenberg's sign)*. These signs, however, are said to be present in fewer than a third of patients with acute deep venous thrombosis (DVT) and are not to be relied on.

The oft-quoted rates of "one-third false-positive" and "one-third false-negative" for diagnosis of thrombophlebitis, when made on clinical grounds alone, apply more to a hospital population of patients at bed rest in whom occult thrombosis is more likely to occur and in whom swelling is more likely to be absent. On the other hand, outpatients with this condition usually present *because of* signs or symptoms, and therefore a higher rate of diagnostic accuracy may be expected in this setting. Nevertheless, this diagnosis can be made confidently on clinical grounds *only* in cases of extensive, major venous thrombosis (e.g., phlegmasia cerulea dolens or phlegmasia alba dolens) or those associated with a marked inflammatory reaction. In contrast, the combination of two simple noninvasive tests (venous plethysmography and venous Doppler examination) or, preferably, examination of the veins with a color duplex scanner, is 95% accurate in diagnoses of DVT (see Chapter 139).

The Swollen Leg

After the painful leg, the swollen leg is the next most common problem on which the vascular surgeon is called to consult. In examining the swollen leg, the consultant should remember another "five Ps":

- Pressure
- Protein
- Permeability
- Paresis
- Pendency

Plasma constituents move into the tissues and return to the vascular space normally during circulation according to Starling's law. The balance of factors influencing this process is a delicate one, particularly in the lower extremity, where gravity provides an additional complicating factor. The valved venomotor pump mechanism is presumably an evolutionary adaptation to the assumption of the upright position by humans, for if a normal person were to stand motionless long enough, venous pressures at the ankle would stabilize in the range of 80 to 100 mmHg and swelling and petechial hemorrhages would appear. With a competent venomotor pump mechanism, however, even modest activity of the calf muscles, such as occurs in intermittently shifting one's weight, reduces this pressure to 20 to 30 mmHg, and what little swelling accumulates during the day usually disappears overnight, when the body is horizontal. Patients who do not take advantage of this respite (e.g., those who sleep night after night with their feet dependent to relieve ischemic pain) experience chronic swelling, as do patients with peroneal palsy or an arthritic or fused ankle who cannot activate the venomotor pump.

Increased permeability secondary to inflammation results in swelling if the extremity is not kept elevated. Similarly, swelling is seen in secondary aldosteronism. The lymphatics are the route by which extravasated protein is returned to the central circulation. If the clearance capacity of this system is restricted because it is congenitally hypoplastic, because it is obliterated by episodes of lymphangitis, or because its outflow is obstructed or interrupted by surgery or irradiation, protein-rich lymph will accumulate in the tissues. A similar mechanism, in reverse, applies in hypoproteinemia, and this occasional cause of swelling should be considered in obscure cases.

High venous pressure is the most common cause of extremity swelling. The source of this increased peripheral venous pressure may be due to (1) a cardiac condition, as in right-sided heart failure or tricuspid valvular disease; or (2) *intrinsic* venous obstruction, as in peripheral venous thrombosis, or (3) *extrinsic* compression, as of the left iliac vein by the right iliac artery. Most commonly, however, the increased pressure is a result of the unrelenting and unopposed transmission, in the upright position, of gravitational pressure through incompetent valves of the deep and communicating veins to the superficial tissues. Venous hypertension secondary to arteriovenous fistulae is rarer and seldom causes swelling in the absence of venous obstruction; however, it does cause changes similar to though more localized than those generally ascribed to venous "stasis" (discussed later).

Clinically, the differential diagnosis of swelling may be difficult when it is of brief duration; in the chronic state, however, characteristic physical findings appear that greatly simplify matters. When a patient presents with a chronically swollen leg, the experienced examiner may make the correct diagnosis in more than 95% of cases simply by noting the distribution of the swelling, its response to elevation, and the associated discomfort and skin changes. These and other diagnostic considerations pertinent to chronically swollen lower extremities are presented in Table 1–2.

If there are no obvious associated skin changes and the edema "pits" readily on pressure, its cause is usually central or systemic (e.g., heart disease, hypoproteinemia, or secondary aldosteronism). The distribution of this type of swelling, sometimes called *orthostatic edema*, is diffuse, but the swelling is greatest peripherally and, to some extent, also involves the foot. The edema associated with peripheral venous disease, even in the acute stage, does not pit readily. In the chronic stage, it is frankly "brawny" and associated with characteristic skin changes caused by chronic venous hypertension. The breakdown of extravasated red blood cells causes the characteristic pigmentation and, together with increased fibrin in the interstitial fluid, leads to inflammation and fibrosis in the subcutaneous tissues. Later, the skin becomes atrophic and breaks down with minor trauma.

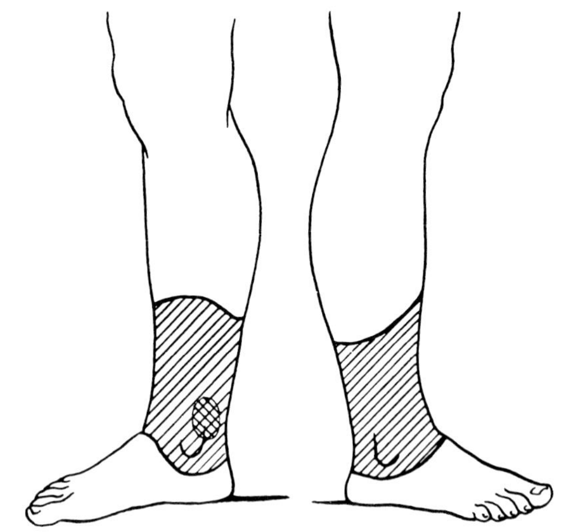

FIGURE 1–3. The "gaiter" distribution of stasis dermatitis and leg ulcers.

These components of so-called stasis dermatitis have a "gaiter" distribution (Figure 1–3), and even in earlier stages, when edema predominates, the feet often are relatively spared compared with the ankles and lower half of the legs. The reason is that this venous hypertension is transmitted to the superficial veins by incompetent perforator veins located in this gaiter area. Eventually, progression of these chronic changes converts the skin and subcutaneous tissues of the lower leg from a diffusely edematous state to a pigmented, atrophic, tightly scarred zone, which, when viewed in contrast to the proximal edema, leads to the descriptive term "inverted-champagne-bottle-leg."

When the vascular surgeon sees a patient with advanced changes of chronic venous insufficiency, it may be impossible, by just looking at the leg, to tell whether these are sequelae of DVT or primary venous valvular incompetence, beginning with varicose veins. A history of DVT or a family history of varicosities is often lacking. A useful approach is to ask which came first. Because it takes considerable time for saphenofemoral venous incompetence to progress downward to involve the perforator and even tibial veins,

TABLE 1–2. DIFFERENTIAL DIAGNOSIS OF CHRONIC LEG SWELLING

CLINICAL FEATURE	VENOUS	LYMPHATIC	CARDIAC ORTHOSTATIC	"LIPEDEMA"
Consistency of swelling	Brawny	Spongy	Pitting	Noncompressible (fat)
Relief by elevation	Complete	Mild	Complete	Minimal
Distribution of swelling	Maximal in ankles and legs, feet spared	Diffuse, greatest distally	Diffuse, greatest distally	Maximal in ankles and legs, feet spared
Associated skin changes	Atrophic and pigmented, subcutaneous fibrosis	Hypertrophied, lichenified skin	Shiny, mild pigmentation, no trophic changes	None
Pain	Heavy ache, tight or bursting	None or heavy ache	Little or none	Dull ache, cutaneous sensitivity
Bilaterality	Occasionally, but usually unequal	Occasionally, but usually unequal	Always, but may be unequal	Always

such patients will admit that they had the varicose veins for many years before swelling and stasis skin changes developed. Patients with post-thrombotic changes may not know they had DVT but they will remember having normal legs before a particular point in time when there was rather abrupt onset of swelling, with stasis skin changes and secondary varicosities coming some time later.

The distribution of *lymphedema* is diffuse, but the swelling is always greater distally, beginning with the toes and moving upward. This swelling is neither pitting nor brawny but firmly "spongy" in character; that is, although it does not significantly resist deformation by pressure, the skin and subcutaneous tissues quickly return to their original position as the pressure is withdrawn. Skin pigmentation and ulceration are rare. If anything, the skin eventually becomes hypertrophic. The end stage of chronic lymphatic insufficiency, *elephantiasis*, with its folds of thickened, lichenified skin hanging over the ankle, is too characteristic to be missed.

Occasionally, patients with the "post-thrombotic syndrome" whose condition progresses to stasis dermatitis and ulceration early may not have typical scarring and contraction of the subcutaneous tissue but instead have an elephantiasis-like appearance. This confusing variant is caused by invasive infection via the chronically ulcerated skin, which obliterates subcutaneous lymphatics and leads to secondary lymphedema.

Not uncommonly, women present with chronically "swollen" legs that have none of the foregoing characteristics. Although often reluctant to admit it, they usually confess that they have always had "thick" ankles. These patients, and often other female relatives, have maldistribution of fat characterized by excessive peripheral deposition in the arms as well as the legs. For unknown reasons, these women are prone to superimposed orthostatic edema and complain of a dull ache and sensitivity of the overlying skin. This swelling, sometimes referred to as *lipedema*, never completely subsides with elevation or diuretics. Furthermore, it is symmetric, with a noticeable sparing of the feet.

Finally, swelling, which always feels greater to the patient than it appears to the examiner, may represent a form of dysesthesia. If such patients also complain of superficial burning discomfort and show signs of autonomic imbalance, a minor form of causalgia or reflex sympathetic dystrophy should be suspected.

The Ulcerated Leg

The third most common problem for which the vascular specialist is likely to be consulted is leg ulcers. There are only three types of chronic ulcers commonly encountered in the lower extremities: (1) ischemic, (2) neurotrophic, and (3) stasis. These forms of ulceration are readily distinguished from one another, as outlined in Table 1–3.

Ischemic ulcers are usually quite painful, and there is likely to be typical ischemic rest pain in the distal forefoot that occurs nocturnally and is relieved by dependency. At first, these ulcers may have irregular edges, but when chronic, they are more likely to be "punched-out." They are commonly located distally over the dorsum of the foot or toes, but may occasionally be pretibial. The ulcer base usually consists of poorly developed, grayish granulation tissue. The surrounding skin may be pale or mottled, and the previously described signs of chronic ischemia are invariably present. Notably, the usual signs of inflammation one would expect surrounding such a skin lesion are absent, for it is the lack of enough circulation to provide the necessary inflammatory response for healing that underlies ischemic ulcers. For the same reason, probing or débriding the ulcer causes little bleeding.

Neurotrophic ulcers, however, are completely painless but bleed with manipulation. They are deep and indolent and are often surrounded not only by acute but also by chronic inflammatory reaction and callus. Their location is typically over pressure points or calluses (e.g., the plantar surface of the first or fifth metatarsophalangeal joint, the base of the distal phalanx of the great toe, the dorsum of the interphalangeal joints of toes with flexion contractures, or the callused posterior rim of the heel pad). The patient usually has long-standing diabetes with a neuropathy characterized by patchy hypesthesia and diminished positional sense, two-point discrimination, and vibratory perception.

The so-called *venous stasis ulcer*, actually due to venous hypertension, is located within the gaiter area (see Fig. 1–3), most commonly near the medial malleolus. It is usually larger than the other types of ulcers and irregular in outline, but also shallower and with a moist granulating base. It is always surrounded by a zone of inflammation and "stasis dermatitis," as already described.

More than 95% of all chronic leg or foot ulcers fit into one of these three recognizable types. The remainder are difficult to distinguish, except that they are not typical of the other three types. Leg ulcers may also be produced by (1) vasculitis, (2) hypertension, and (3) syphilis. Vasculitis often produces multiple punched-out holes and an inflamed indurated base that, on biopsy, suggests fat necrosis or chronic "panniculitis." Hypertensive ulcers represent focal infarcts and are very painful. They may be located around the malleoli, particularly laterally. Although syphilitic ulcers are uncommon today, in any atypical ulcer this or other systemic causes of ulceration, such as chronic ulcerative colitis with pyoderma gangrenosum or tuberculosis, should be suspected. Long-standing ulcers that are refractory to treatment may represent underlying osteomyelitis or a secondary malignant lesion.

Finally, most patients with ulcers of one of the specific types just described name trauma as the initiating agent. Occasionally, trauma may actually be the primary causative factor, with the chronicity of the ulcer being related either to the slow healing that is characteristic of the lower third of the leg or, possibly, to a degree of arterial insufficiency that would otherwise be subclinical. Uncomplicated traumatic ulcers often heal with nonspecific therapy, such as intermittent elevation and application of an Unna boot.

SUMMARY

Good vascular consultation is exemplified by the problem-oriented approach to the painful, swollen, or ulcerated leg;

TABLE 1–3. DIFFERENTIAL DIAGNOSIS OF COMMON LEG ULCERS

TYPE	USUAL LOCATION	PAIN	BLEEDING WITH MANIPULATION	LESION CHARACTERISTICS	SURROUNDING INFLAMMATION	ASSOCIATED FINDINGS
Ischemic	Distally, on dorsum of foot or toes	Severe, particularly at night, relieved by dependency	Little or none	Irregular edge, poor granulation tissue	Absent	Trophic changes of chronic ischemia, absent pulses
Stasis	Lower third of leg (gaiter area)	Mild, relieved by elevation	Venous ooze	Shallow, irregular shape, granulating base, rounded edges	Present	Stasis dermatitis
Neurotrophic	Under calluses or pressure points (e.g., plantar aspect of first or fifth metatarsophalangeal joint)	None	May be brisk	Punched-out, with deep sinus	Present	Demonstrable neuropathy

by careful interrogation; and by thoughtful examination—all guided by experience and an appropriate index of suspicion. Having completed the initial assessment at the bedside or in the office, the vascular surgeon must next consider the need to proceed further diagnostically, either for the sake of diagnosis itself or to provide further objective information on which to base therapeutic decisions. Whether or not the basic diagnosis is obvious, the location and extent of the vascular disease and the degree of circulatory impairment can often be objectively documented by noninvasive diagnostic methods, such as those described in Chapter 2.

Angiographic confirmation is usually obtained *only* if necessary in order to make major therapeutic decisions, including the feasibility of reconstructive vascular surgery or transluminal balloon angioplasty. Because these procedures are not without risk and expense, the choice between interventional and noninterventional (conservative) treatment (see Chapter 2) can and should be made *before* angiographic studies are initiated (see Fig. 1–1).

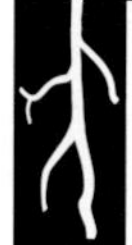

CHAPTER 2

Evaluation and Selection of Patients for Vascular Interventions

Robert B. Rutherford, M.D.

KEY CONSIDERATIONS IN SELECTION OF PATIENTS

The proper selection of patients for interventional treatment, whether it be endovascular or open surgery, is a cornerstone of clinical ability for the vascular surgeon, equal in importance to technical skill. The process can be viewed as a risk:benefit analysis that must always be settled in the patient's favor. The key considerations are outlined in Figure 2–1.

One must weigh carefully both the degree of disability and the natural course of the underlying vascular disorder with optimal medical management against the risk and projected benefits of the intervention under consideration. The benefits of the various interventional options should be considered in terms of both degree and duration; these will vary from patient to patient for the *same* procedure, but we can estimate them by considering specific variables, such as runoff, clinical class, choice of graft, longevity, and other factors known to affect the risk of the procedure and the risk of late failure. The risk of any intervention also clearly varies with the patient. Therefore, this decision process must be *individualized,* and predicted outcomes—in terms of such end points as mortality and major morbidity, initial and late patency, and functional improvement—all must be adjusted to apply to a given procedure being performed on a particular patient by a particular surgeon or other interventionalist.

Typically, this process begins, as depicted in Figure 2–2 (using surgical intervention for peripheral *arterial* occlusive disease as an example), with the initial patient interview and examination, complemented by noninvasive testing, when appropriate. This practice often establishes the nature and severity of the vascular problem and determines whether the patient is likely to be a candidate for intervention. Further studies, such as pulmonary function tests, creatinine clearance, and cardiac stress testing, may be required to evaluate risk, and *only* after these are completed and one is still willing to seriously consider an intervention

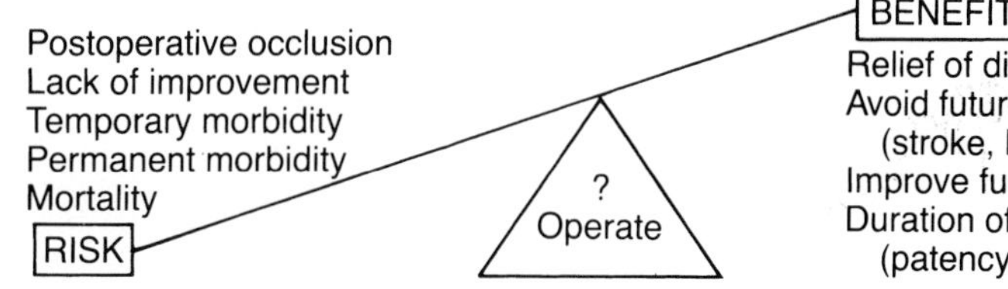

FIGURE 2–1. The risk:benefit analysis that underlies the decision to operate requires accurate assessment of the risks of mortality and morbidity for a given operation, the frequency and consequences of technical and hemodynamic failure (longevity, patency rate), and the likelihood of serious events or sequelae associated with the (medically treated) natural history of the condition.

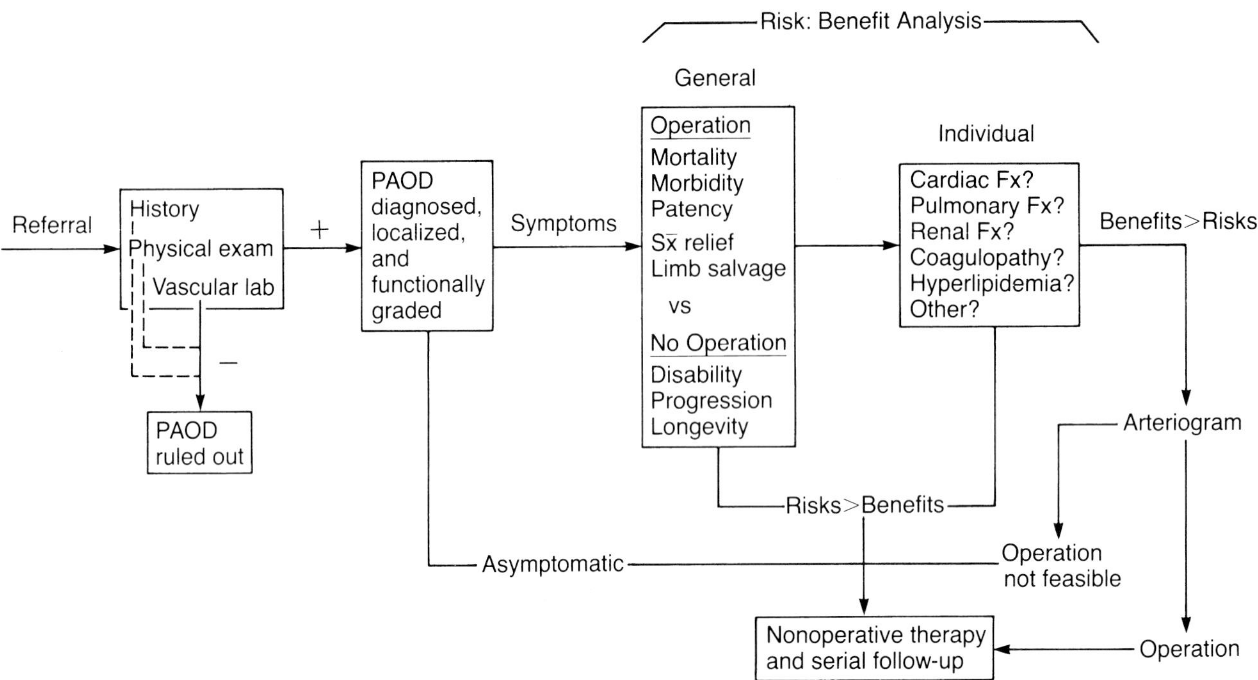

FIGURE 2–2. Stepwise approach to the decision to operate, beginning with initial consultation or outpatient visit and ending, after complete evaluation has confirmed the patient to be a surgical candidate with a reasonable operating risk, with arteriography. PAOD = peripheral arterial occlusive disease.

is an angiogram obtained, to assess the morphologic and anatomic characteristics of the involved vascular segment and, therefore, the most appropriate procedure and its technical feasibility. Obtaining an arteriogram at the *end* of the evaluation is like getting a road map—you don't need it unless you are going to make the trip! However, the development of percutaneous endovascular approaches to deal with many forms of vascular disease has led to some modification of this traditional approach.

Normally, angiography is instrumental in helping one decide between basic treatment options; however, there are certain situations in which, after initial evaluation, one would not recommend an open surgical revascularization but might recommend balloon angioplasty, with or without stenting, as appropriate, if a discrete lesion favorable for the latter treatment were found during arteriography. An example would be a significantly disabled claudicant with a discrete common iliac stenosis. In another example, a similarly disabled claudicant with a femoropopliteal occlusive lesion, duplex scanning can be used to distinguish between short and long occlusive lesions. The latter finding would likely eliminate the need for arteriography because a bypass would not ordinarily be indicated. Conversely, with a short lesion, percutaneous transluminal angioplasty (PTA) would be competing primarily with conservative management (exercise training and possibly pharmacotherapy), not bypass surgery.

Finally, it is important that the preliminary evaluation and investigations be completed before arteriography is performed, because the decision to proceed with balloon angioplasty should be made at the time of arteriography to allow it to be performed during the same session. This practice is in the patient's best interest, and it reduces costs. Needless to say, this requires everyone involved in the decision to be present at the completion of the arteriogram unless they are willing to abrogate their role. This approach is a far cry from a previous era, when one could recommend arteriography and review the findings some time later before making therapeutic recommendations.

The value of considering these factors can best be demonstrated by additional examples drawn primarily from chronic arterial and venous insufficiency of the lower extremities.

Degree of Disability

Disability usually constitutes a relative (rather than a mandatory) indication for intervention, in that the degree of disability must be considered against the background of the patient's work and other normal activities. Claudication that arises after walking one block may not interfere significantly with the sedentary lives of many retired persons, but to one who has worked long and hard in anticipation of a retirement filled with golf, hiking, or travel, that same degree of claudication constitutes a serious restriction. Claudication usually interferes significantly with the lives of most working persons and is an accepted indication for intervention when associated risk factors are reasonable and exercise training has been tried. Persistent ischemic rest pain, however, is an utterly disabling symptom that usually cannot be controlled even with strong analgesics or narcotics and is, therefore, a widely accepted indication for intervention even if it involves arterial reconstructive surgery for almost all patients.

Normal daily activities play as major a role in the choice of the appropriate treatment option for chronic venous insufficiency as for claudication. A homemaker, however busy, can usually arrange duties so that the involved leg can be elevated frequently; an automobile assembly line worker, scrub nurse, barber, or shopkeeper may not be able to follow a strict routine of leg elevation (e.g., for 10 minutes out of every 2 hours) in addition to wearing elastic support hose, which is acknowledged to control all but the severest degrees of chronic venous insufficiency. Other jobs allow patients to use lunch time and morning and afternoon "breaks" for this purpose. We must consider the patients' daily activities and the flexibility allowed by their work before we advise such persons to seek other, less suitable employment or before we recommend one of the procedures designed to combat venous valvular insufficiency or obstruction (see Chapters 148 to 150).

Similarly, one may be willing to intervene promptly in most patients with primary subclavian-axillary vein thrombosis, for the majority of patients suffered this event because of repetitive use of the arm and they will be significantly disabled because of the ongoing need for active use of the involved upper extremity. In contrast, typically chronically ill and debilitated patients with subclavian-axillary vein thrombosis secondary to indwelling catheters experience little long-term disability and, unless there is a desperate need for angioaccess, they can be treated conservatively (see Chapter 85).

Some disabilities are commonly overlooked by clinicians. Considerable discussion of the impact of claudication from aortoiliac occlusive disease on work or recreation may take place without one's even broaching the subject of impotence. Similarly, internists often focus solely on the ability of their drug therapy to control blood pressure in renovascular hypertension without considering the debilitating side effects of multidrug therapy (malaise, asthenia, depression, impotence), eschewing both renal PTA or bypass.

Natural Course of Disease

A further dimension in patient selection is the natural course of the underlying condition. The importance of knowing this is exemplified by atherosclerotic occlusive disease involving the lower extremities. Peabody and associates,[5] in the Framingham study, reported that patients with intermittent claudication ran little more than a 5% risk of major amputation for gangrene within 5 years of the onset of this symptom if treated expectantly, whereas, within the same time frame, 23% had symptoms of coronary insufficiency, 13% suffered cerebrovascular accidents, and 20% died.[5]

From similar experiences, it has been predicted that close to one third of patients undergoing surgery for advanced arteriosclerosis obliterans involving the lower extremity will die of heart disease, stroke, or other consequences of atherosclerosis (ruptured aneurysm, mesenteric ischemia) within 5 years. Even though better medical management, and, in some quarters, more aggressive surgical treatment of coronary and carotid occlusive disease may invalidate these statistics to some degree in the future, the degree of atherosclerosis in the coronary and other circulations must still be seriously considered. However, once arteriosclerosis obliterans has progressed to the point of causing ischemic rest pain, ulcers, or gangrene, the likelihood of an eventual major amputation is great if arterial revascularization is not undertaken. Yet the absolute concept of claudication as a benign form to be treated conservatively and of chronic critical ischemia as an immediate threat to limb viability that demands arterial revascularization has recently been challenged. The ultimate risk of limb loss in the claudicant varies directly with the severity of the occlusive disease and can be stratified according to the level of reduction of the ankle-brachial index (ABI). It is simplistic to say that the risk of limb loss for *all* claudicants is 1% per year, based on the Framingham[5] and other epidemiologic studies that used only clinical assessment. Limb loss, *or the threat of it before successful intervention*, is closer to 5% per year, considering all studies in which there is objective hemodynamic confirmation of the diagnosis.[10]

In reviewing the literature, the author found the risk of limb loss, or the need for intervention to prevent it, to be 3.7% per year in claudicants in reports based on clinical evaluation and 5.8% per year in patients with objective confirmation of diagnosis by noninvasive diagnostic tests. Furthermore, there was a much higher risk of limb loss, or need for intervention to prevent it (8.5% per year), for claudicants with ABIs in the range between that associated with rest pain and with the healing of ischemic lesions (0.40 and 0.60, respectively), based on six studies in the recent literature. This has led to the concept of "chronic *subcritical* ischemia."[11] Conversely, Taylor and Porter[9] have pointed out that in the patient with chronic critical ischemia, one can succeed in preserving limb viability using general supportive measures alone in up to 25% to 40% of cases, a perspective gained from control groups in randomized prospective trials of prostanoids and other nonoperative forms of therapy.

Of course, the prognosis is not as benign for all claudicants, and not all patients with chronic critical ischemia are doomed to limb loss without successful reconstructive arterial surgery. Furthermore, the longevity outlook for patients with arteriosclerosis obliterans (dominated as it is by associated coronary disease) varies with the severity of the disease and also correlates with the ABI level.[12–15] Thus, the temptation to be more aggressive in claudicants with a lower ABI must be tempered by the fact that their risk from coronary disease is relatively higher.

The natural history of untreated deep venous thrombosis (DVT) of the lower extremity, as summarized in Table 2–1 from Bauer's classic study,[1] is one of increasing frequency of stasis dermatitis and ulceration with the passage of time. Although more recent studies suggest that the frequency of these post-thrombotic sequelae is probably less,[4, 7] all recognize that large numbers of potentially productive

TABLE 2–1. NATURAL HISTORY OF UNTREATED DEEP VENOUS THROMBOSIS OF THE LOWER EXTREMITY

Years after phlebitis	5	10	>10
Incidence of stasis dermatitis (%)	45	72	91
Incidence of ulceration (%)	20	52	79

From Bauer GA: A roentgenological and clinical study of the sequels of thrombosis. Acta Chir Scand Suppl 74, p 1, 1942.

members of Western society are significantly disabled by chronic venous insufficiency after phlebitis. The indications for operations designed to mitigate these stasis sequelae must not be considered as much in the light of this inevitability, however, as against the established efficacy of nonsurgical treatment, because it has been shown that stasis dermatitis and ulceration can be *completely* controlled in compliant patients with uncomplicated venous valvular insufficiency who follow a strict postphlebitic routine of intermittent leg elevation and use of proper elastic support. This underlies the point that one must consider not simply the natural history of the vascular condition under consideration in determining the indications for surgical intervention but, rather, its outlook with appropriate nonoperative therapy. The documented effectiveness of exercise therapy in the claudicant (see Chapter 65) and conservative therapy for chronic venous insufficiency (see Chapter 146) are two obvious examples of this modified perspective.

The natural history of chronic arterial and venous insufficiency of the lower extremities tends to be a continuum, albeit subject to episodic exacerbations. In vascular surgery for other conditions, one may not uncommonly be faced with patients with few or no symptoms, in whom the outlook for serious, even lethal, symptomatic progression is sufficient to warrant prophylactic intervention. Conditions for which the outlook is serious include abdominal aortic aneurysms, popliteal aneurysms, splenic aneurysms in women of childbearing age, post-stenotic subclavian aneurysms secondary to cervical rib compression, popliteal artery entrapment, "critical" stenosis of the carotid or mesenteric artery, traumatic arteriovenous fistulae involving central vessels, or large "floating tails" of thrombus after DVT. Because of the element of truth in the adage, "it is difficult to make an asymptomatic patient better," the vascular surgeon must be certain of the projections of the threatening natural history of these and similar conditions and of the *relative* safety of the proposed intervention. The latter is particularly pertinent, now that the era of endovascular intervention has been ushered in.

Operative Risk and Success Rate

The risk of morbidity and death after surgery must be weighed. Even though patients with arteriosclerosis are generally at a higher than average risk for their age, they tolerate operations limited to the extremity, neck, or superficial layers of the trunk relatively well, and vascular procedures confined to these areas carry a relatively small risk if one discounts deaths due to ongoing underlying disease rather than due to new problems precipitated by operation. In patients with limb-threatening ischemia, this risk is no greater than that attending the major amputation that might be required if arterial reconstruction were not undertaken. In fact, statistics gathered from the major series of amputations for "arterial" gangrene suggest that the risk of major amputation is greater than that of peripheral arterial reconstruction.[2, 3] However, if amputations were taken more seriously and were monitored with the same intensity as arterial reconstructions, one would expect mortality rates to be comparable. Thus, although these risks are not truly comparable, because the patient populations are not comparable, the risk of major amputation should not be taken lightly; it is sufficiently significant that peripheral arterial reconstruction should not be abandoned in favor of amputation simply because of a presumed lesser risk.

These same patients, however, would be exposed to a considerably greater magnitude of surgical stress if arterial reconstruction were performed through the abdominal cavity, as in the case of aortoiliac reconstruction. Even so, the mortality rates for those undergoing infrainguinal bypass are *not* significantly less than for those undergoing aortic reconstructions. This is because the former population, often heavily loaded with diabetic patients, has proportionately much more visceral atherosclerosis (e.g., coronary, carotid, renal artery involvement). Most patients with chronic limb-threatening ischemia have multilevel occlusive disease, and typically in this situation one would expect to find superficial femoral artery occlusion in addition to the proximal aortoiliac disease. Parallel experience has also taught us that proximal bypass, performed with a concomitant profundaplasty (thus introducing a full head of systemic arterial pressure into the parallel profunda geniculate collateral bed) obviates the need for dealing with the superficial femoral artery occlusion in most cases (i.e., 85% to 90%). Although this greatly reduces the time and extent of the operation required, it does not reduce the major risk that is associated with the transabdominal reconstruction.

Fortunately, this dilemma has been relieved somewhat by the option now provided by the so-called extra-anatomic bypass procedure—the femorofemoral or axillofemoral bypass. Because of these and other "low-risk" alternatives, such as femoral profundaplasty, it is rare today for the vascular surgeon to have to decline to treat the patient with limb-threatening ischemia (i.e., ischemic rest pain, ulceration, or limited gangrene) because of the risk of reconstructive arterial surgery itself. However, the patency rates of these low-risk alternatives, such as extra-anatomic bypass, do not compare favorably with those for the direct reconstructive procedures and thus are rarely offered for good-risk patients or those with claudication. Furthermore, these low-risk alternatives often carry paradoxically higher mortality rates than those for aortoiliac reconstructions in reported comparisons (see Chapter 68). This is because these procedures are often reserved for patients of prohibitive risk, who, when removed from the ranks of those undergoing direct aortoiliac reconstruction, reciprocally improve the latter's mortality statistics (see Chapters 66 and 68).

When one predicts the risk and success of a vascular operation, the common practice of quoting the "bottom line" results of some major reported series may be misleading for several reasons. First, the surgeon in question may be more or less experienced than those reporting these experiences, depending on the degree to which the procedures were performed or closely supervised by experienced vascular surgeons.

Second, the particular patient to whom this yardstick is being applied is not likely to exactly fit the profile for the average risk of a particular series. The patient's risk with the same operation depends on the coexistence of other significant systemic disorders, such as hypertension, diabetes, and chronic obstructive pulmonary disease, as well as the degree of arteriosclerotic involvement of the coronary and cerebral arteries. The estimation of operative risk clearly must be individualized.

Third, the patient is just as unlikely to have the same severity of occlusive disease reflected in the overall data from reported series. These data reflect a mixture of cases with good and poor runoff; the patient in question is likely to have one or the other. For example, the author has reported an overall 5-year patency rate for axillobifemoral bypass performed for occlusive disease of 47%, but for patients with an open superficial femoral artery this rate was 92% and for those with poor runoff it was 41%.[6]

Finally, it is not uncommon for large series to extend back over a decade or more and, therefore, to fail to reflect accurately more recent technical advances or the subtle but cumulative benefits of experience.

In the 1960s, in what has been referred to as the golden age of vascular surgery, surgeons were obliged to inform patients of a 5% risk of loss of life and a 10% risk of loss of limb for arterial reconstructive procedures on the lower extremity. Furthermore, in an additional 10% of cases, the procedure would fail either to relieve the patient's symptoms or to salvage the limb. The overall initial success rate (survival without major morbidity and a patent arterial reconstruction with symptomatic relief) was then 75%. Today, these risks have been greatly reduced, and the initial success rate, even with all three adverse risks, is closer to 95%.

Although series that include data from the 1960s and 1970s may not reflect it, most major vascular surgery services can now point to operative mortality rates for *elective* aortic aneurysmectomy, aortobifemoral bypass, femoropopliteal bypass, and carotid endarterectomy—four of the most commonly performed vascular operations—in the range of 1% to 3%. These figures reflect (1) the development of methods of avoiding recognized complications, (2) more sophisticated monitoring techniques for directing intravenous fluid and drug therapy during the perioperative period, and (3) more careful patient selection (e.g., not operating for acute stroke and using extra-anatomic bypass rather than direct aortoiliac reconstruction in high-risk patients). The risks of mortality and permanent neurologic morbidity after carotid endarterectomy must now be under 5% for symptomatic patients and under 3% for asymptomatic patients with severe stenosis, to be considered preferable to best medical therapy. Fortunately, most specialized centers now report an overall mortality and permanent neurologic morbidity rate for carotid endarterectomy of less than 2%.

As mentioned earlier, distal arterial reconstructions, which do not invade a major body cavity or cause much blood loss (e.g., femoropopliteal and femorotibial bypasses), and the "low-risk" alternatives, extra-anatomic bypasses and profundaplasty, actually carry a somewhat higher risk of loss of life or limb, in the range of 2% to 5% and 3% to 7%, respectively. This is because the former procedures are performed in patients with more distally distributed atherosclerosis, which in turn is associated with a significantly higher incidence of visceral (coronary and carotid) involvement, and these two procedures are offered *only* to poor-risk patients. Furthermore, both are generally reserved for limb salvage situations, in which multisegmental disease and poor runoff are invariably present.

The 25% to 50% 5-year failure rate commonly cited in the past for arterial prostheses partly reflected a significant incidence of anastomotic aneurysm and occlusion by sloughing pseudointima or intimal hyperplasia. The abandonment of silk sutures and tightly woven Dacron grafts in favor of polypropylene sutures and knitted velour and polytetrafluoroethylene (PTFE) grafts, respectively, and the avoidance of prosthetic grafts in peripheral, small-caliber (<6 mm in diameter) reconstructions in which flexion creases are crossed, runoff is poor, and resting flow rates are slow have contributed to improved results, as have the selective use of antithrombotic drugs and employment of serial graft surveillance protocols. There is no doubt, in the small-caliber, low-flow graft, that saphenous vein grafts (be they in situ, reversed, or translocated in an antegrade orientation after their valves are rendered incompetent) are distinctly superior to any current prosthetic. The rate of failure to use or successfully "harvest" a saphenous vein graft for femoropopliteal bypass used to be reported as between 20% and 40%. Now, with duplex evaluation of prospective veins and the additional use of lesser saphenous or arm veins, this figure is closer to 5% to 10% for primary infrageniculate bypass (see Chapter 35). Similarly, the frequency of late occlusion of these vein grafts—because of stricture, proliferative or degenerative changes, atheromatous degeneration, intimal fibrosis, or paravalvular stenosis—once noted to be as high as 28%,[8] has decreased, now that the causes of damage to the vein during its preparation have been recognized and can be avoided.

Finally, technical developments have allowed in situ bypass to be fully utilized in femorodistal bypass. The suitability of the saphenous vein can be established preoperatively by duplex scanning, and because smaller veins can be used and the aforementioned structural changes are rarer, both vein utilization and patency rates have been significantly improved. The improved results with distal bypass using in situ or reversed saphenous veins, augmented by postoperative surveillance programs (with assisted primary patency rates now approaching those achieved with proximal bypass), are in sharp contrast with those achieved with prosthetic or modified biologic grafts when carried below the knee (<40% for below-knee and <20% for tibial/peroneal [crural] bypass at 5 years). The lack of a small-caliber prosthesis or modified biologic graft that can maintain reasonable patency rates, when anastomosed to the low-flow, high-resistance arteries of the leg, remains the greatest single barrier to successful limb salvage surgery.

The *overall* results in this field do not completely reflect the significant advances that have been made, mainly because more difficult cases are now being subjected to bypass (cases that would have called for primary amputation in the past) and because of the inability of most patients who smoke to refrain from tobacco abuse. Nevertheless, the reconstructive procedures, graft choices, and patency rates have changed significantly since the late 1970s. In recommending appropriate therapy, practicing vascular surgeons need to be as aware of this changing outlook as they are of the technical advances that brought it. Similarly, they must be familiar with changes in other modes of therapy, particularly PTA. Its low risk and cost compensate for its lesser degree and duration of benefit to make it the initial treatment of choice for discrete stenoses, particularly in the larger, proximal arteries. Now used in anywhere from 25% to 40% of patients requiring intervention, PTA tends to be used more in claudicants with isolated disease and good runoff, whereas bypass surgery still dominates in limb salvage settings. Therefore, PTA is not as much in direct competition with arterial reconstructive surgery as one might think, and in many situations it is complementary and adjunctive (see Chapter 72).

Clearly, it is not possible to predict outcome from past experience; neither should one project outcome on the basis of overall results from others' series. Rather, such reports should serve as a frame of reference on which to project one's own results, for all vascular surgeons should regularly analyze their own experiences (see Chapter 3). Furthermore, adjustment should be made not only for the operation and the operator but also for individual considerations, such as associated risk factors, runoff, and types of graft.

DIAGNOSTIC STUDIES

Assessment of Operative Risk

The preoperative evaluation of patients for vascular surgery, including angiography, is deliberately dealt with *after* the discussion of case selection, to emphasize the sequence of events and priorities that should be observed in clinical practice. This tentative decision is upheld in most cases, although occasionally the unexpected discovery of associated disease or a discouraging angiogram will reverse this judgment. Clearly, more is required before surgery than a pertinent history and a physical examination relative to the vascular problem.

The assessment of operative risk is discussed in greater detail in Section VII (see Chapters 40 to 42); only the choice of diagnostic studies required to determine operative risk is considered here. Ordinarily, cardiopulmonary and renal function are carefully evaluated. A complete blood count (CBC), urinalysis, blood urea nitrogen (BUN), and creatinine level determinations, blood glucose, electrocardiogram (ECG), and chest x-ray films are almost routinely ordered. (Special studies for each condition are discussed in detail in the chapters dealing with the individual conditions.) Obviously, if the patient's problem is arteriosclerosis, serum cholesterol and triglyceride levels should be determined and serum lipoprotein electrophoresis should be performed; if the disorder is thromboembolic, a coagulation profile should be obtained. Any intercurrent disease should be investigated on its own merits. More extensive preoperative evaluations may be ordered along the lines indicated by history, physical examination, or the results of the previously mentioned routine tests. In patients with known pulmonary problems, an abnormal chest x-ray, or abnormal blood gas values determined with the patient breathing "room air," formal pulmonary function studies are ordered. In patients with an elevated BUN or creatinine level, a creatinine clearance test is obtained, and contrast urography may be performed simultaneously with angiographic study if the latter is planned. Patients with ECG abnormalities, cardiac symptoms, or evidence of such widespread arteriosclerosis that coronary artery involvement may require radionuclide scanning or Holter's monitoring, or both, to evaluate cardiac perfusion and function—and, in selected cases, cardiac catheterization and coronary angiography—may be performed.

Noninvasive Studies

Special diagnostic procedures are discussed in detail in the later sections of this book, but the value of selectively employing objective, noninvasive methods of preoperative and postoperative monitoring is worthy of emphasis. These studies help one to avoid misdiagnoses and to gauge the extent and severity of the vascular disease before angiography; they determine the hemodynamic significance of the lesions visualized by angiography and allow it to be employed more selectively, and when the physiologic data and angiographic anatomy are considered together, the surgeon not only can better choose the most appropriate operation but also can better predict the hemodynamic outcome.

Duplex scanning, since the superimposition of color-coded velocity information, has been increasingly used to supply anatomic as well as flow information in carotid, venous, and peripheral arterial disease. In most cases, it is used selectively to augment the indirect physiologic tests, but in many instances it can provide all the necessary information with which to plan arterial surgery.

Computed tomography (CT) scans and/or magnetic resonance imaging (MRI) are also being used with increasing frequency to evaluate carotid disease, aortic aneurysms, and congenital vascular disease. Now, in many settings, one or more noninvasive physiologic tests or imaging modalities can characterize the lesions so well that preoperative arteriography may be obviated. This will be seen increasingly as newer, improved forms of vascular imaging become more widely available (see Chapters 10 to 15 for details). Additionally, they provide a readily available means of objectively assessing the initial and continued success of the procedure itself. Noninvasive monitoring of the results of vascular interventions has become an accepted part of overall management.

Furthermore, because newer noninvasive modalities can detect and localize lower extremity occlusive lesions, either singly or in combination, with greater than 95% accuracy, unnecessary "diagnostic" arteriography is eliminated; for all intents and purposes, this study is not obtained until the decision has already been made that the patient needs a revascularization procedure and precise anatomic information is required before determining which is the most appropriate method. The availability of endovascular interventions has caused this position to be modified somewhat, because arteriography is a prelude to these procedures and monitors their technical and anatomic success.

Angiographic Studies

Equally pertinent to this introductory chapter is a discussion of the strategic use of angiography. Arteriographic and phlebographic studies in selected patients provide invaluable information regarding the location and extent of the disease, and occasionally this anatomic information is supplemented by qualitative impressions regarding the rate of blood flow. Now, however, it is often possible to confirm the nature and location of the vascular lesion with reasonable certainty by physical examination, supplemented by some of the newer noninvasive diagnostic methods so that angiography is selectively rather than routinely employed.

Arteriography

Generally, the vascular surgeon obtains an arteriogram to study the condition of the vessels proximal and distal to the lesion. For example, when confronted with superficial femoral artery occlusion, the vascular surgeon wants to ensure that there is not an occult iliac artery stenosis proximally, that the profunda femoris is widely patent and providing maximal collateral flow, and that the condition of the popliteal and infrapopliteal arteries into which a graft may be placed is suitable. Similarly, if an abdominal aortic aneurysm is large enough to be easily felt or if its calcific outline on a cross-table lateral film or ultrasound studies indicates it is 5 to 6 cm in diameter, there is little reason for aortography unless significant proximal (e.g., renal or mesenteric artery) or distal (e.g., iliac or femoral artery) occlusive disease is suspected. In fact, because more abdominal aortic aneurysms are lined by intraluminal clot, their internal diameters often appear misleadingly normal on aortograms. Enhanced CT scans are better for preoperative screening because they reveal most of the associated pathology or anomalies that can complicate repair (e.g., inflammatory aneurysms, horseshoe or ectopic kidney, or vena caval or renal vein anomalies). Ultrasonography is still the most practical method of monitoring for enlargement.

Now that segmental limb pressures and plethysmographic studies are readily obtainable, arteriograms are ordered not for diagnostic curiosity but for therapeutic intent. Good-quality, multiplanar-view arteriograms are absolutely essential in diagnosis of multisegmental disease. Particularly important in this regard are oblique views of the iliac and proximal profunda femoris arteries and adequate visualization of "runoff" vessels distally. By the same token, when one is treating carotid occlusive or ulcerative lesions, angiographic demonstration of disease in the arch vessels, contralateral bifurcation, ipsilateral siphon, or vertebral arteries may be as important as what appears to be the primary lesion.

Phlebography

Phlebography still suffers from indiscriminate use. It was commonly used during the early 80's and before to detect DVT, to rule out deep venous insufficiency in candidates for varicose vein stripping, or to localize incompetent perforators in those with more advanced disease. This can nearly always be determined by duplex scan supplemented by physiologic plethysmographic studies (see Chapters 11 and 13).

SUMMARY

It is only after confirming the existence, nature, and extent of the vascular lesion, and balancing the disability it causes, or is likely to cause despite proper nonoperative management, against the feasibility, risk, and anticipated success of alternative surgical, endovascular, and nonsurgical forms of therapy, that the vascular surgeon is in a position to advise the patient or the referring physician regarding the need for surgical intervention. The manner in which this evaluation is carried out and the judgment that is applied to this stepwise process are the foundation for a successful practice in vascular surgery.

REFERENCES

1. Bauer GA: A roentgenological and clinical study of the sequels of thrombosis. Acta Chir Scand Suppl 74:1, 1942.
2. DeWeese JA, Blaisdell FW, Foster JH: Optimal resources for vascular surgery. Arch Surg 105:948, 1972.
3. Haeger K: Problems of acute deep venous thrombosis: I. The interpretation of signs and symptoms. Angiology 20:219, 1969.
4. Lindner DJ, Edwards JM, Phinney ES, et al: Long term hemodynamic and clinical sequelae of lower extremity deep vein thrombosis. J Vasc Surg 4:436, 1986.
5. Peabody CN, Kannel WB, McNamara PM: Intermittent claudication: Surgical significance. Arch Surg 109:693, 1974.
6. Rutherford RB, Patt A, Pearce WH: Extra-anatomic bypass: A closer view. Presented at the Western Vascular Society, Tucson, Arizona, January 23, 1987. J Vasc Surg 6:437, 1987.
7. Strandness DE, Langlois Y, Cramer M, et al: Long term sequelae of acute venous thrombosis. JAMA 250:1289, 1983.
8. Szilagyi DE, Elliot JP, Hageman JH, et al: Biologic fate of autogenous vein implants of arterial substitutes. Surgery 74:731, 1973.
9. Taylor LM Jr, Porter JM: Natural history of chronic lower extremity ischemia. Semin Vasc Surg 4:181, 1991.
10. McDaniel MM, Cronenwett JL: Natural history of claudication. *In* Porter JM, Taylor LM (eds): Basic Data Underlying Clinical Decision Making in Vascular Surgery. St. Louis, Quality Medical Publishing, 1994, pp 129–133.
11. Rutherford RB, Baker JD, Ernst C, et al: Recommended standards for reports dealing with lower extremity ischemia: Revised version. J Vasc Surg 26:517–538, 1997.
12. Vogt MT, Cauley JA, Newman AB, et al: Decreased ankle/arm blood pressure index and mortality in elderly women. JAMA 270:465, 1993.
13. McDermott MM, Feinglass J, Slavensky R, Pearce WH: The ankle-brachial index as a predictor of survival in patients with peripheral vascular disease. J Gen Intern Med 9:445, 1994.
14. O'Riordain DS, O'Donnell JA: Realistic expectations for the patient with intermittent claudication. Br J Surg 78:861, 1991.
15. Smith I, Franks PJ, Greenhalgh RM, et al: The influence of smoking cessation and hypertriglyceridaemia on the progression of peripheral arterial disease and the onset of critical ischaemia. Eur J Vasc Endovasc Surg 11:402, 1996.

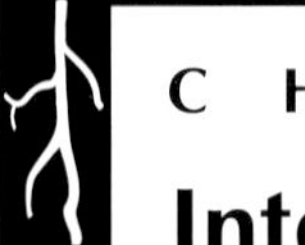

CHAPTER 3

Integrated Assessment of Results: Standardized Reporting of Outcomes and the Computerized Vascular Registry

John V. White, M.D., Darrell N. Jones, Ph.D., and Robert B. Rutherford, M.D.

A BROADENING VIEW OF OUTCOMES ASSESSMENT

The published literature should provide a yardstick against which individual surgical practices and patient outcomes can be measured and serve as a common forum for the comparison of the benefits of different therapeutic approaches. However, unless we use universally accepted standards in reporting the clinical and patient-based outcomes of vascular surgical procedures, one could question whether the yardstick is accurate and whether the forum, in fact, provides any commonality to diverse clinical experiences and patient populations. This consideration begs the larger question of whether published reports provide a true measure of vascular therapy and the benefits derived from it.

Complete assessment of the effectiveness of vascular intervention requires evaluating not only the change in the patient's clinical status but also changes in the patient's functional status and quality of life. Although clinical parameters of therapeutic success, such as graft patency and limb salvage, are essential for the evaluation of vascular surgical intervention, documentation of an improvement in patient quality of life and personal productivity is equally important. The operative treatments of aneurysms and arterial occlusive disease are performed to reduce risk to life and limb and to relieve symptoms but have little direct impact on the underlying pathologic process. The benefit of intervention lies, ultimately, in an improved quality of life. Integrated, complete evaluation of vascular intervention, then, requires the documentation of both clinical and patient-based measures of outcome.

This approach to patient evaluation has been strongly encouraged by the U.S. government. In 1989, Congress created the Agency for Health Care Policy and Research and charged it with the responsibility to conduct research to identify effective health care, develop clinical guidelines based on the findings of effectiveness, and disseminate this information to the public. To evaluate therapeutic effectiveness, the government stresses the use of outcomes measures that assess factors affecting patients directly (e.g., physical and social functioning and pain) rather than intermediate clinical measures (e.g., laboratory test scores).[1] The rising costs of health care in the United States mandate that costly interventions that fail to directly increase the well-being and productivity of patients be eliminated.

This chapter outlines the potential causes of variance and confusion in the literature. A number of suggested clinical and patient-based outcomes reporting standards that might alleviate these problems are offered. Finally, computer-based vascular registries are discussed on the premise that once the manner in which we assess our results is standardized, such registries may provide a more accurate overall view of the practice of vascular surgery as well as a means of studying certain problems cooperatively and with significantly large numbers of cases, larger than would be possible in individual or group experiences.

EVALUATION OF RESULTS: CONFOUNDING FACTORS

When the results of different surgical procedures or practices are compared, a number of potential reasons exist for the observed differences in surgical outcome. Certainly, the most obvious reason and the most commonly offered conclusion is that the particular procedure, graft, or some other feature of the therapeutic approach being studied is intrinsically superior. However, other factors may play a significant, if not the major, role in producing the reported differences. The essential problem lies in identifying these other factors and either avoiding them, when possible (as in a prospective trial), or uniformly reporting them to allow their potential influence to be gauged objectively.

Some of these factors have been identified by category and are listed in Table 3–1. They include:

1. Technical differences (superior surgical skill or experience, use of adjunctive procedures and adjuvant therapies).
2. Statistical artefacts and abuses, particularly with respect to life-table estimates.
3. Differences in patient populations (variations in referral patterns leading to differences in prevalence of disease and associated risk factors, and differences in the indications for surgery producing differences in severity of disease and associated risk factors).
4. Differing criteria for success or failure (e.g., patency, symptomatic relief, hemodynamic improvement, extremity function, mortality, amputation rate.

TABLE 3–1. FACTORS AFFECTING OBSERVED DIFFERENCES IN THE RESULTS OF SURGICAL PROCEDURES

Intrinsically superior approach
Technical differences
- Superior surgical skills or experience
- Differing use of adjunctive and adjuvant therapies

Statistical artefacts and abuses
- Simple misuse or abuse of statistical testing
- Artefacts of the life table

Differences in patient populations
- Duration of follow-up
- Patient exclusions
- Prevalence of disease
- Associated risk factors
- Patient selection and indications for surgery

Differing criteria for success or failure
- Technical and angiographic success
- Hemodynamic success
- Symptomatic and functional success
- Primary or secondary patency

Each of these aspects is illustrated in the following discussion.

Technical Differences

It is very difficult to assess superior surgical skill or judgment by one group that produces better results than those reported by another group. Nevertheless, difference in skill or judgment is a factor that cannot be dismissed. For example, the controversy over the value of carotid endarterectomy is ultimately a risk:benefit analysis that primarily weighs the mortality and morbidity rates of the procedure against the protection offered against stroke, observed from a comparison of the surgical and nonsurgical patients. However, these success rates vary from institution to institution (and from surgeon to surgeon) to such a degree that the surgical skill of individual surgeons or groups of surgeons must be conceded to be an important factor, one that significantly alters the risk:benefit analysis. This is why upper limits of mortality and permanent neurologic morbidity for individual operating surgeons have been recommended for each indication for carotid endarterectomy. Similarly, part of the controversy over the claimed superiority of in situ versus reversed vein graft for femorodistal bypass revolves around significant differences in surgical skill, not only between groups practicing either technique but also between the initial and ultimately acquired skills of the same group.[2, 3]

Factors that are more easily documented include the use of adjunctive procedures and therapeutic adjuvants that might influence outcome. Examples include the use of profundaplasty in association with aortobifemoral bypass performed in the presence of superficial femoral artery occlusion, the routine use of completion arteriography, dextran 40 and antiplatelet drugs, and frequent vascular laboratory surveillance after femorodistal bypass. Such variations may reflect technologic advances more than philosophical differences in technique, making it important to consider the time span covered by each study. Examples are the contrasting results initially reported for extra-anatomic bypass (Table 3–2).

For instance, two articles were published within 4 years of each other by Eugene[4] and Ray[5] and their respective colleagues. Although there are other reasons for the twofold differences in patency and mortality for both axillo-unifemoral and axillobifemoral bypass (see later), the former series covers a period from 1960 to 1975, whereas the latter series reports on the results of operations performed between 1970 and 1979. Thus, there is only a 5-year overlap between the older 15-year and the more recent 9-year experience. Obviously, significant technical advances can emerge during such a time span. In the former series, for example, there was a demonstrated effect on patency of improving arterial prostheses and only seven of the study's 92 extra-anatomic bypasses used the double velour knitted polyester (Dacron) graft, which is in widespread use and which was exclusively used in the latter series. The same can be said for more recent reports.

El Massry and colleagues[6] have reported later results from the same center as Ray and associates.[5] The prosthesis used has *not* significantly changed, although the results have continued to improve. On the other hand, Harris and colleagues[7] have reported very significant improvements with axillofemoral bypass grafting that they credit to the use of a ringed polytetrafluoroethylene (PTFE) prosthesis; yet there are major differences in case selection and, presumably, in technique and postoperative care as well between their earlier and later experiences. The reported results with extra-anatomic bypass are referred to again later to illustrate other reasons for reported differences in surgical procedures.

Statistical Artefacts and Abuses

It is likely that a substantial portion of the medical literature contains errors in the use of statistical methods. This portion has been estimated to range from 40% to 60% ac-

TABLE 3–2. VARIATION IN REPORTED RESULTS FOR EXTRA-ANATOMIC BYPASS

PROCEDURE	AUTHOR	OPERATIVE MORTALITY (%)	FIVE-YEAR PATENCY (%)
Axillounifemoral	El-Massry et al[6]	5	76*
	Ray et al[5]	3	67
	Hepp et al[76]	5	46
	Ascer et al[25]	5	44*
	LoGerfo et al[20]	8	37*
	Chang[73]	NR	33*
	Eugene et al[4]	8	30*
	Rutherford et al[26]	13	19*
Axillobifemoral	El-Massry et al[6]	5	79*
	Ray et al[5]	5	77
	Johnson et al[21]	2	76
	Chang[73]	NR	75*
	LoGerfo et al[20]	8	74
	Hepp et al[76]	5	73
	Rutherford et al[26]	11	62*
	Ascer et al[25]	5	50*
	Eugene et al[4]	8	33*

*Primary patency. All others are secondary patency or not defined.
NR = Not reported.

cording to samples reviewed from American, British, and Canadian medical journals.[8]

The more common abuses include multiple comparisons between population stratifications and the reliance on the *t*-test as a universal "test of significance." Although a critique of statistical techniques is beyond the scope of this discussion, the life-table analysis of survival curves deserves examination. Historically, the methods of the life-table analysis were described in the 1950s[9, 10] but gained a wider appreciation in the medical community when they were described by Peto et al[11, 12] in 1976 to 1977 as a means of measuring survival of patients with cancer and the effect of therapeutic intervention on that survival. The life-table analysis method has subsequently been adopted by vascular surgeons, among others, to measure other outcome criteria, especially patency.

Because it is now common practice to use the life-table method to assess patency, one might assume that two reports employing this method would be comparable. However, a known artefact of this method is the better projected patency rates when a series is "front-loaded" with many recent cases. This results in a characteristic leveling off of the declining patency curve near the end, with the final plateau representing a relatively small number of grafts remaining patent during the later periods. Patency projections during the first 2 to 3 years of a bypass graft experience by the life-table method are notoriously misleading.

Veith and colleagues[13] published a "14-month" comparison of PTFE and autologous saphenous vein (ASV) grafts in "high-risk, limb salvage" cases. There were 45 cases of each type of reconstruction. Figure 3–1 shows projected 14-month patencies that are greater for PTFE than ASV, although admittedly not statistically significant. The mean follow-up times also differed, as might have been suspected from the gradually declining curve for ASV and the flat line for PTFE. Furthermore, it was not stated in the text describing this "comparable series of patients" whether the grafts were performed over the same time span, what proportion were below the knee, whether runoff was comparable, or whether the reported patencies were aided by thrombectomy or revision. Such considerations are addressed later.

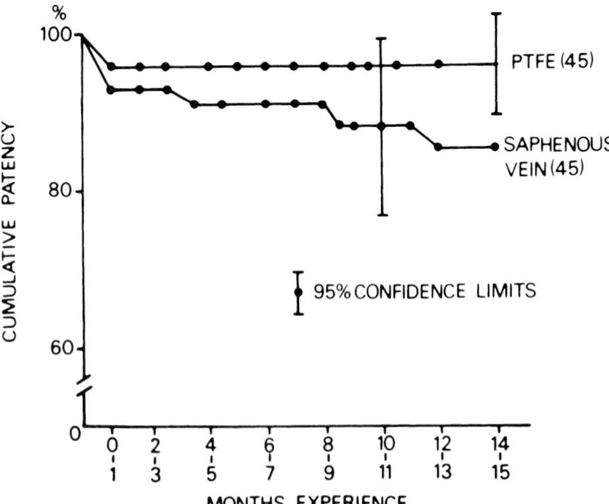

FIGURE 3–1. Life-table comparison of projected 14-month patencies for polytetrafluoroethylene (PTFE) and saphenous vein grafts used in the femoropopliteal position. Comparison of expanded polytetrafluoroethylene and autologous saphenous vein grafts in high risk arterial reconstructions for limb salvage. (From Veith FJ, Moss CM, Fell SC, et al: Surg Gynecol Obstet 147:749, 1978. By permission of Surgery Gynecology & Obstetrics.)

As DeWeese and Robb[14] have pointed out, the life-table method tends to overestimate the actual patency rate (i.e., that measured at the *end* of a given period). In an analysis of "autogenous venous grafts ten years later," they noted that 58% of their femoropopliteal grafts were "patent at the time of death or last follow-up" (once the most common method of projecting patency). The *cumulative* patency of the same grafts using the life-table method was 45% at 10 years, but the *actual* patency of grafts in patients surviving 10 years or beyond graft occlusion was only 38%.

Conversely, the effect of the declining population at risk over the duration of the study can result in secondary patency rates that are lower than the primary patency rates. This results from simply moving an *early* failure, which represents a small percentage of the initial population at risk, to a *later* failure, where it represents a larger percentage of the residual population at risk and thus has a larger effect on the cumulative patency rate. This artefact is a direct result of small populations, limited follow-up, and extrapolation of patency rates beyond what the data will support.

Finally, it is not unusual for comparisons to be made between series of cases with significantly different follow-up. For example, in the previously cited report by Ray and colleagues,[5] 84 axillobifemoral grafts with a mean implant time of 30 months were compared with 105 aortobifemoral grafts with a mean implant time of 44 months. Similarly, comparison was made between axillounifemoral and axillobifemoral grafts based on "mean implant times" of only 20.4 and 9.4 months, respectively, in a study that covered 9 years! The series with the much shorter mean implant times are thus front-loaded compared with the longer series and have a more rapidly declining population at risk.

The preceding observations are not made to impugn the life-table method or to deny the trends it is used to demonstrate but, rather, to show how it may suggest differences that are more apparent than real and to emphasize that the technique provides an estimate, not an actual measure. For a more explicit critique of the method, see the classic article by Underwood and Charlesworth.[15]

Differences in Patient Populations

As noted previously, the declining numbers of patients at risk over the duration of a study can have detrimental effects on the accuracy of the patency estimates. In addition to the simple loss of numbers of patients, lack of diligent follow-up also biases the data. In some cases, one is more likely to receive bad news than good news; that is, patients are more likely to come back or to be referred when the graft fails than when they continue to be asymptomatic. Periodic surveillance of bypass grafts by noninvasive testing has been demonstrated to detect and, by allowing timely intervention, to prevent impending graft failure.[16] Thus, a reasonable degree of follow-up should be required of published reports, and a poorly followed large series, as indicated by those lost to follow-up in the life-table, may not provide as valid an estimate as a well-followed small one.

Patients *excluded* from a report are often as important as (if not more important than) patients *included*. For example, it has been common practice for interventional radiologists to exclude from their projected success rates for transluminal angioplasty patients in whom the procedure was attempted but not successfully completed. Although this technical failure rate is low with proximal dilations, it is much higher with dilations of smaller distal vessels (3% versus 17.5%, respectively, in the authors' experience).[17] Similarly, some vascular surgeons have *eliminated* from their patency projections reconstructions that thrombosed during the immediate postoperative period if patency was not restored and have *included* as patent clotted grafts that were successfully reopened. This may represent a significant proportion of cases; for example, the early postoperative thrombosis rate after "difficult" distal bypasses may exceed 20%.[18]

Also not included in the patency calculations of most bypass series are cases in which the procedure was abandoned because of technical difficulties. This may constitute a significant number of in situ or reverse vein bypasses to tibial or peroneal arteries, being as high as 14% of cases in one early experience with the latter bypass.[19]

In two reports concerning axillobifemoral bypasses from the same affiliated institutions and by mostly the same authors, and appearing within 4 months of each other,[20, 21] mortality rates of 8% and less than 2% were claimed. There were 10 fewer cases and 1 more year covered by the latter study. The apparent explanation for the fourfold difference in mortality reported from the same institutions is the elimination of "emergency" operations from consideration in the second report.

Patient mix is clearly one of the most important contributors to the wide variance in mortality and patency rates between reported series of arterial reconstruction. There may be differences in disease severity and risk factors affecting outcome that reflect intrinsic group differences in disease prevalence, severity, or relative distribution of occlusive lesions. On the other hand, such differences may reflect conscious philosophical differences in indications for operation.

For example, patients undergoing surgery for the indication of claudication are, as a group, younger; have less coronary, carotid, and visceral artery atherosclerotic involvement; and less frequently have diabetes, multilevel disease, or poor "runoff" than patients operated on for limb salvage. This is apparent from Table 3–3, which compares two reports of 100 consecutive femoropopliteal vein bypasses each, performed for claudication and for limb salvage by vascular surgeons at the University of Pennsylvania.[22, 23] Even within the category of limb salvage, results are better for those with ischemic rest pain than for those with nonhealing ulcers, and both, in turn, are better than results for those with digital gangrene. Furthermore, amputation rates are progressively higher in each of these three categories if the bypass graft fails.[24]

Thus, the indications for surgery, represented in different proportions in different series, can, by associated differences in severity of disease and risk factors, significantly influence outcome. In the San Francisco experience with

TABLE 3–3. COMPARISON OF 100 CONSECUTIVE FEMOROPOPLITEAL BYPASSES PERFORMED FOR CLAUDICATION AND FOR "LIMB SALVAGE"

	CLAUDICATION (%)	LIMB SALVAGE (%)
Risk factors		
Cardiac disease	36	56
Diabetes	22	44
Transient ischemic attack, stroke	5	10
Pulmonary disease	19	29
Outcome		
Operative mortality	0	3
Survival (5-year)	74	60
Limb loss	3	30
Patency (5-year)	69	46

extra-anatomic bypass reported by Eugene and coworkers[4] and cited previously, only 12% of patients had surgery for claudication. In contrast, in the Seattle series reported by Ray and colleagues,[5] almost two thirds of patients were claudicants. Similarly, in the San Francisco series, axillofemoral bypass graft was limited, for the most part, to extremely poor-risk patients; in the Boston series, axillobifemoral bypass was liberally applied because the authors "seldom recommended conventional aortoiliac reconstruction in patients over the age of 65, regardless of risk."[21]

Therefore, the higher mortality and lower patency rates reported by the San Francisco group are not surprising. However, an even greater contribution to these differences in patency rates was made by the criteria used in their estimation (see later). Whenever there are major differences in the ratio between claudicants and limb salvage patients, one should also expect differences in survival and patency. In a comparison of recent and earlier experiences with axillofemoral bypass, in which improved results were attributed to changing to an externally supported prosthesis, the proportion of limb salvage cases also changed from 60% to 24%![7]

Differing Criteria for Success or Failure

In some articles, the patency of an arterial bypass or reconstruction is considered to end with its occlusion. Other reports treat as patent any graft that is still open even if patency has been achieved by thrombectomy, thrombolysis, transluminal angioplasty, local revision, extension, or a new inflow source. More recently, these differences have been designated *primary* patency and *secondary* patency, and most reports make this distinction clear. However, the confusion caused by not doing this was tremendous. For example, the "bottom line" 5-year patency rates quoted in the two contrasting reports on axillobifemoral bypass by Ray and Eugene and their colleagues were 77% and 33%, respectively, but the former is a secondary and the latter a primary patency rate.[4, 5]

Johnson and associates,[21] in comparing axillobifemoral with aortobifemoral bypass, noted essentially identical patency rates (76.4% versus 76.9%), but the former was achieved with a 43% rate of thrombectomy or revision compared with 9% for the latter. It is not possible to tell whether any of the 20 successful thrombectomies in the 56 axillobifemoral grafts reported in the companion series by LoGerfo and associates[20] were multiple procedures performed on the same graft, but if they were not (as implied by the term "successful"), the primary 5-year patency rate in this experience from Boston University–affiliated hospitals would not be 76% but would be close to the 33% patency rate reported by Eugene and coworkers[4] from the San Francisco Veterans Hospital.

Why should we argue opposing points of view, which maintain either that a thrombosed graft has clearly failed or that a graft whose patency has been maintained by thrombectomy, dilation, or revision is open and functioning? One reflects the unmodified natural history of the graft or procedure and the other the ultimate utility that can be achieved by the surgeon's close surveillance and persistent efforts. No surgeon likes to report a low patency rate, lest it be considered a personal reflection on his or her ability. Once it becomes more widely appreciated that primary patency reflects mainly the intrinsic merits of the procedure or graft and that secondary patency is more a reflection of the surgeon's skill and persistence, vascular surgeons will accept the stricter definitions of primary patency and should be content to let the secondary patency rate speak for their efforts. Clearly, however, *both rates should be reported*, as in subsequent articles on extra-anatomic bypass by Ascer[25] and Rutherford[26] and their colleagues, in which the large differences between primary and secondary patency rates are readily apparent.

Finally, reports on arterial reconstructive surgery are often unclear about the manner in which patency was determined. The acceptance of the lack of return of limb-threatening ischemia, or clinic notes of "palpable pulses" or "patient not bothered by claudication" by a junior resident or other indirect evidence of graft patency are inappropriate. Scientific articles deserve more objective data, and acceptable criteria are recommended later in this discussion.

Some overall clinical measure of success is needed, commonly the combination of continued relief of symptoms or limb salvage. The former would apply to the claudicant, the latter to patients with ischemic ulcers and digital gangrene, with both applying to patients with ischemic rest pain. Flanigan and associates[27] reported an 81% 5-year success rate for femorofemoral bypass grafts, considering failure to be (1) graft thrombosis, (2) amputation, or (3) failure to relieve symptoms. This dual requirement of clinical improvement *and* patency is admirable, but it brings out the need for objective patency criteria because both symptomatic relief and credit for avoidance of amputation may be quite subjective, and patency has until recently not usually been confirmed arteriographically or by some other direct imaging technique.

The noninvasive vascular laboratory offers objective means of monitoring graft function and supplying confirmatory evidence of both hemodynamic improvement and patency. Because a difference of 0.10 in the ankle-brachial index (ABI) is within the range of observer error, surgeons should demand at least this degree of improvement as evidence of continued graft patency. Currently, this is recommended when associated with categorically improved status but 0.15 as a stand-alone criterion[28] (see later).

When an aortobifemoral bypass or iliac balloon angioplasty is performed for aortoiliac occlusive disease associated with a significant distal lesion (e.g., superficial femoral artery occlusion), the evaluation of success becomes more difficult (Table 3–4). One may have a significantly higher rate of patency, as reflected by persistent elevation of the thigh-brachial index (TBI), than of symptomatic relief, which correlates better with the ABI. Those authors who require both symptomatic relief and an elevate ABI as criteria for success after intervention for aortoiliac occlusive disease, rather than elevation of the TBI, may have contributed to the impression that percutaneous transluminal angioplasty (PTA) for iliac stenoses is not very effective or durable.[29] In contrast are reports in which technical failures are eliminated and an increased TBI is accepted as the ultimate criterion of continued success regardless of the ABI and the patient's symptoms. Using data from a personal experience with PTA, the authors found that, when depending on the criteria chosen, the projected 3-year success rate for iliac dilations varied between 52% and 86%; similarly, with distal dilations, a rate of success as high as 63% or as low as 27% could be claimed.[17]

In fairness, the same can be said for reported experiences with surgical operations for aortoiliac disease, namely that the patency rates do not reflect the degree of hemodynamic improvement or symptomatic relief attained. In a review of 265 aortobifemoral graft limbs in which the initial patency rate was 97.7% and the late patency rate was 88%, the authors found that in spite of excellent patency, 7.3% of grafts failed to bring about improved inflow (a TBI increase < 0.10) because the iliac disease on the better side was not very significant in the first place (a preoperative TBI $>$ 0.95), and 9.4% failed to improve the ABI because of the severity of distal occlusive disease.[30]

In the past, carotid reconstructions have been judged almost exclusively on the basis of continued symptomatic relief; thus, until recently silent restenosis has not been reported. The vascular laboratory and, the use of duplex scanning in particular have changed surgeons' perspective of progression of disease and restenosis of carotid endarterectomies.[31, 32]

Some older examples have been used in the earlier discussion, mainly because they are exemplary of poor reporting practices, which were very prevalent in the past but have been gradually, but not completely, eliminated. From the preceding discussion, however, that although the reader may wish to carry away a simple "bottom line" result from each report, such as a mortality and a patency rate, there are a number of other different but valid measures of

TABLE 3–4. COMPARISON OF "SUCCESS" RATE OF ILIAC DILATIONS AS JUDGED BY DIFFERENT CRITERIA (%)

CRITERION	ALL CASES (n = 66)	INITIAL SUCCESSES ONLY
Thigh-brachial index increased > 0.10	84	89
As above, but sustained	74	79
Ankle-brachial index increased > 0.10	64	68
As above, but sustained	54	58
As above, plus symptomatic improvement	52	54

success or failure, all adding to the overall perspective. These include:

- Primary and secondary patency
- Technical failure and hemodynamic failure
- Postoperative mortality and late survival rates
- Permanent procedure-related morbidity
- Some overall gauge of clinical outcome (i.e., symptomatic relief or "limb salvage")

RECOMMENDED STANDARD REPORTING PRACTICES

Because of the problems outlined previously, the Society for Vascular Surgery (SVS) and the North American Chapter of the International Society for Cardiovascular Surgery (ISCVS) appointed an ad hoc committee on "reporting standards," chaired by the senior author during its first decade. Subcommittees were appointed to recommend reporting standards for lower extremity ischemia,[28, 33] cerebrovascular disease,[34] venous disease,[35] aneurysms,[36] noninvasive testing,[37] and mesenteric and renovascular disease. The first of five subcommittees have reported recommendations that have been published. These reports have several suggestions in common. They define essential terms and make recommendations regarding:

- Clinical classification
- Criteria for improvement, deterioration, and failure
- A grading system for risk factors
- A categorization of operations
- Complications encountered with grades for severity or outcome

Some of the most pertinent recommendations are summarized here.

Estimating Patency Rates

As noted previously, the life-table method has been adopted as the method of choice for estimating graft patency. In the first report of the SVS/ISCVS ad hoc committee, the life-table method for survival (patency) estimation was the only type of analysis recommended for estimating patency rates,[33] but the revised lower extremity ischemia standards[28] also recognized the *Kaplan-Meier method*. Both methods require clear criteria for withdrawal and failure. The point of "lost to follow-up" or "dead with patent revascularization" occurs at the last *objective* evaluation. The committee recommends that patients whose grafts have failed since their last evaluation be treated as having failure dates halfway between the two examination points. This latter criterion is consistent with the spirit of the life-table method, although it does not define the life-table method.

The life-table method has two characteristic features worth noting here. The first is that events on the survival curve (e.g., graft failures) are grouped into intervals. Survival rates are then calculated for each of these intervals and used to generate cumulative patencies that describe the survival curve. The second is the assumption that any withdrawals during an interval occur at the mid-point of the interval. It is this assumption that leads to the characteristic correction to the calculated failure rate in a given interval:

$$\text{failure rate} = \frac{\text{number of failures}}{\text{number at risk} - {}^{1}/_{2}\,(\text{number of withdrawals})}$$

This correction assumes that the individuals who withdraw during an interval contribute to the risk pool for half of the interval but this is *equivalent* to increasing the interval failure rate by the number of expected failures in half of the withdrawal group. Inherent in this correction for censored data is the assumption that the failure rate for each interval is constant over that interval.

With this perspective, the use of the stair-step graphic presentation of the life-table survival curve is, in fact, inappropriate. The life-table graph (but not the Kaplan-Meier graph) is better represented by straight line connections between the patency estimates located at the *end* of each interval. The cumulative patency is the resulting conditional probability at the end of the interval based on the failure rate over the entire interval. In this presentation the only intervals with level lines are those with no failures. The reader is referred to the report of the SVS/ISCVS for details in the calculation of the life-table.[28]

The Kaplan-Meier survival estimate,[38] which is also called the *product-limit method*, is different from the life-table estimate, in that data are *not* grouped into intervals. Events on the survival curve occur only at individual failure points. One can conceptualize the Kaplan-Meier method as a life-table method with intervals containing a single observation and the intervals being very small. Consequently, no corrections are needed for the effect of withdrawals. In contrast to the life-table method, graphic presentation of the Kaplan-Meier survival curve *should* use the stair-step method because, between events on the Kaplan-Meier curve, nothing is really known about the failure rate and it is assumed to be zero.

The life-table method is a technique that makes calculations easier for large amounts of data,[74] and this may have been the main justification for using it rather than the Kaplan-Meier method but desktop computational power would appear to make this distinction moot. Indeed, the Kaplan-Meier method is not valid for numbers of less than 30, whereas the Kaplan-Meier method remains appropriate for any data size.[39] Either method is acceptable if used properly and documented.

Figures 3–2 and 3–3 show a life-table plot and a Kaplan-Meier plot based on the same data set. It can be seen that they give equivalent patency estimates. Complete life-table or Kaplan-Meier data should be submitted with each report, even though it may be the choice of the editor to print only the graph.

Numbers for the patients at risk at the start of each interval (periodically for the Kaplan-Meier method), or the standard error for each estimate of patency, must be displayed. When the standard error of the patency estimate exceeds 10%, the curve should not be drawn or it should be represented by a dotted line or some other means of indicating lack of reliability of the estimate. Comparisons of patency curves should be performed using the log-rank test of significance.[40]

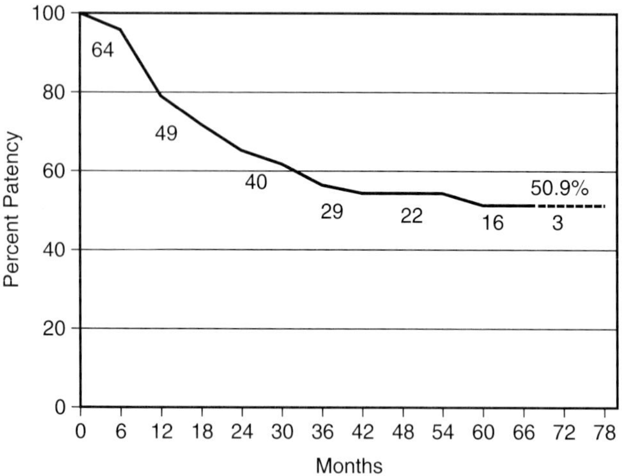

FIGURE 3–2. Patency curve by life-table method. (From Rutherford RB, Baker JD, Ernest C, et al: Recommended standard for reports dealing with lower extremity ischemia: Revised version. J Vasc Surg 26:517–538, 1997.)

Associated Risk Factors

Standardized grading codes for several factors that modify the outcome of procedures performed for arteriosclerotic occlusive disease have been developed, previously published,[33] and recently revised.[28] These factors include (1) diabetes, (2) tobacco use, (3) hypertension, (4) hyperlipidemia and (5) cardiac, renal, and pulmonary status. In every case, although specific and detailed guidelines have been identified, the severity code can be reduced to four simple levels: 0 = absent, 1 = mild, 2 = moderate, and 3 = severe.

Similar severity coding and risk factors have been developed for acute lower extremity deep vein thrombosis (DVT).[35] A system for disease severity scoring has been suggested by the senior author[41] and is the focus of deliberations of the current SVS/ISCVS Committee on Reporting Standards. A detailed analysis of risk factors may not be appropriate for all or even most reports, but it is recommended for any report claiming that such factors do, or do not, affect outcome.

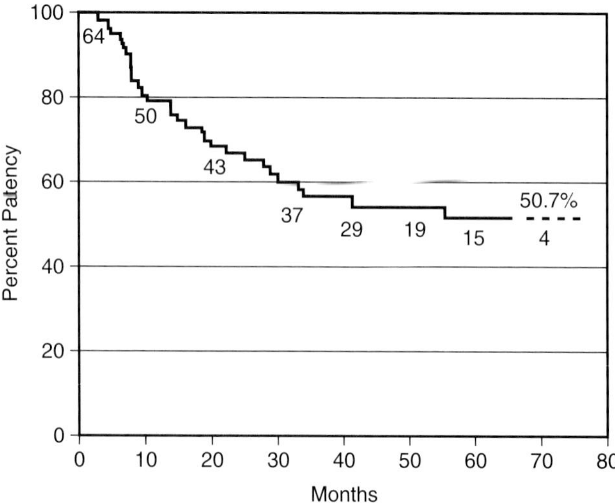

FIGURE 3–3. Kaplan-Meir patency curve. (From Rutherford RB, Baker JD, Ernest C, et al: Recommended standard for reports dealing with lower extremity ischemia: Revised version. J Vasc Surg 26:517–538, 1997.)

Reporting Deaths and Complications

Both early and late mortality rates after revascularization procedures should be reported routinely. The late mortality rates may be included as an additional column in the life table entitled "cumulative mortality." Late deaths should be categorized as due to the underlying disease (e.g., atherosclerosis), to delayed complications of surgical management, or to unrelated factors. In certain peripheral vascular procedures, it may be valuable to include "systemic/remote" and "local nonvascular" complications as well as "local vascular" complications, categorizing them as to type and grading them as to severity and outcome.[28] (For more details, see Section VII, particularly Chapter 39.) In addition, the senior author has published an article on the reporting of complications in vascular surgery that includes (1) a grading of disability, (2) a complications severity grading, and, to (3) to allow comparison between groups or others' experiences, a complications severity score.[42] The comparable reporting practice in cerebrovascular procedures involves reporting stroke-related and non–stroke-related deaths separately as well as separating neurologic morbidity attributable to stroke from that due to cranial nerve injury. For many clinical trials, a stroke severity scale is recommended.[34]

Lower Extremity Arterial Disease

Clinical Classification

The categories, or clinical classifications, recommended for stratifying limbs with *chronic* ischemia are outlined in Table 3–5. The asymptomatic category *(grade 0, category 0)* and a breakdown of claudicants *(grade I)* into three categories (1 to 3) according to duration of treadmill exercise *and* the degree of ankle pressure drop it produces are included to gauge degrees of improvement. These categories are primarily intended for clinical research; for most clinical practices, the classic *grades 0 to III*, similar to Fontaine's classes I to IV, are adequate.

An ankle pressure of 40 mmHg or a toe pressure of 30 mmHg, as an objective criterion of diffuse pedal ischemia, is required to place the patient in category 4 *(grade II)*—ischemic rest pain. Because healing requires an additional inflammatory response, these levels are *increased* to 60 mmHg ankle pressure and 40 mmHg toe pressure in the presence of infection, nonhealing ulceration, loss of tissue, or gangrene (category 5, *grade III*). The term "foot salvage" applies only to the treatment of cases fulfilling both the clinical and the noninvasive testing criteria for categories 4 and 5. Absence of rest pain and no amputation, or, at most, a minor amputation for the designation "limb/foot salvage." Neither a Syme's amputation nor amputation at a below-knee rather than an (anticipated) above-knee level qualifies for inclusion.

Cases of atheroembolism, or the "blue toe syndrome," ordinarily should be considered separately. They should *not* be included in the "threatened" or "limb salvage" categories without objective evidence of diffuse forefoot ischemia.

TABLE 3–5. CLINICAL CATEGORIES OF CHRONIC LIMB ISCHEMIA

GRADE	CATEGORY	CLINICAL DESCRIPTION	OBJECTIVE CRITERIA
0	0	Asymptomatic: no hemodynamically significant occlusive disease	Normal treadmill or stress test
I	1	Mild claudication	Completes treadmill exercise,* AP after exercise > 50 mmHg but 25 mmHg less than BP
	2	Moderate claudication	Between categories 1 and 3
	3	Severe claudication	Cannot complete treadmill exercise; AP after exercise < 50 mmHg
II	4	Ischemic rest pain	Resting AP < 40 mmHg, flat or barely pulsatile ankle or metatarsal PVR; TP < 30 mmHg
III	5	Minor tissue loss: nonhealing ulcer, focal gangrene with diffuse pedal ischemia	Resting AP < 60 mmHg, ankle or metatarsal PVR flat or barely pulsatile; TP < 40 mmHg
	6	Major tissue loss: extending above TM level, functional foot no longer salvageable	Same as Category 5

*Five minutes at 2 miles/hr on a 12% incline.
AP = ankle pressure; BP = brachial pressure; PVR = pulse volume recording; TN = transmetatarsal; TP = toe pressure.

Many of these issues have been addressed in a consensus article on chronic critical ischemia.[43]

Outcome Criteria

The following criteria are recommended for gauging change in limb status:

+3 *Markedly improved*: *no* ischemic symptoms and any foot lesions completely healed; ABI essentially "normalized" (>0.90).

+2 *Moderately improved*: no open foot lesions; still symptomatic but only with exercise and improved by at least one category*; ABI not normalized but increased by more than 0.10.

+1 *Minimally improved*: greater than 0.10 increase in ABI but no categorical improvement or vice versa, an upward categorical shift without an increase in ABI of greater than 0.10.

+0 *No change*: no categorical shift and less than 0.10 change in ABI.

−1 *Mildly worse*: no categorical worsening but ABI decreased more than 0.10 or vice versa, a downward categorical shift with an ABI decrease of less than 0.10.

−2 *Moderately worse*: one category worse or *unexpected* minor amputation (skin intact, preoperatively).

−3 *Markedly worse*: more than one category worse or unexpected major amputation.

*Refers to categories in Table 3–5.

Criteria for Patency

Authors of scientific articles should not accept patency rates that are not based on objective findings; "no evidence of occlusion" cannot be equated with patency for reporting purposes, nor can "palpable pulses" recorded from a clinic visit, considering the inaccuracy of pulse palpation by relatively inexperienced health care professionals. A bypass graft or otherwise reconstructed arterial segment may be considered patent when any of the following criteria are met:

1. Demonstrably patent by conventional arteriography or other established imaging techniques (e.g., digital subtraction arteriography, duplex ultrasonography, contrast-enhanced CT scan, magnetic resonance imaging (MRI), or radionuclide study).

2. Maintenance of the achieved improvement in the appropriate segmental pressure index, (i.e., no more than 0.10 less than the highest postoperative index. Although a greater drop in ABI may occur and the graft or reopened segment may still be patent, *imaging is required in these instances and in any other doubtful circumstances covered under criterion 2, 3, or 4*. To avoid the confusing effects of distal runoff disease, the most appropriate pressure index for this purpose is at the next level beyond the revascularized segment or distal anastamosis.

3. Maintenance of a plethysmographic tracing distal to the reconstruction that is significantly greater in magnitude than the preoperative value (e.g., +5 mm or +50% for pulse volume recording). This criterion is the weakest criterion and acceptable *only* when segmental limb pressures *cannot* be accurately measured, as in many diabetic patients. In most such cases, however, direct imaging is preferable.

4. The presence of a palpable pulse or the recording of a biphasic or triphasic Doppler waveform at two points directly over a superficially placed graft.

5. Direct observation of patency at operation or postmortem examination.

Reporting Patency Status

A graft is considered to have *primary patency* if it has had uninterrupted patency with either no procedures performed on it or a procedure (e.g., transluminal dilation or distal extension from the graft) to manage *disease progression in the adjacent native vessel*. Dilations or minor revisions performed for anastomotic or graft stenoses, graft dilations, or other structural defects *before* occlusion do not constitute exceptions in defining primary patency because they are intended to prevent eventual graft failure. Because the outcome of such interventions to preserve patency of the "failing" graft is markedly different from the outcome of interventions used to restore patency to a thrombosed graft, an *assisted* primary patency rate may be quoted as long as the pure primary patency rate is also noted.

If graft patency is restored *after* occlusion by thrombectomy or thrombolysis, or if problems with the graft itself or one of its anastomoses require PTA revision or reconstruction, it must be listed under *secondary patency.* However, a reoperation, specifically one that does not preserve flow through most of the original graft and at least one of its anastomoses, does *not* contribute to secondary patency. Detailed descriptions and explanations of these and other aspects are provided in the revised version of the recently recommended standards for reports addressing lower extremity ischemia.[28]

Cerebrovascular Disease

Clinical Classification

A scheme for clinical classification of cerebrovascular disease is presented in Table 3–6. This system, called "CHAT," is based on categories of *c*linical status, *h*istory, the responsible *a*rterial lesion, and the pathologic status of the *t*arget organ (brain or eye).

The clinical portion of the system includes both current clinical status and past clinical status or history.[44, 45] The cutoff between current and past has been selected to be 1 year. The primary clinical categories are as follows:

0 Asymptomatic
1 Brief stroke: full recovery in less than 24 hours (internationally more acceptable than transient ischemic attack)
2 Temporary stroke: full recovery in 24 hours to 1 month (often called "resolving ischemic neurologic deficit")
3 Permanent stroke: symptoms or signs lasting longer than 1 month.

In addition to these categories, the category of nonspecific dysfunction (4) allows identification of patients who do not fit into the precise classifications, a regrettable but necessary concession to the realities of clinical medicine. Finally, in the current clinical presentation, a category of changing stroke (formerly stroke-in-evolution) (5) is allowed for patients in whom therapeutic intervention is applied before the outcome of their current episode is known.

In each of the primary clinical classifications 1 to 3, an additional coding can be used to identify the vascular territory involved: carotid-ocular, carotid-hemispheric, vertebrobasilar, other focal, or diffuse. For the changing stroke category, additional coding identifies the nature of the stroke-in-evolution as improving, fluctuating, or deteriorating. After 1 month, a "changing stroke" with residual neurologic signs or symptoms must be reclassified as a "permanent stroke."

The artery and brain (target) involvement is coded simply by whether identifiable lesions are associated with the appropriate territory to match symptoms:

0 = no lesion
1 = appropriate lesion
2 = lesion in other vascular territory
3 = combination of 1 and 2

Subcoding allows identification of the pathology, such as arteriosclerosis or fibromuscular dysplasia, for the artery and hemorrhage or infarct for the brain (or eye) (see Table 3–6).

Diagnostic and Clinical Criteria

The severity of the residual neurologic deficit can be simply classified as either *minor* or *major*, depending on whether independence is maintained. For more detailed classification, the stroke severity scale in Table 3–7 is recommended. This is a graded scale of 1 to 11, depending on the impairment in any one or more of five domains (swallowing, self-care, ambulation, communication, and comprehension). This more detailed classification allows risk-benefit assessments of carotid endarterectomy and the outcome of intervention for stroke.

TABLE 3–6. CLINICAL CLASSIFICATION SCHEME FOR CEREBROVASCULAR DISEASE (CHAT)

C: CURRENT CLINICAL PRESENTATION (<1 YR)	H: PAST HISTORY	A: ARTERY	T: TARGET ORGAN (BRAIN)
		Territory	
0. *Asymptomatic* 1. *Brief* (stroke (<24 hr) a. Carotid-ocular b. Carotid-cortical c. Vertebrobasilar d. Other focal e. Diffuse	0. *Asymptomatic* 1. *Brief* stroke (<24 hr) a. Carotid-ocular b. Carotid-cortical c. Vertebrobasilar d. Other focal e. Diffuse	0. No lesion 1. Appropriate lesion for symptom 2. Lesion only in other vascular territory 3. Combination 1 + 2	0. No lesion 1. Appropriate lesion for symptom 2. Lesion only in other vascular territory 3. Combination 1 + 2
		Pathology	
2. *Temporary* stroke with full recovery (24 hr–1 month); a, b, c, d, e, same as No. 1 3. *Permanent* stroke (>1 month); a, b, c, d, e, same as No. 1 4. *Nonspecific* dysfunction 5. *Changing* stroke a. Improving b. Stable or fluctuating c. Deteriorating	2. *Temporary* stroke with full recovery (24 hr–1 month); a, b, c, d, e, same as No. 1 3. *Permanent* stroke (>1 month); a, b, c, d, e, same as No. 1 4. *Nonspecific* dysfunction	a. Arteriosclerotic plaque c. Cardiogenic (embolic) d. Dissection (spontaneous) e. Aneurysm f. Fibromuscular dysplasia r. Arteritis t. Trauma o. Other	h. Hemorrhage i. Infarct l. Lacuna m. Arteriovenous malformation n. Neoplasm o. Other

TABLE 3–7. NEUROLOGIC EVENT SEVERITY SCALE

SEVERITY GRADE	IMPAIRMENT*	NEUROLOGIC SYMPTOMS	NEUROLOGIC SIGNS
1	None	Present	Absent
2	None	Absent	Present
3	None	Present	Present
4	Minor, in one or more domains	Present	Present
5	Major, in only one domain	NA†	NA
6	Major, in any two domains	NA	NA
7	Major, in any three domains	NA	NA
8	Major, in any four domains	NA	NA
9	Major, in all five domains	NA	NA
10	Reduced level of consciousness	NA	NA
11	Death	NA	NA

From the EC/IC Bypass Study Group: The International Cooperative Study of Extracranial/Intracranial Arterial Anastomosis (EC/IC Bypass Study): Methodology and entry characteristics. Stroke 16:397–406, 1985. By permission of the American Heart Association, Inc.

*Impairment in the domains of swallowing, self-care, ambulation, speech, and comprehension. If independence is maintained despite the impairment, deficit is classified as minor; if independence is lost, it is classified as major.

†Neurologic signs and symptoms are integrated into the higher grades of impairment.

NA = Not applicable.

Contrast arteriography remains the "gold standard" for defining the severity of arterial lesions, but increasingly duplex scanning is being used to provide the same information. Its criteria are standardized against arteriography, and periodic quality assurance testing is required in each institution.

Classification of lesions is based primarily on the per cent diameter reduction *measured* from the view showing the greatest luminal reduction and using the normal outflow vessel as the comparison (e.g., the internal carotid artery beyond the upper extent of disease). The physiologic arguments for using cross-sectional area or residual lumen are valid, but those measures cannot be used as standards as long as current arteriographic methods are widely used. The suggested classification of lesions uses four divisions of stenosis ranges:

- 0% to 19%, normal
- 20% to 59%, mild
- 60% to 79%, moderate
- 80% to 99%, severe
- 100%, occluded

Because of the stratifications used in recent trials, duplex criteria have been developed for other levels of stenosis (e.g., 70%) (see Chapter 130). A second aspect of categorization of lesions is the description of the surface irregularity and ulceration. Recommendations are as follows:

0, normal, smooth surface
1, small ulcer less than 2 mm deep by 5 mm long
2, moderate ulcer
3, large ulcer more than 4 mm deep or 10 mm long
4, complex ulceration

Reporting Results

The results of therapeutic intervention for extracranial arteries are best measured by the occurrence (or absence) of stroke (including transient or temporary cerebrovascular symptoms) in the distribution of the artery operated on and the recurrence (or relief) of preoperative symptoms. If the overall postoperative stroke rate is applied, estimates of benefit can be adversely affected by progression of disease in the contralateral, untreated carotid artery. However, when surgical intervention is intended to relieve hypoperfusion in the contralateral hemisphere, recurrence of those symptoms must also be considered a treatment failure. Carotid patency is not a valid criterion because almost all stenoses are patent preoperatively. Carotid restenosis (>50%) is an appropriate yardstick, but if it is used, the relative incidence of symptomatic versus silent restenosis should be stated. With carotid endarterectomy now being challenged by carotid angioplasty, usually using stenting, it is important that these treatment modalities be judged by the same criteria and end-points. This and the special considerations associated with it have been discussed In detail by the senior author in a recent article.[45]

Additional measures of postoperative status include grading the severity of strokes using the aforementioned stroke severity scale (see Table 3–7) and categorizing the timing of stroke into:

1. Intraoperative stroke.
2. Perioperative stroke: worsening of neurologic status after the initial postoperative evaluation up to a period of 30 days.
3. Late postoperative stroke (after 30 days).

Venous Disease

Deep Venous Thrombosis

The recommended clinical classification of lower extremity venous thrombosis is made on the basis of *location* and *extent* of thrombus. Six segments are identified in the deep venous system affecting the lower extremities: tibial-soleal veins, popliteal vein, common and superficial femoral veins, profunda vein, iliac vein, and the vena cava. (The greater and lesser saphenous veins can also be classified when relevant to the case report.)

Each segment is graded on a 4-point scale of 0 to 3:

0 = patent
1 = nonocclusive thrombus
2 = subsegmental occlusive thrombus
3 = occlusive thrombus throughout the segmental length

Traditionally, this classification required detailed phlebography, but duplex ultrasonography is now used with accuracies equal to or exceeding phlebography, particularly for nonocclusive thrombi.

Associated risk factors for deep venous thrombosis (DVT) differ substantially from those used for other vascular conditions (Table 3–8). Also included in the table is a severity scale for each risk factor. Overall, the maximum point total is 28, and this total score may be used to stratify patients in comparative studies of prophylaxis or therapies.[35] Although this approach may be empirically

TABLE 3–8. ASSOCIATED RISK FACTORS FOR DEEP VENOUS THROMBOSIS (DVT)

RISK FACTOR		SEVERITY SCALE
Prior DVT	0–3	None/suspected/proven/multiple
Immobilization	0–3	None/1–3 days/>3 days/paraplegia
Anesthesia	0–3	Local/45 minutes general/>45 minutes general/>3 hr
Age	0–2	<40 yr/40–70 yr/>70 yr
Malignancy	0–3	None/recurrence/extensive regional tumor/metastatic
Malignant tissue type	0–1	where 1 = adenocarcinoma
Cardiac disease	0–3	New York Heart Association: class 1, class 2, class 3, class 4
Limb trauma	0–4	None/soft tissue injury/fracture of tibia and/or fibula/fracture of femur/ fracture of hip or pelvis
Thrombotic tendency	0–3	None suspected/suspected, proved treated/proved untreated
Hormonal therapy	0–1	No/yes
Pregnancy	0–1	Absent/present
Obesity	0–1	Normal to + 175% ideal body weight/ >175% ideal body weight

useful, the extent to which these risks are "additive" is debatable, and the assignment of relative risk under this scoring system awaits further research. Nevertheless, the consistent identification and grading of individual risk factors allow assessment of population comparability and, indeed, generation of the data necessary for relative risk assessment.

The results of therapy for treatment of DVT (e.g., thrombolytic therapy or thrombectomy) must specify both the patency and the valvular competence using vascular laboratory venous refilling time determinations (see later), except for the larger veins, such as the vena cava, in which valvular competency is irrelevant. There is no benefit to reporting partial clot resolution unless it exceeds 50% and opens up major tributaries.

Chronic Venous Insufficiency

The classification of chronic venous insufficiency (CVI) by clinical severity is outlined in Table 3–9. This system is reminiscent of the CHAT system proposed for cerebrovascular disease, with categories for *c*urrent clinical classification, *h*istory (prior clinical classification) *a*natomic location,

TABLE 3–9. OVERALL CLASSIFICATION FOR CHRONIC VENOUS INSUFFICIENCY

CLINICAL			ANATOMIC	
Class	Current	Prior	LOCATION	ETIOLOGY
0	Asymptomatic	Same	0 unknown	0 Unknown
1	Mild	Same	1 Superficial veins	1 Congenital
2	Moderate	Same	2 Perforators	2 Post-thrombotic
3	Severe (ulceration)	Same	3 Deep calf	
			4 Deep thigh	
			5 Deep iliofemoral	
			6 Deep caval	
			7 Combination of 2–5 (any)	

and *e*tiology. Both current and earlier clinical classifications use a 4-point severity scale:

0 = asymptomatic
1 = mild ankle swelling or painful varicosities, usually limited to superficial veins
2 = moderate CVI with hyperpigmentation in the gaiter area, moderate brawny edema, and subcutaneous fibrosis without ulceration
3 = severe CVI with chronic distal leg pain associated with ulcerated or preulcerative skin changes

The anatomic area is coded as six isolated segments, and code 7 is combined segments. Etiology is coded simply as unknown, congenital, or post-thrombotic.

This scale has been expanded into the *CEAP system*, which categorizes *c*linical, *e*tiologic, *a*natomic, and *p*athophysiologic attributes. The clinical scale has been expanded to a six-level classification, now widely used. The other categories and their subclasses are valuable to separate types of CVI and ordinarily should not be mixed in reporting results. A disability scale and a severity scoring system are also offered, but these have not been used widely. Efforts are under way to further extend the CEAP system's primarily descriptive classifications for more quantifiable severity scoring. Details of the CEAP system and its practical clinical application are provided in Chapter 145.

Functional documentation of CVI historically has used ambulatory venous pressures, which are still considered the standard by many. Normal ambulatory foot venous pressure is less than 50% of standing pressure. One noninvasive correlate of these measures is obtained by photoplethysmographic (PPG) assessment of venous return time (VRT), the time needed for return to baseline PPG levels after venous emptying by plantar flexion (see Chapter 11).[46] Normal VRT is greater than 20 seconds, mild CVI = 15 to 20 seconds, moderate CVI = 5 to 15 seconds, and severe CVI is less than 5 seconds. However, in many patients a normal VRT is considerably longer (e.g., 25 to 40 seconds), and, if one leg is normal, its VRT can be used as that patient's normal value.

A more sophisticated evaluation of venous function can be obtained by air plethysmography (see Chapter 11). Duplex scanning is now frequently used to assess not only segmental venous patency or reflux but also the severity of reflux. The point is that some physiologic measure of venous function is needed to correlate with clinical signs and symptoms in gauging disease severity and its modification by treatment.

Thus, reporting results of therapy and surgical intervention for relief of CVI must include functional as well as symptomatic assessment. One scheme for gauging clinical outcome is outlined in Table 3–10. The major shortcomings of reports on surgical interventions, particularly valvuloplasty and valve interposition, has been the lack of objective venous hemodynamic measurements (see Chapter 11), the lack of other than historical controls, the lack of adjustment for patient compliance or noncompliance with a nonoperative treatment program (e.g., elastic support stockings and intermittent periods of leg elevation), and the lack of assessment of changes in quality of life.

TABLE 3–10. CLINICAL OUTCOME FOR CHRONIC VENOUS INSUFFICIENCY

The final clinical outcome should be classified as follows:

+3	*Asymptomatic*: Improved at least one clinical class. Improvement of VRT and AVP to normal or at least +5 seconds, and −10 torr, respectively.
+2	*Moderate improvement*: Continuing mild symptoms with same clinical and VL improvement as in +3.
+1	*Mild improvement*: Improvement in either clinical class or VL tests, but not both. Unchanged clinically or by laboratory tests.
−1	*Mild worsening*: Worsening of either clinical outcome by one category or VL tests.
−2	*Significant worsening*: Both clinical and VL worsening.
−3	*Marked worsening*: Same as −2 accompanied by either new or worsening ankle ulceration.

VRT = venous refilling time; AVP = ambulatory venous pressure; VL = vascular laboratory.

Arterial Aneurysm

Classification

Arterial aneurysms are defined as focal arterial dilatations with a diameter at least 50% greater than that of the proximal normal arterial segment. Aneurysms may be classified by several factors Including site, etiology, morphology, and clinicopathology. Each of these classifiers may be more appropriate than others, depending on circumstances. For example, etiology is particularly relevant to anastomotic aneurysms but is unknown for arteriosclerotic aneurysms (see also Chapter 22).

Evaluation of Results

Patency is not the most valid measure of long-term success after prosthetic repair of major or central arterial aneurysms. Patient survival and freedom from significant complications are more important factors. The evaluation of complications for lower extremity arterial disease and cerebrovascular disease has been discussed; however, recurrent aneurysm formation should also be included as a major index of long-term success.

It is hoped that (1) adopting precise definitions of essential terms, (2) developing objective criteria by which the various measures of success or failure can be judged, and (3) establishing a standardized scheme by which severity of disease, degrees of improvement or deterioration, and risk factors that affect outcome can be graded will improve the quality of published reports of the results of vascular surgical procedures.[41]

Endovascular Surgery: Special Considerations

Early articles covering endovascular procedures, coming (as many did) from interventional radiology and cardiology sources, did not follow the standards set for open vascular surgical procedures and repeated many of the problems vascular surgeons had encountered earlier. These included:

1. Excluding initial failures from estimates of cumulative success rates.

2. Using varying criteria of success, including anatomic, technical and clinical.

3. Not using objective, hemodynamic criteria to confirm improvement or patency, (e.g., claiming "clinical patency").

4. Not distinguishing between primary and secondary patency (e.g., including redilations without listing their number).

5. Not characterizing or stratifying the anatomic lesions treated.

The publication and adoption of similar reporting standards by the *Journal of Vascular and Interventional Radiology*[47] and the subsequent publication of suggested reporting standards for endovascular procedures by a committee of the SVS/ISCVS[48] have helped immensely, although the latter have been challenged as being too severe by some interventionalists. The recently revised standards for reports on lower extremity ischemia have consolidated this picture somewhat by addressing all interventions, not just open surgical[28]; however, the rapidly increasing use of catheter-directed thrombolysis and other new interventions (particularly endografts, which can be applied to aneurysmal, occlusive, traumatic, and congenital lesions), requires some major adjustments. These have been addressed in some detail by the senior author.[44]

In general, it is recommended that, whenever possible, the revised standards[28] be applied regardless of the method by which occlusive lesions are treated (e.g., classifying acute and chronic ischemia, handling morbidity and mortality, reporting patency, grading risk factors, gauging degrees of change [the +3 to −3 scale], using life-table or Kaplan-Meier methods for plotting outcomes). The original endovascular standards (E) should be retained for lesion characterization and setting the temporal framework for short, intermediate, and long-term reports. The previously mentioned scheme for reporting complications might apply, but additional recommendations are needed to cover puncture site, local entry, and remote complications, such as dissection or rupture. The categories of contrast-related, medication-related, and device-related complications, as proposed by Sacks and colleagues,[49] may also be added. Most of the other standards needed for reports covering the endograft repair of AAAs, which were not included in the original aneurysym reporting standards,[36] have been addressed in a subsequent article by Ahn and coauthors.[50] Adverse events, such as endoleak, graft limb obstruction, device migration, infection, and reasons for explantation or conversion all must be included and reported in a standard way.

Other types of endovascular procedures not yet covered by existing reporting standards are embolotherapy, transjugular intrahepatic portosystemic shunts (TIPS), and caval interuption devices, although a multispecialty consensus statement on the caval interruption devices will soon be published.

Finally, with subcommittees of the SVS/ISCVS Committee on Reporting Standards at work on reporting standards for angioaccess procedures, renal revascularization, mesenteric vascular disease, a vascular surgery operative risk stratification, and carotid duplex criteria, the guidelines for vascular reporting can be expected to change and improve in the future.

CLINICAL AND PATIENT-BASED OUTCOMES PARAMETERS: USE OF QUALITY-OF-LIFE ASSESSMENTS

There are numerous parameters by which the treatment of vascular disease can be evaluated (Table 3–11). An optimal technical result represents a step toward the achievement of an improved functional status and quality of life for the patient. Although the achievement and documentation of an excellent technical outcome are unquestionably important, they are not synonymous with improvement in quality of life. This has been documented in several studies evaluating claudicants by walking distance, ankle-brachial index (ABI), and quality of life. Overall, these comparisons have demonstrated a poor or limited correlation between the clinical parameters and quality-of-life index.

Chetter and colleagues[51] evaluated 235 claudicants with treadmill walking distance, ABI, and the EuroQol generic quality-of-life survey.[75] A poor correlation was found between the clinical parameters of treadmill walking distance and ABI and the measured quality of life.

Similarly, Currie and associates[61] studied 186 patients undergoing treatment for claudication by unsupervised exercise, angioplasty, or surgery. In this study, although angioplasty and surgery improved quality-of-life scores, the improvement did not correlate with relative changes in the ABI. This lack of correlation underscores the difference between clinical and patient-based parameters. Both are essential to determine the impact of vascular disease and its treatment.

Patient-Based Outcomes Parameters

Assessment of the therapeutic risks and benefits associated with treatment of vascular disease requires determination of the following:

1. Manifestations of the condition, as reported by both patient and physician.
2. Impact of the disease on the patient's life and level of functioning.
3. Effect of the treatment and its adverse consequences on the disease and on the patient's life and level of functioning.

TABLE 3–11. COMMON PARAMETERS FOR ASSESSMENT OF VASCULAR INTERVENTION

1. *Clinical parameters*
   a. Physical examination
   b. Symptomatic measures: Rutherford Classification
   c. Objective anatomic and hemodynamic information
      (1) Angiographic information
      (2) Ankle-brachial indices
   d. Technical success
   e. Patency of the treated segment
   f. Limb salvage
   g. Procedural morbidity
   h. Procedural mortality
2. *Patient-based parameters*
   a. Disease—specific functional status
   b. Quality of life/survival
   c. General health status
      (1) Functional status
      (2) Perceived health
      (3) Psychological well-being
      (4) Role functioning

To characterize a disease process or condition, physicians most frequently use physical examination and laboratory data. This information is essential for appropriate diagnosis and treatment, but it does not indicate the manner and severity of the symptoms experienced by the patient. Physical examination and laboratory testing cannot measure these patient effects. Although in broad population studies a reduction of the ABI to the level of 0.30 indicates limb-threatening ischemia, an individual patient with such a degree of circulatory impairment may not experience rest pain and may have no ulcerations or ischemic gangrene. If the patient is sedentary, he or she may not even experience claudication. Conversely, a previously active patient with an ABI of 0.7 and an ambulatory distance of 2 blocks may be functionally very impaired. Thus, documentation of the patient's manifestations of vascular disease through patient-based reporting should greatly improve the physician's understanding of the patient's condition.

Because vascular disease may affect both an end organ, such as the leg, and the overall level of patient function, it is essential that information be collected about the effect of vascular disease on both. The level of functioning may be altered not only by the symptoms of vascular disease but also by the patient's psychologic or emotional response to these physical symptoms. Such responses are unique to individuals and must be directly assessed for each patient. There is evidence that physicians may not be good reporters of symptoms that cannot be easily observed or measured. This was effectively demonstrated by Pell,[52] who asked 201 claudicants to rate their quality of life before their first visit with a vascular surgeon. After the visit, the surgeon was asked to rate the patient's quality of life based on an understanding of the patient's symptoms and examination. The correlation between these two estimates was poor. Only through an understanding of the specific and overall effects of vascular disease on the patient can physicians develop appropriate therapeutic plans.

Both the beneficial and adverse effects of treatment must be recorded in a similar manner. Scientifically sound therapy may not always produce the degree of patient improvement expected by the surgeon. A patent bypass graft and an improved ABI index do not ensure an improved quality of life.

Schneider et al[53] evaluated the functional status and well-being of 60 patients who had undergone successful aortobifemoral bypass grafting at least 6 months earlier. Physical function, role function, and perceived health were found to be worse and bodily pain greater than in those without symptomatic arterial occlusive disease despite a patent bypass. An evaluation of outcomes of patients undergoing distal revascularization for limb-threatening ischemia has documented that limb salvage resulted in greater mobility and independent self-care but also in more patient anxiety and depression.[54] Further analysis of those patients treated by amputation identified a subset of patients (22% of the total) who had less mobility but equivalent independent self-care and lifestyle indices compared with those with successful limb salvage, suggesting that primary amputation may be indicated in some patients. A similar study has documented greater anxieties and less satisfaction among patients requiring repeat vascular surgical interventions compared with those undergoing their first procedure.[55]

These findings indicate that clinical measures (ABI, patency, limb salvage) effectively assess the physiologic impact of vascular intervention but do not adequately describe overall patient benefit or adverse effect. The benefits of any proposed therapy must outweigh the risks to the patient's overall level of function. Only by documenting all of the benefits and adverse effects of a therapy can a physician evaluate the treatment results.

Several outcomes parameters have been defined to permit the acquisition of this patient-based information:

- Functional status
- Perceived health
- Psychologic well-being
- Role function

The *functional status* assessment is directed toward the determination of how well the patient can perform tasks commonly required in daily life, such as climbing stairs, walking across a room, reading a newspaper, and holding a pen. These activities are generic in nature and are independent of gender and occupation.

The *perceived health* evaluation attempts to define how healthy a person believes he or she is and those aspects of ill health that most limit the patient. A patient's perception of his or her health may be adversely affected by disease even after treatment. In a study of 56 patients undergoing successful lower extremity revascularization, Gibbons and coworkers[56] noted that the only independent predictor of improved patient functional status 6 months after surgery was the patient's perception of his or her health status before surgery. Duggan's group,[57] evaluating 17 patients who had successful lower extremity bypass procedures, found that, at a mean of 18 months after surgery, there was a decline in perceived health despite a patent bypass.

Psychologic well-being refers to how worried, anxious, or depressed a patient is about his or her illnesses and treatment. Perceived health and psychologic well-being provide valuable information about the emotional impact of illness and insight into the effects of therapy. Even though claudication is not a directly life-threatening or limb-threatening disorder, Khaira and colleagues[58] documented greater perceived health problems regarding energy, pain, and emotional reactions among claudicants compared with a control group of nonclaudicants.

Role functioning evaluation is directed toward the assessment of the impact of a patient's illness on his or her ability to work and to perform obligatory duties. This dimension provides important information regarding the choice of treatment for claudication, for example.

TABLE 3–12. GENERIC QUALITY-OF-LIFE INSTRUMENTS

Nottingham Health Profile[77]
EuroQol Survey[75]
Sickness Impact Profile[71]
Medical Outcomes Study (MOS) SF-36[80]
Quality of Well-Being Scale[78]

TABLE 3–13. MEDICAL OUTCOMES STUDY 36: ITEM HEALTH SURVEY (SF-36) AREAS OF ASSESSMENT

Perception of health
Psychologic well-being
Role limitations due to physical health problems
Role limitations due to mental health problems
Physical function
Social relations
Pain
Fatigue

GENERIC OUTCOMES ASSESSMENT TOOLS

Several survey instruments are capable of assessing these health dimensions (Table 3–12). Each of these instruments has been broadly applied to large patient populations and has shown both reliability and validity, essential properties for acquiring meaningful information.

Reliability refers to the consistency of measurement of each question within the survey tool. In simplest terms, a reliable question will be answered in the same way by most individuals who have the same overall health condition. *Validity* implies that each question actually measures what is intended and that the answers to similar questions are consistent. In the absence of a change in the patient's condition, answers to specific questions in surveys administered over time should be the same.

The most commonly used health assessment tool in the United States is the Medical Outcomes Study (SF-36).[80] This instrument is subdivided into an eight-index set of questions (Table 3–13). For each health dimension, the response scores are coded, summed, and converted onto a scale from 0 to a high of 100.

As measured by the SF-36, physical function, role function, and pain are significantly affected by peripheral arterial occlusive disease (Fig. 3–4). The eight indices can be used individually or as an overall measure of general health status. Because this is a generic assessment tool, however,

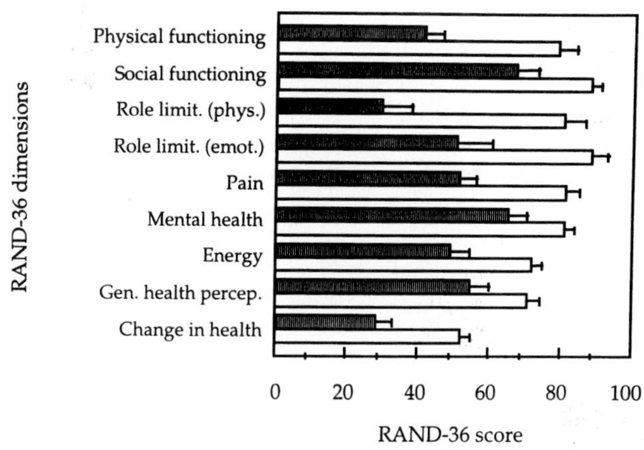

FIGURE 3–4. Impact of claudication on patient quality of life as assessed by the Rand SF-36 health survey, compared with the general population. (From Bosch JL, Hunink MGM: The relationship between descriptive and valuational quality-of-life measures in patients with intermittent claudication. Med Decis Making 16:217–225, 1996).

the subgroups are not disease-specific. Role limitations due to physical health problems, for example, cannot specifically identify the impact of claudication on occupation but manifest the aggregate effect of all co-morbid conditions on the performance of role-related activities.

Disease-Specific Outcomes

Claudication has been the subject of several survey instruments designed to assess the degree of limitation imposed by this symptom on the patient. One of the most widely used assessment instruments at this time is the Walking Impairment Questionnaire (WIQ).[59] This assessment tool has been designed to elicit information regarding the severity of discomfort experienced while walking, the reason for difficulty walking, walking distance and speed, and stair climbing. In studies of exercise therapy for claudication, the WIQ scores for walking distances and speed have improved in conjunction with increased treadmill walking distances. Regensteiner and associates[60] used the WIQ and the SF-20, a derivative of the SF-36, to evaluate patients with severe claudication before and after participation in a supervised exercise training program and compared them with a nonexercised control group. After 24 weeks, WIQ and SF-20 scores improved commensurate with increased treadmill walking distance. The control group failed to show improvement by any testing modality.

Lower Extremity Revascularization

Complete evaluation of the effect of treatment of vascular disease requires a multifactorial assessment of the patient, the disease, and the effect of treatment on each of these. The relationship between various objective clinical parameters, such as ABI and walking distance, and patient-reported outcomes of lower extremity ischemia do not show a high degree of correlation.[53, 56, 57, 61, 62] This is especially true of noninvasive treatments, such as exercise therapy.[63] The assessment of benefit to the patient of an intervention may be altered when both clinical and patient-based parameters are used for evaluation.

Whyman and coauthors[64] used several clinical and patient-based outcomes parameters to evaluate 30 patients undergoing balloon angioplasty and 32 patients treated with aspirin and exercise for claudication. Measures included ABI, treadmill distance to claudication, and quality of life as reported on the *Nottingham Health Profile*.[77] These investigators found that, at 2 years after treatment, patients who had undergone angioplasty had fewer occluded arterial segments than controls, but treadmill distance to claudication and quality of life did not differ significantly. The lack of differences in this and other such studies may arise because quality of life can be significantly affected by co-morbid conditions.[65]

To resolve the confusion in the published literature regarding the benefits of vascular intervention on peripheral arterial occlusive disease, both clinical and patient-based assessments should be reported. Though no formal guidelines have been established, there is now agreement about the most useful information for the evaluation of the treatment of claudication (Table 3–14). Similar guidelines can

TABLE 3–14. RECOMMENDED PARAMETERS FOR THE EVALUATION OF LOWER EXTREMITY ISCHEMIA

1. Standard clinical parameters
   a. Technical success
   b. Morbidity
   c. Mortality
   d. Vascular examination
   e. Ankle-brachial indices
   f. Patency of treated arterial segment
2. Changes in walking distance as measured by a treadmill protocol
3. Changes in symptom severity by Rutherford classification
4. Walking Impairment Questionnaire scores before and after treatment
5. SF-36 Quality of Life scores before and after treatment

be used for the evaluation of the treatment of critical limb ischemia.

The patient-based outcomes information can be obtained by having the patient complete the required questionnaires or by having a nurse administer the forms. The survey tools appear lengthy to some, but the time required for completion is usually less than that required for the corresponding vascular laboratory testing. A more careful evaluation of the outcomes of treatment of peripheral vascular disease permits vascular surgeons to better select appropriate forms of intervention for patients. This integrated approach to critical assessment of the benefit of vascular intervention confirms not only the technical precision of vascular reconstruction but also the long-term improvement in patient status.

COMPUTER-BASED VASCULAR REGISTRY

The need for accurate and uniform reporting standards existed before the advent of computer database techniques, but the microcomputer provides both impetus and a medium for achieving that goal. The requirement by computer data management software for precise, codifiable clinical data should provide some additional impetus to establishing such standards. The availability of powerful but relatively inexpensive hardware and software means that this medium for information is now accessible to the smallest surgical practice.

The clinical databases, or vascular registries, of individuals and well-circumscribed group practices have, in fact, formed the basis of most published reports in vascular surgery.[66] Several groups have advocated the establishment of regional[67] or even national vascular registries (such as the Swedish Vascular Registry). The benefits of such a database can be significant in providing a true picture of vascular surgical practices, prevalence of disease, and prognosis under varying therapies and in the presence of concomitant risk factors. Such a registry may even allow the study of relatively rare problems.

Potential Problems

The use of databases for tracking patients and, in particular, in retrospective studies has the potential for misuse. The major concern is one of scientific method and the associated statistical caveat that such data are indeed retrospective and nonrandomized with respect to any prognostic factors that might be studied.[72] This potential problem is not unique to computer-based "registries"; it is an ongoing issue in clinical research and medicine and is due, in large part, to the fact that the practice of clinical medicine is not performed in a controlled experimental setting.

Ethics and cost are major considerations in conducting prospective randomized trials. Also, a randomized controlled clinical trial does not guarantee unbiased data, and the experimental design cannot balance more than a few important prognostic factors. Considering the cost and effort of the randomized clinical trial and the focus imposed by randomization, the use of (vascular) registries as a source for observational studies should be viewed as a major opportunity not only to improve the design and focus of randomized trials but also to limit the number that need to occur.

The utility of the vascular registry in an observational or retrospective study depends on the quality and uniformity of its data. In addition to the reduction of bias by use of randomization, the randomized controlled trial also benefits from a strict protocol that standardizes definitions and assessment criteria among participating investigators and over time. This standardization allows rational use of stratification by prognostic factors in an attempt to balance the study groups of the experimental population. It is essential that the individual, regional, or national registry use standardized definitions and criteria.

Design Considerations

Collection of data is not synonymous with information. *Information* may be better described as a "process" than as a "commodity"[68] (i.e., the end result of data processing). Philosophically, it can be argued that until data are utilized, information does not exist,[69] but it is certainly true that data that cannot be utilized represent wasted time, effort, and money. Thus, effective retrieval and integration of data begin with an effective storage scheme.

Computer software for data management is usually known as a "database management system" (DBMS).[79] These application software programs perform two separate tasks: (1) data filing (the record-keeper) and (2) data management (the information generator).

The filing structure used in (relational) databases can be conceptualized as a table with rows of records and columns of fields. Data relationships are established by this macrostructure and by "key fields," or unique data items in each record. Commonly used unique keys are Social Security numbers or other assigned patient identifiers. Relationships can be established among separate tables by the use of the key fields (Table 3–15).

Data storage is easy; data management is the difficult part, but the processes are not independent. It may seem obvious that data retrieval and integration are easier when the amount of data is small. Conversely, these processes are meaningless without pertinent data. Which data should be stored is a difficult decision. An all too common approach is the storage of too much data in an attempt to ensure that all the necessary data will be available. The balance between too little and too much is more easily determined if the purpose of collecting the data has been identified.[70]

TABLE 3–15. EXAMPLE OF RELATIONAL TABLE STRUCTURES

File No. 1. Social Security No.	Name	Sex	Date of Birth
111-22-3333	Doe, Jane	F	03/01/39
123-45-6789	Doe, John	M	02/01/39
222-22-2222	Doe, Jack	M	01/01/39
Related Records			
File No. 2. Social Security No.	**Clinic Date**		**CHAT Score**
111-22-3333	01/01/87		2b-1a-1a-li
111-22-3333	01/01/88		0-2b-0-0
222-22-2222	01/01/88		0-0-0-0

CHAT = *c*linical status, *h*istory, *a*rterial lesion, and *t*arget organ.

Over the past several years, numerous commercially designed vascular database products have become available. These products typically use other commercially available DBMSs and provide a predefined data and management structure for the user. This clearly has an advantage for users without the knowledge and time to create their own. However, the considerations in the design have not been fundamentally changed simply because the structure is "prepackaged." Indeed, some of the issues of registry design become more problematic because the commercial package can never fit the user's needs quite as readily as a "custom" database. The buyers of such commercial products should insist on the flexibility to add related tables (files related by key fields) to the commercial product, and never should the buyer be restricted only to queries (reports) written by the commercial concern.

However the registry software is created, the most difficult aspects of a good vascular registry are data entry and maintenance of patient records. For example, when one is interested in follow-up on a 5-year experience with carotid endarterectomy, the registry would not be very useful if 20% of the cases were missing at random—or worse, at some specific biased time over the period of interest.

A major cost of computers in general and databases in particular is the associated labor cost. In this instance, some knowledgeable individual must aid in coding and entering data, or the data will incomplete and unreliable. The vascular surgeon, ideally, participates in the design and creation of the vascular registry but must certainly participate in the ongoing maintenance of the registry.

Multicenter studies are usually the result of either corporate-sponsored research in support of Food and Drug Administration (FDA) applications or government-sponsored research on specific questions (e.g., current Veterans Administration cooperative studies) and occur relatively infrequently. Yet when multicenter reports appear in the literature, they are usually referenced as definitive studies. This perception of the larger importance of multicenter studies, as compared with individual experiences, is a direct result of the increased reliability of larger sample sizes incorporating different patient populations, different surgeons, and so forth, and also of standardizing clinical data, such as clinical classifications, risk factors, and outcome. In effect, the multicenter trial as a well-designed, experimental clinical design benefits from standardized reporting practices.

The vascular registry cannot replace the multicenter or randomized trial, but with the incorporation of standardized reporting practices it provides a means of studying certain problems cooperatively and with larger numbers than would be possible in individual or group experiences. The well-defined vascular registry, at the least, should provide practitioners with a means of assessing their experience and realistically comparing that experience with similarly well-defined published studies.

REFERENCES

1. U.S. Congress, Office of Technology Assessment: Identifying Health Technologies That Work: Searching for Evidence. Pub No. OTA-H-608. Washington DC, U.S. Government Printing Office, 1994.
2. Veith FJ, Gupta SK, Ascer E, et al: Six-year prospective multicenter randomized comparison of autologous saphenous vein and expanded polytetrafluoroethylene grafts in infrainguinal arterial reconstructions. J Vasc Surg 3:104, 1986.
3. Harris PL, Jones D, How T: A prospective randomized clinical trial to compare in situ and reversed vein grafts for femoro-popliteal bypass. Br J Surg 74:252, 1987.
4. Eugene J, Goldstone J, Moore WS: Fifteen-year experience with subcutaneous bypass grafts for lower extremity ischemia. Ann Surg 186:177, 1976.
5. Ray LI, O'Connor JB, Davis CC, et al: Axillofemoral bypass: A critical reappraisal of its role in the management of aortoiliac occlusive disease. Am J Surg 138:117, 1979.
6. El Massry S, Saad E, Sauvage LR, et al: Axillofemoral bypass using externally supported, knitted Dacron grafts: A follow-up through twelve years. J Vasc Surg 17:107, 1993.
7. Harris EJ, Taylor LM, McConnel DB, et al: Clinical results of axillobifemoral bypass using externally supported polytetrafluoroethylene. J Vasc Surg 12:416, 1990.
8. Glantz SA: Primer of Biostatistics. New York, McGraw-Hill, 1981, p 7.
9. Berkson J, Gage RP: Calculation of survival rates for cancer. Mayo Clin Proc 25:270, 1950.
10. Cutler SJ, Ederer F: Maximum utilization of the life table method in analyzing survival. J Chron Dis 8:699, 1958.
11. Peto R, Pike MC, Armitage P, et al: Design and analysis of randomized trials requiring prolonged observations of each patient: I. Introduction and design. Br J Cancer 34:585, 1976.
12. Peto R, Pike MC, Armitage P, et al: Design and analysis of randomized trials requiring prolonged observations of each patient: II. Analysis and examples. Br J Cancer 35:1, 1977.
13. Veith FJ, Moss CM, Fell SC, et al: Comparison of expanded polytetrafluoroethylene and autologous saphenous vein grafts in high risk arterial reconstructions for limb salvage. Surg Gynecol Obstet 147:749, 1978.
14. DeWeese JA, Rob CG: Autogenous venous grafts five years later. Am Surg 174:346, 1971.
15. Underwood CG, Charlesworth D: Uses and abuses of life table analysis in vascular surgery. Br J Surg 71:495, 1984.
16. Berkowitz HD, Hobbs CL, Roberts B, et al: Value of routine vascular laboratory studies to identify vein graft stenosis. Surgery 90:971, 1981.
17. Rutherford RB, Patt A, Kumpe DA: The current role of percutaneous transluminal angioplasty. *In* Greenhalgh KM, Jamieson CW, Nicolaides AN (eds): Vascular Surgery: Issues in Current Practice. London, Grune & Stratton, 1986, pp 229-244.
18. Rutherford RB, Jones DN, Bergentz SE, et al: The efficacy of dextran-40 in preventing early postoperative thrombosis following difficult lower extremity bypass. J Vasc Surg 1:765, 1984.
19. Reichle FA, Tyson RR: Bypasses to tibial or popliteal arteries in severely ischemic lower extremities: Comparison of long-term results in 233 patients. Ann Surg 176:315, 1972.
20. LoGerfo FW, Johnson WC, Corson JD, et al: A comparison of the late patency rates of axillobilateral femoral and axillounilateral femoral grafts. Surgery 81:33, 1977.
21. Johnson WC, LoGerfo FW, Vollman RW: Is axillobilateral femoral graft an effective substitute for aortobilateral iliac femoral graft? Ann Surg 186:123, 1976.
22. Naji A, Barker CF, Berkowitz HD, et al: Femoropopliteal vein grafts for claudication: Analysis of 100 consecutive cases. Ann Surg 188:79, 1978.
23. Naji A, Jennifer C, McCombs PR, et al: Results of 100 consecutive femoropopliteal vein grafts for limb salvage. Ann Surg 188:162, 1978.
24. Sanders RJ: Personal communication.
25. Ascer E, Veith FJ, Gupta SK, et al: Comparison of axillounifemoral and axillobifemoral bypass operations. Surgery 97:169, 1985.
26. Rutherford RB, Patt A, Pearce WH: Extra-anatomic bypass: A closer view. J Vasc Surg 5:437, 1987.
27. Flanigan DP, Pratt DG, Goodreau JJ, et al: Hemodynamic and angiographic guidelines in selection of patients for femoro-femoral bypass. Arch Surg 113:1257, 1978.
28. Rutherford RB, Baker JD, Ernst C, et al: Recommended standards for reports dealing with lower extremity ischemia: Revised version. J Vasc Surg 26:517, 1997.
29. Johnston KW, Colapinto RF, Baird RJ: Transluminal dilation: An alternative. Arch Surg 117:1604, 1982.
30. Rutherford RB, Jones DN, Martin MS, et al: Serial hemodynamic assessment of aortobifemoral bypass. J Vasc Surg 4:428, 1986.
31. Zeirler RE, Bandyk DF, Thiele BL, et al: Carotid artery stenosis following endarterectomy. Arch Surg 117:1408, 1982.
32. Ouriel K, Green RM: Clinical and technical factors influencing recurrent carotid stenosis and occlusion after endarterectomy. J Vasc Surg 5:702, 1987.
33. Rutherford RB, Flanigan DP, Gupta SK, et al: Suggested standards for reports dealing with lower extremity ischemia. J Vasc Surg 4:80, 1986.
34. Baker JD, Rutherford RB, Bernstein EF, et al: Suggested standards for reports dealing with cerebrovascular disease. J Vasc Surg 8:721, 1988.
35. Porter JM, Clagett GP, Cranley J, et al: Reporting standards in venous disease. J Vasc Surg 8:172, 1988.
36. Johnston KW, Rutherford RB, Tilson MD, et al: Suggested standards for reporting on arterial aneurysms. J Vasc Surg 13:444, 1991.
37. Thiele BL, Jones AM, Hobson RW, et al: Standards in noninvasive cerebrovascular testing. J Vasc Surg 15:495, 1992.
38. Kaplan EL, Meier P: Nonparametric estimation from incomplete observations. J Am Stat Assoc 53:457-481, 1958.
39. Lee ET: Statistical Methods for Survival Data Analysis. Belmont, Calif, Wadsworth, 1980, pp 75–92.
40. Lawless JF: Statistical Models and Methods for Lifetime Data. New York, John Wiley & Sons, 1982.
41. Rutherford RB: Presidential Address: Vascular surgery: Comparing outcomes. J Vasc Surg 23:5, 1996.
42. Rutherford RB: Suggested standards for reporting complications in vascular surgery. *In* Towne JB, Bernhard WM (eds): Complications in Vascular Surgery, 3rd ed. St. Louis, Quality Medical Publishing, 1991, pp 1–10.
43. Second European consensus document on chronic critical leg ischaemia. Circulation 84(Suppl 4): IV-1, 1991.
44. Rutherford RB: Reporting standards for endovascular surgery: Should existing standards be modified for newer procedures? Semin Vasc Surg 10:197, 1997.
45. Rutherford RB: Comparing outcomes of carotid interventions: The importance of standardized reporting practices. *In* Branchereau A, Jacobs M (eds): New Trends and Developments in Carotid Artery Disease. Amonk, NY, Futura Publishing Co, 1998, pp 1–8.
46. Barnes RW: Noninvasive techniques in chronic venous insufficiency. *In* Bernstein EF (ed): Noninvasive Diagnostic Techniques in Vascular Disease, 3rd ed. St. Louis, CV Mosby, 1985, p 839.
47. Rutherford RB, Becker GJ: Standards for evaluating and reporting the results of surgical and percutaneous therapy for peripheral vascular disease. J Vasc Interv Radiol 2:169, 1991.
48. Ahn SS, Rutherford RB, Becker GJ, et al: Reporting standards for lower extremity arterial endovascular procedures. J Vasc Surg 17:1103, 1107 1993.
49. Sacks D, Marinelli DL, Martin LG, et al: Reporting standards for clinical evaluation of new peripheral arterial revascularization devices. J Vasc Interv Radiol 8:137, 1997.
50. Ahn SS, Rutherford RB, Johnston KW, et al: Reporting standards for infrarenal endovascular abdominal aorta aneurysm repair. J Vasc Surg 25:405, 1997.

51. Chetter IC, Kester RC, Scott DJ, et al: Correlating clinical indicators of lower-limb ischaemia with quality of life. Cardiovasc Surg 5:361, 1997.
52. Pell JP: Impact of intermittent claudication on quality of life. The Scottish Vascular Audit Group. Eur J Vasc Endovasc Surg 9:469, 1995.
53. Schneider JR, McHorney CA, Malenka DJ, et al: Functional health and well-being in patients with severe atherosclerotic peripheral vascular occlusive disease. Ann Vasc Surg 7:419, 1993.
54. Johnson BF, Evans L, Drury R, et al: Surgery for limb threatening ischemia: A reappraisal of the costs and benefits. Eur J Vasc Endovasc Surg 9:181, 1995.
55. Ronayne R: Feelings and attitudes during early convalescence following vascular surgery. J Adv Nurs 10:435, 1985.
56. Gibbons GW, Burgess AM, Guadagnoli E, et al. Return of well-being and function after infrainguinal revascularization. J Vasc Surg 21:35, 1995.
57. Duggan MM, Woodson J, Scott TE, et al. Functional outcomes in limb salvage vascular surgery. Am J Surg 168:188, 1994.
58. Khaira HS, Shearman CP, Hanger R: Quality of life in patients with intermittent claudication. Eur J Vasc Endovasc Surg 12:511, 1996.
59. Regensteiner JG, Steiner JF, Panzer RJ, Hiatt WR: Evaluation of a walking impairment questionnaire in patients with peripheral arterial disease. J Vasc Med Biol 2:142, 1990.
60. Regensteiner JG, Steiner JF, Hiatt WR: Exercise training improves functional status in patients with peripheral arterial disease. J Vasc Surg 23:104, 1996.
61. Currie IC, Lamont PM, Baird RN, Wilson YG: Treatment of intermittent claudication: The impact on quality of life. Eur J Vasc Endovasc Surg 10:356, 1995.
62. Feinglass J, McCarthy WJ, Slavensky R, et al: Effect of lower extremity blood pressure on physical functioning in patients who have intermittent claudication. J Vasc Surg 24:503, 1996.
63. PACK Claudication Substudy Investigators: Randomized placebo-controlled, double-blind trial of ketanserin in claudicants: Changes in claudication distance and ankle systolic pressure. Circulation 80:1544, 1989.
64. Whyman MR, Ruckley CV, Housley E, et al: Is intermittent claudication improved by percutaneous transluminal angioplasty? A randomized controlled trial. J Vasc Surg 26:551, 1997.
65. Cook TA, Galland RB: Quality of life changes after angioplasty for claudication: Medium-term results affected by co-morbid conditions. Cardiovasc Surg 5:424, 1997.
66. Karmody AM, Fitzgerald K, Branagh BS, et al: Development of a computerized registry for large-scale use. J Vasc Surg 1:594, 1984.
67. Plecha FR, Avellone JC, Beven GC, et al: A computerized vascular registry: Experience of The Cleveland Vascular Society. Surgery 86:826, 1979.
68. Blois MS: Information and Medicine. Berkeley and Los Angeles, University of California Press, 1980, pp 1–17.
69. Blois MS: Information and Medicine. Berkeley and Los Angeles, University of California Press, 1980, pp 22–24.
70. Wasserman AI: Personal computers in the health care environment. *In* Lindberg DAB, Collen MF, Van Brunt EE (eds): Computer Applications in Medical Care. New York, Masson, 1982, pp 51–55.
71. Bergner M, Bobbitt RA, Carter WB, et al: The Sickness Impact Profile: Development and final revision of a health status measure. Med Care 19:787, 1981.
72. Dambrosia JM, Ellenberg JH: Statistical considerations for a medical data base. Biometrics 36:323, 1980.
73. Chang JB: Current state of extra-anantomic bypasses. Am J Surg 152:202, 1986.
74. Colton T: Statistics in Medicine. Boston, Little, Brown, 1974, pp 244–246.
75. EuroQol Group: EuroQol—a new facility for the measurement of health-related quality of life. Health Policy 16:199, 1990.
76. Hepp W, de Jonge K, Pallua N: Late results following extra-anatomic bypass procedures for chronic aortoiliac occlusive disease. J Cardiovasc Surg 29:181, 1988.
77. Hunt SM, McEwen J, McKenna SP (eds): Measuring Health Status. Dover, NH, Croom Helm, 1986.
78. Kaplan RM, Bush JW: Health-related quality of life measurement for evaluation and research and policy analysis. Health Psychol 1:61, 1982.
79. Martin J: Principles of Data-base Management. Englewood Cliffs, NJ, Prentice-Hall, 1976.
80. Ware JE, Sherbourne CD: The MOS 36-item short-form health survey (SF-36)-I: Conceptual framework and item selection. Med Care 30:473, 1992.

SECTION II

BASIC PRINCIPLES IN VASCULAR DISEASE

ANTON N. SIDAWY, M.D.

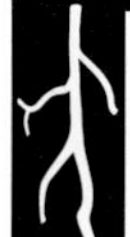

CHAPTER 4

Embryology of the Vascular System

Joseph M. Giordano, M.D.

It is difficult to imagine a more complex structure with all its organs and systems than the human body. Yet within 40 weeks of gestation, the human body develops almost flawlessly from a small clump of cells that appear after conception. To support this rapidly developing embryo, a functional vascular system must be present by the end of the 3rd week of gestation. Up to that point, the embryo receives its nourishment from the yolk sac and through the diffusion of oxygen and nutrients from the maternal circulation.

INITIAL DEVELOPMENT OF THE VASCULAR SYSTEM

The primitive vascular system forms initially from a clump of mesenchymal cells that separate and form channels. These channels eventually unite to form primitive endothelial lined vessels that become a functioning vascular network by the end of the 3rd week (Fig. 4–1). This system then connects to the developing heart that, although it consists only of two tubes, is still capable of effectively circulating blood.

At the beginning of the 4th week, the cardiovascular system consists of two heart tubes connected to a paired dorsal aorta that extends down the entire length of the embryo. The dorsal aortas each have segmental dorsal, lateral, and ventral branches. At the level of the seventh cervical vertebra, the paired dorsal aorta fuse to create the thoracic and abdominal aorta but proximal to the seventh cervical vertebra, the paired dorsal aorta persists. As this is occurring, the heart tubes fuse to form the heart. Cephalad to the developing heart, the truncus arteriosus and the aortic sac form. Six pairs of arteries, called *aortic arches*, develop from the aortic sac, pass laterally around the developing gut, and connect to the paired dorsal aorta.

During the 6th to 8th weeks of gestation, the six aortic arches along with the seventh segmental dorsal artery from each paired dorsal aorta develop into the aortic arch and its major branches. It is interesting that the vascular system of aortic arches present at the beginning of the 6th week of gestation imitates the system found in marine life. Marine animals have a single ventricle. Blood flows from the single ventricular chamber to the aortic sac to the paired aortic arches, which then break up to small capillaries that receive oxygen from the gills. The capillaries re-form to become

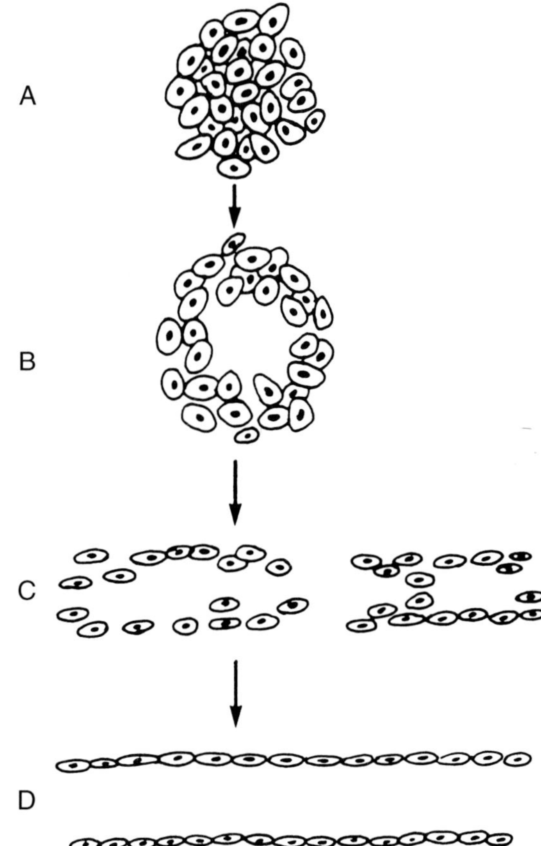

FIGURE 4–1. Initial development of vessels. *A*, Clumps of cells forms. *B*, Cavities develop. *C*, Channels form. *D*, Channels unite to form primitive endothelium-lined vessels.

major vessels again (like the pulmonary veins in the human) that carry the oxygenated blood to the dorsal aorta and the rest of the body.

For the most part, the vascular system in the human is symmetric, with each side of the body a mirror image of the other. One exception to this observation is the aortic arch, which differs on the right side compared with the left. The innominate artery, which divides into the right carotid artery and the subclavian artery, is not present on the left side, which has the left carotid and subclavian arteries originating from the aortic arch. These differences are directly related to the behavior of the left and right aortic arches as they evolve into the mature thoracic aortic arch in humans. The six pairs of arches along with the dorsal aorta, truncus arteriosus, and aortic sac elongate, dilate, regress, and disappear and in general change their configuration to become the fully developed aortic arch. The diagrammatic representation of these changes suggests that the aortic arches are all present at the same time, but this is not the case; some arches are developing while at the same time others are regressing.

Aortic Arch

The first, second, and fifth arches and the distal section of the right sixth arch disappear (Fig. 4–2*A*). The dorsal aorta on both sides between the third and fourth arches also disappears. Blood to the third aortic arch then flows only to the head and neck (Fig. 4–2*B*). The third arch becomes the *common carotid artery,* and the dorsal aorta between the first and third arches becomes the *internal carotid arteries.* The right dorsal aorta distal to the seventh intersegmental artery but proximal to the fused thoracic aorta involutes so that blood entering the right fourth arch flows to the right dorsal aorta and then to the right seventh intersegmental artery. This section eventually becomes the right subclavian and axillary arteries (Fig. 4–2*C*). The section of the aortic sac connected to the right third and fourth aortic arch elongates becoming the innominate artery, with the third arch becoming the right common carotid artery and the fourth arch contributing to the right subclavian artery, as noted above.

The left fourth arch and the left dorsal aorta distal to the left fourth arch dilate and become part of the aortic arch with the left intersegmental artery becoming the left subclavian and axillary artery. The proximal part of both sixth arches becomes the right and left pulmonary artery respectively. The distal part of the right sixth arch disappears, but the distal part of the left sixth arch persists as the ductus arteriosus. This connects the left pulmonary artery to the aorta and in the fetus shunts blood away from the immature fetal lungs to the aorta (Fig. 4–2*D*).

Anomalies

In view of the complex events that occur in the development of the aortic arch and its branches, it is not surprising that anomalies occur.[1–5] Parts of the primitive aortic arch that should disappear actually persist while other parts that should persist actually disappear.

Patent Ductus Arteriosus

Patent ductus arteriosus is the most common vascular anomaly. The ductus arteriosus is formed from the distal part of the left sixth arch. At birth, the ductus constricts, probably as a result of its initial exposure to blood with high oxygen content from the thoracic aorta. By 1 month, the ductus is normally obliterated to become the ligamentum arteriosum. If the ductus arteriosus does not constrict but remains patent, blood is shunted from the high-pressure thoracic aorta to the low-pressure pulmonary system, eventually causing significant pulmonary hypertension.

Coarctation of the Aorta

Aortic coarctation usually occurs at the level of the ligamentum arteriosum. The more common *postductal* type occurs just distal to the ligamentum; the *preductal* type occurs just proximal to the ligamentum.

The etiologic mechanism remains unclear, but the anomaly is thought to result from incorporation of oxygen sensitive muscle tissue from the ductus arteriosum into the wall of the aorta. Normally to close the ductus arteriosus, this muscle constricts when exposed to high oxygen tension. If the muscle is also in the wall of the aorta, the aorta constricts at that level. Eventually, chronic changes occur and the constriction becomes permanent.

Double Aortic Arch

At times, the right dorsal aorta distal to the right seventh intersegmental artery fails to involute. A double aortic arch forms with the right limb passing posterior to the esophagus to join the left limb that passes anterior to the trachea. A vascular ring forms around the esophagus and trachea, sometimes compressing these structures (Figs. 4–3*A* and *B*).

Right Aortic Arch

Involution of the left dorsal aorta distal to the left seventh segmental artery while the right dorsal aorta persists, opposite to the normal sequence, creates a right aortic arch (Figs. 4–4*A* and *B*). The ligamentum arteriosum arises from the distal right sixth arch instead of the distal left sixth arch but still connects to the aorta. If the arch passes to the left side posterior to the esophagus, a vascular ring is formed with the ligamentum arteriosum. If the right aortic arch passes anterior to the esophagus and trachea, a vascular ring is not formed. The right aortic arch with a retroesophageal component may initially be a double aortic arch in which the left dorsal aorta later regresses.

Retroesophageal Right Subclavian Artery

The subclavian artery normally forms from the right fourth aortic arch, the right dorsal aorta distal to the right fourth aortic arch, and the seventh intersegmental artery. A retroesophageal right subclavian artery forms because the right aortic arch and the dorsal aorta distal to the right arch abnormally involute (Figs. 4–5*A* to *C*). The right dorsal aorta distal to the right intersegmental artery then persists instead of involuting, joining the right seventh intersegmental artery to form the right subclavian artery. As the arch of the aorta enlarges and migrates cranially from the aortic sac, the right subclavian in this anomaly also migrates, eventually becoming distal to the left subclavian

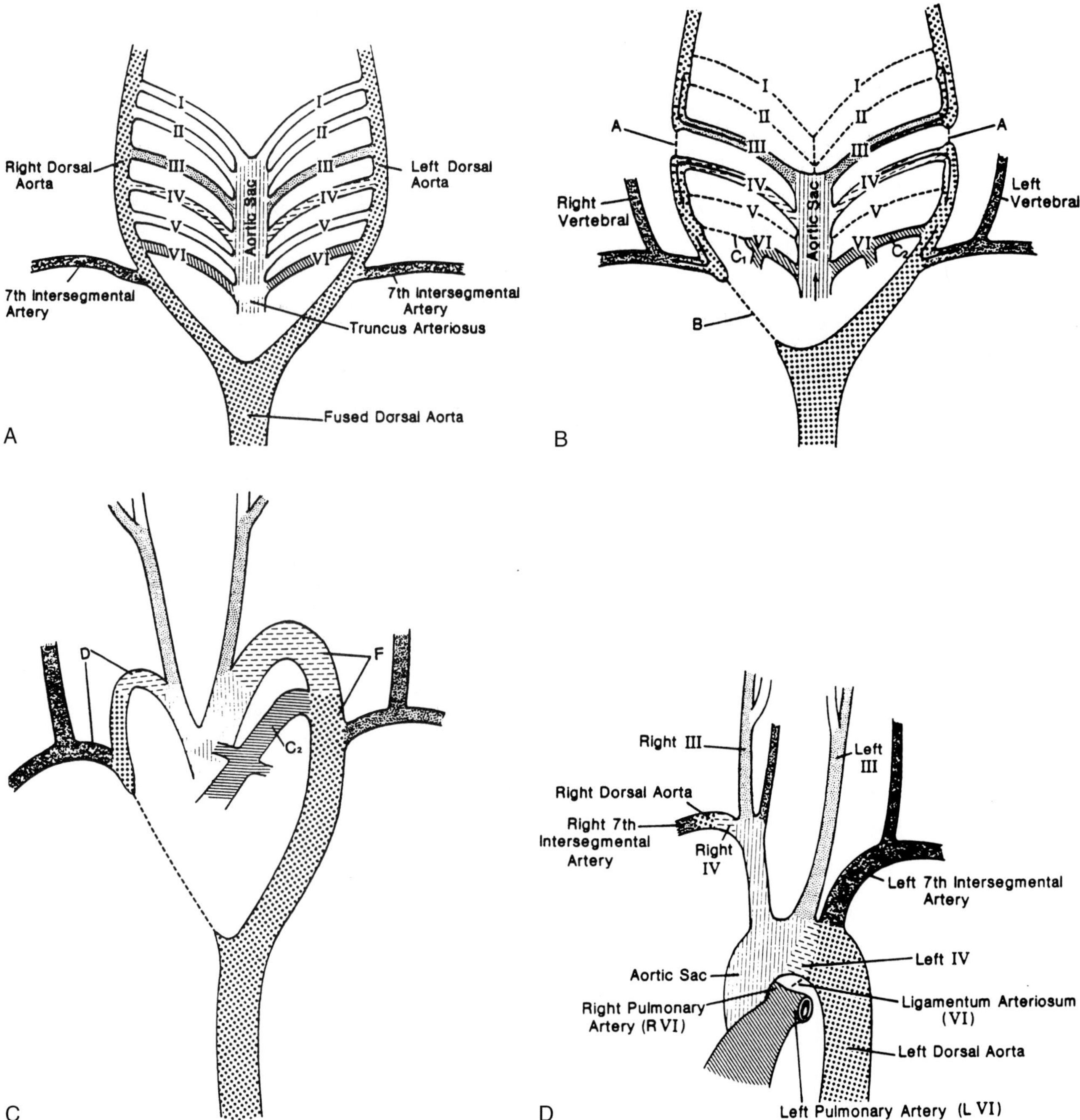

FIGURE 4–2. *A*, The six primitive aortic arches. The first, second, and fifth arches disappear. The paired dorsal aortas fuse at the level of the seventh cervical vertebra to become the thoracic and abdominal aorta. *B*, Differentiation of aortic arches. The dorsal aorta between the third and fourth arches (A) involutes so that blood entering the third arch perfuses the head only. The third arch and its branches become the carotid system. The right dorsal aorta distal to the right seventh intersegmental artery (B) involutes so that blood entering the right fourth arch perfuses the right upper extremity. This system becomes the right subclavian artery. The distal part of the right sixth arch (C-1) involutes, but the distal part of the left sixth arch (C-2) persists, becoming the ductus arteriosus. *C*, Aortic arch development. The right fourth arch, the dorsal aorta distal to the right fourth arch, and the right seventh intersegmental artery become the right subclavian artery (D). The left fourth arch and the left dorsal aorta distal to it becomes part of the aortic arch (F). The left seventh intersegmental artery becomes the left subclavian artery. Pulmonary arteries are forming from the sixth arch with the ductus arteriosus (C-2) present. *D*, Segments of the aortic arches that produce the adult aortic arch. The patent ductus arteriosus has become the ligamentum arteriosum.

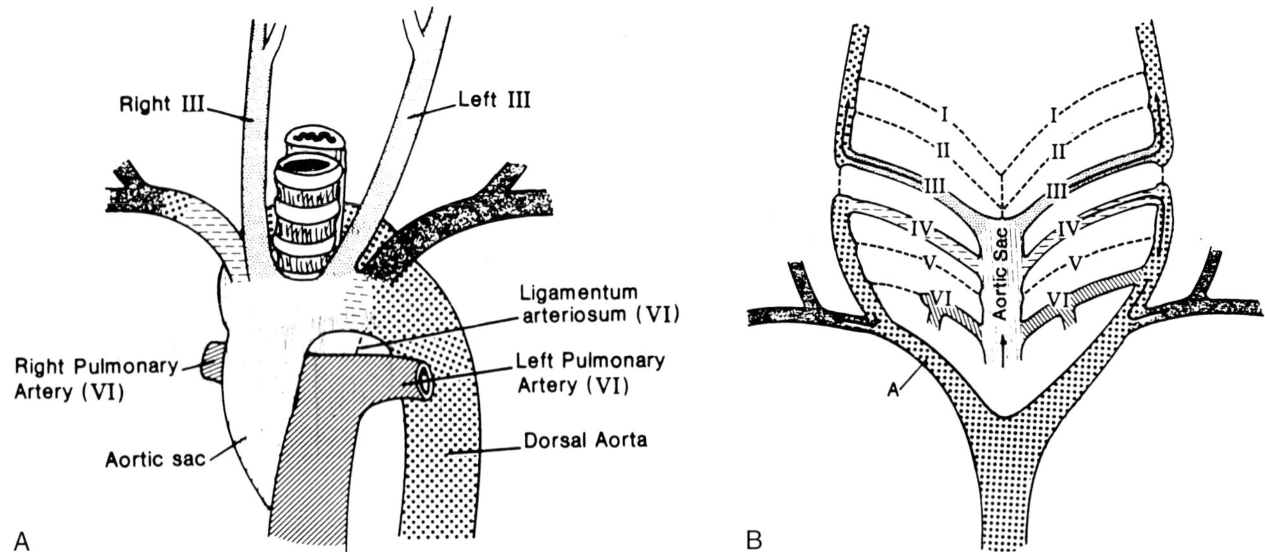

FIGURE 4–3. *A*, Double aortic arch. The aortic arch passes anterior and posterior to the trachea and esophagus, forming a vascular ring. *B*, Double aortic arch. The right dorsal aorta distal to the right seventh intersegmental artery (A) that normally involutes persists to become part of the double aortic arch.

artery. The right subclavian artery then goes from the aorta, which now is on the left side behind the esophagus, to supply the right arm. Most patients with this entity are asymptomatic, but they may have difficulty with swallowing.[2]

Thoracic and Abdominal Aorta

At the 3rd week of gestation, the embryo is developing into a segmental structure throughout its entire length, eventually forming from 36 to 38 segments, or somites. The paired dorsal aorta runs the entire length of the embryo. At each segment, the aorta has dorsal, lateral, and ventral branches.

At the 4th week, the paired dorsal aorta at the level of the seventh cervical vertebra fuse to become the thoracic and abdominal aorta. However, the segmental arteries persist so that each segment of fused aorta has two dorsal, ventral, and lateral branches. These branches involute, dilate, and fuse so that the dorsal branches become the vertebral arteries in the neck, the intercostal arteries in the chest, the lumbar arteries in the abdomen. The fifth lumbar dorsal segmental arteries enlarge to become the common iliac arteries. The paired ventral arteries initially become the *vitelline arteries*, which connect to the yolk sac. As the gastrointestinal tract develops, the vitelline arteries are its blood supply; these arteries eventually fuse to become the celiac, superior mesenteric, and the inferior mesenteric arteries. The ventral arteries at the level of the fifth lumbar segment connect to the dorsal segmental arteries to become

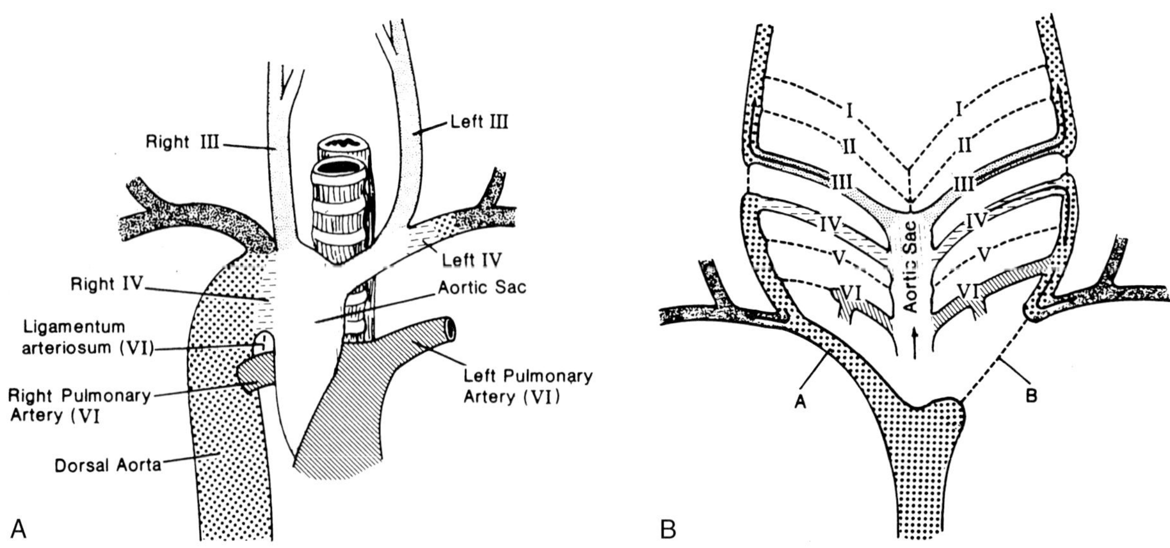

FIGURE 4–4. *A*, The right aortic arch. One of the two types in which the right arch passes anterior to the trachea and esophagus so that no vascular ring is formed. If the right arch passes posterior to the trachea and esophagus, the ligamentum arteriosum and the right arch form a vascular ring. *B*, Right aortic arch. The right dorsal aorta distal to the right seventh intersegmental artery persists (A), while the left dorsal aorta distal to the left seventh intersegmental artery involutes (B), the opposite of the normal occurrence.

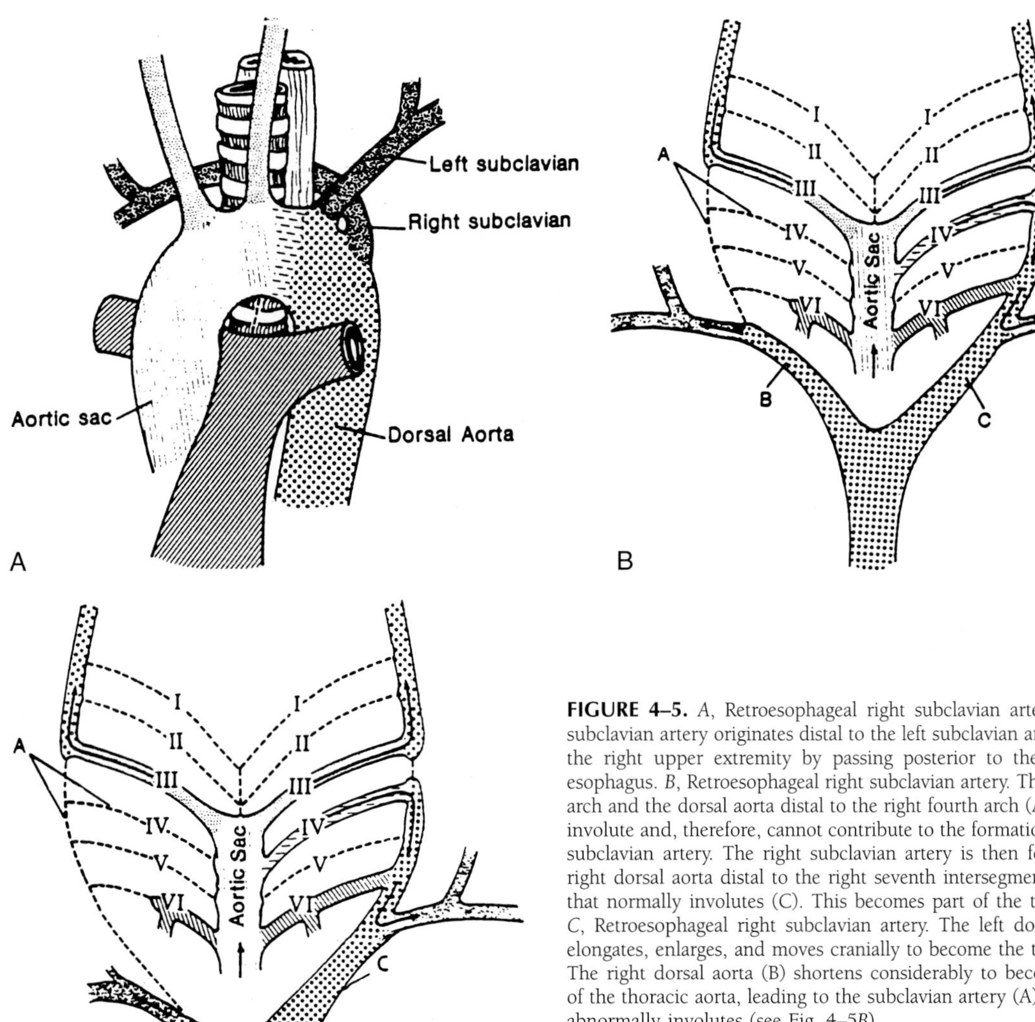

FIGURE 4–5. *A*, Retroesophageal right subclavian artery. The right subclavian artery originates distal to the left subclavian artery, reaching the right upper extremity by passing posterior to the trachea and esophagus. *B*, Retroesophageal right subclavian artery. The right fourth arch and the dorsal aorta distal to the right fourth arch (A) abnormally involute and, therefore, cannot contribute to the formation of the right subclavian artery. The right subclavian artery is then formed by the right dorsal aorta distal to the right seventh intersegmental artery (B) that normally involutes (C). This becomes part of the thoracic aorta. *C*, Retroesophageal right subclavian artery. The left dorsal aorta (C) elongates, enlarges, and moves cranially to become the thoracic aorta. The right dorsal aorta (B) shortens considerably to become a branch of the thoracic aorta, leading to the subclavian artery (A). This section abnormally involutes (see Fig. 4–5*B*).

the internal iliac arteries. The lateral segmental arteries form the renal arteries. Initially, these segmental branches are the blood supply to the primitive urogenital ridge. The pronephros and mesonephros form and then disappear, yielding to the metanephros, which becomes the permanent kidney.

At the seventh week, the metanephros ascends. The caudal segmental arteries disappear; the cranial arteries persist initially but then also disappear, leaving only one segmental artery, on each side, which becomes the renal arteries. Not surprisingly, considerable variations in the arterial supply to the kidney exist.[6, 7] Only 71% of individuals have single arteries to each kidney. The rest have a variety of combinations of hilar and separate branches to the poles of the kidneys. Fusion of the caudad kidney poles arrests the cranial kidney migration. Segmental arteries persist, providing a separate blood supply to the fused kidney. Similarly, ectopic kidneys frequently have multiple segmental arteries instead of a single renal artery. Therefore, evaluation of either a horseshoe or an ectopic kidney prior to a planned surgical procedure must take into account their anomalous arterial blood supply.[8]

The Extremities

Each upper and lower extremity begins as an outgrowth of tissue, a limb bud, off the trunk of the embryo. Initially, the limb bud is nourished by a capillary plexus that coalesces to form a single artery as the limb elongates.

In the *upper extremity*, the development of the arterial supply is relatively simple. The developing single artery becomes the axillary artery, the brachial artery, and the anterior interosseus artery. This system unites with the subclavian artery, formed for the most part in the development of the aortic arch by the seventh intersegmental artery. The radial artery and the ulnar artery form later as branches of the brachial artery and replace the anterior interosseus as the dominant blood supply of the forearm and hand.

The development of the arterial supply to the *lower extremities* is far more complicated (Fig. 4–6). Two systems

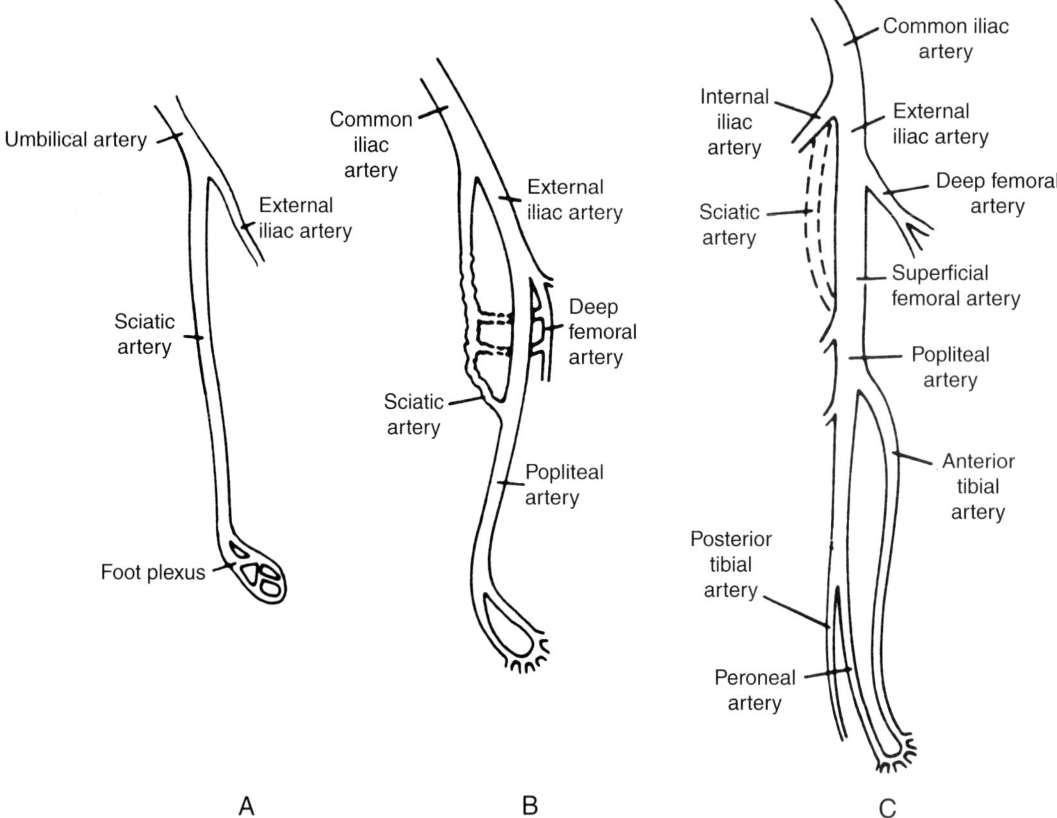

FIGURE 4–6. Arterial supply to the left lower extremity. *A*, Sciatic artery forming as a branch of the umbilical artery initially supplies the entire leg. *B*, The sciatic artery regresses, while the external artery develops into the common femoral artery to supply the thigh. Note that the sciatic artery communicates with the popliteal artery just above the knee. *C*, The sciatic artery disappears, although small portions remain to form the popliteal and peroneal arteries.

develop. The *sciatic* system forms initially.[9] The fifth lumbar dorsal segmental artery becomes the common iliac artery. The umbilical arteries, which are paired ventral segmental arteries, eventually become the internal iliac arteries attaching to the common iliac arteries. The sciatic arteries develop from the internal iliac arteries following the posterior course of the sciatic nerve.

At the 6th week of gestation, the second system of the lower extremity, the *external iliac artery*, develops off the umbilical artery uniting with the femoral system. The iliofemoral system replaces the sciatic system, which completely regresses in the upper thigh. In the lower thigh, the sciatic artery joins the iliofemoral system. In the leg, segments of the sciatic artery persist, forming parts of the popliteal and peroneal artery. In the pelvis, remnants of the sciatic form the internal iliac artery and its branches, the inferior gluteal artery and the superior gluteal artery.

The popliteal artery forms from the union of two arteries: (1) the *deep popliteal artery*, which is part of the sciatic system initially supplying blood to the lower leg, and (2) the later developing *superficial popliteal artery* (Fig. 4–7). The distal section of the deep popliteal artery anterior to the popliteus muscle regresses. The superficial popliteal artery forms posterior to the popliteus muscle and unites with the proximal part of the deep popliteal artery to form the mature popliteal artery.

Lower Extremity Vascular Anomalies

Persistent Sciatic Artery

If the femoral system fails to develop, the sciatic artery may persist instead of regressing, supplying blood to the thigh. The incidence of this rare anomaly is 0.05%.[10] The sciatic artery may be complete from its origin off the internal iliac artery to its union with the popliteal artery. It may also be incomplete, so that its connection with the internal iliac or popliteal artery is through small collaterals. The anomalous persistent sciatic artery is anatomically next to the sciatic nerve, entering the thigh through the sciatic notch, remaining posterior to the adductor magnus until the insertion of that muscle, where it enters the popliteal fossa to join the popliteal artery.

If the artery is complete, the patient with a persistent sciatic artery may present with a palpable popliteal artery but an absent femoral pulse. A persistent sciatic artery in the buttocks is superficial and can be traumatized. Along with immature vascular elements present in the sciatic artery, this condition causes early atherosclerotic changes

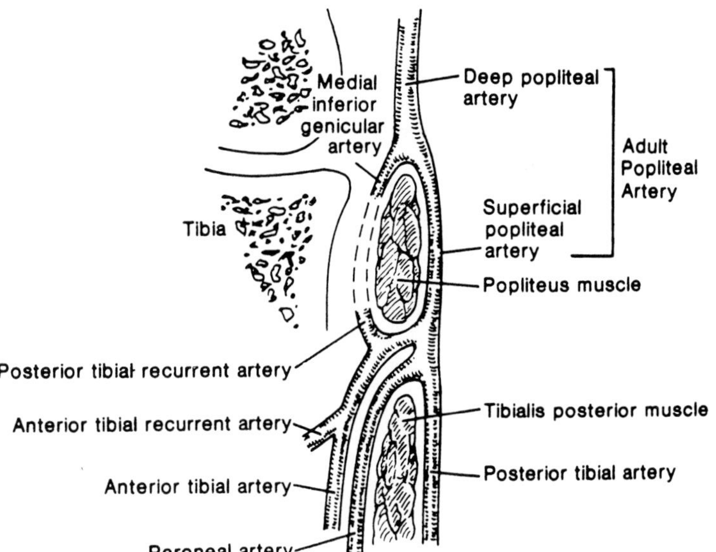

FIGURE 4–7. Embryologic development of the popliteal artery, as modified from Senior (Am J Anat 25:55, 1919[9]). The deep popliteal artery anterior to the popliteus muscle regresses, while the superficial popliteal artery posterior to the popliteus muscle becomes the mature popliteal artery. (From Gibson MHL, Mills JG, Johnson GE, et al: Popliteal entrapment syndrome. Ann Surg 185:341, 1977.)

and, possibly, aneurysm formation in the buttock.[11] The aneurysm may compress the sciatic nerve, causing neurologic symptoms.

Popliteal Entrapment Syndrome

The popliteal entrapment syndrome is an anomaly that results from the delayed attachment of the medial head of the gastrocnemius muscle. The gastrocnemius muscle arises from the calcaneus, migrating cephalad until it divides into a lateral and medial head.[9, 12] The lateral head attaches first to the lateral epicondyle of the femur while the medial head attaches later to the medial epicondyle. At the time of the attachment of the medial head, the popliteal artery has already formed and is in its normal anatomic location.

If the popliteal artery develops late or if the medial head migrates early, the artery is not in its normal location; instead, it is swept medially and impinged against the femur as the medial head attaches to the epicondyle. Actually, no case of the popliteal artery being compressed on the lateral epicondyle has been observed, probably because the lateral head attaches early, well before the popliteal artery forms. Clinically, patients with popliteal entrapment syndrome present at an early age. Claudication and popliteal artery aneurysm formation both result from compression of the artery against the femur by the medial head of the gastrocnemius muscle.

DEVELOPMENT OF THE VENOUS SYSTEM

Like the arterial system, the venous system develops from clumps of cells that form a capillary network. Within 4 weeks of gestation, some of these capillaries enlarge to become the major veins of the embryo. At 4 weeks, three paired venous systems form and drain the yolk sac, the placenta, and the embryo (Fig. 4–8). The vitelline veins drain the yolk sac and intestinal canal, enter the liver, and eventually become the portal vein, the hepatic venous sinusoids, and the hepatic veins. The umbilical vein brings the oxygenated blood from the placenta to the heart. Although only a single vein in the umbilical cord, a paired system of umbilical veins develops initially but regresses, except the portion of the left umbilical vein caudal to the liver, the ductus venosus, which in the mature embryo connects to the right hepatic vein bringing oxygenated blood from the placenta directly to the heart without traversing the liver.

After birth, the ductus venosus atrophies to become the ligamentum teres (round ligament) and the ligamentum venosum of the liver. The paired cardinal veins drain the body of the embryo. The veins cephalad to the heart (the precardinal veins) join the veins caudad to the heart (the postcardinal veins) to form the paired common cardinal veins, which enter the heart. The precardinal veins become the superior vena cava and its major branches; the postcardinal veins below the liver help form the inferior vena cava and its branches.

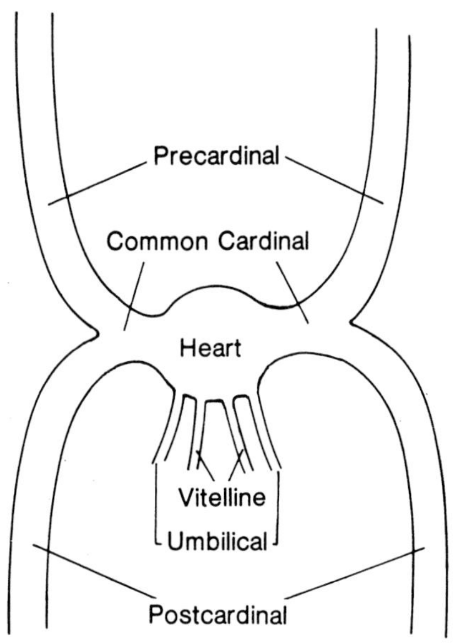

FIGURE 4–8. Venous system of 4-week-old embryo.

Superior Vena Cava

The cephalad portions of the paired precardinal systems become the subclavian and jugular veins. At the 8th week of gestation, the left innominate vein develops obliquely, connecting the left precardinal system to the right precardinal system. At the same time, the section of the left precardinal vein caudal to the developing innominate vein and the left postcardinal vein between the liver and the heart atrophies, so that all the blood from the left side of the head and neck enters the heart through the innominate vein and the superior vena cava. The superior vena cava develops from enlargement of the right precardinal and common cardinal vein. The right postcardinal vein above the liver becomes the *azygos system* (Figs. 4–9*A* and *B*).

Anomalies

Two anomalies can occur from development of the superior vena cava. Neither anomaly is clinically important, except that it produces unusual shadows on chest x-ray studies.

A *double superior vena cava* develops from failure of the caudal section of the left precardinal vein to regress.[13] This may occur with or without the development of the innominate vein.

Left-sided superior vena cava occurs if the caudal section of the right precardinal veins regresses while the caudal section of the left precardinal vein remains open, the opposite of the normal development.[14] An innominate vein forms, but in this anomaly it connects the right precardinal vein to the left precardinal vein, which is becoming a left-sided superior vena cava.

Inferior Vena Cava

The inferior vena cava and the iliac veins develop from three parallel sets of veins that appear at different times during the 6th to 10th weeks of gestation (Figs. 4–10*A* and *B*). The veins appear to go through various changes, but eventually parts of each set coalesce to form the inferior vena cava. The postcardinal veins located on the posterior aspect of the fetus appear first. All of this system regresses except the proximal part of the right postcardinal vein above the liver, which becomes the azygos system, and the most distal section, which becomes the iliac veins.

Next, the subcardinal veins located anterior and medial to the postcardinal veins appear. The left subcardinal completely regresses while the right subcardinal vein becomes the suprarenal inferior vena cava. The supracardinal veins located just posterior to the aorta appear last. The left supracardinal vein disappears while the right supracardinal vein becomes the infrarenal section of the inferior vena cava. The suprarenal portions of the supracardinal veins connect to the proximal portion of the postcardinal veins to become the azygos system and the *hemiazygos system*. The junction of the subcardinal and supracardinal system occurs at the level of the kidney. Small veins form and eventually coalesce to form a large vein anterior and posterior to the aorta at the level of the renal arteries. The posterior vein regresses, but the anterior vein persists to become the left renal vein (Figs. 4–10*C* and *D*).

Anomalies

The anomalies of the inferior vena cava and renal veins include:[15–21]

Duplication: Left-Sided Inferior Vena Cava

Duplication occurs if the left supracardinal vein fails to regress. Both supracardinal veins persist joining at the level of the renal arteries, creating a double inferior vena cava. If the left supracardinal vein persists while the right supracardinal vein regresses (the opposite of normal), a left-sided inferior vena cava occurs. The vein crosses to the right side at the level of the renal arteries. It is a mirror image of the normal anatomy. The right adrenal and gonadal veins, instead of emptying into the inferior vena cava as is normal, empty into the right renal vein; likewise, the left adrenal and gonadal vein empty into the inferior vena cava instead of the left renal vein, as is normal.

Renal Vein Anomalies

The most common venous anomaly occurs in the left renal vein. Retroaortic left renal vein occurs if the posterior left renal vein persists while the anterior left renal vein regresses; this is the opposite of normal. At times, both anterior and posterior left renal veins persist, forming a circumaortic left renal vein. Both veins join just before entering the inferior vena cava so that a venous collar is formed.

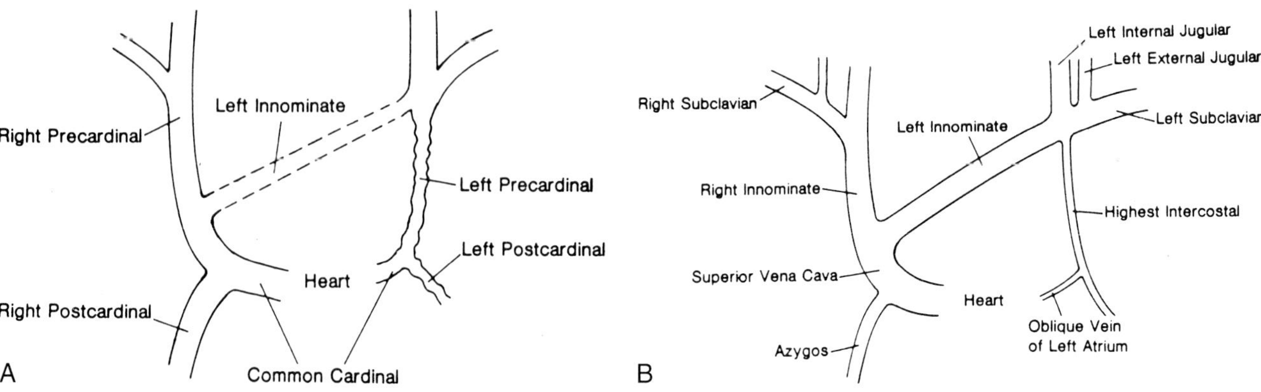

FIGURE 4–9. Development of the superior vena cava and major branches. *B*, Completed development of the superior vena cava and major branches.

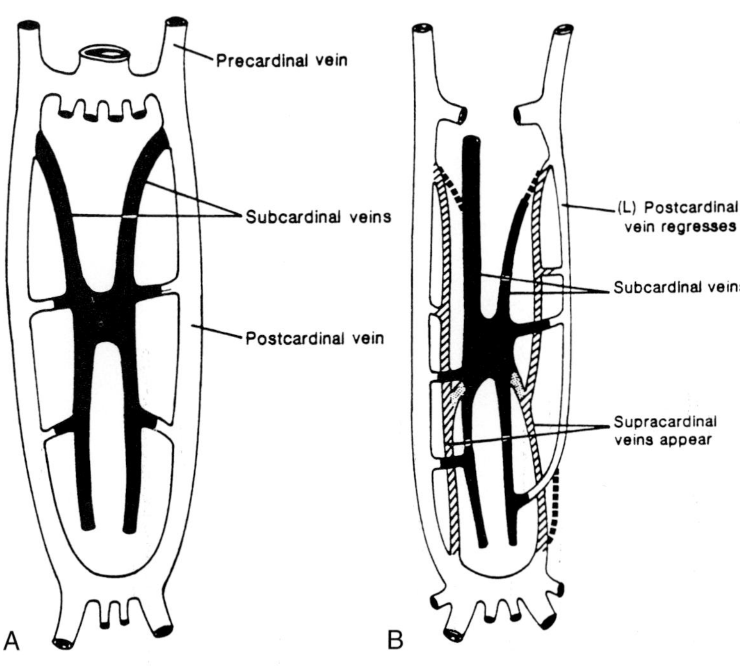

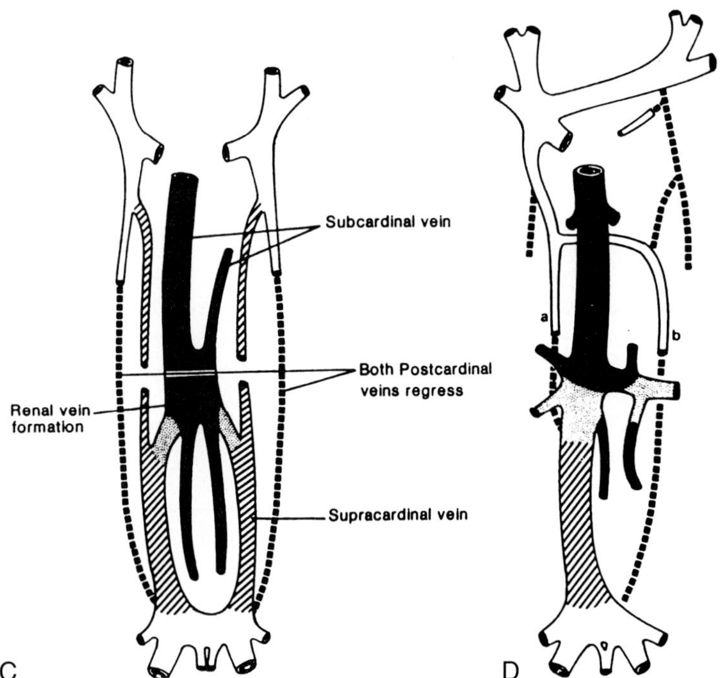

FIGURE 4–10. Development of the inferior vena cava. A. At 6 weeks of gestation, postcardinal veins are dominant with subcaudal system beginning to appear. *B*, At 7 weeks of gestation, subcardinal veins are dominant, and supracardinal system begins to appear. Postcardinal veins are beginning to regress. *C*, At 8 weeks of gestation, subcardinal veins form the suprarenal inferior vena cava. Supracardinal veins form the infrarenal inferior vena cava. Postcardinal veins regress. *D*, The adult inferior vena cava. Portions of the postcardinal veins persist to form the azygos system (A) and the hemiazygos system (B). (From Giordano JM, Trout HH III: Anomalies of the inferior vena cava. J Vasc Surg 3:924, 1986.)

SUMMARY

The arterial and venous systems both begin as a clump of cells that very rapidly develop into the mature vascular system. Anomalies are unusual but interesting. They rarely have a clinical impact. Knowledge of the embryology of the vascular system enables the surgeon to understand the developmental abnormalities. Familiarity with the logic of arterial development enhances our appreciation of the awesome beauty of the human body in general and the vascular system in particular.

REFERENCES

1. Arcinegas E, Hakima M, Hertzler JH, et al: Surgical management of congenital vascular rings. J Thorac Cardiovasc Surg 77:721, 1979.
2. Mahoney EB, Manning JA: Congenital abnormalities of the aortic arch. Surgery 55:1, 1964.
3. Richardson JV, Doty DG, Rossi NP, et al: Operation for aortic arch anomalies. Ann Thorac Surg 31:426, 1981.
4. Binet JP, Langlois J: Aortic arch anomalies in children and infants. J Thorac Cardiovasc Surg 73:248, 1977.
5. Lincoln JCR, Deveall PB, Stark J, et al: Vascular anomalies compressing the esophagus and trachea. Thorax 24:295, 1969.
6. Merklin RJ, Michaels NA: The variant renal and suprarenal blood

supply with data on inferior phrenic, urethral, and gonadal arteries. J Int Coll Surg 29:41, 1958.
7. Gray SW, Skandalokis JE: Embryology for Surgeons. Philadelphia, WB Saunders, 1972, p 486.
8. Anson BJ, Richardson GA, Minear WL: Variations in the number and arrangements of the renal vessels. J Urol 36:211, 1936.
9. Senior HD: The development of the arteries of the human lower extremity. Am J Anat 25:55, 1919.
10. Mayschak DT, Flye WM: Treatment of the persistent sciatic artery. Ann Surg 199:69, 1984.
11. McLellan GL, Morettin LB: Persistent sciatic artery: Clinical, surgical, and angiographic aspects. Arch Surg 117:817, 1982.
12. Gibson MHL, Mills JG, Johnson GE, et al: Popliteal entrapment syndrome. Ann Surg 185:341, 1977.
13. Nandy K, Blair CB Jr: Double superior venae cavae with completely paired azygous veins. Anat Rec 151:1, 1965.
14. Winter FS: Persistent left superior vena cava: Survey of world literature and report of thirty additional cases. Angiology 5:90, 1954.
15. Babian RJ, Johnson DE: Major venous anomalies complicating retroperitoneal surgery. South Med J 72:1254, 1979.
16. Chaung VP, Mena CE, Hoskins PA: Congenital anomalies of the left renal vein: Angiographic consideration. Br J Radiol 47:214, 1974.
17. Dardik H, Loop FD, Cox PA, et al: C-pattern inferior vena cava. JAMA 200:248, 1967.
18. Kolbenstvedt A, Kolmannskog F, Lien HH: The anomalous inferior vena cava: Another structure between the aorta and the superior mesenteric artery. Br J Radiol 54:423, 1981.
19. Berner BJ, Darling C, Fredrick PL, et al: Major venous anomalies complicating abdominal aortic surgery. Arch Surg 108:160, 1974.
20. Mayo J, Gray R, St Louis E, et al: Anomalies of the inferior vena cava. Am J Radiol 140:339, 1983.
21. Giordano JM, Trout HH III: Anomalies of the inferior vena cava. J Vasc Surg 3:924, 1986.

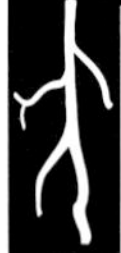

CHAPTER 5

Anatomy of Commonly Exposed Arteries

R. James Valentine, M.D., and Gary G. Wind, M.D.

Vascular surgeons must become intimately acquainted with anatomy of the vascular tree before embarking on correction of vessel pathology. This anatomy is complex and cannot be understood with a superficial overview. A thorough grasp of the anatomic relationships between arteries, veins, and their surrounding structures is fundamental to obtaining adequate operative exposure and avoiding complications. Inadvertent injury to adjacent structures, such as nerves, may be disastrous. Vascular surgeons must also be aware of common anatomic variations and congenital anomalies. Failure to recognize variant anatomy may result in a spectrum of problems ranging from incomplete repair to exsanguination.

The purpose of this chapter is to convey the regional anatomy of arteries that are commonly exposed by vascular surgeons. Developmental anatomy is described in Chapter 4. The continuity of the vascular tree is assumed, but the descriptions are organized by body regions in order to maintain clinical relevancy. A complete and detailed description of all aspects of vascular anatomy is beyond the scope of a single chapter, and the reader is referred to anatomic texts and atlases for study in greater depth.

EXTRACRANIAL CIRCULATION OF THE HEAD AND NECK

Fascial Layers of the Neck

The platysma muscle represents the superficial fascia in the neck covering cutaneous nerves and superficial veins. The deep fascia consists of three specific layers:

1. The investing fascia, the most superficial layer of the deep fascia, extends from the posterior midline and splits to envelop the trapezius and sternocleidomastoid muscles.
2. The middle layer of the deep fascia is also known as the visceral or pretracheal fascia. It encloses the viscera and strap muscles in the central neck.
3. The prevertebral fascia is the deepest layer and covers the paraspinous muscles, the origins of the cervical nerves, the roots of the brachial plexus, and the subclavian artery. Lateral to the first rib, the prevertebral fascia extends to form the axillary sheath.

The deep fascial layers contribute to the aggregation of connective tissue known as the carotid sheath. This sheath is not a discrete fascial sheet. It is bounded by the visceral fascia medially, the prevertebral fascia posteriorly, and the sternocleidomastoid muscle anterolaterally. The contents of the carotid sheath include the carotid artery, the internal jugular vein, and the vagus nerve. The cervical sympathetic chain is embedded within the fibers of the posterior sheath, and the ansa cervicalis is located within the anterior fibers of the sheath.

Carotid Artery

The common carotid artery enters the base of the neck posterior to the sternoclavicular joint and ascends medial to the internal jugular vein. The carotid bifurcation is usually located at the level of the superior border of the thyroid cartilage, but the bifurcation may occur as high as the hyoid bone or as low as the cricoid cartilage. A high bifurcation, which is more common than a low bifurcation,[1] may prompt the surgeon to consider maneuvers such as mandibular subluxation to enhance exposure in the distal neck.[2] The carotid bifurcation is usually crossed anteriorly by the common facial vein, which requires division in order to obtain exposure.

Two small receptors lie intrinsic to the medial wall of the bifurcation: (1) a chemoreceptor known as the *carotid body* and (2) a baroreceptor known as the *carotid sinus*. Nerve twigs to the carotid body from the glossopharyngeal, vagus, and superior cervical sympathetic nerves lie between the internal and external carotid branches. The carotid sinus nerve arises from the baroreceptors at the carotid bifurcation and ascends between the internal and external carotid branches to join the glossopharyngeal nerve. Surgical manipulation of the carotid sinus nerve may cause reflex bradycardia and hypotension.

The external carotid artery supplies the extracranial structures of the head. It gives off several branches before its terminal bifurcation into the maxillary and superficial temporal arteries. These include the superior thyroid, ascending pharyngeal, lingual, facial, occipital, and posterior auricular arteries (Fig. 5–1).

The internal carotid artery ascends vertically in the neck to enter the carotid canal at the base of the skull just anterior to the jugular vein. In its distal ascent, the internal carotid is crossed laterally by pharyngeal tributaries of the internal jugular vein, the hypoglossal nerve, the occipital artery, and the posterior belly of the digastric muscle (Fig. 5–2). Venous tributaries should be carefully controlled and ligated so that troublesome bleeding during internal carotid exposure is avoided. The hypoglossal nerve can be carefully mobilized away from the artery. The sternocleidomastoid branch of the occipital artery tethers the hypoglossal nerve

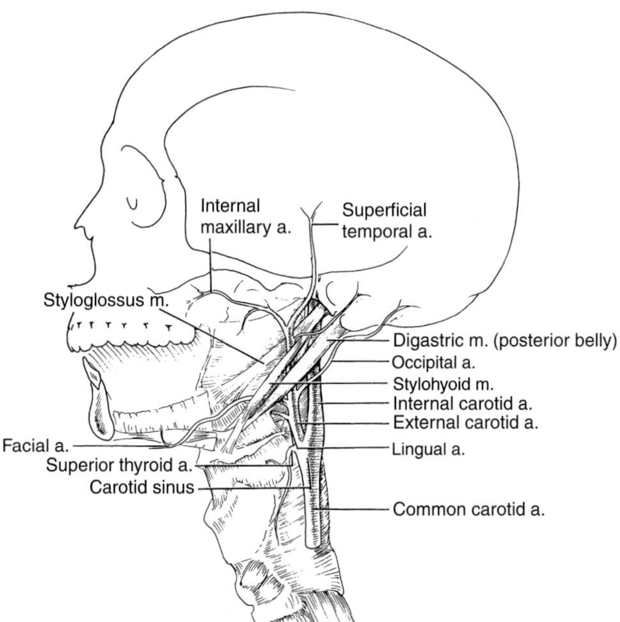

FIGURE 5–1. Relationship between the posterior suspensory muscles of the pharynx and the internal and external carotid arteries. (From Wind GG, Valentine RJ: Anatomic Exposures in Vascular Surgery. Baltimore, Williams & Wilkins, 1990, p 34.)

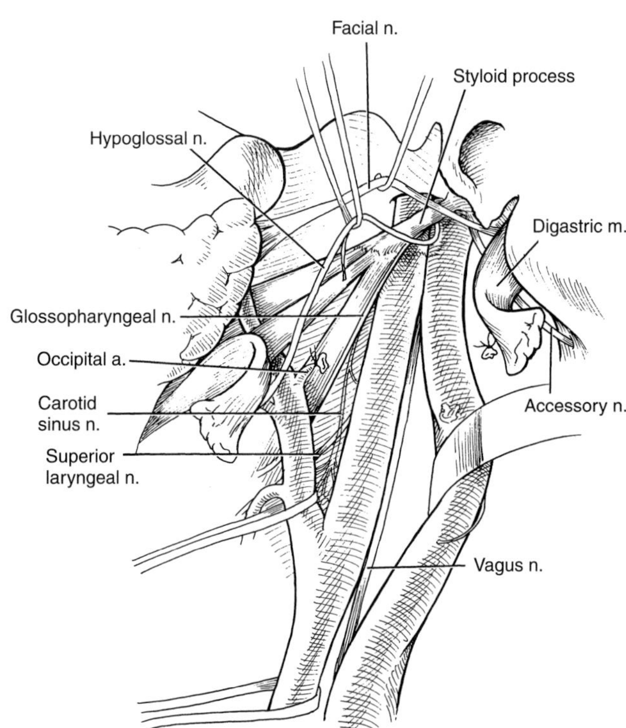

FIGURE 5–2. The internal carotid artery passes deep to the hypoglossal nerve, the occipital artery, and the posterior belly of the digastric muscle. The glossopharyngeal nerve is prone to injury during division of the styloid process. (From Wind GG, Valentine RJ: Anatomic Exposures in Vascular Surgery. Baltimore, Williams & Wilkins, 1990, p 47.)

and should be divided to free the nerve completely. The occipital artery crosses the internal carotid artery at the inferior border of the digastric muscle. Division of the occipital artery and the digastric muscle allows exposure of the internal carotid artery to within 2 cm of the skull base. In its most distal cervical portion, the internal carotid artery passes deep to the styloid process and all associated structures to reach the base of the skull. Exposure of the highest segment of the cervical internal carotid artery is accomplished by dividing the stylohyoid ligament and the stylohyoid, stylopharyngeus, and styloglossus muscles to allow removal of the styloid process.[3]

A number of cranial nerves lie in proximity to the carotid artery and its branches. The *facial nerve* arises posterior to the base of the styloid process and passes anterolaterally to enter the parotid gland, where it is prone to injury during extreme distal exposure of the internal carotid artery. The marginal mandibular branch of the facial nerve, located deep to the platysma, emerges below the angle of the mandible and runs across the ramus of the mandible. It is subject to retractor injury during carotid exposure, causing a visible defect in the ipsilateral orbicularis oris muscle.

The *hypoglossal nerve* descends from the hypoglossal canal and passes lateral to the internal and external carotid arteries before turning anteromedially toward the base of the tongue. Injury to the hypoglossal nerve causes paralysis of the ipsilateral tongue musculature and deviation of the tongue.

The accessory, glossopharyngeal, and vagus nerves exit the skull from the jugular foramen. The *accessory nerve* passes medial to the styloid process and passes obliquely to the upper fibers of the sternocleidomastoid muscle, then to the trapezius muscle. The *glossopharyngeal nerve* runs along the posterior edge of the stylopharyngeus muscle and passes superficial to the internal carotid artery. Loss of its sensory and motor fibers to the tongue and posterior pharynx results in severe complications from inability to swallow and chronic aspiration. The *vagus nerve* descends vertically in the neck between the jugular vein and the internal carotid artery superiorly and the common carotid artery inferiorly.

The *superior laryngeal nerve* originates from the vagus nerve in the neck and runs posterior to the internal and external carotid branches to supply the upper larynx. The *recurrent laryngeal nerve* almost always branches from the vagus nerve within the mediastinum and loops around the subclavian artery on the right side or the ascending aorta on the left, then ascends in the neck in the tracheoesophageal groove. Injury to either the vagus nerve or the recurrent laryngeal nerve produces hoarseness and loss of an effective cough mechanism due to ipsilateral vocal cord paralysis.

In a prospective study of cranial nerve injury during carotid endarterectomy, Hertzer and colleagues[4] documented that recurrent nerve dysfunction (i.e., recurrent or vagal nerve injury) was most common, followed in incidence by hypoglossal nerve injuries (Table 5–1). Fortunately, most nerve injuries are transient.[4, 5]

Vertebral Artery

The vertebral arteries are located beneath the prevertebral fascia in the deep neck. In the proximal third, each artery ascends from its subclavian artery origin to the transverse process of the sixth cervical vertebra, which is known as the carotid, or Chassaignac's, tubercle. In this extraosseous course, the arteries bisect an angle formed by the anterior scalene and longus colli muscles. Under the hood of the inverted "V" formed by these muscles, the vertebral arteries penetrate the prevertebral fascia and enter the transverse process of C6. The phrenic nerves lie on the ventral surfaces of the anterior scalene muscles and are subject to injury during exposure of the vertebral arteries. The distal two thirds of the extracranial vertebral arteries lie within the bony canal formed by the transverse processes of C1 through C6. In this canal, the arteries cross anterior to the roots of the cervical nerves (Fig. 5–3). Extensive venous tributaries accompany the arteries within the canal, making exposure of the interosseous segment somewhat treacherous. To reduce the risk of venous injury, the surgeon should control the vertebral artery by entering the bony canal rather than controlling the artery between the transverse processes.[6] After exiting the transverse processes of the atlas, the arteries enter the cranium through the foramen magnum and converge to form the basilar artery at the lower border of the pons.

TABLE 5–1. CRANIAL NERVE INJURIES DOCUMENTED IN A PROSPECTIVE STUDY OF 240 CAROTID ENDARTERECTOMIES

NERVE	NO. OF PATIENTS	ASYMPTOMATIC*	TRANSIENT DEFECT†
Recurrent laryngeal	14	4 (29%)	8 (57%)
Hypoglossal	13	7 (54%)	9 (69%)
Marginal mandibular	6	—	6 (100%)
Superior laryngeal	5	4 (80%)	4 (80%)
Total	38	15 (39%)	27 (71%)

Adapted from Hertzer NR, Feldman BJ, Beven EG, et al: A prospective study of the incidence of injury to the cranial nerves during carotid endarterectomy. Surg Gynecol Obstet 151:781, 1980.

*Patients without symptoms of nerve injury that would have escaped detection without routine otolaryngologic examination.

†Patients who recovered normal nerve function between 1 and 12 months after operation.

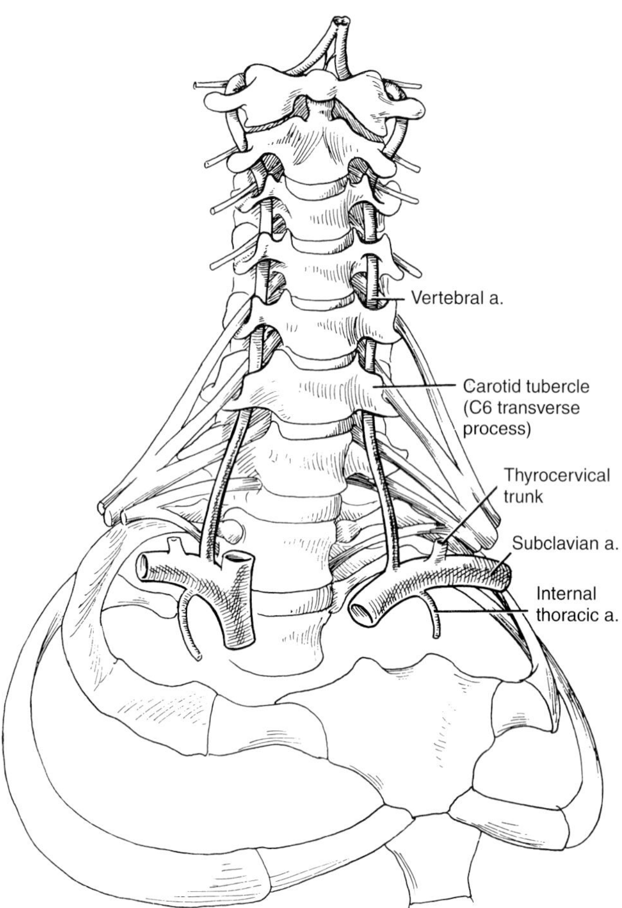

FIGURE 5–3. The vertebral arteries enter the bony canal formed by the transverse processes at the level of C6. (From Wind GG, Valentine RJ: Anatomic Exposures in Vascular Surgery. Baltimore: Williams & Wilkins, 1990, p 49.)

The paired anatomic arrangement of the vertebral arteries provides a well-collateralized circulation to the posterior brain. However, developmental variation may limit collateral flow in some individuals. Hypoplastic vertebral arteries occur in approximately 15% of cases, more commonly on the right side.[7] In the intracranial portion, the arteries do not unite 5% of the time: the vertebral artery terminates as a posterocerebellar artery on the right in 3.1% of individuals, and on the left in 1.8%.[7]

VESSELS OF THE THORACIC OUTLET AND SHOULDER

Anatomy of the Thoracic Outlet

The thoracic outlet is bounded by the bony structures of the superior thorax, which include the spinal column, first ribs, and sternum. Immediately adjacent to the thoracic outlet, the clavicles arch over the medial portions of the first ribs and articulate with the manubrium. Two scalene muscles originate from the vertebral column and insert on the first ribs (Fig. 5–4). The *anterior scalene muscles* originate from the transverse processes of C3–C6 and insert on the inner borders and superior surfaces of the first ribs, just anterior to the grooves for the subclavian arteries. The *middle scalene muscles* arise from the transverse processes of the lower six cervical vertebrae and insert broadly on the posterior aspect of the first ribs. Coursing ventral to the anterior scalene muscles, the subclavian veins constitute the most anterior vascular structures of the superior aperture. The subclavian arteries and the roots of the brachial plexus emerge between the anterior and middle scalene muscles. The entire neurovascular package traverses the costoclavicular passage underneath the middle third of the respective clavicle to reach the axillary space.

A number of developmental anomalies have been associated with neurovascular compression syndromes in the thoracic outlet. In a study of 200 transaxillary surgical procedures performed in 175 patients with symptoms of thoracic outlet compression, Makhoul and Machleder recognized nontraumatic causes in 66%.[8] The distribution of thoracic outlet anomalies is shown in Table 5–2. The most common reported anomalies are related to ligamentous and muscular attachments that insert on the first rib, prompting the rationale for first rib resection to treat all causes of thoracic outlet compression.[9] Cervical ribs are reported to occur in approximately 1% of the normal population, and they are bilateral 50% of the time.[9, 10] Only 5% to 10% of patients with cervical ribs experience symptoms of thoracic outlet compression.[11] Although the majority of cervical ribs are rudimentary or incomplete, most have ligamentous attachments to the first rib. Cervical ribs are most commonly embedded in the fibers of the middle scalene muscle and displace both the subclavian artery and brachial plexus.

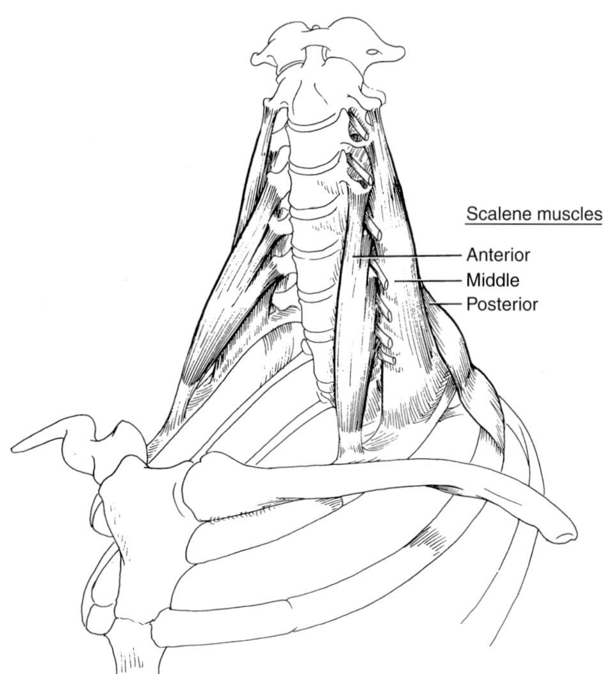

FIGURE 5–4. Two scalene muscles insert onto the first rib. The subclavian vein lies anterior to the anterior scalene muscle, and the subclavian artery lies between the anterior and middle scalene muscles. (From Wind GG, Valentine RJ: Anatomic Exposures in Vascular Surgery. Baltimore: Williams & Wilkins, 1990, p 106.)

TABLE 5–2. ANOMALIES OF THE THORACIC OUTLET FOUND IN 200 TRANSAXILLARY SURGICAL PROCEDURES PERFORMED FOR NEUROVASCULAR COMPRESSION SYNDROMES

ABNORMALITY	NO. OF CASES
None found	68 (34%)
Anomaly of scalene muscle	86 (43%)
Anomaly of subclavius tendon	39 (19.5%)
Scalenus minimus abnormality	20 (10%)
Cervical rib	17 (8.5%)
Fibrous structures or ligamentous abnormalities	15 (7.5%)
Total	200

Adapted from Makhoul RG, Machleder HI: Developmental anomalies at the thoracic outlet: Analysis of 200 consecutive cases. J Vasc Surg 16:534, 1992.

Subclavian Artery

The subclavian arteries ascend in the mediastinum and course over the first ribs behind the anterior scalene muscles. The *right subclavian artery* originates most frequently from the brachiocephalic artery, and the *left subclavian artery* originates as the third branch of the aortic arch. In approximately 1% of the population, the right subclavian artery originates on the left side of the mediastinum as the most distal branch of the aortic arch (Fig. 5–5).[12] Proximal vascular control of the right subclavian artery in its normal position can be obtained via median sternotomy. The trajectory of the aortic arch renders the left subclavian too far posterior to be accessible through a median sternotomy approach; proximal vascular control is best obtained through a lateral thoracotomy. Direct exposure of the subclavian arteries can be obtained through supraclavicular incisions.

The branches of the subclavian artery include the vertebral, internal thoracic, thyrocervical, costocervical, and dorsal scapular arteries:

1. The *vertebral arteries* arise from the superoposterior aspect of the subclavian arteries proximal to the medial border of the anterior scalene muscles.
2. The *internal thoracic arteries* arise opposite the vertebral arteries, on the inferior border of the subclavian arteries.
3. The short, wide *thyrocervical* trunks originate from the subclavian arteries near the medial border of the anterior scalene muscles and branch immediately into the inferior thyroid, superficial cervical, and suprascapular branches.
4. *Costocervical* trunk and *dorsal scapular* artery branches arise from the posterior aspect of both subclavian arteries as they course behind the anterior scalene.

A number of surrounding structures are prone to injury during subclavian artery exposure. The subclavian veins cross ventral to the anterior scalene muscles; large venous tributaries should be carefully ligated during arterial exposure to prevent troublesome bleeding. On the left side, the

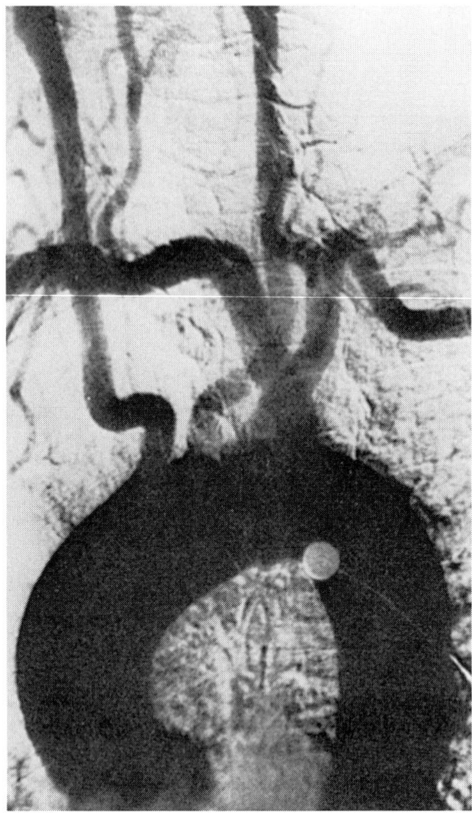

FIGURE 5–5. Arteriogram demonstrating an aberrant right subclavian artery originating as the most distal branch of the aortic arch. (From Valentine RJ, Carter DJ, Clagett GP: A modified extrathoracic approach to the treatment of dysphagia lusoria. J Vasc Surg 5:498–500, 1987. By permission of Journal of Vascular Surgery.)

thoracic duct arches over the subclavian artery to reach the posterior aspect of the subclavian-jugular vein confluence. To prevent chylous leak, the surgeon should identify and ligate this duct. The vagus and phrenic nerves also lie adjacent to the subclavian arteries and must be protected during arterial exposure. The right vagus nerve descends lateral to the right common carotid artery and crosses anterior to the right subclavian artery near its origin. After looping around the inferior border of the subclavian artery, the recurrent laryngeal branch of the right vagus nerve ascends into the neck in the tracheoesophageal groove. The left vagus nerve descends on the lateral border of the left common carotid artery, crosses anterior to the aortic arch, and loops under the arch to ascend posterior to the aorta. The phrenic nerves descend from the neck on the anteromedial surface of the anterior scalene muscles. After crossing anterior to the subclavian arteries, the nerves enter the thorax by passing anteromedial to the internal thoracic arteries. Injury to a phrenic nerve at the time of subclavian artery exposure is most likely during division of the anterior scalene muscle.

Axillary Artery

The lateral border of the first rib is the anatomic boundary marking the transition between the subclavian and axillary arteries. There the artery is joined by divisions and cords of the brachial plexus (Fig. 5–6). As the axillary artery emerges from beneath the costoclavicular passage, it is surrounded by the lateral, posterior, and medial cords. These neural structures exchange fibers around the artery as the neurovascular bundle courses through the axilla under the pectoralis minor muscle, evolving into their final nerve form at the artery's distal third. Throughout their course, the axillary artery and accompanying neural structures are covered by a thin fascia known as the axillary sheath, which is separated from the axillary vein by a fat pad. The distal extent of the axillary artery is marked by the lateral edge of the teres major muscle.

The axillary artery is divided into three anatomic sections:

- The first part extends from the lateral border of the first rib to the medial border of the pectoralis minor.
- The second part is that portion behind the pectoralis minor muscle.
- The third part extends beyond the muscle's lateral border.

The first part of the axillary artery is the simplest to expose because it is medial to the pectoralis muscle and has only one branch, the supreme thoracic artery. Two branches arise from the second part: the thoracoacromial artery and the lateral thoracic artery. Exposure of the second part requires division of the pectoralis minor muscle, risking injury to the medial and lateral pectoral nerves.[13] These nerves are important because they innervate the large pectoralis major muscle, and injury may result in significant cosmetic and functional chest wall defects.

The third part of the axillary artery gives origin to three branches: the subscapular artery, the medial humoral circumflex artery, and the lateral humoral circumflex artery. At this level, the brachial plexus has assumed the final configuration of nerves to the arm. Relative to the axillary artery, the median nerve is located anterior, the radial nerve is posterior, and the ulnar nerve is inferior within the axillary sheath.

ARTERIES OF THE ABDOMEN AND PELVIS

Supraceliac Aorta

The aorta enters the abdomen behind the diaphragm at the level of the lower border of the 12th thoracic vertebra. It is crossed ventrally by the converging diaphragmatic crura at a site known as the median arcuate ligament, deep to the esophagogastric junction. Limited exposure of the aortic segment above the celiac axis can be gained through the lesser sac if one divides the fibers of the median arcuate ligament.[14] This area is usually free of plaque disease and is an excellent alternative site for placement of a proximal anastomosis during bypass construction.[15]

The proximal abdominal aorta is surrounded by a number of visceral and vascular structures. The esophagus enters the abdomen through an opening at the level of the 10th thoracic vertebra, a little to the left and in front of the aortic opening. The cisterna chyli is located on the right posterolateral surface of the aorta, and the connecting thoracic duct ascends into the chest through the aortic aperture in the same plane. More laterally, the inferior vena cava

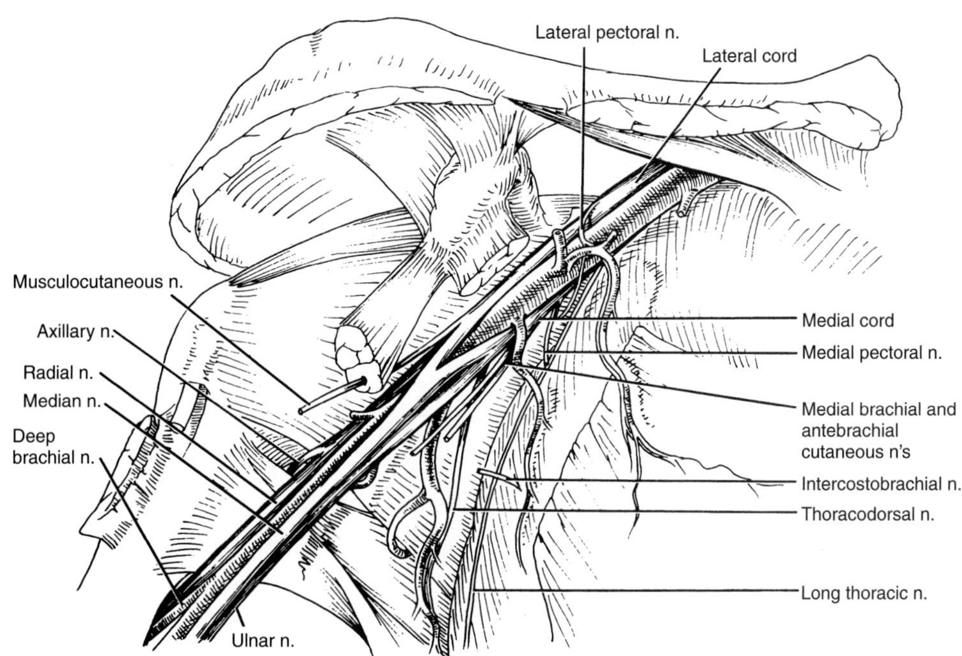

FIGURE 5–6. Divisions and cords of the brachial plexus surround the axillary artery as it emerges beneath the costoclavicular passage. The brachial plexus evolves into its final nerve form at the artery's distal third. (From Wind GG, Valentine RJ: Anatomic Exposures in Vascular Surgery. Baltimore, Williams & Wilkins, 1990, p 142.)

and caudate lobe of the liver limit access to the supraceliac aorta from the right side. Because this aortic segment is covered only by the diaphragmatic crus on the left side, easy access can be obtained by means of a left retroperitoneal approach.[16]

Visceral Aorta and Mesenteric Arteries

The closely spaced and ventrally located visceral arteries prevent ready access to this segment of the abdominal aorta from an anterior approach (Fig. 5–7). The celiac trunk is framed by the median arcuate ligament superiorly and by the superior border of the pancreas inferiorly. It arises directly from the ventral surface of the aorta and is surrounded by tough lymphatic and nerve plexuses. Following a short anterior course, the celiac trunk divides into main arterial branches supplying the circulation of the foregut.

Most commonly, three branches emanate from a trifurcation: the common hepatic artery, the splenic artery, and the left gastric artery. These branches lie deep to the retroperitoneum of the lesser sac. The common hepatic artery passes to the right and enters the hepatoduodenal ligament immediately above the pylorus. The splenic artery passes to the left and follows a serpentine course along the superior border of the pancreas to give off numerous pancreatic and short gastric branches before terminating at the spleen. The right and left gastroepiploic arteries connect the splenic and hepatic circulations, forming a collateral that preserves arterial flow to the spleen when the splenic artery is ligated medial to the left gastroepiploic artery (Fig. 5–8). The left gastric artery ascends beneath the peritoneum to reach the lesser curvature of the stomach.

The origin of the superior mesenteric artery forms a sharp caudal angle with the anterior surface of the aorta. Lying within this angle are the left renal vein, the uncinate process of the pancreas, and the third portion of the duodenum. The proximal part of the superior mesenteric artery is crossed by the neck of the pancreas, and the superior mesenteric vein lies on the right side of the artery at the inferior border of the pancreatic neck. These two structures course over the uncinate process and third portion of the duodenum to run side by side in the small-bowel mesentery. The superior mesenteric artery supplies the intestine from the second part of the duodenum to the midtransverse colon.

The renal arteries arise laterally from the aorta between 2 cm above and below the L1–L2 disc space. Single renal arteries are present in 70% of individuals.[17] Two hilar vessels occur approximately 25% of the time, and three hilar vessels occur in approximately 3%. Among patients with single renal arteries, the left is usually slightly more cephalad than the right. The left renal vein crosses anterior to the aorta in 96% of individuals[18] and is considered to be a reliable marker for locating the left renal artery. In a study of 57 postmortem subjects, the left renal artery was located directly behind the left renal vein in 52%, below (caudal to) the left renal vein in 14%, and above (cephalad to) the left renal vein in 34%.[19] The right renal artery crosses posterior to the inferior vena cava and is usually located directly behind the right renal vein. Both renal veins may receive a lumbar venous tributary, which should be ligated during mobilization to avoid hemorrhage. In addition, the left renal vein receives the left adrenal and gonadal veins.

The inferior mesenteric artery arises on the anterior surface of the aorta approximately 3 to 4 cm above the aortic bifurcation. It is closely applied to the aorta as it courses inferiorly and to the left into the mesentery of the left colon. The inferior mesenteric artery supplies the left third

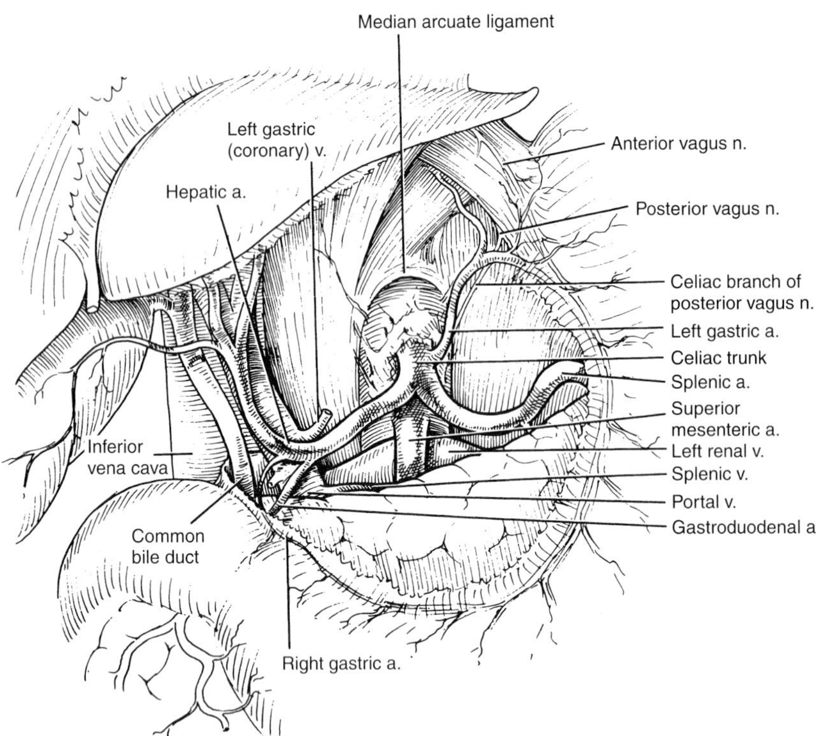

FIGURE 5–7. The celiac trunk and superior mesenteric artery lie deep to the posterior peritoneum of the omental bursa. (From Wind GG, Valentine RJ: Anatomic Exposures in Vascular Surgery. Baltimore, Williams & Wilkins, 1990, p 237.)

of the transverse colon, the descending and sigmoid colon, and most of the rectum.

Collateral Mesenteric Circulation

The three major arteries of the mesenteric circulation are interconnected by a network of branches that form a rich collateral circulation in the event of segmental occlusion.[20] Arising as the second branch of the common hepatic artery, the gastroduodenal artery gives off a retroduodenal branch, which continues as the posterior superior pancreaticoduodenal artery. The gastroduodenal artery then divides into the anterior superior pancreaticoduodenal and right gastroepiploic arteries. The anterior and posterior superior branches anastomose with corresponding branches arising from the superior mesenteric artery. The inferior pancreaticoduodenal vessels arise either separately or as a single trunk from the superior mesenteric artery as it emerges near the inferior border of the pancreas. This collateral network between the celiac axis and superior mesenteric artery is known as the *pancreaticoduodenal arcade* (Fig. 5–9).

A variable collateral circulation between the superior and inferior mesenteric arteries is located in the mesentery of the left colon. This collateral is formed by branches of the

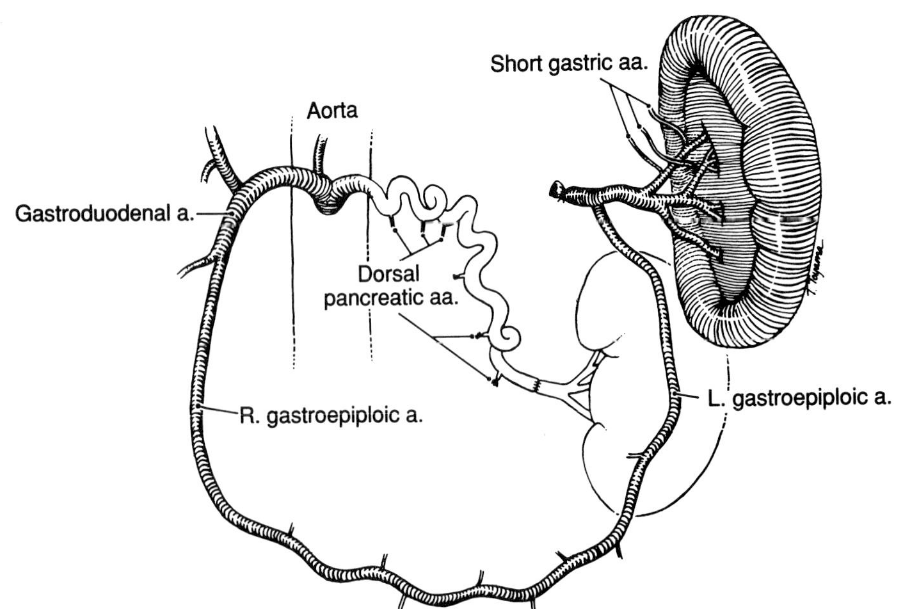

FIGURE 5–8. Collateral circulation to the spleen after splenorenal bypass. (From Valentine RJ, Rossi MB, Myers SI, Clagett GP: Splenic infarction after splenorenal bypass. J Vasc Surg 17:602–606, 1993. By permission of Journal of Vascular Surgery.)

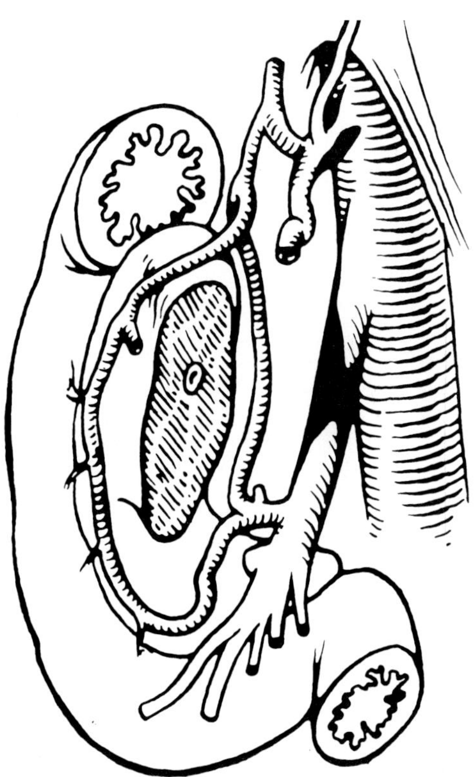

FIGURE 5–9. The pancreaticoduodenal arcade as viewed from a sagittal perspective. This network provides collateral blood flow between the celiac axis and superior mesenteric artery circulations when one or the other is occluded. (From Fisher DF Jr, Fry WJ: Collateral mesenteric circulation. Surg Gynecol Obstet 164:487–492, 1987. By permission of Journal of the American College of Surgeons.

middle colic artery and the left colic artery. The middle colic artery arises as the second branch of the superior mesenteric artery and enters the transverse mesocolon. The left branch of the middle colic artery continues adjacent to the left colon and is usually continuous with the marginal artery, also known as the artery of Drummond. The ascending branch of the left colic artery, a branch of the inferior mesenteric artery, is also usually continuous with the marginal artery and completes the anastomotic network (Fig. 5–10). Normally present medial anastomotic channels between the superior and inferior mesenteric circulations can enlarge into a major vessel in the face of major trunk narrowing. This potential connection (the arc of Riolan) may prevent colon necrosis in individuals with incomplete marginal arteries.[21] It is formed by an early branch of the left colic artery, which ascends directly to join the left branch of the middle colic artery. Known also as the "meandering mesenteric artery," this collateral may enlarge and become tortuous within the mesentery of the left colon in individuals with occlusion of either the inferior or superior mesenteric artery (Fig. 5–11).

Infrarenal Aorta and Iliac Arteries

The distal abdominal aorta below the renal arteries lies slightly to the left of midline and immediately anterior to the vertebral bodies of L1 through L4. The third and fourth portions of the duodenum overlie the aorta and require reflection to the patient's right side during aortic exposure. The surgeon can gain more proximal exposure near the renal arteries by dividing the ligament of Treitz. Anteriorly, the aorta is covered by lymphatic tissue, which the surgeon should ligate to prevent chylous leak.[22] Paired lumbar arteries originate from the posterolateral aortic wall and wrap around the vertebral bodies, dividing into branches supplying the dorsal abdominal wall and spine. A variable plexus of segmental lumbar veins lies between the dorsal surface of the aorta and the anterior surface of the vertebral bodies. These friable venous structures are easily torn and must be carefully avoided during maneuvers to encircle the aorta. A retroaortic left renal vein exists in up to 2.5% of individuals[18] and is also subject to injury during aortic mobilization. Anomalies of the inferior vena cava may also create technical difficulties during aortic exposure (Table 5–3).

The aorta bifurcates at the level of the fourth lumbar vertebra into right and left common iliac arteries. The right common iliac artery crosses anterior to the confluence of the common iliac veins at the inferior vena cava. The right common iliac vein courses posterior to the right common iliac artery, and the left common iliac vein courses deep to the inferior surface of the left common iliac artery (Fig. 5–12). The aortic bifurcation is separated from the fourth vertebra by the left common iliac vein. Adhesions frequently form between the bifurcations of the aorta and vena cava, making manipulation or separation of these structures extremely hazardous. The common iliac arteries give small branches to the psoas major muscle and adjacent nerves. These branches should be ligated at the time of iliac artery mobilization.

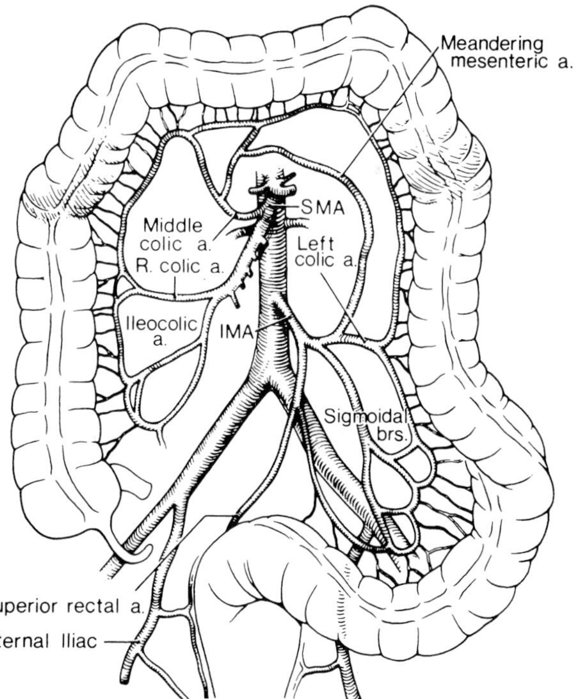

FIGURE 5–10. Arterial circulation of the mesentery. Note the medial anastomotic channels between the superior and inferior mesenteric arteries, which may enlarge to become the meandering mesenteric artery in chronic ischemic states. (From Fisher DF Jr, Fry WJ: Collateral mesenteric circulation. Surg Gynecol Obstet 164:487–492, 1987. By permission of Journal of the American College of Surgeons.)

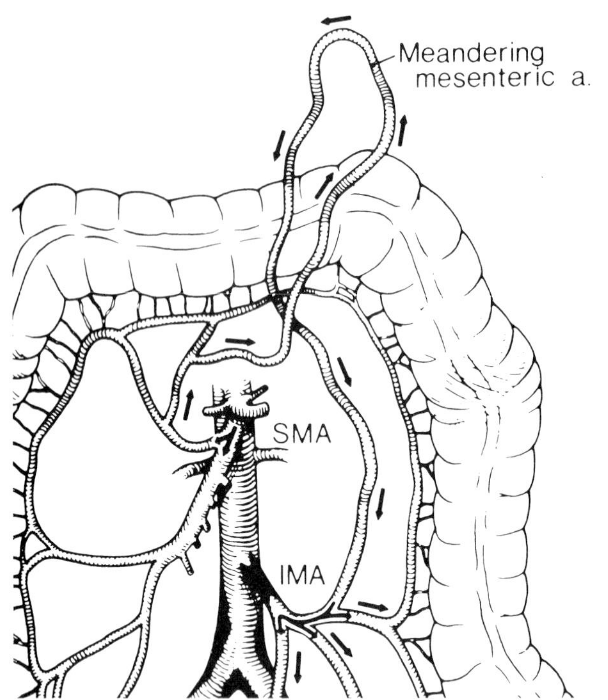

FIGURE 5–11. Chronic ischemia may result in enlargement and tortuosity of the medial anastomotic channel. This serves as an important collateral between the superior and inferior mesenteric arterial circulations. (From Fisher DF Jr, Fry WJ: Collateral mesenteric circulation. Surg Gynecol Obstet 1987; 164:487–492. By permission of Journal of the American College of Surgeons.)

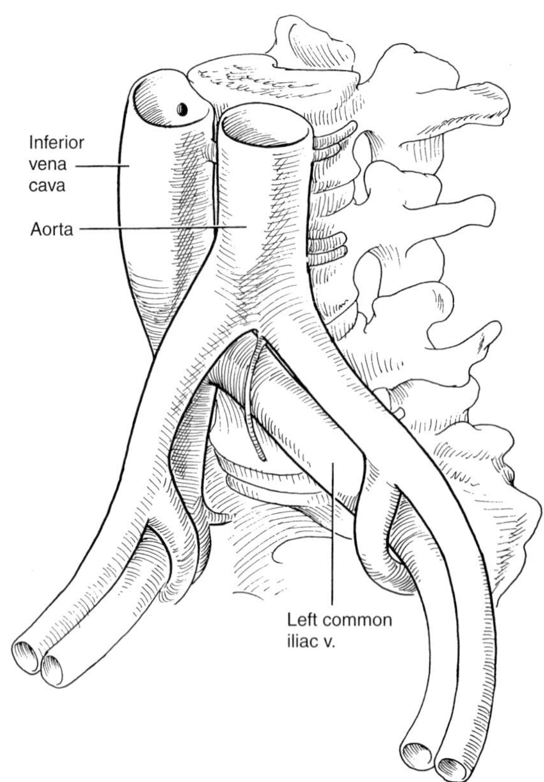

FIGURE 5–12. The aortic bifurcation overrides the bifurcation of the vena cava. (From Wind GG, Valentine RJ: Anatomic Exposures in Vascular Surgery. Baltimore, Williams & Wilkins, 1990, p 271.)

The common iliac arteries bifurcate at the lip of the true pelvis. Crossing on the ventral surface of the iliac bifurcation, the gonadal vessels and ureters enter the pelvis on the anterior surface of the internal iliac arteries. The external iliac arteries pass obliquely along the pelvic brim medial to the psoas muscles, giving off inferior epigastric and deep circumflex iliac branches near the inguinal ligament. The external iliac veins lie medial and deep to the corresponding arteries.

TABLE 5–3. ANOMALIES OF THE INFERIOR VENA CAVA (IVC) AND LEFT RENAL VEIN (LRV)

ANOMALY	INCIDENCE	LOCATION
Duplicated IVC	0.2%–3.0%	Large veins run on both sides of aorta, join anteriorly at level of renal arteries
Left-sided IVC	0.2%–0.5%	Left-sided IVC crosses anterior to aorta at level of renal arteries, then courses on right side of aorta
Absent IVC	Very rare	Veins from lower extremity drain toward diaphragm via ascending lumbar and azygos veins
Retroaortic LRV	1.2%–2.4%	LRV posterior to aorta
Circumaortic LRV	1.5%–8.7%	Venous collar around aorta

Adapted from Giordano JM, Trout HH 3rd: Anomalies of the inferior vena cava. J Vasc Surg 3:924, 1986.

Each internal iliac artery branches into anterior and posterior trunks. Branches of the anterior trunk include (1) the superior and inferior vesicle arteries, (2) the middle rectal artery, (3) the obturator artery, (4) the internal pudendal artery, and (5) the inferior gluteal artery. The posterior trunk branches include (1) the iliolumbar artery, (2) the lateral sacral artery, and (3) the superior gluteal artery.

ARTERIES OF THE LEG

Femoral Arteries

The inguinal ligament marks the boundary between the external iliac and common femoral artery. A fibrous covering, known as the *femoral sheath,* wraps around the common femoral artery and vein, which are separated within the sheath by a well-developed septum. The femoral sheath is perforated by the saphenous vein on the medial aspect. The femoral vessels course within a triangular space defined by muscular boundaries known as *Scarpa's triangle*. This space is bounded on the lateral side by the sartorius muscle, on the medial side by the adductor longus muscle, and on the superior side by the inguinal ligament (Fig. 5–13). Within the triangle, the common femoral vein is located medially, the femoral nerve is located laterally, and the common femoral artery is located in between.

Several branches of the common femoral artery may be encountered during dissection near the inguinal ligament, including the superficial epigastric artery, the superficial circumflex iliac artery, and the superficial external pudendal artery. The deep external pudendal branch arises medially and crosses under the saphenous vein near the saphenofemoral junction. The saphenous vein enters Scarpa's triangle through a medial opening in the fascia lata known as the fossa ovalis. One group of superficial lymph nodes lies directly over the fossa ovalis. Another group of superficial inguinal lymph nodes lies more cephalad in the path of an anterior groin incision to the femoral artery. Ligation of all lymphatics associated with superficial lymph nodes at the time of arterial exposure reduces the risk of a postoperative lymphocele.[22]

The common femoral artery divides into the deep (profunda) and superficial femoral arteries approximately 4 cm distal to the inguinal ligament. Originating on the lateral side of the parent vessel, the deep femoral artery courses posterior to the superficial femoral artery and vein on the medial side of the femur. Near its origin, the deep femoral artery is crossed by the lateral femoral circumflex vein, which can be injured during dissection in the "crotch" that is formed by the origins of the deep and superficial femoral arteries. Early in its course, the deep femoral artery gives medial and lateral femoral circumflex branches (Fig. 5–14). The descending branch of the lateral femoral circumflex artery anastomoses with genicular branches at the knee, providing an important source of collateral blood flow when the superficial femoral artery is occluded. The medial femoral circumflex artery supplies the proximal adductor compartment.

In approximately 20% of cases, the medial or lateral femoral circumflex artery originates directly from the common femoral artery and may be a cause of significant backbleeding from an opened, cross-clamped femoral artery. In its continuation, the deep femoral artery enters the plane posterior to the adductor longus muscle, sending four perforating branches through the adductor magnus along its tendinous insertion to the linea aspera of the femur. These perforators anastomose with each other and provide blood supply to the muscles of the flexor compartment. The second perforator provides a nutrient artery to the femur, and the fourth perforator is the termination of the deep femoral artery.

The superficial femoral artery is the direct continuation of the common femoral artery beyond the deep femoral branch. It enters the aponeurotic tunnel in the thigh, known as the adductor (Hunter's) canal, at the apex of Scarpa's triangle. This tunnel is bounded by the vastus medialis on the anterolateral surface, by the adductor longus on the posterior surface, and by a strong aponeurosis between the adductors and the vastus medialis on the anteromedial surface. Coursing within the canal are the superficial femoral artery and vein, the saphenous nerve, and the nerve to the vastus medialis. The vessels give off a number of variably sized muscular branches, which should be preserved for their potential as collateral vessels during exposure within the adductor canal. The saphenous nerve leaves the canal at the adductor hiatus to course with the saphenous vein to the medial ankle and foot.

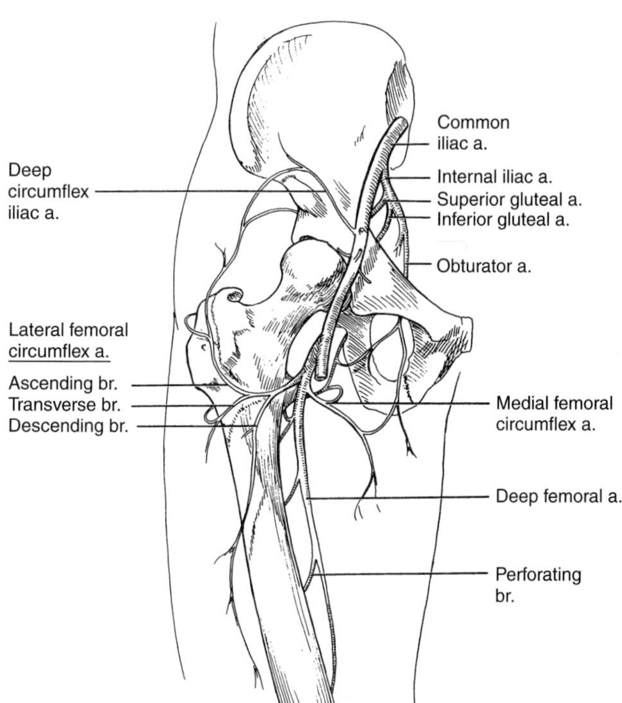

FIGURE 5–14. The deep femoral artery contributes to a rich collateral circulation around the hip joint and proximal femur. (From Wind GG, Valentine RJ: Anatomic Exposures in Vascular Surgery. Baltimore, Williams & Wilkins, 1990, p 349.)

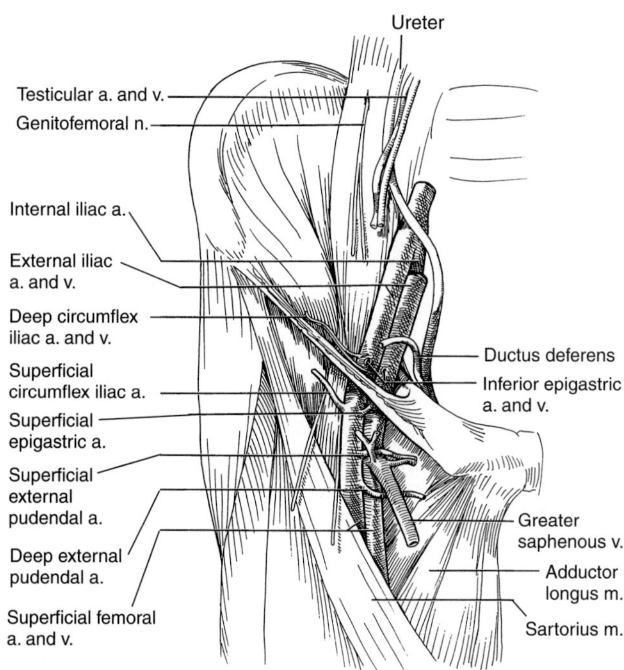

FIGURE 5–13. After passing beneath the inguinal ligament, the femoral vessels course within Scarpa's triangle. Note the relationship of the other retroperitoneal structures to the vessels. From Wind GG, Valentine RJ: Anatomic Exposures in Vascular Surgery. Baltimore, Williams & Wilkins, 1990, p 338.)

Popliteal Artery

The anatomic boundary separating the superficial femoral and popliteal arteries is the adductor hiatus. From this opening in the adductor magnus, the popliteal artery courses distally between the femoral condyles and passes deep to the soleus muscle, where the artery soon gives off an anterior tibial branch. A number of muscular and genicular branches arise from the popliteal artery as it passes through the popliteal fossa. The sural arteries arise at the level of the knee joint and supply the gastrocnemius, soleus, and plantaris muscles. The paired superior, middle, and inferior genicular arteries form a rich collateral anastomosis around the knee.

The popliteal artery is separated from the posterior surface of the femur by a fat pad. The popliteal vein courses around the artery, such that the vein lies posterolateral to the artery at the adductor hiatus, dorsal to the artery between the heads of the gastrocnemius muscle, and medial to the artery in its distal extent. The small saphenous vein joins the popliteal vein in the popliteal fossa between 3 and 7.5 cm above the knee joint.[24] The tibial nerve enters the popliteal fossa between the semimembranosus and biceps femoris muscles. It lies on the lateral aspect of the popliteal vessels at the level of the knee joint, then crosses the vessels posteriorly to become the most superficial midline structure encountered during posterior exposure of the popliteal artery. The peroneal nerve branch follows the medial border of the biceps femoris tendon toward the fibular head (Fig. 5–15).

Infrapopliteal Arteries

The popliteal artery divides into two separate bifurcations below the knee. The term "trifurcation" is a misnomer, because the popliteal artery trunk divides into three separate branches in only 0.4% of cases.[25] The artery first

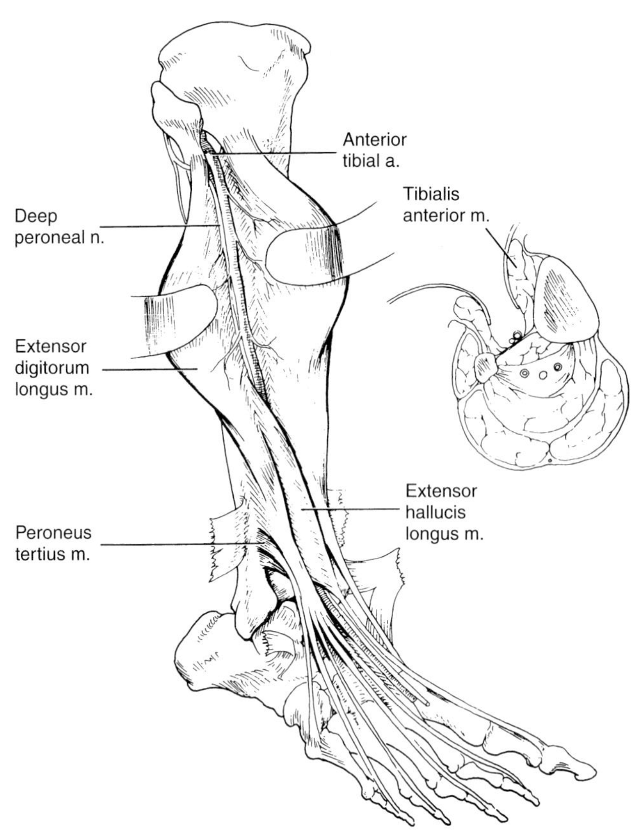

FIGURE 5–16. The anterior tibial artery and deep peroneal nerve lie between the extensor digitorum longus and tibialis anterior muscles in the anterior compartment. (From Wind GG, Valentine RJ: Anatomic Exposures in Vascular Surgery. Baltimore, Williams & Wilkins, 1990, p 418.)

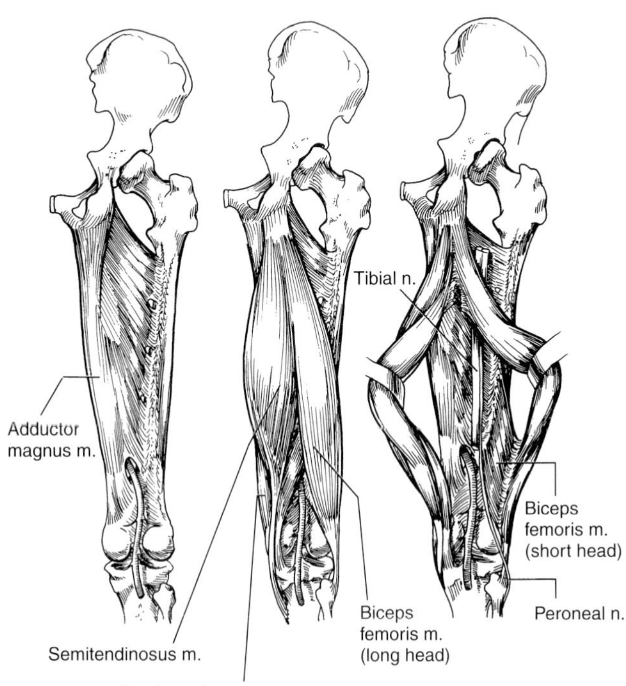

FIGURE 5–15. The peroneal nerve branch of the tibial nerve follows the medial border of the biceps femoris tendon and courses toward the fibular head. (From Wind GG, Valentine RJ: Anatomic Exposures in Vascular Surgery. Baltimore, Williams & Wilkins, 1990, p 377.)

bifurcates into anterior tibial and tibioperoneal branches between 3 and 7 cm below the knee joint. The second bifurcation occurs between 2 and 3 cm more distally, where the tibioperoneal trunk divides into posterior tibial and peroneal branches.

The anterior tibial artery passes anterolaterally and leaves the deep posterior fascial compartment through an opening in the interosseous membrane on the medial side of the fibular neck. The artery enters the anterior compartment between the tibialis anterior and extensor digitorum longus muscles (Fig. 5–16). It is joined early by the deep peroneal nerve, which enters the anterior compartment after winding around the lateral aspect of the fibular head. The neurovascular structures pass through the entire anterior compartment, coursing behind the extensor hallicis longus muscle in their distal extent to reach the dorsum of the foot.

The tibioperoneal trunk lies in the deep posterior compartment on the posterior surface of the tibialis posterior muscle (Fig. 5–17). The anterior tibial vein crosses the tibioperoneal artery and should be divided to enhance exposure from a medial approach. Distal to the bifurcation of the tibioperoneal trunk, the posterior tibial artery branch is accompanied by the tibial nerve and follows an oblique medial course to reach the medial malleolus. In the distal half of the leg, these neurovascular structures lie on the posterior surface of the flexor digitorum longus muscle, just beneath the thin fascia of the deep posterior compartment (Fig. 5–18). The posterior tibial artery is easily ex-

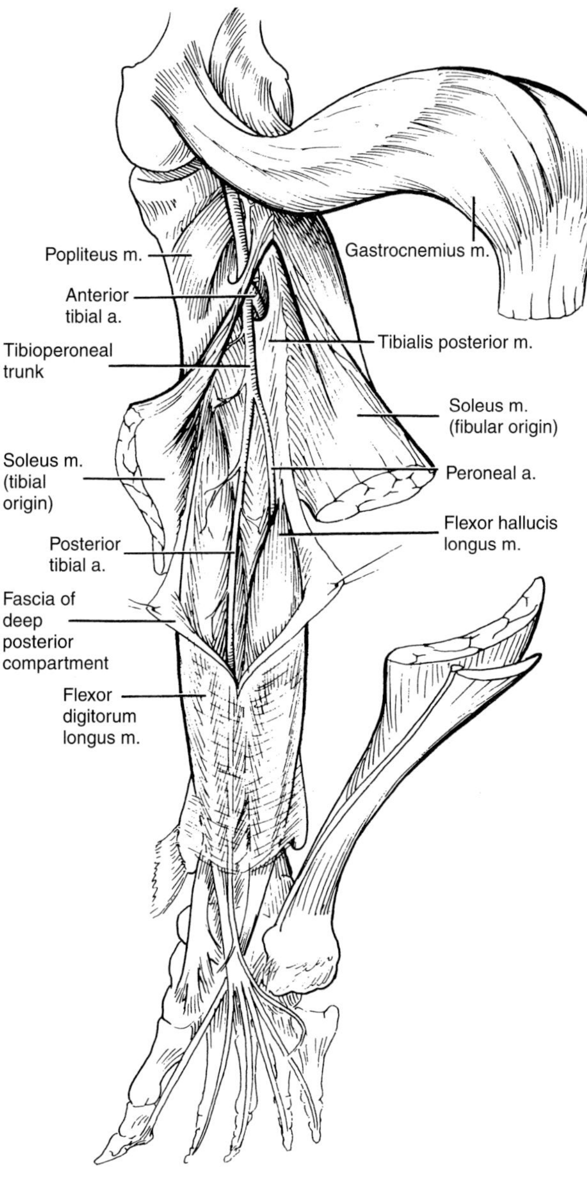

FIGURE 5–17. The peroneal and posterior tibial arteries lie in the deep posterior compartment. The posterior tibial artery courses posterior to the flexor digitorum longus muscle, while the peroneal artery courses flexor hallucis longus muscle. (From Wind GG, Valentine RJ: Anatomic Exposures in Vascular Surgery. Baltimore, Williams & Wilkins, 1990, p 419.)

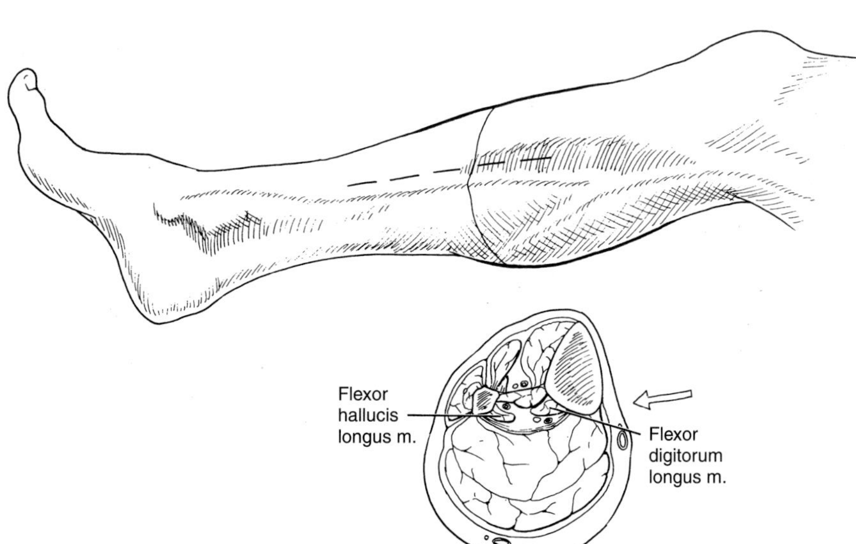

FIGURE 5–18. Relationship of the infrapopliteal arteries to the muscle compartments of the mid-leg. (From Wind GG, Valentine RJ: Anatomic Exposures in Vascular Surgery. Baltimore, Williams & Wilkins, 1990, p 427.)

posed from a medial approach[26] but can also be isolated in its distal extent through a posterior approach.[27]

The peroneal artery courses laterally toward the ankle and lies near the medial surface of the fibula. In its distal extent, the peroneal artery lies between the tibialis posterior and flexor hallicis longus muscles. The peroneal artery can be exposed from a medial approach, but deep dissection behind the tibia sometimes limits exposure.[26] Because the peroneal artery lies just beneath the medial surface of the fibula, fibular resection may yield simpler exposure through a lateral incision.[28] Ouriel[27] has demonstrated that the most distal peroneal artery is readily exposed between the flexor hallicis muscle and the calcaneus tendon through a posterior incision.

REFERENCES

1. Bergman RA, Thompson SA, Afifi AK: Catalogue of Human Variation. Baltimore, Urban & Schwartzenberg, 1984, p 97.
2. Fisher DF Jr, Clagett GP, Parker JI, et al: Mandibular subluxation for high carotid exposure. J Vasc Surg 1:727, 1984.
3. Shaha A, Phillips T, Scalea T, et al: Exposure of the internal carotid artery near the skull: The posterolateral anatomic approach. J Vasc Surg 8:618, 1988.
4. Hertzer NR, Feldman BJ, Beven EG, Tucker HM: A prospective study of the incidence of injury to the cranial nerves during carotid endarterectomy. Surg Gynecol Obstet 151:781, 1980.
5. Schauber MD, Fontenelle LJ, Solomon JW, Hanson TJ: Cranial/cervical nerve dysfunction after carotid endarterectomy. J Vasc Surg 25:481, 1997.
6. Meier DE, Brink BE, Fry WJ: Vertebral artery trauma: Acute recognition and treatment. Arch Surg 116:236, 1981.
7. Thomas GI, Anderson KN, Hain RF, Merendino KA: The significance of anomalous vertebro-basilar artery communications in operations on the heart and great vessels. Surgery 46:747, 1959.
8. Makhoul RG, Machleder HI: Developmental anomalies at the thoracic outlet: An analysis of 200 consecutive cases. J Vasc Surg 16:534, 1992.
9. Pollack EW: Surgical anatomy of the thoracic outlet syndrome. Surg Gynecol Obstet 150:97, 1980.
10. Bergman RA, Thompson SA, Afifi AK: Catalogue of Human Variation. Baltimore, Urban & Schwartzenberg, 1984, pp 201–204.
11. Roos DB: Congenital anomalies associated with thoracic outlet syndrome: Symptoms, diagnosis, and treatment. Am J Surg 132:771, 1976.
12. Valentine RJ, Carter DJ, Clagett GP: A modified extrathoracic approach to the treatment of dysphagia lusoria. J Vasc Surg 5:498, 1987.
13. Moosman DA: Anatomy of the pectoral nerves and their preservation during modified mastectomy. Am J Surg 139:883, 1980.
14. Veith FJ, Gupta S, Daly V: Technique for occluding the supraceliac aorta through the abdomen. Surg Gynecol Obstet 151:426, 1980.
15. Hagino RT, Valentine RJ, Clagett GP: Supraceliac aortorenal bypass. J Vasc Surg 26:482, 1997.
16. Williams GM, Ricotta J, Zinner M, Burdick J: The extended retroperitoneal approach for treatment of extensive atherosclerosis of the aorta and renal vessels. Surgery 88:846, 1980.
17. Wind GG, Valentine RJ: Anatomic Exposures in Vascular Surgery. Baltimore, Williams & Wilkins, 1990, pp 462–463.
18. Trout HH, Giordano JM: Anomalies of the inferior vena cava. J Vasc Surg 3:924, 1986.
19. Valentine RJ, MacGillivray DC, Blankenship CL, Wind GG: Variations in the relationship of the left renal vein to the left renal artery at the aorta. Clin Anat 3:249, 1990.
20. Fisher DF Jr, Fry WJ: Collateral mesenteric circulation. Surg Gynecol Obstet 164:487, 1987.
21. Gonzalez LL, Jaffe MS: Mesenteric arterial insufficiency following abdominal aortic resection. Arch Surg 93:10, 1966.
22. Garrett HE Jr, Richardson JW, Howard HS, Garrett HE: Retroperitoneal lymphocele after abdominal aortic surgery. J Vasc Surg 10:245, 1989.
23. Kwaan JH, Bernstein JM, Connaly JE: Management of lymph fistulas in the groin after arterial reconstruction. Arch Surg 114:1416, 1979.
24. Williams PL, Bannister LH, Berry MM, et al (eds): Gray's Anatomy: The Anatomical Basis of Medicine and Surgery. New York, Churchill Livingstone, 1995, p 1597.
25. Bardsley JL, Staple TW: Variations in branching of the popliteal artery. Radiology 94: 581, 1970.
26. Tiefenbrun J, Beckerman M, Singer A: Surgical anatomy in bypass of the distal part of the lower limb. Surg Gynecol Obstet 141:528, 1975.
27. Ouriel K: The posterior approach to popliteal-crural bypass. J Vasc Surg 19:74, 1994.
28. Dardick H, Dardick I, Veith FJ: Exposure of the tibioperoneal arteries by a single lateral approach. Surgery 75:377, 1974.

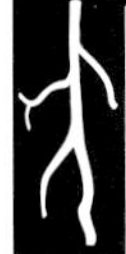

CHAPTER 6

Basic Considerations of the Arterial Wall in Health and Disease

Anton N. Sidawy, M.D., and Marc E. Mitchell, M.D.

A thorough knowledge of cellular components of the arterial wall and atherosclerotic plaque, the role of growth factors in cell cycle control in health and disease, and the role of risk factors in arterial wall injury is of paramount importance in understanding the pathogenesis of vascular disease. Atherosclerotic arterial disease is the main condition leading to arterial insufficiency. Complications resulting from advanced atherosclerosis are the most common indication for vascular reconstructive surgery or endovascular techniques.

Atherosclerosis is a systemic disease affecting the entire arterial tree, but lesions involving the coronary, extracranial cerebral, and lower extremity circulations have the most clinical significance for surgeons. The pathogenesis of atherosclerosis involves a complex series of events with the formation of atherosclerotic plaque as the end result. Injury to the arterial endothelial cell, resulting in endothelial cell dysfunction, is the first step in the process. Activated endothelial cells attract platelets, monocytes, and vascular smooth muscle cells (SMCs), which accumulate and proliferate in the arterial wall. These cellular components produce an excessive amount of connective tissue matrix. The ultimate endpoint is the formation of a mature fibrous plaque. Symptoms occur when advanced lesions are complicated by plaque rupture, hemorrhage into the plaque, emboli, or thrombosis.

The response to injury theory of atherosclerosis was first postulated by Ross in 1973[1] and has become the cornerstone of our current understanding of the pathogenesis of atherosclerosis. The theory states that atherosclerosis is, at least partially, the result of the cellular response to some form of endothelial injury. In many ways, this response to injury is similar to a chronic inflammatory response. Over the last 25 years, the theory has been modified and refined, resulting in a characterization of the events involved in the formation of atherosclerotic plaque.[2]

The process begins with some sort of endothelial cell injury, leading to endothelial dysfunction. This endothelial dysfunction results in changes in endothelial permeability, adhesive characteristics, and responses to various growth and stimulatory factors. Endothelial cells and vascular SMCs interact with monocytes, T lymphocytes, and platelets to form the cellular component of the fibroproliferative response, which ultimately results in the formation of atherosclerotic plaque.

DESCRIPTION AND STAGING OF ATHEROSCLEROTIC LESIONS

Classification

The lesions of atherosclerosis have traditionally been divided into three categories.

The *fatty streak* is the earliest stage of atheroma development and is found in children decades before the development of symptoms. Grossly, fatty streaks appear as slightly raised yellow discolorations on the intimal surface of the vessel, frequently occurring at branch points. Histologically, these lesions consist of lipid-filled macrophages and T-lymphocytes.[3, 4] These lipid-filled macrophages, also known as "foam cells," accumulate in the intima of the vessel wall.

The intermediate or *fibrofatty lesion*, the next stage of plaque development, consists of layers of macrophages and lymphocytes alternating with layers of vascular SMCs. The cells are surrounded by a connective tissue matrix of collagen, elastic fibers, and proteoglycans.[5]

The complicated or *fibrous plaque* is the advanced stage of atherosclerosis. At this stage, the plaque projects into the arterial lumen to a degree that impedes blood flow and produces symptoms. These lesions consist of a dense fibrous cap composed of connective tissue and vascular SMCs. When examined by electron microscopy, the vascular SMCs are seen to occupy a lacuna-like space surrounded by multiple layers of dense basement membrane collagen.[5] Beneath the fibrous cap is a layer containing vascular SMCs and macrophages along with a core of lipid and necrotic debris. Additional layers of vascular SMCs and connective tissue are present underneath the core. Lesions with thick, dense fibrous caps tend to be stable, whereas those with irregular, thin caps are more likely to develop complications such as plaque rupture, ulceration, and hemorrhage, which can cause acute symptoms.

Staging

The American Heart Association has proposed a new staging system (Fig. 6–1 and Fig. 6–2) for human atherosclerotic lesions based on histologic composition and structure.[6, 7] *Type I and II* lesions are considered early lesions. They are the only lesions found in children, but they may also occur in adults.

Type I lesions are microscopically characterized by an increase in the number of intimal macrophages and the accumulation of lipid droplets within the macrophages to form foam cells. Type II lesions include fatty streaks and are the first lesions to be visualized grossly. Not all type II lesions are fatty streaks, with some lesions meeting the microscopic criteria for type II lesions, but still not being

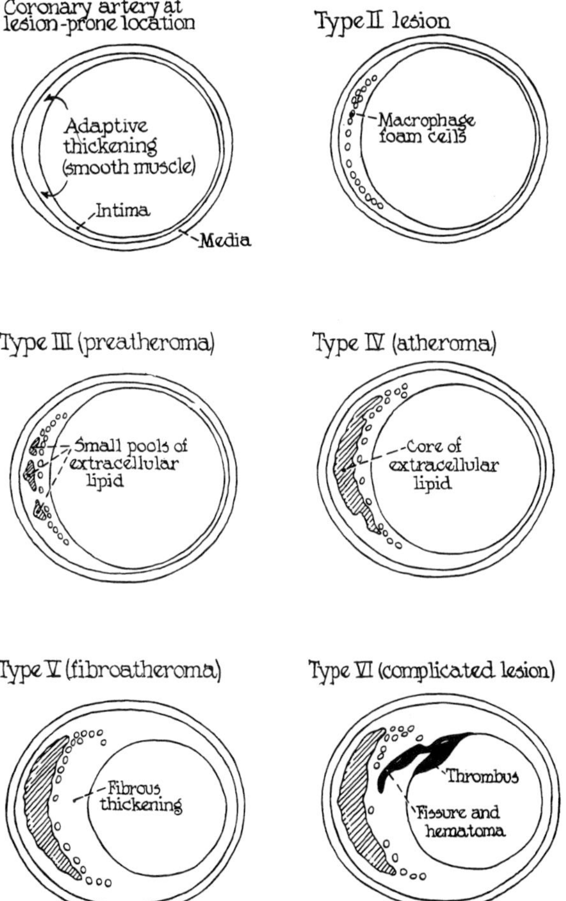

FIGURE 6–1. Cross-sectional drawings of coronary arteries demonstrating the morphology of lesions ranging from adaptive intimal thickening in lesion-prone locations to type VI atherosclerotic lesions. (From Stary HC, Chandler AB, Dinsmore RE, et al: A definition of advanced types of atherosclerotic lesions and a histological classification of atherosclerosis. Circulation 92:1355–1374, 1995.)

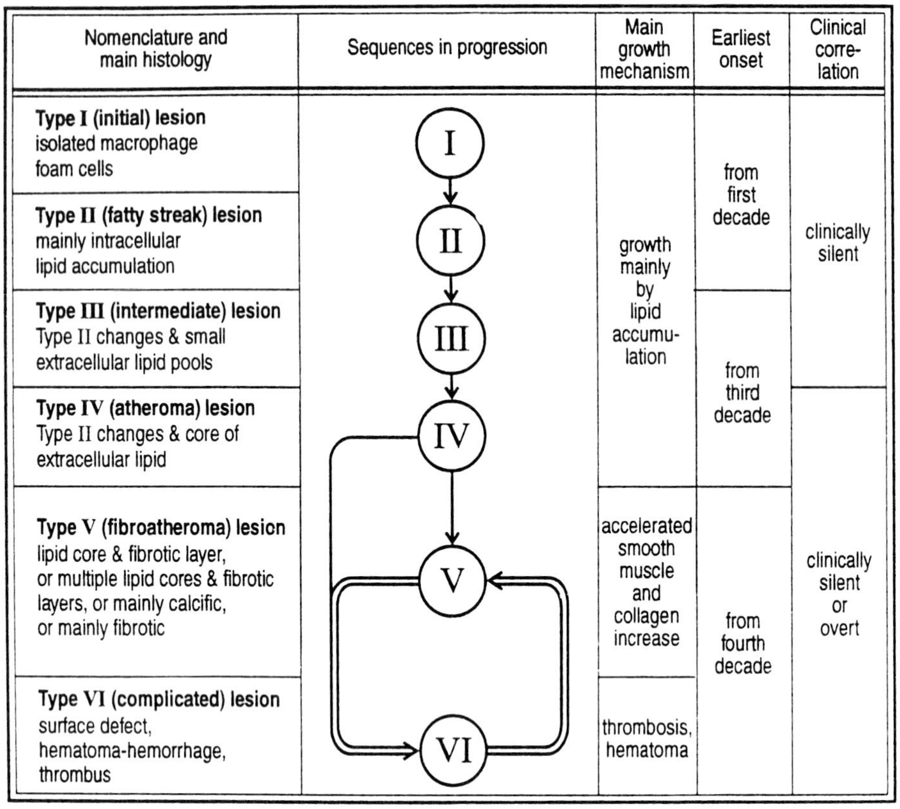

Nomenclature and main histology	Sequences in progression	Main growth mechanism	Earliest onset	Clinical correlation
Type I (initial) lesion isolated macrophage foam cells	I	growth mainly by lipid accumulation	from first decade	clinically silent
Type II (fatty streak) lesion mainly intracellular lipid accumulation	II			
Type III (intermediate) lesion Type II changes & small extracellular lipid pools	III		from third decade	
Type IV (atheroma) lesion Type II changes & core of extracellular lipid	IV			clinically silent or overt
Type V (fibroatheroma) lesion lipid core & fibrotic layer, or multiple lipid cores & fibrotic layers, or mainly calcific, or mainly fibrotic	V	accelerated smooth muscle and collagen increase	from fourth decade	
Type VI (complicated) lesion surface defect, hematoma-hemorrhage, thrombus	VI	thrombosis, hematoma		

FIGURE 6–2. Flow diagram showing the evolution and progression of atherosclerotic lesions. Roman numerals indicate the histologic type of lesion, and the direction of the arrows indicates the usual sequence in which characteristic morphologic changes occur. The loop between types V and VI illustrates how lesions increase in thickness as thrombotic deposits form on their surfaces. (From Stary HC, Chandler AB, Dinsmore RE, et al: A definition of advanced types of atherosclerotic lesions and a histological classification of atherosclerosis. Circulation 92:1355–1374, 1995.)

visible as a fatty streak. Type II lesions consist of layers of foam cells and lipid-containing vascular SMCs. Additionally, there are increased numbers of macrophages not containing lipids present within these lesions. T-lymphocytes and mast cells are also seen in type II lesions. The turnover of foam cells, vascular SMCs, and endothelial cells is increased in type II lesions compared to normal. Most of the lipid in type II lesions is intracellular, primarily within foam cells, but some widely dispersed extracellular droplets are present in some lesions.

Type II lesions may also be *progression-prone (type IIa)* and *progression-resistant (type IIb)*. Type IIa lesions are located in areas of adaptive intimal thickening and contain more foam cells and vascular SMCs compared with type IIb lesions. Adaptive intimal thickening is the result of mechanical forces on the arterial wall, such as shear stress, and occurs in everyone regardless of lipoprotein levels. Atherosclerosis develops preferentially in areas of adaptive intimal thickening.

Type III lesions are intermediaries between the type II lesions and the mature atheromas (type IV lesions). They are similar to type II lesions, but contain characteristic pools of extracellular lipid droplets dispersed among the layers of vascular SMCs. The lipid within the pool is the same as the extracellular lipid seen in type II lesions. These pools are located beneath the layered macrophages and foam cells, disrupting the coherent layer of vascular SMCs. The presence of these lipid pools signifies the progression of type II lesions to type III lesions.

Types IV, V, and *VI* are the advanced atherosclerotic lesions. Type IV lesions are sometimes called *atheromas*. They are characterized by a well-defined collection of extracellular lipid within the intima, known as the "lipid core." The lipid core is formed by the confluence of the lipid pools seen in type III lesions. Particles of calcium are sometimes present within the lipid core. The area between the lipid core and endothelial surface contains macrophages, foam cells, and vascular SMCs along with scattered T-lymphocytes and mast cells. Type IV lesions are frequently eccentric in location, cause a visible thickening of the arterial wall, but usually do not result in a significant narrowing of the arterial lumen and do not produce symptoms.

Type V lesions are characterized by the formation of prominent new fibrous connective tissue, which forms the fibrous cap. These lesions are subdivided based on the make-up of the connective tissue cap. *Type Va* lesions consist of a lipid core, similar to that seen in type IV lesions, covered by a thick fibrous layer composed of extracellular connective tissue matrix. In *type Vb* lesions the lipid core is calcified. Type *Vc* lesions do not have a lipid core and contain little, if any, lipid. Type V lesions are generally present starting in the fourth decade of life and can cause significant narrowing of the arterial lumen, producing symptoms.

Type VI lesions are also known as complicated lesions. They cause the majority of morbidity and mortality from atherosclerosis. Type VI lesions occur when a type IV or V lesion undergoes disruption of the intimal surface, such as with plaque ulceration or hemorrhage into a plaque. Type VI lesions may be the source of emboli or may cause arterial thrombosis. These events frequently result in acute ischemia, which may produce life-threatening or limb-threatening symptoms.

CELLULAR ELEMENTS

Endothelial cells, macrophages, T-lymphocytes, vascular SMCs, and platelets form the cellular component of the atherosclerotic plaque.[5] The interaction of these cells with one another is controlled by the production and release of various chemotactic agents, adhesion molecules, vasoactive agents, growth factors, and cytokines. Once activated, these cells are stimulated to proliferate and produce the connective tissue matrix, which forms the fibrous component of the atherosclerotic plaque.

Endothelial Cells

The response to injury hypothesis postulates that endothelial cell dysfunction is the initial event in the cascade leading to the formation of an atherosclerotic plaque, giving the endothelial cell a central role in atherogenesis. The endothelial cell has many normal physiologic functions. Endothelial cells function as a nonadherent surface for platelets and leukocytes. The endothelium is a nonthrombogenic surface and plays a major role in the modulation of the coagulation system. The endothelium functions as a permeability barrier, controlling the flow of fluids and molecules between the plasma and arterial wall. Vascular tone is modulated by the production and release of nitric oxide (NO), prostacyclin (PGI_2), endothelin, and angiotensin-II by the endothelium. Endothelial cells produce and secrete numerous growth factors and cytokines. The oxidation of lipoproteins, such as low-density lipoprotein (LDL), occurs in the endothelium. Abnormalities in one or more of these endothelial functions occur early in atherogenesis.[2, 5]

Whereas endothelial dysfunction is characteristically seen early in atherogenesis, endothelial disruption is not. Early atherosclerotic lesions tend to develop in areas where the endothelium is morphologically intact.[2] Even though the endothelium can maintain a normal structural integrity, abnormalities in the permeability of the endothelium are seen early in atherogenesis. One manifestation of this abnormality in permeability is the transport of lipoproteins through the endothelium. LDL is oxidized by endothelial cells. Oxidized LDL accumulates in the subendothelial space of the intima.[8] Oxidized LDL has several harmful effects, including stimulation of the production of chemotactic agents and growth factors. Additionally, oxidized LDL has an adverse effect on NO metabolism, causing abnormal vasoconstriction and platelet adherence and aggregation.

The formation of adhesive cell-surface glycoproteins by the endothelium, such as intercellular adhesion molecule-1 (ICAM-1), vascular cell adhesion molecule-1 (VCAM-1), and platelet-endothelial cell adhesion molecule (PECAM), is another early change seen in atherogenesis.[9] These molecules initiate the attachment and adherence of lymphocytes, monocytes, and platelets to the endothelial surface.[10] When activated, the endothelium produces many cytokines and growth factors, including platelet derived growth factor (PDGF), basic fibroblast growth factor (FGF), transforming growth factor-β (TGF-β), insulin-like growth factor I (IGF-I), and interleukin-1 (IL-1).[5] These substances attract and stimulate the proliferation of both vascular SMCs and macrophages. Activated endothelial cells produce abnormal amounts of collagen and connective tissue matrix, contributing to the fibrous proliferation seen in atherogenesis.

Macrophages

Macrophages are found in all atherosclerotic lesions but are most prominent in the early stages of the disease. Their normal function is that of a scavenger, and they present antigens to T-lymphocytes. The macrophage is the primary inflammatory mediator cell of atherogenesis. Monocytes are attracted by adhesion molecules and chemotactic factors produced by endothelial cells. Monocytes migrate to the subendothelial space, becoming macrophages. Early in atherogenesis, these cells take up oxidized LDL and become foam cells. Foam cells are simply macrophages filled with lipid and are characteristically present in early lesions of atherosclerosis. Oxidized LDL causes endothelial cell injury and is one of the main initiators of atherogenesis.

The uptake of oxidized LDL stimulates the productions of growth factors and cytokines by the macrophage. This further stimulates endothelial cells to produce adhesion molecules and chemotactic factors, which attracts more monocytes in a positive feedback loop. Once activated, macrophages produce a number of growth factors and chemotactic agents. The substances known to be produced by macrophages include[5, 11]:

- Monocyte–colony-stimulating factor (M-CSF)
- Granulocyte-monocyte colony-stimulating factor (GM-CSF)
- PDGF
- Epidermal growth factor (EGF)
- Basic FGF
- Transforming growth factor-α (TGF-α)
- TGF-β
- Vascular endothelial cell growth factor (VEGF)
- Monocyte chemoattractant protein-1 (MCP-1)[5, 11]

These substances attract additional monocytes and vascular SMCs, and they stimulate the proliferation of endothelial cells, monocytes, and vascular SMCs.

T-Lymphocytes

T-lymphocytes are present in all atherosclerotic lesions in large numbers. Their precise role in atherogenesis has not been fully determined. Although no specific antigens or antibodies have been clearly linked to atherogenesis, autoantibodies to oxidized LDL have been identified in humans. There appears to be a correlation between titers of these antibodies and the progression of atherosclerosis.[12] T-lymphocytes are known to adhere to atherosclerotic lesions and produce chemotactic agents and cytokines. Tumor necrosis factor-α (TNF-α), alpha-interferon (IFN-α), GM-CSF, and interleukin-2 (IL-2) are produced by activated T-lymphocytes.[5] These substances attract and activate both macrophages and vascular SMCs.

The concept that atherogenesis may be an immune response was postulated more than 30 years ago. The involvement of macrophages and T-lymphocytes in atherogenesis suggests both an immune as well as an inflammatory response. The lymphocytes found in atherosclerotic lesions are polyclonal, indicating that these cells do not develop in response to a single antigen. Several different subclasses of T-lymphocytes have been identified in atherosclerotic plaque, including both CD4 (helper-inducer cells) and CD8 (cytotoxic T cells).[13] There are several indications that T-lymphocytes present in atherosclerotic plaque are activated T-cells. High levels of IL-2 receptors are found on the T-cells, and high levels of IFN-α have been identified in atherosclerotic plaque. IL-2 receptors are markers suggesting the activation of T-lymphocytes, and IFN-α is produced and secreted by activated T-lymphocytes.[14]

Accelerated coronary artery atherosclerosis is a unique variant of atherosclerosis that develops and progresses rapidly in transplanted hearts, suggesting an immunologic cause. The lesions seen in transplanted hearts involve the entire coronary tree and are concentric rather than eccentric in nature. These lesions contain all the cellular elements characteristic of atherosclerosis but have increased numbers of T-lymphocytes and macrophages compared with the typical atherosclerotic lesion.[15] The accelerated progression of these lesions in hearts demonstrating chronic rejection indicates that the immune system may have a role in the progression of atherosclerosis.

Activation of the *complement system* may play a role in both the initiation of atherosclerosis and the acceleration of existing disease. Complement activation may occur by the classical pathway with the deposition of immune complexes in the arterial wall or the binding of specific antibodies to antigens found in vascular tissues. Antibody-independent activation via the alternative pathway may also occur. Cholesterol particles are potent activators of the complement system.[16] Activation of the complement system also results in the production of pro-inflammatory molecules and the terminal membrane attack complex (MAC). Pro-inflammatory molecules (e.g., C5a and C3a) increase vascular permeability, are chemotactic for and activate leukocytes, and cause the expression of adhesion molecules. MAC has been identified in atherosclerotic lesions, particularly fibrous plaque.[17] MAC has been known to increase the production and secretion of many cytokines, growth factors, and adhesion molecules, including:

- Basic FGF
- PDGF
- MCP-1
- P-selectin
- ICAM-1
- TNF-α
- IL-8

Additionally, MAC may stimulate the production of cytokines and growth factors by vascular SMCs and endothelial cells.[16] Complement activation contributes to the stimulation of an inflammatory response, leukocyte recruitment and activation, and proliferation and activation of vascular SMCs and endothelial cells.

Vascular Smooth Muscle Cells

Vascular SMCs are normally located in the media and are a major component of the arterial wall. Their main function is to maintain vascular tone. As humans age, the intima becomes thicker and these cells are found within this layer. The cells tend to accumulate in certain areas, and it is in the intima that atherosclerotic lesions develop. The migration of vascular SMCs to the intima is controlled by the release of various chemotactic agents from endothelial cells, platelets, macrophages, and other vascular SMCs. These cells respond to more than 20 different growth factors.[18] Proliferating vascular SMCs form a significant portion of atherosclerotic plaque and contribute to the narrowing of the vessel lumen by type V lesions.

There are two distinct phenotypes.[19] In the *contractile* state, the cells have more contractile myofilaments in their cytosol and are very responsive to substances that cause vasoconstriction or vasodilation. When stimulated by various cytokines and growth factors, vascular SMCs are transformed into the synthetic phenotype. In the *synthetic* state, there are fewer myofilaments, but a well-developed rough endoplasmic reticulum and Golgi complex are present. These cells are geared for the production of large amounts of proteins. In the synthetic state, vascular SMCs express the genes for the production of several growth factors and cytokines as well as extracellular matrix. These substances are chemotactic for other vascular SMCs, stimulate cell proliferation, and induce other cells to change from the contractile to synthetic phenotype. Cultured vascular SMCs demonstrate a rapid change from the contractile to synthetic state (Fig. 6–3). When stimulated, vascular SMCs in the synthetic state produce excessive amounts of extracellular matrix, which contributes to the volume of the plaque, causing impingement into the lumen of the vessel.

Platelets

The adherence and aggregation of platelets to the endothelial surface occur relatively early in the development of atherosclerosis. As lesions progress, platelet thrombi become more common, particularly at vessel branch points. Advanced atherosclerotic lesions are susceptible to thrombosis or serve as the nidus for platelet emboli, resulting in severe ischemic complications. Thrombosis is frequently the result of platelet adherence to ulcerated or irregular endothelial surfaces. There is evidence that platelets play a role in stimulating the progression of atherosclerotic lesions. Platelets are known to secrete a number of growth factors and vasoactive substances, including[5]:

- PDGF
- TGF-α
- TGF-β
- EGF
- IGF-I
- Thromboxane A_2
- Serotonin
- P-selectin

These substances are important in both recruiting and stimulating the proliferation of leukocytes and vascular SMCs. In animals, platelets have an important role in the progression of atherosclerosis. Rabbits that have been made thrombocytopenic have fewer atherosclerotic lesions compared with animals with normal platelets.[20] Pigs with abnormal von Willebrand factor synthesis are more resistant than normal animals to the development of atherosclerosis when fed a high-cholesterol diet.[21]

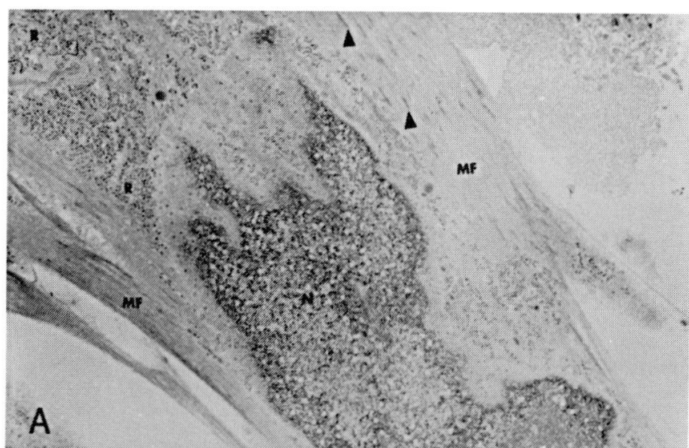

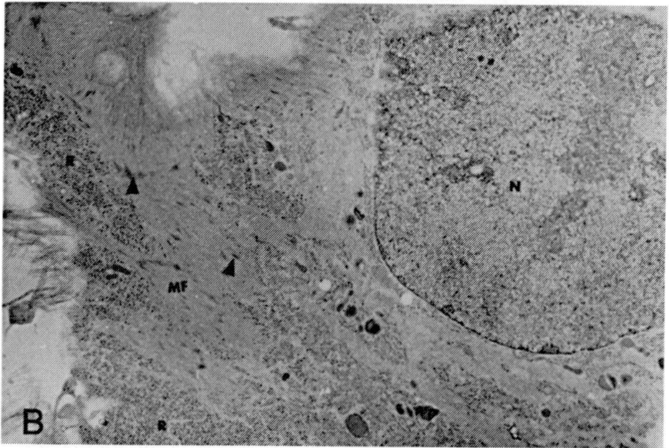

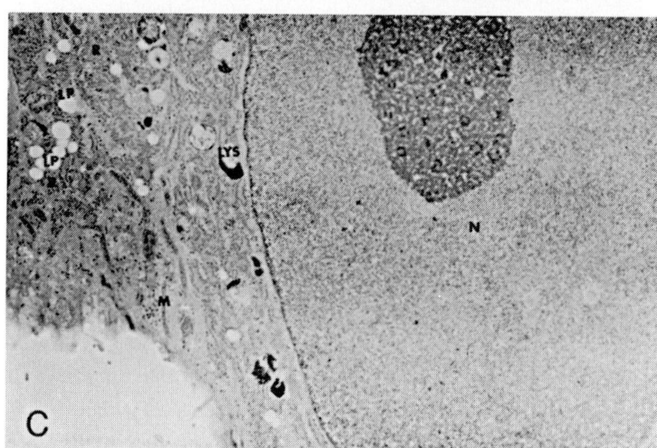

FIGURE 6–3. Composite electron micrograph of cultured tibial vascular smooth muscle cells demonstrating the different phenotypes: *A,* contractile state (passage 3); *B,* intermediate state (passage 5); *C,* synthetic state (passage 7). In *A,* note extent of microfilaments (MF) throughout the cytoplasm and highly irregular nuclear shape (N). *Solid arrowheads* denote dense plaques periodicity along MF. In *B,* there is increase in number of ribosomes and polyribosomes (R). In later passage (*C*), MF disappears. LYS, secondary lyosomes: LP, neural lipids. Magnification: *A*×4150; *B*×3500; *C*×5100. (From Jones BA, Aly HM, Forsyth EA, et al: Phenotypic characterization of human smooth muscle cells derived from atherosclerotic tibial and peroneal arteries. J Vasc Surg 24:883–891, 1996.)

GROWTH FACTORS

Cell differentiation and proliferation are influenced by peptide growth factors.[22] These peptide molecules are important in maintaining the normal development and growth of animal cells; in addition, they play a major role in disease states. The role of growth factors in the development of atherosclerosis and intimal hyperplasia is of great interest to us as physicians taking care of patients with peripheral vascular disease. Factors such as PDGF, FGF, insulin, IGF-I, TGF-α, and TGF-β play important roles in controlling the progression of cells in the cell cycle.[23] Furthermore, various growth factors have been found to influence the motility of cells, particularly vascular SMCs.[24]

Growth factors are mitogens that exert their effects via receptors located in the cell membrane. The interaction of a growth factor with its specific receptor unleashes a series of chemical reactions within the cell that ultimately lead to the specific action of the growth factor.[23] This action can be one of differentiation,[22] proliferation,[25] or chemotaxis.[24] Increased formation and secretion of growth factors and upregulation of their receptors can be found in disease states such as atherosclerosis and intimal hyperplasia.[26] In injury-induced intimal hyperplasia, local production of growth factors is encountered. These growth factors can be secreted by endothelial cells or by vascular SMCs. In addition, macrophages and platelets, which attach themselves to the injured endothelium, also secrete these growth factors.[27] The interaction of these factors with their receptors found on intimal and medial vascular SMCs stimulates the proliferation and migration of these cells through the internal elastic lamina of the arterial wall and their accumulation in the subendothelial layer.[28] The progression of such lesions leads to narrowing or occlusion of the arterial lumen, with resultant ischemia of the organ supplied by the affected artery.

Cell Cycle and Role of Growth Factors

The cell is usually found in a quiescent state called the *G0 phase*.[23] To proliferate, the cell goes through multiple phases that culminate in cell division (mitosis) (Fig. 6–4). The cell

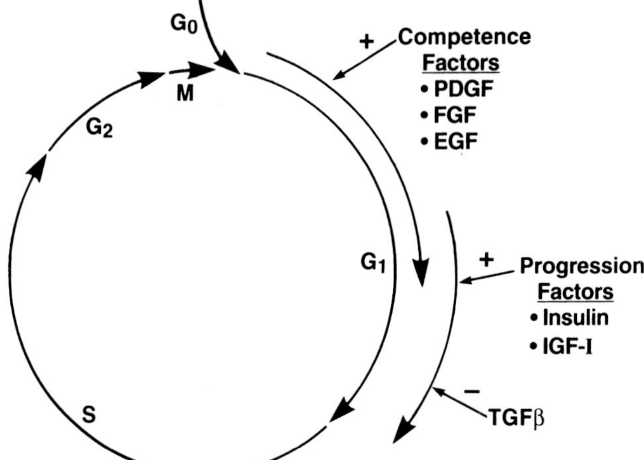

FIGURE 6–4. The cell cycle and the effects that competence and progression growth factors have on the cell while progressing in the G1 phase of the cycle. The cell must be under the influence of both groups in order to progress to the S phase. In addition, transforming growth factor-β (TGFβ) exerts a negative effect on the cell in the later part of the G1 phase. IGF-I, insulin-like growth factor-I; EGF, epidermal growth factor; FGF, fibroblast growth factor; PDGF, platelet-derived growth factor. (From Sidawy AN: Peptide growth factors and their role in the proliferative diseases of the vascular system. *In* Sidawy AN, Sumpio BE, DePalma RG (eds): The Basic Science of Vascular Disease. Armonk, NY, Futura Publishing, 1997, pp 127–149.)

enters the *Gap I phase (GI phase)* under the influence of a group of growth factors called *competence factors*. This group includes PDGF, FGF, and EGF. As the cell progresses in the GI phase, it is subject to the influence of another group of growth factors called *progression factors*. This group includes insulin and IGF-I. During the GI phase, the cell must be under the influence of both groups of factors in order to progress in that phase. If it does not, the cell reverts back to the G0 (quiescent) phase.

If the cell completes the GI phase, it enters the *S phase*, in which deoxyribonucleic acid (DNA) synthesis and chromosome replication take place. After going through the *Gap II phase (GII phase)*, the cell enters the *M phase*, in which mitosis takes place. Some growth factors can play a negative inhibitory role on the progression of the cell cycle. This is illustrated by the negative effect of TGF-β on the progression of the cell in the latter part of the cycle.

Although it has been widely held that specific protein synthesis plays an important role in the progression of the cell cycle, it has been discovered that protein destruction or proteolysis at specific points of the cell cycle triggers different phases of the cycle.[29]

Growth Factor Receptors and Signal Transduction

In order to exert their effects, growth factors interact with specific receptors located in the cell membrane. These receptors belong to a family of peptide receptors called *receptor tyrosine kinases* (RTKs). The peptide structure of these receptors is composed of multiple domains. The extracellular domain is found outside the cell. Once the growth factor interacts with the extracellular domain of its receptor, a signal is transmitted along the receptor molecule. The transmembrane domain anchors the receptor to the cell membrane and transmits the signal to the intracellular cytoplasmic domain. The cytoplasmic tyrosine kinase domain or the intracellular domain plays a major role in translating the signal received into specific cellular responses (Fig. 6–5).[30]

Tyrosine kinase receptors are classified into three subclasses according to their molecular structure (the presence or absence of one or more cysteine-rich residues) and the

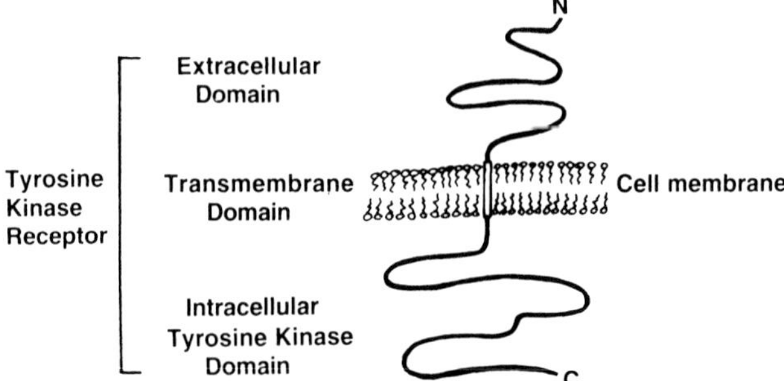

FIGURE 6–5. Depiction of the tyrosine kinase receptor. The N-terminal (N) of the receptor protein molecule is in the extracellular domain, and the C-terminal (C) is located in the intracellular domain. (From Sidawy AN: Peptide growth factors and their role in the proliferative diseases of the vascular system. *In* Sidawy AN, Sumpio BE, DePalma RG (eds): The Basic Science of Vascular Disease. Armonk, NY, Futura Publishing, 1997, pp 127–149.)

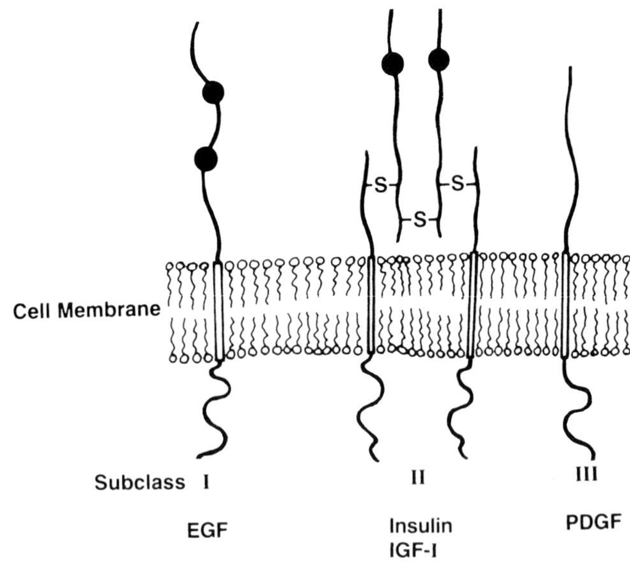

FIGURE 6–6. The three subclasses of the tyrosine kinase receptor. Subclass I is represented by the epidermal growth factor (EGF) receptor containing 2 cysteine-rich residues in its extracellular domain. Subclass II is represented by the insulin and the insulin-like growth factor-I (IGF-I) receptors, which are formed of two α and two β subunits. Each α-subunit contains one cysteine-rich residue in its extracellular domain. Subclass III is represented by the platelet-derived growth factor (PDGF) receptor with no cysteine-rich residue in its extracellular domain. (From Sidawy AN: Peptide growth factors and their role in the proliferative diseases of the vascular system. *In* Sidawy AN, Sumpio BE, DePalma RG (eds): The Basic Science of Vascular Disease. Armonk, NY, Futura Publishing, 1997, pp 127–149.)

number of subunits of which they are formed.[30] For example, the *subclass I* family is represented by the EGF receptor, which contains two cysteine-rich residues in its extracellular domain. The IGF-I and insulin receptors, examples of *subclass II*, are characterized by two α-subunits and two β-subunits, and each of the α-subunits, which form the extracellular domain of the receptor, contains one cysteine-rich residue. In contrast, the PDGF receptor contains no cysteine-rich residue in its extracellular domain, and it is of the *subclass III* family (Fig. 6–6).[30]

The most important events in signal transduction take place in the cytoplasm of the cell (Fig. 6–7).[23, 31] Triggered by growth factor attachment to the extracellular domain, dimerization or polymerization of two or more receptor intracellular domains takes place. The intracellular domains become phosphorylated at multiple locations, and they interact on a molecular level. Intracellular protein molecules belonging to various protein families are then recruited and bind to specific sites along the intracellular cytoplasmic domain of the phosphorylated receptor. These proteins carry specific recognition sites that allow a certain family of proteins to bind to a specific area of the receptor. Thus, various cellular signaling pathways are activated. Each pathway controls a specific function of the growth factor.

The recognition sites found on the cellular proteins are called src homology-2 (SH-2) or src homology-3 (SH-3) domains. In addition, the SH-2 and SH-3 phosphorylated sites of the protein serve to bind them to other cellular

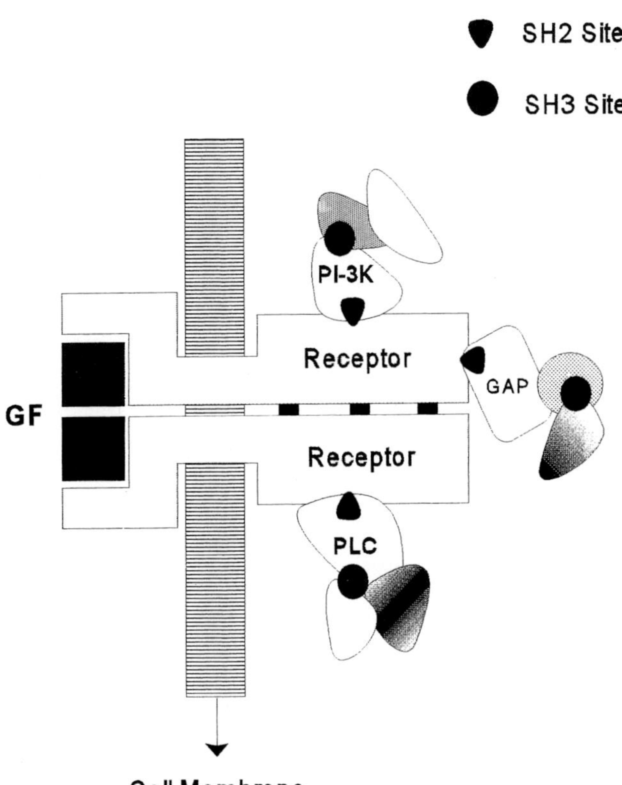

FIGURE 6–7. Once the growth factor (GF) interacts with the extracellular domain of its specific receptor, phosphorylation of the receptor takes place and the intracellular domains of various receptors interact on the molecular level. This in turn phosphorylates the src homology-2 (SH-2) or src homology-3 (SH-3) domains located on certain cellular proteins that belong to the signaling cascade leading to recruitment and binding of proteins carrying these recognition sites. Various proteins that are involved in these pathways include guanosine triphosphatase–activating protein (GAP), phospholipase-C (PLC), and phosphatidylinositol-3 kinase (P1–3K)–binding protein. These cascades of phosphorylation and specific protein binding eventually lead to a specific function of the growth factor.

proteins that belong to the signaling cascade. Various proteins that are involved in these pathways include (1) guanosine triphosphatase activating protein (GAP), (2) phospholipase-C (PLC), and (3) phosphatidylinositol-3 kinase (Pl-3K) binding protein. These cascades of phosphorylation and specific protein binding eventually lead to a specific function of the growth factor; the function may be one of differentiation, proliferation, cell shape change, or motility.[31]

The signaling pathways or cascades rely on the phosphorylation of various proteins for the signal to be transmitted to the nucleus and cause gene activation. One of these pathways is called "Ras pathway." Once the growth factor attaches to its receptor, the receptor phosphorylates itself. Ras, a protein that attaches to the cytoplasmic aspect of the cellular membrane, undergoes phosphorylation and activates Raf-1 protein which in turn phosphorylates mitogen-activated protein kinase (MAPK). MAPK phosphorylates transcription factors inside the nucleus (Myc, jun...) which stimulate gene activity.[31]

"Jak-STAT pathway" is another important signaling pathway.[32, 33] Signal transducers and activators of transcription (STATs) are families of protein that have been found to phosphorylate by Jaks, kinase enzymes activated in response to growth factor interaction with its receptor. The two pathways, Ras and Jak-STAT, may intersect on the way to the nucleus to cause gene activation. The specifics of such interaction are still the subject of intense research. It is believed that MAPK from the Ras pathway enhances STAT activity by causing additional phosphorylation.[34]

Platelet-Derived Growth Factor

The discovery of PDGF was reported by Ross and colleagues in 1974; they showed that platelet-rich serum caused vascular SMCs to proliferate.[25] Although called "platelet-derived" because it was first observed in platelet-rich serum, this growth factor has been found in a variety of cells, including arterial SMCs, fibroblasts, and endothelial cells.[35, 36]

PDGF has three isoforms (AA, BB, and AB), depending on the molecular composition of its two chains (chain A and chain B).[37] In response to balloon catheter injury, PDGF secretion by SMCs is increased.[38] In addition, PDGF messenger ribonucleic acid (mRNA) expression is induced in response to carotid artery injury.[39] PDGF exerts its effects via a specific tyrosine kinase receptor. PDGF receptor is formed of two α-subunits and two β-subunits.[40] This receptor has a very high affinity toward PDGF.

PDGF is a potent mitogen that causes proliferation and tissue remodeling. It is also a potent vasoconstrictor in a concentration-dependent fashion.[41] Whether it is secreted by platelets, endothelial cells, macrophages, or SMCs themselves, PDGF causes proliferation and multiplication of vascular SMCs. Since the half-life of PDGFs is only 2 minutes, it is thought that this growth factor acts near the release site in a paracrine or autocrine fashion.[42] In addition, PDGF plays a role in tissue remodeling. It increases collagen synthesis[43] and stimulates secretion of collagenase by fibroblasts.[44] This effect is important in wound healing and tissue remodeling. Furthermore, PDGF has a chemotactic effect on SMCs and other cells, such as fibroblast and neutrophils.[45]

Fibroblast Growth Factor

In 1974, Gospodarowicz named a material that caused proliferation of fibroblast in culture, FGF.[46] Because that material had a basic isoelectric charge, it was called *basic FGF* (bFGF). It was not until 1980, when Thomas described an acidic isoelectric charge FGF, that it was called *acidic FGF* (aFGF).[47] Many other forms of FGFs were discovered over the years. These growth factors were found to be secreted by a myriad of cells, including fibroblasts, endothelial cells, and SMCs. The same growth factor is given different names, depending on specific characteristics or on the tissue of origin. One FGF, for instance, is heparin-binding growth factor, which is found in the brain.[48] bFGF is a more potent growth factor than aFGF; however, this difference depends on target cells.[49]

The FGFs play an important role in extracellular matrix remodeling. bFGF is found in an insoluble state in the extracellular matrix and participates in tissue regeneration during repair,[50] inducing the fibroblast's production of collagen and proteins, the building blocks of the extracellular matrix.[51, 52] As an angiogenic factor, FGF promotes the formation of new vessels and other factors important in tissue repair. bFGF stimulates the proliferation of endothelial cells and SMCs after catheter-induced arterial injury.[53, 54] An antibody to bFGF has been found to inhibit the proliferation of vascular SMCs after injury.[55]

Insulin and Insulin-like Growth Factors

Although insulin is well known for its metabolic effects, it is also a very important growth factor that stimulates the proliferation of animal cells. In this chapter, we concentrate on the growth-promoting effects of insulin. Although IGFs have metabolic effects similar to those of insulin, our main interest here is their mitogenic effects. Both IGF-I and IGF-II have those effects, but IGF-I is more potent. Insulin is secreted by the pancreas; the IGFs are secreted mainly by the liver. Hepatic secretion of IGFs is growth hormone–dependent. The liver secretion of IGFs is continuous and steady.[56, 57] Once in the circulation, the IGFs travel bound to *IGF-binding proteins,* which are also secreted by the liver.[56] The IGFs are also secreted at the tissue level. Insulin secretion is not continuous; it is usually produced in reaction to serum glucose levels. In addition, insulin travels freely in the circulation, not bound to protein.

Both insulin and the IGFs exert their effects on animal cells via specific receptors. The receptors for IGF-I and insulin are organized as heterotetramers with two α- and two β-subunits (Fig. 6–6). The two receptors can be differentiated by their affinity to the growth factor. The insulin receptor has more affinity for insulin than the IGF-I receptor does, whereas the IGF-I receptor has more affinity to IGF-I than to insulin.

The receptor for IGF-II has a molecular structure differing from that of the IGF-I and insulin receptors. The IGF-II receptor has a very large extracellular domain. Of interest, when insulin exerts its metabolic effects, it does so via the insulin receptor; however, when it exerts its mitogenic effect, it does so via the IGF-I receptor. Using monoclonal antibody against the insulin receptor does not alter the proliferative effect of insulin on human tibial arterial SMCs. In contrast, using monoclonal antibody against the IGF-I receptor prevents insulin from exerting its effect on those cells (unpublished data from our laboratory). Furthermore, IGF-II seems to exert its mitogenic effect via the IGF-I receptor as well.[58]

The mitogenic effects of insulin and IGFs are those of proliferation and differentiation of animal cells. These growth factors induce the proliferation of endothelial and vascular SMCs. In addition, balloon de-endothelialization of rat aorta causes increased IGF-I mRNA, which has been found to peak at 7 days after injury.[59] We have found injury-induced intimal hyperplasia in rabbit aorta to increase IGF-I receptor binding.[26] IGF-I has been found to induce angiogenesis in rabbit corneal model, and the angiogenic effects of IGF-I and bFGF were evidenced in that model.[60] In our as yet unpublished data, we have noted that the mitogenic effects of insulin and glucose on human arterial SMC are synergistic. This mimics the situation in which SMCs are found in non–insulin-dependent diabetic patients, whose serum glucose and insulin levels are found to be increased.

Epidermal Growth Factor and Transforming Growth Factor-α

The term "epidermal growth factor" was coined by Cohen[61, 62] after studies showing that this factor promoted epidermal growth. The EGF molecule consists of 53 amino acids. TGF-α is an analog of EGF. They share sequence homology in about half of their molecular structure. In addition, the EGF receptor has high affinity for TGF-α.[63] The EGF receptor is expressed on most animal cells.

Although the primary target of EGF is epithelial cells, it is a mitogenic factor that stimulates the proliferation and migration of endothelial cells as well. In addition, EGF and TGF-α have been found to induce tube formation by endothelial cells, an important step in angiogenesis.[64] A vasodilator effect has also been shown for EGF upon administration in the femoral artery of the dog.[65]

Transforming Growth Factor-β

First described in the early 1970s, TGF at that time was called "sarcoma growth factor" (SGF).[66] Because this factor could cause morphologic changes in animal cells, it was later named "transforming growth factor."[67] There at least five members in the TGF-β family, numbered from 1 to 5. Each member is composed of 112 to 114 amino acids.[68] The TGF-βs exert their effect via specific receptors. There are four TGF-β receptors, varying in molecular weight. These receptors have been found on most animal cells.[69] TGF-βs are found in great concentration in bone, with the bony skeleton acting as a rich pool for these growth factors. TGF-βs are believed to play an important role in bone metabolism.[70]

TGF-β1 has an interesting effect on the growth and multiplication of cells. Although it can be a stimulator of cell growth, TGF-β1 can also inhibit cell differentiation and proliferation. The type of action exerted by this growth factor on a cell depends on multiple factors, such as the type of cell and the stage of its differentiation.[71] In addition, TGF-β1 may interfere with the growth and proliferation effect of other growth factors, such as insulin. The effect of insulin on arterial SMCs is one of proliferation; however, TGF-β1 has been found to inhibit the proliferative effect of insulin on these cells.[72] Furthermore, TGF-βs play a role in stimulating extracellular matrix protein synthesis and accumulation in bone and other tissues.[73] TGF-βs, especially TGF-β1, interact with multiple growth factors in the proliferation of cells of vascular origin. TGF-β1, as mentioned, inhibits the proliferative effect of insulin in vascular SMCs. It also opposes the proliferative effect of FGF on endothelial cells in culture.[74] This inhibitory effect is not limited to proliferation; TGF-β also inhibits the migratory effect, which is induced by FGF and PDGF.[75]

Vascular Endothelial Growth Factor

VEGF, a peptide growth factor that causes endothelial cell proliferation, has been found to promote the growth of new blood vessels in the myocardium and in the peripheral circulation.[76] VEGF is also known as "vascular permeability factor" (VPF) because it was found to cause vascular leakage in guinea pig skin.[77] It has been suggested that this leakage is important in the process of angiogenesis because it forms a fibrin gel medium that acts as a substrate for endothelial cell proliferation.[78] VEGF exerts its effect via two types of receptors; these receptors are localized to the vascular endothelium.[76]

Although FGF had been found to increase the expression of the 165-amino acid isomer of VEGF, it showed no effect on other VEGF isomers ($VEGF_{121}$, $VEGF_{110}$, $VEGF_{189}$, $VEGF_{206}$).[76, 79] These isomers differ in their isoelectric charge and in their affinity to heparin. These characteristics influence the bioavailability of various isomers and, in turn, influence their effects.[76] By using adenovirus vector expressing the VEGF complementary DNA (cDNA), angiogenesis has occurred, protecting against acute ischemia produced by ligation of the common iliac artery in male Sprague-Dawley rats.[80] Preliminary results have shown that intramuscular injection of naked plasmid DNA encoding the 165-amino acid VEGF isoform induces formation of new blood vessels in patients with chronic ischemia, leading to limb salvage.[81]

Clinical Implications of Growth Factor Physiology

Therapeutic methods can target any step of the signaling pathway, starting from the interaction of the growth factor with its specific receptor and including every subsequent step involved.[82] We have already mentioned some of the important applications in segments dedicated to individual growth factors, and now we describe other, more general methods.

One example that illustrates the efficacy of targeting the signaling pathways is the immunosuppressive drug cyclosporine, which is used to suppress the immune mechanism in organ transplantation.[31] An antibody against FGF has been shown to inhibit the formation of post-injury intimal hyperplasia.[83] Growth factor antagonists can successfully inhibit the binding of the growth factor to its receptor and reversing the progress of the disease. Suramin, a drug that serves as an example of this approach, has been found to be effective in the treatment of some kinds of carcinomas.[84] In addition, antibodies against specific growth factor receptors prevent the interaction between the growth factor and its receptor, leading to inhibition of the growth factor function. SH-2, SH-3, Ras, Raf1, and MAPK blockers are in the process of being developed to interrupt the signaling pathways and to prevent the progression of disease.[31, 82]

RISK FACTORS FOR ATHEROSCLEROSIS

The well-known risk factors for atherosclerosis have all been implicated as contributors to endothelial injury. It is only recently that the pathogenesis of the injury resulting from these risk factors has been determined. Although the underlying mechanism may vary, the resultant endothelial injury is the common initiating factor in the development of atherosclerosis.

Tobacco

Cigarette smoking is well established as an independent risk factor for the development of atherosclerosis, but the mechanism of smoking-induced atherogenesis is not completely understood. There are nearly 5000 chemicals found in cigarette smoke, most of which have yet to be studied. Cigarette smoke has been shown to cause endothelial cell swelling and bleb formation, increased formation of luminal surface projections, subendothelial edema, widening of endothelial junctions, and basement membrane thickening.[85–87] Studies of nicotine alone have demonstrated similar effects[88, 89] along with an increased frequency of endothelial cell death and a decreased rate of cell replication.[90] This abnormal capability for endothelial cell regeneration results in an impaired ability to repair sites of endothelial cell damage. Thus, cigarette smoke not only is toxic to the endothelial cell, causing injury and death, but also inhibits the ability of the endothelium to repair the injury induced by the smoke.

In addition to direct injury to the endothelium, smoking can indirectly damage the endothelium, resulting in endothelial function abnormalities. Smokers have been shown to have abnormal levels of plasma lipoproteins, which return to normal after cessation of smoking.[91] Elevated lipoproteins are another initiator of endothelial cell injury. Cigarette smoking is associated with abnormal prostaglandin production, resulting in an imbalance between prostacyclin and thromboxane A_2.[92] This reduces the antithrombotic potential of the endothelial surface by inducing platelet aggregation and adherence. Smoking inhibits the production of nitric oxide (NO), which has adverse effects on vasomotor regulation, proliferation of vascular SMCs, and platelet and macrophage adhesion.[93] A clinical manifestation of this abnormality in NO metabolism is decreased ability of saphenous vein grafts to dilate in smokers compared with nonsmokers.[94]

Hypertension and Shear Forces

Hypertension, another independent risk factor for the development of atherosclerosis, induces morphologic as well as functional changes in the endothelium. Endothelial cells from hypertensive patients are edematous and project further into the lumen of the vessel than normal.[95] Vessels from hypertensive patients demonstrate vascular SMC proliferation along with thickening of the basement membrane, subendothelial accumulation of fibrin, and increased fibronectin in the extracellular matrix.[96] Growth factors, such as TGF-β and PDGF, are increased, contributing to vascular SMC proliferation.[97] Endothelium-dependent relaxation is impaired in hypertensive patients via abnormalities of NO metabolism.[98] The effect of an acetylcholine infusion on the release of NO is significantly reduced in hypertensive patients.[95] NO production is decreased both in humans with essential hypertension and in animal models of hypertension.[99, 100] Most studies indicate that the endothelial dysfunction seen in hypertensive patients is the *result* of the elevated blood pressure, not the *cause*.[95] It appears that the severity of the endothelial dysfunction associated with hypertension is related to the degree of blood pressure elevation.

Atherosclerosis is seen only in vessels subjected to arterial pressure. Veins do not develop atherosclerosis, but atherosclerosis frequently occurs in vein grafts placed into the arterial circulation. Atherosclerotic lesions tend to occur at certain areas, such as branch points and bends in vessels, indicating that hemodynamic forces other than arterial pressure may have an etiologic role in atherogenesis.

Shear forces appear to have an effect on the development of atherosclerosis. Certain areas of low shear stress, such as the carotid sinus, have a predilection for the development of atherosclerosis.[11] High shear forces at bifurcations may disrupt the endothelium, contributing to the increased frequency of lesions seen in these areas. While it appears likely that shear forces have a part in the development of atherosclerosis, the exact role of shear forces in atherogenesis is not fully understood.

Hyperlipidemia

The relationship between elevated levels of plasma lipoproteins and atherosclerosis has been recognized for many years, but the pathophysiology of lipoprotein-induced endothelial cell injury has been elucidated only recently. It is now known that low-density lipoprotein (LDL) is taken up by the endothelial cells and converted to the oxidized form of LDL, which plays a significant role in the induction of endothelial cell injury. Oxidized LDL blunts endothelium-dependent relaxation by decreasing the production and release of NO by the endothelial cell, and stimulates the endothelium to produce cytokines and growth factors.[8, 11] Additionally, oxidized LDL attracts monocytes and enhances their adhesiveness to the endothelial surface.[10] Subendothelial macrophages ingest oxidized LDL and become foam cells. The role of monocytes and macrophages in the development of atherosclerosis was discussed earlier in this chapter.

Diabetes Mellitus

Diabetes mellitus is another initiator of endothelial cell dysfunction. Using brachial artery vasoactivity to evaluate endothelial cell function, we have found impaired endothelium-dependent relaxation in patients with occult glucose intolerance as well as in those with overt diabetes. Diabetic patients also demonstrate blunting of the normal vasorelaxation seen with hyperemia. This abnormality is exacerbated by an oral glucose load, such as during an oral glucose tolerance test.[101] Endothelin and angiotensin-converting enzyme (ACE) levels, which cause vasoconstriction, are elevated in these patients and may be responsible for this finding.[102, 103]

Several potential mechanisms explain the vascular injury seen in diabetes. Patients with type II diabetes mellitus have elevated levels of both insulin and glucose, which have been shown to be independent stimulants of vascular SMC proliferation[104] (an early step in the development of atherosclerosis). High concentrations of glucose increase the production of endothelial collagen IV and fibronectin as well as the activity of enzymes involved in collagen synthesis.[105] This leads to a thickening of the basement membrane and contributes to the excessive production of extracellular matrix seen in atherosclerosis. Additionally, elevated glucose concentrations have been shown to accelerate cell death and impair cell replication in cultured endothelial cells.[106]

Like smoking, diabetes not only causes endothelial cell injury but also impairs the ability of the endothelial cell to regenerate and repair the injury. Patients with diabetes frequently have associated diseases, such as hypertension or hyperlipidemia, which are also risk factors for development of atherosclerotic vascular disease. The presence of more than one initiator of endothelial injury may have an additive effect on the degree of the injury, the extent of endothelial cell dysfunction, and the rate at which atherosclerosis develops and progresses.

REFERENCES

1. Ross R, Glomset JA: Atherosclerosis and the arterial smooth muscle cell. Science 180:1332–1339, 1973.
2. Ross R: The pathogenesis of atherosclerosis: A perspective for the 1990s. Nature 362:801–809, 1993.
3. Faggiotto A, Ross R, Harker L: Studies of hypercholesterolemia in the nonhuman primate: I. Changes that lead to fatty streak formation. Atherosclerosis 4:323–340, 1984.
4. Stary HC: Evolution and progression of atherosclerotic lesions in coronary arteries of children and young adults. Atherosclerosis 9 (Suppl I):19–32, 1989.
5. Ross R: Cell biology of atherosclerosis. Annu Rev Physiol 57:791–804, 1995.
6. Stary HC, Chandler AB, Glagov S, et al: A definition of intimal, fatty streak, and intermediate lesions of atherosclerosis. Circulation 89:2462–2478, 1994.
7. Stary HC, Chandler AB, Dinsmore RE, et al: A definition of advanced types of atherosclerotic lesions and a histological classification of atherosclerosis. Circulation 92:1355–1374, 1995.
8. Flavahan NA: Atherosclerosis or lipoprotein-induced endothelial dysfunction: Potential mechanisms underlying reduction in EDRF/nitric oxide activity. Circulation 85:1927–1938, 1992.
9. Springer TA: Adhesion receptors of the immune system. Nature 346:425–434, 1990.
10. Berliner JA, Territo MC, Sevanian A, et al: Minimally modified low density lipoprotein stimulates monocyte endothelial interactions. J Clin Invest 85:1260–1266, 1990.
11. Boyle EM, Lille ST, Allaire E, et al: Endothelial cell injury in cardiovascular surgery: Atherosclerosis. Ann Thorac Surg 63:885–894, 1997.
12. Salonen JT, Yla-Harttuala S, Yamamoto R, et al: Autoantibodies against oxidized LDL and progression of carotid atherosclerosis. Lancet 339:883–887, 1992.
13. Libby P, Hansson GK: Biology of disease: Involvement of the immune system in human atherogenesis: Current knowledge and unanswered questions. Lab Invest 64:5–15, 1991.
14. Hansson GK, Holm J, Jonasson L, et al: Detection of activated T lymphocytes in human atherosclerotic plaque. Am J Pathol 135:169–175, 1989.
15. Salomon RN, Hughes CC, Schoen FJ, et al: Human coronary transplantation–associated arteriosclerosis: Evidence for a chronic immune reaction to activated graft endothelial cells. Am J Pathol 138:791–798, 1991.
16. Torzewski J, Bowyer DE, Waltenberger J, et al: Processes in atherosclerosis: Complement activation. Atherosclerosis 132:131–138, 1997.
17. Rus HG, Niculescu F, Constantinescu E, et al: Immunoelectronmicroscopic localization of the terminal C5b-9 complement complex in human aortic fibrous plaque. Atherosclerosis 61:35–42, 1986.
18. Corson MA, Berk BC: Growth factors and the vessel wall. Heart Dis Stroke 2:166–170, 1993.
19. Jones BA, Aly HM, Forsyth EA, et al: Phenotypic characterization of human smooth muscle cells derived from atherosclerotic tibial and peroneal arteries. J Vasc Surg 24:883–891, 1996.
20. Moore S, Freidman RJ, Singal DP, et al: Inhibition of injury induced

thromboatherosclerotic lesions by anti-platelet serum in rabbits. Thromb Haemost 35:70–81, 1976.
21. Fuster V, Bgowie EJW, Lewis JC, et al: Resistance to atherosclerosis in pigs with von Willebrand's disease: Spontaneous and high-cholesterol diet-induced atherosclerosis. J Clin Invest 61:722–730, 1978.
22. Baird A, Bohlen P: Fibroblast growth factors. *In* Sporn MB, Roberts AB (eds): Peptide Growth Factors and Their Receptors. Vol I. New York, Springer-Verlag, 1990, pp 369–418.
23. Aaronson SA: Growth factors and cancer. Science 254:1146–1153, 1991.
24. Zerwes HG, Risau W: Polarized secretion of a platelet-derived growth factor–like chemotactic factor by endothelial cells in vitro. J Cell Biol 105:2037–2041, 1987.
25. Ross R, Glomset JA, Kariya B, Harker L: A platelet-dependent serum factor that stimulates the proliferation of arterial smooth muscle cells *in vitro*. Proc Natl Acad Sci U S A 71:1207–1210, 1974.
26. Sidawy AN, Hakim FS, Jones B, et al: Insulin-like growth factor-I binding in injury-induced intimal hyperplasia of rabbit aorta. J Vasc Surg 23:308–313, 1996.
27. Ross R, Masuda J, Raines EW, et al: Localization of PDGF-B protein in macrophages in all phases of atherogenesis. Science 248:1009–1012, 1990.
28. Ross R: The pathogenesis of atherosclerosis: An update. N Engl J Med 314:488–500, 1986.
29. Baringa M: Research news: A new twist to the cell cycle. Science 269:631–632, 1995.
30. Yarden Y, Ullrich A: Growth factor receptor tyrosine kinase. Ann Rev Biochem 57:443–478, 1988.
31. Brugge JS: New intracellular targets for therapeutic drug design. Science 260:1993.
32. Schindler C, Shuai K, Prezioso VR, Darnell JE: Interferon-dependent tyrosine phosphorylation of a latent cytoplasmic transcription factor. Science 257:809–813, 1992.
33. Zhong Z, Wen Z, Darnell JE: Stat3: A stat family member activated by tyrosine phosphorylation in response to epidermal growth factor and interleukin. Science 264:95–98, 1994.
34. Baringa M: Two major signaling pathways meet at MAP-kinase. Science 269:1673, 1995.
35. Dicorleto PE, Bowen-Pope DF: Cultured endothelial cells produce a platelet-derived growth factor-like protein. Proc Natl Acad Sci U S A 80:1919–1923, 1983.
36. Seifert RA, Schwartz SM, Bowen-Pope DF: Developmentally regulated production of platelet-derived growth factor-like molecules. Nature 311:669–671, 1984.
37. Hammacher A, Hellman U, Johnsson A, et al: A major part of platelet-derived growth factor purified from human platelets is a heterodimer of one A and one B chain. J Biol Chem 263:493–498, 1988.
38. Walker LN, Bowen-Pope DF, Ross R, Reidy MA: Production of platelet-derived growth factor–like molecules by cultured arterial smooth muscle cells accompanies proliferation after arterial injury. Proc Natl Acad Sci U S A 83:7311–7315, 1986.
39. Majesky MW, Reidy MA, Bowen-Pope DF, et al: PDGF ligand and receptor gene expression during repair of arterial injury. J Cell Biol 111:2149, 1990.
40. Seifert RA, Hart CE, Phillips PE, et al: Two different subunits associate to create isoform-specific platelet-derived growth factor receptors. J Biol Chem 264:8771–8778, 1989.
41. Berk BC, Alexander RW, Brock TA, et al: Vasoconstriction: A new activity of platelet-derived growth factor. Science 232:87–90, 1986.
42. Raines EW, Bowen-Pope DF, Ross R: Platelet-derived growth factor. *In* Sporn MB, Roberts AB (eds): Peptide Growth Factors and Their Receptors. Vol I. New York, Springer-Verlag, 1990, pp 173–262.
43. Owen AJ, Geyer RP, Antoniades HN: Human platelet-derived growth factor stimulates amino acid transport and protein synthesis by human diploid fibroblasts in plasma-free media. Proc Natl Acad Sci U S A 79:3203–3207, 1982.
44. Bauer EA, Cooper TW, Huang JS, et al: Stimulation of in vitro human skin collagenase expression by platelet-derived growth factor. Proc Natl Acad Sci U S A 82:4132–4136, 1985.
45. Deuel TF, Sehior RM, Huang SS, et al: Chemotaxis of monocytes and neutrophils to platelet-derived growth factor. J Clin Invest 69:1046–1049, 1982.
46. Gospodarowicz D: Localization of a fibroblast growth factor and its effect alone and with hydrocortisone on cell growth. Nature 249:123–127, 1974.
47. Thomas KA, Riley MC, Lemmon SK, et al: Brain fibroblast growth factor: Nonidentity with mild and basic protein fragment. J Biol Chem 255:5517–5520, 1980.
48. Lobb RR, Fett JW: Purification of two distinct growth factors from bovine neural tissue by heparin affinity chromatography. Biochemistry 23:6295–6299, 1984.
49. Gospodarowicz D: Biological activities of fibroblast growth factors. Ann N Y Acad Sci 638:1–8, 1991.
50. Saksela O, Moscatelli D, Sommer A, Rifkin DB: Endothelial cell–derived heparan sulfate binds basic fibroblast growth factor and protects it from proteolytic degradation. J Cell Biol 107:743–755, 1988.
51. Chua CC, Barritault D, Geiman DE, Ladda RL: Induction and suppression of type I collagenase in cultured human cells. Coll Relat Res 7:277–284, 1987.
52. Davidson JM, Klagsbrun M, Hill KE, et al: Accelerated wound repair, cell proliferation, collagen and accumulation are produced by cartilage-derived growth factor. J Cell Biol 100:1219–1227, 1985.
53. Lindner V, Majack RA, Reidy MA: Basic fibroblast growth factor stimulates endothelial regrowth and proliferation in denuded arteries. J Clin Invest 85:2004–2008, 1990.
54. Lindner V, Lappi DA, Baird A, et al: Role of basic fibroblast growth factor in vascular lesion formation. Circ Res 68:106–113, 1991.
55. Lindner V, Reidy MA: Proliferation of smooth muscle cells after vascular injury is inhibited by an antibody against basic fibroblast growth factor. Proc Natl Acad Sci U S A 88:3739–3743, 1991.
56. Schwander J, Hauri C, Zapf J, Froesch ER: Synthesis and secretion of insulin like growth factor and its binding protein by the perfused rat liver: Dependence on growth hormone status. Endocrinology 113:297–305, 1983.
57. Froesch ER, Schmid C, Schwander J, Zapf J: Actions of insulin-like growth factors. Ann Rev Physiol 47:443–467, 1985
58. Nissley SP, Hasckel JF, Sasaki N, et al: Insulin-like growth factor receptors. J Cell Science 3(Suppl):39–51, 1985.
59. Cercek B, Fishbein MC, Forrester JS, et al: Induction of insulin-like growth factor-I messenger RNA in rat aorta after balloon denudation. Circ Res 66:1755–1760, 1990.
60. Grant MB, Mames RN, Fitzgerald C, et al: Insulin-like growth factor-I acts as an angiogenic agent in rabbit cornea and retina: Comparative studies with basic fibroblast growth factor. Diabetologia 36:282–291, 1993.
61. Cohen S: Isolation and biological effects of an epidermal growth-stimulating protein. Natl Cancer Inst Monogr 13–27, 1964.
62. Cohen S: The stimulation of epidermal proliferation by a specific protein (EGF). Dev Biol 12:394–407,1965.
63. Marquardt H, Hunkapiller MW, Hoot LE, et al: Transforming growth factors produced by retrovirus transformed rodent fibroblast and human melanoma cells: Amino acid sequence homology with epidermal growth factor. Proc Natl Acad Sci U S A 80:4684–4688, 1983.
64. Sato Y, Okamura K, Morimoto A, et al: Indispensable role of tissue-type plasminogen activator in growth factor-dependent tube formation of human microvascular endothelial cells in vitro. Exp Cell Res 204:223–229, 1993.
65. Gan BS, Hollenberg MD, MacCannell KL, et al: Distinct vascular actions of epidermal growth factor–urogastrone and transforming growth factor-α. J Pharmacol Exp Ther 242:331–337, 1987.
66. DeLarco JE, Todaro GJ: Growth factors from murine sarcoma virus–transformed cells. Proc Natl Acad Sci U S A 75:4001–4005, 1978.
67. Roberts AB, Lamb LC, Newton DL, et al: Transforming growth factors: Isolation of polypeptides from viral and chemically transformed cells by acid/ethanol extraction. Prac Natl Acad Sci U S A 77:3494–3498, 1980.
68. Roberts AB, Sporn MB: The transforming growth factor-betas. *In* Sporn MB, Roberts AB (eds): Handbook of Experimental Pharmacology. New York, Springer-Verlag, 1990, pp 419–472.
69. Massague J, Cheifetz S, Boyd FT, Andres JL: TGFβ receptors and TGFβ binding proteoglycans: Recent progress in identifying their functional properties. Ann N Y Acad Sci 593:59–72, 1990.
70. Centrella M, McCarthy TL, Canalis E: Skeletal tissue and transforming growth factor-beta. FASEB J 2:3066–3073, 1988.
71. Sporn MB, Roberts AB, Wakefield LM, deCrombrugghe D: Some recent advances in the chemistry and biology of transforming growth factor-beta. J Cell Biol 105:1039–1045, 1987.
72. Forsyth EA, Aly HM, Najjar SF, et al: Transforming growth factor

β1 inhibits the proliferative effect of insulin on human infragenicular vascular smooth muscle cells. J Vasc Surg 1997; 25:432–6.
73. Centrella M, McCarthy TL, Canalis E: Transforming growth factor beta is a bifunctional regulator of replication and collagen synthesis in osteoblast-enriched cell cultures from fetal rat bone. J Biol Chem 262:2869–7284, 1987.
74. Baird A, Durkin T: Inhibition of endothelial cell proliferation by type beta transforming growth factor: Interactions with acidic and basic fibroblast growth factors. Biochem Biophys Res Commun 138:476–482, 1986.
75. Mii S, Ware JA, Kent KC: Transforming growth factor-β inhibits human vascular smooth muscle cell growth and migration. Surgery 114:464–470, 1993.
76. Ferrara N, Davis-Smyth T: The biology of vascular endothelial growth factor. Endocr Rev 18:4–25, 1997.
77. Senger DR, Galli SG, Dvorak AM, et al: Tumor cells secrete a vascular permeability factor that promotes accumulation of ascites fluid. Science 219:983–985, 1983.
78. Dvorak HF, Harvey VS, Estrella P, et al: Fibrin containing gels induce angiogenesis: Implications for tumor stroma generation and wound healing. Lab Invest 57:673–686, 1987.
79. Seghezzi G, Patel S, Ren CJ, et al: Autocrine regulation of blood vessel formation by fibroblast growth factor-2 and vascular endothelial growth factor: A mechanism for tumor angiogenesis. Surg Forum 48:836–837, 1997.
80. Mack CA, Budendender KT, Polce D, et al: Salvage angiogenesis mediated by an adenovirus vector expressing vascular endothelial growth factor protects against acute arterial occlusion: Physiologic evidence of benefit. Surg Forum 48:447–449, 1997.
81. Isner JM, Pieczek A, Schainfeld R, et al: Clinical evidence of angiogenesis after arterial gene transfer of phVEGF165 in patient with ischemic limb. Lancet 348:370–374, 1996.
82. Levitzki A, Gazit A: Tyrosine kinase inhibition: An approach to drug development. Science 267:1782–1788, 1995.
83. Lindner V, Reidy MA: Proliferation of smooth muscle cells after vascular injury is inhibited by an antibody against fibroblast growth factor. Proc Natl Acad Sci U S A 88:3739–3743, 1995.
84. Gansler T, Vaghmar N, Olson JJ, Graham SD: Suramin inhibits growth factor binding and proliferation of urothelial carcinoma cell cultures. J Urol 148:910–914, 1992.
85. Asmussen I, Kjeldsen K: Intimal ultrastructure of human arteries: Observations on arteries from newborn children of smoking and non-smoking mothers. Circ Res 36:579–589, 1975.
86. Bylock A, Bondjers G, Jansson I, et al: Surface ultrastructure of human arteries with special reference to the effects of smoking. Acta Pathol Microbiol Scand 87A:201–209, 1979.
87. Boutet M, Bazin M, Turcotte H, et al: Effects of cigarette smoke on rat thoracic aorta. Artery 7:56–72, 1980.
88. Booyse FM, Osikowicz G, Quarfoot AJ: Effects of chronic oral consumption of nicotine on the rabbit aortic endothelium. Am J Pathol 102:229–238, 1981.
89. Zimmerman M, McGeachie JK: The effects of nicotine on aortic endothelial cell turnover and ultrastructure. Adv Exp Med Biol 273:79–88, 1990.
90. Lin SJ, Hong CY, Chang MS, et al: Long-term nicotine exposure increases aortic endothelial cell death and enhances transendothelial macromolecular transport in rats. Arterioscler Thromb 12:1305–1312, 1992.
91. Giordano JM: Cigarette smoking and vascular disease. *In* Sidawy AN, Sumpio BE, DePalma RG (eds): The Basic Science of Vascular Disease. Armonk, NY, Futura Publishing, 1997, pp 471–475.
92. Pittilo RM, Mackie JJ, Rowles PM, et al: Effects of cigarette smoking on the ultrastructure of rat thoracic aorta and its ability to produce prostacyclin. Thromb Haemost 48:173–176, 1982.
93. Powell JT, Higman DJ: Smoking, nitric oxide and the endothelium. Br J Surg 81:785–787, 1994.
94. Higman DJ, Greenhalgh RM, Powell JT: Smoking impairs endothelium-dependent relaxation of saphenous vein. Br J Surg 80:1242–1245, 1993.
95. Luscher TF: The endothelium and cardiovascular disease—a complex relation. N Engl J Med 330:1081–1083, 1994.
96. Takasaki I, Chobanian AV, Brecher P: Biosynthesis of fibronectin by rabbit aorta. J Biol Chem 266:17686–17694, 1991.
97. Dzau VJ, Gibbons GH, Cooke JP, et al: Vascular biology and medicine in the 1990s: Scope, concepts, potentials, and perspectives. Circulation 87:705–719, 1993.
98. Panza JA, Quyyumi AA, Brush Jr JE, et al: Abnormal endothelium-dependent vascular relaxation in patients with essential hypertension. N Engl J Med 323:22–27, 1990.
99. Vallance P, Collier J, Moncada S: Effects of endothelium-derived nitric oxide on peripheral arterial tone in man. Lancet 2:997–1000, 1989.
100. Rees D, Ben-Ishay D, Moncada S: Nitric oxide and the regulation of blood pressure in the hypertensive-prone and hypertensive-resistant Sabra rat. Hypertension 28:367–371, 1996.
101. Avena R, Curry KM, Sidawy AN, et al: The effect of occult diabetic status and oral glucose intake on brachial artery vasoactivity in patients with peripheral vascular disease. Cardiovasc Surg 6:584–589, 1998.
102. Takahashi K, Ghatei MA, Lam HC, et al: Elevated plasma endothelin in patients with diabetes mellitus. Diabetologia 33:306–310, 1990.
103. Schernthaner G, Schwarzer C, Kuzmits R, et al: Increased angiotensin converting enzyme activities in diabetes mellitus: Analysis of diabetes type, state of metabolic control and occurrence of diabetic vascular disease. J Clin Pathol 37:307–312, 1984.
104. Avena R, Mitchell ME, Neville RF, Sidawy AN: The additive effects of glucose and insulin on the proliferation of infragenicular vascular smooth muscle cells. J Vasc Surg 28:1033–1039, 1998.
105. Hseuh WA, Anderson PW: Hypertension, the endothelial cell, and the vascular complications of diabetes mellitus. Hypertension 20:253–263, 1992.
106. Lorenzi M, Cagliero E, Toledo S: Glucose toxicity for human endothelial cells in culture: Delayed replication, disturbed cell cycle, and accelerated cell death. Diabetes 34:621–627, 1985.

C H A P T E R 7

Essential Hemodynamic Principles

David S. Sumner, M.D.

Arterial Hemodynamics

Obstruction, or narrowing of the arterial lumen (whether it is the result of atherosclerosis, fibromuscular dysplasia, thrombi, emboli, dissection, trauma, or external compression), interferes with the efficient transport of blood to the peripheral capillary bed. Within the obstructed vessel, the extent of this interference is related to the degree of narrowing and is determined by strict hemodynamic principles. The actual capillary flow deficit depends not only on the severity of the local obstructive lesion but also on its location and on the ability of the body to compensate by increasing cardiac work, by developing collateral channels, and by dilating the peripheral arterioles and precapillary sphincters.

The symptoms and signs of obstructive arterial disease reflect the restriction of blood flow to the capillary bed. With mild obstruction, this restriction is evident only when metabolic demands are increased by exercise, trauma, or infection; with more severe disease, however, capillary perfusion is compromised even during the basal state. Consequently, the disease may be relatively asymptomatic or symptomatic only during exercise, or it may be responsible for continued rest pain and eventual tissue loss.

Except for clot formation and occasional dissection, aneurysms seldom produce symptoms of obstruction. The tendency to rupture is determined by both the intraluminal pressure and the diameter of the aneurysm.

The first part of this chapter deals with the hemodynamic alterations produced by arterial obstruction, the effects of shear, the rationale for surgical intervention, the elastic properties of the arterial wall, and the stresses that lead to rupture of aneurysms.

BASIC HEMODYNAMICS

The flow of blood in the arterial circulation is governed by the fundamental laws of fluid dynamics. Knowledge of these principles permits a better understanding of the physiologic abnormalities associated with arterial obstruction.*

Fluid Energy

We frequently think of pressure as representing the force responsible for the motion of blood. Although pressure is the most obvious and most important of the forces involved, other forms of energy also play a role. With more precision, we can state that blood moves from one point to another in the vascular system in response to differences in *total fluid energy*.[19]

Total fluid energy (E) consists of potential energy and kinetic energy. In turn, the potential energy component can be broken down into intravascular pressure (P) and gravitational potential energy. P represents the pressure produced by contraction of the heart, the hydrostatic pressure, and the static filling pressure of the resting circulation.[58] Hydrostatic pressure is proportional to the weight of the blood and is given by

$$P\ (\text{hydrostatic}) = -\rho g h \qquad (7.1)$$

where ρ is the density of blood (about 1.056 gm · cm^{-3}), g is the acceleration due to gravity (980 cm · sec^{-2}), and h is the distance in centimeters above a given reference point. In the human body, this reference point is roughly at the level of the right atrium.[18] Obviously, hydrostatic pressure may be quite large in comparison with the dynamic pressure and cannot be neglected. For example, at ankle level in a man 5 feet 8 inches tall, this pressure is about 89 mmHg:

$$-(1.056\ \text{gm}\cdot\text{cm}^{-3})\,(980\ \text{cm}\cdot\text{sec}^{-2})\,(-114\ \text{cm}) = 117{,}976\ \text{dynes}\cdot\text{cm}^{-2} \qquad (7.2)$$

$$117{,}976\ \text{dynes}\cdot\text{cm}^{-2} \div 1333\ \text{dynes}\cdot\text{cm}^{-2}/\text{mmHg} = 88.5\ \text{mmHg} \qquad (7.3)$$

In contrast, the static filling pressure is quite low, usually about 7 mmHg.[63] This pressure is related to the interaction between the elasticity of the vascular walls and the volume of blood contained within.

Gravitational potential energy ($+\rho gh$) is calculated in the same as for the hydrostatic pressure but has an opposite sign. It represents the ability of a volume of blood to do work because of its elevation above a given reference point. In many, but not all, circumstances, gravitational potential energy and hydrostatic pressure will cancel each other out.

Finally, kinetic energy represents the ability of blood to do work because of its motion ($\frac{1}{2}\rho v^2$).

If we put these values together, an expression for total fluid energy per unit volume of blood can be obtained:

$$E = P + \rho g h + \tfrac{1}{2}\rho v^2 \qquad (7.4)$$

where E is in ergs per cubic centimeter and v refers to the velocity (cm · sec^{-1}) of a particle of blood moving steadily in a straight line.

*It is interesting that three of the early investigators in the fields of fluid dynamics and elasticity, whose names have been applied to classic laws of hemodynamics, were physicians. These include Daniel Bernoulli (1700–1782) of Switzerland, Thomas Young (1773–1829) of England, and Jean-Leonard-Marie Poiseuille (1799–1869) of France.[69]

Bernoulli's Principle

When fluid flows steadily (without acceleration or deceleration) from one point in a system to another further downstream, its total energy content along any given streamline remains constant, provided there are no frictional losses:

$$P_1 + \rho g h_1 + {}^1\!/_2\, \rho v_1^2 = P_2 + \rho g h_2 + \rho v_2^2 \qquad (7.5)$$

This, the one-dimensional *Bernoulli equation*, is derivable from Newton's laws of motion and is a fundamental formula in fluid mechanics.[35]

Bernoulli's equation is instructive, in that it establishes a relationship between kinetic energy, gravitational potential energy, and pressure in a *frictionless* fluid system. Several apparent paradoxes of fluid flow are readily explained. For example, in Figure 7–1*A*, fluid with the density of blood enters an inclined tube at a pressure of 100 mmHg and flows out at a pressure of 178 mmHg. Thus, fluid moves against the pressure gradient from a point of low pressure to a point where its pressure is high. The total fluid energy remains the same, however, since the gravitational potential energy decreases by an amount exactly equal to the increase in pressure. This situation is analogous to that existing in the arterial tree of a standing person in whom blood pressure in the arteries at ankle level is greater than blood pressure in the aortic arch.

In Figure 7–1*B*, the cross-sectional area of a horizontal tube increases 16 times, resulting in a comparable decrease in fluid velocity. Again, the fluid moves against a pressure gradient, the pressure at the end of the tube being 2.5 mmHg greater than that at the entrance to the tube. The total fluid energy remains the same, however, because of the decrease in kinetic energy. This phenomenon is seldom manifested in the human circulation because associated energy losses effectively mask the slight rise in pressure.

Intravascular pressure measurements made with catheters are subject to errors owing to the effect of kinetic energy. If the catheter faces the oncoming blood end-on, the pressure recorded will be too high by a factor of $\frac{1}{2}\rho v^2$. On the other hand, if the catheter faces downstream, the recorded pressure will be too low by the same factor. At a velocity of 50 cm · sec^{-1}, these errors would equal about 1.0 mmHg and would be inconsequential in a high-pressure system such as the aorta. Nevertheless, they could be of importance in low-pressure, high-flow systems such as the vena cava and pulmonary artery.[19]

Viscosity

The conditions required to fulfill the rigid specifications of Bernoulli's relationship are never met in the human vascular tree or in any other real fluid system. Mechanical energy is always "lost" (converted to heat) in moving fluid from one point to the next.

Energy losses in the peripheral circulation are related principally to the viscosity of blood and to its inertia. In fluids, *viscosity* may be defined as the friction existing between contiguous layers of fluid. The friction is due to strong intermolecular attractions; under these conditions, the fluid layers tend to resist deformation. The familiar equation known as *Poiseuille's law* describes the viscous losses existing in an idealized situation:

$$P_1 - P_2 = \bar{V} \cdot \frac{8L\eta}{r^2} = Q \cdot \frac{8L\eta}{\pi r^4} \qquad (7.6)$$

where $P_1 - P_2$ represents the drop in potential energy (dynes · cm^{-2}) between two points separated by the distance L (cm); Q is the flow (cm^3 · sec^{-1}); and $\bar{V}$ is the mean flow velocity (cm · sec^{-1}) across a tube with an inside radius r (cm). The coefficient of viscosity, η, is expressed in poise (dynes · sec · cm^{-2}).

Under conditions in which Poiseuille's law is operative, the velocities of each concentric layer of fluid describe a *parabolic profile,* with velocity being highest in the center of the stream and becoming progressively lower toward the inner wall. Blood in contact with the wall is stationary. The ratio of the change in velocity (∂v) to the change in the radius (∂r) between each cylindrical laminar layer is known as the *shear rate* (D); the force required to "shear" the fluid is known as the *shear stress* (τ); and the coefficient of viscosity (η) is the ratio of the shear stress to the shear rate:

$$D = -\frac{\partial v}{\partial r} \text{ and } \eta = \frac{\tau}{D} \qquad (7.7)$$

The importance of shear rate and shear stress is discussed later in this chapter.

Because energy losses are inversely proportional to the fourth power of the radius, graphs based on Poiseuille's law are sharply curved (Fig. 7–2). As the diameter of a conduit is reduced, there is little effect on the pressure gradient until a certain degree of narrowing is reached; beyond this point, further reductions in diameter cause the pressure gradient to rise precipitously. Although increasing the rate of flow shifts the curves to the left and linearly increases the pressure gradient at any given radius, these effects are much less marked than those due to changes in radius.

Poiseuille's law applies only to steady (nonpulsatile), laminar flow in a straight cylindrical tube with rigid walls.

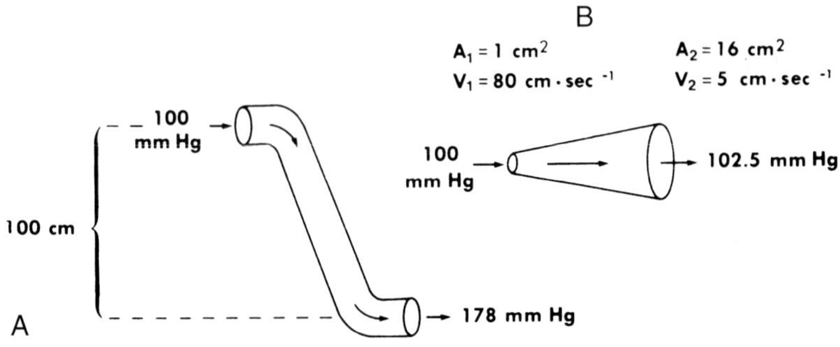

FIGURE 7–1. *A*, Effect of vertical height on pressure in a *frictionless* fluid flowing downhill. *B*, Effect of increasing cross-sectional area on pressure in a *frictionless* fluid system.

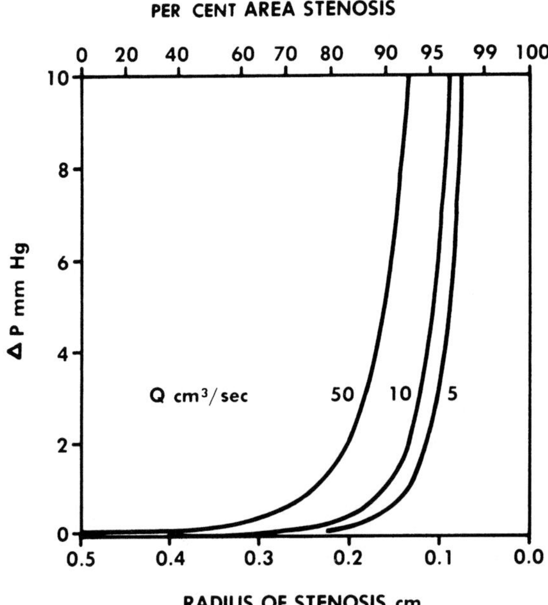

FIGURE 7–2. Curves derived from Poiseuille's law (Eq. 7.6). The stenotic segment is assumed to be 1.0 cm long. Viscosity is 0.035 poise.

Furthermore, the tube must be long enough to allow a parabolic flow profile to develop.

When fluid passes from a large container into a smaller cylindrical tube, the velocity profile at the entrance is essentially flat (same velocity all across the tube diameter). Just beyond the entrance, friction between the stationary outermost layer and the immediately adjacent concentric layer causes the latter to slow down. This layer, in turn, exerts a drag force on the next layer and so on down the tube until the "boundary layer," where fluid is sheared, extends to the center of the tube. At this point, flow is said to be fully "developed," and the profile is truly parabolic. The "entrance length" (L_x) in centimeters required to develop a parabolic profile depends on the radius of the tube and the *Reynolds number* (Re) (see later):

$$L_x = k\, r\, Re \tag{7.8}$$

(The constant, k, varies but approximates 0.16 for Reynolds numbers greater than 50.)

All along the entrance length, the velocity profile is "blunt" rather than parabolic. At each branch point in the arterial tree, a certain distance is needed before flow is developed. Although velocity profiles in smaller arteries (e.g., radial, mesenteric) may be essentially parabolic, in larger arteries (e.g., iliac, common carotid) the entrance length approaches the length of the artery and flow profiles remain blunt. Many investigators have shown that the flow profile in the human abdominal aorta is blunted.[134, 183]

Entrance effects are, of course, only one of many factors modulating the velocity profile. At branch points or in regions where the vessel curves, the momentum of blood near one wall exceeds that on the other side. As a result, velocity profiles are skewed toward one wall and complicated helical flow patterns develop.[107, 153] Thus, the strict conditions required by Poiseuille's law are seldom, if ever, encountered in the living organism. Furthermore, energy losses almost never are totally viscous, and in many cases, viscous losses are less significant than those related to inertia.

Inertia

Inertial losses depend on the mass or density of the blood, ρ, and on the square of the flow velocity, v:

$$\Delta P = k\, {}^1\!/_2\, \rho v^2 \tag{7.9}$$

Because ρ is a constant, the quantity that changes is v. Changes in velocity occur when blood is accelerated or decelerated as in pulsatile flow and when blood passes from a vessel of large lumen (where the velocity is low) to one of small lumen (where the velocity is high)—or vice versa. In addition, v is a vector quantity; that is, any change in direction of flow represents an acceleration.

Flow changes direction whenever the blood vessel forms a curve and at all junctions and branch points. There is also a change in direction when the blood vessel gradually narrows or in pathologic situations in which there is a sudden narrowing and expansion of the flow stream, as in an atherosclerotic stenosis. Moreover, as a result of the expansile nature of the blood vessel wall, velocity vectors must be directed outward during the systolic portion of the pressure wave and inward during the diastolic portion.*

According to the *equation of continuity* (conservation of mass), the product of flow velocity and cross-sectional area is the same at any point along a tube, provided there are no intervening branches to siphon off the fluid:

$$A_1 v_1 = A_2 v_2 \quad \text{or} \quad r_1^2 v_1 = r_2^2 v_2 \tag{7.10}$$

Because kinetic energy losses depend on the square of the velocity (Eq. 7.9) and because the velocity in a stenotic segment is inversely proportional to the square of its radius (Eq. 7.10), kinetic energy losses—like those attributable to viscosity—are inversely proportional to the fourth power of the radius. As illustrated in Figure 7–3, this creates curves that display little sensitivity to reduction in radius until a certain point is reached, beyond which energy losses increase rapidly. Increasing the velocity of flow has a more marked effect on kinetic energy losses than it does on viscous losses (compare Figs. 7–2 and 7–3). This follows from the fact that the velocity term is squared in Equation 7.9 but enters Equation 7.6 only in the first power.

Turbulence

Turbulence, with its random velocity vectors, also depletes the total fluid energy stores. The point at which flow changes from laminar to turbulent is best defined in terms of a dimensionless quantity known as the Reynolds number

---

*Because only flow in the direction of the long axis of the tube is considered in Poiseuille's law, frictional (viscous) energy losses due to molecular interaction involving flow in other directions are neglected in Equation 7.6. Although these losses are difficult to calculate, they are incorporated in a general way in the constant k of Equation 7.9. Thus, *inertial energy loss* is a term of convenience; *all of these losses are ultimately due to viscous effects.*

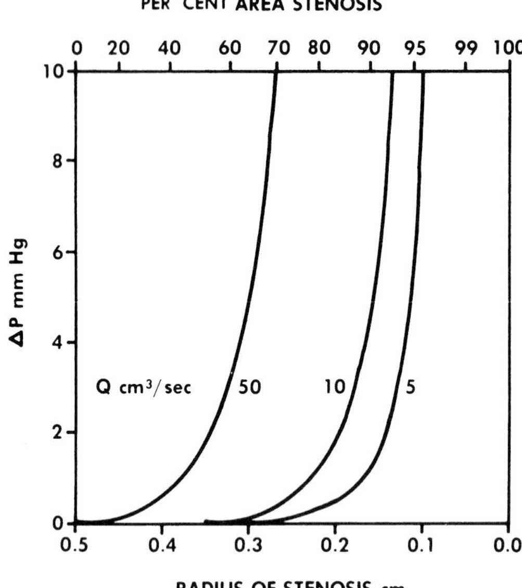

FIGURE 7–3. Effect of increasing stenosis and blood flow on inertial losses at the exit of a stenotic segment that leads into a tube with a radius of 0.5 cm. Curves are based on Equation 7.16. An abrupt exit is assumed.

(Re). Re is proportional to the ratio of inertial forces acting on the fluid to the viscous forces:

$$Re = \frac{\rho v d}{\eta} = \frac{vd}{\nu} \qquad (7.11)$$

where d is the diameter of the conduit, η is the viscosity, and ν is the kinematic viscosity ($\nu = \eta/\rho$). Above a Reynolds number of 2000, local disturbances in the laminar flow pattern result in fully developed turbulence. Below 2000, local disturbances are damped out by the viscous forces.

Since Reynolds numbers are well below 2000 in most peripheral blood vessels, turbulence is unlikely to occur under normal circumstances.[173] However, turbulence does appear to develop in the ascending aorta during the peak systolic ejection phase and may persist during deceleration.[151] These turbulent flashes are short-lived. Yet, in spite of the absence of fully developed turbulence, the pattern of blood flow in a large portion of the circulation may be characterized as "disturbed."[5, 202] Energy losses calculated on turbulent friction factors may more closely approximate experimental results than they do when Poiseuille's law is employed.[174]

Pulsatile Flow

Applying any of these equations to pulsatile blood flow is very difficult. For example, in *steady flow*, kinetic energy can be estimated from the square of the space-averaged velocity of blood flowing past a given point (Eq. 7.9). In *pulsatile flow*, a more complicated expression must be employed that integrates the instantaneous product of the mass flux and the square of the velocity. This method predicts kinetic energies that sometimes are 10 times as great as would be suspected on the basis of the average velocity of blood flow.[15]

In addition, the shape of the velocity profile must be known before the *spatially averaged velocity* across the lumen of a blood vessel can be used to estimate kinetic energy losses (Fig. 7–4). When the profile is nearly flat, as it is with turbulent flow or when the site of flow measurement is within the entrance length of a blood vessel, k in Equation 7.9 will be 1.06.[35] When the profile is parabolic, k becomes 2.0. With pulsatile flow, a parabolic profile is never really attained (Fig. 7–5).[112] As mentioned previously, in larger blood vessels, such as the aorta, the profile may be quite flat and is often skewed. In smaller arteries, a parabolic profile may be approached, especially during the peak forward phase of the flow pulse.

All of these complexities merely add to the energy losses experienced in the circulation. Thus, for a given level of blood flow, the pressure (energy) drop between any two points in the arterial tree may be several times that predicted by Poiseuille's law (Eq. 7.6).[6, 99, 116] Furthermore, the relationship between the pressure gradient and the flow is not linear but defines a curve that is concave to the pressure axis (Fig. 7–6). These nonlinearities are all functions of inertial losses and reflect the effect of the v^2 term. Thus, Poiseuille's law cannot be used to predict pressure-flow relationships in the arterial tree, but it can be used to define the *minimal* energy losses that can be expected under any given flow situation.

Resistance

The concept of hemodynamic resistance is useful when one attempts to understand the physiology of arterial disease. Defined simply as the ratio of the energy drop between two points along a blood vessel ($E_1 - E_2$) to the mean blood flow in the vessel (Q), the equation for hemodynamic resistance (R) is analogous to Ohm's law in electric circuits:

$$R = \frac{E_1 - E_2}{Q} = \frac{P_1 - P_2}{Q} \qquad (7.12)$$

It is often convenient to drop the kinetic energy term ($\frac{1}{2}\rho v^2$) in Equation 7.4, since it seldom contributes appreciably to the total energy. Also, calculations are simplified if the assumption can be made that the subject is supine.

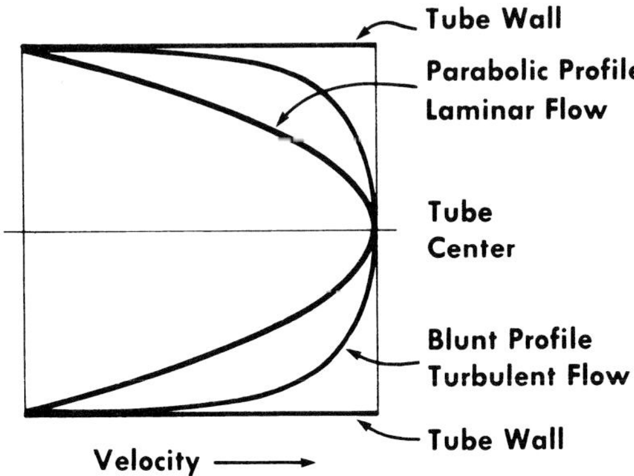

FIGURE 7–4. Velocity profiles of steady laminar and turbulent flow. Velocity is zero at the tube wall and reaches its peak value in the center. A blunt profile is also typical of that seen within the entrance length of a vessel.

FIGURE 7–5. Velocity profiles (*B*) during various phases of a typical femoral arterial flow pulse (*A*). Letters indicate corresponding points in the pulse cycle. In all profiles, the velocity at the wall is zero. At point b, forward flow is nearly maximal and the profile is almost parabolic. At the next point, flow near the wall is reversed while that in the center continues forward. Several profiles, both forward and reverse, are quite blunt. (*A* and *B*, Adapted from McDonald DA: Blood Flow in Arteries, 2nd ed. Baltimore, Williams & Wilkins, 1974.)

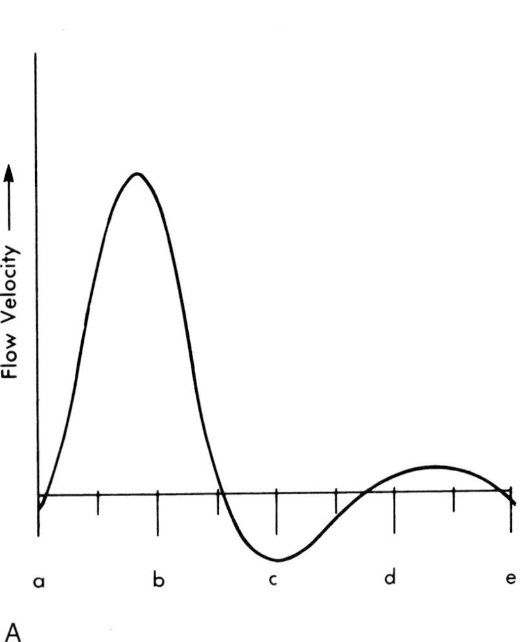

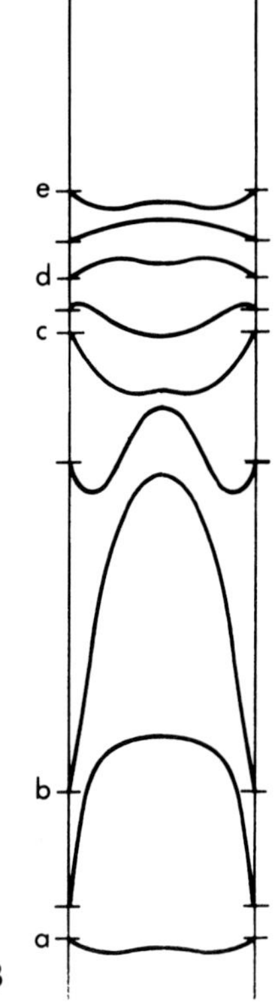

This permits the gravitational terms (ρgh) to cancel. Hence, resistance can be approximated by the ratio of the pressure drop ($P_1 - P_2$) to the flow (Eq. 7.12).

Unlike electric resistance, hemodynamic resistance does not remain constant over a wide range of flows. The minimal possible resistance is given by Poiseuille's law:

$$R_{min} = \frac{8\eta L}{\pi r^4} \tag{7.13}$$

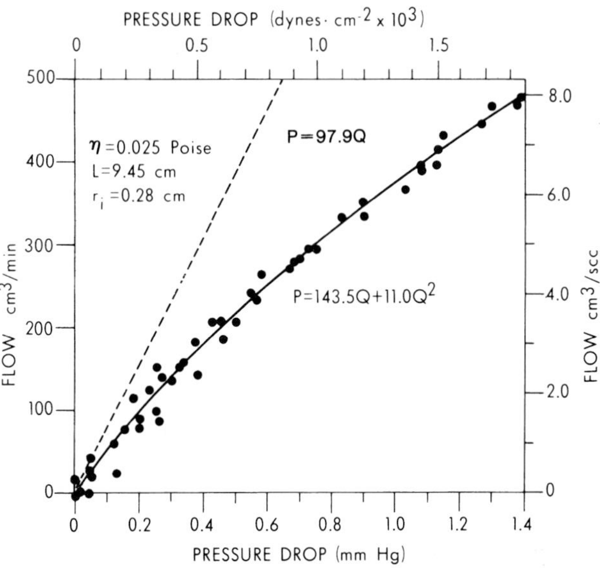

FIGURE 7–6. Pressure drop across a 9.45-cm length of canine femoral artery at varying flow rates. Differential pressure was measured by a specially designed transducer (D. E. Hokanson), and flow, with an electromagnetic flowmeter. Flow rate was varied by constricting a distally located arteriovenous fistula. The line that fits the experimental data best has both a linear and a squared term, corresponding to Poiseuille's law plus kinetic energy losses. The pressure-flow curve predicted from Poiseuille's law (*dashed line*) depicts much less energy loss than actually is the case.

Because of additional energy losses related to acceleration, disturbed flow, and turbulence (all of which are a function of $\frac{1}{2}\rho v^2$), the resistance of a given vascular segment tends to increase as flow velocity increases, provided that there is no concomitant change in vascular diameter (Fig. 7–7).

For the purposes of studying arterial and venous flow dynamics in complex hemodynamic circuitry, resistances in series can be added to obtain the total value:

$$R_{total} = R_1 + R_2 + \cdots + R_n \tag{7.14}$$

When resistances are in parallel, the following relationship may be used:

$$\frac{1}{R_{total}} = \frac{1}{R_1} + \frac{1}{R_2} + \cdots + \frac{1}{R_n} \tag{7.15}$$

The dimensions of hemodynamic resistance are dyne · cm^{-5} · sec. It usually is more convenient, however, to use the *peripheral resistance unit* (PRU), which is millimeters of mercury per milliliter per minute. Thus, 1 peripheral resistance unit is approximately equal to 8×10^4 dyne · cm^{-5} · sec.

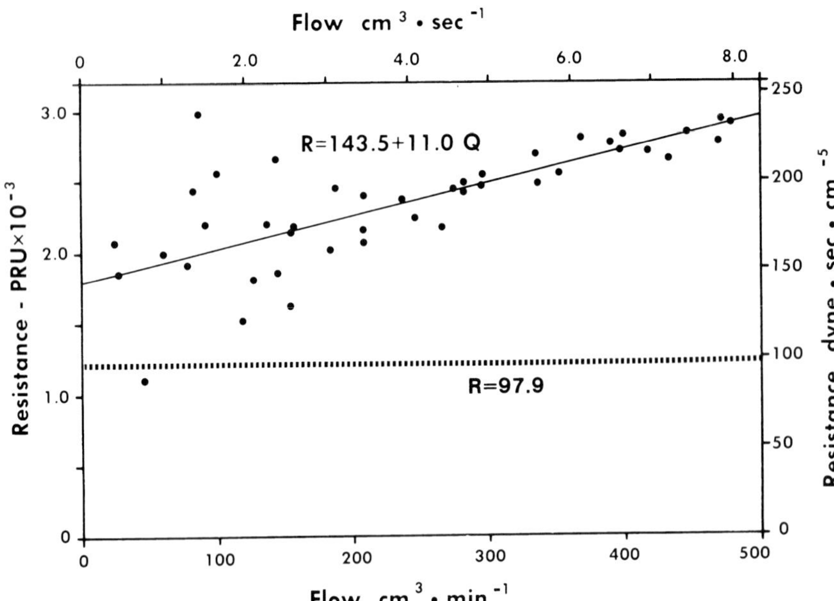

FIGURE 7–7. Resistance derived from pressure-flow curve in Figure 7–6. The constant resistance predicted by Poiseuille's law is depicted by the *dotted line.* Note that the resistance (R) increases with increasing flow. PRV = peripheral resistance unit.

HEMODYNAMICS OF ARTERIAL STENOSIS

Most of the abnormal energy losses in the arterial system result from stenosis or obstruction of the vascular lumen. Because atherosclerosis, the pathologic process in the majority of these lesions, has a predilection for larger arteries, surgical therapy often is possible. Therefore, the study of the hemodynamics of these lesions has a great deal of practical importance.

Energy Losses Associated with Stenoses

In accordance with Poiseuille's law (Eqs. 7.6 and 7.13), so-called viscous energy losses within the stenotic segment are inversely proportional to the fourth power of its radius and directly proportional to its length (see Fig. 7–2). Thus, the radius of a stenosis is of much more significance than its length.[22, 52, 83, 110] In addition, *inertial losses*, which are related to the square of the velocity of blood flow, are encountered both at the entrance to the stenosis and at its exit.[15, 110, 173, 204] The magnitude of these losses varies greatly with the shape of the entrance and exit, being much less for a gradual tapering of the lumen than for an abrupt change. Also, energy losses associated with asymmetric stenoses exceed those associated with axisymmetric stenoses even when the lumen is compromised to the same degree.[203] Although energy losses at the entrance can be appreciable, they are usually greater at the exit, where much of the excess kinetic energy resulting from the increased fluid velocity within the stenosis may be dissipated in a turbulent jet (see Fig. 7–3):

$$\Delta P = k\frac{\rho}{2}(v_s - v)^2 = k\frac{\rho}{2}v^2\left[\left(\frac{r}{r_s}\right)^2 - 1\right]^2 \quad (7.16)$$

In this expression, ΔP represents the energy lost in expansion, v_s refers to the mean flow velocity within the stenotic segment, and v refers to the velocity in the vessel beyond the stenosis. Similarly, r_s and r indicate the radius of the stenotic lumen and that of the uninvolved distal vessel, respectively. The constant, k, varies from about 1.0 for an abrupt orifice to less than 0.2 for one that expands gradually at a 6-degree angle.[37]

These concepts are illustrated graphically in Figure 7–8. This figure emphasizes the relatively small contribution of *viscous losses* to the total decrease in available fluid energy produced by the stenosis. Even if the obstruction were diaphragm-like (L in Eq. 7.6 approaching zero), the energy losses would still be 85% of those with the 1-cm-long stenosis; in other words, most of the energy losses can be attributed to inertial effects.

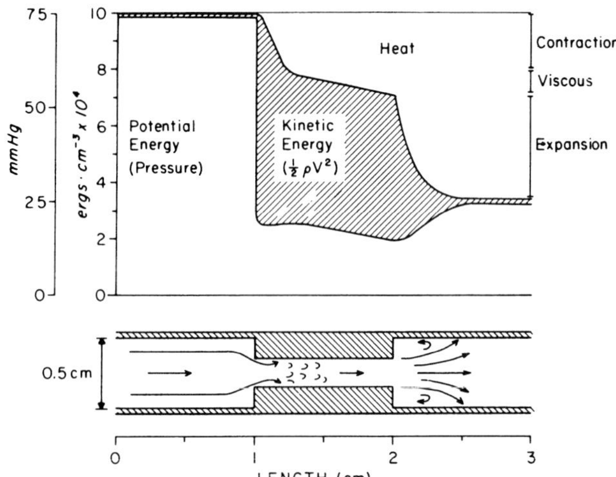

FIGURE 7–8. Diagram illustrating energy losses experienced by blood passing through a stenosis 1 cm long. Flow is assumed to be unidirectional and steady. Very little of the total energy loss is attributable to "viscous" losses. Thus, applications of Poiseuille's law greatly underestimate the pressure drop across an arterial stenosis.

Critical Stenosis

How severe does a stenosis have to be to produce a measurable pressure gradient or a decrease in blood flow, or both? This is an important question for the clinician who attempts to assess the severity of an arterial obstruction from its angiographic appearance. Experimentally, appreciable changes in pressure and flow do not occur until the cross-sectional area of a vessel has been reduced by more than 75% (usually, 80% to 95%).[111, 118] Assuming that the obstructing lesion is symmetric, this reduction in cross-sectional area corresponds to at least a 50% reduction in diameter. The degree of narrowing at which pressure and flow begin to be affected has been called the *critical stenosis.*

Energy losses associated with arterial lesions are inversely proportional to the fourth power of the radius of the stenosis (Eq. 7.6) and to the fourth power of the ratio of the radius of the stenosis to that of the nonstenotic segment (Eq. 7.16). Because these are exponential functions, graphs relating energy losses across a stenosis to the percentage reduction in cross-sectional area are sharply curved, providing theoretical support for the concept of critical stenosis (Fig. 7–9).[15, 22, 110, 119, 204]

Energy losses across stenotic segments also depend on the velocity of blood flow (Eqs. 7.6 and 7.16). In high-flow (low-resistance) systems, significant drops in pressure and flow occur with less severe narrowing than in low-flow systems.[111, 118, 181, 182] Moreover, the curves are less sharply bent when peripheral resistance is low and flow rates are high (see Fig. 7–9). Consequently, critical stenosis varies with the resistance of the runoff bed. When peripheral resistances are low, as in the carotid and coronary systems, critical stenosis may be reached with less narrowing of the lumen than in higher resistance systems, such as the resting lower extremity. Even in the leg, lowering the peripheral resistance sufficiently by exercise or reactive hyperemia may cause a stenosis that is noncritical at rest to become critical.[24, 167, 169] This fact is well worth emphasizing. It accounts for the frequent clinical observation that an iliac lesion may severely restrict the patient during exercise, even though it causes no symptoms at rest and may not appear particularly significant on arteriography.[117, 190]

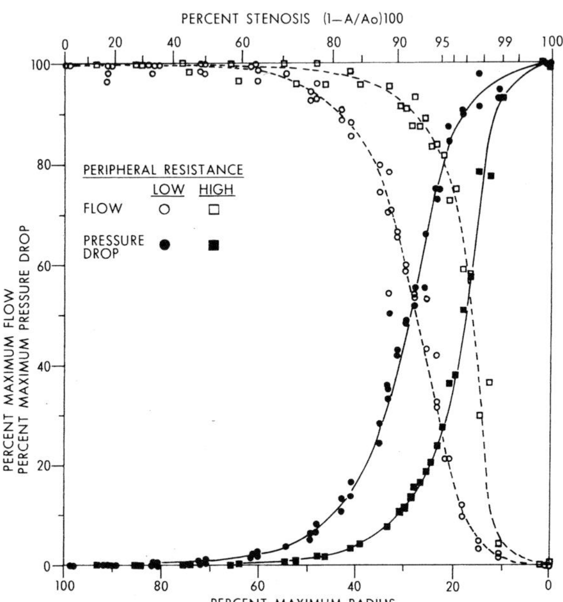

FIGURE 7–9. Relationship of pressure and flow to degree of stenosis in a canine femoral artery. When peripheral resistance is high, the curves are shifted to the right. Percentage change in flow through the stenosis is essentially a mirror image of the percentage of maximal pressure drop across the stenosis.

Precise attempts to relate pressure and flow restriction to per cent stenosis are frustrated by the irregular geometry of the vascular lesions and by the nonlinearities introduced by pulsatile blood flow. Empirical formulas have been devised that fit the experimental data[22]; however, formulas that incorporate known viscous and inertial effects are far more instructive.[15, 110, 204] Nevertheless, for practical purposes *none* of the formulas is very helpful. Thus, any lesion that potentially decreases the arterial lumen by about 75% must be suspect, and its hemodynamic significance must be determined by objective physiologic tests.

Length of Stenosis and Stenoses in Series

Not infrequently, the surgeon is faced with a series of lesions involving a single unbranched arterial segment. The question arises whether repair of one of the lesions will benefit the patient significantly. This question is particularly pertinent when one of the lesions is in an inaccessible location. Such a problem is presented by a stenosis at the origin of the internal carotid artery combined with a similar stenosis in the carotid siphon.

The length of a stenosis principally affects energy losses related to viscosity. Because length enters Poiseuille's equation (Eq. 7.6) only in the first power, whereas radius is elevated to the fourth power, the effect of a change in length on viscous losses is far less than that of a change in radius. Doubling the length of a stenosis would merely double the viscous energy losses, but reducing the radius of the vessel lumen by half would increase the losses by a factor of 16. Moreover, the convective acceleration effects at the exit are independent of the length of the stenosis, and are related to the fourth power of the ratio of the diameters of the unstenosed and stenosed portions of the vessel (Eq. 7.16). Therefore, one would predict that the length of a stenosis is far less important than lesion diameter. These predictions are well supported by experimental observations.[17, 22, 52, 110, 184]

Because entrance and exit effects contribute a large portion of the resistance offered by a stenosis, doubling the length of a lesion without changing its diameter would not double its resistance (see Fig. 7–8). In contrast, the total resistance of two separate lesions of equal length and diameter is approximately double that of the individual lesion, since entrance and exit effects occur at each of the stenoses.[53, 80] Thus, separate stenoses of equal diameter are of more significance than a single stenosis of the same diameter whose length equals the sum of the lengths of the shorter lesions.

When two stenoses of unequal diameter are in series, the tighter of the two has by far the greater effect on resistance (Eqs. 7.6 and 7.16). Total resistance is not affected by the sequence of the stenoses; that is, it makes no difference whether the greater occlusion is proximal or distal.[184] Several practical points emerge from these considerations:

1. The resistances of stenoses in series are roughly additive, although the cumulative effect may be somewhat less than would be anticipated on the basis of the sum of the individual resistances. Therefore, multiple noncritical stenoses may act as a single critical stenosis and result in arterial insufficiency.[53, 80]
2. When two stenotic lesions are of similar caliber, removal of one provides only a modest improvement in blood flow.
3. If the stenoses are of unequal caliber, removal of the less severe results in little increase in blood flow; removal of the more severe may provide significant improvement.

These principles apply only to unbranched arteries; they do not apply to the situation in which the proximal lesion is in an artery feeding a collateral bed that parallels the distal lesion. Thus, endarterectomy of a stenotic iliac artery usually is beneficial even when the superficial femoral artery is completely occluded. In this case, the profunda femoris carries most of the blood to the lower leg, and removal of the proximal iliac obstruction will improve the pressure head at the profunda orifice.[45, 109, 120, 168, 190]

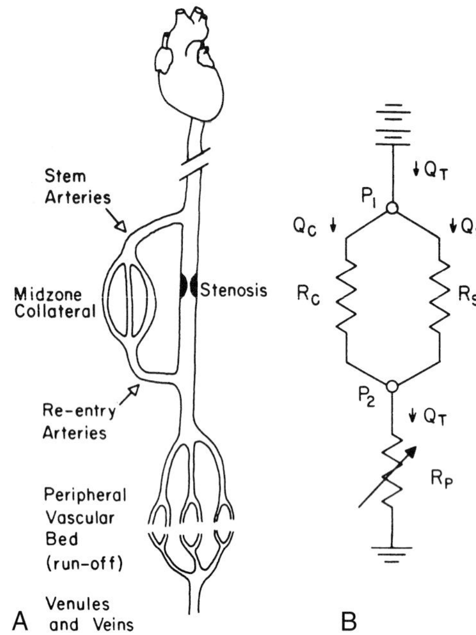

FIGURE 7–10. *A*, The main components of an arterial circuit containing a stenotic major artery. *B*, An electric analogue of this circuit. The battery at the top represents the potential energy source (e.g., the heart); ground potential, at the bottom, indicates the central veins. Q_T is total flow, Q_C is collateral flow, and Q_S is flow through the stenotic artery. Resistances are R_C, collateral; R_S, stenotic artery; and R_P, peripheral "runoff" bed. R_C and R_S are relatively "fixed"; R_P is "variable."

CIRCULATORY PATTERNS IN HUMAN LIMBS

Collateral Circulation and the Peripheral Runoff Bed

Arterial stenoses do not exist in isolation; rather, they are part of a complex hemodynamic circuit.[173, 177] As shown in Figure 7–10, this circuit includes the diseased major artery, a parallel system of collateral arteries, and a peripheral runoff bed.

Dilatation of the involved artery may compensate for the narrowing caused by small or moderate plaques. This compensatory expansion, which has been demonstrated to occur in human coronary arteries and which may also occur in peripheral arteries, is probably mediated by endothelium-derived relaxing factor (nitric oxide) in response to increased shear stress.[59, 218] More severe plaques overwhelm this process and progressively encroach on the residual lumen. To compensate for the increased resistance imposed by a highly stenotic or totally occlusive lesion, two mechanisms are invoked:

- Collateral development
- Dilatation of the resistance vessels in the peripheral bed

Collateral vessels consist of distributing branches of large and medium-sized arteries. Anatomically as well as functionally, it is convenient to divide the collateral bed into (1) stem arteries, (2) mid-zone collaterals, and (3) reentry arteries.[102] For the most part, these vessels are preexisting pathways that enlarge when a stenosis or an occlusion develops in the parallel main arterial supply.[28, 73, 146, 192] Although the mechanism of collateral enlargement is the subject of debate, it appears to be related to an increased pressure gradient across the collateral bed and to an increased velocity of flow (increased shear rate) through the midzone vessels.[28, 68, 73, 81, 192] Again, nitric oxide is the likely mediator.[223]

In spite of continued expansion of the mid-zone vessels, the resistance of the collateral bed always exceeds that of the major artery whose function it has replaced.[104, 177] For example, it would take 256 collaterals, each with a diameter of 2.5 mm or 10,000 collaterals with a diameter of 1.0 mm, to reduce the segmental resistance to that of a major vessel with a diameter of 10 mm (Eqs. 7.13 and 7.15).

Except with gradual dilatation, the resistance of the collateral bed, for practical purposes, is almost fixed. The acute decreases in collateral resistance that occur in response to exercise, sympathectomy, or vasodilator drugs are small and are of relatively little consequence.[10, 26, 44, 104, 177]

In contrast, the peripheral runoff bed has a generally high but quite variable resistance, a large portion of which is concentrated in the terminal arterioles and precapillary sphincters (see Fig. 7–10). Because of their small diameter and heavily muscled walls, these vessels are ideally suited for regulatory function. Their resistance is subject to control by (1) the autonomic nervous system, (2) circulating catecholamines, (3) local metabolic products, and (4) myogenic influences.

Control of Peripheral Vascular Resistance

The cutaneous sympathetic innervation is concerned largely with the regulation of body temperature. Blood vessels within the skin are well supplied with sympathetic vasoconstrictor fibers, especially in the terminal portions such as the fingers, hands, and feet. More proximally (e.g., in the forearm), vasodilator fibers act in conjunction with the

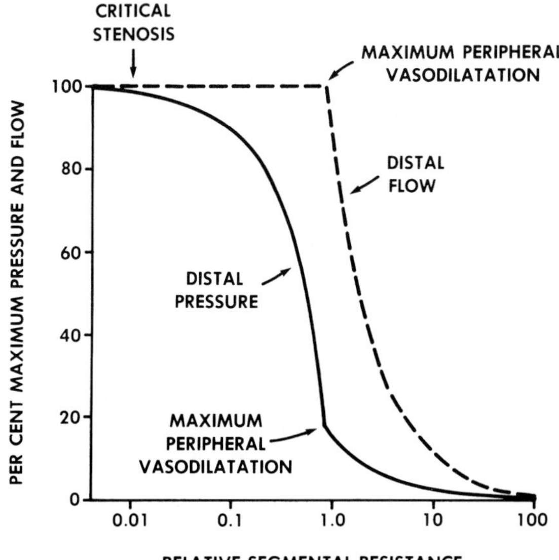

FIGURE 7–11. Although blood pressure distal to a critical stenosis falls progressively with increasing severity of the stenosis, autoregulation maintains normal blood flow to the tissues until maximal peripheral vasodilatation is reached. Beyond this point, pressure and flow are linearly related; increasing stenosis results in a marked decrease in both pressure and flow; and the tissues become ischemic. (Compare with Figure 7–9.) (From Sumner DS: Correlation of lesion configuration with functional significance. *In* Bond MG, Insull W Jr, Glagov S, et al: Clinical Diagnosis of Atherosclerosis: Quantitative Methods of Evaluation. New York, Springer-Verlag, 1983.)

sudomotor apparatus. Nevertheless, most reflex vasodilatation of cutaneous vessels results from the withdrawal of sympathetic impulses.[157] In contrast, blood vessels within skeletal muscles are innervated by both vasodilator and vasoconstrictor fibers. The former respond to emotional stress, and the latter respond to postural changes.[157] These actions, however, are easily overcome by the powerful vasodilator effect of locally produced metabolites that accumulate during exercise or ischemia.[86, 140] Indeed, exercise is perhaps the best single vasodilator of resistance vessels within skeletal muscle.[25, 92, 135]

Arteriolar constriction also occurs in response to dependency (the venoarterial reflex).[11] By restricting arterial inflow, this reflex serves to limit the increase in venous blood volume that accompanies an elevated hydrostatic pressure.

Finally, *autoregulation* deserves mention. This term is used to describe the remarkable ability of most vascular beds to maintain a constant level of blood flow over a wide range of perfusion pressures.[75, 78] In other words, the resistance vessels constrict in response to a rise in blood pressure and dilate in response to a fall. Although the mechanism of autoregulation continues to evoke controversy, it seems to be a myogenic response to stretch that is modified by the local chemical milieu and sympathetic control.[87] Autoregulation is not present when the perfusion pressure drops below a critical level (e.g., about 20 to 30 mmHg for skeletal muscle and about 50 to 60 mmHg for the brain). With pressures below this level, normal blood flow is no longer maintained. Consequently, in these low-pressure situations, flow responds passively to changes in perfusion pressure (Fig. 7–11).

Pressure-Flow Relationships

Normal Limbs

Under resting conditions, blood flow to the normal human leg averages about 300 to 400 ml/min.[25, 54, 97, 139, 185] Calf blood flow hovers around 1.5 to 6.5 ml/min per deciliter (100 ml) of calf, with an average value of about 3.5 ml/dl/min.[64, 166] Blood flow to the gastrocnemius muscle usually is about 2.0 ml/dl/min.[94] This rate of flow is more than adequate to supply all the nutritional needs of the resting limb.

When blood flow is restored to a normal limb that has been rendered ischemic for 5 minutes by means of a proximally placed pneumatic tourniquet, the peripheral arteriolar bed becomes vasodilated. The resulting *reactive hyperemia* reaches peak values of 30 to 40 ml/dl/min and then rapidly subsides to resting levels within a minute or two.[163, 166, 209]

Moderate exercise normally increases total leg blood flow from 5 to 10 times.[25, 92, 135] Muscle blood flow rises to 30 ± 14 ml/dl/min, reaching 70 ml/dl/min during strenuous exercise (Fig. 7–12).[92] On cessation of exercise, blood flow decreases rapidly in an exponential fashion, often reaching pre-exercise levels within 1 to 5 minutes.

The mean blood pressure drop across normal arteries from the heart to the ankle is only a few millimeters of mercury.[19] As the pressure wave travels distally, the systolic pressure increases, the diastolic pressure decreases and the pulse pressure widens (Fig. 7–13).[141] This phenomenon is due to reflection of waves from the high-resistance peripheral arteriolar bed. Under resting conditions, ankle systolic pressures exceed the brachial systolic pressure in normal

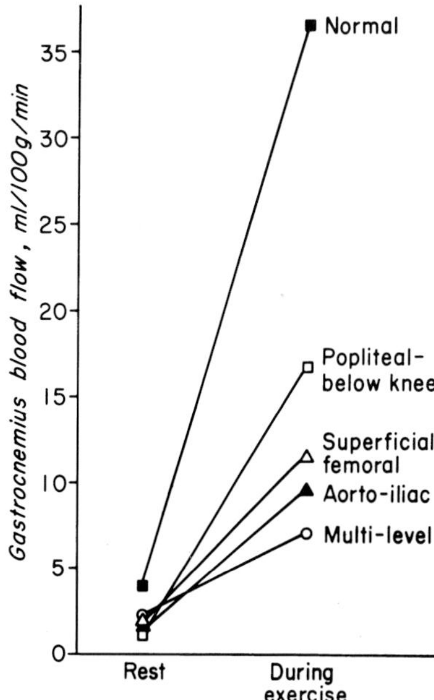

FIGURE 7–12. Mean blood flow at rest and after exercise in normal subjects and in patients with arteriosclerosis obliterans. Location of occlusion is indicated by the labels on the right. Blood flow was measured in the gastrocnemius muscle by the xenon-133 clearance technique. (Data from Wolf EA Jr, Sumner DS, Strandness DE Jr: Correlation between nutritive blood flow and pressure in limbs of patients with intermittent claudication. Surg Forum 23:238, 1972.)

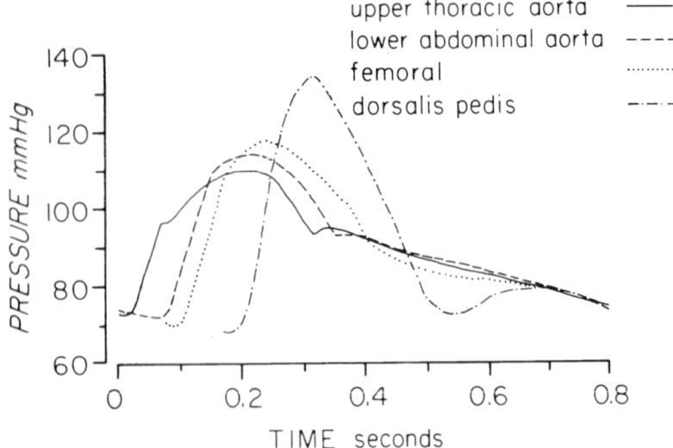

FIGURE 7–13. Pressure pulse contours in a normal subject. (From Standness DE Jr, Sumner DS: Hemodynamics for Surgeons. New York, Grune & Stratton, 1975; redrawn from Remington JW, Wood EH: Formation of peripheral pulse contour in man. J Appl Physiol 9:433, 1956.)

individuals by about 10% (Fig. 7–14).[199] In normal extremities, moderate exercise produces little or no drop in peripheral pressure at ankle level. With very strenuous exercise, the pressure may fall a few millimeters of mercury but rapidly recovers within a minute or so.[165] These findings contrast sharply with the ankle pressure drop that occurs following exercise in limbs with occlusive arterial disease (see Fig. 7–14).

Limbs with Arterial Obstruction

Intermittent Claudication, Ischemic Rest Pain, and Gangrene

Intermittent claudication occurs when blood flow to the exercising muscle mass is unable to meet the requirements of the increased metabolic activity. Apparently, the pain is related to the abnormal accumulation of metabolic products within the muscle.[98] Pain does not develop in normal extremities during exercise, because these metabolic products are rapidly removed by the copious blood flow.

When intermittent claudication is the sole symptom of arterial obstruction, resting blood flow to the involved limbs will be normal (see Fig. 7–12).[54, 64, 97, 135, 166, 176] With further progression of the disease, however, limb blood flow becomes inadequate even when the patient is at rest (see Fig. 7–11).[90] Ischemic rest pain is experienced in the toes and distal portions of the foot, minor trauma may produce painful nonhealing ulcers, and the toes may become gangrenous.[31]

Effect of Reactive Hyperemia and Exercise on Blood Flow

Reactive hyperemia develops in limbs when the circulation is restored after a 5-minute period of ischemia. In limbs with obstructive arterial disease, this response differs significantly from that observed in normal limbs. Not only is peak blood flow lower in obstructed limbs (averaging about 9 to 20 ml/dl/min), but the peak flow may be delayed for from 15 seconds to 2 minutes, and the hyperemia is prolonged for several minutes.[64, 163, 166]

Although blood flow is increased during exercise in limbs with obstructive arterial disease, the increase is far less than that observed in normal limbs undergoing a similar stress (see Fig. 7–12).[55, 92, 135, 194] Flow may even fall below resting levels.[3, 92, 156, 176] After cessation of exercise, the hyperemia is greatly prolonged, subsiding to normal levels in a logarithmic fashion over 4 to 30 minutes (Fig. 7–15). In some limbs with occlusions at two levels (e.g., iliac plus superficial femoral), the peripheral blood flow immediately after exercise may be increased only slightly. Flow then rises for several minutes until a peak level is obtained, before falling gradually to pre-exercise levels (Fig. 7–16). In patients with multilevel occlusions, especially those with rest pain, the flow after exercise may be depressed, peak flow is quite low and very delayed, and the hyperemic state persists for many minutes (Fig. 7–17).[3]

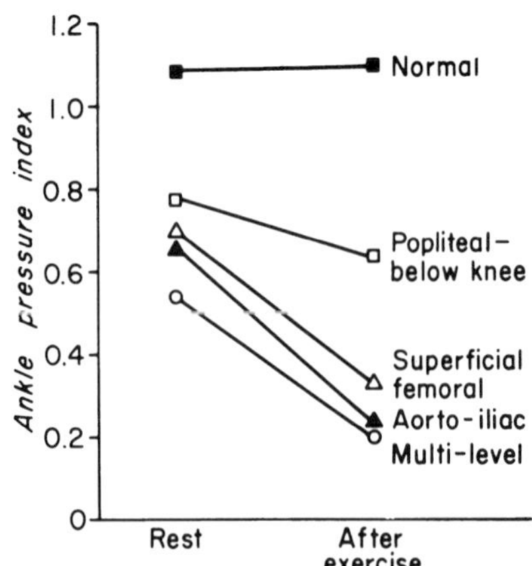

FIGURE 7–14. Mean ankle pressure indices (ankle systolic blood pressure ÷ brachial systolic blood pressure) at rest and after exercise in normal subjects and in patients with arteriosclerosis obliterans. Location of occlusion is indicated by the labels on the right. (Data from Wolf EA Jr, Sumner DS, Strandness DE Jr: Correlation between nutritive blood flow and pressure in limbs of patients with intermittent claudication. Surg Forum 23:238, 1972.)

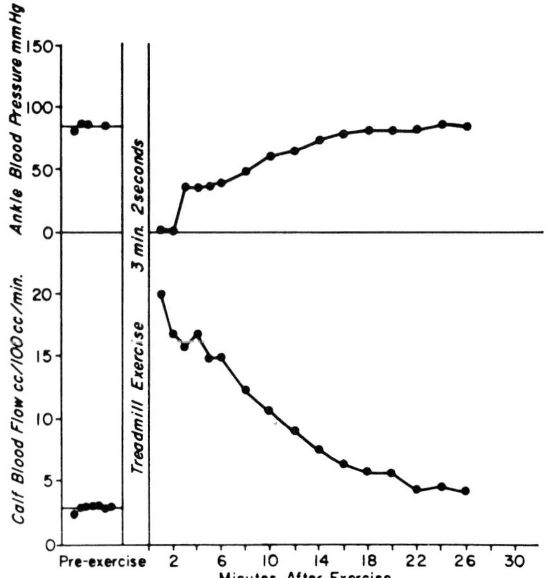

FIGURE 7–15. Ankle blood pressure and calf blood flow before and after exercise in a patient with stenosis of the superficial femoral artery. (From Sumner DS, Strandness DE Jr: The relationship between calf blood flow and ankle blood pressure in patients with intermittent claudication. Surgery 65:763, 1969.)

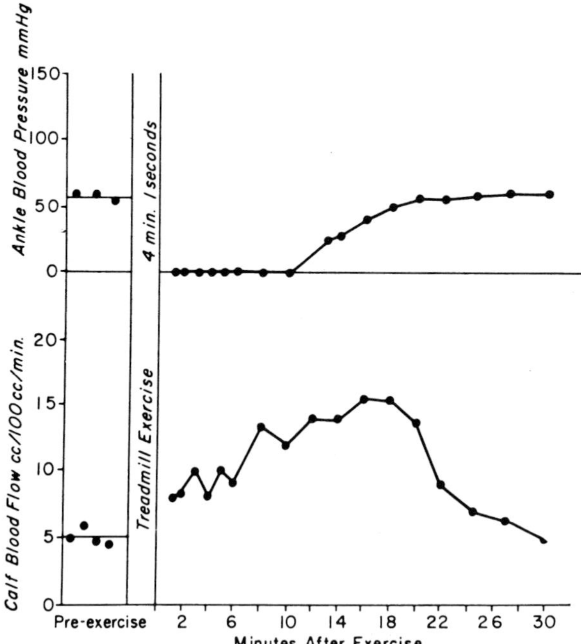

FIGURE 7–16. Ankle blood pressure and calf blood flow before and after exercise in a patient with stenosis of the iliac artery and occlusion of the superficial femoral artery. (From Sumner DS, Strandness DE Jr: The relationship between calf blood flow and ankle blood pressure in patients with intermittent claudication. Surgery 65:763, 1969.)

Blood Pressure at Rest and Following Exercise

Under resting conditions, blood pressure distal to an obstructive arterial lesion is decreased if the lesion is hemodynamically significant at the prevailing level of flow.[103, 108, 123] Ordinarily, most lesions of surgical significance fall into this category (see Fig. 7–14). Measurement of pressures at the ankle by the simple noninvasive techniques described in Chapter 10 provides the clinician with a rapid, accurate, and objective means of assessing the functional severity of the arterial lesion.[23, 57, 171, 176, 193, 194, 199, 201]

When blood flow to the extremity is increased during or after exercise, the blood pressure distal to the arterial lesion falls precipitously (see Fig. 7–14). Recovery to pre-exercise levels requires a prolonged period, usually between 10 and 30 minutes (see Figs. 7–15 to 7–17).[96, 169, 176, 194] Even if the stenosis in a limb is not severe enough to produce a decrease in distal pressure at rest, exercise or reactive hyperemia causes a fall in pressure.[24, 117, 167] Blood pressure begins to recover after peak flows have begun to decline (see Figs. 7–15 to 7–17).[176] These changes account for the disappearance of pedal pulses after exercise in some patients with stenotic lesions.[38, 39]

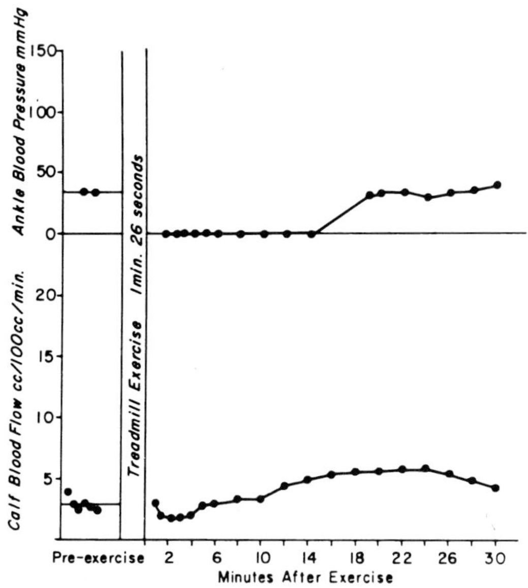

FIGURE 7–17. Ankle blood pressure and calf blood flow before and after exercise in a patient with occlusion of the iliac, common femoral, and superficial femoral arteries. This patient had severe claudication and moderate rest pain. (From Sumner DS, Strandness DE Jr: The relationship between calf blood flow and ankle blood pressure in patients with intermittent claudication. Surgery 65:763, 1969.)

Resistance Changes Accompanying Exercise

Figure 7–18 compares resting and postexercise resistances in normal limbs with those in limbs with occlusive disease of the superficial femoral artery. In normal limbs, *segmental resistance* refers to the resistance of the iliac and femoral arteries. In abnormal limbs, segmental resistance primarily reflects the resistance offered by the collateral arteries bypassing the superficial femoral artery occlusion (parallel resistance; see Eq. 7.15). *Calf resistance* represents the runoff resistance imposed by intramuscular arterioles, capillaries, and venules as well as the veins draining the extremity. The major part of this resistance is contributed by the arterioles. In this example, we can approximate the *total vascular resistance* of the limb by adding the segmental and calf resistances (Eq. 7.14).

At rest, values for the total resistance offered by normal and abnormal limbs are essentially equal; for example, in Figure 7–18, the normal value is 37 peripheral resistance units and the abnormal value is 36. Values for distribution of the resistances, however, are markedly different.[104, 177] Whereas segmental resistance accounts for less than 3% of the total in normal limbs, it makes up about 38% of the

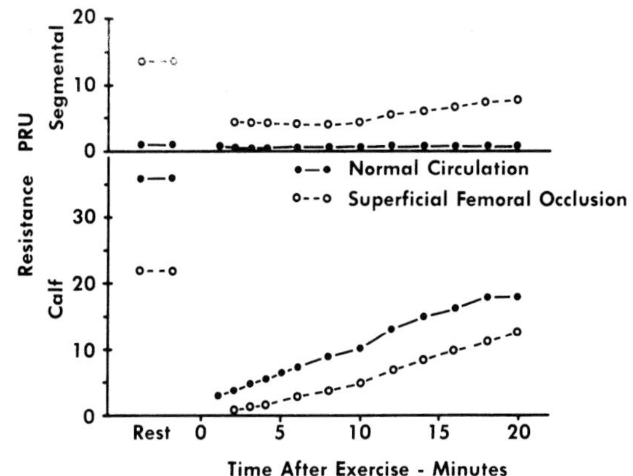

FIGURE 7–18. Segmental (parallel collateral and main channel) resistance and calf (runoff) resistance in normal individuals and in patients with occlusive disease of the superficial femoral artery. Values at rest and after treadmill exercises are shown. PRU = peripheral resistance unit. (Data from Sumner DS, Strandness DE Jr: The effect of exercise on resistance to blood flow in limbs with an occluded superficial femoral artery. Vasc Surg 4:229, 1970.)

total in abnormal limbs. Resting blood flow rates are equal in both groups of limbs only because peripheral arterioles in the abnormal limbs dilate enough to compensate for the elevated segmental resistance. Thus, calf resistance is much less in abnormal limbs than in normal limbs.

During exercise, intramuscular arterioles become widely dilated, thus markedly reducing calf resistance (see Fig. 7–18). After cessation of exercise, calf resistance gradually recovers toward resting values. Recovery is approximately linearly related to time.[177] In normal limbs, there is little change in segmental (collateral) resistance; in abnormal limbs, segmental resistance may remain unchanged or may drop somewhat.[104, 161, 177] Nevertheless, the total drop in resistance (segmental plus calf) is less in abnormal than in normal limbs. This explains why blood flow during exercise is greater in normal limbs than in limbs with occlusive arterial disease.

Although segmental resistance may decrease in limbs with arterial obstruction, it actually constitutes a greater percentage of the total resistance than it does at rest. In Figure 7–18, segmental resistance makes up 82% of the total resistance immediately after exercise. During the same period, segmental resistance in normal limbs makes up less than 14% of total limb resistance. The relative increase in segmental resistance in abnormal limbs explains the decrease in ankle blood pressure after walking.[104, 176] The following discussion clarifies some of these relationships.

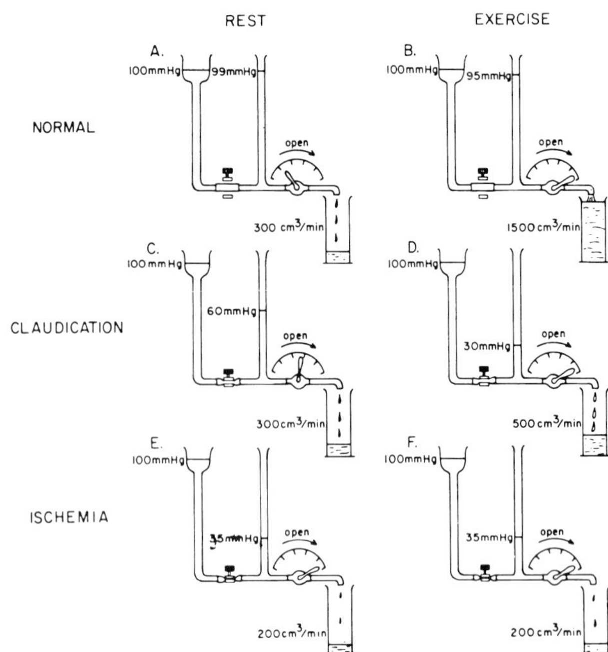

FIGURE 7–19. Hydraulic model of an arterial circuit showing the effect of exercise. See text for details.

Hemodynamics of Arterial Obstruction

Understanding the hemodynamics of intermittent claudication is facilitated by the use of simple models. Figure 7–10 shows a typical vascular circuit containing a stenotic artery. This circuit consists of (1) a proximal fixed (segmental) resistance made up of the stenotic segment and the bypassing collateral and (2) a runoff bed made up of the distal arteries, arterioles, capillaries, and venules as well as the veins that return blood to the heart. As pointed out earlier, the resistance of the runoff bed largely resides in the arterioles and, consequently, is highly variable.

In Figure 7–19, the proximal fixed (segmental) resistance is represented by a compressible tube with a screw-clamp, and the distal runoff resistance is represented by a faucet. The normal situation is depicted in Figure 7–19*A* and *B*. Although at rest the resistance of the distal vascular bed is quite high, the proximal resistance is so low that normal flow is maintained (300 ml/min). During exercise, the intramuscular arterioles dilate, reducing the distal runoff resistance to a remarkable degree. Even though blood flow (Q_t) is increased five times, there is little pressure drop across the proximal (segmental) resistance (see also Eq. 7.12):

$$P_2 = P_1 - Q_t R_{seg} \quad (7.17)$$

Now suppose that an obstruction develops in the proximal vasculature, represented by tightening of the screw-clamp (Fig. 7–19*C* and *D*). The arterioles within the runoff bed dilate enough to compensate for the increased proximal resistance. Because of this autoregulatory process, resting blood flow remains within normal limits. However, the resting blood pressure distal to the obstructed segment is lower than normal (60 mmHg in this example). This is simply a reflection of the increased energy losses that occur across the increased resistance (Eq. 7.17).

With exercise, the intramuscular arterioles dilate fully (see Fig. 7–19*D*). Because of the high proximal resistance, the increase in blood flow is inadequate to meet the metabolic demands of the exercising muscle mass and claudication ensues. In addition, the blood pressure distal to the obstruction experiences a further decrease as a result of the increased rate of flow through the high proximal resistance (see also Fig. 7–15).

Finally, an even worse situation is depicted in Figure 7–19*E* and *F*. Here, the proximal obstruction is so severe that blood flow at rest is only two-thirds the normal value (200 ml/min) despite complete peripheral vasodilatation; consequently, the patient experiences rest pain. Because no further peripheral dilatation is possible, blood flow does not increase with exercise. Blood pressure distal to the obstruction is more profoundly depressed than in the previous examples, because the increase in proximal (segmental) resistance is proportionally greater than the decrease in blood flow (Eq. 7.17; see also Fig. 7–17).

We can summarize these points as follows:

1. At rest, peripheral blood flow is normal in patients with claudication but is decreased in patients with ischemic rest pain.[54, 64, 90, 135, 166, 176]

2. During exercise, peripheral blood flow increases in claudicants, but the increase is less than that occurring in normal limbs.[65, 92, 135, 156, 176, 194] In patients with rest pain, exercise may result in no increase in blood flow.[176]

3. At rest, blood pressure distal to the arterial lesion is decreased in claudicants and even more so in patients with rest pain.[23, 176, 194, 199] Exercise ordinarily results in a further decrease in peripheral pressure.[24, 169, 176, 194]

Multiple Lesions and the Vascular Steal Phenomenon

Obstructing lesions occupying *one* arterial segment (e.g., iliac or superficial femoral artery) commonly cause claudication but seldom result in ischemia at rest. There are, however, certain exceptions. When the lesion is located far distally in the foot or toe, the involved vessel may be an end artery with no adequate collateral branches. Blockage of such a vessel leads to ischemia. In addition, an acute embolic obstruction to the distal aorta, common femoral artery, or popliteal artery may also obstruct stem or reentry collaterals. In effect, this creates a multilevel occlusion that may be responsible for severe peripheral ischemia.

Multilevel occlusions result when lesions involve two or more major arterial segments. Peripheral blood flow is more severely compromised than in single-level occlusions because blood must traverse two or more high-resistance collateral beds before reaching the periphery. If the lesions are chronic and confined to *two* segments (e.g., common iliac and superficial femoral arteries), collateral development usually is adequate to prevent rest pain or ischemic necrosis; claudication, however, is quite severe. Lesions involving *three* segments (e.g., common iliac, femoral, and popliteal arteries) reduce blood flow markedly and frequently cause rest pain.

Figure 7–20 illustrates the effect of exercise on pressure-flow relationships in limbs with two levels of obstruction. In this example, the more proximal fixed resistance (R_I) represents a lesion within the iliac artery, and the distal fixed resistance (R_{SF}) is in the superficial femoral artery. The variable resistances imposed by the peripheral vascular beds of the thigh and calf are represented by R_T and R_C, respectively. Normal resting blood flow to the calf and thigh is maintained by nearly complete vasodilatation in the calf (R_C open) and by partial vasodilatation in the thigh (R_T partly open) (Fig. 7–20*A*). Although exercise causes little change in diameter of the calf vessels, which already were nearly maximally dilated (R_C unchanged), the partial dilatation of the thigh vasculature becomes complete, thereby reducing its resistance to a minimal level (R_T open) (Fig. 7–20*B*). Because the total peripheral resistance is reduced, blood flow through the proximal fixed resistance (R_I) increases, leading to a further drop in pressure P_2 (Eq. 7.17). Because the series of resistances leading to the calf have not changed (R_{SF} + R_C) and because the pressure head (P_2) perfusing the calf drops, blood flow to the calf decreases.

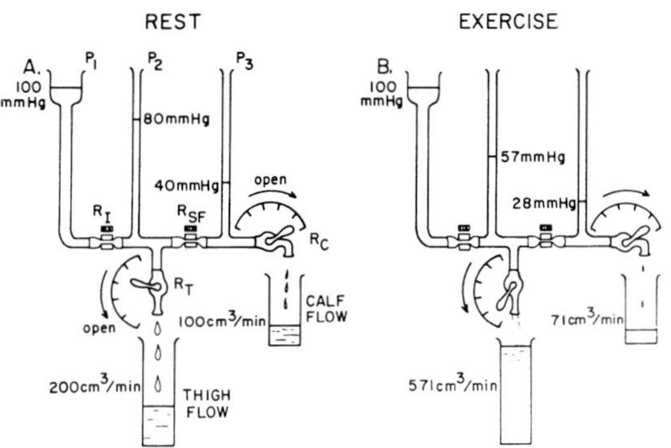

FIGURE 7–20. Hydraulic model illustrating effect of multiple-level arterial obstructive disease. See text for details.

Thus, the effects of exercise are to (1) increase flow to the thigh, (2) decrease flow to the calf, and (3) decrease peripheral blood pressure.[3] Therefore, the proximal vascular bed *steals* blood from the distal. Calf blood flow increases only when thigh blood flow decreases, allowing the distal blood pressure (P_3) to rise (see Fig. 7–16).[3]

In conclusion, exercise or other causes of peripheral vasodilatation have the following effects in limbs with multiple levels of occlusion:

1. Blood flow in the more distal tissues may be normal at rest but may drop to even lower levels during exercise. In fact, the distal tissues may become completely ischemic.[2, 38, 92, 199]
2. Blood pressure below the fixed obstructions is reduced at rest and falls to even lower levels during exercise.[169, 176, 199]
3. One vascular bed can steal from another only when the artery supplying both beds is functionally obstructed.[48, 173, 178]

Normal Arterial Flow and Pressure Waves

A portion of the left ventricular stroke volume is stored in the compliant aorta during systole and is then propelled distally by elastic recoil during diastole. When this surge of blood encounters the high resistance imposed by the arterioles, part is transmitted into the capillaries and part is reflected back up the arterial tree (Fig. 7–21).[173, 191] The magnitude of the reflected wave relative to that of the incident wave is determined by the peripheral resistance, which is greatest when the recipient vascular bed is constricted and least when the bed is dilated.[143]

As the reflected wave moves up the artery, it subtracts from the forward wave. In normal limbs with a high arteriolar tone, this produces a short period of reversed flow in early diastole. As the reflected wave moves proximally beyond the point of observation, a smaller forward flow wave again appears in late diastole. When the arterioles are dilated (as in exercise) or when the baseline resistance of the recipient bed is low (as in the cerebral circulation), the amplitude of the reflected wave is relatively small and shows up only as a transient downward deflection in the diastolic portion of the flow pulse. In this situation, flow remains antegrade throughout the cardiac cycle; there is no reverse flow component.

Although pressure is also reflected at the periphery, the reflected pressure wave—unlike the flow wave—adds to rather than subtracts from the forward wave, producing a characteristic upward deflection on the downslope of the pressure pulse (see Fig. 7–21). As mentioned, the additive nature of the reflected pressure wave accounts for the amplification of systolic pressure and the decrease in diastolic pressure that is observed as blood moves from the aorta to the peripheral arteries (see Fig. 7–13).

Although, as a first approximation, it is convenient to think of reflections as arising primarily from the high-resistance microvascular bed, reflections actually occur all along the arterial system where the vessel narrows, gives

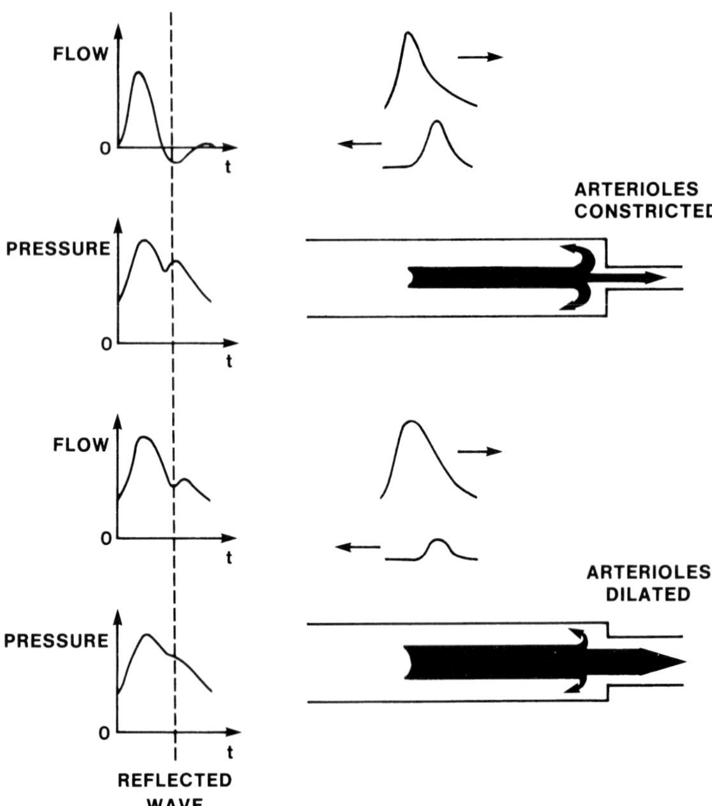

FIGURE 7–21. Effect of reflected waves on the contour of arterial flow and pressure pulses. Reflected waves subtract from forward flow waves but add to pressure waves. Reflection is accentuated by vasoconstriction and attenuated by vasodilatation. t = time. (From Sumner DS: Hemodynamics of abnormal blood flow. *In* Veith FJ, Hobson RW II, Williams RA, Wilson SE [eds]: Vascular Surgery: Principles and Practice, 2nd ed. New York, McGraw-Hill, 1994. Reproduced with permission of McGraw-Hill.)

off branches, or bifurcates. The shape of the pulse is also affected by attenuation of the pressure and flow waves as they move antegrade or retrograde along the artery. Consequently, changes in the waveform attributable to reflections are more clearly seen in peripheral arteries than they are in the proximal aorta, where the amplitude of the reflected wave is greatly diminished.

Fourier analysis permits arterial pressure and flow pulses to be broken down mathematically into a series of harmonics, each having the configuration of a sine wave (Fig. 7–22).[173] These harmonics are characterized by a modulus (amplitude at peak excursion) and a phase angle, which relates the onset of the sine wave to the beginning of the pulse cycle. The fundamental harmonic has the same frequency as that of the arterial pulse, the second harmonic has twice the frequency, and so on to the *n*th harmonic. Most of the pulsatile information is contained in the lower-frequency harmonics, allowing the raw waveform to be reduplicated fairly accurately by a summation of the first five to 10 harmonics. Because the velocity of the various harmonics depends on their frequency, their relative alignment changes as the pulse wave moves distally along the arterial tree. This is another factor that modifies the overall shape of normal flow and pressure waves.

Effect of Stenoses on Waveforms

As illustrated in Figure 7–23, the compliance of the arterial wall and that of any collateral channels constitute hydraulic capacitors, which, together with the stenosis, create a situation analogous to a low-pass filter. Passage of a pressure or flow pulse through this circuit attenuates the high-frequency harmonics and alters phase relationships, resulting in a damped waveform (see Fig. 7–22).

The arterial pulse pressure distal to a stenosis or occlusion is reduced to a greater extent than the mean pressure.[46, 82] This phenomenon is due to energy losses associated with increased velocity flow through high-resistance pathways.[46, 82] Usually, no appreciable decrease in pulse pressure occurs until the stenosis reaches a critical value of 75% to 90% reduction in arterial lumen. Complete absence of pulsation requires a stenosis approaching 99%.[39] The absence of palpable peripheral pulses distal to an arterial occlusion or severe stenosis is due to (1) reduction in the arterial pressure pulse and (2) decreased arterial pressure.

In addition to the reduction in pulse pressure, the contour of the pressure pulse is changed radically. The upslope is delayed, the peak becomes more rounded, the wave on the downslope disappears, and the downslope becomes bowed away from the baseline. These changes are reflected in the plethysmographic pulse, thus providing a sensitive indicator of the presence of arterial disease.[29, 36, 171] Further description of abnormal plethysmographic pulses is found in Chapter 10.

Similar changes are also perceived in the flow pulse distal to an obstructed artery (see Figs. 7–22 and 7–23). In contrast to the normal flow pattern, the wave rises more slowly, has a rounded peak, and declines more gradually toward the baseline during diastole. Almost invariably, the reverse flow component disappears.[57, 60, 172, 199, 200]

A stenosis, even a relatively minor stenosis, disrupts the normal laminar flow pattern, especially in the region of flow separation just beyond the exit (see Fig. 7–8). Because

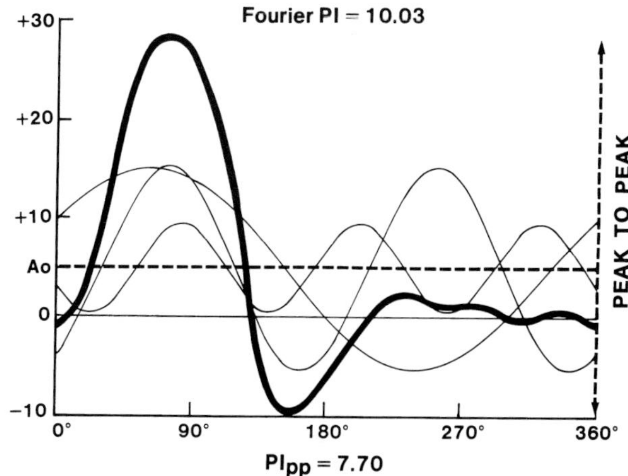

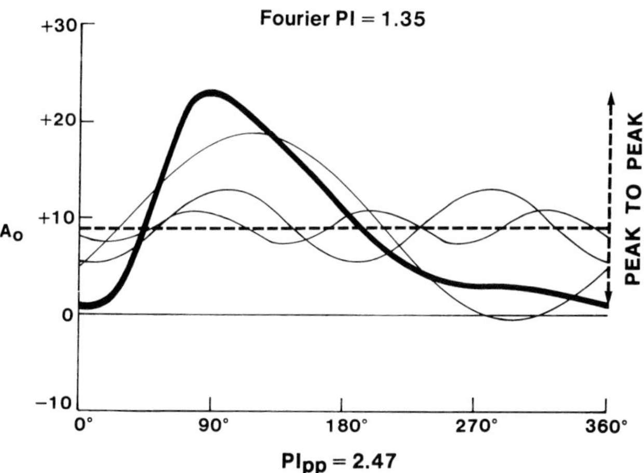

FIGURE 7–22. Fourier analysis of common femoral artery flow waveforms, showing first three harmonics. *Upper panel*: Normal iliac artery. *Lower panel*: Iliac artery obstruction. Ao = mean velocity or amplitude; vertical arrows = maximum "peak to peak" excursion. In comparison with those in the normal pulse, the amplitudes (moduli) of the 2nd and 3rd harmonics in the obstructive pulse are attenuated relative to that of the lst harmonic.

velocity vectors are no longer parallel, multiple frequencies are detected by the Doppler velocimeter, producing a phenomenon known as "spectral broadening." Because the extent of flow disruption is roughly proportional to the degree of stenosis, this finding has proved useful in detecting and grading the severity of stenoses in both carotid and peripheral arteries.[71, 145] Within the stenosis and in the jet just beyond, velocities are accelerated in accordance with the equation of continuity (Eq. 7.10). If mean flow velocities above and within the stenoses are known with certainty, the relative degree of narrowing can be measured with precision—at least theoretically. In actual practice, however, degrees of narrowing are estimated from peak systolic velocity thresholds.[210] Clinical application of flow signals in the diagnosis of arterial disease is discussed in subsequent chapters.

Shear Rate at the Arterial Wall

As mentioned earlier, shear rate (D) is the rate at which the velocity of flow changes between concentric laminae of blood (Eq. 7.7). Although the infinitesimally thin layer of blood in immediate contact with the inner wall of a vessel is static, the contiguous layers are in motion. This creates a shear rate at the wall (D_W) and a corresponding shear stress (τ_W) on the endothelial surface. In terms of mean velocity (V) and mean flow (Q) across a vessel in which the flow profile is parabolic, the shear rate and shear stress at the wall are

$$D_w = 4\frac{V}{R} = 4\frac{Q}{\pi r^3} \qquad (7.18)$$

$$\tau_w = 4\,\eta\frac{V}{r} = 4\,\eta\frac{Q}{\pi r^3} \qquad (7.19)$$

Thus, the shear rate and shear stress at the wall at any instant in the pulse cycle depend on blood viscosity (η) and are directly proportional to the mean velocity of flow and inversely proportional to the inner radius of the vessel. This means that wall shear increases as the mean velocity increases or the radius decreases and that shear decreases as the velocity decreases or the radius increases.

Shear rates at the wall are increased when the velocity profile is blunt, reflecting the decreased radial distance from the wall to the cylindrical plug of maximal velocity flow (see Fig. 7–4). When the profile is skewed (as it is at bifurcations and at areas where the vessel curves), shear is greatest near the wall where the velocity of flow is highest. In these regions, flow may take on a helical pattern, thereby further complicating the pattern of shear.[107] Turbulence not only increases shear stress but also subjects the wall to large oscillatory stresses.[129] At the carotid bulb, shear is greatest near the flow divider and least near the opposite wall, where blood flow may be stagnant or reversed during a large part of the cardiac cycle.[88, 121, 196] In this area of "flow separation," the direction of shear fluctuates during the pulse cycle, corresponding to the direction of the velocity vectors (Fig. 7–24*A*).[88] (Flow is said to be "separated" when the boundary of the main body of flow is no longer attached to the vessel wall but is isolated from the wall by a region in which the velocity vectors have a different orientation.) Similarly, in aneurysms, the axial flow stream is separated from flow in the dilated area near the wall, where velocities are low and flow reversal occurs (Fig. 7–24*B*).[196]

Other regions in which flow separation develops include the lateral walls of the common iliac artery at the aortic bifurcation and just beyond stenoses in atherosclerotic vessels (see Fig. 7–8).[144, 155, 196] In stenotic arteries, the longitudinal extent of flow separation depends on the velocity of flow and the degree of narrowing.[127]

The physiologic and pathophysiologic importance of shear rate and shear stress has been recognized only recently. There is evidence that arteries constrict with decreasing shear[89] and dilate with increasing shear.[70, 79, 115] Teleologically, this may be viewed as an effort to "normalize" shear stress.[207] Apparently, the endothelium in some way senses shear, causing the release of endothelium-derived relaxing factor (nitric oxide), which in turn relaxes the smooth muscles of the arterial wall, allowing the vessel to expand.[62] The classic example of this phenomenon is the increased diameter of arteries feeding an arteriovenous fistula.[70, 207, 218]

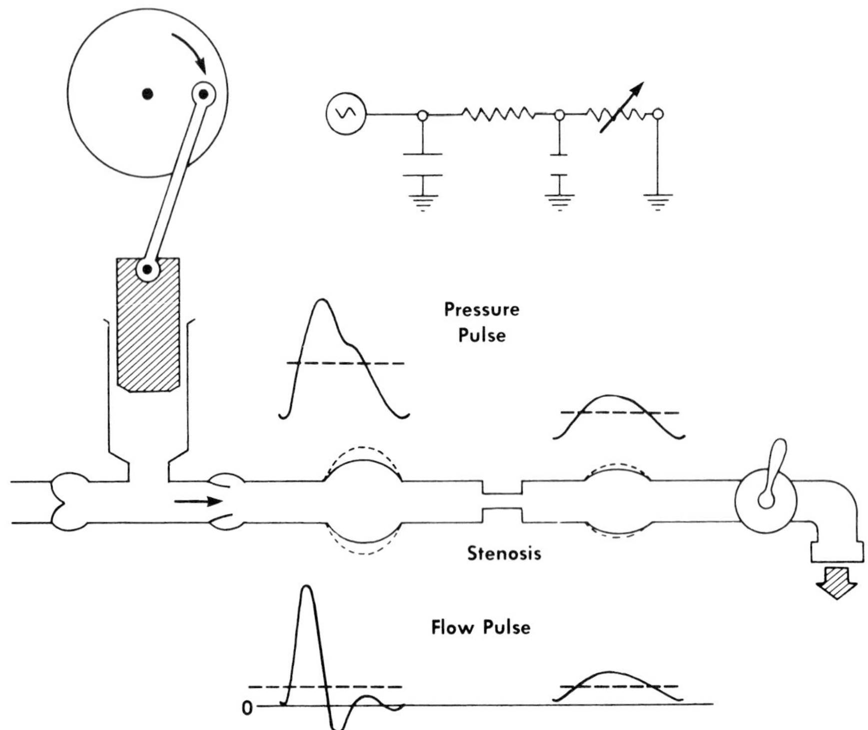

FIGURE 7–23. Effect of a stenosis and compliant vessels on the contour of arterial pressure and flow pulses. Mean pressure *(dashed line)* is reduced, but mean flow *(dashed line)* is unchanged. Faucet represents the variable resistance of the peripheral vascular bed. This, together with the fixed resistance of the stenosis and the compliance of the major arteries, constitutes a model of input impedance. (From Sumner DS: Correlation of lesion configuration with functional significance. *In* Bond MG, Insull W Jr, Glagov S [eds]: Clinical Diagnosis of Atherosclerosis: Quantitative Methods of Evaluation. New York, Springer-Verlag, 1983.)

As mentioned earlier, coronary arteries narrowed by atherosclerotic plaques also tend to dilate, thereby maintaining the lumen at a relatively normal diameter as long as the plaques remain small.[59] This mechanism may be operative in the peripheral circulation as well, where the average diameter of atherosclerotic arteries is usually somewhat larger than that of normal arteries. Post-stenotic dilatation of the axillary artery (frequently observed distal to the site of bony compression in patients with thoracic outlet syndrome) has also been attributed to distorted patterns of shear stress.[129]

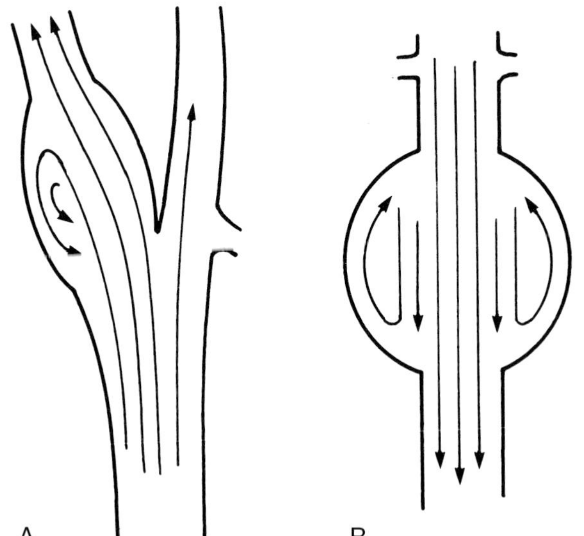

FIGURE 7–24. Diagrammatic representation of flow streamlines in a carotid arterial bifurcation *(A)* and an abdominal aortic aneurysm *(B)*. Flow separation and reversal of flow occur in the carotid bulb and in the distended portion of the aneurysm.

Endothelial cells are aligned and are overlapped (like shingles) in the direction of the wall shear stress.[164] In areas with reduced shear and where the direction of shear oscillates during the pulse cycle, the orientation of these cells is distorted and the pattern of overlap is disrupted. Atherosclerotic plaques tend to form first and develop most rapidly at sites of decreased shear, possibly because the relative stagnation of blood in these regions prolongs the fluid "residence time," modifying mass transport of atherogenic substances from the lumen into the wall and fostering the adherence of platelets and macrophages to the endothelial surface.[88, 121] The endothelial barrier may in turn be more susceptible to penetration owing to the distorted alignment of the cells and the instability of cellular junctions.[88] This explains the preferential location of plaques in the carotid bulb opposite the flow divider and the frequency with which atherosclerotic plaques form at the bifurcations of the terminal aorta, the common femoral artery, and popliteal artery—all areas in which geometry promotes flow separation and decreased shear rates.[88, 155] Once a plaque has formed, further extension may be promoted by the area of stagnant or reversed flow that develops immediately beyond the stenosis (see Fig. 7–8).

Other investigators have observed a positive correlation between shear rate and platelet and fibrin deposition on damaged endothelial surfaces. They have suggested that increased shear rates may be conducive to arterial thrombosis in certain circumstances.[132]

TREATMENT OF ARTERIAL INSUFFICIENCY: PHYSIOLOGIC ASPECTS

On the basis of the arguments presented earlier in this chapter, it is evident that the elevated fixed resistance imposed by obstructed major arteries and by their associated collaterals is the factor responsible for restricting blood flow to the periphery. It follows that intermittent claudication and other symptoms of peripheral ischemia can be alleviated only by reduction of this fixed resistance. Efforts to reduce the resistance of the peripheral vascular bed are seldom beneficial because this resistance either is automatically adjusted to levels adequate to maintain a normal resting blood flow or already is maximally reduced in limbs with ischemia at rest (see Fig. 7–11); it is also maximally reduced during exercise in patients with intermittent claudication (see Fig. 7–18).[30, 66, 140, 147]

Thus, vasodilators may increase the resting blood flow in limbs when resting blood flow is adequate, but they almost never improve flow in an ischemic limb or during exercise.[27, 188] In fact, these agents may cause blood to be diverted from areas of relative ischemia to those where disease is less severe.[93]

Many of these same criticisms can be applied to surgical sympathectomy (Fig. 7–25).[33, 66, 147] Sympathectomy, however, does have the advantage that its effects can be confined to the diseased area. In fact, some relief has been reported in patients with mild rest pain or with superficial ischemic ulcers.[170] Yet even this improvement is difficult to explain, because sympathectomy appears to enhance flow through arteriovenous anastomoses without increasing flow through the nutritive capillary bed (see Chapter 99).[34, 224]

Because no drugs are available that produce appreciable collateral dilatation or cause regression of atherosclerotic plaques, satisfactory reduction of the fixed resistance can be accomplished only by direct surgical means; endarterectomy, replacement grafting, bypass grafting, and balloon angioplasty are all effective (see Fig. 7–25). Exercise therapy is the only nonoperative treatment that consistently affords any objective relief.[90, 162] Although exercise programs extend maximal walking and claudication distances and appear to decrease the flow debt incurred during muscle activity, there is usually little change in ankle pressure.[51, 74] This suggests that the benefits are due in large part to metabolic changes rather than to collateral development. Thus, although exercise is helpful in patients with claudication, it is applicable only when ischemia is absent at rest, and it cannot match the hemodynamic improvement provided by reconstructive surgery.

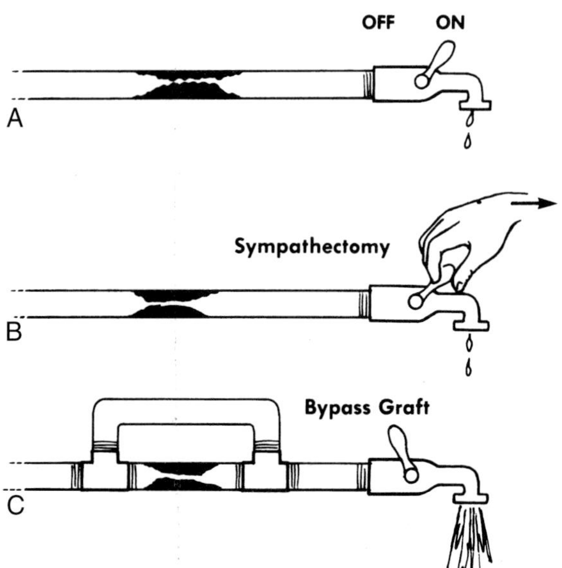

FIGURE 7–25. Hydraulic model contrasting the effects of sympathectomy and bypass grafting on blood flow. *A*, Faucet represents peripheral resistance, which is maximally decreased by exercise. *B*, Resistance cannot be further decreased by sympathectomy. *C*, Bypass graft circumvents the fixed resistance, permitting increased blood flow even with less peripheral vasodilatation. (*A–C*, From Sumner DS: Pathophysiology of arterial occlusive disease. *In* Hershey FB, Barnes RW, Sumner DS [eds]: Noninvasive Diagnosis of Vascular Disease. Pasadena, CA, Appleton Davies, Inc, 1984.)

Temporary relief of severe ischemia at rest sometimes can be obtained by rendering the patient hypertensive, thereby increasing the pressure head perfusing the obstructed vascular circuit.[90, 93] Because of the adverse effects of hypertension, this approach is rarely employed. However, restoring blood pressure to near normal levels by improving cardiac output in hypotensive patients with pump failure and multilevel arterial disease may reverse acute ischemia of the feet and toes.

Hanging the feet over the edge of the bed or walking a few steps often provides complete or partial relief from ischemic rest pain. The temporary improvement in peripheral perfusion that accompanies dependency can be documented objectively with measurement of transcutaneous oxygen tension, which may be increased severalfold compared with levels measured when the patient is supine.[149] According to Equation 7.1, pressure in the dependent arteries, veins, and capillaries is increased by gravity commensurate with the vertical distance from the foot to the heart. Although there is no increase in the arteriovenous pressure gradient, the increased hydrostatic pressure dilates capillaries and microvascular vessels, thereby reducing their resistance, which in turn augments blood flow. Augmentation of blood flow does not occur in nonischemic limbs, because the venoarterial reflex that serves to constrict arterioles in the dependent position remains functional.

Because the viscosity of blood increases with hematocrit, it is possible to augment blood flow by hemodilution.[43, 95, 195] The effects, however, are unpredictable, difficult to control, and not applicable on a long-term basis. Pentoxifylline, a drug that decreases plasma fibrinogen and platelet aggregation and increases erythrocyte flexibility, augments walking tolerance somewhat in patients with claudication, but again the results are variable.[138]

Arterial Grafts

When the decision to use a graft has been made, the surgeon often has some latitude in the choice of graft material, diameter, and anastomotic configuration (end-to-end, side-to-end, or end-to-side). Because of the importance of radius in determining both viscous and inertial energy losses, the graft selected should be large enough to carry all the flow required at rest without causing an evident pressure drop; it should also be large enough to accommodate any increased flow likely to be required during exercise without an appreciable pressure drop. Any limitation of flow should result from the resistance of the peripheral vascular bed and not from the graft.

Table 7–1 lists the pressure gradients that might be expected across a femoropopliteal graft 40 cm long at

TABLE 7–1. CALCULATED MINIMAL PRESSURE GRADIENTS (mmHg) ACROSS A 40-cm GRAFT (η = 0.035 P)

	DIAMETER (cm)				
FLOW (ml/min)	0.2	0.3	0.4	0.5	0.6
60	27	5.3	1.7	0.7	0.3
100	45	8.8	2.8	1.1	0.6
150	67	13	4.2	1.7	0.8
300	134	27	8.4	3.4	1.7
500	223	44	14	5.8	2.8

several levels of flow. Since these calculations were made using Poiseuille's equation (Eq. 7.6), they represent minimal values; the actual pressure drops would be several times as great.[148] Clearly, a graft with an inside diameter less than 3 mm would be of marginal value at flow rates normally observed at rest (60 to 150 ml/min) and would be completely unsatisfactory during exercise (300 to 500 ml/min). This coincides with the clinical observations of many surgeons.[21, 47, 128, 189]

Blood flow in the common femoral artery averages about 350 ml/min at rest and may increase by a factor of 5 to 10 during exercise. According to Poiseuille's equation, a graft 20 cm long with an inside diameter of 7 mm should be able to carry flows of 3000 ml/min with a pressure drop of only 4.5 mmHg. Experimentally, the pressure gradient across similar grafts is much higher, approximating 7 to 10 mmHg at a flow rate of 1200 ml/min.[148, 152] At rest, however, a 7-mm graft should result in a pressure gradient of only a few millimeters of mercury. Therefore, under most physiologic conditions an aortofemoral graft with 7-mm limbs should suffice, restricting flow only during strenuous exercise. Six-millimeter grafts might begin to show some restriction of flow even with mild to moderate exercise.

Under ideal flow conditions, prosthetic grafts develop a thin layer (0.5 to 1.0 mm) of pseudointima. Thus, after implantation a 6-mm prosthetic graft might have an internal diameter of 4 to 5 mm and a 7-mm graft might have a lumen of 5 to 6 mm. For this reason, it seems appropriate, when one performs a femoropopliteal bypass with a prosthetic graft, to select a graft with an original diameter of at least 6 mm. Similarly, the original diameter of an aortofemoral graft should be at least 7 mm.

On the other hand, the diameter of the graft must not be too much larger than that of the recipient arteries.[150] It has been shown, both clinically and experimentally, that irregular clots accumulate on the inner walls of grafts of excessive diameter (much as they do in aneurysms) as the flow stream tries to mold itself to the diameter of the recipient vessels. These clots, which are not densely adherent, tend to separate and may be responsible for graft failure. A high-flow velocity (high shear) is conducive to the formation of a thin, tightly adherent pseudointima. For a given volume of flow, the wall shear rate (or stress) is inversely proportional to the cube of the radius (Eqs. 7.18 and 7.19). Therefore, the shear rate at the wall in a 7-mm graft would be 1.5 times that in an 8-mm graft and 2.9 times that in a 10-mm graft. Thus, the diameter of a prosthetic graft should be small enough to ensure a rapid velocity of flow but large enough to avoid restriction of arterial inflow.

Long-term patency of autogenous vein grafts is compromised by intimal hyperplasia, the development of which has also been associated with low shear rates.[14, 130] Low shear rates cause smooth muscle cells to become secretory and enhance platelet adherence;[130] high shear rates foster continued patency and lessen the tendency for the intima to become hyperplastic. The protective effect of high shear may be due to suppression of the release of endothelin-1, a peptide found in endothelial cells that acts as a vasoconstrictor and a mitogen for smooth muscle cells.[154]

Studies suggest that diameters of human in situ vein grafts change with time to normalize shear stress.[214] Vein grafts with initially high shear rates tend to dilate, but those with low shear rates tend to contract. The diameters of lower extremity vein grafts appear to increase transiently in response to acute increases in blood flow, a response that may be attributed to the release of nitric oxide from the endothelium in response to increased shear stress.[215] However, nitric oxide activity has been shown to be significantly impaired in vein grafts (especially under low-flow conditions), an alteration that may contribute to intimal hyperplasia.[211, 220]

Anastomoses

Because any change in the direction of blood flow increases energy losses due to inertial factors, an end-to-end anastomosis is more hemodynamically efficient than a side-to-end or end-to-side anastomosis.[173] The greater the angle subtended by the graft and host vessels, the greater the energy losses become. Even though energy losses may be increased severalfold by an adverse angle, the increase in pressure drop is only a few millimeters of mercury and is ordinarily of no clinical significance. For example, from the point of view of transmitting blood efficiently, it makes little difference whether the donor anastomosis of a femoral-femoral graft is made with an angle of 135 degrees (requiring flow to reverse itself) or whether it is made with a more hemodynamically satisfactory angle of 45 degrees.[101, 105]

Energy losses, however, are only part of the story. Any time a graft leaves or enters a host vessel at an angle, flow disturbances are created, resulting in zones of flow separation, stagnation, turbulence, and distorted velocity vectors (Figs. 7–26 and 7–27).[9, 32, 101, 128] The "floor" of an end-to-side anastomosis (in the recipient vessel opposite the anastomosis), the "toe" of the anastomosis (on the near wall just beyond the suture line), and the "heel" (on the near wall proximal to the junction) appear to be prominent sites of flow separation where shear is low and shear stress fluctuates.[9, 128] Low shear and oscillatory shear stresses are conducive to platelet adhesion, intimal hyperplasia, and atherosclerosis, and high shear may result in endothelial damage.[32, 101, 113, 205] The ultimate result is endothelial thickening or thrombus formation that may lead to graft failure.[100] Therefore, the goal of a long-term graft patency is best achieved by construction of an end-to-end anastomosis; when this is not feasible, an anastomosis with an acute angle is recommended.

Computer simulations have shown that large shear stress

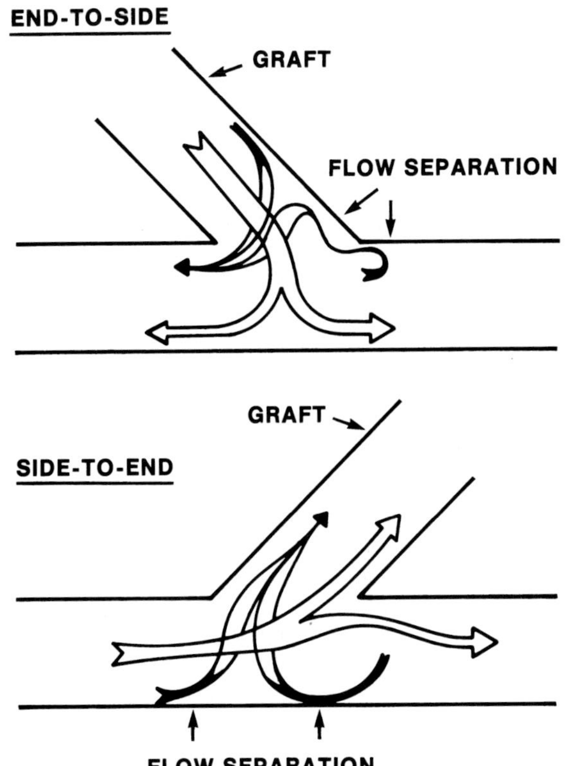

FIGURE 7–26. Flow patterns at end-to-side and side-to-end anastomoses. Near the wall, blood flow may reverse and travel circumferentially to reach the recipient conduit. Areas of flow separation are prone to develop neointimal hyperplasia. (From Sumner DS: Hemodynamics of abnormal blood flow. *In* Veith FJ, Hobson RW, Russell AW, Wilson SE [eds]: Vascular Surgery: Principles and Practice, 2nd ed. New York, McGraw-Hill, 1994. Reproduced with permission of McGraw-Hill.)

gradients at the toe and heel of end-to-side distal anastomoses are associated with the development of myointimal hyperplasia and atheroma.[217] Compared with conventional anastomotic configurations, a Taylor patch decreases these gradients somewhat, especially at high flow rates, but a major (50%) reduction in wall shear stress gradients requires an idealized geometry with a smoothly tapered heel and toe, a graft-to-host diameter ratio of 1.6, and an anastomotic angle of 10° to 15°.

VISCOELASTICITY OF THE ARTERIAL WALL

As intraluminal pressure increases during systole, the arterial wall stretches both circumferentially and longitudinally. During diastole, the process is reversed. The magnitude of the stretch is determined by the stiffness of the arterial wall, which in turn is determined by its composition and thickness.

The stiffness of an elastic material can be described by Young's modulus of elasticity (E), which is the ratio of the applied stress (τ) to the resulting strain (ϵ):

$$E = \tau/\epsilon \qquad (7.20)$$

Compliance (C) is the reciprocal of the elastic modulus (1/E). The circumferential stress applied to an arterial wall is a function of the transmural pressure, P (intraluminal pressure minus the extravascular pressure), the inside radius of the artery, r_i, and its wall thickness, δ[137, 173]:

$$\tau = P\frac{r_i}{\delta} \qquad (7.21)$$

Pressure is in dynes $\cdot$ cm^{-2}, and r_i and d are in centimeters. Circumferential strain, ϵ, is proportional to the ratio of the change in outside radius, Δr_o, to the original outside radius, r_o:

$$\epsilon = \Delta r_o / r_o \qquad (7.22)$$

Therefore, an incremental elastic modulus (E_t) can be obtained by substituting Equations 7.21 and 7.22 in 7.20:

$$E_t = \Delta P\frac{r_o}{\Delta r_o} \cdot \frac{r_i}{\delta} \qquad (7.23)$$

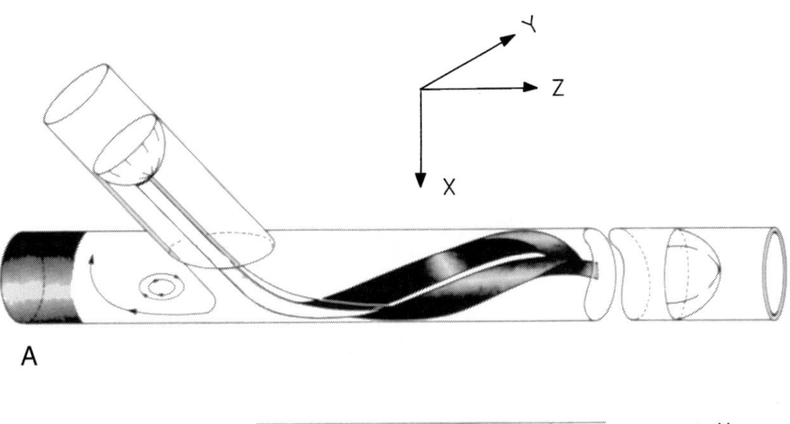

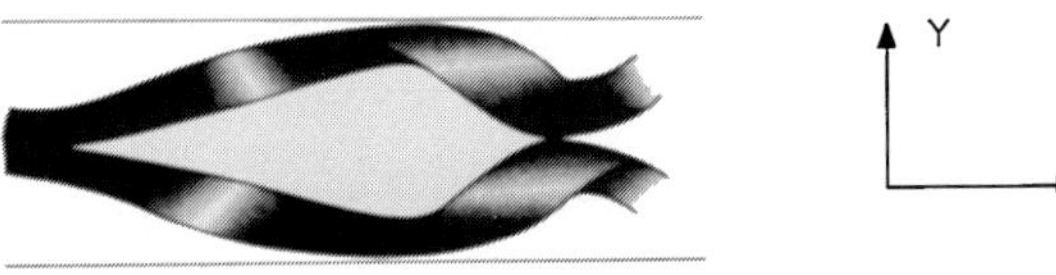

FIGURE 7–27. Flow pattern in a model of an end-to-side anastomosis. Note impingement of high-velocity flow on the "floor" of the anastomosis and the helical pattern that develops beyond the anastomosis. Reversal of flow occurs in the proximal segment of the recipient vessel. *A*, Model tilted toward observer. *B*, Model viewed from above. (From Ojha M, Ethier CR, Johnston KW, Cobbold RSC: Steady and pulsatile flow fields in an end-to-side arterial anastomosis model. J Vasc Surg 12:747–753, 1990.)

Pulse pressure is represented by ΔP. Although this formula allows a first approximation of the stiffness of the materials composing the arterial wall, it does not take into account the variable stress on the different layers (greatest on the inside and least on the outside) and the tendency of the wall thickness to decrease as the radius increases.[173] A more precise formula that incorporates these variables has been devised by Bergel[12]:

$$E = \Delta P \cdot \frac{r_o}{\Delta r_o} \cdot \frac{(1.5)\, r_i^2}{r_o^2 + r_i^2} \qquad (7.24)$$

Because it is often difficult to obtain accurate measurements of arterial wall thickness, several purely descriptive formulas are in common use[137]:

$$E_p = \Delta P \frac{r_o}{\Delta r_o} \qquad (7.25)$$

Compliance (C) is the reciprocal of E_p:

$$C = \frac{\Delta r_o}{\Delta P \cdot r_o} \qquad (7.26)$$

It should be emphasized that Equations 7.25 and 7.26 relate to the behavior of the entire arterial wall, whereas Equations 7.23 and 7.24 describe the stiffness of the materials composing the wall. In other words, two arteries with the same E value (Eq. 7.24) would have different E_p values if their wall thicknesses were different.

In addition to elasticity, viscosity is also a property of the arterial wall.[13] Viscosity causes the expansion of the artery to lag behind the change in pressure. As a result, the elastic modulus of the arterial wall appears to increase with increasing pulse rate. Wall viscosity may also account for some of the energy losses in pulsatile flow because the storage of energy during systole and its release during diastole may be incomplete owing to the friction encountered in expansion and contraction of the arterial wall.

Two fibrous proteins, *elastin* and *collagen,* determine the mechanical properties of the arterial wall. At *low* transmural pressures (<50 to 75 mmHg), most of the circumferential distending force is sustained by lamellae composed of elastin, which is highly extensible. At *higher* pressures, the arterial wall stretches and collagen fibers are gradually recruited to bear an increasingly large portion of the load. Because collagen is about 1000 to 2000 times stiffer than elastin, arteries (and veins) become very stiff at high pressures. Therefore, the typical pressure-diameter curve of arteries has two phases: (1) a low-pressure, compliant part and (2) a high-pressure, stiff part.[40] The elastic modulus of the arterial wall also increases with aging, fibrosis, and calcification—factors that often accompany arteriosclerosis.[122, 173, 222]

Activation of the smooth muscle within the arterial wall has a complex relationship to the elastic modulus but tends to increase stiffness at a given strain.[42, 173] The effect of muscle contraction becomes evident only in the smaller and muscular arteries of the periphery and is most marked in terminal arterioles. In the absence of muscular contraction, all arteries retain a circular cross section even at zero transmural pressure. Therefore, the phenomenon of "critical closure," in which small arteries appear to collapse (occlude) at low perfusion pressures, can occur only when there is an increase in smooth muscle tone.[7]

Table 7–2 lists some of the stress-strain characteristics of atherosclerotic and normal arteries. Most synthetic grafts are stiffer than the arteries they replace, especially after they have been implanted for some time (Table 7–3). This is due to ingrowth of fibrous tissue into the interstices of porous grafts and fibrous encapsulation of the grafts.

Palpable Pulses

Motion of the arterial wall is responsible for the palpable pulses that are so important in the physical examination of the patient in whom arterial disease is suspected. Yet, it is apparent from the values in Table 7–2 that a 7-mm femoral artery in a young subject would expand only 0.2 mm under the influence of a 50-mmHg pulse pressure. Older, stiffer arteries would expand even less. It seems doubtful that the finger could reliably detect this degree of motion. Why, then, are pulses ordinarily so easily felt? When the finger is applied to the skin overlying an artery, the artery is compressed, changing its normally circular cross section into an *ellipse*. It takes much less energy to bend the wall of an elliptically shaped vessel than it does to stretch the wall of a circular vessel.[122] Therefore, when the artery is partially compressed, its expansion in the direction of the

TABLE 7–2. STRESS-STRAIN CHARACTERISTICS OF HUMAN ARTERIES

LOCATION	CHAPTER REFERENCE	REMARKS	ELASTIC MODULUS (E)* (dynes · cm^{-2} · 10^6)	PRESSURE-STRAIN ELASTIC MODULUS† (dynes · cm^{-2} · 10^6)	PER CENT COMPLIANCE (C)‡ NORMALIZED (ΔP = 50 mmHg)
Infrarenal aorta	173	ASO	26.0 ± 14.5	9.8 ± 3.5	0.8 ± 0.3
Terminal aorta	173	ASO	37.7 ± 17.2	15.1 ± 4.1	0.5 ± 0.2
Common iliac artery	173	ASO	24.7 ± 21.5	14.8 ± 15.8	0.8 ± 0.4
Common femoral artery	122	Age <35 yr	—	2.6 ± 1.3	3.0 ± 1.0
	122	Age 35–60 yr	—	3.9 ± 2.0	2.1 ± 0.9
	122	Age >60 yr	—	6.3 ± 4.8	1.2 ± 0.9
	186	—	—	2.3 ± 0.2	3.0 ± 0.3

*Equation 7.24.
†Equation 7.25.
‡Equation 7.26.
ASO, arteriosclerosis obliterans.

TABLE 7–3. STRESS-STRAIN CHARACTERISTICS OF VARIOUS ARTERIAL GRAFTS

GRAFT MATERIAL	CHAPTER REFERENCE	MONTHS IMPLANTED	PRESSURE-STRAIN ELASTIC MODULUS* (dynes · cm^{-2} · 10^6)	PER CENT COMPLIANCE (C)† NORMALIZED (ΔP = 50 mmHg)
Saphenous vein	186	0	3.0 ± 0.6	2.2 ± 0.4
	106	>36	4.9 ± 2.0	1.7 ± 1.0
Umbilical vein	186	0	3.6 ± 0.5	1.9 ± 0.3
Bovine heterograft	186	0	5.1 ± 0.6	1.3 ± 0.2
	67	12	24.2	0.3
Dacron				
Velour	186	0	7.0 ± 1.1	1.0 ± 0.2
Knitted	67	0	17.8	0.4
	67	12	55.5	0.1
Woven	67	0	166.6	0.04
Teflon woven	67	0	148.1	0.05
PTFE	186	0	8.3 ± 1.0	0.8 ± 0.1

*Equation 7.25.
†Equation 7.26.
PTFE, polytetrafluoroethylene.

compression is greatly augmented. In addition, as the artery expands longitudinally, the entire vessel moves toward the skin.

As surgeons, we are accustomed to grading the peripheral pulses on an arbitrary scale (e.g., from 0 to 4+) and to estimating the degree of proximal obstruction based on the magnitude of the pulse. This is predicated on the assumption that the strength of the pulse is directly related to the pulse pressure, which should be decreased distal to an obstruction. Stiff, calcified vessels may display little or no pulse, however, even though there is no decrease in pulse pressure. In contrast, relatively good pulses may be palpated despite a proximal arterial obstruction when the arterial wall is compliant, particularly when the systemic pulse pressure is increased.

Although pulse palpation is a valuable tool for the initial evaluation of the patient with suspected arterial disease, both arteriography and noninvasive tests have repeatedly demonstrated its fallibility.

Stresses at Graft-Artery Anastomoses and False Aneurysms

Coupling a stiff graft to a compliant artery places additional stresses on the suture line, which may lead to intimal hyperplasia or the development of a false aneurysm.[9, 114, 213] With the advent of synthetic sutures, most anastomotic disruptions develop in the arterial wall; the sutures themselves remain intact.[84, 125] On the basis of the data in Tables 7–2 and 7–3, the circumference of a young femoral artery measuring 7 mm in diameter would increase 1.32 mm with each 50-mmHg pressure pulse, whereas the circumference of a woven Dacron graft of the same diameter would increase only 0.02 mm, a disparity of 1.30 mm. Repeated 100,000 times per day, this small difference would result in fatigue of the arterial wall.

Paasche and colleagues have analyzed the stresses produced at an end-to-end anastomosis by a compliance mismatch.[133] Three components of the stress system were identified: axial, hoop, and shear. Of these, shear, which is greatest at the suture lines, is the most disruptive. Both theoretically and experimentally, stresses can be minimized when the ratio of the diameter of a rigid graft to that of a compliant artery is about 1.4.[85, 133]

Because the impedance of a stiff graft is greater than that of a compliant artery, pulsatile energy is reflected at the proximal suture line. When a Dacron graft with an E_p of 55×10^6 dynes · cm^{-2} is sutured to an infrarenal aorta with an E_p of 9.8×10^6 dynes · cm^{-2}, about 41% of the incident pulsatile energy is reflected.[173] Because this augments the pressure pulsations proximal to the graft, additional stresses are placed on the suture line.[124] This may contribute to disruption of the proximal anastomosis.

Shear stresses produced by vibrations generated at end-to-side anastomoses may also contribute to the formation of false aneurysms.

Arterial Wall Stress and Rupture of Aortic Aneurysms

Aneurysms rupture when the tangential stress within their wall exceeds the tensile strength of the wall at any point.

Tangential stress (τ) within the wall of a cylinder is given by Equation 7.21. This equation explains in part why large aneurysms are more likely to rupture than small aneurysms and why rupture is more common in hypertensive patients than in normotensive patients.[16, 56]

Note that Equation 7.21 differs from *Laplace's law,* which usually is stated as

$$T = Pr \qquad (7.27)$$

where r is commonly taken as the outside radius (although more properly it should be the inside radius), and T is tension in dynes per centimeter of cylindrical length. Laplace's law is truly applicable only to very thin-walled structures, such as soap bubbles, and should not be employed to describe stresses in arterial walls.[136]

Because the wall stress in a sphere is one-half that in a cylinder with the same radius and because the typical configuration of an aneurysm is a cross between a sphere and a cylinder, Equation 7.21 actually overestimates the stress in aneurysm walls.[40] Nonetheless, this does not change the essential argument—namely, that wall stress is directly proportional to transmural pressure and to the inner radius of the vessel and is inversely proportional to wall thickness.

Figure 7–28 shows a cylinder with an outside diameter of 2 cm and a wall thickness of 0.2 cm. These dimensions are compatible with those found in atherosclerotic terminal aortas.[173, 179] The circumferential wall stress within this structure would be 8.0×10^5 dynes · cm^{-2} when the internal pressure is 150 mmHg. If this tube were distended without the volume of material increasing in the wall, the wall would simultaneously become thinner. In the case illustrated, the tube has been expanded to aneurysmal dimensions, outside diameter 6 cm, and the wall thickness has decreased to 0.06 cm (Fig. 7–24, *right-hand panel*). Tripling the radius and decreasing the wall thickness cause the circumferential stress in the wall of the expanded cylinder to increase to 98.0×10^5 dynes · cm^{-2}, provided the pressure remains at 150 mmHg (Eq. 7.21). Thus, in this highly artificial model, stress per unit area of wall increases by a factor of 12, even though the arterial diameter has increased only three times.

Owing to the sluggish flow and low shear stress on the inner wall of aneurysms, layers of clot develop that tend to maintain the diameter of the lumen near that of the normal artery (see Fig. 7–24). This thrombus, by increasing the effective thickness of the arterial wall (δ), may reduce wall stress and afford some protection against rupture (Eq. 7.21). On the other hand, the clot might simply transmit pressure undiminished to the wall and have little effect on wall stress. Because thrombi are friable and poorly bonded to the inner surface of the residual wall, they may exert little or no retractive force.[40]

Recently reported computer simulations using the finite element method for analyzing mechanical properties of axisymmetric models of abdominal aortic aneurysms suggest that thrombus may reduce wall stress by as much as 50%.[212, 216, 219] These studies predict that the protective effect is proportional not only to the thickness of the clot relative to the aneurysm diameter but also to the elastic modulus (E_p, Eq. 7.25) of the clot. In other words, the risk of rupture may be less in aneurysms lined with stiff, thick clots.

In real life, aneurysms are never truly axisymmetric. As they elongate, they tend to bow forward at the upper end and deviate to the left. Because posterior expansion is limited by the vertebral column, aneurysms are forced to bulge anteriorly. Asymmetry in the anterior-posterior plane has been shown by finite element analysis to increase wall stress even when the diameter remains unchanged.[225] This effect is particularly evident in the posterior wall adjacent to the vertebral column and in the anterior wall, where the direction of curvature gradually changes from concave outward to concave inward in the vicinity of the aneurysm-normal artery junction. These points appear to be sites of maximal stress in asymmetric aneurysms.

In normal arteries, most of the wall stress imposed by intraluminal pressure is sustained by elastin. It has been suggested that aneurysm formation may be related to degeneration of elastic lamellae caused by atherosclerosis or the action of endogenous elastases.[41, 206, 208] Inflammatory cells may also participate in this process, perhaps by serving as a source of elastases.[4] Rupture, however, is prevented by collagen fibers, which are principally responsible for the integrity of the arterial wall.[41] Although the tensile strength of collagen (about 5 to 7×10^7 dynes · cm^{-2}) far exceeds the wall stress developed in the dilated tube shown in Figure 7–28, it must be pointed out that collagen fibers make up only about 25% of the atherosclerotic arterial wall and only 6% to 18% of the aneurysm wall.[175, 180] Therefore, one would predict that each collagen fiber sustains a greater load than would be expected if the entire wall were composed of collagen. In addition, the aneurysm wall is weakened by fragmentation and other degenerative changes within the fibrous network. (Collagenase activity may play an important role in this process.[20]) On the basis of these considerations, it is not difficult to imagine how an atherosclerotic artery that has become aneurysmal might rupture. Not only is the wall stress greatly increased, but the collagen fibers are more sparsely distributed, disorganized, and fragmented.

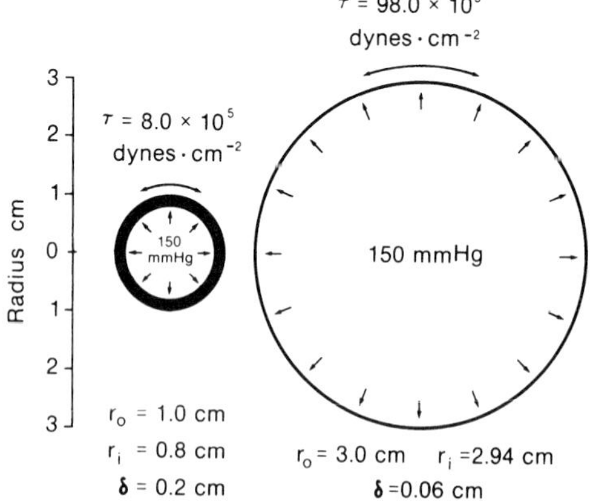

FIGURE 7–28. End-on view of a cylinder 2 cm in diameter before and after expansion to a diameter of 6 cm. Wall area remains the same in the two cases, but wall stress (τ) is greatly increased owing both to the decrease in wall thickness (δ) and to the increase in inside radius (r_i).

Venous Hemodynamics

Venous physiology is, in many respects, more complex than arterial physiology. Veins differ from arteries in a number of ways: they (1) have thinner walls, (2) are collapsible, and (3) contain valves that are oriented to ensure unidirectional flow. There are two large venous systems: superficial and deep, which are connected at intervals by "perforating" or "communicating" veins. *Deep veins* parallel arteries of the same name; *superficial veins* and the large, *saccular veins* (sinusoids) within the calf muscles have no arterial counterparts.

Veins have a larger diameter than that of their accompanying arteries and in the periphery are usually duplicated. Although veins are seldom completely distended, they contain about two thirds of the blood in the body. At corresponding anatomic locations, venous blood pressure is always lower than arterial blood pressure. In veins, the hydrostatic component of the total blood pressure is often proportionately larger than the dynamic component—the opposite of the situation normally prevailing in arteries. Unlike blood flow in arteries, which is pulsatile but relatively constant from one cardiac cycle to the next, blood flow in veins fluctuates with respiration and muscle activity and may cease altogether for brief periods.

BASIC HEMODYNAMICS

In order to understand pressure-flow phenomena in veins, the reader will find it useful to review the effects of gravity on venous pressure, venous pressure-volume relationships, and the peculiarities associated with flow through collapsible tubes.

Venous Pressure

As discussed in the first part of this chapter, venous pressure is composed of dynamic pressure produced by contraction of the left ventricle, hydrostatic pressure produced by the weight of the column of blood, and static filling pressure that is related to the elasticity of the vascular wall. Because a large portion of the fluid energy has been dissipated in the arterioles and capillaries, the dynamic component is relatively low, hovering around 15 to 20 mmHg in the venules and falling to 0 to 6 mmHg in the right atrium. Consequently, in any position other than horizontal, hydrostatic pressure may greatly exceed dynamic pressure. For practical purposes, we can estimate hydrostatic pressure at any point by measuring the distance from that point to the right atrium (Eq. 7.1).

For example, in an individual 6 feet tall (ankle to atrial distance of 131 cm), venous pressure at the ankle would be increased by 102 mmHg in the standing position (Fig. 7–29). If the pressure in the ankle veins were 15 mmHg in a supine position, it would be 15 + 102 = 117 mmHg in the standing position. The intra-arterial pressure would increase by a similar amount. Static filling pressure is so low (only a few mmHg) that it can be neglected.

Because of the increased intravenous pressure, dependent veins dilate, allowing blood to accumulate in the veins of the leg. When a typical individual is tilted from a supine to a standing position, about 250 ml of blood is shifted to each leg.[337] This might produce syncope were it not for the effect of the muscle pump mechanism that ordinarily is operative in the upright position. Active venous constriction does not occur as a reflex response to orthostasis.[341]

At wrist level in the raised arm of an upright individual, the hydrostatic component would be decreased by about 50 mmHg. If venous pressure at the wrist were 15 mmHg in the supine position, the pressure at wrist level might be expected to fall below atmospheric pressure:

$$15\ \text{mmHg} - 50\ \text{mmHg} = -35\ \text{mmHg} \qquad (7.28)$$

Obviously, this is impossible, because the combined effect of the tissue pressure (5 mmHg) and the atmospheric pressure would collapse the veins. Thus, venous pressure in a portion of the body above the heart cannot fall below tissue pressure (see Fig. 7–29).

Venous Pressure-Volume Relationships

Because veins are collapsible tubes, a great variation in venous capacity is possible with little change in venous pressure—a property that adapts veins to their unique role as the major storage facility for blood.

Transmural pressure is the difference in pressure between the intraluminal pressure acting to expand the vein and the tissue pressure acting from the outside to collapse the vein. When venous transmural pressure is increased from 0 to 15 mmHg, the volume of the vein may increase by more than 250%.[316] This vast change in volume is due largely to

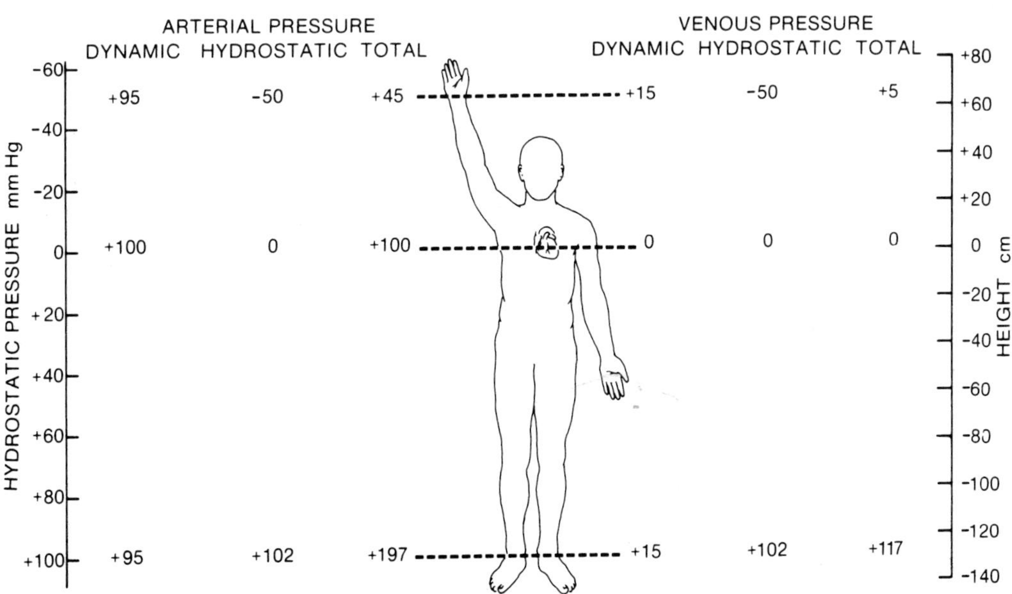

FIGURE 7–29. Effect of standing position on venous and arterial pressures. Zero pressure is at the level of the right atrium. Dynamic pressure represents that produced by the contraction of the left ventricle. If the subject were horizontal, the total intravascular pressure would closely approximate the dynamic pressure because there would be little hydrostatic effect.

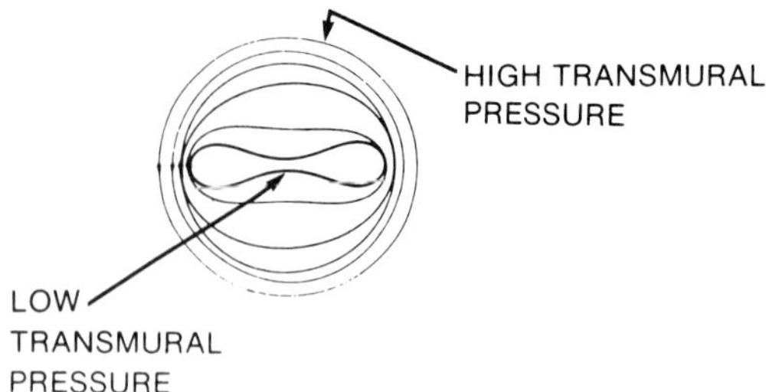

FIGURE 7–30. Cross section of venous lumen at various transmural pressures. At low pressure, the wall collapses into an elliptical configuration; at higher pressures, it becomes circular. Note that the wall also stretches with increasing pressure. (Adapted from Moreno AH, Katz AI, Gold LD, Reddy RV: Mechanics of distention of dog veins and other thin-walled tubular structures. Circ Res 27:1069, 1970. By permission of the American Heart Association, Inc.)

the fact that the cross section of the venous lumen, which is elliptical at low transmural pressures, becomes circular at higher transmural pressures (Fig. 7–30). Little increase in pressure is required to convert a low-volume elliptical tube into a high-volume circular tube, but much more pressure is required to stretch the venous wall once the circular configuration has been reached. In fact, veins are as stiff as arteries when subjected to arterial pressure (Fig. 7–31).[236, 306, 316, 355]

Venous Blood Flow

Like fluid in all hydraulic systems, blood in the veins is propelled from one point to another by an energy gradient and is impeded by multiple factors that constitute resistance to flow. According to Bernoulli's principle, total fluid energy at any point in the venous system consists of (1) the sum of the hydrostatic pressure, (2) the gravitational potential energy, (3) the kinetic energy, and (4) the dynamic pressure produced by contraction of the left ventricle and the surrounding skeletal muscles (Eq. 7.4).

Because hydrostatic pressure and gravitational potential energy are equivalent but have opposite signs, they usually cancel each other; therefore, for most purposes it is sufficient to consider dynamic pressure as the driving force. For example, in the upright individual pictured in Figure 7–29, the energy gradient returning blood from the ankle to the heart is 15 mmHg (the dynamic pressure gradient), not 117 mmHg (the sum of the hydrostatic and dynamic pressures at the ankle). The situation is somewhat different in the raised arm. At wrist level, the pressure is only 5 mmHg (the minimal value necessary to prevent collapse by tissue pressure), but the gradient returning blood to the heart is equivalent to about 50 mmHg because of the positive gravitational positional energy. Thus, blood in the elevated arm essentially "falls" back to the heart. As explained later, a similar situation prevails in the legs when venous valves are incompetent.

Although veins are commonly considered to be low-resistance conduits, the energy gradient from the venules to the right atrium is equal to that from the left ventricle to the arterioles (~15 mmHg). Because veins transport the same amount of blood as arteries and have a potential cross-sectional area three or four times as large, this seems somewhat incongruous. Veins, however, are seldom completely distended. The elliptical cross section assumed in their usual, partially collapsed state offers far more resistance than that dictated by a circular cross section. As veins distend, their resistance falls markedly, allowing increases in blood flow to be accommodated with little increase in the energy gradient.

In the arterial system, pressure, vascular volume, and flow usually change in the same direction. In veins, the opposite frequently occurs; venous pressure and venous volume may decrease as flow increases and may increase as flow decreases or reverses (Fig. 7–32). This apparent paradox is explained by the fact that in the resting state, peripheral venous pressure (P_{pv}) tends to remain relatively constant, whereas central venous pressure (P_{cv}) fluctuates. When central venous pressure falls, the pressure gradient across the intervening segment increases and—provided that the venous resistance (R_v) does not change appreciably—flow (Q_v) increases. At the same time, pressure in the venous segment, which must lie somewhere between peripheral and central pressures, falls. Because venous volume is a function of venous pressure, the volume of the segment also falls. In contrast, when central venous pressure rises, pressure and volume increase while flow ceases or reverses. During exercise, however, contraction of the skeletal muscles momentarily increases peripheral pressure, and venous flow, pressure, and volume are augmented simultaneously.

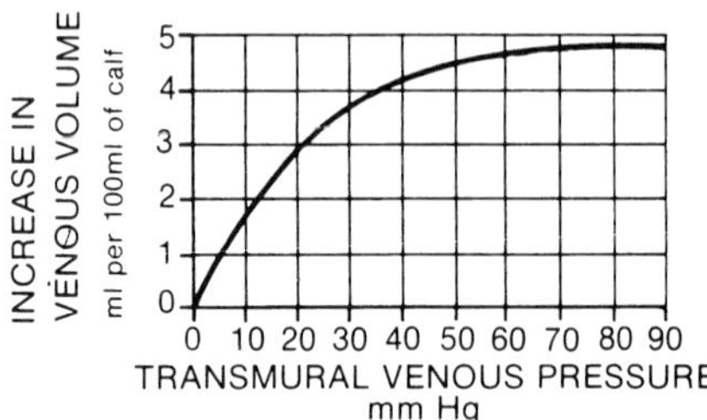

FIGURE 7–31. Relationship of venous volume to transmural pressure. Veins are very compliant at low pressure but are quite stiff at high pressure.

Effect of Cardiac Contraction

The mechanism just described explains how venous flow and pressure are influenced by events occurring in the right side of the heart during the various phases of the cardiac cycle. As shown in Figure 7–33, contraction of the right atrium elevates central venous pressure and causes a transient reversal of venous blood flow. During ventricular systole, the atrium relaxes, venous flow increases, and venous pressure falls. Flow then decreases during diastole until the pressure differential across the tricuspid valve causes the valve to open. At this point, there is again a brief increase in flow, which is followed by a gradual decline to zero.

Although these cardiac-induced flow and pressure pulsations are most easily perceived in the jugular veins, they may be detected with the Doppler flowmeter in the arm veins of resting subjects (Fig. 7–34). Cardiac pulsations are less evident in leg veins, where they tend to be obscured by the large fluctuations in flow produced by respiratory

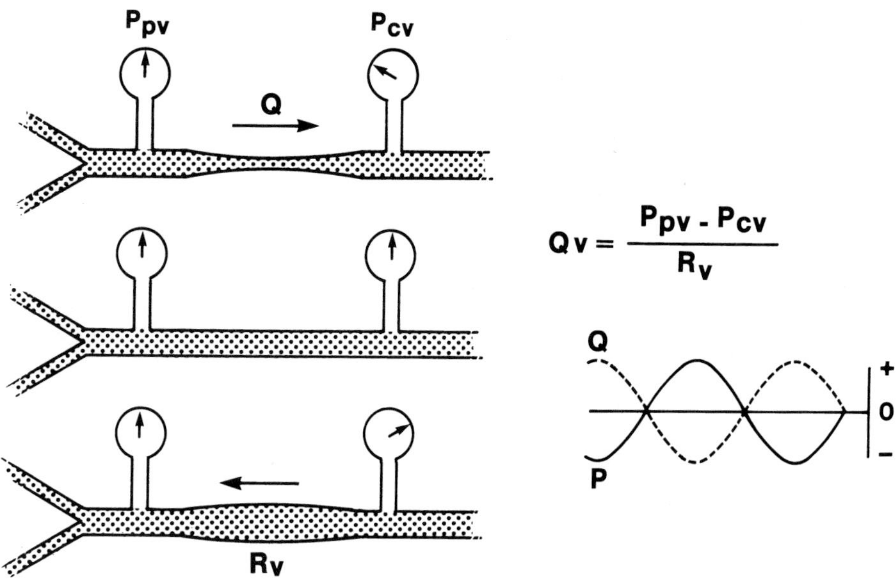

FIGURE 7–32. Relationship of flow (Q_v) in a venous segment to venous resistance (R_v), peripheral venous pressure (P_{pv}), and central venous pressure (P_{cv}). As flow increases, the vein collapses and pressure (P) in the mid-portion of the venous segment decreases. As flow decreases, the opposite occurs: pressure increases and the vein expands. Increasing pressure is indicated by a clockwise movement of the arrows on the meters. (From Sumner DS: Applied physiology in venous problems. *In* Bergan JJ, Yao JST [eds]: Surgery of the Veins. Orlando, Grune & Stratton, 1985, pp 3–23.)

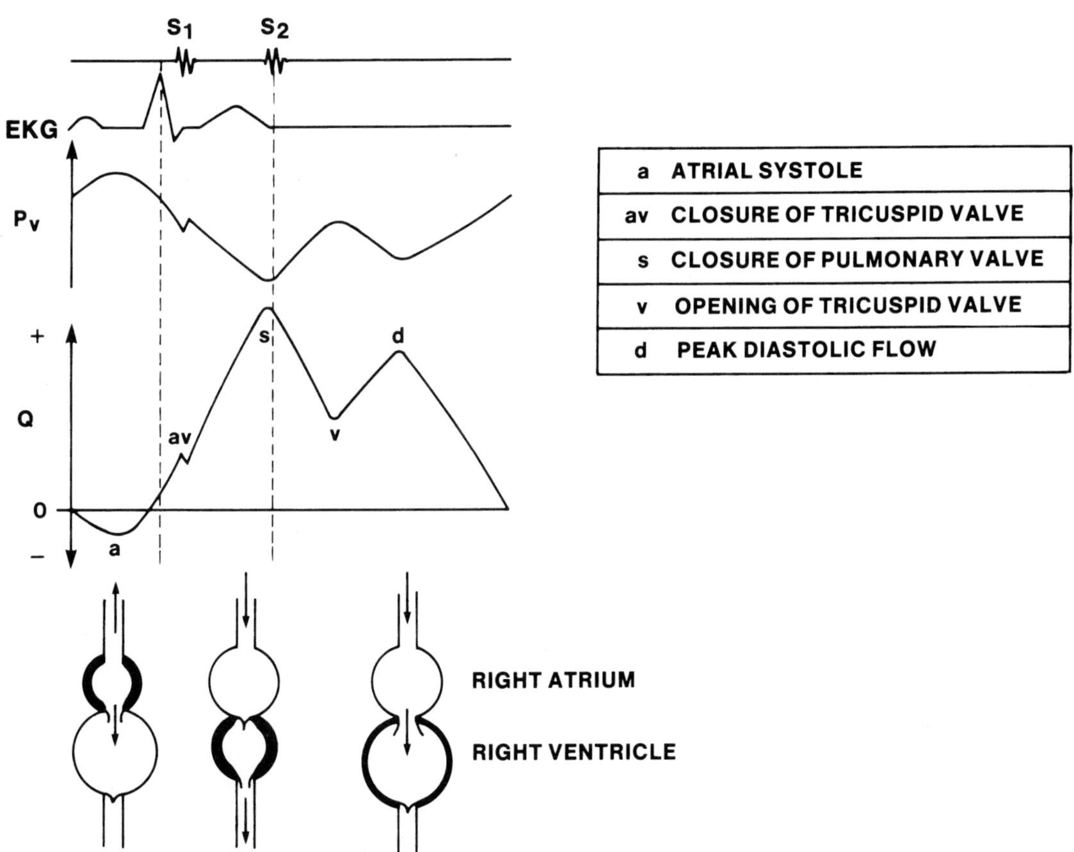

a	ATRIAL SYSTOLE
av	CLOSURE OF TRICUSPID VALVE
s	CLOSURE OF PULMONARY VALVE
v	OPENING OF TRICUSPID VALVE
d	PEAK DIASTOLIC FLOW

FIGURE 7–33. Effect of cardiac contraction on venous pressure (P_v) and venous blood flow (Q). *Vertical dashed lines* define the period of ventricular systole. First and second heart sounds are indicated by S_1 and S_2, respectively. EKG = electrocardiogram. (From Sumner DS: Applied physiology in venous problems. *In* Bergan JJ, Yao JST [eds]: Surgery of the Veins. Orlando, Grune & Stratton, 1985, pp 3–23.)

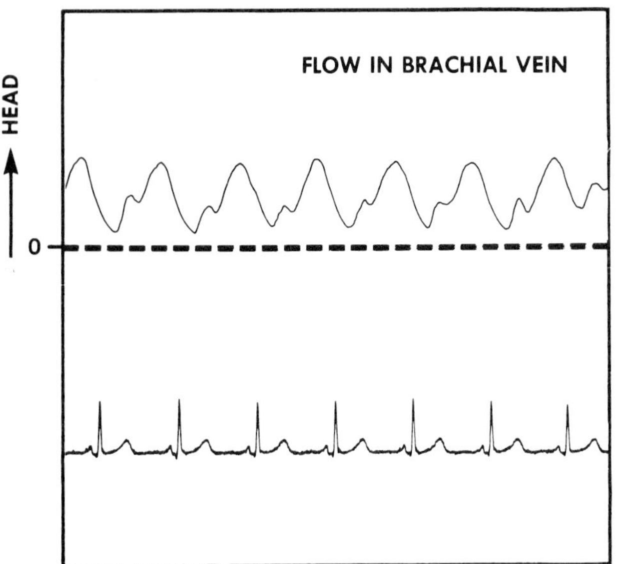

FIGURE 7–34. Doppler recordings of flow in a brachial vein demonstrating pulsations imposed by cardiac contraction. (From Sumner DS: Noninvasive vascular laboratory assessment. *In* Machleder HI [ed]: Vascular Disorders of the Upper Extremity. 3rd ed. Armonk, NY, Futura Publishing Company, 1998, pp 15–62.)

activity. In cases of congestive heart failure, the increased central venous pressure overcomes the respiratory effects, and cardiac pulsations become a prominent feature of the venous flow pattern in the lower extremities.

Flow Through Collapsible Tubes

The collapsible nature of the venous wall is responsible for a peculiar pressure-flow relationship unique to the venous system.[272, 283, 307, 308] These relationships are clarified by the model illustrated in Figure 7–35*A*. In this figure, the energy (15 cm H_2O) driving blood back to the heart is represented by an elevated fluid reservoir. The collapsible tube passes through a closed container that has a certain pressure, in this case, 5 cm H_2O. The end of the tube, representing the right atrium, is open to the atomsphere at baseline level, giving an outflow pressure of 0 cm H_2O.

Pressure in the collapsible tube must rise until it slightly exceeds that within the closed container for the tube to open enough to permit fluid to flow through the system. Thus, flow through the tube depends on the gradient 15 cm H_2O − 5 cm H_2O = 10 cm H_2O rather than on the gradient across the entire length of the tube (15 cm H_2O). It is evident that elevating the driving pressure linearly increases the pressure gradient and, within limits, has the same effect on flow (Fig. 7–35*B*). On the other hand, changes in outflow pressure have no effect on flow unless the outflow pressure rises above the pressure in the closed container, at which point the collapsible tube remains distended (Fig. 7–35*C*). Further increases in outflow pressure decrease the pressure gradient (which now depends on the difference between the driving pressure and the outflow pressure). As a result, flow through the system decreases as the outflow pressure rises above the pressure in the closed container. Clearly, increasing the pressure within the container, while the driving and outflow pressures are maintained at constant levels, decreases flow (Fig. 7–35*D*).

Effect of Respiration

Respiration has a major effect on patterns of venous flow. In a supine subject, the abdominal cavity corresponds to the "closed container" through which the collapsible inferior vena cava must pass (Fig. 7–36). Thus, the pressure gradient driving blood centrally from the legs is the venous pressure in the legs minus the intra-abdominal pressure. When the subject inspires, the diaphragm descends, thereby increasing intra-abdominal pressure. This has the effect of decreasing the pressure gradient and of decreasing blood flow during inspiration. Often the rise in abdominal pressure is sufficient to cause venous outflow from the legs to cease momentarily. During expiration, the diaphragm relaxes, intra-abdominal pressure falls, the inferior vena cava expands, and blood trapped in the leg veins flows cephalad into the abdomen.

These patterns are so consistent that they constitute an important indicator of normal venous flow.[356]

When flow from the upper extremities or the head and neck is considered, the high-pressure "closed container" becomes the extrathoracic tissue pressure, and the "outflow" becomes the intrathoracic venous pressure (see Fig. 7–36). Because the latter ordinarily is lower than the former, respiratory movements have relatively less effect on outflow from the arms and cephalic regions. In general, venous flow *increases* during *inspiration* as the intrathoracic pressure falls and *decreases* during *expiration* as the pressure rises.

As one would predict from the closed container model (see Fig. 7–35), peripheral venous pressures do not reflect the central venous pressure accurately unless the latter is elevated. In cases of congestive heart failure, tricuspid insufficiency, or pulmonary hypertension, central venous pressures rise above tissue pressures and even above abdominal pressures, permitting events of the right side of the heart to be reflected in the peripheral venous flow pattern. As previously discussed, conditions that cause elevated central venous pressure result in a pulsatile flow pattern far distally in the veins of both the upper and the lower extremities.

VENOUS FUNCTION

The primary and most obvious function of the venous system is to return blood to the heart from the capillary beds. In addition, veins play the predominant role in regulating vascular capacity. They also serve as a part of the peripheral pump mechanism, which assists the heart in the transport of blood during exercise. Together with the capillaries, they contribute to the thermoregulatory system of the body.

These vital functions all depend on certain peculiarities of venous anatomy and wall structure and on the presence of venous valves.

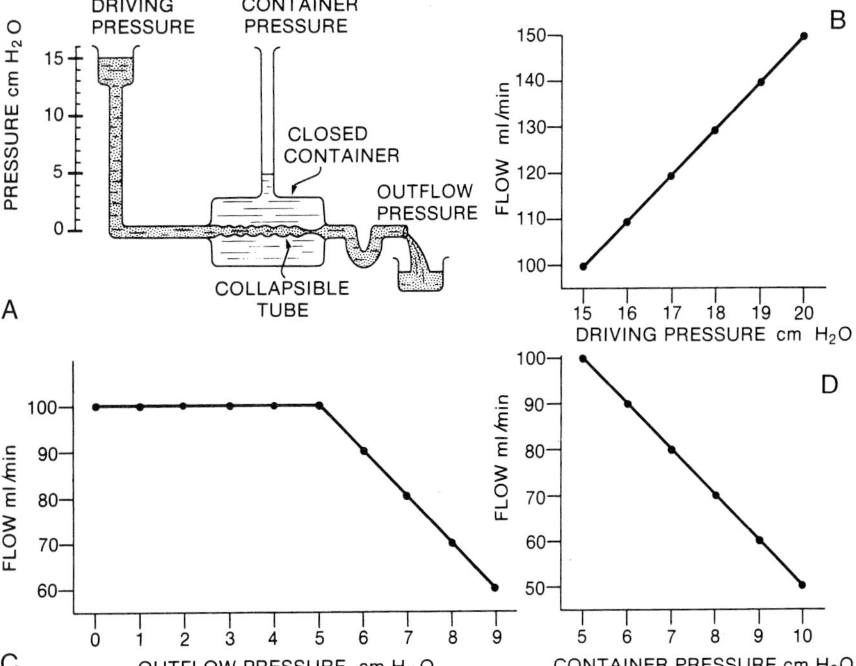

FIGURE 7–35. *A*, Model illustrating "collapsible tube" phenomenon. *B*, Effect of elevating the driving pressure while maintaining container pressure and outflow pressure constant. *C*, Effect of elevating outflow pressure while maintaining driving pressure and container pressure constant. *D*, Effect of elevating container pressure while maintaining driving pressure and outflow pressure constant.

Anatomy and Wall Structures

Superficial veins are relatively thick-walled, muscular structures that lie just under the skin. Among the superficial veins are the greater and lesser saphenous veins of the leg, the cephalic and basilic veins of the arm, and the external jugular veins of the neck. The deep veins are thin-walled and less muscular. They accompany arteries—often as venae comitantes—and bear the same names as the arteries they parallel. The cross-sectional area of these veins is roughly three times that of the adjacent arteries.[257]

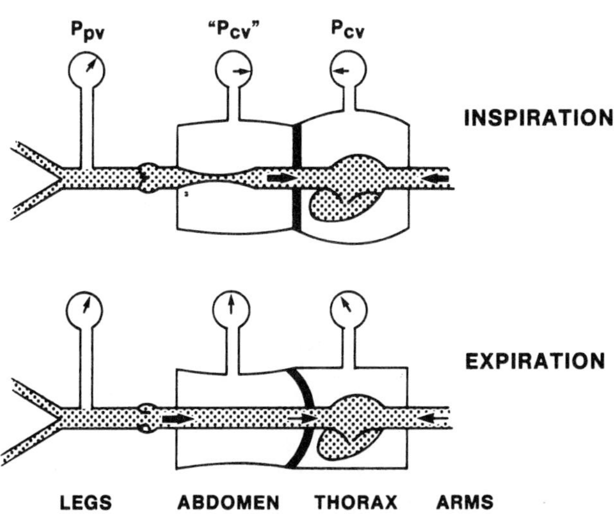

FIGURE 7–36. Effect of respiration on venous blood from the lower extremity, upper abdomen, and brachiocephalic area. Intra-abdominal pressure ("P_{cv}") increases during inspiration and decreases during expiration. (From Sumner DS: Applied physiology in venous problems. *In* Bergan JJ, Yao JST [eds]: Surgery of the Veins. Orlando, Grune & Stratton, 1985, pp 3–23.)

Within the skeletal muscles are large, very thin-walled veins sometimes referred to as *sinusoids.* As part of the "bellows" of the muscle pump mechanism, they serve a particularly important function during exercise. The soleal sinusoids empty into the posterior tibial vein, and the gastrocnemius sinusoids usually drain into the popliteal vein.

In addition to the foregoing, *perforating veins* connect the deep and superficial systems. Of particular interest to the surgeon are a series of about six medial calf perforators that join the posterior tibial vein to the greater saphenous system through a network of superficial veins known as the "posterior arch vein."[349] Other perforators connect the peroneal vein with superficial tributaries of the saphenous vein. Posteriorly, a series of small perforating veins connects the superficial system with the intramuscular veins; these in turn are united at various levels with the posterior tibial vein. Thus, an indirect connection between the superficial and deep systems is provided via the large intramuscular veins.

Perhaps the most important anatomic feature of veins is the presence of *valves* (Fig. 7–37). Each of these delicate but extremely strong bicuspid structures lies at the base of a segment of vein that is expanded into a sinus. This arrangement permits the valves to open widely without coming into contact with the wall, thus permitting rapid closure when flow begins to reverse (within 0.5 second).[311, 366]

There are approximately 9 to 11 valves in the anterior tibial vein, 9 to 19 in the posterior tibial, 7 in the peroneal, 1 in the popliteal, and 3 in the superficial femoral vein. In two thirds of the femoral veins, a valve is present at the upper end within 1 cm of the inguinal ligament. About one quarter of the external iliac veins and one tenth of the internal iliac veins have a valve.[297] The common iliac vein usually has no valves. Superficial veins have fewer valves,

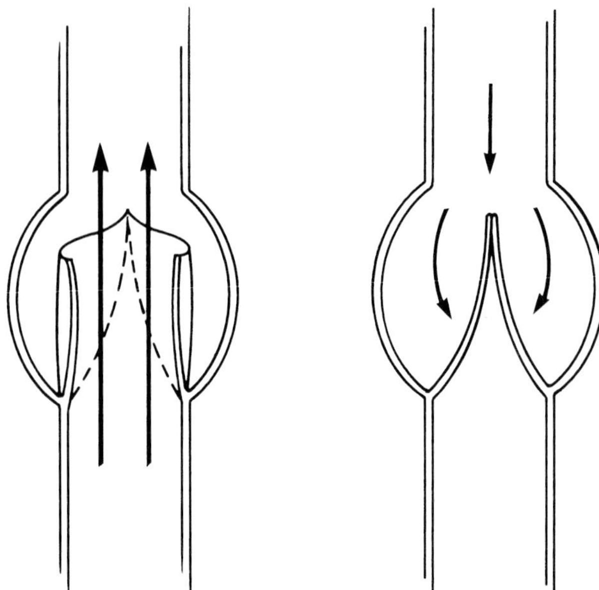

FIGURE 7–37. Representation of a longitudinal section through a venous valve demonstrating the role of sinuses in facilitating opening and closing of valve cusps. (From Sumner DS: Applied physiology in venous problems. *In* Bergan JJ, Yao JST [eds]: Surgery of the Veins. Orlando, Grune & Stratton, 1985, pp 3–23.)

approximately 7 to 9 in the greater and lesser saphenous veins.[242, 275, 303] Valves are present in venules as small as 0.15 mm in diameter.

In all areas of the legs and arms, valve cusps are oriented to direct flow centrally and to prevent reflux. Although the classic teaching is that valves in perforating veins permit blood to flow only from the superficial to the deep venous system, studies have suggested that outward flow occurs in about one fifth of normal limbs under certain conditions.[342] There is also some controversy about the direction of flow in the perforating veins of the foot. Although previous investigators maintained that the foot is unique, in that flow is directed from the deep to the superficial veins,[286, 291] studies by Koslow and DeWeese have suggested that the direction is consistent with that in other segments of the leg (i.e., from superficial to deep).[290]

During the course of the day, there may be some deterioration in valve function, even in normal extremities. About one fifth of otherwise normal legs show evidence of venous reflux after 5 or more hours of upright activity, presumably as a result of venous distention, which renders the valves partially incompetent.[343]

Muscle Pump

The return of blood from the legs to the heart against the force of gravity is facilitated by the muscle pump mechanism. The muscles of the leg act as the power source, and the veins act as the bellows. Although the superficial veins participate, the deep veins and the intramuscular sinusoids play the major role. The presence of competent valves is necessary to ensure that the pump functions efficiently.

When a person with normal leg veins shifts from a horizontal to a vertical position, blood stored in the abdominal and pelvic veins is prevented from "falling" down the leg (in accordance with the gravitational potential energy gradient) by the rapid closure of functioning valves.[358] Capillary inflow gradually fills the calf veins over 70 to 170 seconds until the hydrostatic pressure and gravitational potential energy levels cancel out.[254, 374] From this point on, the dynamic pressure differential again forces blood to flow upward out of the leg. Thus, in the motionless, upright subject, veins simply collect blood from capillaries and transport it passively to the heart, with the energy being supplied totally by left ventricular contraction. Because the venous valves are all open, the column of blood in the veins extends uninterrupted to the right atrium, and the venous pressure at any level equals the sum of the dynamic and hydrostatic pressures (Fig. 7–38*A*). The volume of blood accumulated depends on the total venous pressure and the compliance of the calf veins.

During exercise, skeletal muscle contraction compresses the intramuscular and surrounding veins, raises venous pressure, and forces blood cephalad toward the heart. Closure of valves below the site of compression prevents retrograde flow (Fig. 7–38*B*). On relaxation, the pressure gradient reverses; the valves above the site of compression close, precluding reflux, and the veins remain partially collapsed until they are refilled by inflow from the capillaries. Blood in the partially empty veins is now segregated into short compartments a few centimeters long, within which pressure is diminished in accordance with the venous pressure-volume compliance curve (see Figs. 7–31 and 7–38*C*).[319, 332, 358] (This segregation is seldom visible phlebographically because veins, even at the upper end of each compartment, remain partially filled.) Figure 7–38*C* presents an exaggerated picture to emphasize the reduction in venous pressure.

After a few strong muscular contractions (as in walking

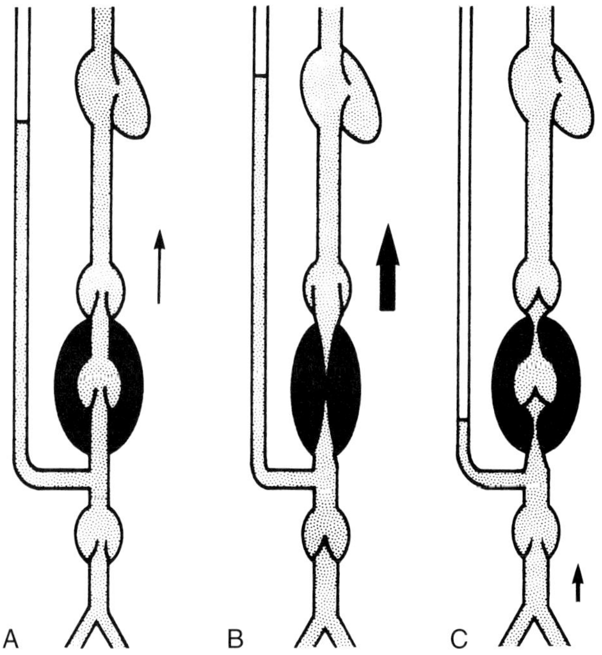

FIGURE 7–38. Operation of the muscle pump. *A*, Resting. *B*, Muscle contraction. *C*, Muscle relaxation. Venous pressure in the distal leg is indicated by the length of the hydrostatic column. (*A–C*, From Sumner DS: Applied physiology in venous disease. *In* Sakaguchi S [ed]: Advances in Phlebology. London, John Libbey and Company, 1987, pp 5–16.)

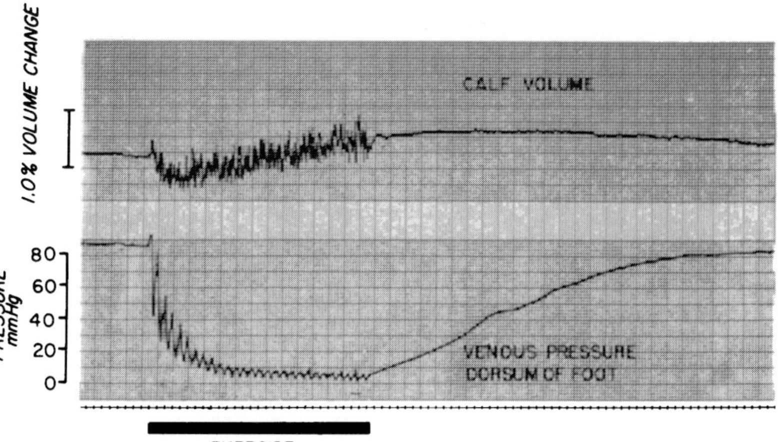

FIGURE 7–39. Effect of exercise on venous pressure at foot level in a subject 5 feet 8 inches tall. (From Strandness DE Jr, Sumner DS: Hemodynamics for Surgeons. New York, Grune & Stratton, 1975.)

or running), venous pressure at the ankle or foot falls to very low levels in normal limbs, often below 20 mmHg (Fig. 7–39).[281, 282, 328, 354, 355] The level reached during exercise is commonly referred to as the *ambulatory venous pressure*.

Valves at the top of each segregated compartment remain closed until the venous pressure just below the valve rises to exceed the pressure at the lower end of the compartment immediately above.[358] Thus, the pressure at the lower end of each compartment usually exceeds the length of the hydrostatic column defined by valve closure.[332] With continued venous refilling, the hydrostatic column is reestablished all the way to the heart.

The muscle pump mechanism is most highly developed in the calf, where the voluminous soleal and gastrocnemial sinusoids compose the major part of the bellows. Contraction of the calf muscles generates extravascular pressures ranging from 40 to 200 mmHg.[229, 302, 303] This produces an equivalent reduction in venous transmural pressure and displaces blood from the compressed venous sinusoids in accordance with the venous volume/transmural pressure compliance curve (see Fig. 7–31).[358] Because of the strong fascial investment of the calf muscles, the intermuscular veins (posterior tibial, anterior tibial, and peroneal) are subjected to similar pressures. Much of the force is also transmitted to the surrounding superficial veins through the connective tissues. Thus, all the veins of the lower leg—both superficial and deep—participate to a greater or lesser degree in the pumping action. All transmit blood centrally with each muscular contraction (Fig. 7–40).[354]

Although pressure in the deep veins exceeds that in the superficial veins during muscle contraction, valves in the perforating veins prevent flow from the deep to the superficial system.[235] (As previously noted, there may be exceptions to this rule.[342]) Valves also prevent the displacement of blood distally toward the foot in the tibial veins. When the muscles relax, the venous sinusoids are refilled by capillary inflow and by flow from the distal deep veins of

FIGURE 7–40. Dynamics of venous blood flow in response to calf muscle contraction in a normal limb. (From Sumner DS: Venous dynamics—varicosities. Clin Obstet Gynecol 24:743, 1981.)

the leg. Some inflow from superficial to deep veins also occurs, but the magnitude of this flow is less than formerly thought (see Fig. 7–40).[230, 354, 355]

Studies suggest that the upward flow of blood in the leg may be initiated by compression of the plantar plexus of veins lying between the deep and superficial intrinsic muscles of the foot. This blood is discharged into the deep veins of the calf, thus priming the muscle pump.[290] The events during normal walking are synchronized in the following order[273]:

1. Dorsiflexion of the foot empties the distal calf veins.
2. Weight bearing empties the foot.
3. Plantar flexion empties the proximal calf veins.

Effects of Venous Pressure Reduction

Reduction of venous pressure facilitates flow through the capillary bed of exercising muscles in the following manner: total pressure in peripheral arteries equals the sum of hydrostatic pressure and pressure generated by left ventricle.

For example, at the arteriolar end of a calf muscle capillary, the total pressure might be 102 mmHg (hydrostatic pressure) plus 95 mmHg (mean dynamic pressure), or 197 mmHg (see Fig. 7–29). During quiet standing, the venous pressure would be 102 mmHg (hydrostatic pressure) plus 15 mmHg (dynamic pressure), or 117 mmHg. This gives a pressure gradient across the muscle arterioles and capillaries of 197 minus 117, or 80 mmHg. With muscle contraction, however, the venous pressure is reduced to 20 mmHg or less. Under these circumstances, the pressure gradient rises to 197 minus 20, or 177 mmHg. Together with the reduction in arteriolar resistance that accompanies exercise, this simple method of increasing the pressure gradient affords a remarkably effective way of augmenting muscle perfusion. Indeed, as much as 30% of the energy required to circulate blood during strenuous exercise may be furnished by the muscle pump, which in a sense acts as a "peripheral heart."[354]

Aside from augmenting blood flow to exercising muscles, the muscle pump, by reducing venous pressure, acts to decrease the volume of blood sequestered in dependent parts of the body. By translocating blood from the peripheral to the central veins, the muscle pump also serves to enhance cardiac function, particularly during exercise.

In addition, reduction of venous pressure decreases the rate of edema formation in the dependent parts of the lower extremities. According to the *Starling concept,* most of the fluid escaping from the arteriolar end of a capillary is returned to the circulation at the venular end (Fig. 7–41).[245, 295, 353, 360] Any excess is removed by lymphatics. The forces acting to drive fluid out of the capillary are the capillary pressure, P_c, and the osmotic pressure of the interstitial fluid, π_{IF}. Acting to return fluid to the circulation are the interstitial fluid pressure, P_{IF}, and the osmotic pressure of the blood, π_c. Therefore, the net pressure, P, moving fluid out of the capillary, is

$$P = P_c + \pi_{IF} - P_{IF} - \pi_c \qquad (7.29)$$

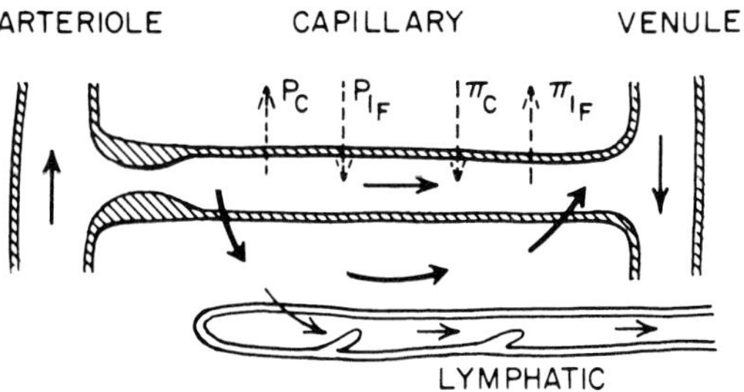

Pressures (mm Hg)

	Arteriolar	Mean capillary	Venular
P_C	35	25	15
P_{IF}	5	5	5
π_C	25	25	25
π_{IF}	5	5	5
P	+10	0	−10

FIGURE 7–41. Fluid exchange in the capillary bed. *Solid arrows* indicate the direction of fluid flow. *Dashed arrows* show the direction of pressure gradients. (From Strandness DE Jr, Sumner DS: Hemodynamics for Surgeons. New York, Grune & Stratton, 1975.)

As shown in Figure 7–41, the mean capillary pressure of +25 mmHg is exactly balanced by the sum of the other pressures:*

$$\pi_{IF} - P_{IF} - \pi_c = +5 - 5 - 25 = -25 \text{ mmHg} \qquad (7.30)$$

Thus, in the supine position, there is little or no net pressure gradient across the capillary wall; however, this equilibrium is disturbed in the dependent parts of an upright individual. For example, if the mean capillary pressure, P_c, is assumed to be 25 mmHg at ankle level in a supine subject, it would rise to about 127 mmHg (25 + 102) in the standing subject (see Fig. 7–29). This creates a pressure gradient of 127 − 25 = 102 mmHg across the capillary wall and encourages the outflow of fluid into the interstitial spaces. The escape of fluid continues until interstitial pressure, P_{IF}, rises sufficiently to balance the high intracapillary pressure. (The rate of fluid transfer is controlled by capillary surface area and permeability.[309]) Because the interstitial tissues are remarkably compliant at low interstitial fluid pressures, a great deal of edema fluid must accumulate before a new equilibrium can be established.[276, 360]

*The magnitude of the interstitial fluid pressure (P_{IF}) has been the subject of considerable debate.[245, 360] Although originally P_{IF} was thought to range between +1 and +5 mmHg, most current evidence suggests that it is actually subatomospheric, on the order of −2 to −7 mmHg. Substituting these negative values for P_{IF} in Equation 7.29 gives a value of +13 to +18 for the intravascular pressure at the mid-point of the capillary (P_c). Thus, some of the numbers in Figure 7–41 and in the accompanying text are changed; however, the basic concepts of transcapillary fluid exchange remain the same.

Total tissue pressure is the sum of the interstitial fluid pressure and the "solid tissue pressure" that is exerted by collagen and ground substance. If the structural elements responsible for solid tissue pressure are compressed, the solid tissue pressure will be positive. Consequently, total tissue pressure commonly ranges between +1 and +5 mmHg. It is this total tissue pressure that determines the transmural pressure across the capillaries and veins. Total tissue pressure and interstitial fluid pressure become equal when edema develops.

Fortunately, if venous valvular function is normal, slight to moderate calf muscle activity markedly reduces venous pressure. In turn, mean capillary pressure falls and the rate of edema formation decreases. Together with arteriolar constriction, which occurs in response to standing, this mechanism keeps edema formation to a minimum.

In summary, the muscle pump serves several important functions:

1. Assists the heart in circulating blood during exercise.
2. Increases central blood volume.
3. Relieves venous congestion in the legs.
4. Decreases peripheral edema.
5. Facilitates flow through exercising muscles.

Although these are not vital functions, their absence creates significant disability.

Control of Venous Capacity

About two thirds of the blood in the body is contained within the venous system. Even so, the total potential venous volume is far from filled. This means that some veins are always partially or completely collapsed. In a state of partial collapse, great fluctuations in venous volume are possible with little change in transmural pressure. This flexibility allows the normal venous reservoir to accept transfusions, intravenous fluids, and blood loss over wide ranges without changing the central venous pressure appreciably. Only when venous pressures are high and veins are filled does excess fluid result in large rises in central venous pressure. Similarly, a nearly empty system may be critically sensitive to sudden blood loss.

Venous capacity is affected not only by fluctuations in transmural pressure but also by the contractile state of the smooth muscle in the venous wall. When transmural pressures are low and veins have collapsed into an elliptical cross section, venomotor tone has little effect on venous capacity; however, when veins are filled sufficiently to assume a circular cross section, venomotor tone plays an important role in regulating venous volume.[324]

Unlike arterioles, which are very sensitive to the local chemical environment, venules and veins are controlled almost exclusively by sympathetic adrenergic activity. In addition, unlike the resting tone of arterioles and arteries, which are almost always partially constricted, the resting tone of veins is minimal under comfortable environmental conditions. Veins within skeletal muscles are devoid of sympathetic innervation, and cutaneous veins are primarily thermoregulatory.[305, 371] Peripheral veins contract more intensely to sympathetic stimuli than the more centrally located veins.

As a rule, veins constrict in response to stimuli that cause an increase in cardiac output.[347] Simultaneously, there usually is a decrease in total peripheral resistance. Because the systemic resistance to blood flow is largely controlled by arterioles, wall tension in veins must increase in conjunction with a decrease in arteriolar tone. Often this disparity of action is related to the vasodilator effect of the local chemical environment on the arterioles that overpowers the systemic adrenergic activity, but sometimes adrenergic activity is directly responsible for simultaneous arteriolar constriction and dilation of the capacitance vessels.[249]

Among the stimuli known to produce venous constriction are pain, emotion, hyperventilation, deep breathing, the Valsalva maneuver, and muscular exercise.[348] The decrease in venous volume that occurs after a deep breath provides a convenient method for assessing the integrity of the sympathetic nerve supply to an extremity. As shown in Chapter 79, Figure 79–7, the volume of a finger or toe, measured plethysmographically, decreases promptly after a deep breath if the sympathetic nerves are intact.

By reducing the peripheral venous volume, venoconstriction during exercise assists the muscular pump mechanism in transferring blood to the central circulation, where it is required to maintain the increased cardiac output. Moreover, the reduced caliber of the veins serves to accelerate venous return. Although venoconstriction increases the hemodynamic resistance of the veins slightly, this effect is more than offset by the accompanying arteriolar dilatation. The intramuscular sinusoids, which are devoid of sympathetic innervation, do not constrict with exercise.[348] Constriction of these veins would not be beneficial because they constitute the major bellows of the muscle pump.

Following hemorrhage, veins constrict both passively, in response to a decreased transmural pressure, and actively, as a result of increased venous tone. With prolonged shock, venoconstriction may give way to dilatation.

Cold causes veins to constrict both directly and as a general reflex response.[367] Although veins do not dilate in response to heat, heat negates the venoconstrictor response to deep breathing, exercise, or other such stimuli. The venous system is particularly important in the regulation of body temperature because superficial veins lie just under the skin, allowing easy transmission of heat from the interior of the body to the skin surface. Within this system, blood flow is slow, giving ample opportunity for the escape of heat. When conservation of heat becomes necessary, the superficial veins constrict, causing venous return to be diverted to the deep veins, which lie in close proximity to the arteries. Not only is the distance to the skin surface increased by this reflex, but the anatomic arrangement of the deep arteries and veins also results in a countercurrent exchange of heat from artery to vein, thus further conserving heat from the interior of the body.

Curiously, venous constriction occurring in response to standing is at best slight and transient and is probably the result of emotional stimuli.[341] Teleologically, leg veins would be expected to constrict in the upright position in order to prevent dependent pooling of blood. Although reflex arteriolar constriction provides some protection against gravitationally induced fluid shifts, the major protection is provided by the muscle pump.

Veins *constrict* in response to epinephrine, norepinephrine, phenylephrine, serotonin, and histamine; they *dilate* in response to phenoxybenzamine, phentolamine, reserpine, guanethidine, nitroglycerin, nitroprusside, barbiturates, and many anesthetic agents. Administration of isoproterenol sometimes appears to cause constriction, but at other times it results in dilatation.

ACUTE VENOUS THROMBOSIS

Small nonocclusive venous thrombi produce no recognizable physiologic defects. When venous obstruction becomes sufficiently extensive, however, physiologic aberrations appear. The resulting changes, all related to an elevation in peripheral venous pressure, include venous congestion and edema. Rarely, shock results from fluid leaking into tissue spaces. In severe cases, the blockage may be so complete that ischemia occurs.

The magnitude of the peripheral venous pressure, P_{pv}, is related to the central venous pressure, P_{cv}; to the blood flow through the part, Q_v; and to the hemodynamic resistance of the intervening veins, R_v (Fig. 7–42):

$$P_{pv} - P_{cv} = Q_v R_v \quad (7.31)$$

or

$$P_{pv} = Q_v R_v + P_{cv}$$

This equation indicates that peripheral venous pressure increases when the central venous pressure rises. Because central venous pressure is usually lower than the intra-abdominal pressure in supine subjects, P_{cv} can be taken to represent the intra-abdominal pressure. This is a manifestation of the *collapsible tube phenomenon,* in which the abdomen acts as a closed container (see Fig. 7–35). As discussed earlier, the inspiratory descent of the diaphragm increases intra-abdominal pressure ("P_{cv}"), decreases blood flow temporarily, and then increases the peripheral pressure, P_{pv}, as blood flow rises to its preinspiratory level (Fig. 7–43). These respiratory fluctuations, so prominent in normal limbs, are partially or completely masked in limbs with deep venous thrombosis (DVT).[356]

Because central venous pressure (P_{cv}) is ordinarily quite low, peripheral venous pressure in limbs with venous obstruction is largely dependent on the product of the blood flow through the limb and the venous resistance ($Q_v R_v$). Thrombotic venous obstruction raises venous resistance but has little effect on total limb blood flow (unless the obstructive process is very extensive and severe). Because blood flow remains unchanged, peripheral venous pressure is elevated commensurate with the increase in venous resistance (Eq. 7.31). *Thus, most significant increases in peripheral venous pressure are related to an increased hemodynamic resistance of the veins.*

In normal limbs, in which venous resistances are low, transient increases in blood flow have little effect on peripheral venous pressure. However, in post-thrombotic limbs or in limbs with acute venous obstruction, an increase in blood flow may elevate the $Q_v R_v$ product significantly. As discussed later, the increase in venous pressure during exercise is responsible for venous claudication. Increases in peripheral pressure in response to reactive hyperemia are useful in the evaluation of chronic venous obstruction.[330]

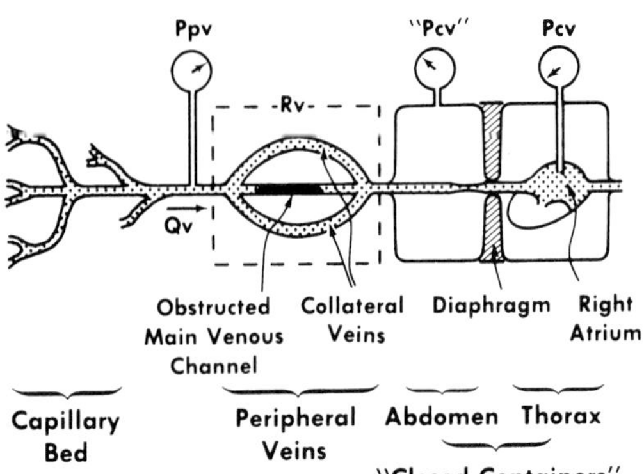

FIGURE 7–42. Major factors involved in venous return from the legs (see text). P_{pv} = peripheral venous pressure; "P_{cv}" = intra-abdominal pressure; P_{cv} = central venous pressure; R_v = peripheral venous resistance; Q_v = venous flow.

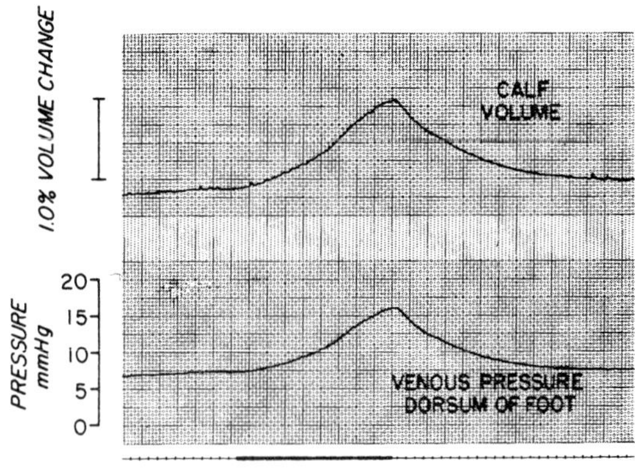

FIGURE 7–43. Effect of a deep breath on the peripheral venous pressure and volume in the lower extremity. The simultaneous increase in pressure and venous volume is caused by a temporary increase in intra-abdominal pressure that interferes with venous outflow from the leg. Volume change was measured with a mercury strain-gauge. (From Strandness DE Jr, Sumner DS: Hemodynamics for Surgeons. New York, Grune & Stratton, 1975.)

Venous resistance depends on:

- Location of the obstructed venous segments
- Length of the obstructions
- Number of veins involved

The immediate effect of an acute venous thrombosis depends on the adequacy of the preexisting collateral channels. A thrombus that blocks large exit or reentry collateral veins elevates the venous resistance more than one that occurs in an isolated venous segment. For example, a thrombus developing in the common femoral vein, where it blocks not only the superficial femoral vein but also reentry of the profunda femoris and saphenous veins (two of the major collaterals from the lower leg), is more devastating than one isolated to the superficial femoral vein.

In limbs with clinically "silent" DVT, there may be no perceptible elevation of venous pressure.[267] Measured at foot level, the average venous pressure in limbs of supine patients with acute phlebitis was found by Husni and colleagues[284] to be 17 mmHg. This was roughly 2.5 times that in normal limbs or in limbs with primary varicose veins (Table 7–4). There was essentially no difference in foot venous pressures between normal subjects and patients with acute phlebitis when they were standing quietly. This reflects the overwhelming contribution of the hydrostatic component, which tends to mask the slight pressure differences produced by the increased venous outflow resistance. On ambulation, however, the venous pressure in normal limbs dropped to about 40% of the pre-exercise value but changed little in the limbs with acute phlebitis (see Table 7–4).

DeWeese and Rogoff[263] found that venous pressures at

TABLE 7–4. VENOUS PRESSURE AT FOOT LEVEL

	PRESSURE (mmHg)*		
	Supine	**Standing**	**Ambulatory**
Control	7 ± 1	90 ± 7	35 ± 9
Varicose veins	7 ± 1	87 ± 5	56 ± 11
Acute phlebitis	17 ± 7	93 ± 4	90 ± 18
Postphlebitic	12 ± 5	90 ± 4	84 ± 16

Adapted from Husni EA, Ximenes JO, Goyette EM: Elastic support of the lower limbs in hospital patients: A critical study. JAMA 214:1456, 1970.

*Values are mean ± standard deviation.

foot level in supine patients ranged from 8 to 18 mmHg when clots were confined to the popliteal or below-knee veins.[263] Pressures were 20 to 51 mmHg when the clots were in the superficial femoral vein and were 32 to 83 mmHg (average, 50 mmHg) in the limbs with iliofemoral thrombosis. Similar values were reported by Ellwood and Lee.[267]

All veins subjected to increased transmural pressure dilate according to the venous pressure-volume curve and become less compliant (see Fig. 7–31). Superficial veins become more prominent, providing an excellent diagnostic sign of DVT. Sometimes this dilatation can so stretch the venous wall that valves cannot coapt properly, resulting in venous insufficiency. Reflux, however, is seldom an impressive finding in acute phlebitis.[340]

Another clinically important result of increased venous pressure is the concomitant increase in mean capillary pressure. This upsets the Starling equilibrium (see Eq. 7.29), leading to the formation of edema. Even subclinical venous thrombi may produce minor swelling that can be detected by careful measurements of limb circumference. In fact, unilateral limb swelling is the best clinical sign of acute venous thrombosis.

The degree of swelling is proportional to the elevation in venous pressure. DeWeese and Rogoff[263] found swelling in only 70% of limbs with popliteal or below-knee thrombosis, and in almost all cases this was less than 1 cm at the ankle.[263] However, swelling was present in 86% of patients with femoral vein thrombosis and in all patients with iliofemoral thrombosis. The increase in circumference exceeded 1.0 cm at the ankle, 2.0 cm at the calf, and 3.0 cm at the thigh in limbs with iliofemoral thrombosis.

Edema formation reaches truly massive proportions in phlegmasia cerulea dolens. In this dreaded condition, which is characterized by near-total thrombosis of all the veins in the involved extremity, together with ipsilateral iliac vein occlusion and obstruction of pelvic collateral veins, fluid loss may reach 6 to 10 L within 5 to 10 days.[278] This massive fluid loss reflects the tremendous elevation in venous pressure, which may reach 16 to 17 times normal values within 6 hours.[351] With the rapid formation of edema, tissue pressures attain values of 25 to 48 mmHg in 1 or 2 days.[247, 351]

Shock caused by fluid loss occurs in about one third of these patients.[246] In addition, a profound circulatory insufficiency develops, characterized by agonizing pain, cyanosis, decreased tissue temperature, absence of pulses, and often gangrene. The exact mechanism of this ischemia is uncertain, but it probably involves shock, increased venous outflow resistance, possible narrowing of the resistance vessels in response to the increased interstitial pressure, and edema (Fig. 7–44).[339, 355]

PRIMARY VARICOSE VEINS

Varicosities of the lower limb that develop spontaneously in the absence of DVT are referred to as "primary varicose

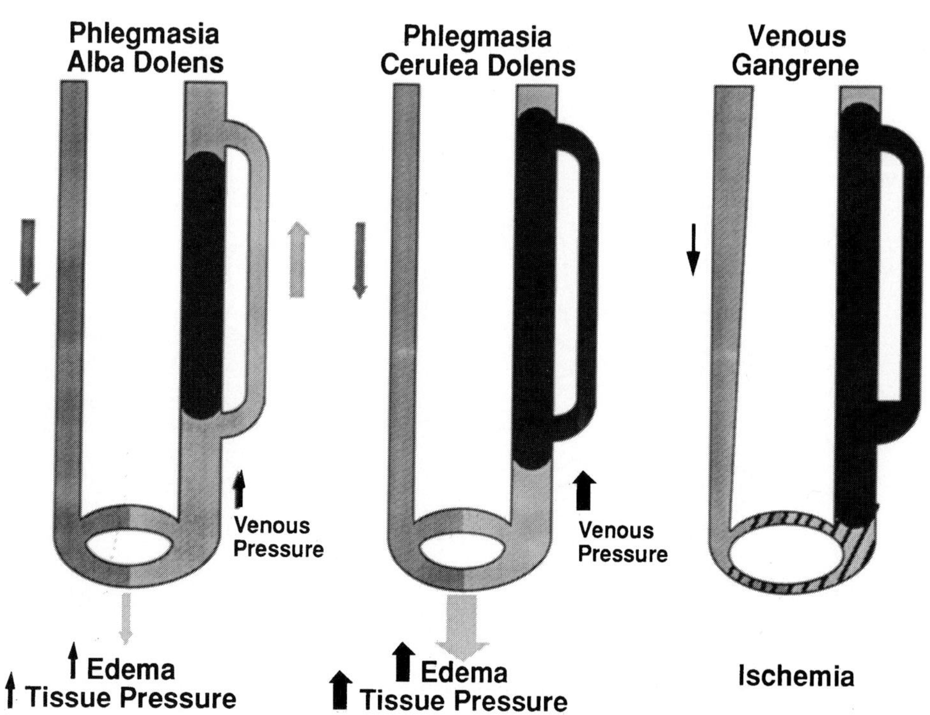

FIGURE 7–44. Pathophysiology of increasing severity of venous obstruction. In each diagram, arterial inflow is shown on the left and venous outflow on the right. *Black areas* indicate the location and extent of thrombus, which is confined to the major venous channels in phlegmasia alba dolens, involves collateral veins as well in phlegmasia cerulea dolens, and extends to the small veins and capillaries in venous gangrene. *Arrow size* indicates the magnitude of arterial and venous flow, venous and tissue pressure, and edema.

veins." The *greater saphenous vein* and its tributaries are the most frequently involved, followed by the lesser saphenous and pelvic veins.

The etiology remains uncertain. Theories include (1) pressure exerted by incompetent perforating veins,[269] (2) increased venous distensibility,[255, 265, 266, 335, 377] (3) increased blood flow through arteriovenous communications,[343, 344] and (4) preexisting abnormalities of smooth muscle and endothelial cells in vein walls.[300] Although these factors undoubtedly play a role, much of the evidence seems to favor progressive descending valvular incompetence in response to congenital absence or incompetence of the common femoral and iliac valves.[270, 301, 304, 333] Under these circumstances, the saphenofemoral valve (which lacks protection not only from hydrostatic pressure but also from episodic pressure increases caused by straining or coughing) becomes incompetent as the vein stretches. Once this valve becomes incompetent, the pressure is transmitted to the next lower valve in the saphenous vein, and so on down the leg. Finally, valves in the *tributary veins* also lose their competence. These subcutaneous veins then elongate, become tortuous, and present as typical varicosities.

Regardless of the etiologic mechanism, the essential physiologic defect is venous valvular incompetence. Although valve leaflets appear to be normal, they fail to coapt properly, perhaps because of the abnormally distensible nature of the venous wall.[258, 266, 362, 377] In the typical patient with extensive greater saphenous varicosities, the iliofemoral valves as well as all the valves in the greater saphenous vein, both above and below knee, are either absent or incompetent.[270, 304, 333] Below the femoral level, the deep venous valves remain competent. Other patterns are common; varicosities may be confined to the above-knee saphenous system or to the below-knee saphenous veins, when the proximal site of venous incompetence is the Hunterian perforator or the popliteal vein. In all cases, there must be continuous column of blood extending to the right atrium that is uninterrupted by the presence of a competent valve.

When a person with varicose veins shifts from a supine to a standing position, blood "falls" down the involved superficial veins uninhibited by functioning valves. Venous reflux fills the calf veins far more rapidly than capillary inflow can, and typically only 5 to 70 seconds is required.[254] Application of a tourniquet to compress the superficial veins normalizes the filling time, confirming the competency of the deep venous valves.[251] With the person in the supine position or during quiet standing, blood flow in varicose veins is sluggish but is directed in the normal cephalad direction (Figs. 7–45 and 7–46).[355] In addition, the presssure at ankle level is no different from that in limbs without venous incompetence (see Table 7–4).[284] When the upright subject with varicose veins begins to walk or otherwise contract the leg muscles, however, a different picture emerges. In this situation, blood flow reverses (during the relaxation phase), flowing distally and quite rapidly toward the feet (see Figs. 7–45 and 7–46).[244, 270] Moreover, the decrease in superficial venous pressure is much less than is normally seen (see Table 7–4).[284, 301, 329]

In response to calf muscle contraction, deep venous pressure drops markedly as a result of the effect of the muscle pump on the normally valved deep veins. Varicose veins also are partially emptied by the muscle contraction, but because of the lack of valvular protection, pressure within these superficial veins experiences only a moderate fall. Therefore, during calf muscle relaxation, a pressure gradient develops that causes blood to flow from the superficial system into the deep system via the perforating veins.[233] As a result, a "private circulation" or circular movement of blood is established in the exercising leg (see Fig. 7–45).[314] Blood pumped through the deep veins of the calf and thigh reaches the common femoral vein, where a portion reverses direction to flow distally down the functionally valveless saphenous vein. On reaching the lower parts of the leg, this blood returns to the deep system through the perforating veins, thereby completing the para-

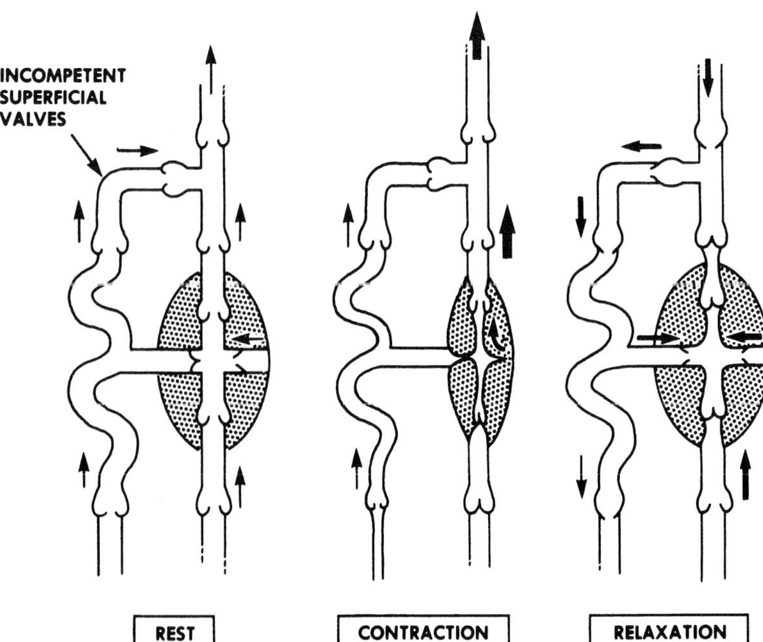

FIGURE 7–45. Primary varicose veins. Dynamics of venous blood flow in response to calf muscle contraction. During relaxation, flow is reversed in the saphenous vein and circular motion is established through the perforating veins. (From Sumner DS: Venous dynamics—varicosities. Clin Obstet Gynecol 24:743, 1981.)

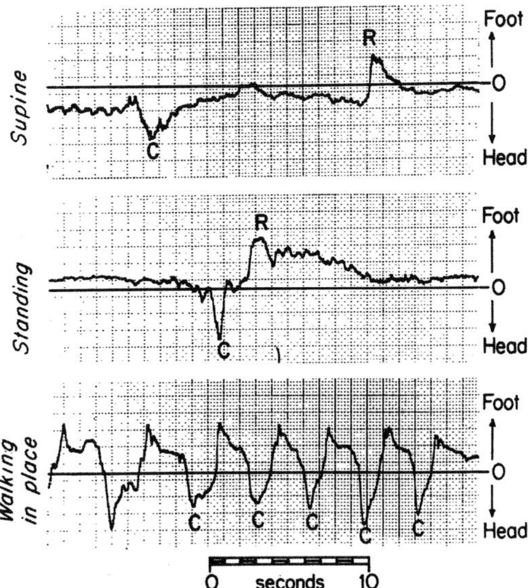

FIGURE 7–46. Blood flow in the greater saphenous vein in a patient with varicose veins. Calf muscle contraction (C) causes blood to flow toward the heart, whereas calf muscle relaxation (R) causes blood to reflux down the leg toward the feet. In the standing position, reflux flow greatly exceeds forward flow. Recordings were made with the Doppler probe pointed cephalad. (From Strandness DE Jr, Sumner DS: Hemodynamics for Surgeons. New York, Grune & Stratton, 1975.)

sitic circuit (Fig. 7–47). During exercise, as much as one fifth to one quarter of the total femoral outflow may be involved in this circular motion.[244]

Surprisingly, this circular motion seems to have little effect on exercise tolerance.[232] Coupled with the chronically increased superficial venous pressure, it does contribute to the progressive distention and elongation of the superficial tributaries of the saphenous vein, producing unsightly varicosities.[352] Clinically, the increased pressure probably contributes to the heaviness and tightness of the lower leg experienced by some patients with varicose veins. Interstitial tissue pressures have been found to be raised.[327]

Compressing the site of the leak (i.e., the saphenofemoral junction) prevents reflux flow during exercise and permits the muscle pump to reduce venous pressure to near-normal levels (see Fig. 7–47).[301, 370] This forms the physiologic basis for high ligation and stripping of varicose veins, the most effective means of treatment.[252] Elastic stockings afford similar protection.[284] The external pressure exerted by the stockings may force the venous valve cusps to come into contact, thereby restoring venous competence.[254]

CHRONIC VENOUS INSUFFICIENCY

Physiologic abnormalities in limbs of patients with chronic venous insufficiency consist of venous outflow obstruction or valvular incompetence, or both (Fig. 7–48). In the individual case, one or the other of the abnormalities may predominate.

As a rule, the obstruction that follows acute venous thrombosis tends to decrease with time. Some thrombi are completely or partially dissolved by the action of thrombolysins; others become organized and recanalized to a variable extent (see Chapter 138). Of equal importance, however, is the progressive enlargement of collateral venous channels, which carry an increasingly large proportion of the venous outflow. The overall effect of these processes is reduced venous resistance. Venous outflow studies suggest that the average venous resistance in postphlebitic limbs is about 1.2 to 1.6 times normal. In contrast, the resistance of postphlebitic limbs is only 0.3 to 0.6 that of limbs with acute thrombosis.[237, 239, 259, 277, 340] At rest, with the person in the supine position, these small elevations in venous resistance usually increase the venous pressure only a few millimeters of mercury at ankle level.[284, 320, 330] Ordinarily, no pressure elevation can be detected in the quietly standing individual (see Table 7–4).[262, 284]

As venous obstruction subsides, venous valvular incompetence increases and is accompanied by progressive hemodynamic deterioration.[289, 310, 373] Organization of thrombi damages venous valves to a variable extent, leaving them incompetent.[264] The small high-resistance channels of recanalized veins, of course, are valveless. Dilatation of collateral veins and the remaining residual channels often prevents their valves from approximating, thus further aggravating the degree of venous incompetence. Plethysmographic studies all show that venous reflux is significantly increased in post-thrombotic limbs and that most of the reflux occurs via deep veins rather than via dilated superficial veins.[238, 253, 340] Post-thrombotic calf veins may also become stiffer (less compliant) than normal veins, possibly due to distention or to changes in wall properties.[319]

Approximately two thirds of patients with chronic venous insufficiency have no history of DVT.[279, 292, 315] There may be no duplex scan or phlebographic evidence of venous thrombosis. In some of these patients, there may have been an unrecognized thrombotic episode; in others, a predisposition to incompetence may have been present since birth.

In patients with chronic deep venous valvular incompe-

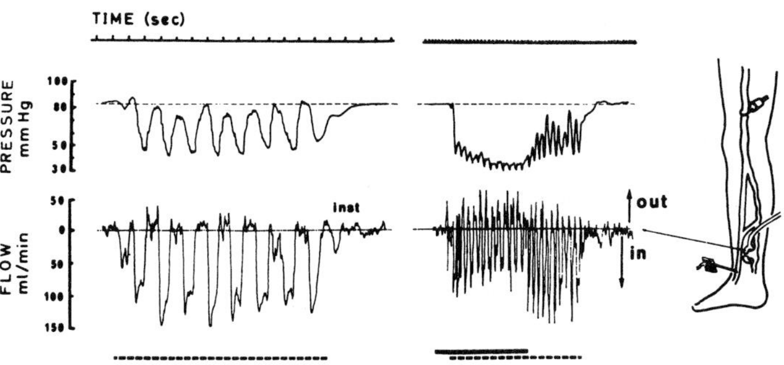

FIGURE 7–47. Flow in an incompetent perforating vein in an erect patient with varicose veins. During walking *(dashed lines)*, flow is directed "in," that is, from the superficial to the deep veins. Pressure in the greater saphenous vein is only slightly reduced. Occluding the greater saphenous vein with a "sling" ligature *(solid line)* causes flow in the perforator to seesaw "in" and "out" and causes the saphenous vein pressure to drop in a nearly normal fashion. (From Bjordal RI: Simultaneous pressure and flow recordings in varicose veins of the lower extremity. A hemodynamic study of venous dysfunction. Acta Chir Scand 136:309, 1970.

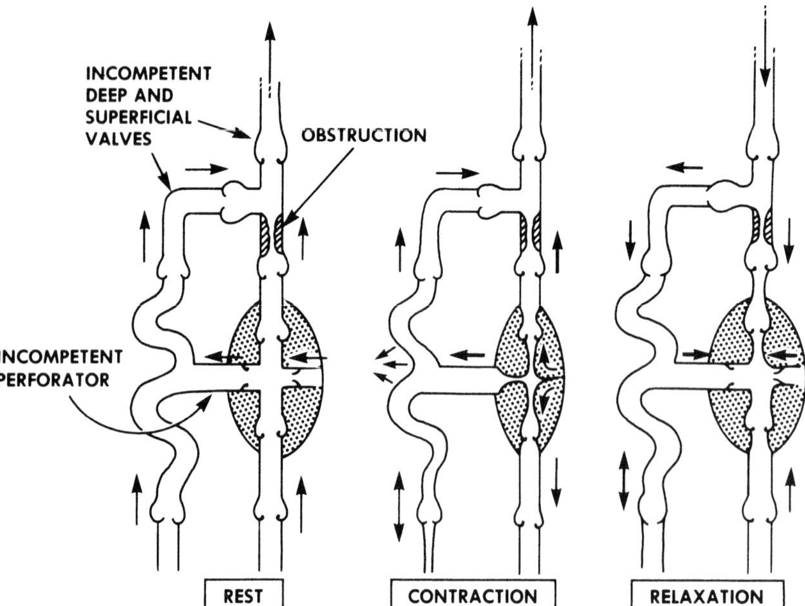

FIGURE 7–48. Chronic venous insufficiency, deep venous incompetence, and secondary varicose veins. Dynamics of venous blood flow in response to calf muscle contraction in a postphlebitic limb with residual deep venous obstruction, incompetent perforating veins, and secondary varicose veins. Note the to-and-fro motion of blood in incompetent perforating veins. (From Sumner DS: Venous dynamics—varicosities. Clin Obstet Gynecol 24:743, 1981.)

tence, changing from a supine to a standing position fills the calf veins even more rapidly (within 5 to 20 seconds) than it does in patients with primary varicose veins.[254, 374] Reflux occurs not only in the deep system but also in any superficial veins that have lost their competence ("secondary varicose veins"). As a rule, application of a tourniquet to prevent reflux in superficial veins does little to prolong venous filling time.[251]

The physiologic aberrations introduced by valvular incompetence and residual obstruction become most evident during exercise (see Fig. 7–48). When calf muscles contract, blood is propelled up the leg in both superficial and deep veins, much as it is in normal limbs. (When valves distal to the site of muscle contraction are incompetent, a small quantity of blood may also be forced retrograde.) The temporary increase in flow exaggerates the effect of even a slight elevation of venous resistance and may actually cause the peripheral venous pressure to rise above resting levels during the phase of active muscle contraction (see Eq. 7.31). If the perforating veins are incompetent (as they often are), blood at high pressure is forced through these veins into the recipient subcutaneous veins. This in turn produces a local increase in capillary pressure.

The overall effect of valvular incompetence and outflow resistance is a reduced quantity of blood ejected with each contraction.[254] Because the volume of blood displaced depends not only on the pressure developed by the calf muscles but also on the compliance of the compressed veins, increased stiffness of the calf veins may play a role in reducing the ejected volume.[319, 332]

When the muscles relax between contractions, incompetent valves allow blood to reflux down the leg, rapidly refilling the empty veins. (Reflux flow rates in limbs with stasis changes average 30 ml/sec and may reach 50 ml/sec.[369]) The hydrostatic column is reestablished to the heart, and peripheral venous pressure rises rapidly between contractions. As a result, the ability of the calf muscle pump to reduce ambulatory venous pressure is severely impaired (Fig. 7–49).[262, 280, 284, 370] The reduction in ambulatory venous pressure tends to be less in limbs with chronic venous insufficiency, in which reflux occurs in both the deep and superficial systems, than it is in limbs with isolated superficial venous incompetence (primary varicose veins), emphasizing the importance of the deep venous valves (see Table 7–4). If, in addition to valvular incompetence, there is a significant element of venous obstruction, there is almost no drop in venous pressure; in some cases, it may even rise.[234, 262, 280, 320] Because ambulatory venous pressure is the parameter that most closely reflects the hemodynamic function of the venous circulation, it is recognized as the "gold standard" for all tests of venous pathophysiology (see Chapter 145).

Owing to the rapid reflux of blood that occurs in the interval between calf muscle contractions, decreased venous

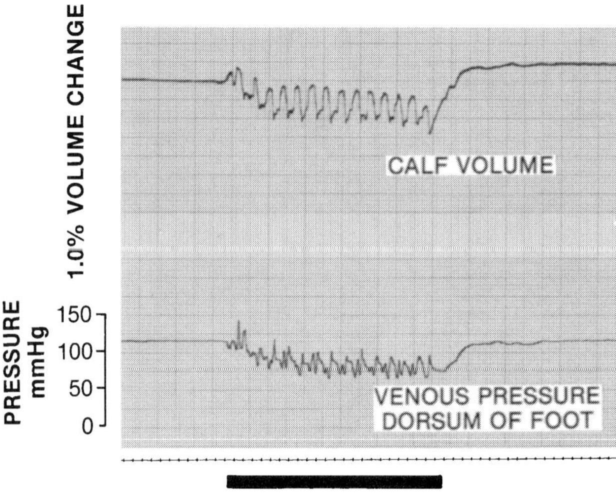

FIGURE 7–49. Effect of exercise on calf volume and venous pressure in a patient with chronic venous insufficiency. (From Strandness DE Jr, Sumner DS: Hemodynamics for Surgeons. New York, Grune & Stratton, 1975.)

TABLE 7–5. CHANGE IN RADIOACTIVITY OF LEG PUMPING AGAINST GRAVITY (45-DEGREE DEPENDENCY)*

	NORMAL	CHRONIC DEEP VENOUS INSUFFICIENCY
Number of legs	21	13
Degree of change (%)	−20.5 (± 6.1)	−10.2 (± 4.8)†
Time required (sec)	0–5.3 (± 2.0)	12.7 (± 7.9)†
Rate of change (%/sec)	−4.6 (± 2.1)	−0.9 (± 0.5)†

From Rutherford JB, Reddy CMK, Walker FG, Wagner HN Jr: A new quantitative method of assessing the functional status of the leg veins. Am J Surg 122:594, 1971.
*Values are mean ± standard deviation.
†Degree of significance of difference from normal: $p < .001$.

compliance, and (when present) increased outflow resistance, evacuation of the calf veins with exercise is less complete in limbs with chronic venous insufficiency than it is in normal limbs. The dependent veins, therefore, are perpetually in a state of partial congestion. Because the veins that constitute the bellows of the muscle pump are primed with an increased volume of blood, the amplitude of the pressure swing that accompanies each contraction of the calf muscle tends to be exaggerated in proportion to the severity of the postphlebitic process.[280, 281] In multilevel disease, the pressure swing may be two or three times that observed in normal limbs.

The efficiency of the venous pump is well demonstrated by radionuclide methods for estimating changes in local blood volume.[338] As shown in Table 7–5, limbs with chronic deep venous insufficiency can pump blood from the calf at only about one-fifth the normal rate. After exercise, the volume reduction is approximately half that achieved in normal limbs. Air plethysmographic studies of limbs with venous valvular incompetence also confirm that an increased amount of blood is left in the calf after exercise (two to four times that remaining in normal limbs).[254] In accordance with the venous pressure-volume compliance curve (see Fig. 7–31), the quantity of blood remaining in the calf after a series of calf contractions, divided by that present at rest in the dependent extremity (residual volume fraction), correlates well with the increased ambulatory venous pressure.[254, 373]

Adverse Effects of Venous Hypertension

Patients with proximal deep venous obstruction sometimes complain of a deep "bursting" pain in the leg during exercise. This pain, which has been called *venous claudication,* is explained by the increased venous pressure and congestion that occur in response to the combination of exercise-induced hyperemia and increased outflow resistance.[363] The distal deep veins in these limbs are often radiologically normal, and valvular insufficiency is not a prominent feature.

In most patients with chronic venous insufficiency, symptoms related to valvular incompetence predominate. Clinically, the most significant functional abnormality is the inability of the venous pump mechanism to provide relief from orthostatic venous hypertension. Capillaries in distal parts of legs are chronically exposed to a high pressure when the patient is upright. This leads to persistent edema. Subcutaneous capillaries and venules elongate and dilate.[248, 268, 271] Blood flow in these dilated and engorged vessels is sluggish compared with blood flow in normal skin.[228] Protein-rich fluid and red blood cells escape into the subcutaneous tissues. As the proteins become organized and the red blood cells disintegrate, the tissues become fibrotic and hyperpigmented, producing a condition known as *lipodermatosclerosis.*[250] Acting on this substrate, trauma (even a mild, often unrecognized injury) may lead to the death of tissue and the development of a chronic ulcer (see Chapter 144).

The frequency with which severe stasis changes and ulcers occur is related to the ambulatory venous pressure. Nicolaides[321] and associates[322] showed that the incidence of ulceration in limbs with ambulatory venous pressures exceeding 80 mmHg is about 80%. In contrast, ulcers seldom develop in limbs with ambulatory venous pressures of less than 30 or 40 mmHg (Table 7–6). Unless measures are taken to counteract edema formation, 50% of limbs with edema present 1 year after an acute DVT become ulcerated within 10 years.[241]

Stasis changes (induration, dermatitis, hyperpigmentation, and ulceration) are limited to the "gaiter area" of the leg, where hydrostatic pressures are high, and are typically worse on the medial aspect of the ankle just above and posterior to the medial malleolus. This distribution suggests that incompetent perforating veins connecting the deep system to the posterior arch vein play a major role by transmitting pressure impulses to fragile superficial veins, causing localized hypoxia and nutritional deficits.[234, 256, 299, 268, 355] The descriptive term *ankle blowout syndrome* was coined to emphasize the importance of incompetent perforating veins to the genesis of venous stasis changes.[256]

Distribution of Valvular Incompetence: Relationship to Stasis Changes

The large number of valves in the infrapopliteal veins and the relative paucity of valves above the knee suggest that these structures have evolved to protect against hydrostatic forces imposed by the assumption of an upright posture. Certainly, the distribution of valves coincides with the hydrostatic pressure to which the veins are subjected. The concentration of valves in the lower leg also implies that they are of major importance to the muscle pump mechanism.

TABLE 7–6. RELATIONSHIP BETWEEN AMBULATORY VENOUS PRESSURE AND THE INCIDENCE OF STASIS ULCERATION

AMBULATORY VENOUS PRESSURE (mmHg)	INCIDENCE OF ULCERS (%)
≤45	0
45–49	5
50–59	15
60–69	50
70–79	75
≥80	80

Data from Nicolaides AN: Noninvasive assessment of primary and secondary varicose veins. *In* Bernstein EF (ed): Noninvasive Diagnostic Techniques in Vascular Disease, 2nd ed. St. Louis, CV Mosby, 1982, pp 575–586.

Unlike venous pressure at the ankle, pressure in the popliteal veins decreases relatively little with exercise and reaches essentially the same level in limbs with gross saphenous varices, in limbs with minimal varicose veins, and in normal limbs (Fig. 7–50).[233, 282, 301] This suggests that the presence or absence of valves above the popliteal vein has little effect on ambulatory venous pressure, whereas valves below the knee play a major role in pressure reduction. These and similar observations prompted earlier investigators to speculate that the absence of valves above the knee may be less detrimental to venous function than the absence of valves below the knee.[233, 282]

Isolated proximal venous valvular incompetence is a relatively benign condition. About 15% of normal limbs and the majority of limbs with primary saphenous varicosities have incompetent common femoral valves as shown by Doppler ultrasonography, yet cutaneous manifestations of chronic venous insufficiency are rarely seen.[270, 333] Furthermore, reflux to the popliteal level during retrograde phlebography commonly occurs in clinically normal limbs.[361]

Investigators using plethysmographic methods or venous pressure measurements have shown that postexercise peripheral venous refilling times* are more likely to be accelerated and ambulatory venous pressures are more likely to be elevated when popliteal or calf veins are incompetent than when incompetence is confined to the above-knee veins (Table 7–7).[274, 293, 294, 298, 326, 336, 350] Because rapid refilling times (Table 7–8) and elevated ambulatory pressures (see Table 7–6) are correlated with stasis changes, these studies explain why popliteal and distal venous incompetence appears to have a more deleterious clinical effect than does isolated proximal venous incompetence.[274, 298, 326, 350] There is even evidence that incompetence of the deep veins at the ankle may be clinically more important than incompetence of the popliteal or proximal calf veins in determining the stage of chronic venous insufficiency.[336]

*Because venous volume depends on venous pressure (see Fig. 7–31), postexercise plethysmographic tracings are roughly correlated with ambulatory venous pressure, and the times required for the venous volume and the venous pressure to return to baseline levels after cessation of exercise are almost identical.[226, 323]

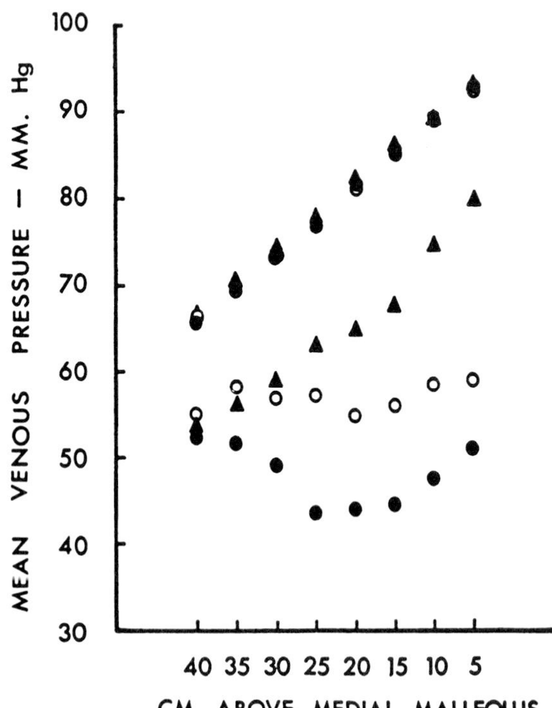

FIGURE 7–50. Pressure in the greater saphenous vein at 5-cm intervals down the leg, starting at the knee (at 40 cm above the medial malleolus) and ending at the ankle (at 5 cm). Symbols indicate normal limbs *(closed circles),* limbs with minimal saphenous varices *(open circles),* and limbs with gross saphenous varices *(triangles).* Pressures at all anatomic levels are superimposed at rest *(upper points).* Ambulatory venous pressures *(lower points)* are identical at the knee but are quite different at the ankle. (From Ludbrook J: Valvular defect in primary varicose veins, cause or effect? Lancet 2:1289, 1963.)

TABLE 7–7. POSTEXERCISE VENOUS RECOVERY TIME VERSUS DISTRIBUTION OF DEEP VENOUS VALVULAR INCOMPETENCE

LOCATION OF INCOMPETENT VALVES*	RECOVERY TIME (sec)†	INTERPRETATION
Distal only	16.4 ± 14.0	Abnormal
Distal and proximal	14.1 ± 8.7	Abnormal
Proximal only	43.5 ± 26.8	Normal
No valvular incompetence	42.8 ± 22.4	Normal

Data from Gooley NA, Sumner DS: Relationship of venous reflux to the site of venous valvular incompetence: Implications for venous reconstructive surgery. J Vasc Surg 7:50, 1988.

*Distal: popliteal and below-knee veins; proximal: common and superficial femoral veins.

†Values are mean ± standard deviation.

Doppler and duplex ultrasonographic studies have been used to study the distribution of venous valvular incompetence in patients with symptoms and signs of chronic venous insufficiency. In limbs with severe stasis changes (ulcers, pigmentation, and induration), combined above-knee and below-knee incompetence is the most common pattern.[292, 231, 279, 315, 365] Isolated below-knee incompetence is less frequent, but most reports indicate that it is somewhat more common than isolated proximal vein incompetence. Combined above-knee and below-knee incompetence was present in 45% of the limbs studied by Moore and colleagues (Fig. 7–51).[315] An additional 23% had isolated below-knee incompetence, for a total of 68% with below-knee involvement.

Van Bemmelen and coworkers[365] reported that 76% of limbs with ulcers had above-knee and below-knee incompetence; an additional 8% had isolated distal incompetence,

TABLE 7–8. POSTEXERCISE VENOUS RECOVERY TIME VERSUS CLINICAL SIGNS IN POSTPHLEBITIC LIMBS

SIGN	RECOVERY TIME (sec)*	LIMBS ABNORMAL (%)
Ulcer, pigmentation	10 ± 7	87
Edema only	26 ± 23	48
None	37 ± 24	27
Varicose veins		
Present	21 ± 19	68
Absent	39 ± 25	21

Data from Gooley NA, Sumner DS: Relationship of venous reflux to the site of venous valvular incompetence: Implications for venous reconstructive surgery. J Vasc Surg 7:50, 1988.

*Values are mean ± standard deviation.

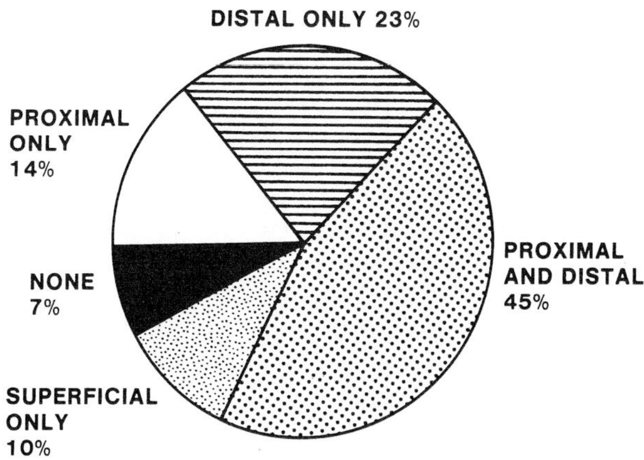

FIGURE 7–51. Distribution of venous valvular incompetence in limbs with stasis ulcers and pigmentation. (From Sumner DS: Pathophysiology of chronic venous insufficiency. Semin Vasc Surg 1:66, 1988.)

for a total of 84% of limbs with below-knee involvement. Thus, in these two studies more than two thirds of limbs with advanced stasis changes had popliteal or below-knee incompetence, either alone or in conjunction with incompetence of the proximal veins.

In limbs with less severe cutaneous manifestations (edema, venous flares), the distribution differs, in that incompetence isolated to the proximal veins is far more common than incompetence confined to the calf veins. In the van Bemmelen series, 59% of limbs with chronic venous disease but no ulcers had isolated proximal vein incompetence; another 29% had combined proximal and distal incompetence; but only 8% had isolated distal incompetence.[365] This suggests that proximal venous incompetence alone is not responsible for the development of ulcers. In contrast, the role of popliteal or below-knee valvular incompetence in the genesis of stasis ulcers is supported by reports that the proportion of limbs with distal incompetence is appreciably higher when ulcers are present (42% to 84%) than when the disease is less severe (3% to 35%).[315, 317, 318, 365]

Although the significance of distal venous incompetence is widely accepted, the relative importance of superficial and deep venous incompetence remains unresolved. Combined superficial and deep venous incompetence, the most common pattern, is found in 20% to 88% of limbs with ulcers or lipodermatosclerosis.[231, 368] In the experience of a number of investigators, incompetence confined to the superficial veins is relatively rare in patients with manifestations of chronic venous insufficiency, occurring in only 0 to 10% of cases (see Fig. 7–51).[231, 315, 318, 336, 365] Others, however, have found incompetence isolated to the superficial veins in the majority (52% to 70%) of patients with severe stasis changes.[296, 346, 368] In most cases, when incompetent superficial veins are associated with deep venous insufficiency, they probably represent secondary varicose veins and are unlikely to be directly responsible for the adverse effects of chronic venous insufficiency. This interpretation does not suffice when the only apparent valvular defects are confined to the superficial system. In these cases, superficial venous incompetence must be solely responsible for stasis changes. Nonetheless, patients with massive, long-standing varicose veins are often asymptomatic and have normal skin and soft, pliable subcutaneous tissues in the gaiter area. This in itself is a strong argument against the theory that superficial venous incompetence alone is sufficient to cause stasis changes.

Analogous to the situation pertaining in the deep system, incompetence of the below-knee greater saphenous vein and lesser saphenous vein, either alone or in conjunction with incompetence of the above-knee saphenous vein, is more strongly associated with ulceration than is incompetence limited to the proximal superficial veins.[279, 292, 293, 317] In one study, only 4% of limbs with isolated above-knee saphenous vein incompetence underwent skin changes and none had an ulcer.[294]

Hypothetical Effects of Different Patterns of Venous Incompetence

A mechanism explaining how the location of venous valvular incompetence may affect ambulatory venous pressure is proposed in Figure 7–52.[310] In normal limbs and in limbs with competent distal but incompetent proximal valves, venous pressures at the ankle are low after exercise because the column of blood extends only to the first competent valve, which is located well below the knee.* However, when the proximal valves are competent but the distal valves are incompetent, the postexercise column is relatively long, extending almost the entire length of the leg. Consequently, ambulatory venous pressures are high, and if the perforating veins are also incompetent, the superficial veins are rapidly refilled, even though their valves may remain competent. When both proximal and distal valves are incompetent, the ankle veins are subjected to the weight of an uninterrupted column of blood extending to the heart, there is little reduction in ambulatory venous pressure, and reflux into the superficial system via incompetent perforating veins is accelerated. Although superficial veins in limbs with superficial venous incompetence are rapidly refilled following exercise, external compression or removal of the saphenous veins relieves venous hypertension as long as the deep valves are competent.

Therapeutic Implications

Because venous valvular incompetence is ultimately responsible for stasis changes in the skin and subcutaneous tissues, it seems logical that restoration of normal valve function should correct the pathophysiologic abnormalities and afford the optimal treatment for this disease. Superficial femoral venous valvuloplasty, transposition of a competent segment of vein into the proximal deep venous system, and autotransplantation of valve-containing venous segments into the superficial femoral or popliteal vein are among the ingenious operations that have been devised for this pur-

*As pointed out earlier, this is admittedly an oversimplification, because venous pressure in each segregated compartment is determined not only by the length of the hydrostatic column but also by venous compliance and the residual content of blood.[332] Therefore, pressures at the lower end of each compartment may correspond to a hydrostatic column that extends several centimeters above the closed valve located at the proximal end of the compartment. The message, however, is unaltered by this simplification.

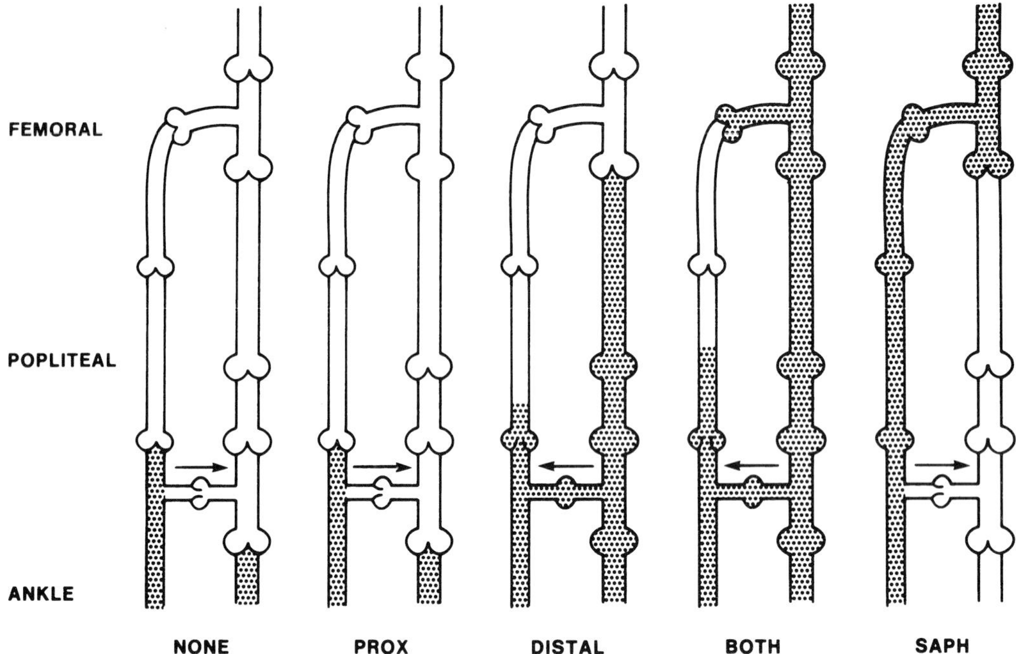

FIGURE 7–52. Comparison of the length of the hydrostatic column of blood measured from the ankle after exercise *(stippled area)* in limbs with no valvular incompetence (NONE), incompetence limited to the proximal deep veins (PROX), incompetence limited to the distal deep veins (DISTAL), incompetence of both proximal and distal deep veins (BOTH), and incompetence limited to the superficial veins (SAPH). In each diagram, saphenous veins are on the left and deep veins are on the right. *Arrows* indicate the direction of flow in perforating veins. (From Gooley NA, Sumner DS: Relationship of venous reflux to the site of venous valvular incompetence: Implications for venous reconstructive surgery. J Vasc Surg 7:50, 1988.)

pose (see Chapter 149). The rationale for all of these procedures is based on the assumption that a single competent valve placed at or above the popliteal level in an otherwise incompetent system will alleviate ambulatory venous hypertension and allow ulcers to heal.

Although clinical results have been encouraging, hemodynamic abnormalities are seldom completely corrected.[260, 287, 325, 331, 345, 359, 372] The models depicted in Figure 7–52 explain this apparent contradiction. When incompetence is confined to the proximal veins and the distal valves remain functional, restoration of proximal venous valvular function is unnecessary. Therefore, valve replacement need be considered only when both proximal and distal veins are incompetent. Although a valve inserted in the proximal superficial femoral vein does interrupt the column of blood to the heart, a long uninterrupted segment of blood remains above the ankle at the cessation of exercise. Ambulatory venous pressure is decreased somewhat but remains high. A popliteal valve replacement would further reduce the length of the hydrostatic column and decrease ambulatory venous pressure but not as efficiently as the multiple competent valves present in normal calf veins, which have the potential of segregating the column of blood into segments only a few centimeters long. Under some circumstances, however, the margin of relief from ambulatory venous hypertension may be sufficient to permit ulcers to heal.

Stripping of incompetent superficial veins would be effective only when the distal deep veins are competent.[252, 261, 279, 312]

PREGNANCY

When a woman in the third trimester of pregnancy lies on her back, the enlarged uterus may compress the inferior vena cava and the common iliac veins.[288, 357] As a result, venous pressure is increased in the legs and venous flow patterns become less responsive to respiration.[285, 313] Interference with venous return reduces cardiac output, sometimes to the extent that hypotension develops.[364] All these effects are relieved if the patient is turned to her side, which allows the uterus to roll away from the pelvic veins.

Early in pregnancy, well before the uterus enlarges significantly, humoral factors cause the veins to become more compliant.[240] Together with the increased venous pressure that occurs later in gestation, these factors cause significant venous distention. Because of these factors, the velocity of blood flow in the leg veins gradually decreases as pregnancy progresses.

Although pregnancy does not cause varicose veins, the increased pressure and venous distensibility exaggerate predisposing factors. Consequently, varicose veins often first appear during pregnancy and become more severe with subsequent pregnancies. In addition, the sluggish venous flow probably contributes to the development of DVT.

SURGICAL VENOUS INTERRUPTION

Ligation of the femoral vein causes a prompt rise in peripheral venous pressure and a significant decrease in femoral artery flow (Fig. 7–53).[375] Although most of this initial resistance to blood flow can be attributed to an increase in venous outflow resistance, an appreciable portion may be due to reflex constriction of arterioles.[355, 376] This information may be pertinent to the treatment of combined trauma to arteries and veins. Although collateral development rapidly alleviates much of the venous outflow obstruction, in

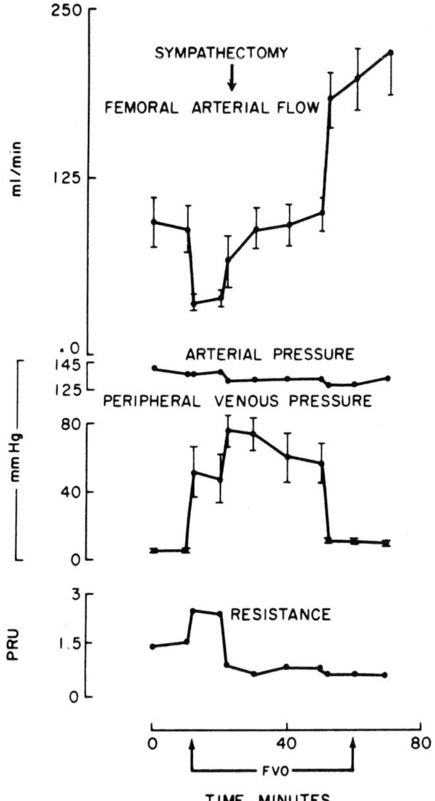

FIGURE 7–53. Effect of femoral vein occlusion (FVO) followed by lumbar sympathectomy on hemodynamics in the canine hindlimb. Peripheral venous pressure was measured from the saphenous vein. Note that occlusion results in a fall in femoral arterial blood flow, a prompt rise in peripheral venous pressure, and a rise in total limb resistance. Sympathectomy increases femoral flow without changing the peripheral venous pressure appreciably, suggesting that the resistance change occurred primarily in the arterioles or venules rather than in the larger venous collaterals. PRU = peripheral resistance unit. (From Wright CB, Sayre JT, Casterline PI, Swan KG: Hemodynamic effects of sympathectomy in canine femoral venous occlusion. Surgery 74:405, 1973.)

the initial period following reconstructive surgery the patency of the arterial repair may be jeopardized if the accompanying vein is ligated.[334]

SELECTED READINGS

Arterial Hemodynamics

Burton AC: Physiology and Biophysics of the Circulation, 2nd ed. Chicago, Year Book Medical Publishers, 1972.

Caro CG, Pedley TJ, Schroter RC, Seed WA: The Mechanics of the Circulation. New York, Oxford University Press, 1978.

Conrad MC: Functional Anatomy of the Circulation to the Lower Extremities. Chicago, Year Book Medical Publishers, 1971.

Dobrin PB: Mechanical properties of arteries. Physiol Rev 58:397, 1978.

Fung YC: Biomechanics: Circulation, 2nd ed. New York, Springer-Verlag, 1997.

Milnor WR: Hemodynamics, 2nd ed. Baltimore, Williams & Wilkins, 1989.

Nichols WW, O'Rourke MF: McDonald's Blood Flow in Arteries: Theoretical, Experimental, and Clinical Principles, 4th ed. London, Arnold, 1998.

Patel DJ, Vaishnav RN: Basic Hemodynamics and Its Role in Disease Processes. Baltimore, University Park Press, 1980.

Shepherd JT: Physiology of the Circulation in Human Limbs in Health and Disease. Philadelphia, WB Saunders Co, 1963.

Strandness DE Jr: Peripheral Arterial Disease: A Physiologic Approach. Boston, Little, Brown & Co, 1969.

Strandness DE Jr, Sumner DS: Hemodynamics for Surgeons. New York, Grune & Stratton, 1975.

Venous Hemodynamics

Bergan JJ, Goldman MP (eds): Varicose Veins and Telangiectasias. St. Louis, Quality Medical Publishing, 1993.

Bergan JJ, Yao JST: Venous Disorders. Philadelphia, WB Saunders, 1991.

Browse NL, Burnand KG, Thomas ML: Diseases of the Veins: Pathology, Diagnosis and Treatment. London, Edward Arnold, 1988.

Dodd H, Cockett FB: The Pathology and Surgery of the Veins of the Lower Limb. 2nd ed. Edinburgh, Churchill Livingstone, 1976.

Gardner AMN, Fox RH: The Return of Blood to the Heart: Venous Pumps in Health and Disease. London, John Libbey Eurotext, 1989.

Gottlob R, May R: Venous Valves: Morphology, Function, Radiology, Surgery. Vienna, Springer-Verlag, 1986.

Guyton AC, Taylor AE, Granger HJ: Circulatory Physiology: II. Dynamics and Control of the Body Fluids. Philadelphia, WB Saunders, 1975.

Johnson HD, Pflug J: The Swollen Leg: Causes and Treatment. Philadelphia, JB Lippincott, 1975.

Ludbrook J: Aspects of Venous Function in the Lower Limbs. Springfield, Ill, Charles C Thomas, 1966.

Raju S, Villavicencio JL: Surgical Management of Venous Disease. Baltimore, Williams & Wilkins, 1997.

Strandness DE Jr, Sumner DS: Hemodynamics for Surgeons. New York, Grune & Stratton, 1975.

Strandness DE Jr, Thiele BL: Selected Topics in Venous Disorders. Pathophysiology, Diagnosis, and Treatment. Mount Kisco, NY, Futura Publishing, 1981.

REFERENCES

Arterial Hemodynamics

1. Abbott WM, Bouchier-Hayes DJ: The role of mechanical properties in graft design. *In* Dardik H (ed): Graft Materials in Vascular Surgery. Miami, Symposia Specialist, 1978, pp 59–78.
2. Allwood MJ: Redistribution of blood flow in limbs with obstruction of a main artery. Clin Sci 22:279, 1962.
3. Angelides NS, Nicolaides AN: Simultaneous isotope clearance from the muscles of the calf and thigh. *In* Puel P, Boccalon H, Enjalbert A (eds): Hemodynamics of the Limbs: 1. Toulouse, France, GEPESC, 1979, pp 547–562.
4. Anidjar S, Dobrin PB, Eichorst M, et al: Correlation of inflammatory infiltrate with the enlargement of experimental aortic aneurysms. J Vasc Surg 16:139, 1992.
5. Attinger EO: Flow patterns and vascular geometry. *In* Pulsatile Blood Flow. New York, McGraw-Hill, 1964, pp 179–200.
6. Attinger EO, Sugawara H, Navarro A, et al: Pressure flow relations in dog arteries. Circ Res 19:230, 1966.
7. Azuma T, Oka S: Mechanical equilibrium of blood vessel walls. Jpn J Physiol 21:1310, 1971.
8. Baird RN, Bird DR, Clifford PC, et al: Upstream stenosis, its diagnosis by Doppler signals from the femoral artery. Arch Surg 115:1316, 1980.
9. Bassiouny HS, White S, Glagov S, et al: Anastomotic intimal hyperplasia: Mechanical injury or flow-induced? J Vasc Surg 15:708, 1992.
10. Beaconsfield PA: A. Effect of exercise on muscle blood flow in normal and sympathectomized limbs. B. Collateral circulation before and after sympathectomy. Ann Surg 140:786, 1954.
11. Beiser GD, Zelis R, Epstein SE, et al: The role of skin and muscle resistance vessels in reflexes mediated by the baroreceptor system. J Clin Invest 49:225, 1970.
12. Bergel DH: The static elastic properties of the arterial wall. J Physiol 156:445, 1961.
13. Bergel DH: The dynamic elastic properties of the arterial wall. J Physiol 156:458, 1961.
14. Berguer R, Higgins RF, Reddy DJ: Intimal hyperplasia: An experimental study. Arch Surg 115:332, 1980.

15. Berguer R, Hwang NHC: Critical arterial stenosis: A theoretical and experimental solution. Ann Surg 180:39, 1974.
16. Bernstein EF, Fischer JC, Varco RL: Is excision the optimum treatment for all abdominal aortic aneurysms? Surgery 61:83, 1967.
17. Brice JG, Dowsett DJ, Lowe RD: Hemodynamic effects of carotid artery stenosis. Br Med J 2:1363, 1964.
18. Burch GE, Winsor T: The phlebomanometer: A new apparatus for direct measurement of venous pressure in large and small veins. JAMA 123:91, 1943.
19. Burton AC: Physiology and Biophysics of the Circulation, 2nd ed. Chicago, Year Book Medical Publishers, 1972.
20. Busuttil RW, Abou-Zamzam AM, Machleder HI: Collagenase activity of the human aorta: Comparison of patients with and without abdominal aortic aneurysms. Arch Surg 115:1373, 1980.
21. Buxton B, Lambert RP, Pitt TTE: The significance of vein wall thickness and diameter in relation to the patency of femoropopliteal saphenous vein bypass grafts. Surgery 87:425, 1980.
22. Byar D, Fiddian RV, Quereau M, et al: The fallacy of applying Poiseuille equation to segmented arterial stenosis. Am Heart J 70:216, 1965.
23. Carter SA: Clinical measurement of systolic pressures in limbs with arterial occlusive disease. JAMA 207:1869, 1969.
24. Carter SA: Response of ankle systolic pressure to leg exercise in mild or questionable arterial disease. N Engl J Med 287:578, 1972.
25. Cobb LA, Smith PH, Lwai S, et al: External iliac vein flow: Its response to exercise and relation to lactate production. J Appl Physiol 26:606, 1969.
26. Coffman JD, Mannick JA: A simple objective test for arteriosclerosis obliterans. N Engl J Med 273:1297, 1965.
27. Coffman JD, Mannick JA: Failure of vasodilator drugs in arteriosclerosis obliterans. Ann Intern Med 76:35, 1972.
28. Conrad MC, Anderson JL III, Garrett JB Jr: Chronic collateral growth after femoral artery occlusion in the dog. J Appl Physiol 31:550, 1971.
29. Conrad MC, Green HD: Hemodynamics of large and small vessels in peripheral vascular disease. Circulation 29:847, 1964.
30. Cousins MJ, Wright CJ: Graft, muscle, skin blood flow after epidural block in vascular surgical procedures. Surg Gynecol Obstet 133:59, 1971.
31. Cranley JJ: Ischemic rest pain. Arch Surg 98:187, 1969.
32. Crawshaw HM, Quist WC, Sarrallach E, et al: Flow disturbance at the distal end-to-side anastomosis: Effect of patency of the proximal outflow segment and angle of anastomosis. Arch Surg 115:1280, 1980.
33. Cronenwett JL, Lindenaur SM: Hemodynamic effects of sympathectomy in ischemic canine hind limbs. Surgery 87:417, 1980.
34. Cronenwett JL, Zelenock GB, Whitehouse WM Jr, et al: The effect of sympathetic innervation on canine muscle and skin blood flow. Arch Surg 118:420, 1983.
35. Daily JW, Harleman DRF: Fluid Dynamics. Reading, Mass, Addison-Wesley, 1966.
36. Darling RC, Raines JK, Brener BJ, et al: Quantitative segmental pulse and volume recorder: A clinical tool. Surgery 72:873, 1973.
37. Daugherty HI, Franzini JB: Steady flow of incompressible fluids in pipes. *In* Fluid Mechanics With Engineering Applications, 6th ed. New York, McGraw-Hill, 1965, pp 191–245.
38. DeWeese JA: Pedal pulses disappearing with exercise: A test for intermittent claudication. N Engl J Med 262:1214, 1960.
39. DeWeese JA, Van deBerg L, May AG, et al: Stenoses of arteries of the lower extremity. Arch Surg 89:806, 1964.
40. Dobrin PB: Mechanics of normal and diseased blood vessels. Ann Vasc Surg 2:283, 1988.
41. Dobrin PB, Baker WH, Gley WC: Elastolytic and collagenolytic studies of arteries. Implications for the mechanical properties of aneurysms. Arch Surg 119:405, 1984.
42. Dobrin PB, Rovick AA: Influence of vascular smooth muscle on contractile mechanics and elasticity of arteries. Am J Physiol 217:1644, 1969.
43. Dormandy JA: Significance of hemorrheology in the management of the ischemic limb. World J Surg 7:319, 1983.
44. Dornhorst AC, Sharpey-Schafer, EP: Collateral resistance in limbs with arterial obstruction: Spontaneous changes and effects of sympathectomy. Clin Sci 10:371, 1951.
45. Dundas P, Hillestad LK: Profunda revascularization: The early postoperative effect upon calf blood flow. Scand J Thorac Cardiovasc Surg 5:275, 1971.
46. Edholm OG, Howarth S, Sharpey-Schafer EP: Resting blood flow and blood pressure in limbs with arterial obstruction. Clin Sci 10:361, 1951.
47. Edwards WS, Holdefer WF, Mohtashemi M: The importance of proper caliber of lumen in femoral-politeal artery reconstruction. Surg Gynecol Obstet 122:37, 1966.
48. Ehrenfeld WK, Harris JD, Wylie EJ: Vascular "steal" phenomenon, an experimental study. Am J Surg 116:192, 1968.
49. Evans DH, Barrie WW, Asher MJ, et al: The relationship between ultrasonic pulsatility index and proximal arterial stenosis in a canine model. Circ Res 46:470, 1980.
50. Farrar DJ, Malindzak GS Jr, Johnson G Jr: Large vessel impedance in peripheral atherosclerosis. Circulation 56(Suppl 2):171, 1977.
51. Feinberg RL, Gregory RT, Wheeler JR, et al: The ischemic window: A method for the objective quantitation of the training effect in exercise therapy for intermittent claudication. J Vasc Surg 16:244, 1992.
52. Fiddian RV, Byar D, Edwards EA: Factors affecting flow through a stenosed vessel. Arch Surg 88:105, 1964.
53. Flanigan DP, Tullis JP, Streeter VL, et al: Multiple subcritical arterial stenoses: Effect on poststenotic pressure and flow. Ann Surg 186:663, 1977.
54. Folse JR: Application of the sudden injection dye dilution principle to the study of the femoral circulation. Surg Gynecol Obstet 120:1194, 1965.
55. Folse R: Alterations in femoral blood flow and resistance during rhythmic exercise and sustained muscular contractions in patients with arteriosclerosis. Surg Gynecol Obstet 121:767, 1965.
56. Foster JH, Bolasny BL, Gobbel WG Jr, et al: Comparative study of elective resection and expectant treatment of abdominal aortic aneurysms. Surg Gynecol Obstet 129:1, 1969.
57. Fronek A, Johansen KH, Dilley RB, et al: Non-invasive physiologic tests in the diagnosis and characterization of peripheral arterial occlusive disease. Am J Surg 126:205, 1973.
58. Gauer OH, Thron HL: Postural changes in the circulation. *In* Hamilton WF, Dow P (eds): Handbook of Physiology. Sect 2, Circulation. Vol III. Washington, DC, American Physiological Society, 1965, pp 2409–2439.
59. Glagov S, Weisenberg E, Zarins CK, et al: Compensatory enlargement of human atherosclerotic coronary arteries. N Engl J Med 316:1371, 1987.
60. Gosling RG, Dunbar G, King DH, et al: The quantitative analysis of occlusive peripheral arterial disease by a nonintrusive ultrasonic technique. Angiology 22:52, 1971.
61. Gosling RG, King DH: Continuous wave ultrasound as an alternative and complement to x-rays in vascular examination. *In* Reneman RS (ed): Cardiovascular Applications of Ultrasound. Amsterdam, North-Holland, 1974, pp 266–282.
62. Griffith TM, Lewis MJ, Newby AC, Henderson AH: Endothelium-derived relaxing factor. J Am Coll Cardiol 12:797, 1988.
63. Guyton AC: Venous return. *In* Hamilton WF, Dow P (eds): Handbook of Physiology. Sect 2, Circulation. Vol II. Washington, DC, American Physiological Society, 1963, pp 1099–1133.
64. Hillestad LK: The peripheral blood flow in intermittent claudication: V. Plethysmographic studies: The significance of the calf blood flow at rest and in response to timed arrest of the circulation. Acta Med Scand 174:23, 1963.
65. Hillestad LK: The peripheral blood flow in intermittent claudication: VI. Plethysmographic studies: The blood flow response to exercise with arrested and free circulation. Acta Med Scand 174:671, 1963.
66. Hoffman DC, Jepson RP: Muscle blood flow and sympathectomy. Surg Gynecol Obstet 127:12, 1968.
67. Hokanson DE, Strandness DE Jr: Stress-strain characteristics of various arterial grafts. Surg Gynecol Obstet 127:57, 1968.
68. Holman E: Problems in the dynamics of blood flow: I. Conditions controlling collateral circulation in the presence of an arteriovenous fistula and following ligation of an artery. Surgery 26:880, 1949.
69. Hopkins RW: Presidential address: Energy, poise, and resilience: Daniel Bernoulli, Thomas Young, J. L. M. Poiseuille, and F. A. Simeone. J Vasc Surg 13:777, 1991.
70. Ingebrigtsen R, Leraand S: Dilatation of a medium-sized artery immediately after local changes of blood pressure and flow as measured by ultrasonic technique. Acta Physiol Scand 79:552, 1970.
71. Jager KA, Phillips DJ, Martin RL, et al: Noninvasive mapping of lower limb arterial lesions. Ultrasound Med Biol 11:515, 1985.

72. James IM, Millar RA, Purves MY: Observations on the extrinsic neural control of cerebral blood flow in the baboon. Circ Res 25:77, 1969.
73. John HT, Warren R: The stimulus to collateral circulation. Surgery 49:14, 1961.
74. Johnson EC, Voyles WF, Atterbom HA, et al: Effects of exercise training on common femoral artery blood flow in patients with intermittent claudication. Circulation 80:III59, 1989.
75. Johnson PC: Review of previous studies and current theories of autoregulation. Circ Res 14:15, 1964.
76. Johnston KW, Maruzzo BC, Cobbold RSC: Errors and artifacts of Doppler flowmeters and their solution. Arch Surg 112:1335, 1977.
77. Johnston KW, Maruzzo BC, Cobbold RSC: Doppler methods for quantitative measurement and localization of peripheral arterial occlusive disease by analysis of the blood velocity waveform. Ultrasound Med Biol 4:209, 1978.
78. Jones RD, Berne RM: Intrinsic regulation of skeletal muscle blood flow. Circ Res 14:126, 1964.
79. Kamiya A, Tagowa T: Adaptive regulation of wall shear stress to flow change in the canine carotid artery. Am J Physiol 239:H14, 1980.
80. Karayannacos PE, Talukder N, Nerem RM, et al: The role of multiple noncritical arterial stenoses in the pathogenesis of ischemia. J Thorac Cardiovasc Surg 73:458, 1977.
81. Keenan RL, Rodbard S: Competition between collateral vessels. Cardiovasc Res 7:670, 1973.
82. Keitzer WF, Fry WJ, Kraft RO, et al: Hemodynamic mechanism for pulse changes seen in occlusive vascular disease. Surgery 57:163, 1965.
83. Kindt GW, Youmans JR: The effect of stricture length on critical arterial stenosis. Surg Gynecol Obstet 128:729, 1969.
84. Kinley CE, Marble AE: Compliance: A continuing problem with vascular grafts. J Cardiovas Surg 21:163, 1980.
85. Kinley CE, Paasche PE, MacDonald AS, et al: Stress at vascular anastomosis in relation to host artery: Synthetic graft diameter. Surgery 75:28, 1974.
86. Kjellmer I: On the competition between metabolic vasodilatation and neurogenic vasoconstriction in skeletal muscle. Acta Physiol Scand 63:450, 1965.
87. Korner PI: Control of blood flow to special vascular areas: Brain, kidney, muscle, skin, liver and intestine. *In* Guyton AC, Jones CE (eds): MTP International Review of Science, Physiology. Series 1. Vol 1. Cardiovascular Physiology. London, Butterworths, 1974, pp 123–162.
88. Ku DN, Giddens DP, Zarins CK, Glagov S: Pulsatile flow and atherosclerosis in the human carotid bifurcation: Positive correlation between plaque location and low and oscillating shear stress. Arteriosclerosis 5:293, 1985.
89. Langille BL, O'Donnell F: Reductions in arterial diameter produced by chronic decreases in blood flow are endothelium-dependent. Science 231:405, 1986.
90. Larsen OA, Lassen NA: Medical treatment of occlusive arterial disease of the legs: Walking exercise and medically induced hypertension. Angiologica 6:288, 1969.
91. Lassen NA: Cerebral blood flow and oxygen consumption in man. Physiol Rev 39:183, 1959.
92. Lassen NA, Kampp M: Calf muscle blood flow during walking studied by the ^{133}Xe method in normals and in patients with intermittent claudication. Scand J Clin Lab Invest 17:447, 1965.
93. Lassen NA, Larsen OA, Sørensen AWS, et al: Conservative treatment of gangrene using mineral corticoid-induced moderate hypertension. Lancet 1:606, 1968.
94. Lassen NA, Lindberg IF, Dahn I: Validity of the xenon 133 method for measurement of muscle blood flow evaluated by simultaneous venous occlusion plethysmography: Observations in the calf of normal man and in patients with occlusive vascular disease. Circ Res 16:287, 1965.
95. LeVeen HH, Moon I, Ahmed N, et al: Lowering blood viscosity to overcome vascular resistance. Surg Gynecol Obstet 150:139, 1980.
96. Lewis JD, Papathanaiou C, Yao ST, et al: Simultaneous flow and pressure measurements in intermittent claudication. Br J Surg 59:418, 1972.
97. Lewis P, Psaila JV, Morgan RH, et al: Common femoral artery volume flow in peripheral vascular disease. Br J Surg 77:183, 1990.
98. Lewis T, Pickering GW, Rothschild P: Observations upon muscular pain in intermittent claudication. Heart 15:359, 1931.
99. Ling SC, Atabek HB, Letzing WG, et al: Non-linear analysis of aortic flow in living dogs. Circ Res 33:198, 1973.
100. LoGerfo FW, Quist WC, Nowak MD, et al: Downstream anastomotic hyperplasia: A mechanism of failure of Dacron arterial grafts. Ann Surg 197:479, 1983.
101. LoGerfo FW, Soncrant T, Teel T, et al: Boundary layer separation in models of side-to-end arterial anastomoses. Arch Surg 114:1369, 1979.
102. Longland CJ: The collateral circulation of the limb. Ann R Coll Surg Engl 13:161, 1953.
103. Lorentsen E, Hoel BL, Hol R: Evaluation of the functional importance of atherosclerotic obliterations in the aorto-iliac artery by pressure/flow measurements. Acta Med Scand 191:399, 1972.
104. Ludbrook J: Collateral artery resistance in the human lower limb. J Surg Res 6:423, 1966.
105. Lye CR, Sumner DS, Strandness DE Jr: Hemodynamics of the retrograde cross-pubic anastomosis. Surg Forum 26:298, 1975.
106. Lye CR, Sumner DS, Strandness DE Jr: The transcutaneous measurement of the elastic properties of the human saphenous vein femoropopliteal bypass graft. Surg Gynecol Obstet 141:891, 1975.
107. Malcome AD, Roach MR: Flow disturbances at the apex and lateral angles of a variety of bifurcation models and their role in the development and manifestations of arterial disease. Stroke 10:335, 1979.
108. Mannick JA, Jackson BT: Hemodynamics of arterial surgery in atherosclerotic limbs: I. Direct measurement of blood flow before and after vein grafts. Surgery 59:713, 1966.
109. Martin P, Frawley JE, Barabas AP, et al: On the surgery of atherosclerosis of the profunda femoris artery. Surgery 71:182, 1972.
110. May AG, DeWeese JA, Rob CA: Hemodynamic effects of arterial stenosis. Surgery 53:513, 1963.
111. May AG, Van deBerg L, DeWeese JA, et al: Critical arterial stenosis. Surgery 54:250, 1963.
112. McDonald DA: Blood Flow in Arteries, 2nd ed. Baltimore, Williams & Wilkins, 1974.
113. McMillan DE: Blood flow and the localization of atherosclerotic plaques. Stroke 16:582, 1985.
114. Mehigan DG, Fitzpatrick B, Browne HI, Bouchier-Hayes DJ: Is compliance mismatch the major cause of anastomotic arterial aneurysms? J Cardiovasc Surg 26:147, 1985.
115. Melkumyants AM, Balashov SA, Veselova ES, Khayutin VM: Continuous control of the lumen of feline conduit arteries by blood flow rate. Cardiovasc Res 21:863, 1987.
116. Milnor WR: Pulsatile blood flow. N Engl J Med 287:27, 1972.
117. Moore WS, Hall AD: Unrecognized aortoiliac stenosis: A physiologic approach to the diagnosis. Arch Surg 103:633, 1971.
118. Moore WS, Malone JM: Effect of flow rate and vessel caliber on critical arterial stenosis. J Surg Res 26:1, 1979.
119. Moore WS, Sydorak GR, Newcomb L, et al: Blood pressure gradient to estimate flow changes with progressive arterial stenosis. Surg Forum 24:248, 1973.
120. Morris GC Jr, Edwards W, Cooley DA, et al: Surgical importance of the profunda femoris artery. Arch Surg 82:32, 1961.
121. Motomiya M, Karino T: Flow patterns in the human carotid artery bifurcation. Stroke 15:50, 1984.
122. Mozersky DJ, Sumner DS, Hokanson DE, et al: Transcutaneous measurement of the elastic properties of the human femoral artery. Circulation 46:948, 1972.
123. Mundth ED, Darling RC, Moran JM, et al: Quantitative correlation of distal arterial outflow and patency of femoropopliteal reversed saphenous vein grafts with intraoperative flow and pressure measurements. Surgery 65:197, 1969.
124. Newman DL, Gosling RG, Bowden NLR, et al: Pressure amplitude increase on unmatching the aorto-iliac junction of the dog. Cardiovasc Res 7:6, 1973.
125. Nichols WK, Stanton M, Silver D, et al: Anastomotic aneurysms following lower extremity revascularization. Surgery 88:366, 1980.
126. Nicolaides AN, Gordon-Smith DC, Dayandas J, et al: The value of Doppler blood velocity tracings in the detection of aortoiliac disease in patients with intermittent claudication. Surgery 80:774, 1976.
127. Ojha M, Cobbold RSC, Johnston KW, Hummel RL: Pulsatile flow through constricted tubes: An experimental investigation using photochromic tracer methods. J Fluid Mech 203:173, 1989.
128. Ojha M, Ethier CR, Johnston KW, Cobbold RSC: Steady and pulsatile flow fields in an end-to-side arterial anastomosis model. J Vasc Surg 12:747, 1990.

129. Ojha M, Johnston KW, Cobbold RSC: Evidence of a possible link between poststenotic dilation and wall shear stress. J Vasc Surg 11:127, 1990.
130. Okadone K, Yukizane T, Mii S, Sugimachi K: Ultrastructural evidence of the effects of shear stress variation on intimal thickening in dogs with arterially transplanted autologous grafts. J Cardiovasc Surg 31:719, 1990.
131. O'Rourke MF: Steady and pulsatile energy losses in the systemic circulation under normal conditions and in simulated arterial disease. Cardiovasc Res 1:313, 1967.
132. Ouriel K, Donayre C, Shortell CK, et al: The hemodynamics of thrombus formation in arteries. J Vasc Surg 14:757, 1991.
133. Paasche PE, Kinley CE, Dolan FG, et al: Consideration of suture line stresses in the selection of synthetic grafts for implantation. J Biomech 6:253, 1973.
134. Pedersen EM, Hjortdal JØ, Hjortdal VE, et al: Three-dimensional visualization of velocity profiles in the porcine abdominal aortic trifurcation. J Vasc Surg 15:194, 1992.
135. Pentecost BL: The effect of exercise on the external iliac vein blood flow and local oxygen consumption in normal subjects, and in those with occlusive arterial disease. Clin Sci 27:437, 1964.
136. Peterson LH: Physical factors which influence vascular caliber and blood flow. Circ Res 18 and 19(Suppl 1):3, 1966.
137. Peterson LH, Jensen RE, Parnell J: Mechanical properties of arteries in vivo. Circ Res 8:622, 1960.
138. Porter JM, Cutler BS, Lee BY, et al: Pentoxifylline efficacy in the treatment of intermittent claudication. Am Heart J 104:66, 1982.
139. Reagan TR, Miller CW, Strandness DE Jr: Transcutaneous measurement of femoral artery flow. J Surg Res 11:477, 1971.
140. Remensnyder JP, Mitchell JH, Sarnoff SJ: Functional sympatholysis during muscular activity. Circ Res 11:370, 1962.
141. Remington JW, Wood EH: Formation of peripheral pulse contour in man. J Appl Physiol 9:433, 1956.
142. Rijsterborgh H, Roelandt J: Doppler assessment of aortic stenosis: Bernoulli revisited. Ultrasound Med Biol 13:241, 1987.
143. Rittenhouse EA, Maxiner W, Burr JW, et al: Directional arterial flow velocity: A sensitive index of changes in peripheral vascular resistance. Surgery 79:359, 1976.
144. Rittgers SE, Shu MCS: Doppler color-flow images from a stenosed arterial model: Interpretation of flow patterns. J Vasc Surg 12:511, 1990.
145. Roederer GO, Langlois YE, Chan AW, et al: Ultrasonic duplex scanning of extracranial carotid arteries: Improved accuracy using new features from the common carotid artery. J Cardiovasc Ultrasonography 1:373, 1982.
146. Rosenthal SL, Guyton AC: Hemodynamics of collateral vasodilatation following femoral artery occlusion in anesthetized dogs. Circ Res 23:239, 1968.
147. Rutherford RB, Valenta J: Extremity blood flow and distribution: The effects of arterial occlusion, sympathectomy, and exercise. Surgery 69:332, 1971.
148. Sanders RJ, Kempczinski RF, Hammond W, et al: The significance of graft diameter. Surgery 88:856, 1980.
149. Scheffler A, Rieger H: A comparative analysis of transcutaneous oximetry ($tcPO_2$) during oxygen inhalation and leg dependency in severe peripheral arterial occlusive disease. J Vasc Surg 16:218, 1992.
150. Schneider JR, Zwolak RM, Walsh DB, et al: Lack of diameter effect on short-term patency of size-matched Dacron aortofemoral grafts. J Vasc Surg 13:785, 1991.
151. Schultz DL: Pressure and flow in large arteries. *In* Bergel DH (ed). Cardiovascular Fluid Dynamics. Vol I. New York, Academic Press, 1972, pp 287–314.
152. Schultz RD, Hokanson DE, Strandness DE Jr: Pressure-flow relations of the end-side anastomosis. Surgery 62:319, 1967.
153. Segadal L, Matre K: Blood velocity distribution in the human ascending aorta. Circulation 76:90, 1987.
154. Sharefkin JB, Diamond SL, Eskin SG, et al: Fluid flow decreases preproendothelin mRNA levels and suppresses endothelin-1 peptide release in cultured human endothelial cells. J Vasc Surg 14:1, 1991.
155. Sharp WV, Donovan DL, Teague PC, Mosteller RD: Arterial occlusive disease: A function of vessel bifurcation angle. Surgery 91:680, 1982.
156. Shepherd JT: The blood flow through the calf after exercise in subjects with arteriosclerosis and claudication. Clin Sci 9:49, 1950.
157. Shepherd JT: Physiology of the Circulation in Human Limbs in Health and Disease. Philadelphia, WB Saunders, 1963.
158. Skidmore R, Woodcock JP: Physiological interpretation of Doppler-shift waveforms: I. Theoretical considerations. Ultrasound Med Biol 6:7, 1980.
159. Skidmore R, Woodcock JP: Physiological interpretation of Doppler-shift waveforms: II. Validation of the Laplace transform method for characterization of the common femoral blood-velocity/time waveform. Ultrasound Med Biol 6:219, 1980.
160. Skidmore R, Woodcock JP, Wells PNT, et al: Physiological interpretation of Doppler-shift waveforms: III. Clinical results. Ultrasound Med Biol 6:227, 1980.
161. Skinner JS, Strandness DE Jr: Exercise and intermittent claudication: I. Effect of repetition and intensity of exercise. Circulation 36:15, 1967.
162. Skinner JS, Strandness DE Jr: Exercise and intermittent claudication: II. Effect of physical training. Circulation 36:23, 1967.
163. Snell ES, Eastcott HHG, Hamilton M: Circulation in lower limb before and after reconstruction of obstructed main artery. Lancet 1:242, 1960.
164. Sottiurai VS, Sue SL, Breaux JR, Smith LM: Adaptability of endothelial orientation to blood flow dynamics: A morphologic analysis. Eur J Vasc Surg 3:145, 1989.
165. Stahler C, Strandness DE Jr: Ankle blood pressure response to gradual treadmill exercise. Angiology 18:237, 1967.
166. Strandell T, Wahren J: Circulation in the calf at rest, after arterial occlusion and after exercise in normal subjects and in patients with intermittent claudication. Acta Med Scand 173:99, 1963.
167. Strandness DE Jr: Abnormal exercise response after successful reconstructive arterial surgery. Surgery 59:325, 1966.
168. Strandness DE Jr: Functional results after revascularization of the profunda femoris artery. Am J Surg 119:240, 1970.
169. Strandness DE Jr, Bell JW: An evaluation of the hemodynamic response of the claudicating extremity to exercise. Surg Gynecol Obstet 119:1237, 1964.
170. Strandness DE Jr, Bell JW: Critical evaluation of the results of lumbar sympathectomy. Ann Surg 160:1021, 1964.
171. Strandness DE Jr, Bell JW: Peripheral vascular disease: Diagnosis and objective evaluation using a mercury strain gauge. Ann Surg 161(Suppl):1, 1965.
172. Strandness DE Jr, Schultz RD, Sumner DS, et al: Ultrasonic flow detection: A useful technique in the evaluation of peripheral vascular disease. Am J Surg 113:311, 1967.
173. Strandness DE Jr, Sumner DS: Hemodynamics for Surgeons. New York, Grune & Stratton, 1975.
174. Streeter VC, Keitzer WF, Bohr DF: Pulsatile pressure and flow through distensible vessels. Circ Res 13:3, 1963.
175. Stromberg DD, Weiderhielm CA: Viscoelastic description of a collagenous tissue in simple elongation. J Appl Physiol 26:857, 1969.
176. Sumner DS, Strandness DE Jr: The relationship between calf blood flow and ankle blood pressure in patients with intermittent claudication. Surgery 65:763, 1969.
177. Sumner DS, Strandness DE Jr: The effect of exercise on resistance to blood flow in limbs with an occluded superficial femoral artery. Vasc Surg 4:229, 1970.
178. Sumner DS, Strandness DE Jr: The hemodynamics of the femorofemoral shunt. Surg Gynecol Obstet 134:629, 1972.
179. Sumner DS, Hokanson DE, Strandness DE Jr: Arterial walls before and after endarterectomy, stress-strain characteristics and collagen-elastic content. Arch Surg 99:606, 1969.
180. Sumner DS, Hokanson DE, Strandness DE Jr: Stress-strain characteristics and collagen-elastic content of abdominal aortic aneurysms. Surg Gynecol Obstet 130:459, 1970.
181. Sydorak GR, Moore WS, Newcomb L, et al: Effect of increasing flow rates and arterial caliber on critical arterial stenoses. Surg Forum 23:243, 1972.
182. Van deBerg L, DeWeese JA, Rob CG: The effect of arterial stenosis and sympathectomy on blood flow and the ergogram. Ann Surg 159:623, 1964.
183. Vieli A, Moser U, Maier S, et al: Velocity profiles in the normal human abdominal aorta: A comparison between ultrasound and magnetic resonance data. Ultrasound Biol Med 15:113, 1989.
184. Vonruden WJ, Blaisdell FW, Hall AD et al: Multiple arterial stenosis: Effect on blood flow. Arch Surg 89:307, 1964.
185. Wahren J, Jorfeldt L: Determinations of leg blood flow during exercise in man: An indicator-dilution technique based on femoral venous dye infusion. Clin Sci Mol Med 45:135, 1973.

186. Walden R, L'Italien GJ, Megerman J, et al: Matched elastic properties and successful arterial grafting. Arch Surg 115:1166, 1980.
187. Walker JR, Guyton AC: Influence of blood oxygen saturation on pressure-flow curve of dog hind leg. Am J Physiol 212:506, 1967.
188. Weissenhofer W, Schenk WG Jr: Hemodynamic response to vasodilation and exercise in "critical" arterial stenosis. Arch Surg 108:712, 1974.
189. Wengerter KR, Veith FJ, Gupta SK, et al: Influence of vein size (diameter) on infrapopliteal reversed vein graft patency. J Vasc Surg 11:525, 1990.
190. Wesolowski SA, Martinez A, Domingo RT, et al: Indications for aortofemoral arterial reconstruction: A study of borderline risk patients. Surgery 60:288, 1966.
191. Westerhof N, Sipkema P, Van Den Bos GC, et al: Forward and backward waves in the arterial system. Cardiovasc Res 6:648, 1972.
192. Winblad JN, Reemtsma K, Vernhet JL, et al: Etiologic mechanisms in the development of collateral circulation. Surgery 45:105, 1959.
193. Winsor T: Influence of arterial disease on the systolic blood pressure gradients of the extremity. Am J Med Sci 220:117, 1950.
194. Wolf EA Jr, Sumner DS, Strandness DE Jr: Correlation between nutritive blood flow and pressure in limbs of patients with intermittent claudication. Surg Forum 23:238, 1972.
195. Wolfe JHN, Waller DG, Chapman MB, et al: The effect of hemodilution upon patients with intermittent claudication. Surg Gynecol Obstet 160:347, 1985.
196. Wong PKC, Johnston KW, Ethier CR, Cobbold RSC: Computer simulation of blood flow patterns in arteries of various geometries. J Vasc Surg 14:658, 1991.
197. Woodcock JP, Gosling RG, Fitzgerald DE: A new non-invasive technique for assessment of superficial femoral artery obstruction. Br J Surg 59:226, 1972.
198. Wyatt MG, Muir RM, Tennant WG, et al: Impedance analysis to identify the at risk femorodistal graft. J Vasc Surg 13:284, 1991.
199. Yao ST: Haemodynamic studies in peripheral arterial disease. Br J Surg 57:761, 1970.
200. Yao ST, Hobbs JT, Irvine WT: Pulse examination by an ultrasonic method. Br Med J 4:555, 1968.
201. Yao ST, Hobbs JT, Irvine WT: Ankle systolic pressure measurements in arterial disease affecting the lower extremities. Br J Surg 56:676, 1969.
202. Yellin EL: Laminar-turbulent transition process in pulsation flow. Circ Res 19:791, 1966.
203. Young DF, Tsai FY: Flow characteristics in models of arterial stenoses. I. Steady flow. J Biomech 6:395, 1973.
204. Young DF, Tsai FY: Flow characteristics of models of arterial stenosis: II. Unsteady flow. J Biomech 6:547, 1973.
205. Zarins CK, Giddens DP, Bharadvaj BK, et al: Carotid bifurcation atherosclerosis: Quantitative correlation of plaque localization with flow velocity profiles and wall shear stress. Circ Res 53:502, 1983.
206. Zarins CK, Xu C, Glagov S: Aneurysmal enlargement of the aorta during regression of experimental atherosclerosis. J Vasc Surg 15:90, 1992.
207. Zarins CK, Zatina MA, Giddens DP, et al: Shear stress regulation of artery lumen diameter in experimental atherogenesis. J Vasc Surg 5:413, 1987.
208. Zarins CK, Glagov S, Vesselinovitch D, Wissler RW: Aneurysm formation in experimental atherosclerosis: Relationship to plaque evolution. J Vasc Surg 12:246, 1990.
209. Zellis R, Mason DT, Braunwald E, et al: Effects of hyperlipoproteinemias and their treatment on the peripheral circulation. J Clin Invest 49:1007, 1970.
210. Zwiebel WJ, Zagzebski JA, Crummy AB, et al: Correlation of peak Doppler frequency with lumen narrowing in carotid stenosis. Stroke 13:386, 1982.
211. Cambria RA, Lowell RC, Gloviczki P, Miller VM: Chronic changes in blood flow alter endothelium-dependent responses in autogenous vein grafts in dogs. J Vasc Surg 20:765, 1994.
212. Di Martino E, Mantero S, Inzoli F, et al: Biomechanics of abdominal aortic aneurysm in the presence of endoluminal thrombus: Experimental characterisation and structural static computational analysis. Eur J Vasc Endovasc Surg 15:290, 1998.
213. Dobrin PB, Mirande R, Kang S, et al: Mechanics of end-to-end artery-to-PTFE graft anastomoses. Ann Vasc Surg 12:317, 1998.
214. Fillinger MF, Cronenwett JL, Besso S, et al: Vein adaptation to the hemodynamic environment of infrainguinal grafts. J Vasc Surg 19:970, 1994.
215. Golledge J, Hicks RCJ, Ellis M, et al: Dilatation of saphenous vein grafts by nitric oxide. Eur J Vasc Endovasc Surg 14:41, 1977.
216. Inzoli F, Boschetti F, Zappa M, et al: Biomechanical factors in abdominal aortic aneurysm rupture. Eur J Vasc Surg 7:667, 1993.
217. Lei M, Archie JP, Kleinstreuer C: Computational design of a bypass graft that minimizes wall shear stress gradients in the region of the distal anastomosis. J Vasc Surg 25:637, 1997.
218. Miller VM, Burnett JC Jr: Modulation of NO and endothelin by chronic increases in blood flow in canine femoral arteries. Am J Physiol 263:H103, 1992.
219. Mower WR, Quiñones WJ, Gambhir SS: Effect of intraluminal thrombus on abdominal aortic aneurysm wall stress. J Vasc Surg 26:602, 1997.
220. Park TC, Harker CT, Edwards JM, et al: Human saphenous vein grafts explanted from the arterial circulation demonstrate altered smooth-muscle and endothelial responses. J Vasc Surg 18:61, 1993.
221. Schwartz LB, Purut CM, Craig DM, et al: Input impedance of revascularized skeletal muscle, renal, and mesenteric vascular beds. Vasc Surg 30:459, 1996.
222. Sonesson B, Hansen F, Stale H, Länne T: Compliance and diameter in the human abdominal aorta: The influence of age and sex. Eur J Vasc Surg 7:690, 1993.
223. Unthank JL, Nixon JC, Dalsing MC: Nitric oxide maintains dilation of immature and mature collateral in the rat hindlimb. J Vasc Res 33:471, 1966.
224. van Dielen FMH, Kurvers HAJM, Dammers R, et al: Effects of surgical sympathectomy on skin blood flow in a rat model of chronic limb ischemia. World J Surg 22:807, 1998.
225. Vorp DA, Raghavan ML, Webster MW: Mechanical wall stress in abdominal aortic aneurysm: Influence of diameter and asymmetry. J Vasc Surg 27:632, 1998.

Venous Hemodynamics

226. Abramowitz HB, Queral LA, Flinn WR, et al: The use of photoplethysmography in the assessment of venous insufficiency: A comparison to venous pressure measurements. Surgery 86:434, 1979.
227. Abu-Own AA, Scurr JH, Coleridge Smith PD: Assessment of microangiopathy of the skin in chronic venous insufficiency by laser Doppler fluxmetry. J Vasc Surg 17:429, 1993.
228. Abu-Own AA, Scurr JH, Coleridge Smith PD: Assessment of microangiopathy of the skin in chronic venous insufficiency by laser Doppler fluxmetry. J Vasc Surg 17:429, 1993.
229. Alimi YS, Barthelemy P, Juhan C: Venous pump of the calf: A study of venous and muscular pressures. J Vasc Surg 20:728, 1994.
230. Almén T, Nylander G: Serial phlebography of the normal lower leg during muscular contraction and relaxation. Acta Radiol 57:264, 1962.
231. Araki CT, Back TL, Padberg FT, et al: The significance of calf muscle pump function in venous ulceration. J Vasc Surg 20:872, 1994.
232. Arenander E: Hemodynamic effects of varicose veins and results of radical surgery. Acta Chir Scand 260(Suppl):1, 1960.
233. Arnoldi CC: Venous pressure in patients with valvular incompetence of the veins of the lower limb. Acta Chir Scand 132:628, 1966.
234. Arnoldi CC, Linderholm H: On the pathogenesis of the venous leg ulcer. Acta Chir Scand 134:427, 1968.
235. Arnoldi CC, Linderholm H: Venous blood pressures in the lower limb at rest and during exercise in patients with idiopathic dysfunction of the venous pump of the calf. Acta Chir Scand 135:601, 1969.
236. Attinger EO: Wall properties of veins. IEEE Trans Biomed Eng 16:253, 1969.
237. Barnes RW, Collicott PE, Mozersky DJ, et al: Noninvasive quantitation of maximum venous outflow in acute thrombophlebitis. Surgery 72:971, 1972.
238. Barnes RW, Collicott PE, Mozersky DJ, et al: Noninvasive quantitation of venous reflux in the postphlebitic syndrome. Surg Gynecol Obstet 136:769, 1973.
239. Barnes RW, Collicott PE, Mozersky DJ, et al: Noninvasive quantitation of venous hemodynamics in postphlebitic syndrome. Arch Surg 107:807, 1973.
240. Barwin BN, Roddie IC: Venous distensibility during pregnancy determined by graded venous congestion. Am J Obstet Gynecol 125:921, 1976.
241. Bauer G: A roentgenological and clinical study of the sequels of thrombosis. Acta Chir Scand 86(Suppl 74):1, 1942.

242. Beecher HK, Field ME, Krogh A: The effect of walking on the venous pressure at the ankle. Skand Arch Physiol 73:133, 1936.
243. Bishara RA, Sigel B, Rocco K, et al: Deterioration of venous function in normal lower extremities during daily activity. J Vasc Surg 3:700, 1986.
244. Bjordal RI: Simultaneous pressure and flow recordings in varicose veins of the lower extremity: A hemodynamic study of venous dysfunction. Acta Chir Scand 136:309, 1970.
245. Brace RA: Progress toward resolving the controversy of positive vs. negative interstitial fluid pressure. Circ Res 49:281, 1981.
246. Brockman SK, Vasko JS: Phlegmasia cerulea dolens. Surg Gynecol Obstet 121:1347, 1965.
247. Brockman SK, Vasko JS: The pathologic physiology of phlegmasia cerulea dolens. Surgery 59:997, 1966.
248. Browse NL: The pathogenesis of venous ulceration: A hypothesis. J Vasc Surg 7:468, 1988.
249. Browse NL, Shepherd JT: Differences in response of veins and resistance vessels in limbs to same stimulus. Am J Physiol 211:1241, 1966.
250. Burnand KG, Whimster I, Naidoo A, et al: Pericapillary fibrin in the ulcer-bearing skin of the leg: The cause of lipodermatosclerosis and venous ulcerations. Br Med J 285:1071, 1982.
251. Christopoulos D, Nicolaides AN: Noninvasive diagnosis and quantitation of popliteal reflux in the swollen and ulcerated leg. J Cardiovasc Surg 29:535, 1988.
252. Christopoulos D, Nicolaides AN, Galloway JMD, Wilkinson A: Objective noninvasive evaluation of venous surgical results. J Vasc Surg 8:683, 1988.
253. Christopoulos D, Nicolaides AN, Szendro G: Venous reflux: Quantification and correlation with the clinical severity of chronic venous disease. Br J Surg 75:352, 1988.
254. Christopoulos DG, Nicolaides AN, Szendro G, et al: Air-plethysmography and the effect of elastic compression on venous hemodynamics of the leg. J Vasc Surg 5:148, 1987.
255. Clarke GH, Vasdekis SN, Hobbs JT, Nicolaides AN: Venous wall function in the pathogenesis of varicose veins. Surgery 111:402, 1992.
256. Cockett FB, Jones DEE: The ankle blowout syndrome, a new approach to the varicose ulcer problem. Lancet 1:17, 1953.
257. Conrad MC: Functional Anatomy of the Circulation to the Extremities. Chicago, Year Book Medical Publishers, 1971.
258. Cotton LT: Varicose veins, gross anatomy and development. Br J Surg 48:549, 1961.
259. Dahn I, Eiriksson E: Plethysmographic diagnosis of deep venous thrombosis of the leg. Acta Chir Scand 398(Suppl):33, 1968.
260. Dalsing MC, Lalka SG, Unthank JL, et al: Venous valvular insufficiency: Influence of a single venous valve (native and experimental). J Vasc Surg 14:576, 1991.
261. Darke SG, Penfold C: Venous ulceration and saphenous ligation. Eur J Vasc Surg 6:4, 1992.
262. DeCamp PT, Schramel RJ, Roy CJ, et al: Ambulatory venous pressure determinations in postphlebitic and related syndromes. Surgery 29:44, 1951.
263. DeWeese JA, Rogoff SM: Phlebographic patterns of acute deep venous thrombosis of the leg. Surgery 53:99, 1963.
264. Edwards EA, Edwards JE: The effect of thrombophlebitis on the venous valve. Surg Gynecol Obstet 65:310, 1937.
265. Edwards JE, Edwards EA: The saphenous valves in varicose veins. Am Heart J 19:338, 1940.
266. Eiriksson E, Dahn L: Plethysmographic studies of venous distensibility in patients with varicose veins. Acta Chir Scand 398 (Suppl):19, 1968.
267. Ellwood RA, Lee WB: Pedal venous pressure: Correlation with presence and site of deep-venous abnormalities. Radiology 131:73, 1979.
268. Fagrell B: Local microcirculation in chronic venous incompetence and leg ulcers. Vasc Surg 13:217, 1979.
269. Fegan WG, Kline AL: The cause of varicosity in superficial veins of the lower limb. Br J Surg 59:798, 1972.
270. Folse R: The influence of femoral vein dynamics on the development of varicose veins. Surgery 68:974, 1970.
271. Franzeck UK, Bollinger A, Huch R, et al: Transcutaneous oxygen tension and capillary morphologic characteristics and density in patients with chronic venous incompetence. Circulation 70:806, 1984.
272. Fry DL, Thomas LJ, Greenfield JC Jr: Flow in collapsible tubes. *In* Patel DJ, Vaishnav RN (eds): Basic Hemodynamics and Its Role in Disease Processes. Baltimore, University Park Press, 1980, pp 407–424.
273. Gardner AMN, Fox RH: The Return of Blood to the Heart. Venous Pumps in Health and Disease. London, John Libbey Eurotext, 1989.
274. Gooley NA, Sumner DS: Relationship of venous reflux to the site of venous valvular incompetence: Implications for venous reconstructive surgery. J Vasc Surg 7:50, 1988.
275. Greenfield ADM: The venous system in cardiovascular functions. *In* Luisada AA (ed): Cardiovascular Functions. New York, McGraw-Hill, 1962.
276. Guyton AC: Interstitial fluid pressure: II. Pressure-volume curves of interstitial space. Circ Res 16:452, 1965.
277. Hallböök T, Göthlin J: Strain gauge plethysmography and phlebography in diagnosis of deep venous thrombosis. Acta Chir Scand 137:37, 1971.
278. Haller JA Jr: Effects of deep femoral thrombophlebitis on the circulation of the lower extremities. Circulation 27:693, 1963.
279. Hanrahan LM, Araki CT, Rodriguez AA, et al: Distribution of valvular incompetence in patients with venous stasis ulceration. J Vasc Surg 13:805, 1991.
280. Hjelmstedt NA: Pressure decrease in the dorsal pedal veins on walking in persons with and without thrombosis. Acta Chir Scand 134:531, 1968.
281. Hjelmstedt NA: The pressure in the veins of the dorsum of the foot in quiet standing and during exercise in limbs without signs of venous disorder. Acta Chir Scand 134:235, 1968.
282. Höjensgård IC, Stürup H: Static and dynamic pressures in superficial and deep veins of the lower extremity in man. Acta Physiol Scand 27:49, 1952.
283. Holt JP: Flow through collapsible tubes and through in situ veins. IEEE Trans Biomed Eng 16:274, 1969.
284. Husni EA, Ximenes JO, Goyette EM: Elastic support of the lower limbs in hospital patients: A critical study. JAMA 214:1456, 1970.
285. Ikard RW, Ueland K, Folse R: Lower limb venous dynamics in pregnant women. Surg Gynecol Obstet 132:483, 1971.
286. Jacobsen BH: The venous drainage of the foot. Surg Gynecol Obstet 131:22, 1970.
287. Johnson ND, Queral LA, Flinn WR, et al: Late objective assessment of venous valve surgery. Arch Surg 116:1461, 1981.
288. Kerr MG, Scott DB, Samuel E: Studies of the inferior vena cava in late pregnancy. Br Med J 1:532, 1964.
289. Killewich LA, Bedford GR, Beach KW, Strandness DE Jr: Spontaneous lysis of deep venous thrombi: Rate and outcome. J Vasc Surg 9:89, 1989.
290. Koslow AR, DeWeese JA: Anatomical and mechanical aspects of a plantar venous plexus. Presented at the Jobst Symposium on Current Issues in Venous Disease, Chicago, 1988.
291. Kuster G, Lofgren CP, Hollinshead WH: Anatomy of the veins of the foot. Surg Gynecol Obstet 127:817, 1968.
292. Labropoulos N, Leon M, Geroulakos G, et al: Venous hemodynamic abnormalities in patients with leg ulceration. Am J Surg 169:572, 1995.
293. Labropoulos N, Leon M, Nicolaides AN, et al: Venous reflux in patients with previous deep venous thrombosis: Correlation with ulceration and other symptoms. J Vasc Surg 20:20, 1994.
294. Labropoulos N, Leon M, Nicolaides AN, et al: Superficial venous insufficiency: Correlation of anatomic extent of reflux with clinical symptoms and signs. J Vasc Surg 20:953, 1994.
295. Landis EM, Pappenheimer JR: Exchange of substances through capillary walls. *In* Hamilton WF, Dow P (eds): Handbook of Physiology. Vol II. Washington DC, American Physiological Society, 1963, pp 961–1034.
296. Lees TA, Lambert D: Patterns of venous reflux in limbs with skin changes associated with chronic venous insufficiency. Br J Surg 80:725, 1993.
297. LePage PA, Villavicencio JL, Gomez FR, et al: The valvular anatomy of the internal iliac venous system and its clinical implications. J Vasc Surg 14:678, 1991.
298. Lindner DJ, Edwards JM, Phinney ES, et al: Long-term hemodynamic and clinical sequelae of lower extremity deep vein thrombosis. J Vasc Surg 4:436, 1986.
299. Linton RR: Post-thrombotic ulceration of the lower extremity: Its etiology and surgical treatment. Ann Surg 138:415, 1953.
300. Lowell RC, Gloviczki P, Miller VM: In vitro evaluation of endothelial

and smooth muscle function of primary varicose veins. J Vasc Surg 16:679, 1992.
301. Ludbrook J: Valvular defect in primary varicose veins, cause or effect? Lancet 2:1289, 1963.
302. Ludbrook J: The musculovenous pumps of the human lower limb. Am Heart J 71:635, 1966.
303. Ludbrook J: Aspects of Venous Function in the Lower Limbs. Springfield, Ill, Charles C Thomas, 1966.
304. Ludbrook J, Beale G: Femoral venous valves in relation to varicose veins. Lancet 1:79, 1962.
305. Ludbrook J, Loughlin J: Regulation of volume in postarteriolar vessels of the lower limb. Am Heart J 67:493, 1964.
306. Lye CR, Sumner DS, Hokanson DE, Strandness DE Jr: The transcutaneous measurement of the elastic properties of the human saphenous vein femoropopliteal bypass graft. Surg Gynecol Obstet 141:891, 1975.
307. Lyon CK, Scott JB, Wang CY: Flow through collapsible tubes at low Reynolds numbers. Circ Res 47:68, 1980.
308. Lyon CK, Scott JB, Anderson DK, Wang CY: Flow through collapsible tubes at high Reynolds numbers. Circ Res 49:988, 1981.
309. Mani R: Venous haemodynamics: A consideration of macro- and microvascular effects. Proc Inst Mech Eng 206:109, 1992.
310. Markel A, Manzo RA, Bergelin RO, Strandness DE Jr: Valvular reflux after deep vein thrombosis: Incidence and time of occurrence. J Vasc Surg 15:377, 1992.
311. Masuda EM, Kistner RL: Prospective comparison of duplex scanning and descending venography in the assessment of venous insufficiency. Am J Surg 164:254, 1992.
312. McEnroe CS, O'Donnell TF Jr, Mackey WC: Correlation of clinical findings with venous hemodynamics in 386 patients with chronic venous insufficiency. Am J Surg 156:148, 1988.
313. McLennan CE: Antecubital and femoral venous pressure in normal and toxemic pregnancy. Am J Obstet Gynecol 45:568, 1943.
314. McPheeters HO, Merkert CE, Lundblad RA: The mechanics of the reverse flow in varicose veins as proved by blood pressure readings. Surg Gynecol Obstet 55:298, 1932.
315. Moore DJ, Himmel PD, Sumner DS: Distribution of venous valvular incompetence in patients with the postphlebitic syndrome. J Vasc Surg 3:49, 1986.
316. Moreno AH, Katz AI, Gold LD, Reddy RV: Mechanics of distention of dog veins and other thin-walled tubular structures. Circ Res 27:1069, 1970.
317. Myers KA, Ziegenbein RW, Zeng GH, Mathews PG: Duplex ultrasonography scanning for chronic venous disease: Patterns of venous reflux. J Vasc Surg 21:605, 1995.
318. Neglén P, Raju S: A rational approach to detection of significant reflux with duplex Doppler scanning and air plethysmography. J Vasc Surg 17:590, 1993.
319. Neglén P, Raju S: Compliance of the normal and post-thrombotic calf. J Cardiovasc Surg 36:225, 1995.
320. Negus D, Cockett FD: Femoral vein pressures in postphlebitic iliac vein obstruction. Br J Surg 54:522, 1967.
321. Nicolaides AN: Noninvasive assessment of primary and secondary varicose veins. *In* Bernstein EF (ed): Noninvasive Diagnostic Techniques in Vascular Disease, 2nd ed. St. Louis, CV Mosby, 1982, pp 575–586.
322. Nicolaides AN, Hussein MK, Szendro G, et al: The relation of venous ulceration with ambulatory venous pressure measurements. J Vasc Surg 17:414, 1993.
323. Nicolaides AN, Miles C: Photoplethysmography in the assessment of venous insufficiency. J Vasc Surg 5:405, 1987.
324. Öberg B: The relationship between active constriction and passive recoil of the veins at various distending pressures. Acta Physiol Scand 71:233, 1967.
325. O'Donnell TF, Mackey WC, Shephard AD, et al: Clinical, hemodynamic, and anatomic follow-up of direct venous reconstruction. Arch Surg 122:474, 1987.
326. Pearce WH, Ricco J-B, Queral LA, et al: Hemodynamic assessment of venous problems. Surgery 93:715, 1983.
327. Pflug JJ, Zubac DP, Kersten DR, Alexander NDE: The resting interstitial tissue pressure in primary varicose veins. J Vasc Surg 11:411, 1990.
328. Pollack AA, Wood EH: Venous pressure in the saphenous vein at the ankle in man during exercise and changes in posture. J Appl Physiol 1:649, 1949.
329. Pollack AA, Taylor BE, Myers TT, Wood EH: The effect of exercise and body position on the venous pressures at the ankle in patients having venous valvular defects. J Clin Invest 28:559, 1949.
330. Raju S: New approaches in the diagnosis and treatment of venous obstruction. J Vasc Surg 4:42, 1986.
331. Raju S, Fredericks R: Valve reconstruction procedures for nonobstructive venous insufficiency: Rationale, techniques, and results in 107 procedures with two- to eight-year follow-up. J Vasc Surg 71:301, 1988.
332. Raju S, Fredericks R, Lishman P, et al: Observations on the calf pump mechanism: Determinants of postexercise pressure. J Vasc Surg 17:459, 1993.
333. Reagan B, Folse R: Lower limb venous dynamics in normal persons and children of patients with varicose veins. Surg Gynecol Obstet 132:15, 1971.
334. Rich NM, Hobson RW II, Wright CB, Fedde CW: Repair of lower extremity venous trauma: A more aggressive approach required. J Trauma 14:639, 1974.
335. Rose SS, Ahmed A: Some thoughts on the aetiology of varicose veins. J Cardiovasc Surg 27:534, 1986.
336. Rosfors S, Lamke L-O, Nordström E, Bygdeman S: Severity and location of venous valvular insufficiency: The importance of distal valve function. Acta Chir Scand 156:689, 1990.
337. Rushmer RF: Effects of posture. *In* Cardiovascular Dynamics, 3rd ed. Philadelphia, WB Saunders, 1970, pp 192–219.
338. Rutherford RB, Reddy CMK, Walker FG, Wagner HN Jr: A new quantitative method of assessing the functional status of the leg veins. Am J Surg 122:594, 1971.
339. Saffle JR, Maxwell JG, Warden GD, et al: Measurement of intramuscular pressure in the management of massive venous occlusion. Surgery 89:394, 1981.
340. Sakaguchi S, Ishitobi K, Kameda T: Functional segmental plethysmography with mercury strain gauge. Angiology 23:127, 1972.
341. Samueloff SL, Browse NL, Shepherd JT: Response of capacity vessels in human limbs to head up tilt and suction on lower body. J Appl Physiol 21:47, 1966.
342. Sarin S, Scurr JH, Coleridge Smith PD: Medial calf perforators in venous disease: The significance of outward flow. J Vasc Surg 16:40, 1992.
343. Schalin L: Arteriovenous communications to varicose veins in the lower extremities studied by dynamic angiography. Acta Chir Scand 146:397, 1980.
344. Schalin L: Arteriovenous communications in varicose veins localized by thermography and identified by operative microscopy. Acta Chir Scand 147:409, 1981.
345. Schanzer H, Pierce EC II: A rational approach to surgery of the chronic venous stasis syndrome. Ann Surg 195:25, 1982.
346. Shami SK, Sarin S, Cheatle TR, et al: Venous ulcers and the superficial venous system. J Vasc Surg 17:487, 1993.
347. Shepherd JT: Role of the veins in the circulation. Circulation 33:484, 1966.
348. Shepherd JT: Reflex control of the venous system. *In* Bergan JJ, Yao JST (eds): Venous Problems. Chicago, Year Book Medical Publishers, 1978, pp 5–23.
349. Sherman RS Sr: Varicose veins: Anatomy, reevaluation of Trendelenburg tests, and an operative procedure. Surg Clin North Am 44:1369, 1964.
350. Shull KS, Nicolaides AN, Fernandes é Fernandes J, et al: Significance of popliteal reflux in relation to ambulatory venous pressure and ulceration. Arch Surg 114:1304, 1979.
351. Snyder MA, Adams JT, Schwartz SI: Hemodynamics of phlegmasia cerulea dolens. Surg Gynecol Obstet 125:342, 1967.
352. Somerville JJF, Byrne PJ, Fegan WG: Analysis of flow patterns in venous insufficiency. Br J Surg 61:40, 1974.
353. Starling EH: On the absorption of fluids from the connective tissue spaces. J Physiol 19:312, 1896.
354. Stegall HF: Muscle pumping in the dependent leg. Circ Res 19:180, 1966.
355. Strandness DE Jr, Sumner DS: Hemodynamics for Surgeons. New York, Grune & Stratton, 1975.
356. Sumner DS: Diagnosis of venous thrombosis by Doppler ultrasound. *In* Bergan JJ, Yao JST (eds): Venous Problems. Chicago, Year Book Medical Publishers, 1978, pp 159–185.
357. Sumner DS: Venous dynamics: Varicosities. Clin Obstet Gynecol 24:743, 1981.

358. Sumner DS: Hemodynamics of the venous system: Calf pump and valve function. *In* Raju S, Villavicencio JL (eds): Surgical Management of Venous Disease. Baltimore, Williams & Wilkins, 1997, pp 16–59.
359. Taheri SA, Heffner R, Meenaghan MA, et al: Technique and results of venous valve transplantation. *In* Bergan JJ, Yao JST (eds): Surgery of the Veins. Orlando, Grune & Stratton, 1985, pp 219–231.
360. Taylor AE: Capillary fluid filtration, Starling forces and lymph flow. Circ Res 49:557, 1981.
361. Thomas ML, Keeling FP, Ackroyd JS: Descending phlebography: A comparison of three methods and an assessment of the normal range of deep vein reflux. J Cardiovasc Surg 27:27, 1986.
362. Thulesius O: Elastizität und Klappenfunktion peripherer Venen bei primarer Varikosis. Phlebol Proktol 8:97, 1979.
363. Tripolitis AJ, Milligan EB, Bodily KC, Strandness DE Jr: The physiology of venous claudication. Am J Surg 139:447, 1980.
364. Ueland K: Pregnancy and cardiovascular disease. Med Clin North Am 61:17, 1977.
365. van Bemmelen PS, Bedford G, Beach K, Strandness DE Jr: Status of the valves in the superficial and deep venous system in chronic venous disease. Surgery 109:730, 1991.
366. van Bemmelen PS, Bedford G, Beach K, Strandness DE: Quantitative segmental evaluation of venous reflux with duplex ultrasound scanning. J Vasc Surg 10:425, 1989.
367. Vanhoutte PM, Shepherd JT: Thermosensitivity and veins. J Physiol (Paris) 63:449, 1970.
368. van Rij AM, Solomon C, Christie R: Anatomic and physiologic characteristics of venous ulceration. J Vasc Surg 20:759, 1994.
369. Vasdekis SN, Clarke GH, Nicolaides AN: Quantification of venous reflux by means of duplex scanning. J Vasc Surg 10:670, 1989.
370. Warren R, White EA, Belcher CD: Venous pressures in the saphenous system in normal, varicose, and postphlebitic extremities. Surgery 26:435, 1949.
371. Webb-Peploe MM, Shepherd JT: Response of large hindlimb veins of the dog to sympathetic nerve stimulation. Am J Physiol 215:299, 1968.
372. Welch HJ, McLaughlin RL, O'Donnell TF Jr: Femoral vein valvuloplasty: Intraoperative angioscopic evaluation and hemodynamic improvement. J Vasc Surg 16:694, 1992.
373. Welkie JF, Comerota AJ, Katz ML, et al: Hemodynamic deterioration in chronic venous disease. J Vasc Surg 16:733, 1992.
374. Welkie JF, Comerota AJ, Kerr RP, et al: The hemodynamics of venous ulceration. Ann Vasc Surg 6:1, 1992.
375. Wright CB, Swan KG: Hemodynamics of venous occlusion in the canine hindlimb. Surgery 73:141, 1973.
376. Wright CB, Sayre JT, Casterline PI, Swan KG: Hemodynamic effects of sympathectomy in canine femoral venous occlusion. Surgery 74:405, 1973.
377. Zoster T, Cronin RFP: Venous distensibility in patients with varicose veins. Can Med Assoc J 4:1293, 1966.

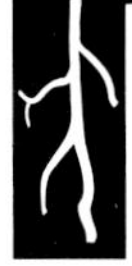

CHAPTER 8

Principles of Hemostasis

John G. Calaitges, M.D.,
and Donald Silver, M.D.

The vascular surgeon, perhaps more than any other physician, must be intimately familiar with the principles of hemostasis and must be able to recognize abnormalities within the system. This chapter reviews the process of hemostasis and situations that contribute to abnormal hemostatic function. Antithrombotic therapy is discussed in Chapter 26. Although the fibrinolytic mechanism is closely related to the coagulation mechanism physiologically and therapeutically, fibrinolysis and thrombolytic therapy are presented in Chapter 28.

HEMOSTASIS

Primary Hemostasis

Primary hemostasis consists of vasoconstriction and the formation of a platelet plug after vessel injury. The interactions of humoral, neurogenic, and myogenic responses lead to vascular smooth muscle cell (SMC) contraction in arteries and arterioles.[1] Once platelets adhere to the injured vessel, they release adenosine diphosphate (ADP), serotonin, and thromboxane A_2, further stimulating SMC contraction. Local production of thrombin also contributes to SMC constriction. Vasoconstriction is additionally potentiated by the loss of endothelium, which produces vasodilating mediators such as prostacyclin (PGI_2) and nitric oxide (NO), formerly referred to as endothelium-derived relaxing factor (EDRF).[2]

Endothelium

The endothelium plays a critical role in the procoagulant and anticoagulant activities of blood.[3] Endothelial cells synthesize PGI_2 in response to thrombin, ADP, adenosine triphosphate (ATP), histamine, and kallikrein.[4, 5] PGI_2 is a vasodilator and inhibits platelet activation by stimulating adenylate cyclase to increase cyclic adenosine monophosphate (cAMP) within the platelet. Nitric oxide, released from the endothelial cells after stimulation by vasoactive peptides, adenine nucleotides, and acetylcholine, also inhibits platelet aggregation.[6]

The liver and the endothelium synthesize antithrombin (AT), the major naturally occurring anticoagulant. Endothelial cells also produce heparan sulfate, a cofactor of AT.[7] Heparan sulfate significantly accelerates AT inactivation of thrombin.

The endothelial cell synthesizes and expresses thrombomodulin, an endothelial cell membrane receptor for thrombin. Protein C activation is greatly accelerated when thrombin binds to thrombomodulin. Activated protein C inhibits activated factors V and VIII and enhances fibrinolytic activity. Protein S, a cofactor for protein C, is synthesized by the liver and endothelial cells. Protein S and factor V potentiate (up to 25-fold) protein C's inactivation of factor Va and VIIIa.[8]

The endothelial cell synthesizes the serine proteases urokinase and tissue plasminogen activator (t-PA). Urokinase and t-PA convert plasminogen to plasmin, the active fibrinolytic enzyme. Endothelial cells synthesize a plasminogen activator inhibitor (PAI-1), which inactivates circulating t-PA.[9]

The endothelium also produces tissue factor pathway inhibitor (TFPI), which inhibits tissue factor–induced thrombus formation by directly inhibiting factor Xa and, in a factor Xa–dependent manner, by inhibiting the prothrombinase complex.[10] Its expression is restricted predominantly to the microvascular circulation. TFPI is released into the plasma following heparin injection.[11] This release of TFPI contributes to the anticoagulant effect of heparin.[12, 13] Infusions of recombinant TFPI have prevented venous and arterial thromboses in animals.[14–18]

Factor V, synthesized by the endothelial cell as well as by the liver, promotes the formation of the prothrombinase complex that leads to the production of thrombin. Endothelial cells are the primary producers of *von Willebrand factor* (factor VIII_{VWF}), which is released into the circulation and the subendothelial matrix. Von Willebrand factor is necessary for platelet binding to subendothelial collagen matrix.

Interleukin-1 (IL-1), endotoxin, and thrombin stimulate the expression of thromboplastin, a tissue factor, on the surface of the endothelial cells.[19] Thromboplastin promotes the activation of factor VII, which contributes to the activation of factor IX, which leads to thrombin formation via the intrinsic pathway.

Platelets

Platelets are produced in the bone marrow by megakaryocytes. These anuclear discoid cells have a volume of 7 to 10 μm^3 and an average circulating life span of 8 to 12 days. The normal platelet count ranges from 200,000 to 400,000 platelets/ml. When platelets are activated (Fig. 8–1), they become spherical, develop pseudopodia, secrete the contents of storage granules, and adhere to each other.

The platelet surface membrane is composed of a bilayer of phospholipids, glycoproteins, and proteins. There are platelet surface receptors for thrombin, serotonin, ADP, collagen, epinephrine, fibronectin, vasopressin, thromboxane A_2, platelet-activating factor (PAF), heparin, and the coagulation proteins factor V, factor VIII, and factor Xa.

The platelet cytoplasm contains several types of storage granules:

1. Alpha granules, which contain factors V and VIII_{VWF}, fibronectin, high-molecular-weight kininogen (HMWK), platelet-derived growth factor (PDGF), beta-thromboglobulin, PAI-1, and platelet factor 4.
2. Dense granules, which contain ADP, serotonin, and calcium.
3. Lysosomes, which contain proteases, acid hydrolases, and glycosidases.

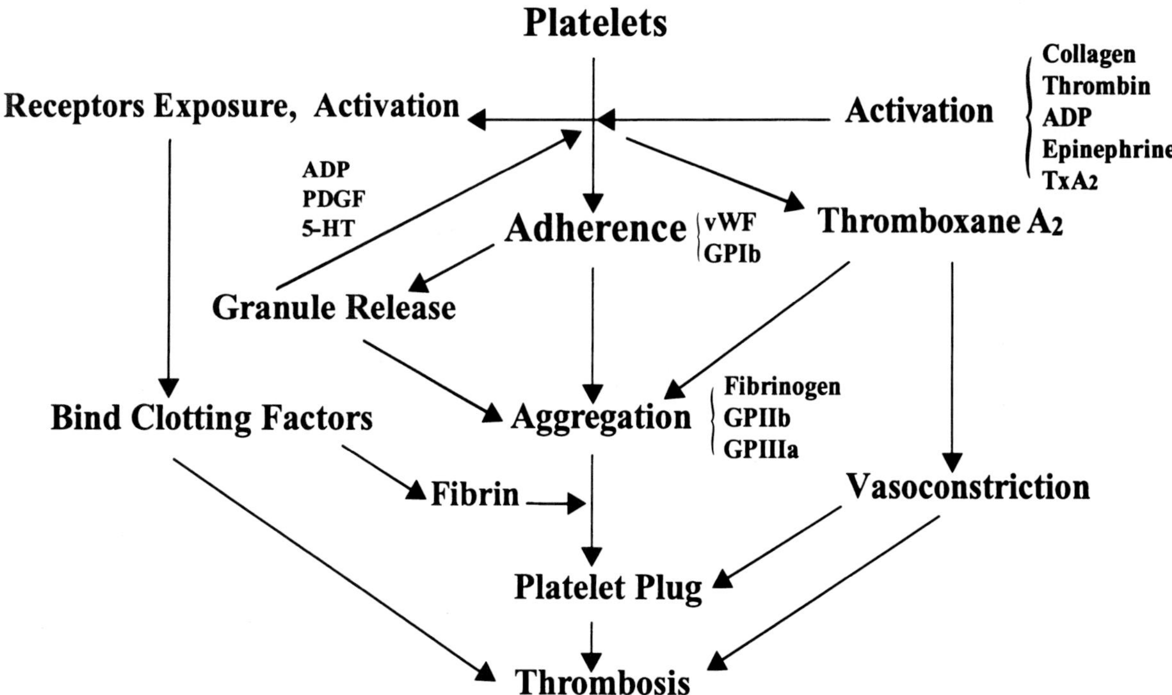

FIGURE 8–1. Mechanism of platelet activation. ADP = adenosine diphosphate; PDGF = platelet-derived growth factor; 5-HT = serotonin (5-hydroxytryptamine); GP = glycoprotein; TxA_2, thromboxane A_2; vWF, von Willebrand factor.

Von Willebrand factor is necessary for the binding of platelets to the areas of disrupted intima. *Glycoprotein* Ib is the primary platelet receptor for this factor. Exposed collagen fibrils are among the initial stimuli for platelet adherence. ADP, thrombin, collagen, and epinephrine interact with specific platelet receptors, resulting in granule content release, and thus stimulate platelet aggregation. ADP released from the dense granules initiates platelet-platelet interaction, which leads to a loose aggregation. Activation of membrane phospholipase results in arachidonic acid release, which stimulates additional platelet aggregation. Platelet cyclooxygenase converts arachidonic acid to the prostaglandin endoperoxides PGG_2 and PGH_2. Thromboxane A_2 is generated by the action of thromboxane synthetase on PGG_2. Thromboxane A_2, PGG_2, and PGH_2 stimulate additional platelet aggregation.[20]

Platelet activation exposes platelet surface fibrinogen receptors, which are instrumental in creating bridges between adjacent platelets. The binding sites consist of glycoproteins factor IIb and factor IIIa on the platelet surface. Binding sites for factor Va are also exposed with platelet activation. Factor Xa complexes with factor Va to form the *prothrombinase complex,* which leads to the final pathway of coagulation.

Coagulation

The Coagulation Cascade

The coagulation cascade consists of a series of reactions in which serine proteases are activated in sequence, the last step resulting in the conversion of fibrinogen to insoluble fibrin (Fig. 8–2).[21, 22] Factor Xa, the active form of factor X, is produced by the action of either the *intrinsic pathway,* which involves the sequential activation of factors XII, XI, and IX and their interaction with factor VIIIa, or the *extrinsic pathway,* which involves the activation of factor VII and a lipoprotein tissue factor (not usually present in blood and hence "extrinsic").

Thrombin is produced from prothrombin by the action of factor Xa, with platelet and endothelial phospholipids providing a surface on which the clotting factor Va and calcium are concentrated. Thrombin cleaves two pairs of peptides (fibrinopeptides A and B) from fibrinogen. The resulting soluble fibrin monomer spontaneously polymerizes and forms a gel. The gel is cross-linked and stabilized by the action of factor XIIIa, which has also been activated by thrombin. The classic division between the extrinsic and the intrinsic pathways is not as sharp as once thought. Several zymogens from either pathway have been found to activate or inhibit aspects of the other.

Activation and Inhibition of Coagulation

Factor XII may be activated in vitro by contact with kaolin or glass, proteolytic enzymes (such as plasmin, kallikrein, and trypsin), endotoxin, low pH, low temperature, and a variety of organic solvents. Factor XIIa initiates the coagulation cascade and contributes to the conversion of prekalli-

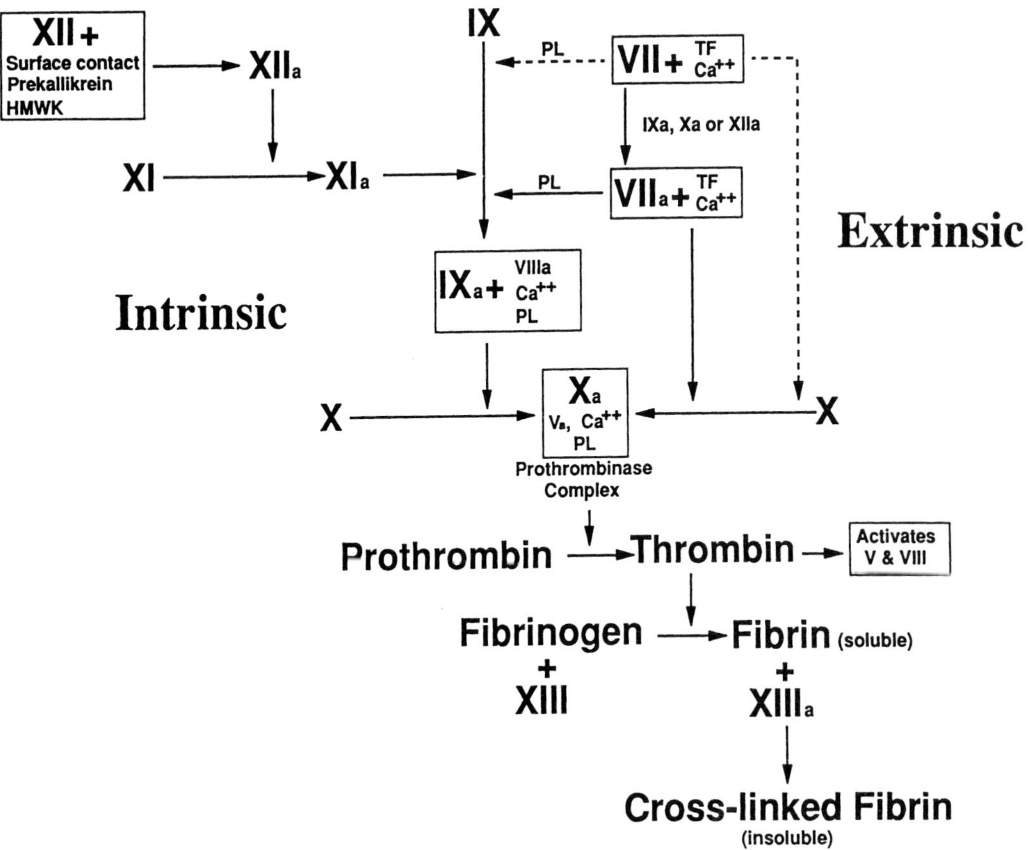

FIGURE 8–2. The two pathways of coagulation operate in conjunction to achieve hemostasis. The intrinsic pathway is initiated by surface contact, whereas the extrinsic pathway is initiated by the release of tissue factor (TF). Phospholipid (PL) is found on activated platelets and endothelial membranes. HMWK = high-molecular-weight kininogen. (From Hoch JR, Silver D: Hemostasis and thrombosis. *In* Moore WS [ed]: Vascular Surgery: A Comprehensive Review. Philadelphia, WB Saunders, 1991.)

krein to kallikrein. Kallikrein cleaves HMWK to form bradykinin and activated HMWK. This latter substance accelerates the activation of both factors XII and XI.

Natural inhibitors of coagulation include alpha$_1$-antitrypsin, TFPI, alpha$_2$-macroglobulin, AT, and protein C. The most important is AT (heparin cofactor), a 65,000-dalton protein present in normal plasma at a concentration of about 300 mg/ml. AT slowly binds and inactivates thrombin; however, this reaction is dramatically accelerated when heparin is present. Heparin induces a conformational change in the AT molecule, which then reacts stoichiometrically with thrombin.[23] AT also binds factors IXa, Xa, XIa, and XIIa. Antithrombin has a major effect in inhibiting coagulation by inhibiting factor Xa. For example, inhibition of 32 units of factor Xa prevents the potential activation of 1600 units of thrombin, a finding that led to trials of low-dose heparin prophylaxis.[24]

AT deficiency occurs as an inherited autosomal disorder. Afflicted individuals exhibit recurrent thrombotic episodes in early adult life. Widespread venous thrombosis is characteristic; thrombosis of the abdominal aorta has been observed.[25, 26] Heparin therapy is ineffective unless AT can be adequately restored by transfusions of fresh frozen plasma, cryoprecipitate, or AT concentrate. AT levels of 75% to 120% are necessary for prophylactic and therapeutic heparin anticoagulation. Normal plasma contains 1 unit of AT/ml, and the intravenous administration of 0.7 U/kg increases the level of AT by 1%. The dose of AT concentrate is calculated by (1) subtracting the patient's AT level from the desired (100% to 120%) level, (2) multiplying this by the patient's weight in kilograms, and (3) dividing the result by 1.4.

Plasma AT levels should be assayed at 12-hour intervals to ensure that the level remains at least 80%.[27] AT replacement should continue until the clinical condition being treated has resolved or until oral anticoagulation has been achieved. Long-term administration of warfarin is recommended for AT-deficient patients who have experienced a thrombotic event.

The *thrombomodulin/protein C–protein S system* has an important role in the regulation of hemostasis in vivo.[28] Protein C is a vitamin K–dependent proenzyme that is activated by thrombin to form a serine protease that inactivates factors Va and VIIIa and blocks platelet receptors for factor Xa. Thrombomodulin, a cofactor on the endothelial surface, enhances the activation of protein C by thrombin up to 20,000-fold. Protein S, a plasma cofactor for the protein C–mediated inactivation of factor Va, has no direct effect on coagulation but forms a complex with activated protein C to enhance the rate of inactivation of factors Va and VIIIa.[28] Activated protein C (APC) also requires factor V as a cofactor to function efficiently as an anticoagulant.

Patients with hereditary deficiencies of either protein C or protein S may have recurrent venous, or, less frequently, arterial thromboembolism. Myocardial infarction in particular has been noted in these patients. Acquired deficiencies of protein C or protein S, or both, can occur in patients with disseminated intravascular coagulation (DIC) or severe hepatic dysfunction and in those taking vitamin K–inhibiting anticoagulants, such as warfarin.

In 1993, the resistance of factor Va to inactivation by APC was recognized as a major risk factor for venous thrombosis. The condition is caused by a single point mutation in the gene for factor V. It is found in 20% to 60% of patients with familial thrombophilia. The factor V mutation is common in whites with a prevalence of 1% to 15%, whereas it is not found in other races.[29, 30] This specific gene mutation renders factor V resistant to inactivation by APC.[31, 32] Inherited APC resistance does not seem to be a significant risk factor for arterial thrombosis.[33] Acquired resistance to APC has been detected in patients with lupus anticoagulants, pregnant patients, and patients taking oral contraceptives.[33–35]

RISK FACTORS FOR THROMBOSIS

Recognition of risk factors remains the most practical method for identifying patients at risk for thrombosis. Patients with acquired risk factors for thrombosis have endothelial injury, stasis, hypercoagulability, or a combination of these. Acquired risk factors and their mechanisms of inducing thrombosis are listed in Table 8–1. Tests have been developed to help detect active thrombosis. These tests demonstrate thrombosis by measurement of fibrinopeptide A, prothrombin fragments 1 and 2, thrombin–antithrombin III complexes, D-dimers, or fibrin monomers, or a combination of these; all are increased during active thrombosis.[36] Platelet activation can be recognized by:

- Measurement of circulating platelet products (e.g., beta-thromboglobulin, platelet factor 4, and thromboxane B_2)
- Demonstration of shortened platelet survival
- In vitro aggregation studies

Increases of platelet activation have been demonstrated in myocardial infarction,[37] unstable angina pectoris,[38] effort-induced angina,[39] transient cerebral ischemic attacks,[40] and recurrent venous thrombosis.[41]

A clear epidemiologic connection between elevated homocyst(e)ine levels and vascular disease has been estab-

TABLE 8–1. ACQUIRED RISK FACTORS FOR THROMBOSIS

FACTOR	PATHOMECHANISM
Soft tissue trauma, thermal injury, operative dissection, stroke	Tissue thromboplastin release
Sepsis	Platelet aggregation, activation of coagulation system
Malignancy	Tumor tissue thromboplastin release, increased coagulation factors, decreased AT III levels
Pregnancy/estrogen use	Increased coagulation factors, low AT III levels, decreased plasminogen activation
Intravascular hemolysis	Activation of intrinsic coagulation pathway by increased phospholipids
Hyperlipidemia, myeloproliferative diseases, diabetes mellitus, hemolytic-uremic syndrome, thrombotic thrombocytopenic syndrome, heparin-induced thrombocytopenia, activated protein C resistance	Platelet aggregation, activation of coagulation

TABLE 8–2. CONGENITAL HYPERCOAGULABLE STATES

Antithrombin deficiency
Activated protein C resistance
Protein C deficiency
Protein S deficiency
Leiden factor
Prothrombin 20210 A
Homocysteinemia
Heparin cofactor II deficiency
Plasminogen and plasminogen activator deficiencies
Increased plasminogen activator inhibitors
Fibrinogen abnormalities

lished.[42, 43] The mechanism appears to be homocyst(e)ine-induced endothelial damage with subsequent thrombus formation and accelerated atherosclerosis. Vitamin supplementation with folate, vitamin B_6, and vitamin B_{12} decreases or even normalizes plasma homocyst(e)ine levels in most cases.[44]

A recently identified mutation in the prothrombin gene (20210 A allele) is associated with elevated prothrombin levels and an increase in venous and arterial thrombosis.[45] The mechanism has not been elucidated, but it is thought that the elevated prothrombin levels lead to increased thrombin production and, consequently, excessive fibrin production.

Some patients are at risk for thrombosis because of congenital hypercoagulable states (Table 8–2). Many of these congenital hypercoagulable states can be detected with appropriate testing.[46] One should test for deficiencies of anticoagulation activities and deficiencies of fibrinolytic activities. When evaluating a patient for hypercoagulability, we usually test for AT, protein C, protein S, APC resistance, homocyst(e)ine concentration, prothrombin levels, anticardiolipin antibody and lupus anticoagulant, and plasminogen and PAIs in addition to the prothrombin time, activated partial thromboplastin time, bleeding time, and platelet count.

REFERENCES

1. Vanhoutte PM: Platelets, endothelium, and vasospasm (Abstract). Thromb Hemost 58:252, 1987.
2. Chesterman CN: Vascular endothelium, haemostasis, and thrombosis. Blood Rev 2:88–94, 1988.
3. Engelberg H: Endothelium in health and disease. Semin Thromb Hemost 15:178–183, 1989.
4. Pearson JD, Carlton JS, Hutchings A: Prostacyclin release stimulated by thrombin or bradykinin in porcine endothelial cells cultured from aorta and umbilical vein. Thromb Res 29:115–124, 1983.
5. Levin RI, Weksler BB, Marcus AJ, et al: Prostacyclin production by endothelial cells. *In* Jaffe EA (ed): Biology of Endothelial Cells. Boston, Martinus Nijhoff, 1984, pp 228–247.
6. Moncada S: Palma RMJ, Higgs EA. Prostacyclin and endothelium-derived relaxing factor: Biological interactions and significance. *In* Verstraete M, Vermylon J, Lijnen HR, Armout J (eds): Thrombosis and Hemostasis. Leuven (Louvain), Belgium, ISTH Leuven University Press, 1985, p 597.
7. Bounassissi V: Sulfated mucopolysaccharide synthesis and secretion in endothelial cell cultures. Exp Cell Res 76:363–, 1973.
8. Suzuki K, Nishioka J, Matsuda M, et al: Protein S is essential for the activated protein C–catalyzed inactivation of platelet-associated factor Va. J Biochem 96:455–460, 1984.
9. Wu KK, Frasier-Scott K, Hatzakis H: Endothelial cell function in hemostasis and thrombosis. Adv Exp Med Biol 242:127–133, 1988.
10. Broze GJ Jr, Warren LA, Novotny WF, et al: The lipoprotein-associated coagulation inhibitor that inhibits the factor VII tissue factor complex also inhibits factor Xa: Insight into its possible mechanism of action. Blood 71:335–343, 1988.
11. Sandset PM, Abildgaard U, Larsen HL: Heparin induces release of extrinsic coagulation pathway inhibitor (EPI). Thromb Res 50:803–813, 1988.
12. Lindahl AK, Abildgarrd U, Staalesen R: The anticoagulant effect in heparinized blood and plasma resulting from interactions with extrinsic pathway inhibitor. Thromb Res 64:155–168, 1991.
13. Lindahl AK, Jacobsen PB, Sandset PM, Abildgaard U: Tissue factor pathway inhibitor with high anticoagulant activity is increased in post-heparin plasma and in plasma from cancer patients. Blood Coagul Fibrinolysis 2:713–721, 1991.
14. Haskel EJ, Torr SR, Day KC, et al: Prevention of arterial reocclusion after thrombosis with recombinant lipoprotein-associated coagulation inhibitor. Circulation 84:948–950, 1991.
15. Khouri RK, Koudsi B, Kaiding F, et al: Prevention of thrombosis by topical application of tissue factor pathway inhibitor in a rabbit model of vascular trauma. Ann Plast Surg 30:398–404, 1993.
16. Lindhal AK, Nordfang O, Wildgoose P, et al: Antithrombotic effects of a truncated tissue factor pathway inhibitor (TFPI) in baboons (Abstract). Thromb Haemost 69:742, 1993.
17. Holst J, Lindblad B, Bergqvist D, et al: Antithrombotic effect of recombinant truncated tissue factor pathway inhibitor ($TFPI_{1-161}$)in experimental venous thrombosis: A comparison with low molecular weight heparin. Thromb Haemost 71:214–219, 1994.
18. Lindahl AK, Wildgoose P, Lumsden AB, et al: Active site-inhibited factor VIIa blocks tissue factor activity and prevents arterial thrombus formation in baboons. Circulation (Suppl) 88:1–417, 1993.
19. Prydz H, Petterson KS: Synthesis of thromboplastin (tissue factor) by endothelial cells. Haemostasis 18(4–6):215–223, 1988.
20. Silver MJ, Smith JB, Ingerman CM, et al: Arachidonic acid–induced human platelet aggregation and prostaglandin formation. Prostaglandins 4:863–875, 1973.
21. Davie EW, Ratnoff OD: Waterfall sequence for intrinsic blood clotting. Science 145:1310, 1964.
22. McFarlane RG: An enzyme cascade in the blood clotting mechanism and its function as a biochemical amplifier. Nature 202:498, 1964.
23. Rosenberg RD: Actions and interactions of antithrombin and heparin. N Engl J Med 292:146–151, 1975.
24. Wessler S: Prevention of venous thromboembolism by low-dose heparin. Mod Concepts Cardiovasc Dis 45:105–109, 1976.
25. Egeberg O: Inherited antithrombin deficiency causing thrombophilia. Thromb Diath Haemorrh 1965;13:516.
26. Shapiro ME, Rodvien R, Bauer KA, Salzman EW: Acute aortic thrombosis in antithrombin III deficiency. JAMA 245:1759–1761, 1981.
27. Schwartz RS, Bauer KA, Rosenberg RD, et al: Clinical experience with antithrombin III concentrate in treatment of congenital and acquired deficiency of antithrombin. Am J Med 87(3B):53S–60S, 1989.
28. Clouse LH, Comp PC: The regulation of hemostasis: The protein C system. N Engl J Med 314:1298–1304, 1986.
29. Dahlbäck B: Resistance to activated protein C as risk factor for thrombosis: Molecular mechanisms, laboratory investigation, and clinical management. Semin Hematol 34:217–234, 1997.
30. Svensson PJ, Dahlbäck B: Resistance to activated protein C as a basis for venous thrombosis. N Engl J Med 330:517–522, 1994.
31. Dahlbäck B: The protein C anticoagulant system: Inherited defects as basis for venous thrombosis. Thromb Res 77:1–43, 1995.
32. Shen L, Dahlbäck B: Factor V and protein S as synergistic cofactors to activated protein C in degradation of factor VIIIa. J Biol Chem 269:18735–18738, 1994.
33. Dahlbäck B, Hillarp A, Rosen S, Zoller B: Resistance to activated protein C, the FV:Q506 allele, and venous thrombosis. Ann Hematol 72:166–176, 1996.
34. Ehrenforth S, Radtke KP, Scharrer I: Acquired activated protein C-resistance in patients with lupus anticoagulants. Thromb Haemost 74:797–798, 1995.
35. Svensson PJ, Zöller B, Dahlbäck B: Evaluation of original and modified APC-resistance tests in unselected outpatients with clinically suspected thrombosis and in healthy controls. Thromb Haemost 77:332–335, 1997.
36. Estivals M, Pelzer H, Sie P, et al: Prothrombin fragment 1 + 2,

thrombin-antithrombin III complexes and D-dimers in acute deep vein thrombosis: Effects of heparin treatment. Br J Haematol 78:421–424, 1991.

37. Guyton J, Willerson JT: Peripheral venous platelet aggregates in patients with unstable angina pectoris and acute myocardial infarction. Angiology 28:695–701, 1977.
38. Sobel M, Salzman EW, Davies GC, et al: Circulating platelet products in unstable angina pectoris. Circulation 63:300–306, 1981.
39. Green LH, Seroppian E, Handin RI: Platelet activation during exercise-induced myocardial ischemia. N Engl J Med 302:193–197, 1980.
40. Steele P, Carroll J, Overfield D, Genton E: Effect of sulfinpyrazone on platelet survival times in patients with transient cerebral ischemic attacks. Stroke 8:396–398, 1977.
41. Steele P, Ellis J, Genton E: Effects of platelet suppressant, anticoagulant and fibrinolytic therapy in patients with recurrent venous thrombosis. Am J Med 64:441–445, 1978.
42. Kang SS, Wong PW, Malinow MR: Hyperhomocyst(e)inemia as a risk factor for occlusive vascular disease. Ann Rev Nutr 12:279–298, 1992.
43. Stampfer MJ, Malinow MR, Willett WC, et al: A prospective study of plasma homocyst(e)ine and risk of myocardial infarction in U.S. physicians. JAMA 268:877–881, 1992.
44. Welch GN, Loscalzo J: Homocysteine and atherothrombosis (Review Article). N Engl J Med 388:1042–1050, 1998.
45. Poort SR, Rosendaal FR, Reitsma PH, Bertina RM: A common genetic variation in the 3′-untranslated region of the prothrombin gene is associated with elevated plasma prothrombin levels and an increase in venous thrombosis. Blood 88:3698–3703, 1996.
46. Corral J, Gonzalez-Conejero R, Lozano ML, et al: The venous thrombosis risk factor 20210 A allele of the prothrombin gene is not a major risk factor for arterial thrombotic disease. Br J Haematol 99:304–307, 1997.
47. Clayton JK, Anderson JA, McNicol GP: Preoperative prediction of postoperative deep vein thrombosis. Br Med J 2:910–912, 1976.

SECTION III

VASCULAR DIAGNOSIS: BASIC TECHNIQUES AND APPLICATIONS

JACK L. CRONENWETT, M.D.

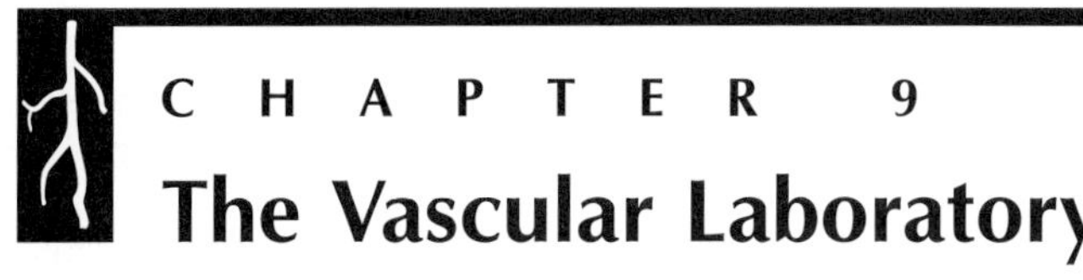

CHAPTER 9

The Vascular Laboratory

J. Dennis Baker, M.D.

THE LABORATORY

The Noninvasive Tests

Like many technical fields in medicine, noninvasive vascular testing had modest origins. The earliest efforts at objective assessment of vascular phenomena date to the days when sympathectomy was the only surgical treatment for vascular insufficiency. Measurement of changes in skin temperature or electrical resistance was used to demonstrate changes in sympathetic activity. The 1940s and 1950s saw the introduction of plethysmographic devices to record pulse pressure waveforms. These early tools were used to measure extremity blood pressures and to estimate blood flow. Methods included application of a variety of pneumatic and strain-gauge sensors. These early devices evolved through the years and in some cases are still utilized. For example, the Winsor pneumatic plethysmograph was followed by the pulse volume recorder (PVR), which continues to be used today. Further applications of pneumatic plethysmography were the Cranley phleborheograph, Gee's ocular pneumoplethysmography (OPG), and, more recently, air plethysmography, as developed by Nicolaides. Other techniques were recording and analysis of vascular bruits, electrical impedance plethysmography (IPG) (such as described by Wheeler for detection of deep vein thrombosis), and photoplethysmography (PPG).

The application of ultrasound techniques to vascular diagnosis has played a major role in the field. In 1958, Satomura reported the use of Doppler signal processing for transcutaneous detection of blood flow. His work led to the development of early nondirectional continuous wave detectors. The initial application of Doppler techniques was in the form of a simple ultrasonic stethoscope, with limited qualitative interpretation of signals. Problems with the subjective nature of this assessment led to the quantitative measurement of extremity systolic pressures and the recording of analog tracings of the Doppler velocity signals. Technical improvements included the design of directional detectors and, later, the evolution of processors to measure the frequency characteristics of the Doppler-shifted signals. More than any other device, the continuous wave (CW) Doppler velocity detector was responsible for the rapid growth of noninvasive testing in the 1970s.

A parallel development was seen in the ultrasound imaging of blood vessels. The initial equipment provided only static, low-resolution images. Technologic improvements provided real-time imaging, analogous to that provided by fluoroscopy. The great leap forward came in 1972, when Strandness and associates developed the duplex scanner, combining both flow and image information in the same examination. By the early 1980s, the duplex scanner became widely used. The initial application was for the examination of the carotid artery and its branch vessels. Subsequently, use of duplex scanning expanded to peripheral arterial and venous applications and, later, investigation of abdominal visceral vessels.

The most important recent development has been color flow encoding, which has simplified or shortened many of the difficult or tedious duplex scanning examinations. Current researchers are investigating the clinical applications of ultrasound contrast agents and three-dimensional image reconstructions.

Evolution of the Vascular Laboratory

The initial noninvasive studies were performed in a few hospitals as part of research efforts. The first identifiable vascular laboratory was set up by Linton at the Massachusetts General Hospital in 1946. Because the focus at that time was on sympathetic activity, one can understand why skin temperature and electrical resistance were the measurements performed.

During the ensuing decade, a few additional pioneering efforts appeared. The growth of arterial reconstructive procedures in the 1960s stimulated interest in clinical investigation among physiologists and vascular surgeons. Publications from research laboratories stimulated interest in the clinical applicability of the techniques, and by the early 1970s there was increasing use of the tests in decisions about patient management. Where research laboratories existed, they expanded to accommodate the growing demand for clinical testing. In institutions where there had been no research efforts, new facilities were established for the primary purpose of providing routine vascular testing. Another phenomenon was the introduction of noninvasive testing into the office setting. As vascular surgeons became acquainted with different testing modalities, office testing became firmly incorporated into routine practice. In 1976, a task force of the American Heart Association, the Intersociety Commission for Heart Disease Resources, published a report on testing for peripheral vascular disease.[6] The group concluded that a clinical vascular laboratory was desirable in institutions treating vascular disease (including venous thromboembolism).

The growth in noninvasive testing required the training of people to carry out the examinations. Much of the work in the original research groups was performed by the physicians who developed the tests. With time, other physicians studied and duplicated the work reported in early publications, but the problem appeared when clinicians decided to create new testing facilities without going through the "learning curve" experienced by early researchers. In some cases, interested physicians visited established laboratories for brief periods to learn techniques and practical tips. Lectures and specific courses helped to school many in the basics of the new field. There was growth in the complexity of tests and the time required for examinations, exceeding the time that physicians could devote to the studies. Increasingly, technologists were recruited from a variety of backgrounds, including nurses, physicians' assistants, catheterization laboratory or operating room technicians, and research assistants. Special courses were developed to help teach these people the relevant vascular anatomy and physiology as well as the specifics of different examinations. By the 1980s, almost all vascular laboratory tests were being performed by technologists under the direction of physicians.

Most of the development of the early physiologic tests was carried out by surgeons and other researchers in the field of vascular disease. As technologic improvements made ultrasound imaging a clinical reality, radiologists showed increasing interest. By the mid-1980s, there was an explosion in noninvasive testing and other specialties became involved, including neurology, neurosurgery, cardiology, and urology.

Currently, testing is performed in many settings, ranging from the solo practitioner conducting the tests alone in an office, to large hospital or clinic departments, to far-ranging mobile units. Although there is no accurate count, I estimate that there are at least 10,000 separate facilities performing noninvasive vascular tests in the United States.

The role of the vascular laboratory has undergone major changes from the original research facilities that started the work in this field five decades ago. The primary goal of noninvasive testing has always been to refine the clinical assessment of vascular disease by providing objective techniques. In the early years, vascular testing assisted the physician in physical assessment and helped identify patients for more complete evaluation, usually involving contrast angiography. Since 1984, improvement in techniques, especially duplex scanning, has resulted in the ability of the noninvasive laboratory to provide the definitive diagnosis for a number of conditions. In the 1980s, the venous scan became the primary test for acute deep vein thrombosis. More recently, it has been a growing practice to recommend carotid endarterectomy solely on the basis of the ultrasound studies, without subjecting the patient to a routine angiogram. A similar approach is currently being studied in patients requiring lower extremity arterial revascularization. These changes have elevated the importance of the vascular laboratory in patient care.

The Quest for Quality

The increasing reliance being placed on the results of vascular laboratory testing demands that the studies have high accuracy. Through the years, reports in the literature from major research centers have emphasized the good correlation that can be obtained when noninvasive tests are compared with angiography or some other reference standard. It is important that every facility strive to achieve similar good results with routine work. The quality of testing depends on several factors: (1) the physicians, (2) the technologists, and (3) the ongoing evaluation of results.

The Physician

All vascular laboratories need a physician to provide direction and supervision. This director has several functions:

- Establishment of the tests to be performed
- Selection of diagnostic criteria
- Interpretation of tests
- Monitoring of the quality of work

In 1988, Rutherford summarized the qualifications needed for a medical director.[43] The most basic is a sound understanding of the clinical principles of vascular disease. Other important areas are (1) knowledge of the principles and the limitations of equipment, (2) familiarity with the testing procedures, (3) understanding of the diagnostic criteria, and (4) experience with the validation of test results. Although other physicians involved with a laboratory may perform only test interpretation, they need similar qualifications.

In the past, vascular surgeons had the clinical knowledge necessary for the vascular laboratory as a result of training and practice, and they acquired much of the technical background from formal courses, books, and articles on the testing procedures and their interpretation. Other specialists, such as radiologists, have the background in ultrasound technique but have needed to learn about peripheral vascular disease. In recent years, most vascular surgery residencies have taught the principles of noninvasive testing together with specific experience in the laboratory. The residents often interpret large numbers of tests under faculty supervision. These efforts were strengthened in 1996, when the Association of Program Directors in Vascular Surgery published a Core Curriculum for Resident Training in the Vascular Diagnostic Laboratory, thus making this experience a formal part of all approved programs. Noninvasive testing techniques still evolve at a rapid pace, so it is important for all physicians in the field to continue to update their knowledge through reading and educational courses.

For a number of years, the issue of physician credentialing or certification for vascular laboratory work has been debated. There are conflicts in some centers about who should be allowed to direct a vascular testing facility or to participate in the interpretation of tests. More often than not, local guidelines for privileging are written to define entry-level knowledge of vascular disease and experience in testing and interpretation. In an effort to establish credibility in noninvasive testing, some physicians have obtained the Registered Vascular Technologist (RVT) credential from the American Registry of Diagnostic Medical Sonographers (ARDMS). Although the examination is not designed to evaluate physician knowledge and skills, passing it at least requires a basic knowledge of ultrasound physics and technology. In 1998, 720 physicians held RVT certificates. Today the only credential designed to identify physician expertise is issued by the American Society of Neuroimaging. This organization has created a written examination, and the certification can be sought by any physician with the requisite education in neuroimaging and prior experience in interpretation of these studies.

The Technologist

The sonographer who performs examinations is also a critical element in the vascular laboratory, especially because many of the tests are very operator-dependent. Knowledge of the relevant anatomy and physiology together with an understanding of the common vascular disease processes is essential. In addition, the examiner needs to understand the physical principles and limitations of the techniques being used. Although vascular testing grew rapidly in the 1980s, there remains a paucity of educational opportunities for people interested in entering the field. After more than two decades of growth of noninvasive testing, only a few associate degree programs and one bachelor-level program are available in the United States. Most of the technologists in the field are still trained by a combination of didactic courses, hands-on instruction, and supervised clinical experience.

In 1977, the Society of Noninvasive Vascular Technologists (later to become the Society for Vascular Technology [SVT]) was formed.[21] One of its goals is to provide relevant courses in the field and to assist members in finding educational opportunities. Unfortunately, there remains great variability in the knowledge and experience of technologists practicing in the field, and some laboratory staff have simply been taught the mechanics of conducting specific examinations.

One of the ways of improving the education of technologists is to define entry-level knowledge and experience. In 1979, the SVT formed a committee to study the issue of voluntary certification.[21] The decision was made to work with the ARDMS to develop a certifying process. This organization had existed since 1975 and had administered examinations for sonographers covering different areas of ultrasound testing. A new examination was developed, and the first RVT credentials were issued in 1983. The basic requirements comprise 2 years of formal education after high school and 24 months of full-time clinical work in a vascular laboratory. The two-part written examination has a clinical section and a technical section on vascular physics and instrumentation. Once credentialed, the technologist is required to accumulate 30 hours of continuing education credits every 3 years in order to maintain active status. In 1998, there were 6740 active RVTs.

More recently, Cardiovascular Credentialing International, an organization that focused primarily on certifying technicians working in invasive and noninvasive cardiac laboratories, extended its process by establishing the credential of Registered Cardiovascular Technician (RCVT) in Vascular Technology. The title of the credential was later changed to Registered Vascular Specialist (RVS).

Credentialing was established as a voluntary process, and technologists have participated for a variety of reasons. In some cases, the certificate has led to higher pay scales. Through the years, only a fraction of those performing vascular testing have been credentialed technologists. This situation is in the process of changing. A recent phenomenon has been the interest of medical insurance providers in the quality of vascular laboratory testing and the perception that credentialed technologists represent proof of adequate entry level experience. As of 1998, seven Medicare carriers require that vascular laboratories employ credentialed technologists either to perform the tests or to directly supervise all tests as a condition for reimbursement. Additional carriers have announced similar requirements starting in 1999. I expect that this trend will continue to grow and will be a strong incentive for vascular laboratory technologists to become credentialed.

Quality Control

From the earliest days, the results of noninvasive vascular tests have been validated by comparison with some accepted reference standard, often the contrast angiogram. It was necessary to determine the criteria for separating normal from "abnormal" or for defining different categories or degrees of disease severity. To a great extent, the acceptance of vascular laboratory testing depended on how well these tests correlated with other diagnostic procedures. In many cases, the early validation work contributed to improvements through refinements in technique and diagnostic criteria.

Once a technique gained acceptance, laboratories would incorporate it, usually buying the same or similar equipment and adopting the published diagnostic criteria. A common problem arose from the fact that laboratories often modified or combined diagnostic criteria from different sources. Any time that criteria are combined or modified, the effects on accuracy need to be confirmed through comparison with a reference standard. Accordingly, laboratory directors need to be familiar with the methodology for comparing test results with reference standards.[4, 46]

A standard assumption is that if one duplicates the equipment and adopts published diagnostic criteria, the clinical accuracies achieved will be similar to those reported in the literature. An inherent problem in many noninvasive procedures is that their accuracy is heavily operator-dependent, particularly for duplex scanning and transcranial Doppler sonography. A great deal of the accuracy potential depends on the knowledge and experience of the examiner and the care with which each examination is conducted. A separate issue is that similar devices may yield somewhat different objective data. It is the responsibility of each laboratory to determine the accuracy of its results through a formal quality assurance program. Comparing the final interpretation of a study with a "gold standard" is the best way to evaluate the quality of work done.

An important problem in evaluating vascular testing is that there are some studies for which we lack a good reference standard. Duplex scanning for the detection of deep vein thrombosis is a good example of this dilemma. Early studies comparing duplex scans with contrast phlebograms showed such good correlation that now the ultrasound study has become the primary diagnostic tool. In most centers, few if any phlebograms are performed to permit contemporary comparisons. Several options are currently being assessed to address this problem, including the possibility of using patient outcome studies to define the accuracy of testing.

Another issue of quality control, especially in larger facilities, is the consistency of testing procedures. The investigators who developed tests recognized the need to minimize variability and went to great efforts to standardize testing procedures. Thus, it is important to have carefully developed written protocols to be followed for each study. Every laboratory should establish a policy to evaluate how closely each examiner adheres to the established instructions. Another way to look for potential testing variability is to have two or more people examine the same patient without knowledge of previous findings. This duplicate test process may help identify weaknesses, especially when the routine quality assurance process has identified problems.

Accreditation

Over the past decade, concern has grown about the variable quality of studies performed in vascular laboratories. Surgeons are constantly confronted with the problem of finding major discrepancies between results of a study performed by an unknown facility and the results obtained when the study is repeated. The Intersocietal Commission for the Accreditation of Vascular Laboratories (ICAVL) was established in 1991 with the goal of creating standards and establishing a voluntary review process for the field.[48] The commission had wide support from specialty groups involved in vascular testing. The initial sponsors were the American Academy of Neurology, American College of Radiology, American Institute of Ultrasound in Medicine, International Society for Cardiovascular Surgery (North American Chapter), Society for Vascular Surgery, Society for Vascular Medicine and Biology, Society of Diagnostic Medical Sonographers, and Society of Vascular Technology. The first group of applications was approved in January 1992, and by January 1998, 878 laboratories had been accredited or reaccredited.

The ICAVL took care, in writing the standards, to be as inclusive as possible. The standards allow application for accreditation by every sort of laboratory, from large ultrasound departments in major medical centers to small laboratories in low-population areas. The emphasis of the accreditation review is on the background and experience of the personnel involved and the quality of the work performed. Some of the problems identified in the review of applications are as follows:

1. Inadequacy of experience or training or lack of appropriate continuing medical education (all personnel are required to have completed 15 hours of courses dedicated to vascular testing every 3 years)
2. Lack of formal examination protocols or failure to adhere to them.
3. Use of multiple sets of diagnostic criteria for a given test.
4. Failure to apply the diagnostic criteria to interpretation of studies.
5. Absence of quality control using comparison studies.

The process of preparing the ICAVL application provides the laboratory with a thorough self-assessment of all aspects of its organization and function and identifies areas for improvement. Accreditation is given for 3 years, and the experience has been that laboratories have shown improvement when reviewed for reaccreditation.

ICAVL accreditation was set up as a voluntary process, and the number of vascular laboratories that have participated is testimony to the interest in ICAVL goals. The accreditation is now being taken to a higher level. Unlike the situation in the past, medical insurance providers are now becoming interested in the quality of medical testing. They regard ICAVL standards as providing entry-level screening for testing facilities. Starting in 1998, the Medicare carrier for the state of Virginia requires ICAVL accreditation as a condition for payment. Six other carriers require either ICVAL or technologists' certification starting in 1998. Four additional carriers are making such a policy effective in 1999. A number of other Medicare carriers together with other large insurance providers are considering similar requirements. So even if there is no current requirement for ICAVL accreditation, directors of vascular laboratories should work toward completing the process both to improve current quality of work and to prepare for future mandates.

Over the last five decades, we have seen the growth of noninvasive testing into a mature part of the evaluation of vascular disease. Many of the early tests have been phased out, replaced by techniques yielding more detailed and more accurate information. Vascular laboratory procedures are not limited to screening tests but often provide the definitive diagnosis upon which the clinician will act. As a result, all involved with this testing must have a strong commitment to the quality of the product. Appropriate training and education of all personnel must be combined with an ongoing quality control program in order to offer the optimal product to the medical community and its patients.

INSTRUMENTATION

Doppler Ultrasound Technology

Velocity Detectors

Transcutaneous detection of blood flow is the most important technique in the noninvasive laboratory. Sato first described the application of the Doppler principle to ultrasound in 1959. The physical principle is that the frequency of sound (or light) emitted by a moving source is shifted up if the source is moving toward the receiver and down if the source is moving away from the receiver. An example from everyday life is the sound of a horn on a fast-moving car or train, which we perceive as being higher pitched as the vehicle approaches and lower pitched as it recedes. In diagnostic ultrasound, a beam of high-frequency ultrasound (usually in the range of 2 to 10 MHz) is transmitted into tissue. Part of the energy is reflected back at each acoustic boundary and detected by the device. Energy reflected off stationary components returns with the same frequency. Moving blood cells in a vessel, however, receive the ultrasound energy at a shifted frequency proportional to the velocity of flow. A part of this energy is reflected back to the detector, and the frequency is further shifted on the return trip. The magnitude of the frequency shift (Δf) is defined by the Doppler equation:

$$\Delta f = \frac{2\, f_0\, V \cos \theta}{C} \tag{9.1}$$

where f_0 = frequency of the transmitted sound, V = velocity of the blood cells, θ = the angle between the axis of the ultrasound beam and the direction of flow of the blood cells, and C = velocity of sound in tissue ($\sim 1.56 \times 10^5$ cm/sec). From this equation, it is important to realize that for a given velocity, Δf is determined by both the angle of insonation and the frequency of transmitted ultrasound.

In most clinical situations, it is helpful to have the highest frequency shift possible. The worst scenario for recording Doppler signals is to have the ultrasound beam at a right angle to the direction of flow ($\cos 90° = 0$), whereas the highest shift is obtained by insonating in the direction of flow. The latter is rarely possible, and typically, attempts are usually made to keep the Doppler insonation angle smaller than 60 degrees. Using higher transmission frequencies would appear to be desirable to increase Δf, but there is an important opposing physical effect. The absorption of sound energy is directly related to the transmission frequency, so that higher frequencies are absorbed more, resulting in a weaker returning signal. Therefore, choice of transmission frequency is a compromise dictated by the desired frequency shift and the tissue depth requirements.

The Doppler equation is commonly rearranged to calculate the velocity of blood flow:

$$V = \frac{C\,(\Delta f)}{2\, f_0 \cos \theta} \tag{9.2}$$

It is this equation that Doppler devices use to convert the detected frequency shifts to estimated velocity. As can be seen, this calculation is valid only if one has an accurate estimate of the Doppler angle θ.

A CW Doppler velocity detector is the simplest design. The probe contains two piezoelectric crystals, one transmitting and the other receiving continuously. The simplest devices detect the shifted frequency but do not distinguish direction. Added circuits allow determination of whether the shifted frequency is above or below the transmitted frequency, indicating whether flow is toward or away from the probe, respectively. A limitation of this system is that signals are detected from all blood vessels insonated by the ultrasound beam. The resulting signal is a sum of the different velocities, often a mixture of arterial and venous flows.

More precise velocity detection is achieved with a pulsed system. In this type of equipment, the probe has a single crystal. A short pulse or burst (0.5 to 1.0 μsec) of ultrasound is transmitted, and after a defined waiting time, the crystal is used in the receive mode for a short period. The duration of the waiting time determines the depth at which sampling occurs, and the duration of the receive period determines the length of the sample volume (the limited space from which velocity information is obtained). The number of times the cycle is repeated per second, or pulse repetition frequency (PRF), varies from 4 to 10 kHz. The pulsed Doppler units allow adjustment of these two time parameters to define the depth (limited by the transmission frequency) and length (often 1 to 15 mm) of the sample volume. A few hand-held velocity detectors have a pulsed Doppler capability, whereas all duplex scanners use this systems.

Data Output and Analysis

The simplest use of a Doppler system is to listen to the audio output. The shifted frequency from blood vessels is within normal hearing range. Nondirectional units produce a single sound output, but directional units have two separate channels for the flow signals toward and away from the probe. Stereo headphones or playback systems allow the examiner to perceive the direction of flow.

In many applications, one needs a graphic record of the frequency data. The simplest signal processor is a zero-crossing detector, which provides a tracing that can be viewed on a screen or printed with a strip chart recorder. The tracing is usually considered to represent the mean of the velocity components at a point in time. With optimal conditions, the tracing is similar to that obtained with an electromagnetic flowmeter. Studies have shown that velocities measured with this technique cannot be used for some quantitative measurements, however, because of inherent errors.[22, 23, 41] The output of the zero-crossing system is actually proportional to the root mean square rather than the mean frequency. In general, the zero-crossing analyzer yields higher than mean frequencies, but under adverse circumstances (e.g., high noise levels in the Doppler signal or when arterial and venous signals are mixed), underestimates of frequency are found. In spite of these limitations, this method of signal processing is still used in most CW units.

Other types of signal processors have been developed that provide tracings specifically representing the instantaneous mean or maximum frequency. Although these systems overcome problems encountered with the zero-crossing method, they are not currently used in commercial systems primarily because of greater cost.

Frequency spectral analysis is the method used in all duplex scanners as well as in some models of CW systems. A computer is used to perform an analysis of the frequency content by the fast Fourier transform (FFT) method. The results are displayed in a sonogram (Fig. 9–1). The frequency is charted on the vertical axis, and time on the horizontal axis. At each point on the graph, the amplitude

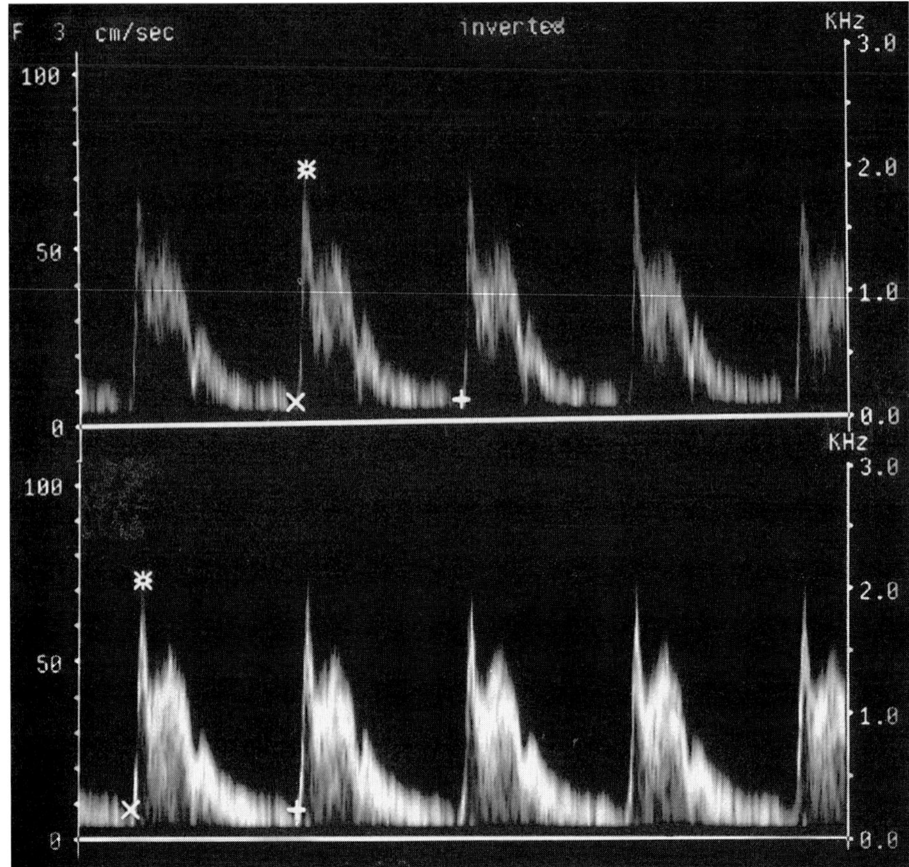

FIGURE 9–1. Sonogram display of the common carotid artery. *Top,* Spectral display of a signal obtained with a small sample volume setting. *Bottom,* Spectral display of a recording from the same artery with a wide sample volume, yielding the sonogram that would be obtained with a continuous wave device. Note filling in of spectral window due to detection of lower velocities near the vessel wall.

of a given frequency is represented by the darkness of the spot.

Figure 9–2 illustrates a sonogram data display and the changes produced by a tight stenosis. With normal flow, most of the cells are traveling at similar velocities, resulting in a narrow spectrum width and a spectral window at the lower velocities. Stenosis yields a wider range of velocities, resulting in a spectral broadening or a decrease in the window. The envelope of the spectral display represents the peak frequency. In addition to the sonogram display, many contemporary spectral analyzers can produce analog traces of the mean and maximum frequencies, which can be helpful in some diagnostic situations.

Despite the greater technical complexity of spectral analysis and its display, its advantages have made it the method of choice for many Doppler applications:

1. It can accurately display situations in which there is simultaneous forward and reverse flow.

2. The complex display often enables differentiation of signals being obtained from two adjacent vessels, especially if these are artery and vein.

3. The effect of noise can usually be distinguished from the underlying velocity signal.

4. The computation program can calculate specific peak, mean, median, mode, and time-averaged-mean frequencies.

Duplex Scanner

Early ultrasound imaging systems provided only low-resolution images, but as technology developed, image quality improved. This led to growing interest in the imaging of superficial vessels. A critical limitation was discovered, however, because fresh thrombus and flowing blood may have the same appearance. Another problem is that advanced atherosclerotic plaques are often calcified, interfering with adequate visualization of the lumen.

The solution came with the creation of the duplex scanner by a team at the University of Washington.[7, 45] This device combined a pulsed Doppler system with a real-time B-mode (brightness-mode) imaging system. The diagnosis of stenosis was based primarily on interpretation of the frequency spectra produced by the pulsed Doppler FFT analyzer. Initially, the image served almost exclusively to identify the correct position for the Doppler sample volume, but as gray scale resolution improved, the image was used in the diagnostic interpretation. The scanner was first used to study the carotid bifurcation because of its superficial location. Over the years, incremental improvements were made, including lower-frequency probes to permit deeper penetration and better probe technology to provide higher image quality.

The greatest improvement in the duplex scanner has been the addition of color encoding.[56] Unlike the conventional systems with a single sample volume, the new scanners have the capability to obtain Doppler signals from a whole region at the same time. Linear array transducer technology is used to create a grid of insonation containing a matrix of small sample volumes (Fig. 9–3). The ultrasound signal returned from each sample volume is analyzed. If there is no change in frequency or phase, the

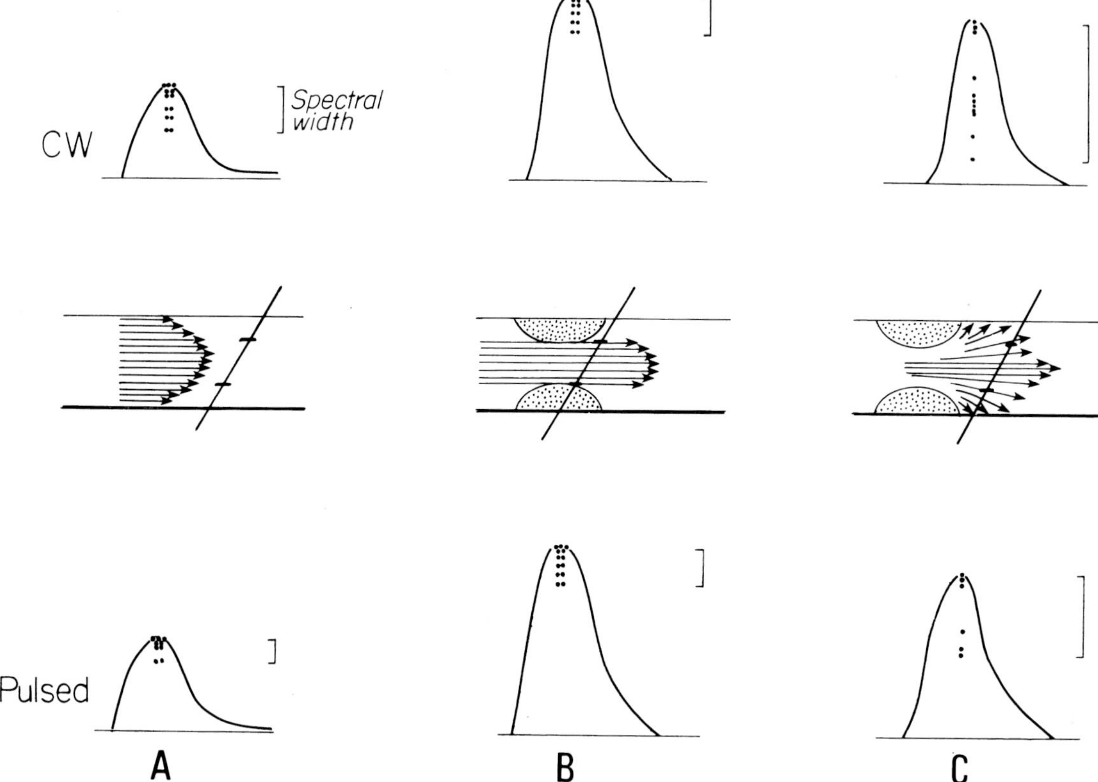

FIGURE 9–2. Schematic representation of sonograms. The velocity vectors at peak systole *(middle row)* are plotted to produce the sonograms produced by continuous wave (CW) and pulsed Doppler systems. Whereas the pulsed system detects only the flow within the sample volume, indicated by the marks on the line representing the ultrasound beam, the CW system detects all the velocities across the vessel. *A,* Normal arterial signal. The CW sonogram has lower frequencies in the signal, thus a wider spectral width. *B,* The signal detected within a stenosis has a higher velocity. Both systems show similar sonograms. *C,* Disturbed flow beyond a stenosis. Again, the spectral width is greater on the CW system. (From Baker JD: The vascular laboratory. *In* Moore WS [ed]: Vascular Surgery: A Comprehensive Review, 5th ed. Philadelphia, WB Saunders, 1998, pp 235–250.)

return signal is from a stationary point and the information is processed to create an element in the gray scale image. A change in phase or frequency indicates motion at that specific point, so the signal is analyzed to determine the magnitude and direction of the motion. A color is assigned to indicate direction toward or away from the probe; red and blue are most commonly used. The hue (darkness or lightness) of the color is used to indicate the magnitude of the velocity—dark for low velocity and lighter for higher velocities. The resulting image shows a real-time color visualization of the flow pattern in the lumen of the vessels, and the vessel wall and the surrounding tissues are shown in the usual gray scale representation.

The advantages offered by color duplex scanners were immediately apparent to the examiners. Normal phenomena, such as the helical flow pattern in the carotid bulb, are well shown. Having a full-color flow map simplifies identification of the site of maximal stenosis. In addition, tortuous vessels are more easily identified and their courses followed.

One must also be aware of the limitations imposed by the technology of color duplex scanning. First, the velocity representations are based on mean velocity values rather than the peak velocity values that have been used in a variety of diagnostic criteria. Whenever specific velocity values are required, they should be obtained using the single sample volume to yield the conventional spectral waveform. Other concerns are (1) lower frame rates, (2) more problems with "aliasing" (improper representation of velocity data), and (3) problems with coding flow signals outside the lumen as a result of improper gain settings on the scanner. Kremkau[29] has written an excellent overview of the pitfalls of color encoding.

Plethysmography

A plethysmograph is a device for measuring or recording variations in (1) the volume of an organ or extremity or (2) the blood contained within or passing through it. A variety of different categories of plethysmographic devices have been used to study the circulation. Mercury-in-Silastic and related strain-gauges can be calibrated to allow measurement of volume changes and calculation of regional blood flow. These have a high-frequency response and can be used for recording pulse volume contours.[47] Volume changes measured by changes in electrical impedance form the basis for IPG, used extensively in the 1970s and 1980s for diagnosis of deep vein thrombosis.[50] The impedance technique was also evaluated for testing of the arterial system.[49] The early pneumatic plethysmographs, such as the Winsor Vasograph, led to the evolution of a variety of tests, some of which are still in use.[51]

Segmental Air Plethysmography

The change in the volume of an extremity between systole and diastole is a reflection of pulsatile blood flow. In the

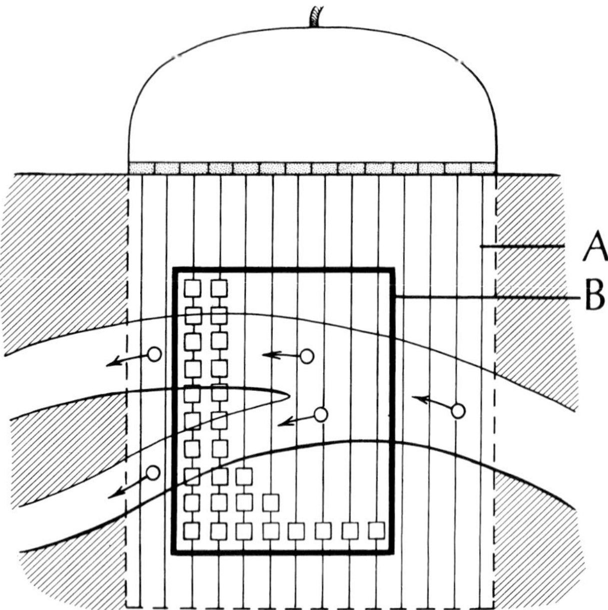

FIGURE 9–3. Color-coded duplex system. A matrix of sample volumes is created. A gray scale image is created within area A. For most examinations, the velocity coding is carried out only in a portion of the whole image, shown by area B. This is done to reduce the amount of data processing, and thus the time, required to create each image. (From Baker JD: The vascular laboratory. *In* Moore WS [ed]: Vascular Surgery: A Comprehensive Review, 5th ed. Philadelphia, WB Saunders, 1998, pp 235–250.)

1970s, the PVR was developed specifically for arterial diagnosis.[12] A recording air plethysmograph is attached to standard blood pressure cuffs. A cuff 18 cm wide is used on the thigh, and cuffs 12 cm wide are used at the upper and lower calf levels. Narrower cuffs can be used to make recordings from the forefoot or from fingers. The cuffs are inflated to 65 mmHg to ensure appropriate contact between the cuff and the extremity. At this pressure, the tracing obtained is very similar to the pressure waveform recorded with an arterial cannula. An important feature of the PVR is the calibration system, which contributes to reproducible results.

Most laboratories rely on qualitative interpretation of the waveforms.[26] A normal trace has a sharp systolic rise and usually displays a prominent dicrotic notch (Fig. 9–4). With increasing proximal occlusive disease, there is loss of the dicrotic notch, prolongation of the downslope, and rounding of the systolic peak. Severe disease produces a flattened wave with slow upstroke and downstroke and low peak amplitude. In patients with unilateral disease, comparisons with waveforms from the normal limb can be made. With bilateral disease, comparison with arm waveforms may be helpful. Raines and colleagues[40] have described using quantitative measurements of the waveforms to establish categories of severity of stenosis, but this approach has not been widely used.

The PVR has been used extensively in vascular laboratories to assess occlusive disease in the legs. Most commonly, the test is used in conjunction with segmental pressure measurements. The plethysmographic recording has an important advantage in that it is not affected by vessel wall stiffness, which can cause erroneously high pressure measurements. Kempczinski[26] and Rutherford and associates[42] have reported excellent diagnostic results from use of the two tests in combination. Another application of the PVR is the assessment of vasculogenic impotence through recording of penile waveforms.[25]

Photoplethysmography

Photoplethysmography is based on measuring the concentration of blood in the cutaneous microcirculation by detecting the reflection of infrared light. The probe contains one or more infrared light sources and a photoelectric cell to measure reflected light. In most applications, the probe is fixed to the skin with transparent, double-sided adhesive tape. The light shines into the skin, and a portion of the beam is reflected back. Blood is more opaque to red light than the other components of the skin and subcutaneous tissue, so the absorption of light is affected by the amount of blood under the source beam. The output of the detector varies with the blood content of the subdermal capillary bed.

The photoplethysmograph can be used in two ways. The more common method is to use the *direct current* (DC) coupling mode. With this mode, the rapid beat-to-beat changes are attenuated so that slower blood volume changes are recorded without major distortion. A common application of the DC coupling mode is the recording of venous refilling after exercise in the evaluation of venous insufficiency. The probe is attached to the foot, and the examination is conducted with the patient standing. After a brief recording is obtained in the resting state, the patient performs five toe rises and then relaxes with no weight-bearing on the leg to be examined. Initially, rapid emptying of the superficial capillary system occurs owing to the calf pump action. Then there is a return to baseline level, gradual in the normal leg and rapid in the leg with venous insufficiency (Fig. 9–5). Studies have shown that the recovery time measured with this noninvasive technique is very close to that obtained by direct measurement of the superficial venous pressure.[1, 37] Several researchers have described methods for calibrating the photoplethysmograph, but these efforts have not been adopted as common practice.[17, 27]

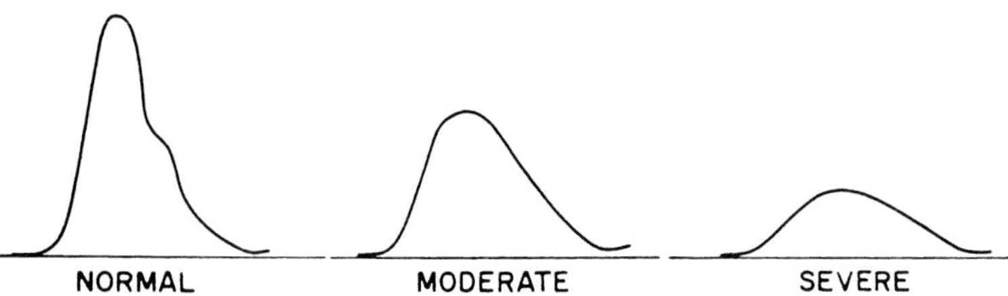

FIGURE 9–4. Pulse volume recordings associated with different degrees of occlusive disease. (From Baker JD: The vascular laboratory. *In* Moore WS [ed]: Vascular Surgery: A Comprehensive Review, 5th ed. Philadelphia, WB Saunders, 1998, pp 235–250.)

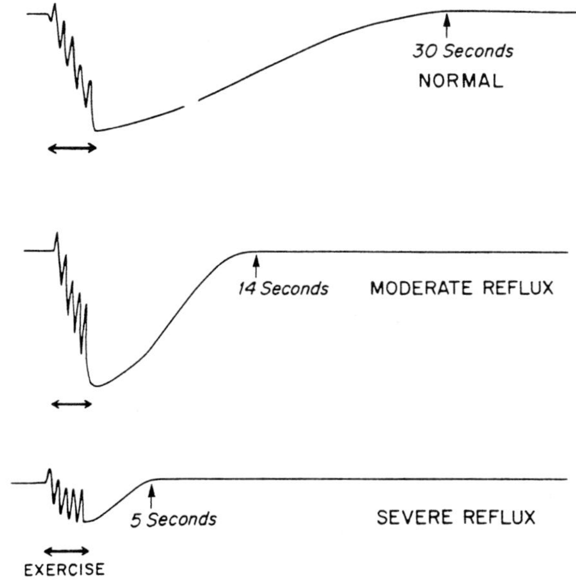

FIGURE 9–5. Evaluation of venous insufficiency with photoplethysmography. Refill times under 20 seconds are abnormal. With severe reflux, there is little initial deflection of the tracing because of ineffectual calf pump action. (From Baker JD: The vascular laboratory. *In* Moore WS [ed]: Vascular Surgery: A Comprehensive Review, 5th ed. Philadelphia, WB Saunders, 1998, pp 235–250.)

The second method is the *alternating current* (AC) coupling mode, which allows display of rapid changes and pulsatile characteristics (Fig. 9–6). The pulses recorded with this mode resemble those obtained with a strain-gauge. The plethysmograph, however, assesses digital flow patterns more quickly and more easily than a strain-gauge. The tracings can be used to show distal disease in the hands or feet. The photoelectric cell is also used to document changes in extremity flow with positional changes of the arm in the evaluation of possible arterial compression at the thoracic outlet.

Transcutaneous Oximetry

The potential value of measurement of intracutaneous oxygen tension (Po_2) was first demonstrated with electrodes inserted into the dermis.[20] The values measured correlated with arterial values; in a patient with hyperemia, the skin Po_2 was close to the Po_2 in the artery. Subsequently, the Clark-type polarographic electrode was modified for use on the skin surface. The values measured at normal skin temperature (2° to 3°C below core temperature) are close to zero. External warming or the induction of hyperemia increases the Po_2 levels detected. The probes that have been used for most clinical investigations contain a heating element to heat the skin under the probe to 43°C, optimizing the gas exchange and capillary blood flow.[16] The probes are small so they can be easily applied to most parts of the body.

The test is performed as follows:

1. The site is cleaned with alcohol to remove grease.
2. A drop of distilled water is placed on the skin, and the probe is attached with a ring of double-sided adhesive tape.
3. A period of about 20 minutes is required for the skin to heat and a plateau to be reached in the Po_2. In an ischemic extremity, 20 to 30 minutes may be required for equilibration.

Early studies evaluating the diagnostic potential of this method in patients with arterial occlusive disease measured the transcutaneous Po_2 ($TcPo_2$) of the foot. Normal subjects had values of 40 to 70 mmHg.[10, 15, 34] The finding of decreasing $TcPo_2$ with age led Cina and associates[10] to recommend concomitant measurement at the upper chest wall. There is considerable overlap in the $TcPo_2$ values detected in normal subjects and in patients with claudication, but the main advantage of the technique is in providing an objective assessment in patients with rest pain and gangrene. Foot $TcPo_2$ measurements in this group range from zero to 30 mmHg. The main applications of transcutaneous oxymetry in the vascular laboratory have been (1)

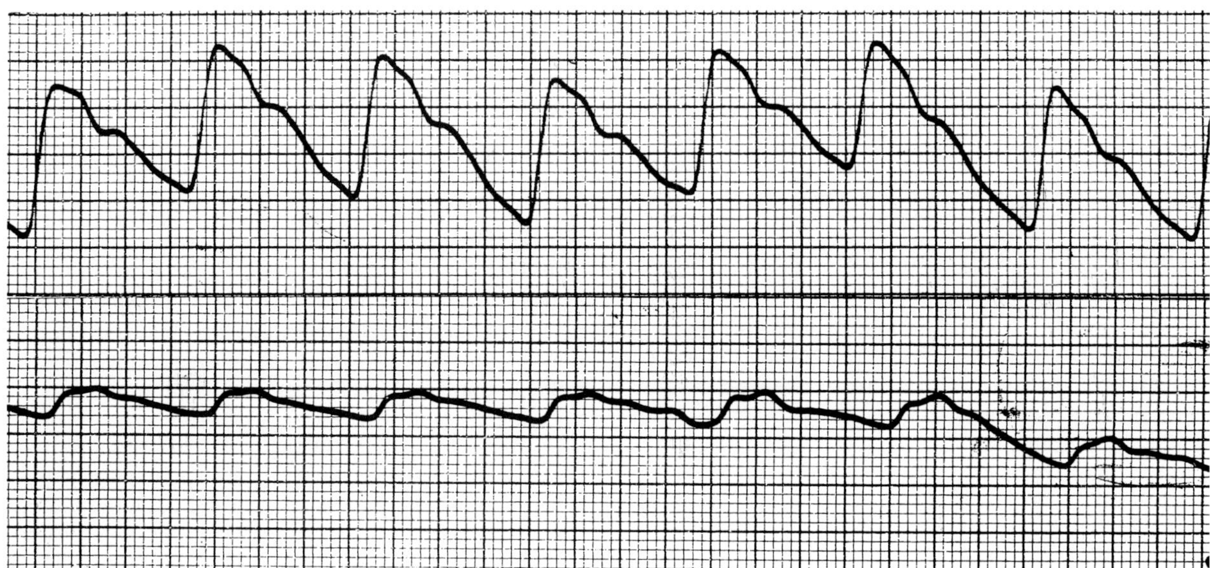

FIGURE 9–6. Photoplethysmograph waveforms recorded from fingers. *Top,* Normal hand. *Bottom,* Marked attenuation of digital flow. Both recordings were made at the same gain.

the determination of healing potential of wounds and (2) the prediction of successful amputation level.[5, 10, 30, 54]

Although measurement of skin oxygen content is an attractive concept, there are a number of practical problems with routine use of the test. The foremost of these is the long time required for equilibration at each recording site. Some manufacturers have made recorders that can accommodate several probes simultaneously, but most devices have a single probe. On average, it takes 25 minutes per site studied. There are also concerns about variability in measurements that might result from differences in body temperature, sympathetic tone, local cellulitis, skin thickness, and edema. Consequently, $TcPO_2$ studies are not performed routinely but are reserved to answer specific questions about wound healing potential.

Intraoperative Flowmeters

Electromagnetic Flowmeter

The electromagnetic flowmeter is based on Faraday's principle, which states that a conductor moving through a magnetic field generates a voltage perpendicular to both the direction of movement and the field.[53, 35] In the clinical setting, the blood is the moving conductor. The voltage produced is defined by

$$V = v \cdot H \cdot d \cdot 10^{-8} \qquad (9.3)$$

where v is the mean velocity in cm/sec, H is the magnetic field strength in gauss, and d is the diameter of the vessel in cm. With a pulsatile flow, the voltage varies directly with the velocity.

The first applications of this principle for measurement of blood flow were tried in 1930, but devices that were practical for clinical measurements were not available until the late 1950s. The typical design for intraoperative use had a perivascular probe containing an electromagnet to generate the field and sensing electrodes to detect the voltage generated. These devices soon became the standard against which other techniques were compared. This type of flowmeter has a number of problems or limitations:

1. The probe must fit snugly on the vessel to ensure good electrical contact between the electrodes on the inside of the probe and the surface of the vessel; this requires a wide range of probe sizes.
2. For optimal accuracy in flow measurement, each probe must be individually calibrated.
3. Many systems require test occlusion of the vessel to provide a "mechanical zero" to adjust the flowmeter.

Limitations include the errors caused by ambient electrical noise and the fact that the recorded output is influenced by hematocrit and vessel wall thickness. The sum of these requirements makes for a system that is tedious to use in most clinical settings, so few vascular surgeons use this type of flow measurement.

Transit Time Flowmeter

The differences in transit time between ultrasound signals traveling upstream and downstream in flowing fluid has been used to measure flow.[31, 35] The probe has two ultrasound transducers, each at 45 degrees to the axis of the vessel, with a reflecting surface that fits behind the vessel. Ultrasound pulses are alternately fired from one crystal, bounce off the reflector, and are received by the second crystal. A given probe is specifically designed for a fixed diameter of artery, so several probes are needed in most applications. Advantages of the transit time flowmeter include:

- No requirement for zeroing
- Fewer problems with electrical interference
- No need to ensure good electrical contact with the vessel wall
- No need for calibration

Intraoperative flow measurement has limited clinical use; however, when it is used, most clinicians prefer the transit time flowmeter over the electromagnetic type.

DERIVED MEASUREMENTS

Noninvasive Extremity Pressure Measurements

Since the 19th century, blood pressure has been measured with a sphygmomanometer using either a stethoscope or palpation of a distal pulse to determine end-points. These techniques are not applicable to smaller vessels, especially for lower pressures in the presence of arterial occlusive disease. In 1950, Winsor described using an air plethysmograph to find the cuff pressure at which pulsation was first recorded.[51] Subsequently, other techniques have been used, including Doppler detectors, mercury strain-gauges, and photoplethysmographs. Detection of flow with a CW Doppler unit is by far the simplest method, for the end-point can be heard with the audio output. In contrast, strain-gauge and photoelectric cell methods require a strip chart or a display system. As a result, the Doppler detector is the most commonly used technique for arterial pressure recording. The plethysmographic methods are reserved for special challenges such as severe ischemia and measurement of digit pressures.

Ankle Pressures

Prior to the test, the patient should rest for 15 minutes to allow for recovery from the effects of walking. The patient is examined in the supine position. A cuff 12 cm wide (standard adult arm cuff) is placed just above the malleolus. Usually, a CW Doppler detector (8 to 10 MHz) is used to detect arterial flow at the ankle level, and the probe position is adjusted to provide the optimal signal. The cuff is inflated until the flow stops and is then slowly deflated until the point at which a signal is again detected. The cuff pressure at this point defines the systolic pressure; diastolic pressure cannot be obtained. The procedure should be repeated several times to ensure accuracy. Measurements are made for both the dorsalis pedis and the posterior tibial branches, and the highest value is used for the ankle pressure. In cases of advanced occlusive disease, sometimes no signal is found in either the dorsalis pedis or the posterior tibial artery; it may be possible to find the anterior branch of the peroneal artery near the lateral malleolus to measure the ankle pressure.

The ankle pressure is usually interpreted in relation to the brachial pressure, with the latter serving as the reference value. The ankle-brachial index (ABI) is the ratio of the ankle pressure to the arm pressure. Both brachial artery pressures are measured with the Doppler detector, and the higher of the two values is chosen for calculation of the ABI. This index is normally in the range of 1.1 to 1.2.[8, 51, 55] A resting ABI of less than 0.95 is considered abnormal. (See Chapter 10 for intererpretation of studies.)

When using pressure measurements, one must recognize sources of error. The most important is the artifact that occurs in patients with advanced arterial calcification. In this situation, the cuff pressure needed to collapse the artery is greater than that required to exceed the intra-arterial pressure. This situation is particularly common in diabetic patients with heavily calcified tibial arteries. The typical vascular laboratory can expect to find this problem in 5% to 15% of patients examined; this rate is higher if diabetic patients are overrepresented in the population studied.

In some cases, arterial stiffness is so severe that blood flow is not stopped even at a cuff pressure of 300 mmHg, in which case the artifact is easily recognized. The problem cases are those in which the a systolic end-point can be detected, for in this situation, one has no idea about the magnitude of the artifact. Recording a PVR or a Doppler waveform often helps to identify a pressure measurement error produced by arterial wall stiffness. Another alternative is to measure pressures in the forefoot or toe, the arteries of which are usually less calcified than tibial arteries. Often, there is less stiffness in the foot vessels. Forefoot pressures are measured with a pediatric cuff, and detection of blood flow with the Doppler probe over a digital branch. Toe pressure measurement requires a special 2-cm cuff, and usually, a photoelectric cell probe is used to detect the systolic end-point. Carter[9] has suggested measuring toe pressures in all patients known to be diabetic.

Segmental Pressures

Because ankle pressures reflect the sum of occlusive disease in the entire limb, segmental pressure measurement has been suggested to (1) identify the level of significant disease and (2) determine whether such disease exists at a single level or multiple levels. For this study, lower leg pressure cuffs are placed just below the knee and just above the malleoli. The thigh examination is performed with either a single cuff 18 cm wide or with two cuffs 10 cm wide, one placed just above the knee and the other as high as possible on the thigh. The Doppler probe is placed over the ankle artery, with the better signal and pressures measured for each level as described previously.

Franzeck and associates[15] have advocated using the popliteal artery as the sensing site for thigh pressures. They found that pressures taken from an ankle sensing site were significantly lower than the pressures taken from a popliteal sensing site in 23% of patients studied. Still, the practice in most laboratories is to use the popliteal artery signal to record thigh pressures only if no ankle signal is found.

The two methods of thigh pressure measurement must be evaluated separately. The single wide cuff is intended to provide the appropriate match to the size of the typical adult thigh. (The recommended cuff width for accurate blood pressure measurement is 1.2 times the diameter of the extremity under the cuff.[28]) The pressure measured in this way can be compared directly with the arm pressure. In general, experience with the single-cuff technique has resulted in accurate identification of aortoiliac or proximal femoral lesions.[14] With this method, however, there are problems separating inflow disease from disease in the superficial femoral artery.

Because of the interest in determining the disease level, many laboratories use two narrow thigh cuffs. The problem with this technique is that an assumption must be made about the magnitude of the artifact due to the use of cuffs widths that are narrower than ideal. In normal subjects, the difference between brachial pressure and thigh pressure measured with a narrow cuff has been reported as 20 to 30 mmHg.[19, 32] This difference requires an assumption to be made about the narrow cuff artifact in the interpretation of results with the double-cuff technique. However, this technique has been shown to be more accurate in separating aortoiliac from superficial femoral disease unless the latter involves the proximal superficial femoral artery, in which case it will affect even measurements taken from cuffs high on the thigh.[13]

Doppler Waveform Analysis

Qualitative Analysis

An arterial velocity waveform is determined by the interaction of many physiologic factors:

- Pulsation generated by the heart
- Viscosity of blood
- Elasticity of the arterial wall in different segments of the arterial tree
- Location and extent of atherosclerosis

Experience has led investigators to associate certain velocity signals with different levels and severity of arterial disease. Consequently, many vascular laboratories assess a Doppler waveform qualitatively and assign it to a category on the basis of simple characteristics. In general, a proximal stenosis damps the waveform with decrease in peak velocity and pulsatility. The simplest method is to characterize a peripheral tracing as normal if it has a reverse flow component in early diastole.[36, 38] This approach has been studied for the detection of hemodynamically significant stenosis in the aortoiliac segment. The presence of a reverse component is highly predictive of normal inflow, but the absence of the reverse flow may often be related to other factors. In general, qualitative waveform categorization may be a first approximation, but it cannot be used for a definitive diagnosis, and more objective, quantitative approaches have been sought.

Pulsatility Index

The most commonly used quantitative analysis is the pulsatility index (PI) described by Gosling and coworkers[18, 52]:

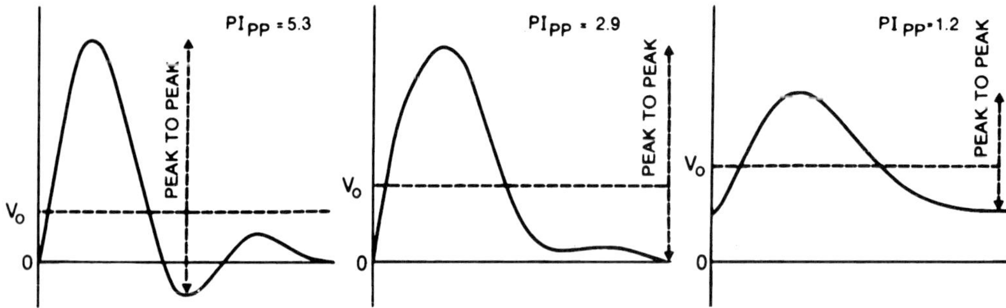

FIGURE 9–7. Calculation of pulsatility index (PI). (From Johnston KW: Processing continuous wave Doppler signals and analysis of peripheral arterial waveforms. *In* Berstein EF [ed]: Vascular Diagnosis. St. Louis, Mosby–Year Book, 1993, pp 149–159.)

$$\text{PI} = \frac{\text{peak-to-peak velocity}}{\text{mean velocity}} \tag{9.4}$$

Figure 9–7 illustrates the PI calculated for different arterial waveforms. The more attenuated a waveform, the lower the PI, and a very flat signal may have a value near zero. PI was not intended as an isolated parameter but was defined in conjunction with Gosling's concept of an arterial damping factor (DF) measured between two points, where

$$\text{DF} = \frac{\text{proximal PI}}{\text{distal PI}} \tag{9.5}$$

In a normal extremity, the more distal one samples in the large arteries, the greater the magnitude of the diastolic reverse flow. This phenomenon is attributed to an increase in the wave reflected from the distal bed. Therefore, DF is less than 1 in a normal extremity and increases to more than 1 as a result of increasing attenuation of the distal wave by occlusive disease.

Most laboratories using PI have employed it as an isolated parameter rather than in the calculation of DF. In part, the reason is that most of the applications of this quantitative analysis have been focused on the definition of aortoiliac disease. Prior to the availability of a duplex scanner suited for abdominal studies, it was not possible to obtain waveforms from the distal aorta in order to calculate the proximal PI required for measuring the DF. Extensive studies have been conducted assessing common femoral artery PI for the evaluation of proximal disease. A considerable limitation has been the extent to which the shape of the femoral tracings can be affected by occlusive disease in the superficial femoral artery. Chapter 10 reviews the major clinical studies to date.

Other Analytic Methods

Experience with PI led some investigators to seek other analytic approaches to the femoral artery waveform. One concern was whether part of the weakness of the method rested in its simplicity. With only two parameters measuring the waveform, a variety of curve shapes may be defined by the same PI. Skidmore and Woodcock[44] developed a new approach that used a curve-fitting program to describe a waveform in terms of the Laplace transform. The third-order equation defining the relationships of the components of the curve yields parameters related to proximal damping, proximal vessel wall stiffness, and the distal runoff. Some investigators have found that this method of analysis yields better diagnostic results than PI calculated for the same waveforms, but other groups have not demonstrated this benefit.[2, 3, 11, 24, 33]

Another method that has been developed uses principal component analysis.[33, 39] Sets of waveforms known to be normal or to have a given degree of stenosis are characterized mathematically. Each new waveform is then compared with the features of each of the categories in the "training set," and the new waveform is assigned to the category of stenosis in the training set that most closely matches. These methods have not had extensive trial because (1) the availability of the necessary equipment is limited and (2) the complex conceptual basis for the analyses has not attracted the interest of enough clinicians.

SELECTED REFERENCES

Baker JD: The vascular laboratory: The past and the future. Am J Surg 164:190–193, 1992.

Beach KW: 1975–2000: A quarter century of ultrasound technology. Ultrasound Med Biol 18:377, 1992.

Sigel B: A brief history of Doppler ultrasound in the diagnosis of peripheral vascular disease. Ultrasound Med Biol 24:169, 1998.

Yao JST: Presidential address: Precision in vascular surgery. J Vasc Surg 5:535,1987.

REFERENCES

1. Abramowitz HB, Queral LA, Flinn WR, et al: The use of photoplethysmography in the assessment of venous insufficiency: A comparison to venous pressure measurements. Surgery 86:434, 1979.
2. Baker JD, Machleder HI, Skidmore R: Analysis of femoral artery Doppler signals by Laplace transform damping method. J Vasc Surg 1:520, 1984.
3. Baker JD, Skidmore S, Cole SEA: Laplace transform analysis of femoral artery Doppler signals: The state of the art. Ultrasound Med Biol 15:13, 1989.
4. Baker JD: Quality assurance in the vascular laboratory. Semin Vasc Surg 7:241, 1994.
5. Ballard JL, Eke CC, Bunt TJ, et al: A prospective evaluation of transcutaneous oxygen measurements in the management of diabetic foot problems. J Vasc Surg 22:485, 1995.
6. Bergan JJ, Darling RC, DeWolfe VG, et al: Report of the Intersociety Commission for Heart Disease Resources: Medical instrumentation in peripheral vascular disease. Circulation 54:A1, 1976.
7. Blackshear WM, Phillips DJ, Thiele BL, et al: Detection of carotid occlusive disease by ultrasound imaging and pulsed Doppler spectrum analysis. Surgery 86:698, 1979.

8. Carter S: Indirect systolic pressure and pulse waves in arterial occlusive disease of the lower extremities. Circulation 37:624, 1968.
9. Carter S: Role of pressure measurements. *In* Berstein EF (ed): Vascular Diagnosis. St. Louis, Mosby–Year Book, 1993, p 486.
10. Cina C, Katsamouris A, Megerman J, et al: Utility of transcutaneous oxygen tension measurements in peripheral arterial occlusive disease. J Vasc Surg 1:362, 1984.
11. Clifford PC, Skidmore R, Bird D, et al: Femoral artery Doppler signal analysis in lower limb ischaemia. J Cardiovasc Surg 23:69, 1982.
12. Darling RC, Raines JK, Brener BJ, et al: Quantitative segmental pulse volume recorder: A clinical tool. Surgery 72:873, 1972.
13. Flanigan DP, Gray B, Schuler JJ, et al: Utility of wide and narrow blood pressure cuffs in the hemodynamic assessment of aortoiliac occlusive disease. Surgery 92:46, 1982.
14. Francfort JW, Bigelow PS, Davis JT, et al: Noninvasive techniques in the assessment of lower-extremity arterial occlusive disease. Arch Surg 119:1145, 1984.
15. Franzeck UK, Bernstein EF, Fronek A: The effect of sensing site on the limb segmental blood pressure determination. Arch Surg 116:912, 1981.
16. Franzeck UK, Talke P, Bernstein EF, et al: Transcutaneous PO_2 measurements in health and peripheral arterial occlusive disease. Surgery 91:156, 1982.
17. Fronek A: Recent developments in venous photoplethysmography. *In* Berstein EF (ed): Vascular Diagnosis. St. Louis, Mosby–Year Book, 1993, p 930.
18. Gosling RG, Dunbar G, King DH, et al: The quantitative analysis of occlusive peripheral arterial disease by non-intrusive ultrasonic technique. Angiology 52:52, 1971.
19. Heintz SE, Bone GE, Slaymaker EE, et al: Value of arterial pressure measurements in the proximal and distal part of the thigh in arterial disease. Surg Gynecol Obstet 146:337, 1978.
20. Huch R, Huch A, Lubbers DW: Transcutaneous Po_2. New York, Thieme Stratton, 1981, p 2.
21. Johnston KW, Kassam M, Koers J, et al: Comparative study of four methods for quantifying Doppler ultrasound waveforms from the femoral artery. Ultrasound Med Biol 10:1, 1984.
22. Johnston, KW, Maruzzo BC, Cobbold RSC: The errors and artifacts of Doppler flowmeters and their solution. Arch Surg 112:1335, 1977.
23. Johnston, KW, Maruzzo BC, Kassam M, Cobbold RSC: Methods for obtaining, processing and quantifying Doppler blood velocity waveforms. *In* Nicolaides AN, Yao JST (eds): Investigation of Vascular Disorders. New York, Churchill Livingstone, 1981, p 532.
24. Jones AM: Education and Certification of the vascular technologist. *In* Bernstein EF (ed): Vascular Diagnosis. St. Louis, Mosby–Year Book, 1993, p 28.
25. Kempczinski RF, Berlatsky Y, Pearce WH: Semi-quantitative photoplethysmography in the diagnosis of lower extremity venous insufficiency. J Cardiovasc Surg 27:17, 1986.
26. Kempczinski RF: Role of the vascular diagnostic laboratory in the evaluation of male impotence. Am J Surg 138:278, 1979.
27. Kempczinski RF: Segmental volume plethysmography: The pulse volume recorder. *In* Kempczinski RF, Yao JST (eds): Practical Noninvasive Vascular Diagnosis. Chicago, Year Book Medical Publishers, 1982, p 105.
28. Kirkendall WM, Burton AC, Epstein FH, et al: Recommendations for human blood pressure determination by sphygmomanometer. Circulation 36:980, 1967.
29. Kremkau FW: Principles and pitfalls of real-time color flow imaging. *In* Berstein EF (ed): Vascular Diagnosis. St. Louis, Mosby–Year Book, 1993, p 90.
30. Lalka SG, Malone JM, Anderson GG, et al: Transcutaneous oxygen and carbon dioxide pressure monitoring to determine outcome of limb ischemia and to predict surgical outcome. J Vasc Surg 7:507, 1988.
31. Lundell A, Bergqvist D, Mattson E, et al: Volume flow measurements with a transit time flowmeter: An in vivo and in vitro variability and validation study. Clin Physiol 13:547, 1993.
32. Lynch TG, Hobson RW, Wright CB, et al: Interpretation of Doppler segmental pressures in peripheral vascular occlusive disease. Arch Surg 119:465, 1984.
33. Macpherson DS, Evans DH, Bell PRF: Common femoral artery Doppler waveforms: A comparison of three methods of objective analysis with direct pressure measurements. Br J Surg 71:46, 1984.
34. Matsen FA, Wyss CR, Pedegana LR, et al: Transcutaneous oxygen tension in peripheral vascular disease. Surg Gynecol Obstet 150:525, 1980.
35. Nicholls SC, Kohler TR, Martin RL, et al: Diastolic flow as a predictor of arterial stenosis. J Vasc Surg 3:498, 1986.
36. Nichols WW, O'Rourke MF: McDonald's Blood Flow in Arteries, 3rd ed. Philadelphia, Lea & Febiger, 1990, p 143.
37. Nicolaides AN, Miles C: Photoplethysmography in the assessment of venous insufficiency. J Vasc Surg 5:405, 1987.
38. Persson AV, Gibons G, Griffey S: Noninvasive evaluation of the aortoiliac segment. J Cardiovasc Surg 22:539, 1981.
39. Prytherch DR, Evans DH, Smith MJ, et al: On-line classification of arterial stenosis severity using principal component analysis applied to Doppler ultrasound signals. Clin Phys Physiol Meas 3:191, 1982.
40. Raines JK, Darling RC, Buth J: Vascular laboratory criteria for the management of peripheral vascular disease in the lower extremities. Surgery 79:21, 1976.
41. Renemen RS, Clarke HF, Simmons N, Spencer MP: In vivo comparison of electromagnetic and Doppler flowmeters: With special attention to the processing of the analogue Doppler signal. Cardiovasc Res 7:557, 1973.
42. Rutherford RB, Lowenstein DH, Klein MF: Combining segmental systolic pressures and plethysmography to diagnose arterial occlusive disease in the legs. Am J Surg 138:211, 1979.
43. Rutherford RB: Qualifications of the physician in charge of the vascular diagnostic laboratory. J Vasc Surg 8:732, 1988.
44. Skidmore R, Woodcock JP: Physiologic interpretation of Doppler-shift waveforms: II. Validation of the LaPlace transform method for characterisation of the common femoral blood-velocity waveform. Ultrasound Med Biol 6:219, 1980.
45. Strandness DE: Duplex Scanning in Vascular Disorders, 2nd ed. New York, Raven Press, 1993, p 1.
46. Sumner DS: Evaluation of noninvasive testing procedures: Data analysis and interpretation. *In* Bernstein EF (ed): Vascular Diagnosis. St. Louis, Mosby–Year Book, 1993, p 39.
47. Sumner DS: Mercury strain-gauge plethysmography. *In* Berstein EF (ed): Vascular Diagnosis. St. Louis, Mosby–Year Book, 1993, p 205.
48. Thiele BL: Accreditation of vascular laboratories. *In* Bernstein EF (ed): Vascular Diagnosis. St. Louis, Mosby–Year Book, 1993, p 36.
49. Van de Water JM, Mount BE, Roettinger WF, et al: Noninvasive assessment of the peripheral vascular system. Arch Surg 112:679, 1977.
50. Wheeler HB, O'Donnell JA, Anderson FA, et al: Occlusive impedance phlebography: A diagnostic procedure for venous thrombosis and pulmonary embolism. Prog Cardiovasc Dis 17:199, 1974.
51. Winsor T: Influence of arterial disease on the systolic blood pressure gradients in the extremity. Am J Med Sci 220:117, 1950.
52. Woodcock JP, Gosling RG, FitzGerald DE: A new non-intrusive technique for assessment of superficial femoral artery obstruction. Br J Surg 59:226, 1972.
53. Woodcock JP: Theory and Practice of Blood Flow Measurement. London, Butterworths, 1975, p 67.
54. Wyss CR, Matsen FA, Simmons CW, et al: Transcutaneous oxygen tension measurements on limbs of diabetic and nondiabetic patients with peripheral vascular disease. Surgery 95:339, 1984.
55. Yao JST: Hemodynamic studies in peripheral arterial disease. Br J Surg 57:761, 1970.
56. Zierler RE, Phillips DJ, Beach KW, et al: Noninvasive assessment of normal carotid bifurcation hemodynamics with color flow ultrasound imaging. Ultrasound Med Biol 13:471, 1987.

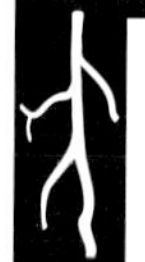

CHAPTER 10

Physiologic Assessment of Peripheral Arterial Occlusive Disease

R. Eugene Zierler, M.D., and David S. Sumner, M.D.

CLINICAL ROLE OF PHYSIOLOGIC TESTING

Interventions for peripheral arterial occlusive disease should be designed to treat a physiologic rather than an anatomic defect. It makes little difference how aesthetically unappealing an arteriosclerotic plaque becomes if it does not restrict blood flow. Therefore, the surgeon who evaluates peripheral arterial disease must concentrate on the physiologic defects that the lesions produce. Although the surgeon gains an appreciation of how these defects limit the patient's activities from the history, the interpretation of symptoms is highly subjective. Beyond an estimate of the physiologic limitations imposed by claudication or the suffering due to ischemic rest pain, the history yields nothing measurable.

The physical examination provides more objectivity, in that pulses can be graded, ulcers measured, gangrenous areas delineated, and pallor, dependent rubor, and skin temperature observed. Even the most skilled surgical diagnostician makes some errors, however, and the nonspecialist physician makes many more.[8, 95, 106] Thus, the physical examination frequently fails to provide an accurate and objective assessment of the severity of arterial disease.

After the history and physical examination, the next logical step in the evaluation of a patient for arterial occlusive disease is physiologic testing.[14] In general, these tests are designed to answer the following questions:

1. Is significant arterial occlusive disease present?
2. If so, how severe is the physiologic impairment?
3. Where are the lesions located?
4. In multilevel disease, which arterial segments are most severely involved?
5. In limbs with tissue loss, what is the potential for primary healing?

Once these questions are answered, the surgeon is better able to decide whether the deficit is severe enough to warrant arteriography as a prelude to intervention. There are also a number of clinical problems that are not easily resolved, even with the help of arteriography. For example, patients with pseudoclaudication may be identified by physiologic testing and spared further vascular evaluation.[31, 53, 82, 150] Patients with demonstrable arterial disease may have concomitant orthopedic or neurologic problems. With the help of physiologic testing, the physician can determine the relative magnitude of the deficit caused by each of these conditions and advise the patient accordingly. In limbs with multilevel disease, it is usually possible to identify which of the lesions is most significant, allowing the surgeon to focus on the more critical lesion.[3, 16, 21, 105, 115, 147, 161]

Physiologic tests are helpful in determining whether an ulcer is due to neuropathy, venous stasis, or ischemia and in deciding whether foot pain is primarily neuropathic or ischemic.[68, 121] They may also enhance the ability of the surgeon to assess the healing potential of a foot lesion or amputation.[11, 20, 66, 100, 159] In cases of suspected vascular trauma, physiologic findings, if negative, may avert an unnecessary vascular exploration or, if positive, may alert the surgeon to the need for immediate operation.[71] Similarly, the recognition and evaluation of suspected iatrogenic vascular injuries, such as those that follow cardiac catheterization or interventional radiologic procedures, are facilitated by physiologic testing.[10] Physiologic tests are uniquely applicable to the diagnosis of intermittent arterial obstructions, such as those arising from entrapment syndromes, and for distinguishing between fixed arterial obstructions and obstructions due to vasospasm. These are but a few of the many areas in which physiologic tests complement the information gleaned from the routine history, physical examination, and arteriogram.

A comprehensive evaluation of peripheral arterial occlusive disease requires the integration of physiologic, anatomic, and clinical information. This chapter reviews the theory, methods, interpretation, and applications of the various physiologic arterial tests available in the vascular laboratory (see Chapter 9). The use of duplex scanning for assessment of arterial disease is considered in Chapter 12.

PRESSURE MEASUREMENT

Measurement of pressure has distinct advantages over measurement of flow for identifying the presence of arterial disease and for assessing its severity. Even though resting flow levels may remain in the normal range, there is almost always a pressure drop across a stenotic lesion, which increases resistance to arterial flow.[27, 145, 155, 164, 166] Pressure measurements can be made more sensitive by augmentation of blood flow through a stenotic segment. This can be accomplished by exercise, the induction of reactive hyperemia, or the intra-arterial administration of vasodilating drugs. With increased blood flow, pressure drops are greater, and even those that were not noticeable under baseline conditions become evident (see Chapter 7).[9, 21, 28, 138, 166]

Ankle Pressure

Of all the noninvasive tests available for evaluating the functional severity of peripheral arterial disease, none is more useful than measurement of systolic blood pressure at the ankle. This test not only provides a simple, reliable means of diagnosing obstructive arterial disease but is also readily applicable to follow-up studies.

Ankle pressure is measured as follows:

1. A pneumatic cuff is placed around the ankle just above the malleoli.
2. A Doppler ultrasonographic probe is placed over the posterior tibial artery, and the pressure is measured at this site.
3. The Doppler probe is placed over the dorsalis pedis artery, and the pressured is measured at this site.

In normal individuals, the pressure measured at these two sites should differ by no more than 10 mmHg. A pressure difference greater than 15 mmHg suggests that there is a proximal occlusion or stenosis in the artery with the lower pressure.[27] The pressure at the site giving the higher value is taken as the ankle pressure.

Occasionally, no audible Doppler flow signal can be obtained over either the posterior tibial or the dorsalis pedis artery. In these cases, a careful search often reveals a peroneal collateral signal anteriorly, near the lateral malleolus. When no Doppler signal can be found, the ankle pressure can often be measured with a plethysmograph placed around the foot or applied to one of the toes.

Normally, the systolic pressure at the ankle exceeds that in the arm by 12 ± 8 to 24 ± 9 mmHg.[18, 28, 92] This difference reflects the augmentation of systolic pressure that occurs as the pressure wave travels peripherally. Distal to a hemodynamically significant lesion, the ankle pressure is almost always decreased.[18, 142, 145, 146] Usually, (1) a single stenosis that decreases diameter by 50% or more or (2) multiple mild irregularities of the arterial lumen reduce the ankle pressure by at least 10 mmHg.[127] Typical ankle-arm pressure gradients are: (1) isolated superficial femoral obstruction, 53 ± 10 mmHg; (2) isolated aortoiliac obstruction, 61 ± 15 mmHg; and (3) multilevel obstruction, 91 ± 23 mmHg.[145]

Ankle-Brachial Index

Because the ankle systolic blood pressure varies with the central aortic pressure, it is convenient to normalize these values by dividing the ankle pressure by the brachial blood pressure.[26, 27, 162, 168] This ratio, which is commonly referred to as the ankle pressure index or *ankle-brachial index* (ABI), normally averages about 1.1 when the well-rested subject is lying supine (Table 10–1). Although the ABI in an occasional patient with functionally significant arterial stenosis exceeds 1.0,[1, 26, 48, 112, 168] the resting index in the vast majority of patients with arterial disease is much lower.[1, 37, 164, 167, 168] In fact, an ABI less than 1.0 is highly suggestive of functional arterial obstruction[26, 27, 37, 166, 167]; only rarely does a normal limb have an index less than 0.92.[58, 112]

As shown in Figure 10–1 and Table 10–2, the ABI varies somewhat with the location of the arterial obstruction.[145, 164, 167] Values tend to be highest when the lesion is confined to the popliteal or below-knee arteries and lowest in limbs with multilevel disease.[90, 126, 164, 168] Carter[27] found that the ABI exceeded 0.50 in 85% of patients with a single level of obstruction but was less than 0.50 in 95% of those with two or more levels. In addition, the ABI decreases as the functional severity of the disease increases, the lowest values being obtained in limbs with impending gangrene and the highest in limbs with mild claudication (Fig. 10–2).[37, 113, 118, 121, 166, 167] The ABI also correlates with arteriographic findings.[127, 168] Values are lowest when there is complete occlusion and highest when there is minimal atheromatous change (Fig. 10–3).[26, 37, 153, 168] As would be predicted on the basis of hemodynamic principles outlined in Chapter 7, the lengths of the occlusive lesion and of the bypassing collateral vessels are less important than their diameters.[39]

Because the ABI is relatively stable from one examination to the next in the same individual, it is an effective means of following the course of a patient's arterial disease over time. A consistent decrease indicates advancing disease or a failure of arterial reconstruction.[15, 101, 102, 111, 148] A spontaneous rise in the ABI is usually attributable to the development of collateral circulation.[131, 132] After successful arterial intervention, there is an increase in the ABI.[37, 140, 147, 148, 168] If all obstructions have been totally removed or bypassed, the ABI exceeds 1.0; however, if there are residual sites of obstruction, the ABI increases but not to normal levels (Fig. 10–4).[147]

Technical Errors

In general, ankle pressure measurements are easily made and are remarkably free of error. The standard deviation between two measurements repeated within a few minutes is about 5 mmHg; the deviation increases to approximately 8 to 9 mmHg between measurements taken a day apart.[108] These figures, however, do not account for variations in the central arterial pressure.

When the ABI rather than the absolute ankle pressure value is considered, the day-to-day results are even more consistent. This test is also subject to interobserver and intraobserver variability as well as to nonpathologic biologic variability. A change in the ABI of 0.15 or more is highly likely to fall outside the 95% confidence limits of normal variation and therefore implies a significant physiologic change.[6, 73]

Medial calcification, which renders the underlying arteries incompressible, is responsible for most of the errors made in measuring ankle pressure with a pneumatic cuff.[48, 65, 118, 139, 149] Because patients with diabetes are particularly prone to this problem, ankle pressure measurements in diabetic patients may be 5% or 10% too high.[118] In these cases, it is sometimes possible to estimate the pressure by elevating the foot and noting the vertical distance of the foot from the bed at the point at which the Doppler signal disappears.[52] Multiplying this distance (in centimeters) by 0.735 gives the pressure in mmHg. Alternatively, the severity of arterial occlusive disease in the lower extremity can be assessed by toe pressure measurements, as discussed later in this chapter.

Inability to distinguish between arterial and venous flow can occur when the arterial flow velocity is decreased and the signal becomes less pulsatile.[1] However, venous signals

TABLE 10–1. SEGMENTAL PRESSURE INDICES IN NORMAL SUBJECTS (MEAN ± SD)*

AUTHOR AND YEAR	THIGH	ABOVE KNEE	BELOW KNEE	ANKLE
Carter (1968)[26]	—	1.16 ± 0.05§	—	1.15 ± 0.08‡
Yao (1970, 1973)[166, 167]	—	—	—	1.11 ± 0.10
Wolf et al (1972)[164]	—	—	—	1.09 ± 0.08†
Fronek et al (1973)[49]	1.34 ± 0.27‖	1.32 ± 0.23‖	1.26 ± 0.24‖	1.08 ± 0.10‡
Cutajar et al (1973)[37]	1.53 ± 0.17†	—	1.17 ± 0.13‡	1.08 ± 0.09‡
Hajjar and Sumner (1976)[58]	1.37 ± 0.20†	1.26 ± 0.11†	1.16 ± 0.10†	1.08 ± 0.08†
Rutherford et al (1979)[126]	1.28 ± 0.17†	1.24 ± 0.17†	1.16 ± 0.17†	1.08 ± 0.17†

*Pressure index equals systolic pressure at site of measurement divided by brachial systolic pressure.
†Cuff 10 × 40 cm.
‡Cuff 12.5 × 30 cm (standard).
§Cuff 15 × 45 cm.
‖Cuff 17 × 50 cm.

can be differentiated from arterial signals with a directional Doppler flowmeter. Moreover, venous signals can be augmented by distal compression, but arterial signals either are not affected or diminish. If doubt still remains, a plethysmograph can be used to sense the return of pulsatile arterial flow as the cuff is deflated.

Segmental Pressure

A decrease in the ankle pressure or ABI indicates that arterial occlusive disease is present, but it does not identify the specific segments involved. Further diagnostic information can be obtained by measuring the pressure gradients down the leg.[63, 81, 139, 162] Only rarely do these measurements need to be made when the ankle pressure is normal.[48]

The following four-cuff method is but one of a number of techniques that have been advocated. Pneumatic cuffs 10 cm in width are placed:

- Around the thigh at groin level
- Around the thigh just above the knee
- Around the calf below the knee
- At ankle level

Blood pressure is measured at each level using a Doppler probe on the posterior tibial or dorsalis pedis artery.

Upper Thigh Pressure

In most normal individuals, blood pressures measured with the four-cuff technique at the upper thigh level exceed those measured at the brachial level by 30 to 40 mmHg.[1, 37, 63, 142] Indices, obtained by dividing the thigh pressure by the brachial pressure, are comparably elevated, averaging around 1.30 to 1.50 (see Table 10–1).

It must be emphasized that these upper thigh pressures do not accurately reflect the true femoral artery pressure. When measured by invasive techniques, the pressure in the common femoral artery is almost identical to the brachial artery pressure.[114] Furthermore, as indicated by the standard deviations given in Table 10–1, upper thigh pressures are highly variable, even in normal subjects. Because of the disparity between cuff width and thigh diameter, higher pressures are obtained in patients with large thighs, and lower, more accurate pressures are obtained in patients with small thighs.[139]

A thigh pressure equal to or lower than the brachial pressure usually indicates hemodynamically significant aortoiliac disease.[37] When the thigh pressure exceeds arm pressure by less than 15 to 30 mmHg, iliac disease may be suspected; but this finding may not indicate iliac disease if the diameter of the thigh is small.[63, 126] Comparison of the pressures obtained from the two thighs is of some value in these cases.[49] A 20-mmHg difference is said to be significant; however, some workers have not found this difference to be a reliable indicator.[120]

Thigh pressure indices associated with aortoiliac obstructive disease are shown in Table 10–2 and Figure 10–5. It is apparent from Figure 10–5 that the upper thigh index may be lower than 1.0 in limbs with superficial femoral

TABLE 10–2. SEGMENTAL PRESSURE INDICES IN PATIENTS WITH OCCLUSIVE ARTERIAL DISEASE OF THE LEGS (MEAN ± SD)*

LOCATION OF OBSTRUCTION	AUTHOR AND YEAR	UPPER THIGH	ABOVE KNEE	BELOW KNEE	ANKLE
Aortoiliac	Fronek et al (1973)[49]	0.72 ± 0.25	0.70 ± 0.24	0.62 ± 0.21	0.57 ± 0.18
	Rutherford et al (1979)[126]	0.81 ± 0.25	0.76 ± 0.25	0.71 ± 0.25	0.68 ± 0.32
	Ramsey et al (1979)[120]	0.81 ± 0.27	0.72 ± 0.25	0.59 ± 0.22	0.54 ± 0.22
Femoropopliteal	Fronek et al (1973)[49]	1.26 ± 0.39	0.92 ± 0.39	0.73 ± 0.30	0.51 ± 0.28
	Rutherford et al (1979)[126]	1.25 ± 0.27	0.86 ± 0.22	0.75 ± 0.18	0.65 ± 0.18
	Ramsey et al (1979)[120]	1.19 ± 0.21	0.87 ± 0.23	0.70 ± 0.18	0.60 ± 0.19
Combined aortoliac and femoropopliteal	Fronek et al (1973)[49]	0.97 ± 0.34	0.79 ± 0.32	0.61 ± 0.28	0.48 ± 0.31
	Rutherford et al (1979)[126]	0.89 ± 0.17	0.72 ± 0.17	0.58 ± 0.17	0.53 ± 0.28
	Ramsey et al (1979)[120]	0.79 ± 0.21	0.62 ± 0.17	0.49 ± 0.15	0.39 ± 0.15

*Pressure index equals systolic pressure at site of measurement divided by brachial systolic pressure.

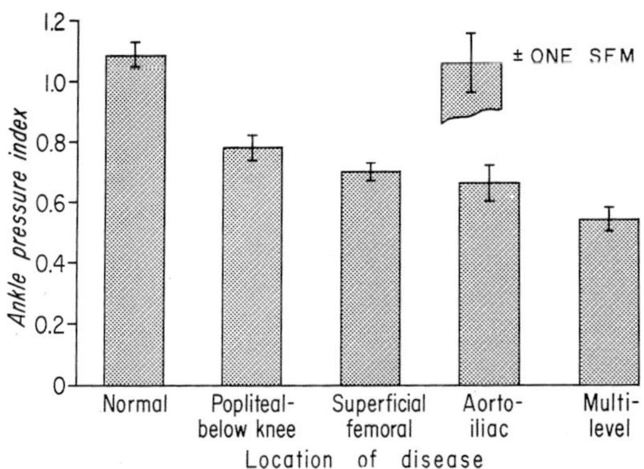

FIGURE 10–1. Resting ankle blood pressure indices (ankle systolic/arm systolic) measured in normal limbs and in limbs with arterial obstruction localized to different anatomic levels. (From Strandness DE Jr, Sumner DS: Hemodynamics for Surgeons. New York, Grune & Stratton, 1975; data from Wolf EA Jr, Sumner DS, Strandness DE Jr: Correlation between nutritive blood flow and pressure in limbs of patients with intermittent claudication. Surg Forum 23:238, 1972.)

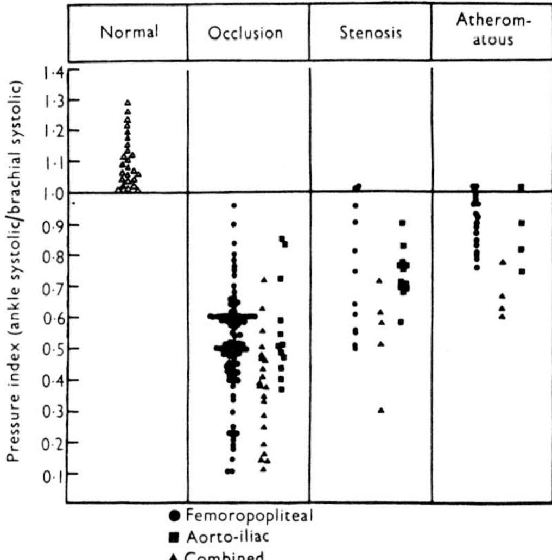

FIGURE 10–3. Relationship of ankle pressure index to the severity of the occlusive process. Note that the index exceeds 1.0 in all normal limbs in this series. (From Yao JST, Hobbs JT, Irvine WT: Ankle systolic pressure measurements in arterial diseases affecting the lower extremities. Br J Surg 56:676, 1969.)

obstructions, even when there is no hemodynamically significant disease in the aortoiliac segment.[17] This situation is somewhat more likely to occur in the presence of concomitant stenosis of the profunda femoris artery. Although the thigh index seldom exceeds 1.0 in limbs with occlusion of the iliac artery, it is not uncommon to find normal indices in limbs with hemodynamically significant stenoses of the iliac arteries.[17] This finding is most likely when the thighs are large; however, there is another possible explanation. Because compression of the upper thigh by the cuff temporarily restricts arterial inflow, the pressure gradient across the external iliac artery is reduced. Consequently, when a stenosis is confined to this artery, the upper thigh pressure reading may be spuriously high.[48]

If an upper thigh index of 1.0 is taken as the lower limit of normal, the data in Figure 10–5 indicate that there would be no mistakes in the normal control group, but in the patient groups, the sensitivity for detecting hemodynamically significant disease would be only 67% and the specificity for identifying the absence of disease would be 90%.[126] Cutajar and coworkers[37] reported that values

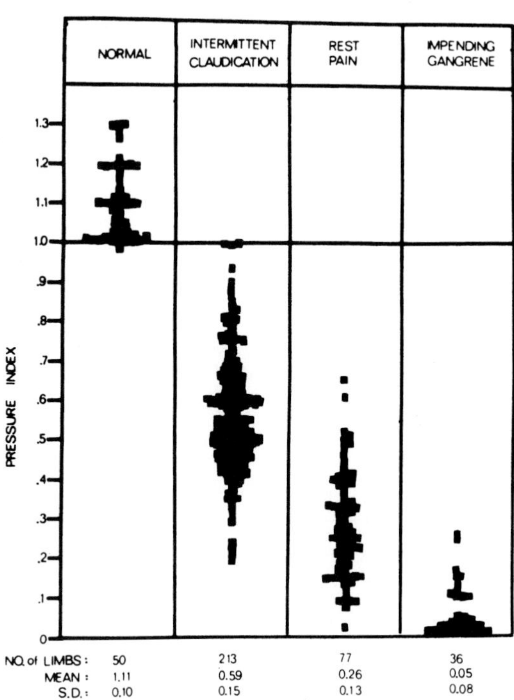

FIGURE 10–2. Relationship of ankle pressure index to functional impairment produced by the occlusive process. (From Yao JST: Hemodynamic studies in peripheral arterial disease. Br J Surg 57:761, 1970.)

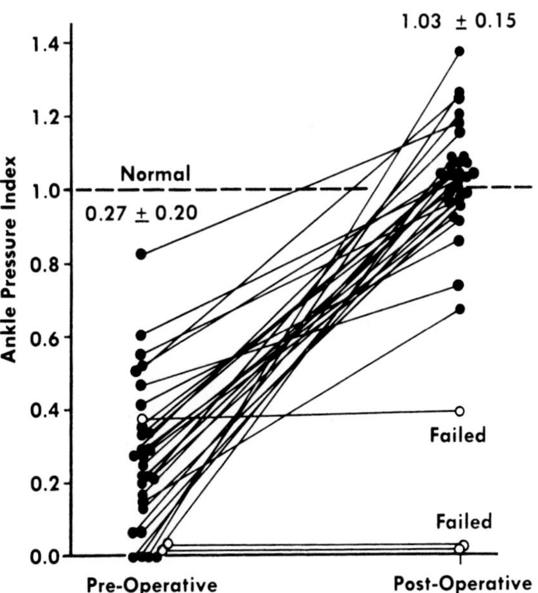

FIGURE 10–4. Results of femorotibial and femoroperoneal grafts. Ankle pressure indices before and after 31 bypass grafts from femoral to tibial, peroneal, or dorsalis pedis arteries. *Open circles* indicate grafts that failed within 30 days. Mean and standard deviations of the patent grafts are indicated. (From Sumner DS, Strandness DE Jr: Hemodynamic studies before and after extended bypass grafts to the tibial and peroneal arteries. Surgery 86:442, 1979.)

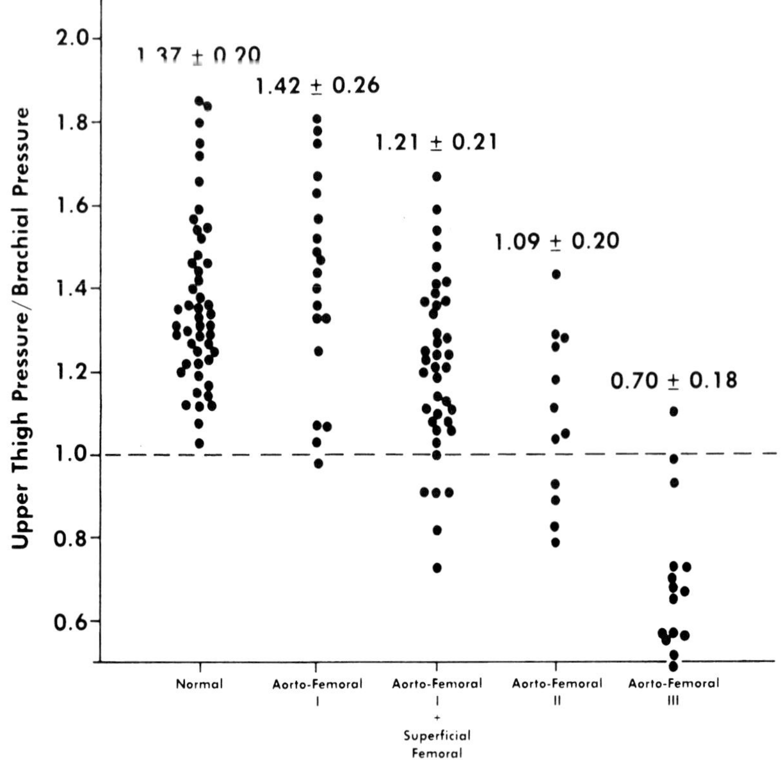

FIGURE 10–5. Identification of aortofemoral obstruction. Upper thigh index in normal limbs and in limbs with arteriosclerotic disease of the aortofemoral segment. Grading of aortofemoral disease is as follows: I, less than 50% diameter stenosis; II, more than 50% diameter stenosis; and III, occlusion. Grades II and III are hemodynamically significant.

exceeding 1.20 are normal, those less than 0.80 suggest occlusion, and those in between usually indicate the presence of aortoiliac occlusive disease. According to these criteria, the data in Figure 10–5 show that only 10% of the studies with indices exceeding 1.20 would be falsely classified as negative results and that only 7% of limbs with indices less than 0.80 would have no hemodynamically significant disease. Between these limits, however, significant disease was found in only 33%. Moreover, 19% of normal control limbs had indices less than 1.20.

Pressure Gradients

The pressure gradient between any two adjacent levels in the normal leg usually is no more than 20 to 30 mmHg (Table 10–3).[1, 139] Gradients greater than 30 mmHg strongly suggest that a significant degree of arterial obstruction is present in the intervening arterial segment.[1, 51, 63] When the artery is occluded, the gradient generally exceeds 40 mmHg.[49, 139] Rutherford and associates[126] found that an upper thigh to above-knee gradient of 15 mmHg best distinguished limbs with superficial femoral artery occlusion from those without. Similar gradients between the above-knee and below-knee levels and between the below-knee and ankle levels were found to have some predictive value related to disease in the popliteal and below-knee segments, respectively.

In addition to measuring "longitudinal" gradients along the leg, it is frequently helpful to compare the pressures in one leg with those at the same level in the other leg. A "horizontal" difference of 20 mmHg in normotensive patients may be significant, implying greater disease at or above this level in the leg with the lower pressure.[49]

The ratio of the pressures in the leg to those in the arm should exceed 1.0 at all levels (see Tables 10–1 and 10–2). Values lower than this at any level in the leg imply significant obstructive disease in the proximal arteries. Theoretically, by making both "longitudinal" and "horizontal" comparisons of the segmental pressures or indices, the examiner should be able to locate the site or sites of arterial obstruc-

TABLE 10–3. PRESSURE GRADIENTS IN NORMAL SUBJECTS (MEAN ± SD)

AUTHOR AND YEAR	ARM–UPPER THIGH	UPPER THIGH–ABOVE KNEE	ABOVE KNEE–BELOW KNEE	BELOW KNEE–ANKLE
Winsor (1950)[162]*	−22	13	11	8
Bell (1973)[13]†	−6 ± 12	2 ± 8	—	—
Hajjar and Sumner (1976)[58]‡	−46 ± 24	13 ± 19	12 ± 4	10 ± 9
Rutherford et al (1979)[126]‡	−35 ± 18	5 ± 12	10 ± 15	11 ± 15

*Cuff 13 cm width.
†Cuff 18 × 60 cm.
‡Cuff 10 × 40 cm.

TABLE 10–4. TYPICAL SEGMENTAL SYSTOLIC ARTERIAL PRESSURES (mmHg)

	NORMAL	ARTERIAL DISEASE			
		Iliac	Superficial Femoral	Iliac and Superficial Femoral	Below Knee
Arm	120	120	120	120	120
Upper thigh	160	110	160	110	160
Above knee	250	100	100	70	150
Below knee	140	90	90	60	140
Ankle	130	80	80	50	90

tion and obtain some idea of their functional significance. Idealized values illustrating this point are shown in Table 10–4.

Isolated disease in the aortoiliac or superficial femoral segments can usually be identified, but in limbs with multilevel disease, identification is frequently less reliable. For example, superficial femoral obstructions may not produce an abnormal gradient in limbs with aortoiliac disease, iliac stenoses may not be recognized in limbs with superficial femoral disease, and below-knee disease is commonly misdiagnosed or overlooked when there is concomitant superficial femoral obstruction (Table 10–5).[63, 126]

Indirect blood pressure measurements have been used in patients with extremity trauma to avoid unnecessary arteriography and determine the need for surgical exploration. Lynch and Johansen[94] obtained Doppler cuff pressures in 100 injured limbs of 93 trauma victims who also underwent arteriography. An arterial pressure index (systolic pressure distal to the site of injury divided by brachial systolic pressure in an uninvolved arm) greater than 0.90 was considered normal. Compared with the arteriographic findings, the arterial pressure index had a sensitivity of 87%, specificity of 97%, and overall accuracy of 95% for detecting arterial injuries. When the results of two false-positive arteriograms were excluded, the sensitivity, specificity, and accuracy of the arterial pressure index increased to 95%, 98%, and 97%, respectively. Using an arterial pressure index of less than 0.90 to select trauma patients with possible occult vascular injuries for arteriography was prospectively evaluated in 100 limbs of 96 patients.[71] Among the 17 limbs with a decreased arterial pressure index, arteriograms were abnormal in 16, and seven underwent arterial repair. For the 83 limbs with a normal arterial pressure index, follow-up evaluation revealed six minor lesions but no major injuries.

Although the arterial pressure index is a simple, rapid, and clinically valuable screening test for arterial injuries, it has several important limitations. This approach cannot be used in cases in which extensive wounds prevent placement of a pneumatic cuff on the injured extremity. In addition, the arterial pressure index does not distinguish between an intrinsic arterial lesion, extrinsic compression, and vasospasm. Finally, distal limb pressure measurement does not detect non–flow-limiting lesions or injuries to nonaxial arteries such as the profunda femoris.

The location and severity of lower extremity arterial lesions can be directly assessed by duplex scanning, as discussed in Chapter 12.

Technical Errors

Cuff width is an important consideration for accurate measurements of limb blood pressure. The use of a cuff that is relatively small compared with the size of the limb results in a falsely high pressure reading or "cuff artifact." This effect is minimized when the cuff width is at least 50% greater than the diameter of the limb where the pressure is being measured. As noted for upper thigh pressure measurements with the four-cuff technique, the magnitude of the cuff artifact can generally be anticipated.

In an effort to achieve a more accurate assessment of the thigh pressure, some investigators have advocated using a

TABLE 10–5. ACCURACY OF SEGMENTAL PRESSURES FOR LOCATING ARTERIAL OBSTRUCTIVE DISEASE

ARTERIOGRAPHIC DIAGNOSIS	DIAGNOSIS BASED ON SEGMENTAL PRESSURE DATA (%)					
	Normal	Aortoiliac	Aortoiliac and Superficial Femoral	Superficial Femoral	Superficial Femoral and Popliteal	Popliteal
Normal	97.2	1.4	—	—	1.4	—
Disease						
Aortoiliac	12.5	75.0	12.5	—	—	—
Aortoiliac and superficial femoral	6.3	6.3	78.0	3.1	6.3	—
Superficial femoral	15.0	—	10.0	55.0	15.0	5.0
Superficial femoral and popliteal*	8.0	—	4.0	24.0	60.0	4.0
Popliteal*	57.0	—	7.0	—	—	36.0

Modified from Rutherford RB, Lowenstein DH, Klein MF: Combining segmental systolic pressures and plethysmography to diagnose arterial occlusive disease of the legs. Am J Surg 138:211, 1979.

*Note: Popliteal includes popliteal artery or two or more of the peroneal-tibial arteries.

single wide (19-cm) cuff rather than two narrower (10-cm) cuffs.[64] Gray and colleagues[55] compared thigh pressures obtained with a wide cuff and direct measurements of femoral arterial blood pressure in an effort to see how accurately the noninvasive pressure predicted the presence of aortoiliac disease. A thigh-brachial index exceeding 0.90 was generally reliable in ruling out inflow disease, with only 13% false-negative results. The thigh pressure was spuriously low in 59% of the studies, however, implying the presence of aortoiliac disease when in fact there was none. All of these false-positive results occurred in limbs with occlusions of the superficial femoral artery. Thus, it would appear that the wide cuff is less accurate than the narrow cuff for diagnosing aortoiliac stenoses.

Moreover, Heintz and associates[63] have shown that detection of superficial femoral disease by means of the "wide cuff to below-knee pressure gradient" is considerably less accurate than it is with the narrow cuff technique, which allows gradients across both the thigh and the knee to be analyzed. Other workers have reached similar conclusions.[45, 125]

Occasionally, the pressure gradient between two adjacent segments of the leg may appear to be reversed. For example, the above-knee pressure may exceed the pressure recorded at the upper thigh or the below-knee pressure may be greater than the pressure recorded at the above-knee level. This reversal of the normal pressure pattern is usually due to local arterial incompressibility or to varying relationships between the size of the cuff and the limb.[1, 48] In hypertensive patients, the gradient between any two adjacent levels may be increased. On the other hand, when the cardiac output is low, the pressure drop may be diminished.[162]

Normal blood pressure gradients may be obtained in limbs with arterial obstructions when collateral channels are quite large. These findings do not really constitute errors because the measurements are designed to reveal *functional* rather than *anatomic* obstruction.[139] For example, the pressure gradient from the below-knee level to the ankle is typically normal when either the anterior tibial or the posterior tibial artery is patent.[1, 67, 93, 129, 139]

Isolated obstructions of arteries that are not directly responsible for perfusion of the distal leg, such as the internal iliac or profunda femoris artery, cannot be detected by segmental pressure measurements.[1, 26] As pointed out earlier in this chapter, occlusions of the profunda femoris artery become evident only if the superficial femoral artery is also occluded. In these cases, the profunda femoris artery constitutes the major collateral channel supplying the lower leg and foot. Therefore, if both of these arteries are obstructed, the upper thigh pressure is abnormally low, even though the aortoiliac segment is completely patent.

Finally, because the ankle is the most distal site of pressure measurement, routine segmental pressures do not detect arterial occlusive lesions distal to the ankle. Lesions involving the plantar or digital arteries, such as vasculitis or microembolism, may be identified by toe pressure measurement or digital plethysmography, as discussed later in the chapter.

Because of the errors inherent in noninvasive assessment of the upper thigh pressure, direct femoral artery pressure measurements, as discussed later in the chapter, are being used more frequently.[9, 21, 43, 99, 157] It should be noted that direct pressure measurements are also subject to errors; most systems, for example, are underdamped, giving spuriously high systolic pressures.[23] Many vascular laboratories also use segmental plethysmography or Doppler flow signal analysis to supplement segmental pressure studies.[118, 126]

Toe Pressure

Toe pressures are measured with a pneumatic cuff of appropriate width (about 1.2 times the diameter of the digit) wrapped around the proximal phalanx, with a flow sensor applied distally.[36, 56, 91, 107] Although mercury strain-gauges work well for this purpose, photoplethysmographs, which are more stable and occupy less space on the tip of the digit, are generally more convenient to use. The systolic blood pressure measured at toe level is usually lower than the brachial or ankle pressure, probably related to measurement techniques. According to Nielsen and associates,[107] pressures in the toes of young normal individuals in the supine position average less than those in the arm. In older subjects, toe pressures are less than arm pressures. Since normal ankle pressure exceeds brachial pressure, normal toe pressures average 24 ± 7 to 41 ± 17 mmHg less than ankle pressures.[13, 30, 107] Ankle to toe gradients that exceed 44 mmHg in young patients or 64 mmHg in older patients are abnormal.[107] The toe-ankle index, obtained by dividing the toe pressure by the ipsilateral ankle pressure, averages 0.64 ± 0.20 in asymptomatic limbs, 0.52 ± 0.20 in limbs with claudication, and 0.23 ± 0.19 in limbs with ischemic rest pain or ulcers.[121] These findings suggest that obstruction of the pedal or digital arteries plays a major role in causing gangrene or ischemic rest pain.[160]

Figure 10–6 shows the distribution of toe pressures in 296 limbs with arteriosclerosis obliterans.[121] No asymptomatic patient had a toe pressure less than 50 mmHg, and only 11% of those whose complaints were limited to claudication had toe pressures less than 30 mmHg. In contrast, 81% of the limbs with ischemic rest pain had toe pressures less than 30 mmHg, and none had toe pressures exceeding 40 mmHg. In 81% of the limbs with toe pressures less than 30 mmHg and in almost all of those with pressures less than 15 mmHg, there were ischemic symptoms at rest. Patients with rest pain usually have toe pressures less than 20 to 30 mmHg.[30, 68, 121, 156]

Toe indices (toe pressure divided by brachial pressure) of patients with arteriosclerosis obliterans are listed in Table 10–6 according to the severity of their symptoms. It is noteworthy that there is little difference between the mean values of diabetic and nondiabetic patients. Spuriously high pressures due to arterial calcification, which are common in diabetic patients, seldom occur at toe level. For this reason, toe indices are reliable indicators of the physiologic severity of arterial occlusive disease and should be used when there is any doubt about the validity of the ankle pressure.[160]

Toe pressures are particularly valuable for demonstrating arterial disease confined to the pedal or digital arteries.[49] In limbs with ischemic ulcers or gangrene, normal ankle pressures and normal ankle pressure indices are often associated with toe pressures in the ischemic range (Fig. 10–7).[67, 121]

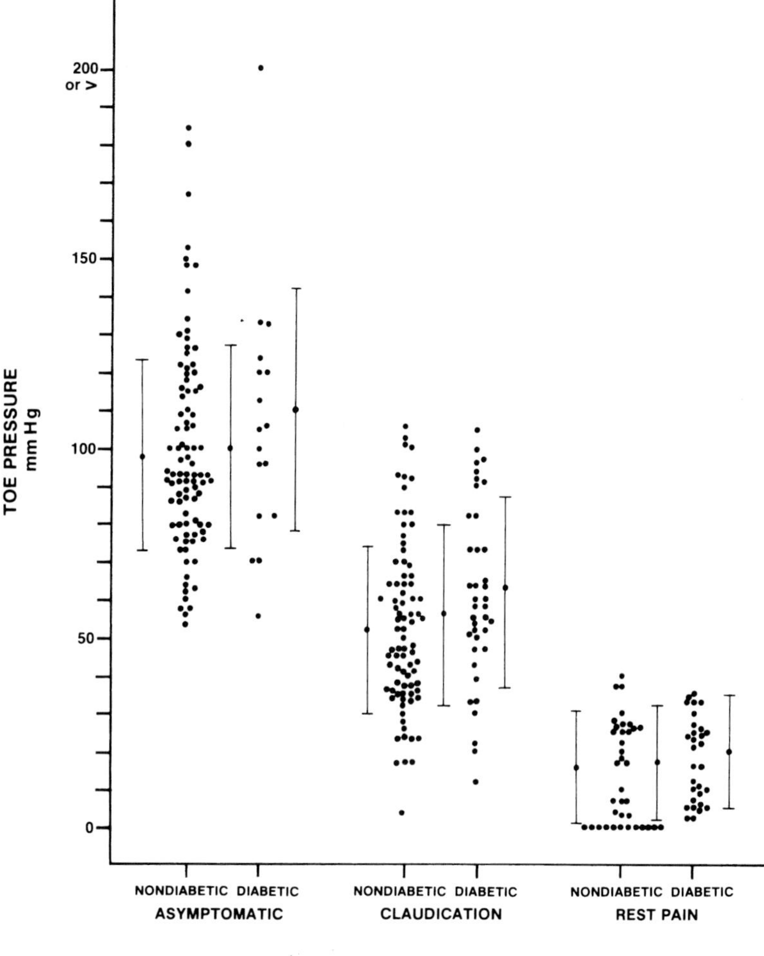

FIGURE 10–6. Toe blood pressures grouped according to symptoms and presence of diabetes in patients with arterial disease. Mean and standard deviations for the nondiabetic and diabetic subgroups and for the two groups combined are indicated by *vertical bars.* (From Ramsey DE, Manke DA, Sumner DS: Toe blood pressure: A valuable adjunct to ankle pressure measurement for assessing peripheral arterial disease. J Cardiovasc Surg 24:43, 1983.)

Carter[29] found that foot lesions usually heal if toe pressures exceed 30 mmHg in nondiabetic patients or 55 mmHg in diabetic patients. In contrast, Holstein and coworkers[68] found no appreciable difference between the two patient groups. In their study, healing occurred in 91% of the limbs in which toe pressures were greater than 30 mmHg, in 50% of limbs in which toe pressures were between 20 and 29 mmHg, and in only 29% of limbs in which toe pressures were less than 20 mmHg. Bone and Pomajzl[20] noted failure of toe amputations in all patients with toe pressures less than 45 mmHg and in 25% of patients with toe pressures between 45 and 55 mmHg; healing occurred in all patients with toe pressures greater than 55 mmHg. Other investigators have reported uniform healing with toe pressures exceeding 10 to 25 mmHg.[12, 128]

In a study by Ramsey and coworkers,[121] toe pressures proved to be of more prognostic value than ankle pressures (see Fig. 10–7). Ulcers and toe amputations failed to heal in 92% of limbs with an ankle pressure less than 80 mmHg, but they also failed to heal in 45% of limbs with higher pressures. There were three cases of failure to heal in limbs with ankle pressures of 150 mmHg; in all three cases, the toe pressures were less than 30 mmHg. With toe pressures less than 30 mmHg, the failure rate was 95%, but with toe pressures more than 30 mmHg, only 14% of the ulcers or amputations did not heal. This experience suggests that toe

TABLE 10–6. TOE INDICES IN PATIENTS WITH ARTERIAL DISEASE (MEAN ± SD)

AUTHOR AND YEAR	NO SYMPTOMS	CLAUDICATION		ISCHEMIA*	
		Nondiabetic	Diabetic	Nondiabetic	Diabetic
Carter and Lezack (1971)[30]	0.91 ± 0.13†	0.43 ± 0.17	0.42 ± 0.16	0.24 ± 0.14	0.19 ± 0.10
Vollrath et al (1980)[160]	0.89 ± 0.16	0.47 ± 0.24	0.60 ± 0.17	0.19 ± 0.15	0.16 ± 0.13‡
Ramsey et al (1983)[121]	0.72 ± 0.19	0.35 ± 0.15	0.38 ± 0.15	0.11 ± 0.10	0.12 ± 0.09

*Ischemic rest pain, ulcers, or gangrene.
†Normal subjects, 52 ± 6 years old; 21 ± 4 years old: 0.86 ± 0.12.
‡Diet-controlled; insulin-dependent: 0.23 ± 0.15.

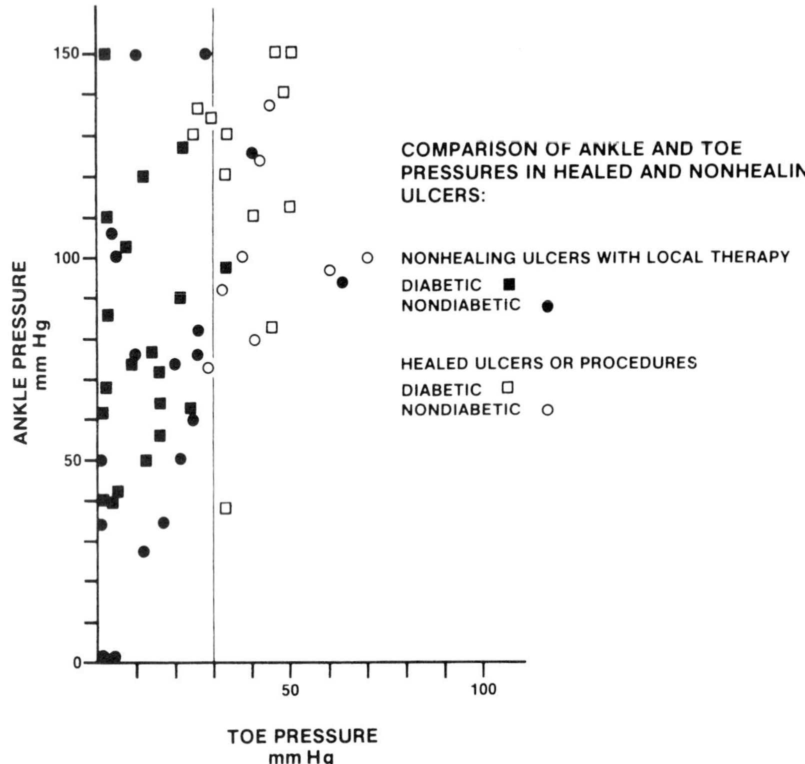

FIGURE 10–7. Comparison of ankle and toe pressures in 58 limbs with healed or nonhealing ischemic ulcers or toe amputations. Note that a toe pressure of 30 mmHg provides good separation between those limbs that healed and those that did not. *Solid symbols* indicate nonhealing ulcers: ■ diabetic, ● nondiabetic. *Open symbols* indicate healed ulcers or procedures: □ diabetic, ○ nondiabetic. (From Ramsey DE, Manke DA, Sumner DS: Toe blood pressure: A valuable adjunct to ankle pressure measurement for assessing peripheral arterial disease. J Cardiovasc Surg 24:43, 1983.)

pressures less than 20 mmHg almost uniformly predict failure of a toe amputation or ulcer to heal.

Penile Pressure

The penis is supplied by three paired arteries: the dorsal penile, the cavernosal (deep corporal), and the urethral (spongiosal) arteries. These arteries are terminal branches of the internal pudendal artery, which originates from the internal iliac artery. The cavernosal artery is most important for erectile function. Obstruction of any of the arteries leading to the corpora cavernosa, including the common iliac artery or terminal aorta, can be responsible for vasculogenic impotence.

Measurement of penile blood pressure is performed with a pneumatic cuff measuring 2.5 cm in width applied to the base of the penis. Return of blood flow when the cuff is deflated can be detected by a mercury strain-gauge plethysmograph, a photoplethysmograph applied to the anterolateral aspect of the shaft, or a Doppler flow probe.[22, 90, 83] Although some investigators have positioned the probe over the dorsal penile arteries, others have emphasized the importance of detecting flow in the cavernosal artery.[104, 116] Because the penile blood supply is paired and obstruction may occasionally be limited to only one side, it has been recommended that pressures be measured on both sides of the penis.[119]

In normal men younger than 40 years, the penile-brachial index (penile pressure divided by brachial systolic pressure) was found by Kempczinski[83] to be 0.99 ± 0.15. Thus, in the absence of any arterial disease, the penile and brachial pressures are roughly equivalent. Older men without symptoms of impotence tend to have lower indices.[83] Penile-brachial indices greater than 0.75 to 0.80 are considered compatible with normal erectile function; an index less than 0.60 is diagnostic of vasculogenic impotence, especially in patients with peripheral vascular disease.[33, 50, 83, 90, 104, 116] A brachial-to-penile pressure gradient less than 20 to 40 mmHg suggests adequate penile blood flow.[22, 83, 90] Gradients in excess of 60 mmHg suggest arterial insufficiency.[83]

Knowledge of the penile pressure can be used to guide the vascular surgeon in planning the operative approach to aneurysmal or obstructive lesions of the aorta and iliac arteries.[104] Maintenance of blood flow to the internal iliac artery preserves potency, and restoration of flow to this artery may improve penile pressure and erectile function if more distal arteries are nondiseased.[116]

Stress Testing

Exercise

As noted in Chapter 7, reducing peripheral vascular resistance by walking exercise is an effective physiologic method for stressing the peripheral circulation. Under such stress, lesions that may not appear to be significant at rest can be evaluated.[28] Exercise testing enables the surgeon to better appreciate the functional disability that the arterial lesions produce.[118] It also permits the surgeon to assess the disability produced by arterial obstruction in relation to the restrictions imposed by orthopedic, neurologic, or cardiopulmonary disease.

It should be emphasized, however, that exercise testing (or other stress testing) is not required for the evaluation of patients with ischemia at rest. Patients with ischemic rest pain, ulcers, or gangrene always have decreased digital artery pressures and usually have low ankle pressures. Moreover, the vast majority of patients with claudication have decreased ankle pressure at rest, and supplementary stress testing is only occasionally necessary to establish the diagnosis.

Although many different exercise protocols are possible, the following protocol has been widely used[143]:

1. After the patient has rested supine for about 20 minutes, baseline ankle and arm pressures are measured.
2. The patient walks on a treadmill at 2 mph up a 10% grade (a) for 5 minutes or (b) until forced to stop because of claudication or other restrictions. The nature of any symptoms and the time at which they appear are recorded. If leg pain occurs, it is important to note which muscle group is first affected. The final walking time is also recorded.[145, 164] However, walking time itself is not a particularly important indicator.[113] The patient's motivation, pain tolerance, and nonvascular symptoms dictate the duration of walking, which tends to correlate poorly with objective hemodynamic measurements.
3. The patient promptly assumes a supine position on the examining table.
4. Ankle and arm pressures are obtained immediately and then every 2 minutes until (a) pre-exercise levels are reached or (b) 20 minutes have elapsed.

A normal individual, regardless of age, is usually able to walk for 5 minutes with little or no drop in ankle pressure.[86, 134, 136, 138, 164] Patients with obstructive arterial disease are seldom able to walk for 5 minutes and always experience an immediate drop in ankle pressure (Fig. 10–8).[138, 145, 164] The magnitude of this drop reflects the extent of the functional disability. Patients with multilevel arterial disease typically walk for a shorter distance and experience a much more extreme drop in ankle pressure.[164, 167] Often in such patients, the ankle pressure is unobtainable for several minutes following cessation of exercise.

Brachial systolic pressure increases after exercise, and this increase is usually much more pronounced in patients with arterial disease than in normal subjects. Although an occasional patient with minimal or no symptoms may not demonstrate a distinct decrease in ankle pressure following exercise, the arm-ankle pressure gradient is increased.[152] Arterial disease may be diagnosed when the post-exercise arm pressure exceeds the ankle pressure by more than 20 mmHg. It is rare for arterial reconstruction to be required for claudication in patients with only mild arm-ankle pressure gradients.

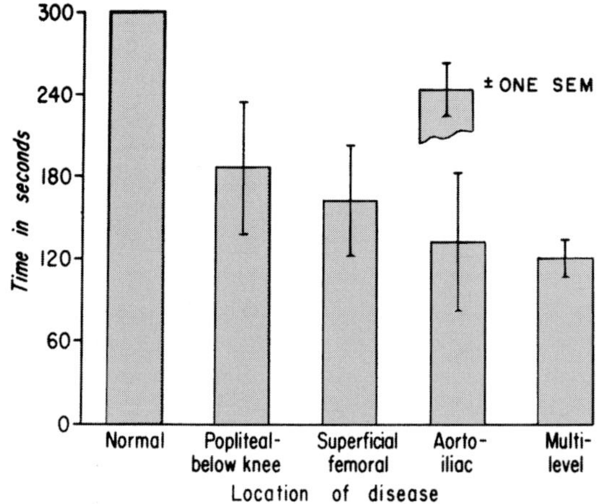

FIGURE 10–8. Treadmill walking times in patients with occlusive arterial disease. Normal subjects almost always can exceed 5 minutes (300 seconds). Treadmill is set at 2 mph, 12% grade. (From Strandness DE Jr, Sumner DS: Hemodynamics for Surgeons. New York, Grune & Stratton, 1975.)

The location of arterial lesions also affects the magnitude of the pressure drop and the time required for the pressure to return to baseline levels. Pressure drops following exercise indicate that the obstruction involves arteries supplying the gastrocnemius and soleus muscles. Because a large portion of the blood supply to these muscles is derived from the sural arteries, which have their origin from the popliteal artery, a drop in ankle pressure following walking exercise signifies an obstruction of the popliteal, superficial femoral, or more proximal vessels. When the obstruction is confined to below-knee vessels, walking exercise seldom causes claudication or a significant drop in ankle pressure.[138, 139]

In general, the more proximal the occlusive disease, the greater its effect on the ankle pressure response to exercise. For example, an isolated aortoiliac lesion usually has more functional significance than a lesion confined to the superficial femoral artery.[145, 167] This phenomenon occurs because the more proximal arteries supply a greater muscle mass than the more distal arteries. Consequently, there is a more severe and prolonged diversion of blood away from the lower leg to the proximal muscle masses.[142, 145]

Reactive Hyperemia

Reactive hyperemia, by increasing the rate of blood flow through stenotic arteries or high-resistance collateral vessels, causes a drop in the ankle pressure similar to that observed after exercise (see Chapter 7).[5, 69, 72, 158] For the reactive hyperemia test, a pneumatic cuff placed around the thigh is inflated to more than systolic pressure for 3 to 7 minutes. After release of the compression, ankle pressures are monitored at 15-, 20-, or 30-second intervals for 3 to 6 minutes or until measurements return to precompression levels.

In normal limbs, ankle pressures decrease immediately to about 80% of precompression levels but then rapidly rise, reaching 90% levels within about 30 to 60 seconds. In limbs with obstructive arterial disease, the magnitude of the pressure decrease coincides well with that seen following exercise, but recovery to resting levels is much faster.[5, 69] The magnitude of the pressure drop depends on the anatomic extent of the disease process and on the extent of functional impairment.[72, 158] Although recovery times are also correlated with the severity of disease (from less than 1 minute to more than 3 minutes), the correlation is not as good as that between severity of disease and the maximal decrease in ankle pressure.[113]

In some laboratories, reactive hyperemia testing has supplanted treadmill exercise for stress testing.[113] In contrast to the treadmill, this test:

1. Is less time-consuming.
2. Can be performed in the patient's room.

3. Uses simple, inexpensive equipment.
4. May result in more standardized stress because the duration of cuff compression can be prescribed and walking time cannot be.
5. Is less dependent on patient motivation.
6. Can be used for patients who cannot walk on the treadmill because of neurologic, cardiac, pulmonary, or orthopedic problems or because of general disability, prior amputation, rest pain, or ischemic ulceration.

However, stress testing is not required to diagnose arterial disease in limbs with rest pain, ulcers, or gangrene; disease of that severity is easily detected and evaluated with resting ankle or toe pressures.[113] In patients who cannot walk because of other problems, disease of sufficient severity to threaten the limb is readily detected without stress testing.

Finally, in contrast to reactive hyperemia testing, treadmill exercise duplicates the physiologic stress responsible for claudication and permits neurologic, cardiopulmonary, and orthopedic problems to be evaluated in relation to the leg arterial disease.[69]

Some disadvantages of the reactive hyperemia test[5, 69, 113] can be listed:

1. It causes mild to moderate discomfort.
2. Thigh compression may be hazardous in limbs with femoropopliteal grafts.
3. Rapid pressure measurements are required to obtain reproducible results.

Ouriel and coworkers[113] found that reactive hyperemia was a less sensitive and less specific indicator than resting ankle pressures or exercise testing. Still, the method has some advantages, and its use may be justified in selected situations in which stress testing is required and treadmill exercise is impossible or impractical.

Direct Measurement of Arterial Pressure

As discussed in Chapter 7, the relationship between arterial pressure, flow, and resistance can be expressed by Poiseuille's law. The degree of narrowing at which pressure and flow begin to decline is called the *critical stenosis*. However, in the intact arterial circulation, autoregulation can maintain normal flow rates distal to a critical stenosis, even when a significant pressure drop is present. Therefore, pressure measurements are more likely than flow measurements to indicate the presence of arterial occlusive disease. Furthermore, measurements of flow rates or peripheral resistance are extremely difficult to perform in the clinical setting.

Direct measurement of arterial pressure in the lower extremity avoids the cuff artifacts and other potential errors associated with noninvasive pressure measurements. Specific approaches include pull-through aortoiliac artery pressures during arteriography, percutaneous measurement of common femoral artery pressures, and intraoperative pressure measurements after arterial exposure. As with the noninvasive methods, direct pressure measurements can be made both in the resting state and following some form of hemodynamic stress. Although a pedal ergometer exercise test has been described for use with percutaneous common femoral artery pressure measurements, a large proportion of patients are unable to perform this test adequately, and it has not been widely used.[133] A simpler technique that does not require strict patient cooperation or any specialized equipment is intra-arterial injection of papaverine to produce peripheral vasodilatation.

Although direct arterial pressure measurements are generally regarded as the reference standard for the physiologic evaluation of peripheral arterial disease, this approach is subject to certain errors that must be recognized. The proper zero level for a particular measurement must be selected, with the relative heights of the patient's heart, the transducer, and the site of measurement taken into account. Underdamping of the needle, transducer, and catheter system is common, especially when air bubbles are present.[23] This tends to augment the pulse pressure and result in excessively high systolic pressure values, although the mean pressure component is less likely to be affected. These problems can be minimized during clinical measurements by (1) the use of stiff tubing with few stopcocks and (2) elimination of fluid leaks and air bubbles.

Percutaneous Pressure Measurement

The direct measurement of arterial pressure is indicated to assess the physiologic severity of aortoiliac disease found on either arteriography or noninvasive testing. Although arteriography is usually adequate to evaluate the significance of infrainguinal arterial disease, it is not adequate for more proximal arterial lesions.[99] Even biplanar arteriography may not allow an accurate assessment of the aortoiliac system.[44]

Because arteriographic procedures are most commonly performed with the use of a femoral puncture site, direct measurements of arterial pressure during arteriography generally assess the aortic, iliac, and femoral segments. Pull-through pressures taken with the arteriogram catheter indicate the hemodynamic significance of any lesions present in the aortoiliac system. Intra-arterial injection of papaverine can be used as a pharmacologic stress test to assess the pressure gradients during high-flow conditions. Studies of hemodynamically normal patients suggest that a hemodynamically significant lesion in the aortoiliac segment is present when the systolic pressure gradient is more than 10 mmHg at rest or 20 mmHg after injection of papaverine hydrochloride (30 mg) into the arteriogram catheter.[151]

Direct measurement of femoral artery pressure is performed by percutaneous puncture of the common femoral artery with a 19-gauge needle attached by rigid fluid-filled tubing to a calibrated pressure transducer. The femoral artery systolic pressure is compared with the brachial artery systolic pressure, and the *femoral-brachial index* (FBI) is calculated. As for the ABI, the brachial artery pressure as measured by Doppler ultrasonography is presumed to represent systemic arterial pressure. A resting FBI greater than or equal to 0.9 is considered normal.[44] Values less than 0.9 indicate the presence of a hemodynamically significant lesion proximal to the common femoral artery.

If the resting FBI is normal, the injection of papaverine can be used to look for less severe lesions that are apparent only at increased flow rates. After direct injection of 30 mg of papaverine hydrochloride through the needle in the common femoral artery, pressures in both the common femoral artery and the brachial artery are monitored. It is particularly important to measure the brachial artery pressure during this test, because papaverine often causes a slight decrease in systemic arterial pressure. The mean decrease in FBI following papaverine injection is 6% for normal subjects, and a decrease of 15% or more indicates a hemodynamically significant lesion.[44] A peak flow increase of 50% or greater is sufficient for a valid test result; reasons for an invalid result include fixed outflow resistance and extravascular injection of papaverine.

Intraoperative Pressure Measurement

The basic principles and techniques for intraoperative pressure measurements are identical to those described for the percutaneous approach. Common femoral artery pressures, taken both before and after papaverine injection, can be used to assess the aortoiliac segment when it is not feasible to obtain these measurements preoperatively. Sequential pressure measurements taken along a native artery or bypass graft can localize areas of hemodynamic abnormality. In this manner, the inflow, graft segment, and distal runoff of an arterial reconstruction can be evaluated, and specific problems identified.

Intraoperative pressure measurements are performed by means of puncture of the exposed artery with a hypodermic needle attached to a length of rigid fluid-filled tubing. A 19-gauge or larger needle provides optimal pressure waveforms, whereas smaller needles are satisfactory for measurement of pressure gradients. The same pressure transducer setup used by the anesthesiologist to monitor radial artery pressure can be used for these measurements. In addition to looking for significant pressure gradients along an arterial reconstruction, one can compare the intraoperative pressures with the systemic pressure, which is typically based on the reading from a radial artery pressure line.

DOPPLER ULTRASONOGRAPHY

Although the absolute magnitude of blood flow measured at rest is of little help in the objective assessment of peripheral arterial occlusive disease, the contour of the velocity pulse wave and disturbances of the flow pattern in individual arteries provide a great deal of important information. Before the development of transcutaneous Doppler ultrasonography, this type of information was essentially unavailable. The presence of a bruit on physical examination signifies a flow disturbance of some type; however, bruits (1) are difficult to quantify, (2) do not appear until the arterial lumen is significantly narrowed, (3) disappear when the stenosis is very severe, and (4) are absent when the artery is totally occluded. Moreover, bruits may arise from arteries adjacent to the vessel of interest, causing additional confusion.

Doppler ultrasonography has become an essential part of the noninvasive evaluation of peripheral arterial disease. Ultrasonography instruments are not only widely available and easy to use but also provide information instantaneously. Many levels of data analysis are available, ranging from the simple to the extremely complex.

Examination Technique

Doppler recordings should be made in a warm room with the patient resting comfortably in a supine position. For most purposes, a pencil-type probe is preferred. Optimal signals are obtained by placing the probe directly over the vessel to be examined at an angle of 45 to 60 degrees. In the lower limb, the common femoral artery is examined at the groin at or slightly above the inguinal crease to avoid confusion with signals arising from the profunda femoris or the proximal superficial femoral artery. Persson and coworkers[115] have emphasized the importance of accurately locating the common femoral artery by using the line drawn between the anterior-superior iliac spine and the pubic tubercle to determine the site of the inguinal ligament. The inguinal skin crease, especially in obese patients, is often well below the inguinal ligament.

Signals from the superficial femoral artery are best detected with the probe positioned medially on the thigh, in the groove between the quadriceps and adductor muscles. When the patient is supine, flexion of the knee and mild external rotation of the leg provide access to the popliteal artery. Alternatively, the popliteal artery can be examined with the patient prone and the feet supported by a pillow to flex the knee. At the ankle level, the posterior tibial arterial signal is obtained just behind the medial malleolus. The dorsalis pedis artery is consistently located slightly lateral to the extensor hallucis longus tendon a centimeter or so distal to the ankle joint. Finally, the lateral tarsal artery (representing the termination of the peroneal artery) can usually be studied by placing the probe anterior and medial to the lateral malleolus.

Although simple nondirectional Doppler devices suffice for many clinical applications, such as measurement of the ABI, direction-sensing instruments supply more information and are necessary for any detailed analysis of the Doppler signal. Even in routine surveys of the peripheral arteries, direction sensing is often a valuable adjunct. The choice of frequency depends on the depth of the vessel being examined. Whereas superficial vessels are best studied with a high-frequency probe (10 MHz), the deeper vessels of the leg require the use of lower frequencies (3 to 5 MHz).

Audible Interpretation

The ear serves as the simplest and most readily available interpreter of the output of the Doppler flowmeter. Skilled observers can derive a great deal of information from the audible signal without resorting to recordings or complex methods of analysis. Because good quality, continuous wave (CW), nondirectional devices meet most of the requirements for audible interpretation, there is no need for bulky, expensive instrumentation. For many purposes, a handheld Doppler flowmeter is sufficient.

Normal peripheral arterial Doppler signals are biphasic or triphasic[141]:

1. The first sound or phase corresponds to the large, high-velocity, forward-flow systolic component of the pulse wave.
2. The second sound or phase is due to the smaller reverse-flow component in early diastole.
3. The third sound or phase is associated with an even smaller, low-velocity, forward-flow component that usually appears in late diastole.

The pitch of the first phase rises rapidly to a peak during systole and then falls abruptly in early diastole. The pitch of the two subsequent phases is always much lower. Finding a clear, crisp, multiphasic signal with a high systolic velocity implies patency of the proximal arteries and almost invariably rules out hemodynamically significant disease.

The characteristics of abnormal Doppler flow signals vary according to whether the probe is positioned proximal to, at, or distal to the site of the occlusive process. Distal to a stenosis or occlusion, flow signals are typically low-pitched and monophasic, because the high-frequency components of the pulse wave have been filtered out by passage through the stenosis or high-resistance collateral channels. As long as the velocity of flow exceeds a certain minimal level (determined by the ultrasound transmission frequency and the cutoff frequency of the high-pass filter used to eliminate extraneous signals arising from wall motion), arterial signals are obtained despite the absence of palpable pulses. Absence of a Doppler signal implies either a flow velocity below the threshold level of the instrument or occlusion of the arterial segment being evaluated. In cases of severe arterial obstruction, the Doppler signal may lose much of its characteristic pulsatility and may be difficult to distinguish from an adjacent venous signal. A directional Doppler ultrasonographic evaluation usually resolves this issue.

Signals detected directly over a stenosis or from an artery immediately distal to a stenosis are high-pitched, noisy, and monophasic. These characteristics reflect the increased velocity of flow within the narrowed lumen and the development of disturbed or turbulent flow patterns in the jet of blood emerging from the stenosis.

Signals obtained from a pulsating artery a few centimeters proximal to an occlusion have a characteristic "to-and-fro" or "thumping" quality. This sound is composed of a low-frequency forward-flow wave followed by a relatively large flow wave reflected from the obstruction. In questionable cases, a directional instrument equipped with frequency meters may aid in the interpretation of the audible signal. When the artery is obstructed distal to the probe and there are no intervening branches to provide outflow, the flowmeters indicate (1) no mean forward flow or (2) low-velocity flows of equal magnitude in both the forward and reverse directions.

Waveform Analysis

The main drawback of the simple audible interpretation of the Doppler flowmeter signal is its inherent subjectivity. Waveform analysis not only is objective but also permits more information to be extracted from the Doppler signal. As discussed in Chapter 9, several methods are available for recording and processing of the Doppler velocity signals. Although the zero-crossing detector output is simple to use, it is often inaccurate and, consequently, is seldom suitable for quantitative work. It does, however, provide a quick method for examining the contour of the waveform, especially in conjunction with segmental pressure measurements. For all quantitative work, spectral analysis of the Doppler signal is the method of choice. In the clinical setting, spectral analysis is most commonly used with the pulsed Doppler component of the duplex scanner (see Chapters 9 and 12).

Qualitative Analysis

Simply inspecting the contour of the velocity waveform obtained from a zero-crossing or audiofrequency spectrum analyzer is often of considerable diagnostic value. As illustrated in Figure 10–9*A*, the normal velocity waveform is triphasic. Velocity increases rapidly in early systole, reaches a peak, and then drops almost equally as rapidly, reversing in early diastole.[79] In late diastole, the velocity tracing again becomes positive before returning to the zero-flow baseline. With increasing peripheral vasoconstriction, the reverse-flow component becomes more exaggerated.[124, 142] When peripheral resistance is reduced after exercise, artificially induced reactive hyperemia, or infusion of vasodilating drugs, the reverse-flow component disappears, the baseline

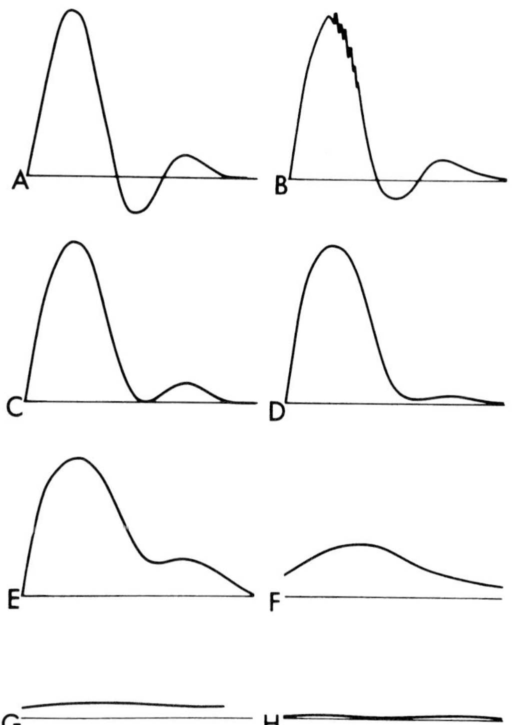

FIGURE 10–9. Different patterns of flow velocity waveforms. *A*, Normal. *B*, Atherosclerotic changes causing turbulence during systolic phase (high frequency). *C* and *D*, Loss of reverse flow due to increasing degree of stenosis. *E–H*, With increasing arterial stenosis, the flow velocity waveform becomes progressively damped. (*A–H*, From Johnston KW, Maruzzo BC, Kassam M, et al: Methods for obtaining, processing and quantifying Doppler blood velocity waveforms. *In* Nicolaides AN, Yao JST [eds]: Investigation of Vascular Disorders. Churchill Livingstone, New York, 1981, p 543.)

TABLE 10–7. TYPICAL PULSATILITY INDICES (PI_{pp}) AND INVERSE DAMPING FACTORS (DF^{-1})

	LOCATION OF ARTERIAL OBSTRUCTION							
	None		Aortoiliac		Superficial Femoral		Aortoiliac and Superficial Femoral	
RECORDING SITE	PI_{pp}	DF^{-1}	PI_{pp}	DF^{-1}	PI_{pp}	DF^{-1}	PI_{pp}	DF^{-1}
Common femoral	13.0		2.4		6.1		3.1	
Popliteal	16.7	1.3	2.7	1.1	4.4	0.7	2.4	0.8
Dorsalis pedis	17.7	1.1	5.6	2.1	5.6	1.3	3.7	1.5
Posterior tibial	18.0		4.6		4.6		3.1	

Data from Johnston KW, Maruzzo BC, Cobbold RSC: Doppler methods for quantitative measurement and localization of peripheral arterial occlusive disease by analysis of the blood velocity waveform. Ultrasound Med Biol 4:209, 1978.

rises above the zero-flow level, and the wave assumes a biphasic rather than a triphasic contour.

Atherosclerotic disease in the arteries proximal to the site of the probe initially produces a subtle change in the contour of the systolic forward-flow wave at the peak or in the early deceleration phase (Fig. 10–9*B*). With increasing proximal stenosis, the reverse-flow component is damped and then disappears entirely (Fig. 10–9*C* and *D*). As the stenosis becomes more severe, progressing to total occlusion, the rate of acceleration of the forward-flow wave decreases, the peak becomes rounded, and the wave becomes continuous and less pulsatile (Fig. 10–9*E* through *H*).[142]

Proximal to a stenosis or occlusion, the waveform may have a nearly normal contour, especially when (1) the disease process is located well below the site being evaluated and (2) there are large outflow branches that serve to reduce the peripheral resistance. However, it is not uncommon to find that the contour is modified perceptibly by increased input impedance and that the resulting wave takes on some of the characteristics commonly associated with proximal stenosis.[106a] For example, recordings made from common femoral arteries proximal to superficial femoral artery occlusions often resemble the waveforms in Figure 10–9*C* and *D*, even in the absence of any significant iliac stenosis. One must keep this fact in mind when attempting to use the contour of the common femoral waveform to detect inflow disease.

By comparing the contours of the Doppler waveforms obtained from the common femoral, popliteal, and pedal arteries, one can usually identify the presence of hemodynamically significant disease and can often localize the disease to the aortoiliac, superficial femoral, or below-knee segment. The presence of multilevel disease is implied when severely dampened waveforms, such as those shown in Figure 10–9*F* through *H*, are recorded from the pedal arteries. Absence of a recordable Doppler signal from any of the pedal arteries indicates severe arterial disease.

Quantitative Analysis

A variety of methods have been proposed for quantitative analysis of Doppler velocity waveforms[3, 4, 70, 75, 130, 161]:

- Peak-to-peak pulsatility index
- Laplace transform
- Power frequency spectrum analysis
- Pulse transit time

Few of these techniques, however, have been widely applied in the clinical setting. Many are little better than simple qualitative analysis, despite the aura of accuracy that numbers convey. A major problem is that most such methods derive their information from sites that are remote from the principal lesion, where flow patterns have reverted toward a more normal configuration. For this reason, direct investigation of the artery at the site of the lesion, as accomplished by duplex scanning, is becoming the preferred noninvasive method for evaluating peripheral arterial disease.[87]

One method that has proved to be of some value is the *peak-to-peak pulsatility index* (PI_{pp}), which can be defined as the peak-to-peak frequency difference of the Doppler waveform divided by the mean frequency. In normal lower extremities, the PI_{pp} increases as the recording site moves from proximal to distal portions of the limb, being greatest in the dorsalis pedis and posterior tibial arteries and least in the common femoral artery.[76, 77] However, when there is an intervening arterial stenosis or occlusion, the PI_{pp} value obtained below the involved segment tends to decrease (Table 10–7).

In order to further quantify these changes in PI_{pp} and permit localization of arterial lesions, the use of a damping factor or inverse damping factor has been proposed.[76, 89] The *damping factor* (DF) is defined as proximal PI_{pp} divided by distal PI_{pp}; the *inverse damping factor* (DF^{-1}) is defined as distal PI_{pp} divided by proximal PI_{pp}. The DF increases and the DF^{-1} decreases across segments with significant arterial disease.

The common femoral PI_{pp} has been advocated as a method for determining the presence or absence of iliac artery or inflow disease. As shown in Table 10–8, mean values obtained by several investigators agree reasonably well for the various categories of disease severity; however, the standard deviations are large, and data from adjacent categories frequently overlap. When arteriography is used as the "gold standard," the sensitivity of the common femoral PI_{pp} for identifying reductions of the iliac artery greater than 50% of the diameter (hemodynamically significant stenoses) varies from 41% to 100%, depending on the laboratory making the measurements and the value of the index chosen as the dividing point between positive and negative results (Table 10–9). Specificities are equally variable. Similar data are reported when the pressure drop

TABLE 10–8. COMMON FEMORAL PULSATILITY INDICES (PI_{pp}) IN LIMBS WITH AORTOILIAC OCCLUSIVE DISEASE (MEAN ± SD)

	SEVERITY OF DIAMETER STENOSIS				
AUTHOR AND YEAR	**Normal**	**Minimal**	**Less Than 50%**	**Greater Than or Equal to 50%**	**Occluded**
Johnston et al (1978)[76]	9.6 ± 2.8	8.1 ± 2.8	4.9 ± 1.3	2.3 ± 1.2	1.6 ± 0.7
Baker et al (1984)[7]	8.3 ± 7.9	7.6 ± 5.0	3.9 ± 1.2	2.4 ± 0.8	1.8 ± 1.1
Harris et al (1974)[59]	7.1 ± 1.8	5.7 ± 3.2		2.8 ± 1.1	1.6 ± 0.9
Ward and Martin (1980)[166]	11.1 ± 5.4	4.1 ± 1.8		3.0 ± 1.0	1.9 ± 0.7
Baird et al (1980)[3]	11.8 ± 5.3	7.4 ± 1.6		3.6 ± 1.6	
Aukland and Hurlow (1982)[2]		6.1 ± 2.3		4.3 ± 2.0	1.3 ± 0.6
Hirai and Schoop (1984)[64]	8.0 ± 2.3	6.1 ± 3.0		3.7 ± 1.6	2.0 ± 0.4

across the aortoiliac segment, a physiologic gold standard, is substituted for the arteriographic image (Table 10–10).

In general, assessment of the hemodynamic status of the iliac artery seems to be more accurate in the absence of concomitant disease in the ipsilateral superficial femoral artery.[41, 122] Distal arterial obstruction tends to lower the femoral pulsatility index in limbs with no stenoses or with low-grade stenoses of the iliac arteries, thereby increasing the number of false-positive results and reducing specificity (see Table 10–10).[7, 41, 75, 122, 151, 161] However, some investigators maintain that distal arterial obstruction has little effect on accuracy.[2, 19, 74, 75, 78]

In theory, simple objective measurements such as the PI_{pp} should be relatively consistent from one laboratory to the next. Since pulsatility indices are independent of heart rate and probe angle, there is no obvious explanation for the observed differences other than biologic variability. It is difficult, therefore, to reconcile the disparate opinions expressed in the literature concerning the value of the PI_{pp} for detecting iliac stenosis.[3, 56, 75, 78, 122] Nonetheless, the assumption that a normal femoral pulsatility index (e.g., greater than 4.0) probably rules out significant iliac stenosis is consistent with many reports.[151] An abnormal index, on the other hand, must be interpreted cautiously, particularly in the presence of infrainguinal obstructive disease.[151]

The mean popliteal artery pulsatility index in normal limbs was found by Harris and associates[59] to be 9.3 ± 3.6, with a range of 4 to 20. In limbs with femoropopliteal disease, mean indices for stenoses less than 50% are reported to be 5.9 ± 3.2 and 7.7 ± 1.1; for hemodynamically significant stenoses, they are 4.7 ± 4.0 and 5.9 ± 1.2; and for occlusion, they are reduced to 1.6 ± 0.9 and 2.3 ± 0.2.[2, 59] Obviously, there is a great deal of overlap between values for different grades of disease, but it is usually possible to distinguish between occlusion and no stenosis.

Calculation of damping factors may provide somewhat better discrimination. Johnston and coworkers[76] found that a DF^{-1} less than 0.9 indicated superficial femoral occlusion. Aukland and Hurlow reported DF values of 0.8 ± 0.1, 1.3 ± 0.2, and 2.1 ± 0.2 for minimal disease, hemodynamically significant stenosis, and occlusion of the superficial femoral artery, respectively.[2]

Pulsatility indices obtained from the dorsalis pedis or posterior tibial arteries at the ankle are probably of little practical value in the assessment of below-knee arterial disease. According to Aukland and Hurlow,[2] the mean index in limbs with patent popliteal-tibial segments (6.5 ± 1.4) did not differ significantly from that in limbs in which these arteries were occluded (4.1 ± 0.8). Although Harris and associates[59] found a significant difference between the pedal indices in normal limbs (8.3 ± 3.1) and in limbs with below-knee disease, there was no statistically significant difference between any of the angiographic grades (less than 50% stenosis, 3.1 ± 2.9; greater than 50% stenosis, 1.9 ± 2.4; occlusion, 1.1 ± 0.6).

TABLE 10–9. ACCURACY OF FEMORAL PULSATILITY INDICES (PI_{pp}) FOR DETECTING ≥50% DIAMETER STENOSES OF THE AORTOILIAC ARTERIAL SEGMENT

AUTHOR AND YEAR	SUPERFICIAL FEMORAL ARTERY	PI_{pp} CRITERION*	SENSITIVITY (%)	SPECIFICITY (%)
Flanigan et al (1982)[42]	—	2.5	70	81
Baird et al (1980)[3]	—	3.0	41	55
Baker et al (1984)[7]	—	3.0	76	81
Johnston et al (1984)[75]	—	3.0	95	97
Baird et al (1980)[3]	—	4.0	55	71
Baker et al (1984)[7]	—	4.0	94	66
Campbell et al (1984)[25]	—	4.0	92	75
Junger et al (1984)[78]	Occluded	5.0	90	95
Baker et al (1984)[7]	—	5.5	100	53
Junger et al (1984)[78]	Patent	7.6	78	89

*PI_{pp} below which ≥50% stenosis is predicted.

TABLE 10–10. ACCURACY OF FEMORAL PULSATILITY INDICES (PI_{pp}) FOR DETECTING HEMODYNAMICALLY SIGNIFICANT PRESSURE DROPS ACROSS THE AORTOILIAC SEGMENT

AUTHOR AND YEAR	CRITICAL PRESSURE DROP (mmHg)	DISTAL ARTERIES	PI_{pp} CRITERION*	SENSITIVITY (%)	SPECIFICITY (%)
Flanigan et al (1982)[42]	5	—	2.5	62	69
Johnston et al	10	Patent	5.5	95	100
(1983)[74]	10	Occluded	5.3	92	92
Thiele et al (1983)[151]	10	Patent	4.0	95	82
	10	Occluded	4.0	96	45
	20 †	Patent	4.0	92	92
	20 †	Occluded	4.0	92	51
Bone (1982)[19]	10%‡	—	4.5	94	100

*PI_{pp} below which pressure drop exceeding the critical value is predicted.
†Critical pressure drop during papaverine-induced hyperemia.
‡Critical drop in femoral/brachial index after reactive hyperemia.

PLETHYSMOGRAPHY

Although direct noninvasive testing by duplex scanning has assumed a more prominent role in recent years, plethysmography remains a valuable noninvasive diagnostic technique. As discussed in Chapter 9, several types of plethysmographic instruments are available, but they all measure the same physiologic parameter: a volume change. Although the division may be somewhat arbitrary, it is convenient to discuss segmental plethysmography and digital plethysmography separately.

Segmental Plethysmography

Although mercury or indium-gallium strain-gauges are quite sensitive and provide excellent recordings of limb volume changes, the air plethysmograph, owing to its rugged construction and the ease with which it is used, has become the standard instrument for segmental plethysmography. The impedance plethysmograph has been useful for diagnosing deep venous thrombosis, but it has not proved to be a reliable tool for studying peripheral arterial disease.

Much of the original work with the air plethysmograph was done by Raines and colleagues,[38, 117] who called their specific instrument the *pulse volume recorder* (PVR); the term has now become almost synonymous with segmental plethysmography. Their approach has been to apply pneumatic cuffs to the upper thigh, calf, and ankle. Larger cuffs are used around the thigh (bladder = 18 × 36 cm) and smaller cuffs around the other two sites (bladder = 12 × 23 cm). The cuffs are inflated to 65 mmHg, a pressure that should require about 400 ± 75 ml of air for the thigh cuff and 75 ± 10 ml of air for each of the other two cuffs. Recordings are then made successively from each site. Measurements may be repeated after the patient has exercised on a treadmill.

Pulse Contour

The normal segmental volume pulse contour is characterized by a steep upstroke, a sharp systolic peak, a downslope that bows toward the baseline, and a prominent dicrotic wave approximately in the middle of the downslope (Fig. 10–10).[38] Significant occlusive disease in arterial segments proximal to the recording cuff is virtually excluded by the presence of a dicrotic wave. The absence of a dicrotic wave, however, is of less diagnostic significance. For example, during the hyperemic period following exercise, the dicrotic wave, which represents the reverse-flow phase of the arterial pulse, may disappear.[85]

Distal to an arterial obstruction, the upslope is less steep, the peak becomes delayed and rounded, the downslope bows away from the baseline, and the dicrotic wave disappears (see Fig. 10–10).[38] As the proximal obstruction becomes more severe, the rise and fall times become more nearly equal and the amplitude decreases. A "mildly abnormal" form has been identified, the contour of which lies between normal and distinctly abnormal.[85] This pulse retains the rapid upslope and sharp systolic peak characteristic of the normal form but loses the dicrotic wave. The downslope tends to bow away from the baseline. Arterial occlusions distal to the recording cuff may produce a "mildly abnormal" waveform in limbs with no proximal disease. Deterioration toward a distinctly abnormal waveform following exercise indicates the presence of significant proximal obstruction.

Pulse Amplitude

According to Darling and associates,[38] the amplitude of the plethysmographic pulse remains highly reproducible in the individual patient provided that constant cuff pressures and volumes are used. Amplitudes, however, vary from patient to patient and are influenced by cardiac stroke volume,

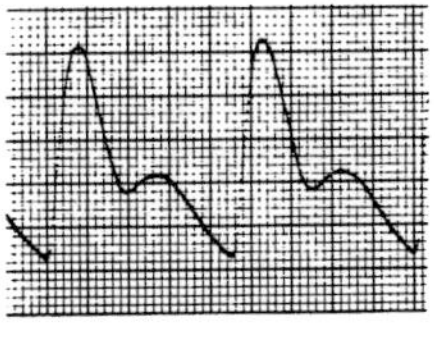

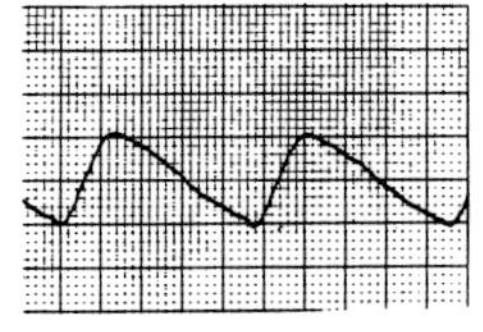

FIGURE 10–10. Normal and abnormal pulse volume contours recorded at ankle level. Normal form shows a prominent dicrotic wave on the downslope. Cuff pressure, 65 mmHg; cuff volume, 75 ml.

TABLE 10–11. DEFINITION OF PULSE VOLUME RECORDER CATEGORIES

PULSE VOLUME RECORDER CATEGORY	CHART DEFLECTION (mm)		DV (mm³)		
	Thigh and Ankle	Calf	Ankle	Calf	Thigh
1	>15*	>200*	>160	>213	>715
2	>15†	>20†	>160	>213	>715
3	5–15	5–20	54–160	54–213	240–715
4	<5	<5	<54	<54	<240
5	Flat	Flat	0	0	0

*With reflected wave.
†No reflected wave.
DV = maximal segmental volume change per heart beat.

blood pressure, blood volume, vasomotor tone, and the size and position of the limb. With progressively severe proximal disease, the pulse amplitude decreases.

Pulses may be classified into five categories that combine amplitude and specific features of the waveform contour (Table 10–11).[118] Category 1 designates a normal pulse contour, and categories 2 through 5 represent waves associated with increasingly severe obstructive disease. Although the actual volume change that occurs during each pulse (DV) is greater in the thigh than it is in the calf, the chart deflection at calf level normally exceeds that at the thigh by 25% or more (see Table 10–11).[84, 126] This so-called augmentation has proved to be an important diagnostic criterion, its absence signifying the presence of superficial femoral artery stenosis.

In normal limbs, pulse amplitude increases after treadmill exercise, reflecting the increased blood flow. Pulse amplitude at the ankle uniformly diminishes after exercise in limbs with arterial disease, however, owing to the diversion of blood to the proximal musculature.[117]

Analysis of Pulses

Pulse volume recordings are generally reported to be reasonably accurate for detecting and localizing arterial obstructions in the lower extremity. Typical tracings from normal limbs and from those with various combinations of peripheral arterial disease are shown in Figure 10–11.[126] When disease is confined to the aortoiliac segment, pulse contours at all levels are abnormal, but the amplitude of the calf pulse exceeds that of the thigh pulse (a manifestation of the augmentation phenomenon). Although pulse contours are also abnormal at all levels when there is combined aortoiliac and superficial femoral arterial disease, the amplitude of the calf pulse is less than that of the thigh pulse. In limbs with isolated superficial femoral arterial obstruction, the thigh pulse is normal but the calf and ankle pulses are abnormal.

The thigh pulse, according to Kempczinski,[84] tends to underestimate the severity of aortoiliac disease. He found, however, that if moderately abnormal waveforms were considered positive, the PVR correctly identified 95% of the significant stenoses in this segment. There were no false-negative results in his series of patients. All false-positive results were obtained in limbs with stenosis of the profunda femoris artery and occlusions of the superficial femoral segment. Limbs with mildly abnormal thigh pulses were subjected to treadmill exercise at 2 mph up a 10% incline. If the contour of the ankle pulse became more abnormal and if its amplitude decreased, significant aortoiliac obstruction was present; if there was no change in the pulse, the abnormal thigh pulse was attributed to superficial femoral disease.[84]

The PVR correctly assessed patency of the superficial femoral artery in 97% of the limbs studied by Kempczinski,[84] but pulse changes did not become evident unless the stenosis exceeded a 90% reduction of the diameter. Isolated mid-popliteal occlusions were associated with normal augmentation of the calf pulse. All false-positive results for superficial femoral disease were obtained in limbs with aortoiliac disease, and all false-negative results in limbs with well-developed collateral vessels bypassing short segmental occlusions of the superficial femoral artery.

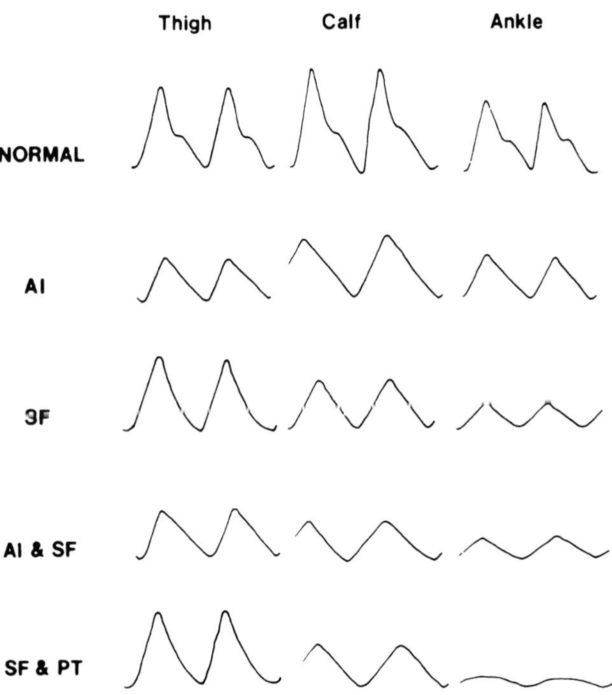

FIGURE 10–11. Pulse volume recorder (PVR) tracings from normal limbs and from limbs with various combinations of peripheral vascular disease. AI, aortoiliac; SF, superficial femoral; PT, popliteal-tibial. (From Rutherford RB, Lowenstein DH, Klein MF: Combining segmental systolic pressures and plethysmography to diagnose arterial occlusive disease of the legs. Am J Surg 138:216, 1979.)

Reidy and colleagues[123] reported that the PVR was 100% sensitive to the presence of aortoiliac stenoses of more than 50% diameter reduction when disease was isolated to that segment; however, the sensitivity fell to 83% in limbs with concomitant superficial femoral artery occlusions. Although negative predictive values were good for aortoiliac stenoses (87%), positive predictive values were low (64%). Therefore, these researchers considered a positive study result to be of little diagnostic value. Negative and positive predictive values were quite acceptable (85% and 91%, respectively), however, when the PVR was used to detect femoropopliteal disease.[84] On the basis of a similar study, Francfort and coworkers[45] concluded that the PVR was inaccurate for detecting aortoiliac disease but that it was highly sensitive to superficial femoral lesions, even in limbs with proximal disease.

Rutherford and associates[126] found that the PVR correctly identified 97% of normal limbs, about 70% of limbs with isolated or combined disease of the aortoiliac and superficial femoral segments, and 100% of limbs with disease confined to the below-knee arteries. When PVR results were considered in conjunction with segmental limb pressures, the accuracy of the combined tests was distinctly better than that of either test alone, ranging between 86% and 100% for all categories of disease. Other investigators have confirmed the complementary roles of the two tests.[45, 84] Therefore, the simultaneous use of PVR and segmental limb pressure measurement is generally advocated. Indeed, this approach was originally recommended by Raines and colleagues.[118] PVR findings are especially important in subjects with calcified arteries, in whom the segmental systolic pressure measurements are often unreliable.[112]

Digital Plethysmography

Although digital plethysmography may be regarded as a form of segmental plethysmography, pulses obtained from the tips of the toes or fingers (see Chapter 79) have special diagnostic significance. Because the recordings are taken from the most distal portions of the extremities, they reflect the physiologic status of all proximal arteries, from the aorta to the arterioles. They are sensitive, therefore, not only to mechanical obstruction but also to vasospasm.

Digit pulse volumes may be recorded with specially designed air plethysmographs that use cuffs with bladders measuring 7 × 2 cm or 9 × 3 cm; however, mercury strain-gauges or photoplethysmographs (PPGs) are usually employed because of their greater sensitivity (Fig. 10–12). Although the PPG does not provide quantitative data, it is the most easily used of the three devices and consequently is preferred by many laboratories.

For optimal recordings to be obtained, studies should be conducted in a warm room (about 72 to 75°F) in which relative humidity is maintained at about 40%. In order to avoid vasospasm, the feet and toes must be warm; this may require immersing the foot in warm water or placing the patient under an electric blanket. At times, it may be necessary to induce postischemic reactive hyperemia, as discussed later.[139]

Pulse Contour

The contour of the digit volume pulse resembles that of the segmental pulses obtained more proximally in the limb

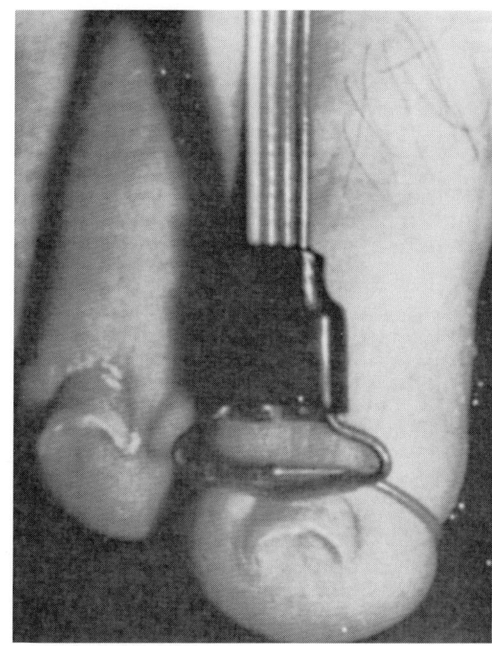

FIGURE 10–12. A mercury strain-gauge applied to the second toe.

(Fig. 10–13).[36, 137, 139, 163, 169] Normally, there is a rapid upslope with a sharp peak and a downslope that bows toward the baseline. A dicrotic wave or notch is usually present on the downslope. Distal to an obstruction, the pulse is considerably more rounded, having a slower upslope, a downslope that bows away from the baseline, and no dicrotic wave. In severe cases of arterial obstruction, no pulse may be perceptible.

Finding a normal toe pulse contour is good evidence that all segments from the heart to the digital arteries are free of functionally significant arterial disease. Similarly, finding an obstructive pulse contour indicates the presence of one or more functionally significant areas of obstruction

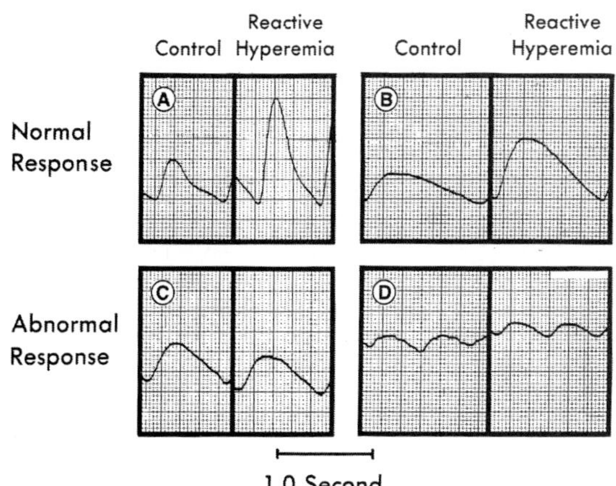

FIGURE 10–13. Reactive hyperemia test; digit pulse, second toe. Digit pulse volume more than doubles in the normal response *(upper panels)*. Little change in pulse volume is evident in abnormal response *(lower panels)*. *A*, Normal circulation (pressure: arm 130, ankle 140). *B*, Superficial femoral occlusion (pressure: arm 100, ankle 80). *C*, Diabetes for 20 years (pressure: arm 135, ankle 135). *D*, Iliac and superficial femoral arterial disease (pressure: arm 118, ankle 46). Attenuation of recorder: *A*, ×10; *B–D*, ×20.

somewhere between the heart and the digital arteries. Thus, digital pulses are especially important in the investigation of ischemia of the toes or forefoot.[144] Pedal or digital artery disease, which may contribute greatly to the ischemic process, may escape detection if the investigation is carried no further than ankle level. Such errors are easily made in diabetic patients, because the ankle arteries are often incompressible and the disease is more likely to involve pedal vessels. As shown in Figure 10–14, perfusion of the toes may be inadequate even in the presence of a relatively normal ankle pressure.

Although more complex methods for describing digital pulse contours have been proposed (including measurements of slope, pulse width at half maximal excursion, and relative amplitudes at various parts of the curve), these measurements have little physiologic meaning and are unnecessary in clinical work.[14, 15]

Reactive Hyperemia

The reactive hyperemia test is valuable as an indicator of the extent of peripheral vascular disease and as a predictor of the efficacy of surgical sympathectomy.[135, 139] A pneumatic cuff (1) is placed around the ankle, calf, or thigh, (2) is inflated to above systolic pressure, (3) is kept at that level for 3 to 5 minutes, and (4) is rapidly deflated. The volume of the toe pulse is then monitored over the next several minutes. In normal limbs, the pulse returns almost immediately, attains half its precompression amplitude within a few seconds, and then rapidly reaches a peak volume (Table 10–12).[47, 57, 144] Maximal excursion is usually more than twice that recorded during the control period (see Fig. 10–13).

The reappearance time of the toe pulse is frequently delayed in legs with arterial occlusive disease, often exceeding 120 seconds in severely involved extremities.[47, 57]

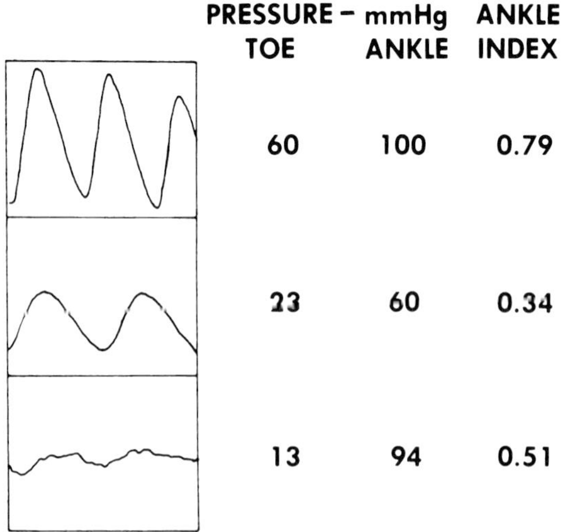

FIGURE 10–14. The configuration of the toe plethysmogram is closely correlated with the toe pressure but is poorly correlated with the ankle pressure or ankle index. *Upper tracing* implies good digital artery perfusion; *middle tracing*, borderline perfusion; *lower tracing*, ischemia. (From Sumner DS: Rational use of noninvasive tests in designing a therapeutic approach to severe arterial disease of the legs. *In* Puel P, Boccalon H, Enjalbert A: Hemodynamics of the Limbs-2. Toulouse, France, GEPESC, 1981, pp 369–376.)

TABLE 10–12. PULSE-REAPPEARANCE TIME AFTER RELEASE OF ARTERIAL OCCLUSION (SEC)

LOCATION OF OCCLUSIVE DISEASE	PULSE-REAPPEARANCE TIME	TIME REQUIRED TO REACH HALF CONTROL VOLUME
No occlusions	0.2 ± 0.1	3.4 ± 0.8
Aortoiliac	7.2 ± 4.0	23.9 ± 6.7
Femoropopliteal	3.7 ± 3.7	26.5 ± 12.7
Popliteal trifurcation	15.2 ± 9.3	23.9 ± 9.4
Multilevel	45.3 ± 5.5	71.2 ± 5.5

Modified from Fronek A, Coel M, Bernstein EF: The pulse-reappearance time: An index of over-all blood flow impairment in the ischemic extremity. Surgery 81:376, 1977.

Because it is difficult to define precisely the time at which the first pulse returns, the time required for the pulse to reach half the precompression volume seems to be a more practical measurement. This value is closely related to the severity of disease and the extent of arterial occlusion (see Table 10–12). Bernstein and colleagues[16] found that the functional results of aortofemoral bypass procedures can be predicted quite well by determining the time required for the pulse to reach half the control volume. Of limbs in which this time was less than 10 seconds, 63% became asymptomatic and 37% were improved. Of limbs in which the time exceeded 90 seconds, however, only 10% became asymptomatic and 50% improved.

The relative increase in pulse volume during reactive hyperemia is an excellent indicator of the functional severity of an arterial obstruction. As discussed in Chapter 7, the peripheral vascular bed is nearly maximally dilated in limbs with severe ischemia, and little further vasodilatation is possible (see Fig. 10–13). Approximately 85% of limbs with obstruction confined to a single segment (e.g., aortoiliac, femoropopliteal, or popliteal trifurcation) display at least a 25% increase in the volume of the toe pulse during reactive hyperemia.[47] In contrast, only about half of the limbs with multilevel disease show a response of this magnitude. Because of preferential flow to the proximal limb, the toe pulse volume in such limbs may remain decreased for a long period after reactive hyperemia and may never exceed the value recorded during the control period.[144]

Experience has shown that surgical sympathectomy is most likely to provide a satisfactory result if the peak reactive hyperemia toe pulse is twice the size of the control pulse. If less dilatation is seen, it is much less likely that sympathectomy would increase peripheral blood flow. Since reactive hyperemia can occur in a fully sympathectomized extremity, the reactive hyperemia test reveals nothing about the integrity of sympathetic innervation; what the test does is to substantiate the ability of the peripheral vessels to dilate in response to a release of vascular tone.

The "deep breath test" or one of its modifications is necessary to demonstrate continued function of the sympathetic nervous system.[40] In response to a deep breath, the pulse volume temporarily decreases provided that sympathetic innervation is intact. Absence of this response implies impairment of sympathetic activity and should be considered a contraindication to surgical sympathectomy.

TRANSCUTANEOUS OXYGEN TENSION

Unlike the methods previously discussed, which are sensitive to hemodynamic changes, transcutaneous oxygen tension ($tcPO_2$) measurements reflect the metabolic state of the target tissues. Although the technique is susceptible to a host of confounding variables, the potential importance of the information derived is so great that the method deserves close attention.

Measurements may be obtained from almost any area of interest, but common locations for assessment of lower extremity arterial perfusion are:

- Dorsum of the foot
- Anteromedial calf about 10 cm below the patella
- Thigh about 10 cm above the patella

The chest in the subclavicular region is often used as a reference site.

In normal limbs, most investigators have observed a modest decrease (5 to 6 mmHg) in $tcPO_2$ from the more proximal parts of the leg to the foot.[24, 34, 96] With increasing age, $tcPO_2$ tends to decrease, paralleling a similar decline in arterial PO_2.[34, 54, 62, 103, 110] For this reason, Hauser and Shoemaker[62] have advocated dividing the $tcPO_2$ measured in the limb by that measured at the subclavicular region to obtain a regional perfusion index (RPI) that is independent of age, cardiac output, and arterial PO_2. Others maintain that this calculation does not significantly enhance the predictive value of the test.[24, 34, 103] Values for $tcPO_2$ also depend on the vertical distance between the measurement site and the heart, decreasing when the limb is elevated and increasing when the limb is dependent.[24, 46, 61, 62, 96] In addition, there may be some increase in $tcPO_2$ with elevations in venous pressure.[46]

Measured $tcPO_2$ values depend on:

- Cutaneous blood flow
- Metabolic activity
- Oxyhemoglobin dissociation
- Oxygen diffusion though the tissues

Changes are not ordinarily perceptible in limbs with mild degrees of arterial disease, because the oxygen supplied far exceeds that required to meet metabolic demands. Under conditions of stress, however, the metabolic demands may utilize a larger portion of the available oxygen, thereby reducing the measured $tcPO_2$. In cases of severe arterial obstruction, oxygen delivery is often marginal, and the quantity of free oxygen reaching the sensor is reduced, leading to an abnormally low $tcPO_2$ value. Thus, $tcPO_2$ is most sensitive to higher grades of arterial obstruction. Even at low levels of perfusion, $tcPO_2$ values are not linearly related to blood flow.[97] The $tcPO_2$ may fall to zero in areas where cutaneous blood flow is still detectable by other methods.[97] This value does not mean that no oxygen is reaching the tissue but rather implies that all available oxygen is being consumed and none remains for diffusion to the sensor.[23, 34, 46]

The most appropriate clinical role for $tcPO_2$ measurements is to assist in the assessment of severe ischemia.[154] Because the results are not affected by arterial calcification, this test is particularly valuable for evaluating diabetic vascular disease.[34, 46, 61, 80]

Resting Values

Representative $tcPO_2$ values obtained from resting supine subjects are given in Table 10–13. The tendency for the values to decrease from the more proximal to the more distal parts of the lower limb is minimal in normal limbs but becomes more pronounced with increasing severity of disease. Irrespective of the site of measurement, normal $tcPO_2$ values are approximately 60 mmHg. Measurements in normal younger subjects are usually about 10 mmHg higher than those given in Table 10–13, which correspond to the values observed for patients in the age groups most susceptible to atherosclerosis.[34, 62, 103] In general, a $tcPO_2$ greater than 55 mmHg may be considered normal at any measurement site regardless of age.[34] The average normal RPI is about 90%.[62]

Peripheral measurements reflect the deleterious effects of increasing obstructive disease more dramatically than more proximal measurements. For example, there is little difference among the thigh $tcPO_2$ values for any of the disease groups listed in Table 10–13. Although statistically significant differences are often demonstrated between the values of normal extremities and extremities with claudication, and between extremities with claudication and those with rest pain, there is enough overlap to prevent individual tests from discriminating accurately among the various disease

TABLE 10–13. REPRESENTATIVE TRANSCUTANEOUS OXYGEN TENSION ($tcPO_2$) VALUES AT REST, SUPINE POSITION (mmHg, MEAN ± SD)

AUTHOR AND YEAR	NORMAL*			CLAUDICATION			REST PAIN		
	Foot	Calf	Thigh	Foot	Calf	Thigh	Foot	Calf	Thigh
Clyne et al (1982)[35]	59 ± 4	63 ± 5	64 ± 6	51 ± 10	64 ± 9	67 ± 9	36 ± 16	50 ± 16	55 ± 18
Hauser and Shoemaker (1983)[62]	59 ± 10	56 ± 10	64 ± 7	46 ± 12	49 ± 9	57 ± 9	—	—	—
Cina et al (1984)[34]†	64 ± 4	64 ± 4	—	46 ± 5	55 ± 4	—	17 ± 4	42 ± 6	—
Byrne et al (1984)[24]	60 ± 7	63 ± 8	66 ± 8	56 ± 4	59 ± 5	66 ± 7	4 ± 4	29 ± 20	50 ± 14
				37 ± 12	48 ± 10	54 ± 7‡			
Kram et al (1985)[89]	47 ± 12	53 ± 15	—	33 ± 14	37 ± 13	—	20 ± 16	29 ± 20	—

*Older subjects.
†Values estimated from published graphs.
‡More severe claudication.

categories.[34] Many patients with claudication have resting $tcPO_2$ values in the normal range, even at foot level.[24] However, values in limb-threatening ischemia are significantly reduced. At foot level, $tcPO_2$ values are usually less than 20 mmHg in legs with severe rest pain, ischemic ulcers, or gangrene.[24, 34, 109] In the series reported by Wyss and coworkers,[165] 46% of nondiabetic limbs with $tcPO_2$ values less than 20 mmHg required amputation.

Enhancement Procedures

Recordings of $tcPO_2$ may be made:

- After exercise
- Following a period of ischemia
- During oxygen inhalation
- With the legs in a dependent position

These are among the various modifications of the basic measurement procedure that have been advocated to enhance the discriminatory ability of $tcPO_2$ values.

Dependent Position

Franzeck and colleagues[46] observed an average increase of 15 ± 7 mmHg in the $tcPO_2$ on the dorsum of the foot in normal subjects when they moved from a supine to a sitting position. In the sitting position, the sensor was 54 cm below the heart. With standing, which extended the distance to 84 cm, the $tcPO_2$ rose by an average of 28 ± 14 mmHg. The increase in $tcPO_2$ that accompanies standing occurs at all levels of the leg but is most evident at foot level, where the hydrostatic pressure is greatest.

In general, this augmentation in $tcPO_2$ is directly proportional to the severity of limb ischemia. Byrne and associates[24] noted an average increase of 20 mmHg in limbs with rest pain compared with an average increase of 10 mmHg in normal limbs. On the basis of their data, $tcPO_2$ rises by about 18% in normal limbs; by 22% in limbs with claudication and normal resting $tcPO_2$ values; by 58% in limbs with claudication and abnormal resting $tcPO_2$ values; and by 88% in limbs with rest pain. Oh and associates[109] retrospectively separated severely ischemic extremities into two groups according to the change in $tcPO_2$ that occurred with standing: Group I was defined by a $tcPO_2$ increase of less than 15 mmHg (average 4 ± 5 mmHg), and group II by an increase of more than 15 mmHg (average 36 ± 11 mmHg). Despite the fact that both groups had similar supine $tcPO_2$ values (4 ± 5 mmHg and 6 ± 5 mmHg, respectively), the manifestations of disease were more severe in group I limbs (61% ulcers or gangrene, 48% rest pain, and 39% claudication) than in group II limbs (29% ulcers or gangrene, 46% rest pain, and 68% claudication).

The increase in oxygen tension that occurs when a patient with an ischemic limb sits or stands may explain how dependency relieves rest pain. As discussed in Chapter 7, elevation of the hydrostatic pressure dilates capillaries and other resistive vessels, thereby permitting more blood to flow at the same arteriovenous pressure gradient. In addition, any muscular activity with the leg dependent may decrease venous pressure and increase the arteriovenous pressure gradient. With the increase in capillary blood flow, more oxygen is delivered to the tissues. In the most severely ischemic extremities, these physiologic compensatory mechanisms are nearly exhausted, and the increase in blood flow is inadequate to provide relief.

Exercise

In limbs with restricted arterial inflow, the dilatation of intramuscular vessels induced by exercise diverts blood away from cutaneous vascular beds, causing $tcPO_2$ to fall. In normal limbs, this "steal" is not evident because arterial inflow is adequate to supply both vascular beds. Therefore, it is not surprising to find that post-exercise:pre-exercise ratios of ankle pressures and ankle $tcPO_2$ values are highly correlated (r = .918), as demonstrated by the treadmill studies of Matsen and associates.[98]

Byrne and associates[24] observed that $tcPO_2$ values measured on the dorsum of the foot during treadmill exercise remained at about the same level as those obtained during quiet standing; however, during the period following exercise, after the subjects had resumed a supine position, the $tcPO_2$ values fell in all patients with significant arterial obstruction, even in those with normal resting values (Table 10–14). No fall in $tcPO_2$ values was evident in normal subjects. Similar but less marked changes occurred at calf level. These researchers concluded that post-exercise $tcPO_2$ measurements accurately distinguished between subjects with intermittent claudication and those who were normal.

Hauser and Shoemaker[62] found that the chest $tcPO_2$ value increased during exercise in patients with claudication, perhaps explaining the failure of limb values to decrease. However, the RPI (limb $tcPO_2$/chest $tcPO_2$) at foot level did decrease during exercise, even in normal extremities. When RPI values obtained during exercise were compared with values obtained when the patient was standing, a decrease

TABLE 10–14. EFFECT OF EXERCISE ON FOOT TRANSCUTANEOUS OXYGEN TENSION ($tcPO_2$) (mmHg, MEAN ± SD)

TYPE OF OBSTRUCTION	$tcPO_2$ VALUES			
	Supine	**Standing**	**Exercise**	**Postexercise***
Normal	60 ± 7	71 ± 7	75 ± 9	69 ± 7
Claudication†	56 ± 4	58 ± 8	53 ± 10	33 ± 16
Claudication	37 ± 12	58 ± 12	49 ± 18	23 ± 20
Rest pain	4 ± 4	25 ± 20	26 ± 26	5 ± 7

Data from Byrne P. Provan JL, Ameli FM, et al: The use of transcutaneous oxygen tension measurements in the diagnosis of peripheral vascular insufficiency. Ann Surg 200:159, 1984.

*Postexercise measurements made with patient supine.

†Claudicators with normal resting $tcPO_2$ values.

TABLE 10–15. POSTISCHEMIC TRANSCUTANEOUS OXYGEN TENSION ($tcPo_2$) RECOVERY RATE ($T_{1/2}$) (SEC)

AUTHOR AND YEAR	NORMAL		CLAUDICATION		REST PAIN	
	Foot	Calf	Foot	Calf	Foot	Calf
Franzeck et al (1982)[46]	87 ± 27	60 ± 15	136 ± 73	131 ± 69	—	—
Cina et al (1984)[34]	49 ± 6	—	114 ± 2	—	—	—
Kram et al (1985)[89]*	66 ± 18	48 ± 18	156 ± 60	126 ± 42	204 ± 78	126 ± 66

*Based on limb : chest $tcPo_2$ ratio.

of more than 10% at the thigh or more than 15% at the calf was found to be highly specific for intermittent claudication. Normal limbs measured at these levels demonstrated no fall in RPI. After exercise, the RPI at the foot in normal limbs always returned to pre-exercise values within 1 minute. In limbs with claudication, the average time to recover one half of the exercise drop was about 4 minutes.

Reactive Hyperemia

In the reactive hyperemia test for $tcPo_2$, inflation of a pneumatic cuff to more than systolic pressure is followed by a rapid decline in the $tcPo_2$ measured more distally on the leg. When the cuff is deflated after a period of ischemia (usually about 4 minutes), the $tcPo_2$ rapidly returns to precompression levels in normal extremities. In limbs with occlusive arterial disease, the rate of recovery is much slower. Recovery rates are usually expressed as the time required for the $tcPo_2$ to return to one half of the precompression value ($T_{1/2}$).

Representative results are shown in Table 10–15. Cina and coworkers[34] reported a range of 43 to 60 seconds in normal limbs and 75 to 150 seconds in limbs with claudication; there were no overlapping values. Kram and associates[88] found that postischemic recovery times based on the RPI (limb $tcPo_2$/chest $tcPo_2$) were more diagnostic of arterial disease than toe pulse recovery times. Values for $T_{1/2}$ in excess of 84 seconds at the calf and 102 seconds at the foot were considered to indicate disease.[88, 89]

Oxygen Inhalation

Inhalation of pure oxygen markedly augments the $tcPo_2$ in normal limbs but has less effect in limbs with severe arterial occlusion. Ohgi and associates[110] reported that pretibial values increased from (1) 70 ± 9 to 365 ± 87 mmHg in normal legs, (2) 34 ± 33 to 115 ± 109 mmHg in legs with chronic occlusion, and (3) 23 ± 30 to 96 ± 57 mmHg in legs with acute occlusion. According to Harward and colleagues,[60] the prediction of amputation healing based on $tcPo_2$ determinations may be enhanced by oxygen inhalation.

LASER DOPPLER VELOCIMETRY

A relative index of cutaneous blood flow can be obtained with the laser Doppler velocimeter. The output of this instrument, which is expressed in millivolts (mV), is roughly proportional to the average blood flow in a 1.5-mm^3 volume of skin lying 0.8 to 1.5 mm below the skin surface. According to Karanfilian and associates,[79] tracings from normal skin exhibit three major characteristics:

1. Pulse waves that coincide with the cardiac cycle.
2. Vasomotor waves that occur four to six times per minute.
3. A mean blood flow velocity that is represented by the elevation of the tracing above a zero baseline.

In the leg, the highest velocities are obtained from the skin of the big toe, followed, in descending order, by velocities from the skin of the plantar surface of the foot, dorsal foot, distal leg, thigh, and proximal leg.

In limbs with peripheral vascular disease, pulse waves are attenuated, mean velocities are decreased, and vasomotor waves may disappear (Table 10–16).[80] The reactive hyperemic response to a period of cuff-induced ischemia is diminished, and the time to reach maximal hyperemia is markedly delayed (see Table 10–16).[80] Karanfilian and associates[80] investigated the ability of laser Doppler studies to predict healing of ulcers or forefoot amputations in a series of ischemic limbs. In limbs in which the mean velocity recorded from the plantar aspect of the foot or big toe exceeded 40 mV and the pulse wave amplitude exceeded 4 mV, 96% of the lesions or amputations healed. In contrast, in limbs in which these criteria were not met, 79% of the lesions or amputations failed to heal. These

TABLE 10–16. LASER DOPPLER MEASUREMENTS FROM THE BIG TOE (MEAN ± SD)

	BASELINE VALUES		REACTIVE HYPEREMIA TEST	
	Velocity (mV)	Pulse Amplitude (mV)	Peak/Baseline Ratio*	Time to Maximal Velocity (sec)
Normal	197 ± 174	77 ± 63	3.1 ± 0.9	18 ± 7
Ischemic	67 ± 42	5 ± 4	1.7 ± 1.6	150 ± 48

Data from Karanfilian RG, Lynch TG, Lee BC, et al: The assessment of skin blood flow in peripheral vascular disease by laser Doppler velocimetry. Am Surg 50:641, 1984.
*Ratio of peak postischemic velocity to preischemic velocity.

results were not quite as good as those obtained in the same extremities through the use of $tcPo_2$.

The laser Doppler velocimeter can also be used in conjunction with a pneumatic cuff to estimate skin blood pressure at almost any level of the upper or lower extremities. These measurements are made with the probe (which merely serves as a flow sensor) placed under the pneumatic cuff. Castronuovo and associates[32] obtained cutaneous pressure in normal subjects averaging 47 ± 28 mmHg in forearms and thighs and 73 ± 28 mmHg in the plantar skin of the big toe; these pressures are similar to those in precapillary vessels. Much lower values were found in the plantar skin of the toe (17 ± 15 mmHg) and in the dorsal skin of the foot (10 ± 10 mmHg) in limbs with rest pain, ulceration, or gangrene.

Although laser Doppler velocimetry is a valid physiologic test, it has not been widely used in vascular laboratories. Results cannot be calibrated in terms of actual blood flow, and much of the information that the test provides can be obtained with more established techniques.

SUMMARY

Although many different methods for studying the arterial circulation have been discussed in this chapter, not all are indicated in the evaluation or follow-up for every patient.[14] Some tests are not as accurate as others, some are more difficult to perform, and many provide overlapping information or information that is not pertinent to the clinical questions being asked. The best policy is to select those modalities that (1) supply the most information, (2) have been shown to be reliable by critical prospective evaluation, and (3) are known to be economical in terms of both time and cost.

REFERENCES

1. Allan JS, Terry HJ: The evaluation of an ultrasonic flow detector for the assessment of peripheral vascular disease. Cardiovasc Res 3:503, 1969.
2. Aukland A, Hurlow RA: Spectral analysis of Doppler ultrasound: Its clinical application in lower limb ischemia. Br J Surg 69:539, 1982.
3. Baird RN, Bird DR, Clifford PC, et al: Upstream stenosis: Its diagnosis by Doppler signals from the femoral artery. Arch Surg 115:1316, 1980.
4. Baker AR, Evans DH, Prytherch DR, et al: Haemodynamic assessment of the femoropopliteal segment: Comparison of pressure and Doppler methods using ROC curve analysis. Br J Surg 73:559, 1986.
5. Baker JD: Poststress Doppler ankle pressures: A comparison of treadmill exercise with two other methods of induced hyperemia. Arch Surg 113:1171, 1978.
6. Baker JD, Dix D: Variability of Doppler ankle pressures with arterial occlusive disease: An evaluation of ankle index and brachial-ankle gradient. Surgery 89:134, 1981.
7. Baker JD, Machleder HI, Skidmore R: Analysis of femoral artery Doppler signals by Laplace transform damping method. J Vasc Surg 1:520, 1984.
8. Baker WH, String ST, Hayes AC, et al: Diagnosis of peripheral occlusive disease: Comparison of clinical evaluation and noninvasive laboratory. Arch Surg 113:1308, 1978.
9. Barnes RW: Noninvasive methods to evaluate acute vascular problems. *In* Haimovici H (ed): Vascular Emergencies. New York, Appleton-Century-Crofts, 1982, pp 7–26.
10. Barnes RW, Hafermann MD, Petersen J, et al: Noninvasive assessment of altered limb hemodynamics and complications of arterial catheterization. Radiology 107:505, 1973.
11. Barnes RW, Shanik GD, Slaymaker EF: An index of healing in below-knee amputation: Leg blood pressure by Doppler ultrasound. Surgery 79:13, 1976.
12. Barnes RW, Thornhill B, Nix L, et al: Prediction of amputation wound healing: Roles of Doppler ultrasound and digit photoplethysmography. Arch Surg 116:80, 1981.
13. Bell G: Systolic pressure measurements in occlusive vascular disease to assess run-off preoperatively. Scand J Clin Lab Invest 31(Suppl 128):173, 1973.
14. Bergan JJ, Yao JST: Invited overview: Role of the vascular laboratory. Surgery 88:9, 1980.
15. Berkowitz HD, Hobbs CL, Roberts B, et al: Value of routine vascular laboratory studies to identify vein graft stenosis. Surgery 90:971, 1981.
16. Bernstein EF, Rhodes GA, Stuart SH, et al: Toe pulse-reappearance time in prediction of aortofemoral bypass success. Ann Surg 193:201, 1981.
17. Bernstein EF, Witzel TH, Stotts JS, et al: Thigh pressure artifacts with noninvasive techniques in an experimental model. Surgery 89:319, 1981.
18. Bollinger A, Mahler F, Zehender O: Kombinierte Druck- und Durchflussmessungen in der Beurteilung arterieller Durchblutungsstörungen. Dtsch Med Wochenschr 95:1039, 1970.
19. Bone GE: The relationship between aorto-iliac hemodynamics and femoral pulsatility index. J Surg Res 32:228, 1982.
20. Bone GE, Pomajzl MJ: Toe blood pressure by photoplethysmography: An index of healing in forefoot amputation. Surgery 89:569, 1981.
21. Brener BJ, Raines JK, Darling RC, et al: Measurement of systolic femoral arterial pressure during reactive hyperemia. Circulation 49–50(Suppl II):259, 1974.
22. Britt DB, Kemmerer WT, Robison JR: Penile blood flow determination by mercury strain gauge plethysmography. Invest Urol 8:673, 1971.
23. Bruner JMR, Krenis LJ, Kunsman JM, et al: Comparison of direct and indirect methods of measuring arterial blood pressure. Med Instrum 15:11, 1981.
24. Byrne P, Provan JL, Ameli FM, et al: The use of transcutaneous oxygen tension measurements in the diagnosis of peripheral vascular insufficiency. Ann Surg 200:159, 1984.
25. Campbell WB, Cole SEA, Skidmore R, et al: The clinician and the vascular laboratory in the diagnosis of aorto-iliac stenosis. Br J Surg 71:302, 1984.
26. Carter SA: Indirect systolic pressure and pulse waves in arterial occlusive disease of the lower extremities. Circulation 37:624, 1968.
27. Carter SA: Clinical measurement of systolic pressures in limbs with arterial occlusive disease. JAMA 207:1869, 1969.
28. Carter SA: Response of ankle systolic pressure to leg exercise in mild or questionable arterial disease. N Engl J Med 287:578, 1972.
29. Carter SA: The relationship of distal systolic pressures to healing of skin lesions in limbs with arterial occlusive disease, with special reference to diabetes mellitus. Scand J Clin Lab Invest 31(Suppl 128):239, 1973.
30. Carter SA, Lezack JD: Digital systolic pressures in the lower limb in arterial disease. Circulation 43:905, 1971.
31. Castronuovo JJ, Flanigan DP: Pseudoclaudication of neurospinal origin. Vasc Diagn Ther 5:21, 1984.
32. Castronuovo JJ Jr, Pabst TS, Flanigan DP, et al: Noninvasive determination of skin perfusion pressure using a laser Doppler. J Cardiovasc Surg 28:253, 1987.
33. Chiu RC-J, Lidstone D, Blundell PE: Predictive power of penile/brachial index in diagnosing male sexual impotence. J Vasc Surg 4:251, 1986.
34. Cina C, Katsamouris A, Megerman J, et al: Utility of transcutaneous oxygen tension measurements in peripheral arterial occlusive disease. J Vasc Surg 1:362, 1984.
35. Clyne CAC, Ryan J, Webster JHH, et al: Oxygen tension on the skin of ischemic legs. Am J Surg 143:315, 1982.
36. Conrad MC, Green HD: Hemodynamics of large and small vessels in peripheral vascular disease. Circulation 29:847, 1964.
37. Cutajar CL, Marston A, Newcombe JF: Value of cuff occlusion pressures in assessment of peripheral vascular disease. Br Med J 2:392, 1973.

38. Darling RC, Raines JK, Brener BJ, et al: Quantitative segmental pulse volume recorder: A clinical tool. Surgery 72:873, 1972.
39. Delius W, Erikson U: Correlation between angiographic and hemodynamic findings in occlusions of arteries of the extremities. Vasc Surg 3:201, 1969.
40. Delius W, Kellerova E: Reactions of arterial and venous vessels in the human forearm and hand to deep breath or mental strain. Clin Sci 40:271, 1971.
41. Evans DH, Barrie WW, Asher MJ, et al: The relationship between ultrasonic pulsatility index and proximal arterial stenosis in a canine model. Circ Res 46:470, 1980.
42. Flanigan DP, Collins JT, Schwartz JA, et al: Hemodynamic and arteriographic evaluation of femoral pulsatility index. J Surg Res 32:234, 1982.
43. Flanigan DP, Ryan TJ, Williams LR, et al: Aortofemoral or femoropopliteal revascularization? A prospective evaluation of the papaverine test. J Vasc Surg 1:215, 1984.
44. Flanigan DP, Williams LR, Schwartz JA, et al: Hemodynamic evaluation of the aortoiliac system based on pharmacologic vasodilatation. Surgery 93:709, 1983.
45. Francfort JW, Bigelow PS, Davis JT, et al: Noninvasive techniques in the assessment of lower extremity arterial occlusive disease: The advantages of proximal and distal thigh cuffs. Arch Surg 119:1145, 1984.
46. Franzeck UK, Talke P, Bernstein EF, et al: Transcutaneous Po_2 measurements in health and peripheral arterial occlusive disease. Surgery 91:156, 1982.
47. Fronek A, Coel M, Bernstein EF: The pulse-reappearance time: An index of over-all blood flow impairment in the ischemic extremity. Surgery 81:376, 1977.
48. Fronek A, Coel M, Bernstein EF: The importance of combined multisegmental pressure and Doppler flow velocity studies in the diagnosis of peripheral arterial occlusive disease. Surgery 84:840, 1978.
49. Fronek A, Johansen KH, Dilley RB, et al: Noninvasive physiologic tests in the diagnosis and characterization of peripheral arterial occlusive disease. Am J Surg 126:205, 1973.
50. Gaylis H: The assessment of impotence in aorto-iliac disease using penile blood pressure measurements. S Afr J Surg 16:39, 1978.
51. Gibbons GE, Strandness DE Jr, Bell JW: Improvements in design of the mercury strain gauge plethysmograph. Surg Gynecol Obstet 116:679, 1963.
52. Gilfillan RS, Leeds FH, Spotts RR: The prediction of healing in ischemic lesions of the foot: A comparison of Doppler ultrasound and elevation reactive hyperemia. J Cardiovasc Surg 26:15, 1985.
53. Goodreau JJ, Creasy JK, Flanigan DP, et al: Rational approach to the differentiation of vascular and neurogenic claudication. Surgery 84:749, 1978.
54. Gothgen I, Jacobsen E: Transcutaneous oxygen tension measurement: I. Age variation and reproducibility. Acta Anaesthesiol Scand Suppl 67:66, 1978.
55. Gray B, Kmiecik JC, Spigos DD, et al: Evaluation of Doppler-derived upper thigh pressure in the assessment of aorto-iliac occlusive disease. Bruit 4:29, 1980.
56. Gundersen J: Segmental measurement of systolic blood pressure in the extremities including the thumb and great toe. Acta Chir Scand Suppl 426:1, 1972.
57. Gutierrez IZ, Gage AA, Makuta PA: Toe pulse study in ischemic arterial disease of the legs. Surg Gynecol Obstet 153:889, 1981.
58. Hajjar W, Sumner DS: Segmental pressures in normal subjects 16 to 32 years of age. Unpublished observations, 1976.
59. Harris PL, Taylor LA, Cave FD, et al: The relationship between Doppler ultrasound assessment and angiography in occlusive arterial disease of the lower limbs. Surg Gynecol Obstet 138:911, 1974.
60. Harward TRS, Volny J, Golbranson F, et al: Oxygen inhalation-induced transcutaneous Po_2 changes as a predictor of amputation level. J Vasc Surg 2:220, 1985.
61. Hauser CJ, Klein SR, Mehringer CM, et al: Superiority of transcutaneous oximetry in noninvasive vascular diagnosis in patients with diabetes. Arch Surg 119:690, 1984.
62. Hauser CJ, Shoemaker WC: Use of a transcutaneous Po_2 regional perfusion index to quantify tissue perfusion in peripheral vascular disease. Ann Surg 197:337, 1983.
63. Heintz SE, Bone GE, Slaymaker EE, et al: Value of arterial pressure measurements in the proximal and distal part of the thigh in arterial occlusive disease. Surg Gynecol Obstet 146:337, 1978.
64. Hirai M, Schoop W: Hemodynamic assessment of the iliac disease by proximal thigh pressure and Doppler femoral flow velocity. J Cardiovasc Surg 25:365, 1984.
65. Hobbs JT, Yao ST, Lewis JD, et al: A limitation of the Doppler ultrasound method of measuring ankle systolic pressure. Vasa 3:160, 1974.
66. Holstein P, Dovey H, Lassen NA: Wound healing in above-knee amputations in relation to skin perfusion pressure. Acta Orthop Scand 50:59, 1979.
67. Holstein P, Sager P: Toe blood pressure in peripheral arterial disease. Acta Orthop Scand 44:564, 1973.
68. Holstein P, Noer I, Tønnesen KH, et al: Distal blood pressure in severe arterial insufficiency. Strain-gauge, radioisotopes, and other methods. *In* Bergan JJ, Yao JST (eds): Gangrene and Severe Ischemia of the Lower Extremities. New York, Grune & Stratton, 1978, pp 95–114.
69. Hummel BW, Hummel BA, Mowbry A, et al: Reactive hyperemia vs treadmill exercise testing in arterial disease. Arch Surg 113:95, 1978.
70. Humphries KN, Hames TK, Smith SWJ, et al: Quantitative assessment of the common femoral to popliteal arterial segment using continuous wave Doppler ultrasound. Ultrasound Med Biol 6:99, 1980.
71. Johansen K, Lynch K, Paun M, et al: Noninvasive vascular tests reliably exclude occult arterial trauma in injured extremities. J Trauma 31:515, 1991.
72. Johnson WC: Doppler ankle pressure and reactive hyperemia in the diagnosis of arterial insufficiency. J Surg Res 18:177, 1975.
73. Johnston KW, Hosang MY, Andrews DF: Reproducibility of noninvasive vascular laboratory measurements of the peripheral circulation. J Vasc Surg 6:147, 1987.
74. Johnston KW, Kassam M, Cobbold RSC: Relationship between Doppler pulsatility index and direct femoral pressure measurements in the diagnosis of aortoiliac occlusive disease. Ultrasound Med Biol 9:271, 1983.
75. Johnston KW, Kassam M, Koers J, et al: Comparative study of four methods for quantifying Doppler ultrasound waveforms from the femoral artery. Ultrasound Med Biol 10:1, 1984.
76. Johnston KW, Maruzzo BC, Cobbold RSC: Doppler methods for quantitative measurement and localization of peripheral arterial occlusive disease by analysis of the blood velocity waveform. Ultrasound Med Biol 4:209, 1978.
77. Johnston KW, Maruzzo BC, Kassam M, et al: Methods for obtaining, processing and quantifying Doppler blood velocity waveforms. *In* Nicolaides AN, Yao JST (eds): Investigation of Vascular Disorders. London, Churchill Livingstone, 1981, pp 532–558.
78. Junger M, Chapman BLW, Underwood CJ, Charlesworth D: A comparison between two types of waveform analysis in patients with multisegmental arterial disease. Br J Surg 71:345, 1984.
79. Karanfilian RG, Lynch TG, Lee BC, et al: The assessment of skin blood flow in peripheral vascular disease by laser Doppler velocimetry. Am Surg 50:641, 1984.
80. Karanfilian RG, Lynch TG, Zirul VT, et al: The value of laser Doppler velocimetry and transcutaneous oxygen tension determination in predicting healing of ischemic forefoot ulcerations and amputations in diabetic and nondiabetic patients. J Vasc Surg 4:511, 1986.
81. Karpman HL, Winsor T: The plethysmographic peripheral vascular study. J Int Coll Surg 30:425, 1958.
82. Kavanaugh GJ, Svien HJ, Holman CB, et al: "Pseudoclaudication" syndrome produced by compression of the cauda equina. JAMA 206:2477, 1968.
83. Kempczinski RF: Role of the vascular diagnostic laboratory in the evaluation of male impotence. Am J Surg 138:278, 1979.
84. Kempczinski RF: Segmental volume plethysmography in the diagnosis of lower extremity arterial occlusive disease. J Cardiovasc Surg 23:125, 1982.
85. Kempczinski RF: Segmental volume plethysmography: The pulse volume recorder. *In* Kempczinski RF, Yao JST (eds): Practical Noninvasive Vascular Diagnosis, 2nd ed. Chicago, Year Book Medical Publishers, 1987, pp 140–153.
86. King LT, Strandness DE Jr, Bell JW: The hemodynamic response of the lower extremity to exercise. J Surg Res 5:167, 1965.
87. Kohler TR, Nance DR, Cramer MM, et al: Duplex scanning for diagnosis of aortoiliac and femoropopliteal disease: A prospective study. Circulation 76:1074, 1987.
88. Kram HB, Appel PL, White RA, et al: Assessment of peripheral

vascular disease by postocclusive transcutaneous oxygen recovery time. J Vasc Surg 1:628, 1984.
89. Kram HB, White RA, Tabrisky J, et al: Transcutaneous oxygen recovery and toe pulse-reappearance time in the assessment of peripheral vascular disease. Circulation 72:1022, 1985.
90. Lane RJ, Appleberg M, Williams WA: A comparison of two techniques for the detection of the vasculogenic component of impotence. Surg Gynecol Obstet 155:230, 1982.
91. Lassen NA, Tuedegaard E, Jeppesen FI, et al: Distal blood pressure measurement in occlusive arterial disease strain gauge compared to xenon-133. Angiology 23:211, 1972.
92. Lorentsen E: Calf blood pressure measurements: The applicability of a plethysmographic method and the result of measurements during reactive hyperemia. Scand J Clin Lab Invest 31:69, 1973.
93. Lorentsen E: The vascular resistance in the arteries of the lower leg in normal subjects and in patients with different degrees of atherosclerotic disease. Scand J Clin Lab Invest 31:147, 1973.
94. Lynch K, Johansen K: Can Doppler pressure measurement replace "exclusion" arteriography in the diagnosis of occult extremity arterial trauma? Ann Surg 241:737, 1991.
95. Marinelli MR, Beach NW, Glass MJ, et al: Noninvasive testing vs clinical evaluation of arterial disease: A prospective study. JAMA 241:2031, 1979.
96. Matsen FA III, Wyss CR, Pedegana LR, et al: Transcutaneous oxygen tension measurement in peripheral vascular disease. Surg Gynecol Obstet 150:525, 1980.
97. Matsen FA III, Wyss CR, Robertson CC, et al: The relationship of transcutaneous Po_2 and laser Doppler measurements in a human model of local arterial insufficiency. Surg Gynecol Obstet 159:418, 1984.
98. Matsen FA III, Wyss CR, Simmons CW, et al: The effect of exercise upon cutaneous oxygen delivery in the extremities of patients with claudication and in a human laboratory model of claudication. Surg Gynecol Obstet 158:522, 1984.
99. Moore WS, Hall AD: Unrecognized aortoiliac stenosis. Arch Surg 103:633, 1971.
100. Moore WS, Henry RE, Malone JM, et al: Prospective use of xenon-133 clearance for amputation level selection. Arch Surg 116:86, 1981.
101. Mozersky DJ, Sumner DS, Strandness DE Jr: Long-term result of reconstructive aortoiliac surgery. Am J Surg 123:503, 1972.
102. Mozersky DJ, Sumner DS, Strandness DE Jr: Disease progression after femoropopliteal surgical procedures. Surg Gynecol Obstet 135:700, 1972.
103. Mustapha NM, Redhead RG, Jain SK, et al: Transcutaneous partial oxygen pressure assessment of the ischemic lower limb. Surg Gynecol Obstet 156:582, 1983.
104. Nath RL, Menzoian JO, Kaplan KH, et al: The multidisciplinary approach to vasculogenic impotence. Surgery 89:124, 1981.
105. Nicholls SC, Kohler TR, Martin RL, et al: Use of hemodynamic parameters in the diagnosis of mesenteric insufficiency. J Vasc Surg 3:507, 1985.
106. Nicolaides AN: Value of noninvasive tests in the investigation of lower limb ischemia. Ann R Coll Surg Engl 60:249, 1978.
106a. Nicolaides AN, Gordon-Smith IC, Dayandas J, et al: The value of Doppler blood velocity tracings in the detection of aortoiliac disease in patients with intermittent claudication. Surgery 80:774, 1976.
107. Nielsen PE, Bell G, Lassen NA: The measurement of digital systolic blood pressure by strain gauge technique. Scand J Clin Lab Invest 29:371, 1972.
108. Nielsen PE, Bell G, Lassen NA: Strain gauge studies of distal blood pressure in normal subjects and in patients with peripheral arterial diseases: Analysis of normal variation and reproducibility and comparison to intraarterial measurements. Scand J Clin Lab Invest 31(Suppl 128):103, 1973.
109. Oh PIT, Provan JL, Amelie FM: The predictability of the success of arterial reconstruction by means of transcutaneous oxygen tension measurements. J Vasc Surg 5:356, 1987.
110. Ohgi S, Ito K, Mori T: Quantitative evaluation of the skin circulation in ischemic legs by transcutaneous measurement of oxygen tension. Angiology 32:833, 1981.
111. O'Mara CS, Flinn WR, Johnson ND, et al: Recognition and surgical management of patent but hemodynamically failed arterial grafts. Ann Surg 193:467, 1981.
112. Osmundson PJ, Chesebro JH, O'Fallon WM, et al: A prospective study of peripheral occlusive arterial disease in diabetes: II. Vascular laboratory assessment. Mayo Clin Proc 56:223, 1981.
113. Ouriel K, McDonnell AE, Metz CE, et al: A critical evaluation of stress testing in the diagnosis of peripheral vascular disease. Surgery 91:686, 1982.
114. Pascarelli EF, Bertrand CA: Comparison of blood pressures in the arms and legs. N Engl J Med 270:693, 1964.
115. Persson AV, Gibbons G, Griffey S: Noninvasive evaluation of the aorto-iliac segment. J Cardiovasc Surg 22:539, 1981.
116. Queral LA, Whitehouse WM Jr, Flinn WR, et al: Pelvic hemodynamics after aorto-iliac reconstruction. Surgery 86:799, 1979.
117. Raines JK: Diagnosis and analysis of arteriosclerosis in the lower limbs from the arterial pressure pulse. Doctoral Thesis, Massachusetts Institute of Technology, Boston, 1972.
118. Raines JK, Darling RG, Buth J, et al: Vascular laboratory criteria for the management of peripheral vascular disease of the lower extremities. Surgery 79:21, 1976.
119. Ramirez C, Box M, Gottesman L: Noninvasive vascular evaluation in male impotence: Technique. Bruit 4:14, 1980.
120. Ramsey DE, Johnson F, Sumner DS: Anatomic validity of segmental pressure measurement. Unpublished observations, 1979.
121. Ramsey DE, Manke DA, Sumner DS: Toe blood pressure—a valuable adjunct to ankle pressure measurement for assessing peripheral arterial disease. J Cardiovasc Surg 24:43, 1983.
122. Reddy DJ, Vincent GS, McPharlin M, et al: Limitations of the femoral pulsatility index with aortoiliac stenosis: An experimental study. J Vasc Surg 4:327, 1986.
123. Reidy NC, Walden R, Abbott WA, et al: Anatomic localization of atherosclerotic lesions by hemodynamic tests. Arch Surg 116:1041, 1981.
124. Rittenhouse EA, Maixner W, Burr JW, et al: Directional arterial flow velocity: A sensitive index of changes in peripheral vascular resistance. Surgery 79:350, 1976.
125. Rutherford RB, Jones DN, Martin MS, et al: Serial hemodynamic assessment of aortofemoral bypass. J Vasc Surg 4:428, 1986.
126. Rutherford RB, Lowenstein DH, Klein MF: Combining segmental systolic pressures and plethysmography to diagnose arterial occlusive disease of the legs. Am J Surg 138:211, 1979.
127. Sanchez SA, Best EB: Correlation of plethysmographic and arteriographic findings in patients with obstructive arterial disease. Angiology 20:684, 1969.
128. Schwartz JA, Schuler JJ, O'Connor RJA, et al: Predictive value of distal perfusion pressure in the healing of amputations of the digit and the forefoot. Surg Gynecol Obstet 154:865, 1982.
129. Siggard-Anderson J, Ulrich J, Engell HC, et al: Blood pressure measurements of the lower limb: Arterial occlusions in the calf determined by plethysmographic blood pressure measurements in the thigh and at the ankle. Angiology 23:350, 1972.
130. Skidmore R, Woodcock JP, Wells PNT, et al: Physiological interpretation of Doppler-shift waveforms. III: Clinical results. Ultrasound Med Biol 6:227, 1980.
131. Skinner JS, Strandness DE Jr: Exercise and intermittent claudication. I: Effect of repetition and intensity of exercise. Circulation 36:15, 1967.
132. Skinner JS, Strandness DE Jr: Exercise and intermittent claudication. II: Effect of physical training. Circulation 36:23, 1967.
133. Sobinsky KR, Williams LR, Gray G, et al: Supine exercise testing in the selection of suprainguinal versus infrainguinal bypass in patients with multisegmental arterial occlusive disease. Am J Surg 152:185, 1986.
134. Stahler C, Strandness DE Jr: Ankle blood pressure response to graded treadmill exercise. Angiology 18:237, 1967.
135. Strandness DE Jr: Long-term value of lumbar sympathectomy. Geriatrics 21:144, 1966.
136. Strandness DE Jr: Abnormal exercise responses after successful reconstructive arterial surgery. Surgery 59:325, 1966.
137. Strandness DE Jr: Peripheral Arterial Disease: A Physiologic Approach. Boston, Little, Brown & Co, 1969.
138. Strandness DE Jr, Bell JW: An evaluation of the hemodynamic response of the claudicating extremity to exercise. Surg Gynecol Obstet 119:1237, 1964.
139. Strandness DE Jr, Bell JW: Peripheral vascular disease, diagnosis and objective evaluation using a mercury strain gauge. Ann Surg 161(Suppl 4):1, 1965.
140. Strandness DE Jr, Bell JW: Ankle pressure responses after reconstructive arterial surgery. Surgery 59:514, 1966.

141. Strandness DE Jr, Schultz RD, Sumner DS, et al: Ultrasonic flow detection: A useful technic in the evaluation of peripheral vascular disease. Am J Surg 113:311, 1967.
142. Strandness DE Jr, Sumner DS: Hemodynamics for Surgeons. New York, Grune & Stratton, 1975.
143. Strandness DE Jr, Zierler RE: Exercise ankle pressure measurements in arterial disease. *In* Bernstein EF (ed): Noninvasive Diagnostic Techniques in Vascular Disease, 4th ed. St. Louis, Mosby–Year Book, 1993, p 547.
144. Sumner DS: Rational use of noninvasive tests in designing a therapeutic approach to severe arterial disease of the legs. *In* Puel P, Boccalon H, Enjalbert A (eds): Hemodynamics of the Limbs—2. Toulouse, France, GEPESC, 1981, pp 369–376.
145. Sumner DS, Strandness DE Jr: The relationship between calf blood flow and ankle blood pressure in patients with intermittent claudication. Surgery 65:763, 1969.
146. Sumner DS, Strandness DE Jr: The effect of exercise on resistance to blood flow in limbs with an occluded superficial femoral artery. J Vasc Surg 4:229, 1970.
147. Sumner DS, Strandness DE Jr: Aortoiliac reconstruction in patients with combined iliac and superficial femoral arterial occlusion. Surgery 84:348, 1978.
148. Sumner DS, Strandness DE Jr: Hemodynamic studies before and after extended bypass grafts to the tibial and peroneal arteries. Surgery 86:442, 1979.
149. Taguchi JT, Suwangool P: Pipe-stem brachial arteries: A cause of pseudohypertension. JAMA 228:733, 1974.
150. Tait WF, Charlesworth D, Lemon JG: Atypical claudication. Br J Surg 72:315, 1985.
151. Thiele BL, Bandyk DF, Zierler RE, et al: A systematic approach to the assessment of aortoiliac disease. Arch Surg 118:477, 1983.
152. Thulesius O: Systemic and ankle blood pressure before and after exercise in patients with arterial insufficiency. Angiology 29:374, 1978.
153. Thulesius O, Gjöres JE: Use of Doppler shift detection for determining peripheral arterial blood pressure. Angiology 22:594, 1971.
154. Tønneson KH: Transcutaneous oxygen tension in imminent foot gangrene. Acta Anaesthesiol Scand 68:107, 1978.
155. Tønneson KH, Noer I, Paaske W, et al: Classification of peripheral occlusive arterial diseases based on symptoms, signs, and distal blood pressure measurements. Acta Chir Scand 146:101, 1980.
156. Turnipseed WD, Acker CW: Postoperative surveillance: An effective means of detecting correctable lesions that threaten graft patency. Arch Surg 120:324, 1985.
157. Udoff EJ, Barth KH, Harrington DP, et al: Hemodynamic significance of iliac artery stenosis: Pressure measurements during angiography. Radiology 132:289, 1979.
158. Van De Water JM, Indech CDV, Indech RB, et al: Hyperemic response for diagnosis of arterial insufficiency. Arch Surg 115:851, 1980.
159. Verta MJ Jr, Gross WS, vanBellen B, et al: Forefoot perfusion pressure and minor amputation for gangrene. Surgery 80:729, 1976.
160. Vollrath KD, Salles-Cunha SX, Vincent D, et al: Noninvasive measurement of toe systolic pressures. Bruit 4:27, 1980.
161. Ward AS, Martin TP: Some aspects of ultrasound in the diagnosis and assessment of aortoiliac disease. Am J Surg 140:260, 1980.
162. Winsor T: Influence of arterial disease on the systolic blood pressure gradients of the extremity. Am J Med Sci 220:117, 1950.
163. Winsor T, Sibley AE, Fisher EK, et al: Peripheral pulse contours in arterial occlusive disease. Vasc Dis 5:61, 1968.
164. Wolf EA Jr, Sumner DS, Strandness DE Jr: Correlation between nutritive blood flow and pressure in limbs of patients with intermittent claudication. Surg Forum 23:238, 1972.
165. Wyss CR, Matsen FA III, Simmons CW, et al: Transcutaneous oxygen tension measurements on limbs of diabetic and nondiabetic patients with peripheral vascular disease. Surgery 95:339, 1984.
166. Yao JST: Hemodynamic studies in peripheral arterial disease. Br J Surg 57:761, 1970.
167. Yao JST: New techniques in objective arterial evaluation. Arch Surg 106:600, 1973.
168. Yao JST, Hobbs JT, Irvine WT: Ankle systolic pressure measurements in arterial diseases affecting the lower extremities. Br J Surg 56:676, 1969.
169. Zetterquist S, Bergvall V, Linde B, et al: The validity of some conventional methods for the diagnosis of obliterative arterial disease in the lower limb as evaluated by arteriography. Scand J Clin Lab Invest 28:409, 1971.

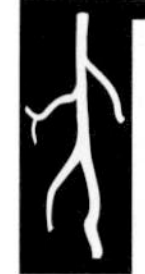

CHAPTER 11

Physiologic Assessment of the Venous System

Enrique Criado, M.D., and Marc A. Passman, M.D.

The diagnosis of venous disease requires a thorough understanding of the capabilities and limitations of the different diagnostic tests available and a knowledge of the disease process under investigation. The physiologic assessment of venous disease offers information about the presence of venous obstruction, and about thrombus or reflux in the limb as a whole or in individual venous segments.

Most current physiologic tests for venous disease rely on the evaluation of limb volume changes using different techniques that measure extremity venous emptying and venous refill patterns. Direct venous imaging using ultrasonography has an advantage over physiologic testing, in that it eliminates the uncertainty regarding the location and extent of the obstruction or valvular incompetence. Duplex ultrasonography provides anatomic information regarding size, location and number of main venous trunks, presence of lumen obstruction, and possible sources of external compression. Additionally, duplex ultrasonography provides physiologic information of venous flow patterns and functional integrity of valves in individual venous segments.

Duplex ultrasonography, therefore, is the most reliable tool for the diagnosis of venous disease and, without doubt, the most widely used and accurate test for the diagnosis of deep venous thrombosis (DVT) and valvular incompetence. For these reasons, most physiologic tests for the diagnosis of DVT have been abandoned in favor of duplex scanning and are of historical or academic interest. On the other hand, physiologic venous testing has gained an important role in the evaluation of chronic venous insufficiency in combination with duplex scanning. Venous duplex scanning is discussed separately in Chapter 13.

In this chapter, we focus on the various physiologic tests for venous disease and mention only some aspects of the physiologic assessment of venous disease using duplex scanning. Our discussion of physiologic testing is in two parts: (1) application in the diagnosis of deep vein thrombosis and (2) application in the diagnosis of chronic venous insufficiency.

DEEP VENOUS THROMBOSIS

The physiologic evaluation of DVT can be divided into two general areas:

1. Venous hemodynamic tests, including continuous wave Doppler ultrasound, venous plethysmography, phleborheography, and thermography.
2. Tests based on thrombus detection, including radionuclide tests and D-dimer testing.

Although venous duplex scanning has replaced most of these tests, these physiologic studies provide important understanding of the pathophysiologic alterations caused by venous thrombosis. The use of venous duplex scanning, computed tomographic (CT) imaging, magnetic resonance imaging (MRI), and venography is discussed in Chapters 13, 14, 15, and 17, respectively.

Continuous Wave Doppler Ultrasonography

The application of transcutaneous Doppler ultrasound for the diagnosis of DVT is based on the measurement of venous flow patterns. With a continuous wave Doppler device, a transducer containing two piezoelectric crystals mounted side by side is coupled to the skin with ultrasonic gel over the vein under investigation. One crystal transmits a continuous ultrasonic signal in the range of 5 to 12 MHz, and the second crystal receives the reflected sound waves. A shift in the transmitted frequency occurs when the initial signal is reflected from the moving red blood cells within the vein, allowing detection of blood flow. The reflected frequency is *increased* if motion is toward the probe and *decreased* if motion is away, by an amount that is linearly related to red blood cell velocity. This difference is expressed as an audible signal or recorded graphically and allows detection of the direction of the blood flow.

Studies are performed with the patient relaxed in the supine, reversed Trendelenburg position to facilitate venous dilation of the dependent extremity. Slight external rotation and abduction of the hip or shoulder and flexion of the knee or elbow allow access to veins and avoid venous compression by normal anatomic structures. Coupled to the skin through an ultrasonic gel medium, the Doppler probe is placed lightly over the vein being studied. During examination of the superficial veins, pressure on the skin is avoided to prevent collapse of the underlying vein and only moderate pressure is applied during study of the deep veins. In the lower extremity, the deep venous system, including the common femoral, femoral, popliteal, and posterior tibial veins, are insonated and differentiated from adjacent arteries. The superficial veins, including the greater saphenous vein in the thigh and calf, and the lesser saphenous vein are also studied. In the upper extremity, the subclavian, axillary, brachial, cephalic, and basilic veins are examined.

Normal venous flow has spontaneous variability and is phasic with respiration, corresponding to a low-pitched phasic Doppler signal, which can be detected in each vein segment of the lower extremity down to the greater saphenous vein at the ankle or the upper extremity down to the cephalic vein in the forearm. In the lower extremity, venous flow decreases with inspiration and increases with expiration (Fig. 11–1*A*). During *inspiration,* intra-abdominal pressure increases with compression of the inferior vena cava, resulting in decreased lower extremity venous outflow. During *expiration,* intra-abdominal pressure falls, with emptying of the lower extremity veins into the inferior vena cava. A Valsalva maneuver causes cessation of spontaneous phasic venous flow, with initial flow augmentation on release, followed by a return to normal phasic flow. The opposite occurs in the upper extremity veins, with increased venous flow during early inspiration owing to increased negative intra-thoracic pressure, whereas decreased flow occurs during expiration when intrathoracic pressure increases.

Additional retrograde cardiac pulsations may also be detected, superimposed on the phasic venous flow, and are more prominent in the upper than lower extremity (Fig. 11–1*A*). However, these respiratory variations are dependent on the patient's position, with venous flow increasing on inspiration and decreasing on expiration in both the upper and lower extremities for a person in the upright position (Fig. 11–1*B*).

Obstruction of a vein is characterized by absence of normal spontaneous venous flow or by loss of phasic variation with respiration. If the Doppler probe is placed directly over an obstruction, there is complete absence of spontaneous flow (Fig. 11–2*B*). If the probe is placed below the site of obstruction, there is loss of phasic changes in venous flow with respiration, corresponding to a monophasic, low-frequency signal (Fig. 11–2*C*). Several maneuvers (including deep breathing, Valsalva, active plantar flexion or hand squeezing, and manual distal compression of the calf or forearm) produce augmentation of venous flow. Compression of a normal vein distal to a probe produces flow augmentation; compression proximal to a probe decreases or stops flow, with flow augmentation on release. In the presence of venous thrombosis, compression of the vein distal to the obstruction results in no augmentation of flow (Fig. 11–2*D*).

Venous Doppler ultrasound examination is safe, portable, inexpensive, and reasonably accurate. Validation studies of continuous wave Doppler ultrasound, in contrast to phle-

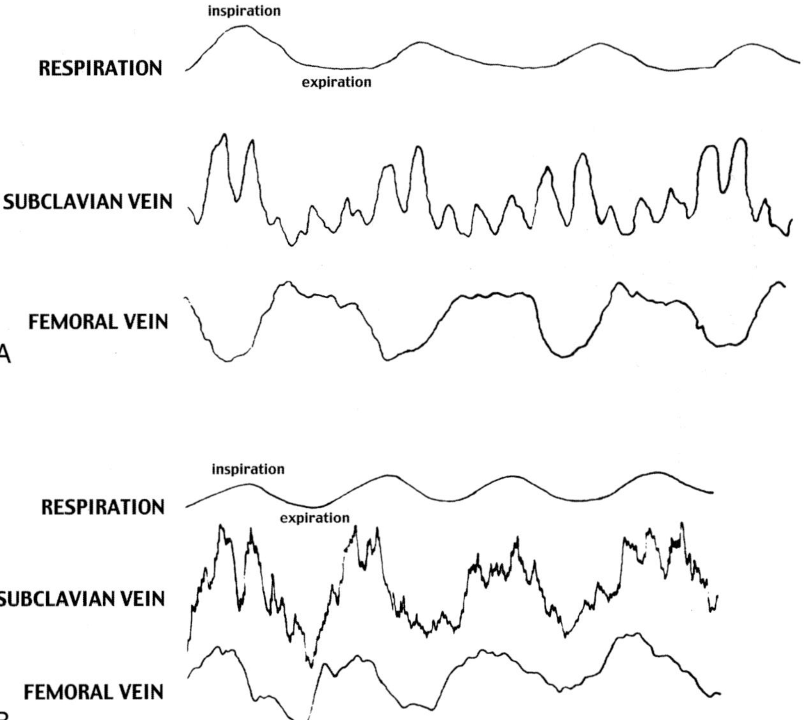

FIGURE 11–1. Doppler signal in the subclavian and femoral veins recorded simultaneously with respiration in the horizontal (*A*) and vertical (*B*) positions. (Adapted from Lewis JD: Venous occlusions and incompetence in the lower limb: A study with a directional Doppler. *In* Reneman RS [ed]: Cardiovascular Applications of Ultrasound. New York, Elsevier North Holland-Biomedical Press, 1974, p 371.)

bography, for lower extremity DVT report a sensitivity of 31% to 96% and a specificity of 51% to 94%.[11, 36, 39, 67, 81, 116, 121, 123, 139] This wide variation may reflect different study populations and techniques as well as duration of the thrombotic process. Although most studies suggest that Doppler ultrasound is more accurate for femoral and popliteal DVT than for calf vein thrombosis, Sumner and Lambeth[123] reported a sensitivity and specificity of 94% and 90% for above-knee DVT and 91% and 84% for below-knee DVT, respectively. Similarly, Barnes and associates[11] reported a sensitivity of 94% and specificity of 78% for below-knee thrombosis.

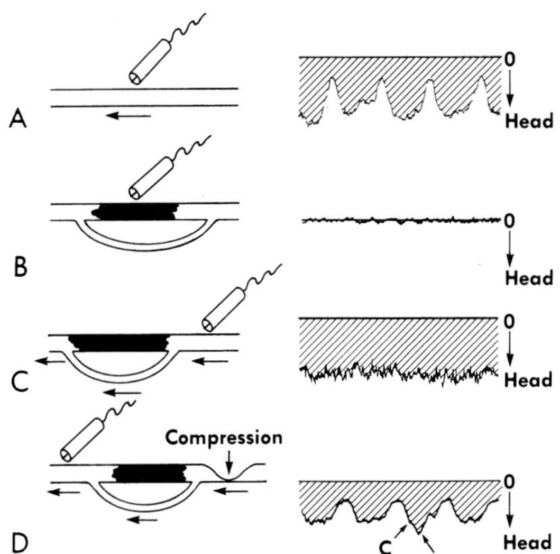

FIGURE 11–2. Changes in venous flow pattern produced by an obstructing thrombus. *A,* No obstruction, normal flow pattern. *B,* Probe over the obstruction. *C,* Probe distal to the obstruction. *D,* Lack of augmentation when the vein is obstructed distal to the probe.

Several other limitations are present with venous Doppler ultrasound:

1. Improved accuracy and reproducibility require the examiner to possess expertise and experience with the venous Doppler techniques.[78]
2. Doppler ultrasound can detect only thrombi in the major deep veins that are in continuity from the distal extremity to the heart. Tributaries such as the internal iliac, deep femoral, peroneal, gastrocnemius, and soleal veins are inaccessible, and isolated thrombi will be missed.
3. For a thrombus to be detected, the thrombus must sufficiently occlude the lumen to produce a flow disturbance; therefore, nonocclusive thrombi may be missed because venous flow is still present.[36, 52, 78]
4. Anatomically adjacent collateral or duplicate veins can be mistaken for normal, occluded deep veins.
5. Doppler techniques cannot distinguish external compression from internal thrombosis.[73, 106]
6. Venous flow is altered in patients with conditions such as severe congestive heart failure or tricuspid valve insufficiency, with increased cardiac pulsations superimposed on the venous signal.[73]

Because of these limitations, continuous wave Doppler ultrasound for the diagnosis of DVT has largely been replaced with venous duplex scanning, which combines many of the same Doppler principles and criteria, already discussed, with real time B-mode and color flow ultrasound imaging (see Chapter 13).

Venous Plethysmography

Plethysmography is a noninvasive method of detecting blood volume changes in an extremity. It is dependent on hemodynamic principles of volume displacement and venous capacitance. Although several techniques have been described, including strain-gauge plethysmography, impedance plethysmography, segmental air plethysmography, and photoplethysmography (light reflection rheography), they are all based on these same physiologic principles.

With the patient in the supine position, lower extremity veins are not completely filled and are able to accommodate increased blood volume before reaching maximal capacitance. With normal venous outflow, positional change or release of an externally inflated cuff will result in rapid emptying of the leg veins (Fig. 11–3*A*). In the presence of venous obstruction, the peripheral venous pressure is already elevated with an increased baseline venous volume, and maximal venous capacitance is reached with smaller volume changes. With increased venous outflow resistance, venous emptying with leg elevation or rapid release of the cuff results in slower emptying of leg veins (Fig. 11–3*B*). Resistance to venous outflow is also dependent on the relationship between venous filling and the percentage of normal venous cross section that is patent (Fig. 11–4).

Strain-Gauge Plethysmography

Strain-gauge plethysmography uses a polymeric silicone (Silastic) conductor tube filled with mercury or indium-gallium. This tube is connected to a plethysmograph via electrical contacts at each end through which a small electrical current is applied (Fig. 11–5). As the strain-gauge is stretched by a change in calf circumference, resistance through the alloy conductor tube increases and voltage change is recorded.

The strain-gauge is automatically calibrated with an electrical signal so that a 1% change in gauge resistance corresponds to a 1% change in limb volume (corresponding to milliliters per 100 milliliters of calf volume). With the patient in the supine position, the lower extremity is slightly elevated to facilitate venous drainage and externally rotated at the hip and flexed at the knee. The leg is supported under the thigh and foot so that the calf is approximately 30 degrees above the examination table. The strain-gauge is placed circumferentially around the calf at the point of maximal diameter. A wide pneumatic cuff is placed around the thigh and is inflated to 50 mmHg for approximately 2 minutes or until the recorded tracing reaches a plateau. The cuff is rapidly deflated, and the decrease in limb volume is recorded.

Venous volume (VV) is defined as the increase in limb volume above the baseline value with cuff inflation, and *maximal venous outflow* (MVO) is measured as the tangent to the steepest portion of the downslope of the venous outflow curve that is recorded after cuff deflation. An alternate method for calculating MVO involves measuring the segment of venous outflow curve during the 0.5- to 2.0-second interval after cuff deflation to avoid measurement error from rapid emptying of venous collaterals in patients with DVT.[28] Although increase in VV averages approximately 2% to 3% above baseline for normal limbs, compared with less than 2% for limbs with acute DVT, VV is unreliable as a single diagnostic criterion, with MVO being more reliable and accurate.[9, 50]

Barnes and associates[9, 10] reported a MVO for normal volunteers of 45 ± 18 ml/100 ml/min compared to 13 ± 7 ml/100 ml/min for iliofemoral DVT, 11 ± 4 ml/100 ml/min for femoropopliteal DVT, and 20 ± 16 ml/100 ml/min for calf DVT. With a MVO of less than 20 ml/100 ml/min used as a diagnostic criterion, sensitivity was 90% for above-knee DVT and 66% for below-knee DVT and the overall specificity was 81%. Pini and associates[99] reported a sensitivity of 97% for proximal DVT and 60% for distal DVT. The overall specificity was 96% using similar MVO

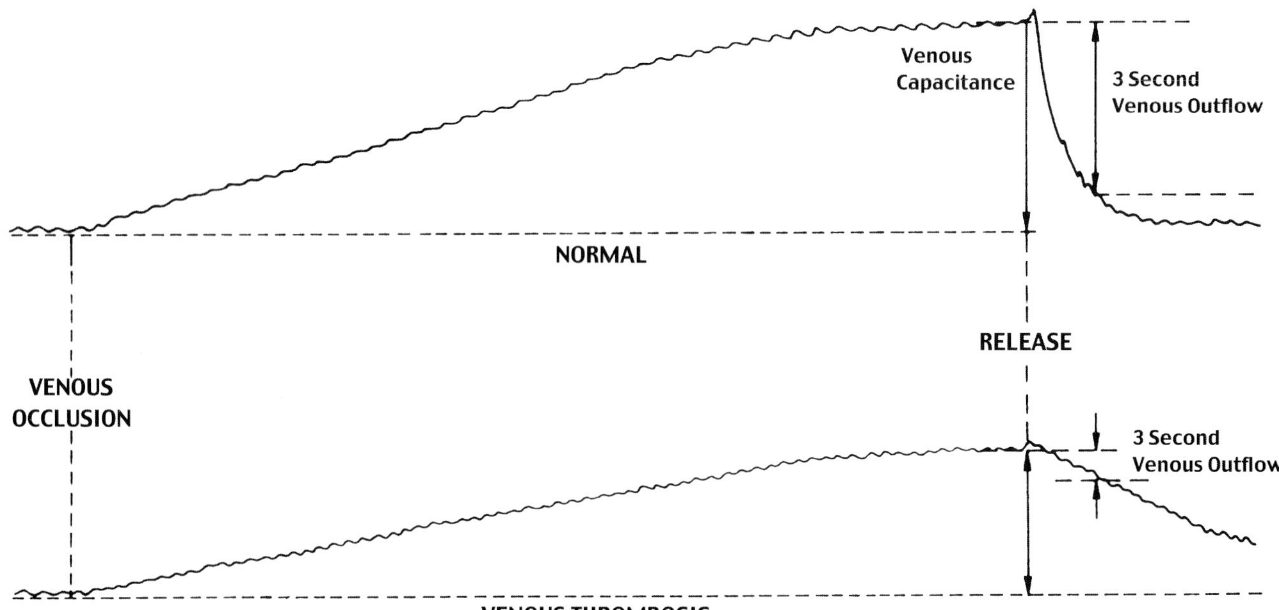

FIGURE 11–3. Impedance plethysmography tracing with difference in venous capacitance and 3-second venous outflow for normal extremities *(upper)* and in the presence of deep venous thrombosis *(lower)*. (From Wheeler HB, Anderson FA Jr: Diagnosis of deep vein thrombosis by impedance plethysmography. *In* Bernstein EF [ed]: Vascular Diagnosis, 4th ed. St. Louis, Mosby–Year Book, 1993, pp 820–829.)

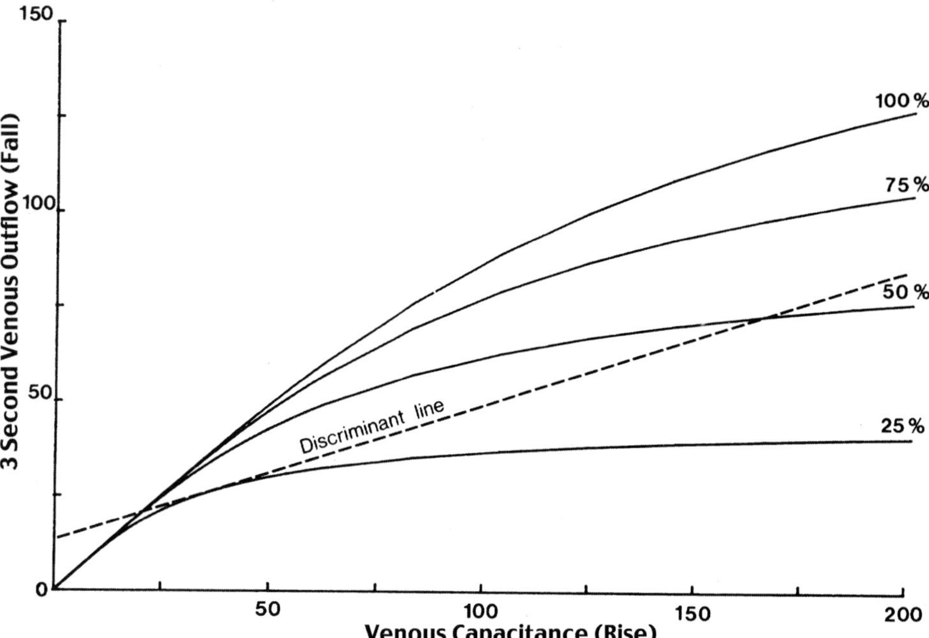

FIGURE 11–4. Relationship between 3-second venous outflow and venous capacitance with different percentages of venous outflow obstruction. (From Wheeler HB, Anderson FA: Detection of deep vein thrombosis by impedance plethysmography. *In* Aburahma AF, Diethrich EB [eds]: Current Noninvasive Vascular Diagnosis. Littleton, Mass, PSG Publishing Company, 1988, pp 283–296.)

criteria and a calculated MVO multiplied by venous capacitance (VC) index.

Another method uses a discriminate line chart plotting *venous capacitance* (VC), which is defined as the maximum height in millimeters above the calibrated baseline of the tracing prior to deflation, against *venous outflow* (VO), the difference in height of the tracing at 0.5 second and at 2.0 seconds after deflation divided by time elapsed (min). Using this method, Cramer and associates[14] showed that the VO/VC ratio maintained a sensitivity of 100% and specificity of 92% for acute DVT.

Use of strain-gauge plethysmography for upper extremity DVT has also been described. Zufferey and colleagues[143] reported a mean MVO of 162 ± 52 ml/100 ml/min in normal upper extremities compared to 79 ± 30 ml/100 ml/min in arms with acute DVT, suggesting a diagnostic limit of 110 ml/100 ml/min.

Inaccuracies with strain-gauge plethysmography result from the presence of nonocclusive thrombi or well-developed collaterals, which tend to increase venous outflow and falsely elevate MVO. Prolonged recumbency, postural changes, muscle wasting, arterial disease, or cardiac failure tend to alter venous filling, leading to measurement error.

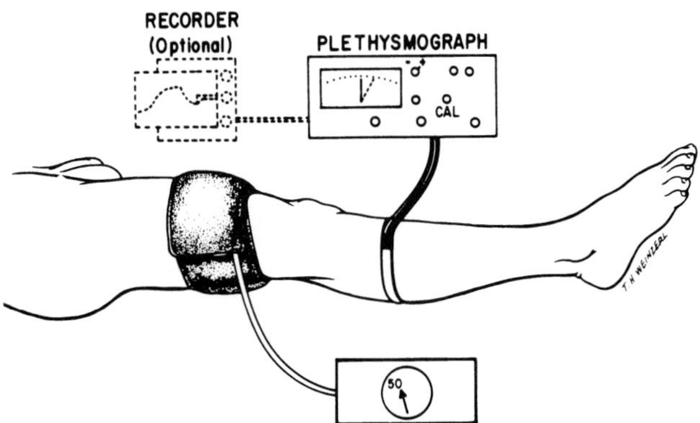

FIGURE 11–5. Venous plethysmography with mercury strain-gauge applied to the calf to measure limb volume changes after inflation of a proximal thigh cuff.

Impedance Plethysmography

Impedance plethysmography measures changes in the electrical resistance (impedance) of the extremity, which indirectly reflects changes in limb fluid volume. When the blood volume of the extremity is increased, the resistance to an electrical current decreases proportionately and is measured by the voltage change between two electrodes applied to the limb, with resistance calculated according to Ohms' Law:

$$\text{voltage} = \text{current} \times \text{resistance}$$

For examination of the lower extremity, patient position is similar to that used for strain-gauge plethysmography, with external rotation at the hip and flexion at the knee and 30-degree leg elevation to facilitate venous drainage. Two electrodes attached to a plethysmograph are placed 10 to 15 cm apart on the calf, and a pneumatic cuff is placed on the thigh (Fig. 11–6). For examination of the upper extremity, a standard pneumatic cuff is placed around the middle of the upper arm and electrodes are placed around the forearm. After calibration, the cuff is inflated to 50 mmHg for 45 seconds and then rapidly deflated, although improved accuracy may be seen with increased cuff pressure[113] or with prolonged venous occlusion times of up to 120 seconds.[63] Changes in impedance during cuff inflation and deflation are recorded and plotted as "rise" and "fall" corresponding to venous outflow over a 3-second period after cuff release (see Fig. 11–3). Comparison with an empirically derived discriminant line determines the presence or absence of venous obstruction (Fig. 11–7).[64]

Impedance plethysmography has been found to be a reliable, reproducible, and accurate test for the detection of

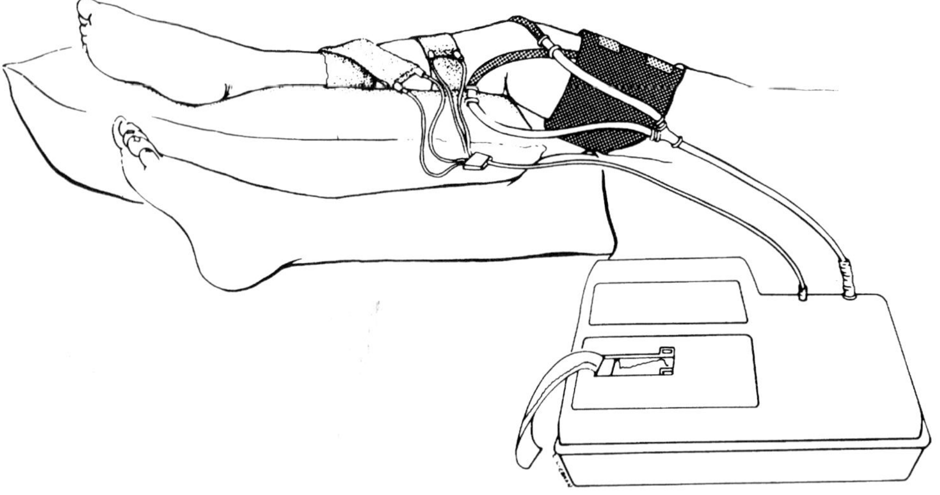

FIGURE 11–6. Impedance plethysmography measures change in electrical resistance between two electrodes applied on the calf, which reflects changes in venous volume produced by inflation of a proximal thigh cuff. (From Wheeler HB, Anderson FA Jr: Impedance plethysmography. *In* Kempczinski RF, Yao JST [eds]: Practical Noninvasive Diagnosis, 2nd ed. Chicago, Year Book Medical Publishers, 1987.)

acute DVT, especially in symptomatic patients with proximal DVT. Hull and associates[63] reported a sensitivity of 93% and specificity of 97% for impedance plethysmography, compared with phlebography for proximal DVT. Diagnostic accuracy fell to 83% for asymptomatic patients, and was relatively insensitive for calf vein thrombosis.

Based on a compilation of published reports, Wheeler[138] compared impedance plethysmography and phlebography from 2561 limbs and reported an overall sensitivity and specificity of 94% for proximal DVT, with an increased sensitivity of 96% in symptomatic patients compared to 90% in asymptomatic patients. There is further evidence suggesting that impedance plethysmography misses a significant number of DVTs in high-risk asymptomatic patients.

Comerota and associates reported a sensitivity of 83% for proximal DVT in patients after clinical diagnosis in contrast to only 33% for surveillance of high-risk patients.[25] This difference can be attributed to the increased presence of nonocclusive thrombi and calf vein thrombosis in asymptomatic patients undergoing postoperative surveillance.[4] Serial testing at 1, 2, 5, and 10 days after an initial normal test may improve accuracy, with increased venous occlusion from propagation of a calf vein thrombosis into the proximal veins or increasing venous thrombus load.[60] Sequential studies can also be used to quantify resolution of thrombus in patients whose initial abnormal impedance plethysmography result has become normal.[61, 66]

Inaccuracies with impedance plethysmography are similar to those with strain-gauge plethysmography. They in-

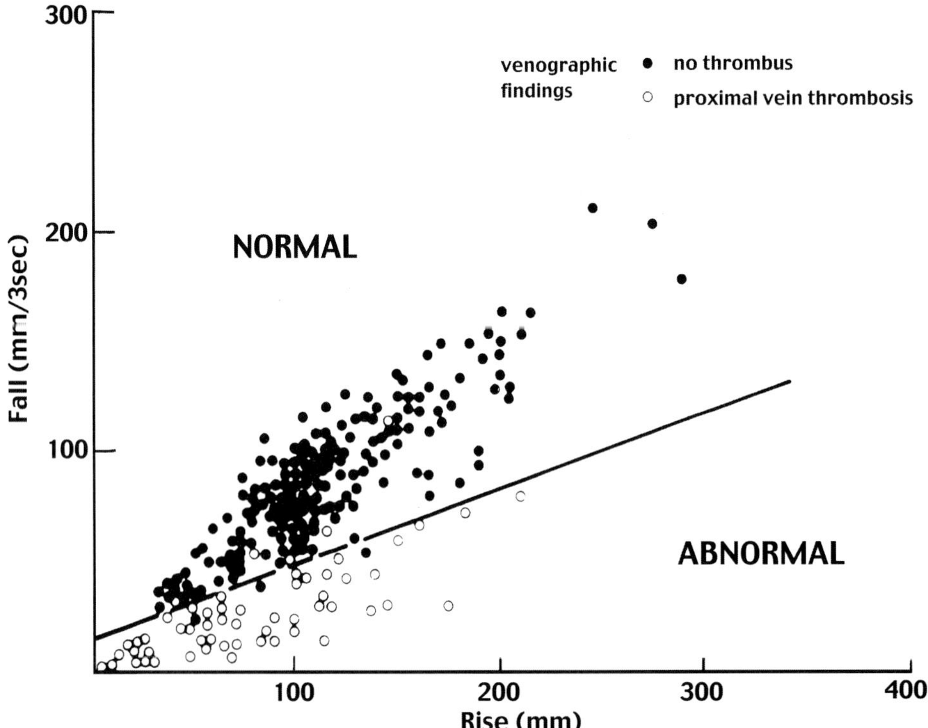

FIGURE 11–7. Plot of impedance plethysmographic results as a function of venous capacitance (rise) and 3-second venous outflow (fall). A discriminant line distinguishes normal limbs from those with proximal deep venous thrombosis. (From Hull R, van Aken WG, Hirsh J, et al: Impedance plethysmography using the occlusive cuff technique in the diagnosis of venous thrombosis. Circulation 53:696, 1976. Reprinted by permission of the American Heart Association, Inc.)

clude any condition limiting venous outflow or causing elevated venous pressure, such as extrinsic compression, severe congestive heart failure, and previous DVT with inadequate collateralization or recanalization. Inadequate venous filling from reduced arterial inflow in patients with arterial obstructive disease or poor cardiac output may also contribute to inadequate study results. Skeletal traction, plaster casts or bandages, obesity, lack of patient cooperation, muscle spasms, or incomplete patient relaxation may further limit examination.

Segmental Air Plethysmography

Segmental air plethysmography, which uses a pulse volume recorder, is another method of measuring changes in venous limb volume. Patient position is similar to that for other types of venous plethysmographic studies. An air-filled plastic sleeve is wrapped circumferentially around the calf or forearm, inflated to a pressure of 6 to 10 mmHg to maintain contact with the limb, and connected to a pressure recorder. Changes in limb volume are reflected as pressure changes within this pneumatic sleeve and are produced after sequential timed inflation and deflation of a proximal cuff to 50 mmHg, allowing measurement of venous capacitance and MVO.

Various diagnostic criteria have been proposed. Nicholas and associates,[86] using a MVO of less than 50% over 2 seconds as diagnostic of DVT, reported a 83% accuracy. Hanel and coworkers,[52] measuring MVO over a 1-second interval after deflation, reported a sensitivity of 77% and specificity of 62%. With a venous scoring system proposed by Raines and associates,[102] which assigns points based on segmental venous capacitance, MVO, venous Doppler signals, and presence or absence of respiratory waves, sensitivity between 76% and 90% and specificity between 66% and 100% have been reported.[59, 109, 115] With discriminant analysis, van Rijn and associates[134] reported a sensitivity of 94% for proximal occlusive DVT but 33% for proximal nonocclusive DVT and 17% for calf vein thrombosis. Gardner and associates described criteria for upper extremity DVT in which a percentage of venous outflow less than 45% during the 1-second interval after deflation accurately predicted the presence of venous thrombosis.[45] With variable diagnostic criteria and inconsistent validation, the clinical usefulness of segmental air plethysmography for detecting DVT of the upper or lower extremity has not been clearly established.

Photoplethysmography (Light Reflection Rheography)

In photoplethysmography, infrared light is transmitted through a diode placed on the skin and reflected light is detected by a photoelectric sensor. The transmitted light penetrates 1 to 2 mm into the skin, is scattered by tissue, and is absorbed by red blood cells. The reflected light varies in intensity and is inversely proportional to the amount of blood contained in the subcutaneous microcirculation, which is indirectly related to the venous volume of the limb.

Light reflection rheography is a modification of photoplethysmography that incorporates three light-emitting diodes centrally arranged around the photoelectric sensor and transmits an infrared wavelength (940 nm) not affected by skin pigmentation. A thermistor allows more accurate measurement of skin temperature, which reduces the variability related to thermoregulatory changes in the subcutaneous microcirculation. The probe is placed on the skin approximately 10 cm above the medial malleolus. The patient is seated in a chair, with legs dependent and feet flat on the floor for 5 minutes. After this interval, the patient performs 10 dorsiflexions over a 15-second period. The test is repeated after a rest period of 3 to 5 minutes.

In the absence of venous obstruction, calf muscle contraction causes a decrease in venous pressure as blood is ejected into the proximal deep veins from the subcutaneous microcirculation, thereby decreasing light reflectivity. In patients with DVT, venous outflow resistance is increased, and the subcutaneous microcirculation fails to empty with calf contraction, resulting in minimal change in light reflectivity (Fig. 11–8). The rate of venous emptying is calculated from the change in light reflection with exercise (R) divided by time (T). A value of $\Delta R/T \leq 0.35$ mm/sec is considered positive for DVT.[82]

On the basis of these criteria, sensitivity for light reflection rheography between 92% and 96% and specificity between 82% and 84%, respectively, have been reported.[8, 83, 128] In a prospective validation study, however, light reflection rheography more accurately predicted the absence of DVT than its presence, suggesting that this technique

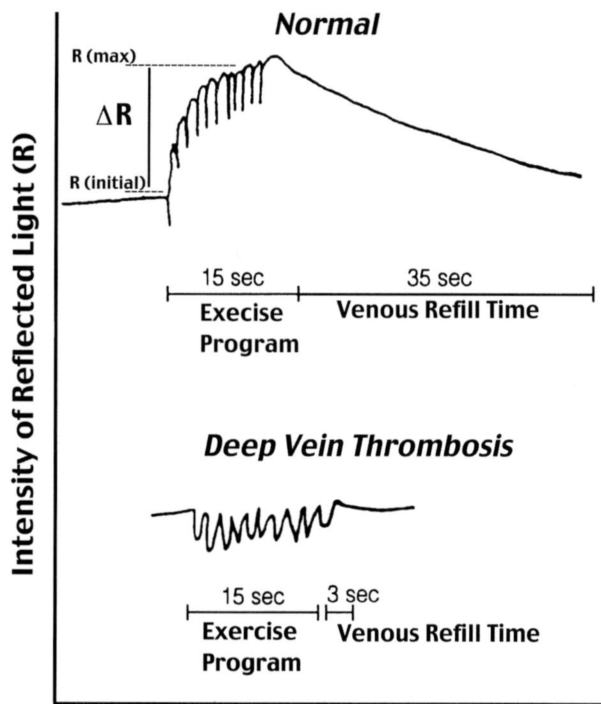

FIGURE 11–8. Light reflection rheography showing light reflectivity for normal limbs *(above)* and in the presence of deep venous thrombosis *(below)*. (From Arora S, Lam DJK, Kennedy C, et al: Light reflection rheography: A simple noninvasive screening test for deep vein thrombosis. J Vasc Surg; 18:767–772, 1993. Reprinted by permission of The Society for Vascular Surgery and International Society for Cardiovascular Surgery, North American Chapter.)

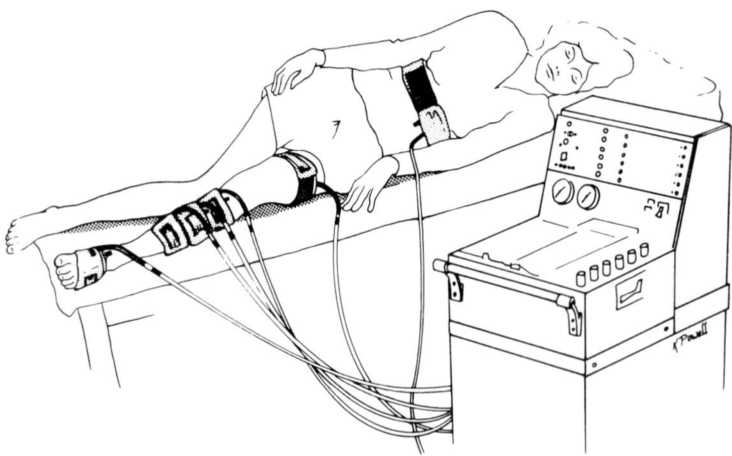

FIGURE 11–9. Phleborheography cuffs applied to the thorax, thigh, upper calf, mid-calf, lower calf, and foot to measure venous volume change in response to respiration and compression of the foot and calf.

may be more useful for surveillance.[1] Although light reflection rheography has also been described for diagnosis of axillary and subclavian thrombosis, reproducible criteria have not yet been validated.[84]

Phleborheography

Phleborheography is a variation of venous plethysmography; it measures phasic volume changes in the lower extremity that occur with the normal respiratory cycle. A normal breathing pattern produces a cyclic decrease in lower limb volume with expiration and increase with inspiration, related to the effect on venous outflow of intra-abdominal pressure from the rising and falling diaphragm. In the presence of deep venous obstruction, these respiratory waves are decreased or absent.

With the patient in the supine, reverse Trendelenburg position, pneumatic cuffs connected to a pressure transducer are placed around the foot, lower calf, mid-calf, upper calf, mid-thigh, and lower thorax. The cuffs are inflated to a pressure of 10 mmHg to maintain contact with the skin (Fig. 11–9).[30] Compression of the foot is produced by repeated rapid inflations of the cuff to 100 mmHg for 0.5 seconds every 20 seconds for three cycles, and this results in emptying of blood from the foot, with no resistance to venous outflow in the normal limb. When venous obstruction is present, foot compression increases limb volume distal to the obstruction and resistance to outflow is noted. With repeated inflation of the mid-calf cuff to 50 mmHg using the same inflation sequence, blood is propelled up the normal extremity and emptied from the foot. Increased volume in the foot and absence of proximal wave propagation indicates venous obstruction (Fig. 11–10).

For upper extremity phleborheography, pneumatic cuffs are placed on the wrist, mid-forearm, upper forearm, and upper arm. Compression sequences are performed at the wrist, and volume changes are measured through the more proximal cuffs. However, because of increased retrograde cardiac pulsations and more extensive collateralization in the upper extremity, interpretation of respiratory waves and compression is more difficult.[118, 122]

Overall sensitivity for phleborheography in the lower extremity has ranged from 79% to 93%, and specificity has ranged from 87% to 97%. Phleborheography is most accurate for proximal DVT in symptomatic patients.[23, 24, 26, 92] Phleborheography is least sensitive for calf vein thrombosis and in asymptomatic patients.[25] Validation of phleborheography in the upper extremity is not as well documented,

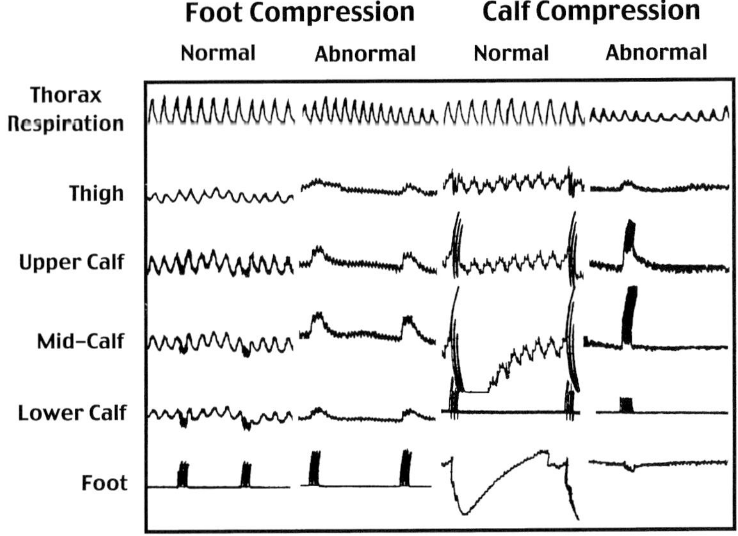

FIGURE 11–10. Phleborheographic tracings from normal limbs and in the presence of deep venous thrombosis with foot and calf compression. (From Cranley JJ, Canos AJ, Sull WJ, et al: Phleborheographic technique for diagnosis of deep venous thrombosis of the lower extremities. Surg Gynecol Obstet 141:331, 1975. Reprinted by permission of Surgery, Gynecology & Obstetrics.)

although sensitivity between 84% and 88% and specificity between 75% and 92% have been reported.[118, 122]

Phleborheography is technically demanding and calls for more experience in performance and interpretation than other venous plethysmographic techniques. It is also limited by the same sources of error as other venous plethysmographic tests, including patient cooperation, muscle spasm, and extrinsic venous compression.

Thermography

Venous thrombosis produces an inflammatory reaction with release of vasoactive substances, causing a microcirculatory hyperemic response and increase in local skin temperature of up to 2°C.[27, 28] This temperature change may not be evident clinically, but it can be detected with thermographic techniques.

A scanning camera with an indium antimonid or cadmium mercury telluride infrared detector is used. The patient is examined in both supine and prone positions, with the legs slightly elevated to prevent venous pooling. The patient's temperature is allowed to equilibrate to ambient room temperature, which should not exceed 20°C, to decrease artifact from vasodilation or sweating, and the examination should be performed in a place absent of air currents. The lower extremities are imaged segmentally with the thermographic camera, which records gray scale images on a video monitor.[27, 28] An alternative method uses liquid crystal detectors applied directly to the leg that respond to different temperatures by emitting light of different wavelengths.[110]

A normal scanning thermogram shows an even distribution of temperature throughout the limb, with anatomic cool zones noted over the patella and surface of the tibia. A gradual temperature gradient is noted moving toward the warmer proximal portion of the extremity. In the presence of DVT, a diffuse area of elevated temperature is observed in the calf or thigh, with loss of patellar and tibial cooling.[14, 27, 28] Liquid thermograms are considered abnormal if an area of increased temperature is noted in the symptomatic limb compared with the normal side.[110]

Validation of thermography with both infrared scanning and liquid crystal techniques has yielded variable results; sensitivity has ranged from 75% to 95%, specificity from 20% to 90%.[5, 14, 28, 51, 58, 107, 110, 117] Any condition that raises the skin temperature (e.g., trauma, infection, malignancy, hematoma, arthritis, superficial thrombophlebitis, ruptured Baker's cyst) will raise the skin temperature and yields a false-positive result. Conditions such as muscle weakness, paralysis, or arterial insufficiency may lower the temperature, and chronic thrombosis may produce no temperature change. The expensive, bulky equipment and need for ambient temperature control further limits the clinical utility of thermography for routine diagnosis of DVT.

Radionuclide Tests

Iodine 125–Fibrinogen Uptake

The detection of thrombus by uptake of radiolabeled fibrinogen was first described by Hobbs and Davies in 1960[57] and was introduced to clinical use by Kakkar and associates[68] in 1970. The matrix of fresh thrombus is composed largely of fibrin, which is formed from its soluble precursor fibrinogen. The ^{125}I-fibrinogen uptake test is performed with intravenous injection of 100 μCi of ^{125}I-fibrinogen into a peripheral vein, followed by interval measurement along the lower extremity for radiolabeled fibrin incorporation into fresh thrombus.

Thyroid uptake of radiolabeled iodine is blocked with oral potassium iodide, administered 24 hours prior to the test, or with intravenous sodium iodide infused 1 hour before the radioactive tracer is injected. Four hours after ^{125}I-fibrinogen injection, the patient is placed in the supine position with 30-degree elevation of the legs. The radioactivity is recorded via a scintillation counter over the precordium and is adjusted to read 100% and at 5-cm intervals along the femoral vein in the thigh, the popliteal vein across the knee, and tibial veins down the calf to the ankle. Repeated readings are made at 24-hour intervals. The ^{125}I-fibrinogen uptake test result is considered abnormal if activity along the vein relative to the precordium is increased by 20% or more at the same or adjacent point on the leg and findings are persistent for more than 24 hours.

Validation studies have determined ^{125}I-fibrinogen uptake to be a more accurate test for calf vein thrombosis than for proximal DVT. Comerota and associates[25] reported a sensitivity of 81% for calf vein thrombosis in contrast to 63% for proximal DVT in patients who had undergone total joint replacement. As a surveillance test in asymptomatic patients undergoing orthopedic procedures, however, ^{125}I-fibrinogen uptake is not as reliable, with a sensitivity of 49% to 79%.[25, 54, 68, 74, 96, 114] As a test for symptomatic patients, ^{125}I-fibrinogen uptake is also inferior to Doppler ultrasound, venous plethysmography, and venous duplex scanning, with a variable sensitivity of 21% to 83%, although specificity remains higher—between 54% and 97%.[17, 62, 68] Clinical use is further limited by:

1. Failure to detect thrombus in the proximal thigh or pelvic veins because of scatter from the bladder or attenuation from the overlying tissue in the upper thigh.
2. Delay in diagnosis because of the time needed for incorporation of fibrinogen by the thrombus.
3. Risk of donor blood products.

Thrombus Scintigraphy

The ideal radiotracer should bind specifically and rapidly to clot, and it should have a rapid clearance rate so that detection can be made a few hours after injection.[20] Several other experimental methods of thrombus imaging using various radiolabeled tracers deserve brief mention, although few have been promising enough to be available for routine clinical use. A more detailed discussion is beyond the scope of this chapter.

Other forms of fibrinogen uptake imaging include fibrinogen labeled with iodine 131,[19] iodine 123,[35] or technetium 99m,[56] none of which offers an advantage to ^{125}I-fibrinogen, except that ^{123}I-labeled fibrinogen is more accurate for proximal DVT.[35] Antifibrin monoclonal antibody, which binds to circulating fibrinogen before incorporation into clot, has also been developed, but detection of DVT can be delayed more than 48 hours.[119] Fibrin fragments (^{131}I-labeled fragment E1), which bind to fibrin dimers and polymers but not fibrin monomers or fibrinogen, allow imaging of old thrombus, but they may also show some delay in incorporation.[72] Fibrinolysis-based imaging using ^{131}I-labeled or ^{111}In-labeled recombinant tissue plasminogen activator, ^{99m}Tc-labeled streptokinase, or urokinase may also allow visualization of thrombi that are not actively incorporating fibrinogen.[69, 79]

Platelets labeled with ^{111}In have also been used in imaging of thrombi. However, the thrombus must be less than 6 hours old, and successful imaging usually requires a delay of up to 72 hours for adequate platelet deposition.[40] Anticoagulation with heparin may also inhibit platelet deposition, leading to decreased accuracy.[41] Future use of a radiolabeled antiplatelet monoclonal antibody injected intravenously may avoid the tedious preparation required for standard radiolabeled platelets.

Radionuclide Venography

The technique of radionuclide venography uses ^{99m}Tc-labeled microspheres or macroaggregated albumin injected through the small veins on the dorsum of both feet. The patient is supine with legs elevated, and the progression of the tracer is followed up the extremity with a gamma camera. A normal radionuclide phlebogram has a well-defined continuous column of radioactivity converging in the pelvis. Nonfilling areas, delayed progression of tracer, visualization of collateral channels, or residual radioactivity may indicate venous obstruction. When these criteria are used, overall sensitivity has been between 73% and 90% and specificity has been between 70% and 99%, with improved accuracy for proximal DVT than calf vein thrombosis.[13, 37]

An alternative method using ^{99m}Tc-labeled red blood cells involves blood pool measurement, with selective visualization of veins because of their increased capacitance compared to arteries. Although sensitivity and specificity with this technique have been reported as 90% and 93%, respectively, the clinical applicability of this type of radionuclide venography has not been established.[141]

D-Dimer Testing

D-dimer is a plasmin-mediated degradation product of fibrin, in which elevated titers indicate increased fibrin formation and active fibrinolysis. In addition to DVT, conditions such as disseminated intravascular coagulation (DIC), trauma, arterial thrombosis, surgery, or sickle cell crisis can cause an elevated D-dimer level.

Most laboratory assays for D-dimer use a monoclonal antibody against epitopes on the D-dimer fragment that are absent on fibrinogen, fibrin, or other fibrin degradation products (FDPs). The enzyme-linked immunosorbent assay (ELISA) tests use both a monoclonal antibody to D-dimer and a second antibody to either fibrin or fibrinogen to quantitate D-dimer concentrations as low as 30 to 80 ng/mL. Latex agglutination assays use a single monoclonal antibody attached to latex beads to detect D-dimer concentration in the range of 200 to 500 ng/mL but take only a few minutes to perform in contrast to the several hours for ELISA.[12]

Overall sensitivity for D-dimer testing has ranged from a sensitivity of 73% to 100% and a specificity of 10% to 100%.[18, 47, 55, 95, 120, 130] This wide variation reflects the many different techniques available, some of which are operator-dependent, with no consensus for a cutoff point between normal and abnormal. Lack of standardization has made extrapolation and comparison of results difficult. In general, ELISAs are more sensitive than latex agglutination assays, although two newer rapid methods, which use immunofiltration and whole blood agglutination, have sensitivities exceeding 94%.[34, 48] Furthermore, accuracy improves with increasing D-dimer levels corresponding to increasing extent of DVT on venograms.[18] The clinical role of D-dimer testing, alone or in combination with other diagnostic studies for DVT, has yet to be determined, but it is limited principally by its low specificity.

CHRONIC VENOUS INSUFFICIENCY

The fundamental pathophysiologic derangement found in patients with chronic venous insufficiency is persistent elevation of the venous pressure at rest and during exercise. This sustained increase in venous pressure is secondary to failure of the calf muscle pump mechanism to empty the lower extremity veins adequately. Failure of the calf muscle pump function may be caused by valvular incompetence, venous obstruction, calf muscle impairment, or a combination of these factors. The diagnosis of chronic venous insufficiency, therefore, should be directed toward the evaluation of these problems and determination of how each one contributes to the severity of chronic venous insufficiency.

The diagnostic evaluation is both functional and anatomic. The investigation should (1) determine whether the patient has valvular reflux, venous outflow obstruction, or both; (2) quantitate the severity of each; and (3) precisely localize which venous segments are involved in each problem. Valvular incompetence is the prevailing physiologic problem in patients presenting with chronic venous insufficiency. The majority of patients (>90%) with advanced venous insufficiency who present with skin changes or ulceration (class IV, V, and VI chronic venous insufficiency, according to the Society for Vascular Surgery/International Society for Cardiovascular Surgery [SVS/ISCVS] reporting standards on venous disease[101]) have valvular incompetence as the prevailing problem, whereas only a minority have venous obstruction as an isolated underlying cause.[53, 70, 77]

The old, widespread concepts that chronic venous insufficiency leading to skin ulceration is always secondary to deep vein pathology and that superficial venous incompetence is rarely the cause are no longer sustainable. It has been shown that more than one third of patients with skin ulceration from chronic venous insufficiency have valvular incompetence confined to the superficial veins, the perforating veins, or both, without evidence of deep vein involvement, and in 50% of those patients, valvular incompetence is isolated to the superficial system.[53] Patients with reflux confined to the superficial and communicating systems can be treated surgically, with predictably good results, whereas patients with deep venous valvular incompetence require complex venous reconstructions, which carry lower success rates and worse long-term prognoses. Therefore, because of the significant therapeutic and prognostic implications, it is important to determine whether the venous reflux involves the deep, superficial, or communicating veins.

Unfortunately, no single diagnostic tool can deliver all of the information required to completely understand the pathophysiology of chronic venous insufficiency. To obtain this information, we currently rely on several diagnostic tests that in combination can provide both anatomic and quantitative functional data. Some tests are purely qualitative (e.g., Doppler venous examination, photoplethysmography), some incorporate precise anatomic and functional information (e.g., duplex ultrasonography), and others assess venous function in a global quantitative fashion (e.g., ambulatory venous pressure measurement, air plethysmography). The physiologic approach to the treatment of the patient with chronic venous insufficiency requires one to know whether there is venous obstruction or valvular incompetence and to what extent the deep, superficial, and communicating systems are involved. The ability to conduct an appropriate workup in a patient with chronic venous insufficiency and to reach a correct diagnosis that will enable optimal treatment depends on the clinician's understanding of the capabilities and limitations of all tests available.

The laboratory evaluation insufficiency has evolved significantly. However, despite the improvements made in the available technology, reliable and accurate quantitation of venous obstruction and reflux remain elusive.

Ambulatory Venous Pressure

Venous hypertension, the main pathophysiologic consequence of chronic venous insufficiency, is the net result of venous outflow obstruction, valvular incompetence, or their combination. In 1949, Pollack and Wood[100] observed that muscle contraction during exercise increases the blood return from the lower limbs, thus reducing lower extremity venous pressure. They also noted that when walking ceases, there is a gradual return to the resting venous pressure level. Arnoldi and associates[7] demonstrated that variations in venous pressure are identical in the deep and superficial venous systems, which validated the use of superficial foot vein pressure monitoring for the investigation of deep venous hemodynamics.

The *ambulatory venous pressure* (AVP) is defined as the venous pressure in the superficial foot veins after 10 tiptoe exercises performed by the patient in the standing position. Measurement of the AVP reflects the basic hemodynamic derangement present in patients with chronic venous insufficiency and is considered, to some extent, the hemodynamic gold standard for validating the results of noninvasive venous testing and for substantiating the results of venous surgery. The measurement of AVP quantitates the net effect of all hemodynamic factors involved in venous insufficiency, but it does not give any information about the individual components contributing to the problem.

Unfortunately, AVP measurement is an invasive procedure not practical for repeated use or as a screening test. A noninvasive method for estimating AVP has been developed by Zamboni and associates[141] based on a significant linear correlation found between AVP values measured invasively in incompetent greater saphenous veins at the thigh and the vein diameter measured by ultrasonography with and without proximal venous occlusion. In this study, the investigators found that at venous pressures over 20 mmHg, changes in greater saphenous vein diameter closely correlated with changes in AVP before and after 10 tiptoe exercises. By calculating the hydrostatic pressure at rest (distance to the third intercostal space) at the point where the venous diameter was measured, they estimated the AVP based on the change in greater saphenous vein diameter after exercise. This sound approach to the noninvasive estimation of the AVP, however, appears to be observer-dependent and requires further validation of its reproducibility before it can be clinically applied.

We can obtain the AVP by cannulating a superficial foot vein with a 21- to 23-gauge butterfly needle and by connecting it to a pressure transducer and a pen recorder. The resting baseline venous pressure is measured with the patient standing and holding on to a frame to avoid calf muscle contraction. The patient performs 10 tiptoe exercises at a rate of 1 per second and returns to the original resting position, remaining steady as the venous refilling time is recorded. To determine the influence of the superficial and perforating veins on the refilling time, the examiner can repeat the procedure with tourniquets or thin cuffs to occlude the superficial system above the knee, below the knee, or at the ankle. Correction of the refill time with a tourniquet implies the presence of an incompetent saphenous system, perforators above the level of the tourniquet, or both. Failure of the tourniquet application to improve refilling time is interpreted as incompetence of deep veins, communicating veins, or both. Deep venous obstruction may manifest as an increase, rather than a decrease, in venous pressure during exercise or when the resting baseline pressure is exceeded during the hyperemic phase after exercise.

AVP values in normal patients and in patients with venous disease are presented in Table 11–1. Nicolaides and Zukowski[91] found that the highest venous pressure levels are associated with perforator and deep venous incompetence and that competence of the popliteal vein is a major factor in determining the severity of venous hypertension. They also demonstrated the existence of a progression in

TABLE 11–1. RANGE OF AMBULATORY VENOUS PRESSURE VALUES IN NORMAL LIMBS AND IN LIMBS WITH VENOUS DISEASE

TYPE OF LIMB	AMBULATORY VENOUS PRESSURE (mmHg)
Normal	15–30
Varicose veins with competent perforators	25–40
Varicose veins with incompetent perforators	40–70
Deep valvular incompetence	55–85
Deep valvular incompetence with proximal obstruction	60–110
Proximal obstruction with a competent popliteal vein	25–60

Adapted from Nicolaides AN, Zukowski AJ: The value of dynamic venous pressure measurements. World J Surg 10:919, 1986.

the incidence of skin ulceration with increasing levels of AVP (Table 11–2). However, a substantial overlap of AVP values exists between normal limbs and limbs with different clinical categories of chronic venous insufficiency. Despite the value of this test, AVP values are within normal limits in approximately 20% to 25% of patients with venous stasis ulceration.[105] Furthermore, there is poor correlation between AVP measurements and the results of deep valvular reconstruction. These problems imply that other factors may be involved in the origin of skin ulceration in patients with chronic venous insufficiency.

Even with its limitations, measurement of the AVP is now used for validation of new diagnostic techniques, for hemodynamic assessment of the results of deep venous surgery, and for clinical investigation. To improve the predictive value of venous pressure measurement, Raju and Fredericks[105] introduced the concept of a *reflux index*, defined as the product of multiplying the AVP by the venous pressure elevation that occurs in the supine position during a sustained Valsalva maneuver at 30 to 40 mmHg. Using a reflux index of 150 as the discriminant point, these investigators found that 98% of patients with ulcers fell beyond this level, implying that a reflux index below 150 has a 98% predictive value in determining the absence of skin ulceration. Furthermore, they showed that patients with successful valvular reconstructions experienced a significant decrease in the reflux index, whereas those who did not show clinical improvement had increased reflux indices.

The Valsalva-induced foot venous pressure elevation may represent the degree of transmission of venous pressure from the deep to the superficial system. If the communications between the deep and superficial systems are large and incompetent, the potential for pressure transmission is undampened, whereas with small and competent communications, the pressure transmission would be dampened.

In general, although AVP measurement is the most accurate hemodynamic parameter to study venous physiology and venous hypertension, it is only one factor of the complex and still incompletely understood pathophysiology of chronic venous insufficiency.

Valvular Incompetence

Venous valvular incompetence, or *venous reflux*, is produced by the presence of pathologic reverse venous flow that occurs when vein valves are congenitally absent or, more commonly, when valves are damaged by acquired processes, such as the recanalization of venous thrombosis or undue venous dilatation. Reflux can involve any of the valves of the superficial, deep, or communicating veins, and its severity is proportional to the number of valves and venous territories involved and to the amount of blood that refluxes in each vein.

To evaluate venous valvular function appropriately, we must understand the physiology of valve closure. Because venous reflux is, in great part, the result of gravity, it should be measured with the patient in the standing position. A certain degree of physiologic valvular reflux, by the way, is found in normal subjects, and this reflux may become more pronounced during prolonged daily physical activity.[16] On the other hand, our experience suggests that in normal individuals, prolonged standing does not produce significant deterioration in valvular competence or calf muscle pump function.[31] Valve closure does not occur with antegrade flow cessation alone; it requires reversal of flow to a minimum velocity of 30 cm/sec.[131] For this reason, venous valves remain open in patients in the supine position and deep breathing causes valve leaflet wobbling without closure. Reverse flow velocity above 30 cm/sec results in valve closure within 100 msec.

With the patient in the supine position, manual compression of the thigh cannot generate reverse flow velocities high enough to produce valve closure in many cases. Similarly, the Valsalva maneuver generates sufficiently high reverse flow velocities to produce closure of the iliofemoral valves only, but in the limb this maneuver rarely produces enough reflux velocity to elicit valve closure unless the proximal valves are severely incompetent.[131] Therefore, proximal manual compression and Valsalva maneuvers in supine patients are not entirely reliable methods for the assessment of venous reflux. In this regard, Foldes and associates[43] demonstrated that in the supine position, duplex scanning detected reflux in fewer than 30% of 66 venous segments in which reflux was evident during examination in the standing position.

Several tests are widely available to detect the presence of deep and superficial vein valvular incompetence and to quantitate its degree, including:

- Venous refill time measured by photoplethysmography or direct venous pressure monitoring
- Continuous wave Doppler ultrasound examination
- Venous filling index (VFI) measured with air plethysmography
- Descending and ascending phlebography
- Duplex scanning

The ideal test for the assessment of valvular reflux should (1) be noninvasive, (2) precisely define the anatomic location of the incompetent venous segments, (3) measure the degree of reflux in each individual vein, (4) quantitate the global hemodynamic effect of venous reflux on the limb in question, and (5) be technically simple and inexpensive. Obviously, no single test is currently available with all these features; thus, several of these studies must be combined, depending on the questions to be answered in each individual patient.

Ideally, to confirm the validity of a noninvasive test for

TABLE 11–2. INCIDENCE OF SKIN ULCERATION (ACTIVE OR HEALED) IN RELATION TO THE AMBULATORY VENOUS PRESSURE LEVEL IN 251 LIMBS

NO. OF LIMBS	AMBULATORY VENOUS PRESSURE (mmHg)	INCIDENCE OF ULCERATION (%)
34	<30	0
44	31–40	12
51	41–50	22
45	51–60	38
34	61–70	57
28	71–80	68
15	>80	73

From Nicolaides AN, Sumner DS: Investigation of Patients with Deep Vein Thrombosis and Chronic Venous Insufficiency. Los Angeles, Med-Orion, 1991, p 30.

the evaluation of valvular incompetence, one should compare it with a known standard. Unfortunately, descending phlebography, considered as such, has limited value in the assessment of reflux, for reasons explained later. Duplex scanning, and color flow imaging in particular, have become the most valuable tools for evaluating valvular incompetence and are becoming the new standards.

Photoplethysmography

Photoplethysmography (PPG) is an indirect, qualitative, noninvasive method of assessing the presence of venous reflux. It is very popular because of its simplicity, low cost, and ease of performance. Photoplethysmography is based on the emission of infrared light by a diode into the skin and the reception of the backscattered light by an adjacent photoreceptor. It allows continuous recording of instantaneous changes in cutaneous capillary network blood content, identifying reflux by measuring the time required for the skin capillaries to refill after they are emptied.

The procedure involves the application of a phototransducer with double-sided tape to the anteromedial aspect of the lower leg above the medial malleolus. The test is performed as the patient sits with the legs hanging freely. Recording is accomplished, with the patient at rest, to obtain a baseline tracing during five consecutive foot flexion-extensions and, finally, until the tracing returns to baseline level again (Fig. 11–11). The venous *refill time* (RT), or venous recovery time, obtained with PPG tracings measures the time taken to return to baseline capillary fullness at rest after capillary emptying with a standardized calf muscle exercise. The refill time obtained with PPG tracings depends on (1) the efficiency of dermal venous emptying with exercise, (2) the arterial capillary inflow, and mainly, (3) the degree of venous valvular competence. The refill time obtained with PPG tracings correlates closely with the refill time procured by direct venous pressure monitoring; however, it does not correlate with the AVP of the limb in question and therefore lacks quantitative value in terms of gauging the severity of venous reflux.[2, 87]

In the past, attempts to quantitate venous reflux with a calibrated PPG technique showed improved correlation of the refill time with the AVP, but the technique was cumbersome and never gained widespread use.[93] More recent efforts to quantitate reflux using computer analysis of PPG refill time with duplex scanning as the standard were unsuccessful in obtaining good separation between different clinical categories. Furthermore, the best criterion found to separate normal limbs from incompetent limbs was a 95% refill time of 15 seconds, which provided only a 50% sensitivity and an 80% specificity in identifying deep reflux.[112] Venous reflux, as assessed by PPG, is determined primarily by the presence of valvular incompetence in the saphenous system and distal deep calf veins, whereas proximal deep vein incompetence (i.e., incompetence of the common and superficial femoral veins) has little influence on the PPG refill time.[49, 98] The PPG refill time is susceptible to variation, depending on the transducer position in the lower leg and on the type and amount of limb exercise performed during the recording.[108] Furthermore, there is substantial variability in repeated refill times in the same individual and the refill time is related more to the presence of superficial than of deep venous reflux. Therefore, PPG refill time appears to reflect local, rather than global, venous dysfunction.

Despite its limitations, PPG refill time has value as a screening test for venous valvular incompetence. A normal refill time in an asymptomatic limb is a good predictor of venous competence in the superficial, calf communicating, and distal deep venous territories.[87, 98] A shortened refill time that normalizes with a limb tourniquet occluding the superficial system implies incompetence of the superficial system alone or in combination with perforators located proximal to the tourniquet (see Fig. 11–11). If the refill time does not correct with tourniquet application to the limb, it implies the presence of valvular incompetence in the deep system, in perforators located distal to the tourniquet, or in both. The normal value for PPG venous refill time varies from 18 to 23 seconds among different laboratories and depends on the individual exercise protocol and

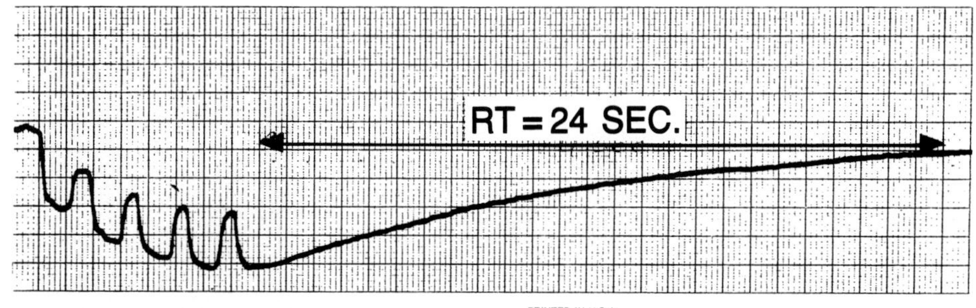

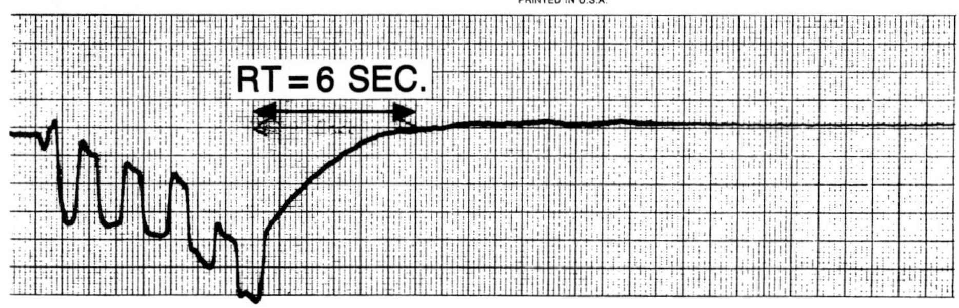

FIGURE 11–11. Photoplethysmographic tracing. After a baseline tracing is obtained, the patient performs five tiptoe movements *(descending sawtooth tracing)*. The recording continues until the initial baseline is reached again. The refill time (RT) is measured from the lowest point of the tracing to the point at which the baseline level is regained. *A,* The recovery time corrects after placement of an above-knee tourniquet to occlude the superficial system, implying reflux confined to the superficial system. *B,* Shortened refill time after five tiptoe exercises.

instrumentation used.[2, 87] For this reason, every laboratory should develop its own data to obtain the value that distinguishes normal patients from patients with venous reflux.

With the advent of duplex scanning, which allows direct assessment of valvular incompetence in combination with anatomic localization of the venous segments involved, the value of PPG for the diagnosis of venous reflux has been restricted. Its main role is in the evaluation of patients with varicose veins, in whom a shortened refill time that corrects with an above-knee or a below-knee tourniquet predicts good results with superficial venous surgery.

Continuous Wave Doppler Ultrasound Evaluation of Reflux

Continuous wave Doppler evaluation of venous reflux is based on the detection of the flow direction in the veins of the lower extremity.[44] Its main advantages are the speed of the technique and the low cost of the instrument. Doppler ultrasound evaluation offers merely a qualitative assessment of venous reflux; it cannot quantitate the severity of valvular incompetence and does not give any anatomic information. It is most suitable for the office evaluation of reflux at the saphenofemoral and saphenopopliteal junctions.

The examination is performed with the patient standing, holding on to a rail to ensure immobility, and bearing weight on the opposite leg to avoid muscle contraction. The saphenofemoral junction is examined with the physician facing the patient, whereas the saphenopopliteal junction is examined from behind, with the patient's leg slightly flexed. The Doppler probe is placed at a 45-degree angle to the skin, and the probe position is adjusted to obtain the optimal venous signal. The venous signal is confirmed by forward flow augmentation elicited with distal manual compression. Reverse flow is assessed during a Valsalva maneuver and coughing, and with the sudden release of distal manual compression.

If no flow, or flow lasting less than 0.5 second, is detected during these maneuvers, one may infer valvular competence in that venous segment; the detection of prolonged flow (>0.5 second) on release denotes the presence of reflux.[90] When reflux is documented with this maneuver, the examination can be repeated with finger or tourniquet compression of the greater or lesser saphenous vein a few centimeters distal to the examination site. If the reflux disappears, it means that the superficial vein is incompetent but the deep vein is competent. If the reflux does not disappear, one may infer that the deep system is incompetent.

This method, in expert hands, has a very high sensitivity and specificity in detecting popliteal vein reflux. However, continuous wave Doppler evaluation of venous valvular incompetence is a very limited test because the probe detects flow in all the vascular structures located in the path of the sound wave, making it impossible to determine in which vessel the reflux signal originated. For these reasons, the use of continuous wave Doppler ultrasound should be restricted to the screening of valvular reflux at the level of the saphenofemoral and saphenopopliteal junctions, and therapeutic decisions regarding reflux should be based on further testing.

Duplex Scanning

The success and experience that have been accumulated with duplex scanning in the diagnosis of DVT since the early 1980s have prompted its application to the evaluation of valvular incompetence. Duplex scanning permits direct detection of valvular reflux in individual veins and allows visualization of valve leaflet motion (Fig. 11–12); it can also quantitate the degree of incompetence by measuring vein cross-sectional area, reverse flow velocity, and duration of reflux, which allows the calculation of the amount of reflux in milliliters per second (Fig. 11–13):

$$\text{flow} = \text{velocity} \times \text{cross-sectional area}$$

Reflux duration in the popliteal vein, measured with the patient standing and with the use of rapid-deflation cuffs in normal limbs, is usually less than 0.5 second.[131] Although 0.5 second of valve closure time is the accepted cut-off value for the presence of reflux, we found[31] that 98.7% of 308 valve closure time measurements in individual venous segments, of normal limbs, under baseline conditions were under 0.33 seconds. The reflux volume at peak reflux velocity, average reflux flow, and mean peak reflux velocity have been shown to be significantly higher in patients with skin changes than in patients without them.[135]

The early experience with duplex scanning for the assessment of venous reflux was based on the identification of individual veins with B-mode ultrasonography and on the detection of pathologic reflux by placing the pulsed Doppler sample volume at multiple sites along the venous segment while performing limb compression and release maneuvers. The initial experience by pioneers in the field was encouraging and revealed an 84% sensitivity and an 88%

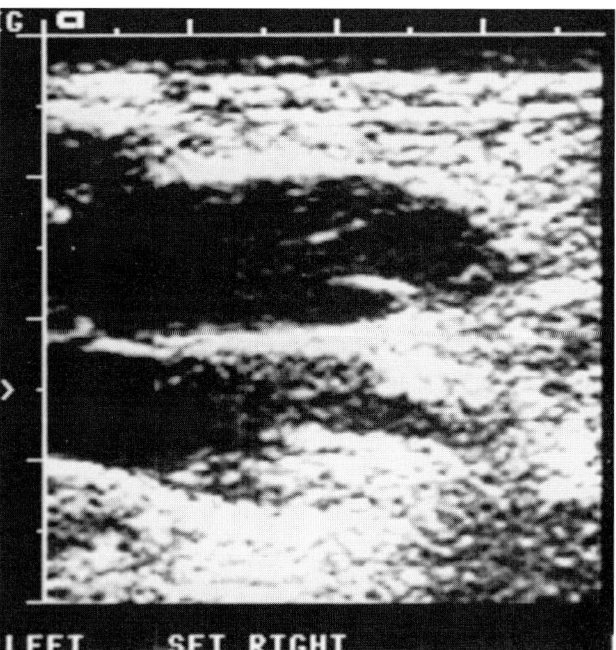

FIGURE 11–12. B-mode ultrasound image of a deep vein with an open valve. Real-time visualization of this segment would allow assessment of valve leaflet motion. (Courtesy of Patty Daniel, R.N., R.V.T.)

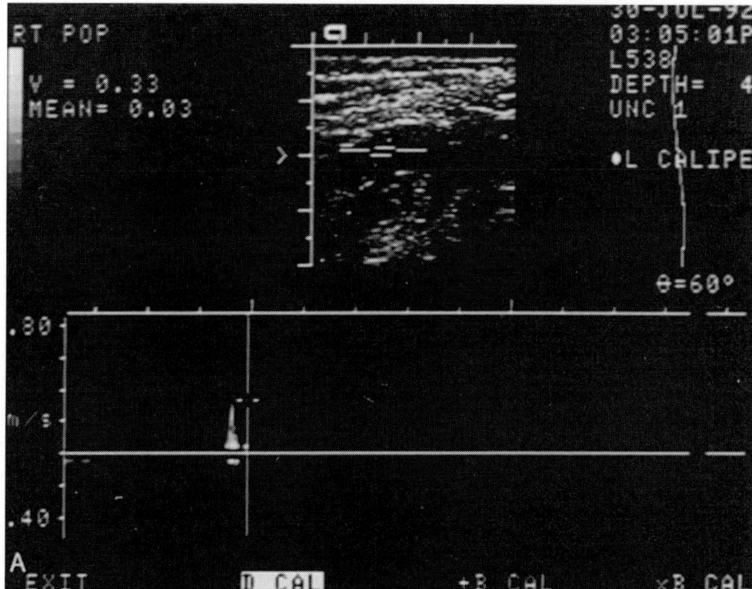

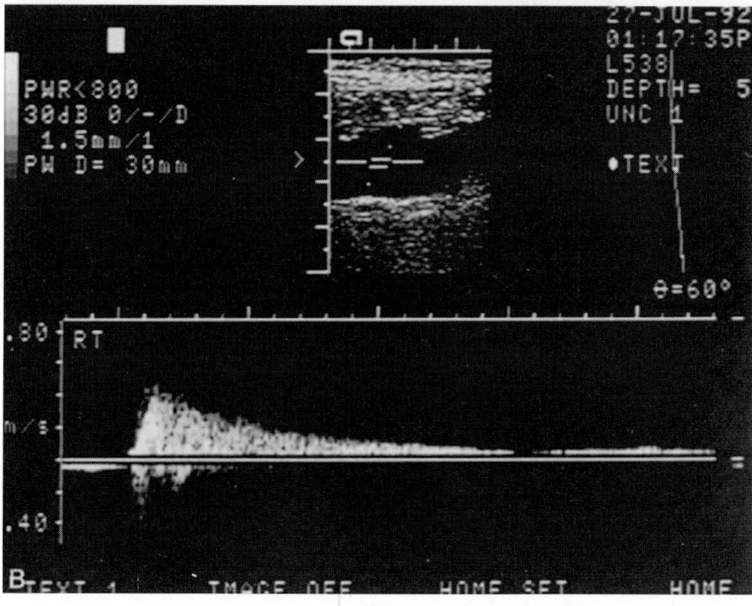

FIGURE 11–13. Popliteal vein reflux flow velocity spectra recorded in the standing position, with reflux elicited with a rapid-deflation cuff inflated to 100 mmHg at mid-calf (reflux flow above the zero line). *A,* Reflux spectrum in a normal popliteal vein in a subject without a history of venous disease. The peak reflux velocity is 33 cm/sec, and the reflux time is 72 milliseconds. *B,* Reflux spectrum of a severely incompetent popliteal vein in a subject with class III chronic venous insufficiency and venographically documented grade IV reflux. The reflux peak velocity is over 50 cm/sec, and the reflux time approaches 3 seconds.

specificity in the diagnosis of common femoral and popliteal vein incompetence.[125] However, the complete examination of all venous systems in both limbs with the use of this technique is time-consuming and inadequate for screening purposes. The advent of color flow duplex scanning has dramatically reduced the time required for this evaluation by allowing real-time visualization of the flow direction without the need for repeated pulsed Doppler sampling (Figs. 11–14 and 11–15; see Color Plate).

Duplex scanning–derived reflux velocity correlates with the clinical severity of insufficiency, as classified according to the Joint Council of the SVS/ISCVS reporting standards on venous disease.[135] Bergan and coauthors[15] showed a promising correlation between reflux quantitation in individual veins and the clinical severity of venous insufficiency. However, duplex scanning does not allow hemodynamic quantitation of overall limb reflux; this requires supplemental testing with air plethysmography and AVP measurement.

The maneuvers used to elicit valve closure during the evaluation of venous reflux are as important as the method employed to document the reversed flow. The standard physical methods of eliciting venous reflux are carried out with the patient in either the supine or the erect position. They include manual compression proximal to the insonation site, release of manual compression distal to the insonation site, and the sudden increase of intra-abdominal pressure with the Valsalva maneuver or coughing. However, these maneuvers have been found inadequate for eliciting reflux.[27] Proximal manual compression of the horizontal limb results not in valve closure but, rather, in prolonged reflux followed by flow cessation. Furthermore, manual proximal and distal limb compression produce such vari-

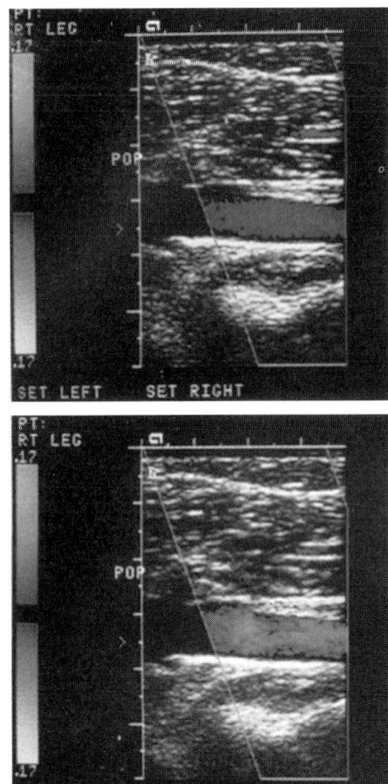

FIGURE 11–14. Real-time imaging with color flow duplex scanning allows quick assessment of venous incompetence by identifying bidirectional flow. In color flow images of an incompetent popliteal (POP) vein, blue hue *(top)* represents flow away from the transducer and red hue *(bottom)* represents flow toward the transducer (reversed flow). See Color Plate.

ability in reflux duration that they do not allow quantitative interpretation.[132] The Valsalva maneuver in the supine position allows physiologic reflux down to the knee level, but when the iliofemoral valves are competent, it does not produce flow reversal at more distal sites.

In regard to the evaluation of reflux in the supine position, valves that clearly reflux with the patient standing may appear competent when the patient is supine and the duration of reflux with the patient in the erect position is shorter than that with the patient supine.[132] It has also been suggested that the reflux assessed with the patient in the erect position correlates better with the clinical severity of chronic venous insufficiency than does that evaluated with the patient recumbent.[85]

The use of rapid-inflation and deflation cuffs with the patient in the standing position provides standardization in the evaluation of reflux, avoiding the variability inherent in the use of manual compression or the Valsalva maneuver. Rapid distal cuff deflation simulates physiologic muscle relaxation and is the most reproducible method available for eliciting valve closure. Pressures of 80 mmHg in the thigh, 100 mmHg in the calf, and 120 mmHg in the foot, with 3 seconds of inflation time and 0.3 second of deflation time, have been suggested as adequate for this examination.[132]

The methodology for the investigation of venous reflux with duplex scanning is currently evolving; nevertheless, it appears essential that the evaluation be performed with the patient standing and with reproducible means used to elicit valve closure. More data are needed on the significance of the duration and the velocity of reflux in individual veins in the evaluation and treatment of patients with chronic venous insufficiency. Despite this, duplex scanning and color flow imaging are the most valuable and promising tools for the assessment of venous incompetence.

Descending Phlebography

The reliability of noninvasive studies in the localization and quantitation of venous valvular incompetence has made phlebography rarely necessary in the evaluation of patients with chronic venous insufficiency. Descending phlebography offers morphologic information on the venous system, assesses valve function, and can identify residual postthrombotic changes and the occasional cases of valvular aplasia. However, it allows visualization of the lumen of only those venous segments that contrast reaches in sufficient concentration, and it can reliably assess the competence of those valves only when contrast is injected in conjunction with maneuvers that produce enough retrograde flow velocity to elicit physiologic valve closure.

The technical aspects of descending phlebography are discussed in Chapter 17. It is important to recognize that because venous reflux is a dynamic phenomenon, static radiographs have limited diagnostic value. To avoid this problem, one can record descending phlebographic images on videotape to permit review of the reverse flow dynamics.

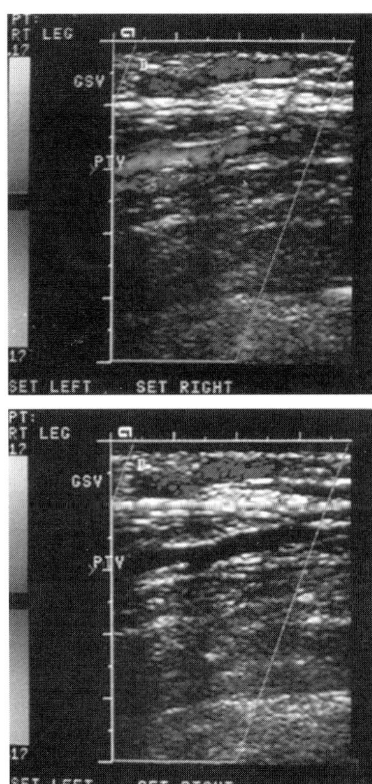

FIGURE 11–15. Simultaneous color flow real-time images of the posterior tibial vein (PTV) and the greater saphenous vein (GSV). *Top,* Both veins show flow toward the transducer (blue hue). *Bottom,* Greater saphenous vein shows no color because flow has ceased, which implies valvular competence in the posterior tibial vein. See Color Plate.

TABLE 11–3. PHLEBOGRAPHIC GRADING OF VALVE REFLUX

Normal valve	Closes completely; no leakage regardless of Valsalva maneuver effort
Minimal leakage	Wisp of contrast goes through the valve with a forced Valsalva maneuver
Moderate leakage	Obvious retrograde flow during a Valsalva maneuver
Severe leakage	Contrast cascades distally without a Valsalva maneuver

Adapted from Kistner RL, Ferris EB, Randhawa G, et al: A method of performing descending venography. J Vasc Surg 4:464, 1986.

The proximal valves located in the common femoral, superficial femoral, deep femoral, and greater saphenous veins are evaluated, and if any of them allows reflux, the distal extent is documented.

Following Kistner and associates,[71] the findings are categorized according to (1) individual valve function (Table 11–3) and (2) the overall extent of reflux (Table 11–4). It is noteworthy that the presence of a competent valve in the distal superficial femoral or popliteal vein that prevents reflux into the calf minimizes the clinical significance of the degree of valvular incompetence.[71] The observation of intraluminal septations and valvular scarring suggests that the cause of the valvular incompetence is post-thrombotic, whereas the absence of luminal abnormalities in a patient without a history of DVT is consistent with the diagnosis of primary valvular incompetence. The evaluation of reflux in the deep femoral vein may have important therapeutic implications because it has been suggested that valvular reconstruction of the superficial femoral and popliteal veins may fail to produce hemodynamic improvement in the presence of uncorrected reflux in the deep femoral vein.[38]

The quantitation of venous reflux based on descending phlebography has shown poor correlation with the clinical severity of chronic venous insufficiency in the limb. In this regard, Ackroyd and coworkers[3] found that 67% of limbs with chronic venous insufficiency that had skin changes, ulceration, or both had no evidence of pathologic reflux and that only 31% of limbs with post-thrombotic changes documented by ascending phlebography had significant reflux on the descending venogram. In contrast, studies done with duplex scanning showed that 87% to 93% of limbs with skin changes, ulceration, or both had valvular reflux in at least one venous system.[49, 53] This discrepancy illustrates the inherent shortcoming of descending phlebography. Descending phlebography is limited by the presence of competent valves in a proximal venous segment because they prevent the passage of contrast, precluding evaluation of the distal segments. Furthermore, in patients without any evidence of deep venous disease, descending phlebography performed in the semi-erect and supine positions, with or without a Valsalva maneuver, demonstrates physiologic reflux into the proximal or distal superficial femoral vein in most cases (grades I and II reflux).[3, 127] This is probably due to the inability of the Valsalva maneuver to elicit effective valve closure in many individuals and to the higher specific gravity of the contrast material (compared with blood) that trickles through relaxed valves by gravity.

TABLE 11–4. PHLEBOGRAPHIC CLASSIFICATION OF REFLUX

Grade 0	No evidence of reflux
Grade 1	Minimal reflux through one or more valves during a Valsalva maneuver
Grade 2	Considerable reflux in the thigh, but a competent valve is present in the distal femoral or popliteal vein
Grade 3	Considerable reflux in the thigh, with leakage through the popliteal vein into the proximal calf
Grade 4	Cascading reflux from the proximal femoral veins into the popliteal and calf veins

Adapted from Kistner RL, Ferris EB, Randhawa G, et al: A method of performing descending venography. J Vasc Surg 4:464, 1986.

Descending phlebography still remains an essential part of the evaluation of reflux for the planning of deep venous reconstruction, and for this purpose optimal anatomic information is obtained by combining both ascending and descending phlebography. Descending phlebography is also indicated in those rare instances when noninvasive studies fail to provide details of valvular competence.

Air Plethysmography

Air plethysmography (APG) is a noninvasive technique that allows detection of lower extremity volume changes in relation to gravity and exercise. Its application to the diagnosis of venous disease is based on the premise that acute changes in limb volume are almost entirely secondary to changes in venous blood content. Although this technique has been available for several decades, it was not until Christopoulos and Nicolaides[21, 22] introduced calibrated air plethysmography in the 1980s that it became useful for the quantitative evaluation of venous hemodynamics.

The air plethysmograph is a fairly simple device consisting of a 14-inch-long inflatable plastic sleeve with a capacity of 5 L. The device is placed around the patient's leg from below the knee to the ankle. The air chamber is connected with plastic tubing to a pressure transducer, an amplifier, and a pen recorder. With the patient supine, the heel resting on a support, and the leg externally rotated and slightly flexed to facilitate venous emptying, the chamber is inflated to a pressure of 6 mmHg to obtain good contact between the sleeve and the limb (Fig. 11–16). With the patient in this position, the examiner calibrates the plethysmograph by injecting a standard volume of air (100 ml) into the chamber, measuring the change in pressure, and withdrawing the same volume again. Once the calibration is satisfactory, the volume changes are recorded during a sequence of exercises to elicit leg emptying with 45 degrees of elevation, leg refill in the standing non–weight-bearing position, calf blood ejection during one bilateral tiptoe exercise and during 10 consecutive tiptoe exercises, and finally refill again in the standing non–weight-bearing position (Fig. 11–17).

The performance of the test requires patient cooperation and fastidious technique to avoid artifacts derived from contact of the air chamber with any object or from muscle contraction in the standing position. A small number of patients cannot undergo testing with air plethysmography because of their extreme leg size or their inability to perform the exercise routine.

From the volume recording, measurements of venous

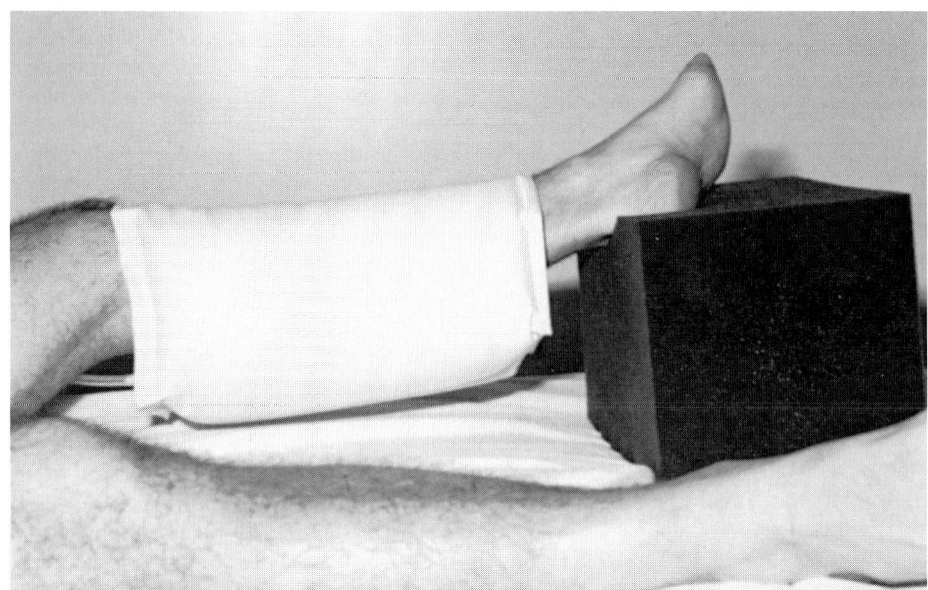

FIGURE 11–16. Calibration of the air plethysmograph. With the patient supine, the heel resting on a support, and the leg slightly flexed and externally rotated, the air chamber is filled to a pressure of 6 mmHg. Calibration is performed by injecting and withdrawing a standard volume of air in the system (100 ml) and observing the variation in pressure on the recording.

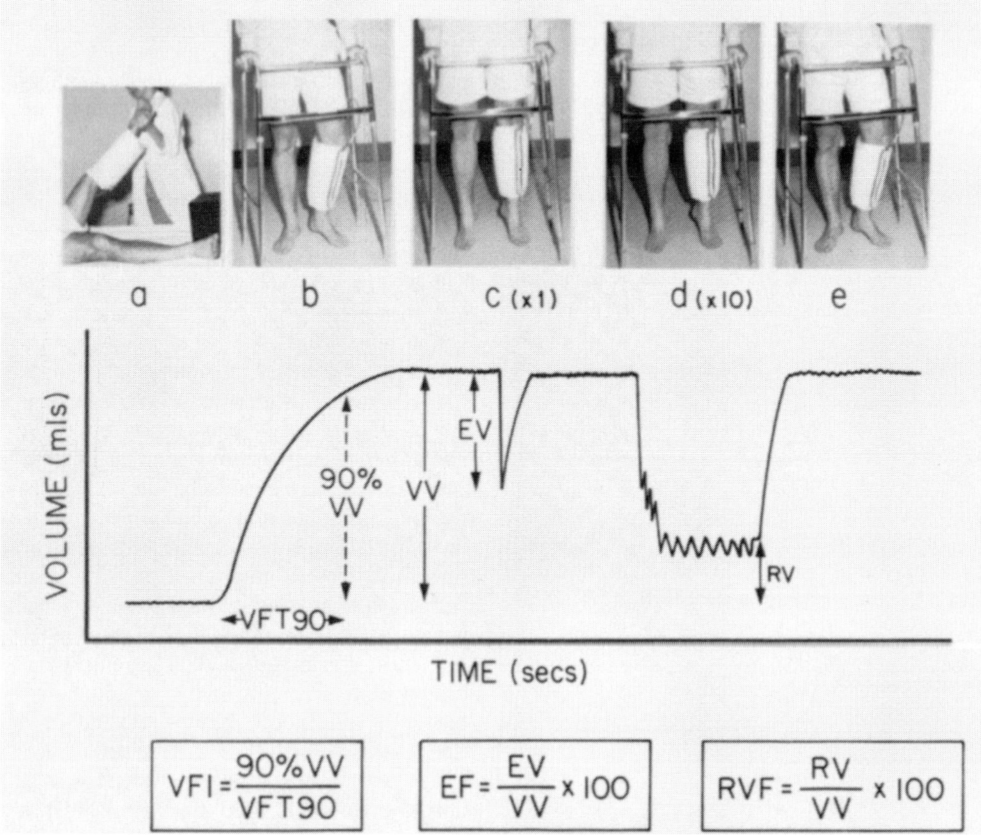

FIGURE 11–17. Limb volume changes recorded during the standard sequence of postural changes and tiptoe exercises performed with calibrated air plethysmography. After calibration, the patient lies supine with 45-degree passive leg elevation with slight knee flexion and external rotation until maximal venous emptying occurs (*a*). The patient stands up without bearing weight on the leg under examination until maximal venous filling occurs (first plateau of the tracing) (*b*). The patient performs a single tiptoe exercise with both legs and returns to non–weight-bearing (*c*). After reaching the second complete venous filling plateau, the patient performs 10 consecutive tiptoe exercises (*d*) and again returns to the non–weight-bearing position as in *b* (*e*). VV, functional venous volume; VFT, venous filling time; VFI, venous filling index; EF, ejection fraction; EV, ejected volume; RV, residual volume; RVF, residual volume fraction. (Courtesy of Cynthia Burnham, R.N., R.V.T.)

hemodynamics are obtained directly or they are calculated. The functional venous volume, venous filling time, calf ejection volume, and residual venous volume are direct measurements; the VFI, calf ejection fraction, and residual volume fraction are calculated values.

- The functional venous volume (VV) represents the increase in leg venous volume from supine leg elevation to the standing position and is given in milliliters. VV evaluates venous capacitance, which tends to be elevated in limbs with chronic venous insufficiency.
- The venous filling index (VFI) is a measure of the rate of venous refill of the limb expressed in milliliters per second, and it evaluates overall valvular competence. The VFI is calculated by dividing 90% of the VV by the time taken to reach 90% of the VV (VFT90).
- The ejection volume (EV) measures the decrease in venous volume (in milliliters) achieved with one tiptoe exercise and represents the volume of blood expelled by the calf with a single calf muscle contraction.
- The ejection fraction (EF) is calculated by dividing the EV by the VV and multiplying the result by 100. This percentage represents the emptying power of one calf contraction.
- The residual volume (RV) measures the amount of blood left in the calf at the end of 10 consecutive tiptoe exercises, given in milliliters.
- The residual volume fraction (RVF) is calculated by dividing the RV by the VV and multiplying by 100 to express the percentage of the total calf blood volume that remains in the calf after 10 tiptoe exercises, which evaluates overall calf muscle pump function.

When the VFI is elevated, the test is repeated with an above-knee tourniquet to assess the influence of the superficial system on the degree of reflux. The coefficient of variability in the measurement on different days of VFI, EF, and RVF is lower than that for VV, VFT, EV, and RV because the latter depend on the daily fluctuations of venous compliance, whereas the former are normalized values not affected by daily variations.[22] The variability of air plethysmography parameters in repeated measurements is significant however, and has been found to range from 7.5% to 27%.[139] It is important to understand, therefore, the inherent variations of these measurements when applied to patient evaluation and to assessing hemodynamic changes following treatment for venous insufficiency.

The initial reports using air plethysmography found a direct correlation between RVF and AVP.[22, 137] Unfortunately, the correlation between RVF and AVP has been poor in other laboratories.[97] Christopoulos and coworkers[22] found that 80% of limbs with venous disease had increased VV and that the VFI was less than 1.7 ml/sec in normal limbs, between 2 and 30 ml/sec in limbs with superficial incompetence, and 7 to 28 ml/sec in limbs with evidence of deep venous disease. Furthermore, they suggested an increasing incidence of skin ulceration with increasing levels of RVF.

Unfortunately, the large amount of overlap in the VFI values does not allow good discrimination between patients with different severities of venous disease.[65, 133] The VFI, however, is a good screening test for the presence of any type of reflux and has been found to have a 100% sensitivity and 90% specificity in identifying venous reflux.[46] An increase in the incidence of ulceration was observed by Christopoulos and associates[21] with increasing levels of reflux and decreasing values of calf EF. However, our experience[32] and that of van Bemmelen and associates[133] suggest that although the VFI offers some prediction of the incidence of venous ulceration, the EF and RVF have no clear effect on the incidence of venous ulceration (Figs. 11–18 and 11–19). On the other hand, Araki and associates[6] found, in a small population, that the presence of an abnormal EF and/or RVF were strong determinants of the presence of ulceration. Welch and associates[136] reported that VFI values obtained with air plethysmography could differentiate normal limbs from those with reflux but could not differentiate between limbs with mild reflux and those with severe reflux as assessed with descending phlebography. In our experience, 82% of the limbs with VFI greater than 5 ml/sec had deep and or perforator reflux, 7% of limbs with a normal VFI (≤2 ml/sec) had evidence of deep and/or perforator reflux by duplex evaluation, while limbs with intermediate VFI levels (between 2 and 5 ml/sec) have a 45% incidence of deep and/or perforator reflux (Fig. 11–20).[32]

In conclusion, the combination of hemodynamic parameters obtained with air plethysmography offers quantitative information about the presence of reflux (VFI), the integrity of the calf muscle pump mechanism (EF), and the overall venous function (RVF).

The application of calibrated air plethysmography to the evaluation of chronic venous insufficiency appears scientifically and medically sound. The experience with this test suggests that the VFI is a useful parameter to quantitate the overall degree of limb reflux. Yet, the EF and RVF obtained with air plethysmography do not have a clear role in the evaluation of patients with chronic venous insufficiency.

Evaluation of Perforator Vein Incompetence

The clinical significance of the presence of *incompetent calf perforating veins* (ICPVs) was initially recognized by Linton.[75, 76] The hemodynamic relevance of ICPVs was documented by Zukowski and associates,[144] who found that in an unselected population of patients with chronic venous insufficiency, 40% of the patients presenting with varicose veins and no evidence of deep venous disease had ICPVs. In 70% of these patients, perforator incompetence had moderate to severe hemodynamic significance whereas in one third, perforator incompetence appeared to be of no hemodynamic consequence. In this study, none of the patients with inconsequential ICPVs had skin changes or ulceration, whereas 68% of those with moderate and 100% of those with severe perforator incompetence had skin changes or ulceration. The normal direction of flow in perforating veins occurs during muscle relaxation and is from the superficial to the deep venous system. However, small perforating veins (<1 mm) that may not harbor valves may allow physiologic bidirectional flow.[111] Calf perforating veins follow a quite constant anatomic distribution and bear one to three valves, which are located deep to the muscle fascia.[33, 129]

The evaluation of calf perforator vein incompetence is

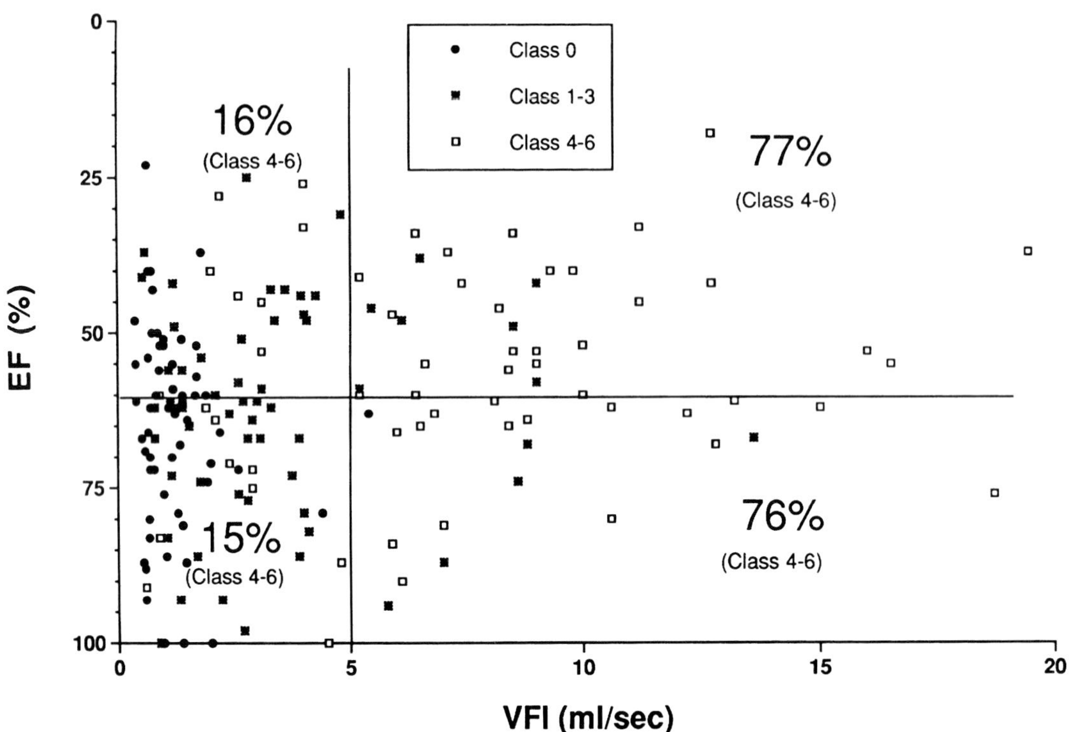

FIGURE 11–18. Combined effect of venous filling index (VFI) and ejection fraction (EF) on the clinical severity of disease. Although the incidence of severe disease is significantly higher ($p < .05$) in limbs with VFI values of more than 5 ml/sec, an abnormal EF value did not produce a significant difference in the incidence of severe venous disease (classes 4, 5, and 6), regardless of whether the VFI was above or below 5 ml/sec ($p > .9$). The percentages represent the limbs with severe venous disease (classes 4, 5, and 6) among limbs falling in that section of the scattergram. (From Criado E, Farber MA, Marston WA, et al: The role of air plethysmography in the diagnosis of chronic venous insufficiency. J Vasc Surg; 27:660, 1998. Reprinted by permission of The Society for Vascular Surgery and International Society for Cardiovascular Surgery, North American Chapter.)

based on the identification of reverse flow from the deep to the superficial system. However, it appears that outward flow in otherwise normal perforating veins can be elicited with proximal limb compression, and it has been suggested that a reliable demonstration of perforator vein incompetence is that of outward flow following the release of distal compression.[111] Therefore, any evaluation method should take these factors into consideration.

Continuous wave Doppler detection of ICPVs was pioneered by Miller and Foote.[80] With the patient in the supine position, tourniquets are placed to occlude the superficial system proximal and distal to the area being examined. The medial aspect of the calf is scanned systematically while distal manual compression and relaxation are performed at each insonation site to elicit bidirectional flow. The presence of a Doppler flow signal during both compression and relaxation of the distal limb would correspond to the location of an ICPV. Using intraoperative assessment of perforator incompetence as the standard, O'Donnell and colleagues showed that Doppler examination is very sensitive in identifying limbs with ICPVs.[94] Unfortunately, this method has a very high false-positive rate in identifying individual incompetent perforators and is not more accurate than physical examination in predicting the presence or individual location of ICPVs.

Ascending phlebography has been a popular method used for the diagnosis of ICPVs and was considered the standard. The examiner injects contrast material into a superficial vein of the foot and forces the contrast into the deep system by applying a tourniquet as low as possible around the ankle.[41] With the patient supine or with the feet slightly down, contrast is injected under fluoroscopy and the study is recorded for later review. The presence of incompetent perforators is indicated by the passage of contrast from the deep to the superficial veins and by the presence of dilatation, irregularity, and tortuosity, which are common features of ICPVs. A tourniquet is placed just proximal to each ICPV that is identified to avoid further filling of the superficial system, which would obscure the evaluation of the more proximal segments. Despite the use of careful technique, as the ascending venogram progresses proximally, most of the superficial and deep systems is opacified by contrast material, making determination of the direction of flow difficult, if not impossible. Using this method, Thomas and coworkers[127] were able to identify preoperatively 81% of the incompetent perforators found at the time of surgery.

Ascending phlebography is associated with a significant rate of false-negative findings in determining the overall presence or absence of ICPVs, an incidence that is even higher at the time of localization of the ICPV site.[40] Although phlebography demonstrates a significantly lower incidence of false-positive findings than does Doppler ultrasound evaluation, neither phlebography nor Doppler evalu-

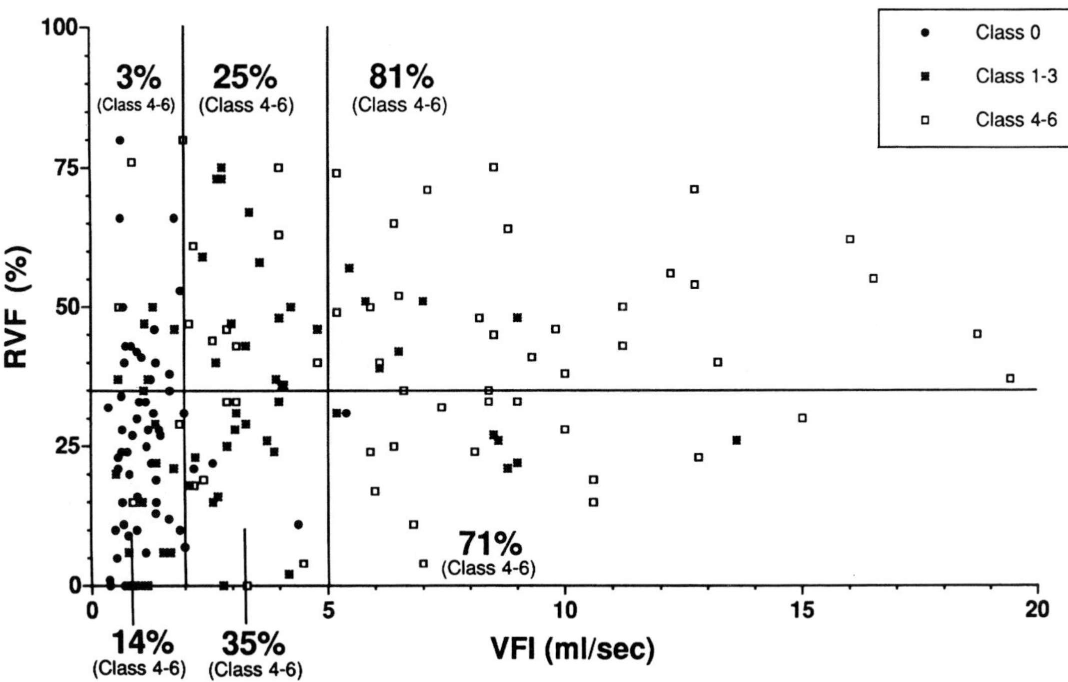

FIGURE 11–19. Influence of the residual volume fraction (RVF) on the severity of disease in relation to the venous filling index (VFI). An abnormal RVF (>35%) did not produce a significant increase in the incidence of severe venous disease (classes 4, 5, and 6) in combination with high (>5 ml/sec) or low VFI values (>2 and <5 ml/sec; $p = .3$ and $p = .67$, respectively). The percentages represent the limbs with severe venous disease disease (classes 4, 5, and 6) among limbs falling in that section of the scattergram. (From Criado E, Farber MA, Marston WA, et al: The role of air plethysmography in the diagnosis of chronic venous insufficiency. J Vasc Surg 27:660, 1998. Reprinted by permission of The Society for Vascular Surgery and International Society for Cardiovascular Surgery, North American Chapter.)

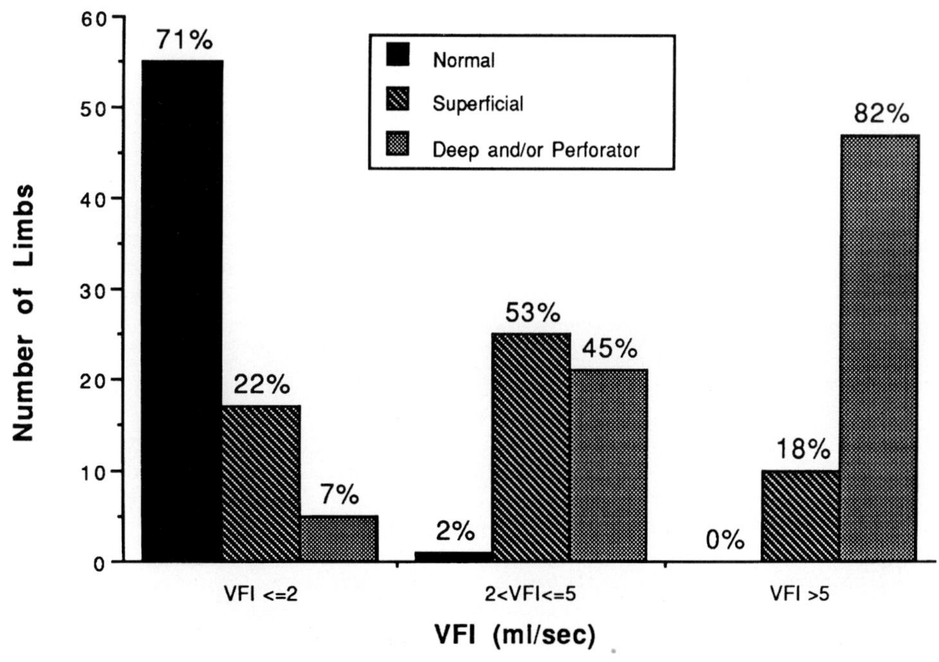

FIGURE 11–20. Type of reflux stratified by level of venous filling index for 186 limbs studied with air plethysmography. The numbers above the columns represent the percentage of limbs with each type of reflux. (From Criado E, Farber MA, Marston WA, et al: The role of air plethysmography in the diagnosis of chronic venous insufficiency. J Vasc Surg 27:660, 1998. Reprinted by permission of The Society for Vascular Surgery and International Society for Cardiovascular Surgery, North American Chapter.)

ation is superior to clinical examination in the diagnosis of the presence or localization of the site of an ICPV.[94]

Duplex imaging can identify both competent and incompetent perforating veins, whereas ascending phlebography cannot visualize most competent perforators. Hanrahan and associates[93] found that duplex scanning identified all perforators seen on phlebography, but duplex scanning classified as incompetent a smaller number of veins than phlebography. This discrepancy was probably produced by the use in this study of vessel size as the sole phlebographic criterion of incompetence; however, a good correlation between duplex identification of competent and incompetent perforators and operative findings was found.

The diagnosis of ICPVs with conventional duplex scanning is time-consuming because it requires placement of the pulsed Doppler sample volume in each vein identified by B-mode ultrasonography to ascertain the flow characteristics of the vessel. Perforating veins are sometimes small and tortuous, and the sample volume size of the pulsed Doppler may exceed the diameter of the vein in question, which may lead to errors in determination of flow direction. The use of color flow duplex imaging overcomes this uncertainty to a great extent and expedites the procedure dramatically. We are unaware of any data comparing color flow duplex imaging with other diagnostic modalities or with operative findings. However, in our experience, color flow duplex scanning can identify ICPVs reliably; unfortunately, the sensitivity of this test has not yet been determined.

The identification of bidirectional flow (red hue alternating with blue) during calf or foot compression maneuvers in a vein traveling fairly horizontally from the superficial to the deep system is diagnostic of an ICPV (Fig. 11–21; see Color Plate). At the onset of calf muscle contraction, flow through ICPVs is from deep to superficial veins; as muscle contraction progresses, flow is partially or completely interrupted. During passive muscle compression and release, outward flow is not interrupted in ICPVs; it is interrupted in competent perforators. Color flow duplex scanning is superior to conventional duplex scanning for the evaluation of ICPVs and is currently the most useful test for this purpose.

Evaluation of Venous Outflow Obstruction

The assessment of venous outflow obstruction is an essential part of the evaluation of chronic venous insufficiency. Screening for venous obstruction should be performed with noninvasive methods, with duplex scanning the test of choice. The evaluation of venous obstruction with the use of duplex scanning is conducted in a fashion similar to that used for the evaluation of DVT.

Duplex scanning (1) directly visualizes and locates intraluminal obstruction, (2) assesses the characteristics of venous flow distal to the inguinal ligament, and (3) identifies the presence of collateral veins around the obstructed venous segments. However, duplex ultrasonography does not give any quantitative information about the degree of obstruction and cannot help the examiner to appraise obstruction in obese patients or when excess bowel gas or inflammatory changes are present in the pelvic region.

When duplex scanning is not available, an alternative method for the screening of venous obstruction is the use of the Doppler ultrasound venous survey. It is the simplest screening test for venous obstruction, and cost of instrumentation is minimal. The patient is erect or recumbent; the deep veins are located by their anatomic relation to major arteries, and the venous system is interrogated systematically from the groin to the ankle. The absence in the venous signal of flow spontaneity or phasicity with respiration and the lack of augmentation with distal limb compression are indirect signs of venous obstruction. Unfortunately, Doppler evaluation (1) cannot identify double femoral or popliteal veins, (2) cannot discern partial obstruction from no obstruction, (3) may interpret well-developed collaterals as patent axial veins, and (4) cannot evaluate pelvic, deep thigh, or calf veins. All of these limitations are surmounted by duplex scanning. Furthermore, Doppler ultrasonography does not give accurate information about the location and extent of venous obstruction and cannot quantitate the degree of obstruction present.

Ascending phlebography has long been considered the standard for the evaluation of venous obstruction. It offers accurate anatomic information regarding the extent and location of venous obstruction and the presence of collateral venous return; however, it does not quantitate the hemodynamic severity of venous outflow obstruction and is an invasive procedure that is inappropriate as a screening tool. With the advent of duplex scanning, the phlebographic evaluation of venous obstruction has been restricted to the preoperative assessment of patients undergoing venous reconstruction and to the diagnosis of pelvic vein obstruction in areas that duplex ultrasonography cannot access or in which its findings appear ambiguous. Pelvic vein patency is in many cases best evaluated with descending phlebography, mainly when more distal obstruction is present.

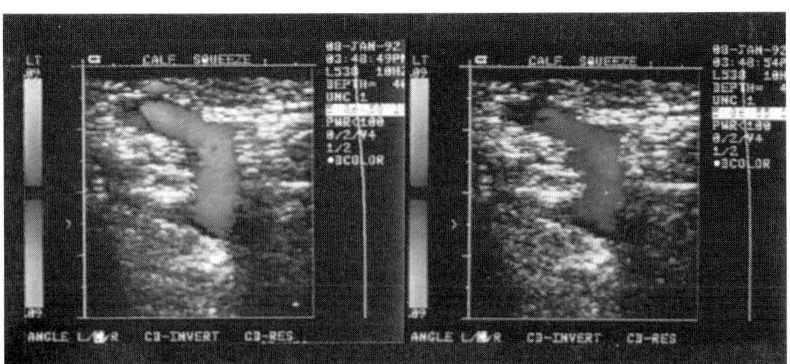

FIGURE 11–21. Color flow images of an incompetent calf perforating vein. *Right,* Transverse calf insonation demonstrating flow from the greater saphenous vein to the deep calf vein. *Left,* Flow reversal (red hue) after the release of distal calf compression. See Color Plate.

Quantitative Evaluation

Quantitation of the degree of venous outflow obstruction is necessary to determine the impact of the obstructive component on the overall severity of chronic venous insufficiency. It is most important for assessing the results of different treatment modalities and for understanding hemodynamic changes in patients with chronic venous insufficiency. Venous pressure measurement and determination of the venous emptying rate are currently used for appraising the degree of venous obstruction.

The severity of venous outflow obstruction is determined by the degree of blockage of the main axial veins and by the effectiveness of the development of collateral venous channels. The anatomic evaluation of venous outflow obstruction does not provide any assessment of the hemodynamic impact of the obstruction. When severe chronic venous insufficiency is thought to be secondary to venous outflow obstruction, quantitative evaluation is essential to correlate the degree of obstruction with the clinical status. Quantification of outflow obstruction is now possible with the use of functional studies that measure volume changes after the release of proximal venous occlusion, the venous pressure differential between the foot and the arm, venous pressure changes following reactive hyperemia, and the combination of simultaneous pressure and volume change that permits the calculation of venous outflow resistance.

The studies that measure pressure changes are invasive; they are not suitable for screening purposes and are more appropriate for the preoperative and postoperative evaluation of patients undergoing venous reconstructive surgery and for clinical research.

Arm-Foot Venous Pressure Differential

Measurement of the arm-foot pressure differential was described by Raju.[103] With the patient supine, the procedure involves cannulating the superficial veins of the foot and hand with butterfly needles. Pressure transducers are placed at the level of the puncture sites, and the pressures are recorded simultaneously. Using ascending phlebography to assess the presence of venous obstruction, Raju[103] found that the arm-foot pressure differential was 4 mmHg or less in patients without evidence of obstruction, whereas differentials greater than 4 mmHg in most patients with phlebographic evidence of obstruction had arm-foot pressure. A normal arm-foot pressure differential found in several patients with deep venous obstruction was attributed to the presence of well-developed venous collaterals.

To elucidate the contribution of collateral circulation to the venous outflow, Raju[104] measured the increase in foot venous pressure following reactive hyperemia and found better separation between normal patients and patients with phlebographically proven obstruction.[104] Normal patients exhibited an increase in venous pressure of less than 6 mmHg, whereas patients with proven obstruction had an increase of 8 mmHg or more. The combination of these two tests was 90% sensitive and 93% specific in diagnosis of venous obstruction in the quoted study. The false-negative results found with this test were in patients who had phlebographic obstruction with good functional collateral channels in whom the obstruction produced few, if any, hemodynamic repercussions.

On the basis of these two tests, Raju classifies the severity of outflow obstruction into four categories:

- Group 1 patients have fully compensated obstruction from collateralization; they have a normal arm-foot pressure differential and a normal venous pressure response to hyperemia despite proven phlebographic obstruction.
- Patients in group 2 have partially compensated obstruction; collateral veins are adequate at rest (normal arm-foot pressure differential) but become insufficient during reactive hyperemia (elevated hyperemia-induced foot venous pressure).
- Group 3 patients have minimal compensation of venous return with collateral flow; they have an abnormal arm-foot pressure differential and an abnormal hyperemic foot pressure elevation.
- Patients in group 4 have the most severe form of outflow obstruction, with an elevated arm-foot pressure differential but no pressure elevation during reactive hyperemia because they have such a high degree of obstruction and fixed flow that reactive hyperemia cannot be induced.

Although the described methods are fairly simple, their invasive nature makes them more suitable for the evaluation of patients with severe symptoms of obstruction, for the interpretation of results of deep venous reconstructions, and for investigational purposes.

Measurement of Venous Outflow Rate and Resistance

The rate of lower extremity venous emptying after the sudden release of venous occlusion reflects the net resistance of the limb venous outflow. The rate of venous outflow is directly proportional to the pressure gradient present between the calf veins and the inferior vena cava.[124] The venous emptying rate can be measured by the decrease in leg venous volume over a period of time after the release of venous occlusion. The rate can be monitored with strain-gauge, impedance, air, or any other plethysmographic instrument.

All tests that measure the venous outflow rate are performed with a similar technique. The patient lies supine, with the leg slightly elevated (10 to 15 degrees), externally rotated, and flexed to facilitate venous emptying. The volume monitoring device is placed on the calf, and a venous occlusion cuff is placed around the upper thigh and inflated to 50 to 70 mmHg. Maximal venous filling is allowed with the cuff inflated, and the cuff is suddenly deflated with the aid of a rapid-deflation valve. From the volume tracing recorded during the entire sequence, the maximal venous outflow and the 1-, 2-, or 3-second outflow fraction can be calculated. The rate of venous emptying is given by the maximal venous outflow, which is calculated from the slope of the tangent to the initial downslope tracing. The outflow fraction is calculated by measuring the volume decrease during the first 1, 2, or 3 seconds from the onset of deflation (Fig. 11–22). Using mercury-in-Silastic strain-gauge plethysmography, Fernandes[42] and coworkers found good separation of the maximal venous outflow between limbs with phlebographically proven deep venous obstruction and those without obstruction (Fig. 11–23). In the same study, limbs with incompetent superficial or deep

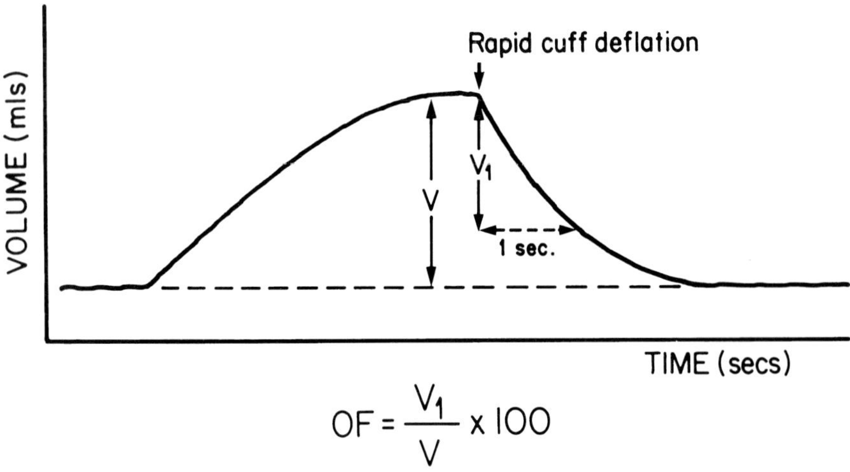

FIGURE 11–22. Typical outflow fraction tracing obtained with air plethysmography. After complete venous filling with a thigh tourniquet, rapid deflation *(arrow)* allows venous emptying. The outflow fraction (OF) is obtained by dividing the amount of venous volume emptied in 1 second (V1) by the venous volume (V) and multiplying by 100.

veins had maximal venous outflow values that overlapped with those of normal limbs but not with those of limbs that had obstruction.

The 1-second outflow fraction determined with air plethysmography is a rapid, noninvasive method of assessing outflow obstruction that can be obtained as part of the standard air plethysmography study. With the patient supine, the leg is slightly elevated and the instrumentation set in the same manner as for standard air plethysmography. A venous occlusion cuff is inflated on the upper thigh to 70 mmHg, and the leg is allowed to fill until a volume plateau is reached on the tracing; the cuff is then suddenly deflated, and the outflow fraction is calculated from the volume drop observed during the first second of the outflow curve (Fig. 11–22). The volume emptied in 1 second is divided by the total leg volume and multiplied by 100, which expresses the percentage of leg blood volume passively emptied in 1 second. Using this test, Nicolaides and Sumner[90] found the following:

1. Limbs without evidence of obstruction have outflow fractions of greater than 38% of the venous volume measured with the occlusion cuff inflated.
2. Limbs with moderate obstruction have fractions of 30% to 38%.
3. Limbs with severe obstruction have outflow fractions of less than 30%.

The 1-second outflow fraction permitted good discrimination between extremities with a normal arm-foot pressure differential and those with an increased arm-foot pressure differential (>5 mmHg).

Venous outflow resistance can be calculated by simultaneously monitoring foot venous pressure and leg volume changes. A standard AVP monitoring device is connected to a butterfly needle inserted into a superficial foot vein while the venous outflow is recorded with air plethysmography. The outflow resistance can be calculated from the formula

$$\text{resistance} = \text{pressure} \div \text{flow (mmHg/ml/min)}$$

At any given point of the outflow, the pressure is obtained from the pressure curve and the flow is calculated from the tangent of the corresponding point in the volume curve.[9] By plotting the resistance against the pressure obtained at multiple points of the outflow curve from a large number of patients with different degrees of venous obstruction, Nicolaides and Sumner[89] found good separation between the pressure-resistance curves at various degrees of obstruc-

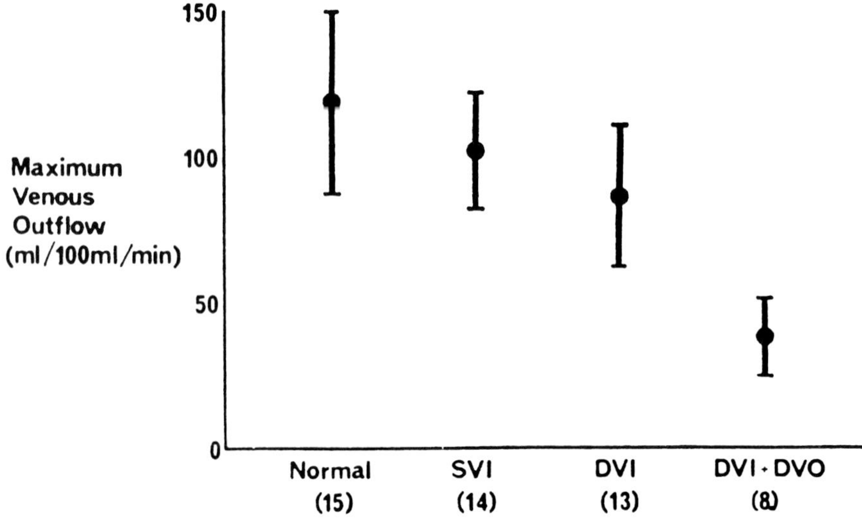

FIGURE 11–23. Maximal venous outflow measured with strain-gauge plethysmography in patients with chronic venous insufficiency. The maximal venous outflow in patients with deep venous incompetence and obstruction (DVI+DVO) is clearly lower than that in normal patients and in those with superficial venous incompetence (SVI) and deep venous incompetence (DVI). Note the overlapping between normal patients and patients with SVI and DVI. (From Fernandes e Fernandes J, Horner J, Needham T, et al: Ambulatory calf volume plethysmography in the assessment of venous insufficiency. Br J Surg 66:327, 1979. Reprinted by permission of Butterworth-Heineman Ltd.)

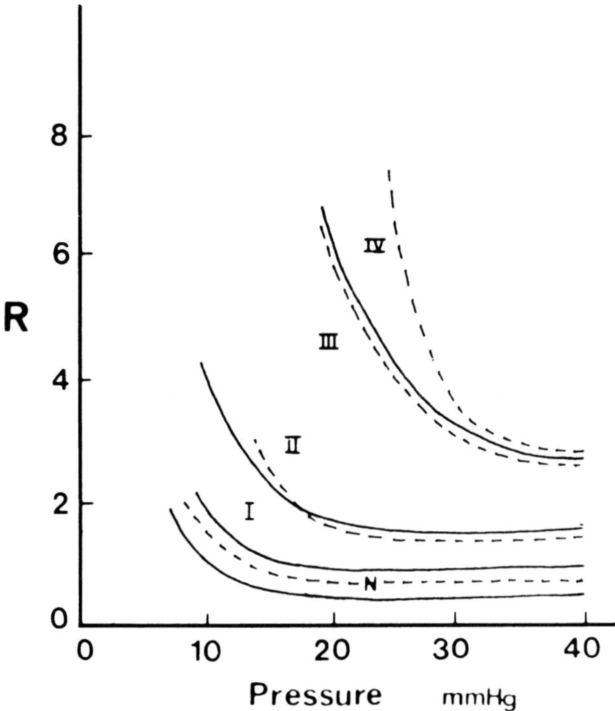

FIGURE 11–24. Relationship between outflow resistance curves and Raju's classification (grades I to IV) of outflow obstruction. With more severe forms of outflow obstruction, the resistance (R) is higher at any given venous pressure. The slope in the increase of outflow resistance with decreasing venous pressure levels is more pronounced in patients with severe outflow obstruction (grades III and IV). (From Nicolaides AN, Sumner DS: Investigation of Patients with Deep Vein Thrombosis and Chronic Venous Insufficiency. Los Angeles, Med-Orion, 1991, p 59.)

tion, corresponding with the arm-foot pressure gradient classification established by Raju[104] (Fig. 11–24).

REFERENCES

1. Abbott GT, Diggory RT, Harris I: Comparison of light reflection rheography with ascending venography in the diagnosis of lower limb deep venous thrombosis. Br J Radiol 68(810):593, 1995.
2. Abramowitz HB, Queral LA, Flinn WR, et al: The use of photoplethysmography in the assessment of venous insufficiency: A comparison to venous pressure measurements. Surgery 86:434, 1979.
3. Ackroyd JS, Lea Thomas M, Browse NL: Deep vein reflux: An assessment by descending phlebography. Br J Surg 73:31, 1986.
4. Agnelli G, Cosmi B, Radicchia S, et al: Features of thrombi and diagnostic accuracy of impedance plethysmography in symptomatic and asymptomatic deep vein thrombosis. Thromb Haemost 70(2):266, 1993.
5. Anderson S: Thermography and plethysmography in the diagnosis of deep venous thrombosis: A comparison with phlebography. Acta Med Scand 219(4):359, 1986.
6. Araki CT, Back TL, Padberg FT, et al: The significance of calf muscle pump function in venous ulceration. J Vasc Surg 20:872, 1994.
7. Arnoldi CC, Greitz T, Linderholm H: Variations in the cross sectional area and pressure in the veins of the normal human leg during rhythmic muscular exercise. Acta Chir Scand 132:507, 1966.
8. Arora S, Lam DJK, Kennedy C, et al: Light reflection rheography: A simple noninvasive screening test for deep vein thrombosis. J Vasc Surg 18:767, 1993.
9. Barnes RW, Collicott PE, Mozersky DJ, et al: Noninvasive quantitation of maximum venous outflow in acute thrombophlebitis. Surgery 72:971, 1972.
10. Barnes RW, Hokanson DE, Wu KK, et al: Detection of deep vein thrombosis with an automatic electrically calibrated strain gauge plethysmograph. Surgery 83:219, 1977.
11. Barnes RW, Russell HE, Wu KK, et al: Accuracy of Doppler ultrasound in clinically suspected venous thrombosis in the calf. Surg Gynecol Obstet 143:425, 1976.
12. Becker DM, Philbrick JT, Bachhuber TL, et al: D-dimer testing and acute venous thromboembolism: A shortcut to accurate diagnosis? Arch Intern Med 156:939, 1996.
13. Bentley PG, Hill PL, DeHass HA, et al: Radionuclide venography in the management of proximal venous occlusion: A comparison with contrast venography. Br J Radiol 52:289, 1979.
14. Bergqvist D, Efsing HO, Hallbrook T: Thermography: A non-invasive method for diagnosis of deep venous thrombosis. Arch Surg 112:600, 1977.
15. Bergan JJ, Moulton S, Beeman S, et al: Quantification of venous reflux in lower extremity venous stasis. J Vasc Surg 15:442, 1992.
16. Bishara RA, Sigel B, Rocco K, et al: Deterioration of venous function in normal lower extremities during daily activity. J Vasc Surg 3:700, 1986.
17. Browse NL, Clapham WF, Croft DN, et al: Diagnosis of established deep vein thrombosis with the ^{125}I-fibrinogen uptake test. Br Med J 4:325, 1971.
18. Chapman CS, Akhtar N, Campbell S, et al: The use of D-dimer assay by enzyme immunoassay and latex agglutination techniques in the diagnosis of deep vein thrombosis. Clin Lab Haematol 12:37, 1990.
19. Charkes ND, Dugan MA, Maier WO, et al: Scintigraphic detection of deep-vein thrombosis with I-131–fibrinogen. J Nucl Med 15:1163, 1974.
20. Chaudhuri TK, Fink, S, Farpour A: Physiologic considerations in imaging of lower extremity venous thrombosis. Am J Physiol Imaging 6:90, 1991.
21. Christopoulos D, Nicolaides AN, Cook A, et al: Pathogenesis of venous ulceration in relation to the calf muscle pump function. Surgery 106:829, 1989.
22. Christopoulos DG, Nicolaides AN, Szendro G, et al: Air-plethysmography and the effect of elastic compression on venous hemodynamics of the leg. J Vasc Surg 5:148, 1987.
23. Classen JH, Richardson JB, Koontz: A three year experience with phleborheography: A noninvasive technique for the diagnosis of deep venous thrombosis. Ann Surg 195:800, 1982.
24. Collins GJ, Rich, NM, Anderson CA, et al: Phleborheographic diagnosis of venous obstruction. Ann Surg 189:25, 1979.
25. Comerota AJ, Katz ML, Grossi RJ, et al: The comparative value of noninvasive testing for diagnosis and surveillance of deep venous thrombosis. J Vasc Surg 7:40, 1988.
26. Comerota AJ, White JV, Katz ML: Diagnostic methods for deep vein thrombosis: Venous Doppler examination, phleborheography, iodine-125 fibrinogen uptake, and phlebography. Am J Surg 150(4A):14, 1985.
27. Cooke ED, Pilcher MF: Thermography in diagnosis of deep venous thrombosis. Br Med J 2:523, 1973.
28. Cooke ED, Pilcer, MF: Thrombosis: Preclinical diagnosis by deep vein thermography. Br J Surg 61:971, 1974.
29. Cramer M, Langlois Y, Beach K, et al: Standardization of venous flow measurement by SGP in normal subjects. Bruit 7:33, 1983.
30. Cranley JJ, Canos AJ, Sull WJ, et al: Phleborheographic technique for diagnosis of deep venous thrombosis of the lower extremities. Surg Gynecol Obstet 141:331, 1975.
31. Criado E, Daniel PF, Marston WA, et al: Physiologic variations in lower extremity venous valvular function. Ann Vasc Surg 9:102, 1995.
32. Criado E, Farber MA, Marston WA, et al: The role of air plethysmography in the diagnosis of chronic venous insufficiency. J Vasc Surg 27:660, 1998.
33. Criado E, Johnson G Jr: Venous disease. Curr Probl Surg 28:343, 1991.
34. Dale S, Gogstad GO, Brosstad F, et al: Comparison of three D-dimer assays for the diagnosis of DVT: ELISA, latex, and immunofiltration assay (NycoCard D-dimer), Thromb Haemost 71:270, 1994.
35. DeNardo SJ, Bogren HG, DeNardo GL: Detection of thrombophlebitis in the lower extremities: A regional comparison of I-123 fibrinogen scintigraphy and contrast venography. AJR 145:1045, 1985.
36. Dosick SM, Blakemore WS: The role of Doppler ultrasound in acute deep venous thrombosis. Am J Surg 136:265, 1978.

37. Ennis JT, Elmes RJ: Radionuclide venography in the diagnosis of deep vein thrombosis. Radiology 125:441, 1977.
38. Eriksson I, Almgren B: Influence of the profunda femoris vein on venous hemodynamics of the limb. J Vasc Surg 4:390, 1986.
39. Evans DS: The early diagnosis of deep vein thrombosis by ultrasound. Br J Surg 57:726, 1970.
40. Ezekowitz MD, Pope CF, Sostman HD, et al: Indium-111 platelet scintigraphy for the diagnosis of acute venous thrombosis. Circulation 73:668, 1986.
41. Fedullo PF, Moser KM, Moser KS, et al: Indium-111–labeled platelets: Effect of heparin on uptake by venous thrombi and relationship to activated partial thromboplastin time. Circulation 66:632, 1982.
42. Fernandes E, Fernandes J, Horner J, et al: Ambulatory calf volume plethysmography in the assessment of venous insufficiency. Br J Surg 66:327, 1979.
43. Foldes M, Blackburn M, Hogan J, et al: Standing versus supine positioning in the evaluation of venous reflux. J Vasc Technol 15:321, 1991.
44. Folse R, Alexander RH: Directional flow detection for localizing venous valvular incompetency. Surgery 67:114, 1970.
45. Gardner GP, Cordts PR, Gillespie DL, et al: Can air plethysmography accurately identify upper extremity deep venous thrombosis? J Vasc Surg 18:808, 1993.
46. Bays RA, Healy DA, Atnip RG, et al: Validation of air plethysmography, photoplethysmography, and duplex ultrasonography in the evaluation of severe venous stasis. J Vasc Surg 20:721, 1994.
47. Ginsberg JS, Brill-Edwards PA, Demers C, et al: D-dimer in patients with clinically suspected pulmonary embolism. Chest 104:1679, 1993.
48. Ginsberg JS, Wells PS, Brill-Edwards P, et al: Application of a novel and rapid whole blood assay for D-dimer in patients with clinically suspected pulmonary embolism. Thromb Haemost 73:35, 1995.
49. Gooley NA, Sumner DS: Relationship of venous reflux to the site of venous valvular incompetence: Implications for venous reconstructive surgery. J Vasc Surg 7:50, 1988.
50. Hallbook T, Gothlin J: Strain gauge plethysmography and phlebography in diagnosis of deep venous thrombosis. Acta Chir Scand 137:37, 1971.
51. Hamberg O, Madsen G, Hansen PB, et al: Segmental mean temperature differences in the diagnosis of acute venous thrombosis in the legs. Scand J Clin Lab Invest ; 47:191, 1987.
52. Hanel KC, Abbott WM, Reidy NC, et al: The role of two noninvasive tests in deep venous thrombosis. Ann Surg 1981; 194:725.
53. Hanrahan LM, Araki CT, Rodriguez AA, et al: Distribution of valvular incompetence in patients with venous stasis ulceration. J Vasc Surg 13:805, 1991.
54. Harris WH, Athanasoulis C, Waltman AC, et al: Comparison of ^{125}I-fibrinogen scanning with phlebography for detection of venous thrombi after elective hip surgery. N Engl J Med 292:665, 1975.
55. Heaton DC, Billings JD, Hickton CM: Assessment of D dimer assays for the diagnosis of deep vein thrombosis. J Lab Clin Med 110:588, 1987.
56. Higashi S, Kuniyasu Y: An experimental study of deep-vein thrombosis using Tc-99m fibrinogen. Eur J Nucl Med 9:548, 1984.
57. Hobbs JT, Davies JWL: Detection of deep venous thrombosis with ^{131}I-labelled fibrinogen in the rabbit. Lancet 2:134, 1960.
58. Holmgren K, Jacobsson H, Johnson H, et al: Thermography and plethysmography, a non-invasive alternative to venography in the diagnosis of deep vein thrombosis. J Intern Med 228(1):29, 1990.
59. Howe HR, Hansen KJ, Plonk GW: Expanded criteria for the diagnosis of deep venous thrombosis. Arch Surg 119:1167, 1984.
60. Huisman MV, Buller HR, ten Cate JW, et al: Serial impedance plethysmography for suspected deep venous thrombosis in outpatients: The Amsterdam General Practitioner Study. N Engl J Med 314(13):823, 1986.
61. Huisman MV, Buller HR, ten Cate JW: Utility of impedance plethysmography in the diagnosis of recurrent deep-vein thrombosis. Arch Intern Med 148:681, 1988.
62. Hull R, Hirsh J, Sackett DL, et al: Replacement of venography in suspected venous thrombosis by impedance plethysmography and ^{125}I-fibrinogen leg scanning. Ann Intern Med 94:12, 1981.
63. Hull R, Taylor DW, Hirsh J: Impedance plethysmography: The relationship between venous filling and sensitivity and specificity for proximal vein thrombosis. Circulation 53:696, 1978.
64. Hull R, van Aken WG, Hirsh J, et al: Impedance plethysmography using occlusive cuff technique in the diagnosis of venous thrombosis. Circulation 53:696, 1976.
65. Iafrati MD, Welch H, ODonell TF, et al: Correlation of venous noninvasive tests with the Society for Vascular Surgery/International Society for Cardiovascular Surgery clinical classification of chronic venous insufficiency. J Vasc Surg 19:1001, 1994.
66. Jay R, Hull R, Carter C, et al: Outcome of abnormal impedance plethysmography results in patients with proximal-vein thrombosis: Frequency of return to normal. Thromb Res 36:259, 1984.
67. Johnson WC: Evaluation of newer techniques for the diagnosis of venous thrombosis. J Surg Res 16:473, 1974.
68. Kakkar VV, Nicolaides AN, Renny JTG, et al: ^{125}I-labelled fibrinogen test adapted for routine screening of deep vein thrombosis. Lancet 1:540, 1970.
69. Kempi V, Van der Linden W, Von Scheele C: Diagnosis of deep vein thrombosis with Tc-99m–streptokinase: A clinical comparison with phlebography. Br Med J 4:748, 1974.
70. Killewich LA, Martin R, Cramer M, et al: An objective assessment of the physiologic changes in the postthrombotic syndrome. Arch Surg 120, 1985.
71. Kistner RL, Ferris EB, Randhawa G, et al: A method of performing descending venography. J Vasc Surg 4:464, 1986.
72. Knight LC, Abrams MJ, Schwartx DA, et al: Tc-99m–labeling of fragment E1 for thrombosis imaging. J Nucl Med 31:776, 1990.
73. Kupper C, Shugart R, Burnham S: Errors of Doppler ultrasound in diagnosis of deep venous thrombosis. Bruit 3(12):15, 1979.
74. Linblad B, Bergqvist D, Fredin H, et al: The accuracy of 125-I–radioactive uptake test for detection of deep venous thrombosis using different labelled proteins (fibrinogen, albumin) and compared to phlebography in hip surgery patients. Vasa 16:251, 1987.
75. Linton RR: The communicating veins of the lower leg and the operative technic for their ligation. Ann Surg 107:582, 1938.
76. Linton RR: The post-thrombotic ulceration of the lower extremity: Its etiology and surgical treatment. Ann Surg 138:415, 1953.
77. McEnroe CS, O'Donnell TF Jr, Mackey WC: Correlation of clinical findings with venous hemodynamics in 386 patients with chronic venous insufficiency. Am J Surg 156:148, 1988.
78. Meadway J, Nicolaides AN, Walker CJ, et al: Value of Doppler ultrasound in diagnosis of clinically suspected deep vein thrombosis. Br Med J 4:552, 1975.
79. Millar WT, Smith JFB: Localization of deep-venous thrombosis using technetium 99m-labeled urokinase. Lancet 2:695, 1974.
80. Miller SS, Foote AV: The ultrasonic detection of incompetent perforating veins. Br J Surg 61:653, 1974.
81. Milne RM, Griffiths JMT, Gunn AA, et al: Postoperative deep venous thrombosis. Lancet 2:445, 1971.
82. Mitrani AA, Gonzales ML, Blake D, et al: Light reflection rheography: A new non-invasive method for evaluation of deep vein thrombosis (Abstract). Clin Res 37:8A, 1989.
83. Mitrani AA, Gonzales ML, O'Connell MT, et al: Detection of clinically suspected deep vein thrombosis using light reflection rheography. Am J Surg 161(6):646, 1991.
84. Mukherjee D, Anderson CA, Sado AS, et al: Use of light reflection rheography for diagnosis of axillary or subclavian venous thrombosis. Am J Surg 161(6):651, 1991.
85. Neglen P, Raju S: Should duplex Doppler scanning replace descending phlebography as the gold standard in evaluation of venous reflux? J Vasc Surg 15:442, 1992.
86. Nicholas GG, Miller FJ, Demuth WE, et al: Clinical vascular laboratory diagnosis of deep venous thrombosis. Ann Surg 186:213, 1977.
87. Nicolaides AN, Miles C: Photoplethysmography in the assessment of venous insufficiency. J Vasc Surg 5:405, 1987.
88. Nicolaides AN, Sumner DS: Investigation of Patients with Deep Vein Thrombosis and Chronic Venous Insufficiency. Los Angeles, Med-Orion, 1991, p 31.
89. Nicolaides AN, Sumner DS: Investigation of Patients with Deep Vein Thrombosis and Chronic Venous Insufficiency. Los Angeles, Med-Orion, 1991, p 59.
90. Nicolaides AN, Sumner DS: Investigation of Patients with Deep Vein Thrombosis and Chronic Venous Insufficiency. Los Angeles, Med-Orion, 1991, p 61.
91. Nicolaides AN, Zukowski AJ: The value of dynamic venous pressure measurements. World J Surg 10:919, 1986.
92. Nolan T, Ordonez C, Rosen AJ, et al: Diagnostic accuracy of phleborheography in deep venous thrombosis. Am J Surg 48:77, 1982.

93. Norris CS, Beyrau A, Barnes RW: Quantitative photoplethysmography in chronic venous insufficiency: A new method of noninvasive estimation of ambulatory venous pressure. Surgery 94:758, 1983.
94. O'Donnell TF Jr, Burnand KG, Clemenson G, et al: Doppler examination vs clinical and phlebographic detection of the location of incompetent perforating veins. Arch Surg 112:31, 1977.
95. Ott P, Astrup L, Hartvig J, et al: Assessment of D-dimer in plasma: Diagnostic value in suspected deep venous thrombosis of the leg. Acta Med Scand 116:505, 1988.
96. Paiement G, Wessinger SJ, Waltman AC, et al: Surveillance of deep venous thrombosis in asymptomatic total hip replacement patients: Impedance phlebography and fibrinogen scanning versus roentgenographic phlebography. Am J Surg 155:400, 1988.
97. Payne SPK, Thrush AJ, London NJM, et al: Venous assessment using air plethysmography: A comparison with clinical examination, ambulatory venous pressure measurement and duplex scanning. Br J Surg 80:967, 1993.
98. Pearce WH, Ricco J-B, Queral LA, et al: Hemodynamic assessment of venous problems. Surgery 93:715, 1983.
99. Pini M, Poti R, Poli T, et al: Accuracy of strain-gauge plethysmography as a diagnostic test in clinically suspected deep venous thrombosis. Thromb Res 35(2):149, 1984.
100. Pollack AA, Wood EH: Venous pressure in the saphenous vein at the ankle in man during exercise and changes in posture. J Appl Physiol 1:649, 1949.
101. Porter JM, Moneta GL, and An International Consensus Committee on Chronic Venous Disease. J Vasc Surg 21:635, 1995.
102. Raines JK, Jaffrin MY, Rao S: A noninvasive pressure-pulse recorder: Development and rationale. Med Instrum 7:245, 1973.
103. Raju S: New approaches to the diagnosis and treatment of venous obstruction. J Vasc Surg 4:42, 1986.
104. Raju S: A pressure-based technique for the detection of acute and chronic venous obstruction. Phlebology 3:207, 1988.
105. Raju S, Fredericks R: Hemodynamic basis of stasis ulceration: A hypothesis. J Vasc Surg 13:491, 1991.
106. Ramirez C, Box M, Gottesman L: Characteristics of extrinsic compression noted in plethysmographic and Doppler techniques for deep venous thrombosis. Bruit 4(9):42, 1980.
107. Ritchie WGM, Soulen RL, Lapayowker MS: Thermographic diagnosis of deep venous thrombosis. Radiology 131:341, 1979.
108. Rosfors S: Venous photoplethysmography: Relationship between transducer position and regional distribution of venous insufficiency. J Vasc Surg 11:436, 1990.
109. Russell JC, Becker DR: The noninvasive venous vascular laboratory. Arch Surg 118:1024, 1983.
110. Sandler DA, Martin JF: Liquid crystal thermography as a screening test for deep vein thrombosis. Lancet I:665, 1985.
111. Sarin S, Scurr JH, Coleridge Smith PD: Medial calf perforators in venous disease: The significance of outward flow. J Vasc Surg 16:40, 1992.
112. Sarin S, Shields DA, Scurr JH, et al: Photoplethysmography: A valuable noninvasive tool in the assessment of venous dysfunction? J Vasc Surg 16:154, 1992.
113. Satiani B, Paoletti D, Henry M, et al: A critical appraisal of impedance plethysmography in the diagnosis of acute deep venous thrombosis. Surg Gynecol Obstet 161(1):25, 1985.
114. Sautter RD, Larson DE, Bhattacharyya SK, et al: The limited utility of fibrinogen I-125 leg scanning. Arch Intern Med 139:148, 1979.
115. Schroeder PJ, Dunn E: Mechanical plethysmography and Doppler ultrasound. Arch Surg 117:300, 1982.
116. Sigel B, Popky GL, Wagner DK, et al: Comparison of clinical and Doppler ultrasound evaluation of confirmed lower extremity venous disease. Surgery 64:332, 1968.
117. Soini IH: Thermography in suspected deep venous thrombosis of lower leg. Eur J Radiol 5:281, 1985.
118. Sottiurai VS, Towner K, McDonnell AE, et al: Diagnosis of upper extremity deep venous thrombosis using noninvasive technique. Surgery 91:582, 1982.
119. Spar IL, Goodland RL, Schwartz DA, et al: Detection of preformed thrombi in dogs by means of I-131–labeled antibodies to dog fibrinogen. Circ Res 17:322, 1965.
120. Speiser W, Mallek R, Koppensteiner R, et al: D-dimer and TAT measurement in patients with deep venous thrombosis: Utility in diagnosis and judgement of anticoagulant treatment effectiveness. Thromb Haemost 64:196, 1990.
121. Strandness DE Jr, Sumner DS: Ultrasonic velocity detector in the diagnosis of thrombophlebitis. Arch Surg 104:180, 1972.
122. Sullivan ED, Peter DJ, Cranley JJ: Phleborheography of the upper extremity. Arch Surg 118:1134, 1983.
123. Sumner DS, Lambeth A: Reliability of Doppler ultrasound in the diagnosis of acute venous thrombosis both above and below the knee. Am J Surg 138:205, 1979.
124. Sumner D: Strain-gauge plethysmography. *In* Bernstein EF (ed): Noninvasive Diagnostic Techniques in Vascular Disease, 3rd ed. St. Louis, CV Mosby, 1985, p 746.
125. Szendro G, Nicolaides AN, Zukowski AJ, et al: Duplex scanning in the assessment of deep venous incompetence. J Vasc Surg 4:237, 1986.
126. Thomas ML, McAllister V, Rose DH, et al: A simplified technique of phlebography for the localisation of incompetent perforating veins of the legs. Clin Radiol 23:486, 1972.
127. Thomas ML, Keeling FP, Ackroyd JS: Descending phlebography: A comparison of three methods and an assessment of the normal range of deep vein reflux. J Cardiovasc Surg 27:27, 1986.
128. Thomas PR, Butler CM, Bowman J, et al: Light reflection rheography: An effective non-invasive technique for screening patients with suspected deep venous thrombosis. Br J Surg 78(2):207, 1991.
129. Thomson H: The surgical anatomy of the superficial and perforating veins of the lower limb. Ann R Coll Surg Engl 61:198, 1979.
130. van Beek EJR, van den Ende B, Berckmans RJ, et al: A comparative analysis of D-dimer assays in patients with clinically suspected pulmonary embolism. Thromb Haemost 70:408, 1993.
131. van Bemmelen PS, Beach K, Bedford G, et al: The mechanism of venous valve closure. Arch Surg 125:617, 1990.
132. van Bemmelen PS, Bedford G, Beach K, et al: Quantitative segmental evaluation of venous valvular reflux with duplex ultrasound scanning. J Vasc Surg 10:425, 1989.
133. van Bemmelen PS, Mattos MA, Hodgson KJ, et al: Does air plethysmography correlate with duplex scanning in patients with chronic venous insufficiency? J Vasc Surg 18:796–807, 1993.
134. van Rijn ABB, Heller I, Van Zijl J: Segmental air plethysmography in the diagnosis of deep vein thrombosis. Surg Gynecol Obstet 165:488, 1987.
135. Vasdekis SN, Clarke GH, Nicolaides AN: Quantification of venous reflux by means of duplex scanning. J Vasc Surg 10:670, 1989.
136. Welch HJ, Faliakou EC, McLaughlin RL, et al: Comparison of descending phlebography with quantitative photoplethysmography, air plethysmography, and duplex quantitative valve closure time in assessing deep venous reflux. J Vasc Surg 16:304, 1992.
137. Welkie JF, Kerr RP, Katz ML, et al: Can noninvasive venous volume determinations accurately predict ambulatory venous pressure? J Vasc Technol 15:186, 1991.
138. Wheeler HB: Diagnosis of deep vein thrombosis. Review of clinical evaluation and impedance plethysmography. Am J Surg 150:7, 1985.
139. Yang D, Vandogen YK, Stacey MC: Variability and reliability of air plethysmographic measurements for the evaluation of chronic venous disease. J Vasc Surg 26:638, 1997.
140. Yao JST, Gourmos C, Hobbs JT: Detection of proximal vein thrombosis by Doppler ultrasound flow-detection method. Lancet 1:1, 1972.
141. Zamboni A, Portaluppi F, Marcellino MA, et al: Ultrasonographic assessment of ambulatory venous pressure in superficial venous incompetence. J Vasc Surg 26:796, 1997.
142. Zorba J, Schier D, Posituck G: Clinical value of blood pool radionuclide venography. AJR 146:1051, 1986.
143. Zufferey P, Pararas C, Monti M, et al: Assessment of acute and old deep venous thrombosis in upper extremity by venous strain gauge plethysmography. Vasa 21:263, 1992.
144. Zukowski AJ, Nicolaides AN, Szendro G, et al: Haemodynamic significance of incompetent calf perforating veins. Br J Surg 78:625, 1991.

C H A P T E R 1 2

Arterial Duplex Scanning

Robert M. Zwolak, M.D., Ph.D.

Duplex ultrasound scanning celebrates its 25th birthday coincident with publication of this fifth edition of Rutherford's *Vascular Surgery*.[10, 11] The technology continues to gain sophistication, and rapid growth persists in technical refinement, diagnostic accuracy, and clinical utility. Carotid artery duplex scanning is now the standard initial evaluation of patients with extracranial cerebrovascular disease; in fact, many surgical authorities use duplex scanning as the only preoperative examination prior to carotid endarterectomy.[152]

Since publication of the previous edition, duplex scanning of the renal and mesenteric arteries has earned more widespread acceptance as screening studies for arterial occlusive disease. An increasing number of technologists and surgeons have gained expertise with the performance and interpretation of these sophisticated examinations. Clinicians have come to rely on duplex scanning for postprocedural evaluation of surgical and interventional procedures performed on the carotid, renal, and mesenteric vessels. Use of duplex scanning of aortoiliac and femoropopliteal arteries is becoming more widespread as investigators test the accuracy of the technique and the overall ability to plan percutaneous intervention or even bypass surgery on the basis of these examinations. Finally, as experience accrues with endovascular aneurysm surgery, surgeons have found duplex ultrasound scanning to be one means of evaluating the hemodynamic integrity of these reconstructions. Overall, arterial duplex scanning is an increasingly important tool for the vascular surgeon. This chapter provides basic principles, currently accepted diagnostic thresholds, and indications for study.

PRINCIPLES OF SCANNERS

Most current duplex scanners actually provide three types of information:

- Gray-scale B-mode (ultrasound) imaging
- Color flow imaging
- Pulsed Doppler spectral waveform analysis (see Chapter 9)

Although a great deal of information may be gained from review of the B-mode and color flow images, most recently published duplex algorithms for estimation of arterial stenosis are based on blood flow velocity. The pulsed Doppler flow detector has the ability to sample a very small volume of tissue, guided in real time by the B-mode and color flow images. Velocity values are derived from the Doppler frequency shift of the reflected ultrasound waves, and current scanners automatically convert the frequency shift data to blood flow velocity if the angle between the transmitted ultrasound beam and the blood flow channel ("Doppler angle" or "beam-to-vessel angle") is known (see Chapter 9). Thus, duplex scanning provides a remarkably complementary package of anatomic and physiologic information that is unrivaled by other modalities. The value is even more striking because instrument cost is only a fraction of most sophisticated radiologic imaging systems.

Since velocity measurements derived from duplex scanning depend on accurate real-time estimation of the Doppler angle, accuracy of these methods remains significantly operator-dependent. Determination of the Doppler angle is crucial. Several researchers have argued that operators should always attempt to maintain a 60-degree angle, whereas others reason that angle correction is acceptable so long as the angle between the beam and the flowing blood remains less than 60 degrees.[118] Although this is not a settled issue, authorities agree that accurate velocity results are unlikely with an angle more than 60 degrees.

The mathematical explanation rests on the relationship between frequency shift and velocity calculated by using the Doppler equation. The velocity is a function of the cosine of the angle between the ultrasound beam and the blood flow. At angles between 60 and 90 degrees, the cosine value changes rapidly; thus, an increasingly greater potential for error in calculated velocity results for even a small error in angle. For example, an error in angle measurement of 2 degrees would produce a 6% velocity error if a 58-degree angle were incorrectly estimated as a 60-degree angle. In contrast, a 17% velocity error would result if that same 2-degree measurement error were made with an angle of 80 degrees (estimated at 78 degrees).

Duplex ultrasound scanning remains an operator-dependent technology, and any treatise on this topic would be incomplete without comment about the skill required to perform this specialized vascular ultrasound examination. Vascular technologists must understand the traditional imaging concepts of B-mode ultrasound and the strengths and weaknesses of color flow interpretation. They must also be familiar with the more complex hemodynamic issues and the pathophysiology of vascular disease. In order to provide the interpreting physician with accurate data, every technologist must have a working knowledge and familiarity with the Doppler equation and a special respect for collection of appropriate Doppler angle corrected blood flow velocities.

Efforts to ensure this high level of competence at the technologist level are found in the Registered Vascular Technologist (RVT) credentialing process. Acknowledgment that an entire laboratory is well schooled in these issues is demonstrable by certification from the Intersocietal Commission for the Accreditation of Vascular Laboratories (ICAVL). Because credentialing has been addressed in more detail in Chapter 9, it is sufficient to say here that a great deal of the variability in the quality of duplex scanning would be eliminated if technologists and laboratories universally achieved these levels of achievement.

In order to determine the degree of arterial stenosis from duplex scanning data, investigators have drawn correlations between duplex scanning–derived velocities and measurements of stenosis made on angiograms. Studies of this type define the core values of duplex scanning, and many will be cited in this chapter. The implications of this relationship between new technology and the established "gold standard" are manifold. One of the most important has to do with the two-dimensional nature of angiographic images, which limits stenosis measurements to diameter reduction rather than area reduction. All major duplex scanning publications express results in terms of diameter reduction, although the velocity information obtained by the duplex scanner is ideally suited to the more important parameter of cross-sectional area reduction.

In the clinical setting, this issue is more than a trivial mathematical relationship because atherosclerotic plaque accumulates in an asymmetric pattern. Thus, when duplex scanning and arteriographic categories of stenosis disagree, the reason may be inherent limitations of the arteriogram rather than inaccuracy of the duplex scan. This point is established early because many accuracy figures are cited in the following sections. At each step, the reader must recall that the ultimate standard is the patient, and a quoted accuracy rate of 90% for duplex scanning does not necessarily mean that duplex scanning is wrong 10% of the time. Unfortunately, investigators are only beginning to determine how to measure absolute, true stenosis percentage in vivo.

EVALUATION OF CEREBROVASCULAR ARTERIES

Extracranial Carotid Arteries

Noninvasive evaluation of extracranial cerebrovascular disease was the first remarkable achievement of duplex scanning, and the initial diagnostic criteria published by investigators at the University of Washington have withstood the test of time (Table 12–1).[123, 124] However, publication of the North American Symptomatic Carotid Endarterectomy Trial (NASCET) in 1991 and the Asymptomatic Carotid Atherosclerosis Study (ACAS) results in 1995 created new challenges for the carotid artery duplex scan[37, 111]:

1. The NASCET study adopted a technique for interpretation of angiographic stenosis severity not commonly employed prior to publication of that trial; this meant that all duplex scanning criteria published before that date used a different angiographic scale by which to correlate stenosis categories.
2. Both NASCET and ACAS identified surgical benefit at stenosis thresholds not routinely identified by existing duplex scanning algorithms.

These issues are addressed in the following discussions.

TABLE 12–1. ORIGINAL UNIVERSITY OF WASHINGTON INTERNAL CAROTID ARTERY STENOSIS GRADING CRITERIA*

DIAMETER REDUCTION (%)	DOPPLER FREQUENCY SHIFT (kHz)†
0	Peak systolic frequency < 4 kHz; no spectral broadening
1–15	Peak systolic frequency < 4 kHz; spectral broadening only in deceleration phase of systole
16–49	Peak systolic frequency < 4 kHz; spectral broadening throughout systole
50–79	Peak systolic frequency > 4 kHz; end-diastolic frequency < 4.5 kHz
80–99	End-diastolic frequency > 4.5 kHz
Occlusion	No internal carotid flow signal; flow to zero in common carotid artery

*Expressed in frequency shift and based on European method of angiographic stenosis measurement.

†Criteria based on a pulsed-Doppler transducer with a 5-MHz transmitting frequency, a small sample volume relative to the internal carotid artery, and a 60-degree beam-to-vessel angle. Approximate angle-adjusted velocity equivalents are 4 kHz = 125 cm/sec and 4.5 kHz = 140 cm/sec.

Technique

For the routine carotid artery duplex scanning examination, Doppler probes with transmitting frequencies from 4 to 7.5 MHz are appropriate. Starting in a transverse plane, the technologist uses B-mode and color flow scanning to identify the common carotid artery (CCA) at the base of the neck, and then follows the vessel distally to the bifurcation. Occasionally, the carotid bifurcation may be seen in its entirety as the classic "tuning fork" image (Fig. 12–1; see Color Plate).

Next, the technologist identifies the internal carotid artery (ICA) and the external carotid artery (ECA) branches. Although the identification is usually straightforward, the technologist must be totally confident of the distinction between the ICA and ECA in every study. The ICA is usually the posterior branch and reflects a low-resistance Doppler signal, whereas the ECA is typically anterior with a high-resistance signal. In unusual cases, both the relative locations and the Doppler signal characteristics of these vessels may vary.

When stenosis of both the ICA and ECA is severe, establishing their identity becomes more difficult. Two characteristics can be used to identify the ECA:

1. The presence of branches; the ICA almost never has extracranial branches.
2. The "temporal tap" maneuver; tapping the temporal artery near the zygomatic arch causes a reflected wave that is visible in the ECA Doppler spectrum.

Color flow imaging may also be helpful when the internal carotid is tortuous, kinked, or coiled (Fig. 12–2; see Color Plate). The ICA should be followed as far distally as possible.

Once a preliminary survey of the bifurcation has been completed and an appreciation of the anatomy gained, the technologist repeats the examination in sagittal and transverse imaging planes for collection of Doppler velocity data and representative images. Doppler signals are re-

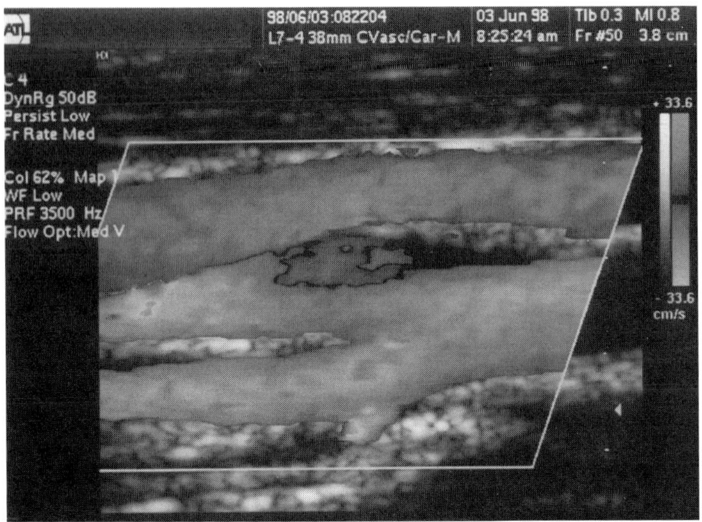

FIGURE 12–1. Color flow duplex image of normal carotid bifurcation. The superior thyroid branch is visible, originating from the external carotid. Small region of color flow reversal in the carotid bulb is a normal finding in patients entirely free of carotid atherosclerosis. See Color Plate.

corded from a segment of relatively straight, nondiseased CCA and from any regions that harbor stenoses. The CCA is examined as far centrally as possible, with special attention to the intrathoracic portion of the artery if the Doppler signal suggests a proximal stenosis. The Doppler sample volume probe is then "swept through" the bifurcation and the ICA, and spectra are recorded in areas demonstrating the highest peak systolic and end-diastolic velocities. Care is taken to maintain a Doppler angle of 60 degrees or less. Color flow imaging may be used to help identify regions of maximal stenosis for Doppler sampling, but plaque characteristics can best be appreciated in gray scale imaging.

In the preoperative patient, identification of a relatively normal distal segment of ICA beyond the region of plaque accumulation is a finding of import for the surgeon. Also, it is helpful to the surgeon for the technologist to note whether the patient has an unusually high or low carotid artery bifurcation. Examination of the ECA may be relatively brief, with recording of a representative image and Doppler signal.

Interpretation

Accurate interpretation of carotid duplex scanning data is a complex issue, and only a brief summary is presented here. The typical carotid duplex scan report includes angle-corrected peak systolic velocity (PSV) and end-diastolic velocity (EDV) within the tightest portion of an ICA stenosis, or representative values if there is no stenosis (Fig. 12–3; see Color Plate). PSV in the CCA is usually reported as well, especially since several stenosis-grading scales employ the ratio of PSV in the ICA to PSV in the CCA to determine stenosis category. A description of plaque characteristics is included, and careful note is made of unusual anatomy. The NASCET grading scale may indicate a 0% stenosis when the patient may actually have very significant plaque accumulation in the carotid bulb (see later). For this reason, it is especially important to note bulky plaque because a report of minimal stenosis may mislead the referring physician to believe that no atherosclerotic disease is present (Fig. 12–4; see Color Plate).

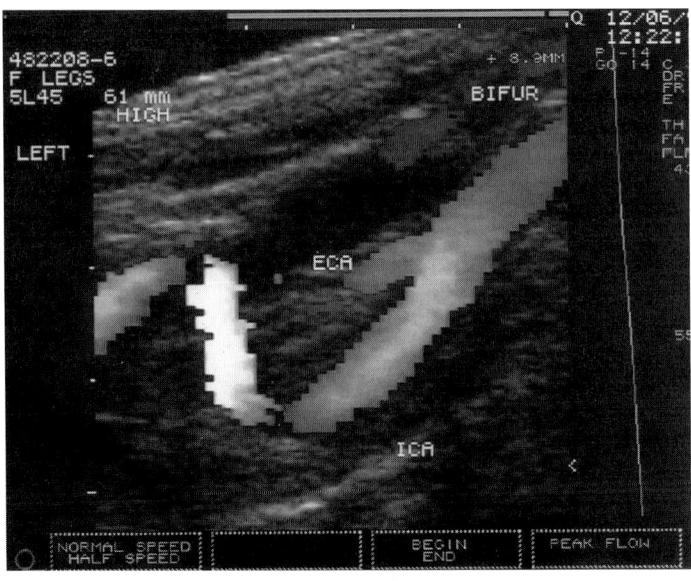

FIGURE 12–2. Color flow facilitated anatomic definition and Doppler angle correction of this tortuous internal carotid artery (ICA). Subsequent Doppler sampling through the entire length of the ICA failed to identify significant stenoses. ECA = external carotid artery. See Color Plate.

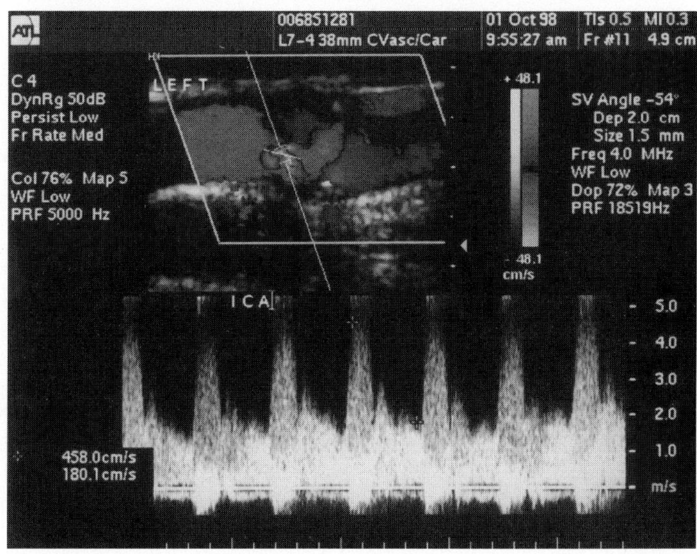

FIGURE 12–3. Identification of carotid stenosis is best performed using angle-corrected Doppler velocity and spectral analysis. In this study, the sample volume is placed in a region of disordered blood flow, indicated by the focal color variation in the color flow inset. Recorded peak systolic velocity (PSV) of 458 cm/sec and end-diastolic volume of 180 cm/sec fall well above thresholds for 70% stenosis on all published grading scales. Common carotid artery (CCA) PSV of 65 cm/sec (not shown) produced calculated ICA:CCA ratio of 7.0, also indicating greater than 70% stenosis by all published grading scales. ICA = internal carotid artery. See Color Plate.

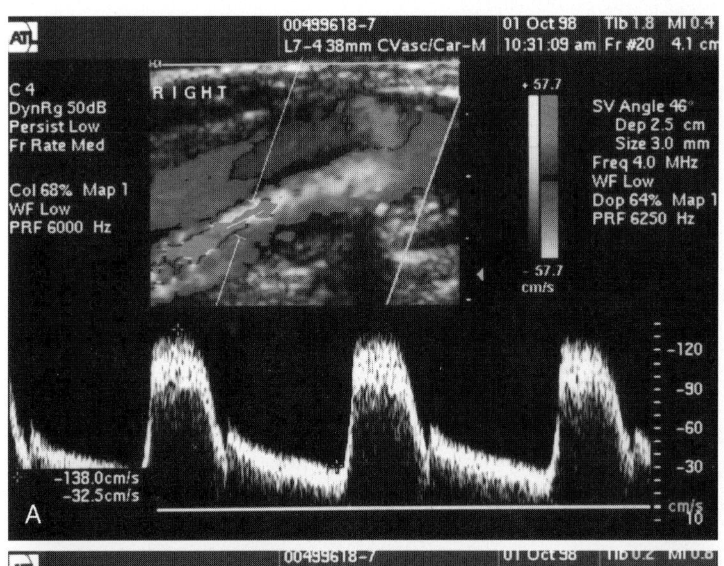

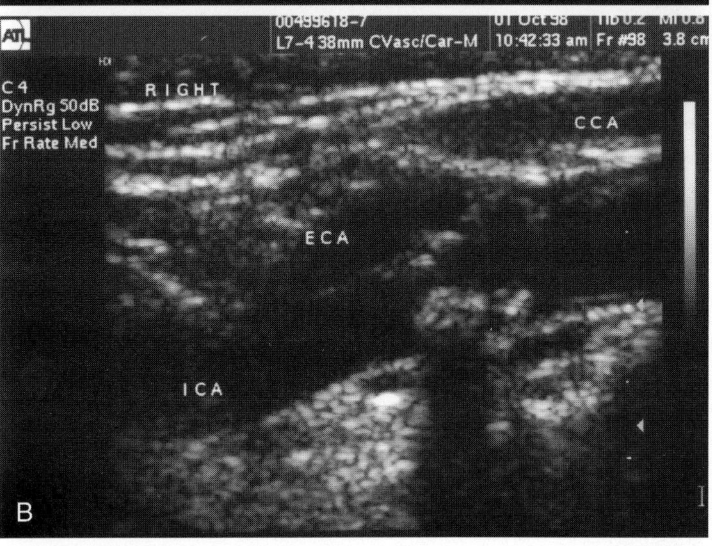

FIGURE 12–4. Examination of the carotid bifurcation with gray scale B-mode imaging is the best method for evaluating atherosclerotic plaque characteristics. *A*, The Doppler spectral window is clear, and velocities are minimally elevated. Color flow gain is well adjusted, and by visual interpretation the far wall plaque is unremarkable. *B*, The same carotid bifurcation is examined using magnified B-mode without color flow. A focal, bulky plaque is apparent. Even in the absence of severe stenosis, a plaque of this magnitude may occasionally be the source of atheroembolic symptoms. CCA = common carotid artery; ECA = external carotid artery; ICA = internal carotid artery. See Color Plate.

Findings suggestive of intrathoracic CCA or innominate artery occlusive disease, or of distal ICA or intracranial disease, should also be noted on the report.

Accurate estimation of ICA stenosis is crucial. The estimate must be based either on each laboratory's locally developed and tested criteria or on criteria adopted from the literature and verified locally with comprehensive quality assurance correlation. Both angiographic and surgical stenosis measurements should be sought for correlation. The importance of verifying duplex scan–based stenosis estimates cannot be overemphasized.

Development of interpretive duplex scanning criteria may be best understood when considered in historical perspective. Contrast arteriography was the gold standard chosen by early ultrasound investigators to confirm the accuracy of carotid duplex scanning. Duplex scan studies published prior to 1990 used what has come to be known as the "ECST method" after the European Carotid Surgery Trial.[10, 17, 36, 122, 123, 151] With this method, the carotid artery stenosis is calculated by comparing arteriographic measurement of the smallest diameter in the stenosis to an estimate of the normal diameter of the carotid bulb. Since the stenosis is often in the bulb, the normal diameter is truly an estimate based on the angiographer's sense of how large the bulb was prior to plaque accumulation. The NASCET and ACAS trials institutionalized a new convention for angiographic measurement of carotid stenosis with a technique that used the diameter of the distal ICA rather than the carotid bulb as the "normal" diameter.[37, 111]

The NASCET carotid measurement technique achieves better measurement reproducibility but simultaneously introduces an illogical element. Because the normal carotid bulb is substantially larger than the normal distal ICA, a bulky plaque may accumulate within the bulb but a residual diameter greater than the distal ICA may be maintained. This situation results in a "negative" stenosis calculation by the NASCET method for a lesion that may be as much as 50% as calculated by the ECST method. At moderate degrees of stenosis, the difference between ECST and NASCET methods remains significant. A 50% stenosis measured by the NASCET method corresponds roughly to a 70% stenosis by the ECST method. At higher degrees of stenosis, the measurements begin to converge. Thus, carotid stenosis estimations based on the early duplex scanning grading schemes systematically overestimate the degree of narrowing compared with angiograms read according to the NASCET method. Most publications since 1990 that establish duplex scanning stenosis grading scales are based on the NASCET method of angiogram measurement.[24, 38, 40, 59, 76, 93, 94, 104] However, the original criteria developed at the University of Washington, and thus widely used in many laboratories, are based on the ECST method of angiogram measurement.

The second major issue for carotid duplex scanning related to publication of NASCET and ACAS results was the establishment of surgical benefit at percentages of ICA stenosis (70% for NASCET and 60% for ACAS) that did not correspond to previously determined thresholds in early duplex classification schemes. Not surprisingly, a number of publications appeared that identified duplex scanning velocity criteria, first for a 70% stenosis[38, 59, 76, 93, 104] and later for a 60% stenosis.[24, 40, 94] All studies used contrast arteriograms measured by the NASCET method as the standard.

In general, high levels of diagnostic accuracy were identified in these single-institution reports. Unfortunately, the threshold values varied more than would be expected given the uniformly high level of accuracy (Tables 12–2 to 12–4). Few duplex scanning studies have been published that identify a 50% stenosis threshold using the NASCET method of angiogram measurement,[38] but focus on this issue is certain to be renewed now that the final results of the NASCET study have revealed a surgical benefit for patients with symptomatic disease at a 50% ICA stenosis.

Caveats, Pitfalls, and Special Issues

Instrument Variation

As indicated in Tables 12–2 to 12–4, different researchers identified strikingly different threshold velocity values for

TABLE 12–2. CAROTID ARTERY DUPLEX SCANNING PEAK SYSTOLIC VELOCITY (PSV) DIAGNOSTIC THRESHOLDS BASED ON NASCET ANGIOGRAM MEASUREMENTS*

PERCENTAGE STENOSIS	AUTHORS	PSV VELOCITY THRESHOLD (cm/sec)	INSTRUMENT	ACCURACY (%)
50	Faught et al[38]	130	Siemans	97
60	Carpenter et al[24]	170	Hewlett-Packard	92
60	Fillinger et al[40]	220	Siemans	95
60	Fillinger et al[40]	240	ATL	91
60	Moneta et al[94]	260	Acuson/ATL	90
70	Faught et al[38]	210	Siemans	93
70	Kuntz et al[76]	229	Acuson	87
70	Hunink et al[59]	230	Acuson	>85
70	Neale et al[104]	270	Acuson	88
70	Moneta et al[93]	325	Acuson	88
70	Kuntz et al[76]	340	ATL	92

*Reported only for studies listing overall accuracy rate greater than 65%, and listed in order of ascending PSV.

†Moneta et al[94] required addition of end-diastolic velocity (EDV) > 70 cm/sec to reach maximum accuracy of 90%. PSV > 260 cm/sec (without additional EDV data) produced highest PSV accuracy of 88%.

ATL = Advanced Technology Laboratories; NASCET = North American Symptomatic Carotid Endarterectomy Trial.

TABLE 12–3. CAROTID ARTERY SCANNING DUPLEX DIAGNOSTIC THRESHOLDS USING ICA:CCA PEAK SYSTOLIC VELOCITY RATIO AND ANGIOGRAM MEASUREMENTS PERFORMED BY NASCET CONVENTION*

STENOSIS (%)	AUTHOR	VELOCITY RATIO THRESHOLD	INSTRUMENT	ACCURACY (%)
60	Fillinger et al[40]	2.6	Siemans	96
60	Fillinger et al[40]	3.3	ATL	93
70	Moneta et al[93]	4.0	Acuson	88

*Presented in order of ascending ratio.
ATL = Advanced Technology Laboratories; CCA = common carotid artery; ICA = internal carotid artery; NASCET = North American Symptomatic Carotid Endarterectomy Trial.

the same degree of ICA stenosis. This issue is important because the randomized trials focus almost exclusively on ICA stenosis in determining which patients should undergo endarterectomy. Commonly obtained ICA velocities may be interpreted as lying above or below the threshold for surgical consideration, depending on the grading scale used by the interpreting physician (Fig. 12–5; see Color Plate).

Although ultrasonography is known to be an operator-dependent technology, several publications have also documented machine-to-machine variation as contributing to variability of results.[31, 40, 58, 76] For example, Howard and colleagues[58] studied the individual accuracy results of 63 duplex scanning instruments used in the ACAS trial. They determined a velocity or frequency shift threshold for each machine to detect a 60% stenosis at a 90% positive predictive value threshold. For 20 scanners using peak systolic velocity for threshold determination, the median value was 198 cm/sec for 60% stenosis with a wide range of 151 to 407 cm/sec. Only 21% of these instruments achieved what the authors called "excellent" sensitivity of 80% or better. The authors concluded that duplex scanner performance is likely overstated in the literature but that specific devices perform satisfactorily. They emphasized the importance of local standardized series and aggressive quality control if duplex scanning is to be used in the selection of patients for carotid surgery.

Fillinger and associates[40] tested the accuracy of four individual duplex scanners at two ICAVL-approved vascular laboratories. All four scanners produced criteria resulting in accuracy of more than 90% for detecting a 60% ICA stenosis, but the criteria varied between machines. The log regression equation relating duplex scanning values with angiographic stenosis value was statistically different for one of the four scanners. In a similar single-institution study, Kuntz and colleagues[76] found markedly different optimal duplex scanning criteria for detection of a 70% ICA stenosis with duplex scanners from two manufacturers.

The general conclusion from these studies is unmistakable: Duplex scanning can be an extremely accurate means to evaluate carotid stenosis, but diagnostic threshold velocities must be verified for at least each model of scanner and, perhaps, for each machine. Although duplex scanning interpretation may be and should be standardized, such is not yet the case. Even in the hands of skilled technologists, diagnostic thresholds vary substantially, and an important underlying cause may be incorporated in the electronics or the software of the ultrasound instrumentation.

What Is the True Gold Standard?

Another perspective on the vexing problem of the accuracy of carotid artery duplex scanning has been to question the validity of the presumed gold standard, that is, measurement of ICA stenosis by contrast angiography. Pan and coworkers[114] hypothesized that the two-dimensional nature of angiography measurement limits its accuracy. They compared duplex scanning velocity, conventional angiography, and magnetic resonance angiography (MRA) measurements for the evaluation of carotid artery stenosis. For the gold standard, they measured excised plaques, calculating stenosis by comparison of the residual lumen with the outer diameter of the specimen; thus, their stenosis results were analogous to measurement by the ECST technique. They found that duplex scanning and MRA correlated more closely to the actual operative specimens than conventional angiogram measurements. Angiography measurements

TABLE 12–4. CAROTID ARTERY DUPLEX SCANNING DIAGNOSTIC THRESHOLDS USING INTERNAL CAROTID ARTERY END-DIASTOLIC VELOCITY AND ANGIOGRAM MEASUREMENTS PERFORMED BY NASCET CONVENTION*

STENOSIS (%)	AUTHOR	EDV VELOCITY THRESHOLD (cm/sec)	INSTRUMENT	ACCURACY (%)
50	Carpenter et al[24]	40	Hewlett-Packard	86
70	Kuntz et al[76]	63	Acuson	88
70	Faught et al[38]	100†	Siemans	95
70	Neale et al[104]	110	Acuson	93
70	Moneta et al[93]	130	Acuson	86
70	Kuntz et al[76]	131	ATL	89

*Presented in order of ascending EDV.
†Faught also required PSV >130 cm/sec in addition to stated EDV value to reach stated accuracy.
ATL = Advanced Technology Laboratories; EDV = end-diastolic velocity; ICA = internal carotid artery; NASCET = North American Symptomatic Carotid Endarterectomy Trial; PSV = peak systolic velocity.

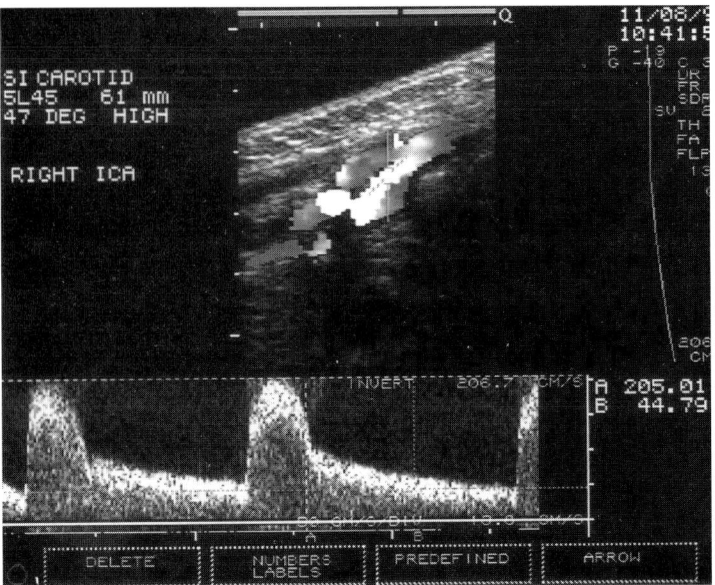

FIGURE 12–5. The Doppler spectrum in this image was obtained at the region of highest internal carotid artery velocity. With an angle-corrected peak systolic velocity (PSV) of 205 cm/sec and end-diastolic volume of 45 cm/sec, this lesion would be interpreted as greater than 60% stenotic by at least one published scale,[24] but less than 60% by several others.[40, 94] The example reinforces the need for local validation of whichever scale is chosen for interpretation. ICA = internal carotid artery. See Color Plate.

tended to underestimate actual stenosis far more often than the other techniques.

In a similar effort, Suwanwela and associates[139] used residual ICA lumen diameter from en bloc endarterectomy specimens as their gold standard and arbitrarily defined a residual lumen of 1.5 mm or less as severe stenosis. In this setting, a PSV greater than 360 cm/sec produced a maximum accuracy of 82% (85% sensitivity, 78% specificity) for identification of an ICA lumen of 1.5 mm or less. Combined parameters were identified that resulted in 96% sensitivity but low (61%) specificity, and another combination had 100% specificity but low (72%) sensitivity.

This approach is attractive because it provides flexibility for the noninvasive laboratory. First, laboratories may continue quality assurance efforts in the absence of angiographic correlation data using a more valid gold standard, namely, surgical specimens. Second, it is appealing to be able to adjust diagnostic thresholds according to whether high sensitivity or high specificity is desired. Without varying far from a point of maximum accuracy, one could potentially apply criteria with higher sensitivity in the clinical setting of symptomatic disease, a situation in which a false-negative duplex scanning result might have dire clinical consequences. In contrast, higher specificity would be desirable in the clinical setting of an asymptomatic stenosis, in which a more benign natural history demands a lack of false-positive studies that could lead to inappropriate endarterectomies.

Carotid Endarterectomy Based on Duplex Scanning

In many centers, a major shift in preoperative carotid artery imaging strategies has occurred since publication of the previous edition of this text. Carotid endarterectomy is now performed commonly without prior contrast arteriography, on the basis of information from duplex scanning alone or in combination with magnetic resonance angiography. This practice is desired to avoid the stroke risk associated with angiography and is supported by a large body of clinical literature.[25, 33, 46, 47, 49, 55, 57, 72, 85, 88, 90, 101, 102, 115, 119, 133, 144, 150, 152] A smaller number of articles cite the hazards of this approach, focusing on the occasional misinterpretation of duplex scanning results even among experienced technologists and the lack of stenosis measurement accuracy among various centers.[48, 58, 129] At least two later studies addressed specific technical issues to be considered when the duplex scan may be the only preoperative imaging study.[145, 150]

Measurement of Stenosis with Contralateral Internal Carotid Artery Occlusion

When one ICA is occluded, brain perfusion is maintained by compensatory flow increases in the contralateral ICA and the vertebral arteries. Since flow and velocity are linked, it is not surprising that the remaining patent ICA may have elevated velocities in this setting even in the absence of stenosis. Several researchers have made the observation that velocity-based grading scales may overestimate stenosis in a patent ICA when the opposite side is occluded.[43, 136, 146] This is an important caveat and should be recalled during interpretation of results when the situation is encountered.

Many variables enter the determination of exactly how much the patent ICA velocities will increase, including:

1. Contribution of compensatory flow from the vertebral arteries.
2. Adequacy of the circle of Willis.
3. The possibility that little increased flow is required if the patient suffered a significant stroke coincident with ICA occlusion.

Thus, it remains to be determined whether accurate duplex scanning stenosis grading scales can be developed for use in the patient in whom the contralateral ICA is occluded.

Intraoperative Carotid Artery Duplex Scanning

Failure to recognize technical errors of surgery, such as residual flaps, suture line stricture, and plaque dissection, can result in vessel thrombosis or distal embolization. In no circumstance can this failure be more devastating than during carotid endarterectomy. The practice of evaluating surgical results with angiography (completion angiography) has been used for decades, and proponents continue to publish data supporting the utility of this technique.[147] Subjective evaluation using continuous-wave Doppler ultrasonography has also been used for many years, but extensive documentation of the sensitivity and specificity of this method is lacking.

In 1988, Bandyk and associates[8] described the utility of pulsed-wave Doppler velocity and spectrum analysis for evaluation of carotid endarterectomy sites in 1988. Intraoperative duplex scanning of the carotid endarterectomy site was described by Sawchuk and coworkers in 1989.[125] This group focused on real-time B-mode evaluation and observed that small residual flaps (<3 mm) and minor stenoses identified during completion duplex scans did not appear to result in major postoperative complications.[125]

Baker and colleagues[5] re-explored 3% of 316 carotid endarterectomies on the basis of intraoperative duplex scanning when large flaps, residual plaques, and severe turbulence were encountered. They did not repair a much larger group of minor defects, including flaps less than 2 to 3 mm, and there was no difference in perioperative complications in the group with unrepaired minor defects. These authors concluded that routine use of intraoperative completion duplex scanning resulted in more precise performance of the operation, because they refined their surgical technique according to expectation of the duplex scan findings. They also encountered a higher incidence of late restenosis in the group with unrepaired minor defects, but this observation is not universal.[84]

In follow-up studies, Bandyk and associates[9, 66] continued to emphasize elevated velocities and abnormalities in Doppler velocity spectrum in addition to anatomic defects in the decision whether to reopen carotid endarterectomy sites. They considered a site to be abnormal when spectral broadening and PSV greater than 150 cm/sec were found, but most of the lesions they repaired had PSV values of 200 to 250 cm/sec.[9]

The technique of intraoperative carotid duplex scanning is straightforward. Most often, linear array probes with transmitting frequencies of 7 to 10 MHz are employed. Several manufacturers have developed miniaturized transducers with small footprints for this purpose. The literature strongly supports duplex scanning for intraoperative evaluation of carotid endarterectomy. When duplex scanning is used for this purpose, the decision to reopen the site is challenging because the study is very sensitive, and a proportion of very minor abnormalities may be safely left in place. For instance, residual flaps less than 2 mm probably may be safely left in place, unless they (1) cause substantial turbulence or high velocities or (2) lie in a small ICA. The literature supports intervention for larger flaps, major turbulence, and high velocities in the CCA or ICA.

Brachiocephalic Arteries

Occlusive disease of the supra-aortic trunks is infrequent, but in patients undergoing evaluation for carotid endarterectomy it is very important to know whether these vessels harbor a severe stenosis. Research on the use of duplex scanning in this area has not been extensive, but it gains importance as an increasing number of surgeons perform endarterectomy on the basis of duplex scanning without other imaging studies. Initial reports suggest that duplex scanning has good sensitivity for identification of severe great vessel stenoses within the mediastinum.[3, 19, 82, 143] The routine duplex scanning examination, however, does not evaluate arch vessels, and in many situations, the origins of these vessels cannot be seen by current duplex scanner technology. Thus, diagnosis of arch vessel stenosis or occlusion often must be made on the basis of indirect duplex scan findings in the distal cervical extensions of these arteries.

When the point of maximal great vessel stenosis is seen during the routine examination, the following generic Doppler criteria for stenosis identification probably apply: (1) a pre-stenotic, stenotic, and post-stenotic Doppler waveform pattern with (2) at least a two-fold step-up in PSV. Indirect findings indicative of a more central great vessel stenosis are (1) post-stenotic turbulence with spectral broadening and disorganization of the waveform envelope or (2) a markedly diminished and nonpulsatile waveform. Similarly, (1) a notched vertebral waveform, (2) pendular flow, (3) systolic deceleration, and (4) reverse flow with diastolic antegrade flow are signs of more central supra-aortic trunk stenosis.[82]

Vertebral Arteries

The vertebral arteries undergo evaluation during a routine extracranial cerebrovascular duplex scan. These vessels can be imaged between the transverse processes of the cervical vertebrae, posterior and slightly medial to the CCA. They can usually be followed centrally to their origins at the subclavian artery, but this portion of the study is more difficult.

Ackerstaff and colleagues[3] and Bendick and Jackson[15] published early reports comparing duplex scanning and angiography of the vertebral arteries. Bendick and Jackson[15] found that duplex scanning adequately evaluated the vertebral arteries in 93% of 900 vessels. There was good correlation with angiographic findings in normal, stenotic, and occluded arteries. Reversed flow in the vertebral was readily identifiable by duplex scanning and was a reliable indicator of anatomic subclavian steal. Doppler flow abnormalities were identified in 95% of severely stenotic or occluded vessels, but duplex scanning was insensitive to moderate stenosis of the vertebral artery origin. The finding of unusually strong flow signals in one vertebral artery was associated with (1) severe occlusive disease in the opposite side, (2) subclavian steal with reversed vertebral flow direction on the opposite side, or (3) hemodynamically significant carotid disease.

The objective findings in these early reports of vertebral artery duplex scanning have withstood the test of time, but no quantitative grading scales for vertebral stenosis have been generally accepted. In most laboratories, interpretation of vertebral artery duplex scanning consists of:

- Comments on successful identification of the vessel
- Patency
- Flow direction
- Subjective interpretation of Doppler flow signals

Findings that deserve special comment include:

- Hyperemic flow

- Damped signal suggesting proximal stenosis
- Highly resistive signal suggesting intracranial stenosis or occlusion
- A pre-stenotic, stenotic, post-stenotic pattern suggesting a focal cervical stenosis

Later publications have suggested that application of color flow imaging to vertebral duplex scanning allows accurate diagnosis of dissection.[13] Another suggests that color flow imaging improves accuracy in the diagnosis of subclavian steal, although determination of vertebral flow direction based on traditional gray scale duplex scanning is relatively straightforward.[69] Finally, power Doppler imaging has been suggested as a complementary technique for evaluation of the vertebral artery, especially at the origin where the traditional study may be less accurate.[120]

Doppler and Duplex Scanning Evaluation of the Transcranial Arteries

In 1982, Aaslid and coworkers[1] introduced "transcranial Doppler" (TCD), the use of a low-frequency (2-MHz) Doppler device to penetrate the skull and measure blood flow velocity and direction in the intracranial arteries. They identified evaluation of vasospasm after subarachnoid hemorrhage as the primary indication for TCD, and it remains the best noninvasive test to establish that diagnosis. TCD instruments employed during the initial decade were "blind" pulsed Doppler machines without accompanying B-mode or color flow imaging. Thereafter, many duplex scanner manufacturers offered low-frequency transducers that added B-mode and color flow imaging to the information obtained with the TCD approach.

Both the original Doppler devices and the newer duplex transcranial scanning devices have been referred to as "TCD," causing some ambiguity. Workers in the field have now begun to use the term "transcranial imaging" (TCI) to distinguish the combination color flow Doppler imaging modality. The two approaches remain complementary. TCI allows more rapid and confident identification of intracranial vessels, and the learning curve is less challenging. The original TCD may retain the advantage for evaluation through very small transtemporal windows.

Indications

Evaluation of cerebral vasospasm remains the predominant and best-established indication for TCD. Intraoperative monitoring during carotid endarterectomy holds more interest for vascular surgeons, and the technique continues to undergo a critical appraisal for use in:

- Monitoring for emboli[2, 44, 80]
- Determining the need for shunt placement[1, 4, 22]
- Confirming adequate shunt function[127]
- Detecting intraoperative carotid artery thrombosis[45]

Results thus far are inconclusive for most of these indications. For instance, in the studies on the use of TCD monitoring to determine the need for shunt placement, authors reached contradictory conclusions.[1, 4, 22] Some authors have been frustrated by the inability to achieve and maintain an adequate transtemporal window during surgery. Technical failure rate on this basis ranges from approximately 15% to 40%.[2, 14]

Despite technical limitations and the potentially cost-intensive nature of intraoperative TCD monitoring, this technique holds substantial promise. Spencer[137] described a state-of-the-art effort monitoring 500 carotid endarterectomies with intraoperative TCD. Embolism, hyperperfusion, and hypoperfusion were identified by TCD and correlated with cerebrovascular complications. He argued that the perioperative stroke rate may be reduced when the surgeon takes appropriate measures on the basis of the findings of TCD monitoring.

Another important question for vascular surgeons is whether TCD should accompany routine extracranial duplex scanning in the evaluation of patients with carotid atherosclerosis. Several publications discuss this topic, again with mixed conclusions. Cantelmo and associates[21] and Comerota and coworkers[27] examined the issue and concluded that TCD had no material effect on diagnostic or treatment plans in patients with extracranial carotid artery disease. In contrast, Can and colleagues[20] found that both reversed flow in the ipsilateral ophthalmic artery identified through a transorbital window and a side-to-side difference in distal intracranial ICA PSVs of more than 50% were 100%-specific markers for identifying a severe ICA stenosis. They concluded that the specificity of extracranial duplex scanning could be enhanced if TCD were added to the routine examination.

Perhaps the most compelling argument for preoperative TCD resides in its ability to identify patients at risk for postoperative hyperperfusion syndrome.[65, 67, 103] Several publications associate high postoperative middle cerebral artery (MCA) velocities with onset of hyperperfusion headaches, seizures, and intracranial hemorrhage. The best determinant of what constitutes an elevated velocity is probably the preoperative baseline value, although intraoperative or early postoperative velocities may suffice. Unfortunately, very many preoperative studies would need to be performed in order to have such a baseline for the few patients who have headaches after surgery. Thus, the approach is likely to lack cost-effectiveness. Investigators continue to study and debate this issue, but practicing surgeons have not embraced preoperative TCD. A 1997 survey of expert vascular surgeons found that only 3% believed that TCD was an indicated preoperative test in the routine evaluation of extracranial atherosclerosis.[152]

Technique

The typical TCD study begins with identification of the best transtemporal window through identification of bony landmarks, including the petrous ridge and sphenoid bone. The MCA is identified first as having blood flow toward the TCD probe. Velocities and sampling depths are recorded at three sites along this artery. The anterior cerebral artery (ACA) ordinarily flows away from the TCD probe, slightly deeper than the MCA. Often the bidirectional MCA-ACA bifurcation signal serves as a landmark. The first (P1) segment of the posterior cerebral artery (PCA) is found slightly posterior to the MCA-ACA complex. P1 flows toward the transducer, but the second (P2) segment of the PCA curves to flow away from the transducer.

The transoccipital approach is used to sample the vertebral arteries. These vessels traverse the foramen magnum with flow direction away from the probe. The vertebral arteries are often tortuous, but they eventually converge to form the basilar artery, which also has flow away from the TCD probe. Mean velocities, sample depth, and flow direction are recorded at each sampling site. Special attention is given to areas of unusual flow velocity or direction.

Interpretation

By convention, TCD blood flow is recorded as mean velocity rather than the angle-corrected PSV used in extracranial carotid duplex scanning. The rationale stems from inability of the original "blind" Doppler technique to determine the angle between the artery and the incoming ultrasound beam; mean velocity is less dependent upon the angle. The assumption is reasonable for the MCA and ACA because the actual angle approximates zero, making the magnitude of angle correction relatively small. Angle-corrected normal velocity ranges based on color flow duplex scanning analysis have also been published,[128] but to date, most investigators continue to use mean values.

The range of normal mean blood flow velocity in the MCA is between 30 and 80 cm/sec, and vasospasm or stenosis confirmed angiographically correlates with velocities of 120 cm/sec or greater.[1, 109] Comparison of mean velocity in the MCA with that in the distal extracranial ICA can help distinguish hyperemia from vasospasm when MCA velocity is elevated.[108]

Interpretation of TCD signals for emboli monitoring during carotid surgery relies upon a distinctive, harmonic, chirping or whistling signal that must be distinguished from sounds indicating probe motion artifact.[138, 142] Accurate definition of TCD embolic signals has been the subject of a multicenter review.[86] For identification of patients at risk for post–carotid endarterectomy hyperperfusion syndrome, a threshold level appears to be approximately a 100% increase in MCA velocity.[65, 67, 103] Comparison with the contralateral MCA may also be useful in these patients.

EVALUATION OF ABDOMINAL VISCERAL ARTERIES

Renal Arteries

The ability to achieve a surgical or interventional cure for renovascular hypertension distinguishes it from essential hypertension, which affects a vastly greater number of patients. For several decades, contrast arteriography was the only modality useful in making the diagnosis of renovascular hypertension. The magnitude, risks, and expense of this procedure often discouraged physicians from obtaining the study, so the diagnosis was frequently overlooked. The unfortunate result of untreated renovascular occlusive disease is ultimate progression to renal failure, even if the multitude of other hypertension-induced complications are avoided through aggressive blood pressure control.

Duplex ultrasound scanning of the renal arteries was described in 1984 by Norris and colleagues[110] in a study that combined data from an experimental canine model and an initial human trial. The authors pointed out that transducers with lower transmitting frequencies were necessary to sample arteries deep in the abdomen. They recorded the frequency of returned echoes and found that with increasing arterial stenosis, the ratio of end-diastolic frequency to peak systolic frequency (end-diastolic ratio [EDR]) decreased. They also described diagnostic parameters that have become standard in the search for arterial stenosis by duplex scanning:

1. Elevated peak frequency shift.
2. Irregular Doppler profile outline.
3. Systolic spectral broadening.
4. Locally increased velocity within the stenosis compared to pre-stenotic and post-stenotic regions.

It should be pointed out that renal duplex scanning is probably the most difficult duplex ultrasound examination, and the excellent published results described in the following paragraphs have been obtained by very skilled technologists. Most reports cite a 5% to 12% incidence of technically unsatisfactory examinations, primarily due to bowel gas or patient obesity. Nevertheless, this study can be mastered by most technologists given the proper equipment and adequate training.

Indications

Renovascular disease in the United States is caused primarily by atherosclerosis and fibromuscular dysplasia. Clinical manifestations are hypertension, ischemic nephropathy, or both. The classic patient with atherosclerotic renovascular disease is older than 50 years, has typical atherogenic risk factors, and may have long-standing mild or moderate essential hypertension. Blood pressure suddenly becomes difficult to control, and serum creatinine level may begin to increase.

Patients with fibromuscular dysplasia are much younger and almost always female. They rarely have preexisting hypertension, and the diagnosis is often made fortuitously or during evaluation for nonspecific symptoms.

Renal duplex scanning is an appropriate test in both settings. Clinical decision-making based on the study results depends on the patient's pre-test probability of disease and the established accuracy of the laboratory performing the examination.

Technique

Patients are best examined after an overnight fast to minimize interference by bowel gas. A low-frequency (2.25- to 3.0-MHz) transducer is employed. The examination begins with the patient in supine position. Using an anterior midline approach, the technologist obtains a center stream suprarenal aortic velocity in a long axis view at a 60-degree Doppler angle. The technologist then rotates the probe 90 degrees to obtain a transverse image and identifies the left renal vein as it crosses anterior to the aorta (Fig. 12–6; see Color Plate); this is usually an excellent landmark for the renal artery origins. In order to achieve a technically complete duplex scan examination, the technologist should evaluate the arteries along their entire length from the aorta

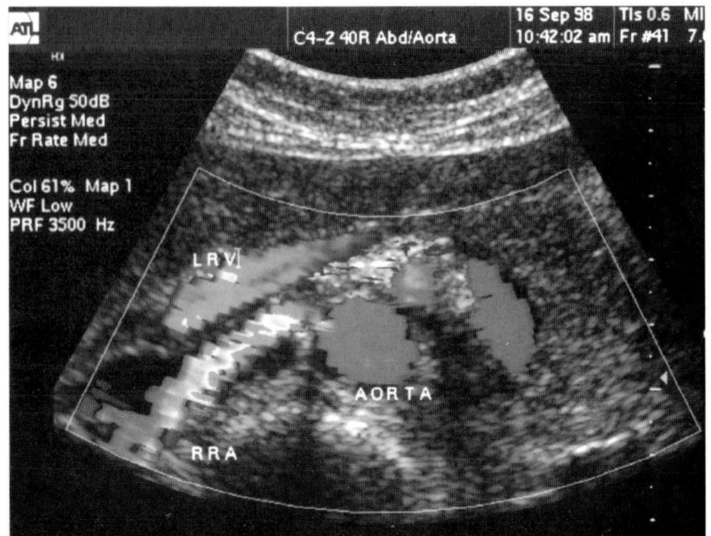

FIGURE 12–6. Transverse view of aorta, right renal artery (RRA), left renal vein (LRV), and origin of left renal artery (unlabeled). This is a typical color flow landmark enabling the examiner to begin Doppler spectral data collection in the renal arteries. See Color Plate.

to the renal pelvis (Fig. 12–7; see Color Plate). Angle-corrected Doppler velocity spectral waveforms are recorded at the origin and at proximal, middle, and distal locations, with special attention to any focal site where abnormal velocities are found. It should be recalled that patients with atherosclerosis tend to have lesions near the renal origins whereas young women are more likely to have focal mid-renal stenoses caused by fibromuscular disease.

If overlying bowel gas prevents visualization, turning the patient to the lateral decubitus position frequently allows visualization of the renal artery at the kidney. This may then be followed back to the aorta. Typically, a combination of supine and lateral decubitus positions is necessary for thorough evaluation of the entire renal artery. The technologist searches the aorta for accessory renal arteries, which are examined in detail when identified. Peak systolic velocities and Doppler spectra are recorded, and renal-aortic PSV ratios are calculated. The technologist images the kidneys with the patient in the lateral decubitus position, using a lateral axillary approach to obtain coronal and long axis views. Pole-to-pole length of each kidney is measured, with an attempt to maintain a consistent approach for reproducible values.[62] Doppler signals are also obtained from interlobar and arcuate renal arteries. If indirect tests are used to supplement the direct examination (see later), the technologist obtains Doppler spectra from the renal hilum for determination of acceleration time and acceleration index.

Interpretation and Accuracy

Normal renal arteries have a low-resistance Doppler waveform with PSV less than 180 cm/sec (Fig. 12–8; see Color Plate). Kohler and associates[75] introduced the concept of using a ratio of the PSV in the renal artery to the PSV in the aorta (renal-aortic ratio [RAR]) as a diagnostic criterion for identification of clinically significant renal artery occlusive disease. In a retrospective comparison of duplex scanning with angiographically graded stenosis, an RAR greater than 3.5 corresponded to a diameter-reducing stenosis of 60% or larger (Fig. 12–9; see Color Plate). Application of this diagnostic threshold resulted in a sensitivity of 91%

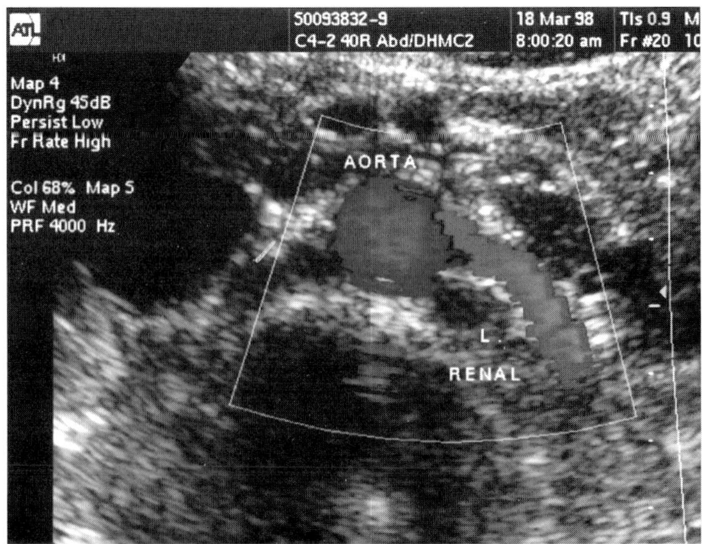

FIGURE 12–7. Color flow image of left renal artery from aorta to renal pelvis. After the artery is located, its entire length is sampled for Doppler velocities and spectra. See Color Plate.

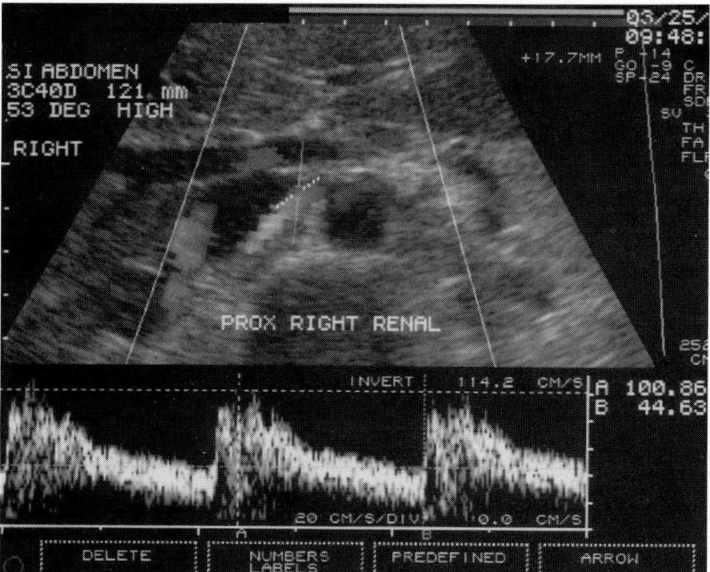

FIGURE 12–8. Normal Doppler spectrum sampled from proximal right renal artery. Waveform has rapid upstroke and high flow throughout diastole. This low resistance morphology indicates normal low resistance of the renal parenchyma. See Color Plate.

and a specificity of 95%. Kohler and associates[75] also calculated the EDR, as described earlier by Norris and coworkers.[110] They found that EDR tended to be lower in patients who had elevated serum creatinine levels but did not have renal artery stenosis. This analysis led to the suggestion that EDR is a marker for end-stage renal parenchymal disease.

Taylor and colleagues[141] published a prospective validation of the original University of Washington RAR threshold of 3.5. Overall agreement of these results with those of angiography was 93%. Duplex scanning identified 38 of 39 arteries with stenosis of less than 60%, 11 of 14 arteries with stenosis of 60% to 99%, and 4 of 5 arteries with total occlusion. This technique therefore had an 84% sensitivity, a 97% specificity, and a positive predictive value of 94%, just slightly less accuracy than found by the original retrospective analysis.[75]

Independent prospective validation in a series of 74 patients was reported by Hansen and coworkers[53] from Bowman Gray School of Medicine in 1990. The duplex scanning technique used in this study was also very thorough, consisting of 10 Doppler probe sampling sites per artery with the use of both an abdominal and a flank approach. An RAR of 3.5 or greater was used as a threshold indicator of stenosis of 60% or greater only if the elevated velocities were identified in the presence of a turbulent waveform. An occlusion was diagnosed if the artery was identified by B-mode imaging yet no Doppler signal could be obtained. This patient cohort had a high incidence of disease, with 10% of the arteries occluded and more than 25% stenotic. Twenty kidneys had multiple renal arteries, several of which were stenotic. Duplex scanning was technically inadequate in only 6 of 74 cases; 4 of the patients concerned had normal arteries and 2 had stenoses. For the remaining scanning studies, the authors found a sensitivity of 88%, a specificity of 99%, a positive predictive value of 98%, and a negative predictive value of 92%. Accuracy was

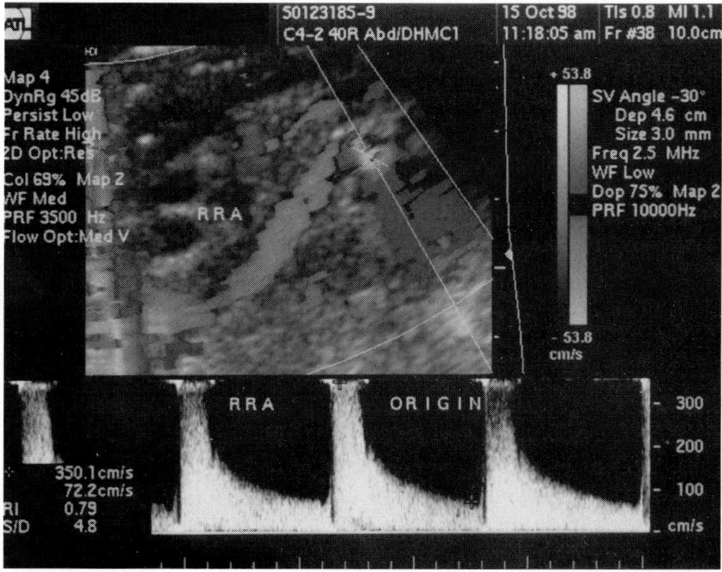

FIGURE 12–9. Abnormal right renal artery (RRA) with a peak systolic velocity (PSV) of 350 cm/sec. Aortic PSV was 70 cm/sec, resulting in a renal-aortic ratio of 5.0. Stenosis was subsequently confirmed by angiography. The image demonstrates the importance of accurate angle correction in tortuous renals. See Color Plate.

influenced by the presence of diseased accessory arteries, but not by concomitant aortoiliac disease or renal insufficiency.

Hansen and coworkers[53] also examined the use of a PSV of 200 cm/sec or higher as a marker for stenosis of 60% or greater. They found that the accuracy of this isolated renal artery velocity equaled that of the RAR threshold. This report emphasized the presence of multiple renal arteries as a major pitfall of renal artery evaluation by duplex scanning. Sensitivity was only 67% in the subset of patients with multiple renal arteries. These authors also found that a low EDR was statistically associated with increased creatinine levels. There was no correlation of EDR with blood pressure normalization or return of renal function after revascularization. Finally, these authors concluded that a patient with significant hypertension should undergo an arteriogram if the renal duplex scan is negative. Their conclusion was based on the negative predictive value of 92%, a value that they judged was inadequate to confidently rule out renovascular occlusive disease in a patient with a high pre-test probability of disease.

Hoffman and associates[56] tested the accuracy of a PSV of 180 cm/sec or higher in the identification of any degree of renal artery stenosis. They found a 95% sensitivity and 90% specificity for this threshold. These researchers also tested an RAR of 3.5 or higher for identification of stenosis of 60% or greater; they found a 92% sensitivity but only a 62% specificity in this cohort.

On the basis of an amalgamation of the results of these three studies, the University of Washington group now suggests the diagnostic algorithm reported in the previous version of this text. They recommend reporting a renal artery as:

1. Normal if the PSV is below 180 cm/sec and the RAR is below 3.5.
2. Having stenosis under 60% if the PSV above 180 cm/sec but the RAR below 3.5.
3. Having stenosis over 60% if the RAR > 3.5, regardless of whether the PSV is below or above 180 cm/sec.

A prospective trial of this specific algorithm has not been published.

Olin and colleagues[113] from the Cleveland Clinic, however, tested an algorithm whereby either a PSV of 200 cm/sec or higher or a RAR of 3.5 or higher indicated the presence of renal artery stenosis of 60% or greater. This is perhaps the largest prospective series comparing duplex scanning and angiography for renal artery stenosis published to date. Their patient cohort also had a high incidence of renal disease. Accuracy in this series was excellent, with a sensitivity of 98%, specificity of 98%, positive predictive value of 99%, and negative predictive value of 97%.

In conclusion, most researchers found the RAR threshold of more than 3.5 to be accurate using a variety of instrumentation. Likewise, a PSV threshold of greater than 200 cm/sec was accurate in two large studies. As noted, the Cleveland Clinic algorithm diagnoses a greater than 60% renal artery stenosis if either of these thresholds is identified. As a starting point for laboratories undertaking this examination, either threshold or the combination seems reasonable. As noted in the discussion on carotid artery duplex scanning, however, individual laboratory results are likely to vary. Ongoing quality assessment must be performed with renal duplex scanning to determine whether published thresholds are accurate in individual laboratories.

Indirect Renal Artery Evaluation

Intrarenal sampling has been proposed as a rapid and easy method to determine the presence of a renal artery stenosis without actually having to study the main renal artery directly. Martin and associates[87] suggested that a prolonged hilar acceleration time indicated the presence of a more proximal renal artery stenosis. Sampling was done at the interlobar branches within the hilum with a Doppler angle defined as zero. Time was recorded to the initial or "compliance" peak. An acceleration time longer than 0.100 sec indicated a proximal arterial stenosis. This finding has not been widely validated.

Handa and colleagues[52] suggested that a decreased slope of frequency change over time, defined as the acceleration index, indicated a proximal renal artery stenosis. The threshold they used was a value less than 3.78 kHz shift/sec. These authors found a sensitivity of 100% and a specificity of 93% for the test. Once again, this method has not been validated extensively.

Schwerk and coworkers[130] measured the intrarenal resistive index:

$$\frac{\text{PSV} - \text{EDV}}{\text{PSV}} \times 100$$

They then compared one side with the other. A difference in resistive index of more than 5% was indicative of a 50% renal artery stenosis. These researchers found a sensitivity of 82% and specificity of 92% with this technique. They pointed out that the method loses accuracy in patients with bilateral stenoses and is not applicable in those with only one patent renal artery.

"Pulsus tardus" and "pulsus parvus" are old terms used to describe waveforms with slow and delayed upstrokes. In general, these terms may describe the intraparenchymal signals found in kidneys beyond a renal artery stenosis. In particular, they have been identified as signs of thoracoabdominal aortic coarctation in the pediatric age group.[91]

Overall, the indirect methods take less time to perform than direct duplex scanning of the renal arteries, and they are certainly easier. Unfortunately, none has undergone a truly rigorous prospective trial. The indirect methods have been summarized in more detail by Isaacson and Neumyer.[62]

Evaluation After Renal Revascularization

Eidt and colleagues[35] pointed out that duplex scanning techniques can be used effectively for evaluation of renal revascularizations, both surgical and percutaneous. They tested the same parameters used for native renal artery stenosis and found reasonable accuracy. A major point of their report was the observation that renal artery bypass grafts may originate from many places, including the infrarenal aorta, supraceliac aorta or the splenic, gastroduodenal, hepatic, or iliac arteries. To save time and improve study yield, the technologist should be informed of the source of the bypass inflow. In a later publication, Taylor and associates[140] made essentially the same observations regarding the utility of duplex scanning after renal revascularization.

Renal Transplant Evaluation

Use of duplex scanning to evaluate renal transplants has been reviewed by many workers and is summarized in the publications of Neumyer and colleagues.[105–107] In brief, the transplant renal artery and vein may be evaluated by duplex ultrasonography for patency and the presence of stenosis.[135] Neumyer suggests using a transplanted artery to external iliac artery PSV ratio of 3.0 as a threshold to identify significant stenosis.[107] Increased PSV and spectral broadening are also findings associated with stenosis of the transplant artery. Most workers agree that the ability of duplex scanning to distinguish acute rejection from acute tubular necrosis using resistive indices or other measures is controversial at best and perhaps not efficacious.[42]

Mesenteric Arteries

Diagnosis of chronic mesenteric ischemia is difficult because the symptoms are nonspecific. Prior to the mid-1980s, the only means to confirm the clinical suspicion of chronic mesenteric ischemia was contrast angiography. One of the earliest reports of noninvasive diagnosis of this entity was a case study published by Jager and coworkers[63] in 1984. These authors described elevated PSV obtained by duplex scanning in the superior mesenteric artery (SMA) of a woman with a 6-month history of postprandial epigastric pain, diarrhea, and a 30-pound weight loss.[63] Subsequent digital subtraction aortography confirmed the suspicion of mesenteric occlusive disease.

In 1991, two large retrospective comparisons identified duplex scanning–derived blood flow velocities that provided accurate identification of severe mesenteric arterial stenosis.[18, 97] Since then, the examination has been adopted by many laboratories, and several prospective studies have been published confirming the accuracy of the velocity thresholds. Like renal artery duplex scanning, mesenteric artery examination by duplex scanning entails a substantial learning curve. Once mastered, however, this is an important and rewarding study.

Indications

Most commonly, mesenteric duplex scanning is a screening test for the elderly patient with symptoms of chronic mesenteric ischemia. Although evaluation of the elderly atherosclerotic patient with postprandial abdominal pain, “food fear,” and weight loss should proceed directly to diagnostic angiography, many patients with mesenteric ischemia have less classic signs and symptoms. Patients in this latter group benefit from the duplex scanning examination because it either confirms the necessity for angiography, if positive, or defers angiography in favor of other diagnostic studies, if negative.

Less common indications for this study include evaluation of possible median arcuate compression syndrome and follow-up evaluation of patients who have undergone surgical or interventional mesenteric revascularization.[140] When performed by a technologist with general knowledge of the mesenteric vascular anatomy, duplex scanning may also be utilized for evaluation of the portal and hepatic vasculature.[50, 112, 134] Unfortunately, patients with acute mesenteric ischemia usually have too much air-filled bowel to allow accurate duplex imaging.

Technique

It is important that mesenteric duplex scanning be performed after the patient has fasted at least 6 hours because the SMA waveform changes from a low-flow, high-resistance morphology to a high-flow, low-resistance form after the subject has eaten (Fig. 12–10; see Color Plate). Examinations are generally performed with the patient supine or in a slight reverse Trendelenburg position. Low-frequency transducers are required to perform this study, typically with Doppler transmitting frequencies ranging from 2.0 to 3.0 MHz and imaging frequencies from 2.0 to 4.0 MHz. Initial transducer positioning is just below the xiphoid, but a right lateral approach, with the liver used as an acoustic window, may also offer an excellent view.

The technologist examines the celiac, common hepatic, and superior mesenteric arteries thoroughly (Fig. 12–11; see Color Plate). Doppler waveforms and velocities are recorded with careful attention to angle correction because each of these vessels may be very tortuous.[121] The technologist attempts to identify the splenic, gastroduodenal, and inferior mesenteric arteries. Knowledge of common mesenteric anatomic anomalies is important because they are found in approximately 20% of patients.[68, 153]

Interpretation and Accuracy

Moneta and colleagues[97] found that either a PSV of 275 cm/sec or higher or the absence of a flow signal predicted a 70% to 100% stenosis of the SMA with sensitivity and specificity of 89% and 92%, respectively. They identified a PSV of 200 cm/sec or higher as the most accurate celiac artery threshold with a sensitivity of 75% and a specificity of 89%.

My colleagues and I found end-diastolic velocity (EDV) to be more accurate for diagnosis of SMA stenosis.[18] We identified an EDV of 45 cm/sec or higher to be the best indicator of a 50% or greater stenosis of the SMA, with a sensitivity of 100% and a specificity of 92%. We also found a PSV of 300 cm/sec or higher to be highly specific but less sensitive for severe stenosis in the SMA. In that initial study, we found no accurate diagnostic velocity threshold for severe stenosis in the celiac artery and postulated that the generous collateral circulation in this region might limit the pathophysiologic requirement for high-velocity flow across a narrowed celiac axis. LaBombard and coworkers,[77] in the same laboratory, subsequently identified retrograde flow in the common hepatic artery as a reliable indicator of severe celiac artery stenosis or occlusion.

Moneta and colleagues[95] published a prospective validation analysis of their diagnostic criteria in 1993. They confirmed excellent accuracy in the SMA and good accuracy in the celiac artery for the criteria noted previously. Subsequently, we tested our original mesenteric duplex scanning criteria and confirmed excellent sensitivity and

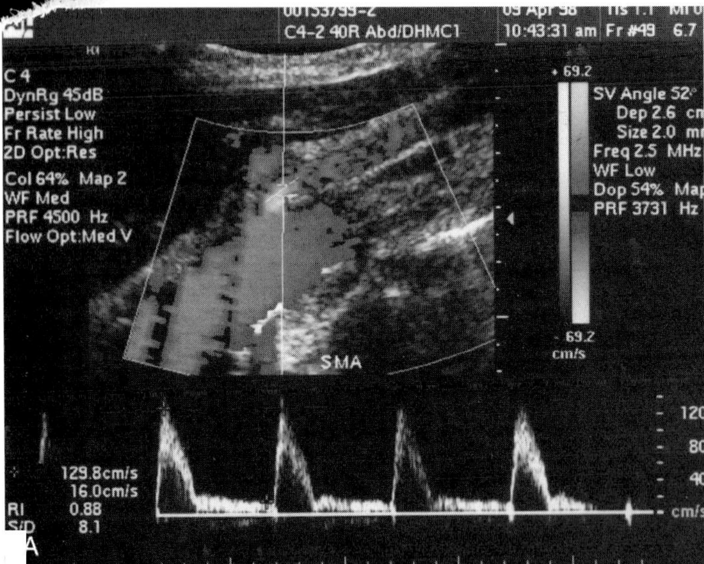

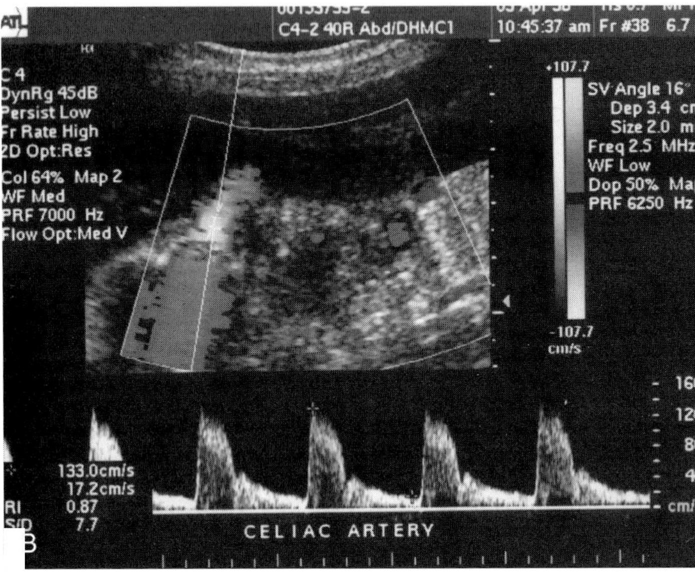

FIGURE 12–10. *A*, Normal, fasting, high-resistance waveform in the superior mesenteric artery (SMA). Angle correction is crucial as the SMA curves sharply beyond its origin from the aorta. *B*, The celiac origin has a low-resistance Doppler waveform. See Color Plate.

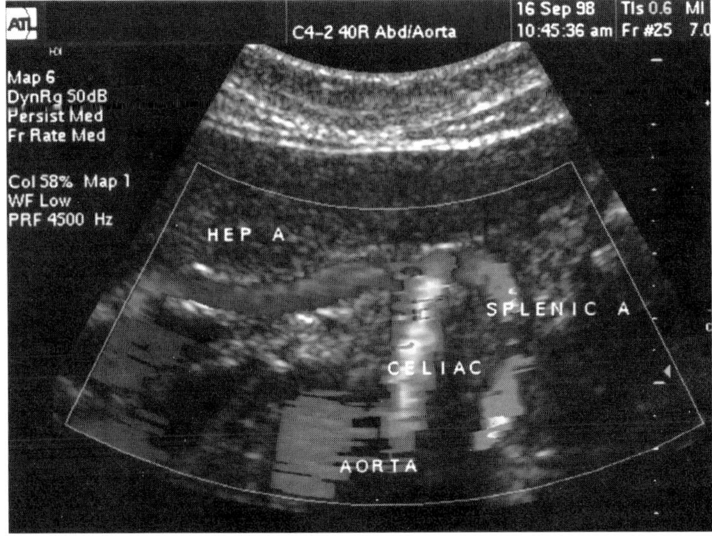

FIGURE 12–11. Color flow appearance of the celiac axis and bifurcation into the splenic and common hepatic arteries. Common hepatic artery flow direction may be retrograde if the celiac artery is severely stenotic or occluded. Visual impression of flow direction based on color flow must be confirmed by Doppler sampling. See Color Plate.

specificity for EDV of 45 cm/sec or higher for identification of either a 50% or greater stenosis or an occlusion of the SMA.[153] Diagnostic accuracy for celiac artery stenosis was excellent with the use of an EDV of 55 cm/sec or higher or a PSV of 200 cm/sec or higher. Retrograde blood flow direction in the common hepatic artery was 100% predictive of severe celiac stenosis or occlusion.

Independent confirmation of mesenteric duplex scanning accuracy was provided in a report by Perko and associates.[117] These authors compared duplex scanning results with angiographic measurement of stenosis in a cohort of symptomatic patients. The manuscript emphasizes end-diastolic velocities as the more accurate means by which to diagnose significant mesenteric stenosis, but review of their data indicates that both PSV and EDV were remarkably accurate (>90%) for this purpose.

A final important issue in mesenteric duplex scanning involves identification of anatomic anomalies. These are found in approximately 20% of the population and may substantially affect accurate interpretation of the study. For example, a replaced right hepatic artery arising from the SMA may increase velocities and change the SMA waveform from triphasic to biphasic in the absence of stenosis.[153] With attention to detail, most anomalies can be correctly identified by duplex scanning. Thus, it is important for sonographers and interpreters to be familiar with the more common variants to avoid interpretation pitfalls.

Summary

Mesenteric duplex scanning is an accurate, noninvasive method to diagnose chronic mesenteric arterial disease. Once the technique of this study has been mastered, it may be applied with confidence in the evaluation of possible chronic mesenteric ischemia and other abdominal vascular disorders. As with all other arterial duplex scanning examinations, more than one set of diagnostic criteria has been published. For mesenteric duplex scanning, the discrepancy between the published thresholds is not excessive. Individual laboratories must choose their own best-fit criteria on the basis of angiographic and clinical correlation.

EVALUATION OF LOWER EXTREMITY ARTERIAL DISEASE

Aortoiliac, Femoropopliteal, Tibial, and Pedal Arteries

The potential role of duplex scanning in the evaluation and management of lower extremity arterial disease has undergone substantial investigation. Studies published in the late 1980s and early 1990s indicated the ability of duplex scanning to identify stenotic lesions from the aorta to the pedal vessels, and several described the potential for duplex scanning to replace arteriography in the planning of lower extremity revascularization.[28, 64, 73, 74] Later investigations comparing the accuracy of color flow duplex scanning with angiography in patients undergoing lower extremity revascularization reached similar conclusions, finding the accuracy of duplex scanning equal to[83] or better than[149] angiography for prediction of adequate outflow targets.

Indications

Arterial mapping with duplex scanning may be of assistance in the evaluation and treatment of patients with symptomatic lower extremity arterial insufficiency in at least three ways. First, aortoiliac and femoropopliteal duplex scanning may be used to identify percutaneous intervention targets in patients with intermittent claudication.[28] Patients found to have focal iliac or femoral stenoses may be advised regarding the potential suitability of angioplasty, whereas those with long occlusions may be counseled that surgery would likely be required to relieve symptoms. This information may help the patient and physician decide whether to proceed with angiography.[30] In addition, the duplex scanning information will help in planning the optimal approach for treatment of the target lesion.

The second, more encompassing role for duplex scanning lies in its potential as a substitute for angiography in patients requiring aortofemoral or infrainguinal reconstruction. Several small series published in the 1990s have reached increasingly positive results about this application.[73, 83, 149]

The third potential role for duplex scanning in the evaluation of the lower extremities lies in its potential to find suitable distal revascularization targets when none are visualized by angiography.[71] In these circumstances, performance of duplex arterial mapping requires a skilled technologist and is labor-intensive.

Technique

Duplex scanning evaluation of the aorta and iliac arteries employs the same 2- to 3-MHz transducers employed for evaluation of mesenteric and renal arteries. Patients are best studied after an overnight fast. Initial positioning is supine, but right and left lateral decubitus positions may be helpful to accomplish a complete study. The technologist begins the examination with the transducer placed just below the xiphoid, where the aorta is imaged in a sagittal plane. The evaluation proceeds along to the bifurcation and each iliac artery through the pelvis to the groin.[29]

A 5- or 7.5-MHz transducer is typically used to study the femoral, popliteal, and tibial vessels. Evaluation of the popliteal and tibial arteries is best performed with a combination of prone and supine patient positioning. The tibial arteries are usually scanned from the infrageniculate popliteal artery distally, but the technologist may facilitate this portion of the study in patients with advanced disease by starting at the ankle and scanning cephalad. Color flow imaging is useful to identify all vessels initially and to search for regions of color flow disturbance indicative of stenosis. Subsequently, the technologist "sweeps" the pulsed Doppler probe through all segments. Representative images and Doppler velocity spectra are recorded in all regions. The technologist should pay special attention to areas of stenosis; images and spectra should be recorded within, proximal to, and immediately beyond the narrowed region. Technical adequacy of this examination for identification of all vessels exceeds 90% in most reports, although evaluation of the peroneal artery may be somewhat less successful.[96]

Interpretation and Accuracy

The most widely recommended criterion for diagnosis of peripheral artery stenosis is a 100% PSV step-up (velocity ratio ≥ 2.0) compared with a normal segment of artery proximal to the stenosis. Several investigators determined that this finding correlated closely with a 50% or greater reduction of angiographic diameter.[28, 64, 74, 96] A small number of studies found best accuracy at higher velocity ratios of 2.5[78] and 3.0.[79] Most studies indicate that spectral broadening and loss of a previously present end-systolic reverse-flow component should also be identified for confident diagnosis of a 50% or greater stenosis. Although a number of early studies attempted to establish multiple stenosis categories in a manner similar to carotid disease categorization,[28, 73, 74] most contemporary publications have not pursued that concept, limiting duplex scanning categorization of peripheral arteries[83, 96, 98] to the following:

- Patent without significant stenosis
- Patent with stenosis ≥ 50%
- Occluded

Identification of peripheral stenoses by color Doppler imaging without Doppler velocity data has been studied, and the results were predictably poor.[54]

Accuracy data have been compiled using both angiography and determination of best lower extremity bypass target as gold standards. In the aorta and iliac segments, sensitivities from 81% to 91% and specificities from 90% to 99% have been determined in blinded comparisons of duplex scanning with angiography.[28, 30, 74, 78, 96, 98] For identification of femoral and popliteal stenoses, reported accuracy covers a wider range, with sensitivities from 67% to 91% but specificities from 94% to 99%.[28, 74, 96]

Fewer studies compare duplex scanning evaluation of tibial lesions with angiography. Moneta and colleagues evaluated the ability of duplex scanning to determine interruption of patency of the tibial artery from origin to ankle.[96] They found sensitivity and specificity of 90% and 93%, respectively, for anterior and posterior tibial artery stenosis, but lower values of 82% and 74%, respectively, for identification of stenosis in the peroneal artery. Sensier and coworkers[132] found substantial agreement between color flow duplex scanning and arteriography at all arterial levels, but the correspondence was less good for tibial vessels.

Two later reports examined the ability of duplex scanning to predict the optimal revascularization procedure. Wilson and associates[149] performed 44 femorocrural reconstructions for critical ischemia following contrast angiography and duplex scanning. Angiography correctly identified a suitable target artery in 73% of cases but was indeterminate, failed to identify any target, or identified an inferior target in the remainder. Duplex scanning correctly identified a suitable runoff vessel in all patients. The authors concluded that duplex scanning was superior to angiography for preoperative assessment of runoff vessels during femorocrural reconstruction. Ligush and colleagues[83] performed a similar prospective analysis in 36 patients whose eventual treatment included 34 vascular reconstructions, 4 amputations, and 2 nonoperative treatments. Five of the revascularizations were inflow procedures, and the remainder were infrainguinal. Duplex scanning allowed correct prediction of surgical treatment in 83% of cases, whereas angiography was correct in 90%; these accuracy rates were not statistically different. The researchers concluded that duplex scanning can be used reliably to predict vascular reconstruction strategies.

An important question in duplex scanning of lower extremity arterial disease is the ability of the technique to identify distal stenoses in the presence of multilevel disease. Sensier and coworkers[131] addressed this question directly by comparing the accuracy of duplex scanning and angiography in (1) regions of isolated stenosis and (2) regions where adjacent stenoses were present. They found that duplex scanning was not adversely affected by adjacent stenosis. Ligush and colleagues[83] made a similar observation, although their study was not designed to directly test this question.

On the basis of these observations as well as the individual accuracy values presented in the preceding sections, it is somewhat surprising that duplex scanning has not supplanted arteriography on a more widespread basis in the evaluation of lower extremity arteries.

Ultrasound-Guided Compression Repair of Postcatheterization Pseudoaneurysms

Pseudoaneurysm formation after percutaneous femoral artery catheterization has become a common occurrence in most medical centers. In 1991, ultrasound-guided compression repair of this problem was described, making it perhaps the first therapeutic maneuver in noninvasive vascular technology.[39] Since then, a large number of series have proved the safety and efficacy of this technique.[32, 100, 116, 126]

The process begins with identification of the neck of the pseudoaneurysm (Fig. 12–12; see Color Plate). The probe is placed over the neck, and compression is applied until flow ceases. Many algorithms for this procedure include application of a Doppler probe over the ankle for constant monitoring of blood flow to the foot, allowing the operator to eliminate flow through the pseudoaneurysm neck without applying enough force to block femoral artery flow. Compression is applied for 10- to 15-minute intervals, and the pseudoaneurysm is checked for thrombosis. Multiple compressions are occasionally required for successful thrombosis. In patients who experience pain from the procedure, intravenous sedation and analgesia may be administered as long as appropriate cardiopulmonary monitoring is performed. A new development in this field is the injection of thrombin into the pseudoaneurysm under duplex scanning guidance. Initial reports suggest that this is a safe and effective technique that substantially reduces the physical effort and time requirements of the procedure.[70, 81]

Arterial Bypass Graft Surveillance

Duplex surveillance of infrainguinal arterial bypass grafts has become a major component of postoperative care following vascular reconstructions performed with autogenous conduit. Identification of the failing bypass graft is crucial

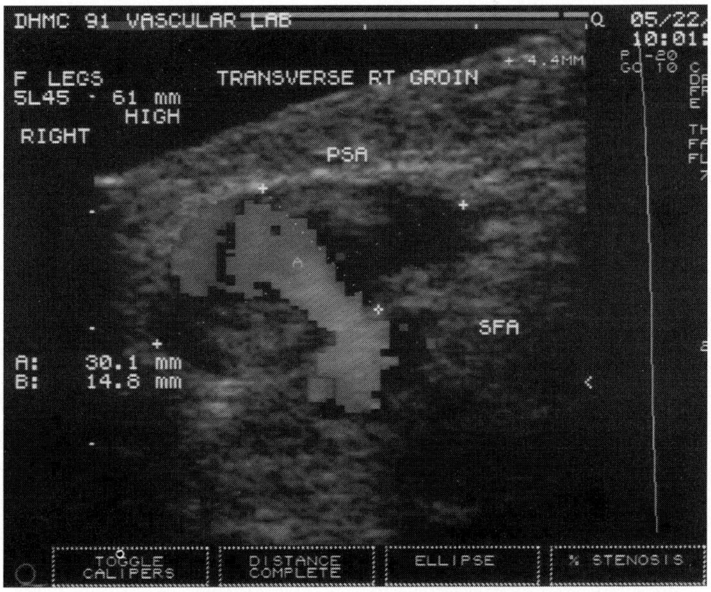

FIGURE 12–12. Pseudoaneurysm arising from the superficial femoral artery (SFA) just beyond the femoral bifurcation. Pseudoaneurysm (PSA) is partially thrombosed. Swirling blood is seen in the remainder. Compression over the PSA neck is frequently successful in achieving complete thrombosis (see also Fig. 48–6). See Color Plate.

because meaningful long-term graft salvage is often not possible once thrombosis occurs. Clinical parameters such as return of ischemic symptoms and reduction of ankle pulse quality are insensitive markers for hemodynamically significant stenoses within failing grafts. Several studies revealed that only one third of hemodynamically significant graft stenoses can be diagnosed from the history and physical examination alone.[34,60,99]

Early publications argued for and against the benefit of the Doppler-derived ankle-brachial pressure index (ABI) to detect failing vein grafts, but at best, the ABI is an insensitive parameter to follow.[12,16] Bandyk and associates[6] reported that Doppler-derived low PSV (<45 cm/sec) and absence of diastolic forward flow were predictive of impending graft failure. Mills and colleagues[92] confirmed the predictive utility of a low PSV in a much larger cohort of reversed vein grafts. This parameter may be used as a rapid surveillance technique that involves sampling the graft in only one or two areas. This sampling approach may be insensitive to focal stenosis, however, and it is nonspecific in that the low PSV may be due to inflow stenosis, graft stenosis, or even poor runoff. A more contemporary technique involves scanning the entire graft to search for flow disturbances, loss of the typical flow pattern, unusually low or high PSVs, and regions of PSV step-up.

Technique

The study is typically performed with use of transmitting frequencies from 4.0 to 7.5 MHz. Knowledge of the origin, insertion, and route of the bypass aids performance and speed of examination. In situ grafts are usually easy to identify and follow along their subcutaneous route, whereas grafts in anatomic or extra-anatomic tunnels are more challenging.

Scanning begins at the inflow artery, crosses the proximal anastomosis, and proceeds distally along the body of the graft to include the distal anastomosis. Scanning with color flow imaging may expedite the examination by allowing rapid identification of regions with high velocity or disturbed flow patterns. Doppler spectra may be obtained at areas where the color map identifies turbulence or a velocity step-up. For calculation of a velocity ratio, a Doppler spectrum must also be recorded proximal to the stenosis in a region of undisturbed flow (Fig. 12–13; see Color Plate). Careful Doppler angle adjustment is required at the distal anastomosis, where the graft may approach the outflow artery at a steep angle. If low PSVs (<45 cm/sec) are identified throughout the graft, a search may be undertaken for inflow and outflow disease. Low PSVs may be normal findings in a graft with a very large diameter; these findings are typical when basilic vein has been used as the conduit.

Diagnostic Thresholds and Accuracy

Results of graft surveillance protocols similar to the technique just described were published simultaneously in 1993 by two teams of workers.[60,89] Both reports concluded that surveillance by color flow duplex scanning successfully detected graft-threatening stenoses and that elective repair of stenotic lesions within saphenous vein arterial bypass grafts significantly prolonged patency. Although these studies were not prospective, randomized trials, their results were thoroughly analyzed. The two studies identified an improvement in assisted primary patency of approximately 20% at 3 to 5 years in grafts that were revised after duplex scanning surveillance detected problems, in comparison with grafts that were not revised when stenoses were identified and with grafts undergoing only clinical follow-up.

In 1994, Fillinger and associates[41] employed duplex scanning surveillance techniques to evaluate in situ grafts that remained free of stenosis. They found that normally functioning conduits remodel over time such that diameter, volume flow rate, PSV, and shear stress tend to stabilize at uniform values regardless of the initial vein graft diameter. Grafts with initially small diameters enlarged, whereas those with large diameters eventually reduced in flow-channel caliber, such that no significant difference in diameter was present at 1 year after placement. Of the hemodynamic variables studied, shear stress was most strongly associated

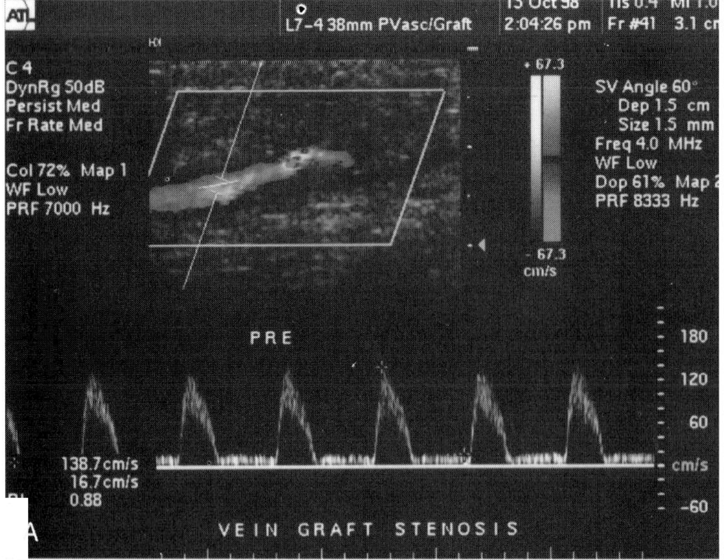

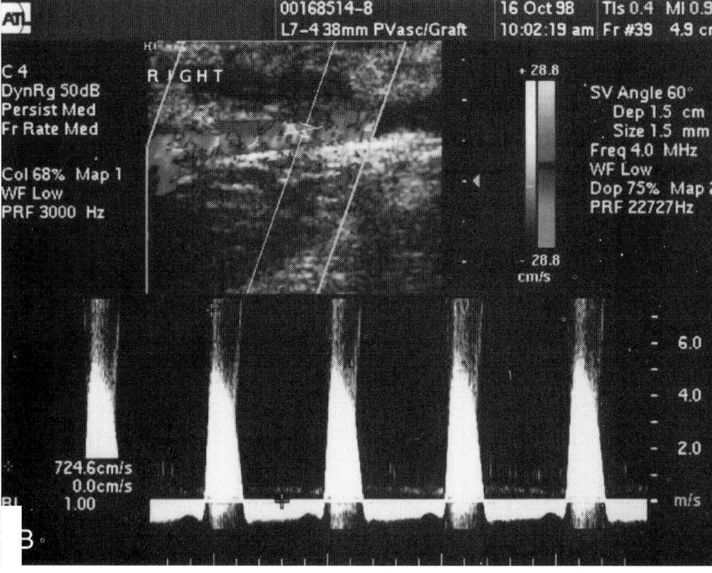

FIGURE 12–13. *A*, Bypass graft Doppler spectrum proximal to a vein graft stenosis reveals a peak systolic velocity (PSV) of 139 cm/sec with a clear systolic window. *B*, Region of bypass stenosis with markedly elevated PSV (725 cm/sec), spectral broadening, and tissue vibration causing color pixels outside the flow channel. See Color Plate.

with the change in diameter over time. Thus, in the absence of focal graft-threatening stenosis, human saphenous vein appears capable of adapting to its hemodynamic environment by modulating diameter to normalize shear stress.

For arterial bypass grafts with developing stenosis, the optimal threshold for intervention is an area of intense investigation. Diagnostic criteria have evolved primarily toward use of the *PSV ratio*, defined as the highest PSV within a stenosis divided by the PSV within a nonstenotic, adjacent section of the bypass. Recommended threshold values in the literature range from 1.5 to 4.0, with the higher values found in later reports.[7, 23, 26, 51, 60, 61, 89, 148] Bandyk's group[51] now recommends intervention thresholds consisting of both a velocity ratio greater than 3.4 and a PSV value higher than 300 cm/sec.

Similarly, Westerband and coworkers[148] successfully tested a velocity ratio of 3.5 and a PSV higher than 300 cm/sec for identification of graft-threatening stenoses. These authors found it additionally important to retain consideration of low-velocity criteria in the search for failing grafts. Although both groups tested some of the highest recommended thresholds in the literature, very few bypass grafts in their series failed while under active surveillance, and the graft patency rates were excellent. The highest PSV ratio threshold (>4.0) was published by Idu and colleagues.[61] In a prospective analysis, these authors recommended surgical revision without angiography when such a PSV ratio is encountered.

Although this area is still undergoing active investigation, the current literature supports the relative safety of deferring graft revision until a stenosis reaches a PSV ratio of at least 3.4. As with all other areas of duplex scanning interpretation, each laboratory should track clinical and angiographic results to determine the optimal thresholds for vein bypass graft revision at its own institution.

REFERENCES

1. Aaslid R, Markwalder T, Nornes H: Noninvasive transcranial Doppler ultrasound recording of flow velocity in basal cerebral arteries. J Neurosurg 57:769–774, 1982.

2. Ackerstaff RG, Jansen C, Moll FL, et al: The significance of microemboli detection by means of transcranial Doppler ultrasonography monitoring in carotid endarterectomy. J Vasc Surg 21:963–969, 1995.
3. Ackerstaff RGA, Hoeneveld H, Slowikowski JM: Ultrasonic duplex scanning in atherosclerotic disease of the innominate, subclavian, and vertebral arteries: A comparative study with angiography. Ultrasound Med Biol 10:409–418, 1984.
4. Arnold M, Sturzenegger M, Schaffler L, Seiler RW: Continuous intraoperative monitoring of middle cerebral artery blood flow velocities and electroencephalography during carotid endarterectomy: A comparison of the two methods to detect cerebral ischemia. Stroke 28:1345–1350, 1997.
5. Baker WH, Koustas G, Burke K, et al: Intraoperative duplex scanning and late carotid artery stenosis. J Vasc Surg 19:829–833, 1994.
6. Bandyk DF, Cato RF, Towne JB: A low flow velocity predicts failure of femoropopliteal and femorotibial bypass grafts. Surgery 98:799–809, 1985.
7. Bandyk DF, Johnson BL, Gupta AK, Esses GE: Nature and management of duplex abnormalities encountered during infrainguinal vein bypass grafting. J Vasc Surg 24:430–438, 1996.
8. Bandyk DF, Kaebnick HW, Adams MB, Towne JB: Turbulence occurring after carotid bifurcation endarterectomy: A harbinger of residual and recurrent carotid stenosis. J Vasc Surg 7:261–274, 1988.
9. Bandyk DF, Mills JL, Gahtan V, Esses GE: Intraoperative duplex scanning of arterial reconstructions: Fate of repaired and unrepaired defects. J Vasc Surg 20:426–433, 1994.
10. Barber FE, Baker DW, Nation AWC, Strandness DEJ: Ultrasonic duplex echo Doppler scanner. IEEE Trans Biomed Eng 21:109–115, 1974.
11. Barber FE, Baker DW, Strandness DEJ, et al: Duplex scanner: II. For simultaneous imaging of artery tissues and flow. 1974 Ultrasonic Symposium Proceedings. IEEE Cat. No. 74CH0896–ISU:744–748, 1974.
12. Barnes RW, Thompson BW, MacDonald CM, et al: Serial noninvasive studies do not herald postoperative failure of femoropopliteal or femorotibial bypass grafts. Ann Surg 210:486–492, 1989.
13. Bartels E, Flugel KA: Evaluation of extracranial vertebral artery dissection with duplex color-flow imaging. Stroke 27:290–295, 1996.
14. Bass A, Krupski WC, Schneider PA, et al: Intraoperative transcranial Doppler: Limitations of the method. J Vasc Surg 10:549–553, 1989.
15. Bendick PJ, Jackson VP: Evaluation of the vertebral arteries with duplex sonography. J Vasc Surg 3:523–530, 1986.
16. Berkowitz J, Hobbs C, Roberts B, et al: Value of routine vascular laboratory studies to identify vein graft stenoses. Surgery 90:971–979, 1981.
17. Blackshear WM, Phillips DJ, Chikos PM, et al: Carotid artery velocity patterns in normal and stenotic vessels. Stroke 11:67–71, 1980.
18. Bowersox JC, Zwolak RM, Walsh DB, et al: Duplex ultrasonography in the diagnosis of celiac and mesenteric artery occlusive disease. J Vasc Surg 14:780–790, 1991.
19. Brunholzl C, von Reutern GM: Hemodynamic effects of innominate artery occlusive disease: Evaluation by Doppler ultrasound. Ultrasound Med Biol 15:201–204, 1989.
20. Can U, Furie KL, Suwanwela N, et al: Transcranial Doppler ultrasound criteria for hemodynamically significant internal carotid artery stenosis based on residual lumen diameter calculated from en bloc endarterectomy specimens. Stroke 28:1966–1971, 1997.
21. Cantelmo NL, Babikian VL, Johnson WC, et al: Correlation of transcranial Doppler and noninvasive tests with angiography in the evaluation of extracranial carotid disease. J Vasc Surg 11:786–791, 1990; discussion, 791–792.
22. Cao P, Giordano G, Zannetti S, et al: Transcranial Doppler monitoring during carotid endarterectomy: Is it appropriate for selecting patients in need of a shunt? J Vasc Surg 26:973–979, 1997; discussion, 979–980.
23. Caps MT, Cantwell-Gab K, Bergelin RO, Strandness DE Jr: Vein graft lesions: Time of onset and rate of progression. J Vasc Surg 22:466–474, 1995; discussion, 475.
24. Carpenter JP, Lexa FJ, Davis JT: Determination of sixty percent or greater carotid artery stenosis by duplex Doppler ultrasonography. J Vasc Surg 22:697–705, 1995.
25. Cartier R, Cartier P, Fontaine A: Carotid endarterectomy without angiography: The reliability of Doppler ultrasonography and duplex scanning in preoperative assessment. Can J Surg 36:411–416, 1993.
26. Chalmers RT, Hoballah JJ, Kresowik TF, et al: The impact of color duplex surveillance on the outcome of lower limb bypass with segments of arm veins. J Vasc Surg 19:279–286, 1994; discussion, 286–288.
27. Comerota AJ, Katz ML, Hosking JD, et al: Is transcranial Doppler a worthwhile addition to screening tests for cerebrovascular disease? J Vasc Surg 21:90–95, 1995; discussion, 95–97.
28. Cossman DV, Ellison JE, Wagner WH, et al: Comparison of contrast arteriography to arterial mapping with color-flow duplex imaging in the lower extremities. J Vasc Surg 10:522–528, 1989; discussion, 528–529.
29. Cramer MM: Color flow duplex examination of the abdominal aorta: Atherosclerosis, aneurysm, and dissection. J Vasc Technol 19:249–260, 1995.
30. Currie IC, Jones AJ, Wakeley CJ, et al: Non-invasive aortoiliac assessment. Eur J Vasc Endovasc Surg 9:24–28, 1995.
31. Daigle RJ, Stavros AT, Lee RM: Overestimation of velocity and frequency values by multielement linear array Dopplers. J Vasc Technol 14:206–212, 1990.
32. Davies AH, Hayward JK, Irvine CD, et al: Treatment of iatrogenic false aneurysm by compression ultrasonography. Br J Surg 81:1230–1231, 1995.
33. Dawson DL, Zierler RE, Kohler TR: Role of arteriography in the preoperative evaluation of carotid artery disease. Am J Surg 16:619–624, 1991.
34. Disselhoff B, Bluth J, Jakimowicz J: Early detection of stenosis of femoral-distal grafts: A surveillance study using color-duplex scanning. Eur J Vasc Surg 3:43–48, 1989.
35. Eidt JF, Fry RE, Clagett GP, et al: Postoperative follow-up of renal artery reconstruction with duplex ultrasound. J Vasc Surg 8:667–673, 1988.
36. European Carotid Surgery Trialists' Collaborative Group: MRC European carotid surgery trial: Interim results for symptomatic patients with severe (70–99%) or with mild (0–29%) carotid stenosis. Lancet 337:1235–1243, 1991.
37. Executive Committee for the Asymptomatic Carotid Atherosclerosis Study: Endarterectomy for asymptomatic carotid artery stenosis. JAMA 273:1421–1428, 1995.
38. Faught WE, Mattos MA, van Bemmelen PS, et al: Color-flow duplex scanning of carotid arteries: New velocity criteria based on receiver operator characteristic analysis for threshold stenoses used in the symptomatic and asymptomatic carotid trials. J Vasc Surg 19:818–828, 1994.
39. Fellmeth BD, Roberts AC, Bookstein JJ, et al: Postangiographic femoral artery injuries: Nonsurgical repair with US-guided compression. Radiology 178:671–675, 1991.
40. Fillinger MF, Baker RJ, Zwolak RM, et al: Carotid duplex criteria for a 60% or greater angiographic stenosis: Variation according to equipment. J Vasc Surg 24:856–864, 1996.
41. Fillinger MF, Cronenwett JL, Besso S, et al: Vein adaptation to the hemodynamic environment of infrainguinal grafts. J Vasc Surg 19:970–979, 1994.
42. Frauchiger B, Bock A, Eichlisberger R, et al: The values of different resistive parameters in distinguishing biopsy-proved dysfunction of renal allografts. Nephrol Dial Transplant 10:527–532, 1995.
43. Fujitani RM, Mills JL, Wang LM, Taylor SM: The effect of unilateral internal carotid artery occlusion upon contralateral duplex study: Criteria for accurate interpretation. J Vasc Surg 16:459–468, 1992.
44. Gaunt ME, Martin PJ, Smith JL, et al: Clinical relevance of intraoperative embolization detected by transcranial Doppler ultrasonography during carotid endarterectomy: A prospective study of 100 patients. Br J Surg 81:1435–1439, 1994.
45. Gaunt ME, Ratliff DA, Martin PJ, et al: On-table diagnosis of incipient carotid artery thrombosis during carotid endarterectomy by transcranial Doppler scanning. J Vasc Surg 20:104–107, 1994.
46. Gelabert HA, Moore WS: Carotid endarterectomy without angiography. Surg Clin North Am 70:213–223, 1990.
47. Gertler JP, Cambria RP, Kistler JP, et al: Carotid surgery without arteriography: Noninvasive selection of patients. Ann Vasc Surg 5:253–256, 1991.
48. Geuder JW, Lamarello PJ, Riles TS, et al: Is duplex scanning sufficient evaluation before carotid endarterectomy? J Vasc Surg 9:193–201, 1989.
49. Goodson SF, Flanigan DP, Bishara RA, et al: Can carotid duplex scanning supplant arteriography in patients with focal carotid artery symptoms? J Vasc Surg 5:551–557, 1987.

50. Grant EG, Melany M: Doppler imaging of the liver. J Vasc Technol 19:277–284, 1995.
51. Gupta AK, Bandyk DF, Cheanvechai D, Johnson BL: Natural history of infrainguinal vein graft stenosis relative to bypass grafting technique. J Vasc Surg 25:211–220, 1997; discussion, 220–225.
52. Handa N, Fukunaga R, Etani H: Efficacy of echo-Doppler examination for the evaluation of renovascular disease. Ultrasound Med Biol 14:1–5, 1988.
53. Hansen KJ, Tribble RW, Reavis SW, et al: Renal duplex sonography: Evaluation of clinical utility. J Vasc Surg 12:227–236, 1990.
54. Hatsukami TS, Primozich JF, Zierler RE, et al: Color Doppler imaging of infrainguinal arterial occlusive disease. J Vasc Surg 16:527–531, 1992; discussion, 531–533.
55. Hill JC, Carbonneau K, Baliga PK, et al: Safe extracranial vascular evaluation and surgery without preoperative arteriography. Ann Vasc Surg 4:34–38, 1990.
56. Hoffmann U, Edwards JM, Carter S, et al: Role of duplex scanning for the detection of atherosclerotic renal artery disease. Kidney Int 39:1232–1239, 1991.
57. Horn M, Michelini M, Greisler HP, et al: Carotid endarterectomy without arteriography: The preeminent role of the vascular laboratory. Ann Vasc Surg 8:221–224, 1994.
58. Howard G, Baker WH, Chambless LE, et al: An approach for the use of Doppler ultrasound as a screening tool for hemodynamically significant stenosis (despite heterogeneity of Doppler performance). Stroke 26:1951–1957, 1996.
59. Hunink MGM, Polak JF, Barlan MM, O'Leary DH: Detection and quantification of carotid artery stenosis: Efficacy of various Doppler velocity parameters. AJR Am J Roentgenol 160:619–625, 1993.
60. Idu MM, Blankenstein JD, de Gier P, et al: Impact of a color-flow duplex surveillance program on infrainguinal vein graft patency: A five-year experience. J Vasc Surg 17:42–52. 1993; discussion. 52–53.
61. Idu MM, Buth J, Hop WC, et al: Vein graft surveillance: Is graft revision without angiography justified and what criteria should be used? J Vasc Surg 27:399–411. 1998; discussion. 412–413.
62. Isaacson J, Neumyer MM: Direct and indirect renal arterial duplex and Doppler color flow evaluations. J Vasc Technol 19:309–316, 1995.
63. Jager KA, Fortner GS, Thiele BL, Strandness DE Jr: Noninvasive diagnosis of intestinal angina. J Clin Ultrasound 12:588–591, 1984.
64. Jager KA, Phillips DJ, Martin RL, et al: Noninvasive mapping of lower limb arterial lesions. Ultrasound Med Biol 11:515–521, 1985.
65. Jansen C, Sprengers AM, Moll FL, et al: Prediction of intracerebral hemorrhage after carotid endarterectomy by clinical criteria and intraoperative transcranial Doppler monitoring: Results of 233 operations. Eur J Vasc Surg 8:220–225, 1994.
66. Johnson BL, Gupta AK, Bandyk DF, et al: Anatomic patterns of carotid endarterectomy healing. Am J Surg 172:188–190, 1996.
67. Jorgensen LG, Schroeder TV: Defective cerebrovascular autoregulation after carotid endarterectomy. Eur J Vasc Surg 7:370–379, 1993.
68. Kadir S: Celiac, superior, and inferior mesenteric arteries. *In* Kadir S (ed): Atlas of Normal and Variant Angiographic Anatomy. Philadelphia, WB Saunders, 1991, pp 297–364.
69. Kaneko A, Ohno R, Hattori K, et al: Color-coded Doppler imaging of subclavian steal syndrome. Intern Med 37:259–264, 1998.
70. Kang SS, Labropoulos N, Mansour A, Baker WH: Percutaneous ultrasound guided thrombin injection: A new method for treating postcatheterization femoral pseudoaneurysms. J Vasc Surg 27:1032–1038, 1998.
71. Karacagil S, Lofberg AM, Granbo A, et al: Value of duplex scanning in evaluation of crural and foot arteries in limbs with severe lower limb ischaemia—a prospective comparison with angiography. Eur J Vasc Endovasc Surg 12:300–303, 1996.
72. Kent KC, Kuntz KM, Patel MR, et al: Perioperative imaging strategies for carotid endarterectomy. JAMA 274:888–893, 1995.
73. Kohler TR, Andros G, Porter JM, et al: Can duplex scanning replace arteriography for lower extremity arterial disease? Ann Vasc Surg 4:280–287, 1990.
74. Kohler TR, Nance DR, Cramer MM, et al: Duplex scanning for diagnosis of aortoiliac and femoropopliteal disease: A prospective study. Circulation 76:1074–1080, 1987.
75. Kohler TR, Zierler RE, Martin RL, et al: Noninvasive diagnosis of renal artery stenosis by ultrasonic duplex scanning. J Vasc Surg 4:450–456, 1986.
76. Kuntz KM, Polak JF, Whittemore AD, et al: Duplex ultrasound criteria for the identification of carotid stenosis should be laboratory specific. Stroke 28:597–602, 1997.
77. LaBombard FE, Musson A, Bowersox JC, Zwolak RM: Hepatic artery duplex as an adjunct in the evaluation of chronic mesenteric ischemia. J Vasc Technol 16:7–11, 1992.
78. Legemate DA, Teeuven C, Hoeneveld H, Eikelboom BC: Value of duplex scanning compared with angiography and pressure measurement in the assessment of aortoiliac arterial lesions. Br J Surg 78:1003–1008, 1991.
79. Leng GC, Whyman MR, Donnan PT, et al: Accuracy and reproducibility of duplex ultrasonography in grading femoropopliteal stenoses. J Vasc Surg 17:510–517, 1993.
80. Lennard N, Smith J, Dumville J, et al: Prevention of postoperative thrombotic stroke after carotid endarterectomy: The role of transcranial Doppler ultrasound. J Vasc Surg 26:579–584, 1997.
81. Liau C, Ho F, Chen M, Lee Y: Treatment of iatrogenic femoral artery pseudoaneurysm with percutaneous thrombin injection. J Vasc Surg 26:18–23, 1997.
82. Ligush J Jr, Burnham CB, Burnham SJ, et al: Accuracy of the duplex scan in occlusive disease of the supraaortic trunks. J Vasc Technol 20:81–86, 1996.
83. Ligush J Jr, Reavis SW, Preisser JS, Jansen KJ: Duplex ultrasound scanning defines operative strategies for patients with limb-threatening ischemia. J Vasc Surg 28:482–491, 1998.
84. Lipski DA, Bergamini TM, Garrison RN, Fulton RL: Intraoperative duplex scanning reduces the incidence of residual stenosis after carotid endarterectomy. J Surg Res 60:317–320, 1996.
85. Lustgarten JH, Solomon RA, Quest DO, et al: Carotid endarterectomy after noninvasive evaluation by duplex ultrasonography and magnetic resonance angiography. Neurosurgery 34:612–619, 1994.
86. Markus HS, Ackerstaff R, Babikian V, et al: Intercenter agreement in reading Doppler embolic signals: A multicenter international study. Stroke 28:1307–1310, 1997.
87. Martin RL, Nanra RS, Wlodarczyk J: Renal hilar Doppler analysis in the detection of renal artery stenosis. J Vasc Technol 15:173–180, 1989.
88. Mattos MA, Hodgson KJ, Faught WE, et al: Carotid endarterectomy without angiography: Is color-flow duplex scanning insufficient? Surgery 116:776–783, 1994.
89. Mattos MA, van Bemmelen PS, Hodgson KJ, et al: Does correction of stenoses identified with color duplex scanning improve infrainguinal graft patency? J Vasc Surg 17:54–66, 1993.
90. McKittrick JE, Cisek PL, Pojunas KW, et al: Are both color-flow duplex scanning and cerebral arteriography required prior to carotid endarterectomy? Ann Vasc Surg 7:311–316, 1993.
91. McLeary MS, Rouse GA: Tardus-parvus Doppler signals in the renal arteries: A sign of pediatric thoracoabdominal aortic coarctations. Am J Radiol 167:521–523, 1996.
92. Mills JL, Harris EJ, Taylor LM Jr, et al: The importance of routine surveillance of distal bypass grafts with duplex scanning: A study of 379 reversed vein grafts. J Vasc Surg 12:379–386, 1990; discussion, 387–389.
93. Moneta GL, Edwards JM, Chitwood RW, et al: Correlation of North American Symptomatic Carotid Endarterectomy Trial (NASCET) angiographic definition of 70% to 99% internal carotid artery stenosis with duplex scanning. J Vasc Surg 17:152–159, 1993.
94. Moneta GL, Edwards JM, Papanicolaou G, et al: Screening for asymptomatic internal carotid artery stenosis: Duplex criteria for discriminating 60% to 99% stenosis. J Vasc Surg 21:989–994, 1995.
95. Moneta GL, Lee RW, Yeager RA, et al: Mesenteric duplex scanning: A blinded prospective study. J Vasc Surg 17:79–86, 1993.
96. Moneta GL, Yeager RA, Antonovic R, et al: Accuracy of lower extremity arterial duplex mapping. J Vasc Surg 15:275–283, 1992; discussion, 283–284.
97. Moneta GL, Yeager RA, Dalman R, et al: Duplex ultrasound criteria for diagnosis of splanchnic artery stenosis or occlusion. J Vasc Surg 14:511–520, 1991.
98. Moneta GL, Yeager RA, Lee RW, Porter JM: Noninvasive localization of arterial occlusive disease: A comparison of segmental Doppler pressures and arterial duplex mapping. J Vasc Surg 17:578–582, 1993.
99. Moody P, Gould DA, Harris PL: Vein graft surveillance improves patency in femoropopliteal bypass. Eur J Vasc Surg 4:117–121, 1990.

100. Mooney MJ, Tollefson DFJ, Andersen CA, et al: Duplex-guided compression of iatrogenic femoral pseudoaneurysms. J Am Coll Surg 181:155–159, 1995.
101. Moore WS, Ziomek S, Quinones-Baldrich WJ, et al: Can clinical evaluation and noninvasive testing substitute for arteriography in the evaluation of carotid artery disease? Ann Surg 208:91–94, 1988.
102. Muto PM, Welch HJ, Mackey WC, O'Donnell TF: Evaluation of carotid artery stenosis: Is duplex ultrasonography sufficient? J Vasc Surg 24:17–24, 1996.
103. Naylor AR, Whyman MR, Wildsmith JAW, et al: Factors influencing the hyperaemic response after carotid endarterectomy. Br J Surg 80:1523–1527, 1993.
104. Neale ML, Chambers JL, Kelly AT, et al: Reappraisal of duplex criteria to assess significant carotid stenosis with special reference to reports from the North American Symptomatic Carotid Endarterectomy Trial and the European Carotid Surgery Trial. J Vasc Surg 20:642–649, 1994.
105. Neumyer MM: Ultrasonographic assessment of renal and pancreatic transplants. J Vasc Technol 19:321–329, 1991.
106. Neumyer MM, Gifford RRM, Thiele BL: Identification of early rejection in renal allografts with duplex ultrasound. J Vasc Technol 12:19–25, 1988.
107. Neumyer MM, Gifford RRM, Yang HC, Thiele BL: Applications of duplex ultrasound/color flow imaging for the evaluation of renal allografts. J Vasc Technol 15:156–160, 1991.
108. Newell DW, Aaslid R: Transcranial Doppler: Clinical and experimental uses. Cerebrovasc Brain Metab Rev 4:122–143, 1992.
109. Newell DW, Winn HR: Transcranial Doppler in cerebral vasospasm. Neurosurg Clin North Am 1:319–328, 1990.
110. Norris CS, Pfeiffer JS, Rittgers SE, Barnes RW: Noninvasive evaluation of renal artery stenosis and renovascular resistance. J Vasc Surg 1:192–201, 1984.
111. North American Symptomatic Carotid Endarterectomy Trial Collaborators: Beneficial effect of carotid endarterectomy in symptomatic patients with high-grade carotid stenosis. N Engl J Med 325:445–453, 1991.
112. O'Connor SE, LaBombard E, Musson AM, Zwolak RM: Duplex imaging of distal splenorenal shunts. J Vasc Technol 15:28–31, 1991.
113. Olin JW, Piedmonte MR, Young JR, et al: The utility of duplex ultrasound scanning of the renal arteries for diagnosing significant renal artery stenosis. Ann Intern Med 122:833–837, 1995.
114. Pan XM, Saloner D, Reilly LM, et al: Assessment of carotid artery stenosis by ultrasonography, conventional angiography, and magnetic resonance angiography: Correlation with ex vivo measurement of plaque stenosis. J Vasc Surg 21:82–89, 1995.
115. Patel MR, Kuntz KM, Klufas RA, et al: Preoperative assessment of the carotid bifurcation: Can magnetic resonance angiography and duplex ultrasonography replace contrast arteriography? Stroke 26:1753–1758, 1995.
116. Paulson EK, Kliewer MA, Hertzberg BS, et al: Color Doppler sonography of groin complications following femoral artery catheterization. AJR Am J Roentgenol 165:439–444, 1995.
117. Perko MJ, Just S, Schroeder TV: Importance of diastolic velocities in the detection of celiac and mesenteric artery disease by duplex ultrasound. J Vasc Surg 26:288–293, 1997.
118. Primozich JF, Daigle RJ: Should a constant 60 degree angle or multiple angles be used in carotid duplex imaging? J Vasc Technol 17:307–313, 1993.
119. Ricotta JJ, Holen J, Schenk E, et al: Is routine angiography necessary prior to carotid endarterectomy? J Vasc Surg 1:96–102, 1984.
120. Ries S, Steinke W, Devuyst G, et al: Power Doppler imaging and color Doppler flow imaging for the evaluation of normal and pathological vertebral arteries. J Neuroimaging 8:71–74, 1998.
121. Rizzo RJ, Sandager G, Astleford P, et al: Mesenteric flow velocity variations as a function of angle of insonation. J Vasc Surg 11:688–694, 1990.
122. Roederer GO, Langlois YE, Chan AW, et al: Ultrasonic duplex scanning of extracranial carotid arteries: Improved accuracy using new features from the common carotid artery. J Cardiovasc Ultrasonography 1:373–380, 1982.
123. Roederer GO, Langlois YE, Jager KA, et al: A simple spectral parameter for accurate classification of severe carotid disease. Bruit 8:174–178, 1984.
124. Roederer GO, Langlois YE, Jager KA, et al: The natural history of carotid arterial disease in asymptomatic patients with cervical bruits. Stroke 15:605–613, 1984.
125. Sawchuk AP, Flanigan DP, Machi J, et al: The fate of unrepaired minor technical defects detected by intraoperative ultrasonography during carotid endarterectomy. J Vasc Surg 9:671–675, 1989; discussion, 675–676.
126. Schaub F, Theiss W, Heinz M, et al: New aspects in ultrasound-guided compression repair of postcatheterization femoral artery injuries. Circulation 90:1861–1865, 1994.
127. Schneider PA, Rossman ME, Torem S, et al: Transcranial Doppler in the management of extracranial cerebrovascular disease: Implications in diagnosis and monitoring. J Vasc Surg 7:223–231, 1988.
128. Schoning M, Niemann G, Hartig B: Transcranial color duplex sonography of basal cerebral arteries: Reference data of flow velocities from childhood to adulthood. Neuropediatrics 27:249–255, 1996.
129. Schwartz SW, Chambless LE, Baker WH, et al: Consistency of Doppler parameters in predicting arteriographically confirmed carotid stenosis. Stroke 28:343–347, 1997.
130. Schwerk WB, Restrepo IK, Stellwaag M, et al: Renal artery stenosis: Grading with image-directed Doppler US evaluation of renal resistive index. Radiology 190:785–790, 1994.
131. Sensier Y, Hartshorne T, Thrush A, et al: The effect of adjacent segment disease on the accuracy of colour duplex scanning for the diagnosis of lower limb arterial disease. Eur J Vasc Endovasc Surg 12:238–242, 1996.
132. Sensier Y, Hartshorne T, Thrush A, et al: A prospective comparison of lower limb colour-coded Duplex scanning with arteriography. Eur J Vasc Endovasc Surg 11:170–175, 1996.
133. Shifrin EG, Bornstein NM, Kantarovsky A, et al: Carotid endarterectomy without angiography. Br J Surg 83:1107–1109, 1996.
134. Sorrell K: The role of color flow duplex ultrasonography in portosystemic shunts. J Vasc Technol 19:285–293, 1995.
135. Sorrell K, Blackshear B, Fogle M: Diagnosis of occlusive renal vein thrombosis in renal allografts by duplex ultrasonography. J Vasc Technol 16:119–123, 1992.
136. Spadone DP, Barkmeier LD, Hodgson KJ, et al: Contralateral internal carotid artery stenosis or occlusion: Pitfall of correct ipsilateral classification—a study performed with color-flow imaging. J Vasc Surg 11:642–649, 1990.
137. Spencer MP: Transcranial Doppler monitoring and causes of stroke from carotid endarterectomy. Stroke 28:685–691, 1997.
138. Spencer MP, Thomas GI, Nicholls SC, Sauvage LR: Detection of middle cerebral artery emboli during carotid endarterectomy using transcranial Doppler ultrasonography. Stroke 21:415–423, 1990.
139. Suwanwela N, Can U, Furie FL, et al: Carotid Doppler ultrasound criteria for internal carotid artery stenosis based on residual lumen diameter calculated from en bloc carotid endarterectomy specimens. Stroke 27:1965–1969, 1996.
140. Taylor DC, Houston GTM, Anderson C, et al: Follow-up of renal and mesenteric artery revascularization with duplex ultrasonography. Can J Surg 39:17–20, 1996.
141. Taylor DC, Kettler MD, Moneta GL, et al: Duplex ultrasound scanning in the diagnosis of renal artery stenosis: A prospective evaluation. J Vasc Surg 7:363–369, 1988.
142. van Zuilen EV, Moll FL, Vermeulen FEE, et al: Detection of cerebral microemboli by means of transcranial Doppler monitoring before and after carotid endarterectomy. Stroke 26:210–213, 1995.
143. Verlato F, Grego F, Avruscio GP, et al: Diagnosis of high-grade stenosis of innominate artery. Angiology 44:845–851, 1993.
144. Wagner WH, Treiman RL, Cossman DV, et al: The diminishing role of diagnostic arteriography in carotid artery disease: Duplex scanning as definitive preoperative study. Ann Vasc Surg 5:105–110, 1991.
145. Wain RA, Lyon RT, Veith FJ, et al: Accuracy of duplex ultrasound in evaluating carotid artery anatomy before endarterectomy. J Vasc Surg 27:235–242, 1998; discussion, 242–244.
146. Walters GK, Jescovitch AJ, Jones CE: The influence of contralateral carotid stenosis on duplex accuracy: The role of collateral cerebral flow. J Vasc Technol 19:111–114, 1995.
147. Westerband A, Mills JL, Berman SS, Hunter GC: The influence of routine completion arteriography on outcome following carotid endarterectomy. Ann Vasc Surg 11:14–19, 1997.
148. Westerband A, Mills JL, Kistler S, et al: Prospective validation of threshold criteria for intervention in infrainguinal vein grafts undergoing duplex surveillance. Ann Vasc Surg 11:44–48, 1997.

149. Wilson YG, George JK, Wilkins DC, Ashley S: Duplex assessment of run-off before femorocrural reconstruction. Br J Surg 84:1360–1363, 1997.
150. Zaweski JE, Musson AM, Zwolak RM: Carotid endarterectomy without angiography: Guidelines for duplex evaluation. J Vasc Technol 20:151–156, 1996.
151. Zwiebel WJ, Austin CW, Sackett JF, Strother CM: Correlation of high-resolution, B-mode and continuous-wave Doppler sonography with arteriography in the diagnosis of carotid stenosis. Radiology 149:523–532, 1983.
152. Zwolak RM: Expert commentary: Carotid endarterectomy without angiography: Are we ready? Vasc Surg 31:1–9, 1997.
153. Zwolak RM, Fillinger MF, Walsh DB, et al: Mesenteric and celiac duplex scanning: A validation study. J Vasc Surg 27:1039–1047, 1998.

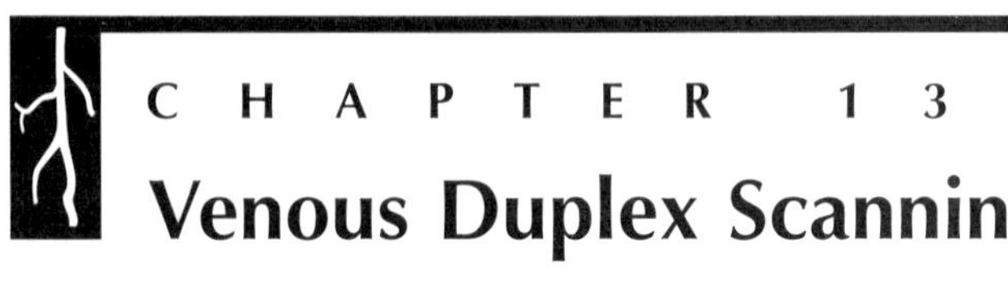

CHAPTER 13
Venous Duplex Scanning

Mark H. Meissner, M.D.

Approximately 1 million patients annually undergo investigation for suspected acute deep venous thrombosis (DVT) in North America.[62, 133] Accurate diagnosis of DVT is important since improper withholding of anticoagulation is associated with the well-recognized risk of pulmonary embolism, and inappropriate treatment carries the inconvenience, expense, and risks of anticoagulation. Unfortunately, clinical diagnosis of DVT is inaccurate: the classic findings of pain, swelling, and tenderness are equally as common in limbs with and without objectively confirmed thrombosis.[8, 25, 44, 61] The diagnosis of DVT therefore requires confirmatory testing, and several diagnostic modalities have been used clinically.

Ascending venography has historically been the "gold standard" for diagnosis for acute DVT.[55] However, venography is invasive, not easily repeatable, may be impossible to perform or interpret in 9% to 14% of patients, and may be associated with interobserver disagreements in 4% to 10% of studies.[31, 35, 98, 128, 151] All venous segments are not visualized in 10% to 30% of studies, and the profunda femoris and iliac veins are frequently not seen.[21] In the upper extremity, venography does not demonstrate the internal jugular vein and frequently fails to identify venous segments beyond an obstruction.[11, 34] Furthermore, the use of contrast agents is associated with occasional allergic reactions and may induce thrombosis in up to 8% of cases.[18] Impedance plethysmography (IPG), which correlates a reduced rate of venous outflow with proximal thrombosis, was previously the most widely used noninvasive test. However, since IPG is insensitive to isolated calf vein and nonocclusive proximal thromboses, negative test results require serial follow-up examination. Furthermore, IPG cannot provide precise anatomic localization of an occluding thrombus.

The use of real-time ultrasonography, as described by Talbot in 1982,[136] has overcome many of these limitations and provides an accurate, noninvasive, and portable means of confirming venous thrombosis in the upper and lower extremities. Uniformly high sensitivities of 93% to 97% and specificities of 94% to 99% have been reported for the ultrasound diagnosis of proximal DVT.[14, 62, 72, 155] Accurate localization of thrombus to specific venous segments has also enabled the course of thrombosis to be serially followed, permitting more precise characterization of the natural history of acute DVT. Furthermore, since both anatomic obstruction and valvular reflux can be evaluated with duplex ultrasonography, similar techniques can be used in the diagnosis of acute DVT and the characterization of chronic venous disease.

ULTRASOUND APPLICATIONS IN ACUTE DEEP VENOUS THROMBOSIS

Instrumentation

Continuous wave Doppler ultrasound has been used in the diagnosis of acute DVT since the early 1970s.[132] Although acute and chronic venous disease can be diagnosed based on aberrant venous flow, continuous wave Doppler does not allow selective interrogation of vessels within a large sample volume.[70] Real-time B-mode ultrasonography relies on gray scale imaging and the absence of venous compressibility as the primary diagnostic criteria for acute DVT. Although accurate in the diagnosis of proximal thromboses, compression ultrasonography provides no information regarding venous flow. Real-time gray scale imaging and Doppler flow are combined in duplex and color flow instruments. Duplex instruments include a range-gated pulsed Doppler allowing flow to be characterized at precise anatomic locations defined by the B-mode image, whereas color flow Doppler superimposes a color map of the Doppler shift on the real-time gray scale image.[70] Modern equipment for venous applications includes high-resolution B-mode ultrasound with "slow flow" color Doppler ultrasound capable of detecting low venous flow velocities. These technologic advances have made the study less operator dependent and have improved the identification of difficult-to-visualize venous segments. Color flow Doppler may permit identification of flow in vessels smaller than the limits of gray scale resolution[157] and is particularly useful in imaging the calf and iliac veins.[92]

Because axial resolution and tissue penetration are inversely related,[70] the highest frequency transducer capable of visualizing the venous segment under study should be utilized. The iliac veins require a 3- to 3.5-MHz ultrasound probe capable of imaging the depths of the pelvis, whereas a 5- to 7.5-MHz imaging transducer is adequate for the deep veins of the upper and lower extremities. A higher frequency probe (10 MHz) is helpful for imaging the superficial veins of the lower extremity as well as the upper extremity veins. A pulsed Doppler frequency of 3 MHz is suitable for the iliac veins and 5 MHz is acceptable for the upper and lower extremity veins. The dynamic range, gray scale gain, and time gain compensation should be adjusted to minimize intraluminal artifacts while providing good definition of the venous walls. The color velocity scale and gain should maximize the detection of low-venous-flow velocities while confining color flow within the sample box to the vessel lumen. A low wall filter setting facilitates detection of low-flow velocities. As a convention, many laboratories adjust the spectral display to show prograde venous flow below the baseline.

Examination Technique

Although more limited examinations have been proposed,[24, 73, 115, 153] complete examination involves interrogation of the lower extremities from the inferior vena cava to the tibial veins. At each site, venous compressibility and the presence of echogenic thrombus are evaluated on the B-mode image, while the Doppler is used to assess venous flow characteristics. The deep veins are assessed in transverse and then longitudinal views. Initial transverse scanning allows identification of the superficial and deep veins in relation to adjacent arterial structures and facilitates recognition of duplicated veins.[104] Gentle pressure on the scanhead is required to avoid venous occlusion, particularly in evaluation of the superficial veins. Compression maneuvers, performed in transverse view to avoid lateral displacement of the transducer,[146] are performed every one to two cm from the inguinal ligament to the calf. Complete coaptation of the venous walls with gentle probe pressure excludes the presence of a thrombus. Moving to a longitudinal view, spectral Doppler signals and color flow images are obtained from the venous segment being interrogated. Color flow Doppler may assist in longitudinal tracking and in identifying the luminal encroachment of echolucent thrombus.

To facilitate lower extremity venous filling, the venous duplex examination is performed with the head elevated in 10- to 20-degree reverse Trendelenburg position. The examination is begun in the lower abdomen and pelvis, where Doppler flow evaluation is often possible, even though compressibility may be limited and bowel gas may obscure complete visualization of the inferior vena cava and iliac veins. On crossing the inguinal ligament, the origins of the greater saphenous and profunda femoris veins can be identified in transverse section. The veins of the thigh are examined with the leg slightly flexed and externally rotated to avoid compression of the popliteal vein. The superficial femoral vein is imaged from an anteromedial approach and followed to the distal third of the thigh, where it moves deeply through the adductor canal. The superficial femoral vein is frequently duplicated[104] and requires a critical assessment of the Doppler spectrum and color flow image at the adductor canal, where it may be incompressible. The popliteal vein is most easily examined with the patient prone or resting on the side opposite that being examined with the hip and knee slightly flexed. The lesser saphenous vein is identified as it courses from the saphenopopliteal junction to a position just above the fascia, whereas the gastrocnemial veins can be observed to penetrate the muscle.

After examination of the distal popliteal vein, the patient is returned to the supine position for examination of the posterior tibial and peroneal veins. The calf veins may alternatively be studied with the patient sitting, a technique that may facilitate venous filling and visualization.[9, 32] The paired posterior tibial veins are identified adjacent to the artery between the medial malleolus and the Achilles tendon at the level of the ankle. Moving cephalad, the paired peroneal veins are identified along the medial border of the fibula, although a posterior approach may be necessary in a large calf.[139] In the presence of thrombus, the soleal veins may be distended and readily apparent. Isolated calf vein thrombosis most often involves the peroneal veins followed by the posterior tibial veins; isolated anterior tibial thrombosis is distinctly unusual.[86, 87, 111, 123] Visualization of both the posterior tibial and peroneal veins is required to achieve acceptable sensitivity, although routine scanning of the anterior tibial veins may be unnecessary.

Examination of the upper extremity and the thoracic inlet is performed with the patient supine, the neck turned slightly away from the side being examined and the upper extremity abducted to facilitate access to the axilla. The internal jugular vein is identified in the neck and followed centrally to image the medial subclavian and innominate veins from a supraclavicular approach. The lateral subclavian vein and axillary vein are then visualized from an infraclavicular approach. Overlying bone and muscle prevent routine use of compression in evaluating the innominate, subclavian, and medial axillary veins; color flow Doppler and the venous response to inspiration may be particularly useful in these areas.[41, 42] If required, examination then proceeds down the medial aspect of the arm, with evaluation of the axillary, paired brachial, basilic, and cephalic veins. The paired radial and ulnar veins are then assessed in the forearm.

Diagnostic Criteria for Acute Deep Venous Thrombosis

A complete venous ultrasound evaluation incorporates information from the B-mode image, Doppler spectrum, and color flow image. Diagnostic criteria for acute DVT are shown in Table 13–1 and include an evaluation of venous compressibility, intraluminal echoes, venous flow characteristics, and luminal color filling. Venous incompressibility is the most widely used diagnostic criterion for acute DVT. Normal venous walls completely coapt, obliterating the

TABLE 13–1. VENOUS DUPLEX ULTRASOUND CRITERIA FOR ACUTE DEEP VENOUS THROMBOSIS

DIAGNOSTIC CRITERIA	ADJUNCTIVE CRITERIA
Venous incompressibility	Increased venous diameter
Thrombus visualization	<50% diameter increase with Valsalva maneuver
Absent or diminished spontaneous venous flow	Immobile venous valves
Absence of respiratory phasicity	
Absent or incomplete color filling of lumen	

venous lumen, with gentle probe compression (Fig. 13–1). Adjunctive gray scale findings include the appearance of echogenic thrombi within the vein lumen and dilation of an acutely thrombosed segment.[48] However, acute thrombus is usually less echogenic than older thrombus[137] and may be visible in only 50% to 90% of acute DVTs.[32, 64, 107]

The Doppler spectrum and color flow image serve to further support the diagnosis, increase accuracy in regions that are ordinarily difficult to compress, and permit differentiation of occlusive from nonocclusive thrombi. Above the popliteal vein, normal lower extremity venous flow is spontaneous, varies with respiration, and augments with distal compression or release of proximal compression (Fig. 13–2) (see Color Plate). Spontaneous flow should also diminish during and augment after a Valsalva maneuver. Although spontaneous flow may normally be absent in the tibioperoneal veins, augmented flow should be present with distal compression of the foot or calf. The absence of flow, either spontaneously or with augmentation, suggests occlusive thrombosis.

Respiratory variation reflects diminished or absent flow with increases in intra-abdominal pressure during the respiratory cycle. Continuous flow signals without respiratory variation, lack of augmentation with release of proximal compression, and continuous flow during a Valsalva maneuver suggest a proximal obstruction, whereas diminished or absent augmentation with distal compression implies an obstruction in the intervening caudal venous segments.[5, 134] The observation of cardiac pulsatility in the lower extremity Doppler signal suggests congestive heart failure or another cause of increased central venous pressure.[8] Color flow Doppler may be particularly helpful in areas where compression is limited by anatomy, edema, obesity, or pain. In the absence of thrombus, the color flow map within the sample box should completely fill the venous lumen (Fig. 13–3) (see Color Plate).[74] Complete color filling of the lumen, however, may be absent in patent calf veins.[9]

Normal upper extremity venous flow shows more cardiac and respiratory variability than does lower extremity venous flow with subclavian flow increasing and diameter decreasing 41% to 78% during rapid inspiration (the sniff maneuver).[34, 49] Flow is interrupted or diminished while diameter increases during the Valsalva maneuver. In evaluating the veins of the thoracic inlet, the internal jugular vein is assessed using B-mode criteria similar to those for the lower extremity veins. However, visualization and compressibility of the subclavian vein are limited by the clavicle, and assessment relies on thorough evaluation of indirect flow criteria.[148] Patency of the subclavian vein is confirmed by complete color filling of the lumen, normal respiratory phasicity and cardiac pulsatility of the Doppler signal, and venous collapse with the sniff maneuver. Direct visualization of thrombus, absent or incomplete color filling of the lumen, and an absent diameter response to rapid inspiration suggest thrombosis.[22, 41] Although the lung and thoracic cage usually obscure direct visualization, the absence of respiratory phasicity, cardiac pulsatility, and inspiratory venous collapse may also suggest innominate or superior vena cava obstruction.[11, 34, 54] Such a diagnosis may be supported by the observation of numerous venous collaterals on the color flow image. However, these indirect observations cannot distinguish central thrombosis from intrinsic stenosis or extrinsic compression.

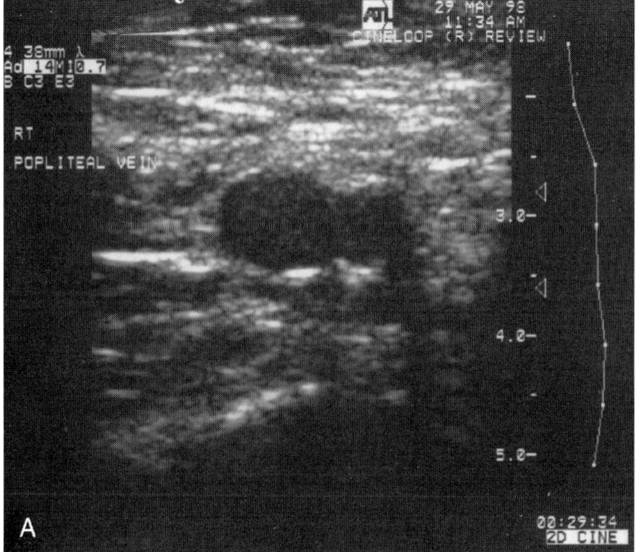

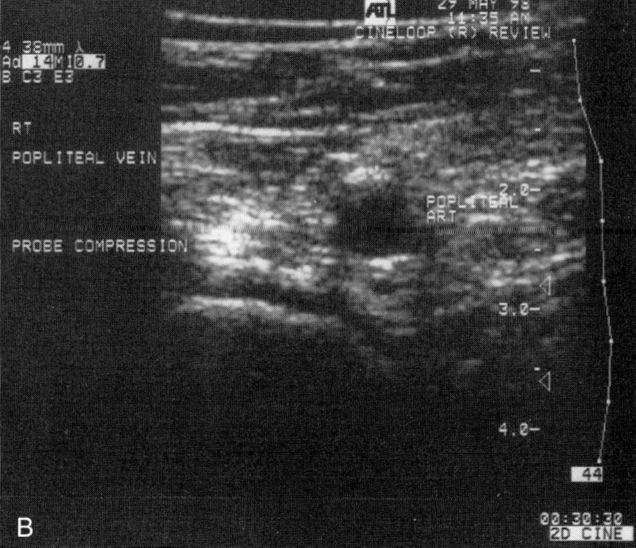

FIGURE 13–1. Compression ultrasonography. A transverse image of a normal popliteal artery and vein is shown in *A*. The normal popliteal vein is larger than the corresponding artery. With gentle probe compression (*B*), the lumen of the normal vein is obliterated while the popliteal artery remains uncompressed.

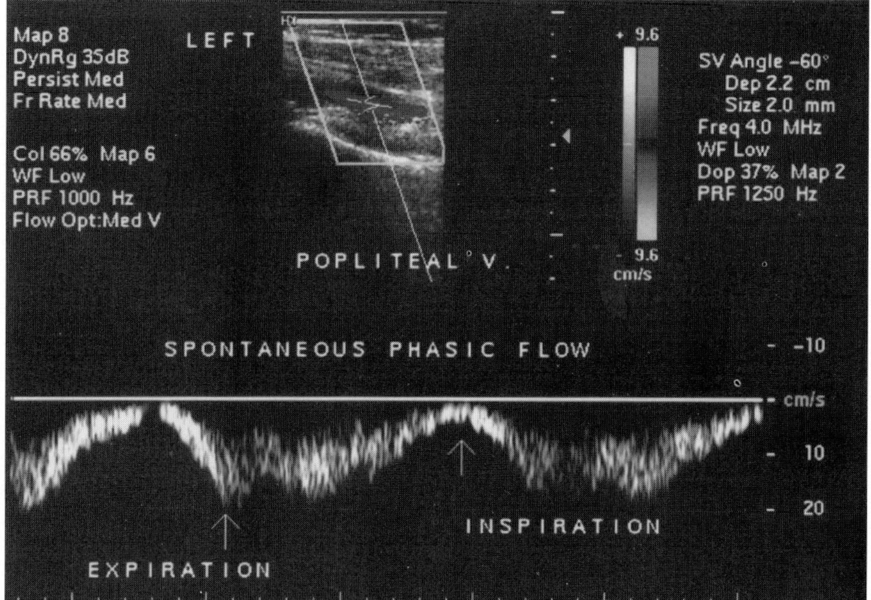

FIGURE 13–2. Doppler spectrum popliteal vein. Antegrade flow in the popliteal vein is displayed below the baseline. Unobstructed venous flow in the proximal veins is spontaneous with respiratory variation. Flow velocity increases with a reduction in intra-abdominal pressure during expiration and is damped or ceases during inspiration. (See Color Plate.)

In contrast to other noninvasive modalities, occlusive and nonocclusive thrombi can be differentiated on the basis of these criteria. Although it does not influence initial treatment, this distinction is important in following the course of a thrombus and defining recurrent thrombotic events. A patent segment is fully compressible, has no pathologic intraluminal echoes, demonstrates complete color filling of the lumen, and has spontaneous flow that varies with respiration and augments with distal compression. A segment with nonocclusive thrombus may have a visible thrombus within the lumen and is not completely compressible, but has flow present either spontaneously or with augmentation. A segment with an occlusive thrombus has similar B-mode characteristics but has no flow present either spontaneously or with augmentation. Seventy-three per cent to 94% of thrombi are occlusive at the time of presentation.[78]

Although the American Institute of Ultrasound in Medicine recommends evaluation of both the real-time image and venous flow signals,[1] utilization of these diagnostic criteria varies between laboratories. Venous incompressibility is the most widely used criteria and has excellent sensitivity and specificity for the detection of DVT in the common femoral and popliteal veins. It is also among the most objective of these criteria, with interobserver agreement reported to be 100%.[73] However, neither venous compressibility nor the other diagnostic elements are equally sensitive in detecting acute venous thrombus at all levels of the venous system. In considering B-mode incompressibility, visualization of thrombus, absence of spontaneous flow, and absence of phasic flow across all venous segments, only the absence of phasic flow has both a sensitivity and a specificity higher than 90% (Table 13–2).[64] Venous incompressibility is nonspecific in areas such as the adduc-

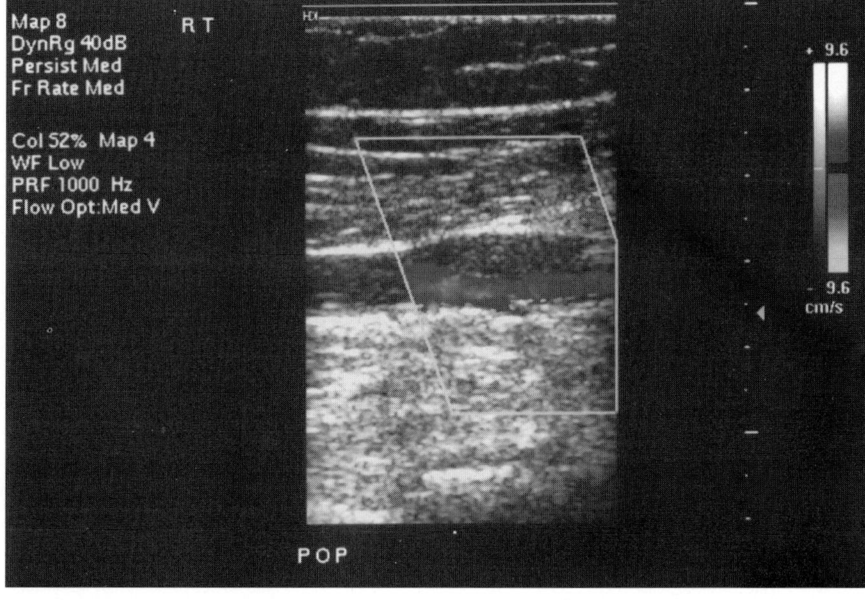

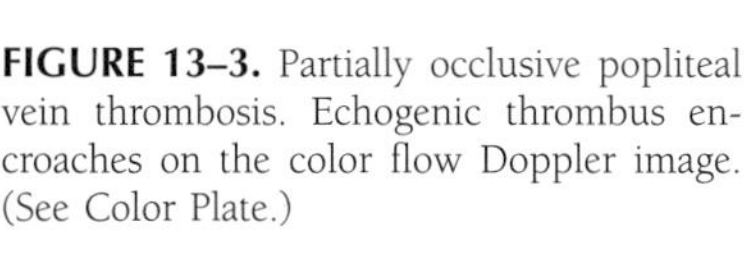
FIGURE 13–3. Partially occlusive popliteal vein thrombosis. Echogenic thrombus encroaches on the color flow Doppler image. (See Color Plate.)

TABLE 13–2. ANALYSIS OF VENOUS DUPLEX CRITERIA*

CRITERIA	SENSITIVITY (%)	SPECIFICITY (%)	PPV (%)	NPV (%)
Thrombus visualized	50 (34–66)	92 (62–98)	95 (69–100)	37 (14–59)
Incom-pressibility	79 (66–92)	67 (40–93)	88 (67–95)	50 (18–82)
Absent spontaneous flow	76 (63–90)	100 (88–100)	100 (85–100)	57 (29–85)
Absent phasic flow	92 (79–97)	92 (62–98)	97 (81–99)	79 (41–92)

From Killewich LA, Bedford GR, Beach KW, Strandness DE: Diagnosis of deep venous thrombosis: A prospective study comparing duplex scanning to contrast venography. Circulation 79:810–814, 1989.

*Values in parentheses are 95% confidence intervals.

PPV = positive predictive value; NPV = negative predictive value.

tor canal, whereas spontaneous flow is insensitive to nonocclusive thrombus. Sensitivity is markedly improved when these criteria are used in combination, with a visible thrombus in the absence of spontaneous flow and the absence of spontaneous, phasic flow having the best overall sensitivity and specificity (Table 13–3).[64] Although instrumentation has improved and color flow Doppler has become available since this study, these observations caution against using isolated criteria for the diagnosis of DVT and suggest that complete assessment requires integration of the B-mode image and Doppler spectra.

Other thrombus characteristics that may be identified with duplex include the presence of a free-floating thrombus tail. Based on venography, a *free-floating thrombus* has been defined as a greater than 5-cm segment of proximal thrombus surrounded by contrast agent.[95, 105] Duplex definitions of a free-floating thrombus have varied but can be identified by color imaging when flow is observed completely surrounding a central filling defect. This definition requires that such thrombi be differentiated from thrombus fragmentation occurring during the course of recanalization.[30] It has also been suggested that movement of the unattached segment within the flow stream be included in the definition.[43, 145] Free-floating elements have been observed in 6% to 69% of DVTs,[7] and the sensitivity and specificity of color flow duplex scanning in comparison

TABLE 13–3. SENSITIVITY AND SPECIFICITY OF COMBINED DIAGNOSTIC VARIABLES*

VARIABLES	SENSITIVITY (%)	SPECIFICITY (%)
T + P	95 (82–98)	83 (52–95)
T + F + P	95 (82–98)	83 (52–95)
T + F + P + VC	95 (82–98)	58 (30–86)
F + P	92 (79–97)	92 (62–98)
F + T	87 (76–98)	92 (62–98)
T + F + VC	87 (76–98)	67 (40–93)
F + VC	84 (73–96)	67 (40–93)
T + VC	82 (69–94)	67 (40–93)

From Killewich LA, Bedford GR, Beach KW, Strandness DE: Diagnosis of deep venous thrombosis: A prospective study comparing duplex scanning to contrast venography. Circulation 79:810–814, 1989.

*Values in parentheses are 95% confidence limits.

T = visualization of thrombus; F = absence of spontaneous flow; P = absence of phasic flow with respiration; VC = venous incompressibility.

with venography have been reported to be 68% and 86%, respectively.[110] Among patients followed with duplex ultrasonography for a mean of 7 days after identification of a free-floating thrombus, 55% demonstrated attachment of the free-floating tail; 24% showed partial or complete resolution of the tail; 9% showed an increase in the size of the free-floating component; and 12% had no change in thrombus characteristics.[7] Some have suggested that these nonadherent thrombi are associated with an increased risk of pulmonary embolism and warrant placement of a vena cava filter,[43, 105] whereas others have recommended anticoagulation alone[110] or filter placement only for patients failing to demonstrate thrombus attachment within 10 days.[17] In a small venographic series including 5 free-floating thrombi, the risk of embolism following anticoagulation was significantly higher in patients with free-floating ileofemoral thrombi (60%) than in those with occlusive thrombi (5.5%).[105] However, others have reported that the majority of emboli associated with free-floating thrombi occur prior to therapy.[7, 17, 145] Among these patients, most of whom received anticoagulation, only 3% to 10% sustained a pulmonary embolus after institution of treatment. Two prospective series employing routine lung scanning have also reported conflicting results. Monreal and associates[95] found recurrent pulmonary embolism despite anticoagulation in 21% of patients with free-floating ileofemoral thrombosis in comparison with 5% of patients with adherent thrombus. However, a more benign prognosis was suggested by Pacouret and colleagues,[110] the incidence of pulmonary embolism after the institution of therapeutic anticoagulation being similar in patients with (3.3%) and without (3.7%) free-floating elements. The clinical relevance of these findings remains controversial, and no randomized trials comparing management options have been performed.

Limitations of Venous Ultrasonography

Despite its utility, duplex ultrasonography does have some well-recognized limitations in the diagnosis of acute DVT. Among studies limited to the proximal veins, the results are indeterminate or nondiagnostic in 1% to 6% of patients.[74, 138] Anatomic factors that may limit visualization of the pelvic, superficial femoral, calf, and thoracic inlet veins must be considered when interpreting the results of venous ultrasound. Imaging of the inferior vena cava and iliac veins may be precluded by overlying bowel gas, and their deep location often prevents assessment of compressibility. Difficult compressibility may similarly limit evaluation of the superficial femoral vein at the adductor canal. Adequate evaluation of the tibial and peroneal veins may be impeded by large calf size, edema, or operator inexperience. Compression of the medial axillary, subclavian, and innominate veins may be prevented by overlying musculoskeletal structures, whereas acoustic shadowing may prevent visualization of the subclavian vein directly beneath the clavicle. Although occasionally visible with a small footprint transducer in the suprasternal notch, the central innominate vein and superior vena cava are often not routinely imageable with ultrasound. Interpretation of indirect Doppler evidence also has some limitations, since the absence of respiratory phasicity and augmentation may be due to proximal extrinsic compression rather than thrombosis.

Color flow technology has improved the evaluation of these segments, although assessment of the calf and iliac veins does require more time and technologist experience. Messina and colleagues[92] reported adequate visualization of both the common and external iliac veins in 47% of patients and of the external iliac alone in 79%. Despite being incompressible in most cases, the color flow and Doppler spectra are frequently sufficient to exclude occlusive thrombus in these segments. As important, the absence of complete iliac obstruction can be inferred by a spontaneous and phasic common femoral Doppler signal in more than 90% of cases. Continuous common femoral vein flow that does not change with a Valsalva maneuver is highly specific for proximal iliac or caval obstruction, although this finding cannot differentiate occlusive DVT from external compression by adenopathy, pelvic masses, or postoperative changes.[5] Spectral flow characteristics are also unable to exclude a nonocclusive proximal thrombus. Using color flow Doppler with slow-flow capabilities, technically adequate studies of all three paired tibial veins have been reported in 72% to 94% of symptomatic extremities.[86, 92]

Recurrent symptoms of pain and edema are common after an episode of acute DVT and are a challenge for most diagnostic tests.[56] Such symptoms may result from persistent obstruction early after an acute event, late manifestations of valvular incompetence, or recurrent DVT. Identification of recurrent thrombosis is particularly important since the risks of pulmonary embolism and more severe post-thrombotic manifestations[89, 119] may require a change in treatment. Unfortunately, variable degrees of residual occlusion, partial recanalization, intimal thickening, and collateral formation may mask new intraluminal filling defects on venography and also limit the utility of duplex ultrasonography in this setting.[29, 78, 97]

Despite early recanalization in most patients,[66, 90, 97, 117, 143] compression ultrasound studies may remain abnormal in 50% of patients after 6 months and in 27% to 70% of patients after 1 year.[12, 78, 97, 117] Thrombus echogenicity and heterogeneity do tend to increase with thrombus age. However, marked variation in thrombus echogenicity occurs, and this has not proved consistently useful for differentiating acute from chronic thrombus.[97] Despite these limitations, color flow ultrasonography may be more useful than venography in identifying some characteristics of chronic thrombosis versus recurrent acute DVT (Table 13–4).[15] Acutely thrombosed segments tend to be dilated, whereas the diameter of chronically thrombosed segments is reduced.[48, 97, 108] A free-floating tail, if present, also tends to suggest an acute thrombus.[134] In contrast, the presence of venous collaterals and multiple flow channels within the lumen is more consistent with chronic thrombosis.

TABLE 13–4. ULTRASOUND CHARACTERISTICS OF ACUTE VERSUS CHRONIC THROMBUS

DIAGNOSTIC CRITERIA	ACUTE THROMBUS	CHRONIC THROMBUS
Incompressibility	Spongy	Firm
Vein diameter	Dilated	Decreased
Echogenicity	Echolucent	Echogenic
Heterogeneity	Homogenous	Heterogeneous
Luminal surface	Smooth	Irregular
Collaterals	Absent	Present
Flow channel	Confluent	Multiple
Free-floating tail	May be present	Absent

Several strategies have been proposed to increase the utility of venous ultrasonography in the setting of recurrent symptoms. A baseline venous duplex examination obtained 3 to 6 months after an acute event may be useful in defining recurrent episodes of acute DVT.[12, 97, 117] In comparison with previous examinations, a 2-mm or greater increase in compressed thrombus thickness has been reported to have a sensitivity and specificity of 100% for recurrent proximal venous thrombosis.[117] Demonstration of activated coagulation or new fibrin deposition may also be useful as an adjunct to indeterminate ultrasound findings. Imaging with ^{125}I-labeled fibrinogen has previously been useful in this regard,[8, 56] although its use is limited by the risk of viral transmission. Strategies incorporating markers of acute intravascular thrombosis, such as D-dimer cross-linked fibrin degradation products, may be a useful alternative[39] but have not been evaluated in the setting of recurrent DVT.

Extent of Examination

Despite anatomic limitations, the frequency of multisegmental involvement affords duplex ultrasound a high sensitivity for the diagnosis of acute DVT. The sensitivity of ultrasound in detecting thrombus within an entire limb is higher than the sensitivity in an individual venous segment. These considerations, as well as the operator experience and time required to perform a complete venous duplex examination, have prompted some laboratories to limit examination to the common femoral and popliteal veins in symptomatic patients. Abbreviated studies often include compression in the region of the saphenofemoral junction, including the deep and superficial femoral vein confluences, and the popliteal vein, including the saphenopopliteal junction and tibial vein confluences.[115] Spectral and color flow Doppler analysis is not routinely performed. Although shorter complete examination times are achievable,[99, 133] in direct comparison these abbreviated studies reduced examination time from between 18 (unilateral proximal examination) and 57 minutes (bilateral examination including iliac and tibial veins) to between 5 and 10 minutes.[113, 115, 153] In comparison with a complete color flow duplex examination, Poppiti and coworkers[115] reported a sensitivity of 100% and specificity of 98% for limited compression examination of the proximal veins. Others have achieved nearly identical levels of sensitivity and specificity for limited compression studies.[24, 73, 153]

However, despite reports that more than 99% of proximal thrombi involve segments examined by limited compression ultrasonography,[113] other data suggest that this approach may overlook thrombi isolated to the iliac veins in 2% to 5% of cases and to the superficial femoral vein in 5% of patients.[31, 38, 79, 92, 127, 146] As untreated proximal vein thrombosis is associated with a 20% to 50% risk of recurrent venous thromboembolism,[121] this small percentage cannot be entirely discounted as insignificant. The clinical relevance of thrombosis confined to the calf veins remains more controversial. Most early postoperative thrombi begin in the calf veins,[61] while clinical series of largely symptomatic patients have reported isolated calf vein thrombosis to account for 12% to 33% of ultrasound-documented thromboses[26, 86, 88, 106] and 9% to 46% of those diagnosed with venography.[21, 31, 91, 119] Although the incidence of major pulmonary embolism and late post-thrombotic symptoms is less than after proximal venous thrombosis, isolated calf vein thrombi may not be clinically insignificant. Concurrent pulmonary embolism has been reported in approximately 10% of patients when clinical suspicion is supplemented by objective tests[88, 91, 111] and in up to 33% of patients when routine ventilation-perfusion (V/Q) lung scans have been obtained.[68, 96] Furthermore, approximately one fourth of patients with isolated calf vein thrombosis have persistent symptoms of pain and edema during follow-up.[87, 88] More important, approximately 20% of such thrombi propagate proximally[61, 71, 77, 88] with an associated increase in the risk of symptomatic pulmonary embolism. Although management of isolated calf vein thrombosis remains controversial, many authors have concluded that the benefits of treatment exceed the risks and inconvenience of anticoagulation in patients without contraindications.[53, 57, 121] These considerations would favor routine color flow evaluation of the calf veins. Restricting studies to the proximal veins requires that calf vein thrombi be considered clinically insignificant and that serial testing be performed to exclude proximal propagation. A single, technically adequate examination including the calf veins could potentially eliminate the need for serial studies in many patients, although the safety of this approach has not been prospectively evaluated.

As many as 32% of venous thrombi may be bilateral, a finding that has prompted many laboratories to perform bilateral studies on all patients referred for suspected acute DVT.[30, 76] Bilateral examination is clearly appropriate for those with bilateral symptoms, undergoing postoperative screening, and with suspected pulmonary embolism. However, a positive venous ultrasound in an asymptomatic extremity contralateral to a symptomatic extremity without DVT is uncommon. Strothman and associates[133] found a contralateral thrombus in 22% of patients with acute DVT in a unilaterally symptomatic extremity, although thrombi in asymptomatic extremities were always associated with DVT in the symptomatic extremity. Since identification of thrombus in the asymptomatic limb does not change the management, the need for routine bilateral ultrasonography has been questioned[27, 130, 133] Other authors have reached the opposite conclusion, finding a thrombus isolated to the contralateral limb in 1% of patients referred for unilateral symptoms and in 5% of those with unilateral symptoms and documented thrombosis.[99] A selective approach to the issue has been recommended by some, with bilateral scans limited to those with bilateral symptoms, pulmonary embolism, and ongoing thrombotic risk factors.[27, 104] However, such approaches do not consider the potential value of a complete baseline study in the event of future thromboembolic symptoms.[56]

Accuracy of Venous Ultrasonography

The potential morbidity of pulmonary embolism and recurrent thrombosis mandates a high sensitivity for any diagnostic test for DVT, whereas the risks of inappropriate anticoagulation require that specificity also be high. Despite its shortcomings, ascending venography remains the diagnostic reference standard for DVT. Evaluation of the sensitivity and specificity of venous ultrasound therefore requires comparison with venography according to precise criteria for evaluation of a new diagnostic test.[14, 72] To eliminate bias, these criteria require that consecutive patients with suspected DVT prospectively undergo both ultrasonography and venography with independent, blinded interpretation of the results according to explicitly defined standards.[62, 152, 155] Although not uniformly conforming to these criteria, more than 60 published studies have evaluated the sensitivity and specificity of ultrasound, with or without spectral Doppler and color flow imaging, for the detection of DVT.[30] The results clearly suggest that the sensitivity and specificity of venous ultrasound depend on the population studied. The sensitivity for evaluation of symptomatic patients is substantially higher than for surveillance screening of asymptomatic high-risk patients. Even among symptomatic patients, the sensitivity of venous ultrasound depends on the pretest probability of disease. A sensitivity of 91% may be achieved in patients with a high pretest probability of disease, in whom thrombi are presumably larger and more frequently proximal in extent, in comparison with a sensitivity of only 67% among those with a low pretest probability.[40, 151] Similar factors presumably account for the reduced sensitivity in asymptomatic patients undergoing screening examinations.[53, 85]

More than 80% of symptomatic venous thrombi involve the easily interrogated proximal veins,[62] and the sensitivity and specificity for symptomatic proximal venous thrombosis are uniformly high. In reviewing 15 early studies, Becker and colleagues[14] reported a mean sensitivity of 96% and a mean specificity of 99% for the detection of thigh and popliteal thromboses. Among 4 studies enrolling consecutive patients with blinded interpretation of diagnostic tests, White and colleagues[155] noted a sensitivity of 93%, a specificity of 98%, a positive predictive value of 97%, and a negative predictive value of 93%. In an analysis of 18 studies using a variety of ultrasound techniques, Kearon and coworkers[62] reported a weighted mean sensitivity and specificity of 97% and 94%, respectively with mean positive and negative predictive values of 97% and 98%, respectively for proximal DVT. The sensitivity and specificity for the detection of proximal DVT in selected studies with prospective enrollment of consecutive patients and blinded interpretation are shown in Table 13–5. The sensitivity and specificity of compression, duplex, and color Doppler ultrasound for proximal DVT are similar.[14, 74, 133]

Since duplex ultrasonography is less sensitive for isolated calf vein thrombosis than for femoropopliteal thrombosis, the sensitivity of ultrasonography within an entire lower extremity is less than for proximal DVT alone. Depending on the incidence of isolated calf vein thrombosis, the sensitivity of proximal venous ultrasonography for detection of DVT within an entire extremity is reduced to between 68% and 91%.[4, 73, 74, 94, 123] However, few studies have systematically evaluated the calf veins beyond their confluence, and many of these have employed only B-mode compression or duplex.[62] In contrast to the proximal veins, adequate evaluation of the calf veins is difficult without color imaging. Limited data suggest that normal calf veins

TABLE 13–5. DUPLEX ULTRASOUND FOR SYMPTOMATIC PROXIMAL DEEP VENOUS THROMBOSIS (DVT)

AUTHOR	YEAR	METHOD	*n* (% POSITIVE*)	SENSITIVITY (%)	SPECIFICITY (%)
Cronan et al[28]	1987	Compression	51 (47)	93	100
Appelman et al[2]	1987	Compression	112 (46)	96	97
O'Leary et al[107]	1988	Duplex	50 (48)	92	96
Lensing et al[73]	1989	Compression	220 (30)	100	99
Rose et al[123]	1990	Color Doppler	75 (35)	96	100
Mitchell et al[94]	1991	Duplex	64 (35)	96	85
Cogo et al[24]	1993	Compression	158 (30)	100	100
Aronen et al[4]	1994	Compression	119 (29)	97	100
Lewis et al[74]	1994	Color Doppler	103 (20)	95	99

*Percentage of venograms positive for proximal DVT.

are more reliably visualized by color flow duplex than by venography.[10] In color flow duplex studies of symptomatic patients, the sensitivity and specificity have varied from 95% and 100% in patients with both proximal and distal thromboses[9] to 88% and 96% among patients with isolated calf thrombosis.[156] However, edema, calf size, collateral veins, and anatomic inaccessibility may limit visualization of the tibial veins,[86, 123] and sensitivity in this region is highly dependent on the technical adequacy of the study. Sensitivity and specificity for calf vein thrombosis may be as high as 95% to 100% for technically adequate studies in comparison with 30% to 70% for technically limited studies.[123] In laboratories experienced in color flow Doppler, technically adequate studies of the paired tibial veins have been reported in up to 100% of normal extremities[9, 139] and 60% to 94% of symptomatic limbs.[86, 123]

Because ultrasound is noninvasive and easily repeatable, it has also been used to screen asymptomatic patients at high risk for DVT. Populations considered for routine screening have included those undergoing elective orthopedic[152] and neurosurgical[36] procedures, those hospitalized in the intensive care unit,[46, 52] and high-risk trauma patients.[20] Unfortunately, the accuracy of duplex ultrasonography in screening asymptomatic patients is substantially less than for symptomatic patients. This is not surprising, since such thrombi are presumably smaller, more often nonocclusive, confined to fewer segments, and more frequently isolated to the calf veins than those that give rise to symptoms.[85] Postoperative swelling and wounds may also limit ultrasound access to all venous segments.

Most screening studies have been performed following elective orthopedic surgical procedures, and this literature has been critically reviewed in a meta-analysis by Wells and associates.[152] Among studies enrolling consecutive patients and using blinded interpretation, the sensitivity and specificity of ultrasound for proximal DVT were 62% and 97%, respectively. This was substantially worse than the sensitivity of 95% and specificity of 100% reported in less methodologically rigorous trials. Others have noted similar differences between studies.[72] The clinical relevance of asymptomatic thrombi overlooked by ultrasound is unknown. It is possible that small, nonocclusive thrombi confined to the calf veins may never cause clinical symptoms. Such thrombi may be analogous to those detected by ^{125}I-labeled fibrinogen, 35% of which spontaneously resolve within 72 hours.[61] However, pending prospective studies regarding the outcome of negative examinations in asymptomatic patients, the sensitivity and specificity of ultrasound must be regarded as only moderate.[152]

Duplex ultrasonography has also proved to be sensitive for the diagnosis of upper extremity thrombosis. Among 13 patients with effort thrombosis, Grassi and Polak[42] reported no false-negative or false-positive findings with color flow imaging. An overall sensitivity and specificity of 89% and 100%, respectively, for axillary-subclavian stenosis or occlusion has also been reported among symptomatic dialysis patients with previous central venous catheterization.[11] In a prospective evaluation of 58 symptomatic patients, Prandoni and colleagues[118] reported sensitivities and specificities of 96% and 93.5%, respectively, for compression ultrasonography and 100% and 93%, respectively, for color flow imaging. Reports of lower sensitivity and specificity have been associated with errors due to superior vena cava or central innominate vein thrombosis, inadequate imaging of the subclavian vein, and the inability to differentiate extrinsic compression from thrombosis.[69] Venography may thus be warranted when clinical suspicion or indirect evidence such as abnormal respiratory variation or prominent venous collaterals suggests a proximal thrombosis despite an otherwise negative ultrasound examination.

Clinical Utility of Venous Ultrasonography

The high specificity of ultrasonography allows anticoagulation to be instituted without confirmatory venography,[94] whereas the high sensitivity for proximal thrombosis makes it possible to withhold anticoagulation if serial examinations are negative. However, 3% to 7% of documented thromboses have an initial study that is negative for proximal thrombosis and, if limited to the proximal veins, serial examinations are required.[23, 47] Initial diagnostic failure rates may be higher among inpatients and those with persistent symptoms.[131, 138] The incidence of thromboembolism within 6 months of serially negative ultrasound examinations is less than 2%,[47, 62] and withholding anticoagulation in symptomatic patients with two negative ultrasound examinations 5 to 7 days apart has proved safe.[19, 23]

Venous duplex ultrasonography may also be more cost-effective than other diagnostic strategies.[16] In a cost-effectiveness analysis of several strategies, venous duplex of the proximal veins was associated with an average of 4.53 deaths per 1000 patients at an average cost of $2138 per patient in comparison with 4.44 deaths and $2437 for routine venography.[51] Addition of a second duplex 5 to 7 days following a negative study decreased the death rate to 3.79 per 1000, but at a high incremental cost of $390,000 per life saved. Strategies employing venous ultrasound were more cost-effective than venography as long as the sensitivity and specificity remained greater than 93%. Alternatives to serial duplex scanning have been proposed, but their cost-effectiveness is unknown. Among these, the combined use of D-dimer measurements and noninvasive studies may safely eliminate the need for serial studies if both are negative.[39] A complete, technically adequate examination including the calf veins might also be more cost-effective if the safety of withholding anticoagulation after a single negative study were known.

Indications for Venous Ultrasonography

The accuracy, availability, and noninvasive nature of venous duplex ultrasonography have led to its widespread clinical application in a variety of symptomatic and asymptomatic patients. In comparison with historical requests for venography, Glover and Bendick[40] noted a sixfold increase in the yearly number of lower extremity venous duplex studies. Criado and Burnham[26] have further estimated that approximately 7 venous duplex scans are performed for each DVT diagnosed. Despite the recognized inaccuracy of clinical presentation, concerns about overutilization and misuse of limited vascular laboratory resources have forced some consideration of the appropriate indications for venous duplex scanning. Although clinical evaluation cannot confirm or exclude the diagnosis of DVT with absolute accuracy, it can be used to stratify patients into those with a high or low pretest probability of disease. Based on the presence of thrombotic risk factors, clinical signs and symptoms, and the possibility of alternative diagnoses, high-risk and low-risk groups can be defined with an 85% and 5% prevalence of DVT, respectively.[151]

The value of clinical screening prior to duplex scanning appears to be more clearly defined for symptomatic outpatients than for inpatients. The overall prevalence of acute lower extremity DVT in outpatient vascular laboratory referrals varies from 12% to 25%.[26, 40, 50, 80, 99, 106] The prevalence of positive outpatient studies increases from 2.1% among patients without swelling or thrombotic risk factors to 13% in those with thrombotic risk factors but no swelling, to approximately 50% in patients with acute unilateral swelling.[40] Among outpatients, the negative predictive value of the absence of unilateral swelling or an existing thrombotic risk factor is greater than 97%.[26, 40] Chronic unilateral swelling and bilateral swelling are associated with a significant prevalence of chronic findings, although an acute DVT may be found in less than 1%.[40] Other common indications for vascular laboratory referral, such as joint pain or cellulitis in the absence of thrombotic risk factors, are associated with an exceedingly low prevalence of acute DVT.[40] The prevalence of positive studies is higher among inpatient referrals, ranging from 16% to 31%.[26, 40, 50, 106] Bilateral DVT, accounting for 35% of positive inpatient studies,[26] and comorbid medical problems are also more common in this population. Not surprisingly, it is more difficult to define those factors that are associated with a negative inpatient study.[106] Among symptomatic inpatients, acute DVT has been identified in 55% of patients with the acute onset of unilateral swelling, but also in 20% of those with bilateral swelling.

Although the absence of acute unilateral limb swelling and recognized risk factors may identify an outpatient population with a low prevalence of positive scan findings, restricting studies to those meeting this criteria misses 2% to 5% of patients with an acute DVT.[40, 151] Furthermore, ultrasound is also useful for the identification of chronic DVT in 5% to 10%[37, 40, 74] and findings such as a Baker's cyst, muscle hematoma, popliteal aneurysm, joint effusion, or lymphadenopathy in 5% to 18% of symptomatic outpatients, which may explain their clinical presentation and assist in management.[14, 30, 131, 138, 155] The true utility of such clinical criteria may be in selecting studies and maximizing the efficiency of scarce vascular laboratory resources. Furthermore, the positive and negative predictive value of any diagnostic test depends on the probability of disease in a population.[154] High negative predictive value in populations with a low probability of disease and high positive predictive value among those with a high probability of disease justify management of negative and positive findings in these respective groups based on noninvasive studies alone. However, ultrasound findings that contradict clinical impressions must be regarded with suspicion.

Venous duplex ultrasonography is also frequently employed in the evaluation of patients with suspected pulmonary embolism. Although most pulmonary emboli do arise from the deep veins of the lower extremities, there are little data to support ultrasound as the initial diagnostic test for suspected pulmonary embolism. Venous duplex is not sufficiently accurate to be used as the sole diagnostic test for pulmonary embolism. In comparison with pulmonary angiography, the sensitivity and specificity of lower extremity venous duplex are only 44% and 86%, respectively.[65] Such figures are similar to the 38% sensitivity of other noninvasive lower extremity studies (pulse-volume plethysmography and continuous wave Doppler) for the diagnosis of pulmonary embolism.[129] Thrombus associated with a documented pulmonary embolism may have completely embolized or involved segments such as the upper extremity, abdominal, iliac, or profunda veins that were not interrogated. Although a normal duplex scan cannot reliably exclude pulmonary embolism, initial identification of an acute DVT could theoretically avoid further diagnostic evaluation in some patients. However, only 9% to 14% of venous duplex studies disclose an acute DVT in this setting.[33, 37, 40, 75, 84] Positive duplex scans may be present in as many as 40% of patients with unilateral leg symptoms but only 5% of those without leg symptoms[33] and 1.6% of those with neither leg symptoms nor thrombotic risk factors.[40] In contrast, 25% to 35% of pulmonary V/Q scans are either high probability or normal and require no further diagnostic testing unless clinical suspicion is low.[33, 84] Most investigators have thus recommended V/Q scanning as the initial diagnostic test for suspected pulmonary embolism,[63] with lower extremity ultrasound reserved for nondiagnostic scintigraphy. Initial V/Q scanning followed by venous duplex for nondiagnostic studies, and pulmonary angiography if the ultrasound is normal, is theoretically associated with the lowest morbidity, mortality, and number of patients in whom anticoagulation is inappropriately withheld.[109] Initial venous duplex might be appropriate for those with concurrent unilateral leg symptoms, although this presentation accounts for less than 10% of patients with suspected pulmonary embolism.[33] Although noninvasive venous testing after a diagnostic (high probability or normal) V/Q scan may be useful as a baseline for future events, this approach changes management in only 4% of patients and has been questioned as a routine measure.[75]

ULTRASOUND APPLICATIONS IN CHRONIC VENOUS DISEASE

Chronic venous disease may result from primary venous valvular insufficiency or a previous episode of acute DVT and includes a spectrum of clinical problems ranging from telangiectasias and varicose veins to venous ulceration.[116] However, the hemodynamics underlying the severe manifestations of swelling, hyperpigmentation, and ulceration are similar: valvular reflux or retrograde flow through damaged or absent valves leads to the development of ambulatory venous hypertension.[67] Residual venous obstruction also plays a role in the post-thrombotic syndrome, a combination of reflux and obstruction being more common than either abnormality alone in patients with skin changes and ulceration.[59, 60] However, despite the well-characterized hemodynamics, clinical manifestations such as pain, swelling, and ulceration are not specific for venous disease. Only two thirds of patients with chronic leg ulcers have objective evidence of venous disease,[125] while edema occurring after an episode of DVT may be due to either residual venous obstruction or the development of valvular incompetence and ambulatory venous hypertension. Evaluation of the venous system may be important in establishing an etiology for such nonspecific complaints, as well as in defining the severity and anatomic location of reflux and obstruction, selecting patients for extirpative or reconstructive procedures, assessing hemodynamic improvement after such procedures, and establishing the natural history of chronic venous disease.

Diagnostic Tests for Chronic Venous Disease

The ideal diagnostic test for chronic venous disease should be capable of defining the presence of both residual venous obstruction and valvular incompetence, localizing these abnormalities to precise segments of the superficial and deep venous systems, and quantifying the degree of abnormality in a manner that correlates with the clinical severity of disease. The ideal test should thus provide both anatomic and hemodynamic information, for which descending phlebography and ambulatory venous pressure (AVP) measurements are considered the standard reference test. However, in addition to their invasive nature, both of these studies have limitations. Competent proximal valves may prevent venographic assessment of distal reflux, while hyperbaric contrast medium may stream past normal valves in the relaxed leg. Evaluation of the greater and lesser saphenous veins may also be limited with this technique.[6] AVP measurements reflect the global hemodynamics within an extremity and show a linear relationship with the prevalence of ulceration.[103, 112] However, AVP cannot localize the hemodynamic aberrations beyond the superficial or deep venous systems and is influenced by both reflux and obstruction. Photoplethysmography and air plethysmography are the most widely utilized noninvasive tests for the evaluation of chronic venous disease, but they have their own specific limitations.[13, 102, 120, 142, 149, 150] However, all provide only an indirect assessment of global venous hemodynamics without precise characterization of the underlying abnormalities. Furthermore, since reflux at multiple levels may be required to be hemodynamically significant, these measurements may be insensitive to isolated segmental reflux.[120]

In contrast, duplex ultrasonography has the potential to provide both anatomic and physiologic information. Valvular reflux can be identified by Doppler spectral analysis, while the B-mode image allows localization of both anatomic obstruction and reflux to precise segments of the venous system. Duplex scanning not only provides the anatomic information lacking in global hemodynamic tests but also avoids the venographic limitations of proximal valve competence and hyperbaric contrast medium while permitting valve function to be evaluated under conditions that simulate normal calf muscle pump function.[100] Accordingly, it may be the most accurate test for identification of isolated but hemodynamically significant reflux in the distal deep venous segments.[6, 124]

Duplex Scanning for Chronic Venous Disease

Duplex scanning is capable of characterizing partial and complete anatomic obstruction as well as valvular incompetence in the deep, superficial, and perforating veins. The criteria for the diagnosis of obstruction are similar to those described for the evaluation of acute DVT. Several methods of assessing valvular incompetence in the deep and superficial venous systems have been proposed, and selection of an appropriate technique requires consideration of the mechanism of valvular closure.

As described by van Bemmelen and associates,[140, 141] the lower extremity valve cusps remain open while the patient is resting in the supine position. Valve closure is a passive event initiated by reversal of the resting antegrade transvalvular pressure gradient. As the pressure gradient is reversed, there is a short period of retrograde flow, or reflux, until the gradient becomes sufficient to cause valve closure. Valve closure requires not only the cessation of antegrade flow but also a brief retrograde flow interval of sufficient velocity to completely coapt the cusps. At reverse flow velocities greater than 30 cm/sec, valve closure occurs within 100 msec and produces a sharp Doppler spectrum with a clear end-point (Fig. 13–4). At velocities less than 30 cm/sec, reverse flow may persist for longer intervals even in the presence of competent valves. The determination of valvular incompetence therefore requires that pathologic retrograde flow be demonstrated in response to maneuvers that consistently generate an adequate reverse flow velocity. Furthermore, since clinically relevant reflux occurs during calf muscle contraction and relaxation in the erect position, these maneuvers should approximate the conditions of upright exercise as closely as possible.

Methods used to elicit reflux with duplex ultrasonogra-

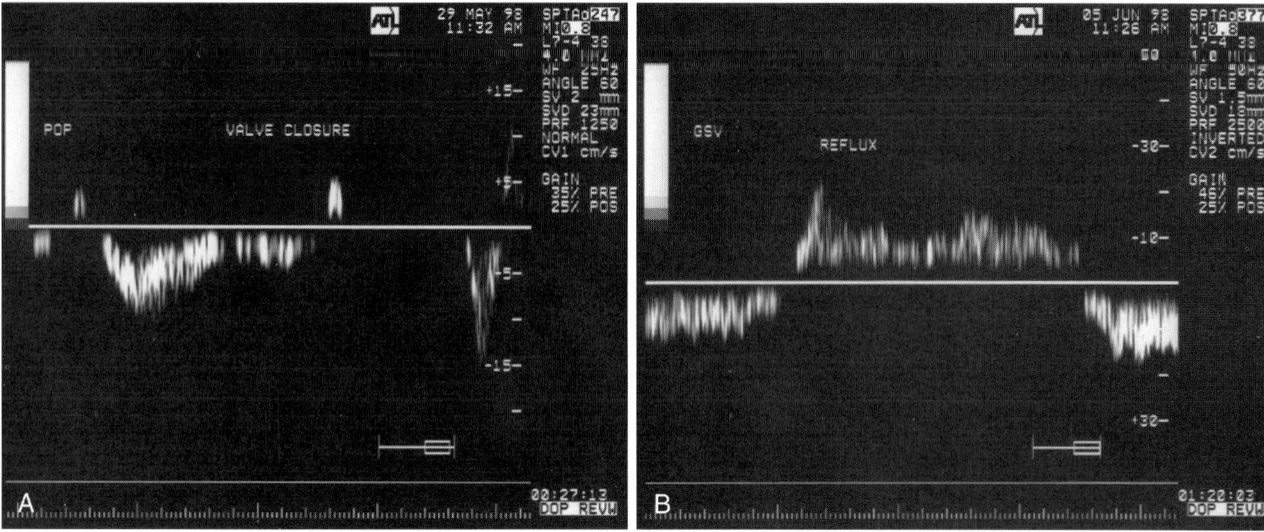

FIGURE 13–4. Duplex detection of valvular reflux. With reversal of normal antegrade flow, there is a brief interval of retrograde flow prior to valve closure. In the presence of a competent valve, valve closure appears as a clearly demarcated period of retrograde flow (above the baseline) of less than 0.5 seconds' duration *(A)*. In the presence of valvular incompetence *(B)*, the duration of reverse flow is prolonged.

phy include the Valsalva maneuver, manual proximal compression or distal compression release, and standardized cuff compression proximal to or cuff deflation distal to the venous segment of interest. In addition to the theoretical considerations discussed earlier, the ideal method of eliciting reflux would clearly distinguish competent from incompetent venous segments by providing a short duration of reverse flow in normal subjects and a prolonged duration of reflux in symptomatic patients with incompetent valves. Although all techniques may be performed either supine or standing, the upright position is preferred since the time required for valve closure in normal subjects is greater in the supine position.[3, 141] With respect to the individual maneuvers, acceptable results have been achieved with a Valsalva maneuver,[83] although diminished sensitivity below proximal competent valves and in the distal deep venous segments has also been reported.[6, 81, 82] The duration of reverse flow across venographically competent valves is also more variable with the Valsalva maneuver.[82] Proximal compression methods are inferior to release of distal compression, producing variable results with a poor separation between normal and diseased limbs.[3, 141] Deflation of a cuff distal to the imaged segment in the standing position gives the shortest, most reproducible duration of reverse flow in normal subjects with a sensitivity of 91% and specificity of 100% for the detection of popliteal reflux.[3] Although diligent efforts may produce acceptable results with manual distal compression in the standing position, cuff deflation provides a more consistent and standardized approach.

The accuracy of standing distal cuff deflation has been compared with reflux determination in the supine position using manual limb compression and Valsalva maneuvers.[81, 100] Considering standing cuff deflation as the reference standard within individual venous segments, the supine maneuvers are less sensitive than cuff deflation in identifying reflux at all levels (Table 13–6). The Valsalva maneuver is more sensitive in the proximal segments, whereas manual compression is more sensitive in the distal segments. The best sensitivity for the supine maneuvers is achieved when the presence of reflux is defined as a positive result with either limb compression or a Valsalva maneuver. Similarly, when quantified using a multisegment scoring system applied to the entire limb, standing distal cuff deflation provided a sensitivity of 77% and specificity of 85% for the

TABLE 13–6. SENSITIVITY AND SPECIFICITY OF SUPINE MANEUVERS VERSUS STANDING DISTAL CUFF DEFLATION FOR DETECTING VENOUS REFLUX

	METHOD (%)					
	Valsalva		Manual Compression		Combined*	
SEGMENT*	*Sensitivity*	*Specificity*	*Sensitivity*	*Specificity*	*Sensitivity*	*Specificity*
CFV	75	86	21	98	79	86
GSV	67	100	10	100	67	100
SFV	83	97	50	97	88	93
PPV	49	98	73	88	76	88
PTV	20	99	30	92	30	92

From Markel A, Meissner MH, Manzo RA et al: A comparison of the cuff deflation method with Valsalva's maneuver and limb compression in detecting venous valvular reflux. Arch Surg 129:701–705, 1994. Copyright 1994 American Medical Association.

*Combined Valsalva and manual compression maneuvers. Reflux is considered to be present if the result of either individual maneuver is positive.

CFV = common femoral vein; GSV = greater saphenous vein; SFV = superficial femoral vein; PPV = popliteal vein; PTV = posterior tibial vein.

differentiation of clinically mild and severe venous disease in comparison with 61% and 60%, respectively, for supine duplex and 50% and 41%, respectively, for descending phlebography.[100]

Standardized Standing Cuff Deflation

In evaluating reflux using the technique of standing cuff deflation,[100, 101, 141] the patient stands supported by a frame, with the leg slightly flexed and weight borne by the contralateral extremity. Pneumatic cuffs are placed distal to the segment of interest and inflation pressure is varied according to the hydrostatic pressure at that level. The common femoral, proximal superficial femoral, profunda femoris, and proximal greater saphenous veins are evaluated with a 24-cm thigh cuff inflated to 80 mmHg; the distal superficial femoral and popliteal veins with a 12-cm calf cuff inflated to 100 mmHg; and the posterior tibial veins using a 7-cm foot cuff inflated to 120 mmHg (Fig. 13–5). A rapid cuff inflator (Hokanson, Bellevue, Wash.) is used to provide inflation over approximately 3 seconds and rapid deflation within 0.3 seconds. The spectral display is adjusted to show antegrade flow below the baseline and reverse flow, or reflux, above the baseline. Each segment is then sequentially imaged in a longitudinal plane at a distance less than 5 cm from the cuff. Doppler signals are recorded as the cuff is inflated until antegrade flow ceases and then as the cuff is rapidly deflated. Ninety-five percent of normal valves will close within 0.5 seconds of cuff deflation (Fig. 13–6),[141] a value that provides complete separation between normal volunteers and those with clinical manifestations of chronic venous disease.[3] Although the duration of retrograde flow can also be determined using color flow Doppler, this may underestimate the duration of reflux in comparison with spectral measurements.[3]

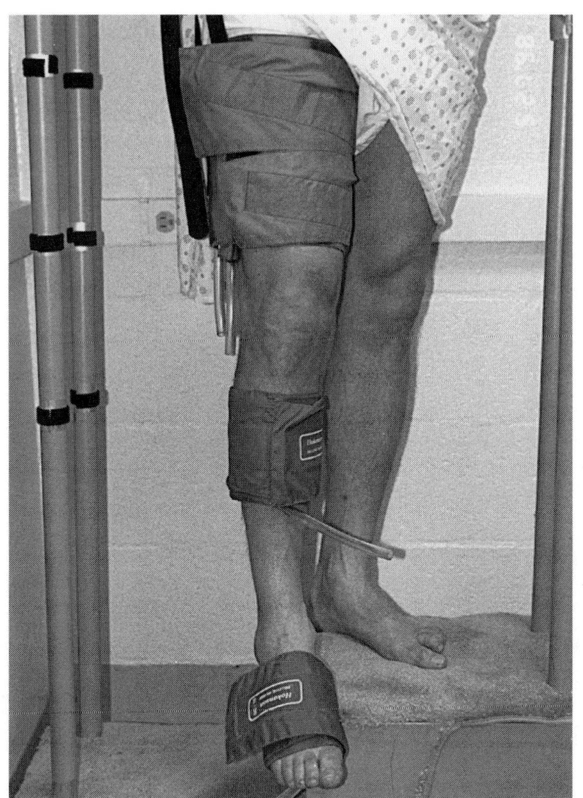

FIGURE 13–5. Reflux determination using standing distal cuff deflation. The patient stands with his weight supported on the contralateral extremity. Inflation pressure is adjusted according to the hydrostatic pressure at the level of the segment being imaged using a 24-cm cuff (Hokanson, Bellevue, Wash.) inflated to 80 mmHg for the thigh, a 12-cm cuff inflated to 100 mmHg for the calf, and a 7-cm cuff inflated to 120 mmHg for the foot.

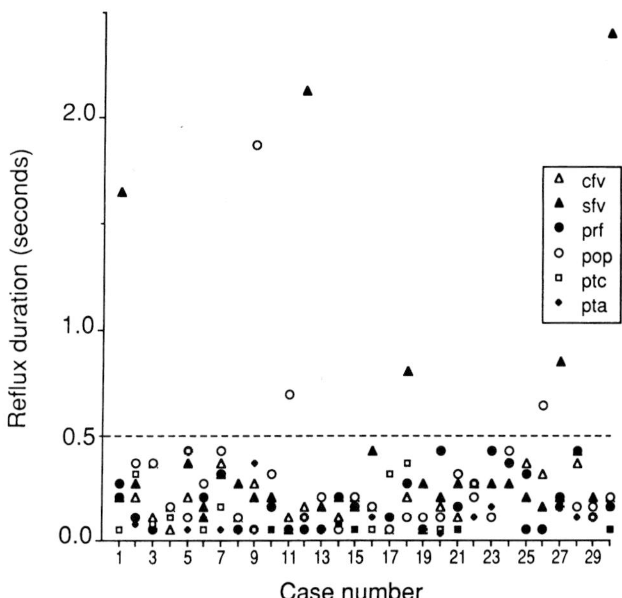

FIGURE 13–6. Duration of reflux in individual venous segments of 30 normal extremities in response to distal cuff deflation in the standing position. The duration of retrograde flow, or reflux, is less than 0.5 seconds in 95% of venous segments. cfv, common femoral vein; sfv, superficial femoral vein; prf, profunda femoris vein; pop, popliteal vein; ptc, posterior tibial vein, calf; pta, posterior tibial vein, ankle. (From van Bemmelen PS, Bedford G, Beach K, et al: Quantitative segmental evaluation of venous valvular reflux with duplex ultrasound scanning. J Vasc Surg 10:425–431, 1989.)

Standing distal cuff deflation for the detection of reflux does have some disadvantages in comparison with alternative maneuvers. Although a well-trained technologist can perform the entire study, assigning different technologists to scan and operate the pneumatic cuff inflator facilitates the learning process. The technique also requires additional equipment and a patient capable of standing for approximately 30 minutes. However, the results of these studies reflect pathologic refiux and its clinical severity better than either supine duplex studies or descending phlebography.[81, 100]

Quantitative Applications of Duplex Scanning

Although duplex ultrasonography accurately identifies and localizes segmental venous reflux, the relationship of these findings to global venous hemodynamics is less well-defined. Abnormal direct venous pressure measurements are present in only 80% of those with common femoral or popliteal venous reflux detected by duplex.[135] Theoretically, the magnitude of duplex-detected reflux should correlate with the severity of hemodynamic and clinical derangements, and several methods to quantify reflux have been proposed. Neglen and Raju[100, 101] have suggested anatomic scoring systems, analogous to those used for descending phlebography, based on either the axial extent or segmental distribution of reflux. Alternatively, duplex-derived valve closure times may be determined from the duration of reverse flow on the Doppler spectral tracing. Total valve closure times can be calculated as the sum of segmental closure times in the entire extremity or within the superficial and deep venous systems.[122, 147] Finally, reflux flow volumes can be calculated from duplex-determined reflux velocities and venous cross-sectional area.[122, 144]

Among these, methods of quantifying the anatomic extent of reflux have been more consistent than hemodynamic quantification. Neglen and Raju[100] found the quantitative extent of reflux determined by duplex to better reflect the clinical severity of disease than does standard phlebographic scoring. Quantitative anatomic scores were also correlated with invasive and noninvasive indices of reflux. Other authors[6] have similarly found abnormal foot volumetry findings to correlate more closely with the extent of reflux determined by duplex than with that determined by phlebography. Attempts to quantify global venous hemodynamics with duplex have yielded inconsistent results. Segments included in the calculation of total valve closure times have varied between studies, as has the relationship to clinical manifestations and noninvasive measurements of global reflux. No studies have directly correlated duplex-derived valve closure times with AVP.[13] Although a relationship between total valve closure times, air plethysmographic indices of reflux, and the presence of venousulceration has been noted by some,[147] others have noted a poor correlation with both air plethysmography[122] and severe clinical manifestations.[58, 122] Valve closure times in individual venous segments are poorly correlated with reflux volume, since large volumes may reflux over short intervals or small volumes over long intervals.[122] Measurements of peak reflux volume flow, however, may have some utility, with peak volume flows above 10 ml/sec defining a group with a 66% prevalence of skin changes.[144]

Pending further evaluation of these quantitative duplex methods, there may be no ideal noninvasive study for the evaluation of chronic venous insufficiency. The inherent dichotomy between global assessment of hemodynamics and accurate localization of segmental reflux and obstruction may require a combination of tests in some circumstances. This has been viewed as analogous to lower extremity arterial assessment in which physiologic measurements such as the ankle-brachial index and anatomic studies such as arteriography provide complementary information.[149] For the present, it may be necessary to combine the unique ability of duplex scanning to assess and localize both obstruction and reflux, with measurements of hemodynamic severity determined by tests such as air plethysmography.[101] A combination of these studies may obviate the need for invasive tests in all but those requiring precise visualization of valvular anatomy in anticipation of venous reconstruction.

Evaluation of Perforator Incompetence

The perforating veins are evaluated in the upright position, scanning along the course of the superficial femoral vein in the mid-thigh and the posterior tibial and posterior arch veins in the calf. One to five perforating veins are usually traceable as they penetrate the fascia between the superficial and deep venous systems.[114] Perforating veins may occur anywhere along the medial calf, most commonly just below the malleolus and 15 to 19 cm and 30 to 34 cm proximally.[93, 126] Unfortunately, the direction of normal flow and the definition of perforating vein reflux remain controversial.[126] Flow in normal perforating veins is unidirectional and occurs only during distal compression of the foot or calf, whereas incompetent segments are identified by bidirectional flow with reverse flow during the relaxation phase after compression.[93] Duplex identifies more perforating veins than does ascending venography,[45] and in comparison with surgical findings, has been reported to have a sensitivity of 82% and specificity of 100% for the identification of competent and incompetent perforating veins.[114]

SUMMARY

Although duplex ultrasonography has facilitated the investigation of many areas of vascular disease, it has arguably had one of its greatest impacts in the evaluation of acute and chronic venous disease. For the diagnosis of proximal venous thrombosis, sensitivities and specificities approaching 95% in comparison with contrast venography have been well documented. Serial compression ultrasonography has largely supplanted contrast venography for the diagnosis of proximal DVT in symptomatic patients, and withholding anticoagulation in those with negative studies 5 to 7 days apart has been shown to be safe and cost-effective. The use of color flow Doppler has facilitated DVT diagnosis in areas such as the calf and iliac veins that are difficult to evaluate with compression ultrasound. Although these advantages may make it theoretically possible to exclude acute DVT on the basis of a single, technically adequate and complete color flow study, the safety of such an approach has not been validated prospectively. Similarly, the value of duplex ultrasound in screening high-risk asymptomatic patients for acute DVT will remain unclear until the natural history of patients with overlooked thrombi has been established. Duplex ultrasonography has also become the noninvasive standard for defining valvular incompetence and persistent venous occlusion in chronic venous disease. Erect evaluation using distal cuff deflation allows standardized physiologic assessment of reflux in individual segments. Although global measurements of venous hemodynamics and descending venography will continue to have some role in the evaluation of patients before and after reconstructive procedures, duplex ultrasound is capable of providing precise diagnosis and anatomic localization of the abnormalities underlying chronic venous disease.

REFERENCES

1. American Institute of Ultrasound in Medicine: Guidelines for the Performance of Vascular/Doppler Ultrasound Examination. Laurel, Md, American Institute of Ultrasound in Medicine, 1992.

2. Appelman PT, De Jong TE, Lampman LE: Deep venous thrombosis of the leg: US findings. Radiology 163:743, 1987.
3. Araki CT, Back TL, Padberg FT, et al: Refinements in the ultrasonic detection of popliteal vein reflux. J Vasc Surg 18:742, 1993.
4. Aronen RJ, Svedstrom E, Yrjana J, et al: Compression sonography in the diagnosis of deep venous thrombosis of the leg. Ann Med 26:377, 1994.
5. Bach AM, Hahn LE: When the common femoral vein is revealed as flattened on spectral Doppler sonography: Is it a reliable sign for diagnosis of proximal venous obstruction? AJR Am J Roentgenol 168:733, 1997.
6. Baker SR, Burnand KG, Sommerville KM, et al: Comparison of venous reflux assessed by duplex scanning and descending phlebography in chronic venous disease. Lancet 341:400, 1993.
7. Baldridge ED, Martin MA, Welling RE: Clinical significance of free-floating venous thrombi. J Vasc Surg 11:62, 1990.
8. Barnes RW, Wu KK, Hoak JC: Fallibility of the clinical diagnosis of venous thrombosis. JAMA 234:605, 1975.
9. Baxter GM, Duffy P: Calf vein anatomy and flow: Implications for color Doppler imaging. Clin Radiol 46:84, 1992.
10. Baxter GM, Duffy P, Partridge E: Colour flow imaging of calf vein thrombosis. Clin Radiol 46:198, 1992.
11. Baxter GM, Kincaid W, Jeffrey RF, et al: Comparison of colour Doppler ultrasound with venography in the diagnosis of axillary and subclavian vein thrombosis. Br J Radiol 64:777, 1991.
12. Baxter GM, Duffy P, MacKechnie S: Colour Doppler ultrasound of the post-phlebitic limb: Sounding a cautionary note. Clin Radiol 43:301, 1991.
13. Bays RA, Healy DA, Atnip RG, et al: Validation of air plethysmography, photoplethysmography, and duplex ultrasonography in the evaluation of severe venous stasis. J Vasc Surg 30:721, 1994.
14. Becker DM, Philbrick JT, Abbitt PL: Real-time ultrasonography for the diagnosis of lower extremity deep venous thrombosis. Arch Intern Med 149:1731, 1989.
15. Belcaro G: Evaluation of recurrent deep venous thrombosis using color duplex scanning—comparison with contrast venography. Vasa 21:22, 1992.
16. Bendayan P, Boccalon H: Cost-effectiveness of noninvasive tests including duplex scanning for diagnosis of deep venous thrombosis. Vasa 20:348, 1991.
17. Berry RE, George JE, Shaver WA: Free-floating deep venous thrombosis: A retrospective analysis. Ann Surg 211:719, 1990.
18. Bettmann MA, Robbins A, Braun SD, et al: Contrast venography of the leg: Diagnostic efficacy, tolerance, and complication rates with ionic and nonionic contrast media. Radiology 165:113, 1987.
19. Birdwell BG, Raskob GE, Whitsett TL, et al: The clinical validity of normal compression ultrasonography in outpatients suspected of having deep venous thrombosis. Ann Intern Med 128:1, 1998.
20. Brasel KJ, Borgstrom DC, Weigelt JA: Cost-effective prevention of pulmonary embolus in high-risk trauma patients. J Trauma 42:456, 1997.
21. Browse NL, Thomas ML: Source of nonlethal pulmonary emboli. Lancet 1:258, 1974.
22. Burbidge SJ, Finlay DE, Letourneau JG, et al: Effects of central venous catheter placement on upper extremity duplex US findings. J Vasc Interv Radiol 4:399, 1993.
23. Cogo A, Lensing AWA, Koopman MMW, et al: Compression ultrasonography for diagnostic management of patients with clinically suspected deep vein thrombosis: Prospective cohort study. BMJ 316:617, 1998.
24. Cogo A, Lensing AWA, Prandoni P, et al: Comparison of real-time B-mode ultrasonography and Doppler ultrasound with contrast venography in the diagnosis of venous thrombosis in symptomatic outpatients. Thromb Haemost 70:404, 1993.
25. Cranley JJ, Canos AJ, Sull WJ: The diagnosis of deep venous thrombosis: Fallability of clinical symptoms and signs. Arch Surg 111:34, 1976.
26. Criado E, Burnham CB: Predictive value of clinical criteria for the diagnosis of deep vein thrombosis. Surgery 122:578, 1997.
27. Cronan JJ: Deep venous thrombosis: One leg or both legs. Radiology 200:323, 1996.
28. Cronan JJ, Dorfman GS, Scola FH, et al: Deep venous thrombosis: US assessment using vein compression. Radiology 162:191, 1987.
29. Cronan JJ, Leen V: Recurrent deep venous thrombosis: Limitations of US. Radiology 170:739, 1989.
30. Dauzat M, Laroche J-P, Deklunder G, et al: Diagnosis of acute lower limb deep venous thrombosis with ultrasound: Trends and controversies. J Clin Ultrasound 25:343, 1997.
31. de Valois JC, van Schaik CC, Verzibergen F, et al: Contrast venography: From gold standard to "golden backup" in clinically suspected deep vein thrombosis. Eur J Radiol 11:131, 1990.
32. Elias A, Le Corff G, Bouvier JL, et al: Value of real-time B-mode ultrasound imaging in the diagnosis of deep vein thrombosis of the lower limbs. Int Angiol 6:175, 1987.
33. Eze AR, Comerota AJ, Kerr RP, et al: Is venous duplex imaging an appropriate initial screening test for patients with suspected pulmonary embolism? Ann Vasc Surg 10:220, 1996.
34. Falk RL, Smith DF: Thrombosis of upper extremity thoracic inlet veins: Diagnosis with duplex Doppler sonography. Am J Roentenol 149:677, 1987.
35. Fletcher JP, Kershaw LZ, Barker DS, et al: Ultrasound diagnosis of deep venous thrombosis. Med J Aust 153:453, 1990.
36. Flinn WR, Sandager GP, Cerullo LJ, et al: Duplex venous scanning for the prospective surveillance of perioperative venous thrombosis. Arch Surg 124:901, 1989.
37. Fowl RJ, Strothman GB, Blebea J, et al: Inappropriate use of venous duplex scans: An analysis of indications and results. J Vasc Surg 23:881, 1996.
38. Frederick MG, Hertzberg BS, Kliewer MA, et al: Can the US examination for lower extremity deep venous thrombosis be abreviated? A prospective study of 755 examinations. Radiology 199:45, 1996.
39. Ginsberg JS, Kearon C, Douketis J, et al: The use of D-dimer testing and impedance plethysmographic examination in patients with clinical indications of deep vein thrombosis. Arch Intern Med 157: 1077, 1997.
40. Glover JL, Bendick PJ: Appropriate indications for venous duplex ultrasonic examinations. Surgery 120:725, 1996.
41. Gooding GAW, Hightower DR, Moore EH, et al: Obstruction of the superior vena cava or subclavian veins: Sonographic diagnosis. Radiology 159:663, 1986.
42. Grassi CJ, Polak JF: Axillary and subclavian venous thrombosis: Follow-up evaluation with color flow US and venography. Radiology 175:651, 1990.
43. Greenfield LJ: Free-floating thrombus and pulmonary embolism [letter]. Arch Intern Med 157:2661, 1997.
44. Haeger K: Problems of acute deep venous thrombosis. Part 1. The interpretation of signs and symptoms. Angiology 20:219, 1969.
45. Hanrahan LM, Araki CT, Fisher JB, et al: Evaluation of the perforating veins of the lower extremity using high-resolution duplex imaging. J Cardiovasc Surg 32:87, 1991.
46. Harris LM, Curl GR, Booth FV, et al: Screening for asymptomatic deep vein thrombosis in surgical intensive care patients. J Vasc Surg 26:764, 1997.
47. Heijboer H, Buller HR, Lensing AWA, et al: A comparison of real-time compression ultrasonography with impedance plethysmography for the diagnosis of deep vein thrombosis in symptomatic outpatients. N Engl J Med 329:1365, 1993.
48. Hertzberg BS, Kliewer MA, DeLong DM, et al: Sonographic assessment of lower limb vein diameter: Implications for the diagnosis and characterization of deep venous thrombosis. AJR Am J Roentgenol 168:1253, 1997.
49. Hightower DR, Gooding GA: Sonographic evaluation of the normal respiratory response on subclavian veins to respiratory maneuvers. Invest Radiol 20:517, 1985.
50. Hill S, Holtzman G, Martin D, et al: Selective use of the duplex scan in diagnosis of deep venous thrombosis. Am J Surg 170:201, 1995.
51. Hillner BE, Philbrick JT, Becker DM: Optimal management of suspected lower extremity deep venous thrombosis: An evaluation with cost assessment of 24 management strategies. Arch Intern Med 152:165, 1992.
52. Hirsch DR, Ingenito EP, Goldhaber SZ: Prevalence of deep venous thrombosis among patients in medical intensive care. JAMA 274:335, 1995.
53. Hirsh J, Lensing AWA: Natural history of minimal calf vein deep venous thrombosis. *In* Bernstein EF (ed): Vascular Diagnosis, 4th ed. St. Louis, Mosby–Year Book, 1993, pp 779–781.
54. Hubsch PJ, Stigbauer RL, Schwaighofer BW, et al: Internal jugular and subclavian vein thrombosis caused by central venous catheters. J Ultrasound Med 7:629, 1988.
55. Hull R, Hirsh J, Sackett DL, et al: Clinical validity of a negative

venogram in patients with clinically suspected venous thrombosis. Circulation 64:622, 1981.
56. Hull RD, Carter CJ, Jay RM, et al: The diagnosis of acute, recurrent, deep venous thrombosis: A diagnostic challenge. Circulation 67:901, 1983.
57. Hyers TM, Hull RD, Weg JG: Antithrombotic therapy for venous thromboembolic disease. Chest 108 (Suppl):335S, 1995.
58. Iafrati MD, Welch H, O'Donnell TF, et al: Correlation of venous noninvasive tests with the Society for Vascular Surgery/International Society for Cardiovascular Surgery clinical classification for chronic venous insufficiency. J Vasc Surg 19:1001, 1994.
59. Johnson BF, Manzo RA, Bergelin RO, et al: The site of residual abnormalities in the leg veins in long-term follow-up after deep venous thrombosis and their relationship to the development of the post-thrombotic syndrome. Int Angiol 15:14, 1996.
60. Johnson BF, Manzo RA, Bergelin RO, et al: Relationship between changes in the deep venous system and the development of the post-thrombotic syndrome after an acute episode of lower limb deep vein thrombosis: A one- to six-year follow-up. J Vasc Surg 21:307, 1995.
61. Kakkar VV, Flanc C, Howe CT, et al: Natural history of postoperative deep vein thrombosis. Lancet 2:230, 1969.
62. Kearon C, Julian JA, Math M, et al: Noninvasive diagnosis of deep venous thrombosis: McMaster Diagnostic Imaging Practice Guidelines Initiative. Ann Intern Med 128:663, 1998.
63. Kelley MA, Carson JL, Palevsky HI, et al: Diagnosing pulmonary embolism: New facts and strategies. Ann Intern Med 114:300, 1991.
64. Killewich LA, Bedford GR, Beach KW, et al: Diagnosis of deep venous thrombosis: A prospective study comparing duplex scanning to contrast venography. Circulation 79:810, 1989.
65. Killewich LA, Nunnelee JD, Auer AI: Value of lower extremity venous duplex examination in the diagnosis of pulmonary embolism. J Vasc Surg 17:934, 1993.
66. Killewich LA, Bedford GR, Beach KW, et al: Spontaneous lysis of deep venous thrombi: Rate and outcome. J Vasc Surg 9:89, 1989.
67. Killewich LA, Martin R, Cramer M, et al: An objective assessment of the physiological changes in the postthrombotic syndrome. Arch Surg 120:424, 1985.
68. Kistner RL, Ball JJ, Nordyke RA, et al: Incidence of pulmonary embolism in the course of thrombophlebitis of the lower extremities. Am J Surg 124:169, 1972.
69. Knudson GJ, Wiedmeyer DA, Erickson SJ, et al: Color flow sonographic imaging in the assessment of upper extremity deep venous thrombosis. AJR Am J Roentgenol 154:399, 1990.
70. Kremkau FW: Doppler Ultrasound: Principles and Instrumentation. Philadelphia, WB Saunders, 1990.
71. Lagerstedt CI, Olsson C, Fagher BO, et al: Need for long-term anticoagulant treatment in symptomatic calf vein thrombosis. Lancet 2:515, 1985.
72. Lensing AWA, Davidson BL, Prins MH, et al: Diagnosis of deep vein thrombosis with ultrasound imaging in symptomatic patients and asymptomatic high-risk patients. *In* Hull R, Raskob G, Pineo G (eds): Venous Thromboembolism: An Evidence-Based Atlas. Armonk, NY: Futura Publishing Co, 1996, p 115.
73. Lensing AW, Prandoni P, Brandjes D, et al: Detection of deep vein thrombosis by real-time B-mode ultrasonography. N Engl J Med 320:342, 1989.
74. Lewis BD, James EM, Welch TJ, et al: Diagnosis of acute deep venous thrombosis of the lower extremities: Prospective evaluation of color Doppler flow imaging versus venography. Radiology 192:651, 1994.
75. Lipski DA, Shepard AD, McCarthy BD, et al: Noninvasive venous testing in the diagnosis of pulmonary embolism: The impact on decision making. J Vasc Surg 26:757, 1997.
76. Lohr JM, Hasselfeld KA, Byrne MP, et al: Does the asymptomatic limb harbor deep venous thrombosis? Am J Surg 168:184, 1994.
77. Lohr JM, Kerr TM, Lutter KS, et al: Lower extremity calf thrombosis: To treat or not to treat? J Vasc Surg 14:618, 1991.
78. Mantoni M: Deep venous thrombosis: Longitudinal study with duplex US. Radiology 179:271, 1991.
79. Markel A, Manzo RA, Bergelin R, et al: Acute deep vein thrombosis: Diagnosis, localization, and risk factors. J Vasc Med Biol 3:432, 1991.
80. Markel A, Manzo R, Bergelin R, et al: Pattern and distribution of thrombi in acute deep venous thrombosis. Arch Surg 127:305, 1992.
81. Markel A, Meissner MH, Manzo RA, et al: A comparison of the cuff deflation method with Valsalva's maneuver and limb compression in detecting venous valvular reflux. Arch Surg 129:701, 1994.
82. Masuda EM, Kistner RM: Prospective comparison of duplex scanning and descending venography in the assessment of venous insufficiency. Am J Surg 164:254, 1992.
83. Masuda EM, Kistner RL, Eklof B: Prospective study of duplex scanning for venous reflux: Comparison of Valsalva and pneumatic cuff techniques in the reverse Trendelenburg and standing positions. J Vasc Surg 20:711, 1994.
84. Matteson B, Langsfeld M, Schermer C, et al: Role of venous duplex scanning in patients with suspected pulmonary embolism. J Vasc Surg 24:768, 1996.
85. Mattos MA, Londrey GL, Leutz DW, et al: Color-flow duplex scanning for the surveillance and diagnosis of acute deep venous thrombosis. J Vasc Surg 15:366, 1992.
86. Mattos MA, Melendres G, Sumner DS, et al: Prevalence and distribution of calf vein thrombosis in patients with symptomatic deep venous thrombosis: A color flow duplex study. J Vasc Surg 24:738, 1996.
87. McLafferty RB, Moneta GL, Passman MA, et al: Late clinical and hemodynamic sequelae of isolated calf vein thrombosis. J Vasc Surg 27:50, 1998.
88. Meissner MH, Caps MT, Bergelin RO, et al: Early outcome after isolated calf vein thrombosis. J Vasc Surg 26:749, 1997.
89. Meissner MH, Caps MT, Bergelin RO, et al: Propagation, rethrombosis, and new thrombus formation after acute deep venous thrombosis. J Vasc Surg 22:558, 1995.
90. Meissner MH, Manzo RA, Bergelin RO, et al: Deep venous insufficiency: The relationship between lysis and subsequent reflux. J Vasc Surg 18:596, 1993.
91. Menzoian JO, Sequeira JC, Doyle JE, et al: Therapeutic and clinical course of deep venous thrombosis. Am J Surg 146:581, 1983.
92. Messina LM, Sarpa MS, Smith MA, et al: Clinical significance of routine imaging of iliac and calf veins by color flow duplex scanning in patients suspected of having acute lower extremity deep venous thrombosis. Surgery 114:921, 1993.
93. Miller SS, Foote AV: The ultrasonic detection of incompetent perforating veins. Br J Surg 61:653, 1974.
94. Mitchell DC, Grasty MS, Stebbings WS, et al: Comparison of duplex ultrasonography and venography in the diagnosis of deep venous thrombosis. Br J Surg 78:611, 1991.
95. Monreal M, Ruiz J, Salvador R, et al: Recurrent pulmonary embolism: A prospective study. Chest 95:976, 1989.
96. Moreno-Cabral R, Kistner RL, Nordyke RA: Importance of calf vein thrombophlebitis. Surgery 80:735, 1976.
97. Murphy TP, Cronan JJ: Evolution of deep venous thrombosis: A prospective evaluation with US. Radiology 177:543, 1990.
98. Naidich JB, Feinberg AW, Karp-Harman H, et al: Contrast venography: Reassessment of its role. Radiology 168:97, 1988.
99. Naidich JB, Torre JR, Pellerito JS, et al: Suspected deep venous thrombosis: Is US of both legs necessary? Radiology 200:429, 1996.
100. Neglen P, Raju S: A comparison between descending phlebography and duplex Doppler investigation in the evaluation of reflux in chronic venous insufficiency: A challenge to phlebography as the "gold standard." J Vasc Surg 16:687, 1992.
101. Neglen P, Raju S: A rational approach to detection of significant reflux with duplex Doppler scanning and air plethysmography. J Vasc Surg 17:590, 1993.
102. Nicolaides AN, Christopoulos D: Quantification of venous reflux and outflow with air plethysmography. *In* Bernstein EF (ed): Vascular Diagnosis, 4th ed. St. Louis, Mosby–Year Book, 1993, p 915.
103. Nicolaides AN, Hussein MK, Szendro G, et al: The relationship of venous ulceration with ambulatory venous pressure measurements. J Vasc Surg 17:414, 1993.
104. Nix ML, Troilett RD, Nelson CL, et al: Is bilateral duplex examination necessary for unilateral symptoms of deep venous thrombosis? J Vasc Technol 15:296, 1991.
105. Norris CS, Greenfield LJ, Herrmann JB: Free-floating ileofemoral thrombus: A risk of pulmonary embolism. Arch Surg 120:806, 1985.
106. Nypaver TJ, Shepard AD, Kiell CS, et al: Outpatient duplex scanning for deep vein thrombosis: Parameters predictive of a negative study result. J Vasc Surg 18:821, 1993.
107. O'Leary DH, Kane RA, Chase BM: A prospective study of the efficacy of B-scan sonography in the detection of deep venous thrombosis in the lower extremities. J Clin Ultrasound 16:1, 1988.

108. Ohgi S, Ito K, Tanaka K, et al: Echogenic types of venous thrombi in the common femoral vein by ultrasonic B-mode imaging. Vasc Surg 25:253, 1991.
109. Oudkerk M, van Beek EJR, van Putten WLJ, et al: Cost-effectiveness analysis of various strategies in the diagnostic management of pulmonary embolism. Arch Intern Med 153:947, 1993.
110. Pacouret G, Alison D, Pottier J-M, et al: Free-floating thrombus and embolic risk in patients with angiographically confirmed proximal deep venous thrombosis. Arch Intern Med 157:305, 1997.
111. Passman MA, Moneta GL, Taylor LM, et al: Pulmonary embolism is associated with the combination of isolated calf vein thrombosis and respiratory symptoms. J Vasc Surg 25:39, 1997.
112. Payne SP, London NJ, Newland CJ, et al: Ambulatory venous pressure: Correlation with skin condition and role in identifying surgically correctable disease. Eur J Endovasc Surg 11:195, 1996.
113. Pezullo JA, Perkins AB, Cronan JJ: Symptomatic deep vein thrombosis: Diagnosis with limited compression US. Radiology 198:67, 1996.
114. Pierik EG, Toonder IM, van Urk H, et al: Validation of duplex ultrasonography in detecting competent and incompetent perforating veins in patients with venous ulceration of the lower leg. J Vasc Surg 26:49, 1997.
115. Poppiti R, Papanicolaou G, Perese S: Limited B-mode venous imaging versus complete color flow duplex venous scanning for detection of proximal deep venous thrombosis. J Vasc Surg 22:553, 1995.
116. Porter J, Moneta G: Reporting standards in venous disease: An update. International Consensus Committee on Chronic Venous Disease. J Vasc Surg 21:635, 1995.
117. Prandoni P, Cogo A, Bernardi E, et al: A simple ultrasound approach for detection of recurrent proximal vein thrombosis. Circulation 88 (4 part 1):1730, 1993.
118. Prandoni P, Polistena P, Bernardi E, et al: Upper extremity deep vein thrombosis: Risk factors, diagnosis, and complications. Arch Intern Med 157:57, 1997.
119. Prandoni P, Villalta S, Polistena P, et al: Symptomatic deep vein thrombosis and the post-thrombotic syndrome. Haematologica 80(2 Suppl):42, 1995.
120. Raju S, Fredericks R: Evaluation of methods for detecting venous reflux: Perspectives in venous insufficiency. Arch Surg 125:1463, 1990.
121. Raskob G: Calf vein thrombosis. *In* Hull R, Raskob G, Pineo G (eds): Venous Thromboembolism: An Evidence-Based Atlas. Armonk, NY, Futura Publishing Co, 1996, p 307.
122. Rodriguez AA, Whitehead CM, McLaughlin RL, et al: Duplex-derived valve closure times fail to correlate with reflux flow volumes in patients with chronic venous insufficiency. J Vasc Surg 23:606, 1996.
123. Rose SC, Zwiebel WJ, Nelson BD, et al: Symptomatic lower extremity deep venous thrombosis: Accuracy, limitations, and role of color duplex flow imaging in diagnosis. Radiology 175:639, 1990.
124. Rosfors S, Bygdeman S, Nordstrom E: Assessment of deep venous incompetence: A prospective study comparing duplex scanning with descending phlebography. Angiology 41:463, 1990.
125. Ruckley CV: Does venous reflux matter. Lancet 341:411, 1993.
126. Sarin S, Scurr JH, Coleridge Smith PD: Medial calf perforators in venous diseases: The significance of outward flow. J Vasc Surg 16:40, 1992.
127. Sarpa MS, Messina LM, Smith M, et al: Reliability of venous duplex scanning to image the iliac veins and to diagnose iliac vein thrombosis in patients suspected of having acute deep venous thrombosis. J Vasc Technol 15:299, 1991.
128. Sauerbrei E, Thomson JG, McLachlan MS, et al: Observer variation in lower limb venography. J Can Assoc Radiol 32:28, 1981.
129. Schiff MJ, Feinberg AW, Naidich JB: Noninvasive venous examinations as a screening test for pulmonary embolism. Arch Intern Med 147:505, 1987.
130. Sheiman RG, McArdle CR: Bilateral lower extremity US in the patient with unilateral symptoms of deep venous thrombosis: Assessment of need. Radiology 194:171, 1995.
131. Sluzewski M, Koopman MMW, Schuur KH, et al: Influence of negative ultrasound findings on the management of inpatients and outpatients with suspected deep vein thrombosis. Eur J Radiol 13:174, 1991.
132. Strandness DE, Sumner DS: Ultrasonic velocity detector in the diagnosis of thrombophlebitis. Arch Surg 104:180, 1972.
133. Strothman G, Blebea J, Fowl RJ: Contralateral duplex scanning for deep venous thrombosis is unnecessary in patients with symptoms. J Vasc Surg 22:543, 1995.
134. Sumner DS, Mattos MA: Diagnosis of deep vein thrombosis with real-time color and duplex scanning. *In*: Bernstein EF (ed): Vascular Diagnosis, 4th ed. St. Louis, Mosby–Year Book, 1993, p 785.
135. Szendro G, Nicolaides AN, Zukowski AJ, et al: Duplex scanning in the assessment of deep venous incompetence. J Vasc Surg 4:237, 1986.
136. Talbot SR: Use of real-time imaging in identifying deep venous obstruction: A preliminary report. Bruit 6:41, 1982.
137. Talbot SR: B-mode evaluation of peripheral veins. Semin Ultrasound CT MR 9:295, 1988.
138. Vaccaro JP, Cronan JJ, Dorfman GS: Outcome analysis of patients with normal compression US exams. Radiology 175:645, 1990.
139. van Bemmelen PS, Bedford G, Strandness DE: Visualization of calf veins by color flow imaging. Ultrasound Med Biol 16:15, 1990.
140. van Bemmelen PS, Beach K, Bedford G, et al: The mechanism of venous valve closure—its relationship to the velocity of reverse flow. Arch Surg 125:617, 1990.
141. van Bemmelen PS, Bedford G, Beach K, et al: Quantitative segmental evaluation of venous valvular reflux with duplex ultrasound scanning. J Vasc Surg 10:425, 1989.
142. van Bemmelen PS, van Ramshorst B, Eikelboom BC: Photoplethysmography reexamined: Lack of correlation with duplex scanning. Surgery 112:544, 1992.
143. van Ramshorst B, van Bemmelen PS, Honeveld H, et al: Thrombus regression in deep venous thrombosis: Quantification of spontaneous thrombolysis with duplex scanning. Circulation 86:414, 1992.
144. Vasdekis SN, Clarke GH, Nicolaides AN: Quantification of venous reflux by means of duplex scanning. J Vasc Surg 10:670, 1989.
145. Voet D, Afschrift M: Floating thrombi: Diagnosis and follow-up by duplex ultrasound. Br J Radiol 64:1010, 1991.
146. Vogel P, Laing FC, Jeffrey RB, et al: Deep venous thrombosis of the lower extremity: US evaluation. Radiology 163:747, 1987.
147. Weingarten MS, Czeredarczuk M, Scovell S, et al: A correlation of air plethysmography and color flow–assisted duplex scanning in the quantification of chronic venous insufficiency. J Vasc Surg 24:750, 1996.
148. Weissleder R, Elizondo G, Stark DD: Sonographic diagnosis of subclavian and internal jugular vein thrombosis. J Ultrasound Med 6:577, 1987.
149. Welch HJ, Faliakou EC, McLaughlin RL, et al: Comparison of descending phlebography with quantitative photoplethysmography, air plethysmography, and duplex quantitative valve closure time in assessing deep venous reflux. J Vasc Surgery 16:913, 1992.
150. Welkie JF, Comerota AJ, Katz ML, et al: Hemodynamic deterioration in chronic venous disease. J Vasc Surg 16:733, 1992.
151. Wells PS, Hirsh J, Anderson DR, et al: Accuracy of clinical assessment of deep vein thrombosis. Lancet 345:1326, 1995.
152. Wells PS, Lensing AW, Davidson BL, et al: Accuracy of ultrasound for the diagnosis of deep venous thrombosis in asymptomatic patients after orthopedic surgery: A meta-analysis. Ann Intern Med 122:47, 1995.
153. Wester JP, Holtkamp M, Linnebank ER, et al: Noninvasive detection of deep venous thrombosis: Ultrasonography versus duplex scanning. Eur J Vasc Surg 8:357, 1994.
154. Wheeler HB, Hirsh J, Wells P, et al: Diagnostic tests for deep venous thrombosis: Clinical usefulness depends on probability of disease. Arch Intern Med 154:1921, 1994.
155. White RH, McGahan JP, Daschbach MM, et al: Diagnosis of deep vein thrombosis using duplex ultrasound. Ann Intern Med 111:297, 1989.
156. Yucel EK, Fisher JS, Eggin TK, et al: Isolated calf venous thrombosis: Diagnosis with compression US. Radiology 179:443, 1991.
157. Zwiebel WJ: Color-encoded blood flow imaging. Semin Ultrasound CT MR 9:320, 1988.

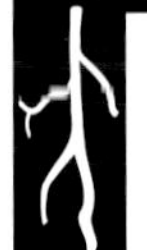

CHAPTER 14

Computed Tomography and Three-Dimensional Reconstruction in Evaluation of Vascular Disease

Mark F. Fillinger, M.D.

Preoperative imaging for vascular surgery is steadily becoming less invasive. For example, many surgeons are now comfortable performing carotid endarterectomy based on duplex ultrasound examination alone, with selective use of angiography.[1] Similarly, it was once thought that preoperative angiography was necessary for repair of abdominal aortic aneurysms (AAAs),[2] but technologic advances have lead many surgeons to perform AAA repair on the basis of computed tomography (CT) alone.[3, 4]

As with many technologic advances, the process of image creation continues to become more difficult for the average end-user to understand. A knowledge of the basic principles behind CT imaging remains important, however, so that the limitations, artefacts, and opportunities for image optimization will not be overlooked. A better grasp of the image creation process and terminology should also aid collaboration between those creating the images and those who use the images to plan surgical intervention.

BASIC CONCEPTS AND TECHNOLOGY

Conventional Computed Tomography

Computed tomography is aptly named; that is, a structure is mapped and displayed as graphical "slices" with the assistance of computer technology. Work in the 1960s by Godfried Hounsfield eventually led to production of the first clinical CT scanner, produced by Elector-Musical Instruments, Ltd, and installed in Atkinson Morleys Hospital, Wimbledon, England, in 1971.[5] Many of the principles used in this *first-generation* CT scanner still apply today and provide a framework for understanding the technology.

As with most imaging modalities, the fundamental unit for this CT scanner consists of an *emitter* and a *detector*; an x-ray beam is transmitted through the tissue and is detected on the other side. The emitter produces a very thin (highly collimated) x-ray beam that sweeps in linear fashion across the body cross section (Fig. 14–1). The detector moves simultaneously with the emitter as a unit, recording data from 160 separate, parallel, and immediately adjacent beams. The emitter and detector units are mounted within a *gantry*, which is rotated 1 degree before another linear, transverse sweep takes place. This process is repeated through 180 degrees of rotation, producing the data necessary to form a 160 × 160 *matrix* for a single cross-sectional image.

The information collected by the detector is the *attenuation* of the x-ray beam. Attenuation is the rate of reduction of x-ray energy recorded at the detector. Attenuation increases with increased thickness, density, or atomic number of the material the beam passes through, and attenuation decreases with increased peak kilovoltage (kVp) of the x-ray beam. The x-ray energy interacts with tissue to produce attenuation by means of atomic ionization events via the photoelectric and Compton effects. Although the importance of these effects is beyond the scope of this text, the energy levels used in CT imaging indicate that soft tissue interactions involve primarily the Compton effect. Images are therefore mostly a result of the physical density and electron density of the tissue being imaged and the energy of the x-ray beam.

The *CT number* was defined to simplify quantification of the linear attenuation coefficient (μ) produced by a tissue at a given x-ray beam energy by normalizing it against the attenuation coefficient of water. The CT number is therefore defined as $K(\mu - \mu_{H2O})/\mu_{H2O}$, where K is a constant, μ is the attenuation coefficient of the tissue, and μ_{H2O} is the attenuation coefficient of water. When a scaling constant (K) of 1000 is used, the CT number is said to be expressed in *Hounsfield units* (H).

Clinically, CT numbers range from the extremes of air (−1000 H) to dense bone (1000 H), but fat (−20 to −100 H), water (0 H), and muscle/blood (40 to 60 H) tend to lie in a much narrower range.[6] Differences in such factors as the energy level of the beam and tissue thickness prevent the density in Hounsfield units from being absolutely uniform from one CT scan to another, but the ranges are similar.

Once the range of CT numbers for a scan is determined, the range can be broken up into smaller ranges for graphical display by a set of gray scale values. For example, in the chest, CT numbers approaching 1000 H (bone) are typically assigned values close to pure white and CT numbers approaching −1000 H (air) are typically assigned values close to pure black. CT numbers between −1000 H to +1000 H would then be displayed as graduated shades of gray.

This concept appears simple until one realizes that the x-ray emitter/detector combination is similar in operation to conventional x-ray film. The detector measures the attenuation of x-rays through the *entire path traversed by the*

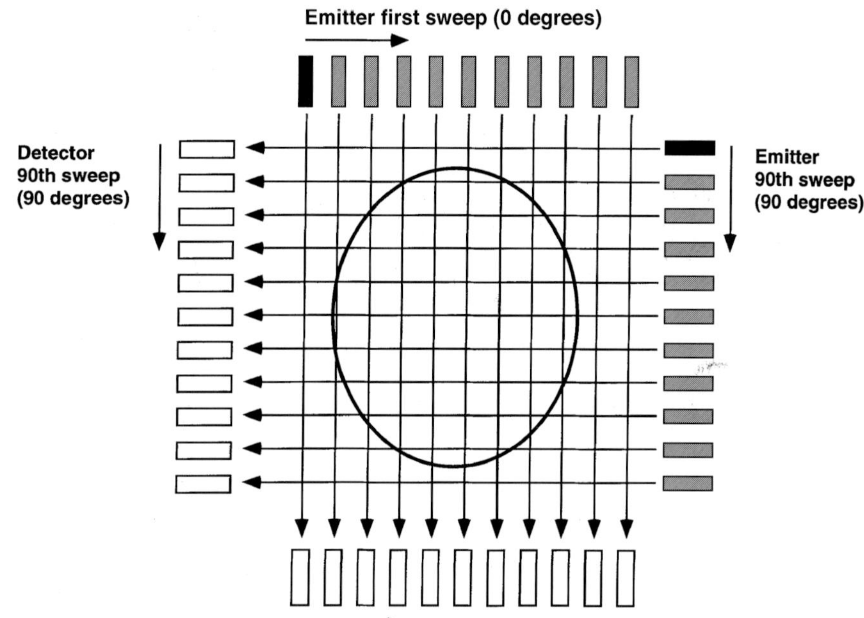

FIGURE 14–1. Principle of operation for a first-generation CT scanner.

beam. This being the case, how can the attenuation coefficient for each small area on the matrix be calculated and displayed separately for each of the 160 × 160 = 25,600 data points in the matrix? This problem is solved by a computer. Digital data are collected from the attenuation of multiple x-ray beams traversing the same point in the matrix from different angles. An ingenious method is then used to calculate *backward* to the density, which must be present at each location in the matrix. A combination of hardware, mathematical algorithms, and computer software results in the cross-sectional images of CT scans. This method was such a leap forward in imaging technology that Hounsfield and Cormack shared the Nobel Prize in 1980.

Thus, a first-generation CT scanner is capable of producing a cross-sectional image with a 160 × 160 matrix. Each data point in the matrix is mapped to a gray scale for display and is known as a *pixel* because it represents a "picture element." When displayed as a whole, this matrix of gray squares becomes an interpretable image, just as different densities of black and white dots are used to create photographs in a newspaper. In this manner, the first-generation CT scanner was able to create a cross-sectional image of the human body—an impressive accomplishment. Unfortunately, this process required approximately 5 minutes to create a single cross section. Early CT scans were thus applicable only to parts of the body with limited motion (e.g., the head) because the back-calculation algorithm depends on the subject's remaining in one position while data are collected for the entire cross section.

To obtain useful scans in areas such as the chest and abdomen, engineers designed subsequent generations of CT scanners that would decrease the time required to obtain a complete cross-sectional image. The *second-generation* CT scanner used an emitter that produced a broader, fan-shaped x-ray beam and an array of 30 detectors instead of a single detector. This greatly reduced the number of emitter locations required to complete a single transverse sweep and also reduced the number of transverse sweeps (1-degree increments were no longer required for a complete cross-sectional image). The time for a single cross-sectional scan was thus reduced to approximately 15 seconds.

Present-day CT uses *third-generation* and *fourth-generation* scanners. With a third-generation scanner, the emitter produces a wider, fan-shaped x-ray beam. Hundreds of detectors are arranged in an arc (Fig. 14–2). Because the beam/detector combinations cover the entire patient, no transverse sweep is required; both emitter and detector array rotate in a continuous 180- or 360-degree arc to produce a complete cross-sectional scan in 1 second. With the fourth-generation CT scanner, the detector array covers the entire 360-degree arc and only the emitter rotates. Today, scan times are similar for third-generation and fourth-generation scanners, and there is no clear clinical advantage for either type.[7]

Advances in hardware and computer software technology have also greatly improved the graphical image display despite the reduced scan times. A first-generation CT scanner produced a cross-sectional image with a 160 × 160 matrix, but current scanners typically generate a 512 × 512 or 1024 × 1024 matrix. Each data point in the matrix is mapped to a gray scale for display, so that the size of the matrix and the *field of view* directly affect the resolution of the *display* (the smallest distinguishable element). Data points are *displayed* as a two-dimensional (2-D) picture, and each point in the display matrix is a pixel (picture element). Data points are *acquired* in three dimensions, however, and each data point in the matrix actually represents a *voxel* (volume element) whose thickness is equal to that of the x-ray beam (Fig. 14–3).

One advantage of CT over magnetic resonance imaging (MRI) is that CT data are typically displayed in a 512 × 512 matrix or greater, with resolutions of 0.2 to 1.0 mm^2 for each pixel. MRI data display is generally limited to a

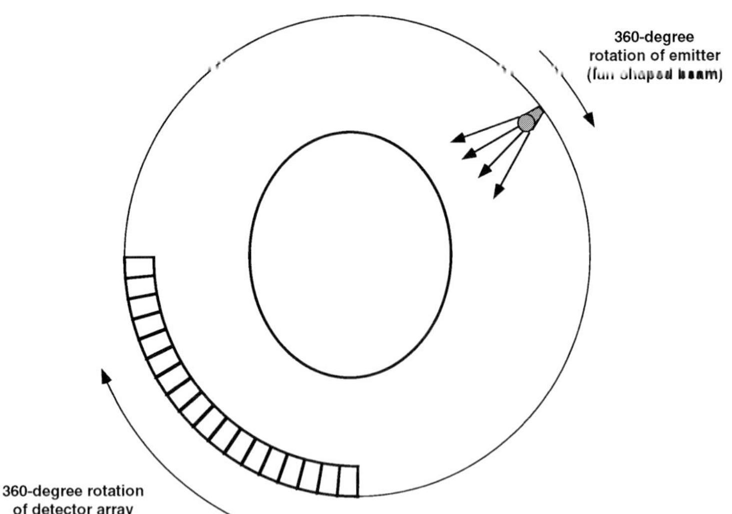

FIGURE 14–2. Principle of operation for a third-generation CT scanner.

256 × 256 matrix, and resolution in the axial plane is roughly half that of CT. The pixel for a CT display, however, represents a voxel that may be 1 to 10 mm thick, and MRI typically has better resolution along the longitudinal axis.

Spiral CT

The most recent advance to achieve widespread clinical application is spiral or helical CT technology. Although the scan time needed to produce a single cross-sectional image is greatly reduced in third-generation and fourth-generation CT scanners, the rotating elements on the gantry (the detector array and/or the emitter) are still limiting if they are attached to power cables. Power cables attached to the rotating elements force the unit to perform a cross-sectional scan in one direction, stop, and then scan in the reverse direction for the next cross section (in order to unwind the cables). This increases the time needed to scan the volume of interest and makes *motion artefact* more likely. The development of the *slip-ring gantry* eliminated cables by allowing the rotating elements to receive power via sliding rings that make electrical contact with stationary brushes. Thus, the emitter and detector array can rotate continuously in the same direction. More important, the computer can acquire data continuously because there is no need to stop and reverse direction. With conventional CT, there would still be a pause in data acquisition while the table (patient) moves to a new position for the next cross section to be scanned. However, if the table moves in a continuous linear motion through the gantry while the x-ray emitter and detector rotate continuously over 360 degrees, data can be acquired in a single sweep over the entire volume of interest. With this technique, the emitter traces out a spiral relative to the patient (i.e., a *spiral CT* or *helical CT* scan) (Fig. 14–4).

Spiral or helical CT technology has several important ramifications beyond a simple decrease in scan time. A spiral CT scan collects data over a continuous *volume* rather than for discontinuous *slices* (Fig. 14–5). The most obvious advantage of acquiring data over a continuous volume is that thin axial slices can be reconstructed from the digital dataset at arbitrarily small intervals *without additional radiation exposure*. Conventional CT can produce similar overlapping or adjacent axial slices, but the tradeoff is increased scan time and additional radiation exposure. Cross-sectional images are therefore typically produced at 10-mm intervals in conventional CT but at 3- to 5-mm intervals with spiral CT. In spiral CT terminology, this is typically

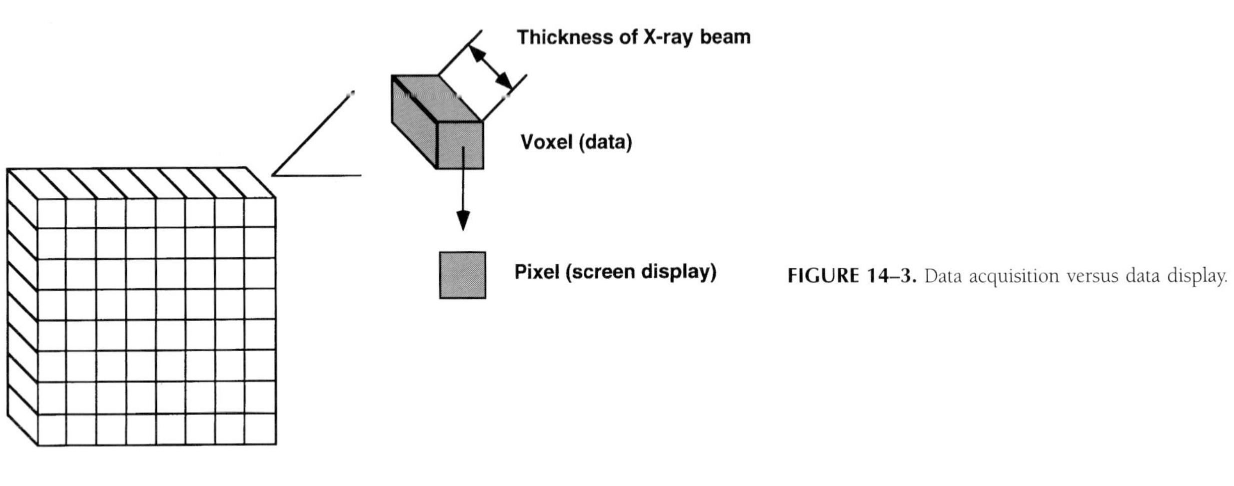

FIGURE 14–3. Data acquisition versus data display.

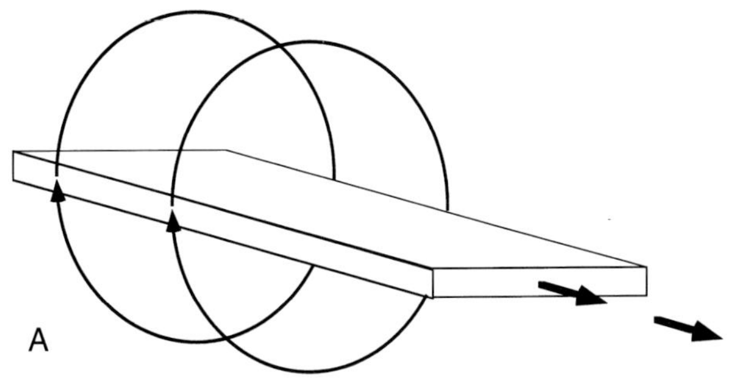

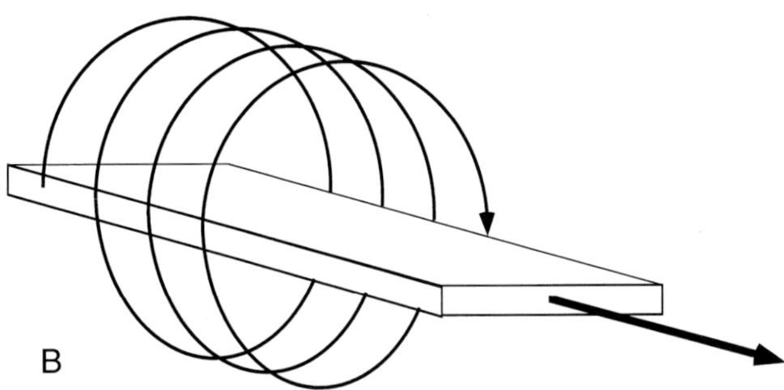

FIGURE 14–4. Conventional *(A)* versus spiral *(B)* CT scan gantry motion.

referred to as the "reconstruction interval." When the attempt is made to ascertain fine detail, such as a potential renal artery stenosis, a reconstruction interval as small as 1 mm might be used.

Multiplanar Reformats and Computed Tomography Angiography

Another advantage of data acquisition over an entire volume is the ability to reconstruct, or *reformat*, the data in arbitrary planes. Reformatting CT data into coronal, sagittal, or other nonaxial planes is often referred to as *multiplanar reformatting* or *multiplanar reconstruction* (MPR). A schematic representation of this process is shown in Figure 14–6. Although this process is theoretically possible with conventional CT, it is not practical because of considerations of scan time, motion artefact, and radiation exposure. In many cases, a spiral CT scan covers the volume of interest during a single breath-hold. Because structures in the volume of interest have not moved during the scan, MPRs produce useful images with minimal motion artefact (Fig. 14–7).

The ability of spiral CT to view the data in coronal, sagittal, or arbitrarily defined planes often yields more insight into vascular anatomy than is possible with axial views alone. For example, evaluation of potential renal artery occlusive disease is best performed in axial and coronal sections, whereas the celiac and superior mesenteric arteries are best seen in axial and sagittal planes. Reformats along curved planes may also be useful for evaluation of tortuous iliac arteries or aortic branch vessels but should be interpreted with caution because such images are in an arbitrary and unnatural "warped" plane (Fig. 14–7*C* and *D*). Spiral CT reveals far more anatomic detail than conventional CT by combining rapid CT data acquisition during a single breath-hold, a focus on vascular structures during a single intravenous contrast bolus, small reconstruction intervals, and multiplanar reformatting. The resulting images sometimes resemble those seen with angiography, and the process is often referred to as *CT angiography* (CTA). This modality has greatly enhanced the ability of CT to evaluate vascular occlusive disease of aortic branches and iliac arteries (see Clinical Applications).[8, 9]

Three-Dimensional Reconstruction

The combination of rapid scanning over the volume of interest, new software algorithms, and advances in computer technology have made it possible to create striking three-dimensional (3-D) reconstructions from spiral CT data. If CT creates images by a process analogous to slicing a loaf of bread, 3-D reconstruction is like putting the slices in the loaf of bread back together. In this case, however, the reconstruction can be limited to individual structures that meet certain parameters, such as density and location within the scan volume. If bony structures are of primary interest, the computer algorithm can reconstruct only those elements of the CT (voxels) that are of bone density (i.e., CT numbers or attenuation coefficients of bone). For vascular structures, CTA produces contrast density within the vessel lumen at the appropriate time, so that 3-D recon-

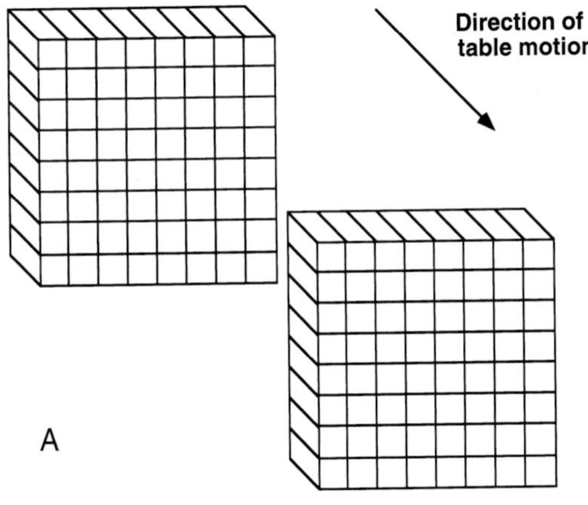

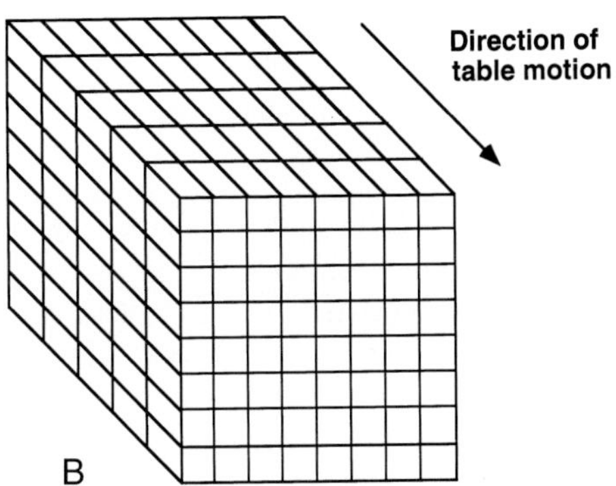

FIGURE 14–5. Discontinuous *(A)* versus continuous *(B)* data for conventional and spiral CT.

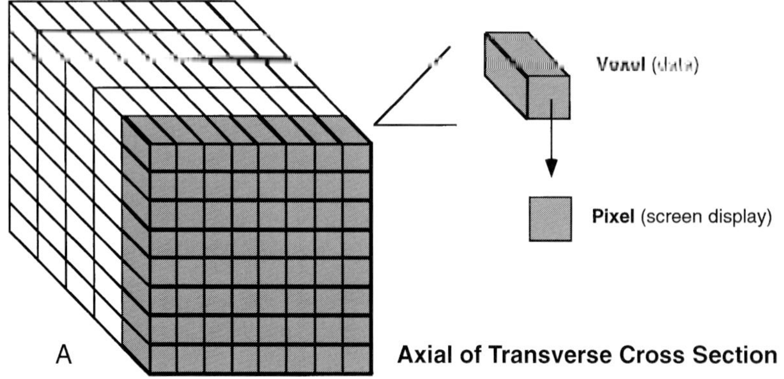

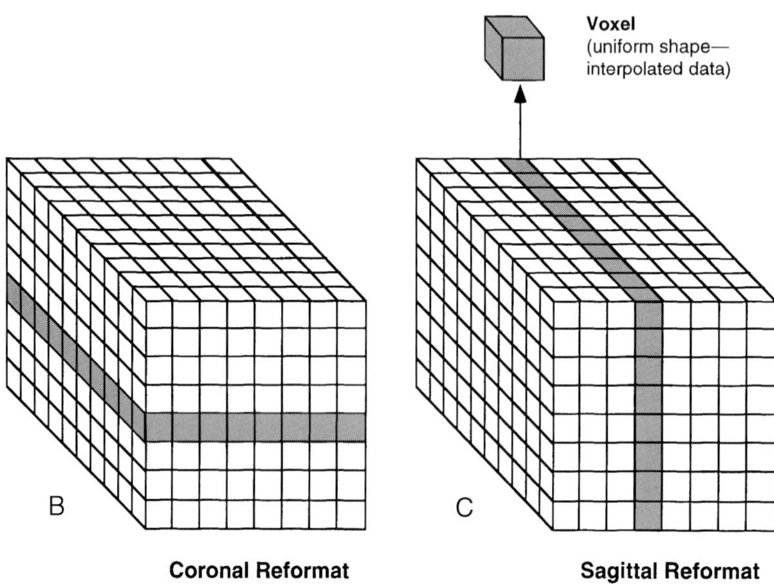

FIGURE 14–6. Because spiral CT data are acquired and stored over a continuous volume, they can be used to create axial *(A)* coronal *(B)*, and sagittal *(C)* sections. For display purposes, the non-uniform voxel is interpolated into a cube, but the quality of the data still depends on the length of the original voxel, which is determined by the collimation. Reformatting CT data into coronal, sagittal, or other nonaxial planes is often referred to as multiplanar reformatting.

struction of the vessel lumen can be performed. When this type of 3-D reconstruction (or 3-D model) is created, the density (CT numbers) of vascular contrast and bone may overlap.

Therefore, bony structures are either included in the model or "cut away" using a tool sometimes referred to as an "electronic scalpel." Calcium within the vessel wall cannot be easily cut away, however; it is usually included in a reconstruction of the contrast-enhanced vessel lumen. This produces the typical computer-generated 3-D reconstruction, which is most often displayed as a *surface-shaded display* (SSD). In a surface-shaded display, the exterior of the structure is opaque and shaded to provide an appreciation of depth (Fig. 14–8). The 3-D reconstruction can greatly aid the interpretation of difficult anatomy. Although such reconstructions lack the detail of the CT images, morphologic features within the 3-D image are easily recognizable in far less time than it takes to review the CT data. This depiction of 3-D relationships is probably most helpful in surgical planning for complicated open procedures or endovascular procedures.[4, 10–12]

One problem with SSD of 3-D models is that the bulk of structures, such as calcified plaque, cannot be fully appreciated because all CT numbers (physical densities) included in the model are given the same opaque color in the display. One method that better displays different physical densities is called *maximum intensity projection* (MIP). MIP images display the 2-D projection that would result if one could see only the densest structures (structures that project the maximum intensity). Although a MIP image is created from the 3-D volume data, it is a projection—similar to an angiogram—and must be defined from a particular point of view (Fig. 14–9). MIP images are relatively familiar to surgeons and interventional radiologists, and although they display calcified plaque well, adequate evaluation of the structure requires a large number of views; even then, a heavily calcified vessel may obscure important details regarding the vessel lumen and the degree of stenosis.

Another method to improve the display of structures with different physical densities involves SSD of multiple objects simultaneously. This process is based on (1) determining which densities are relevant to interpretation of the image and (2) coding, or *segmentation*, of those CT densities as separate objects. This allows separate 3-D reconstructions and/or color-coded display of the pertinent CT densities.

In vascular surgery, the most clinically relevant structures

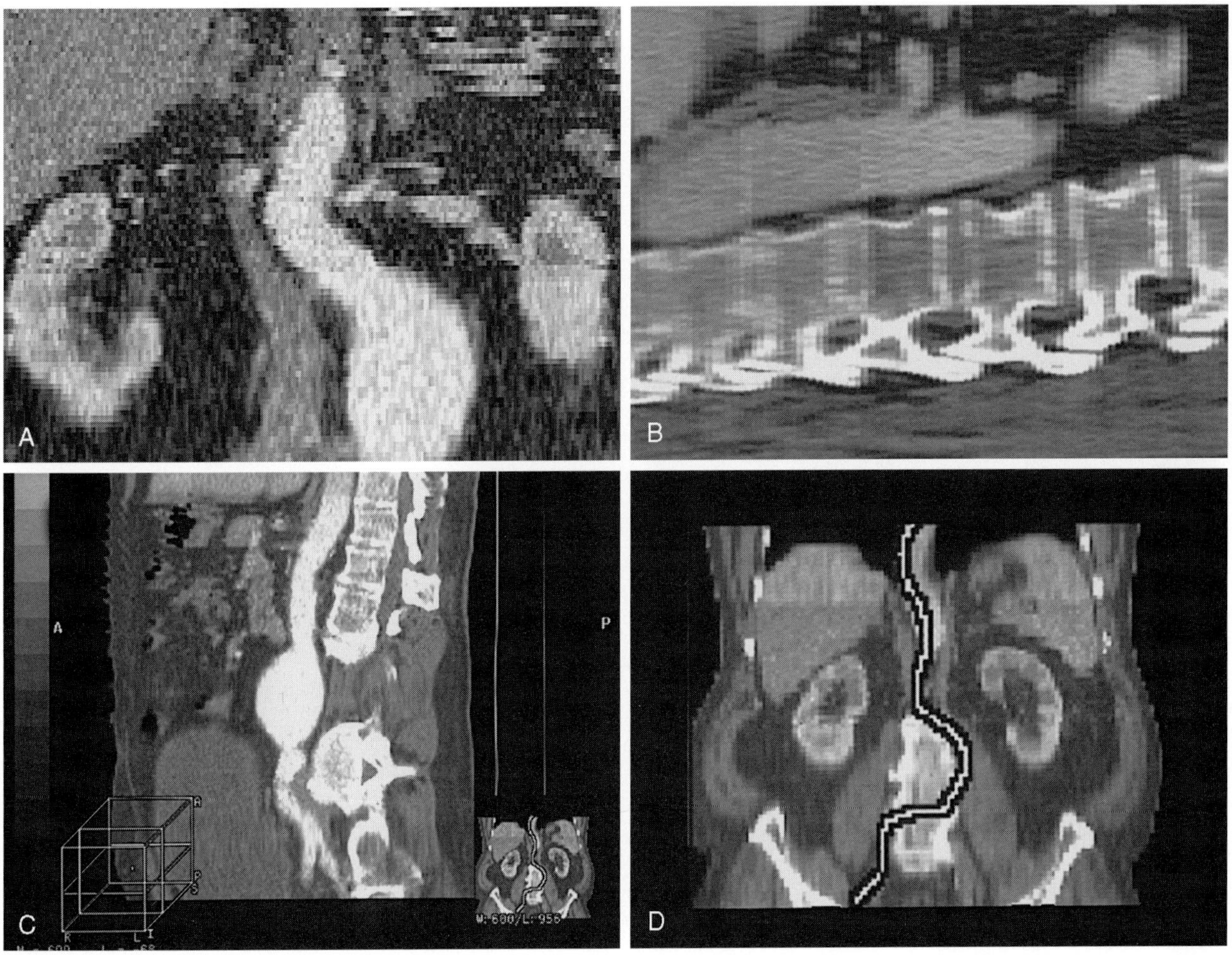

FIGURE 14–7. Clinical examples of multiplanar reformatting.

A, Coronal reformat displaying the aorta of a patient with an infrarenal aneurysm. The more proximal aorta is not seen because it is out of the plane of this CT slice. The renal arteries are seen, but it is unclear whether they are stenotic or whether the origin of both renal arteries would be seen in a different section (thus the need to view multiple coronal and axial CT slices). The left renal artery origin is actually stenotic, but the right is not.

B, Sagittal reformat of the abdominal aorta, demonstrating the celiac artery. The superior mesenteric artery is seen in a different sagittal section.

C, Curvilinear reformat. For a long segment of the aorta and the right iliac artery to be seen together on one CT slice, the data are reformatted along a warped plane corresponding to the lumen. A cursor is used to plot a line through the tortuous lumen of the aorta seen in *A*, and the data are reformatted along this highly curved plane *(inset)*.

D, Magnified view of the inset from panel C, demonstrating how tortuous the reformatted CT plane would appear if seen "end on" from a coronal section. The curvilinear reformat can produce a helpful display, but it must be interpreted with caution because tortuous structures appear to be relatively straight and surrounding structures are distorted. Note the lumbar spine moving in and out of the reformatted plane.

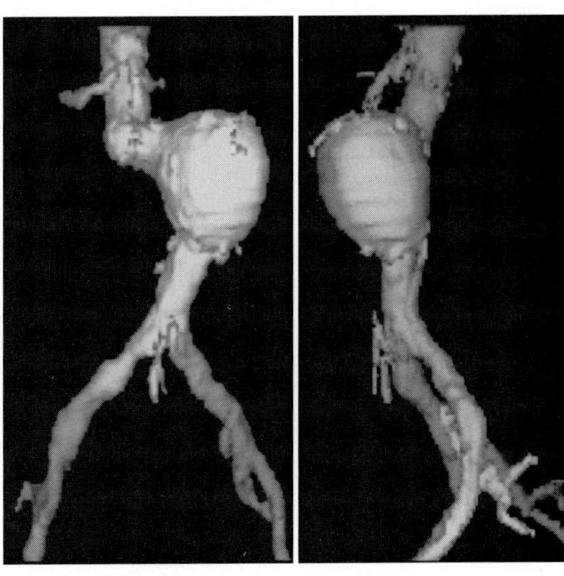

FIGURE 14–8. Computer-generated surface-shaded display (SSD) of CT data. The three-dimensional (3-D) relationships of the aneurysm and surrounding structures are immediately apparent in these anteroposterior *(left)* and left lateral *(right)* views. In this typical single-object 3-D SSD, the threshold for reconstruction is the density of contrast-enhanced blood. Because calcified plaque is denser than contrast-enhanced blood, it is included in the reconstruction. The spine was removed electronically before the 3-D reconstruction was made. An infinite number of views are possible on the computer screen used to create the views, but a limited number of views are printed as hard copy to demonstrate the anatomy.

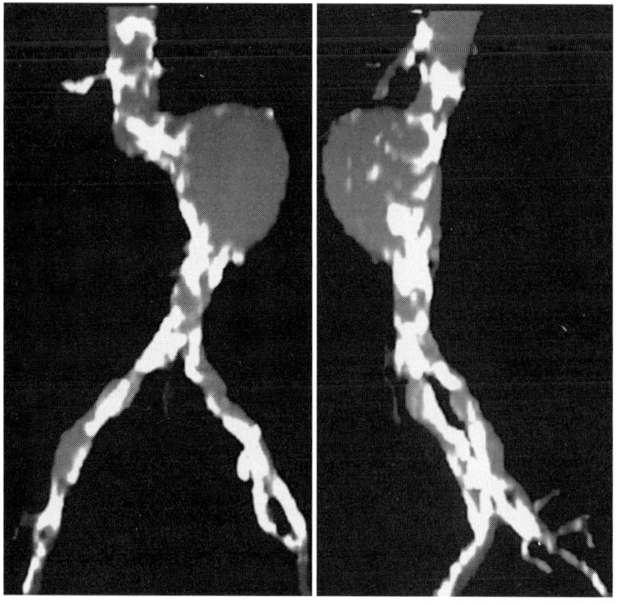

FIGURE 14–9. Maximum intensity projection (MIP) images of the same abdominal aortic aneurysm shown in Figure 14–8, anteroposterior *(left)* and left lateral *(right)* views. Because this reconstruction represents a two-dimensional projection of the structure along a line defined in three-dimensional space, the MIP image appears similar to an arteriogram. Only the structure with maximum intensity is projected, so that calcified plaque is displayed prominently. MIP images display calcified plaque well, but this same feature can obscure the residual lumen in locations where the vessel is heavily calcified (the iliac arteries in particular).

are the contrast-enhanced vessel lumen, calcified plaque, noncalcified plaque, and thrombus. Noncalcified atherosclerotic plaque and thrombus have essentially identical CT numbers and cannot be distinguished as separate objects. However, the last two structures are distinct from contrast-enhanced blood flow, and blood flow can be distinguished from calcified plaque to a reasonable degree. With proper CT protocols and software algorithms, these structures can be displayed separately on the basis of density.

Because there is some density overlap and since the edge-detection abilities of the human eye are far superior to computer algorithms at present, the "segmentation" process used to create a multiple-object SSD is usually semi-automated (i.e., some human intervention and review are required in order for ensuring accurate segmentation on the computer). Although the multiple-object segmentation process is more time-consuming, the resulting 3-D reconstructions display information not available with any other imaging modality (Fig. 14–10) (see Color Plate). Because the separate elements can be viewed in combination or separately, this type of reconstruction has the advantages of single-object SSD and MIPs without most of their disadvantages. This 3-D method can best display the extent of an aneurysm (because thrombus is visible), degree of calcification, and lumen narrowing due to plaque, especially if structures of differing density can be made invisible or transparent (Fig. 14–11) (see Color Plate). Plaque can be made invisible electronically to simulate an angiogram or may be included for planning of a surgical procedure. As with any 3-D reconstruction, however, the 3-D model must

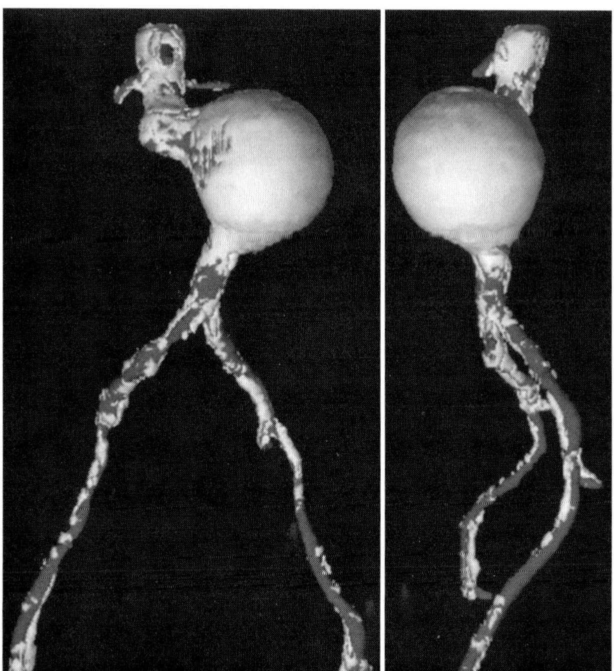

FIGURE 14–10. Multiple-object surface-shaded display (SSD), anteroposterior *(left)* and left lateral *(right)* views of the same abdominal aortic aneurysm seen in Figures 14–8 and 14–9. Contrast-enhanced blood flow is displayed in red, thrombus and noncalcified plaque are displayed in yellow, and calcified plaque is white. In this type of three-dimensional reconstruction, all of the components of the aneurysm are seen. Multiple views are helpful, and it is preferable if the display can be rotated and viewed at will on a computer screen. This type of display is most helpful in determining the true extent of an aneurysm, since thrombus is clearly visible. (See Color Plate.)

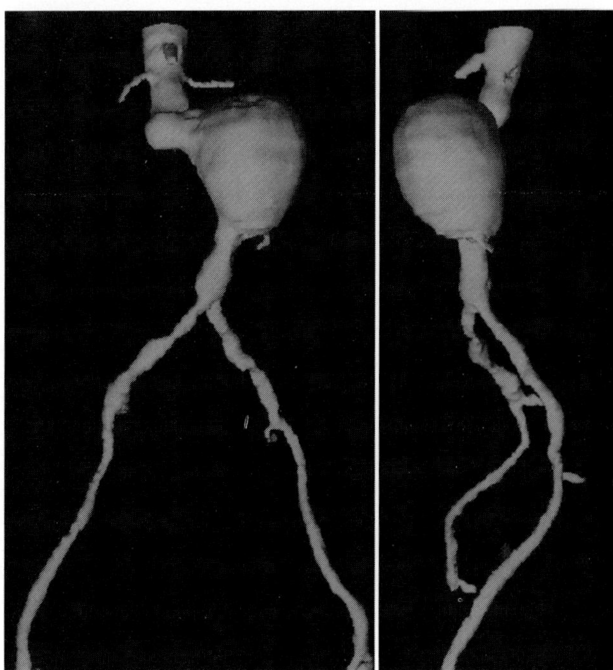

FIGURE 14–11. Multiple-object, surface-shaded display (SSD) from Figure 14–10 with all structures made invisible except blood flow, using the same anteroposterior *(left)* and left lateral *(right)* views. With calcified plaque made invisible, the degree of occlusive disease becomes apparent in the iliac arteries. A key point is that calcified plaque was modeled separately and has been made invisible; thus, this three-dimensional reconstruction does *not* have the same appearance as that of the typical one-object SSD shown in Figure 14–8. For surgical planning, it is preferable if the objects can be made visible or invisible at will on a computer screen. An alternative is to print hard copy images in multiple views with the various components sequentially highlighted, transparent, or invisible. (See Color Plate.)

always be interpreted in the context of the actual CT data and the potential artefacts that may occur. With some types of software, CT slices can even be displayed simultaneously within the 3-D reconstruction, which may help provide context for the data (Fig. 14–12) (see Color Plate). Depending on availability, this capacity to demonstrate the CT slice within the 3-D model can also be used to verify the accuracy of the 3-D reconstruction and can demonstrate that it is an accurate representation of the data.

Image Optimization and Common Artefacts Related to Spiral Computed Tomography Imaging

Knowledge of the physical concepts behind creation of CT images allows an understanding of concepts related to image optimization and image artefacts. These concepts are a concern to radiologists on a daily basis, and they are useful for surgeons interested in improving routine vascular CT imaging, CT protocols for unique situations, and differentiation of artefacts from pathology.

Although spiral CT technology has led to a number of advances in imaging, it is not without drawbacks. Because the data are acquired in one continuous sweep, tube overheating limits the distance that can be covered with each "spiral." This is probably the single most limiting factor for spiral or helical CT in the abdomen and pelvis and drives most of the image optimization strategies for aortic applications. The distance covered during a CT spiral is determined by:

- Duration of the scan (~30 to 60 sec)
- Speed of rotation (usually 1 rotation/sec)
- *Collimation* (beam thickness or slice thickness, 1 to 10 mm but usually 3 to 7 mm)
- *Pitch* (ratio of table speed to slice thickness)

Balancing these factors is essentially a compromise between data quality and the distance that can be covered in a single spiral. For example, one way to increase the distance covered during a single spiral scan is to decrease power so that the tube heats less quickly and the duration of the scan can be maximized. The problem is that the image

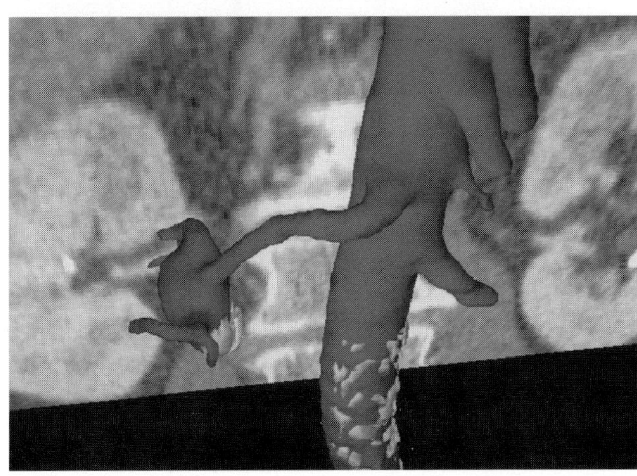

FIGURE 14–12. Multiple-object, surface-shaded display with a CT slice displayed in the context of the model in three-dimensional space. Thus, the right renal artery aneurysm is displayed with its branches heading toward the CT display of the right kidney. The central branch exiting the aneurysm is cut off as it disappears into the CT slice. (See Color Plate.)

may degrade if power is inadequate (a problem known as *photopenia*).

Another way to cover more distance during the time it takes for a tube to reach its heat capacity is to widen the collimation (slice thickness). Unfortunately, increasing the slice thickness compromises the longitudinal resolution and the quality of MPRs and 3-D reconstructions (Fig. 14–13). Increased slice thickness also compromises the ability to detect small structures, such as accessory renal arteries, because of *averaging artefact*. With this type of artefact, the attenuation from contrast within a 1-mm accessory renal artery is averaged with the attenuation from surrounding soft tissue. If the slice is thick, the attenuation from the artery is lost because it represents only a small portion of the slice. The small vessel is less likely to be missed with a thinner slice (Figs. 14–14 and 14–15). Thin slices, however, decrease the volume covered by the scan. During a typical 30-second scan (1 rotation/sec, pitch of 1), using a collimation of 3 mm translates into only 9 cm covered along the longitudinal axis.

One strategy for resolving this problem is to use fine collimation for portions of the scan where it is needed to detect small vessels (e.g., in the visceral segment of the aorta) and "thicker" collimation for areas where it is less

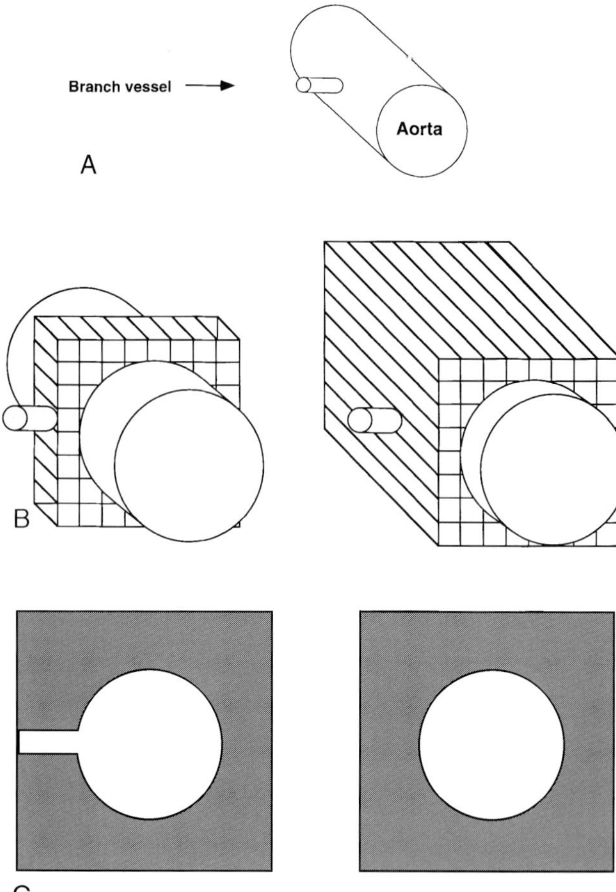

FIGURE 14–14. Importance of slice thickness with regard to detection and display of small vessels. *A,* Schematic diagram of a branch vessel arising from the aorta. *B,* The same vessels depicted during data acquisition using thin collimation *(left)* or thicker collimation *(right)*. *C,* Axial display of the data acquired in *B*. The branch vessel is seen clearly when it is in the center of a CT slice with thin collimation *(left)* because there is minimal averaging with data from low-density soft tissue in the same slice *(right)*.

noticeable (e.g., in the iliac arteries). One should keep in mind that "collimation" and "reconstruction interval" are *not* interchangeable terms; collimation is the width of the x-ray beam (slice thickness over which data are collected), and reconstruction interval is the interval at which cross sections are created for display. Once the volume is scanned and the data are stored, axial cross sections can be reconstructed at arbitrary intervals. Up to a point, increasing the reconstruction interval improves the quality of a scan because it creates overlapping slices, increases longitudinal resolution, and decreases some types of artefact. The optimal ratio of reconstruction interval to collimation is at least 2:1, and 3:1 is preferable for MPRs and 3-D reconstruction.[13]

Another way to cover more distance over the duration of the scan is to increase pitch (the ratio of table speed to slice thickness). The best image quality is obtained with a pitch of 1 (e.g., 3 mm/sec table speed and 3-mm collimation), but this limits the distance that can be covered. With the use of 180-degree linear interpolation algorithms instead of the original 360-degree interpolation algorithms, images of relatively good quality can still be obtained with a pitch greater than 1.[13–15] Longitudinal resolution is also improved by 180-degree linear interpolation algorithms. Of

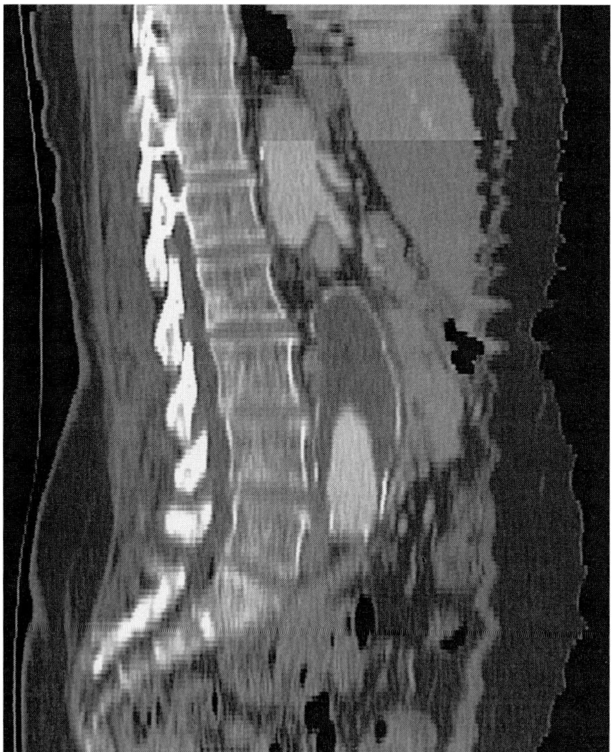

FIGURE 14–13. Importance of slice thickness (collimation) with regard to quality of multiplanar reformat (MPR). In this sagittal section, three "spirals" are apparent. The spiral in the central third of the scan has 3-mm collimation, and the spiral in the proximal third of the scan has 7-mm collimation (in the thoracic aorta, where the longitudinal resolution is less crucial in this patient). Note the difference in resolution and clarity for the spine and disc spaces. The transition point between these two spiral acquisitions was planned above the celiac axis so that potential motion artefact would be less likely to affect the quality of MPRs in a key location. Also note the motion artefact at the skin surface, which does not affect the relatively fixed aorta. The celiac and superior mesenteric artery origins are well visualized, and the apparent narrowing at the celiac artery origin is not artefact; it is also seen in other CT slices.

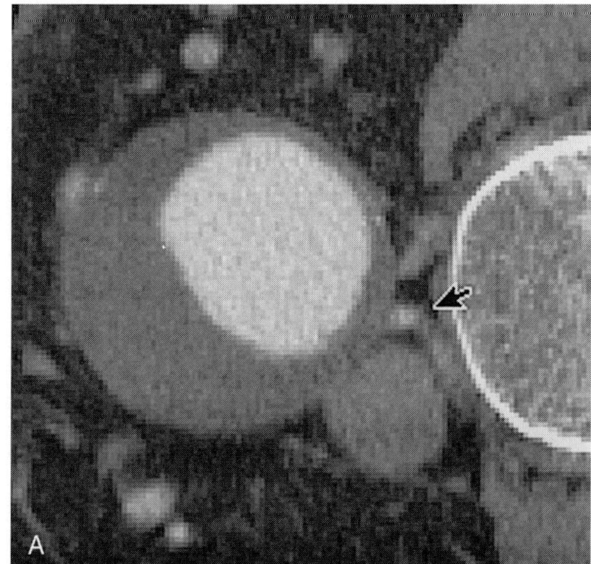

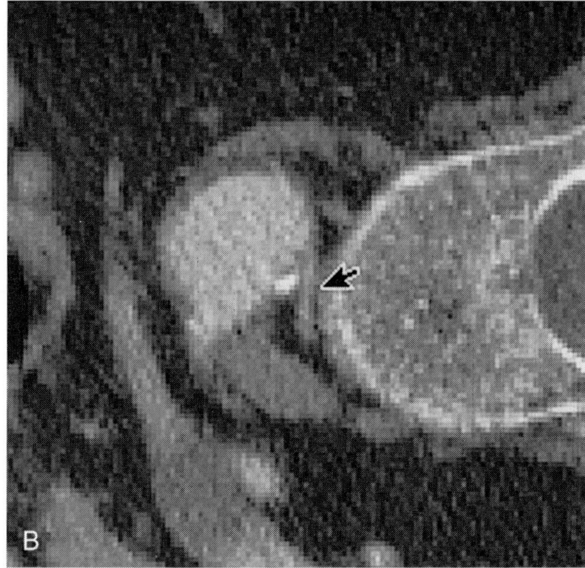

FIGURE 14–15. Clinical example of the effects of collimation for the display of small vessels. *A,* Small lumbar artery is easily seen in a CT slice at a location where the collimation is 3 mm *(arrow).* The contrast density is similar to that of the aorta. *B,* This larger lumbar artery *(arrow)* should be more prominent relative to the contrast within the aortic lumen, but at this location the collimation is 7 mm. With 7-mm or thicker collimation, a small lumbar artery or a small accessory renal artery can easily be missed.

course, there are tradeoffs. Noise is increased somewhat by 180-degree interpolation algorithms and higher pitch ratios. Fortunately, the degradation in image quality is relatively slight. The current upper limit on pitch is 2, also designated 2:1 (e.g., 6 mm/sec table speed and 3-mm collimation).

Ultimately, one can do only so much to maximize the distance covered during a single spiral scan. Fortunately, many scanners have the capacity to combine multiple spirals (i.e., multiple acquisitions) with a short interval to allow patient breathing between scans. This technique can increase the total duration of the scan and, therefore, the distance covered (e.g., from a single 30-second spiral to three 15-second spirals). Many scanners also permit different parameters for each spiral, so that pitch, power, and collimation can be optimized for each spiral. Combining multiple spiral scans is the only way to obtain adequate coverage of both the thoracic and abdominal aortas; it is also useful when coverage is desired from the celiac artery to the femoral arteries (e.g., for evaluation prior to endovascular AAA repair when the access path anatomy is nearly as important as the AAA anatomy). One disadvantage of this technique is that the patient is more likely to move between spirals and may find it difficult to resume breath-hold at the same position for each spiral. Both of these scenarios make motion artefact more likely (Fig. 14–16).

Although these types of motion artefact might not affect the quality of axial reformats, they may create obvious

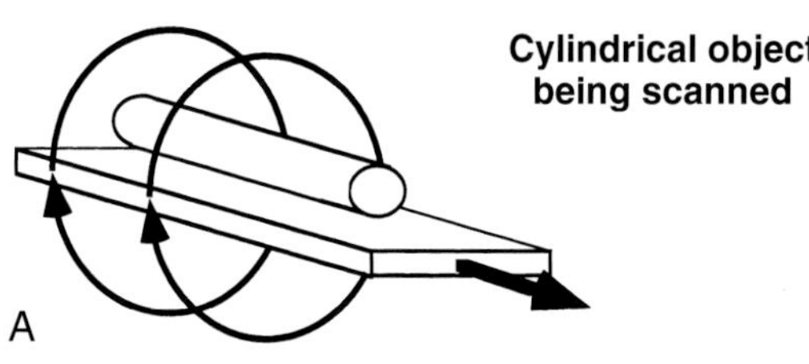

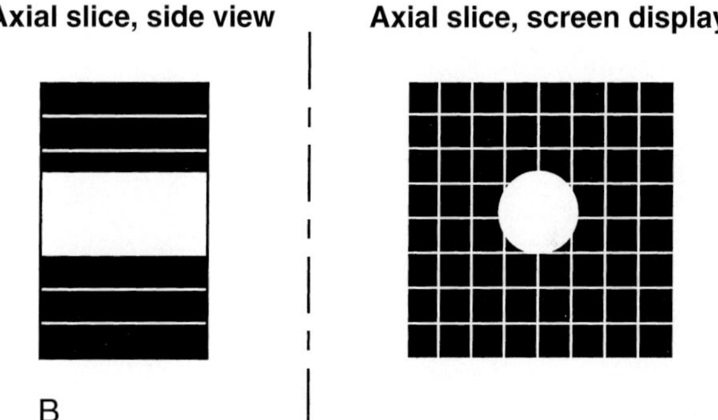

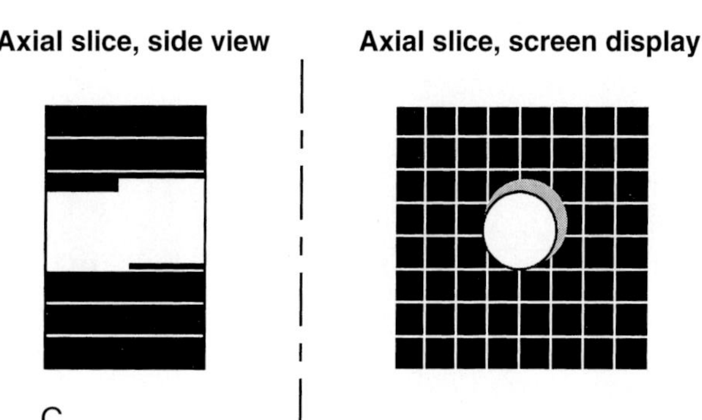

FIGURE 14–16. *A,* The decrease in the time needed for a spiral CT scan to cover the volume of interest decreases *motion artefact,* which distorts the object of interest. *B,* Without motion, the structure of interest is depicted clearly. *C,* If motion occurs, overlapping slices are less helpful because the organ, tumor, or vessel of interest has moved from one cross-sectional scan to the next, resulting in a distorted representation of the object. For example, this type of motion can create a distortion of the aorta that can be mistaken for an intimal flap or dissection.

discontinuities in multiplanar reformats (MPRs) or 3-D reconstructions. For this reason, it is important to plan the transition point between breath-holds so that it will not be in a crucial area (see Fig. 14–13). It is important to educate patients and obtain their cooperation to reduce motion artefact. Fortunately, most vascular structures are in areas that allow shallow breathing for patients who cannot hold their breath for an entire spiral acquisition. In most vascular patients, the vessels are also quite stiff and move very little during a cardiac cycle. However, the aortic arch of a young patient is a notable exception, and motion artefact can sometimes simulate the appearance of a traumatic injury or aortic dissection owing to distortion of the lumen.[16] These artefacts may be greatly reduced or eliminated when ultrafast *fifth-generation* scanners become available.[16]

Other Common Artefacts

Streak artefact or *scatter artefact* arises from interfaces between materials with large differences in density from the surrounding structures. This artefact is commonly seen with dense materials, such as prosthetic hips and metallic stents in endografts. Scatter may also occur as a result of dense intravenous contrast in the subclavian or brachiocephalic veins because dense contrast is often infused rapidly into these veins during the scan and they may be adjacent to air-filled lung parenchyma. Because this phenomenon can complicate CT scans for evaluation of aortic arch vessels, the contrast infusion should come from the arm opposite the vessel of interest or from a lower extremity.

Averaging artefact has already been mentioned with regard to "missing" a small vessel because of surrounding soft tissue, but it can also work in the opposite fashion. With this artefact, the large attenuation from a small piece of calcified plaque within a CT slice "averages" with thrombus-density material to produce a display with an intermediate density, similar to the density of intraluminal contrast. This often occurs within aortic aneurysms and should be suspected when contrast-density material appears with no apparent inflow or outflow vessel and when a piece of calcium or metal is nearby. This type of artefact is reduced by use of a small reconstruction interval.

Stairstep artefact results when the reconstruction interval on spiral CT is too large, creating a stepped appearance in the vessels. This artefact is most likely to occur in vessels oriented away from the direction of the scan (e.g., renal and iliac arteries). If such an appearance is noted in a multiplanar reformat, it is difficult to evaluate potential occlusive disease. Some of these artefacts are displayed in Figure 14–17.

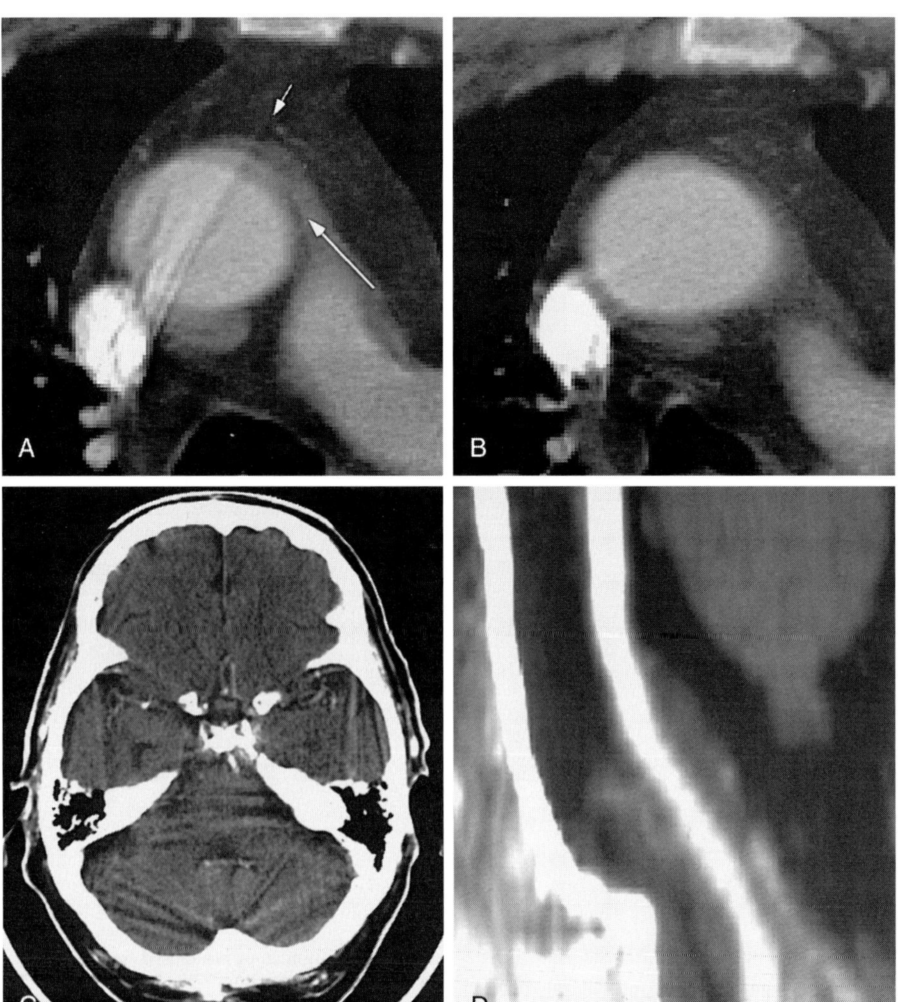

FIGURE 14–17. CT artefacts.

A, Motion artefact, described schematically in Figure 14–16, is shown here in the thoracic aorta, creating the impression of an intimal flap or dissection *(longer arrow)*. The position of these artefacts is usually due to aortic motion from the left anterior to the right posterior position. Streak artefact is also seen arising from dense contrast within the superior vena cava. The longer streak is clearly artefact because it extends beyond the vessel wall *(shorter arrow),* but the shorter streak could be misinterpreted as an intimal flap. One clue is the appearance of an obvious streak artefact in the same vessel. Another clue is the interface between structures with large differences in density. Other clues to the true nature of the aorta come from the benign patient history and the immediately adjacent CT slice.

B, The apparent pathologic features (artefacts) shown in *A* are not present in this immediately adjacent CT slice.

C, Intracranial streak artefact can make it difficult to detect infarcts in locations surrounded by dense bone. Beam hardening artefact is also common on head CT scans and occurs when low-energy portions of the x-ray beam are absorbed by thick, dense structures such as the skull. The residual beam that proceeds through the dense bone has a higher energy and may cause a small area of adjacent tissue to appear less dense (darker) than it should be. This can create an artefact resembling an ischemic infarct immediately adjacent to the skull.

D, Stairstep artefact creates a stepped appearance in the vessel (see text). This artefact is unique to spiral or helical CT.

Field of View

The last important parameter in relation to image optimization is field of view (FOV). As mentioned previously, the size of the display matrix and the field of view have a direct impact on the axial resolution of the display. If the field of view is kept to the minimum necessary, pixel size is decreased. For example, if the field of view is 30 cm and the matrix size is 512 × 512, each pixel in the display of axial slices is 0.6 mm. If the field of view is reduced to 20 cm, pixel size is improved to 0.4 mm.

In general, this degree of refinement is not an important consideration, except possibly when detailed measurements are necessary (e.g., in endovascular surgery or calculation of carotid artery stenosis). However, post hoc image optimization and CT scan protocols more strongly affect one's ability to distinguish different structures and the edges of those structures (see Post hoc Image Optimization and Computed Tomography Scan Protocols).

Post hoc Image Optimization

As described earlier, the CT number can range from −1000 to +1000 H. For convenience, however, workstations typically display the range of CT numbers as a positive integer ranging from 0 to 4096. (With a 12-bit digital computer display, 2^{12} = 4096 possible shades of gray.) Ideally, the area of interest will not encompass an extremely wide range of CT numbers because the number of gray scale values detectable by the human eye is limited to approximately 40 shades of gray.[17] Thus, the boundaries between fat (−20 to −100 H) and muscle (40 to 60 H) would be much more difficult to detect if the entire gray scale display (from white to black) spanned from −1000 H to +1000 H instead of −100 H to +100 H.

For an ideal display, the center of the gray scale display range is set to the average of the CT numbers in the structure of interest and the limits of gray scale representation are set to the smallest possible range of CT numbers. This can be done after the fact by the CT technician or radiologist. The range of values for gray scale representation is known as the *window width* for the display, and the center of this range is called the *window level*. The window level and width are adjusted on the CT workstation before hard copies are printed, but they can still be altered on the workstation as long as the dataset is retained in electronic format. Although this may seem clinically unimportant, adjustment of the window level with visual feedback in real time can be very useful in areas with wide variations in contrast density. For example, this often occurs when the clinician is attempting to determine the true lumen in a calcified vessel or attempting to determine whether there is perigraft flow around or through dense metallic areas of an endovascular stent-graft. Review of magnified images on a workstation with a radiologist may help the clinician to see detail that is far beyond the capabilities of the traditional small hard copy images.

Computed Tomography Scan Protocols

All of the concepts and considerations so far described are ultimately used to form a scan protocol. Following is a CT scan protocol that might be used for CT of the abdomen and pelvis for evaluation of an AAA prior to endovascular repair. This protocol covers the distance from the celiac artery to the distal external iliac arteries and still maintains good image quality and contrast. This protocol is modified from the one used in the Department of Radiology, Dartmouth-Hitchcock Medical Center, Hanover, N.H.

1. *Scan parameters:* 120 kVp, 280 mA (minimum), 1 sec
2. *Length of helical exposure:* 30+ seconds
3. *Pitch:* 1:1
4. *Collimation and sequence:* First scan with no contrast, 7-mm collimation, 100 mA to localize celiac artery
   a. 3 mm, celiac artery to below renal arteries (90-mm distance)
   b. 7 mm, distal aorta to common femoral or external iliac arteries
   c. 7 mm, thoracic aorta above celiac artery (optional)
5. *Patient instructions*
   a. Patient is coached with hyperventilation
   b. Patient performs a breath-hold in mid-inspiration
   c. Patient breathes slowly if necessary (with a breathing pause mid-scan when split helix used)
6. *Contrast:* non-ionic, 300 mg/ml
7. *Contrast volume:* 140 ml (more may be acceptable)
8. *Route of administration:* intravenous, arm vein
9. *Rate of infusion:* 2 to 2.5 ml/sec
10. *Scan delay*: 25 sec (or use SmartPrep or similar utility)
11. *Reconstruction algorithm:* standard
12. *Reconstruction interval:* 1 or 2 mm
13. *Field of view*
    a. 28 cm or greater for entire scan
    b. Both external iliac and common femoral arteries distally to be included

An alternative might be to use a pitch of 2:1 with 3-mm collimation to scan from the celiac artery to the pelvis. If necessary, a second spiral at 5-mm collimation could be added at a pitch of 1.5 to 2.0, and lower power (e.g., 200 to 220 mA). The field of view can also be reduced to 22 cm but would likely need to increase to 28 cm on the distal (second) spiral to ensure inclusion of both external iliac arteries.

Contrast

Notably, the rapid infusion of contrast and the large distances covered for CTA generally require a significant infusion of contrast. A typical CTA study from the celiac artery to the external iliac arteries may require 120 to 180 ml of 60% ionic or 300 mgI/ml non-ionic contrast,[7] which is similar to the dose of contrast for an aortogram with runoff. Although the risk of renal damage may be less than for direct aortic injection of full-strength contrast through a catheter positioned adjacent to the renal arteries, it is nonetheless a limitation for patients with significant renal impairment. If the creatinine level is twice normal, the protocol can be performed in a well-hydrated patient with lower doses of low-osmolar contrast, and less clarity can be accepted in the iliac arteries, where adjunctive duplex ultrasonography can be used if necessary. More caution is needed if the patient has diabetes or a history of congestive heart failure.

If the creatinine level is 2.5 to 3 times normal, a "screening" CT scan can be performed without contrast, or magnetic resonance angiography (MRA) with gadolinium contrast is used. CT can be performed with gadolinium, but the large volume of contrast can be expensive. MRA cannot be used if the patient is claustrophobic or has an implanted device. The distance covered is limited with current MR technology, and resolution is approximately half that of CT, but good delineation of anatomy and useful 3-D reconstructions can usually be obtained. Dialysis patients can have contrast CT if it is timed with the dialytic procedure to prevent problems from the volume load. Fortunately, the limitation of impaired renal function is not a frequent problem.

The other limitation of iodinated contrast is allergy, but true allergic reactions to contrast are rare. Severe reactions (hypotension, dyspnea, loss of consciousness) occur at a rate of approximately 0.22% with ionic contrast and 0.04% with non-ionic contrast.[18] Reactions requiring hospitalization or the care of an anesthesiologist are even less frequent (0.04%, ionic contrast; 0.004%, non-ionic contrast). Patients with allergies to other substances or with asthma are about twice as likely to have a reaction to contrast, and patients with a previous contrast reaction have roughly five times the average risk. Clinical judgment is required, but in most cases of suspected allergy, pretreatment with antihistamines and corticosteroids can reduce the incidence of reactions significantly, even if non-ionic contrast is used.[19] With these techniques, most patients can safely undergo contrast-enhanced CT.

CLINICAL APPLICATIONS

Head and Neck

Intracranial Hemorrhage versus Infarction

The first clinical application of CT was for the evaluation of intracranial structures, and CT continues to have an important role in this area. Differentiation of cerebral infarction from intracranial hemorrhage has important diagnostic and therapeutic implications for patients presenting with acute neurologic symptoms. The treatment of stroke as a "brain attack" that might benefit from treatment with thrombolytic therapy or other minimally invasive therapy is gaining favor. Most of these potential therapeutic agents must be given as quickly as possible, making rapid diagnosis crucial. For example, thrombolytic therapy must be administered within 3 hours to achieve a favorable balance between decreased rates of infarction versus increased intracranial hemorrhage.[20] Acute intracranial hemorrhage is a contraindication to thrombolytic therapy, however, and must be ruled out prior to initiation of therapy. Intracranial hemorrhage must also be ruled out when a neurologic deficit occurs following carotid endarterectomy.

CT has a diagnostic accuracy of approximately 90% in the evaluation of acute intracranial hemorrhage, whereas the changes associated with intracranial hemorrhage on MRI take several days to develop.[21, 22] Conversely, CT changes associated with acute ischemic infarction may take several days to develop, and only larger infarcts are apparent within the first 24 hours. The relative sensitivity for infarction within the first 24 hours after the clinical event is approximately 50% for CT and 80% for MRI.[23] MRI also appears to be more sensitive to late changes associated with infarction and hemorrhage[22–24] and is less affected by bone-related artefacts in evaluation of lesions in the brain stem or cerebellum. For acute presentations, however, CT remains a more rapid and less expensive diagnostic test that is applicable in most clinical situations.

No matter which test is used, diagnosis of acute hemorrhage can be difficult in some situations, and expert interpretation should be utilized whenever feasible.[25] We should remember that acute hemorrhage is determined on a CT *without* intravenous contrast and should not be confused with "luxury perfusion" around an infarct or contrast enhancement of a tumor (Fig. 14–18). Acute intracranial hemorrhage is detected on CT scans without intravenous contrast because the intact red blood cells initially have a high protein content, are more dense than the surrounding structures, and produce a high-density lesion (see Fig. 14–18). In later stages following the acute hemorrhage, the red blood cells lyse and lose hemoglobin and the area becomes isodense with the surrounding tissue on CT. MRI would be more useful at this point.

Intracranial and Extracranial Vasculature

Although MRA has been more popular for imaging intracranial vasculature, the advent of spiral CT with CTA and 3-D reconstruction has made it possible to obtain useful images of intracranial and extracranial vessels as well.[7] Imaging of the intracranial circulation with CT is made more difficult by contrast timing and interference from dense bone in some areas; with some effort, however, useful images can be produced. Spiral CT is extremely accurate in detecting cerebral aneurysms larger than 3 mm[26, 27] and can be useful in intracranial dissections over time.[28]

For extracranial vessels, excellent CT images can be obtained without much difficulty. CT imaging for extracranial vessels is easier than for intracranial vessels because:

1. The carotid arteries are not contained within dense bony structures.
2. Contrast timing for scans from the upper thorax to the skull base is not too difficult.
3. The field of view is small.
4. The vessels are oriented perpendicular to the axial plane.

MRA has been relatively popular for the evaluation of extracranial cerebrovascular occlusive disease, but it tends result in an overestimate of the severity of stenoses.[29] For evaluation of carotid occlusive disease, CT has not been studied as extensively, although as early as 1982 Riles and colleagues demonstrated that spiral CT could be more accurate than angiography for carotid occlusions.[30] More recently, spiral CT has shown a high degree of accuracy in determining the degree of carotid stenosis,[31] and this accuracy may be enhanced using CT reformats perpendicular to the vessel lumen.[32]

In addition to providing a familiar display, 3-D reconstruction portrays more than just the vessel lumen, making it easy to rapidly assess the extent of disease at the carotid

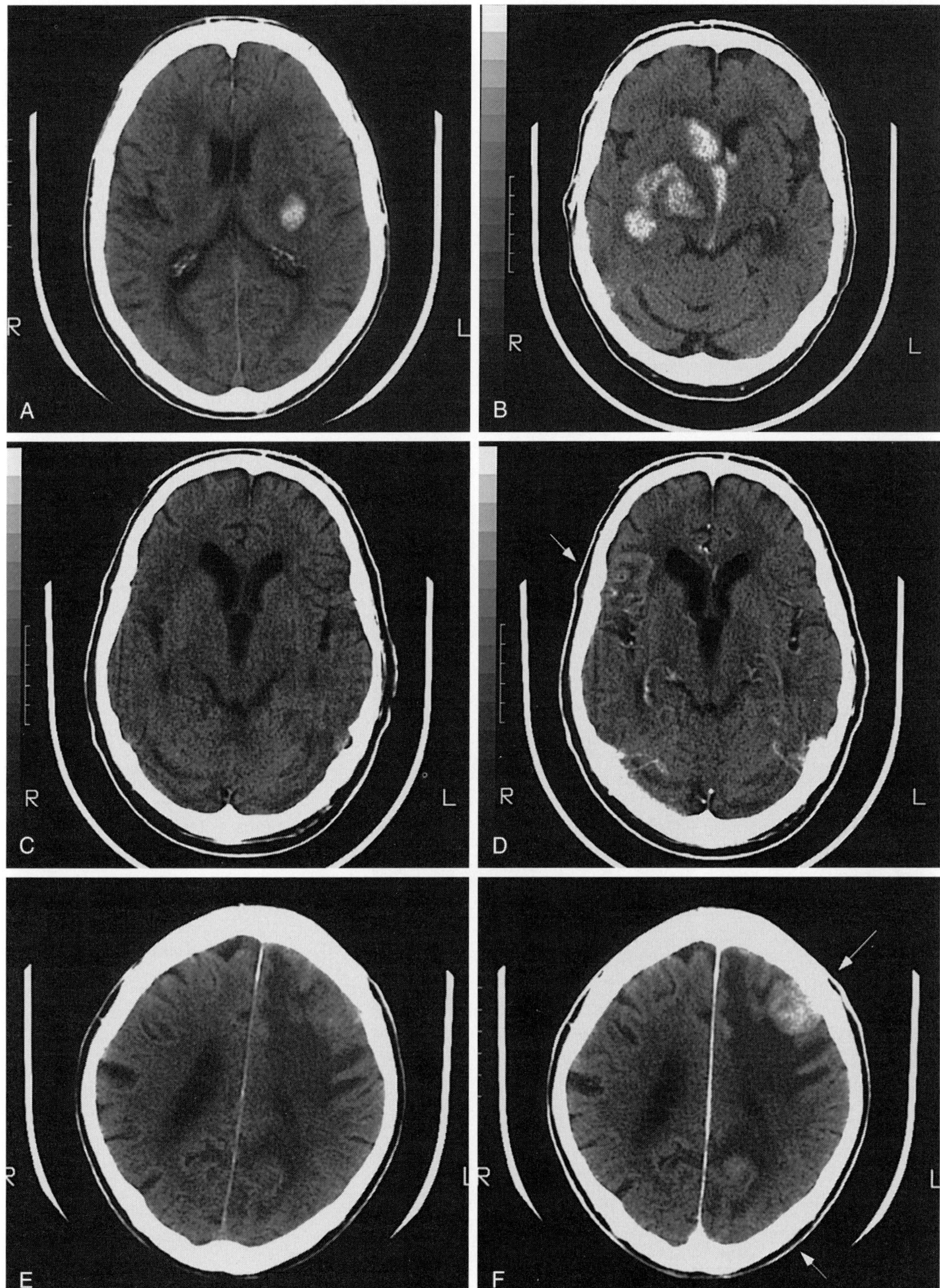

FIGURE 14–18. Demonstration of lesions on head CT scan that can be misinterpreted without expert help.

A, CT scan of the head without intravenous contrast demonstrates hemorrhage in a patient with severe hypertension.

B, A much larger intracranial hemorrhage with a midline shift and blood in the ventricle on a CT, again without intravenous (IV) contrast. A CT scan without IV contrast is the imaging modality of choice when acute hemorrhage is suspected.

C, Right middle cerebral artery distribution ischemic infarct on a head CT scan with no IV contrast. The lesion is relatively subtle.

D, The same infarct shown in *C,* but this time IV contrast was used. This contrast enhancement is characteristic of an ischemic infarction and is classically gyriform. It is generally thought to be secondary to breakdown of capillary barriers with leakage of contrast or due to "luxury perfusion" around the infarct itself. This feature is usually absent 3 to 6 months after the infarction.

E, Another hypodense lesion on a noncontrast CT. This is not an ischemic infarction but, rather, edema from a tumor.

F, IV contrast enhancement of the tumor *(longer arrow)* helps to demonstrate the large amount of edema characteristic of an intracranial neoplasm. The *shorter arrow* points to another lesion in this patient with metastatic lung cancer. This lesion is less dense in this CT slice because it is smaller and not in the center of the slice (it is clearly visible in an adjacent slice).

bifurcation (Fig. 14–19) (see Color Plate). Despite the utility of the images, 3-D reconstructions should be used to enhance, not replace, evaluation and measurements from the source (CT) images.[33]

Although many investigators are using duplex ultrasonography as the sole preoperative imaging modality prior to carotid endarterectomy, there are some limitations in this area. CT can be used to evaluate pathologic features that are difficult to evaluate by duplex scanning, such as intrathoracic lesions, intracranial disease (including tumors), calcified vessels, total internal carotid artery occlusions, high bifurcations, and internal carotid artery plaques that extend to the base of the skull. The relationship of the carotid bifurcation to bony structures (e.g., cervical vertebrae) can preoperatively reveal potential difficulties with surgical exposure,[34, 35] and this relationship can be readily displayed by means of 3-D reconstructions or concurrent display of MPRs (Fig. 14–20) (see Color Plate).

MRA is also somewhat limited in this capacity relative to CT. Misdiagnosis of low flow as occlusion is lessened by the use of gadolinium enhancement, but this adds to the expense of MRA, which is already higher than that for CTA. MR also shows some limitation in identifying calcifications within vessels. Although this problem is decreasing as technology improves,[36] significant lesions can be missed because calcified plaque does not provide an intense signal in MR images.

Proximal Lesions (Arch Vessel Disease)

Although angiography remains the standard for evaluating intracranial and aortic arch occlusive disease, improvement in CT (and MR) is leading to strategies that provide a more thorough vascular evaluation than is possible with duplex ultrasonography without the morbidity or cost of angiography.[37] As a result of improvements in noninvasive imaging

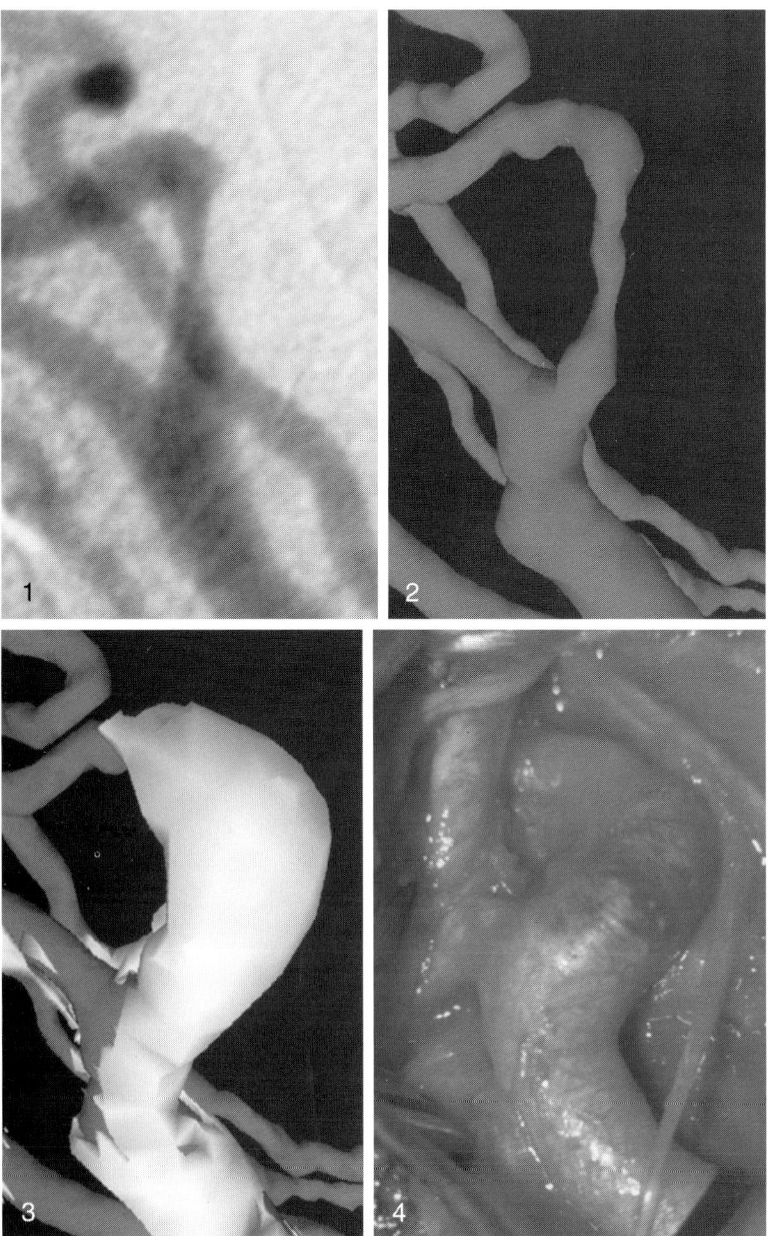

FIGURE 14–19. Demonstration of carotid artery disease. From *left* to *right: 1,* Angiogram of an internal carotid artery stenosis; *2,* three-dimensional (3-D) reconstruction of blood flow (red) in the same location; *3,* 3-D reconstruction of blood flow and plaque or thrombus (yellow); and *4,* intraoperative photograph of the same location. There is obviously a striking similarity despite rotation of the head and neck in the operative photograph. (See Color Plate.)

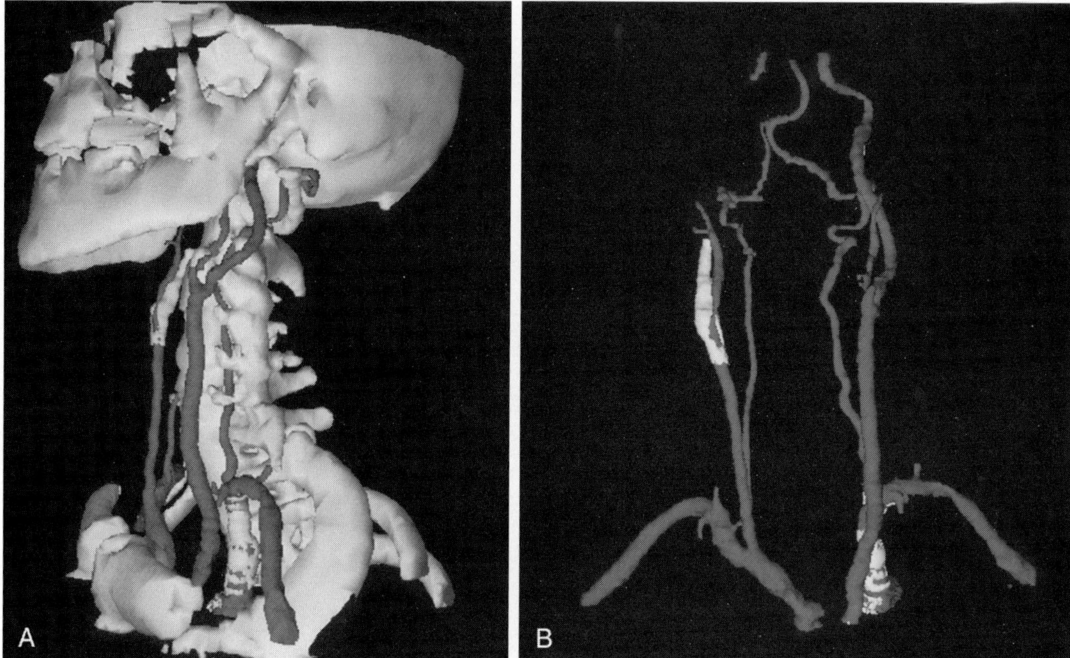

FIGURE 14–20. Multiple-object, three-dimensional reconstruction can demonstrate the relationship of the extracranial vessels and the bony structures as an aid to surgical planning. *A*, With bony structures. *B*, Without bony structures. (See Color Plate.)

modalities and a stroke risk of 0.6% to 1.2% with angiography,[38, 39] the role of diagnostic angiography prior to carotid endarterectomy is becoming limited.[1]

Figure 14–21 provides a comparison of arteriography, MR, and CT with 3-D reconstruction for an innominate artery lesion and demonstrates some of the potential benefits of CT for arch lesions. The problem of detecting calcified lesions on MRI and MRA is also shown. Nonetheless, one should use caution when evaluating arch lesions on CT scans because of the potential for motion artefact from aortic pulsation and streak artefact from concentrated contrast infusion in veins immediately adjacent to suspected occlusive disease. Some of these problems can be avoided with the use of lower concentrations of contrast and infusions into the upper extremity opposite from the suspected arterial lesion. Infusion of contrast into a lower extremity vein can be used, if necessary, but is less desirable.

Thorax

Aortic Arch Vessels

Clinical applications for CT of the thorax include evaluation of every major vessel in the chest. Imaging of the aortic arch vessels can be useful for the evaluation of occlusive disease (see Fig. 14–21), and CT can also demonstrate important arch anomalies. The utility of such imaging continues to improve with refinement of scanning protocols for these vessels. We have found that CT can demonstrate relatively subtle lesions, such as arteritis of the subclavian arteries, if caution is used to avoid artefact from intravenous infusions of contrast. Because the subclavian arteries generally travel perpendicular to the direction of table movement, spiral CT is needed to evaluate these lesions using multiplanar formats or 3-D reconstructions. Some newer CT protocols for evaluation of the thoracic outlet have demonstrated the arterial and venous deformation that occurs with upper extremity abduction, and this may become a useful study for patients with suspected thoracic outlet syndrome (Fig. 14–22) (see Color Plate).[40]

Aortic Dissections

With the advent of fast scanners and spiral techniques, CT has become the study of choice in most cases of thoracic dissection.[41, 42] The sensitivity and specificity of spiral CT for dissection of the thoracic aorta appear to be equal to or better than those of transesophageal echocardiography and MRA, and it is superior for diagnosis of dissection of the arch vessels.[42] With proper timing of the contrast bolus, the true and false lumens are both opacified and can be seen to spiral down along the thoracic aorta (Fig. 14–23) (see Color Plate). Curvilinear artefacts simulating an aortic dissection most commonly occur in the ascending aorta (up to 35% of cases have some artefact in this location). Fortunately, these artefacts can usually be distinguished from genuine pathology (see Fig. 14–17). With CT, the false lumen can be visualized even if it is thrombosed, with evidence provided by a spiraling crescent of thrombus density within the aorta. Other evidence of thoracic dissection includes displacement of calcium with the vessel wall, aneurysm, atelectasis, and hemothorax. Because MRI is limited in depicting calcifications and thrombus density material, it does not demonstrate aortic dissection well if one lumen is thrombosed.

Traumatic Aortic Injury

Evidence of traumatic aortic injury, such as an intimal flap, dissection, or mediastinal hematoma, can be visualized with

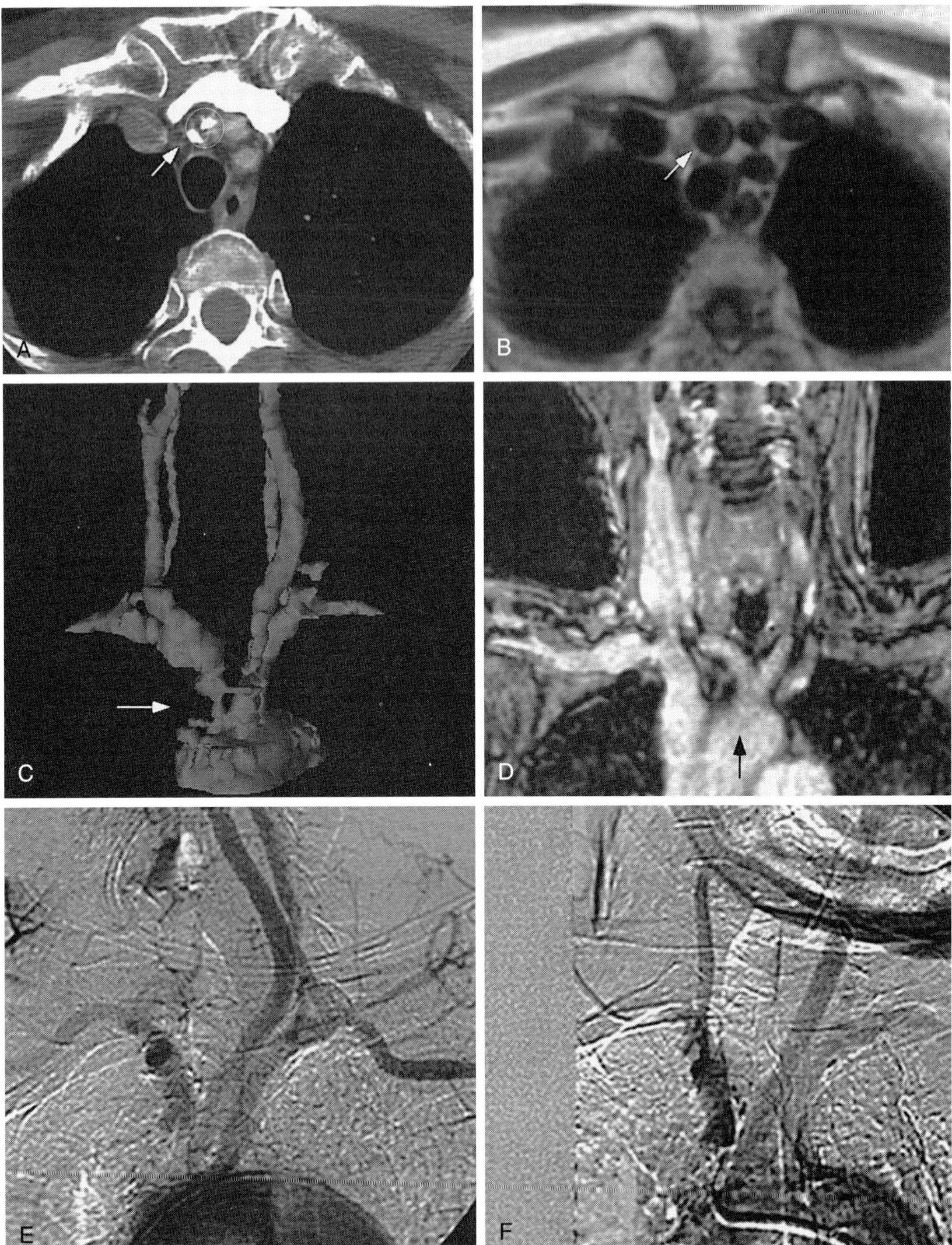

FIGURE 14–21. Comparison of CT, MR, CT with three-dimensional (3-D) reconstruction, and arteriography for an innominate artery lesion. *A,* Axial CT image demonstrates two areas of dense calcification within the innominate artery (*arrow* and *thin circle*). The contrast-enhanced lumen at this location is extremely small. *B,* Axial MR at the same location illustrates the problem of detecting the calcified lesions at the same location on the MR image (arrow). Note the density of surrounding bony structures. *C,* Multiple-object 3-D reconstruction, with all objects invisible except contrast-enhanced blood flow. The innominate artery stenosis is nicely demonstrated. The irregularity of the adjacent arch is mostly due to defects from plaque, which was made invisible on the computer-generated display. *D,* The resolution and location of the plane of reconstruction on gadolinium-enhanced MRA result in a less accurate depiction of the anatomy. *E,* Arch aortogram demonstrates the innominate lesion with such slow flow that the carotid bifurcation cannot be visualized well despite selective injection *(F)*. The carotid bifurcation is better visualized in *C* and is, in fact, relatively free of disease, as depicted on the 3-D reconstruction.

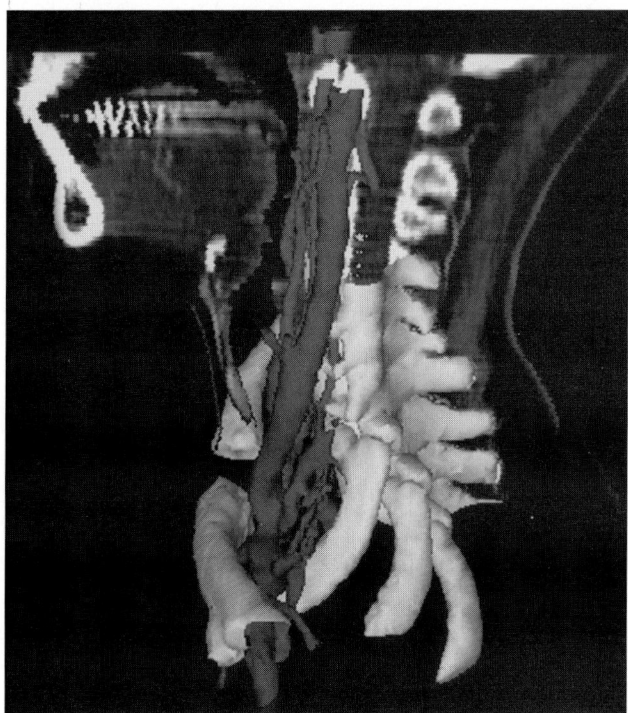

FIGURE 14–22. Three-dimensional reconstruction of the bony and vascular structures of the thoracic outlet. (See Color Plate.)

spiral CT. As technology advances, the diagnostic accuracy of CT continues to improve and large series have now demonstrated diagnostic accuracy of 75% to 99% for CT in traumatic aortic injury.[43–45] CT is probably the primary study of choice in pediatric patients owing to vessel size and time considerations.[46] In some cases, the CT evidence is definitive enough to operate without aortography[45]; in general, however, aortography is still required to rule out traumatic aortic injury requiring intervention. Even in centers with less than optimal imaging, CT continues to have a role in traumatic aortic injury; CT of the head or abdomen is often needed urgently, and aortography sometimes causes a significant delay in treatment. However, the diagnostic accuracy of CT should be established in an individual center before the role of aortography diminishes significantly (Fig. 14–24).

Thoracic Aneurysms

Traditionally, thoracic aneurysms have been evaluated by a combination of CT and angiography, but advances in CT imaging technology are beginning to change this area as well. Depiction of the aneurysm as a 3-D reconstruction can make interpretation of the extent of aneurysm more rapid and accurate.[10, 11, 41] With the advent of spiral CT and protocols using thin slices, it is also possible to identify the number and location of patent intercostal arteries. This capacity can be useful for planning the cross-clamp location and the potential for reimplantation of intercostal arteries (Fig. 14–25) (see Color Plate).

Pulmonary Vessels

The diagnosis of pulmonary embolus is a promising new CT application that is made possible by the dynamic contrast bolus and rapid acquisition of volume data provided in spiral CT. Spiral CT can detect pulmonary emboli even in patients without clinically suspected disease[47] and may be more accurate and more specific than ventilation-perfusion scans.[48, 49] With several centers reporting promising results, spiral CT may become the primary noninvasive imaging study for pulmonary embolus. The reader should keep in mind that a workstation-based search, "scrolling" through the dataset in cinematic fashion, can improve the pulmonary embolus detection rate over that possible with traditional hard copy review.[47]

The role of 3-D reconstruction in pulmonary applications[50] remains to be determined, but it appears helpful in the following:

- Treatment of pulmonary arteriovenous malformations
- Enhancing the understanding of the postoperative reorientation of the pulmonary vessels
- Surgical planning for pulmonary tumors
- Diagnosis of marginated thromboembolic disease

An example is shown in Figure 14–26 (see Color Plate).

Abdomen and Pelvis

One of the most important roles of CT in vascular surgery is evaluation prior to AAA repair. Optimal imaging before repair involves a great deal of anatomy, such as:

- The precise proximal and distal extent of the aneurysm
- Occlusive or aneurysmal disease in the visceral, renal, and iliac arteries
- Multiple renal arteries or accessory renal arteries
- Venous structures, such as retroaortic renal veins
- Duplicate or left-sided vena cava
- Vascular anomalies, including horseshoe kidney
- Aortic dissections

Even "minor" anatomic features, such as patency of the inferior mesenteric artery (IMA), the number and location of patent lumbar arteries, and the degree of calcified or noncalcified plaque at the sites of intended anastomoses, can alter the operative plan or the risk-benefit ratio of the procedure.

Whereas most of these anatomic features can be dealt with at the time of AAA repair, it is generally safer and more efficient if the surgeon has full knowledge of the anatomy prior to the procedure. Traditionally, delineation of all the aforementioned anatomic features required a combination of conventional CT and angiography; today, state-of-the-art spiral CT with the potential addition of 3-D reconstruction is all that is required in most cases.

Extent and Nature of Abdominal Aortic Aneurysms

Perhaps the single most important morphologic consideration for repair of an aortic aneurysm is the proximal and distal extent of disease. Evaluating the extent of an aneurysm is difficult with angiography because of the potential for a thrombus-filled lumen. MRA findings can also be misleading because thrombus and calcified plaque are generally not displayed prominently with currently available equipment.

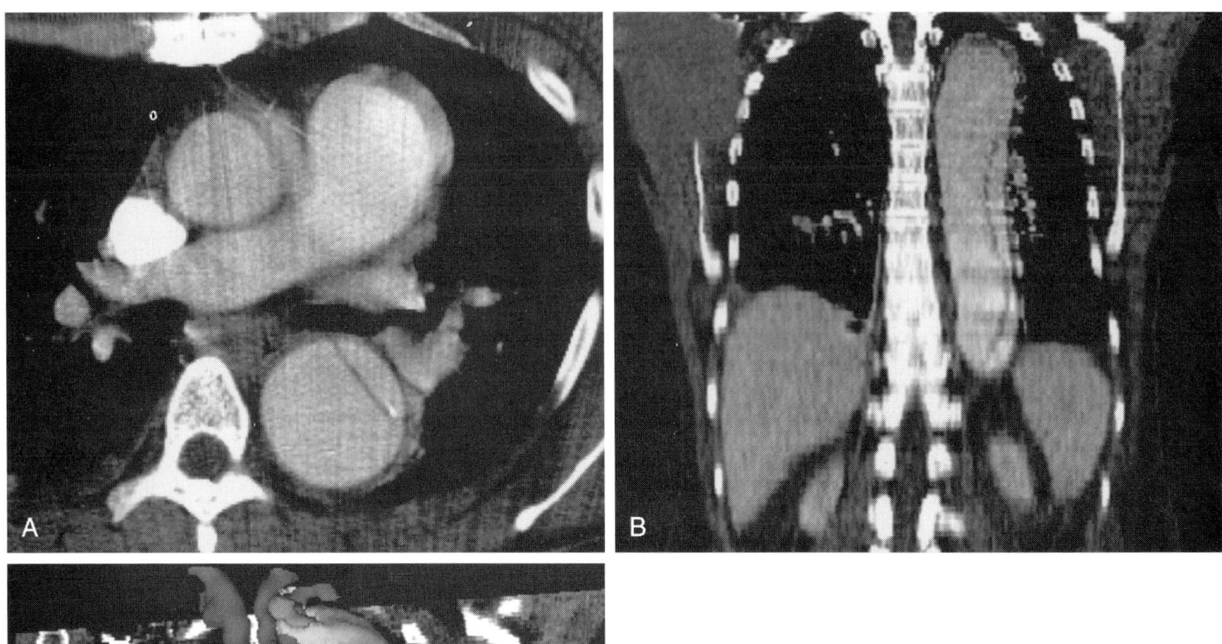

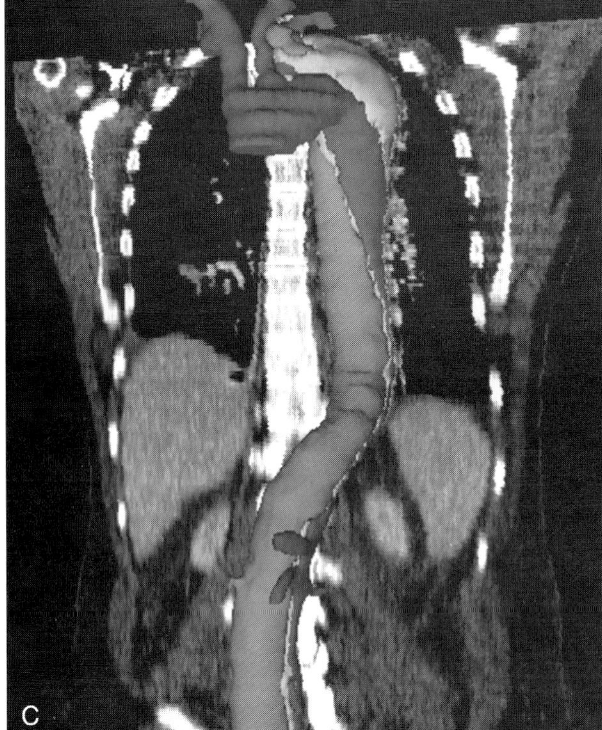

FIGURE 14–23. Dissection of the thoracic aorta. *A,* Axial CT demonstrates dissection within the descending thoracic aorta. Compare this picture with the artefacts in Figure 14–17. CT artefacts can create the impression of a dissection, but these can usually be distinguished from genuine pathology. *B,* Coronal reformat demonstrates the dissection in a consistent manner over a long segment of aorta. *C,* Three-dimensional (3-D) reconstruction depicts (1) the blood from the true lumen supplying the celiac, superior mesenteric artery, and left renal artery (red); (2) blood from the false lumen involving the left subclavian artery and supplying the right renal artery (magenta); and (3) thrombus (yellow). This illustration demonstrates how a 3-D reconstruction can rapidly convey a large amount of information. A coronal CT slice has been placed within the model at the appropriate location to lend context. (See Color Plate.)

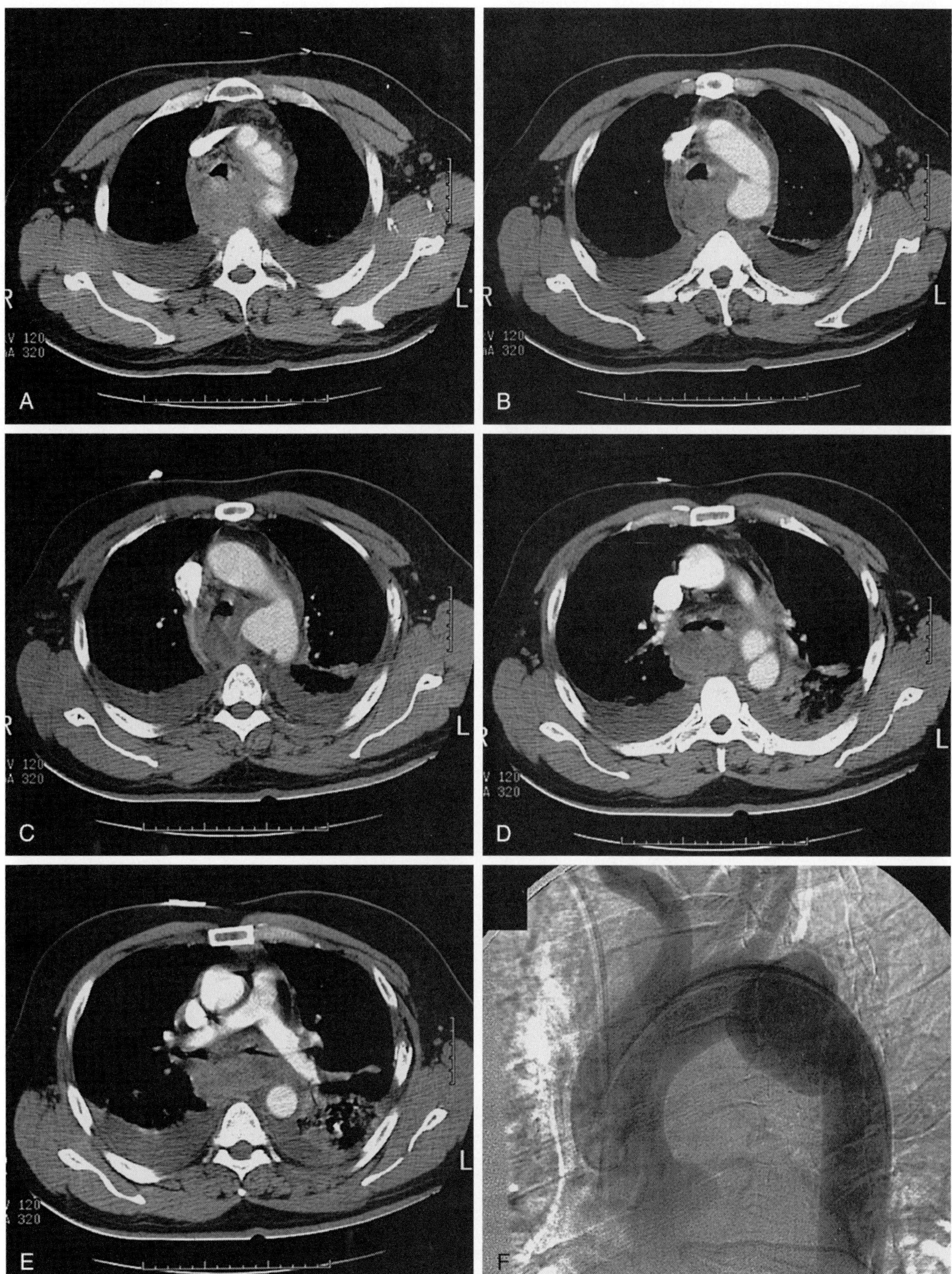

FIGURE 14–24. Traumatic aortic injury. *A*, Dissection beginning at the level of the left subclavian artery. *B–D*, Continuation of the dissection or transection and apparently abnormal dilation of the aorta (especially inferomedially). The more distal descending aorta appears relatively normal in *E*, although the associated atelectasis, effusion, and mediastinal hematoma are still present. *F*, Aortogram demonstrates the aneurysmal portion of the injury.

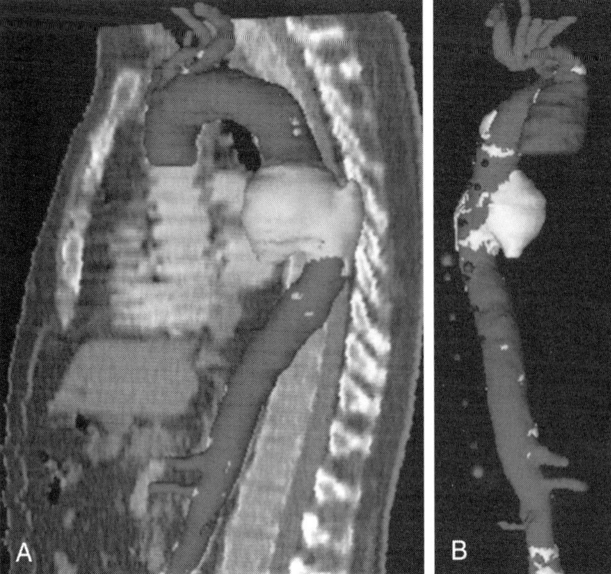

FIGURE 14–25. *A,* Aneurysm of the thoracic aorta demonstrated using three-dimensional (3-D) reconstruction with simultaneous display of a sagittal CT slice to lend context. Motion artefact is much greater around the heart and proximal ascending aorta. The focal blebs displayed in the model were verified at the time of surgery. *B,* Intercostal arteries are marked on the CT slices and are displayed on the 3-D model using interactive software (blue marks). The red marks were placed to denote the top of the eighth thoracic vertebra (T8) and the bottom of the 12th thoracic vertebra. The large intercostal artery near the top of T8 was identified and preserved at the time of operation. (See Color Plate.)

The use of CT avoids both of these problems (Fig. 14–27) (see Color Plate). It is apparent from this figure that an angiogram of the contrast-filled lumen does not reveal the aneurysmal nature of the aorta at the level of the renal arteries because much of the aneurysm is occupied by thrombus. Thus, CT is generally recognized as the best imaging modality for ascertaining the proximal and distal extent of an aortic aneurysm. Spiral CT offers distinct advantages over conventional CT in this respect because the data may be viewed from different perspectives via MPR and 3-D reconstructions (see Fig. 14–27). These reconstructions can be especially helpful in determining the extent of aneurysmal disease and the locations for optimal cross-clamp placement.[10, 11]

At our center (Dartmouth-Hitchcock Medical Center), patients with AAAs are evaluated with spiral CT, including MPR and 3-D reconstruction, and the aneurysm frequently involves the suprarenal aorta. Many of these patients have already undergone conventional CT and angiography, or they have had adjunctive arteriography. In this subset of patients with suprarenal aneurysms, conventional CT and angiography often fail to predict the true extent of the aneurysm and the optimal cross-clamp location. In our experience, however, preoperative spiral CT with 3-D reconstruction has revealed the correct proximal and distal extent of the aneurysm compared with operative findings. Spiral CT with 3-D reconstruction also appears to be superior to spiral CT alone, and this does not appear to be a finding unique to our center.[10, 11] It has been suggested that CT sometimes overestimates the extent of aneurysmal disease, but in our experience CT has not predicted a suprarenal aneurysm when only an infrarenal AAA was present.

Iliac Artery Aneurysms

Determining the extent of an aneurysm includes evaluation for a potential iliac artery aneurysm, either as an extension of an aortic aneurysm or as isolated disease. In many cases, conventional CT has been poor in this regard, and even relatively recent series have reported error rates of 16% in detection of iliac aneurysms.[51] However, groups using spiral CT with MPRs alone have noted an accuracy above 90% for detection of iliac aneurysms.[8] In our series of AAAs evaluated by spiral CT with MPRs and 3-D reconstruction, we have not missed an iliac artery aneurysm confirmed during open repair.

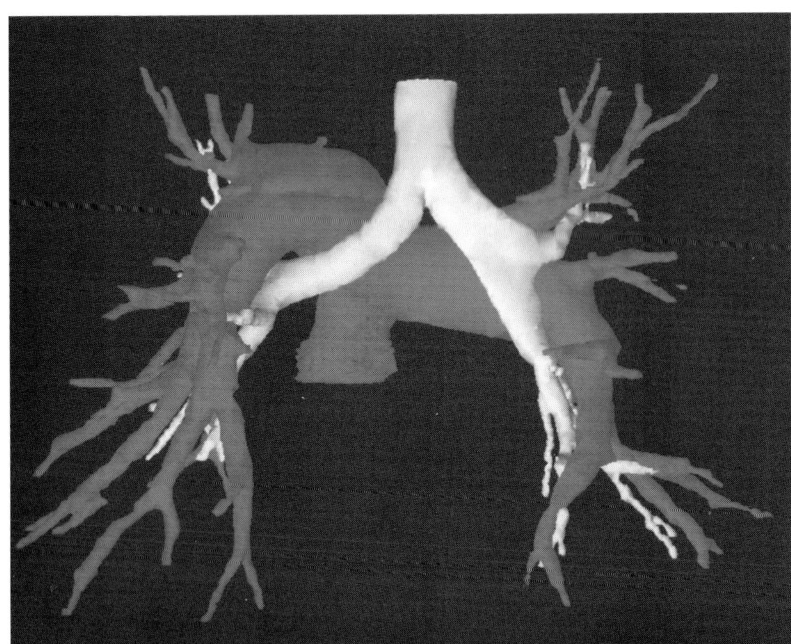

FIGURE 14–26. Three-dimensional reconstruction of the pulmonary arteries (in blue to represent non-oxygenated blood) and the tracheobronchial tree (in yellow). (See Color Plate.)

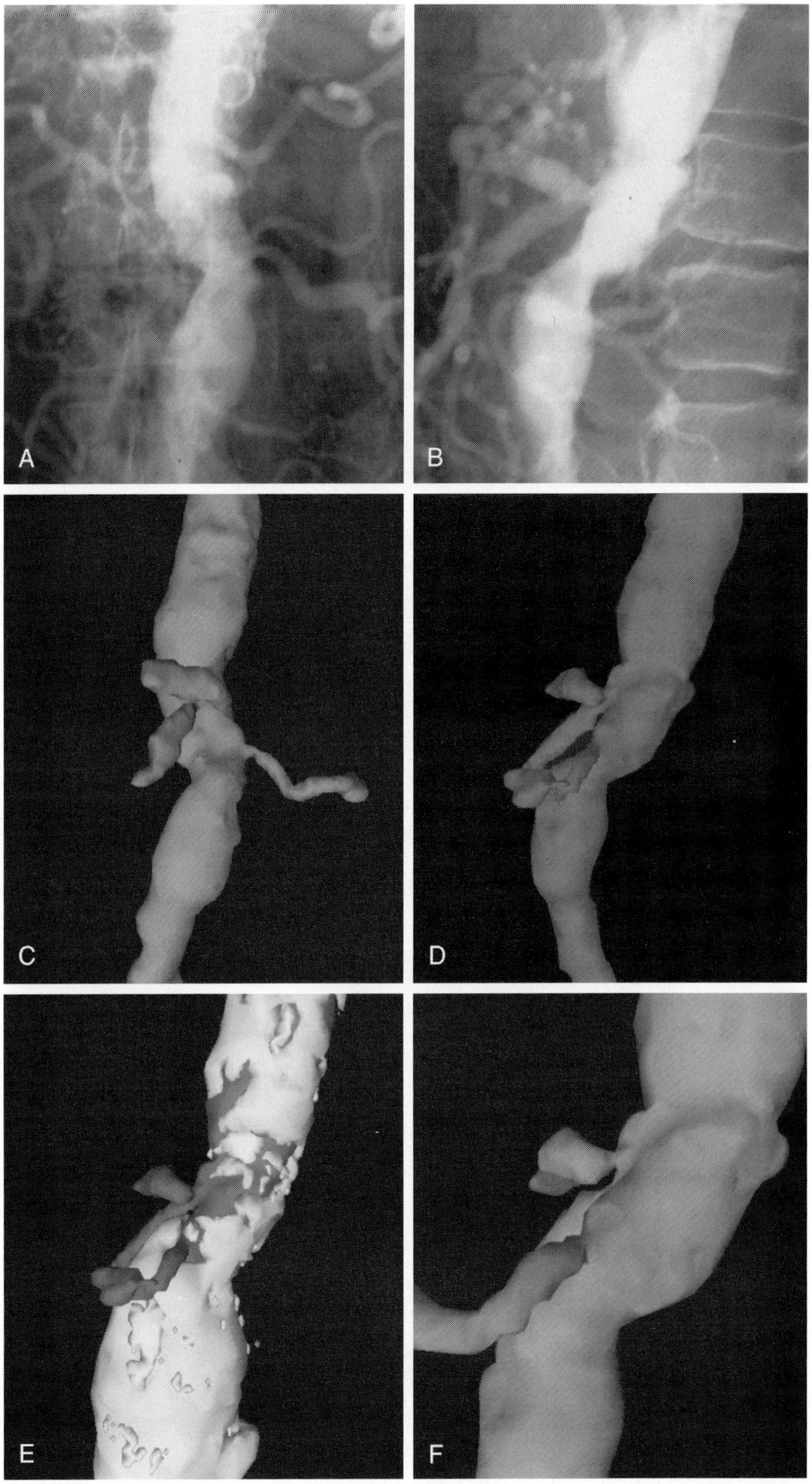

FIGURE 14–27. Anteroposterior (AP) *(A)* and lateral aortographic views *(B)* of what appears to be an infrarenal abdominal aortic aneurysm (AAA). The right renal artery is occluded and the left renal artery has a mild stenosis. *C* and *D,* AP and lateral three-dimensional (3-D) reconstruction images of only the contrast-enhanced blood flow demonstrate the same findings. *E,* Multiple-object 3-D reconstruction with calcified plaque (white) and thrombus (yellow) made visible demonstrates that the AAA actually involves the suprarenal aorta, including the origin of the superior mesenteric artery. This was confirmed at operation. This view of the reconstruction was very useful for determining a good location for the aortic cross-clamp (proximal to the celiac artery) and for determining that beveled anastomosis could be performed along the relatively normal aorta. The left renal artery was reimplanted on an aortic patch following endarterectomy of the plaque at the renal artery origin. *F,* Celiac artery stenosis is demonstrated on a magnified and rotated 3-D reconstruction image with only blood flow made visible. The lesion was confirmed at operation. The celiac stenosis was missed by angiography because it overlapped the superior mesenteric artery on the lateral view. *(C–F,* See Color Plate.)

Unusual Aneurysm Pathology

Occasionally, it may be important to detect the pathology of an aneurysm in addition to its extent. CT has traditionally been an excellent study for demonstrating *ruptured, inflammatory,* and *mycotic aneurysms*. Clinical history and physical examination are important to differentiate these symptomatic aneurysms (clinical aspects are discussed in Chapters 89, 91, and 97). For more subtle presentations, however, CT frequently aids the diagnosis.

Inflammatory aneurysms typically have a thickened wall described as an outer "rind" that is enhanced by the uptake of intravascular contrast (Fig. 14–28*A*). *Mycotic aneurysms* may also have inflammatory aspects, but these are less

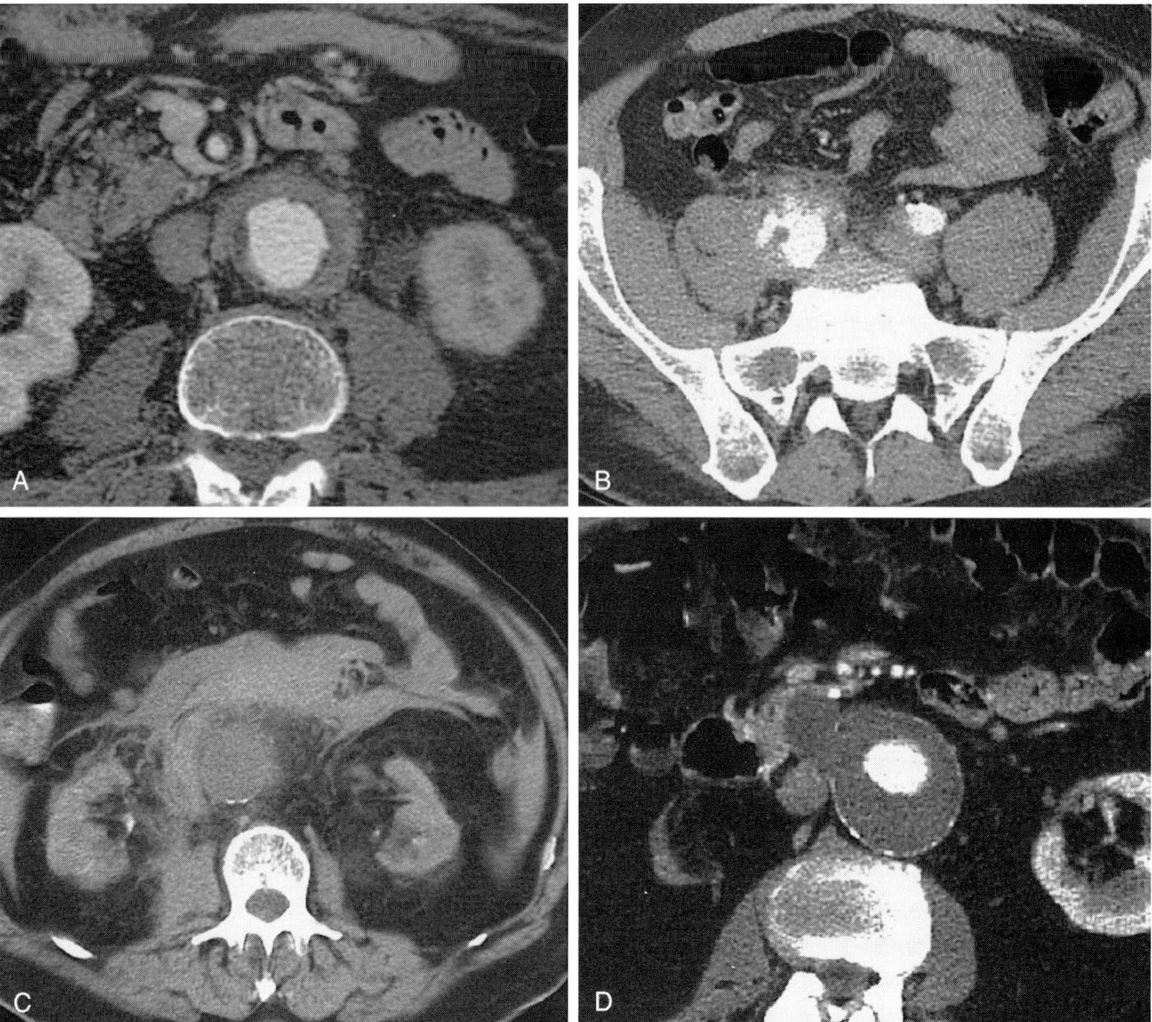

FIGURE 14–28. Variations in aneurysm pathology. *A*, Inflammatory abdominal aortic aneurysm (AAA). In this case, there is a clearly outlined, thickened wall (or rind) that demonstrates mild contrast enhancement. Even when the rind is only mildly enhanced as in this case, it is distinctly different from the intraluminal thrombus within the AAA. *B*, Mycotic right common iliac artery aneurysm. There is also inflammation around mycotic aneurysms, but in this case it is more diffuse and blurs the surrounding tissue planes. Note the irregular, ulcerated lumen. *C*, Ruptured AAA. Blood and water-density material associated with a ruptured aneurysm may also blur soft tissue planes, but frequently the blood dissects extensively through the soft tissue. A focal rupture of the aortic wall may be seen if there is calcification within the wall of the AAA, but often the precise point of rupture is not easily identified. *D*, Focal outpouching from an aneurysm wall, commonly called a "bleb" or blister. Absence of calcification is noted in this portion of the aortic wall, but this patient was completely asymptomatic at elective referral more than 1 week following the CT scan.

circumscribed and tend to extend into adjacent soft tissues. Mycotic aneurysms are also more likely to have an irregular shape or a focal ulceration with a "punched-out" appearance (Fig. 14 28*B*).

Ruptured aneurysms usually have clear extravasation of water or blood-density material that obscures the vessel wall, but this extravasation is usually not contrast-enhanced in a stable patient (Fig. 14–28*C*). While a ruptured aneurysm may have an obvious break in the aortic wall demonstrated by calcifications, discontinuity within the wall can occur in asymptomatic aneurysms without evidence of infection. These focal aortic outpouchings are also known as "blebs," or blisters. Aortic blebs on an AAA have a thinner wall than the surrounding aneurysm or normal aorta and may represent a higher risk for rupture (Fig. 14–28*D*).[52] Infrarenal aortic dissections and isolated iliac artery dissections are uncommon, but we have been able to demonstrate this pathologic feature on more than one occasion using spiral CT with MPR and 3-D models. For iliac artery dissections, standard MPR as well as reformats perpendicular to the vessel are especially helpful (Fig. 14–29).

Pathology in Other Organs

CT demonstrates pathology in the abdomen that is evident in nonvascular structures. An abnormally small kidney with poor contrast enhancement should direct attention to possible renal artery occlusive disease. Aortic emboli might be detected as renal or splenic infarction.

Hepatic air is often a sign of serious disease elsewhere, and CT is the best imaging study for the detection and differentiation of hepatic air.[53]

Air in the portal vein usually extends to the periphery of the liver and may be due to ischemic bowel or an intra-abdominal abscess. Portal venous air should be differentiated from air in the biliary tree, which is usually more

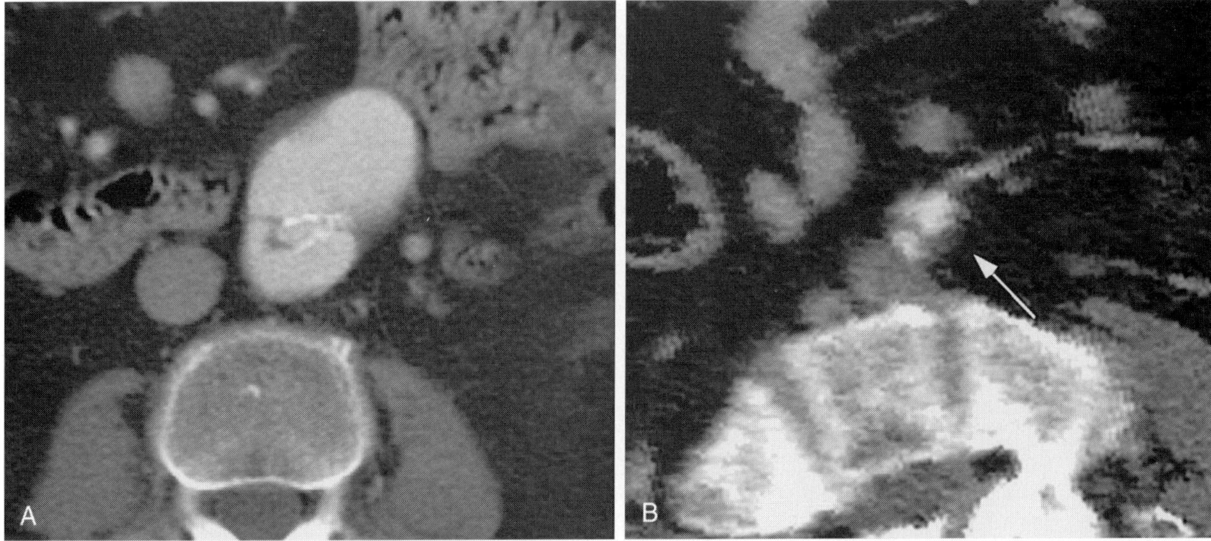

FIGURE 14–29. *A,* Infrarenal aortic dissection with calcified web demonstrated on axial CT scan. This dissection extended into both common iliac arteries. *B,* Isolated left common iliac artery dissection *(arrow)* on a CT slice reformatted perpendicular to the vessel. There was no aortic dissection in this patient, and the isolated iliac artery dissection was not seen on standard CT reformats. The dissection was confirmed at the time of operation. If a reformat perpendicular to the vessel had not been obtained, the patient would have had an aortic tube graft abdominal aortic aneurysmal repair instead of an aortoiliac repair.

centrally located and typically arises from a pathologic or surgically created connection between the biliary tree and the bowel.[53, 54]

Postoperative air within the abdominal cavity itself can be present in the postoperative period for up to 4 weeks,[55, 56] but air in the early postoperative period is not always benign (Fig. 14–30).

Air around an aortic graft at later time points likely represents a graft infection. An aortoenteric fistula may result in CT findings of periaortic inflammation, air, or a focal aortic pseudoaneurysm, and the likelihood of positive findings on CT is extremely high when a graft infection, graft-enteric fistula, or primary aortoenteric fistula from an AAA is present.[57]

Pathology After Open Aneurysm Repair

CT is useful in asymptomatic patients for surveillance at late time points after open AAA repair. In a large population-based study, approximately 10% of patients experienced a major graft complication at a mean follow-up of 6 years after elective open repair.[58] The incidence of late graft complications after ruptured AAA repair is approximately twice the incidence of late graft complications after elective

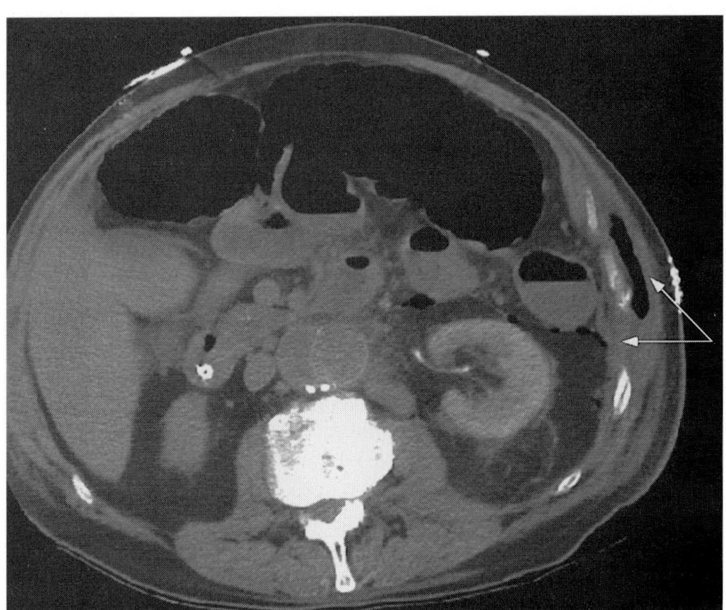

FIGURE 14–30. Abdominal air 1 week following suprarenal abdominal aortic aneurysmal (AAA) repair via a left retroperitoneal approach (arrows). This finding may represent trapped air in the early postoperative period after an AAA repair, but it should be taken seriously. In this case, it was due to a perforation in the sigmoid colon. The air surrounding Gerota's fascia anterior to the kidney is in a tissue plane that was not dissected at the time of initial surgery.

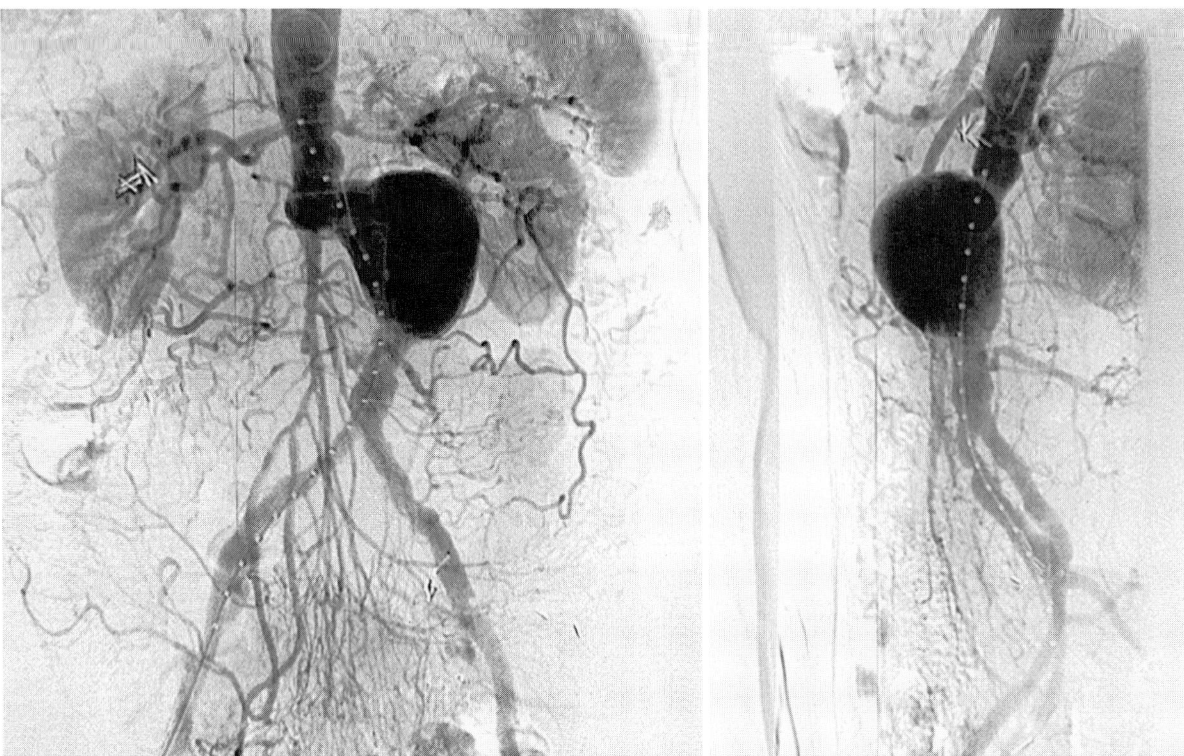

FIGURE 14–31. Demonstration of iliac artery occlusive disease. Compare the right common iliac artery occlusive disease demonstrated on this arteriogram to the multiple-object three-dimensional (3-D) reconstruction from a CT scan of the same patient (see Fig. 14–11). The angiogram catheter is in the right common iliac artery, and the lesion can also be seen on the lateral view. The right common iliac artery occlusive disease is displayed appropriately using the 3-D reconstruction technique in Figure 14–11, but the inclusion of calcified plaque in a single-object surface-shaded display produces a less accurate representation of the anatomy (see Fig. 14–8).

repair.[59] CT is important for follow-up because the most common late graft complication after elective or emergent AAA repair is an asymptomatic pseudoaneurysm.[58, 59]

Occlusive Disease in Aortic Branches

Another key aspect in the preoperative evaluation of AAAs is the extent of occlusive disease in aortic branch vessels. Patients with suspected iliac, renal, or visceral occlusive disease have always required angiography prior to AAA repair because evaluation of occlusive disease has been a traditional downfall of conventional CT.[60] With conventional CT, tube overheating problems limited the number of slices that were able to be obtained and the volume of the body that could be covered by the scan. Therefore, fewer axial slices were obtained in the visceral and renal segments and very few slices were obtained in the iliac segment. The paucity of slices and the tortuosity of the vessels thus made evaluation of occlusive disease difficult.

Spiral CT, however, can cover a large volume and still provide large numbers of thin multiplanar reformats. This ability is key to the evaluation of occlusive disease. Large numbers of thin axial slices make it more likely that a stenosis will be clearly seen on axial slices alone and also improve the quality of MPRs and 3-D reconstructions. Thus, with appropriate scan protocols and adequate timing of the vascular contrast bolus, evaluation of iliac occlusive disease with spiral CT is far superior to conventional CT, rivaling angiography.[8, 9] In our institution, spiral CT with MPRs and 3-D reconstruction is more accurate than spiral CT with axial slices alone or even angiography for evaluation of iliac artery occlusive disease. The accuracy of angiography, of course, is enhanced when multiple views are available, but even so, a multiple-object 3-D reconstruction can reveal details about plaque and relative stenosis with viewpoints from any desired angle. Compare the occlusive disease demonstrated on an angiogram (Fig. 14–31) to the multiple-object 3-D reconstruction from a CT of the same patient (see Figs. 14–10 and 14–11). The principal advantages of angiography for iliac artery occlusive disease include the ability to (1) perform pull-back pressure, (2) measure enhanced gradients, and (3) accomplish therapeutic maneuvers that are impossible with the less invasive CT study.

Renal and Mesenteric Artery Pathology

The evaluation of occlusive disease in the renal and mesenteric vessels is more difficult than evaluation of iliac occlusive disease. The vessels are smaller, the stenotic areas are often short, and the vessels may be oriented perpendicular to conventional axial slices. Again, spiral CT is superior to conventional CT because of the availability of extremely thin (1 to 2 mm) axial slices and multiplanar reconstructions. We generally use a protocol that consists of 3-mm collimation, with 1-mm axial reconstructions (reformats) through the visceral segment. These arteries are best evaluated by views or slices perpendicular to the long axis of the vessel. Thus, the renal arteries are best evaluated with axial, coronal, and 3-D reconstructions, but the celiac and superior mesenteric arteries are best depicted in axial, sagittal, and 3-D reconstructions. CT artefacts are possible, including motion artefacts and partial volume averaging artefact (e.g., signal averaging from dense structures, such as calcium, causes a small rim of adjacent thrombus to have the appearance of contrast-enhanced blood flow). Multiplanar reconstructions are often helpful in this regard, and confidence is increased when a stenosis appears consistently in multiple views.

The utility of spiral CT with 3-D reconstruction for the evaluation of renal artery stenosis is illustrated in Figure 14–32. We have found spiral CT with 3-D reconstruction to be quite accurate compared with angiography and direct inspection at the time of surgery. In a pilot study evaluating the renal and visceral arteries for stenoses greater than 50%, spiral CT with MPRs and interactive 3-D reconstructions had an accuracy of 97% relative to operative findings, which compared well with the 93% accuracy of angiography (unpublished data). Other investigators have also found a high degree of accuracy for evaluation of renal artery stenoses using spiral CT or MPR alone,[8, 61–63] although sensitivities in the 90% range are not universal.[64, 65]

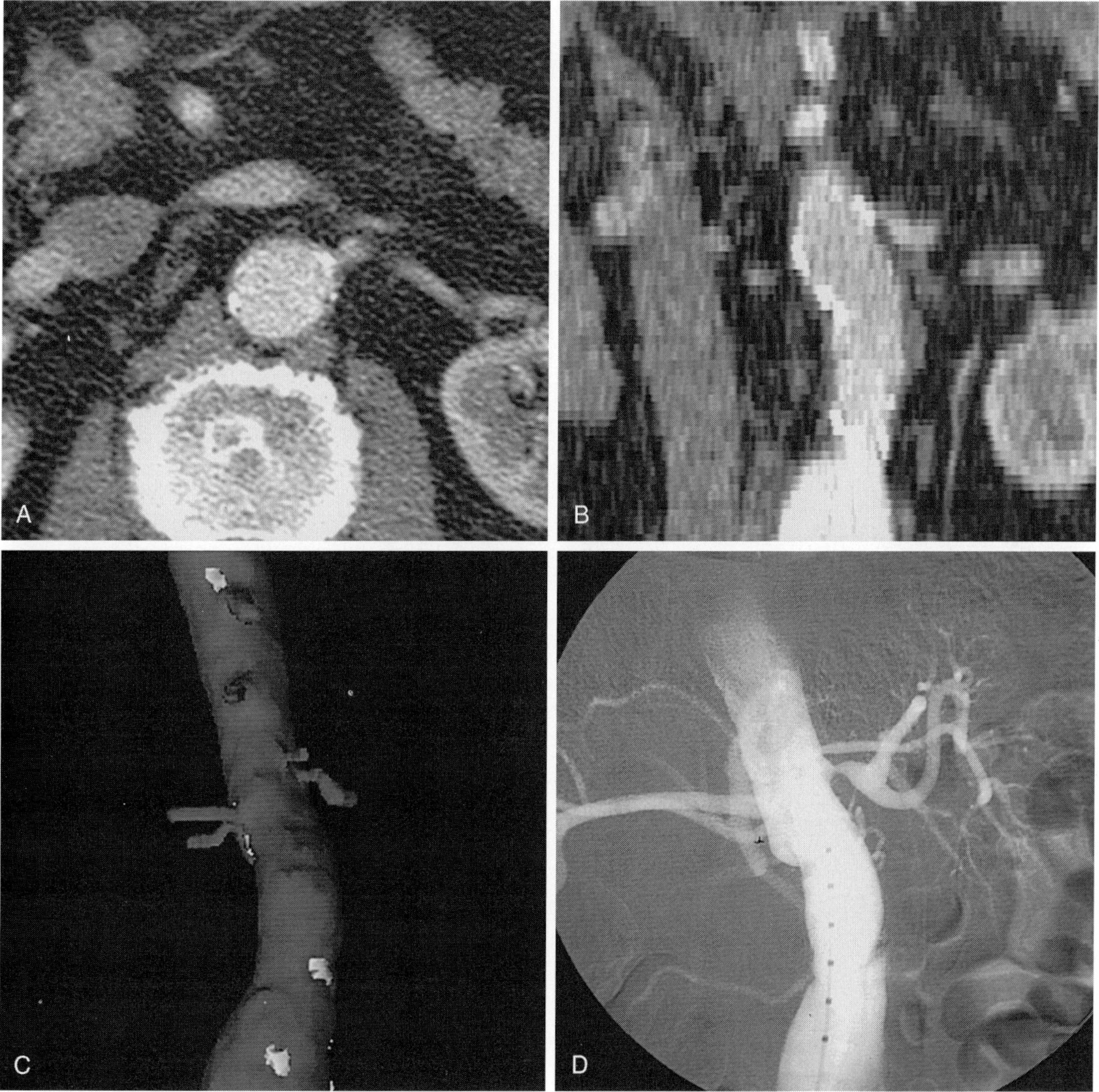

FIGURE 14–32. Spiral CT with three-dimensional (3-D) reconstruction for the evaluation of renal artery stenosis. *A,* Axial CT suggests a left renal artery stenosis, but multiple slices above and below this location must be reviewed because the apparent discontinuity might also be caused by a tortuous artery moving in and out of the plane of the axial CT slice. *B,* Coronal reformat also suggests stenosis, but again multiple slices must be reviewed because the apparent stenosis could be caused by the artery moving in and out of the plane of the reformatted CT slice. *C,* A 3-D reconstruction demonstrates a stenosis in the lower left renal artery near its origin. A left upper pole accessory renal artery and two right renal arteries are also seen. The stenosis and the multiple renal arteries were confirmed by reviewing the entire set of CT slices, as would normally be done in evaluation of this type of stenosis. The depiction of the stenosis cannot be assumed to be accurate until it is confirmed by the CT review; once this is accomplished, the 3-D reconstruction is excellent for preoperative planning because it can be viewed from any desired angle on the computer screen. *D,* Angiogram depicts the left lower renal artery stenosis, the left upper pole accessory renal artery, and two right renal arteries.

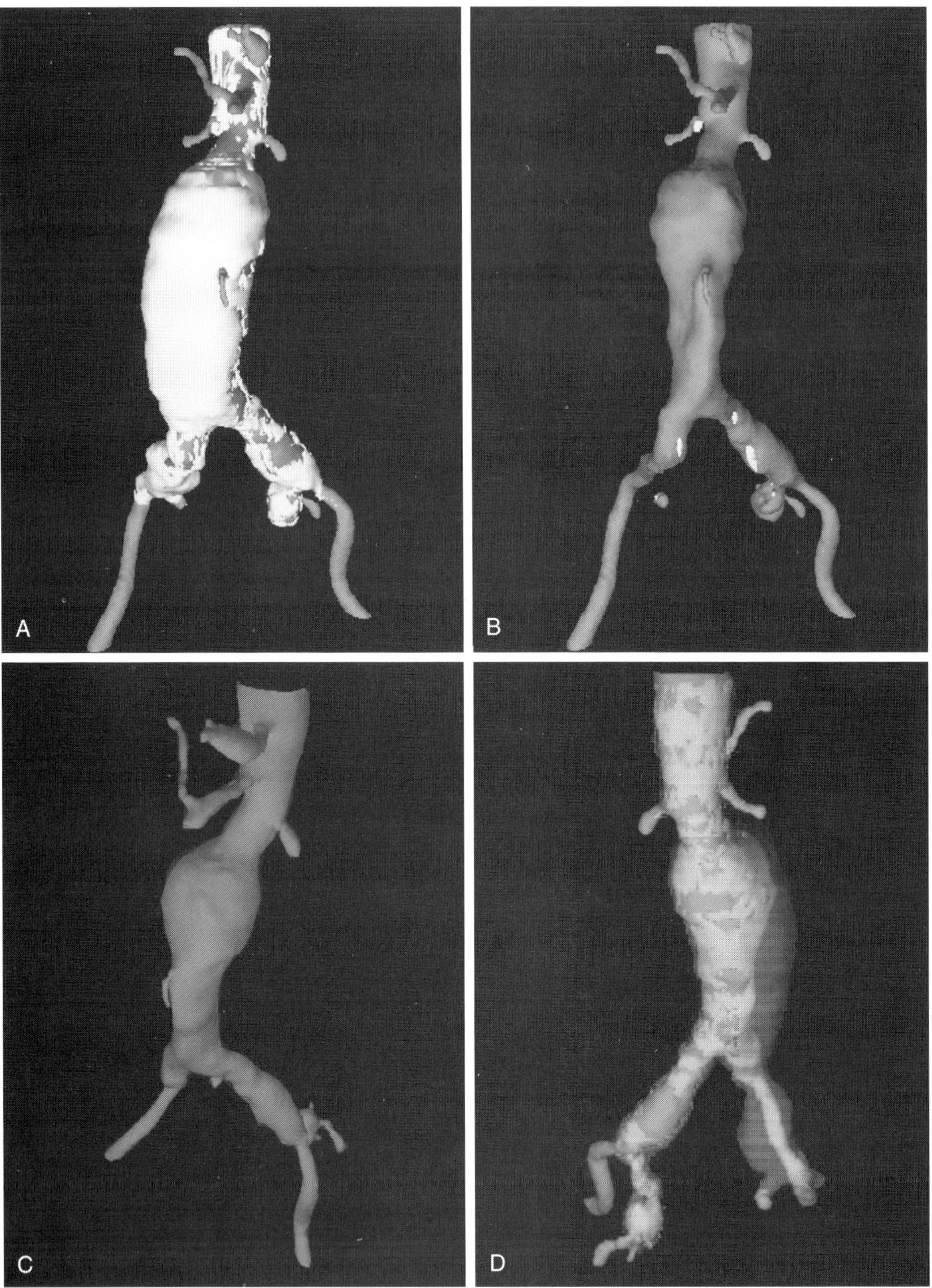

FIGURE 14–33. Demonstration of several abnormalities on one 3-D reconstruction, highlighting the utility of multiple views and a multiple-object display. This study was obtained to evaluate a possible infrarenal abdominal aortic aneurysm (AAA) and also revealed a celiac artery aneurysm, a replaced right hepatic artery arising from the superior mesenteric artery, multiple iliac artery aneurysms, and a right internal iliac artery occlusion. We can best understand the various abnormalities by rotating the model and changing the visibility of thrombus, which can be done in real time on a workstation or a personal computer with specialized software. *A*, Anteroposterior (AP) view of a multiple-object 3-D reconstruction with blood flow (red), thrombus or noncalcified plaque (yellow), and calcified plaque (white) all included in the model. *B*, A 3-D reconstruction with thrombus made invisible demonstrates the right internal iliac artery occlusion. *C*, Oblique view of the 3-D reconstruction demonstrates the celiac artery aneurysm and the replaced right hepatic artery better than other views. *D*, The outflow branches of the left internal iliac artery aneurysm are best seen on a posterior view with thrombus made transparent. (See Color Plate.)

In general, however, the accuracy of spiral CT is uniformly superior to reported values for conventional CT.[60] The depiction of visceral artery stenosis also appears to be accurate in most studies.[8, 64]

Typically, arteriography has also been necessary in evaluation of atypical pathology, such as a replaced right hepatic artery arising from the superior mesenteric artery or visceral artery aneurysms. Current technology has made CT very useful in these areas also. Anatomy that once required angiography can be clearly depicted by 3-D reconstruction of CT data (Fig. 14–33) (see Color Plate). Clearly, 3-D reconstructions for assessment of renal or visceral artery pathology should not be interpreted in the absence of the actual CT data.[65] Any abnormality on the 3-D model should be correlated with the CT images at the same location.

It should be emphasized that a complete CT evaluation of visceral or renal artery occlusive disease includes a thorough study of all available axial slices and MPRs, preferably with magnified views in a "scrolling" or "movie" format on a workstation computer or a personal computer. If 3-D reconstructions are available, magnified and rotated views with and without plaque highlighted are helpful (see Figs. 14–27 and 14–33). Software that allows the CT slice to be inserted into the appropriate location on the 3-D model (for simultaneous viewing) makes correlation easier. One should take care when evaluating single-object SSDs, which may include calcified plaque as part of the contrast-enhanced blood flow (compare Fig. 8–11 and Fig. 14–31 for iliac artery occlusive disease). Appropriate scanning protocols and detailed evaluation are needed to obtain high-quality results, and adjunctive studies, such as duplex scanning, can be helpful. If this latest-generation technology continues to produce excellent results, however, angiography will rarely be necessary for the preoperative evaluation of AAAs and pathology near the origin of the visceral arteries.

Detection of Accessory Renal Arteries and Inferior Mesenteric Artery Patency

It has traditionally been difficult to gain consistent results with conventional CT in detecting accessory renal arteries and the inferior mesenteric artery (IMA). With appropriate protocols, however, spiral CT is fairly effective in detecting the presence and patency of these vessels. A 3-D reconstruction is also helpful in this regard, but the key to accuracy in imaging these vessels involves very thin axial reconstructions and the ability to scroll through every axial slice to look for the presence of these small vessels. With 1- to 2-mm reconstructions, a typical spiral CT scan for AAA evaluation generates hundreds of axial slices. It is not enough to review only the 20 to 40 hard copy images that might be printed from a single scan; the radiologist or surgeon must use the CT workstation to review every axial slice. In our institution, the surgeon uses special software to review each individual slice on a personal computer. Automated 3-D reconstruction algorithms are unreliable for these small vessels because the contrast enhancement may be poor (another form of partial volume averaging) (see Figs. 14–14 and 14–15).

Our current CT scan protocol uses the following:

- Collimation (3 mm) through the visceral-renal segment
- Axial (1-mm) reconstructions
- Scrolling through each of the axial sections (including magnified views)
- Use of multiplanar reformatting to view the vessels in two or three planes
- Usually, 3-D reconstructions capable of displaying the blood flow, thrombus, and calcified plaque as separate objects

The separate objects in the multiple-object 3-D models can also be viewed individually and rotated to view the structure from any angle. We have found this technique to be extremely accurate for detecting the number, location, and patency of accessory renal arteries. When 3-D construction is compared with operative findings, we have identified patent accessory renal arteries with nearly 100% accuracy. Other groups have noted an accuracy of 96% to 100% for the detection of accessory renal arteries.[62, 65, 66] The accuracy of these techniques is now sufficient to use CTA with 3-D reconstruction as the sole preoperative imaging modality for the evaluation of living related transplant donors.[67, 68]

The 3-D reconstructions can also display end-organ parenchyma, which can be useful for living related renal donors or other renal applications (see Fig. 14–12). We have found this technique to be more accurate than angiography in the determination of inferior mesenteric artery patency.

Evaluation of Other Abdominal and Pelvic Pathology

CT has traditionally been found to aid in the detection of unusual structures such as horseshoe kidney (Fig. 14–34) (see Color Plate), retroaortic renal vein, circumaortic renal vein, and duplicate or left-sided vena cava (Fig. 14–35).[51] Owing to technical advantages, spiral CT is excellent for detection of these anomalies. For more complex anomalies, 3-D reconstruction is particularly useful because one can quickly gain a large amount of information about spatial relationships using this technology. Tortuous vessels, and venous pathology in particular, are much more obvious with 3-D reconstruction than with CT alone (Fig. 14–36) (see Color Plate).

Because of the dynamic nature of spiral CT, it can also demonstrate an *aortocaval fistula*, which is usually seen in association with an AAA or a history of back surgery.[69, 70] Preoperative diagnosis of aortocaval fistula is important because of the high mortality rate when the diagnosis is not made before surgery.[71] In the presence of an aortocaval fistula, aortic contrast suddenly decreases distal to the fistula. A sudden decrease in aortic contrast can also occur as a result of poor timing of the contrast infusion, however.

The key to detection of an aortocaval fistula is to appreciate the dramatic density of contrast within the inferior vena cava at the site of the fistula and at more proximal locations. Because of the fistula, the aorta and the vena cava have similar levels of intravascular contrast, and *both* display a sudden decrease in intravascular contrast at precisely the

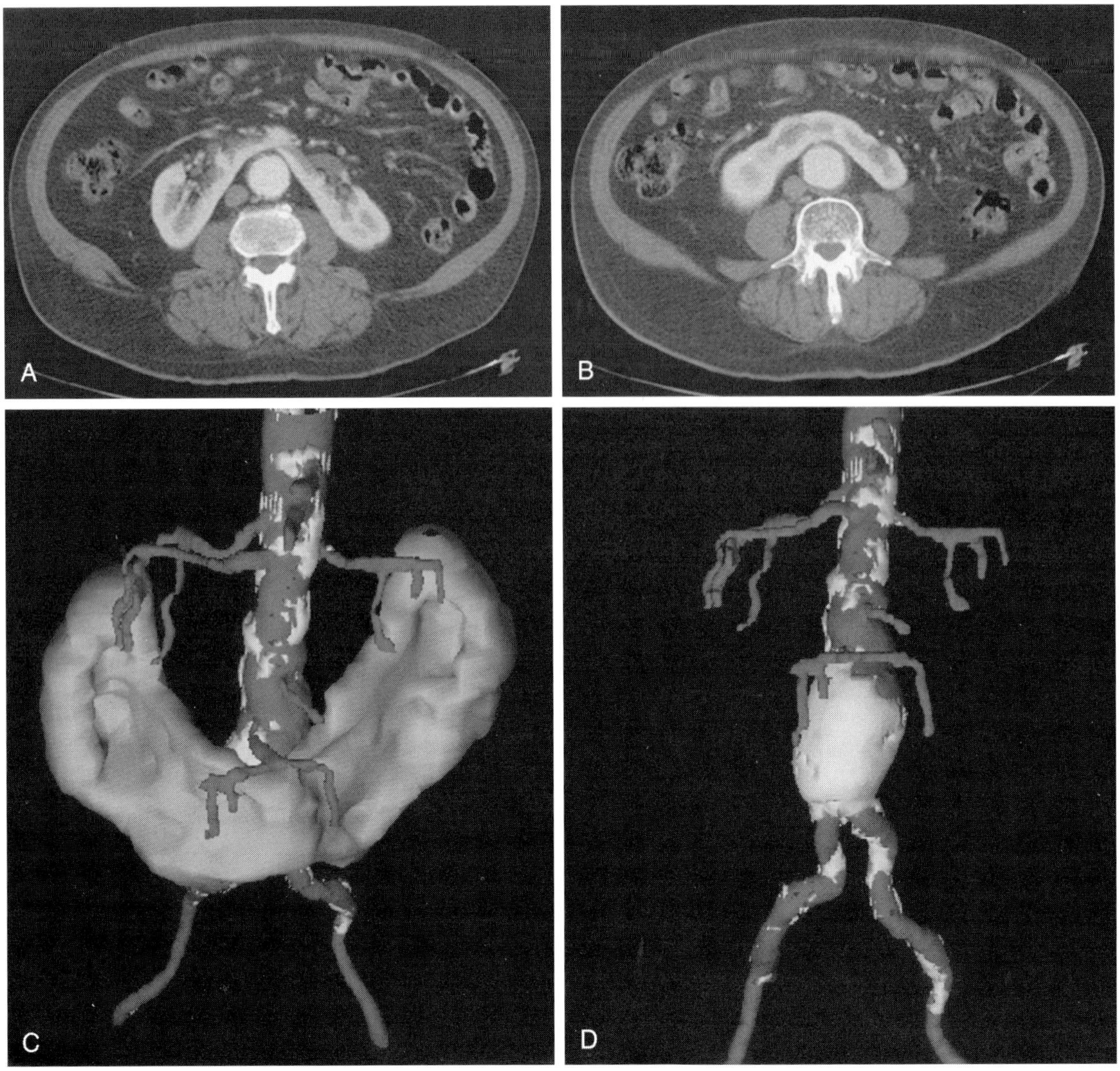

FIGURE 14–34. *A*, Horseshoe kidney on axial CT scan. *B*, The portion of the horseshoe kidney that crosses the midline is often relatively thin, but in this case the parenchyma does not appear to be attenuated. *C*, A 3-D reconstruction with the horseshoe kidney and associated complex blood supply clearly visible. The reconstruction is rotated slightly to demonstrate a stenosis in the lowest midline renal artery near its origins. A very large amount of information is gained rapidly using this technology, as it would be extremely difficult to trace the renal arteries through their course on CT slices. Angiography does not provide a 3-D perspective of the renal parenchyma. *D*, Anteroposterior view of the 3-D reconstruction with the kidney made invisible, demonstrating a small abdominal aortic aneurysm arising just distal to the lowest renal artery (which is in the midline). (*C* and *D*, See Color Plate.)

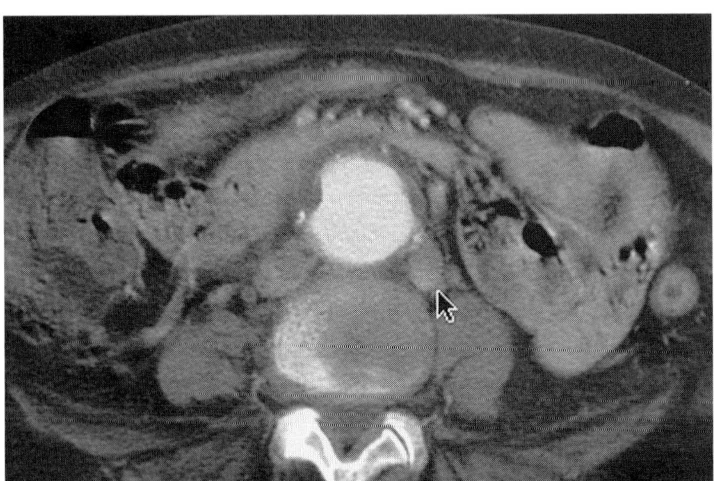

FIGURE 14–35. Duplicate vena cava (*arrow*) seen on axial CT slice.

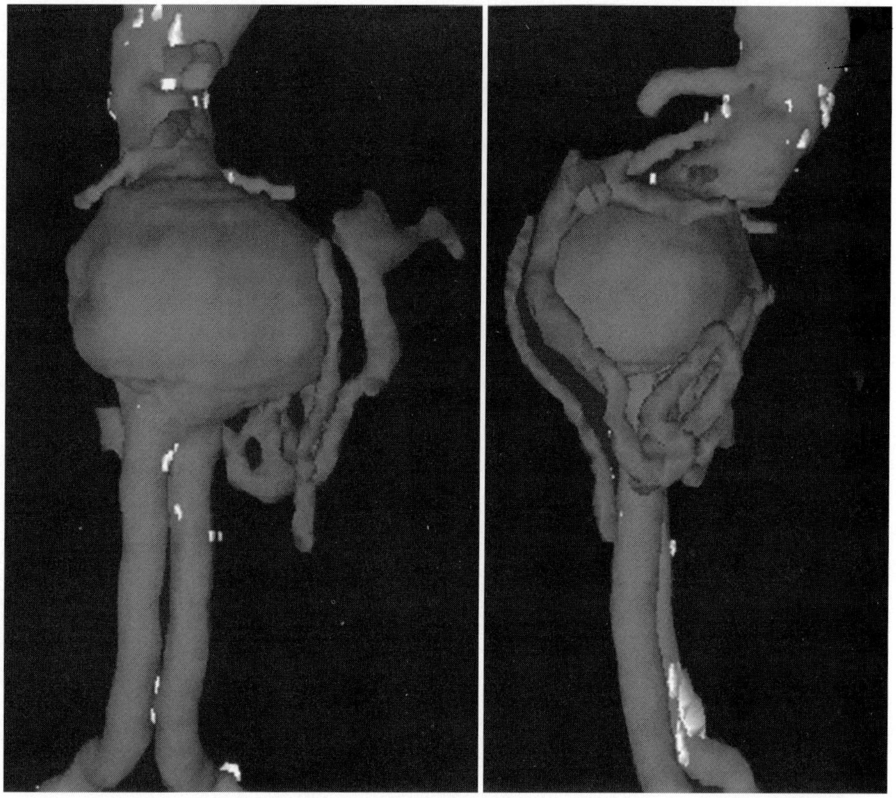

FIGURE 14–36. Three-dimensional (3-D) reconstruction of image occlusion of the left renal vein by an 8-cm aneurysm, which developed proximal to an infrarenal abdominal aortic aneurysm (AAA) repair many years earlier. Huge left-sided venous collaterals and their 3-D relationship to the AAA are easily seen. In this case, 3-D reconstruction changed the operative approach from retroperitoneal to transabdominal. (See Color Plate.)

same location (Fig. 14–37). Spiral CT with MPRs and interactive 3-D reconstructions can also accurately identify infrarenal aortic dissections, iliac artery dissections, the number and location of patent lumbar arteries, and the degree of calcified or noncalcified plaque at the sites of potential anastomoses.

Computed Tomography for Patient Selection and Graft Sizing Before Endovascular Abdominal Aortic Aneurysm Repair

With the advent of endovascular surgery, CT evaluation of aortic aneurysms has gained great importance. Of course, many of the key aspects of preoperative imaging for standard "open" AAA repair and endovascular AAA repair overlap. Clearly, one must be able to evaluate the extent of the aneurysm, any unusual pathology, and the extent of visceral and iliac artery occlusive disease. The degree of imaging accuracy required for endovascular repair, however, is much greater than that required for open repair. A standard open procedure can be modified while it is in progress in order to account for unexpected extension of an aneurysm, accessory renal arteries, or a large patent IMA; in endovascular AAA repair, such corrections are not possible.

Another crucial difference is that graft length and diameter for endovascular repair must be determined *prior* to graft deployment, with a potentially dramatic impact on short-term and long-term outcomes if the measurements are incorrect. Some endograft sizing errors can be corrected without conversion to open repair, but many cannot. Numerous measurements must be performed accurately prior to endovascular AAA repair, including:

- Diameter and length of the aortic "neck"
- Diameter and length of the aortic or iliac "cuffs"
- Length of the graft in relation to the "seal zones"
- Diameter of the access vessels

Even small errors in any one of these measurements can lead to major problems, such as:

- Inability to deploy the endograft
- Graft migration
- Inappropriate occlusion of branch vessels
- Inadequate sealing (endoleak) and subsequent aneurysm rupture

Because of these stringent requirements, preoperative imaging algorithms for endovascular AAA repair at many centers include both CT and angiography. CT scans are used to screen candidates for endovascular repair, to determine the extent of the aneurysm, and to obtain diameter measurements. Angiograms are used for length measurements and evaluation of occlusive disease. While this system has been used successfully in centers of excellence, it has potential pitfalls. Simple axial CT slices often do not cut through planes perpendicular to the vessel, resulting in elliptical cross sections that can make diameter measurements difficult (Fig. 14–38).

Generally, the narrowest diameter of the elliptical cross section is the "true" arterial diameter, but this is not always the case because the aorta does not always have a simple cylindrical or conical shape. Thus, conventional CT may lead to a slight overestimation of diameter on axial slices, while spiral CT slices reconstructed perpendicular to the vessel tend to be more accurate.[12, 72] Simply using sagittal or coronal reconstruction is not always adequate, because

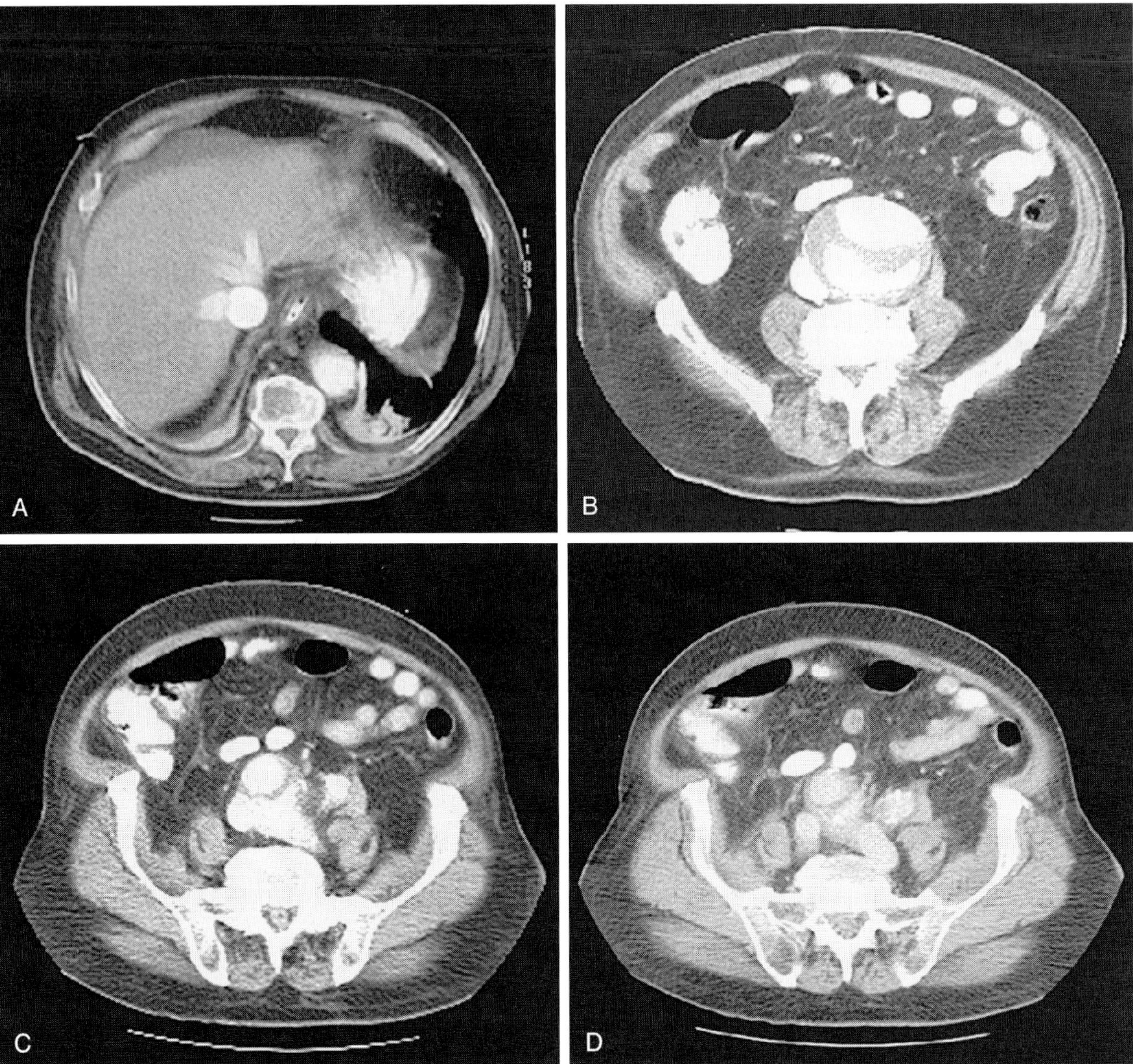

FIGURE 14–37. Aortocaval fistula associated with an abdominal aortic aneurysm (AAA), seen here on axial CT scans. The key to detection of an aortocaval fistula is to appreciate the dramatic change in contrast within the inferior vena cava at the site of the fistula and at more proximal locations. *A,* The vena cava is dramatically enhanced by intravascular contrast, even at locations quite proximal to the fistula. *B,* Central portion of the AAA demonstrating continued bright enhancement of the vena cava and and an aortic web or dissection. *C,* Axial CT scan just proximal to the site of the fistula. The aortic web is still present, and the contrast enhancement of the vena cava is still similar to that of the aorta. *D,* Axial CT scan just distal to the fistula. Since the bowel opacification has not changed, the dramatic change in intraluminal contrast is not due to a change in the CT window level. If the change in contrast were simply due to poor timing of the intravenous contrast bolus, the aortic contrast might suddenly decrease, but there would not be a simultaneous change from dense contrast to dilute contrast within the vena cava at the same location.

these sections may not be perpendicular to the vessel either or may not cut through the center of the vessel over an adequate length. Curvilinear reformats make length measurements difficult and straighten out angles that may affect an endovascular repair.

Owing to length measurement difficulties associated with conventional and even spiral CT, the current standard is to perform angiography with a graduated marker catheter for length measurements and simultaneous evaluation of occlusive disease prior to endovascular repair. Unfortunately, angiography provides a 2-D projection of a 3-D structure, making interpretation of the true anatomic dimensions more difficult. Moreover, the catheter does not usually follow the proposed graft path, since its diameter is not the same as that of the endograft. Thus, one must estimate how far the catheter deviates from the likely graft path in order to make adjustments to the proposed graft length. It has also become clear that angiography tends to *systematically* underestimate diameter measurements by 6% to 17%, even with orthogonal views using a marker catheter and appropriate calibration.[12, 72] Thus, even with a combination of conventional CT and angiography, measurements are still difficult and sometimes inaccurate. Spiral CT with 3-D reconstruction and CT reformats perpendicular to the vessel lumen eliminate the diameter measurement problems associated with the other techniques (see Fig. 14–38).[12, 72]

CTA with 3-D reconstruction offers several other important benefits that are crucial for imaging prior to endovascular surgery.[4, 12, 72] In conjunction with spiral CTA and

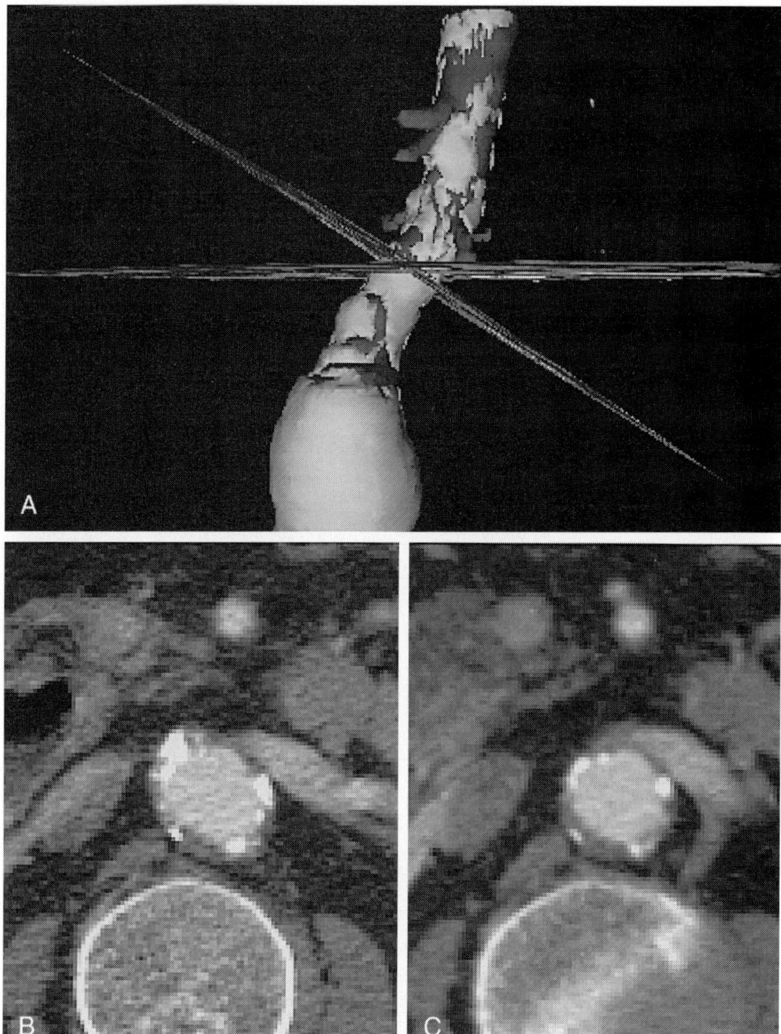

FIGURE 14–38. Diameter measurement issues and solutions using CT. *A,* Three-dimensional (3-D) reconstruction with simultaneous display of CT slices in 3-D space. The CT slices shown here are a standard axial reformat and a reformat perpendicular to the aorta. The 3-D model was rotated to demonstrate the intersection of the two CT slices at the same location on the aorta. *B,* The same axial CT slice shown in *A.* The axial slice does not intersect the aortic neck perpendicular to its axis, thus creating an elliptical cross section. Although the smaller diameter (minor axis of the ellipse) is usually very similar to the true diameter, elliptical cross sections also occur in noncylindrical vessels and at the margins of aneurysms. Viewing multiple cross sections in sequence can help with this problem, but evaluation is still difficult. *C,* The CT slice reformatted perpendicular to the aorta (shown in *A*) accurately depicts the essentially circular lumen and provides a diameter measurement without ambiguity. This cross section of the aorta also provides a more correct impression of thrombus thickness, which is artefactually enhanced on an elliptical cross section. Note the renal vein and vertebrae, which help verify the magnification, location, and orientation of the slices.

multiplanar reformats, 3-D reconstruction speeds assimilation of the CT data and makes the extent of the aneurysm rapidly apparent.[10, 11] More important, specialized measurement software and unique aspects of the 3D reconstruction can eliminate most of the measurement problems associated with conventional techniques. Software algorithms can be used to display the center line of the blood flow channel in the infrarenal aorta and iliac arteries, allowing length measurements along the vessel center line in tortuous aortic or iliac segments. In some systems, graft paths along a line other than the center line can also be defined by the user, which is necessary because an endovascular graft may not follow the center line of the blood flow channel throughout its entire course. We have used such a system for a large number of endovascular AAA repairs and found it to be extremely accurate. In test phantoms and in our clinical experience, the center line and user-defined graft path innovations described herein have eliminated length measurement problems.[72, 73] Several similar systems are commercially available or in development, and at least two have reported success using this type of specialized software for length measurements.[12, 72–74]

In a comparative study using life-size models with shapes similar to actual AAAs, we have compared (1) spiral CT alone, (2) angiography with a 1-cm graduated catheter, (3) intravascular ultrasonography (IVUS), and (4) CTA with interactive 3-D reconstructions and specialized measurement software.[72] Although all of these methods produced reasonable results in experienced hands, with care taken to avoid pitfalls, CTA with interactive 3-D reconstructions was the only imaging method that was accurate for *both* diameter and length measurements, thus allowing it to be used reliably as the sole preoperative imaging modality. This technique (CTA/3-D) is also less invasive and less expensive than the combination of other techniques that would otherwise be necessary.

Another unique innovation made possible by CTA with interactive 3-D reconstructions and specialized software is a technique that we have termed "virtual graft," in which the diameter, length, and path of a proposed endograft can be simulated in 3-D space.[74] This simulated graft can be displayed within the 3-D model of the AAA and used to investigate potential problems with endograft sizing, kinking, and stenosis (Fig. 14–39) (see Color Plate). It is also useful for determining the diameter, length, extent of overlap, and number of components needed for modular endografts. We have used other aspects of this system to evaluate the proposed access path for the delivery system (including

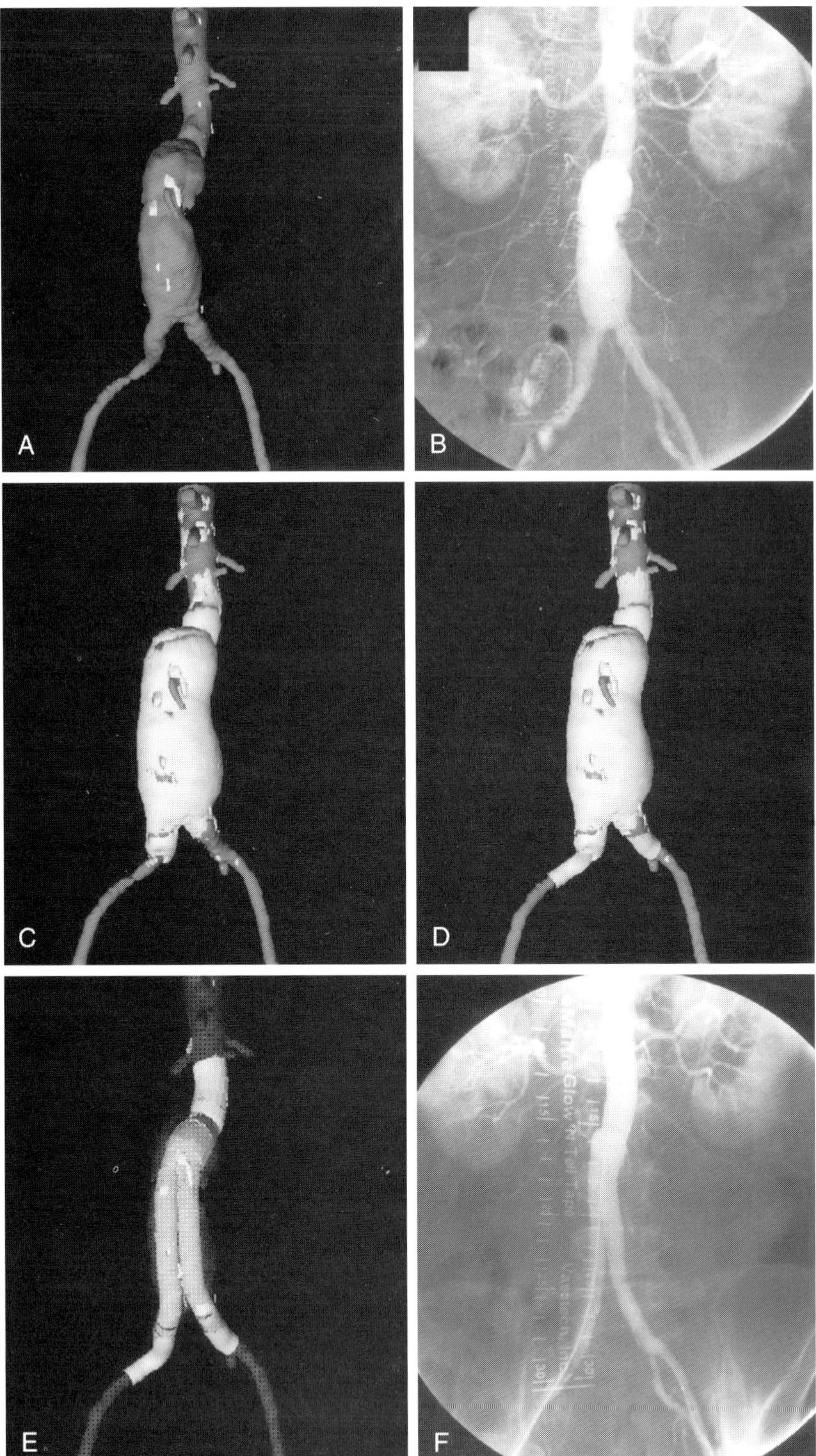

FIGURE 14–39. *See legend on opposite page*

iliac artery tortuosity, diameter, and calcification) and have found it extremely helpful. Other institutions have also demonstrated that CTA alone can be accurate for the evaluation of iliac artery occlusive disease.[8, 9]

In our institution, spiral CTA with interactive 3-D reconstruction has almost entirely eliminated the need for angiography prior to endovascular AAA repair. This method has reliably demonstrated important anatomic features that were either unclear or not demonstrated on conventional CT or angiographic imaging. We also found graft sizing to be accurate and reliable with this method and angiographic measurements to be misleading.

Even though the technique does require special software and a dedicated team, including a radiologist, technologist, and surgeon, to produce quality results, it appears that spiral CT with 3D reconstruction and specialized software is emerging as the standard for the preoperative evaluation of patients prior to endovascular AAA repair for the following reasons:

- Unique imaging capabilities
- Superior measurement accuracy
- Lower cost
- Decreased radiation dose
- Reduced patient morbidity

The key with this modality is to have good CT imaging protocols, 3-D reconstruction software that has been validated in phantoms and in clinical use, and proper training in the use of the software. Specialized software and 3-D reconstructions can also be used in this fashion with MRI/MRA, but MR evaluations of this type are currently limited by generally lower resolution, difficulty in imaging calcified plaque, limitations in volume covered, patient claustrophobia, and expense. Many of these limitations are being addressed for MR, but currently CT has significant advantages in this area if the patient has adequate renal function to tolerate the contrast load.

Postoperative Follow-up for Endovascular Abdominal Aortic Aneurysm Repair

Unlike the case with standard open aortic aneurysm repair, follow-up is crucial for endovascular AAA repair. If there is no perigraft flow or endoleak following endograft placement, the natural history is a decrease in aneurysm size.[75–77] However, an aneurysm occasionally enlarges without apparent endoleak, and ruptures can occur in this situation.[78, 79] A late, secondary endoleak, which can lead to rupture, is also a possibility.[80, 81] Late stent-graft deformation is an important issue for long-term follow-up because it can also lead to late secondary endoleak, aneurysm rupture, or graft thrombosis.[80, 81]

Spiral CT is a primary imaging modality after endovascular AAA repair. It is generally considered to be more sensitive to endoleak than duplex scanning, and CT provides more accurate and reproducible diameter measurements than duplex does.[82, 83] Spiral CT is strongly preferred over conventional CT; spiral CT is capable of small reconstruction intervals and multiplanar reconstructions.[4] Using a CT workstation or specialized software, one can look at highly magnified views of axial reconstructions or multiplanar reconstructions in rapid sequence to "follow" a suspected endoleak to potential inflow and outflow sources. The latter technique is strongly recommended over simple review of selected small hard copy images, in which subtle endoleaks may be missed. Delayed scans following contrast infusion also improve accuracy when one is trying to detect an endoleak.[84] When specialized software is available for 3-D reconstruction of spiral CT data, it is helpful for visualization of aneurysm and endograft deformation. The 3-D reconstructions also aid the examiner to characterize endoleak by demonstrating the inflow and outflow sources in a single image, even if the endoleak is subtle or difficult to interpret on individual CT images (Fig. 14–40) (see Color Plate).

Volume Measurements

A 3-D reconstruction can be used to calculate the volume of any structure in the 3-D model, and data regarding imaging for tumors and other 3-D structures indicate volume measurements are much more sensitive to a change in size than maximal diameter measurements.[85, 86] We have found that volume data appear to be much more sensitive than maximum diameter for the detection of AAA size changes following endovascular AAA repair.[87] The early detection of aneurysm enlargement can be crucial in follow-up for endovascular repair because it indicates the aneurysm is still at risk for rupture and usually precedes evidence of endoleak or overt rupture.[75–79] Thus, CT volume measurements may become a standard postoperative test for aneurysm exclusion or risk of rupture.

FIGURE 14–39. Use of CT with three-dimensional (3-D) reconstruction and specialized software in endovascular abdominal aortic aneurysmal repair.

A, Preoperative 3-D reconstruction showing contrast-enhanced blood flow (red) and calcified plaque (white). Owing to the accuracy of this technique, preoperative angiograms are not necessary.

B, Angiogram performed on the operating table at the time of the procedure, which is necessary to deliver the device even if a preoperative angiogram had been performed. Note the similarity to the 3-D reconstruction.

C, Preoperative 3-D reconstruction including thrombus, demonstrating the need for CT prior to endovascular repair. The iliac arteries are aneurysmal proximally, especially on the left. The endograft cannot be implanted into thrombus and must be long enough to achieve a seal in the normal common iliac artery.

D, Preoperative planning with a "virtual graft," which is displayed in bright yellow. The brighter yellow of the simulated endograft protrudes beyond the red blood flow and the lighter yellow of the thrombus for sufficient lengths proximally and distally; thus, this 3-D reconstruction demonstrates that the proposed graft is appropriately oversized to achieve a seal at the neck of the infrarenal aorta and in the iliac arteries. This view rapidly provides a check to be sure that the proposed endograft is not too small or excessively oversized. It also graphically demonstrates the quality and length of the "seal zone."

E, Preoperative stimulation using the virtual endograft, in this case with thrombus invisible and blood flow made transparent to better demonstrate the anticipated course of the proposed endograft. The prediction here is that the endograft will dilate as it exits the aortic neck (consistent with the degree of oversizing) and deviate slightly at the same location because it must follow the aortic lumen. It is anticipated that some deviation and constriction of the limbs will occur at the aortic bifurcation, but this does not appear to be excessive. This same technology and display is used to evaluate graft length along the center line of the lumen or along a user-defined path. In this case, the length and diameter of the endograft were simulated to coincide with an available graft size. An endograft of this length is anticipated to end just above the left internal iliac artery origin and extend beyond the right iliac artery stenosis if it is deployed appropriately (with the proximal endograft just below the renal arteries).

F, Completion angiogram at the time of the procedure verifies the accuracy of the preoperative computer simulation. The endograft was deployed just below the renal arteries and ends just above the left internal iliac artery origin. The endograft also extends beyond the right iliac stenosis, which is no longer apparent. (*A, C, D,* and *E,* See Color Plate.)

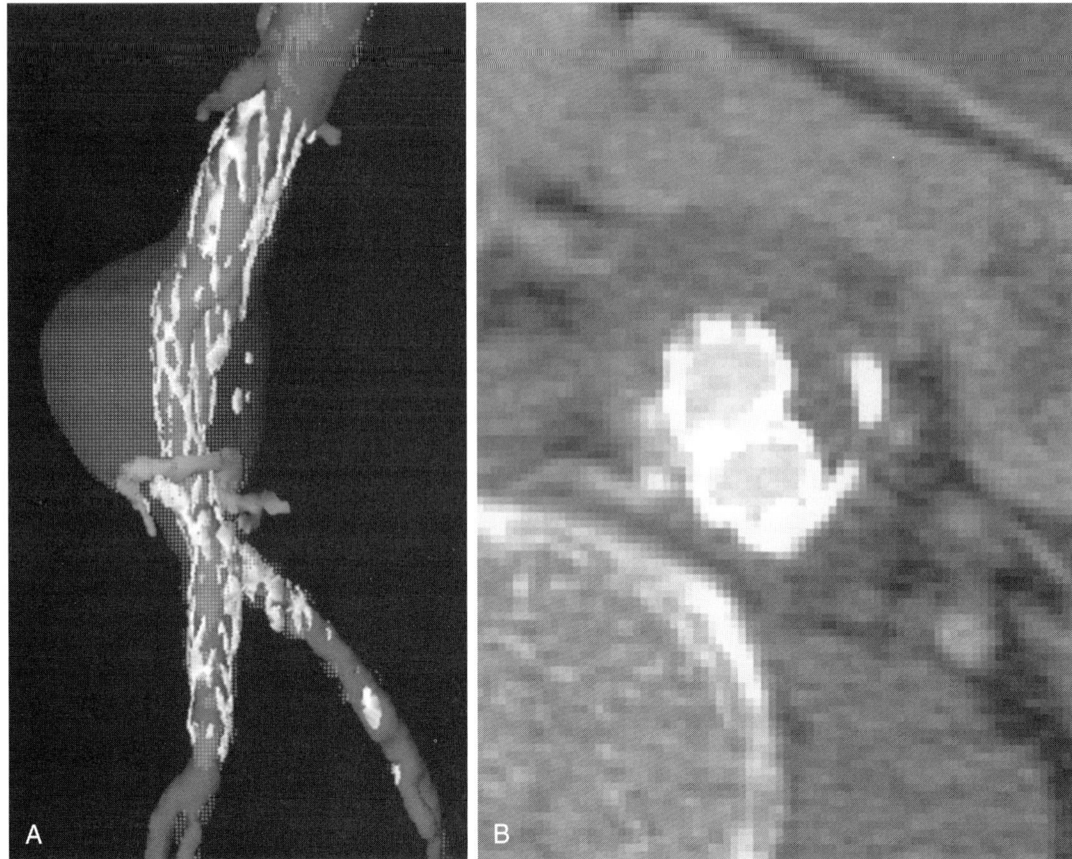

FIGURE 14–40. Perigraft flow (endoleak) following endovascular abdominal aortic aneurysmal repair, as displayed on three-dimensional (3-D) reconstruction *(A)* and axial CT *(B)* images. The 3-D reconstruction (created from the CT data) is rotated to a posterolateral view. Multiple-object 3-D display includes the densities consistent with contrast-enhanced lumen (red); thrombus and noncalcified plaque (yellow, made transparent to display the endoleak); calcified plaque and metallic stent (white); and contrast-enhanced endoleak (magenta). The 3-D display demonstrates that the endoleak is associated with a patent lumbar artery and a patent inferior mesenteric artery (IMA). The axial CT cross section shows the endograft; contrast enhancement outside the lumen of the endograft (endoleak); the patent lumbar artery connecting to the endoleak; and a contrast-enhanced IMA. From a single axial slice, it is impossible to decipher the connection to the IMA, which could be filling via collateral flow. The 3-D reconstruction immediately conveys the relationship of the endoleak to the other structures in a much more intuitive fashion than that obtainable by scrolling through multiple CT slices. (*A*, See Color Plate.)

Lower Extremity

With the introduction of spiral CT and CTA, the use of CT for evaluation of infrainguinal vascular disease has been increasing. Although duplex scanning and MRA have dominated noninvasive imaging of the lower extremities, CT still has a role in selected cases. CT is quite useful for the evaluation of femoral and popliteal artery aneurysms. With the use of CTA and 3-D reconstructions, CT can effectively demonstrate the location and extent of aneurysmal disease (Fig. 14–41) (see Color Plate). In conjunction with the history and physical examination, CT can rule out significant occlusive disease in the superficial femoral or popliteal artery, but it is not the most cost-effective study in this regard unless it is used in conjunction with aneurysm localization.

CT can be very helpful for detecting unusual pathology, such as popliteal entrapment syndrome[88, 89] and adventitial cystic disease (Fig. 14–42).[88, 90] In fact, spiral CT evaluation of vascular disease in the thigh and popliteal fossa—including occlusive disease—appears to be more accurate than angiography.[88, 90] CT evaluation of tibial-level disease is much more difficult, however, because it is difficult to time the intravenous contrast delivery in a manner that enhances the arteries sufficiently without also enhancing the adjacent veins to a similar extent. Arteriovenous malformations in the lower extremity present similar difficulties; they can be imaged by CT but are usually better delineated by MRA.

Venous Pathology

Throughout our text on clinical applications, we have documented the use of CT to evaluate venous pathology. CT is most useful for demonstrating venous anomalies around arterial structures of interest (e.g., a retroaortic renal vein, a circumaortic renal vein, a duplicate vena cava, a left-sided vena cava, or an aortocaval fistula). The utility of spiral CT for demonstrating pulmonary embolus appears promising.

Although MR generally delineates arteriovenous malformations better than CT does, spiral CT can be useful in

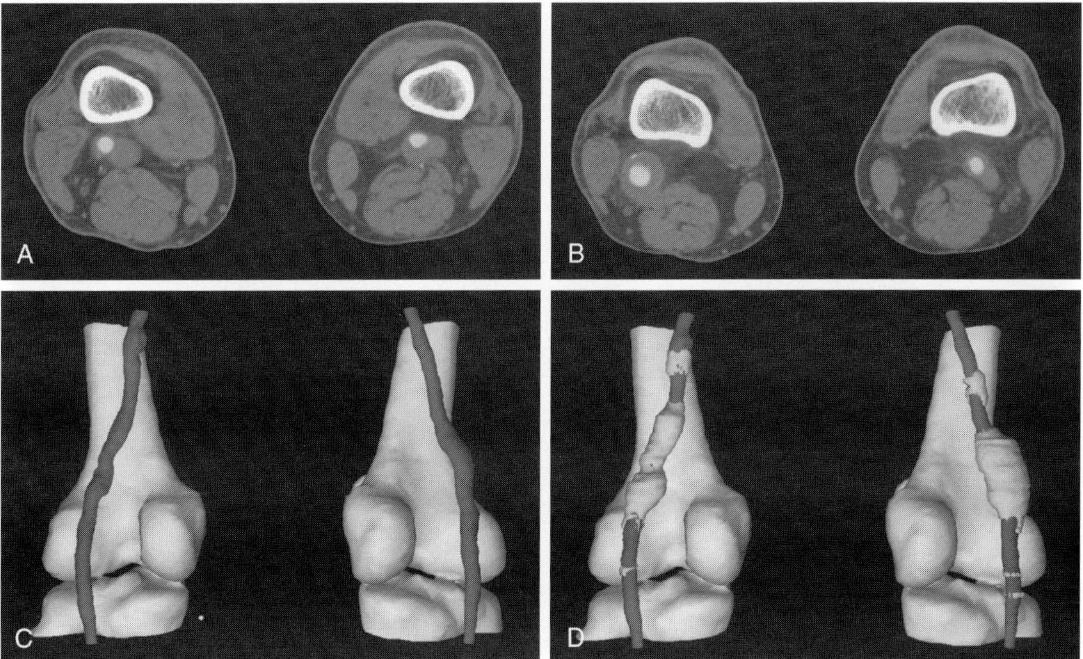

FIGURE 14–41. Bilateral popliteal aneurysms. *A,* The lumen can have a variable appearance, as demonstrated by the eccentric cross section on the patient's left *(right). B,* This axial CT cross section demonstrates a more characteristic circular lumen with circumferential thrombus on the patient's right *(left).* As with other aneurysms, the diameter of the contrast-enhanced lumen does not correlate with the outer diameter of the vessel, thus making angiography a poor diagnostic modality. *C,* Posterior view of the 3-D reconstruction with only the contrast-enhanced blood flow (red) and bones (white) made visible. This view is similar to an angiogram and would not depict the full extent of the aneurysms. The patient had no occlusive disease on ultrasound examination or ankle-brachial indices. *D,* This posterior view of the 3-D reconstruction, with thrombus and plaque added, nicely depicts the full extent of the aneurysms. In this case, bypass of the lesions could be performed without angiography. (*C* and *D,* See Color Plate.)

selected cases (Fig. 14–43) (see Color Plate).[91, 92] CT has a sensitivity of 85% in detection of esophageal varices compared to endoscopy and has the advantage of demonstrating collateral pathways and large portosystemic shunts with greater sensitivity than angiography does.[93] In selected cases, CT is also useful for the evaluation of portal, mesenteric, caval, or iliac vein thrombosis.[94–96]

The Future

"Fifth-generation" CT scanners have been developed, and eventually they may see widespread commercial use. With such scanners, the x-ray beam is moved electronically and the detector array encompasses 360 degrees; thus, there are no physical components to rotate in the gantry. These scanners offer the promise of scan times so rapid that even cardiac motion is not problematic. Because of the speed of beam movement, tube overheating should also be less problematic, since as many as 32 complete (360-degree) cross sections can be performed in 1 second. Other advances may include adding detectors in the Z direction to improve longitudinal resolution.

Three-dimensional reconstruction is already commonplace, and this method will continue to become more sophisticated and easier to perform. Interactive 3-D reconstruction is now available, and research is being performed that incorporates these interactive models into fluoroscopic images in real time. This form of "enhanced reality" may be used to enhance angiography and other invasive procedures. The 3-D reconstructions are also being studied in advanced simulators ("virtual reality"), which may be useful for teaching or learning new techniques. The extent to which these advances will be clinically useful remains to be seen, but current computer technology is allowing rapid advancement in these elements of imaging technology.

Despite advances in CT, MR will continue to have a role in certain conditions, such as intracranial lesions and arteriovenous malformations. However, MR is limited by patient tolerance, implanted devices, resolution, display of calcified plaque, display of thrombus, availability, and expense. CT will thus remain the imaging modality of choice for pathology that is displayed in a similar manner on both CT and MR (except for the few patients with severe renal insufficiency who are not receiving dialysis treatment).

SUMMARY

Spiral CT, CTA, and 3-D reconstruction techniques continue to increase the clinical role of CT in vascular surgery. Techniques such as multiplanar reformatting and 3-D reconstruction are helpful in many cases and crucial in others. Traditionally, delineation of key anatomic features has required a combination of conventional CT and angiography, but only state-of-the-art spiral CT with MPRs is necessary in many cases. When "basic" CTA is not sufficient, more recent advances increase the utility even further. Reformats perpendicular to the vessel lumen are helpful when precise measurements of vessel diameter are needed.

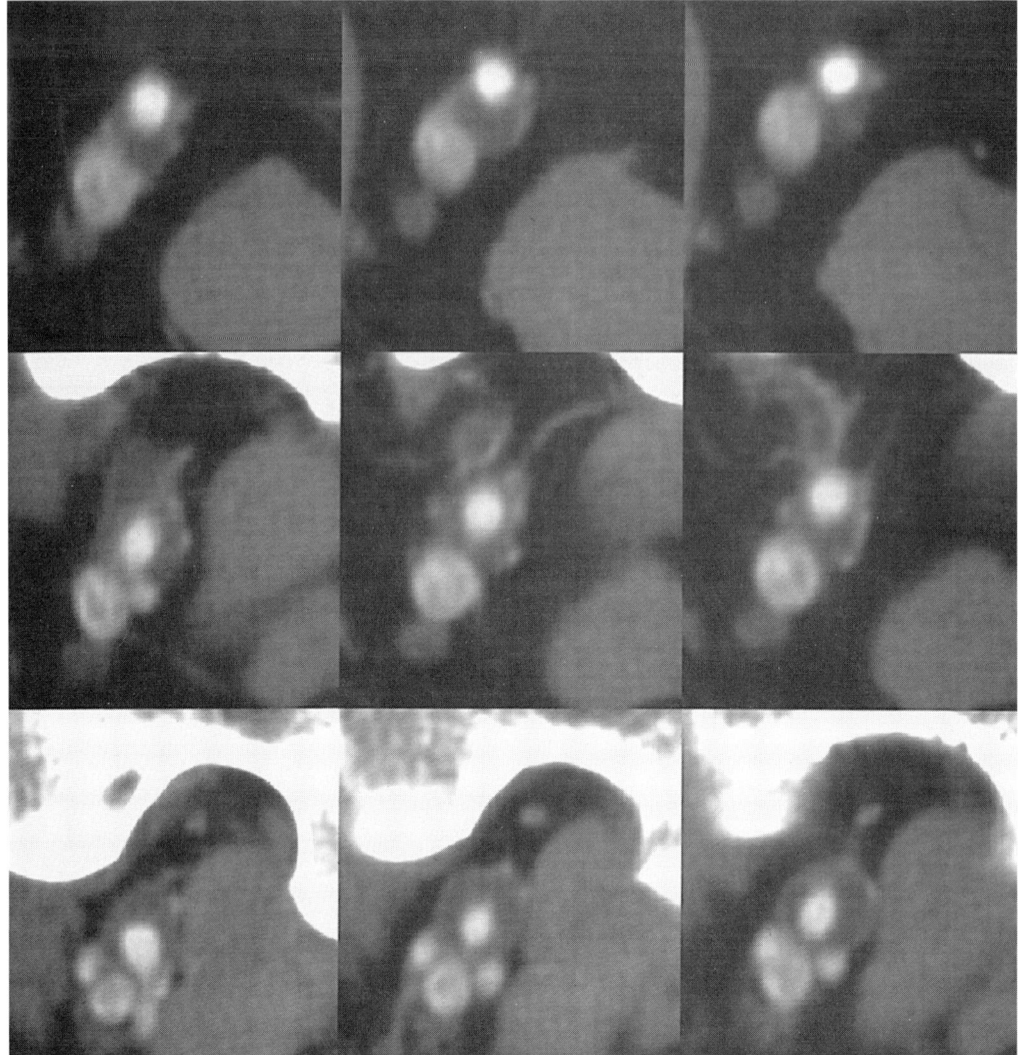

FIGURE 14–42. Adventitial cystic disease. Sequential axial CT slices through the popliteal fossa reveal the varied appearance of adventitial cystic disease in a single patient. Some locations have a circular cross section with the cyst surrounding the entire circumference, giving the appearance of a popliteal artery aneurysm. In other locations, however, the cysts have a characteristic multiloculated appearance. The panel in the second row, *far right*, demonstrates a portion of the cyst extending toward the joint space. Bony structures and the joint space are at the *top* in each panel.

The addition of 3-D reconstruction can provide further insight, especially if thrombus and calcified plaque are depicted as separate objects. Access to a CT workstation or specialized software is helpful for delineating many anatomic features, and crucial for evaluations such as visceral artery occlusive disease, patency of the accessory renal arteries and inferior mesenteric artery, and preoperative planning in endovascular surgery.

With appropriate protocols, spiral CT with MPRs and 3-D reconstruction appears to be more accurate than conventional CT or angiography in the evaluation of (1) suprarenal aortic aneurysms, (2) the potential for endovascular aneurysm repair, (3) endograft sizing, and (4) suspected occlusive disease as well as in delineation of complex anatomy. As this technology becomes more widely available and more thoroughly evaluated, it will continue to decrease or eliminate the need for preoperative angiography. Angiography will be reserved for highly selected patients and will become oriented toward a therapeutic rather than a diagnostic role.

Acknowledgments: I would like to thank Robert F. Jeffery, M.D., and John Weaver, M.D. (Department of Radiology, Dartmouth-Hitchcock Medical Center), who have diligently worked on optimizing spiral CT protocols for our institution and have provided technical assistance in formatting spiral CT data for 3-D reconstruction. I would also like to acknowledge Medical Media Systems, West Lebanon, N.H. (including Peter J. Robbie, MFA; S. D. Pieper, Ph.D.; Michael A. McKenna, Ph.D.; and David T. Chen, Ph.D.) for providing grant and research support, novel software, and technical assistance, which enabled construction of many of the 3-D images displayed here. Last, I would like to thank those who helped provide CT data and images for illustrations, including Richard A. Morse, M.D., White River Junction Veterans Affairs Hospital, White River Junction, Vt.; Robert F. Jeffrey, M.D., David Langdon, M.D., and Christopher J. Kuhn, M.D., from Dartmouth-Hitchcock Medical Center, Lebanon, N.H.;

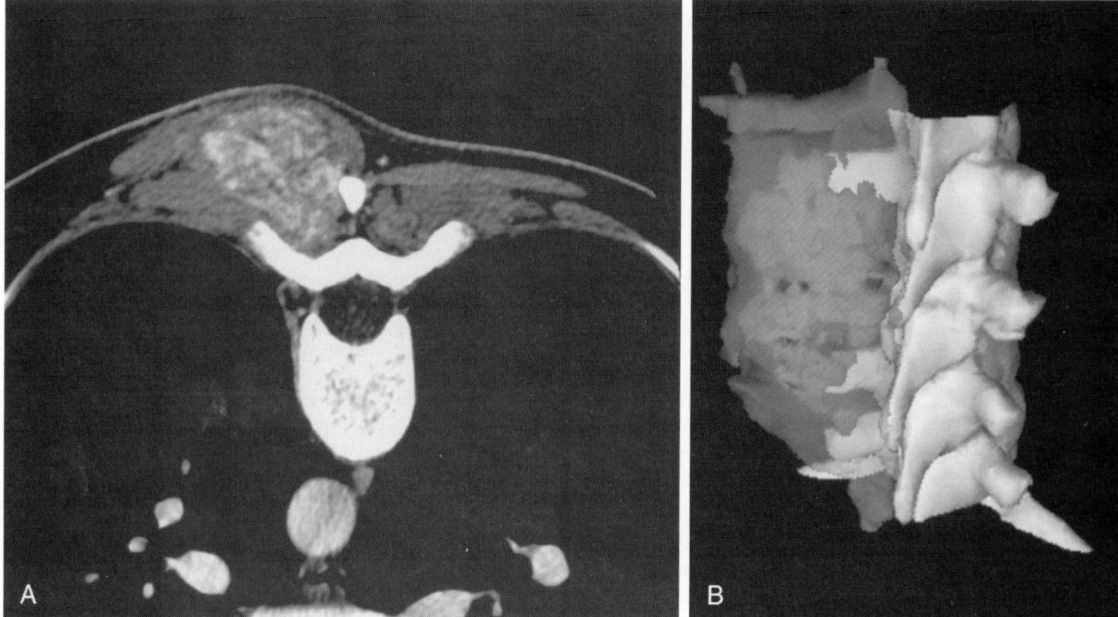

FIGURE 14–43. Arteriovenous malformation adjacent to the spine on axial CT *(A)* and three-dimensional (3-D) reconstruction derived from the CT data *(B)*. On the 3-D reconstruction, the spine is white, the contrast-enhanced vessels are red and the surrounding structures are yellow (made transparent to reveal the vasculature). *(B,* See Color Plate.)

John Edwards, M.D., University of Cincinnati; and Werner Lang, M.D., Friedrich-Alexander Universitat, Erlangen, Germany.

REFERENCES

1. Zwolak RM: Carotid endarterectomy without angiography: Are we ready? Vasc Surg 31:1–9, 1997.
2. Brewster DC, Retana A, Waltman AC, Darling AC: Angiography in the management of aneurysms of the abdominal aorta: Its value and safety. N Engl J Med 292:822–825, 1975.
3. Simoni G, Perrone R, Cittadini G, et al: Helical CT for the study of abdominal aortic aneurysms in patients undergoing conventional surgical repair. Eur J Vasc Endovasc Surg 12:354–358, 1996.
4. Fillinger MF: Utility of spiral CT in the preoperative evaluation of patients with abdominal aortic aneurysms. *In* Whittemore AD (ed): Advances in Vascular Surgery. Vol 5. St. Louis, Mosby–Year Book, 1997, pp 115–131.
5. Hounsfield GN: Computerized transverse axial scanning (tomography): I. Description of system. Br J Radiol 46:1016–1022, 1973.
6. Webster J: Encyclopedia of Medical Devices and Instrumentation. New York, John Wiley & Sons, 1988, p 834.
7. Zeman RK, Brink JA, Costello P, et al: Helical/Spiral CT: A Practical Approach. New York, McGraw-Hill, 1995, p 300.
8. Raptopoulos V, Rosen MP, Kent KC, et al: Sequential helical CT angiography of aortoiliac disease. AJR Am J Roentgenol 166:1347–1354, 1996.
9. Rieker O, Düber C, Neufang A, et al: CT angiography versus intra-arterial digital subtraction angiography for assessment of aortoiliac occlusive disease. AJR Am J Roentgenol 169:1133–1138, 1997.
10. Rubin GD, Walker PJ, Dake MD, et al: Three-dimensional spiral computed tomographic angiography: An alternative imaging modality for the abdominal aorta and its branches. J Vasc Surg 18:656–665, 1993.
11. Balm R, Eikelboom BC, van Leeuwen MS, Noordzij J: Spiral CT-angiography of the aorta. Eur J Vasc Surg 8:544–551, 1994.
12. Broeders I, Blankensteijn J, Olree M, et al: Preoperative sizing of grafts for transfemoral endovascular aneurysm management: A prospective comparative study of spiral CT angiography, arteriography, and conventional CT imaging. J Endovasc Surg 4:252–261, 1997.
13. Wang G, Vannier MW: Optimal pitch in spiral computed tomography. Med Phys 24:1635–1639, 1997.
14. Wang G, Vannier MW: Spatial variation of section sensitivity profile in spiral computed tomography. Med Phys 21:1491–1497, 1994.
15. Brink JA, Heiken JP, Wang G, et al: Helical CT: Principles and technical considerations. RadioGraphics 14:887–893, 1994.
16. Duvernoy O, Coulden R, Ytterberg C: Aortic motion: A potential pitfall in CT imaging of dissection in the ascending aorta. J Comput Assist Tomogr 19:569–572, 1995.
17. Castleman KR: Digital Image Processing. Englewood Cliffs, NJ: Prentice-Hall, 1979.
18. Katayama H, Yamaguchi K, Kozuka T,et al: Adverse reactions to ionic and nonionic contrast media: A report from the Japanese Committee on the Safety of Contrast Media. Radiology 175:621–628, 1990.
19. Lasser EC, Berry CC, Mishkin MM, et al: Pretreatment with corticosteroids to prevent adverse reactions to nonionic contrast media. AJR Am J Roentgenol 162:523–526, 1994.
20. Tong DC, Yenari MA, Albers GW: Intravenous thrombolytic therapy in acute stroke. Vasc Med 2:51–60, 1997.
21. Lim ST, Sage DJ: Detection of subarachnoid blood clot and other thin flat structures by computed tomography. Radiology 123:79–84, 1977.
22. Meyer JR, Gorey MT: Differential diagnosis of nontraumatic intracranial hemorrhage. Neuroimaging Clin North Am 8:263–293, 1998.
23. Yuh WT, Crain MR, Loes DJ, et al: MR imaging of cerebral ischemia: Findings in the first 24 hours. AJNR Am J Neuroradiol 12:621–629, 1991.
24. Crain MR, Yuh WT, Greene GM, et al: Cerebral ischemia: Evaluation with contrast-enhanced MR imaging. AJNR Am J Neuroradiol 12:631–639, 1991.
25. Schriger DL, Kalafut M, Starkman S, et al: Cranial computed tomography interpretation in acute stroke: Physician accuracy in determining eligibility for thrombolytic therapy. JAMA 279:1293–1297, 1998.
26. Strayle-Batra M, Skalej M, Wakhloo AK, et al: Three-dimensional spiral CT angiography in the detection of cerebral aneurysm. Acta Radiol 39:233–238, 1998.
27. Young N, Dorsch NW, Kingston RJ, et al: Spiral CT scanning in the detection and evaluation of aneurysms of the circle of Willis. Surg Neurol 50:50–60, 1998; discussion 60–1.
28. Lanzino G, Kaptain G, Kallmes DF, et al: Intracranial dissecting aneurysm causing subarachnoid hemorrhage: The role of computerized tomographic angiography and magnetic resonance angiography. Surg Neurol 48:477–481, 1997.
29. Riles TS, Eidelman EM, Litt AW, et al: Comparison of magnetic resonance angiography, conventional angiography, and duplex scanning. Stroke 23:341–346, 1992.
30. Riles TS, Posner MP, Cohen WS, et al: The totally occluded internal

carotid artery: Preliminary observations using rapid sequential computerized tomographic scanning. Arch Surg 117:1185–1188, 1982.
31. Cinat M, Lane CT, Pham H, et al: Helical CT angiography in the preoperative evaluation of carotid artery stenosis. J Vasc Surg 28:290–300, 1998.
32. Wise SW, Hopper KD, Ten Have T, Schwartz T: Measuring carotid artery stenosis using CT angiography: The dilemma of artifactual lumen eccentricity. AJR Am J Roentgenol 170:919–923, 1998.
33. Papp Z, Patel M, Ashtari M, et al: Carotid artery stenosis: Optimization of CT angiography with a combination of shaded surface display and source images. AJNR Am J Neuroradiol 18:759–763, 1997.
34. Fisher DF Jr, Clagett GP, Parker JI, et al: Mandibular subluxation for high carotid exposure. J Vasc Surg 1:727–733, 1984.
35. Mock CN, Lilly MP, McRae RG, Carney WI Jr: Selection of the approach to the distal internal carotid artery from the second cervical vertebra to the base of the skull. J Vasc Surg 13:846–853, 1991.
36. Wildy KS, Yuan C, Tsuruda JS, et al: Atherosclerosis of the carotid artery: Evaluation by magnetic resonance angiography. J Magn Reson Imaging 6:726–732, 1996.
37. Patel MR, Kuntz KM, Klufas RA, et al: Preoperative assessment of the carotid bifurcation: Can magnetic resonance angiography and duplex ultrasonography replace contrast arteriography? Stroke 26:1753–1758, 1995.
38. Brott T, Toole JF: Medical compared with surgical treatment of asymptomatic carotid artery stenosis. Ann Intern Med 123:720–722, 1995.
39. Carotid endarterectomy for patients with asymptomatic internal carotid artery stenosis: National Institute of Neurological Disorders and Stroke. J Neurol Sci 129:76–77, 1995.
40. Matsumura JS, Rilling WS, Pearce WH, et al: Helical computed tomography of the normal thoracic outlet. J Vasc Surg 26:776–783, 1997.
41. Bradshaw KA, Pagano D, Bonser RS, et al: Multiplanar reformatting and three-dimensional reconstruction for pre-operative assessment of the thoracic aorta by computed tomography. Clin Radiol 53:198–202, 1998.
42. Sommer T, Fehske W, Holzknecht N, et al: Aortic dissection: A comparative study of diagnosis with spiral CT, multiplanar transesophageal echocardiography, and MR imaging. Radiology 199:347–352, 1996.
43. Fabian TC, Richardson JD, Croce MA, et al: Prospective study of blunt aortic injury: Multicenter Trial of the American Association for the Surgery of Trauma. J Trauma 42:374–380; 1997; discussion, 380–383.
44. Gavant ML, Menke PG, Fabian T, et al: Blunt traumatic aortic rupture: Detection with helical CT of the chest. Radiology 197:125–133, 1995.
45. Wicky S, Capasso P, Meuli R, et al: Spiral CT aortography: An efficient technique for the diagnosis of traumatic aortic injury. Eur Radiol 8:828–833, 1998.
46. Trachiotis GD, Sell JE, Pearson GD, et al: Traumatic thoracic aortic rupture in the pediatric patient. Ann Thorac Surg 62:724–731, 1996; discussion, 731–732.
47. Gosselin MV, Rubin GD, Leung AN,et al: Unsuspected pulmonary embolism: Prospective detection on routine helical CT scans. Radiology 208:209–215, 1998.
48. Garg K, Welsh CH, Feyerabend AJ, et al: Pulmonary embolism: Diagnosis with spiral CT and ventilation-perfusion scanning: Correlation with pulmonary angiographic results or clinical outcome. Radiology 208:201–208, 1998.
49. Cross JJ, Kemp PM, Walsh CG, et al: A randomized trial of spiral CT and ventilation perfusion scintigraphy for the diagnosis of pulmonary embolism. Clin Radiol 53:177–182, 1998.
50. Remy J, Remy-Jardin M, Artaud D, Fribourg M: Multiplanar and three-dimensional reconstruction techniques in CT: Impact on chest diseases. Eur Radiol 8:335–351, 1998.
51. Todd GJ, Nowygrod R, Benvenisty A, et al: The accuracy of CT scanning in the diagnosis of abdominal and thoracoabdominal aortic aneurysms. J Vasc Surg 13:302–310, 1991.
52. Faggioli GL, Stella A, Gargiulo M, et al: Morphology of small aneurysms: Definition and impact on risk of rupture. Am J Surg 168:131–135, 1994.
53. Schulze CG, Blum U, Haag K: Hepatic portal venous gas: Imaging modalities and clinical significance. Acta Radiol 36:377–380, 1995.
54. Sisley JF, Miller DM, Nesbit RR Jr: Computerized axial tomography (CT) as an aid in the diagnosis of hepatic portal venous gas: A case report. Surgery 101:376–379, 1987.
55. O'Hara PJ, Borkowski GP, Hertzer NR, et al: Natural history of periprosthetic air on computerized axial tomographic examination of the abdomen following abdominal aortic aneurysm repair. J Vasc Surg 1:429–433, 1984.
56. Qvarfordt PG, Reilly LM, Mark AS, et al: Computerized tomographic assessment of graft incorporation after aortic reconstruction. Am J Surg 150:227–231, 1985.
57. Mark A, Moss AA, Lusby R, Kaiser JA: CT evaluation of complications of abdominal aortic surgery. Radiology 145:409–414, 1982.
58. Hallett JW Jr, Marshall DM, Petterson TM, et al: Graft-related complications after abdominal aortic aneurysm repair: Reassurance from a 36-year population-based experience. J Vasc Surg 25:277–284,1997; discussion, 285–286.
59. Cho JS, Gloviczki P, Martelli E, et al: Long-term survival and late complications after repair of ruptured abdominal aortic aneurysms. J Vasc Surg 27:813–819, 1998; discussion, 819–820.
60. Salaman RA, Shandall A, Morgan RH, et al: Intravenous digital subtraction angiography versus computed tomography in the assessment of abdominal aortic aneurysm. Br J Surg 81:661–663, 1994.
61. Galanski M, Prokop M, Chavan A, et al: Renal arterial stenoses: Spiral CT angiography. Radiology 189:185–192, 1993.
62. Van Hoe L, Baert AL, Gryspeerdt S, et al: Supra- and juxtarenal aneurysms of the abdominal aorta: Preoperative assessment with thin-section spiral CT. Radiology 198:443–448, 1996.
63. Kaatee R, Beek FJ, Verschuyl EJ, et al: Atherosclerotic renal artery stenosis: Ostial or truncal? Radiology 199:637–640, 1996.
64. Cikrit DF, Harris VJ, Hemmer CG, et al: Comparison of spiral CT scan and arteriography for evaluation of renal and visceral arteries. Ann Vasc Surg 10:109–116, 1996.
65. Rubin GD, Dake MD, Napel S, et al: Spiral CT of renal artery stenosis: Comparison of three-dimensional rendering techniques. Radiology 190:181–189, 1994.
66. Costello P, Gaa J: Spiral CT angiography of abdominal aortic aneurysms. RadioGraphics 15:397–406, 1995.
67. Rubin GD, Alfrey EJ, Dake MD, et al: Assessment of living renal donors with spiral CT. Radiology 195:457–462, 1995.
68. Pozniak MA, Balison DJ, Lee FT Jr, et al: CT angiography of potential renal transplant donors. RadioGraphics 18:565–587, 1998.
69. Brewster DC, Cambria RP, Moncure AC, et al: Aortocaval and iliac arteriovenous fistulas: Recognition and treatment. J Vasc Surg 13:253–264, 1991; discussion, 264–265.
70. Davis PM, Gloviczki P, Cherry KJ Jr, et al: Aorto-caval and ilio-iliac arteriovenous fistulae. Am J Surg 176:115–118, 1998.
71. Schmidt R, Bruns C, Walter M, Erasmi H. Aorto-caval fistula—an uncommon complication of infrarenal aortic aneurysms. Thorac Cardiovasc Surg 42:208–211, 1994.
72. Farber A, Fillinger MF, Connors J, et al: Comparison of angiography, intravascular ultrasound and three dimensional CT for morphologic evaluation in a three dimensional aneurysm model. Submitted.
73. Fillinger MF, McKenna MA, Pieper SD, et al: CT angiography with three-dimensional reconstruction: Measurement accuracy and clinical utility. Submitted.
74. Fillinger MF, Robbie PJ, McKenna MA, et al: The "virtual" graft: Preoperative simulation of endovascular grafts using spiral CT with interactive three-dimensional reconstructions. J Endovasc Surg 4(Suppl I):10, 1997.
75. Balm R, Kaatee R, Blankensteijn JD, et al: CT-angiography of abdominal aortic aneurysms after transfemoral endovascular aneurysm management. Eur J Vasc Endovasc Surg 12:182–188, 1996.
76. Matsumura JS, Pearce WH, McCarthy WJ, Yao JS, EVT Investigators: Reduction in aortic aneurysm size: Early results after endovascular graft placement. J Vasc Surg 25:113–23, 1997.
77. May J, White GH, Yu W, et al: A prospective study of changes in morphology and dimensions of abdominal aortic aneurysms following endoluminal repair: A preliminary report. J Endovasc Surg 2:343–347, 1995.
78. May J, White G, Yu W, et al: A prospective study of anatomico-pathological changes in abdominal aortic aneurysms following endoluminal repair: Is the aneurysmal process reversed? Eur J Vasc Endovasc Surg 12:11–17, 1996.
79. Torsello G, Klenk E, Kasprzak B, Umscheid T: Rupture of abdominal aortic aneurysm previously treated by endovascular stentgraft. J Vasc Surg 28:184–187, 1998.
80. Matsumura JS, Moore WS, Endovascular Technologies Investigators: Clinical consequences of periprosthetic leak after endovascular repair of abdominal aortic aneurysm. J Vasc Surg 27:606–613, 1998.

81. Alimi YS, Chafke N, Rivoal R, et al: Rupture of an abdominal aortic aneurysm after endovascular graft placement and aneurysm size reduction. J Vasc Surg 28:178–183, 1998.
82. Thomas PR, Shaw JC, Ashton HA, et al: Accuracy of ultrasound in a screening programme for abdominal aortic aneurysms. J Med Screening 1:3–6, 1994.
83. Lederle FA, Wilson SE, Johnson GR, et al: Variability in measurement of abdominal aortic aneurysms: Abdominal Aortic Aneurysm Detection and Management Veterans Administration Cooperative Study Group. J Vasc Surg 21:945–952, 1995.
84. Schurink GWH, Aarts NJM, Wilde J, et al: Endoleakage after stent-graft treatment of abdominal aortic aneurysm: Implications on pressure and imaging—an in vitro study. J Vasc Surg 28:234–241, 1998.
85. Riccabona M, Nelson TR, Pretorius DH, Davidson TE: In vivo three-dimensional sonographic measurement of organ volume: Validation in the urinary bladder. J Ultrasound Med 15:627–632, 1996.
86. Wheatley JM, Rosenfield NS, Heller G, et al: Validation of a technique of computer-aided tumor volume determination. J Surg Res 59:621–626, 1995.
87. Fillinger MF, Dookeran NM, Robbie PJ, et al: Volume measurements using three-dimensional reconstruction of spiral CT data: Validation and clinical utility compared to measurement of maximum aneurysm diameter. Submitted.
88. Beregi JP, Djabbari M, Desmoucelle F, et al: Popliteal vascular disease: Evaluation with spiral CT angiography. Radiology 203:477–483, 1997.
89. Takase K, Imakita S, Kuribayashi S, et al: Popliteal artery entrapment syndrome: Aberrant origin of gastrocnemius muscle shown by 3D CT. J Comput Assist Tomogr 21:523–528, 1997.
90. Rizzo RJ, Flinn WR, Yao JS, et al: Computed tomography for evaluation of arterial disease in the popliteal fossa. J Vasc Surg 11:112–119, 1990.
91. Kurihashi A, Tamai K, Saotome K: Peroneal arteriovenous fistula and pseudoaneurysm formation after blunt trauma: A case report. Clin Orthop Issue 304, 218–221, 1994.
92. Rauch RF, Silverman PM, Korobkin M, et al: Computed tomography of benign angiomatous lesions of the extremities. J Comput Assist Tomogr 8:1143–1146, 1984.
93. Taylor CR: Computed tomography in the evaluation of the portal venous system. J Clin Gastroenterol 14:167–172, 1992.
94. Kuszyk BS, Osterman FA Jr, Venbrux AC, et al: Portal venous system thrombosis: Helical CT angiography before transjugular intrahepatic portosystemic shunt creation. Radiology 206:179–186, 1998.
95. Baldt MM, Zontsich T, Kainberger F, et al: Spiral CT evaluation of deep venous thrombosis. Semin Ultrasound CT MR 18:369–375, 1997.
96. Rijs J, Depreitere B, Beckers A, et al: Mesenteric venous thrombosis: Diagnostic and therapeutic approach. Acta Chir Belg 97:247–249, 1997.

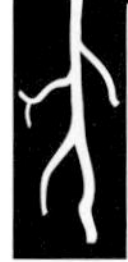

CHAPTER 15

Magnetic Resonance Imaging and Angiography

Omaida C. Velázquez, M.D.,
Richard A. Baum, M.D.,
and Jeffrey P. Carpenter, M.D.

Magnetic resonance imaging (MRI) and magnetic resonance angiography, which includes magnetic resonance arteriography (MRA) and magnetic resonance venography (MRV), have evolved as noninvasive, sensitive, accurate, and cost-effective methods of preoperative evaluation of peripheral arterial vascular disease, renal artery stenosis, popliteal artery entrapment syndrome, diseases of the venous system, and arteriovenous malformations. Perhaps the most dramatic impact of MRI and MRA in vascular disease has been noted in the diagnosis, assessment, and preoperative planning for patients with arterial peripheral vascular disease of the lower extremities, endeavors in which these modalities can often replace contrast angiography.

MRA is accurate and reliable, compared with conventional contrast angiography, in the preoperative imaging of inflow vessels[14] and the preoperative grading of stenosis severity in peripheral arteries.[27] MRA accurately identifies patent runoff vessels not always visualized by conventional contrast angiography.[13, 40] The recent addition of non-nephrotoxic contrast agents, such as gadolinium, has further improved accuracy and expanded applications of MRA.[10, 30, 38, 46–48, 53] MRA is also cost-effective[8, 37, 61] compared with contrast arteriography. MRI and MRA can be easily performed as outpatient procedures.[52] When MRA findings are properly interpreted by an experienced team, this modality may be used as the sole preoperative test for planning peripheral bypass procedures in the lower extremities[7, 8] or for endovascular interventions.[37] MRV accurately reveals deep venous thrombosis (DVT) in lower extremity veins and pelvic veins, which are often inaccessible for duplex scanning.[11]

Although many technical and practical limitations remain to be explored and solved before the widespread acceptance and application of MRI and MRA/MRV in vascular diseases, some centers have already replaced conventional contrast angiography with MRA in the preoperative evaluation of patients with some common vascular diseases, such as aortic aneurysm[43, 48] and peripheral arterial disease of the lower extremities.[3, 4, 7, 8, 37]

TECHNIQUE

MRI is based on the reactions of various tissues to a magnetic field followed by a radiofrequency (RF) radiation pulse. The magnetic resonance (MR) signal is generated by hydrogen nuclei (protons), which exist within tissues. Therefore, the signal emitted is related to the proton density of the specific tissue. The MR signal is captured by an array of detectors surrounding the tissue in the scanner. The protons within tissue spin under the influence of the magnetic force within the MR scanner. The spinning protons, in turn, generate a magnetic field, which may be assigned a vector indicating its direction.

Normal tissue, unexposed to the MR scanner magnet, contains protons whose magnetic vectors are arranged randomly. However, tissue that is exposed to the strong magnet of the MR scanner contains protons with magnetic fields aligned along the axis of the applied magnetic force. An externally applied radiofrequency radiation pulse then disturbs the alignment. The protons absorb the energy from this radiation pulse and their alignment becomes disturbed, leading to a temporary "excited" state. As the protons realign with the applied magnetic field within the scanner, the energy released generates a radiofrequency signal, or echo, which can be detected by the MR receiver. It is this detected signal that is used to create the "spin echo" MR image.

MRA is a physiologic method for vascular imaging, physiologic rather than the anatomic method of conventional contrast angiography. The images are generated by taking advantage of the effects related to the flow of blood relative to the stationary surrounding soft tissue. This fundamental principle is the basis for understanding the two primary techniques of MRA currently used[52]:

- Time of flight (TOF) angiography
- Phase-contrast (PC) angiography

TOF angiography relies on differences in saturation of tissue protons in the surrounding stationary soft tissue versus moving tissue (flowing blood). Soft tissue repeatedly exposed to radiofrequency pulses within the MR scanner becomes saturated and yields a weak echo signal, since protons lack sufficient time to realign with the magnetic field between repeated radiofrequency pulses. However, fresh protons from flowing blood, having not been exposed to the radiofrequency pulses within the imaging plane of the scanner, produce a large echo signal in response to a radiofrequency pulse (Figs. 15–1 and 15–2).

Protons undergo a change in the phase of their rotation as they move through a magnetic field. Phase contrast angiography takes advantage of these physical properties of protons. The magnitude of the phase change for these protons is proportional to the velocity of the moving protons and to the size of the magnetic field gradient. The background can be eliminated by a complex method of subtraction of the applied gradient. Both an image of flow and the velocity of the blood flow can be calculated because the phase change is proportional to the velocity of the blood flow. Background suppression is greater for phase contrast than for TOF angiography because only moving protons can generate a signal. This makes phase contrast angiography very sensitive to slow flow. Information can be acquired in the form of either two-dimensional (2-D) or three-dimensional (3-D) volume acquisition images.

MRA is specifically programmed to detect only forward flow in order to avoid imaging veins. Therefore, arterial retrograde filling via collateral arteries, which can usually be seen by conventional contrast angiography, may be missed by MR arteriography without the use of contrast. Imaging of venous blood flow or MRV can be accomplished by simply reversing the direction of the saturating radiofrequency pulses.

The method of selecting either arterial or venous blood flow depends on which pulse sequence has been chosen. With TOF techniques, the addition of saturation pulses to tissues superior or inferior to the imaging plane allows for the selective elimination of the signal from blood flow traveling in one direction. However, just because an inferior saturation pulse has been applied in the legs, there is no assurance that all of the visible flow will be arterial. Only

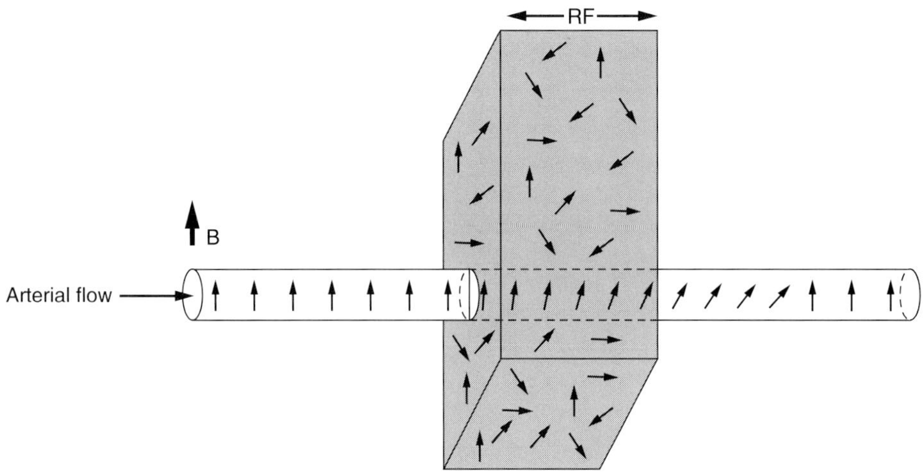

FIGURE 15–1. Time-of-flight effects. Soft tissue within the magnetic resonance (MR) scanner, which has been repeatedly irradiated with radiofrequency (RF) pulses, has become saturated and yields a weak echo signal, causing it to appear dark on MR images. However, fresh protons that are fully aligned with the externally applied magnetic field (B), having not been exposed to the RF pulses within the side imaging plane of the scanner, produce a large echo signal in response to an RF pulse. This fully magnetized blood produces a bright signal in contrast to the saturated surrounding soft tissue, selectively imaging blood flow. This is known as flow-related enhancement. (From Calow A, Ernst CB [eds]: Vascular Surgery: Theory and Practice. Stamford, Conn, Appleton & Lange, 1995, pp 405–419.)

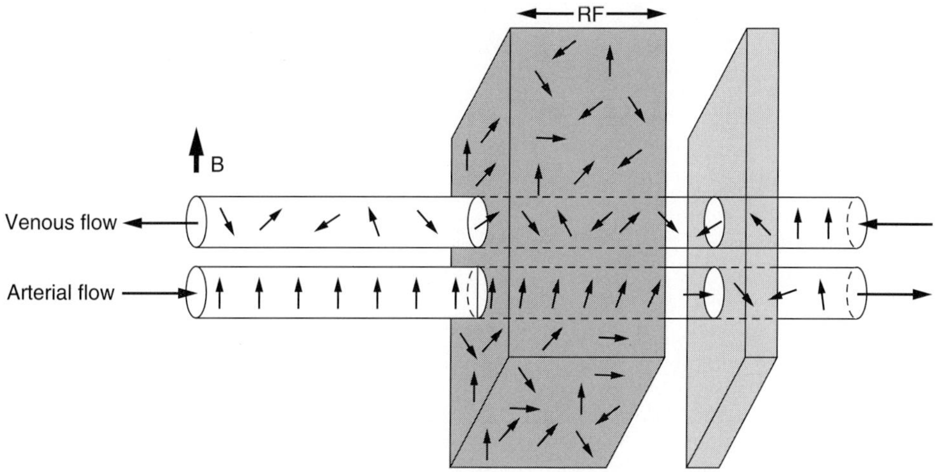

FIGURE 15–2. Presaturation. Selective imaging of the arteries and veins is accomplished by the use of presaturation with the radiofrequency (RF) either inferior or superior to the imaging plane. To image arteries selectively, one chooses inferior saturation to suppress the magnetization of venous blood flowing from superior to inferior to reach the imaging plane. The venous blood, which is fully magnetized before reaching the presaturation band, becomes saturated in the presaturation band before entering the imaging plane. Thus, it yields little or no signal in the imaging plane side itself. On the other hand, arterial blood flowing from superior to inferior is fully magnetized on entering the imaging plane and still yields a strong echo signal in response to RF pulses in the imaging plane. (From Calow A, Ernst CB [eds]: Vascular Surgery: Theory and Practice. Stamford, Conn, Appleton & Lange, 1995, pp 405–419.)

flow moving in the head-to-foot direction is displayed with an inferior saturation band, and on occasion the flow is venous.

Four parameters influence the various echo pulse sequences[52]:

1. The *repetition time* is an important component of MRA because it helps to determine (a) the amount of stationary tissue suppression there will be, (b) how sensitive the sequence will be to slow flow, (c) the overall examination time, and (d) the frequency of pulsatility artefacts.
2. *Slice thickness* plays a key role in MRA in that thicker slices have a better signal-to-noise ratio and allow the study to be completed more quickly but result in decreased image resolution.
3. The *flip angle* is also an important parameter in MRA, since the larger it is, the greater the magnitude of the signal intensity from flow within the vessel lumen. Conversely, the smaller the flip angle for volume acquisitions, the smaller the contribution of saturation to signal loss in three-dimensional TOF MRA.
4. *Time to echo* affects the image quality of MRA; a shorter time to echo results in less spin dephasing and therefore yields more accurate information about post-stenotic jets.

CLINICAL APPLICATION

Peripheral Vascular Disease of the Lower Extremities

Conventional Arteriography

Contrast angiography has been viewed as the conventional standard for preoperative evaluation in patients requiring revascularization of the lower extremities. However, conventional contrast angiography is associated with an overall minor and major complication rate of approximately 8%, with a risk of severe contrast reaction varying from 0.04% to 0.22%.[18, 24, 29, 55, 60]

The arterial puncture necessary for the study may be associated with bleeding, hematoma, pseudoaneurysm, and pain at the site. In addition, there is a modest risk of contrast allergy, which can be associated with anaphylactoid reaction (1 in 2000) and death (1 in 40,000). In patients older than 60 years, the risk for idiosyncratic reactions increases fourfold (1 in 10,000).[1, 60] Moreover, since 29% of patients with peripheral vascular disease may show some evidence of baseline renal insufficiency, contrast-induced worsening of renal function[18, 24] continues to be an important issue of concern. Conventional contrast angiography also shows a low sensitivity for detecting patent runoff vessels compared with intraoperative arteriography. The ability to visualize distal runoff vessels by this technique is hindered by lack of filling with enough contrast in up to 70% of cases.[21, 42, 50, 51] Even when performed with the digital subtraction arteriography (DSA) technique, more runoff vessels are seen on intraoperative than on preoperative arteriograms.[56]

MRA is an alternative noninvasive imaging modality that avoids the complications of arterial puncture, eliminates the risk of contrast-induced renal failure, and has greater sensitivity than contrast angiography for identifying patent distal vessels in patients with severe peripheral arterial occlusive disease.[13, 40]

Imaging of Inflow Vessels

When MRA is compared with conventional contrast angiography in preoperative studies of the aorta, iliac artery and femoral artery, the two imaging modalities are concordant in almost all cases.[14] MRA was found to have a sensitivity of 99.6%, a specificity of 100%, a positive predictive value of 100%, and a negative predictive value of 98.5% for detecting patent segments, occluded segments, and hemodynamically significant stenoses. The therapeutic plans re-

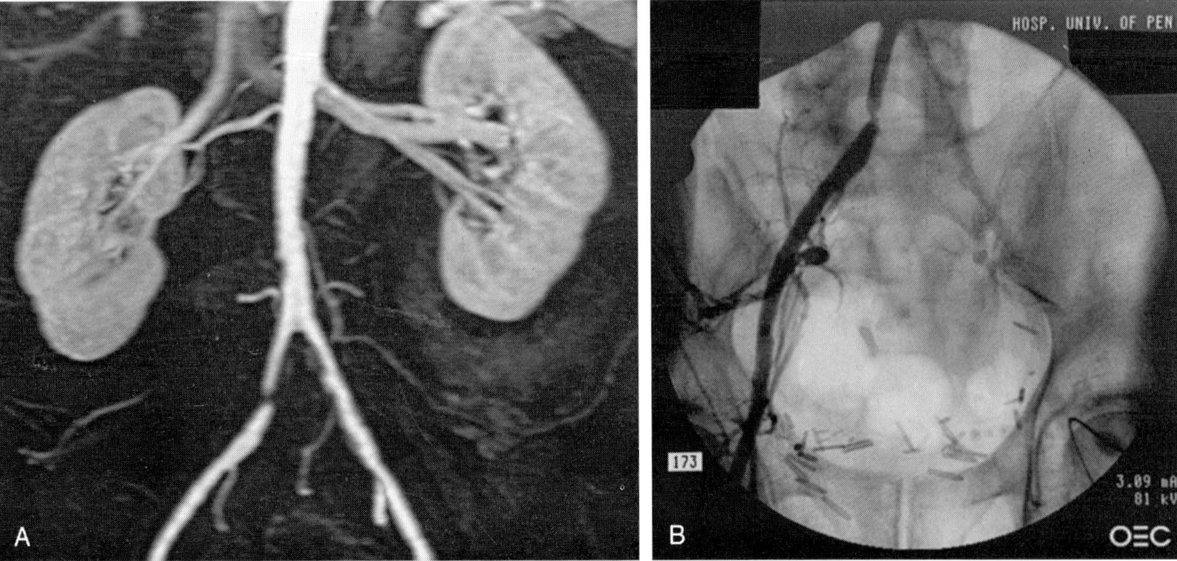

FIGURE 15–3. Preoperative magnetic resonance angiographic (MRA) study *(A)* from patients with right leg claudication shows right common iliac artery stenosis. Intraoperative arteriogram *(B)* prior to angioplasty confirms the presence of the lesion.

garding inflow based on either MRA or conventional angiography have been noted to be 100% concordant (Fig. 15–3).[14]

Evaluating the Degree of Arterial Stenosis

Compared with preoperative conventional contrast angiography as the reference gold standard, MRA is highly accurate for evaluating and grading the degree of arterial stenosis in patients with peripheral arterial disease of the lower extremities.[5, 13, 14, 27] In a study of 19 patients in whom the arterial vasculature (from the distal aorta through the crural vessels) was evaluated by MRA, the magnitude of 48 arterial stenoses were measured with a high degree of accuracy ($r = 0.83$; $p < .001$) when compared to contrast angiography (Fig. 15–4).[27] It has been noted that the combination of cross-sectional views, multiple projection planes, three-dimensional reconstruction, and rotational views of stacked axial images in MRA studies, can provide a superior view of the spatial relationship of blood flow and plaque morphology.[27, 61]

Imaging Suitable Target Vessels

MRA yields a sensitivity of 100% for detecting patent runoff vessels[5, 13, 40] compared with intraoperative arteriography. In a study of 23 patients (25 legs) that compared the imaging results from MRA and conventional angiography, discrepancies were noted in 18 of 25 limbs.[40] These discrepancies universally involved superior detection of distal runoff vessels by MRA. MRA never failed to demonstrate flow in a segment of vessel that was identified as patent on conventional preoperative, post-interventional or intraoperative arteriograms.[40] All vessels found to be patent by MRA were confirmed to be patent by operative exploration and intraoperative arteriograms.[40] These results have been confirmed in a larger study of 51 patients (55 limbs)[13] as well as by a blinded, prospective, multicenter trial that included 155 patients from six American hospitals.[5] MRA is significantly more sensitive than conventional angiography in identifying patent runoff vessels, with 24% to 48%[13, 40] additional patent vessel segments noted with MRA but not conventional contrast angiography (Figs. 15–5 and 15–6).[40] The increased sensitivity of MRA for detection of patent runoff vessels is most evident in the more distal segments (Fig. 15–7).[13, 40]

The explanation for the increased sensitivity of MRA over conventional preoperative angiography is based on the mechanism of image formation in each of the two techniques. Since contrast angiography requires a bolus injection of contrast material to opacify the vessel lumen, multiple segmental occlusions between the site of the injection

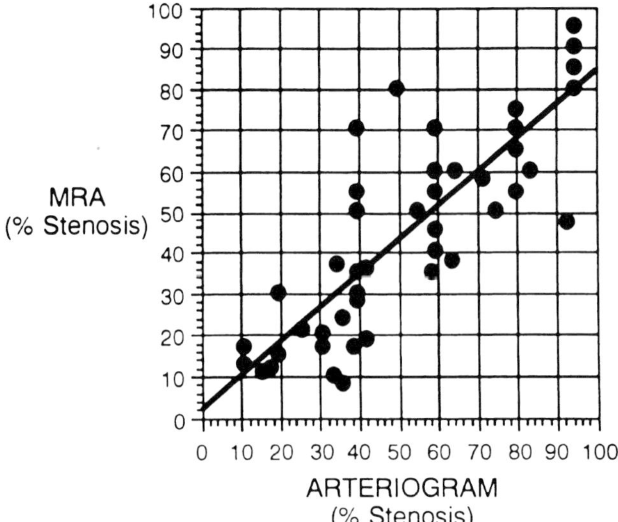

FIGURE 15–4. Correlation of magnetic resonance angiographic (MRA) and arteriographic measurements of stenosis. Pearson correlation coefficient = 0.83 ($p < .001$). Linear regression line: y = 1.87 + 0.81 (x), 95% confidence intervals intercept, 7.6, 11.4; slope, 0.6, 1.0. (From Hertz SM, Baum RA, Owen RS, et al: Comparison of magnetic resonance and contrast arteriography in peripheral arterial stenosis. Am J Surg 166:112–116, 1993. With permission from Excerpta Medica, Inc.)

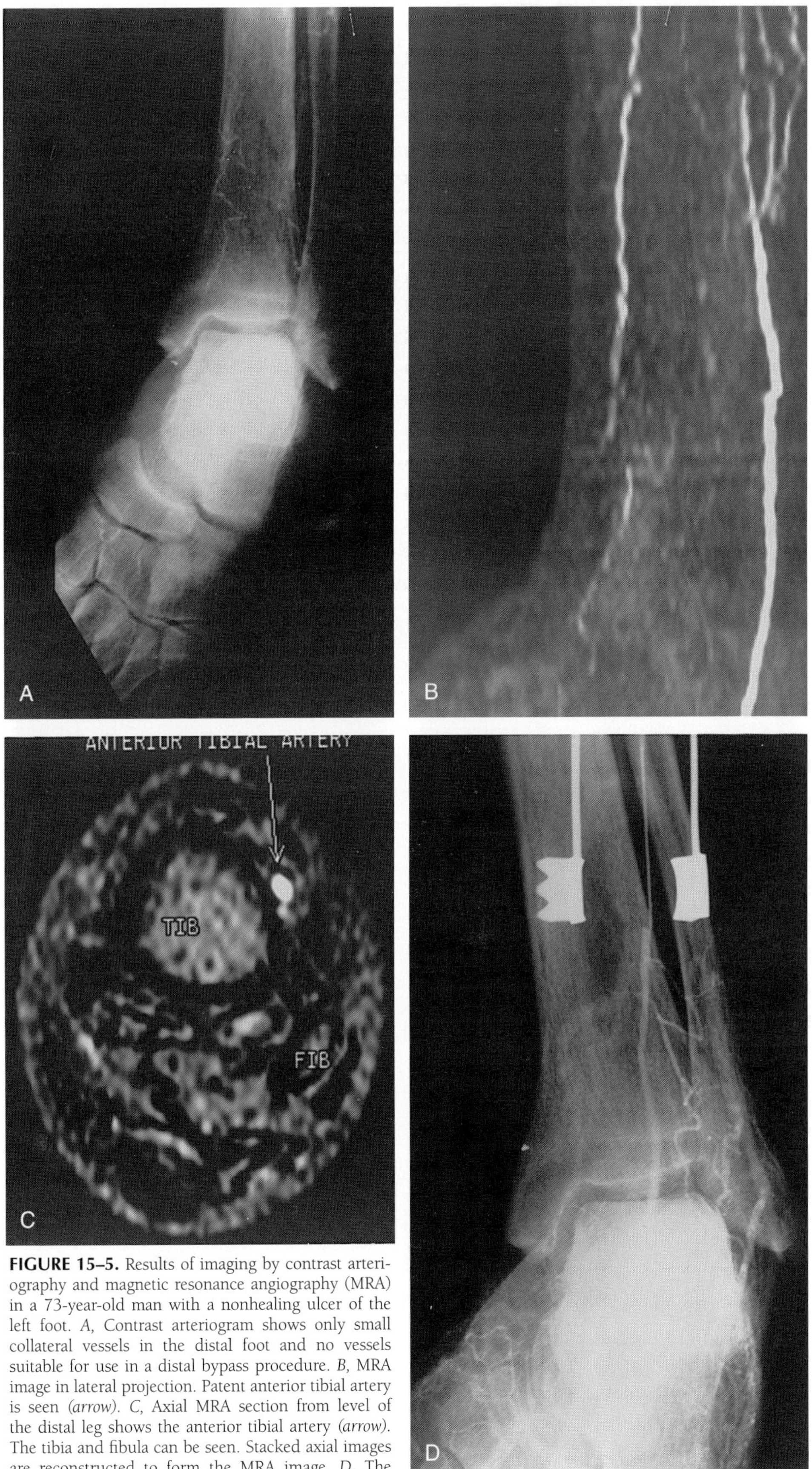

FIGURE 15–5. Results of imaging by contrast arteriography and magnetic resonance angiography (MRA) in a 73-year-old man with a nonhealing ulcer of the left foot. *A*, Contrast arteriogram shows only small collateral vessels in the distal foot and no vessels suitable for use in a distal bypass procedure. *B*, MRA image in lateral projection. Patent anterior tibial artery is seen *(arrow)*. *C*, Axial MRA section from level of the distal leg shows the anterior tibial artery *(arrow)*. The tibia and fibula can be seen. Stacked axial images are reconstructed to form the MRA image. *D*, The anterior tibial artery was explored operatively and found to be patent. Successful limb-salvage procedure was performed on the basis of these findings. TIB = tibia; FIB = fibula. (From Owen RS, Carpenter JP, Baum RA, et al: Magnetic resonance imaging of angiographically occult runoff vessels in peripheral arterial occlusive disease. N Engl J Med 326:1577, 1992.)

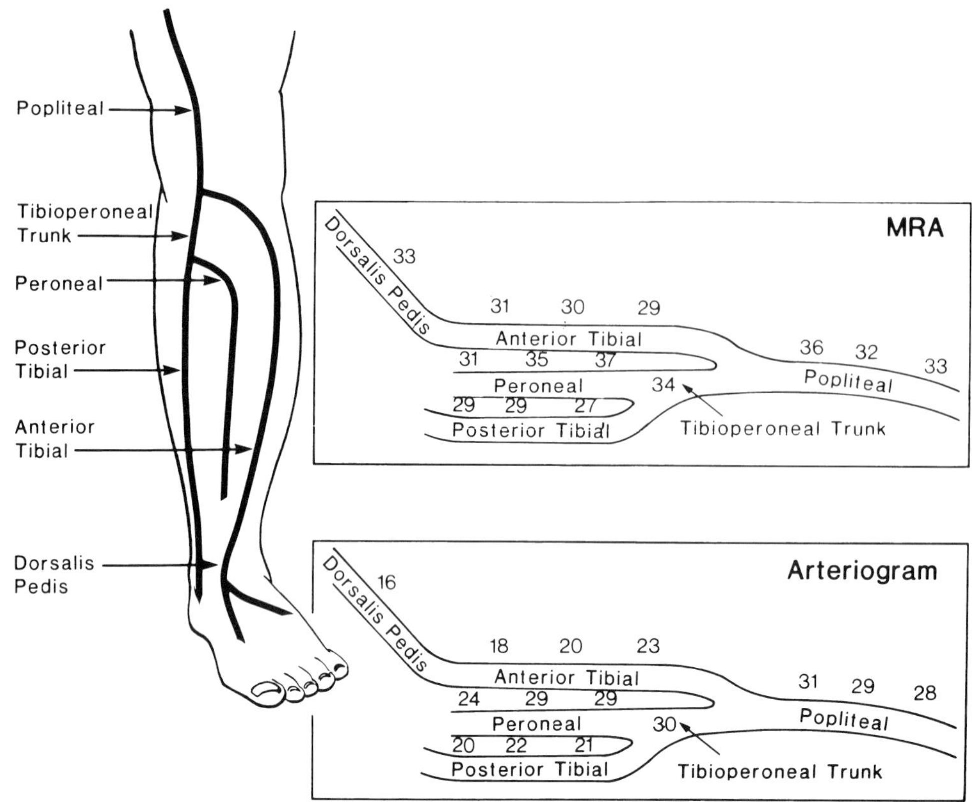

FIGURE 15–6. Comparison of patent vessel segments imaged by magnetic resonance angiography (MRA) and by contrast arteriography. The lower leg arteries were divided into 14 segments, which were scored as patent or occluded. The number of patent segments imaged by each technique is shown for each location. MRA identified every patent vessel segment seen by arteriography (sensitivity, 100%). An additional 106 segments (24%) that were unseen by arteriography were found to be patent on MRA. These patent vessel segments were scored further for the presence of hemodynamically significant stenoses. (From Carpenter JP, Owen RS, Baum RA, et al: Magnetic resonance angiography of peripheral runoff vessels. J Vasc Surg 16:807–115, 1992.)

and the distal target vessel can dilute the contrast as it goes through collateral arteriolar and capillary beds. Patients with severe symptomatic ischemia often have multiple segmental occlusions, which can lead to several dilutions and reconstitutions of the contrast bolus. Conversely, image formation in MRA depends only on the presence of local

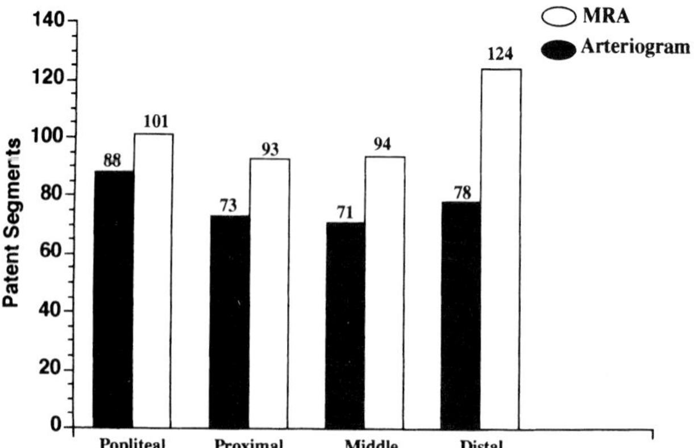

FIGURE 15–7. Comparison of patent vessel segments imaged by magnetic resonance angiography (MRA) and arteriography by location. The increased sensitivity of MRA is noted at every location but is greatest in distal segments (49% greater sensitivity). (From Carpenter JP, Owen RS, Baum RA, et al: Magnetic resonance angiography of peripheral runoff vessels. J Vasc Surg 16:807–815, 1992.)

flow with velocity as low as 2 cm/sec.[52] Furthermore, although cortical bone is "transparent" on MRA, cortical bone may obscure vessels that overly bony structures in conventional contrast angiography.[13]

The improved detection by MRA of patent runoff vessels not identified by conventional angiography or the identification of better-suited target vessels led to improved limb salvage in 13% to 22% of cases.[5, 13, 40] In the setting of contrast arteriograms as the only available preoperative imaging modality, patients in whom no patent runoff vessel can be visualized often undergo blind exploration of potential distal target vessels combined with intraoperative angiography. Either a bypass or an amputation follows, depending on the findings at exploration. In the absence of preoperative identification of a target vessel for the distal vascular anastomoses, blind exploration usually necessitates multiple skin incisions, which in the setting of an ischemic limb increases the likelihood of poor wound healing.

Magnetic Resonance Arteriography as the Sole Preoperative Imaging Technique

MRA can be used as the sole preoperative imaging technique for successful planning of vascular reconstructions.[7, 8] In a study of MRA as the sole preoperative imaging modality, 80 consecutive patients evaluated for lower extremity bypass, presenting with either ischemic rest pain or tissue

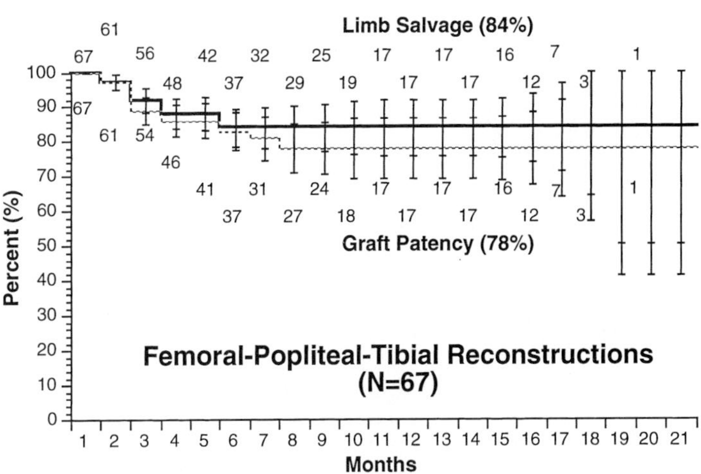

FIGURE 15–8. Results of infrainguinal bypasses, with MRA as the sole preoperative imaging modality. Life-table analysis of 67 infrainguinal bypass procedures revealed an 84% limb salvage rate *(solid line)* and a 78% primary graft patency rate *(dashed line)* at 21 months of follow-up. The number of grafts at risk for each interval as well as the standard error for each interval is shown. (From Carpenter JP, Baum RA, Holland GA, et al: Peripheral vascular surgery with magnetic resonance angiography as the sole preoperative imaging modality. J Vasc Surg 20:861–871, 1994.)

loss, were imaged by outpatient MRA of the juxtarenal aorta through the foot.[8] MRA findings were confirmed by intraoperative intra-arterial pressure measurements for proximal vessels and post-bypass arteriography for runoff vessels.[8] Life-table analysis of graft patency and limb salvage was performed (Fig. 15–8).[8] Two patients could not tolerate MRA and required contrast arteriography, but all others underwent reconstructive procedures on the basis of MRA alone (11 aortobifemoral and 67 infrainguinal reconstructions). Intraoperative findings regarding suitability of inflow and outflow vessels confirmed the accuracy of MRA in every case.

MRA indicated that none of the patients undergoing infrainguinal bypass had significant inflow occlusive disease. This was confirmed at operation with pressure measurements of inflow vessels that were all within 10 mmHg of peak systolic systemic pressure. Intraoperative completion arteriography and preoperative MRA results were identical (Figs. 15–9 and 15–10) for all except two patients with minor discrepancies. All aortobifemoral reconstruc-

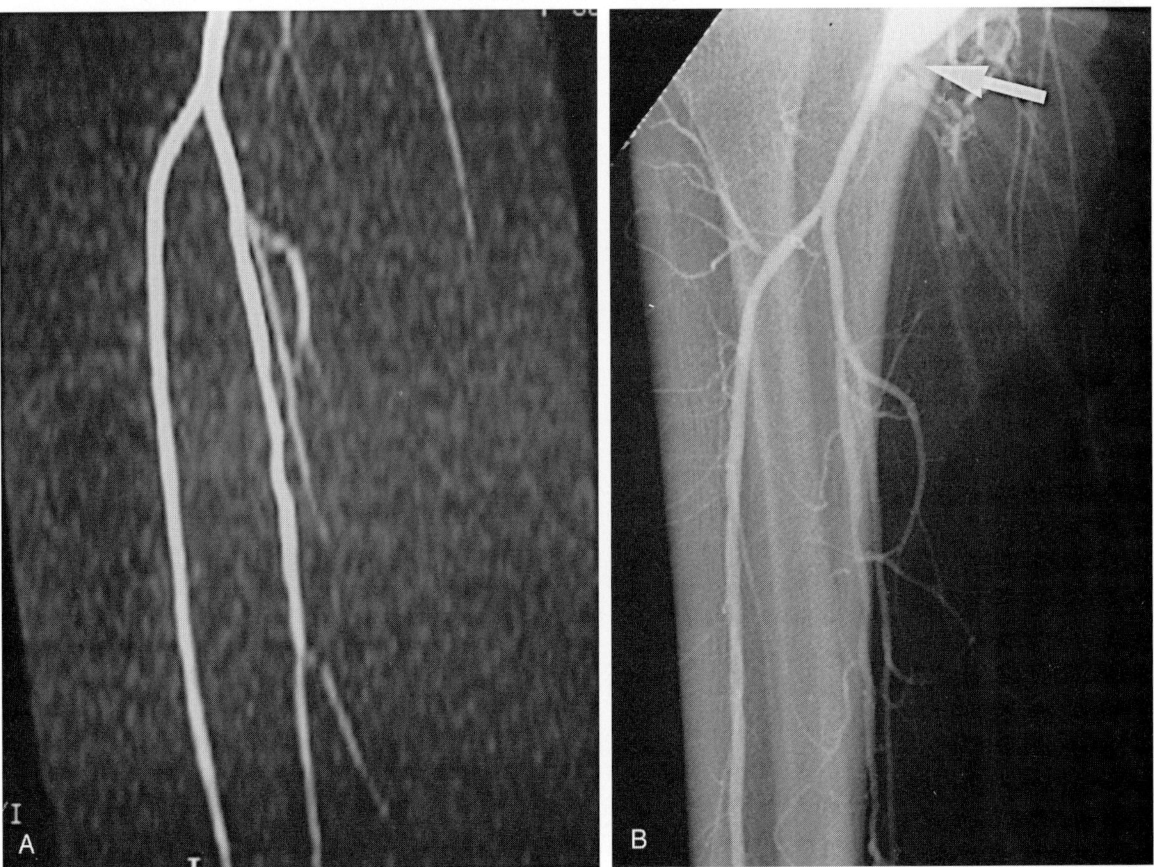

FIGURE 15–9. Preoperative and intraoperative imaging studies from a patient undergoing infrageniculate femoropopliteal bypass. *A,* Preoperative MR arteriogram of the infrageniculate popliteal artery and runoff vessels is shown. *B,* Intraoperative post-bypass arteriogram demonstrates infrageniculate femoropopliteal bypass anastomosis *(arrow)* and comparable imaging of runoff. (From Carpenter JP, Baum RA, Holland GA, et al: Peripheral vascular surgery with magnetic resonance angiography as the sole preoperative imaging modality. J Vasc Surg 20:861–871, 1994.)

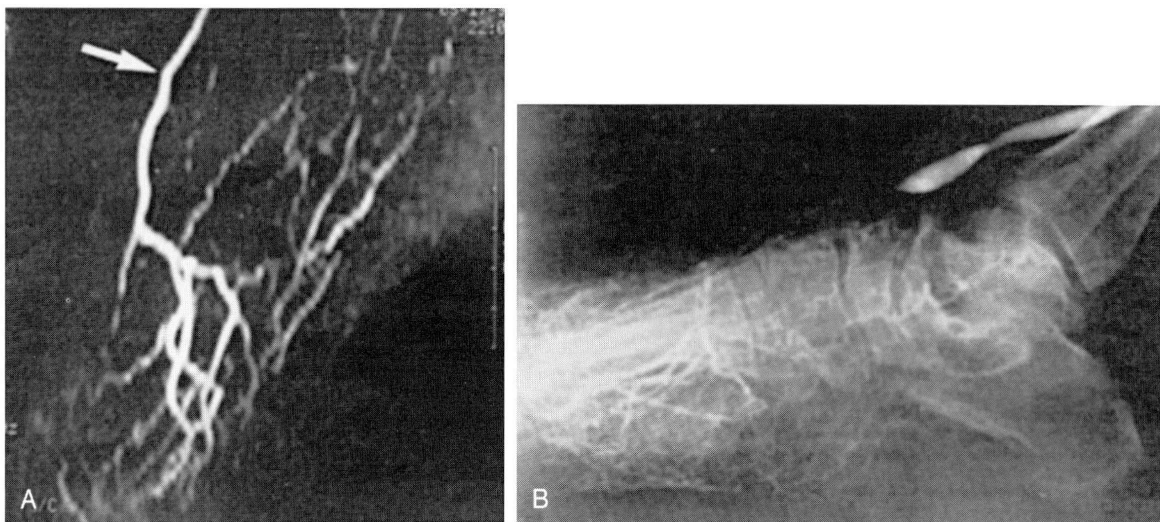

FIGURE 15–10. Preoperative and intraoperative imaging of a patient undergoing a femorodorsalis pedis bypass. Preoperative MR arteriogram of the foot (*A*) shows the dorsalis pedis artery (*arrow*) in continuity with incomplete pedal arch. This finding is confirmed by the post-bypass intraoperative arteriogram (*B*). (From Carpenter JP, Baum RA, Holland GA, et al: Peripheral vascular surgery with magnetic resonance angiography as the sole preoperative imaging modality. J Vasc Surg 20:861–871, 1994.)

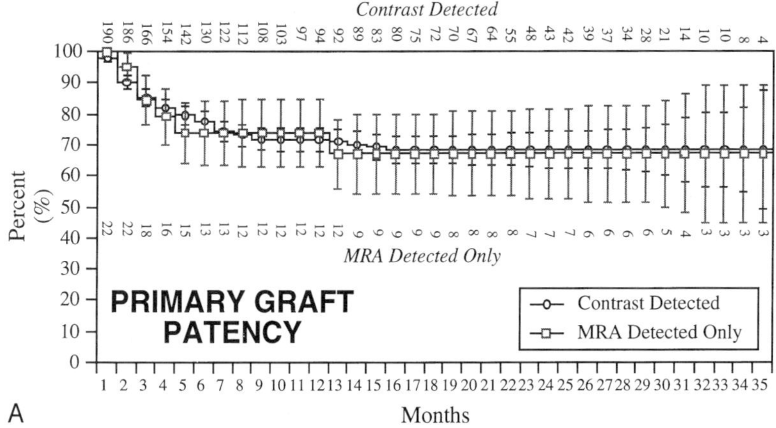

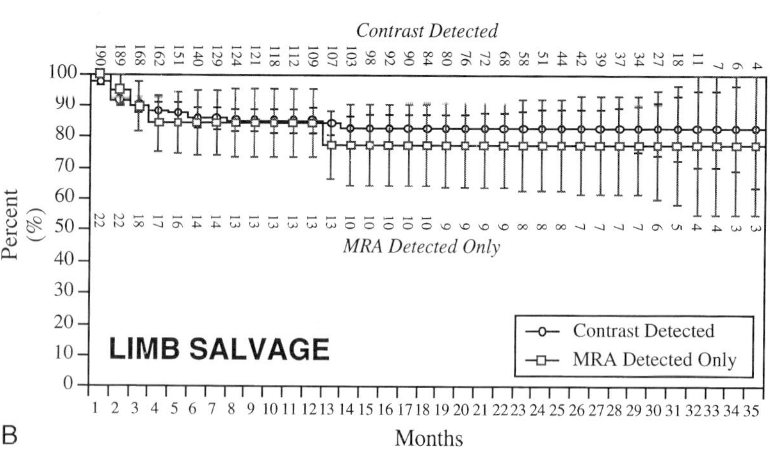

FIGURE 15–11. Survival curves depicting primary graft patency rate (*A*) and limb salvage rate (*B*) for patients receiving bypasses to "angiographically occult" runoff vessels compared with patients receiving bypasses to contrast arteriography (CA)–detected runoff vessels. A1 bypasses were to infrageniculate outflow. Thirty-five months after surgery the primary graft patency rate was 68% for bypasses to CA-detected vessels and 67% for MRA-detected vessels. The limb salvage rate was 83% for patients with CA-detected vessel bypass and 78% for patients with angiographically occult runoff. There were no statistically significant differences between the groups for graft patency (p = .92) and limb salvage (p = .84) rates. (From Carpenter JP, Golden MA, Barker CF, et al: The fate of bypass grafts to angiographically occult runoff vessels detected by magnetic resonance angiography. J Vasc Surg 23:483–489, 1996.)

tions remained patent, and all limbs were salvaged. The infrainguinal reconstructions carried an 84% limb salvage rate and a 78% primary graft patency rate at 21 months.[8] This rate was identical to that of a cohort of similar surgical patients consecutively undergoing contrast arteriography.

Angiographically Occult Runoff Vessels

MRA has facilitated the performance of bypass procedures in patients who were considered not to be bypass candidates because of the absence of a suitable target vessel on the preoperative conventional contrast arteriogram. In a study of 212 autogenous vein infragenicular bypasses performed for limb salvage, 22 (12%) were anastomosed to "angiographically occult" runoff vessels.[9] Life-table analysis of these bypasses to angiographically occult vessels was comparable to bypasses to contrast angiography–detected runoff vessels, with no significant difference in primary graft patency or limb salvage rates. The accuracy of MRA in predicting patency of angiographically occult vessels was confirmed in every case by intraoperative findings. At 35 months after surgery, the primary graft patency rate was 68% for bypasses to contrast angiography–detected vessels and 67% for MRA-detected vessels. The limb salvage rate was 83% for contrast angiography–detected vessel bypass patients and 78% for patients with angiographically occult runoff vessels (Fig. 15–11). It is recommended that MRA be performed when conventional preoperative contrast angiography fails to reveal runoff vessels suitable for use in a limb salvage procedure, as the greater sensitivity of MRA may facilitate successful bypass surgery and improve the overall limb salvage rate.

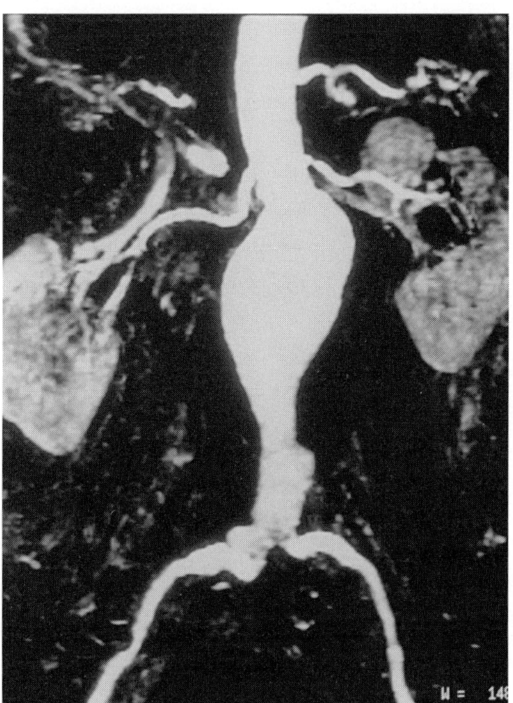

FIGURE 15–12. Gadolinium-enhanced magnetic resonance angiography (MRA) of an abdominal aortic aneurysm. Note left renal artery stenosis. MRA, may be used as a sole preoperative imaging technique for patients with abdominal aortic aneurysms. The technique accurately both depicts the arteriographic image of the aneurysm and, in combination with conventional MR images, shows its dimensions. The three-dimensional rotational views provide information about the geometry of the aneurysm that may be valuable for planning endovascular aneurysm repairs.

Cost-Effectiveness

MRA is more cost-effective than contrast arteriography.[8, 37, 61] The cost of a contrast arteriogram exceeds that of MRA, and MRA may be performed on an outpatient basis without the use of a short-stay unit. A cost savings of $1288 has been noted for each patient treated with preoperative MRA alone compared with contrast arteriography when MRA is used as the sole preoperative imaging modality.[8] The potential savings from reduced morbidity, given the noninvasive and non-nephrotoxic nature of MRA, were not taken into account in these cost analyses.

Aorta and Branch Arteries: Improved Accuracy with Gadolinium

Visceral Arteries

The advent of the non-nephrotoxic contrast agent gadolinium (Gd) has broadened the accuracy and applications of MRA as a vascular imaging technique. Turbulence and motion artefacts[14, 30, 46–48] can hamper the accuracy of MRA for imaging renal and visceral abdominal arteries as well as the aortic arch. The use of gadolinium greatly enhances the accuracy of imaging these arteries.[30, 43, 46–48, 53] Currently, gadolinium-enhanced three-dimensional TOF MRA is employed for preoperative imaging prior to aortic surgery, including thoracoabdominal and infrarenal aneurysm repair and occlusive disease of the aorta, as well as for renal and visceral artery reconstructions (Fig. 15–12).

In a prospective study of 63 patients with suspected visceral aortic branch occlusive disease, breath-hold ultrafast three-dimensional gadolinium-enhanced MRA techniques, combined with two-dimensional TOF MRA techniques, accurately identified and graded all (51 of 51) renal, celiac, superior mesenteric, and inferior mesenteric artery stenoses or occlusions. The combination of these MRA imaging techniques resulted in 100% sensitivity, specificity, and accuracy compared with conventional contrast angiography.[53]

Renal Artery Stenosis

MRA can accurately assess the main renal arteries for the presence of critical stenoses[23, 30, 47, 53] (Fig. 15–13). Traditional TOF MRA compared favorably with conventional angiography with a 91% sensitivity, a 94% negative predictive value, and an overall accuracy of 81%.[28] In this early study, however, accessory renal arteries were not well visualized and the morphology of arteries (e.g., fibromuscular disease) could not be appreciated. Yet, this study suggested that MRA is a highly sensitive screening test for the presence of renal artery stenosis compared with conventional contrast arteriography. More recently, gadolinium-enhanced MRA and breath-holding MRA techniques have been employed with greater accuracy, allowing for routine detection of accessory renal arteries and fibromuscular disease[23, 43, 46–48, 53] (Fig. 15–14).

In a prospective study of the abdominal aorta and the

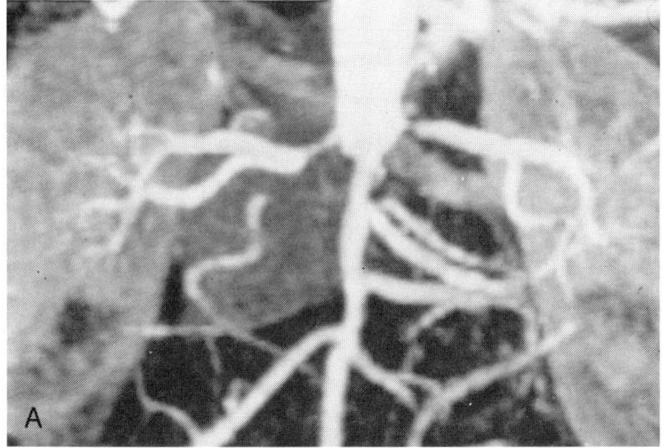

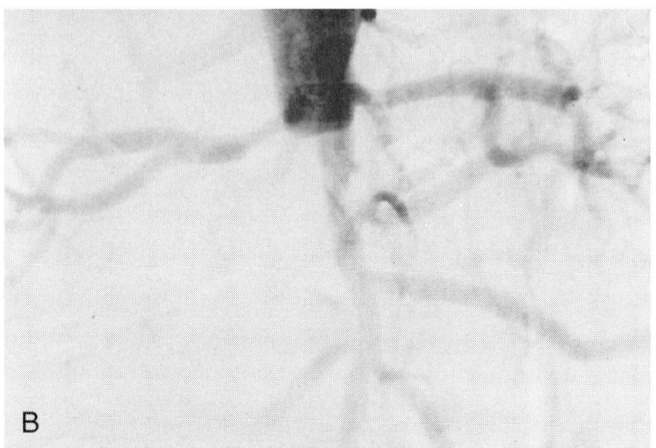

FIGURE 15–13. Bilateral renal artery stenosis in a 52-year-old man with suspected renovascular hypertension and Leriche's syndrome. *A,* Coronal enhanced breath-hold three-dimensional spoiled gradient-echo maximum-intensity-projection image shows bilateral proximal renal artery stenoses *(arrows)* and occlusion of the infrarenal abdominal aorta. *B,* On a conventional arteriogram, the superior mesenteric artery obscures left renal artery stenosis. (From Siegelman ES, Gilfeather M, Holland GA, et al: Pictorial essay: Breath-hold ultrafast three-dimensional gadolinium-enhanced MR angiography of the renovascular system. AJR Am J Roentgenol 168(4): 1035, 1997.)

renal arteries that compared traditional two-dimensional TOF and other MRA techniques with breath-hold ultrafast three-dimensional spoiled gradient-echo (SPGR) gadolinium-enhanced MRA, the latter resulted in superior specificity and sensitivity for detecting renal artery stenoses and accessory renal arteries.[30] With breath-hold ultrafast three-dimensional SPGR, eight of nine (89%) accessory renal arteries and 100% of 31 renal artery stenoses studied were accurately identified and graded. Studies using other Gd-enhanced three-dimensional MRA methods without breath-holding have reported 50% to 70% sensitivity in identifying accessory renal arteries (Fig. 15–15) and 71% to 85% sensitivity for renal artery stenoses.[43, 46] In breath-hold ultrafast three-dimensional SPGR gadolinium-enhanced MRA, the improved image quality and the ability to detect vascular lesions and to identify vessels not seen with two-dimensional TOF, or other three-dimensional Gd-enhanced MRA imaging methods, results from the elimination of respiratory motion artefact.[30] The three-dimensional volume acquisition obtained from a single 18- to 32-second patient breath hold can be reformatted at a workstation, and the vascular anatomy may be viewed in any projection and with a variety of section thicknesses.[23, 53] Therefore, this MR imaging technique can be particularly useful in the evaluation of aberrant arteries, vascular stenoses, aneurysms, and aortic dissections (Fig. 15–16).[23, 53]

Aortic Arch and Great Vessels

Gadolinium-enhanced MRA techniques have been applied to imaging the aortic arch and its branches.[10] The utility and accuracy of gadolinium-enhanced MRA imaging of the aortic arch (Figs. 15–17 to 15–20) have been prospectively evaluated and compared with conventional contrast arteriography in 28 patients thought to have carotid or arch vessel disease.[10] A total of 196 arch vessels containing 58 stenoses and four occlusions were examined. Substantial

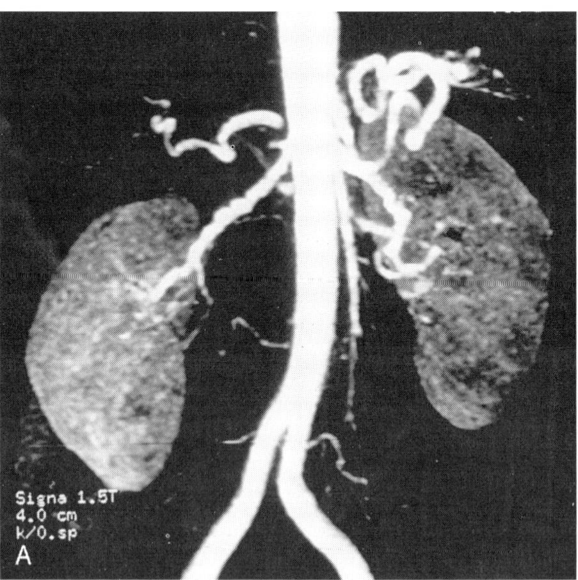

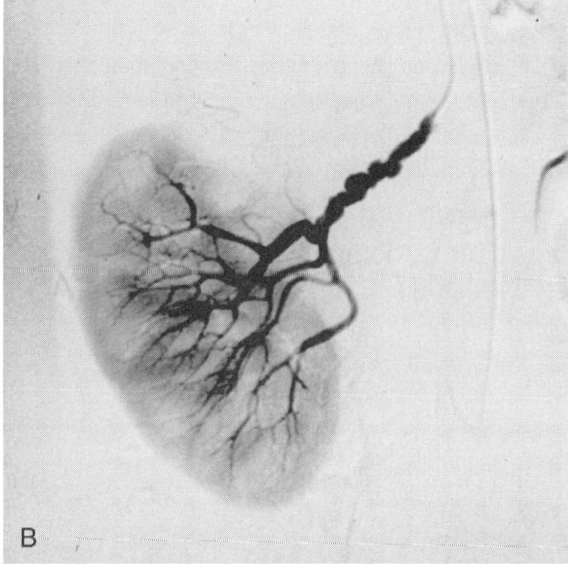

FIGURE 15–14. Fibromuscular dysplasia in a 53-year-old woman with suspected renovascular hypertension. *A,* Right posterior oblique enhanced breath-hold three-dimensional spoiled gradient-echo maximum-intensity projection images shows characteristic distribution and appearance of fibromuscular dysplasia. *B,* Conventional arteriogram shows similar findings. (From Siegelman ES, Gilfeather M, Holland GA, et al: Pictorial essay: Breath-hold ultrafast three-dimensional gadolinium-enhanced MR angiography of the renovascular system. AJR Am J Roentgenol 168(4):1035, 1997.)

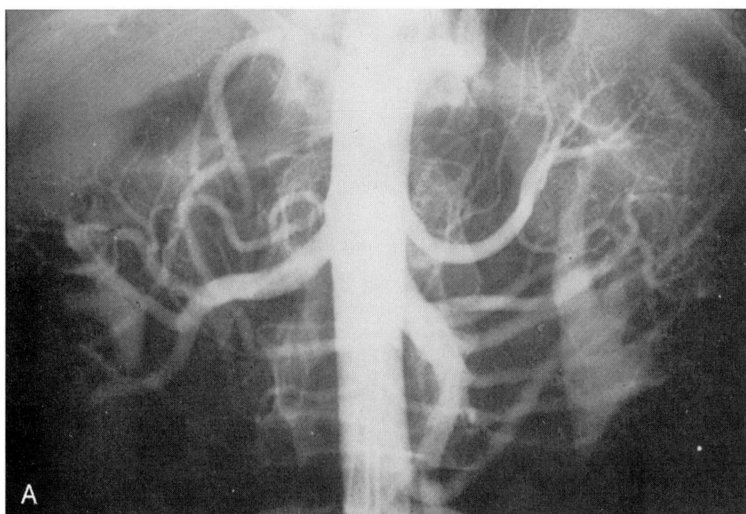

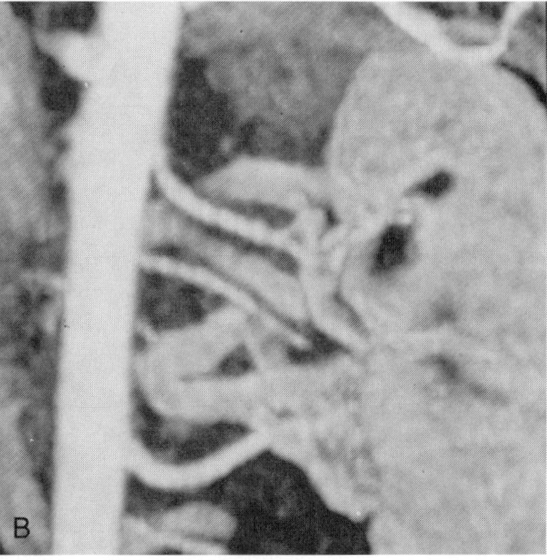

FIGURE 15–15. Multiple accessory left renal arteries in a 33-year-old man who was a potential renal transplant donor. *A,* Conventional aortogram shows three left renal arteries *(arrows)* and a patent main right renal artery. *B,* Left posterior oblique enhanced breath-hold three-dimensional spoiled gradient-echo maximum-intensity-projection image created from limited imaging volume shows three normal left renal arteries *(straight arrows)* seen in *A.* Note draining veins *(curved arrows).* (From Siegelman ES, Gilfeather M, Holland GA, et al: Pictorial essay: Breath-hold ultrafast three-dimensional gadolinium-enhanced MR angiography of the renovascular system. AJR Am J Roentgenol 168(4):1035, 1997.)

interobserver agreement in interpretation of the MRA studies was noted. The fast gadolinium-enhanced MRA accurately identified all anatomic variants (Fig. 15–18) and provided an arteriographic image of the aortic arch that is superior to any obtained by other noninvasive imaging methods.[10] Fast gadolinium-enhanced MRA can detect significant stenotic lesions of the aortic arch with a 97% accuracy and a 98% predictive value (see Figs. 15–19 and 15–20).[10] A normal result on MRA strongly predicts a normal contrast arteriographic study result.

Popliteal Entrapment

MRI and MRA techniques can demonstrate the anatomic relationships between the popliteal artery and the muscles within the popliteal fossa, thereby constituting ideal noninvasive screening modalities for the diagnosis of *popliteal artery entrapment syndrome* (PAES) prior to angiography or surgery.[16, 20, 25, 49] The combination of MRI and MRA allows for detailed evaluation of the relationships between the gastrocnemius muscle and the popliteal artery at rest as well as during stress, when evidence of popliteal artery occlusion may be demonstrated. This combined morphologic and functional evaluation of both soft tissues and vasculature makes the MRI and MRA modalities ideally suited for assessment of young adults with intermittent claudication thought to have PAES.[16, 20, 25, 49]

One study of 17 patients (33 limbs) was conducted to assess the efficacy of dynamic MRA as an alternative to conventional contrast angiography in patients with surgically proven PAES.[22] Nine patients (17 limbs) with known PAES underwent positional-provocation DSA and two-dimensional TOF dynamic MRA of the popliteal fossae. In addition, 8 normal volunteers (16 limbs) underwent dynamic MRA. Two observers blinded to the known surgical findings and the results of the DSA independently evaluated the 33 limbs of the 17 subjects on the basis of maximum-intensity projection images and transverse MRA source images. A grading of the stenosis by MRA was compared with that indicated by DSA. MRA correctly identified 13 of 17 limbs (76%) from patients with surgically proven PAES, correctly indicating greater than 50% stenosis of the popliteal artery. Dynamic MRA also indicated stenosis of 1% to 50% in four of the 16 normal limbs (25%) and no stenosis in the other 12 normal limbs.

This study suggested that conventional contrast angiography may not be necessary when dynamic MRA indicates stenosis greater than 50% in patients with clinical suspicion of PAES. Stenoses between 1% and 50% noted by dynamic MRA, however, may need confirmation from contrast arteriography, when clinically indicated.[22] MRA is also accurate for diagnosis of bypass graft entrapment syndromes (Fig. 15–21).[12]

Venous Disease

In the diagnosis of DVT, MRI and MRV can provide more information than other traditional tests, such as ultrasound, computed tomography (CT), and contrast venography.[11, 44] In some areas of the body, such as the neck and pelvis, MRI and MRV may now be considered the imaging modality of choice for identifying collateral venous channels and diagnosing the underlying cause of the thrombosis.[11, 34, 41, 44, 57]

In a study of 101 lower extremity, abdominal, and pelvic venous systems, MRV was compared with duplex ultrasound and contrast venography and was found to be nearly perfect in detection of DVT (Fig. 15–22).[11] MRV compared favorably with duplex scanning of the lower extremities and consistently imaged the pelvic veins and vena cava, which are often inaccessible to duplex scanning. In addition, the hypogastric and deep femoral veins, not normally visualized by contrast venography without selection catheterization, were routinely seen. MRV may be the test of choice for detection of DVT in the abdominal or pelvic veins. MRA of the pulmonary arteries appears promising for the noninvasive diagnosis for pulmonary embolus.[38]

The accuracy of MRI and MRV in the diagnosis of venous

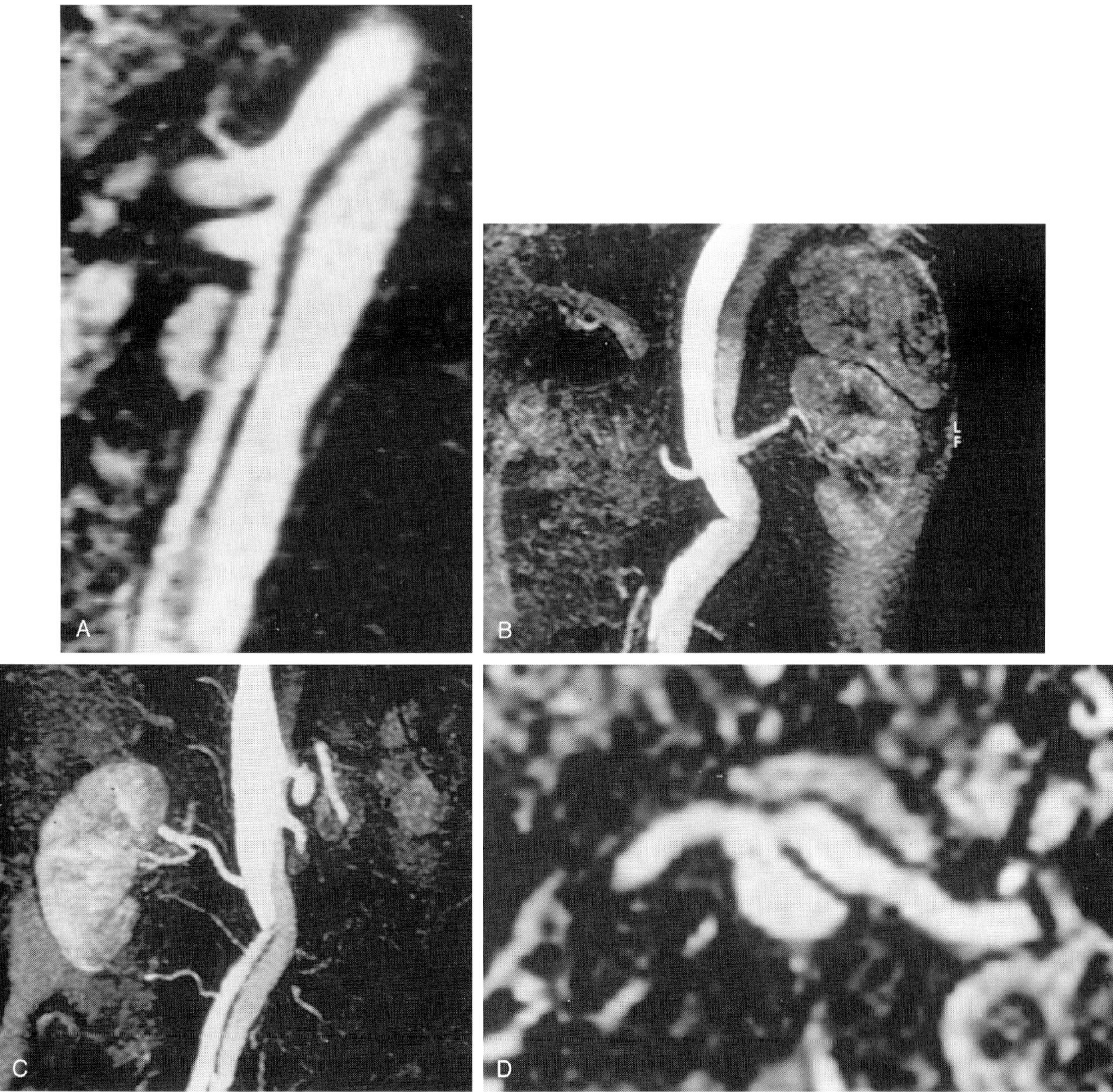

FIGURE 15–16. Renal artery visualization in a 64-year-old man with type B aortic dissection. *A–C*, Coronal *(A)*, axial *(B)*, and sagittal *(C)* enhanced breath-hold dimensional spoiled gradient-echo maximum-intensity-projection images show dissection of abdominal aorta. Left renal artery is supplied mostly from anterior lumen, as are celiac axis and superior mesenteric artery. Right renal artery is supplied by both anterior and posterior lumina. (From Siegelman ES, Gilfeather M, Holland GA, et al: Pictorial essay: Breath-hold ultrafast three-dimensional gadolinium-enhanced MR angiography of the renal vascular system. AJR Am J Roentgenol 168:1035, 1997.)

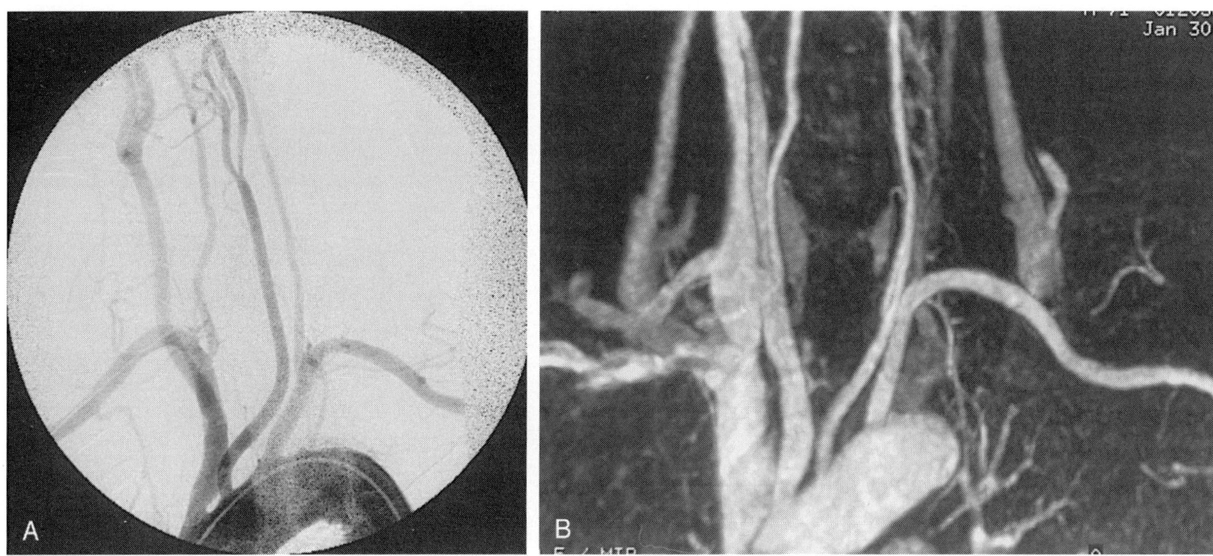

FIGURE 15–17. Normal anatomy of aortic arch depicted by contrast arteriography *(A)* and magnetic resonance angiography (MRA) *(B)*. Central veins filled with gadolinium are seen on MRA of the arch as well as arteries. (From Carpenter JP, Holland GA, Barker CF, et al: Magnetic resonance angiography of the aortic arch. J Vasc Surg 25:145, 1997.)

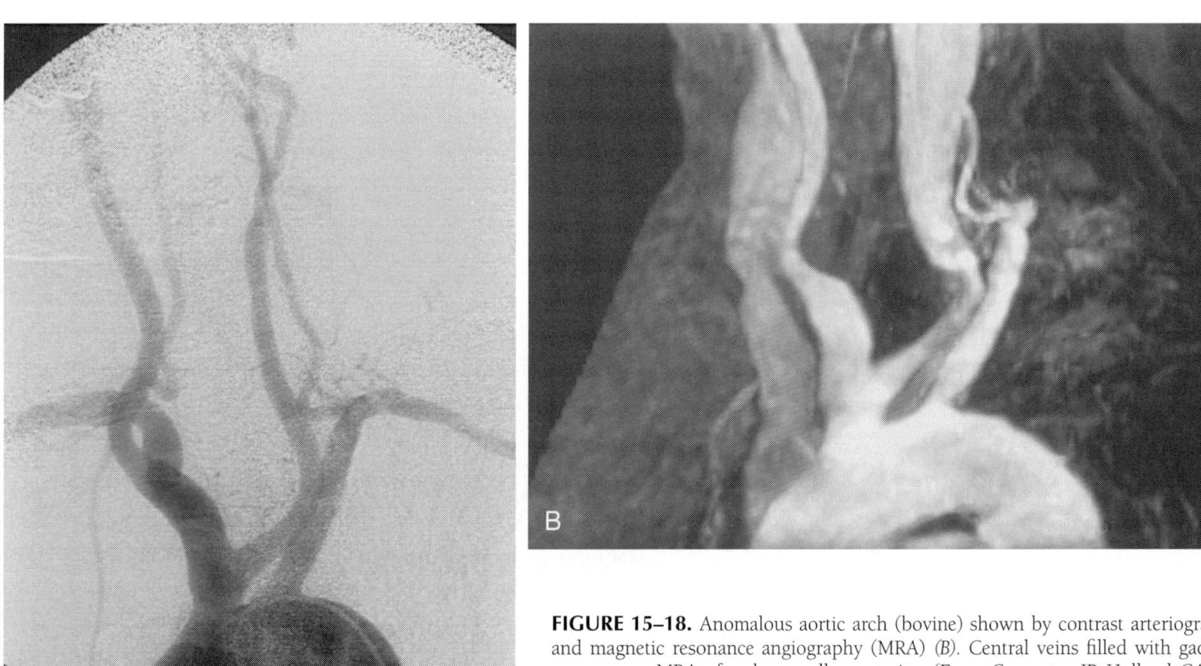

FIGURE 15–18. Anomalous aortic arch (bovine) shown by contrast arteriography *(A)* and magnetic resonance angiography (MRA) *(B)*. Central veins filled with gadolinium are seen on MRA of arch as well as arteries. (From Carpenter JP, Holland GA, Barker CF, et al: Magnetic resonance angiography of the aortic arch. J Vasc Surg 25:145, 1997.)

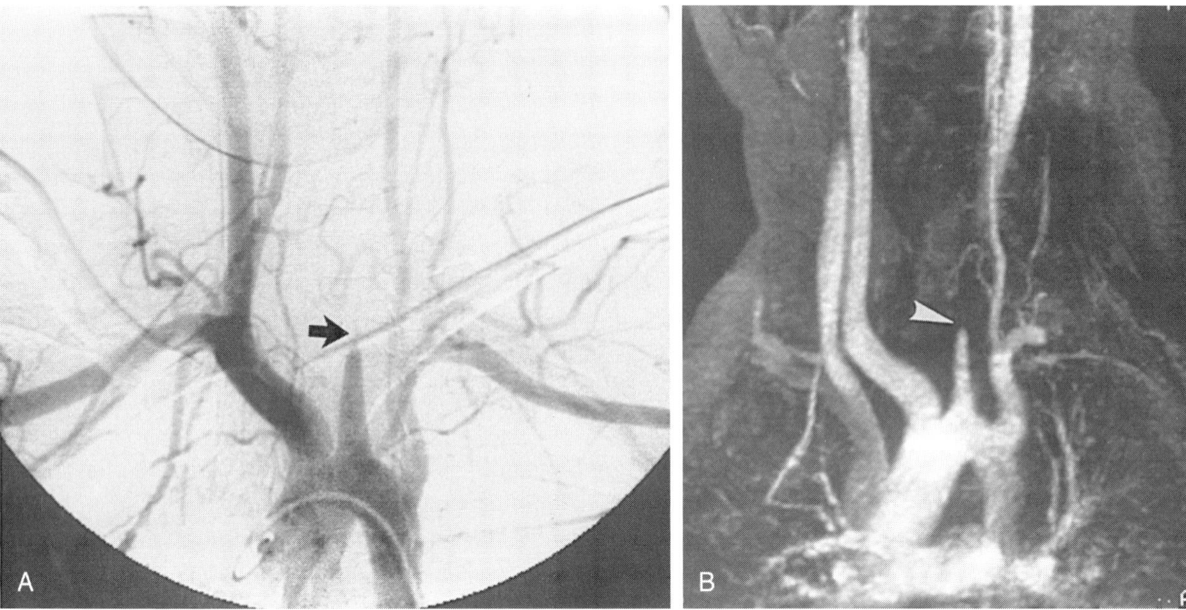

FIGURE 15–19. Dissection and occlusion of the left common carotid artery *(arrow)* seen by arteriography *(A)* and magnetic resonance angiography *(arrowhead) (B)*. (From Carpenter JP, Holland GA, Barker CF, et al: Magnetic resonance angiography of the aortic arch. J Vasc Surg 25:145, 1997.)

thrombosis of the cervical or mediastinal veins has been reported to be as high as 100%.[34] MRV has proved extremely reliable and accurate in the diagnosis of thoracic venous obstructions.[15] With digital subtraction venography used as the gold standard, the sensitivity and specificity of MRV (with three orthogonal planes) have been 94% and 100%, respectively, for detecting venous patency within the thoracic cavity.[15] The sensitivity and specificity of MRV for detecting complete venous obstruction within the thoracic cavity were 100% and 98%, respectively.[15] In the shoulder region, MRV demonstrated a sensitivity and specificity of 93% and 100%, respectively, for detecting venous patency and 100% and 97% for detecting venous obstruction.[15] MRV with three orthogonal planes can, therefore, provide a relatively complete and reliable venous map in the thoracic and shoulder regions without the need for contrast.[15]

MRI/MRV not only accurately identifies the site of DVT but also allows the identification of conditions that may cause, mimic, or be associated with venous thrombosis, such as ruptured Baker's cysts, cellulitis, muscle tears, hematomas, and external venous compression from tumors or other anatomic anomalies.[11, 44] MRI may be useful in accurately detecting DVT in pregnant women in whom thrombosis of the pelvic veins is clinically suspected.[11, 57] Duplex ultrasonography is suboptimal in this clinical setting because it does not easily visualize pelvic veins. CT has the disadvantage of radiation exposure in the setting of pregnancy.

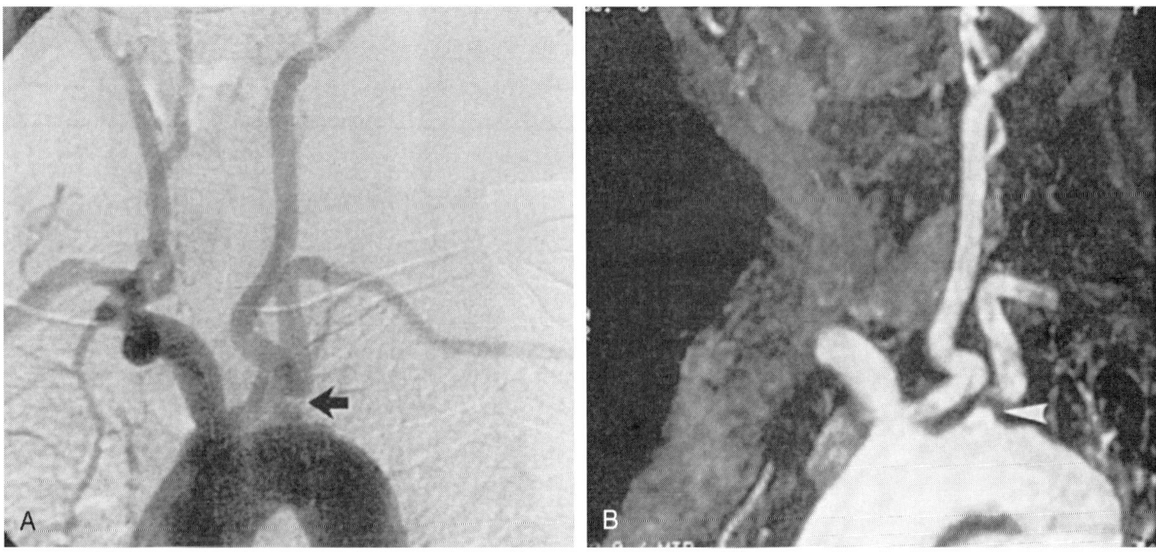

FIGURE 15–20. Stenotic lesion of left subclavian artery origin *(arrow)* demonstrated by contrast arteriography *(A)* and magnetic resonance angiography (MRA) *(arrowhead) (B)*. The amount of stenosis was 75% by arteriography and 80% by MRA. (From Carpenter JP, Holland GA, Barker CF, et al: Magnetic resonance angiography of the aortic arch. J Vasc Surg 25:145, 1997.)

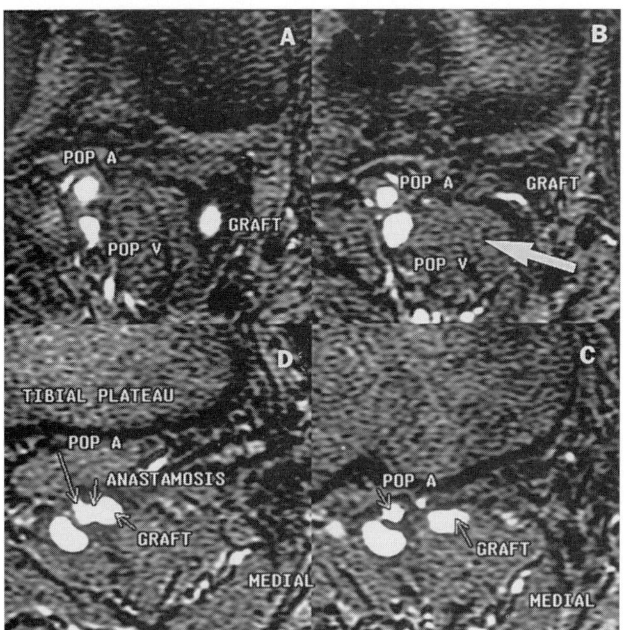

FIGURE 15–21. Magnetic resonance angiogram from a patient with iatrogenic entrapment of a below-knee femoropopliteal bypass graft. *A–D,* Proximal *(A)* to distal *(D)* axial images demonstrate the course of the graft passing superficial to the medial head of the gastrocnemius muscle *(arrow)* *(B)* and compression between the gastrocnemius and the tendons of the semitendinosus and gracilis muscles. Entrapment was relieved by division of the medial head of the gastrocnemius muscle.

MRI and MRV technology can serve as a useful adjuvant imaging modality that offers a noninvasive approach to the difficult diagnostic problem of assessing non-neoplastic venous thrombosis of the renal veins.[58] MRI and MRV can also accurately depict normal and abnormal portal and hepatic venous anatomy in relation to the hepatic parenchyma and thus may be useful in planning transjugular intrahepatic portosystemic shunts (TIPSs).[36] Fast-spin-echo MRV offers a reliable, accurate depiction of venous anatomy in the evaluation of slow-flow systems, such as the calf and forearm veins.[6] MRV also has proved to be extremely useful in the confirmation of the traditionally difficult-to-diagnose entity of cerebral venous thrombosis.[41] Brain MRV has a major role in the diagnosis and follow-up of dural venous thrombosis.[34] High-resolution MRV of the intracranial subependymal veins is as effective as conventional cerebral angiography.[39]

Vascular Malformations

Although conventional contrast angiography can demonstrate the components of a vascular malformation, the technique may be technically challenging in small patients with complex venous anomalies. The role of MRV in the evaluation of children with predominantly low-flow, vascular malformations of the extremities has been studied and compared with conventional contrast angiograms as the standard.[35] It has been noted that MRI/MRV accurately visualizes all significant vascular anomalies seen with contrast angiography.[35] In addition, MRV demonstrates some veins not opacified by the conventional contrast study.[35] MRV visualizes both superficial and deep conducting veins, whereas contrast angiography is a more directed study, evaluating only vascular channels that are intentionally opacified.[35] The combination of MRI and MRV imaging is a noninvasive method that can form the basis for determining the prognosis and choosing the individual treatment for children with low-flow congenital vascular malformations of the extremities.[31, 35] MRI/MRV is now considered to be the initial diagnostic test of choice for vascular malformations.[31] Further investigations are not necessary in low-flow lesions.[31, 35] In cases of high-flow and combined-flow lesions, angiography is indicated, following MRI and MRV,

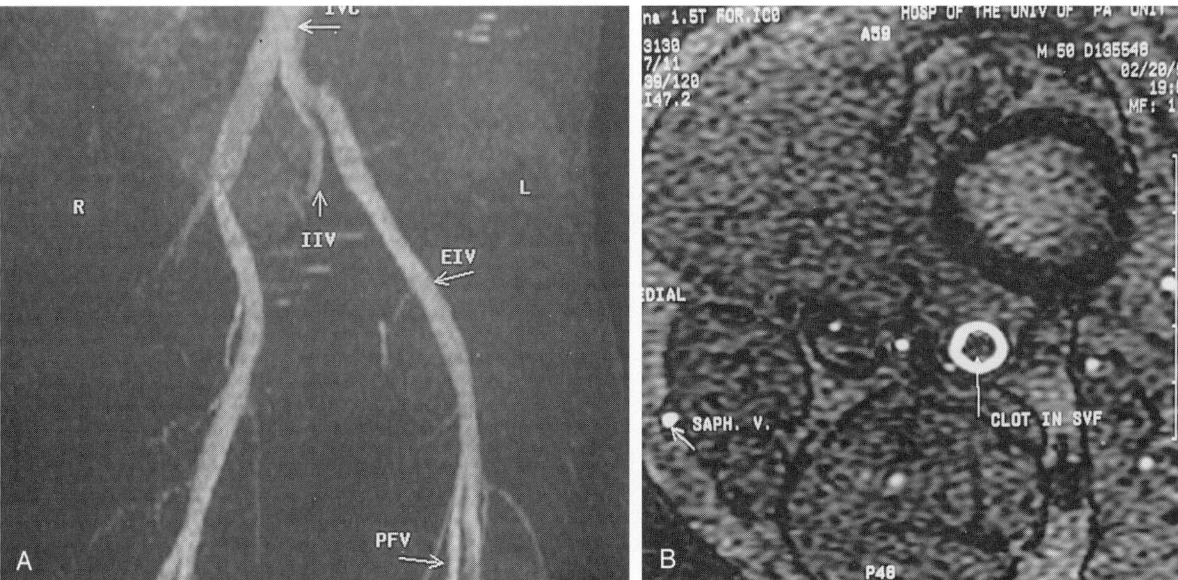

FIGURE 15–22. Magnetic resonance venograms of projectional reconstruction of normal venous system *(A)* and cross-sectional transaxial image *(B)* show partially occlusive thrombus. The inferior vena cava (IVC), internal iliac vein (IIV), external iliac vein (EIV), superficialis femoris vein (SFV), and profunda femoris vein (PFV) can be seen.

for showing the exact angioarchitecture, which is essential for treatment planning.[19, 31]

For congenital vascular malformations of the hand, MRI/MRV can clearly define the anatomic extent of the lesion, its relationship to surrounding tissues, and the flow characteristics in each patient.[17] The imaging information obtained is concordant with that obtained from conventional arteriography in these patients,[17] such that MRI/MRV is now considered an effective imaging modality in the management of vascular malformations of the hand. Resectability of the lesion can be assessed on the basis of extent of tissue involvement and flow characteristics, information that may be accurately obtained from the MRI/MRV images.[17] This technique provides detailed images of the arterial and venous components of the lesions while obviating the requirement for intravenous contrast, ionizing radiation, or an invasive procedure.

MRI/MRV is useful as a noninvasive modality for evaluating pulmonary vascular malformations as small as 1 cm in diameter.[54] However, the specificity, sensitivity, and accuracy of MRI/MRV for the diagnosis of vascular malformations of the extremities, hands, trunk, and pulmonary tree remain to be prospectively studied and validated against conventional contrast angiography as the standard imaging test. At least one report has indicated that preoperative conventional arteriography and venography remain essential in planning surgical treatment for patients with vascular malformations.[33]

MRI, MRA, and MRV technology may also be a useful, noninvasive modality for diagnosis of malformations of cerebral cortical development, which are a significant cause of epilepsy in adults and of developmental delay and epilepsy in children.[2, 32] MRI, MRA, and MRV are particularly useful in the evaluation of angiographically occult vascular malformations in patients with neurologic symptoms and negative findings on a conventional contrast brain angiogram.[59] In a comparison study of CT, MRI/MRA/MRV, and cerebral angiography, MRI/MRA/MRV was superior to CT in detecting cerebral arteriovenous malformations (AVMs).[45] The strength of MRI, MRA, and MRV over CT scan lies in the ability of the technology to detect abnormal vessels, even in the presence of fresh or older hematoma, and to precisely identify the size and location of the AVM.[45] Although MRI, MRA, and MRV can provide accurate and reliable three-dimensional images of blood vessels, further studies validating the technique are required before it may be viewed as a potential substitute for conventional contrast angiography prior to surgical treatment of cerebral AVMs.

Indications for MR Imaging, MRV, and MR Arteriography in Vascular Disease

MRI/MRA/MRV technology has proved useful in an increasing number of clinical applications. Although some indications remain under study and require extensive validation, many are widely accepted. MRI/MRA/MRV is emerging as the study of choice for diagnosis and preoperative planning in many patients with peripheral vascular disease of the lower extremities; aortic aneurysm; DVT of the neck, chest, lower extremities, and pelvis; and low-flow vascular malformations of the hands and extremities in children. MRA is a useful screening test for carotid artery disease; pathology of the aortic, visceral, and renal arterial branches; and cerebral vascular malformations. MRA needs to be compared with and validated against the reference standard—contrast angiography—as with any other noninvasive vascular imaging modality.

SUMMARY

Improvements in vascular techniques have greatly expanded the treatment options for many patients suffering from vascular diseases. Detailed and accurate vascular imaging is essential for preoperative planning. Although conventional contrast angiography has been the time-honored standard imaging technique for vascular diseases, the method is invasive with attendant limitations and risks. MRI, MRA, and MRV represent new, noninvasive vascular techniques that may be added to the preoperative assessment options, with the potential for improved sensitivity, avoidance of morbidity, and cost savings. MRA and MRV are rapidly developing as vascular imaging techniques. Individual centers must validate their MR results and interpretations against standard contrast angiography to ensure accuracy equivalent to that reported from centers of excellence. With new developments in hardware, software, and MR non-nephrotoxic contrast agents, the applicability of MR to vascular surgery will continue to expand. MRA already has a major role and in some cases has supplanted the need for conventional contrast angiography in preoperative vascular surgical evaluation.

REFERENCES

1. Ansell G, Tweedle MCK, West CR, et al: The current status of reactions to intravenous contrast media. Invest Radiol 15:S32–S39, 1980.
2. Barkovich AJ: Malformations of neocortical development: Magnetic resonance imaging correlates. Curr Opin Neurol 9(2):118–121, 1996.
3. Baum RA, Carpenter JP: Can magnetic resonance angiography replace contrast arteriography in the patient with arterial occlusive disease? Postgrad Rad 14:95, 1994.
4. Baum RA, Carpenter JP: Can magnetic resonance angiography replace contrast arteriography in the patient with arterial occlusive disease? Postgrad Rad 14:95, 1994.
5. Baum RA, Rutter CM, Sunshine JH, et al, for the American College of Radiology New Technology Assessment Group: Multicenter trial to evaluate peripheral vascular magnetic resonance angiography. JAMA 274:875–880, 1995.
6. Bluemke DA, Wolf RL, Tani I, Tachiki S, et al: Extremity veins: Evaluation with fast-spin-echo MR venography. Radiology 204(2):562–565, 1997.
7. Cambria RP, Yucel EK, Brewster DC, et al: The potential for lower extremity revascularization without contrast arteriography: Experience with magnetic resonance angiography. J Vasc Surg 17:1050–1057, 1993.
8. Carpenter JP, Baum RA, Holland GA, et al: Peripheral vascular surgery with magnetic resonance angiography as the sole preoperative imaging modality. J Vasc Surg 20:861–871, 1994.
9. Carpenter JP, Golden MA, Barker CF, et al: The fate of bypass grafts to angiographically occult runoff vessels detected by magnetic resonance angiography. J Vasc Surg 23:483–489, 1996.
10. Carpenter JP, Holland GA, Barker CF, et al: Magnetic resonance angiography of the aortic arch. J Vasc Surg 25:145–151, 1997.
11. Carpenter JP, Holland GA, Baum RA, et al: Magnetic resonance venography for the detection of deep venous thrombosis: Comparison with contrast venography and duplex Doppler ultrasound. J Vasc Surg 18:734–741, 1993.

12. Carpenter JP, Lieberman MD, Shlansky-Goldberg R, et al: Infrageniculate bypass graft entrapment. J Vasc Surg 18:81–89, 1993.
13. Carpenter JP, Owen RS, Baum RA, et al: Magnetic resonance angiography of peripheral runoff vessels. J Vasc Surg 16:807–115, 1992.
14. Carpenter JP, Owen RS, Holland GA, et al: Magnetic resonance angiography of the aorta, iliac and femoral arteries. Surgery 116:17–23, 1994.
15. Chang YC, SU CT, Yang PC, et al: Magnetic resonance angiography in the diagnosis of thoracic venous obstruction. J Formos Med Assoc 97(1):38–43, 1998.
16. Dicesare E, Simonetti C, Morettini G, et al: Popliteal artery entrapment: MR findings. J Comput Assist Tomogr Mar-Apr 16(2):295–2957, 1992.
17. Dissa JJ, Chunk KC, Gellad FE, et al: Efficacy of magnetic resonance angiography in the evaluation of vascular malformations of the hand. Plast Reconstr Surg 99:136; discussion 145–147, 1997.
18. D'Elia JA, Gleason RE, Alday M: Nephrotoxicity from angiographic contrast material: A prospective study. Am J Med 72(5):719–725, 1982.
19. Dobson MJ, Hartley RW, Ashleigh R, et al: MR angiography and MR imaging of symptomatic vascular malformations. Clin Radiol 52(8):595–602, 1997.
20. Erdoes LS, Devine JJ, Bernhard VM, et al: Popliteal vascular compression in a normal population. J Vasc Surg 20:978–986, 1994.
21. Flanigan DP, Williams LR, Keifer T, et al: Pre-bypass operative angiography. Surgery 92:627–633, 1982.
22. Forster BB, Houston, JG, Macham LS, et al: Comparison of two-dimensional time-of-flight dynamic magnetic resonance angiography with digital subtraction angiography in popliteal artery entrapment syndrome. Can Assoc Radiol J 48(1):11–18, 1997.
23. Gilfeather M, Holland GA, Siegelman ES, et al: Gadolinium enhanced ultrafast three-dimensional spoiled gradient echo imaging of the abdominal aorta and visceral and iliac vessels: Technique and pictorial review. RadioGraphics 17:423–432, 1997.
24. Goldman K, Salvesen S, Hegedus V: Acute renal failure after contrast medial injection. Invest Radiol S19:S125, 1984.
25. Hayashi S, Hamanaka Y, Sueda T, et al: A case of adventitial cystic disease of the popliteal artery preoperatively diagnosed by magnetic resonance imaging. Nippon Geka Gakkai Zasshi March 94(3):314, 1994.
26. Hertz SM, Baum RA, Holland GA, Carpenter JP: Magnetic resonance angiographic imaging of angioplasty and atherectomy sites. J Cardiovasc Surg 35:1–6, 1994.
27. Hertz SM, Baum RA, Owen RS, et al: Comparison of magnetic resonance and contrast arteriography in peripheral arterial stenosis. Am J Surg 166:112–116, 1993.
28. Hertz SM, Holland GA, Baum RA, et al: Evaluation of renal artery stenosis by magnetic resonance angiography. Am J Surg 168:140, 1994.
29. Hessel SJ, Adams DF, Abrams HL: Complications of angiography. Radiology 138:273, 1981.
30. Holland GA, Dougherty L, Carpenter JP, et al: Breath-hold ultrafast three dimensional gadolinium-enhanced MR angiography of the aorta, the renal, and other visceral abdominal arteries. AJR Am J Roentgenol 166:971, 1996.
31. Hovius SE, Borg DH, Paans PR, et al: The diagnostic value of magnetic resonance imaging in combination with angiography in patients with vascular malformations: A prospective study. Ann Plast Surg 37:278–285, 1996.
32. Huber G, Henkes H, Hermes M, et al: Regional association of developmental venous anomalies with angiographically occult vascular malformations. Eur Radiol 6(1):30–37, 1996.
33. Huch Boni RA, Brunner U, Bollinger A, et al: Management of congenital angiodysplasia of the lower limb: Magnetic imaging and angiography versus conventional angiography. Br J Radiol 68(816):1308–1315, 1995.
34. Laissy JP, Dell'Isola B, Petitjean C, et al: Magnetic resonance angiography: Fields of exploration, main indications and limitations. J Mal Vasc 22(5):287–302, 1997.
35. Laor T, Burrows PE, Hoffer FA: Magnetic resonance venography of congenital vascular malformations of the extremities. Pediatr Radiol 26(6):371–380, 1996.
36. Lee JP: Variation in portal and hepatic venous anatomy as shown by magnetic resonance imaging: Implications for transjugular intrahepatic portosystemic shunt. Clin Radiol 50(2):108–110, 1995.
37. Levy MM, Baum RA, Carpenter JP: Endovascular surgery based solely upon noninvasive preprocedural imaging. J Vasc Surg 28(6):995–1003, 1998.
38. Meaney JFM, Weg JG, Chenevert TL, et al: Diagnosis of pulmonary embolism with magnetic resonance angiography. N Engl J Med 336:1422–1427, 1997.
39. Ohkawa M, Fujiwara N, Katoh T, et al: Detection of subependymal veins using high resolution magnetic resonance venography. Acta Med Okayama 51:321, 1997.
40. Owen RS, Carpenter JP, Baum RA, et al: Magnetic resonance imaging of angiographically occult runoff vessels in peripheral arterial occlusive disease. N Engl J Med 326:1577–1581, 1992.
41. Patel MR, Edelman RR: MR angiography of the head and neck. Top Magn Reson Imaging 8:345–365, 1996.
42. Patel PR, Semel L, Clauss RH: Extended reconstruction rate for limb salvage with intraoperative pre-reconstruction angiography. J Vasc Surg 7:531–537, 1988.
43. Petersen MJ, Cambria RP, Kaufman JA, et al: Magnetic resonance angiography in the preoperative evaluation of abdominal aortic aneurysms. J Vasc Surg 21:891–898, 1995.
44. Pope CF, Dietz MJ, Ezekowitz MD, et al: Technical variables influencing the detection of acute deep vein thrombosis by magnetic resonance imaging. Magn Reson Imaging 9:379–388, 1991.
45. Pott M, Huber M, Assheuer J, et al: Comparison of MRI, CT and angiography in cerebral arteriovenous malformations. Bildgebung 59(2):98–102, 1992.
46. Prince MR: Gadolinium-enhanced MR aortography. Radiology 191:155–164, 1994.
47. Prince MR, Narasimham DL, Stanley JC, et al: Breath-hold gadolinium-enhanced MR angiography of the abdominal aorta and its major branches. Radiology 197:785, 1995.
48. Prince MR, Narasimham DL, Stanley JC, et al: Gadolinium-enhanced magnetic resonance angiography of abdominal aortic aneurysms. J Vasc Surg 21:656, 1995.
49. Rosset E, Hartung O, Brunet C, et al: Popliteal artery entrapment syndrome: Anatomic and embryologic bases, diagnostic and therapeutic considerations following a series of 15 cases with a review of the literature. Surg Radiol Anat 17:161–169, 23–27, 1995.
50. Ricco JB, Pearce WH, Yao JST, et al: The use of operative pre-bypass arteriography and Doppler ultrasound recordings to select patients for extended femorodistal bypass. Ann Surg 198:646, 1983.
51. Scarpato R, Gembarowicz R, Farber S, et al: Intra-operative pre-reconstruction arteriography. Arch Surg 116:1053–1055, 1981.
52. Schiebler ML, Listerud J, Baum RA, et al: MR arteriography of the pelvis and lower extremities. Magn Reson Q 9(3):152–187, 1993.
53. Siegelman ES, Gilfeather M, Holland GA, et al: Pictorial essay: Breath-hold ultrafast three-dimensional gadolinium-enhanced MR angiography of the renovascular system. AJR Am J Roentgenol 168:1035–1040, 1997.
54. Silverman JM, Julien PJ, Herfkens RJ, et al: Magnetic resonance imaging evaluation of pulmonary vascular malformations. Chest 106:1333–1338, 1994.
55. Sjejado WJ, Toniolo G: Adverse reactions to contrast media: A report from the Committee on Safety of Contrast Media of the International Society of Radiology. Radiology 137:299, 1980.
56. Smith TP, Cragg AH, Berbaum KS, Nakagawa N: Comparison of the efficacy of digital subtraction and filmscreen angiography of the lower limb: Prospective study in 50 patients. AJR Am J Roentgenol 158:431–436, 1992.
57. Spritzer CE, Evans AC, Kay HH: Magnetic resonance imaging of deep venous thrombosis in pregnant women with lower extremity edema. Obstet Gynecol 85(4):603–607, 1995.
58. Tempany CM, Morton RA, Marshal FF: MRI of the renal veins: Assessment of nonneoplastic venous thrombosis. J Comput Assist Tomogr 16(6):929–934, 1992.
59. Tomlinson FH, Houser OW, Scheithauer BW, et al: Angiographicaly occult vascular malformations: A correlative study of features on magnetic resonance imaging and histological examination. Neurosurgery 34:792–799; discussion 799–800, 1884.
60. Waugh JR, Sacharias N: Arteriographic complications in the DSA era. Radiology 182:243, 1992.
61. Yin D, Baum RA, Carpenter JP, et al: The cost-effectiveness of magnetic resonance angiography in symptomatic peripheral vascular disease. Radiology 194:757–764, 1995.

CHAPTER 16

Principles of Arteriography

Kim J. Hodgson, M.D.

Despite significant advances in less invasive methods of imaging the vascular system, such as duplex ultrasonography and magnetic resonance angiography, arteriography remains the "gold standard" by which all vascular imaging modalities are judged. Furthermore, although screening for vascular disease is best undertaken with these noninvasive techniques, contrast arteriography continues to be the imaging technique most commonly employed to plan vascular reconstructions, especially those involving long segments of diseased vessels. Moreover, preprocedure and postprocedure arteriography is an essential part of practically all of the ever-expanding number of endovascular therapeutic procedures that vascular surgeons are increasingly incorporating into their practices. Consequently, it is imperative that vascular surgeons appreciate both the techniques involved in performing arteriography and the incumbent complications and sources of error that might mislead the diagnosis and thereby compromise the treatment rendered to the patient.

This chapter reviews the general principles applicable to arteriography, including the design and operation of radiographic equipment, angiographic contrast agents and filming procedures, and the related topic of radiation safety. Specific endovascular techniques relevant to angiographic procedures, such as obtaining vascular access, use of catheters and guide wires, and associated interventional procedures, are reviewed in Chapter 32.

BASIC CONCEPTS OF RADIOGRAPHIC IMAGE RECORDING

In its most basic form, the "cut-film" radiograph, arteriographic imaging is achieved by means of radiographic exposure of a sheet of x-ray film through an anatomic region placed between the x-ray source and the film while a relatively radiopaque contrast agent is within the vessel of interest. The disparate radiodensities of the contrast-filled vessel and the surrounding tissues yield an image of the contours and characteristics of the inside of the vessel. Although surgeons frequently perform "single-shot" completion arteriograms to evaluate newly created bypass grafts, comprehensive diagnostic arteriography requires the recording of a series of images obtained while the contrast agent passes through the vessel of interest. To achieve this with cut-film recording requires a mechanism to move a series of x-ray films under the anatomic area of interest as the x-ray exposure is made. Such rapid-sequence film changers can transport up to 30 individual films at rates of up to six films per second.

Unfortunately, viewing the results of the series of angiographic images requires waiting for the films to be developed, which considerably prolongs the angiographic examination, particularly if subsequent interventions are performed and further angiographic reevaluation is needed. Furthermore, the patient must be repositioned over the film changer after catheter placement has been accomplished under the fluoroscopic x-ray source and image intensifier. This additional step adds time, complexity, and potential for catheter dislodgment to the examination.

Other methods of recording angiographic images during contrast passage include *videoradiography*, whereby the fluoroscopic images are recorded on videotape for later review, and *cineradiography*, in which the recording medium is motion picture film. Both methods suffer from inferior image resolution compared with cut-film radiography and the newer technique of *digital subtraction angiography* (DSA) (to be discussed shortly) and are generally considered inadequate peripheral vascular imaging modalities by today's standards. Cineradiography, however, continues to be the mainstay of coronary angiography archival imaging because its high-speed filming produces the best possible images of the heart and its vessels, which are in constant motion. Review of each injection of coronary contrast agent during the procedure to determine whether adequate visualization occurred, however, typically utilizes videoradiography because it would be impractical to develop the cineradiographic film after each filming run.

Digital Subtraction Angiography

Advances in computer data processing power have led to the development of DSA, a recording technique in which the fluoroscopic image is amplified and digitized, allowing for subsequent processing by a number of methods that can enhance visualization of the structures of interest.

Perhaps the most powerful of these methods is the *subtraction* of the radiodensities of the surrounding tissues and vessel wall from the images obtained after a contrast agent has been introduced into the lumen of the vessel. Typically, the computer subtracts the pixels of the first image of the series (the *mask image*), from the subsequent images. As long as there has been no movement between the time the mask image was obtained and the time contrast agent filled the vessel, the result is an image derived solely from the column of contrast agent within the lumen of the vessel without the image degradation frequently caused by the contrasting radiodensities of the surrounding tissues.

Unfortunately, any movement that has occurred, be it skeletal or visceral, can degrade the image substantially.

Fortunately, however, any image of the series can be designated as the mask image, frequently allowing the undesirable consequences of movement occurring prior to the arrival of the contrast agent to be mitigated by the selection of a new mask image that had been exposed after the movement occurred but either before or after the contrast agent was within the vessel of interest (Fig. 16–1*A* and *B*). Consequently, when movement is observed during the filming process, filming should be continued until after the contrast agent has cleared the vessel so that these late

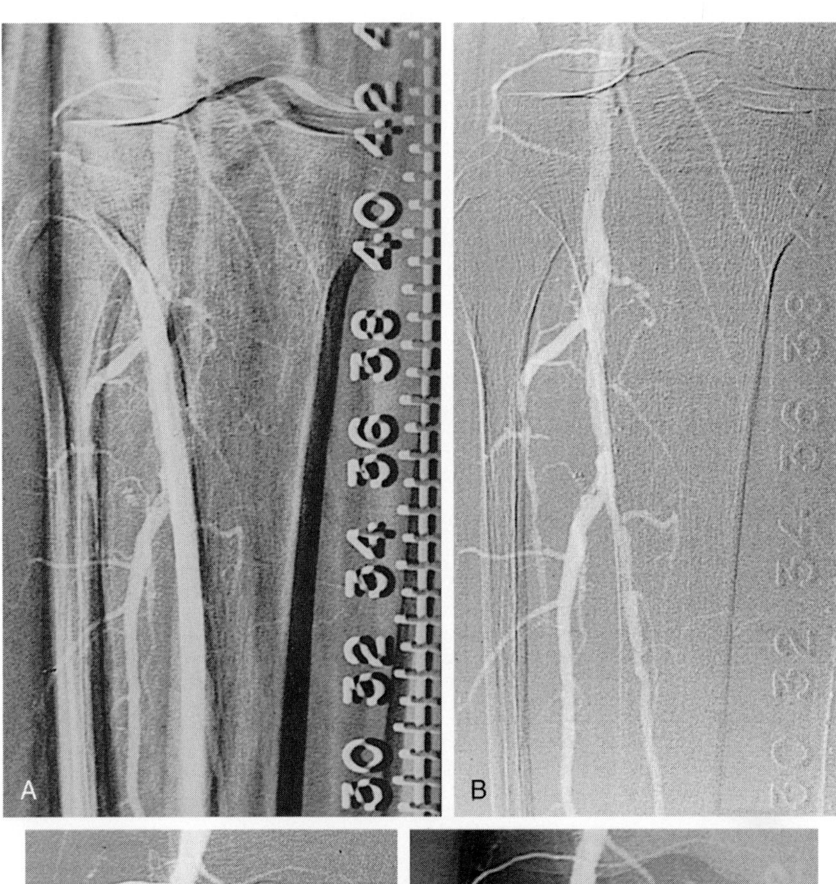

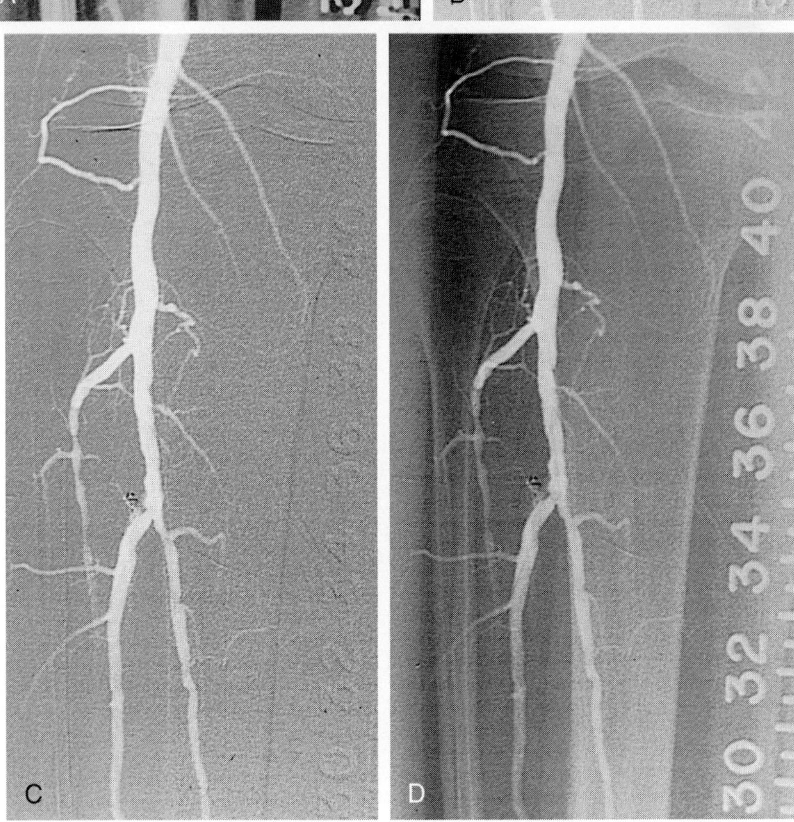

FIGURE 16–1. *A,* Image degradation caused by patient movement, most of which occurred prior to the arrival of contrast, permitting selection of a new mask image to minimize the effect of the movement. *B,* Image improvement due to new mask image selection, choosing one closer in time to the arrival of the contrast agent. *C,* Further improvement obtained by pixel shifting of the image. *D,* Subtraction can be turned off to reveal anatomic landmarks.

images are also available to be used as mask images to be subtracted from the contrast-enhanced images.

A variety of other postprocessing capabilities are now commonplace on DSA equipment, permitting the trained operator to substantially "clean up" the angiographic images to yield the best possible angiographic visualization. One such capability is the combination of multiple images to show contrast agent throughout the length of a vessel even though any single image alone would have demonstrated contrast agent within only a limited area (Fig. 16–2). The effect of movement occurring after the contrast agent has entered the field of view can often be minimized by *pixel shifting* the image, whereby the mask image is slid vertically or horizontally (or both) over the contrast-enhanced image to realign the two, thereby negating the degrading effect of movement (see Fig. 16–1*B* and *C*). Subtraction can also be turned off so that radiographic landmarks are easily visible, a technique that aids in the performance of subsequent selective catheterizations or interventions (see Fig. 16–1*D*).

The technique called *road mapping* allows an image of the contrast-filled vessel (the "road map") to be displayed on the fluoroscopy monitor while a real-time image of any changing radiodensities, such as the passage of a guide wire, is visualized within the road map. This can facilitate the passage of catheters and guide wires through diseased or tortuous vessels but is very sensitive to any movement of the patient, which severely degrades the image. Some equipment allows the operator to switch in and out of the road mapping function. The operator can then use the road map function to verify the location needed without having to endure the sometimes confounding effects of even minor movement throughout the manipulation.

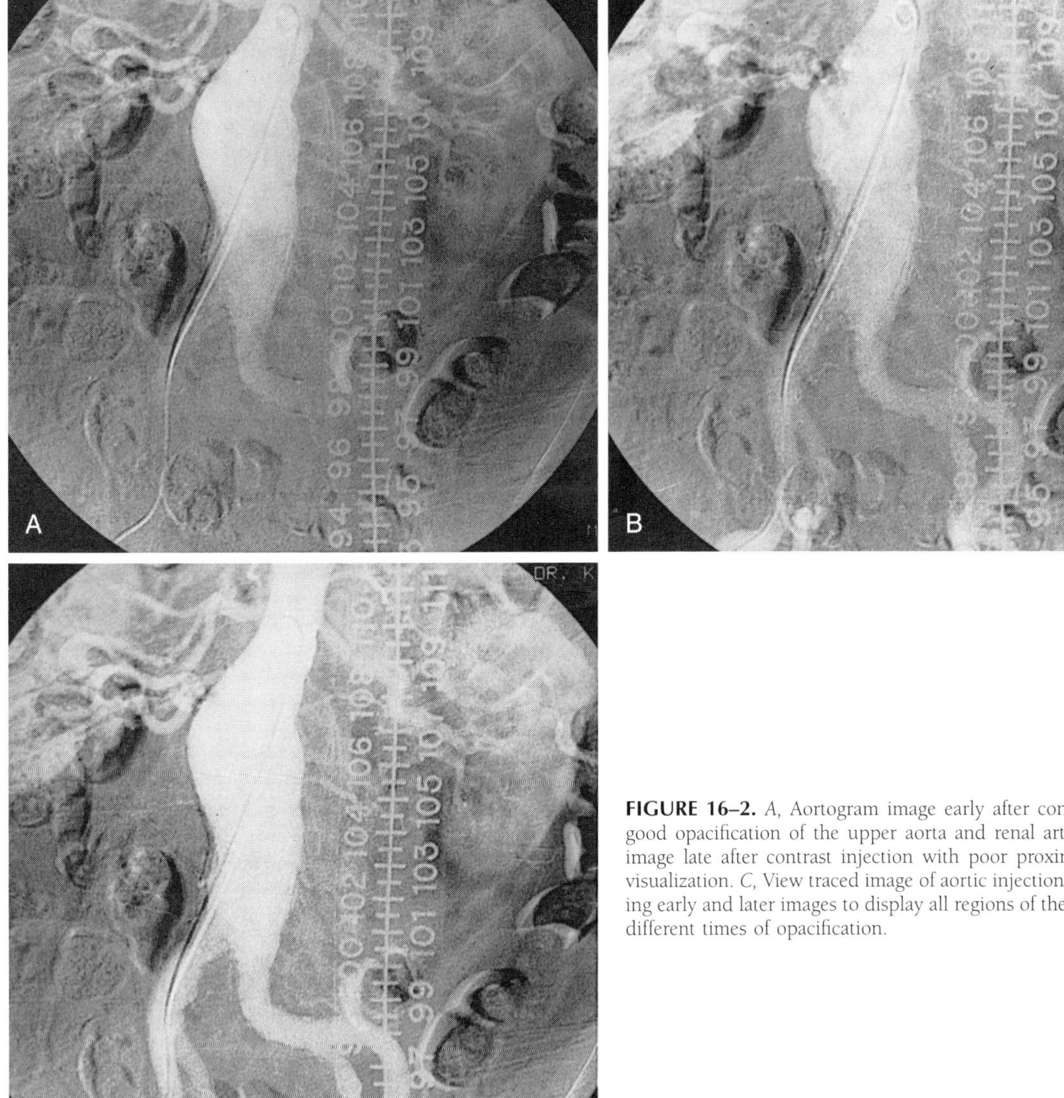

FIGURE 16–2. *A,* Aortogram image early after contrast injection with good opacification of the upper aorta and renal arteries. *B,* Aortogram image late after contrast injection with poor proximal but good distal visualization. *C,* View traced image of aortic injection created by combining early and later images to display all regions of the vasculature despite different times of opacification.

Last, with DSA, image contrast, brightness, edge enhancement, sharpness, and even the coloration of the contrast agent can all be modified before the image is printed on x-ray film. Laser film printers are essential for high-quality archival images and provide a variety of film formats, from one large to up to 15 smaller images on a standard 14- by 17-inch sheet of film. Consequently, because only the most revealing of the images are printed, there is considerable savings in film and storage costs compared with traditional cut-film angiography.

In addition to the myriad postprocessing capabilities, a number of other advantages of DSA have resulted in its supplanting cut-film angiography as the standard format in use for peripheral vascular angiographic imaging today. Because filming for DSA uses the same x-ray source and image intensifier as fluoroscopy, there is no need to reposition the patient between catheter placement and image acquisition. This feature significantly expedites the examination, as does the fact that the images obtained can be viewed immediately, with no waiting for the films to be developed. Furthermore, any dislodgment of the catheter is immediately apparent and can often be corrected before the contrast agent is injected, avoiding unnecessary repetition of filming runs and injection of more contrast agent. Additionally, digital amplification combined with image subtraction allows for adequate opacification with smaller quantities of contrast agent, frequently diluted to half-strength, reducing both patient discomfort (by way of lower contrast agent osmolality) and cost. Although the spatial resolution typically found in DSA units today is slightly less than that obtained with cut-film angiography, this difference is rarely clinically relevant and is more than compensated for by the superior opacification seen with DSA, particularly in small vessels with minimal flow.

A final advantage of DSA is the ability to obtain images with variable levels of magnification, depending on the needs of the examination. A typical DSA suite used for peripheral vascular work consists of an image intensifier that can be set to a range of sizes, usually from 7 to 15 inches. Whereas renal arteries are often first evaluated with a flush aortogram filmed at the 12- or 15-inch setting, subsequent selective catheterization runs are usually performed with an image intensifier size of 7 or 8 inches, allowing better visualization of anatomic detail. Similarly, a unilateral lower extremity runoff series can be obtained with five to seven injections of contrast agent if filming is performed with the image intensifier on the 9-inch setting, but the same evaluation might require only three or four runs at the 15-inch setting. Furthermore, with an image intensifier setting of 15 inches, both legs of most patients can be imaged simultaneously, further reducing the number of runs needed to perform the evaluation, though not necessarily the amount of contrast agent infused.

Intravenous Digital Subtraction Angiography

Although there was initial enthusiasm that DSA could be performed with the use of relatively small volumes of contrast agent injected intravenously, thereby eliminating the expense and risk of arterial catheterization and minimizing contrast toxicity, the limitations of this approach soon became apparent, and this method has largely been abandoned.[1, 6, 18] Foremost among the problems is that the contrast agent is usually too diluted by the time it reaches the arterial region of interest to provide adequate resolution. Furthermore, with all of the vessels in the region filling at the same time, overlapping vessels often obscure the vessel of interest and provide a confusing and uninterpretable image. Filming in multiple projections may allow all segments of the artery to be evaluated without overlapping interference; doing so, however, requires multiple injections of contrast agent, negating the promise of minimizing the volume of contrast agent infused. Conversely, although intra-arterial DSA poses the risks and expense of arterial catheterization, it derives the maximal benefit of the digital technique in terms of image quality and can be performed with the infusion of comparable or even smaller volumes of contrast agent.

Single-Injection, Multiple-Field Digital Subtraction Angiography

The advent of image intensifiers suitably large to permit simultaneous bilateral lower extremity imaging stimulated interest in the development of a means to enable DSA of the entire length of both legs with one bolus of contrast agent delivered into the infrarenal abdominal aorta. The principal obstacle that had to be overcome was the means by which multiple mask images could be obtained for subsequent subtraction from the corresponding contrast-enhanced images. Two slightly different approaches to this problem have emerged.

In the first method, films are obtained in *stages*, utilizing four image intensifier positions pre-set by the operator, that cover the entire length of the lower extremities with some overlap of the images. Once the procedure is set up, the run is initiated by the automated procurement of the mask images from each stage (mask run) as the image intensifier moves to each pre-set position, starting at the feet and ending in the abdomen. A bolus of contrast agent is then injected with the camera filming at the uppermost position, typically the lower abdomen. As the bolus of contrast agent begins to fill the femoral arteries, the operator triggers movement of the camera to the exact position where the next mask image was obtained, and filming continues with this new field of view. As the contrast agent nears the distal aspect of each subsequent stage, the camera is moved again, until the entire area of interest has been covered (contrast run). Because the mask images were obtained prior to the contrast run, the progress of contrast agent through the bed of distribution is viewed in subtraction mode, facilitating both visualization and the decision about when to move the camera to the next stage of the series. Once the run is completed, images from the various film stages are electronically "seamed" together and can be viewed with or without subtraction of their corresponding masks.

The second approach to long-segment DSA maintains a fixed image intensifier position, moving the table, and therefore the patient, instead. A larger number of smaller incremental movements, referred to as *steps*, are used than in the staged system. This approach allows the operator to follow the progress of the bolus of contrast agent down the leg more closely. However, because the mask images are obtained after the contrast run, visualization during filming is in a nonsubtracted format. The rate of movement of the table can be slowed, or even stopped, in areas where opacification is delayed. Once the entire area of interest has been covered, the table returns to the beginning position and the mask run is performed, with the table automatically being advanced through the same step sequence that was used during the contrast run. The mask images are then subtracted from the contrast-enhanced images, yielding a DSA image of the entire length of the lower extremities. As with the staged format, the images may be viewed with or without digital subtraction and may also undergo postprocessing in many of the ways previously discussed to improve the quality of the raw image.

As with single-field DSA, the principal limitation of both of these multiple-field DSA techniques is the need for the patient to keep absolutely still during the aquisition of both the mask images and contrast-enhanced images. Whereas the typical single-field filming run lasts for less than 15 seconds, long-segment runs and mask image aquisition often last for up to 2 minutes. Patient cooperation is therefore an absolute necessity. Because the duration of the contrast run is largely a function of the transit time of the contrast agent, it is identical in the two techniques. The mask run, however, is performed more quickly with the staged technique, which may be less prone to motion-related image degradation. In contrast, the stepped technique allows for finer movements of the subject and can often achieve superior vessel opacification because movement of the field of view can more closely track the progress of the bolus of contrast agent. In practice, both techniques work reasonably well, with little advantage of one over the other.

Bilateral imaging may be compromised with both techniques when more severe disease on one side results in significantly different transit times on the two sides. In such situations, it may not be possible to step or stage the contrast run in such a fashion that adequate opacification is present on both sides simultaneously. This problem can be overcome by performing unilateral filming of each side separately (Fig. 16–3). Additionally, since unilateral filming is typically performed through a selective unilateral catheterization positioned more distally in the arterial tree, it has the added advantage of superior vascular opacification by virtue of injection of the contrast agent closer to the area of interest, resulting in less dilution of contrast agent during transit.

Such unilateral examinations can be performed with either (1) the use of a single injection of a bolus of contrast agent and the multiple-field format already described or (2) sequential single-field filming and repeated injections of contrast agents. Typical injection volumes for single-injection multiple-field filming range from 80 to 100 ml of full-strength contrast agent for bilateral leg filming and 50 to 60 ml for unilateral filming. For comparison, multiple-injection single-field lower extremity filming usually utilizes 10 ml of half-strength contrast agent per injection, with complete coverage of the extremity requiring between four and six filming runs, depending on the size of the image intensifier. Consequently, single-injection multiple-field DSA does not result in the use of a smaller volume of contrast agent than that used for sequential single-field filming.

EQUIPMENT AND PERSONNEL REQUIREMENTS

The requisite equipment to perform angiographic evaluation depends greatly on the nature and scope of the evaluation being undertaken. Whereas direct-exposure single-shot intraoperative angiography may be suitable for bypass planning or for completion evaluation of bypass grafts or embolectomy procedures, DSA is a practical requirement for almost all other vascular diagnostic or therapeutic procedures. Furthermore, fluoroscopic visualization can substantially aid in the performance of many standard surgical procedures, allowing them to be performed more safely, expeditiously, and effectively.

Therefore, every effort should be made to gain access to equipment and facilities suitable for the task at hand in order to achieve the best possible visualization in the most convenient manner under given clinical circumstances. At minimum, this requires access to digital subtraction radiographic equipment with instantaneous digital playback. It is also incumbent on the surgeon to become familiar with the features and mode of operation of the available equipment so as to ensure that the best possible imaging is achieved.

Currently available DSA equipment can be broadly divided into two categories: fixed, ceiling-mounted units with remote power generators and portable self-contained units. The merits of each of these types of systems are discussed in the next section. Regardless of which type of system is used, however, certain accessory equipment is highly recommended to optimize the utility of the system. Many of the postprocessing and image-enhancing DSA features previously reviewed are now available on portable units, though they are not always standard equipment and are not necessarily as convenient to use as those on fixed-mount units. Nonetheless, they should all be considered essential to performance of the broad range of endovascular diagnostic and therapeutic procedures. Also commonplace today are dual video monitors, which allow the display of a reference image on one screen and the active fluoroscopic image on the other. With intravascular ultrasound (IVUS) playing an increasing role in endovascular interventions, particularly endoluminal grafting, the ability to display the IVUS image on the fluoroscopy monitor as a "picture in picture" (PIP) can be a helpful feature.

Although the single-injection, multiple-field angiography previously discussed is a highly convenient feature, it is far from essential, even if full-leg angiography is commonly performed in a surgeon's practice. However, an image intensifier of 9 inches would be the minimum practical size for performing full lower extremity angiography, and a 12- or 15-inch image intensifier would be even better because it would allow the full length of the limb to be filmed with fewer contrast injections and radiographic runs.

A pair of x-ray sources (and their corresponding film changers or image intensifiers) positioned at orthogonal angles allows for the simultaneous filming in two different planes during one injection of contrast agent (biplanar angiography). Such a system is both expensive and cumbersome, and the ability to conveniently alter the filming angles is limited. With the reduced volumes of contrast

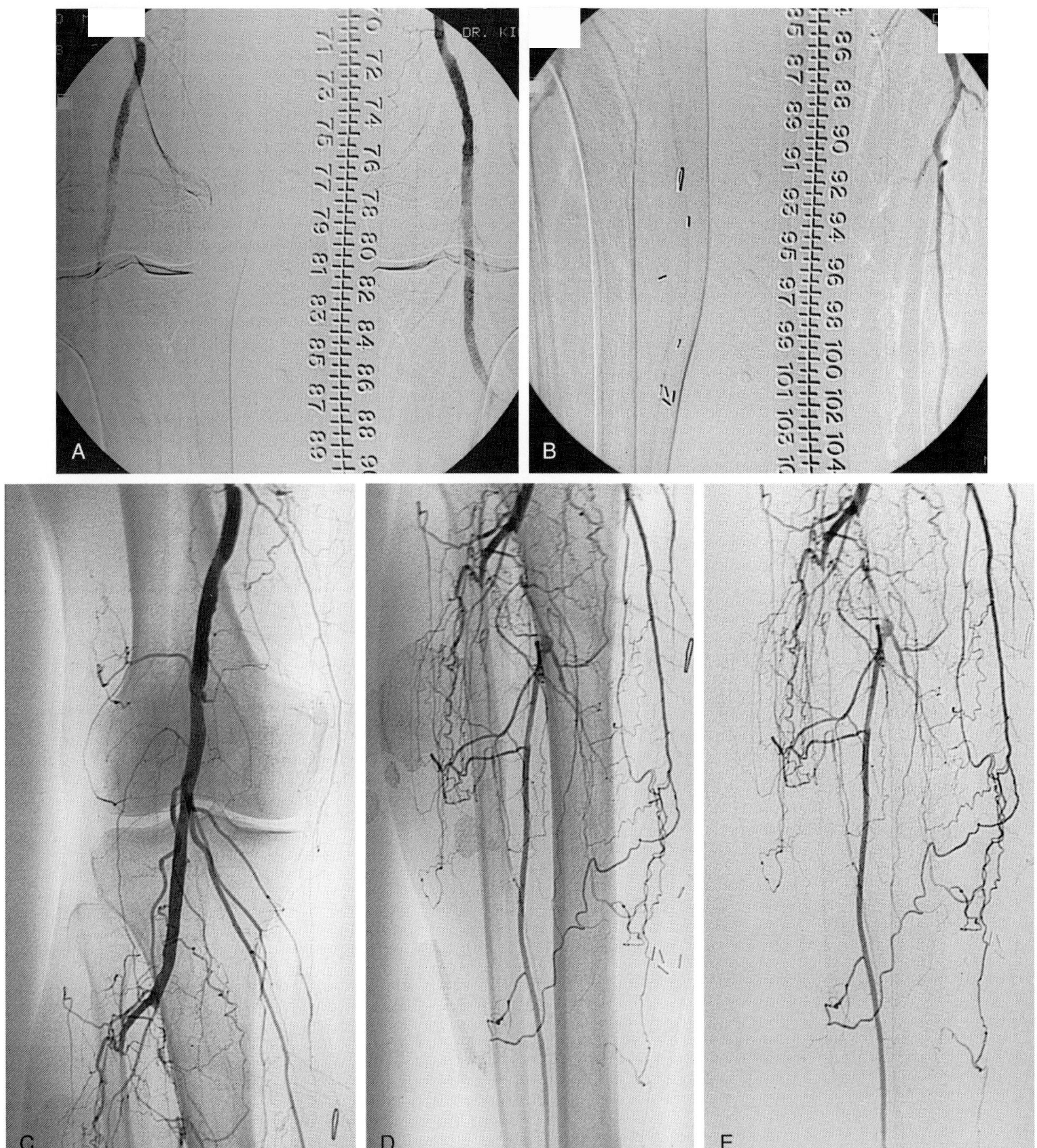

FIGURE 16–3. *A,* Single-injection, multiple-field digital subtraction angiography showing delayed opacification of the right popliteal region compared with that of the left. *B,* Differential opacification becomes a severe impediment to adequate visualization of the trifurcation region on both sides. *C,* Selective catheterization of the external iliac artery with hand injection of contrast material produces the greatest degree of opacification, as well as the greatest detail. Shown here is the popliteal region. *D,* Selective injection of trifurcation region. *E,* Selective injection of trifurcation region with digital subtraction turned on.

agent required with DSA, there is currently little application for biplanar capability in the evaluation of peripheral vascular disease, and it should not be considered a necessary component of a vascular angiography facility.

An often overlooked piece of radiographic equipment that can have significant effect on the quality and convenience of radiographic imaging is the fluoroscopy table. In its most basic form, a fluoroscopy table serves to provide adequate support for the patient while allowing x-rays to penetrate without significant distortion. The more open the undercarriage, the more flexibility there is to move the C-arm to different fields of view. The ultimate in an open undercarriage is a table that is supported at only one end, leaving the other end, and the patient on it, completely suspended and unobstructed. This type of table permits the angiographer to pan the x-ray tube from head to toe of the patient without repositioning around table supports. Such tables are often constructed of carbon fiber technology, allowing them to be strong enough to support the patient yet sufficiently radiolucent to permit good imaging.

Unfortunately, with all of these types of tables, the patient's position remains stationary and the C-arm is moved to change the field of view, a somewhat cumbersome maneuver. It is substantially more convenient for the C-arm to remain relatively stationary and the table to move. This allows the angiographer to have much more control over the selected field of view without having to work through an intermediary who moves the C-arm, because the table controls are typically on the side of the table and can be operated by the surgeon without breaking the sterile field. Changing the field of view with a movable table is a much more fluid operation than moving the C-arm assembly to a new position.

One limitation of all fluoroscopy tables is the range of positioning options available. Although most tables can be raised and lowered, and some can be tilted to put the patient in Trendelenburg or reverse Trendelenburg position, few tables can be rotated side-to-side or moved to put the patient in flexion or extension positions.

Monitoring of patients during angiographic procedures is important, to ensure their comfort, cooperation, and safety during the procedure. Real-time electrocardiographic (ECG) monitoring and automated blood pressure measurements would be considered standard capabilities for contemporary endovascular suites. Once arterial access has been achieved, monitoring of blood pressure directly from the angiographic sheath is preferable; this capability also has great utility to assess the hemodynamic significance of occlusive disease and the results of intervention. Whereas the ability to measure intra-arterial pressures from one source at a time is generally sufficient, it is often helpful to be able to evaluate two sources simultaneously, allowing for the comparison of the pressure in a vessel of interest with that in the aorta.

Appropriate personnel to attend to the needs of both the patient and the angiographer generally consists of three radiology technicians:

1. One who has scrubbed for surgery at the table and is assisting.
2. One circulating in the room to provide necessary supplies.
3. One running the radiographic equipment.

Furthermore, a nurse is typically present to monitor the patient and to administer any sedative, analgesic, or other medications or fluids requested by the angiographer.

FIXED-MOUNT VERSUS PORTABLE RADIOGRAPHIC EQUIPMENT

Radiographic equipment can be generally divided into two basic categories:

- Fixed-mount units in rooms typically dedicated to radiographic procedures
- Portable C-arm fluoroscopy units with digital capabilities that can be used in a variety of locations

The advent of endoluminal grafting procedures that require operative vascular access has created interest in equipping operating rooms with fixed-mount quality equipment or creating angiographic suites with operating room sterility and supplemental lighting. Clearly, the goal is to have the imaging quality and convenience of an angiographic suite in a room suitably equipped to perform operative procedures. For the foreseeable future, however, most surgeons will have to choose one aspect or the other as their primary concern and accept the compromises entailed. Because angiography is performed principally as a stand-alone procedure via the percutaneous route of access, the superior imaging environment of the dedicated angiographic suite is the obvious choice unless a concomitant surgical procedure is mandatory.

The distinction between these two types of systems lies in the portability of the power-generating units, not in the portability of the x-ray tube and image intensifier component. Fixed-mount units have significantly larger and more powerful generators that, although producing superior imaging, exact a price in terms of the space required to house them and systems designed to keep them cool. These generators typically occupy a room of their own adjacent to the angiographic suite. Despite these apparent drawbacks, such units provide significantly greater power output, which translates into better imaging and improved ability to penetrate large and dense objects. Furthermore, although the focal spot size on portable units usually ranges from 0.3 to 1.4 mm in diameter, the greater power output available with fixed-mount units allows for focal spot sizes as small as 0.15 mm, resulting in substantially better resolution.

Other differences between the two types of units pertain to the C-arm gantry component, which contains the x-ray source below and the image intensifier above. Fixed-mount units are available with image intensifiers measuring up to 17 inches, but image intensifiers in most portable units are no larger than 12 inches. Furthermore, fixed-mount units enable the operator to vary the distance between the x-ray tube and the image intensifier, an adjustment not available with portable units. This adjustment allows the image intensifier to be placed closer to the patient, not only improving the image quality but also enlarging the field of view and minimizing radiation scatter.

Another advantage of fixed-mount units is the ability to alter the orientation of the C-arm via electromechanical drives, the controls for which are available to the angiographer at tableside without violation of the sterile field. This is a much more fluid and efficient operation than required with portable units, for which the operator must physically unlock and then move the C-arm assembly. The latter situation usually requires working through a radiography technician, removing the surgeon from direct control of the process of field selection.

Although overheating is no longer a significant problem with the newer portable fluoroscopy units available today, older units, many of which are still in service, tend to overheat during fluoroscopy-intensive procedures. Newer equipment has largely overcome this problem through advances in cooling technology as well as power usage algorithms that switch to pulsed fluoroscopy as the x-ray tube begins to overheat. Although this power usage algorithm may prevent the tube from overheating and shutting down, it does so by reducing the "frame rate" of fluoroscopy, resulting in somewhat choppy fluoroscopic visualization. For these reasons, these older fluoroscopy units are not well suited to endovascular procedures but may be acceptable for angiography alone.

As would be expected, the advantages of fixed-mount fluoroscopic units come at significantly higher prices than portable units, with the former costing between $750,000 and $1,500,000 and the latter $150,000 to $200,000. Furthermore, installation of ceiling-mounted units often requires structural modifications to the room, such as reinforced mounting plates, under-floor electrical conduit, and lead lining in the walls of the room, all of which further increase the cost. Some workers would advocate installing fixed-mount units in the operating room. This arrangement may be practical, however, only if the volume of endovascular surgical procedures is high because use of these rooms for nonangiographic procedures may be somewhat encumbered by the radiographic equipment, which can be only moved aside, not removed from the room entirely. Therefore, portable C-arm units remain a more versatile option with regard to operating room utilization, especially when one considers that they can be moved to other rooms to provide imaging for other procedures once the imaging aspects of a given procedure have been completed.

CHOOSING THE VENUE: OPERATING ROOM OR ANGIOGRAPHIC SUITE?

The choice of working environment should be based entirely on the needs of the patient and the intended procedure, not on "turf" considerations or interdisciplinary rivalries. Despite significant advances in the image quality available with portable digital fluoroscopy units, angiography performed in a dedicated angiographic facility provides uniformly superior image quality and convenience of image aquisition. Therefore, in the absence of a true angiographic operating room, the only reason to consider performing angiography or any other endovascular procedure in the operating room is when the superior sterile environment present in that venue is necessary for a concomitant procedure. This situation may occur when:

1. Surgical revascularization is being performed with the guidance of immediate preprocedure angiography.
2. A revascularization is assessed at conclusion by intraoperative (completion) angiography.

Although some surgeons might choose to perform inflow dilatations in the operating room concomitant with distal revascularizations, this approach has many disadvantages that render it ill advised unless access to the lesion being dilated is available only through an operative exposure, a rarely encountered situation. Foremost among the disadvantages is the fact that performing the procedure in the operating room generally involves the suboptimal imaging available from a portable fluoroscopy unit, complicating the procedure and compromising assessment of the outcome. Furthermore, the hemodynamic and functional success of the intervention cannot be determined prior to basing a bypass graft on it, potentially jeopardizing the longevity of the bypass if the intervention is a short-term failure.

Additionally, if the intervention is immediately unsuccessful, the patient may have to undergo a much more extensive operative revascularization than had been planned, perhaps even mandating a change in anesthetic or both inflow and outflow operative revascularizations in the same operation. Lastly, in many patients in need of inflow interventions, supplemental perfusion from the angioplasty is sufficient and distal revascularization is not needed. For all of these reasons, inflow interventions are best performed in a dedicated angiographic facility prior to performance of a distal surgical revascularization, as long as the lesion can be safely accessed percutaneously or through a minor operative exposure. This sequence allows both procedures to be performed in facilities optimal for each.

In patients with vascular trauma and coexisting life-threatening injuries that mandate prompt surgical treatment, it is often best to perform arteriography in the operating room once the higher-priority problems have been addressed. This approach is relatively simple and efficacious with extremity vascular trauma because these areas are fairly simple to visualize and can usually be accessed directly at the site of injury or percutaneously more proximal to the anticipated vascular defect. Intraoperative angiographic evaluation of central vascular trauma, however, can be more problematic because both catheter position and quality imaging are more difficult to obtain. Considering the potential magnitude of the possible problems, the need for power injection of contrast agent, and the importance of superior image quality, such patients are generally best studied with fixed-mount, dedicated angiographic equipment. Furthermore, the angiographic suite is usually better equipped to address issues that can be treated endoluminally, such as with embolization coils or other devices.

A final scenario for which operative angiography is useful is in the evaluation of patients undergoing thromboembolectomy. Though many surgeons obtain simple single-shot radiographs of the distal vasculature following embolectomy, the procedure itself can be greatly facilitated and performed more safely under fluoroscopic guidance (Fig. 16–4). Fluoroscopic visualization during catheter passage, for example, can detect deviations in the course of the catheter that might signify either passage down a collateral vessel or subintimal dissection, either of which would contraindicate inflation of the balloon. The use of half-strength contrast agent in the embolectomy balloon enables the surgeon to observe its return passage through the vascular system and minimize potentially injurious overdistention. Furthermore, sites of occlusive lesions can be detected and traction on them minimized if the surgeon can observe the deformation of the balloon as it passes through the region. If subsequent angiographic evaluation reveals retained thrombus in the trifurcation vessels, selective catheter passage can be performed, using a leading guide wire if needed, to extract as much thrombus as possible. Lastly, any significant focal occlusive lesions that are identified and are suitable for endovascular treatment can be subsequently dilated at the same setting. If the lesions are not so suited, the angiogram can at least demonstrate the anastomotic

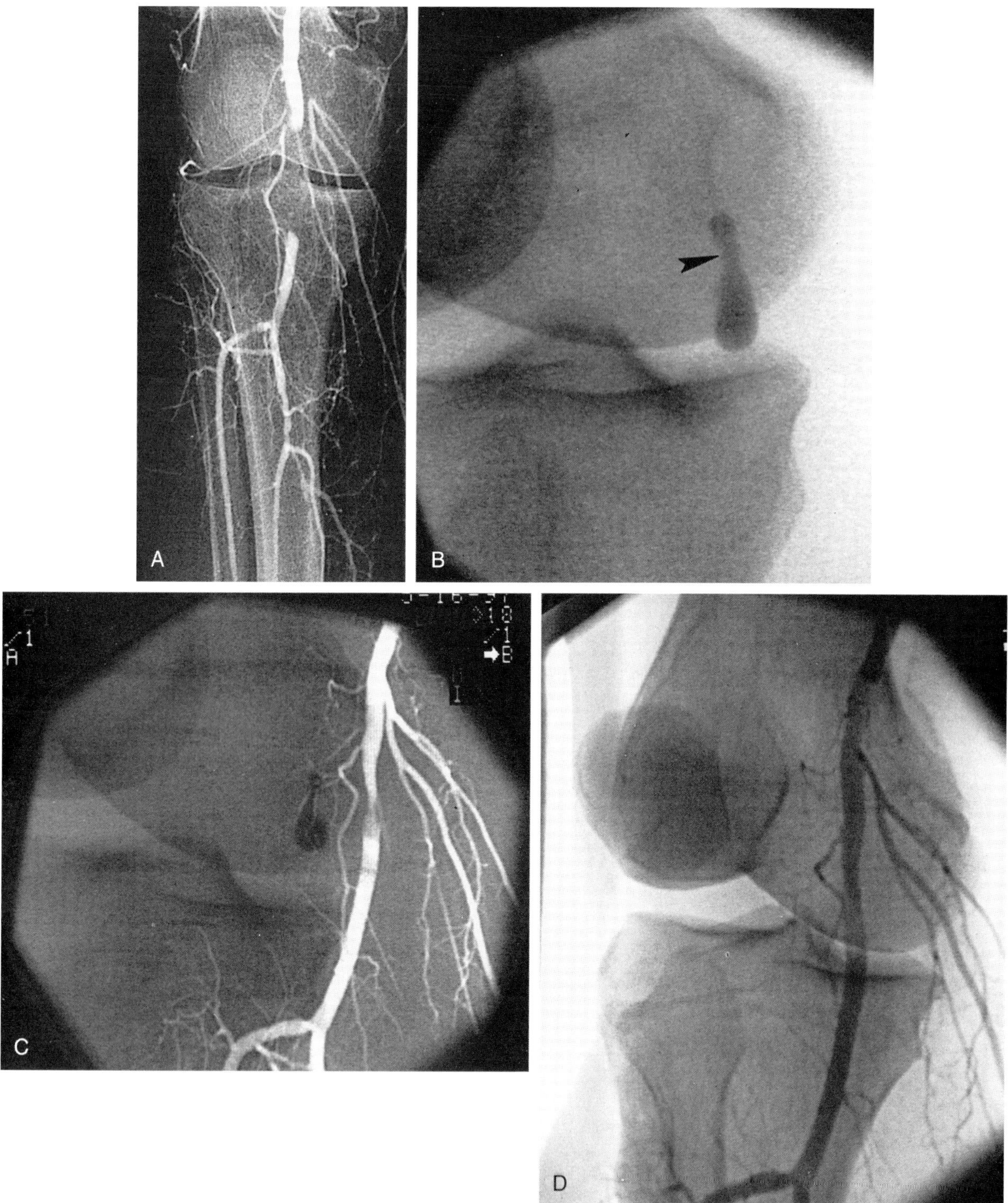

FIGURE 16–4. *A,* Preoperative angiogram revealing abrupt occlusion of the mid-popliteal artery in a patient with acute ischemic symptoms suggestive of embolization. *B,* Deformation of the embolectomy balloon is noted in the popliteal region during extraction of the thrombus, suggesting an underlying stenotic lesion. *C,* On-table digital subtraction angiogram following embolectomy revealing the suspected mid-popliteal artery stenosis. *D,* Completion arteriogram following balloon dilatation of the mid-popliteal artery stenosis. (From Yao JS, Pearce WH [eds]: Techniques in Vascular and Endovascular Surgery. Stamford, Conn, Appleton & Lange, 1997.)

options available and can be of help in the planning of the optimal revascularization procedure.

The more appropriate venue in which to perform endovascular procedures that require insertion of devices too large to be achieved percutaneously, such as endoluminal aortic aneurysm grafts, remains a topic of debate. Surgeons generally prefer to perform these procedures in the operating room, which has the advantage of a seamless conversion of the procedure to open repair in the event of complications or failure of implantation. Furthermore, proponents of this approach cite the superior sterile environment present in the operating room as a major deciding factor. In fact, full conversion of implantation procedures to open surgery have been relatively rare, and most often, all that is needed is access to the external iliac artery for repair or bypass of insertion-related trauma, exposure that can readily be obtained in an angiographic suite. Graft infections have not, to date, been a major issue; this is not surprising if one considers that most endoluminal devices are completely enclosed in their delivery systems prior to release within the body and are, therefore, not easily contaminated. Consequently, though concerns about sterility persist, the superior imaging environment of a dedicated angiographic suite or a true operating angiographic facility is preferred by most surgeons.

CONTRAST AGENTS

For intravascular anatomic detail to be apparent on radiographic imaging, an agent with a radiodensity that contrasts with that of the surrounding tissues must be present within the vessel at the time of the radiographic exposure. Although the contrast agent utilized for the evaluation is typically of greater radiodensity than the surrounding tissues, intraluminal visualization can also be achieved by injection of an agent that is less radiopaque than the adjacent tissues, such as carbon dioxide gas.[9, 21] This technique may be useful in a very select group of patients, most notably those with compromised renal function for whom the nephrotoxicity of standard contrast agents might be problematic, but it is considerably more complicated and usually results in images that lack sufficient detail for many clinical situations. For these reasons, and because contrast agent–related nephropathy is usually a self-limited problem, carbon dioxide angiography remains a rarely used imaging modality in most vascular practices and is not discussed further here.

All currently available angiographic contrast agents achieve their radiopacity by virtue of iodine atoms attached to one or more benzene rings. Conventional angiographic contrast agents are compounds of one fully substituted benzene ring (with three iodine atoms) acting as an anion and a cationic component (either sodium, methylglucamine, or a combination of the two). In solution they dissociate, effectively doubling the osmolality of the contrast agent.

The osmolality of contrast agents can be reduced by linking two benzene rings with each cation (*dimeric* formulation), effectively doubling the number of iodine atoms for the same level of osmolality. Another way to lessen the osmolality of contrast agents is to formulate the benzene ring so that it does not dissociate at all; such a formulation is known as a *non-ionic* contrast agent. Both of these modifications result in agents with osmolalities approximately half those of conventional contrast agents. Thus, although conventional contrast agents range from 1500 to 1700 mOsm at 300 mg/ml of iodine, non-ionic and dimeric compounds range from 580 to 880 mOsm at 300 mg/ml of iodine. Non-ionic dimeric formulations have also been created with osmolalities of about 320 mOsm. Some of the more commonly used contrast agents and their specifications are listed in Table 16–1.

Toxicity

Systemic

The toxicity of iodinated contrast agents is principally due to their hyperosmolality; hence the interest in formulating agents with reduced osmolality. Other factors, however, such as the side chains on the benzene ring, do exert an influence on various toxic effects of these agents. In general practice, however, these differences have fairly minor effects when the agents are injected into peripheral arteries.

The most common side effects of contrast agent injection are:

TABLE 16–1. COMMONLY USED CONTRAST AGENTS

CONTRAST AGENT	MANUFACTURER	STRUCTURE	IODINE CONTENT (mg/ml)	OSMOLALITY (mOsm/kg)	AVERAGE WHOLESALE COST ($/50 ml)
Conray 30	Mallinckrodt Medical	Ionic	141	681	4.36
Conray 60	Mallinckrodt Medical	Ionic	282	1539	10.23
Hexabrix	Mallinckrodt Medical	Ionic dimer	320	600	54.00
Isovue-128	Bracco Diagnostics	Non-ionic	128	290	46.87
Isovue-200	Bracco Diagnostics	Non-ionic	200	413	53.75
Isovue-300	Bracco Diagnostics	Non-ionic	300	524	56.33
Isovue-370	Bracco Diagnostics	Non-ionic	370	796	88.75*
Omnipaque 140	Nycomed, Inc.	Non-ionic	140	322	38.94
Omnipaque 300	Nycomed, Inc.	Non-ionic	300	672	54.00
Omnipaque 350	Nycomed, Inc.	Non-ionic	350	844	58.81
Optiray 160	Mallinckrodt Medical	Non-ionic	160	355	33.00
Optiray 320	Mallinckrodt Medical	Non-ionic	320	702	48.00
Oxilan 350	Cook Corporation	Non-ionic	350	695	50.00
Renografin-60	Bracco Diagnostics	Ionic	292	1549	11.77
Renografin-76	Bracco Diagnostics	Ionic	370	2188	16.41
Ultravist 150	Berlex Laboratories	Non-ionic	150	774	27.00
Ultravist 300	Berlex Laboratories	Non-ionic	300	774	36.00
Visipaque 270	Berlex Laboratories	Non-ionic	270	290	56.70
Visipaque 320	Berlex Laboratories	Non-ionic	320	290	61.75

Adapted from Drug Topics Red Book. Montvale, NJ, Medical Economics Publishers, 1998.
*Price given for 75 ml.

- Nausea
- Vomiting
- Discomfort in the distribution of the vascular bed into which the contrast agent is infused

The last condition is largely related to the osmolality of the contrast agent, with hyperosmolar agents causing greater discomfort.[20] With an osmolality below a threshold level of 400 to 500 mOsm, patients usually do not experience any significant discomfort. Although nausea and vomiting are also related to the osmolality of the agent used, other less well-defined factors also play a role.[3] For a given osmolality, for example, non-ionic agents tend to produce less nausea and vomiting than ionic agents do.

Contrast agents also have several histamine-related side effects, ranging in severity from minor, such as urticaria, to life-threatening, such as cardiorespiratory arrest. The former are usually treated with antihistamines, whereas the latter may require full hemodynamic and respiratory support with vasopressors and mechanical ventilation. It is important to distinguish cardiorespiratory arrest from the more common vagally mediated hypotension, with or without bradycardia, because the treatment for these two conditions is vastly different: Cardiac arrest requires the use of vasopressors while a vasovagal reaction is best treated with intravenous saline and atropine, 0.5 to 1.0 mg given intravenously (IV).

Factors predisposing to the development of these systemic side effects include[2, 17]:

- A history of contrast reactions
- Asthma
- Other allergies
- Anxiety

Consequently, reasonable efforts should be made to keep patients calm and comfortable. Intravenous analgesic and sedative agents are commonly administered as needed to achieve the desired degree of patient comfort, for example, midazolam (Versed), 1 to 2 mg IV, and nalbuphine (Nubain), 5 to 10 mg IV. Although antihistamines are commonly used to treat the symptoms of cutaneous reactions, such as urticaria, they have not prevented the development of such conditions. Administration of corticosteroids *prior to* injection of contrast agent (hydrocortisone, 100 mg IV, or methylprednisolone, 32 mg PO [by mouth]; 12 and 2 hours prior), however, has proved effective at decreasing the rates of new and recurrent contrast-related side effects.[8, 11] Although the use of non-ionic contrast media does not eliminate these risks entirely, Katayama[10] has demonstrated a reduction in the rates of all adverse reactions (from 12.6% to 3.1%) and of severe reactions (from 0.22% to 0.04%) in patients receiving intravenous non-ionic, low-osmolality agents compared with those who received ionic, high-osmolality contrast agents.

Cardiac Toxicity

All contrast agents have the potential to affect cardiac function by disturbing intracardiac conduction, myocardial function, or coronary artery tone. This effect is generally manifested as a fall in both heart rate and blood pressure. It is markedly lessened, but not eliminated, by the use of one of the low-osmolality agents. Cardiac toxicity is not usually a clinically significant factor, however, except perhaps in patients with greatly reduced cardiac function. Some of the older contrast agent preparations contained additives capable of binding calcium, leading to sudden drops in ionized calcium that could produce electromechanical dissociation. This problem is not a major concern with the contrast agents commonly in use today.

Hematologic Side Effects

Although conventional contrast agents can retard coagulation when in contact with blood, this effect may be less with the non-ionic contrast agents. The clinical significance of this difference, if any, is not well established. Nonetheless, since red blood cell aggregates are known to occur when blood is in contact with any type of contrast agent,[3] it is advisable to minimize contact between the contrast agent and blood. Fundamental measures that will minimize the risk are:

- Judicious flushing of catheters with saline after contrast agent injection
- Avoidance of blood back-up into the syringe

Nephrotoxicity

All contrast agents are cleared from the body by glomerular filtration with no appreciable tubular reabsorption. Although numerous risk factors for the development of contrast agent nephropathy have been suggested, only the presence of preexisting renal dysfunction has been directly correlated with the development of this complication.[16] Furthermore, despite popular belief, neither the type of contrast agent used nor the volume infused has been demonstrated to play a role.[7, 14, 16, 19] Consequently, in patients with normal renal function, infusion volumes need not be limited for fear of causing contrast agent nephropathy, although maintenance of adequate hydration and urine flow rates is generally advisable.

In patients with diminished renal function or hyperosmolar states (e.g., multiple myeloma), however, administration of contrast agents should be minimized and adequate hydration and urine flow rates should be carefully monitored. Diabetes per se is not a risk factor for contrast agent–related nephrotoxicity, but the frequent presence of coexisting renal insufficiency, whether clinically apparent or not, increases the risk of unmasking occult renal insufficiency after administration of contrast agents. Since maintenance of a good urine output is especially desirable in patients with preexisting renal insufficiency, either mannitol or a diuretic as well as intravenous hydration is often given to such patients. Furthermore, because a motionless patient is essential for good angiographic image acquisition, it may be helpful to place a Foley catheter for patients who receive diuretics, especially those about to undergo prolonged procedures. Patients with complete renal failure, of course, are principally at risk for hyperosmolar volume overload and therefore generally undergo dialysis shortly after angiography.

Choosing a Contrast Agent

Clearly, given an informed choice, patients would prefer to undergo angiography with a non-ionic contrast agent, primarily owing to the lessened discomfort involved. Unfortunately, non-ionic contrast agents are considerably more expensive than ionic agents (see Table 16–1). Health care providers, including Medicare, are becoming more insistent about documentation of "need" to justify the use of non-ionic agents. Although acceptable indications may vary from provider to provider, Table 16–2 lists conditions generally believed to justify the use of non-ionic contrast preparations, even though, as previously discussed, scientifically sound evidence is lacking for many of them.

From the clinician's perspective, non-ionic agents are also the agents of choice because patient comfort during the procedure translates to an easier and less stressful examination all around. Contrast-related pain, "hot flashes," and muscle spasm often cause patient movement with resultant image degradation. This effect can be particularly problematic during filming of distal lower extremity vasculature, where transit times are slow. Movement occurring once contrast agent has entered the field of view is difficult to negate by remasking or pixel shifting. Furthermore, stepped or staged multiple-field DSA, by virtue of the span of time between procurement of the contrast-enhanced images and mask images, may be impossible to perform because of excessive movement. Last, the reduction in serious and overall adverse reaction rates with non-ionic media simplifies the physician's role and facilitates the conduct of an expeditious examination.

Administering a Contrast Agent

Angiographic evaluation of large high-flow vessels, such as the aortic arch, abdominal aorta, or vena cava, requires relatively large volumes of contrast agent infused over a brief period. Furthermore, full-strength contrast agent is typically required in these locations owing to the dilutional effect of the bloodstream. Consequently, it is not generally feasible to inject the necessary quantities of relatively viscous contrast agent by hand and, therefore, a power injector is used. Power injectors allow infusion of pre-set volumes of contrast agent over selected periods, typically, large volumes within several seconds. Pressure limits can also be set to ensure that an inappropriately forceful and potentially injurious jet of contrast agent is not injected or to prevent catheter rupture in the event of a kink in the catheter.

TABLE 16–2. MEDICARE-ACCEPTED INDICATIONS FOR USE OF NON-IONIC CONTRAST MEDIA

- Previous history of contrast reaction (beyond a sensation of heat, flushing, or a single episode of nausea or vomiting)
- History of asthma
- History of other allergies (e.g., foods, drugs, pollens)
- Presence of significant cardiac dysfunction (e.g., recent cardiac decompensation, unstable angina, severe arrhythmia, recent myocardial infarction, pulmonary hypertension)
- Presence of generalized severe debilitation (e.g., diabetes mellitus, renal failure, multiple myeloma, shock, respirator dependency, paralysis, cachexia, dehydration, leukemia, chronic obstructive pulmonary disease)
- Presence of sickle cell anemia

Adapted from the Medicare Hospital Manual, Section 443. Washington, DC, Government Printing Office: 1997 HCFA Pub No. 10.

In contrast to angiography of high-flow vessels, for which power injection of contrast agent is typically required, the reduced volume and concentration of contrast agent needed for selective catheter studies makes hand injection feasible and offers several advantages. Chief among these is the efficiency of accomplishing catheter placement and proceeding directly with filming rather than having to switch from the hand-held syringe to the power injector each time a filming run is performed. This is particularly advantageous with tenuous catheterizations, in which delays and extraneous movements may result in dislodgment of the catheter. Furthermore, hand injection allows the volume and infusion rate of the contrast agent to be varied during the run as needed to achieve the desired opacification. An additional advantage is the ability to vary the concentration of contrast agent used with each injection by mixing different proportions of contrast agent and saline when refilling the syringe (Fig. 16–5). Power injectors generally hold 200 ml of contrast solution, and once they are filled, it is more difficult to alter the concentration from run to run.

As with all selective catheter injections, care must be taken during hand injections to ensure that the force of the stream of contrast agent exiting the end of the catheter does not propel the catheter out of the selected vessel or cause injury to the vessel from the jet effect of fluid exiting the distal end hole. The chief disadvantage of hand injection for angiography in situations suitable for either power or hand injection is the greater radiation exposure for the physician, who is in closer proximity to the x-ray source than would be necessary with the power injection technique. Typical contrast agent injection volumes, methods, and rates are detailed in Table 16–3.

For very distal evaluations that use a proximally placed catheter, pre-injection of contrast agent before the actual filming run is begun can reduce radiation exposure by eliminating pointless filming prior to the arrival of the contrast agent. The delay between injection of contrast agent and initiation of filming depends greatly on the severity of intervening occlusive disease and the cardiac output of the patient. The location of the catheter relative to the area of interest is another variable to take into consideration, with more selective (distal) catheterizations resulting in earlier and more complete vascular opacification. Ultimately, judgment about the significance of each of these factors and their effect on contrast agent transit time develops with experience and guides the angiographer's decisions about proper timing of the injection and filming.

Even with selective catheterization, however, more concentrated contrast agent may be required to achieve adequate opacification of distal vessels, particularly if significant upstream occlusive disease slows transit and permits greater dilution of the contrast agent during its transit through collateral vessels. If opacification remains suboptimal despite use of full-strength contrast agent and a selectively positioned catheter, pharmacologic vasodilatation by direct injection of a vasodilator through the diagnostic catheter may enhance visualization. Agents commonly used for this include nitroglycerin (100 to 300 μg) and papaverine (10 to 30 mg), both of which are also useful in treating

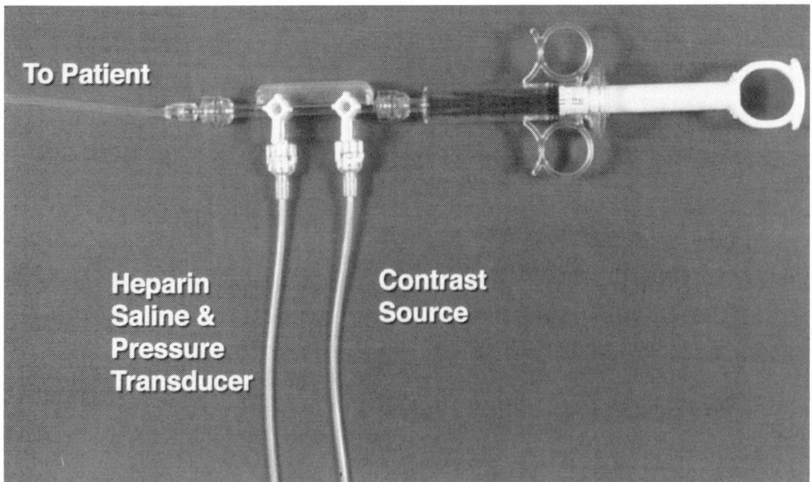

FIGURE 16–5. Rapid and convenient setup for selective angiography contrast mixing and delivery. The control syringe and manifold setup facilitates reloading after each contrast injection. One hand operates the syringe, and the other regulates the proportions of contrast material and saline in the final mixture via the stopcocks on the manifold. Between injections, the saline line can be left on flush to keep the catheter irrigated or transduced to monitor blood pressure.

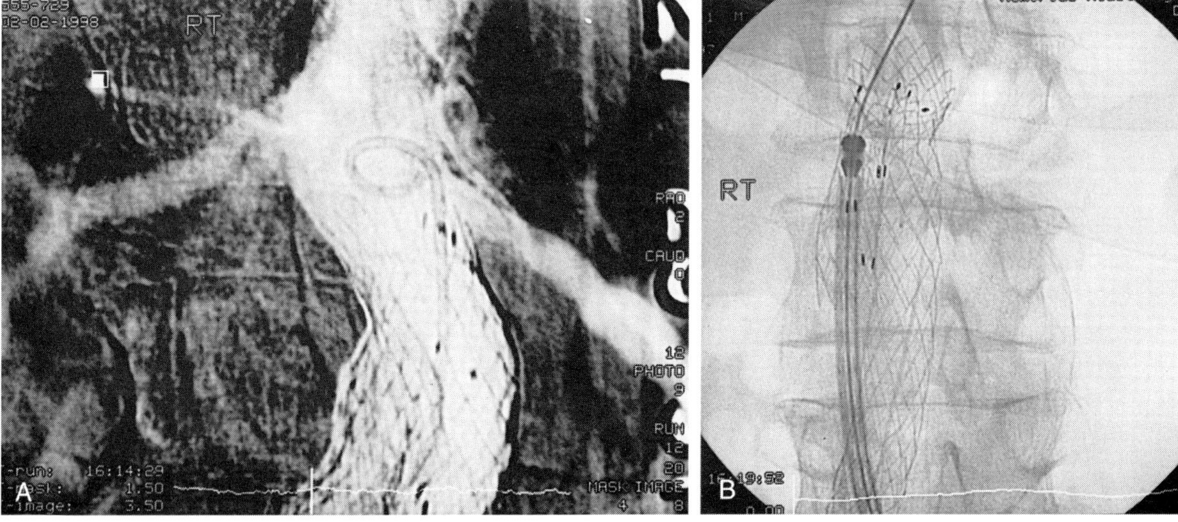

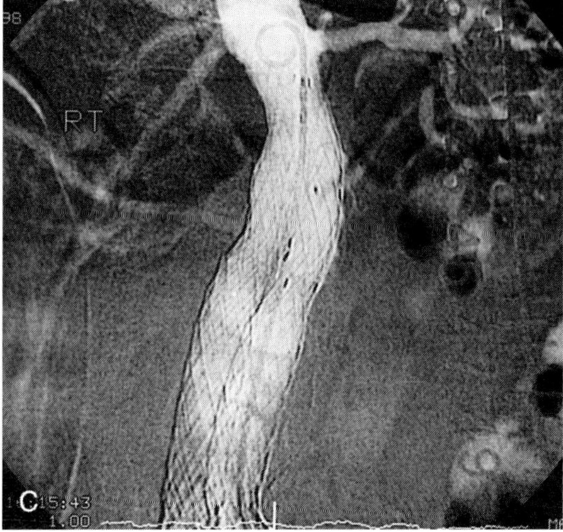

FIGURE 16–6. *A*, Completion aortic endograft angiogram in the anteroposterior projection, giving the appearance of overriding of the endograft on the left renal artery. *B*, Unsubtracted visualization of the endograft stent rings revealing them to be out of alignment, consistent with anterior angulation of the aortic neck. *C*, Completion angiogram obtained in the 36-degree cranial projection, which aligns the front and back apices of the endograft and reveals that the endograft is well clear of the left renal artery.

TABLE 16–3. TYPICAL CONTRAST INJECTION VOLUMES, METHODS, AND RATES USED FOR VARIOUS VASCULAR REGIONS

LOCATION	SUGGESTED INJECTION METHOD	INJECTION RATE (ml/sec)	TOTAL VOLUME (ml)
Aortic arch	Power	20	40
Selective carotid artery	Hand or power	5–10	10
Selective vertebral artery	Hand	3–4	5
Selective subclavian/brachial arteries	Hand or power	5–10	10
Abdominal aorta	Power	20	40
Renal and mesenteric arteries	Hand	5–10	10
Iliac artery	Hand or power	10	10
Infrainguinal segments	Hand or power	5–10	10
Aorta to pedal arteries, stepped run	Power	20	90*

*Full-strength contrast agent; for all other locations, half-strength contrast agent is typically used for digital subtraction angiography.

catheterization-associated vasospasm. Other vasodilatory measures, such as warming of the extremity and use of reactive hyperemia, may also assist in visualizing the distal vascular tree.[5]

SOURCES OF ERROR WITH ANGIOGRAPHY

The detrimental effect of patient movement on image quality and the methods to correct for it have already been thoroughly discussed. Motion artefacts remain, however, the most common source of image degradation encountered during angiography. Nonetheless, other factors can also lead to confounding images and associated errors.

First and foremost, the presence of tissues similar in radiodensity to the contrast agent in use frequently compromises the quality of the rendered image. The tissue most commonly responsible for this degradation of image quality is bone, and calcified plaque can have a similar effect. Although filming at different angles may succeed in separating the bone from the vessel, and thereby negating the interference of the bone, this maneuver may not be possible with calcified plaque or in areas with multiple or diffuse osseous structures, such as the pelvis or lower leg. Usually, however, a combination of views can succeed in minimizing the artefact and demonstrating the luminal characteristics of the vessel of interest.

Contrast agent in superimposed vessels can obscure visualization of luminal irregularities in the overlapping regions. This problem commonly occurs near vascular bifurcations, where occlusive lesions are also common. Therefore, it is incumbent upon the angiographer to search for views that separate the vessels and allow visualization of all areas. Although this goal is usually achieved through the use of different oblique projections, the use of cranial or caudal rotation is often helpful, particularly in areas of anterior or posterior angulation (Fig. 16–6). The typical configuration of the iliac and femoral bifurcations is best splayed out in the contralateral and ipsilateral anterior oblique projections, respectively (Fig. 16–7). The aortic arch is best viewed in the left anterior oblique projection, whereas the celiac axis and superior mesenteric arteries are visualized best in the lateral projection. The renal arteries can arise directly lateral or slightly anterior or posterior to the aorta (Fig. 16–8). Therefore, the angiographer must determine the most appropriate view to visualize the origin of the vessel of interest so that an orificial lesion is not missed (Table 16–4).

An additional source of error that has been encountered quite frequently since the advent of endoluminal grafting procedures is the artefact produced when tortuous vessels are straightened by stiff guide wires (Fig. 16–9). The size and rigidity of these devices require the use of very stiff guide wires in order for the device to track through the iliac system. Angiograms obtained when these wires are in place may give the appearance of luminal stenoses or dissections produced by the unnatural course the vessel is forced into by the stiff guide wire. This finding can be particularly worrisome at the completion of a procedure, when it is conceivable that passage of the device has indeed damaged the vessel. Although the appearance is somewhat characteristic, it is best to exchange the stiff guide wire for a softer one and then reevaluate the situation to be sure of the diagnosis.

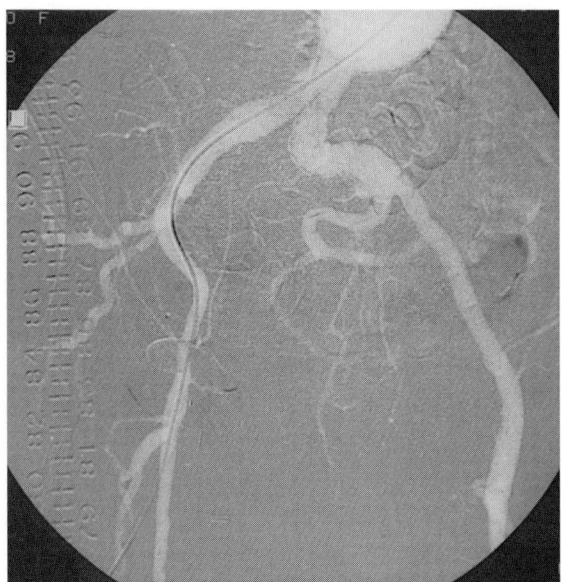

FIGURE 16–7. Pelvic arteriogram taken in the 30-degree right anterior oblique position, which splays out the contralateral iliac and ipsilateral femoral bifurcations.

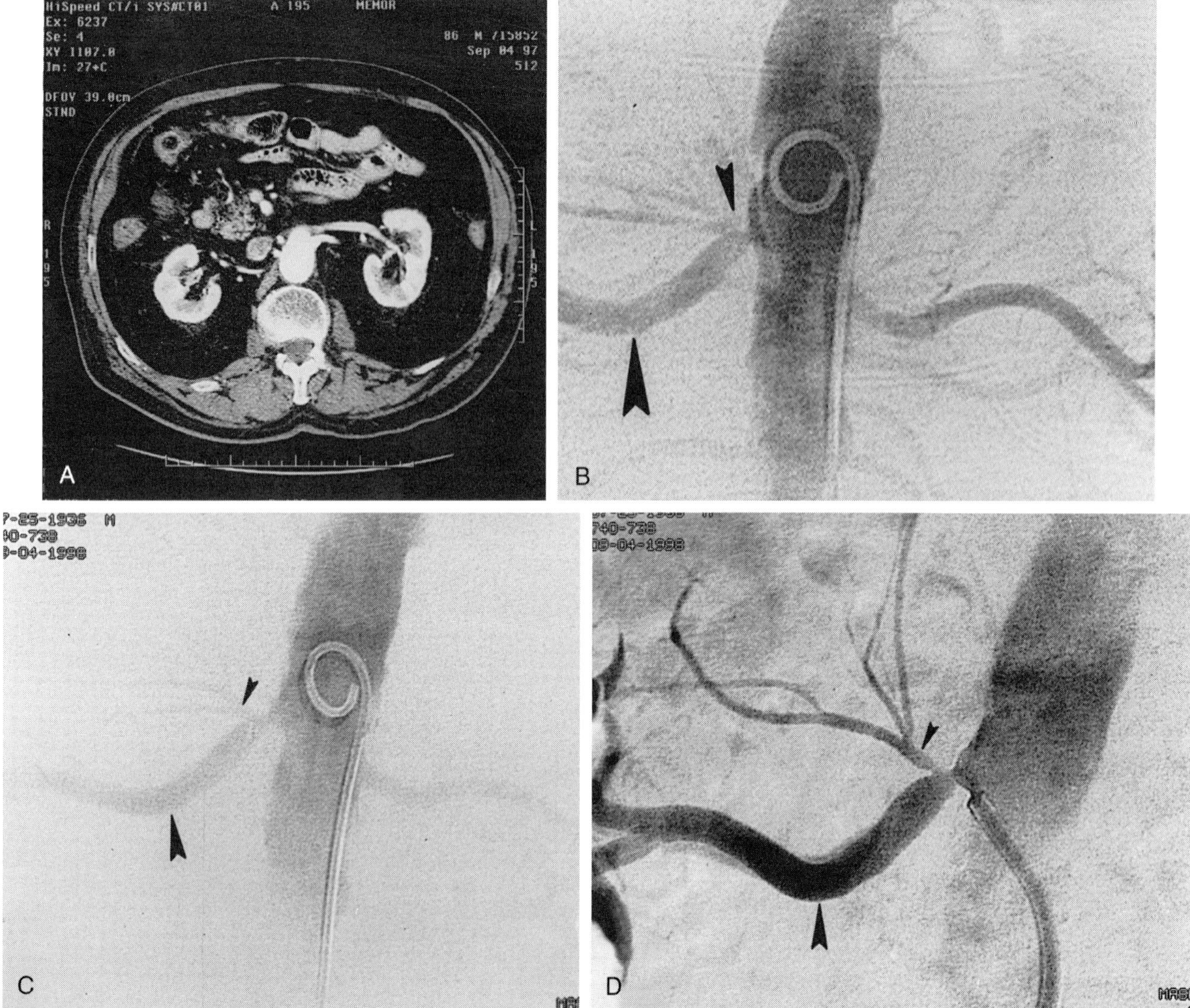

FIGURE 16–8. *A,* CT scan showing both right and left renal arteries arising from the anterior surface of the aorta. The best radiographic view for each of these will be the 10- to 15-degree contralateral anterior oblique projection. *B,* Flush aortogram in the anteroposterior projection, suggesting a right renal artery (*large arrow*) stenosis at the renal orifice. Also noted is a branch vessel (*small arrow*) which, in this view, appears to arise from the aorta itself. *C,* Flush aortogram in the 15-degree left anterior oblique projection allows better evalution of the origin of the right renal artery. This projection reveals that the right renal artery (*large arrow*) stenosis is not truly orificial and suggests that the branch vessel (*small arrow*) arises from the renal artery directly. *D,* Selective right renal angiogram obtained in the 15-degree left anterior oblique projection. This projection offers the best opacification and characterization of the renal artery stenosis as well as delineation of the origin of the branch vessel.

BASICS OF RADIATION SAFETY

Because exposure to ionizing radiation is an unavoidable aspect of angiography, no review of the topic would be complete without a discussion of means of minimizing this hazard. Two basic mechanisms exist for achieving this goal:

- Reducing the output of radiation
- Shielding the operator from exposure

The requisite close proximity of the operator to the x-ray source during fluoroscopy-guided catheter and guide wire manipulation makes fluoroscopy the single greatest source of occupational radiation exposure in medicine today.[4, 12, 15] With more complex endoluminal grafting, stent, and thrombolytic procedures being performed more frequently, fluoroscopy times have increased substantially and so has the potential for excessive radiation exposure.

Perhaps the simplest means of reducing radiation produced during fluoroscopy is judicious attention to its use. Inattentive and inexperienced operators tend to continue fluoroscopy long after completing the technical maneuver at hand. Clearly, if the operator is not looking at the video monitor, there is no need for the fluoroscopy to be "on." Similarly, when performing radiographic imaging, the operator should terminate the run as soon as the relevant information has been obtained. Also, it is not uncommon for an inexperienced operator to "study" the fluoroscopic image in real time even though a static image on the monitor from a quick "flash" of fluoroscopy would suffice and would substantially reduce radiation output.

When the anatomic area of interest is substantially

TABLE 16–4. RECOMMENDED RADIOGRAPHIC FILMING PROJECTIONS FOR OPTIMAL SEPARATION OF ARTERIAL BRANCHES

LOCATION	RECOMMENDED FILMING PROJECTION
Aortic arch	30-degree left anterior oblique
Cervical carotid arteries	Anteroposterior (AP) and lateral
Intracranial carotid arteries	AP and lateral
Vertebrobasilar system	AP and lateral
Renal artery origin	AP ± 10 degrees
Celiac or superior mesenteric artery origin	Lateral
Iliac bifurcation	20-degree contralateral anterior oblique
Femoral bifurcation	20-degree ipsilateral anterior oblique
Trifurcation and tibial arteries	Anatomic AP (or 20-degree ipsilateral anterior oblique with feet in the neutral supine position)

smaller than the overall field of view, using a smaller image intensifier size reduces the amount of radiation produced, with the added benefit of improving the image quality. For rectangular areas of interest, such as in extremity evaluations, it is possible to narrow the sides of the beam of radiation to reduce radiation output. This technique, termed *collimation*, has no detrimental effect on image quality and simplifies the radiographic exposure by eliminating areas with large variations in radiodensity.

A final mechanism for reducing radiation output is the use of *pulsed* rather than *continuous* fluoroscopy. Unfortunately, the image quality in this mode is definitely degraded and noticeably choppy, for which reason it is not often used in most practices.

Despite reductions in excessive radiation output, there is always a need to shield the operator and other personnel from hazardous ionizing radiation produced during the conduct of endovascular procedures. Lead aprons and thyroid shields are universally utilized to shield the most radiation-sensitive organs: the thyroid, gonads, breasts, and red bone marrow. It has been well documented that the thickness of lead aprons worn is the only variable that significantly affects the amount of radiation recorded on monitoring badges worn underneath them; the best protection is provided by aprons with a 1.0-mm thickness of lead in front.[13] The use of leaded glass screens and collimation would be expected to reduce radiation exposure, but in actual clinical practice no statistically significant effect on over-lead or under-lead monitoring badge doses were found for these variables.[13] Finally, many endovascular therapists who perform large numbers of procedures wear leaded glasses with side shields during endovascular procedures to reduce the risk of cataract formation from exposure to ionizing radiation.

SUMMARY

Although the role of arteriography in the diagnosis of vascular disease may be diminished by new technology under development, it remains the standard and an integral component of all of the rapidly developing endovascular procedures. Therefore, it is incumbent upon vascular surgeons (1) to understand the basic principles of radiographic imaging and arteriographic evaluation and (2) to safely and effectively apply the principles to their practices and evolving methods. The information presented in this chapter should enable vascular surgeons to make informed decisions about radiographic equipment and techniques and to

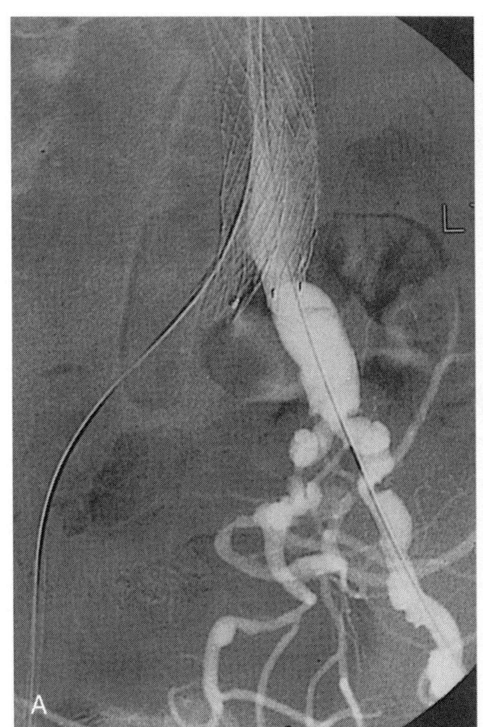

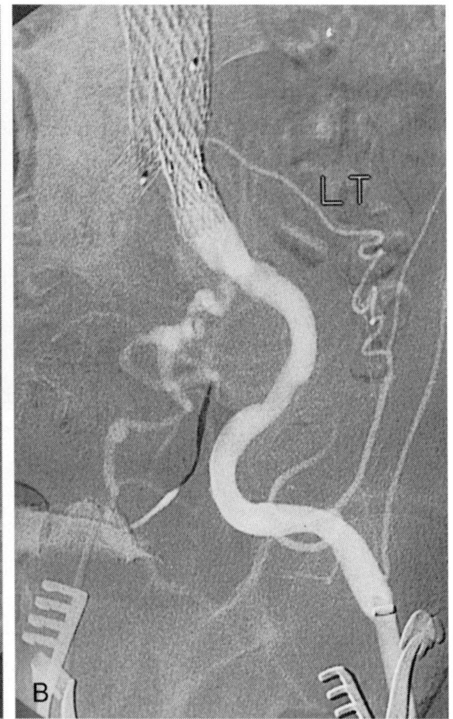

FIGURE 16–9. Left iliac angiogram obtained after aortic endografting, with an Amplatz super-stiff guide wire in place through the iliac system. Forced straightening of the external iliac artery produces the appearance of multiple luminal stenoses. *B,* Same left iliac angiogram immediately after removal of the guide wire. Once the iliac arteries resume their natural configuration, the "stenoses" are seen to resolve.

avoid the common pitfalls of these procedures. However, to put this information to good use, vascular surgeons must persevere in the pursuit of access to the best available radiographic facilities. With this combination of knowledge and facilities, vascular surgeons are well positioned to render the best available endovascular and surgical care to their patients and to participate actively in the development and evaluation of new techniques.

REFERENCES

1. Aaron JO, Hesselink JR, Oot R, et al: Complications of intravenous DSA performed for carotid artery disease: A prospective study. Radiology 153:675–678, 1984.
2. Bettmann MA: Ionic versus nonionic contrast agents for intravenous use: Are all the answers in? Radiology 175:616–618, 1990.
3. Bettmann MA: Contrast agents. *In* Kim D, Orron DE (eds): Peripheral Vascular Imaging and Intervention. St. Louis, Mosby–Year Book, 1992.
4. Bush WH, Jones D, Brannen GE: Radiation dose to personnel during percutaneous renal calculus removal. AJR 145:1261–1264, 1985.
5. Cohen MI, Vogelzang RL: A comparison of techniques for improved visualization of the arteries of the distal lower extremity. AJR 147:1021–1024, 1986.
6. Crummy AB, Stieghorst MF, Turski PA, et al: Digital subtraction angiography: Current status and use of intra-arterial injection. Radiology 145:303–307, 1982.
7. Gomes AS, Lois JF, Baker JD, et al: Acute renal dysfunction in high-risk patients after angiography: Comparison of ionic and nonionic contrast media. Radiology 170:65–68, 1989.
8. Greenberger PA, Patterson R, Tapio CM: Prophylaxis against repeated radiocontrast media reactions in 857 cases. Arch Intern Med 145:2197–2200, 1985.
9. Hawkins IF: Carbon dioxide digital subtraction angiography. AJR 139:19–24, 1982.
10. Katayama H: Report of the Japanese Committee on the Safety of Contrast Media. Presented to the Radiological Society of North America, 1988.
11. Lasser EC, Berry CC, Talner, et al: Pretreatment with corticosteroids to alleviate reactions to intravenous contrast material. N Engl J Med 317:845–849, 1987.
12. Lowe FC, Auster M, Beck TJ, et al: Monitoring radiation exposure to medical personnel during percutaneous nephrolithotomy. Urology 28:221–226, 1986.
13. Marx MV, Niklason L, Mauger EA: Occupational radiation exposure to interventional radiologists: A prospective study. J Vasc Interv Radiol 3:597–606, 1992.
14. Miller DL, Chang R, Wells WT, et al: Intravascular contrast media: Effect of dose on renal function. Radiology 167:607–611, 1988.
15. National Council on Radiation Protection and Measurements (NCRP): Implementation of the Principle of as Low as Reasonably Achievable (ALARA) for Medical and Dental personnel. NCRP Report No. 107. Bethesda, Md, NCRP, 1990.
16. Parfrey PS, Griffiths SM, Barrett BJ, et al: Contrast material-induced renal failure in patients with diabetes mellitus, renal insufficiency, or both: A prospective controlled study. N Engl J Med 320:143–149, 1988.
17. Podrid PJ: Role of higher nervous activity in ventricular arrhythmia and sudden cardiac death: Implication for alternative antiarrhythmic therapy. Ann N Y Acad Sci 432:296–313, 1984.
18. Reilly LM, Ehrenfeld WK, Stoney RJ: Carotid digital subtraction angiography: Comparative roles of intra-arterial and intravenous imaging. Surgery 96:909–917, 1984.
19. Schwab SJ, Hlatky MA, Pieper KS, et al: Contrast nephrotoxicity: A randomized controlled trial of a nonionic and an ionic radiographic contrast agent. N Engl J Med 320:149–153, 1989.
20. Smith D, Yahiku PY, Maloney MD, et al: Three new low-osmolality contrast agents: A comparative study of patient discomfort. Am J Neuroradiol 9:137–139, 1988.
21. Weaver FA, Pentecost MJ, Yellin AE, et al: Clinical applications of carbon dioxide/digital subtraction angiography. J Vasc Surg 13:266–273, 1991.

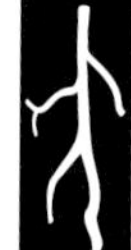

CHAPTER 17

Principles of Venography

Michael A. McKusick, M.D., and
Peter Gloviczki, M.D.

LOWER EXTREMITIES

Ascending Venography

The diagnosis of lower extremity deep vein thrombosis (DVT) was largely a clinical one until the 1960s, when contrast venography became a part of standard medical practice.[19] First introduced by Berberich and Hirsch[7] in 1923, lower extremity venography was used by dos Santos[17] in 1938 to confirm a clinically suspected diagnosis of DVT. The technique evolved over many years and became the "gold standard" for the diagnosis of DVT.[35] In 1940, Bauer[5] published details of normal venographic anatomy and of the venographic appearance of acute and chronic DVT (Figs. 17–1 to 17–6). Early leg venography required venous cutdown for access to the deep system, but this technique was modified by Welch and coworkers, who recommended contrast injection into a superficial vein in the foot with a tourniquet applied above the ankle to prevent filling of the superficial veins, which often obscured the deep system.[39] Diagnostic criteria for DVT were established in 1963 by De Weese and Rogoff,[16] who reported their review of 100 positive leg venograms.

In past decades, the technique used for lower extremity

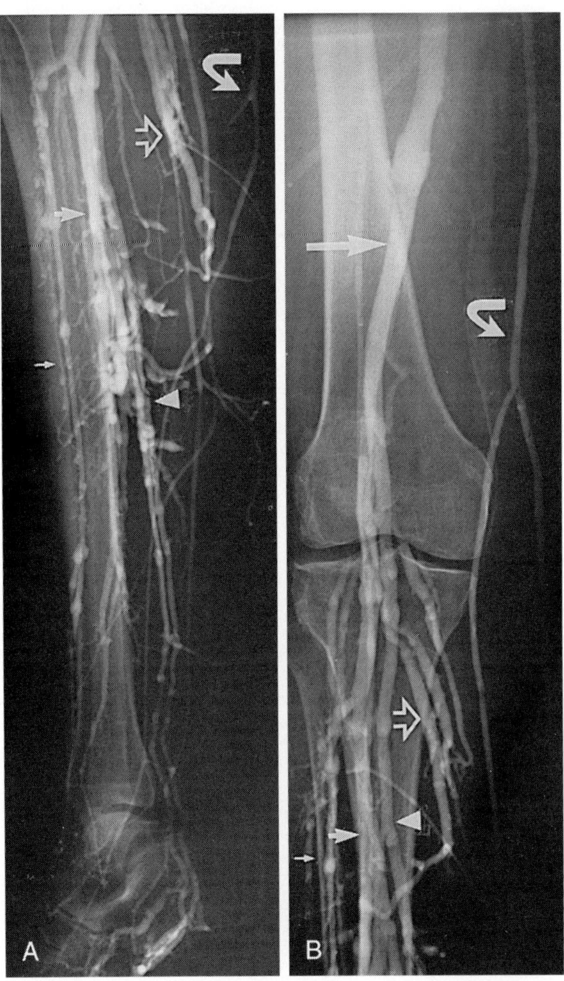

FIGURE 17–1. Normal right leg venogram. *A,* Lateral calf projection. *B,* Anteroposterior knee. Anterior tibial veins *(small arrow)*; peroneal veins *(short arrow)*; posterior tibial veins *(arrowhead)*; gastrocnemius veins *(open arrow)*; greater saphenous vein *(curved arrow)*; and popliteal vein *(long arrow)*.

ascending venography has been modified many times.[18, 23, 26, 27, 32, 35] However, even as the technique has been refined and the examination has been made safer and less painful with the use of modern contrast agents, it remains a relatively invasive study that requires an often painful venipuncture, injection of iodine-based contrast agents, and exposure of the patient to ionizing radiation. For this reason, venous duplex imaging with compression was developed as a noninvasive alternative to venography for the diagnosis of acute DVT. With sensitivities and specificities of greater than 95% in symptomatic patients with acute DVT, it is no wonder that venous duplex imaging has overtaken contrast venography as the study of choice for evaluating patients with suspected leg vein thrombosis.[10, 14] Even in suspected calf vein thrombosis, ultrasonography has shown sensitivities of 95% and specificities of 100% in experienced hands and is now trusted by many clinicians as the diagnostic test of choice.[6, 9, 10]

With the emergence of ultrasonography as the primary diagnostic tool for evaluation of acute leg DVT, the number of lower extremity venograms performed in our practice has decreased from a high of 450 patients in 1982 to only 40 patients in 1997. Because of this dramatic decrease in patient numbers, it is difficult to train residents in the performance and interpretation of leg venography, a fact that will further decrease the availability and accuracy of the examination for future practitioners.

Indications and Accuracy

Properly performed and interpreted, lower extremity venography remains a powerful tool in the evaluation of both acute and chronic DVT and is unsurpassed in its vivid depiction of venous anatomy and morphology. Ascending leg venography is clearly indicated when a high clinical suspicion of thrombosis is present in the setting of negative or equivocal noninvasive tests.[40] With very high diagnostic accuracy, a leg venogram is immediately useful for evaluation of the presence of deep venous disease. However, this so-called gold standard is uninterpretable in 5% to 15% of patients because of poor technique.[27] The number of poor-quality examinations will likely increase in the future as patient numbers continue to decline, and this will only further diminish the utility of the examination.

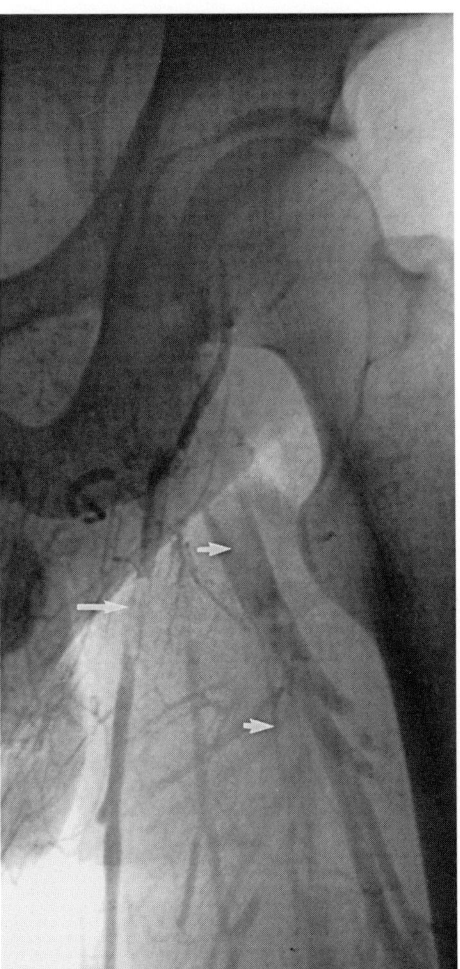

FIGURE 17–2. Acute thrombus in the deep femoral and greater saphenous veins. The deep femoral vein *(short arrows)* and greater saphenous vein *(long arrow)* are shown. The superficial femoral vein is occluded.

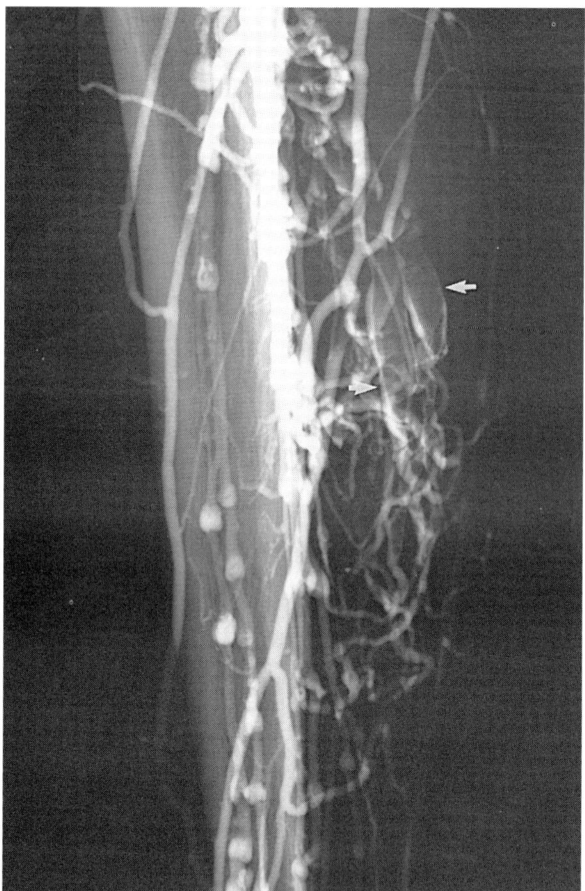

FIGURE 17–3. Acute thrombosis of the soleal veins. *Arrows* indicate fresh thrombus filling the soleal veins.

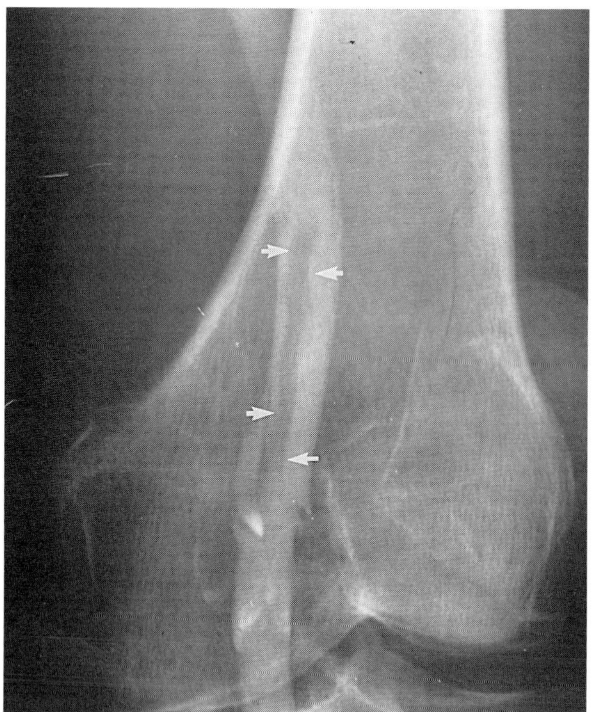

FIGURE 17–4. Subacute thrombus in the popliteal vein. *Arrows* denote retracted thrombus indicating subacute thrombosis.

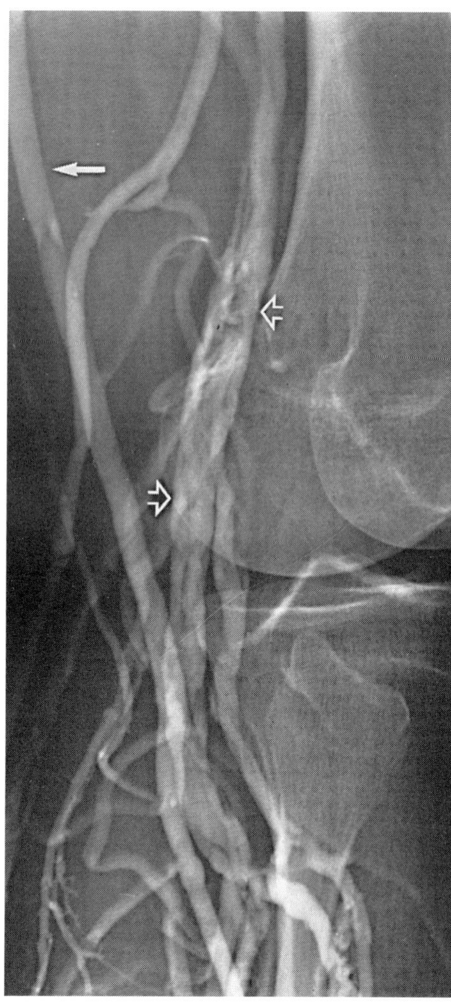

FIGURE 17–5. Chronic popliteal vein thrombosis. Note extensive recanalization of the popliteal vein *(open arrows)* and relatively large caliber of the greater saphenous vein *(arrow)*.

Technique

Good-quality ascending venography is not difficult to accomplish, but it does call for a relatively cooperative patient. Patients should fast for 3 to 4 hours and should be well hydrated to avoid the risks of emesis and renal toxicity, which can be associated with intravenous contrast administration. Patients with significant leg swelling may benefit from an Ace wrap to displace edema fluid and to make venous cannulation easier. Warm packs to the dorsum of the foot may also facilitate venous access.

A 22-gauge plastic intravenous cannula is placed into a dorsal vein of the foot. The saphenous vein can also be used, but a tourniquet is then essential to drive contrast into the deep system. The patient is positioned on a radiographic fluoroscopy table with tilt capability and a foot rest to enable positioning in the 40- to 60-degree upright position. The contralateral leg is supported with a small platform so that no weight is borne on the leg to be examined. Side grip handles are placed on the table so that the patient feels secure in the semi-upright position. Either digital spot films or regular cut films can be used for acquisition.

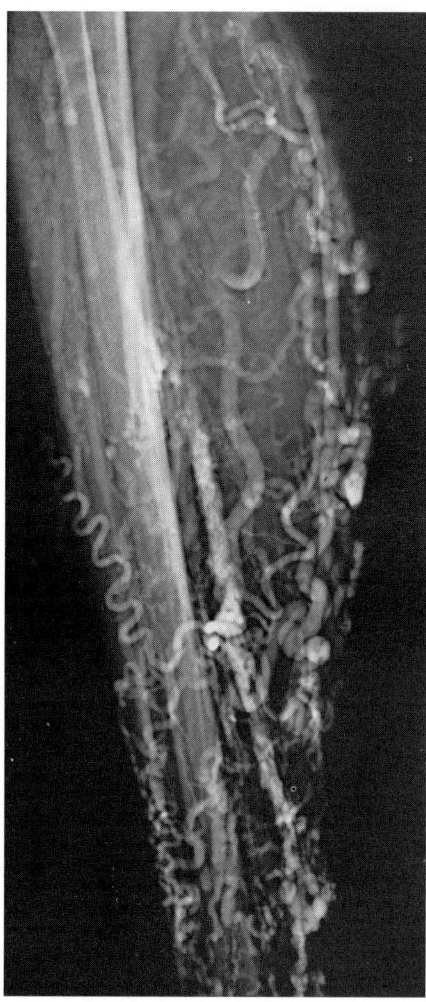

FIGURE 17–6. Chronic deep vein thrombosis. Note extensive collateral channels and nonvisualization of normal deep venous structures.

If the patient is examined for venous valvular incompetence, a 100-cm ruler with opaque markers is placed along the lateral aspect of the leg to determine the correct distance of incompetent perforating veins from the ankle. A tourniquet above the ankle is needed in these cases to prevent filling of the superficial veins, and fluoroscopic evaluation with videotaping is performed to capture the location of incompetent perforating veins. In the patient with acute DVT, we do not routinely use the marker system and fluoroscopy is used to optimize visualization of the presence and location of thrombus. Because the anterior tibial, sural, and gastrocnemius veins fill better without a tourniquet, this is not applied in the setting of acute DVT unless no deep filling occurs.[22]

The examination is begun with the patient in the 40- to 60-degree semi-upright position. Intravenous contrast material with an organically bound iodine concentration of 200 mgI/ml is used to decrease pain and to minimize endothelial damage by the hypertonic contrast agent.[1] As contrast is injected, fluoroscopic evaluation is performed to ensure against extravasation and to optimize deep vein opacification. Spot films are taken as the deep system fills. At least two projections are needed in the tibial and popliteal locations.

As contrast ascends, additional filming of the deep and superficial femoral veins is performed. About 60 to 80 ml of contrast is needed to fill the deep venous system adequately from the ankle to the groin. For visualization of the ileocaval region, the fluoroscopy table is lowered to a flat position and the patient is asked to hold the breath while the leg is elevated 6 inches from the table top. Fluoroscopy is performed to determine maximum opacification of the veins, and a spot film is obtained. In most patients, it is easy to visualize from the low inferior vena cava (IVC) down to the common femoral bifurcation on one image.

With completion of the examination, the veins are flushed with 50 ml of 0.45 normal saline to minimize contrast contact with the venous endothelium. In most patients, this technique yields beautiful, diagnostic-quality images. Additional contrast material can be injected, as needed, to visualize problem areas, and if any questions remain, a focused ultrasound study is ordered to complement venography.

In patients undergoing evaluation primarily for venous valvular incompetence, the fluoroscopic examination is recorded on videotape rather than spot films (Fig. 17–7). This medium lends itself to a graphic demonstration of incompetent perforating veins. With marker ruler in place, it is simple to translate information from the recorded image to location on the leg, in centimeters, from the ankle. We have found this a most satisfactory way to study patients who need presurgical diagnostic imaging before ligation of incompetent perforating veins is considered.

Descending Venography

As with ascending venography, lower extremity descending venography has been largely replaced by duplex scanning in the evaluation of patients with suspected deep vein incompetence. Color duplex sonography has shown good agreement with descending venography in the grading of

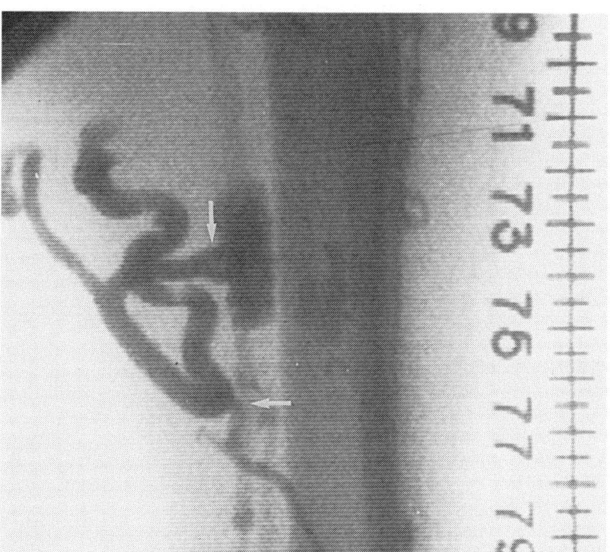

FIGURE 17–7. Incompetent medial calf perforating veins. Single-frame image of a videotape shows free flow of contrast from the posterior tibial vein through the incompetent perforating veins *(arrows)* into the superficial varicose veins.

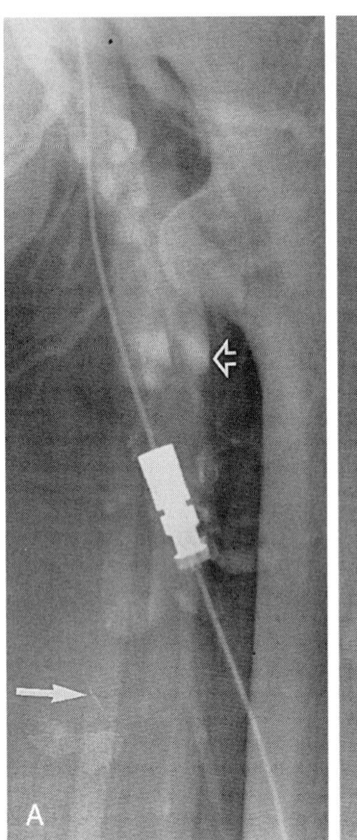

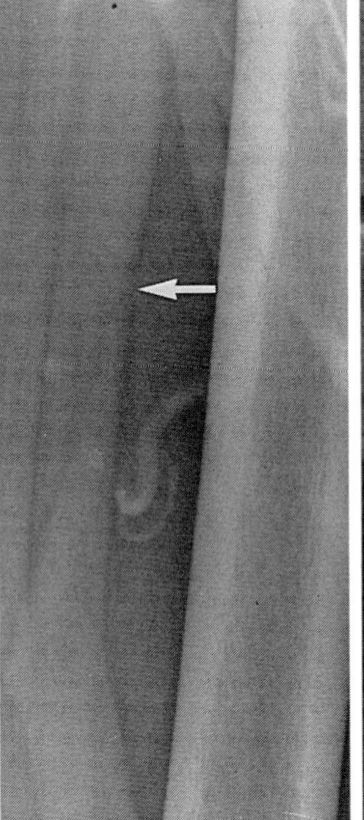

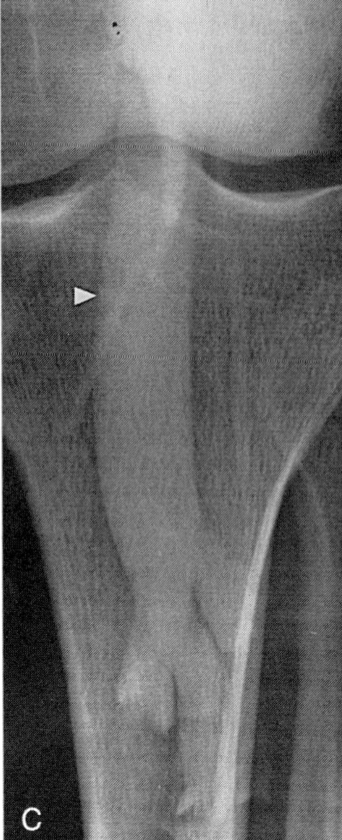

FIGURE 17–8. *A–C,* Descending left leg venogram demonstrates grade 4 reflux. Note lack of valves in the superficial femoral vein *(arrow)* and the large caliber of the popliteal vein *(arrowhead)*. The deep femoral vein *(open arrow)* is shown.

deep and superficial vein reflux.[3] For this reason, we perform descending contrast venography only in patients with significant deep vein occlusive disease who are candidates for venous bypass, vein valve repair, or valve transplantation.

Indications and Interpretation

Descending venography is used in concert with ascending venography to distinguish primary valvular incompetence from thrombotic disease. The ascending venogram demonstrates the location and extent of post-thrombotic disease, as manifested by occlusion, venous recanalization, collateral channels, and superficial varicosities. The descending venogram identifies the level of deep vein reflux and morphology of the venous valves (Fig. 17–8). We use the classification outlined by Kistner and colleagues[25] to categorize the severity of deep vein reflux (Table 17–1).

TABLE 17–1. VENOGRAPHIC CATEGORIES OF DEEP VEIN REFLUX

Grade 0	Normal valvular function with no reflux.
Grade 1	Minimal reflux confined to the upper thigh.
Grade 2	More extensive reflux, which may reach the lower thigh; a competent valve is present in the popliteal vein and there is no reflux to the calf level.
Grade 3	Reflux as above but associated with popliteal valvular incompetence and leakage of contrast into the calf veins.
Grade 4	Virtually no valvular competence with immediate and dramatic reflux distally into the calf. This type of reflux often opacifies incompetent calf perforators.

From Kistner RL, Ferris EB, Rawdhawa G, et al: A method of performing descending venography. J Vasc Surg 4:464–468, 1986.

Although reflux may occur into the saphenous vein, isolated superficial venous reflux is relatively uncommon in symptomatic patients with advanced chronic venous disease.[30] Most patients with symptoms of chronic venous insufficiency who undergo venography in our practice have reflux into the deep venous system with or without associated saphenous vein reflux. With the use of descending venography, candidates are selected for deep vein valve repair or transplant, which is offered to patients with grade 3 or 4 reflux who have recurrent symptoms of venous insufficiency after treatment of superficial varicosities and perforator vein incompetence.

Technique

Descending venography is performed on a tilt radiographic table to allow for examination in the 40- to 60-degree upright position. Venous access is obtained via sterile Seldinger technique through the common femoral vein. A short 4 or 5 French (Fr.) straight catheter with multiple side holes is positioned in the external iliac vein. If both legs are to be studied, the contralateral leg is imaged by means of a 65-cm Simmons II catheter (Cordis Corp., Miami, Fla.) with side holes. The Simons II catheter can be easily negotiated over a guide wire across the iliac bifurcation into the opposite external iliac vein. The catheter is fixed to the groin with sterile adhesive strips to prevent dislodgment when the patient is upright. The contralateral leg is supported with a small platform, as with ascending venography, so that no weight is borne on the limb to be examined.

With the patient in the semi-upright position, contrast material is injected by hand through the femoral catheter. Iodinated contrast, 20 to 30 ml, with a concentration of

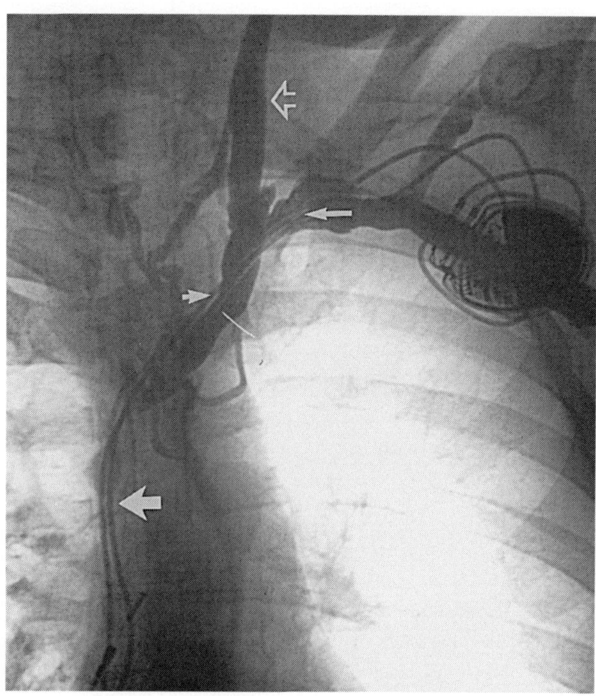

FIGURE 17–9. Chronic thrombosis of the superior vena cava, the innominate veins, and the subclavian veins caused by cardiac pacer wires. Chronic subclavian vein thrombosis *(long arrow)*; innominate vein *(short arrow)*; and expected location of the superior vena cava *(large arrow)*. Note reflux of contrast up the left internal jugular vein *(open arrow)*.

200 mgI/ml is used. As the contrast material is injected, the patient is asked to perform a sustained Valsalva maneuver to enhance evidence of valvular incompetence. We record the study by videotaping the live fluoroscopic examination as the patient undergoes evaluation from the femoral region to the knee and below. Specific areas of interest can be studied further with sequential contrast injections to optimize image capture of valve location and function as well as extent of reflux. The videotape format is ideal for this examination, and we no longer take spot films during descending venography.

UPPER EXTREMITY VENOGRAPHY

Venography of the upper extremity is normally performed for evaluation of the central veins of the arms and chest. Although primary axillary-subclavian vein thrombosis is relatively uncommon (<2% of all DVT), the incidence of central venous occlusion is still rising because of the increasing use of long-term central venous catheters and transvenous cardiac pacers (Fig. 17–9).[15,33,38]

Upper extremity venography remains the procedure of choice for most clinicians in the evaluation of central thoracic venous disease, especially in the setting of axillary-subclavian vein thrombosis caused by thoracic outlet compression.[36] In these cases, venography is performed in conjunction with thrombolytic therapy. Pre-lysis venography establishes the extent and location of the disease, and the post-lysis examination demonstrates residual thrombosis and extrinsic compression requiring further treatment. In patients with signs and symptoms of upper extremity thrombosis caused by neoplasm, central venous catheters, or thrombophilic state, however, both compression ultrasound and magnetic resonance angiography (MRA) have proved accurate in establishing a diagnosis.[34,20] MRA is especially helpful in demonstrating patency of the central veins and allows planning of central venous catheter placement in patients with a history of central vein occlusion.

Indications

We are currently performing upper extremity venography in patients with primary axillary-subclavian vein thrombosis who are candidates for thrombolytic therapy. The examination is performed to show the extent of thrombosis and to guide placement of infusion catheters for administration of the lytic agent (Fig. 17–10). The post-lysis study, as mentioned, is needed to detect the presence of residual thrombus and, when performed with thoracic outlet maneuvers, to determine the degree of extrinsic compression. This information is crucial to determine the need for additional therapy for prevention of recurrent thrombosis.

Patients with suspected central vein occlusion who are not candidates for MRA, because of a cardiac pacemaker or claustrophobia, for example, are also studied with upper extremity venography. By far, however, the major indication for upper extremity venography at our institution is placement of a peripherally inserted central catheter (PICC) using fluoroscopic and intravenous contrast guidance.

Technique

Originally described by Lea Thomas and Andress in 1971, the technique used for upper extremity venography has

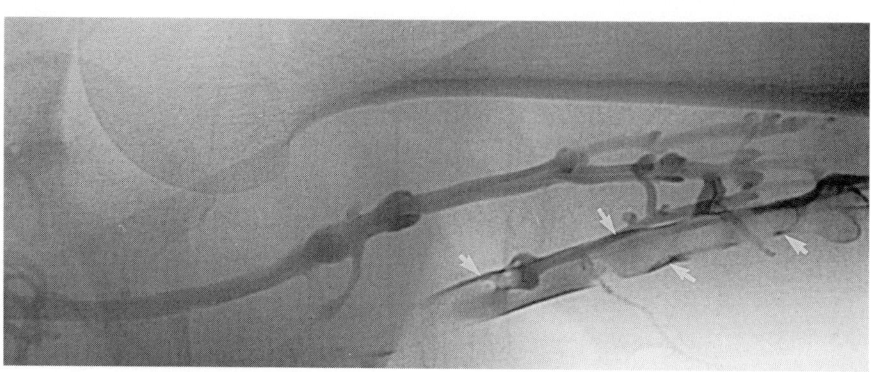

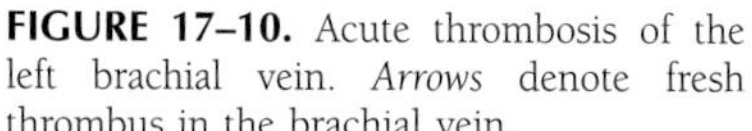

FIGURE 17–10. Acute thrombosis of the left brachial vein. *Arrows* denote fresh thrombus in the brachial vein.

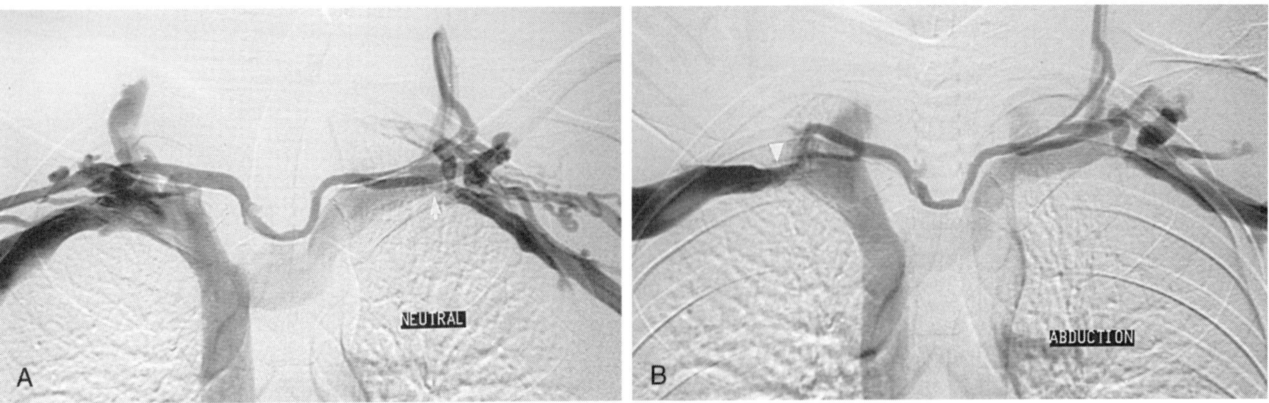

FIGURE 17–11. Bilateral upper extremity venogram in a patient with bilateral thoracic outlet syndrome. *A*, Neutral position. Note chronic thrombosis of left subclavian vein *(arrow)*. *B*, Abduction view. *Arrowhead* denotes impingement of the right subclavian vein at level of the first rib.

changed significantly with the dissemination of digital subtraction equipment.[2, 28, 31] Digital techniques allow the examination to be performed more quickly and with less contrast material than is used with cut-film studies. We are doing all upper extremity venography procedures using digital imaging equipment and firmly believe that this is the current standard of practice.

For evaluation of the central veins of the thorax, we perform venography by injecting through an intravenous site in the antecubital fossa or forearm with the arm in a neutral position at the patient's side. Contrast material, 20 to 30 ml, with a concentration of 200 mgI/ml is injected by hand for each projection needed. Digital imaging of the axillary region and mediastinum is acquired at one image per second as the patient suspends respiration. Adequate imaging of the superior vena cava (SVC) in some patients requires bilateral injections. This helps to compensate for contrast washout in the SVC by unopacified blood from the opposite innominate vein. Alternatively, although somewhat less effective, the arm being studied can be elevated slightly during the injection to facilitate contrast inflow to the SVC.

For evaluation of extrinsic compression of the axillary-subclavian junction, the patient is studied in both neutral and abducted positions (Fig. 17–11). The arm is abducted by bending it at the elbow and by tucking the hand behind

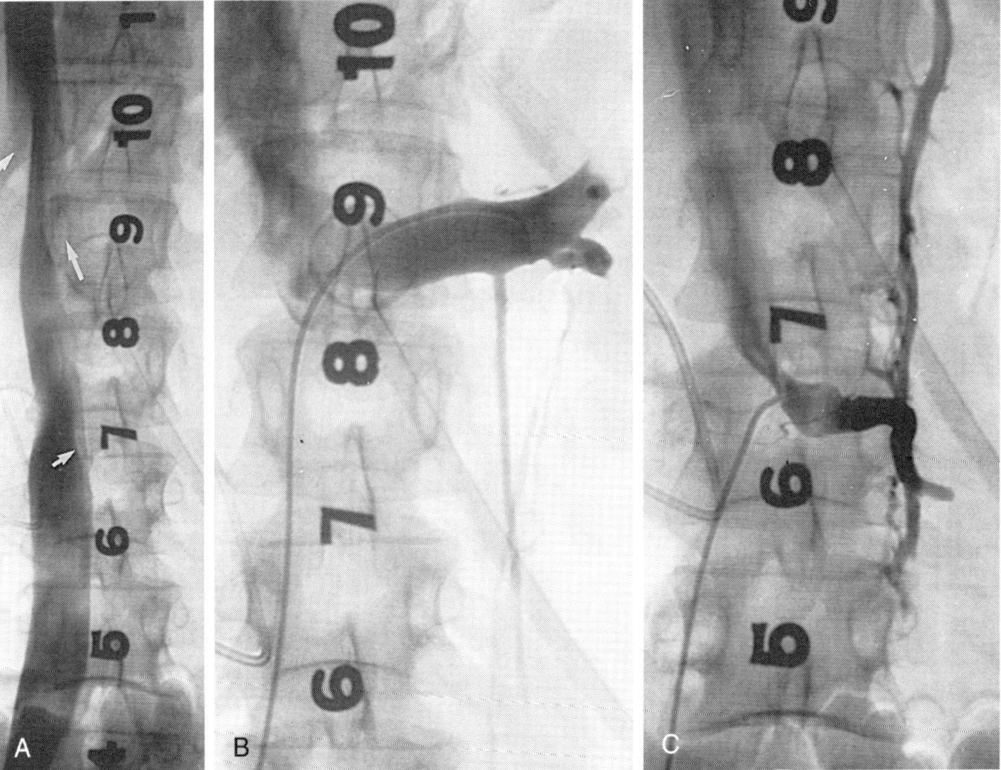

FIGURE 17–12. Normal inferior vena cavogram. *A*, Note wash-in of unopacified blood from the renal veins *(large arrows)* and the left ascending lumbar veins *(small arrow)*. *B*, Selective left renal venogram confirms location of the renal vein. *C*, Selective left lumbar venogram.

the patient's head. Imaging of the axillary and subclavian vein regions is thus obtained during maximal thoracic outlet compression.

During fluoroscopic placement of a PICC, a small intravenous cannula in the patient's hand or forearm is injected with contrast material to opacify the deep veins in the arm. Fluoroscopy is then used to guide needle puncture of a deep vein suitable for catheter placement. Before a PICC is placed, the central veins of the thorax are evaluated with this technique to confirm patency and suitability for catheter advancement into the SVC.

CENTRAL ABDOMINAL VENOGRAPHY

Venography of the central veins of the abdomen has largely been replaced by cross-sectional imaging techniques, such as ultrasound study, computed tomography (CT), and magnetic resonance imaging (MRI). These noninvasive modalities not only are less costly but also usually provide a great deal more diagnostic information than catheter venography can. For this reason, the number of central venographic studies performed in our practice for diagnostic purposes has dwindled markedly in recent years.

Indications

The most common central abdominal venographic examination that we perform is a contrast study of the IVC prior to placement of an IVC filter. This is done to provide details of renal vein anatomy to allow for proper positioning of the filter in the infrarenal cava. Often, selective renal venography is performed in addition to the cavography to distinguish ascending lumbar veins from anomalous circumaortic left renal veins (Fig. 17–12).[21] Theoretically, it is important to place the caval filter below the origin of a large anomalous renal vein to prevent pulmonary emboli from propagating around the filter through this potential collateral vessel.[37]

Hepatic venography is also commonly performed in conjunction with wedge and free pressure measurements in patients with suspected portal hypertension or Budd-Chiari syndrome.[13]

Technique

Most venographies of the central veins of the abdomen are performed from either a common femoral or internal jugular vein approach using standard Seldinger technique. Real-time ultrasound guidance is helpful for the internal jugular approach in patients with poorly palpable carotid pulses or obesity. To image the IVC, a catheter with multiple side holes is inserted into the cava and positioned at the iliac bifurcation. Contrast material with an iodine concentration of 370 mgI/ml is administered with a power injector at a rate of 20 ml/sec for 2 seconds. Digital image acquisition is at two per second for 5 seconds with centering over the area of interest (Figs. 17–13 and 17–14).

Selective renal or hepatic vein catheterization is performed by means of a variety of catheter shapes according to the anatomy at hand and the approach. For example, if hepatic venography is done in conjunction with a biopsy, the transjugular route is chosen; if no biopsy is needed, femoral access is adequate. The downward acute angle of the origins of the hepatic veins from the IVC from the femoral approach is markedly different from the obtuse angle generated by jugular access and catheters for selective injections are chosen appropriately. The same is true for renal vein catheterization. Although the amount of contrast used for imaging depends on vein size and flow, a total of 20 ml at 5 to 8 ml/sec generally opacifies most renal or hepatic venous structures (Figs. 17–15 and 17–16). Again, digital images are obtained at a rate of two per second.

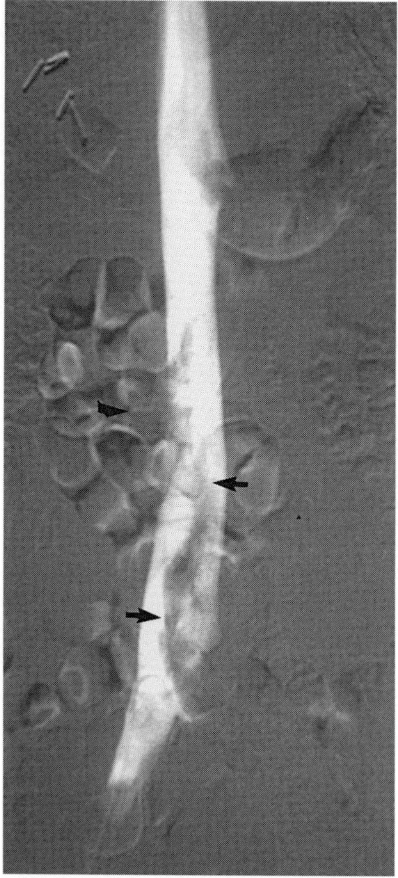

FIGURE 17–13. Inferior vena cavogram. *Arrows* indicate extension of a thrombus from the left common iliac vein into the inferior vena cava.

COMPLICATIONS

Most of the complications of venography result from the side effects of the iodinated contrast material used for the examination; few complications arise from catheter placement. These complications can be grouped into three categories:

- Problems related to the toxic effect of the contrast material on vascular endothelium
- Allergic reactions to administration of contrast material
- Nephrotoxicity of iodine-based contrast agents

High-osmolar contrast material (HOCM) is hypertonic, with

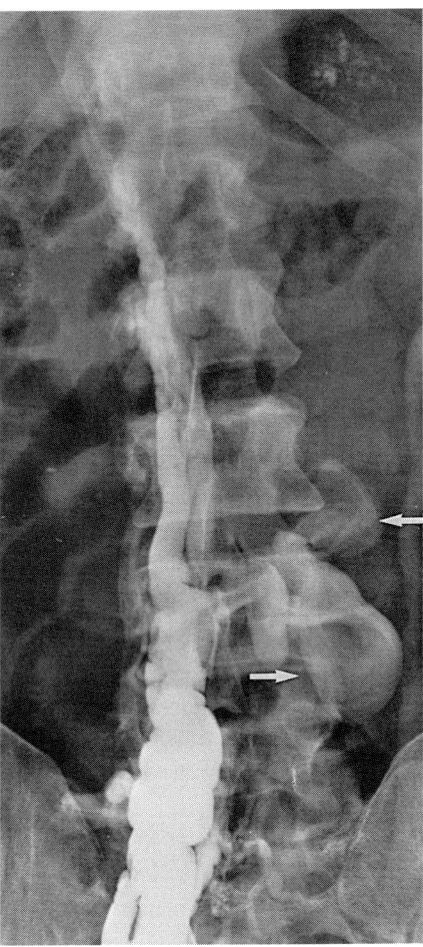

FIGURE 17–14. Chronic occlusion of the inferior vena cava. Note extensive recannalization of the inferior vena cava and large ascending lumbar collateral channels *(arrows)*.

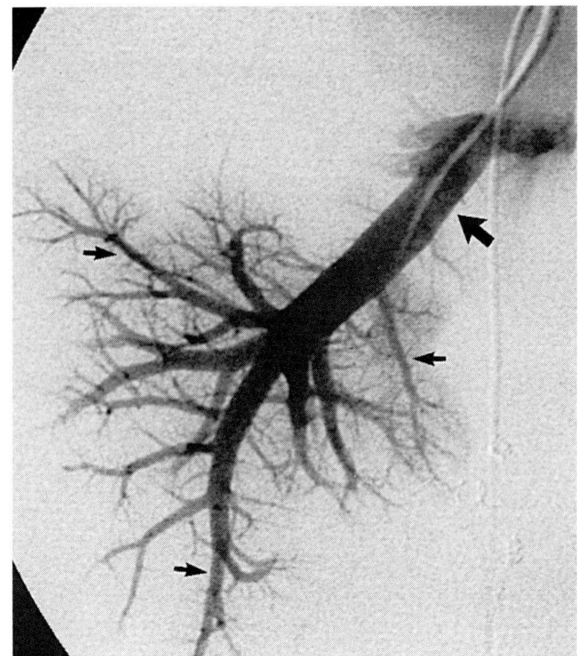

FIGURE 17–15. Digital subtraction right hepatic venogram. Note the main right hepatic vein *(large arrow)* and detail of the hepatic vein branches *(small arrows)*.

a concentration of up to six times the osmolality of human plasma. When used for lower extremity venography, this agent causes patient discomfort at the injection site. This contrast material is also thought to induce endothelial cell damage, which may result in venous thrombosis. The reported incidence of post-venography phlebitis caused by use of HOCM ranges from 9% to 31%.[8] This incidence has been decreased by (1) dilution of the contrast with saline solution (thereby reducing the agents osmolality) or (2) use of modern *low-osmolar contrast material* (LOCM).

Low-osmolar agents have an osmolality of about one-third that of HOCM but are still hypertonic, with a concentration of about double that of plasma. A prospective study using LOCM for ascending leg venography reported no postvenography DVT in 102 consecutive patients who underwent follow-up duplex ultrasonography.[1] In this same study, minor adverse reactions such as nausea, local pain, or dizziness occurred in 11 (7%) of 157 patients examined.

Allergic reactions to contrast material administration are uncommon but are potentially severe and can lead to cardiopulmonary collapse and death. Reactions to contrast material are categorized as mild, moderate, or severe. Most reactions require no treatment; non–life-threatening reactions (e.g., urticaria, mild laryngeal edema, bronchospasm) can be easily treated.

Severe contrast reactions are true medical emergencies. They are defined as anaphylaxis, hypotension, or hypertension requiring intervention, angina, cardiac arrhythmia, pulmonary edema, or laryngeal edema/spasm or bronchospasm sufficient to cause airway obstruction. These reactions are related, in part, to the contrast material used and are known to be less severe with the use of LOCM. A meta-analysis of the risks of severe reactions, including death, comparing high- versus low-osmolar agents found a rate of severe reaction of 157 per 100,000 patients with HOCM

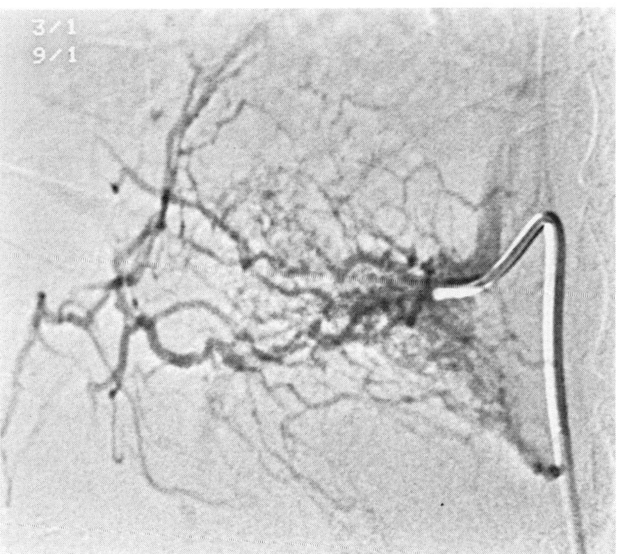

FIGURE 17–16. Budd-Chiari syndrome. Right hepatic venogram shows occlusion of the central hepatic venous channel with multiple intrahepatic collaterals.

and a rate of 31 per 100,000 patients with LOCM.[12] The use of low-osmolar contrast thus reduces the risk of a severe reaction by approximately 80%. The rate of death remains identical with either agent at about 0.9 per 100,000 patients.

In our practice, patients with known contrast allergies undergo a pretreatment regimen of 50 mg of prednisone by mouth 13, 7, and 1 hour before the study. 50 mg of diphenhydramine hydrochloride (Benadryl) and 25 mg of ephedrine are also given 1 hour before the exam. LOCM agents are always used in these patients. Patients who experience a severe contrast reaction are given appropriate intravenous doses of hydrocortisone sodium succinate (Solu-Cortef), epinephrine, and antihistamines and are admitted to hospital for observation and supportive therapy.

Iodine-based contrast material is known to be nephrotoxic, also apparently because of its hypertonicity. Patients with preexisting renal insufficiency, diabetes, or dehydration are at most risk for contrast-induced renal failure. Although the matter is controversial, the data suggest that LOCM is less nephrotoxic than HOCM, as demonstrated by decreased changes in serum creatinine or glomerular filtration rate after administration of LOCM.[4, 24, 29] Patients with preexisting renal insufficiency of any cause appear to be at higher risk for nephrotoxicity with HOCM than with LOCM.[29] This may justify the use of low-osmolar agents in this patient population.

It is the relatively high cost of LOCM compared with HOCM that prevents these newer agents from being used exclusively in everyday practice. Many insurance carriers do not reimburse for the use of LOCM; in fact, the medical literature partially supports this stance on a cost-benefit analysis basis. One study showed that a total substitution of LOCM for HOCM would not decrease mortality rates at all and that each severe reaction would be prevented at a cost of $62,000 per event.[11] Thus, most radiologists have concluded that LOCM use should be restricted to patients at high risk for an untoward event from contrast administration. In our practice, this category includes the following situations:

- A documented allergy to contrast material
- A history of iodine intolerance
- Advanced cardiac, pulmonary, or renal disease
- Asthma requiring steroid use

In addition, pediatric patients and older patients would be excluded.

It is hoped that with technologic improvements, manufacturers' costs will diminish and that these savings will be passed on to hospital and physician consumers in the form of less expensive contrast agents. Until it makes economic sense to totally switch to LOCM, each practitioner must determine which patients should receive these admittedly superior contrast agents.

REFERENCES

1. Abu Rahma AF, Powell M, Robinson PA: Prospective study of safety of lower extremity phlebography with nonionic contrast medium. Am J Surg 171:255–257, 1996.
2. Andrews JC, Williams DM, Cho KJ: Digital subtraction venography of the upper extremities. Clin Radiol 38:423–424, 1987.
3. Baldt MM, Bohler K, Zontsich T, et al: Preoperative imaging of lower extremity varicose veins: Color coded duplex sonography or venography? J Ultrasound Med 15:143–154, 1996.
4. Barrett BJ, Carlisle EJ: Meta-analysis of the relative nephrotoxicity of high- and low-osmolality iodinated contrast media. Radiology 188:171–178, 1993.
5. Bauer G: A venographic study of thromboembolic problems. Acta Chir Scand Suppl 61, 1940.
6. Baxter GM, Duffy P, Partridge E: Colour flow imaging of calf vein thrombosis. Clin Radiol 46:198–201, 1992.
7. Berberich J, Hirsch S: Die rontgenographische Darstellung der Arterien und Venen am lebenden Menschen. Klin Wschr 2:2226, 1923.
8. Bettman MA, Salzman EW, Rosenthal D, et al: Reduction of venous thrombosis complicating phlebography. AJR 134:1169–1172, 1980.
9. Bradley MJ, Spencer PA, Alexander L, et al: Colour flow mapping in the diagnosis of calf deep vein thrombosis. Clin Radiol 47:399–402, 1993.
10. Burn PR, Blunt DM, Sanson HE, et al: The radiological investigation of suspected lower limb deep vein thrombosis. Clin Radiol 52:626–628, 1997.
11. Caro JJ, Trindade E, McGregor M: The cost-effectiveness of replacing high-osmolality with low-osmolality contrast media. AJR Am J Roentgenol 159:869–874, 1992.
12. Caro JJ, Trindade E, McGregor M: The risks of death and severe nonfatal reactions with high- vs low-osmolality contrast media: A meta-analysis. AJR Am J Roentgenol 156:825–832, 1991.
13. Cavaluzzi JA, Sheff R, Harrington DP, et al: Hepatic venography and wedge pressure measurements in diffuse liver disease. AJR 129:441–446, 1977.
14. Comerota AJ, Katz ML, Hashemi HA: Venous duplex imaging for the diagnosis of acute deep venous thrombosis. Haemostasis 23 (Suppl) 1:61–71, 1993.
15. Coon WW, Willis PW: Thrombosis of axillary and subclavian veins. Arch Surg 94:657–663, 1967.
16. DeWeese JA, Rogoff SM: Phlebographic patterns of acute deep venous thrombosis of the leg. Surgery 53:99–108, 1963.
17. dos Santos JC: La phlebographie directe. J Int Chir 3:625, 1938.
18. Greitz T: The technique of ascending phlebography of the lower extremity. Acta Radiol 42:421–441, 1954.
19. Hager K: Problems of acute deep venous thrombosis: I. The interpretation of signs and symptoms. Angiology 20:219–223, 1969.
20. Hartnell GG, Hughes LA, Finn JP, et al: Magnetic resonance angiography of the central chest veins: A new gold standard? Chest 107:1053–1057, 1995.
21. Hicks ME, Malden ES, Vesely TM, et al: Prospective anatomic study of the inferior vena cava and renal veins: Comparison of selective renal venography with cavography and relevance in filter placement. J Vasc Interv Radiol 6:721–729, 1995.
22. Kalebo P, Anthmyr B-A, Eriksson BI, et al: Optimization of ascending phlebography of the leg for screening of deep vein thrombosis in thromboprophylactic trials. Acta Radiol 38:320–326, 1997.
23. Kamida CB, Kistner RL, Eklof B, Masuda EM: Lower extremity phlebography. *In* Gloviczki P, Yao JS (eds): Handbook of Venous Disorders. London, Chapman and Hall, 1996, pp 152–167.
24. Katholi RE, Taylor GJ, Woods WT, et al: Nephrotoxicity of nonionic low-osmolality versus ionic high-osmolality contrast media: A prospective double blind randomized comparison in human beings. Radiology 186:183–187, 1993.
25. Kistner RL, Ferris EB, Rawdhawa G, et al: A method of performing descending venography. J Vasc Surg 4:464–468, 1986.
26. Kistner RL, Kamida CB: 1994 Update on phlebography and varicography. Dermatol Surg 21:71–76, 1995.
27. Lea Thomas M: Techniques of phlebography: A review. Eur J Radiol 11:125–130, 1990.
28. Lea Thomas M, Andress MR: Axillary phlebography. AJR 113:713–721, 1971.
29. Moore RD, Steinberg EP, Powe NR, et al: Nephrotoxicity of high-osmolality versus low-osmolality contrast media: Randomized clinical trial. Radiology 182:649–655, 1992.
30. Morano JU, Raju S: Chronic venous insufficiency: Assessment with descending venography. Radiology 174:441–444, 1990.
31. Natu JC, Sequeira JC, Weitzman AF: An improved technique for axillary phlebography. Radiology 142:529–530, 1982.
32. Nicolaides AN: Diagnosis of venous thrombosis by phlebography. *In* Bergan JJ, Yao JS (eds): Venous Problems. Chicago, Year Book Medical Publishers, 1978, pp 123–140.

33. Phibbs B, Marriot HJL: Complications of permanent transvenous pacing. N Engl J Med 3112:1428–1432, 1985.
34. Prandoni P, Polistena P, Bernardi E, et al: Upper-extremity deep vein thrombosis: Risk factors, diagnosis and complications. Arch Intern Med 157:57–62, 1997.
35. Rubinov K, Paulin S: Roentgen diagnosis of venous thrombosis of the leg. Arch Surg 104:134–144, 1972.
36. Rutherford RB, Hurlbert SN: Primary subclavian-axillary vein thrombosis: Consensus and commentary. Cardiovasc Surg 4:420–423, 1996.
37. Vesely T: Interventional radiologist at work: Question and answer. J Vasc Interv Radiol 2:225–226, 1997.
38. Warden GD, Wilmore DW, Pruitt BA: Central venous thrombosis: A hazard of medical progress. Trauma 13:620, 1973.
39. Welch CE, Faxon HH, McGahey CE: The application of phlebography to the therapy of thrombosis and embolism. Surgery 12:162, 1942.
40. Wheeler HB, Hirsch J, Wells, et al: Diagnostic tests for deep vein thrombosis: Clinical usefulness depends on probability of disease. Arch Intern Med 154:1921–1928, 1994.

SECTION IV

ARTERIAL DISEASES

ROBERT B. RUTHERFORD, M.D.

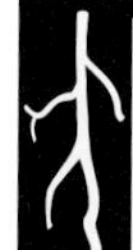

CHAPTER 18

Artery Wall Pathology in Atherosclerosis

Christopher K. Zarins, M.D., and
Seymour Glagov, M.D.

Atherosclerosis is the principal pathologic process affecting the large arteries. Atherosclerosis is a degenerative disease characterized by the accumulation of cells, matrix fibers, lipids, and tissue debris in the intima, which may result in narrowing of the lumen and obstruction of blood flow or ulceration, embolization, and thrombosis. Intimal plaque deposition may be accompanied by arterial enlargement and thinning of the underlying artery wall. Such enlargement may compensate for the enlarging intimal plaque and prevent lumen stenosis. It may also, under certain circumstances, lead to aneurysm formation with eventual artery wall rupture. Dissection, arteritis, and other degenerative conditions may also result in similar clinical complications, but these are rare compared with atherosclerosis and are dealt with elsewhere.

This chapter discusses the problem of atherosclerosis as it relates to the functional biomechanical properties of the artery wall. Both normal and pathologic responses of the artery wall are considered, as are differences in the evolution of atherosclerotic lesions. Local differences that may account for the propensity of certain areas to form extensive and complex plaques or aneurysms are also discussed.

STRUCTURE AND FUNCTION OF THE ARTERY WALL

Arteries are not simply a passive system of tubes of uniform and fixed composition that distribute blood to organs. Investigation has revealed that the major arteries are intricate biomechanical structures well suited to carry out their metabolic and mechanical functions under a wide range of conditions.[1] Arteries respond to acute hemodynamic alterations by changing caliber, by either constriction or dilatation.[2] Several mechanisms operate to limit hemorrhage in the event of disruptive injury and to restore wall integrity without long-term sequelae.[3] Arteries also adapt to gradual changes in local hemodynamic stresses and to systemic environmental conditions in order to maintain optimal diameter and mechanical characteristics and to ensure continued adequate blood flow.[4] The following brief review of the functional microanatomy of the artery wall indicates the range and limits of artery wall adaptability.

Intima

The intima, the innermost layer of the artery wall, extends from the luminal surface to the internal elastic lamina. The luminal surface is lined by the endothelium, a continuous monolayer of flat, polygonal cells. Between the endothelium and the internal elastic lamina, the intima is normally very narrow, with the endothelium lying directly on the internal elastic lamina and containing only a few scattered leukocytes, smooth muscle cells, and connective tissue fibers. It is in this region that atherosclerotic lesions develop.

Endothelium

The endothelium rests on a basal lamina that provides a continuous, pliable, and compliant substrate. Changes in cell shape and in the extent of junctional overlap among adjacent endothelial cells occur in relation to (1) changes in artery diameter associated with pulsatile wall motion, (2) changes in configuration associated with bending or stretching, and (3) the intimal accumulation of cells and matrix fibers during the development of intimal atherosclerotic plaques.[5] These changes act to prevent the development of discontinuities in the endothelial lining.

The endothelium also has numerous focal attachments to the underlying internal elastic lamina.[6] These relatively tight and rigid junctions contribute to stability by preventing slippage, telescoping, or detachment of endothelial cells and disruption or denudation by elevations in shear stress or by other mechanical forces. The endothelium presents a thromboresistant surface as well as a selective interface for diffusion, convection, and active transport of circulating substances into the underlying artery wall.[7]

Endothelial cells play a critical role in the physiology and pathophysiology of vascular disorders.[8] They respond to hemodynamic stresses and may transduce an atheroprotective force[9] by regulating the ingress, egress, and metabolism of lipoproteins and other agents that may participate in the initiation and progression of intimal plaques.[3, 5]

Endothelial Injury

The endothelial surface can be injured or disrupted by various means but regenerates rapidly after focal denudation. The healing response, if extensive, may be accompanied by smooth muscle cell proliferation and migration and intimal thickening.[10, 11] A series of reactions set into motion by focal endothelial denudation has been proposed as the initiating event in the pathogenesis of atherosclerosis.

According to this hypothesis, endothelial injury and desquamation may be caused by (1) mechanical forces, such as elevated wall shear stress and hypertension; (2) metabolic intermediates, such as those that characterize hyperlipidemia; (3) immunologic reactions; and (4) increased exposure to vasoactive agents. Such endothelial desquamation would expose subendothelial tissues to the circulation and stimulate platelet deposition, the release of a platelet-derived growth factor, cellular proliferation, and eventual lipid deposition and plaque formation.[12] Focal, repeated disruptive endothelial injuries and responses to those injuries would account for the localized nature of plaque deposition.

There is little evidence, however, to support the belief that endothelial injury or disruption in the form of desquamation, with or without platelet adhesion, occurs in regions of the vascular tree at highest risk for future lesion development.[13] In addition, there is no direct evidence that experimentally induced endothelial damage or removal results in eventual sustained lesion formation,[14] even in the presence of hyperlipidemia. On the contrary, evidence has been advanced that the formation of experimental intimal plaques may require the presence of an endothelial covering.[15, 16] Although platelets may play a role in the transition of early plaques to more complex and advanced forms,[17] their effect on plaque initiation remains questionable. Platelet-derived growth factor has been isolated from other cellular elements that participate in plaque formation,[18] and smooth muscle cell proliferation may be an aspect of an overall healing reaction of arteries rather than the underlying primary event in atherosclerosis. Later studies have attempted to define injury in terms of functional alterations that may predispose to the formation of atherosclerotic lesions.[19, 20]

Under normal circumstances, the vascular endothelium functions as an antithrombotic surface and contributes to the regulation of vascular tone and artery lumen diameter through the secretion of vasoconstrictors (e.g., angiotensin II) and vasodilators and inhibitors of platelet aggregation (e.g., prostacyclin and endothelium-derived relaxing factor).[21, 22] Such factors maintain the smooth muscle cells of the media in a contractile, nonproliferative phenotype with low cholesterol ester content. In response to endothelial cell activation or injury, endothelial cells become increasingly permeable to low-density lipoprotein, have higher replicative rates, develop prothrombotic properties, and express surface glycoproteins that promote the adhesion and ingress of neutrophils, monocytes, and platelets.[23] Endothelial cells and monocytes release cytokines, growth factors, and leukotrienes inducing prostacyclin production, which further promotes monocyte adhesion and diapedesis. The net effect of cytokine and growth factor production is the stimulation of smooth muscle cell proliferation and migration. As a result of these changes, extracellular lipid as well as foam cells containing cholesterol esters accumulate in the intima.

These observations suggest that humoral mediators, growth factors, and cytokines from altered endothelial cells and from inflammatory cells interacting with other arterial cells are important mediators of macrophage infiltration, smooth muscle cell proliferation, and lipid deposition. Although physical and mechanical endothelial disruption and denudation may not be reactions that initiate or precipitate events in atherosclerotic plaque formation, biologic reactions of the endothelium and artery wall during injury and repair may play important roles in the proliferative and lipid deposition stage of plaque formation.

Media

The media extends from the internal elastic lamina to the adventitia. Although an external elastic lamina demarcates the boundary between the media and adventitia in many vessels, a distinct external elastic lamina may not be present, particularly in vessels with a thick and fibrous adventitial layer. The outer limit of the media can nevertheless be distinguished in nearly all intact arteries because, in contrast to the adventitia, the media consists of closely packed layers of smooth muscle cells in close association with elastin and collagen fibers.

The *smooth muscle cell* layers are composed of groups of similarly oriented cells, each surrounded by a common basal lamina and a closely associated interlacing basketwork of type III collagen fibrils arranged so as to tighten about the cell groups as the media is brought under tension; this configuration tends to hold the groups of cells together and prevent excessive stretching or slippage. In addition, each cellular subgroup or fascicle is encompassed by a system of similarly oriented *elastic fibers* such that the effective unit of structure is a musculoelastic fascicle. In relation to the curvature of the artery wall, each fascicle is oriented in the direction of the imposed tensile stress. Focal tight attachment sites between smooth muscle cells and elastic fibers are normally abundant.[24]

The aorta and its immediately proximal, larger branches are called *elastic arteries* because of the prominence of their elastic fibers. In such vessels, the elastin fiber systems of the musculoelastic fascicles are thick and closely packed, resulting in an appearance on transverse cross section of elastin lamellae alternating with smooth muscle layers. Thicker, crimped, type I collagen bundles are woven between adjacent large elastic lamellae.[25] The elastin fibers are relatively extensible and allow for compliance and recoil of the artery wall in relation to pulse propagation during the cardiac cycle. The extensive interconnected transmural arrangement of the elastic fibers of the musculoelastic fascicles tends to ensure uniform distribution of tensile mural stresses and prevent the propagation of flaws that develop in the media with age. The thick, crimped collagen fiber bundles provide much of the tensile strength of the media and, because of their high elastic modulus, limit distention and prevent disruption even at very high blood pressures (Fig. 18–1).[26]

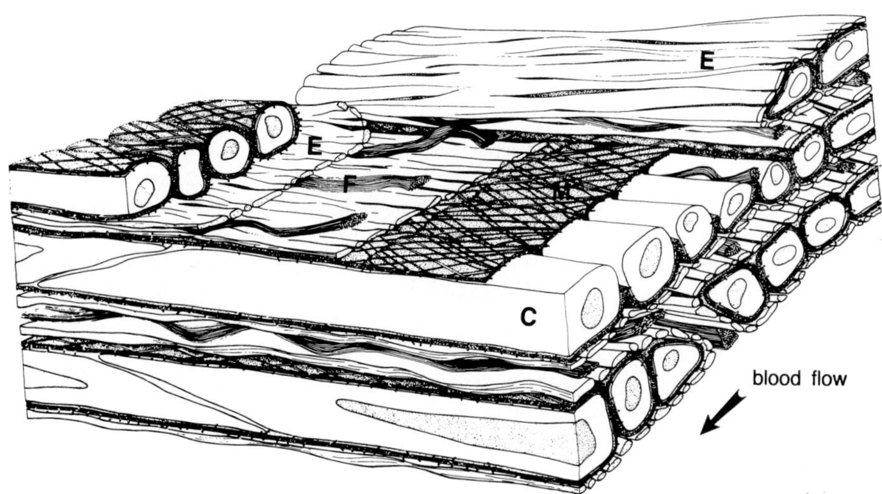

FIGURE 18–1. Transmural organization of the media of large elastic arteries such as the aorta. Groups of smooth muscle cells (C), oriented with their long axes perpendicular to the longitudinal axis of the artery (axis of blood flow), are surrounded by a network of fine type III collagen fibrils within a matrix of basal lamina (M). They are surrounded by a closely associated system of elastic fibers (E) oriented in the same direction as the smooth muscle cells. Wavy bundles or fibers (F) of type I collagen are woven between the adjacent large elastic lamellae and provide much of the tensile strength of the media. Elastin fibers allow for compliance and recoil of the artery during the cardiac cycle. (From Clark JM, Glagov S: Transmural organization of the arterial wall: The lamellar unit revisited. Arteriosclerosis 5:19, 1985.)

The smaller-caliber *muscular arteries* contain relatively less collagen and elastin and more smooth muscle cells than elastic arteries and can therefore alter their diameter rapidly by constricting or dilating. The musculoelastic fascicles, which are most clearly evident in elastic arteries, are also the structural unit of muscular arteries and, as in elastic arteries, are generally aligned in the direction of the tensile forces. However, because of the preponderance of smooth muscle cells relative to elastin and collagen fibers, they are less prominent and the layering of the media is therefore less distinct (Fig. 18–2).[26]

Medial thickness and the number of musculoelastic layers, or *lamellar units,* are closely related to the lumen radius and to mural tangential tension. Tangential tension on the artery wall is, in general, proportional to the product of pressure and radius (Laplace's law), whereas the actual tensile stress per unit of cross-sectional area is inversely proportional to the wall thickness. The average tension per lamellar unit tends to be constant for homologous vessels in mammals. With increasing species size, mammalian adult aortic radius enlarges, with corresponding increases in medial thickness and in the number of musculoelastic layers, or lamellar units.[27] Because (1) aortic pressure is similar for most adult mammals and (2) individual medial layers tend to be of similar thickness regardless of species, there is a very nearly linear relationship between adult aortic radius and the number of medial fibrocellular lamellar units. On the average, the tangential tension per aortic lamellar unit is close to 2000 dynes/cm. For the pulmonary trunk, wall tension is about 1000 dynes/cm.

For muscular arteries, such as the coronary and renal vessels, total tangential tension and the number of transmural layers are also linearly related.[27] In addition, the relative proportions of collagen and elastin differ between muscular and elastic arteries. The media of the proximal aorta and that of the major brachiocephalic elastic arteries contain a

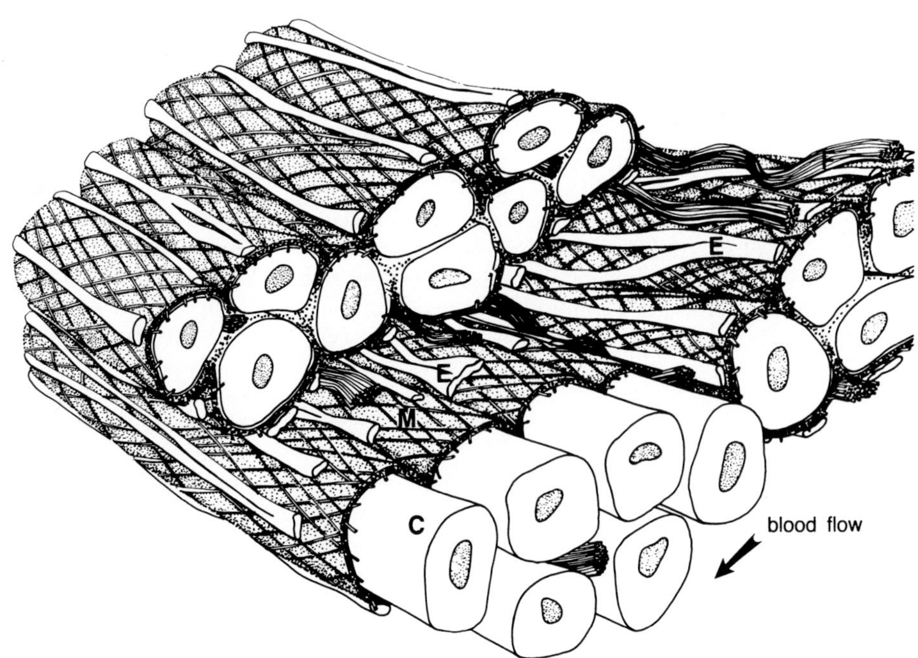

FIGURE 18–2. Transmural organization of a muscular artery. Smooth muscle cells (C) are more numerous and prominent and are organized in groups oriented with their long axes perpendicular to the long axis of the artery. Contraction or relaxation of smooth muscle cells allows for rapid alterations in lumen diameter. Smooth muscle cells are surrounded by a basal lamina matrix containing a meshwork of type III collagen fibrils (M). Elastin fibers (E) and type I collagen fibers (F) are present but are less prominent than in elastic arteries. (From Clark JM, Glagov S: Transmural organization of the arterial wall: The lamellar unit revisited. Arteriosclerosis 5:19, 1985.)

larger proportion of elastin and a lower proportion of collagen than the media of the abdominal aorta or of the distal peripheral vessels.[28] The proximal major vessels are therefore more compliant than the abdominal aorta but are also more fragile and prone to tear when sutured.

Medial smooth muscle cells, in addition to synthesizing the collagen and elastin fibers that determine the mechanical properties of the aortic wall, are actively engaged in metabolic processes that contribute to wall tone and may be related to susceptibility to plaque formation.[29] Under conditions of increased pulse pressure, wall motion, and wall tension, such as exist proximal to an aortic coarctation, medial smooth muscle cell metabolism is higher, as is plaque formation.[30] Conversely, when wall motion, pulse pressure, and smooth muscle cell metabolism are decreased, as in areas distal to a severe arterial stenosis, intimal plaque formation is inhibited, despite the continued presence of strong atherogenic stimuli such as marked hyperlipidemia.[31] In vitro studies have revealed that cyclic stretching of smooth muscle cells grown on elastin membranes results in greater biosynthetic activity,[32] and acute arterial injury experiments have revealed that an intact, metabolically active media may be required for intimal plaque formation.[33] The composition and microarchitecture of the media are designed to ensure stability, whereas the metabolic state of the media appears to be an important factor in the pathogenesis of atherosclerotic lesions.

Adventitia

The adventitia is composed of fibrocellular connective tissue and contains a network of vasa vasorum composed of small arteries, arterioles, capillaries, and venous channels as well as nerves that mediate smooth muscle tone and contraction. The adventitia varies in thickness and organization. In some arteries, such as the proximal renal and mesenteric trunks, the adventitia is a layered structure composed of both collagen and elastic fibers and may be thicker than the associated media. In the normal aorta, removal of the adventitia has little effect on static pressure-volume relationships.[34] In atherosclerotic arteries, however, increasing intimal plaque thickness may be associated with atrophy of the underlying media.[35] Under these circumstances, a thickened adventitia may contribute to tensile support. The tensile strength and adequacy of the adventitia to provide such support are well demonstrated following carotid or aortoiliac endarterectomy. In these procedures, the entire intima and most or all of the media are usually removed, leaving only the adventitia to provide support, and aneurysmal degeneration after endarterectomy is very rare.

Vasa Vasorum

The inner layers of the aortic media are nourished by diffusion from the lumen. Diffusion of nutrients is apparently sufficient to nourish the inner 0.5 mm of the adult mammalian aortic media, which corresponds to approximately 30 medial fibrocellular lamellar units.[36] When the aorta is thicker than 30 medial lamellar layers, the outer layers of the media are nourished by vasa vasorum that penetrate into the media. Vasa vasorum usually arise from the parent artery at branch junctions and arborize in the adventitia. In thick-walled arteries, mural stresses and deformations may affect vasa vasorum blood flow, and hypertension may impair vasal flow.[37]

Intimal plaque formation increases intimal thickness and may thereby enlarge the diffusion barrier between the lumen and the smooth muscle cells of the media. This increase in wall thickness may be accompanied by an ingrowth of vasa vasorum, and vasa vasorum have been identified in atherosclerotic lesions. Both intraplaque hemorrhage and plaque breakdown or disruption may be potentiated by changes in the vascular supply of the artery wall and plaque.

ADAPTIVE RESPONSES OF THE ARTERY WALL

Adaptive responses of arteries and the healing response to arterial injuries serve to maintain the structural and functional integrity of the arterial tree. Normal responses to altered biomechanical and hemodynamic conditions result in compensatory changes in artery wall thickness, lumen diameter, or both, whereas abnormal or pathologic conditions may engender alterations in wall thickness and lumen diameter that proceed to lumen stenosis, aneurysm formation, or obstructive intimal hyperplasia.[1, 38, 39]

Wall Thickness

Artery wall thickness and composition are closely related to *tangential tension* and strain in the wall. During normal growth and development, arteries adapt to rises in tangential tension by increasing the number of medial lamellar units and by the accumulation of matrix fibers to increase wall thickness.[40]

For example, at birth, the ascending aorta and pulmonary trunk are equal in diameter, in wall thickness, and in the concentration of elastin and collagen. In the immediate postnatal period, however, with expansion of the lungs, pressure in the pulmonary artery falls and pressure in the aorta rises. Volume flow and diameter remain equivalent in the two vessels, but a marked difference in blood pressure develops, resulting in profound alterations in medial growth and development. The high-pressure aortic media becomes thicker with an greater number of medial lamellae.

The differences can be attributed to different rates of collagen and elastin accumulation, which correspond closely to the differences in total tangential tension for the two vessels.[41] At any given interval during early postnatal growth, however, the number of cells is the same for the two vessel segments. Thus, smooth muscle cells of the media are apparently capable of a remarkable range of biosynthetic activity in response to imposed tensile stress.

In adult life, arterial wall thickening also occurs in response to increases in tangential tension, but this thickening occurs not through increases in the number of medial lamellar units but by means of intimal thickening and changes in matrix volume and composition. In patients with hypertension, arterial and arteriolar intimal thickening develops as an adaptive response to the increase in wall tension, and the relative proportion of matrix fiber changes in favor of collagen.[42] Similarly, the performance of a distal arterial bypass increases wall tension by raising pressure as well as by producing a large rise in lumen radius at the anastomotic site. The resulting increase in tangential wall tension can stimulate intimal thickening as an adaptive response to the rise in tension.

Quantitative morphologic studies of human carotid bifurcations have demonstrated greater intimal thickness in association with lumen enlargement with resultant preservation of normal tangential mural tension.[43, 44] The factors that differentiate a normal adaptive intimal thickening from an inappropriate intimal hyperplastic response resulting in lumen stenosis at a vascular anastomosis are not well understood. Techniques to precisely measure stresses in the artery wall are now available and will help define the role of mechanical forces in artery wall response.[45, 46]

Lumen Diameter

Under normal conditions, adaptive alterations in lumen diameter are determined by *blood flow* in the artery. During embryologic development, arteries with high-volume flow enlarge, and those with low flow become smaller.[47] When parallel flow channels exist, the one with higher flow enlarges and persists, whereas the one with lesser flow atrophies and disappears. During extrauterine growth, increases in artery lumen diameter also keep pace with changes in flow.[48] Arteries exposed to abnormal increases in flow, such as those feeding an arteriovenous fistula, may also increase in size, whereas arteries exposed to abnormal decreases in flow, such as vessels supplying an amputated limb, adapt with a decrease in size.[49]

The mechanism for adjustment of lumen diameter appears to be mediated by wall *shear stress,* which is the effective velocity gradient at the endothelium-blood interface.[4] Because shear stress is inversely related to the cube of the radius, small alterations in radius have a major effect on wall shear stress. In mammals, wall shear stress normally ranges between 10 and 20 dynes/cm^2 at all levels of the arterial tree.[50] In experimentally produced arteriovenous fistulae, the afferent artery has been shown to enlarge just enough to restore shear stress to baseline levels.[51] Wall shear stress thus appears to act as a regulating signal to determine artery size, and this response depends on the presence of an intact endothelial surface.[52–55] The response is mediated by the release of endothelium-derived relaxing factor or nitric oxide (NO).[56, 57] Thus, the endothelium functions as a mechanically sensitive signal transduction interface between the blood and the artery wall.[58, 59] NO plays an important role in both the acute and chronic increases in vessel caliber that occur in response to greater flow.[60, 61] Inhibition of NO synthesis by means of long-term oral administration of L-NAME can inhibit flow-induced arterial enlargement.[62, 63]

Atherosclerotic arteries are also capable of enlarging in response to increases in blood flow and wall shear stress, but this process may be limited.[64] Atherosclerotic artery enlargement is further discussed later in this chapter. The nature and mechanisms of the artery wall adaptive processes that allow arteries to adjust lumen diameter are currently being actively investigated. Understanding the mechanism and limits of the adaptive process and identifying the consequences for the vessel wall of shear stress that is persistently higher or lower than normal will be of value in clinical efforts to maintain normal lumen caliber.

FUNCTIONAL PATHOLOGY OF ATHEROSCLEROSIS

The features that distinguish normal arterial adaptation in response to changing hemodynamic and mechanical conditions from pathologic processes affecting the artery wall are not well defined. Intimal thickening and changes in wall thickness and lumen diameter occur as functions of both age and atherosclerosis. A prominent feature distinguishing atherosclerotic plaques is the presence of lipid in intimal lesions. However, it is unclear whether all lesions containing lipids are necessarily precursors of clinically significant atherosclerotic plaques.

Intimal Thickening

Intimal thickening may represent an adaptive response acting to reduce lumen caliber in reaction to conditions of chronically reduced blood flow, or it may be a response designed to augment wall thickness under conditions of chronically increased wall tensile stress.[65, 66] Focal intimal thickenings have been observed at or near branch points in the arteries of infants and fetuses and probably represent local remodeling of vessel wall organization related to growth and the associated redistribution of tensile stress.[67] Diffuse fibrocellular intimal thickening can occur as a more generalized phenomenon without a clear relationship to branches or curves and may result in a diffusely thickened intima that is considerably thicker than the media. Lipid accumulation is not a prominent feature in such intimal thickening, and the lumen remains regular and normal or slightly larger than normal in diameter.[68]

Although there is little direct evidence that diffuse intimal thickening is a precursor of lipid-containing atherosclerotic plaques, both intimal thickening and plaques tend to occur in similar locations, and intimal thickening is most evident in vessels that are especially susceptible to atherosclerosis.[69, 70] Evidence has also been presented that diffuse forms of intimal thickening do not develop uniformly and that foci of relatively rapid thickening undergo dystrophic changes, which give rise to necrosis and other features characteristic of plaques.[71] The relationship of these findings to usual atherosclerosis remains to be defined.

Fatty Streaks

Fatty streaks are flat yellow focal patches or linear streaks seen on the lumen surface of arteries. They correspond to the accumulation of lipid-laden foam cells in the intima. Fatty streaks are evident in most individuals older than age 3 years. They are found with increasing frequency between the ages of 8 and 18 years, after which many apparently resolve despite the frequent presence of matrix materials among the characteristic cells. Fatty streaks may be seen in the arteries of persons of any age and may be noted adjacent to or even superimposed on advanced atherosclerotic plaques. Fatty streaks and atheromata, however, do not have identical patterns of localization, and fatty streaks usually do not compromise the lumen or ulcerate.[72]

In experimental animals, diet-induced lesions resembling fatty streaks occur early, before characteristic atherosclerotic lesions prevail. These lesions are characterized by foam cells under a preserved and intact endothelial surface with no evidence of disruption.[73] Some evidence has been presented that endothelial cells covering experimental fatty streak–type lesions are attenuated and fragile and may predispose to endothelial disruption, platelet adhesion, and possible transformation into a fibrous plaque.[74] Attachment of endothelial projections to underlying basal lamina and elastin, however, remains prominent in early fatty streak lesions. Although morphologic studies have identified transitional features, a firm line of evidence linking fatty streaks to fibrous plaque formation has not yet been established.

Fibrous Plaques

Fibrous plaque is the term used to identify the characteristic and unequivocal atherosclerotic lesion. Such intimal deposits appear in the second decade of life but usually do not become predominant or clinically significant until the fourth decade. Fibrous plaques are usually eccentric, and most are covered by an intact endothelial surface.

Although there is considerable variation in the composition and configuration of plaques, a characteristic architecture prevails for manifest advanced plaques. The immediate subendothelial region usually consists of a compact and well-organized stratified layer of smooth muscle cells and connective tissue fibers known as the *fibrous cap* (Fig. 18–3). This structure may be quite thick and may have architectural features resembling those of the media, including the formation of a subendothelial elastic lamina. The fibrous cap may provide structural support or may function as a barrier to sequester thrombogenic debris in the underlying necrotic core of the plaque from the lumen. Its lumen surface is regular and maintains a concave contour corresponding to the circular or oval cross-sectional lumen contour of the uninvolved vessel wall segment.

The *necrotic core* usually occupies the deeper central regions of the plaque and contains amorphous as well as crystalline and droplet forms of lipid. Cells with morphologic and functional characteristics of smooth muscle cells or macrophages are noted about the necrotic core and at the edges or shoulders of the plaques.[75] Both cell types may contain lipid vacuoles. In addition, calcium salts and myxoid deposits, as well as matrix fibers, including collagen, elastin, fine fibrillar material, structures resembling basal lamina, and amorphous ground substance, are evident.

Atherosclerotic plaques show evidence of uneven or episodic growth, including dense fibrocellular regions adjacent to organizing thrombus and foci of atheromatous debris. Intermittent ulceration and healing may occur, and there is evidence that thrombi formed on lesions are incorporated into them and resurfaced with a fibrocellular cap and an intact endothelial layer.

Vasa vasorum penetrate from the adventitia or possibly from the lumen to supply the plaque and fibrous cap

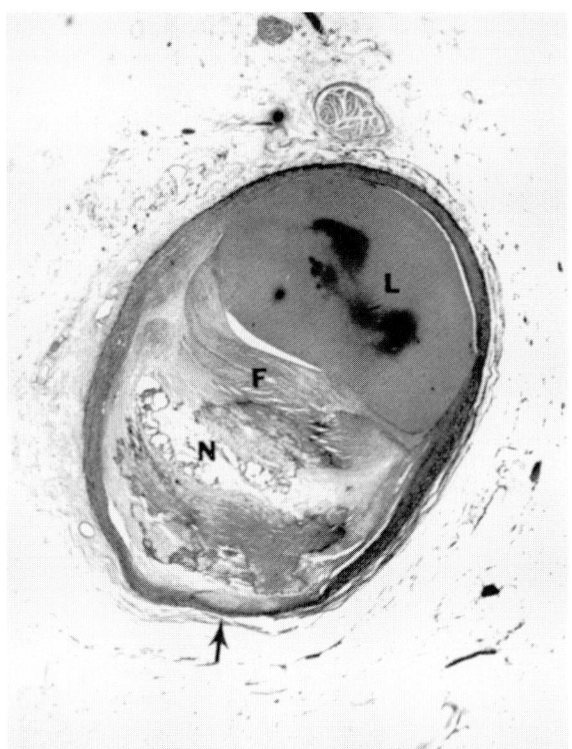

FIGURE 18–3. Cross section of a human artery with an advanced atherosclerotic plaque. The fibrous cap (F) is a well-organized layer of smooth muscle cells and fibrous tissue that separates the necrotic core (N) of the plaque from the lumen (L). The media beneath the plaque may become thin and atrophic *(arrow)*. The lumen contains a gelatin cast used to redistend and maintain lumen contour.

and serve to organize thrombotic deposits.[76] The *media* underlying an atherosclerotic plaque may become thin and attenuated, with bulging of the plaque toward the adventitia (see Fig. 18–3), but the tissue between the necrotic core and the media is usually densely fibrotic. Support of the artery wall may also be taken up by the fibrous cap or a thickened adventitial layer.

Some *advanced lesions,* particularly those associated with aneurysms, may appear to be atrophic and relatively acellular, consisting of dense fibrous tissue, prominent calcific deposits, and only minimal evidence of a necrotic center. *Calcification* is a prominent feature of advanced plaques and may be quite extensive, involving both the superficial and deeper reaches of the plaques. Although there is no consistent relationship between plaque size or complexity and the degree of calcification, calcific deposits are most prominent in plaques in older individuals and in areas such as the abdominal aortic segment and coronary arteries, where plaques form earliest.[77]

Advanced lesions are called fibrocalcific, lipid-rich, fibrocellular, necrotic, myxomatous, and so forth, depending on their morphologic features. The presence of large quantities of lipid, necrotic material, and cells tends to make a lesion *soft* and friable, in contrast to the *hard,* rubbery, or brittle consistency of a mainly fibrocalcific lesion.

Plaque Morphology

The common perception that atherosclerotic plaques bulge into the lumen of arteries reflects the fact that most often, plaques are evaluated by angiography, which reveals the lumen contour in a longitudinal or axial projection. A narrowing of the lumen thus is usually perceived as a protrusion of plaque into the lumen (Fig. 18–4). This perception is supported by the gross observations of vascular surgeons and pathologists, who usually examine the luminal surface of atherosclerotic arteries en face or on cross section with the arteries collapsed. Without distending intraluminal pressure, the relatively uninvolved sector of the artery wall recoils, and the eccentric plaque is usually thrown up as a protrusion or bulge. Viewed en face in vessels laid open by longitudinal section, the fibrous or complex plaque is seen as an elevation, with either smooth or irregular surface contours (see Fig. 18–4). The purely descriptive term *raised plaque* has been used to contrast this appearance with that of the fatty streak, which usually does not appear to be elevated in such preparations.

Restoration of in vivo configuration can be achieved by redistending the artery during fixation at controlled levels of intraluminal pressure.[78] Under these circumstances, the cross-sectional lumen contour is usually regular and round or oval, even in the presence of very large and extensive atherosclerotic lesions.[79] The usual eccentric atherosclerotic plaque therefore presents a concave luminal contour on transverse section, does not protrude into the lumen, and instead tends to bulge outward from the lumen. Thus, the external cross-sectional contour of an atherosclerotic artery tends to become oval, whereas the lumen tends to remain circular.

Although plaques may appear as focal or segmental projections into the lumen on longitudinal angiographic or ultrasonic images, cross-sectional views reveal rounded lumen contours. Cross-sectional lumen contours in pressure perfusion–fixed arteries that are irregular or slit-like, with protrusions of the plaque or its contents into the lumen, usually signify that a complication of plaque evolution such as ulceration, hemorrhage, dissection, or thrombosis has occurred. Circumferential, rigid fibrocalcific plaques may retain an in vivo circular lumen configuration, however, even when dilating pressure is absent.

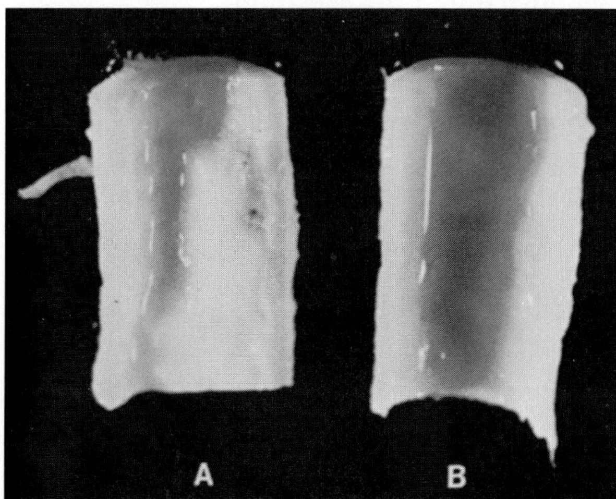

FIGURE 18–4. Effect of vessel collapse on the luminal surface appearance of atherosclerotic plaques. *A,* The artery was fixed while collapsed with no distending intraluminal pressure. Note the apparent bulge of the plaque into the lumen. *B,* The vessel was fixed while distended with an intraluminal pressure of 100 mmHg. Note that there is no visible protrusion of plaque into the lumen and that the lumen contour is rounded. Both segments are from the same human superficial femoral artery, and multiple histologic sections confirm that both segments have the same volume of intimal plaque.

Atherosclerotic Arterial Enlargement

As intimal plaques enlarge, a closely associated enlargement of the affected artery segment tends to limit the stenosing effect of the enlarging intimal plaque (Fig. 18–5). Such enlargement of atherosclerotic arteries has been demonstrated in experimental atherosclerosis,[80–84] as well as in human coronary,[64, 85–88] carotid,[89–91] and superficial femoral[92, 93] arteries and the abdominal aorta.[94, 95] Enlargement may proceed by mechanisms suggested by the demonstrated adaptive response to altered flow or by direct effects of the plaque on the artery wall.[96] Focal intimal plaque deposition would tend to decrease lumen diameter, thereby raising local blood flow velocity and wall shear stress and inducing dilatation of the artery to restore baseline shear stress levels. Atrophy of the media underlying the plaque could also result in outward bulging of the artery in the region of the plaque in order to maintain an adequate lumen caliber. Thus, an increase in intimal plaque volume appears to induce an increase in artery size.

In the human left main coronary artery, such enlargement keeps pace with increases in intimal plaque and is effective in preventing lumen stenosis until plaque area occupies, on the average, approximately 40% of the cross-sectional area encompassed by the internal elastic lamina area (i.e., the potential lumen area if a plaque were not present) (Fig. 18–6). Continued plaque enlargement or complication apparently exceeds the ability of the artery to enlarge, and lumen stenosis may then develop.[64]

Individual segments of the arterial tree, however, may respond differently to increasing intimal plaque.[97] In the distal left anterior descending coronary artery, arterial enlargement occurs more rapidly than intimal plaque deposition. This may result in a net increase in lumen area rather than lumen stenosis in the most severely diseased arteries.[85] Individual variation has also been demonstrated in the superficial femoral artery.[98] Thus, it appears that the development of lumen stenosis, the maintenance of a normal lumen cross-sectional area, or the development of an increase in lumen diameter is determined by the relative rates of plaque growth and artery enlargement.[99] Reduction in artery size can also result in the development of lumen stenosis, and this phenomenon has been demonstrated in vivo with intravascular ultrasound.[100] Further study of this phenomenon of artery enlargement, or reduction in size, particularly in regions associated with great morbidity related to plaque deposition, is needed for a full understanding of the processes involved in the development of atherosclerotic stenoses and aneurysms.

LOCALIZATION OF ATHEROSCLEROTIC PLAQUES

Atherosclerosis is a generalized disorder of the arterial tree, and epidemiologic studies have identified a number of

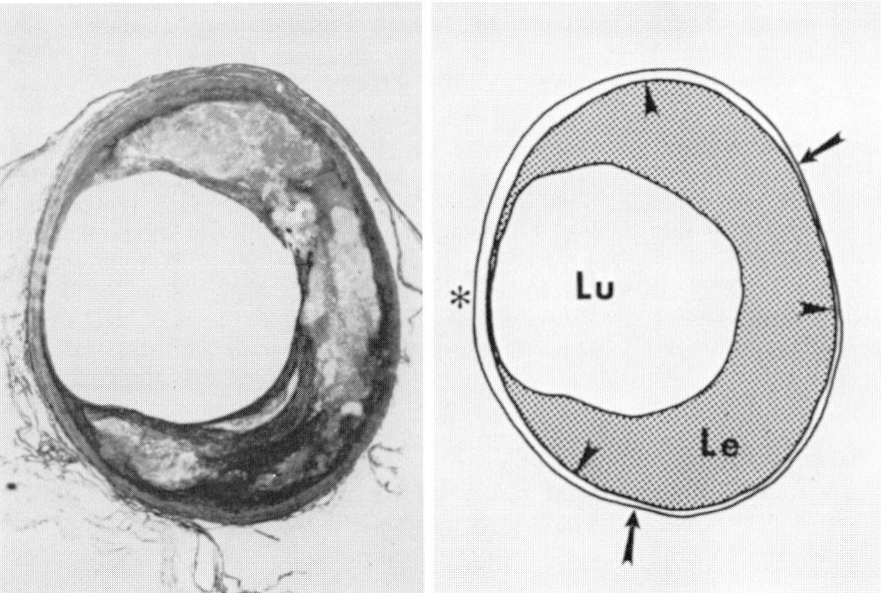

FIGURE 18–5. Cross section of a human left main coronary artery demonstrating atherosclerotic arterial enlargement. Despite an enlarging lesion (Le) area, the lumen (Lu) area is preserved owing to artery enlargement. The lumen contour remains rounded, but the external artery contour becomes oval because of the eccentric nature of the plaque. When intimal plaque area exceeds 40% of internal elastic lumina area *(arrowheads)*, compensatory enlargement apparently fails and stenosis develops. Enlargement may occur by dilatation of the uninvolved artery wall segment *(asterisk)* or atrophy of the media underlying the plaque *(arrows)*. (From Glagov S, Weisenberg E, Zarins CK, et al: Compensatory enlargement of human atherosclerotic coronary arteries. Reprinted by permission of The New England Journal of Medicine, 316:1371, 1987.)

clinical risk factors associated with the development and complication of plaques[101]:

- Cigarette smoking
- Elevated serum lipid levels
- Hypertension
- Obesity
- Diabetes mellitus
- Physical inactivity
- Emotional stress
- Genetic predisposition

Some of these factors appear to be more closely associated with atherosclerosis in certain arterial beds than in others. For example, serum levels of cholesterol and low-density lipoprotein are strongly related to coronary heart disease but only moderately related to cerebrovascular or peripheral occlusive disease. Cerebrovascular disease is closely related to hypertension,[102] but cigarette smoking is the principal risk factor for peripheral occlusive disease.[103]

In addition to differences in systemic risk factor associations, variations in local hemodynamic and artery wall properties appear to exert major selective effects on plaque formation.[104, 105] Certain regions of each vascular bed are especially prone to plaque formation, whereas others are usually spared.[106] For example, the coronary arteries, carotid bifurcation, infrarenal abdominal aorta, and iliofemoral arteries are particularly susceptible to plaque formation, but the thoracic aorta and the common carotid, distal internal carotid, renal, mesenteric, and upper extremity arteries are particularly resistant. Such differences have been associated with variations in the distribution of shear and tensile stresses produced by variations in geometry and flow in differing segments of the arterial tree.[1] Although plaques may occur in straight vessels away from branch points, they are usually located at bifurcations or bends, where variations in hemodynamic conditions are especially likely to occur.[107]

Hemodynamic Considerations

A number of hemodynamic variables have been proposed to account for the selective distribution of plaques:

- Shear stress
- Flow separation and stasis
- Oscillation of shear stress vectors
- Turbulence
- Hypertension

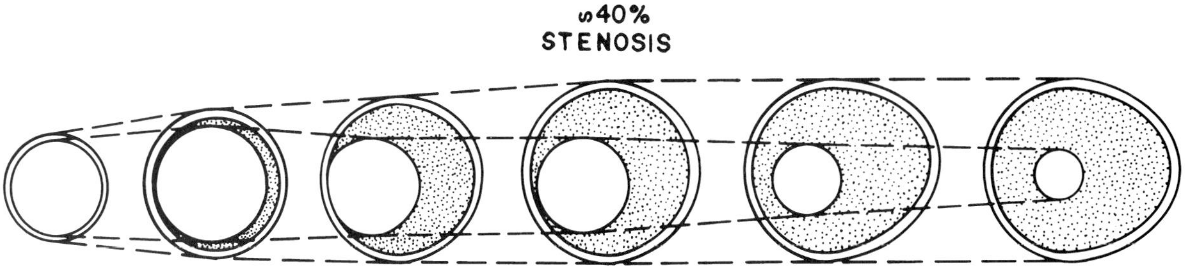

∽40%
STENOSIS

FIGURE 18–6. Possible sequence of changes in atherosclerotic arteries in response to enlarging atherosclerotic plaques. In the early stages of intimal plaque deposition, the lumen remains normal or enlarges slightly *(left)*. When intimal plaque enlarges to involve the entire circumference of the vessel and produces more than 40% stenosis, the artery can no longer enlarge at a rate sufficient to prevent narrowing of the lumen. (From Glagov S, Weisenberg E, Zarins CK, et al: Compensatory enlargement of human atherosclerotic coronary arteries. Reprinted by permission of The New England Journal of Medicine, 316:1371, 1987.)

Several texts have provided detailed, in-depth consideration of the relevant fluid dynamic principles.[1, 4]

Wall Shear Stress

Wall shear stress is the tangential drag force produced by blood moving across the endothelial surface. It is a function of the velocity gradient of blood near the endothelial surface. Its magnitude is directly proportional to blood flow and blood viscosity and inversely proportional to the cube of the radius. Thus, a small change in the radius of a vessel has a large effect on wall shear stress.

High shear stress was implicated in atherogenesis when endothelial desquamation and smooth muscle proliferation were considered to be prime factors in plaque initiation,[12] and experimental studies showed that short-term experimental elevations of shear stress could cause endothelial disruption.[108] Long-term elevations of shear stress were not associated with endothelial injury, however, and regions of relatively high shear stress appeared to be selectively spared from plaque formation.[109]

It is now evident that atherosclerotic plaques localize preferentially in regions of *low shear stress* and not in regions of high shear stress. This fact has been demonstrated in quantitative studies correlating early plaque formation in pressure perfusion–fixed human carotid bifurcations with wall shear stress determinations in analogous geometrically precise flow models (Fig. 18–7).[110] Plaques form where shear stress values are near zero (i.e., at the lateral wall opposite the flow divider), and it has been suggested that a threshold value may exist below which plaque deposition tends to occur.[111] Similar quantitative studies of the human aortic bifurcation have also shown that plaques localize in regions of low rather than high shear stress.[112]

Low shear rates may retard the transport of atherogenic substances away from the wall, resulting in a greater accumulation of lipids.[113] In addition, low shear stress may interfere with endothelial surface turnover of substances essential both to artery wall metabolism and to the maintenance of optimal endothelial metabolic function.[9, 114] Low wall shear stress has also been shown to be a factor in the development of intimal hyperplasia.[115]

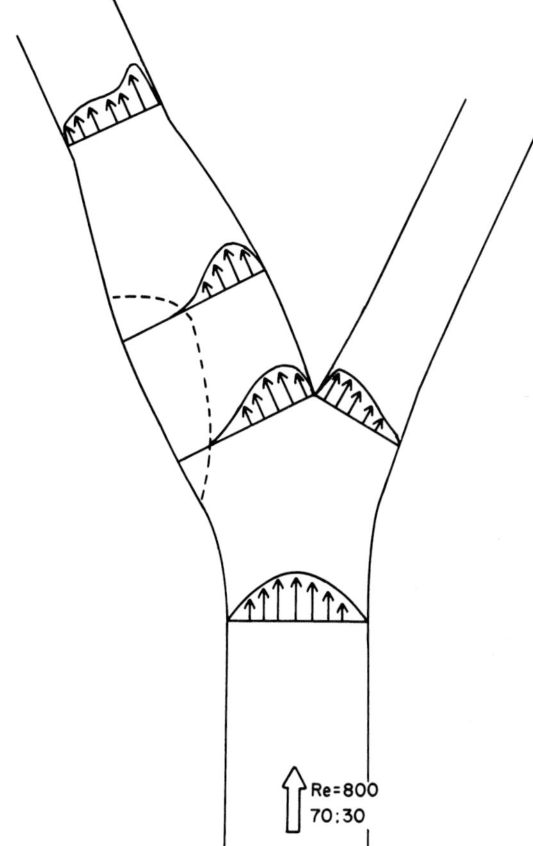

FIGURE 18–7. Axial velocity profiles measured with laser Doppler anemometry in a glass model carotid bifurcation under conditions of steady flow (Reynolds number, 800; flow division ratio of internal carotid:external carotid, 70:30). The velocity profile is skewed toward the inner wall of the carotid bifurcation, resulting in a steep velocity gradient and high wall shear stress. Along the outer wall of the internal carotid sinus, the velocity profile is flat and there is an area of flow separation with very low flow velocities (*dotted line*) and very low wall shear stress. It is in this region of the human carotid bifurcation that intimal plaques form. (From Zarins CK, Giddens DP, Bharadvaj BK, et al: Carotid bifurcation atherosclerosis: Quantitative correlation of plaque localization with flow velocity profiles and wall shear stress. Circ Res 53:502, 1983.)

Flow Separation and Stasis

In especially susceptible areas, such as the outer wall of the carotid bifurcation, where flow velocity is reduced and flow separation occurs, fluid and particles are cleared slowly (Fig. 18–8) and have an *increased residence time*.[4, 111, 116, 117] The vessel wall would therefore have a prolonged exposure to atherogenic particles. Time-dependent lipid particle–vessel wall interactions would thus be facilitated and would favor plaque formation. In addition, blood-borne cellular elements that may play a role in atherogenesis would have a greater probability of deposition, adhesion, or diapedesis into the vessel wall in such regions.[118] Flow separation has, for example, been shown to favor deposition of platelets in vitro,[119] which may contribute to plaque induction and complication. Radiographic and ultrasound studies confirm the presence of flow separation and stasis in this outer wall region of the carotid bifurcation.[120] Not only do early intimal thickenings and plaques localize in this region, but complications, stenoses, and ulcerations also predominate here.

Oscillation of Flow

Blood velocity varies markedly during the course of the cardiac cycle, resulting in a fluctuation in the magnitude of wall shear stress that is a normal feature at the blood-artery interface. Along the inner wall of the carotid bifurcation on the side of the flow divider, blood flow and shear stress vary but the vector is always in the forward direction. Along the outer wall of the carotid bifurcation, opposite the flow divider where intimal plaques form, there is a reversal of axial flow direction during systole and phasic retrograde flow along the wall (Fig. 18–9). This results in a directional oscillation of the shear stress vector during the cardiac cycle.[111]

Variations in shear stress direction associated with pulsatile flow may favor greater endothelial permeability by

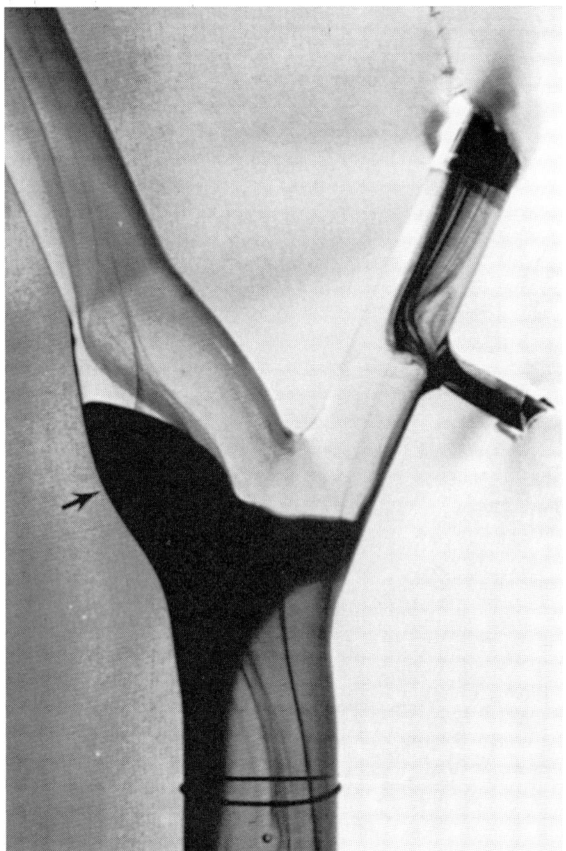

FIGURE 18–8. Flow visualization with dye injection in a glass model carotid bifurcation illustrating slow clearance from the separated flow region along the outer wall of the internal carotid sinus (*arrow*). Dye remains along the outer wall and within the separation zone long after it has been convected away from the region of the flow divider and distal internal carotid artery. (From Zarins CK, Giddens DP, Bharadvaj BK, et al: Carotid bifurcation atherosclerosis: Quantitative correlation of plaque localization with flow velocity profiles and wall shear stress. Circ Res 53:502, 1983.)

direct mechanical effects on cell junctions, whereas relatively high unidirectional shear stresses may not be injurious[121] and may even favor endothelial mechanical integrity.[122] Endothelial cells are normally aligned in the direction of flow[123] in an overlapping arrangement.[124] Cyclic shifts in the relationship between shear stress direction and the orientation of intercellular overlapping borders may disturb the relationships between ingress and egress of particles through junctions. This hypothesis agrees well with reports of (1) increased permeability of cultured, confluent endothelial cells subjected to changes in shear stress[125] and (2) greater permeability to Evans blue dye in relation to differences in endothelial cell orientation,[126] which may be associated with different flow patterns. Oscillatory shear stress has also been shown to influence endothelium and nitric oxide synthase expression[127] as well as stimulate adhesion molecule expression in cultured human endothelial cells.[128]

Because oscillation of shear stress direction at susceptible sites occurs during systole, the number of such oscillations over time is directly related to the number of systoles (i.e., to heart rate). Heart rate has been implicated as an independent risk factor in coronary atherosclerosis and is discussed further in the section dealing with the coronary arteries. Reduction in heart rate in experimental atherosclerosis has been shown to retard carotid plaque progression.[81, 129]

Turbulence

Turbulence, defined as random, disordered flow, is rarely seen in the normal vascular tree. Turbulent flow has often been implicated as a factor in the pathogenesis of plaque.[130, 131] However, in vitro observations and experimental atherosclerosis studies fail to support this concept. In model studies of the carotid bifurcation, a zone of complex secondary and tertiary flow patterns including counterrotating helical trajectories is demonstrable in regions of plaque formation, but turbulence does not occur (Fig. 18–10).[132] In vivo pulsed Doppler ultrasound studies of carotid arteries have confirmed this finding in normal human subjects.[133]

Turbulence may develop in association with stenoses and irregularities of the flow surface caused by atherosclerotic

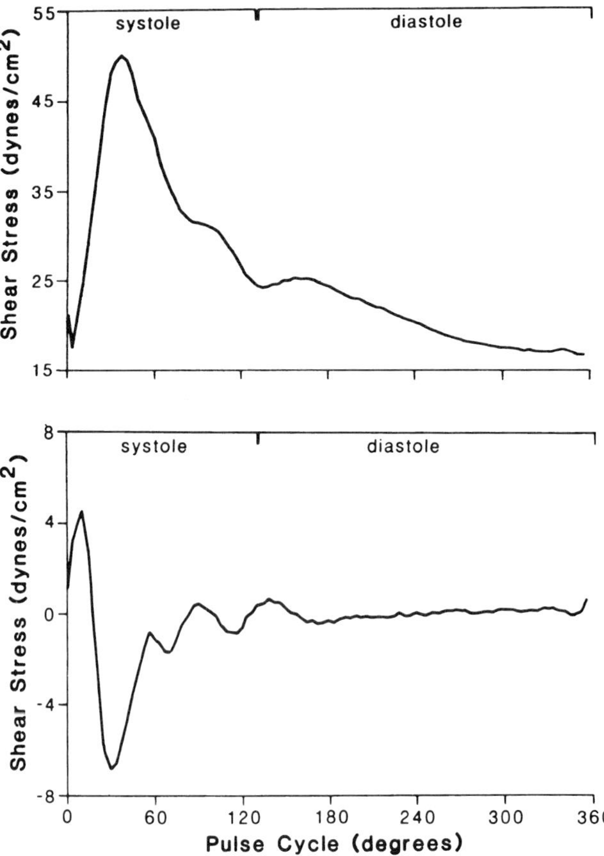

FIGURE 18–9. Shear stress alterations in the carotid bifurcation during the cardiac cycle. *Top,* Along the inner wall of the internal carotid sinus, shear stress is high and always in the forward direction (18 to 50 dynes/cm²). Plaque does not form in this area. *Bottom,* Along the outer wall of the sinus, shear stress is low (+5 to −6 dynes/cm²) and changes direction during the cardiac cycle from a forward to a reverse vector with multiple oscillations. This oscillation in the shear stress vector is highly correlated with early plaque formation. (From Ku DN, Giddens DP, Zarins CK, et al: Pulsatile flow and atherosclerosis in the human carotid bifurcation: Positive correlation between plaque location and low and oscillating shear stress. Arteriosclerosis 5:293, 1985.)

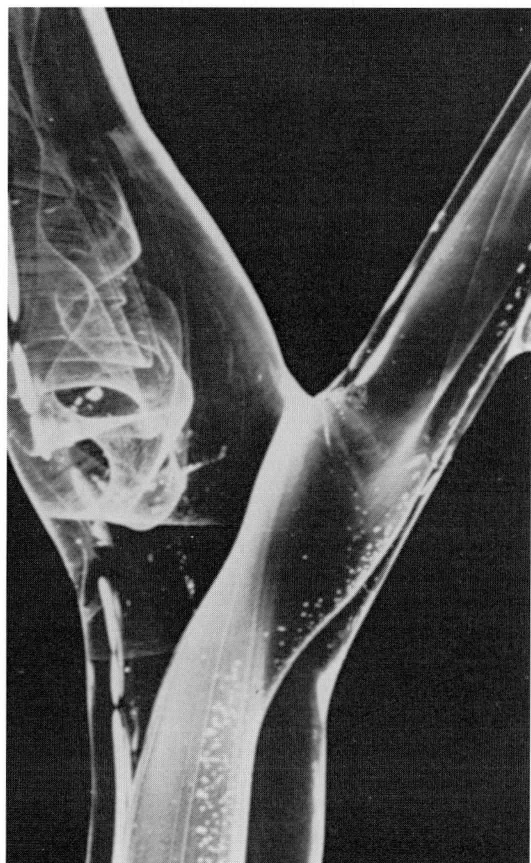

FIGURE 18–10. Hydrogen bubble flow visualization in a glass model carotid bifurcation. Streamlines are skewed toward the apex of the carotid flow divider, and in the outer wall of the carotid sinus, there is a zone of complex secondary and tertiary flow patterns, including flow reversal and counterrotating helical trajectories. However, no random, disordered flow or turbulence is present.

plaques, although the turbulence is located distal to rather than at the lesion. Experimentally produced stenoses reveal that turbulence is greatest two to four vessel diameters distal to the stenosis in an area in which post-stenotic dilatation frequently develops but diet-induced plaques do not readily occur.[134–136] Thus, turbulence per se has not been shown to be an initiating factor in atherogenesis. Nevertheless, turbulence may play a role in plaque disruption or thrombogenesis. Further investigation is needed to establish these relationships.

Hypertension

Hypertension has been identified as an important risk factor in the development of clinical complications of atherosclerosis, such as myocardial infarction and stroke.[137] Postmortem studies have revealed that hypertension is associated with an increase in both the extent and the severity of atherosclerosis.[106] Elevated blood pressure alone does not induce atherosclerosis in experimental animals. In the presence of hyperlipidemia, however, hypertension enhances plaque formation.[138–140] Yet atherosclerotic plaque does not form despite the presence of hypertension and severe hyperlipidemia when pulse pressure, wall motion, or both are decreased.[141, 142]

Although hypertension does enhance experimental plaque formation, it also inhibits plaque regression when cholesterol levels are reduced.[143] Hypertension also results in enhanced coronary artery plaque progression despite the reduction of hypercholesterolemia.[144] These observations suggest that factors other than blood pressure per se may be of primary importance in plaque pathogenesis. However, hypertension may play an important role in the evolution and clinical complications of atherosclerotic plaques.

Artery Wall Motion

In addition to the role of shear forces in the localization of atherosclerotic lesions, the amplitude of the stretching movements of the arterial wall associated with the excursion in blood pressure during the cardiac cycle may also be implicated in the pathogenesis of atherosclerosis. The relationship between localization of diet-induced lesions and the extent of cyclic arterial wall stretching has been examined, and the data suggest a direct relationship between increased wall motion and plaque deposition. Conversely, reduced cyclic arterial stretching results in sparing from atherosclerosis.[141]

Further evidence for such an interpretation has been obtained in experiments in which cyclic stretching of short segments of aorta was restricted by encirclement, without narrowing, by a surrounding rigid tube.[145] The intimal surface in the immobilized segment remained free of atherosclerotic lesions. Pulse pressure and intraluminal flow were presumably unchanged. Other studies have reported similar findings in less than critical constrictions by rigid collars.[146] Clinically, calcification of arteries due to atherosclerosis may diminish wall motion and reduce the rate of subsequent plaque deposition.

Sparing of the artery distal to a stenosis is seen clinically in patients with long-standing chronic occlusions of the abdominal aorta. Whether restoration of arterial wall motion to normal by removal of a proximal obstruction would accelerate the distal atherosclerotic process or enhance intimal hyperplasia at an anastomotic site is unknown. Experimental data suggest that restoration of aortic wall motion to normal after 3 months of stenosis returns the rate of distal lesion formation to control levels but does not accelerate it.[146a] Further investigations of the relationships among wall composition, wall compliance, pulse pressure, and plaque localization in both human vessels and experimental models could provide information of practical value with regard to the likely effects on distal segments of the relief of proximal stenosis.

Effects of Exercise

Exercise results in a significant increase in cardiac output and heart rate and a reduction in peripheral resistance. This increase markedly alters the hemodynamic condition in the vascular tree. The adverse hemodynamic conditions that exist in the carotid bifurcation and abdominal aorta under resting flow conditions are transiently eliminated during exercise. Low flow velocity and low wall shear stress are increased, particle residence time is reduced, and oscillatory shear becomes unidirectional. These changes have been studied in model flow systems in the abdominal aorta[147] and at simulated vascular anastomoses.[148, 149] The effects of exercise in the abdominal aorta have been studied with the use of computational flow techniques.

We developed a computer model of the human abdominal aorta to evaluate aortic blood flow quantitatively under rest and graded exercise conditions. Figure 18–11 (see Color Plate) shows the velocity field in a computer model of the abdominal aorta under simulated resting and exercise conditions at mid-diastole along the mid-plane of the aorta. It should be noted that under resting conditions, a large vortex develops along the posterior wall of the aorta. This region of flow stasis and high particle residence time disappears with moderate levels of simulated lower limb exercise, such as might be obtained with a brisk walk. Wall shear stress and vortex flow patterns were measured and the lesion-prone infrarenal aorta was compared with the lesion-resistant suprarenal aorta. At rest, the posterior wall of the infrarenal aorta demonstrated negative, low wall shear stress, flow reversal, and vortex flow patterns, whereas the suprarenal aorta showed higher, positive, shear stress with uniform flow and no vortex formation. Because the suprarenal aorta is less prone to atherosclerotic lesions than the abdominal aorta, the shear stress at this site, 1.2 dynes/cm^2 under resting conditions, was assumed to be the minimum needed to inhibit atherosclerosis.

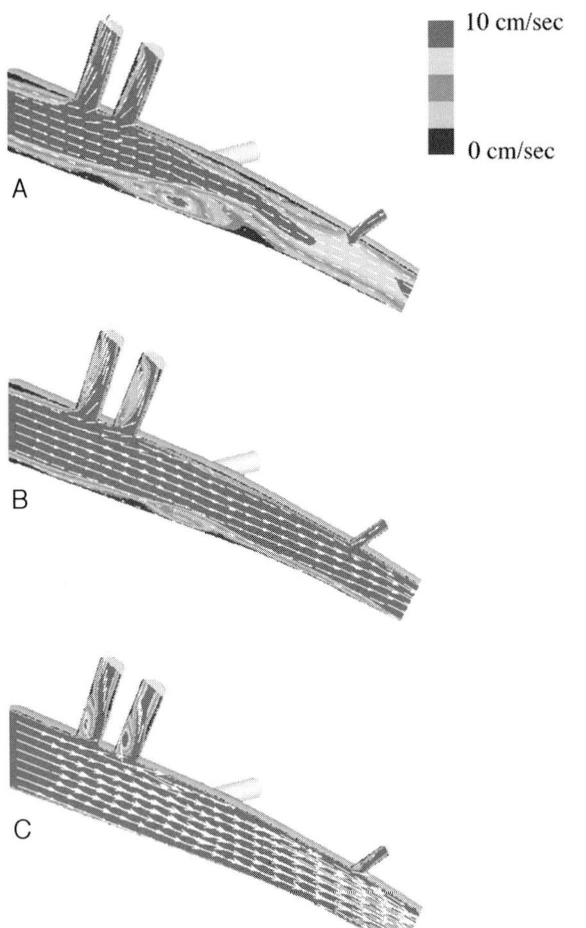

FIGURE 18–11. Mid-plane slice of the abdominal aorta model displaying contours of axial velocity and the velocity vector field at mid-diastole for (*A*) resting conditions, (*B*) moderate exercise conditions, and (*C*) vigorous exercise conditions. (See Color Plate.)

Moderate exercise increases infrarenal aortic blood flow and normalizes the shear stress in the lesion-prone infrarenal aorta. An increase of only 2.3 L/min of blood flow to the legs changes the infrarenal blood flow from a complex, recirculating flow to a uniform, unidirectional flow. In addition, under these moderate exercise conditions, the shear stress in the infrarenal aorta exceeds the shear stress in the suprarenal aorta. These data support the increasing body of evidence that low levels of exercise have a beneficial effect in limiting atherosclerosis. The duration or frequency of exposure to higher than resting levels of shear stress necessary to inhibit atherosclerosis is, at present, unknown.[148, 150–154]

Susceptible Regions of the Vascular Tree

Carotid Arteries

The carotid bifurcation is particularly prone to plaque formation, with focal plaque deposition occurring principally at the origin of the internal carotid artery, whereas the proximal common carotid artery and the distal internal carotid artery are relatively spared. The geometry of the carotid bifurcation is an important determinant of the hemodynamic conditions that favor plaque formation. The internal carotid sinus has a cross-sectional area twice that of the immediately distal internal carotid segment. This configuration, in combination with the branching angle, results in a large area of flow separation and low and oscillating shear stress along the outer wall of the sinus and a region of laminar flow and high unidirectional shear stress along the inner wall of the sinus.[110, 111] The manner in which these differences may determine plaque localization at the outer wall of the sinus has been discussed.

As plaques enlarge at the outer wall, however, the geometric configuration of the lumen is modified so that other flow patterns may develop that favor plaque formation on the side and inner walls. In its most advanced and stenotic form, atherosclerotic disease of the carotid bifurcation may therefore involve the entire circumference of the sinus, including the region of the flow divider, but the plaques are nevertheless largest and most complicated at the outer and side walls of the proximal internal carotid bifurcation.[155] When there is a severe stenosis, the modified hemodynamic conditions that exist at the carotid bifurcation, including the turbulence that may underlie the characteristic bruit, may also compromise integrity of existing carotid plaques and contribute to their tendency to fissure, ulcerate, and form thromboemboli.

Coronary Arteries

Velocity profile and wall shear stress measurements in model human coronary arteries reveal that low wall shear stress, flow separation, and oscillation occur at sites susceptible to plaque localization.[156] These near-wall flow field characteristics are similar to those found in susceptible regions of the carotid bifurcation.

Several special hemodynamic features of the coronary arteries may explain their particular propensity for development of clinically significant plaques. The epicardial coronary tree has a complex geometric configuration of branchings and curves. Mechanical torsions and flexions of the vessels are evident during the cardiac cycle as the configuration of the cardiac chambers changes. In addition, there are marked variations in flow rate during the cardiac cycle.[157] The coronary arteries experience two different systolic pulses of flow during each cardiac cycle.[158] If oscillation in the direction of the shear stress vector during systole is indeed a major factor in plaque localization,[159] the coronary arteries would be expected to be more vulnerable to plaque formation than other systemic arteries in which only a single systolic pulse is present.

In experimental atherosclerosis, a 20% reduction in mean heart rate resulted in a 50% reduction in diet-induced coronary artery atherosclerotic plaques.[160] Similarly, there was a significant reduction in carotid bifurcation atherosclerosis with reduction in heart rate.[81, 161] In humans, a number of major prospective clinical studies have found high heart rates in men at rest to be predictors of future clinical coronary heart disease, whereas low heart rates had a protective effect.[162, 163] The beneficial effects of exercise on limiting coronary atherosclerosis may result from a reduction in resting heart rate, an intermittent increase in coronary flow and wall shear stress, or a combination of the two.

Abdominal Aorta

Atherosclerotic plaques in humans are found throughout the length of the aorta but are rarely clinically significant in the thoracic segment. In contrast, the infrarenal abdominal aorta is particularly prone to the development of clinically significant lesions, with the formation of obstructive plaques, ulcerations, thrombi, and aneurysmal degeneration. The differences in susceptibility between the thoracic and abdominal portions of the aorta may be related to differences in (1) flow conditions, (2) mural architecture, and (3) vasa vasorum blood supply.[164]

The thoracic aorta is the main conduit carrying blood flow to the viscera and extremities. Much of the cardiac output is delivered to the cerebral and upper extremity vessels as well as to the visceral organs; the renal arteries alone take up to 25% of the cardiac output.[165] Levels of flow in the infrarenal aorta, in contrast, largely depend on the muscular activity of the lower extremities. With mechanized transportation and an increasingly sedentary lifestyle, reduced physical activity may result in an overall reduction in flow velocity in the abdominal aortic segment. As previously described, Figure 18–11 displays the velocity field in a computer model of the abdominal aorta under simulated resting exercise conditions at mid-diastole along the mid-plane of the aorta. This region of flow stasis and high particle residence time disappears with moderate levels of simulated lower limb exercise, such as might be obtained with a brisk walk.

The long-term effect of reduced flow velocity may be further accentuated by the tendency of the aorta to enlarge with age. Although the human thoracic aortic media is furnished with intramural vasa vasorum, the abdominal aorta is relatively avascular.[104] Thus, reduced and marked variations in luminal flow rate as well as discrepancies between medial thickness and medial nutrition may combine to enhance the accumulation of atherogenic substances in the abdominal aortic intima.

Conversely, increased flow velocity such as occurs with exercise increases wall shear stress, reduces particle residence time, and eliminates oscillation of shear in the infrarenal aorta. [149, 152, 166] These factors may be important in plaque formation in the infrarenal aorta and may explain the beneficial effects of exercise in preventing plaque formation.

Superficial Femoral Artery

The arteries of the lower extremities are frequently affected by atherosclerotic plaques, whereas vessels of similar size in the upper extremities are usually spared. In addition to differences in hydrostatic pressure, the arteries of the lower extremities are subjected to more marked variations in flow rate, depending on the level of physical activity. As in the abdominal aorta, a sedentary lifestyle would tend to favor low flow rates and lead to increased plaque deposition in vessels of the lower extremities.

Cigarette smoking and diabetes mellitus are the risk factors most closely associated with atherosclerotic disease of the lower extremities.[167] The manner in which these factors and the special hemodynamic conditions are mutually enhancing in the vessels of the lower extremities remains to be elucidated. The arterial media in the lower extremities may be rendered more dense by the greater smooth muscle tone induced by nicotine.[168] Such a change could interfere with transmural transfer of materials entering the intima and favor accumulation of atherogenic materials, as has been suggested by pharmacologic experiments.[169]

Of the arteries of the lower extremity, the superficial femoral artery is the most common site of multiple stenotic lesions, and the profunda femoris tends to be spared. Plaques in the superficial femoral artery have not been shown to occur preferentially at branching sites, but stenotic lesions tend to appear earliest at the adductor hiatus, where the vessel is straight and branches are few. Increased susceptibility to plaque formation because of mechanical trauma caused by the closely associated adductor magnus tendon has been proposed to explain the selective localization of occlusive disease in this area.[170] However, studies have suggested that the adductor canal segment of the superficial femoral artery is not more prone to plaque formation but rather is limited in its ability to dilate or enlarge in response to increasing intimal plaque. Thus, an equivalent volume of intimal plaque results in more stenosis at the adductor canal.[92]

EVOLUTION OF ATHEROSCLEROTIC LESIONS

Atherosclerosis is not necessarily a continuous process leading inexorably to artery stenosis or other clinically significant complications. Plaque formation involves an interaction among systemic risk factors and local conditions in the lumen and artery wall in the context of a living tissue capable of healing and remodeling. The evolution of atherosclerotic lesions therefore involves initiating and sustaining processes as well as adaptive responses and involutional changes. The natural history of atherosclerotic lesions in humans is poorly understood despite the available experimental data concerning the progression and regression of plaques.

Plaque Initiation

Plaque initiation refers to the earliest detectable biochemical and cellular events leading to or preceding the formation of atherosclerotic lesions. Possible mechanisms of plaque initiation have received a great deal of attention. Research has centered principally on several possibilities, including altered endothelial function or turnover resulting in increased permeability, oxidative alteration of insudated lipids by endothelium, and subsequent ingress of macrophages.[171] Other possibilities are various stimuli to smooth muscle proliferation, including circulating mitogens,[172] and limitations of transmural transfer or egress related to the composition and organization of subendothelial tissues and media.[173] High levels of specific lipoprotein cholesterol fractions have also been implicated.[174] Although each of these possibilities can be related to early lesion development in experimental models and may be related to one or another of the epidemiologically identified risk factors, none has as yet been demonstrated to underlie the mural disturbance that leads to plaque formation. Some or several of these changes may well prove to be significant.

It is not clear, however, that inhibiting the possible initiating injury to the artery wall is of primary importance in the clinical control of atherosclerosis. Later research has focused principally on several possibilities, including (1) altered endothelial function linked to an inflammatory response to injury with leukocyte adhesion and diapedesis, and (2) cell proliferation, smooth muscle cell migration, and macrophage foam cell formation with lipid accumulation in both cell types. The lipids accumulated include cholesterol, cholesterol esters, and triglycerides. Greater lipoprotein infiltration coupled with disregulation of the cholesterol ester cycle activity and cholesterol efflux processes has been proposed to explain the pathobiology of this lipid accumulation process. Moreover, T-cells, macrophages, and smooth muscle cells may release specific biologic response modifiers that may participate in the disregulation of lipid metabolism, thereby enhancing lipid accumulation.[23, 29]

It is well recognized that very old people with no clinically manifest atherosclerotic disease during life are found at autopsy to have substantial and advanced atherosclerotic plaques. Longevity and good health in these people were associated not with the prevention of plaque initiation or formation but with (1) the stable nature of the plaque, (2) control of progression, (3) adequate artery adaptation, and (4) prevention of the complications of such lesions.

Plaque Progression

Plaque progression refers to the continuing increase in intimal plaque volume, which may result in narrowing of the lumen and obstruction of blood flow. Progression may be rapid or slow, continuous or episodic. Rates of accretion may also vary with the stage of plaque development, plaque composition, and cell population of the lesion. Some of these factors may be modulated by clinical risk factors, whereas others are related to the changes in circulation and wall composition associated with lesion growth.

At the tissue level, plaque progression involves:

1. Cellular migration, proliferation, and differentiation.
2. Intracellular and extracellular accumulation of lipids.
3. Extracellular matrix accumulation.
4. Degeneration and cell necrosis.

Progression also implies evolution and differentiation of plaque organization and stratification. In general, these features are designed to maintain an adequate lumen channel for as long as possible. The formation of a fibrous cap, the sequestration of necrotic and degenerative debris, and the persistence of a regular and round lumen cross section, as well as adaptive enlargement of the artery, reflect an overall healing process. In the long term, these reactive processes may prove inadequate, but they may also retard or arrest the atherogenic process. If plaque enlargement occurs under these conditions, plaque progression is well tolerated. Lumen diameter and blood flow are maintained even in the presence of advanced and extensive lesions.

Plaque modeling also includes incorporation and organization of mural thrombi and healing and reendothelialization of ulcerations, suggesting further means of restoring and preserving optimal conditions for adequate laminar flow. Plaque disruptions that undergo remodeling may leave defects corresponding to healed or restructured walls without the development of clinical symptoms.

One must understand the processes that regulate plaque development, differentiation, and healing in order to comprehend why one plaque progresses unfavorably with stenosis, ulceration, or thrombosis and another progresses without obstruction or complication. It is likely that rates of cell proliferation, lipid deposition, fibrous cap formation, necrosis and healing, calcification, and inflammation vary over time and may differ with location at the same point in time. Such differences probably account for the spectrum of morphologic changes in plaques in a given patient at the same time.

Changes in local hemodynamics that occur during plaque progression may also alter plaque composition and the rate of progression. Increases in shear stress in a developing stenosis may inhibit further plaque formation but may also favor erosion of the fibrous cap and ulceration. Developing stenoses may also alter hemodynamic conditions to enhance lesion formation and complication distally.[175] Severe, hemodynamically significant stenoses, however, enhance plaque formation in the proximal arterial segments[176] and inhibit it distally[143] because of changes in pulse pressure, wall motion, and medial smooth muscle metabolism.[177]

Plaque Regression

Plaque regression refers to a discernible decrease in intimal plaque volume; this may occur through (1) resorption of lipids or extracellular matrix, (2) cell death, and (3) cell migration out of the plaque.

Significant reduction in lesion volume has been demonstrated in a number of animal models in which experimentally elevated serum lipid levels have been markedly reduced by an alteration in diet or administration of lipid-lowering drugs.[178–180] Lesions previously induced by an atherogenic diet respond readily, although not uniformly. Coronary and aortic lesions in monkeys tend to regress, but carotid lesions appear to be resistant.[181] Severe, long-standing lesions in swine are much more resistant to regression than early foam cell lesions.[182] Animal studies usually involve induction and regression periods of several months. Whether human lesions, which may have accumulated over decades, also decrease significantly in volume is as yet unclear.

Just as local hemodynamic conditions exert a profound influence on plaque progression, so they are important in regression. Severe proximal stenosis inhibits plaque formation[176] but also inhibits plaque regression in the distal arterial tree.[143] Hypertension promotes continued experimental plaque progression in the coronary arteries despite the reduction of hypercholesterolemia.[144] Despite both plaque regression elsewhere and the reversal of hypercholesterolemia, experimental plaque formation and complication can continue in the arteries distal to a stenosis, indicating that local hemodynamic factors and metabolic conditions in the artery wall may greatly modify systemic influences on plaque function during both progression and regression.[143]

Plaque Regression Studies in Humans

Apparent regression of atherosclerosis has been documented by serial contrast arteriography in humans. Angiographic regression of atherosclerotic lesions has been demonstrated in humans in coronary[183–185] and peripheral[81] arteries. Each of these trials has demonstrated luminal changes on angiography rather than by direct evidence of plaque regression. It should be noted that each trial to date has demonstrated simultaneous angiographic evidence of lesion progression *and* regression of different lesions during the treatment, indicating the complexity of the process.

Although plaque regression is usually thought of as simply a resorption of plaque material, it may proceed by different mechanisms. A decrease in intimal plaque volume may occur owing to a change in plaque metabolism, resulting in dissolution of the fibrous cap, ulceration and erosion, and embolization of the necrotic core.

Apparent regression may also take place when the rate of artery wall enlargement exceeds the rate of plaque deposition. Most human plaque regression studies performed to date have used angiography to document lesion regression.[186] However, angiography provides information only on lumen diameter and contour, not on the volume and composition of the atherosclerotic lesion itself. Thus, if intimal plaque deposition and artery wall dilatation keep pace, no change is noted on arteriography despite continued plaque progression. Conversely, if dilatation exceeds plaque deposition, this change noted on arteriography is taken as evidence of regression even if plaque deposition continues.[187] Such a phenomenon occurs at the outset of plaque formation in some vessels and is quite prominent in some locations. Certainty with regard to reduction in lesion volume or regression of atherosclerosis in humans must be based on a direct assessment of the plaque and artery wall as well as of lumen caliber.

Although plaque regression may a priori seem desirable, regression regimens could alter the composition and organization of plaques, especially those with soft, semifluid, or pultaceous contents, leading to plaque ulceration or disruption, release of plaque debris, and thrombosis and embolism. In certain circumstances, particularly with well-organized sclerotic plaques, the plaque may provide mechanical support to the artery wall. This may be especially significant if medial atrophy has occurred underneath the plaque. Plaque dissolution under these circumstances could leave a weakened artery wall and potentiate aneurysm formation. Experimental studies have revealed aneurysm formation in monkeys undergoing cholesterol-lowering regression regimens.[188, 189]

Further studies of the direct effects of regression regimens on plaques and the artery wall are needed, and plaque regression must be defined in terms of its specific effects on well-established atherosclerotic plaques. An alternative therapeutic goal may be arrest or control of progression, plaque stabilization, and enhancement of artery wall adaptation.

Plaque Complications and Stability

Clinical sequelae of atherosclerotic lesions are usually caused by the complications of plaques. Complications such as plaque disruption or ulceration may result in embolization of plaque materials or the exposure of plaque components to the circulation, thereby causing occlusive or embolizing thrombi. Critical lumen narrowing or the presence of plaque complications at a few critical locations in the vascular tree is the predominant determinant of clinical symptoms, rather than plaque size per se.

Susceptibility of plaques to disruption, fracture, or fissuring is likely to be associated with their structure, composition, and consistency.[190] Plaque fracture and disruption are important features in the development of clinical symptoms.[191, 192] Plaques may be of various types:

- Relatively soft and pliable
- Friable or cohesive
- Densely sclerotic
- Calcific and brittle

A plaque may have a well-formed fibrous cap, similar in architecture and thickness to a normal artery wall, which thereby effectively sequesters the plaque and its contents from the lumen. The necrotic interior of other plaques, however, may be separated from the lumen only by a narrow zone of connective tissue or by endothelium alone.[193, 194]

Advanced plaques with intact, well-organized fibrous caps would be expected to present smooth and regular lumen surfaces to the bloodstream. Abnormal levels of wall shear stress and departures from laminar, unidirectional flow may favor local accumulation, adhesion, and deposition of thrombocytes, monocytes, and fibrin. These hemodynamic disturbances are likely to occur distal to stenoses, at foci of endothelial surface irregularity or extrinsic mechanical trauma, and in regions of softened plaque consistency.[195] Local mechanical stresses resulting from (1) sudden changes in pressure, flow, or pulse rate or (2) torsion and bending in relation to organ movements may precipitate disruption of friable or brittle plaques. Conversely, changes in vessel configuration associated with plaque progression and stenosis may create conditions favoring the development of hemodynamic shear forces that can cause plaque rupture.[196]

Although vessel segments distal to tight stenoses tend to be spared, degrees of stenosis not tight enough to prevent distal plaque formation may nevertheless engender unstable flow conditions that could modify plaque composition and configuration. In experimental animals, plaques located immediately distal to a region of moderate narrowing have been shown to be more complex in structure and composition than those that occur in the same region in the absence of a proximal stenosis.[175] The likelihood of turbulence is also enhanced as significant stenoses develop and as vessels enlarge and become tortuous with age or when multiple plaques occur in the same vessel in close axial proximity.

Because regions of high flow velocity tend to be spared, increasing flow velocity at progressive narrowings could also conceivably be associated with local slowing of the atherogenic process. Decreased flow velocity due to distal obstruction, reduced pressure, or greater peripheral resistance would have the opposite effect. Further information is needed concerning the factors that determine plaque complication or stability in human atherosclerosis.

ANEURYSM FORMATION

The association between atherosclerosis and aneurysm formation has long been recognized in humans. The demonstrations of increased proteolytic enzyme activity[197–199] and of a familial tendency for abdominal aortic aneurysm formation[200] have led some investigators to suggest that aneurysm formation is primarily a genetically controlled connective tissue dysfunction with little or no relation to atherosclerosis. However, experimental evidence reveals that (1) aneurysms can be induced in animals by feeding them high-cholesterol atherogenic diets for prolonged periods and (2) aneurysm formation is associated with destruction of the medial lamellar architecture of the aortic wall.[201, 202] Furthermore, aneurysm formation has been noted to be related to plaque regression in both controlled[189] (Fig. 18–12) and uncontrolled[188, 203] trials.

Increasing intimal plaque is associated with arterial enlargement and atrophy of the underlying arterial media, as described earlier in this chapter. Under these circumstances, the atherosclerotic plaque may contribute to the structural support of the artery wall. Significant plaque regression by resorption of lipid and extracellular matrix can reduce plaque volume. Further reduction in plaque volume can occur by erosion of the fibrous cap, elution of the necrotic core, and plaque ulceration. The net effect may be a thinned artery wall incapable of supporting the greater mural tension brought about by earlier atherosclerotic arterial enlargement. This increase in wall stress, together with the biologic interaction between metabolic plaque resorption and proteolytic enzyme activity on the arterial wall, can result in progressive arterial dilatation and aneurysm formation. Histologic examination of the aorta in animals with experimentally induced aneurysms and in humans with aneurysms reveals similar atrophic characteristics of atherosclerotic plaque, with loss of the elastin lamellar architecture of the artery wall (Fig. 18–13). Loss of elastin is a prominent feature, along with the loss of collagen and thinning of the aortic wall.

In humans, a strong association exists between atherosclerosis and aneurysm formation, which have common risk factors. Aneurysms form in the same distributions as atherosclerotic plaques, but the greatest vulnerability to aneurysm formation is in the abdominal aorta. The abdominal aorta is particularly susceptible to plaque formation and may be particularly vulnerable because of its medial lamellar architecture and limited aortic wall nutrition, as discussed earlier. These considerations suggest that abdominal aortic aneurysm formation may complicate the atherosclerotic process under special experimental and human clinical conditions. It appears at a relatively late phase of plaque evolution, when plaque regression and media atrophy predominate, rather than in earlier phases, when cell proliferation, fibrogenesis, and lipid accumulation characterize plaque progression.

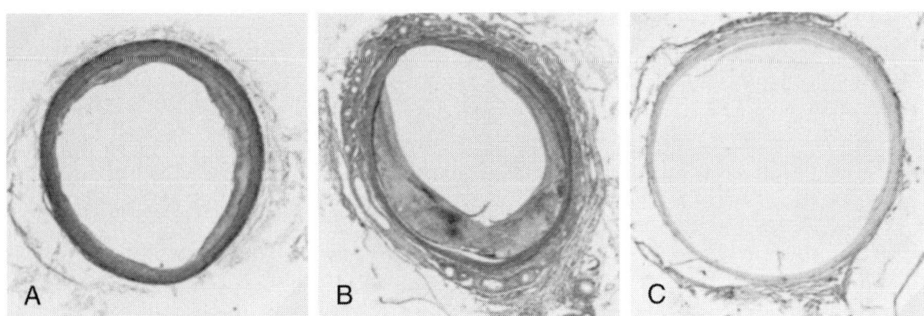

FIGURE 18–12. Aneurysmal enlargement of the abdominal aorta in a controlled trial of regression of experimental atherosclerosis. Transverse sections of the abdominal aorta from three groups of monkeys are shown. In group I (*A*), there was moderate plaque formation after a 6-month diet containing 2% cholesterol and 25% peanut oil. In group II (*B*), plaques were much larger and the media was slightly thinner after 12 months of the atherogenic diet, but the artery size (internal elastic lumina area) did not change significantly (*B*). After 6 months of the atherogenic diet, followed by a low-cholesterol regression diet (group III, *C*), plaques were significantly smaller and were absent in some regions. The media was thin, and the artery size (internal elastic lumina area) was increased twofold. (Weigert-van Gieson, original magnification ×10.) (*A–C*, From Zarins CK, Xu C-P, Glagov S: Aneurysmal enlargement of the aorta during regression of experimental atherosclerosis. J Vasc Surg 15:90, 1992.)

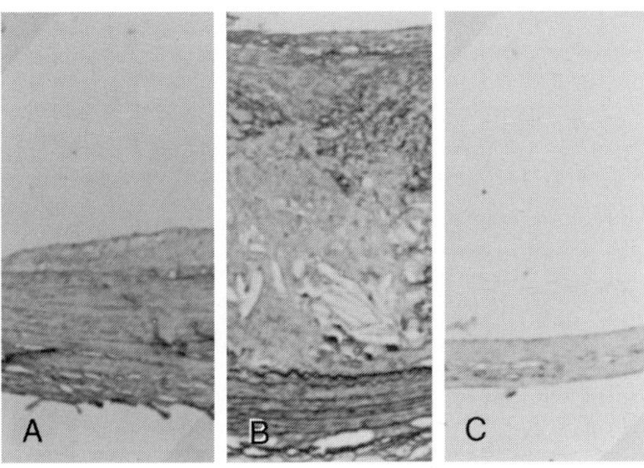

FIGURE 18–13. Histologic changes in the abdominal aorta of the sections shown in Figure 18–12. After 6 months of the atherogenic diet (group I, *A*), a moderate amount of plaque formed, with characteristic foamy cell prevalence and little change in the media. After 12 months of the atherogenic diet (group II, *B*), plaques were complex, with the formation of fibrous caps and evidence of necrosis and cholesterol accumulation. The media appeared normal, with clearly stained elastic lamellae and smooth muscle cells. After 6 months of the atherogenic diet and 6 months of the regression diet (group III, *C*), plaques were much smaller and largely fibrotic. The media was thinned, and elastic lamellae were largely inapparent. These histologic changes are similar to those seen in human aneurysms. (Weigert-van Gieson, original magnification ×75.) (*A–C*, From Zarins CK, Xu C-P, Glagov S: Aneurysmal enlargement of the aorta during regression of experimental atherosclerosis. J Vasc Surg 15:90, 1992.)

SUMMARY

Atherosclerosis is a systemic disorder with localized plaque deposition in selected sites on the arterial tree. Low or oscillatory wall shear stress, or both, and prolonged particle residence time due to flow stasis are the hemodynamic conditions associated with plaque formation. Alterations in local hemodynamic conditions also result in adaptive changes in the artery wall to maintain an adequate lumen caliber for blood flow. The primary adaptive response to enlarging intimal plaque is compensatory artery enlargement. Other responses, such as sequestering the plaque to one side and walling it off with a fibrous cap, can permit long-term clinical stability despite extensive atherosclerotic plaque formation.

Clinical complications of atherosclerosis occur when the normal adaptive and compensatory mechanisms fail and complications such as stenosis, ulceration, embolization, and thrombosis develop. A better understanding is needed of (1) the normal adaptive responses of arteries, (2) the processes and evolution of atherosclerotic lesions, and (3) the means by which plaques can be stabilized to prevent local plaque complications and subsequent clinical consequences.

Acknowledgments: This work was supported by the National Heart, Lung, and Blood Institute NHLBI grant HL-15062 and National Science Foundation NSF grant CME 7921551.

REFERENCES

1. Glagov S, Zarins CK, Giddens DP, Ku DN: Hemodynamics and atherosclerosis. Arch Pathol Lab Med 112:1018, 1988.
2. Zarins CK: Adaptive responses of arteries. J Vasc Surg 9:382, 1989.
3. Schwartz S, Heimark R, Majesky M: Developmental mechanisms underlying pathology of arteries. Physiol Rev 70:1177, 1990.
4. Giddens DP, Zarins CK, Glagov S: Response of arteries to near-wall fluid dynamic behavior. Appl Mech Rev 43:S96, 1990.
5. Taylor KE, Glagov S, Zarins CK: Preservation and structural adaptation of endothelium over experimental foam cell lesions. Arteriosclerosis 9:881, 1989.
6. Tsao CH, Glagov S: Basal endothelial attachment: Tenacity at cytoplasmic dense zone in the rabbit aorta. Lab Invest 23:520, 1970.
7. Jaffe EA: Biology of Endothelial Cells. Boston, Martinus Nijhoff, 1984.
8. Cines, DB, Pollak ES, Buck CA, et al: Endothelial cells in physiology and in the pathophysiology of vascular disorders. Blood 91:3527, 1998.
9. Traub O, Berk BC: Laminar shear stress: Mechanisms by which endothelial cells transduce an atheroprotective force. Arterioscler Thromb Vasc Biol 18:677, 1998.
10. Clowes AW, Clowes MM, Reidy MA: Kinetics of cellular proliferation after arterial injury: III. Endothelial and smooth muscle growth in chronically denuded vessels. Lab Invest 54:295, 1986.
11. Clowes AW, Reidy MA: Prevention of stenosis after vascular reconstruction: Pharmacological control of intimal hyperplasia—a review. J Vasc Surg 13:885, 1991.
12. Ross R, Glomset JA: The pathogenesis of atherosclerosis. N Engl J Med 295:369, 1976.
13. Zarins CK, Taylor KE, Bomberger RA, et al: Endothelial integrity at aortic ostial flow dividers. Scanning Electron Microsc 3:249, 1980.
14. Reidy MA: Biology of disease: A reassessment of endothelial injury and arterial lesion formation. Lab Invest 53:513, 1985.
15. Chidi CC, Klein L, DePalma R: Effect of regenerated endothelium on collagen content in the injured artery. Surg Gynecol Obstet 148:839, 1979.
16. Falcone DJ, Hajjar DP, Minick CR: Lipoprotein and albumin accumulation in reendothelialized and deendothelialized aorta. Am J Pathol 114:112, 1984.
17. Faggiotto A, Ross R: Studies of hypercholesterolemia in the nonhuman primate: II. Fatty streak conversion to fibrous plaque. Arteriosclerosis 4:341, 1984.
18. DiCorleto PE, Bowen-Pope DF: Cultured endothelial cells produce a platelet-derived growth factor–like protein. Proc Natl Acad Sci U S A 80:1919, 1983.
19. Bevilacqua MP, Pober JS, Majeau GR, et al: Interleukin 1 (IL-1) induces biosynthesis and cell surface expression of procoagulant activity in human vascular endothelial cells. J Exp Med 160:618, 1984.
20. Einhorn S, Eldor A, Vladavsky I, et al: Production and characterization of interferon from endothelial cells. J Cell Physiol 122:200, 1985.
21. Whatley R, Zimmerman G, McIntyre T, Prescott S: Lipid metabolism and signal transduction in endothelial cells. Prog Lipid Res 29:45, 1990.
22. Gimbrone MA Jr, Resnick N, Nagel T, et al: Hemodynamics, endothelial gene expression, and atherogenesis. Ann N Y Acad Sci 811:1, 1997.
23. Hajjar DP, Pomerantz KB: Signal transduction in atherosclerosis: Integration of cytokines and the eicosanoid network. FASEB J 6:2933, 1992.
24. Clark JM, Glagov S: Structural integration of the arterial wall: I. Relationships and attachments of medial smooth muscle cells in normally distended and hyperdistended aortas. Lab Invest 40:587, 1979.
25. Gay S, Miller EJ: Collagen in the Physiology and Pathology of Connective Tissue. Stuttgart, New York, Gustav Fischer, 1978.
26. Clark JM, Glagov S: Transmural organization of the arterial wall: The lamellar unit revisited. Arteriosclerosis 5:19, 1985.
27. Wolinsky H, Glagov S: A lamellar unit of aortic medial structure and function in mammals. Circ Res 20:99, 1967.
28. Fischer GM, Llaurado JG: Collagen and elastin content in canine arteries from functionally different vascular beds. Circ Res 19:3984, 1966.
29. Pomerantz K, Hajjar D: Eicosanoids in regulation of arterial smooth muscle cell phenotype, proliferative capacity, and cholesterol metabolism. Arteriosclerosis 9:413, 1989.
30. Davis HR, Runyon-Hass A, Zarins CK, et al: Interactive arterial effects of hypertension and hyperlipidemia. Fed Proc 43:711, 1984.

31. Lyon RT, Zarins CK, Glagov S: Artery wall motion proximal and distal to stenoses. Fed Proc 44:1136, 1985.
32. Leung DYM, Glagov S, Mathews MB: Cyclic stretching stimulates synthesis of matrix components by arterial smooth muscle cells in vitro. Science 191:475, 1976.
33. Bomberger RA, Zarins CK, Glagov S: Medial injury and hyperlipidemia in development of aneurysms or atherosclerotic plaques. Surg Forum 31:338, 1980.
34. Wolinski H, Glagov S: Structural basis for the static mechanical properties of the aortic media. Circ Res 14:400, 1964.
35. Crawford T, Levene CI: Medial thinning in atheroma. J Pathol 66:19, 1953.
36. Wolinsky H, Glagov S: Nature of species differences in the medial distribution of aortic vasa vasorum in mammals. Circ Res 20:409, 1967.
37. Heistad DD, Marcus ML, Law EG, et al: Regulation of blood flow to the aortic media in dogs. J Clin Invest 62:133, 1978.
38. Glagov S, Bassiouny HS, Giddens DP, Zarins CK: Pathobiology of plaque modeling and complication. Surg Clin North Am 7:545, 1995.
39. Glagov S: Intimal hyperplasia, vascular modeling and the restenosis problem. Circulation 8:2888, 1994.
40. Wolinsky H, Glagov S: Zonal differences in modeling of the mammalian aortic media during growth. Fed Proc 26:357, 1967.
41. Leung DYM, Glagov S, Mathews MB: Elastin and collagen accumulation in rabbit ascending aorta and pulmonary trunk during postnatal growth: Correlation of cellular synthetic response with medial tension. Circ Res 41:316, 1977.
42. Wolinsky H: Long-term effects of hypertension on the rat aortic wall and their relation to concurrent aging changes. Circ Res 30:301, 1972.
43. Masawa N, Glagov S, Zarins CK: Quantitative morphologic study of intimal thickening at the human carotid bifurcation: I. Axial and circumferential distribution of maximum intimal thickening in asymptomatic uncomplicated plaques. Atherosclerosis 107:137, 1994.
44. Masawa N, Glagov S, Zarins CK: Quantitative morphologic study of intimal thickening at the human carotid bifurcation: II. The compensatory enlargement response and the role of the intima in tensile support. Atherosclerosis 107:147, 1994.
45. Vito RP, Choi HS, Seifferth TA, et al: Measurement of strain in soft biological tissue. *In* Hanagud S, Kamat M (eds): Developments in Theoretical and Applied Mechanics, Proceedings, Society of Engineering Science, 1990.
46. Vito RP, Whang MC, Giddens DP, et al: Stress analysis of the diseased arterial cross-section. ASME Adv Biomed Eng 17:273, 1990.
47. Thoma R: Untersuchungen über die Histogenase and Histomechanik des Gefass Systems. Stuttgart, F Enke, 1893.
48. Mulvihill DA, Harvey SC: The mechanism of the development of collateral circulation. N Engl J Med 104:1032, 1931.
49. Holman E: Problems in the dynamics of blood flow: I. Condition controlling collateral circulation in the presence of an arteriovenous fistula, following the ligation of an artery. Surgery 26:889, 1949.
50. Kamiya A, Togawa T: Adaptive regulation of wall shear stress to flow change in the canine carotid artery. Am J Physiol 239:H14, 1980.
51. Masuda H, Bassiouny HS, Glagov S, Zarins CK: Artery wall restructuring in response to increased flow. Surg Forum 40:285, 1989.
52. Langille BL, O'Donnell F: Reductions in arterial diameter produced by chronic decreases in blood flow are endothelium-dependent. Science 231:405, 1986.
53. Pohl U, Holtz J, Busse R, Bassenge E: Crucial role of endothelium in the vasodilator response to increased flow in vivo. Hypertension 8:37, 1986.
54. Hull SSJ, Kaiser L, Jaffe MD, Sparks HVJ: Endothelium-dependent flow-induced dilatation of canine femoral and saphenous arteries. Blood Vessels 23:183, 1986.
55. Rubanyi GM, Romero CJ, Vanhoutte PM: Flow induced release of endothelium-derived relaxing factor. Am J Physiol 250:H1145, 1986.
56. Furchgott RF: Role of endothelium in responses of vascular smooth muscle. Circ Res 53:557, 1983.
57. Koller S, Sun D, Huang A, Kaley G: Corelease of nitric oxide and prostaglandins mediates flow-dependent dilation of rat gracilis muscle arterioles. Am J Physiol 267:H326, 1994.
58. Davies PF: Flow-mediated endothelial mechanotransduction. Physiol Rev 75:519, 1995.
59. Cooke JP, Rossitch EJ, Andon NA, et al: Flow activates an endothelial potassium channel to release an endogenous nitrovasodilator. J Clin Invest 88:1663, 1991.
60. Holtz J, Fostermann U, Pohl U, et al: Flow-dependent, endothelium-mediated dilatation of epicardial coronary arteries in conscious dogs: Effects of cyclooxygenase inhibition. J Cardiovasc Pharmacol 6:1161, 1984.
61. Miller VM, Burnett JCJ: Modulation of NO and endothelin by chronic increases in blood flow in canine femoral arteries. Am J Physiol 263:H103, 1992.
62. Tronc F, Wassef M, Esposito B, et al: Role of NO in flow-induced remodeling of the rabbit common carotid artery. Arterioscler Thromb Vasc Biol 16:1256, 1996.
63. Guzman RJ, Abe K, Zarins CK: Flow-induced arterial enlargement is uninhibited by suppression of nitric oxide synthase activity in vivo. Surgery 122:273, 1997.
64. Glagov S, Weisenberg E, Zarins CK, et al: Compensatory enlargement of human atherosclerotic coronary arteries. N Engl J Med 316:1371, 1987.
65. Glagov S, Bassiouny HS, Giddens DP Zarins CK: Intimal thickening: Morphogenesis, functional significance and detection. J Vasc Invest 1:2, 1995.
66. Glagov S, Zarins CK, Masawa N, et al: Mechanical functional role of non-atherosclerotic intimal thickening. Front Med Biol Eng 5:37, 1993.
67. Wilens SL: The nature of diffuse intimal thickening of arteries. Am J Pathol 27:825, 1951.
68. Movat HZ, More TH, Haust MD: The diffuse intimal thickening of the human aorta with aging. Am J Pathol 34:1023, 1958.
69. Tejada C, Strong JP, Montenegro MR, et al: Distribution of coronary and aortic atherosclerosis by geographic location, race and sex. Lab Invest 18:5009, 1968.
70. Glagov S, Bassiouny H, Masawa N, et al: Induction and composition of intimal thickening and atherosclerosis. *In* Boccalon H (ed): Vascular Medicine. Paris, Elsevier Science Publishers, 1993, pp 13–18.
71. Tracy RE, Kissling GE: Age and fibroplasia as preconditions for atheronecrosis in human coronary arteries. Arch Pathol Lab Med 111:957, 1987.
72. McGill HC Jr: Atherosclerosis: Problems in pathogenesis. *In* Paoletti R, Gotto AM (eds): Atherosclerosis Reviews. New York, Raven Press, 1977, pp 27–65.
73. Taylor KE, Glagov S, Zarins CK: Preservation and structural adaptation of endothelium over experimental foam cell lesions. Arteriosclerosis 9:881, 1989.
74. Faggiotto A, Ross R: Studies of hypercholesterolemia in the nonhuman primate: II. Fatty streak conversion to fibrous plaque. Arteriosclerosis 4:341, 1984.
75. Stary HO: The intimal macrophage in atherosclerosis. Artery 8:205, 1980.
76. Paterson JC: Vascularization and haemorrhage of the intima of arteriosclerotic coronary arteries. Arch Pathol 22:312, 1936.
77. Rifkin RD, Parisi HF, Follard E: Coronary calcification in the diagnosis of coronary artery disease. Am J Cardiol 44:141, 1979.
78. Glagov S, Eckner FAO, Lev M: Controlled pressure fixation apparatus for hearts. AMA Arch Pathol 76:640, 1963.
79. Zarins CK, Zatina MA, Glagov S: Correlation of postmortem angiography with pathologic anatomy: Quantitation of atherosclerotic lesions. *In* Bond MG, Insull W Jr, Glagov S, et al (eds): Clinical Diagnosis of Atherosclerosis. New York, Springer-Verlag, 1983, pp 283–303.
80. Bond MG, Adams MR, Bullock BC: Complicating factors in evaluating coronary artery atherosclerosis. Artery 9:21, 1981.
81. Beere PA, Glagov S, Zarins CK: Experimental atherosclerosis at the carotid bifurcation of the cynomolgus monkey. Atherosclerosis Thromb 12:1245, 1992.
82. Armstrong ML, Heistad DD, Marcus MI, et al: Structural and hemodynamic responses of peripheral arteries of macaque monkeys to atherogenic diet. Arteriosclerosis 5:336, 1985.
83. Holvoet P, Theilmeier G, Shivalkar B, et al: LDL hypercholesterolemia is associated with accumulation of oxidized LDL, atherosclerotic plaque growth, and compensatory vessel enlargement in coronary arteries of miniature pigs. Arterioscler Thromb Vasc Biol 18:415, 1998.
84. Clarkson TB, Prichard RW, Morgan TM, et al: Remodeling of coronary arteries in human and nonhuman primates. JAMA 271:289, 1994.

85. Zarins CK, Weisenberg E, Kolettis G, et al: Differential enlargement of artery segments in response to enlarging atherosclerotic plaques. J Vasc Surg 7:386, 1988.
86. Losordo DW, Rosenfield K, Kaufman J, et al: Focal compensatory enlargement of human arteries in response to progressive atherosclerosis: In vivo documentation using intravascular ultrasound. Circulation 9:2570, 1994.
87. Vavuranakis M, Stefanadis C, Toutouzas K, et al: Impaired compensatory coronary artery enlargement in atherosclerosis contributes to the development of coronary artery stenosis in diabetic patients: An in vivo intravascular ultrasound study. Eur Heart J 18:1090, 1997.
88. Nakamura Y, Takemori H, Shiraishi K, Inoki I, et al: Compensatory enlargement of angiographically normal coronary segments in patients with coronary artery disease: In vivo documentation using intravascular ultrasound. Angiology 47:775, 1996.
89. Masawa N, Glagov S, Bassiouny H, Zarins CK: Intimal thickness normalizes mural tensile stress in regions of increased intimal area and artery size. Arteriosclerosis 8:621a, 1988.
90. Bonithon-Kopp C, Touboul PJ, Berr C, et al: Factors of carotid arterial enlargement in a population aged 59 to 71 years: The EVA study. Stroke 27:654, 1996.
91. Crouse JR, Goldbourt U, Evans G, et al: Risk factors and segment-specific carotid arterial enlargement in the Atherosclerosis Risk in Communities (ARIC) cohort. Stroke 27:69, 1996.
92. Blair JM, Glagov S, Zarins CK: Mechanism of superficial femoral artery adductor canal stenosis. Surg Forum 41:359, 1990.
93. Pasterkamp G, Borst C, Post MJ, et al: Atherosclerotic arterial remodeling in the superficial femoral artery: Individual variation in local compensatory enlargement response. Circulation 93:1818, 1996.
94. Zarins CK, Xu CP, Glagov S: Clinical correlations of atherosclerosis: Aortic disease. *In* Fuster V (ed): Syndromes of Atherosclerosis: Correlations of Clinical Imaging and Pathology. Armonk, NY, Futura Publishing, 1996, pp 33–42.
95. Zarins CK, Xu CP, Glagov S: Aneurysmal and occlusive atherosclerosis of the human abdominal aorta. J Vasc Surg 18:526, 1993.
96. Zarins CK, Zatina MA, Giddens DP, et al: Shear stress regulation of artery lumen diameter in experimental atherogenesis. J Vasc Surg 5:413, 1987.
97. Birnbaum Y, Fishbein MC, Luo H, et al: Regional remodeling of atherosclerotic arteries: A major determinant of clinical manifestations of disease. J Am Coll Cardiol 30:1149, 1997.
98. Wong CB: Atherosclerotic arterial remodeling in the superficial femoral artery: Individual variation in local compensatory enlargement response. Circulation 95:279, 1997.
99. Keren G: Compensatory enlargement, remodeling, and restenosis. Adv Exp Med Biol 430:187, 1997.
100. Smits PC, Bos L, Quarles van Ufford MA, et al: Shrinkage of human coronary arteries is an important determinant of de novo atherosclerotic luminal stenosis: An in vivo intravascular ultrasound study. Heart 79:143, 1998.
101. Strong JP, Eggen DA: Risk factors and atherosclerotic lesions. *In* Jones RJ (ed): Atherosclerosis. II. New York, Springer-Verlag, 1970, pp 355–364.
102. Wolfe PA, Kannel WB, Verter J: Epidemiologic appraisal of hypertension and stroke risk. *In* Guthrie GP Jr, Kotchen TA (eds): Hypertension and the Brain. Mt. Kisco, NY, Futura Publishing Company, 1984, pp 221–246.
103. Greenhalgh RM: Biochemical abnormalities and smoking in arterial ischemia. *In* Bergan JJ, Yao JST (eds): Gangrene and Severe Ischemia of the Lower Extremities. New York, Grune & Stratton, 1978, pp 39–60.
104. Glagov S: Hemodynamic risk factors: Mechanical stress, mural architecture, medial nutrition and the vulnerability of arteries to atherosclerosis. *In* Wissler RW, Geer JC (eds): The Pathogenesis of Atherosclerosis. Baltimore, Williams & Wilkins, 1972, pp 164–199.
105. Texon M: The hemodynamic concept of atherosclerosis. Bull N Y Acad Med 36:263, 1960.
106. Glagov S, Rowley DA, Kohut R: Atherosclerosis of human aorta and its coronary and renal arteries. Arch Pathol Lab Med 72:558, 1961.
107. Ravensbergen J, Ravensbergen JW, Krijger JK, et al: Localizing role of hemodynamics in atherosclerosis in several human vertebrobasilar junction geometries. Arterioscler Thromb Vasc Biol 18:693, 1998.
108. Fry DL: Acute vascular endothelial changes associated with increased blood velocity gradients. Circ Res 22:165, 1968.
109. Bassiouny HS, Lieber BB, Giddens DP, et al: Quantitative inverse correlation of wall shear stress with experimental intimal thickening. Surg Forum 39:328, 1988.
110. Zarins CK, Giddens DP, Bharadvaj BK, et al: Carotid bifurcation atherosclerosis: Quantitative correlation of plaque localization with flow velocity profiles and wall shear stress. Circ Res 53:502, 1983.
111. Ku DN, Giddens DP, Zarins CK, et al: Pulsatile flow and atherosclerosis in the human carotid bifurcation: Positive correlation between plaque location and low and oscillating shear stress. Arteriosclerosis 5:293, 1985.
112. Friedman MH, Hutchins GM, Bargeron CB, et al: Correlation between intimal thickness and fluid shear in human arteries. Atherosclerosis 39:425, 1981.
113. Caro CG, Fitz-Gerald JM, Schroter RC: Atheroma and arterial wall shear: Observation, correlation and proposal of a shear dependent mass transfer mechanism for atherogenesis. Proc R Soc Lond 117:109, 1971.
114. Robertson AJ Jr: Oxygen requirements of the human arterial intima in atherogenesis. Prog Biochem Pharmacol 4:305, 1968.
115. Singh TM, Zhuang YJ, Masuda H, Zarins CK: Intimal hyperplasia in response to reduction of wall shear stress. Surg Forum 48:445, 1997.
116. Talukder N, Giddens DP, Vito RP: Quantitative flow visualization studies in a carotid artery bifurcation model. *In* 1983 Biomechanics Symposium, Applied Mechanics Division, Vol. 56; and Fluids Engineering Division, Vol. 1. New York, American Society of Mechanical Engineers, 1983, pp 165–168.
117. Tsao R, Jones SA, Giddens DP, et al: Measurement of particle residence time and particle acceleration in an arterial model by an automatic particle tracking system. Proceedings of the 20th International Congress on High Speed Photography and Photonics, September 21–25, 1992, Victoria, BC, Canada.
118. Gerrity RG, Goss JA, Soby L: Control of monocyte recruitment by chemotactic factor(s) in lesion-prone areas of swine aorta. Arteriosclerosis 5:55, 1985.
119. Parmentier EM, Morton WA, Petschek HE: Platelet aggregate formation in a region of separated blood flow. Phys Fluids 20:2012, 1981.
120. Fox JA, Hugh AE: Static zones in the internal carotid artery: Correlation with boundary layer separation and stasis in model flows. Br J Radiol 43:370, 1976.
121. Fry DL: Hemodynamic forces in atherogenesis. *In* Scheinberg P (ed): Cerebrovascular Disease. New York, Raven Press, 1976, pp 77–95.
122. DeKeulenaer GW, Chappell DC, Ishizaka N, et al: Oscillatory and steady laminar shear stress differentially affect human endothelial redox state: Role of a superoxide-producing NADH oxidase. Circ Res 82:1094, 1998.
123. Nerem RM, Levesque MJ, Cornhill JF: Vascular endothelial morphology as an indicator of the pattern of blood flow. J Biomech Eng 103:171, 1981.
124. Clark JM, Glagov S: Luminal surface of distended arteries by scanning electron microscopy: Eliminating configurational artifacts. Br J Exp Pathol 57:129, 1976.
125. Dewey CF, Bussolari SR, Gimbrone MA, et al: The dynamic response of vascular endothelial cells to fluid shear stress. J Biomech Eng 103:177, 1981.
126. Fry DL: Responses of the arterial wall to certain physical factors. Ciba Found Symp 12:93, 1973.
127. Ziegler T, Bouzourene K, Harrison VJ, et al: Influence of oscillatory and unidirectional flow environments on the expression of endothelin and nitric oxide synthase in cultured endothelial cells. Arterioscler Thromb Vasc Biol 18:686, 1998.
128. Chappell DC, Varner SE, Nerem RM, et al: Oscillatory shear stress stimulates adhesion molecule expression in cultured human endothelium. Circ Res 82:532, 1998.
129. Bassiouny HS, Lee DC, Zarins CK, Glagov S: Low diurnal heart rate variability inhibits experimental carotid stenosis. Surg Forum 46:334, 1995.
130. Davies PF, Remuzzi A, Gordon EJ, et al: Turbulent fluid shear stress induces vascular endothelial cell turnover in vitro. Proc Natl Acad Sci U S A 83:2114, 1986.
131. Gutstein WH, Farrell GA, Armellini C: Blood flow disturbance and endothelial cell injury in pre-atherosclerotic swine. Lab Invest 29:134, 1973.
132. Bharadvaj BK, Mabon RF, Giddens DP: Steady flow in a model of the human carotid bifurcation: Part II. Laser Doppler anemometer measurements. J Biomech Eng 15:363, 1982.
133. Ku DN, Giddens DP: Pulsatile flow in a model carotid bifurcation. Arteriosclerosis 3:31, 1983.

134. Ku DN, Zarins CK, Giddens DP, et al: Reduced atherogenesis distal to stenosis despite turbulence and hypertension (Abstract). Circulation 74(Suppl II):457, 1986.
135. Khalifa AMA, Giddens DP: Characterization and evolution of poststenotic flow disturbances. J Biomech 14:279, 1981.
136. Coutard M, Osborne-Pellegrin MJ: Decreased dietary lipid deposition in spontaneous lesions distal to a stenosis in the rat caudal artery. Artery 12:82, 1983.
137. Kannel WB, Schwartz MJ, McNamara PM: Blood pressure and risk of coronary heart disease: The Framingham study. Dis Chest 56:43, 1969.
138. Hollander W, Madoff I, Paddock J, et al: Aggravation of atherosclerosis by hypertension in a subhuman primate model with coarctation of the aorta. Circ Res 38(Suppl 2):63, 1976.
139. McGill HC Jr, Carey KD, McMahan CA, et al: Effects of two forms of hypertension on atherosclerosis in the hyperlipidemic baboon. Arteriosclerosis 5:481, 1985.
140. Folkow BL: Physiological aspects of primary hypertension. Physiol Rev 62:347, 1982.
141. Lyon RT, Runyon-Hass A, Davis HR, et al: Protection from atherosclerotic lesion formation by inhibition of artery wall motion. J Vasc Surg 5:59, 1987.
142. Bomberger RA, Zarins CK, Taylor KE, et al: Effect of hypotension on atherogenesis and aortic wall composition. J Surg Res 28:402, 1980.
143. Zarins CK, Bomberger RA, Taylor KE, et al: Artery stenosis inhibits regression of diet-induced atherosclerosis. Surgery 88:86, 1980.
144 Xu C-P, Glagov S, Zatina MA, Zarins CK: Hypertension sustains plaque progression despite reduction of hypercholesterolemia. Hypertension 18:123, 1991.
145. Tropea BI, Schwarzacher S, Chang A, et al: Reduction of artery wall motion inhibits plaque formation. Surg Forum 47:350–35, 1996.
146. Suzuki K: Experimental studies on morphogenesis of arteriosclerosis, with special reference to relation between hemodynamic change and developments of cellulofibrous intimal thickening and atherosclerosis. Gunma J Med Sci 16:185, 1967.
146a. Lyon RT, Davis HR, Runyon-Hass A, Glagov S: Does relief of critical arterial stenosis accelerate distal atherosclerosis? J Vasc Surg 30:191, 1996.
147. Ku DN, Glagov S, Moore JE, Zarins CK: Flow patterns in the abdominal aorta under simulated postprandial and exercise conditions: An experimental study. J Vasc Surg 9:309, 1989.
148. Giddens EM, Giddens DP, White SS, et al: Exercise flow conditions eliminate stasis at vascular graft anastomoses. Proceedings of the Third Mid-Atlantic Conference in Biofluid Mechanics. New York, New York University Press, 1990, pp 255–267.
149. Taylor CA, Tropea BI, Hughes TJR, Zarins CK: Effect of graded exercise on aortic wall shear stress. Surg Forum 46:331, 1995.
150. Bassiouny HS, Zarins CK, Choi E, et al: Hemodynamic stress and experimental aortoiliac atherosclerosis. J Vasc Surg 19:426, 1994.
151. Taylor CA, Hughes TJR, Zarins CK: Computational investigations in vascular disease. Computers in Physics 10:224, 1996.
152. Schalet BJ, Taylor CA, Harris EJ, et al: Quantitative assessment of human aortic blood flow during exercise. Surg Forum 48:359, 1997.
153. Taylor CA, Hughes TJR, Zarins CK: Finite element modeling of blood flow in arteries. Int Assoc Computational Mechanics "Expressions" 3:4, 1997.
154. Jones SA, Giddens DP, Loth F, Zet al: In-vivo measurements of blood flow velocity profiles in canine ilio femoral anastomotic bypass grafts. J Biomech Eng 119:30, 1997.
155. Bassiouny HS, Davis H, Masawa N, et al: Critical carotid stenoses: Morphologic and biochemical similarity of symptomatic and asymptomatic plaques. J Vasc Surg 9:202, 1989.
156. Tang TD, Giddens DP, Zarins CK, Glagov S: Velocity profile and wall shear measurements in a model human coronary artery. ASME Adv Biomed Eng 17:261, 1990.
157. Klocke FJ, Mates RE, Canty JM, et al: Coronary pressure-flow relationships: Controversial issues and probable implications. Circ Res 56:310, 1985.
158. Granata L, Olsson RA, Huvos A, et al: Coronary inflow and oxygen usage following cardiac sympathetic nerve stimulation in unanesthetized dogs. Circ Res 16:114, 1965.
159. Ku DN, Giddens DP: Pulsatile flow in a model carotid bifurcation. Arteriosclerosis 3:31, 1983.
160. Beere PA, Glagov S, Zarins CK: Retarding effect of lowered heart rate on coronary atherosclerosis. Science 226:180, 1984.
161. Bassiouny HS, Zarins CK, Hovanessian A, Glagov S: Heart rate and experimental carotid atherosclerosis. Surg Forum 48:373, 1992.
162. Dyer AR, Persky V, Stamler J, et al: Heart rate as a prognostic factor for coronary heart disease and mortality: Findings in three Chicago epidemiologic studies. Am J Epidemiol 112:736, 1980.
163. Williams PT, Wood PD, Haskell WL, et al: The effects of running mileage and duration on plasma lipoprotein levels. JAMA 247: 2674, 1982.
164. Wolinsky H, Glagov S: Comparison of abdominal and thoracic aortic medial structure in mammals: Deviation from the usual pattern in man. Circ Res 25:677, 1969.
165. Guyton AC: Textbook of Medical Physiology, 2nd ed. Philadelphia, WB Saunders, 1961, p 356.
166. Moore JE, Xu CP, Glagov S, et al: Fluid wall shear stress measurements in a model of the human abdominal aorta: Oscillatory behavior and relationship to atherosclerosis. Atherosclerosis 110:225, 1994.
167. Gordon T, Kannel WB: Predisposition to atherosclerosis in the head, heart and legs: The Framingham Study. JAMA 221:661, 1972.
168. Winniford MD, Wheelan KR, Kremers MS, et al: Smoking-induced coronary vasoconstriction in patients with atherosclerotic coronary artery disease: Evidence for adrenergically mediated alterations in coronary artery tone. Circulation 73:662, 1986.
169. Caro CG, Fish PJ, Jay M, et al: Influence of vasoactive agents on arterial hemodynamics: Possible relevance to atherogenesis. Abstr Biorheol 23:197, 1986.
170. Balaji MR, DeWeese JA: Adductor canal outlet syndrome. JAMA 245:167, 1981.
171. Ross R: The pathogenesis of atherosclerosis—an update. N Engl J Med 314:488, 1986.
172. Benditt EP, Barrett T, McDougall JK: Viruses in the etiology of atherosclerosis. Proc Natl Acad Sci U S A 80:6388, 1983.
173. Caro CG: Transport of material between blood and wall in arteries. Ciba Found Symp 12:127, 1973.
174. Ross R, Harker L: Hyperlipidemia and atherosclerosis. Science 193:1094, 1976.
175. Bomberger RA, Zarins CK, Glagov S: Subcritical arterial stenosis enhances distal atherosclerosis (Resident Research Award). J Surg Res 30:205, 1981.
176. Davis HR, Runyon-Hass A, Zarins CK, et al: Interactive arterial effects of hypertension and hyperlipidemia. Fed Proc 43:711, 1984.
177. Cozzi PJ, Lyon RT, Davis HR, et al: Aortic wall metabolism in relation to susceptibility and resistance to experimental atherosclerosis. J Vasc Surg 7:706, 1988.
178. Malinow MR: Experimental models of atherosclerosis regression. Atherosclerosis 48:105, 1983.
179. Wissler RW, Vesselinovitch D: Combined effects of cholestyramine and probucol on regression of atherosclerosis in rhesus monkey aortas. Appl Pathol 1:89, 1983.
180. Stary HC: Regression of atherosclerosis in primates. Virchows Arch 383:117, 1979.
181. Clarkson TB, Bond MG, Bullock BC, et al: A study of atherosclerosis regression in *Macaca mulatta*: V. Changes in abdominal aorta and carotid and coronary arteries from animals with atherosclerosis induced for 38 months and then regressed for 24 or 48 months at plasma cholesterol concentrations of 300 or 200 mg/dl. Exp Mol Pathol 41:96, 1984.
182. Daoud AS, Jarmolych J, Augustyn JM, et al: Sequential morphologic studies of regression of advanced atherosclerosis. Arch Pathol Lab Med 105:233, 1981.
183. Blankenhorn DH, Nessim SA, Johnson BL, et al: Beneficial effects of combined colestipol-niacin therapy on coronary atherosclerosis and coronary venous bypass grafts. JAMA 257:3233, 1987.
184. Brown G, Albert JJ, Fisher LD, et al: Regression of coronary artery disease as a result of intensive lipid-lowering therapy in men with high levels of apolipoprotein B. N Engl J Med 323:1290, 1990.
185. Buchwald H, Varco RL, Matts PJ, et al: Effect of partial ileal bypass surgery on mortality and morbidity from coronary heart disease in patients with hypercholesterolemia: Report of the Program on the Surgical Control of the Hyperlipidemias (POSCH). N Engl J Med 323:946, 1990.
186. Barndt R, Blankenhorn DH, Crawford DW, et al: Regression and progression of early femoral atherosclerosis in treated hyperlipoproteinemic patients. Ann Intern Med 86:139, 1977.
187. Zarins CK, Zatina MA, Glagov S: Correlation of postmortem angiog-

raphy with pathologic anatomy: Quantitation of atherosclerotic lesions. *In* Bond MG, Insull W Jr, Glagov S, et al (eds): Clinical Diagnosis of Atherosclerosis: Quantitative Methods of Evaluation. New York, Springer-Verlag, 1983, pp 283–306.
188. Zarins CK, Glagov S, Wissler, RW, Vesselinovitch D: Aneurysm formation in experimental atherosclerosis: Relationship to plaque evolution. J Vasc Surg 12:246, 1990.
189. Zarins CK, Xu C-P, Glagov S: Aneurysmal enlargement of the aorta during regression of experimental atherosclerosis. J Vasc Surg 15:90, 1992.
190. Glagov S, Bassiouny HS, Sakaguchi Y, et al: Mechanical determinants of plaque modeling, remodeling and disruption. Atherosclerosis 131:S13, 1997.
191. Falk E, Shah P, Fuster V: Coronary plaque disruption. Circulation 92:657, 1995.
192. Fuster V, Badimon L, Badimon IJ, Chesebro JH: The pathogenesis of coronary artery disease and the acute coronary syndromes, parts I and II. N Engl J Med 326:242, 1992.
193. Glagov S, Zarins CK, Giddens DP, et al: Atherosclerosis: What is the nature of the plaque? *In* Strandness DE Jr, Didisheim P, Clowes AW, et al (eds): Vascular Diseases: Current Research and Clinical Applications. Orlando, Fla, Grune & Stratton, 1987, pp 15–33.
194. Bassiouny HS, Sakaguchi Y, Mikucki SA, et al: Juxtaluminal location of plaque necrosis and neoformation in symptomatic carotid stenosis. J Vasc Surg 26:585, 1997.
195. Felton CV, Crook D, Davies MJ, Oliver MF: Relation of plaque lipid composition and morphology ro the stability of human aortic plaques. Arterioscler Thromb Vasc Biol 17:1337, 1997.
196. Gertz SD, Roberts WC: Hemodynamic shear force rupture of coronary arterial atherosclerotic plaques. Am J Cardiol 66:1368, 1990.
197. Campa JS, Greenhalgh RM, Powell JT: Elastin degradation in abdominal aortic aneurysms. Atherosclerosis 65:13, 1987.
198. Dobrin PB, Baker WH, Gley WC: Elastolytic and collagenolytic studies of arteries: Implications for the mechanical properties of aneurysms. Arch Surg 119:405, 1984.
199. Menashi S, Campa JS, Greenhalgh RM, Powell JT: Collagen in abdominal aortic aneurysm: Typing, content and degradation. J Vasc Surg 6:578, 1987.
200. Johansen K, Koepsell T: Familial tendency for abdominal aortic aneurysm. JAMA 256:1934, 1986.
201. Bomberger RA, Zarins CK, Glagov S: Medial injury and hyperlipidemia in development of aneurysms or atherosclerotic plaques. Surg Forum 31:338, 1980.
202. Zatina MA, Zarins CK, Gewertz BL, Glagov S: Role of medial lamellar architecture in the pathogenesis of aortic aneurysms. J Vasc Surg 1:442, 1984.
203. DePalma RG, Koletsky S, Bellon EM, Insull W Jr: Failure of regression of atherosclerosis in dogs with moderated cholesterolemia. Atherosclerosis 27:297, 1977.

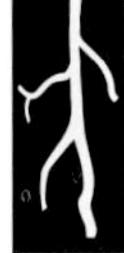

CHAPTER 19

Atherogenesis and the Medical Management of Atherosclerosis

William R. Hiatt, M.D., and
John P. Cooke, M.D., Ph.D.

Atherosclerosis is the cause of peripheral arterial disease and of vascular disease affecting the coronary, cerebral, and other vital circulations. Patients with peripheral arterial occlusive disease (PAOD) commonly present for treatment because of symptoms of intermittent claudication or critical leg ischemia. However, there is such significant overlap, in patients with PAOD, of concomitant and severe coronary and cerebrovascular disease that treatment goals need to focus on both the effects of atherosclerosis in the peripheral circulation and the systemic nature of the disease, which is associated with a much increased risk of cardiovascular events that lead to cardiovascular morbidity and mortality. Therefore, all patients presenting for treatment of their extremity atherosclerosis should have their risk factors rigorously assessed, and appropriate therapies should be instituted to decrease the risks of both peripheral progression and cardiovascular mortality. In this chapter, we discuss the risk factors for peripheral and systemic atherosclerosis, the pathogenesis of atherosclerosis, and the medical management of this disorder.

EPIDEMIOLOGIC CONSIDERATIONS

PAOD affects 12% of the general population and 20% of persons older than 70 years.[42, 75] As mentioned earlier, PAOD is a marker for systemic atherosclerosis and thus is associated with a markedly increased risk of cardiovascular events.[43] The systemic nature of this disease and the increased risk of cardiovascular events emphasize the importance of aggressive risk factor modification and of antiplatelet therapies.

Table 19–1 lists certain natural history studies that evaluated risk of all-cause and cardiovascular disease (CVD) mortality rates in patients with PAOD.[43, 106, 107, 140, 187] In all of these studies, cases of PAOD were identified using the ankle/brachial index (ABI) as a screening tool, or an other appropriate objective hemodynamic measure. Patients were then observed for the occurrence of cardiovascular events. Table 19–1 demonstrates that, on average, an age-matched control group has an all-cause mortality rate of 1.6% per year. This rate increases to 4.8% per year for patients with

TABLE 19–1. MORTALITY RISK IN PERIPHERAL ARTERIAL OCCLUSIVE DISEASE

AUTHOR (YEAR)	NO.	GROUP	ALL MORTALITY (EVENT RATE/YR) Control	PAOD	RR (95% CI)	CVD MORTALITY (EVENT RATE/YR) Control	PAOD	RR (95% CI)
Criqui (1992)	565	Men	1.7	6.2	3.1 (1.9–4.9)	0.8	4.2	5.9 (3.0–11.4)
		Women	1.2	3.3		0.4	1.8	
Vogt (1993)	1492	Women	1.1	5.4	3.1 (1.7–5.5)	0.4	3.0	4.0 (1.7–9.1)
Leng (1996)	1498	Symptomatic	2.0	3.8	1.6 (0.9–2.8)	0.7	2.7	2.7 (1.3–5.3)
		Asymptomatic	2.0	6.1	2.4 (1.6–3.7)	0.7	2.3	2.1 (1.1–3.8)
Leng (1996)	1582	All patients	2.1	4.4	1.8 (1.3–2.4)	0.1	2.4	2.3 (1.5–3.6)
Newman (1997)	1537	Men	1.5	5.3	3.0 (2.8–5.3)	0.5	2.2	3.4 (1.3–8.9)
		Women	1.3	3.8	2.7 (1.6–4.6)	0.4	1.6	3.3 (1.3–8.6)
Total/Average	6674		1.6	4.8	2.5	0.5	2.5	3.4

CI = confidence interval; CVD = cardiovascular disease; N = sample size; PAOD = peripheral arterial occlusive disease; RR = relative risk.

PAOD, a 2.5-fold increase. Cardiovascular mortality rates are similarly affected, with an overall event rate of 0.5% per year in controls and of 2.5% per year in patients with PAOD. This is a 3.4-fold increased relative risk. Importantly, women are at only slightly less risk than men, and even asymptomatic individuals have a markedly greater risk of cardiovascular events. The presence of PAOD is an *independent* risk factor for mortality, even when other known risk factors are controlled for.

This increased event rate in patients with PAOD underscores the importance of intensive medical management to reduce the risks of cardiovascular morbidity and mortality. Importantly, patients with PAOD are underrecognized by primary care physicians and thus are generally undertreated for their risk factors.[122] All vascular specialists and primary care physicians must increase their awareness of the problem and become more aggressive in this aspect of patient management.

RISK FACTORS

Table 19–2 lists the major and minor risk factors for PAOD. The major risk factors have been determined from large epidemiologic studies and are highly concordant with the risk factors for coronary and cerebrovascular disease. The minor risk factors have been determined from smaller observational studies but are important to clinicians who desire comprehensive risk assessment in this patient population. When evaluated together using multivariate modeling techniques, the following risk factors emerge as primarily important in the development and progression of PAOD: age, diabetus mellitus, current smoking status, alterations in lipid metabolism, hypertension, elevated plasma homocysteine levels, and elevated fibrinogen levels. Also, for any number of risk factors in an individual patient, the presence of cigarette smoking nearly doubles the risk of progression of PAOD, independent of other associated risk factor.[137] Further discussions of these risk factors follow.

TABLE 19–2. RISK FACTORS FOR PERIPHERAL ARTERIAL OCCLUSIVE DISEASE

Major
Age
Diabetes
Cigarette smoking
Hyperlipidemia
Hypertension
Homocysteinemia
Fibrinogenemia
Minor
Male gender
Nonwhite race
High-fat diet
Hypercoagulable states
Excessive alcohol
Asymmetric dimethylarginine (ADMA)
C-reactive protein

Age

All forms of CVD become more prevalent with age, and thus it is not surprising that PAOD is more frequent in the elderly population. In several studies, the risk of PAOD increased 1.5- to 2-fold for every 10-year increase in age.[75, 137, 186]

Diabetes Mellitus

Diabetes has been long recognized as a major risk factor for PAOD. In the Framingham Trial with 16-year follow-up, the age-adjusted risk ratio for intermittent claudication in diabetic patients, compared with controls, was five times greater for men and four times greater for women.[94–96] In other epidemiologic studies where PAOD was defined by the ABI, diabetes increased the risk approximately threefold.[75] The peripheral atherosclerosis observed in patients with diabetes is typically more distal in distribution and often more extensive. Diabetes is also associated with peripheral neuropathy and inadequate response to infections, leading to complicated and serious compromise of the lower extremities, including diabetic foot ulcers.

While diabetes is strongly associated with peripheral atherosclerosis, the degree of glycemic control, as defined by blood sugar concentration or hemoglobin A_{1c} at any given time point, has not been closely associated with the severity of the peripheral atherosclerosis.[10] Thus, diabetes is a critical risk factor for development of PAOD, particularly in conjunction with other risk factors.

Cigarette Smoking

Cigarette smoking and diabetes are generally considered to be the most potent risk factors for peripheral atherosclerosis.[97, 98, 101, 102] In general, cigarette smoking is associated with an approximately threefold increase in risk for peripheral atherosclerosis.[75, 137, 139, 186] Current smokers are at higher risk than former smokers, and the number of pack-years is associated with the severity of disease. For example, former smokers had a sevenfold greater risk of PAOD, whereas current smokers had a 16-fold increased risk.[37]

In addition to being a major risk factor for PAOD, current cigarette smoking also significantly affects PAOD outcomes. Table 19–3 lists several of these major outcomes. For example, progression from intermittent claudication to ischemic rest pain occurs significantly more frequently in patients who use tobacco than in those who do not.[80, 90, 153] Graft patency results are also significantly affected by cigarette smoking, in terms of prosthetic as well as vein conduits.[80, 138] Amputation rates are also driven by current smoking status and are approximately twice to three times those of nonsmokers.[170] Finally, patient survival is significantly worse for those who continue to smoke than for those who quit.[80]

TABLE 19–3. EFFECTS OF TOBACCO ON OUTCOMES OF PERIPHERAL ARTERIAL OCCLUSIVE DISEASE (PAOD)

CLINICAL EVENT	TOBACCO USE (%)	ABSTINENCE (%)
PAOD Clinical Progression		
Claudication to rest pain: 5-yr progression	18	0
Revascularization Procedure Success Rates		
Vein graft patency at 1 yr	70	90
"Reconstruction success"	19	81
Vein graft patency at 3 yr	50	90
Patency rate at 3 yr	78	94
Prosthetic bypass patency rate at 1 yr	65	85
Cumulative patency rate		
1–12 mo	66.7	75.4
1–2 yr	55.2	65.5
2–3 yr	52.6	63.6
3–4 yr	48.6	60.8
4–5 yr	48.6	55.7
Secondary graft patency		
1 mo	70	91
12 mo	40	75
Vein graft patency (femoropopliteal) at 2 yr	60	90
Vein/Dacron graft patency (aortofemoral) at 4 yr	75	90
Vein graft patency at 1 yr	63	84
Amputation Rates		
Amputation rate	23	10
Cumulative limb loss rate		
1–12 mo	2.7	2.0
1–2 yr	14.9	3.3
2–3 yr	22.8	6.5
3–4 yr	28.1	6.5
4–5 yr	28.1	10.9
Patient Survival		
1 yr	85	100
3 yr	40	67
5 yr	36	66

Adapted from Hirsch AT, Treat-Jacobson D, Lando HA, et al: The role of tobacco cessation, antiplatelet and lipid-lowering therapies in the treatment of peripheral arterial disease. Vasc Med 2:243–251, 1997. (Summarizes literature.)

Hyperlipidemia

Alterations in lipid metabolism are a major risk factor for all forms of atherosclerosis. Several large epidemiologic trials have conclusively shown that elevations in total cholesterol and in low-density lipoprotein (LDL) cholesterol levels and decreases in high-density lipoprotein (HDL) cholesterol levels are significantly and independently associated with cardiovascular mortality.[64, 121, 151] For example, a 1-mg/dl increase in HDL cholesterol concentration is associated with a 2% to 3% decrease in coronary artery disease (CAD) risk and a 4% to 5% decrease in CVD mortality.[64] The role of triglyceride elevations has been debated, but more recent studies have conclusively shown that elevated *fasting* levels of triglycerides are also a strong and independent predictor of ischemic heart disease and PAOD.[28, 50, 88]

In PAOD, several lipid fractions are individually important in determining the presence and progression of peripheral atherosclerosis. Independent risk factors for PAOD include elevations of total cholesterol, LDL cholesterol, triglycerides, and lipoprotein(a) [LP(a)].[75, 89, 137] Protective against PAOD are HDL cholesterol and apolipoprotein A_1 (APO A_1).[89] For every 10-mg/dl increase in total cholesterol concentration, the risk of PAOD increases approximately 10%.[75]

Elevations in LP(a) constitute a newly recognized independent risk factor for CAD and PAOD.[21, 115, 183] In studies of CAD, elevations in LP(a) increase the risk approximately twofold. In patients with PAOD, LP(a) is considered elevated when levels are above 30 mg/dl.[183] Treatment options for modifying this lipid fraction are limited, but its role in peripheral atherosclerosis is now well established (see later).

Hypertension

Hypertension is also a well-recognized risk factor for atherosclerotic diseases, particularly stroke and ischemic heart disease.[171] In patients with PAOD, hypertension increases risk approximately two to three times.[75, 137, 159, 172, 186] Hypertension has also been found to be an independent risk factor, but it is probably less important than the other ones listed earlier.[92]

Homocysteine

Alterations in homocysteine metabolism are a newly recognized, independent risk factor for all forms of atherosclerosis, particularly PAOD.[22, 34, 83, 118, 131, 173] In epidemiologic studies, elevations in homocysteine levels are strongly associated with the premature development of coronary, carotid, and peripheral atherosclerosis. The relative risk is increased approximately twofold.

Homocysteine works through a variety of putative mechanisms.[189] Homocysteine is an amino acid that can react with LDL cholesterol to form oxidized LDL cholesterol, which is often found in foam cells and early atherosclerotic lesions. Through the formation of reactive oxygen species, homocysteine can promote endothelial dysfunction, proliferation of vascular smooth muscle cells, lipid peroxidation, and, as discussed earlier, oxidation of LDL cholesterol.[189] An elevated homocysteine level is also a well-recognized risk factor for thrombophlebitis and thus promotes both venous and arterial thrombosis. All of these mechanisms accelerate the development of atherosclerosis. Elevation in homocysteine levels may be due to genetic defects of homocysteine metabolism, typically caused by cystathionine β-synthase deficiency. The homozygous form of the disease is quite rare, but it results in life-threatening manifestations of arterial and venous thrombosis at an early age. Heterozygotes have homocysteine concentrations approximately 2 to 4 times greater than those of unaffected individuals. Alterations in vitamin B_{12} metabolism are also associated with increases in homocysteine levels. Perhaps the most common cause of homocysteine elevation is dietary deficiency in B vitamins, particularly folic acid and vitamins B_6 and B_{12}.

Fibrinogen and Alterations in Blood Rheology

Elevations of fibrinogen concentration have only recently been recognized as a cardiovascular risk factor. In a meta-analysis, an elevation in fibrinogen level was associated with an approximately twofold to fourfold risk of myocardial infarction or stroke.[52] Increased blood fibrinogen level is also associated with increased blood viscosity. Thus, in patients with PAOD, increased fibrinogen (and thus increased viscosity) was an independent predictor of peripheral atherosclerosis.[49, 104] In addition to their relationships to the presence of PAOD, increased fibrinogen level and blood viscosity are associated with more severe claudication.[114] This risk factor is associated with increased viscosity and microcirculatory defects in oxygen delivery. Thus, greater fibrinogen elevations are associated with more severe claudication symptoms. The effect of treatment for increased blood viscosity and fibrinogen elevation has not yet been determined.

Hypercoagulable States

Alterations in coagulation are commonly associated with the development of venous thrombosis and thromboembolism; however, except for changes in homocysteine metabolism, hypercoagulable states have been less thoroughly evaluated in patients with PAOD. In one study, presence of the lupus anticoagulant was associated with peripheral atherosclerosis.[47] Also, markers of platelet activation, such as increases in beta-thromboglobulin levels, are associated with PAOD.[32] However, the prevalence of these abnormalities is very low, and the role of each risk factor is not fully substantiated. Therefore, there are no recommendations for routine screening for hypercoagulable states.

Alcohol

Alcohol use is well known variously to decrease and to increase risks for CVD and cardiovascular events. Taken in small amounts (less than one drink per day), ethanol is associated with increased HDL cholesterol levels, which may be protective against atherosclerosis.[169] Taken in large amounts, however (four or more drinks per day), alcohol increases blood pressure substantially and predisposes the affected person to cardiac arrhythmias. This, then, increases the risk of cardiovascular events.[142] Thus, the effects of alcohol vary widely with the level of use.

The Physician's Health Study was conducted as a primary prevention trial of the effectiveness of aspirin and antioxidants in preventing CVD in physicians. One of the findings of this study was that moderate alcohol consumption (approximately one drink per day) was associated with a slightly decreased risk of PAOD.[29]

Other Risk Factors

Several small series have identified some perhaps interesting and surprising risk factors for peripheral atherosclerosis. It has been observed that diet may be a risk factor for PAOD. For example, increased consumption of fiber-containing foods was associated with higher ABIs and increased consumption of meat products with lower ABIs.[48] In another trial, the O blood type was found to protect against the development of claudication.[60] Increased excretion of urinary albumin is an independent predictor of PAOD.[193]

In persons with CAD, markers of inflammation have been associated with the development of atherosclerosis and with plaque rupture. Elevation of C-reactive protein is a marker of systemic inflammation. In the Physician's Health Study, elevated C-reactive protein was a risk factor for the development of symptomatic PAOD and a risk factor for peripheral revascularization.[155]

The formation of nitric oxide (NO) is critical to maintaining normal endothelial function, and alterations in endothelial function are well documented in patients with atherosclerosis. In patients with PAOD, NO synthesis can be inhibited by the endogenous compound asymmetric dimethylarginine (ADMA). The levels of ADMA in patients with PAOD are directly correlated with inhibition of NO synthesis and the severity of claudication symptoms.[19] Potentially, this inhibition of NO synthesis can be reversed by dietary supplementation with L-arginine.

PATHOGENESIS OF ATHEROSCLEROSIS

Risk Factors and Atherogenesis

In Europe, the United States, and, increasingly, Asia, atherosclerosis affecting the coronary or carotid arteries is the most prevalent cause of morbidity and annual mortality. Elevated levels of serum cholesterol correlate with the clinical prevalence of atherosclerosis. Myocardial infarctions are much less common in countries where dietary intake of cholesterol and serum cholesterol levels are low than in countries where a typical Western diet is consumed and cholesterol levels are higher.[93, 103] The recent "westernization" of diets in Asia, together with the popularity of tobacco, has been associated with a dramatic increase in atherosclerotic vascular disease. In some Asian countries (e.g., the Philippines), coronary events are now the greatest cause of mortality. Other major risk factors for atherosclerotic disease are hypertension, diabetes mellitus, and family history of premature atherosclerosis. Additional determinants include sedentary lifestyle, LP(a), hyperhomocysteinemia, elevated fibrinogen levels, increased C-reactive peptide, and the constellation of metabolic abnormalities associated with insulin resistance. What follows is the authors' current view of atherogenesis. This subject is also covered, including other related aspects, in Chapters 6 and 18.

Atherosclerosis has been said to be a "response to injury" of the endothelium; however, the one or several mechanisms by which hypercholesterolemia and the other risk factors alter the endothelium have not yet been described. Recent studies suggest that there may be a common pathway by which these risk factors affect endothelial function. Experimental models of hypertension, hypercholesterolemia, diabetes mellitus, and tobacco exposure are characterized by common endothelial abnormalities: increased generation of superoxide anion and reduced bioactivity and/or synthesis of endothelium-derived NO.[143, 154, 174, 180]

Role of Endothelial Dysfunction

Aberrations in endothelial function from oxidative stress to the cells can occur within minutes to hours of exposure to noxious stimuli. Oxidative stress perturbs the cell membrane and increases endothelial permeability. Moreover, the increased endothelial elaboration of oxygen-derived free radicals activates oxidant-sensitive transcriptional proteins such as nuclear factor κB (NFκB). Activated NFκB translocates to the nucleus, where it induces expression of adhesion molecules (e.g., vascular cell adhesion molecule [VCAM-1]) and chemokines (e.g., monocyte chemoattractant peptide [MCP-1]) that participate in monocyte adhesion and infiltration (Fig. 19–1).[13, 44, 156, 179, 182] The expression of these adhesion molecules and chemokines may explain the observation that, within several days of consuming a high-cholesterol diet, monocytes adhere to the endothelium, particularly at intercellular junctions.[156] Therefore, the endothelial injury that triggers atherosclerosis may be intracellular oxidative stress (precipitated by hypercholesterolemia and other risk factors).

The monocytes migrate into the subendothelium, where they begin to accumulate lipid and become foam cells. This is the earliest event in the formation of the fatty streak. The activated monocytes (macrophages) release mitogens and chemoattractants that recruit additional macrophages and vascular smooth muscle cells into the lesion. In addition, they generate reactive oxygen species that increase oxidative stress in the vessel wall and accelerate oxidation of LDL cholesterol trapped in the subintimal space.

The oxidation of LDL particles in the subintimal space promotes foam cell formation[13, 156] because the oxidized LDL is taken up via the scavenger receptor. Unlike the receptor for native LDL, the scavenger receptor is not downregulated by intracellular cholesterol levels. Accordingly, oxidized LDL continues to be taken up by the macrophages via the scavenger receptor, with the result that the macrophages become grossly swollen with lipid, giving them a characteristic "foamy" appearance on microscopy.

As foam cells accumulate in the subendothelial space, they distort the overlying endothelium and eventually may even rupture through the endothelial surface.[156] In these areas of endothelial ulceration, platelets adhere to the vessel wall, releasing epidermal growth factor (EGF), platelet-derived growth factor (PDGF), and other mitogens and cytokines that contribute to smooth muscle cell migration and proliferation. These factors induce smooth muscle cells in the vessel wall to proliferate and to migrate into the area of the lesion. These vascular smooth muscle cells undergo a change in phenotype from "contractile" cells to "secretory" cells. These secretory vascular smooth muscle cells elaborate extracellular matrix (e.g., elastin), which transforms the lesion into a fibrous plaque.

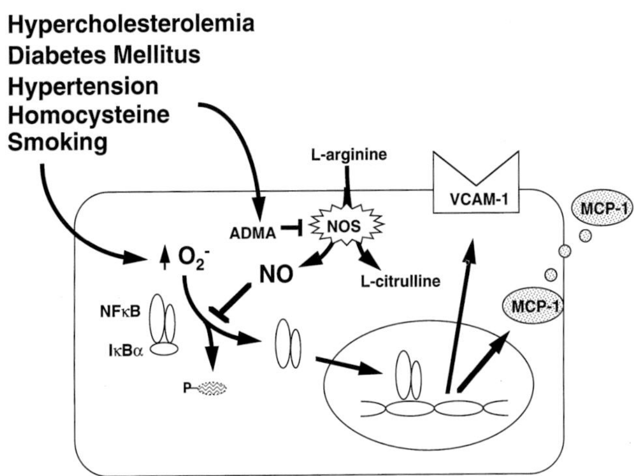

FIGURE 19–1. Atherosclerotic risk factors such as hypercholesterolemia, hypertension, tobacco use, and diabetes mellitus lead to increased free radical production and decreased nitric oxide (NO) activity in endothelial cells. This endothelial dysfunction has not only acute effects on vascular tone but also chronic effects on vessel structure. Increased superoxide anion leads to activation of nuclear factor κB (NFκB) via phosphorylation and degradation of the inhibitor protein (IκBα). NFκB is then free to translocate into the nucleus to initiate transcription of pro-atherogenic genes such as vascular cell adhesion molecule (VCAM-1) and monocyte chemoattractant peptide (MCP-1). NO can inhibit these processes by inhibiting superoxide production, directly scavenging superoxide anions, and increasing the transcription and activity of IκBα. Moreover, since NO is a paracrine factor, it can have important inhibitory effects on circulating leukocytes and underlying smooth muscle cells. NOS = nitric oxide synthase. ADMA = asymmetric dimethylarginine.

Extracellular matrix may contribute significantly to growth of the lesion. Indeed, a genetic variant of the stromelysin promoter that causes reduced degradation of extracellular matrix is associated with accelerated progression of atherosclerosis.[192] In addition to elaborating extracellular matrix, the smooth muscle cells may also become engorged with lipid to form foam cells.

The lesion grows with the recruitment of more cells, the elaboration of extracellular matrix, and the accumulation of lipid until it is transformed from a fibrous plaque to a complex one. The complex plaque typically is characterized by a fibrous cap that overlies a necrotic core. (*Necrotic* core may be a misnomer, since apoptosis undoubtedly contributes in a significant way to cell death and likely is involved in the formation of the cell-free, lipid-rich area in the interior of a complex plaque.) The necrotic core is composed of cell debris and cholesterol and contains a high concentration of the thrombogenic tissue factor, which is secreted by macrophages. In later-stage lesions, calcification may occur. Calcifying vascular cells in the vessel wall can transform into osteoblast-like cells and secrete bone proteins such as osteopontin.[146] Microscopic examination of these areas reveals a histologic appearance very similar to that of bone. Oxidized lipoprotein stimulates the elaboration of bone protein by these vascular cells. By contrast, oxidized lipoprotein reduces bone formation by osteoblasts.[146] This intriguing finding may account for the clinical observation that in some patients with atherosclerosis (typically older women), radiographs show nearly as much calcium in the aorta as in the spine.

Cellular Mechanisms That Oppose Atherogenesis

Most of the research into the pathophysiology of atherosclerosis has focused on the factors that precipitate or worsen vascular disease; however, a number of endogenous mechanisms oppose atherogenesis. HDL cholesterol may participate in reverse cholesterol transport (from the vessel to the liver), and it contains enzymes that metabolize platelet-activating factor (PAF) (i.e., paraoxonase and acetylhydrolase).[194] Tissue plasminogen activator (t-PA) is produced by endothelial cells[185] and, by inducing fibrinolysis, may reduce the accretion for thrombus onto the vessel wall. Intracellular superoxide dismutase detoxifies oxygen-derived free radicals. Endothelium-derived NO and prostacyclin (PGI_2) inhibit several processes that promote development of an atherosclerotic plaque.[39] NO and PGI_2 are vasodilators and inhibit adherence of platelets and leukocytes to the endothelium. In addition, NO and PGI_2 inhibit the proliferation of vascular smooth muscle cells and macrophages and suppress the generation of oxygen-derived free radicals. The reduction in oxidative stress turns off the oxidant-responsive genes (e.g., MCP-1 and VCAM-1) that mediate monocyte binding and infiltration into the vessel wall.[185]

It is well known that hypercholesterolemia reduces the bioactivity of endothelium-derived NO[72, 123] (see later). In parallel, the endothelium begins to generate superoxide anion.[143] In rabbit models, this increased generation of superoxide anion induced by hypercholesterolemia can be reversed by placing the animal on a low-cholesterol diet.[144] The reduction in superoxide anion generation is associated with improvement in endothelium-dependent vasodilator function. In addition to inducing generation of superoxide anion, hypercholesterolemia causes a decline in tissue glutathione levels and thus increases susceptibility to oxidative damage.[116]

Multiple mechanisms may account for the abnormalities in the L-arginine/NO pathway induced by hypercholesterolemia. These include (1) reduced availability of L-arginine, (2) abnormalities of endothelial receptor–G protein coupling, (3) decreased levels of cofactors such as tetrahydrobiopterin, (4) reduced NO synthase expression and activity, (5) increased degradation of NO by superoxide anion or oxidized lipoproteins, and (6) circulating inhibitors of NO synthase.[38] Accumulating evidence indicates that endogenous methylarginines inhibit the activity of NO synthase. One of these, ADMA, is a competitive inhibitor of NO synthase, and its level is elevated in patients who have atherosclerosis or risk factors for atherosclerosis.[17, 19] The elevation in ADMA probably explains the observation that administering L-arginine to individuals with atherosclerosis (or risk factors for atherosclerosis) restores endothelial vasodilator function and can even reduce symptoms of CAD or PAOD.[16, 35, 41, 51, 109]

Chronic L-arginine supplementation enhances vascular NO production, reduces superoxide anion generation, suppresses monocyte adherence, and inhibits (and even reverses) intimal lesion formation in hypercholesterolemic rabbits.[18, 30, 40, 181, 188] By contrast, pharmacologic inhibition of NO synthase or genetic deletion of the enzyme accelerates atherogenesis in animal models.

Plaque Vulnerability and Rupture

Plaque rupture is accepted as the major cause of acute coronary syndromes[58] and likely plays an important role in the progression of PAOD. A role for plaque rupture as a cause of acute coronary syndromes, in aortic atheroembolism, and in symptomatic CAD is well described. That plaque rupture contributes to acute exacerbations of PAOD, or to its gradual progression, is very likely but has not yet been definitively demonstrated. Plaque rupture (and subsequent thrombosis) is often asymptomatic, but it contributes to the rapid growth of lesions as the thrombus undergoes fibrosis. Histopathologic studies reveal that, at the site of a coronary thrombosis, plaque rupture is noted in two thirds of cases.[58, 184] The remaining cases appear to be due to thrombosis at the site of endothelial denudation.[184]

Areas of endothelial denudation in the coronary arteries of hypercholesterolemic rabbits are typically associated with collections of macrophages subjacent to the injured endothelium (Fig. 19–2, *left*). Moreover, in adjacent areas, single macrophages or collections of them may be observed to be emerging through microulcerations in the endothelial surface (Fig. 19–2, *right*).

A number of characteristics distinguish stable plaque from plaque that is likely to rupture or that has ruptured. A common feature of the ruptured plaque is thinning of the overlying fibrous cap, which is composed largely of vascular smooth cells and extracellular matrix. In ruptured plaques, the fibrous cap appears to be eroded at the shoulder of the lesion, where the cap meets the intima of the normal segment of the vessel wall. This is the area that is subjected to the greatest hemodynamic stress and where rupture typically occurs.[54]

Another typical feature is a large necrotic core filled with lipid and cell debris. The lipid core has a semi-fluid consistency at body temperature, which likely plays a role in plaque stability; that is, the more fluid the core is, the more mechanical stress the fibrous plaque must bear.[113] Another characteristic of the ruptured plaque is intraplaque and intraluminal thrombosis.[168] Angioscopic studies have revealed that patients with unstable angina characteristically have complex ulcerated lesions with associated thrombosis, whereas those with stable angina typically have obstructed lesions with an unperturbed endothelial surface.[164]

Finally, another common feature of ruptured plaque is intense infiltration of the plaque with macrophages (Fig. 19–3).[184] It is now evident that macrophages in the plaque play a key role in determining many of the characteristic features of vulnerable plaque and in predisposing the lesion to rupture.

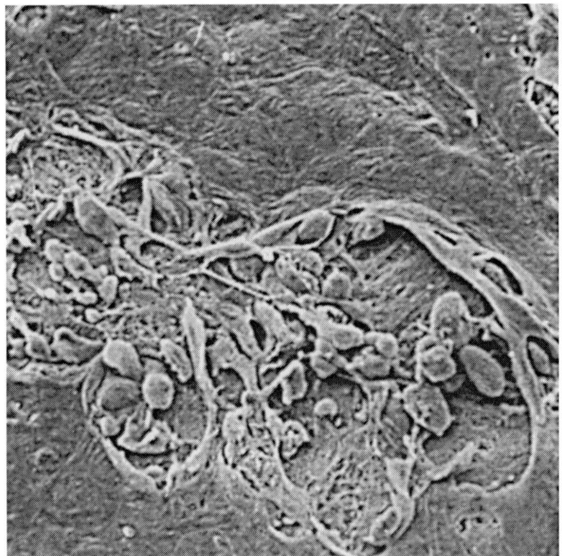
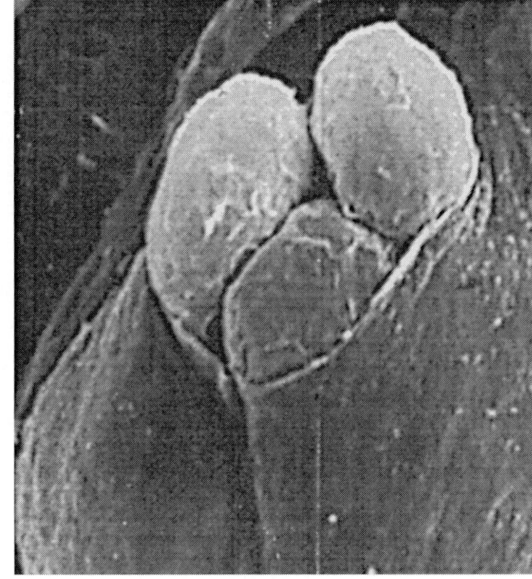

FIGURE 19–2. Scanning electron microphotographs from the coronary artery of a rabbit fed a high-cholesterol diet for 10 weeks. *Left*, Area of endothelial ulceration. *Right*, Lipid-laden macrophage, apparently emerging from the subintimal space.

Role of Macrophages

Accumulating evidence indicates that macrophages are responsible for some key features of the vulnerable plaque, including endothelial denudation, thin fibrous cap, large acellular core, and thrombogenicity of the plaque's contents. In normal vessels, the synthesis and degradation of extracellular matrix are remarkably slow, collagen turnover being measured in years.[176] In the diseased vessels, however, extracellular matrix degradation is accelerated, and this can lead to structural weakening of the fibrous cap. Intense infiltration of macrophages is invariably observed at the site of plaque rupture where the fibrous cap appears to be undermined. In addition to cathepsins, these macrophages are synthesizing abundant amounts of metalloproteinases (MMP-1, MMP-3, and MMP-9).[26, 74, 141] These MMPs degrade extracellular matrix, weakening the fibrous cap.[59, 105, 162]

In addition to increased degradation of extracellular matrix, inflammatory cells may reduce collagen synthesis by vascular smooth muscle cells. T cells in the region of the fibrous cap elaborate interferon gamma (IFN-γ), a potent inhibitor of collagen synthesis.[62] Furthermore, IFN-γ is known to induce apoptosis of vascular smooth muscle cells.[62] The vascular smooth muscle cells may also be under attack from hydrochlorous acid and peroxynitrate anion produced by the macrophages, both of which free radicals may induce apoptosis.[11, 61, 71, 85] The increased apoptosis may account for the observation that fibrous caps that have ruptured have half as many smooth muscle cells as

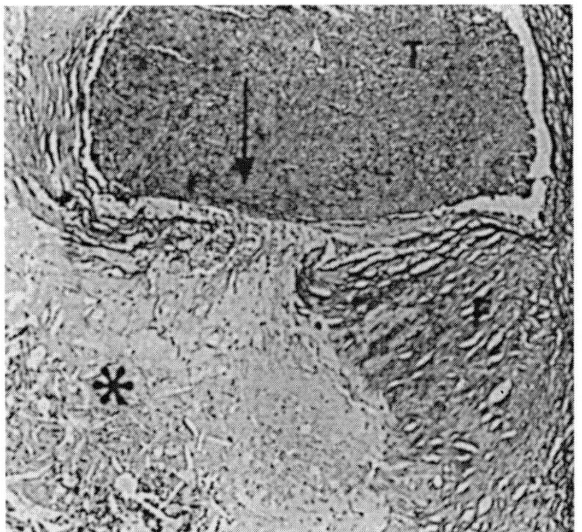

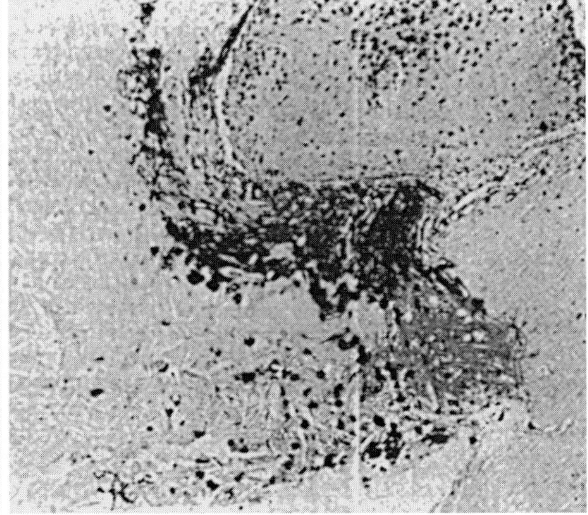

FIGURE 19–3. *Left*, A microphotograph of a cross section through a ruptured plaque in a human coronary artery. Note the thrombus in the lumen (T) and the point of plaque rupture (*arrow*). At this point, the fibrous cap appears to have been thinned, exposing the lumen to the contents of the necrotic core (*asterisk*). *Right*, An adjacent cross section has been stained using a monoclonal antibody directed at macrophage antigen. Note the intense accumulation of macrophages in the area of rupture. (From van der Wal AC, Becker AE, van der Loos CM, Das PK: Site of intimal rupture or erosion of thrombosed coronary atherosclerotic plaques is characterized by an inflammatory process irrespective of the dominant plaque morphology. Circulation 89:36–44, 1994.)

unruptured fibrous caps.[54] Macrophages contribute to the thrombotic nature of the vulnerable plaque. The macrophages in the lesion are a rich source of tissue factor, which can be found in the acellular core as well as in the vascular smooth muscle of the fibrous cap.[120, 132] Macrophage content and expression of tissue factor correlate with rupture of the human atherosclerotic plaque.[6, 111, 132] Macrophage and tissue factor constituents are greater in coronary atherectomy specimens from patients with unstable angina than in those from persons with stable angina.[6]

Role of Infection

The causative factors initiating inflammation of the fibrous cap are unknown; however, mounting circumstantial evidence implicates infection in the progression of atherosclerosis.[12, 110] There is seroepidemiologic and immunohistochemical evidence that infectious agents such as cytomegalovirus (CMV), herpesviruses, and *Chlamydia pneumoniae* are associated with atherosclerotic vascular disease and vascular events.[66, 126, 128, 160] Such infections may trigger plaque rupture by increasing hemodynamic stress (e.g., via tachycardia and increased cardiac output that may accompany a febrile illness) or may directly affect the vascular biology of the plaque. Infection localizing to the plaque may activate endothelial cells to express adhesion molecules, may stimulate vascular cells to undergo proliferation, or may induce resident inflammatory cells to elaborate cytokines that promote further local inflammation.[110]

Imaging Modalities for Detecting Vulnerable Plaque

It is apparent, from the preceding discussion, that an imaging modality to detect vulnerable plaques would be useful so as to identify (and appropriately manage) those patients at the greatest risk for a catastrophic vascular event. Unfortunately, currently there are no adequate imaging modalities for detecting vulnerable plaque. Angiography can detect stenoses, but this information is not useful in predicting vulnerability to rupture. Indeed, some 50% to 75% of plaque ruptures that lead to coronary thrombosis occur at sites where the plaque caused less than 50% narrowing of the lumen.[5, 45, 111] Furthermore, intravascular ultrasound studies reveal that the volume of intimal lesions is often underestimated by angiography.[152] Intravascular ultrasonography is superior to angiography in assessing plaque burden and can provide some information on characteristics of the lesion; however, the currently available two-dimensional images cannot provide the tissue characterization necessary to reproducibly differentiate stable atheromas from unstable ones.

Whereas angioscopy and intravascular ultrasonography can identify thrombosis and some of the lipid-rich plaques, these techniques are invasive and not practical for evaluating the prognosis in the majority of persons who have minimal symptoms or none. Noninvasive tests are needed to determine risks for acute coronary syndromes; however, current noninvasive tests are neither sensitive nor specific.

In one study, patients with CAD were prospectively evaluated with angiography, exercise testing, and ambulatory monitoring; however, none of these tests or combinations of them were effective in predicting acute events.[133] This is probably because severity of stenosis (which is assessed by these measures) is to a significant degree unrelated to acute events.[119]

Ultra-fast computed tomography is noninvasive and is useful in measuring calcium content in vessel walls, but more information is needed relating calcium content to risk of clinical events. Indeed, in patients with stroke, the risk of recurrent vascular events is negatively correlated with aortic calcium content.[36] Magnetic resonance angiography (MRA) may replace angiography for detecting stenoses, but currently it is ineffective at detecting vulnerable plaques. The study of carotid artery lesions prior to endarterectomy using magnetic resonance imaging (MRI) may be capable of effectively discriminating lipid core, fibrous caps, calcifications, and normal media and adventitia.[177]

Triggers of Acute Vascular Events

There is a circadian pattern of acute myocardial infarction and sudden death, with most heart attacks occurring in the morning, during arousal from sleep or shortly thereafter.[135, 190] A similar circadian pattern is observed in certain physiologic parameters, with increases in heart rate, blood pressure, and platelet aggregability during the morning hours.[136] The circadian variations in hemodynamic stress and blood coagulability probably account for the increased frequency of vascular events in the morning hours and are probably driven by increased sympathetic nerve flow during arousal from sleep.[136] In addition to this circadian variation, there is also a weekly variation, with increased events occurring on Mondays in workers but not in retired persons.

The sympathetic nervous system is also activated by fear, anger, and strenuous exertion, a fact that may account for the increased risk of myocardial infarction associated with emotional or physical stress. The Onset study revealed that the risk of myocardial infarction was elevated about 200% after an outburst of anger, heavy exertion, or sexual activity.[129, 130, 134] Several other external events have been reported as possible triggers, including earthquakes, blizzards, heat waves, and missile strikes.[63, 108, 125, 161, 178] All of these triggers likely exert their effects via the sympathetic nervous system, which may explain the observation that β-adrenergic antagonists confer longevity on patients with atherosclerotic CAD. Since most patients with PAOD also have CAD, β-adrenergic agents are often useful in treating attendant myocardial ischemia, hypertension, or arrhythmia. Beta-adrenergic antagonists do not exacerbate PAOD.

TREATMENT

Overview

Patients with peripheral atherosclerosis who present for evaluation and treatment of their leg complaints must first be considered for aggressive risk factor modification. These patients are at high risk for cardiovascular events because of the systemic nature of their disease. The following topics address specific approaches to risk factor modification. Many of the data presented here have been derived from larger clinical trials in treating patients who have coronary disease or are at high risk for coronary and cerebral vascular events. Few data are available that specifically address the effects of risk factor modification on the peripheral circulation or in patients presenting specifically with PAOD.

Thus, our approach is to review both the literature that addresses key points regarding risk factor modification in patients with coronary and cerebral atherosclerotic disease and the facts about risk factor modification for PAOD. Since much information has been obtained from populations who did not have PAOD, our current recommendations are based on extrapolations from these larger populations.

Diabetes

Aggressive control of blood sugar and treatment of insulin resistance are essential in the management of diabetes. Several strategies are well established and are not discussed in detail here. Caloric restriction and exercise are the most important lifestyle changes that can be made. Patients with type II diabetes that is not controlled with these measures typically are given oral hypoglycemic medications and newer agents such as metformin or troglitazone to improve insulin sensitivity. Insulin therapy is reserved for patients who cannot be managed successfully with these therapies. Unfortunately, there are no concrete data on the effects of improved glycemic control on peripheral atherosclerosis. Excellent glycemic control alone may not be sufficient to treat atherosclerosis. Therefore, the clinician must address the other cardiovascular risk factors (smoking, hypertension, hyperlipidemia) in the diabetic patient, in addition to treating the diabetes itself.

Hypertension

A critical factor in the management of diabetes is control of hypertension. In patients with diabetes, hypertension significantly increases the risk of PAOD and of several other cardiovascular complications.[124] Treatment of hypertension should be addressed in all patients with diabetes, with the goal of achieving the lowest blood pressure the patient can tolerate. The recommended agents are diuretics and angiotensin-converting enzyme (ACE) inhibitors. Calcium channel blockers should be avoided because they may increase the risk of cardiac events.[53] Improved cardiovascular outcomes have been observed in patients with diabetes in lipid-lowering trials. Lowering cholesterol in these patients reduces mortality from coronary heart disease. These results are discussed later.

Foot Care

In addition to treatment of the diabetes and attendant risk factors, another important aspect is good foot care. This is dealt with in detail in Chapter 76. It has recently been demonstrated that establishing foot care programs in primary care medical clinics helps to prevent infections, and even amputations, in persons with diabetes. Such interventions can prevent the progression to foot ulceration in patients with diabetes.[112]

Smoking Cessation Strategies

Several approaches have been advocated to modify smoking behavior in patients with CVD. These have ranged from physician advice to nicotine replacement to specific drug therapies; the results are summarized in Table 19–3. It is well known that the rate of spontaneous smoking cessation in the population remains low because tobacco is addicting. Thus, more structured programs have been recommended that focus on behavior modification and physician advice, measures associated with abstinence rates of approximately 15% after 1 year. In general however, these "quit rates" are considered inadequate.[55, 80] In one large study involving 16,000 men at high risk for CAD, enrollment in a clinical trial and the recommendation to stop smoking resulted in a 25% quit rate in the intervention group over 4 years, as compared with 17% in the control group.[81]

Nicotine Replacement

Nicotine replacement therapy in combination with behavior modification is slightly more effective than behavior modification alone. A meta-analysis of several placebo-controlled trials revealed cessation rates of 23% to 27% over 6 to 12 months with a nicotine patch and of 13% to 18% with placebo.[91] Also, transdermal nicotine patches have been shown to be safe in patients with medical diseases, even high-risk populations. Thus, this is a strategy that should be considered for patients with PAOD.

Antidepressant Therapy

Recent observations suggest that there is an association between tobacco dependence and depression. Antidepressant therapy may help patients to quit smoking. Several studies have evaluated the antidepressant bupropion as an aid to smoking cessation in combination with the established therapies discussed earlier. In one large study, bupropion was associated with a cessation rate of 50% at 1 year.[147] These results suggest that combined therapy with behavior modification, nicotine replacement, and antidepressants may be necessary to obtain acceptable quit rates in smokers with PAOD.

In conclusion, an aggressive and multifaceted approach must be implemented to help patients with PAOD to quit smoking. Table 19–3 presents the benefits of tobacco cessation as compared with its continued use in regard to both life and limb. At a minimum, treatment should consist of a behavior modification program and nicotine replacement. Other pharmacologic interventions may be warranted for this powerfully addicted population.

Hyperlipidemia

Several effective therapies have been developed for hyperlipidemia. Dietary restriction of cholesterol and saturated fats has only a modest effect on LDL cholesterol levels; however, caloric restriction and weight loss can lead to substantial decreases in triglyceride levels, and this is important in the management of PAOD. Low-cholesterol diets can also be supplemented with large amounts of soluble fiber. In particular, when fiber is ingested in the form of psyllium, additional small but significant decreases in total and LDL cholesterol levels (in the range of 5% to 7%) are realized.[87, 166] This effect is independent of those produced by other macronutrients in the diet. In patients with mild elevations in cholesterol, these dietary interventions may be sufficient to reduce cholesterol levels.

The statin drugs have become a well-established means of reducing LDL cholesterol levels. In general, large decreases in LDL cholesterol concentration can be achieved with this form of therapy. In addition to statin drugs, gemfibrozil has been shown to lower LDL cholesterol and triglycerides, and to confer the added benefit of increase in HDL cholesterol concentration. Another means for modifying HDL cholesterol is niacin, but this is associated with a high incidence of side effects, including abnormalities of liver function, glucose intolerance, and increased uric acid concentration. In one large study of veterans with dyslipoproteinemias, controlled-release niacin reduced LDL cholesterol levels by 24% and increased HDL levels by 6%. Unfortunately, almost half of the patients discontinued therapy because of side effects.[67] Thus, although niacin is effective, side effects limit its usefulness. For patients with refractory elevations in LDL cholesterol, stepped care should include a statin drug (such as pravastatin) and then the addition of other agents, such as niacin, cholestyramine, and gemfibrozil. The practicality of this approach is well established, and such treatment may be necessary in a minority of patients, although it often produces significant side effects.[148]

Effect of Cholesterol Decreases on Risk of Cardiovascular Events

Several very large, well-controlled trials have been conducted in patients who have underlying CAD or are at increased risk for coronary events to determine the benefits of cholesterol lowering. The major compounds tested were simvastatin and pravastatin. The study populations included patients with CAD and established hyperlipidemia and patients with CAD whose cholesterol levels were in the "normal" range. In patients with CAD, reducing cholesterol levels with the therapies discussed earlier has been clearly associated with improvements in coronary event rates.

One of the early large trials of lipid-lowering therapy, the Helsinki Heart Study, looked at 4081 men at risk for coronary events. Treatment with gemfibrozil was associated with increases in HDL cholesterol levels and decreases in LDL levels. The study also showed a 34% reduction in the incidence of coronary heart disease events but no effect on total mortality.[56]

The Scandinavian Simvastatin Survival Study (the 4S Trial) was the first lipid-lowering trial that demonstrated very significant decreases in both total mortality and CAD mortality.[3, 99] The trial enrolled patients who had experienced a myocardial infarction and whose total cholesterol levels were elevated. More than 4000 patients participated in this secondary prevention trial and were followed for an average of 5.4 years. Total cholesterol was decreased in the "active drug" arm by 25% and LDL cholesterol by 35%, and HDL cholesterol increased by 8%. The results of the study showed a 30% reduction in total mortality and 42% reduction of risk for major coronary events. The benefits were closely correlated with on-treatment reductions in levels of total and LDL cholesterol and of apolipoprotein B (apoB).[150]

In the Cholesterol And Recurrent Events (CARE) Trial, patients were studied who had experienced a myocardial infarction but whose lipid values were in the normal range.[158] More than 4000 patients were included, and their total cholesterol levels were below 240 mg/dl and LDL cholesterol levels ranged from 115 to 174 mg/dl. Pravastatin was used in this trial and was associated with significant improvements in lipid profiles (20% decrease in total cholesterol and 28% decrease in LDL cholesterol; mean LDL cholesterol concentration on therapy <100 mg/dl). Treated patients experienced a 24% decrease in fatal and nonfatal infarctions but showed no difference in total mortality. Additional benefits were reductions in the need for coronary bypass surgery and in the rate of strokes. The major benefits of pravastatin were seen in patients whose LDL cholesterol level at baseline was above 125 mg/dl, with less additional benefit seen in those with levels lower than 125 mg/dl at baseline.[157]

The results of all the cholesterol-lowering trials have been evaluated by several meta-analyses.[65, 68] These meta-analyses have clearly established that patients with CVDs such as CAD and PAOD should have a target LDL cholesterol level lower than 100 mg/dl. In these trials, for every 10-percentage-point reduction in total cholesterol, CAD mortality risk was reduced by 15% and total mortality risk by 11%.[65] This benefit has also been shown to be rather universal and not restricted to any particular group of patients. For example, a subanalysis of the 4S study has shown that cholesterol-lowering therapy is effective in both women and elderly patients and, therefore, that these therapies should not be restricted to any particular subgroup.[127]

Based on these studies and others, the National Cholesterol Education Program recommends that patients with underlying PAOD begin cholesterol-lowering therapy if their LDL level is above 130 mg/dl, with the goal of 100 mg/dl or lower. These data have been driven particularly by the finding that patients with a beginning LDL level of 125 mg/dl or higher realize significant benefit from cholesterol-lowering therapy.

Cholesterol Reduction in Peripheral Arterial Occlusive Disease

In patients with PAOD, cholesterol-lowering therapies have been associated with stabilization or regression of peripheral atherosclerosis. For example, in the carotid circulation, carotid wall thickness (as measured by ultrasonography) has been shown to be affected positively by reductions in cholesterol levels.[57, 82] In patients with PAOD, the use of colestipol combined with niacin therapy was also shown to stabilize or regress femoral atherosclerosis.[14]

The observation that cholesterol lowering had the potential to improve the peripheral circulation prompted several clinical trials. The Surgical Control of Hyperlipidemias (POSCH) study used ileal bypass surgery to lower lipid concentrations and included a 10-year follow-up.[27] This trial showed that lowering cholesterol was associated with slower progression of PAOD. Specifically, the risk for development of an abnormal ABI (i.e., <0.95) was reduced by 44%, and the risk of developing clinical manifestations of PAOD was reduced by 30%, both as compared with rates in the control group. In the 4S Trial, the reduction in cholesterol concentration with simvastatin therapy was associated with a 38% reduction in the risk of new or more severe symptoms of intermittent claudication, as compared with placebo.[149] Thus, cholesterol lowering has been associated with major reductions in cardiovascular morbidity and mortality and in less progression of PAOD symptoms in patients with systemic atherosclerosis. These results clearly indicate the critical need for cholesterol-lowering therapy for all patients with atherosclerosis.

As discussed above, LP(a) is also an independent risk factor for PAOD, but no effective drug therapies are available to treat this lipid abnormality. In a recent study, patients with CAD plus PAOD who had elevations in total cholesterol and in LP(a) were randomized to receive either simvastatin alone or simvastatin with biweekly apheresis in an attempt to further lower the LP(a) level.[100] The apheresis therapy (consisting of withdrawal and partial reinfusion of blood) used a system to selectively absorb lipoproteins that contain apoB, which was expected to reduce the levels of very-low-density lipoprotein, LDL cholesterol, and LP(a). This study clearly showed that treatment with simvastatin alone had no effect on LP(a) levels, whereas patients randomized to the simvastatin with apheresis arm had a 19% overall reduction in LP(a) levels. Changes in PAOD were assessed with duplex imaging of the femoral and tibial vessels. Patients randomized to simvastatin therapy alone experienced an increase in the number of occlusive lesions in their peripheral circulations, whereas those randomized to simvastatin plus apheresis experienced a decrease. Thus, while apheresis is not a practical means of treating hyperlipidemia, this study does suggest that LP(a) levels are critically important in the development of peripheral atherosclerosis and that when LP(a) concentration is reduced, peripheral arterial circulation improves.

In general, patients with PAOD are at high risk for myocardial infarction and ischemic strokes. Cholesterol-lowering therapies based primarily on statin drugs can be expected to produce significant reductions in cardiovascular event rates. Furthermore, they may have positive effects on the peripheral circulation, though such effects are less firmly established. A number of therapies are available for patients with PAOD: diet and soluble fiber supplements for those with modest elevations in LDL cholesterol concentration, and simvastatin and other agents for those who need more intensive therapy.

Hypertension Therapy

CVD and associated hypertension always warrant aggressive measures to lower both systolic and diastolic blood pressures. Initial management should include behavior modification strategies. Dietary modification with restrictions of sodium, alcohol, and fat intake and increases in fruits and vegetables, along with exercise, are associated with modest reductions in blood pressure.[8] In addition to lifestyle modification, detailed guidelines have been published for the detection and treatment of hypertension by the Joint National Committee.[1, 163] These guidelines provide clinicians an approach to pharmacologic treatment of hypertension and are not repeated in this chapter. It is important, however, to recognize that many effective medications are available to lower blood pressure in patients with CVD.

A number of very large clinical trials have been performed to establish the benefits of antihypertensive therapy. Perhaps the best summary of these trials is a published meta-analysis of results in 20,820 women and 19,975 men.[69] The principal treatments were thiazide diuretics and beta-adrenergic blockers. In women, lowering blood pressure reduced cardiovascular deaths by 14%, fatal and nonfatal strokes by 38%, and major cardiovascular events overall by 26%. In men, lowering blood pressure reduced cardiovascular deaths by 29%, fatal and nonfatal strokes by 34%, and all major cardiovascular events by 22%. Another meta-analysis summarized data for 15,559 patients older than 59 years whose main treatments were thiazide diuretics and beta-adrenergic blockers.[84] The treatment reduced mortality of all causes by 12%, stroke mortality by 36%, and coronary heart disease mortality by 25%. These results are important, since most patients with PAOD fall within this age range.

Historically, in patients with PAOD there has been concern that beta-adrenergic blockers might possibly worsen the symptoms of claudication; however, several studies have shown that this class of drugs is safe in claudicants and are an acceptable choice for lowering blood pressure.[77] Large reductions in systolic pressure and leg perfusion by any class of antihypertensive agent may, however, result in modest exacerbation of claudication symptoms.[165]

The goals of treating hypertension in patients with PAOD should be similar to those for patients who have other CVDs. Any class of antihypertensive therapy would be appropriate, and the choice of agent would be guided by the individual patient's needs. The ideal blood pressure goals for patients with PAOD are similar to those for persons with other CVDs. Again, the individual patient's needs guide the clinician, particularly in avoiding both side effects and extreme blood pressure reduction that produces symptoms of hypotension. Should a patient complain of slightly worsening claudication with lower blood pressure, this should not deter the clinician from achieving ideal blood pressure goals. This is true because new and effective treatments for claudication are available that do not interfere with lowering blood pressure.

Treatment of Elevated Homocysteine Levels

Most patients with elevated homocysteine levels can easily be treated by supplementation with B vitamins. In fact, folic acid was recently approved as a supplement in cereal grain products. Levels of folic acid achieved by this means are sufficient to significantly reduce plasma homocysteine levels, an effect that may have therapeutic efficacy.[117] Older patients with vitamin B_{12} deficiencies should not be treated with folic acid alone because this can precipitate peripheral neuropathy unless vitamin B_{12} is also provided.

Despite the ease of therapy, no clinical trials have demonstrated efficacy of B vitamins in reducing ischemic events.[167] Clinicians may consider screening for elevated homocysteine levels in young patients who present with PAOD and who have no other cardiovascular risk factors for premature peripheral atherosclerosis. These patients may be candidates for B vitamin supplementation if their homocysteine levels are elevated; however, clinical recommendations on treatment of homocysteine elevation should await clinical trial results. This aspect is also discussed in some detail in Chapter 65.

Estrogen Treatment

Estrogen is a hormone that is cardioprotective, and this may partly explain the higher incidence of CVD in males as compared with females. The protective mechanisms may include increasing HDL cholesterol levels and improving vascular endothelial function. The effects of estrogen replacement in postmenopausal women with PAOD have not been specifically investigated, but estrogen treatment would seem reasonable. Importantly, PAOD often develops later in life than CAD does, so that women are likely go through menopause before PAOD develops. Therefore, administration of estrogen to women, particularly those at high risk for atherosclerosis, should be considered after menopause unless this is contraindicated.

Exercise Therapy

Exercise clearly has a role in improving the symptoms and walking ability of patients with claudication.[76, 78] The effects of routine exercise on cardiovascular mortality have not been studied in PAOD; however, other studies have shown a positive association between physical activity and reduced mortality.[70] Thus, exercise may have multiple benefits for patients with PAOD (see Chapter 65).

Antiplatelet Therapy

In addition to risk factor modification, other therapies have been used to slow the progression of peripheral atherosclerosis and to decrease cardiovascular morbidity and mortality. The role of platelets in thrombus formation has led to many studies of the effectiveness of various antiplatelet agents, particularly aspirin, in preventing thrombus formation and subsequent acute ischemic events.

A comprehensive overview of the efficacy and safety of antiplatelet agents in the prevention of ischemic events in high-risk patients was performed via a meta-analysis conducted by the Antiplatelet Trialists' Collaboration (ATC).[2, 7] This meta-analysis included 145 randomized trials with more than 100,000 patients at risk for vascular events, 70,000 at high risk (i.e., because of clinically evident atherosclerosis). The results show conclusively that when compared with placebo, antiplatelet therapy reduces the risk of ischemic events by approximately 25%. Unfortunately, very few patients with PAOD were included in the ATC analysis. Thus, there is no conclusive evidence yet that aspirin is effective in preventing ischemic events in patients with PAOD. Despite the lack of evidence, it nevertheless seems prudent to treat patients with PAOD with low-dose aspirin.

Ticlopidine, an inhibitor of adenosine diphosphate–induced platelet aggregation, has been reported to be more effective than aspirin in preventing cardiovascular events in patients with atherosclerosis.[2] In patients with PAOD, ticlopidine has been shown to be more effective than placebo at reducing the risk of fatal and nonfatal myocardial infarction and stroke.[9, 20, 86] Thus, there is good evidence that antiplatelet agents of the thienopyridine class are effective in PAOD. This observation has led to the development of other drugs in the ticlopidine class, including the new agent clopidogrel, which lacks many of the side effects of ticlopidine.

The Clopidogrel versus Aspirin for the Prevention of Ischemic Events (CAPRIE) trial was a large, randomized, controlled trial conducted in 16 countries, including the United States, to compare the benefits of two different antiplatelet agents in the prevention of ischemic events.[31] More than 19,000 patients participated in this trial. Patients were included who had recently had a myocardial infarction or an ischemic stroke or who had established PAOD. The primary outcome of this study was a composite end-point, including first occurrence of fatal or nonfatal ischemic stroke, myocardial infarction, or other vascular death. In the CAPRIE trial, overall risk of ischemic events was reduced 8.7% ($p < .05$) more with clopidogrel than with aspirin.

More than 6000 patients were enrolled in the CAPRIE trial because they had PAOD. A subgroup analysis of the PAOD patients showed 23.8% risk reduction with clopidogrel in this group. Thus, the benefit of clopidogrel in the PAOD group was substantially greater than that of aspirin in terms of reducing risk for ischemic events. The large benefit of clopidogrel over aspirin in the subgroup with PAOD has not yet been explained. It is unlikely that this occurred merely by chance, because the statistical test for heterogeneity was positive, which suggests that the benefit of clopidogrel was not equal across the three clinical subgroups. Perhaps patients with PAOD respond differently to clopidogrel than do patients with coronary or carotid atherosclerosis. Another possibility is that patients with PAOD have a cluster of other risk factors that predict greater response to clopidogrel than to aspirin. Further analyses from this important trial will be necessary to clarify these questions.

Aspirin, ticlopidine, and clopidogrel all can cause side effects. Aspirin causes gastrointestinal disturbances in some patients, although it is well tolerated by the majority. Patients taking ticlopidine require extensive hematologic monitoring, because the side effect profile includes neutropenia as well as the more common findings of rash and diarrhea. Patients who took clopidogrel had a higher incidence of diarrhea, rash, and pruritus than those who took aspirin but a lower incidence of gastrointestinal disturbances and upper gastrointestinal tract bleeds. This was true even though aspirin-intolerant patients were excluded from the trial. Clopidogrel, although closely related to ticlopidine, does not carry the increased risk of neutropenia; therefore, no hematologic monitoring is required with this new drug.

Given that PAOD is a systemic atherosclerotic disease and that affected patients have strong and independent risks of cardiovascular morbidity and mortality, PAOD patients should be treated with antiplatelet agents unless they are contraindicated. Specifically, clopidogrel may be more effective than aspirin in patients with PAOD.

Complementary Therapies

Certain health supplements may be useful for PAOD. Those that have the greatest scientific documentation are L-carnitine, L-arginine, and the antioxidants. A number of descriptive and case-control studies have shown an association between antioxidant vitamin intake and reductions in cardiovascular events.[46] Antioxidants may render LDL cholesterol resistant to oxidation, which should make that lipid fraction less atherogenic. In addition, the effects on LDL cholesterol and other mechanisms may improve endothelium-dependent vasodilatation by reducing oxidative degradation of NO.[46]

Vitamins C and E and beta-carotene have been the most popular of the antioxidant supplements. Beta-carotene has, however, fallen out of favor, because several large trials failed to show a benefit in reducing cardiovascular events. Moreover, there was an excess of lung cancer events.[73, 145] By contrast, in patients with CAD, vitamin E (400 to 800 IU/day) reduced the risk of non-fatal myocardial infarctions.[100] Further work must be done to define the formulation and dosing of antioxidant vitamins, but on the basis of the current evidence, it seems reasonable to recommend antioxidant therapy for patients with PAOD, preferably vitamin E (200 to 400 IU/day) and vitamin C (250 to 500 mg/day).

L-Carnitine and propionyl-L-carnitine are natural substances and cofactors for fatty acid transport into mitochondria.[23] Free fatty acids cannot enter the mitochondria but, when esterified to L-carnitine, are transported by carnitine translocase into the mitochondria for oxidation and energy generation. With PAOD an alteration in carnitine homeostasis occurs that is related to the severity of ischemia.[24, 79] In affected persons, administration of L-carnitine increases total carnitine content in the ischemic muscle, reduces lactate production during exercise, and improves walking capacity.[25] Accordingly, some patients may benefit from the addition of L-carnitine (500 mg twice daily) to their regimen.

As previously mentioned, the semiessential amino acid L-arginine is the precursor of the potent vasodilator endothelium-derived NO. Individuals with PAOD appear to synthesize less NO, possibly owing to elevated levels of ADMA, the endogenous NO synthase inhibitor.[19] In patients with critical limb ischemia, an infusion of L-arginine (30 mg) increases urinary nitrogen oxides and urinary cyclic guanosine monophosphate (both reflective of increased NO synthesis), and it is as effective as prostaglandin E_1 at increasing limb blood flow.[19] In patients with PAOD, twice-

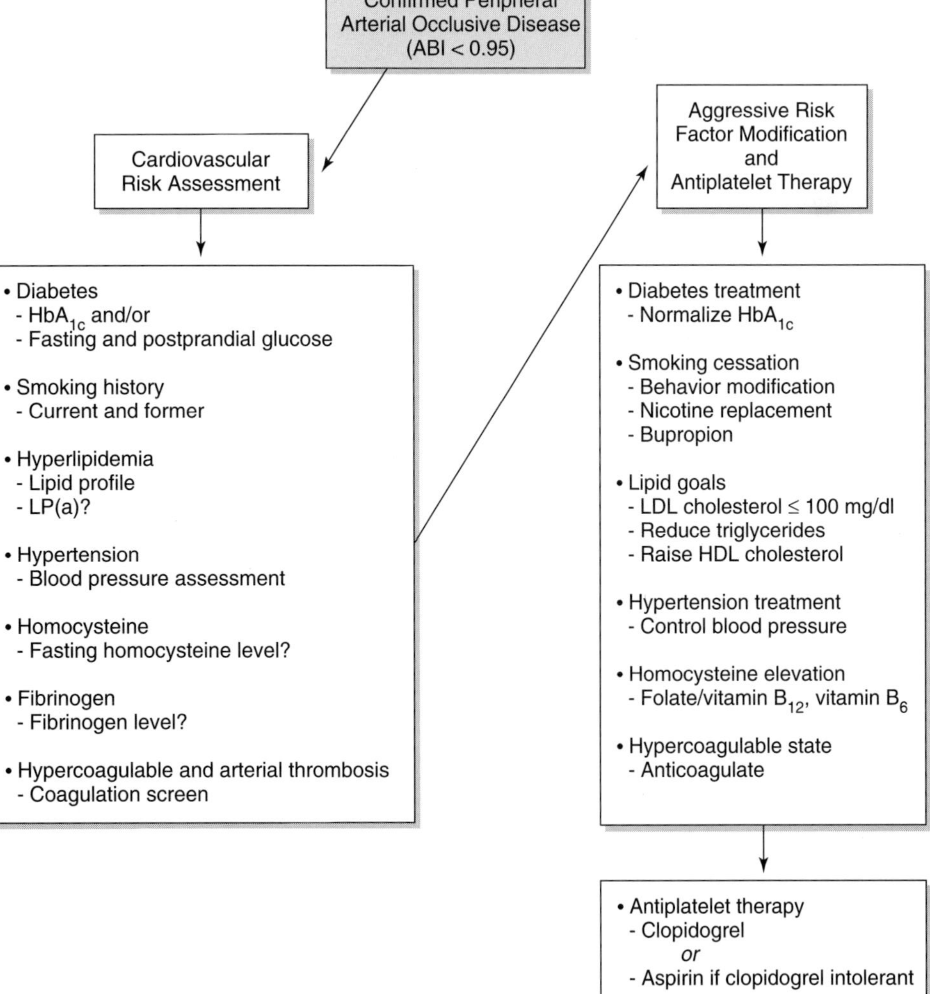

FIGURE 19–4. An overall strategy for reducing risk of peripheral arterial occlusive disease. ABI = ankle-brachial index; Hb = hemoglobin; LP(a) = lipoprotein A; LDL = low-density lipoprotein; HDL = high-density lipoprotein; ? = insufficient data to recommend.

daily infusion of L-arginine (8 mg) increases walking distance.[15] In patients with CAD, oral L-arginine (6 to 9 gm/day) improves coronary blood flow response to acetylcholine by 150%, reduces angina, and significantly increases walking time on the treadmill before ST segment depression is observed.[33, 109] Oral L-arginine also has antiplatelet effects and reduces monocyte adhesiveness.[4, 175] Therefore, 4 to 8 mg/day of oral L-arginine may benefit these patients.

SUMMARY

Patients with peripheral atherosclerosis are at very high risk for CVD morbidity and mortality. A reduced ABI is an independent predictor of mortality and an indicator of systemic atherosclerosis. The primary causes of death in patients with PAOD are cardiovascular and are due to myocardial infarctions and strokes. Despite these alarming figures, few studies have looked at the specific benefits of risk factor modification and of antiplatelet therapy in reducing the risk of these systemic events in patients with PAOD.

Despite the lack of group-specific data, patients with PAOD should not be ignored. In the preceding discussion, we have advocated an aggressive approach to risk factor modification, including normalization of LDL cholesterol levels, smoking cessation, treatment of diabetes and associated risk factors, and lowering of blood pressure. These guidelines were derived primarily from large studies of patients at risk for CAD, and the results were extrapolated to the PAOD population.

Finally, all patients with PAOD should receive antiplatelet therapy. Clopidogrel is the preferred agent, but if it is not available, at minimum, aspirin should be given. An overall strategy for risk reduction is presented in Figure 19–4.

REFERENCES

1. 1988 Joint National Committee: The 1988 report of the Joint National Committee on detection, evaluation, and treatment of high blood pressure. Arch Intern Med 148:1023–1038, 1988.
2. Collaborative overview of randomized trials of antiplatelet therapy: I: Prevention of death, myocardial infarction, and stroke by prolonged antiplatelet therapy in various categories of patients. Antiplatelet Trialists Collaboration. BMJ 308:81–106, 1994.
3. Randomized trial of cholesterol lowering in 4444 patients with coronary heart disease: The Scandinavian Simvastatin Survival Study (4S). Lancet 344:1383–1389, 1994.
4. Adams MR, McCredie R, Jessup W, et al: Oral L-arginine improves endothelium-dependent dilatation and reduces monocyte adhesion to endothelial cells in young men with coronary artery disease. Atheroselerosis 129:261–269, 1997.
5. Ambrose JA, Winters SL, Arora RR, et al: Coronary angiographic morphology in myocardial infarction: A link between the pathogenesis of unstable angina and myocardial infarction. J Am Coll Cardiol 6:1233–1238, 1985.
6. Annex BH, Denning SM, Channon KM, et al: Differential expression of tissue factor protein in directional atherectomy specimens from patients with stable and unstable coronary syndromes. Circulation 91:619–622, 1995.
7. Antiplatelet Trialists' Collaboration: Secondary prevention of vascular disease by prolonged antiplatelet treatment. BMJ 296:320–331, 1988.
8. Appel LJ, Moore TJ, Obarzanek E, et al: A clinical trial of the effects of dietary patterns on blood pressure. DASH Collaborative Research Group. N Engl J Med 336:1117–1124, 1997.
9. Arcan JC, Blanchard J, Boissel JP, et al: Multicenter double-blind study of ticlopidine in the treatment of intermittent claudication and the prevention of its complications. Angiology 39:802–811, 1988.
10. Beach KW, Strandness DE: Arteriosclerosis obliterans and associated risk factors in insulin-dependent and non–insulin-dependent diabetes. Diabetes 29:882–888, 1980.
11. Beckman JS, Koppenol WH: Nitric oxide, superoxide, and peroxynitrite: The good, the bad, and ugly. Am J Physiol 271:C1424–C1437, 1996.
12. Benditt EP, Barrett T, McDougall JK: Viruses in the etiology of atherosclerosis. Proc Natl Acad Sci U S A 80:6386–6389, 1983.
13. Berliner JA, Navab M, Fogelman AM, et al: Atherosclerosis: Basic mechanisms. Oxidation, inflammation, and genetics. Circulation 91:2488–2496, 1995.
14. Blankenhorn DH, Azen SP, Crawford DW, et al: Effects of colestipol-niacin therapy on human femoral atherosclerosis. Circulation 83:438–447, 1991.
15. Boger RH, Bode-Boger SM, Thiele W, et al: Restoring vascular nitric oxide formation by L-arginine infusion therapy improves the symptoms of intermittent claudication in patients with peripheral arterial disease. J Am Coll Cardiol 32:1336–1344, 1998.
16. Bode-Boger SM, Boger RH, Alfke H et al: L-Arginine induces nitric oxide–dependent vasodilation in patients with critical limb ischemia: A randomized, controlled study. Circulation 93:85–90, 1996.
17. Boger RH, Bode-Boger SM, Szuba A, et al: Asymmetric dimethylarginine (ADMA): A novel risk factor for endothelial dysfunction: Its role in hypercholesterolemia. Circulation 98:1842–1847, 1998.
18. Boger RH, Bode-Boger SM, Mugge A, et al: Supplementation of hypercholesterolaemic rabbits with L-arginine reduces the vascular release of superoxide anions and restores NO production. Atherosclerosis 117:273–284, 1995.
19. Boger RH, Bode-Boger SM, Thiele W, et al: Biochemical evidence for impaired nitric oxide synthesis in patients with peripheral arterial occlusive disease. Circulation 95:2068–2074, 1997.
20. Bokissel JP, Peyrieux JC, Destors JM: Is it possible to reduce the risk of cardiovascular events in subjects suffering from intermittent claudication of the lower limbs? Thromb Haemost 62:681–685, 1996.
21. Bostom AG, Cupples LA, Jenner JL, et al: Elevated plasma lipoprotein(a) and coronary heart disease in men aged 55 years and younger. A prospective study. JAMA 276:544–548, 1996.
22. Brattstrom L, Israelsson B, Norrving B, et al: Impaired homocysteine metabolism in early-onset cerebral and peripheral occlusive arterial disease. Atherosclerosis 81:51–60, 1990.
23. Bremer J: Carnitine—metabolism and functions. Physiol Rev 63:1420–1480, 1983.
24. Brevetti G, Angelini C, Rosa M, et al: Muscle carnitine deficiency in patients with severe peripheral vascular disease. Circulation 84:1490–1495, 1991.
25. Brevetti G, Chiariello M, Ferulano G, et al: Increases in walking distance in patients with peripheral vascular disease treated with L-carnitine: A double-blind, cross-over study. Circulation 77:767–773, 1988.
26. Brown DL, Hibbs MS, Kearney M, et al: Identification of 92-kD gelatinase in human coronary atherosclerotic lesions: Association of active enzyme synthesis with unstable angina. Circulation 91:2125–2131, 1995.
27. Buchwald H, Bourdages HR, Campos CT, et al: Impact of cholesterol reduction on peripheral arterial disease in the Program on the Surgical Control of the Hyperlipidemias (POSCH). Surgery 120:672–679, 1996.
28. Burchfiel CM, Laws A, Benfante R, et al: Combined effects of HDL cholesterol, triglyceride, and total cholesterol concentrations on 18-year risk of atherosclerotic disease. Circulation 92:1430–1436, 1995.
29. Camargo CAJ, Stampfer MJ, Glynn RJ et al: Prospective study of moderate alcohol consumption and risk of peripheral arterial disease in U.S. male physicians. Circulation 95:577–580, 1997.
30. Candipan RC, Wang BY, Buitrago R, et al: Regression or progression: Dependency on vascular nitric oxide. Arterioscler Thromb Vasc Biol 16:44–50, 1996.
31. CAPRIE Steering Committee: A randomized, blinded, trial of clopidogrel versus aspirin in patients at risk of ischaemic events (CAPRIE). Lancet 348:1329–1339, 1996.

32. Catalano M, Russo U, Libretti A: Plasma beta-thromboglobulin levels and claudication degrees in patients with peripheral vascular disease. Angiology 37:339–342, 1986.
33. Ceremuzynski L, Chamiec T, Herbaczynska-Cedro K: Effect of supplemental oral L-arginine on exercise capacity in patients with stable angina pectoris. Am J Cardiol 80:311–333, 1997.
34. Clarke R, Daly L, Robinson K, et al: Hyperhomocysteinemia: An independent risk factor for vascular disease. N Engl J Med 324:1149–1155, 1991.
35. Clarkson P, Adams MR, Powe AJ, et al: Oral L-arginine improves endothelium-dependent dilation in hypercholesterolemic young adults. J Clin Invest 97:1989–1994, 1996.
36. Cohen A, Tzourio C, Bertrand B, et al, FAPS Investigators: Aortic plaque morphology and vascular events: A follow-up study in patients with ischemic stroke. French Study of Aortic Plaques in Stroke. Circulation 96:3838–3841, 1997.
37. Cole CW, Hill GB, Farzad E, et al: Cigarette smoking and peripheral occlusive disease. Surgery 114:753–757, 1993.
38. Cooke JP, Dzau VJ: Derangements of the nitric oxide synthase pathway, L-arginine, and cardiovascular diseases. Circulation 96:379–382, 1997.
39. Cooke JP, Dzau VJ: Nitric oxide synthase: Role in the genesis of vascular disease. Annu Rev Med 48:489–509, 1997.
40. Cooke JP, Singer AH, Tsao P, et al: Antiatherogenic effects of L-arginine in the hypercholesterolemic rabbit. J Clin Invest 90:1168–1172, 1992.
41. Creager MA, Gallagher SJ, Girerd XJ, et al: L-Arginine improves endothelium-dependent vasodilation in hypercholesterolemic humans. J Clin Invest 90:1248–1253, 1992.
42. Criqui MH, Fronek A, Barrett-Connor E, et al: The prevalence of peripheral arterial disease in a defined population. Circulation 71:510–515, 1985.
43. Criqui MH, Langer RD, Fronek A, et al: Mortality over a period of 10 years in patients with peripheral arterial disease. N Engl J Med 326:381–386, 1992.
44. Cybulsky MI, Gimbrone MAJ: Endothelial expression of a mononuclear leukocyte adhesion molecule during atherogenesis. Science 251:788–791, 1991.
45. Davies MJ, Thomas A: Thrombosis and acute coronary-artery lesions in sudden cardiac ischemic death. N Engl J Med 310:1137–1140, 1984.
46. Diaz MN, Frei B, Vita JA, Keaney JFJ: Antioxidants and atherosclerotic heart disease. N Engl J Med 337:408–416, 1997.
47. Donaldson MC, Weinberg DS, Belkin M, et al: Screening for hypercoagulable states in vascular surgical practice: A preliminary study. J Vasc Surg 11:825–831, 1990.
48. Donnan PT, Thomson M, Fowkes FGR, et al: Diet as a risk factor for peripheral arterial disease in the general population: The Edinburgh Artery Study. Am J Clin Nutr 57:917–921, 1993.
49. Dormandy JA, Hoare E, Khattab AH, et al: Prognostic significance of rheological and biochemical findings in patients with intermittent claudication. Br Med J 4:581–583, 1973.
50. Drexel H, Steurer J, Muntwyler J, et al: Predictors of the presence and extent of peripheral arterial occlusive disease. Circulation 94(Suppl I):II-199–II-205, 1996.
51. Drexler H, Fischell TA, Pinto FJ, et al: Effect of L-arginine on coronary endothelial function in cardiac transplant recipients: Relation to vessel wall morphology. Circulation 89:1615–1623, 1994.
52. Ernst E, Resch KL: Fibrinogen as a cardiovascular risk factor: A meta-analysis and review of the literature. Ann Intern Med 118:956–963, 1993.
53. Estacio RO, Jeffers BW, Hiatt WR, et al: The effect of nisoldipine as compared with enalapril on cardiovascular outcomes in patients with non–insulin-dependent diabetes and hypertension. N Engl J Med 338:645–652, 1998.
54. Falk E: Why do plaques rupture? Circulation 86:III30–III42, 1992.
55. Fiore MC, Jorenby DE, Baker TB: Smoking cessation: Principles and practice based upon the AHCPR Guideline, 1996. Ann Behav Med 19:213–219, 1997.
56. Frick MH, Elo O, Haapa K, et al: Helsinki Heart Study: Primary-prevention trial with gemfibrozil in middle-aged men with dyslipidemia: Safety of treatment, changes in risk factors, and incidence of coronary heart disease. N Engl J Med 317:1237–1245, 1987.
57. Furberg CD, Adams HPJ, Applegate WB, et al: Effect of lovastatin on early carotid atherosclerosis and cardiovascular events. Asymptomatic Carotid Artery Progression Study (ACAPS) Research Group. Circulation 90:1679–1687, 1994.
58. Fuster V: Lewis A. Conner Memorial Lecture: Mechanisms leading to myocardial infarction: Insights from studies of vascular biology. Circulation 90:2126–2146, 1994.
59. Galis ZS, Sukhova GK, Libby P: Microscopic localization of active proteases by in situ zymography: Detection of matrix metalloproteinase activity in vascular tissue. FASEB J 9:974–980, 1995.
60. Garrison RJ, Havlik RJ, Harris RB, et al: ABO blood group and cardiovascular disease: The Framingham study. Atherosclerosis 25:311–318, 1976.
61. Geng YJ, Libby P: Evidence for apoptosis in advanced human atheroma. Colocalization with interleukin-1 beta–converting enzyme. Am J Pathol 147:251–266, 1995.
62. Geng YJ, Wu Q, Muszynski M, et al: Apoptosis of vascular smooth muscle cells induced by in vitro stimulation with interferon-gamma, tumor necrosis factor- alpha, and interleukin-1 beta. Arterioscler Thromb Vasc Biol 16:19–27, 1996.
63. Glass RI, Zack MM Jr: Increase in deaths from ischemic heart disease after blizzards. Lancet 1:485–487, 1979.
64. Gordon DJ, Probstfield JL, Garrison RJ, et al: High-density lipoprotein cholesterol and cardiovascular disease: Four prospective American studies. Circulation 79:8–15, 1989.
65. Gould AL, Rossouw JE, Santanello NC, et al: Cholesterol reduction yields clinical benefit: Impact of statin trials. Circulation 97:946–952, 1998.
66. Grattan MT, Moreno-Cabral CE, Starnes VA, et al: Cytomegalovirus infection is associated with cardiac allograft rejection and atherosclerosis. JAMA 261:3561–3566, 1989.
67. Gray DR, Morgan T, Chretien SD, Kashyap ML: Efficacy and safety of controlled-release niacin in dyslipoproteinemic veterans. Ann Intern Med 121:252–258, 1994.
68. Grundy SM: Statin trials and goals of cholesterol-lowering therapy. Circulation 97:1436–1439, 1998.
69. Gueyffier F, Boutitie F, Boissel JP, et al: Effect of antihypertensive drug treatment on cardiovascular outcomes in women and men: A meta-analysis of individual patient data from randomized, controlled trials. The INDANA Investigators. Ann Intern Med 126:761–767, 1997.
70. Hakim AA, Petrovitch H, Burchfiel CM, et al: Effects of walking on mortality among nonsmoking retired men. N Engl J Med 338:94–99, 1998.
71. Heinecke JW: Mechanisms of oxidative damage of low density lipoprotein in human atherosclerosis. Curr Opin Lipidol 8:268–274, 1997.
72. Heistad DD, Armstrong ML, Marcus ML, et al: Augmented responses to vasoconstrictor stimuli in hypercholesterolemic and atherosclerotic monkeys. Circ Res 54:711–718, 1984.
73. Hennekens CH, Buring JE, Manson JE, et al: Lack of effect of long-term supplementation with beta carotene on the incidence of malignant neoplasms and cardiovascular disease. N Engl J Med 334:1145–1149, 1996.
74. Henney AM, Wakeley PR, Davies MJ, et al: Localization of stromelysin gene expression in atherosclerotic plaques by in situ hybridization. Proc Natl Acad Sci U S A 88:8154–8158, 1991.
75. Hiatt WR, Hoag S, Hamman RF: Effect of diagnostic criteria on the prevalence of peripheral arterial disease: The San Luis Valley diabetes study. Circulation 91:1472–1479, 1995.
76. Hiatt WR, Regensteiner JG, Hargarten ME, et al: Benefit of exercise conditioning for patients with peripheral arterial disease. Circulation 81:602–609, 1990.
77. Hiatt WR, Stoll S, Nies AS: Effect of β-adrenergic blockers on the peripheral circulation in patients with peripheral vascular disease. Circulation 72:1226–1231, 1985.
78. Hiatt WR, Wolfel EE, Meier RH, Regensteiner JG: Superiority of treadmill walking exercise vs. strength training for patients with peripheral arterial disease: Implications for the mechanism of the training response. Circulation 90:1866–1874, 1994.
79. Hiatt WR, Wolfel EE, Regensteiner JG, Brass EP: Skeletal muscle carnitine metabolism in patients with unilateral peripheral arterial disease. J Appl Physiol 73:346–353, 1992.
80. Hirsch AT, Treat-Jacobson D, Lando HA, Hatsukami DK: The role of tobacco cessation, antiplatelet and lipid-lowering therapies in the treatment of peripheral arterial disease. Vasc Med 2:243–251, 1997.
81. Hjermann I, Velve BK, Holme I, Leren P: Effect of diet and smoking

intervention on the incidence of coronary heart disease: Report from the Oslo Study Group of a randomised trial in healthy men. Lancet 2:1303–1310, 1981.
82. Hodis HN, Mack WJ, LaBree L, et al: Reduction in carotid arterial wall thickness using lovastatin and dietary therapy: A randomized controlled clinical trial. Ann Intern Med 124:548–556, 1996.
83. Hoogeveen EK, Kostense PJ, Becks PJ, et al: Hyperhomocysteinemia is associated with an increased risk of cardiovascular disease, especially in non–insulin-dependent diabetes mellitus: A population-based study. Arterioscler Thromb Vasc Biol 18:133–138, 1998.
84. Insua JT, Sacks HS, Lau TS, et al: Drug treatment of hypertension in the elderly: A meta-analysis. Ann Intern Med 121:355–362, 1994.
85. Isner JM, Kearney M, Bortman S, Passeri J: Apoptosis in human atherosclerosis and restenosis. Circulation 91:2703–2711, 1995.
86. Janzon L, Bergqvist D, Boberg J, et al: Prevention of myocardial infarction and stroke in patients with intermittent claudication: Effects of ticlopidine. Results from STIMS, the Swedish Ticlopidine Multicenter Study. J Intern Med 227:301–308, 1990.
87. Jenkins DJ, Wolever TM, Rao AV, et al: Effect on blood lipids of very high intakes of fiber in diets low in saturated fat and cholesterol. N Engl Med 329:21–26, 1993.
88. Jeppesen J, Hein HO, Suadicani P, Gyntelberg F: Triglyceride concentration and ischemic heart disease: An eight-year follow-up in the Copenhagen Male Study. Circulation 97:1029–1036, 1998.
89. Johansson J, Egberg N, Hohnsson H, Carlson LA: Serum lipoproteins and hemostatic function in intermittent claudication. Arterioscler Thromb 13:1441–1448, 1993.
90. Jonason T, Bergstrom R: Cessation of smoking in patients with intermittent claudication. Acta Med Scand 221:253–260, 1987.
91. Joseph AM, Norman SM, Ferry LH, et al: The safety of transdermal nicotine as an aid to smoking cessation in patients with cardiac disease. N Engl J Med 335:1792–1798, 1996.
92. Juergens JL, Barker NW, Hines EA: Arteriosclerosis obliterans: A review of 520 cases with special reference to pathogenic and prognostic factors. Circulation 21:188–195, 1960.
93. Kannel WB, Castelli WP, Gordon T: Cholesterol in the prediction of atherosclerotic disease: New perspectives based on the Framingham study. Ann Intern Med 90:85–91, 1979.
94. Kannel WB, D'Agostino RB, Wilson PW, et al: Diabetes, fibrinogen, and risk of cardiovascular disease: The Framingham experience. Am Heart J 120:672–676, 1990.
95. Kannel WB, McGee DL: Diabetes and cardiovascular disease. The Framingham Study. JAMA 241:2035–2038, 1979.
96. Kannel WB, McGee DL: Update on some epidemiologic features of intermittent claudication: The Framingham study. J Am Geriatr Soc 33:13–18, 1985.
97. Kannel WB, McGee DL, Castelli WP: Latest perspectives on cigarette smoking and cardiovascular disease: The Framingham study. J Cardiac Rehabil 4:267–277, 1984.
98. Kannel WB, Shurtleff D, National Heart and Lung Institute, National Institutes of Health: The Framingham study: Cigarettes and the development of intermittent claudication. Geriatrics 28:61–68, 1973.
99. Kjekshus J, Pedersen TR: Reducing the risk of coronary events: Evidence from the Scandinavian Simvastatin Survival Study (4S). Am J Cardiol 76:64C–68C, 1995.
100. Kroon AA, van Asten WN, Stalenhoef AF: Effect of apheresis of low-density lipoprotein on peripheral vascular disease in hypercholesterolemic patients with coronary artery disease. Ann Intern Med 125:945–954, 1996.
101. Krupski WC: The peripheral vascular consequences of smoking. Ann Vasc Surg 5:291–304, 1991.
102. Krupski WC, Rapp JH: Smoking and atherosclerosis. Perspect Vasc Surg 1:103–134, 1988.
103. Kugiyama K, Kerns SA, Morrisett JD, et al: Impairment of endothelium-dependent arterial relaxation by lysolecithin in modified low-density lipoproteins. Nature 344:160–162, 1990.
104. Lee AJ, Lowe GDO, Woodward M, Tunstall-Pedoe H: Fibrinogen in relation to personal history of prevalent hypertension, diabetes, stroke, intermittent claudication, coronary heart disease, and family history: The Scottish Heart Health Study. Br Heart J 69:338–342, 1993.
105. Lendon CL, Davies MJ, Born GV, Richardson PD: Atherosclerotic plaque caps are locally weakened when macrophage density is increased. Atherosclerosis 87:87–90, 1991.
106. Leng GC, Fowkes FG, Lee AJ, et al: Use of ankle brachial pressure index to predict cardiovascular events and death: A cohort study. BMJ 313:1440–1444, 1996.
107. Leng GC, Lee AJ, Fowkes FG, et al: Incidence, natural history and cardiovascular events in symptomatic and asymptomatic peripheral arterial disease in the general population. Int J Epidemiol 25:1172–1181, 1996.
108. Leor J, Poole WK, Kloner RA: Sudden cardiac death triggered by an earthquake [see comments]. N Engl J Med 334:413–419, 1996.
109. Lerman A, Burnett JCJ, Higano ST, et al: Long-term L-arginine supplementation improves small-vessel coronary endothelial function in humans. Circulation 97:2123–2128, 1998.
110. Libby P, Egan D, Skarlatos S: Roles of infectious agents in atherosclerosis and restenosis: An assessment of the evidence and need for future research. Circulation 96:4095–4103, 1997.
111. Little WC, Constantinescu M, Applegate RJ, et al: Can coronary angiography predict the site of a subsequent myocardial infarction in patients with mild-to-moderate coronary artery disease? Circulation 78:1157–1166, 1988.
112. Litzelman DK, Slemenda CW, Langefeld CD, et al: Reduction of lower extremity clinical abnormalities in patients with non–insulin-dependent diabetes mellitus. A randomized, controlled trial. Ann Intern Med 119:36–41, 1993.
113. Loree HM, Tobias BJ, Gibson LJ, et al: Mechanical properties of model atherosclerotic lesion lipid pools. Arterioscler Thromb 14:230–234, 1994.
114. Lowe GDO, Fowkes FGR, Dawes J, et al: Blood viscosity, fibrinogen, and activation of coagulation and leukocytes in peripheral arterial disease and the normal population in the Edinburgh Artery Study. Circulation 87:1915–1920, 1993.
115. Lupattelli G, Siepi D, Pasqualini L, et al: Lipoprotein(a) in peripheral arterial occlusive disease. Vasa 23:321–324, 1994.
116. Ma XL, Lopez BL, Liu GL, et al: Hypercholesterolemia impairs a detoxification mechanism against peroxynitrite and renders the vascular tissue more susceptible to oxidative injury. Circ Res 80:894–901, 1997.
117. Malinow MR, Duell PB, Hess DL, et al: Reduction of plasma homocyst(e)ine levels by breakfast cereal fortified with folic acid in patients with coronary heart disease. N Engl J Med 338:1009–1015, 1998.
118. Malinow MR, Kang SS, Taylor LM, et al: Prevalence of hyperhomocyst(e)inemia in patients with peripheral arterial occlusive disease. Circulation 79:1180–1188, 1989.
119. Mann JM, Davies MJ: Vulnerable plaque: Relation of characteristics to degree of stenosis in human coronary arteries. Circulation 94:928–931, 1996.
120. Marmur JD, Thiruvikraman SV, Fyfe BS, et al: Identification of active tissue factor in human coronary atheroma. Circulation 94:1226–1232, 1996.
121. Martin MJ, Hulley SB, Browner WS, et al: Serum cholesterol, blood pressure, and mortality: Implications from a cohort of 361,662 men. Lancet 2:933–936, 1986.
122. McDermott MM, Mehta S, Ahn H, Greenland P: Atherosclerotic risk factors are less intensively treated in patients with peripheral arterial disease than in patients with coronary artery disease. J Gen Intern Med 12:209–215, 1997.
123. McLenachan JM, Williams JK, Fish RD, et al: Loss of flow-mediated endothelium-dependent dilation occurs early in the development of atherosclerosis. Circulation 84:1273–1278, 1991.
124. Mehler PS, Jeffers BW, Estacio R, Schrier RW: Associations of hypertension and complications in non–insulin-dependent diabetes mellitus. Am J Hypertens 10:152–161, 1997.
125. Meisel SR, Kutz I, Dayan KI, et al: Effect of Iraqi missile war on incidence of acute myocardial infarction and sudden death in Israeli civilians. Lancet 338:660–661, 1991.
126. Melnick JL, Adam E, DeBakey ME: Possible role of cytomegalovirus in atherogenesis. JAMA 263:2204–2207, 1990.
127. Miettinen TA, Pyorala K, Olsson AG, et al: Cholesterol-lowering therapy in women and elderly patients with myocardial infarction or angina pectoris: Findings from the Scandinavian Simvastatin Survival Study (4S). Circulation 96:4211–4218, 1997.
128. Minick CR, Fabricant CG, Fabricant J, Litrenta MM: Atheroarterio sclerosis induced by infection with a herpesvirus. Am J Pathol 96:673–706, 1979.
129. Mittleman MA, Maclure M, Sherwood JB, et al: Triggering of acute

myocardial infarction onset by episodes of anger: Determinants of Myocardial Infarction Onset Study Investigators. Circulation 92:1720–1725, 1995.
130. Mittleman MA, Maclure M, Tofler GH, et al: Triggering of acute myocardial infarction by heavy physical exertion. Protection against triggering by regular exertion. Determinants of Myocardial Infarction Onset Study Investigators [see comments]. N Engl J Med 329:1677–1683, 1993.
131. Molgaard J, Malinow MR, Lassvik C, et al: Hyperhomocyst(e)inaemia: An independent risk factor for intermittent claudication. J Intern Med 231:273–279, 1992.
132. Moreno PR, Bernardi VH, Lopez-Cuellar J, et al: Macrophages, smooth muscle cells, and tissue factor in unstable angina. Implications for cell-mediated thrombogenicity in acute coronary syndromes. Circulation 94:3090–3097, 1996.
133. Mulcahy D, Husain S, Zalos G, et al: Ischemia during ambulatory monitoring as a prognostic indicator in patients with stable coronary artery disease. JAMA 277:318–324, 1997.
134. Muller JE, Mittleman A, Maclure M, et al: Triggering myocardial infarction by sexual activity: Low absolute risk and prevention by regular physical exertion. Determinants of Myocardial Infarction Onset Study Investigators. JAMA 275:1405–1409, 1996.
135. Muller JE, Stone PH, Turi ZG, et al: Circadian variation in the frequency of onset of acute myocardial infarction. N Engl J Med 313:1315–1322, 1985.
136. Muller JE, Tofler GH, Stone PH: Circadian variation and triggers of onset of acute cardiovascular disease. Circulation 79:733–743, 1989.
137. Murabito JM, D'Agostino RB, Silbershatz H, Wilson WF: Intermittent claudication: A risk profile from The Framingham Heart Study. Circulation 96:44–49, 1997.
138. Myers KA, King RB, Scott DF, et al: The effect of smoking on the late patency of arterial reconstructions in the legs. Br J Surg 65:267–271, 1978.
139. Newman AB, Sutton-Tyrrell K, Rutan, GH, et al: Lower extremity arterial disease in elderly subjects with systolic hypertension. J Clin Epidemiol 44:15–20, 1991.
140. Newman AB, Tyrrell KS, Kuller LH: Mortality over four years in SHEP participants with a low ankle-arm index. J Am Geriatr Soc 45:1472–1478, 1997.
141. Nikkari ST, O'Brien KD, Ferguson M, et al: Interstitial collagenase (MMP-1) expression in human carotid atherosclerosis. Circulation 92:1393–1398, 1995.
142. Notzon FC, Komarov YM, Ermakov SP, et al: Causes of declining life expectancy in Russia. JAMA 279:793–800, 1998.
143. Ohara Y, Peterson TE, Harrison DG: Hypercholesterolemia increases endothelial superoxide anion production. J Clin Invest 91:2546–2551, 1993.
144. Ohara Y, Peterson TE, Sayegh HS, et al: Dietary correction of hypercholesterolemia in the rabbit normalizes endothelial superoxide anion production. Circulation 92:898–903, 1995.
145. Omenn GS, Goodman GE, Thornquist MD, et al: Effects of a combination of beta carotene and vitamin A on lung cancer and cardiovascular disease. N Engl J Med 334:1150–1155, 1996.
146. Parhami F, Morrow AD, Balucan J, et al: Lipid oxidation products have opposite effects on calcifying vascular cell and bone cell differentiation: A possible explanation for the paradox of arterial calcification in osteoporotic patients. Arterioscler Thromb Vasc Biol 17:680–687, 1997.
147. Pasternak M: Sustained-release bupropion for smoking cessation. N Engl J Med 338:619–620, 1998.
148. Pasternak RC, Brown LE, Stone PH, et al: Effect of combination therapy with lipid-reducing drugs in patients with coronary heart disease and "normal" cholesterol levels. A randomized, placebo-controlled trial. Harvard Atherosclerosis Reversibility Project (HARP) Study Group. Ann Intern Med 125:529–540, 1996.
149. Pedersen TR, Kjekshus J, Pyorala K, et al: Effect of simvastatin on ischemic signs and symptoms in the Scandinavian Simvastatin Survival Study (4S). Am J Cardiol 81:333–335, 1998.
150. Pedersen TR, Olsson AG, Faergeman O, et al: Lipoprotein changes and reduction in the incidence of major coronary heart disease events in the Scandinavian Simvastatin Survival Study (4S). Circulation 97:1453–1460, 1998.
151. Pekkanen J, Linn S, Heiss G, et al: Ten-year mortality from cardiovascular disease in relation to cholesterol level among men with and without preexisting cardiovascular disease. N Engl J Med 322:1700–1707, 1990.
152. Pinto FJ, Chenzbraun A, Botas J, et al: Feasibility of serial intracoronary ultrasound imaging for assessment of progression of intimal proliferation in cardiac transplant recipients. Circulation 90:2348–2355, 1994.
153. Quick CRG, Cotton LT: The measured effect of stopping smoking on intermittent claudication. Br J Surg 69(Suppl):S24–S26, 1982.
154. Rajagopalan S, Kurz S, Munzel T, et al: Angiotensin II–mediated hypertension in the rat increases vascular superoxide production via membrane NADH/NADPH oxidase activation: Contribution to alterations of vasomotor tone. J Clin Invest 97:1916–1923, 1996.
155. Ridker PM, Cushman M, Stampfer MJ, et al: Plasma concentration of C-reactive protein and risk of developing peripheral vascular disease. Circulation 97:425–428, 1998.
156. Ross R: Cellular and molecular studies of atherosclerosis. Atherosclerosis 131:S3–S4, 1997.
157. Sacks FM, Moye LA, Davis BR, et al: Relationship between plasma LDL concentrations during treatment with pravastatin and recurrent coronary events in the Cholesterol And Recurrent Events trial. Circulation 97:1446–1452, 1998.
158. Sacks FM, Pfeffer MA, Moye LA, et al: The effect of pravastatin on coronary events after myocardial infarction in patients with average cholesterol levels. N Engl J Med 335:1001–1009, 1996.
159. Safar ME, Laurent S, Asmar RE: Systolic hypertension in patients with arteriosclerosis obliterans of the lower limbs. Angiology 38:287–295, 1987.
160. Saikku P, Leinonen M, Mattila K et al: Serological evidence of an association of a novel *Chlamydia,* TWAR, with chronic coronary heart disease and acute myocardial infarction. Lancet 2:983–986, 1988.
161. Semenza JC, Rubin CH, Falter KH, et al: Heat-related deaths during the July 1995 heat wave in Chicago. N Engl J Med 335:84–90, 1996.
162. Shah PK, Falk E, Badimon JJ, et al: Human monocyte–derived macrophages induce collagen breakdown in fibrous caps of atherosclerotic plaques. Potential role of matrix-degrading metalloproteinases and implications for plaque rupture. Circulation 92:1565–1569, 1995.
163. Sheps SG, Dart RA: New guidelines for prevention, detection, evaluation, and treatment of hypertension: Joint National Committee VI. Chest 113:263–265, 1998.
164. Sherman CT, Litvack F, Grundfest W, et al: Coronary angioscopy in patients with unstable angina pectoris. N Engl J Med 315:913–919, 1986.
165. Solomon SA, Ramsay LE, Yeo WW, et al: β Blockade and intermittent claudication: Placebo controlled trial of atenolol and nifedipine and their combination. Br Med J 303:1100–1104, 1991.
166. Sprecher DL, Harris BV, Goldberg AC, et al: Efficacy of psyllium in reducing serum cholesterol levels in hypercholesterolemic patients on high- or low-fat diets. Ann Intern Med 119:545–554, 1993.
167. Stampfer MJ, Malinow MR: Can lowering homocysteine levels reduce cardiovascular risk? N Engl J Med 332:328–329, 1995.
168. Stary HC, Chandler AB, Dinsmore RE, et al: A definition of advanced types of atherosclerotic lesions and a histological classification of atherosclerosis. A report from the Committee on Vascular Lesions of the Council on Arteriosclerosis, American Heart Association. Arterioscler Thromb Vasc Biol 15:1512–1531, 1995.
169. Steinberg D, Pearson TA, Kuller LH: Alcohol and atherosclerosis. Ann Intern Med 114:967–976, 1991.
170. Stewart CP: The influence of smoking on the level of lower limb amputation. Prosthet Orthot Int 11:113–116, 1987.
171. Stokes J, Kannel WB, Wolf PA, et al: The relative importance of selected risk factors for various manifestations of cardiovascular disease among men and women from 35 to 64 years old: 30 years of follow-up in the Framingham Study. Circulation 75:V65–V73, 1987.
172. Sutton KC, Wolfson SKJ, Kuller LH: Carotid and lower extremity arterial disease in elderly adults with isolated systolic hypertension. Stroke 18:817–822, 1987.
173. Taylor LM, DeFrang RD, Harris EJ, Porter JM: The association of elevated plasma homocyst(e)ine with progression of symptomatic peripheral arterial disease. J Vasc Surg 13:128–136, 1991.
174. Tesfamariam B, Cohen RA: Free radicals mediate endothelial cell dysfunction caused by elevated glucose. Am J Physiol 263:H321–H326, 1992.
175. Theilmeier G, Chan JR, Zalpour C, et al: Adhesiveness of mononuclear cells in hypercholesterolemic humans is normalized by dietary L-arginine. Arterioscler Thromb Vasc Biol 17:3557–3564, 1997.
176. Tikkanen MJ, Laakso M, Ilmonen M, et al: Treatment of hypercholes-

terolemia and combined hyperlipidemia with simvastatin and gemfibrozil in patients with NIDDM: A multicenter comparison study. Diabetes Care 21:477–481, 1998.
177. Toussaint JF, Lamuraglia GM, Southern JF, et al: Magnetic resonance images lipid, fibrous, calcified, hemorrhagic, and thrombotic components of human atherosclerosis in vivo. Circulation 94:932–938, 1996.
178. Trichopoulos D, Katsouyanni K, Zavitsanos X, et al: Psychological stress and fatal heart attack: The Athens (1981) earthquake natural experiment. Lancet 1:441–444, 1983.
179. Tsao PS, Buitrago R, Chan JR, Cooke JP: Fluid flow inhibits endothelial adhesiveness. Nitric oxide and transcriptional regulation of VCAM-1. Circulation 94:1682–1689, 1996.
180. Tsao PS, Buitrago R, Chang H, et al: Effects of diabetes on monocyte-endothelial interactions and endothelial superoxide production in fructose-induced insulin-resistant and hypertensive rats (Abstract). Circulation 92:A2666, 1995.
181. Tsao PS, McEvoy LM, Drexler H, et al: Enhanced endothelial adhesiveness in hypercholesterolemia is attenuated by L-arginine. Circulation 89:2176–2182, 1994.
182. Tsao PS, Wang B, Buitrago R, et al: Nitric oxide regulates monocyte chemotactic protein-1. Circulation 96:934–940, 1997.
183. Valentine RJ, Kaplan HS, Green R, et al: Lipoprotein(a), homocysteine, and hypercoagulable states in young men with premature peripheral atherosclerosis: A prospective, controlled analysis. J Vasc Surg 23:53–61, 1996.
184. van der Wal AC, Becker AE, van der Loos CM, Das PK: Site of intimal rupture or erosion of thrombosed coronary atherosclerotic plaques is characterized by an inflammatory process irrespective of the dominant plaque morphology. Circulation 89:36–44, 1994.
185. Vaughan DE: The renin-angiotensin system and fibrinolysis. Am J Cardiol 79:12–16, 1997.
186. Vogt MT, Cauley JA, Kuller LH, Hulley SB: Prevalence and correlates of lower extremity arterial disease in elderly women. Am J Epidemiol 137:559–568, 1993.
187. Vogt MT, Cauley JA, Newman AB, et al: Decreased ankle/arm blood pressure index and mortality in elderly women. JAMA 270:465–469, 1993.
188. Wang BY, Singer AH, Tsao PS, et al: Dietary arginine prevents atherogenesis in the coronary artery of the hypercholesterolemic rabbit. J Am Coll Cardiol 23:452–458, 1994.
189. Welch GN, Loscalzo J: Homocysteine and atherothrombosis. N Engl J Med 338:1042–1050, 1998.
190. Willich SN, Linderer T, Wegscheider K, et al: Increased morning incidence of myocardial infarction in the ISAM Study: Absence with prior beta-adrenergic blockade: ISAM Study Group. Circulation 80:853–858, 1989.
191. Willich SN, Lowel H, Lewis M, et al: Weekly variation of acute myocardial infarction: Increased Monday risk in the working population. Circulation 90:87–93, 1994.
192. Ye S, Eriksson P, Hamsten A, et al: Progression of coronary atherosclerosis is associated with a common genetic variant of the human stromelysin-1 promoter which results in reduced gene expression. J Biol Chem 271:13055–13060, 1996.
193. Yudkin JS, Forrest RD, Jackson CA: Microalbuminuria as predictor of vascular disease in non-diabetic subjects: Islington Diabetes Survey. Lancet 2:530–533, 1988.
194. Zimmerman GA, McIntyre TM, Prescott SM: Adhesion and signaling in vascular cell-cell interactions. J Clin Invest 100:S3–S5, 1997.

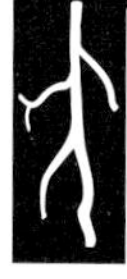

CHAPTER 20

Thromboangiitis Obliterans (Buerger's Disease)

Jeffrey W. Olin, D.O.

Thromboangiitis obliterans (TAO) is a nonatherosclerotic segmental inflammatory disease that most commonly affects the small and medium-sized arteries and veins in the upper and lower extremities. It is classified in the miscellaneous category of vasculitis. It differs from the more commonly encountered vasculitides in that there is often a highly inflammatory thrombus with relative sparing of the blood vessel wall. In many of the earlier published reports, TAO was most commonly encountered in young men. However, in the more recent Western literature, the incidence of TAO seems to be increasing in women. Virtually all patients are heavy users of tobacco, usually cigarette smoking.

In 1879, von Winiwarter reported the pathologic findings of a 57-year-old man with a 12-year history of foot pain that eventually resulted in gangrene and amputation. The pathologic specimen demonstrated intimal proliferation, thrombosis, and fibrosis.[86] von Winiwater was the first to suggest that the *endarteritis* and *endophlebitis* that were present in the amputated specimen were distinct from atherosclerosis.[86] Twenty-nine years later Leo Buerger (born the same year as von Winiwarter's original report) provided a detailed and accurate description of the pathology of the endarteritis and endophlebitis in 11 amputated limbs.[7] Based on his pathologic examination, Buerger called the disease *thromboangiitis obliterans*. He made a point to differentiate the clinical and pathologic findings of TAO from those of atherosclerosis, and this distinct clinical pathologic entity was later called *Buerger's disease*. However, in a subsequent monograph,[8] it is probable that many of the patients described with TAO may have had atherosclerosis instead.

Shortly after the publication of Buerger's comprehensive monograph,[8] Allen and Brown[3] reported on 200 cases of TAO evaluated at the Mayo Clinic from 1922 to 1926. Most of their patients were Jewish men who were heavy cigarette smokers. They noted that these patients developed foot claudication as well as trophic changes "such as excessive callosities in the weight bearing areas, or . . . gangrenous ulcers of the digits or gangrene involving the toes or the entire foot."[3] Pathologically, the description was identical to that of Buerger's original report, although Allen and Brown suggested that TAO was a disease of infectious origin, a hypothesis that has never been proved.

EPIDEMIOLOGY

Although Buerger's disease has a worldwide distribution, it is now more prevalent in the Middle, Near, and Far East than in North America and Western Europe.[45, 50] The incidence of Buerger's disease has declined in the United States and Europe, possibly owing to the adoption of stricter diagnostic criteria. A number of the cases of TAO identified at Mount Sinai Hospital (the location of Leo Buerger's original work) were later considered to have been diagnosed incorrectly.[27]

At the Mayo Clinic, the prevalence rate of patients with the diagnosis of Buerger's disease steadily declined from 104 per 100,000 patient registrations in 1947 to 12.6 per 100,000 patient registrations in 1986.[45, 49]

At the International Symposium on Buerger's Disease in Bad Gastein, Austria, in 1986, Cachovan[9] reported widely varying prevalence rates of Buerger's disease in patients with peripheral arterial occlusive disease in Europe and other countries: 0.5% to 5.6% in Western European countries, 3% in Poland, 6.7% in East Germany, 11.5% in Czechoslovakia, 39% in Yugoslavia, 80% in Israel (Ashkenazim), 45% to 63% in India, and 16% to 66% in Korea and Japan. These rates were calculated from highly selected series of patients treated at specialized institutions and not from the general population.

In Asia, a much higher proportion of patients with limb ischemia has been attributed to Buerger's disease than that in the United States and Europe. In a series from Delhi,[60] Buerger's disease accounted for 63%, arteriosclerosis obliterans for 15%, and miscellaneous causes for 22% of 169 cases of limb ischemia during a 3-year period. In a report from South India in 1989,[6] 186 (53%) of 352 patients with peripheral vascular disease were diagnosed as having Buerger's disease and the remaining 166 (47%) as having arteriosclerosis obliterans.

In 1973, Hill and colleagues[29] described an analysis of 106 patients with Buerger's disease in Java, Indonesia: All the patients were cigarette smokers, and only one was a woman. The patients were from the lowest socioeconomic sector of the community. The authors concluded that the environmental factors of significance in this disease as it occurred in Java appeared to be tobacco, cold injury, and a past history of mycotic infection.

In 1976, the Buerger's Disease Research Committee of the Ministry of Health and Welfare of Japan[4] analyzed 3034 patients (2930 men and 104 women) with the disease from all over Japan and estimated its incidence to be about 5 per 100,000 population. In 1986, the Epidemiology of Intractable Disease Research Committee of the Ministry of Health and Welfare of Japan[61] estimated that there were 8858 patients with the disease who were treated at various medical institutions (5 per 100,000 population); they found no significantly greater prevalence among manual laborers. The number of new patients with Buerger's disease in Japan seems to be decreasing slightly, but the number of the patients under the care of a physician remains almost unchanged due to recurrences.[61, 78, 79] Shionoya[79] stated that according to unofficial estimates, there are 60,000 to 80,000 patients with Buerger's disease in China.

Buerger's Disease in Women

The reported incidence of Buerger's disease in women was 1% to 2% in most published series of cases before 1970. Several recently published series showed a much higher incidence of women with the disease. The author and colleagues have demonstrated that 26 (23%) of 112 patients with Buerger's disease from 1970 to 1987 at the Cleveland Clinic Foundation were women.[65] In an additional 40 patients with Buerger's disease evaluated at the author's institution from 1988 to 1996, 30% were women.[66] Other series have shown an increased prevalence of TAO in women: twelve (11%) of 109 cases of the disease from 1981 to 1985 in Rochester, Minnesota[49]; 5 (19%) of 26 in 1987 a University of Oregon Study[59]; 48 (14%) of 355 from 1975 to 1984 in Yugoslavia[71]; and 12 (22.6%) of 53 patients in a Swiss study.[42] The reason for the apparent increase in the number of women with Buerger's disease is unknown. It is possible that the increased number of women smokers accounts for the increased prevalence. The prevalence of Buerger's disease in Japanese women remains relatively low compared with the increased number of women smokers,[78, 79] and a recent study group of 89 patients from Hong Kong were all men.[39] The reported incidence varies, depending on the diagnostic criteria used to diagnose TAO.

ETIOLOGY AND PATHOGENESIS

The etiology of Buerger's disease is unknown. Although TAO is a type of vasculitis,[44] there are two major distinguishing features of Buerger's disease compared with the other forms of vasculitis. Pathologically, the thrombus in TAO is highly cellular, with much less intense cellular activity in the wall of the blood vessel. In addition, TAO differs from many other types of vasculitis in that the usual immunologic markers (elevation of acute-phase reactants such as Westergren sedimentation rate and C-reactive protein, the presence of circulating immune complexes, and the presence of commonly measured autoantibodies [such as antinuclear antibody, rheumatoid factor, and complement levels]) are usually normal or negative.

Smoking

There is an extremely strong association between heavy tobacco use and TAO.[65, 68] Kjeldsen and Mozes[36] have demonstrated that patients with TAO have higher tobacco consumption and carboxyhemoglobin levels than do patients with atherosclerosis or a control group of patients. There have been occasional cases of TAO in users of smokeless tobacco or snuff.[34, 46, 57] It is possible that there is an abnormal sensitivity or allergy to some component of tobacco and that this sensitivity in some way leads to an inflammatory small vessel occlusive disease.[25, 87] The incidence of TAO is higher in countries in which the consumption of tobacco is large. There is a higher incidence of TAO in India among people of a low socioeconomic class who smoke *bidis* (homemade cigarettes with raw tobacco).[22, 33]

It is not known if cigarette smoking is causative or contributory to the development of Buerger's disease. However, tobacco use is a major factor in the activity of the disease. The progression and continued symptoms associated with TAO are closely linked with continued use of tobacco. Although passive, or "involuntary," smoking (secondary smoke) has not been shown to be associated with the onset of TAO, it may be an important factor in the continuation of symptoms in patients during the acute phase of Buerger's disease. Matsushita and associates[53] have shown that there is a close relationship between active smoking and an active course of Buerger's disease, using the level of cotinine (a metabolite of nicotine) as a measurement of active smoking.

Lie[51] described one case of pathologically proven Buerger's disease affecting the upper extremities of a 62-year-old man who had allegedly discontinued smoking 15 years earlier. However, this report did not contain urinary nicotine cotinine, or carboxyhemoglobin measurements. Therefore, it is possible that this person was still smoking.

It has been suggested that purified tobacco glycoprotein (TGP) could be related to changes in vascular reactivity that may occur in cigarette smokers.[5] Papa and colleagues[69] demonstrated that there was no difference in the humoral response and that patients with TAO and healthy smokers had the same cellular response to TGP antigen, whereas nonsmokers did not respond at all.

Most investigators believe that tobacco is an important etiologic factor in patients who develop TAO. However, only a small number of smokers worldwide eventually develop TAO; therefore, other factors must be involved in the pathogenesis of TAO.

Genetics

Although no gene associated with TAO has been identified, there may be a not yet identified genetic predisposition to developing the disease. There is no consistent pattern in human leukocyte antigen (HLA) haplotypes among patients with Buerger's disease. In the United Kingdom, there was a preponderance of HLA-A9 and HLA-B5 antigens, whereas other HLA haplotypes were increased in patients with TAO from Japan, Austria, and Israel.[56, 62, 63, 68, 82] This finding may be based on genetic differences in various populations as well as methodologic differences in each of the studies cited.[68] Mills and colleagues[59] performed HLA testing in 11 patients with TAO and found no distinctive pattern that was identifiable.

Hypercoagulability and Endothelial Function

Although some studies have failed to identify a specific hypercoagulable state in patients with Buerger's disease,[10, 14, 80] others have shown one or more abnormalities.[12, 80] Chaudhury and colleagues[12] demonstrated that the level of urokinase plasminogen activator was twofold higher and free plasminogen activator inhibitor 1 was 40% lower in patients with TAO compared with healthy volunteers. After venous occlusion, tissue plasminogen activator antigen was increased in patients with Buerger's disease and in healthy volunteers, but the increase was much more pronounced in the control group. This suggests that there is some form of endothelial derangement characterized by increased urokinase plasminogen activator release and decreased plasminogen activator inhibitor 1 release in patients with Buerger's disease. In addition, there is an increased platelet response to serotonin in patients with Buerger's disease.[71]

Eichhorn and associates[19] measured several autoantibodies (cANCA, pANCA, antinuclear antibodies, anti-Ro, anticardiolipin antibodies) in 28 patients with TAO. These autoantibody measurements were negative in all patients. However, 7 patients with active disease had antiendothelial cell antibody (AECA) titers of 1857 ± 450 arbitrary units (AU) compared with 126 ± 15 AU in 30 normal control subjects ($p < .001$) and 461 ± 41 AU in 21 patients in remission ($p < .01$). Antibodies from the sera of patients with active disease reacted not only with surface epitopes but also with sites within the cytoplasm of human endothelial cells. If these findings are corroborated, assays that measure AECA titers may prove to be useful in following the disease activity of patients with Buerger's disease.

Makita and colleagues[52] demonstrated that there was impaired endothelium-dependent vasorelaxation in the peripheral vasculature of patients with Buerger's disease. Forearm blood flow (FBF) was measured plethysmographically in the *nondiseased* limb (1) after the infusion of acetylcholine (endothelium-*dependent* vasodilator), (2) after the infusion of sodium nitroprusside (endothelium-*independent* vasodilator), and (3) after occlusion-induced reactive hyperemia. The increase in FBF response to intra-arterial acetylcholine was lower in patients with TAO than in healthy controls (14.1 ± 2.8 ml/min per dl of tissue volume vs. 22.9 ± 2.9 ml/min per dl, $p < .01$). There was no significant increase in FBF response to sodium nitroprusside (13.1 ± 4 ml/min per dl vs. 16.3 ± 2.5 ml/min per dl), and there was no significant difference between the two groups after reactive hyperemia. These data indicate that endothelial-dependent vasodilation is impaired even in the nondiseased limb of patients with TAO.

Immunologic Mechanisms

Several studies have examined the immunologic mechanisms in patients with TAO. Adar and colleagues[1] studied 39 patients with Buerger's disease and measured the cell-mediated sensitivity for types I and III collagen by an antigen-sensitive thymidine incorporation assay. There was an increased cellular sensitivity to types I and III collagen (normal constituents of human arteries) in patients with TAO compared with patients with arteriosclerosis obliterans or healthy male controls. There was a low but significant level of anticollagen antibody in 7 of 39 serum samples from patients with TAO, whereas this antibody was not detected in the control group of patients. Circulating immune complexes have been found in the peripheral arteries of some patients with TAO.[15, 23, 24, 73]

In summary, there is no single etiologic mechanism present in all patients with TAO. Tobacco seems to play a central role in the initiation and the continuance of the disease. Other etiologic factors such as genetic predisposition, immunologic mechanisms, endothelial dysfunction, and abnormalities in coagulation may play a role in some patients.

PATHOLOGY

In Buerger's disease there is an inflammatory thrombosis that affects the arteries and the veins, and the histopathology of the involved blood vessels varies according to the chronologic age of the disease at which the tissue sample is obtained for examination. The histopathology is most likely to be diagnostic at the acute phase of the disease. It evolves to changes being consistent with or suggestive of the disease in the appropriate clinical setting at the immediate stage or subacute phase, and becomes virtually indeterminate at the end-stage or chronic phase when all that remains is organized thrombus and fibrosis of the blood vessels.[7, 17, 41–43, 50, 88]

Dible[17] stated that the pathologic diagnosis of Buerger's disease was by no means always secure.

> *There is so much variation from case to case, depending upon the stage of the disease and the characteristic capriciousness of the lesions, that it is difficult to give a succinct account of the histology.*[17]

Nevertheless, Dible[17] believed that the histologic distinction between Buerger's disease and atherosclerosis was so clear-cut that a differentiation could be made with a high degree of accuracy by simply examining tissue sections containing digital arteries and veins. The small blood vessels in the hand and foot are not usually affected by atherosclerosis.

The acute-phase lesion is characterized by acute inflammation involving all coats of the vessel wall, especially of the veins, in association with occlusive thrombosis. Around the periphery of the thrombus there are often polymorphonuclear leukocytes with karyorrhexis, the so-called microabscesses, in which one or more multinucleated giant cells may be present (Fig. 20–1). This histologic finding in thrombophlebitis is most characteristic of, but may not be specific for, Buerger's disease.[40] This striking inflammatory thrombotic lesion occurs with greater regularity in veins than in arteries (Fig. 20–2).

It is not known whether the vascular lesions of Buerger's disease are primarily thrombotic or primarily inflammatory. In either event, the intense inflammatory infiltration and cellular proliferation seen in the acute-stage lesions are distinctive, especially when the veins are involved. If a biopsy of the acute and often tender nodular subcutaneous phlebitic lesion is obtained at an early stage, one may observe several coexisting lesions in different segments of the same affected vein. There may be acute phlebitis without thrombosis, acute phlebitis with thrombosis, and acute phlebitis with thrombus containing microabscesses and giant cells.

The acute phase is followed by an intermediate phase,

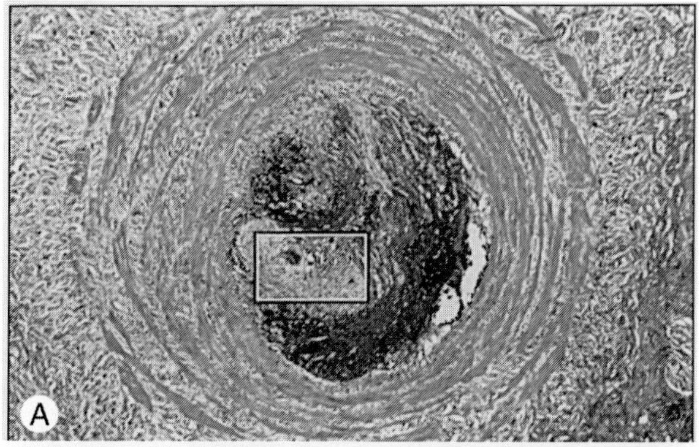

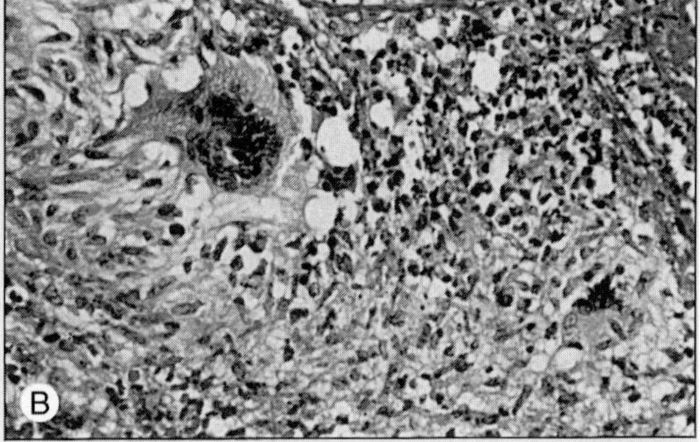

FIGURE 20–1. *A*, Typical acute histologic lesion of Buerger's disease in a vein with intense thromboangiitis. (×64.) *B*, Close-up view of the boxed area in *A*, showing a microabscess in the thrombus and two multinucleated giant cells. (×400.) (H&E.) (From Lie JT: Thromboangiitis obliterans [Buerger's disease] revisited. Pathol Annu 23 [Part 2]:257–291, 1988.)

in which there is progressive organization of the occlusive thrombus in the arteries and veins (see Fig. 20–2). At this stage there is often a prominent inflammatory cell infiltrate within the thrombus and much less inflammation in the vessel wall. The chronic phase, or end-stage lesions, is characterized by completed organization of the occlusive thrombus with extensive recanalization, prominent vascularization of the media, and adventitial and perivascular fibrosis (Fig. 20–3).

> *In all three stages, the normal architecture of the vessel wall subjacent to the occlusive thrombus and including the internal elastic lamina remains essentially intact. These findings distinguish thromboangiitis obliterans from arteriosclerosis and from other systemic vasculitides in which there is usually more striking disruption of the internal elastic lamina and the media, disproportional to those attributable to aging change.*[67]

Buerger's disease is segmental in distribution: "skip" areas of normal vessels between diseased ones are common, and the intensity of the periadventitial reaction may be quite variable in different segments of the same vessel. These skip lesions may be observed angiographically and histopathologically.

The histopathology of Buerger's disease is often inconclusive in the intermediate or chronic lesions. A characteristic finding in TAO, however, is the marked cellular proliferation and inflammatory infiltrate in the thrombus. This is unique to Buerger's disease and is rarely seen in other etiologies of arterial or venous thrombosis. Lymphohistiocytic cells and, to a much lesser extent, granulocytic leuko-

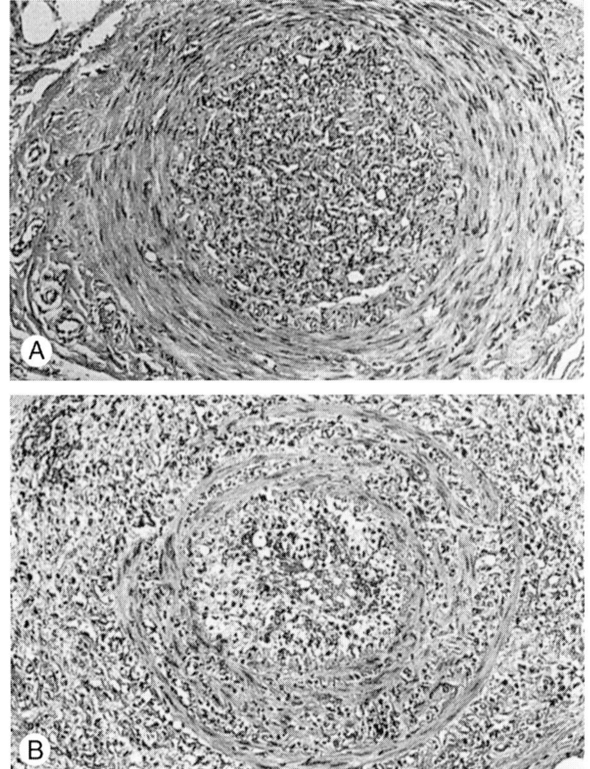

FIGURE 20–2. Digital artery (A) and digital vein (B) of the intermediate stage of Buerger's disease. Note the prominent inflammatory infiltrate and early organization of the thrombus. (H&E, ×64.) (From Lie JT: Thromboangiitis obliterans [Buerger's disease] revisited. Pathol Annu 23 [Part 2]:257–291, 1988.)

cytes contribute to the inflammatory infiltrates. Eosinophils may be present but seldom in excess number.[47] Another unique feature of Buerger's disease is that the elastic lamina usually remains intact, whereas there may be disruption of the elastic lamina in other forms of vasculitis.

The end-stage chronic lesions are the least distinctive of the three morphologic stages of Buerger's disease. In some patients, especially those older than 40 years of age, Buerger's disease and arteriosclerosis may coexist and thus create further diagnostic uncertainty and controversy. Buerger's disease does not confer an immunity to atherosclerosis or arteriosclerosis that is aging related. In fact, the history of heavy tobacco use in most patients with TAO may actually increase the likelihood of eventually developing atherosclerosis.

The process of thrombus organization in TAO is essentially identical to that in ordinary thrombosis, but with an added inflammatory component. The invasion of organizing smooth muscle cells from the media of the blood vessel appears more intensified, resulting in a hypercellular thrombus with rapid organization. Prominent inflammatory cell infiltrate in thrombus organization is a hallmark of Buerger's disease. Initial preservation of the internal elastic lamina is another distinguishing feature from arteriosclerosis or atherosclerosis and necrotizing vasculitis.

Buerger's Disease of Blood Vessels in Unusual Locations

Buerger's disease, as already noted, is almost exclusively a disease of the small and medium-sized blood vessels in the lower and upper limbs. There have been only occasional reports, usually without adequate histologic proof, of involvement of large elastic arteries such as the aorta, the iliac arteries, and the pulmonary artery. Although Buerger[8] had noted that vascular obliteration could affect blood vessels other than those of the limbs, the involvement of the cerebral, coronary, renal, and mesenteric arteries has been documented in an occasional patient, almost all as single case reports.[16, 18, 74] Although rare, there have been reports of multiple organ involvement in Buerger's disease.[26] An extreme example of Buerger's disease with combined peripheral and visceral involvement was that of an 18-year-old male cigarette smoker who, in a span of 15 years, underwent bilateral lumbar and dorsal sympathectomies, two bowel resections, and 13 amputations, including bilateral above-elbow and above-knee amputations, before he succumbed at age 33 to another episode of bowel infarction from recurrent Buerger's disease of the mesenteric arteries and veins.[11]

The histopathology of visceral TAO is identical to that observed in blood vessels of the limbs with involvement of both arteries and veins. There are even rarer instances of Buerger's disease in a saphenous vein arterial graft,[48] or in the temporal arteries of young smokers, in some preceded by peripheral ischemia ending in amputations.[47] Also not widely known is the occurrence of Buerger's disease in

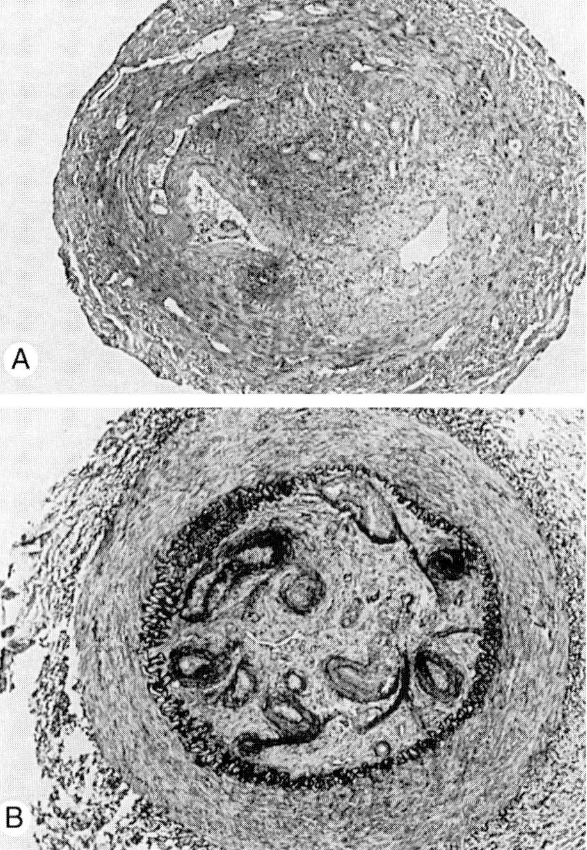

FIGURE 20–3. Chronic-stage lesion of Buerger's disease in a radial artery. Note the extensive recanalization of the organized thrombus with prominent vascularization of the media, intact internal elastic lamina, and some residual lymphomononuclear cell infiltrate. (A, H&E, ×64; B, Elastic Van Gieson stain, ×64.) (From Lie JT: Thromboangiitis obliterans [Buerger's disease] revisited. Pathol Annu 23[Part 2]:257–291, 1988.)

TABLE 20–1. PRESENTING SIGNS AND SYMPTOMS IN THROMBOANGIITIS OBLITERANS

SIGNS AND SYMPTOMS	NO. (%)
Intermittent claudication	70 (63)
Rest pain	91 (81)
Ischemic ulcers	85 (76)
Upper extremity	24 (28)
Lower extremity	39 (46)
Upper and lower extremities	22 (26)
Thrombophlebitis	43 (38)
Raynaud's phenomenon	49 (44)
Sensory findings	77 (69)
Abnormal Allen's test	71 (63)

Modified from Olin JW, Young JR, Graor RA, et al: The changing clinical spectrum of thromboangiitis obliterans (Buerger's disease). Circulation 82 (Suppl IV): IV-3–IV-8, 1990.

testicular and spermatic arteries and veins, as was originally described by Buerger.[8] These reports of Buerger's disease in unusual locations are looked at with skepticism by some investigators. A diagnosis of TAO in unusual locations should be made only when the histopathologic findings are classic for the acute lesion *and* the clinical presentation is consistent with Buerger's disease. Although TAO occurs most frequently in the infrapopliteal and infrabrachial arteries, it is not uncommon to see involvement of the superficial femoral artery. Less commonly, Buerger's disease affects the brachial artery. Iliac artery involvement is occasionally seen.[77] Involvement of the other arteries mentioned earlier is exceedingly rare.

CLINICAL FEATURES

The classic presentation of Buerger's disease is in a young male smoker with the onset of symptoms before the age of 40 to 45 years. There appears to be an increased incidence of TAO in women, according to some reports.[49, 59, 65] This does not appear to be the case, however, in the Japanese literature.[39, 78, 79] Buerger's disease usually begins with ischemia of the distal small arteries and veins. As the disease progresses, it may involve more proximal arteries. Large artery involvement has been reported in TAO, but this is unusual and rarely occurs in the absence of small vessel occlusive disease.[77]

Patients may present with claudication of the feet, the legs, and occasionally the arms and hands. Foot or arch claudication may be the presenting manifestation and is often mistaken for an orthopedic problem, resulting in a considerable delay before the correct diagnosis is made. Later in the course of the disease patients may develop ischemic ulcerations in the distal portion of the toes and/or fingers.

At the Cleveland Clinic Foundation, 112 patients with Buerger's disease were evaluated between 1970 and 1987.[65] The presenting clinical signs and symptoms are shown in Table 20–1. Intermittent claudication occurred in 70 patients (63%). The age and gender distribution and the presenting signs and symptoms were virtually identical in a follow-up series of an additional 40 patients evaluated from 1988 to 1996.[66] The initial location of claudication was the arch of the foot in many patients. As the disease progressed, claudication often moved proximally to cause typical calf claudication.

Seventy-six per cent of patients had ischemic ulcerations at the time of presentation.[65] However, if there was heightened awareness of the early manifestations of TAO (foot or arch claudication), many patients could be identified sooner and treated before they developed ischemic ulcerations (Figs. 20–4 and 20–5).

Two or more limbs are almost always involved in Buerger's disease.[34, 79] Shionoya[79] noted that two limbs were affected in 16% of patients, 3 limbs in 41%, and all four limbs in 43% of patients. Because of the proclivity to involve more than one limb, it has been the author's practice to perform an arteriogram of both upper and/or lower extremities in patients who clinically present with involvement of only one limb. It is not uncommon to see angiographic abnormalities consistent with Buerger's disease in limbs that are not yet clinically involved.

In patients with lower extremity ulceration in whom Buerger's disease is a consideration, an Allen's test should be performed to assess the circulation in the hands and fingers (Fig. 20–6).[2, 64] An abnormal Allen's test in a young smoker with lower extremity ulcerations is highly suggestive of TAO since it demonstrates small vessel involvement in both the upper and lower extremities. In the Cleveland Clinic series, 63% of all patients demonstrated an abnormal

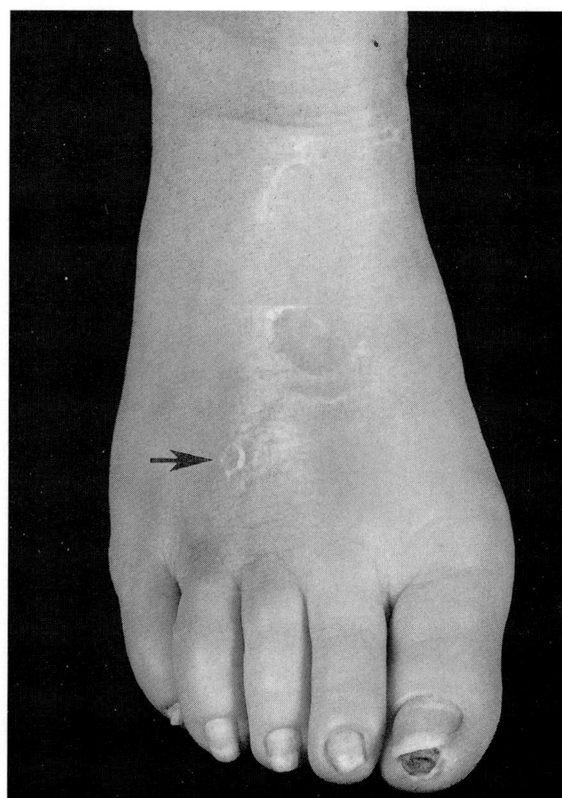

FIGURE 20–4. Ischemic ulcer on the distal portion of the right great toe in a young man with acute Buerger's disease. Note the superficial thrombophlebitis on the dorsum of the foot *(arrow)* with marked erythema around the phlebitis. (From Olin JW, Lie JT: Thromboangiitis obliterans. *In* Cooke JP, Frohlich ED [eds]: Current Management of Hypertension and Vascular Disease. Philadelphia, BC Decker, 1992, pp 265–271.)

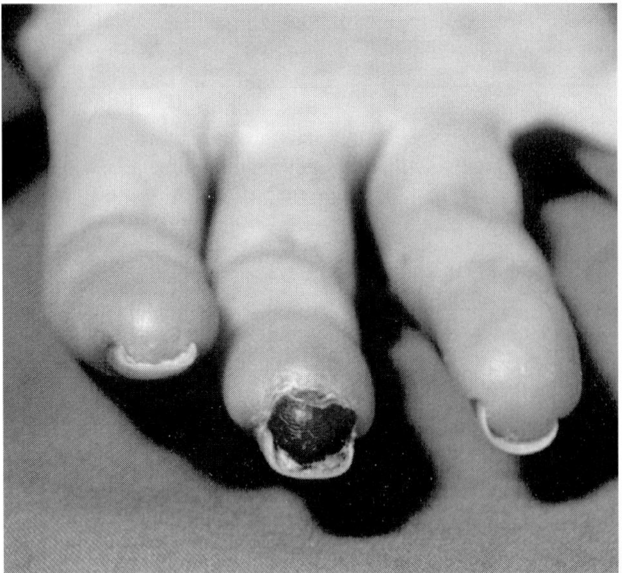

FIGURE 20–5. Ischemic ulcers on the index and middle fingers of a patient with Buerger's disease.

Allen's test.[65] The distal nature of TAO and the involvement of the lower and upper extremities help differentiate TAO from atherosclerosis. Except in patients with end-stage renal disease and diabetes, atherosclerosis does not occur in the hand and rarely occurs distal to the subclavian artery.

Superficial thrombophlebitis occurred in approximately 40% of patients with TAO in the Cleveland Clinic series.[65] The thrombophlebitis may be migratory and may parallel disease activity.[68] Biopsy of an acute superficial thrombophlebitis often demonstrates the typical histopathologic lesions of acute Buerger's disease.

Cold sensitivity is common and may be one of the earliest manifestations of TAO. This may be related to ischemia or to markedly increased muscle sympathetic nerve activity, as has been demonstrated in patients with TAO compared with a control group.[89] Typical Raynaud's phenomenon has been reported in approximately 40% of patients. The extremities of patients with Buerger's disease often have an erythematous or cyanotic appearance.[35]

Sensory findings are common in TAO, occurring in 69% of cases in the Cleveland Clinic series.[65] Much of these sensory abnormalities are due to ischemic neuropathy, which occurs late in the course of TAO. It has been demonstrated on gross and microscopic pathology that the nerve fibers may be encased with the inflammatory or fibrotic material in Buerger's disease, thus accounting for some of the sensory abnormalities.

Diagnostic Criteria

There have been several different diagnostic criteria proposed for the diagnosis of TAO. Papa and Adar[68] have proposed various clinical, angiographic, histopathologic, and exclusionary criteria for the diagnosis of TAO. A recent report by these investigators suggested a point scoring system to help establish the diagnosis of Buerger's disease.[70] Mills and Porter[57] have proposed major and minor diagnostic criteria for Buerger's disease. Their major criteria include the following: onset of distal extremity ischemic symptoms before the age of 45 years; tobacco abuse; undiseased arteries proximal to the popliteal or brachial level; objective documentation of distal occlusive disease by four-limb plethysmography; and arteriography and/or histopathology and exclusion of proximal embolic sources, trauma and local lesions, autoimmune diseases, hypercoagulable states, and atherosclerosis (diabetes, hyperlipidemia, renal failure, hypertension). Their minor criteria include migratory superficial phlebitis, Raynaud's syndrome, upper extremity involvement, and instep claudication.

Classifying the criteria as major and minor serves no

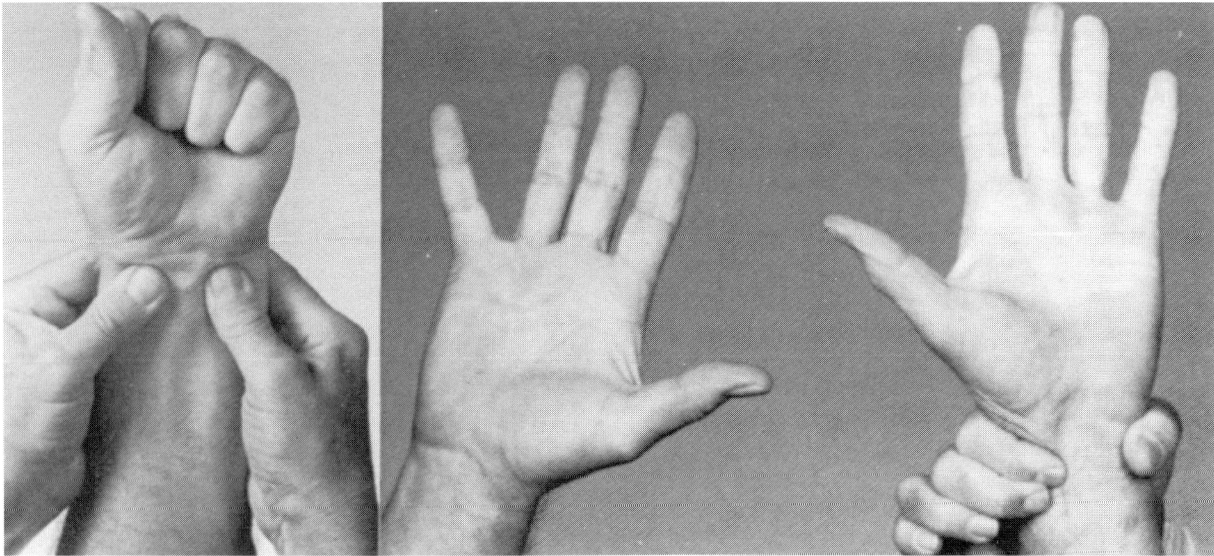

FIGURE 20–6. Allen's test with occlusion of the radial and ulnar pulse by compression *(left side)*. The pressure on the ulnar pulse is released while the radial pulse is still compressed. The hand does not fill with blood; note the paleness of the hand on the right compared with the left, indicating occlusion of the ulnar artery *(right side)*. (From Olin JW, Lie JT: Thromboangiitis obliterans. *In* Cooke JP, Frohlich ED [eds]: Current Management of Hypertension and Vascular Disease. Philadelphia, BC Decker, 1992, pp 265–271.)

useful purpose. It does not help diagnose TAO, nor is it helpful in understanding the pathophysiology or in formulating a treatment plan. In addition, there are an increasing number of patients who fulfill all the major criteria for TAO but also have the exclusionary criteria of hypertension or hyperlipidemia. Some of these patients develop typical atherosclerosis 15 or 20 years after the original diagnosis of TAO. Therefore, if patients meet the criteria of distal extremity involvement, tobacco use, exclusion of a proximal source of emboli or atherosclerosis, in the absence of a definable hypercoagulable state, hyperlipidemia and/or hypertension should not be exclusionary for the diagnosis of TAO.

Laboratory and Arteriographic Findings

There are no specific laboratory tests to aid in the diagnosis of TAO. A complete serologic profile to exclude other diseases that can mimic TAO should be obtained. These include the following: complete blood count with differential, liver function, renal function, fasting blood sugar, urinalysis, acute-phase reactants (Westergren sedimentation rate and C-reactive protein), antinuclear antibody, rheumatoid factor, complement measurements, serologic markers for CREST syndrome (*c*alcinosis, *R*aynaud's phenomenon, *e*sophageal disease, *s*clerodactyly, *t*elangiectasia) and scleroderma (anticentromere antibody and Scl-70), and a complete hypercoagulability screen to include antiphospholipid antibodies.

A proximal source of emboli may be excluded by performing echocardiography (two-dimensional and/or transesophageal) and arteriography. The angiographic features of Buerger's disease are well known.[38, 54, 55, 83] Although the findings on arteriography may be suggestive, there are no pathognomonic angiographic findings in TAO.

The usual arteriographic findings are shown in Table 20–2 and Figures 20–7 to 20–9. Proximal arteries should be normal, demonstrating no evidence of atherosclerosis, aneurysm, or other source of proximal emboli. Although the disease has been rarely reported in the proximal arteries,[77] in most cases the proximal arteries should be normal. A pathologic specimen is necessary to diagnose Buerger's disease with proximal artery involvement. The disease is confined most often to the distal circulation and is almost always infrapopliteal in the lower extremities and distal to the brachial artery in the upper extremities. There is small and medium-sized vessel involvement, such as the digital arteries in the fingers and toes, the palmar and plantar arteries in the hand and foot, as well as the tibial, peroneal, radial, and ulnar arteries.[67, 68] Isolated disease below the popliteal artery almost never occurs in atherosclerosis. Even the patient with diabetes mellitus often has multisegment disease with some evidence of proximal artery involvement. However, since diabetes is exclusionary for the diagnosis of TAO (in the absence of a pathologic specimen), there should be no confusion between these two diseases.

TABLE 20–2. CHARACTERISTIC ARTERIOGRAPHIC FINDINGS IN THROMBOANGIITIS OBLITERANS

1. Involvement of small and medium-sized vessels
   a. Digital arteries of fingers and toes
   b. Palmar, plantar, tibial, peroneal, radial, and ulnar arteries
2. Segmental occlusive lesions: diseased arteries interspersed with normal-appearing arteries
3. More severe disease distally
4. Collateralization around areas of occlusion: "corkscrew collaterals"
5. Normal proximal arteries: no atherosclerosis
6. No source of embolus

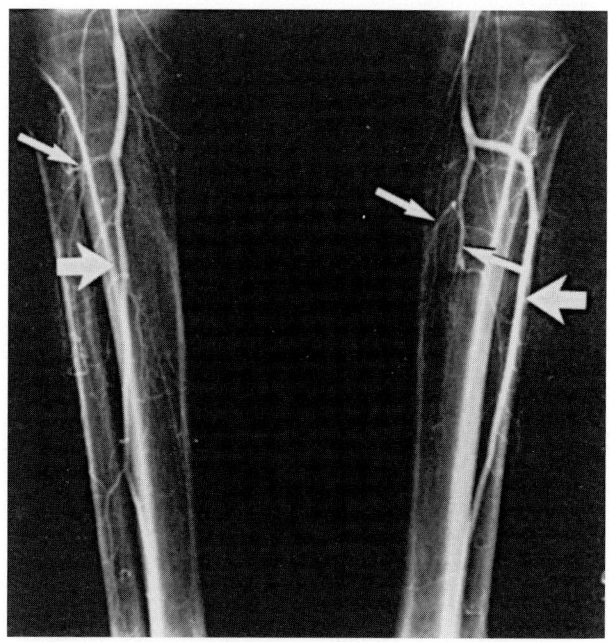

FIGURE 20–7. There is disease of the popliteal and infrapopliteal arteries bilaterally in a patient with thromboangiitis obliterans. In the right leg the anterior tibial artery *(small arrow)* and the posterior tibial artery are occluded at their origin. The peroneal artery is patent *(large arrow)*. In the left leg the anterior tibial artery is patent *(large arrow)*, but the posterior tibial and peroneal arteries *(small arrows)* are occluded proximally. (From Olin JW, Lie JT: Thromboangiitis obliterans. *In* Cooke JP, Frohlich ED [eds]: Current Management of Hypertension and Vascular Disease. Philadelphia, BC Decker, 1992, pp 265–271.)

Arteriographically (and pathologically), TAO is a segmental disorder, demonstrating areas of diseased vessels interspersed with normal blood vessel segments (see Figs. 20–8 and 20–9A). There is often evidence of multiple vascular occlusions with collateralization around the obstructions ("corkscrew collaterals") (see Fig. 20–8). Corkscrew collaterals are not pathognomonic of Buerger's disease because they may be present in other small vessel occlusive diseases such as CREST syndrome and scleroderma. In fact, the arteriographic appearance of Buerger's disease may be identical to that seen in patients with scleroderma, CREST syndrome, systemic lupus erythematosus, rheumatoid vasculitis, mixed connective tissue disease, and antiphospholipid antibody syndrome. However, the clinical and serologic manifestations of these other immunologic diseases should help differentiate them from TAO. Irregularity or calcification of the blood vessel wall should be exclusionary for the diagnosis of Buerger's disease.[68] The author has found the algorithm shown in Figure 20–10 to be helpful in the diagnosis of TAO.[67]

Differential Diagnosis

The diagnosis of TAO should not be difficult if diseases that mimic TAO are excluded. The most important diseases

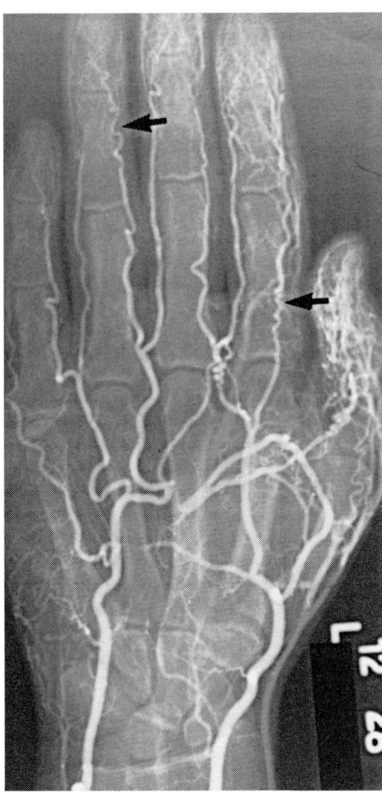

FIGURE 20–8. Multiple digital artery occlusions with evidence of collateralization ("corkscrew collaterals") *(arrows)* around the areas of occlusion. (From Olin JW, Lie JT: Thromboangiitis obliterans. *In* Cooke JP, Frohlich ED [eds]: Current Management of Hypertension and Vascular Disease. Philadelphia, BC Decker, 1992, pp 265–271.)

to exclude are atherosclerosis, emboli, and autoimmune diseases, as discussed earlier. Under most circumstances, with the use of echocardiography and arteriography, atherosclerosis and emboli can be excluded with a high degree of clinical certainty.

The diagnosis in patients who have scleroderma or CREST syndrome is usually obvious from a clinical examination of the skin, a history of other systemic features that occur in these diseases, and the presence of serologic markers such as Scl-70 or anticentromere antibodies. Nailfold capillaroscopy is usually quite distinctive in patients with CREST syndrome or scleroderma.

A careful search should be undertaken for the presence of systemic lupus erythematosus, rheumatoid arthritis, mixed connective tissue disease, antiphospholipid antibody syndrome and other types of vasculitis. Serologic markers often help eliminate the presence of these conditions. Patients with antiphospholipid antibody syndrome may present with evidence of both arterial and venous thrombotic events. These patients may have a prolonged activated partial thromboplastin time, a positive circulating "lupus type" anticoagulant, and/or the presence of high-titer anticardiolipin antibodies. Several cases of typical Buerger's disease with the presence of elevated anticardiolipin antibodies have been encountered at our institution and elsewhere, but this is an uncommon occurrence.[10, 66] A pathologic specimen would clearly differentiate these two entities since antiphospholipid antibody syndrome is, in reality, a vasculopathy (the presence of thrombus with no inflammatory components) as opposed to the typical pathologic findings in Buerger's disease (a highly inflammatory thrombus). We have also demonstrated that some patients with Buerger's disease have markedly elevated levels of plasma homocysteine.[66] Preliminary data suggest that elevated homocysteine levels may be a poor prognostic sign and may predict those patients who ultimately require amputation.

It should not be difficult to differentiate patients with TAO from those with Takayasu's arteritis or giant cell arteritis. Whereas patients with TAO manifest distal extremity ischemia, patients with Takayasu's arteritis or giant cell arteritis present with proximal vascular involvement. The arteriographic features of Takayasu's disease or giant cell arteritis are distinctive. Many patients with Takayasu's arteritis have elevations in the acute-phase reactants (erythrocyte sedimentation rate and C-reactive protein), but this finding is not invariable and may not correlate with disease activity.[32]

In the presence of lower extremity involvement, the possibility of popliteal artery entrapment syndrome or cystic adventitial disease should be considered, both of which should be readily apparent on arteriography, computed tomography scan, or magnetic resonance imaging. An aneurysm of the popliteal artery should be easily diagnosed by physical examination.

A careful history should be taken for the possibility of ergotamine use (abuse) because this may cause severe ischemia in multiple limbs. Ergotamine ingestion and TAO may cause both lower and upper extremity ischemia. Even if the patient denies a history of migraine headaches or previous ergotamine use, ergotamine blood levels should be obtained in some patients to exclude this condition. If there is isolated involvement of the upper extremity, occupational hazards such as vibratory tool use and hypothenar hammer syndrome should be considered.

THERAPY

Various therapies available for TAO are shown in Table 20–3. However, *the cornerstone of therapy is the complete discontinuation of cigarette smoking or the use of tobacco in any form*. It has been demonstrated in many case reports and series that complete abstinence from tobacco is the only way to halt the progression of Buerger's disease and to avoid future amputations.[13, 21, 65] Even one or two cigarettes a day is enough to keep the disease active. In patients with documented TAO, smokeless tobacco (chewing tobacco or snuff) has also been reported to cause Buerger's disease and to keep it active once it has already occurred.[34, 46] Marijuana smoking may also cause progression. Of 152 patients with Buerger's disease treated at the Cleveland Clinic from 1970 to 1996, adequate long-term follow-up was obtained in 120 patients (Fig. 20–11). Fifty-two patients (43%) discontinued cigarette smoking. If gangrene was not present at the time the patient discontinued smoking, amputation did not occur. Overall, 49 patients (94%) avoided amputation in the ex-smoking group. In the 68 patients who continued smoking, 29 patients (43%) required one or more amputations. The mean follow-up in the original series was

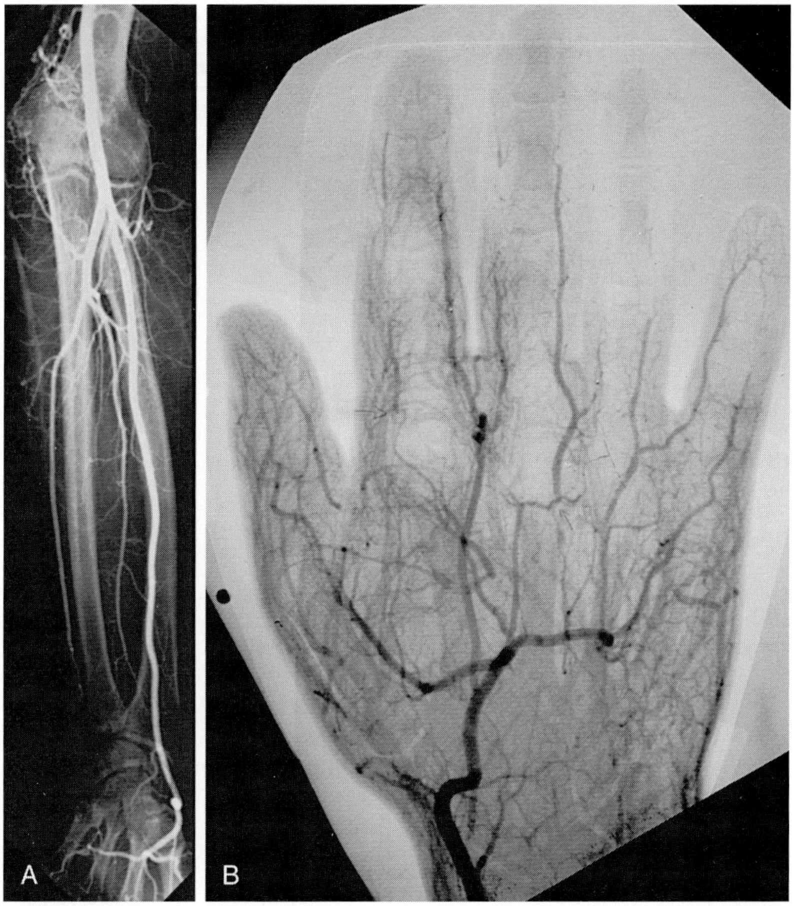

FIGURE 20–9. *A,* Arteriogram demonstrating a normal brachial artery with a radial artery that supplies the hand. The interosseous artery ends just above the wrist. The ulnar artery is diseased and occludes above the wrist. *B,* Note the occluded ulnar artery. There are multiple digital artery occlusions. Some digits have multiple "skip" areas, with patent arteries interspersed with occluded arteries.

91.6 ± 84 months (range, 1 to 460 months), and the follow-up in the additional 40 patients was a mean of 31 months (range, 1.6 to 89.7 months). Using Chi-square analysis, these data were highly significant. In the most recent series, there was also a relationship between elevated plasma homocysteine levels and amputation.[66]

Some authors have suggested that it is extremely difficult to get patients with TAO to discontinue smoking.[57] The

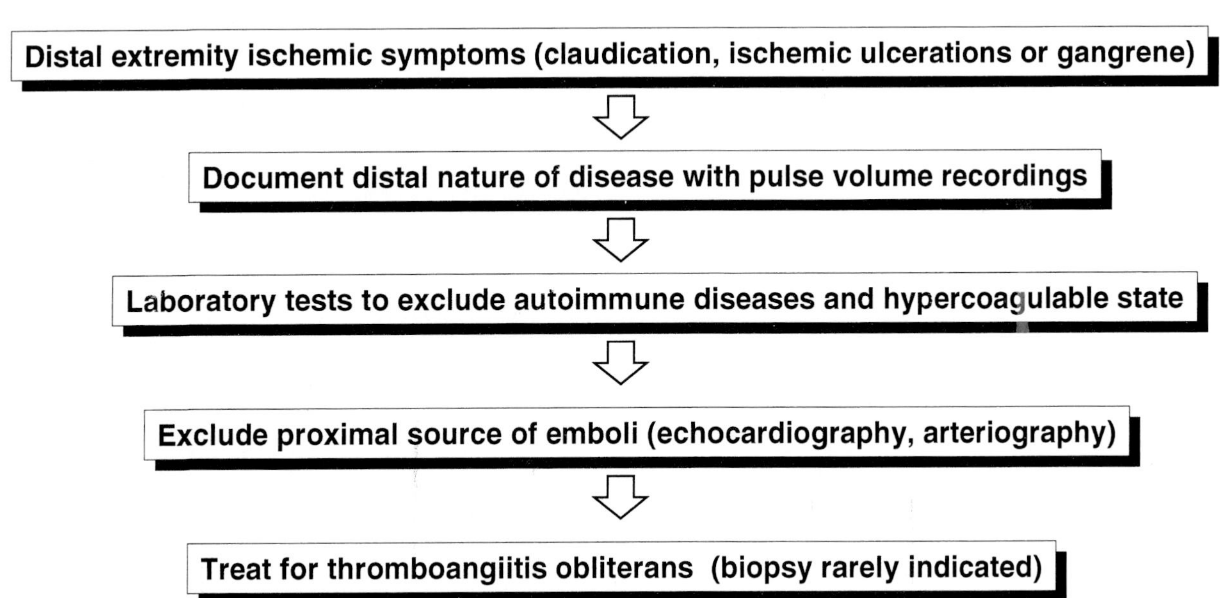

FIGURE 20–10. Algorithm for the diagnosis of thromboangiitis obliterans. (From Olin JW, Lie JT: Thromboangiitis obliterans (Buerger's disease). *In* Loscalzo J, Creager MA, Dzau VJ [eds]: Vascular Medicine. Boston, Little, Brown, 1996, pp 1033–1049.)

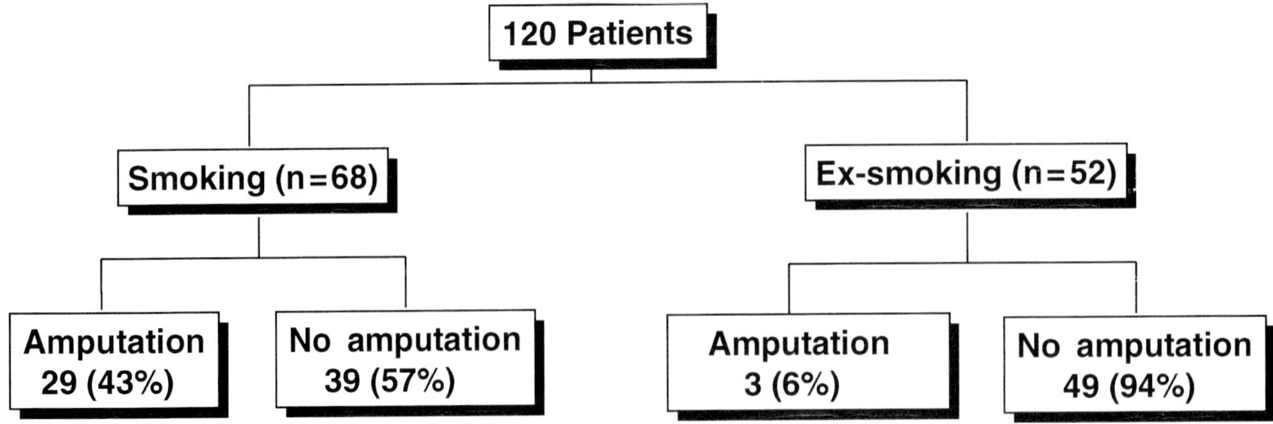

FIGURE 20–11. Smoking status related to amputation. (Adapted from Olin JW, Young JR, Graor RA, et al: The changing clinical spectrum of thromboangiitis obliterans [Buerger's disease]. Circulation 82 [Suppl IV]: IV-3–IV-8; and Olin JW, Childs MB, Bartholomew JR, et al: Anticardiolipin antibodies and homocysteine levels in patients with thromboangiitis obliterans. Presented at the American College of Rheumatology, Orlando, September 1997.)

author and colleagues have found that it may be easier to convince patients with Buerger's disease to stop smoking compared with those with atherosclerosis. Among 120 patients followed long term, 43% of the patients with TAO were able to discontinue smoking.[65, 66] The correlation of smoking cessation to disease activity (healing of ischemic ulcerations and avoidance of amputation) is so strong that if patients state that they have stopped using tobacco products and the disease is still active, a urine nicotine and cotinine level should be measured to determine if they are telling the truth, or if they are using other nicotine products such as nicotine gum and patches or are being exposed to large amounts of environmental (secondary) tobacco smoke.[53]

Since smoking cessation is so closely tied to disease activity and future amputation, it is extremely important for the physician to educate and counsel the patient on the importance of discontinuing the use of all tobacco products (Fig. 20–12). Some investigators have recommended using anecdotes or photographs of patients who had prior amputations, or using group meetings with other patients with TAO as a means to get the patient to stop smoking.[34] Education is probably the most important aspect. Patients can be reassured that if they are able to discontinue tobacco use, the disease will remit and amputations will not occur as long as critical limb ischemia (gangrene and tissue loss)

TABLE 20–3. TREATMENT OF THROMBOANGIITIS OBLITERANS

1. Have the patient stop smoking or using tobacco in any form
2. Advise the patient to avoid passive smoking (at least until healed)
3. Treat local ischemic ulcerations and pain:
   a. Foot care
      (1) Lubricate skin with lanolin-based cream
      (2) Lamb's wool between toes
      (3) Avoid trauma (heel protectors, bed cradle)
   b. Trial of calcium channel blockers, antiplatelet agents, and/or pentoxifylline
   c. Iloprost (not currently available in the United States)
   d. Analgesics, to control pain
   e. Sympathectomy
   f. Bypass surgery, if anatomically feasible and patient has stopped smoking
   g. Implantable spinal cord stimulator (last resort before amputation)
4. Treat cellulitis with antibiotics and superficial phlebitis with nonsteroidal anti-inflammatory agents
5. Amputate when all else fails*

*While still investigational, vascular endothelial growth factor may prove to be helpful in ulcer healing and relief of rest pain.

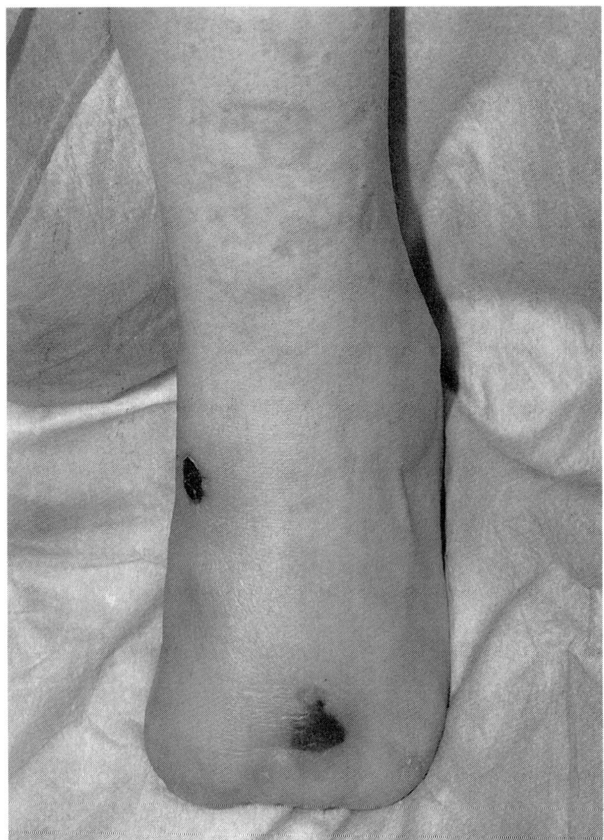

FIGURE 20–12. This patient underwent a transmetatarsal amputation in the past. He continued to smoke and has developed several areas of ischemic ulceration on the foot. (From Olin JW, Lie JT: Thromboangiitis obliterans [Buerger's disease]. *In* Loscalzo J, Creager MA, Dzau VJ [eds]: Vascular Medicine. Boston, Little, Brown, 1996, p 1047.)

Table 20–4. ASPIRIN VERSUS ILOPROST FOR CRITICAL LIMB ISCHEMIA IN THROMBOANGIITIS OBLITERANS

OUTCOME VARIABLES	ILOPROST (*n* [%])	ASPIRIN (*n* [%])
At Day 28	$n = 68$	$n = 65$
Responders	58 (85)*	11 (17)
Relief of rest pain	43 (63)	18 (28)
Ulcer healing	18/52 (35)	6/46 (13)
At 6 Months	$n = 51$	$n = 44$
Responders	45 (88)	12 (21)
Amputations	3 (6)	8 (18)

From Fiessinger JN, Schafer M, for the TAO Study Group: Trial of iloprost versus aspirin treatment for critical limb ischaemia of thromboangiitis obliterans. Lancet 335:555–557, 1990. © by The Lancet, 1990.
*$p < .05$.

has not already occurred. However, if significant arterial segments are occluded, the patient may continue to have intermittent claudication and/or Raynaud's phenomenon.

It is unclear whether involuntary smoking (secondary smoke) can cause TAO. The author recommends that patients with active TAO avoid as much involuntary smoking as possible until the disease becomes quiescent.

Other than discontinuation of cigarette smoking, all other forms of therapy are palliative. Fiessinger and Schafer conducted a prospective, randomized, double-blind trial comparing a 6-hour daily infusion of iloprost (a prostaglandin analogue) with aspirin (Table 20–4).[20] All patients entered into the study had critical limb ischemia defined as ischemic rest pain in a limb with or without tissue necrosis for which continuous analgesics in the hospital were required for at least 7 days. Iloprost was superior to aspirin at 28 days in achieving total relief of rest pain and complete healing of all trophic changes. In addition, at 6 months 88% of the patients receiving iloprost responded to therapy as compared with 21% of the aspirin group. Only 6% ended with amputations compared with 18% in the aspirin group. It appears that iloprost is also a useful modality in helping patients with critical limb ischemia get through the early period when they first discontinue cigarette smoking. Iloprost is not yet available for use in the United States, although it is available in several European countries.

It has been shown that an oral extended-release preparation of iloprost is equivalent to the intravenous form.[28] Based on these findings, the European TAO Study Group recently completed a double-blind, randomized trial comparing *oral* iloprost with placebo.[85] Three-hundred nineteen patients from six European countries were randomized to oral iloprost (100 or 200 μg) or placebo twice a day for 8 weeks. All patients had rest pain or trophic lesions. There was an additional 6-month follow-up period. The primary end-point was total healing of the most important lesion. The secondary end-point was total relief of rest pain without the need for analgesics. The combined end-point consisted of the patient being alive without major amputation, no lesions, no rest pain, and no analgesic use. The results of this study were as follows: (1) total healing of lesions was not significantly different between treatment groups at any time; (2) for total relief of rest pain without the need of analgesics, low-dose iloprost was significantly more effective than placebo at the end of follow-up (low-dose iloprost 63%, placebo 49%, $p = .020$); (3) for the combined end-point, iloprost (50%) was superior to placebo (35%) ($p = .016$); and (4) high-dose iloprost failed to show a significant treatment effect over placebo. Oral iloprost was safe. Both doses of iloprost showed no effect versus placebo on *total healing of all lesions*. It appears that the intravenous form of iloprost is more effective than the oral form in ulcer healing.

There is no substitute for good general vascular care in the treatment of patients with severe ischemia. A reverse Trendelenburg (vascular) position should be used in patients who have severe ischemic rest pain. Adequate narcotics should be made available during the period of severe ischemia. Anticoagulation has never been demonstrated to be effective in TAO. However, if other options are not available, some investigators use anticoagulants in an attempt to "buy time" and improve collateral flow in a severely ischemic limb. Good foot and hand care should be undertaken. If significant vasospasm is present, calcium channel blocking agents such as nifedipine, nicardipine, or amlodipine should be used.[64] Pentoxifylline has not been adequately studied in patients with TAO. Since this drug increases the red blood cell membrane flexibility and allows red blood cells to fit through a smaller vascular space, it is not unreasonable to try pentoxifylline in the severely ischemic patient.

The role of sympathectomy in preventing amputations or in treating pain is unclear. Twenty-three patients from the author's institution underwent sympathectomy, and there was no difference in the amputation rate between those undergoing sympathectomy and those not undergoing the procedure.[65] Occasionally sympathectomy may help the healing of superficial ischemic ulcerations and relieve rest pain.[82a]

There are a few anecdotal reports in the literature on the use of implantable spinal cord stimulators in patients with Buerger's disease. The author's group has recently treated one patient with this modality, resulting in complete healing of all upper extremity ulcerations. It may be worthwhile to consider a spinal cord stimulator to help decrease pain and avoid amputation in patients for whom surgical revascularization is not an option and when other forms of therapy are not effective. A recently published paper shows that vascular endothelial growth factor was very effective in healing the ischemic ulcers and relief of rest pain in patients with TAO.[31a]

There is little information regarding the use of intra-arterial thrombolytic therapy as an adjunct for the treatment of Buerger's disease. In one series,[30] selective low-dose intra-arterial streptokinase (10,000-U bolus followed by 5000 U/hr) was administered to 11 patients with long-standing Buerger's disease who had gangrene or pregangrenous lesions of the toes or feet. Many of these patients had previously had lumbar sympathectomies. The investigators reported an overall success rate (defined as amputation being avoided or altered) of 58.3%.

Kubota and coworkers[37] recently treated a patient with a "superselective" infusion of urokinase into the dorsalis pedis artery and demonstrated recanalization of this artery and healing of an ischemic toe ulcer. The patient has remained asymptomatic for four years. The author's experience with the use of thrombolytic therapy has not been as successful as that reported by Hussein and el Dorri[30] and Kubota and coworkers.[37] Thrombi in the superficial femoral artery have been successfully lysed, but the severe distal occlusive disease is often resistant to thrombolysis. From a pathologic standpoint, there is a highly inflammatory thrombus that quickly becomes encased with connective tissue and fibrous material. Therefore, thrombolytic therapy may not be effective in many of these patients. However, if the patient is facing amputation, it is not unreasonable to give a short trial of catheter-directed thrombolytic therapy as long as no contraindications exist.

Surgical revascularization for Buerger's disease is not usually a viable alternative owing to the diffuse segmental involvement and extreme distal nature of the disease. There is often not a distal blood vessel available for bypass surgery. However, if the patient is severely ischemic and has a distal patent artery available for terminal anastomosis, then bypass surgery should be considered with the use of autogenous vein.[57] Inada and associates[31] demonstrated that of 236 patients with Buerger's disease, only 11 (4.6%) patients had lesions that were amicable to surgical revascularization. In the 11 patients who underwent surgical revascularization, the bypass remained patent for 4 months to 7 years, with a mean time of 2.8 years. Other investigators have reported an early success rate of 29% for arterial reconstruction in patients with TAO.[58]

Sayin and colleagues[76] recently reported on the surgical treatment of 216 patients with Buerger's disease. This total number represented 9.7% of all of the patients treated in the Department of Cardiovascular Surgery at Istanbul University Cerrahpasa Medical School from 1981 to 1991. Lumbar sympathectomy was performed in 183 (85%) of the 216 patients. Twenty-one patients underwent direct arterial reconstruction consisting of thromboendarterectomy with patch angioplasty (5), aortofemoral or iliofemoral bypass grafting (5), femoropopliteal bypass grafting (6), and femorocrural bypass grafting (5). Thirty-three patients underwent amputation. They noted that 4 of the 5 endarterectomized segments had occluded by the 7-year follow-up. One iliofemoral, 3 femoropopliteal, and 2 femorocrural bypasses were also occluded. These authors suggested that the long-term patency of these grafts was not good, but in many instances the short-term patency was sufficient to allow healing of the ulcerations associated with TAO.

The most recent surgical series reported by Sasajima and associates[75] evaluated the role of infrainguinal bypass over an 18-year period in patients with Buerger's disease. Seventy-one autogenous vein bypasses were performed in 61 patients. Fifty-nine per cent of patients were operated on for an ischemic ulcer or gangrene, but 41% were operated on for claudication. Virtually all patients were heavy smokers. Eighty-five per cent of the bypasses were to the crual arteries or arteries below the ankle. There were 38 graft failures, the main causes being poor distal vessels, progression of disease, or vein graft stenosis. Of the 38, 10 were restored to patency with surgical revision. The primary patency was 48.8% and secondary patency was 62.5% at 5 years. At 10 years the primary and secondary patency rates were 43% and 56%, respectively. The patency rates were 66.8% in the group that stopped smoking and 34.7% ($p <$ .05) in the group that continued to smoke. Of the 28 secondary failures, 11 underwent amputation and 14 had disabling claudication. Some of the patients in this series may not have actually had TAO. Ten patients were older than 50 years of age and 41% were operated on for claudication.

The only other surgical approach in patients with Buerger's disease is that of omental transfer.[81, 84] Singh and Ramteke[81] reported on 50 patients with TAO who underwent omental transfer for rest pain and/or nonhealing ischemic ulcers. All patients showed an improvement in skin temperature, rest pain decreased in 36 patients, and claudication distance increased in 48 patients. The ulcers healed in 32 of 36 patients.

SUMMARY

TAO is a nonatherosclerotic, segmental, inflammatory disease that affects the small and medium-sized arteries and veins in the lower and upper extremities. In some way, it is causally related to tobacco use. Discontinuation of tobacco is the mainstay of treatment. In patients who successfully stop smoking, amputation almost never occurs. Other forms of therapy are palliative.

REFERENCES

1. Adar R, Papa MC, Halperin Z, et al: Cellular sensitivity to collagen in thromboangiitis obliterans. N Engl J Med 308:1113–1116, 1983.
2. Allen EV: Thromboangiitis obliterans: Methods of diagnosis of chronic occlusive arterial lesions distal to the wrist with illustrative cases. Am J Med Sci 178:237–244, 1929.
3. Allen EV, Brown GE: Thromboangiitis obliterans: A clinical study of 200 cases. Ann Intern Med 1:535–549, 1928.
4. Annual Report of the Buerger's Disease Research Committee of the Ministry of Health and Welfare of Japan. K Ishikawa (ed). Tokyo, 1976, pp 3–15, 86–97.
5. Becker CG, Dublin T, Wiedman A: Hypersensitivity to tobacco antigen. Proc Soc Nat Acad Sci USA 73:1712–1716, 1976.
6. Booshanam VM: Role of sympathectomy in Buerger's disease. Presented at the 7th Congress of the Asian Surgical Association in Penang, 1989.
7. Buerger L: Thromboangiitis obliterans: A study of the vascular lesions leading to presenile spontaneous gangrene. Am J Med Sci 136:567–580, 1908.
8. Buerger L: The Circulatory Disturbance of the Extremities, Including Gangrene, Vasomotor, and Trophic Disorders. Philadelphia, WB Saunders, 1924.
9. Cachovan M: Epidemiologie und geographisches Verteilungsmuster der Thromboangiitis obliterans. *In* Heidrich H (ed): Thromboangiitis Obliterans Morbus Winiwarter-Buerger. Stuttgart, Georg Thieme, 1988, pp 31–36.
10. Casellas M, Perez A, Cabero L: Buerger's disease and antiphospholipid antibodies in pregnancy. Ann Rheum Dis 52:247–248, 1993.
11. Cebezas-Moya R, Dragstedt LR III: An extreme example of Buerger's disease. Arch Surg 101:632–634, 1970.
12. Chaudhury NA, Pietraszek MH, Hachiya T, et al: Plasminogen activators and plasminogen activator inhibitor 1 before and after venous occlusion of the upper limb in thromboangiitis obliterans (Buerger's disease). Thromb Res 66:321–329, 1992.
13. Corelli F: Buerger's disease: Cigarette smoker disease may always be cured by medical therapy alone—uselessness of operative treatment. J Cardiovasc Surg 14:28–36, 1973.
14. Craven JL, Cotton RC: Haematological differences between thromboangiitis obliterans and atherosclerosis. Br J Surg 54:862–867, 1967.
15. De Albuquerque RR, Delgado L, Correia P, et al: Circulating immune

complexes in Buerger's disease–endarteritis obliterans in young men. J Cardiovasc Surg 30:821–825, 1989.
16. Deitch EA, Sikkema WW: Intestinal manifestation of Buerger's disease. Am Surg 47:326–328, 1981.
17. Dible JH: The Pathology of the Limb Ischaemia. Edinburgh, Oliver & Boyd, pp 79–96, 1966.
18. Donatelli F, Triggiani M, Nascimbene S, et al: Thromboangiitis obliterans of coronary and internal thoracic arteries in a young woman. J Thorac Cardiovasc Surg 113:800–802, 1997.
19. Eichhorn J, Sima D, Lindschau C, et al: Antiendothelial cell antibodies in thromboangiitis obliterans. Am J Med Sci 315:17–23, 1998.
20. Fiessinger JN, Schafer M: Trial of iloprost versus aspirin treatment for critical limb ischaemia of thromboangiitis obliterans. The TAO Study. Lancet 335:555–557, 1990.
21. Gifford RW, Hines EA: Complete clinical remission in thromboangiitis obliterans during abstinence from tobacco: Report of a case. Proc Staff Meet Mayo Clin 26:241–245, 1951.
22. Grove WJ, Stansby GP: Buerger's disease and cigarette smoking in Bangladesh. Ann R Coll Surg Engl 74:115–118, 1992.
23. Gulati SM, Madhra K, Thusoo TK, et al: Autoantibodies in thromboangiitis obliterans. Angiology 33:642–650, 1982.
24. Gulati SM, Saha K, Kant L, et al: Significance of circulating immune complexes in thromboangiitis obliterans (Buerger's disease). Angiology 35:276–281, 1984.
25. Harkavy J: Tobacco sensitivities in thromboangiitis obliterans, migratory phlebitis, and coronary artery disease. Bull N Y Acad Med 9:318–322, 1933.
26. Harten P, Muller-Huelsbeck S, Regensburger D, Loeffler H: Multiple organ manifestations in thromboangiitis obliterans (Buerger's disease). Angiology 47:419–425, 1996.
27. Herman BE: Buerger's syndrome. Angiology 26:713–716, 1975.
28. Hildebrand M: Pharmacokinetics and tolerability of oral lloprost in thromboangiitis obliterans. Eur J Clin Pharmacol 53:51–56, 1997.
29. Hill GL, Moeliono J, Tumewu F, et al: The Buerger syndrome in Java: A description of the clinical syndrome and some aspects of its aetiology. Br J Surg 60:606–613, 1973.
30. Hussein EA, el Dorri A: Intra-arterial streptokinase as adjuvant therapy for complicated Buerger's disease: Early trials. Int Surg 78:54–58, 1993.
31. Inada K, Iwashima Y, Okada A, Matsumoto K: Non-atherosclerotic segmental arterial occlusion of the extremities. Arch Surg 108:663–667, 1974.
31a. Isner JM, Baumgartner I, Rauh G, et al: Treatment of thromboangiitis obliterans (Buerger's disease) by intramuscular gene transfer of vascular endothelial growth factor: Preliminary clinical results. In press.
32. Jaff M, Olin JW, Young JR: Failure of acute-phase reactants to predict disease activity in Takayasu's arteritis. J Vasc Med Biol 4:223–227, 1994.
33. Jindal RM, Patel SM: Buerger's disease in cigarette smoking in Bangladesh. Ann R Coll Surg Engl 74:436–437, 1992.
34. Joyce JW: Buerger's disease (thromboangiitis obliterans). Rheum Dis Clin North Am 116:463–470, 1990.
35. Kimura T, Yoshizaki S, Tsushima N, et al: Buerger's colour. Br J Surg 77:1299–1301, 1990.
36. Kjeldsen K, Mozes M: Buerger's disease in Israel: Investigations on carboxyhemoglobin and serum cholesterol levels after smoking. Acta Chir Scand 135:495–498, 1969.
37. Kubota Y, Kichikawa K, Uchida H, et al: Superselective urokinase infusion therapy for dorsalis pedis artery occlusion in Buerger's disease. Cardiovasc Intervent Radiol 20:380–382, 1997.
38. Lambeth JT, Yong NK: Arteriographic findings in thromboangiitis obliterans with emphasis on femoropopliteal involvement. AJR 109:553–562, 1970.
39. Lau H, Cheng SWK: Buerger's disease in Hong Kong: A review of 89 cases. Aust NZ J Surg 67:264–269, 1997.
40. Leu HJ, Bollinger A: Phlebitis saltans sive migrans. Vasa 7:440–442, 1978.
41. Leu HJ: Early inflammatory changes in thromboangiitis obliterans. Pathol Microbiol 43: 151–156, 1975.
42. Leu HJ: Thromboangiitis obliterans Buerger: Pathologisch-anatomische Analyse von 53 Fallen. Schweiz Med Wschr 115:1080–1086, 1985.
43. Shionoya S, Leu HJ, Lie JT: Buerger's disease (thromboangiitis obliterans). *In* Stehbens WE, Lie JT (eds): Vascular Pathology. London, Chapman & Hall, 1995, pp 657–678.
44. Lie JT: Diagnostic histopathology of major systemic and pulmonary vasculitic syndromes. Rheum Dis Clin North Am 16:269–292, 1990.
45. Lie JT: The rise and fall and resurgence of thromboangiitis obliterans (Buerger's disease). Acta Pathol Jpn 39:153–158, 1989.
46. Lie JT: Thromboangiitis obliterans (Buerger's disease) and smokeless tobacco. Arthritis Rheum 31:812–813, 1988.
47. Lie JT, Michet CJ Jr: Thromboangiitis obliterans with eosinophilia (Buerger's disease) of the temporal arteries. Hum Pathol 19:598–602, 1988.
48. Lie JT: Thromboangiitis obliterans (Buerger's disease) in a saphenous vein arterial graft. Hum Pathol 18:402–404, 1987.
49. Lie JT: Thromboangiitis obliterans (Buerger's disease) in women. Medicine 64:65–72, 1987.
50. Lie JT: Thromboangiitis obliterans (Buerger's disease) revisited. Pathol Annu 23 (Part 2):257–291, 1988.
51. Lie JT: Thromboangiitis obliterans (Buerger's disease) in an elderly man after cessation of cigarette smoking—a case report. Angiology 38:864–867, 1987.
52. Makita S, Nakamura M, Murakami H, et al: Impaired endothelium-dependent vasorelaxation in peripheral vasculature of patients with thromboangiitis obliterans (Buerger's disease). Circulation 94(Suppl II): II-211–II-215, 1996.
53. Matsushita M, Shionoya S, Matsumoto T: Urinary cotinine measurements in patients with Buerger's disease: Effects of active and passive smoking on the disease process. J Vasc Surg 14:53–58, 1991.
54. McKusick VA, Harris WS, Ottsen OE, et al: Buerger's disease: A distinct clinical and pathologic entity. JAMA 181:93–100, 1962.
55. McKusick VA, Harris WS, Ottsen OE, Goodman RM: The Buerger syndrome in the United States: Arteriographic observations with special reference to involvement of the upper extremities and the differentiation from atherosclerosis and embolism. Bull Johns Hopkins Hosp 110:145–176, 1962.
56. McLoughlin GA, Helsby CR, Evans CC, et al: Association of HLA-A9 and HLA-B5 with Buerger's disease. Br Med J 2:1165–1166, 1976.
57. Mills JL, Porter JM: Buerger's disease: A review and update. Semin Vasc Surg 6:14–23, 1993.
58. Mills JL, Porter JM: Buerger's disease (thromboangiitis obliterans). Ann Vasc Surg 5:570–572, 1991.
59. Mills JL, Taylor LM, Porter JK: Buerger's disease in the modern era. Am J Surg 154:123–154, 1987.
60. Nigam R, Naraynan PS, Sharma SR, et al: Thromboangiitis obliterans and arteriosclerosis obliterans as cause of limb ischemia in Delhi. Ind J Surg 42:9–15, 1980.
61. Nishikimi N, Shionoya S, Mizuno S, et al: Result of national epidemiological study of Buerger's disease. J Jpn Coll Angiol 27:1125–1130, 1987.
62. Numano F, Sasazuki T, Koyama T, et al: HLA in Buerger's disease. Exp Clin Immunogenet 3:195–200, 1986.
63. Otawa T, Juji I, Kawano N, et al: HLA antigen in thromboangiitis obliterans. JAMA 230:1126, 1974.
64. Olin JW, Lie JT: Thromboangiitis obliterans (Buerger's disease). *In* Cooke JP, Frohlich ED (eds): Current Management of Hypertension and Vascular Disease. Philadelphia, BC Decker, 1992, pp 265–271.
65. Olin JW, Young JR, Graor RA, et al: The changing clinical spectrum of thromboangiitis obliterans (Buerger's disease). Circulation 82(Suppl IV): IV-3–IV-8, 1990.
66. Olin JW, Childs MB, Bartholomew JR, et al: Anticardiolipin antibodies and homocysteine levels in patients with thromboangiitis obliterans. Presented at the American College of Rheumatology, Orlando, Fla, September 1997.
67. Olin JW, Lie JT: Thromboangiitis obliterans (Buerger's disease). *In* Loscalzo J, Creager MA, Dzau VJ (eds): Vascular Medicine. Boston, Little, Brown, 1996, pp 1033–1049.
68. Papa MZ, Adar R: A critical look at thromboangiitis obliterans (Buerger's disease). Vasc Surg 5:1–21, 1992.
69. Papa M, Bass A, Adar R, et al: Autoimmune mechanisms in thromboangiitis obliterans (Buerger's disease): The role of tobacco antigen and the major histocompatibility complex. Surgery 111:527–531, 1992.
70. Papa MZ, Rabi I, Adar R: A point scoring system for the clinical diagnosis of Buerger's disease. Eur J Vasc Endovasc Surg 11:335–339, 1996.
71. Pietraszek MH, Chaudhury NA, Koyano K, et al: Enhanced platelet response to serotonin in Buerger's disease. Thromb Res 60:241–246, 1990.
72. Pirnat L, Simic LJ: Epidemiologie und geographisches Verteilungs-

muster der Endangiitis obliterans. *In* Heidrich H (ed): Thromboangiitis Obliterans Morbus Winiwarter-Buerger. Stuttgart, Georg Thieme, 1988, pp 36–38.

73. Roncon A, Delgado L, Correia P, et al: Circulating immune complexes in Buerger's disease. J Cardiovasc Surg 30:821–825, 1989.
74. Rosen N, Sommer I, Knobel B: Intestinal Buerger's disease. Arch Pathol Lab Med 109:962–963, 1985.
75. Sasajima T, Kubo Y, Inaba M, et al: Role of infrainguinal bypass in Buerger's disease: An eighteen-year experience. Eur J Vasc Endovasc Surg 13:186–192, 1997.
76. Sayin A, Bozkurt AK, Tuzun H, et al: Surgical treatment of Buerger's disease: Experience with 216 patients. Cardiovasc Surg 1:377–380, 1999.
77. Shionoya S, Ban I, Nakata Y, et al: Involvement of the iliac artery in Buerger's disease (pathogenesis and arterial reconstruction). J Cardiovasc Surg 19:69–76, 1978.
78. Shionoya S: Buerger's Disease: Pathology, Diagnosis and Treatment. Nagoya, University of Nagoya Press, 1990, p 261.
79. Shionoya S: Buerger's Disease (thromboangiitis obliterans). *In* Rutherford RB (ed): Vascular Surgery. Philadelphia, WB Saunders, 1989, pp 207–217.
80. Siguret V, Alhenc-Gelas M, Aiach M, et al: Response to DDAVP stimulation in thirteen patients with Buerger's disease. Thromb Res 86:85–87, 1997.
81. Singh I, Ramteke VK: The role of omental transfer in Buerger's disease: New Delhi's experience. Aust N Z J Surg 66:372–376, 1996.
82. Smolen JS, Youngchaiyud U, Weidinger T, et al: Autoimmunological aspects of thromboangiitis obliterans (Buerger's disease). Clin Immunol Immunopathol 11:168–177, 1978.

82a. Swigris JJ, Olin JW, Mekhail NA: Implantable spinal cord stimulator to treat the ischemic manifestations of thromboangiitis obliterans (Buerger's disease). J Vasc Surg (in press).

83. Szilagi D, DeRusso FJ, Elliot JP: Thromboangiitis obliterans: Clinico-angiographic correlations. Arch Surg 88:824–835, 1964.
84. Talwar S, Jain S, Porwal R, et al: Free versus pedicled omental grafts for limb salvage in Buerger's disease. Aust N Z J Surg 68:38–40, 1998.
85. The European TAO Study Group: Oral iloprost in the treatment of thromboangiitis obliterans (Buerger's disease): A double-blind, randomized, placebo-controlled trial. Eur J Vasc Endovasc Surg 16:300–307, 1998.
86. von Winiwarter F: Ueber eine eigenthumliche Form von Endarteritis und Endophlebitis mit Gangran des Fusses. Arch Klin Chir 23:202–226, 1879.
87. Westcott FN, Wright IS: Tobacco allergy and thromboangiitis obliterans. J Allerg 9:555–564, 1938.
88. Williams G: Recent view on Buerger's disease. J Clin Pathol 22:573–578, 1969.
89. Yamamoto K, Iwase S, Mano T, Shionoya S: Muscle sympathetic outflow in Buerger's disease. J Autonom Nerv Sys 44:67–76, 1993.

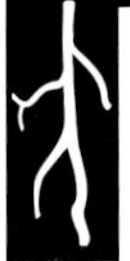

CHAPTER 21

Takayasu's Disease: Nonspecific Aortoarteritis

Joseph M. Giordano, M.D., and
Gary S. Hoffman, M.D.

Takayasu's disease is an arteritis of unknown etiology affecting primarily the aorta and its main branches, resulting in segmental stenosis, occlusion, dilatation, and aneurysm formation in arteries. The stenotic and occlusive lesions, in the absence of adequate collateral flow, may cause regional ischemia. Although the majority of reported cases are from the Far East, the disease occurs worldwide.[1–11] In addition, Takayasu's arteritis affects females predominantly but has also been described in males.[1–8, 10, 11] Patients who have the disease can present with a systemic illness with acute or chronic ischemia, the asymptomatic absence of pulses, or a combination of these presentations. Takayasu's arteritis is a rare disease that requires both long-term medical and surgical care to achieve improved survival and quality of life. This chapter reviews the current literature on Takayasu's arteritis and focuses primarily on clinical features of the disease, diagnostic modalities, and the treatment of this complex disorder.

INCIDENCE AND ETIOLOGY

Takayasu's arteritis occurs most frequently in the Far East.[1] A postmortem series in Japan demonstrated evidence of Takayasu's arteritis in approximately 1 of every 3000 autopsy cases.[12] A population study of Olmsted County, Minnesota, revealed a yearly incidence rate of 2.6 cases per 1 million inhabitants, and a hospital-based study in a defined area of Sweden estimated the yearly incidence of this disease to be 6.4 cases per 1 million inhabitants.[8, 13] The last figure might be high because the series included several older patients who may actually have had giant cell (temporal) arteritis.[10]

The cause of Takayasu's arteritis remains unclear. Because of the known association of microorganisms and aortitis, an infectious etiology has long been considered.[14] There have been reports of a relationship between tuberculosis and Takayasu's arteritis, with one series reporting active tuberculous infection in 60% of autopsy cases of nonspecific aortitis and other series noting a high incidence of tuberculin-positive skin hypersensitivity.[6, 10, 11, 15] However, other analyses of similar groups of patients have not borne out this association.[8–11] Several studies have proposed various human leukocyte antigen (HLA) associations, suggesting a genetic predisposition for the disease.[16–22] The strong predilection for women, the geographic incidence, and the occasional familial occurrence also suggest the role of genetic factors. However, investigators have not consistently found the same genetic associations, and further studies need to be performed. Using the technique of restriction fragment length polymorphism, investigators have demonstrated an association between Takayasu's arteritis and the HLA-D gene at the genomic level.[21] Another report proposed a negative association between this disease and HLA-DR1, implying a protective effect of this antigen.[22] The tendency for the disease to affect women of reproductive age has suggested a potential role for hormonal influences in the pathogenesis of the disorder.[7]

The bulk of evidence favors autoimmune mechanisms. However, the antigens responsible for inciting these events have remained elusive. The production of a variety of antibodies to endothelial cells in some, but not all, patients with systemic vasculitis suggests that these are secondary events and not etiologic factors.[23, 24]

CLINICAL FEATURES

Takayasu's arteritis occurs in females seven to eight times more frequently than in males.[1–13] It generally occurs in patients younger than 40 years of age, but older patients may be affected.[2, 5, 11, 23, 25] It has been called a "great imitator" in medicine because of its nonspecific and varied clinical presentations.[26, 27]

The disease has been subdivided into an *early* (systemic inflammatory, "prepulseless") phase and a *late* (occlusive, "pulseless") phase.[6, 8, 9, 11, 14, 27, 28] Although these phases are not distinct and may overlap, awareness of the varied presentations of Takayasu's arteritis may enable the diagnosis to be established early in the course of the illness. Some patients present with nonspecific signs and symptoms of a systemic inflammatory illness, such as fever, myalgias, arthralgias, and weight loss; other patients complain of pain over a presumably inflammed artery, such as carotodynia. Clues to the diagnosis during this phase include hypertension, vascular bruits, asymmetric arm blood pressures, and early ischemic symptoms. The disease can be very difficult to diagnose during this stage. Some patients present with both systemic inflammatory disease and ischemic manifestations simultaneously. Many patients present in the late, occlusive stage of disease and never manifest a recognized systemic inflammatory component.[14]

Most patients present with symptoms of arterial insufficiency.[6–11, 14] Takayasu's arteritis is a diffuse aortitis that may affect the entire aorta and its branches as well as the pulmonary arteries.[6–10, 26, 29] The disease has been divided into types based on sites of involvement[6]:

- Type I, localized to the aortic arch and its branches
- Type II, involving the descending and abdominal aorta and its branches, also called "a typical coarctation of the aorta"
- Type III, manifesting features of types I and II
- Type IV, combining features of types I through III with pulmonary artery disease

Most reported cases fall into the category of type III disease, emphasizing the diffuse nature of the aortitis.[6, 11] The most commonly affected arteries are the subclavian artery, descending aorta, renal artery, carotid artery, mesenteric arteries, ascending aorta, and abdominal aorta,[6–11] although the vertebral, splenic, pulmonary, coronary, iliac, femoral, brachial, and tibial arteries may also be involved.[6–10] Symptoms referable to vascular disease may vary widely and include syncope, dizziness, claudication, and angina; stroke or myocardial infarction may occur. In the North American experience, aneurysms were uncommon but in a surgical experience from South Africa, 70% of 81 patients with Takayasu's disease underwent surgery for aneurysmal degeneration.[30]

This disease was first described by an ophthalmologist, and ocular signs such as blurred vision, amaurosis fugax, and diplopia have been reported. Hypertension due to renal artery stenosis or coarctation of the aorta may occur. Dilatation of the proximal aorta may lead to aortic insufficiency. Congestive heart failure may result from hypertension, aortic insufficiency, and coronary ischemia.[10, 31] Coronary artery involvement may cause angina; the coronary ostia are more frequently affected than distal sites.[10, 31, 32]

Pulmonary artery disease is often asymptomatic. Pulmonary artery stenoses have been found in up to 70% of patients when the pulmonary vasculature was systematically evaluated. Occasionally, patients may present with severe pulmonary hypertension or even hemoptysis.[10, 33–37] The disease can mimic chronic pulmonary thromboembolic disease.[38] Perfusion lung scans may be useful in screening and observation of these patients.[39] Although obstructive lesions are commonly seen in the visceral arteries, they are rarely symptomatic because of the development of collateral vessels.[40, 41] However, mesenteric infarction secondary to such lesions has been reported in several patients.[40, 41]

Physical findings generally associated with this disorder include vascular bruits, absent or diminished pulses, hypertension, and asymmetry of the blood pressure between the right and the left arms and between the upper and the lower extremities. The retinopathy commonly noted in early reports but not in the more recent series is believed to be secondary to ischemia leading to neovascularization.[2, 6–10]

Cutaneous diseases, such as erythema nodosum and pyoderma gangrenosum, occur in up to 16% of patients.[10, 42, 43] Various forms of glomerulonephritis have been noted but are uncommon.[10, 44, 45] Takayasu's arteritis has also been reported in association with juvenile rheumatoid arthritis, sarcoidosis, and inflammatory bowel disease.[10, 46–48]

No specific laboratory markers are associated with Takayasu's arteritis. During the systemic inflammatory phase, patients commonly present with an elevated erythrocyte sedimentation rate (ESR), anemia of chronic disease, and leukocytosis.[3, 8–10] However, neither these nor other surrogate markers of endothelial injury have been sufficiently sensitive or specific to be the principal tool for treatment decision making.[49, 50]

IMAGING STUDIES

Angiography

Angiography remains the most valuable technique in the diagnosis and evaluation of patients with Takayasu's disease.

Several distinctive angiographic findings have been described,[5, 51] including:

- Narrowing of the aorta and other major arteries, which may be short and segmental, long and diffuse, or progress to complete occlusion
- Arterial dilatation and aneurysm formation, both fusiform and saccular
- Any combination of these findings

The majority of patients have both aneurysmal and stenotic lesions. This combination of radiographic findings is usually diagnostic, especially when other supportive clinical data are present. Occasionally, however, a single lesion is identified in an asymptomatic patient, or angiographic findings suggest atherosclerotic changes and the diagnosis can be established only by careful observation of the patient. We believe that serial angiography should be part of the initial evaluation of all patients with suspected Takayasu's arteritis regardless of the clinical assessment of disease activity. Angiograms obtained at 3- to 6-month intervals, correlated with clinical features of disease, provide a good assessment of disease activity.[52] Refinements in magnetic resonance angiography (MRA) have made this technique a popular alternative to invasive angiography. New vascular lesions suggest active arteritis, whereas progressive vessel stenosis in a previously diseased area may be a result of either scarring or active disease. The potential complications associated with angiography require that each arteriogram be carefully considered. Because of the diffuse nature of this disease, the angiographer should attempt to visualize as much of the arterial tree as possible, particularly the *brachiocephalic vessels*; the entire *aorta*; and the *renal*, *celiac*, and *mesenteric arteries*. In the absence of suggestive symptoms, we do not routinely perform coronary or pulmonary angiography.

At the time of angiography, blood pressure should be measured directly in the ascending aorta; this value should be compared with measurements obtained in the extremities.[53] Subclavian and axillary artery disease can interfere with accurate peripheral measurements and may make the assessment of systemic hypertension difficult in these patients. This is important to remember because hypertension leads to significant long-term morbidity associated with Takayasu's arteritis.[54]

Other Modalities

Although angiography remains the principal modality to establish the diagnosis, other noninvasive imaging techniques, such as ultrasound and magnetic resonance imaging (MRI), are playing an increasing role in the diagnosis and management of patients with this disease.[55–60] Computed tomography (CT) and MRA scans demonstrate distinctive wall changes including thickening, crescents, and indistinct outline peculiar to this disease and may actually be used for diagnosis and determination of disease activity.[61, 62] These techniques have the disadvantage of not providing intravascular pressure measurements. In the setting of innominate, subclavian, aortoiliac, and femoral stenoses, knowledge of the aortic root pressure is essential to medical and surgical management.

PATHOLOGY

Histologically, the formation of stenotic lesions is secondary to intimal proliferation and fibrotic contraction of the media and adventitia, whereas aneurysms may form in areas where there is inflammation of the media and disruption of the elastic lamina.[4, 40, 63] Active lesions are characterized by granulomatous vasculitis, leading to disruption of the media; a lymphocytoplasmic infiltrate is initially seen in the vasa vasorum of the adventitia and, in the later stages, in the media.[64] Langhans' and foreign body giant cells are often present, whereas neutrophils are uncommon. Adventitial fibrosis and intimal proliferation occur in more chronic lesions. This may evolve to transmural sclerosis with little or no inflammatory infiltrate. Thrombosis may occur, and areas of turbulent flow may lead to secondary atherosclerosis.[26] The diagnosis of Takayasu's arteritis is usually based on the combination of clinical features and compatible angiographic findings.

Pathology specimens are sometimes obtained at surgery or from autopsy examinations. We suggest specimens be obtained from affected vessels at the time of revascularization procedures. Histologic proof of inflammation may be found in normal-appearing vessels serving as the origin or insertion of bypass grafts.[40, 53]

MEDICAL THERAPY

The management of Takayasu's arteritis is directed at:

1. Relieving the systemic manifestations of the disease and decreasing the inflammation in affected vessels.
2. Identifying and treating the complications of the vascular disease both medically and surgically.[52, 65, 66]

Glucocorticosteroid therapy, prednisone given at 1 mg/kg/day, is generally effective in controlling clinical manifestations and disease progression in patients with active disease.[8–10, 52, 65, 66] The authors maintain patients on this initial dose of daily prednisone for 1 to 3 months. After this period, in the absence of any evidence of active disease, we attempt to taper and discontinue prednisone over 6 months to a year. However, some patients do not respond to prednisone therapy and either have signs of active disease while they are receiving high doses of daily prednisone or are unable to be weaned from the drug.[3, 9, 52] Because there is certainty of severe side effects from sustained high-dose prednisone over long periods, treatment is always tapered after initial improvement.

Cyclophosphamide has been effective in treating some patients with Takayasu's arteritis who have had progressive disease while receiving daily glucocorticosteroids or who have experienced relapse in the course of tapering treatment.[9] However, cyclophosphamide is associated with a number of toxic effects, including infertility, cystitis, bladder carcinoma, and lymphoma.[67] Several groups have successfully treated these patients with low-dose weekly oral methotrexate at a dose of 0.15 to 0.35 mg/kg/week.[68, 69] Patients who manifest convincing features of active disease, such as systemic symptoms, progressive or new angiographic lesions, and an elevated ESR despite aggressive therapy, may need to be maintained on a daily prednisone regimen at the lowest effective dose. We do not think that long-term glucocorticosteroid therapy is warranted in a patient with the isolated finding of an elevated ESR. Likewise, the appropriate treatment of patients with clinically and angiographically quiescent disease who have an inflammatory lesion on biopsy performed during surgery remains controversial. This is not an unusual occurrence and has been reported in 44% of biopsy specimens in Takayasu's patients obtained during bypass operations to clinically normal arteries.[62] Although symptoms of acute inflammation often abate with glucocorticosteroid therapy, it is not clear that therapy totally eradicates the inflammatory process in the aorta.[3, 6] The value of antiplatelet drugs, such as aspirin, dipyridamole, and vasodilators, has not been formally studied.

The vasculitis section at the National Institute of Allergy and Infectious Disease has reported on the results of medical therapy in the largest series of North American patients with Takayasu's disease.[66] Patients were treated with glucocorticoids either alone or in combination with cytotoxic therapy; 80% of patients required medical treatment, and 25% of those treated did not achieve remission. Of those patients who responded with remission, 50% later experienced relapse. The authors also concluded that current laboratory markers are often inadequate to guide clinical management.

The cause of death in the patient with Takayasu's arteritis is usually related to the vascular complications of the disease, including hypertension, aortic insufficiency, and stroke.[10, 54] Patients should be followed up expectantly for secondary complications and treated aggressively, both medically and surgically.[70]

Later studies have indicated improved survival rates compared with those of older studies; one series reported an overall 5-year survival rate of 94%.[7–10, 54, 65] This result is probably due to earlier detection of the disease, anti-inflammatory therapy, and recognition and treatment of disease complications that have been associated with poor outcomes.[7–10, 52, 65] However, many questions about treatment remain unanswered and await future clinical studies.

PERCUTANEOUS TRANSLUMINAL ANGIOPLASTY

Percutaneous transluminal angioplasty (PTA) is an accepted modality for the treatment of patients with peripheral vascular disease due to atherosclerosis. Excellent results have been obtained in arteries involved with short-segment stenoses, particularly in the iliac and renal arteries, less impressive results have been reported for longer or occluded lesions in the more distal arterial segments. Because Takayasu's arteritis affects arteries that would be treated with PTA if they had atherosclerotic occlusive disease involvement, it is not surprising that angioplasty is advocated as a primary form of treatment in arterial segments affected with Takayasu's arteritis.[71–74]

Takayasu's arteritis presents the angiographer with unique technical problems not found in atherosclerosis. The disease is a panarteritis with active and chronic phases that may involve all three arterial wall layers. Whether the trauma of balloon dilatation in the active phase of the disease exacerbates inflammation and restenosis is unclear. Although this theory remains unproven, some angiographers recommend PTA *only* if the disease is in an inactive phase, as determined clinically.[71, 72]

In the chronic phase, extensive periarterial wall fibrosis, intimal thickening, and widespread transmural chronic changes produce a stenotic artery that is rigid and noncompliant. Dilatation may not be possible, or three to five attempts at balloon dilatation may be necessary before the "waist" of the stenosis is eliminated. Restenosis in these noncompliant vessels can occur quickly. The introduction of arterial stents may reduce the incidence of restenosis. However, long-term follow-up for arterial stents in Takayasu's disease has not been reported. Distal embolization resulting from PTA in an artery involved with Takayasu's arteritis is unusual because the intima is thickened, and unlike an artery in atherosclerosis, the artery is relatively smooth and not calcified or ulcerated.

Hypertension due to renal artery stenosis from Takayasu's arteritis is commonly treated with PTA. A short-segment narrowing just beyond the orifice is technically advantageous for PTA. If the adjacent aortic wall is not involved, the stenosis can be traversed with a catheter. Multiple attempts at dilatation may be necessary before the stenosis is eliminated. A growing experience with PTA for renal arteries suggests an initial success rate of 85% to 95%.[73–75] Provided that overdistention of the artery with the balloon is not attempted, complications, including dissection and occlusion, are unusual. Restenosis occurs in 15% to 20% of cases and is most likely to occur in renal arteries that have a residual stenosis or 20% to 30% after the initial dilatation.[73]

Reports of successful balloon dilatation of the aorta, subclavian artery, and mesenteric vessels have been published, with encouraging initial results mentioned for the descending and abdominal aorta.[71, 72, 76–78] The common carotid and the iliac arteries often have long-segment stenoses that preclude PTA.

These reports suggest that short-segment stenoses of arteries affected with Takayasu's arteritis can be dilated. The good long-term results of PTA on arteries affected with arteriosclerotic occlusive disease should not be extrapolated to arteries with Takayasu's disease. Even after only 6 months of follow-up, restenosis of dilated arteries has been reported.[79] This is not surprising, given the nature of the arterial pathology, the effects of trauma from balloon dilatation, and the poor compliance of arteries with Takayasu's disease. However more recent studies suggest better long-term results. Therefore with the low complication rate and improved results, it appears reasonable to attempt balloon dilatation on renal arteries and other branches of the aorta.

PRINCIPLES OF SURGICAL TREATMENT

The following are general principles of surgical treatment:

1. Patients with Takayasu's arteritis present the surgeon with problems that differ from the clinical problems of atherosclerosis. Treatment must be individualized, and

there must be careful coordination between medical and surgical treatment and provision for long-term follow-up.

2. The surgeon should not assume that, because most patients with Takayasu's arteritis are young, complications from systemic medical problems are uncommon. These patients may have significant cardiac problems, including a low but definite incidence of coronary artery involvement.[20, 31, 32, 80] In 54 patients studied in India, 35 had hypertension, 24 had congestive heart failure, and 27 had ejection fractions under 45%.[31] Of 32 North American patients, 5 had ischemic heart disease and 18 eventually had significant hypertension.[8] Systemic hypertension is frequently unrecognized and untreated because of subclavian involvement and misleading arm blood pressure measurements, resulting in left ventricular hypertrophy and congestive heart failure.

3. Most patients do not need urgent or emergency surgery but can undergo elective surgical procedures, allowing time for a complete evaluation and even control of active disease.

4. Although it is not always possible, avoiding surgical procedures during the acute phase of the disease is preferred. Reports have suggested, but not proved, that fewer surgical complications occur if medical treatment has initially controlled the acute phase of the illness.[79] The use of the ESR to determine disease activity is not reliable.[56]

5. Bypass of obstructive lesions is the preferred surgical approach. To minimize anastomotic complications, the surgeon performs proximal and distal anastomoses in arteries free of disease as shown on the arteriogram. It is advisable, if possible, to avoid arteries for anastomotic sites that have a high incidence of involvement.[40, 81] These arteries may later become involved, causing stenoses of the anastomotic site. Again, even arteries that appear normal on arteriography may have microscopic evidence of disease. One study reported a 44% incidence of microscopic involvement.[40, 53, 66] Endarterectomy with patch grafting is technically difficult because involvement of all three arterial layers may be present. Even if endarterectomy is possible, suturing arteries affected with disease may cause anastomotic and other local problems later.

CEREBROVASCULAR SYSTEM

Cerebrovascular symptoms in the young patient population affected by Takayasu's disease are common because of the high incidence of involvement of the major branches of the aortic arch. The lateralizing cerebrovascular symptoms of stroke, transient ischemic attacks, and amaurosis fugax occur in 8% to 35% of patients.[8, 40, 79, 80] The incidence of stroke alone has been reported to be 14%.[81] A high incidence of nonlateralizing symptoms, such as dizziness and syncope, has also been reported.[8, 40, 79, 81] Although it is easy to postulate that these symptoms are consistent with extensive involvement of the aortic arch arteries that limits cerebral blood flow, documentation of this is lacking. Not all patients with dizziness allegedly due to cerebrovascular involvement demonstrate a reduction in ocular pressures, indicating that hemodynamically significant carotid arterial disease may not always be present.[8] Nonlateralizing symptoms may be due to causes other than stenoses of aortic arch arteries, such as accelerated hypertension, arrhythmias, and congestive heart failure.

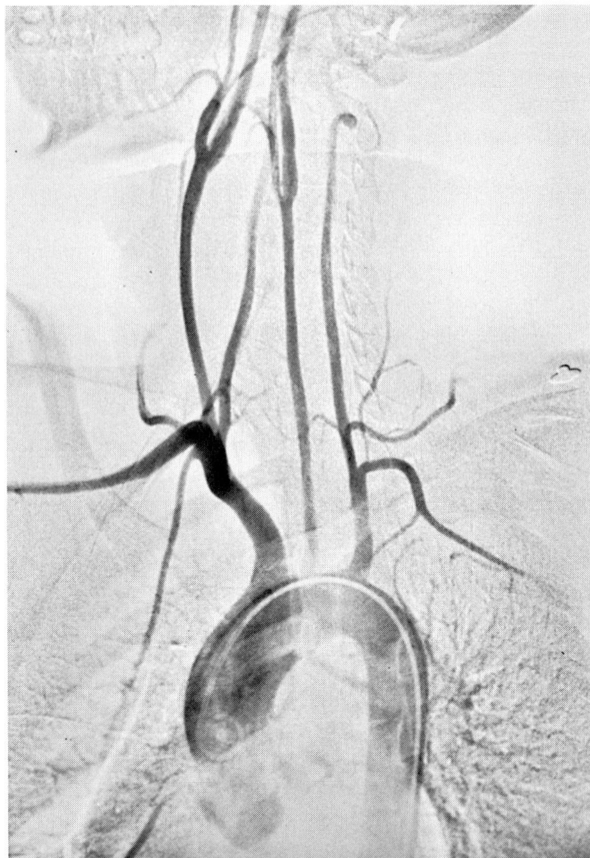

FIGURE 21–1. Characteristic long tapered stenosis of the left common carotid artery, with sparing of the carotid bifurcation.

Arteriograms of the aortic arch and its branches usually show a long area of stenosis involving the common carotid artery while usually sparing the carotid bifurcation and the internal carotid artery (Fig. 21–1). The intima of the involved artery appears smooth, without evidence of ulcerations or segmental narrowing that can cause local turbulence; therefore, it is unlikely to be a source of major emboli. More likely, stroke occurs from total occlusion of one or more aortic arch arteries. Because the common carotid and subclavian arteries are frequently involved, blood flow is restricted to not only the internal carotid but also the external and vertebral arteries, reducing collateral blood flow. The innominate artery itself is at times occluded. If one or all of these involved vessels suddenly become occluded, the patient may sustain a stroke from the marked reduction in cerebral blood flow. In our series, all four patients who sustained a major stroke had occlusion of one or more thoracic aortic arch arteries, suggesting that the stroke occurred from a reduction in cerebrovascular blood flow.[81]

Bypass is recommended to prevent stroke in patients who have hemodynamically significant stenoses of either the innominate or carotid arteries. These bypasses should originate from the ascending aorta, *not* the more commonly involved subclavian artery. The ascending aorta has only a

5% incidence of involvement, reducing the potential for proximal anastomotic problems. The distal anastomosis can be placed at the carotid bulb, which along with the external and internal carotid artery is usually open and spared of disease even if the common carotid is occluded. Strokes did not occur in the seven patients who underwent bypass.[81]

RENOVASCULAR HYPERTENSION

The incidence of hypertension in patients with Takayasu's arteritis is high, ranging from 20% to 72%.[6, 8, 9, 10] This diagnosis is important because the major morbidity and mortality from the disease (i.e., that caused by congestive heart failure, cardiomyopathy, hemorrhagic stroke, hypertensive encephalopathy, and myocardial infarction) are due to the effects of uncontrolled hypertension. However, the frequent involvement of both subclavian arteries may mask the diagnosis of hypertension, leaving patients with significantly elevated blood pressure that is both undiagnosed and untreated. Most cases of hypertension are due to renal artery stenosis. Some reviews report a high incidence of mid-abdominal aortic coarctation that can also cause renovascular hypertension.[6, 40] It is not clear from these reports whether this mid-abdominal aortic coarctation is due to developmental abnormalities or to Takayasu's disease.

Correction of renal artery stenosis is recommended for renovascular hypertension and kidney salvage. PTA has assumed a more important role in the management of patients with renovascular hypertension. If PTA is unsuccessful or is technically not possible, renal artery bypass should be performed. For this young patient population, we recommend an aggressive approach rather than prolonged periods of antihypertensive medication.

Renal artery disease is usually confined to the proximal segment, leaving an uninvolved segment available for the distal anastomosis (Fig. 21–2). The frequent involvement of the infrarenal aorta may preclude the use of this artery for the proximal anastomosis. Therefore, it may be necessary to use the hepatic, splenic, or supraceliac abdominal aorta as the inflow site only if there is no evidence of disease in these arteries. A vein is the preferred conduit for the bypass.

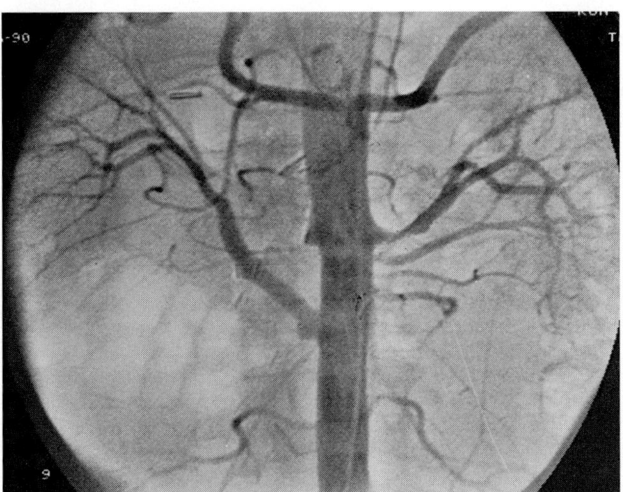

FIGURE 21–2. Classic involvement of the left renal artery with Takayasu's arteritis. Note the bypass of the right renal artery.

Stenotic involvement of the descending thoracic or mid-abdominal aorta has been reported in European studies to be a common cause of renovascular hypertension.[40, 82] This requires a more extensive procedure: revascularization of the distal abdominal aorta combined with bypass to both renal arteries. Surgical treatment of renovascular hypertension due to Takayasu's arteritis has been reported in only a small number of series, but follow-up has been extensive.[8, 40, 79] In general, results are comparable to those of the larger series of surgical treatment for renovascular hypertension due to atherosclerosis.

VISCERAL ARTERY INVOLVEMENT

The incidence of celiac and superior mesenteric artery involvement varies from 5% to 66%.[8, 9, 40] Arterial blood flow to the visceral circulation can also be compromised by stenoses of the thoracic or suprarenal aorta. Despite this high incidence of disease, clinical problems are unusual, with few indications for surgical corrections.[40, 41] An aggressive approach to visceral artery involvement was reported from Russia.[82] In a large series of 300 patients, 25% had visceral artery involvement; nine had chronic visceral ischemia. Forty-one patients underwent visceral artery reconstruction, which included 13 graft bypasses and 28 transaortic endarterectomies. Surgical correction of the visceral circulation was recommended even if patients are asymptomatic. This experience is not consistent with that reported in series from North America.[8, 79, 81] In addition, endarterectomy of these lesions can be difficult because of inflammatory disease and severe fibrosis in the arterial wall. We recommend observation of asymptomatic patients with visceral artery involvement. A bypass originating from the uninvolved abdominal aorta is recommended only for the rare patients with symptoms of *chronic* intestinal ischemia.

UPPER AND LOWER EXTREMITY ARTERIAL DISEASE

Symptoms of upper extremity ischemia are common because of the frequent involvement of the subclavian and axillary arteries. Unlike atherosclerosis, which is characterized by short-segment proximal stenosis or occlusion, Takayasu's arteritis involves much longer segments of these arteries (Fig. 21–3). Because the subclavian artery is usually involved both proximal and distal to the origin of the vertebral artery, the *subclavian steal syndrome* is rare. With long-segment arterial involvement, symptoms of upper extremity ischemia tend to be more severe in patients with Takayasu's arteritis than in those with atherosclerosis. Because these patients are young and active, bypass for upper arm ischemia is sometimes necessary. Measurement of blood pressure in the upper arm may be inaccurate because of involvement of both subclavian arteries. In view of the potentially devastating morbidity of uncontrolled hypertension, it is appropriate to consider upper extremity revascu-

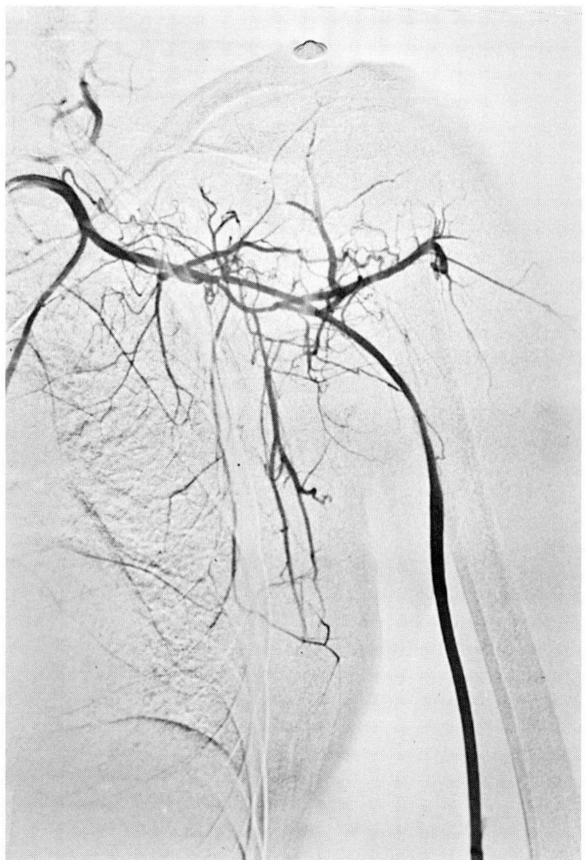

FIGURE 21–3. Long-segment involvement of the subclavian and axillary arteries, classic for Takayasu's disease.

larization in otherwise asymptomatic patients with bilateral involvement in order to provide access for accurate determination of systemic blood pressure.

Bypass with grafts originating from the ascending aorta is the preferred method for revascularization of the upper extremity. The use of the common carotid artery as the inflow vessel, even if it is uninvolved, should be discouraged. The high incidence of disease in the common carotid arteries places the patient at increased risk for graft occlusion at a later date. Revascularization of the subclavian artery is frequently done concomitantly with a bypass of one or both common carotid arteries with hemodynamically significant stenosis or total occlusion. Two common clinical approaches include the use of a bifurcation graft from the ascending aorta with limbs to both subclavian arteries and the use of a bifurcation graft, with one limb to the subclavian artery and one to the carotid artery, at the bulb.

Claudication of the lower extremity is considerably less common than upper extremity ischemic symptoms.[8, 79] This is due to less frequent involvement of the iliac arteries and the low incidence of the disease in the femoral and distal arterial circulation. Most cases of lower extremity claudication result from abdominal aortic involvement, particularly in the infrarenal abdominal aorta. It is peculiar that the disease may cause marked narrowing of the aorta below the renal arteries but spares the distal aorta (Fig. 21–4). Rest pain, gangrene, and nonhealing ulcerations occur but are unusual.

Claudication symptoms can be severe, and it is not clear whether a conservative measure, such as a walking program, increases exercise tolerance. Because the patients are young and have severe symptoms, a more aggressive approach is warranted at times. Most cases involve bypass of the stenotic abdominal aorta. Because the disease usually affects the aorta below the renal arteries, the proximal anastomosis of a bifurcation graft is placed in the supraceliac aorta. Another approach is bypass with a 10-mm tube graft from the lower thoracic aorta retroperitoneally to the left external iliac artery. Both legs are then perfused through the spared lower distal abdominal aorta.[83]

ANEURYSMS

The incidence of aneurysm formation from Takayasu's arteritis varies in reports from different parts of the world. Large series of aneurysms were reported in Japan[84] and India,[85] where aneurysms occurred in 31.9% (36 of 113) and 22.2% (30 of 135) of cases, respectively. Both studies reported that the aneurysms were multiple, saccular and fusiform, associated with stenotic lesions, and most commonly found in the ascending, thoracic, and abdominal aorta. Other arteries (e.g., subclavian and brachiocephalic) were less commonly involved. These studies reported a low incidence of aneurysm resection and rupture, with each study noting only one ruptured aneurysm. Aneurysms were more common in Japanese patients older than 40 years of age, but this finding was not confirmed in the report from India.

A more recent series from South Africa reported that 70% of 81 patients with Takayasu's disease underwent an operation for aneurysmal degeneration.[30] Two patients died after surgery for a ruptured aneurysm involving the thoracic abdominal aorta. Other studies reported a lower incidence of aneurysms, with a 10% occurrence in a large series from Russia and an even lower incidence from North America (Fig. 21–5).[8, 81, 82]

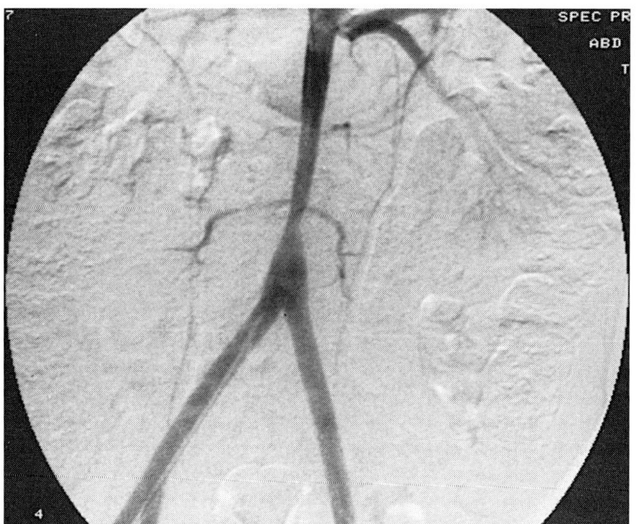

FIGURE 21–4. Involvement of the infrarenal abdominal aorta. Note the sparing of the distal aorta. Bypass from the thoracic aorta to the left iliac artery perfuses both legs.

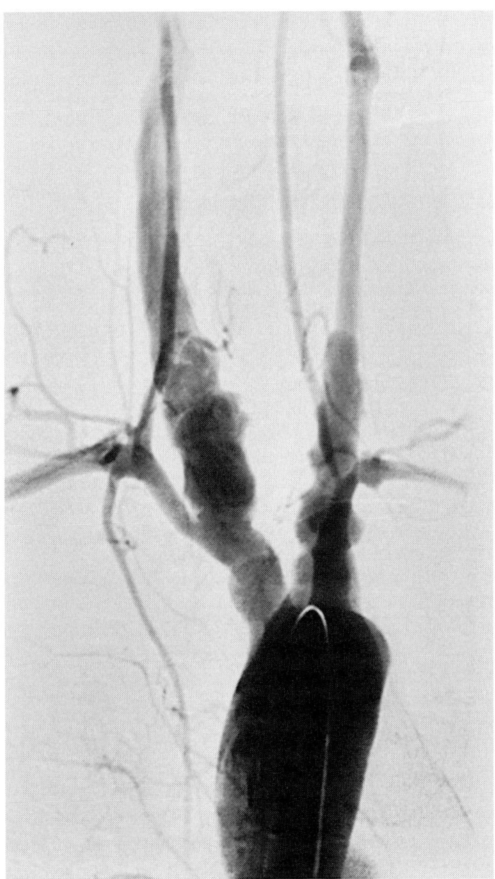

FIGURE 21–5. Extensive aneurysmal involvement of the ascending aorta and its main branches in a 17-year-old patient.

The incidence of aneurysm rupture is low. Nevertheless, localized fusiform or saccular aneurysms in a medically stable patient should be treated surgically. These patients are young and can anticipate a long life. The risk of aneurysm "repair" is probably lower than the risk of rupture in patients observed for a long period. Resection and aortic valve replacement are also recommended for aneurysms of the ascending aorta causing clinically significant aortic insufficiency.

SURGICAL RESULTS

Reports of surgical series have emphasized that patients with Takayasu's arteritis can undergo revascularization with minimal morbidity and mortality.[30, 40, 79, 81] These excellent results are due to careful preoperative evaluation, avoidance of procedures in patients with active disease, careful patient selection, and the use of maximal medical therapy to control the disease process. None of these series is large, and the follow-up on all patients has been limited. Because these patients have a much longer life expectancy than older patients surgically treated for atherosclerosis, 20- to 30-year follow-up may yield less impressive results.

The available evidence suggests that these patients have a low incidence of anastomotic problems. Although one series reported the development of 5 false aneurysms in 90 patients undergoing procedures over 35 years, other series reported that false aneurysms did not occur.[79, 81, 86]

In a large series of Takayasu's disease reported from Japan, 91 patients with 259 anastomoses observed for up to 37 years developed 22 anastomotic aneurysms, an incidence of 8.5%.[87] The formation of aneurysms was related to the presence of true aneurysms from the disease itself and the type of suture material. Of the 22 anastomotic aneurysms, 18 occurred in cases in which silk was used for the anastomosis. When synthetic suture material was used, only 1.8% demonstrated anastomotic aneurysms, at 10 years and 3.5% at 20 years.

With that length of follow-up, these rates of anastomotic aneurysms with synthetic suture are acceptable and compatible with anastomotic aneurysms that develop after an operation for atherosclerotic occlusive disease. Although anastomotic stenoses have been reported, the incidence is reasonable and their occurrence is not necessarily related to the activity of disease at the time of surgery.[79, 81] Anastomotic stenoses may be related to the development of intimal hyperplasia from compliance mismatch of synthetic grafts and may not necessarily be a result of local recurrence. Because patients with Takayasu's arteritis should undergo periodic arteriography to assess disease activity, the opportunity to document anastomotic problems exists.

Although the surgical series are small, good clinical results have been reported. Aggressive surgical therapy can be performed in these patients with minimal morbidity and mortality. Patients with significant carotid lesions have had successful bypass procedures, reducing the incidence of stroke during follow-up. Renal artery bypass has cured or decreased hypertension. The long-term results of procedures to relieve upper to lower extremity ischemia have been successful in most cases.

SUMMARY

Takayasu's disease is a complex arteritis of unknown etiology that affects a young predominantly female patient population. Stenoses and occlusion of the major arteries create the life-threatening sequelae of this disease. Surgeons are consulted to assess, and to recommend treatment for, the clinical consequences of arterial involvement, but few surgeons have significant experience with this unusual disease. It is important for surgeons to appreciate the differences between arterial problems due to atherosclerosis and those due to Takayasu's disease and not treat them exactly the same. It is equally important for the treating physicians to coordinate medical and surgical therapy carefully. Follow-up must be comprehensive and long term. Thoughtful medical and surgical therapy should be combined to produce excellent long-term results.

REFERENCES

1. McKusick VA: A form of vascular disease relatively frequent in the Orient. Am Heart J 63:57, 1962.
2. Judge RD, Currier RD, Gracie WA, et al: Takayasu's arteritis and the aortic arch syndrome. Am J Med 32:379, 1962.
3. Nakao K, Ikeda M, Kimata S-I, et al: Takayasu's arteritis: Clinical

report of eighty-four cases and immunological studies of seven cases. Circulation 35:1141, 1967.
4. Vinijchaikul K: Primary arteritis of the aorta and its main branches (Takayasu's arteriopathy): A clinicopathologic autopsy study of eight cases. Am J Med 43:15, 1967.
5. Hachiya J: Current concepts of Takayasu's arteritis. Semin Roentgenol 5:245, 1970.
6. Lupi-Herrera E, Sanchez-Torres G, Marcushamer J, et al: Takayasu's arteritis: Clinical study of 107 cases. Am Heart J 93:94, 1977.
7. Ishikawa K: Natural history and classification of occlusive thromboaortopathy (Takayasu's disease). Circulation 57:27, 1978.
8. Hall S, Barr W, Lie JT, et al: Takayasu arteritis: A study of 32 North American patients. Medicine 64:89, 1985.
9. Shelhamer JH, Volkman DJ, Parrillo JE, et al: Takayasu's arteritis and its therapy. Ann Intern Med 103:121, 1985.
10. Hall S, Buchbinder R: Takayasu's arteritis. Rheum Dis Clin North Am 16:411, 1990.
11. Procter CD, Hollier LH: Takayasu's arteritis and temporal arteritis. Ann Vasc Surg 6:195, 1992.
12. Nasu T: Takayasu's truncoarteritis in Japan: A statistical observation of 76 autopsy cases. Pathol Microbiol 43:140, 1975.
13. Waern AU, Anderson P, Hemmingsson A: Takayasu's arteritis: A hospital-region based study on occurrence, treatment and prognosis. Angiology 34:311, 1983.
14. Lande A, Berkmen YM: Aortitis. Pathologic, clinical and arteriographic review. Radiol Clin North Am 14:219, 1976.
15. Kinare SG: Aortitis in early life in India and its association with tuberculosis. J Pathol 100:69, 1970.
16. Isohisa I, Numano F, Maezawa H, et al: Takayasu disease. Tissue Antigens 12:246, 1978.
17. Naito S, Arakawa K, Saito S, et al: Takayasu's disease: Association with HLA-B5. Tissue Antigens 12:143, 1978.
18. Sasazuki T, Ohta N, Isoshisa I, et al: Association between Takayasu disease and HLA-DHO. Tissue Antigens 14:177, 1979.
19. Volkman DJ, Mann DL, Fauci AS: Association between Takayasu's arteritis and a B-cell alloantigen in North Americans. N Engl J Med 306:464, 1982.
20. Numano F, Isohisa I, Maezawa H, et al: HL-A antigens in Takayasu's disease. Am Heart J 98:153, 1979.
21. Takeuchi Y, Matsuki K, Saito Y, et al: HLA-D region genomic polymorphism associated with Takayasu's arteritis. Angiology 41:421, 1990.
22. Khraisis MM, Gladman DD, Dagenais P, et al: HLA antigens in North American patients with Takayasu arteritis. Arthritis Rheum 35:573, 1992.
23. Eichhorn J, Sima D, Thiele B, et al: Anti-endothelial cell antibodies in Takayasu arteritis. Circulation 94:2396, 1996.
24. Navarro M, Cervera R, Font J, et al: Anti-endothelial cell antibodies in systemic autoimmune disease: Prevalence and clinical significance. Lupus 6:521, 1997.
25. Morales E, Pineda C, Martinez-Lavin M: Takayasu's arteritis in children. J Rheumatol 18:1081, 1991.
26. Lie JT: The classification and diagnosis of vasculitis in large and medium-sized vessels. Pathol Annu 22(Pt 1):125, 1987.
27. Strachan RW: The natural history of Takayasu's arteriopathy. Q J Med 33:57, 1964.
28. Volkman DJ, Fauci AS: Takayasu's arteritis. *In* Lichtenstein L, Fauci AS (eds): Current Therapy in Allergy and Immunology 1983–1984. Philadelphia, BC Decker, 1983, p 143.
29. Lande A, Gross A: Total aortography in the diagonsis of Takayasu's arteritis. Am J Roentgenol 116:165, 1972.
30. Robbs JV, Abdoll-Carrim A, Kadwa AM. Arterial Reconstruction for nonspecific arteritis (Takayasu's disease). Eur J Vasc Surg 8:401, 1994.
31. Panja M, Kar AK, Dutta AL, et al: Cardiac involvement in non-specific aorto-arteritis. Int J Cardiol 34:289, 1992.
32. Amano J, Suzuki A: Coronary artery involvement in Takayasu's arteritis. J Thorac Cardiovasc Surg 102:554, 1991.
33. Lupi E, Sanchez G, Horwitz S, et al: Pulmonary artery involvement in Takayasu's arteritis. Chest 67:69, 1975.
34. Haas A, Stiehm ER: Takayasu's arteritis presenting as pulmonary hypertension. Am J Dis Child 140:372, 1986.
35. Yamada I, Shibuya H, Matsubara O, et al: Pulmonary artery disease in Takayasu's arteritis: Angiographic findings. Am J Roentgenol 159:263, 1992.
36. Rocha MP, Guntupalli KK, Moise KJ, et al: Massive hemoptysis in Takayasu's arteritis during pregnancy. Chest 106:1619, 1994.
37. Koyabu S, Isaka N, Yada T, et al: Severe respiratory failure caused by recurrent pulmonary hemorrhage in Takayasu's arteritis. Chest 104:1905, 1993.
38. Kerr KM, Auger WR, Fedullo PF, et al: Large vessel pulmonary arteritis mimicking chronic thromboembolic disease. AM J Respir Crit Care Med 152(1):367, 1995.
39. Umehara I, Shibuya H, Nakagawa T, et al: Comprehensive analysis of perfusion scintigraphy in Takayasu's arteritis. Clin Nucl Med 16:352, 1991.
40. Lagneau P, Michel JB, Vuong PN: Surgical treatment of Takayasu's disease. Ann Surg 205:157, 1987.
41. Nussaume O, Bouttier S, Duchatelle J-P, et al: Mesenteric infarction in Takayasu's disease. Ann Vasc Surg 4:117, 1990.
42. Pernidiaro CV, Winkelmann RK, Hunder GG: Cutaneous manifestations of Takayasu's arteritis. J Am Acad Dermatol 17:998, 1987.
43. Frances C, Boisnic S, Bletry O, et al: Cutaneous manifestations of Takayasu arteritis. Dermatologica 181:266, 1990.
44. Hellmann DE, Hardy K, Lindenfeld S, et al: Takayasu's arteritis associated with crescentic glomerulonephritis. Arthritis Rheum 30:451, 1987.
45. Koumi S-I, Endo T, Okumura H, et al: A case of Takayasu's arteritis associated with membranoproliferative glomerulonephritis and nephrotic syndrome. Nephron 54:344, 1990.
46. Hall S, Nelson AM: Takayasu's arteritis and juvenile rheumatoid arthritis. J Rheumatol 13:431, 1986.
47. Rose CD, Eichenfield AH, Goldsmith DP, et al: Early onset sarcoidosis with aortitis: "Juvenile systemic granulomatosis?" J Rheumatol 17:102, 1990.
48. Achar KN, Al-Nakib B: Takayasu's arteritis and ulcerative colitis. Am J Gastroenterol 81:1215, 1986.
49. Akazawa H, Ikeda H, Yamamoto K, et al: Hypercoagulable state in patients with Takayasu's arteritis. Thromb Hemost 75:72, 1996.
50. Hoffman GS, Ahmed AE. For the international network for the study of the systemic vasculitides: Surrogate markers of disease activity in patients with Takayasu's arteritis. A preliminary report. Int J Cardiol 66:191, 1998.
51. Lande A, Rossi P: The value of total aortography in the diagnosis of Takayasu's arteritis. Radiology 114:287, 1975.
52. Leavitt RY, Fauci AS: Takayasu's arteritis. *In* Lichtenstein LM, Fauci AS (eds): Current Therapy in Allergy, Immunology and Rheumatology, 4th ed. Philadelphia, BC Decker, 1992, p 218.
53. Kieffer E, Piquois AL, Bertal A, et al: Reconstructive surgery of the renal arteries in Takayasu's disease. Ann Vasc Surg 4:156, 1990.
54. Ishikawa K: Survival and morbidity after diagnosis of occlusive thromboaortopathy (Takayasu's disease). Am J Cardiol 47:1026, 1981.
55. Buckley A, Southwood T, Culham G, et al: The role of ultrasound in evaluation of Takayasu's arteritis. J Rheumatol 18:1073, 1991.
56. Maeda H, Handa N, Matsumoto M, et al: Carotid lesions detected by B-mode ultrasonography in Takayasu's arteritis: "Macaroni sign" as an indicator of the disease. Ultrasound Med Biol 17:695, 1991.
57. Dashefsky SM, Cooperberg PL, Harrison PB, et al: Total occlusion of the common carotid artery with patent internal carotid artery: Identification with color flow Doppler imaging. J Ultrasound Med 10:417, 1991.
58. Oneson SR, Lewin JS, Smith AS: MR angiography of Takayasu arteritis. J Comput Assist Tomogr 16:478, 1992.
59. Tanigawa K, Eguchi K, Kitamura Y, et al: Magnetic resonance imaging detection of aortic and pulmonary artery wall thickening in the acute stage of Takayasu's arteritis. Arthritis Rheum 35:476, 1992.
60. Yamada I, Numano F, Suzuki S: Takayasu arteritis: Evaluation with MR imaging. Radiology 188:89, 1993.
61. Park JH, Chung JW, IM JG et al: Takayasu arteritis evaluation of mural changes in the aorta and pulmonary artery with CT angiography. Radiology 196:89, 1995.
62. Sharma S, Sharma S, Taneja K, et al: Morphologic mural changes in the aorta revealed CT in patients with non-specific aortoarteritis (Takayasu's arteritis). AJR AM J Roentogenol 167:1321, 1996.
63. Nasu T: Pathology of pulseless disease. Angiology 14:225, 1963.
64. Seko Y, Minota S, Kawasaki A, et al: Perforin secreting killer cells infiltration and expression of the 6s-kd heat shock proteins in aortic tissue of patients with Takayasu's arteritis. J Clin Invest 93:750, 1994.
65. Fraga A, Mintz G, Valle L, et al: Takayasu's arteritis: Frequency of systemic manifestations (study of 22 patients) and favorable response to maintenance steroid therapy with adrenocorticosteroids (12 patients). Arthritis Rheum 15:617, 1972.

66. Kerr GS, Hallahan CW, Giordano J, et al: Takayasu arteritis. Ann Intern Med 120:919, 1994.
67. Hoffman GS, Kerr GS, Leavitt RY, et al: Wegener's granulomatosis: A prospective analysis of 158 patients. Ann Intern Med 116:488, 1992.
68. Hoffman GS, Leavitt RY, Kerr GS, et al: Treatment of Takayasu's arteritis with methotrexate. Arthritis Rheum 34(Suppl):74, 1991.
69. Liang GC, Nemickas R, Madayag M: Multiple percutaneous transluminal angioplasties and low-dose pulse methotrexate for Takayasu's arteritis. Rheumatology 16:1370, 1989.
70. Hoffman GS: Treatment of resistent Takayasu's arteritis. Rheum Dis Clin North Am 21:73, 1995.
71. Sharma S, Rajani M, Kaul U, et al: Initial experience with percutaneous transluminal angioplasty in the management of Takayasu's arteritis. Br J Radiol 63:517, 1990.
72. Park JH, Han MC, Kim SH, et al: Takayasu's arteritis: Angiographic findings and results of angioplasty. Am J Radiol 153:1069, 1989.
73. Sharma S, Saxena A, Talwar KK, et al: Renal artery stenosis caused by non-specific arteritis (Takayasu's disease): Results of treatment with percutaneous transluminal angioplasty. Am J Radiol 158:417, 1982.
74. Sharma S, Thatai D, Saxena A, et al: Renovascular hypertension resulting from non-specific aortoarteritis in children: Midterm results of percutaneous transluminal renal angioplasty and predictors of restenosis. Am J Roentgenol 166:157, 1966.
75. Tyagi S, Singh B, Kaul UA, et al: Balloon angioplasty for renovascular hypertension in Takayasu's arteritis. Am Heart J 125:1386, 1993.
76. Rao SA, Mandalam KR, Rao VR, et al: Takayasu arteritis: Initial and long-term follow-up in 16 patients after percutaneous transluminal angioplasty of the descending throacic and abdominal aorta. Radiology 189:173, 1993.
77. Tyagi S, Kaul UA, Nair M, et al: Balloon angioplasty of the aorta in Takayasu's arteritis: Initial and long-term results. Am Heart J 124:876, 1992.
78. Kumar S, Mandalam R, Rao VRK, et al: Percutaneous transluminal angioplasty in non-specific aortoarteritis (Takayasu's disease): Experience in 16 cases. Cardiovasc Intervent Radiol 12:321, 1990.
79. Weaver FA, Yellin AE, Campen DH, et al: Surgical procedures in the management of Takayasu's arteritis. J Vasc Surg 12:429, 1990.
80. Talwar KD, Kumar K, Chopra P, et al: Cardiac involvement in nonspecific aortoarteritis (Takayasu's arteritis). Am Heart J 122:1666, 1991.
81. Giordano J, Leavitt RY, Hoffman G, et al: Experience with surgical treatment of Takayasu's disease. Surgery 109:252, 1991.
82. Prokrovsky AV: Nonspecific aortoarteritis. *In* Rutherford RB (ed): Vascular Surgery, 3rd ed. Philadelphia, WB Saunders, 1989, p 217.
83. Giordano J: Surgical treatment of Takayasu's disease. *In* Ernst CB, Stanley JC (eds): Current Therapy in Vascular Surgery, 2nd ed. Philadelphia, BC Decker, 1991, p 169.
84. Matsumura K, Hirano T, Takeda K, et al: Incidence of aneurysms in Takayasu's arteritis. Angiology 42:308, 1991.
85. Kumar S, Subramanyan R, Ravi Mandalam K, et al: Aneurysmal form of aortoarteritis (Takayasu's disease): Analysis of thirty cases. Clin Radiol 42:342, 1990.
86. Takagi A, Tada J, Sato O: Surgical treatment for Takayasu's arteritis. J Cardiovasc Surg 30:553, 1989.
87. Miyata T, Osamu S, Deguchi J, et al: Anastomotic aneurysms after surgical treatment of Takayasu's arteritis: A 40 year experience. J Vasc Surg 27:438, 1998.

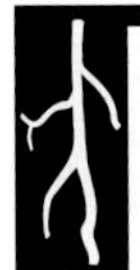

CHAPTER 22

Arterial Aneurysms: Etiologic Considerations

Bobby S. Glickman, M.D., Jason P. Rehm, M.D., and B. Timothy Baxter, M.D.

CLASSIFICATION

The classification of aneurysms is controversial and has been the subject of attempts to introduce uniformity and agreement. The authors use a modification of the scheme devised by the Society of Vascular Surgery/International Society of Cardiovascular Surgery (SVS/ISCVS) Subcommittee on Reporting Standards for Arterial Aneurysms.[1] (Table 22–1) As the details of genetic predisposition become apparent for many aneurysm types, including *degenerative* ones, the distinction between diseases previously considered inherited (e.g., Marfan's syndrome) and those considered acquired (e.g., degenerative) is becoming blurred. Thus, a previously employed heading of *congenital aneurysm* is not used in this scheme. Similarly, as the role of inflammation is elucidated in nearly all aneurysm types, this term is not included here as an etiologic category except for its traditional use in designating the *inflammatory variant* of degenerative aneurysms. Arguments contesting this distinction that favor grouping the inflammatory variant as a manifestation of the more common *nonspecific degenerative aneurysm* are introduced later.

Along with *traumatic* and *anastomotic*, *dissection* is categorized under the broad category of *pseudoaneurysms* (false aneurysms). Although dissection is not considered in detail in this chapter, it does not ordinarily lead to a true aneurysm even when the affected vessel reaches aneurysmal proportions because not all layers of the vessel wall are involved. Instead, an acute dissection with communication between the true and false lumen resembles a pulsatile pseudoaneurysm contained intramurally. In the wall of a chronic healed dissection, the intima and inner media are separated from the outer media and adventitia by intramural hematoma. Rarely, dissection of the arterial wall occurs de novo in an existing true aneurysm. A *miscellaneous*

TABLE 22–1. ETIOLOGIC CLASSIFICATION OF ARTERIAL ANEURYSMS

Primary connective tissue disorders
Marfan's syndrome
Ehlers-Danlos syndrome
Miscellaneous
Focal medial agenesis
Tuberous sclerosis
Turner's syndrome
Menkes' syndrome
Mechanical (hemodynamic)
Post-stenotic
Arteriovenous fistula and postamputation-related
Pseudoaneurysms
Traumatic
Dissection
Pancreatitis-related
Anastomotic
Arteritis-related
Takayasu's disease
Giant cell arteritis
Systemic lupus erythematosus
Behçet's syndrome
Kawasaki's disease
Infectious (mycotic)
Bacterial
Fungal
Spirochetal
Pregnancy-related
Degenerative
Nonspecific (historically called "arteriosclerotic")
Inflammatory variant
Graft failure

category groups diseases associated with known chromosomal abnormalities with *focal medial agenesis*, which would otherwise stand alone.

Vascular remodeling is a fundamental feature of all true aneurysms. This remodeling may result from the interplay of hemodynamic forces and primary structural weakness or as a primary response to inflammatory influences. Furthermore, the complexity of interaction between native components of the vessel wall and the transient residents, carried in by the circulation, such as components of the inflammatory, coagulation, and possibly autoimmunogenic cascades, is being uncovered by intense research. Included among the goals of this effort are the elucidation of the pathways of aneurysm formation and critical regulating points where intervention might slow, halt, or reverse the process. Currently, surgical or endovascular intervention is the only accepted definitive therapy, although control of blood pressure and smoking cessation are believed to be efficacious measures.

Before we discuss each type of aneurysm, a brief review of arterial wall architecture is important for understanding the processes that cause structural failure in aneurysm development. Collagen and elastin are the major structural proteins in the arterial wall. Collagen imparts tensile strength to the vessels, whereas elastin is responsible for its recoil capacity.

Arteries have three distinct layers: intima, media, and adventitia. The *intima* consists of a layer of endothelial cells that adhere to a basement membrane to form the lumen flow surface. In the *media*, elastic fibers are arranged in layers between smooth muscle cells to form lamellar units. The number of units is a function of arterial wall tension; this relationship is well preserved throughout mammalian species, with the exception of the human abdominal aorta, which contains fewer units than expected for the load it bears.[2] This interesting fact may be one of the reasons that the abdominal aortic aneurysm (AAA) is common in humans. Furthermore, as an early example of its stability, the average life span of alveolar elastin fibers may be about 70 years.[2a] The majority of elastin is produced in the late fetal and early neonatal periods, with limited ability for repair or replacement in the adult period.[2b] Thus, the critical step of elastolysis in AAA formation may be irreversible. The *adventitia* is a layer of investing connective tissue that also contains elastin, along with most of the load-bearing collagen. Studies have suggested that failure of the collagen in this important zone is a pivotal event in aneurysm development.[3]

PRIMARY DISORDERS

Marfan's Syndrome

Nearly a century ago, Marfan described features of the syndrome that bears his name, but not until about 1950 did skeptics become convinced that the disease was due to a single mutant gene.[4] The identification of this gene has resulted from a combination of classic and reverse genetics. The classic approach is to begin with a candidate protein and to pursue it to the gene level, whereas the reverse approach is to start with genomic deoxyribonucleic acid (DNA) of members of affected families and to study the segregation of different chromosomes (or their fragments) with the phenotype by analysis of marker restriction fragment length polymorphisms (RFLPs) within the family. The reverse approach initially led to the exclusion of most chromosomes other than 15 and eventually led to the assignment of the Marfan gene to the long arm of chromosome 15 in several Finnish families.[5]

Along the classic line, McKusick is credited with suggesting that an understanding of the biochemical feature that the aorta and the suspensory ligament of the lens have in common might lead to characterization of the underlying defect.[6] Fibrillin, a microfibrillar protein of connective tissue discovered by Sakai and coworkers in 1986, was such a candidate.[7] In 1990, Hollister and coworkers described abnormalities of fibrillin in both skin and cultured fibroblasts from patients with Marfan's syndrome.[8] Other investigators mapped genes for the fibrillins to chromosomes 5 and 15, and it has now been shown that the gene on chromosome 15 is linked to the Marfan phenotype.[9] Closing the loop, Dietz and colleagues demonstrated identical point mutations in the fibrillin gene in two patients with Marfan's syndrome; this mutation changed the codon for arginine at residue 239 to a glycine.[10] This story is a paradigm for the power of new biologic techniques in uncovering the molecular basis of vascular diseases.

Ehlers-Danlos Syndrome

A prototype of the classic form of Ehlers-Danlos syndrome (EDS) was described by vanMeekeren in the 17th century.[11]

A young Spanish man could stretch the skin from his right chest to his left ear. Barabas noted that the heterogeneity of the syndrome is implied even by its name,[12] and multiple phenotypic variations of the syndrome are now recognized. Ehlers described a case with excess bruising, and Danlos described a case with excess scarring. Each patient had hyperextensibility of the skin and hypermobility of the joints. The eponym *Ehlers-Danlos* was coined by Weber in 1936.[13]

Ten clinical types of this syndrome have been assigned (I through X). EDS-I and EDS-IV are the types associated with life-threatening vascular catastrophies. EDS-I and EDS-II result from type V collagen mutations and are the most common forms of this syndrome. EDS-I (gravis) is an autosomal dominant disorder with severe joint hypermobility and hyperextensibility of skin. Arterial ruptures may occur in type I disease, but they are not common.

In 1967, Barabas described two patients with severe arterial complications who had soft, thin skin with an extreme tendency to bruise.[14] This ecchymotic variant was subsequently classified as type IV. Spontaneous perforations of the colon also occur in type IV disease. Tears of peripheral arteries occur spontaneously or after trivial trauma, and visceral branches are also prone to disruptions. Gentle application of vascular clamps may result in uncontrollable hemorrhage, and surgery under such conditions has been described by Wesley and associates as a "surrealistic" experience.[15]

The first abnormalities of collagen in ED-IV were discovered in 1975, when Pope and coworkers reported deficiency of type III collagen in tissue and cultured fibroblasts.[16] This group subsequently suggested that there were both clinical and molecular heterogeneities among the ED-IV patients.[17] Both Pope and coworkers[18] and Barabas[14] have taken the position that the patient should not be classified as having ED-IV, even with proven abnormalities in type III collagen, unless the classic skin changes are present.

A family in which several members have had abdominal aortic aneurysms associated with a point mutation in the type III procollagen gene has been described, but members of this family do not have the classic changes of ED-IV.[19]

MISCELLANEOUS FORMS

Several other systemic disorders are associated with aneurysm development:

- Focal medial agenesis
- Tuberous sclerosis
- Gonadal dysgenesis (Turner's syndrome)
- Menkes' kinky-hair syndrome

Focal medial agenesis has been mainly responsible for intracranial berry aneurysms, with rare reports of peripheral aneurysms.[20]

Tuberous sclerosis, an autosomal dominant developmental abnormality of the central nervous system associated with seizures, mental retardation, and adenoma sebaceum in infants and children, has been associated with thoracic and abdominal aneurysms. Possible etiologic contributors to these disorders include aortic medial defects (i.e., elastin fragmentation and fibromuscular dysplasia) and hypertension.[21]

Patients with gonadal dysgenesis (*Turner's syndrome*; 45, XO karyotype) can manifest skeletal and connective tissue abnormalities.[22, 23] The aneurysms are often associated with stenotic aortic segments (coarctations); however, infrarenal aneurysms have been reported.

Menkes' kinky-hair syndrome, a rare X-linked syndrome manifested by rapid central nervous system (CNS) and arterial degeneration, is caused by an abnormality in copper transport.[24] The blotchy mouse is believed to represent the animal counterpart of this disease.[25, 27]

Lysyl oxidase, a copper-dependent metalloenzyme, promotes the formation of stable cross-links in elastin (desmosine cross-links) and fibrillar collagen (pyridinoline cross-links). Once these cross-links are formed, elastin and collagen are remarkably resistant to proteolytic degradation.

MECHANICAL (HEMODYNAMIC) FACTORS IN ANEURYSM FORMATION

Post-stenotic aneurysms begin as post-stenotic dilatations but become true aneurysms when the diameter criterion is met and when the ectasia becomes permanent and fixed. These aneurysms have historically been thought to occur in a normal arterial wall purely as a result of mechanical factors. Coarctation of the aorta is a classic example. Other disease entities included in this category are pulmonary and aortic valvular disease, cervical rib, and impingement on peripheral arteries caused by any abnormally situated anatomic structures (e.g., popliteal entrapment secondary to an abnormal insertion of the medial head of the gastrocnemius).

Mechanical factors postulated as initiators of post-stenotic dilatation include:

- Elevated lateral wall pressures
- Turbulence
- Abnormal shear stress
- Vibratory forces

Application of Bernoulli's principle predicts, in rigid-walled cylinders with laminar flow, an increase in the post-stenotic lateral pressures created by the acceleration of flow past the stenosis.

In vitro and in vivo studies have documented significant turbulence in the flow exiting a stenotic segment. Trauma secondary to arterial wall vibration generated by the turbulence may be responsible for the post-stenotic dilatation.

The development of elevated shear stress has also been reported in the post-stenotic segment. The abnormal shear stress has been suggested to produce a cyclic pulling on the arterial wall, causing local weakening and dilatation. In addition, endothelial cells exposed to abnormal shear stress can secrete vasoactive substances and other factors that may lead to remodeling and dilatation of the vessel.

An increase in the collagenase activity of aortic tissue distal to a stenosis has been shown in the cynomolgus monkey. This finding suggests that factors other than purely mechanical forces may be associated with the initiation and progression of post-stenotic aneurysm development.[28]

PSEUDOANEURYSMS

Traumatic Aneurysms

Full-thickness traumatic disruption of the normal arterial wall is the leading cause of pseudoaneurysms. They are false aneurysms because the wall lacks all three layers of a normal artery. The capsule is composed of the surrounding compacted periadventitial tissue. This type of false aneurysm is basically a pulsatile hematoma. Both penetrating and blunt trauma can cause pseudoaneurysm. Penetrating injuries occurring outside the hospital are most commonly related to gunshot and stab wounds. Repeated arterial punctures in drug addicts may also cause pseudoaneurysm. Other etiologic factors in this category that have been noted with increasing frequency include iatrogenic injuries from invasive techniques.

After the injury, a hematoma forms within the surrounding tissues and a fibrous wall develops. If a communication persists between the artery and the hematoma sac, a pseudoaneurysm develops. Common examples of blunt trauma resulting in the formation of pseudoaneurysms include *deceleration* injuries of the descending thoracic aorta and *compression* injuries of the abdominal aorta from seat belts. *Blunt* injuries generally produce linear transverse tears in the artery similar to those seen with aortic dissections. The tear tends to be full thickness resulting in a contained rupture.

Periarterial inflammation of a noninfectious nature may cause pseudoaneurysm by digestion of the arterial wall from an extrinsic source. The prototypical example is digestion of the adventitia and outer media of the splenic artery from pancreatitis or the contents of a pseudocyst.

Anastomotic Aneurysms

When grafts are inserted to replace or bypass occluded or aneurysmal segments of the arterial tree, aneurysms can form at the junction between the graft and the host artery as well as in the body of the graft itself. The former (anastomotic aneurysms) are essentially false aneurysms containing no elements of the original arterial wall. They are, in essence, a connective tissue sac that communicates with the defect between graft and host artery. The fibrous capsule surrounding the anastomosis lacks the inherent strength to withstand the mechanical stresses of systemic arterial flow. Anything that causes a separation between graft and host artery can produce an anastomotic aneurysm. The use of silk sutures, suture line infection, inadequate suture purchase, and abnormal shearing forces bearing on the suture line because of joint flexion, compliance mismatch between prosthesis and artery, and turbulence due to junctional flow disturbances have all been implicated.

ARTERITIS

In *Takayasu's disease* occlusive or stenotic changes in the aorta and its major branches are the most frequently identified lesions, but aneurysms have been reported in up to 31% of patients.[29] These patients are more commonly female and tend to be younger than patients with nonspecific aneurysms. Aneurysms are found at almost any level of the aorta and in many visceral arteries. Aneurysmal degeneration has traditionally been attributed to post-stenotic changes, but evidence now suggests that primary arterial wall abnormalities may also be present. Recently, investigators have demonstrated a probable autoimmune link to Takayasu's disease; T-cell receptor expression showed restriction in the regions responsible for immunologic recognition, suggesting that a single antigen is targeted in the aorta of patients with Takayasu's disease.[30]

Giant cell or *temporal arteritis* is characterized by panarteritis with mononuclear and giant cell infiltration, similar to the lesion of Takayasu's disease.[31] Occurring in elderly patients, aneurysms associated with this disorder can involve any portion of the aorta and its branches, with a particular propensity for the ascending aorta and the axillary-brachial segment. *Behçet's syndrome* may be associated with aortitis of the ascending aorta, which may extend to the sinuses of Valsalva and may produce aneurysmal degeneration. There have been rare reports of aneurysms associated with *systemic lupus erythematosus*, and along with the aneurysms associated with *periarteritis nodosa*, these tend to be visceral.

Kawasaki's disease, or mucocutaneous lymph node syndrome, is a multisystem disease of children. Common manifestations include skin rash, conjunctivitis, lymphadenopathy, myocarditis, and aneurysms. Aneurysms most commonly occur in the coronary arteries but have been reported throughout the arterial tree.[31]

The arteritides are discussed in further detail in Chapters 21 and 25.

INFECTIOUS (MYCOTIC) ANEURYSMS

Although the association between bacterial endocarditis and distal arterial disruptions had already been noted by Koch, Osler was the first to use the term *mycotic aneurysm* in his Gulstonian lectures of 1884. Osler used the term to describe multiple aortic aneurysms laden with fungal vegetations in a patient with bacterial endocarditis. Since then, the term "mycotic" has been applied to any aneurysm believed to have developed secondary to any infectious process, although this term is a misnomer in the sense that a true fungal etiology is rare. Historically, bacterial endocarditis and syphilis were the most common causes of mycotic aneurysms. The advent of antibiotics has reduced the incidence of these entities, so that an initial traumatic event is now considered the leading cause.

There are several mechanisms of infection.

Direct extension from a contiguous septic focus causing arterial disruption with aneurysm formation is the rarest mode of development, demonstrating the exceptional resistance of the normal arterial wall to extravascular infection. *Embolomycotic aneurysms* are thought to result from septic emboli lodging within vessel orifices or their vasa vasorum. Bacterial endocarditis remains the most common etiologic factor in this category. *Cryptogenic mycotic aneurysms* form when microbes from an unknown primary site infect a segment of vessel wall. The syphilitic (luetic) aneurysm, which is the classic type, was responsible for more than 50% of all aneurysms in the preantibiotic era and usually affected the ascending aorta.

Ozsvath and coworkers described a possible autoimmune etiology for syphilitic aneurysms based on molecular mimicry of an aortic protein by the *Treponema pallidum* organism.[32] The abdominal aorta is now the most common location for cryptogenic mycotic aneurysms.[33] Older series reported predominantly gram-positive organisms, including *Streptococcus* species and *Staphylococcus* species, with *Salmonella* species being the most common gram-negative organisms. *Salmonella* species seem to have a special affinity for normal arterial walls. More recent series have reported *Staphylococcus aureus* to be the predominant isolate from mycotic aneurysms.[33] In addition, gram-negative and anaerobic infections are now more commonly encountered, with unusual species such as fungi, yeasts, and mycobacteria found in immunocompromised patients.

Juvonen and coworkers have identified *Chlamydia pneumoniae* in 12 of 12 consecutive AAA specimens and in none of 9 controls. This newly recognized pathogen has been proposed as a possible source of smoldering inflammation in the aortic wall with ensuant aneurysmal degeneration.[34] The additional data showing a strong association between *C. pneumoniae* and AAAs suggest that antibiotics might inhibit progression of AAAs.

Penetrating arterial trauma is the most common cause of mycotic aneurysms; the aneurysm results from the introduction of an inoculum at the site of arterial injury or adjacent hematoma. The large increase in the incidence of this type of aneurysm can be attributed to an increase in the use of invasive techniques and the current epidemic of substance abuse with intra-arterial injections of illicit drugs. This kind of infected aneurysm was one of the earliest forms of aneurysmal disease clearly recognized, during the preantiseptic era, when bloodletting was commonplace.

Infection of a preexisting aneurysm occurs occasionally. Although it is not proper to consider such aneurysms mycotic in origin, infection may occur from bacteremia, resulting in sepsis, fever, and rapid expansion of the aneurysm. Interestingly, organisms can be cultured from approximately 10% of routine abdominal aortic aneurysms[35]; this suggests that simple colonization is much more common and less virulent than a true invasive infection.

PREGNANCY-ASSOCIATED ANEURYSMS

Arterial rupture is a leading cause of maternal death. Vessels that have been reported to be the site of aneurysmal rupture during pregnancy most commonly include the splenic artery, cerebral artery, and aorta, followed by the renal, iliac, coronary, and ovarian arteries. More than 50% of ruptured aneurysms suffered by women under the age of 40 years are pregnancy-related.[36, 37] Manalo-Estrella and Barker described decreased levels of acid mucopolysaccharides and fragmentation of reticular fibers in the aortic walls of 16 patients dying of other causes during pregnancy.[38] Twelve age-adjusted nonpregnant control subjects did not manifest these changes. Thus, in addition to obvious connective tissue changes during pregnancy, such as the relaxation of pelvic ligaments before parturition, the effects of hormonal changes on other connective tissue structures (e.g., vascular) may be a generalized phenomenon. Furthermore, Zucker and associates have found a doubling of plasma levels of matrix metalloproteinase-2 (MMP-2), a protease capable of degrading both elastin and fibrillar collagen, in the latter half of pregnancy.[39]

DEGENERATIVE ANEURYSMS

Nonspecific Aneurysms

The most common form of aneurysmal disease, which usually affects the infrarenal abdominal aorta as well as the popliteal, femoral and iliac arteries, has historically been called the *atherosclerotic aneurysm*. Although these aneurysms show gross and microscopic evidence of atheromatous disease, the notion that atherosclerosis is the underlying cause of the arterial dilatation has become controversial. An alternative scenario is that as the vessel dilates, boundary layer separation occurs along the surface and hemodynamic forces stimulate subintimal proliferative changes resulting in plaque formation. Although difficult to refute, this suggestion—that dilatation may precede and be the cause of atheromatous change—is problematic, considering the advanced complex plaque present, particularly on the posterior wall, even in small AAAs.

The nature of the relationship between atheromatous disease and degenerative aneurysms is controversial. Still, some trials have borne out the association between AAAs and some epidemiologic factors known to be associated with atherosclerosis. The landmark Aneurysm Detection and Management (ADAM) study included 73,451 United States veterans who underwent ultrasound screening and tracking of epidemiologic variables. Aneurysms 4.0 cm or larger were detected in 1031(1.4%) of participants. Smoking was the risk factor most strongly associated with AAA (odds ratio, 5.57).[40] Female gender, African American race, and diabetes mellitus were negatively associated with AAA in the ADAM trial.[40] The Honolulu Heart Study found that increased cholesterol levels were also associated with AAA.[41] As in the ADAM trial, diabetes mellitus is the only risk factor for atherosclerosis not associated with AAA. Hypertension proved to be a weaker positive correlate of AAA in the ADAM study.

Watt and colleagues[41a] showed that elevated serum triglyceride was strongly related to death from ruptured AAA in a prospective cohort of 21,520 men attending a London clinic. Smoking and elevated LDL, blood pressure and body mass index were also positive correlates but did not reach statistical significance for risk of death from ruptured AAA.

Cronenwett and associates[42, 43] described a predictive value of diastolic hypertension for rupture and elevated pulse pressure for expansion of aneurysms. Interestingly, the same investigators found emphysema to be a strong predictor of rupture and suggested that a systemic increase in proteinase activity may account for both phenomena. This theory is corroborated by Rao and coworkers[43a] who found that plasma from 14 AAA patients had significantly less capacity to inhibit elastase than matched controls.

A phenomenon cited in support of the concept that

aneurysms are simply the result of a lifetime of wear and tear is the steady increase in the incidence of the disease with aging. However, an autopsy study of 45,838 individuals found that in men the incidence peaks at age 80 and then declines.[44] This observation suggests that environmental factors may be important in the accumulated risk for AAAs, but a point is reached at which the pool of genetically susceptible individuals has been exhausted. As with atherosclerosis in general, women show a delay in the age of onset of AAAs and the rate increases throughout a woman's life span. This observation may explain why the dramatic male predominance in the sixth and seventh decades of life is not seen in the eighth decade.

Several investigators have mentioned a true increase in the incidence of AAA over the last several decades. Melton and colleagues reported an increased incidence of approximately sevenfold in a well-studied Minnesota community.[45] The phenomenon cannot be explained on the basis of the fact that more people are living long enough to reach the age of risk, because the increase in prevalence is age-specific.[44, 46] While there is no currently accepted explanation for this observed increase in prevalence, the regression model of Zarins and coauthors (see experimental models)[47] suggests one possible explanation of increasing AAA incidence: aggressive dietary restriction and lipid-lowering medication.

Martin was among the first to question whether dilating disease of the aorta was fundamentally different from stenosing disease.[48] Tilson and Stansel observed that in comparison with patients with atherosclerotic occlusive disease, the patients with aneurysms were older, represented a higher ratio of males to females, had less distal peripheral vascular disease, and showed a superior long-term graft patency rate.[49] Baxter and associates demonstrated generalized matrix changes throughout the aorta of patients with aneurysm.[50] In addition, the generalized arteriomegaly of nonatherosclerotic segments,[51] the association with aneurysms of minimally atherosclerotic arteries (e.g., the popliteal), and the association with complex inguinal hernias[52] suggest that the disease involves unknown systemic or constitutional factors in addition to atherosclerotic stimuli. Investigators have recently demonstrated a correlation between carotid artery stiffness and the presence of AAAs, further implicating a systemic vascular abnormality.[53]

Experimental Models

Models of aneurysmal disease may be divided into the following categories:

- Spontaneous
- Pharmacologic
- Dietary
- Surgical

Spontaneous aneurysms occur consistently in the blotchy mouse, which has a mutation on the X chromosome, and rarely in other species, such as horses (usually stallions) and turkeys. The blotchy mouse mutation interferes with copper metabolism, and copper is a cofactor for lysyl oxidase, the enzyme that forms stable cross-links in collagen and elastin. Aneurysms of the blotchy mouse have been described in detail,[26, 27] but attempts to make correlations with the disease in humans have been disappointing. After Tilson presented preliminary data with the suggestion that copper deficiency might be important in patients,[54] two studies reported that copper levels were normal[55, 56] and one study reported that copper levels were elevated.[57]

A promising new category of experimental animals includes those with known genetic alterations. These *transgenic* or "knockout" (i.e., certain gene products have been effectively eliminated or knocked out from the genome) animals are predominantly mice. Carmeliet and colleagues utilized the apolipoprotein E knockout mouse, in which aortic aneurysms develop in association with atherosclerosis, to explore the role of the serine proteases, tissue-type plasminogen activator (t-PA) and urokinase-type plasminogen activator (u-PA). Using double knockouts (apolipoprotein E plus t-PA or apolipoprotein E plus u-PA) they showed an important role for u-PA in aneurysm formation and speculated that this is related to u-PA's ability to activate metalloproteinases.[58]

Pharmacologic aneurysms may be induced by lathyrism or by steroid use. The most common lathyrogen in experimental use is beta-aminopropionitrile, which has been studied extensively in turkeys.[59, 60] Corticosteroids have been used to induce aortic aneurysms or aortic ruptures in hamsters[61] and mice.[62]

Dietary models fall into two categories: copper deficiency and variations in cholesterol intake. On a regimen of strict copper restriction, aneurysms develop diffusely in the pig.[63] The induction of aneurysms by high-cholesterol feeding appears to occur only rarely, and it is not entirely clear whether this incidence is significantly greater than that due to chance alone.[64, 65] However, the feeding of atherogenic diets to predisposed surgical and genetic models has been more fruitful.[58, 66] DePalma and colleagues were the first to report aneurysms in association with experimental regression of atherosclerosis in dogs.[67] More recently, Zarins and associates reported an increase of approximately twofold in the internal elastic lamella area (a 38% increase in diameter) in the abdominal aorta of six monkeys receiving regression diets.[47] The diet used for induction of atherosclerosis contained 25% peanut oil, which tends to induce an inflammatory variant of atherosclerosis. This factor may also be important in aneurysm pathogenesis. In a hypertensive mouse model that overproduces angiotensin II, frequent aneurysms and rupture of the thoracic and abdominal aortae have developed when a high salt intake was provided.[67a]

The *surgical models* are a mixed group, including (1) ex vivo preparations, (2) transplantation (immunologic), (3) hemodynamic types, and (4) direct injuries. A xenograft model in the rat provides insight into the role of enzymes capable of digesting elastin and collagen in AAA formation and rupture.[67b] Allografts of the aorta in inbred rats provide an interesting model for studying the relative importance of immunologic variables versus hemodynamic factors such as hypertension.[68] Post-stenotic dilatations are also being studied. Anidjar and colleagues have shown that elastase infusion under superphysiologic pressures produced aneurysms in the rat aorta.[69] The theoretical basis for this model was direct elastin degradation, but recent investigations have shown that specific elastase activity may not be the actual mechanism.[69a] In fact, the dilatation corresponded temporally, not with the early elastin degradation, but with the ensuing inflammatory response.[70, 71]

A variation on the Anidjar/Dobrin theme is described by Nackman, who demonstrated that infusion of elastin degradation products alone in the form of six amino acid chains produces adventitial angiogenesis accompanied by modest dilatation in the rat aorta.[72] This further validates the concept of the inflammatory response as the pivotal event in the original Anidjar/Dobrin model. (For further discussion, see Role of Inflammation.) Investigators have applied calcium chloride to rabbit periaortic tissues, creating an animal prone to aneurysm formation when subject to combined high-cholesterol feeding and periaortic thioglycolate administration.[73]

Finally, a group from Leicester University described an ex vivo porcine aortic model of aneurysm pathogenesis that employed the elastin-related injury developed by Anidjar and Dobrin. The convenience of the in vitro preparation simplifies the task of modifying multiple experimental conditions[74]; still, results need to be validated by reproducing these measures in aortic aneurysms in vivo. Many observations gleaned from human aortic tissue studies, regarding the roles of proteolysis and inflammation have been further tested and validated by these animal models during the past several years.

Genetic Susceptibility and Candidate Genes

In 1977, Clifton reported three brothers who had ruptured AAAs during the seventh decade of life.[75] Tilson and Seashore reported on 50 families in 1984 with two or more first-order relatives affected with AAAs.[76] Because about 25% of the families had father-son patterns, the investigators concluded that if there was only one aneurysm gene, it would have to be autosomal. Interestingly, when this series was extended to 94 families, the male:female ratio of affected offspring of the 22 affected fathers was 62:2.[77]

Johansen and Koepsell also confirmed the familial incidence of AAA in their study of 250 patients and 250 atherosclerotic control subjects. They reported a sixfold increase in the risk: the odds ratio for an AAA among first-degree relatives of probands (19%) versus control patients.[78] Numerous other studies support the concept of an important genetic susceptibility factor.[79–84] Powell and Greenhalgh calculated the genetic component to be approximately 70% in a multifactorial model.[82] Subsequently, Powell and coworkers suggested an association between AAA and polymorphisms of two genes on the long arm of chromosome 16.[85]

About 25% of AAA patients are aware of another first-order relative with the disease, and if the male siblings of a proband are screened with ultrasonography, approximately 20% to 30% have positive findings.[86–88] Because one must live a long time to pass through the age of risk, it has been speculated that the true lifetime incidence in a sibling surviving to old age might approach 50%, which would be compatible with a single dominant gene. However, the most extensive genetic analysis reported to date, by Majumder and colleagues,[89] proposed an autosomal recessive mode.

The first conclusive evidence of mutation in a gene for structural protein in a family with AAA disease was presented by Kontusaari and coworkers.[19] There was a point mutation in the type III procollagen gene, which resulted in the substitution of an arginine for the glycine at position 691. The presence of the small amino acid glycine at every third position in the helical portion of the fibrillar collagens is essential to permit normal coiling, so that the substitution resulted in a collagen that was thermally unstable, with a lowered melting point. The family was not typical of most with clustering of AAAs, because in two patients AAAs were detected at young ages. Several mutations in type III collagen have been linked to late-onset AAA.[90] A systematic search for other fibrillar collagen mutations in 50 cases of adult-onset AAA did not identify another structurally significant mutation.[91]

Fibrillin, a microfibrillar protein, is part of the elastin molecule. Mutations in fibrillin cause Marfan's syndrome. Two fibrillin mutations have been found in association with infrarenal AAA.[92] Given the strong association of fibrillin with elastin and the markedly higher levels of elastin in the proximal compared to the distal aorta, it would be unlikely that fibrillin or elastin mutations would be manifested primarily in the distal aorta. For example, a mutation of the fibrillin I gene different from Marfan's syndrome has been identified in 9 members of a kindred with an autosomal dominant inheritance pattern manifesting aortic root enlargement and ascending aortic aneurysm and dissection.[93] Another family has been found to have a mutation in the type III procollagen gene that causes a splicing error.[94]

On the theme of mutations that might stimulate aneurysm formation by promoting proteolysis, Powell and colleagues[85] reported the association of AAA with an allele of the haptoglobin gene on chromosome 16, the product of which appears to promote elastolysis in vitro. This illustrates the hypothesis that entry into the loop may occur at some site other than a structural abnormality of a matrix protein. The finding has not as yet been confirmed.

A subset of patients (in the range of 10%) may have a deficiency allele of alpha$_1$-antitrypsin, as reported by Cohen and colleagues,[95] illustrating the concept that the genetic predisposition is at the level of failure of protease inhibition. However, this finding also remains unconfirmed.

Researchers have now identified a genetic predisposition to the development of the inflammatory variant of degenerative aneurysm. The locus of the predisposition is mapped to the human leukocyte antigen (HLA-DR) molecule where the B$_1$ allele conveys an increased risk. The investigators suggest the association indicates a role for antigen recognition in the pathogenesis of the inflammatory aortic aneurysm.[96]

Despite considerable efforts, no mutation of the major aortic connective tissue proteins have been found to account for the frequency of adult-onset degenerative aortic aneurysm. Given the apparently significant role of the inflammatory process in the pathogenesis of AAAs, a better understanding of the genes regulating the relationship between the inflammatory cells and the mesenchymal cells of the vascular wall may prove helpful in elucidating a genetic basis for this disease.

Matrix Changes in the Aneurysmal Aorta

Elastin and collagen are the main matrix components of the aortic wall. The role of each in aneurysm formation appears complex. Early studies suggested that loss of elastin and collagen content in the aortic walls was adequate to explain the formation of aneurysms by mechanical principles.[97] While multiple subsequent studies have confirmed the destruction of normal elastin structure in aneurysmal aorta and a relative decrease in its concentration,[85, 87, 88, 98–102] other investigators have demonstrated an increase in the total mass of elastin.[103] The paradox is explained next.

Tropoelastin, the fundamental unit of the elastin fiber, forms a complex around a framework of microfibrillar proteins to form the elastin fiber. The majority of elastin is formed before birth, with relatively little production for growth and repair in the adult. Still, low levels of synthesis in the adult aorta are suggested by the presence of small amounts of tropoelastin messenger ribonucleic acid (mRNA) and the stability of elastin concentration with normal aortic growth.[104, 105] One of the consistent histologic features of aneurysmal tissue is fragmentation of the medial elastic lamellae and decreased elastin staining.[106, 107] Minion and colleagues have shown that the absolute mass of elastin is increased in the aneurysmal aorta compared to the normal aorta.[103] The apparent discrepancy between this observation and the marked decrease in elastin staining of AAA tissue may relate to poor uptake of the stain by newly synthesized unorganized fibrils within the plaque as well as a general redistribution of the medial elastin over a larger aortic diameter. Thus, the increase in total elastin does not keep pace with aortic expansion, and its concentration is markedly decreased relative to collagen.[103]

White and coauthors have demonstrated a reduction of both the adventitial elastic lamellae and the number of fibers per lamellae in aneurysm tissue compared to normal aortic tissue.[108] Work in animal models indicates that elastin degradation may in fact be important in AAA pathogenesis. It appears less likely that this is a direct mechanical effect of elastin degradation but, rather, a secondary effect of elastin degradation products stimulating a destructive immune response.[72]

Collagen has also been examined extensively. Types I and III are the main types found in both the normal and aneurysmal aorta. The absolute mass of collagen in aneurysmal aorta is increased but to a greater degree than elastin.[93, 103, 109] Because the tensile strength of collagen is four orders of magnitude greater than that of elastin,[110] it is logical to infer that destruction of collagen would be required for aneurysm formation. This is in contrast to the evidence of increased collagen mass.

Several explanations may satisfy this conflict:

1. The total mass of the collagen measured may include partially degraded fibers, which would not contribute to circumferential integrity.
2. The increase in collagen mass may not be commensurate with the increasing wall stress of the expanding aneurysm.
3. The loss of elastic recoil may increase stress on the collagen. An interesting observation in this regard is the description of a soluble factor regulating collagen synthesis in AAA,[111] which differs from the usual regulation at the level of transcription.[112]

Finally, R.W. Thompson and colleagues have demonstrated smooth muscle cell *apoptosis* (programmed cell death) in the absence of signs of necrosis in the media of human AAA. These findings were associated with a significant decrease in medial smooth muscle cell density and increased production of p53, a potential mediator of cell cycle arrest and programmed cell death.[113] Henderson and colleagues[113a] add that macrophages and T-lymphocytes appear to be elaborating the mediators which produce the apoptosis in AAA smooth muscle cells. These investigators point out the important role of the smooth muscle cell in maintenance of medial architecture and matrix remodeling.

Proteolytic Enzymes and Their Inhibitors

The role of collagenolytic and elastolytic enzymes found in aneurysmal tissue has been the subject of a number of important studies. Busuttil and coworkers[114] and Cannon and Read[115] were the first to report increased elastolytic activity in AAAs. Dubick and colleagues also implicated a serine protease showing a twofold to threefold increase in elastolytic activity that they attributed to pancreatic elastase.[116] Enzymes for which elastin is a substrate include the serine protease, neutrophil elastase, and the matrix metalloproteinases (MMPs), 92 kD (MMP-9), 72 kD (MMP-2) gelatinase, matrilysin (MMP-8), and macrophage metalloelastase (MMP-12). Both of the gelatinases (MMP-2 and MMP-9) effectively degrade elastin and type IV collagen and MMP-2 has been shown to have true collagenolytic activity.[117]

Cohen et al,[118] in their extensive work on neutrophil elastase, reported that peripheral neutrophils from patients with AAAs exhibit increased neutrophil elastase activity. Although neutrophils are not seen in significant numbers in advanced aneurysmal tissue, this observation does not preclude their potential role in the initiation of the disease process. The authors have also shown that smooth muscle cells from AAA explants secrete increased amounts of proteolytic enzymes in response to stimulation by elastin degradation products.[119]

Nackman, Karkowski, and Tilson showed similar results in a rat model.[72] Studies suggest that the proteolytic activities of MMP-2 and MMP-9 are predominant in aortic matrix degradation while a new role for plasmin and the plasminogen activators has been identified in increasing MMP activation.

Studies using zymography, Northern blot, substrate assay, and immunoblot techniques confirm that MMP-9 is elevated in AAA compared with normal controls.[120–126] Animal models validate this result as well.[74] Other investigations have shown an increase in MMP-9 activity or detection in AAA compared to atherosclerotic aortas.[125–127] These findings do not yet enjoy universal agreement. Other investigators specifically demonstrated the presence of activated MMP-9 in AAA walls, a finding not observed in normal controls.[124] Macrophages are believed to be the primary source of MMP-9 in AAAs[125] but the evidence suggests that smooth muscle cells may also be a source of this enzyme. The normal aorta appears to express MMP-9 in the absence of invading inflammatory cells,[128] and smooth muscle cells derived from AAA secrete MMP-9 in culture.[126] In addition, cultured aneurysmal smooth muscle cells demonstrate increased expression of metalloproteinases in response to products secreted by inflammatory cells.[111]

MMP-2 also appears to be involved in AAA pathogenesis. Several studies demonstrate increased tissue levels of MMP-2 in AAA compared to atherosclerotic aortas and even greater increases compared to normal controls.[112, 124, 126, 129, 130] In addition to its ability to degrade elastin, MMP-2 can also degrade intact fibrillar collagen.[117] Other investigators have shown that thrombin can stimulate vascular smooth muscle cells to produce activated MMP-2.[131]

The precise role of the various MMPs in different phases of matrix destruction is not known with certainty. Studies by Freestone and coworkers, however, have shown that MMP-2 is the principal proteolytic enzyme present in smaller aneurysms measuring 4 to 5.5 cm, whereas MMP-9 is the principal proteolytic enzyme in aneurysms larger than 5.5 cm.[132] Using the polymerase chain reaction (PCR) to amplify mRNA, McMillan and colleagues confirmed the increased MMP-9 expression in aneurysms measuring 5.0 to 6.9 compared to those measuring 4.0 to 5.0 cm or greater than 7.0 cm.[133] These interesting findings are interpreted by the study authors as suggesting that MMP-2 is possibly involved in initial elastolysis, whereas MMP-9 is a delayed contributor to aneurysm expansion up to a certain diameter, at which time other mechanical or biochemical influences predominate.

Enzymes involved in coagulation and fibrinolysis have been shown to possess a regulatory capability for MMP production and activation.[58] Increased levels of plasmin have been described in AAAs.[134, 135] Examining AAA, atherosclerotic and normal aortas, Shireman and associates[136] found a threefold elevation of t-PA activator in AAAs and atherosclerotic aortas compared to normal aortas. Furthermore, they found levels of u-PA in AAAs that were double those found in atherosclerotic aortas and eightfold higher than normal.[11] The investigators suggest that u-PA, known to play a role in tissue remodeling, may be responsible for the differential elevation of plasmin seen in AAAs. Newman and coauthors have localized u-PA synthesis to the macrophage in AAAs using immunohistochemistry.[137]

Work by Carmeliet and colleagues using transgenic knockout mice has validated and advanced the concept of an important interaction between serine and metalloproteinases.[58] This group used apolipoprotein E–deficient mice that were prone to AAAs (see animal models). The animals in this study also were engineered to lack combinations of u-PA or t-PA. Animals deficient in u-PA were found to be protected against aneurysm formation. Since u-PA cannot directly degrade collagen or elastin, the authors suggested an indirect effect through MMP activation. Deficiency of t-PA did not confer protection.[58] The group also used macrophages from mice deficient (i.e., knockout mice) in MMP-3, MMP-9 or MMP-12 in combination with apolipoprotein E and u-PA. In vitro elastin degradation was inhibited in the MMP-12 knockout mice but not in mice lacking MMP-3 or MMP-9. This model suggests that the protective effect seen in vivo in the u-PA knockout mouse was associated with MMP-12 activity. This observation strengthens the finding of Curci and coworkers, who propose a key role for MMP-12 as the pathophysiologically important enzyme in AAA formation in human aortas.[137a]

The possibility of failure of antiproteolytic systems as a mechanism of disease in AAAs was suggested by Cannon and Read in 1982.[115] Cohen and colleagues suggested that an imbalance between serine elastase and alpha$_1$-antitrypsin levels may cause AAA in some patients.[138] Similarly, Brophy and coworkers showed a relative deficiency in immunoreactive tissue inhibitor of MMPs (TIMP) in AAA tissue, suggesting such an imbalance between the metalloproteinase systems and TIMP, their most important physiologic inhibitors, predisposes to AAA.[139] Allaire and associates showed that local overexpession of TIMP-1 in their rat xerotransplant model could prevent aneurysm development and that the aneurysms were caused specifically by MMPs, but the mechanism of inhibition is not fully understood.[67b]

Role of Inflammation

Beckman, reviewing 156 specimens of AAA tissue, found that more than two thirds had a notable infiltration of chronic inflammatory cells in the adventitia.[140] Interestingly, this zone is the site of most of the structural collagen. It is well known clinically that aneurysms are uncommon after endarterectomy if the adventitia (and external elastic lamella) remain intact. Brophy and coworkers confirmed a significant infiltration of the adventitia in AAA with inflammatory cells,[141] and Koch and colleagues took initial steps to identify these cells immunohistochemically.[142] They reported significant numbers of macrophages and T-cells, and this finding has been confirmed by another technique based on fluorescence-activated cell sorting.[143] In addition, Brophy and associates demonstrated an increase in immunoglobulin by Western blot assay in the aneurysmal tissue.[141]

Complementing this descriptive evidence, experimental evidence is available linking inflammation to aneurysm formation. Ricci and colleagues[144] used an anti CD-18 monoclonal antibody to inhibit leukocyte adhesion in an elastase-infusion rat model; observations included a decreased inflammatory process and attenuation of AAA expansion. Hingorani and coauthors have used the same rat model to demonstrate that a tumor necrosis factor–blocking agent attenuates the inflammatory response, whereas an interleukin-1 blocking agent does not show an effect.[144a] Similar experiments have demonstrated attenuation of AAA expansion using prednisone or cyclosporine.[145]

Other animal models have implicated the inflammatory process as a key event in aneurysm pathogenesis. The short peptide molecules that result from elastin degradation are well-known chemotactic mediators for inflammatory cell migration. Nackman and coauthors observed that the elastin degradation products alone, infused into the rat infrarenal aorta, produced histologic features of aneurysmal disease in the setting of the characteristic inflammatory infiltrate.[72] This result presents the question of whether structural changes of elastolysis are as important as the ensuant inflammatory response. Freestone and colleagues used periaortic application of calcium chloride to induce aneurysm formation. Again, the key event appears to be macrophage infiltration into the adventitia.[73]

Investigators have worked to define a role for autoimmunity in *degenerative* AAAs; however, the data are conflicting. In favor of a role for autoimmunity, Gregory and coworkers extracted immunoglobulin (Ig) from 11 of 14 AAA specimens that would bind to the matrix fibers of normal aortas.

Such immunoglobulins were present in only one of nine organ donor aortas.[146] Hirose's group pursued the nature of the isolated IgG using sophisticated techniques suggesting that the antibody target may be a microfibril-associated glycoprotein.[147] Sequencing and comparative homology studies also prompted the investigators to speculate regarding a virus-induced molecular mimicry mechanism of autoimmunity, but this hypothesis remains unproven. Other investigators have compiled evidence against an autoantigenic process in AAA disease. Walton and associates demonstrated that B-cells from AAA tissue expressed an unrestricted range of their variable regions, suggesting that the inflammatory infiltrate is not an autoimmune response to a limited repertoire of tissue antigens.[148] Another group performed the complementary experiment, evaluating T-cell receptor variable expression from the AAA adventitial infiltrate. Again, the T-cell repertoire was polyclonal and not restricted.[149]

Potential Pharmacologic Interventions

The crescendo of interest in the basic biology of aneurysmal disease may have significant practical consequences in the near future. If a gene were discovered that accounted for a large subset of patients with AAAs, it could quickly become routine to screen for an etiologic mutation in the gene with a simple blood test. If patients were identified to be at risk, they could be advised to have periodic ultrasound examinations to detect potential problems before there was any risk of rupture. In addition, pharmacologic interventions may be developed to prevent the disease in patients shown to be susceptible by the previously described approach or to stabilize the connective tissue matrix and prevent aneurysm enlargement in those with small AAAs.

One such potential intervention has already received some attention in experimental animals. Simpson and coworkers found that propranolol reduced the incidence of AAAs in the β-aminopropionitrile–induced turkey model by some mechanism other than its hemodynamic effects on pulse and blood pressure.[59] Additional studies suggested a direct stimulatory effect on the cross-linking of connective tissue components.[60] Similar findings have been reported in the aneurysm-prone blotchy mouse,[150, 151] although a more recent study in this model found propranolol-mediated aneurysm attenuation related to decreased heart rate with no effect on the lysyl oxidase enzyme, believed to be important in collagen and elastin cross-linking.[152] The literature suggests that some beta-blocking agents may have direct connective tissue effects.[153–155]

Clinical studies of propranolol show a decreased growth of AAA in retrospective series.[122, 156] Furthermore, selective β_1-adrenergic antagonists were not effective when compared with the nonselective agent propranolol.[157] This finding is in contrast to that of Cronenwett and coauthors, who did not find an inhibitory effect on aortic aneurysm growth in their cohort of patients with an AAA.[158]

Holmes and associates have found that indomethacin, an inhibitor of macrophage MMP production, reduces aneurysm growth in the rodent elastase-infusion model. The mechanism is believed to be inhibition of MMP-9. This same group noted a relationship between prostaglandin E_2 (PGE_2) production and aneurysm development in human aortas. These investigators further localized the PGE_2 production to macrophages and discovered its regulation by cyclooxygenase type II (Cox II).[160] Cox II is a potential target for pharmacologic intervention.

Doxycycline and other tetracyclines act as nonspecific inhibitors of the MMPs. Proposed mechanisms include binding to the enzyme's active zinc sites[161] or inactive calcium sites causing conformational change or by direct transcriptional downregulation.[162] Other mechanisms have been proposed as well.[163] Animal studies of doxycycline show potential for use in the treatment of aneurysm. Petrinec and colleagues observed suppression of aneurysm formation by high-dose doxycycline in the elastase-infusion rodent model accompanied by significantly decreased MMP-9 production.[164] Furthermore, Boyle and colleagues used an elastase-treated porcine aortic organ culture model to show significantly decreased elastin degradation and MMP-9 production mediated by doxycycline.[163] Considering the safety and long-term clinical experience with doxycycline, one can anticipate clinical trials for small AAAs in the near future.

Inflammatory Aneurysms

The term "inflammatory aneurysm" was first used by Walker and colleagues[165] to describe AAAs in 19 patients who showed excessive thickening of the walls and perianeurysmal adhesions to adjacent organs.[165] Numerous reports thereafter suggested that these aneurysms represented a variant of nonspecific aneurysms with distinct clinical, operative, and pathologic features.[166, 167] Most commonly involving the abdominal aorta, inflammatory aneurysms account for 5% of AAAs. Clinically, most of these aneurysms are associated with symptoms of back pain and weight loss along with an elevation in the erythrocyte sedimentation rate. At laparotomy, the aneurysms are encased in a dense, shiny fibrotic reaction with frequent involvement of the duodenum, ureters, and inferior vena cava. Pathologic analysis of the wall demonstrates marked thickening of the media and adventitia. Varying degrees of infiltration into these two layers with lymphocytes, plasma cells, and mononuclear cells, along with endarteritis of the vasa vasorum, are usually present.

The etiology of this variant of nonspecific aneurysms is unknown. Advocates of the theory that distinct etiologic factors are responsible for inflammatory aneurysm development have offered trauma, chronic leakage of blood or urine, intramural hemorrhage, and primary autoimmune disorder as possible initiators. Other investigators believe that the characteristic inflammatory process represents an extension of the inflammation observed in the nonspecific aneurysms.[168] In support of this latter theory is the regression of the fibrotic process in the retroperitoneum after graft placement. Why these patients respond with greater intensity and extension of the inflammatory response, however, remains enigmatic. There must be a biochemical basis for this heightened response. One possibility might be the liberation of an elastin-derived degradation product with unique chemotactic characteristics; another might be the abundant production by the inflammatory cells present of a cytokine with intense angiogenic properties. As described earlier (see Genetic Susceptibility and Candidate Genes), investigators have proposed an autoimmunologic mechanism in the formation of inflammatory aneurysms.[96]

GRAFT ANEURYSMS

Aneurysms have developed in the body of almost every arterial substitute used to date.[169] Aneurysmal development was one of the main reasons for abandonment of the arterial *homograft*. Subsequently, *heterografts* (or more specifically, ficin-digested, formaldehyde-treated bovine carotid arteries) also showed a propensity for aneurysm formation.[170] The similarly modified human umbilical vein graft had to be reinforced with a circumferential Dacron mesh to prevent aneurysmal development. Despite this, up to 65% of aneurysmal degeneration is being reported in unsupported umbilical vein grafts patent at 5 years,[171] and histologic examination suggests that the collagen cross-linking process used is inadequate to prevent tissue digestion to a degree that can be compensated for even by an improved Dacron mesh.

Arterial autografts do not usually become aneurysmal, but vein autografts placed in the systemic arterial tree may become aneurysmal. The saphenous vein, because it must withstand gravitational pressures, is thicker-walled. After implantation, it becomes even thicker by increased connective tissue deposition. Nevertheless, when used in extremity arterial reconstruction, the reported incidence of aneurysm development is 4%.[172] In addition, when this graft is placed in the aortorenal position, where the flows are generally higher, the rate of aneurysmal development is even higher. This complication has been partly attributed, although without proof, to forceful dilatation of the vein graft during its removal and preparation for implantation. This is no longer common practice, but no reports have yet reflected any decrease in the development of these aneurysms.

Prosthetic grafts have been made of a number of materials, including Vinyon, nylon, Orlon, Teflon, Dacron, and polytetrafluoroethylene. The first three were quickly abandoned because of frequent complications, not the least of which was loss of tensile strength and aneurysm formation. The overwhelming preference today in prosthetic grafts is Dacron or polytetrafluoroethylene.

Knitted Dacron is more compliant than *woven* Dacron and may be less likely to contribute to anastomotic aneurysm formation. In addition, the knitted fabric has larger interstices through which capillary ingrowth can reach, nourish, and secure the neointima. In an effort to improve this ingrowth, knitted grafts were made progressively more porous until reports began to appear of diffuse dilatation or fragmentation and aneurysm formation.[173] Adoption of a *velour* construction and a tighter-wrap knit may have solved this problem, for it has not been reported to date with any frequency with third-generation prostheses. Even the relatively solid expanded grafts, as originally constructed, were associated with a significant incidence of aneurysm formation.[174] This problem has since been combatted either by adding an outer helical wrap or by increasing the thickness of the graft wall.

SUMMARY

Surgery is an effective treatment for AAAs, and less invasive approaches should reduce the morbidity and mortality of repair. Knowledge of the pathogenesis of AAA is steadily increasing and may lead to effective medical therapy at the molecular level to prevent matrix changes characteristic of AAA. Our tools used to detect genetic predisposition to AAA are also improving, and this may permit therapy at the level of gene expression. Smoking cessation continues to be a modality of prevention for some.

REFERENCES

1. Johnston KW, Rutherford RB, Tilson MD, et al: Suggested standards for reporting on arterial aneurysms. J Vasc Surg 13:452, 1991.
2. Wolinsky H, Glagov S: A lamellar unit of aortic medial structure and function in mammals. Circ Res 20:99, 1967.
2a. Shapiro SD, Endicott SK, Campbell EJ, et al: Marked longevity of human lung parenchymal elastic fibers deduced from prevalence of D-aspartate and nuclear weapons-related radiocarbon. J Clin Invest 87:1828, 1991.
2b. Powell JT, Vine N, Crossman M: On the accumulation of D-asparate in elastin and other proteins of the ageing aorta. Atherosclerosis 97:201, 1992.
3. Tilson MD, Elefteriades J, Brophy CM: Tensile strength and collagen in abdominal aortic aneurysm disease. *In* Greenhalgh RM, Mannick JA, Powell JT (eds): The Cause and Management of Aneurysms. London, WB Saunders, 1990, pp 97–104.
4. Pyeritz RE: Marfan syndrome. N Engl J Med 323:987, 1990.
5. Kainulainen K, Pulkkinen L, Savolainen A, et al: Location on chromosome 15 of the gene defect causing Marfan syndrome. N Engl J Med 323:935, 1990.
6. McKusick VA: Mendelian Inheritance in Man, 5th ed. Baltimore, Johns Hopkins University Press, 1978.
7. Sakai LY, Keene DR, Engvall E: Fibrillin, a new 350-kD glycoprotein component of extracellular microfibrils. J Cell Biol 103:2499, 1986.
8. Hollister DW, Godfrey M, Sakai LY, Pyeritz RE: Immunohistologic abnormalities of the microfibrillar-fiber system in the Marfan syndrome. N Engl J Med 323:152, 1990.
9. Lee B, Godfrey M, Vitale E, et al: Linkage of Marfan syndrome and phenotypically related disorder to two different fibrillin genes. Nature 352:330, 1991.
10. Dietz HC, Cutting GR, Pyeritz RE, et al: Marfan syndrome caused by a recurrent de novo missense mutation in the fibrillin gene. Nature 352:337, 1991.
11. vanMeekeren JA: De delatabilitate extraordinaria cutis. As quoted by Sheiner NM, Miller N, Lachance C: Arterial complications of Ehlers-Danlos syndrome. J Cardiovasc Surg 26:291, 1985.
12. Barabas AP: Ehlers-Danlos syndrome. *In* Greenhalgh RM, Mannick JA, Powell JT (eds): The Cause and Management of Aneurysms. London, WB Saunders, 1990, pp 57– 67.
13. Weber FP: The Ehlers-Danlos syndrome. Br J Dermatol 48:609, 1936.
14. Barabas AP: Heterogeneity of the Ehlers-Danlos syndrome. Br Med J 2:612, 1967.
15. Wesley Jr, Mahour GH, Wooley MM: Multiple surgical problems in two patients with Ehlers-Danlos syndrome. Surgery 86:319, 1980.
16. Pope FM, Martin GR, McKusick VA: Patients with type IV EDS lack type III collagen. Proc Natl Acad Sci U S A 72:1314, 1975.
17. Pope FM, Nicholls AC, Jones PM, et al: EDS IV (acrogeria): New autosomal dominant and recessive types. J R Soc Med 73:180, 1980.
18. Pope FM, Child AH, Nicholls AC, et al: Type III collagen deficiency with normal phenotype. J R Soc Med 76:518, 1983.
19. Kontusaari S, Tromp G, Kuivaniemi H, et al: A mutation in the gene for type III procollagen (COL3A1) in a family with aortic aneurysms. J Clin Invest 86:1465, 1990.
20. O'Hara PJ, Ratcliff NB, Grove RA, et al: Medical agenesis associated with multiple extracranial, peripheral and visceral arterial aneurysms. J Vasc Surg 2:298, 1985.

21. Hagood CA, Garvin DD, Lachina FM, et al: Abdominal aortic aneurysm and renal hamartoma in an infant with tuberous sclerosis. Surgery 79:713, 1976.
22. Allen DB, Hendricks SA, Levy JM: Aortic dilation in Turner syndrome. J. Pediatr 109:302, 1986.
23. Lin AE, Lippe BM, Geffner ME, et al: Aortic dilation, dissection, and rupture in patients with Turner syndrome. J Pediatr 109:820, 1986.
24. Danks DM, Campbell PE, Walker-Smith G, et al: Menkes' kinky-hair syndrome. Lancet 1:1100, 1972.
25. Hunt DM: Primary defect in copper transport underlies mottled mutants in the mouse. Nature 249:852, 1974.
26. Andrews EJ, White WJ, Bullock LP: Spontaneous aortic aneurysms in blotchy mice. Am J Pathol 78:199, 1975.
27. Brophy CM, Tilson JE, Braverman IM, Tilson MD: Age of onset, pattern of distribution and histology of aneurysm development in a genetically predisposed mouse model. J Vasc Surg 8:45, 1988.
28. Zarins CK, Runyon-Hass A, Zatina MA, et al: Increased collagenase activity in early aneurysmal dilation. J Vasc Surg 3:238, 1986.
29. Takagi A, Kajiura N, Tada Y, Ueno A: Surgical treatment of non-specific inflammatory arterial aneurysms. J Cardiovasc Surg 27:117, 1986.
30. Seko Y, Sato O, Tagaki A, et al: Restricted usage of T cell receptor V alpha and V beta genes in infiltrating cells in aortic tissue of patients with Takayasu's arteritis. Circulation 93:1788, 1996.
31. Fukushige J, Bill MR, McNamara DG: Spectrum of cardiovascular lesions in mucocutaneous lymph node syndrome: Analysis of eight cases. Am J Cardiol 45:98, 1980.
32. Ozsvath KJ, Horose H, Xia S, Tilson MD: Molecular mimicry in human aortic aneurysmal diseases. Ann N Y Acad Sci 800:288, 1996.
33. Brown CB, Busuttil RW, Baker JD, et al: Bacteriologic and surgical determinants of survival in patients with mycotic aneurysms. J Vasc Surg 1:541, 1984.
34. Juvonen J, Juvonen T, Saikku P, et al: Demonstration of *Chlamydia pneumoniae* in the walls of abdominal aortic aneurysms. J Vasc Surg 25:499, 1997.
35. Ernst CB, Campbell C, Daugherty ME, et al: Incidence and significance of intra-operative bacterial cultures during abdominal aortic aneurysmectomy. Ann Surg 185:626, 1977.
36. Barrett JM, Van Hooyclonk JE, Boehm FH: Pregnancy related rupture of arterial aneurysms. Obstet Gynecol Surg 37:557, 1982.
37. Williams GM, Gott VL, Brawley RK, et al: Aortic disease associated with pregnancy. J Vasc Surg 8:470, 1988.
38. Manalo-Estrella P, Barker AE: Histopathologic findings in human aortic media associated with pregnancy. Arch Pathol 83:336, 1967.
39. Zucker S, Lysik RM, Gurfinkel M, et al: Immunoassay of type IV collagenase/gelatinase (MMP-2) in human plasma. Immunol Methods 148:189, 1992.
40. Ledesle FA, Johnson GR, Ballard DJ, et al: Prevalence and associations of abdominal aortic aneurysm detected through screening. Aneurysm Detection and Management (ADAM) Veterans Affairs Cooperative Study Group. Ann Intern Med 126:441, 1997.
41. Suorez BK: Honolulu heart study: Review of genetic analyses. Prog Clin Biol Res 147:105, 1984.
41a. Watt HC, Law MR, Wald NJ, et al: Serum triglyceride: A possible risk factor for ruptured AAA. Int J Epidemiol 27:949, 1999.
42. Cronenwett JL, Murphy TF, Zelenock GB, et al: Actuarial analysis of variables associated with rupture of small abdominal aortic aneurysms. Surgery 98:472, 1985.
43. Cronenwett JL, Sargent SK, Wall MH, et al: Variables that affect the expansion rate and outcome of small abdominal aortic aneurysms. J Vasc Surg 11:260, 1990.
43a. Rao SK, Mathrubuthan M, Sherman D, et al: Reduced capacity to inhibit elastase in AAA. J Surg Res 82:24, 1999.
44. Bengtsson H, Bergquist D, Sternby NH: Increasing prevalence of abdominal aortic aneurysms: A necropsy study. Eur J Surg 158:19, 1992.
45. Melton L, Bickerstaff L, Hollier L, et al: Changing incidence of abdominal aortic aneurysms: A population based study. Am J Epidemiol 120:379, 1984.
46. Fowkes FGR, MacIntyre CCA, Ruckley DV: Increasing incidence of aortic aneurysms in England and Wales. Br Med J 298:33, 1989.
47. Zarins CK, Xu C, Glagov S: Aneurysmal enlargement of the aorta during regression of experimental atherosclerosis. J Vasc Surg 15:90, 1992.
48. Martin P: On abdominal aortic aneurysms. J Cardiovasc Surg 19:597, 1978.
49. Tilson MD, Stansel HC: Differences in results for aneurysms vs. occlusive disease after bifurcation grafts: Results of 100 elective grafts. Arch Surg 115:1173, 1980.
50. Baxter BT, Davis VA, Minion DJ, et al: Abdominal aortic aneurysms are associated with altered matrix proteins of the nonaneurysmal aortic segments. J Vasc Surg 19:797, 1994.
51. Tilson MD, Dang C: Generalized arteriomegaly: A possible predisposition to formation of abdominal aortic aneurysms. Arch Surg 116:1030, 1981.
52. Cannon DJ, Casteel L, Reed RD: Abdominal aortic aneurysms, Leriche's syndrome, inguinal hernation and smoking. Arch Surg 119:387, 1984.
53. Sonesson B, Hansen F, Lanne T, et al: Abdominal aortic aneurysm: A general defect in the vasculature with focal manifestations in the abdominal aorta? J Vasc Surg 26:247, 1997.
54. Tilson MD: Decreased hepatic copper levels: A possible chemical marker for the pathogenesis of aortic aneurysms in man. Arch Surg 117:1212, 1982.
55. Senapati A, Carsson L, Fletcher C, et al: Is tissue copper deficiency associated with abdominal aortic aneurysms? Br J Surg 72:352, 1985.
56. Dubick MA, Hunter GC, Casey SM, Keen CL: Aortic ascorbic acid, brace elements, and superoxide dismutase activity in human aneurysmal occlusive disease. Proc Soc Exp Biol Med 184:138, 1987.
57. Alston J, Fody E, Couch L, et al: A prospective study of hepatic and skin copper levels in patients witn abdominal aortic aneurysms. Surg Forum 24:466, 1983.
58. Carmeliet P, Moons L, Collen D, et al: Urokinase-generated plasmin activates matrix metalloproteinases during aneurysm formation. Nat Genet 17:439, 1997.
59. Simpson CF, Kling JM, Palemer RF: The use of propranolol for the protection of turkeys from the development of beta-aminoproprionitrile induced aortic rupture. Angiology 19:414, 1968.
60. Boucek RJ, Gunia-Smith Z, Noble NL, Simpson CF: Modulation by propranolol of the lysyl cross-links in aortic elastin and collagen of the aneurysm-prone turkey. Biochem Pharmacol 32:275, 1983.
61. Steffee CH, Snell KC: Dissecting aortic aneurysms in hamsters treated with cortisone acetate. Proc Soc Exp Biol Med 90:712, 1955.
62. Reilly JM, Brophy CM, Tilson MD: Hydrocortisone rapidly induces aortic rupture in genetically susceptible mouse. Arch Surg 125:707, 1990.
63. Coulson WF, Cranes WH: Cardiovascular studies on copper-deficient swine. Am J Pathol 43:945, 1963.
64. Zarins CK, Glagov S, Vesselinovitch D, Wissler RW: Aneurysm formation in experimental atherosclerosis: Relation to plaque evolution. J Vasc Surg 12:246, 1990.
65. Stickland HL, Bond MG: Aneurysms in a large colony of squirrel monkeys (*Samimi sciureus*). Lab Anim Sci 33:589, 1983.
66. Freestone T, Turner RJ, Powell JT, et al: Influence of hypercholesterolemia and adventitial inflammation on the development of aortic aneurysm in rabbits. Arterioscler Thromb Vasc Biol 17:10, 1997.
67. DePalma R, Koletsky S, Bullon E, et al: Failure of regression of atherosclerosis in dogs with moderate cholesterolemia. Atherosclerosis 27:297, 1977.
67a. Nishije N, Sujiyama F, Kimoto K, et al: Salt-sensitive aortic aneurysm and rupture in hypertensive transgenic mice that overproduce angiotensis II. Lab Invest 78:1059, 1988.
67b. Allaire E, Forough R, Clowes AW, et al: Local overexpression of TIMP-1 prevents aortic aneurysm degeneration and rupture in a rat model. J Clin Invest 102:1413, 1998.
68. Schmitz-Rixen T, Colnin RB, Megerman J, et al: Immunosuppressive treatment of aortic allografts. J Vasc Surg 7:82, 1988.
69. Anidjar S, Salzmann JL, Genetric D, et al: Elastase induced experimental aneurysms in rats. Circulation 82:973, 1990.
69a. Curci JA, Thompson RW: Variable induction of experimental AAA with different preparations of porcine pancreatic elastase. J Vasc Surg 29:385, 1999.
70. Dobrin P, Baker W, Gley W: Elastolytic and collagenolytic studies of arteries. Arch Surg 119:405, 1984.
71. Anidjar S, Dobrin PB, Chejfec G: Progressive enlargement of experimental aortic aneurysms is associated with iniltration of inflammatory cells. J Cardiovasc Surg 32(Suppl):39, 1991.
72. Nackman GB, Karkowski FJ, Tilson MD, et al: Elastin degradation

products induce adventitial angiogenesis in the Anidjar/Dobrin rat aneurysm model. Surgery 122:39, 1997.
73. Freestone T, Turner RJ, Powell JT, et al: Influence of hypercholesterolemia and adventitial inflammation on the development of aortic aneurysms in rabbits. Arterioscler Thromb Vasc Biol 17:10, 1997.
74. Wills A, Thompson MM, Bell PR, et al: Elastase-induced matrix degradation in arterial organ cultures: An in vitro model of aneurysmal disease. J Vasc Surg 24:667, 1996.
75. Clifton M: Familial abdominal aortic aneurysms. Br J Surg 64:765, 1977.
76. Tilson MD, Seashore MR: Fifty families with abdominal aortic aneurysms in two or more first-order relatives. Am J Surg 147:551, 1984.
77. Tilson MD, Seashore MR: Ninety-four families with clustering of abdominal aortic aneurysms (AAA). Part II. Circulation 70:II-14, 1984.
78. Johansen K, Koepsell T: Familial tendency for abdominal aortic aneurysms. JAMA 256:1934, 1986.
79. Tilson MD, Seashore MR: Human genetics of the abdominal aortic aneurysm. Surg Gynecol Obset 119:792, 1984.
80. Norrgard O, Rais O, Angquist KA: Familial occurrence of abdominal aortic aneurysms. Surgery 95:650, 1984.
81. Cole CW, Barber GG, Bouchard AG, et al: Abdominal aortic aneurysm: Consequences of a positive family history. Can J Surg 32:117, 1988.
82. Powell JT, Greenhalgh RM: Multifactorial inheritance of abdominal aortic aneurysm. Eur J Vasc Surg 1:29, 1987.
83. Darling RC III, Brewster DC, Darling RC, et al: Are familial abdominal aortic aneurysms different? J Vasc Surg 10:39, 1989.
84. Collin J, Walton J: Is abdominal aortic aneurysm a familial disease? Br Med J 299:493, 1989.
85. Powell JT, Bashir A, Dawson S, et al: Genetic variation on chromosome 16 is associated with abdominal aortic aneurysm. Clin Sci 78:13, 1990.
86. Collin J, Walton J, Araujo L, Lindsell D: Oxford screening programme for abdominal aortic aneurysm in men aged 65–74 years. Lancet 1:613, 1988.
87. Bengtsson H, Norrgard O, Angquist KA, et al: Ultrasonographic screening of the abdominal aorta among siblings of patients with abdominal aortic aneurysms. Br J Surg 76:589, 1989.
88. Webster MW, Ferrell RE, St. Jean PL, et al: Ultrasound screening of first-degree relatives of patients with an abdominal aortic aneurysm. J Vasc Surg 13:9, 1991.
89. Majumder PP, St. Jean PL, Ferell RE, et al: On the inheritance of abdominal aortic aneurysm. Am J Hum Genet 48:164, 1991.
90. Deak S, Ricotta JJ, Mariani TJ: Abnormalities in the biosynthesis of type III procollagen in cultured skin fibroblasts from two patients with multiple aneurysms. Matrix 12:92, 1992.
91. Tromp G, Wu Y, Prockop DJ, et al: Sequencing of cDNA from 50 unrelated patients reveals that mutations in the triple-helical domain of type III procollagen are an infrequent cause of aortic aneurysms. J Clin Invest 19:2539, 1993.
92. Dietz HC: New insights into the genetic basis of aortic aneurysms. Monogr Pathol 37:144, 1995.
93. Francke U, Berg MA, Tynan K, et al: A Gly 1127 ser mutation in an EGF-like domain of the fibrillin-I gene is a risk factor for ascending aortic aneurysm and dissection. Am J Hum Genet 56:1287, 1995.
94. Kontusaari S, Tromp G, Kuivaniemi H, et al: Inheritance of an RNA splicing mutation (G+1 IVS200) in the type III procollagen (COL3AI) in a family having aortic aneurysms and easy bruisability: Phenotypic overlap between familial arterial aneurysms and Ehlers-Danlos syndrome type IV. Am J Hum Genet 47:112, 1990.
95. Cohen JR, Sarfati I, Ratner L, Tilson MD: Alpha-1 antitrypsin phenotypes in patients with abdominal aortic aneurysms. J Surg Res 49:319, 1990.
96. Rasmussen TE, Hallett JW Jr, Weyand CM, et al: Genetic risk factors in inflammatory abdominal aortic aneurysms: Polymorphic residue 70 in the HLA-DR b_1 gene as a key genetic element. J Vasc Surg 25:356, 1997.
97. Sumner DS, Hokanson DE, Strandness DE: Stress-strain characteristics and collagen-elastin content of abdominal aortic aneurysms. Surg Gynecol Obstet 130:459, 1970.
98. Rizzo RJ, McCarthy WJ, Dixit SN, et al: Collagen types and matrix protein content in human abdominal aortic aneurysms. J Vasc Surg 10:365, 1989.
99. Campa JS, Greenhalgh RM, Powell JT: Elastin degradation in abdominal aortic aneurysms. Atherosclerosis 65:13, 1987.
100. Gandhi R, Keller S, Cantor J, et al: Analysis of elastin crosslinks in the insoluble matrix of aneurysmal abdominal aorta. FASEB J 6:A1914, 1992.
101. Tilson MD: Histochemistry of aortic elastin in patients with nonspecific aortic aneurysmal disease. Arch Surg 123:503, 1988.
102. White JV, Haas K, Phillips S, Comerato AJ: Adventitial elastolysis is a primary event in aneurysm formation. J Vasc Surg 17:371, 1993.
103. Minion D, Davis VA, Najezchleb PA, et al: Elastin is increased in abdominal aortic aneurysms. J Surg Res 57:443, 1994.
104. Mesh C, Baxter BT, Pearce W: Collagen and elastin gene expression in arotic aneurysms. Surgery 112:256, 1992.
105. Baxter B, Halloran B: Matrix protein metabolism in abdominal aortic aneurysms. *In* Aneurysms: New Findings and Treatment. Norwalk, Conn, Appleton & Lange, 1994, p 25.
106. Rizzo RJ, McCarthy WJ, Dixit SN, et al: Collagen types and matrix protein content in human abdominal aortic aneurysms. J Vasc Surg 10:365, 1989.
107. Baxter BT, McGee GS, Shively VP, et al: Elastin content, cross-links and mRNA in normal and aneurysmal human aorta. J Vasc Surg 16:192, 1992.
108. White JV, Haas K, Philips S, et al: Adventitial elastolysis is a primary event in aneurysm formation. J Vasc Surg 17:371; discussion 380, 1993.
109. Menashi S, Campa JS, Greenhalgh RM, et al: Collagen in abdominal aortic aneurysm: Typing, content, and degradation. J Vasc Surg 6:578, 1987.
110. Dorbrin PB: Mechanical properties of arteries. Physiol Rev 58:397, 1978.
111. Keen RR, Nolan KD, Cipollone M, et al: Interleukin-1 beta induces differential gene expression in aortic smooth muscle cells. J Vasc Surg 20:774; discussion 784, 1994.
112. McMillan WD, Patterson BK, Keen RR, et al: In situ localization and quantification of seventy-two-kilodalton type IV collagenase in aneurysmal, occlusive and normal aorta. J Vasc Surg 22:295, 1995.
113. Lopez-Candales A, Homles DR, Thompson RW, et al: Decreased vascular smooth muscle cell density in medial degeneration of human abdominal aortic aneurysms. Am J Pathol 150:993, 1997.
113a. Henderson EL, Gend YJ, Sukhova CK, et al: Death of smooth muscle cells and expression of mediators of apoptosis by T lymphocytes in human AAA. Circulation 99:96, 1999.
114. Busuttil RW, Rinderbriecht H, Flesher A, Carmack C: Elastase activity: The role of elastase in aortic aneurysm formation. J Surg Res 32:214, 1982.
115. Cannon DJ, Read RC: Blood elastolytic acitivity in patients with aortic aneurysms. Ann Thorac Surg 34:10, 1982.
116. Dubick MA, Hunter GC, Perez-Lizano E, et al: Assessment of the role of pancreatic proteases in human abdominal aortic aneurysms and occlusive disease. Clin Chem Acta 1771:1, 1988.
117. Aimes RT, Quigley JP: Matrix metalloproteinase-2 is an interstitial collagenase. Biol Chem 270:5872, 1995.
118. Cohen J, Mandell C, Chang JB, et al: Elastin metabolism of the infrarenal aorta. J Vasc Surg 7:210, 1988.
119. Cohen J, Sarfati I, Danna D, Wise L: Smooth muscle cell elastase, atherosclerosis and abdominal aortic aneurysms. Ann Surg 216:327, 1992.
120. Herron GS, Unemori E, Wong M, et al: Connective tissue proteinases and inhibitors in abdominal aortic aneurysms. Arterioscler Thromb 11:1667, 1991.
121. Newman KM, Malon AM, Tilson MD, et al: Matrix metalloproteinases in abdominal aortic aneurysm: Characterization, purification and their possible sources. Connect Tissue Res 30:265, 1994.
122. Vine N, Powell JT: Metalloproteinases in degenerative aortic disease. Clin Sci 81:233, 1991.
123. McMillan WD, Patterson BK, Pearce WH, et al: *In situ* localization and quantification of mRNA for 92-kD type IV collagenase and its inhibitor in aneurysmal, occlusive and normal aorta. Arterioscler Thromb Vasc Biol 15:1139, 1995.
124. Sakalihasan N, Delvenne P, Lapiere CM, et al: Activated forms of MMP-2 and MMP-9 in abdominal aortic aneurysms. J Vasc Surg 24:127, 1996.
125. Thompson RW, Holmes DR, Mertens RA, et al: Production and localization of 92-kilodalton gelatinase in abdominal aortic aneurysms: An elastolytic metalloproteinase expressed by aneurysm-infiltrating macrophages. J Clin Invest 96:318, 1995.
126. Patel MI, Melrose J, Ghosh P, Appleberg J: Increased synthesis of

matrix metalloproteinases by aortic smooth muscle cells is implicated in the etiopathogenesis of abdominal aortic aneurysms. J Vasc Surg 24:82, 1996.
127. Webster MW, McAuley CE, Steed DL, et al: Collagen stability and collagenolytic acitivity in the normal and aneurysmal human abdominal aorta. Am J Surg 161:635, 1991.
128. Newman KM, Jean-Claude J, Li H, et al: Cellular localization of matrix metalloproteinases in the abdominal aortic aneurysym wall. J Vasc Surg 20:814, 1994.
129. Davis V, Persidskaia R, Baxter BT, et al: Matrix metalloproteinase-2 production and its binding to the matrix are increased in abdominal aortic aneurysms. Arterioscler Thromb Vasc Biol 18:1625, 1998.
130. Li Z, Li L, Zielke HR, et al: Increased expression of 72-kd type IV collagenase (MMP-2) in human aortic atherosclerotic lesions. Am J Pathol 148:121, 1996.
131. Galis ZS, Kranzhofer R, Libby P, et al: Thrombin promotes activation of matrix metalloproteinase-2 produced by cultured smooth muscle cells. Arterioscler Thromb Vasc Biol 17:483, 1997.
132. Freestone T, Turner RJ, Powell JT, et al: Inflammation and matrix metalloproteinases in the enlarging abdominal aortic aneurysm. Arterioscler Thromb Vasc Biol 15:1145, 1995.
133. McMillan WD, Tamarina NA, Pearce WH, et al: Size matters: The relationship between MMP-9 expression and aortic diameter. Circulation 96:2228, 1997.
134. Jean-Claude J, Newman KM, Tilson MD, et al: Possible key role for plasmin in the pathogenesis of abdominal aortic aneurysms. Surgery 116:472, 1994.
135. Murphy G, Atkinson S, Ward R, et al: The role of plasminogen activators in the regulation of connective tissue metalloproteinases. Ann N Y Acad Sci 667:1, 1992.
136. Shireman PK, McCarthy WJ, Pearce WH, et al: Elevations of tissue-plasminogen activator and differential expression of urokinase-type plasminogen activator in diseased aorta. J Vasc Surg 25:157, 1997.
137. Newman KM, Jean-Claude J, Tilson MD, et al: Cellular localization of matrix metalloproteinases in the abdominal aortic aneurysm wall. J Vasc Surg 20:814, 1994.
137a. Curci J, Liao S, Thompson RW, et al: Expression and localization of macrophage elastase (matrix metalloproteinase-12) in abdominal aortic aneurysms. J Clin Invest 102:1900, 1998.
138. Cohen JR, Mandell C, Margolis I, et al: Altered aortic protease and antiprotease activity in patients with ruptured aortic aneurysms. Surg Gynecol Obstet 164:335, 1987.
139. Brophy CM, Sumpio B, Reilly JM, Tilson MD: Decreased tissue inhibitor of metalloproteinases (TIMP) in abdominal aortic aneurysm tissue: A preliminary report. J Surg Res 50:653, 1991.
140. Beckman EN: Plasma cell infiltrates in abdominal aortic aneurysm. Am J Clin Pathol 85:21, 1986.
141. Brophy CM, Reilly JM, Smith GJW, Tilson MD: The role of inflammation in nonspecific abdominal aortic aneurysm disease. Ann Vasc Surg 5:299, 1991.
142. Koch AE, Haines GK, Rizzo RJ, et al: Human abdominal aortic aneurysms: Immunophenotypic analysis suggesting an immune-mediated response. Am J Pathol 137:1199, 1990.
143. Newman KM, Malon AM, Shin R, et al: Matrix metalloproteinases in abdominal aortic aneurysm disease. FASEB J 6:A1914,1992.
144. Ricci MA, Stindberg G, Pilcher DB, et al: Anti-CD 18 monoclonal antibody slows experimental aortic aneurysm expansion. J Vasc Surg 23:301, 1996.
144a. Hingorani A, Ascher E, Salles-Cunha S: The effect of tumor necrosis factor binding protein and interleukin-1 receptor antagonist on the development of abdominal aortic aneurysms in a rat model. J Vasc Surg 28:522, 1998.
145. Dobrin PB, Baumgartner N, Anidjar S, et al: Inflammatory aspects of experimental aneurysms: Effect of methylprednisolone and cyclosporine. Ann N Y Acad Sci 800:74, 1996.
146. Gregory AK, Yin NX, Tilson MD, et al: Features of autoimmunity in the abdominal aortic aneurysm. Arch Surg 131:85, 1996.
147. Hirose H, Ozsvath KJ, Tilson MD, et al: Molecular cloning of the complementary DNA for an additional member of the family of aortic aneurysm antigenic proteins. J Vasc Surg 26:313, 1997.
148. Walton LJ, Powell JT, Parums DV: Unrestricted usage of immunoglobulin heavy chain genes in B cells infiltrating the wall of atherosclerotic abdominal aortic aneurysm. Atherosclerosis 135:65, 1997.
149. Yen HC, Lee FY, Chau LY: Analysis of the T cell receptor V beta repertoire in human aortic aneurysms. Atherosclerosis 135:29,1997.
150. Brophy CM, Tilson JE, Tilson MD: Propranolol delays the formation of aortic aneurysms in the male blotchy mouse. J Surg Res 44:687, 1988.
151. Brophy CM, Tilson JE, Tilson MD: Propranolol stimulates the cross-linking of matrix components in the skin from the aneurysm-prone blotchy mouse. J Surg Res 46:330, 1989.
152. Moursi MM, Beebe HG, Stanky JC, et al: Inhibition of aortic aneurysm development in blotchy mice by beta adrenergic blockade independent of altered lysyl oxidase activity. J Vasc Surg 21:792, 1995.
153. Harty RF: Sclerosing peritonitis and propranolol. Arch Intern Med 1438:1424, 1978.
154. Tilson MD: Propranolol versus placebo for small abdominal aortic aneurysms. J Vasc Surg 5:872, 1992.
155. Reilly JM, Tilson MD: The effects of pharmacologic agents on aortic aneurysm disease. *In* Veith FJ (ed): Current Critical Problems in Vascular Surgery. St. Louis, Quality Medical Publishing, 1990, pp 222–226.
156. Englund R, Hudson P, Stanton A, et al: Expansion rates of small abdominal aortic aneurysms. Aust N Z J Surg 68:21, 1998.
157. Gadowski GR, Pilcher DB, Ricci MA: Abdominal aortic expansion rate: Effect of size and beta adrenergic blockade. J Vasc Surg 19:727, 1994.
158. Cronenwett JL, Sargent SK, Wall MH, et al: Variables that affect the expansion rate and outcome of small abdominal aortic aneurysms. J Vasc Surg 11:260, discussion 268, 1990.
159. Holmes DR, Petrinec D, Reilly JM, et al: Indomethacin prevents elastase-induced abdominal aortic aneurysms in the rat. J Surg Res 63:305, 1996.
160. Holmes DR, Wester W, Reilly JM, et al: Prostaglandin E_2 synthesis and cyclooxygenase expression in abdominal aortic aneurysm. J Vasc Surg 25:810, 1997.
161. Sorsa T, Ding Y, Salo T, et al: Effects of tetracyclines on neutrophil, gingival, and salivary collagenases: A functional and Western blot assessment with specific reference to their cellular source in periodontal disease. Ann N Y Acad Sci 732:112, 1994.
162. Lovejoy B, Clearsby A, Hassell AM, et al: Structural analysis of the catalytic domain of human fibroblast collagenase. Ann N Y Acad Sci 732:375, 1994.
163. Boyle JR, McDermott E, Thompson MM, et al: Doxycycline inhibits elastin degradation and reduces metalloproteinase activity in a model of aneurysmal disease. J Vasc Surg 27:354, 1998.
164. Petrinec D, Liac S, Thompson RW, et al: Doxycycline inhibition of aneurysmal degeneration in an elastase-induced rat model of abdominal aortic aneurysms: Preservation of aortic elastin associated with suppressed production of 92 kd gelatinase. J Vasc Surg 23:336, 1996.
165. Walker DI, Bloor K, Williams G, Gillie I: Inflammatory aneurysms of the abdominal aorta. Br J Surg 83:425, 1978.
166. Goldstone J, Malone JM, Moore WS: Inflammatory aneurysms of the abdominal aorta. Surgery 83:425, 1978.
167. Rose AG, Dent DM: Inflammatory variant of abdominal atherosclerotic aneurysm. Arch Pathol Lab Med 105:409, 1981.
168. Rasmussen TE, Hallet JW Jr: Inflammatory aortic aneurysms: A clinical review with new perspectives in pathogenesis. Ann Surg 225:155, 1997.
169. Edwards WS: Arterial grafts: Past, present and future. Arch Surg 113:1225, 1978.
170. Dale WA, Lewis MR: Further experiences with bovine arterial grafts. Surgery 80:711, 1976.
171. Karkow WS, Cranley JJ, Cranley RD, et al: Extended study of aneurysm formation in umbilical vein grafts. J Vasc Surg 4:486, 1986.
172. Szilagyi EE, Elliot JP, Hageman JH, et al: Biologic fate of autogenous vein implants as arterial substitutes. Ann Surg 178:232, 1973.
173. Ottinger LW, Darling RC, Wirthlin LS, et al: Failure of ultra-light-weight knitted Dacron grafts in arterial reconstruction. Arch Surg 111:146, 1976.
174. Campbell CD, Brooks DH, Webster MW, et al: Aneurysm formation in expanded polytetrafluoroethylene prostheses. Surgery 74:491, 1976.

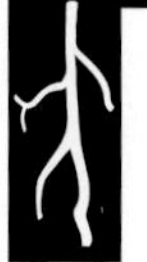

CHAPTER 23
Arterial Fibrodysplasia

James C. Stanley, M.D., and
Thomas W. Wakefield, M.D.

Arterial fibrodypsplasia encompasses a heterogeneous group of nonatherosclerotic vascular occlusive and aneurysmal diseases. Principal forms of arterial fibrodysplastic stenoses include (1) intimal fibroplasia, (2) medial hyperplasia, (3) medial fibroplasia, and (4) perimedial dysplasia.[121] The first two entities represent distinctly different pathologic processes, whereas the latter two appear to represent a continuum of disease. Compounding this classification are hypoplastic dysplastic vessels occurring as true developmental lesions. Various combinations of dysplastic lesions exist, as do other less easily categorized vessel wall derangements. It is important to distinguish primary arterial disease from secondary fibrodysplasia occurring in vessels subjected to earlier inflammatory events, physical insults, and other distinct disease entities.

Dysplastic diseases are known to affect the following:

- Renal arteries
- Extracranial and intracranial cerebral arteries
- Axillary, subclavian, and brachial arteries
- Celiac, superior mesenteric, and inferior mesenteric arteries and a number of their branches
- Iliac, femoral, popliteal, tibial, and peroneal arteries
- Aorta

Venous involvement has been rare, having been reported in the superficial veins of the lower extremity as well as in the renal vein.[30, 49, 97] However, the existence of primary venous fibrodysplasia is controversial.

Complications of arterial fibrodysplasia, namely macroaneursyms, dissections, and arteriovenous fistulae, should be classified as "secondary" events and differentiated from the primary fibrodysplastic lesion. Arterial dysplasia represents a systemic arteriopathy in most instances, although discussions on this subject usually focus on the specific vessels involved.[65, 66]

RENAL ARTERIES

The precise incidence of renal artery dysplastic disease in the general population is unknown, but it is less than 0.5%. The frequency among black hypertensive patients appears to be even lower. Renal artery dysplasia, first described in 1938,[56] is second only to atherosclerosis as the most common cause of surgically correctable hypertension. The entire spectrum of dysplastic stenoses affects the renal artery.[115, 116] The specific types of renal artery fibrodysplasia warrant separate consideration.

Forms of Renal Artery Fibrodysplasia

Intimal fibroplasia of the renal artery affects male and female patients with equal frequency. This lesion accounts for approximately 5% of all dysplastic renal artery stenoses and is observed in infants, adolescents, and young adults more often than in older people. Primary intimal fibroplasia most often affects the main renal artery, usually occurring as a smooth focal stenosis (Fig. 23–1*A*). Segmental vessel involvement is a more uncommon manifestation of intimal disease. The latter usually present as web-like lesions (Fig. 23–1*B*).

Irregularly arranged subendothelial mesenchymal cells within a loose matrix of fibrous connective tissue projecting into the vessel lumen characterize primary intimal fibroplasia (Fig. 23–2). The internal elastic lamina, although occasionally disrupted, is always identifiable. Primary intimal proliferation is usually circumferential. The cause of primary intimal fibroplasia is unknown. In some cases, it appears to represent persistent fetal arterial musculoelastic cushions, similar to the intimal cushions occurring at cerebral artery bifurcations in adults.[137] Lipid-containing foam cells and inflammatory cells are not part of this disease. Medial and adventitial tissues are usually normal in these dysplastic vessels.

Secondary intimal fibroplasia is often difficult to differentiate from primary intimal disease. Certain secondary lesions occur with developmental ostial lesions or advanced medial dysplasia as a likely consequence of altered flow through these stenoses (Fig. 23–3). Blunt vascular trauma or intraluminal insults following thrombosis may contribute to other secondary lesions, with medial and adventitial structures in such cases appearing relatively uninvolved (Fig. 23–4). Long, tubular stenoses may be evidence of secondary disease occurring as a consequence of recanalization of a previously thrombosed artery (Fig. 23–5). In this regard, certain cases of intimal fibroplasia have been suggested to represent a resolved arteritis, such as might occur with rubella.[125] In certain instances, an infectious-immunologic cause has been supported by evidence of immunoglobulin deposition within intimal tissues of the stenotic vessels.[22]

Once a hemodynamically important arterial stenosis develops, progression of intimal fibroplasia appears a likely consequence of abnormal surface blood flow, even if the initiating etiologic factors have resolved. The specific cellular messengers responsible for this tissue proliferation have not been identified. Intimal lesions appear to progress at a much slower rate than do medial fibroplastic stenoses.[76]

Medial hyperplasia without associated fibrosis is an un-

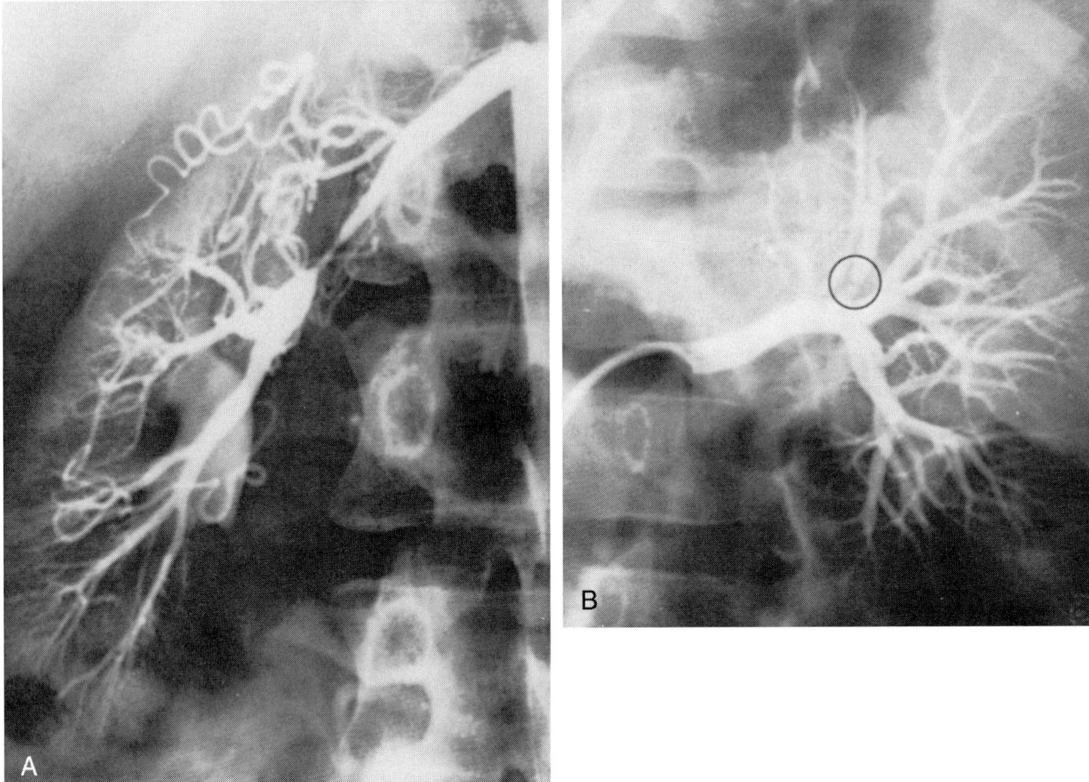

FIGURE 23–1. Primary intimal fibroplasia. *A*, Focal stenosis of the mid-portion of the main renal artery in a young adult. *B*, Intraparenchymal web-like stenosis of a segmental artery in a child. (*A*, From Stanley JC, Fry WJ: Renovascular hypertension secondary to arterial fibrodysplasia in adults: Criteria for operation and results of surgical therapy. Arch Surg 110:922–928, 1975. Copyright 1975, American Medical Association. *B*, From Stanley JC, Fry WJ: Pediatric renal artery occlusive disease and renovascular hypertension: Etiology, diagnosis and operative treatment. Arch Surg 116:669–676, 1981. Copyright 1981, American Medical Association.)

usual cause of renal artery stenosis. In fact, the existence of this particular dysplastic disease is subject to debate. In certain instances, oblique sections of the arterial wall or specimens near bifurcations may misleadingly portray an increase in medial thickness. Similarly, unusually large amounts of smooth muscle separated by recognizable excesses of ground substance represent medial fibrodysplasia,[15] not medial hyperplasia. Medial hyperplasia of the renal artery has been most often described in women during their fourth and fifth decades of life. If indeed this type of lesion actually exists, it will certainly account for fewer than 1% of dysplastic renovascular lesions. Focal stenoses caused by medial hyperplasia usually involve the mid-portion of the renal artery, not its branchings or segmental vessels (Fig. 23–6). Increases in smooth muscle cell numbers with minimal disorganization and the absence of ground substance excesses characterize medial hyperplasia (Fig. 23–7). Intimal and adventitial structures are usually normal, although in severe stenoses intimal fibroplasia may occur as a secondary event. Medial hyperplasia of the renal artery has not been associated with any clearly recognized cause. Contributing to the controversy surrounding this lesion is the fact that a non-neoplastic increase in smooth muscle elsewhere within the vascular system is unusual.

Medial fibrodysplasia accounts for nearly 85% of dysplastic renovascular disease. More than 90% of patients with medial fibrodysplasia are female. This dysplastic lesion is exceedingly uncommon among African Americans. The disease is diagnosed most often during the fourth decade of life. Although medial fibrodysplasia is considered to be a systemic arteriopathy, clinically overt arterial involvement is usually limited to the renal, extracranial internal carotid, and external iliac vessels.

The morphologic appearance of renal artery medial fibrodysplasia ranges from a solitary focal stenosis to its more common presentation as a series of stenoses with intervening aneurysmal outpouchings (Fig. 23–8). The latter, which causes a string-of-beads appearance, has not been observed in female patients before menarche, with the exception of a single case report.[88] The thin-walled mural aneurysms are usually evident grossly, as are distinct webs projecting internally (Fig. 23–9). Medial fibrodysplasia most commonly affects the distal main renal artery, with extensions into first-order segmental branches occurring in approximately 25% of cases.

Progression of medial fibrodysplasia appears to occur in 12% to 66% of patients with main renal artery lesions.[34, 76, 108, 118] Some have suggested that the initial changes of this disease represent smooth muscle changes and that over time a fibrotic process occurs that has a more ominous prognosis than the earlier changes.[2] Progression is generally thought to be more likely to affect premenopausal women, but some authors have noted no differences related to age.[106] Among a group of 71 potential kidney donors with angiographic evidence of renal artery fibrodysplasia, hypertension developed in 26% over an average follow-up of 7½

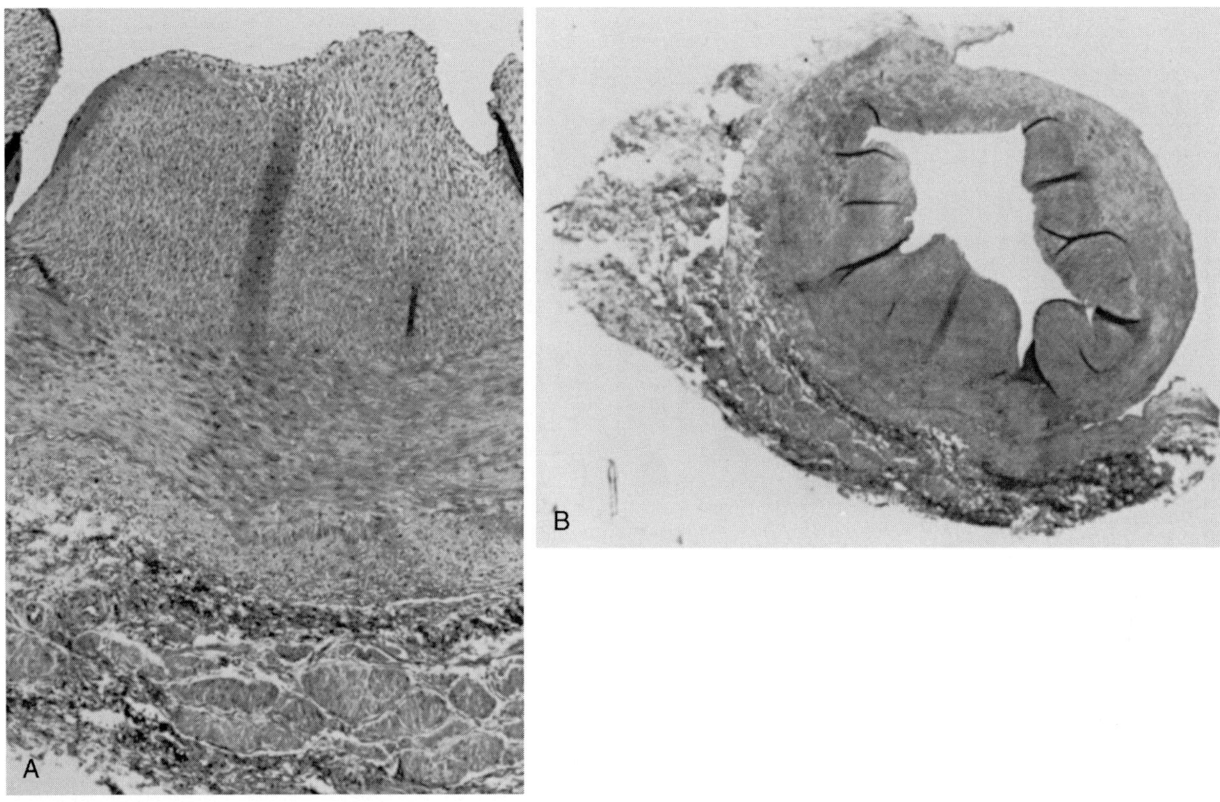

FIGURE 23–2. Primary intimal fibroplasia. *A*, Subendothelial mesenchymal cells within a loose fibrous connective tissue matrix are noted above an intact internal elastic lamina, a normal media, and normal adventitial tissues. (×100.) *B*, Luminal encroachments by this primary form of intimal fibroplasia are usually circumferential. (×35.) (*A* and *B*, H&E.) (*A*, From Stanley JC: Morphologic, histopathologic and clinical characteristics of renovascular fibrodysplasia and arteriosclerosis. *In* Bergan JJ, Yao JST [eds]: Surgery of the Aorta and Its Body Branches. New York, Grune & Stratton, 1979, pp 355–376. *B*, From Stanley JC: Pathologic basis of macrovascular renal artery disease. *In* Stanley JC, Ernst CB, Fry WJ [eds]: Renovascular Hypertension. Philadelphia, WB Saunders, 1984, pp 46–74.)

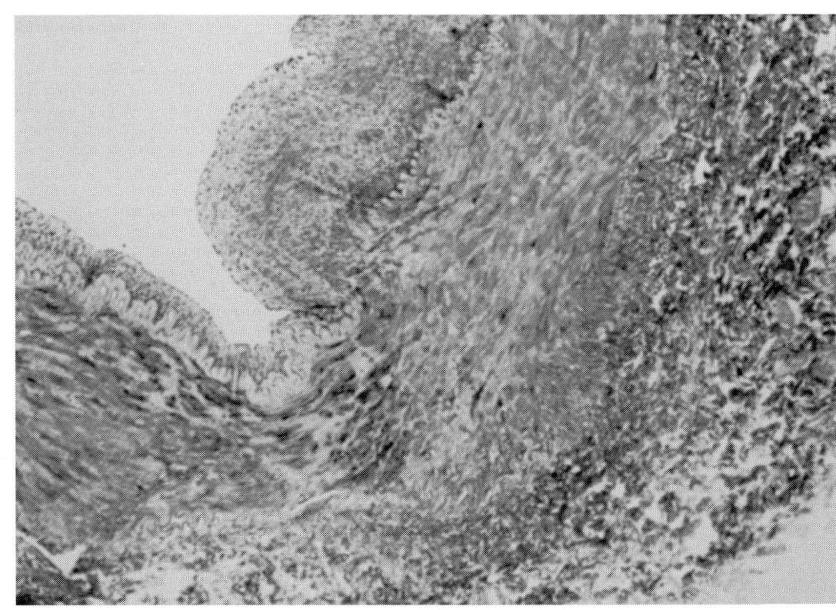

FIGURE 23–3. Secondary intimal fibroplasia. Cellular subendothelial tissue in an artery exhibiting advanced medial fibroplasia. (Masson, ×80.) (From Stanley JC: Pathologic basis of macrovascular renal artery disease. *In* Stanley JC, Ernst CB, Fry WJ [eds]: Renovascular Hypertension. Philadelphia, WB Saunders, 1984, pp 46–74.)

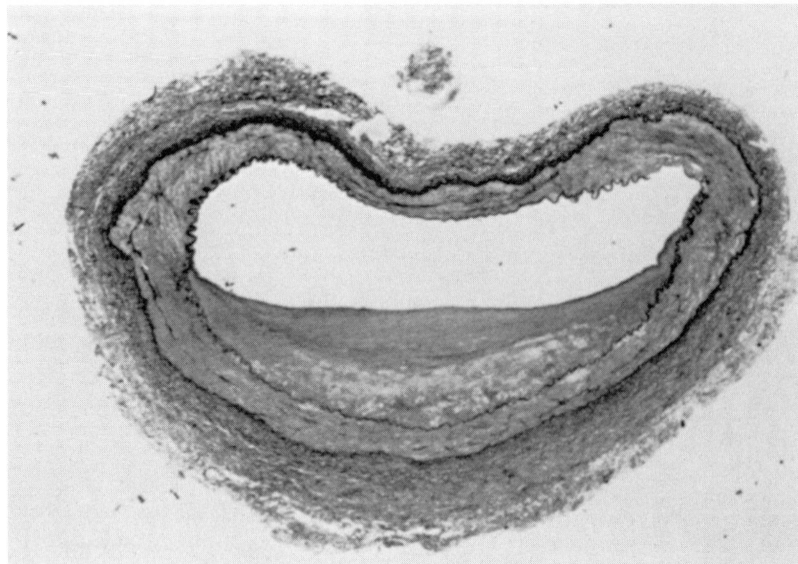

FIGURE 23–4. Secondary intimal fibrodysplasia. Marked intimal thickening in an otherwise relatively normal vessel, consistent with the organization of prior intraluminal thrombus. (Movat, ×40.)

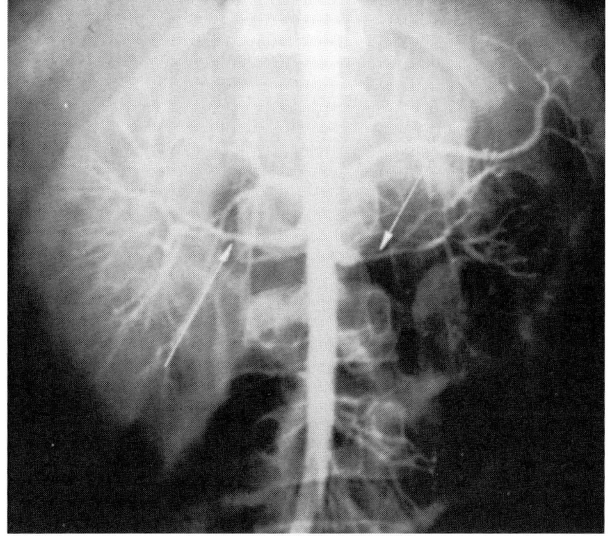

FIGURE 23–5. Secondary intimal fibroplasia. Long tubular stenoses *(arrows)* in the main distal renal arteries of an infant. (From Whitehouse WM Jr, Cho KJ, Coran AS, Stanley JC: Pediatric arterial disease. *In* Neiman HL, Yao JST [eds]: Angiography of Vascular Disease. New York, Churchill Livingstone, 1985, pp 289–306.)

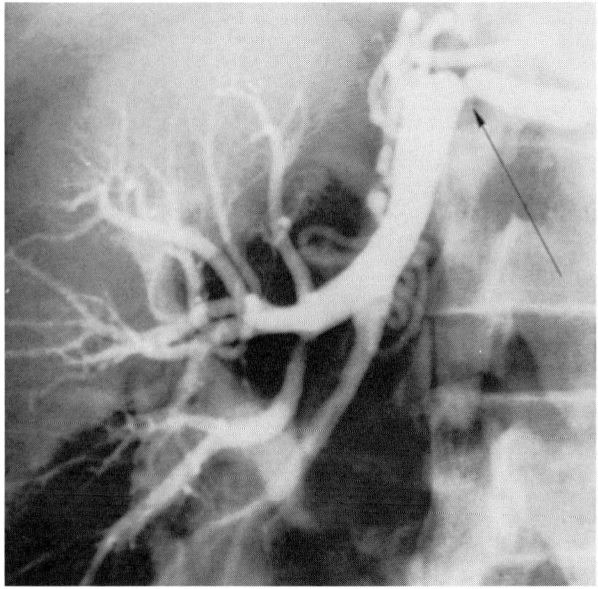

FIGURE 23–6. Medial hyperplasia. Focal stenosis *(arrow)* affecting the mid-portion of the main renal artery.

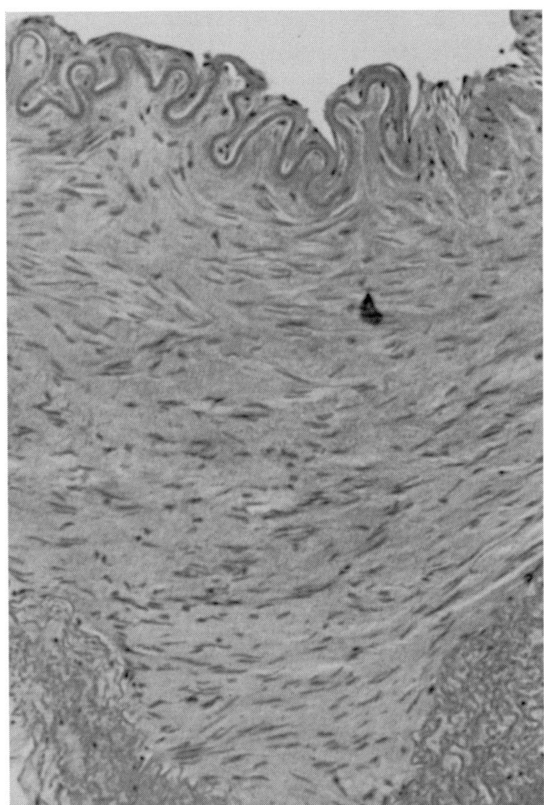

FIGURE 23–7. Medial hyperplasia. Unusual dysplastic lesion with excessive medial smooth muscle in an otherwise normal vessel. (H&E, ×120.) (From Stanley JC: Morphologic, histopathologic and clinical characteristics of renovascular fibrodysplasia and arteriosclerosis. *In* Bergan JJ, Yao JST [eds]: Surgery of the Aorta and Its Body Branches. New York, Grune & Stratton, 1979, pp 355–376.)

years.[16] Hypertension developed in only 6% of an age-matched and sex-matched group of control patients. In these instances, blood pressure increases were considered to be a reflection of progressive renal artery disease. Acute changes in fibrodysplastic renal vessels are relatively uncommon, although in one series 18% had progressed to complete occlusion.[25] Regression of renal artery dysplastic stenoses has been reported,[82] although the validity of such an event has been challenged.[74]

Two histologic forms of renal artery medial fibrodysplasia are well recognized (Fig. 23–10): The first is evident by disease to the outer media (*peripheral* form) and the second exhibits disease throughout the entire media (*diffuse* form). The second form is noted twice as often as the former. Gradations between these extremes have been observed in the same vessel, supporting the tenet that they represent the same disease process. The peripheral form of medial fibrodysplasia is usually encountered in younger patients. It is possible that with the passage of time, more advanced disease evolves to affect the entire media. Consistent with this hypothesis are observed changes in the arteriographic appearance of these lesions, with multiple severe stenoses in series and true macroaneurysms developing in many patients who initially had a solitary lesion or a few stenoses of minimal severity.

Peripheral medial fibrodysplasia is characterized by compact fibrous connective tissue replacing smooth muscle in the outer media. Less obvious findings are moderate accumulations of collagen and ground substances separating disorganized smooth muscle within the inner media. Intimal tissues and the internal elastic lamina are rarely affected in these peripheral lesions. Although continuity of the external elastic lamina is frequently lost, the adventitia is usually normal. Certain peripheral forms of medial fibrodysplasia were previously thought to represent perimedial or subadventitial disease.[39, 72, 73]

Diffuse medial fibrodysplasia is characterized by more severe disorganization and disruption of normal smooth muscle architecture. Occasionally, the diffuse form of dysplasia results in an amorphous-like media (Fig. 23–11). In other vessels, excessive medial accumulations of fibrous tissue alternate with areas of marked medial thinning (Fig. 23–12). In some instances, the media is nearly absent; these regions account for the vessel's mural aneurysmal dilatations. Internal elastic lamina fragmentation and subendothelial fibrosis may also be evident. These latter two changes are considered secondary events in instances of

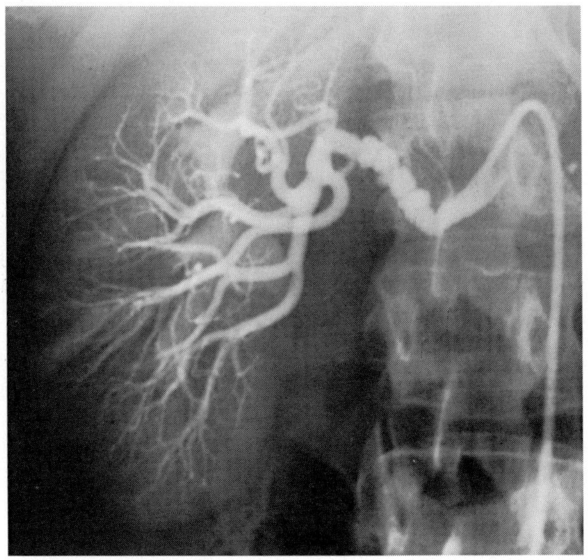

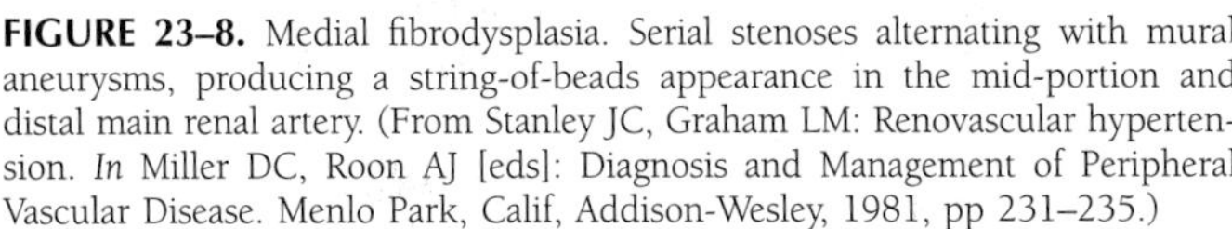

FIGURE 23–8. Medial fibrodysplasia. Serial stenoses alternating with mural aneurysms, producing a string-of-beads appearance in the mid-portion and distal main renal artery. (From Stanley JC, Graham LM: Renovascular hypertension. *In* Miller DC, Roon AJ [eds]: Diagnosis and Management of Peripheral Vascular Disease. Menlo Park, Calif, Addison-Wesley, 1981, pp 231–235.)

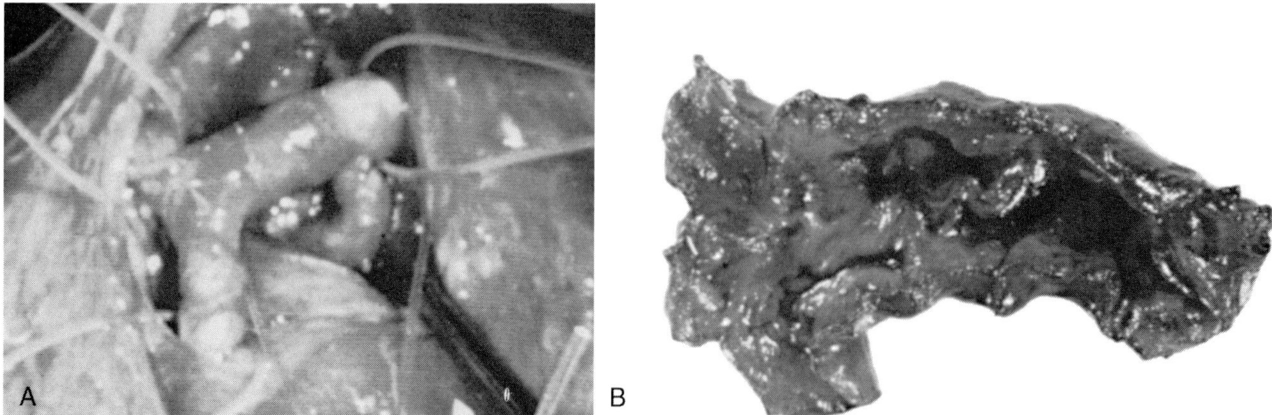

FIGURE 23–9. Medial fibrodysplasia. *A*, Gross appearance of mural aneurysms characteristic of this type of renal artery dysplasia. *B*, Internal appearance of webs projecting into the lumen of an excised main renal artery specimen. (*A* and *B*, From Stanley JC: Pathologic basis of macrovascular renal artery disease. *In* Stanley JC, Ernst CB, Fry WJ [eds]: Renovascular Hypertension. Philadelphia, WB Saunders, 1984, pp 46–74.)

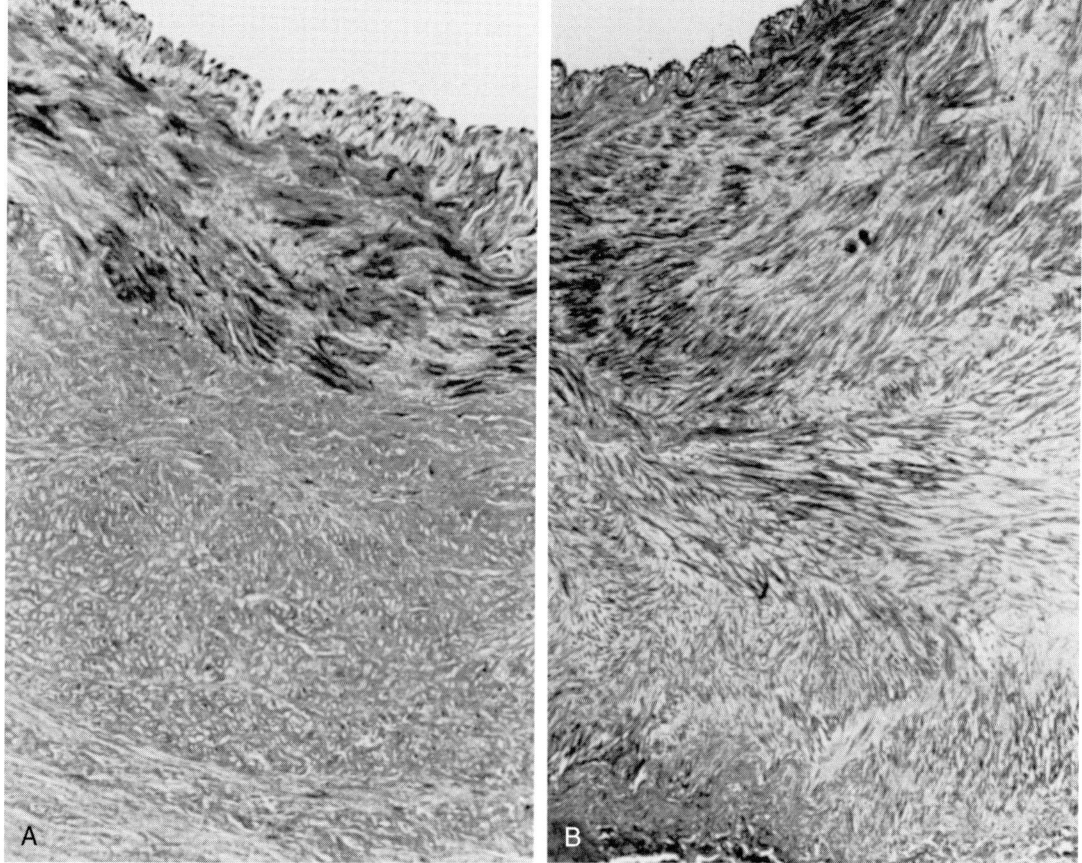

FIGURE 23–10. *A*, Peripheral form of medial fibrodysplasia. Dense fibrous connective tissue in the outer media, with disordered inner medial smooth muscle and normal intimal tissues. *B*, Diffuse form of medial fibrodysplasia. Total replacement of the media by disorganized cellular tissue (myofibroblasts) surrounded by fibrous connective tissue. (Masson, ×120.) (*A* and *B*, From Stanley JC: Morphologic, histopathologic and clinical characteristics of renovascular fibrodysplasia and arteriosclerosis. *In* Bergan JJ, Yao JST [eds]: Surgery of the Aorta and Its Body Branches. New York, Grune & Stratton, 1979, pp 355–376.)

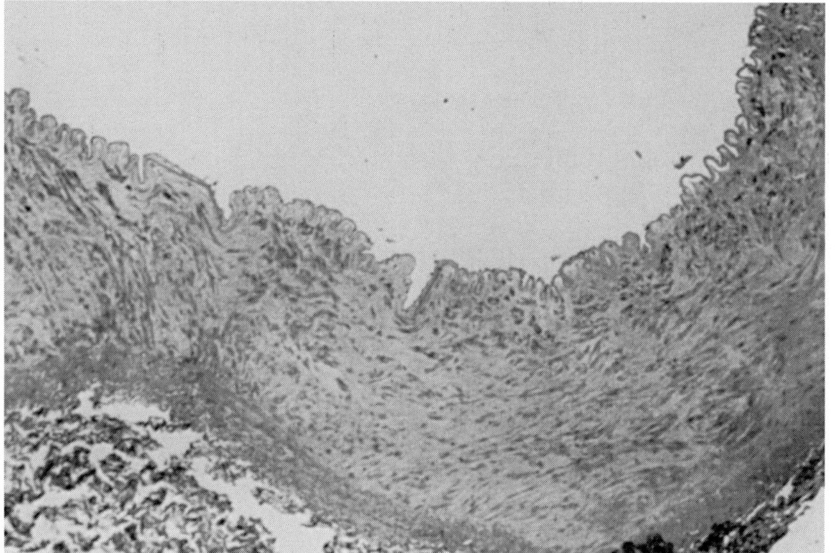

FIGURE 23–11. Diffuse form of medial fibrodysplasia. Amorphous appearance of excessive ground substances and fibrous connective tissue throughout the media. (Masson, ×80, longitudinal section.) (From Stanley JC: Pathologic basis of macrovascular renal artery disease. *In* Stanley JC, Ernst CB, Fry WJ [eds]: Renovascular Hypertension. Philadelphia, WB Saunders, 1984, pp 46–74.)

more advanced medial fibrodysplasia. Adventitial tissues are relatively uninvolved in medial fibrodysplasia.

Extensive fragmentation and distortion of the internal elastic lamina occur in some renal arteries (Fig. 23–13). Deeper dissections may extend into middle and outer medial structures as limited dissections (Fig. 23–14*A*), or they may progress as large intramural hematomas that compress the vessel lumen (Fig. 23–14*B*).[38] Loss of vessel integrity at bifurcations, with alterations in elastic tissue, is thought to lead to the development of renal artery macroaneurysms (Fig. 23–15).[123]

Perimedial dysplasia is the dominant abnormality affecting approximately 10% of dysplastic renal arteries. It may coexist with medial fibrodysplasia. Most patients exhibiting perimedial dysplasia have been female, usually in their fourth or fifth decade of life. These lesions present as either focal stenoses or multiple constrictions involving the midportion of the main renal artery without mural aneurysms (Fig. 23–16*A*). Excessive elastic tissue at the junction of the media and the adventitia is the distinguishing feature of perimedial dysplasia (Fig. 23–16*B*). Minimal increases in medial ground substance surrounding intact smooth muscle cells, with little alteration of intimal tissues, characterize inner portions of the vessel wall in many of these dysplastic lesions whose dominant feature is a homogeneous collar of elastic tissue adjacent to the outer media (Fig. 23–17).

Certain ultrastructural features are common to medial fibrodysplasia and perimedial dysplasia.[114] Both exhibit accumulations of ground substance and fibrous elements. Perimedial dysplasia is differentiated by collections of amorphous material and elastic tissue at the adventitial-medial border. Most important, both manifest a spectrum of change within the cellular composition of the media, ranging from near-normal smooth muscle to myofibroblasts. Fibroblasts are not a usual component of the media and are infrequently observed in these diseased

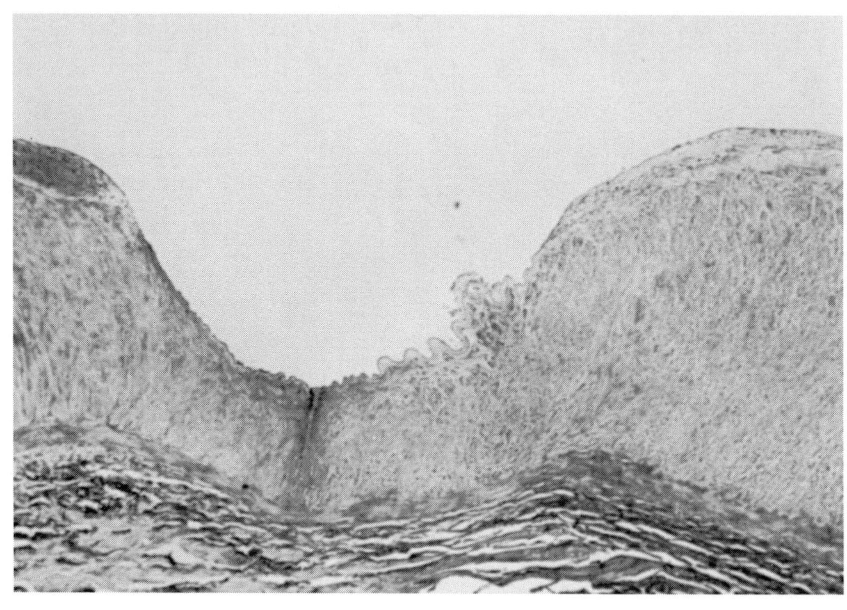

FIGURE 23–12. Diffuse form of medial fibrodysplasia. Regions of excessive fibroproliferation with intervening area of medial thinning. (Masson, ×60, longitudinal section.) (From Stanley JC: Morphologic, histopathologic and clinical characteristics of renovascular fibrodysplasia and arteriosclerosis. *In* Bergan JJ, Yao JST [eds]: Surgery of the Aorta and Its Body Branches. New York, Grune & Stratton, 1979, pp 355–376.)

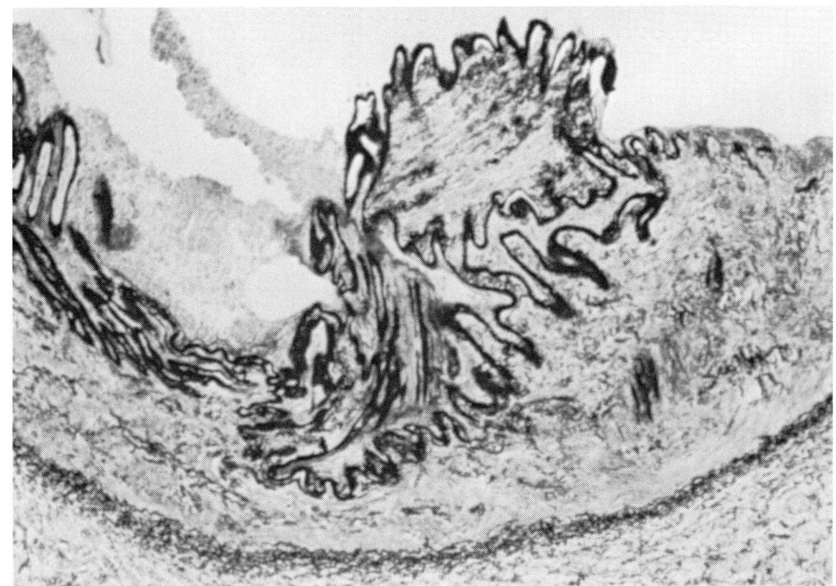

FIGURE 23–13. Medial fibrodysplasia. Extensive fragmentation and distortion of the internal elastic lamina with dissection. (Movat, ×160.)

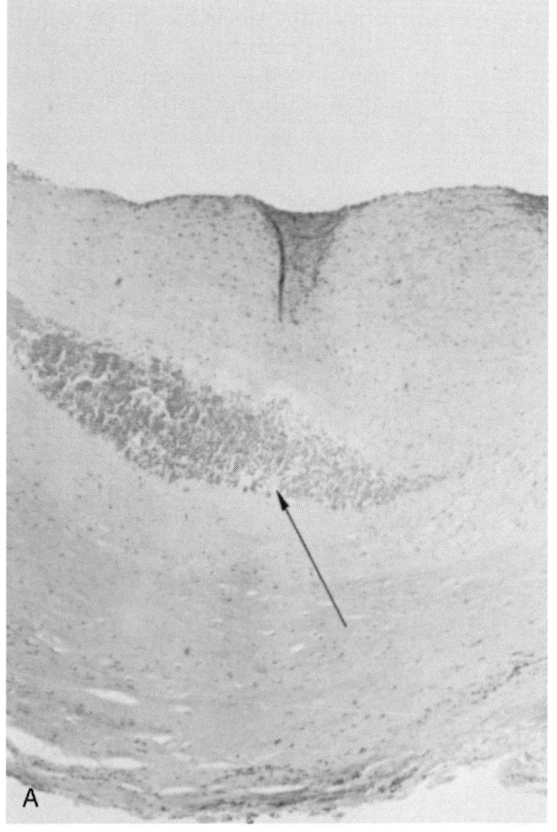

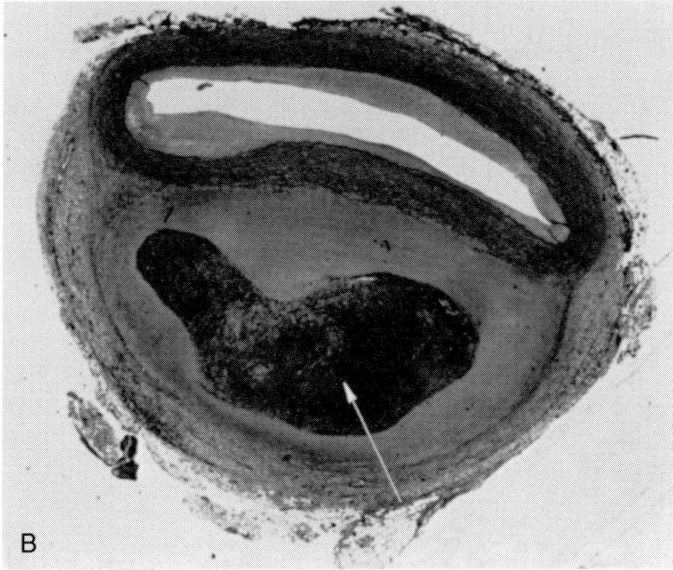

FIGURE 23–14. Dissections complicating medial fibrodysplasia. *A*, Intramedial dissection with limited hemorrhage *(arrow)*. (×120.) *B*, Deep medial dissection with large intramural hematoma *(arrow)* compressing the vessel lumen. (×60.) (*A* and *B*, H&E.) (*A* and *B*, From Stanley JC: Pathologic basis of macrovascular renal artery disease. *In* Stanley JC, Ernst CB, Fry WJ [eds]: Renovascular Hypertension. Philadelphia, WB Saunders, 1984, pp 46–74.)

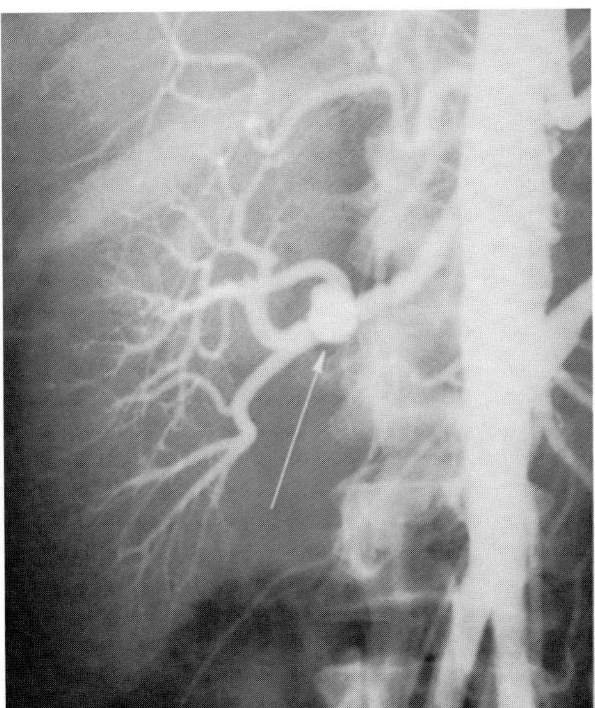

FIGURE 23–15. Macroaneurysms and medial fibrodysplasia. Large macroaneurysm *(arrow)* at a bifurcation of the renal artery. (From Ernst CB, Stanley JC, Fry WJ: Multiple primary and segmental renal artery revascularization utilizing autogenous saphenous vein. Surg Gynecol Obstet 137:1023, 1973.)

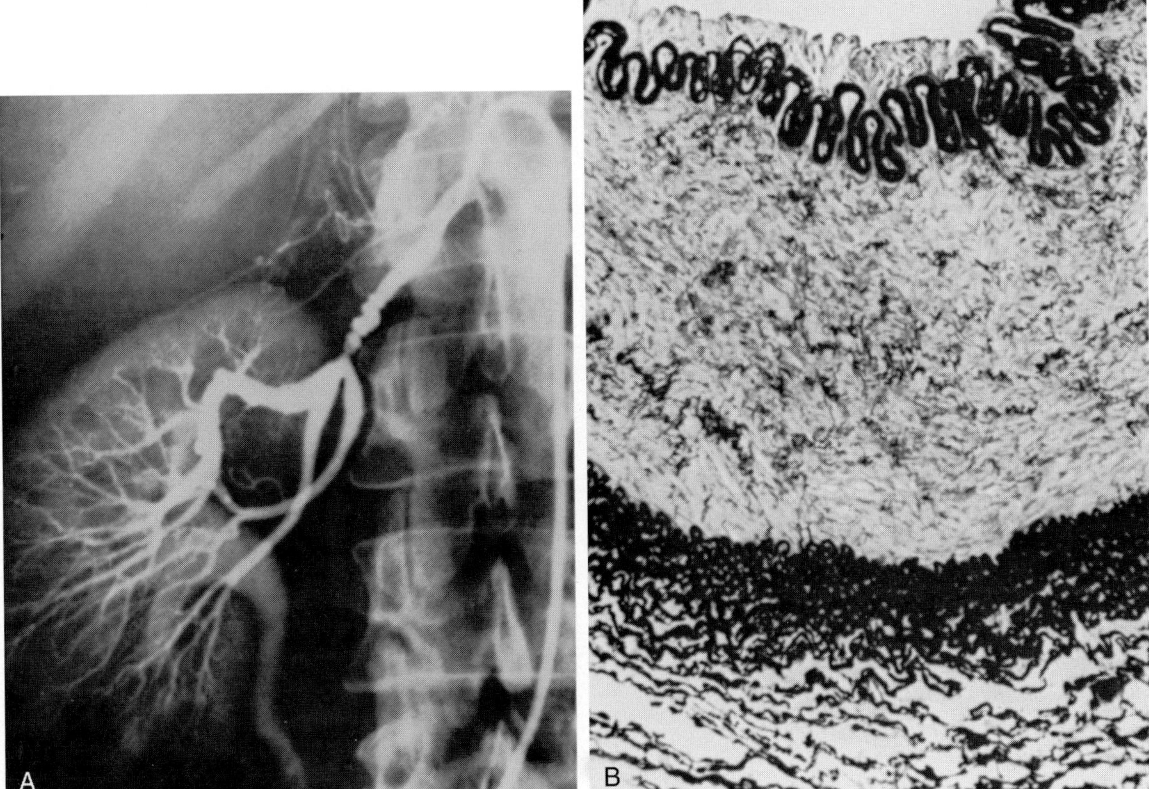

FIGURE 23–16. Perimedial dysplasia. *A*, Multiple stenoses without mural aneurysms in the mid-portion of the renal artery are characteristic of these lesions. *B*, These stenoses are due to excessive accumulations of elastic tissue at the medial-adventitial junction. (Verhoeff, ×120.) (*A* and *B*, From Stanley JC: Morphologic, histopathologic and clinical characteristics of renovascular fibrodysplasia and arteriosclerosis. *In* Bergan JJ, Yao JST [eds]: Surgery of the Aorta and Its Body Branches. New York, Grune & Stratton, 1979, pp 355–376.)

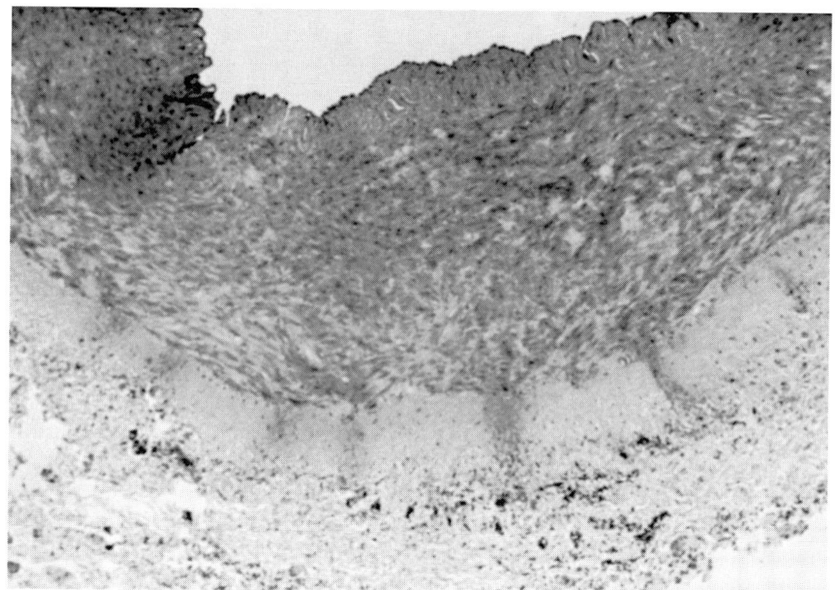

FIGURE 23–17. Perimedial dysplasia. Homogeneous collar of elastic tissue adjacent to the outer media is the dominant feature of this lesion. (H& E, ×80.) (From Stanley JC: Pathologic basis of macrovascular renal artery disease. *In* Stanley JC, Ernst CB, Fry WJ [eds]: Renovascular Hypertension. Philadelphia, WB Saunders, 1984, pp 46–74.)

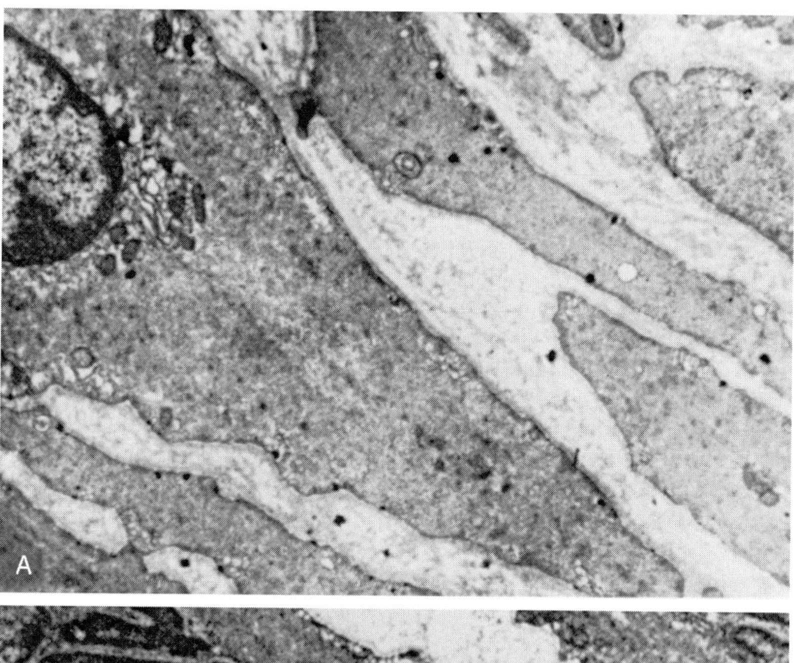

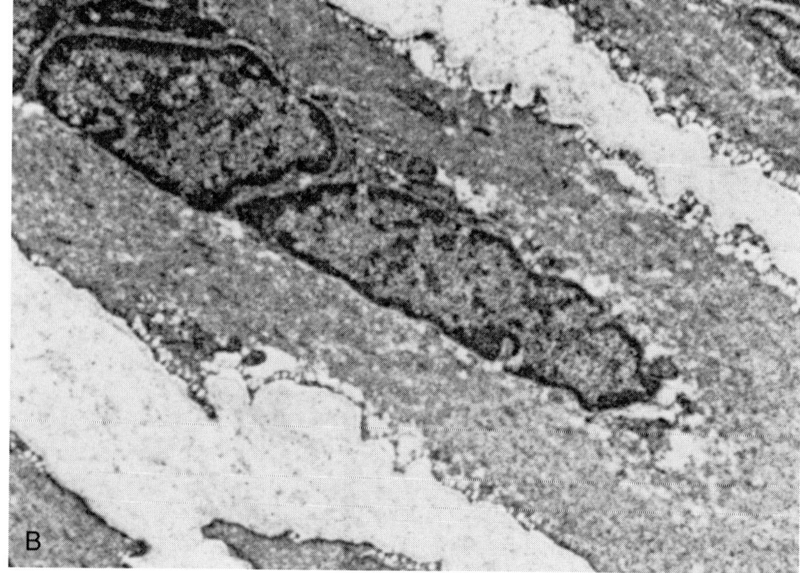

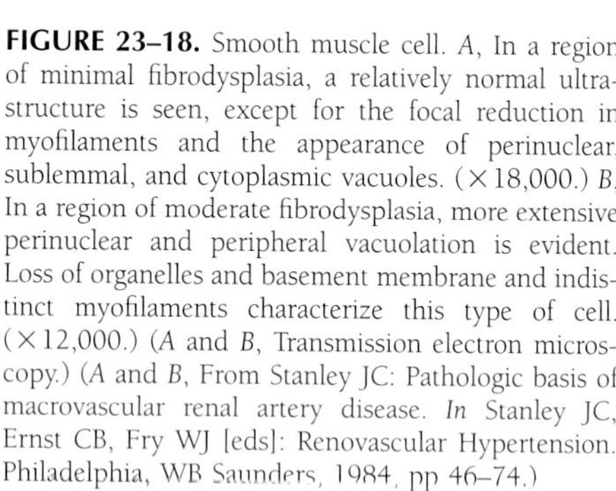

FIGURE 23–18. Smooth muscle cell. *A*, In a region of minimal fibrodysplasia, a relatively normal ultrastructure is seen, except for the focal reduction in myofilaments and the appearance of perinuclear, sublemmal, and cytoplasmic vacuoles. (×18,000.) *B*, In a region of moderate fibrodysplasia, more extensive perinuclear and peripheral vacuolation is evident. Loss of organelles and basement membrane and indistinct myofilaments characterize this type of cell. (×12,000.) (*A* and *B*, Transmission electron microscopy.) (*A* and *B*, From Stanley JC: Pathologic basis of macrovascular renal artery disease. *In* Stanley JC, Ernst CB, Fry WJ [eds]: Renovascular Hypertension. Philadelphia, WB Saunders, 1984, pp 46–74.)

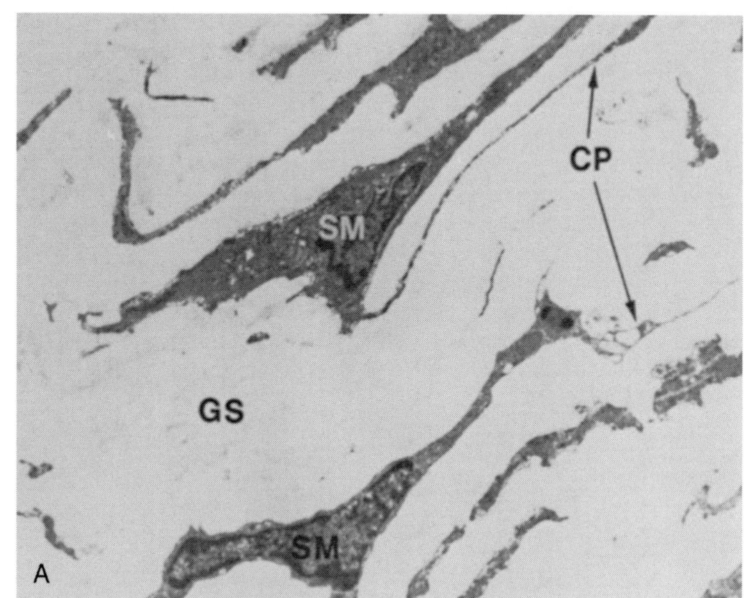

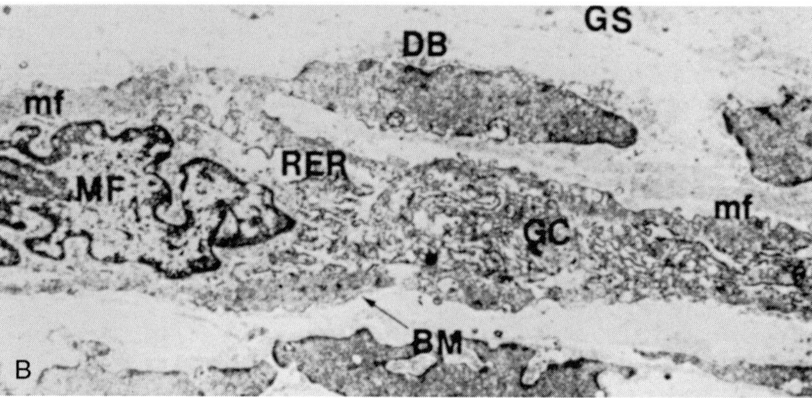

FIGURE 23–19. *A*, Smooth muscle cell in an area of advanced fibrodysplasia. Isolation of slender cytoplasmic processes by excesses in ground substances, and pyknotic nuclei were typical of these markedly abnormal cells. (×6000.) *B*, Myofibroblast associated with medial fibroplasia. The convoluted nucleus is typical of smooth muscle, but increased numbers of centrally located organelles reflect the change in function from one of contractility to secretion. (×8000.) (*A* and *B*, Transmission electron microscopy.) SM, smooth muscle; GS, ground substance; CP, cytoplasmic processes; mf, myofilament; DB, dense body; RER, rough endoplasmic reticulum; MF, myofibroblast; GC, Golgi complex; BM, basement membrane. (*A* and *B*, From Sottiurai VS, Fry WJ, Stanley JC: Ultrastructure of medial smooth muscle and myofibroblasts in human arterial dysplasia. Arch Surg 113:1280–1288, 1978. Copyright 1978, American Medical Association.)

tissues. Similarly, macrophages and leukocytes, suggesting an inflammatory process, are not a relevant component of either medial fibroplasia or perimedial dysplasia. Normal smooth muscle cells are characterized by (1) close apposition of cytoplasmic processes; (2) a deeply indented and convoluted ovoid nucleus surrounded by a modest number of cellular organelles; (3) orderly arranged thick and thin myofilaments parallel to the longitudinal cell axis, with electron-dense bodies at their attachment to the plasma lamina; (4) basal laminations; and (5) scattered micropinocytotic vesicles.

The earliest alterations in the smooth muscle ultrastructure of dysplastic vessels are focal myofilament reductions as well as perinuclear sublemmal and cytoplasmic vacuolations (Fig. 23–18). In areas of advanced dysplasia, certain smooth muscle cells exhibit extreme deterioration, whereas others become fibroblast-like in appearance. The former are invariably isolated from surrounding cells by excessive amounts of ground substance (Fig. 23–19*A*). In these tissues, long, slender cytoplasmic processes reflect decreased cell volumes. Cell membranes are often indistinct, and the nucleus is usually pyknotic, containing dense chromatin material. Confluences of micropinocytotic vesicles are common, and subcellular organelles are sparse. Myofilaments appear dense and homogeneous in these cells. Modification of medial smooth muscle cells to fibroblast-type cells represents a continuum within dysplastic tissues. Alterations in nuclear contour, loss of myofilaments, and increases in free ribosomes, rough endoplasmic reticulum, Golgi's complexes, and mitochondria seemingly parallel altered function from one of contractility to one of secretion.

Myofibroblasts are the end-product of smooth muscle tranformation. Typical of these cells is a convoluted nucleus with numerous indentations and evaginations (Fig. 23–19*B*). Major juxtanuclear increases in subcellular organelles and the presence of peripherally located cytoplasmic filaments are characteristic of myofibroblasts. Myofilaments are scant and poorly defined. Active exopinocytotic deposition of proteinaceous matter may be evident in some cells (Fig. 23–20).

Vasa vasorum within the media of diseased arteries are usually widely separated from adjacent cellular tissue by fibrous material and homogeneous mucoid substances. The type of surrounding connective tissue appears to be related to the category of arterial dysplasia. Vasa vasorum within medial fibrodysplasia are predominantly surrounded by collagen bundles, whereas those in perimedial dysplasia are usually surrounded by amorphous mucoid substances consistent with elastic tissue.

The pathogenesis of *medial fibrodysplasia* and *perimedial dysplasia* has been the subject of much speculation.[53, 121] Hormonal effects on smooth muscle, mechanical stresses

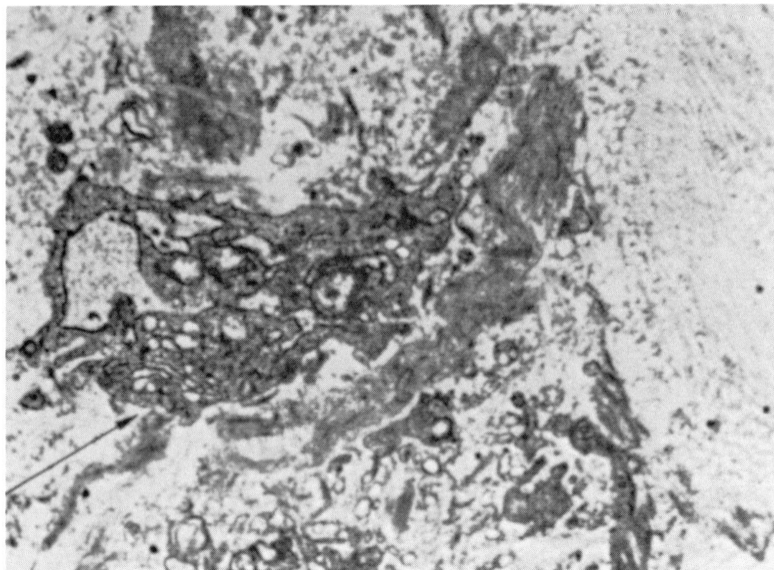

FIGURE 23–20. Myofibroblast in a region of extensive fibroplasia, exhibiting exopinocytotic secretion of proteinaceous matter *(arrow)*. (Transmission electron microscopy, ×25,000.) (From Stanley JC: Pathologic basis of macrovascular renal artery disease. *In* Stanley JC, Ernst CB, Fry WJ [eds]: Renovascular Hypertension. Philadelphia, WB Saunders, 1984, pp 46–74.)

on vessel walls, and the peculiar distribution of vasa vasorum in arteries exhibiting these lesions are all considered to be contributing factors. The exact relation of these factors to each other, or their association with other unrecognized pathogenic mechanisms, remains unknown. Because of the familial nature of this disease, a genetic-related autosomal dominant etiology with incomplete penetrance has been suggested; however, confirmatory arteriographic or histologic evidence to firmly establish such a contention has not been presented.[33, 69, 81, 99, 102] In fact, the absence of a female predilection in much of the data generated by those supporting a genetic etiology lessens the validity of their contention. Nevertheless, the familial frequency of those lesions that are multifocal suggests a genetic predisposition or cause.[87]

Hormonal influences seem likely in view of arterial dysplasia's unusual female predilection. More than 95% of patients exhibiting medial and perimedial disease are women. Pregnancy, although known to cause rather profound vascular wall changes, including alterations in medial structures (especially elastic tissue), is not an obvious etiologic factor in arterial fibrodysplasia. The reproductive histories of patients in a large series with this arteriopathy did *not* reveal gravity or parity rates different from those in the general population.[121]

Antiovulants are also known to affect the arterial wall. However, the use of such drugs by fewer than half the female patients in the Michigan series does not support any obvious cause-and-effect association of progestins with arterial dysplasia.[121] A similar lack of association with oral contraceptive use has been reported in a case-control study.[102] Certain smooth muscle cells and fibroblasts exposed to estrogens demonstrate increased synthesis of proteinaceous substances, including collagen.[98] It is speculated that physiologic preconditioning of vascular smooth muscle cells to a secretory state by normal circulating estrogens associated with the reproductive cycle may account for the more frequent occurrence of medial dysplastic disease in females.

Unusual physical stresses due to ptosis of the kidneys may be associated with fibrodysplastic changes in the renal arteries (Fig. 23–21). Comparable stretch or traction forces are less likely to occur in similar-sized vessels unaffected by this disease. Ptotic kidneys are known to be common among patients with renal artery dysplastic lesions.[17, 52] In some cases, positional changes causing greater ptosis have been correlated with increases in blood pressure.[130] The fact that the right kidney is usually more ptotic than the left may account for the known greater severity of right-sided disease in the majority of adults wth bilateral medial fibroplasia. In addition, in the case of unilateral lesions, 80% involve the right renal arteries. Cyclic stretching of smooth muscle cells in tissue culture causes an unusually large synthesis of collagen and certain acid mucopolysaccharides.[59]

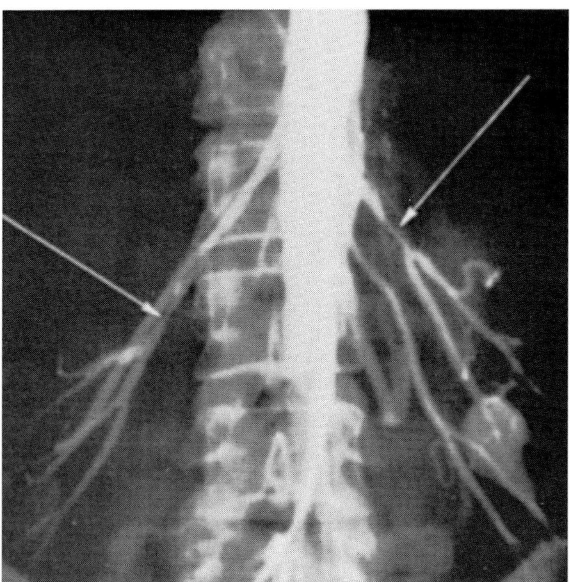

FIGURE 23–21. Medial fibrodysplasia manifesting as irregular narrowings *(arrows)* affecting the mid-portion of the main renal arteries to ptotic kidneys, which appear stretched during upright aortography.

Although the existence of similar mechanisms in vivo is speculative, the predilection for dysplastic disease to occur most often in vessels subjected to peculiar mechanical forces may reflect an important pathogenic phenomenon. It is cautionary to note that in one case-control study, renal mobility was not greater in patients with renovascular fibrodysplasia.[102]

A final etiologic factor may be related to mural ischemia in dysplastic arteries. Vasa vasorum of muscular arteries usually originate from branchings of parent vessels.[5, 55] The renal, extracranial internal carotid, and external iliac arteries are the three vessels most likely to develop medial fibrodysplasia. The latter two arteries, in particular, have relatively few branches compared with similar-sized vessels. Compromise of vasa vasorum in these vessels, in which a sparsity of these nutrient channels may already exist, may lead to significant mural ischemia. Vasospasm may occur in these cases and further exacerbate vessel wall ischemia.[28, 89, 111] Destruction of the media may be a consequence of such an ischemic injury and account for certain of the histologic changes present in arterial fibrodysplasia.[61, 111] The concept that insufficient vessel wall nourishment causes dysplastic changes is supported by the common involvement of the outermost part of the media in peripheral medial fibroplasia. It is precisely in this region that ischemia from inadequate vasa vasorum blood flow would be predictably greatest. Fibrodysplasia limited to the inner part of the media has never been reported. Vasa vasorum in these vessels have exhibited both dilatation[40] and isolation from adjacent medial smooth muscle cells.[68] Experimental occlusion of the vasa vasorum produces a dysplastic lesion in animals similar to that seen in humans, which supports the tenet that mural ischemia is a factor in the evolution of arterial dysplasia.[113]

Tissue hypoxia per se may be the inciting event in stimulating fibroplasia, but altered tissue pH, accumulation of metabolites, and other factors may be just as important. Cigarette smoking has been implicated as an important etiologic factor in this disease, although the mechanism has not been defined.[102] Smooth muscle cells are central to the dysplastic process. Medial smooth muscle cells are considered by some investigators to represent multifunctional mesenchymal cells. The duration and exact degree of ischemia necessary to stimulate myofibroblasts are unknown. Myofibroblasts have been observed to develop in other tissues after very brief hypoxic events.[67] No evidence exists that myofibroblasts evolve from dormant mesenchymal cells, although this is a remote possibility. Some investigators believe that myofibroblasts represent contractile fibroblasts rather than modified smooth muscle cells[32]; however, fibroblasts are not a normal part of artery media.

Developmental Renal Artery Stenoses

Developmental renal artery stenoses are a unique form of renal artery dysplasia. There is no apparent gender predilection for this entity, and its exact frequency is unknown. Among patients with pediatric renovascular hypertension, nearly 40% appear to have developmental renal artery lesions.[119, 124] Among adults with intimal fibroplastic renal artery disease, approximately 20% have stenoses that appear to represent growth or developmental defects. Similarly, certain adults with isolated renal arteriosclerosis may have had preexisting developmentally narrowed vessels.

Thus, developmental renal artery occlusive disease appears to be an uncommon, but not rare, entity in the general hypertensive population. Conversely, nearly 80% of patients with abdominal aortic developmental lesions have coexisting renal artery stenoses and renovascular hypertension.[27] Developmental stenoses of the renal arteries are usually hypoplastic in character. As such, they have an external appearance of an hourglass constriction. Most developmental lesions occur at the origin of the vessel (Fig. 23–22).

The histologic character of the majority of these lesions, especially when they are recognized in pediatric patients, usually reveals abnormalities in more than one of the three layers of the vessel.[19, 119, 122, 124] Sparse medial tissue and intimal fibroplasia are the most common histologic characteristics of these stenoses (Fig. 23–23*A*). Fragmentation with duplication of the internal elastic lamina is a frequent finding, and excesses in adventitial elastic tissue may be present (Fig. 23–23*B*). Similarly, irregular deficiencies in medial tissue may be observed in these diminutive vessels (Fig. 23–23*C*). In some cases, especially those associated with neurofibromatosis, abnormal proliferative changes within the media are apparent.[37, 78, 107] Occasionally, rather amorphous post-stenotic aneurysms affect the main renal artery in patients exhibiting central aortic coarctations and renal artery occlusive disease.

Developmental renal artery narrowings appear to be related to certain in utero events. Under normal circumstances, the paired dorsal aortas fuse and usually all but one of their lateral branches to each kidney regress during the same period of embryonic development, leaving a solitary renal artery. Events that alter transition of mesenchyme to medial smooth muscle tissue at this time, or its latter condensation and growth, may cause aortic or renovascular anomalies. This may explain the unusual occurrence of these lesions in neurofibromatosis as well as in other genetic disorders occasionally encountered in isolated kindred.[36, 124]

Several theories exist with regard to the cause of these lesions. One proposes that the constrictive lesions follow lack of, or unequal fusion of, the two dorsal aortas,[71] with subsequent obliteration of one of these channels and constriction of the associated renal artery. The basis for such an event is unknown. It may follow an acquired insult in utero or an event during early life that arrests the growth of an otherwise normal aorta. In some instances, this insult may be viral. The fact that certain viruses, including the rubella virus, are cytocidal as well as inhibitory to cell replication supports this theory.[92] Examples of aortic hypoplasia and renal artery stenosis associated with gestational rubella have been observed.[110] In such instances, inhibition of smooth muscle cell mitoses may preclude normal aortic growth and produce renal artery ostial stenoses.

Renal arteries originate within mesenchymal tissue near the two dorsal aortas. They are initially represented by a caudally located group of vessels to the mesonephros that are replaced during fetal growth with a more cephalic group of vessels to the metanephros. A solitary artery to the primitive kidney usually evolves from each of these lateral vessel groups. Development of a single dominant vessel apparently occurs because of its obligate hemodynamic advantage over adjacent channels. Flow changes due to an evolving aortic coarctation in the region in which single renal arteries might normally arise may give coexisting polar channels hemodynamic advantages that cause their persistence. In support of such a hypothesis of renal artery occlusive disease in this subgroup of patients is the fact that central abdominal aortic coarctation and hypoplasia are frequently associated with multiple stenotic renal arteries.[35, 122, 124]

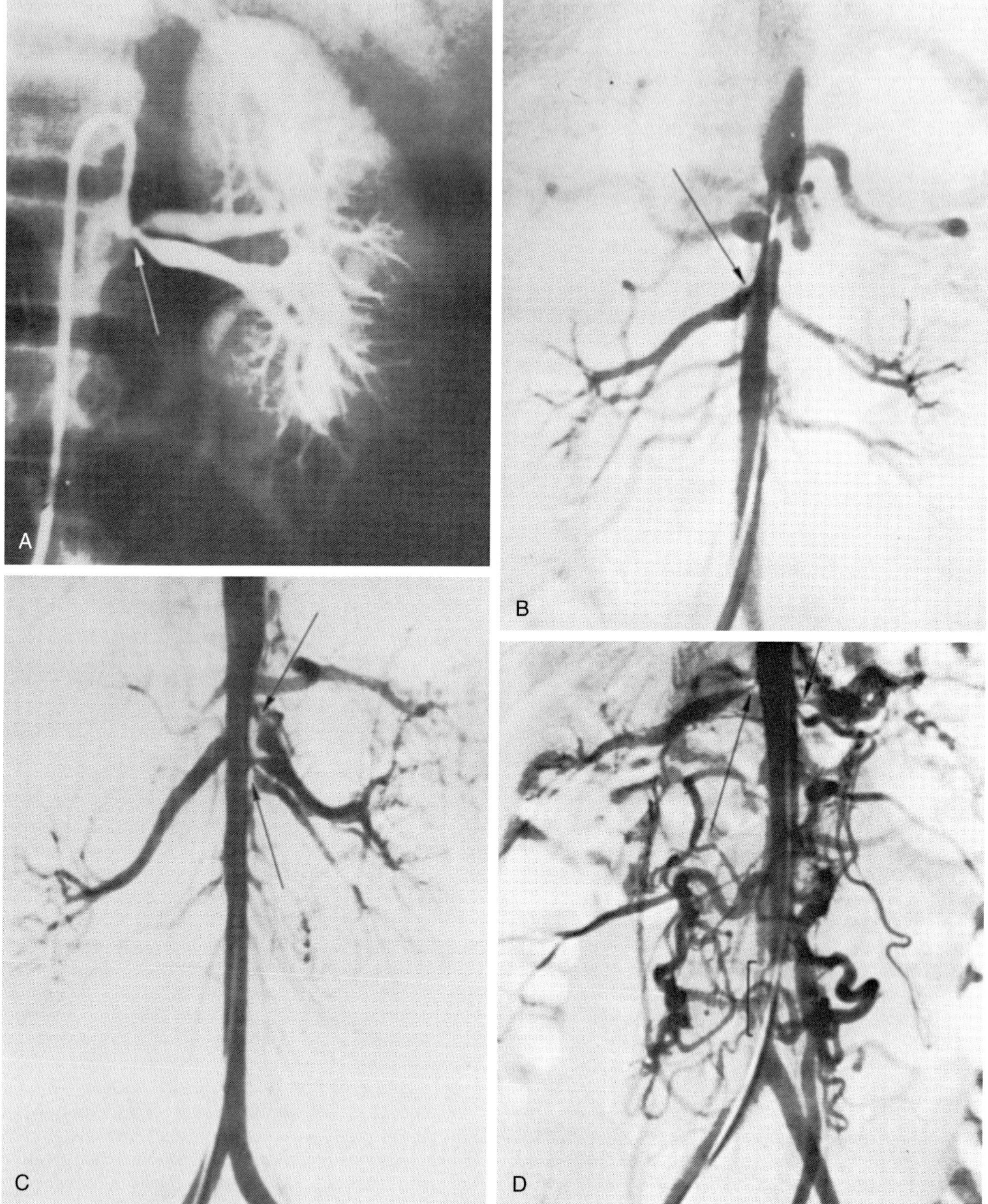

FIGURE 23–22. Developmental renal artery stenoses. *A*, Proximal stenosis *(arrow)* in a patient with neurofibromatosis. *B*, Proximal stenosis *(arrow)* in a patient with multiple renal arteries and mid-abdominal coarctation. *C*, Multivessel stenoses *(arrows)* in a patient with aortic hypoplasia. *D*, Bilateral proximal stenoses *(arrows)* in a patient with focal infrarenal aortic coarctation *(bracket)*. (*A*, From Stanley JC, Fry WJ: Pediatric renal artery occlusive disease and renovascular hypertension: Etiology, diagnosis and operative treatment. Arch Surg 116:669–676, 1984. Copyright 1984, American Medical Association. *B* and *C*, From Graham LM, Zelenock GB, Erlandson EE, et al: Abdominal aortic coarctation and segmental hypoplasia. Surgery 86:519, 1979.)

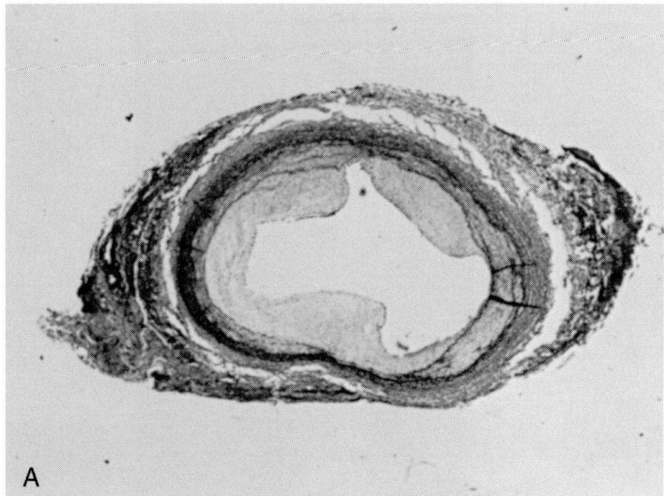

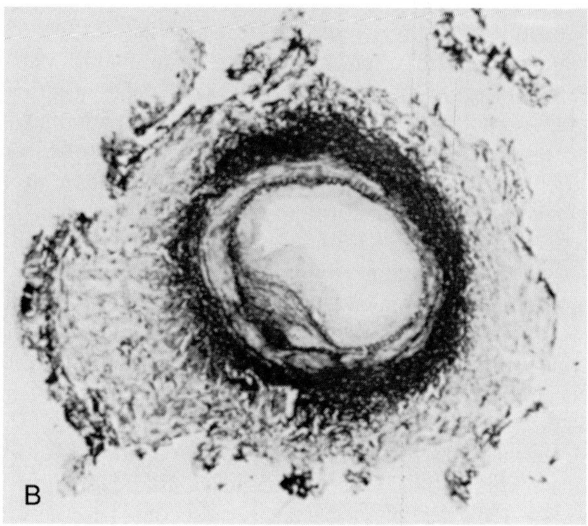

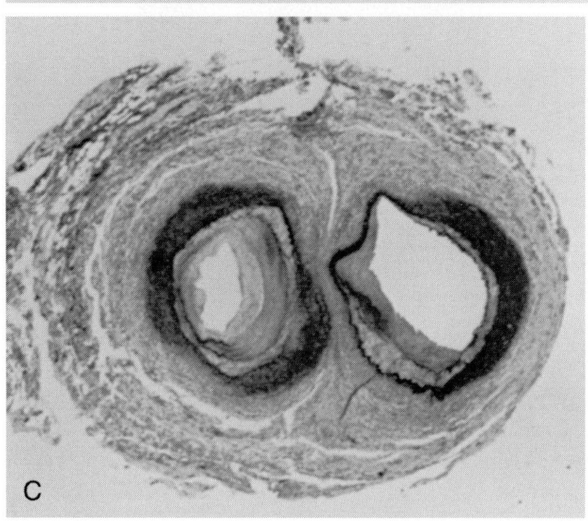

FIGURE 23–23. Hypoplastic developmental renal artery stenoses. *A*, Secondary intimal fibroplasia, fragmentation of the internal elastic lamina, and diminutions in medial tissue are typical features of this stenotic lesion. The greatest luminal dimension is 2 mm. (×80.) *B*, Marked fragmentation and duplication of the internal elastic lamina and attenuation of medial tissues characterize this vessel. Intimal fibroplasia encroaches on the vessel lumen, which is less than 1 mm in diameter. Adventitial elastic tissues appear excessive. (×100.) *C*, Diminutive paired renal arteries at their aortic origin exhibiting deficient media. (×100.) (*A–C*, Movat.) (*A* and *B*, From Stanley JC, Graham LM, Whitehouse WM Jr, et al: Developmental occlusive disease of the abdominal aorta, splanchnic and renal arteries. Am J Surg 142:190, 1981.)

EXTRACRANIAL AND INTRACRANIAL CEREBRAL ARTERIES: CAROTID AND VERTEBRAL ARTERIES

Arterial fibrodysplasia of the extracranial and intracranial cerebral vasculature is a clinical entity of potential importance, although controversy exists beyond the simple assertion that certain lesions cause cerebral ischemic symptoms. The precise incidence of this disease is poorly defined, although lesions of the extracranial internal carotid artery (ECICA) were noted in 0.42% of 3600 patients undergoing cerebral arteriographic examinations.[120] This finding was nearly identical to the 0.4% reported from the Mayo Clinic.[104] Many of these examinations were for suspected cerebrovascular disease, and thus the true frequency of ECICA fibrodysplasia in the general population would be expected to be lower. Unfortunately, the much lower 0.02% incidence of this disease among necropsy examinations is likely to be too low because of the uncommon removal of distal segments of the ECICA during routine autopsies.[104] Vertebral artery disease is even less common, having been noted in approximately 20% of patients manifesting ECICA fibrodysplasia.[112, 120]

Various pathologic processes have been categorized as ECICA fibrodysplasia.[84, 104] This fact makes interpretation of the existing literature difficult. The two major subgroups of cerebrovascular lesions include (1) intimal fibroplasia and (2) medial fibrodysplasia. The intimal form is often associated with elongation, kinking, and coiling of the carotid artery and appears for the most part to be a secondary rather than a primary dysplastic process. This seems particularly to be true of intracranial intimal fibroplasia.[43] Occasional atypical lesions appear as isolated webs of the ECICA.[136]

Medial fibrodysplasia of the ECICA was first documented arteriographically and histologically more than three decades ago.[14, 86] These lesions invariably occur in female patients, with a mean patient age at the time of recognition being approximately 55 years.[13, 112, 120] Classic lesions of this type in childhood have been rare,[64] and when present, they often affect intracranial vessels.[57, 109] If previous definitions of medial fibrodysplasia are rigidly applied, this particular subgroup has rarely been described in men.[1] Similarly, these lesions, like those of the renal artery, have been infrequently recognized among African American patients.[60, 79]

Medial fibrodysplasia of the ECICA typically involves a 2- to 6-cm segment of the mid-carotid artery adjacent to the second and third cervical vertebrae (Fig. 23–24). The serial stenoses are often evident on examination of the external surface of the artery (Fig. 23–25). Bilateral disease has been reported to occur in 35% to 85% of patients with these lesions, with an average incidence of approximately 65%.[10, 13, 15, 112, 120, 126] Involvement of the ECICA at its origin with the classic form of this dysplastic lesion has not been described. Carotid arteries affected by medial fibrodysplasia are often elongated, and kinking occurs in approximately 5% of cases (Fig. 23–26). Typical medial fibrodysplastic lesions of the anterior intracranial arteries are uncommon.[31, 57, 95] Similar lesions of the external carotid artery or its branches have been reported, but they are exceedingly rare.[42]

Vertebral artery disease, in the form of either multiple stenoses (Fig. 23–27) or nonocclusive mural aneurysms (Fig. 23–28), has often been overlooked. These lesions develop in the lower vertebral artery at the level of the fifth cervical vertebra, or higher, at the level of the second cervical vertebra. They exhibit marked irregularities and are often accompanied by eccentric mural aneurysms, but they do not manifest the typical string-of-beads appearance noted in other muscular vessels affected with medial fibrodysplasia. Dysplastic lesions of the basilar artery are an uncommon form of intracranial medial fibrodysplasia.[103]

Noncerebrovascular medial fibrodysplasia occurs in many patients with ECICA lesions. Renal artery involvement affects as many as 25% of these individuals.[24, 120] The frequency of simultaneous ECICA and renal artery dysplasia may be even higher, and it has been reported to be 50% in patients who underwent arteriographic assessments of both vessels.[26] Similar lesions have also been observed in the external iliac and superior mesenteric arteries.[24]

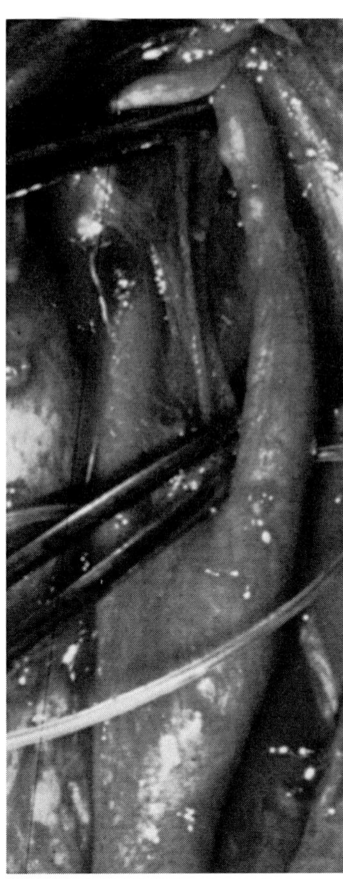

FIGURE 23–25. Medial fibrodysplasia of the extracranial internal carotid artery. Operative exposure of the artery reveals an external beaded appearance due to serial narrowings.

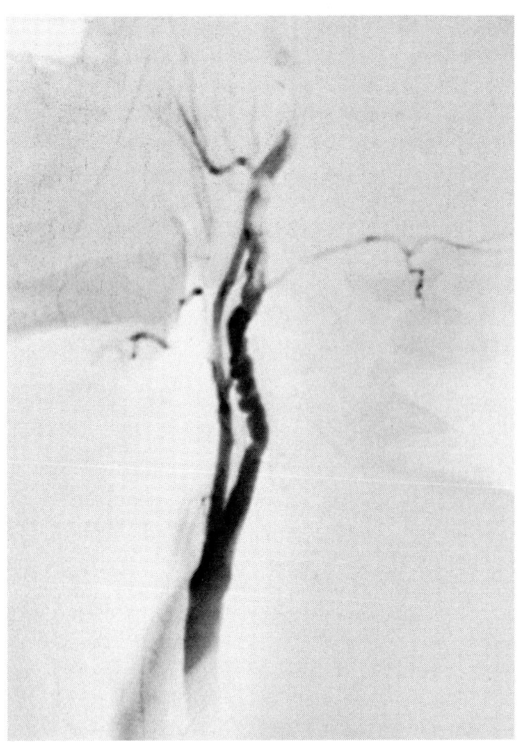

FIGURE 23–24. Medial fibrodysplasia of the extracranial internal carotid artery adjacent to the second and third cervical vertebrae, with characteristic serial stenoses alternating with mural aneurysms. (From Stanley JC, Fry WJ, Seeger JF, et al: Extracranial internal carotid and vertebral artery fibrodysplasia. Arch Surg 109:215–222, 1974. Copyright 1974, American Medical Association.)

Coexistent intracranial aneurysms have been documented in 12% to 25% of patients with ECICA medial fibrodysplasia.[10, 15, 31, 79, 120, 135] Solitary intracranial aneurysms are present in 80% of these patients, with multiple aneurysms occurring in the remaining 20% of cases. A meta-analysis of 18 series, excluding those with subarachnoid hemorrhage, revealed a 7.3% prevalence of cerebral aneurysms in patients with carotid or vertebral fibrodysplasia.[12] Although intracranial arteries are occasionally the site of dysplastic disease, aneurysms seemingly do not develop in the involved vessel.[12, 51] Instead, they may appear to evolve as a generalized dysplastic arteriopathy, manifested by weakening in arterial branches, which increases the likelihood of berry aneurysm formation.[70, 85, 116, 123] These aneurysms tend to occur on the same side as the ECICA disease.[80] The anatomic distribution of aneurysms in patients with medial fibrodysplasia is the same as that in patients not affected with dysplastic ECICA.[120] Hypertension may contribute to the evolution of these aneurysms, but it has not been identified as a dominant factor in their pathogenesis.

Complications occurring with medial fibrodysplasia of the ECICA appear to be related to (1) encroachment on the lumen that causes flow reductions, (2) occasional collection of thrombi[60, 91] within the cul-de-sacs, (3) potential distal embolization, and (4) dissections and rupture with arteriovenous fistula formation.[7, 93] The precise incidence of these complications has not been determined, but they appear to occur in fewer than 10% of cases. Frequently, dissections obliterate clear evidence of the underlying fibrodysplastic process, and many individuals experiencing this complication are thought to have suffered from spontaneous dissections.[3] Progression of ECICA medial fibrodysplasia may approach 30%, but the exact rate has yet to be defined.[101, 112, 120, 125, 139] Complications occurring with medial fibrodysplasia of the vertebral arteries are rare and are usually related to thromboembolism or dissections.[90, 133]

The pathogenesis of ECICA medial fibrodysplasia is poorly understood, but it appears to be similar to that occurring in the renal vessels. The role of mural ischemia may be greater because very few muscular branches have origins from the extracranial portion of the internal carotid artery, thus reducing the number of intrinsic vasa vasorum in this vessel. Certainly, unusual traction or stretch stresses that occur with hyperextension and rotation of the neck appear to be another dominant factor in the development of these lesions.

Trauma has been cited as an etiologic factor in instances of vertebral artery fibrodysplasia.[46] In fact, unrecognized adventitial bleeding due to vertebral artery injury during birth may be important in the later development of these dysplastic lesions.[140]

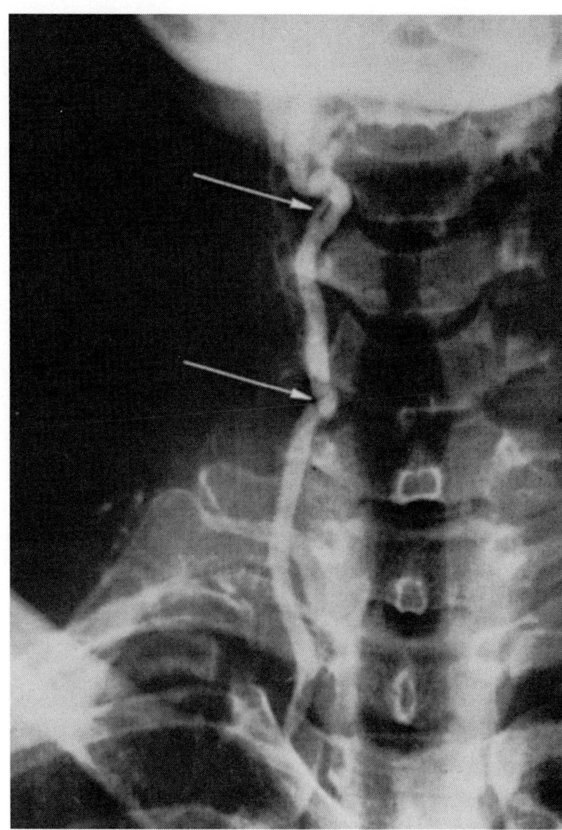

FIGURE 23–27. Medial fibrodysplasia of the vertebral artery with irregular stenoses *(arrows)*.

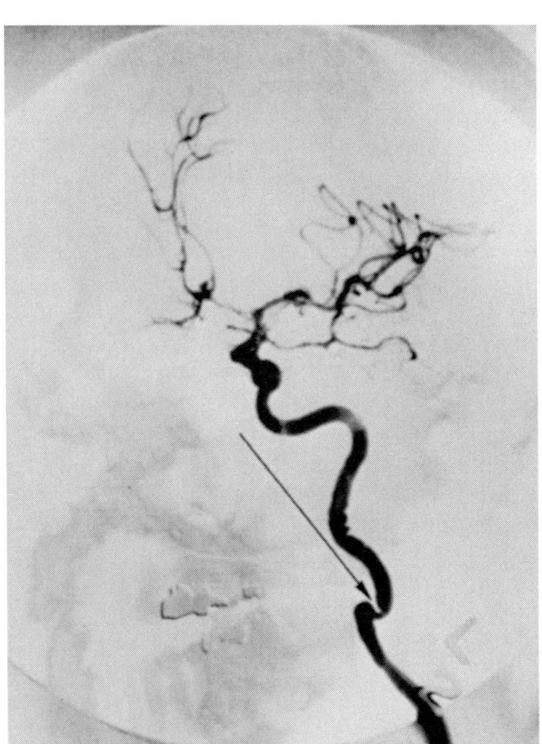

FIGURE 23–26. Medial fibrodysplasia of the extracranial internal carotid artery with angulation *(arrow)* affecting a tortuous elongated segment. (From Stanley JC, Fry WJ, Seeger JF, et al: Extracranial internal carotid and vertebral artery fibrodysplasia. Arch Surg 109:215–222, 1974. Copyright 1974, American Medical Association.)

ILIAC, FEMORAL, POPLITEAL, AND TIBIAL ARTERIES

The third vessel most commonly affected with medial fibrodysplasia is the external iliac artery.[134] Serial stenoses with intervening mural aneurysms typically affect the proximal third of this vessel (see Fig. 23–28). These lesions are similar to those of the renal and ECICA vessels and may in fact occur in patients with these other lesions.[24, 129, 131, 134] Fibroproliferative processes primarily involve the medial tissue adjacent to areas of relative thinning (Fig. 23–29). Occasional fibrodysplastic lesions of the iliac vessels appear as solitary dilatations. Complications of external iliac artery fibrodysplasia usually reflect encroachment on the lumen, with restriction of blood flow or the development of microthrombi that embolize peripherally.[77] Acute dissection may occur with these lesions, but it is not common.[6, 129] Most individuals with medial fibrodysplasia of the iliac vessels have been women patients in their 5th or 6th decade of life (~10 years older than those presenting with similar renovascular disease).[44, 45] This same pathologic lesion has been observed in an adolescent African American male, albeit in association with a peculiar shortening of the affected lower extremity.[68]

Although exceedingly rare, similar lesions reflecting the systemic nature of medial fibroplasia have been reported to affect the femoral, popliteal, and tibial vessels of the lower extremity.[49, 105, 132] In some instances, these extremity lesions have thrombosed[132]; in others they have been associated

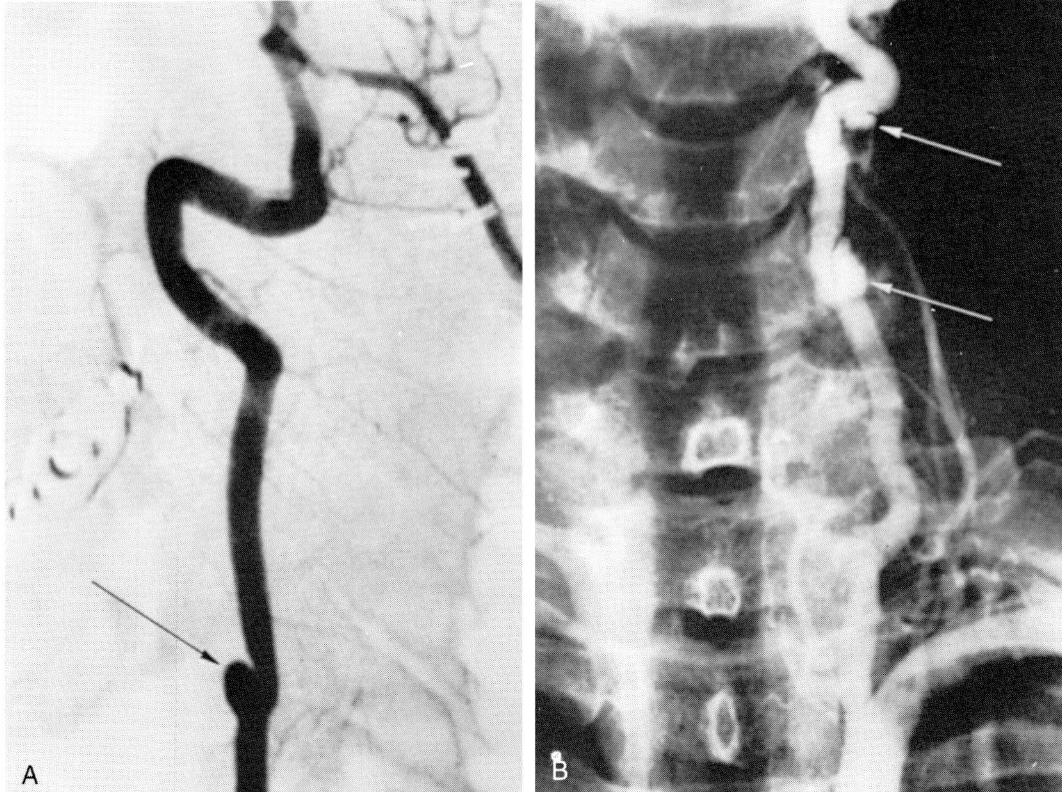

FIGURE 23–28. Medial fibrodysplasia of the vertebral artery. *A*, Isolated saccular intramural aneurysm *(arrow)*. *B*, Multiple lesions *(arrows)* suggesting dissection and aneurysm formation. (*A* and *B*, From Stanley JC, Fry WJ, Seeger JF, et al: Extracranial internal carotid and vertebral artery fibrodysplasia. Arch Surg 109:215–222, 1974. Copyright 1974, American Medical Association.)

with aneurysmal changes.[28, 41, 83, 96, 127] The etiology of dysplastic lesions of the iliac or femoral arteries may be related more to the paucity of vasa vasorum than to any physical stretch or traction stresses. Indeed, the latter causes would be unlikely to affect any of these lower extremity muscular vessels. The incidence of external iliac artery fibrodysplasia in the general population is unknown, but this condition has been reported to occur in 1% to 6% of patients with renal artery arterial fibrodysplasia.

Intimal fibroplasia of the external iliac artery, as well as

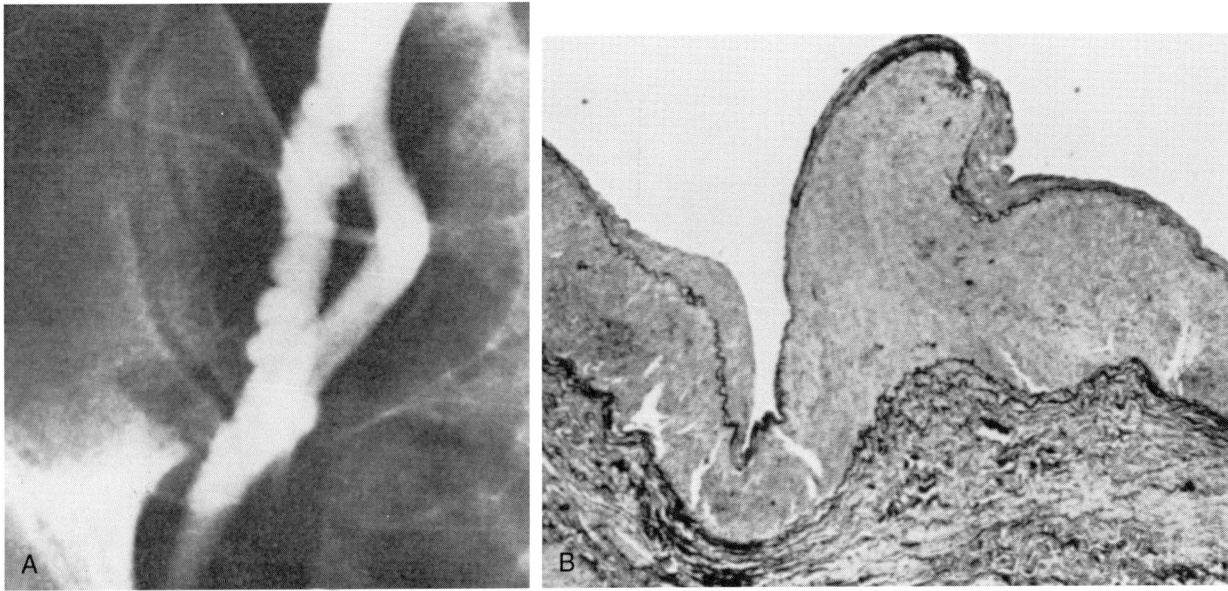

FIGURE 23–29. Medial fibrodysplasia of the external iliac artery. *A*, Multiple stenoses with intervening mural dilatations. *B*, Irregular proliferative changes within the media and minimal intimal fibroplasia. (Elastic van Gieson, ×20, longitudinal section.) (*A* and *B*, From Walter JF, Stanley JC, Mehigan JT, et al: External iliac artery fibrodysplasia. Am J Roentgenol 131:125, 1978.)

that of the femoral, popliteal, and tibial vessels, is usually considered to be a secondary pathologic phenomenon rather than a primary etiologic process. Although most instances of intimal disease affecting these vessels may be the consequence of prior trauma, the result of thromboembolism with recannulation of intraluminal thrombus, or the sequela of a prior arteritis, certain cases appear to represent primary intimal fibroplasia.[27]

AXILLARY, SUBCLAVIAN, AND BRACHIAL ARTERIES

The most common dysplastic lesion affecting upper extremity vessels appears to be *intimal fibroplasia*, which is usually manifested by smooth focal or long tubular stenoses. There is a slight predominance of women among patients with these dysplastic lesions. Speculation exists as to the etiology, although the most likely underlying cause is related to an arteritis, frequently affecting all mural elements. The difficulties in differentiating some of these lesions from resolved Takayasu's arteritis are considerable. Indeed, only in the presence of obvious aortic arch, brachiocephalic, or more distal abdominal aortic disease consistent with an inflammatory aortoarteritis can the existence of this secondary form of transmural disease be easily considered. Other intimal fibroplastic lesions affecting the subclavian and axillary vessels may be a consequence of injury (that associated with repetitive subclavian trauma at the thoracic outlet from costoclavicular entrapment) or of abnormal flow associated with anatomic bands causing vascular narrowing in the same region. Axillary artery involvement may also be the consequence of blunt trauma, with manifestations occurring many years after the actual vascular injury.

Dysplastic disease compatible with medial fibroplasia, with characteristic dilatations and constrictions or histologic confirmation of this form of dysplasia, may affect the subclavian,[8, 23] brachial,[9, 11, 21, 49, 63, 94] and radial and ulnar arteries.[54] However, these particular lesions of the upper extremity arteries are too uncommon to be rigorously classified as to type and clinical importance.

SPLANCHNIC ARTERIES: CELIAC AND MESENTERIC ARTERIES

Intimal fibroplasia may affect the origins of the three principal splanchnic vessels: the (1) celiac artery, (2) the superior mesenteric artery, and (3) the inferior mesenteric artery. The basis of these lesions is unknown, but this fibrodysplasia may reflect a secondary phenomenon occurring in developmentally narrowed vessels. Ostial fibrodysplastic lesions are quite common in patients with intestinal angina and often exhibit associated atherosclerotic changes.[48] Intimal fibroplasia tends to occur more often in women than in men, with nearly equal involvement of the celiac and superior mesenteric arteries. The hepatic as well as the splenic and iliac vessels have all demonstrated fibrodysplastic tubular stenoses, which may represent the outcome of prior arteritis or resolved thrombosis. Occasional patients demonstrate more distal disease in the celiac or superior mesenteric circulatory beds. A dilated appearance of the celiac artery just beyond an eccentric stenosis due to median ligament compression of this vessel is relatively common. Although earlier reports attributed this particular lesion to medial fibrodysplasia, it may simply represent chronic fibrosis of the "trapped" proximal vessel with poststenotic dilatation.

Characteristic medial fibrodysplasia is rare within the splanchnic circulation, although histologic evidence of it has been reported.[75] When present, this form of splanchnic vascular disease is often associated with similar renal or carotid lesions.[75, 100] Histologic evidence of medial dysplasia is also common among patients having splenic artery aneurysms.[117] In fact, the development of these aneurysms may be a reflection of compromised vascular integrity due to the disruptive dysplastic process. Similar aneurysms have been noted in other splanchnic vessels, including the superior mesenteric artery.[18] The proximal superior mesenteric artery may exhibit medial fibrodysplastic occlusive disease a few centimeters beyond its origin as it exists beneath the pancreas over the top of the duodenum. The basis of these latter lesions has not been established, although unusual stretch forces at the root of the mesentery may contribute to dysplastic changes. Involvement of smaller mesenteric branches has been reported but is considered exceedingly rare.[138]

Intestinal branch narrowings that have been considered dysplastic in character usually represent intimal lesions resulting from an earlier inflammatory process, be it part of the spectrum of an earlier arteritis or an adjacent inflammatory process, such as pancreatitis. The occurrence of splanchnic arterial fibrodysplasia is so uncommon as to prevent any firm conclusions about its natural history.

OTHER VESSELS

Most other vessels affected with dysplastic disease involve intimal fibroplasia. Exceptions exist; medial fibrodysplasia also affects the coronary arteries, exhibiting dissections as well as thromboses.[4, 47, 62, 128] Other dysplastic lesions have been noted among patients ranging from neonates to the elderly, in large arteries the size of the aorta to very small vessels, such as the coronary sinus node artery.[20, 42, 50] Certain aortic lesions may represent developmental webs or consequences of a prior intraluminal thrombotic event. Many of the latter lesions do not appear arteriographically to be very distinct from focal arteriosclerosis.[58] It is unlikely that the changes in these vessels represent a systemic arteritis in its active stage, although they may represent an end stage of an earlier arteritis. Again, experience with these rare forms of arterial dysplasia is so meager as to preclude rendering of any firm conclusions about their etiology or clinical relevance.

REFERENCES

1. Abdul-Rahman AM, Salih A, Brun A, et al: Fibromuscular dysplasia of the cervico-cephalic arteries. Surg Neurol 9:216, 1978.
2. Alimi Y, Mercier C, Pellissier J-F, et al: Fibromuscular disease of the

renal artery: A new histopathologic classification. Ann Vasc Surg 6:220–224, 1992.
3. Andersen CA, Collins GJ Jr, Rich NM, McDonald PT: Bilateral internal carotid arterial occlusions associated with fibromuscular dysplasia. Vasc Surg 13:349, 1979.
4. Arey JB, Segal R: Fibromuscular dysplasia of intramyocardial coronary arteries. Pediatr Pathol 7:97, 1987.
5. Bader H: The anatomy and physiology of the vascular wall. *In* Hamilton WF (ed): Handbook of Physiology. Vol 2. Washington, DC, American Physiological Society, 1963, pp 865–889.
6. Burri B, Fontolliet C, Ruegsegger C-H, Mosimann R: External iliac artery dissection due to fibromuscular dysplasia. Vasa 12:76, 1983.
7. Canova A, Esposito S, Patricolo A, et al: Spontaneous obliteration of a carotid-cavernous fistula associated with fibromuscular dysplasia of the internal carotid artery. J Neurosurg Sci 31:37, 1987.
8. Chambers JL, Neale ML, Appleberg M: Fibromuscular hyperplasia in an aberrant subclavian artery and neurogenic thoracic outlet syndrome: An unusual combination. J Vasc Surg 20:834,1994.
9. Cheu HW, Mills JL: Digital artery embolization as a result of fibromuscular dysplasia of the brachial artery. J Vasc Surg 14:225,1991.
10. Chiche L, Bahnini A, Koskas F, et al: Occlusive fibromuscular disease of arteries supplying the brain: Results of surgical treatment. Ann Vasc Surg 11:496, 1997.
11. Ciocca RG, Madson DL, Wilkerson DK, et al: Fibromuscular dysplasia of the brachial artery: An endovascular approach. Am Surgeon 61:161, 1995.
12. Cloft HJ, Kallmes DF, Kallmes MH, et al: Prevalence of cerebral aneurysms in patients with fibromuscular dysplasia: A reassessment. J Neurosurg 88:436, 1998.
13. Collins GJ Jr, Rich NM, Clagett GP, et al: Fibromuscular dysplasia of the internal carotid arteries: Clinical experience and follow-up. Ann Surg 194:89, 1981.
14. Connett M, Lansche JM: Fibromuscular hyperplasia of the internal carotid artery: Report of a case. Ann Surg 162:59, 1965.
15. Corrin LS, Sandok BA, Houser OW: Cerebral ischemic events in patients with carotid artery fibromuscular dysplasia. Arch Neurol 38:616, 1981.
16. Cragg AH, Smith TP, Thompson BH, et al: Incidental fibromuscular dysplasia in potential renal donors: Long-term clinical follow-up. Radiology 172:145, 1989.
17. de Deeuw D, Donker AJM, Burema J, et al: Nephroptosis and hypertension. Lancet 1:213, 1977.
18. den Butter G, Bockel JH, Aarts JCNM: Arterial fibrodysplasia: Rapid progression complicated by rupture of a visceral aneurysm into the gastrointestinal tract. J Vasc Surg 7:449, 1988.
19. Devaney K, Kapur SP, Patterson K, Chandra RS: Pediatric renal artery dysplasia: A morphologic study. Pediatr Pathol 11:609, 1991.
20. Dominguez FE, Tate LG, Robinson MJ: Familial fibromuscular dysplasia presenting as sudden death. Am J Cardiovasc Pathol 2:269, 1988.
21. Dorman RL Jr, Kaufman JA, LaMuraglia GM: Digital emboli from brachial artery fibromuscular dysplasia. Cardiovasc Intervent Radiol 17:95, 1994.
22. Dornfeld L, Kaufman JJ: Immunologic considerations in renovascular hypertension. Urol Clin North Am 2:285, 1975.
23. Drury JK, Pollock JG: Subclavian arteriopathy in the young patient. Br J Surg 68:617, 1981.
24. Effeney DJ, Ehrenfeld WK, Stoney RJ, Wylie EJ: Why operate on carotid fibromuscular dysplasia? Arch Surg 115:1261, 1980.
25. Ekelund L, Gerlock J, Molin J, Smith C: Roentgenologic appearance of fibromuscular dysplasia. Acta Radiol [Diagn] 19:433, 1978.
26. Ehrenfeld WK, Wylie EJ: Fibromuscular dysplasia of the internal carotid artery. Arch Surg 109:676, 1974.
27. Esfahani F, Rooholamini SA, Azadeh B, Daneshbod K: Arterial fibrodysplasia: A regional cause of peripheral occlusive vascular disease. Angiology 40:108, 1989.
28. Fiche M, Patra P, Chaillou P: Medial fibrodysplasia and aneurysm of the popliteal artery. Ann Vasc Surg 5:456, 1991.
29. Fievez ML: Fibromuscular dysplasia of arteries: A spastic phenomenon? Med Hypotheses 13:341, 1984.
30. Finley JL, Dabbs DJ: Renal vascular smooth muscle proliferation in neurofibromatosis. Hum Pathol 19:107, 1988.
31. Frens DB, Petajan JH, Anderson R, Deblanc HJ Jr: Fibromuscular dysplasia of the posterior cerebral artery: Report of a case and review of the literature. Stroke 5:161,1974.
32. Gabbiani G, Majno G, Ryan GB: The fibroblast as a contractile cell. The myo-fibroblast. *In* Kulonen E, Pikkarainen J (eds): Biology of Fibroblast. New York, Academic Press, 1973, pp 139–154.
33. Gladstien K, Rushton AR, Kidd KK: Penetrance estimates and recurrence risks for fibromuscular dysplasia. Clin Genet 17:115, 1980.
34. Goncharenko V, Gerlock AJ, Shaff MI, Hollifield SW: Progression of renal artery fibromuscular dysplasia in 42 patients as seen on angiography. Radiology 139:45, 1981.
35. Graham LM, Zelenock GB, Erlandson EE, et al: Abdominal aortic coarctation and segmental hypoplasia. Surgery 86:519, 1979.
36. Grange DK, Balfour IC, Chen SC, et al: Familial syndrome of progressive arterial occlusive disease consistent with fibromuscular dysplasia, hypertension, congenital cardiac defects, bone fragility, brachysyndactyly, and learning disabilities. Am J Med Genet 75:469, 1998.
37. Halperin M, Currarino G: Vascular lesions causing hypertension in neurofibromatosis. N Engl J Med 273:248, 1965.
38. Harrison EG Jr, Hunt JC, Bernatz PE: Morphology of fibromuscular dysplasia of the renal artery in renovascular hypertension. Am J Med 43:97, 1967.
39. Harrison EG, McCormack LJ: Pathologic classification of renal artery disease in renovascular hypertension. Mayo Clin Proc 46:161, 1971.
40. Hata J-I, Hosoda Y: Perimedial fibroplasia of the renal artery: A light and electron microscopy study. Arch Pathol Lab Med 103:220, 1979.
41. Herpels V, Van de Voorde W, Wilms G, et al: Recurrent aneurysms of the upper arteries of the lower limb: An atypical manifestation of fibromuscular dysplasia—a case report. Angiology 38:411, 1987.
42. Hill LD, Antonius JI: Arterial dysplasia. Arch Surg 90:585, 1965.
43. Hirsch CS, Roessmann U: Arterial dysplasia with ruptured basilar artery aneurysm: Report of a case. Hum Pathol 6:749, 1975.
44. Horne TW: Fibromuscular hyperplasia of the iliac arteries. Aust N Z J Surg 45:415, 1975.
45. Houston C, Rosenthal D, Lamis PA, Stanton PE Jr: Fibromuscular dysplasia of the external iliac arteries: Surgical treatment by graduated internal dilatation technique. Surgery 85:713, 1979.
46. Hugenholtz H, Pokrupa R, Montpetit VJA, et al: Spontaneous dissecting aneurysm of the extracranial vertebral artery. Neurosurgery 10:96, 1982.
47. Imamura M, Yokoyama S, Kikuchi K: Coronary fibromuscular dysplasia presenting as sudden infant death. Arch Pathol Lab Med 121:159, 1997.
48. Insall RL, Chamberlain J, Loose HWC: Fibromuscular dysplasia of visceral arteries. Eur J Vasc Surg 6:668, 1992.
49. Iwai T, Konno S, Hiejima K, et al: Fibromuscular dysplasia in the extremities. J Cardiovasc Surg 26:496, 1985.
50. James TN: Morphologic characteristics and functional significance of focal fibromuscular dysplasia of small coronary arteries. Am J Cardiol 65:12G, 1990.
51. Kalyanaraman UP, Elwood PW: Fibromuscular dysplasia of intracranial arteries causing multiple intracranial aneurysms. Hum Pathol 11:481, 1980.
52. Kaufman JJ, Maxwell MH: Upright aortography in the study of nephroptosis, stenotic lesions of the renal artery, and hypertension. Surgery 53:736, 1963.
53. Kelly TF Jr, Morris GC: Arterial fibromuscular dysplasia: Observations on pathogenesis and surgical management. Am J Surg 143:232, 1982.
54. Khatri VP, Gaulin JC, Amin AK: Fibromuscular dysplasia of distal radial and ulnar arteries: Uncommon cause of digital ischemia. Ann Plast Surg 33:652, 1994.
55. Lang J: Mikroskopische Anatomie der Arterien. Angiologica 2:225, 1965.
56. Leadbetter WF, Burkland CE: Hypertension in unilateral renal disease. J Urol 39:611, 1938.
57. Lemahieu SF, Marchau MMB: Intracranial fibromuscular dysplasia and stroke in children. Neuroradiology 18:99, 1979.
58. Letsch R, Kantartzis M, Sommer T, Garcia M: Arterial fibromuscular dysplasia: Report of a case with involvement of the aorta and review of the literature. Thorac Cardiovasc Surg 28:206, 1980.
59. Leung DYM, Glagov S, Matthews MB: Cyclic stretching stimulates synthesis of matrix components by arterial smooth muscle cells in vitro. Science 191:475, 1976.
60. Levien LJ, Fritz VU, Lurie D, et al: Fibromuscular dysplasia of the extracranial carotid arteries. S Afr Med J 65:261, 1984.
61. Lie JT: Segmental mediolytic arteritis: Not an arteritis but a variant

of arterial fibromuscular dysplasia. Arch Pathol Lab Med 116:238–241, 1992.
62. Lie JT, Berg KK: Isolated fibromuscular dysplasia of the coronary arteries with spontaneous dissection and myocardial infarction. Hum Pathol 18:654, 1987.
63. Lin WW, McGee GS, Patterson BK, et al: Fibromuscular dysplasia of the brachial artery: A case report and review of the literature. J Vasc Surg 16:66, 1992.
64. Llorens-Terol J, Sole-Llelnas J, Tura A: Stroke due to fibromuscular hyperplasia of the internal carotid artery. Acta Paediatr Scand 72:299, 1983.
65. Luscher TF, Keller HM, Imhof HG, et al: Fibromuscular hyperplasia: Extension of the disease and therapeutic outcome. Results of the University Hospital Zurich cooperative study on fibromuscular hyperplasia. Nephron 44:109, 1986.
66. Luscher TF, Lie JT, Stanson AW, et al: Arterial fibromuscular dysplasia. Mayo Clin Proc 62:931, 1987.
67. Madden JW, Carlson EC, Hines J: Presence of modified fibroblasts in ischemic contracture of the intrinsic musculature of the hand. Surg Gynecol Obstet 140:509, 1975.
68. Madiba TE, Robbs JV: Fibromuscular dysplasia of the external iliac artery in association with congenital short leg and mesodermal malformation: A case report. S Afr J Surg 27:139, 1989.
69. Major P, Genest J, Cariter P, Kuchel O: Heredity fibromuscular dysplasia with renovascular hypertension. Ann Intern Med 86:583, 1977.
70. Masuzawa T, Nakahara N, Kobayashi S: Intracranial multiple berry aneurysms associated with fibromuscular dysplasia and mixed connective tissue disease. Neurol Med Chir (Tokyo) 27:42, 1987.
71. Maycock Wd'A: Congenital stenosis of the abdominal aorta. Am Heart J 13:633, 1937.
72. McCormack LJ, Noto TJ Jr, Meaney TF, et al: Subadventitial fibroplasia of the renal artery: A disease of young women. Am Heart J 73:602, 1967.
73. McCormack LJ, Poutasse EF, Meaney TF, et al: A pathologic arteriographic correlation of renal arterial disease. Am Heart J 73:602, 1967.
74. McGrath TW: Fibromuscular dysplasia vs catheter-induced renal artery spasm [Letter]. Am J Roentgenol 148:651, 1987.
75. Meacham PW, Brantley B: Familial fibromuscular dysplasia of the mesenteric arteries. South Med J 80:1311, 1987.
76. Meaney TF, Dustan HF, McCormack LJ: Natural history of renal arterial disease. Radiology 91:881, 1968.
77. Mehigan JT, Stoney RJ: Arterial microemboli and fibromuscular dysplasia of the external iliac arteries. Surgery 81:484, 1977.
78. Mena E, Bookstein JJ, Holt JF, Fry WJ: Neurofibromatosis and renovascular hypertension in children. Am J Roentgenol 118:39, 1973.
79. Mettinger KL: Fibromuscular dysplasia and the brain: II. Current concept of the disease. Stroke 13:53, 1982.
80. Mettinger KL, Ericson K: Fibromuscular dysplasia and the brain: Observations on angiographic, clinical and genetic characteristics. Stroke 13:46, 1982.
81. Morimoto S, Kuroda M, Uchida K, et al: Occurrence of renovascular hypertension in two sisters. Nephron 17:314, 1976.
82. Nemcek AA, Holmburg CE: Reversible renal fibromuscular dysplasia. Am J Roentgenol 147:737, 1986.
83. Neukirch C, Bahnini A, Delcourt A, et al: Popliteal aneurysm due to fibromuscular dysplasia. Ann Vasc Surg 10:578, 1996.
84. Osborn AG, Anderson RE: Angiographic spectrum of cervical and intracranial fibromuscular dysplasia. Stroke 8:617, 1977.
85. Ouchi Y, Tagawa H, Yamakado M, et al: Clinical significance of cerebral aneurysm in renovascular hypertension due to fibromuscular dysplasia: Two cases in siblings. Angiology 40:581, 1989.
86. Palubinskas AJ, Ripley HR: Fibromuscular hyperplasia in extra-renal arteries. Radiology 82:451, 1964.
87. Pannier-Moreau I, Grimbert P, Fiquet-Kempf B, et al: Possible familial origin of multifocal renal artery fibromuscular dysplasia. J Hypertension 15:1797, 1997.
88. Park SH, Chi JG, Choi Y: Primary intimal fibroplasia with multiple aneurysms of renal artery in childhood. Child Nephrol Urol 10:51, 1990.
89. Paulson GW: Fibromuscular dysplasia, antiovulant drugs, and ergot preparations. Stroke 9:172, 1978.
90. Perez-Higueras A, Alvarez-Ruiz F, Martinez-Bermejo A, et al: Cerebellar infarction from fibromuscular dysplasia and dissecting aneurysm of the vertebral artery. Stroke 19:521, 1988.
91. Perry MO: Fibromuscular dysplasia of the carotid artery. Surg Gynecol Obstet 134:57, 1972.
92. Plotkin SA, Boue A, Boue JG: The in vitro growth of rubella virus in human embryo cells. Am J Epidemiol 81:71, 1965.
93. Reddy SV, Karnes WE, Earnest F IV, Sundt TM Jr: Spontaneous extracranial vertebral arteriovenous fistula with fibromuscular dysplasia. J Neurosurg 54:399, 1981.
94. Reilly JM, McGaw DJ, and Sicard GA: Bilateral brachial artery fibromuscular dysplasia. Ann Vasc Surg 7:483, 1993.
95. Rinaldi I, Harris WO Jr, Kopp JE, Legier J: Intracranial fibromuscular dysplasia: Report of two cases, one with autopsy verification. Stroke 7:511, 1976.
96. Ritota P, Quirke TE, Keys RC, et al: A rare association of fibromuscular dysplasia of the femoral artery with aneurysm and occlusion treated alternatively. J Cardiovasc Surg 35:239, 1994.
97. Rosenberger A, Adler O, Lichtig H: Angiographic appearance of the renal vein in a case of fibromuscular dysplasia of the artery. Radiology 118:579, 1976.
98. Ross R, Klebanoff SJ: Fine structural changes in uterine smooth muscle and fibroblasts in response to estrogen. J Cell Biol 32:155, 1967.
99. Rushton AR: The genetics of fibromuscular dysplasia. Arch Intern Med 140:233, 1980.
100. Salmon PJM, Allan JS: An unusual case of fibromuscular dysplasia. J Cardiovasc Surg 29:756, 1988.
101. Sandok BA: Fibromuscular dysplasia of the internal carotid artery. Neurol Clin 1:17, 1983.
102. Sang CN, Whelton PK, Hamper UM, et al: Etiologic factors in renovascular fibromuscular dysplasia. Hypertension 14:472, 1989.
103. Saygi S, Bolay H, Tekkok IH, et al: Fibromuscular dysplasia of the basilar artery: A case with brain stem stroke. Angiology 41:658, 1990.
104. Schievink WI, Bjornsson J: Fibromuscular dysplasia of the internal carotid artery: A clinicopathological study. Clin Neuropathol 15:2, 1996.
105. Schneider PA, LaBerge JM, Cunningham CG, et al: Isolated thigh claudication as a result of fibromuscular dysplasia of the deep femoral artery. J Vasc Surg 15:657, 1992.
106. Schreiber MJ, Pohl MA, Novick AC: The natural history of atherosclerotic and fibrous renal artery disease. Urol Clin North Am 11:383, 1984.
107. Schurch W, Messerli FH, Genest J, et al: Arterial hypertension and neurofibromatosis: Renal artery stenosis and coarctation of abdominal aorta. Can Med Assoc J 113:878, 1975.
108. Sheps SG, Kincaid OW, Hunt JC: Serial renal function and angiographic observations in idiopathic fibrous and fibromuscular stenoses of the renal arteries. Am J Cardiol 30:55, 1972.
109. Shields WD, Ziter FA, Osborn AG, Allen J: Fibromuscular dysplasia as a cause of stroke in infancy and childhood. Pediatrics 59:899, 1977.
110. Siassi B, Glyman G, Emmanouilides GC: Hypoplasia of the abdominal aorta associated with the rubella syndrome. Am J Dis Child 120:476, 1970.
111. Slavin RE, Saeki K, Bhagavan B, et al: Segmental arterial mediolysis: A precursor to fibromuscular dysplasia? Modern Pathol 8:287, 1995.
112. So EL, Toole JF, Dalal P, Moody DM: Cephalic fibromuscular dysplasia in 32 patients: Clinical findings and radiologic features. Arch Neurol 38:619, 1981.
113. Sottiurai VS, Fry WJ, Stanley JC: Ultrastructural characteristics of experimental arterial medial fibrodysplasia induced by vasa vasorum occlusion. J Surg Res 24:169, 1978.
114. Sottiurai VS, Fry WJ, Stanley JC: Ultrastructure of medial smooth muscle and myofibroblasts in human arterial dysplasia. Arch Surg 113:1280, 1978.
115. Stanley JC: Morphologic, histopathologic and clinical characteristics of renovascular fibrodysplasia and arteriosclerosis. *In* Bergan JJ, Yao JST (eds): Surgery of the Aorta and Its Body Branches. New York, Grune & Stratton, 1979, pp 355–376.
116. Stanley JC: Pathologic basis of macrovascular renal artery disease. *In* Stanley JC, Ernst CB, Fry WJ (eds): Renovascular Hypertension. Philadelphia, WB Saunders, 1984, pp 46–74.
117. Stanley JC, Fry WJ: Pathogenesis and clinical significance of splenic artery aneurysms. Surgery 76:898, 1974.
118. Stanley JC, Fry WJ: Renovascular hypertension secondary to arterial

fibrodysplasia in adults: Criteria for operation and results of surgical therapy. Arch Surg 110:922, 1975.
119. Stanley JC, Fry WJ: Pediatric renal artery occlusive disease and renovascular hypertension: Etiology, diagnosis and operative treatment. Arch Surg 116:669, 1981.
120. Stanley JC, Fry WJ, Seeger JF, et al: Extracranial internal carotid and vertebral artery fibrodysplasia. Arch Surg 109:215, 1974.
121. Stanley JC, Gewertz BC, Bove EL, et al: Arterial fibrodysplasia: Histopathologic character and current etiologic concepts. Arch Surg 110:561, 1975.
122. Stanley JC, Graham LM, Whitehouse WM Jr, et al: Developmental occlusive disease of the abdominal aorta, splanchnic and renal arteries. Am J Surg 142:190, 1981.
123. Stanley JC, Rhodes EL, Gewertz BL, et al: Renal artery aneurysms: Significance of macroaneurysms exclusive of dissections and fibrodysplastic mural dilatations. Arch Surg 110:1327, 1975.
124. Stanley JC, Zelenock GB, Messina LM, et al: Pediatric renovascular hypertension: A thirty-year experience of operative treatment. J Vasc Surg 21:212, 1995.
125. Stewart DR, Price RA, Nebesar R, Schuster SR: Progressing peripheral fibromuscular hyperplasia in an infant: A possible manifestation of the rubella syndrome. Surgery 73:374, 1973.
126. Stewart MT, Moritz MW, Smith RB III, et al: The natural history of carotid fibromuscular dysplasia. J Vasc Surg 3:305, 1986.
127. Stinnett DM, Graham JM, Edwards WD: Fibromuscular dysplasia and thrombosed aneurysm of the popliteal artery in a child. J Vasc Surg 5:769, 1987.
128. Tanaka M, Watanabe T, Tomaki S, et al: Revascularization in fibromuscular dysplasia of the coronary arteries. Am Heart J 125:1167, 1993.
129. Thevenet A, Latil JL, Albat B: Fibromuscular disease of the external iliac artery. Ann Vasc Surg 6:199, 1992.
130. Tsukamoto Y, Komuro Y, Akutsu F, et al: Orthostatic hypertension due to coexistence of renal fibromuscular dysplasia and nephroptosis. Jpn Circ J 52:1408, 1988.
131. Twigg HL, Palmisano PJ: Fibromuscular hyperplasia of the iliac artery: A case report. Am J Roentgenol 95:418, 1965.
132. Van den Dungen JJAM, Boontje AH, Oosterhuis JW: Femoropopliteal arterial fibrodyplasia. Br J Surg 77:396, 1990.
133. Vles JSH, Hendriks JJE, Lodder J, Janevski B: Multiple vertebrobasilar infarctions from fibromuscular dysplasia-related dissecting aneurysm of the vertebral artery in a child. Neuropediatrics 21:104, 1990.
134. Walter JF, Stanley JC, Mehigan JT, et al: External iliac artery fibrodysplasia. Am J Roentgenol 131:125, 1978.
135. Wesen CA, Elliott BM: Fibromuscular dysplasia of the carotid arteries. Am J Surg 151:448, 1986.
136. Wirth FP, Miller WA, Russell AP: Atypical fibromuscular hyperplasia: Report of two cases. J Neurosurg 54:685, 1981.
137. Wright I: Age changes in the peripheral arteries in man. Cardiovasc Anat Pathol 11:157, 1964.
138. Yamaguchi R, Yamaguchi Q, Isogai M, et al: Fibromuscular dysplasia of the visceral arteries. Am J Gastroenterol 91:1635, 1996.
139. Yamamoto I, Kageyama N, Usui K, Yoshida J: Fibromuscular dysplasia of the internal carotid artery: Unusual arteriographic changes with progression of clinical symptoms. Acta Neurochir (Wien) 50:293, 1979.
140. Yates PO: Birth trauma to the vertebral arteries. Arch Dis Child 109:215, 1974.

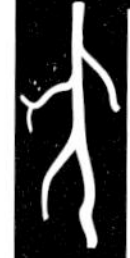

CHAPTER 24

Pathologic Intimal Hyperplasia as a Response to Vascular Injury and Reconstruction

Alexander W. Clowes, M.D.

Since 1950, reconstruction has become the rule rather than the exception for the treatment of occlusive disease of major arteries. Techniques previously limited to the aorta and large branch vessels have been improved and extended to small vessels of the brain, heart, viscera, and extremities. These reconstructions cannot be expected to last indefinitely, because stenosis and, ultimately, spontaneous thrombosis frequently develop. Exactly why arterial reconstructions are unsuccessful is not known, although one possibility is that narrowing of the lumen of a graft or endarterectomized artery is in essence a form of recurrent or continuing atherosclerosis superimposed on normal wound healing.[1, 2] It is known, from the studies of wound healing in humans and animals, that luminal narrowing is caused by two processes: (1) smooth muscle cell (SMC) and matrix accumulation and (2) shrinkage (vasoconstriction) associated with pathologic remodeling of the vessel.[3]

This chapter first defines a number of clinical conditions in which smooth muscle proliferation and intimal thickening play a significant part in the failure of vascular reconstructions. The mechanisms controlling smooth muscle growth are then considered in more detail. Finally, the operative and nonoperative approaches available for prevention and treatment of intimal thickening and luminal narrowing are evaluated.

EXAMPLES OF PATHOLOGIC INTIMAL HYPERPLASIA

A number of surgical procedures are themselves disruptive of the normal vascular architecture. Simply passing an inflated *balloon embolectomy catheter* along a vessel denudes

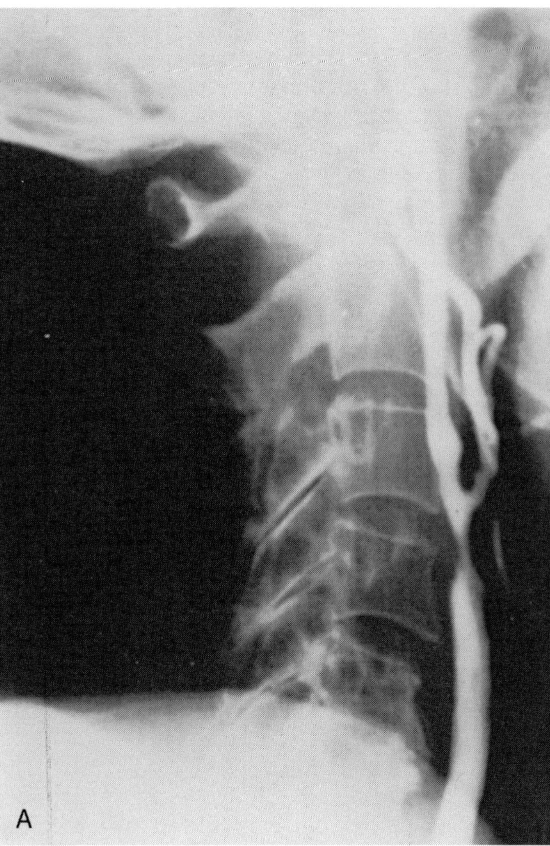

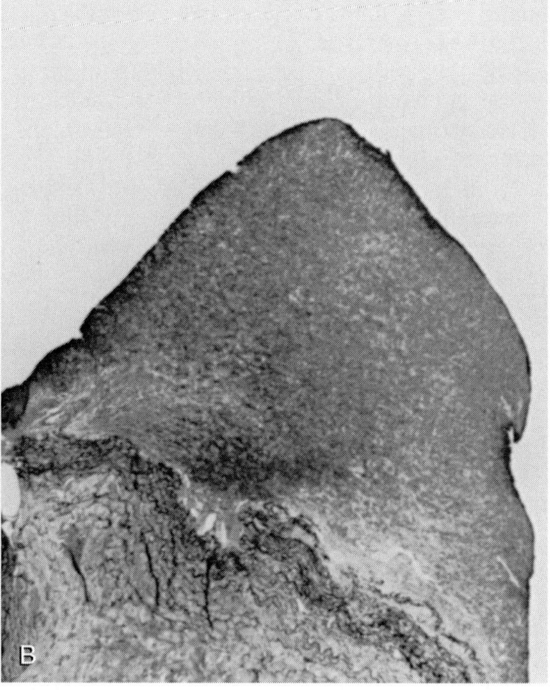

FIGURE 24–1. *A*, Arteriogram showing stenosis in common carotid 6 months following endarterectomy. (Courtesy of R.E. Zierler, M.D.) *B*, Histologic cross section of a recurrent carotid stenosis demonstrating massive accumulation of connective tissue. (Courtesy of D. Gordon, M.D.)

the surface of its endothelium, stretches the wall, and destroys some of the SMCs in the media.[4, 5] In animal models (described later), platelets accumulate in a thin layer on the denuded surface; in turn, they are displaced by regenerating endothelium and proliferating intimal SMCs. Ultimately, the intima thickens as a consequence of the accumulation of SMCs and extracellular matrix. In small vessels in humans, this embolectomy catheter–induced intimal thickening can cause diffuse narrowing of the lumen[6]; in larger vessels, this process seems not to be of clinical importance.

Percutaneous transluminal angioplasty with or without a stent is used to dilate stenotic segments of atherosclerotic arteries. In so doing, this produces a rent in the plaque and disruption of the intimal elastic lamina; the outer media and adventitia stretch but are not disrupted and maintain the structural integrity of the conduit.[7–9] Thrombus forms in the disrupted portion of the plaque and over a period of weeks is remodeled into a fibrous lesion by tbe invasion of myofibroblasts derived from the adventitia.[10–12] As might be expected, this procedure yields the best results when the stenoses are discrete and are located in large vessels with high blood flow.[13–15] Although significant restenosis is only a modest problem in large vessels (e.g., iliac arteries), it is an important cause of ischemia and reduction in blood flow in small vessels such as the coronary and femoropopliteal arteries.

Approximately 30% of dilated coronary arteries develop marked restenosis by 6 months.[16, 17] This figure comes from studies of patients who complain of new or recurrent symptoms and show ischemic changes on the electrocardiogram during treadmill testing performed prior to coronary angiography. Hence, the actual incidence of restenosis is likely to be even greater than 30%. The lesions causing restenosis are largely fibrous and contain mostly SMCs. In superficial arteries, restenosis is often adjacent to but not at the site of the dilation.[18, 19]

Although intimal thickening contributes to restenosis, pathologic remodeling with reduction in the cross-sectional area inside the external elastic lamina is the most important factor. The importance of this form of vascular shrinkage has been documented in animal and human vessels subjected to balloon angioplasty.[20–24] It does not occur in stented vessels where the dimensions of the vessel are rigidly maintained by the stents. In this circumstance, luminal narrowing is due entirely to intimal hyperplasia.

Endarterectomy is an equally traumatic form of vascular reconstruction and is also associated with the development of a hyperplastic intimal lesion that in some instances is sufficient to narrow the reconstructed lumen and reduce blood flow. The development of recurrent stenosis has been described in some detail in patients undergoing carotid endarterectomy.[25–30] Although the incidence of symptomatic recurrent stenosis appears to be low (~1%), the actual incidence of greater than 50% stenosis, as documented by duplex scanning or angiography, is between 10% and 20%.

These lesions exhibit at least two kinds of morphology (Fig. 24–1); if examined within the first two years after surgery, they are smooth, white, firm, and fibrous and contain SMCs and extracellular matrix. At later times, the lesions often have a friable and rubbery layer of thrombus at the luminal surface, with some underlying regions showing accumulations of lipid, calcium, and hemorrhage as well as foci of smooth muscle.

These results suggest that repair in severely traumatized vessels is brought about by proliferation of SMCs or myofibroblasts derived perhaps from remnants of media, adjacent undamaged vessel, or even the adventitia. The new intimal lesion is further enlarged by synthesis and deposition of extracellular matrix by smooth muscle, including elastin, collagen and proteoglycans. To what extent endothelium reestablishes a luminal surface is not known. Some of the details of this healing process have been defined in animal models and are reviewed later in the chapter.

All the examples of intimal hyperplasia complicating the restorative and reconstructive procedures just described appear to be associated with extensive endothelial denudation and destruction of at least a part of the artery wall. In healing *vascular grafts*, the relationship between injury and intimal hyperplasia is not as obvious. It is certain that vigorous distention of a vein graft already in spasm or passage of a valvulotome can damage the endothelium and the graft wall, but because these defects are relatively small, endothelium should regenerate within a few days.[31–33] Nevertheless, such grafts may develop intimal thickening over a period of months. Significant stenosis in peripheral reconstructions develops in approximately 10% of vein grafts and is usually apparent within 6 to 24 months.[34–36] These lesions can be diffuse or limited and have been reported to be associated with scarring at the sites of vein valves or trauma. They have also been described in the less traumatized in situ vein grafts.[37] The lesions in these grafts are fibrous and smooth and resemble morphologically the early lesions of carotid restenosis.

At later times, some vein grafts develop frank atherosclerosis. These lesions are particularly prevalent in coronary artery bypass grafts (Fig. 24–2).[38, 39] A study of patients over 10 years following surgery at the Montreal Heart Institute demonstrated by serial angiography that 50% of the grafts eventually manifested thrombosis and 50% of the remaining grafts exhibited the angiographic appearance of advanced atherosclerosis.[40] There was a significant correlation between plasma low-density lipoprotein (LDL), apoprotein B levels, and graft atherosclerosis.[41] Why these grafts steadily deteriorate over time is not known. It is possible that the scarring process associated with adaptation of vein grafts to the arterial circulation makes the grafts more susceptible to exogenous atherogenic stimuli. This hypothesis is supported by the observation that coronary grafts made of internal mammary arteries, which do not need to adapt to the arterial circulation, also do not develop atherosclerotic plaques and do not exhibit the same high failure rates as vein grafts.[40]

In *synthetic grafts*, significant intimal thickening develops at the anastomoses or, just beyond, in the distal vessels (Fig. 24–3).[42–45] These lesions are similar to those found early on in vein grafts and usually appear within the first two years after surgery. In humans, coverage of the inner surface of synthetic grafts by endothelium and subendothelial connective tissue is limited to the first few centimeters at either end, although occasional islands of endothelium have been reported, perhaps derived from circulating endothelial precursors.[46–49] It appears, then, that the adjacent artery serves as the primary source of covering cells and that those cells have only a limited capacity to migrate along the graft. In contrast, lesions in vein grafts appear to be the result of proliferation of cells already residing in the graft.

To what extent injury plays a role in the healing of vascular grafts and the development of excessive intimal hyperplasia is not known. In part, this is because it is extremely difficult to document in humans the extent of endothelial denudation, wall disruption, and the sequence of reparative events. In addition, from animal studies it is now known that there may be a wide range of injurious insults; some cause disruption of the vascular architecture and others cause subtle loss of endothelium that is repaired before denudation becomes apparent.

EXPERIMENTAL STUDIES

Large undiseased arteries are made of layers of SMCs alternating with layers of elastin and collagen in the media

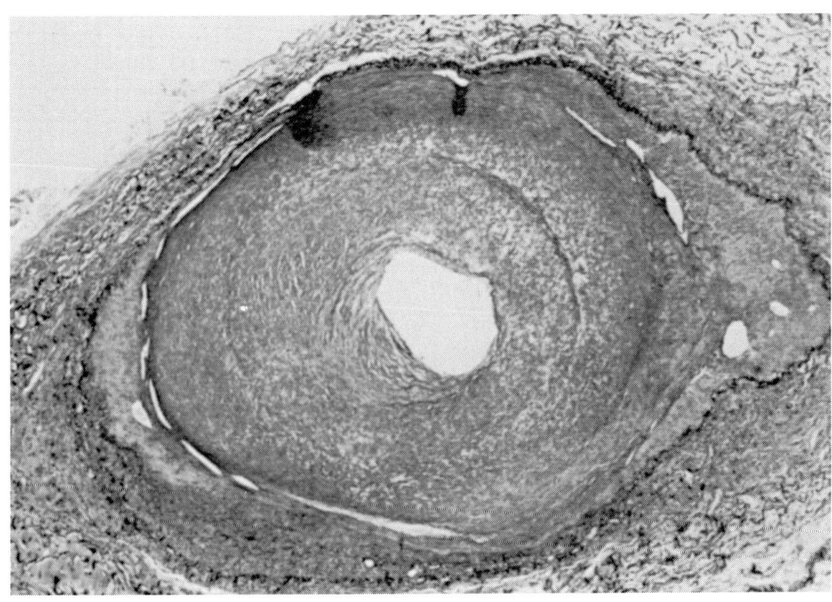

FIGURE 24–2. Histologic cross section demonstrating massive arteriosclerotic plaque in a saphenous vein coronary artery bypass graft. The patient had undergone bypass grafting 6 years previously. (×45.) (Courtesy of D. Gordon, M.D.)

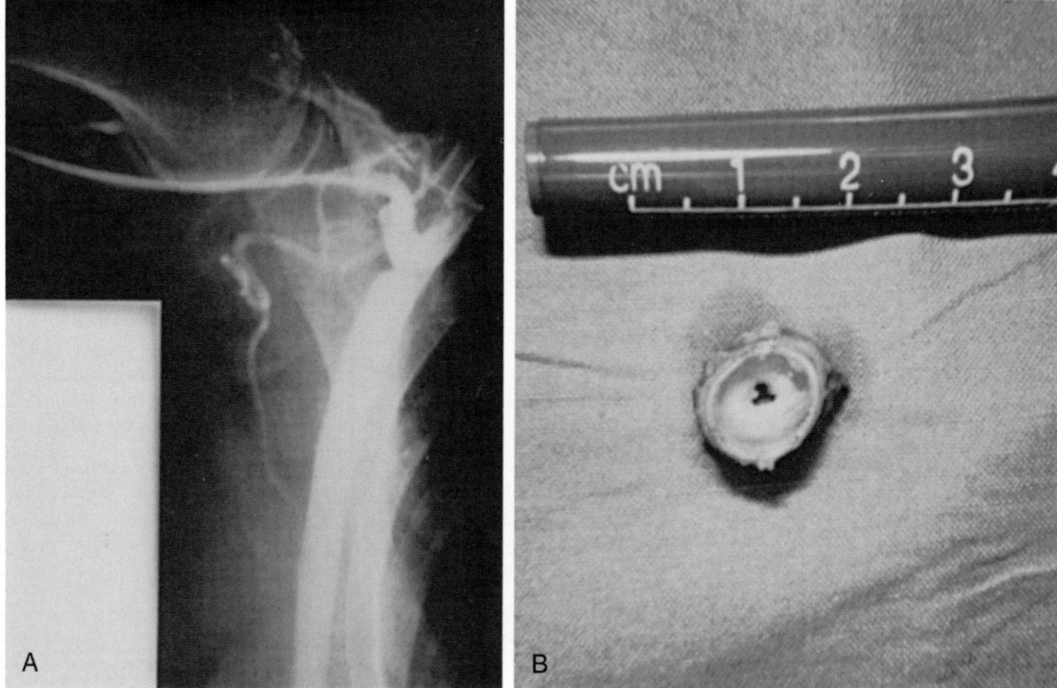

FIGURE 24–3. An elderly woman had symptomatic decrease in right ankle blood pressure 2 years after right axillofemoral bypass with a Dacron graft. *A*, Right transaxillary arteriogram showed a buckle in the axillary artery and a thin, diaphragm-like stenosis at the anastomosis. The stenotic portion of the graft was resected. *B*, End-on view showed a pinhole opening. The lesion was composed of smooth muscle cells covered by endothelium. (*A* and *B*, From Clowes AW: Current theories of arterial graft failure. Vasc Diagn Ther 3:41–52, 1982.)

and are covered on the luminal surface by a continuous monolayer of endothelium. In adult animals, endothelium and SMCs are in a state of quiescence, and turnover of these cells is barely detectable; in the rat, this figure is approximately 0.06%/day.[4] After the surface has been denuded of endothelium, a stereotyped sequence of events ensues and leads to intimal thickening (Fig. 24–4). The denuded regions are immediately covered by a carpet of platelets. The platelets are then displaced by an advancing front of regenerating endothelium over a period of days. At the same time, SMCs in the media begin to proliferate. They then migrate into the intima and continue to proliferate as well as to synthesize and to secrete large amounts of extracellular matrix.

Even as the endothelial cells are being stripped away, platelets begin to adhere to the exposed subendothelium and to spread.[50, 51] The adherence and spreading are mediated by glycoproteins present in the platelet membranes and exogenous substrate molecules, such as von Willebrand's factor, fibrin, collagen and thrombospondin.[52] It is surprising that the accumulation of platelets on the denuded surface of normal artery is a limited process, and if inhibited for a period of 8 hours by the infusion of prostacyclin (PGI_2), it does not occur at all.[53, 54] The reason for this change is not known; it might be related to some form of chemical adaptation that renders the denuded wall nonthrombogenic. Synthetic arterial surfaces lacking an endothelial covering do not exhibit this property and remain thrombogenic for years.[55]

As part of the process of adhesion, platelets release their granules. These granules contain not only vasoactive and thrombotic factors, such as serotonin, adenosine diphosphate, fibrinogen, and von Willebrand's factor, but also growth factors, such as platelet-derived growth factor (PDGF), transforming growth factor beta (TGF-β), and epidermal growth factor[56]; in theory, these growth factors might be the mitogenic stimulus for the initiation of smooth muscle growth since they are potent activators of SMC growth in vitro.

Endothelial cells regenerate from untraumatized sources adjacent to the damaged vessel and advance as a broad-growing edge.[57, 58] In damaged thoracic aorta, endothelial cells derived from intercostal vessel artery orifices migrate not only longitudinally but also transversely around the perimeter of the aorta. In vessels subjected to endarterectomy, transected vasa vasorum can serve as sources of endothelium.[59] Migration begins within hours of injury and proliferation begins by 24 hours. In most circumstances, the process goes to completion. If the distance between sources of endothelium is large, however, the denuded region may never become covered with endothelium.[60] The reason for the limited ability of endothelium to cover a denuded surface has yet to be identified.

SMCs respond to the injury stimulus by first proliferating in the media, then migrating from the media to the intima, and finally proliferating in the intima to form an intimal thickening. In the balloon-injured rat carotid, SMCs synthesize deoxyribonucleic acid (DNA) (s phase) approximately 27 hours after injury.[61] They then continue to proliferate for 7 to 14 days before stopping spontaneously (Fig. 24–5). A limited cohort of cells enter the growth fraction (between 20% and 40%) and do so shortly after injury.[62] The apparent growth fraction does not change after the first few days.

Once committed to proliferation, these cells appear to

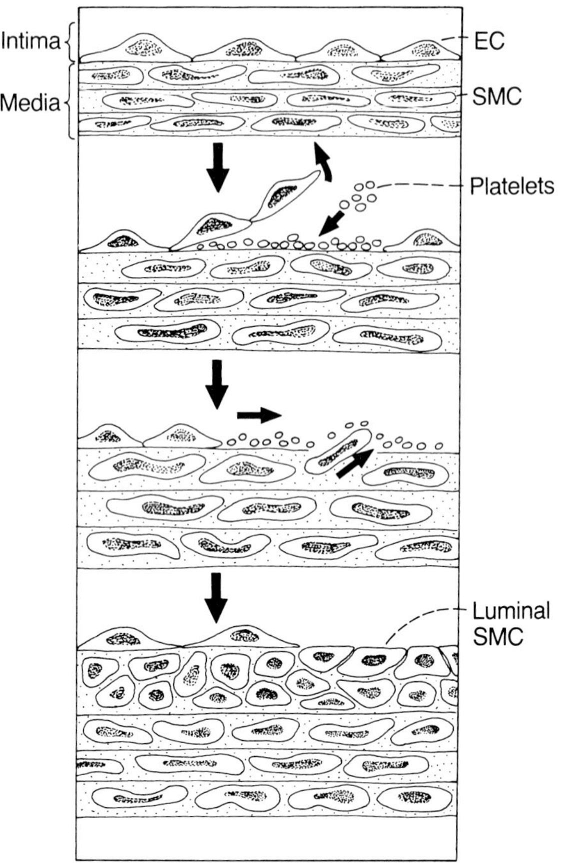

FIGURE 24–4. Schematic representation of arterial reaction to injury. *Upper panel,* A normal elastic artery is shown in cross section with endothelium (EC) on the luminal surface and smooth muscle cells (SMC) in the media. When the endothelial layer is disrupted, platelets accumulate in the denuded region (*second panel*). The surface layer is regenerated by an advancing endothelial front even as smooth muscle cells begin to proliferate in the media and migrate into the intima (*third panel*). Smooth muscle cells continue to proliferate to form an intimal thickening. They also form a luminal surface (luminal SMC) where endothelium is absent (*bottom panel*).

undergo three to four rounds of division and then stop dividing despite the absence of an overlying endothelium. In injured rat carotid artery, the central portion of the artery remains without endothelium for more than 12 months. In this region, SMCs form a surface that is relatively nonthrombogenic. Unlike endothelium, however, it is incapable of forming a layer of limited permeability for large molecules. SMCs located at the luminal surface of chronically denuded regions continue to proliferate at levels (~10- to 100-fold) above background, even as late as 1 year after injury.[60] This proliferation of surface SMCs appears to be matched by cell death because there is no net accumulation of smooth muscle within the wall after 2 weeks.

In the injured rat carotid artery, although the SMC content of the wall is the same at 2 and 12 weeks, nevertheless the amount of intimal thickening doubles between 2 and 12 weeks (Fig. 24–6).[5] The increase in intimal volume can be accounted for entirely by an increase in extracellular matrix, including elastin, collagen, and proteoglycan. In some circumstances, massive lipid accumulation is observed, particularly underneath the regenerated endothelium.[63]

Considered all together, these observations support the concept that the process of injury-induced intimal thickening involves early thrombosis on the denuded wall followed by SMC proliferation and, finally, deposition of matrix by SMCs. Hence, smooth muscle proliferation plays a central role in the development of the intimal lesion. Endothelium, in this model of intimal thickening, appears to modulate smooth muscle proliferation, accumulation of lipid, and to some extent vasomotor activity in the artery.[64] The "reaction-to-injury" hypothesis suggests that the initial injury and the final intimal thickening might be linked by the early thrombotic events and the release of smooth muscle growth factors from adherent platelets into the damaged artery.[64] This hypothesis is supported by early studies of arterial injury in animals. Injured aortas from rabbits rendered thrombocytopenic by administration of antiplatelet antibody appeared to develop smaller intimal thickenings.[65, 66] The reduction in intimal thickening in the ballooned rat carotid model of arterial injury is due to inhibition of SMC migration, and the magnitude of the first wave of SMC proliferation is the same in control and thrombocytopenic animals.[67] These somewhat unexpected results indicate that factors from thrombus are chemoattractants for SMCs and fibroblasts. These factors are now being defined.

One of the factors released from platelets, PDGF, stimulates SMC migration from the media when infused in pharmacologic doses.[68] Injection of an antibody to PDGF or the

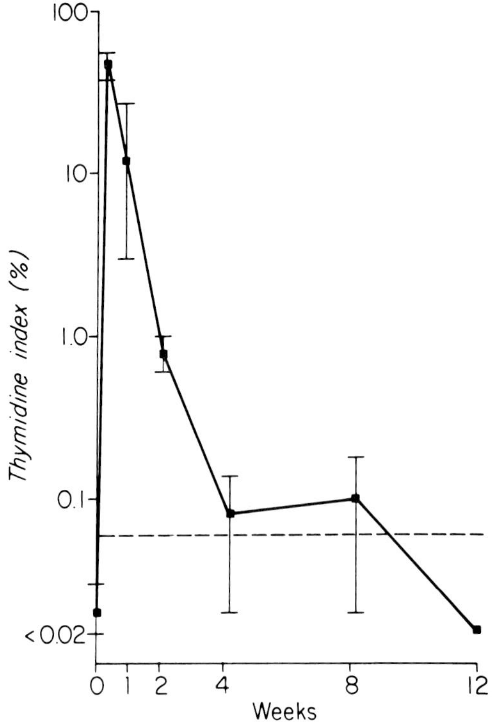

FIGURE 24–5. Schematic representation of the pattern of smooth muscle cell proliferation (thymidine index) as a function of time after injury. These cells start in the resting state with a labeling index of approximately 0.06% per day (*dashed line*). After injury, the fraction of proliferating cells increases to 20% to 50% per day and then returns to background levels by 4 weeks.

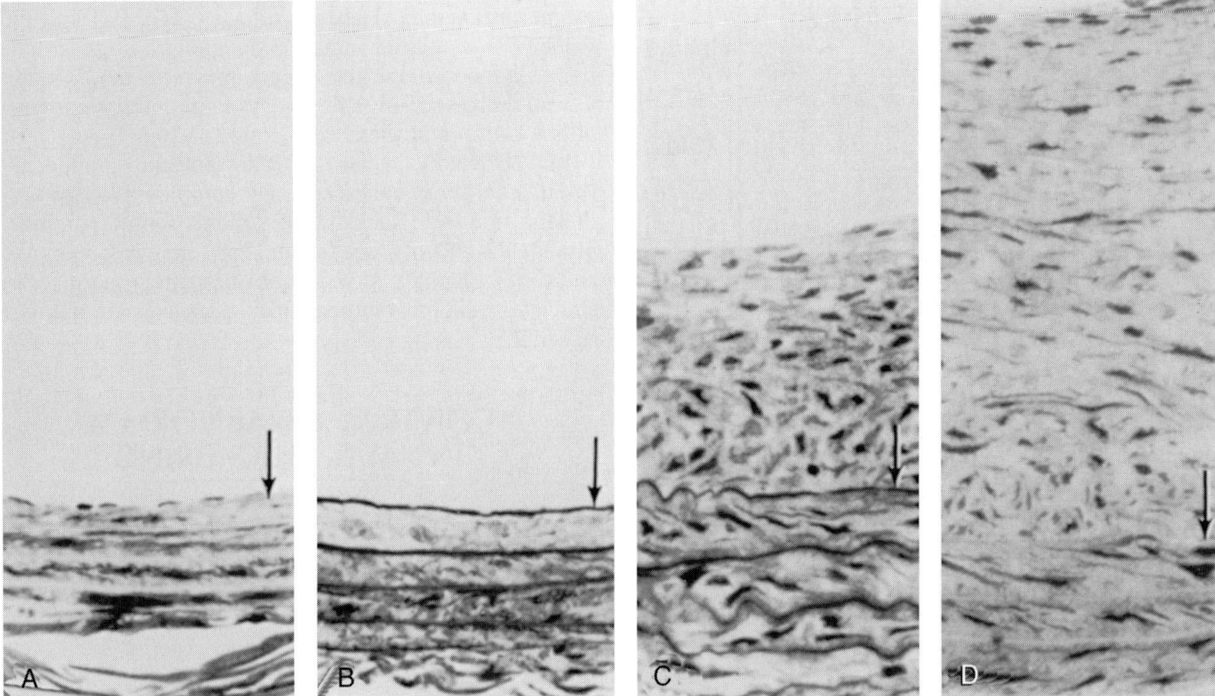

FIGURE 24–6. Histologic cross sections of rat carotid artery before injury (*A*), immediately after endothelial denudation with a balloon catheter (*B*), 2 weeks after injury (*C*), and 12 weeks after injury (*D*). Note the marked intimal thickening at 2 and 12 weeks. *Arrows* indicate elastic lamina. The lumen is at top. (*A–D*, From Clowes AW, Reidy MA, Clowes MM: Kinetics of cellular proliferation after arterial injury: I. Smooth muscle growth in the absence of endothelium. Lab Invest 49:327–333, 1983. © U.S. and Canadian Academy of Pathology, Inc, 1983.)

beta form of the PDGF receptor or antisense oligonucleotide release against the PDGF receptor blocks intimal thickening but not SMC proliferation (E. Owens and A. Clowes, unpublished results).[69, 70] Thus, it appears that platelets and PDGF from platelets (or possibly vascular wall cells) regulate SMC movement and, thereby, intimal thickening in damaged arteries. However, studies using pharmacologic inhibitors of platelet aggregation have *not* provided convincing support for the role of platelets in the intimal thickening process except in circumstances associated with massive accumulation of thrombus.[54, 71–76] An explanation for these negative results is that most antithrombotic drugs do not block platelet adhesion.

The thrombocytopenia experiments raise several disturbing questions. If platelet factors affect only SMC migration, what regulates SMC proliferation in injured arteries and vascular grafts? Furthermore, what is the importance, if any, of vessel and cellular injury in this process? Answers to these questions come from studies of different animal models of vascular repair.

Selective removal of endothelium with a fine-filament loop produces detectable gaps, which are healed by migration and proliferation of adjacent endothelial cells. Nevertheless, even in examples of this kind of injury, which requires seven days or more for full repair, little SMC proliferation in the underlying media is evident,[57] although some intimal thickening can develop.[77] Infusion of endotoxin also produces endothelial injury, but a form of injury that can be repaired by local migration and proliferation at sufficient speed to allow repair before dead and dying endothelial cells actually are liberated from the surface. In this latter circumstance, no gaps are apparent and therefore no platelet accumulation is observed on the affected arteries. As well, no SMC proliferation is observed.

Several models have become available in which SMCs proliferate in the absence of endothelial denudation. It is apparent that they do so in response to hypertension, in the presence of a remote indwelling arterial catheter producing thrombosis, and over healing vascular grafts.[78–81] In all of these examples, there has been no evidence of actual denudation, although the endothelial cells exhibit increased thymidine labeling. There has also been a rough correlation between medial smooth muscle and overlying endothelial proliferation. In each case, SMCs proliferate *only* where endothelium is present. In the grafts, the endothelium is unlike regenerated endothelium in injured artery, and it continues to proliferate even though no gaps are apparent in the monolayer; this observation suggests that the endothelium may be subjected to a chronic but non-denuding form of injury.

In general, these experiments suggest that SMCs can proliferate whether or not endothelial cells are present. Furthermore, there may be a correlation between the extent of injury and the magnitude of the proliferative responses.[82] Medial damage and SMC proliferation are greater in balloon-injured than in filament loop–injured rat carotid arteries, even though the endothelium is stripped completely in the two situations. Denudation alone is not sufficient to drive SMC proliferation, and effects of balloon catheter injury other than denudation (such as injury to the underlying media and distention of the vessel) must be important. In models of chronic endothelial proliferation without denudation, the factors responsible for stimulating SMC growth must come from the vascular wall cells them-

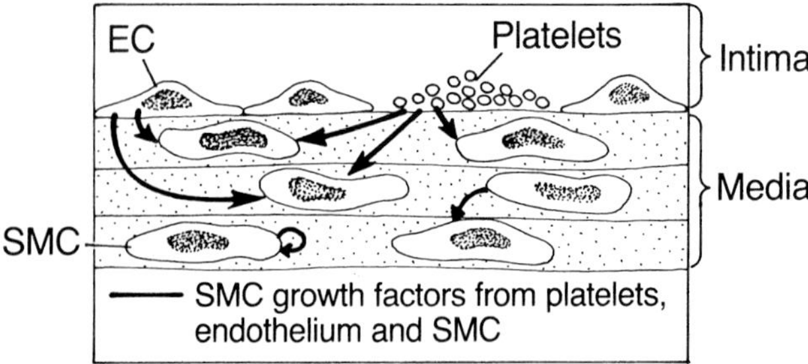

FIGURE 24–7. Diagrammatic representation of an injured artery suggests that a variety of cell types, including platelets, endothelium (EC), and smooth muscle cells (SMC), might secrete growth factors for smooth muscle cells. Macrophages (not shown) also synthesize and secrete smooth muscle mitogens.

selves, since platelets do not adhere to the endothelial lining.

It thus appears that something more than factors from platelets is required for smooth muscle growth. As suggested earlier, the vascular wall cells themselves or possibly small resident populations of macrophages appear to be the logical sources (Fig. 24–7).[83–85] At present, it is known that endothelial cells, SMCs, and macrophages in culture can synthesize and secrete several defined growth factors, one of which resembles PDGF.[86, 87]

Another such factor is basic fibroblast growth factor (bFGF). bFGF is stored in endothelial and smooth muscle cells, is released in response to injury, and is stored in the matrix.[88] It is a potent mitogen for endothelium and SMCs. When administered to rats in pharmacologic amounts, it stimulates SMC and endothelial proliferation; medial SMC proliferation is markedly inhibited by an antibody to bFGF.[89–91] These experiments indicate that the injury process itself and the factors released from dead and damaged cells stimulate the first wave of SMC proliferation while factors from platelets stimulate migration of SMCs into the intima (Fig. 24–8). The factors regulating proliferation in the intima have yet to be defined and may include angiotensin II,[92] thrombin,[93] endothelin,[93] insulin-like growth factor I,[94] and PDGF.[95, 96] Other factors, such as gamma interferon,[97] heparan sulfate,[98] TGF-β,[99] and nitric oxide[100, 101] may limit intimal SMC growth. Physical forces, such as blood flow and blood pressure, may modulate vascular structure by altering the local cellular expression of one or more of these biochemical factors.[80, 102, 103]

In conclusion, repair in even the simplest model of vascular injury is an exceedingly complex process; nevertheless, studies in such simple systems should continue to provide insights of value for understanding vascular growth and development[104] as well as for designing pharmacologic strategies to control intimal thickening after arterial reconstruction.

CONTROL OF ABNORMAL INTIMAL THICKENING

The formation of a thickened intima is part of the normal reparative response of an artery and graft to injury. As noted earlier, under some circumstances the amount of intima becomes excessive and produces marked luminal narrowing. This occurs in coronary arteries subjected to balloon angioplasty (30% in 6 months),[16, 17] vein grafts used for peripheral arterial bypass (10% in 6 to 24 months),[35] and coronary bypass grafts (52 to 75% in 10 years)[40, 41] and is an important cause of low flow and eventual thrombosis. In large measure, the therapy for prevention or correction of excessive intimal thickening has taken one of two approaches:

1. Antiplatelet and anticoagulant drugs have been given based on the assumption that the accumulation of platelets and clotting factors plays a role in early and late thrombosis and might play a role in the development of intimal thickening.[73, 76, 105]
2. Further surgical reconstruction has been undertaken based on the assumption that renewed or continued intimal thickening is unlikely.

Aspirin and dipyridamole have been effective in reducing coronary bypass graft failure by approximately 10% in several clinical series.[73] However, these drugs are effective

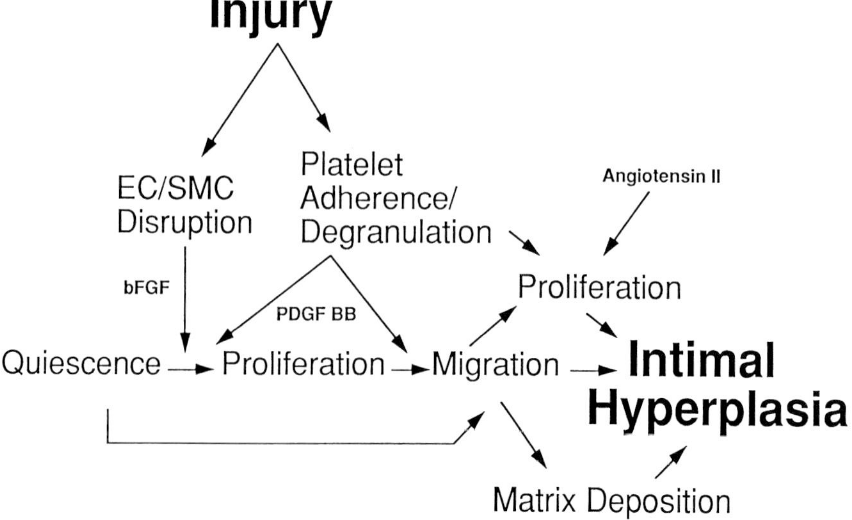

FIGURE 24–8. Diagram representing how injury to the artery might cause endothelial (EC) and smooth muscle cell (SMC) disruption and release of intracellular mitogens such as basic fibroblast growth factor (bFGF). FGF then stimulates medial smooth muscle proliferation. Factors from platelets, such as platelet-derived growth factor (PDGF), regulate movement of the smooth muscle cells from the media to the intima. Angiotensin II also affects the intimal thickening process. (From Clowes AW, Reidy MA: Prevention of stenosis after vascular reconstruction: Pharmacologic control of intimal hyperplasia—a review. J Vasc Surg 13:885–891, 1991.)

only if given at or within a short time of the surgery; if therapy is delayed more than two days the drugs are of no benefit when the grafts are evaluated by angiography at late times. This observation suggests that these drugs are preventing either acute graft occlusion or the early accumulation of thrombus, which might later be remodeled into a fibrous lesion. Similar studies in patients receiving peripheral bypass grafts have shown a negative or a weak effect.[73, 76] In animal studies, the effects of antithrombotic drugs on intimal thickening in injured arteries and in vascular grafts have been both positive and negative.[71–75, 106] In view of what is known about smooth muscle proliferation and intimal thickening, it seems logical that aspirin and related drugs affect only wound healing events associated with platelet aggregation and accumulation of large thrombi.

Newer forms of antithrombotic therapy (inhibitors of platelet glycoprotein IIb/IIIa, ticlopidine) appear to provide long-term benefit in coronary arteries subjected to angioplasty or peripheral vein bypass grafts.[50, 107] Although the drugs probably exert their effects by inhibiting platelet activation, they may also block SMC directly. For example, the SMC integrin $\alpha_v\beta_3$ is structurally related to platelet glycoprotein IIb/IIIa and, together with other integrins, is utilized for cell attachment and migration.[108]

Further vascular reconstruction has remained the principal form of therapy for salvage of failing grafts and other vascular reconstructions. Several groups have demonstrated that assiduous follow-up of patients undergoing vein bypass reconstruction of femoropopliteal disease allows stenoses due to intimal hyperplasia to be discovered before these lesions actually cause graft thrombosis.[35, 37, 109] If these lesions are reconstructed before they cause thrombosis, the long-term outcome is extremely good; if the grafts go on to thrombosis and the stenotic lesions are identified by arteriography only after the grafts have been subjected to thrombectomy, however, the reconstructions generally fail.

These results tend to support the conclusion that the stenotic process, at least in peripheral bypass grafts, is limited and, if corrected, does not recur; this conclusion fits very well with the observations in animal models indicating that arterial intimal thickening in response to injury is a self-limited process. The difference in humans relates to the presence of significant atherogenic risk factors, which have a marked impact on the atherosclerotic process in proximal and distal vessels as well as in the grafts.

The clinical experience with recurrent carotid stenosis is similar to the experience with the peripheral bypass grafts; the carotid arteries, when treated with vein patch grafts, remain patent. Stenotic lesions at anastomoses between synthetic grafts and arteries have proved more difficult to correct because they tend to recur. No satisfactory approach has been developed to deal with these problems. In general, it appears that frequent follow-up assessments of surgical reconstructions followed by appropriate further reconstruction provides optimal treatment for intimal hyperplastic lesions causing luminal stenosis of vascular reconstructions. Antithrombotic therapy seems to reduce the rate of occlusion in coronary bypass grafts and in arteries subjected to angioplasty. The benefit of these drugs in preventing carotid restenosis and peripheral graft occlusion is not certain.

Several interesting forms of therapy are being developed. As has been obvious throughout this chapter, endothelium plays a pivotal and complicated role in the function of the normal artery and the artery undergoing repair. Regenerating endothelium over injured artery suppresses SMC proliferation and inhibits platelet accumulation on the artery wall.[110] Because of these observations, a number of investigators have been studying the behavior of grafts deliberately seeded with endothelium.[111] These grafts, at least in animal models, tend to resist thrombosis and to have lesser amounts of intimal thickening. Endothelial seeding also appears to improve graft patency in humans.[112, 113] We have pursued an alternative approach to solving the problem of endothelialization of synthetic grafts. By changing the porosity of polytetrafluoroethylene (PTFE) grafts (from 30 to 60 μm internodal distance), we have been able to produce spontaneous rapid endothelialization in animal experiments. This endothelial layer develops from multiple transmural capillaries arising from the granulation tissue surrounding the graft.[114] It is unfortunate that when the 60 μm PTFE grafts are placed in humans as femoropopliteal bypasses, they do not appear to develop an endothelial lining, although occasional intramural capillaries are seen.[47] Adjuvant pharmacology is necessary to stimulate capillary ingrowth and endothelial coverage. Some form of endothelial chemoattractant (e.g., bFGF) might be inserted into the interstices of the graft. This approach to enhancing spontaneous endothelialization is being pursued actively in a number of laboratories.[115, 116]

Another alternative is to employ specific inhibitors of SMC proliferation since, as already shown, proliferation of SMC and subsequent deposition by SMC of extracellular matrix are central to the development of intimal hyperplasia. A number of drugs have been tried in animal models of arterial injury and in patients undergoing transluminal angioplasty of the coronary arteries. Although many drugs are inhibitory in the animal models, none have proved successful in preventing coronary restenosis in humans.[117–120]

Cytotoxic and cytostatic strategies are being developed to destroy or suppress proliferative SMCs and thereby limit intimal hyperplasia. For example, local irradiation has been used in animals and, to a limited extent, in humans.[121–123] The long-term impact of radiation is not known. Arteries treated in this way might remain patent, or they might develop fibroproliferative lesions.

Cytostatic strategies may prove to be of greater value, since the problem is to restrict SMC growth while still permitting repair of the vascular injury. In addition, it is now understood that luminal narrowing may be the consequence of vascular constriction as well as intimal hyperplasia.[124] Inhibitors that block both aspects of this process would be potentially valuable. Several factors possess vasodilator and growth inhibitor properties; for example, nitric oxide released by the endothelial nitric oxide gene transferred to the wall or by local administration of nitric oxide analogues dilates vessels and suppresses intimal thickening.[101]

Gene therapy has the potential to introduce inhibitor genes into the site of injury and thereby produce a local pharmacologic effect without causing systemic toxicity. Gene transfer is accomplished using various viral or nonviral vectors containing DNA encoding the inhibitor gene, and the expression of the gene can last for a short or long time, depending on the vector.[125] However, no trials have yet been conducted to establish proof of efficacy.

SUMMARY

SMC proliferation and the formation of a thickened intima is part of normal wound healing in injured arteries and vascular grafts. At times, this process becomes excessive and leads to luminal stenosis and eventual failure of vascular reconstructions. Many of the growth factors and inhibitors that regulate the balance between normal healing and pathologic stenosis have been defined. Nevertheless, the treatment of vascular stenosis due to intimal hyperplasia remains largely surgical. A detailed understanding of the biology of SMC growth and intimal hyperplasia should eventually lead to new forms of preventive adjuvant therapy.

REFERENCES

1. Ross R, Glomset JA: The pathogenesis of atherosclerosis. N Engl J Med 295:369–377, 420–425, 1976.
2. Clowes AW, Gown AM, Hanson SR, Reidy MA: Mechanisms of arterial graft failure: I. Role of cellular proliferation in early healing of PTFE prostheses. Am J Pathol 118:43–54, 1985.
3. Libby P: Lesion versus lumen. Nature Med 1:17–18, 1995.
4. Clowes AW, Reidy MA, Clowes MM: Kinetics of cellular proliferation after arterial injury: I. Smooth muscle growth in the absence of endothelium. Lab Invest 49:327–333, 1983.
5. Clowes AW, Reidy MA, Clowes MM: Mechanisms of stenosis after arterial injury. Lab Invest 49:208–215, 1983.
6. Chidi CC, DePalma RG: Atherogenic potential of the embolectomy catheter. Surgery 83:549–557, 1978.
7. Mondy JS, Williams JK, Adams MR, et al: Structural determinants of lumen narrowing after angioplasty in atherosclerotic nonhuman primates. J Vasc Surg 26:875–883, 1997.
8. Steele PM, Chesebro JH, Stanson AW, et al: Balloon angioplasty: Natural history of the pathophysiological response to injury in a pig model. Circ Res 57:105–112, 1985.
9. Zarins CK, Lu CT, Gewertz BL, et al: Arterial disruption and remodeling following balloon dilatation. Surgery 92:1086–1095, 1982.
10. Geary RL, Williams JK, Golden D, et al: Time course of cellular proliferation, intimal hyperplasia, and remodeling following angioplasty in monkeys with established atherosclerosis: A nonhuman primate model of restenosis. Arterioscler Thromb Vasc Biol 16:34–43, 1996.
11. Scott NA, Cipolla GD, Ross CE, et al: Identification of a potential role for the adventitia in vascular lesion formation after balloon overstretch injury of porcine coronary arteries. Circulation 93:2178–2187, 1996.
12. Shi Y, O'Brien JE, Jr, et al: Adventitial myofibroblasts contribute to neointimal formation in injured porcine coronary arteries. Circulation 94:1655–1664, 1996.
13. Gallino A, Mahler F, Probst P, Nachbur B: Percutaneous transluminal angioplasty of the arteries of the lower limbs: A 5-year follow-up. Circulation 70:619–623, 1984.
14. Lally ME, Johnston KW, Andrews D: Percutaneous transluminal dilatation of peripheral arteries: An analysis of factors predicting early success. J Vasc Surg 1:704–709, 1984.
15. Tegtmeyer CJ, Hartwell GD, Selby JB, et al: Results and complications of angioplasty in aortoiliac disease. Circulation 83(Suppl)I53–I60, 1991.
16. Holmes DR, Vlietstra RE, Smith HC, et al: Restenosis after percutaneous transluminal coronary angioplasty (PCTA): A report from the PTCA Registry of the National Heart, Lung, and Blood Institute. Am J Cardiol 53:77C–81C, 1984.
17. Fanelli C, Aronoff R: Restenosis following coronary angioplasty. Am Heart J 119:357–368, 1990.
18. Kumpe DA, Jones DN: Percutaneous transluminal angioplasty: Radiological viewpoint. Vasc Diagn Therapy 3:19–22, 1982.
19. Spence K, Freiman DB, Gatenby R: Long-term results of transluminal angioplasty of the iliac and femoral arteries. Arch Surg 116:1377–1384, 1981.
20. Lafont A, Guzman LA, Whitlow PL, et al: Restenosis after experimental angioplasty: Intimal, medial, and adventitial changes associated with constrictive remodeling. Circ Res 76:996–1002, 1995.
21. Hoffmann R, Mintz GS, Dussaillant GR, et al: Patterns and mechanisms of in-stent restenosis: A serial intravascular ultrasound study. Circulation 94:1247–1254, 1996.
22. Post MJ, De Smet BJGL, Van der Helm Y, et al: Arterial remodeling after balloon angioplasty or stenting in an atherosclerotic experimental model. Circulation 96:996–1003, 1997.
23. Mintz GS, Popma JJ, Pichard AD, et al: Arterial remodeling after coronary angioplasty: A serial intravascular ultrasound study. Circulation 94:35–43, 1996.
24. Kakuta T, Usui M, Coats WD, Jr, et al: Arterial remodeling at the reference site after angioplasty in the atherosclerotic rabbit model. Arterioscler Thromb Vasc Biol 18:47–51, 1998.
25. Callow AD: Recurrent stenosis after carotid endarterectomy. Arch Surg 117:1082–1085, 1982.
26. Clagett GP, Robinowitz M, Youkey JR, et al: Morphogenesis and clinicopathologic characteristics of recurrent carotid disease. J Vasc Surg 3:10–23, 1986.
27. Nicholls SC, Phillips DJ, Bergelin RO, et al: Carotid endarterectomy: Relationship of outcome to early restenosis. J Vasc Surg 2:375–381, 1985.
28. Stoney RJ, String ST: Recurrent carotid stenosis. Surgery 80:705–710, 1976.
29. Thomas M, Otis SM, Rush M, et al: Recurrent carotid artery stenosis following endarterectomy. Ann Surg 200:74–79, 1984.
30. Zierler RE, Bandyk DF, Thiele BL, Strandness DE Jr: Carotid artery stenosis following endarterectomy. Arch Surg 117:1408–1415, 1982.
31. Cambria RP, Megerman J, Abbott WM: Endothelial preservation in reversed and in situ autogenous vein grafts. Ann Surg 202:50–55, 1985.
32. Fuchs JC, Mitchener JS, 3d, Hagen PO: Postoperative changes in autologous vein grafts. Ann Surg 188:1–15, 1978.
33. LoGerfo FW, Quist WC, Cantelmo NL, Haudenschild CC: Integrity of vein grafts as a function of initial intimal and medial preservation. Circulation 68:II-117–II-124, 1983.
34. Szilagyi DE, Elliott JP, Hageman JH, et al: Biologic fate of autogenous vein implants as arterial substitutes. Ann Surg 178:232–245, 1973.
35. Whittemore AD, Clowes AW, Couch NP, Mannick JA: Secondary femoropopliteal reconstruction. Ann Surg 193:35–42, 1981.
36. Gentile AT, Mills JL, Gooden MA, et al: Identification of predictors for lower extremity vein graft stenosis. Am J Surg 174:218–221, 1997.
37. Bandyk DF, Kaebnick HW, Stewart GW, Towne JB: Durability of the in situ saphenous vein arterial bypass: A comparison of primary and secondary patency. J Vasc Surg 5:256–268, 1987.
38. DePalma RG: Atherosclerosis in vascular grafts. Atheroscler Rev 6:146–177, 1979.
39. Spray TL, Roberts WC: Changes in saphenous veins used as aortocoronary bypass grafts. Am Heart J 94:500–516, 1977.
40. Grondin CM, Campeau L, Lesperance J, et al: Comparison of late changes in internal mammary artery and saphenous vein grafts in two consecutive series of patients 10 years after operation. Circulation 70:I-208–I-212, 1984.
41. Campeau L, Enjalbert M, Lesperance J, Bourassa MG: The relation of risk factors to the development of atherosclerosis in saphenous-vein bypass grafts and the progression of disease in the native circulation. N Engl J Med 311:1329–1332, 1984.
42. Echave V, Koornick AR, Haimov M, Jacobson JH: Intimal hyperplasia as a complication of the use of the polytetrafluoroethylene graft for femoral-popliteal bypass. Surgery 86:791–798, 1979.
43. LoGerfo FW, Quist WC, Nowak MD, et al: Downstream anastomotic hyperplasia: A mechanism of failure in Dacron arterial grafts. Ann Surg 197:479–483, 1983.
44. Selman SH, Rhodes RS, Anderson JM, et al: Atheromatous changes in expanded polytetrafluoroethylene grafts. Surgery 87:630–637, 1980.
45. Szilagyi DE, Smith RF, Elliott JP, Allen HM: Long-term behavior of a Dacron arterial substitute: Clinical, roentgenologic and histologic correlations. Ann Surg 162:453–477, 1965.

46. Berger K, Sauvage LR, Rao AM, Wood SJ: Healing of arterial prostheses in man: its incompleteness. Ann Surg 175:118–127, 1972.
47. Clowes AW, Kohler T: Graft endothelialization: The role of angiogenic mechanisms. J Vasc Surg 13:734–736, 1991.
48. Shi Q, Wu MH-D, Hayashida N, et al: Proof of fallout endothelialization of impervious Dacron grafts in the aorta and inferior vena cava of the dog. J Vasc Surg 20:546–557, 1994.
49. Wu MH-D, Shi Q, Wechezak AR, et al: Definitive proof of endothelialization of a Dacron arterial prosthesis in a human being. J Vasc Surg 21:862–867, 1995.
50. Coller BS, Anderson KM, Weisman HF: The anti–GPIIb-IIIa agents: Fundamental and clinical aspects. Haemostasis 26:285–293, 1996.
51. LeBreton H, Topol E, Plow EF: Evidence for a pivotal role of platelets in vascular reocclusion and restenosis. Cardiovasc Res 31:235–236, 1996.
52. George JN, Nurden AT, Phillips DR: Molecular defects in interactions of platelets with the vessel wall. N Engl J Med 311:1084–1098, 1984.
53. Groves HM, Kinlough-Rathbone RL, Richardson M, et al: Platelet interaction with damaged rabbit aorta. Lab Invest 40:194–200, 1979.
54. Groves HM, Kinlough-Rathbone RL, Mustard JF: Development of nonthrombogenicity of injured rabbit aortas despite inhibition of platelet adherence. Arteriosclerosis 6:189–195, 1986.
55. Stratton JR, Thiele BL, Ritchie JL: Platelet deposition on Dacron aortic bifurcation grafts in man: Quantitation with indium 111 platelet imaging. Circulation 66:1287–1293, 1982.
56. Bowen-Pope DF, Ross R, Seifert RA: Locally acting growth factors for vascular smooth muscle cells: Endogenous synthesis and release from platelets. Circulation 72:735–740, 1985.
57. Reidy MA: A reassessment of endothelial injury and arterial lesion formation. Lab Invest 53:513–520, 1985.
58. Schwartz SM, Haudenschild CC, Eddy EM: Endothelial regeneration: I. Quantitative analysis of initial stages of endothelial regeneration in rat aortic intima. Lab Invest 38:568–580, 1978.
59. Shi Q, Wu H-D, Sauvage LR, et al: Reendothelialization of isolated segments of the canine carotid artery with reference to the possible role of the adventitial vasa vasorum. J Vasc Surg 12:476–487, 1990.
60. Clowes AW, Clowes MM, Reidy MA: Kinetics of cellular proliferation after arterial injury: III. Endothelial and smooth muscle growth in chronically denuded vessels. Lab Invest 54:295–303, 1986.
61. Majesky MW, Schwartz SM, Clowes MM, Clowes AW: Heparin regulates smooth muscle S phase entry in the injured rat carotid artery. Circ Res 61:296–300, 1987.
62. Clowes AW, Schwartz SM: Significance of quiescent smooth muscle migration in the injured rat carotid artery. Circ Res 56:139–145, 1985.
63. Falcone DJ, Hajjar DP, Minick CR: Lipoprotein and albumin accumulation in reendothelialized and deendothelialized aorta. Am J Pathol 114:112–120, 1984.
64. Ross R: Pathogenesis of atherosclerosis: An update. N Engl J Med 314:488–500, 1986.
65. Friedman RJ, Stemerman MB, Wenz B, et al: The effect of thrombocytopenia on experimental atherosclerotic lesion formation in rabbits: Smooth muscle cell proliferation and re-endothelialization. J Clin Invest 60:1191–1201, 1977.
66. Moore S, Friedman RJ, Singal DP, et al: Inhibition of injury-induced thromboathero-sclerotic lesions by antiplatelet serum in rabbits. Thromb Haemost 35:70–81, 1976.
67. Fingerle J, Johnson R, Clowes AW, et al: Role of platelets in smooth muscle cell proliferation and migration after vascular injury in rat carotid artery. Proc Natl Acad Sci U S A 86:8412–8416, 1989.
68. Jawien A, Bowen-Pope DF, Lindner V, et al: Platelet-derived growth factor promotes smooth muscle migration and intimal thickening in a rat model of balloon angioplasty. J Clin Invest 89:507–511, 1992.
69. Ferns GAA, Raines EW, Sprugel KH, et al: Inhibition of neointimal smooth muscle accumulation after angioplasty by an antibody to PDGF. Science 253:1129–1132, 1991.
70. Sirois MG, Simons M, Edelman ER: Antisense oligonucleotide inhibition of PDGFR-β receptor subunit expression directs suppression of intimal thickening. Circulation 95:669–676, 1997.
71. Bomberger RA, DePalma RG, Ambrose TA, Manalo P: Aspirin and dipyridamole inhibit endothelial healing. Arch Surg 117:1459–1464, 1982.
72. Clowes AW, Karnovsky MJ: Failure of certain antiplatelet drugs to affect myointimal thickening following arterial injury. Lab Invest 36:452–458, 1977.
73. Clowes AW: The role of aspirin in enhancing arterial graft patency. J Vasc Surg 3:381–385, 1986.
74. Faxon DP, Sanborn TA, Haudenschild CC, Ryan TJ: Effect of antiplatelet therapy on restenosis after experimental angioplasty. Am J Cardiol 53:72C–76C, 1984.
75. Radic ZS, O'Mallery MK, Mikat EM, et al: The role of aspirin and dipyridamole on vascular DNA synthesis and intimal hyperplasia following deendothelialization. J Surg Res 41:84–91, 1986.
76. Clagett GP, Genton E, Salzman EW: Antithrombotic therapy in peripheral vascular disease. Chest 95:128S–139S, 1989.
77. Fingerle J, Au YPT, Clowes AW, Reidy MA: Intimal lesion formation in rat carotid arteries after endothelial denudation in absence of medial injury. Arteriosclerosis 10:1082–1087, 1990.
78. Owens GK, Reidy MA: Hyperplastic growth response of vascular smooth muscle cells following induction of acute hypertension in rats by aortic coarctation. Circ Res 57:695–705, 1985.
79. Reidy MA, Chao SS, Kirkman TR, Clowes AW: Endothelial regeneration: VI. Chronic nondenuding injury in baboon vascular grafts. Am J Pathol 123:432–439, 1986.
80. Kohler TR, Kirkman TR, Kraiss LW, et al: Increased blood flow inhibits neointimal hyperplasia in endothelialized vascular grafts. Circ Res 69:1557–1565, 1991.
81. Geary RL, Kohler TR, Vergel S, et al: Time course of flow-induced smooth muscle cell proliferation and intimal thickening in endothelialized baboon vascular grafts. Circ Res 74:14–23, 1994.
82. Clowes AW, Clowes MM, Fingerle J, Reidy MA: Regulation of smooth muscle cell growth in injured artery. J Cardiovasc Pharmacol 14(Suppl 6):S12–S15, 1989.
83. Landry DB, Couper LL, Bryant SR, Lindner V: Activation of the NF-kappa B and I kappa B system in smooth muscle cells after rat arterial injury: Induction of vascular cell adhesion molecule-1 and monocyte chemoattractant protein-1. Am J Pathol 151:1085–1095, 1997.
84. Stadius ML, Gown AM, Kernoff R, Collins CL: Cell proliferation after balloon injury of iliac arteries in the cholesterol-fed New Zealand White rabbit. Arterioscler Thromb 14:727–733, 1994.
85. Hancock WW, Adams DH, Wyner LR, et al: $CD4^+$ mononuclear cells induce cytokine expression, vascular smooth muscle cell proliferation, and arterial occlusion after endothelial injury. Am J Pathol 145:1008–1014, 1994.
86. Raines EW, Ross R: Platelet-derived growth factor in vivo. Cytokines 5:74–114, 1993.
87. Claesson-Welsh L: Mechanism of action of platelet-derived growth factor. Int J Biochem Cell Biol 28:373–385, 1996.
88. D'Amore PA: Modes of FGF release in vivo and in vitro. Cancer Metastasis Rev 9:227–238, 1990.
89. Lindner V, Majack RA, Reidy MA: Basic fibroblast growth factor stimulates endothelial regrowth and proliferation in denuded arteries. J Clin Invest 85:2004–2008, 1990.
90. Lindner V, Lappi DA, Baird A, et al: Role of basic fibroblast growth factor in vascular lesion formation. Circ Res 68:106–113, 1991.
91. Lindner V, Reidy MA: Proliferation of smooth muscle cells after vascular injury is inhibited by an antibody against basic fibroblast growth factor. Proc Natl Acad Sci USA 88:3739–3743, 1991.
92. Daemen MJAP, Lombardi DM, Bosman FT, Schwartz SM: Angiotensin II induces smooth muscle cell proliferation in the normal and injured rat arterial wall. Circ Res 68:450–456, 1991.
93. McNamara CA, Sarembock IJ, Bachhuber BG, Stouffer GA, et al: Thrombin and vascular smooth muscle cell proliferation: Implications for atherosclerosis and restenosis. Semin Thromb Hemost 22:139–144, 1996.
94. Bornfeldt KE, Arnqvist HJ, Capron L: In vivo proliferation of rat vascular smooth muscle in relation to diabetes mellitus insulin-like growth factor I and insulin. Diabetologia 35:104–108, 1992.
95. Majesky MW, Reidy MA, Bowen-Pope DF, et al: PDGF ligand and receptor gene expression during repair of arterial injury. J Cell Biol 111:2149–2158, 1990.
96. Golden MA, Au YPT, Kirkman TR, et al: Platelet-derived growth factor activity and mRNA expression in healing vascular grafts in baboons: Association in vivo of platelet-derived growth factor mRNA and protein with cellular proliferation. J Clin Invest 87:406–414, 1991.
97. Hansson GK, Jonasson L, Holm J, et al: Gamma interferon regulates

vascular smooth muscle proliferation and Ia expression in vitro and in vivo. Circ Res 63:712–719, 1988.
98. Castellot JJ, Jr, Addonizio ML, Rosenberg R, Karnovsky MJ: Cultured endothelial cells produce a heparin-like inhibitor of smooth muscle cell growth. J Cell Biol 90:372–379, 1981.
99. Majesky MW, Lindner V, Twardzik DR, et al: Production of transforming growth factor β_1 during repair of arterial injury. J Clin Invest 88:904–910, 1991.
100. Cooke JP, Dzau VJ: Nitric oxide synthase: Role in the genesis of vascular disease. Annu Rev Med 48:489–509, 1997.
101. Von der Leyen HE, Gibbons GH, Morishita R, et al: Gene therapy inhibiting neointimal vascular lesion: *In vivo* transfer of endothelial cell nitric oxide synthase gene. Proc Natl Acad Sci U S A 92:1137–1141, 1995.
102. Kraiss LW, Kirkman TR, Kohler TR, et al: Shear stress regulates smooth muscle proliferation and neointimal thickening in porous polytetrafluoroethylene grafts. Arterioscler Thromb 11:1844–1852, 1991.
103. Kraiss LW, Geary RL, Mattsson EJR, et al: Acute reductions in blood flow and shear stress induce platelet-derived growth factor-A expression in baboon prosthetic grafts. Circ Res 79:45–53, 1996.
104. Schwartz SM, Heimark RL, Majesky MW: Developmental mechanisms underlying pathology of arteries. Physiol Rev 70:1177–1210, 1990.
105. Le Breton H, Plow EF, Topol EJ: Role of platelets in restenosis after percutaneous coronary revascularization. J Am Coll Cardiol 28:1643–1651, 1996.
106. Lovaas ME, Gloviczki P, Hollier LH, Kaye MP: Quantitative effects of antiplatelet therapy on healing of the endarterectomized canine aorta. Am J Surg 146:164–169, 1983.
107. Becquemin JP: Effect of ticlopidine on the long-term patency of saphenous-vein bypass grafts in the legs. N Engl J Med 337:1726–1731, 1997.
108. Luscinskas FW, Lawler J: Integrins as dynamic regulators of vascular function. FASEB J 8:929–938, 1994.
109. Bandyk DF, Bergamini TM, Towne JB, et al: Durability of vein graft revision: The outcome of secondary procedures. J Vasc Surg 13:200–210, 1991.
110. Bush HL, Jr, Jakubowski JA, Sentissi JM, et al: Neointimal hyperplasia occurring after carotid endarterectomy in a canine model: Effect of endothelial cell seeding vs perioperative aspirin. J Vasc Surg 5:118–124, 1987.
111. Graham LM, Vinter DW, Ford JW, et al: Endothelial cell seeding of prosthetic vascular grafts: Early experimental studies with cultured autologous canine endothelium. Arch Surg 115:929–933, 1980.
112. Magometschnigg H, Kadletz M, Vodrazka M, et al: Prospective clinical study with in vitro endothelial cell lining of expanded polytetrafluoroethylene grafts in crural repeat reconstruction. J Vasc Surg 15:527–535, 1992.
113. Zilla P, Deutsch M, Meinhart J, et al: Clinical in vitro endothelialization of femoropopliteal bypass grafts: An actuarial follow-up over three years. J Vasc Surg 19:540–548, 1994.
114. Clowes AW, Kirkman TR, Reidy MA: Mechanisms of arterial graft healing: Rapid transmural capillary ingrowth provides a source of intimal endothelium and smooth muscle in porous PTFE prostheses. Am J Pathol 123:220–230, 1986.
115. Desgranges F, Barritault D, Caruelle JP, Tardieu M: Transmural endothelialization of vascular prostheses is regulated in vitro by fibroblast growth factor 2 and heparan-like molecule. Int J Artif Organs 20:589–598, 1997.
116. Gray JL, Kang SS, Zenni GC, et al: FGF-1 affixation stimulates ePTFE endothelialization without intimal hyperplasia. J Surg Res 57:596–612, 1994.
117. Popma JJ, Califf RM, Topol EJ: Clinical trials of restenosis after coronary angioplasty. Circulation 84:1426–1436, 1991.
118. Mak KH, Topol EJ: Clinical trials to prevent restenosis after percutaneous coronary revascularization. Ann N Y Acad Sci 811:255–288, 1997.
119. Herrman J-PR, Hermans WRM, Vos J, Serruys PW: Pharmacological approaches to the prevention of restenosis following angioplasty: The search for the Holy Grail? (Part II). Drugs 46:249–262, 1993.
120. Herrman J-PR, Hermans WRM, Vos J, Serruys PW: Pharmacological approaches to the prevention of restenosis following angioplasty: The search for the Holy Grail? (Part I). Drugs 46:18–52, 1993.
121. Verin V, Urban P, Popowski Y, et al: Feasibility of intracoronary β-irradiation to reduce restenosis after balloon angioplasty: A clinical pilot study. Circulation 95:1138–1144, 1997.
122. Teirstein PS, Massullo V, Jani S, et al: Catheter-based radiotherapy to inhibit restenosis after coronary stenting. N Engl J Med 336:1697–1703, 1997.
123. Serruys PW, Levendag PC: Intracoronary brachytherapy: The death knell of restenosis or just another episode of a never-ending story? Circulation 96:709–712, 1997.
124. Libby P, Ganz P: Restenosis revisited: New targets, new therapies. N Engl J Med 337:418–419, 1997.
125. Clowes AW: Vascular gene therapy in the 21st century. Thromb Haemost 78:605–610, 1997.

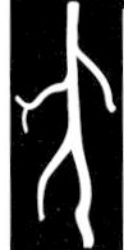

CHAPTER 25

Uncommon Arteriopathies

Thom W. Rooke, M.D., and
John W. Joyce, M.D.

Logical approaches to common arterial and venous diseases are based on an understanding of the usual etiology and behavior of well-defined entities and are constantly refined by experience and literature review. In contrast to the common vascular conditions are the infrequently encountered problems that occur at random, seen perhaps only once or twice in a physician's career. Fortunately, such challenges often announce themselves by departing from the expected in tempo, location, age, setting, or particular clinical or laboratory features. Thus, one is best prepared for these uncommon diseases by a sound knowledge of common problems and their variations.

Until recently, knowledge of fibromuscular dysplasia, popliteal and thoracic entrapments, femoral and popliteal cystic disease, thromboangiitis obliterans, nonspecific aortoarteritis, and atherothrombotic microemboli was scattered throughout the medical literature. All are now well delineated and are discussed elsewhere in this text. Three additional diverse disease groups with vascular manifestations are presented in this chapter: the vasculitides, heritable disorders, and a selection of uncommon acquired lesions. Congenital and acquired clotting disorders warrant a separate chapter.

VASCULITIS

The term *arteritis* generically includes any arterial inflammatory response that either radiation or direct, embolic, or contiguous infection may induce. In common usage, however, the term is usually applied to a diverse group of diseases of unknown or immunologic origin. Indeed, the term *vasculitis* is preferable because veins as well as arteries are involved in many entities.

The vasculitides can be classified according to:

- Vessel size
- Microscopic features of tissue reaction (i.e., necrotizing, granulomatous, giant cell, infectious, radiation)
- Clinical features

Table 25–1 lists the vasculitides as specific clinical entities, although it should be noted that the manifestations of periarteritis and the various hypersensitivity syndromes may overlap.

Acute or chronic inflammatory changes of small, medium, and large arteries or veins are the hallmarks of vasculitis. Most of the entities (those listed without asterisks in Table 25–1) involve small vessels. They manifest as characteristic, often multiple organ system dysfunctions, accompanied by systemic signs of fever, malaise, and weight loss. Associated rheumatologic and cutaneous lesions are common.

Immune mechanisms are implicated in almost all entities involving the small vessels. Known triggers of the reactions include:

TABLE 25–1. CLINICAL CLASSIFICATION OF THE VASCULITIDES

Periarteritis nodosa*
Hypersensitivity angiitis
Scleroderma*
Systemic lupus erythematosus*
Serum sickness
Henoch-Schönlein purpura
Essential mixed cryoglobulinemia
Malignancy
Churg-Strauss syndrome
Wegener's granulomatosis
Lymphomatoid granulomatosis
Thromboangiitis obliterans*
Giant cell arteritis
Temporal arteritis*
Nonspecific aortoarteritis*
Miscellaneous
Relapsing polychondritis*
Behçet's disease*
Mucocutaneous lymph node syndrome (Kawasaki's syndrome)*
Erythema nodosum
Hypocomplementemic vasculitis
Rheumatoid syndromes*

*Denotes entities that involve larger blood vessels.

1. Drugs, such as hydralazine, sulfonamides, procainamide, and amphetamines.
2. Infections, such as gonococcus, streptococcus, and hepatitis B.
3. Inflammation, such as ulcerative colitis, biliary cirrhosis, and serum sickness.
4. Neoplasia, such as lymphoma, myeloma, cancer, and chronic leukemia.

In most instances, however, an inciting factor is not identified. Most are treated by steroids and cytotoxic or immunosuppressive agents, and the role of surgery is limited to biopsy and removal of necrotic tissue. Several excellent reviews consolidate the scattered literature on these diverse microcirculatory diseases, known immunologic observations, and their therapy.[1–6]

Major occlusive and aneurysmal diseases of the aorta and its branches are hallmarks of several of the syndromes (marked by asterisks in Table 25–1). Thromboangiitis obliterans is discussed in Chapter 20, nonspecific aortoarteritis in Chapter 21, and scleroderma in Chapter 82. The remaining entities are presented in this chapter.

Giant Cell Arteritis

Some writers consider the term *giant cell arteritis* synonymous with *temporal arteritis,* but the authors of this chapter share with others[1] a more generic usage that includes both temporal arteritis and nonspecific aortoarteritis (Takayasu's disease). The histology of each disorder is identical in the acute phase, and both have as major manifestations (1) the insidious development of occlusive disease of limb, carotid, visceral, and renal arteries and (2) inflammation, aneurysm, or dissection of the thoracic and abdominal parts of the aorta. They also share angiographic, laboratory, and systemic features. However, Takayasu's disease occurs predominantly in females younger than 50 years of age, whereas temporal arteritis is rare before 50 years of age and the female distribution is less.

Arterial lesions occur in all patients with Takayasu's arteritis; aortic involvement is typical, and branch vessel stenosis is universal, usually occurring near the aortic takeoff. In contrast, occlusive extracranial arterial lesions occur in about 9% to 14% of patients with temporal arteritis; the lesions are usually more peripheral, and the aorta is involved only occasionally. Of importance, steroids suppress systemic symptoms and can reverse or arrest arterial lesions in the acute phase of both diseases.[7–10] The aneurysmal and stenotic lesions of Takayasu's arteritis, however, frequently require operative management, whereas surgery is indicated only occasionally in temporal arteritis.

Temporal Arteritis

The name *temporal arteritis* does not fully describe the disease as it is now understood, yet other names, such as cranial, granulomatous, Horton's, or systemic giant cell arteritis, also lack specificity or overlap with other conditions. The original term is preferred by the authors because of its historical origin[11] and common use.

A careful population-based study defined the average annual incidence of temporal arteritis as 17.4 cases per

100,000 persons older than 50 years of age.[12] The incidence increases with age: 1.4 times the average for ages 50 to 59 years, 10.7 times for ages 60 to 69 years, 29.6 times for ages 70 to 79 years, and 28.9 times after 80 years. Females predominate by ratios of 2:1 to 4:1.

Arterial Lesions

Arterial lesions of the limbs in temporal arteritis are clinically quite characteristic. An insidious, bilaterally symmetric stenosis or occlusion occurs at a steady pace over only 1 to 3 months, producing limb claudication and absence of distal pulses. Tissue necrosis is rare and usually reflects trauma superimposed on advanced occlusive disease. Raynaud's phenomenon is noted on occasion. When treated during the acute phase with adequate steroids, the lesions may clear or improve significantly.

The most common site of arterial involvement is the subclavian-axillary-brachial system. Indeed, it is axiomatic that patients older than 50 years in whom bilateral arm claudication develops over a few weeks have temporal arteritis (Fig. 25–1). The second most common pattern is bilateral involvement of the profunda and superficial femoral arteries, with similar clinical behavior (Fig. 25–2). Presentation with symptoms in both upper and lower extremities (in stages), or of the legs alone, also occurs. On occasion, additional focal lesions occur at the elbow and knee and in the arteries of the forearm and calf.[7, 12–14]

Rare sites of involvement include the celiac, superior mesenteric, iliac, renal, and coronary arteries. Myocardial infarction and death have been documented.[15] The common and internal carotid arteries, the latter chiefly in the petrous and cavernous portions, have shown modest, patchy lesions.[16] Extensive involvement of the vertebral artery to a point just above its dural entry can cause posterior circulation stroke from secondary thrombosis. A 12% incidence of transient ischemic attack or stroke was noted in 166 cases of biopsy-proven temporal arteritis, 4% involving events in the vertebrobasilar system and 8% occurring in the carotid distribution.[17] Angiographic evidence of arteritis in the proximal portions of the anterior, middle, and posterior cerebral arteries has been documented.[18] Aneurysms of the ascending aorta (often with dissection and occasionally with aortic valve incompetence) and aneurysms of the proximal descending infrarenal abdominal aorta occur occasionally.[7, 15]

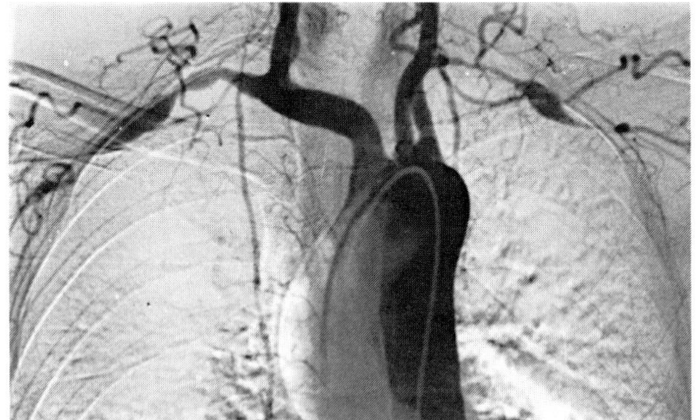

FIGURE 25–1. Focal tapered stenosis and post-stenotic dilatation in the axillary-subclavian system. The patient is a 67-year-old woman who experienced 2 weeks of disabling occipital and neck pain; arm claudication was noted 15 weeks later. The erythrocyte sedimentation rate was 101 mm/hr. Blood pressure and pulses returned during the 10th week of steroid therapy.

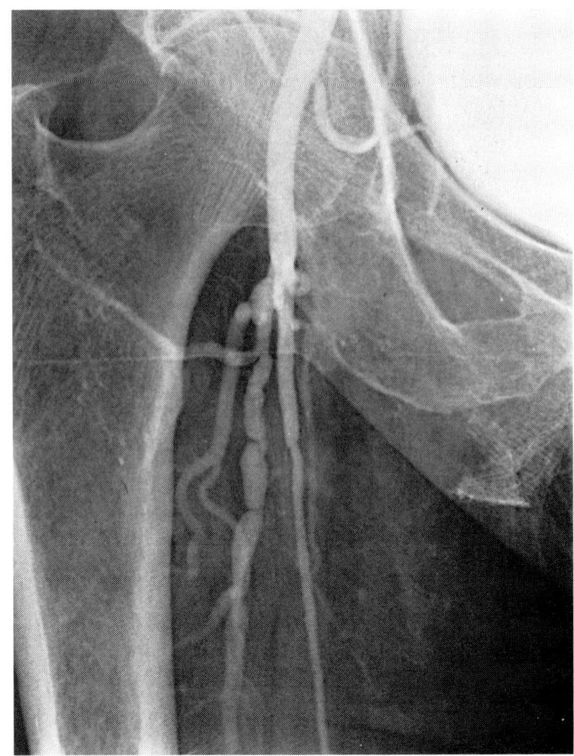

FIGURE 25–2. Arteritis of the right superficial and profunda femoral arteries. A similar lesion was seen on the left and in both subclavian arteries. Bilateral calf claudication developed in a 65-year-old woman following 2 months of malaise and arthralgias, and bilateral arm claudication developed subsequently. Temporal artery biopsy results were positive. Steroid therapy restored pulses and full function in three limbs and improved the left leg.

Angiographic Findings

Angiography demonstrates typical findings in temporal arteritis. Affected arteries show multiple stenotic areas that are almost always bilateral (in paired arteries) and often are associated with post-stenotic dilatation (see Fig. 25–1). Stenotic segments may be short, or long and tapering (Fig. 25–3). Occlusions occur at the end of a tapered area. The chronic nature of the occlusive process usually allows the development of generous collateral vessels, particularly in the upper extremity (Fig. 25–4).

The same angiographic features are found in distal limb vessels involved with Takayasu's arteritis; the diagnosis is clarified by the difference in patient age and the associated proximal arterial and aortic lesions common to Takayasu's arteritis. Ergotism may also cause similar focal or long, tapered lesions. Proper inquiry about use of ergot and the absence of laboratory and clinical findings typical of arteritis establish the diagnosis.[19]

Clinical Picture

A typical case begins with a "flu-like" illness characterized by malaise, fever of 100° to 101°F, weight loss, scalp tender-

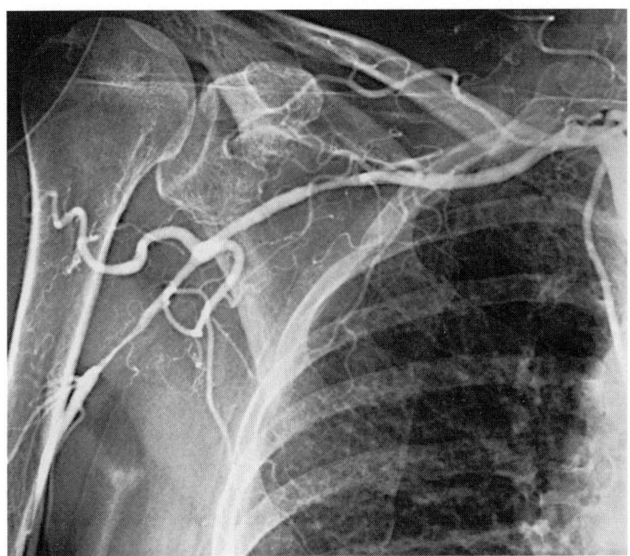

FIGURE 25–3. Multiple tapering stenosis and post-stenotic dilatation in the right brachial and axillary arteries. There is a similar distribution of lesions on the left. The temporal artery biopsy results were positive.

ness or headache, and myalgias, chiefly of the shoulder and hip girdles. After a period of 1 to 3 weeks, some of these symptoms may become quiescent or may intensify. Tender, red, and elevated temporal or occipital arteries or the disappearance of their pulses occurs in 45% to 60% of patients. The girdle stiffness and pain may intensify (polymyalgia rheumatica) and dominate the symptoms. Jaw claudication develops in about two thirds of patients. Frank synovial reaction of wrist and knee joints occurs in a few.

Major eye complications occur at about 3 months but may develop over a span ranging from 3 days to 5 months after onset. These symptoms (which may be unilateral or bilateral) include partial or total blindness, amaurosis fugax, and, on occasion, extraocular muscle dysfunction of sudden onset. Such complications are explained by (1) arteritis of the ophthalmic or posterior ciliary vessels and, to a lesser extent, (2) occlusion of the central retinal artery or vein.[16, 20]

Involvement of large arteries occurs in about 9% to 14% of patients at a median time of 8 months from onset (range, 0 to 84 months).[7] The untreated disease is self-limited to a course of 1 to 3 years and has a mortality of less than 10%,[21] death being caused by aortic dissection, aneurysm rupture, myocardial infarction, or stroke.[7, 15, 21] Death and the significant morbidity of the ocular and arterial complications can be prevented, however, by adequate steroid therapy.[7, 20, 22]

In patients with such a typical course and an abnormal temporal artery, temporal arteritis is readily diagnosed. The usual tempo of the disease should allow early diagnosis and therapy, preventing the later ocular and vascular complications. However, the disease may be a diagnostic challenge. In rare instances, the disease tempo is accelerated; blindness has been seen within 3 days,[17] and fatal aortic dissection has been noted within 2 weeks of onset.[7]

Because the symptoms mimic those of other common illnesses and are scattered over several weeks' time, their correct correlation by the patient or physician may not be made. Many older patients do not recall all events unless they and family members are carefully questioned. Most noteworthy is the fact that any single feature of the syndrome may be so dominant that the presentation suggests obscure fever, occult malignancy, lymphoma, or various rheumatic diseases. Fevers of 103° to 104°F, shaking chills, drenching sweats, rapid loss of 20 to 30 pounds, and depression can contribute to the diagnostic problem.

Laboratory Findings

Elevation of the erythrocyte sedimentation rate (ESR) in the range of 40 to 140 mm/hr is characteristic of active temporal arteritis. A normal ESR is rarely found, but one must be careful to exclude instances in which the ESR has been suppressed by anti-inflammatory agents given for the

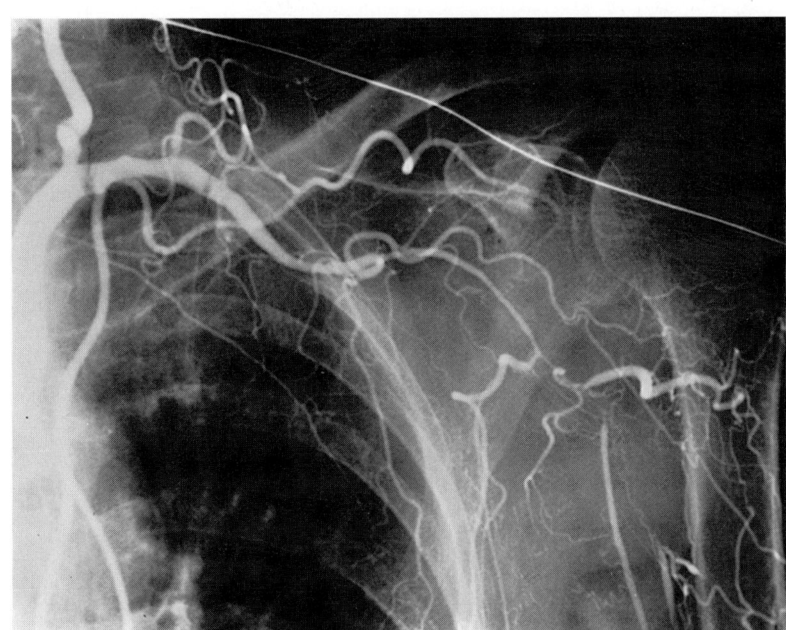

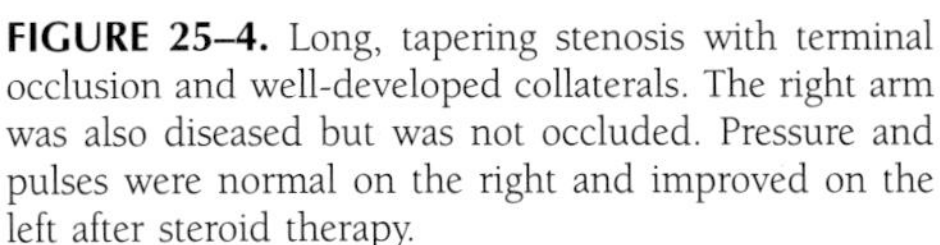

FIGURE 25–4. Long, tapering stenosis with terminal occlusion and well-developed collaterals. The right arm was also diseased but was not occluded. Pressure and pulses were normal on the right and improved on the left after steroid therapy.

musculoskeletal or systemic symptoms.[23] Most patients have a mild normocytic anemia, and both mild hypochromic anemia and intravascular coagulopathy can occur. The leukocyte count and differential blood count are normal in most patients, but in about a quarter of cases, mild leukocytosis is seen.[24] Mild thrombocytosis is not uncommon. Additional mild and nonspecific findings that clear promptly with treatment include increased alpha$_2$-globulin, transaminase elevation to one to two times normal, prothrombin time elevation of 1.2 to 1.5 times control, and elevation of alkaline phosphatase values to twice normal.[25]

Polymyalgia Rheumatica

Polymyalgia rheumatica is defined as a significant, often crippling pain and stiffness *without local tenderness,* involving the muscles of the neck, shoulder, and hip girdles in varying combinations. It has been present for at least 1 month in patients older than 50 years of age, is accompanied by a high ESR, and responds dramatically to steroids. Its incidence is almost four times that of temporal arteritis,[12, 26] yet it is a component of more than half of cases of temporal arteritis.[5, 10]

Although arteritis is not part of polymyalgia by definition, it is found to be present silently in 5% to 40% of patients when routine biopsy of the temporal arteries is performed.[14, 27] The presence of arteritis is a critical question; high-dose steroids are essential to prevent the ocular and arterial complications of arteritis, whereas the complications of steroid therapy can be minimal with the low-dose schedules that suffice to control uncomplicated polymyalgia.[26, 27] Of note, polymyalgia rheumatica on occasion may also be the prodrome of rheumatoid arthritis, periarteritis nodosa, systemic lupus erythematosus (SLE), occult infection, malignancy, or infectious endocarditis.[28]

Biopsy

Biopsy should be considered in most cases of polymyalgia rheumatica in view of the preceding observations and because a palpably abnormal artery is found in only 45% to 60% of biopsy-proven cases of temporal arteritis.[14, 29] Biopsy is recommended when typically inflamed arteries are noted, to preclude the all too frequently late challenge of the initial diagnosis once steroid withdrawal causes confusing symptoms.

Biopsy is performed with the patient under local anesthesia, and a 2- to 3-cm segment is adequate when the vessel is visibly diseased. As discussed, "blind" biopsy, without identification of a palpably abnormal artery, is often called for; in such cases, a generous segment of 4 to 7 cm is advised. Also, multiple sections are examined because the pathology can be quite focal, with multiple, long skip areas. For patients in whom such a biopsy specimen yields negative results, a similar contralateral biopsy is helpful in 10% to 15% of cases. In one study employing these guidelines in a carefully observed population, temporal artery biopsy was 94% predictive of the need for high-dose steroids.[29]

Therapy

The major achievement of steroid therapy in temporal arteritis is the rapid suppression of symptoms and the prevention of blindness. Blindness does not occur after adequate steroids have been given.[20–22]

Because (1) the time between onset of arteritis and visual loss may be as little as 3 days and (2) the interval between involvement of a second eye after damage to the first may be 2 to 7 days, the authors consider temporal arteritis a medical emergency.[20] Once the diagnosis is suspected, blood samples are taken and steroids begun immediately. Biopsy is accomplished on subsequent days, and steroid doses are tapered if the biopsy result is negative. It is noteworthy that the incidence of blindness cited in early reports (40% to 50%) has now dropped (10% to 20%), an improvement attributable to early diagnosis and effective therapy.[13, 20, 29]

In the authors' protocol, 60 mg of prednisone in divided, twice-daily doses is given for a week and is then reduced to 45 mg/day given in divided doses for a month. With this program, systemic symptoms are suppressed in 24 to 72 hours, and the ESR normalizes in 1 to 2 weeks. When pulse deficits are present, improvement in Doppler systolic pressures begins after 4 to 6 weeks. The daily dose is subsequently reduced by 5-mg increments at intervals of 2 to 3 weeks; when a level of 15 mg/day is reached, 1-mg reductions are made at similar intervals. The clinical status and ESR are monitored at each dose change. Ten per cent to 15% of patients require therapy into a second or even a third year. Steroid therapy is eventually stopped in all patients. Recrudescence of disease is treated by doubling of the dosage for 3 to 4 weeks and assessment of disease suppression by means of the ESR and the presence of symptoms.

The anticipated steroid side effects must be explained to the patient. A no-added-salt diet is advised, and acid suppression is given to the patient with a history of peptic disease or if dyspepsia develops during treatment. Calcium and vitamin D supplementation should be considered to offset the risk of steroid-induced osteoporosis. A prospective, randomized trial of alternate-day steroid therapy showed reduction of steroid side effects but incomplete suppression of disease; daily dosage is therefore advised.[13]

The need for surgery in temporal arteritis occurs occasionally. Indications are significant aortic valve incompetence, aneurysmal disease, aortic dissection, and those rare cases in which claudication remains limiting after adequate steroid therapy has been given.[30, 31] The authors have seen bypass grafts that had been placed in two patients become occluded during the active phase of arteritis.[32]

Periarteritis Nodosa

Periarteritis nodosa may be seen from childhood on but is most common in the fourth through sixth decades of life. Men predominate by a ratio of 2:1. Lesions are characteristically focal, with skip zones, and affect the small and medium-sized arteries of almost all organs. The sequence of damage is:

1. Acute inflammation.
2. Necrosis.
3. Secondary thrombosis.
4. Late fibrosis.

About 20% of patients experience small aneurysms of visceral, renal, or distal limb vessels. Lesions in different stages of evolution in a given organ or artery are typical, in contrast to the uniform age of lesions seen in hypersensitivity angiitis.[1, 2, 6]

Presentation in periarteritis nodosa is usually characterized by an insidious progression of multiple accumulating manifestations, but on occasion it is fulminant with death occurring in days or weeks. Systemic symptoms of fever, malaise, and weight loss are common. Many combinations of organ involvement occur; the more common are:

- Mononeuritis multiplex (60% to 70% of cases)
- Renal disease (microhematuria, glomerulitis; 50% to 60%)
- Gastrointestinal problems (50%)
- Arthralgias (50%)
- Hypertension (40%)

Less common manifestations include severe myalgia, stroke, rash, skin infarctions, and orchitis. Pulmonary infiltrates and nodules, hemoptysis, and pleurisy occur, but the incidence is modest when those cases better classified as Churg-Strauss granulomatosis are excluded. Pericarditis, myocarditis, and inflammation of the coronary arteries are often noted at autopsy but are usually clinically silent. Elevation of the ESR, mild anemia, and moderate leukocytosis are usual.[1, 2, 33–35]

Raynaud's phenomenon occurs in a few patients. Digital arteritis (which may progress to infarction), livedo vasculitis of the legs (which often ulcerates), and arteriolar ulcerations occur in less than 5%; steroids often suppress these lesions.[33, 34]

The major surgical challenge in periarteritis nodosa is in the gastrointestinal and renal circulations, where lesions of the secondary and tertiary branches of the visceral, renal, and hepatic arteries cause occlusion or become aneurysmal.[34, 36–38] Occlusions result in cholecystitis, appendicitis, gut perforation, gastrointestinal hemorrhage, or ischemic obstruction. Technical problems with concern for gut viability in this multifocal disease often dictate second-look surgery.[36, 39] Aneurysmal lesions can rupture, causing intrahepatic, perinephric, and intraperitoneal hemorrhage. These aneurysms often regress with vigorous steroid and cyclophosphamide therapy, and they should therefore be treated even when asymptomatic.[37, 40]

Steroid therapy has increased the 5-year survival from less than 15% of untreated patients to more than 50% of treated patients.[1, 2, 34, 37] Cyclophosphamide is a valuable adjunct in acute, severe cases.[31] Vasculitis of the kidneys and gastrointestinal tract is the prime cause of mortality in the acute phase; cardiovascular and cerebral events can occur in long-standing cases, often from severe hypertension.[34]

Systemic Lupus Erythematosus

SLE is best considered an autoimmune disease that deposits damaging biologic substances via the microcirculation of specific tissues. Antibodies to deoxyribonucleic acid (DNA) and other cellular components have been clearly identified.[41, 42] The resulting disease occurs chiefly in women in the second through fourth decades of life. Multisystem manifestations, such as arthritis, nephritis, pericarditis, pleuritis, cerebritis, lymphadenopathy, and hepatosplenomegaly, occur in varying combinations. A characteristic facial rash occurs in 20% of cases. The ESR is significantly elevated, and leukopenia is common. The tempo of disease may be smoldering, intermittent, or fulminant. A small subset of patients have additional findings suggesting periarteritis, scleroderma, or dermatomyositis, the so-called overlap syndromes. Antimalarial agents, nonsteroidal anti-inflammatory drugs, steroids, and both azathioprine and cyclophosphamide supplements can be effective in suppressing the disease, depending on its intensity.[1, 37]

Arteritis of small and medium-sized vessels is an additional component of the basic mechanism in a significant number of patients with SLE. Major sites of vasculitis are the skin (livedo, nodules, infarcts), the intestinal tract (ischemic perforation and hemorrhage of gut, pancreas, gallbladder, and appendix), and the renal, pulmonary, and coronary circulations.

Although arteritis is not seen in larger vessels, the vascular surgeon may be the first to encounter certain cases of SLE. A circulating anticoagulant, or inhibitor, occurs in 5% to 10% of cases, causing thrombosis of major arteries and veins, often as an early or even the presenting sign of SLE. Major thrombosis can occur in[43–46]:

1. The inferior vena cava.
2. Renal, retinal, and leg and arm veins.
3. Pulmonary arteries.
4. Arteries of the aortoiliac, femoral, axillary, carotid, cerebral, coronary, and retinal systems.

In a study of 205 patients with the lupus anticoagulant, 26% experienced approximately equal incidences of arterial or venous thrombosis.

The diathesis can be controlled by heparin and warfarin. The response of the circulating anticoagulant to steroids is unpredictable and slow; anticoagulation is therefore continued until the anticoagulant is suppressed.[46] Vascular surgery can be performed when indicated, with the use of anticoagulant protection. Of note, hemorrhage is not a feature of the circulating anticoagulant in SLE. Further, the anticoagulant is not specific to SLE nor diagnostic of it and can be seen in association with Behçet's disease, periarteritis, and other vasculitides.[43, 46]

Behçet's Disease

Recurrent aphthous ulcers of the mouth and genitalia, uveitis and recurrent hypopyon, and a variety of skin lesions, including erythema nodosum, pustules, acne, and hypersensitivity to needle puncture, are the major manifestations of Behçet's disease, an unusual disorder. Additional lesions are nonerosive synovitis, recurrent meningoencephalitis, inflammatory bowel disease, and major arterial and venous problems. At least four classification schemes exist, each calling for various combinations of major or minor criteria to establish the diagnosis. Also, except for aphthous lesions and ocular disease, there is disagreement about what constitute the major criteria.

Behçet's disease is seen worldwide but occurs more commonly in Asian and Mediterranean countries. Blindness occurs in up to 25% of patients with ocular involvement.[47, 48] The pathology is that of a vasculitis affecting large or small arteries and veins. Immune complexes have been found in vessel walls. Cyclosporine, azathioprine, and chlorambucil have reduced the frequency of ocular attacks, and chlorambucil has proved beneficial in treatment of meningoencephalitis. No agents (including steroids, indomethacin, and colchicine), however, have been predictable in suppressing the disease completely.[49–51, 51a]

Major arterial and venous lesions occur in 6% to 25% of cases and are the leading cause of death. Thrombosis can occur in almost any superficial or deep vein. Anticoagulation is effective in preventing further events, in the authors' limited experience, but the duration of treatment is indeterminate and is guided by the quiescence of other manifestations of the disease.[52, 56]

Both focal arterial thrombosis and aneurysm formation can occur and may coexist in a given patient. Almost all named arteries have been involved in either process. The aneurysms in Behçet's disease are usually saccular and are often multiple.[47, 48, 52, 53, 56] Pulmonary arteries are often aneurysmal and can cause fatal hemoptysis with rupture.[54, 55]

Tissue analysis has uniformly reported intimal hyperplasia, fragmentation of the internal elastic membrane, adventitial plasmacytosis, and infiltrates of the vasa vasorum. The lesions are random and focal. Bypass grafts or interposition grafts have been successful when they are sutured into healthy tissue. Anastomotic aneurysms and thromboses are not uncommon, however. Further, false aneurysm formation at sites of catheterization and needle puncture is a hazard.[51–53, 57, 58] Whether the medical agents listed here suppress the vascular manifestations of Behçet's disease has not been shown.

Kawasaki's Disease (Mucocutaneous Lymph Node Syndrome)

A unique syndrome of unknown origin, Kawasaki's disease affects, chiefly, infants in the first year of life and small children and, rarely, a few patients older than 9 years. More than 63,000 patients had been diagnosed in Japan by 1984, the first description by Kawasaki having appeared in 1967.[59, 60] Significant endemic groups have been studied in other parts of Asia, Europe, and North America.

The illness begins with a week or more of high spiking fever, followed by conjunctivitis, truncal erythema, cricopharyngeal edema, cervical adenopathy, and erythema of the soles and palms. In the second phase, arthralgias, dry and cracking lips, and desquamation of involved skin occur. Laboratory findings are not specific and include mild anemia, neutrophilia, high ESR, and often marked thrombocytosis. Aseptic meningitis, hepatitis, pleurisy, and diarrhea may occur.[59]

Kawasaki's disease is self-limited, but about 0.5% of patients die in the acute phase of an intense vasculitis, which has a distribution in the small and medium-sized arteries and veins indistinguishable from that of periarteritis nodosa.[61] The most common lethal lesions, however, are multiple coronary artery aneurysms that undergo thrombosis or rupture. The incidence of coronary aneurysm formation is about 15%[62]; it occurs usually in the first month but sometimes 6 to 48 months later. Echocardiography in the first month is highly sensitive in recognizing aneurysm formation.[63]

No specific treatment has been identified. Aspirin suppresses systemic symptoms but has not been proven to reduce the vasculitis. Steroids may be life-saving for patients with myocarditis and shock but have failed to reduce the incidence of coronary artery stenosis and aneurysm.[64] However, studies have documented that high-dose gamma globulin given intravenously in the acute phase has had a significant impact on the occurrence of coronary disease.[66, 67] Coronary artery angiography and surgery are fully incorporated into management.[61, 65] Spontaneous regression of aneurysms as well as late coronary occlusion occurs.[68]

Aneurysms of the abdominal aorta and brachial, axillary, iliac, renal, hepatic, and mesenteric arteries have been observed as occasional late sequelae of Behçet's disease. When symptomatic or expanding, such aneurysms can be successfully operated upon using standard techniques of end-to-end anastomosis or saphenous interposition grafting.[65, 69, 70] Just what the late incidence of arterial aneurysms will be, or whether acute-phase gamma globulin therapy will minimize this risk, is still unknown.

Rheumatoid Disease with Vasculitis

A noninflammatory endarteritis occurs in patients with rheumatoid arthritis and may cause Raynaud's phenomenon, periungual infarcts, digital pad ulcers, or gangrene. In addition, an active vasculitis indistinguishable from periarteritis nodosa may be seen with rheumatoid arthritis, causing extensive digital gangrene, arteriolar ulcers of the legs, and mesenteric ischemia or bowel infarction. The syndrome occurs late in the course of rheumatoid arthritis, when patients have advanced joint changes, cutaneous nodules, positive antinuclear antibody test results, and high rheumatoid titers.[71, 72] High-dose steroids often help such patients, unless mononeuritis is present.[73] Cyclophosphamide can be a valuable adjunct to steroids.[74] Gastrointestinal vascular catastrophes and renal disease are the usual terminal events.[73]

In a small percentage of patients with rheumatoid arthritis, ankylosing spondylitis, Reiter's syndrome, juvenile rheumatoid arthritis, or the arthritis of inflammatory bowel disease, a proximal aortitis may develop, causing aneurysms of the ascending aorta or aortic valve incompetence. This is a late event in such diseases. Aneurysms of the descending and thoracoabdominal aorta have also been noted. The lesions can be surgically treated.[75–79] The role of adjunctive steroids is not clear.

Relapsing Polychondritis

Relapsing polychondritis, a rare disease, is easily diagnosed from a cluster of readily apparent defects. Unfortunately, the associated vascular problems that are a major source of mortality are often overlooked, and an opportunity for corrective surgery is lost.[80, 81]

Presentation is characterized by several major findings, all of which occur with a frequency of 50% or higher in major reviews:

- Auricular chondritis
- Nasal chondritis

- Respiratory tract chondritis
- Seronegative polyarthritis
- Ocular inflammation (episcleritis, conjunctivitis, uveitis)
- Audiovestibular damage

Malaise and fever are common, and the ESR is markedly elevated in most patients. Age of onset ranges from 13 to 84 years with a median of 51 years, and the sex ratio is about equal.[82]

Tissue changes seen in the aorta in relapsing polychondritis include an increased level of collagen in the media, lymphocytic reaction of the adventitia, a decrease in mucopolysaccharide content, and inflammatory cells around the vasa vasorum.[80–82] Aneurysms of the ascending, descending, thoracoabdominal, or infrarenal aorta occur in about 10% of cases. Aortic valve incompetence or dissection is common with ascending aortic aneurysms. All of the listed lesions have been successfully operated on,[80, 81] suggesting that regular screening for aortic lesions is justified.

Other forms of vasculitis overlap with relapsing polychondritis in 20% to 30% of cases. They include periarteritis, SLE, discoid lupus, Behçet's disease, and Reiter's syndrome; several of these are responsive to medical therapy.[82, 83]

Michet and colleagues[82] report 5- and 10-year survival probabilities from the time of diagnosis as 74% and 55%, respectively. Of 41 deaths in the 112 patients these researchers observed, 7 resulted from vasculitis and 5 from cardiovascular disease. Steroids, aspirin, dapsone, and other agents suppress many manifestations of relapsing polychondritis, but it is not clear from the small populations described whether any agent prevents aortic damage.

CONGENITAL DISEASES WITH ARTERIAL INVOLVEMENT

Congenital diseases with arterial involvement are diverse disorders, each with multifaceted presentations, and fortunately rare. Major components of all of these disorders are, however, dramatic and often devastating cardiovascular complications (including spontaneous rupture, dissection, and aneurysm formation in the aorta and its major branches, and occlusive disease of the distal arteries). These vascular events occur in a young population, in the second through fifth decades, but the age spectrum ranges from childhood through the 70s, depending on the intensity of expressivity of a specific deficit in a given patient.

Several of the diseases discussed here are not only congenital but also hereditary. They include the Marfan syndrome, Ehlers-Danlos syndrome, pseudoxanthoma elasticum, homocystinurea, neurofibromatosis, and tuberous sclerosis. The genetic behavior of these diseases is well understood and detailed. Specific knowledge of their cellular and molecular deficits continues to emerge.[84–88]

Other well-defined arterial lesions that are congenital but not hereditary are cystic disease of the popliteal and femoral arteries (see Chapter 74), popliteal artery entrapment syndromes (see Chapter 75), thoracic outlet arterial compression (see Chapter 84), aortic coarctation, and persistent sciatic artery.

The Marfan Syndrome

Marfan's syndrome is characterized by an autosomal dominant defect in the cross-linking of collagen, caused by mutations of type I procollagen or its processing enzymes.[86–88] About 15% of cases are from de novo mutations. Defects in elastin have also been described, and studies have identified a mutation of the fibrillin gene on chromosome 15 as the cause of the syndrome.[89] At autopsy, tissue changes are confined to the ascending aorta, which is thickened but weakened, and show irregular muscle bundle patterns, increased collagen, decreased elastin, and, sometimes, vacuoles in the media.[84]

The diagnosis is clinical and is based on combinations of musculoskeletal, ocular, and hereditary features (all exceeding the 80th percentile in incidence) and on the cardiovascular findings that occur in 95% of patients.[84–91] Musculoskeletal abnormalities are multiple, but the most important involve limb length and proportions. Most but not all patients are tall, and critical measurements of proportion show that the arm span exceeds height and that upper segment length (pubes to crown) is 0.86 or less than lower segment length. The distal limbs tend to be more severely affected, resulting in arachnodactyly. Body habitus changes of lesser specificity but considerable frequency include kyphoscoliosis, pectus carinatum and pectus excavatum, genu recurvatum, pes planus, and hypermobile joints; recurrent patellar and hip dislocations; hernias; reduced body fat; and muscular hypotonia. At least 80% of patients have ectopic lenses (sometimes requiring slit-lamp examination to identify) caused by redundant or broken suspensory ligaments. Significant myopia is common, and spontaneous retinal detachment occurs in some cases.[84–91]

Mitral valve prolapse, ascending aortic aneurysm and dissection, and aortic valve incompetence are major cardiovascular manifestations. Mitral valve prolapse occurs in more than 90% of cases; it may be diagnosed only by echocardiography and is rarely florid enough to cause congestive heart failure and warrant repair. Aneurysms of the ascending aorta are seen in at least 80% of patients. The syndrome causes aortic valve incompetence in many, leading to congestive heart failure, and on occasion produces angina pectoris. Dissection in these aneurysms is the major cause of death in patients with the Marfan syndrome. Sometimes aneurysm formation is confined to the sinuses of Valsalva, where rupture and cardiac or pulmonary fistulae can follow. There have been a few documented cases of abdominal aortic aneurysm, both with and without involvement of the ascending aorta. Bacterial endocarditis may occur in the damaged valves. The average life expectancy of the patient with the Marfan syndrome is to the mid-40s, and cardiovascular dysfunction causes most deaths. Fatalities have been recorded in the first 2 years of life, and few patients survive past age 70 years.[84–91]

Initial diagnosis and management of the acute or chronic complications of aortic dissections can involve the cardiovascular surgeon. Dissection is typically a major event with (1) severe chest or abdominal pain, (2) shock, (3) aortic branch vessel deficits, and (4) findings of altered mediastinal or tracheal anatomy. Involvement of branch vessels may consist merely of reduction or absence of pulses, but in a third of cases it is manifested by significant target organ dysfunction, such as stroke, visceral or limb ischemia, accelerated hypertension, and, occasionally, myocardial ischemia.

Dissection of the aorta may occur, however, without recent diagnostic pain, or the sequence of events can be obscured by a cerebral deficit. Under these circumstances, aortic dissection may first be diagnosed at the time of angiography or surgery for ischemia of the brain, limbs, viscera, or kidney. At this juncture, the cardiovascular surgeon must determine whether a local repair is necessary and must then direct medical or surgical efforts toward the primary tear to enhance survival.

In dissection of the ascending aorta (a common event in the Marfan syndrome), resection and graft of the primary site usually restore flows to the occluded limb vessels, and the need for direct revascularization or aortic fenestration is rare.[92, 93] Focal stroke does not contraindicate life-protecting primary repair of the ascending aorta.[93, 94] Visceral and partial renal ischemia may also improve when repair is prompt.

Although rare in patients with the Marfan syndrome, dissection of the descending aorta is problematic. In many hands, medical therapy has equaled or bettered the survival achieved by primary surgical repairs.[94] However, residual limb and partial visceral or renal ischemia may require urgent fenestration or a bypass procedure. Surgical salvage of an ischemic limb is reasonable, but mortality from visceral and renal ischemia is very high with this combined approach. For these reasons, and to eliminate the basic danger of aortic rupture, primary repair of the descending aorta is preferred by other physicians.[92, 93]

In patients with chronic dissection, significant (1) aortoiliac and descending aortic aneurysms and (2) renovascular lesions warrant repair. Renovascular lesions may respond to revascularization or reimplantation, but nephrectomy may be required.[94, 95]

There is evidence that (1) beta-blocker therapy started before aortic incompetence develops can retard the incompetence and aneurysm growth[96] and (2) the incidence of fatal dissection is reduced by elective replacement of the aortic valve and ascending aorta when the transverse diameter exceeds 6 cm in patients with the Marfan syndrome.[97]

Ehlers-Danlos Syndrome

The clinical features of Ehlers-Danlos syndrome (ED) as commonly described include:

1. Joint laxity with a potential for recurrent effusions and dislocation.
2. Hyperextensible skin.
3. Fragility of the skin that allows wide splitting or gross ecchymosis, producing "cigarette paper" scars after minor trauma.

Fragility of the ocular globe, kyphoscoliosis, a tendency toward spontaneous rupture or large diverticula of the gut, and, finally, catastrophic arterial complications in about 4% of patients are additional uncommon components of the disease.[84, 85, 98, 99]

Accumulating observations, however, have defined eight and probably ten clinical types of ED, each with one or more features predominating.[88] Further, current knowledge of the genetics and biochemistry of collagen formation has delineated at least nine faults in gene formation or in the multiple enzymatic sequences that convert procollagen to collagen. These specific molecular defects now explain a few, but not all, of the variants of ED. Continued use of the clinical classification of ED, types I to X, remains appropriate until definitive biochemical data allow a complete etiologic nosology. ED is an autosomal dominant disorder, and an X-linked variant has been identified.[85, 86]

Type I ED has varying combinations of the classic skin and joint findings, a modest incidence of mitral valve prolapse, and occasional dilatation of the sinuses of Valsalva. The same lesions are randomly reported in all other types; the actual incidence awaits prospective, noninvasive screening of the small groups of affected patients over a prolonged period. Of note, an instance of aortic rupture has occurred in type VI ED, the ocular-coliotic variant.[85]

Major arterial defects are the dominant findings in type IV ED, representing about 4% of all cases of ED.[99] At least three molecular defects in the formation of collagen III have been defined, but these findings have still not been clearly correlated with specific arterial syndromes.[88] In type IV ED, joint hypermobility may be absent or mild and may be confined to the fingers when present. Skin hyperelasticity is also minimal or absent, although translucent, thin truncal skin and premature aging of the facial and hand skin are typical when this sign is present. Easy, extensive bruisability from minor trauma is common, and type IV ED is often called the arterial-ecchymotic type.[84, 85, 99]

Spontaneous arterial rupture, multiple aneurysms, and dissection of the aorta and arteriovenous fistulae result from a diffuse thinning of the media with reduced elastin and fragmented internal elastic membranes (Fig. 25–5).[85] An excellent report of five affected families and a careful literature review have summarized the vascular findings in ED. Spontaneous hemorrhage occurred 38 times in the 36

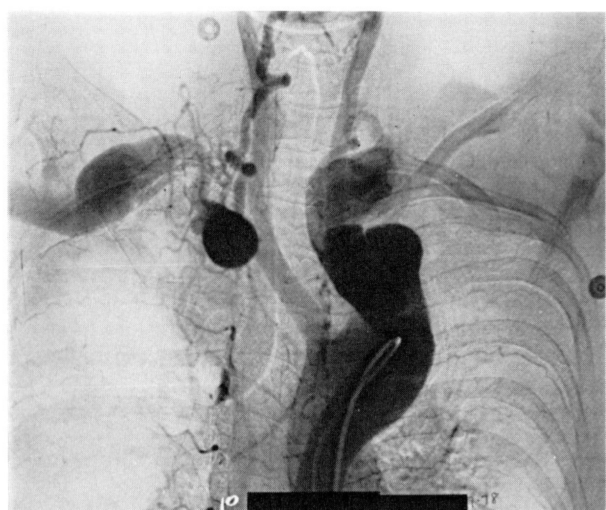

FIGURE 25–5. Bizarre, extensive ectasia and aneurysmal changes of the subclavian arteries. The patient was a 36-year-old woman with the long limbs, kyphoscoliosis, hyperelastic skin, and extensible joints typical of Ehlers-Danlos syndrome. There was a lesser degree of ectasia and aneurysm formation of the ascending and thoracoabdominal aorta and the iliac and superior mesenteric arteries. Sudden death from dissection of the ascending aorta occurred 1 year later.

patients analyzed, chiefly in the aorta and the visceral, carotid, and calf arteries, but also in the iliac, femoral, and subclavian-axillary arteries, and occasionally in the coronary arteries. Twenty-nine aneurysms (including aortic dissection) were found in 15 patients at all the listed sites except the femoropopliteal segment; visceral, carotid, and aortic lesions were most common. Eight instances of arteriovenous fistulae, five at the carotid-cavernous site, were noted.[98]

The 36 patients in this report underwent 29 vascular operations: ligation of 15 bleeding vessels, five aneurysms, and four carotid-cavernous fistulae; one thrombectomy; and four bypass procedures (only the last-named one was successful).[98] Other successful aortic grafts have been reported.[100, 101] There were seven surgical deaths, and 21 deaths were attributed to hemorrhage. Arteriography, performed in 12 patients, was complicated by significant hematoma in five patients, femoral artery occlusion in one, and death from bleeding in two.[98] Thus, the intrinsic arterial fragility of type IV ED frustrates both diagnostic and surgical efforts.[98]

Ligation is the procedure of choice, when feasible, and reconstruction can be offered when essential only after the patient has been duly cautioned about the risks; reinforcement of sutures and ligation sites is essential.[102] For evaluation, the use of intravenous digital subtraction angiography, computed tomography, and magnetic resonance imaging (MRI) is preferred to direct, cautious angiography when possible. Specific therapy of the enzymatic defects is not to be expected. Genetic counseling and regular follow-up are of paramount importance for patients and family.

Pseudoxanthoma Elasticum

Pseudoxanthoma elasticum (PXE) is the least common of the congenital disorders with arterial involvement, and affected patients rarely need vascular surgery. PXE is an autosomal recessive disorder, differing from ED in that the primary defect is in elastin rather than in collagen. The constellation of signs includes cutaneous, ocular, and cardiovascular manifestations and a significant incidence of upper intestinal and uterine hemorrhage. Diagnosis is usually made in patients in the fourth through sixth decades of life, but the disease can be apparent before age 10 years.[84, 103–105] Although the disorder predominates in females in most reports, this statistic may reflect a greater concern with cosmetic signs in women; the incidence of PXE with no skin lesions is higher in men.[103]

Ninety per cent or more of patients with PXE have the characteristic skin lesion or angioid retinal streaks. Elevated plaques similar to xanthomas develop in the folds of the neck and axillae and, to a lesser extent, in those of the groin, cubital, popliteal, submammary, and umbilical areas. Reticulations and lax, redundant folds develop in time (Fig. 25–6). Biopsy findings are specific and demonstrate varying degrees of fragmentation and clumping of elastin.[84, 103–105]

Angioid streaks are dark brown or red channels, usually wider than retinal vessels, that surround and radiate from the optic disc. They represent fractures in Bruch's membrane and may proceed to focal hemorrhages with late chorioretinal scarring and varying degrees of central blindness, usually bilateral. (*Note:* Angioid streaks also occur with Paget's disease of bone, sickle cell anemia, and hyperphosphatemia.) Upper intestinal hemorrhage occurs in up to one third of patients and is associated with marked thinning of vessels in the gastric mucosa and submucosa; 7 of 11 women in one PXE population experienced significant uterine bleeding, leading to hysterectomy in 6.[105]

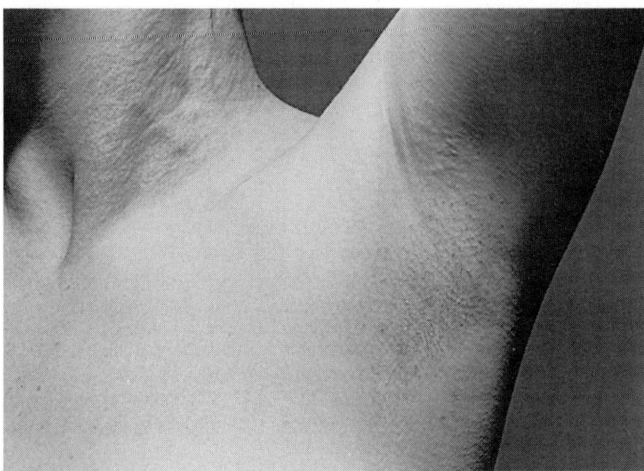

FIGURE 25–6. Soft, chamois-colored papules with the linear and reticular pattern typical of pseudoxanthoma elasticum seen in the neck and axillary folds of a 30-year-old woman. Similar lesions were seen across the popliteal spaces and in the groin folds. Angioid streaks in the retina were noted. The left radial and right posterior tibial pulses were not palpable. No arterial symptoms were noted. Angiography was not performed.

Cardiovascular problems of PXE include occlusive peripheral arterial disease, coronary occlusive disease, atrial subendocardiofibrosis, and renovascular hypertension.[103–105] From 15% 50% of patients experience angina, and a few infarcts are seen in patients at an average age of 38 years and occasionally in teenagers. Diffuse coronary calcification and triple-vessel disease are common, for which surgery has been successfully accomplished. The renal lesion is noted in intrarenal arteries, and most researchers attribute stroke in patients with PXE to long-standing hypertension.[105]

Reduction or absence of limb pulses and premature arterial calcification have been noted in PXE for almost a century and have an incidence of 15% to 50%. The distal third of the radial and ulnar vessels is the most common site for occlusion (usually with preservation of the interosseous artery). Less common locations are the tibioperoneal, celiac, popliteal, and superficial femoral arteries. Contemporary studies utilizing noninvasive testing with exercise would be useful to more fully define the extent of peripheral arterial involvement.* Leg claudication is common, but ischemia of the hand or foot is rare. Of note, the aorta and its primary branches are spared.[103–106]

Standard techniques of reconstructive surgery can be successfully employed when indicated for rest pain, ische-

**Editor's note:* This traditionally accepted distribution of lesions in pseudoxanthoma elasticum (PXE) is, to some extent, based on angiographic follow-up of symptoms and pulse deficits. Routine screening of a large cohort of patients with PXE by noninvasive methods (segmental limb pressures and plethysmography) indicates that partially occlusive lower extremity lesions, especially of the femoropopliteal segment, are more common than has been realized and may even be more common than the more obvious, totally occlusive lesions of the distal upper extremity arteries (R. B. Rutherford, unpublished data).

mic ulceration, or advanced claudication.[107] Patients presenting with modest claudication warrant regular follow-up to detect the coronary artery disease that develops with significant frequency.

Homocystinurea

Homocystinurea is an autosomal recessive error of methionine metabolism caused by a deficiency of cystathionine synthetase, homocysteine methyltransferase, or other enzymes that allows homocystine to accumulate in body tissues and fluids. Early in life, affected patients demonstrate a high rate of ocular defects (ectopic lens, acute glaucoma, retinal detachment, and cataract), mental retardation of varying severity (up to 40% of patients), and skeletal defects similar to those seen in the Marfan syndrome. In addition, accelerated fibrous arteriosclerosis causing arterial occlusive disease in the first three decades of life occurs, complicated by a propensity for acute thrombotic events in the arterial and venous systems. These events are almost equally divided among acute venous thrombosis, peripheral occlusions, myocardial infarction, and stroke, and there is a significant incidence of premature death due to pulmonary embolism, myocardial infarction, and stroke.[108–112] Of importance, the defect can be corrected by administration of cofactors such as pyridoxine, folate, and cobalamin in up to half of affected patients, retarding subsequent progression of disease.[112, 114]

Increased levels of plasma homocystine have been noted in patients with premature occlusive disease of the heart, brain, and peripheral systems, particularly after methionine loading. Ongoing studies suggest that plasma homocystine levels are an independent risk factor for vascular disease.[112–114, 114a, 114b]

Neurofibromatosis

Neurofibromatosis is an autosomal dominant defect linked to chromosome 17 that is expressed in a broad mosaic of clinical patterns:

1. Almost universal involvement of the skin and eyes.
2. Involvement of the brain and spinal cord in up to half of patients.
3. Occasional (but distinctive) involvement of the long bones by dysplasia.
4. Stenotic lesions and sometimes aneurysm formation in the major arteries.

Cutaneous lesions may be subtle or extensive and include café au lait spots (six or more), neurofibromas, hypopigmentation or hyperpigmentation, and freckling in the axillary or groin region. Small hamartomas are detected by MRI of the brain in almost 50% of patients. Cerebral neurofibromas, optic gliomas, and both paraspinal and intradural neurofibromas and astrocytomas occur in 2% to 14% of patients.[115]

The incidence of vascular involvement in neurofibromatosis is unknown, but an evolving appreciation of arterial lesions is suggested by an increasing number of case reports. The most commonly documented lesion is tubular coarctation of the pararenal aorta and proximal stenosis of the renal arteries, usually occurring in combination but occasionally seen independently.

Affected patients present in their second or third decade of life with significant hypertension and sometimes claudication. Aneurysm of the renal artery and its branches may occur. When available, tissue may show only intimal proliferation; more commonly, however, neurogenic cells are found in the media and adventitia. Standard bypass procedures are effective.[116] Stenotic and aneurysmal lesions of the internal carotid artery and stenosis of the anterior and middle cerebral, superior mesenteric, and celiac arteries have also been reported.[117]

Tuberous Sclerosis

Tuberous sclerosis is an autosomal dominant defect characterized by multiple small angiofibromas involving almost any organ but chiefly the brain, face, and kidneys. It manifests in the first decade of life with facial lesions, varying degrees of mental retardation, or seizures. Death can result from[118]:

- Extensive replacement of the renal parenchyma and renal failure
- Malignant brain tumor
- Rhabdomyoma of the heart with conduction disturbance
- Pneumonia and sepsis following status epilepticus

Aneurysm formation is a rare manifestation of the disease. Fewer than a dozen such aneurysms have been reported, most in the infrarenal abdominal aorta. Prosthetic graft replacement has been successful and durable.[119, 120] An axillary artery aneurysm has been associated with the disease,[121] and at the authors' institution, a solitary ruptured thoracic aneurysm occurred in a series of more than 350 patients.[118] An abdominal aneurysm has been successfully repaired (Fig. 25–7).

Most aneurysms of childhood are secondary to infection following umbilical artery catheterization.[119] Kawasaki's disease and nonspecific aortoarteritis are other causes of childhood aneurysms. Aneurysms caused by heritable connective tissue disorders and neurofibromatosis manifest during the second decade of life or later.

Coarctation of the Abdominal Aorta

Abdominal aortic coarctation or hypoplasia is a nonhereditary lesion that is seen randomly and accounts for only 0.5% to 2% of all coarctations. The stenosis may be quite focal or may involve the entire intra-abdominal aorta. Most lesions occur above or at the level of the renal arteries. The proximal renal arteries are involved in about 80% of cases, and the celiac and superior mesenteric arteries are affected on occasion (Fig. 25–8).

Lesions are commonly detected in the second or third decade of life because of hypertension or claudication.[122–124] Hypertension is caused by activation of the renin-angiotensin system.[123, 124] Physical examination may show hypertension, an abdominal bruit, reduced or delayed femoral pulses, and, sometimes, palpable collateral arteries on the abdominal wall. Like patients with classic thoracic aortic coarctation, patients with abdominal aortic coarctation are subject to cerebrovascular accidents, coronary disease, and

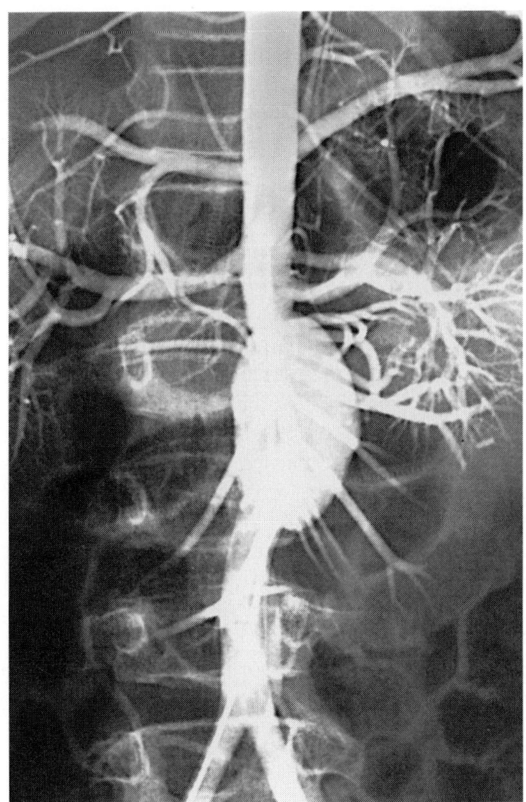

FIGURE 25–7. A 3-cm abdominal aortic aneurysm in a 9-year-old girl with tuberous sclerosis. The aneurysm was discovered during ultrasound imaging for assessment of a ventriculoperitoneal shunt placed because of recurrent astrocytoma. The aorta distal to the lesion measures 0.9 cm. The aneurysm was treated by conventional tube graft repair.

congestive heart failure in the third and fourth decades of life if control of hypertension is not timely.[123]

Repair follows established surgical principles. Depending on the extent of the lesion, hypertension can be treated by aortorenal bypass, splenorenal or hepatorenal shunts, reimplantation of the kidney, or nephrectomy (with or without aortic replacement as required by hypertension or claudication). The durability of autogenous vein or hypogastric artery grafts makes them preferable to prosthetic bypass in these youthful patients. Staging of renal and aortic procedures is sometimes a prudent choice.[124]

Abdominal coarctation (the "mid-aortic syndrome") may also be associated with neurofibromatosis, radiation therapy (Fig. 25–9), focal atherosclerosis of the thoracic or abdominal aorta (all discussed in this chapter), and nonspecific aortoarteritis (see Chapter 21).

Persistent Sciatic Artery

Persistence of the sciatic artery (axial artery) is rare, with fewer than 100 reported cases and a prevalence of 0.25 per 1000 patients studied by angiography.[125] Knowledge of the lesion is important because it provides both a diagnostic and a therapeutic challenge.

During early embryonic development, the femoral plexus is supplied both *ventrally* by the internal iliac artery, later to evolve into the femoropopliteal system, and *dorsally* by the axial artery, which later normally regresses to become the gluteal (sciatic) artery. In the *complete* form of this syndrome, the large embryonic sciatic vessel communicates directly with the popliteal artery, with or without an intact femoropopliteal vessel. In the *incomplete* form, the anomalous artery may terminate anywhere in the pelvis or thigh. Pillet and colleagues[126] have provided a useful classification of the various variations. An apparent paradox is created when the femoral pulse is absent yet distal pulses are full, being supplied by the persistent sciatic artery, which enters the leg deeply through the sciatic notch; this is known as *Cowie's sign*.[127, 128]

The syndrome is usually diagnosed in patients 50 years of age but may be noted throughout life. Sex distribution is almost equal, and the lesions are bilateral in a third of cases. More than a third of these lesions are found incidental to angiographic or necropsy studies. Aneurysm forma-

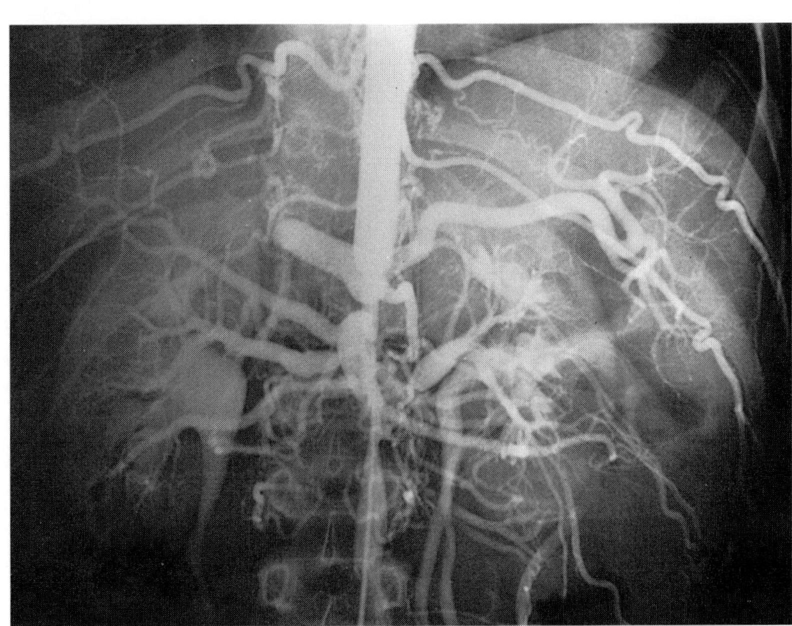

FIGURE 25–8. Multiple congenital stenoses of the abdominal aorta, the celiac and superior mesenteric arteries, two right renal arteries, and one left renal artery in a young male patient. When seen at age 11, the boy had reduced and delayed femoral and distal pulses bilaterally, claudication, and accelerated hypertension with serial values of 160–170/115–120 mmHg. Aortoaortic, renal, hepatic, and superior mesenteric Dacron bypass grafting were performed. The patient was normotensive and well at age 26 years, and all grafts were patent. Note the enlarged intercostal arteries that contributed to palpable collateral arteries for the legs.

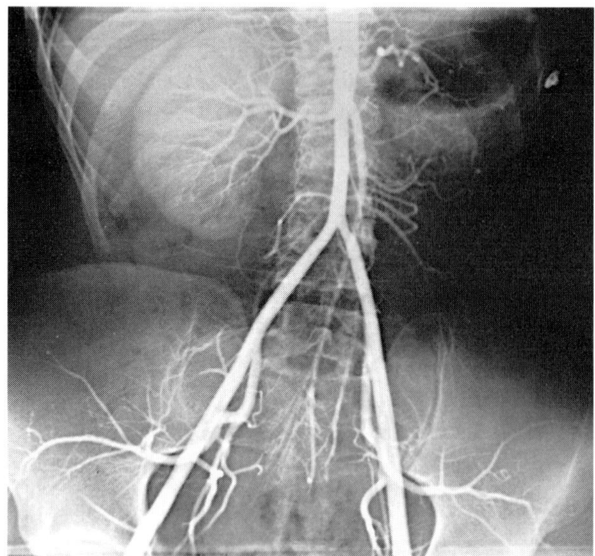

FIGURE 25–9. Hypoplastic abdominal aorta, solitary right renal artery, and splenic artery in a 24-year-old man who had received radiation therapy for left renal neuroblastoma at 6 months of age. The atrophic left kidney was removed, and the patient's hypertension decreased at age 11 years. When seen at age 24 years, the patient described bilateral buttock, thigh, and calf claudication since age 6 years, and he had never run without experiencing claudication. He declined surgery and was normotensive and well at age 37 with antihypertensive drug therapy.

tion, chiefly in the pelvic portion of the artery, accounts for most clinical signs. Manifestations include a pulsatile buttock mass, distal embolization, rupture, and compression of the sciatic nerve.[128] On occasion, aneurysm formation in an incomplete sciatic artery in the thigh may mimic a soft tissue tumor.[129]

Surgery is indicated for rupture, symptomatic aneurysms, and ischemic complications. Both ligation and embolization are effective.[128, 130] Angiography of both legs is essential for diagnosis and surgical planning; bypass procedures must be added when the femoropopliteal system is not intact.

UNCOMMON ACQUIRED ARTERIOPATHIES

The effects of trauma, drugs, and occupational hazards on the arterial system are detailed in Chapters 58 to 61 and 87. The microcirculation is subject to an additional diverse group of mechanisms that includes atheroembolism and environmental, hematologic, and immune processes (see Chapters 56 and 82). Four other uncommon problems warrant discussion here.

Tumor

Only a few hundred primary vascular tumors have been recognized. Most are leiomyosarcomas and leiomyomas of the venous system, and only 20%, numbering a few dozen cases, involve the arteries.[131–135] These are almost exclusively various sarcomas, including fibrosarcoma, myxosarcoma, fibroxanthoma, spindle cell and giant cell sarcoma, and leiomyosarcoma. Isolated instances of benign myxoma and fibromyxoma have been reported.[136] The sarcomas are located most commonly in the pulmonary arteries or any portion of the aorta, and occasionally in the femoral, popliteal, splenic, mesenteric, internal mammary, and other arteries.[133, 135] Local spread is usual, and metastases are common, chiefly to the skin, pleura, bones, lungs, adrenals, kidneys, liver, and spleen. Males are predominantly affected[133–135] by all except malignant fibrous histiocytoma,[132] and the diagnosis is usually made between the ages of 40 and 80 years.

Tumors may be intraluminal, intimal, or adventitial. Clinical presentation may be a mass found incidental to imaging or examination, claudication, acute ischemia from local thrombosis, distal embolization of tumor or thrombus, or a false aneurysm. Significant renovascular hypertension from aortic coarctation or renal artery involvement is not uncommon.[135]

Survival in all forms of sarcoma is usually measured in months, and recurrence is common after resection. Arterial repair is feasible for palliation. Aggressive adjunctive chemotherapy, currently evolving, offers hope of better survival in selected cases.[132] The importance of careful histologic examination of resected material or emboli for identification of both primary tumors and tumors embolizing from other sources is self-evident.

Radiation

Massive radiation therapy from any source occasionally causes early or late arterial lesions of clinical significance. These occur predominantly when the dosage has exceeded 5000 rads.[137–139] Radiation-induced arterial injury[137, 138, 140–142] can be expressed many ways:

1. Acute thrombosis or arterial rupture (in the early months of radiation arteritis).
2. Arterial fibrosis and stenosis (later signs).
3. Accelerated local atherosclerosis (usually 3 to 10 years after treatment).

Almost any artery can sustain damage. Presenting symptoms include exsanguinating hemorrhage, acute carotid or peripheral arterial occlusion, claudication, transient ischemic attacks, stroke, and hypertension (see Fig. 25–9).[137, 139, 143]

Standard techniques of carotid endarterectomy and bypass, as well as replacement or bypass of other arteries, can be safely accomplished with some greater technical challenge in patients with inflamed or fibrosed tissues.[139, 143] Of importance is the potential for late graft infection (up to 25%) in the area of prior radiation. When possible, the irradiated area should be avoided, autologous grafts used when feasible, and regular surveillance of grafts performed in zones of radiation.[139] In some cases, angioplasty with or without stenting is preferred to surgery.[143a, 143b]

Focal Calcific Aortic Obstruction

A unique localized manifestation of atherosclerosis, focal calcific obstruction causes significant obstruction of the abdominal or thoracic aorta and manifests as advanced coarctation.[144–147] It is estimated to account for less than 1% of operable aortic disease.[145] The lesion is only a few centimeters in length and consists of a heavily calcified thrombus that reduces the aortic lumen and produces a pressure gradient. The lesion is usually associated with other manifestations of atherosclerosis. Patients are more commonly female, are almost always heavy smokers, and present between 30 and 60 years of age. Calcific obstructive disease of both the thoracic and abdominal aorta is easily overlooked when angiographic or ultrasound examination is used to assess a more obvious disorder and is not extended to include these lesions.[146]

The abdominal form, often called "coral reef" atherosclerosis, predominates and is located in the celiac or (rarely) infrarenal aorta. Renal and visceral artery stenoses may coexist, but the hemodynamics of the calcific lesion cause hypertension in almost all patients and claudication in most. Fatal acute thrombotic occlusion has been reported, but distal embolization (large emboli) is rare.[145] Thromboendarterectomy or bypass procedures eliminated the pressure gradient in 18 reported cases.[146]

Fewer than 10 cases of the thoracic form have been reported. The lesion is just distal to the left subclavian artery, and dense, speckled calcification of the aortic knob is seen with chest radiographs or other images. Transesophageal echocardiography allows indirect measurement of the pressure gradient. Affected patients all present with severe hypertension and often with recurrent congestive heart failure or coronary events. Surgical resection with prosthetic replacement is the most common procedure; it has been used in six reported cases with favorable results.[146] Severe calcification of the aortic arch and left subclavian artery may preclude this procedure, and successful bypass grafting was recently utilized at the authors' institution.

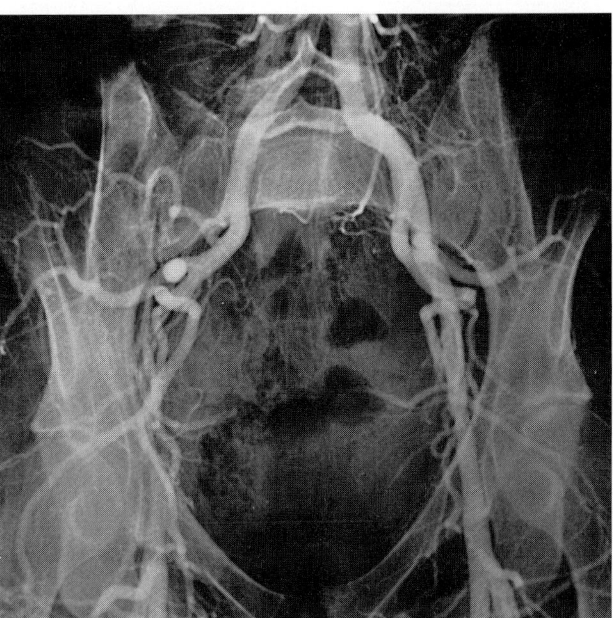

FIGURE 25–10. Complete occlusion of the right external iliac artery and remarkable collateral development in a 30-year-old woman. The patient, who was a high-level competitive cyclist for many years, experienced thigh and calf claudication during heavy workloads for 4 years and could identify an acute reduction in exercise capacity 6 months before diagnosis. Ten minutes on the treadmill at 4 mph and with a 15% grade was required to duplicate her symptoms: ankle brachial indices were 0.71 at rest and 0.31 immediately after exercise. She was asymptomatic following bypass repair. Note, however, the early stenosis of the left external iliac artery, which became symptomatic at higher workloads after repair of the right.

Iliac Syndrome in Cyclists

An arterial lesion peculiar to competitive cyclists has been described and carefully analyzed.[148, 149] A review of 23 cases is uniform in reporting clinical, angiographic, surgical, and pathologic observations that define a new entity.

The affected cyclists had accumulated 50,000 to 150,000 km of high-level training and competition over several years, and symptoms began between the ages of 20 and 42 years. All complained of claudication, 21 characterizing it as buttock and thigh pain followed by numbness of the entire limb, and two as only heaviness and numbness. Symptoms often occurred only under maximal stress, such as "hill climbing" or sprinting, and quick relief was obtained as the pace was reduced. All but one of the patients were men, and only one patient had bilateral symptoms. Pulse and ankle systolic pressures were normal at rest but dropped when symptoms were reproduced by strenuous ergometric cycling. A lower quadrant bruit was noted at rest in eight patients but only with the thigh flexed. Thus, both the history and physical examination are compatible with a subcritical stenosis that becomes hemodynamically significant only with maximal stress.[149]

Arteriography has demonstrated modest narrowing of the mid-portion of the external iliac artery over 5 to 6 cm, with some lengthening and tortuosity when the thigh was flexed. At surgery, direct and angioscopic examinations have shown intimal hyperplasia, confirmed by microscopy, that was eccentrically located at the greatest curves produced in the artery by the cycling position. The stenoses were in the range of 40% to 60%.

All patients underwent (1) segmental resection to shorten the artery, (2) endarterectomy, and (3) ligation of a prominent psoas arterial branch (believed to enhance iliac artery lengthening), when present, in this series. All patients returned to cycling,[149] but we are aware of patients who have needed to discontinue cycling because of this problem.

A solitary case in our experience differs in that complete thrombotic occlusion was superimposed on the basic lesion, and a contralateral lesion has become symptomatic since the initial repair (Fig. 25–10). Since the original description of this disease, additional cases caused by endofibrosis[150] as well as dissection[151, 152] have been reported.

REFERENCES

1. Fauci AS, Haynes BF, Katz P: The spectrum of vasculitis: Clinical, pathologic, immunologic, and therapeutic considerations. Ann Intern Med 89:660, 1978.
2. Sheps SG, McDuffie FC: Vasculitis. *In* Juergens JL, Spittell JA, Fairbairn JF (eds): Peripheral Vascular Disease. Philadelphia, WB Saunders, 1980, p 493.
3. Hunder GG, Lie JT: The vasculitides. *In* Spittell JA Jr (ed): Clinical Vascular Disease. Philadelphia, FA Davis, 1983, p 261.
4. Paulus H, Kono D: Upper extremity manifestations of systemic vascular disorders. *In* Machleder HA (ed): Vascular Disorders of the Upper Extremity. Mount Kisco, NY, Futura Publishing, 1989, p 305.
5. Churg A, Churg J: Systemic Vasculitides. New York, Igaku-Shoin, 1991.

6. Calabrese LH, Clough JD: Systemic vasculitis. *In* Young JR, Graor RA, Olin JW, et al (eds): Peripheral Vascular Disease. St. Louis, Mosby–Year Book, 1991, p 339.
7. Klein RG, Hunder GG, Stanson AW, Sheps SG: Large artery involvement in giant cell (temporal) arteritis. Ann Intern Med 83:806, 1975.
8. Fraga A, Mintz G, Valle L, Flores-Izquierdo G: Takayasu's arteritis: Frequency of systemic manifestations (study of 22 patients) and favorable response to maintenance steroid therapy with adrenocorticosteroids (12 patients). Arthritis Rheum 15:617, 1972.
9. Hall S, Barr W, Lie JT, et al: Takayasu's arteritis: A study of 32 North American patients. Medicine 64:89, 1985.
10. Shelhamer JH, Volkman DJ, Parrillo JE, et al: Takayasu's arteritis and its therapy. Ann Intern Med 103:121, 1985.
11. Horton BT, Magath TB, Brown GE: An undescribed form of arteritis of the temporal vessels. Proc Staff Meet Mayo Clin 7:700, 1932.
12. Huston KA, Hunder GG, Lie JT, et al: Temporal arteritis: A 25-year epidemiologic, clinical and pathologic study. Ann Intern Med 88:162, 1978.
13. Hunder GG, Sheps SG, Allen GL, Joyce JW: Daily and alternate-day corticosteroid regimens in treatment of giant cell arteritis: Comparison in a prospective study. Ann Intern Med 82:613, 1975.
14. Fauchald P, Rygvold O, Sytese B: Temporal arteritis and polymyalgia rheumatica: Clinical and biopsy findings. Ann Intern Med 77:845, 1972.
15. Save-Soderbergh J, Malmvall BE, Andersson R, et al: Giant cell arteritis as a cause of death: Report of nine cases. JAMA 255:493, 1986.
16. Wilkinson IMS, Russell RWR: Arteritis of the head and neck in giant cell arteritis: A pathologic study to show the pattern of arterial involvement. Arch Neurol 27:378, 1972.
17. Caselli RJ, Hunder GG, Whisnant JP: Neurologic disease in biopsy-proven giant cell (temporal) arteritis. Neurology 38:352, 1988.
18. Enzmann D, Scott WR: Intracranial involvement of giant-cell arteritis. Neurology 27:794, 1977.
19. Stanson AW, Klein RG, Hunder CG: Extracranial angiographic findings in giant cell (temporal) arteritis. Am J Roentgenol 127:957, 1976.
20. Hollenhorst RW, Brown JE, Wagener HP, et al: Neurologic aspects of temporal arteritis. Neurology 10:490, 1967.
21. Anderson T: Arteritis temporalis (Horton): A symptom of generalized vascular disease. Acta Med Scand 128:153, 1947.
22. Birkhead NC, Wagener HP, Shick RM: Treatment of temporal arteritis with adrenal corticosteroids: Results of fifty-five cases in which lesion was proved at biopsy. JAMA 163:821, 1957.
23. Wong RL, Korn JH: Temporal arteritis without an elevated erythrocyte sedimentation rate: Case report and review of the literature. Am J Med 80:959, 1986.
24. Whitaker JJ, Hagedorn AB, Pease GL: Anemia in temporal arteritis. Postgrad Med 40:35, 1966.
25. Dickson ER, Maldonado JE, Sheps SG, et al: Systemic giant cell arteritis with polymyalgia rheumatica: Reversible abnormalities of liver function. JAMA 224:1496, 1973.
26. Chuang TY, Hunder GG, Ilstrup DM, et al: Polymyalgia rheumatica: A 10-year epidemiologic and clinical study. Ann Intern Med 97:672, 1982.
27. Hunder GG, Allen GL: The relationship between polymyalgia rheumatica and temporal arteritis. Geriatrics 28:134, 1973.
28. Hunder GG, Disney TF, Ward LE: Polymyalgia rheumatica. Mayo Clin Proc 44:849, 1969.
29. Hall S, Lie JT, Kurland LT, et al: The therapeutic impact of temporal artery biopsy. Lancet 2:1217, 1983.
30. Austen WG, Blennerhassett JB: Giant cell aortitis causing an aneurysm of the ascending aorta and aortic regurgitation. N Engl J Med 272:80, 1965.
31. Halpin DP, Moran KT, Jewell ER: Arm ischemia secondary to giant cell arteritis. Ann Vasc Surg 2:381, 1988.
32. Joyce JW, Hollier LH: The giant cell arteritis: Temporal and Takayasu's arteritis. *In* Bergan JJ, Yao JST (eds): Evaluation and Treatment of Upper and Lower Extremity Circulatory Disorders. New York, Grune & Stratton, 1984, p 465.
33. Frohnert PP, Sheps SG: Long-term follow-up study of periarteritis nodosa. Am J Med 43:8, 1967.
34. Cohen RD, Conn DL, Ilstrup DM: Clinical features, prognosis, and response to treatment in polyarteritis. Mayo Clin Proc 55:146, 1980.
35. Rose GE, Spencer H: Polyarteritis nodosa. Q J Med 26:43, 1957.
36. McCauley RL, Johnston MR, Fauci AS: Surgical aspects of systemic necrotizing vasculitis. Surgery 97:104, 1985.
37. Fauci AS, Katz P, Haynes BF, et al: Cyclophosphamide therapy of severe systemic necrotizing vasculitis. N Engl J Med 301:235, 1979.
38. Wold LE, Baggenstoss AH: Gastrointestinal lesions of periarteritis nodosa. Mayo Clin Proc 24:28, 1949.
39. Selke FW, Williams GB, Donovan DL, et al: Management of intraabdominal aneurysms associated with periarteritis nodosa. J Vasc Surg 4:294, 1986.
40. Mogle P, Hallerin Y, Kobrin K, et al: Rapid regression of aneurysms in polyarteritis nodosa. Br J Radiol 55:536, 1982.
41. Decker JL, Steinberg AD, Reinersten JL: Systemic lupus erythematosus: Evolving concepts. Ann Intern Med 91:587, 1979.
42. Donadio JV Jr, Holley KE, Ferguson RH, et al: Treatment of diffuse proliferative lupus nephritis with prednisone and combined prednisone and cyclophosphamide. N Engl J Med 299:1151, 1978.
43. Boey ML, Colaco CB, Gharavi AE, et al: Thrombosis in systemic lupus erythematosus: Striking association with the presence of circulating lupus anticoagulant. Br Med J 287:1021, 1983.
44. Gluek HI, Kent KS, Weiss MA, et al: Thrombosis in systemic lupus erythematosus: Relation to the presence of circulating anticoagulants. Arch Intern Med 145:1389, 1985.
45. Bowie EJW, Thompson JH, Cascuzzi PA, et al: Thrombosis in SLE despite circulating anticoagulants. J Lab Clin Med 62:416, 1963.
46. Gastineau DA, Kazmier FJ, Nichols WL, et al: Lupus anticoagulant: An analysis of the clinical and laboratory features of 219 cases. Am J Hematol 19:265, 1985.
47. Shimizu T, Ehrlich GE, Inaba G, et al: Behçet disease (Behçet syndrome). Semin Arthritis Rheum 8:223, 1979.
48. O'Duffy JD: Vasculitis in Behçet's disease. Rheum Dis Clin North Am 16:423, 1990.
49. O'Duffy JE, Robertson DM, Goldstein NP: Chlorambucil in the treatment of uveitis and meningoencephalitis of Behçet's disease. Am J Med 76:75, 1984.
50. Masuda K, Nakajima A, Urayama A, et al: Double-masked trial of cyclosporin versus colchicine and long-term open study of cyclosporin in Behçet's disease. Lancet 1:1096, 1989.
51. Yazici H, Pazarli H, Barnes CG, et al: A controlled trial of azathioprine in Behçet's syndrome. N Engl J Med 322:281, 1990.
51a. Avci O, Gurler N, Gunes AT: Efficacy of cyclosporine on mucocutaneous manifestations of Behçet's disease. J Am Acad Dermatol 36:796, 1997.
52. Plotkin GR: Cardiac, vascular, renal and pulmonary features. *In* Plotkin GR, Calabro JJ, O'Duffy JD (eds): Behçet's Disease: A Contemporary Synopsis. Mt. Kisco, NY, Futura Publishing, 1988, p 203.
53. Du LTH, Bletry O, Wechsler B, et al: Arterial manifestations in Behçet's disease: Fifteen cases in a series of 250 patients. *In* O'Duffy JD, Kokmen Emre (eds): Behçet's Disease: Basic and Clinical Aspects. New York, Marcel Dekker, 1991, p 145.
54. Durieux P, Bletry O, Huchon G, et al: Multiple pulmonary artery aneurysms in Behçet's disease and Hughes-Stovin syndrome. Am J Med 71:736, 1981.
55. Grenier P, Bletry O, Cornud F, et al: Pulmonary involvement in Behçet disease. Am J Radiol 137:565, 1981.
56. Enoch BA, Castillo-Olivares JD, Khoo TCL, et al: Major vessel complications in Behçet's syndrome. Postgrad Med J 44:453, 1968.
57. Little AG, Zarins CG: Abdominal aortic aneurysm and Behçet's disease. Surgery 91:359, 1982.
58. Shefir A, Stewart P, Mendes DM: The repetitive vascular catastrophes of Behçet's disease: A case report with review of the literature. Ann Vasc Surg 6:85, 1992.
59. Yanagawa H, Kawasaki T, Shigematsu I: Nationwide survey on Kawasaki disease in Japan. Pediatrics 80:58, 1987.
60. Kawasaki T: Mucocutaneous lymph node syndrome: Clinical observation of 50 cases. Jpn J Allergy 16:178, 1967.
61. Nakamura Y, Yanagawa H, Kawasaki T: Mortality among children with Kawasaki disease in Japan. N Engl J Med 326:1246, 1992.
62. Kato H, Ichinose E, Yoshioka F, et al: Fate of coronary aneurysms in Kawasaki disease: Serial coronary angiography and long-term follow-up study. Am J Cardiol 49:1758, 1982.
63. Capannari TE, Daniels SR, Meyer RA, et al: Sensitivity, specificity and predictive value of two-dimensional echocardiography in detecting coronary artery aneurysms in patients with Kawasaki disease. J Am Coll Cardiol 7:355, 1986.
64. Bierman FZ, Gersony WM: Kawasaki disease: Clinical perspective. J Pediatr 111:789, 1987.

65. Sethi S, Ott DA, Nihill M: Surgical management of the cardiovascular complications of Kawasaki's disease. Texas Heart Inst J 10:343, 1983.
66. Newburger JW, Takahashi M, Burns JC, et al: The treatment of Kawasaki syndrome with intravenous gamma globulin. N Engl J Med 315:341, 1986.
67. Neuberger JW, Takahashi M, Beiser AS, et al: A single intravenous infusion of gamma globulin as compared with four infusions in the treatment of acute Kawasaki syndrome. N Engl J Med 324:1633, 1991.
68. Takahashi M, Mason W, Lewis AB: Regression of coronary aneurysms in patients with Kawasaki syndrome. Circulation 75:387, 1987.
69. Fukushige J, Nhill MR, McNamara DG: Spectrum of cardiovascular lesions in mucocutaneous lymph node syndrome: Analysis of eight cases. Am J Cardiol 45:98, 1980.
70. Caputo AE, Roberts WN, Yee YS, et al: Hepatic artery aneurysm in corticosteroid-treated, adult Kawasaki's disease. Ann Vasc Surg 5:533, 1991.
71. Rao SL, Misra RC, Chugh SK: Digital arteriopathy in rheumatoid arthritis. J Chronic Dis 29:205, 1976.
72. Scott DGI, Bacon PA, Tribe CR: Systemic rheumatoid vasculitis: A clinical and laboratory study of 50 cases. Medicine 60:288, 1981.
73. Ferguson RH, Slocumb CH: Peripheral neuropathy in rheumatoid arthritis. Bull Rheum Dis 11:251, 1961.
74. Abel T, Andrews BS, Cunningham PH, et al: Rheumatoid vasculitis: Effect of cyclophosphamide on the clinical course and levels of circulating immune complexes. Ann Intern Med 93:407, 1980.
75. Gruickshank B: Pathology of ankylosing spondylitis. Bull Rheum Dis 10:211, 1960.
76. Ansell BM, Bywaters EGL, Doniach I: The aortic lesions of ankylosing spondylitis. Br Heart J 20:507, 1958.
77. Paulus HE, Pearson CM, Pitts W Jr: Aortic insufficiency in five patients with Reiter's syndrome: A detailed clinical and pathologic study. Am J Med 53:464, 1972.
78. Kean WF, Anastassiades TP, Ford PM: Aortic incompetence in HLA B27-positive juvenile arthritis. Ann Rheum Dis 39:294, 1980.
79. Duvernoy WFC, Schatz IJ: Rheumatoid spondylitis associated with aneurysmal dilation of the entire thoracic aorta. Henry Ford Hosp Med Bull 14:309, 1966.
80. Cipriano PR, Alonso DR, Baltaxe HA, et al: Multiple aortic aneurysms in relapsing polychondritis. Am J Cardiol 37:1097, 1976.
81. Esdaile J, Hawkins D, Gold P, et al: Vascular involvement in relapsing polychondritis. Can Med Assoc J 116:1019, 1977.
82. Michet CJ, McKenna CH, Luthra HS, et al: Relapsing polychondritis: Survival and predictive roles of early disease manifestations. Ann Intern Med 104:74, 1986.
83. Hughes RAC, Berry CL, Seifert M, et al: Relapsing polychondritis: Three cases with a clinico-pathological study and literature review. Q J Med 41:363, 1972.
84. McKusick VA (ed): Heritable Disorders of Connective Tissue, 4th ed. St. Louis, CV Mosby, 1972.
85. Steinberg AG, Bearn AC, Motulsky AG, et al (eds): Progress in Medical Genetics, New Series, Vol 5, Genetics of Cardiovascular Disease. Philadelphia, WB Saunders, 1983.
86. Prockop DJ, Kivirikk KI: Heritable disease of collagen. N Engl J Med 311:376, 1984.
87. McKusick VA: Mendelian Inheritance in Man, 6th ed. Baltimore, John Hopkins University Press, 1982.
88. Peyritz R: Ehlers-Danlos syndromes. *In* Steinberg AG, Bearn AC, Motulsky AG, et al (eds): Progress in Medical Genetics, New Series, Vol 5, Genetics of Cardiovascular Disease. Philadelphia, WB Saunders, 1983.
89. Sarfarazi M, Tsipouras P, Del Mastro R, et al: A linkage map of 10 loci flanking the Marfan syndrome locus on 15q: Result of an international consortium study. Med Genet 29:75, 1992.
90. Abraham PA, Pereida AJ, Carnes WH, et al: Marfan syndrome: Demonstration of abnormal elastin in aorta. J Clin Invest 70:1245, 1982.
91. Peyritz RE, McKusick VA: The Marfan syndrome: Diagnosis and management. N Engl J Med 300:772, 1979.
92. DeBakey ME, McCollum CH, Crawford ES, et al: Dissecting aneurysms of the aorta. *In* Bergen J, Yao J (eds): Aneurysms: Diagnosis and treatment. New York, Grune & Stratton, 1982, p 97.
93. Miller DC: Surgical management of aortic dissection: Medications, preoperative management, and long-term results. *In* Doroghazi RM, Slater EE (eds): Aortic Dissection. New York, McGraw-Hill, 1983, pp 197–243.
94. Cambria RP, Brewster DC, Gertler J, et al: Vascular complications associated with spontaneous aortic dissection. J Vasc Surg 7:199, 1988.
95. Adib K, Belzer FO: Renal autotransplantation in dissecting aortic aneurysm with renal artery involvement. Surgery 84:686, 1978.
96. Peyritz RE: Propranolol retards aortic root dilation in the Marfan syndrome. Circulation Suppl 3:111, 1983.
97. Gott VL, Pyeritz RE, Cameron DE, et al: Composite graft repair of Marfan aneurysm of the ascending aorta: Results in 100 patients. Ann Thorac Surg 52:38, 1991.
98. Cikrit DF, Miles JH, Silver D: Spontaneous arterial perforation: The Ehlers-Danlos specter. J Vasc Surg 5:248, 1987.
99. Beighton P: Lethal complications of the Ehlers-Danlos syndrome. Br Med J 3:656, 1968.
100. Luscher TF, Essandon LK, Lie JT, et al: Renovascular hypertension: A rare cardiovascular complication of the Ehlers-Danlos syndrome. Mayo Clin Proc 62:223, 1987.
101. Sherry C, Agomuoh OS, Goldin MD: Review of Ehlers-Danlos syndrome: Successful repair of rupture and dissection of abdominal aorta. J Cardiovasc Surg 29:530, 1988.
102. Bellenot F, Boisgard S, Kantelip B, et al: Type IV Ehlers-Danlos syndrome with isolated arterial involvement. Ann Vasc Surg 4:15, 1990.
103. Connor PJ Jr, Juergens JL, Perry HO, et al: Pseudoxanthoma elasticum and angioid streaks: A review of 106 cases. Am J Med 30:537, 1961.
104. Altman LK, Fialkow PJ, Parker F, et al: Pseudoxanthoma elasticum: An underdiagnosed genetically heterogeneous disorder with protean manifestations. Arch Intern Med 134:1048, 1974.
105. Mendelsohn G, Buckley BH, Hutchins GM: Cardiovascular manifestations of pseudoxanthoma elasticum. Arch Pathol Lab Med 102:298, 1978.
106. Carlborg V, Ejrup B, Gronglad E, et al: Vascular studies in pseudoxanthoma elasticum and angioid streaks. Acta Med Scand 350(Suppl 166):3, 1959.
107. Carter DJ, Vince FP, Woodword DAK: Arterial surgery in pseudoxanthoma elasticum. Postgrad Med J 52:291, 1976.
108. Carson NAJ, Cusworth DC, Dent CE, et al: Homocystinurea: A new inborn error of metabolism associated with mental deficiency. Arch Dis Child 38:425, 1963.
109. Gibson JB, Carson NAJ, Neil DW: Pathologic findings in homocystinuria. J Clin Pathol 17:427, 1964.
110. Harker LA, Slichter SJ, Scott CR, et al: Homocystinemia: Vascular injury and arterial thrombosis. N Engl J Med 291:537, 1974.
111. Muss SH, Skouby F, Levy HL. The natural history of homocystinurea due to cystathionine beta synthetase deficiency. Am J Hum Genet 37:1, 1985.
112. Boers GHL, Smals AGH, Trijbels FJM: Heterozygote for homocystinuria in premature peripheral and cerebral arterial disease. N Engl J Med 313:709, 1985.
113. Clarke R, Daly L, Robinson K, et al: Hyperhomocystinemia: An independent risk factor for vascular disease. N Engl J Med 324:1149, 1991.
114. Harris EJ Jr, Taylor LM Jr, Malinow MR, et al: The association between elevated plasma homocysteine and symptomatic peripheral arterial disease. Surg Forum 40: 307, 1989.
114a. Singh H: Selections from current literature: Homocysteine: A modifiable risk factor for cardiovascular disease. Fam Pract 14:335, 1997.
114b. Ray M, Kumar L, Prasad R: Homocysteineuria with early thromboembolic episodes and rapid response to high dose pyridoxine. Indian Pediatr 34:67, 1997.
115. Mulvihill JJ, Parry DM, Sherman JL, et al: Neurofibromatosis I (Recklinghausen disease) and neurofibromatosis II (bilateral acoustic neurofibromatosis): An update. Ann Intern Med 113:39, 1990.
116. Halpern M, Currarino G: Vascular lesions causing hypertension in neurofibromatosis. N Engl J Med 273:248, 1965.
117. Riccardi VM: Neurofibromatosis: Phenotype, Natural History, and Pathogenesis. Baltimore, John Hopkins University Press, 1992, p 124.
118. Shepherd CW, Gomez MR, Lie JT, et al: Causes of death in patients with tuberous sclerosis. Mayo Clin Proc 66:792, 1991.
119. Roques X, Choussat A, Bourdeaud'hui A, et al: Aneurysms of the abdominal aorta in the neonate and infant. Ann Vasc Surg 3:335, 1989.
120. Van Reedt-Dortland RW, Bax NM, Huber J: Aortic aneurysm in a 5-year-old boy with tuberous sclerosis. J Pediatr Surg 26:1420, 1991.

121. Libby PA, Maitem AN, Strauss EB: Axillary artery aneurysm in a patient with tuberous sclerosis. Pediatr Radiol 20:94, 1989.
122. DeBakey MF, Garrett E, Howell JF, et al: Coarctation of the abdominal aorta with renal arterial stenosis: Surgical considerations. Ann Surg 165:830, 1967.
123. Onat T, Zeren E: Coarctation of the abdominal aorta: Review of 91 cases. Cardiology 54:140, 1969.
124. Hallett JW, Brewster DC, Darling RC, et al: Coarctation of the abdominal aorta: Current options in surgical management. Ann Surg 191:430, 1980.
125. Greebe J: Congenital anomalies of the iliofemoral artery. J Cardiovasc Surg 18:317, 1977.
126. Pillet J, Cronier P, Mercier PH, et al: The ischiopopliteal trunk: A report of two cases. Anat Clin 3:329, 1982.
127. Cowie TN, McKeller NJ, McLean, et al: Unilateral congenital absence of the external iliac and femoral arteries. Br J Radiol 33:520, 1960.
128. Noblet D, Gasmi T, Mikati A, et al: Persistent sciatic artery: Case report, anatomy and review of the literature. Ann Vasc Surg 2:390, 1988.
129. Simon MA, Scully RE, Springfield DS, et al: Case records of the Massachusetts General Hospital: Case 32, 1992. N Engl J Med 327:412, 1992.
130. Becquemin JP, Gaston A, Caubret P, et al: Aneurysm of persistent sciatic artery: Report of a case treated by endovascular occlusion and femoropopliteal bypass. Surgery 98:605, 1985.
131. Kevorkian Y, Cento DP: Leiomyosarcoma of large arteries and veins. Surgery 73:390, 1972.
132. Busby JR, Ochsner JL, Emory WB, et al: Malignant fibrous histiocytoma arising from descending thoracic aorta. Ann Vasc Surg 4:185, 1990.
133. Becquemin JP, Lebbe C, Saada F, et al: Sarcoma of the aorta: Report of a case and review of the literature. Ann Vasc Surg 2:225, 1988.
134. Briggs PJ, Poolry J, Malcolm AJ, et al: Popliteal artery leiomyosarcoma: A case report and review of the literature. Ann Vasc Surg 4:365, 1990.
135. Josen AS, Khine M: Primary malignant tumor of the aorta. J Vasc Surg 9:493, 1989.
136. Kattus AA, Longmire WP, Cannon JA, et al: Primary intraluminal tumor of the aorta producing malignant hypertension. N Engl J Med 262:694, 1960.
137. Marcial-Rojas RA, Castro JR: Irradiation injury to elastic arteries in the course of treatment for neoplastic disease. Ann Otol 71:945, 1962.
138. Poon TP, Kanshepolsky J, Tchertkoff V: Rupture of the aorta due to radiation injury. JAMA 205:875, 1968.
139. Phillips G, Peer RM, Upson JF, et al: Complications of bypass operations for radiation-induced arterial disease. J Vasc Surg 16:305, 1992.
140. Butler M, Lane R, Webster J: Irradiation injury to large arteries. Br J Surg 67:341, 1980.
141. Conomy J, Kellermeyer R: Delayed cerebrovascular consequences of therapeutic radiation. Cancer 36:1702, 1975.
142. Silverberg G, Britt R, Goffinet D: Radiation-induced carotid artery disease. Cancer 41:130, 1978.
143. Francfort JW, Gallager JF, Penmann E, et al: Surgery for radiation-induced symptomatic carotid atherosclerosis. Ann Vasc Surg 3:16, 1989.
143a. McBride KD, Beard JD, Gaines PA: Percutaneous intervention for radiation damage to axillary arteries. Clin Radiol 49:630, 1994.
143b. Hinchcliffe M, Ruttley MS, Carolan-Rees G: Case report: Percutaneous transluminal angioplasty of irradiation induced bilateral subclavian artery occlusions. Clin Radiol 50:804, 1995.
144. Axilrod HD: Obstruction of the aortic isthmus by a calcified thrombus. Arch Pathol 41:63, 1946.
145. Qvarfordt PG, Reilly LM, Sedwitz MM, et al: "Coral reef" atherosclerosis of the supra-renal aorta: A unique clinical entity. J Vasc Surg 1:903, 1989.
146. Peillon C, Morlet C, Laissy JP, et al: Endoaortic calcific proliferation of the upper abdominal aorta. Ann Vasc Surg 3:181, 1989.
147. Coffin O, Maiza D, Alsweis S: Calcified obstructive disease of the aortic isthmus. Ann Vasc Surg 4:147, 1990.
148. Mosimann R, Walder J, VanMelle G: Stenotic intimal thickening of the external iliac artery: Illness of the competition cyclist. Vasc Surg 19:258, 1985.
149. Rousselet MC, Saint-Andre JP, L'Hoste P, et al: Stenotic intimal thickening of the external iliac artery in competition cyclists. Hum Pathol 21:524, 1990.
150. Abraham P, Leftheriotis G, Bourre Y, et al: Echography of external iliac artery endofibrosis in cyclists. Am J Sports Med 21:861, 1993.
151. Scheerlinck TA, Van den Brande P: Popliteal: Post-traumatic intima dissection and thrombosis of the external iliac artery in sportsman. Eur J Vasc Surg 8:645, 1994.
152. Cook PS, Erdoes LS, Selzer PM, et al: Dissection of the external iliac artery in highly trained athletes. J Vasc Surg 22:173, 1995.

SECTION V

FUNDAMENTAL THERAPEUTIC AND TECHNICAL CONSIDERATIONS

ROBERT B. RUTHERFORD, M.D.

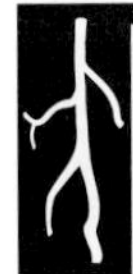

CHAPTER 26

Antithrombotic Therapy

John G. Calaitges, M.D.,
and Donald Silver, M.D.

The vascular specialist must be intimately familiar with ways to alter the hemostatic process to benefit the patient. The vascular surgeon should be able to reduce a patient's rate of coagulation, to render a patient's blood totally incoagulable, and to enhance the patients's coagulation process when necessary. This chapter describes how the hemostatic process can be altered with antithrombotic therapy to reduce the potential for arterial or venous thromboembolism. The process of hemostasis (i.e., normal and abnormal coagulation mechanisms) is reviewed in detail in Chapter 8.

PHARMACOLOGIC MEASURES

Heparin

Heparin is an effective agent for the prevention and management of thromboembolic disorders. Unfractionated heparin is a negatively charged, helical sulfated polysaccharide with a molecular weight (MW) that ranges between 4000 and 40,000 daltons. Commercial heparin is obtained from pork or beef lung or intestine. The greater part of pharmaceutical heparin is devoid of anticoagulant activity; only about 30% of a heparin preparation is able to bind to antithrombin (AT).[1]

Heparin is administered either subcutaneously or intravenously. Intramuscular injection is associated with an unacceptably high rate of hematoma formation. Slow absorption from subcutaneous sites may prolong the "heparin effect" to 8 to 12 hours.[2] Lower blood levels have been observed after subcutaneous administration of the heparin calcium salt compared with the sodium salt.[2] Heparin is bound by the plasma proteins and has a circulating half-life of approximately 90 minutes. Heparin clearance occurs primarily through the reticuloendothelial system. Secondary renal clearance occurs when the reticuloendothelial system becomes saturated with heparin.

Heparin has no anticoagulant activity; its anticoagulant effect depends on the presence of adequate amounts of functionally active AT. Heparin binds to AT in a 1:1 ratio and induces a conformational change in the AT that makes its active centers more available for binding to thrombin and the other serine proteases. The heparin-AT complex irreversibly inhibits the active serine proteases IIa, IXa, Xa, XIa, and XIIa. After the serine proteases are bound to the heparin-AT complex, heparin dissociates and is available to bind to other AT-binding sites.

Low-molecular-weight heparins (LMWHs) are 4000- to 8000-dalton derivatives of unfractionated heparin produced by controlled enzymatic or chemical depolymerization processes. They have fewer saccharide units (<18 to 20 saccharides), resulting in an inability to bind to AT and thrombin simultaneously. However, these saccharide units can interact with AT and factor Xa, and cause the release of tissue factor pathway inhibitor (TFPI) from the endothelium.[3] The antithrombotic effect of the LMWHs is due to their inhibition of factor Xa. LMWHs produce a more predictable anticoagulant response because of their better bioavailability, longer half-life, and dose-independent renal clearance.[4] Consequently, laboratory monitoring is unnecessary except in patients with renal insufficiency.[5] LMWHs are associated with less bleeding than unfractionated heparin in laboratory animals because they (1) produce less inhibition of platelet function, (2) do not increase microvascular permeability, and (3) are less likely to inferfere with the interaction between platelets and vessel walls.[6]

Large amounts of heparin are required to interfere with the coagulation process in patients with extensive thrombosis. Ineffective responses to heparin therapy may also occur in patients with congenital or acquired deficiencies of AT. AT levels are decreased in patients with intravascular coagulation or hepatic insufficiency and during heparin therapy. Patients who are deficient in AT require fresh frozen plasma, cryoprecipitate, or AT concentrate to raise the AT level to at least 80% of normal if the blood is to be anticoagulated with heparin. Platelet factor 4, released during platelet activation, may interfere with the binding of heparin to AT.[7]

Administration

Intravenous (IV) heparin is administered either by continuous infusion or, less preferably, by intermittent injection.

Prospective trials have indicated htat there are fewer hemorrhagic complications when heparin is given by continuous infusion and that smaller doses are required for "adequate" anticoagulation.[8–10] When heparin is administered by continuous infusion, a loading dose of 75 to 100 U/kg is given to initiate therapy; this is usually followed by an infusion of approximately 1000 U/hr. The rate of infusion is adjusted to maintain the monitoring test value within a prescribed range. If the activated partial thromboplastin time (aPTT) is used as the monitor, the recommended range for patients with active thrombosis is 1.7 to 2.0 times the control value. Spontaneous bleeding rarely occurs if the aPTT remains less than twice the control value.

When subcutaneous heparin is given prophylactically to surgical patients to prevent venous thromboembolism, it is injected in doses of 5000 units every 8 to 12 hours, starting 2 hours preoperatively. Therapeutic subcutaneous heparin usually requires 10,000 to 20,000 units every 8 to 12 hours; the dose is adjusted so that the aPTT will be 1.5 to 1.8 times the control value 30 minutes before the next dose. When heparin is given subcutaneously, concentrated solutions should be used to limit the administered volume. The injections are given carefully with a short needle in the subcutaneous tissue of the anterior abdominal wall or the anterior thigh.

Other tests available to regulate heparin therapy include (1) the whole blood clotting time (two to three times control value), (2) whole blood activated decalcification time (two to three times control value), and (3) calcium thrombin time (two to six times control value). The therapeutic range of heparin as assayed by protamine titration or anti-Xa assay is 0.5 to 1.5 U/ml (0.5 U/ml usually provides adequate anticoagulation).

Before heparin therapy or heparin prophylaxis is begun, a simple assessment of hemostasis should be performed, including prothrombin time (PT), partial thromboplastin time (PTT), and platelet count, because hemorrhagic complications are common when preexisting coagulation defects are present.

LMWHs may be administered by subcutaneous, IV, or intra-arterial routes. The dose per weight varies according to the LMWH preparation utilized. If the standard doses are used, no special monitors are required.

Prophylaxis

The inhibition of factor Xa by AT and heparin prevents the potential generation of a considerably large amount of thrombin. Thus, small doses of heparin should have a major antithrombotic effect. Sharnoff and DeBlasio first suggested that prophylactic small doses of heparin could reduce the incidence of fatal pulmonary embolism.[11] Many controlled studies have subsequently confirmed the efficacy of this method but have also shown the limitations of low-dose (5000 units subcutaneously every 8 to 12 hours) heparin prophylaxis. These studies have been summarized by Salzman and Davies.[12] Small subcutaneous doses of heparin reduced the incidence of venous thrombosis as detected by labeled fibrinogen in general surgical patients. In aggregate, the incidence of venous thrombosis was reduced from around 27% (1173 of 4373 patients) to about 6% (168 of 2570 patients) with a range of 0.8% to 13.5%. Laboratory monitoring (apart from initial screening for bleeding disorders) does not appear to be required. The incidence of bleeding complications is low: 0.2% of patients given low-dose heparin died of bleeding, the same rate as in the control group.[13]

The effect of low-dose heparin on the incidence of pulmonary embolism has been more difficult to study because of the lack of standardized criteria for diagnosis. Kakkar and associates[13] studied 4121 general surgical patients over 40 years of age who were randomized to receive either 5000 units of heparin or a placebo subcutaneously every 8 hours, starting 2 hours preoperatively and continuing for 7 days. There were 80 postopertive deaths in the heparin-treated group, of which two were attributed to pulmonary embolism; 16 of the 100 deaths in the control group were attributed to pulmonary embolism.[13] The study has been criticized because of a lower autopsy rate in the heparin-treated group (66% versus 72% in the control group) and because of lax criteria for determining whether an embolus was the cause of death. Despite these criticisms, the results support the use of heparin in venous thromboembolism prophylaxis.

Low-dose heparin has been disappointing in patients undergoing hip surgery or open prostatectomy; however, heparin given in a dose that is titrated to a therapeutically prolonged aPTT, rather than one that is arbitrarily fixed, has been effective in these patients.[14, 15] Although there are reports of its use in neurosurgical patients, heparin has not gained wide acceptance because of the potential for disastrous bleeding complications.

Heparin is routinely used in vascular surgery to prevent clotting in vessels and grafts during and after "clamping." Usually, 5000 to 7000 units of heparin is administered intravenously porior to the appplication of the vascular clamps. Porous vascular grafts are "preclotted" prior to heparin administration. Many vascular surgeons are now using grafts that are impregnated with albumin or collagen to reduce the graft "leakage" and to eliminate the need for preclotting. For each hour that the vascular clamps are in place, a dose of 1000 to 2000 units of additional heparin is given. Heparin reversal is rarely necessary when adequate mechanical hemostasis has been achieved. Patients who have grafts that are at risk for early thrombosis (e.g., below-knee prosthetic grafts) are maintained on a heparin regimen intravenously (aPTT 1.5 to 1.7 times control value) until warfarin anticoagulation is satisfactory. In the postoperative period, for prophylaxis of deep venous thrombosis (DVT), our vascular patients who are immobile are maintained on a subcutaneous heparin regimen (usually 5000 units every 8 to 12 hours) or one of the LMWH preparations until they are ambulatory.

Prior to the insertion of arterial and venous cannulas for cardiopulmonary bypass, patients receive 300 units/kg heparin. Additional heparin is administered periodically to maintain an activated coagulation time (ACT) of at least 400 seconds. The effect of heparin is often reversed at the end of cardiopulmonary bypass. The cardiopulmonary bypass pump return lines should be removed before the protamine is administered. The adequacy of heparin reversal is determined by the ACT, thrombin time (TT), aPTT, or protamine titration test. Protamine sulfate administered intravenously in a dose of 1.0 mg per 100 units of heparin immediately reverses the anticoagulant effect of heparin. One third to one half of the calculated protamine dose should be infused slowly to avoid the risks of hypotension, bradycardia, and vasodilatation.[16] Protamine binds to heparin and interferes with its reaction with AT. When large doses of heparin are given, as during cardiopulmonary bypass, "heparin rebound" may occur because of the dissociation of the heparin-protamine complex or because of further release of heparin from the microcirculation or extravascular sources. Additional protamine sulfate may be required in these instances. Excessive protamine administration may cause an anticoagulant effect because of the interaction of protamine with platelets and serum proteins.

Hemorrhage may also occur from an overdose of LMWH. The overdose may be partially neutralized by the IV injection of protamine sulfate. The dose of protamine varies according to the LMWH preparation. The recommended dosage of protamine sulfate is 1 mg of protamine sulfate for each milligram of enoxaparin or 1 mg of protamine per every 100 anti–factor Xa international units (IU) of dalteparin sodium (Fragmin). Generally, it is not possible to completely neutralize, with protamine, the anti–factor Xa activity of the LMWH.

Complications

Hemorrhagic complications have been observed in 10% to 20% of patients who had normal hemostasis before receiving heparin and in up to 50% of patients with thrombocytopenia or uremia.[17] Patients with active bleeding, intracranial hemorrhage, a recent neurosurgical proceduce, or malignant hypertension may experince major bleeding complications during heparin therapy. Patients who have had recent operative procedures or a stroke are also at risk for bleeding if they receive heparin. Therapeutic doses of heparin in other patients are not likely to be associated with bleeding unless there is an underlying bleeding tendency. Bleeding complications can be reduced by close monitoring of the aPTT. The aPTT should be kept in the range of 1.7 to 2.0 times control. Concomitant administration of aspirin or other antiplatelet function–inhibiting drugs increases the risk of hemorrhage.

Approximately 2% to 3% of patients receiving heparin develop heparin-associated antiplatelet antibodies (HAAbs). The incidence in patients undergoing vascular reconstruction is 21% (authors' unpublished data). These antibodies lead to thrombocytopenia and thrombohemorrhagic complications. The *heparin-induced thrombocytopenia syndrome* (HIT) occurs after 4 to 15 days of therapy in patients exposed to heparin for the first time. HIT may occur on the first day of reexposure to heparin; therefore, daily platelet counts should be obtained in all patients receiving heparin.

The development of HIT is independent of the type, dose, or route of administration of heparin. LMWH is associated with a lower incidence of HAAb production compared with unfractionated heparin.[18] HIT should be considered when a patient receiving any form of heparin has a falling platelet count or a platelet count less than 100,000/mm^3, increasing resistance to anticoagulation with heparin, or new or progressive thrombohemorrhagic complications. HIT has been associated with a 23% mortality and a 61% morbidity.[19] Mortality and morbidity can be reduced to 12% and 22.5%, respectively, if the diagnosis is promptly established and heparin administration is stopped.[20]

When the diagnosis is suspected, all heparin sources, including heparin-coated catheters, should be discontinued and platelet function inhibited. We administer aspirin 325 mg by mouth or 600 mg per rectum as soon as the diagnosis is suspected and then daily. A LMWH may be used if HAAbs do not cross-react with the agent. The cross-reactivity rate with LMWH varies from 20% to 61%, depending on the LMWH product.[18, 21]

The diagnosis is confirmed by an increasing platelet count following cessation of heparin, cessation of the thrombohemorrhagic complications, and positive platelet aggregometry or ^{14}C-serotonin release studies. Patients with HAAbs should not receive the heparin to which they have been sensitized; alternate forms of anticoagulation (warfarin, dextran, or heparin substitutes) are administered if needed. The antibodies may be present for a few weeks or, in our experience, up to 13 years. For all patients with a history of HIT, test results must be negative for the antibodies before patients receive additional heparin to which they have been sensitized.

Sensitivity reactions occur in 2% to 5% of patients receiving heparin. Bronchiole constriction, urticaria, lacrimation, and anaphylaxis in rare instances may occur. Alopecia and osteoporosis occur in fewer than 1% of patients receiving long-term (>6 months) heparin. Hair growth resumes with cessation of heparin therapy.

Warfarin

Oral anticoagulants interfere with the utilization of vitamin K by the liver during the synthesis of factors II, VII, IX, and X. Vitamin K is a cofactor in the reaction that converts glutamyl residues of clotting factor precursors to the carboxyglutamyl residues required for the binding of calcium. When oral anticoagulants are given, antigenically similar clotting factors are produced that are inactive because of their abnormal calcium binding characteristics.

The rate at which anticoagulation occurs depends on the circulating half-lives of the factors. Although factor VII has a half-life of 6 hours, prothrombin has a half-life of 3 days. Anticoagulation is thus not complete for several days, although the PT may be in the therapeutic range within 36 hours because of a reduced level of factor VII. For this reason, therapy with heparin is advised for the first 2 to 4 days of anticoagulation with warfarin. An additional reason for a few days of heparin therapy when warfarin therapy is initiated is that warfarin suppresses the vitamin K–dependent protein C level (half-life, 4 to 6 hours), resulting in a transient procoagulant state, thus supporting the need for heparin anticoagulation during the first 2 to 4 days of anticoagulation with warfarin.

Administration

Warfarin is readily absorbed from the intestine, with peak plasma concentrations being reached in 2 to 12 hours. Ninety-seven per cent of warfarin is bound to albumin and has a circulating half-life of 36 to 40 hours. The unbound fraction is responsible for the anticoagulant effect.

Warfarin therapy is usually initiated with a daily dose of 7.5 to 10 mg. An IV warfarin preparation is available and can be administered before oral intake is begun. The IV dose is the same as the enteral dose. A reduced dose is given to the older patients, patients with hepatic insufficiency, and patients receiving parenteral nutrition or broad-spectrum antibiotics. The maintenance dose of warfarin is determined by the PT, which should be maintained at an International Normalized Ratio (INR) of 2.0 to 2.5. Hemorrhagic complications are infrequent when PT is maintained at this level. The PT should be monitored frequently until it stabilizes and then can be monitored infrequently (e.g., every 4 to 8 weeks).

It is a misconception that patients receiving warfarin should not receive aspirin. Aspirin provides additional protection to the patient through its platelet inhibiting-function; the regulation of PT is not affected by aspirin.

Prophylaxis

Warfarin anticoagulation during and after surgery is effective in preventing venous thrombosis and fatal pulmonary embolism. Sevitt and Gallagher's study[22] of 300 patients with hip fractures demonstrated a reduced incidence of clinically diagnosed DVT from 29% in control patients to 3% in patients who received prophylactic warfarin anticoagulation. At autopsy, the incidence of thrombosis was 83% in the control group and 14% in the group receiving anticoagulants. Pulmonary embolism was thought to be the cause of death in 10% of the control patients but in none of those receiving anticoagulant therapy.[22]

Several other studies have confirmed these findings. In the aggregate, warfarin reduces the rate of venographically detected thrombosis from 47.3% to 23.4% and decreases the frequency of fatal pulmonary embolism from a range of about 2% to 10% to approximately 0.4% in patients undergoing hip surgery.

Long-term postoperative warfarin therapy may enhance infrapopliteal polytetrafluoroethylene (PTFE) graft patency. Flinn and colleagues[23] reviewed a series of patients who had femorotibial or femoropopliteal bypass with PTFE grafts while receiving perioperative heparin and postoperative warfarin anticoagulation. The authors noted a significant improvement in graft patency rates in the infrapopliteal position (37% of patients had patent grafts after 4 years) compared with historical controls (who had a 12% 4-year graft patency rate).[24] The PTs were maintained at twice the control values.

Complications

Bleeding occurs in 4% to 22% of patients receiving warfarin. Fatal hemorrhage has been reported in 1.8% of patients with arterial disease who received warfarin.[25] In the studies in which warfarin was used as the sole prophylactic agent during hip replacement, there was a 0.3% incidence of fatal bleeding. The incidence of bleeding is less if the warfarin dosage is adjusted to cause less elevation of the PT (to 1.3 to 1.5 times control value).[26] Warfarin anticoagulation can be reversed and bleeding controlled with intramuscular or IV vitamin K in approximately 24 hours. If rapid reversal is needed, fresh frozen plasma should be given.

Less common complications of warfarin therapy include urticaria, dermatitis, alopecia, fever, nausea, diarrhea, abdominal cramping, and hypersensitivity reactions. Dermal gangrene of the breast, thigh, or buttocks is a rare complication. The dermal venous thrombosis and dermal gangrene have been related to the hypercoagulable state, which can occur with warfarin-induced decreases of protein C. It is not known why this event is limited to the skin.[27] For the first 2 to 4 days of warfarin therapy, heparin should be administered to avoid this complication. Patients with protein C deficiency are particularly at risk for warfarin-induced thrombosis.

Responsiveness to warfarin may be altered by drugs (Table 26–1) or by circumstances that:

1. Interfere with its absorption (e.g., cholestyramine).
2. Displace it from albumin (e.g., aspirin, indomethacin, sulfinpyrazone, phenylbutazone, chloral hydrate, clofibrate, sulfonamides, and anabolic steroids).
3. Reduce its metabolism in the liver, thus increasing its effect (e.g., chloramphenicol and tricyclic antidepressants).
4. Enhance its metabolism, thus decreasing its effect (e.g., alcohol, glutethimide, and barbiturates).
5. Alter vitamin K absorption or availability (e.g., obstructive jaundice, diarrhea, parenteral nutrition, cholestyramine, neomycin, laxatives, or broad-spectrum antibiotics).

Warfarin should not be given during pregnancy, especially in the first trimester, because it has a teratogenic effect. The risk of hemorrhagic birth injuries precludes its use near term. If antithrombotic therapy is required during pregnancy, heparin is usually chosen.

Dextran

Dextran is a polysaccharide that was developed as a plasma expender in the early 1940s. Its antithrombotic properties

TABLE 26–1. DRUG INTERACTIONS WITH ORAL ANTICOAGULANTS

POTENTIATING EFFECT	ANTAGONIZING EFFECT
Allopurinol	Antihistamine
Aminoglycosides	Carbamazepine
Anabolic steroids	Cholestyramine
Chloramphenicol	Glutethimide
Clofibrate	Griseofulvin
Clorpromazine	Haloperidol
Cimetidine	Oral contraceptives
Cotrimoxazol	Phenobarbital
Dipyridamole	Phenytoin
Disulfiram	Spironolactone
Metronidazole	Vitamin K
Oral hypoglycemic drugs	
Phenylbutazone	
Quinidine	
Salicylate	
Tricyclic antidepressants	

From Humphrey PW, Hoch JR, Silver D: Hemostasis and thrombosis. *In* Moore WS (ed): Vascular Surgery: A Comprehensive Review, 4th ed. Philadelphia, WB Saunders, 1993.

were noted in the 1960s and led to its use in the management of thromboembolic disorders in the 1970s. Two preparations are available for clinical use in the United States:

- Dextran 70 (average MW 70,000 daltons, with 90% in the range of 20,000 to 115,000 daltons)
- Dextran 40 (average MW 40,000 daltons, with 90% in the range of 10,000 to 80,000 daltons)

The two preparations seem to have equivalent antithrombotic effects.

Dextran decreases platelet aggregation and adhesiveness and causes prolongation of the bleeding time. Formation of a dextran complex with von Willebrand's factor has been demonstrated and may contribute to the decreased platelet function. The antithrombotic effect of dextran is enhanced by its interference with fibrin polymerization.

Administration

The dosage of dextran for antithrombosis is 500 ml given immediately preoperatively or intraoperatively, followed by 500 to 1000 ml given daily during the postoperative period.

Prophylaxis

Dextran has been used to prevent venous and arterial thromboses. Pooled results of several randomized clinical trials using dextran as a prophylactic agent have demonstrated reductions in DVTs (15.6% with dextran versus 24.2% in controls) and pulmonary emboli (1.2% with dextran versus 2.8% in controls).[28] Dextran has provided effective DVT prophylaxis in patients undergoing hip surgery (resulting in a rate of approximately 6.5% DVT).[29–33]

In an international multicenter prospective study of general surgical, gynecologic, urologic, and orthopedic petients undergoing elective operations lasting at least 30 minutes, prophylaxis with dextran 70 (given as three 500-ml doses, the first dose given during surgery) was compared with low-dose subcutaneous heparin (5000 units given every 8 hours, starting 2 hours before surgery and continuing for 6 days or until full mobility). There was no difference in the incidence of fatal pulmonary embolism in the two groups.[34] An equal number of bleeding complications occurred with both regimens, and serious allergic reactions occurred in 1.1% of patients receiving dextran.

Complications

The most common complications of dextran infusions are hemorrhage and volume overload. These are reduced when the volume of dextran infused is limited to less than 10% of the patient's blood volume daily. Other less common complications include allergic reactions (~1% of patients) and, rarely, anaphylactoid-type reactions (<0.1% of patients). The preinfusion of short-chain dextrans (MW 3000 to 6000 daltons) to patients known to be sensitive to dextran prevents or diminishes allergic or anaphylactic reactions. Major complications, such as volume overload and hemorrhage, are more frequent with dextran 70 than with dextran 40.[35]

Ancrod

Ancrod, an amino acid compound (MW, 37,000 daltons) is derived from the venom of the Malayan pit viper (*Agkistrodon rhodostoma*). The circulating half-life of ancrod ranges from 3 to 5 hours. Ancrod is excreted unchanged in the urine. Ancrod cleaves the A-fibrinopeptides (A, AY, and AP) from circulating fibrinogen. The resultant fibrin does not undergo cross-linking and therefore is more susceptible to fibrinolytic activity and to phagocytosis by the reticuloendothelial system than is normal fibrin. In addition to interfering with coagulation, the lowered fibrinogen concentration reduces the blood's viscosity and improves rheology. Platelets and the other coagulation proteins are unaffected by ancrod.

Ancrod is administered by the subcutaneous or IV route. The level of hypofibrinogenemia is more readily controlled by the IV route. It has been demonstrated that plasma fibrinogen concentrations of 0.2 to 0.6 g/L are adequate for hemostasis but effectively prevent spontaneous thrombosis. Anticoagulation can be achieved by the infusion of 70 to 100 units (1 to 2 U/kg) over 12 to 36 hours; this usually results in a decline of fibrinogen to the level of 0.4 to 0.6 g/L. Surgery can be safely performed with fibrinogen concentrations in this range. Serum fibrinogen levels should be measured every 12 hours for the initial 48 hours and then daily; the infusion rate is adjusted to maintain the fibrinogen level in the desired range. Resistance to ancrod may occur after 4 to 6 weeks of therapy through the occurrence of serum proteinase inhibitors that bind and inactivate it.[36]

Ancrod is well suited for use in patients with heparin-induced thrombocytopenia who continue to require anticoagulation. Ancrod has been effective in patients with AT deficiency who are resistant to the effects of heparin and require anticoagulation.[37] Ancrod has been used successfully to manage patients with stroke, DVT, pulmonary embolism, and central retinal thrombosis. It has also been used as an anticoagulant in patients requiring hemodialysis, cardiopulmonary bypass, and peripheral vascular surgery.

Complications

The complications associated with ancrod are fever, minor allergic reactions, and hemorrhage. If uncontrollable hemorrhage occurs, the administration of cryoprecipitate effectively reverses ancrod's effects. Surgical procedures can be performed while the patient is receiving ancrod with minimal risk of significant hemorrhage.

Thrombin Inhibitors: Hirudin and Argatroban

Hirudin is a water-soluble, heat-resistant, single-peptide chain derived form the salivary glands of the leech (*Hirudo medicinalis*). Hirudin blocks thrombin instantaneously and irreversibly at multiple sites without the interaction of AT.[38] Its small size allows it to inhibit thrombin within clots. It has no effect on platelets. The half-life of hirudin's effect on the aPTT is about 2 hours. A recombinant form (desirudin) has been produced in sufficient quantities for therapeutic use.

Hirudin is aministered by the subcutaneous or IV route. Applications of hirudin or derivatives thereof may be indicated for (1) prophylaxis and treatment of postoperative venous thrombosis and diffuse microthrombosis, (2) prevention of arterial thrombosis, and (3) enhancement of fibrinolytic therapy or angioplasty to prevent reocclusion. There is no specific antidote for reversing the effects of hirudin.

Argatroban is an arginine derivative that binds competitively to the catalytic (active) site of thrombin; it is also able to block fibrin-bound thrombin. Argatroban has been used as an adjunctive to thrombolytic therapy. It can reduce intimal hyperplasia and prevent restenosis after percutaneous transluminal angioplasty (PTA) by 30% versus control.[39–42] It is administered intravenously as a drip either with or without a bolus; the aPTT should be maintained 1.5 to 2.0 times normal.

Hirudin and argatroban may be particularly useful as alternative anticoagulatory agents in patients sensitized to heparin or in patients with hereditary or acquired AT deficiency.

PLATELET FUNCTION INHIBITION

Many drugs alter platelet activity. Several have been evaluated in clinical trials as antithrombotic agents. Aspirin, dipyridamole, and ticlopidine have been investigated most extensively.

Aspirin

Aspirin (ASA) irreversibly acetylates the cyclooxygenase of platelets, thus interfering with the conversion of arachidonic acid to the prostaglandin endoperoxides and inhibiting platelet synthesis of thromboxane A_2. Because platelets are anucleate and cannot synthesize new enzymes, their functional inhibition is permanent. A single dose of aspirin results in defective platelet function that can be detected for several days.[43] The altered cyclooxygenase also reduces the production of prostacyclin in the endothelium. However, new cyclooxygenase is readily synthesized by the nucleated endothelial cells; hence, prostacyclin production by endothelial cells is restored within a few hours.

The net result of the administration of modest doses of aspirin (e.g., 600 mg or less once or twice a day) is an inhibition of thromboxane A_2 synthesis. It is possible that larger doses of aspirin might tilt the balance in favor of thrombosis by blocking endothelial prostacyclin production. However, no evidence of a thrombotic effect of aspirin has been documented in humans.

Administration

For platelet function inhibition, we prescribe enteric-coated aspirin, 325 mg daily, with a meal. A few of our patients take 80 mg of aspirin twice daily for this purpose.

Prophylaxis

Although aspirin is ineffective in the management of ongoing thrombosis, it is helpful in maintaining vascular graft patency and in reducing the incidence of transient ischemic attacks (TIAs), stroke, myocardial infarction, and death.

Significant improvement in the early patency of both saphenous and polytetrafluoroethylene (PTFE) grafts has been demonstrated in two randomized clinical trials when patients were given preoperative aspirin and dipyridamole.[44, 45] No proven difference in femoropopliteal bypass patency was found when aspirin and dipyridamole were begun 24 hours postoperatively.[46] We prescribe aspirin (325 mg daily) in the preoperative period for most patients undergoing vascular reconstructive surgery, and we continue it indefinitely.

Improved graft patency has also been reported in patients receiving aspirin after coronary artery bypass. One clinical trial reported graft thrombosis in 10% of patients submitting to coronary artery bypass who received a placebo, whereas graft thrombosis occurred in only 3% of patients receiving aspirin and dipyridamole at the time of bypass.[47] Follow-up at 1 year revealed a 25% occlusion rate in the placebo group and an 11% occlusion rate in the treated group. Aspirin alone has proved to be as effective as a combination of aspirin and dipyridamole in patients undergoing coronary artery bypass.[48]

A significant reduction in the incidence of TIAs, stroke, and death in men taking aspirin was demonstrated by the Canadian Cooperative Study Group.[49] Several other clinical trials of aspirin alone or aspirin in combination with dipyridamole have shown reductions in the incidences of stroke and death.[50–52] A reduced incidence of fatal myocardial infarctions has also been demonstrated in studies in which patients received either aspirin alone or aspirin in combination with dipyridamole. The effective doses of aspirin for reducing graft thrombosis, TIAs, stroke, myocardial infarction, and progression of atherosclerotic occlusive disease have ranged from 80 mg once daily to 625 mg twice daily.[45, 53–55]

Complications

Contraindications to the use of platelet function–inhibiting agents include a bleeding tendency, peptic ulceration, and sensitivity to the agent. Care should be exercised when these agents are combined with warfarin or heparin because this combination results in an increased tendency toward bleeding. Chronic aspirin administration may be associated with elevation of blood urea and uric acid concentrations, but gout rarely occurs.

Ticlopidine

Ticlopidine irreversibly alters the platelet membrane, inhibiting platelet aggregation induced by collagen, platelet-activating factor (PAF), adrenaline, and adenosine diphosphate (ADP).[56] It is administered orally in a dose of 250 mg twice a day. Ticlopidine reduces the combined event rate per year for stroke, myocardial infarction, or vascular death by 23% in patients who have had a previous stroke.[57] A trial of ticlopidine in patients with intermittent claudication demonstrated only a 10% improvement in distances walked when compared to a placebo.[58] A randomized trial evaluating the effect of ticlopidine on long-term patency of saphenous vein bypass grafts in the leg demonstrated a significant improvement (82% versus 63%, $p = .02$) in 2-year patency when matched against a placebo.[59]

Complications of ticlopidine therapy, which include neutropenia, pancytopenia, and agranulocytosis, have been described in 2% of patients.[57] These complications usually resolve when the medication is stopped.

Ticlopidine and Aspirin

In an effort to increase antiplatelet activity and decrease postprocedural thrombosis, the combined use of ticlopidine and aspirin has been investigated. The efficacy and potency of antiplatelet activity of ticlopidine is increased by aspirin.[60] In patients with coronary artery stents, combined antiplatelet therapy reduced clinical cardiovascular events, stent thrombosis, and hemorrhagic events in contrast to anticoagulant therapy.[61]

Dipyridamole

Dipyridamole suppresses platelet aggregation by inhibiting platelet phosphodiesterase, which causes an increase in intracellular cyclic adenosine monophosphate (cAMP). Elevated cAMP results in a decrease in cytoplasmic calcium with platelet aggregation inhibition. Other actions of dipyridamole may include inhibition of the synthesis of thromboxane A_2 and potentiation of the inhibition of platelet function by adenosine. The hypothesis that dipyridamole is synergistic with aspirin in its antithrombotic effect has not been supported by clinical trials.

Administration

Dipyridamole, 25 to 50 mg, is usually given by mouth three to four times daily.

Prophylaxis

Dipyridamole's effectiveness as a prophylactic vascular or cardiovascular agent alone or in combination with aspirin has yet to be confirmed.

Complications

Headache is the most common complication of dipyridamole administration, occurring in approximately 10% of patients. Other complications include diarrhea, flushing, and rash.

Glycoprotein IIb/IIIa Inhibitors

Glycoprotein (GP) IIb/IIIa antagonists (e.g., abciximab, lamifiban, eptifibatide [Integrelin]) prevent platelet aggregation by inhibiting the binding of fibrinogen to the platelet GP IIb/IIIa receptor. Clinical trials have demonstrated a decreased death and myocardial infarction rate at 6 months (6.6% versus 1.8%; $p = .018$ and 11.1% versus 2.4%; $p = .002$, respectively) in patients with unstable angina and myocardial infarctions undergoing angioplasty either alone or with stent placement.[62, 63] Indications for use of this class of drugs may include stroke prevention, myocardial and peripheral vascular occlusive disease, and heparin-induced thrombocytopenia.

These agents are used as a bolus of 0.25 mg/kg followed by continuous infusion of 10 μg/min to maintain a bleeding time of 30 minutes. Bleeding times return to near normal 12 hours after the medication is discontinued.

The major risk of GP IIb/IIIa administration receptor antagonists is bleeding. Platelet suppression can be partially reversed by administration of fresh platelets.[64]

PHYSICAL MEASURES FOR THROMBOEMBOLISM PROPHYLAXIS

Physical measures for the prevention of thromboembolism are an attractive alternative to drug prophylaxis. They are noninvasive and are without major side effects or risks for bleeding. Early and aggressive mobilization provides a modest reduction, as determined by labeled fibrinogen studies, in the incidence of thrombosis in the elderly population. Elastic stockings and venous pneumatic compression with inflatable leggings have successfully reduced the incidence of DVT.[65] A review of four randomized clinical trials evaluating the effectiveness of elastic stockings revealed a 9.3% incidence of DVT in patients wearing stockings and a 24.5% incidence in controls.[26]

The rate of postoperative DVT in surgical patients using pneumatic compression is about 8% (25 of 270 patients), a rate comparable to that achieved with low-dose heparin.[12] Venous pneumatic compression has also been effective in preventing DVT in neurosurgical patients and in patients undergoing open prostatectomy.[14, 65] In patients undergoing hip operations who have had previous thromboembolic events, pneumatic compression "stockings" have been as effective as warfarin if the preoperative venogram is normal.[66] In one clinical trial,[12] the rate of clinically diagnosed pulmonary embolism in surgical patients using pneumatic compression was 0.9%. A combination of low-dose heparin and pneumatic compression stockings may be more effective than either used alone for preventing DVT.[67]

The regimen of prophylaxis should give the patient the most satisfactory protection with the least number of side effects. Young patients (<40 years of age) with no risk factors who undergo general surgery usually do not require specific measures. Low-dose subcutaneous heparin, LMWH, or pneumatic compression stockings are effective prophylactic measures in general surgical patients.[66] Pneumatic compression stockings are effective in neurosurgical and open prostatectomy patients in whom heparin is contraindicated or ineffective.

Warfarin or dextran may be used in patients who are at a high risk for the occurrence of a thrombotic event. Patients in this category include those with prior thromboembolism, malignant disease, or hip fractures. A meta-analysis comparing LMWH and standard heparin administered subcutaneously demonstrated no benefit difference between the two agents in general surgical patients, but LMWH demonstrated a larger absolute risk reduction for venous thrombosis in orthopedic patients.[68]

Thromboembolism is a serious problem in patients with major trauma. A reasonable approach to treatment of these patients includes pneumatic compression stockings or dextran, or both, in the immediate post-injury period. When the hazard of hemorrhage has abated, low-dose heparin or LMWH may be prescribed in addition to pneumatic compression stockings if the risk of thromboembolism remains significant. If the trauma patient has bilateral lower extremity fractures prohibiting the use of pneumatic stockings and a contraindication to the use of low-dose heparin, duplex scanner surveillance (every 2 to 3 days) of the deep venous systems of the lower extremities is indicated. If DVT occurs under these circumstances and anticoagulation is prohibited, the insertion of a vena caval filter should be considered.

ANTITHROMBOTIC THERAPY IN DIFFERENT CLINICAL SETTINGS

Major Arterial Embolism

The management and prognosis of peripheral arterial embolism depend on the vessels that are occluded and the source of the emboli. The goals of management are to restore the circulation to normal and to prevent recurrences.

Heparin is administered promptly to patients with acute arterial thromboembolism to prevent thrombus propagation and to maintain the patency of collateral vessels. The patient is usually given a 5000 to 10,000 unit bolus of IV heparin while diagnostic or therapeutic measures are in process. If the patient has an embolectomy, additional IV heparin is usually given. In the postoperative period, heparin is infused at a rate that will maintain the aPTT at 1.5 to 1.7 times control value. The heparin infusion should be continued for 3 to 4 days in the postoperative period while endothelial healing occurs. Postoperative bleeding complications are minimal if the aPTT is not allowed to exceed twice the control value. If warfarin therapy is indicated, it should be started in the immediate postoperative period to allow for a 3- to 4-day overlap with the heparin therapy.

Three retrospective studies compared reembolism and mortality rates in patients receiving and not receiving anticoagulation. The rate of reembolization was reduced by approximately 30%, and this was associated with a lower overall mortality in patients receiving anticoagulants.[69–71]

Anticoagulation with warfarin appears to reduce the incidence of recurrent cerebral emboli in patients with mitral valve stenosis.[72] Myocardial mural thromboses are common sources of peripheral emboli, and patients with these thromboses usually receive anticoagulation therapy first with heparin and then with warfarin. The threat of embolization from a mural thrombus associated with a myocardial infarct decreases with time, and it has been suggested that anticoagulants can be discontinued after one year.[73] Peripheral embolization related to ulcerated aortic plaques with thrombus is treated by endarterectomy or replacement of the involved segment of aorta.

The role of thrombolytic therapy in acute thromboembolic occlusions of the extremities is discussed in Chapter 28.

Cerebrovascular Disease

Antithrombotic therapy has been evaluated in the management of completed stroke, stroke-in-evolution, and TIAs. Anticoagulation is of no benefit in patients with a completed stroke. The value of anticoagulation in nonhemorrhagic evolving strokes is not clear. Anticoagulation does not reduce the number of deaths, but it may be of benefit in reducing the size of the infarction. Studies have suggested that anticoagulants reduce the frequency of TIAs, but this suggestion remains controversial.[72, 74] Anticoagulation may be useful in patients who have cerebral emboli from a cardiac source because of the approximately 15% chance of a second embolism within 2 weeks of the ischemic event.[72] Anticoagulant therapy may reduce the risk of early (within 2 weeks) recurrent cerebral embolism by two thirds.[75]

Attention has focused on inhibition platelet function in the management of TIAs. Fields and coworkers reported a randomized double-blind trial of aspirin for the treatment of TIAs. Although there was no significant difference in the rates of death or cerebral or retinal infarction, there was a significant difference in favor of aspirin when death, cerebral infarction, and the occurrence of TIAs were considered together as an end-point.[76]

The Canadian Cooperative Study Group studied the effects of placebo versus aspirin alone or in combination with sulfinpyrazone in 585 patients who had TIAs. They found a striking reduction (48%) in the ensuing risk of stroke or death in men treated with aspirin. No benefit was seen with aspirin in women or with sulfinpyrazone in either sex.[49] These studies and others have clearly established that aspirin therapy results in a 20% to 30% reduction in the incidence of stroke among men with TIAs and minor strokes.[77, 78]

The accepted dose of aspirin varies from 325 to 1300 mg/day. We currently use 325 mg daily. A British study showed that 325 mg/day compared with 1300 mg/day offered equal protection with few side effects from the occurrence of a stroke after a TIA.[77]

The North American Symptomatic Carotid Endarterectomy Trial (NASCET) and Asymptomatic Carotid Artery Stenosis (ACAS) study firmly documented the beneficial effect of carotid endarterectomy compared with medical (antiplatelet) therapy in symptomatic and asymptomatic patients with at least 60% carotid stenosis. In the NASCET study, patients who underwent carotid endarterectomies showed significant reductions in the occurrence of minor, major, and fatal ipsilateral strokes. The cumulative risk of any ipsilateral strokes at 2 years was 26% for the medically treated group and 9% for the surgically treated group, a 17% risk reduction. There was a 10.6% reduction in the occurrence of major or fatal ipsilateral strokes with surgical therapy compared with medical therapy.[79] In the ACAS study, the aggregate risk over 5 years for ipsilateral stroke, any perioperative stroke, and death was 5.1% for surgical patients and 11% for patients treated medically. This difference was highly significant.[80]

Deep Venous Thrombosis

The therapeutic options available for the treatment of venous thrombosis include anticoagulation, fibrinolytic therapy, and surgery (venous filters with venous interruption or thrombectomy). Only anticoagulation therapy is discussed here.

The management of an asymptomatic calf vein thrombosis is controversial. Surveillance alone, either by impedance plethysmography or by duplex scanning,[81] has been advocated when a thrombus is confined to the calf because only 20% of untreated calf thrombi propagate proximally to a point at which they pose the threat of a major pulmonary embolism.[82] However, one study has documented a 10% incidence of pulmonary emboli originating from the deep calf veins.[83] A controlled prospective study of patients on a medical service also documented a 29% recurrence of calf DVT within 90 days after a 5-day course of heparin, an 18% rate of proximal extension of the calf thrombi, and a 3.6% incidence of pulmonary emboli. In comparison, patients who received anticoagulant therapy for 3 months had none of these complications.[84]

We recommend a minimum of 3 months of anticoagulation (initial IV heparin therapy, or LMWH followed by warfarin or subcutaneous heparin or LMWH) for patients with calf DVT unless anticoagulation therapy is contraindicated. When such therapy is contraindicated, close surveillance with duplex scanning is recommended to identify patients with proximal extension of the thrombotic process. These patients may require a vena caval filter.

For a deep venous thrombus, especially one that extends above the calf, a bolus of heparin (100 to 200 U/kg body weight) is given, followed by a continuous infusion of heparin (~1000 U/hr). The infusion is adjusted to maintain the aPTT at 1.7 to 2.0 times the control value. The continuous IV infusion method, compared with intermittent IV infusion or the subcutaneous administration of heparin, carries a smaller incidence of hemorrhagic complication, is easier to monitor, requires less heparin, and provides a "stable level" of incoagulability.

A study comparing subcutaneous LMWH to continuous intravenous heparin in the treatment of DVT reported that LMWH was as effective and safe as the continuous infusion of heparin. Six of 213 patients (2.8%) who received LMWH and 15 of 219 patients (6.9%) who received continuous IV heparin experienced new episodes of venous thromboembolism. Initial therapy resulted in major bleeding in 1 (0.5%) patient receiving LMWH and in 11 (5.0%) patients receiving continuous heparin.[85]

We recommend 5 to 7 days of IV heparin therapy for DVT. The heparin is continued longer if the symptoms do not resolve during this time. Warfarin therapy is begun on the first day of heparin therapy. Heparin is discontinued when the INR is 2.5 to 3.0. The optimal duration of oral anticoagulation therapy is not known. However, the recurrence rate of thrombosis is higher in patients who have received anticoagulation treatment for less than 3 months. We recommend at least 3 to 6 months of anticoagulant therapy.

Recurrent thromboembolism occurs in 2% to 3% of patients who are "adequately" treated with anticoagulants and is more common in patients with proximal thrombi than in those with thrombi confined to the calf.[25, 86] A comparison of LMWH administered at home and unfractionated heparin administered in the hospital for proximal DVT demonstrated the safety and efficacy of LMWH. A dose of 1 mg/kg of enoxaparin was administered twice daily.[87, 88]

Heparin is the drug of choice for the treatment of DVT during pregnancy because heparin does not cross the placenta. After 7 to 10 days of IV heparin therapy, the pregnant patient is managed with 10,000 to 15,000 units/day of subcutaneous heparin, given in divided doses, or an equivalent dose of LMWH, for continued inhibition of the coagulation mechanism. The heparin, or LMWH is usually stopped prior to delivery. Anticoagulation with heparin is continued after delivery.

Placement of an inferior vena caval filter is indicated in patients with DVT if anticoagulation is not possible because of active bleeding, intracranial hemorrhage, a recent neurosurgical procedure, or malignant hypertension or if extension of thrombosis occurs despite "adequate" anticoagulation (see Chapter 142).

Pulmonary Embolism

Anticoagulation, unless contraindicated (as in active bleeding), is the standard method of management for both major and minor emboli. Support for this practice was initiated by a randomized controlled trial undertaken by Barritt and Jordan.[89] After a diagnosis of pulmonary embolism by clinical signs, electrocardiogram, and chest x-ray, patients were randomized to receive heparin in addition to an oral anticoagulant or to receive no treatment. Of the first 19 control patients, 5 died from recurrent embolism and 5 others had nonfatal recurrences. Among the first 16 patients receiving anticoagulants, there was 1 death from pneumonia and a bleeding duodenal ulcer. Among an additional 38 patients studied, all of whom received anticoagulation, 1 developed a nonfatal recurrent embolism. Despite its shortcomings, this trial emphasized the value of anticoagulation therapy in the management of uncomplicated pulmonary embolism.

In patients with suspected pulmonary embolism, heparin is given promptly even before the diagnosis is confirmed by arteriogram or ventilation-perfusion scanning. Once the diagnosis is established, anticoagulation is provided in a fashion similar to that employed for managing DVT. We continue warfarin or self-administered subcutaneous standard or LMWH anticoagulation for 6 months in patients who have had a pulmonary embolism. If a patient has recurrent pulmonary embolism after discontinuation of anticoagulant therapy, a longer period (12 months) of warfarin anticoagulation is recommended.

Vena caval filter placement is considered for patients who have recurrent pulmonary emboli despite adequate oral anticoagulation or if anticoagulation is contraindicated.

REFERENCES

1. Coon WW: Some recent developments in the pharmacology of heparin. J Clin Pharmacol 19:337–349, 1979.
2. Bentley PG, Kakkar VV, Scully MF, et al: An objective study of alternative methods of heparin administration. Thromb Res 18:177–187, 1980.
3. Lane DA, Denton J, Flynn AM, et al: Anticoagulant activities of heparin oligosaccharides and their neutralization by platelet factor 4. Biochem J 218:725–732, 1984.

4. Handeland GF, Abildgaard U, Holm HA, Arnesen KE: Dose adjusted heparin treatment of deep venous thrombosis: A comparison of unfractionated and low molecular weight heparin. Eur J Clin Pharmacol 39:107–112, 1990.
5. Cadroy Y, Pourrat J, Baladre MF, et al: Delayed elimination of enoxaparin in patients with chronic renal insufficiency. Thromb Res 63:385–390, 1991.
6. Weitz JI. Low-molecular-weight heparins. N Engl J Med 337:688–698, 1997.
7. Handin RI, Cohen HJ: Purification and binding properties of human platelet factor four. J Biol Chem 251:4273–4282, 1976.
8. Glazier RL, Crowell EB: Randomized prospective trial of continuous versus intermittent heparin therapy. JAMA 236:1365–1367, 1976.
9. Hull RD, Raskob GE, Hirsh J, et al: Continuous intravenous heparin compared with intermittent subcutaneous heparin in the initial treatment of proximal-vein thrombosis. N Engl J Med 315:1109–1114, 1986.
10. Salzman EW, Deykin D, Shapiro R, et al: Management of heparin therapy: Controlled prospective trial. N Engl J Med 292:1046–1050, 1975.
11. Sharnoff JG, DeBlasio G: Prevention of fatal postoperative thromboembolism by heparin prophylaxis. Lancet 2:1006–1007, 1970.
12. Salzman EW, Davies GC: Prophylaxis of venous thromboembolism: Analysis of cost effectiveness. Ann Surg 191:207–218, 1980.
13. Prevention of fatal postoperative pulmonary embolism by low doses of heparin. An International Multicentre Trial. Lancet 2:45–51, 1975.
14. Coe NP, Collins RE, Klein LA, et al: Prevention of deep vein thrombosis in urological patients: A controlled, randomized trial of low-dose heparin and external pneumatic compression boots. Surgery 83:230–234, 1978.
15. Harris WH, Salzman EW, Athanasoulis C, et al: Comparison of warfarin, low-molecular-weight dextran, aspirin, and subcutaneous heparin in prevention of venous thromboembolism following total hip replacement. J Bone Joint Surg (Am) 56:1552–1562, 1974.
16. Hoch JR, Silver D: Complications and failures of anticoagulant therapy. *In* Bernhard VM, Towne JB (eds): Complications in Vascular Surgery. St. Louis, Quality Medical Publishing, 1991, p 118.
17. Pitney WR, Pettit JE, Armstrong L: Control of heparin therapy. Br Med J 4:139–141, 1970.
18. Slocum MM, Adams JG Jr, Teel R, et al: Use of enoxaparin in patients with the heparin-induced thrombocytopenia syndrome. J Vasc Surg 23:839–843, 1996.
19. Silver D, Kapsch D, Tsoi EK: Heparin induced thrombocytopenia, thrombosis, and hemorrhage. Ann Surg 198:301–306, 1983.
20. Laster J, Cikrit D, Silver D: The heparin-induced thrombocytopenia syndrome: An update. Surgery 102:763–770, 1987.
21. Kikta MJ, Keller MP, Humphrey PW, Silver D: Can low molecular weight heparins and heparinoids be safely given to patients with heparin-induced thrombocytopenia syndrome? Surgery 114:705–710, 1993.
22. Sevitt S, Gallagher N: Prevention of venous thrombosis and pulmonary embolism in injured patients. Lancet 2:981–989, 1959.
23. Flinn WR, Rohrer MJ, Yao JS, et al: Improved long-term patency of infragenicular polytetrafluoroethylene grafts. J Vasc Surg 7:685–690, 1988.
24. Veith FJ, Gupta SK, Ascer E, et al: Six-year prospective multicenter randomized comparison of autologous saphenous vein and expanded polytetrafluoroethylene grafts in infrainguinal arterial reconstruction. J Vasc Surg 3:104–114, 1986.
25. Gallus AS, Hirsh J: Treatment of venous thromboembolic disease (Review). Semin Thromb Hemost 2:291–331, 1976.
26. Hull R, Hirsh J, Jay R, et al: Different intensities of oral anticoagulant therapy in the treatment of proximal vein thrombosis. N Engl J Med 307:1676–1681, 1982.
27. Clouse LH, Comp PC: The regulation of hemostasis: The protein C system. N Engl J Med 314:1298–1304, 1986.
28. Clagett GP, Reisch JS: Prevention of venous thromboembolism in general surgical patients: Results of a meta-analysis (Review). Ann Surg 208:227–240, 1988.
29. Fearnley GR, Chakrabarti R, Hocking ED: Fibrinolytic effects of diguanides plus ethylestrenol in occlusive vascular disease. Lancet 2:1008–1011, 1967.
31. Harris WH, Salzman EW, Athanasoulis C, et al: Aspirin prophylaxis of venous thromboembolism after total hip replacement. N Engl J Med 297:1246–1249, 1977.
32. Bergqvist D: Prevention of postoperative thromboembolism in Sweden: The development of practice during five years. Thromb Haemost 53:239–241, 1985.
33. Ljungstrom KG: Prophylaxis of postoperative thromboembolism with dextran 70: Improvements of efficacy and safety. Acta Chir Scand Suppl 514:1–40, 1983.
34. Gruber UF, Saldeen T, Brokop T, et al: Incidences of fatal postoperative pulmonary embolism after prophylaxis with dextran 70 and low dose heparin: An international multicentre study. Br Med J 280:69–72, 1980.
35. Ring J, Messmer K: Incidence and severity of anaphylactoid reactions to colloid volume substitutes. Lancet 1:466–469, 1977.
36. Pitney WR, Bray C, Holt PJ, Bolton G: Acquired resistance to arvin. Lancet 1:79–81, 1969.
37. Cole CW, Bormanis J: Ancrod: A practical alternative to heparin. J Vasc Surg 8:59–63, 1988.
38. Grutter MG, Priestle JP, Rahuel J, et al: Crystal structure of the thrombin-hirudin complex: A novel mode of serine protease inhibition. EMBO J 8:2361–2365, 1990.
39. Jang IK, Gold HK, Ziskind AA, et al: Prevention of platelet-rich arterial thrombosis by selective thrombin inhibition. Circulation 81:219–225, 1990.
40. Jang IK, Gold HK, Leinbach RC, et al: Persistent inhibition of aterial thrombosis by a 1-hour intravenous infusion of argatroban, a selective thrombin inhibitor. Coronary Artery Dis 3:407–414, 1992.
41. Gold HK, Torres FW, Garabedian HD, et al: Evidence for a rebound coagulation phenomenon after cessation of a 4-hour infusion of specific thrombin inhibitor in patients with unstable angina pectoris (see comments). J Am Coll Card 21:1039–1047, 1993.
42. Imanishi T, Arita M, Tombuchi Y, et al: Effects of locally administered argatroban on restenosis after balloon angioplasty: Experimental and clinical study. Clin Ex Pharm Phys 24:800–806, 1997.
43. O'Brien JR: Effects of salicylates on human platelets. Lancet 1:779–783, 1968.
44. Goldman M, Hall C, Dykes J, et al: Does ^{111}indium-platelet deposition predict patency in prosthetic arterial grafts? Br J Surg 70:635–638, 1983.
45. Green RM, Roedersheimer LR, DeWeese JA: Effects of aspirin and dipyridamole on expanded polytetrafluoroethylene graft patency. Surgery 92:1016–1026, 1982.
46. Kohler TR, Kaufman JL, Kacoyanis G, et al: Effect of aspirin and dipyridamole on the patency of lower extremity bypass grafts. Surgery 96:462–646, 1984.
47. Chesebro JH, Fuster V, Elveback LR, et al: Effect of dipyridamole and aspirin on late vein-graft patency after coronary bypass operation. N Engl J Med 310:209–214, 1984.
48. Lorenz RL, Schacky CV, Weber M, et al: Improved aortocoronary bypass patency by low-dose aspirin (100 mg daily): Effects on platelet aggregation and thromboxane formation. Lancet 1:1261–1264, 1984.
49. A randomized trial of aspirin and sulfinpyrazone in threatened stroke: Canadian Cooperative Study Group. N Engl J Med 299:53–59, 1978.
50. Turpie AG: Antiplatelet therapy. Clin Hematol 10:497–520, 1981.
51. Bousser MG, Eschwege E, Haguenau N, et al: "AICLA" controlled trial of aspirin and dipyridamole in the secondary prevention of atherothrombotic cerebral ischemia. Stroke 14:5–14, 1983.
52. Ramirez-Lassepas M: Platelet inhibitors for TIAs: A review of prospective drug trial results (Review). Postgrad Med 75:52–62, 1984.
53. Harlan JM, Harker LA: Hemostasis, thrombosis, and thromboembolic disorders: The role of arachidonic acid metabolites in platelet-vessel wall interactions (Review). Med Clin North Am 65:855–880, 1981.
54. Mustard JF, Kinlough-Rathbone RL, Packham MA: Aspirin in the treatment of cardiovascular disease: A review. Am J Med 74:43–49, 1983.
55. Lewis HD Jr, Davis JW, Archibald DG, et al: Protective effects of aspirin against acute myocardial infarction and death in men with unstable angina: Results of a Veterans Administration Cooperative Study. N Engl J Med 309:396–403, 1983.
56. Bruno JJ: The mechanism of action of ticlopidine. Thromb Res Suppl 4:59–67, 1983.
57. Gent M, Blakely JA, Easton JD, et al: The Canadian American Ticlopidine Study (CATS) in thromboembolic stroke (see comments). Lancet 2:442–443, 1989.
58. Arcan JC, Blanchard J, Boissel JP, et al: Multicenter double-blind study of ticlopidine in the treatment of intermittent claudication and the prevention of its complications. Angiology 39:802–11, 1988.

59. Becquemin JP: Effect of ticlopidine on the long-term patency of saphenous-vein bypass grafts in the legs. N Engl J Med 337:1726–1731, 1997.
60. Splawinska B, Kuzniar J, Malinga K, et al: The efficacy and potency of antiplatelet activity of ticlopidine is increased by aspirin. Int J Clin Pharmacol Ther 34:352–356, 1996.
61. Hobson AG, Sowinski KM: Ticlopidine and aspirin therapy following implantation of coronary artery stents (Review). Ann Pharmacother 31:770–772, 1997.
62. Rao AK, Pratt C, Berke A, et al: Thrombolysis in myocardial infraction (TIMI) trial—Phase I: Hemorrhagic manifestations and changes in plasma fibrinogen and the fibrinolytic system in patients treated with recombinant tissue plasminogen activator and streptokinase. J Am Coll Cardiol 11:1–11, 1988.
63. Landefeld CS, Cook EF, Flatley N, et al: Identification and preliminary validation of predictors of major bleeding in hospital patients starting anticoagulant therapy. Am J Med 82:703–713, 1987.
64. Tcheng JE, Ellis SG, George BS, et al: Pharmacodynamics of chimeric glycoprotein IIb/IIIa integrin antiplatelet antibody Fab 7E3 in high-risk coronary angioplasty. Circulation 90:1757–1764, 1994.
65. Skillman JJ, Collins RE, Coe NP, et al: Prevention of deep vein thrombosis in neurosurgical patients: A controlled randomized trial of external pneumatic compression boots. Surgery 83:354–358, 1978.
66. Harris WH, Raines JK, Athanasoulis C, et al: External pneumatic compression versus warfarin in reducing thrombosis in high risk hip patients. *In* Madden J, Hume M (eds): Venous Thromboembolism: Prevention and Treatment. New York, Appleton-Century-Crofts, 1976, pp 51–60.
67. Torngren S: Optimal regimen of low dose heparin prophylaxis in gastrointestinal surgery. Acta Chir Scand 145:87–93, 1979.
68. Nurmohamed MT, Rosendaal FR, Buller HR: Low-molecular-weight heparin versus standard heparin in general and orthopaedic surgery: A meta-analysis. Lancet 340:152–156, 1992.
69. Eriksson I, Holmberg JT: Analysis of factors affecting limb salvage and mortality after embolectomy. Acta Chir Scand 143:237–240, 1977.
70. Green RM, DeWeese JK, Rob CG: Arterial embolectomy before and after the Fogarty catheter. Surgery 77:24–33, 1975.
71. Holm J, Schersten T: Anticoagulant treatment during and after embolectomy. Acta Chir Scand 138:683–687, 1972.
72. Genton E, Barnett HJ, Fields WS, et al: Cerebral ischemia: The role of thrombosis and antithrombotic therapy: Study group on antithrombotic therapy. Stroke 8:150–175, 1977.
73. Carter AB: Prognosis of cerebral embolism. Lancet 2:514–519, 1965.
74. Millikan CH, McDowell FH: Treatment of transient ischemic attacks. Stroke 9:299–308, 1978.
75. Cerebral Embolism Task Force: Cardiogenic brain embolism. Arch Neurol 43:71–84, 1986.
76. Fields WS, Lemak NA, Frankowski RF, Hardy RJ. Controlled trial of aspirin in cerebral ischemia. Stroke 8:301–314, 1977.
77. Riekkinen PJ, Lowenthal A, Googers FA: Main results of the European Stroke Prevention Study. Neurology 37 (Suppl 1):103, 1987.
78. Grotta JC: Current medical and surgical therapy for cerebrovascular disease. N Engl J Med 317:1505–1516, 1987.
79. Beneficial effect of carotid endarterectomy in symptomatic patients with high-grade stenosis: North American Symptomatic Carotid Endarterectomy Trial Collaborators. N Engl J Med 325:445–453, 1991.
80. The Executive Committee for the Asymptomatic Carotid Atherosclerosis Study: Endarterectomy for asymptomatic carotid artery stenosis. JAMA 273:1421–1428, 1995.
81. Mattos MA, Londrey GL, Leutz DW, et al: Color-flow duplex scanning for the surveillance and diagnosis of acute deep venous thrombosis. J Vasc Surg 15:366–375, 1992.
82. Clayton JK, Anderson JA, McNicol GP: Preoperative prediction of postoperative deep vein thrombosis. Br Med J 2:910–912, 1976.
83. Kakkar VV, Howe CT, Nicolaides AN, et al: Deep vein thrombosis of the legs: Is there a high risk group? Am J Surg 120:527–530, 1970.
84. Lagerstedt CI, Olsson CG, Fagher BO, et al: Need for long term anticoagulant treatment in symptomatic calf-vein thrombosis. Lancet 2:515–518, 1985.
85. Hull RD, Raskob GE, Pineo GF, et al: Subcutaneous low-molecular-weight heparin compared with continuous intravenous heparin in the treatment of proximal-vein thrombosis (see comments). N Engl J Med 326:975–982, 1992.
86. Hull R, Delmore T, Genton E, et al: Warfarin sodium versus low-dose heparin in the long-term treatment of venous thrombosis. N Engl J Med 301:855–858, 1979.
87. Levine M, Gent M, Hirsh J, et al: A comparison of low-molecular-weight heparin administered primarily at home with unfractionated heparin administered in the hospital for proximal deep-vein thrombosis (see comments). N Engl J Med 334:677–681, 1996.
88. Koopman MM, Prandoni P, Pivoella F, et al: Treatment of venous thrombosis with intravenous unfractionated heparin administered in the hospital as compared with subcutaneous low-molecular-weight heparin administered at home: The Tasman Study. N Engl J Med 334:682–687, 1996.
89. Barritt DW, Jordan SC: Anticoagulant drugs in the treatment of pulmonary embolism. Lancet 1:1309–1312, 1960.

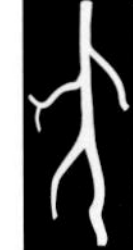

CHAPTER 27

Circulation-Enhancing Drugs

John A. Dormandy, D.Sc., F.R.C.S.

SCOPE

Drugs of greatest benefit and most widely used in patients with impaired circulation to the legs are antiplatelets and anticoagulants. Antiplatelets are the only group of drugs that have been shown to significantly improve the outlook for these patients in terms of fatal and nonfatal cardiovascular events, such as myocardial infarction or ischemic stroke. Patients with peripheral arterial occlusive disease (PAOD) in the leg have been shown to have a two- to threefold increased risk of such events, even if the arterial disease is asymptomatic.[1] Antiplatelet drugs decrease the incidence of nonfatal cardiovascular events by about 25% and of fatal cardiovascular events by about 15%. Specific contraindication to the use of antiplatelet drugs, such as gastrointestinal hemorrhage, excludes only about 10% of patients, and the need for all other patients to receive this type of therapy is now widely recognized (see Chapters 19 and 26).

Although long-term oral anticoagulation may also affect

the development of cardiovascular complications, the potential dangers of their use over prolonged periods are much greater compared with antiplatelets, and these drugs are used only occasionally for this indication. They are indicated, however, when the risk of arterial thrombosis is particularly great, in patients with deep venous thrombosis or in the immediate treatment of patients with acute arterial occlusions. The use of anticoagulants in these specific circumstances is considered elsewhere (see Chapter 26 and Section V, which describe acute ischemia).

This chapter focuses specifically on drugs primarily used to treat localized disease in patients with PAOD. Some of these drugs also have a role in the management of ischemia in the cerebral, renal, and mesenteric circulations. The use of drugs in Raynaud's syndrome is discussed in Chapter 82.

Despite the long history of drug therapy for PAOD, so far there has been no spectacular breakthrough comparable to the drug treatment of myocardial ischemia. Many drugs have been available for a long time that can successfully control the symptoms of angina or offer significant control of congestive cardiac failure due to myocardial ischemia. No drug of comparable efficacy has yet been marketed for the symptoms of *intermittent claudication* or *critical leg ischemia* (CLI). This is particularly surprising, since drugs with a wide range of mechanisms of action have been tried. The lack of effective drugs, however, may change in the near future with a number of new agents now under investigation. PAOD is an area of pharmacologic wilderness. At the same time we are developing third and fourth generations of effective drugs for hypertension, there are still no drugs of proven *significant* efficacy for PAOD.

This chapter highlights all drugs specifically used for PAOD, many licensed in only some countries, and new drugs under active investigation with encouraging early results, suggesting that licensure may be expected in the next 2 to 3 years. The two main topics are (1) drugs to be considered for intermittent claudication and (2) drugs used for CLI. Although the underlying pathologic features in the large arteries is identical, the final pathophysiology giving rise to the symptoms and signs differ. Intermittent claudication is caused by short, completely reversible episodes of muscle ischemia; CLI is the result of continuous, and often irreversible, underperfusion of the skin of the foot.

The pharmacologic strategies are thus usually quite different, although some drugs have been advocated for use in all degrees of severity of PAOD. In this chapter, the various mechanisms of pharmacologic action that have been tried are followed by an assessment of the clinical efficacy of specific agents. The separation of consideration of possible mechanisms of action from the clinical evidence for specific drugs is necessary because most drugs currently used in this indication have a large range of possible mechanisms and usually no clinical benefit can be attributed to a particular mechanism.

DRUGS USED TO TREAT INTERMITTENT CLAUDICATION

Possible Mechanisms of Action

Vasodilators

It is understandable that vasodilators should have been the first class of drugs to be investigated for PAOD. A variety of classic pharmacologic approaches exist for bringing about vasodilatation. These include (1) direct-acting agents (e.g., papaverine), (2) alpha-adrenergic antagonists (e.g., phenoxybenzamine), and (3) ganglion blockers (e.g., guanethidine). Newer types of agents include angiotensin-converting enzyme (ACE) inhibitors (such as enalapril) and calcium channel blockers (such as nifedipine). Unfortunately, the problem is that all these vasodilators affect only vessels capable of normal pharmacologic reaction and have no effect on the fixed occlusions or stenosis—the problems in PAOD.

In 1959, Gillespie was the first to demonstrate that such vasodilators can actually cause a deterioration in the symptoms of PAOD by causing vasodilatation in the relatively normal parts of the circulation. The decrease in the vascular resistance in these areas can actually cause a "steal" of blood away from the already ischemic legs, where the resistance remains unaltered.[2] This pharmacologic steal phenomenon has subsequently been confirmed by other workers.[3]

The issue of vasodilatation may yet become important as we learn more about the effect of drugs on collateral vessels. Their pharmacology may be different from that of normal arteries of similar size. It has been assumed that the collateral vessels will be maximally dilated in response to the local consequences of ischemia, such as a decrease in the oxygen tension and acidosis. A number of newer drugs used for PAOD also have some vasodilator effect, particularly the prostaglandins. Because of the belief that vasodilatation may be counterproductive, there has been a strategy to classify many drugs used for intermittent claudication under another mechanism of action. Frequently, such other mechanisms are ill defined and unproven. This has led to the use of the term "vasoactive" to describe any drugs believed to have an effect on peripheral ischemia, although it is to be noted that the drug is not simply a vasodilator. The term vasoactive does not define a mechanism of action, and its use should be confined to that of an umbrella term for all drugs having a peripheral vascular effect.

Rheologic Drugs

Hemorrheology is the study of the physical flow properties of blood. It began to be widely studied in the 1970s with the availability of viscometers, which could be used clinically on small samples. Previously, the science of viscometry had been almost wholly confined to commercial areas like the oil industry. Soon the concept of rheologically active drugs that would lower the viscosity of blood, and therefore increase blood flow through the same narrow channels, was espoused by the pharmaceutical industry as the obvious answer to developing drugs for treatment of atherosclerotic diseases. Much of this early enthusiasm was misplaced because of an imperfect understanding of the peculiarities of blood rheology, but the term "rheologically active drug" is still occasionally used, often incorrectly.

Blood, unlike water or oil, is non-Newtonian and does not obey Poiseuille's equation, suggesting a linear inverse relationship between flow and viscosity. The non-Newtonian behavior of blood is largely due to the presence of red blood cells (RBCs) and their tendency to aggregate at low shear rates (flow rates) due to the binding of adjacent RBCs by long protein molecules, principally fibrinogen. Blood thus becomes abnormally viscous at low shear rates. The viscosity of blood at any given shear rate is therefore principally dependent on hematocrit and plasma fibrinogen concentration.[4] Both of these variables can critically influence whole blood viscosity. For instance, an increase in hematocrit from 45% to 55% increases the viscosity of whole blood at high shear rates by almost 100%.[4] Whole blood viscosity, however, only influences blood flow in larger vessels, such as arteries. In arterioles, a number of other mechanisms (such as plasma skimming) come into play, determining blood flow velocity.

Much less is known about *microrheology*, the flow properties of blood in the microcirculation, and this is probably the level at which hemorrheology has the greatest impact on the pathophysiology of ischemia. In 1976, a simple filtration technique was described in which whole blood was filtered through 5-μm diameter pores as an analogy to what was thought to happen in a microcirculation.[5] The results were interpreted to reflect RBC deformability. In this and subsequent publications, the filterability of whole blood was shown to be decreased in a range of cardiovascular diseases, including PAOD. It ultimately became clear that the decreased filterability was almost wholly due to the effect of white blood cells (WBCs), which even in the passive state are about 1000 times more rigid than RBCs. It is now widely accepted that the decreased whole blood filterability in patients with PAOD largely depends on the number of WBCs and their level of activation; active WBCs are several times more rigid than passive WBCs.[6]

Thus, abnormal hemorrheology in patients with PAOD is now believed to be due, at a *macrocirculatory* level, to an increase in plasma fibrinogen and hematocrit[7]; at the *microcirculatory* level, the decreased blood filterability[5, 8] is probably due to the increased number of WBCs and to increased WBC cell activation.[9]

The simplest and most obvious method for decreasing whole blood viscosity is lowering hematocrit, and haemodilution has been widely investigated in a number of circulatory diseases (see next topic). At the macrorheologic level, lowering plasma fibringen is, theoretically, an attractive approach. This method almost certainly decreases whole blood viscosity and increases blood flow. Moderate decreases in plasma fibrinogen have been achieved with clofibrate, which is orally active and relatively safe, although it has not been widely tested for use in intermittent claudication.[10] Much more dramatic decreases in plasma fibrinogen have been achieved with defibrinogenating drugs, such as ancrod (Arvin). When such agents are used, the plasma fibrinogen concentration has been lowered to 25% to 50% of that in normal inpatients without any adverse side effects. This has been accompanied by the expected drop in whole blood viscosity.[11]

In the past, such agents have been available only for administration by injection and only small, limited trials have been performed in patients with intermittent claudication. Defibrinogenation would seem a more reasonable approach in patients with critical leg ischemia but, perhaps surprisingly, initial clinical trials in both these types of PAOD have yielded negative results.[12]

The most widely used drug for the treatment of intermittent claudication, pentoxifylline, is now believed to act in part by a microrheologic mechanism. This agent was originally thought to be a vasodilator, but subsequently it was shown to decrease whole blood viscosity probably by increasing whole blood filterability.[13] This occurs presumably by the effect on WBCs and, possibly, on plasma fibrinogen and platelet aggregation.[14, 15] Ehrly has also demonstrated an increase in muscle oxygen tension in claudicants taking pentoxifylline,[16] although this finding has not been duplicated by others.

Hemodilution

Hemodilution, lowering hematocrit, and decreasing the whole blood viscosity increase blood flow in animals as well in humans.[17] At the same time, however, it decreases the oxygen-carrying capacity of the blood. There has been an ongoing theoretical and practical debate about the optimum hematocrit, in which the balance between increased flow due to decreased hematocrit on the one hand and decreased oxygen-carrying capacity of the blood on the other hand provides the optimal oxygen delivery.[18] With strain-gauge plethysmography, an inverse relationship between whole blood viscosity and total leg blood flow has been demonstrated in humans.[19] The consensus seems to be that in patients with narrowed arteries the optimal hematocrit is about 40%, at the lower end of the normal range. In patients with cardiovascular disease, the hemodilution probably has to be normovolemic; (e.g., removing 1 unit of blood at a time and replacing it with a plasma expander). Such normovolemic dilution has been of some benefit to patients with intermittent claudication in short-term trials, but there are obvious problems, such as iron deficiency, in proposed long-term use.

Low-molecular-weight dextran (mean, 40,000) is widely used clinically as a plasma expander. The consequent hemodilution decreases whole blood viscosity and increases blood flow. Studies in humans have shown that the rheologic effect of dextran 40 is no different from that of other plasma expanders, such as saline.[19] Because of the need for long-term effect, it has never come into use for the treatment of intermittent claudication. Its most dramatic clinical benefit seems to be as adjuvant therapy for small-caliber high-risk arterial anastomoses. In a randomized trial, Rutherford and colleagues showed a definite benefit for this use, at least in the early postoperative period.[20] This result has not been tested in other randomized trials, but dextran 40 is nevertheless frequently used on an empirical basis perioperatively. However, dextran 40 may interfere with blood typing and cross-matching,[21] may produce occasional anaphylactic reactions, and sometimes causes increased bleeding.

Serotonin Antagonists

Serotonin has a marked platelet-aggregating effect. Some serotonin antagonists also possibly have a rheologic effect, which may be secondary to decreasing platelet aggregation.

Ketanserin, a serotonin receptor 2 (S2) antagonist, was tested in a large double-blind, randomized prospective study of 4000 patients with intermittent claudication.[22] It was hoped that ketanserin might have a beneficial effect on nonfatal and fatal cardiovascular events, but this could be demonstrated only retrospectively in a subgroup of the patients. Ketanserin had no effect on intermittent claudication.[23]

Naftidrofuryl (Praxilene) is widely used in Europe for the treatment of intermittent claudication. It has been said to have some serotonin antagonist effects,[24] but some claim that it increases production of adenosine triphosphate (ATP) and decreases lactate accumulation in ischemic tissues.[25]

Muscle Metabolism–Enhancing Drugs

Apart from naftidrofuryl, which has long been available, some newer agents may enhance the metabolism in ischemic tissues and therefore have a favorable effect on intermittent claudication. An example is *carnitine*, a cofactor for skeletal muscle intermediary metabolism during exercise. Carnitine helps in maintaining normal metabolism under hypoxic stress.[26] Patients with PAOD accumulate acylcarnitines in skeletal muscle.[27] The supplementation of carnitine in patients with claudication would seem logical and has recently been the subject of clinical trials.

Cilostazol, a possible phosphodiesterase inhibitor, has also been used in clinical trials. Like many vasoactive "compounds" cilostazol has a number of potential mechanisms of action, which also include vasodilation and antiplatelet activity (see also later discussion).[28]

Clinical Efficacy

Readers should keep a number of issues in mind when assessing the evidence for clinical efficacy in drugs used specifically for the treatment of intermittent claudication:

1. The spontaneous clinical course of intermittent claudication is exceedingly variable from patient to patient. Epidemiologic evidence suggests that approximately 75% of such patients will become stable or will even show improvement of symptoms without any specific medication. The course followed by an individual patient, however, is unpredictable. Symptomatic progression presumably depends on the extent to which collaterals are developed and, possibly, the patient's ability to alter his or her walking pattern so as to protect ischemic muscle.

2. For many years now, all patients with intermittent claudication have received standard advice about modifying their lifestyle in terms of eliminating risk factors (e.g., smoking) and maximizing exercise. Most claudicants are now given antiplatelet therapy and treated for any lipid abnormality. Similarly, coexisting diseases (e.g., diabetes) must be treated. These interventions will also modify the progression of symptoms in intermittent claudication, and it is thus incorrect to think of a pure "placebo effect" in controlled drug trials. Any benefit in the control group receiving placebo may well be due to other measures rather than a true placebo effect. Almost all well-designed trials of drug therapy for claudication show a significant improvement in claudication distance in the control group receiving placebo. In large studies, this figure has been about 15% increase in claudication distance during the first 6 months of treatment and another 15% during the second 6 months.[29] Therefore, it is absolutely essential to have a placebo control group when any drug is tested for an effect on claudication distance.

3. Consideration of the difference between statistical significance and clinical significance is inescapable in claudicants. If the number of patients is sufficiently large, a mean increase in claudication distance of as little as 10% can be *statistically* significant but is clearly not *clinically* significant. Regulatory authorities are particularly focused on statistical significance, but physicians are more concerned with clinical significance.

4. In all drug trials for intermittent claudication, there is a tremendous variation in response, with some patients having an apparently dramatic improvement with drug treatment. It has therefore been occasionally argued that if a drug produces no side effects, is safe and relatively cheap, physicians should be encouraged to administer it because some patients may improve dramatically. This is illogical, because the same random dramatic response also occurs with placebo.

5. It is widely accepted by experts and regulatory authorities that the only appropriate primary end-point in trials for intermittent claudication is the measured walking distance on a treadmill. Although such wide agreement is to be welcomed, there are special problems with treadmill testing. First, most of these patients are older and find it difficult to become accustomed to walking on a treadmill. There is therefore a learning process that varies from patient to patient. Second, there has been considerable controversy about the relative merits of a *constant* gradient versus an *increasing* gradient for the treadmill exercise. There is little to choose between these two methods in terms of reproducibility. Initial claims that the graded exercise program abolished most of the placebo effects have not been substantiated by later trials. Although both pain-free distance and absolute walking distance are usually recorded, it is now believed that the latter is more reproducible.

6. It has been argued that any improvement in absolute claudication distance on a treadmill is insufficient to characterize drugs for intermittent claudication. It is suggested that a patient's perception of changes in quality of life are really more relevant. More recent studies have included some quality-of-life instrument, although it is not agreed as to which questionnaire is most appropriate for use in claudicants. Until a specialized instrument for use in these cases has become established, validated, and widely accepted, changes in treadmill walking distance will have to remain the primary measure of success.

From this discussion of possible mechanisms of action, it is clear that most of the drugs advocated may have multiple mechanisms of action and on occasion new mechanisms have been discovered after the introduction of the drug. From the clinical point of view, it is more practical to group these drugs according to the weight and quality of clinical trial evidence of benefit in intermittent claudication. Individual drugs should thus be considered according to:

- Established drugs with proven but small benefit
- Established drugs with minimal or no benefit
- Newer incompletely studied drugs with potential benefit

Table 27–1 summarizes the results of published, placebo-

TABLE 27–1. RANDOMIZED, PLACEBO-CONTROLLED, DOUBLE-BLIND TRIALS OF PHARMACOTHERAPY IN INTERMITTENT CLAUDICATION

DRUG	AUTHOR	YEAR	NO. OF PATIENTS	DOSE	DURATION	PLACEBO (%)	DRUG (%)	*p* VALUE	FUNCTIONAL ASSESSMENT[2]	COMMENT
Pentoxifylline	Porter[31]	1982	128	1.2 gm/day	6 mo	38	56	.19	No	
	Lindgarde[32]	1989	150	1.2 gm/day	6 mo	29	50	.09	No	
	(subset)		109	1.2 gm/day	6 mo	30	63	<.05	No	
Naftidrofuryl	Adhoute[34]	1986	94	633 mg	6 mo	28	60	<.001	Yes	
	Adhoute[35]	1990	118	600 mg	6 mo	46	93	<.05	No	Data given for initial claudication distance
	Kriessmann[36]	1988	136	633 mg	3 mo	35	78	<.05	No	Data given for initial claudication distance
	Trübestein[38]	1984	104	600 mg	3 mo	40	55	NS	No	
	Moody[37]	1984	180	633 mg	6 mo	25	31[3]	.045	Yes	Data given for initial claudication distance
Ticlopidine	Balsano[40]	1989	151	500 mg/day	21 mo	38	71	<.01	No	
Dextran	Ernst[44]	1990	20	500 ml	6 wk	0	39	<.001	No	Crossover trial
Nicotinic acid (Hexopal)	Kiff[48]	1988	80	4 gm/day	3 mo	87	50	NS	Yes	
Cinnarizine	Staessen[46]	1977	26	200 mg	4 mo	30[4]	75[4]	<.05	Yes	Placebo = phenobarbitone
	Barber[47]	1980	45	225 mg	4 mo	11	142	—	No	Data given for initial claudication distance
	Donald[91]	1979	40	225 mg	3 mo	34	113	NS	No	Data given for initial claudication distance
Propionyl-L-carnitine	Brevetti[51]	1995	245	1–3 gm/day	6 mo	46	73	<.05	No	Crossover trial
	Brevetti[52]	1997	173	2 gm/day	12 mo	55	102	<.01	No	
Beraprost	Lievre[57]	1996	83	60–120 μg/day	3 mo	41[6]	91[6]	NS	No	
Prostaglandin E_1	Belch[55]	1997	80	3 doses	2 mo	−14	53	<.01	Yes	
	Diehm[56]	1997	213	60 μg/day	2 mo	60	101	<.05	No	
Cilostazol	Money	1998	239	200 mg/day	4 mo	13%	47%	<0.001	Yes	
	Dawson	1998	81	200 mg/day	3 mo	10%	63%	<0.01	Yes	

[1]ACD = % change in absolute claudication distance compared to baseline value.
[2]Functional status defined by the Walking Impairment Questionnaire and Medical Outcomes Study SF-36.
[3]Percentage of subjects improving walking distance by 50% compared with baseline value.
[4]Percentage of subjects improving walking distance by 100% compared with baseline value.
[5]Unpublished data.
[6]Only the subset of patients at the optimal dose is reported.
NS = not significant.

controlled, double-blind randomized prospective studies of changes in absolute claudication distance.

Established Drugs with Proven but Small Benefit in Claudication

Pentoxifylline

Pentoxifylline is probably the most widely prescribed drug for improving claudication distance. Pentoxifylline improves whole blood filterability, lowers plasma fibrinogen levels, and decreases whole blood viscosity and platelet aggregation. In the 1970s, there were a number of small trials in Europe. The duration of most of these trials was only 4 to 8 weeks, now thought to be less than appropriate for this condition. In many of the trials, suboptimal doses of pentoxifylline were used.

In 1982, the result of a large United States placebo-controlled trial in 128 patients treated for 6 months was published.[31] The optimal dose of 1200 mg/day was used. This showed a 56% improvement in absolute claudication disease in contrast to 38% improvement in the placebo group ($p = .19$).[30] Side effects included relatively mild symptoms of nausea, vomiting, and dizziness, symptoms that required discontinuation of the drug in only 3% to 5% of the patients. The percentage of improvements was expressed as a mean difference between weeks 2 and 24. The actual improvement over placebo from entry to 6 months in absolute claudication distance was 18% (not statistically significant).

A more recent and larger study, also over 6 months, showed a 20% improvement over placebo ($p = .09$).[32] This study demonstrated that a subgroup of patients with symptoms for longer than a year and an ankle-bronchial-pressure index (ABPI) of less than 0.8 responded better to the drug.

No trials with pentoxifylline published so far have attempted to assess any change in quality of life. In general, therefore, it seems reasonable to accept that pentoxifylline does produce a real, if modest, improvement in treadmill claudication distance, but its greater benefit in a subgroup of claudicants remains to be established, as does any overall benefit to quality of life.

Naftidrofuryl

Naftidrofuryl is licensed and has been widely prescribed for claudication in Europe for more than 20 years. It is believed to have an anti-serotonin effect as well as a metabolic mechanism.[33] In four placebo-controlled studies lasting 3 to 6 months, naftidrofuryl was significantly more effective than placebo in improving walking distances,[34–37] although a later study showed no significant difference.[38] The magnitude of the benefit obtained is comparable to that of pentoxifylline.

Established Drugs with Minimal or No Benefit in Claudication

Antiplatelet Drugs

Aspirin

As mentioned later, all patients with intermittent claudication should receive low-dose aspirin or another antiplatelet agent unless specifically contraindicated because of its ability to modify the high risk of nonfatal and fatal cardiovascular events in these patients. However, no studies of aspirin have shown a benefit in terms of improving claudication distance. One study published in 1985 suggested that aspirin slowed the progression of atherosclerosis in the femoral artery, as assessed by serial arteriograms.[39]

Thienopyridine

A newer group of antiplatelet agents are the thienopyridine derivatives, which act by selectively and irreversibly inhibiting the binding of ATP to its receptor on platelets. *Ticlopidine* belongs to this group and is well established as an antiplatelet agent with benefits similar to low-dose aspirin in terms of atherothrombotic complications. Only one study, however, has examined its effect on claudication distance; a statistically significant improvement ($p = < .01$) was noted.[40]

Vasodilators

Although vasodilators were the first class of agents used to treat claudication, they have not shown any clinical efficacy in randomized controlled trials.[41–43]

Normovolemic Hemodilution

Although theoretically lowering the hematocrit should improve blood flow by lowering whole blood viscosity, it is uncertain whether the increase in blood flow compensates for the decrease in oxygen-carrying capacity of the blood. There is also the practical problem associated with repeated hemodilution, which might be necessary if it were used to treat claudication. However, one double-blind, placebo-controlled trial of dextran hemodilution did show a significant efficacy in selected patients.[44]

Other "Vasoactive" Drugs

Some placebo-controlled trials using ketanserin, a serotonin antagonist, nicotinic acid (Hexopal) and cinnarizine, a calcium channel blocker, had failed to show consistent improvement. Other drugs that have been tried for this claudication include aminophylline, gingko biloba, and buflomedil,[45–49] which have shown no effect. All of these drugs have been available and intermittently tested for claudication over many years.

Chelation Therapy

Chelation therapy has been advocated for the treatment of atherosclerosis and intermittent claudication. Four randomized, double-blind, multicenter trials of edetate disodium (EDTA) have been reviewed.[50] The technique was not effective in treating the symptoms of claudication in any of these studies; furthermore, frequent infusions of EDTA tend to produce severe hypocalcemia and may be actually dangerous.

Newer, Incompletely Studied Drugs with Potential Benefit in Improving Claudication

Carnitine

Two large trials of propionyl-L-carnitine have shown that the optimal dose is 2 gm/day and that there is a statistically significant improvement in absolute claudication distance.[51, 52]

Cilostazol

Cilostazol is a phosphodiesterase inhibitor that has vasodilator and antiplatelet activities.[28] Two fully published controlled randomized studies have shown a statistically significant improvement in walking distance compared to placebo.[53, 53a]

Prostaglandins

Until recently, prostaglandins (PGs) have had to be given intravenously, and for many years they were tested only in patients with critical leg ischemia (CLI); however, there have been a few studies in claudicants. In one open study, 44 patients were treated either with intravenous pentoxifylline (control group) or with intravenous PGE_1 (alprostadil) for 4 weeks.[54] All patients also underwent an exercise rehabilitation program. The exercise program alone resulted in a 99% increase in maximum walking distance; pentoxifylline, a 119% increase; and PGE_1 perfusion, a very dramatic 371% increase.

A placebo-controlled, double-blind dose-ranging study of a pro-drug of PGE_1 (AS-013) given intravenously was studied in 80 claudicants over 8 weeks. There was a significantly greater increase ($p = < .101$) in absolute walking distance in the combined active treatment groups (53%) compared to placebo group (−14%). There was also a dose-related improvement in the response to the quality-of-life questionnaire.[55]

In another study, intravenous PGE_1 was given over 8 weeks to 213 claudicants. Pain-free walking distance increased by 60% in the placebo group but to 101% in the treated group ($p = < .05$). These improvements remained virtually unchanged over 3 months of follow-up without treatment.[56]

Orally active prostaglandins have also been developed, such as beraprost, a PGI_2 (epoprostenol) analogue. In a dose-ranging study with the drug, increased claudication distance was found to be statistically not significant.[57] There is an ongoing placebo-controlled, double-blind study of oral iloprost, another prostacyclin analogue. As drug concentrations are reached with intravenous preparations, all prostaglandins elicit side effects in a significant number of patients. Side effects are usually headache, flushing, and nausea, but no significant adverse reactions have been found. In the treatment of claudicants, the presence of side effects, even if they are not important medically, are probably unacceptable.

Other New Agents

A number of other new approaches are under active investigation, but most are still at the stage of animal models. These include drugs that open potassium channels in vascular smooth muscle[58] and vascular endothelial growth factor (VEGF).[91]

Conclusion

At present, the principal use of drugs in patients with intermittent claudication is in modifying the serious systemic cardiovascular risk from nonfatal and fatal myocardial infarction and ischemic strokes (see also Chapter 19). Despite three decades of trials with a range of medications, the pharmacologic treatment of claudication itself is still limited to a few drugs of uncertain efficacy. This lack of success stories is particularly surprising when contrasted with the large number of drugs that effectively control the symptoms of ischemia in the heart. Therefore, all patients with intermittent claudication should be prescribed antiplatelet therapy, unless specifically contraindicated, but none of the drugs considered in this chapter would be justifiably used as *first-line* treatment for the actual symptom of claudication. These drugs should be given only when some evidence of objective efficacy has been demonstrated in terms of walking distance in placebo-controlled, double-blind studies of sufficient duration. These drugs may be used as *second-line* therapy in selected patients.

The initial treatment of claudication must continue to rely on the well-established principles of appropriate lifestyle modifications and elimination of risk factors when possible. The most important advice that a physician can offer is to discontinue smoking and to participate in a regular walking exercise program. The prescription of any drug that might improve claudication would only detract from the impact of this crucial advice. Fortunately, the majority of claudicants observe a marked benefit after 6 to 12 months if they follow this advice. The current drugs for improving claudication may then possibly be tried to achieve further improvement, or they may be tried in patients who have repeatedly been unwilling or unable to follow the usual advice. It is to be hoped that one of the newer drugs in development may fill the present serious gap in our armamentarium for dealing with intermittent claudication.

DRUGS USED TO TREAT CRITICAL LEG ISCHEMIA

Mechanism of Action

In this chapter, the term "critical leg ischemia" (CLI) is used to characterize all patients with ischemic symptoms at rest by contrast to intermittent claudication. Patients may have either rest pain or trophic skin changes, such as ulcers and gangrene. CLI differs from intermittent claudication most importantly in terms of pathophysiology and natural history. In claudication, the final pathologic event is transient ischemia of the skeletal muscle; in CLI, the final pathologic event is long-standing, often continuous, ischemia of the microcirculation in the skin.

Second, the natural history of intermittent claudication is a gradual improvement or stabilization in the majority of patients without the need for interventional treatment. In contrast, most patients with CLI require a major amputation in the absence of successful revascularization.

The risk of fatal or nonfatal cardiovascular events is also even greater in CLI than in claudication. Although the underlying primary lesion in both claudicants and CLI patients is PAOD, the difference in the secondary pathology affects the possible pharmacologic treatment modalities.

The magnitude of the necessary effect of any pharmacologic intervention also needs to be much greater than that required in claudicants. A quite modest increase in skeletal muscle blood flow may produce a detectable and possibly significant improvement in claudication distance. To some degree, this may also be true in patients with ischemic rest pain, but it is generally accepted that the improvement in blood flow necessary to prevent progression of gangrene or to bring about healing of an ischemic ulcer needs to be considerable.

The pathophysiology of the nutritive microcirculation in ischemic skin probably differs greatly from that of the intermittent short-lasting ischemia of skeletal muscle. In CLI, it is thought that there is a dysfunction of the microcirculatory flow regulatory mechanism in the skin manifested by abnormal vasomotion and resulting in an uneven distribution of the already decreased blood flow, which can easily be visualized on capillary microscopy.[59] This functional disturbance is thought to be associated with inappropriate activation of the microcirculatory defense mechanisms manifested by microthrombosis. This is believed to be principally due to a vicious circle involving activated platelets, WBCs and endothelium in the skin microcirculation.[60]

The criticisms already discussed in relation to the use of vasodilators and hemodilution apply equally to patients with CLI (see Vasodilators and Hemodilution). Serotonin antagonists and metabolism-enhancing drugs (discussed earlier) probably have no role in the different pathophysiology of CLI.

Pharmacotherapy for CLI has mostly been targeted against inappropriate activation of the WBCs, downregulation of platelet activation, and inappropriate endothelial function particularly in relation to nitric oxide. Particular interest is focused on the role of inappropriate WBCs. The hypothesis suggests that the inappropriately activated WBC becomes abnormally rigid, clogging the microcirculation. The WBC then releases a number of noxious substances, causing local damage. This includes proteolytic enzymes, damaging the capillary membrane; leukocyte-derived oxygen free radicals; and platelet-activating factor (PAF).[61]

Clinical Efficacy

As with intermittent claudication, some problems are associated with the clinical testing of pharmacotherapy in patients with CLI.

1. There is ongoing controversy about the type of patients who should be entered into such trials and a question regarding the definition of CLI. Much of the controversy would disappear if more understood the distinction between a clinical definition for everyday use in the treatment of individual patients and the definition for large double-blind, placebo-controlled trials. The former definition should include all patients who have rest pain or trophic skin changes predominantly due to arterial disease. It is acceptable to include in this clinical definition patients with milder disease who may well not lose their leg even in the absence of successful revascularization. For clinical trials, it is much more important to have an exclusive definition resulting in a reasonably homogeneous group of patients who would probably require a major amputation in the absence of successful revascularization. Such a definition usually includes an ankle or toe systolic pressure below a certain limit, which is less (e.g., 40 mmHg) in patients with only rest pain than in patients with trophic skin changes (e.g., 70 mmHg).

2. The issue of stratification, particularly for patients only with rest pain compared with patients with trophic skin changes, and diabetic versus nondiabetic patients, has not been resolved. It seems logical to avoid stratification unless there is good prior evidence that a particular drug is likely to have significantly different benefits in the various strata.

3. As with trials involving intermittent claudication, the term "placebo response" is inappropriate. In all trials of pharmacotherapy and CLI, all patients are given standard therapy, including local foot care, infection control, optimization of cardiac output, and analgesia as necessary. Some patients respond favorably to this standard background therapy, which should not properly be termed a placebo response.

4. Because of the greater potency required and the acceptability of some side effects, many drugs examined for the treatment of CLI, most notably the prostaglandins, have side effects that are sometimes obvious to both the patient and the physician. It may therefore be argued that some trials cannot be truly "double-blind."

5. The issue of primary end-point is more difficult in trials studying CLI than in trials studying intermittent claudication. In patients with CLI, there are three levels at which response can be assessed: (a) at the level of the *local lesion* in the foot, in terms of relief of rest pain and healing of ulcers; (b) in terms of *limb salvage*, to examine the need for major amputation; and (c) in terms of *patient survival*, because inevitably there will be a significant mortality in any trial of CLI patients lasting several months. This problem has not been fully resolved. The current tendency is to use a global primary end-point to represent the optimal outcome for the patient—being alive—without an amputation, without rest pain, and without trophic skin changes.

6. As with patients with intermittent claudication, it would be unethical to withhold additional treatment from CLI patients during the course of a drug trial if this is clinically indicated. Patients who deteriorate may need surgical or endovascular intervention, and on an intention-to-treat analysis of the trial an increased number of interventions in one group may falsely give the impression that patients assigned to that group had a more favorable outcome from the placebo or drug.

7. One of the biggest problems in trials of drug therapy for CLI has been the possibly quite proper reluctance of investigators to enter patients who might also be suitable for some form of intervention. The tendency has been to study patients who have already undergone a number of failed interventions and these patients will inevitably be at the most severe end of the spectrum of CLI. In some patients, the pathologic changes will have become irreversible, and no treatment (pharmacologic or otherwise) can prevent a major amputation.

Prostanoids

Apart from producing vasodilatation, prostanoids also have a powerful antiplatelet effect and possibly modifying effect

TABLE 27–2. COMPARATIVE LONG-TERM (7–28 DAYS' TREATMENT) TRIALS OF PROSTANOIDS IN PATIENTS WITH CRITICAL LIMB ISCHEMIA (CLI)

AUTHOR	NO. OF PATIENTS (% WHO WERE DIABETIC)	DRUG AND ROUTE OF ADMINISTRATION	DOSAGE	FOLLOW-UP	END-POINTS	RESULTS	*p*	TRIAL DESIGN
Sakaguchi[66]	65	PGE_1 (IA) vs. niacinate oral (200 mg 6 × daily)	0.05 or 0.15 ng/kg/min × 24 continuous infusion × 2–6 wk	End of infusion	Ulcer size Pain	Reduced by higher dose vs. niacinate + lower dose	.039	DB
Böhme[67]	34	PGE_1 (IA) vs. ATP (IA)	10–20 μg/60 min × 23 days	End of infusion	Ulcer size Rest pain	Reduced Reduced	NS NS	O
Trübestein[68]	57	PGE_1 vs. 30 mg ATP (IA)	20 μg over 60 min daily × 3 wk	3 wk	Analg. cons. Ulcer size Amputation	Reduced Reduced Reduced	<.04 <.02 .02	O
Diehm[69]	46	PGE_1 vs. placebo (IV)	60 μg/4 hr/day × 3 wk	1 mo	Pain Analg. cons. Clinical stage	Reduced Reduced Improved	<.04 <.02 .007	DB
Ciprostene Study Group 1991[70]	211	PGE_1 vs. placebo (IV)	120 ng/kg/min × 8 hr/daily × 7 days	4 mo	Ulcer size	Reduced by 50%	<.005	DB
Diehm 1997[71]	213	PGE_1 vs. placebo (IV)	60 μg × 2 hr × 4 weeks	3 mo	Walking distance on treadmill	Improved	<.005	DB
ICAI Study Group 1998[72]	1560	PGE_1 (IV) vs routine treatment	60 μg daily × 28 days	6 mo	CLI disappearance	Reduced odds ratio, 0.73	.002	O
Trübestein[73]	70	PGE_1 (IV) vs. pentoxifylline	2 × 40 μg over 2 hr daily × 4 wk	6 mo	Rest pain Analg. cons. Ulcer size	Reduced Reduced Reduced	NS <.005 <.05	O
Balzer[74]	113 (34%)	Iloprost vs. placebo (IV)	0.5–2 ng/kg/min × 6 hr × 14 days	End of infusion	Analg. cons.	Reduced	<.05	DB
Diehm[75]	101	Iloprost vs. placebo (IV)	Up to 2 ng/kg/min × 6 hr × 28 days	End of infusion	Ulcer size	Reduced	<.05	DB
Norgren[76]	103 (32%)	Iloprost vs. placebo (IV)	0.5–2 ng/kg/min × 6 hr × 14 days	End of infusion	Ulcer size	Reduced	NS	DB
Brock[77]	109 (100%)	Iloprost vs. placebo (IV)	0.5–2 ng/kg/min × 6 hr × 28 days	End of infusion	Ulcer size Rest pain	Reduced Reduced	<.05 <.05	DB
U.K. Study Group[78]	151 (31%)	Iloprost vs. placebo (IV)	Up to 2 ng/kg/min × 6 hr daily × 28 days	1 mo 6 mo	Ulcer healing Ulcer healing	Reduced Reduced	<.05 <.01	DB
Guilmot[79]	128 (58%)	Iloprost vs. placebo (IV)	Up to 2 ng/kg/min × 6 hr daily × 21 days	1 mo 2 mo	Rest pain Rest pain	Reduced Reduced	<.05 NS	DB

NS = not statistically significant; PGE_1 = prostaglandin E_1; analg. cons. = analgesic consumption; CLI = critical limb ischemia; O = open; DB = double-blind; ATP = adenosine triphosphate; IV = intravenous; IA = intra-arterial; ICAI = Ischemia Cronica Critica Degli Arti Inferiori.

on leukocyte activation and endothelial damage.[62] This is probably why prostanoids have become the most widely tested group of drugs for CLI. Initially PGE_1 was mainly evaluated by intra-arterial administration because of its rapid pulmonary inactivation.[63] Intravenous studies with PGE_1 were subsequently undertaken when it was demonstrated that after a temporary inactivation by the lung metabolites having a similar biologic activity to the parent compound PGE_1.[64]

Since the first report of the effects of intra-arterial infusion of PGE_1 given to four patients with unreconstructable leg ischemia in 1979,[65] there have been 14 randomized controlled double-blind trials, with the medication administered for at least a week using PGE_1 or PGI_2 (Table 27–2).[66–79] Iloprost, a more stable prostacyclin analogue, has been tested in six of these 14 randomized controlled trials.[77–82] When prostanoids were administered for more than 7 days, six of the seven trials with PGE_1 and six of the seven trials with iloprost had a statistically significant favorable difference in at least one of the end-points. This response seemed to be greater when the prostanoids were administered for 4 weeks compared to shorter periods.

Data on major amputation at 3 to 6 months follow-up were available in three studies.[76, 78, 79] Patients who received iloprost were much less likely to have undergone a major amputation than patients in the placebo group (23% versus 39%; $P < .05$) during the treatment and follow-up period. More important, patients who received iloprost had a much greater probability of completing the follow-up period alive with both legs than patients who received placebo (35% versus 55%; $P < .05$).[80] As mentioned earlier, there may have been a bias in these trials introduced by the frequent side effects of prostanoids, thereby jeopardizing the blindness of the trials; however, results in terms of major amputation are difficult to ignore.

Currently, there are three ongoing trials of an oral formulation of iloprost in patients with CLI. In each of these trials, the inclusion criteria specify that patients should not be suitable for any type of reconstruction; therefore, the patient population tends to be at the severe end of the CLI spectrum. So far, it has not been thought ethically acceptable to randomize patients to prostanoids (or any other form of medication) and interventional treatment by surgery or angioplasty. One trial using intravenous iloprost showed significant pain relief and healing of ischemic ulcers in patients with Buerger's disease.[81] A smiliar study has now been completed with orally active iloprost.[82]

Drugs Used Primarily to Treat Intermittent Claudication

Many of the drugs previously described in the context of treatment of intermittent claudication have also been tried intermittently for the treatment of CLI. There is little substantial evidence to support their use in this indication.[83] Intravenous pentoxifylline has been investigated in patients with CLI in two double-blind, placebo-controlled studies involving treatment for 3 weeks. In one, the severity of the rest pain was significantly less in the pentoxifylline group.[84] The second study, using oral pentoxifylline, showed a similar trend in terms of rest pain but did not reach statistical significance.[85] There were no beneficial results in terms of avoiding major amputation. There have been no trials specifically examining the effect of antiplatelet drugs on the progression of CLI. Similarly, there have been no trials with the use of long-term anticoagulant agents. Despite many open trials reporting promising results with the use of defibrinogenating agents,[86, 87] two placebo-controlled, double-blind studies using ancrod showed no benefit in terms of healing of ischemic ulcers or reducing the need for amputation.[88]

Conclusion

There have been no randomized, controlled studies of any drug treatment in CLI comparing pharmacotherapy to conventional revascularization. Thus, although pharmacotherapy cannot be recommended as primary treatment in these patients, it may have a role when revascularization is technically impossible or when it has failed, leaving the patient with continuing symptoms and the risk of a major amputation. Some prostanoids are now licensed in some countries, but not in the United States, for this indication. It appears reasonable to try a short course of intravenous prostanoid in such patients because there is some evidence of efficacy. It is essential to monitor patients carefully, however, so that an amputation is not unduly delayed if the ischemia progresses.

The advent of orally active prostanoids will considerably improve the ease of treatment and its possible duration. These preparations may therefore prove valuable in the future. No other type of drug should be considered for CLI in the absence of any positive, properly controlled trials indicating efficacy.

Possibly the most exciting prospect is gene-induced angiogenesis. Most work so far has been done with VEGF, which increases collateral flow and capillary density in animal models.[89] There have also been encouraging results in an open clinical trial using naked plasmid deoxyribonucleic acid, including VEGF, injected directly into ischemic muscles in patients with CLI.[90]

REFERENCES

1. Dormandy J, Mahir M, Ascady G, et al: Fate of the patient with chronic leg ischemia. J Cardiovasc Surg 30:50–57, 1989.
2. Gillespie G: The case against vasodilator drugs in occlusive vascular disease of the legs. Lancet 1:995–997, 1959.
3. Coffman JD: Pathophysiology of intermittent claudication. *In* Spittell JA Jr (ed): Pharmacologic Approach to Treatment of Limb Ischemia. Philadelpia, American College of Clinical Pharmacology, 1983, pp 43–52.
4. Chien S, Dormandy J, Ernst E, Matrai A (eds): Clinical Haemorrheology. Boston. Martinus Nijhoff, 1987.
5. Reid JL, Dormandy JA, Barnes AJ, et al: Impaired red cell deformity in peripheral vascular disease. Lancet 1:666–668, 1976.
6. Ernst E, Hammerschmidt DE, Bagge U, et al: Leukocytes and the risk of ischemic disease. JAMA 257:2318–2324, 1987.
7. Dormandy JA, Hoare E, Colley J: Clinical hemodynamic and biochemical findings in 126 patients with intermittent claudication. Br Med J 4:576–581, 1973.
8. Ehrly AM, Kohler HJ: Altered deformability of erythrocytes from patients with chronic occlusive arterial disease. Vasa 5:319–322, 1976.
9. Ernst E, Hammerschmidt D, Bagge U, et al: Leukocytes and risk of ischemic disease. JAMA 257:2318–2324, 1987.

10. Dormandy J, Hoare E, Dormandy T: Effects of clofibrate on blood viscosity in intermittent claudication. Br Med J 4:259–262, 1974.
11. Dormandy J, Goyle K, Reid H: Treatment of severe intermittent claudication by controlled defibrinogenation. Lancet i:625–626, 1977.
12. Lowe G, Dunlop D, Lawson D, et al: Double blind controlled clinical trial of ancrod for ischaemic rest pain of the leg. Angiology 33:46–50, 1982.
13. Angelkort B, Doppelfield E: Treatment of chronic arterial occlusive disease: Clinical study with a new galenic preparation of pentoxifylline. Trental 400. Pharmatherapeutica 3(Suppl I):18–29, 1983.
14. Muller R: Hemorrheology and peripheral vascular disease: A new therapeutic approach. J Med 12:209–235, 1981.
15. Schumalzer EA, Chien S: Filterability of subpopulations of leukocytes: Effects of pentoxifylline. Blood 64:542–546, 1984.
16. Ehrly AM, Salger-Lorenz K: Influence of pentoxifylline on muscle tissue oxygen tension of patients with intermittent claudication before and after pedal ergometry exercise. Angiology 38:93–100, 1987.
17. Yates C, Berent A, Dormandy J: Increase in leg blood flow by normovolaemic haemodilution in intermittent claudication. Lancet ii:166–168, 1979.
18. Dormandy J: Fahreus Lecture: The dangerous red cell. Clin Haemorrheol 4:115–132, 1984.
19. Dormandy J: Influence of blood viscosity on blood flow and the effects of low molecular weight dextran. Br Med J 4:716–719, 1971.
20. Rutherford RB, Jones DN, Bergentz SE, et al: The efficacy of dextran 40 in preventing early postoperative thrombosis following difficult lower extremity bypass. J Vasc Surg 1:765–773, 1984.
21. Rothermel JE, Wessinger JB, Stichfield FE: Dextran 40 and thromboembolism in total hip replacement surgery. Arch Surg 106:135–137, 1973.
22. Prevention of atherosclerotic complications with Ketanserin Trial Group: Prevention of atherosclerotic complications: Controlled trial of ketanserin. Br Med J 298:424–430, 1989.
23. Prevention of atherosclerotic complications with Ketanserin Trial Group. Randomised placebo controlled double blind trial of ketanserin in claudicants. Circulation 80:1544–1548, 1989.
24. Hollenberg N, Nie Q: The effect of naftidrofuryl, a 5-HT_2 antagonist, on collateral vascular response to serotonin antiplatelet activation. J Cardiovasc Pharmacol 16(Suppl 3):S36–S39, 1990.
25. Shaw S, Johnson R: The effect of naftidrofuryl on the metabolic response to exercise in men. Acta Neurol Scand 52:231–237, 1975.
26. Bieber LL: Carnitine. Ann Rev Biochem 57:261–283, 1988.
27. Hiatt WR, Wolfel EE, Regensteiner JG, Brass EP: Skeletal muscle carnitine metabolism in patients with unilateral peripheral arterial disease. J Appl Physiol 73:346–353, 1992.
28. Okuda Y, Kimura Y, Yamashita K: Cilostazol. Cardiovasc Drug Rev 11:451–465, 1993.
29. PACK Claudication Substudy Investigators: Randomized placebo-controlled, double-blind trial of ketanserin in claudicants: Changes in claudication distance and ankle systolic pressure. Circulation 80:1544–1548, 1989.
30. AbuRahma AF, Woodruff BA: Effects and limitations of pentoxifylline therapy in various stages of peripheral vascular disease of the lower extremities. Am J Surg 160:266–270, 1990.
31. Porter JM, Cutler BS, Lee BY, et al: Pentoxifylline efficacy in the treatment of intermittent claudication: Multicenter controlled double-blind trial with objective assessment of chronic occlusive arterial disease patients. Am Heart J 104:66–72, 1982.
32. Lindgarde F, Jelnes R, Bjorkman H, et al: Scandinavian Study Group: Conservative drug treatment in patients with moderately severe chronic occlusive peripheral arterial disease. Circulation 80:1549–1556, 1989.
33. Waters KJ, Craxford AD, Chamberlain J: The effect of naftidrofuryl (Praxilene) on intermittent claudication. Br J Surg 67:349–351, 1980.
34. Adhoute G, Bacourt F, Barral M, et al: Naftidrofuryl in chronic arterial disease: Results of a six month controlled multicenter study using naftidrofuryl tablets 200 mg. Angiology 37:160–169, 1986.
35. Adhoute G, Andreassian B, Boccalon H, et al: Treatment of stage II chronic arterial disease of the lower limbs with the serotonergic antagonist naftidrofuryl: Results after 6 months of a controlled, multicenter study. J Cardiovasc Pharmacol 16(Suppl 3):S75–S80, 1990.
36. Kriessmann A, Neiss A: Demonstration of the clinical effectiveness of naftidrofuryl in intermittent claudication Vasa 24:27–32, 1988.
37. Moody AP, Al-Khaffaf HS, Lehert P, et al: An evaluation of patients with severe intermittent claudication and the effect of treatment with naftidrofuryl. J Cardiovasc Pharmacol 23(Suppl 3):S44–S47, 1984.
38. Trübestein G, Bohme H, Heidrich H, et al: Naftidrofuryl in chronic arterial disease: Results of a controlled multicenter study. Angiology 35:701–708, 1984.
39. Hess H, Mietaschk A, Deichsel G: Drug-induced inhibition of platelet function delays progression of PAOD: A prospective double-blind arteriographically controlled trial. Lancet 1:415–419, 1985.
40. Balsano F, Coccheri S, Libretti A, et al: Ticlopidine in the treatment of intermittent claudication: A 21-month double-blind trial. J Lab Clin Med 114:84–91, 1989.
41. Solomon SA, Ramsay LE, Yeo WW, et al: β Blockade and intermittent claudication: Placebo controlled trial of atenolol and nifedipine and their combination. Br Med J 303:1100–1104, 1991.
42. Coffman JD: Vasodilator drugs in peripheral vascular disease. N Engl J Med 300:713–717, 1979.
43. Spence JD, Arnold JMO, Munoz CE, et al: Angiotensin-converting enzyme inhibition with cliazapril does not improve blood flow, walking time, or plasma lipids in patients with intermittent claudication. J Vasc Med Biol 4:23–28, 1993.
44. Ernst E, Kollar L, Matrai A: A double-blind trial of dextran: Haemodilution versus placebo in claudicants. J Intern Med 227:19–24, 1990.
45. Picano E, Testa R, Pogliani M, et al: Increase of walking capacity after acute aminophylline administration in intermittent claudication. Angiology 40:1035–1039, 1989.
46. Staessen AJ: Treatment of peripheral circulatory disturbances with cinnarizine: A multi-centre, double-blind, placebo-controlled evaluation. Proc Soc Med 70(Suppl 8):S17–S20, 1977.
47. Barber JH, Reuter CA, Jageneau AHM, Loots W: Intermittent claudication: A controlled study in parallel time of the short-term and long-term effects of cinnarizine. Pharmatherapeutica 2:400–407, 1980.
48. Kiff RS: Does inositol nicotinate (Hexopal) influence intermittent claudication? A controlled trial. Br J Clin Pract 42:141–145, 1988.
49. Trübestein G, Balzer K, Bisler H, et al: Buflomedil in arterial occlusive disease: Results of a controlled multicenter study. Angiology 35:500–505, 1984.
50. Ernst E: Chelation therapy for peripheral arterial occlusive disease: A systematic review. Circulation 96:1031–1033, 1997.
51. Brevetti G, Perna S, Sabba C, et al: Propionyl-L-carnitine in intermittent claudication: Double-blind, placebo-controlled, dose titration, multicenter study. J Am Coll Cardiol 26:1411–1416, 1995.
52. Brevetti G, Diehm C, Lambert D: European multicenter study on propionyl-L-carnitine in intermittent claudication. Vol 96. Abstracts from the 70th Scientific Sessions, 1997.
53. Money SR, Herd JA, Isaacsohn JL, et al: The effect of cilostazol on walking distance in patients with intermittent claudication caused by peripheral vascular disease. J Vasc Surg 27:267–275, 1998.
53a. Dawson DL, Cutler BS, Meissner MH, et al: Cilostazol has beneficial effects in the treatment of intermittent claudication. Circulation 98:678–686, 1998.
54. Scheffler P, de la Hamette D, Gross J, et al: Intensive vascular training in stage IIb of peripheral arterial occlusive disease: The additive effects of intravenous prostaglandin E_1 or intravenous pentoxifylline during training. Ciculation 90:818–822, 1994.
55. Belch JJF, Bell PRF, Creissen D, et al: Randomised, double-blind study evaluating the efficacy and safety of AS-013, a prostaglandin E_1 prodrug, in patients with inermittent claudication. Circulation 95:2298–2302, 1997.
56. Diehm C, Balzer K, Bisler H, et al: Efficacy of a new prostaglandin E_1 regimen in outpatients with severe intermittent claudication: Results of a multicenter placebo-controlled double-blind trial. J Vasc Surg 25:537–544, 1997.
57. Liervre M, Azoulay S, Lion L, et al: A dose-effect study of beraprost sodium in intermittent claudication. J Cardiovasc Pharmacol 27:788–793, 1996.
58. Cook NS, Rudin M, Pally C, et al: Effects of the potassium channel openers SDZ-PCO 400 and cromakalim in an in vivo rat model of occlusive arterial disease assessed by 31P-NMR spectroscopy. J Vasc Med Biol 4:14–22, 1993.
59. Ubbink D, Jacobs M, Tangelder G, et al: The usefulness of capillary microscopy, transcutaneous oximetry and laser Doppler fluxmetry in the assessment of the severity of lower limb ischaemia. J Microcirc 14:34–44, 1994.
60. Lowe G: Pathophysiology of critical leg ischaemia. *In* Dormandy J, Stock G (eds): Critical Leg Ischaemia. Berlin, Springer-Verlag, 1990, p 17.

61. Bradbury A, Murie J, Ruckley C: Role of the leucocyte in the pathogenesis of vascular disease. Br J Surg 80:1503, 1993.
62. Lowe GDO: Pathophysiology of critical limb ischemia. *In* Dormandy J, Stock G (eds): Critical Leg Ischemia: Its Pathophysiology and Management Berlin, Springer-Verlag 1990, pp 17–38.
63. Piper PJ, Vane JR, Wyllie JH: Inactivation of prostaglandins by the lungs. Nature 225:600–604, 1970.
64. Peskar BA, Hesse WH, Rogatti W, et al: Formation of 13, 14-dihydroprostaglandin E_1 during intravenous infusion of prostaglandin E_1 in patients with peripheral arterial disease. Prostaglandins 41:225–228, 1991.
65. Szczeklik A, Nizankowski R, Slawinski S: Successful therapy of advanced arteriosclerosis obliterans with prostacyclin. Lancet 1:1111–1114, 1979.
66. Sakaguchi S: Prostaglandin E_1 intra-arterial infusion therapy in patients with ischemic ulcer of the extremities. Int Angiol 3:39–42, 1984.
67. Böhme H, Brülsaver M, Härtel U, Bollinger A: Kontrollierte Studie zur Wirnsamkeit von I.A. PGE, Infusionen bei Peripherer Arterieller Verschlusskrankheit in Stadium and IV. Vasa 20(Suppl):206–208, 1987.
68. Trübestein G, Diehm C, Gruss JD, Horsch S: Prostaglandin E_1 in advanced occlusive arterial disease: Results of a multicentre study. Vasa 17(Suppl):39–43, 1987.
69. Diehm C, Hübsch-Müller C, Stammler F: Intravenöse Prostaglandin E_1: Therapie bei Patienten mit peripherer arterieller Verschlusskrankheit (AVK) im Stadium Ili: Eine doppelblinde, placebo-kontrollierte Studie. *In* Heinrich H, Böhme H, Rogatti W (eds): Prostaglandin E_1 Wirkungen und therapeutische Wirksamheit. Heidelberg, Springer-Verlag, 1988, pp 133–143.
70. Ciprostene Study Group: The effect of ciprostene in patients with peripheral vascular disease (PVD) characterized by ischemic ulcers. J Clin Pharmacol 31:81–87, 1991.
71. Diehm C, Balzer K, Bisler H, et al: Efficacy of a new prostaglandin E_1 regimen in outpatients with severe intermittent claudication: Results of a multicenter placebo-controlled double-blind trial. J Vasc Surg 254:537–544, 1997.
72. Ischemia Cronica Critica Degli Arti Inferiori (ICAI) Study Group: Prostanoids in chronic leg ischaemia: The results of a large randomised trial with prostaglandin E_1. Submitted.
73. Trübestein G, von Bary S, Breddin K, et al: Intravenous prostaglandin E_1 versus pentoxifylline therapy in chronic arterial occlusive disease: A controlled randomised multicenter study. Vasa 28:44–49, 1989.
74. Balzer K, Bechara G, Bisler H, et al: Placebo-kontrollierte, doppelblinde Multicenterstudie zur Wirksamkeit von Iloprost bei der Behandlung ischämischer Ruheschmerzen von Patienten mit periphereren arterieller Durchblutungsstörungen. Vasa 20(Suppl):379–381, 1987.
75. Diehm C, Abri O, Baitsch G, et al: Iloprost, ein stabiles Prostacyclinderivat bei arterieller Verschlüsskrankheit im Stadium IV. Dtsch Med Wochenschr 114:783–788, 1989.
76. Norgren L, Alwmark A, Ängqvist KA, et al: A stable prostacyclin analogue (iloprost) in the treatment of ischaemic ulcers of the lower limb: A Scandinavian-Polish placebo-controlled, randomised multicenter study. Eur J Vasc Surg 4:463–467, 1990.
77. Brock FE, Abri O, Baitsch G, et al: Iloprost in der Behandlung ischaemischer Gewebsläsionen bei Diabetikern. Schweiz Med Wochenschr 120:1477–1482, 1990.
78. United Kingdom Severe Limb Ischemia Study Group: Treatment of limb threatening ischemia with intravenous iloprost: A randomised double-blind placebo controlled study. Eur J Vasc Surg 5:511–516, 2991.
79. Guilmot JL, Diot E for the French Iloprost Study Group: Treatment of lower limb ischaemia due to atherosclerosis in diabetic and nondiabetic patients with iloprost, a stable analoque of prostacyclin: Results of a French Multicentre trial. Drug Invest 3:351–359, 1991.
80. Dormandy JA, Loh A: Critical limb ischemia. *In* Tooke JE, Lowe GDO (eds): A Textbook of Vascular Medicine. London, Arnold, 1996, pp 221–236.
81. Fiessinger JN, Schafer M, and the Thromboangitis Obliterans Study Group: Trial of iloprost versus aspirin treatment for critical limb ischemia of thromboangiitis obliterans. Lancet 335:555–557, 1990.
82. Verstraete M: Oral iloprost in the treatment of thromboangitis obliterans (Buerger's disease): A double blind randomised placebo controlled trial. Eur J Vasc Endovasc Surg 16:300–307, 1998.
83. Lowe GDO: Drugs in cerebral and peripheral arterial disease. Br Med J 300:524–528, 1990.
84. The European Study Group: Intravenous pentoxifylline for the treatment of chronic critical limb ischaemia. Eur J Vasc Endovasc Surg 9:426–436, 1995.
85. The Norwegian Pentoxifylline Multicenter Trial Group: Efficacy and clinical tolerance of parenteral pentoxifylline in the treatment of critical lower limb ischemia: A placebo controlled multicenter study. Int Angiol 15:75–80, 1996.
86. Lowe GDO: Defibrination, blood flow and blood rheology. Clin Hemorrheol 4:15–28, 1984.
87. Lowe GDO, Dunlop DJ, Lawson DH, et al: Double-blind controlled trial of ancrod in the relief of ischemic rest pain of the leg. Angiology 33:46–50, 1982.
88. Tønnessen KH, Sager P, Gormsen J: Treatment of severe foot ischemia by difibrination with ancrod: A randomised blind study. Scand J Clin Lab Invest 38:431–435, 1978.
89. Takeshita S, Zheng L, Brogi E, et al: Therapeutic angiogenesis. J Clin Invest 93:662–670, 1994.
90. Isner JM, Pieczek A, Schainfeld R, et al: Clinical evidence of angiogenesis following arterial gene transfer of phVEGF165. Lancet 348:370–374, 1996.
91. Donald JF: A multicentre general practice study of cinnarizine in the treatment of peripheral vascular disease. J Int Med Res 7:502–506, 1979.

CHAPTER 28

Principles of Thrombolytic Therapy

Vikram S. Kashyap, M.D., and William J. Quiñones-Baldrich, M.D.

The most common indication for intervention in the practice of vascular surgery is occlusion of a vessel segment or bypass graft by a thrombus or clot. Vascular surgical techniques have evolved to the point at which most arterial occlusions and some venous thromboses can be successfully managed. Since the early 1980s, however, pharmacologic dissolution of these occlusive thrombi has become a clinical reality and is being used successfully with increasing frequency. An understanding of the fibrinolytic system and how plasminogen activation affects both physiologic and pathologic thrombi is important for the appropriate use of thrombolytic therapy.

In both arterial and venous thrombosis the body's own system fails to maintain fluidity of the blood in the affected vessel. The imbalance resulting in thrombosis may be the result of multiple factors, including vessel injury or other intrinsic vessel wall lesion, a low-flow state, hypercoagulability of blood, or, more frequently, a combination of these. Disordered progressive coagulation of blood in vivo is prevented during normal conditions by an intricate system of checks and balances that primarily involves the coagulation and fibrinolytic systems. To maintain homeostasis, abnormal depositions of fibrin (the end-product of the coagulation cascade) is rapidly followed by local stimulation of the fibrinolytic system. Nevertheless, the fibrinolytic system is easily overwhelmed in pathologic states, resulting in clinical thrombosis.

With the development of drugs capable of stimulating the fibrinolytic system, together with a better understanding of the components and interactions leading to fibrinolysis, it is now possible to treat pathologic intravascular thrombi with the goal of complete dissolution. The drugs available, although lacking precise control, have proved valuable, and they represent a significant advance in treating patients with difficult thrombotic problems. It is likely that newer, more specific fibrinolytic agents, combined with advanced drug delivery systems, will improve still further the outcome of appropriately selected patients.

This chapter focuses on the fibrinolytic system and available lytic agents. We discuss current experimental and clinical experience with the use of fibrinolytic therapy for peripheral arterial and venous disease; the reader should keep in mind that fibrinolytic therapy is still evolving. This chapter should provide the clinician with not only an understanding of the fibrinolytic system and the available fibrinolytic agents but also guidelines for patient selection.

THE FIBRINOLYTIC SYSTEM

Since the early 1980s, substantial progress has occurred that has expanded our understanding of the intricate feedback control and activity mechanisms of the fibrinolytic system. This has led to safer and more effective use of fibrinolytic drugs. The fibrinolytic system's vital function involves maintenance of blood fluidity, and enhancement of that function allows resolution of pathologic thrombi. In 1958, Astrup proposed the concept of dynamic equilibrium for the coagulation and fibrinolytic systems.[9] In this delicate balance, the fibrinolytic process breaks down fibrin, which is continuously being deposited throughout the cardiovascular system as the result of limited activation of the coagulation system. This baseline fibrinolytic activity is under both local and systemic control mechanisms involving circulating inhibitors, cell-bound receptors, and other components of both the coagulation and the fibrinolytic systems. Under normal physiologic conditions, the process allows local, but not systemic, fibrinolysis. The coagulation and fibrinolytic systems interact through feedback mechanisms that are not fully understood. Nevertheless, some important feedback mechanisms have been elucidated, most of which may have clinical implications.

The key enzyme in the fibrinolytic system and the final common pathway is plasminogen (Fig. 28–1). This glycoprotein, produced in the liver, consists of a heavy amino-terminal region made up of five homologous but distinct triple-disulfide–bonded domains (*kringles*) joined to a lighter catalytic carboxy-terminal domain. Activation of plasminogen occurs by the cleavage of an arginine-valine bond, producing changes in conformation, leading to an increased affinity for both substrate (fibrin) and activator.

Four forms of human plasminogen have been identified that depend on variation in the N-terminus and the degree of glycosylation. The two main forms in plasma are collectively known as *Glu-plasminogen*; the other two forms, found mostly absorbed or bound to fibrin, are collectively known as *Lys-plasminogen*. Lys-plasminogen is formed rapidly from Glu-plasminogen by the catalytic action of plasmin.[20] Treatment of either Glu-plasminogen or Lys-plasminogen with various proteases results in lower-molecular-weight forms of human plasminogen. These have been observed in vivo in septic patients.[63]

The heavy chain of plasminogen (nonenzymatic portion) is composed of an activation peptide and five homologous domains known as kringles.[94] These kringles have a high degree of sequence homology with each other and with domains found in prothrombin, tissue plasminogen activator (t-PA), urinary plasminogen activator (u-PA), and factor XII. A repeating unit in a unique protein called *apolipoprotein a*, Lp(a), has significant homology to kringle 4 of plasminogen. This may help to explain why patients with abnormalities of Lp(a) may exhibit a hypercoagulable condition. Kringles are responsible for the binding of plasmino-

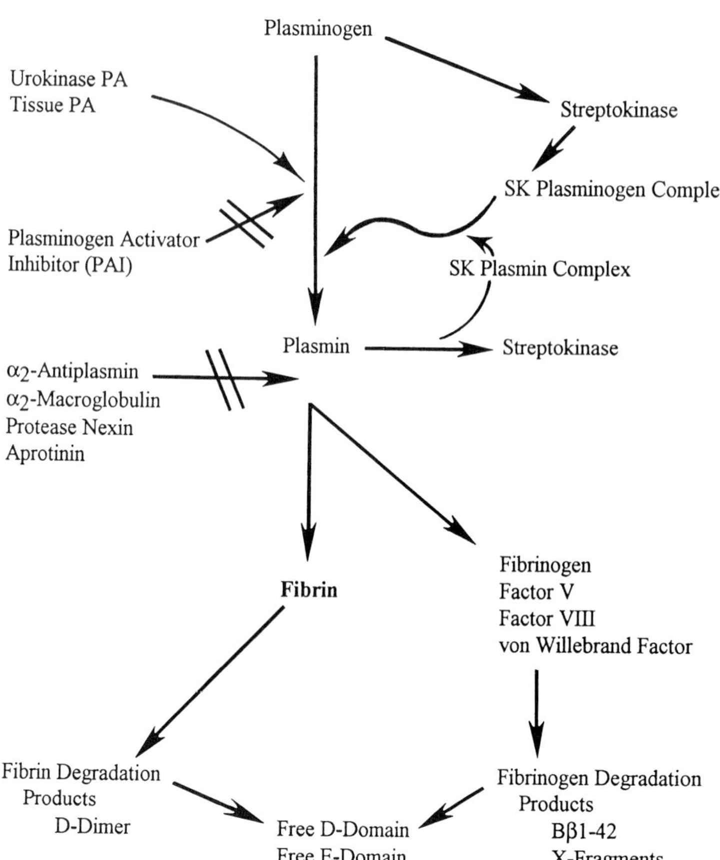

FIGURE 28–1. Simplified scheme of the fibrinolytic system. PA = plasminogen activator; SK = streptokinase.

gen or plasmin to fibrin, alpha$_2$-antiplasmin, and other important macromolecules necessary for the process of fibrinolysis.[116, 148] In addition, the kringles of plasminogen have been implicated in mediating neutrophil adherence to endothelial cells.[70]

Plasminogen in its Glu form usually exists in a closed structure. This conformation becomes open on the binding of lysine or lysine analogues. This conformational change produces a Glu-plasminogen with properties similar to those of Lys-plasminogen and, in many instances, is referred to as the *pseudo-Lys-form*. The main difference is that Lys-plasminogen continues to have lysine-binding sites that have a stable open conformation.[143] The open conformation of plasminogen renders the molecule much more readily cleaved, forming the active enzyme plasmin. The open conformation also binds more readily to the fibrin surface. The major binding of plasminogen to fibrin occurs through a strong lysine-binding site in the first kringle.[135, 136] Lysine analogues, such as tranexamic acid and ε-aminocaproic acid, promote the open conformation of Glu-plasminogen, thus potentially increasing fibrinolysis. In vivo, however, they also prevent the binding of the open conformation of plasminogen to fibrin and, therefore, exert a predominant antifibrinolytic effect.[123]

The primary substrates of plasmin are fibrinogen and fibrin. Circulating fibrinogen is composed of two identical subunits, each composed of three protein chains known as A (α), B (β), and gamma (γ) chains.[28] The two subunits of fibrinogen are joined to form the E-domain of the molecule. Two arms extending from this E-domain form the D-domains of the molecule. D-domains have binding sites for plasminogen and plasmin. Fibrinogen in the circulation is complexed to various degrees with plasminogen through these binding sites. Small peptides also extend from the E-domain, forming part of the α, β, and γ chains. The peptides from the A alpha and B beta chains are known as *fibrinopeptides A* and *B* and are cleaved from the molecule by thrombin during conversion of fibrinogen to fibrin. Once these fibrinopeptides have been removed by thrombin, a fibrin monomer is formed. These monomers remain soluble until polymers are formed from the interaction between the E-domain of one monomer and the D-domains of two other monomers. These fibrin polymers have little strength or stability until factor XIII, activated by thrombin, cross-links adjacent fibrin monomers through adjacent D-domains. Thus, plasminogen originally bound to fibrinogen becomes incorporated in the thrombus as this conversion occurs.

Plasmin cleaves both fibrin and fibrinogen between the D-domain and the E-domain. The result of this degradation is free D- and E-domains. Free D- and E-domains in plasma can be the result of degradation of both fibrinogen and fibrin monomers. The presence of D-dimers, however, implies degradation of cross-linked fibrin. D-dimers can be assayed, documenting fibrinolysis instead of fibrinogenolysis.[107] In contrast, attacks of plasmin on fibrinogen can produce end-terminal peptide-B beta 1-42, which is a measure of plasmin action on fibrinogen.[102]

An understanding of the action of plasmin on fibrinogen may help to clarify the clinical responses noted during thrombolytic therapy. As cleavage of fibrinogen proceeds, residual polypeptides, collectively known as *X-fragments*, are formed. These fragments are not distinguishable by standard laboratory assays for fibrinogen. Loss of sites responsible for cross-linking leads to formation of fibrin that is relatively weak. These X-fragments may be incorporated into both newly forming and existing thrombi, causing them to be more fragile and sensitive to the action of plasmin. Large amounts of these X-fragments can be produced during thrombolytic therapy. The newly formed fibrin, which contains these fragments, is more sensitive to the action of plasmin. This may help to explain why a decrease in bleeding complications has not been seen with fibrin-specific agents such as t-PA. Clinical evidence suggests that bolus therapy, as opposed to continuous intravenous infusion, of t-PA may be associated with a decrease in bleeding tendencies. Incorporation of these X-fragments into newly formed fibrin may represent a lower bleeding risk during intermittent bolus therapy[2] because of the lower plasma levels of the activator compared with the constant high levels seen during continuous intravenous infusion.

Fibrinogen is somewhat protected from the actions of plasmin in circulation by powerful and fast-acting plasmin inhibitors. These inhibitors neutralize free plasmin but are not as effective on fibrin-bound plasmin. During thrombolytic therapy, however, circulating plasmin levels exceed the capacity of plasmin inhibitors and fibrinogenolysis thus occurs.

Plasmin attacks other proteins in the plasma and extracellular spaces. The list of substrates for plasmin continues to increase and includes coagulation factors (e.g., factors V and VIII, von Willebrand's factor). In addition, plasmin may reduce the effect of thrombin intermediates, further interfering with the coagulation cascade.[52]

Plasmin can also lead to the release of kinin from high-molecular-weight kininogen. It can activate prekallikrein, both directly and indirectly,[17] and this may also induce further kinin formation. Plasmin attacks the protein components of the basement membrane and also activates other proteases within the extracellular matrix. Therefore, it may affect fibronectin, collagen, and laminin. Many of these secondary effects of plasmin are not fully understood, and their clinical implications are unknown. Understanding the control mechanisms of this protease requires a familiarity with its activators and inhibitors.

Activators of Plasminogen

Two main types of plasminogen activator have been identified in humans. The first one was isolated from human urine by MacFarlane and Pilling in 1946.[74] It was named *urokinase*, or urinary plasminogen activator (u-PA). It is a serine protease with a limited substrate specificity. It consists of a serine protease region B-chain and a short A-chain. The protease portion, known as *single-chain* u-PA (scu-PA), is responsible for the activation of plasminogen to plasmin. This portion of the activator has homology to domains on t-PA and other proteins involved in coagulation. It does not, however, contain lysine-binding sites and thus has no fibrin-binding properties.[69] High-affinity receptors for u-PA that recognize the molecule have been demonstrated in several cell types,[10, 12, 91] and its focal concentration on cell surfaces might be a mechanism by which cells invade the intracellular matrix and play a role in both normal and pathologic states. Both u-PA (urokinase) and pro-urokinase plasminogen activator (pro-urokinase) are available commercially (see later).

u-PA rapidly activates plasminogen through its susceptible cleavage site when it is in the open conformation (Lys-plasminogen), but it is much less efficient with the closed form of plasminogen (Glu-plasminogen).[119] Physiologic concentrations of chloride ions stabilize the closed conformation of Glu-plasminogen and therefore may inhibit activation.[131] Pro-urokinase is activated by plasminogen to form a two-chain activator. Questions remain about the intrinsic activity of pro-urokinase before its conversion to the two-chain form. The low intrinsic activity of pro-urokinase may be sufficient to act as a primer for the fibrinolytic system, particularly by activation of fibrin-bound plasminogen. Although without intrinsic fibrin-binding ability, pro-urokinase may be converted to the two-chain form by fibrin-bound plasmin. Because this activation most likely occurs on the surface of the clot, the apparent fibrin specificity of pro-urokinase may be explained. In addition, pro-urokinase appears to have enhanced activity in the presence of Lys-plasminogen, mostly found bound to thrombus.

A second plasminogen activator distinct from u-PA was discovered in melanoma cells in 1980 and was found to be the product of vascular endothelial cells.[66] t-PA has been cloned and found to have a structure similar to that of u-PA.[37] It is secreted as a single-chain protein with activity equal to the two-chain t-PA formed by the action of its own substrate, plasmin. In circulation, t-PA is found mostly in the single-chain form.[124]

t-PA seems to bind to the clot surface in the presence of fibrin, enhancing the affinity of t-PA for plasminogen by 1000-fold.[54] This affinity is significantly affected by removal of the second kringle from the plasminogen molecule, suggesting a role for this kringle.[56]

t-PA binds to other surfaces in addition to fibrin. Extracellular matrix components such as collagen and gelatin can activate t-PA in the absence of fibrin.[114] t-PA is also bound and activated on the surface of platelets, which may help target the action of t-PA, leading to cleavage of glycoprotein-Ib (GPIb) and loss of platelet binding. This antiplatelet effect has been observed with t-PA administration. Others have suggested that platelet aggregation is inhibited by affecting GPIIb/GPIIIa receptors. In contrast, increased platelet aggregability has been observed early in therapy, followed by reduced aggregation later in therapy.[106]

Partly digested fragments (X-fragments) and clots incorporating these fragments bind more aggressively with t-PA than do fresh undigested clots.[53] This may be the result of conformational changes that optimize the presentation of the stimulator region of fibrin.

Inhibitors of Fibrinolysis

Inhibitors of fibrinolysis are composed of two main groups: (1) proteins that exhibit antiactivator activity and (2) proteins that exhibit antiplasmin activity. Both play a significant role in controlling otherwise disordered lytic activity. Whereas plasminogen activator inhibitors (PAIs) occur both in plasma and at the cellular level, antiplasmins occur mostly in circulating plasma.

PAI-1 controls the physiologic activity of both u-PA and t-PA. PAI-1 is synthesized in the liver and vascular endothelial cells and is normally present in trace amounts in plasma. Plasma insulin appears to be the major physiologic regulator of PAI-1 activity in plasma.[4, 134] Plasma insulin levels correlate with PAI activity and body mass index. In addition, experimental studies suggest that release of platelet-derived growth factors (PDGFs) may attenuate fibrinolysis in vivo by augmenting endothelial cell syntheses and release of PAI-1 locally in the vicinity of thrombi and by increasing the hepatic secretion of PAI-1 into the circulation.[38, 39, 73] In plasma, PAI-1 circulates in a stable complex with a binding protein, recently identified as vitronectin. Platelet activation may falsely elevate PAI-1 antigen levels because of release of inactive PAI from platelets.[31, 113, 133]

Diurnal fluctuations of both t-PA and PAI-1 have been described. t-PA activity is lowest in the early morning and highest in the afternoon. Plasma PAI activity peaks in the early morning and passes through a trough in the afternoon. Overall, there is decreased fibrinolytic activity in the morning.[5, 6, 19, 46] Differences in patterns have also been seen between men and women, suggesting a hormonal influence.[132] PAI activity may also vary with diet.[90] Caffeine-containing beverages may enhance fibrinolytic activity; however, smoking induces an acute increase in t-PA. This increase in t-PA induced by smoking may deplete normal stores, paradoxically decreasing fibrinolytic activity. Increased levels of PAI-1 are frequently combined with a decreased capacity to release t-PA, are probably related to depleted stores,[50] and can be demonstrated in up to 40% of patients with deep vein thrombosis (DVT).[48, 59, 89, 149] Increased plasma PAI activity may also be part of an acute phase reaction seen in postoperative patients, which in part may explain the propensity of DVT to develop. Impaired fibrinolytic function caused by elevated plasma PAI activity is the most commonly observed disturbance of the hemostatic system in patients with thrombotic disease, both venous and arterial.[146]

The other group of important inhibitors of the fibrinolytic system is plasmin inhibitors. Plasmin inhibitors include alpha$_2$-antiplasmin, alpha$_2$-macroglobulin, protease nexin, and aprotinin. These proteins inhibit plasmin once it is formed.

Alpha$_2$-antiplasmin is a protease inhibitor single-chain glycoprotein and is a member of the serpin family. It is the main physiologic inhibitor of plasmin. Inhibition of plasmin by alpha$_2$-antiplasmin is a two-step process. The first step is reversible and is followed by formation of a covalent complex involving the active sites of plasmin. The half-life of alpha$_2$-antiplasmin and plasmin complex is approximately 12 hours.[23] Abnormal concentrations of alpha$_2$-antiplasmin have been documented in some clinical disorders[24, 76] and have been found useful in the evaluation of patients with disseminated intravascular coagulation (DIC).[120]

Alpha$_2$-macroglobulin is a nonspecific inhibitor of endoproteases. It forms a covalent complex with plasmin at various ratios.[25] The most important mechanism of alpha$_2$-macroglobulin inhibition is a molecular trap process. Cell surface receptors for clearance of the complex have been demonstrated in fibroblasts.[86, 141]

Protease nexin is also a member of the *serpin* family and is secreted by anchored human fibroblasts. Protease nexin has been categorized according to its affinity for heparin. High-affinity protease nexin is the major form found in human fibroblasts.[109] It is a broad-spectrum inhibitor of trypsin-like serine proteases, which include trypsin, thrombin, urokinase, plasmin, and one-chain and two-chain t-PA. Once the proteases are bound to protease nexin, degradation occurs through internalization via nexin receptors on the cell surface.[72]

Aprotinin is a serine protease inhibitor obtained from bovine organs. It is also known as *basic pancreatic trypsin inhibitor* and is a potent inhibitor of trypsin, plasma kallikrein, urinary kallikrein, and plasmin. Aprotinin is thought to play an important physiologic role in the maintenance of hemostasis.[35] It does not appear to be a major inhibitor of plasmin. However, clinical grade material is now commercially available under the name of Trasylol (Bayer, West Haven, Conn.). This compound reduces postoperative bleeding after cardiac surgery and other major operations.[105] In animal models, it has been shown to serve as an antidote for bleeding induced by administration of recombinant t-PA.[21] Because aprotinin acts as a direct inhibitor of plasmin and not of plasminogen activators, it is postulated that aprotinin may serve as an antidote for other plasminogen activators.

Other inhibitors of fibrinolysis exert their antifibrinolytic effect by blocking the binding of plasmin to fibrin. These antifibrinolytic agents are lysine analogues and are commercially available as ϵ-aminocaproic acid and tranexamic acid. As mentioned earlier, conformational changes are produced by these agents on plasmin, inducing an increased affinity for fibrin. Sufficient amounts of the antifibrinolytic agent, however, block the lysine-binding sites, thus exerting their antifibrinolytic effect.

Other Biologic Roles

Biologic functions other than those involving coagulation have now been firmly established for several components of the fibrinolytic system. These components are thought to be actively involved in biologic functions at the cellular level, such as embryogenesis, neuronal growth, ovulation, muscle regeneration, wound healing, angiogenesis, and tumor growth and invasion. Expression of certain components of the system have been observed both in vitro and in vivo.

In certain malignancies, expression of u-PA has been correlated with an unfavorable clinical prognosis. Tumor cell invasion as well as migration may be specifically linked to the expression of u-PA, t-PA, and their inhibitors in endothelial cells and smooth muscle cells. This observation may be relevant, not only in thrombosis and atherogenesis but also specifically during reparative processes following vascular injury.[64] Expression of these components is modulated by transcriptional regulation of cytokines, interferon, tumor necrosis factor (TNF), and hormones (e.g., corticosteroid and gonadotropins).[41, 67, 92, 115, 140] Growth factors, including those found in fibroblasts, platelets, and endothelial cells, may also control the expression of certain components of the fibrinolytic system at the cellular level.

Cell movement through the extracellular membrane is

a pivotal step in many physiologic and pathophysiologic processes. Focal proteolysis of the extracellular components may be accomplished in part by metalloproteinases that are activated primarily by plasmin.[26, 108, 122] Thus, generation of u-PA or t-PA is an important step in cell migration. Although both t-PA and u-PA are plasminogen activators, their cellular function may be different owing to their respective inhibition by PAI. u-PA, for example, is secreted in a single-chain form, which is resistant to inhibition by PAI. u-PA has been found to be a growth stimulant for epidermal tumor cell lines and is mitogenic for malignant renal cells.[61] Its mitogenic potential may have implications in the proliferation of endothelial and smooth muscle cells during both repair of vascular injury and atherogenesis. Receptors for u-PA may allow this protein to be localized on the cell surface in high concentrations at focal points where activation of plasminogen takes place during cell migration. PAI is present on cell surfaces and is uniformly distributed in the cell substratum.[68, 98] This differential distribution may allow focal points of proteolysis on the cell surface with inhibition in the cell substratum, providing a foothold for the migrating cell.

It is evident that the fibrinolytic system has now been identified as playing an increasingly pivotal role in both physiologic and diseased states. With the development of a specific inhibitor, it may well be possible to utilize some of these mechanisms to favor resolution of pathologic processes. These appear to encompass a large variety of pathologic states, well beyond those limited to thromboembolic disorders.

It is now recognized that certain specific thromboembolic disorders are a result of impaired fibrinolysis. Congenital disturbances of the fibrinolytic system associated with DVT and pulmonary embolism have been described. These are generally caused by plasminogen deficiencies, including both dysplasminogenemias and hypoplasminogenemias.[146] The genetic defect responsible for these variants seems to be more common in Japan but is virtually absent among white Americans.[7] In addition, approximately 15% of patients with dysfibrinogenemias appear to have an increased risk of thrombosis. This may also involve impaired fibrinolytic function. The abnormal fibrin formed may not stimulate t-PA–mediated plasminogen activation, or it may not be readily degraded by plasmin.

Lipoprotein-a, also known as Lp(a), is a low-density lipoprotein (LDL)–like protein with apolipoprotein-a. There is a striking homology between apolipoprotein-a and one of the kringles of the plasminogen molecule.[79] It has been postulated that Lp(a) might mediate a prothrombotic function by interfering with the physiologic functions of plasminogen. It competitively inhibits the binding of plasminogen to fibrinogen or fibrin[51, 71] and to plasminogen receptors on endothelial cells.[43, 49, 83] Elevated levels of Lp(a) have been associated with thrombotic disorders.

A relationship between PAI and thrombotic disorders has also been suggested. Experimentally, release of platelet-associated growth factors may decrease fibrinolysis in vivo by increasing endothelial cell synthesis and release of PAI and increasing hepatic secretion of PAI into the circulation.

Impaired fibrinolytic function is the most common biochemical or hemostatic disturbance seen in patients with idiopathic DVT. It has been shown that 30% to 40% of patients with idiopathic DVT have impaired fibrinolytic function.[146] This impairment seems to be related to increased plasma levels of PAI combined with a decreased capacity to release t-PA. It has been postulated that continuous release of t-PA, perhaps induced by increased PAI activity, may lead to depleted endothelial stores of t-PA, thus hampering fibrinolytic response.[50]

Well-established risk factors for coronary heart disease (e.g., cigarette smoking, diabetes, obesity, age, hypertension, and hyperlipoproteinemia) are associated with decreased fibrinolytic activity.[147] There is also a negative association between the intake of vegetables, fruits, and root vegetables and plasma PAI activity.[90] There is a strong relationship between serum triglycerides and PAI levels in plasma.[50, 58, 82] This raises the possibility that hypertriglyceridemia may lead to a predisposition to thrombosis through an increase in PAI concentration.

PAI activity is increased in plasma in the postoperative period. This appears to be part of an acute phase reaction and may be secondary to platelet release of PAI.[42]

Syndrome X, a cluster of hypertriglyceridemia, hypertension, central obesity, and insulin resistance with hyperinsulinemia, has gained interest because of its potential association with impaired fibrinolytic function. PAI activity is increased in plasma, probably as a result of the hyperinsulinemic state.[146] This suggests that insulin may be an added risk factor for coronary heart disease, exerting its effects through modification of other risk factors, including triglyceride-rich lipoproteins and plasma PAI activity

FIBRINOLYTIC AGENTS

Drugs used to activate the fibrinolytic system pharmacologically may be classified as *direct* and *indirect* activators. Indirect activators achieve increased fibrinolytic activity in vivo without acting directly in vitro on plasminogen. These activators include a long list of drugs whose mechanisms of action are variable and have not been elucidated. Chronic enhancement of fibrinolytic activity is theoretically attractive, although of unproven clinical value. Most indirect fibrinolytic drugs lose their effectiveness with time, as with nicotinic acid and adrenalin. Both of these substances cause an abrupt but transient increase in activity by release of endothelial t-PA.

Antidiuretic hormone (ADH) is capable of stimulating the fibrinolytic system at the expense of severe cardiovascular side effects. A more prolonged response may be obtained with desamino-*D*-arginine vasopressin (DDAVP), although this response seems clinically insignificant compared with the procoagulant effects of this agent. Steroids and diguanides (phenformin) have been the most promising of these compounds. Stanozolol, an anabolic steroid, is capable of producing sustained stimulation of the fibrinolytic system for periods of more than 5 years with daily administration.[144]

Evidence of the clinical usefulness of indirect fibrinolytic agents is mostly anecdotal. The long-term benefits of an enhanced fibrinolytic system remain to be established. Increased fibrinolytic activity may occur in patients whose baseline activity is depressed. In other instances, no clinical benefit is observed despite a sustained drug effect. Importantly, fibrinolytic capacity may be decreased by chronic stimulation, thus rendering the system incapable of responding adequately to a thrombotic stimulus.[148] Further investigation is necessary before the value of chronic manipulation of the fibrinolytic system is established.

Direct fibrinolytic agents are capable of converting plasminogen to plasmin, thus exerting their lytic activity through the final common pathway of the fibrinolytic system. They do not have fibrinolytic activity themselves and require plasminogen to exert their lytic action. These direct fibrinolytic activators, of which streptokinase and urokinase are prime examples, achieve their lytic effect to a great extent by overwhelming the circulating plasmin inhibitors and generating an abundance of plasmin (exogenous fibrinolysis).

It is known that thrombus contains plasminogen within its substance. Activation of thrombus-bound plasminogen to plasmin results in local fibrinolysis, and, importantly, this process is partially protected from circulating inhibitors (endogenous fibrinolysis). Thrombolysis without systemic lytic activity can thus be achieved. Investigators are now concentrating on producing agents with a high affinity for thrombus-bound plasminogen with little activation of the circulating proenzyme. t-PA obtained from melanoma cell lines and, more recently, through use of recombinant deoxyribonucleic acid (rDNA) technology has undergone initial clinical and experimental trials with encouraging results.[45, 78, 126] Systemic fibrinolysis still occurs with these agents but to a lesser extent than with streptokinase and urokinase.

Streptokinase

Streptokinase is a *nonenzymatic* protein produced by Lancefield's group C strains of beta-hemolytic streptococci. The fibrinolytic activity of a filtrate of beta-hemolytic streptococci was discovered in 1933 by Tillett and Garner.[125] It initially combines with plasminogen on an equimolar basis (1:1 stoichiometric ratio) to form the activator complex. This streptokinase–plasminogen complex then activates the fibrinolytic mechanism by converting uncomplexed plasminogen to plasmin. As the process evolves, the streptokinase–plasminogen complex is gradually converted to the streptokinase–plasmin form, which can also activate and convert plasminogen. Because this conversion takes place slowly, initial activity is due to the streptokinase–plasminogen complex, whereas later activity is due to the streptokinase–plasmin form. With streptokinase, the supply of fibrin-bound plasminogen may be exhausted by combining it with streptokinase to form the activator complex. As a result, insufficient plasminogen may remain to be activated. Thus, there is a decrease in thrombolytic effect with concentrations of streptokinase above 2500 to 5000 U/ml.[85]

The kinetics of these reactions have been studied mostly in vitro. A more complicated series of reactions occurs in vivo following an infusion of streptokinase. Initially, the drug is neutralized by circulating antistreptococcal antibodies. Any remaining drug combines with circulating plasminogen, forming the activator complex, which converts plasminogen to plasmin. Plasmin combines with excess free streptokinase, is neutralized by circulating antiplasmin, or binds to preformed fibrin. The latter effect produces the desired thrombolytic action. The two half-lives that are detected at 16 and 83 minutes underscore the complexity of these reactions and have a significant effect on the concentration and activity of the drug.

Streptokinase is a foreign protein and therefore is antigenic. Human plasma usually contains antibodies directed against streptokinase that have developed as a result of previous infections with beta-hemolytic streptococci. When streptokinase is infused, an antigen-antibody complex is formed, thus rendering it biochemically inert. Therefore, sufficient amounts of streptokinase must be infused to neutralize the antibodies before fibrinolytic activation is obtained.[57] Minor (and occasionally major) allergic reactions to streptokinase are not uncommon and have been reported at a frequency range of 1.7% to 18%.[110] Serum sickness, with leukocytoclastic vasculitis, is another potential rare complication and is attributed to a delayed hypersensitivity reaction to the foreign protein streptokinase.[130]

Urokinase

Urokinase is a direct activator that is capable of initiating fibrinolysis without forming an activator complex. It is a trypsin-like serine protease that was originally isolated from human urine by MacFarlane and Pilling in 1946.[74] In 1967, urokinase was successfully isolated from tissue cultures of human embryonic kidney cells.[14] Urokinase is nonantigenic, and its pyrogenicity is low. Urokinase requires an initial high loading dose, and, like streptokinase, it possesses little specific affinity for fibrin[78] and therefore does not discriminate between circulating plasminogen and fibrin-bound plasminogen.

Urokinase cleaves plasminogen (its only known protein substrate) by first-order reaction kinetics to plasmin. Its pH and temperature are relatively stable. No neutralizing antibodies are present, and its direct mechanism of action allows for a better dose-response relationship compared with streptokinase. Urokinase does not contain lysine-binding sites, which explains its lack of affinity for fibrin.[69] Receptors for urokinase have been demonstrated in several cell types, as mentioned earlier, and these are postulated as a mechanism for cellular movement in the extracellular matrix.

Activation of plasminogen by urokinase occurs through proteolysis. On intravenous administration, urokinase is rapidly removed from the circulation via hepatic clearance. The half-life of urokinase in humans is about 14 minutes. Urokinase also reacts with other proteins, including fibrinogen. The Lys form of plasminogen is much more readily cleaved by urokinase, and this activation may be enhanced by the presence of fibrin.[145]

Laboratory findings in patients receiving urokinase have shown a lesser fibrinogenolytic response than streptokinase,[81] although results in clinical practice have paralleled those of streptokinase. A decreased incidence of bleeding complications has been suggested by several investigators and may be explained by a reduction in plasminemia.[13, 121, 138]

Tissue Plasminogen Activator

t-PA, a serine protease present in most body tissues,[3, 8] can cause in vivo activation of the fibrinolytic system. It is similar in nature to plasminogen activator produced by human vascular endothelial cells.[1, 16] t-PA is a poor enzyme in the absence of fibrin, but the presence of fibrin strikingly enhances the activation rate of plasminogen by t-PA. The high affinity of t-PA for plasminogen in the presence of fibrin allows efficient activation on the fibrin clot without significant conversion by t-PA of plasminogen in circulating plasma.[100, 101] Under normal physiologic conditions, fibrin-bound t-PA activates the conversion of fibrin-bound plasminogen to plasmin. The plasmin thus formed on the fibrin surface rapidly induces thrombolysis. t-PA circulating in the blood has a low affinity for circulating plasminogen; therefore, plasmin is not formed in the circulation. Circulating alpha$_2$-antiplasmin is not consumed, fibrinogen is not degraded, and a systemic lytic state is avoided.

Although t-PA was identified in the 1940s, its isolation and purification proceeded slowly until the 1980s, when it became possible to extract it from uterine tissue. Subsequently, the Bowes melanoma cell line was found to secrete a plasminogen activator similar to human uterine t-PA.[22] Through the use of recombinant DNA technology, the human t-PA gene has been cloned. The recombinant human tissue-type plasminogen activator (rt-PA) appears to be biologically identical to plasminogen activator derived from the melanoma cell line.

t-PA is a direct plasminogen activator. Commercially available rt-PA (alteplase) is a combination of two types of t-PA. A single-chain form is cleaved by plasminogen to yield two-chain t-PA. Both the one-chain and two-chain forms of t-PA are comparable in activity, the one-chain activator being quickly converted to the two-chain type as lysis proceeds. The half-life of t-PA has been estimated at between 4 and 7 minutes in vivo.[111]

Because it is a fibrin-selective agent, most of the thrombolytic effect of t-PA is secondary to fibrin-bound plasminogen converted to plasmin, although the importance of a fresh supply of plasminogen to maintain the fibrin-bound plasminogen pool has been emphasized. Experimental studies suggest that clot lysis induced by activation of plasminogen is dependent on clot-associated plasminogen, which in turn depends on the concentration of plasminogen in plasma. Depletion of both contributes to a lower frequency and rapidity of recanalization, which is more noticeable with nonfibrin-selective agents compared with fibrin-selective agents, probably as the result of depletion of plasminogen induced by nonselective agents.[128]

Despite a milder hemostatic defect demonstrated by laboratory evaluation and the theoretical benefit of being a fibrin-selective agent, systemic bleeding complications in clinical trials of t-PA have been similar to those seen with other lytic agents.[126] Determining the optimum dosage and administering t-PA continue to be refined, with bolus infusion of t-PA suggested as a method of decreasing bleeding complications.

t-PA may also bind and be activated on platelet surfaces through binding to platelet receptors. The action of t-PA on platelet surfaces may lead to rapid cleavage of GPIb and loss of platelet binding to von Willebrand's factor. This may explain why concentrations of t-PA achieved early in therapy may inhibit platelet aggregation.

Results of the limited experience available with the use of rt-PA in patients with peripheral vascular occlusions have suggested the occurrence of fewer systemic complications with increased effectiveness of therapy and decreased infusion times. Several controlled randomized trials of t-PA compared with other fibrinolytic agents in the acute phase of myocardial infarction have suggested a slight but important increase in intracranial bleeding. The incidence appears to be increased in patients who have been receiving oral anticoagulants prior to therapy, patients weighing less than 70 kg, and patients older than 65 years of age.[27]

Acylated Streptokinase–Plasminogen Complex

Attempts to produce fibrin-specific agents have led to derivatives of streptokinase that change not only its biologic activity but also the duration of such activity. *p*-Anisoylated human plasminogen–streptokinase activator complex (APSAC) is the most studied and the most frequently used derivative of streptokinase. It is an acylated complex of streptokinase with human Lys-plasminogen. Acylation of the catalytic site of the plasminogen molecule delays the formation of the active fibrinolytic enzyme plasmin but leaves the lysine-binding sites necessary to bind the complex to fibrin. Acylation also prevents activation of circulating plasminogen by streptokinase, delaying such activation for the interval necessary for the complex to bind to fibrin. Deacylation of the molecule then leads to activation of the streptokinase moiety, a large percentage of the drug being bound to fibrin at the time of deacylation. Any deacylation occurring in the circulation is rapidly deactivated by antiplasmins.[84]

The potency of APSAC has been found to be 10 times that of streptokinase in vivo. This increased activity is dependent on both fibrin binding and the deacylation process. The half-life of APSAC is about 105 minutes. This prolonged half-life is desirable in patients with acute myocardial infarction and, combined with its increased fibrin selectivity, is a welcomed improvement over the parent drug, streptokinase. It shares, however, the same side effects characteristic of streptokinase because antistreptococcal antibodies have a significant inhibitory effect on APSAC. Antibodies form in patients given APSAC, and therefore re-treatment with either the parent drug (streptokinase) or APSAC should not be instituted within 6 months.

The prolonged half-life of APSAC may be a disadvantage in patients needing regional infusion. In patients with peripheral vascular disease, the possibility of having to proceed with surgical intervention shortly after failed fibrinolytic therapy is an important consideration in the selection of the appropriate lytic agent. Thus, shorter-acting drugs may be preferable in the treatment of arterial thrombosis.

Plasmin B-Chain–Streptokinase Complex

When the smallest derivative of plasmin that retains enzymatic activity (plasmin B-chain) is utilized, another derivative of streptokinase is produced, known as the *plasmin B-chain–streptokinase complex*. The half-life of this preparation is estimated at 4.5 hours, which is prolonged compared with that of streptokinase. Its efficiency in lysing fibrin is four times that of streptokinase, its activity falling somewhere between that of streptokinase and that of urokinase.[117] This complex may have certain advantages over streptokinase because of its prolonged half-life and its increased affinity for fibrin-bound plasminogen. Its advantages over other available lytic agents, such as u-PA or t-PA, must await clinical trials.

Pro-Urokinase

Different molecular weight forms of urokinase with variable activity are recognized. A single-chain form of urokinase of about 55,000 daltons was isolated by Husain and colleagues in 1983.[55] It has superior fibrin specificity and lytic activity compared with urokinase.

Pro-urokinase is highly effective in the conversion of Lys-plasminogen to plasmin. It has little or no activity in the conversion of Glu-plasminogen to plasmin. High concentrations of Lys-plasminogen are present in thrombus, which gives pro-urokinase fibrin-specific properties. Plasminogen that has been absorbed in thrombus changes its configuration to a pseudo-Lys form that is also attacked by pro-urokinase, converting it to Lys-plasmin. Circulating pro-urokinase is stable in plasma because of its resistance to plasma inhibitors and ionized calcium.[93]

Pro-urokinase has a prolonged half-life that, in some instances, has been estimated to be several days.[47] Such a prolonged half-life may have disadvantages in clinical situations in which patients may require surgery shortly after unsuccessful lytic therapy. Furthermore, in vitro studies have failed to demonstrate a benefit of pro-urokinase to urokinase with respect to thrombolytic activity.[151] Further clinical studies must be conducted to evaluate whether the fibrin specificity of pro-urokinase translates to a clinical advantage.

Immunofibrinolysis

In an attempt to develop fibrin-specific agents, investigators have bonded monoclonal antifibrin antibodies to urokinase or streptokinase, rendering these agents fibrin selective. A marked increase in in vitro fibrinolysis has been demonstrated compared with unmodified drug. These monoclonal antibodies do not appear to cross-react with fibrinogen, which may explain the enhanced activity.[15] Repeated therapy, however, would require different monoclonal antibodies to avoid adverse immunologic reactions. The clinical applicability of these agents remains to be determined.

t-PA Mutants

In the attempt to produce lytic agents that are more effective with a decreased potential for bleeding complications, the native t-PA molecule has been modified. One such modification is *reteplase*, a third-generation t-PA mutant produced with recombinant technology. Compared with t-PA, reteplase has improved clot penetration, a longer half-life, and a faster initiation of thrombolysis.[152] Other t-PA mutants have been developed to alter the regulatory interaction with PAI-1. Changing amino acids in a specific area of t-PA decreases the rate of inhibition by PAI-1 and thus leads to a longer half-life.[153] The use of these and other t-PA mutants may play a significant role in coronary thromboses. Any role that these t-PA mutants may play in peripheral thromboses remains to be seen.

THROMBOLYTIC (FIBRINOLYTIC) THERAPY

Guidelines

Generally, two clinical approaches are used in modern practice for the administration of lytic agents: systemic and regional. *Systemic* lytic therapy involves intravenous administration of the drug, the goal being establishment of a systemic lytic state capable of dissolving fibrin wherever deposited. *Regional* administration of thrombolytic agents appears to enhance effectiveness of some agents and to decrease systemic complications by local targeted instillation. This is accomplished by catheter-directed administration into the thrombotic material.

Systemic thrombolytic therapy has been used to treat peripheral arterial occlusions, but results have been disappointing owing to a significant incidence of bleeding complications. Today, systemic therapy is usually used for venous thromboembolic states. Regional intravascular infusion of the lytic agent avoids some of the systemic complications and is largely used for peripheral arterial thromboses and graft occlusions. Occasionally, localized venous thrombotic disorders, such as axillosubclavian vein thrombosis, may be treated by local intravenous instillation of the lytic agent. Collateral pathways rapidly develop following venous thrombosis, making local infusion less advantageous, and systemic therapy remains the delivery method of choice for the treatment of infrainguinal deep venous thrombosis and pulmonary embolism.

Patient selection is important in order to obtain favorable results with either systemic or regional thrombolytic therapy. The following topics include guidelines for selecting patients for lytic therapy, administering and monitoring therapy, and dealing with complications as well as some perspective on the expected outcomes. Most of the available clinical experience has been with streptokinase and urokinase, and the discussion thus emphasizes these two agents. Experience with t-PA is also presented, emphasizing its differences from streptokinase and urokinase.

The principles of systemic and regional fibrinolytic therapy are discussed separately. The reader should remember that complications and side effects may be similar, regardless of the method of administration, because of the systemic effects that may be seen, even with regional administration. The discussion is limited to general principles of both systemic and regional thrombolytic therapy for the treatment of venous and peripheral arterial occlusions. Thrombolytic treatment of acute coronary thromboses and acute stroke is specifically omitted. (For more details, see specific chapters covering the various clinical entities for which thrombolytic therapy may be recommended.)

Systemic Thrombolytic Therapy

Patient Selection

The goal of systemic thrombolytic therapy is to establish a systemic lytic state characterized by a prolongation of the thrombin time (twice normal) and the presence of detectable fibrin degradation products. During a systemic lytic state, fibrin is degraded wherever it has been deposited throughout the body. Hemostatic plugs are as vulnerable to lysis as the clot and thrombus for which therapy has been initiated. Selection of patients for systemic lytic therapy is based on the documented presence of an accepted indication and the absence of absolute contraindications (Table 28–1).

Careful evaluation for the presence of contraindications to systemic lytic therapy is of paramount importance in avoiding serious bleeding complications. Contraindications to systemic thrombolytic therapy[88] are listed in Table 28–1. *Absolute* contraindications include (1) active internal bleeding and (2) recent (within 2 months) cerebrovascular accident or other intracranial pathology. *Relative* major contraindications include (1) left heart thrombus, (2) recent (<10 days) major surgery, (3) trauma, (4) obstetric delivery, (5) organ biopsy or puncture of a noncompressible vessel, (6) recent gastrointestinal bleeding, and (7) severe uncontrolled hypertension. In these circumstances, patients are at a significant risk for peripheral embolization or bleeding, and thus the indication for thrombolytic therapy must be carefully weighed against the hazards of bleeding. The use of systemic thrombolytic therapy under these circumstances should essentially be reserved for life-threatening pulmonary emboli.

Relative minor contraindications carry a higher risk of complications, but the benefits of therapy may still outweigh the hazards. Peripheral embolization from a central source is a potential hazard of systemic lytic therapy. Therefore, valvular heart disease or atrial fibrillation without demonstrable left heart thrombus on echocardiography and a previous history of emboli represents a minor contraindication to systemic lytic therapy. Severe liver disease delays metabolism of the drug and, in addition, may compound a preexisting coagulopathy. This makes the response to thrombolytic drug infusion less predictable.

TABLE 28–1. CONTRAINDICATIONS FOR SYSTEMIC LYTIC THERAPY

Absolute
Active internal bleeding
Recent (<2 mo) cerebrovascular accident
Intracranial pathology
Relative: Major
Recent (<10 days) major surgery, obstetric delivery, or organ biopsy
Left heart thrombus
Active peptic ulcer or gastrointestinal pathology
Recent major trauma
Uncontrolled hypertension
Relative: Minor
Minor surgery or trauma
Recent cardiopulmonary resuscitation
Atrial fibrillation with mitral valve disease
Bacterial endocarditis
Hemostatic defects (e.g., renal or liver disease)
Diabetic hemorrhagic retinopathy
Pregnancy
Contraindications for Streptokinase
Known allergy
Recent streptococcal infection
Previous therapy within 6 mo

Data from NIH [National Institutes of Health] Consensus Development Conference: Thrombolytic therapy in treatment. Ann Intern Med 93:141, 1980.

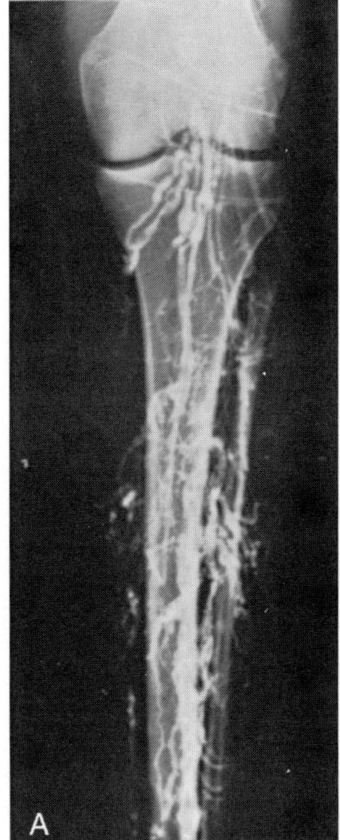

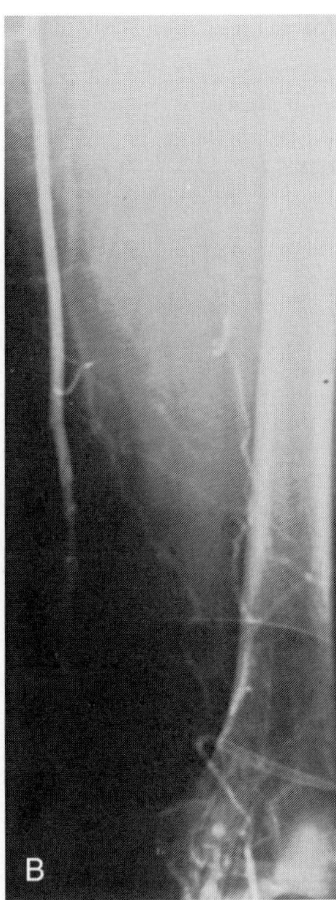

FIGURE 28–2. Phlegmasia cerulea of the left lower extremity in a 57-year-old woman. Venogram after streptokinase therapy. *A*, Incomplete clearance of calf thrombi. *B*, Persistent occlusion of the deep femoral system. The superficial system is patent. This treatment was sufficient to achieve limb salvage (see text).

During pregnancy, a systemic lytic state may precipitate abruptio placentae or may lead to hypofibrinogenemia in the fetus with an increased risk of bleeding. Antistreptococcal antibodies can neutralize streptokinase, blocking the formation of the activator complex. For these reasons, streptokinase is specifically contraindicated in patients with recent streptococcal infection, previous streptokinase therapy within 6 months, known allergy to streptokinase, or high titers of antistreptococcal antibodies. In these situations, urokinase is the agent of choice.

Systemic administration of thrombolytic agents in current clinical practice is usually limited to the management of DVT (Fig. 28–2) or pulmonary embolism. (See chapters that deal specifically with these entities.) Doses of the three agents more commonly used for this purpose are shown in Table 28–2.

Systemic administration of fibrinolytic drugs creates a significant hemostatic defect. Thus, patients should be monitored appropriately and invasive procedures should be avoided. Intramuscular injections are contraindicated. Fibrinogen levels are usually monitored not only to document the presence of a systemic lytic state but also to alert the clinician of levels that may predispose the patient to significant bleeding. Although fibrinogen levels do not correlate precisely with the risk of bleeding, bleeding more frequently occurs when fibrinogen levels fall below 100 mg/dl.

In view of the significant contraindications to lytic ther-

TABLE 28–2. SYSTEMIC ADMINISTRATION OF COMMON THROMBOLYTIC AGENTS

	DOSE	
DRUG	**Systemic**	**Regional**
Streptokinase	250,000 U IV/30 min 100,000 U IV/hr	5000–10,000 U/hr
Urokinase	4400 U/kg/10 min 4400 U/kg/hr	1000–4000 U/min
Tissue-type plasminogen activator	40–50 mg IV/2 hr	0.05–0.1 mg/kg/hr

apy frequently encountered in patients presenting with DVT or pulmonary embolism, the impact of lytic therapy in the management of these patients is limited. Documentation of the diagnosis is essential before thrombolytic therapy is initiated for either DVT or pulmonary embolism. Noninvasive studies during therapy are useful. Patients with severe cardiopulmonary compromise are the most appropriate candidates for thrombolytic therapy. The duration of therapy is best guided by the clinical response, and noninvasive studies with repeated invasive angiographic studies are best reserved to evaluate the final outcome. As a rule, if no improvement is seen within 24 hours, it may be best to either discontinue therapy or use an alternative agent.

Method

The goal of intravenous administration of thrombolytic agents is to establish a lytic state. This is evidenced by prolongation of the thrombin time or partial thromboplastin time (PTT) and by the presence of fibrin degradation products. Once the diagnosis is objectively established and the patient is thought to be a suitable candidate for lytic therapy, informed consent should be obtained. Pretreatment fibrinogen level, thrombin time, prothrombin time, PTT, hematocrit, and platelet count should be obtained. If heparin is being administered, it is discontinued.

The thrombolytic agent is then given intravenously with a loading dose (urokinase 4400 U/kg given over 10 minutes or streptokinase 250,000 U given over 30 minutes) aimed at establishing a lytic state rapidly. These doses have been estimated to establish such a state in approximately 95% of patients. The lytic state is then maintained by a continuous infusion of the agent (urokinase, 4400 U/kg/hr, or streptokinase, 100,000 U/hr). When streptokinase is chosen, we prefer to administer 100 mg of hydrocortisone prior to initiation of therapy to prevent or decrease some of the allergic reactions that may occur.

Invasive procedures, intramuscular injections, and cutdowns should be avoided. When arterial blood gas determinations are needed, they should be obtained from the wrist, followed by at least a 20-minute compression of the artery. Puncture of noncompressible arteries is contraindicated.

Three to 4 hours after the infusion is started, thrombin time (or PTT if thrombin time is not available), fibrinogen level, and fibrin degradation products are obtained. These measurements document the presence of a systemic lytic state. A drop in the fibrinogen level is to be expected and, in the absence of bleeding complications, is accepted. However, the hematocrit should be observed every 6 hours. If a lytic state is not seen after the initial 4 hours, another bolus dose is given and the hourly dose is increased. Alternatively, if streptokinase has been used, a change to urokinase may be advisable.

After completion of therapy, anticoagulants should be started 2 to 3 hours after discontinuation of the lytic agent. No heparin loading dose is necessary and should be avoided. Warfarin therapy should follow in a conventional manner.

Complications of Systemic Lytic Therapy

Clearly, bleeding is the most feared and frequent complication of systemic thrombolytic therapy. The incidence of major bleeding (requiring discontinuation of therapy or blood transfusions) has been estimated at between 7% and 45%.[30, 87] The number and type of invasive procedures and the duration of therapy appear to influence significantly the incidence of bleeding complications. Superficial bleeding at invaded sites is easily controlled with pressure. Avoidance of unnecessary procedures with preservation of an intact vascular system is the best preventive measure.

Internal bleeding, evidenced by an unexplained reduction in hematocrit, is usually localized to the gastrointestinal tract. This may be the result of poor patient selection or unknown risk factors. Intracranial bleeding is the most serious hemorrhagic complication. As a rule, any change in the neurologic status of a patient receiving thrombolytic therapy should be considered an intracranial bleed until proved otherwise. The infusion should be discontinued immediately and appropriate diagnostic and therapeutic measures instituted. Reversal of the lytic state by rapid administration of fresh frozen plasma or cryoprecipitate is advisable. Administration of ϵ-aminocaproic acid (plasmin inhibitor) is *not* recommended and carries a significant risk of aggravating the process for which lytic therapy was instituted. Increasing the dose of streptokinase to decrease its proteolytic effect is theoretically correct but has been abandoned as a clinical option.

Superficial bleeding, which can be controlled by local measures, can be tolerated in the final stages of therapy. If it occurs at the beginning of therapy or if bleeding is significant enough to require transfusion, the drug should be discontinued and the systemic lytic state reversed.

Bleeding can occur during the lag period between the termination of lytic therapy and the administration of anticoagulant.[30, 34] Thus, it is advisable to delay heparin administration until the thrombin time or the PTT is less than twice normal, and heparin should be initiated without a loading dose. It is unclear why bleeding might occur with urokinase. With streptokinase, however, as plasma levels of the drug decrease, more plasminogen is available for activation of the already formed streptokinase-plasminogen complex.

Intermittent administration of the lytic agent, allowing for plasminogen repletion, has been advocated by some investigators but is cumbersome and has not been shown to improve the results of continuous administration.

Generally, laboratory parameters correlate poorly with the risk of bleeding. However, extremely low fibrinogen levels (<20% of baseline) in the presence of an otherwise minor bleeding complication increase the chance of significant bleeding enough to require cessation of therapy. An alternative, in these instances, is to discontinue the drug, correct the coagulopathy, and restart the infusion several hours later.

Pulmonary embolism can occur during treatment for DVT; however, its occurrence may be more frequent than with conventional heparin therapy. In the absence of bleeding complications, continuation of therapy appears advisable. If recurrent emboli are observed, discontinuation of the fibrinolytic agent, heparin administration, and insertion of a caval filter may be life-saving.

Serious allergic reactions can occur rarely with streptokinase, but they are extremely rare with urokinase. However, febrile allergic reactions can occur in up to 30% of patients receiving streptokinase and have been increasingly recognized in patients receiving urokinase. These allergic reactions are well tolerated and generally are of no clinical consequence; however, if a serious allergic reaction is evident, immediate discontinuation of the drug is mandatory. Pretreatment of patients with antihistamines, steroids, or meperidine usually prevents allergic and pyretic side effects.

Regional Thrombolytic Therapy

Systemic thrombolytic therapy has been utilized for the treatment of thrombosis and emboli in the arterial tree. It is effective in acute arterial thromboses that have been present for less than 10 days.[110] The results of intravenous infusion of thrombolytic agents in patients with chronic arterial thrombotic occlusions have not been encouraging.[97, 142] Martin, using a titrated loading dose of streptokinase and a 72-hour infusion of 100,000 U/hr, reported successful treatment in only 8.9% of patients with chronic femoral occlusions, 19.5% of those with chronic iliac occlusions, and 24.4% of those with chronic aortic occlusions.[77] Enthusiasm for this approach was further dampened by the high incidence of hemorrhagic complications.

In an attempt to circumvent the hemorrhagic problems, Dotter and coworkers[29] proposed the administration of low-dose thrombolytic therapy through an angiographically placed intra-arterial catheter. The purpose of this technique was to increase the rate of fibrinolysis and decrease the systemic effect and its associated complications. Katzen and Van Breda[60] and others have evaluated and recommended this regimen. Presently, the indications for regional thrombolytic therapy include thrombosis following percutaneous angioplasty, native or graft occlusion, arteriovenous fistula thrombosis, and perhaps visceral ischemia secondary to native vessel thrombosis.

The contraindications to regional thrombolytic therapy are similar to those for systemic therapy (Table 28–1). In addition, intolerable ischemia with neurologic impairment should be viewed as an absolute contraindication to regional thrombolytic therapy because prompt revascularization is needed to prevent further neurologic deterioration.

In the standard technique, a No. 5 French angiographic catheter is advanced so that its tip is near or just within the thrombus. Streptokinase, usually in a dose of 5000 to 8000 U/hr, or urokinase in a dose of 1000 to 4000 U/min, is then infused. Patients are restudied at varying intervals of 6 to 12 hours. Treatment times vary from 1 to 48 hours, with occasional patients requiring longer infusion times. The concomitant use of heparin is controversial but is often used to avoid pericatheter thrombosis (Fig. 28–3).

The results of several early series are summarized in Table 28–3. Despite localized infusion, systemic fibrinolysis occurs within 12 to 24 hours with degradation of fibrinogen, plasminogen, factor V, and factor VIII. Major or minor complications have occurred in 15% to 30% of patients in most series.[85] If the catheter does not properly penetrate the thrombus, lysis is slowed and inefficient because the lytic agent is "washed out" through collateral vessels, the fibrinolytic effect is the result of the systemic lytic state.

McNamara and Fischer,[80] using a high-dose intra-arterial urokinase regimen, reported complete clot lysis in 75% of patients. The method involves making a passageway through the clot with a guide wire or catheter and then instilling urokinase at 4000 U/min for 2 hours. If patency is restored, the catheter is withdrawn proximal to the remaining clot and the urokinase is infused at 1000 to 2000 U/min until complete lysis is accomplished. With this technique, the mean infusion time was 18 hours and the incidence of bleeding complications was low even with the use of heparin to prevent pericatheter thrombosis. The higher cost of urokinase in relation to streptokinase can be justified on the basis of the shorter infusion time and fewer bleeding complications.

In general, with both the low-dose regimen and the high-dose urokinase regimen, the likelihood of serious bleeding increases if the fibrinogen dose is decreased to less than 100 mg/dl.[80, 129] When heparin is used with low-dose streptokinase, the PTT should be limited to two times normal.[11, 85] With the shorter duration, high-dose urokinase technique, a PTT of three to five times normal prevented new thrombus formation effectively without increased risk of bleeding. Most applications of regional thrombolytic therapy have been in the management of extremity arterial disease.[62]

Acute thrombosis occurring immediately following percutaneous transluminal angioplasty usually is a result of fresh thrombi. These thrombi respond well to thrombolytic therapy, and the success rate for treatment is high in this situation.[75, 129, 137]

Local low-dose streptokinase or urokinase thrombolytic therapy has also been used successfully in the treatment of occluded grafts (Fig. 28–4).[11] The catheter tip should be inserted into the clot or as close to it as possible. With the catheter in such a position, there are no collaterals to bypass the occlusion: thus all of the fibrinolytic agent is directed into the thrombus. Becker and coworkers[11] reported complete lysis in 71% of grafts, Van Breda and associates[139] in 60%, and Gardiner and colleagues in 59%.[40] Perler and associates[95] obtained successful lyses in only 3 of 10 (33%) patients. Concomitant heparin was used sporadically in the Perler and associates[95] series. In the series reported by McNamara and Fischer,[80] one third of the thrombotic occlusions treated were graft thrombi.

Thrombolytic agents may dissolve fibrin in the interstices of knitted Dacron or, less commonly, polytetrafluoroethylene grafts.[99, 104, 139] This can lead to perigraft extravasation, which does not usually cause significant symptoms[99] but may result in marked bleeding.[139]

Acute and subacute hand ischemia resulting from thromboembolic events has also been treated successfully with

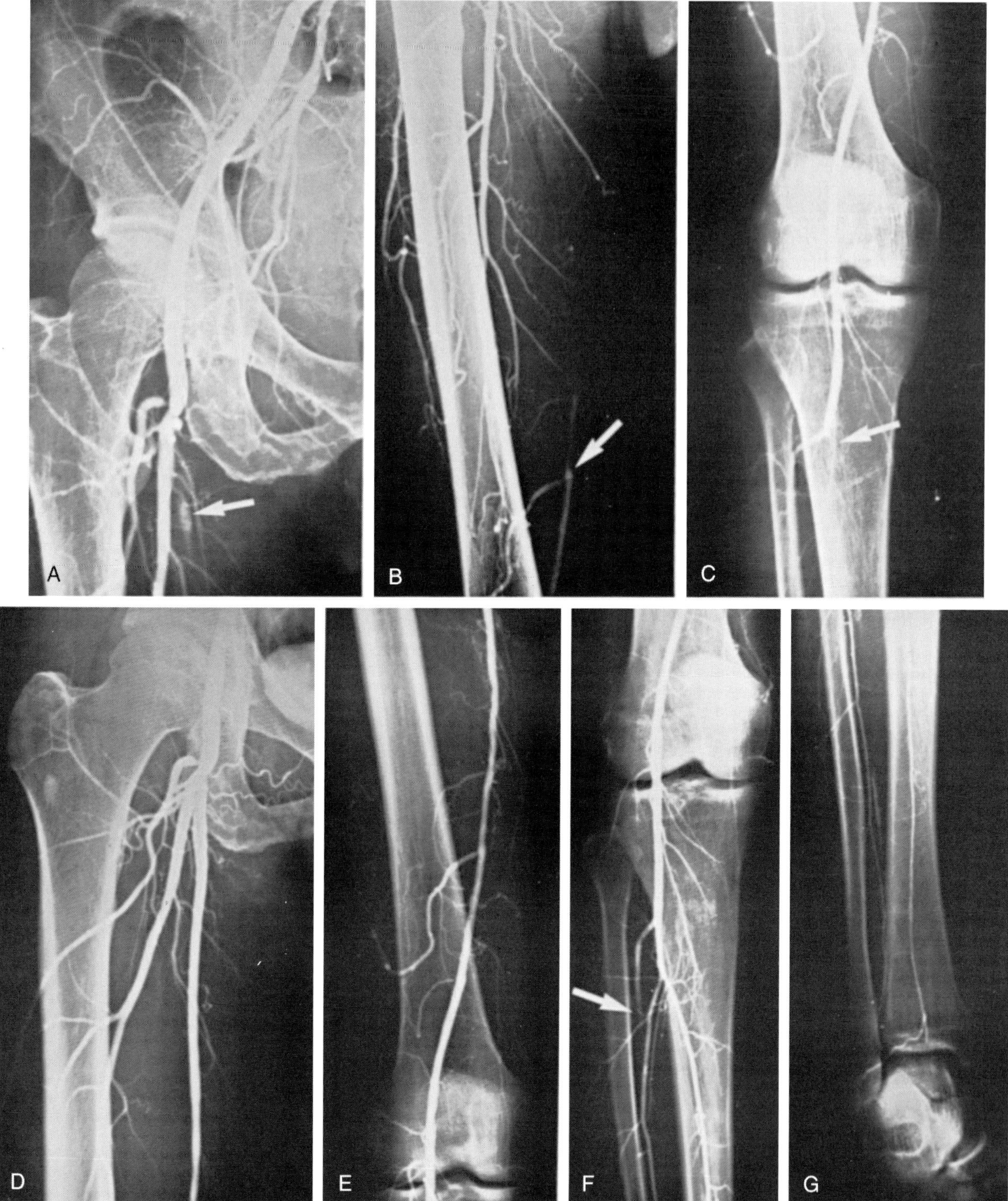

FIGURE 28–3. The patient is a 54-year-old man who was admitted to the hospital with rest pain and ischemic changes in his right foot and a history suggestive of embolic episodes. An aortogram showed moderate atherosclerotic changes. Runoff study shows the following. *A*, Occlusion of the right superficial femoral artery (SFA) at its origin with delayed filling of a short interrupted segment of the right SFA proximally (*arrow*). *B*, The right SFA reconstitutes at the adductor hiatus (*arrow*). *C*, There is abrupt occlusion of the tibioperoneal trunk proximally, suggesting embolic occlusion (*arrow*). The anterior tibial artery terminated abruptly in the mid-calf. A catheter was advanced to the level of the thrombus, and low-dose intra-arterial streptokinase infusion was started. After 24 hours of therapy, the right SFA and tibioperoneal trunk were patent; however, there was evidence of extensive thrombus sheathing in the infusion catheter proximally. Despite the presence of fever, the streptokinase infusion was increased to systemic doses for 16 additional hours, at which time major bleeding developed from the catheter entry site, with a drop in hematocrit necessitating transfusion and cessation of lytic therapy. An arteriogram was performed at cessation of thrombolytic therapy. Recanalization of the right SFA (*D*) and patency of the popliteal artery (*E*). *F*, The tibioperoneal trunk is patent. The anterior tibial artery remained occluded proximally (*arrow*). *G*, In the calf, the posterior tibial and peroneal arteries are patent to the ankle. A short, interrupted segment of the anterior tibial artery is seen in the mid-calf. One week later, the patient underwent an aortoiliac bypass to remove the site of embolism and subsequently did well.

TABLE 28–3. RESULTS OF THROMBOLYTIC THERAPY

REFERENCE	TOTAL NO. INFUSIONS	COMPLETE LYSIS (%)	DURATION INFUSION (HR)	MAJOR BLEEDING (%)
Low-Dose Streptokinase				
Dotter[29]	17	35	71	24
Katzen[60]	12	92	7	17
Totty[129]	19	38	44	19
Becker[11]	57	47	—*	12
Mori[85]	50	44	38	8
High-Dose Urokinase				
McNamara[80]	93	83	18	4

*Duration of infusion not reported.

low-dose intra-arterial regional thrombolytic therapy. Favorable results were reported in 9 of 10 patients in one series.[127] Becker and coworkers[11] reported successful thrombolysis in 71% of patients with renal dialysis shunts but in none of five patients with fistulae. The better results with shunts were attributed to the lack of collateral pathways through which fibrinolytic therapy is washed away.

Occlusions of the celiac, superior mesenteric, and renal arteries have also been successfully treated with intra-arterial fibrinolytic therapy.[36, 96, 150] The technique has not gained widespread use because the poor tolerance of these organs to ischemia imposes time limitations, and changes in their circulatory status cannot be easily monitored. When fibrinolytic therapy is used, frequent angiographic surveillance of clot dissolution is required because clinical parameters alone are unreliable in detecting worsening visceral ischemia.

Because a systemic lytic state may occur with prolonged regional intravascular thrombolytic therapy, patient selection is guided by criteria similar to those used for systemic therapy. *Absolute* contraindications include (1) active internal bleeding, (2) recent surgery or trauma to the area to be perfused, (3) recent cerebrovascular accident, and (4) documented left heart thrombus. *Relative* contraindications include (1) recent surgery, (2) gastrointestinal bleeding or trauma, (3) severe hypertension, (4) mitral valve disease, (5) endocarditis, (6) hemostatic defects, (7) and pregnancy.[129] Patients who have had recent vascular surgery can be treated in the postoperative setting[18]; however, because of perigraft extravasation, Dacron graft occlusions should not be treated in the early postoperative period (less than 4 to 6 weeks).[118, 139]

In addition, and of particular importance, thrombolysis should *not* be attempted in any patient whose ischemia has been of sufficient severity or duration to cause severe motor or sensory impairment or in patients whose ischemia cannot be tolerated for the anticipated duration of the infusion. Serious sequelae and high mortality, similar to those associated with operative revascularization of a limb with advanced ischemia, can also occur with thrombolytic therapy.[80, 85]

It was initially thought that thrombotic occlusions more than 1 to 2 weeks old were unlikely to respond to thrombolytic therapy. However, intrathrombotic injections of streptokinase or urokinase can bring about complete fibrinolysis in occlusions up to several years old. Lammer and coworkers[65] reported success in 75% of 47 patients with chronic occlusions. Still, earlier thrombi are more sensitive to lysis, as evidenced by the experience with postangioplasty thrombosis.

There is no consensus regarding laboratory monitoring during local thrombolytic therapy. The therapeutic effect of regional thrombolytic therapy is most accurately determined by serial angiography.[62] Hemorrhagic complications occur primarily at sites of vascular cannulation as a result of lysis of hemostatic thrombi but cannot be correlated or predicted from specific laboratory values. Bleeding complications are usually associated with increasing duration of therapy rather than with the dose of the agent. Baseline studies to identify existing hemostatic defects should be performed. These include hemoglobin, hematocrit, platelet count, PTT, prothrombin time, bleeding time, serum fibrinogen level, and fibrin degradation products. During therapy, in order of decreasing value, the fibrinogen level, thrombin time, fibrinogen degradation products, and PTT may be monitored at intervals. If heparin is used, the thrombin time is inaccurate and the PTT may be used to determine heparin dose.[62] Although hematologic monitoring cannot regularly predict the safety or efficacy of thrombolytic infusion, a low fibrinogen level (i.e., $<$100 mg/dl) correlates sufficiently well with the occurrence of bleeding complications that it should not be ignored, even if there is no evidence of active bleeding.

Local thrombolytic therapy with streptokinase or urokinase has several major drawbacks:

1. It does not always result in complete lysis.
2. There is no predictor of successful infusion.
3. It is not possible to predict how long an infusion may be necessary to restore patency.

Ease of passage of the guide wire through the occlusion remains the best predictor of potential success.

The approach chosen for access to the arterial system needs to maximize access to the occluding segment and minimize morbidity. Arterial punctures distal to the presumed occlusion and sites where bleeding may cause serious morbidity (e.g., the axillary or translumbar approach), should be avoided. Contralateral puncture with the catheter passed around the aortic bifurcation is preferred and is associated with a lower risk of complications compared with antegrade ipsilateral puncture. Occlusions distal to the mid-superficial femoral artery may be approached with an antegrade ipsilateral puncture. Infusions into the upper extremity or aortic branches are best carried out through a

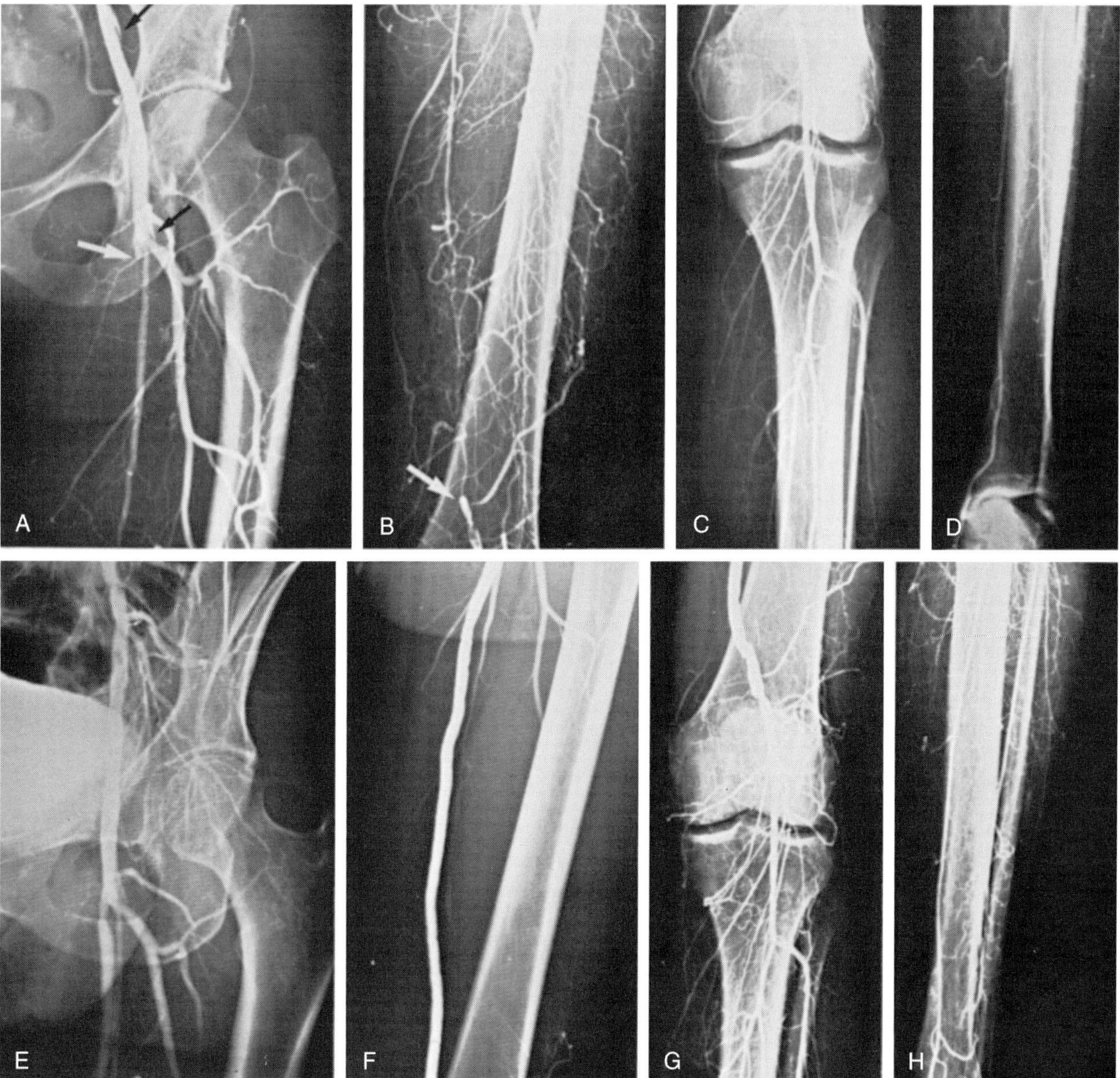

FIGURE 28–4. The patient is a 56-year-old woman who had recently undergone thrombectomy of her femoropopliteal bypass graft and returned with recurrent ischemic symptoms in the left lower extremity. *A*, An arteriogram shows complete occlusion of the graft at its proximal anastomosis (*white arrow*). Also noted is an incidental post-thrombectomy dissection of the left common femoral artery (*black arrows*). *B*, The left superficial femoral artery is occluded in the mid-thigh. Multiple collaterals reconstitute the proximal popliteal artery, which contains a thrombus (*arrow*). *C*, The distal popliteal artery is patent as is the anterior tibial artery and the tibioperoneal trunk. A small thrombus is seen in the tibioperoneal trunk. *D*, Three-vessel runoff is present in the lower leg. The catheter was advanced to the level of the graft and urokinase infusion was instituted at 4000 U/min for several hours followed by 1000 U/min with concomitant low-dose heparin. Total infusion time was 19 hours. The postinfusion arteriogram shows that the graft is patent proximally (*E*). Residual postoperative narrowing is seen at the proximal anastomosis. *F*, The graft is widely patent in the thigh. *G*, The distal graft anastomosis is recanalized, and the previously seen thrombus in the popliteal artery is lysed. *H*, Three-vessel runoff to the ankle is present. No hemorrhagic complications occurred, and the patient did well.

transfemoral approach. End-hole catheters are usually used for infusion with the tip embedded in the thrombus. Multiple-hole catheters are preferred for longer occlusions.

The dosage chosen depends largely on the length and volume of the thrombus and on the location and clinical importance of the vascular territory. Small-volume, short thrombi in important territories (e.g., renal) are best treated with high-dose infusions aimed at rapid resolution. Creation of a channel into the thrombus with the angiographic guide wire is of prognostic significance and is technically necessary. Inability to pass the guide wire through the occlusion suggests either plaque or a well-organized thrombus, which may be resistant to fibrinolysis; yet, easy passage of the guide wire through the occlusion not only establishes a channel in which the thrombolytic agent will have the opportunity to concentrate but also suggests a soft lysable thrombus. Lacing the thrombus with 50,000 U of urokinase, so that the agent is distributed within the thrombus itself and then retrieving the catheter for infusion, is frequently practiced and seems effective.

Switching to a low-dose regimen is appropriate when prolonged infusions seem necessary; however, angiography is repeated within 12 to 16 hours to document progress. Bleeding complications appear to correlate most closely with duration of therapy rather than with the total dosage of the agent. Thus, high-dose, short-term infusions are better tolerated than long-term, low-dose infusions.

Administration of heparin during regional thrombolytic therapy remains controversial. Patients with profound ischemia who are found to have very low flow in the extremity and those in whom pericatheter thrombus formation is significant (e.g., when 3 to 4 cm of the catheter extends into a vessel with low or no flow) can benefit from heparin administration. Heparin may have an enhancing effect in increasing thrombolysis and minimizing the adverse consequences of a potential episode of distal clot migration or embolization. Heparin therapy, however, may result in an increased incidence and severity of pericatheter bleeding during lytic therapy and a higher risk of distant bleeding.

When heparin is administered, it is usually best to use it as a continuous infusion to maintain a prolonged PTT of 1.5 to 2.0 times the control value. A bolus infusion prior to initiation of continuous therapy is used in the presence of acute severe ischemia or when low-flow states are identified. In a coaxial system, a lower dose of heparin may be administered through the larger sheath, usually 500 U/hr. The PTT must not exceed 60 seconds at the time of catheter and sheath removal. Heparin may then be restarted without a bolus. The procedure is technically demanding and requires substantial labor and resource commitment.[137]

The fibrin-specific thrombolytic agent rt-PA has been used in clinical trials. Risius and coworkers[103] reported the use of this agent in 25 patients with thrombosed peripheral arteries or bypass grafts. The age of the occlusions ranged from 1 hour to 21 days (mean, 6.5 days). Thrombolysis occurred in 23 of 25 patients (92%). The failures occurred in two patients with thrombosed femoropopliteal grafts in whom the grafts could not be catheterized. Time to lysis ranged from 1 to 6.5 hours (mean, 3.6 hours), with the total dose ranging from 4.5 to 58 mg. Thrombus age had no effect on the infusion time or on the total dose infused. Six patients (24%) experienced profound decreases in plasma fibrinogen levels, and absolute values were less than 100 mg/dl. Complications occurred in three patients (12%). Decreases in plasma fibrinogen, plasminogen, and $alpha_2$-antiplasmin indicative of a systemic lytic state occurred with longer infusion times, suggesting that the fibrin specificity of rt-PA is relative. Nonetheless, with the total doses and infusion durations employed, rt-PA exerted a lesser systemic lytic effect than did streptokinase or urokinase. rt-PA appears to be a potent and potentially highly effective thrombolytic agent, but additional clinical studies are necessary to determine the ultimate role of rt-PA and other new fibrinolytic agents.

Despite results of thrombolytic therapy from a multitude of retrospective studies, a number of questions remained unanswered. Results from randomized trials have more precisely delineated the role of thrombolytic therapy in peripheral vascular disease. The STILE trial (Surgery Versus Thrombolysis for Ischemia of the Lower Extremity) compared optimal surgical therapy with intra-arterial catheter-directed thrombolysis for native arterial or bypass graft occlusions.[154] Stratification by duration of ischemic symptoms revealed that patients with ischemia of less than 14 days' duration had lower amputation rates with thrombolysis and shorter hospital stays, whereas patients with ischemia for longer than 14 days who were treated surgically had less ongoing or recurrent ischemia and showed a trend toward lower morbidity. At 6 months, amputation-free survival was improved in patients with acute ischemia treated with thrombolysis, but patients with chronic ischemia had lower amputation rates when treated surgically. Fifty-five per cent of patients treated with thrombolysis had a reduction in magnitude of their surgical procedure. Of note, no difference was seen between the use of rt-PA and urokinase.

Analysis of a subgroup of patients in the STILE trial with native, nonembolic arterial thrombosis in the lower extremities has been completed.[155] Similar to the original study, a large percentage of patients (22%) could not receive thrombolytic therapy because of an inability to position the infusion catheter. Factors associated with a poor outcome in the lytic group included femoropopliteal occlusion, diabetes, and critical ischemia. At 1 year, the incidences of both recurrent ischemia and amputation were higher in the thrombolytic group, causing the investigators to conclude that surgical revascularization was more effective and durable.

Based on these and other results, a multicenter, randomized, prospective trial comparing thrombolysis with surgery for acute lower extremity ischemia of less than 14 days' duration has been carried out (TOPAS study).[156] The most effective dose for urokinase was determined to be 4000 U/min with complete thrombolysis in 71% of patients. After successful thrombolytic therapy, either surgical or endovascular intervention was performed on the lesion responsible for the occlusion if found. When compared with the surgical arm, the 1-year limb salvage and mortality rates were not statistically different.

From the results already detailed, it is evident that thrombolytic therapy is an important and effective part of the armamentarium in treating patients with relatively acute ischemia. However, one must use considerable judgment in patient selection, and careful planning of anticipated surgical intervention must be done. Regardless of the type of agent used, fibrinolytic therapy should not be considered as curative. Although lysis alone can be quite successful in initially restoring patency to a vessel or graft, more often lysis allows delineation of an underlying arterial stenosis or graft abnormality that then must be treated by operation or angioplasty to maintain patency.[118, 129] Long-term patency of native arteries managed in this manner is reasonably good, as is patency of proximal grafts, but late patency in infrainguinal bypasses is disappointing (i.e., $<20\%$).

The intraoperative use of thrombolytic agents is now supported by both experimental and clinical experience. (See chapters that describe this potentially valuable method of administration.)

Complications of Regional Lytic Therapy

Complications of local thrombolytic therapy include hemorrhage, distal embolization, pericatheter thrombosis, graft extravasation, fever, and allergic reactions. In addition, all complications discussed earlier under Systemic Thrombolytic Therapy may be seen when prolonged regional infusions are necessary.

Distal embolization of clot fragments may cause temporary worsening of symptoms in the treated region. The emboli often disappear with continued thrombolytic therapy; however, occasionally embolectomy may be required.[80] Pericatheter thrombosis is common and may be avoided by the use of heparin, either systemically or through coaxial systems.[11, 33]

Fever is common with streptokinase and may occur in up to 30% of patients, however, severe allergic reactions are rare. Re-treatment with streptokinase within 6 months should be avoided.

As with any form of lytic therapy, bleeding is the most feared and frequent complication of regional fibrinolytic therapy. The risk of major bleeding (requiring cessation of therapy or blood transfusions) ranges from 5% to 15%, even when appropriate precautions are observed.[44, 80] Bleeding is usually related to systemic effects of the drug, and management is discussed earlier under Complications of Systemic Lytic Therapy.

The most recent experience seems to indicate that the risk of bleeding correlates more with the duration of therapy than with the actual dose of the agent used. It is preferable to use higher-dose protocols, especially in circumstances in which a shortened duration of infusion may be anticipated. Although specific coagulation parameters do not correlate with the risk of bleeding, the presence of a systemic lytic state decidedly increases this risk. The presence of such systemic effects may help determine the most appropriate course of action in the presence of a minor bleeding complication. A systemic lytic state is heralded by a 50% drop in fibrinogen from baseline or a prolongation of the thrombin time to two times normal, or both.

If significant progress is being made in the presence of systemic effects, continuation of therapy is warranted. If no significant improvement is noted within the last interval of observation, reassessment should be based on weighing the risks and benefits of continuing thrombolytic therapy versus alternative interventions, including operative revascularization.

Treatment of hemorrhagic complications depends on the severity of the process and progress made during lytic therapy. Oozing around the catheter entry site without hematoma formation during the late stages of the infusion may be locally controlled, keeping the patient under observation. A similar situation in the early stages of the infusion, when more than 12 to 24 hours of therapy are anticipated, should lead to discontinuation of the drug. Development of a significant hematoma or bleeding at a remote site requires cessation of therapy. Replacement of fibrinogen with components (e.g., cryoprecipitate or fresh frozen plasma) usually suffices because the half-lives of urokinase, streptokinase, and t-PA are relatively short.

Pseudoaneurysm formation is rare but may occur secondary to bleeding from an arterial puncture site. Current methods of management of pseudoaneurysm are applicable.

Intracranial bleeding is perhaps the most feared complication of any form of lytic therapy. This is discussed under Systemic Thrombolytic Therapy, but any change in the neurologic status of a patient during thrombolytic therapy should be viewed as a complication of treatment and the agent discontinued.

Fatal pulmonary emboli have been reported during intra-arterial fibrinolytic therapy.[112] A potential mechanism for this complication implies decreased venous circulation in the ischemic extremity with formation of clot, partial lysis, and eventual embolization. Treatment options include cessation of lytic therapy with heparinization and maintaining or increasing the dose of the plasminogen activator. If the latter course is chosen, leaving the intra-arterial catheter in place may decrease the risk of bleeding though the puncture site.

Conversion of an ischemic myocardial infarction into a hemorrhagic infarct has been reported as a complication of lytic therapy. No relationship between the lytic agent and the few reported cases can be made. Nevertheless, deterioration of cardiac function in the presence of an acute myocardial infarction during thrombolytic therapy should lead the clinician to consider this possibility. Therapy may need to be discontinued until the cause of the cardiac decompensation has been determined.

SUMMARY

The fibrinolytic system is the body's intricate system that maintains fluidity of blood in the vascular tree. An imbalance in both local and systemic factors may result in thrombosis and clinical evidence of ischemia. Both direct and indirect activation of plasminogen leads to fibrinolysis and resolution of thrombotic occlusions. A knowledge and understanding of the fibrinolytic system are likely to improve the clinical results obtained with thrombolytic drugs. Furthermore, development of more effective agents relies on enhancing an agent's specific affinity to fibrin and therefore the fibrin-bound plasminogen.

Thrombolytic agents are delivered either systemically or regionally with catheter-directed instillation into thrombotic material. The latter modality, often in conjunction with surgical revascularization, is used frequently for arterial thromboses and has the advantage of targeted therapy. This may reduce the most dreaded complication of thrombolytic therapy, which is hemorrhage remote to the offending thrombotic occlusion. It is evident that the powerful fibrinolytic system, which ensures the fluidity of blood under physiologic conditions, may be harnessed as part of the treatment in patients with thromboembolic disorders.

REFERENCES

1. Aastad B: Purification and characterization of human vascular plasminogen activator. Biochim Biophys Acta 621:241, 1980.
2. Agnelli G, Parise P: Bolus thrombolysis in venous thromboembolism. Chest 101:172S, 1992.
3. Albrechtson OK: The fibrinolytic activity of human tissue. Br J Haematol 3:284, 1957.
4. Alessi MC, Juhan-Vague I, Kooistra T, et al: Insulin stimulates the synthesis of plasminogen activator inhibitor 1 by hepatocellular cell line Hep G2. Thromb Haemost 60:491, 1988.
5. Andreotti F, Davies GJ, Hackett DR, et al: Major circadian fluctuations in fibrinolytic factors and possible relevance to time of onset

of myocardial infarction, sudden cardiac death and stroke. Am J Cardiol 62:635, 1988.
6. Angleton P, Chandler WL, Schmer G: Diurnal variation of tissue-type plasminogen activator and its rapid inhibition. Circulation 79:101, 1989.
7. Aoki N, Takeno K, Sakata Y: Differences of frequency distributions of plasminogen phenotypes between Japanese and American populations: New methods for the detection of plasminogen variants. Biochem Genet 22:871, 1984.
8. Astrup T: Stage A: Isolation of a soluble fibrinolytic activator from animal tissue. Nature 170:929, 1952.
9. Astrup T: The haemostatic balance. Thromb Diath Haemost 2:347, 1958.
10. Barnathan ES, Kuo A, Rosenfeld L, et al: Interaction of single-chain urokinase-type plasminogen activator with human endothelial cells. J Biol Chem 265:2865, 1990.
11. Becker GJ, Rabe FE, Richmond BD, et al: Low-dose fibrinolytic therapy. Radiology 148:663, 1983.
12. Behrendt N, Ronne E, Plough M, et al: The human receptor for urokinase plasminogen activator. NH_2-terminal amino acid sequence and glycosylation variants. J Biol Chem 265:6453, 1990.
13. Belkin N, Belkin B, Bucknam CA, et al: Intraarterial fibrinolytic therapy: Efficacy of streptokinase versus urokinase. Arch Surg 121:769, 1986.
14. Bernik MB, Kwaan HC: Origin of fibrinolytic activity in cultures of the human kidney. J Lab Clin Med 70:650, 1967.
15. Bode C, Matsueda G, Haber E: Targeted thrombolysis with a fibrin-specific antibody urokinase conjugate. Circulation 72:111, 1985.
16. Booyse FM, Scheinbuks JR, Radek J, et al: Immunological identification and comparison of plasminogen activator forms in cultured normal human endothelial cells and smooth muscle cells. Thromb Res 24:495, 1981.
17. Burrowes CE: Activation of human prekallikrein by plasmin. Fed Proc 30:451, 1971.
18. Chaise L, Comerota AJ, Soulen RC, et al: Selective intraarterial streptokinase in the immediate postoperative period. JAMA 247:2397, 1982.
19. Chandler WL, Trimble SL, Loo S-C, Mornin D: Effect of PAI-1 levels on the molar concentrations of active tissue plasminogen activator (t-PA) and t-PA/PAI-1 complex in plasma. Blood 76:930, 1990.
20. Claeys H, Molla A, Verstraete M: Conversion of NH_2-terminal glutamic acid to NH_2-terminal lysine human plasminogen by plasmin. Thromb Res 3:515, 1973.
21. Clozel JP, Banken L, Roux S: Aprotinin: An antidote for recombinant tissue-type plasminogen activator (rt-PA) active in vivo. J Am Coll Cardiol 16:507, 1990.
22. Collen D: Human tissue type plasminogen activator: From the laboratory to the bedside. Circulation 72:18, 1985.
23. Collen D, Wiman B: Turnover of antiplasmin, the fast-acting plasmin inhibitor of plasma. Blood 53:313, 1979.
24. Cucuianu N, Crisnic I, Knauer O, et al: Severe bleeding in heterozygous a_2 plasmin inhibitor deficiency. Rev Roum Biochim 26:273, 1989.
25. Cummings H, Castellino F: Interaction of human plasmin with human a_2-macroglobulin. Biochemistry 23:105, 1984.
26. Dairbairn S, Gilbert R, Ojakian G, et al: The extracellular matrix of normal chick embryo fibroblasts. Its effect on transformed chick fibroblasts and its proteolytic degradation by the transformation. J Cell Biol 101:1790, 1985.
27. De Jaegere PP, Arnold AA, Balk AH, Simoons ML: Intracranial hemorrhage in association with thrombolytic therapy: Incidence and clinical predictive factors. J Am Coll Cardiol 19:289, 1992.
28. Doolittle RF: Fibrinogen and fibrin. Annu Rev Biochem 53:195, 1984.
29. Dotter CT, Rosch J, Seaman AJ: Selective clot lysis with low-dose streptokinase. Radiology 11:31, 1974.
30. Elliot MS, Immelman EJ, Jeffery P, et al: A comparative randomized trial of heparin vs. streptokinase in the treatment of acute proximal venous thrombosis. An interim report of a prospective trial. Br J Surg 66:838, 1979.
31. Erickson LA, Hekman CM, Loskutoff DJ: The primary plasminogen-activator inhibitors in endothelial cells, platelets, serum and plasma are immunologically related. Proc Natl Acad Sci USA 82:8710, 1985.
32. Eskridge JM, Becker GJ, Rabe FE, et al: Carotid occlusion in a canine model. Semin Intervent Radiol 2:405, 1985.
33. Eskridge JM, Becker GJ, Rabe FE, et al: Catheter related thrombosis and fibrinolytic therapy. Radiology 149:429, 1983.
34. Feissinger JN, Vayssiairat M, Juillet Y, et al: Local urokinase in arterial thromboembolism. Angiology 31:715, 1980.
35. Fioretti E, Angeletti M, Citro G, et al: Kunitz-type inhibitors in human serum. Identification and characterization. J Biol Chem 262:3586, 1987.
36. Flickinger EG, Jonnsrude IS, Osburn HL, et al: Local streptokinase infusion for superior mesenteric artery thromboembolism. AJR 140:771, 1983.
37. Friezner Degen SJ, Rajput B, Reich E: The human tissue activator gene. J Biol Chem 261:6972, 1986.
38. Fujii S, Lucore CL, Hopkins WE, et al: Potential attenuation of fibrinolysis by growth factors released from platelets and their pharmacologic implications. Am J Cardiol 63:1505, 1989.
39. Fujii S, Sobel BE: Induction of plasminogen activator inhibitor by products released from platelets. Circulation 82:1485, 1990.
40. Gardiner GA, Koltun W, Kandarpa K, et al: Thrombolysis of occluded femoropopliteal grafts. AJR 147:621, 1986.
41. Gelehrter TD, Sznycer-Laszuk R, Zeheb R, et al: Dexamethasone inhibition of tissue-type plasminogen activator (t-PA) activity; paradoxical induction of both t-PA antigen and plasminogen activator inhibitor. Mol Endocrinol 1:97, 1987.
42. Gomez MJ, Carroll RC, Hansard MR, et al: Regulation of fibrinolysis in aortic surgery. J Vasc Surg 8:348, 1988.
43. Gonzales-Gronow M, Edelberg JM, Pizzo SV: Further characterization of the cellular plasminogen binding site: Evidence that plasminogen 2 and lipoprotein(a) compete for the same site. Biochemistry 28:2374, 1989.
44. Graor RA, Risius B, Denny KM, et al: Local thrombolysis in the treatment of thrombosed arteries, bypassed grafts, and arteriovenous fistulas. J Vasc Surg 2:406, 1985.
45. Graor RA, Risius B, Young JR, et al: Peripheral artery and bypass graft thrombolysis with recombinant human tissue type plasminogen activator. J Vasc Surg 3:115, 1986.
46. Grimaudo V, Hauert J, Bachmann F, et al: Diurnal variation of the fibrinolytic system. Thromb Haemost 59:495, 1988.
47. Gurewich V, Pannell R, Louie S, et al: Effective and fibrin specific clot lysis by a zymogen precursor form of urokinase (pro-urokinase): A study in vitro and two animal species. J Clin Invest 73:1731, 1984.
48. Häggroth L, Mattson C, Felding P, et al: Plasminogen activator inhibitors in plasma and platelets from patients with recurrent venous thrombosis and pregnant women. Thromb Res 42:585, 1986.
49. Hajjar KA, Gavish D, Breslow JL, et al: Lipoprotein(a) modulation of endothelial cell surface fibrinolysis and its potential role in atherosclerosis. Nature 339:303, 1989.
50. Hamsten A, Wiman B, de Faire U, Bömback M: Increased plasma levels of a rapid inhibitor of tissue plasminogen activator in young survivors of myocardial infarction. N Engl J Med 313:1557, 1985.
51. Harpel PC, Gordon BR, Parker TS: Plasmin catalyzes binding of lipoprotein(a) to immobilized fibrinogen and fibrin. Proc Natl Acad Sci U S A 86:3847, 1989.
52. Henkin J, Marcotte P, Yang H: The plasminogen-plasmin system. Prog Cardiovasc Dis 34(2):135, 1991.
53. Higgins D, Vehar G: Interaction of one-chain tissue plasminogen activator with intact and plasmin-degraded fibrin. Biochemistry 26:7786, 1987.
54. Hoylaerts M, Rijken DC, Lijnen HR, et al: Kinetics of the activation of plasminogen by human tissue plasminogen activator. J Biol Chem 257:2912, 1982.
55. Husain SS, Gurewich V, Lipinski B: Purification and partial characterization of a single-chain, high-molecular-weight form of urokinase from human urine. Arch Biochem Biophys 220:31, 1983.
56. Ichinose A, Takio K, Fujikawa K: Localization of the binding site of tissue-type plasminogen activator in fibrin. J Clin Invest 78:163, 1986.
57. Johnson AJ, McCarty WR: The lysis of artificially induced intravascular clots in man by infusions of streptokinase. J Clin Invest 38:1624, 1959.
58. Juhan-Vague I, Vague PH, Alessi MC, et al: Relationships between plasma insulin, triglyceride, body mass index, and plasminogen activator inhibitor 1. Diabetes Metab 13:331, 1987.
59. Juhan-Vague I, Valadier J, Alessi M-C, et al: Deficient t-PA release and elevated PA inhibitor levels in patients with spontaneous deep venous thrombosis. Thromb Haemost 57:67, 1987.

60. Katzen BT, Van Breda A: Low-dose streptokinase in treatment of arterial occlusions. AJR 136:1171, 1981.
61. Kirchheimer JC, Wojta J, Christ G, et al: Proliferation of a human epidermal tumor cell line stimulated by urokinase. FASEB J 1:125, 1987.
62. Klatte EC, Becker GJ, Holden RE, et al: Fibrinolytic therapy. Radiology 159:619, 1986.
63. Kordich L, Porterie V, Lago O, et al: Mini-plasminogen–like molecule in septic patients. Thromb Res 47:553, 1987.
64. Kwaan HC: The biologic role of components of the plasminogen-plasmin system. Prog Cardiovasc Dis 34(5):309, 1992.
65. Lammer J, Pilger E, Justich E, et al: Fibrinolysis in chronic arteriosclerotic occlusions: Intrathrombotic injection of streptokinase. Radiology 157:45, 1985.
66. Levin EG: Latent tissue plasminogen activator produced by human endothelial cells in culture: Evidence for an enzyme–inhibitor complex. Proc Natl Acad Sci U S A 80:6804, 1983.
67. Levin EG, Loskutoff DJ: Regulation of plasminogen activator production by cultured endothelial cells. Ann N Y Acad Sci 401:184, 1982.
68. Levin EG, Santell L: Association of a plasminogen activator inhibitor (PAI-1) with the growth substratum and membrane of human endothelial cells. J Cell Biol 105:2543, 1987.
69. Lijnen HR, Zamarron C, Blaber M, et al: Activation of plasminogen by pro-urokinase. I. Mechanism. J Biol Chem 261:1253, 1986.
70. Lo SK, Ryan TJ, Gilboa N, et al: Role of catalytic and lysine-binding sites in plasmin-induced neutrophil adherence to endothelium. J Clin Invest 84:793, 1989.
71. Loscalzo J, Weinfeld M, Fless GM, et al: Lipoprotein (a), fibrin binding and plasminogen activation. Arteriosclerosis 10:240, 1990.
72. Low DA, Baker JB, Koonce WC: Released protease–nexin regulates cellular binding, internalization, and degradation of serine proteases. Proc Natl Acad Sci U S A 78:2340, 1981.
73. Lucore CL, Fujii S, Wun T-C, et al: Regulation of the expression of type 1 plasminogen activator inhibitor in Hep G2 cells by epidermal growth factor. J Biol Chem 263:15845, 1988.
74. MacFarlane RG, Pilling J: Observations on fibrinolytic plasminogen, plasmin and antiplasmin content of human blood. Lancet 2:562, 1946.
75. Marder VJ, Soulen RL, Atichartakarn V, et al: Quantitative venographic assessment of deep vein thrombosis in the evaluation of streptokinase and heparin therapy. J Lab Clin Med 89:1018, 1977.
76. Marongiu F, Conti M, Mameli G, et al: Is the imbalance between thrombin and plasmin activity in diabetes related to the behavior of antiplasmin activity? Thromb Res 58:91, 1990.
77. Martin M: Thrombolytic therapy in arterial thromboembolism. Prog Cardiovasc Dis 21:351, 1979.
78. Matsuo O, Rijken DC, Cullen D: Thrombolysis by human tissue plasminogen activator and urokinase in rabbits with experimental pulmonary embolus. Nature 291:590, 1981.
79. McLean JW, Tomlinson JE, Kuang W-J, et al: cDNA sequence of human apolipoprotein (a) is homologous to plasminogen. Nature 300:132, 1987.
80. McNamara TO, Fischer JR: Thrombolysis of peripheral arterial and graft occlusions: Improved results using high dose urokinase. AJR 144:769, 1985.
81. McNicol GP, Gale SB, Douglas AS: In vitro and in vivo studies of a preparation of urokinase. Br Med J 1:909, 1963.
82. Mehta J, Mehta P, Lawson D, et al: Plasma tissue plasminogen activator inhibitor levels in coronary artery disease: Correlation with age and serum triglyceride concentrations. J Am Coll Cardiol 9:263, 1987.
83. Miles LA, Fless GM, Levin EG, et al: A potential basis for the thrombotic risks associated with lipoprotein(a). Nature 339:301, 1989.
84. Monk JP, Heel RC: Anisoylated plasminogen streptokinase activator complex (APSAC): A review of its mechanism of action, clinical pharmacology, and therapeutic use in acute myocardial infarction. Drugs 34:25, 1987.
85. Mori KW, Bookstein JJ, Heeney DJ, et al: Selective streptokinase infusion: Clinical and laboratory correlates. Radiology 148:677, 1983.
86. Mosher DF, Vaheri A: Binding and degradation of a_2-macroglobulin by cultured fibroblasts. Biochim Biophys Acta 627:113, 1980.
87. National Heart and Lung Institute Cooperative Study Group: Urokinase pulmonary embolism trial: Phase I results. JAMA 214(12): 2163, 1970.
88. NIH Consensus Development Conference: Thrombolytic therapy in treatment. Ann Intern Med 93:141, 1980.
89. Nilsson IM, Ljungner H, Tengborn L: Two different mechanisms in patients with venous thrombosis and defective fibrinolysis: Low concentrations of plasminogen activator or increased concentration of plasminogen activator inhibitor. Br Med J 290:1453, 1985.
90. Nilsson TK, Sundell B, Hellsten G, et al: Reduced plasminogen activator inhibitor activity in high consumers of fruits, vegetables and root vegetables. J Intern Med 227:267, 1990.
91. Nykjaer A, Petersen CM, Christensen EI, et al: Urokinase receptors in human monocytes. Biochim Biophys Acta 1052:399, 1990.
92. Ohlsson M, Peng XR, Liu YX, et al: Hormone regulation of tissue-type plasminogen activator gene expression and plasminogen activator–mediated proteolysis. Semin Thromb Hemost 17:286, 1991.
93. Pannell R, Gurewich V: Pro-urokinase: A study of its stability in plasma and of a mechanism for its selective fibrinolytic effect. Blood 67:1215, 1986.
94. Patthy L, Trexler M, Vali Z, et al: Kringles: Modules specialized for protein binding. Homology of the gelatin-binding region of fibronectin with the kringle structures of proteins. FEBS Lett 171:131, 1984.
95. Perler BA, White RI, Ernst CG, et al: Low-dose thrombolytic therapy for infrainguinal graft occlusions: An idea whose time has passed? J Vasc Surg 2:799, 1986.
96. Pillari G, Doscher W, Fierstein J, et al: Low-dose streptokinase in the treatment of celiac and superior mesenteric artery occlusion. Arch Surg 118:1340, 1983.
97. Poliwoda H, Alexander K, Buhl V, et al: Treatment of chronic arterial occlusions with streptokinase. N Engl J Med 280:689, 1969.
98. Pollanen J, Saksela O, Salonen EM, et al: Distinct localizations of urokinase-type plasminogen activator and its type 1 inhibitor under cultured human fibroblasts and sarcoma cells. J Cell Biol 104:1085, 1987.
99. Rabe FE, Becker GJ, Richmond BD, et al: Contrast extravasation through Dacron grafts: A sequela of low-dose streptokinase therapy. AJR 138:917, 1982.
100. Rijken DC, Collen D: Purification and characterization of the plasminogen activator secreted by human melanoma cells in culture. J Biol Chem 256:7035, 1981.
101. Rijken DC, Hoylaerts M, Collen D: Fibrinolytic properties of one-chain and two-chain human extrinsic (tissue type) plasminogen activator. J Biol Chem 257:2920, 1982.
102. Ring M, Butman S, Bruck D, et al: Fibrin metabolism in patients with acute myocardial infarction during and after treatment with tissue-type plasminogen activator. Thromb Haemost 60:428, 1988.
103. Risius B, Graor RA, Geisinger MA, et al: Recombinant human tissue-type plasminogen activator for thrombolysis in peripheral arteries and bypass grafts. Radiology 60:183, 1986.
104. Rosner NH, Dous PE: Contrast extravasation through Dacron grafts: A sequela of low-dose streptokinase therapy. AJR 148:668, 1984.
105. Royston D: Review paper: The serine antiprotease aprotinin (Trasylol™): A novel approach to reducing postoperative bleeding. Blood Coagul Fibrin 1:55, 1990.
106. Rudd MA, George D, Amarante P, et al: Temporal effects of thrombolytic agents in platelet function in vivo and their modulation by prostaglandins. Circ Res 67:1175, 1990.
107. Rylatt DB, Blake LE, Cottis DA, et al: An immunoassay for human D-dimer using monoclonal antibodies. Thromb Res 31:767, 1983.
108. Salo T, Liotta LA, Keski-Oja J, et al: Secretion of basement membrane collagens degrading enzyme and plasminogen activator by transformed cells—role in metastasis. Int J Cancer 30:669, 1982.
109. Scott RW, Bergman BL, Bajpai A, et al: Protease nexin: Properties and a modified purification procedure. J Biol Chem 260:7029, 1985.
110. Sharma GV, Cella G, Parisi AF, et al: Thrombolytic therapy. N Engl J Med 306:1268, 1982.
111. Sherry S: Tissue plasminogen activator (t-PA): Will it fulfill its promise? N Engl J Med 313:1014, 1985.
112. Sicard GA, Schier JJ, Totty WG, et al: Thrombolytic therapy for acute arterial occlusion. J Vasc Burg 2:65, 1985.
113. Sprengers ED, Akkerman JWN, Jansen BG: Blood platelet plasminogen activator inhibitor: Two different pools of endothelial cell type plasminogen activator inhibitor in human blood. Thromb Haemost 55:325, 1986.
114. Stack S, Gonzalez-Gronow M, Pizzo S. Regulation of plasminogen activation by components of the extracellular matrix. Biochemistry 29:4966, 1990.

115. Strickland S, Beers WH: Studies on the role of plasminogen activator in ovulation. J Biol Chem 18:5694, 1976.
116. Sugiyama N, Iwamoto M, Abiko A: Effects of kringles derived from human plasminogen on fibrinolysis in vitro. Thromb Res 47:459, 1987.
117. Summaria L: The plasmin β-chain streptokinase complex. *In* Comerota AJ (ed): Thrombolytic Therapy. Orlando, Fla, Grune & Stratton, 1988.
118. Sussman B, Dardik H, Ibrahim IM, et al: Improved patient selection for enzymatic lysis of peripheral arterial and graft occlusions. Am J Surg 148:244, 1984.
119. Takada A, Sugawara Y, Takada Y: Enhancement of the activation of Glu-plasminogen by urokinase in the simultaneous presence of tranexamic acid or fibrin. Haemostasis 1:26, 1989.
120. Takahashi H, Hanano M, Takizawa S, et al: Plasmin-α_2-plasmin inhibitor complex in plasma of patients with disseminated intravascular coagulation. Am J Hematol 28:162, 1988.
121. Tennant SN, Dixon J, Venable TC, et al: Intracoronary thrombolysis in patients with acute myocardial infarction: Comparison of the efficacy of urokinase versus streptokinase. Circulation 69:756, 1984.
122. Testa JE, Quigley JP: The role of urokinase-type plasminogen activator in aggressive tumor cell behavior. Cancer Metastasis Rev 9:355, 1990.
123. Thorsen S: Differences in the binding to fibrin of native plasminogen and plasminogen modified by protolytic degradation influence of ϵ-aminocarboxylic acids. Biochim Biophys Acta 393:55, 1975.
124. Thorsen S, Philips M, Selmer J, et al: Kinetics of inhibition of tissue-type and urokinase-type plasminogen activator by plasminogen-activator inhibitor type 1 and type 2. Eur J Biochem 175:33, 1988.
125. Tillett WS, Garner RL: The fibrinolytic activity of hemolytic streptococci. J Exp Med 58:485, 1933.
126. TIMI Study Group: Thrombolysis in myocardial infarction (TIMI) trial. Phase I findings. N Engl J Med 312:932, 1985.
127. Tisnado J, Cho S, Beachley MC, et al: Low-dose fibrinolytic therapy in hand ischemia. Semin Intervent Radiol 2:367, 1985.
128. Torr SR, Nachowiak DA, Fujii S, Sobel BE: "Plasminogen steal" and clot lysis. J Am Coll Cardiol 19(5):1085, 1992.
129. Totty WG, Gilula LA, McClennan BL, et al: Low-dose intravascular fibrinolytic therapy. Radiology 143:59, 1982.
130. Totty WG, Romano T, Benian GM, et al: Serum sickness following streptokinase therapy. AJR 138:143, 1982.
131. Urano T, Chibber B, Castellino F: The reciprocal effects of ϵ-aminohexanoic acid and chloride ion on the activation of human plasminogen by human urokinase. Proc Natl Acad Sci U S A 84:4031, 1987.
132. Urano T, Sumiyoshi K, Nakamura M, et al: Fluctuation of tPA and PAI-1 antigen levels in plasma: Difference in their fluctuation patterns between male and female. J Thromb Res 60:55, 1990.
133. Urden G, Chmielewska J, Carlsson T, et al: Immunological relationship between plasminogen activator inhibitors from different sources. Thromb Haemost 57:29, 1987.
134. Vague P, Juhan-Vague I, Alessi MC, et al: Metformin decreases the high plasminogen activator inhibition capacity, plasma insulin and triglyceride levels in non-diabetic obese subjects. Thromb Haemost 57:326, 1987.
135. Vali Z, Patthy L: Locations of the intermediate and high-affinity ϵ-aminocarboxylic acid-binding sites in human plasminogen. J Biol Chem 257:2104, 1982.
136. Vali Z, Patthy L: The fibrin-binding site of human plasminogen. Arginines 32 and 34 are essential for fibrin affinity of the kringle 1 domain. J Biol Chem 259:13690, 1984.
137. Van Breda A, Katzen BT: Thrombolytic therapy of peripheral vascular disease. Semin Intervent Radiol 2:354, 1985.
138. Van Breda A, Katzen BT, Deutsch AS: Urokinase versus streptokinase in local thrombolysis. Radiology 165:109, 1987.
139. Van Breda A, Robison JC, Feldman L, et al: Local thrombolysis in the treatment of arterial graft occlusions. J Vasc Surg 1:103, 1984.
140. Van Hinsberg VWM, van den Berg EA, Fiers W, et al: Tumor necrosis factor induces the production of urokinase-type plasminogen activator by human endothelial cells. Blood 75:1991, 1990.
141. Van Leuven F, Cassiman JJ, Van Den Berghe H: Demonstration of an α_2-macroglobulin receptor in human fibroblasts, absent in tumor-derived cell lines. J Biol Chem 254:5155, 1970.
142. Verstraete M, Vermylen J, Donati MB: The effect of streptokinase infusion on chronic arterial occlusion and stenoses. Ann Intern Med 74:377, 1971.
143. Violand BN, Sodetz JM, Castellino FJ: The effect of ϵ-amino caproic acid on the gross conformation of plasminogen and plasmin. Arch Biochem Biophys 170:300, 1975.
144. Walker ID, Davidson JF: Long-term fibrinolytic enhancement with anabolic steroid therapy: A five-year study. *In* Davidson JF, Rowan RM, Samama MM, Desnoyers PC (eds): Progress in Chemical Fibrinolysis and Thrombolysis. Vol 3. New York, Raven Press, 1978, pp 491–500.
145. Watahiki Y, Takeda Y, Takeda A: Kinetic analyses of the activation of Glu-plasminogen by urokinase in the presence of fibrin, fibrinogen or its degradation products. Thromb Res 46:9, 1987.
146. Wiman B, Hamsten A: Impaired fibrinolysis and risk of thromboembolism. Prog Cardiovasc Dis 34(3):179, 1991.
147. Wiman B, Hamsten A: The fibrinolytic enzyme system and its role in the etiology of thromboembolic disease. Semin Thromb Hemost 16:207, 1990.
148. Wiman B, Lijnen HR, Collen D: On the specific interaction between the lysine-binding sites in plasminogen and complementary sites in α_2-antiplasmin and in fibrinogen. J Biochim Biophys Acta 579:142, 1979.
149. Wiman B, Ljungberg B, Chmielewska J, et al: The role of the fibrinolytic system in deep vein thrombosis. J Lab Clin Med 105:267, 1985.
150. Zajko AB, McLean GK, Grossman RA, et al: Percutaneous transluminal angioplasty and fibrinolytic therapy for renal allograft arterial stenoses and thrombosis. Transplantation 33:447, 1982.
151. Fox D, Ouriel K, Green RM, et al: Thrombolysis with prourokinase versus urokinase. An in vitro comparison. J Vasc Surg 23:657, 1996.
152. Smalling RW: Pharmacologic and clinical impact of the unique molecular structure of a new plasminogen activator. Eur Heart J 18(Suppl F):F11, 1997.
153. Tachias K, Madison EL: Variants of tissue-type plasminogen activator that displays extraordinary resistance to inhibition by the serpin plasminogen activator inhibitor type 1. J Biol Chem 272:14580, 1997.
154. The STILE Investigators: Results of a prospective randomized trial evaluating surgery versus thrombolysis for ischemia of the lower extremity. Ann Vasc Surg 220:251, 1994.
155. Weaver FA, Comerota AJ, Youngblood M, et al: Surgical revascularization versus thrombolysis for nonembolic lower extremity native artery occlusions: Results of a prospective randomized trial. J Vasc Surg 24: 513, 1996.
156. Ouriel K, Veith FJ, Sasahara AA: Thrombolysis or Peripheral Arterial Surgery: Phase 1 results. TOPAS investigators. J Vasc Surg 23:64, 1996.

CHAPTER 29

Basic Vascular Surgical Techniques

Robert B. Rutherford, M.D.

To avoid unnecessary repetition elsewhere in this book, this chapter reviews some of the basic technical principles on which vascular surgery is based, for example (1) dissection, exposure, and control of vessels; (2) intraoperative hemostasis and anticoagulation; (3) vascular incisions and closure; and (4) basic anastomotic techniques. The fundamental aspects of the more specialized techniques thromboembolectomy and endarterectomy as well as of endovascular techniques are covered in Chapters 30 to 32.

HISTORICAL BACKGROUND

Everyone's view of the history of the development of vascular surgical techniques is different. This personal view is presented for the reader's appreciation of what we now take for granted: how difficult the early days must have been and how far we have come.

The first recorded vascular reconstruction was reported by Lambert in 1762. He described Hallowell's closure, in 1759, of a small opening in a brachial artery, performed with a pin around which a thread was twisted. This was a historic step; before that time, restoration of flow had always been sacrificed for the sake of hemostasis, and ligation was essentially the only vascular procedure practiced. Unfortunately, Asman's subsequent failures to achieve patency after vascular repair with similar techniques in experimental animals discouraged the surgeons of the day, and for almost a century it was believed that suture material entering the lumen of a vessel would invariably produce an obliterating thrombosis.

By 1882, Schede had accomplished the first successful lateral vein repair. The first direct vascular anastomosis probably was Nicolai Eck's lateral anastomosis, in 1877, between the inferior vena cava and the portal vein in dogs. The opposing surfaces of the two vessels were sutured together by two rows of interrupted sutures. A suture at one corner was left untied temporarily to allow a special instrument to be inserted to slit open each vessel and allow cross-flow through the anastomosis. Although this was technically a lateral, or side-to-side, anastomosis, it was converted into an end-to-side portacaval shunt by subsequent ligation of the hepatic limb of the portal vein. It is interesting to reflect on Eck's enduring fame as a result of this experiment, considering that he had only one survivor and made no other significant contributions to surgery.

In 1899, Kummell performed the first end-to-end anastomosis of an artery in a human—if one discounts Murphy's invagination anastomosis 2 years earlier. As a background to these and other sporadic clinical successes, the decades following the beginning of the 20th century witnessed numerous experimental studies evaluating almost every conceivable suture technique. Absorbable versus nonabsorbable sutures and continuous versus interrupted, simple versus mattress, and everting versus edge-to-edge approximation techniques all were tried. These endeavors culminated in the classic studies by Carrel and Guthrie that established the principles and techniques of the modern vascular anastomosis.[1, 2] These investigators also were the first to achieve significant experimental success with fresh and preserved homografts and heterografts for vascular replacement and bypass.[3]

In 1906, Goyanes used a segment of popliteal vein to bridge a defect caused by the excision of an aneurysm of the accompanying artery. The next year, Lexer used the saphenous vein for arterial reconstruction following excision of an axillary artery aneurysm. Although the stage appeared to be set by the aforementioned experimental studies and by continuing, though sporadic, clinical successes such as these, widespread clinical application of these principles and techniques did not occur for almost 40 years. The reasons for this delay are not entirely clear, but the innovation of better diagnostic techniques (especially angiography and cardiac catheterization), the evolution of vascular prostheses and homograft storage methods, the development of techniques that allowed thoracotomy to be performed at reasonable risk, and the availability of heparin and type-specific, cross-matched blood were probably all important in the final launching of the "golden era of cardiovascular surgery," which began after World War II.

Before the technical explosion that followed in the 1950s, the mainstays of surgery for peripheral vascular disease were (1) arterial ligation for vascular trauma, arteriovenous fistulae, or aneurysm, (2) simple vascular repair with or without local thrombectomy for acute occlusion, (3) sympathectomy for chronic ischemia, and (4) a variety of amputations. The implantation, first of arterial homografts, then of a succession of plastic prostheses culminating in the porous, knitted polyester (Dacron) graft of today; the emerging preference for fresh venous and arterial autografts for replacement of smaller arteries; and, finally, the additional availability of the human umbilical vein allograft and the expanded polytetrafluoroethylene (Teflon) graft have now provided the vascular surgeon with an adequate array of arterial substitutes for most situations. Unfortunately, the concomitant development and refinement of vascular suture materials, atraumatic vascular clamps, and other mechanical devices, such as vena caval filters and embolectomy catheters, have received almost better cover-

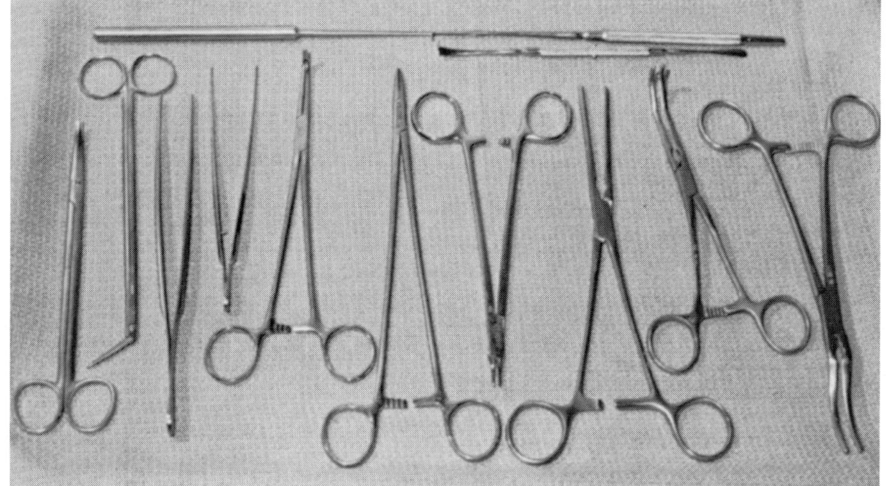

FIGURE 29–1. Some basic vascular instruments, including, from left to right: Metzenbaum and angled Potts scissors; DeBakey and Swan-Brown forceps; a right-angle clamp; long and short vascular needle holders; straight, Satinsky, and spoon-shaped vascular clamps; and (at *top*) a blunted nerve hook and Penfield and Freer dissectors for endarterectomy.

age in manufacturers' brochures than in the formal surgical literature.

INSTRUMENTS AND SUTURE MATERIAL

The instruments essential for simple vascular procedures, in addition to the standard instruments used in any operative dissection, comprise only the following:

- Vascular forceps
- Fine-pointed diamond-jawed needle holder
- Right-angled clamp
- Vascular scissors
- An assortment of atraumatic vascular clamps

Vascular forceps usually have fine teeth or serrations that interdigitate, allowing them to grip the vessel wall without crushing, as exemplified by the DeBakey or Swan-Brown forceps shown in Figure 29–1. Similar requirements pertain to vascular clamps, and although many different designs are available, most achieve their nonslipping, noncrushing, occlusive grip by means of several longitudinal rows of serrations or teeth on the inside of the jaw or clamp, which are offset so that they interdigitate, as shown in Figure 29–2. An assortment of such vascular clamps, of different sizes and shapes, is necessary to accommodate differences in extent of exposure, depth of wound, size of vessel, and angle of application (i.e., transverse, oblique, or tangential) (Fig. 29–3).

In addition to these vascular clamps, which have handles that allow them to be held and with which vessel position can be manipulated, there are smaller vascular clamps without handles, the jaws of which are held in the occlusive position by a spring. These so-called bulldog clamps, or large neurosurgical aneurysm clips, are useful for working on smaller vessels or controlling branches or tributaries, particularly when the exposure is limited (Fig. 29–4).

Moistened umbilical tapes, polymeric silicone (Silastic) loops, or thin rubber catheters are used to encircle vessels and their major tributaries during dissection and manipulation. A heavy silk suture, doubly looped around a small branch or tributary, can, by the weight of a hemostat clamped to its end, control intraoperative bleeding from these branches without crowding the operative field with additional vascular clamps. During maneuvers to dissect, free, and encircle vessels, a right-angled clamp with fine (but not too pointed) tips is invaluable.

Small Metzenbaum scissors or (on smaller, more delicate vessels) plastic or even iris scissors are particularly suitable for dissection on or around the vessels because they do not have sharp-pointed tips and are less likely to injure the vessel inadvertently. Curved, straight, or angled Potts scissors, however, are preferable for incision or excision of the vessel wall itself because they have delicately pointed tips. An assortment of balloon and irrigating catheters is useful

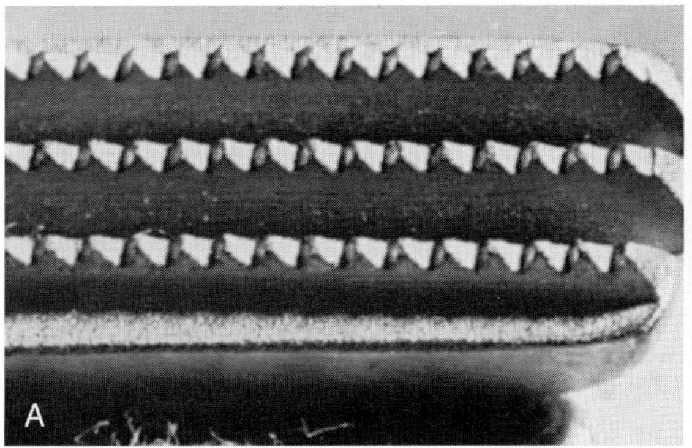

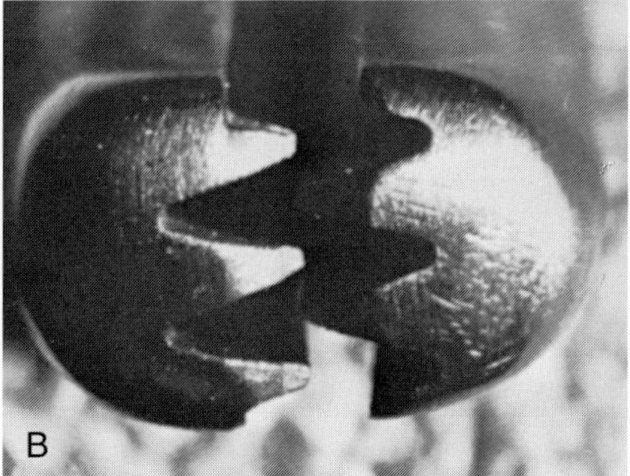

FIGURE 29–2. Magnified views show the multiple "teeth" of a typical vascular clamp. *A*, Side view of one jaw. *B*, End-on view of the jaws interdigitating.

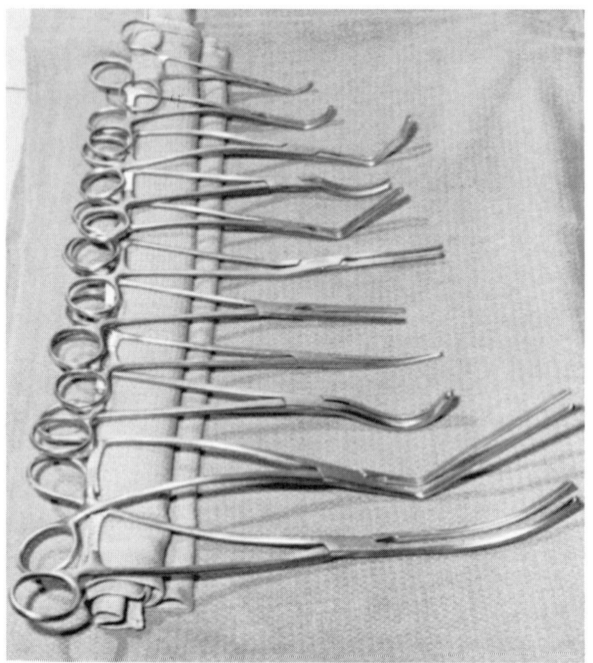

FIGURE 29–3. An assortment of vascular clamps demonstrating the variety of shapes and sizes.

for many purposes in addition to that of removing intravascular thrombus (see Chapter 30).

To some extent, the selection of vascular suture material, like that of vascular instruments, is an individual matter, and every surgeon has favorites. The caliber of the suture used should be as fine as possible, short of risking suture line disruption (and anastomotic aneurysm formation), to minimize hemorrhage through suture holes and the amount of suture material in contact with the vessel lumen. As a frame of reference, a range from 2-0 to 7-0 is used in most clinical practice as the surgeon progresses from the aorta centrally to the radial or crural arteries peripherally. For most peripheral anastomoses, 5-0 or 6-0 sutures usually are preferred. All vascular sutures should be swaged onto fine, one-half-circle or three-eighths-circle, round needles with tapered or slightly beveled tips. Flattening of the body of such a fine needle parallel with the radius of its curve and placing of a tapered cutting edge on the side of its tip facilitate penetration through hard arteriosclerotic plaques and avoid bending the body of the needle during the anastomosis.

Braided fine silk, lubricated with sterile mineral oil or bone wax, handles well and is satisfactory for autogenous tissues, especially venous anastomoses, but polytetrafluoroethylene-coated Dacron and monofilament polypropylene usually are preferred for arterial work because of their greater strength and durability and their reduced tissue reactivity. Absorbable monofilament suture with a long half-life (e.g., polydioxanone suture) is now being used instead of interrupted sutures in pediatric vascular surgery to allow anastomotic growth. It is common practice to use doubled swaged-on vascular suture (i.e., with a needle on each end) to allow more flexibility and speed in performing vascular anastomoses.

VASCULAR EXPOSURE AND CONTROL

Vascular exposure and control usually constitute the first order of business during any vascular operation. They are attained before systemic anticoagulation is instituted, to facilitate the dissection and minimize blood loss. A clear knowledge of the anatomic relationships among the involved vessels, their major collaterals or tributaries, and the surrounding structures is essential, since the procedure often is performed for occlusive disease and the luxury of dissecting toward a palpable pulse is not afforded the surgeon. In such a situation, however, the surgeon may be able to detect the location of an arteriosclerotic artery that is hardened or contains firm thrombosis by rolling it with the fingertip from side to side in the underlying tissues. A patent, though pulseless, artery can be located with a sterile Doppler probe; this device may be particularly helpful for dissecting through scarred or inflamed tissues.

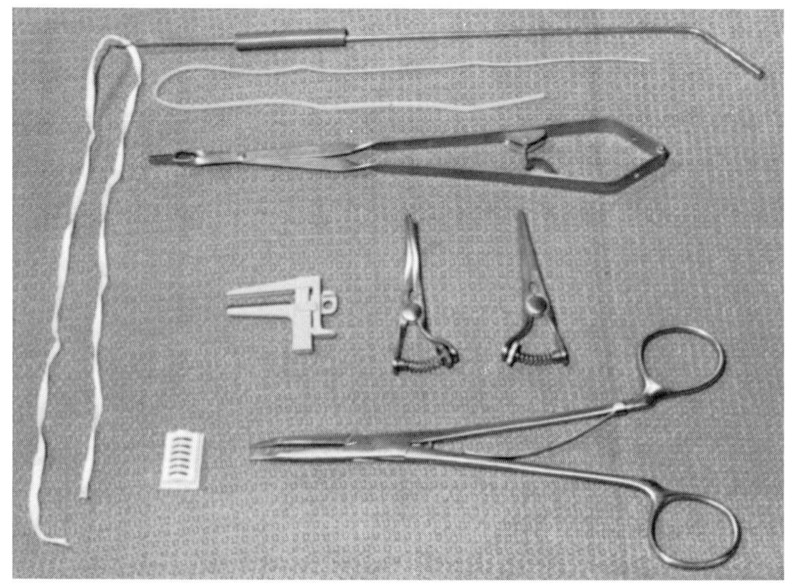

FIGURE 29–4. A variety of instruments used to control or occlude smaller arterial branches. Shown (from *top* down) are a modified Rummel tourniquet that uses umbilical tape, a polymeric silicone rubber (Silastic) "loop," a Heifitz aneurysm clip with applicator, a Fogarty clamp, two DeBakey bulldog clamps, and metal surgical clips (Ligaclips) with applicator.

Major vessels usually are enclosed in an identifiable fascial envelope or sheath, incision of which normally is the final step in obtaining exposure because (1) the characteristic pattern of the vasa vasorum immediately identifies an exposed artery and (2) the bluish white color and the almost ballotable sensation (imparted by the rapid refilling following the quick application and release of pressure) usually makes the accompanying vein easy to recognize.

Smaller, more peripheral vessels, such as may be encountered at the wrist or ankle, may go into spasm during the dissection. This event, or the lack of arterial pulsations below an obstructive lesion, may make the distinction between an adjacent artery and vein difficult. Observing the direction of blood flow after temporary occlusion or comparing the color of microaspirates of blood taken with a tuberculin syringe and 25-gauge needle can be helpful maneuvers in these situations.

In the presence of arterial or venous occlusive disease, considerable inflammatory reaction and connective tissue may surround the vessels. In this situation, the standard advice to dissect off the looser outer adventitial layers and "stay close" to the artery is particularly worthwhile. Arteries are usually approached from the direction of their closest proximity to the skin, and because they rarely give off major branches in that direction, the nearest, or uppermost, surface of the artery normally is devoid of branches, or "free." Once in the correct plane inside the loose outer investiture of the artery and after its upper surface has been exposed fully, the surgeon should dissect a convenient segment of the artery free circumferentially in this same plane by gently spreading the tissues with a right-angle clamp, taking care not to puncture the accompanying vein, which may be closely adherent to the opposite surface, especially near bifurcations.

Next, the surgeon passes an umbilical tape or Silastic loop around the artery and clamps its loose ends with a hemostat. Traction on this tape and on each additional encircling tape progressively draws the arterial structures up out of their bed, allowing restricting points of fixation and major branches to be identified, thus making the dissection progressively easier. The surgeon should proceed in this manner until an adequate length of arterial segment and all its major branches are completely free and encircled with tapes. Small branches may represent potentially significant future collateral vessels; therefore, rather than divide them, the surgeon should control such branches temporarily with a double loop of heavy braided silk or a small cerebral aneurysm clip.

To obtain control of the vessels, even in elective procedures, the surgeon does best to dissect out first the major inflow vessels and then the main outflow vessels before proceeding with lesser collaterals. Depending on the operative procedure planned, exposure and control of one or more such arterial segments may be necessary, and if a bypass graft between such segments is to be constructed, the surgeon should prepare the intervening "tunnel" or passage for the graft before heparin is given.

HEMOSTASIS AND ANTICOAGULATION

The processes of hemostasis and anticoagulation lie at the very foundation of vascular surgery. Only the simplest, most abbreviated vascular surgical procedures can be undertaken without the need to interrupt the flow of blood temporarily. In performing such interruption, the surgeon must avoid the two opposing complications of vascular surgery: exsanguinating hemorrhage and intravascular thrombosis.

Hemostasis

Hemostasis, produced spontaneously by spasm and platelet thrombi in smaller vessels and by clamping and ligature in larger vessels, is an integral part of almost every surgical dissection. Whenever the operation involves the direct transgression of major blood vessels, however, as is characteristic of vascular surgery, blood flow must be either temporarily or permanently interrupted. Temporary interruption requires the application of atraumatic vascular clamps or double-looped Silastic tapes after exposure and control of the vessels have been achieved, as illustrated in Figure 29–5. A valuable alternative during bypass to small calcified distal arteries, to avoid crushing or otherwise traumatizing them, is the application of a sterile pneumatic tourniquet during the distal anastomosis.

Anticoagulation

With ligation or division of major vessels, the surgeon does not ordinarily need to take any measures to prevent thrombus formation in the interrupted vessel. Thrombus formation usually occurs eventually within the blind end of the vessel and propagates back as far as the takeoff of the last major collateral. In most vascular procedures, however, the vessels are not simply divided but are explored, replaced, or bypassed; also, to ensure restoration of flow *after* an arteriotomy or venotomy has been closed or an anastomosis has been performed, the surgeon must either (1) prevent intravascular thrombus formation while flow is interrupted or (2) remove the accumulated thrombus immediately before completion of the final suture line. If a vessel, such as the external jugular vein of the dog, is occluded temporarily between two adjacent vascular clamps or nooses, the blood trapped in the intervening segment ordinarily does not clot. If the same vessel is simply opened and then closed with fine silk sutures, thrombosis commonly does occur. Understandably, such segmental vascular thrombosis is even more likely to occur

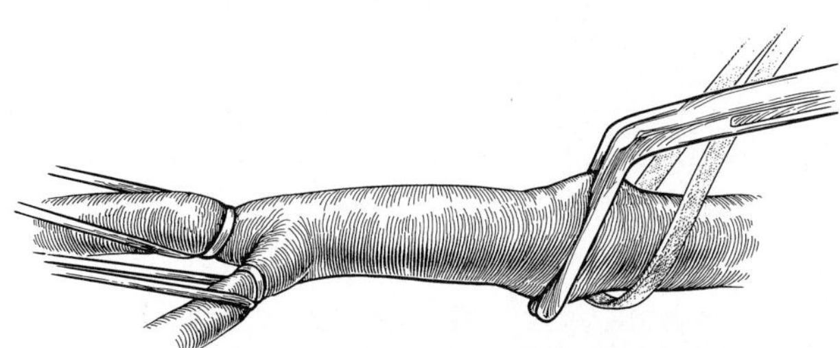

FIGURE 29–5. Two methods for obtaining temporary vascular control. A standard vascular clamp occludes the proximal inflow vessel, while less traumatic polymeric silicone (Silastic) loops are adequate for the smaller distal branches. (From Rutherford RB: Basic vascular techniques. *In* Atlas of Vascular Surgery: Basic Techniques and Exposures. Philadelphia, WB Saunders, 1993, p 16.)

in diseased vessels during the more extensive manipulations required in vascular surgery.

If the procedure is relatively simple, accumulated thrombus may be extracted with forceps or balloon catheters just before placement of the final sutures, and flow is thus restored before further clotting occurs. Although this practice is still used as an expedient in selected circumstances, it carries a small but definite risk of failure that has been made unnecessary by the introduction of heparin anticoagulation. This step is used in all but the simplest vascular procedures; the only major exception is thoracoabdominal aneurysm repair, in which timely flushing and irrigation are preferred to heparinization because of large anastomoses, high flows, and the risk of creating a bleeding diathesis.

Although spontaneous clotting may be retarded by aspirin, dextran, dipyridamole, and other drugs that reduce platelet aggregation, and by coumarin drugs that reduce the circulating levels of clotting factors II, VII, IX, and X, none of these drugs are reliable for preventing intravascular thrombosis during the performance of a major vascular procedure. In sufficient dosage, however, heparin does render blood incoagulable at normal temperatures and pH. The action of heparin is complex, affecting platelet adhesiveness, the endothelial cells' negative charge (or zeta potential), and the early phases of clotting by inhibiting the activation of factors IX and X. The major action of heparin is believed to result from its union with a cofactor in the blood to form an antithrombin that inhibits the conversion of fibrinogen to fibrin. Given intravenously, it has an effective action for up to 3 to 4 hours, or even longer with higher or repeated dosage.

A satisfactory level of anticoagulation may be achieved within 5 minutes after the intravenous injection of 100 units (~1.0 mg) per kg body weight of aqueous sodium heparin. For continued, sustained anticoagulation, as required during longer vascular procedures, one third to one half of this dose may be repeated at hourly intervals. During procedures in which the blood will be exposed to large surface areas of foreign material, as during cardiopulmonary bypass, larger doses of heparin (up to 300 units/kg) usually are advisable. Using larger doses also significantly lengthens the half-life of heparin.

Rendering the blood completely incoagulable, however, is not without its disadvantages. Wound surfaces that would remain naturally hemostatic may bleed profusely, and spontaneous bleeding may occur elsewhere in the body. Fortunately, these complications are extremely rare during most vascular operations, a common exception being repair of a thoracoabdominal aortic aneurysm.

Although the greatest risk of segmental thrombosis during a vascular procedure lies in the static circulation distal to the point of occlusion, regional heparinization cannot be achieved practically. Therefore, after dissection and exposure of the vessel has been carried out, including "tunneling," and after a porous knitted Dacron graft (if it is to be used) has been preclotted, the appropriate systemic dosage of heparin (usually 100 units/kg) is injected intravenously by the anesthesiologist at the direction of the surgeon. The time is noted so that half of this dose can be repeated in 1 to 1½ hours during longer procedures.

Whenever large tissue surfaces have been exposed during the course of the dissection or whenever there is extensive oozing of blood from the tissues or prosthesis after completion of the anastomosis, the heparin effect may be reversed before wound closure with an equivalent dose of protamine sulfate, that is, milligram for milligram, allowing for the temporal decay of heparin that was given earlier. It is important to remember that protamine (1) may cause hypotension if it is injected too rapidly and (2) may produce the opposite of the intended effect, namely, hypocoagulability, if it is administered in a dose in excess of that needed to counteract the heparin. For this reason, the surgeon usually asks the anesthesiologist to give half of the calculated dose over the first 5 minutes, and then an additional 5 mg every few minutes until the surgeon notes a decrease in oozing or the appearance of clots in the operative field. In most vascular procedures, however, protamine need not be given; instead, the effects of administered heparin are simply allowed to wear off.

VASCULAR INCISIONS AND CLOSURES

Entering a vessel through a simple lateral incision ranks only slightly above vessel ligature in complexity. The maneuver is used clinically to introduce catheters or cardiac bypass cannulas and to remove thrombi, emboli, or atheromatous deposits. Only two aspects deserve special consideration here:

- Manner of closure
- Direction of the incision

Closure of either longitudinal or transverse incisions usually produces some reduction in the cross-sectional area of the vessel. At normal systemic pressures, a reduction of almost 50% in diameter is required to produce a significant hemodynamic effect or gradient in most peripheral arteries. There may be some turbulence with lesser degrees of stenosis, however, particularly in low-flow, high-resistance situations. Furthermore, there is a tendency toward hypercoagulability in the immediate postoperative period, and these factors, combined with the break in intimal continuity and the presence of foreign (suture) material at the site of closure, may lead to thrombosis. For these reasons, care must be taken to minimize this narrowing.

Longitudinal incisions offer good exposure and can be extended readily (Fig. 29–6). They have the additional advantage of being convertible into an end-to-side anastomosis. Closure of a longitudinal incision in *smaller* (<4 mm) vessels, however, probably narrows the lumen over a greater distance than occurs with a transverse incision and therefore is more likely to produce significant stenosis and turbulence and lead to thrombosis. For this reason, a transverse arteriotomy or venotomy usually is preferable in smaller vessels (Fig. 29–7). When a longitudinal incision is necessary, narrowing of its closure may be obviated by the insertion of an elliptical patch graft of vein or Dacron into the arteriotomy (Fig. 29–8).

Placement of Vascular Sutures

Regardless of the manner in which the vascular suture is placed, two rules always should be observed:

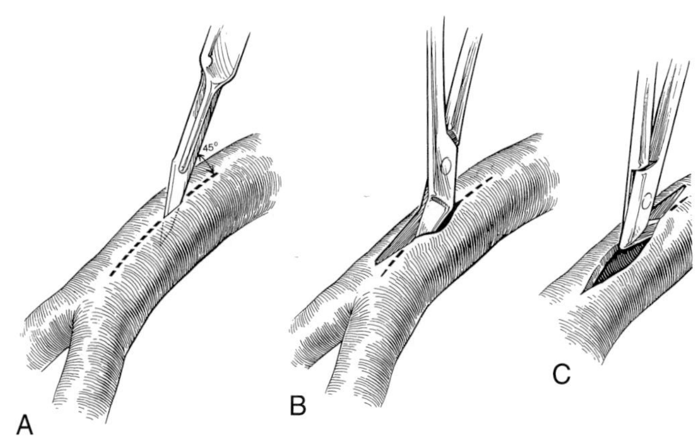

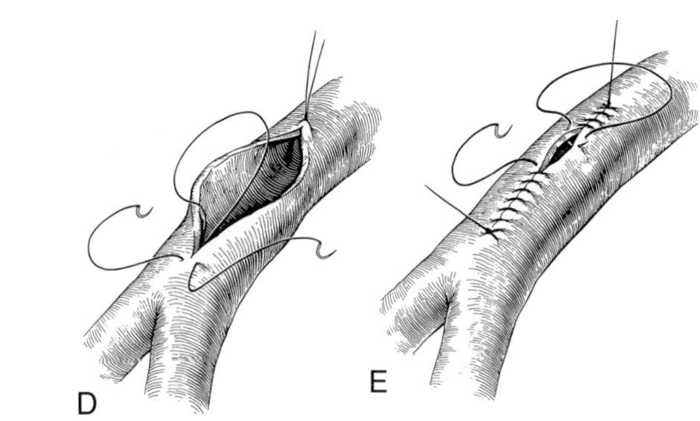

FIGURE 29–6. *A–E*, Longitudinal arteriotomy is begun with a sharp scalpel blade and completed with Potts scissors. Closure is accomplished with continuous suture, run from each end toward the middle. (From Rutherford RB: Basic vascular techniques. *In* Atlas of Vascular Surgery: Basic Techniques and Exposures. Philadelphia, WB Saunders, 1993, p 31.)

1. Excess adventitial tissue should be excised from the outer surface of the vessel so that it will not be dragged into the anastomosis and promote suture line thrombus formation.
2. The suture should pass through all layers, particular care being taken always to include the intima.

Interrupted sutures are still popular for very small anastomoses and in growing children to allow anastomotic growth. A simple over-and-over suture usually is chosen for most arterial closures or anastomoses, with "bites" taken 1 mm apart and 1 mm from the edges, unless the vessels are large, thick-walled, or diseased. Eversion of the edges

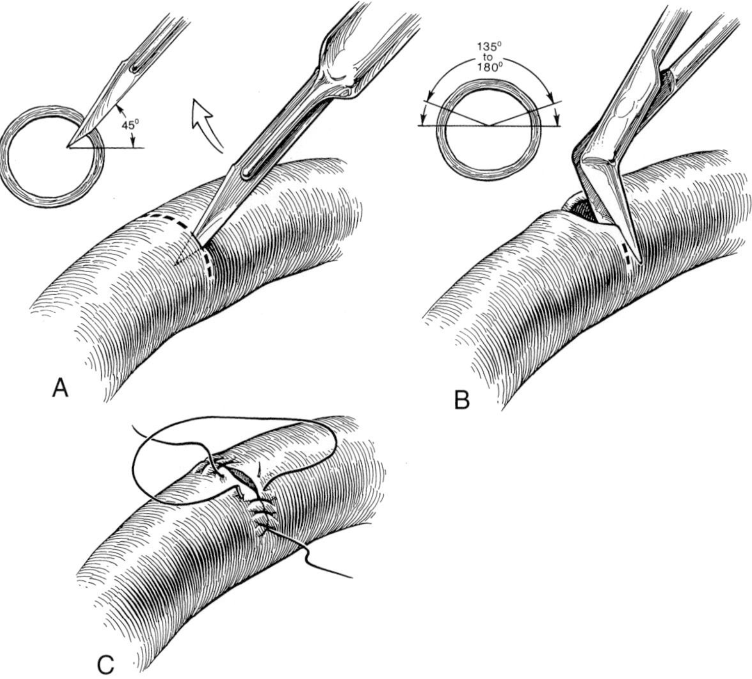

FIGURE 29–7. *A–C*, Transverse arteriotomy is performed first with a scalpel blade followed by enlargement to 135 to 180 degrees of the circumference using Potts scissors. Continuous closure, from both ends toward the middle, is most commonly employed. (From Rutherford RB: Basic vascular techniques. *In* Atlas of Vascular Surgery: Basic Techniques and Exposures. Philadelphia, WB Saunders, 1993, p 30.)

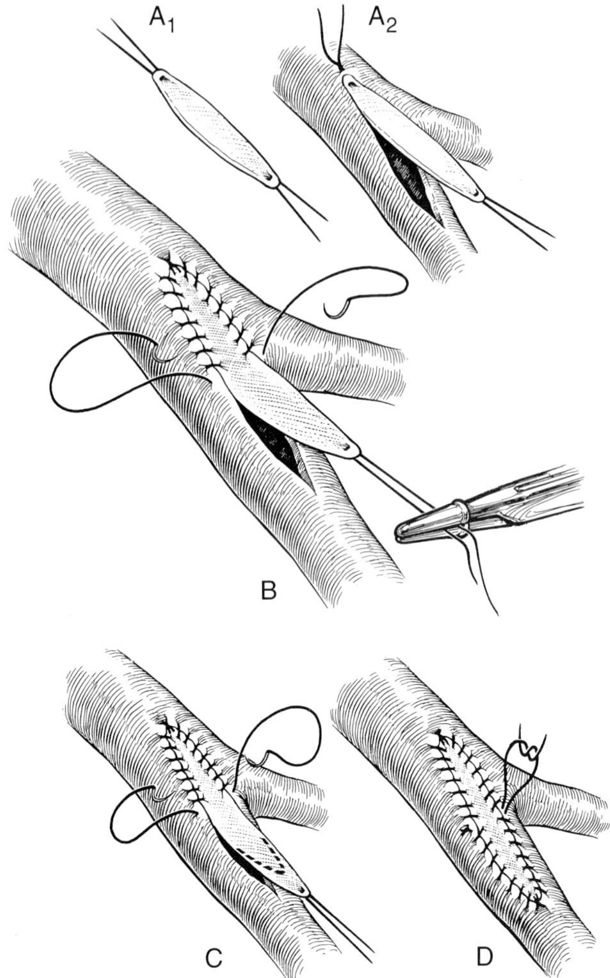

FIGURE 29–8. *A–D*, Patch angioplasty. A thin elliptical patch is fashioned, and mattress sutures are placed in both tips. One suture is carried into the corner of the arteriotomy and is tied to begin closure, aided by traction on the other suture. The closure is continued from each end, along the sides of the arteriotomy, toward the middle, where the sutures are tied to each other. Before the second corner is begun, the tip may need to be trimmed for better fit. (From Rutherford RB: Basic vascular techniques. *In* Atlas of Vascular Surgery: Basic Techniques and Exposures. Philadelphia, WB Saunders, 1993, p 33.)

to produce a smooth, sutureless internal surface by the placement of continuous or interrupted horizontal mattress sutures has lost much of its original popularity, mainly because the theoretical advantages have not been manifested in major arterial reconstructions and because the technique tends to produce a greater narrowing at the closure or anastomosis. Even with the simpler, over-and-over continuous suture, the surgeon can achieve some eversion in most anastomoses by starting each "corner" with a horizontal mattress suture (Kunlin's technique) and then gently holding out the edges of the vessel or graft with forceps as they are being sutured together.

Whenever possible, the direction of penetration of vessels should be from the inside out, with care being taken to include the intima. This issue is particularly important in suturing of arteriosclerotic arteries, in which penetration in the reverse direction may push a hard plaque inward rather than penetrate it, creating an intimal flap that may be dissected further by arterial flow and thus lead to occlusion. The vascular suture must be pulled taut continuously to avoid suture line bleeding at slack points. In this regard, vascular suture line bleeding can be stopped, in most cases, with finger tamponade, a little patience, and, occasionally, the help of a fine, superficially placed suture that draws more adventitia over the leak. If deeper sutures are required, flow should be interrupted again while they are placed; otherwise, new suture holes are created that may bleed more vigorously than the old.

The surgeon must take care as suturing nears the corner, or end, of an anastomosis to ensure that the opposite side of the vessel or graft is not being caught by the suture. Inserting a fine nerve hook with blunted point through the opening in the anastomosis as each stitch is placed is a useful precaution against this error. Another safeguard is the practice of always beginning at and sewing away from the corners and toward the "middle" of each suture line, using two separate sutures that are tied together there.

Methods of Vascular Interruption

The permanent interruption of flow through a major vessel may be accomplished in several ways (Fig. 29–9). Smaller arteries or veins may be divided between two hemostats before ligature and release of the clamps or, preferably, if there is adequate exposure, doubly ligated before division. In the latter approach, a curved or right-angle clamp usually is passed under the vessel after it has been dissected free, and a ligature, held taut by a clamp at its distal end,

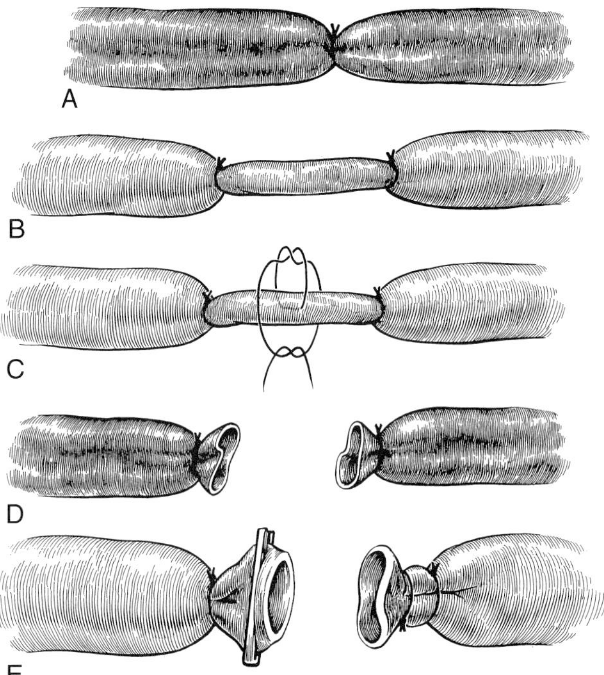

FIGURE 29–9. Vascular interruption techniques for small arteries and veins. *A*, Single ligation. *B*, Double ligation in continuity. *C*, Double ligation with intervening transfixion suture. *D*, Double ligation and division. *E*, Reinforcement of ligatured ends with a transfixion suture or metal clip. (From Rutherford RB: Basic vascular techniques. *In* Atlas of Vascular Surgery: Basic Techniques and Exposures. Philadelphia, WB Saunders, 1993, p 26.)

is "fed" into the grasp of the right-angle clamp and pulled around the vessel as the latter is withdrawn. This maneuver is repeated, the two ligatures then are tied, and the vessel between them is divided.

Because of the potential danger that pulsations, thrusting against the blind end of an artery that has been simply ligated and divided, eventually may force the ligatures off, it usually is advisable to ligate larger arteries doubly on *both* sides of the point of division, with the central one of each of these pairs of ligatures being a "transfixion" or "suture ligature" that is placed through the lumen of the vessel and tied on either side of it. Another alternative, which usually is reserved for the largest of vessels, is division between vascular clamps, followed by a formal closure of the cut ends by continuous vascular suture.

If, however, interruption of flow is all that is desired and division of the vessel is not required, ligation-in-continuity is an acceptable alternative to the maneuvers just mentioned; furthermore, if the vessel in question is short and difficult to control with vascular clamps, this may be not only the most expedient but also the safest approach. The recommended technique for ligation-in-continuity is to place two heavy ligature circumferences around the vessel, thereby interrupting flow, and then to place a transfixion suture between them to destroy intimal continuity and promote an organized thrombotic occlusion of that segment. This precaution is designed to prevent later recanalization, the major objection to simple ligation-in-continuity.

The clinical situation that best illustrates the application of the foregoing principles is that used in correcting a patent ductus arteriosus. Indeed, the early history of cardiovascular surgery was enriched and enlivened by studies and debates centering on the most appropriate technical approach for closing this congenital anomaly.

VASCULAR ANASTOMOSES

End-to-End Anastomosis

The end-to-end anastomosis is performed as follows:

1. It is usually begun with two corner sutures placed 180 degrees apart. Although they may be placed as simple sutures, a horizontal mattress suture results in slight eversion of the suture line and facilitates intima-to-intima approximation. If double-ended vascular sutures are used, these corner sutures are tied, both ends being left at equal length.
2. One needle from each corner is used to "run" the suture line in a simple over-and-over fashion to the middle of each side of the anastomosis, where the ends of the two sutures are tied together, completing the anterior half of the anastomosis.
3. The surgeon then rotates the vessel ends 180 degrees by moving the vascular clamps to expose the previous "posterior" half of the anastomosis.
4. The suture line is continued in an identical fashion to complete the anastomosis (Fig. 29–10).

If the vessel ends are not sufficiently mobile for this technique, the surgeon may perform the "posterior" half of the suture line transluminally or place the corner sutures directly anteriorly and posteriorly, instead of laterally, and sew from the posterior midline around each side to the anterior midline. With this approach, only minimal rotation of the vascular clamps is necessary to make the suture line readily visible.

A final option is "triangulation," in which the surgeon places three stay sutures 120 degrees apart and sews from one to the other much as described for the corner sutures,

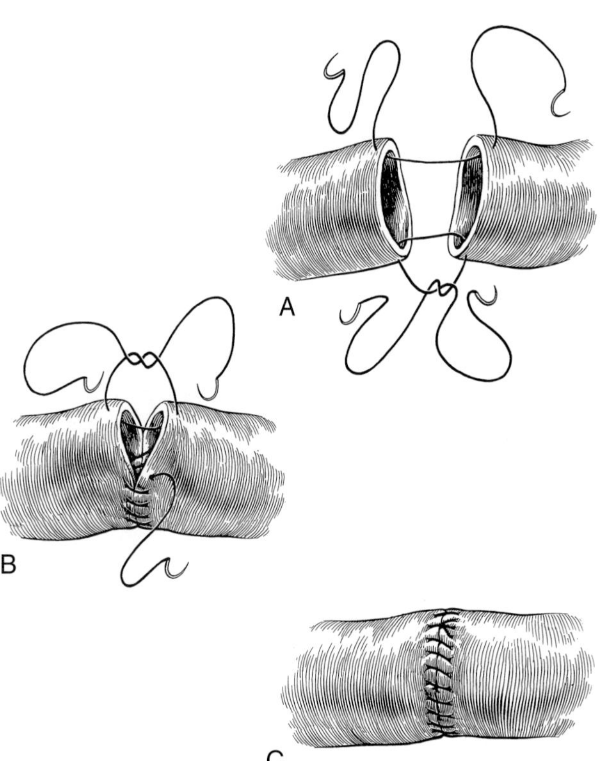

FIGURE 29–10. *A–C,* A simple perpendicular end-to-end anastomosis begun with two sutures 180 degrees apart and run continuously toward each other. (From Rutherford RB: Basic vascular techniques. *In* Atlas of Vascular Surgery: Basic Techniques and Exposures. Philadelphia, WB Saunders, 1993, p 35.)

rotating the vessel with the clamps so that the segment being sutured is always directly anterior. This maneuver avoids catching opposite walls in the tight corners that may be created with the use of two stay sutures 180 degrees apart. Unfortunately, it is usually most needed when there is limited exposure in small vessels, and in these circumstances the clamps may have to be reapplied rather than rotated.

If the vessels to be joined are relatively small (e.g., 2 to 5 mm in diameter), the surgeon may enlarge the anastomosis by beveling the ends 45 degrees in opposite directions. If the vessel is thin-walled and flexible, the surgeon can slit the opposing ends longitudinally for a length approximating the vessel's diameter but 180 degrees out of phase from each other and then round off the corners (Fig. 29–11). These flanged or beveled anastomoses are designed to avoid the circumferential, constricting effect that may be produced by a simple perpendicular end-to-end anastomosis in smaller vessels.

In addition, because a continuous suture, when used for end-to-end anastomosis, may result in "purse-stringing," or circumferential narrowing of the anastomosis, interrupted sutures may be preferred for end-to-end anastomosis of smaller vessels. If smooth, monofilament vascular sutures with doubled swaged-on needles are used, the sutures can be placed and left untied before completion of the anastomosis. The vascular clamps can then be slowly released, allowing the lumen to expand and the suture to slide slightly to accommodate this expansion (Fig. 29–12). The sutures are then tied while the clamps are briefly reapplied. These techniques apply as well to the direct interposition of a segment of vein or prosthetic graft as they do to a direct end-to-end anastomosis.

End-to-Side Anastomosis

The end-to-side anastomosis has wide clinical use in placement of arterial bypass grafts. The side of the "recipient" vessel may be prepared by elliptical excision or simple longitudinal incision, and the end of the donor vessel usually is beveled to produce an acute angle of entry and to minimize turbulence. Although the optimal angle of entry for an end-to-side anastomosis depends on the velocity of flow across it, this angle should be 30 to 45 degrees or less for arterial anastomosis. Such an acute angle results in a functional approximation and minimal turbulence.

As illustrated in Figure 29–13, end-to-side anastomosis is performed as follows:

1. The end of the donor vessel (vein or prosthetic graft) is fashioned (cut, beveled, or trimmed) to fit into the lateral opening in the recipient artery or vein, whose length is at least twice the diameter of the donor vessel.
2. The "heel" of the anastomosis is started first, with a running suture carried part way along each side.
3. The "toe" of the anastomosis is started, with continuous sutures brought along each side to meet the other sutures in the middle on both sides.

This heel-first, toe-last technique is the safest end-to-side technique. It ensures good hemostasis at the most inaccessible aspect (the heel), allows accurate suture placement at the most critical point to avoid narrowing (the

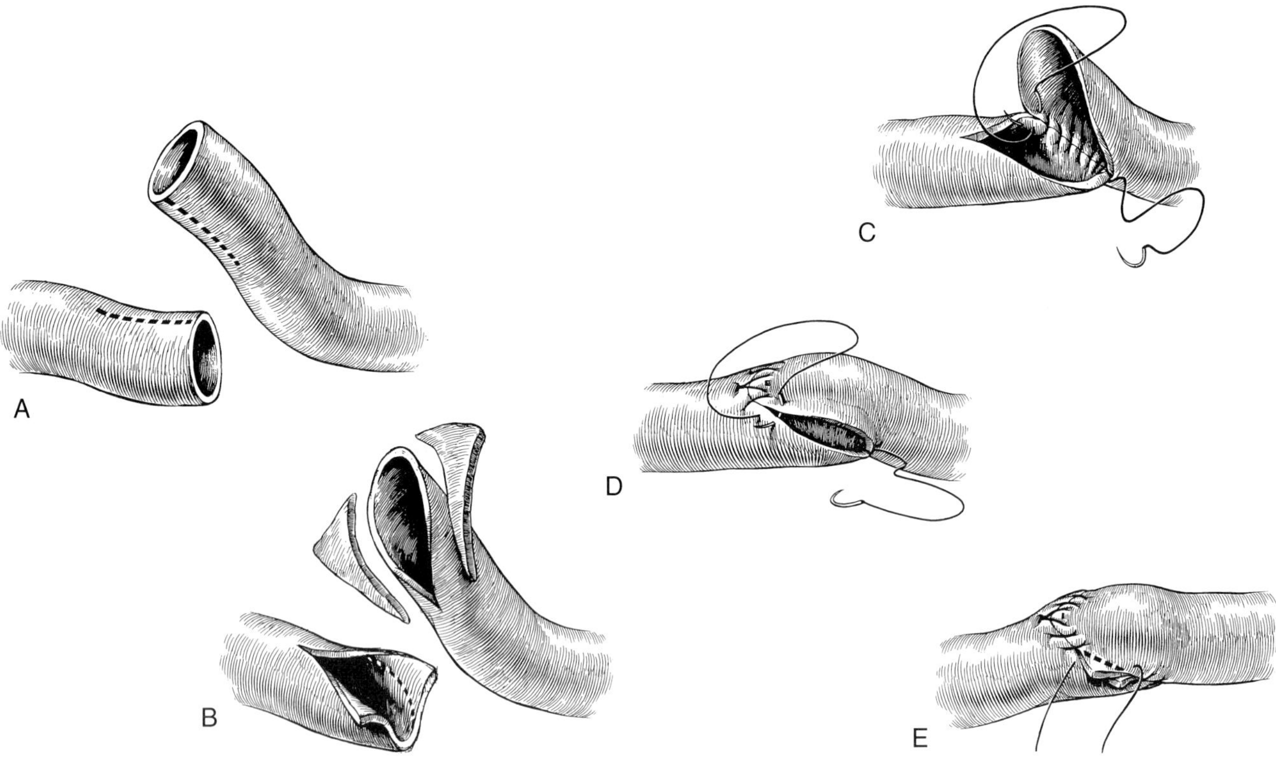

FIGURE 29–11. Technique of oblique end-to-end anastomosis. *A*, The two ends are slit 180 degrees apart. *B*, The resultant corners and adjacent lateral edges are trimmed conservatively. Anastomosis is (*C*) begun in one corner (head-to-toe) and (*D*) run to and around the opposite end and back toward the starting point. *E*, The other suture is run up to meet it in the middle, trimming any remaining "angles" to avoid "dog ears." (From Rutherford RB: Basic vascular techniques. *In* Atlas of Vascular Surgery: Basic Techniqes and Exposures. Philadelphia, WB Saunders, 1993, pp 40–41.)

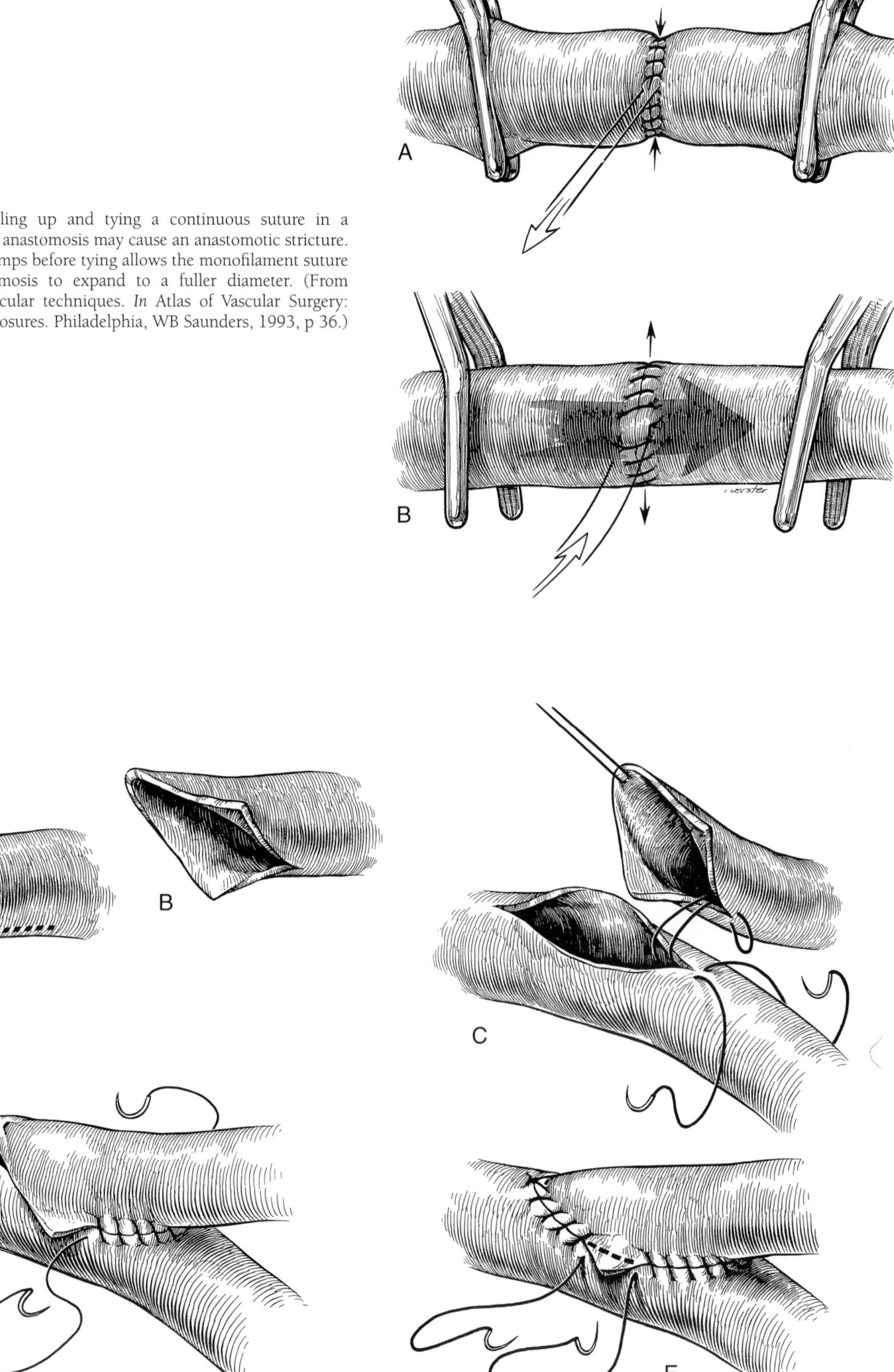

FIGURE 29–12. *A*, Pulling up and tying a continuous suture in a perpendicular end-to-end anastomosis may cause an anastomotic stricture. *B*, Briefly releasing the clamps before tying allows the monofilament suture to slide and the anastomosis to expand to a fuller diameter. (From Rutherford RB: Basic vascular techniques. *In* Atlas of Vascular Surgery: Basic Techniques and Exposures. Philadelphia, WB Saunders, 1993, p 36.)

FIGURE 29–13. Typical end-to-side, prosthesis-to-recipient artery anastomosis. *A* and *B*, The graft is trimmed. *C*, The "heel" of the anastomosis is started with a mattress suture. *D*, With the heel completed, the "toe" is begun with another horizontal mattress suture. *E*, Excess edges require trimming before completion. (From Rutherford RB: Basic vascular techniques. *In* Atlas of Vascular Surgery: Basic Techniques and Exposures. Philadelphia, WB Saunders, 1993, pp 50–51.)

toe), permits adjustments to be made in the fit of the anastomosis by trimming of the graft tip or lengthening of the arteriotomy (Fig. 29–14), and enables the final sutures to be placed quickly and accurately along the sides. Although the end to side anastomosis must be modified, depending on the nature of the host and donor vessels, it is equally applicable to the anastomosis of prosthesis to artery, vein to artery, vein to vein, and artery to artery. It is one of the most commonly used techniques in reconstructive vascular surgery.

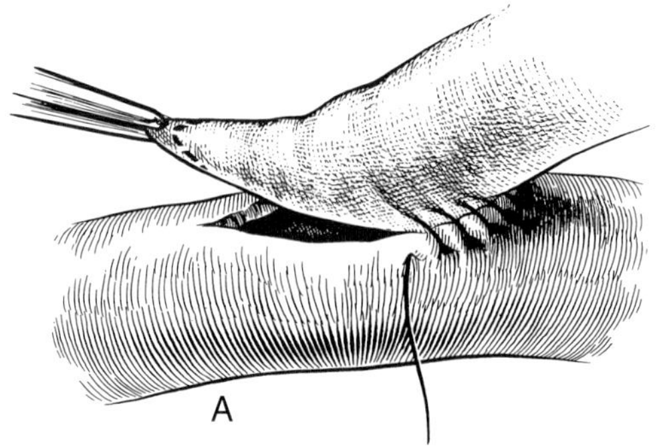

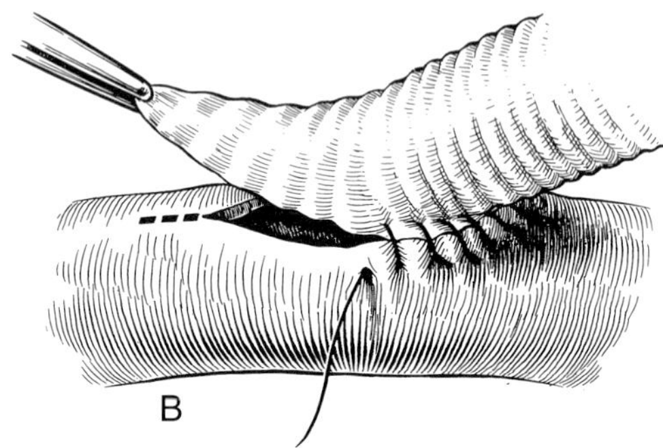

FIGURE 29–14. The advantages of the heel-first, toe-last sequence is illustrated. This method allows a final length adjustment by either trimming the tip (toe) (*A*) or extending the arteriotomy (*B*). (From Rutherford RB: Basic vascular techniques. *In* Atlas of Vascular Surgery: Basic Techniques and Exposures. Philadelphia, WB Saunders, 1993, p 53.)

Side-to-Side Anastomosis

Although the side-to-side anastomosis is not commonly used in clinical vascular surgery, the best-known examples of this technique probably are the side-to-side portacaval shunt, the Potts and Waterston aortopulmonary anastomosis, and arteriovenous fistulae. For this anastomosis:

1. A curved, spoon-shaped, or angled Satinsky's vascular clamp is placed laterally on adjacent segments of the two vessels to be anastomosed.
2. Matching longitudinal incisions are made in (or equal ellipses removed from) each segment.
3. The adjacent openings are sutured together with continuous suture, the posterior line being performed intraluminally.

There are many varieties of each of these basic techniques. Knowledge of them and of vascular exposures are the two major foundations of operative technique in vascular surgery. For further details of these and other basic techniques, the reader is referred to the companion volume, *Atlas of Vascular Surgery: Basic Techniques and Exposures.*[4]

REFERENCES

1. Carrel A: The surgery of blood vessels. Johns Hopkins Med J 18:18, 1907.
2. Guthrie CG: Heterotransplantation of blood vessels. Am J Physiol 19:482, 1907.
3. Carrel A: Heterotransplantation of blood vessels preserved in cold storage. J Exp Med 9:226, 1907.
4. Rutherford RB: An Atlas of Vascular Surgery: Basic Techniques and Exposures. Philadelphia, PA, WB Saunders, 1993.

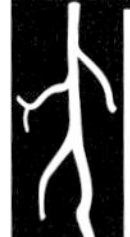

CHAPTER 30

Techniques for Thromboembolectomy of Native Arteries and Bypass Grafts

Ricardo T. Quintos II, M.D., and Frank J. Veith, M.D.

The need for thromboembolectomy of both native arteries and arterial bypass grafts almost always arises in current practice in patients who have advanced arteriosclerosis and who present with acute limb or organ ischemia (see also Chapters 28, 54, 55, 71, 79, 109, and 126). In the past, many patients with this presentation had an embolus arising from the heart and lodging at a bifurcation within a relatively disease-free arterial tree. Surgical removal of the embolus, either directly or with the aid of balloon catheters, was deemed one of the simplest of modern-day vascular operations. This is no longer the case because the elimination of rheumatic heart disease and atrial fibrillation means that almost all patients who currently present with acute limb ischemia have advanced underlying atherosclerosis. This results in atypical localization of emboli, difficulty in clearly differentiating embolization from thrombosis, greater difficulty in restoring adequate distal circulation, and the need for more complex vascular surgical procedures to do so. Moreover, these procedures must often be performed in patients who are quite ill from medical comorbidities.

Arterial embolectomy to treat acute occlusions was first attempted more than 100 years ago by Szabanajeff,[1] but it was only in 1911 when Einar Key in Stockholm and Georges Labey in Paris independently performed the first successful femoral embolectomies.[2] Labey's procedure[2] required extensive dissection to remove the embolus and its propagated thrombus. The associated morbidity and mortality did not generate much enthusiasm for the procedure, and over the next half century techniques of arterial embolectomy were sporadically reported in the literature with variable results.

The introduction of the balloon catheter technique in 1963[3] heralded an era of arterial thromboembolectomy with reduced morbidity. This technique permitted removal of thromboembolic material from sites proximal and distal to the arteriotomy with a minimum of invasiveness and tissue dissection. As the devices and the procedure became standardized, balloon thromboembolectomy became a suitable, safe, and effective method for the revascularization of an acutely occluded vessel.

Over the next three decades, changing trends in the etiology of acute occlusions have led to a demonstrated decline in the effectiveness of simple balloon catheter embolectomy.[4, 5] Because of this change in results, various methods have been developed either to replace or to serve as an adjunct to simple balloon catheter embolectomy. Nevertheless, balloon catheter embolectomy by itself or with adjunctive techniques continues to be a valuable tool in the treatment of acute arterial occlusion. In this chapter, we describe both established and newer techniques for performing surgical thromboembolectomy when indicated in the patient population. Most of the established techniques depend on use of the single-lumen balloon thromboembolectomy catheter, although a variety of newer catheters are also described. In standard practice, all of these catheters are passed blindly through the lumen of the arterial tree, a maneuver that can be difficult or impossible when extensive arteriosclerotic plaque is present. The newer techniques use catheters, guide wires, balloons, and stents placed under digital fluoroscopic control to improve and simplify thromboembolectomy of both native arteries and grafts.

GENERAL CONSIDERATIONS

The first important consideration in regard to a thromboembolectomy is determining the underlying cause of the acute occlusion. Since about 1960, and especially since 1970, this etiologic mechanism has changed from cardiac emboli from rheumatic heart disease to cardiac emboli from myocardial infarction or atrial fibrillation and in situ thrombotic events secondary to generalized atherosclerosis.[5, 6] The typical patient with acute arterial occlusion has changed from a young person with rheumatic heart disease to an older, medically ill person with diffuse arterial disease.[7] Although some authors claim that an occlusion arising from atherosclerotic thrombus has many characteristics in common with true emboli and therefore the intervention should basically be the same,[8] the etiology of the acute ischemic event (whether true embolism or thrombosis in the setting of severe peripheral vascular disease) significantly influences the success or failure of a simple embolectomy.[5]

Obtaining a complete history and physical examination, including bilateral ankle-brachial indices (ABIs) and segmental pressures, gives an indication of the underlying presence of chronic disease. Full *arteriography* should generally be performed before operation for several reasons. Precise arteriographic localization of the occlusion helps the surgeon to place the incision in the optimal site. In addition, unexpected inflow disease may be detected and appropriate sites of inflow and outflow may be selected should a bypass be required. Nonocclusive ischemia may be ruled out.[9] Finally, unsuspected second emboli may be detected and treated. Indeed, multiplicity of occlusions in locations not usually sites of chronic disease is one of the most certain pieces of evidence to support embolization as the etiologic mechanism of the acute ischemic event. The arteriogram can thus provide important information about the occlusive event and delineate the management plan accordingly.

A simple balloon embolectomy may be limb- and lifesaving in most cases of true embolism; however, for an acute thrombotic event superimposed on chronic progressive occlusive disease, this procedure by itself usually does not suffice for revascularization, and adjunctive techniques or a well-planned and well-executed bypass operation may be required to achieve a successful outcome.

Another issue concerns the choice of instrumentation. Since its introduction in 1963, the embolectomy catheter has undergone minor modifications, but the general concept behind its use has remained relatively constant.[10, 11] The catheter consists of a hollow, pliable shaft with a compliant, distensible balloon at the distal end (Fig. 30–1, top). The compliant balloon is effective in extracting true emboli and the acute clot formed from stasis at a critically narrowed segment. The compliance of the balloon, while having the advantage of minimizing intimal trauma, proves disadvantageous for removal of the occlusion due to plaque from atherosclerotic disease (Fig. 30–2). For managing more adherent clots, a latex-covered spiral cable catheter has been developed that is more effective in extracting the dense, adherent, mature thrombus (see Fig. 30–1, middle). A spiral cable catheter without the latex covering is advocated for use in synthetic grafts (see Fig. 30–1, bottom). This graft thrombectomy catheter works as a ringed variable diameter device that strips out densely adherent fibrinous material associated with graft healing. Additional discussions of the causes, methods, and instrumentation for managing arterial thromboembolism are presented in Chapters 28 and 55.

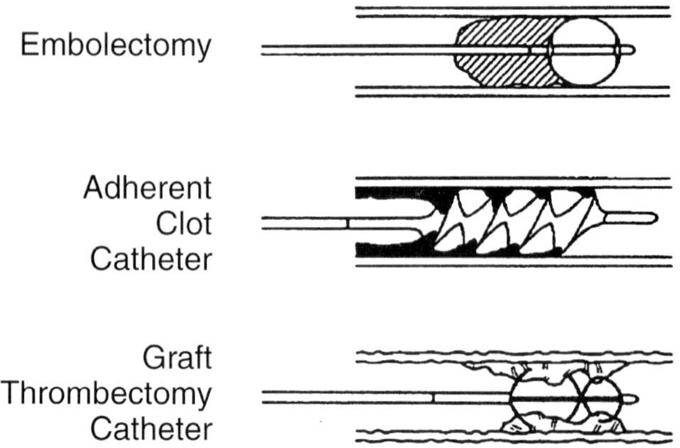

FIGURE 30–1. Types of thromboembolectomy catheters. (From Fogarty TJ, White JV: Thrombectomy, Pharmacological and Mechanical Thrombolysis. *In* Ahn SS, Hodgson KJ [eds]: Handbook on Endovascular Procedures. Coursebook for NA-ISCVS/SVS Third Annual Endovascular Surgery Workshop, San Diego, June 1998.)

A third consideration is ensuring the least amount of arterial injury. Balloon catheter embolectomy is not without its complications and injurious effects.[12] The correlation between shear forces applied to the arterial wall during instrumentation and the degree of intimal injury resulting in intimal hyperplasia is well recognized.[13–15] Some authors compared the different brands of balloon embolectomy catheters and their potential for injury and intimal damage.[8, 9] Although differences among the various brands have been described, these differences are slight. Moreover, freedom from underlying chronic disease and the use of the proper technique may have more to do with preventing intimal damage than the choice of any particular brand of balloon catheter.[16]

ESTABLISHED BALLOON CATHETER THROMBOEMBOLECTOMY TECHNIQUE

Operative catheter thromboembolectomy begins with exposure of an adequate length of artery to allow control both proximal and distal to the catheter introduction site. A transverse arteriotomy was used in the past, but we now prefer a *longitudinal incision* to allow for the possibility of converting the arteriotomy to a graft anastomotic site if a bypass is required. Careful closure with or without a patch does not produce luminal narrowing, even in small diseased arteries. After opening the artery, we inspect the lumen to ensure that catheter passage does not take place subintimally.

The balloon catheter is inspected and prepared for use. The balloon is inflated with saline and checked for concentricity and leaks. Concentricity is important because an eccentric balloon will displace the catheter tip and body toward one side of the arterial wall and will produce increased drag and friction.[17] Inflation and deflation of the balloon are repeated to make the balloon more pliable. This increases balloon control during the procedure. Small-bore syringes are recommended for balloon inflation, but some find that the smaller stroke distance resulting from the use of larger-bore syringes affords finer control. For smaller-diameter catheters (1 Fr. and 2 Fr.), air is used to inflate the balloon because the inflation lumen of these catheters is too tiny to permit quick adjustments in balloon size if saline inflation is performed. When even small amounts of air may be hazardous, as in the cerebral vasculature, carbon dioxide can be used for inflation.

Before occluding arteries and introducing the balloon catheter, we give systemic heparin (1 to 1.5 mg/kg). Catheter advancement must be performed with great care. Although the pliable embolectomy catheter is designed to facilitate passage, cannulation may be difficult at times because of arterial disease or tortuosity. A common site of difficulty is the popliteal artery. Varying the angle of knee flexion may allow the catheter to pass. Persistent inability to pass the catheter indicates atherosclerotic obstruction or narrowing of the vessel, and it is more prudent to assess the area using intraoperative arteriography rather than persist in potentially damaging attempts at catheter passage. It may be advantageous to place the incision below the knee and the arteriotomy at the distal popliteal artery to perform safe embolectomy of the distal popliteal and its branches.[18]

Catheter retrieval must be performed in a gentle manner with the least possible amount of shear force, repeated the least possible number of times that ensures complete clot extraction. When a large amount of pull force is required to remove the catheter, either the balloon has been overinflated, or the lumen of the artery is being narrowed by plaque. In these cases, balloon inflation should be diminished. On the other hand, when the balloon embolectomy catheter is withdrawn from a vessel with an increasing diameter, addition of saline may be required for the balloon to maintain arterial wall contact. Balloon overinflation causes an inordinate amount of shear force to be exerted on the arterial endothelium. Endothelial injury and plaque dislodgment may occur. Certain techniques for decreasing shear force and friction have been described. These include slowly inflating the balloon in the first half centimeter of catheter motion during withdrawal and allowing a small amount of heparinized blood in the lumen proximal to the point of embolic obstruction.[19]

The importance of distal catheter passage cannot be overemphasized. Distal thrombus may be discontinuous with proximal thrombus. Vigorous backflow resulting from proximal thromboembolectomy can give false assurance of

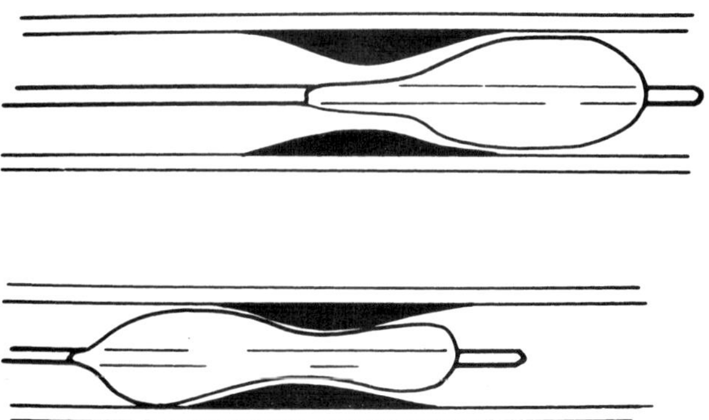

FIGURE 30–2. Compliance of the embolectomy balloon.

distal patency. Failure to remove the distal thrombus results in the retained thrombus propagating proximally to cause reocclusion. Patency of the distal vasculature must always be confirmed by completion arteriography or return of distal pulses (pedal or radial).

EMBOLECTOMY IN SPECIFIC VESSELS

Aortoiliac Embolectomy

Bilateral groin incisions are made, and the common, superficial, and deep femoral arteries are isolated and controlled with vessel loops or clamps (Fig. 30–3). Prior to arteriotomy, the common femoral artery is palpated to determine the location of plaque. A longitudinal arteriotomy is made proximal to the bifurcation to allow visualization when the superficial and deep femoral arteries are cannulated. Distal exploration is carried out first through the superficial and deep femoral arteries. Passage of a long (15 to 20 cm) length of a No. 2 or No. 3 Fr. embolectomy catheter ensures that the deep femoral artery, rather than one of the large circumflex branches that arise from this vessel, has been cannulated.

Following distal embolectomy, heparin-saline solution is infused into the femoral system and the common femoral artery is clamped. Embolectomy of the aorta and the ipsilateral iliac artery with a No. 6 Fr. catheter is carried out while the contralateral common femoral artery is occluded in order to prevent clot dislodgment into the opposite distal arterial tree. The contralateral side is explored in a smaller manner to rule out embolization that may have occurred to either side (Fig. 30–3). After flow is restored, complete clearing of the arterial tree must be confirmed by the detection of pedal pulses. If these cannot be detected, completion arteriography is mandatory, and a bypass may be required.

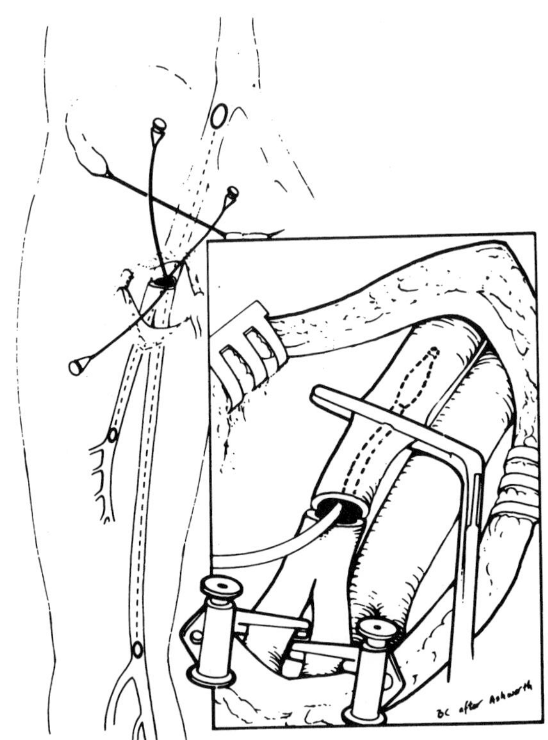

FIGURE 30–3. Cannulation of both proximal and distal vessels in aortoiliac embolectomy. Although a transverse arteriotomy may be used, a longitudinal arteriotomy is preferred.

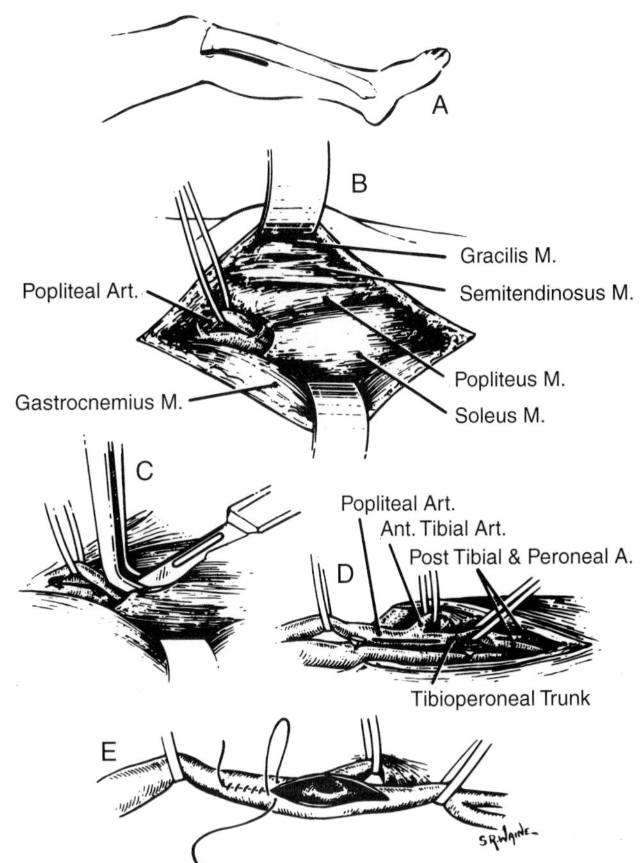

FIGURE 30–4. Embolectomy of the distal popliteal artery. *A*, Incision for exposure of the distal popliteal artery. *B*, Exposure of the vascular bundle after incision of the deep fascia and retraction of gastrocnemius muscle posteriorly. *C*, Division of overlying soleus muscle fibers. *D*, Mobilized distal popliteal artery, anterior tibial artery, and tibioperoneal trunk and position of longitudinal incision in the artery. *E*, Ostia of anterior tibial artery as seen through the arteriotomy and closure of the arteriotomy with fine vascular sutures without producing any stenosis. *M* = muscle; Art. = artery; Ant. = anterior. (From Gupta SK, Samson RH, Veith FJ: Embolectomy of the distal part of the popliteal artery. Surg Gynecol Obstet 153:254, 1981.)

Infrainguinal Embolectomy

Infrainguinal occlusions are approached through a groin incision. Catheter explorations through the superficial and deep femoral systems are carried out as just described. Two catheters No. 2 or No. 3 Fr. are sequentially passed into the distal lower extremity. The first catheter usually passes into the peroneal or posterior tibial artery. Inflating the balloon may allow the subsequent catheter to pass into the anterior tibial artery.[20] When occlusions involve the popliteal artery and its trifurcated branches, it is best to approach the arterial tree with a below-knee incision.[18] The arteriotomy is placed opposite the origin of the anterior tibial artery (Fig. 30–4). With this approach, it is easier to pass the catheter into all three crural arteries, and damage to a slightly diseased superficial femoral artery is avoided.

Upper Extremity Occlusions

An arteriotomy is performed in the brachial artery just proximal to the bifurcation at the antecubital fossa to allow access and control of all three arteries.[21, 22] Emboli in the proximal subclavian artery can be removed by retrograde extraction, although one must continually be aware of the possibility of fragmentation of emboli during extraction with displacement to the cerebral circulation.

Renal and Mesenteric Occlusions

The techniques for management of renal and mesenteric embolic occlusions (see Chapters 109 and 126) are similar to those described for management for peripheral occlusions, albeit with two major differences. First, because the external support provided by adjacent tissue is significantly less in the vessels supplying the viscera than in those of the peripheral vasculature, the risk of perforation is higher in these vessels. Therefore, catheter advancement and manipulations should be performed with greater care and gentleness. Second, procedures in these arterial systems must be accomplished under angiographic or fluoroscopic control and never as a blind procedure, as has been done in the past.

Graft Thrombectomy

Prosthetic graft thrombectomy (see Chapter 71) is performed in a similar manner to that done on native arteries. An initial extraction using the balloon catheter is accomplished with the extraction of soft clots, followed by passage of special catheters, described previously, that address the problem of removing the adherent thrombus that is frequently encountered in artificial conduits. The catheter is passed in the low-profile configuration until it is positioned within the region of the adherent material within the graft. The pitch of the spiral retrieval element is then adjusted to engage the adherent material, and the catheter is withdrawn through the arteriotomy or graftotomy.

Intraoperative Monitoring and Postprocedure Assessment and Evaluation

The aim of surgical embolectomy is to restore the peripheral circulation to its preocclusive state. Evaluation of results must be based on restoration of pulses or completion arteriography. Complete extraction of the embolus and the propagated thrombus is absolutely necessary for the success of the procedure. One clue to the completeness of extraction is the appearance of the extracted thrombus. Usually, although not always, a smooth, tapering clot indicates adequate removal; a sharp cutoff suggests that additional thrombotic material remains. As mentioned previously, vigorous back-bleeding is not an indicator of the completeness of thromboembolectomy. The presence of a water-hammer pulse suggests distal obstruction. Even with these clues and arteriography, however, it may still be difficult to assess results in atherosclerotic patients.

Completion arteriography or fluoroscopy remains the standard for the evaluation of procedural success. It has been reported that up to 68% of thromboembolectomies clinically deemed successful required reinterventions for residual lesions detected by radiographic means.[23] Digital fluoroscopy is a valuable newer adjunct that, in addition to demonstrating the success of the procedure, can facilitate the accurate identification, localization, and treatment of significant underlying arterial lesions during the procedure.[24, 25]

NEWER TECHNIQUES AND PROCEDURES FOR THROMBOEMBOLECTOMY

The traditional methods of thromboembolectomy have the disadvantage of being performed blindly. Information is not provided to the surgeon regarding the extent of clot removal or the localization of underlying disease. Techniques employing fluoroscopically guided catheters and guide wires eliminate the blind aspects of the procedure. These techniques allow the operator to (1) manipulate and direct the catheter through difficult, diseased arteries and branches, (2) monitor and control balloon inflation, (3) detect and retrieve any residual clot, and (4) detect and treat underlying hemodynamically significant atherosclerotic plaque.

Fluoroscopically Assisted Thromboembolectomy

Fluoroscopically guided catheter and guide wire thromboembolectomy has been used and described by our group.[25] This method uses digital cinefluoroscopy with a mobile C-arm unit (Philips BV 212) and catheter-based endovascular techniques to facilitate balloon catheter passage and the accurate identification, localization, and treatment of the underlying arterial lesions. It also reduces the risk of arterial damage and intimal injury. With the use of a directional catheter and guide wires, even tortuous diseased arteries can be traversed under fluoroscopic guidance (Fig. 30–5). The balloon catheter can be inflated with contrast and withdrawn to remove the clot while the balloon configuration is visualized fluoroscopically. This prevents overdistention of the balloon and allows identification of stenosing lesions as they distort the image of the balloon.

After the clot is removed, these lesions may be confirmed angiographically by injection into a catheter or the sidearm of the hemostatic sheath. Once identified, the lesion can be treated by an angioplasty balloon or stent placement. This technique, therefore, provides immediate feedback and allows immediate interventional elimination of uncovered lesions.

To perform retrograde iliac thrombectomy, the surgeon inserts a hemostatic vascular sheath into the artery and uses a guide wire and directional catheter to cross the occluded or diseased arterial segments (Fig. 30–6; see Fig. 30–5). The sheath is then advanced over the wire; the dilator is removed, and a standard balloon catheter is passed (see Fig. 30–5). The sheath is retracted, and the

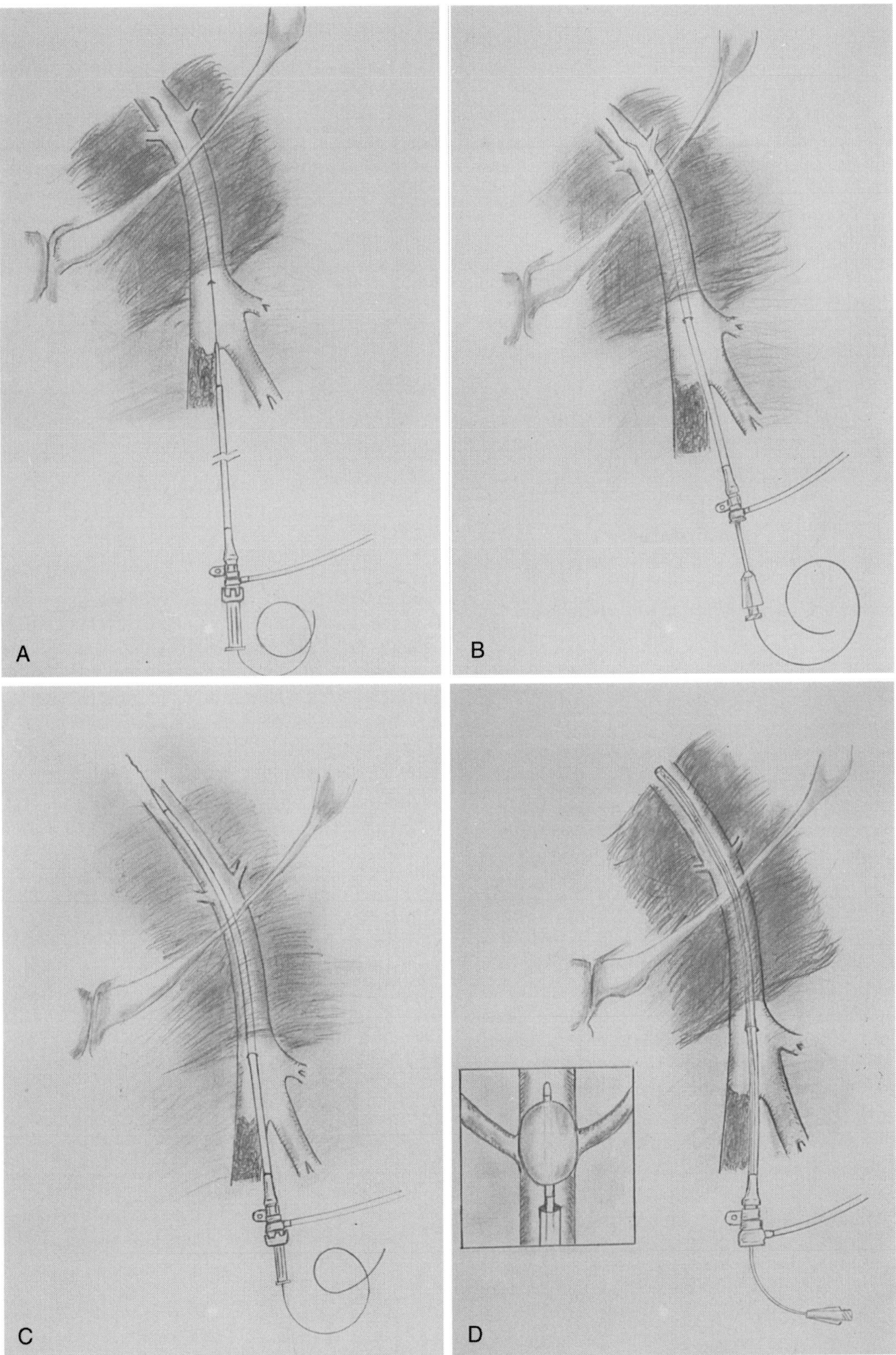

FIGURE 30–5. Diagrams illustrating fluoroscopically assisted thromboembolectomy using over-the-wire technique I. *A*, Guide wire has been inserted a short distance through a needle. Needle has been removed, and hemostatic sheath and its dilator are being advanced over the guide wire. Entrance through arterial wall is facilitated by rotating sheath and dilator as they are advanced as a unit. *B*, After removal of dilator, directional catheter (Berenstein) is inserted through sheath over wire. Under fluoroscopic guidance, wire is advanced well into external iliac artery. *C*, Catheter is removed, leaving wire and sheath in place. Dilator is replaced, and sheath and dilator are advanced over wire well into external iliac artery. *D*, Dilator is removed along with guide wire, leaving sheath within iliac artery. Balloon catheter is advanced within sheath. After retracting the sheath, the balloon is inflated with dilute contrast and withdrawn under fluoroscopic guidance to remove clot and identify lesions (*inset*). (Adapted from Veith FJ, Sanchez LA, Ohki T: Technique for obtaining proximal intraluminal control when arteries are inaccessible or unclampable because of disease or calcification. J Vasc Surg 27:582, 1998.)

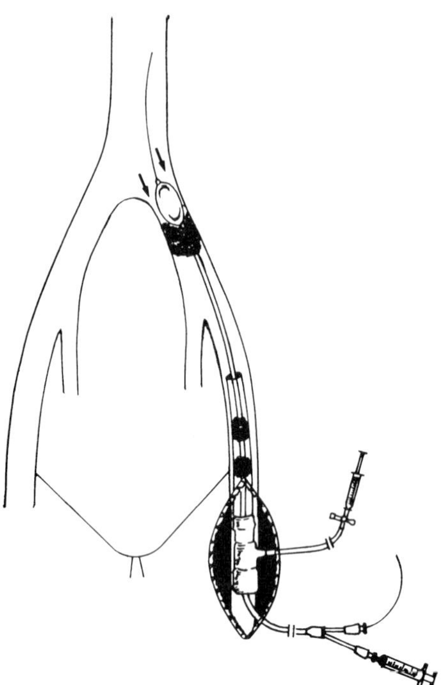

FIGURE 30–6. Diagram illustrating fluoroscopically assisted thromboembolectomy using over-the-wire technique II. Following passage of a radiographic guide wire, a balloon thrombectomy catheter equipped with two lumens is passed through a hemostatic valve in a previously placed vascular sheath. Under fluoroscopic control, the balloon is withdrawn through the vessel containing the clot, and the clot is advanced into the introducer sheath. Several passes of the balloon thrombectomy catheter may be made prior to the removal of the sheath containing the thrombectomized clot. (From Parsons RE, Marin ML, Veith FJ, et al. Fluoroscopic assisted thromboembolectomy: An improved method for treating acute arterial occlusions. Ann Vasc Surg 10:201, 1996.)

inflated balloon is withdrawn to remove the clot. Alternatively, a double-lumen balloon catheter may be inserted over the wire and passed through the occlusion (see Fig. 30–6). Under fluoroscopic guidance, the balloon is filled with dilute contrast medium until the balloon profile approaches the size of the underlying vessel lumen. Gentle withdrawal of the balloon catheter is then undertaken under fluoroscopic control. Deformities of the balloon profile caused by underlying arterial lesions are identified and the locations noted. These lesions can be treated by repeated thrombectomy, angioplasty with or without stent placement, or surgical revascularization.

Intraoperative Thrombolysis

Certain situations may arise in which the distal outflow tract is occluded by clots that cannot be retrieved by mechanical means. In these instances, intraoperative thrombolysis may offer a viable option for revascularization.[26, 27] After removal of as much thrombus as possible using mechanical extraction devices, the inflow artery is occluded and boluses of urokinase are instilled distally. After 20 minutes, angiography and the urokinase bolus are repeated until the distal bed is cleared of clot. This procedure and the use of percutaneous catheter-directed urokinase to treat acute thromboembolic occlusions are discussed further in Chapters 28 and 55.

Aspiration Thromboembolectomy

A possible adjunct or alternative to thrombolysis and surgical embolectomy is aspiration thromboembolectomy.[28, 29] This method may be performed percutaneously or via an open arteriotomy. The technique involves passage of a No. 8 Fr. sheath through which a No. 5 or No. 8 Fr. aspiration catheter is advanced along a guide wire to the site of the occlusion. A 50-ml syringe is then used to apply suction to the end of the aspiration catheter. Withdrawal of the aspiration catheter is carried out while suction is maintained. Repeated aspirations are performed to clear the occlusion. The limitation of the technique is that it can only be used in distal peripheral acute occlusions and not in the larger arterial branches, such as the iliac arteries, because of the large volumes of material that would require aspiration in these vessels.

SUMMARY

The changing trends in etiology and patient population in acute arterial occlusion dictate that the treatments be modified accordingly in order to achieve optimum results. Although simple balloon catheter thromboembolectomy has greatly improved the management of acute arterial occlusion, the occurrence of thromboembolic problems in patients with increasingly advanced underlying arteriosclerosis means that patients will be increasingly difficult to treat. This mandates that we improve our diagnostic and therapeutic techniques to improve results in this challenging group of patients. To this end, the use of digital cinefluoroscopy and catheter–guide wire techniques combined with endovascular treatments, such as angioplasty and stents, are important technical adjuncts that can simplify and improve balloon thromboembolectomy procedures in the future.

Acknowledgments: U.S. Public Health Service (Grant No. HL02990-04), the James Hilton Manning and Emma Austin Manning Foundation, the Anna S. Brown Trust, and the New York Institute for Vascular Studies.

REFERENCES

1. Szabanajeff: On the question of blood vessel suture. Russk Khir Arkh 11:625, 1895.
2. Labey, cited by Mesney M, Dumont NJ: Embolie femorale au cours d'um retrecissement mitral pur. Arteriotomie. Guerison Bull Acad Med 66:358, 1911.
3. Fogarty TJ, Cranley JJ, Krause RJ, et al: A method for extraction of arterial emboli and thrombi. Surg Gynecol Obstet 116:241, 1963.
4. Hight DW, Tilney NL, Couch NP: Changing clinical trends in patients with peripheral arterial emboli. Surgery 79:172, 1976.
5. Hill SL, Donato AT: The simple Fogarty embolectomy: An operation of the past? Am Surgeon 60:907, 1994.
6. Braithwaite BD, Earnshaw JJ: Arterial embolectomy: A century and out. Br J Surg 81:1705, 1994.
7. Haimovici H, Moss CM, Veith FJ: Arterial embolectomy revisited. Surgery 78:(4)409, 1975.
8. Fogarty TJ, Hermann GD: New techniques for clot extraction and managing acute thromboembolic limb ischemia. *In* Veith FJ (ed): Current Critical Problems in Vascular Surgery. Vol 3. St. Louis, Quality Medical Publishing, 1991, pp 197–203.

9. Dardik H, Dardik I, Spreyregen S, Veith FJ: Asymmetrical nonocclusive ischemia of the lower extremities. JAMA 227:1417, 1974.
10. Niblet PG, Fleischl JM, Campbell WB: Which balloon embolectomy catheter? Br J Surg 77:930, 1990.
11. Schwarcz TH, Dobrin PB, Mrkvicka R, et al: Balloon embolectomy catheter-induced arterial injury: A comparison of four catheters. J Vasc Surg 11:382. 1990.
12. Foster JH, Carter JW, Edwards WH, et al: Arterial injuries secondary to the use of the Fogarty catheter. Ann Surg 171:971, 1970.
13. Goldberg EM, Goldberg MC, Chowdhury LN, et al: The effects of balloon embolectomy-thrombectomy catheters on vascular architecture. J Cardiovasc Surg 24:74, 1983.
14. Chidi C, DePalma R: Atherogenic potential of the embolectomy catheter. Surgery 83:549, 1987.
15. Jorgensen RA, Drobin PB: Balloon embolectomy catheters in small arteries: IV. Correlation of shear forces with histologic injury. Surgery 93:798, 1983.
16. Bowles CR, Olcott C, Pakter RL, et al: Diffuse arterial narrowing as a result of intimal proliferation: A delayed complication of embolectomy with the Fogarty balloon catheter. J Vasc Surg 7:487, 1988.
17. Dobrin PB, Jorgensen RA: Balloon embolectomy catheters in small arteries: III. Surgical significance of eccentric balloons. Surgery 93:402, 1983.
18. Gupta SK, Samson RH, Veith FJ: Embolectomy of the distal part of the popliteal artery. Surg Gynecol Obstet 153:254, 1981.
19. Dobrin PB, Jorgensen RA: Balloon embolectomy catheters in small arteries: A technique to prevent excessive shear forces. J Vasc Surg 2:692, 1985.
20. Santiago O, Diethrich EB, Bahadir I, et al: A double balloon occlusion technique for embolectomy in the trifurcation vessels. Surg Gynecol Obstet 174:164, 1992.
21. Haimovici H: Cardiogenic embolism of the upper extremity. J Cardiovasc Surg 23:209, 1982.
22. Dregelid E: Diameter of the brachial artery: The selection of arteriotomy site for embolectomy. Ann Chir Gynaecol 76:222, 1987.
23. Crolla RM, van de Pavoordt ED, Moll FL: Intraoperative digital subtraction angiography after thromboembolectomy: Preliminary experience. J Endovasc Surg 2:168, 1995.
24. Robicsek F: Dye-enhanced fluoroscopy-directed catheter embolectomy. Surgery 95:622, 1984.
25. Parsons RE, Marin ML, Veith FJ, et al: Fluoroscopically assisted thromboembolectomy: An improved method for treating acute arterial lesions. Ann Vasc Surg 10:201, 1996.
26. Quinones-Baldrich WJ, Zierler RE, Hiatt JC: Intraoperative fibrinolytic therapy: An adjunct to catheter thromboembolectomy. J Vasc Surg 2:319, 1985.
27. Beard JD, Nyanekye I, Earnshaw JJ, et al: Intraoperative streptokinase: A useful adjunct to balloon catheter embolectomy. Br J Surg 80:21, 1993.
28. Murray JG, Brown AL, Wilkins RA: Percutaneous aspiration thromboembolectomy: A preliminary experience. Clin Radiol 49:553, 1994.
29. Cleveland TJ, Cumberland DC, Gaines PA: Percutaneous aspiration thromboembolectomy to manage the embolic complications of angioplasty and as an adjunct to thrombolysis. Clin Radiol 49:549, 1994.

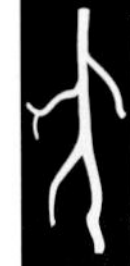

CHAPTER 31
Endarterectomy

Louis M. Messina, M.D., and Ronald J. Stoney, M.D.

The possibility of directly removing occlusive arterial lesions that impair blood flow became a clinical reality a half a century ago, when Dos Santos of Lisbon successfully restored patency to the superficial femoral artery of a man with a threatened limb.[6] He named this operation "arterial disobstruction," or "disobliteration," and attributed its feasibility to the use of the new anticoagulant drug heparin. Bazy and Reboul[1] later described this procedure as *endarterectomy,* and Leriche and Kunlin[12] chose the more comprehensive term *thromboendarterectomy* to indicate removal of obstructing thrombus as well as the diseased arterial intima. There is no truly precise term to describe this technique completely because, when it is properly performed, the inner media is also removed; however, the terms endarterectomy and thromboendarterectomy, which are interchangeable, are used most often.

Four years after Dos Santos' operation, Wylie of San Francisco performed the first thromboendarterectomy in the United States in an epic operation to relieve aortoiliac obstruction.[19] Shortly thereafter, Wylie reported a large experience with this technique at the University of California Medical Center in San Francisco (UCSF).[17] Since the 1950s, at UCSF, continued use of endarterectomy as one of the preferred therapeutic options for patients with occlusive vascular disease has resulted in a significant experience with this operative technique in all arterial sites where such lesions occur.

The critical features that make endarterectomy feasible are the pathologic localization of atherosclerotic plaques to the intima and subjacent media of the diseased artery as well as the segmental distribution of plaques at areas of turbulent flow within the arterial tree. The outer media and adventitia are spared by atherosclerosis; therefore, a cleavage plane can be readily developed between the diseased and nondiseased zones of the arterial wall. Such a cleavage plane is marked by poor adherence between the two zones, and it is macroscopically continuous throughout the length of the lesion. With localized segmental regions of atherosclerotic stenosis, the tapering distal termination of the lesion, or "end-point," coincides with a transition of plaque involvement of the intima and media to involvement of the intima alone. This allows removal of the plaque smoothly or with only a minimal residual ledge of slightly thickened intima that is adherent to the underlying media.

When such an intimal ledge is present, it can be transected on a bevel to minimize the risk of an obstructing flap becoming elevated after restoration of flow. If the distal end-point is not adherent to the underlying media, it can be secured with fine "tacking" sutures tied externally (rarely required). Nearly all anatomic patterns of occlusive atherosclerosis are suitable for endarterectomy, whether the disease is localized, diffuse, calcific, or otherwise degenerative.

The immediate success of endarterectomy also depends on the characteristics of the residual arterial wall that resist dilation and eventual disruption following restoration of pulsatile flow at systemic blood pressures. It has always been of great interest that the residual outer media and adventitia left after endarterectomy have sufficient tensile strength to support the vessel wall; this is true even in the aorta, where the medial myoelastic lamellae are thought to be very important to vascular integrity. However, this arterial function is destroyed if any degree of dilation or aneurysmal degeneration is present. Current information suggests that aneurysmal degeneration involves an imbalance of degradative metalloproteases and metalloprotease inhibitors throughout the arterial wall, perhaps most importantly in the adventitia, and that this process may be biochemically distinct from the atherosclerotic changes evident in occlusive disease patterns (see Chapters 18 and 22). Endarterectomy of such an artery, even if initially successful, predictably leads to aneurysmal dilation of the endarterectomized segment over time. For this reason, the presence of aneurysmal disease is the only specific and absolute contraindication to endarterectomy for the management of occlusive arterial disease.

PATTERNS OF ATHEROSCLEROSIS

There are three distinct patterns of occlusive atherosclerosis, which can be characterized according to (1) site in the arterial tree, (2) relation to sites of arterial fixation, and (3) proximity to sites of turbulence. Each pattern is associated with specific arterial lesions amenable to endarterectomy.

Sites Within The Arterial Tree

Lesions in the 10 major aortic branches are predictably located near the origin of the vessel from the aorta, are short, and terminate with a smooth transition to a nearly normal lumen within the arterial branch. Only rarely is the aortic ostia of an involved aortic branch spared, with the obstructing lesion developing within the proximal artery itself and extending distally for a variable length.

These features of aortic branch atherosclerosis make transaortic endarterectomy an important technique for improving perfusion in all vascular beds supplied by these branches, except for the three branches of the transverse aortic arch. In this location, a proximal aortic cross-clamp cannot be applied without producing intolerable cardiac strain. Therefore, transvessel retrograde endarterectomy is necessary, but the proximal occluding clamp must include the orifice of the branch (e.g., the innominate artery). The five major abdominal aortic branches (three viscerals, two renals) are ideally suited for transaortic endarterectomy. Disease affecting the two terminal aortic branches, the iliac arteries, consistently extends to the iliac bifurcation or further. Therefore, in addition to the transaortic approach, transiliac endarterectomy is necessary to facilitate safe and complete removal of these lengthy lesions.

Sites of Arterial Fixation

The superficial femoral artery traverses the adductor canal in the lower third of the thigh. At this site, it is confined by the adductor magnus muscle and is locally fixed by the adductor tendon at the hiatus through which it passes as it enters the popliteal space. This normal anatomic configuration favors the development of atherosclerotic disease at this particular site in the femoropopliteal arterial segment. Osseous or myofascial anomalies may also cause fixation of arteries in other locations, particularly near active joints. The subclavian artery near the thoracic outlet and the popliteal artery adjacent to the knee are typical examples. A cervical rib or gastrocnemius muscle entrapment produces arterial compression and eventually injury.

Repeated arterial injury of the subclavian artery produces post-stenotic aneurysm or focal atherosclerotic intimal ulceration. These can produce upper extremity microembolization or macroembolization. The focal occlusive and ulcerated lesions of the subclavian arterial tree are quite amenable to thromboendarterectomy through the affected artery; however, when either subclavian or popliteal aneurysms are present, it is preferred that they be replaced with a graft.

Sites of Turbulence

Turbulent blood flow produces areas of low shear stress that enhance the deposition of intimal atheromatous lesions. The carotid bifurcation may be the most common example, although the bifurcations of the infrarenal aorta, common femoral, and popliteal arteries are also important in relation to lower extremity ischemia. The carotid bifurcation is the undisputed site for preferential use of open endarterectomy in vascular surgery as it is now practiced, and in many surgeons' practices it is the *only* place where this technique is employed! Currently, however, carotid stenting is being evaluated in trials with endarterectomy to treat symptomatic carotid atherosclerosis.

TECHNIQUE

When we analyze atheromatous lesions carefully, we see that they comprise a heterogeneous spectrum of disease. Most vascular surgeons are familiar with the lesion in the carotid bifurcation and perhaps portions of lesions removed to facilitate the implantation of grafts in other sites in the arterial tree. The pathologist dutifully reports the segment of atherosclerotic plaque and describes the microscopic features in relatively bland terms. To the surgeon who regularly uses the technique of endarterectomy, however, it becomes obvious that different lesions require different endarterectomy techniques.

The variation in the composition of these lesions is in

part the result of metabolism of the arterial wall and the response to injury and repair and certainly the result of systemic and local factors currently unknown. Activity within an atherosclerotic plaque, such as hemorrhage, alters the composition of the lesion and its intimal surface. Finally, the location, distribution, luminal size, and contour of the atheroma vary significantly and affect not only the conduct of the endarterectomy but also the short-term and long-term results.

Five specific techniques of endarterectomy are available to the surgeon, depending on the type, extent, and location of the lesion to be removed and on his or her experience.

Open Endarterectomy

Open endarterectomy is the most commonly employed technique, originally advocated by Bazy and Reboul[1] and performed through a longitudinal arteriotomy. The procedure exposes the extent of the lesion to be removed and allows direct separation of the disease from the subjacent arterial wall. A dural elevator or clamp is the instrument usually selected to separate the atheroma from the arterial wall. The most common example is carotid bifurcation endarterectomy (Fig. 31–1).

Semi-closed Endarterectomy

The semi-closed technique was originally performed by Dos Santos.[7] Either transverse or longitudinal arteriotomies are placed at the proximal and distal extents of the lesion within the artery. A distal end-point is established, and retrograde separation of the atheromatous plaque or core from the uninvolved artery proceeds in a proximal direction through the unopened vessel (Fig. 31–2). One or more

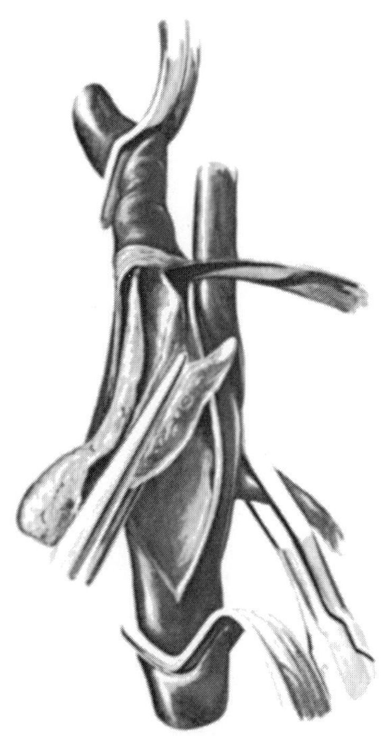

FIGURE 31–1. Eversion endarterectomy of distal internal carotid lesion beyond end of the arteriotomy.

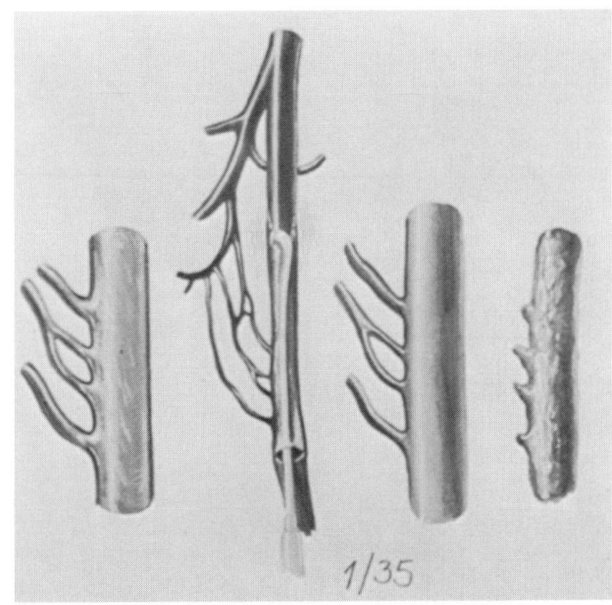

FIGURE 31–2. Semi-closed endarterectomy. Retrograde separation of plaque with loop stripper yields atheromatous core with branch artery orifices.

intervening arteriotomies may be used to disobliterate long arterial segments. This procedure is continued to the proximal arteriotomy, where the lesion is detached and then removed; a hand-held loop stripper[2] or gas-powered or electric-powered strippers that oscillate[13] are available and may be used to traverse long distances between arteriotomies. These devices maintain the separation plane between the atheroma and the residual arterial wall. The semi-closed technique is commonly used in the iliac or superficial femoral artery. It avoids the use of a long segmental patch, which would generally be required if the endarterectomy were performed in an open manner through a longitudinal arteriotomy.

Extraction Endarterectomy

The technique of extraction endarterectomy requires either retrograde or antegrade removal of an atheroma through a single arteriotomy, either transverse or longitudinal, in the involved vessel. It is performed using straight or slightly curved long-jawed clamps or a dural elevator. If the endarterectomy is performed retrograde, the proximal end-point is separated by clamping the artery, which fractures or crushes the plaque. This technique is used in performing common femoral and distal external iliac endarterectomies. If the endarterectomy is performed in an antegrade direction, the distal end-point is identified by external palpation of the artery. The surgeon gently controls and removes the atheromatous termination by grasping it in the jaws of the clamp—in effect, operating *beyond* his or her direct vision. This technique may be particularly useful in endarterectomies of lesions of hypogastric or profunda femoris origin (Fig. 31–3).

When transaortic endarterectomy (open) involves the removal of lesions from the orifices of major arterial branches (renal or visceral), the portion of the endarterec-

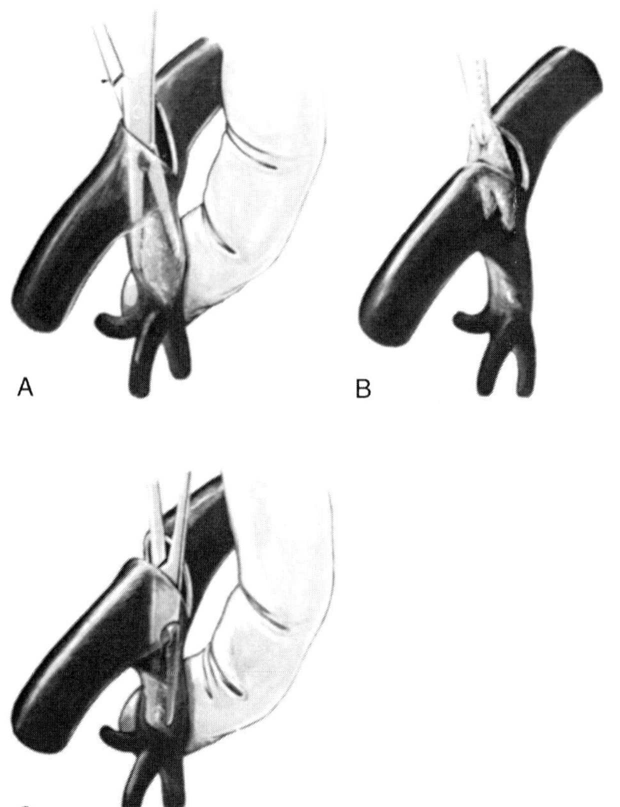

FIGURE 31–3. Hypogastric endarterectomy. *A*, Development of intimal core with hemostat. *B*, Extraction of specimen (incomplete). *C*, Removal of residual fragments.

tomy conducted in the branch artery uses the extraction principle. The dissection plane is carried from the aorta into the branch circumferentially and is extended beyond the orifice. Within 1.5 to 3 cm, the thickened intima returns to a normal thin layer and separates cleanly. The well-mobilized branch is prolapsed toward the aorta, and simultaneous traction on the specimen permits visualization of the end-point. Special angled extraction clamps (Figs. 31–4 and 31–5) facilitate the endarterectomy and removal of the occlusive lesion in the proximal aortic branch (Figs. 31–6 and 31–7).

Eversion Endarterectomy

The eversion technique, originally described by Harrison and associates,[9] requires distal transection of the artery beyond the site of disease and eversion or turning back of the residual proximal arterial wall upon itself as traction is applied to the atheromatous core. The core of disease can be transected at its origin after the eversion is complete and the atheroma removed. The arterial wall is then drawn back distally into a normal position, restoring the now patent artery to its normal location, where it can be reanastomosed to the distal arterial segment. This technique can also be used to disobliterate totally occluded excised arterial segments, which can then be employed in remote sites as arterial autografts. Common examples are the use of the internal or external iliac arteries and the occluded superficial femoral artery.

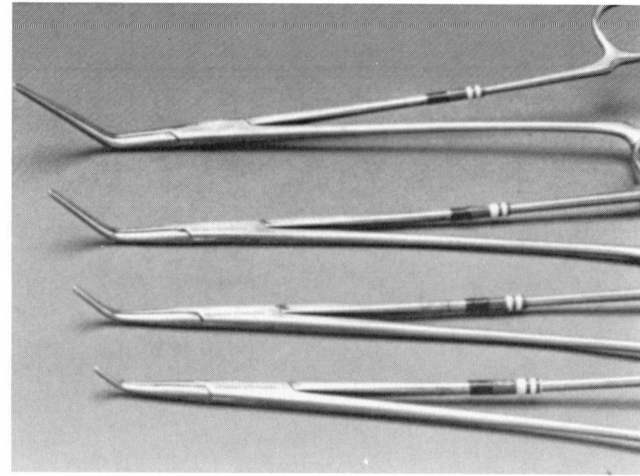

FIGURE 31–4. Special angled extraction clamps facilitate extraction endarterectomy.

Selective Endarterectomy

This selective technique is a modification of the semiclosed endarterectomy and is used to remove discontinuous atheromatous lesions in one arterial segment. It is performed in a retrograde manner through a distal arteriotomy. The procedure requires precise sizing of the arterial loop stripper to the artery to be treated. The operator is guided during careful retrograde advancement of this instrument by the *feel* of resistance as the loop engages, separates, and then disengages the discontinuous lesion in the artery. This type of endarterectomy is often suitable in the external iliac artery.

Selective endarterectomy can be performed within the diseased arterial segment itself (e.g., superficial femoral artery), through the parent artery (e.g., the aortorenal region), or both (e.g., the carotid or common femoral bifurcation). In endarterectomy performed from the parent artery, the disease in the parent artery should always be separated

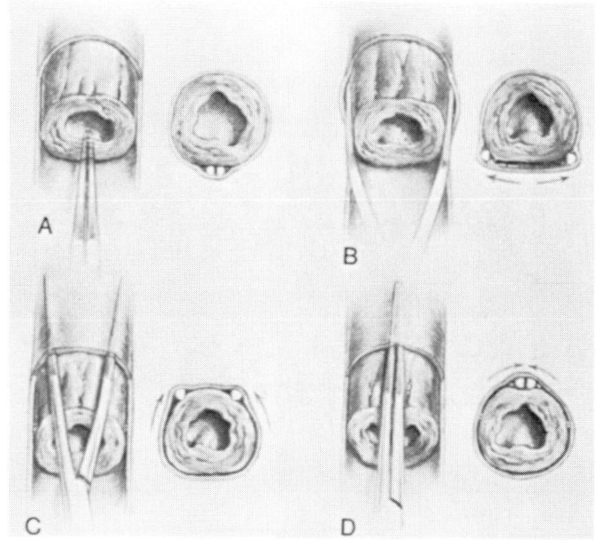

FIGURE 31–5. *A–D*, Use of angled extraction clamp to separate atheromatous core from arterial wall circumferentially during extraction endarterectomy.

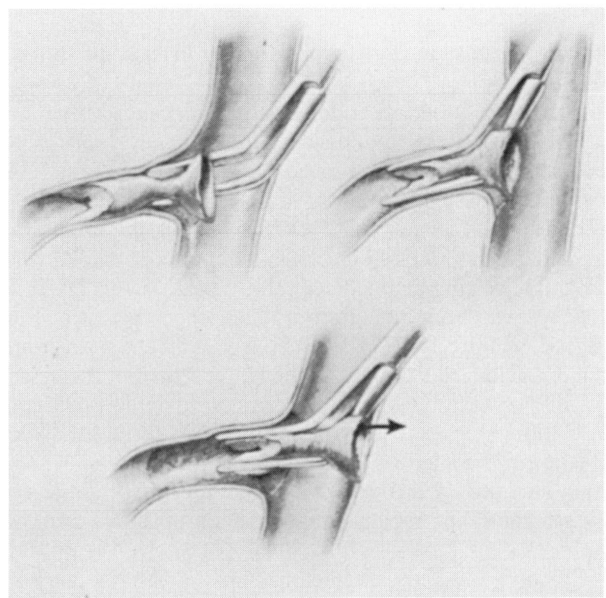

FIGURE 31–6. Angled extraction clamps allow endarterectomy of branch vessels to a disease-free end-point.

before the endarterectomy plane is extended into the diseased branch (e.g., transaortic renal thromboendarterectomy) (Fig. 31–7). In cases of disease contained in both the parent artery and its bifurcation branches, it is usually preferable to separate the disease first from the parent (proximal artery) and next from the less critical bifurcation branch, completing the endarterectomy finally in the critical bifurcation branch. An example of this is carotid bifurcation endarterectomy.

RESULTS

The results of endarterectomy depend, above all, on the experience of the vascular surgeon with this method of revascularization. The pattern of disease, the clinical consequences of the flow-obstructing lesion, and the characteristics of the atheroma are less important determinants of the outcome. Localized lesions with short terminations or transitions to normal or nearly normal distal arteries are ideal for endarterectomy. As in every method of revascularization, a normal inflow capable of delivering high-energy blood flow to the reconstructed vascular bed and a patent distal arterial tree that perfuses the organ or extremity provide the best characteristics for a durable endarterectomy. High-flow vascular beds (i.e., visceral, renal) are ideal for endarterectomy because their high flow rates result in extended patency.[15, 16, 18]

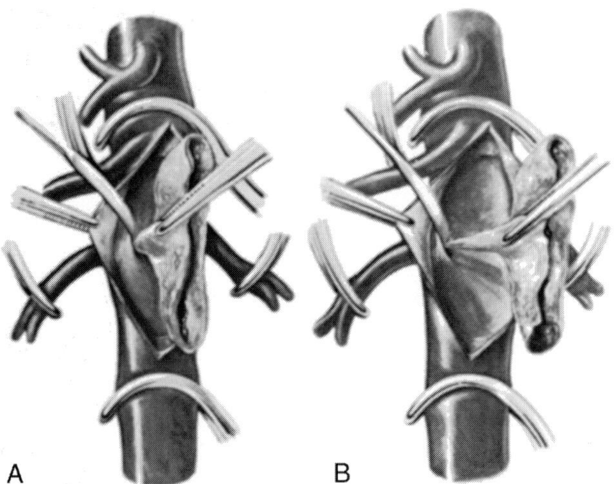

FIGURE 31–7. Removal of renal lesions. *A,* Dissection in endarterectomy plane in right renal artery after aortic portion has been completed. *B,* End-point of renal endarterectomy.

Endarterectomy, once the preferred method of revascularization in most medical centers, has gradually been replaced by bypass graft techniques. Prosthetic grafts are generally preferred for bypass of occlusive disease of the abdominal aorta and the iliac branches, and autologous vein grafts are favored for the infrainguinal arteries supplying the lower extremities. Aortofemoral and femoropopliteal bypass procedures replaced endarterectomy for lower extremity revascularization in the early 1960s, and by the mid-1970s femorotibial bypass was developed to revascularize ischemic limbs with distal tibial disease.

Lengthy endarterectomy procedures were abandoned for several reasons: (1) to minimize the dissection, (2) to shorten the procedure, and (3) to use the now available reliable autogenous and prosthetic grafts. The original technique of long endarterectomy was less than ideal. Crude devices were designed to disobliterate diseased vessels, but no standardized technique or training was available to new vascular surgeon trainees in acquiring the skill to perform such procedures. Only reports by Inahara[11] in Oregon and Imparato and colleagues[10] in New York emphasized the excellent results that could be achieved by endarterectomy when the technique was precisely performed in the superficial femoral and popliteal arterial segments. However, early and late patency rates of femoropopliteal endarterectomies performed by others were found to be inferior to comparable bypass grafts, and the bypass graft became firmly established as the preferred method for revascularization in these arterial beds.

Although prosthetic textile grafts have performed admirably in proximal sites, namely the aorta and its terminal branches, the results with prosthetics remain inferior to those achieved with autogenous saphenous vein grafts in the lower extremity itself. Because the greater saphenous vein is suitable in only about 80% of patients, other autogenous revascularization techniques must frequently be sought. The use of autologous cephalic or lesser saphenous veins (see Chapter 35) is one alternative, and another is superficial femoropopliteal endarterectomy performed by an open or semi-closed technique (see Chapter 67).

It is therefore appropriate to consider new technologic contributions that may overcome those factors reported to cause poor results. Extensive circumferential mobilization of long segments of the arterial tree has been considered mandatory to facilitate semi-closed endarterectomy when these long occlusions are disobliterated. Circumferential fibrosis can develop throughout the length of the endarterectomized segment, causing narrowing and eventual occlusion, and this has contributed to the low late patency rate of endarterectomy. Because endarterectomy is a controlled arterial injury that ideally heals by intimal regrowth, an optimal environment is necessary for this healing to occur. Extensive mobilization of the entire length of the artery to be treated may in fact devascularize the artery, stimulating postoperative periarterial fibrosis, impaired metabolism of the arterial wall, and therefore compromised arterial healing.

To eliminate these possible local problems arising from previous endarterectomy techniques, we have begun to evaluate new instruments and exposures that minimize trauma during semi-closed endarterectomy of long arterial segments. Although the air-driven oscillating loop device developed by Lerwick and Amsco-Hall has certain attractive features,[13] it is unwieldy and awkward because of its weight, inflexibility, and immobility. Its air hose tethers the instrument and makes its use somewhat restrictive. We have designed and developed an electric loop endarterectomy stripper that is light and flexible and adapts to various anatomic sites in the arterial tree. This device is battery-powered and can be sterilized.

Studies are now under way to assess the immediate and long-term patency rates of these technologic modifications for superficial femoropopliteal semi-closed endarterectomy. Minimal dissection and the reduced intimal trauma using the power-driven loop to create the endarterectomy cleavage plane are obvious immediate benefits of this method compared with older techniques that use the hand-held or even the oscillating Lerwick loop instruments. The early results are encouraging, and the regulation of arterial healing and the myointimal response to injury may support increasing future use of this potentially valuable technique.

As noted earlier, the healing of arteries subjected to endarterectomy involves a number of favorable and unfavorable cellular responses. In the past, the late development of neointimal hyperplasia was responsible for the occlusive failure of many long-segment endarterectomy techniques. Research into the cellular and molecular biology of arterial healing may now make it feasible to consider novel pharmacologic adjuncts to the performance of endarterectomy to modulate these events. For example, investigation using a well-established animal model of intimal injury has allowed Clowes and Reidy[3] to categorize arterial healing into three phases of myointimal cell response: (1) cellular *migration* into the neointimal layer, (2) myointimal cell *proliferation,* and (3) deposition of *extracellular matrix* (also see Chapter 24).

The precise factors regulating each of these phases are now becoming more clear, and this may allow the use of pharmacologic adjuncts such as heparin,[4] angiotensin-converting enzyme (ACE) inhibitors,[5] and growth factor antagonists[8, 14] to improve the results of endarterectomy. Limited clinical trials are now under way to evaluate the potential of heparin-like agents to limit myointimal cell migration and proliferation, ACE inhibitors to modulate myointimal cell proliferation, and other agents to limit the deposition of matrix materials. It may also be possible, owing to the exciting developments in gene transfer technology currently under way, to use these methods to manipulate the healing response of the arterial wall following endarterectomy. With the availability of these new adjunctive therapies, it would not be surprising to see endarterectomy become a more widely applied technique of arterial reconstruction for occlusive disease during the next decade.

A technically perfect endarterectomy depends on a number of instruments and new techniques now available to the vascular surgeon. Improved illumination of the field by fiberoptic headlights aids in detection and elimination of technical defects that may adversely affect the healing of the endarterectomy site. The use of angioscopy may further aid in inspecting segments of the disobliterated artery at sites remote from the arteriotomies and, therefore, may improve the precision with which a smooth endarterectomy plane is achieved throughout the entire length of the vessel. Finally, we have now accumulated considerable experience with intraoperative duplex scanning with spectral analysis to confirm the adequacy of endarterectomy in various locations and are pleased with its accuracy in intraoperative assessment of the repair compared with operative arteriography.

The benefits of endarterectomy for the vascular surgeon who has mastered the technique and has the knowledge and skill to utilize it appropriately in the practice of vascular surgery are immeasurable. It expands the individual's understanding of atherosclerotic occlusive disease and its potential for management. This knowledge extends the vascular surgeon's ability to improve perfusion for any patient, even when the alternative, the bypass graft procedure, is either contraindicated or impossible.

Dos Santos[6] knew the problems he faced in the battle to manage occlusive arterial disease successfully with this technique when he wrote, "At the beginning failure was usual, success occasional." The proper use of endarterectomy, after more than 50 years, is still not without controversy. However, as technical refinements, improved instrumentation, training programs offering technical opportunities in endarterectomy, and pharmacologic modification of the arterial response to injury and healing are perfected, it is our opinion that endarterectomy will assume an increasingly important role for the vascular surgeon.

REFERENCES

1. Bazy L, Reboul H: Technique de l'endarterectomie desobliterate. J Int Chir 65:196, 1950.
2. Cannon JA, Barker WF: Successful management of obstructive femoral atherosclerosis by endarterectomy. Surgery 38:48, 1955.
3. Clowes AW, Reidy MA: Prevention of stenosis after vascular reconstruction: Pharmacologic control of intimal hyperplasia:A review. J Vasc Surg 13:885, 1991.
4. Clowes AW, Clowes MM: Kinetics of cellular proliferation after arterial injury: IV. Heparin inhibits rat smooth muscle mitogenesis and migration. Circ Res 58:839, 1986.
5. Clowes AW, Clowes MM, Vergel SC, et al: Heparin and cilazapril together inhibit injury-induced intimal hyperplasia. Hypertension 18 (Suppl):II-65, 1991.
6. Dos Santos JC: Sur la desobstuction des thrombus arterielles anciennes. Mem Acad Chir 73:409, 1947.
7. Dos Santos JC: Late results of reconstructive arterial surgery (restoration, disobliteration, replacement with the establishment of some operative principles). J Cardiovasc Surg 5:445, 1964.
8. Ferns GAA, Raines EW, Sprugel KH, et al: Inhibition of neointimal smooth muscle accumulation after angioplasty by an antibody to PDGF. Science 253:1129, 1991.
9. Harrison JH, Jordan WD, Perez AR: Eversion thromboendarterectomy. Surgery 61:26, 1967.

10. Imparato AM, et al: Comparison of three techniques for femoropopliteal arterial reconstruction. Ann Surg 117:375, 1973.
11. Inahara T: Eversion endarterectomy for aorto-ilio-femoral occlusive disease. Am J Surg 138:196, 1979.
12. Leriche R, Kunlin J: Essais de desobstruction des enteres thromboses suivant la technique de Jean Cid Dos Santos. Lyon Chir 42:475, 1947.
13. Lerwick ER: Oscillating loop endarterectomy for peripheral vascular reconstruction. Surgery 97:574, 1985.
14. Lindner V, Reidy MA: Proliferation of smooth muscle cells after vascular injury is inhibited by an antibody against basic fibroblast growth factor. Proc Natl Acad Sci USA 88:3739, 1991.
15. Rapp JH, Reilly LM, Quarfordt PG, et al: Durability of endarterectomy and antegrade grafts in the treatment of chronic visceral ischemia. J Vasc Surg 3:799, 1986.
16. Stoney RJ, Ehrenfeld WK, Wylie EJ: Revascularization method in chronic visceral ischemia. Ann Surg 186:468, 1977.
17. Wylie EJ: Thromboendarterectomy for arteriosclerotic thrombosis of major arteries. Surgery 23:275, 1952.
18. Wylie EJ: Endarterectomy and autogenous arterial grafts in the surgical treatment of stenosing lesions of the renal artery. Urol Clin North Am 2:351, 1975.
19. Wylie EJ, Kerr E, Davis O: Experimental and clinical experiences with the use of fascia lata applied as a graft about major arteries after thromboendarterectomy and aneurysmorrhaphy. Surg Gynecol Obstet 93:257, 1951.

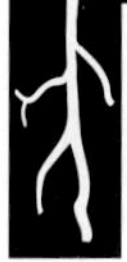

C H A P T E R 3 2

Fundamental Techniques in Endovascular Surgery

Kim J. Hodgson, M.D.

Endovascular therapies for peripheral vascular occlusive disease have evolved over the past several decades to become viable alternative approaches to surgical revascularization for many patients with peripheral vascular disease. More recently, endoluminal grafting of abdominal aortic aneurysms has been progressing through clinical trials, and U.S. Food and Drug Administration (FDA) approval for some of these devices appears imminent. Consequently, if vascular surgeons wish to remain on the forefront of the diagnosis and treatment of peripheral vascular disease, they need to add these techniques to their armamentarium. By doing so, they can offer comprehensive multimodality diagnostic and therapeutic care to vascular patients, a position that allows for objective treatment decisions without the bias inherently present when the controlling physician can only perform some of the possible therapeutic procedures.

Unfortunately, although most vascular surgeons have a general familiarity with the concepts related to endovascular procedures, concepts are not the same as skills. For example, all too often surgeons try to equate central venous catheter placement with percutaneous arterial catheterization in an attempt to gain credentials to perform percutaneous endovascular interventions. In practice, however, most are quickly humbled by how challenging this seemingly simple aspect of percutaneous endovascular procedures can sometimes be. Furthermore, although the concepts of the Seldinger technique utilized in both procedures are analogous, neither the skills required nor the risks to the patient are comparable. Vascular surgeons need to transform concepts into skills, a feat that can be accomplished only through actual experience performing endovascular procedures.

This chapter reviews the fundamental concepts related to the performance of the broad spectrum of diagnostic and therapeutic endovascular procedures, with the aforementioned caveat that this is no substitute for actual human hands-on training. Specific indications, results, and complications are addressed elsewhere (see Chapters 16, 38, 53, 72, and 90).

The guidelines concerning the characteristics and attributes of certain catheters, wires, and devices are generalizations to be considered only when one approaches a given clinical situation, each of which is unique and possessed of its own nuances. The ability to anticipate how a given catheter or guide wire will likely perform is based on analysis of the situation that must take into account multiple variables, including the extent of tortuosity and angulation present, the working distances involved, the characteristics of the target vessel or lesion, and many others. Ultimately, this boils down to judgment, which itself can come only from experience with similar situations. Once these basic techniques are mastered, however, innovative applications become possible and allow increasingly complex situations to be successfully addressed.

GAINING AND MAINTAINING PERCUTANEOUS VASCULAR ACCESS

By definition, all endovascular procedures require the surgeon to gain access to the lumen of the arterial or venous system in order to proceed. Although this can be performed percutaneously or by direct surgical exposure of the access vessel, the majority of endovascular procedures can and should be performed via the percutaneous route of vascular access. While conceptually simple, percutaneous access is actually the most uncontrolled component of any endovascular procedure, since it is performed with minimal benefit of any imaging guidance. The potential for mishap is real and can preclude performance of the intended endovascular procedure, limit the therapeutic options available, or actually render the patient worse off than before.

Vessel Puncture Equipment and Techniques

There are basically two types of entry needles to choose from: "single-wall" and "double-wall" puncture needles. The single-wall puncture needle is most familiar to surgeons and the one most commonly used. It is basically a bevel-tipped hollow needle large enough to accommodate a 0.035-inch guide wire. The needle is advanced toward the palpated pulse until the anterior wall of the vessel is punctured and pulsatile blood flow returns. A J-tipped guide wire is advanced through the needle into the vessel and threaded toward the target region.

Theoretically, blood return out of the hub of the needle may occur while the beveled area is still within the wall of the vessel, and subsequent wire passage may then dissect any plaque in the region. Therefore, it is crucial to evaluate the characteristics of blood return through the needle to ensure that a central position of the needle in the vessel is likely. If blood return is inconsistent or less than would be expected on the basis of the patient's symptoms and the quality of the pulse, the surgeon should subtly manipulate the needle to try to improve the quality of the blood return before attempting to pass the guide wire. Furthermore, fluoroscopic observation of guide wire passage, routine for many interventionalists, should definitely be performed if any resistance to advancement is met to ensure that the guide wire is not dissecting the wall of the vessel (Fig. 32–1). The importance of this cannot be overemphasized because it minimizes vascular injury not only at the insertion site but also farther along the course of the guide wire. Similarly, the sheath should never be advanced over the entry guide wire until radiographic evaluation has confirmed that the wire is properly positioned and without kinks.

The double-wall puncture needle is a two-component system that combines a blunt-tipped hollow needle with a bevel-tipped stylet, which projects slightly out the end of the needle. The double-wall puncture technique involves the intentional passage of the needle-stylet assembly through both walls of the vessel until it contacts the underlying bone. The stylet is then removed, and the needle is slowly withdrawn until blood return is noted (assuming that the target vessel was actually punctured). The needle angle is then flattened somewhat so that the surgeon can direct the subsequently passed guide wire more centrally within the lumen of the vessel.

Theoretically, there is less chance of plaque dissection with this approach, although insufficient withdrawal or premature angulation of the needle can still result in dissection of the posterior wall. Because this technique affords little protection against dissection and creates an unnecessary puncture of the posterior wall of the vessel, it has not

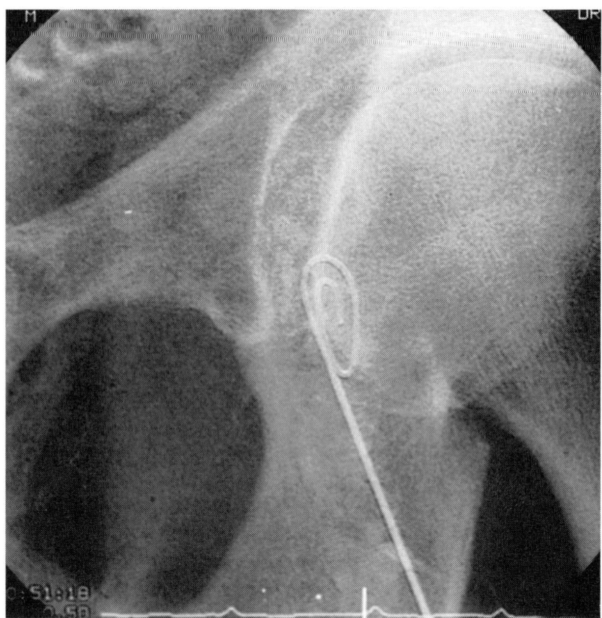

FIGURE 32–1. Extreme curling of the entry guide wire as it emerges from the puncture needle, indicating likely subintimal passage. (From Hodgson KJ, Mattos MA, Sumner DS: Access to the vascular system for endovascular procedures: Techniques and indications for percutaneous and open arteriotomy approaches. Semin Vasc Surg 10[4]:206–221, 1997.)

gained a large following among vascular surgeons, who generally prefer the less traumatic single-wall puncture technique with its instantaneous feedback at the time the vessel is punctured.

Although rarely used, a third type of vessel puncture system has particular advantages when the target vessel is pulseless, especially if it is in close proximity to sensitive structures that may be injured by multiple needle passages. This two-component needle (*Smart*Needle, CardioVascular Dynamics, Inc., Irvine, Calif.) is designed for single-wall puncture but is constructed like a double-wall needle; however, its inner stylet is a Doppler probe that can assist in directing the needle to the intended vessel puncture site. Once below the skin, the needle is panned side to side to locate arterial flow signals that allow the needle to be advanced directly toward the target vessel. Vessel puncture is accompanied by a significant increase in amplitude of the Doppler signal, at which time the Doppler stylet is removed, blood return is observed, and an entry guide wire is advanced as previously described.

Although the *Smart*Needle may be helpful for common femoral artery punctures below iliac artery occlusions, anatomic and radiographic landmarks are usually sufficient guidance in this situation and avoid the extra expense. Some interventionists have reported using this system to puncture the popliteal artery for retrograde approaches to the superficial femoral artery[1]; others have advocated its use for puncturing a pulseless axillary artery, in which the risks of brachial plexus injury from misdirected needle passages or from a puncture-related axillary sheath hematoma can be high.

Maintaining Vascular Access

After vascular access has been achieved, one must consider how best to maintain it. If a purely diagnostic procedure is planned and multiple catheter and guide wire exchanges are not likely, the surgeon can minimize the size of the puncture wound by using a full-length guide wire as the entry wire and simply advancing the diagnostic catheter directly into the vessel over the guide wire. This is a reasonable approach when all imaging can be performed through flush aortography (or vena cavography) without the need for selective catheterizations, which generally requires exchanging out the pigtail catheter for one or more selective catheters.

Each catheter or guide wire exchange has the potential to traumatize the vessel puncture site by enlarging it, lifting an intimal flap, or both. Furthermore, during each exchange, some blood escapes from the puncture, forming a localized hematoma that may compromise effective compression after completion of the case. Therefore, unless the desired study can be accomplished with just one catheter and without much manipulation, an indwelling sheath should be used. Because of the higher profile and irregular surface characteristics of balloon angioplasty catheters and stents, use of a sheath is absolutely mandatory for interventional procedures.

Sheaths are essentially access ports to the vascular system placed at the time initial vascular access is achieved and removed after completion of the diagnostic study or intervention. Subsequent exchanges of guide wires, diagnostic catheters, and interventional catheters or devices are all performed through the lumen of the sheath, which functions to minimize trauma to the vessel wall, as well as extravasation of blood from the puncture site during exchanges. Back-bleeding from the sheath itself is prevented by a hemostatic valve located in its hub, which also maintains hemostasis when catheters or guide wires are in place by sealing around these devices.

There are limits, however, to how effective the hemostatic valve can be, particularly when very small guide wires or noncoaxial *intravascular ultrasound* (IVUS) catheters are in place. In the former case, leakage is a function of difficulty in sealing around such a small device; in the latter case, a seal is difficult to obtain because the profile of the IVUS catheter alongside the guide wire presents an irregular shape for the valve to seal against. Very-large-diameter sheaths (in the 22 French [Fr.] range) designed to accommodate large-diameter endoluminal aortic aneurysm devices may have a clamping chamber instead of a hemostatic valve because it is problematic to design a hemostatic valve that can effectively seal around a range of sizes as great as that encountered in this situation, from the 0.035-inch guide wire to the 7-mm diameter endograft delivery system.

Sheaths come in a variety of diameters and lengths, but the diameters most commonly used are in the 5 to 6 Fr. range (1 Fr. = 3 mm) because most diagnostic and balloon catheters are of this size. Placement of stents requires the use of sheaths in the 7 to 10 Fr. range, iliac and superficial femoral artery endografts require approximately 10 Fr. sheaths, and aortic endografts require a sheath as large as 22 to 25 Fr. if a sheath is even used at all. The size designation denotes the *internal* diameter of the sheath as opposed to catheters, which are sized in French by their *external* diameters. Accordingly, the maximal size catheter that can be placed through a 5 Fr. sheath is a 5 Fr. catheter. A standard 5 Fr. sheath has an outside diameter of approximately 6 to 7 Fr., which represents a 1 to 2 Fr. increase in the size of the puncture than would be made if a sheath was not used. In practice, this is not a clinically significant issue, and the benefits of sheaths far outweigh this consideration or their relatively modest cost.

There are four basic lengths for sheaths: 3 to 5 cm, 10 to 12 cm, 22 to 25 cm, and 30 to 40 cm. The two longer-length ranges are generally needed only for Palmaz stent or endograft placement and contralateral work. The 10- to 12-cm length is standard for most peripheral vascular diagnostic and interventional procedures, and the 3- to 5-cm length is used mostly for dialysis graft work. Some long sheaths, referred to as *crossover sheaths,* have preshaped curved tips or kink-resistant internal support to facilitate their use over the aortic bifurcation. Some manufacturers place a radiopaque marker on the end of their sheaths to facilitate their visualization under fluoroscopic imaging. This is particularly valuable during interventional work, especially stent placement, when it is crucial to know that the stent is completely outside of the sheath before deployment is begun.

Another useful feature of sheaths is the *side-port connection,* which allows for blood sampling, pressure monitoring, vasodilator administration, and contrast injection during the procedure. For example, if the entry guide wire cannot be passed all of the way up the vessel at the time of initial vascular access, visualization of the cause of the problem can be helpful (Fig. 32–2). Although injecting contrast directly through the entry needle may elucidate the nature of the obstruction, the obstruction is often better visualized if the sheath is inserted a limited distance into the vessel and a diagnostic study is done through the sheath because the small-diameter needle may not allow a sufficient volume of contrast to be infused rapidly enough for adequate visualization. If direct injection through the needle is undertaken, however, attaching the dye-loaded syringe to the entry needle via a segment of intravenous extension tubing can minimize movement of the needle and, therefore, possible arterial injury during injection.

VASCULAR ACCESS SITES AND TECHNIQUES

Access to the arterial system is typically obtained through one of three approaches:

- Retrograde common femoral puncture
- Antegrade common femoral puncture
- Retrograde axillary-brachial puncture

Occasionally, access may be gained through the superficial femoral or popliteal arteries or by direct puncture of a graft, such as an axillobifemoral bypass (Fig. 32–3), whereas puncture of dialysis grafts is commonplace. On the venous side of the circulation, the retrograde femoral and antegrade jugular approaches are standard approaches well known to vascular surgeons and are not further described here.

In general, selecting the site in closest proximity to the target lesion provides the greatest number of therapeutic

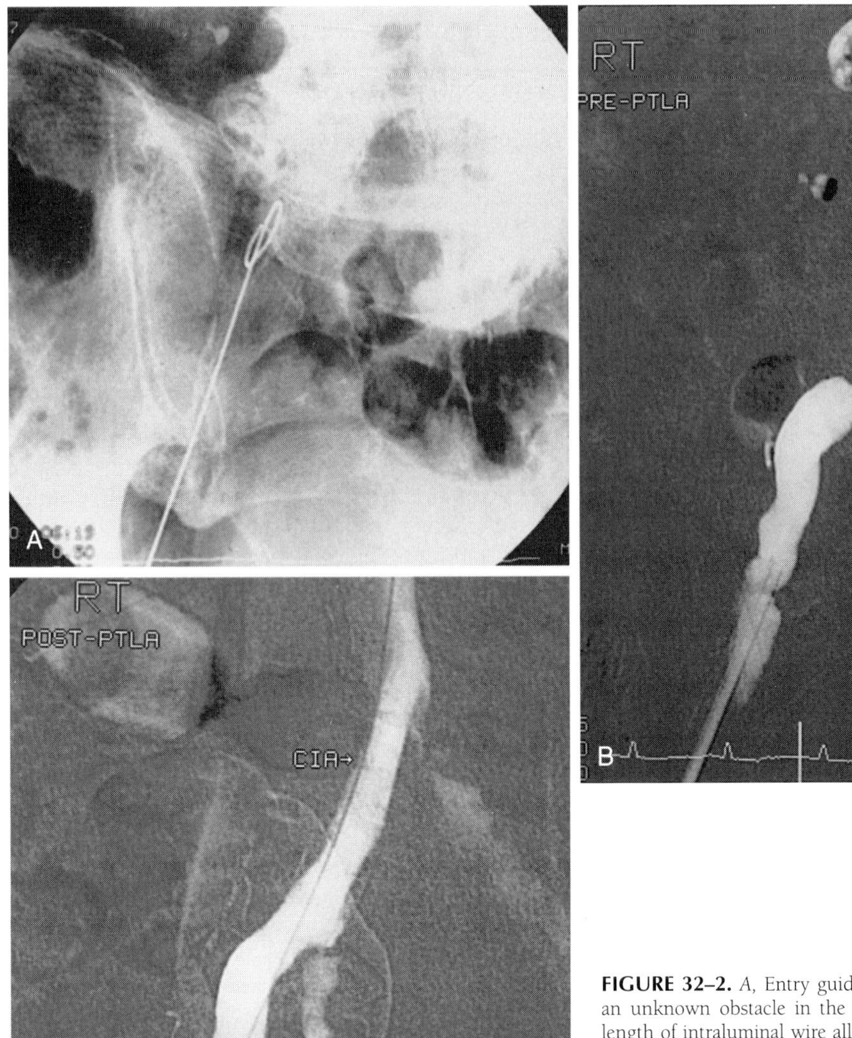

FIGURE 32–2. *A,* Entry guide wire advancement is impeded by an unknown obstacle in the iliac artery region. *B,* An adequate length of intraluminal wire allows placement of a sheath, through which this diagnostic study was performed, revealing the nature of the problem to be a stenosis in the external iliac artery (EIA). *C,* Controlled guide wire passage is now possible and subsequent dilatation is performed. PTLA = percutaneous transluminal angiography; CIA = common iliac artery.

options and best catheter response as long as there is adequate working room between the puncture site and the lesion to safely inflate balloons and deploy stents. Although a common concern among surgeons, direct puncture of vascular grafts, even in their anastomotic regions, is not generally problematic. However, the associated scar tissue may hinder sheath placement, requiring predilatation of the track with a dilator one or two French sizes larger than the intended sheath. If this measure fails, switching to a stiff guide wire or sheath may be required. Scarred groins can be advantageous, however, because postprocedure hematoma formation is uncommon—a consequence of the absence of a tissue space in which blood collects.

Retrograde Common Femoral Artery Cannulation

The retrograde femoral artery puncture is the most common approach and the one with the least risk because of its relatively large size and because it can be effectively compressed against the underlying osseous structures. A thorough understanding of the anatomic relationship of the femoral artery and the surrounding bony and ligamentous structures is essential, particularly if the femoral pulse is weak or absent, because the risk of puncture-site bleeding is significantly increased if the puncture occurs above the inguinal ligament or on the side of the artery. A lateral puncture is rarely a problem if there is a good pulse to guide the way, but an appreciation of the location of the inguinal ligament is crucial.

Difficulty in compressing the femoral artery cephalad to the inguinal ligament is responsible for the increased risk of bleeding complications, particularly retroperitoneal bleeding, observed with suprainguinal punctures.[2, 3] Punctures overly distal in the common femoral artery can also be problematic because the smaller size of the artery in this location and the more abundant plaque commonly found in the distal common femoral and proximal superficial femoral arteries results in a greater risk of thrombosis and dissection. Furthermore, the relative abundance of arterial and venous branches and the less adherent perivascular tissues found distal to the femoral bifurcation result in an increased risk of hematomas, false aneurysms, and arteriovenous fistulae with low punctures.[4]

Palpation of the pubic tubercle and the anterior superior iliac crest is not always helpful because many older patients are too obese to allow for definitive localization of the structures. Furthermore, both anatomic and radiographic landmarks for the location of the inguinal ligament are poor predictors of its actual location.[5] The most medial cortex of the femoral head, on the other hand, has been found to average 14.8 mm (range, 7 to 35 mm) below the inguinal ligament[5] and 33 mm (range, 2 to 66 mm) above the femoral bifurcation.[6] In 79% of patients, at least part of the common femoral artery lumen is located over the medial third of the femoral head.[6] Consequently, puncturing the femoral artery 1 cm lateral to the most medial cortex of the femoral head, as assessed radiographically, appears to be best for both retrograde and antegrade femoral artery catheterizations.

When the surgeon does this, the femoral head should be centered in the field of view to avoid parallax errors that might otherwise occur. Additionally, any rotation of the patient's pelvis on the angiographic table distorts the relationship between the artery and the femoral head. If the femoral pulse is weak or absent, the artery can often be visualized radiographically by calcium deposits in the vessel wall, further aiding its successful puncture.

Once the site of intended needle insertion is ascertained, the skin and subcutaneous tissues are anesthetized with 1% lidocaine, and a small skin nick is made with a No. 11 knife blade. The entry needle is then advanced through the skin nick toward the pulse at an angle of about 45 to 60 degrees. Keeping one finger on the pulse as one advances the needle can help to guide the needle and may also stabilize the artery somewhat. If the patient experiences discomfort as the needle approaches the artery, one may inject more lidocaine through the entry needle into that region. "Shooting" pains down the anterior thigh may indicate femoral nerve stimulation from a laterally positioned needle that should be redirected. Although some interventionists attach a syringe to the needle and apply suction as they advance the needle, I prefer to use an "open" needle because this allows assessment of the "quality" of the puncture and needle position by the force of the stream of blood that is expelled.

Once good blood return is obtained, the **J**-end of an entry guide wire (typically packaged with the sheath) is advanced through the needle. If *any* resistance is encountered, further advancement under fluoroscopic guidance is mandatory. Once the wire is beyond the tip of the needle and advancing smoothly, it is generally best to "fluoro it up" the iliac artery. This ensures smooth passage, and areas where the wire "hangs up" can be noted for further assessment. It is not uncommon for the wire to curl in the common femoral or iliac artery as it is being advanced. This can usually be resolved by slight rotation or repositioning of the needle and re-advancement of the guide wire under fluoroscopic visualization. In some instances, one can switch to the straight "floppy" end of the wire (testing with the hand first to ensure that it is a floppy wire) and attempt to pass it. One can place a slight angle on the straight end of the wire by gently bending it over the tip of the thumbnail, giving the wire some steerability.

If the entry guide wire becomes kinked or damaged it is best to replace it. Although the surgeon can switch to a full-length diagnostic guide wire (because one will generally already be open and ready to use), it must be a metal wire. Plastic-coated guide wires, such as the Turemo glide wire

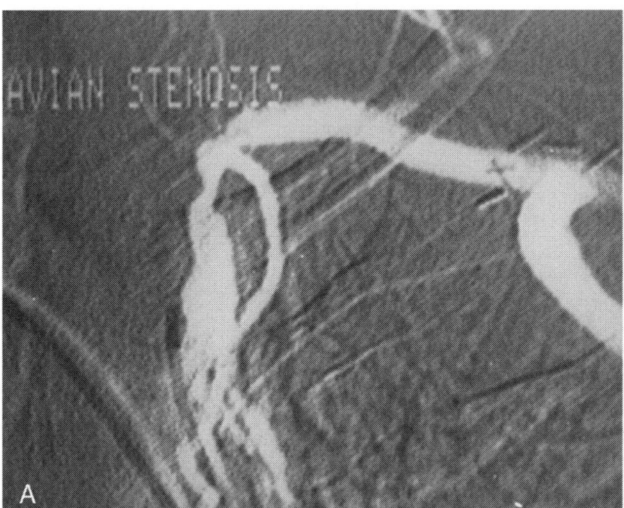

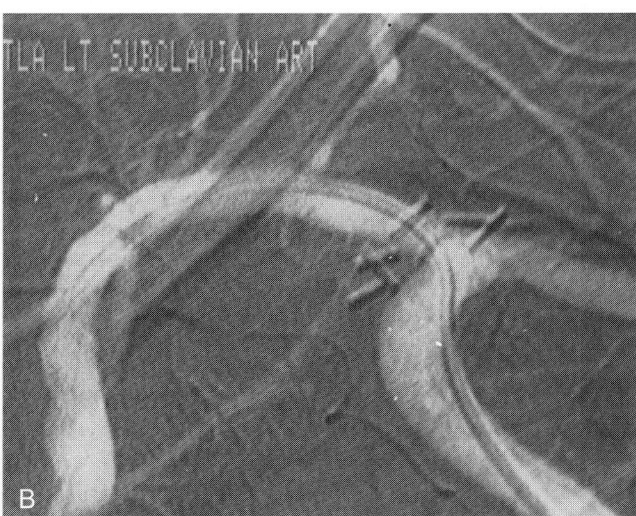

FIGURE 32–3. *A,* Stenosis of the left subclavian artery providing inflow to an axillobifemoral bypass approached via direct puncture of the graft over the anterior chest wall to avoid the risks of an axillary or brachial puncture. *B,* Completion arteriogram after balloon dilatation of the left subclavian artery.

(Boston Scientific Corp., Nadick, Mass.) should *never* be used through an entry needle because the plastic coating can be shaved off by the bevel of the needle.[7, 8]

Once the wire is successfully positioned in the iliac artery or distal aorta and there has been radiographic confirmation that there are no kinks, loops, or significant deviations in the course of the wire, the sheath may be inserted. The needle is withdrawn off of the wire, and pressure is held over the puncture site while an assistant threads the dilator-sheath assembly onto the wire for its subsequent advancement over the wire into the iliac artery. A firm, smooth motion is employed to advance the sheath over the wire. If resistance is met, fluoroscopy can be used to ascertain the reason. It is most important to try to advance the sheath in line with the wire because any angulation or arching creates resistance that may hinder passage.

Once the sheath is advanced to the hub, it is important to evaluate the situation again radiographically before the wire is withdrawn because, particularly in obese patients, the sheath may not have advanced into the artery but may be curled in the subcutaneous tissue. If the tip of the guide wire is up against a stenosis, the wire (and possibly the dilator) may have to be withdrawn a bit while the sheath is being advanced so as not to traumatize the stenotic lesion. However, the sheath should never be advanced on its own without a wire and a tapering dilator leading the way.

In patients who have undergone numerous femoral catheterizations or previous femoral artery dissections, significant resistance to advancement of the sheath may be encountered. In such instances, it is advisable to pass a dilator one French size larger than the intended sheath size over the wire to create a larger track through the scar before attempting to re-advance the sheath. If continued resistance is encountered, one can go up yet another French size or reinsert the previous dilator into the vessel and exchange out the guide wire for a stiffer wire that will allow the sheath to track better through the scar and into the vessel. Perisheath bleeding from "overdilatation" is rarely a problem, and postprocedure hematomas are uncommon because the scar does not allow a place for blood to collect.

Antegrade Common Femoral Artery Cannulation

The antegrade femoral artery puncture is considerably more difficult for two basic reasons:

1. Body contours tend to interfere with access to the artery.
2. The close proximity of the puncture site to the origin of the superficial femoral artery (SFA) or lower extremity bypass grafts limits available "working room" between the needle puncture and the first bifurcation.

The second consideration mandates as high a puncture as possible (still entering the artery below the inguinal ligament), whereas the first often renders this quite difficult. Access can sometimes be facilitated if a roll of towels is placed under the ipsilateral hip to extend it or if an assistant retracts the abdomen up and out of the way. In most cases, it is necessary to cannulate the SFA or a bypass graft at the time of the initial sheath placement because having to retract the sheath out of the profunda femoris artery and to manipulate it into the SFA later risks inadvertent sheath removal and loss of vascular access.

Consequently, passage of the entry guide wire must be carefully observed fluoroscopically, and the wire must be seen to follow the anticipated course of the SFA or graft before the sheath is advanced over the wire (Fig. 32–4*A* and *B*). When in doubt, one should perform a scout angiogram through the entry needle to identify the origin of the vessel of interest and its course (Fig. 32–5).

Alternatively, a small (4 Fr.) dilator can be advanced into the artery and an angiogram performed through it. If the dilator turns out to be in the SFA, it can be rewired and the sheath placed. If it is in the profunda femoris artery (PFA) and the puncture site is proximal enough on the common femoral artery (CFA) to allow for guide wire manipulation, the dilator can be slowly withdrawn while an angled guide wire is manipulated through the dilator and into the SFA (Fig. 32–4*C*). Any movement of the angiographic table or image intensifier between performance of the scout study and attempted wire passage should be avoided because it alters the relationships between the anatomic and radiographic landmarks, thereby confusing the situation.

Angiographic evaluation sometimes reveals that the puncture is in the SFA itself. If there is still sufficient working room to address the lesion of interest, there is no need to withdraw and repuncture. If, however, the puncture is in the PFA or too distal in the CFA to allow wire manipulation, the needle needs to be removed, pressure held for 5 to 10 minutes, and the puncture attempt repeated.

On occasion, disease in the SFA prevents the standard entry J-wire from passing into or far enough down the SFA. In such situations the floppy end of the wire can be used, usually after placing a slight angle (~60 degrees) on it, as described earlier. The remainder of the sheath placement procedure is the same as outlined earlier. One must remember to check sheath placement radiographically prior to removing the guide wire, however, because subcutaneous curling of the sheath rather than intravascular positioning is most common with the antegrade CFA puncture.

Axillary Artery Cannulation

On occasion, such as when bilateral iliac artery occlusions are present, arterial access must be obtained via the axillary approach. More accurately termed a *high-brachial puncture* (as it is most commonly performed today), this site of access also provides a straighter path of approach to acutely angled renal arteries, which is very important if there is orificial disease that may need to be stented. Unless there is evidence of coexisting subclavian-axillary disease, the left axillary artery is the preferred site to puncture. This is because it is generally easier to manipulate the wire or catheter into the descending aorta from the left than the right. This is particularly so if the innominate artery originates low on the arch (Fig. 32–6). Furthermore, when the aorta is approached from the right side, the catheter and wire reside in the flow path to the right common carotid artery and may, therefore, increase the risk of stroke.

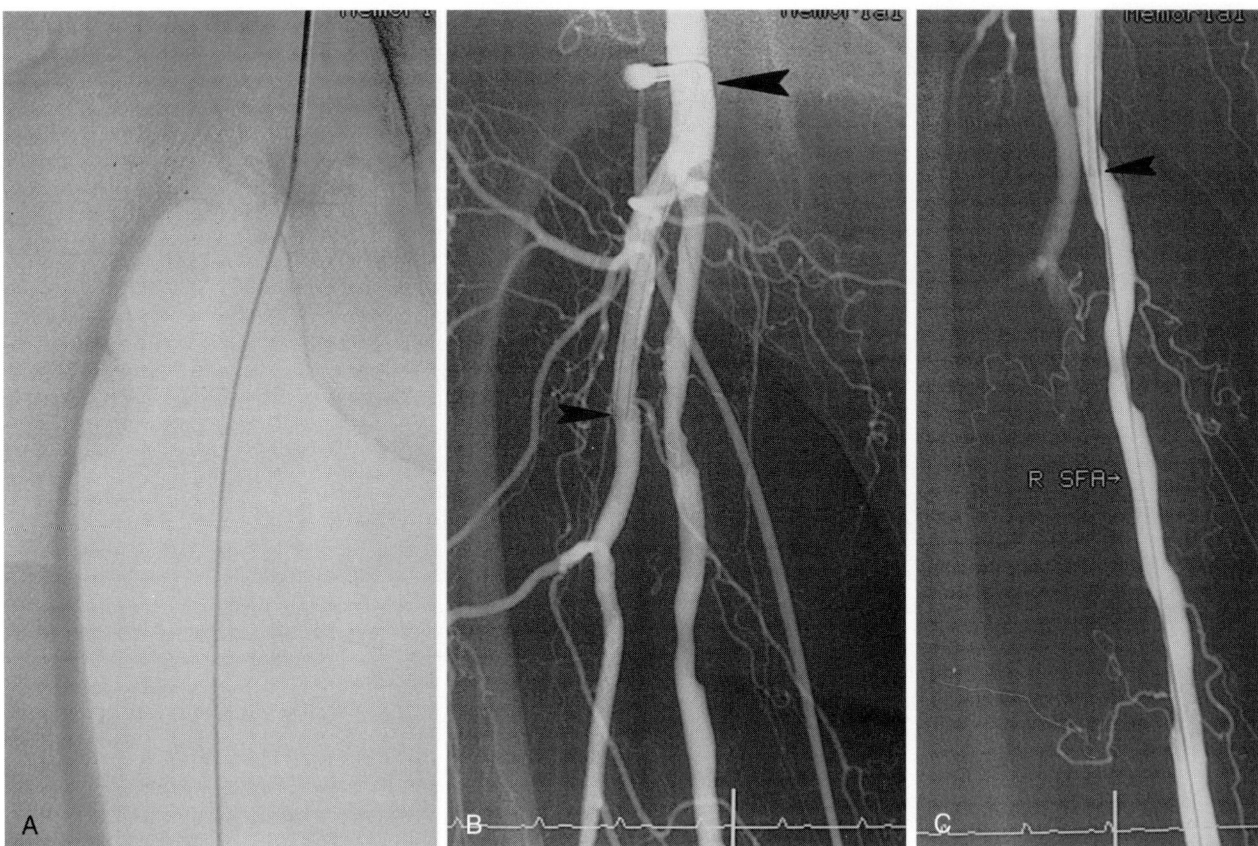

FIGURE 32–4. *A,* Initial guide wire passage during antegrade femoral artery catheterization demonstrates medial deviation of the guide wire suggestive of passage into the profunda femoris artery. *B,* Failing to appreciate this, the sheath was inserted over the guide wire, and subsequent angiography confirms its placement in the profunda femoris artery. *Upper arrowhead* = puncture site; *lower arrowhead* = distal tip of sheath in profunda femoris artery. *C,* Nonetheless, because the puncture was sufficiently proximal to the femoral bifurcation, there was adequate working room to allow the sheath to be retracted, the guide wire redirected and advanced into the superficial femoral artery, and the sheath re-advanced over the guide wire into the intended position in the superficial femoral artery. *Arrowhead* = distal tip of sheath in superficial femoral artery. (From Hodgson KJ, Mattos MA, Sumner DS: Access to the vascular system for endovascular procedures: Techniques and indications for percutaneous and open arteriotomy approaches. Semin Vasc Surg 10[4]:206–221, 1997.)

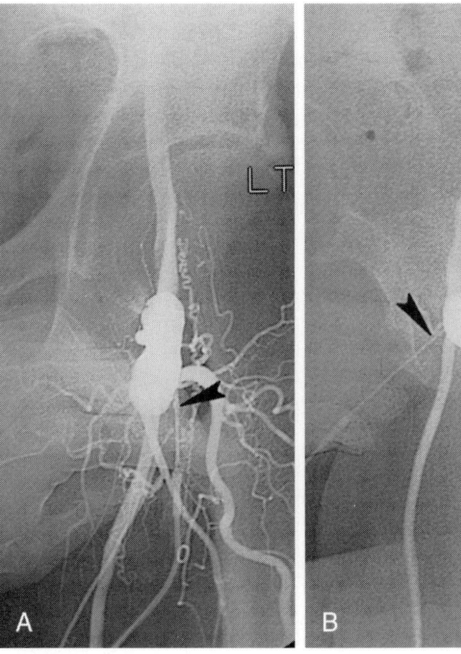

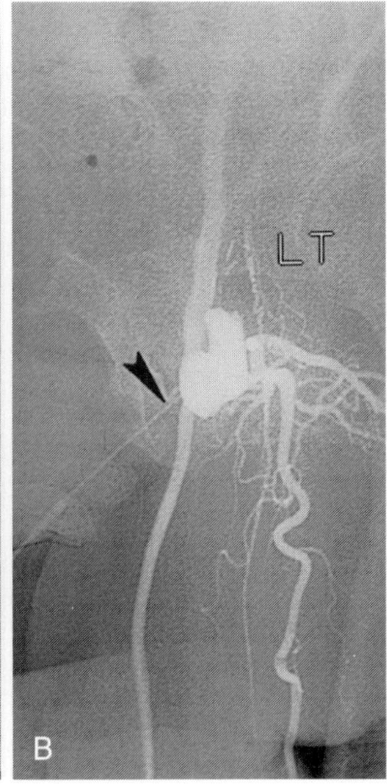

FIGURE 32–5. *A,* Multiple unsuccessful attempts to advance the guide wire into the superficial femoral artery from this needle puncture (*arrowhead*) prompted performance of a direct injection arteriogram. This demonstrated the needle puncture location to be in the hood of an old graft, but still in communication with the inflow iliac artery. Nonetheless, the guide wire repeatedly coiled in this region and was unable to be advanced up the iliac artery. *B,* Angiography performed in a different projection reveals that the puncture is in the cul de sac of an occluded graft, explaining the difficulty experienced advancing the guide wire into the iliac artery. LT = left femoral. *Arrow* = puncture needle.

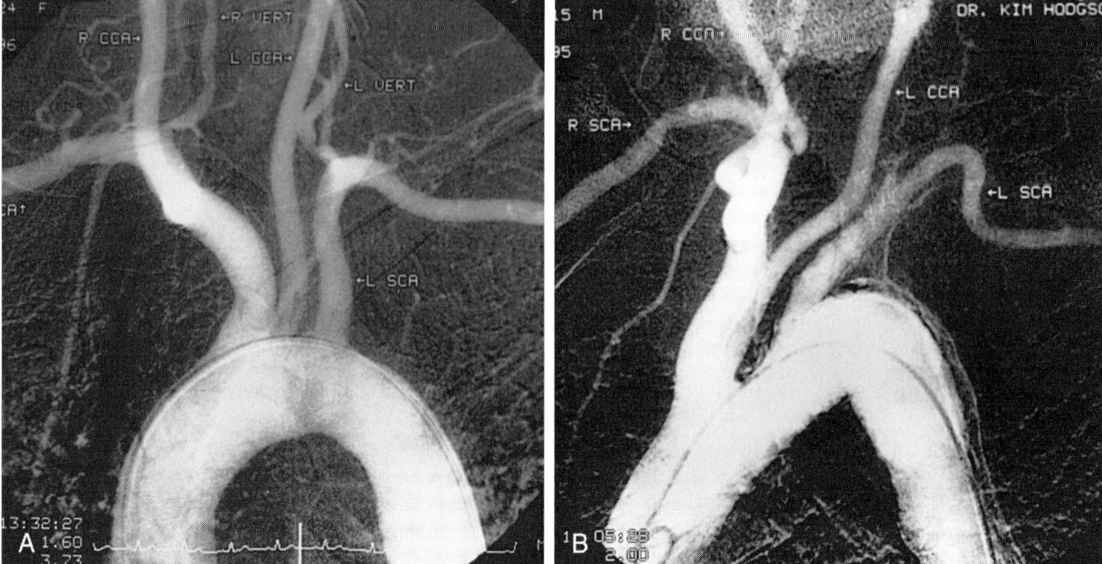

FIGURE 32–6. *A,* Aortic arch angiogram revealing the origins of all of the brachiocephalic vessels to be located high on the arch, which would allow for abdominal aortic access via either the right or the left axillary approach. *B,* Aortic arch angiogram revealing more proximal orgins of all of the brachiocephalic vessels, especially the innominate artery, which would impair abdominal aortic catheterization and manipulation from the right axillary approach. CCA = common carotid artery; SCA = subclavian artery. (From Hodgson KJ, Mattos MA, Sumner DS: Access to the vascular system for endovascular procedures: Techniques and indications for percutaneous and open arteriotomy approaches. Semin Vasc Surg 10[4]:206–221, 1997.)

Proper positioning of the patient is important and is best achieved by having the patient place his or her ipsilateral hand palm upward behind the head. The axillary (high-brachial) artery pulse is palpated lateral to the pectoralis major muscle, and the overlying skin is anesthetized. The close proximity of the brachial plexus trunks mandates a careful deliberate passage of the needle, although direct nerve injury from the needle is uncommon, occurring in fewer than 1% of axillary punctures.[9, 10] A patient's complaints of shooting pain down the arm should prompt retraction followed by redirection of the needle. The highly mobile axillary-brachial artery often benefits from manual fixation by the surgeon's second hand.

Once good arterial blood return is encountered, the guide wire is advanced into the artery, after which the sheath is advanced over the entry wire, as previously outlined. A full-length angiographic guide wire (preferably a J-wire) is then advanced through the sheath under fluoroscopic guidance and manipulated down the descending aorta, a maneuver best observed in the left anterior oblique orientation. If the wire repeatedly courses into the ascending aorta, an angled diagnostic catheter (e.g., Bernstein, Cobra) can be used to direct the wire down the descending aorta. From here, the remainder of the particular procedure is performed in the usual fashion.

In general, it is advisable to use the smallest sheath possible in the axillary and brachial arteries because their relatively small size increases the risk of vessel thrombosis. Furthermore, puncture-related hemorrhage, more common with larger punctures, raises the additional risk of axillary sheath hematoma with neurologic compromise, which is reported to occur in 2% to 3% of axillary artery catheterizations.[11, 12] This complication requires immediate recognition and surgical decompression if permanent neurologic dysfunction is to be avoided. The development of peripheral paresthesias warrants close observation, whereas any loss of motor function mandates emergent surgical attention to minimize the risk of permanent neurologic deficit.[12, 13] Despite attempts to minimize the puncture size, on occasion it is necessary to stent via the axillary approach and the sheath must be upsized to a 7 or 8 Fr., usually a well-tolerated situation.

The axillary (high-brachial) approach is considered preferable to an antecubital brachial artery puncture because the latter artery tends to go into spasm easily. This problem, in combination with its smaller diameter, greatly increases the risk of puncture-related thrombosis. Consequently, I have had little experience with this approach and do not recommend it. Furthermore, the translumbar approach to the arterial system is not used; it is essentially limited to diagnostic procedures and we prefer the axillary approach when the common femoral arteries are unsuitable access sites.

Venous Cannulation

The only other approaches that one needs to know are those that provide access to the venous system for the performance of renal vein renin sampling or vena caval filter placement. The technique of femoral venous puncture parallels that of its corresponding artery. Basically, the femoral vein is located just medial to the artery, the pulsation of which is typically used as its landmark. If arterial pulsation is absent, the vein can be found approximately 2 cm lateral to the pubic tubercle. As with arterial punctures, one advances the guide wire up the iliac vein under fluoroscopic visualization to ensure against any inadvertent misplacement of the sheath. Although vena caval filters can be inserted via the contralateral femoral approach, the jugular vein is preferred as an access site because it reduces the risk of instrumentation through thrombus or potential venous injury from the filter carrier, which may predispose to development of deep venous thrombosis on the unaffected side.

Catheterization of the jugular vein for insertion of a vena caval filter is best performed on the right side because this provides a straight shot to the infrarenal vena cava. The jugular vein is punctured just lateral to the carotid artery either anterior or posterior to the sternocleidomastoid muscle. I prefer to place a standard 5 Fr. sheath initially through which to perform an inferior vena cavagram to ensure that the inferior vena cava is not too large for a percutaneous caval filter (<29 mm). If the location of the renal veins is not apparent, the veins are selectively catheterized to ensure that the filter is positioned appropriately.

ANGIOGRAPHIC GUIDE WIRES

Despite differences in materials and handling characteristics, all guide wires serve the same basic function: to facilitate the positioning of catheters in particular locations by providing guidance and support for the catheter being advanced over them. The characteristics required to achieve this depend on the unique anatomic circumstances present as well as on the nature of the task.

To address these varying requirements, guide wires are available with a variety of diameters, lengths, tip shapes, tip and shaft stiffnesses, and antifriction coatings. Small-diameter wires are difficult to see under fluoroscopy, although radiopaque material, such as gold or platinum, can be used in the tip to address this problem. Similarly, radiopaque markers can be placed at fixed distances from each other to allow calibration of the computer for subsequent measurement of vessel diameters (Fig. 32–7). *Steerability,* or the degree of correlation between rotation of the shaft of the guide wire ex vivo and that of the guide wire tip in vivo, can also vary between different types of wires. Disposable "torque" devices designed to grip guide wires and facilitate their manipulation are frequently necessary, especially with hydrophilic coated wires, which are difficult to grip.

Classic guide wires are constructed of two different wire components: an inner wire called a *mandrel,* which tapers toward the tip to produce a floppier tip than shaft and an outer stainless steel coil wrap. Typically, a safety wire connects the mandrel to the tip of the outer coil to prevent their separation. In some wires, the inner mandrel, which is responsible for most of the stiffness of the wire, can be moved within the outer coil to vary the stiffness and shape of the tip of the wire. With infusion guide wires, the inner core wire can be removed, allowing its channel to be used to infuse contrast or thrombolytic agents.

The Turemo glide wire (Boston Scientific Corp.) is a relatively new instrument that has become popular because of its excellent torque response and low-friction coating. It is constructed of a nitinol (nickel-titanium) inner core with a polyurethane outer coating, and the surface is further coated with a hydrophilic polymer, making it extremely slippery when wet. This characteristic facilitates guide wire advancement, particularly through tortuous areas, as well as catheter–guide wire exchanges.

To successfully serve its function, the guide wire itself, alone or with directional catheter assistance, must be able to be manipulated into the desired location without traumatizing the vessel. Tip shape plays a major role in this function, with **J**-tipped configurations being the least traumatic and least likely to dissect or perforate blood vessels but also the least likely to negotiate tight stenoses. The most common **J**-wires have either 1.5- or 3-mm arc radii, resulting in wires that lead with 3- or 6-mm prows, respectively.

Guide wires also come with angled or straight tips, and most metal guide wire tips can be shaped as desired if they are bent over a thumbnail. Having a shaped tip gives the guide wire directionality and facilitates its being directed into branch vessels. At times, complex anatomic curves are best negotiated with a combination of a directional catheter and guide wire, using the catheter to direct the wire into branch vessels, after which the catheter is advanced over the guidewire. Regardless of configuration, most guide wire tips are fairly floppy over a distance of 3 to 8 cm to minimize the risk of dissection and perforation.

Most guide wires in use today have some type of antifriction coating, often polytetrafluoroethylene (Teflon), to facilitate guide wire placement and catheter-wire exchanges. Nonetheless, one can keep guide wires clean by wiping them down after each catheter exchange. This prevents blood from drying on the wire and hindering catheter passage. The hydrophilic coating of the Turemo glide wire renders it extremely slippery when it is wet, but "tacky" when it starts to dry out. These types of wires should be wet wiped before each new catheter passage to minimize friction between the wire and the catheter, thereby reducing the risk of losing the guide wire position during the catheter exchange. As previously mentioned, such hydrophilic coatings can be shaved off if wires are used with them through entry needles; therefore, these types of wires are not used for initial vascular access.

The ability of a guide wire to support subsequent catheter passage, particularly around multiple turns, depends greatly on the stiffness of the shaft of the wire. To some extent, this is a function of guide wire diameter; even within the same size category however, several guide wire stiffnesses are available. In general, the most flexible shafted guide wire that provides sufficient support to achieve the desired catheter position should be used, bearing in mind that larger and stiffer devices, such as stents and endoluminal grafts, require stiffer wires to reliably track over. Different devices have various maximum guide wire sizes, with standard diagnostic and balloon catheters typically accepting up to a 0.035- or 0.038-inch guide wire, whereas small-vessel angioplasty catheters often accept only up to an 0.018-inch guide wire. If the guide wire alone is insufficient to provide the necessary support to achieve the desired catheter position, supplemental external support can be provided by an appropriately shaped guiding catheter (see later).

Guide wires are generally available in two length ranges. The standard lengths range from 145 to 180 cm and are useful for positioning catheters, but they are not long enough to allow "exchanging out" a catheter unless the lesion crossing to be maintained is within about 30 to 40 cm from the site of vascular access. This maneuver, in which the guide wire is left in its final desired position

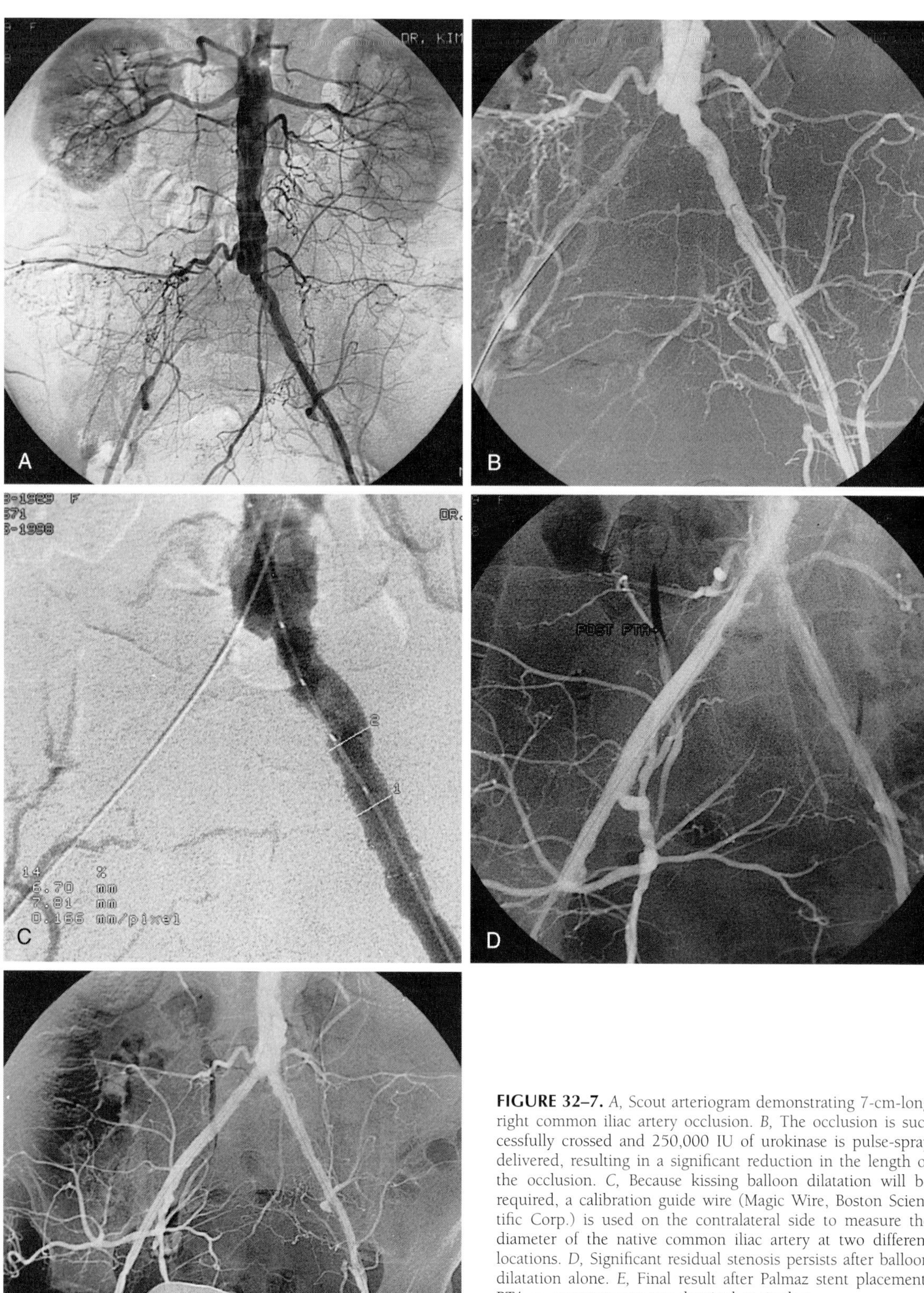

FIGURE 32–7. *A*, Scout arteriogram demonstrating 7-cm-long right common iliac artery occlusion. *B*, The occlusion is successfully crossed and 250,000 IU of urokinase is pulse-spray delivered, resulting in a significant reduction in the length of the occlusion. *C*, Because kissing balloon dilatation will be required, a calibration guide wire (Magic Wire, Boston Scientific Corp.) is used on the contralateral side to measure the diameter of the native common iliac artery at two different locations. *D*, Significant residual stenosis persists after balloon dilatation alone. *E*, Final result after Palmaz stent placement. PTA = percutaneous transluminal angioplasty.

while one catheter is removed from over the wire and replaced with another, requires a sufficient length of wire to allow complete withdrawal of the initial catheter without having to relinquish the desired position of the guide wire or lose contact with the ex vivo tail of the wire. Wires long enough to permit this exchange (*exchange-length guide wires*) are typically in the range of 240 to 300 cm in length. Some guide wires have a "docking" feature, which allows a standard wire to be transformed into an exchange-length wire by attaching an extension onto the standard length wire.

Guide wire diameters are specified in fractional inches, ranging from 0.012 to 0.052 inch, with 0.035 inch the most commonly used size for peripheral work. As previously noted, given the same material and method of construction, guide wire diameter is the primary variable influencing the stiffness of the wire.

Clearly, a guide wire is just one component of the instrumentation system used for a particular task, and it is important to ensure that the guide wire and catheter or device to be tracked over it have compatible sizes. Although guide wires with smaller diameters than the maximal lumen size of a catheter can be used through that catheter, the resultant diminution of support generally renders this an undesirable combination. Furthermore, when coil embolization is performed, the guide wire diameter, catheter lumen size, and embolization coil diameter must be closely matched before one attempts to push the coil through the catheter with the guide wire so that the coil does not begin to take its shape prematurely within the catheter, resulting in jamming of the coil inside the catheter.

A smaller than maximum allowable guide wire has sometimes been used when a larger catheter is being exchanged for a smaller catheter that would accommodate only the smaller guide wire. Additionally, when radiographic contrast (or another liquid) must be infused through a catheter while the guide wire is in place, use of a smaller than maximal guide wire allows some of the catheter lumen to remain open to transmit the contrast agent, although achievable flow rates will be small and resultant opacification frequently suboptimal. Unfortunately, compensating for this by infusion of full-strength contrast rarely improves the situation because the increased viscosity of the contrast inhibits its flow through the small residual lumen.

Ultimately, guide wire selection is a function of the task at hand and the given anatomic configuration. Initial evaluation is generally performed with a guide wire least likely to cause injury to the vessel wall, such as a J-wire. If target lesions are identified, it may be appropriate to switch to a calibrated wire for accurate sizing or to an angled or straight-tipped wire to traverse stenotic lesions. Working with relatively large or stiff devices or through tortuous vessels may mandate the use of a stiffer shafted wire in order to get the device to track the wire without dislodging it. Despite these general guidelines, wire selection is often based on operator familiarity and experience, and the use of multiple wires to address different challenges during a given case is not uncommon.

DIAGNOSTIC CATHETERS

Diagnostic catheters are designed to facilitate the delivery of radiographic contrast to specific areas of the vascular system to permit radiographic opacification of the flow channel of these vessels. Catheters intended for contrast infusion in the aorta and vena cava are typically advanced to that location from the site of vascular access over a guide wire and are referred to as *nonselective* catheters. In contrast, *selective* catheters are designed to engage the orifices of branch vessels and may or may not be advanced further out the selected vascular tree before contrast infusion.

Generally, optimal visualization occurs when the catheter position is close to the area of interest, thereby maximizing contrast density in this region while minimizing opacification of adjacent overlapping vessels that may obscure detail in the area of interest. Although some nonselective catheters can be used in conjunction with a guide wire support and direction to perform selective catheterizations (Fig. 32–8), this is not their primary function. Ancillary uses for selective catheters include:

- Instillation of pharmacologic agents (e.g., vasodilators or sclerosants)
- Delivery of embolic material
- Sampling of blood from specific locations (e.g., renal vein renin sampling)

Nonselective catheters are not generally suitable for these uses.

Catheter Construction and Characteristics

A variety of characteristics of diagnostic catheters determine how they will behave and to what use they are best suited. Principal among these variations is the shape a catheter assumes (or can be made to assume) once it is intravascular and the leading guide wire has been removed. Other important characteristics include catheter stiffness, tip design, torque response, antifrictional properties, radiopacity, and the presence of multiple side holes in addition to the end hole. Most selective catheters available today are made of polyethylene, which has good *torquability* (i.e., twisting of the ex vivo portion of the catheter produces a similar degree of rotation of the in vivo tip of the catheter) and *pliability* and holds its shape well. Nylon is often used in the construction of high-flow catheters (e.g., pigtail) because nylon can withstand higher infusion pressures than polyethylene. Polyurethane is a softer, more pliable material that yields catheters with poor torquability but that tracks guide wires well, although the higher coefficient of friction often mandates a friction-reducing coating on either the guide wire or catheter lumen. To improve torquability of polyurethane catheters, a fine wire mesh is often incorporated into the catheter wall. Experience with various catheters is necessary to learn which ones work best in various settings.

Catheter length also needs to be considered to ensure that the catheter can reach the target vessel from the selected site of vascular access. Catheters are typically available in 65- and 100-cm working lengths, with the shorter lengths suitable for abdominal and proximal contralateral lower extremity catheter placements and the longer lengths for arch, brachiocephalic, and distal contralateral lower extremity work if there is a common femoral artery site of access.

In contrast to sheaths, diagnostic catheter diameters are

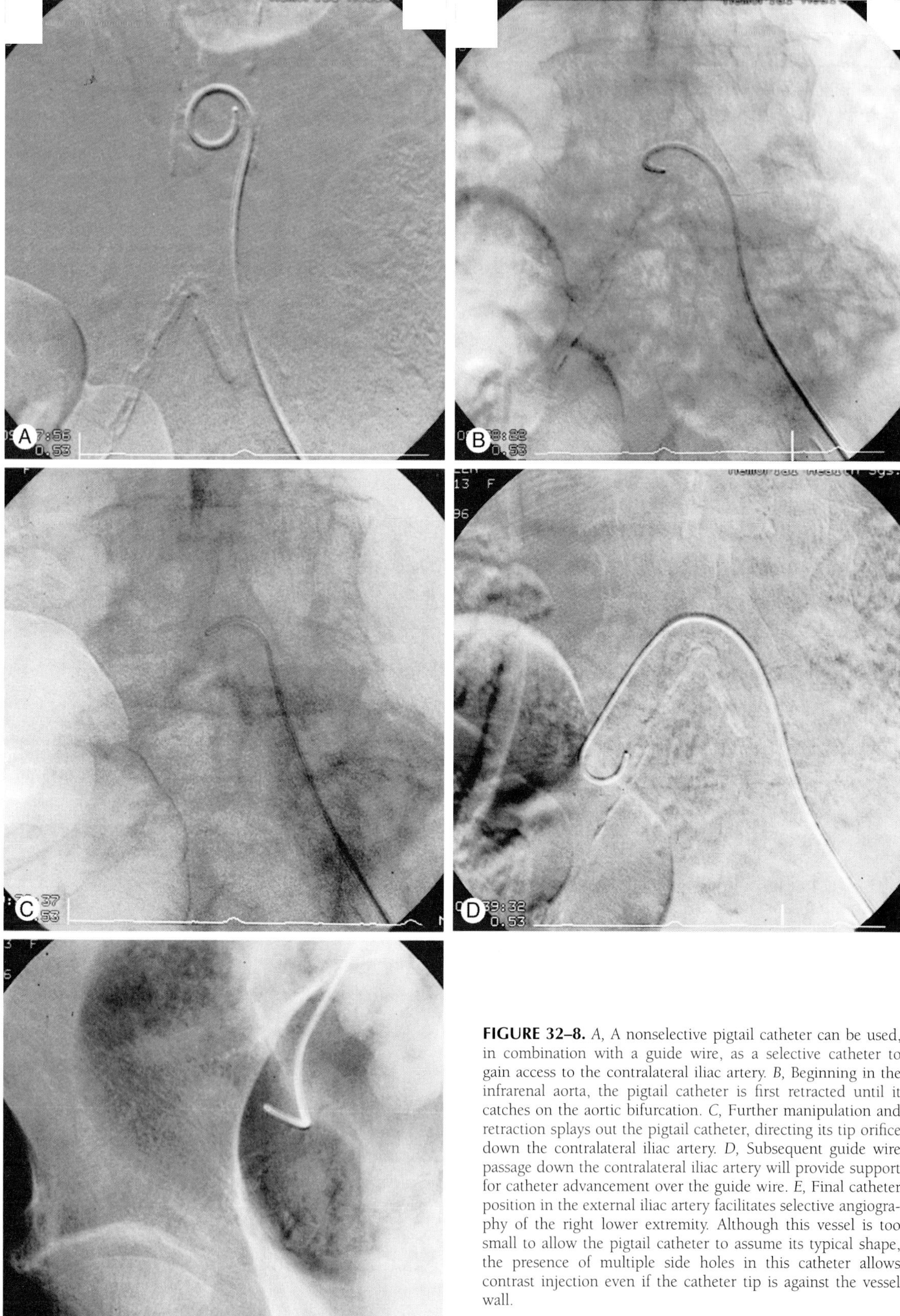

FIGURE 32–8. *A,* A nonselective pigtail catheter can be used, in combination with a guide wire, as a selective catheter to gain access to the contralateral iliac artery. *B,* Beginning in the infrarenal aorta, the pigtail catheter is first retracted until it catches on the aortic bifurcation. *C,* Further manipulation and retraction splays out the pigtail catheter, directing its tip orifice down the contralateral iliac artery. *D,* Subsequent guide wire passage down the contralateral iliac artery will provide support for catheter advancement over the guide wire. *E,* Final catheter position in the external iliac artery facilitates selective angiography of the right lower extremity. Although this vessel is too small to allow the pigtail catheter to assume its typical shape, the presence of multiple side holes in this catheter allows contrast injection even if the catheter tip is against the vessel wall.

sized (in French units) by their *outside* diameter, with their lumen (*inside*) diameters determined by the thickness of the catheter wall. Diagnostic catheter sizes commonly used for peripheral work range from 4 to 6 Fr. and typically have inside diameters (specified in fractional inches) of 0.035 or 0.038 inch, the former being the most common. Catheters as small as 2 to 3 Fr. are available and can be advanced through standard diagnostic catheters, acting as "guiding" catheters (to be discussed shortly), for superselective work. Obviously, the lumen of such small catheters can accommodate only a commensurately smaller guide wire and allows only relatively low-contrast infusion rates.

Shape is by far the most crucial characteristic to be considered in catheter selection. Shaped catheters can be subcategorized in several ways according to their many characteristics. Multiple side-hole catheters are used to infuse relatively high volumes of contrast into high-flow vessels, where injection under higher pressure is required to achieve adequate opacification. The multiple holes dissipate the flow of contrast, minimizing the potentially injurious "jet effect" of the injectate on the vessel wall if it were all injected out of a single end hole. Furthermore, the multiple sites of injection into the flow stream provide more uniform opacification of the vessel. The "pigtail" and "tennis racquet" catheters have further improved on this aspect with shapes that maximize contrast dispersion. These catheters are typically used for aortic and vena caval studies and do not "form" (i.e., assume their shape) in smaller vessels (Fig. 32–8D). Virtually all multiple side-hole catheters are "self-forming"; that is, they assume their shape spontaneously after removal of the guide wire in the intended vessel size.

Forming and Using Catheters

Catheters whose curves have an overall radius less than the diameter of the blood vessel are generally self-forming and are useful for selecting the origins of a number of branch vessels. Advancement of the catheter farther into the branch vessel is usually performed over a guide wire, although this is not always so. Selection of tip shape largely depends on the angulation of the branch of interest.

In contrast, catheters with too large a curve to form spontaneously need to be manipulated into their shape, usually by engaging the tip in a side branch while advancing the body of the catheter, effectively "folding" the catheter over on itself. These catheters usually form U-turn configurations. Typically, one can advance them within the side branch several centimeters by withdrawing the body of the catheter once the tip has engaged the branch vessel. This improves the quality of the angiogram by minimizing contrast reflux and washout in the aorta.

The technique of forming catheters is crucial to master (Fig. 32–9). Generally, the catheter is supported by a guide wire inserted to the point of the dominant curve in the catheter. With the tip engaged in a side branch or "caught" on some plaque, the catheter body is advanced while the tip stays fixed, effectively manipulating the catheter into its designed shape. There is a definite risk of embolization during such manipulation; consequently, forming catheters in the ascending aorta is ill advised. Instead, when used for brachiocephalic catheterization, the catheters are usually formed in the distal arch or proximal descending aorta and then advanced into the ascending aorta in their formed state.

Although some catheters are shaped to engage side branches while they are being pushed forward, others are designed to be most effective when being withdrawn. The endovascular surgeon must carefully analyze the orientation of the aorta and its relevant branches and should perform all catheter manipulations under fluoroscopic guidance to reduce the risk of plaque dissection or perforation. During the selection process, one should remember to consider the geometry of all of a catheter's curves and to envision the shape the catheter will take when confined by the walls of the vessel. Although the Cobra 2 (C-2) and internal mammary (IMA) catheters can cross the aortic bifurcation, the nonselective pigtail catheter can usually be manipulated across as well (see Fig. 32–8), saving on cost if the pigtail catheter was already used for the aortogram. The guide wire is used to partially open the curve of the pigtail so that it can be engaged in the contralateral common iliac artery. The guide wire is then advanced down the iliac, followed by the catheter. Table 32–1 lists catheters commonly used to access different vessels.

Diagnostic catheters are also important for interventional procedures because they facilitate access to branch artery lesions. For diagnostic studies, it is usually necessary only that the catheter tip be engaged in the vessel origin in order to obtain good images; however, interventional work frequently requires guide wire support well beyond the lesion being treated. Using the curve of the catheter to select a branch vessel allows for the passage of a guide wire into that branch and beyond the lesion, facilitating its subsequent treatment. Furthermore, diagnostic catheters are also used to perform coil embolization of branch vessels into which they have been manipulated. Finally, in a fashion similar to that of marker guide wires, catheters with fixed distance radiopaque markers are available to facilitate computer calibration and subsequent vessel diameter or length measurements.

TABLE 32–1. COMMONLY USED SELECTIVE CATHETERS

VESSEL	CATHETER SHAPE	CATHETER NAME
Contralateral iliac	Self-forming	Cobra 1, 2, or 3; internal mammary; pigtail
	Manual forming	Simmons 1, 2, or 3; Chuang C; crossover
Renal/mesenteric	Self-forming	Cobra 1, 2, or 3; renal double curve (RDC, short or long); superior mesenteric artery (SMA)/celiac curve
	Manual forming	Simmons 1, 2, or 3; Shepherd Hook
	Axillary approach	Berenstein; Weinberg; Cobra 1 or 2
Subclavian/carotid	Self-forming	Berenstein; Weinberg; right Judkins (JR4)
	Manual forming	Simmons 1, 2, or 3; Headhunter H3

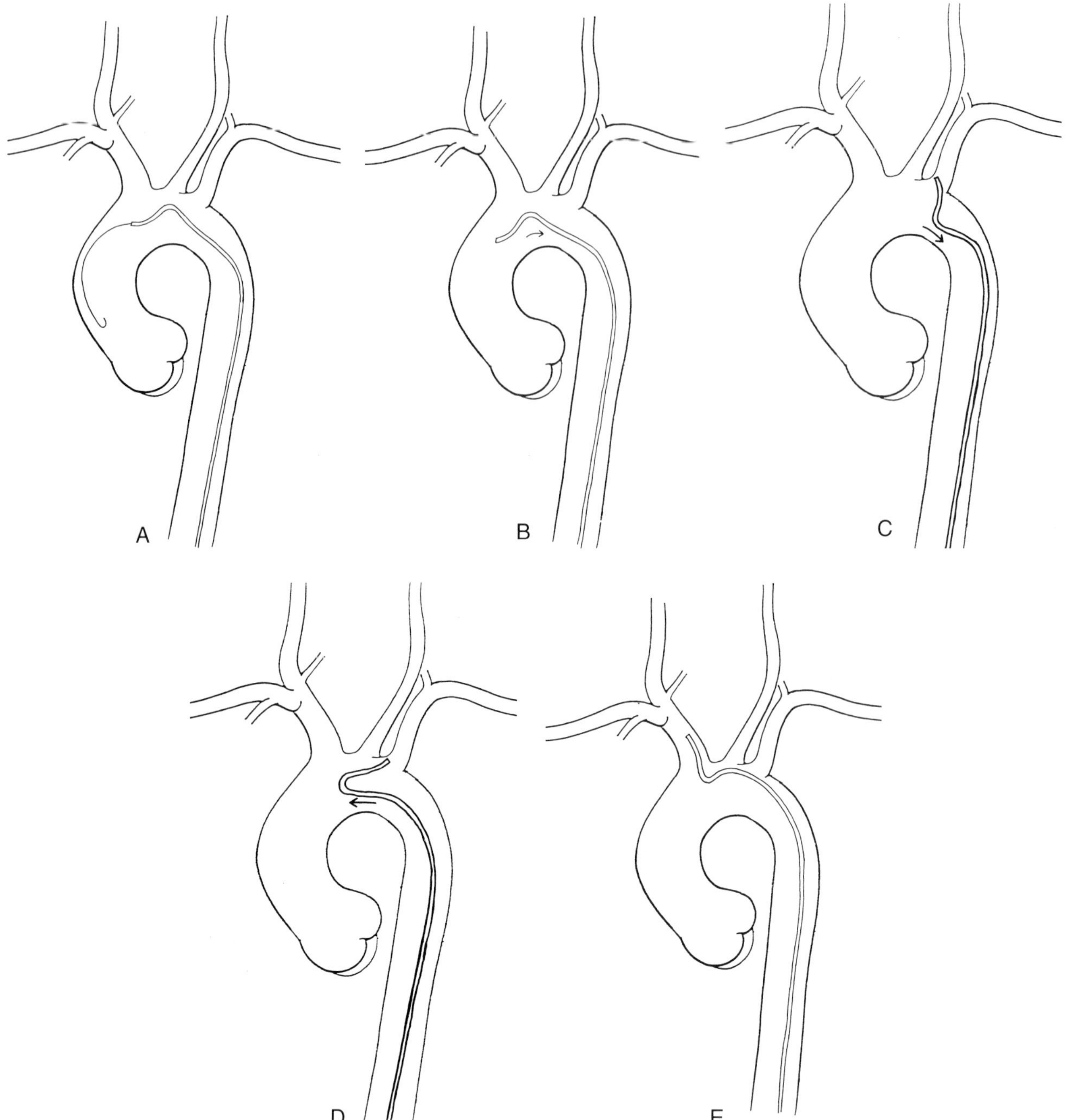

FIGURE 32–9. This series of drawings depicts how a Simmons catheter is manually formed into its pre-set shape. *A,* The catheter is first advanced over a guide wire into the aortic arch. *B,* The guide wire is removed, but the catheter does not spontaneously assume its U-turn shape because the aortic diameter is insufficient to allow for this. *C,* The catheter is rotated and retracted so that it engages the orifice of the left subclavian artery. *D,* The catheter is then advanced with the tip engaged, resulting in a "folding over" of the catheter, which is now in its pre-set shape. *E,* The catheter is then advanced beyond the origin of the innominate artery and retracted to engage the tip well up into the innominate artery for subsequent angiography or further advancement over a guide wire. *Arrows* in *B, C,* and *D* denote direction of movement described.

GUIDING CATHETERS

Guiding catheters are large-diameter catheters, usually pre-shaped to one of the self-forming curves through which balloon catheters or other interventional devices are passed. Their use has several advantages and few limitations except for the requisite larger vessel puncture necessary to accommodate the larger sheath through which they are used. One use of these catheters during endovascular interventions is to provide a mechanism to angiographically evaluate the results of the intervention without losing access to the treated area (Fig. 32–10*A* and *B*) because a lesion undergoing treatment should remain traversed by a guide wire or catheter maintaining *lesion crossing* at all times until an interventional result has succeeded.

Guiding catheters, by virtue of their oversized lumens,

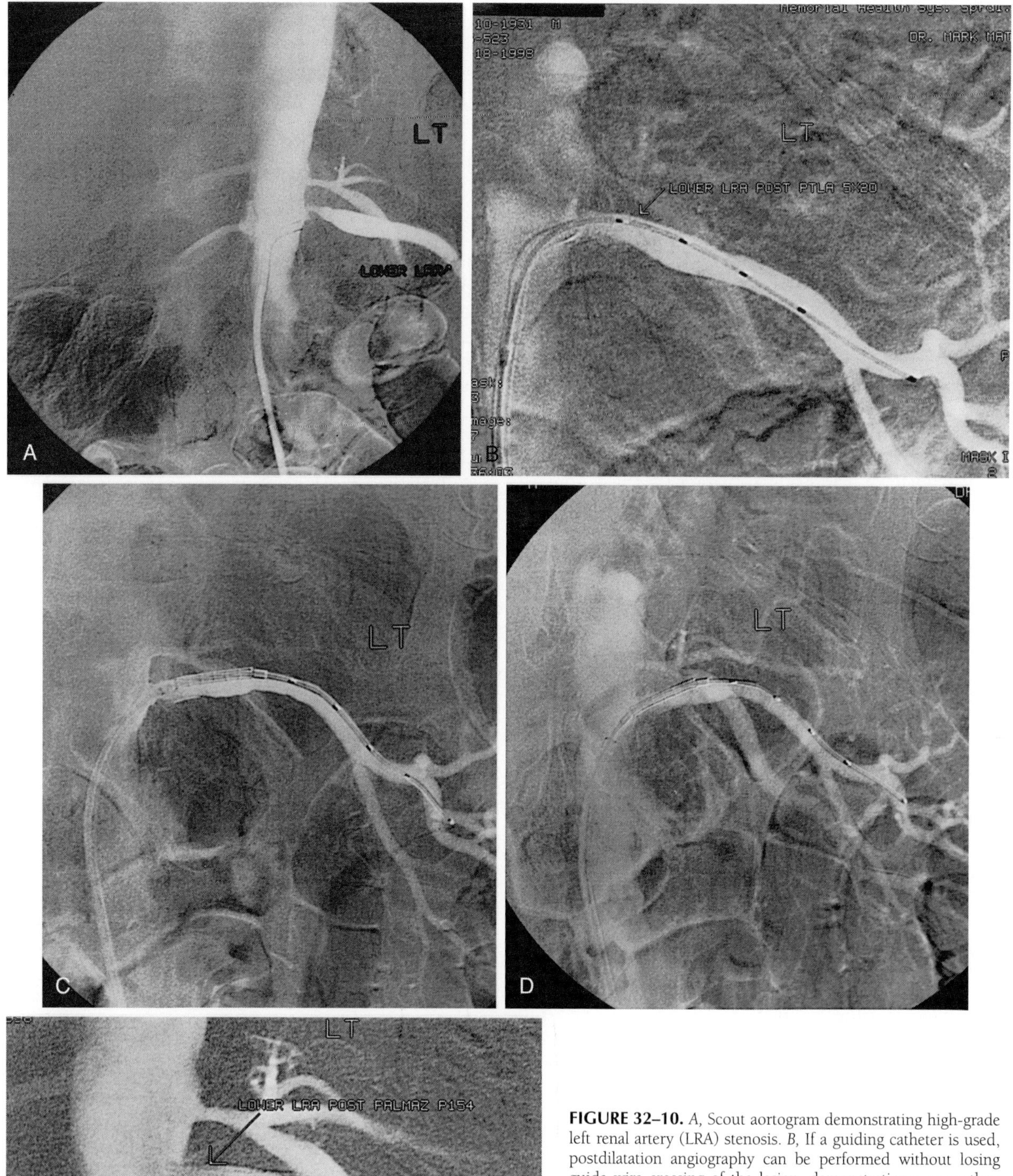

FIGURE 32–10. *A,* Scout aortogram demonstrating high-grade left renal artery (LRA) stenosis. *B,* If a guiding catheter is used, postdilatation angiography can be performed without losing guide wire crossing of the lesion, demonstrating a more than 30% residual stenosis. PTLA = percutaneous transluminal angioplasty. *C,* Contrast injection through the guiding catheter allows final positioning of the Palmaz stent prior to its deployment. In this image the stent is too far into the artery, missing the area of residual stenosis. *D,* Following retraction of the stent, repeated angiography demonstrates the stent to be in good position. *E,* Final completion arteriogram showing well-positioned stent at the renal artery origin. LT = left.

allow for contrast injection while the balloon and/or guide wire remains in position across the lesion. This is analogous to the use of crossover sheaths (see earlier) for contralateral iliac and lower extremity interventions. Because the balloon material can distort the image and alter flow dynamics, it is usually withdrawn or, at least retracted into the catheter away from the area of vessel undergoing evaluation before contrast injection.

Clinical Applications

Without the use of a crossover sheath or guiding catheter; angiographic evaluation of an intervention site without losing lesion crossing requires leaving the tip of the catheter just beyond the most distal aspect of the dilated area, removing the guide wire, and forcefully injecting through the guide wire channel of the balloon catheter. Usually, a sufficient volume of contrast refluxes proximally and allows a general assessment of the adequacy of the intervention, although the balloon material may degrade the image somewhat. If all proceeds well, the catheter can be withdrawn to a position upstream of the lesion and formal completion angiography can be performed. If a problem is revealed that requires another dilatation after the lesion crossing has been relinquished, the lesion must be re-crossed. This procedure carries a significant risk of plaque dissection and subintimal wire passage. If this maneuver is attempted, it is performed under fluoroscopic guidance and is best accomplished with a J-wire.

An alternative to prematurely relinquishing guide wire crossing of the angioplasty site is to switch the standard guide wire for an undersized one, which may make it possible to inject dye through a slightly withdrawn balloon with the lesion crossing maintained by the undersized guide wire. In general, this requires use of a wire smaller than usually necessary to accomplish the other technical requirements of the procedure. Both the "contrast reflux" and "small wire" angiography techniques may provide adequate imaging in relatively small, low-flow vessels, but obtaining adequate opacification in larger, high-flow vessels can be problematic. The use of a guiding catheter in this situation overcomes these difficulties.

A related use of guiding catheters is for determining appropriate positioning of a balloon catheter or stent prior to its inflation or deployment (Fig. 32–10*C* and *D*). Because contrast injection can be performed while the device is across the lesion, there is the opportunity to make any final adjustments in its position prior to completing the intervention. This is particularly crucial when stents are deployed at the orifice of branch vessels (e.g., for renal or subclavian artery lesions), because the risk of an excessive amount of the stent projecting into the aorta can be minimized. Furthermore, if the length of guide wire that can be positioned beyond the lesion is restricted (e.g., with renal artery stenoses), there may not be enough of the stiff part of the wire through the lesion for the interventional device to track to its intended site. In this situation, guiding catheters can provide substantial external support and guidance to the interventional device. This is particularly valuable when acute vascular angulation is present.

Guiding catheters also have the capability of facilitating performance of balloon angioplasty of distant contralateral sites or through tortuous arteries by reducing the arterial wall friction effect on the interventional catheter passing through them. In essence, the guiding catheter acts as a reduced friction sleeve through which the interventional catheter is passed. When used over the aortic bifurcation, for example, both crossover sheaths and guiding catheters redirect the force vector of the interventional catheter being passed through them so that it is as if it were being introduced from the aorta itself, resulting in improved torquability and pushability of the interventional catheter.

In a similar fashion, guiding catheters provide a smooth pathway to a lesion when implanting Palmaz stents (Johnson & Johnson, New Brunswick, N.J.). Without them, or a sheath performing a similar function, there would be excessive risk of either vessel wall trauma or stent dislodgment from the catheter during passage of the stent to its intended site of deployment.

Finally, guiding catheters are used for passage of snares and graspers to protect the walls of the vessel along the way to the target lesion.

Sizing and Usage

Guiding catheters are sized by the minimum size of the sheath through which the catheter will pass. Typical sizes range from 7 to 10 Fr. Therefore, the French size of the catheter refers to its maximal *outside diameter* (OD). Also crucial, of course, is the *inside diameter* (ID) because this determines the size of the device that can be passed through it and how much additional channel is available for injection of contrast.

In a situation analogous to that of diagnostic catheters, the ID is expressed in fractional inches. These characteristics vary slightly among manufacturers but are usually detailed on the package, which should be reviewed prior to selection. Because of the increased diameter of these catheters, large volumes of contrast can be injected easily. Unlike sheaths, however, guiding catheters do not have hemostatic valves, mandating the use of a hemostatic plug or *Y-adapter* on the guiding catheter so that significant volumes of blood do not leak out alongside the guide wire or balloon catheter.

In contrast to sheaths that come with tapered dilators, which create a smooth transition from the size of the guide wire to that of the sheath, most guiding catheters have no similar tapered obturator. Consequently, there is typically a significant step-off between the wire and the guide catheter (e.g., from the 0.035-inch OD of the guide wire to the 0.105-inch OD of a typical 8 Fr. guide catheter), which can easily snag atheromatous plaque or debris during passage.

Although most guiding catheters have soft pliable tips designed to minimize vascular trauma, it is still advisable to observe their passage under fluoroscopy to minimize this risk. Manufacturers have started to provide long tapering obturators with some of their guiding catheters, similar to the dilators used with sheaths during insertion, to address this concern.

BALLOON ANGIOPLASTY CATHETERS

Balloon angioplasty catheters may differ with regard to several factors, including the following:

- Balloon material
- Presence of friction-reducing coatings on the balloon or catheter shaft
- Mechanism of balloon inflation
- Length of catheter tip extending beyond the balloon
- Length of the "shoulder" of the balloon (that part of the balloon at each end that does not achieve the rated balloon diameter but tapers to its attachment site on the shaft of the balloon)

The last two factors—tip and shoulder length—are relevant in dilatatation near branch points or where the amount of balloon or catheter shaft extending beyond the balloon must be limited.

Construction Variables

Differences in balloon construction have a great effect on performance. Early balloons were made of polyvinyl chloride but were overly compliant, resulting in both lower burst pressures and a tendency to dilate beyond their rated size. Less compliant materials, such as polyethylene (and its derivatives), polyester and woven Dacron, have essentially replaced polyvinyl chloride for peripheral angioplasty. Differences between these materials relate to the balloon's maximal inflation pressure, profile (how closely the balloon wraps around the catheter shaft), pliability, compliance, and resistance to perforation by calcified plaque or stents. Polyester and woven Dacron balloons are "high-pressure" balloons, usually rated to 17 atmospheres (atm), whereas most polyethylene balloons are rated to 12 atm. Balloons capable of withstanding higher inflation pressures are often needed for dilating heavily calcified plaques and bypass grafts stenoses.

The Olbert balloon (Boston Scientific Corp.) is unique, having a dual coaxial shaft construction that results in a very low-profile balloon both before and after inflation. Furthermore, the Olbert's woven Dacron balloon material is pliable, which makes it good for dilating curved arterial segments and is durable, making it less likely to be perforated by exophytic calcified plaques or projecting edges of stents. The tradeoff with this balloon is that, for a given guide wire size, the balloon catheter shaft is one French size larger than a standard balloon, requiring a proportionally larger introducer sheath or guiding catheter.

Some manufacturers have begun to apply a hydrophilic coating to the outside of the balloon that may aid in advancing the balloon through tight stenoses, occlusions, or guiding catheters. Unfortunately, such coatings also make it difficult to securely affix Palmaz stents to these balloons, and many a stent has been dislodged or lost because of them. For this reason, and because such coatings were probably not necessary in the first place, their use on the balloons themselves is declining, although the catheter shaft may still be coated in this way. If it is necessary to mount a stent on a coated balloon, one should make every effort to remove the coating by rubbing the balloon vigorously with a gauze sponge before mounting the stent.

Angioplasty Balloon Selection

Having identified a lesion for dilatation and selected the appropriate type of balloon, one must consider balloon diameter and length, usable catheter length, catheter shaft diameter, and the maximum size guide wire accepted by that the catheter. Balloon diameters range from 1.5 to 18 mm, in 0.5-mm increments for balloons less than 5 mm in diameter and 1.0-mm increments for larger balloons. Ideally, balloon diameter should be 10% to 20% greater than the adjacent "normal" vessel diameter.

When measuring off a conventional arteriogram, one must size the balloon to the actual measurement because the magnification factor of the filming technique generally provides this level of overdilatation. If digital subtraction angiography (DSA), is used, it may be necessary to calculate the "normal" vessel diameter by calibrating the computer with a marker wire or another standardization device (see Fig. 32–7). With experience comes the ability to judge vessel size from the DSA image without performing measurements, although caution should always be exercised in crucial situations.

Balloon lengths vary but generally include lengths approximating 2.0, 4.0, and 10.0 cm. Although the length selected is usually gauged to allow complete dilatation with a single positioning of the balloon, it is sometimes necessary to perform overlapping dilatations to cover the entire lesion if the balloon length is shorter than the lesion and a longer balloon cannot be used. One reason to perform overlapping dilatations rather than use a longer balloon would be when the next longer size would necessitate the balloon extending into a smaller diameter branch vessel that would be at risk for overdilatation. Another situation to avoid is the use of a long balloon on a curved arterial segment, such as the external iliac artery because the balloon tends to straighten out the artery when it is inflated, which may result in injury at the relatively fixed end-points of the dilatation.

Angioplasty catheters are available in several lengths (e.g., 40, 75, and 120 cm). Selection depends on the location of the lesion to be treated and the site of vascular access. The shortest catheter that will reach the lesion is usually best because longer catheters are more difficult to manipulate. This is particularly true with smaller shaft-sized catheters because they are inherently more floppy and cannot accept the larger guide wires (0.035 to 0.038 inch) that provide the support necessary to negotiate tortuous vessels over long distances. When it is necessary to use a smaller catheter and wire over a long distance, a stiff-shaft guide wire may be helpful by providing supplemental internal support, or a guiding catheter may be used for additional external support. Larger shaft balloon catheters are generally more "pushable" because of their inherent rigidity, but this may work against their negotiation of tight turns, such as in dilatatation of an iliac artery contralateral to the site of vessel puncture.

TECHNIQUE OF BALLOON ANGIOPLASTY

Selecting the Approach

With vascular access obtained and the target lesion identified, the patient generally receives heparin anticoagulation therapy, 3000 to 5000 IU given intravenously or intra-arterially. Depending on the location and nature of the lesion to be dilated, a guiding catheter or crossover sheath may be selected to facilitate performance of the procedure. Switching to a different site of access may be indicated because the best approach to a lesion to be dilated is usually from the closest point of vascular access that allows adequate working room to complete the procedure. This optimizes catheter tracking (pushability), the lack of which can be a problem, especially with acutely angled aortic bifurcations or tortuous iliac arteries.

Lesions of the common femoral artery or very distal external iliac artery can be treated only from the contralateral femoral or axillary approach because an ipsilateral puncture cannot provide adequate working room for the balloon, even without a sheath. If a contralateral iliac artery occlusion precludes an over-the-top approach, a potential alternate approach might be the axillary artery puncture, the retrograde ipsilateral superficial femoral puncture, or the popliteal artery puncture.

Certain situations require special consideration during balloon angioplasty. Atherosclerotic plaques occurring at bifurcations are essentially single plaques with extensions into both vessels. Dilatation of only one aspect of the plaque can result in fracture of the plaque in the other branch with the potential for dissection and occlusion. The aortic bifurcation is a common location for this situation, with atherosclerotic plaque involving the origins of both of the common iliac arteries.

Dilatation is best accomplished with the "kissing balloon" technique, whereby both proximal common iliac arteries are dilated simultaneously from bilateral femoral artery punctures with the balloons "kissing" in the distal aorta (Fig. 32–11). This approach supports both sides during dilatation and is recommended for proximal common iliac lesions, even if only one of them is severe enough to warrant therapeutic dilatation. At the least in a situation such as this, access to the "contralateral" vessel should be preserved by placement of a guide wire across the region prone to dissection. That way, if balloon dilatation of a proximal iliac artery stenosis causes a dissection into the contralateral iliac artery, a balloon angioplasty catheter can be advanced over the contralateral guide wire to remedy the situation. Similarly, when a stenosis is in close proximity to a branch vessel, such as in a mid-renal artery stenosis, passage of two guide wires across the stenosis, with one out each branch, ensures access to both branches should a dissection occur after treatment of the proximal lesion (Fig. 32–12).

Dilatation across major branch vessel origins must be approached with caution because the process may result in occlusion of the branch vessel. This this may be of little consequence for some vessels, such as the hypogastric artery, but loss of a vertebral artery during dilatation of a subclavian lesion may have more severe consequences.

Accessing the Lesion

After the lesion to be treated is identified and the best approach is formulated, achieving guide wire crossing is the next step before balloon dilatation. For ipsilateral iliac or lower extremity lesions, the guide wire can simply be advanced through the introducer sheath and manipulated across the lesion Although a **J**-tipped guide wire has the lowest potential for injuring the vessel, many lesions are too severely stenotic, or the path to them too tortuous, to allow passage of such a wire because the wire has a large-profile, nondirectional leading element. The standard 3-mm radius **J**-wire leads with a 6-mm-wide prow, but smaller radius **J**-wires such as the 1.5-mm (3-mm prow) may be able to negotiate moderately tight stenoses with the minimized risk of dissection afforded by a **J**-tip configuration.

Alternatively, a straight or angled floppy-tipped wire (e.g., Benson, Wholey, or Turemo) can be used with care and under fluoroscopic guidance. The Turemo wire has a hydrophilic coating that renders it so slippery that extreme care must be taken to ensure that the guide wire does not create a dissection, which may result in dilatation within the wrong plane, with resultant occlusion of the vessel. At times, these floppy-tipped wires benefit from the additional support afforded by advancing a diagnostic catheter to within 1 or 2 cm of the end of the wire. An angulated catheter can also help to direct the wire through tortuous segments or angulated lesions.

During dilatation of renal, subclavian, or other branch vessels, it is often necessary to use specially shaped diagnostic or guiding catheters to direct the guide wire toward the origin of the vessel of interest. If a guiding catheter is used to provide additional catheter support or to facilitate completion angiography, guide wire passage is followed simply by advancing the balloon over the wire through the catheter. Use of a **Y**-adapter allows this procedure to be performed with minimal blood leakage through the guiding catheter because the balloon catheter is not usually large enough to fully obturate the lumen of the guiding catheter.

If a diagnostic catheter has been used to direct a guide wire across a stenosis, it must be removed before the balloon catheter can be advanced into position over the wire. Great care must be taken during this catheter exchange to ensure that wire crossing of the lesion is maintained without letting the wire travel too far beyond the lesion where it might cause damage to branch vessels. When vessel angulation is steep or if there is limited room beyond the lesion to gain guide wire "purchase," use of a stiff-shafted guide wire may be instrumental in getting the balloon catheter to follow the wire into the branch vessel and across the lesion. Otherwise, the catheter tends to dislodge the guide wire out of the branch. Alternatively, a guiding catheter can be used to support and direct the balloon catheter into the area to be dilated.

Special Considerations for Total Occlusions

Dilating arterial occlusions poses another challenge to the endovascular therapist. Often the occlusion has a soft thrombotic core that allows guide wire passage, thereby making balloon dilatation feasible. This generally mandates use of an angled or floppy-tipped guide wire, though sometimes the 1.5-mm radius J-wire can be pushed through an occlusion with less chance of a dissection. Resistant occlusions may require support of the guide wire by a catheter, with only the distal 1 to 3 cm of the wire projecting out the end of the catheter. This allows the flexible tip to probe the lesion while preventing the wire from buckling under

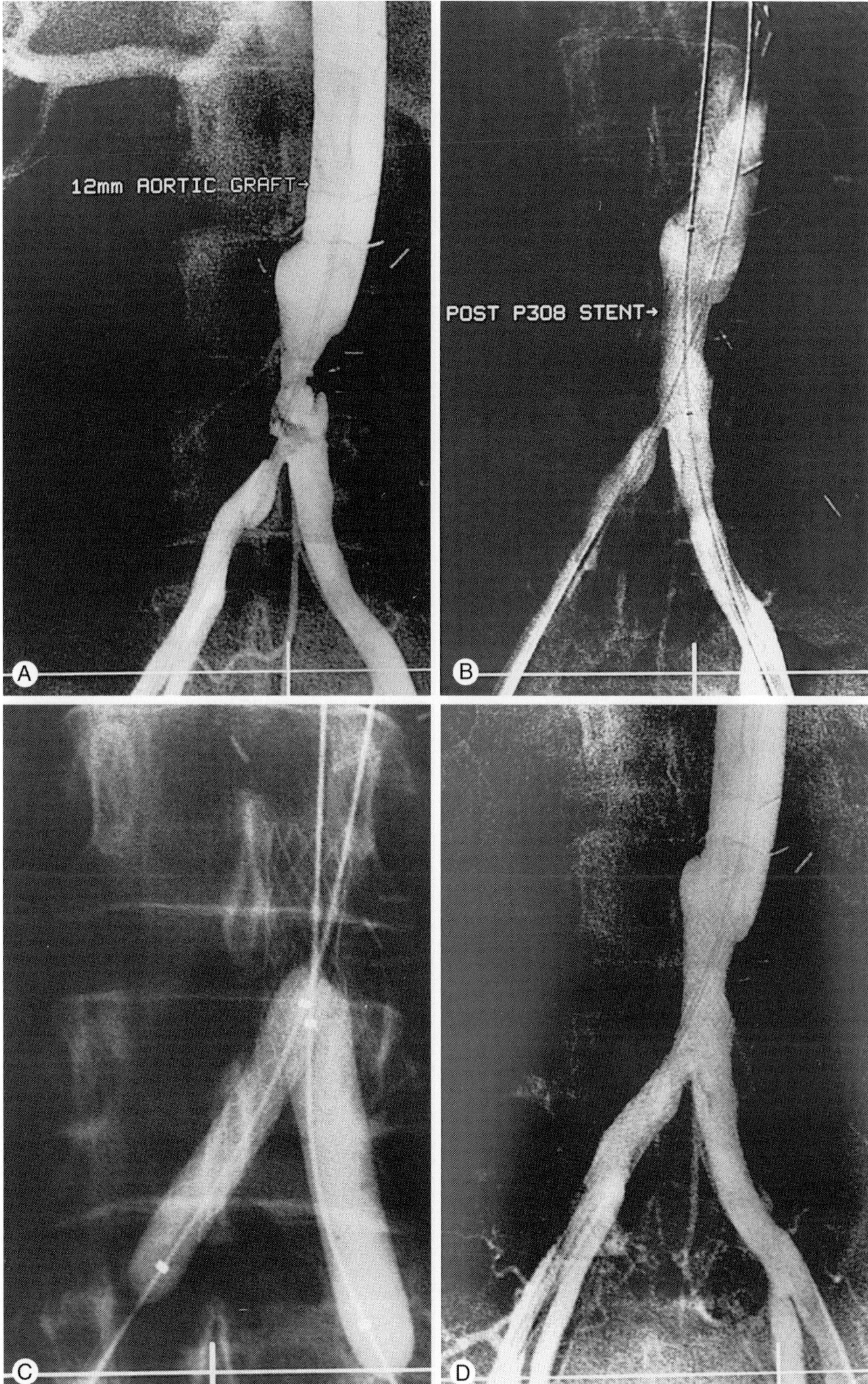

FIGURE 32–11. *A*, Complex atheromatous plaque just distal to the distal anastomosis of a descending thoracic to infrarenal abdominal aorta bypass (performed with a 12-mm Dacron graft) and extending into the iliac arteries, most notably on the right. *B*, Endovascular repair begins with dilatation and primary Palmaz stenting of the distal aorta with a 12 mm × 4 cm balloon and a P308 stent. *C*, The iliac arteries are then dilated (8 mm × 4 cm on right; 10 mm × 4 cm on left) with primary Palmaz stenting of the right common iliac artery (P294) using the kissing balloon technique. *D*, Final angiographic result. Resting ankle-brachial index (ABIs) and exercise treadmill test scores normalized.

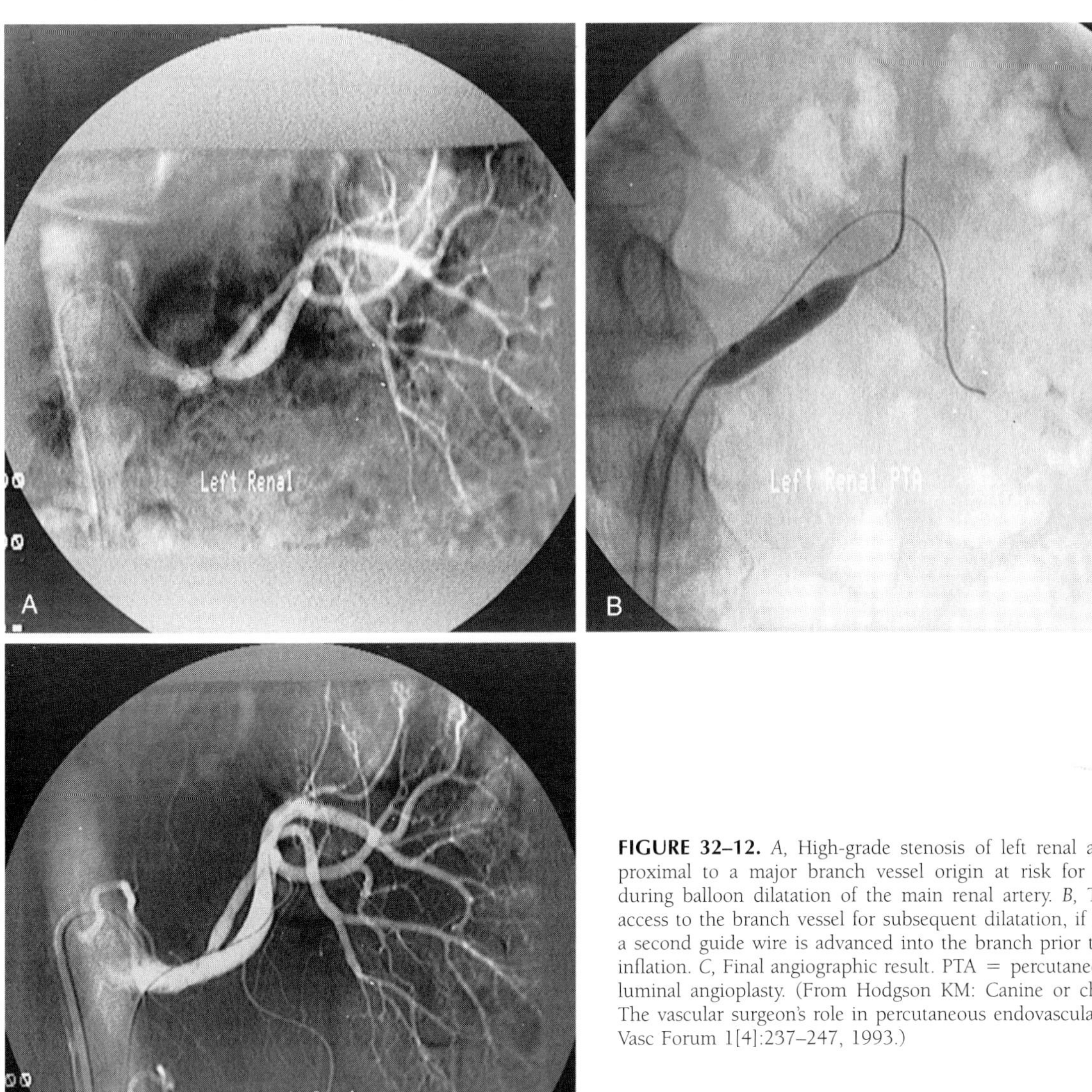

FIGURE 32–12. *A,* High-grade stenosis of left renal artery just proximal to a major branch vessel origin at risk for occlusion during balloon dilatation of the main renal artery. *B,* To protect access to the branch vessel for subsequent dilatation, if necessary, a second guide wire is advanced into the branch prior to balloon inflation. *C,* Final angiographic result. PTA = percutaneous transluminal angioplasty. (From Hodgson KM: Canine or chameleon: The vascular surgeon's role in percutaneous endovascular therapy. Vasc Forum 1[4]:237–247, 1993.)

the stress of firm forward pressure. Guide wire passage through occlusions often occurs, not surprisingly, in a subintimal plane. Therefore, reentry of the guide wire into the lumen of the vessel must be confirmed to ensure that dilatation reestablishes continuity of the flow channel rather than extends the occlusion.

When an angled or **J**-tipped wire is used, reentry into the lumen of the vessel can be confirmed by spinning the wire and observing free rotation of the tip in its angled or **J**-form. Otherwise, careful inspection of the course of the wire in several projections may provide adequate assurance of intraluminal location, particularly if the vessel can be opacified with contrast or is sufficiently calcified to be visible under fluoroscopy. Better yet, advancing a small catheter over the guide wire and into the reentered vessel allows for injection of contrast to confirm that reentry has occurred.

Many interventionists advocate a trial of thrombolysis after traversal of an occlusion because a significant component of the occlusion may be thrombotic in nature and, therefore, amenable to dissolution (Fig. 32–13). Thrombolysis reduces the overall length of the vessel requiring subsequent dilatation, and therefore the risks of injury to this area, and minimizes the chance of embolization of unstable thrombus during the dilatation. Although the chances of successful clot lysis are significantly enhanced if the thrombus is less than 2 weeks old,[14–16] even a substantially older clot can be successfully lysed, though less predictably so.[16] The inherent instability of acute thrombus mandates a trial of lysis before dilatation in these circumstances, but the need to attempt lysis in clinical situations suggestive of more chronic occlusions is debated.

The usual approach is to perform pulse-spray thrombolysis with 250,000 IU (one vial) of urokinase administered

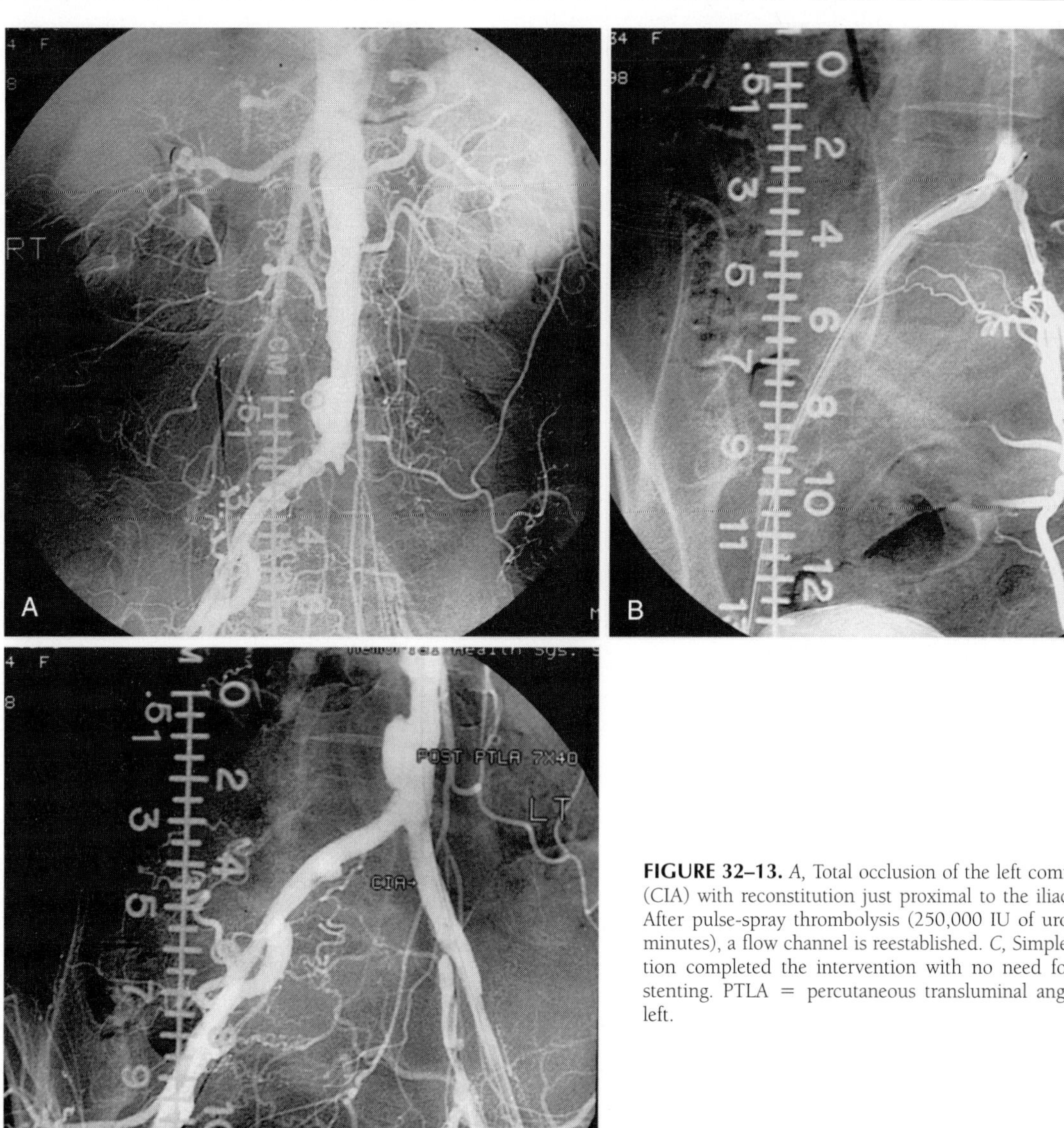

FIGURE 32–13. *A,* Total occlusion of the left common iliac artery (CIA) with reconstitution just proximal to the iliac bifurcation. *B,* After pulse-spray thrombolysis (250,000 IU of urokinase over 25 minutes), a flow channel is reestablished. *C,* Simple balloon dilatation completed the intervention with no need for supplemental stenting. PTLA = percutaneous transluminal angioplasty; LT = left.

over 20 to 30 minutes, after which a follow-up angiogram is performed. If no significant thrombolysis has occurred and the clinical situation is consistent with a chronic occlusion, it is generally safe to proceed with dilatation. If some lysis is apparent but residual thrombus appears to be present, however, another round or two of pulse-spray thrombolysis or a 4- to 8-hour infusion is indicated before dilatation. If the signs and symptoms suggest acute thrombosis, however, inability to achieve significant clot lysis after the initial round of pulse-spray administration should not be taken to indicate that the occlusion has only stable thrombus present, and an additional round of pulse-spray urokinase or a 4- to 8-hour infusion is generally indicated. Such continuous infusions are generally run at 4000 IU/min for the first 4 hours and then decreased to 2000 IU/min thereafter because these dosages have the greatest thrombolytic efficacy for an acceptable complication risk.[17]

Angioplasty Balloon Preparation and Usage

After the lesion has been crossed with the guide wire and all questions of unstable thrombus have been resolved, it is possible to proceed with balloon angioplasty with the sizing guidelines previously reviewed. Except for the Olbert angioplasty catheter, which can be used directly out of the package, balloon angioplasty catheters must undergo a preparation process referred to as a "negative preparation" prior to their first usage. This involves the application of suction to the catheter with a syringe partially filled with contrast diluted to 30% to 50%. Higher concentrations of contrast are excessively viscous and result in slow inflation and deflation times.

Suction is generally applied for 30 seconds, after which it is slowly released with the syringe held upright so that radiographic contrast is drawn back into the shaft of the catheter, replacing most of the air that had been present. This procedure minimizes the presence of air bubbles in the balloon, which can embolize if a balloon ruptures and ensures the lowest possible balloon profile. The mechanism of deployment of the Olbert balloon makes such preparation unnecessary and, in fact, may actually worsen its profile.

Balloon angioplasty catheters are generally not test-inflated before use because the inflation would enlarge the profile of the balloon, possibly complicating its passage across a lesion. As with all catheters, the lumen of the balloon catheter is irrigated with heparinized saline before it is used. Although pressure-monitored inflation devices are commonly used, some interventionists advocate simple hand inflation with a 10-ml syringe. After the angioplasty is completed, the balloon is again placed under suction, after which it is withdrawn from the region and out the introducer sheath. This minimizes, as best as possible, the profile of the balloon as it is withdrawn from the vascular system.

The balloon can be correctly positioned across the lesion to be dilated by fluoroscopic reference to anatomic structures or radiopaque marker systems that were in place at the time of the scout angiogram. The marker system must not be moved, and the alignment of the scout and positioning images must be identical; otherwise, parallax effects result in improper positioning of the balloon.

When angioplasty is performed through a guiding catheter, downstream of an indwelling sheath, or upstream but within approximately 15 cm of a sheath, contrast can be injected alongside the balloon catheter to confirm correct balloon position, provided that the sheath or guiding catheter has been adequately oversized to provide an adequate residual luminal space within the sheath. Alternatively, with a smaller-diameter guide wire than the maximum size that the catheter can accommodate, it is possible to inject contrast out the end of the catheter as it is being advanced toward the lesion. This alternative procedure mandates the use of a Y-adapter and is limited by the requisite use of a wire that may be too small to provide adequate guidance for the angioplasty catheter. Furthermore, the amount of contrast that can be injected by this method is limited as is, therefore, the resultant opacification.

Although balloon angioplasty can be performed with relative safety without inflation pressures being monitored, the syringe used should be no smaller than 10 ml so that excessive pressures are not generated, causing increased risk of balloon rupture. It is preferable to inflate with a pressure-monitoring device to ensure that safe limits are not exceeded. The optimal number and duration of inflations are not known, but most endovascular therapists inflate for 30 to 60 seconds at a time, two to three times. Inflations of 2 minutes or more may reduce the risk of restenosis by inducing greater medial smooth muscle dysfunction.[18]

The patient commonly feels pain during dilatation that generally resolves with deflation of the balloon. The pain is thought to be related to stretching of the adventitial nerve fibers, and absence of pain may, in fact, indicate insufficient dilatation. Persistent pain after deflation of the balloon should prompt reevaluation of the situation by contrast injection because it may indicate arterial rupture with extravasation.

ASSESSMENT OF RESULTS

When to conclude endovascular therapy and when to continue, perhaps with a larger balloon or placement of a stent, can be difficult to determine. Dilatation-associated dissections can, at times, produce a worrisome-appearing angiogram even though the therapeutic result is excellent (Fig. 32–14). As long as the dissection does not extend beyond the dilated area and does not obstruct flow, it need not be considered a significant problem and should not increase the risk of restenosis. Yet on the other hand, a satisfactory angiographic result may actually be hemody-

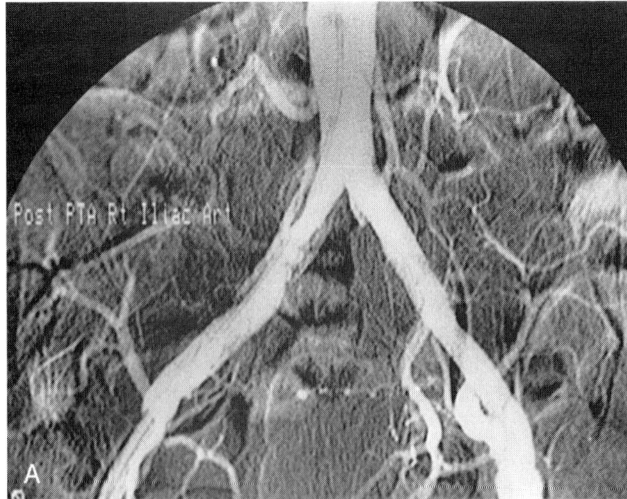

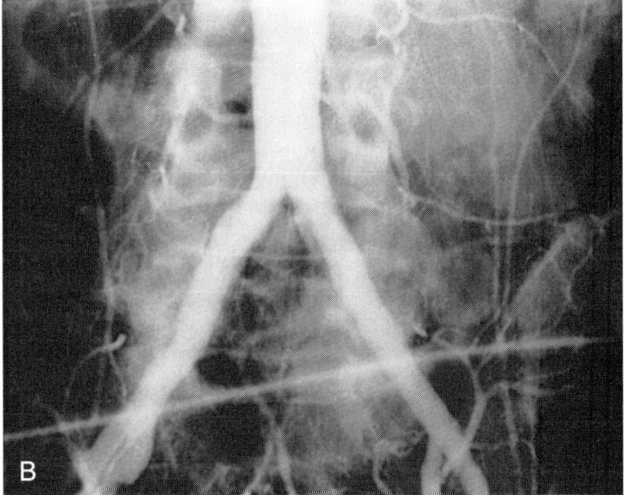

FIGURE 32–14. *A*, Severe dissection of the right common iliac artery following balloon dilatation of a high-grade stenosis performed for claudication at a time prior to the availability of stents. Nonetheless, the patient's symptoms resolved, and ankle-brachial index normalized. PTA = percutaneous transluminal angioplasty. *B*, Same artery 6 months later at the time of an unrelated angiogram. The patient maintained his clinical and hemodynamic successes as well.

namically suboptimal because of the limitations of the angiographic method of assessment.

IVUS may allow better evaluation of the angioplasty results, but discussion of this method is beyond the scope of this chapter. Most angioplasties performed today are evaluated solely on the basis of completion angiography despite some potential shortcomings of this technique. The accuracy of angiography can be improved when several different planes are viewed and the catheter is selected and positioned to ensure adequate opacification without the introduction of contrast injection artifacts. The catheter must be large enough to deliver an adequate volume of contrast and positioned proximal enough to the region under study to ensure thorough mixing of the contrast within the bloodstream before it reaches the area of interest. When a lesion is dilated from the retrograde approach, contrast can be injected through the deflated balloon catheter (left in position across the dilated lesion to maintain lesion crossing) after removal of the guide wire. Although the wings of balloon material may degrade the image somewhat, this technique is generally adequate for a reasonable assessment of the result of the intervention and to allow a decision to be made about the need for further intervention.

In antegrade intervention situations, the tip of the balloon catheter is downstream of the dilated lesion. In such instances, use of a guiding catheter or sheath allows for contrast infusion from above, which provides the best opacification. Otherwise, there are only two other means of assessing the interventional result without losing "lesion crossing." The best alternative is to leave the deflated balloon catheter in place across the lesion, remove the guide wire, and forcefully inject through the balloon catheter, the goal being to get sufficient reflux of contrast to opacify the area of interest. High-flow situations compromise opacification with this technique, and there is always a risk of embolization because of the "jet effect" of forceful injection through a small-diameter end-hole catheter. Alternatively, a significantly undersized guide wire may allow for injection of enough contrast through the proximally retracted balloon catheter with the wire left in place through the balloon catheter and across the lesion.

In general, a balloon dilatation procedure is considered technically successful if there is less than a 30% residual stenosis after the procedure is completed. Greater residual stenoses, although often not hemodynamically significant, correlate with early recurrence of the stenosis. Sometimes hemodynamic assessment may be possible and is considered a more reliable measure of success than the angiographic appearance alone. Dilatation of an iliac lesion from the ipsilateral approach, for example, allows for measurement of a "pull-through pressure" whereby the distal aspect of an end-hole catheter is placed proximal to the dilated area and the blood pressure is measured through the catheter as it is withdrawn through the lesion.

Ordinarily, there should be no discernible decrement in pressure within or on the downstream side of the dilated area, although a drop of 5 to 10 mmHg is probably not significant. For such a determination to be performed from a contralateral puncture, the catheter must actually be positioned across the lesion at the time that the downstream pressure is measured. Because the catheter itself may partially obstruct the flow channel, thereby producing a pressure drop, this technique has an increased false-positive rate. If no significant pressure differential is detected by this approach, however, it can generally be assumed that dilatation has been successful. For SFA dilatations performed from either an ipsilateral or a contralateral common femoral puncture, this approach is the only way to perform a hemodynamic assessment. Unfortunately, obstruction of flow from the catheter becomes even more significant as the size of the artery decreases, introducing an even greater level of error with this approach in the superficial femoral and renal arteries than in the iliac system.

When bilateral retrograde femoral sheaths are in place, it is possible to display simultaneous waveforms from both external iliac arteries. This allows comparison of the pressure below an iliac dilatation with an index arterial pressure obtained from the contralateral iliac artery. If there is coexisting contralateral iliac disease, a catheter can be advanced into the aorta on that side to provide a true measure of "normal" arterial pressure. This method of assessing the result of intervention is particularly useful when "kissing" balloon dilatation has been performed because bilateral sheaths will already be present.

Finally, pharmacologic provocation can be used to assess the significance of any residual stenosis by continuous pressure monitoring downstream from a treated area after injection of 100 to 200 μg of nitroglycerin or 10 to 20 mg of papaverine into the ipsilateral extremity intra-arterial circulation. A drop in pressure exceeding 20 mmHg is evidence that the residual stenosis was hemodynamically significant. Although these doses do not usually produce a measurable drop in systemic blood pressure, this source of error is negated by measurement of the contralateral iliac or aortic pressure to detect a pressure differential of 20 mmHg or greater. Measurement of ankle-brachial indices in the early post-treatment period may not be helpful because maximal improvement in pressure is typically not seen for at least several days. Furthermore, coexisting occlusive disease often obscures significant improvement in the treated area.

INTRAVASCULAR STENTS

When dilatation is performed with an appropriately sized balloon, treatment of a more than 30% residual stenosis, a persistent pressure gradient with or without pharmacologic provocation, or a severe dissection is generally achieved by placement of a stent. There are only two stents with FDA approval for use in the peripheral vascular system, and they are approved only for use in iliac arteries. Nonetheless, off-label use of stents is rampant and includes approved iliac stents in noniliac locations as well as stents approved only for use in the biliary system in any number of vascular locations.

FDA approval for intravascular use is anticipated for a number of these stents, as is the introduction of even more new iterations of the stent theme. Therefore, it is impossible to provide detailed descriptions of or specific instructions for all of the stents that will be available in the foreseeable future. Consequently, this discussion reviews only the gen-

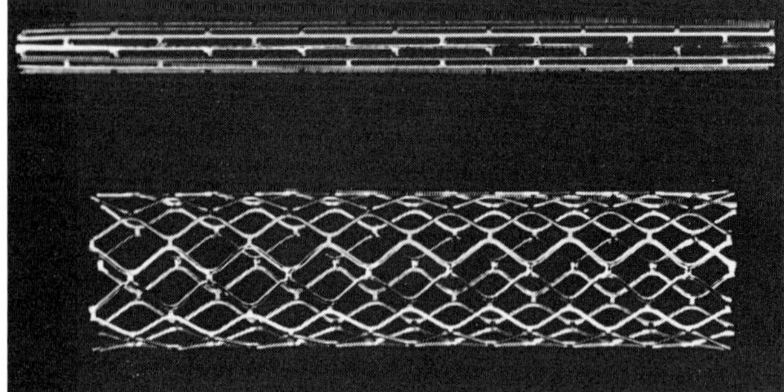

FIGURE 32–15. Palmaz P308 stent in undeployed *(top)* and deployed *(bottom)* states.

eral characteristics of intravascular stents, their modes of deployment, and relevant differences between categories of stents.

Stent Characteristics

Stents can be classified by a number of characteristics, but the most relevant include their (1) method of deployment, (2) flexibility, (3) ability to be crushed by external pressure, (4) radial strength, (5) radiopacity, (6) predictability of final deployment location and length, (7) ability to be repositioned prior to complete deployment, and (8) the material they are constructed of. Each type of stent is available in different sizes and varies in both diameter and length. Requisite sheath sizes vary among stents and among stent sizes within a stent family, but most stents need sheaths ranging from 7 to 10 Fr. Furthermore, some stents can be advanced through the vascular system without a covering sheath or guiding catheter, while others cannot.

Perhaps the most dichotomous characteristic of stents is their method of deployment: *self-expanding* or *balloon-expanded*. The Palmaz stent (Johnson & Johnson) (Fig. 32–15) is the prototype and the only stent in use that requires balloon expansion to bring about deployment, although it is advisable to balloon-dilate all stents after their deployment to ensure full expansion and vessel wall contact.

Balloon-Expanded Stents

Because of its balloon expandability, the Palmaz stent comes in only a few diameters, the final stent diameter being dependent on the size of the balloon used to deploy it. This balloon expandability also permits subsequent dilatation to a larger size if the original assessment of the necessary diameter proves to be too small; however, this balloon expandability restricts the ability to use a stent in areas where the vessel size changes, such as when one goes from the common to the external iliac artery, unless different diameter balloons are used in each of these areas. When different diameter balloons are used, the procedure becomes significantly more complex and the risk of overdistention of the smaller of the two arteries is greater. Furthermore, optimal vessel wall contact may not be achievable near the transition zone.

Because the Palmaz stent must be delivered to its intended site mounted on an angioplasty balloon, the risk of dislodgment of the undeployed stent from the balloon is present. This situation usually occurs when the stent is advanced to its intended site of deployment, most often when one is negotiating turns in the vascular system. It is for this reason that Palmaz stents are passed through delivery sheaths or guiding catheters instead of being advanced through the vascular system bare, where contact with the vessel wall may dislodge the stent or traumatize the vessel.

Once in position across the lesion, the sheath or guiding catheter is retracted to allow balloon inflation. When properly positioned on the angioplasty catheter, balloon expansion occurs at both ends of the stent first (Fig. 32–16), ensuring that the stent remains centered on the balloon and deploys at its intended site. It is critical to ensure that the stent remains reasonably centered on the balloon before initiating deployment, however, so that subsequent balloon inflation does not propel the stent forward or backward off of the balloon (Fig. 32–17). This can be a challenging situation to address because, in its undeployed state, the balloon is difficult to reposition into the stent to permit its deployment not only because of the stent's small internal channel but also because it is not fixed in space.

A related failure of complete deployment can occur if the balloon ruptures during deployment. Although this can often be addressed by rapid hand or power inflation of the balloon to overwhelm the leak, essentially filling the balloon faster than the fluid can leak out, at times this may be unsuccessful and a free-floating or marginally secured stent is the result. As long as the stent has achieved a reasonable degree of fixation, the leaking balloon can usu-

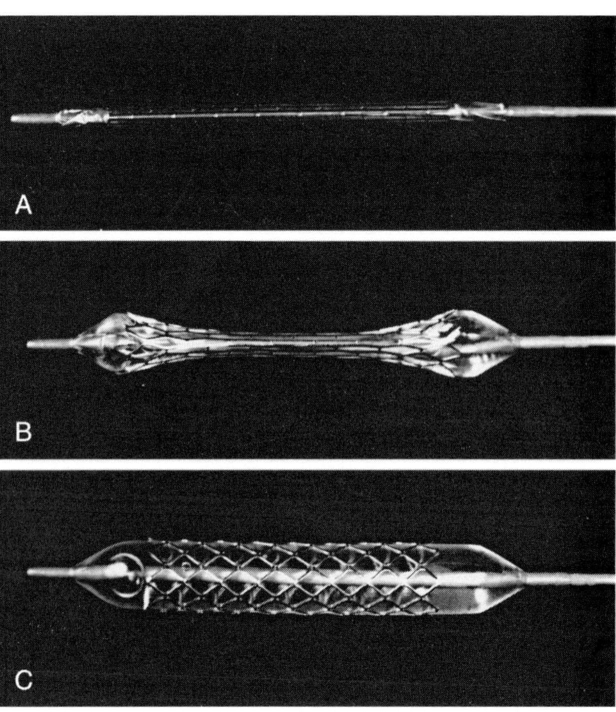

FIGURE 32–16. *A,* Expansion sequence of a Palmaz stent. The predeployed stent is centered on the balloon at the start of deployment. *B,* The balloon first inflates at the ends of the stent. *C,* Complete expansion of the stent occurs last in the center.

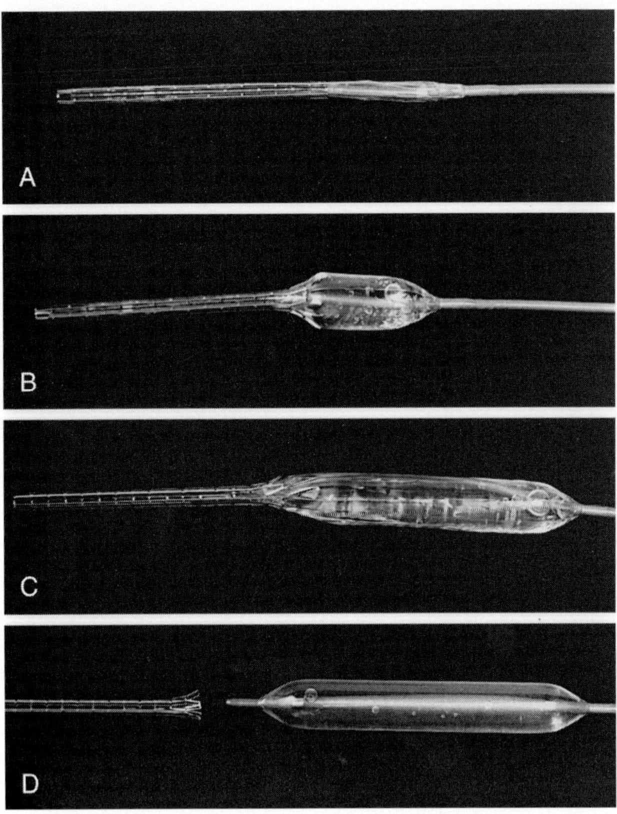

FIGURE 32–17. *A,* A pre-deployment Palmaz stent malpositioned on the balloon catheter. *B,* As inflation proceeds, the balloon inflates proximally first. *C* and *D,* Further inflation progressively propels the unexpanded stent off of the end of the catheter.

ally be exchanged for a new balloon that can be carefully advanced into the stent to complete the deployment.

Self-Expanding Stents

Self-expanding stents differ because they spontaneously expand once the containing delivery system is retracted; therefore, if properly sized, they will immediately achieve secure fixation within the vessel. If undersized for the vessel in which they are deployed, however, they may not make adequate wall contact (Fig. 32–18). In contrast to the Palmaz stent, self-expanding stents cannot be overdilated to achieve secure fixation unless an oversized stent is placed within them to maintain their dilatation beyond their rated diameter. This limitation makes accurate size selection much more critical than with Palmaz stents and requires a much larger inventory of stents because a given self-expanding stent has a much narrower range of expansion than a Palmaz stent.

Typically, self-expanding stents are available in 1-mm diameter increments up to 8 mm, after which subsequently larger sizes increase in 2-mm increments. In contrast, Palmaz stents come in two basic diameter ranges, 4 to 9 mm and 8 to 12 mm.

Another difference between these two categories of stents is in the conformability to changing vessel diameters, a particular asset of the self-expanding variety of stent. Furthermore, the self-expanding stents tend to be much more flexible, accommodating tortuous vessels without imparting kinks at the end-points of the stent. This flexibility extends to the undeployed state as well easily and permits self-expanding stents (compared with Palmaz stents) to be manipulated through tortuous vessels and over the aortic bifurcation. Although deploying a Palmaz stent from across the aortic bifurcation is restricted to relatively short stent lengths, typically 2 cm or less, self-expanding stents of 10 cm or more can easily be used to perform this maneuver.

Although self-expanding stents are advanced through the vascular system without requisite sheath or guiding catheter access to the lesion, they are encased by an outer catheter of their own. This outer catheter is an integral component of their delivery system that maintains their collapsed state until it is retracted and the stent is allowed to expand. This feature also protects the vessels being traversed from being traumatized during passage of the catheter. Although the size of the vascular access sheath varies between stent brands and within the size range of each type of stent, most peripheral vessels can be approached through sheaths ranging from 7 to 10 Fr.

Two different mechanisms are responsible for expansion of self-expanding stents: (1) the method of fabrication and (2) the material used in their construction. Although the Wallstent (Schneider, Boston Scientific Corp., Nadick, Mass.) achieves its expansion by virtue of its stainless steel braid construction (Fig. 32–19), most of the newer stents being developed rely on the self-expansion properties of the thermal memory metal nitinol (Fig. 32–20). This alloy of nickel and titanium can be manufactured to assume a specific size and shape when unconstrained at body

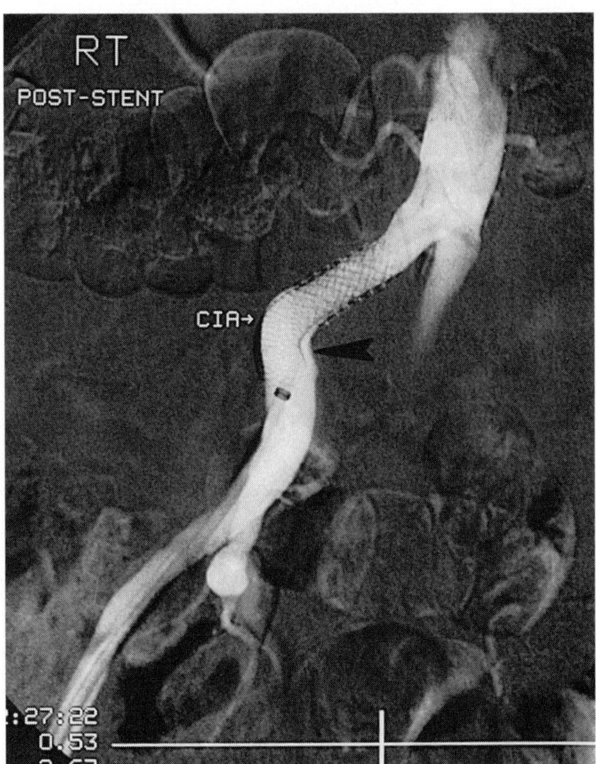

FIGURE 32–18. An undersized Wallstent not in contact with the vessel wall. CIA = common iliac artery.

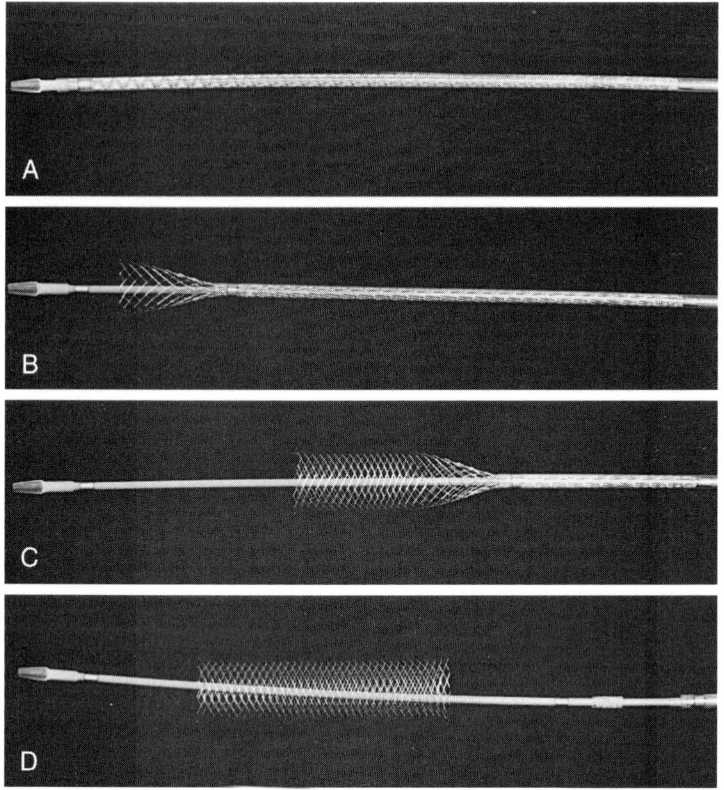

FIGURE 32–19. *A*, Sequence of deployment of a Wallstent. The collapsed Wallstent can be seen mounted on its delivery catheter over a length about twice the stent's rated length. *B*, As the outer covering component of the delivery system is retracted the stent begins to expand, in a funnel configuration that permits repositioning of the stent distally, but not proximally, once deployment has begun. *C*, After further deployment, the stent is fully expanded distally so this end-point is now known and is still changeable by virtue of the reconstraining feature of the new Wallstent delivery system. *D*, After complete retraction of its outer covering, the stent is fully expanded and no longer recapturable. Note the degree of shortening of the stent from its predeployment length.

temperature, yet it is conformable enough when chilled to be compressed into a relatively small-diameter delivery system.

The principal advantage of the generic stents over the braided stainless steel construction is the predictability of the final overall length once deployed in the body. With the braided construction the stent is longer when constrained in a smaller vessel, rendering its final length of coverage difficult to predict in even uniformly sized vessels and virtually impossible to foresee in vessels with a lack of uniformity in their diameter.

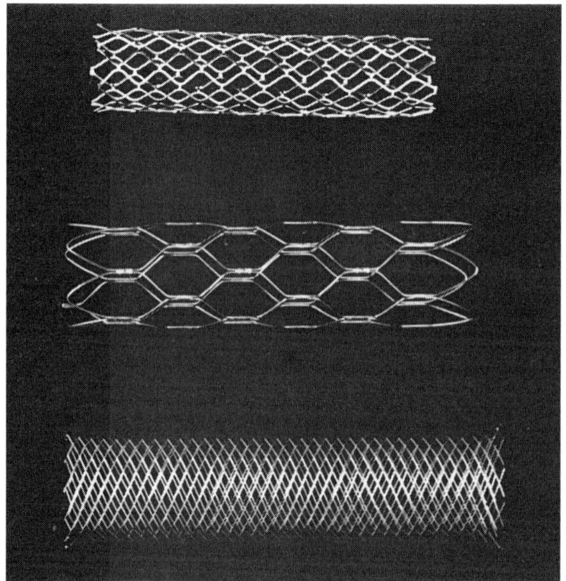

FIGURE 32–20. Comparison of stent reconstruction. From *top* to *bottom* are the balloon-expanded Palmaz stent, the self-expanding nitinol Symphony stent, and the self-expanding stainless steel Wallstent.

At its longest when still contained in its delivery system, the Wallstent shortens as it is deployed and its diameter expands (see Fig. 32–19). In contrast, nitinol stents exhibit minimal foreshortening with deployment and, therefore, have a much more predictable final length (see Fig. 32–20). Although the Palmaz stent also shortens as it is dilated to larger diameters, this action is much less pronounced than with the Wallstent (see Fig. 32–15). For this reason, Wallstents are rarely used when the final length and stent position are critical, such as near the origins of aortic branch vessels or across the origins of critical branch vessels (Fig. 32–21).

Because Wallstents deploy from distal to proximal (with regard to the catheter shaft), it is the proximal stent end-point location that is problematic. Furthermore, the radial strength of Wallstents at their end-points is much less than that of the Palmaz or nitinol stent, rendering the Palmaz and nitinol the preferred stents for branch vessel origins. However, Wallstents are the only available stents that can be recaptured during deployment (up to about 85% deployment), a feature that can facilitate repositioning of the stent if the apparent destined final position appears to be problematic.

Other Relevant Stent Characteristics

An additional advantage of the self-expanding stents is their resistance to being permanently deformed by external

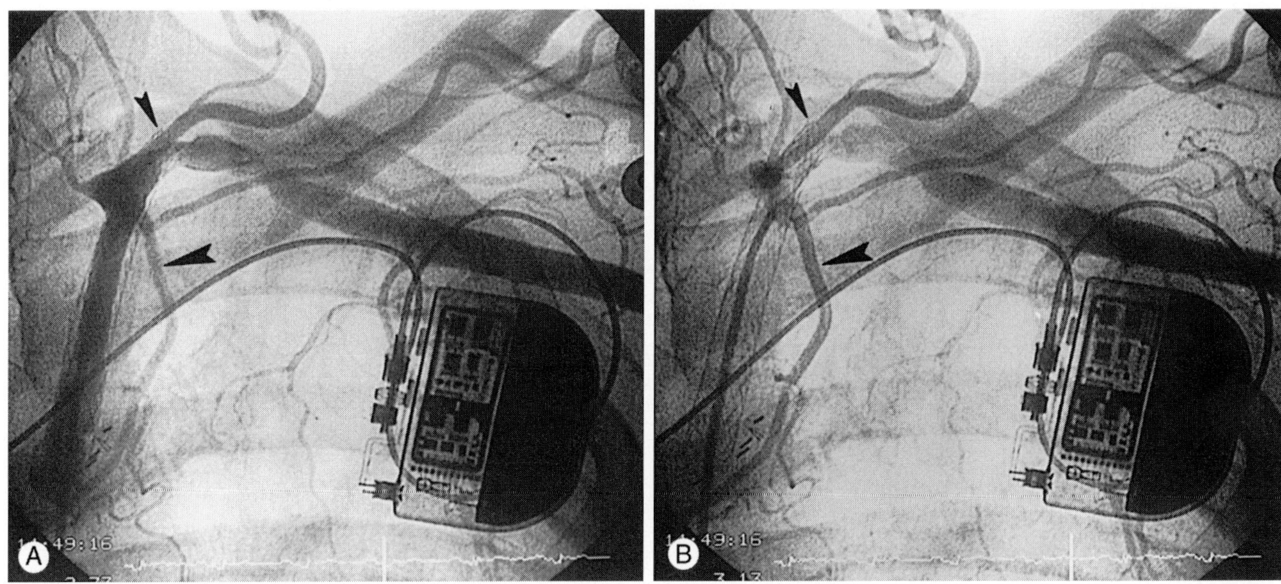

FIGURE 32–21. *A,* Patient underwent Wallstent placement (at an outlying institution) in the left subclavian artery, which is providing inflow to a mammary artery coronary graft *(bottom arrowhead). Top arrowhead* indicates the distal extent of the stent, which was presumably placed via the ipsilateral brachial-axillary approach. Although possibly of no consequence, placing the coronary graft at risk by overlying a stent should generally be avoided. Although this was likely purely a mistake in sizing the stent, the unpredictability of the final length of the Wallstent contributes significantly to the risk of this complication and may contraindicate use of the Wallstent in situations such as this, when critical branch vessels are in close proximity to the lesion being treated. *B,* A late-phase view of the same patient provides better visualization of the stent. *Arrowheads* are as in *A.*

forces such as manual pressure or flexion forces across a joint. For this reason, Palmaz stents are not generally recommended for use in the region of the inguinal ligament or at the knee. Furthermore, care must be taken when one operates in the vicinity of a Palmaz stent because vascular clamping near or within such a stent would likely result in a sustained collapse of the lumen of the vessel even after removal of the clamp.

A final significant difference between stents pertains to their radiopacity. Although stainless steel stents are usually relatively easy to visualize, nitinol stents, particularly those with an open architecture, can be extremely difficult to see, particularly with portable fluoroscopy units. If they cannot be seen clearly, they cannot be positioned accurately during deployment and their very existence may not be appreciated during subsequent radiographic evaluations. This problem has been recognized by nitinol stent manufacturers, and efforts are under way to address this issue.

SUMMARY

The explosive growth in endovascular techniques in the 1980s and 1990s now provides a multitude of options to patients with vascular disease. Although some options will likely not pass the test of time and will be discarded, others have already proved their worth and become standards of care. To keep current with the emerging technology is a challenge in itself.

This chapter reviews the fundamental techniques and instrumentation relevant to presently available technology but in no way constitutes a mechanism for the reader to become proficient in these techniques without supplemental training. Once mastered, however, the basic skills should help one in moving forward to implement existing methods and to investigate promising new developments.

REFERENCES

1. Whitely MS, Magee TR, Torrie EP, Galland RB: Minimally invasive superficial femoral artery endarterectomy: Early experience with a modified technique. Eur J Vasc Endovasc Surg 16:254–258, 1998.
2. Hessel SJ, Adams DF, Abrams HL: Complications of angiography. Radiology 138:273–281, 1981.
3. Illescas FF, Baker ME, McCann R, et al: CT evaluation of retroperitoneal hemorrhage associated with femoral arteriography. AJR 146:1289–1292, 1986.
4. Altin RS, Flicker S, Naidech HJ: Pseudoaneurysm and arteriovenous fistula after femoral artery catheterization: Association with low femoral punctures. AJR Am J Roentgenol 152:629–631, 1989.
5. Rupp SB, Vogelzang RL, Nemcek AA, et al: Relationship of the inguinal ligament to pelvic radiographic landmarks: Anatomic correlation and its role in femoral arteriography. J Vasc Interv Radiol 4:409–413, 1993.
6. Dotter CT, Rosch J, Robinson M: Fluoroscopic guidance in femoral artery puncture. Radiology 127:266–267, 1978.
7. Reagan K, Matsumoto AH, Teitelbaum GP: Comparison of the hydrophilic guidewire in double- and single-wall entry needles: Potential hazards. Cathet Cardiovasc Diagn 24:205–208, 1991.
8. Kim JK, Kang HK: Percutaneous retrieval of the peeled-off plastic coating from a guide wire (Letter). J Vasc Interv Radiol 5:657–658, 1994.
9. McIvor J, Rhymer JC: Two hundred forty-five transaxillary arteriograms in arteriopathic patients: Success rate and complications. Clin Radiol 45:390–394, 1992.
10. Westcott JL, Taylor PT: Transaxillary selective four-vessel arteriography. Radiology 104:277–281, 1972.
11. Kinney EV, Fogarty TJ, Newman CE: Catheter skills. *In* White RA,

Fogarty TJ (eds). Peripheral Endovascular Interventions. St. Louis, Mosby-Year Book, 1996, pp 235–247.
12. Chitwood RW, Shepard AD, Shetty PC, et al: Surgical complications of transaxillary arteriography: A case controlled study. J Vasc Surg 23:844–850, 1996.
13. O'Keefe DM: Brachial plexus injury following axillary arteriography. J Neurosurg 53:853–857, 1980.
14. Ouriel K, Veith FJ, Sasahara AA, and the Thrombolysis or Peripheral Arterial Surgery (TOPAS) Investigators: A comparison of recombinant urokinase with vascular surgery as initial treatment for acute arterial occlusion of the legs. N Engl J Med 338:1105–1111, 1998.
15. Ouriel K: Thrombolysis or operation for peripheral arterial occlusion. Vasc Med 1:159–161, 1996.
16. Wholey MH, Maynar MA, Wholey MH, et al: Comparison of thrombolytic therapy of lower-extremity acute, subacute, and chronic arterial occlusions. Cathet Cardiovasc Diagn 44:159–169, 1998.
17. Ouriel K, Veith FJ, Sasahara AA, and the TOPAS Investigators: Thrombolysis or peripheral arterial surgery: Phase I results. J Vasc Surg 23:64–73, 1996.
18. Consigny PM, LeVeen RF: Effects of angioplasty balloon inflation time on arterial contractions and mechanics. Invest Radiol 23:271–276, 1988.

SECTION VI

VASCULAR GRAFTS

RICHARD F. KEMPCZINSKI, M.D.

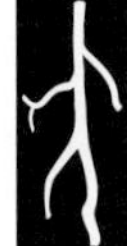

CHAPTER 33

Vascular Conduits: An Overview

Richard F. Kempczinski, M.D.

Although an arterial aneurysm was successfully repaired by Matas in 1888 and a functioning vascular anastomosis was performed by Murphy in 1897, most vascular surgeons feel that the real birth of their specialty occurred more than 50 years later, with the introduction of the first practical arterial prosthesis. In the intervening half century, a variety of potential vascular grafts had been tested and rejected.

During these early years of vascular prosthetic development, the characteristics of the *ideal graft* were defined.[30] This ideal graft must be readily available in a variety of sizes and lengths and suitable for use throughout the body. It must be durable upon long-term implantation in humans, nonreactive, and free of toxic or allergic side effects. It must also be appropriately elastic, conformable to body surfaces, pliable, and easy to suture. Its cut ends should not fray, and it should not kink at flexion points. The luminal surface must be smooth, minimally traumatic to formed blood elements, resistant to infection, and nonthrombogenic. The graft must be available at a reasonable cost and should be capable of being repeatedly sterilized without alteration.

Although no current prosthetic material satisfies all these requirements, a number of satisfactory alternatives are available. This chapter and the next five (Chapters 34 to 38) review the characteristics and biologic behavior of various arterial substitutes, the clinical considerations in their handling, and the complications encountered with their use.

HISTORICAL BACKGROUND

Table 33–1 briefly summarizes the history of materials that have been used as vascular grafts. Although Carrel and Guthrie[5] initially demonstrated that homologous and heterologous artery and vein were effective arterial substitutes in dogs and Goyanes[14] confirmed that autologous vein transplants in humans could serve as a suitable arterial replacement, most early graft development focused on the use of impervious nonbiologic tubes. Although these functioned adequately as short-term passive conduits, they were never incorporated by the host and ultimately suture line disruption, distal embolization, or thrombosis developed.

In 1948, Gross and colleagues[16] returned to the arterial allograft and launched the modern era of vascular surgery. With the introduction of Vinyon-N in 1952, porous, fabric arterial prostheses emerged and soon dominated the market.[3] Three years later, the introduction of "crimping" brought added flexibility and elasticity to the fabric grafts and extended their use.[10] Over the years, stronger and more durable textiles, such as polyester (Dacron), were developed, and numerous modifications of fabrication were introduced, but the basic principle that so revolutionized vascular surgery has stood the test of time (see Chapter 37).[6]

In 1966, the *bovine heterograft* ushered in a new generation of vascular prostheses (i.e., the tanned collagen tube).[24] Although this particular graft has been abandoned because

TABLE 33–1. HISTORY OF VASCULAR GRAFTS

AUTHOR	TYPE OF GRAFT
Carrel et al, 1906	Homologous and heterologous artery and vein transplant in dogs
Goyanes, 1906	First autologous vein transplant in man
Tuffier, 1915	Paraffin-lined silver tubes
Blakemore, 1942	Vitallium tubes
Hufnagel, 1947	Polished methyl methacrylate tubes
Gross et al, 1948	Arterial allografts
Donovan, 1949	Polyethylene tubes
Voorhees, 1952	Vinyon-N, first fabric prosthesis
Egdahl, 1955	Siliconized rubber
Edwards and Tapp, 1955	Crimped nylon
Edwards, 1957	Polytetrafluoroethylene (Teflon)
DeBakey, 1960	Polyester (Dacron)
Rosenberg, 1966	Bovine heterograft
Sparks, 1968	Dacron-supported autogenous fibrous tubes
Soyer et al, 1972	Expanded polytetrafluoroethylene (ePTFE)
Dardik, 1975	Human umbilical cord vein (HUCVAG)
Parodi, 1991	Stented endograft

of its tendency to aneurysmal dilation and thrombosis, it was the prototype for the *human umbilical cord vein allograft* (HUCVAG). The HUCVAG is available in several lengths, but it is useful only for the replacement of small to medium-sized vessels because it is available only in diameters of 5 to 8 mm.

Because all its living elements are killed during the fixation process, the HUCVAG gradually loses compliance as it is replaced by host collagen. The original HUCVAG was reinforced with a thin external Dacron mesh to prevent aneurysmal dilatation. However, virtually all such grafts have become dilated or have developed frank aneurysm if they remained patent for more than 5 years.[17] The graft has recently been modified by increasing the strength of its surrounding Dacron mesh, but only long-term follow-up will determine whether this has corrected the problem (see Chapter 36).

Polytetrafluoroethylene (Teflon [PTFE]) was first used as a vascular prosthesis in 1957.[9] It was found to be extremely durable and has been widely used as a woven arterial substitute. In the late 1960s, a process was developed for extruding PTFE (ePTFE) to create a nonfabric graft that enjoyed all the advantages of Teflon without several of its disadvantages. This prosthesis was first used clinically in 1972 and has subsequently been widely applied as a small and medium-sized vessel replacement (see Chapter 37).[31]

In 1991, the vascular endograft was introduced by Parodi and initiated a minor revolution within vascular surgery that continues today. Both Dacron and ePTFE have been used for the graft material, and fixation has been either incorporated as an integral part of the graft or has been achieved using arterial stents. The endograft is rapidly evolving, and it is unclear which, if any, of the current experimental prototypes will eventually be considered preeminent (see Chapter 38).

BIOLOGIC BEHAVIOR OF VASCULAR GRAFTS

Although most discussions of vascular grafts emphasize their physical characteristics, numerous factors other than a graft's composition are equally important in regard to determining its clinical success. Paramount among these is the realization that bypass grafts fail to halt progression of the underlying disease process, which ultimately appears responsible for most graft failure. In addition, patient selection and choice of operative procedures are tremendously important in determining long-term clinical success and may explain some of the variation in reported results.

Interspecies Variations

Furthermore, because most grafts are initially tested in various experimental animal models, there are wide interspecies variations in the host response to an implanted vascular graft that influence its biologic behavior. In humans, spread of the endothelial pannus that originates at the anastomoses is very limited when compared with its extent in the pig, calf, or baboon. Furthermore, the ingrowth of fibroblasts through the wall of the prosthesis and the ability to "heal" the inner lining is rudimentary compared with healing in various other species in which it occurs rapidly and may be complete in 4 to 8 weeks.[29] The behavior of prostheses in dogs most closely parallels that in humans, thus explaining the emergence of the dog as the favorite animal model for studying vascular grafts. The reader should keep these differences in mind when reviewing reported results.

Fabric Prostheses

Fabric prosthetic grafts represented a radical departure from the rigid metal and plastic tubes that preceded them. Virtually all arterial prostheses develop a layer of fibrin of varying thickness on their luminal surfaces. In addition, endothelium grows across each anastomosis in an attempt to bridge the defect and cover the graft's luminal surface. In nonporous prostheses, this luminal fibrin cannot be organized by the ingrowth of connective tissue, and the spreading endothelial pannus does not become adherent, thus predisposing to distal embolization of fibrin fragments or intimal proliferation and graft occlusion.

In contrast, the porous fabric prostheses develop a thin layer of luminal fibrin that is gradually replaced by mature collagen growing in from the outer surface of the prosthesis, resulting in a stable, relatively nonthrombogenic luminal surface. In many experimental animals, this layer is then rapidly covered by endothelium spreading from the anastomoses. The advantages of such "healing" of prosthetic grafts, in addition to those already described, include an increased resistance to late hematogenous infection and improved patency in low-flow situations (see Chapter 37).[21, 27]

Unfortunately, increasing the porosity of grafts to facilitate this healing was accompanied by an increased incidence of both early and late hemorrhage as well as increased fiber fragmentation and aneurysm formation.[4] Thus, it is necessary in the design of any prosthesis to strike a balance between a relatively low *implantation porosity* and a high *biologic porosity* to tissue ingrowth.

Velour Knitting

Some modifications of graft construction have improved graft healing by employing a loose, filamentous yarn throughout the entire graft or by adding a textured velour surface to standard Dacron grafts.[28] Such velour-knitted Dacron prostheses develop a thinner fibrin lining and are more likely to undergo transmural healing, thus creating the most favorable situation for endothelialization of the luminal surface. Despite these modifications, complete endothelialization of long grafts has not yet been observed in the human subject.[2]

Protein Coating

Still another technique used to achieve low implant and high biologic porosity is the coating of a high-porosity knitted Dacron graft with bovine collagen or human albumin. Such grafts require no "preclotting" with the patient's own blood at the time of implantation but still permit the ingrowth of tissue into and around the graft fibers as the coating is gradually replaced by autologous collagen.[11] In addition to facilitating graft placement and reducing perioperative blood loss, such grafts may provide a better substrate for ingrowth of host endothelium.

There are two major unresolved problems with the clinical use of prosthetic arterial grafts:

1. A persistently higher thrombosis rate compared with autologous grafts when they are used for small vessel replacement in a low-flow runoff bed.
2. An increased risk of graft infection, especially when they are sutured to the common femoral artery.

Endothelial Seeding

One of the major differences between prosthetic vascular grafts and autologous grafts is the absence of a living endothelial layer on the luminal surface. Despite all previous efforts to modify the structure and composition of vascular prostheses to foster the ingrowth of an endothelial lining, no vascular prosthesis implanted in a human being has ever developed an intact, continuous endothelial layer. Because endothelium poses unique thromboresistant properties and may also help to protect the underlying vascular wall from secondary infection, a large body of research has focused on techniques designed to foster the development of such a lining.

The most promising of these involves the "seeding" of autologous endothelial cells into the graft prior to implantation.[15] Host endothelial cells are harvested from a small segment of vein and are either added to the blood used to "preclot" the graft prior to implantation or are used to coat grafts that would not otherwise require preclotting. Although such seeded endothelial cells have been shown to replicate and completely cover the flow surface of both fabric and ePTFE grafts in a number of different animal models, human endothelial cells are much more easily traumatized and may behave differently. Thus far, no "endothelium-seeded" vascular prosthesis has developed a confluent endothelial lining in the human subject.

Colloidal Graphite

Other physical modifications being studied to render the flow surface of small-diameter vascular prostheses thromboresistant involve coating the luminal surface of such grafts with colloidal graphite.[7] Although this approach appears to increase the thromboresistance of various grafts in animal models, its clinical applicability remains to be proved. When such a colloidal graphite surface is rinsed with a cationic, surface-active agent, it is capable of bonding heparin, which may further increase its thromboresistance. This ability to bind heparin to its surface may be the most important anticoagulant property of a carbon-lined graft. At the moment, no carbon-coated graft is approved for clinical use.

Antibiotic Bonding

Finally, because infection of a vascular prosthesis is an extremely disastrous and feared complication, a new procedure for the bonding of antibacterial agents directly to the graft has been developed.[22] In the past, attempts to coat grafts directly with antibiotics failed because of the poor penetration of drugs into the graft material. Furthermore, because no antibiotic is effective against all bacterial strains, any antibiotic chosen for bonding to the graft might be ineffective against a particular bacterial pathogen or might select for organisms that are resistant to its therapeutic spectrum. No antibiotic-coated vascular grafts have yet been approved for use in humans.

Graft Compliance

One additional characteristic of prosthetic grafts that may significantly influence their long-term function is *compliance.* Although many current prostheses have an initial compliance that is similar to that of the host artery, virtually all of them undergo fibrous ingrowth and become rigid. The exceptions to this generalization are the autograft artery and vein, which maintain essentially normal compliance even on long-term implantation. This decrease in compliance has been implicated in the loss of the graft's ability to "self-clean" its intimal surface and may be responsible for the progressive deposition of luminal fibrin that occurs in most grafts.[8] In addition, the disparity in compliance that develops between the implanted graft and the host artery creates stress at the anastomoses, which has been implicated in the formation of anastomotic false aneurysms and the development of neointimal fibroplasia.[8, 13]

SELECTION AND HANDLING OF VASCULAR GRAFTS

No graft currently available is suitable for every clinical application, and grafts must be selected on an individual basis for each case. Table 33–2 lists vascular grafts in current use and indicates the preferred and alternate choices for various clinical applications.

Autogenous artery is an almost ideal vascular replacement (see Chapter 34).[33] Few large arteries in the body are expendable, however, and thus its limited availability makes autogenous artery suitable only for short segmental replacements of small and medium-sized arteries. *Autogenous vein,* specifically the greater saphenous vein, is usually available in longer segments. Although subject to some medial fibrous intimal proliferation and long-term degeneration, it has proved to be a durable and amazingly serviceable replacement, especially for extremity bypass grafting.[32] Unfortunately, in 20% to 30% of patients, the reversed saphenous vein will be either unavailable, of inadequate caliber, or of poor quality, and alternate substitutes must be found.[19] The resurgence of interest in using the *saphenous vein* in situ for lower extremity bypass grafting has resulted in a much greater utilization (>90%) of the vein and may also improve long-term patency (see Chapter 35).[20]

The bovine heterograft was initially used for a variety of clinical applications. Because of frequent late complications, however, its usefulness is presently limited to vascular access. The HUCVAG was reinforced with an external mesh of Dacron to prevent aneurysmal dilatation, and it func-

TABLE 33–2. CLINICAL APPLICATION OF AVAILABLE VASCULAR GRAFTS IN USE

	TYPE OF GRAFT						
	Biologic			Prosthetic			
	Autograft		*Allograft*	*Dacron*¶		*Teflon*¶	
CLINICAL APPLICATION	*Artery*	*Vein*	*(HUCVAG)*	*Knitted*	*Woven*	*Woven*	*ePTFE*
Thoracic aorta					P	P	A
Ruptured aneurysm				A†‡#	P	A	A
Infrarenal aorta and aortoiliofemoral bypass				P‡			A
Aortovisceral bypass	P	P		A			A
Femoropopliteal bypass		P	A	A			A
Femorotibial bypass		P	A§				A‖
Axillofemoral bypass				P			P
Femorofemoral bypass							P
Extrathoracic bypass*				P			A
Arteriovenous shunt				A			P
Venous replacement		P		A			A

*Extrathoracic bypass for arch vessel occlusion.
†Albumin-coated.
‡Possibly as endovascular graft.
§With distal arteriovenous fistula.
‖With cuff of autogenous vein.
¶Dacron and Teflon are trade names for polyester and polytetrafluoroethylene, respectively.
#When more than one "preferred" or "alternate" choice is listed, there is rarely compelling reason to pick one over the other and selection is usually based on the bias or training of the surgeon.
P = preferred; A = alternate; ePTFE = expanded polytetrafluoroethylene; HUCVAG = human umbilical cord vein allograft.

tioned quite satisfactorily as a replacement for small and medium-sized vessels. However, as long-term clinical experience with this graft has accumulated, it now appears that more than a third of such *patent* grafts have become significantly dilated or frankly aneurysmal, thus raising serious questions regarding their future clinical application (see Chapter 36).

Although PTFE has been used most widely in replacement of small to medium-sized extremity vessels, it is also available as a bifurcated prosthesis for aortic replacement that appears particularly suitable for the management of ruptured aneurysms. It has also become popular for vascular access.

Graft Size

The choice of a graft is based not only on its physical characteristics but also on clinical considerations. The size of the vessel to be bypassed or replaced is obviously of importance. Because no autograft is large enough to replace the aorta or vena cava, prosthetic grafts are necessary, and as a result of their large caliber and high flow, they have performed satisfactorily. Conversely, because of the frequent thrombosis of most prosthetic grafts in small-vessel replacement, autogenous tissue is generally preferable for such situations.

Placement of oversized grafts results in an exuberant layer of luminal fibrin, impaired healing, and ultimately an increased frequency of graft thrombosis.[25] The aim of surgery, therefore, should be to choose a graft large enough to deliver the increased blood flows that will be required during reactive hyperemia but still small enough to maintain the velocity of blood flow at rest that will prevent the formation of excessive luminal fibrin. Sauvage and colleagues[27] demonstrated that this "thrombotic threshold velocity" varies, depending on the graft material and the time after implantation. No prosthetic flow surface yet developed can remain patent at the low flow rates possible with endothelium-lined autogenous grafts; this is the rationale behind their use when outflow is limited.

The patient's age must also be considered. Grafts used in children or young adults must be capable of growth. Under such circumstances, autogenous tissue should be used whenever possible, and interrupted sutures should be employed for at least a portion of the anastomosis.

Local Considerations

In the presence of infection or heavy contamination, such as frequently occurs in arterial trauma, prosthetic grafts should be avoided because of the risk of infection. It may be necessary in such cases to harvest a viable artery from a remote, clean field, replace it with a prosthetic graft, and then use the autograft within the contaminated field to restore arterial continuity (see Chapters 34 and 36).

Given the effectiveness of modern perioperative support, expediency and reduced operating time are rarely considerations in the selection of graft materials. However, an occasional older patient with limited life expectancy and with a serious medical condition may not tolerate a prolonged operation. Under such circumstances, one might choose a prosthetic graft to avoid the additional time required to harvest an autogenous saphenous vein, especially if arm veins or vein fragments would have to be used.

Once the graft has been selected, the surgeon must create the most favorable environment for its incorporation. This includes the avoidance of perigraft hematoma, which would prevent fibrous ingrowth and coverage of the graft with viable tissue. The graft must not be placed in proximity to the serosal surface of the bowel, since this may result in vascular enteric fistula formation. In addition, the perioperative use of prophylactic antibiotics for 24 to 72 hours is generally advised to minimize the risk of graft infection.

When the procedure is completed, the operating surgeon should carefully record the precise type and lot number of the implanted graft. If complications later develop, this information will be vital in determining whether failure of the graft represented an isolated occurrence or was part of a widespread pattern, suggesting a flaw in graft design.

Because atherosclerosis is a progressive disease and since bypass grafting does not alter its course, the vascular surgeon must accept responsibility for closely observing the patient indefinitely. One must be alert not only to the early detection of impending graft failure—and act promptly to prevent it—but also to the development of arterial occlusions in sites remote from the original surgery.

COMPLICATIONS

The history of vascular grafts is replete with examples of prostheses that initially functioned well, only to develop late complications. Graft failure may not occur for several years after implantation, and all new grafts should be tested and proved durable for at least 5 years before widespread clinical acceptance. Two basic categories of graft complications occur:

- *Direct* complications involving failure of the graft itself
- *Indirect* complications related to the graft but not impairing its function

Direct Complications

The most common direct graft complication is thrombosis. Although this development is occasionally idiopathic and responsive to simple thrombectomy, it is usually a consequence of disease progression, technical problems, or atheroembolism and will require some form of remedial surgery. Most grafts undergo some dilation in response to arterial pressure.[23] Occasionally, this reaches the proportions of a true aneurysm and may rarely result in graft disruption.[1] Autogenous vein undergoes gradual medial fibrosis as well as intimal proliferation in response to arterial pressure.[12] In addition, atherosclerosis may develop, which can lead to graft stenosis and thrombosis.

Indirect Complications

Indirect complications may call for additional surgery despite continued graft patency. Perhaps the most common of these is a false aneurysm at one or more suture lines (see Chapter 48). Graft infection is usually a disastrous complication and requires removal of the entire graft if suture lines are involved (see Chapter 47). Late infection in the midbody of a graft may occasionally respond to local therapy thus allowing salvage of the graft.[18] Distal emboli may result from either poor fixation of the luminal fibrin or aneurysmal dilatation of the graft. If the graft has not been adequately covered by viable tissue, it can erode into adjacent hollow viscera, such as the bowel or bladder, causing septicemia or bleeding (see Chapter 49).

SUMMARY

Although a variety of suitable prosthetic grafts are available for nearly every clinical situation, clearly no ideal prosthesis has yet been developed. Large-diameter grafts with high flow have excellent patency rates but remain subject to infection. On the other hand, smaller diameter prostheses, as used in the lower extremity, continue to become thrombosed at unacceptable rates. In addition to the search for newer graft materials, current prosthetic research has centered on the creation of infection-resistant conduits by binding antibiotics to the graft itself and to rendering small grafts less thrombogenic by the addition of endothelial cells to the preclot used to prepare them for implantation.[15, 22] Modification of the graft's luminal surface by pretreating it with various substances, such as fibronectin and basement membrane gel, is also being explored as another approach to facilitate endothelial cell coverage of these grafts. Such work offers hope that a prosthetic material will be found that is readily available in a variety of sizes, resistant to both infection and thrombosis, and suitable for replacement of large to small arteries throughout the body.

REFERENCES

1. Berger K, Sauvage LR: Late fiber deterioration in Dacron arterial grafts. Ann Surg 193:477, 1981.
2. Berger K, Sauvage LR, Rao AM, et al: Healing of arterial prostheses in man: Its incompleteness. Ann Surg 175:118, 1972.
3. Blakemore AH, Voorhees AB Jr: Use of tubes constructed from Vinyon "N" cloth in bridging arterial defects: Experimental and clinical. Ann Surg 140:324, 1954.
4. Blumenberg RM, Gelfand ML: Failure of knitted Dacron as an arterial prosthesis. Surgery 81:493, 1977.
5. Carrel A, Guthrie CG: Uniterminal and biterminal venous transplantations. Surg Gynecol Obstet 2:266, 1906.
6. DeBakey ME, Cooley DA, Crawford ES, et al: Clinical application of a new flexible knitted Dacron arterial substitute. Am Surg 24:862, 1958.
7. Debski R, Borovetz H, Haubold A, Hardesty R: Polytetrafluoroethylene grafts coated with ULTI carbon. Trans Am Soc Artif Intern Organs 28:456, 1982.
8. Edwards WS: Arterial grafts. Past, present, and future. Arch Surg 113:1225, 1978.
9. Edwards WS, Lyons C: Three years' experience with peripheral arterial grafts of crimped nylon and Teflon. Surg Gynecol Obstet 107:62, 1958.
10. Edwards WS, Tapp JS: Chemically treated nylon tubes as arterial grafts. Surgery 38:61, 1955.
11. Freischlag JA, Moore WS: Clinical experience with a collagen-impregnated knitted Dacron vascular graft. Ann Vasc Surg 4:449, 1990.
12. Fuchs JCA, Mitchener JS, Hagen P: Postoperative changes in autologous vein grafts. Ann Surg 188:1, 1978.
13. Gaylis H: Pathogenesis of anastomotic aneurysms. Surgery 90:509, 1981.
14. Goyanes DJ: Substitution plastica de las arterias por las venas: Aao arterioplastia venosa, aplicada, como nuevo metodo, al tratamiento de los aneurismas. El Siglo Medico, September 1, 1906, p 346; September 8, 1906, p 561.
15. Graham LM, Burkel WE, Ford JW, et al: Immediate seeding of enzymatically derived endothelium in Dacron vascular grafts. Arch Surg 115:1289, 1980.
16. Gross RE, Hurwitt ES, Bill AH Jr, et al: Preliminary observations on the use of human arterial grafts in the treatment of certain cardiovascular defects. N Engl J Med 239:578, 1948.
17. Karkow WS, Cranley JJ, Cranley RD, et al: Extended study of aneurysm formation in umbilical vein grafts. J Vasc Surg 4:486, 1986.

18. Kwaan JHM, Connolly JE: Successful management of prosthetic graft infection with continuous povidone-iodine irrigation. Arch Surg 116:716, 1981.
19. Leather RP, Shah DM, Karmody AM: Infrapopliteal arterial bypass for limb salvage: Increased patency and utilization of the saphenous vein used "in situ." Surgery 90:1000, 1981.
20. Leather RP, Shah DM, Buchbinder D, et al: Further experience with the saphenous vein used in situ for arterial bypass. Am J Surg 142:506, 1981.
21. Malone JM, Moore WS, Campagna G, et al: Bacteremic infectability of vascular grafts: The influence of pseudointimal integrity and duration of graft function. Surgery 78:211, 1975.
22. Moore WS, Chvapil M, Seiffert G, et al: Development of an infection-resistant vascular prosthesis. Arch Surg 116:1403, 1981.
23. Nunn DB, Freeman MH, Hudgins PC: Postoperative alterations in size of Dacron aortic grafts. Ann Surg 189:741, 1979.
24. Rosenberg N, Gaughran ERL, Henderson J, et al: The use of segmental arterial implants prepared by enzymatic modification of heterologous blood vessels. Surg Forum 6:242, 1955.
25. Sanders RJ, Kempczinski RF, Hammond W, et al: The significance of graft diameter. Surgery 88:856, 1980.
26. Sauvage LR, Berger K, Beilin LB, et al: Presence of endothelium in an axillary femoral graft of knitted Dacron with an external velour surface. Ann Surg 182:749, 1975.
27. Sauvage LR, Berger K, Mansfield PB, et al: Future directions in the development of arterial prostheses for small and medium caliber arteries. Surg Clin North Am 54:213, 1974.
28. Sauvage LR, Berger K, Nakagawa Y, et al: An external velour surface for porous arterial prostheses. Surgery 70:940, 1971.
29. Sauvage LR, Berger K, Wood SJ, et al: Interspecies healing of porus arterial prostheses: Observations, 1960–1974. Arch Surg 109:698, 1974.
30. Scales JT: Tissue reactions to synthetic materials. Proc R Soc Med 46:647, 1953.
31. Soyer T, Lempinen M, Cooper P, et al: A new venous prosthesis. Surgery 72:864, 1972.
32. Szilagyi DE, Elliott JP, Hageman JH, et al: Biologic fate of autogenous vein implants as arterial substitutes: Clinical, angiographic and histopathologic observations in femoro-popliteal operations for atherosclerosis. Ann Surg 178:232, 1973.
33. Wylie EJ: Vascular replacement with arterial autografts. Surgery 57:14, 1965.

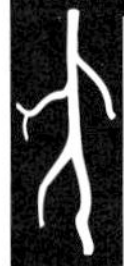

C H A P T E R 3 4

The Arterial Autograft

Rishad M. Faruqi, M.B.B.S., F.R.C.S. (Eng.), F.R.C.S. (Ed.)
and Ronald J. Stoney, M.D.

The superiority of arterial autografts over other forms of vascular conduits is now widely accepted. This is made evident by the increasing use of arterial autografts in coronary revascularization procedures, which started with the use of the internal mammary artery and has now moved to the use of the gastroepiploic and radial arteries in preference to saphenous vein as the conduit of choice. Arterial autografts for peripheral vascular replacement were introduced in 1964 at the University of California Medical Center in San Francisco.[1] The past 35 years have provided an opportunity to examine the usefulness and durability of this graft, which has been employed for a wide range of arterial problems.[2–5] Experimental data show that arterial autograft implants grow along with the native artery, making it ideal for arterial substitution in children and growing adolescents.[6, 7] The results of more than 400 autograft reconstructions indicate that it is the ideal arterial graft because it:

- Retains its viability
- Demonstrates proportional arterial growth when used in children
- Does not degenerate with time
- Heals in an infected field
- Exhibits normal flexibility at points of joint motion

Experimental results showing that an optimal compliance match at an arterial graft anastomosis leads to a reduction in graft thrombosis may help to explain the excellent patency seen with arterial autograft reconstruction.[8]

PROCUREMENT

Autografts can be procured from various donor sites in the arterial system (Fig. 34–1). Whenever possible, the auto-

TABLE 34–1. ARTERIAL AUTOGRAFT SIZES AND RECIPIENT ARTERIAL SITES

	SIZE		
AUTOGRAFT	Length (cm)	Diameter (mm)	RECIPIENT SITE
Internal iliac	4–5	7–8	Renal Visceral
External iliac	7–10	6–8	Carotid Renal Common femoral Popliteal
Superficial femoral	10–20	5–6	Common femoral Profunda Cross-femoral subcutaneous bypass

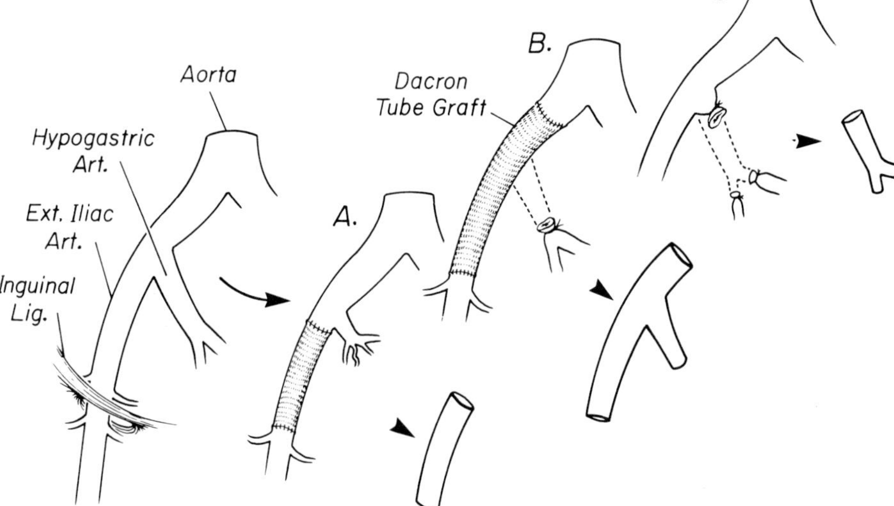

FIGURE 34–1. Procurement of iliac autografts. As depicted here, the iliac arteries are the best source of arterial autografts that can be obtained in grafts of various diameters and lengths, with or without distal branches.

graft selected should closely approximate the size of the artery being replaced (Table 34–1). Often the autograft can be obtained from a donor site within the same surgical field in which the arterial reconstruction is to be performed. The splenic artery should be avoided for use as an autograft in older patients because it is frequently kinked or coiled, making it unsuitable for transplantation (Fig. 34–2).

Reconstruction of the donor site when the common or external iliac artery segments are used may be performed satisfactorily with prosthetic grafts. Excised internal iliac arterial segments, frequently used as renal artery grafts, do not need to be replaced. Arterial autografts also may be constructed from an arterial segment previously occluded by atherosclerosis. The thrombosed superficial femoral artery has been the most commonly used donor vessel of this type (Fig. 34–3). Normal patency is restored by an eversion or semi-closed endarterectomy. Such a segment can be used as a conduit for revascularization after removal of an infected synthetic graft. The vessel is also suitable for use as a patch or bypass graft for distal reconstruction of the profunda femoris artery (Fig. 34–4).

Although most arterial autografts are used in the abdomen or groin, more remote arteries (e.g., carotid, popliteal) occasionally may require an autograft for repair. When arterial autografts are used in these positions, a donor artery is seldom available within the same operative field. In these cases, a donor artery may be harvested from the iliac vessels via an oblique lower abdominal incision and a retroperitoneal approach. This incision is well tolerated by the patient and allows for harvest of 4 to 7 cm of internal

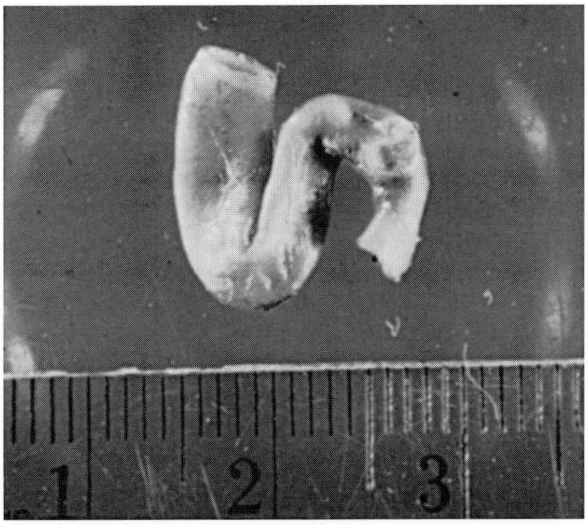

FIGURE 34–2. Photograph of a harvested splenic artery. The obvious tortuosity makes this an unacceptable vessel for use as an autograft.

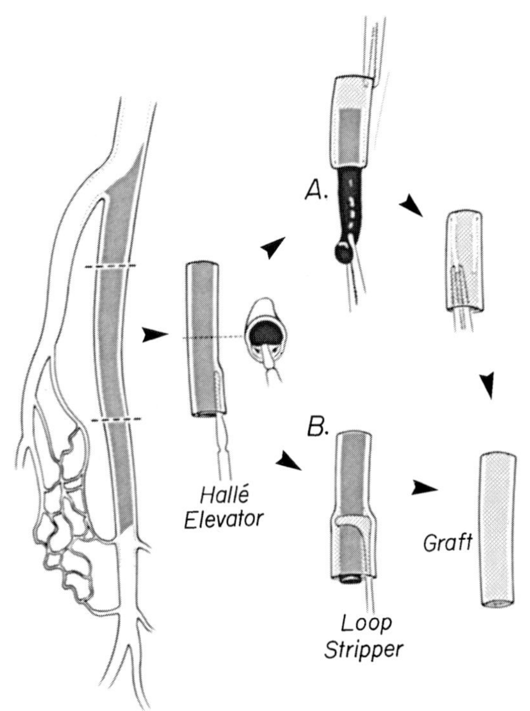

FIGURE 34–3. An occluded superficial femoral artery is an alternative source of arterial autograft, which can be prepared by either of the techniques depicted here. *A*, Eversion endarterectomy. *B*, Loop endarterectomy.

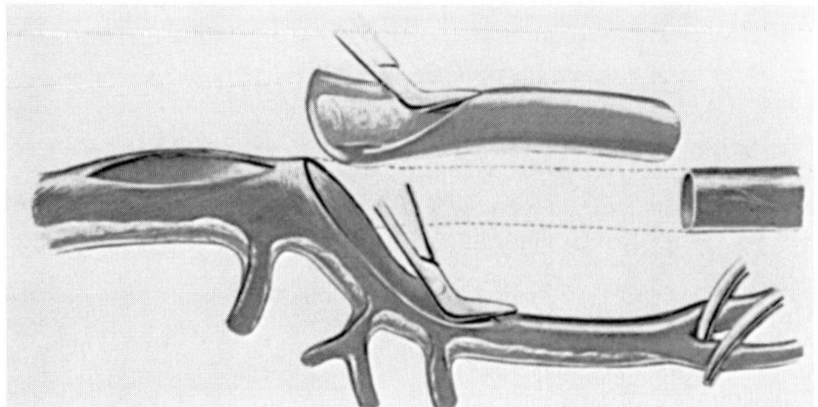

FIGURE 34–4. A chronically thrombosed superficial femoral artery has been removed and is being prepared for placement as a patch onto the profunda femoris artery. (From Wylie EJ, Stoney RJ, Ehrenfeld WK, et al: Manual of Vascular Surgery. Vol 2. New York, Springer-Verlag, 1986, p 15.)

iliac artery. One may obtain increased conduit length by removing the common and external iliac arteries and reconstructing these vessels with synthetic material (see Table 34–1).

In patients with internal carotid artery occlusion and symptomatic ipsilateral external carotid artery disease, the occluded internal carotid artery may be used to facilitate external carotid endarterectomy. This can be accomplished by harvesting the internal carotid artery and using it as a patch angioplasty, similar to the procedure described for profundoplasty (see Fig. 34–4) or by leaving the internal carotid artery attached and rolling it over onto the external carotid artery as a patch (Fig. 34–5).[9]

PLACEMENT

End-to-end autograft anastomoses, with the use of interrupted sutures, are recommended whenever circumferential arterial defects are repaired. Partial defects in the circumference of an artery are covered with an opened arterial autograft used as a patch or gusset, and the anastomosis is performed with a continuous suture (see Fig. 34–5). When coverage of the autograft is not possible because of infection or inadequate skin flaps, secondary wound healing consistently occurs, leading to granulation over the exposed functioning autograft. No thrombosis, impairment in autograft healing, or secondary hemorrhage has occurred under these circumstances of delayed wound healing.

INDICATIONS

Although an arterial autograft is the ideal arterial substitute, size and availability preclude its use in most circumstances requiring aortic replacement (i.e., abdominal aortic aneurysm or aortoiliac femoral occlusive disease). Nevertheless, autografts are used preferentially for certain primary vascular repairs as well as in secondary repairs to reconstruct defects in arterial continuity following removal of an infected prosthesis.

PRIMARY ARTERIAL RECONSTRUCTIONS

Renal Artery Fibrous Dysplasia

Renal artery occlusive lesions involving portions of the main renal artery and its branches produce renovascular hypertension. The fibromuscular dysplastic lesions of the renal arteries are particularly amenable to arterial autograft

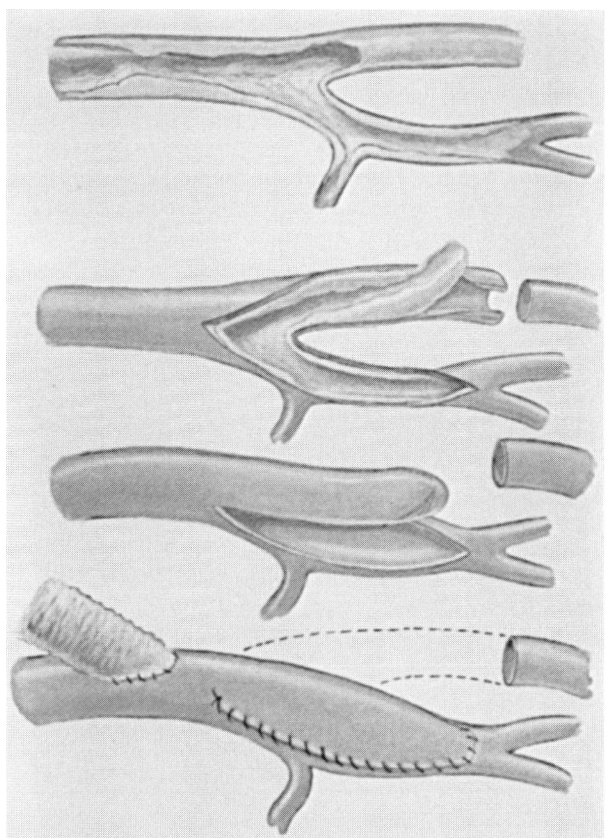

FIGURE 34–5. Profunda femoral endarterectomy utilizing the occluded superficial femoral artery as a transposed patch angioplasty. This method allows autogenous hinge-flap closure. (From Stoney RJ, Effeney DJ: Wylie's Atlas of Vascular Surgery: Basic Considerations and Techniques. Philadelphia, JB Lippincott, 1992.)

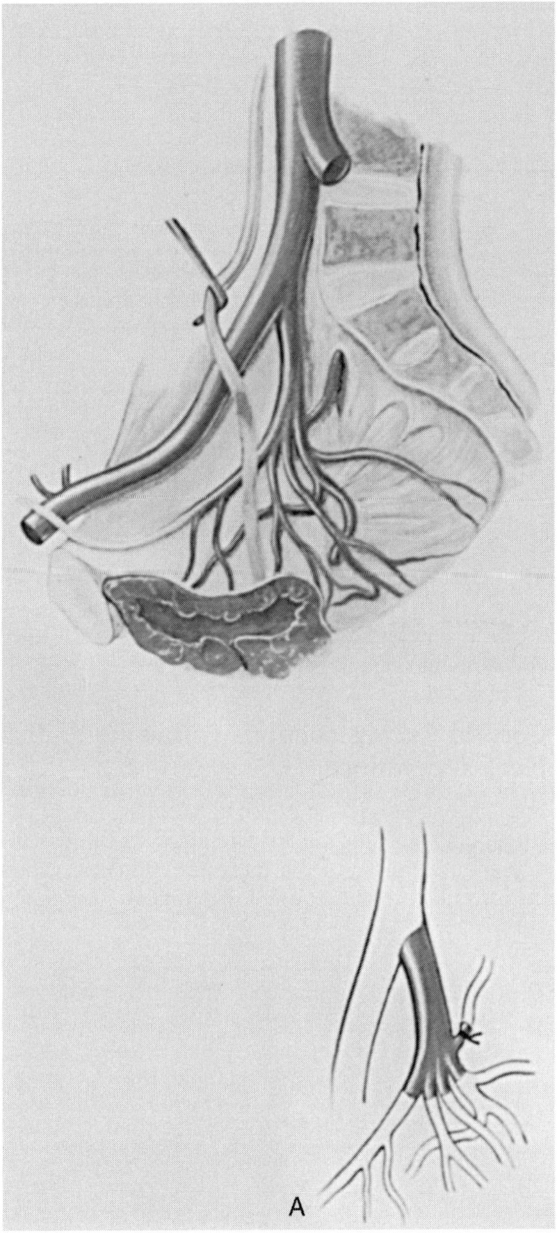

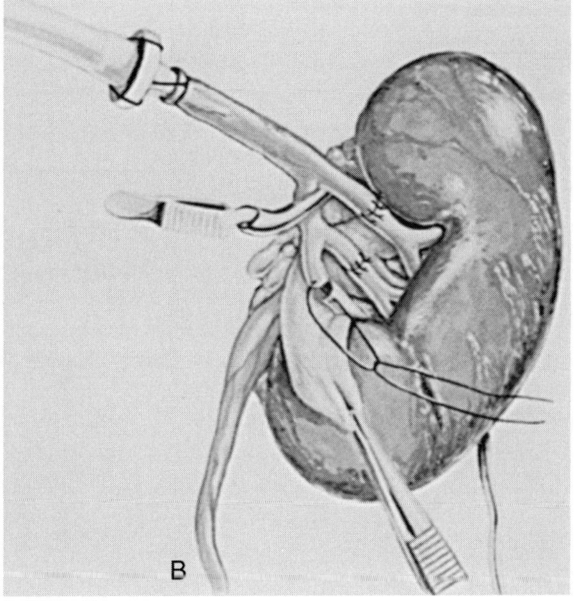

FIGURE 34–6. Illustration of a hypogastric artery demonstrating its terminal branches (*A*), which make this vessel ideal for use when branched renal artery reconstruction is required (*B*). (*A* and *B*, From Wylie EJ, Stoney RJ, Ehrenfeld WK, et al: Manual of Vascular Surgery. Vol 2. New York, Springer-Verlag, 1986, p 221.)

reconstruction. The hypogastric artery is the same diameter as the renal artery, and its branches closely approximate those of the renal artery branches in size and configuration (Fig. 34–6). Durable results have been achieved in 135 patients who underwent 143 aortorenal arterial autograft reconstructions.[3, 10, 11] Arteriographic follow-up over 20 years has revealed only one late graft occlusion, one anastomotic stenosis, and one aneurysmal dilatation; this aneurysm has remained arteriographically stable for more than 10 years. Hypertension was cured or improved in 96% of the patients, supporting our view that this is the preferred graft for patients with nonatherosclerotic renal artery lesions of the primary, secondary, or tertiary branches causing renovascular hypertension.

Peripheral Aneurysms

Carotid, popliteal, and femoral artery aneurysms are ideal sites for arterial autografts because (1) the lengths of the diseased segments are short and (2) their normal diameter closely approximates that of the external iliac artery (Fig. 34–7). For common femoral artery aneurysms, the donor external iliac artery segment is frequently tortuous and can be mobilized and extended to the femoral bifurcation for repair of these aneurysms (Fig. 34–8).[12]

Renal and Visceral Aneurysms

The internal iliac artery is an ideal replacement for renal or visceral aneurysms requiring resection (Fig. 34–9).

Arterial Trauma

Prosthetic grafts should not be used to restore arterial continuity after trauma if the wound has been heavily contaminated and infection appears likely. In such circumstances, an autogenous graft of artery or vein may be

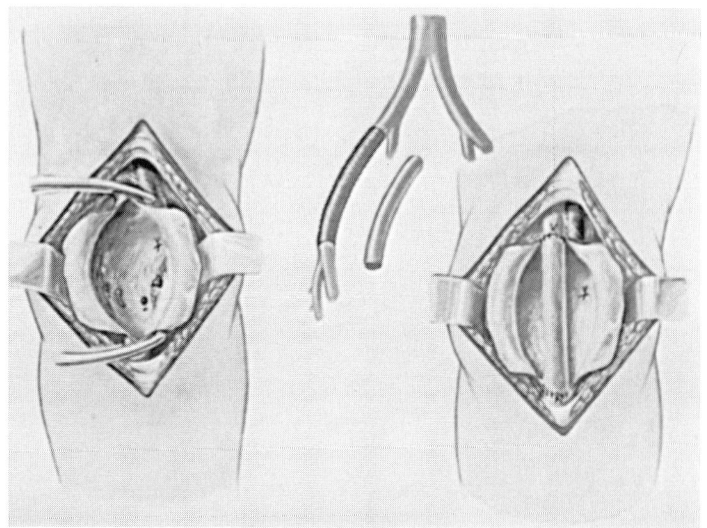

FIGURE 34–7. An exposed and opened popliteal artery aneurysm is being replaced with an external iliac artery autograft. The harvest site is reconstructed with a prosthetic graft. (From Wylie EJ, Stoney RJ, Ehrenfeld WK, et al: Manual of Vascular Surgery. Vol 2. New York, Springer-Verlag, 1986, p 58.)

harvested from a remote clean field and used as a satisfactory substitute. The resulting defect in donor arterial continuity is repaired with a suitable prosthetic conduit.

Limb Salvage Surgery for Cancer

With the passage of time, the more radical disfiguring operations for bone and soft tissue malignancies of the extremities have given way to operations involving complex reconstructions following excision of the tumor and its environs.[13] Given the ability of arterial autografts to grow, avoid kinking across joints, and resist infections, it serves as the ideal conduit for these reconstructions, especially in children and growing adolescents.

Carotid Reconstructions Following Radical Neck Operations

For reasons similar to those mentioned for limb salvage surgery, some surgeons have resorted to the use of arterial autografts in place of the more traditional saphenous vein in carotid reconstruction after radical neck surgery for

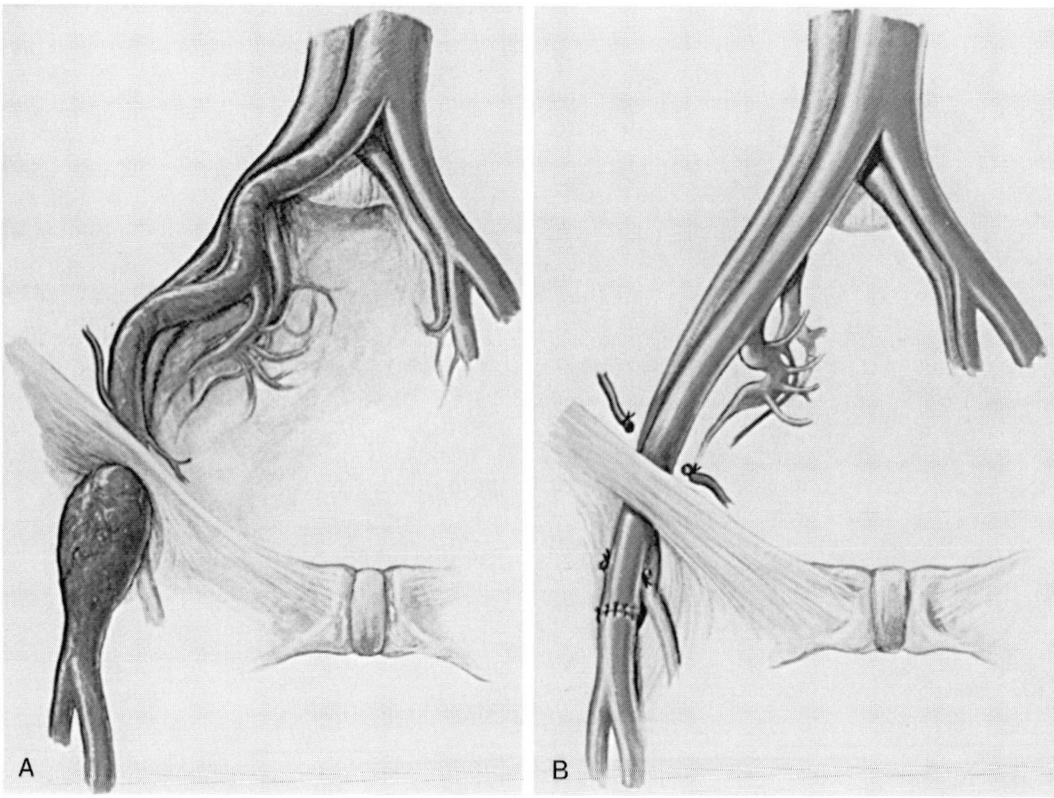

FIGURE 34–8. A femoral artery aneurysm before (*A*) and after (*B*) reconstruction with external iliac artery. (*A* and *B*, From Wylie EJ, Stoney RJ, Ehrenfeld WK, et al: Manual of Vascular Surgery. Vol 2. New York, Springer-Verlag, 1986, p 61.)

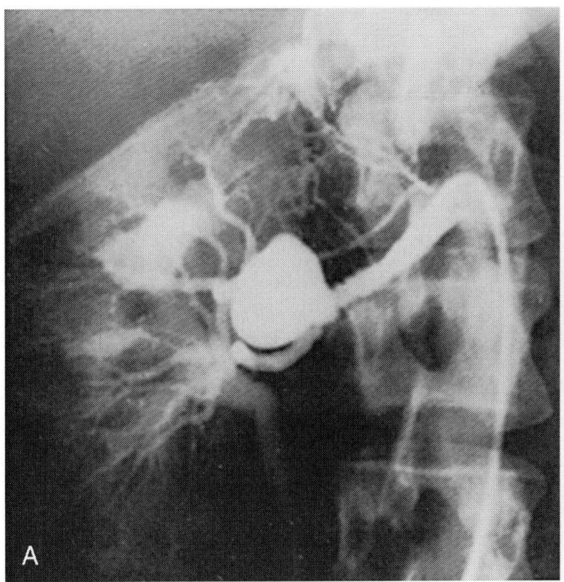

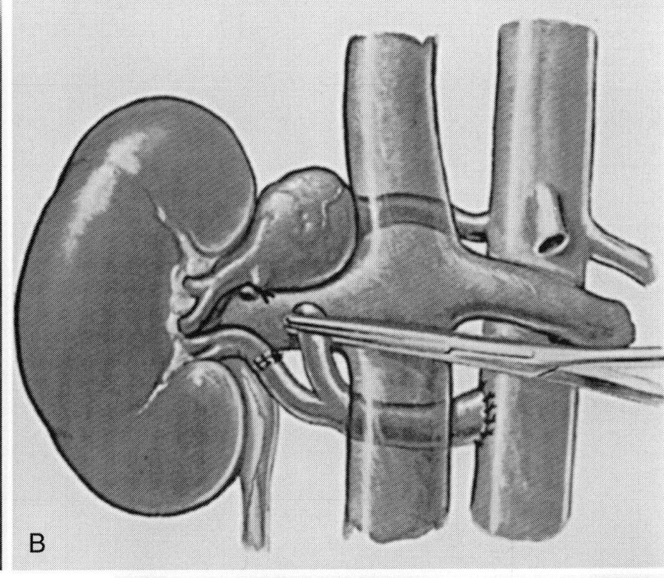

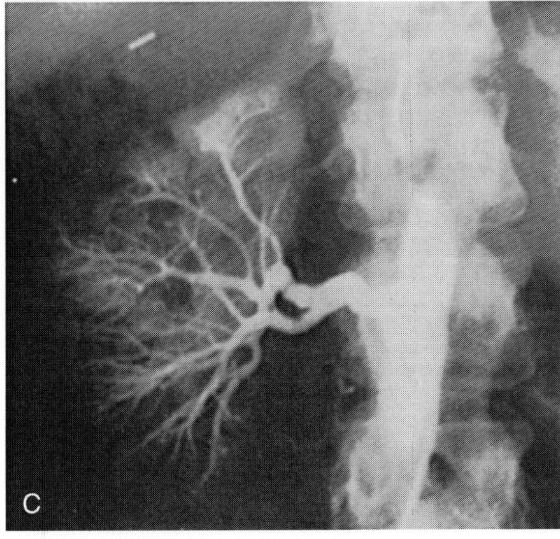

FIGURE 34–9. *A,* Arteriogram demonstrating a renal artery aneurysm at the bifurcation of the renal artery. *B,* In situ branched autograft repair. *C,* Postoperative arteriogram demonstrating a patent reconstruction. (A–C, From Wylie EJ, Stoney RJ, Ehrenfeld WK, et al: Manual of Vascular Surgery. Vol 2. New York, Springer-Verlag, 1986, p 61.)

cancers that involve this vessel.[14] The superficial femoral or the external iliac artery serves as an ideal conduit for this purpose. Given the size-match of these vessels, they may be used for common or internal carotid artery reconstruction when these arteries have been resected *en bloc* with the tumor. On occasion, we have used the hypogastric artery for this purpose if the segment to be replaced is short. Donor site reconstruction may then be performed with a prosthetic graft or with saphenous vein in the case of the superficial femoral artery.

SECONDARY ARTERIAL RECONSTRUCTIONS

Infected Prostheses

When removal of a patent infected prosthesis is planned, another source of perfusion is usually necessary to supply the limbs. Although extra-anatomic bypass techniques that avoid the septic field are available, in our experience the infected graft-artery segment in the groin can be reconstructed in situ by an autogenous cross-femoral graft. We prefer a conduit of arterial autograft obtained from either occluded superficial femoral artery or, if needed, the previously bypassed external iliac artery (Fig. 34–10). No patients have experienced subsequent infections of the cross-femoral autograft repair when this technique has been used.[15]

Mycotic aneurysms or primarily infected arterial repairs in other sites (e.g., popliteal artery-carotid bifurcation) occur rarely; however, when they do occur, they can be excised and replaced with arterial autograft. Thus, when excision of any infected arterial segment produces distal ischemia and remote bypass is not feasible, autografts from the iliac arteries can be used and may be expected to heal without failure.

Anastomotic False Aneurysms

A complication of graft healing, the anastomotic pseudoaneurysm is often caused by suture or arterial wall degeneration. It usually appears at sites of active motion near a major joint. Autogenous artery segments can be useful as

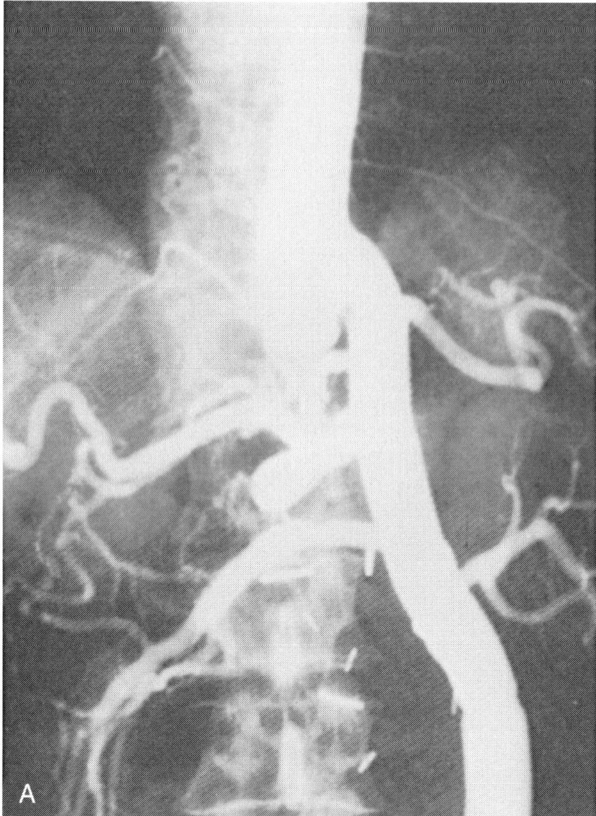

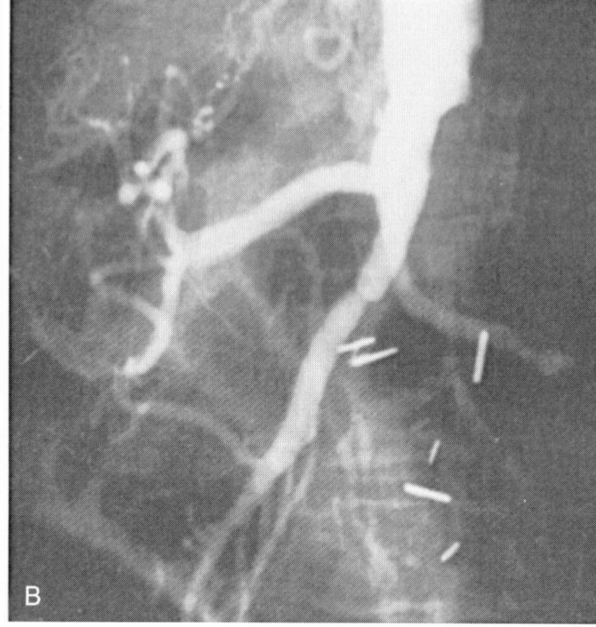

FIGURE 34–10. *A,* Radiograph of an infected aortobifemoral bypass graft originating from the thoracic aorta. Contaminated synthetic grafts to the visceral circulation originated from this prosthesis. *B,* Radiograph showing the completed reconstruction after graft excision. Harvested right common, internal, and external iliac arteries were utilized to reconstruct the visceral circulation. The proximal anastomosis originates from the stump of the aorta. The origin of the excised graft was repaired using a patch from the residual common iliac artery. (*A* and *B,* From Stoney RJ, Effeney DJ: Wylie's Atlas of Vascular Surgery: Complications Requiring Reoperation. Philadelphia, JB Lippincott, 1991.)

interposition grafts to repair the defect after excision of the aneurysms.[16]

LATE FAILURE OF ARTERIAL RECONSTRUCTION

Any late complication following an arterial reconstruction may threaten its function or may contribute to its subsequent failure. Therefore, reoperative arterial repairs are indicated to manage late complications of arterial reconstruction. These complications include:

- Progression of the original disease
- False aneurysm formation, whether anastomotic or primary
- Altered healing of the arterial repair or prosthetic implant
- Deterioration of the host artery or prosthesis

The goal of a reoperative arterial repair is to reestablish or preserve arterial or prosthetic graft patency. Patch and conduit arterial autografts have proved suitable for accomplishing these objectives. Since many reoperative arterial repairs are required because of late failure of an original revascularization of the lower extremity, repair in the limb (usually the groin region) is common. Conduit or patch autografts are easily harvested from the chronically occluded superficial femoral artery within the same operative field (see Figs. 34–3 and 34–4). A suitable length of the artery can be reclaimed, as illustrated, to provide an autograft for a variety of revascularization requirements. Of more than 400 arterial autograft reconstructions performed at the University of California Medical Center in San Francisco over the past 34 years, nearly a quarter (98) were used in cases of late failure of a previous arterial repair.[17] Most of these were either combined with in situ thromboendarterectomy or used alone to repair defects in vascular continuity. Successful secondary repairs with durable results were achieved in nearly every patient.

SUMMARY

The arterial autograft is an ideal arterial substitute because it retains its function as an artery despite its transplantation to a new site. The suitability of the arterial autograft for certain primary aortic branch reconstructions, arterial repair in growing children, complex distal renal artery reconstructions, and complications of vascular reconstructions, including sepsis, makes it an essential part of the armamentarium of the complete vascular surgeon.

Acknowledgments: This chapter was supported in part by the Pacific Vascular Research Foundation, San Francisco, California.

REFERENCES

1. Wylie EJ: Vascular replacement with arterial autografts. Surgery 57:14, 1965.
2. Stoney RJ, Wylie EJ: Arterial autografts. Surgery 67:18, 1970.
3. Lye CR, String ST, Wylie EJ, et al: Aortorenal arterial autografts. Arch Surg 110:1321, 1975.
4. Stoney RJ, DeLuccia N, Ehrenfeld WK, et al: Aortorenal arterial autografts. Arch Surg 116:1416, 1981.
5. Ehrenfeld WK, Stoney RJ, Wylie EJ: Autogenous arterial grafts. *In* Stanley JC, et al (eds): Biologic and Synthetic Vascular Prostheses. New York, Grune & Stratton, 1982.
6. Kreitman B, Riberi A, Zeranska M, et al: Growth potential of aortic autografts and allografts: Effects of cryopreservation and immunosuppression in an experimental model. Eur J Cardiothoracic Surg 11:943, 1997.
7. Kreitman B, Riberi A, Jimeno MT, Metras D: Experimental basis for autograft growth and viability. J Heart Valve Dis 4:379, 1995.
8. Abbott WM, Megerman J, Hasson JE, et al: Effect of compliance mismatch on vascular graft patency. J Vasc Surg 5:376, 1987.
9. Wylie EJ, Stoney RJ, Ehrenfeld WK, et al: Manual of Vascular Surgery. Vol II. New York, Springer-Verlag, 1986.
10. Kent KC, Salvatierra O, Reilly LM, et al: Evolving strategies for the repair of complex renovascular lesions. Ann Surg 206:272, 1987.
11. Murray SP, Kent KC, Salvatierra O, Stoney RJ: Complex branch renovascular disease: Management options and late results. J Vasc Surg 19:338, 1994.
12. Inahara T: Aneurysms of the common femoral artery: Reconstruction with the mobilized external iliac artery. Am J Surg 111:795, 1966.
13. Upton J, Kocher MS, Wolfort MS: Reconstruction following resection of malignancies of the upper extremities. Surg Oncol Clin North Am 5:847, 1996.
14. Jacobs JR, Arden RL, Marks SC, et al: Carotid artery reconstruction using superficial femoral arterial grafts. Laryngoscope 104(6 pt 1): 689, 1994.
15. Qvarfordt PG, Reilly LM, Ehrenfeld WK, et al: Surgical management of vascular graft infections: Local treatment, graft excision, and methods of revascularization. *In* Bernhard VM, Towne JB (eds): Complications in Vascular Surgery. New York, Grune & Stratton, 1985, pp 499–511.
16. Stoney RJ, Albo RJ, Wylie EJ: False aneurysms occurring after arterial grafting operations. Am J Surg 110:157, 1965.
17. Qvarfort PG, Stoney RJ: Arterial autografts. Acta Chir Scand 529(Suppl):37, 1985.

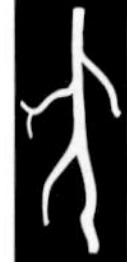

C H A P T E R 3 5

The Autogenous Vein

Jonathan B. Towne, M.D.

For revascularization of the lower extremity, the autogenous vein is the conduit of choice for small caliber arterial bypass. This superiority of autogenous conduits has been repeatedly documented in the vascular surgical literature.[1–4] Since the 1970s, there has been a progressive improvement in the results of lower extremity bypass, which is attributed to better vein harvest techniques; improvements in operative technique, including the use of small caliber sutures; and optical magnification. Intraoperative assessment of the vascular repair with angiography, duplex imaging, and Doppler flow studies has become routine, and patients are studied with postoperative surveillance protocols. As a result of these improvements, the type of conduit now remains the primary determinant of long-term graft patency.

With the development of cellular biology research techniques, a new understanding is evolving about the function of the autogenous vein. Instead of serving as a passive conduit, the vein graft actively participates in keeping blood fluid as it passes over the endothelium. This chapter reviews the structure and function of the autogenous vein and the reasons for its superior performance as a conduit for lower limb arterial reconstruction.

ANATOMY

The *greater saphenous vein* is the longest vein in the body; it begins at the medial aspect of the dorsum of the foot and terminates in the femoral vein just distal to the inguinal ligament. Classically, it ascends anterior to the medial malleolus along the medial side of the leg in relationship to the saphenous nerve.[5] It passes posterior to the medial condyle of the tibia and femur and usually traverses the medial thigh, gaining access to the common femoral vein at the fossa ovalis. The significant variations from normal saphenous vein anatomy should be familiar to all surgeons who use the vessel for arterial reconstruction.

In a classic study from Albany, Shah and his group evaluated the greater saphenous venous system in 385 legs of 331 patients.[6] Their findings comprise the most detailed account of the greater saphenous vein anatomy and its variations that is available in the literature. Only 38.2% of their venograms demonstrated a conventional saphenous vein that had a continuous trunk arising anterior to the ankle and ending in the common femoral vein. The other 61.8% of venograms demonstrated significant variations which the authors studied by anatomic region.

In the thigh, the vein presented as single trunk in 65% of patients. This was the classical medially located trunk in 60%. In 5%, however, the trunk of the saphenous vein was located in a more lateral position. A complete double system was present in 11%, and an additional 15% had portions of a double system. Less common variations occurred in 9%. Usually, the double trunks in the thigh rejoined and formed a single trunk within 10 cm of the knee joint, although occasionally the junction occurred more proximally.

In the leg, the saphenous vein had a single trunk in only 45% of the patients. The usual location of the saphenous vein was 1 to 2 cm posterior to the medial border of the tibia. The vein also occurred in a more posterior position, which Shah and colleagues defined as 4 to 6 cm posterior to the medial border of the tibia.[6] In 46% of patients, a well-defined double trunk was present, of which the anterior branch was the most dominant. The bifurcation of the saphenous vein usually occurred within 5 cm of the knee joint, but occasionally occurred at the mid-thigh level.

Veith and associates, in an earlier study using the preoperative saphenous venography in 100 extremities in 60 patients, noted an absence of the saphenous vein in 4%.[7] The exact incidence of total absence of the saphenous vein is not known, but it is important to realize that anomalies can occur, and the surgeon needs to be prepared to deal with them.

The valves in the saphenous vein are classically bicuspid, although on occasion they may have only one cusp. The valve cusps are oriented parallel to the surface of the skin. The physiologic basis of this feature was detailed by Edwards, who demonstrated that if the valves are parallel to the surface of the skin, they remain competent when external pressure is applied to the leg.[8] Shah and colleagues encountered an average of 6.3 valves in each saphenous vein bypass that they performed.[6] There usually is a valve at the fossa ovalis and one 5 cm distally. The number of valves in the remainder of the vein varies and ranges from as few as one and to as many as 13.

Knowledge of the vagaries of the saphenous system is particularly important for surgeons who plan to prepare the vein for in situ bypass using angioscopic guidance to avoid exposing the entire vein. When a segment of identified vein does not appear to be of adequate caliber for a bypass, it may often be found in parallel with a totally or partially double system. With the best-quality segments of the saphenous system used, an autogenous conduit can usually be constructed.

ALTERNATE SOURCES OF AUTOGENOUS VEIN

The saphenous vein may be unusable for many reasons. Most commonly, it has been harvested previously for coronary artery bypass or peripheral vascular surgery. On occasion, it can be congenitally absent or may have suffered the ravages of superficial phlebitis. In a series by Taylor and coworkers,[2] the incidence of patients without an intact usable saphenous vein was 22%. However, by using alternative sources for autogenous vein, these authors were able to perform lower extremity revascularization with all autogenous material in 94% of their patients.

Contralateral Saphenous Vein

Although the most obvious alternative source of a missing or inadequate saphenous vein is the contralateral leg, some surgeons are reluctant to use the contralateral saphenous vein. Such use removes the potential to use that vein for bypass vascular surgery in that limb, and these surgeons believe that for limb salvage each leg should contribute its own autogenous conduit.

Lesser Saphenous Vein

Another source of autogenous vein is the lesser saphenous vein, which originates posterior to the lateral malleolus as a continuation of the lateral marginal vein.[5] It ascends proximally along the lateral margin of the Achilles tendon, coursing medially to reach the middle of the popliteal fossa, where it perforates the fascia and joins the popliteal vein. The lesser saphenous vein is accompanied through much of its course by the sural nerve.

Multiple variations are present in the lesser saphenous vein. It can perforate the fascia in the middle portion of the calf and then proceed in the proximal third of the calf in the subfascial position. This vein may also be unusable for bypass because of previous episodes of phlebitis. The patency, size, and course of the lesser saphenous can be determined with duplex scanning prior to harvesting of the vein.

In the operating room, the patient is initially placed prone on the operating table to allow both lesser saphenous veins to be removed simultaneously. The incisions are closed, and the patient is turned to the supine position, reprepared, and draped. Although this approach takes more time, it allows the precise and gentle vein dissection that is necessary to obtain the optimum conduit. If the lesser saphenous vein is patent in both lower extremities, these two segments can be spliced together to perform most distal tibial bypasses.

Cephalic Vein and Basilic Vein

The *cephalic vein* is a favored alternative among some practitioners (Fig. 35–1).[9] It courses from the anatomic "snuff box" on the radial side of the wrist to the deltopectoral groove, where it joins the axillary vein. As with the saphenous vein in the leg, there are many anatomic variations in the arm veins (Figs. 35–2 and 35–3).[10] A dominant secondary branch may arise on the dorsum of the hand, joining the primary cephalic vein in the forearm. Double cephalic veins in the forearm may course in parallel and join together proximal to the antecubital fossa. Occasionally, there may be an accessory cephalic vein that remains on the radial side of the cephalic vein and usually joins it at the elbow.

The *basilic vein* begins in the ulnar part of the dorsal venous network of the hand and runs proximally on the posterior surface of the ulnar side of the forearm, inclining toward the anterior surface distal to the elbow, where it is joined by the medial antecubital vein. Proximal to the elbow it ascends obliquely, crossing in the groove between the biceps and the pronator teres. It then crosses the brachial artery from which it is separated by the bicipital aponeurosis. The basilic vein then runs proximally along the medial border of the biceps brachia, perforating the deep fascia distal to the middle of the arm. It ascends to

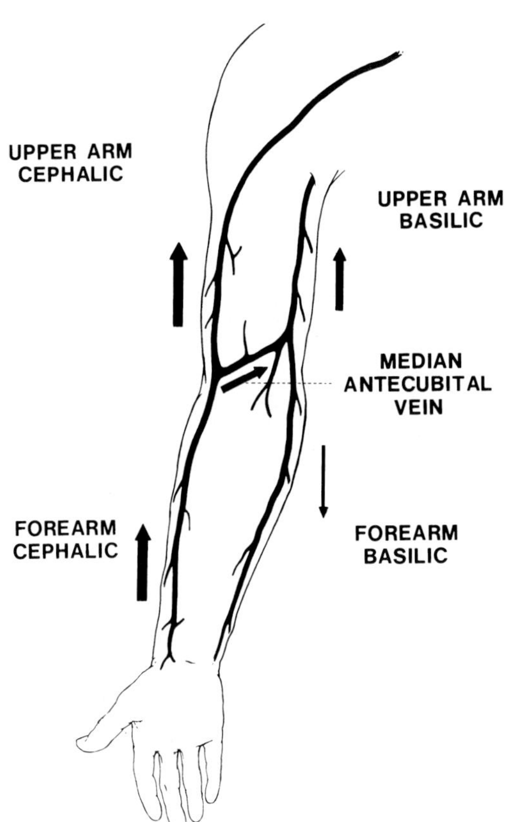

FIGURE 35–1. Order of preference of arm veins for alternative antogenous grafts: 1, cephalic (forearm and arm); 2, forearm cephalic–median antecubital–arm basilic; 3, basilic (forearm and arm); 4, composite (lower and upper extremity veins).

the distal border of the teres major muscle, where it joins the brachial vein to form the axillary vein.

There is a great variation in the superficial veins of the forearm, and often a reciprocal relationship exists between the cephalic and basilic veins. One or the other may predominate, and the other may be absent. Because many patients with vascular occlusive disease have had multiple prior hospitalizations, the cephalic and basilic veins and their branches in the arm are often damaged because of previously place intravenous lines and the need for many venipunctures for drawing blood.

Other Sources

Other potential sources of autogenous vein are the *internal jugular vein*, which can be used when a short segment of large-caliber conduit is needed, as in injuries of the common femoral vein. The internal jugular vein is a better size match than the contralateral saphenous vein.

The *superficial femoral vein* can be used as a conduit. Because of its large size, it is often ideal for autogenous replacement of aortofemoral segments when infected prosthetic grafts must be removed. Work by Clagett and coauthors has demonstrated its durability for this approach, and their long-term studies show that the venous sequelae are reasonable.[11, 12] The harvest of this conduit is tedious.

MICROSCOPIC ANATOMY

The intima is a thin endothelial layer on the luminal surface of the vessel, lying on a fenestrated basement membrane.[13] In cross section, the intimal layer lies in folds along the inner surface of the vessel. As a result of poor cytoplasmic uptake of histologic stains, only the nuclei are seen distinctly. With en face sectioning, the orderly distribution of the nuclei in the endothelial cells can be appreciated. The smooth muscle cells are arranged in an inner longitudinal and outer circumferential directions and are interlaced with collagen and elastic fibrils. Elastic fibrils appear to be oriented predominantly in the longitudinal direction.[13] The adventitia forms the outer layer of the vein wall and is frequently thicker than the media; it consists of a loose collagen network interspersed with vasa vasorum. Longitudinal or spirally arranged smooth muscle cells may appear in the portion of the adventitia adjacent to the media.[13]

PHYSIOLOGY

The autogenous vein serves as a superior conduit because it is a living structure that actively participates in keeping the flowing stream of blood liquid as it crosses its surface. A variety of molecules secreted by the vein wall have been identified, including (1) the glycosaminoglycans, which serve as cofactors for antithrombin III, and (2) heparin cofactor II.[14] Thrombomodulin, protein C, and protein S are also secreted and together participate in inactivation of coagulant antihemophilic factor (factor VIII) and proaccelerin (factor V).[15] The endothelial cells also synthesize pros-

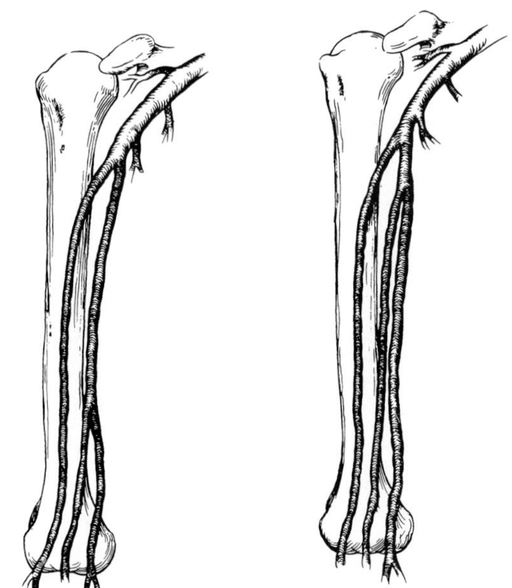

FIGURE 35–2. Variations in the confluence of the basilic and brachial veins. (From Andrus G. Harris RW: The place of arm veins in arterial revascularization. *In* Bergen J, Yao JST [eds]: Arterial Surgery: New Diagnostic and Operative Techniques. Orlando, Fla, Grune & Stratton, 1988, p 526.)

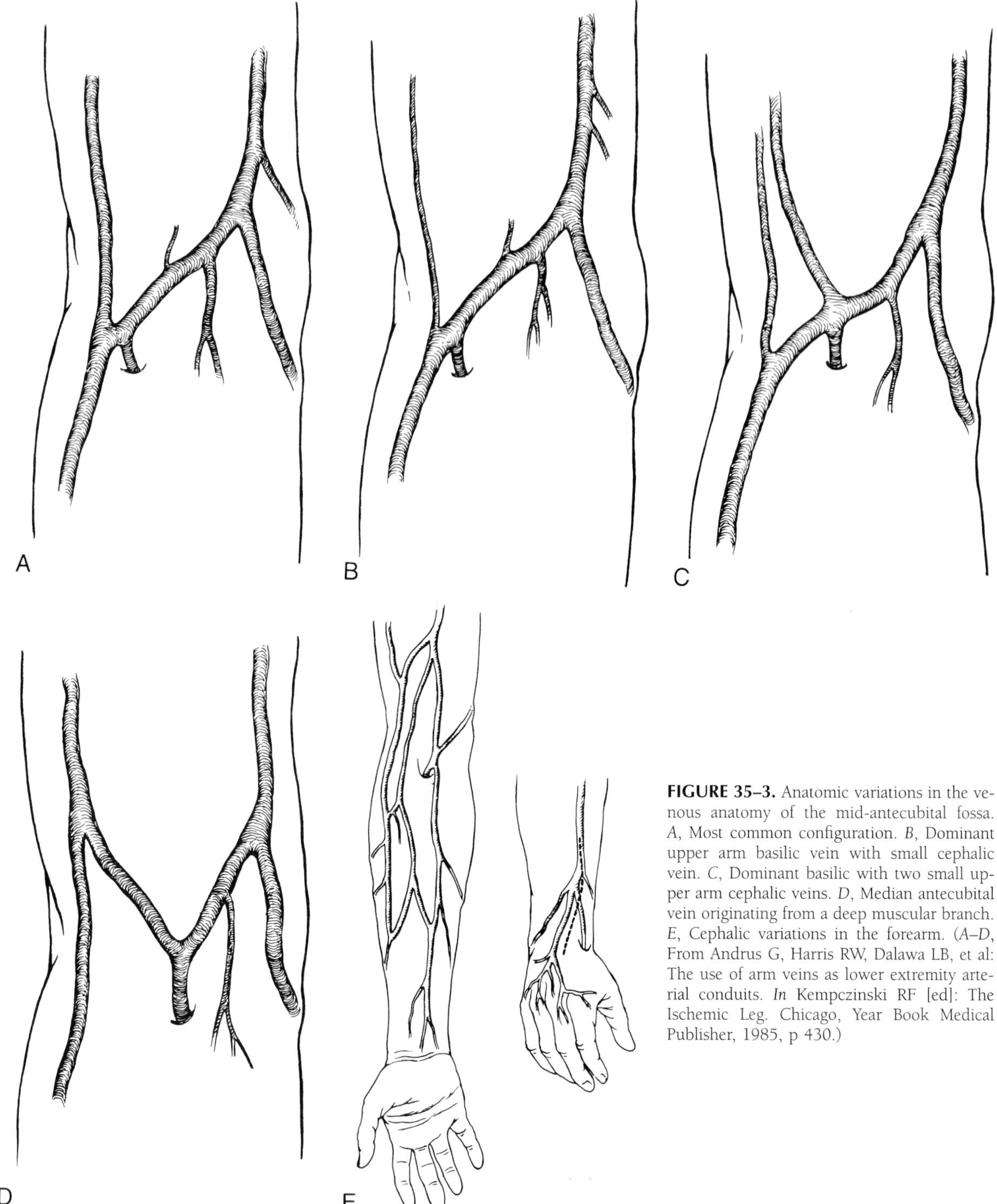

FIGURE 35–3. Anatomic variations in the venous anatomy of the mid-antecubital fossa. *A*, Most common configuration. *B*, Dominant upper arm basilic vein with small cephalic vein. *C*, Dominant basilic with two small upper arm cephalic veins. *D*, Median antecubital vein originating from a deep muscular branch. *E*, Cephalic variations in the forearm. (*A–D*, From Andrus G, Harris RW, Dalawa LB, et al: The use of arm veins as lower extremity arterial conduits. *In* Kempczinski RF [ed]: The Ischemic Leg. Chicago, Year Book Medical Publisher, 1985, p 430.)

tacyclin, a potent inhibitor of platelet aggregation and a stimulus for platelet disaggregation.[16, 17]

Ratnoff and his group have demonstrated that endothelial cells secrete in addition a substance that inactivates Hageman factor, which prevents the first steps of the intrinsic pathway of thrombus formation.[14] Additional work has identified another potent, locally vasoactive substance known as endothelium-derived relaxing factor (EDRF).[18, 19] EDRF mediates vascular relaxation tonically in response to increased flow and to a variety of agonists (adenosine triphosphate [ATP], 5-hydroxytryptamine [5-HT]) that may be released by activated platelets. EDRF is also a potent inhibitor of platelet aggregation and adhesion. The chief function of EDRF is to restrict vasoconstriction and thrombus propagation at sites of vascular injury. Iba and associates have evaluated the ability of the vein endothelium to secrete tissue plasminogen activator (t-PA), which triggers the fibrolytic cascade to maintain blood in a fluid state.[20]

TECHNIQUES OF VEIN HARVEST AND PREPARATION

There are three variables to be evaluated in the harvesting of autogenous veins:

1. The pressure at which the vein is distended.
2. The use of vasoactive agents to dilate the vein.
3. The temperature at which the vein is stored.

Pressure

A variety of reports have demonstrated the deleterious effect of high pressures in distending the saphenous vein prior to bypass. Kurusz and colleagues showed that the morphology of the endothelium of venous specimens was preserved when the distending pressure was limited to 200 mmHg.[21] In contrast, veins distended without pressure controls showed massive endothelial disruption. The control of pressure was a greater factor in endothelial preservation than the type of distending solution (blood, saline, cardioplegic solution).

Bonchek, in a similar study, demonstrated in a primate model that veins distended at high pressures (700 mmHg) showed severe damage to the endothelium and increased lipid uptake by the vein wall.[22] He stated that the upper limit of pressures used for vein distention and preparation should be in the range of 300 to 400 mmHg. It is universally accepted that pressure needs to be carefully controlled in the distention of veins. Lawrie and associates also showed that pressurization of veins to 400 mmHg lessened the EDRF relaxation compared with control veins.[18] This work basically provides functional evidence that substantiates the morphologic findings of the previous investigators.

Malone's group detected changes in the venous endothelial fibrolytic activity with increased pressures.[23] As the pressure increased from control levels to 700 mmHg, fibrolytic activity progressively decreased, demonstrating the adverse effects of pressure on venous function.[23] Abbott and colleagues also demonstrated that hydrostatic dilatation is associated with a stiffening of the vein wall.[24]

Vasoactive Agents

The second factor affecting vein harvest is the use of papaverine to dilate veins either prior to or after vein harvest. LoGerfo and coworkers recommended percutaneous infiltration with papaverine along the course of the vein before making an incision to dissect the vein.[25] Endothelial morphology was best preserved when veins were treated with papaverine before they were excised and when a warm solution was used for the dilatation of the vein grafts. In addition to preservation of intimal morphology, dilation of the veins with papaverine made them resistant to adverse effects of pressure up to 500 mmHg.

Similar findings were noted by Baumann and colleagues, who demonstrated that veins preserved with a combination of plasmalyte and papaverine showed the least degree of endothelial cell contraction, the best endothelial preservation, and no microaggregates of leukocytes on the surface.[26] They hypothesized that the vigorous prolonged contracture of a vein leads to endothelial protrusion and sloughing. As the vein wall continues to contract beyond a certain critical limit, the total area of luminal surface upon which the endothelial lining rests becomes reduced to less than the total area of the endothelial cell layer. Because of their tight interendothelial junctions, endothelial cells cannot reorient themselves or slide over one another as do the smooth muscle cells in the media of the contracting wall, and they herniate into the lumen as they are disrupted from the vessel wall.

Sottiurai and colleagues studied the effect of high and low pressure vein distention and the effect of papaverine on a long-term canine jugular vein model.[27] They noted that mechanical distention of the vein to 150 mmHg or more induced endothelial damage, subendothelial leukocyte infiltration, and excessive intimal and medial fibroplasia. Papaverine protected the mural myoblast during mechanical distention, reduced medial fibroplasia, and enhanced intimal hyperplasia and elastic tissue formation in the media. Papaverine was useful in vein preparation because it protected the endothelium and smooth muscle cells and prevented leukocyte infiltration and medical fibrosis.

Temperature

The temperature at which an excised vein should be stored is controversial. LoGerfo and coworkers suggested that optimum storage should be 4°C.[25] In more recent studies of vein graft function, either through elaboration of molecules (such as prostacyclin) or by the graft's ability to dilate in response to a variety of agonists, cold storage appears to be deleterious. Gundry and colleagues initially demonstrated that cold blood or saline immersion fully preserved the endothelium and that cold saline immersion produced medial edema.[28]

Using prostacyclin as a metabolic marker of endothelial functional capacity, Bush and associates noted that normothermia (37°C) during vein graft storage was the optimal temperature for preserving the prostacyclin production.[17] Hypothermic storage markedly impaired the subsequent capacity of the endothelium to produce prostacyclin. A progressive decrease in storage temperature resulted in a stepwise decrease in prostacyclin production following ex vivo storage. This work suggests that hypothermia induced direct and persistent metabolic injury in the endothelial cell.

Lawrie and colleagues studied the effect of storage solution on the activity of EDRF using an open ring preparation of fresh human saphenous veins.[18] They noted that veins stored at 2° to 4°C demonstrated severe depression of EDRF relaxation compared to those stored at 37°C. At this time, the author recommends careful distention of the harvested veins with papaverine and storage at room temperature until the veins are inserted into the circulation.

OPERATIVE TECHNIQUES

In the harvesting of veins, it is essential to use meticulous delicate techniques. Multiple incisions can be made in

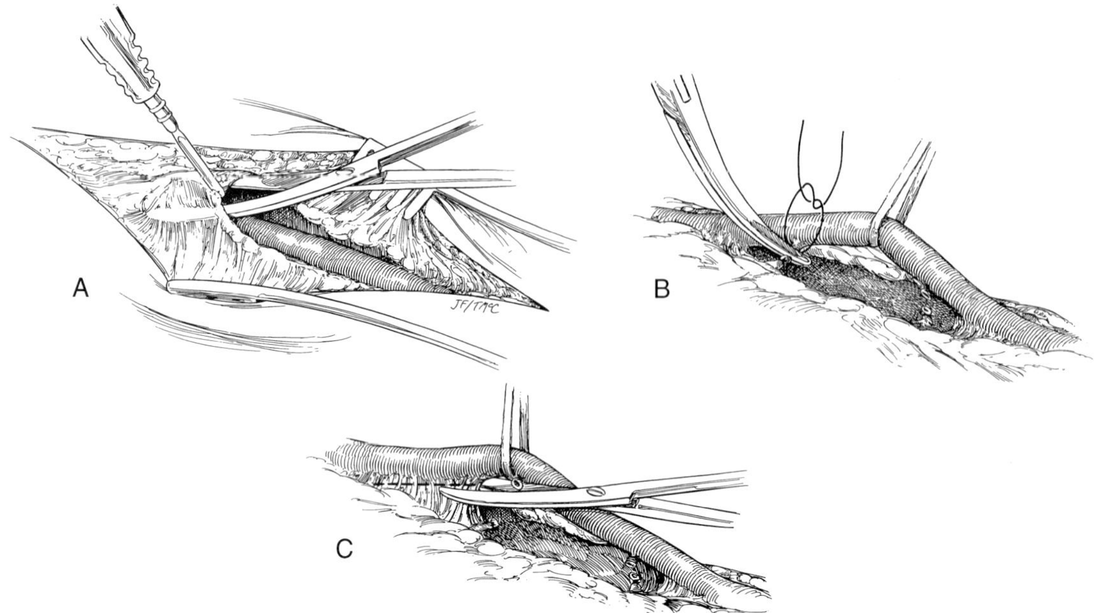

FIGURE 35–4. Vein harvest. *A*, the vein is exposed through the use of upward traction on the overlying tissues by spread scissor blades (or clamp) to protect the underlying vein from injury. *B*, Traction with a polymeric silicone (Silastic) loop often reveals the location of tributaries, which are then ligated and divided with 1-mm ends. *C*, Trimming away tissue 2 to 3 mm from the vein allows small tributaries inadvertently cut to be later clamped and tied. (*A–C*, From Rutherford R: Atlas of Vascular Surgery. Philadelphia, WB Saunders, 1993, p 75.)

harvesting the saphenous vein if care is taken not to exert undue traction or pressure in moving the vein from beneath the skin bridges. When a lesser saphenous vein and arm veins are being harvested, a continuous incision seems to make the process easier. This is particularly true for arm veins, which are thin and easily injured. Before dissection, papaverine is injected along the course of the vein. Side branches are carefully mobilized and ligated so that the ligature does not impinge on the lumen of the vessel (Figs. 35–4 and 35–5). Previous mapping of the veins by duplex ultrasonography helps in placement of incisions. One should close vein harvest sites meticulously, avoiding suture techniques that create skin ischemia. Particularly in diabetic patients, these wounds can become necrosed and slough, resulting in prolonged convalescence after the arterial bypass.

CONTROVERSIES IN GRAFTING

There is probably no greater area of disagreement among vascular surgeons than that concerning the selection of techniques for lower extremity bypass. For patients who have intact saphenous veins, the surgeon has three options:

- Perform a reverse vein graft, usually tunneled anatomically
- Perform an in situ bypass
- Remove the vein, incise the valves, and place the vein in an antegrade fashion

The difficulty in resolving this issue deals with the fact that comparing various series is difficult owing to several common variables: (1) the smallest size of vein that is

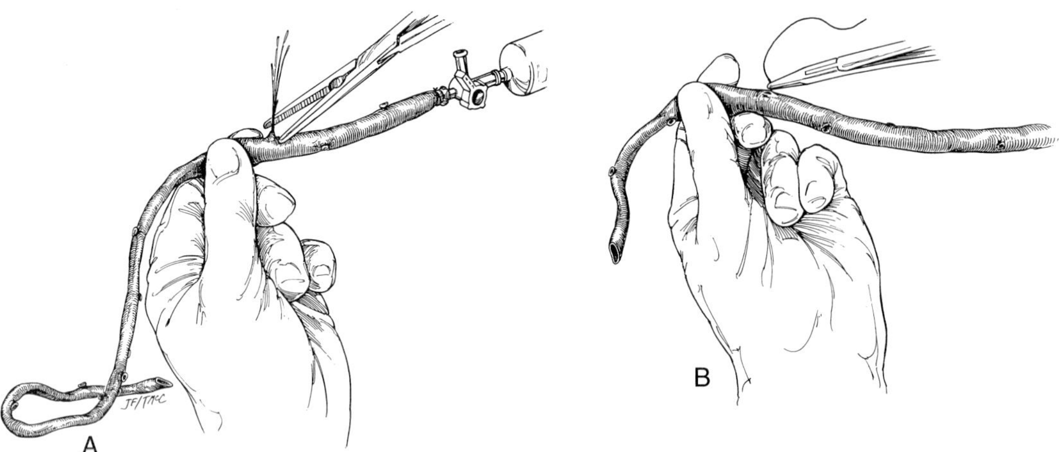

FIGURE 35–5. *A*, Gentle segmental dilatation of the vein may reveal leaks from small tributaries that were inadvertently cut. *B*, Avulsed tributaries must be repaired with fine sutures. (*A* and *B*, From Rutherford R: Atlas of Vascular Surgery. Philadelphia, WB Saunders, 1993, p 77.)

considered usable, (2) the different proportion of limb salvage and claudication patients, and (3) differences in operative technique. Excellent results have been reported with all techniques.

Several reports indicated that the in situ technique was superior because it allowed better endothelial preservation. Buchbinder and colleagues published the results of canine carotid bypasses with jugular vein using both the *in situ* technique and the *reverse technique*.[29] With the reverse technique, there was extensive endothelial sloughing and denuding of the flow surface; with the in situ technique, a normal endothelium was retained. The biochemical basis of this finding was presented by Bush and coworkers who, also with a canine model, noted higher levels of prostacyclin from in situ grafts compared to veins that were reversed.[30]

Cambria and associates compared in situ grafts with atraumatically dissected, nondistended reverse grafts and with grafts that were distended to a pressure of 500 mmHg. They noted that endothelial denudation was least, on average in the in situ grafts, intermediate in the reverse grafts, and most severe in the reversed and distended grafts.[31] Perhaps of greater significance, there was no difference in endothelial fibrolytic activity between the in situ and gently handled reverse grafts at 24 hours or 6 weeks after surgery. Batson and Sottiurai, also using a canine model, compared nonreversed, reversed, and in situ grafts. They could distinguish no discernible morphologic differences in the translocated and in situ grafts.[32]

To date, no clinical study has shown conclusively which bypass technique is better. Selection of one technique over another involves a series of tradeoffs. With the in situ technique, there is a learning curve during which the unique techniques of the procedure must be mastered. The valves need to be incised, and patent side branches need to be ligated. There is an inherent incidence of reoperation because of residual competent valve cusps and missed arteriovenous fistulae. The advantages are that the large end of the saphenous vein is anastomosed to the common femoral artery and the small end, which is a better size match, is anastomosed to the distal artery. With the in situ technique, the smaller veins have a potential use as bypass conduits. In the author's experience, conduits as small as 2 mm in diameter have been used in situ and excellent long-term patency has been obtained. With the in situ technique, 2 mm is the lower limit of venous diameter that is usable for long bypasses owing to technical problems with valve ablation in the small veins.

Precise data on vein diameter are currently absent in the literature originating from the major centers that champion the use of the reverse vein. Once this information is forthcoming, this disparity in results can be resolved. Whichever technique is used, the procedure must be done well and the vein must be of good quality.

Stratification of vein graft patency based on vein diameter has failed to consistently demonstrate statistically significant differences in early and long-term patency rates. The author noted that veins with a diameter of less than 3 mm had a 30-day patency (86%), which was lower than veins 3 to 3.9 mm (97%), or of those greater than 4 mm in diameter (98%).[33] Sonnenfeld and Cronestrand, in a study of reversed veins used for femoral popliteal bypass, noted no difference in patency between veins less than 3 mm and those greater that 3 mm.[34] Because 82% of their grafts were with above-knee popliteal artery, and 70% were in patients whose operative indication was claudication, it is difficult to compare their results with the author's series.

In a series in which all grafts were made to infrapopliteal arteries in limb salvage patients, Wengerter and colleagues noted decreased patency in reverse vein grafts less than 3.5 mm in diameter.[35] It is the author's impression that the in situ technique allows the use of smaller diameter veins for distal bypass.

It is very difficult to evaluate the quality of the vein. Small-diameter veins may be the result of previous phlebitic processes that have caused thickening of the valve wall, scarring of the vein endothelium, and loss of distensibility. These poor-quality veins are not suitable for use as arterial conduits. Small veins that can be used for arterial bypasses must be thin-walled and distensible. Some of the poor results reported by previous authors using small veins may have been due to the fact that the veins were of poor quality.

When small veins are used for the in situ bypass, meticulous surgical technique is required to prevent vein injury. Early in the author's experience, the endothelium of small veins was lacerated during valve lysis because the small vein contracted around the valvotome. To prevent vein spasm in small conduits, the author now infuses a solution of 500 ml of dextran, 60 mg of papaverine and 500 IU of heparin into the distal vein to dilate it prior to insertion of the valvotome. This technique prevents the smooth muscle of the vein from constricting around the valvotome.

Two-, three-, and four-year patency rates of small-diameter veins in the author's series were no different from the rates reported with larger-diameter conduits, demonstrating the durability of small conduits.[33] Patients with small-diameter conduits may not have hemodynamically normal limbs. The function and flow characteristics of a graft can be quantitated by measuring graft flow velocity. For smaller-diameter grafts to carry the same volume of blood, the velocity of flow must be increased proportionally.

In a previously reported study, the author noted that 23% of bypasses had flow-restrictive venous conduits.[36] These were characterized by small-diameter vein grafts, increased graft flow velocity, and smaller postoperative increases in ankle brachial indices, which average 0.67 on the first postoperative day and increase to 0.89 at 1 week. Because these bypass grafts are utilized for patients who have limb-threatening ischemia, there is, nonetheless, sufficient blood flow to heal ulcers and prevent rest pain. The good-quality small saphenous vein is a suitable conduit and should be considered for use in lower limb bypasses, particularly with the in situ technique.

The principal determinant of success with vein bypass surgery is the quality of the conduit. Portions of the vein may be absent because of previous coronary artery bypass or arterial bypass surgery, or the vein may have suffered previous phlebitic processes, rendering portions of it unusable. Regardless of which technique is used, modification of the conduit is necessary, ranging from localized repair of short stenotic segments to imposition of long segments to have sufficient graft for the autologous bypass. In addition, technical errors that may occur during vein harvest or graft preparation by valve lysis can necessitate vein modification.

In a series of 361 consecutive bypasses, modifications were required in 23% of the grafts[37]; of these, 10% were needed because of a sclerotic segment, a small-diameter vein, the presence of varicosities, or previous utilization. In 13%, modification was necessitated by technical errors related to the in situ technique; these included vein injury, anastomotic stenosis, retained valves, and torsion of the graft. It is significant that this modification affected both the short-term and long-term patency of the grafts. The primary patency at 3 months was 20% better in the unmodified group. These data emphasize the need for meticulous dissection of the veins to avoid technical errors, and they illustrate the fact that if multiple repairs of the vein are required, results are still reasonable but not as good as if an unmodified, continuous length of vein had been used.

LONG-TERM CHANGES IN VEIN GRAFTS

Because the vein is a biologic conduit, it has a dynamic life. Deterioration of the vein graft can occur throughout its life and is related to specific processes at various time intervals. Most changes that occur in a graft in the first 30 days after implantation are related to (1) technical errors in the construction of the bypass, (2) patient selection, or (3) quality of the conduit (Fig. 35–6). Problems that occur in

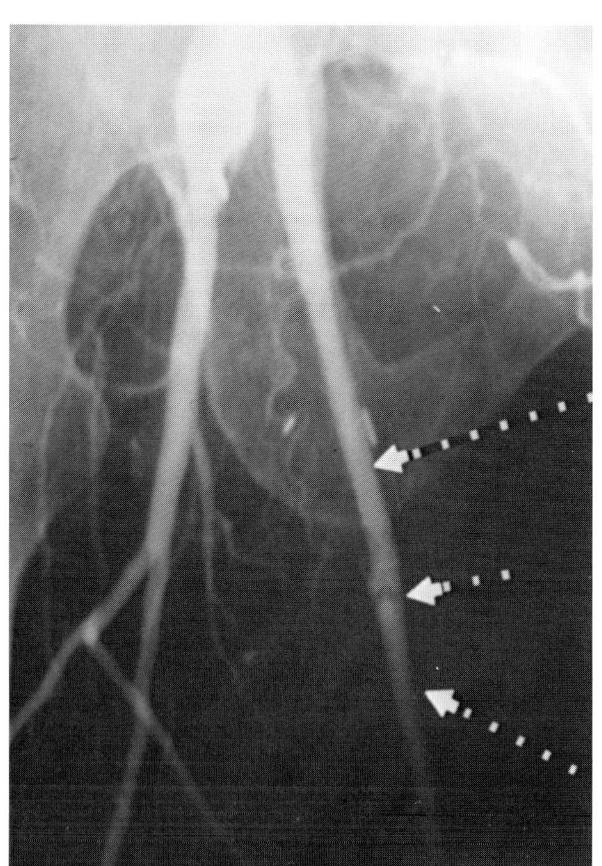

FIGURE 35–6. Retained valve *(arrows)* following in situ bypass.

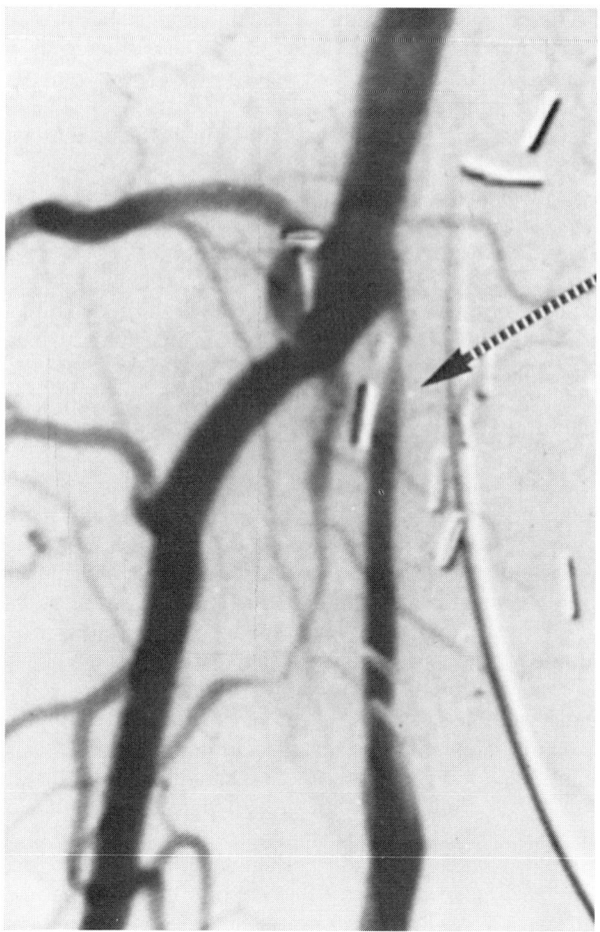

FIGURE 35–7. Postoperative stenosis *(arrow)* occurring in vein graft 8 months after operation.

the interval between 30 days and 2 years are usually attributed to (1) fibrointimal hyperplasia, which occurs at sites of anastomosis; (2) areas of vein repair; and (3) sites of valve incisions (Fig. 35–7). After 24 months, changes are primarily due to the progression of atherosclerosis. Excellent short-term and long-term patency rates and limb salvage rates are now achievable.[38] Technical success has outpaced physiologic and anatomic knowledge of the mature arterialized vein graft.

Using color duplex ultrasonography, the author found that only 43% of lower extremity bypass grafts, patent for a median of 79 months, were normal; nearly half the normal grafts had needed either conduit revisions or correction of inflow or outflow disease progression to maintain patency. In addition, nearly one in five grafts harbored lesions that would pose a threat to continued long-term patency.[38]

Atherosclerotic degeneration of saphenous vein grafts was first described in 1947, when a femoral interposition graft, which had been in place for 22 years, was removed and found to contain atheromatous plaques.[39] In 1973, Szilagyi and associates reported their experience with lower extremity saphenous vein grafts that had been studied by arteriography.[40] These authors described eight different morphologic findings in grafts of varying ages. Several of these related to surgical technique, including suture stenosis caused by tying side branches too closely, long venous side branch stump, and traumatic stenosis caused by clamps. They also described the changes that occur later, including intimal thickening, mild intimal hyperplasia at valve sites, arterial sclerotic irregularity, and aneurysmal dilatation.

In our study, autogenous grafts were examined at least 4½ years after construction. The early postoperative changes noted by Szilagyi's group were not detectable. However, our group did find three distinct atherosclerotic abnormalities: wall plaque, aneurysmal dilatation, and discrete stenosis.[38] The most prevalent finding was wall plaque, which was present in all the abnormal grafts, although it was frequently overshadowed by more impressive stenosis or aneurysms. Typically, plaques were several centimeters long, multicentric, echogenic, and slightly raised from the normal wall. These are a mild form of atherosclerotic degeneration. In the Szilagyi series, atherosclerotic changes developed in approximately 45 months.

Atkinson and colleagues examined coronary artery saphenous vein grafts at autopsy and found atherosclerotic changes in 21%, which had been in place an average of 62.7 months.[41] However, when DeWeese and Rob followed long-term grafts using arteriography, they noted atherosclerotic changes in only three of 18 patients studied after 5 years, and two grafts did not develop changes until after 10 years.[42] The author's group used color duplex ultrasonography to interrogate the grafts and were able to visualize changes in the arterial wall,[38] such as thickening and wall plaque that are not necessarily seen on contrast arteriography, which defines only the column of flowing blood. Thus, this group found a high incidence of atherosclerotic changes with evidence of it in more than 50% of the grafts at a median postoperative follow-up time of 74 months.

Aneurysmal degeneration in saphenous vein grafts is a more dramatic late development (Fig. 35–8). It is infrequent, with only 29 cases described in the literature.[43] The author's group found eight grafts harboring 16 segments with aneurysmal change.[38] Five (63%) of these grafts had become occluded and had undergone either a thrombectomy or thrombolysis many months prior to diagnosis of the vein graft aneurysm. For three grafts with aneurysms, there had been no history of occlusion and two of these were reversed saphenous vein grafts.

The author postulates that transmural ischemic injury occurs at the time of graft thrombosis or vein harvest. This alters the integrity of the vein graft wall, allowing subsequent aneurysm formation. Vein graft aneurysms have been described to be atherosclerotic in nature, but this may be a result of the ongoing reparative changes rather than the cause of the aneurysm.

The site of the autogenous graft affects its tendency to develop aneurysm degeneration. Stanley and coworkers, studying aortorenal vein grafts, noted that one third exhibited uniform expansion, with an 18% mean increase in diameter.[43] Eight of these grafts expanded 25% to 47%, and six grafts showed aneurysmal dilatation manifested by concentric dilatations averaging 114% and ranging from 62% to 150%.

Vein grafts are susceptible to atherosclerotic changes. The development of these lesions is accelerated because vein graft changes occur over several years, whereas native vessels show the same result over decades. Changes in long-term vein grafts are usually combinations of both fibrointimal hyperplasia and atherosclerosis.

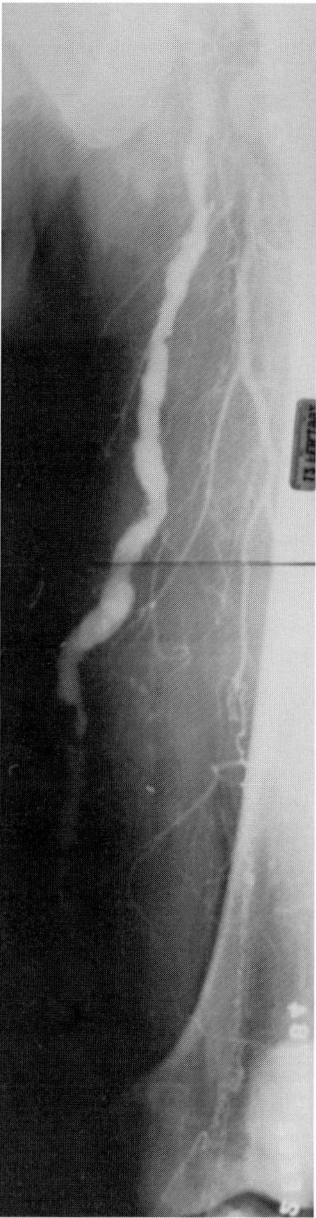

FIGURE 35–8. Arteriogram of aneurysmal vein graft. Stenotic areas and aneurysmal areas exist in same graft. (From Reifsnyder T, Towne JB, Seabrook GR, et al: Biology of long-term autogenous vein grafts. J Vasc Surg 17:207, 1993.)

In the author's study, atherosclerotic changes that threatened graft survival were noted in 11 extremities. These lesions were always very discrete and short and were surrounded by a normal vein graft proximally and distally. Half of these stenoses were at the site of previous defect, and the other half developed in the undisturbed segments de novo. One of the author's patients had undergone nine different procedures in an attempt to correct recurrent stenosis in the distal third of the femoral anterior tibial graft. Even when the stenosis plus 10 cm of normal graft on either side was replaced, new stenosis in the mid-portion of replacement graft occurred within a few months. Why stenosis developed in some grafts while only wall plaque developed in others is unknown.

The relationship between risk factors and the development of vein graft atherosclerosis has been examined. Campeau and colleagues studied saphenous vein grafts in the coronary circulation and documented the development of new stenoses or changes in stenoses older than 10 years.[44] They found that new or changing stenoses developed in patients with significantly higher lipid levels. In their necropsy study, Atkinson and colleagues found that atherosclerotic lesions in coronary saphenous vein grafts were related to hypercholesterolemia.[41] In this study, there were no risk factors (hypertension, coronary artery disease, diabetes mellitus, smoking, treated hyperlipidemia) that significantly predicted the occurrence of graft lesions, but lipid levels were not prospectively evaluated.

A prospective study correlating lipids and lower extremity graft morphology would help further elucidate the natural history of autogenous bypasses. Vein grafts used for lower extremity bypass are ideally suited for this kind of study. Unlike grafts used in the coronary circulation, lower extremity bypasses can be sequentially studied noninvasively by the color duplex scanner without risk or discomfort to the patient.

Long-term graft morphology is affected by postoperative revisions. In the author's study, 38 (53%) of the grafts underwent at least one revision either to repair the conduit or to protect inflow and outflow. Revised conduits contained 12 of the 15 graft-threatening lesions, whereas the grafts that had never been modified tended to be normal in appearance. During the early postoperative period, revisions involved the conduit and were necessary to correct technical errors, such as retained valves, missed arteriovenous fistulae, a twisted graft, and the use of an unsuitable vein segment. These revisions did not invariably condemn the graft, because seven of 11 (64%) were normal at the time of long-term follow-up.

Between 1 and 24 months postoperatively, grafts were most commonly revised because of stenotic lesions at the anastomoses and valve sites, which microscopically demonstrated fibrointimal hyperplasia. This tended to portend future problems, and only 17% of these conduits were normal, as shown by color duplex scanning at late follow-up. After 2 years, the grafted extremities were affected more by the ongoing atherosclerotic process. Inflow and outflow disease progression necessitated two thirds of the late revisions. Thus, the cause of impending graft failure varies with the length of time the graft has been in place.

In a study of 550 consecutive lower extremity autogenous vein bypasses to determine the incidence and causes of abnormalities that threaten graft patency beyond 2 years, the authors noted that of the 236 grafts in which surveillance abnormalities developed, 50 (21%) demonstrated the first abnormality more than 2 years after the primary bypass.[45] Of the grafts free of abnormalities at 24 months, 30% subsequently went on to develop at least one abnormality during the remaining life of the graft. Thirty primary interventions occurred more than 24 months after the initial bypass, of which 63% involved the conduit or its anastomosis, 17% were inflow procedures, 17% were outflow procedures, and 3% were for graft replacement. For grafts remaining primarily patent longer than 24 months, the incidence of subsequent primary graft failure during the remaining life of the graft was 11%. This value was calculated by dividing the summation of primary graft failures occurring after 2 years by the number of primary patent grafts at risk at the beginning of the third year of follow-up. Of grafts remaining primarily patent at the beginning of any given 1-year interval, 10% went on to primary graft failure at some point in the life of the graft. More important, the ravages of atherosclerosis are incessant.

The necessity for perpetual graft surveillance cannot be overemphasized. Our surveillance protocol now consists of seeing patients with mature grafts twice yearly. The 6-month visit is brief, consisting of a physical examination, an ankle-brachial index, and a single graft flow velocity. Each year, in addition to these measures, we now scan the entire graft.

When a good vein conduit is used and no intraoperative problems are encountered, the grafts do not develop intrinsic conduit lesions that threaten patency. Nonetheless, atherosclerotic changes are seen, as evidenced by the high incidence of wall plaque. In less than optimal circumstances, graft-threatening lesions in the conduit and in the inflow and outflow vessels occur continually. If the lesion is identified and corrected in a timely manner, prolonged patency is obtained. The autogenous lower extremity bypass can be durable, but diligent surveillance is required by the vascular surgeon.

REFERENCES

1. Bergamini TM, Towne JB, Bandyk DF, et al: Experience with in situ saphenous vein bypasses during 1981–1989: Determinant factors of long-term patency. J Vasc Surg 13:137–49, 1991.
2. Taylor LM, Edwards JM, Porter JM: Present status of reversed vein bypass grafting: Five-year results of a modern series. J Vasc Surg 11:193–206, 1990.
3. Leather RP, Shah DM, Chang BB, Kaufman JL: Resurrection of the in situ saphenous vein bypass: 1000 cases later. Ann Surg 208:435–442, 1988.
4. Veith FJ, Gupta SK, Ascer E, Flores-White S, Towne JB, et al: Six year prospective multicenter randomized comparison of autologous saphenous vein and expanded PTFE grafts in infrainguinal arterial reconstructions. J Vasc Surg 3:104–114, 1886.
5. Goss CM (ed): Gray's Anatomy of the Human Body, 29th ed. Philadelphia, Lea & Febiger, 1975, pp 717–719.
6. Shah DM, Chang BB, Leopold PW, et al: The anatomy of the greater saphenous venous system. J Vasc Surg 3:273–283, 1986.
7. Veith FJ, Moss CM, Sprayregen S, Montefusco C: Preoperative saphenous venography in arterial reconstructive surgery of the lower extremity. Surgery 85:253–256, 1979.
8. Edwards EA: The orientation of venous valves in relation to body surfaces. Anat Rec 64:369–385, 1986.
9. Andrus G, Harris RW, Salles-Cunha SX, et al: Arm veins for arterial revascularization of the leg: Arteriographic and clinical observations. J Vasc Surg 4:416–427, 1986.
10. CM Goss (ed): Gray's Anatomy of the Human Body, 29th ed., Philadelphia, Lea & Febiger, 1975, pp 700–703.
11. Clagett GP, Valentine RJ, Hagino RT: Autogenous aortoiliac/femoral reconstruction from superficial femoral-popliteal veins: Feasibility and durability. J Vasc Surg 25:255–270, 1997.
12. Hagino RT, Bengtson TD, Fosdick DA, et al: Venous reconstructions using the superficial femoral-popliteal vein. J Vasc Surg 26:829–837, 1997.
13. Fuchs JCA, Mitchener JS III, Hagen P: Postoperative changes in autologous vein grafts. Ann Surg 188:1–15, 1978.
14. Ratnoff OD, Everson B, Embury P, et al: Inhibition of the activation

of Hageman factor (factor XII) by human vascular endothelial cell culture suppurates. Proc Natl Acad Sci U S A 88:10740–10743, 1991.
15. Marlar RA: Protein C in thromboembolic disease. Semin Thromb Hemost 2:387–393, 1985.
16. Eldor A, Falcone DJ, Hajjar DP, et al: Recovery of prostacyclin production by de-endothelialized rabbit aorta. J Clin Invest 67:735–741, 1981.
17. Bush HL, McCabe ME, Nabseth DC: Functional injury of vein graft endothelium. Arch Surg 119:770–774, 1984.
18. Lawrie GM, Weilbacher DE, Henry PD: Endothelium-dependent relaxation in human saphenous vein grafts. J Thorac Cardiovasc Surg 100:612–620, 1990.
19. Angelini GD, Christie MI, Bryan AJ, Lewis MJ: Surgical preparation impairs release of endothelium-derived relaxing factor from human saphenous vein. Ann Thorac Surg 48:417–420, 1989.
20. Iba T, Shin T, Sonoda T, et al: Stimulation of endothelial secretion of tissue-type plasminogen activator by repetitive stretch. J Surg Res 50:457–460, 1991.
21. Kurusz M, Christman EW, Derick JR, et al: Use of cold cardioplegic solution for vein graft distention and preservation: A light and scanning electron microscopic study. Ann Thorac Surg 32:68–74, 1981.
22. Bonchek LI: Prevention of endothelial damage during preparation of saphenous veins for bypass grafting. J Thorac Cardiovasc Surg 79:911–915, 1980.
23. Malone JM, Kischer CW, Moore WS: Changes in venous endothelial fibrinolytic activity and histology with in vitro venous distention and arterial implantation. Am J Surg 142:178–182, 1981.
24. Abbott WM, Wieland S, Austin WG: Structural changes during preparation of autogenous venous grafts. Surgery 76:1031–1040, 1973.
25. LoGerfo FW, Quist WC, Crawshaw HM, Haudenschild C: An improved technique for preservation of endothelial morphology in vein grafts. Surgery 90:1015–1024, 1981.
26. Baumann FG, Catinella FP, Cunningham JN Jr, Spencer FC: Vein contraction and smooth muscle cell extensions as causes of endothelial damage during graft preparation. Ann Surg 194:199–211, 1981.
27. Sottiurai VS, Sue SL, Batson RC, et al: Effects of papaverine on smooth muscle cell morphology and vein graft preparation. J Vasc Surg 2:834–842, 1985.
28. Gundry SR, Jones M, Ishihara T: Optimal preparation techniques for human saphenous vein grafts. Surgery 88:785–794, 1980.
29. Buchbinder D, Singh JK, Karmody AM, et al: Comparison of patency rate and structural change of in situ and reversed vein arterial bypass. J Surg Res 30:213–218, 1981.
30. Bush HL, Jakubowski JA, Curl GR, et al: The natural history of endothelial structure and function in arterialized vein grafts. J Vasc Surg 3:204–215, 1986.
31. Cambria RP, Megerman J, Abbott WM: Endothelial preservation in reversed and in situ autogenous vein grafts. Ann Surg 202:50–55, 1985.
32. Batson RC, Sottiurai VS: Nonreversed and in situ vein grafts. Ann Surg 201:771–779, 1985.
33. Towne JB, Schmitt DD, Seabrook GR, Bandyk DF: The effect of vein diameter on patency of in situ grafts. J Cardiovasc Surg 32:192–196, 1991.
34. Sonnenfeld T, Cronestrand R: Factors determining outcome of reversed saphenous vein femoropopliteal bypass grafts. Br J Surg 67:642–648, 1980.
35. Wengerter KR, Veith FJ, Gupta SK, Ascer E: Influence of vein size (diameter) on intrapopliteal reversed vein graft patency. J Vasc Surg 11:525–531, 1990.
36. Bandyk DF, Kaebnick HW, Bergamini TM, Moldenhauer PK, Towne JB: Hemodynamics of in situ saphenous vein arterial bypass. Arch Surg 123:477–482, 1988.
37. Bergamini TM, Towne JB, Bandyk DF, et al: Experience with in situ saphenous vein bypasses during 1981 to 1989: Determinant factors of long term patency. J Vasc Surg 13:137–149, 1991.
38. Reifsnyder T, Towne JB, Seabrook GR, et al: Biology of long-term autogenous vein grafts: A dynamic evolution. J Vasc Surg 17:207–217, 1993.
39. Batzner IC: Uber die Chirurgie der Arterien Verlotzungen und die Frage des Venentransplantats. Der Chirurg 17:345, 1947.
40. Szilagyi DE, Elliott JP, Hageman JH, et al: Biologic fate of autogenous vein implants as arterial substitutes. Ann Surg 178:232–244, 1973.
41. Atkinson JB, Forman MB, Vaughn WK, et al: Morphologic changes in long-term saphenous vein bypass grafts. Chest 88:341–348, 1985.
42. DeWeese JA, Rob C: Autogenous venous grafts ten years later. Surgery 82:775–784, 1977.
43. Stanley JC, Ernst CB, Fry WJ: Fate of 100 aortorenal vein grafts: Characteristics of late graft expansion, aneurysmal dilatation, and stenosis. Surgery 74:931–944, 1973.
44. Campeau L, Enjulbert M, Lesperance J, et al: The relation of risk factors to the development of atherosclerosis in saphenous vein bypass grafts and the progression of disease in the native circulation. N Engl J Med 311:1329–1332, 1984.
45. Erickson CA, Towne JB, Seabrook GR, et al: Ongoing vascular laboratory surveillance is essential to maximize long-term in situ saphenous vein bypass patency. J Vasc Surg 23:18–27, 1996.

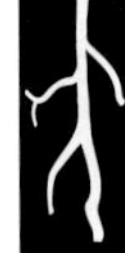

CHAPTER 36

Biologic Grafts for Lower Limb Revascularization

Herbert Dardik, M.D., and Kurt Wengerter, M.D.

The *autologous saphenous vein* is the standard against which the performance of all other vascular grafts is measured. However, even autologous saphenous vein is far from ideal. It may be absent or diseased or too small or too short, and time is required for procurement and preparation. Finally, after implantation as an arterial conduit, it may undergo various forms of biodegradation. Therefore, an alternative vascular conduit is still needed when revascularization is mandatory but the saphenous vein is inadequate, for any reason.

For decades, alternatives to the autologous saphenous vein have been studied by surgeons, engineers, and textile personnel. Some of these alternatives have proved more useful than others, although still others have been discarded. For example, unmodified heterografts are no longer used because of accelerated biodegradation. Unmodified allograft saphenous veins enjoyed brief popularity, but despite apparent low immunogenicity, most were ultimately rejected. Perhaps pretreatment of allografts or even xenografts with chemical agents, freezing techniques, or lyophilization might result in biologic materials that retain durable function. Clinical experience with aldehyde-processing and cryopreservation has, in fact, provided unique insights into the usefulness, liabilities, and challenges of biologic materials deployed as vascular conduits.

MODIFIED UMBILICAL VEIN GRAFT

Human umbilical cords average approximately 50 cm in length and normally contain one vein and two arteries in a mucopolysaccharide matrix called "Wharton's jelly" (Fig. 36–1). At birth, the vessels are collapsed but the vein can easily be dilated up to 7 mm in diameter and the arteries can be dilated up to 4 mm. Roentgenographic studies have shown that the vessels are of uniform diameter. They have no branches, valves, or vasa vasorum. Manometric studies in vitro have shown that these vessels can tolerate pressures in excess of 600 mmHg.

Initially, we implanted unmodified segments of human umbilical cord veins in the aorta of baboons.[23] Although early patency was achieved, predictable rejection occurred within several weeks of implantation. On gross histologic examination, aneurysm formation and thrombosis were present; on microscopy, necrosis, microabscesses, and macrophage and plasma cell infiltration were seen. Previous attempts to use unmodified umbilical cord vessels had met with similar failure.[2, 48, 72]

Inspired by the pioneering work of Carpentier[16] and Rosenberg[55] and their co-workers, we studied the effects of both dialdehyde starch and glutaraldehyde tanning on umbilical cord vessels prior to their implantation as vascular conduits. Unlike the previous failed attempts that occurred predictably without aldehyde processing, success was now routinely achieved, first in the laboratory and later in a small pilot clinical study.[22, 26] The superiority of glutaraldehyde as a tanning agent compared with dialdehyde starch was apparent histologically and was confirmed by immunologic studies.[51]

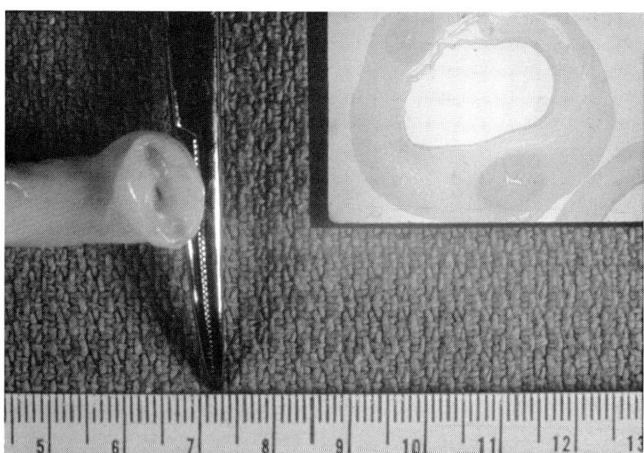

FIGURE 36–1. Umbilical cord obtained at delivery. *Inset,* Larger umbilical vein at center and two smaller umbilical arteries are visualized clearly by microscopy.

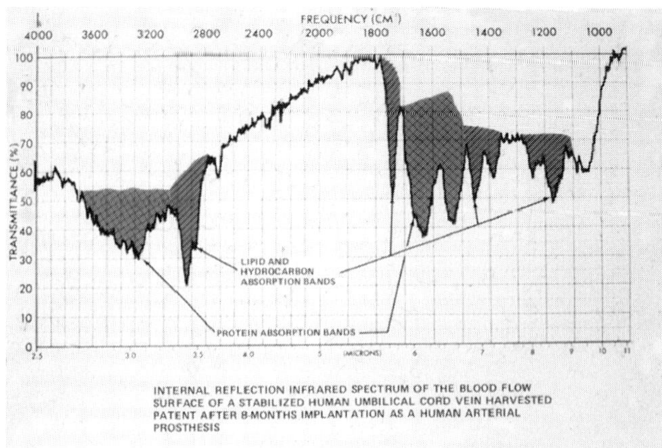

FIGURE 36–2. Internal reflection infrared spectrum of the blood flow surface of a stabilized human umbilical cord vein, harvested patent after 8 months of implantation as a human arterial prosthesis. Lipid deposition reflects accelerated progression of this patient's generalized atherosclerosis.

In addition, chemical and physical analyses of the interface, including internal reflection spectroscopy and contact angle determinations, were used to characterize the intimal surface and to compare it with that of natural blood vessels, bovine heterografts, and synthetic materials.[4, 5] The former method "fingerprinted" the flow surface and provided important information regarding the presence and amount of lipid deposition (Fig. 36–2); the latter measured critical surface tension and, therefore, surface energy as a marker for thrombogenicity (Fig. 36–3).

Mechanical tests have also been employed to ensure the adequacy of the cross-links produced by aldehyde tanning. Light, scanning, and transmission electron microscopy have yielded much information regarding structure, function, and durability following implantation. Long-term studies

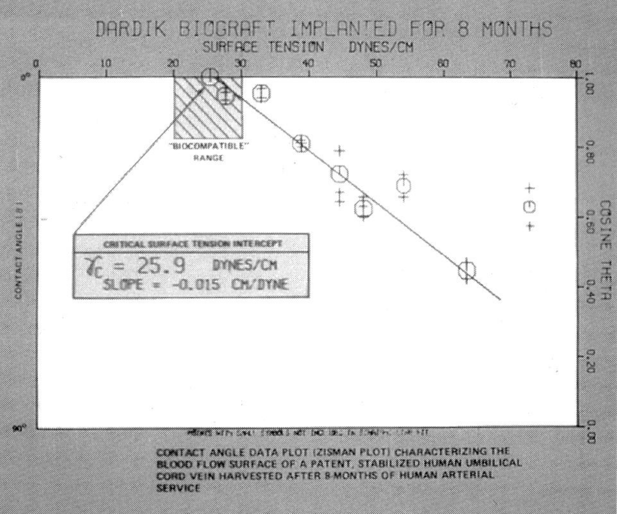

FIGURE 36–3. Contact angle data plot (Zisman Plot) characterizing the blood flow surface of a patent, glutaraldehyde-stabilized human umbilical cord vein harvested after 8 months of human arterial service. Values of 25 ± 5 dynes/cm reflect thromboresistance.

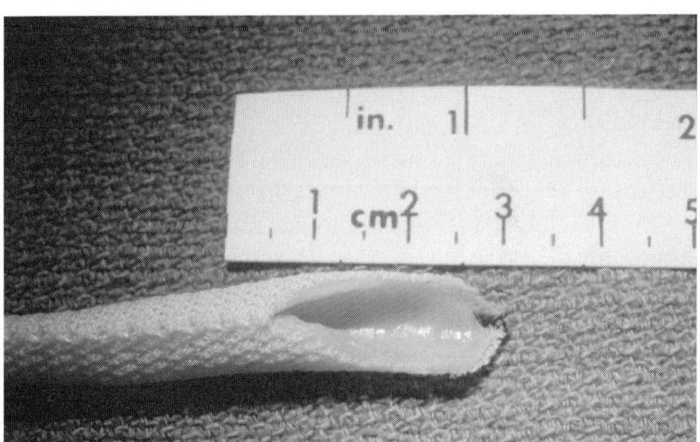

FIGURE 36–4. Umbilical vein graft employed for lower extremity revascularization. The inner diameter is 5 mm, and the outer surface is covered with an elastic polyester mesh. Recently manufactured grafts have a uniform thin wall with a dense mesh on the outer surface, including a guideline.

have shown that the glutaraldehyde-stabilized umbilical vein graft retains its basic architecture even though instances of aneurysmal biodegradation have been noted.[24, 29] On the basis of improved manufacturing and quality control, this graft has now proved remarkably stable and resistant to, but certainly not immune to, the forces of biodegradation.

Current umbilical grafts consist of manually stripped and prepared veins that have been stabilized with glutaraldehyde under optimal pH and temperature control (Fig. 36–4). Aldehyde cross-linkage of the protein moieties increases tensile strength and masks antigenicity. A polyester (Dacron) mesh is placed about the vein, which is then sterilized and stored in 50% ethanol. Most important, processing with glutaraldehyde sterilizes the tissue of bacteria, viruses, and fungi and renders it nonantigenic (Table 36–1).

Clinical Indications

The glutaraldehyde-stabilized human umbilical vein graft (Biograft, BioVascular, Inc., St. Paul, Minn.) is used for revascularization of the ischemic lower limb when autologous vein is unavailable or unsuitable. In 1972, when the work on this prosthesis began, the superiority of saphenous vein was not thoroughly appreciated, the bovine graft was being abandoned, polytetrafluoroethylene (PTFE) was not available and Dacron was not widely used for small/medium vessel replacement. During the ensuing quarter-century, the saphenous vein confirmed its superiority, PTFE developed a loyal following despite its recognized shortcomings, Dacron was revisited and appeared to earn new supporters, and the umbilical vein graft filled a small but definite niche.

TABLE 36–1. EFFECTS OF GLUTARALDEHYDE ON BIOLOGIC MATERIAL

Reduces antigenicity
Increases strength via cross-linking
Inhibits degradation
Sterilizes tissue

Traditionally, femoral-popliteal implantation has been the standard site for clinical evaluation of new grafts. It has become apparent, however, that this particular focus may be far less demanding than heretofore appreciated. The crural vessels present a far greater challenge to the various bypass materials because of their smaller size, lower rate of blood flow, remoteness from the inflow source, length of graft required, and the potentially deleterious effect of knee flexion (except for grafts placed subcutaneously along the lateral or medial aspect of the knee). Clinical investigation of the glutaraldehyde-treated umbilical vein graft was initiated in those patients requiring crural reconstruction but lacking suitable autogenous veins.[27] With increasing experience and confidence in the use of this material in peroneal and tibial reconstructions, its applicability to the popliteal artery became obvious and was reinforced by subsequent clinical results.

Glutaraldehyde-stabilized umbilical veins have been employed in other areas of vascular reconstruction (e.g., axillofemoral, aortorenal, aortocoronary, and carotid-subclavian bypass) and as patch material for post-endarterectomy angioplasty. Although clinically effective, umbilical vein grafts appear to offer no clear advantage in these sites. They have also been used to establish arteriovenous fistulae for dialysis and chemotherapy. Experience in these areas, although promising, has been limited.[8, 25, 56]

Vascular surgeons generally agree that the *ipsilateral autologous saphenous vein* is the graft of choice for lower limb revascularization. If it is unavailable or unsuitable, consideration is given to contralateral saphenous vein and lesser saphenous and upper extremity veins, which may require composite or sequential construction. Because of the effort required to carry out such an "all-autologous policy," there has been movement in some circles toward prosthetics, which are easier to deploy and which decrease operative time. It is essential that vascular surgeons know the outcomes of their operations, which includes risk factors and site and quality of the runoff, so that the appropriate graft material will be selected in a particular setting. In general, biologic tissue outperforms synthetic material in medium-sized and small vessel replacement, but the gap may be narrowed with adjunctive measures.[3, 31, 47, 65, 67]

Operative Technique

With the glutaraldehyde-stabilized human umbilical vein graft, several important technical maneuvers must be observed. Foremost is the gentleness with which the graft must be handled. Intimal fracture and extensive mural dissection of blood can occur if the graft is handled roughly or if standard clamps are applied. Before implantation, alcohol and aldehyde residues are thoroughly rinsed out. The variable thickness of the wall may present some difficulty to the novice, which can easily be overcome with a little practice. The critical aspect of performing an anastomosis with the umbilical vein graft is to pass the needle through the intimal surface. This step can be easily missed in a thicker section of the graft. Some surgeons prefer to reflect the polyester mesh while performing the anastomosis tissue to tissue and then simply tack the mesh down later; others perform the anastomosis by placing the needle through mesh and graft at the same time.

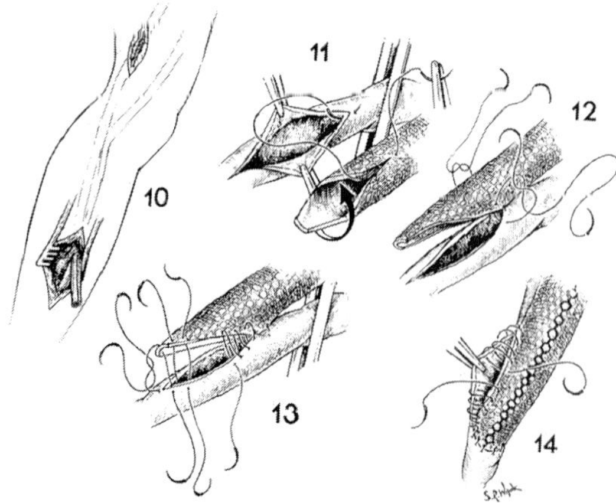

FIGURE 36–5. Interrupted suture technique is generally employed at the heel and toe of all crural anastomoses and many popliteal anastomoses. Continuous parachute techniques are often employed at the femoral level.

These technical matters, as well as the choice of which anastomosis to do first, the type of suture material, and specific anastomotic techniques, are best left to the preference of the experienced surgeon. *Interrupted suture technique* is advocated at the toe and heel of distal anastomosis, particularly at tibial and peroneal sites (Fig. 36–5). During tunneling of the graft, it is essential to pass the graft through a metallic or plastic tube. If the unprotected graft is pulled through tissue planes, damage may occur because of the high friction between the polyester mesh and the host tissues. We prefer to place all grafts to the anterior tibial and peroneal arteries in the lateral subcutaneous position. Similarly, a *medial subcutaneous position* is employed for distal posterior tibial bypasses. The *anatomic position* is employed for all popliteal and proximal posterior tibial bypasses. Systemic heparinization is employed and monitored intraoperatively by the activated clotting time test.

Patients threatened with imminent limb loss and requiring reconstruction to a tibial or peroneal artery and where a prosthetic graft is necessary should be considered for an adjunctive, distal arteriovenous fistula, which produces an increased velocity of blood flow through the graft above the thrombotic threshold level.[44, [illegible]] Although most of the augmented graft flow is diverted into the low-resistance venous circuit, distal arterial flow is maintained, albeit at low pressure and decreased velocity.

Most fistulae are constructed by the common ostium technique. Parallel arteriotomy and venotomy incisions (~25 mm long) are anastomosed to create a posterior suture line. This permits the bypass graft to be anastomosed end to side to a common ostium (Fig 36–6). Several variations of this technique are possible. The success of this operation depends not only on the quality of the venous circuit but also on the skill, patience, and commitment by the vascular surgeon in performing technically demanding procedures. Using a tourniquet in this type of operation helps to simplify the procedure and to decrease the time required for its performance. This method has become routine in our practice.

Most of the lower extremity revascularization procedures that we perform are with epidural anesthesia. Benefits often include the following:

1. The surgical stress response is inhibited.
2. Cardiorespiratory depression may be decreased.
3. Intubation may be avoided.
4. Earlier ambulation and hospital discharge are more likely.

The main disadvantage in patients undergoing vascular procedures is the risk of epidural hematoma. This complication is extremely rare, and in view of the benefits, we consider epidural anesthesia as the method of choice for securing analgesia. In addition, postoperative epidural morphine permits a postoperative pain-free continuum that is unmatched by any other method.

Completion intraoperative arteriography has proved successful, and we believe that it should be routine along with the performance of completion duplex sonography for all lower extremity bypass operations. With these techniques, technical errors or unsuspected pathology is often detected, and, just as important, it is possible to obtain a clear record that provides an accurate short-term prognosis and guide to future direction of care (Fig. 36–7).

During the operation, the patient, of course, receives

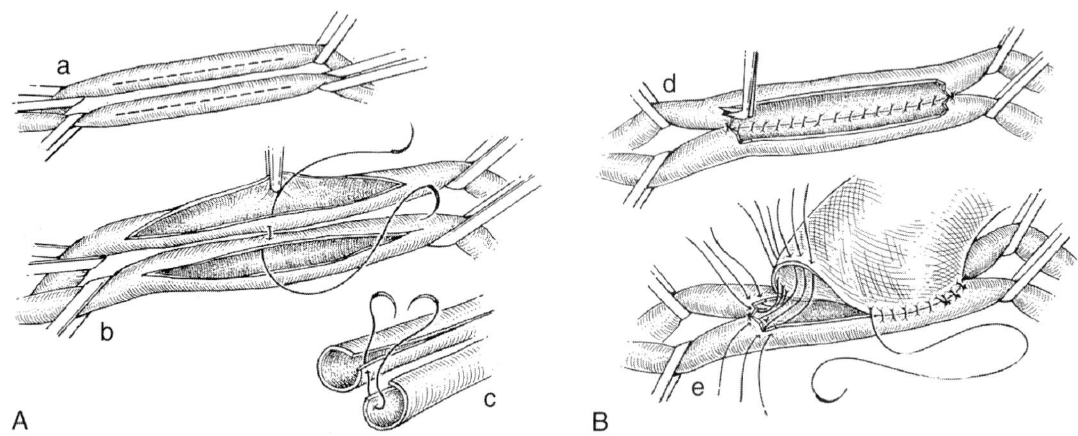

FIGURE 36–6. *A*, Technique of a distal arteriovenous fistula involves parallel arteriotomy and venotomy incisions (a), approximately 20 to 25 mm in length and anastomosing the apposing walls with a continuous 7-0 polypropylene suture (b, c). *B*, The ovoid ostium (d) is converted to a rectangle (e), and the umbilical vein graft is sewn end-to-side with interrupted sutures at the heel and toe, continuous along the lateral margins.

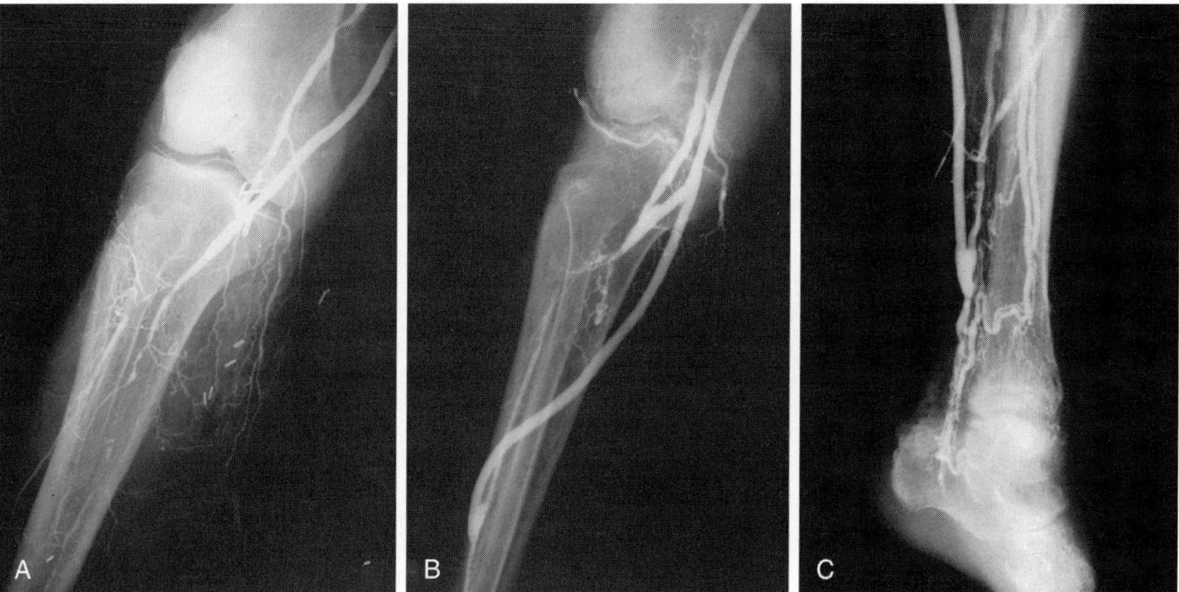

FIGURE 36–7. *A–C,* Completion angiograms depicting a femoropopliteal below bypass into a blind segment (*A*), a femoropopliteal sequential anterior tibial bypass (*B*), and a femoroposterior tibial bypass with an adjunctive distal arteriovenous fistula (*C*).

therapeutic doses of heparin. If the patient does not have significant cardiac or renal disease, we also employ low-molecular-weight dextran during surgery and for an additional 2 days postoperatively we give 500 ml/day for 3 days.[57] Postoperatively, the patients continue to take heparin until they can be switched to sodium warfarin (Coumadin). The dose of warfarin is usually adjusted to maintain the patient within an appropriate therapeutic range, but on occasion we employ an empirical low-dose regimen (2.5 mg/day) for patients who are noncompliant or when the anticoagulation level is difficult to control. Aspirin is generally not used for umbilical vein grafts, although in exceptional circumstances we have combined aspirin, low-dose Coumadin, and subcutaneous heparin.

Patients are generally immobilized for several days with a foam knee immobilizer. This is kept on the patient while the patient is in bed, but it is removed when the patient starts to walk. Length of hospitalization is dependent on the status of the foot; hospitalization is prolonged when the presence of lesions or gangrenous sites necessitates care.

Results

Since the first clinical trials with umbilical vein grafts for lower-limb revascularization were initiated in 1974, doubt and skepticism with regard to their efficacy have coexisted with reports demonstrating superior performance as a prosthetic alternative to autologous vein. Most of these studies comparing the performance of vascular grafts are flawed by (1) short-term to medium-term follow-up, (2) varying indications for operation, and (3) differences in underlying pathology. Few prospective randomized studies exist; of those that do, practically all are flawed by poor case selection, bias, or unfair interpretation of results.[1, 32, 42]

Our total experience with the glutaraldehyde-stabilized umbilical vein graft now exceeds 1200 cases. We documented our first decade of experience (1975 to 1985) to show half-life patencies for popliteal, tibial, and peroneal bypasses of 6.5, 2.3, and 1.7 years, respectively.[30] Some authors have expressed concern regarding the latter two numbers and also with the finding of a 36% incidence of aneurysm and 21% incidence of dilation after 5 years of implantation. Despite these concerns about graft degeneration, only 6% of patients have actually required surgical intervention because of aneurysmal graft dilation within 5 years after implantation.

A follow-up report during the second decade of experience with the umbilical vein graft (1985 to 1995) confirmed improving secondary patency rates at 5 years: 65% and 45% for popliteals and crurals, respectively, during this latter period compared with 57% and 33%, as reported during the first decade of experience.[19] Furthermore, only two graft aneurysms were discovered during the 1985 to 1995 period, suggesting an improvement in cord vein selection and processing.

Our current data confirm the trend toward better primary and secondary patency rates as well as better control of biodegradation. Interestingly, surveillance studies of autologous vein grafts are also showing a 30% rate of morphologic change during the first year after implantation and lesser percentages during subsequent years. When added, the total percentage of duplex demonstrated changes in morphology in autologous vein reconstruction approaches 50%! Admittedly, most of these changes do not require intervention, but this is also true of all biologic grafts, a fact rarely acknowledged by critics of the umbilical vein graft.

For the years 1990 to 1997, the most recent data for primary and secondary cumulative graft patency and limb salvage rates are shown in Figures 36–8 and 36–9. There were no statistically significant differences between any of the primary and secondary patency rates of a particular reconstruction. Secondary patency rates for popliteal and crural reconstruction at 5 years were 67% and 51%, respectively. These figures were 6% and 12% better than their respective primary patency rates. Cumulative limb salvage rates at 5 years were 80% and 68%, respectively, for popli-

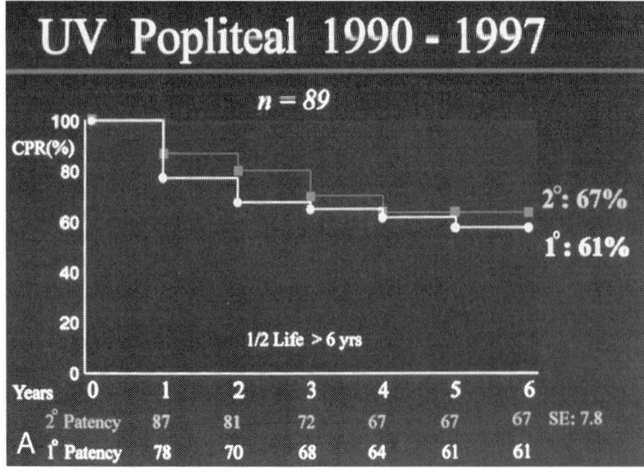

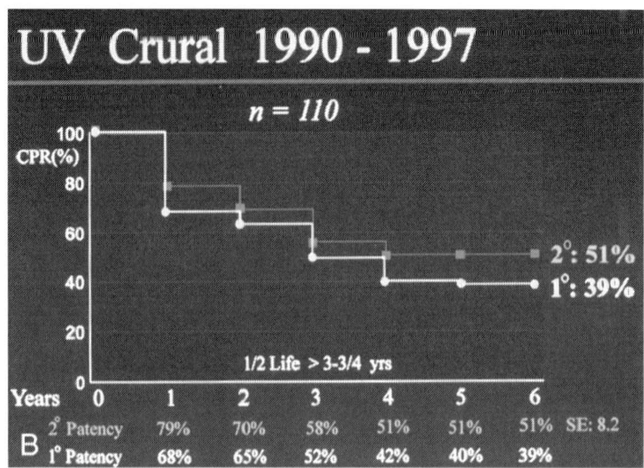

FIGURE 36–8. *A*, Cumulative primary and secondary patency rates for umbilical vein grafts placed distally into the popliteal artery (predominantly below the knee) from 1990 through 1997. *B*, Results for crural bypasses performed during this same period.

teal and crural reconstructions. The marked improvement in the crural data is, we believe, due to the creation of an adjunctive distal arteriovenous fistula.[20, 31]

Factors relating to graft failure include (1) quality of the artery at the site of distal anastomosis and, more important, (2) distal runoff. Calcification, reduced diameter, presence of thrombus, and absence of the pedal arch are additional factors associated with early graft thrombosis, but none is absolute. In fact, durable patency can be achieved in some of these cases, a reflection of multiple factors and especially technical skill. Case selection is therefore critical, but currently available evaluation modalities, both angiographic and noninvasive, can be misleading.

Intraoperative angiography may be helpful, but arterial exploration with direct manual injection of heparinized saline provides the simplest and fastest answer regarding the functional status of the distal circulation. High resistance, as measured by this method, albeit crude and subjective, is associated with predictable early failure. Most of the causes of the high resistance can be confirmed by arteriography. Under these circumstances, one should consider abandoning the bypass procedure particularly if, in the case of a crural bypass, an adjunctive distal arteriovenous fistula cannot be constructed.[31] These are obviously desperate circumstances, and we must consider the general clinical status of the patient before proceeding with reconstructive, rather than ablative, surgery.

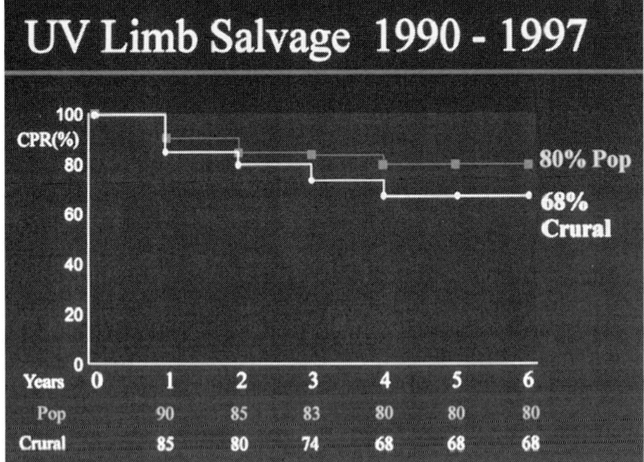

FIGURE 36–9. Cumulative limb salvage rates for umbilical vein (UV) popliteal and crural bypasses performed from 1990 through 1997.

Complications

Thrombosis

Thrombosis is the most common complication associated with any vascular graft. With the umbilical vein, thrombosis can result from faulty technique, unfamiliarity with the graft's unique handling characteristics, or poor case selection. Thrombosis resulting from the graft itself occurs where the flow surface is damaged, thereby permitting blood to dissect intramurally. Defective grafts are possible, of course, but these are almost always detected during the manufacturing process by a number of quality control tests.

If the intraoperative arteriogram shows poor runoff or absence of runoff and if a more distal anastomosis would be impossible to perform, early postoperative thrombosis is accepted as a failure and reoperation is not considered. In all other situations, early and unanticipated thrombosis should be immediately reexplored and its cause should be searched for and corrected. Because a distal arteriovenous fistula is routinely constructed with all of our crural bypasses employing an umbilical vein graft, reexploration for early thrombosis is performed if the venous outflow is good (size and quality), regardless of the state of the arterial runoff.

The most important aspect of successful thrombectomy of an umbilical vein graft is extreme gentleness in its performance.[18] Overinflation of a balloon catheter can easily disrupt the graft. It is preferable to evacuate most of the thrombus by gentle external massage or by direct saline irrigation through proximal and distal arteriotomies prior to passage of a balloon catheter. In fact, we omit the use of the balloon catheter for the graft itself if the other maneuvers are clearly effective. Late graft thrombosis can be similarly managed, but preoperative arteriography should be performed to evaluate proximal and distal disease progression. Thrombolysis is an option and can be an effective alternative to surgery. Lesions responsible for thrombosis may be discovered with clot lysis and treated by endovascular or direct means. Placement of a new graft, even to areas remote from the original bypass, may be preferable, particularly when an intense desmoplastic response has occurred at the anastomoses and an endovascular approach is not feasible or predictably successful.

Late graft thrombosis does not inevitably lead to amputation, particularly when digital or forefoot amputations or ulcerations have already healed. The rate of limb salvage following tibial bypass is similar to that obtained with popliteal reconstructions. Although peroneal reconstruction is associated with the lowest salvage rate, the preservation of more than half of such limbs for 2 to 4 years emphasizes the importance of continuing peroneal artery reconstruction in appropriately selected cases.[27]

Infection

Infection represents one of the most serious complications of any vascular prosthesis. Although the umbilical vein graft is not immune to infection, the glutaraldehyde tanning employed during its manufacture seems to impart some degree of increased resistance. This is unlike the bovine heterograft which, tanned with dialdehyde starch, would often dissolve when infected, resulting in life-threatening hemorrhage. The umbilical vein graft is able to maintain structural integrity under these adverse conditions to permit appropriate preparation and revision.

The incidence of infection for umbilical vein grafts is similar to the incidence with saphenous vein grafts ($<3\%$). Although most infected grafts must be removed to cure the sepsis and prevent bleeding, some grafts may be salvaged by intensive antibiotic therapy combined with wide local drainage, muscle transposition, or flap advancement to cover the graft.

Aneurysms

True aneurysm of the umbilical vein graft is extremely uncommon today. This is in contradistinction to the bovine heterograft. Superior tanning achieved with glutaraldehyde, use of an outer polyester mesh, and preservation of the umbilical vein's intrinsic anatomy by avoiding ficin digestion are all believed to contribute to greater resistance to biodegradation. The development of an aneurysm probably reflects a combination of host metabolic factors and inadequate or reversal of aldehyde cross-links. Aneurysms involving the umbilical vein graft should be resected, if they are symptomatic or larger than 2 to 3 cm, and replaced with an interposition or new bypass graft.

Because almost all *false aneurysms* that occur at anastomotic sites are due to faulty technique, the incidence of this complication has fallen dramatically with increasing experience. Some false aneurysms still occur because of excessive mural thinning following endarterectomy of the recipient vessel. Correction of false aneurysms may require patch angioplasty or interposition grafting. If infection is present, wide drainage, graft excision, and extra-anatomic bypass may all be necessary.

Intimal Hyperplasia

Because the glutaraldehyde-stabilized umbilical vein graft is not viable, it is intrinsically incapable of developing intimal hyperplasia. Hyperplasia may, however, originate in the host vessels near the anastomosis and may extend into the graft lumen. This is believed to be due in part to local turbulence, which in turn, is due to residual disease, compliance mismatch, wide angulation of the anastomosis, and size disparity between the graft and host vessels. Surgical trauma is also a key ingredient. Correction of these factors, when possible, may decrease the incidence of intimal hyperplasia but does not eliminate it; this problem must be resolved at the molecular level.

CRYOPRESERVED SAPHENOUS VEIN GRAFTS

Since the first attempts at revascularization, vein and artery allografts have been considered prime sources of graft material. Although Carrel[17] reported the successful long-term use of arterial allograft in the aorta nearly 90 years ago, clinical application did not begin until after Gross[36] documented the successful use of allografts to treat aortic coarctation in 1948. This led the way for arterial allograft placement in the 1950s by surgeons performing newly introduced lower extremity bypass procedures for limb salvage. These grafts were harvested from cadavers, and they were either fresh or frozen for later use at the same institution. Preservation procedures varied, with storage at 0°C to −50°C in various buffered solutions. It soon became evident that the arterial allograft was subject to significant degeneration, with high rates of calcification, aneurysm formation, rupture, and occlusion.[45, 64] It was recognized that immunologic mechanisms played an important role in the degeneration of these grafts, and within 10 years arterial allografts were largely abandoned in favor of autologous vein and prosthetics.

The reports of Ochsner[49] and Tice[66] in the early 1970s renewed interest in the venous allograft. These optimistic early reports held that veins were less antigenic than arteries and would be less susceptible to the degradation seen with arterial allografts. Although the thick cellular media of the artery underwent degeneration without fibrosis, the media of the vein was thinner and more resistant to ischemia.[49] The media of the venous allograft transforms into a strong fibrous layer with large amounts of collagen deposition, and it is associated with less aneurysmal degeneration than the arterial allograft.

Cryopreservation

Frozen storage of veins without cryopreservation uniformly results in death of the cells. Cryopreservation involves the use of techniques to ensure tissue viability upon thawing. This method was made possible by the discovery of cryoprotectants, such as dimethylsulfoxide (DMSO), which rapidly diffuse through cell membranes and prevent formation of lethal intracellular ice crystals.[10] Cryopreservation techniques include atraumatic harvest of the vessel, low temperature storage during transport, and treatment in 10% to 15% DMSO followed by controlled ultra-low-temperature freezing to −196°C with liquid nitrogen. Variations in the rate of cooling and other aspects of the technique, including

TABLE 36–2. EFFECTS OF CRYOPRESERVATION ON VEIN GRAFTS

AUTHOR	YEAR	FINDING
Barner et al[7]	1966	Medial smooth muscle degeneration and collagen deposition; plasma cell infiltrate in media
Weber et al[69]	1975	80% of endothelium viable
Calhoun et al[13]	1977	Scanning electron microscopy: intimal disruption, exposure of collagen loss of intima by 30 days after implantation, cellular infiltrate in media
L'Italien et al[41]	1979	No change in compliance or elastic modulus
Malone et al[43]	1980	Endothelial fibrinolytic activity decreased
Sachs et al[58]	1982	Endothelial cells not viable in culture
Passani et al[50]	1988	Prostacyclin production maintained when slow freezing employed
Showalter et al[62]	1989	Endothelium disrupted at 3 mo, intact at 9 mo after implantation; prostacyclin production decreased at 3 mo, normal at 9 mo after implantation; compliance decreased by 50%, restored by 3 mo after implantation
Brockbank et al[12]	1990	Smooth muscle tension reduced to 52% of normal; connective tissue synthesis reduced to 44% of normal
Elmore et al[33]	1991, 1992	Platelet deposition increased; normal thromboxane A_2 release; prostacyclin and prostaglandin F_2 production increased; decreased contraction in response to potassium chloride
Miller et al[46]	1993	Poor response to prostacyclin and nitrous oxide
Faggioli et al[34]	1994	No endothelial cell growth in culture; endothelium on scanning electron microscopy abnormal after cryopreservation
Bambang et al [6]	1995	Higher release of thrombomodulin from endothelium

the use of chondroitin sulfate as an added cryopreservative, may affect the results achieved.[10, 11, 50] Some reports,[11] but not all,[7, 35] indicate that the cryopreserved graft can be stored for long periods of time (months, possibly years) without deterioration. The availability of cryopreservation has thus enabled the establishment of tissue banks to collect, process, store, and disseminate allografts.[10] The cryopreserved vein graft has the added benefit of being grossly indistinguishable from fresh autogenous vein, with similar handling and suturing characteristics. Cost remains an issue, as it is significantly more expensive than prosthetic and human umbilical vein graft.

The first clinical use of cryopreservation of vascular grafts was reported by Tice and Zerbino[66] in 1970. Their initial results were favorable and led to the speculation that cryopreservation not only maintained a viable endothelium with low thrombogenicity but also might reduce antigenicity of the endothelium.[9, 66] Weber and colleagues[70] and other authors[12] later confirmed that cryopreserved endothelium did maintain 80% of its viability. Further experimental work during the 1970s[13] and later[34] led to the recognition that although some of the graft function was intact at implantation, significant alterations had occurred during the cryopreservation process (Table 36–2).[34]

Calhoun and coworkers [13] also showed that significant deterioration of cryopreserved autograft veins, which could not be explained by rejection alone, occurred after implantation. These changes included intimal disruption and loss within 30 days of implantation, luminal fibrin deposition, and cellular infiltrates in the media. By the second month after implantation, the intima had been repopulated with endothelium from the host.[54, 63, 71]

The cryopreserved vein graft may be the most susceptible to thrombosis during this interval—prior to the replacement of the endothelium. This concept is supported by evidence that prostacyclin levels fall to a low shortly after implantation (but return to normal after 4 to 6 months[50, 62]) and provides a rationale for the use of antiplatelet agents, which have been effective early after implantation of cryopreserved vein grafts.[46, 53, 54]

Graft Patency and Clinical Experience

The advent of cryopreservation techniques has led to increased availability and renewed interest in both vein and artery allografts. Although early experimental studies documented that cryopreservation does not completely protect allografts from the rejection process,[7, 13] the continued need for an alternative graft when autogenous vein is not available has driven some clinical centers to examine the use of cryopreserved vein grafts.[37, 44, 61, 68] Unfortunately, the results of these studies (see Table 36–2) mirror earlier experiences with allografts, yielding patency rates at 1 year that are generally less than 50%. As a result, most authors recommend only cautious use when saphenous vein is not available (Table 36–3).[14, 40, 44, 68] Similar conclusions have been found in studies assessing the use of cryopreserved veins in coronary artery bypass surgery.[38, 39, 60]

The poor results with these grafts has been attributed to

TABLE 36–3. MAJOR STUDIES OF CRYOPRESERVED SAPHENOUS VEIN LOWER EXTREMITY (INFRAINGUINAL) BYPASS GRAFT PATENCY RESULTS SINCE 1993

AUTHOR	YEAR	NO. OF GRAFTS	ONE-YEAR PATENCY (%)
Harris et al[37]	1993	25	36 (S)
Shah et al[61]	1993	43	66 (P)
Walker et al[68]	1993	39	28 (P), 46 (S)
Martin et al[44]	1994	115	37 (P)
Leseche et al[40]	1997	25	52 (S)
Carpenter and Tomaszewski[15]	1998	40	13 (P)
TOTAL		287	

P = primary; S = secondary.

both rejection and the effects of the cryopreservation process. Loss of endothelium occurs shortly after implantation of the cryopreserved graft[13, 71] and increases graft thrombogenicity.[53, 54] Treatment with antiplatelet agents, such as aspirin, has been somewhat successful.[53, 54, 63] Evidence of rejection has been demonstrated in experimental[13, 34, 52, 71] and clinical[15, 37, 40, 61] reports of cryopreserved vein allografts and has recently been associated specifically with T-lymphocyte infiltration of all layers of the graft wall.[15] Successful use of the allograft may depend on immunosuppression; however, this adjunct has achieved only partial success[14, 15, 52, 59] and is associated with significantly increased morbidity.[52]

SUMMARY

The glutaraldehyde-stabilized umbilical vein graft is a musculocollagenous tube lined by a thromboresistant basement membrane and covered with a polyester mesh. Its use for lower extremity vascular reconstruction has been clinically assessed since 1975. On the basis of some long-term studies of patency and durability, this conduit does have a role in revascularization of the lower limb. Experience, judgment, and meticulous technique are prerequisites for securing long-term graft patency. No graft material can compensate for failure to adhere to these principles. The use of glutaraldehyde-stabilized umbilical vein facilitates these operations by providing a reliable, nonantigenic material that is mechanically equivalent to normal arteries and physically and chemically biocompatible. By studying the umbilical vein graft, we have gained new insights in the use of biologic material as a conduit for lower limb revascularization. An immediate advantage has been the observation of the efficacy of the umbilical vein graft in reversing ischemia and achieving limb salvage. Nonetheless, prospective randomized studies are necessary to access the comparative role of this graft with others currently available.

Cryopreserved veins have been extensively studied, and the general consensus has been largely negative. Despite cryopreservation and immunosuppression, these grafts remain immunologically active, a factor probably responsible for their high failure rate. Continuing concerns about their high cost and unacceptable early failure rate severely limit the clinical indications for their use.

REFERENCES

1. Aalders GJ, Van Vroonhoven JMV, Lobach, JHC, et al: PTFE versus human umbilical vein in clinical trial. J Cardiovasc Surg 29:186, 1988.
2. Anzola J, Palmer TH, Welch S: Long femoral and iliofemoral grafts. Surg Forum 2:223, 1951.
3. Ascer E, Gennaro M, Pollina RM, Ivanov M, et al: Complementary distal arteriovenous fistula and deep vein interposition: A five-year experience with a new technique to improve infrapopliteal prosthetic bypass patency. J Vasc Surg 24:134, 1996.
4. Baier RE, Abbott WM: Comparative biophysical properties of the flow surfaces of contemporary vascular grafts. *In* Dardik H (ed): Graft Materials in Vascular Surgery. Miami, Fla, Symposia Specialists, 1978, p 79.
5. Baier RE, Akers CH, Perlmutter S, et al: Processed human umbilical cord veins for vascular reconstructive surgery. Trans Am Soc Artif Intern Organs 22:514, 1976.
6. Bambang LS, Mazzucotelli JP, Moczar M, et al: Effects of cryopreservation on the proliferation and anticoagulant activity of human saphenous vein endothelial cells. J Thorac Cardiovasc Surg 110:998–1004, 1995.
7. Barner HB, DeWeese J, Schenk EA: Fresh and frozen homologous venous grafts for arterial repair. Angiology 17:389–401, 1966.
8. Baur GM, Porter JM, Gletcher WS: Human umbilical cord vein allograft arteriovenous fistula for chemotherapy access. Am J Surg 138:238, 1979.
9. Boren CH, Roon AJ, Moore WS: Maintenance of viable arterial allografts by cryopreservation. Surgery 83:382–391, 1978.
10. Brockbank KGM: Basic principles of viable tissue preservation. *In* Clark DR (ed): Transplantation Techniques and Use of Cryopreserved Allograft Cardiac Valves and Vascular Tissue. Boston, Adams Publishing Group, Ltd, 1989, pp. 9–23.
11. Brockbank KGM: Effects of cryopreservation upon vein function *in vivo*. Cryobiology 31:71–81, 1994.
12. Brockbank KGM, Donovan TJ, Ruby ST, et al: Functional analysis of cryopreserved veins: Preliminary report. J Vasc Surg 11:94–102, 1990.
13. Calhoun AD, Baur GM, Porter JM, et al: Fresh and cryopreserved venous allografts in genetically characterized dogs. J Surg Res 22:687–697, 1977.
14. Carpenter EW, Lindenauer SM: Immunosuppression in arterial and venous allografts. Arch Surg 106:75, 1973.
15. Carpenter JP, Tomaszewski JE: Human saphenous vein allograft bypass grafts: Immune response. J Vasc Surg 27:492–499, 1998.
16. Carpentier A, Blondeau P, Laurens P: Replacement des valvules mitales et tricuspides pare des heterogrefes. Ann Chir Thorac Cardiovasc 7:33, 1968.
17. Carrel A: Ultimate results of aortic transplantation. J Exp Med 15:389–398, 1912.
18. Dardik H: Technical aspects of umbilical bypass to the tibial vessels. J Vasc Surg 1:916, 1984.
19. Dardik H: The second decade of experience with the umbilical vein graft for lower-limb revascularization. Cardiovasc Surg 3:265, 1995.
20. Dardik H: The threatened limb. Sci Med 4:44, 1997.
21. Dardik H: The use of an adjunctive arteriovenous fistula in distal extremity bypass grafts with outflow obstruction. *In* Kempczinski RF (ed): The Ischemic Leg. Chicago, Year Book Medical Publishers, 1985.
22. Dardik H, Dardik I: Successful arterial substitution with modified human umbilical vein. Ann Surg 183:252, 1976.
23. Dardik H, Dardik I: The fate of human umbilical cord vessels used as interposition arterial grafts in the baboon. Surg Gynecol Obstet 140:567, 1975.
24. Dardik H, Baier RE, Weinberg S, et al: Morphologic and biophysical assessment of long-term human umbilical cord vein implants employed as vascular conduits. Surg Gynecol Obstet 154:17, 1982.
25. Dardik H, Hessler K, Ibrahim IM, et al: Arteriovenous fistulas: Preliminary clinical experience employing glutaraldehyde tanned human umbilical cord vein. Trans Am Soc Artif Intern Organs 4:64, 1981.
26. Dardik H, Ibrahim IM, Dardik I: Modified and unmodified umbilical vein allografts and xenografts employed as arterial substitutes: A morphologic assessment. Surg Forum 26:286, 1976.
27. Dardik H, Ibrahim IM, Dardik I: The role of the peroneal artery for limb salvage. Ann Surg 189:189, 1979.
28. Dardik H, Ibrahim IM, Sprayregen S, et al: Clinical experience with modified human umbilical cord vein for arterial bypass. Surgery 79:618, 1976.
29. Dardik H, Ibrahim IM, Sussman B, et al: Biodegradation and aneurysm formation in umbilical vein grafts: Observation and realistic strategy. Ann Surg 199:61, 1984.
30. Dardik H, Miller N, Dardik A, et al: A decade of experience with the glutaraldehyde-tanned human umbilical cord vein graft for revascularization of the lower limb. J Vasc Surg 7:336, 1988.
31. Dardik H, Silvestri R, Alasio T, et al: Improved method to create the common ostium variant of the distal arteriovenous fistula for enhancing crural prosthetic graft patency. J Vasc Surg 24:240, 1996.
32. Eickhoff JH, Broome A, Ericsson BF, et al: Four years' results of a prospective, randomized clinical trial comparing polytetrafluoroethylene and modified human umbilical vein for below-knee femoropopliteal bypass. J Vasc Surg 6:506, 1987.
33. Elmore JR, Gloviczki P, Brockbank KGM, Miller VM: Cryopreservation affects endothelial and smooth muscle function of canine autogenous saphenous vein grafts. J Vasc Surg 13:584–592, 1991.

34. Faggioli GL, Gargiulo M, Giardino R, et al: Long-term cryopreservation of autologous veins in rabbits. Cardiovasc Surg 2:259–265, 1994.
35. Fujitani R M, Bassiouny HS, Gewertz BL, et al: Cryopreserved saphenous vein allogenic homografts: An alternative conduit in lower extremity arterial reconstruction in infected fields. J Vasc Surg 15:519–526, 1992.
36. Gross RE, Huwitt ES, Bill AH Jr, Pierce EC II: Preliminary observations on the use of human arterial grafts in the treatment of certain cardiovascular defects. N Engl J Med 239:578–579, 1948.
37. Harris RW, Schneider PA, Andros G, et al: Allograft vein bypass: Is it an acceptable alternative for infrapopliteal revascularization? J Vasc Surg 18:553–560, 1993.
38. Iaffaldano RA, Lewis BE, Johnson SA, et al: Patency of cryopreserved saphenous vein grafts as conduits for coronary artery bypass surgery. Chest 108:725–729, 1995.
39. Laub GW, Muraldharan S, Clancy R, et al: Cryopreserved allograft veins as alternative coronary artery bypass conduits: Early phase results. Ann Thorac Surg 54:826–831, 1992.
40. Leseche G, Pena C, Bouttier S, et al: Femorodistal bypass using cryopreserved venous allografts for limb salvage. Ann Vasc Surg 11:230–236, 1997.
41. L'Italien GJ, Maloney RD, Abbott WM: The preservation of the mechanical properties of venous allografts by freezing. J Surg Res 27:239–243, 1979.
42. McCollum C, Kenchington G, Alexander C, et al: PTFE or HUV for femoro-popliteal bypass: A multi-centre trial. Eur J Vasc Surg 5:435, 1990.
43. Malone JM, Moore WS, Kischer CW, et al: Venous cryopreservation: Endothelial fibrinolytic activity and histology. Ann Surg Res 29:209–222, 1978.
44. Martin RS III, Edwards WH, Mulherin JL Jr, et al: Cryopreserved saphenous vein allografts for below-knee lower extremity revascularization. Ann Surg 219:664–672, 1994.
45. Meade JW, Linton RR, Darling RC, Menendez CV: Arterial homografts. Arch Surg 93:392–399, 1966.
46. Miller VM, Bergman RT, Gloviczki P, Brockbank KG: Cryopreserved venous allografts: Effects of immunosuppression and antiplatelet therapy on patency and function. J Vasc Surg 18:216–226, 1993.
47. Miller JH, Foreman RK, Ferguson L, et al: Interposition vein cuff for anastomosis of prosthesis to small artery. Aust N Z J Surg 54:283, 1984.
48. Nabseth DC, Wilson JT, Tan B, et al: Fetal arterial heterografts. Arch Surg 81:929, 1960.
49. Ochsner JL, DeCamp PT, Leonard GL: Experience with fresh venous allografts as an arterial substitute. Ann Surg 173:933–939, 1971.
50. Passani SL, Angelini GD, Breckenridge IM, Newby AC: Endothelial function can be preserved during cryo-storage of human saphenous vein. Eur J Cardiothorac Surg 2:233–236, 1988.
51. Perloff LJ, Christie BA, Ketharanathan V, et al: A new replacement for small vessels. Surgery 89:31, 1981.
52. Posner MP, Makhoul RG, Altman M, et al: Early results of infrageniculate arterial reconstruction using cryopreserved homograft saphenous conduit (CADVEIN) and combination low-dose systemic immunosuppression. J Am Coll Surg 183:208–216, 1996.
53. Ricotta JJ, Collins GJ, Rich NM: Effects of aspirin and dextran on patency of bovine heterografts in the venous system. Ann Surg 189:116–119, 1978.
54. Ricotta JJ, Schaff HV, Gadacz TR: The effects of aspirin and dipyridamole on the patency of allograft veins. J Surg Res 26:262–269, 1979.
55. Rosenberg N, Martinez A, Sawyer PN, et al: Tanned collagen arterial prosthesis of bovine carotid origin in man: Preliminary studies of enzyme-treated heterografts. Ann Surg 164:247, 1966.
56: Rubio PA, Farrell EM: Modified human umbilical vein graft arteriovenous fistulae as a source of angioaccess in maintenance hemodialysis. Cardiovasc Dis Bull Texas Heart Inst 7:51, 1980.
57. Rutherford R, Jones DN, Bergentz SE, et al: The efficacy of Dextran 40 in preventing early postoperative thrombosis following difficult lower extremity bypass. J Vasc Surg 1:765, 1984.
58. Sachs SM, Ricotta J, Scott DE, DeWeese JA: Endothelial integrity after venous cryopreservation. J Surg Res 32:218–227, 1982.
59. Schmitz-Rixen T, Megerman J, Colvin RB, et al: Immunosuppressive treatment of aortic allografts. J Vasc Surg 7:82–92, 1988.
60. Selke FW, Stanford W, Rossi NP: Failure of cryopreserved saphenous vein allografts following coronary artery bypass surgery. J Cardiovasc Surg 32:820–823, 1991.
61. Shah RM, Faggioli GL, Mangione S, et al: Early results with cryopreserved saphenous vein allografts for infrainguinal bypass. J Vasc Surg 18:965–971, 1993.
62. Showalter D, Durham S, Sheppeck R, et al: Cryopreserved venous homografts as vascular conduits in canine carotid arteries. Surgery 106:652–659, 1989.
63. Sitzmann JV, Imbembo AL, Ricotta JJ, et al: Dimethylsulfoxide-treated, cryopreserved venous allografts in the arterial and venous systems. Surgery 95:154–159, 1984.
64. Szilagyi DE, McDonald RT, Smith RF, et al: Biological fate of human arterial homografts. Arch Surg 75:506–529, 1957.
65. Taylor RS, Loh A, McFarland RJ, et al: Improved technique for polytetrafluoroethylene bypass grafting: Long-term results using anastomotic vein patches. Br J Surg 79:348, 1992.
66. Tice DA, Zerbino VR: Clinical experience with preserved human allografts for vascular reconstruction. Surgery 72:260–267, 1972.
67. Tyrrell MR, Wolfe JHN: New prosthetic venous collar anastomotic technique: Combining the best of other procedures. Br J Surg 78:1016, 1991.
68. Walker PJ, Mitchell S, McFadden PM, et al: Early experience with cryopreserved saphenous vein allografts as a conduit for complex limb-salvage procedures. J Vasc Surg 18:561, 1993.
69. Weber TR, Dent TL, Lindenauer SM, et al: Viable vein graft preservation. J Surg Res 18:247, 1975.
70. Weber TR, Lindenauer SM, Dent TL, et al: Long-term patency of vein grafts preserved in liquid nitrogen in dimethylsulfoxide. Ann Surg 184:709–712, 1976.
71. Williams GM, Krajewski CA, Dagher FJ, et al: Host repopulation of endothelium. Transpl Proc 3:869–872, 1971.
72. Yong NK, Eiseman B: The experimental use of heterologous umbilical vein grafts as aortic substitutes. Singapore Med J 3:52, 1962.

CHAPTER 37

Prosthetic Grafts

David C. Brewster, M.D.

Although autogenous arterial and venous grafts represent the nearest approximations of the ideal blood vessel substitute and are acknowledged to provide the best results of vascular reconstruction, it is evident that such autologous grafts may not always be expendable, are often difficult to procure, and may in fact be unavailable due to prior use or a diseased condition of their own. Similarly, autogenous tissue conduits may be inadequate in size or length for use in a particular anatomic position or clinical situation. Examples of such circumstances are the unsuitability of saphenous vein grafts for aortoiliac reconstruction for aneurysmal or occlusive disease and the not uncommon difficulty of obtaining a vein graft of adequate length and caliber for long distal small-vessel bypass procedures. Modified biografts, as described in Chapter 36, are appealing in concept, but their structural stability and functional durability are uncertain.

For these reasons, the need for substitute vascular grafts is a continuing concern in the field of vascular surgery. Indeed, development of a variety of prosthetic grafts has been a vital factor in the extraordinary advances and achievements in vascular reconstructive surgery made since the early 1950s, along with other notable achievements such as the control of blood coagulation, the study of diseased vessels by angiography, and so on.[1, 2]

Although the available synthetic grafts are generally satisfactory for large-vessel reconstruction of the aortoiliac segment of the arterial tree, the limitations and less than optimal results of prosthetic grafts utilized for medium-vessel and small-vessel (less than 6 mm) procedures below the inguinal ligament are well recognized and continue to represent a major challenge. Recurring problems related to prosthetic grafts, principally thrombosis, anastomotic problems such as anastomotic aneurysm and intimal hyperplasia, potential of structural deterioration, healing abnormalities, and susceptibility to infection continue to occur and result in the need for reoperation.

Intensive laboratory and clinical research since the 1950s has led to a wealth of data on the basic biologic mechanisms of blood and tissue reactions to foreign materials in replacement grafts. Yet much remains unknown about such interactions and the consequences of these interactions within the graft itself and the vascular bed downstream. Although it is now appreciated that a successful vascular graft is far more than an inert conduit carrying blood from one area to another, there is continuing controversy about the importance and relevance of specific structural, mechanical, and electrochemical features of the graft and its flow surface that ultimately determine its long-term behavior and clinical effectiveness.

A lack of consensus about the optimal design features of the ideal vessel substitute has led to an often bewildering array of vascular grafts of different materials, as well as frequent modifications of grafts of even the same prosthetic material by means of alterations in the specific composition and production techniques utilized in their manufacture. Such alterations have been proposed to improve the performance and characteristics of the graft, usually in terms of patency, durability, healing and incorporation within host tissues, resistance to infection, reduced blood loss through the graft, and better handling qualities.

Various claims about the benefits of one type of prosthetic graft over another have been made, although it is often difficult to discern science from salesmanship. Past clinical studies have often lacked adequate controls to allow accurate conclusions to be reached, leading to confusing, often conflicting results. Laboratory investigation is frequently hampered by species variability and recognized differences in the behaviors of grafts in humans and in various laboratory animals.[3] Commercial pressures and interests often result in the clinical availability of new prostheses before adequate experience with its anticipated performance and behavior is available. Hence, it is often difficult for the practicing vascular surgeon who is not a chemical engineer, polymer chemist, or laboratory biologic scientist to evaluate the vast amount of data and claims and to make informed choices regarding the proper use of prosthetic grafts.

In this chapter a broad classification of prosthetic grafts is outlined, and some design concepts and principles important to a basic understanding of vascular grafts are discussed briefly. The specific features, physical properties, and known biologic behaviors of various blood vessel substitutes in common usage are examined, with emphasis on the particular advantages and potential limitations unique to each type of graft. The applicability and recommended use of specific prosthetic grafts for various clinical problems are summarized, and, finally, the potential direction of future development is examined.

CLASSIFICATION

A *prosthesis* is defined as an artificial device meant to replace a missing or malfunctioning body part. With vascular prosthetic grafts, the intent is to substitute the graft for a segment of an arterial tree whose function is compromised by injury, occlusive disease, or aneurysmal degenerative changes. The prosthetic graft provides a substitute conduit for blood flow, allowing the diseased segment to be repaired, excised, or bypassed.

TABLE 37–1. CLASSIFICATION OF PROSTHETIC GRAFTS

SYNTHETIC	BIOLOGIC	COMPOSITE
Textile	Allografts	End-to-end straight grafts
Woven Dacron	Arterial homografts	Sequential grafts
Knitted Dacron	Venous allografts	
Velour	Umbilical vein	
Biologically coated	Xenografts	
Nontextile	Bovine carotid	
Teflon (ePTFE)	Canine carotid	
Polyurethane	Fibrocollagenous tubes	
Bioabsorbable	Autogenous	
	Heterogenous	

ePTFE = expanded polytetrafluoroethylene.

As shown in Table 37–1, prosthetic grafts can be classified according to their method of construction and basic component. The blood vessel substitute can be entirely manufactured or synthetic, or it can be derived from various naturally occurring tissues (biologic grafts). Almost all currently available synthetic grafts are constructed from polymers. In textile or fabric grafts, typically varieties of polyester (Dacron) prostheses, the basic polymer is first made into a yarn, which is then used to construct a graft by various methods of knitting or weaving.

Nontextile grafts, for example, polytetrafluoroethylene (PTFE) and polyurethane, are manufactured by techniques of precipitation or extrusion of the polymer from solutions or sheets of the material. In contrast to synthetic grafts, biologic prosthetic grafts (discussed in Chapter 36) are composed of actual tissues, most often blood vessels (arteries and veins) themselves, taken from other humans (allografts or homografts) or other animal species (xenografts or heterografts). Although vascular grafts made from the patient's artery or vein can certainly be considered biologic grafts, they are not discussed in this chapter. Such autogenous (autologous) conduits are discussed in earlier chapters and are not pertinent to this section concerning prosthetic substitutes.

A third broad category of vascular conduits appropriate to a discussion of prosthetic grafts is composite grafts. Such grafts are constructed by combining segments of a prosthetic with autogenous material to form a substitute vessel conduit, which is occasionally done when the available length of an autogenous tissue graft is inadequate for the required reconstruction.

GRAFT DESIGN CONCEPTS AND PRINCIPLES

There is general agreement about the desirable characteristics of a vessel substitute that contribute to its function as an optimal vascular graft (Table 37–2). As initially enumerated by Scales in 1953, a primary prerequisite is for the prosthesis to be biocompatible with the host into which it is implanted.[4] Its material must be free of significant toxic, allergic, and carcinogenic side effects. Because all prosthetic grafts are foreign material to the body, some tissue reaction is expected and, in fact, is probably desirable in terms of generating a healing response leading to incorporation within host tissue. Yet this tissue reactivity and subsequent "healing" response must not be excessive or otherwise detrimental in terms of excessive thickness of perigraft fibrous tissue formation or the inner graft cellular or tissue lining. Similarly, overly reactive responses at graft-host vessel anastomoses are undesirable because they may progressively compromise graft flow and ultimately result in graft closure.

A graft should be physically durable and free from deleterious dimensional instability over time, which would result in significant dilatation, aneurysm formation, rupture, or excessive elongation that could promote tortuosity, kinking, and eventual thrombosis. The graft should be as resistant to infection as possible and be capable of being adequately sterilized without deterioration and conveniently stored in a sterilized condition for prolonged periods. A graft should be readily available in a variety of sizes and lengths as required by different clinical situations.

From a surgeon's perspective, a graft should be easy to implant. This characteristic is principally determined by various properties that, in aggregate, determine the so-called handling characteristics of the conduit. The graft should have adequate flexibility or pliability, that is, the ability to bend without significant kinking, a quality that is especially important in long grafts across joints or grafts that must follow curved or irregular pathways. In addition, the graft should be sufficiently conformable or able to coapt satisfactorily to diseased irregular vessel ends or arteriotomies at anastomotic sites. Similarly, the graft should have good suturability; that is, suture needles should be able to penetrate the graft without undue resistance, and the graft should retain sutures adequately without their pulling through the wall and should not fray when cut to required

TABLE 37–2. CHARACTERISTICS OF IDEAL PROSTHETIC GRAFT

Biocompatible with host
Physically durable
Resistant to infection
Easy to sterilize and store
Available in variety of sizes
Easy to implant
Impervious to blood leakage
Nonthrombogenic
Compliant
Low cost
Ease of manufacturing

lengths or shapes. Handling characteristics of a graft are closely related to and determined by the material used to construct the graft and, in the case of textile grafts, the material's porosity.

When implanted, a vascular graft clearly needs to be relatively impervious to blood leakage through the graft wall to prevent potentially life-threatening hemorrhage and limit perigraft hematoma formation, which may not only hinder the desired healing responses by the host but also foster possible graft infection. Imperviousness is closely related to graft porosity. All grafts may be thought of as a combination of a porous scaffold or framework and a material that closes the interstices of the framework if they are large enough to allow blood to escape.

Macroporous interstices of autografts or biologic prostheses are closed by nature with a cellular parenchyma that is viable in autografts and preserved in a nonviable state by aldehyde processing or a similar method in various biologic prosthetic grafts.[5] In microporous grafts, the interstices are so small owing to the manufacturing method or nature of the graft material that the cohesive forces of the blood (viscosity and surface tension) are stronger than intraluminal pressure, thereby preventing or limiting significant perigraft bleeding.

Examples of such microporous grafts are those composed of expanded PTFE (ePTFE) or tightly woven Dacron, in which no preclotting is necessary. In contrast, macroporous synthetic grafts, typically knitted Dacron or more loosely woven Dacron, have porosities that require preclotting by the surgeon before implantation. Graft interstices can be closed by a fibrin matrix deposited during the preclotting process or by application of various "coatings" such as collagen, albumin, or gelatin during the graft manufacturing process itself.

Since the early phases of textile synthetic graft development, porosity has been considered an important characteristic of a successful vascular substitute. The concepts of porosity and "healability" of vascular grafts are closely intertwined. The cellular response by which the host attempts to incorporate (heal) a foreign body (the graft) has two components: (1) pannus ingrowth of smooth muscle cells and endothelial cells from the ends of the artery itself and (2) vascularized fibrous tissue invading the wall of the prosthesis. Pannus ingrowth is closely limited to the area of anastomotic union, but fibrous encapsulation of the graft occurs along the entire outer surface of the conduit from perigraft areolar tissue.

Awareness of the potential value of porous grafts followed observation of the high failure rate of impermeable synthetic conduits. It was thought that porous grafts would allow autogenous tissue ingrowth through such pores that would initiate and provide adherence for a stable intimal lining. This hypothesis was strengthened experimentally by Edwards in 1957, who showed a higher rate of thrombosis in dogs with tightly woven polytetrafluoroethylene (Teflon) grafts than with knitted or more porous woven Teflon prostheses.[6] This correlated with clinical observations of higher failure rates of low-porosity, tightly woven aortic Teflon grafts owing to separation and dissection of their poorly adherent pseudointimal lining.[7, 8]

The concept that larger pore size correlates well with improved patency and long-term function was emphasized by Weslowski and colleagues.[9] Rapid and unencumbered ingrowth of areolar tissue from perigraft sources through the interstices of porous grafts during the process of incorporation and encapsulation of the graft by the host was thought to be a vital component in achieving a "healed" graft with an organized cellular, hypothrombogenic flow surface.[10, 11] The stability of such an inner lining was enhanced by nourishment of its cells not only by diffusion from luminal blood but also by its own vasa vasorum, and its attachment improved by actual connection to the invading fibrous tissue.

The greater the porosity or the thinner the graft wall, the better such a process could be achieved, and the more favorable the handling characteristics of the graft. Extension of this "gossamer" concept led eventually to creation of a highly porous, very-thin-walled Dacron graft. Such ultralightweight grafts, however, proved to have other negative features such as structural deterioration (discussed later).

Acceptable limits of porosity are dictated by the increased time requirements and the difficulty required to preclot a high porosity graft adequately and by the occasional but potentially disastrous loss of an initially adequate preclot leading to transgraft hemorrhage, perhaps related to a fibrinolytic reaction. Although woven Dacron grafts are easier to preclot and some very-low-porosity woven grafts require no effort in this regard, their handling characteristics are recognized to be less desirable, and their healing potential is thought to be reduced as compared with higher-porosity knitted grafts. Therefore, as with most prosthetic grafts, the mechanical properties of the end-product often represent a compromise between engineering and design concepts and functional requirements. In the case of currently used textile grafts, ease of preclotting is balanced against handling qualities and healing potential, with different varieties of textile grafts favoring one consideration over another by virtue of different components and fabrication techniques. This diversity, of course, provides the surgeon with various options of graft selection in different clinical circumstances.

Increasing laboratory and clinical experience with newer grafts, however, has led to reexamination of the importance of graft porosity. With ePTFE grafts it has been shown that, in fact, smaller pore sizes correlate with better patency.[12, 13] Sustained patency and generally adequate healing of other varieties of grafts have therefore challenged the traditional idea that porosity of the graft is an indispensable quality for satisfactory function. Although mechanical porosity may be desirable for fabric grafts, this type of porosity is not necessary to the same extent for ePTFE grafts, autogenous tissue grafts, and other forms of biologically derived grafts. Hence, obligatory porosity for all types of grafts does not seem to be an absolute graft design concept. The conclusion is inevitable that the degree of thrombogenicity of the inner graft surface is a more important functional determinant.[14]

The concept of graft thrombogenicity is obviously of pivotal importance in the design of a clinically useful and successful prosthetic graft, but it is incompletely understood and difficult to measure or quantify. The key to understanding graft thrombogenicity is appreciation of the extremely complex and dynamic biologic events occurring at the blood-graft interface. A requirement of a successful graft is that its inner flow surface not provoke a significant thrombotic reaction to blood flowing over it. Many characteristics of the material used to construct the prosthesis, including its chemical composition, electrical charge, surface texture, elasticity, and porosity, cause many complex responses at the interfaces with blood, adjacent artery, and surrounding tissue.[15, 16]

On exposure to blood flow after implantation, the luminal surface of a vascular prosthesis is immediately coated with a layer of serum proteins, principally fibrinogen. The characteristics of the particular graft surface, both chemical and physical, affect protein absorption. Differences in fibrinogen absorption are related to the characteristics of a graft surface; surfaces that are irregular and have many electrochemically active sites tend to absorb proteins more rapidly than do relatively smooth and inert surfaces.[16] Within minutes, platelets adhere to the flow surface, usually to a degree directly proportional to the concentration of adherent fibrinogen.[15]

With platelet adhesion, contact "activation" rapidly occurs with release of various bioactive substances such as adenosine diphosphate and thromboxane A_2. These in turn cause aggregation and activation of other platelets, deposition of leukocytes, and activation of the intrinsic coagulation system with deposition of fibrin and red blood cells. When this process is controlled or limited, the graft surface remains patent and becomes lined with a relatively thin layer of proteinaceous material and compacted fibrin, traditionally referred to as *neointima* or *pseudointima*. When the process is not controlled, graft thrombosis occurs as the graft lumen is obliterated by continued deposition of cellular elements and fibrin.

If a graft flow surface has little platelet contact-activating capacity, it is said to be *passive*. If it has the additional ability, like that of endothelium-lined native vessels, to deactivate platelets, neutralize thrombin, and lyse fibrin, it is said to possess *antithrombotic capacities*.[5] The confluent, living, and functioning endothelial surface of a vascular autograft, when properly and atraumatically procured, has enormous advantages over the flow surface of any synthetic prosthesis because of its powerful antithrombotic capabilities. These antithrombotic characteristics of endothelial cells result from the generation of prostacyclin, plasminogen activators, antithrombin III, and other antithrombotic compounds. To emphasize the differences between autografts with a living endothelial surface and any current graft, it is useful to recall that the endothelial surface maintains the patency of human capillaries at a caliber of 4 μm (smaller than the caliber of red blood cells that must elongate to traverse them). In contrast, no truly satisfactory prosthetic graft below a caliber of 6 mm (6000 μm) currently exists.[5]

Although the luminal surfaces of prosthetic grafts in various laboratory animal species do ultimately become covered with a confluent layer of viable endothelial cells, this process unfortunately has not been demonstrated to occur in the human with any available prosthetic graft.[17] In humans, endothelialization is seen only within 1 to 2 cm of the ends of the graft from transanastomotic pannus ingrowth or occasionally in focal patches within the body of a graft.[18] This observation of "incomplete healing" in humans has keyed interest in endothelial cell seeding of grafts (discussed later).

The likelihood of thrombosis of a vascular graft is related not only to the inherent thrombogenicity of the material from which it is constructed but also to the velocity and nature of blood flow (e.g., turbulent versus laminar) over its surface. Differences in the propensities for thrombus formation also undoubtedly vary among individual patients, but our ability to determine high-risk and low-risk patient profiles preoperatively by a battery of tests is currently ill defined and quite limited.[19] Regardless of the thrombotic potential of the graft or patient, the faster blood flows through a graft, the less opportunity there is for thick fibrin deposition and platelet adherence and aggregation to occur on the flow surface. Sauvage and associates termed this the *thrombotic threshold velocity*.[20] The lower the thrombogenicity of a surface, the lower the flow a graft can tolerate.

This is a crucial factor in the long-term superior patency of autogenous vein grafts for long lower extremity revascularization extending below the knee, where hemodynamic conditions are often unfavorable. At low flow rates, or as sheer stresses and exposure times increase, thrombotic consequences limit the applicability of many materials. The size of the conduit is a related factor because deposition of a relatively thick graft lining (Fig. 37–1) will logically have a greater adverse impact on a small-caliber substitute than on a large-sized graft utilized for aortoiliac reconstruction.

The interplay of thrombogenicity, graft size, and flow rates is dramatically illustrated by the marked difference in results with the same prosthetic material when utilized in different anatomic positions. For instance, Sauvage and colleagues, using similar Dacron grafts, reported after 5 years a 99% patency in the aortoiliac position, about 50% patency in the femoropopliteal position, and only 15% to 20% patency in a location distal to the calf.[21] Long-term function of low-porosity, tightly woven, crimped Dacron prostheses is generally good in a position such as the thoracic aorta. In this high-flow location, the importance of transmural healing and thrombogenicity of the flow surface is minimal. Similarly, the relationship and importance of graft caliber and flow velocity are important in understanding the potential adverse effects of late graft dilation and the generally inferior results with initial implantation of too large a prosthesis in comparison to native vessels.[22]

The mechanical properties of vascular grafts have also received considerable attention. Logically, it would seem

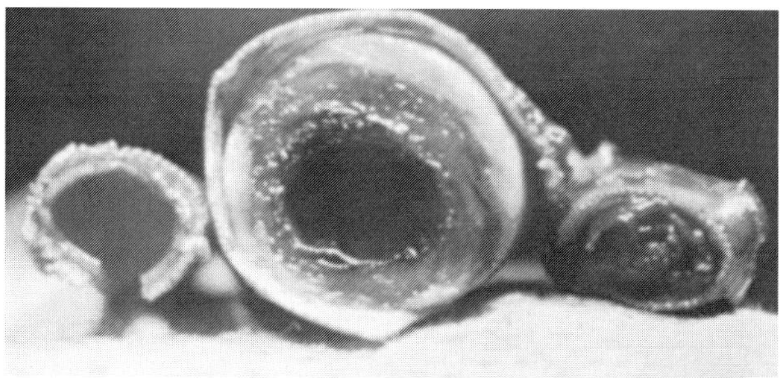

FIGURE 37–1. Deposition of chronic thick pseudointima in a polyester (Dacron) graft in response to reduced flow and small capacity of the diseased outflow tract.

to be appropriate to attempt to match the biophysical characteristics of the graft and the artery that the graft is meant to replace. There is considerable controversy about the issue of compliance and its importance. Compliance may be defined as the percentage of radial change per unit of pressure. It is a convenient index of vessel wall distensibility as a reflection of a pressure pulse.[23] The viscoelastic nature of arteries is derived principally from their structural proteins collagen and elastin, with other components such as smooth muscle, endothelium, and ground substance contributing to a lesser extent.

The disadvantage of noncompliant materials that lack such viscoelastic components is loss of elastic recoil that normally occurs during diastole and thereby provides energy to maintain prograde flow during the diastolic portion of the cardiac cycle. The consequence of a compliance mismatch at artery-graft interfaces is thought to be regional hemodynamic disturbances, which result in turbulent blood flow and shear forces that are imparted to adjacent flow surfaces. Such flow disruption has been implicated in the pathophysiologic mechanisms of perianastomotic intimal hyperplasia, anastomotic aneurysms, and acceleration of downstream atherosclerotic changes.[24–26] These factors, and hence compliance, may therefore play a significant part in graft thrombosis and may explain, in part, the inferior performance of prosthetic grafts for medium-vessel and small-vessel replacements.

All currently available prosthetic grafts are less compliant than host arteries, with arterial or venous autografts most nearly approaching normal values, modified biologically derived grafts such as human umbilical vein and bovine heterografts in the intermediate range, and Dacron and ePTFE grafts relatively noncompliant. Abbott and coworkers have demonstrated a close relationship between compliance and patency of grafts in both the laboratory and in the human.[23, 27, 28]

It is difficult to separate the biophysical effects of compliance from other factors related to graft thrombogenicity, and experimental models are therefore sometimes imperfect. Certainly events occurring at the anastomotic interface are complex, and to establish a cause and effect relationship with a single variable such as compliance may not be possible. For instance, it is recognized that the pathogenesis of intimal hyperplasia is very complex indeed, with a host of biomechanical, hemodynamic, and biochemical mediators contributing to the cellular proliferation characteristic of this lesion. In addition, diseased arteries are not necessarily compliant, and although a graft may have desirable compliance upon implantation, the inevitable stiffening that occurs with the healing process likely alters its compliance. Nonetheless, it seems reasonable to conclude that approximating the compliance of native arteries is, in general, a valuable graft design concept.

A final mechanical factor suggested to be potentially important in graft design is external support. By the use of relatively stiff rings or coils placed around the outside of the graft, it is hoped to eliminate or minimize potential adverse events such as kinking or mechanical compression that might compromise graft flow and function. Such external supports may be constructed of the same material as the graft or from other biocompatible substances. Evidence of the potential benefit of this concept is discussed later.

TEXTILE SYNTHETIC GRAFTS

Development of prosthetic grafts was spawned in 1952 with the seminal observation by Voorhees and colleagues that a silk thread lying loose within the right ventricle of a dog being used for investigation of homograft valve leaflets had become covered over its entire length with a smooth, glistening, endothelial-like coating, free of macroscopic thrombi, within a period of several months.[29] This observation led the investigators to reason that fine-mesh synthetic fabrics might therefore be used to bridge arterial defects, with fibrin plugs in the fabric interstices preventing initial hemorrhage and the material ultimately becoming covered with a similar tissue coating.

Tubes 1 to 6 cm in length, constructed from Vinyon-N cloth, were placed in the abdominal aorta of dogs. At sacrifice within several months, it was noted that the luminal surfaces of these grafts were indeed covered by a thin, shiny layer that on histologic examination was seen to be composed of collagen fibers and flattened fibroblasts, without significant foreign body reaction or giant cell formation. Fibroblasts growing into and through the interstices of the graft wall were evident. The architecture of the graft lining was strikingly similar to that of the normal aorta except for the absence of elastic and smooth muscle elements.[29] Within 2 years, in 1954, they reported implantation of such synthetic grafts in 18 patients to treat 17 abdominal aneurysms and one popliteal aneurysm, and the development of prosthetic grafts was launched.[30]

A variety of synthetic materials were investigated as possible fabric grafts, including Vinyon-N, nylon, Teflon, Ivalon, Orlon, and Dacron.[31–35] Many of these basic materials lost significant tensile strength following implantation or exhibited other problems for manufacturing or sterilization. The tensile strengths of Dacron (polyethylene terephthalate) and Teflon (PTFE), however, remain essentially unchanged long after implantation.[36] Hence, these polymers became predominant in clinical and commercial application and development of textile prostheses. Although Teflon is slightly less reactive than Dacron, this property may in fact be less desirable because it reduces tissue incorporation.[37] The important contributions of DeBakey and others eventually led to the emergence of Dacron as the standard material for virtually all textile synthetic grafts in current usage.[38] Teflon is no longer used as a fabric, but rather in its nontextile extruded form, ePTFE.

Fabrication

Dacron yarn may be made into a prosthetic graft by weaving, knitting, or braiding methods. The yarn is a multifilament yarn that contains many small, continuous filaments and is generally texturized with spiral and coil-spring shapes to impart greater elasticity and softness and better handling qualities than can be achieved by nontexturized or monofilament yarns.

In woven grafts, fabric threads are interlaced in a simple over-and-under pattern (Fig. 37–2) in both lengthwise (warp) and circumferential (weft) directions. Many variations are possible; for example, the weft yarn can go over two or three warp yarns and then under only one warp

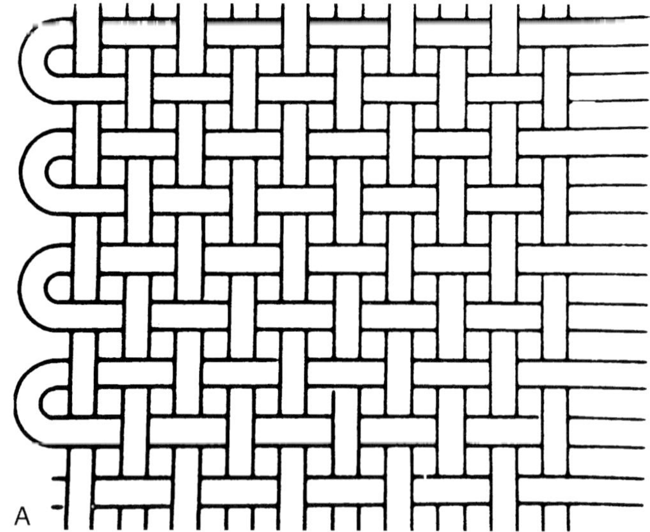

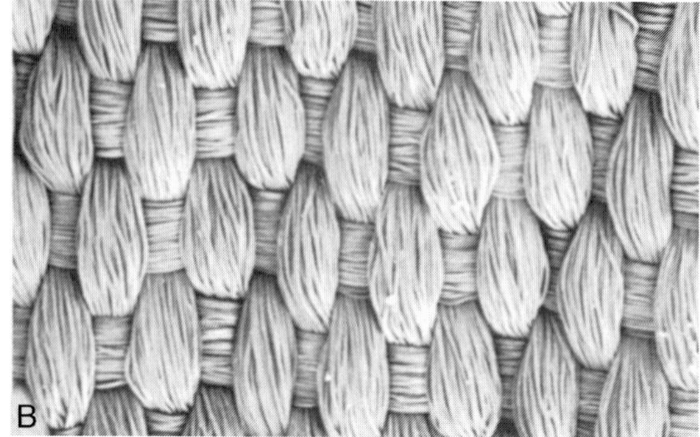

FIGURE 37–2. Woven Dacron graft. *A*, Schematic drawing of a typical over-and-under interlacing weave pattern of woven vascular grafts. *B*, Scanning electron micrograph of the surface of a woven Dacron graft. (Original magnification, ×50.)

fiber before the pattern is repeated. Such variations in the weave pattern, however, have not been shown to yield any significant advantage or difference compared with the common simple structure.[39] Woven fabric grafts, in general, have little to no stretch in any direction. Because loosely woven cloth tends to fray when cut, and the yarn tends to slide and gather, woven grafts are generally tightly constructed because the permissible looseness of the weave is limited. Therefore, woven grafts are typically of low porosity, very strong, and relatively stiff.

The advantages of such grafts are reduced bleeding through the smaller interstices and less likelihood of dilatation or structural deformation over time. These features are a trade-off for the disadvantages of less desirable handling features, reduced compliance, and a tendency to fray at cut edges. It is often recommended that woven vascular grafts be cut with a cautery to prevent unraveling of the cut edge. Because of their reduced porosity, woven grafts have a potential for reduced tissue incorporation, transmural tissue ingrowth, and less cellular organization and secure attachment of the inner flow surface.

In a knit structure, the yarns can be oriented in either a predominantly longitudinal (warp knitting) or circumferential (weft knitting) direction. Warp-knitted grafts have more dimensional stability, and most knit grafts are manufactured in the longitudinal direction. Knit fabrics are constructed by yarns looped around a needle to form a continuous interlocking chain of loops (Fig. 37–3). The spacing of the yarns and therefore the pore dimensions are related to the size of the needles used and the radius of the curvature taken by the yarn as it bends around the needles.[39] Thus knitted grafts have a greater range of possible porosities than woven grafts and possess, in general, a higher porosity than woven grafts. The ability of the loops to rotate with respect to one another also produces more stretch in all directions.

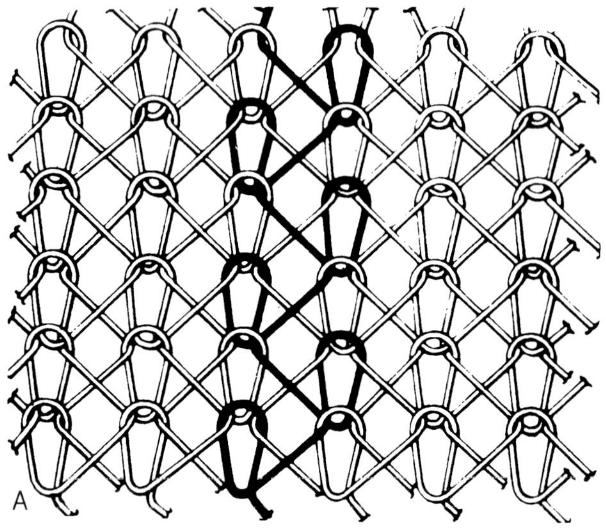

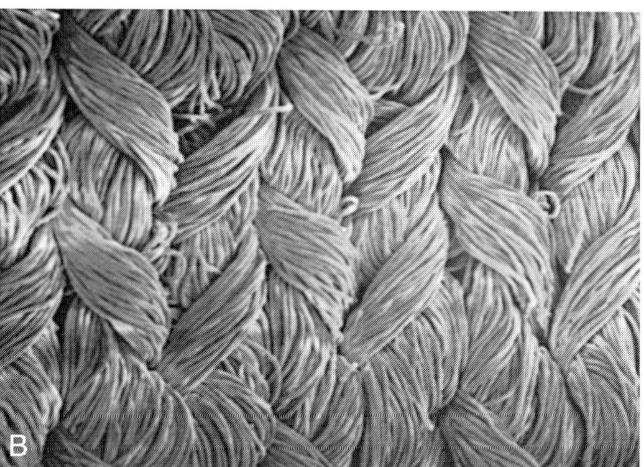

FIGURE 37–3. Knitted polyester (Dacron) graft. *A*, Schematic drawing of a yarn configuration for warp knitting with interlocking loops. *B*, Scanning electron micrograph of the surface of a graft knitted from texturized Dacron yarn. (Original magnification, ×50.)

These features create the recognized advantages and disadvantages of knitted Dacron grafts. Better theoretical healing characteristics owing to greater porosity, greater mechanical compliance, and acknowledged superior handling features such as suturability, flexibility, conformability, and a lesser tendency to fray are balanced against the time requirement and potential difficulty of the need to preclot the graft to make it impervious to blood loss through the graft wall upon implantation. In addition, knitted grafts are less strong than woven textile grafts and hence are subject to more frequent structural changes following implantation. Braided fabrics are no longer used because they require heavier yarn, fray easily, and are bulky and relatively nonporous.[40]

A frequently employed modification of textile synthetic grafts is the addition of a velour finish to the inner or outer graft surface or to both graft surfaces. Velour fabrics are constructed with loops of yarn extending upward at right angles to the fabric's surface, giving it a plush, velvety texture (Fig. 37–4). As first described by Hall and colleagues[41] and Lindenauer and coworkers[42] and later emphasized by Sauvage and associates,[43] velour can be formed on a woven or knitted structure. The porosity and thickness of the pile surface can be varied with the choice of yarn, the number of loops, whether the loops are uncut or cut, and so on. It is also possible to fabricate a velour-like surface with vigorous brushing of a standard knit or woven textile, resulting in broken or cut filaments rather than loops on the surface.[39]

Velour fabrication improves the elasticity and handling features of knitted and woven grafts, but its primary purpose is to provide a superior environment of lattices, or a so-called trellis, to which fibrin can adhere and fibroblasts can attach to and "crawl on."[44] This process is intended to facilitate initial preclotting, thereby enabling more porous grafts to be used, and subsequently to promote healing of the prosthesis by the host as well.[5] Grafts with external velour surfaces are thought to produce a graft that is better incorporated by adjacent host fibrous tissue and to achieve better tissue ingrowth into the graft wall (Fig. 37–5). Internal velour surfaces are thought to yield better cellular organization and a firmer anchorage for the fibrinothrombus material that initially lines a synthetic graft.

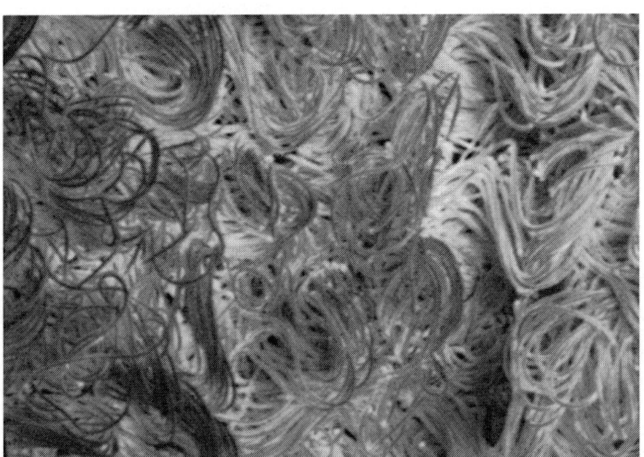

FIGURE 37–4. Scanning electron micrograph of the outer surface of a velour, knitted Dacron graft. Note the thick, rough, plush surface achieved by loops of yarn extending perpendicular to fabric's surface. (Original magnification, ×50.)

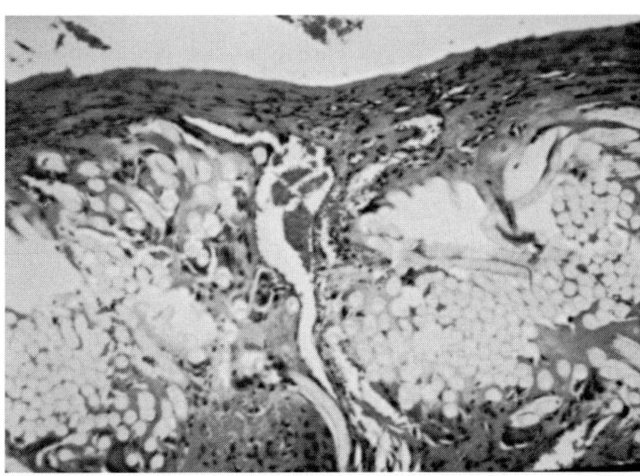

FIGURE 37–5. Light micrograph of a velour Dacron prosthesis 13 months after implantation in a human. Tissue ingrowth through graft interstices is seen, with the luminal surface *(top)* covered by a relatively thin, well-organized layer of fibrin and collagen, synthesized by fibroblasts present within the tissue. Capillaries, such as the one in the center of this photomicrograph, are clearly evident and contribute to the organization and maintenance of the pseudointimal tissue. (H&E, original magnification, ×40.)

No internal, external, or "double" velour grafts have been conclusively shown to result in differences in thrombogenicity or long-term performance, however, compared with standard Dacron grafts.[45] The uncertainty of the benefit of velour surfaces is illustrated by the fact that even advocates of external velour grafts such as Sauvage and associates believe that internal velour surfaces are undesirable owing to their tendency to promote formation of a thicker inner lining with its potentially increased thrombogenicity.[5, 44, 46]

All standard and velour knitted Dacron grafts require preclotting before insertion to seal the interstices of the porous fabric and to decrease implantation bleeding. Higher-porosity grafts are more difficult to preclot than many woven low-porosity grafts, which require little or no preclotting in normal circumstances. Although it has been suggested that, from a healing perspective, grafts with a porosity of 10,000 ml/cm^2/min would be ideal,[9, 37] this level of porosity is unrealistic because of the inordinate difficulties of satisfactorily preclotting such a graft. Grafts with a porosity of approximately 4000 ml/cm^2/min can be used, but most knitted grafts commonly employed in clinical practice have porosities in the range of 1200 to 1900 ml/cm^2/min. In addition to rendering the graft impervious to bleeding, proper preclotting, as emphasized by Sauvage, renders the flow surface of a raw Dacron graft less thrombogenic by depositing a compacted hypothrombogenic fibrin layer.[5]

Surgeons use a variety of methods of preclotting. For relatively low-porosity grafts, the surgeon can simply wet the external surface of the graft or place it in a basin with 50 to 60 ml of blood obtained from a convenient vessel before administering heparin. For more porous grafts, many surgeons prefer to flush the graft repeatedly with the nonheparinized withdrawn blood, forcing it through the graft interstices until they tighten up with fibrin. Any excess clotted blood should be carefully suctioned out, but further flushing with saline tends to negate the effects of preclotting and is not recommended.

The surgeon may find preclotting with heparinized blood to be difficult and tedious. The addition of a small amount of thrombin to the withdrawn blood can help considerably. Yates and colleagues have recommended a more complex three-stage process, emphasizing the need for a terminal flushing with heparinized blood to neutralize thrombin on the flow surface.[47] The benefits of this technique are uncertain, however, and it is more complex and time-consuming than other widely utilized preclotting methods.

Crimping of fabric grafts is done to impart flexibility, elasticity, and shape retention (kink resistence) with bending. Almost all current textile grafts employ this feature. It is recognized, however, that much of the initial elasticity is lost with the stretching that occurs during implantation as well as the inevitable stiffening that occurs with later tissue incorporation.

Crimping has a number of potential disadvantages. It increases the thickness of the graft wall and reduces the effective internal diameter of the prosthesis. Furthermore, the unevenness of the inner graft surface interferes with smooth laminar flow and leads to increased fibrin deposition in convexities of the graft and a potential increase in surface thrombogenicity.[40] Although such considerations may not cause problems in large-caliber grafts, significant adverse consequences can result in small-diameter arterial replacements. This has prompted some investigators to abandon crimping and use noncrimped grafts to which external support has been added to avoid kinking with bending and to foster dimensional stability.[48] Such external support is usually achieved by added rings or coils of prosthetic material to the external surface of the conduit. Perhaps the smooth noncrimped surface of ePTFE grafts, supported or not, is advantageous in this respect as well.

There has been a tremendous shift toward the use of biologically coated Dacron grafts. The manufacturer can render porous textile grafts impervious by coating or impregnating them during the manufacturing process with various absorbable biodegradable materials, such as xenogenic bovine dermal collagen, allogeneic albumin, and gel. This process has the appealing feature of providing grafts with zero or low implantation porosity without the time needed for preclotting while retaining the subsequent potential healing advantages of relatively high-porosity fabrics.[49] Although the process may stiffen the graft slightly, the favorable handling characteristics of the basic material, generally knitted Dacron, are largely retained and are superior to low-porosity woven grafts. The protein matrix is gradually resorbed within several months, permitting normal or even enhanced healing responses.[50–52]

Some evidence suggests that early thrombogenicity and possibly infectibility of the graft surface may be lessened by such graft coatings.[49, 53–55] Although concern about possible immune reponses or allergic reactions to the coating substances exists, low antigenicity and no evidence of clinically adverse effects have been noted.[52, 56, 57] Although implantation of a Dacron aortic prosthesis has been found to activate the complement system significantly, collagen-impregnated grafts have not been found to provoke any greater complement activation than their nonsealed conventional Dacron counterparts.[58]

The surgeon can apply albumin or fibrin glue in the operating room to render porous grafts impervious,[59] but most interest currently centers on commercially produced collagen-coated or albumin-coated grafts with "off-the-shelf" availability. Early clinical experience with collagen-impregnated grafts (Hemashield-Meadox Medicals, Oakland, NJ) for thoracic and abdominal aortic reconstructions has been favorable, with no apparent graft-related problems reported.[60–62] Good experimental and clinical results have been reported with albumin-coated prostheses (Bard Cardiovascular, Billerica, Mass.).[51, 63–66] Gelatin has been similarly used as a sealant in Dacron grafts, such as Gelsoft prostheses (Sulzer Vascutek USA, Inc., Austin, Texas), with favorable results.[67–70]

The principal advantages of this design concept are expediency (in terms of eliminating the need for preclotting) and reducing the operative blood loss related to transgraft bleeding. Most clinical experience has been obtained with large vessel reconstructions; whether the possible laboratory evidence of lower flow surface thrombogenicity in the early post-implant period is in fact real or will translate into improved long-term patency in medium-vessel or small-vessel reconstructions cannot be determined without further experience and data.

These grafts appear to be safe, although one must realize that resorption of the protein matrix will eventually unmask the underlying basic fabrication of the graft. If this is prone to dilatation or adverse performance in any other fashion, the initial implantation advantages of biologically coated grafts will obviously be dissipated. In addition, all such grafts are more expensive (approximately double the price) than standard textile grafts. With the current pressures for cost control and economic constraints in medicine, one wonders if the expediency of such grafts justifies their greater expense, especially in large vessel reconstructions, where conventional textile synthetic grafts have provided generally satisfactory long-term results.

The most common inherent complication of fabric Dacron prostheses is the propensity for some varieties of such grafts to dilate over time. Dilatation may be diffuse and may involve the entire graft, or it may be confined to more limited portions of the graft, resulting in enlargement of the graft body, limb, or areas of focal aneurysmal change.[71–78] Generalized dilation is by far the most prevalent manifestation.

The incidence of structural deterioration in Dacron grafts was formerly thought to be low (1% to 3%). The data are undoubtedly inaccurate, however, because much of the data predate the availability of comprehensive imaging of grafts during late follow-up and they often were gathered only from symptomatic patients who were studied.[79] The changes in dilatation have been increasingly observed and reported. Dilatation has been noted to occur immediately, with implantation and restoration of arterial pressure to the graft, and may possibly be progressive at later follow-up intervals.

A variety of knitted Dacron grafts have been shown to measure 10% to 20% more than the manufacturers' alleged box size at the time of declamping in the operating room.[80, 81] Progressive dilatation may continue, although the rate of change decreases with the passage of time.[82, 83] Late studies by ultrasound or CT scan follow-up 1 to 20 years after implantation have shown mean increases of 23% to 94% compared with initial implant size.[81, 84]

The likelihood of such altered dimensional stability has been closely related to the method of fabrication. Woven grafts with interlacing yarns have a high initial modulus and strength and therefore exhibit little to no dilatation. Because of their looped structure, knitted fabrics have much less resistance to extension because their interlocking loops straighten in the line of highest stress. Weft-knitted grafts are less dimensionally stable than warp-knitted constructions.[84, 85] Very thin, highly porous, ultra-lightweight knitted grafts have been noted to manifest the greatest structural problems.[86]

In addition to simple structural slippage of the knit pattern, other factors have occasionally been implicated to cause dilatation.[79, 87] These include mechanical fatiguing or actual fracture of yarn fibers; damage to the material by the manufacturing process (heating, crimping, and so on); improper or excessively frequent sterilization procedures; and traumatic handling, clamp applications to the graft, use of cutting-tipped needles, and so on. Although generally considered biologically stable, some evidence suggests that biodegradation of Dacron fibers can occur over time owing to the degradative effects of tissue fluids and enzymes.[82] Nunn and colleagues have noted an increased incidence of dilatation in hypertensive patients.[80]

Although a considerable number of reported instances involved varieties of grafts that are no longer manufactured, the potential dimensional instability of knitted Dacron grafts appears to be a consideration even in current generations of such prostheses.[81] The clinical impact of graft dilatation remains uncertain but is a concern. Modest dilatation does not necessarily imply graft failure, and no clear association between graft dilatation and graft complications has been directly established.[81] Nonetheless, structural defects have led on occasion to delayed bleeding through the graft or to actual rupture. More important, dilatation has been imputed as a major etiologic factor in the subsequent development of anastomotic aneurysms.[88, 89]

Finally, deposition of mural thrombus and the lower velocity of flow through such dilated conduits may well contribute to an increased frequency of thrombosis. Perhaps it is advisable for the surgeon to select a slightly "undersized" graft when he uses a knitted Dacron prosthesis. Because evidence suggests that dimensional alterations may be progressive and may lead to potentially serious late complications, lifetime patient follow-up with periodic CT scan evaluation of the entire graft appears advisable.[84]

NONTEXTILE SYNTHETIC GRAFTS

Expanded Teflon (ePTFE) Grafts

Despite generally satisfactory functioning of early synthetic grafts for aortoiliac reconstruction, the frequently disappointing long-term performance of Dacron grafts for more peripheral procedures involving smaller arteries, particularly those below the inguinal ligament, was a strong impetus for the development of other prosthetic materials and fabrication methods. Although textile Teflon grafts had been largely abandoned and replaced with Dacron as the material of choice for fabric prostheses, a method of extruding the Teflon polymer was discovered in 1969 by Robert W. Gore.[90] It was used only for industrial purposes until 1972, when Soyer and colleagues used ePTFE to replace the inferior vena cava in experimental animals.[91] Shortly thereafter, Matsumoto and coworkers reported good patency of such grafts as an arterial substitute in dogs.[92] Campbell and colleagues reported the first clinical use of ePTFE arterial grafts in 1976.[93]

The expanded polymer is manufactured by a heating and mechanical stretching process and extruded through a die, producing a porous material of a characteristic structure that has solid nodes interconnected by fine fibrils (Fig. 37–6). Fibril length can be varied and determines the pore size, which in standard ePTFE grafts currently available measures 30 μm. (The result is a unique nontextile material that can be fashioned into a tubular vascular graft. The material is chemically inert, highly electronegative, and hydrophobic. Initial observation of aneurysmal change in early grafts[94] led manufacturers to add a thin outer reinforcing wrap of ePTFE material to provide circumferential strength, increase wall thickness, or add external coil support. Such modifications have eliminated the structural instability of current ePTFE prostheses.

Although ePFTE is considered a porous material, the behavior of ePTFE grafts in terms of implantation bleeding through the graft wall is considerably different from that of conventional porous textile prostheses. The node-fibril structure of ePTFE material occupies only about 15% to 20% of the total volume of the expanded polymer. The void space is filled with air. Although the porosity (ratio of pores to material) of ePTFE is greater than that of textile Dacron grafts, the void spaces are smaller than the voids between the fiber bundles of fabric materials. The hydrophobicity of ePTFE material also limits bleeding. For these reasons, porosity is difficult to determine by methods such as the Weslowski water porosity test, which is used to characterize the porosity of textile grafts.[90] In essence, ePTFE grafts can be thought of as a microporous framework that requires no material to close its tiny interstices and can be used without preclotting.

Although the luminal surface of ePTFE grafts is negatively charged, immediately on exposure to blood events

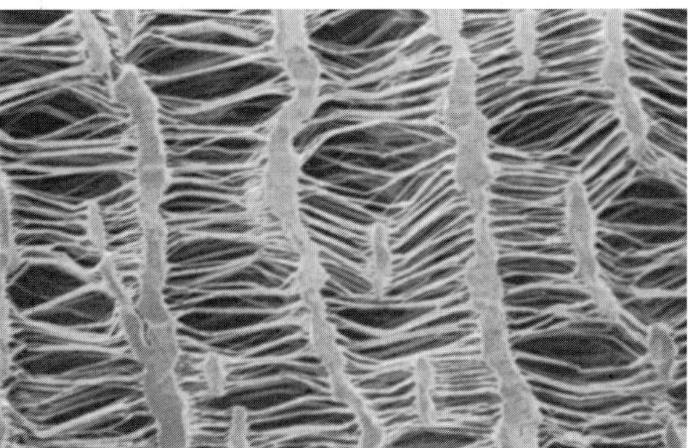

FIGURE 37–6. Scanning electron micrograph of the luminal surface of a Gore-Tex extruded polytetrafluoroethylene (ePTFE) graft demonstrating the characteristic node-fibril microstructure. (Original magnification, ×1000.)

and interactions occur that are common to other synthetic polymers. Proteins adhere rapidly to the surface within 30 to 60 seconds, followed by platelet aggregation. If the process is limited and flow is sufficient, the graft eventually becomes lined with a thin, relatively acellular protein film. Although the graft is incorporated by the surrounding tissues, little tissue grows into the PTFE wall even after 6 months in the dog.[5, 95] This is probably due to the microporous nature of the material and to the external reinforcing wrap.[96] As a consequence, in ePTFE grafts any endothelialization is restricted to pannus ingrowth within 1 to 2 cm of each anastomosis.

In the baboon model, Clowes and associates were able to demonstrate improved capillary ingrowth from surrounding granulation tissue and production of an endothelial lining in ePTFE grafts by making the grafts more porous.[97, 98] Such experimental, higher-porosity ePTFE grafts (mean internodal distance, 60 μm), however, lack an external wrap and are not available for clinical use.

The relationship of pore size to graft performance remains uncertain. Early work on ePTFE grafts by Campbell and colleagues actually correlated increasing fibril length (pore size) with inferior patency in dogs, which was thought to be due to development of a thicker neointima.[12] Indeed, the general success of microporous ePTFE as an arterial substitute has seriously challenged the previously accepted Weslowski concept of higher porosity as a desirable if not indispensable quality for function of an arterial substitute.[14]

A variety of modified ePTFE grafts have become available. In addition to the standard ePTFE prosthesis, some grafts now have a thinner wall construction (still retaining the outer wrap, however), resulting in easier handling characteristics, better conformability, and perhaps improved compliance. Recently, processing alterations have also produced a "stretch" ePTFE graft, which has some inherent elasticity not in the original grafts. Longitudinal extensibility, the stretch feature of the graft, is achieved by a "microcrimping" of the fibrils of the tube (Fig. 37–7). Despite such microcrimping of the fibrils, the luminal surface remains smooth. No additional materials, such as elastomers, are used to produce the stretch characteristic.

The actual internodal spacings, or fibril lengths, are similar in nonstretch and extended stretch ePTFE grafts. When the stretch graft is extended, with tension achieved either manually or by arterial pressure distention, the tented fibrils are extended to their full length. At that point, no further elongation is possible, and the microstructure of the stretch graft is identical to that of a standard ePTFE prosthesis. This has provided a conduit with a softer, more conformable wall and excellent handling qualities, possibly less tendency to kink across joints, and less necessity for the surgeon to cut the graft to precise required lengths. However, there are no data to suggest improved patency or any other outcome benefits other than improved handling features and ease of implantation.

A variety of externally supported ePTFE grafts are currently available (Fig. 37–8). It is thought that external support rings or coils may lessen possible mechanical compression, particularly in subcutaneously placed extra-anatomic grafts. Early studies that examined the importance of external graft compression as a cause of graft thrombosis

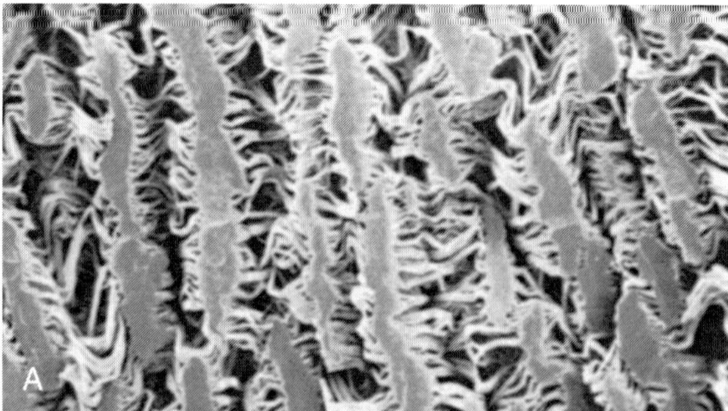

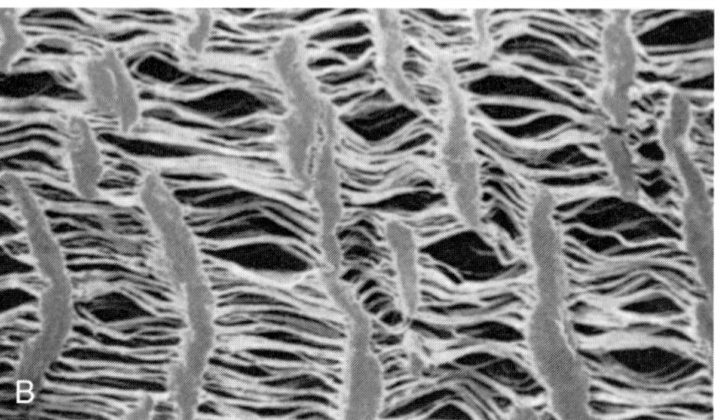

FIGURE 37–7. Scanning electron photomicrograph of the luminal surface of a Gore-Tex expanded polytetrafluoroethylene (ePTFE) stretch vascular graft. (×1000.) *A*, Relaxed microstructure demonstrating "microcrimping" of internodal fibrils. *B*, Moderately tensioned graft, with longitudinal extensibility achieved by extending crimped or tented fibrils. Microstructure is now identical to that of conventional ePTFE graft (see Fig. 37–6), with internodal spacing (fibril length) of approximately 25 μm.

gave conflicting results.[99–101] Newer, much improved results (compared with historic controls) of externally supported Dacron and ePTFE grafts in the axillofemoral and femoropopliteal positions, however, suggest that this concept may indeed be valuable for these types of reconstructions.[102, 103]

In addition, external support may help to reduce the possible kinking of ePTFE grafts across the knee joint, which has been suggested to be a contributing factor in the less-than-optimal performance of below-knee ePTFE grafts.[48, 99, 104] Several reports [48, 105–107] have suggested that improved patency occurs when externally supported ePTFE grafts are used for femoropopliteal or tibial revascularization, although results of a randomized prospective study by Gupta and colleagues[108] did not demonstrate any statistically significant benefit.

In addition to external support, several other treatment adjuncts or technical modifications have been suggested to improve the late results of ePTFE grafts. Flinn and coworkers reported improved late patency of infrageniculate ePTFE grafts when patients were maintained indefinitely on postoperative warfarin.[109] There is also increasing evidence that patency of ePTFE grafts to the below-knee popliteal and particularly the infrageniculate level may be improved by insertion of a vein cuff or patch at the distal anastomosis.[110–117] Although variations of the specific technique exist, the study results suggest that the general method may be a useful adjunct when long ePTFE is grafted to distal vessels. Furthermore, laboratory evidence suggests that this technique may help to reduce the potential of compliance mismatch to stimulate neointimal hyperplasia, lessen mechanical distortions at the anastomosis, and improve hemodynamics and blood flow through anastomoses constructed in such a manner.

Although most clinical experience with ePTFE has involved relatively small-caliber tubular grafts for infrainguinal or extra-anatomic arterial reconstructions, ePTFE aortic bifurcation grafts have been available since approximately 1980. Subsequent technologic changes in production have resulted in a stretch bifurcation prosthesis that has a thinner wall and some longitudinal extensibility, considerably reducing the stiffness of the graft that was previously noted by many surgeons. The current prosthesis is softer and more flexible and has improved handling characteristics and conformability.

Several reports of the clinical use of ePTFE aortic grafts have been favorable. Corson and colleagues described its use in aortic aneurysm repair in 216 patients from 1980 to 1987.[118] Thirty-one per cent of the grafts were carried to the femoral level. Although no significant difference in short-term patency or complication rates between ePTFE and a concurrent equal number of Dacron grafts was detected during a mean follow-up period of 22 months, the authors stressed the lack of any graft dilatation or anastomotic false aneurysms and the advantages associated with the implantation imperviousness of the ePTFE grafts. In a somewhat later follow-up report extending the experience of this group, no graft limb thromboses or false aneurysms were noted with ePTFE grafts, and only one infection occurred.[119]

Cintora and colleagues compared ePTFE with Dacron grafts in a nonrandomized, nonprospective series of 312 patients undergoing aortofemoral bypass graft for aortoiliac occlusive disease.[120] They found no significant difference in patency (cumulative 4-year patency, Dacron 90% versus ePTFE 97%) but noted that complications affected 13% of the Dacron group and only 4% of the ePTFE group. All six graft infections and all seven double-limb thromboses occurred in Dacron grafts. Anastomotic aneurysms, amputations, and late graft revisions were more frequent with Dacron grafts. Forty-four per cent of the patients with Dacron grafts required blood transfusion compared with 7% of the ePTFE group.

Burke and associates retrospectively reviewed Dacron and ePTFE aortic bifurcation grafts in 42 patients with a hypoplastic aorta (external diameter of infrarenal aorta, less than 14 mm).[121] They found much better patency with the ePTFE grafts than with the Dacron grafts of a similar size used in a historic control group and concluded that ePTFE bifurcation grafts were preferred for patients with small aortic and iliac vessels. Other studies have reported favorable results with ePTFE aortic grafts as well.[122–125]

These reports seem to suggest an established role for ePTFE grafts for aortic reconstruction as well as for more standard applications. One prospective randomized study from Vienna, however, reported no difference in patency between Dacron and ePTFE aortic grafts and a higher complication rate in the PTFE group, thus failing to confirm the alleged advantage of ePTFE grafts in terms of infection, frequency of anastomotic aneurysm, and so on.[126] Further experience must be accumulated.

There are several potential advantages of ePTFE grafts as a prosthetic vessel substitute. They do not require preclotting, do not leak, are resistant to dilatation in their current form, and are biocompatible. Most surgeons believe that ePTFE grafts are easier to thrombectomize than vein grafts or Dacron conduits if graft thrombosis has occurred.[127] There is some clinical and laboratory evidence that ePTFE grafts are more resistant to infection,[128–130] perhaps due to their smoother surfaces, which have less chance of bacterial adherence.[131, 132] Several investigators have reported less platelet deposition, and hence potentially less thrombogenicity of the flow surface, with ePTFE than with Dacron grafts.[133–136] Grafts of ePTFE have also been shown by Shepard and associates to cause substantially less complement activation than Dacron grafts following implantation, with less corresponding polymorphonuclear leukocyte infiltration and release of potent and potentially damaging inflammatory mediators.[137] Such mechanisms may better foster potential endothelial cell growth and contribute to a less thrombogenic flow surface, which is necessary for successful smaller vessel grafting.

Healing at ePTFE-native vessel anastomoses has also been demonstrated to result in a stronger bond with greater anastomotic tensile strength than that achieved with Dacron

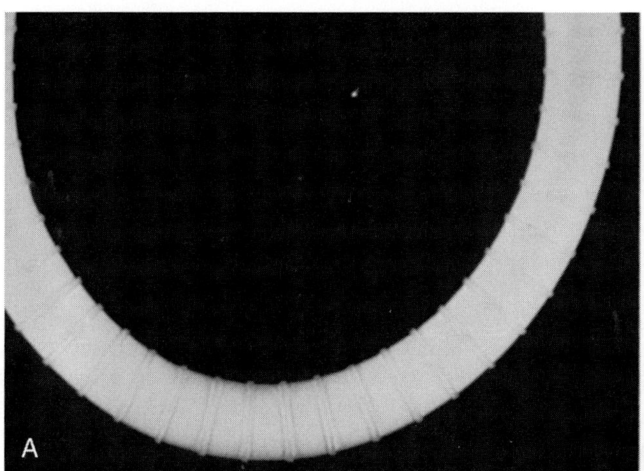

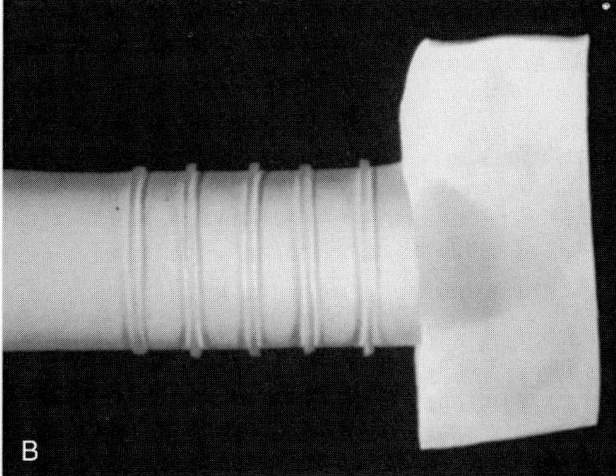

FIGURE 37–8. *A*, Example of an externally supported polytetrafluoroethylene (ePTFE) graft. *B*, Close-up view of detachable external rings; the end of the prosthesis has been opened, demonstrating standard smooth inner graft surface. (*A* and *B*, Courtesy of Gore-Tex, W.L. Gore and Associates.)

grafts[138]; this has implications for a potentially lower rate of anastomotic aneurysm formation and may explain why the observed incidence of such pseudoaneurysms has been low with ePTFE grafts.

Finally, ePTFE grafts are clearly easier to use than autogenous vein grafts. Reduced operating time, more limited incisions and dissection, and similar considerations may be a factor in some elderly high-risk patients.[139]

The principal disadvantage of ePTFE grafts is their less compliant nature than that of autogenous materials or even other prosthetic grafts, including Dacron. As emphasized by several groups of investigators, such viscoelastic mechanical discrepancies between a prosthetic material and the native artery to which it is attached may foster development of energy and flow disturbances at the interface, potentially contributing to graft failure or anastomotic aneurysm formation.[23, 25, 27, 28, 140] Compliance mismatch may play an important role in the frequent development of perianastomotic healing abnormalities, neointimal hyperplasia, and acceleration of distal arteriosclerosis, which are so often causative factors in failure of ePTFE grafts.[26, 141–143]

Although such processes are common modes of graft failure in general, ePTFE grafts appear to be particularly vulnerable, most likely due to their poor compliance (Fig. 37–9). Experimental studies have shown that anastomotic narrowing may occur with ePTFE grafts owing to surface thrombus formation or chronic endothelial injury.[144, 145] Antiplatelet agents have been demonstrated to reduce platelet adherence to ePTFE grafts and decrease intimal hyperplasia in experimental models, but the clinical utility of such pharmaceutical agents in enhancing the long-term function of ePTFE grafts has not been as promising.[146–148]

A propensity for troublesome bleeding through needle holes at sutured anastomoses of ePTFE grafts is also commonly recognized by many vascular surgeons. This bleeding may be obviated to a substantial degree by using fine-caliber suture material with small needles. Topical hemostatic agents such as oxidized cellulose, powdered collagen, and fibrin glue may also be applied after completion of anastomoses to hasten sealing of needle holes with fibrin and platelets.[149] Use of sutures made of ePTFE by W.L. Gore and Associates, which are especially designed for this problem and have a near 1:1 suture:needle diameter ratio, may also help to minimize such bleeding.[150] There are also anecdotal comments by some vascular surgeons that stretch ePTFE grafts may have less propensity to needle hole bleeding, perhaps due to the ability of this modified material to constrict around suture material to a greater degree than the standard nonextensible graft.

The higher cost of ePTFE grafts than vein grafts or standard Dacron synthetic grafts is also a relative disadvantage. However, the moderately increased expense of the prosthesis itself does not reflect the possible savings of expensive operating room time with the use of ePTFE grafts rather than vein grafts or the potentially improved long-term patency compared with standard Dacron conduits for lower limb revascularization if a vein graft is not possible. A recent comparative study by Abbott and coworkers, however, suggests that the patencies of Dacron and ePTFE femoropopliteal grafts are quite similar.[151]

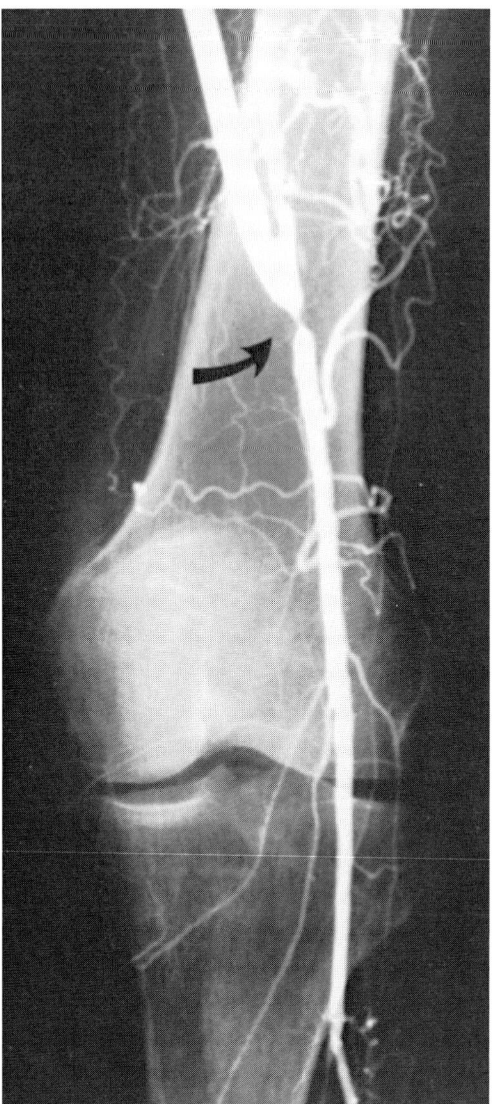

FIGURE 37–9. Neointimal hyperplasia *(arrow)*, just beyond distal anastomosis of above-knee polytetrafluoroethylene (ePTFE) femoropopliteal bypass graft, threatens graft function and patency 9 months after implantation.

COMPOSITE GRAFTS

It is well established that 20% to 30% of patients undergoing primary infrainguinal revascularization procedures do not have a suitable ipsilateral greater saphenous vein for the entire bypass.[152–154] In some of these patients, the saphenous vein has been used in prior cardiac or peripheral vascular procedures or has been previously stripped because of varicosities. In others, intrinsic vein abnormalities, including small size, early multiple branching, areas of sclerosis, and varicosities, limit the length of usable vein. The problem is of even greater magnitude in patients who require reoperation and secondary revision procedures, in whom a suitable vein is not available in 40% to 50% of cases.[155]

In such situations, the contralateral saphenous vein may

be employed, but it often has the same problems of size, quality, and length that have afflicted the ipsilateral vein. In addition, clinically significant occlusive disease in the contralateral limb may be a cause of concern about taking the vein from this leg. The lesser saphenous vein or arm veins are valuable alternatives, but often such veins are too short for a long below-knee popliteal or tibial pulse.

The acknowledged inferior performance of prosthetic conduits for such long grafts is believed to reflect the consequences of the greater thrombogenicity of the prosthetic graft flow surface and the lower flow rates in grafts to those smaller vessels with frequently compromised runoff. In addition, the adverse effects of possible kinking of the stiffer prosthetic material as it crosses the knee joint, and the potentially greater impact of neointimal hyperplasia developing at the distal anastomosis of a prosthetic graft to a small distal vessel, may also pose important limits to sustained function of infrageniculate prosthetic bypasses.[24, 28, 99, 104, 141]

Composite grafts have been suggested to help overcome some of these problems. Such grafts are defined as vascular conduits made up of two or more distinct portions. Although some authors[156–158] have used the term *autogenous composite graft* to refer to a graft constructed by splicing together two or more segments of autogenous vein, composite grafts are commonly understood to refer to a combination of both prosthetic material and autogenous vein composing a vascular graft of adequate length. Typically, the proximal segment is a prosthetic material such as Dacron or ePTFE, while the distal segment of the graft utilizes an available portion of autologous vein (greater saphenous, lesser saphenous, arm vein). In direct composite grafts (Fig. 37–10*A*), the prosthetic and vein components are joined by some type of end-to-end anastomosis.

As originally suggested by Edwards and associates,[159] a "sequential graft" implies use of a single graft with several points of distal anastomoses to different runoff beds. A *composite sequential graft* (Fig. 37–10*B*) refers to a graft composed of a proximal prosthetic conduit inserted into an isolated segment of patent popliteal artery, above or below the knee, that possesses some runoff of its own via geniculate collateral branches. The distal portion of the graft is a vein graft, usually arising end to side from the distal portion of the proximal prosthetic graft, which continues distally to a patent tibial or peroneal vessel in the calf or, on occasion, in the ankle or foot. Such a configuration suggests that even if the distal vein segment occludes, the proximal prosthetic bypass to the isolated popliteal segment might retain patency on its own. The addition of the second distal bypass segment is designed to increase flow through the prosthetic component, thereby improving its patency and augmenting the extent of overall revascularization of the extremity.[159–161]

The theoretical advantage of either form of composite graft is the use of the more flexible and kink-resistant vein segment to traverse the knee joint. Even if the length of available autogenous tissue is insufficient for this purpose, a distal vein segment may facilitate anastomosis to a small diseased distal vessel, potentially reducing the chance of later compromise due to perianastomotic intimal hyperplasia. This is similar to the rationale for the use of an interposition vein cuff with prosthetic grafts, which has been suggested by many authors to improve significantly the late patency of below-knee or tibial ePTFE grafts.[110–117]

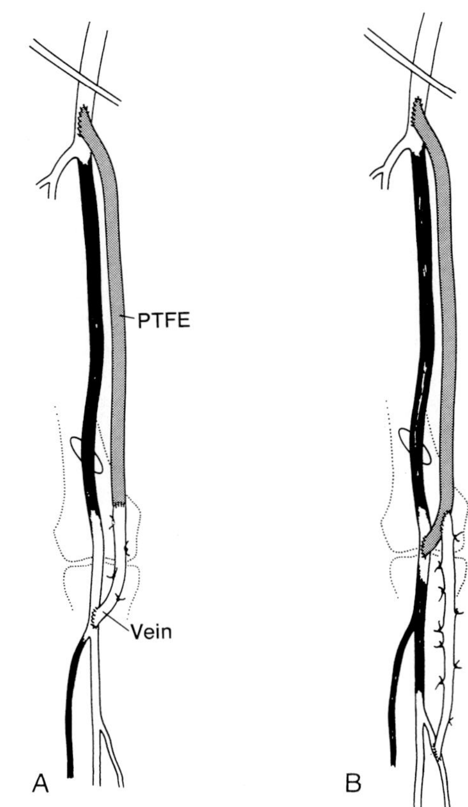

FIGURE 37–10. Types of composite grafts. *A*, Direct composite graft, with end-to-end anastomosis of graft components. *B*, Composite sequential bypass graft, with insertion of proximal prosthetic graft into isolated popliteal artery segment and continuation of distal vein segment to a tibial artery.

Potential disadvantages of composite grafts are the time and difficulty involved in obtaining a suitable vein segment from some other remote area as well as the need to perform a third anastomosis to join the prosthetic vein segments. This composite anastomosis may be difficult owing to a size discrepancy between the two graft segments, and difficulties with kinking, rotation, or excessive angulation may occur at this point. Compliance mismatch and turbulent flow may also occur at this junction, although the greater caliber of the two conduits at this point may lessen its potential impact compared with the smaller distal anastomosis. Finally, anastomotic aneurysms may develop over time at this location; we have seen several.

Conflicting results regarding the benefits of composite grafts have been reported. Some early investigators[162–165] found no better patency rates than those achieved with standard all-prosthetic grafts, while other authors[166, 167] suggested improved results with composite grafts. Our own results at the Massachusetts General Hospital have been described by LaSalle and colleagues.[168] There was no statistical difference in long-term patency between 39 composite grafts and 79 prosthetic grafts of various types to the below-knee popliteal artery. The length of vein relative to prosthesis did not appear to influence the long-term function of composite grafts. The results of both alternative grafts were markedly inferior to the results of vein grafts (73% cumulative patency at 5 years). Because of the added difficulties of constructing such grafts and the lack of conclusive evidence of better performance compared with currently available prosthetic grafts, we found little support for the use of composite graft reconstructions. Femorotibial grafts were not included in this analysis, however.

The controversy continues. The long-term results of composite grafts were improved compared with all prosthetic grafts in a number of more recent studies,[169–175] although, as Karacagil and colleagues[176] point out, the composite grafts are equivalent to those prosthetic grafts emphasizing a vein cuff. Indeed, whether a composite construction is superior to use for a vein cuff is uncertain. Theoretically, if a long enough vein segment is available to cross the knee joint, a composite bypass seems more appealing. If only a short vein segment is available, it seems logical that results with a vein cuff would likely be the same. Other studies of composite grafts fail to show benefit, however.[177, 178]

Most favorable results are reported with the composite sequential grafts. Flinn and colleagues obtained an 80% cumulative patency rate at 2 years for 30 composite PTFE-vein femoropopliteal-tibial sequential grafts, which is indistinguishable from the rate for a group of 12 similar grafts done entirely with vein and much superior to the 47% 2-year patency of sequential grafts done with PTFE grafts alone.[161] The investigators found that such grafts utilizing an otherwise inadequate segment of saphenous vein were a sound alternative in the revascularization procedure if the arteriographic configuration was suitable for sequential grafting. McCarthy and associates reported longer-term follow-up data on such grafts performed at Northwestern University, noting generally acceptable results that are superior to results obtained with all-prosthetic tibial bypass grafts.[179]

Similarly, Verta reported excellent long-term results of 54 composite sequential bypass grafts of PTFE and saphenous vein to the distal tibial or pedal vessels.[180] Patency rates by the life-table method were 81.4% at 2 years and 72.4% at 4 years. Verta believed that the use of vein distally allowed the creation of anastomoses to delicate distal vessels with a graft material of more appropriate viscoelastic properties that is better able to tolerate low-flow states (34.8 ml/min in his series).[180] The major drawback to the technique noted in Verta's report was the additional time required (an average of 51 minutes) compared with that needed for direct femorotibial vein grafts. Again, a patent segment of popliteal artery is required for construction of a composite sequential graft.

Firm conclusions about the utility of composite grafts are difficult to arrive at based on available clinical data. Early series are hard to compare owing to variability in factors such as severity of ischemia, primary versus redo operations, popliteal versus tibial anastomoses, and differences in techniques and actual materials used in fashioning the composite grafts. Overall, it seems fair to acknowledge the often unsatisfactory performance of prosthetic grafts in distal revascularizations, and therefore composite grafts remain a reasonable alternative. Although fairly equivalent results in the femoropopliteal position may not justify the additional time and difficulty of composite grafts compared with straight prosthetic bypasses, real advantages may well exist for tibial bypass, especially if a composite sequential configuration is possible.

GRAFT SELECTION

When selecting a graft for a particular vascular reconstructive procedure, the surgeon considers the performance characteristics of various conduits in relation to the requirements imposed by the specific clinical problem. After such variables are weighed, a rational choice of a graft appropriate for the circumstances unique to the individual patient can be made. No single graft is always optimal for a certain operation, and there is no consensus of opinion about the available options in many situations. Considerable controversy exists about certain aspects of graft selection partly because of the substantial variation in reported long-term performances of grafts in the literature and partly because of the personal preferences of individual surgeons.

From a surgeon's perspective, certain features are most important. These include (1) patency, (2) convenience, (3) absence of complications, and (4) cost. Desire for long-term patency is obvious. Although the patency in part reflects the thrombogenicity of the graft, sustained graft function is also heavily dependent on its position as well as design. The term *convenience* refers to the presence of desirable handling qualities that facilitate graft implantation, ease of preclotting or lack of such a need entirely, and the ready availability of a graft in the needed size and configuration. The surgeon also wants a graft to be free of subsequent complications, such as structural degeneration, infection, and healing abnormalities.

Finally, if anticipated performance of a graft is thought to be relatively equivalent to another option in all these aspects, the less expensive alternative may be the most appropriate choice in this cost-conscious era.

Although uncertainty and controversy are acknowledged, the attributes and weaknesses of currently available blood vessel substitutes can be considered for general areas of application, and several preferred alternatives can be identified.

Aortic Reconstruction

Size and length requirements preclude the use of autogenous venous or arterial grafts, and aortic allografts are unsatisfactory for elective aortic reconstruction given the existing methods of procurement and preservation as well as continued immunologic phenomena. Hence, a prosthetic graft is required. Fortunately, a variety of prostheses are available that function quite adequately in these large-diameter, high-flow positions, in which graft thrombogenicity is a consideration of much lower priority.

For procedures on the thoracic aorta and for extensive thoracoabdominal aortic reconstructions, bleeding is often a prime consideration, particularly if the patient requires cardiopulmonary bypass, high-dose systemic heparinization, and so on. In these instances, tightly woven Dacron grafts of relatively low porosity are an appropriate choice. Their long-term patency and dimensional stability have been highly satisfactory, overcoming their chief drawbacks of poor surgical handling characteristics, tendency to fray, and limited tissue ingrowth.

These disadvantages become more important, however, in complex thoracoabdominal aortic reconstructions performed with the method of Crawford[181] as opposed to simple tube grafts for large vessel aneurysm repair. In the complex reconstructions, "buttons" must be cut in the graft and sutured from within the aneurysm around orifices of critical visceral or intercostal vessels. The stiffness and poor conformability of conventional low-porosity woven Dacron grafts may be a significant impediment in this regard. Therefore, use of one of the biologically coated "zero-porosity" knitted Dacron grafts may be advantageous. ePTFE tubular grafts have similar appeal. Similar considerations regarding the desirability of an impervious graft apply to patients with ruptured abdominal aortic aneurysms and to those with a coagulation disorder of some sort.

For elective infrarenal aortoiliac replacement or bypass, Dacron prostheses have long been a conventional and successful choice and have excellent, well-documented long-term results. [21, 182–186] Many surgeons prefer knitted grafts owing to their better handling and healing characteristics. Such features are thought by many to be particularly important for aortofemoral grafts done for occlusive disease that must cross the inguinal ligament, often with anastomoses made to a diseased femoral artery or profunda femoris branch alone.[182] The long-term patency advantages of knitted versus woven grafts, however, have not been conclusively established, and several currently manufactured, more porous woven Dacron grafts have acceptable handling qualities.

In current practice, biologically coated Dacron grafts dominate the market, constituting 80% to 90% of sales in 1997.[187] This no doubt reflects the expedience and convenience of their low implant porosity, which eliminates the need for preclotting, and their retained flexibility, conformability, suturability, and so forth. ePTFE aortic grafts have similar potential attributes. In addition to its imperviousness, ePTFE has adequate handling features and may be more resistent than Dacron to infection or development of late anastomotic aneurysm formation.[118–123, 128–132, 138]

The greater cost of either coated or ePTFE grafts, approximately two to three times that of a conventional Dacron prosthesis, is a relative drawback. The reduction in blood loss and likely shorter operating room times associated with use of ePTFE grafts, however, probably offsets their greater expense. Other surgeons think that the less expensive conventional grafts should be used unless hemorrhagic complications are anticipated.[188] Generally, the good function of many varieties of available prosthetic grafts for aortic reconstruction make it unlikely that patency will be a primary discriminating feature for graft selection for such procedures; issues of cost, convenience, and diminished late complications will probably assume greater importance.

Infrainguinal Reconstruction

It is well established that for lower extremity bypass grafts autogenous saphenous vein is the preferred choice, particularly for long distal bypasses.[139, 152, 189–192] Two major areas of disagreement remain, however. First, some authorities propose that prosthetic grafts are, in fact, the graft of choice when bypass to the above-knee popliteal level is feasible. Second, if a below-knee bypass is required and no autogenous vein is available, controversy persists as to the best material for the prosthetic conduit and whether prosthetic grafts are in fact superior to primary amputation. These topics are covered in more detail in the chapters dealing specifically with these procedures.

Proponents of preferential use of prosthetic grafts for above-knee femoropopliteal reconstruction emphasize that numerous studies, including some well-controlled, randomized, and prospective series, have not detected statistically significant differences in patency or limb salvage rates between vein and prosthetic grafts in this position, particularly at shorter follow-up intervals and in patients undergoing operation for claudication.[139, 193–200] The advantages of initial use of prosthetic grafts are the shorter operative time and the need for less dissection and for only two small incisions—factors that may be advantageous in the high-risk elderly patient population.

The compromised long-term survival of many of these patients may also reduce the importance of truly long-term graft patency. It is reasoned that even if patency rates with prosthetic conduits are slightly lower, the saphenous vein will still be available for use in reoperation if this is required.[201] Graft failure is also anticipated in a significant number of patients who have primary vein grafts. It is well recognized that reoperations using autogenous vein result in much higher long-term patency rates than reoperations using prosthetic grafts.[155, 198, 202, 203]

Hence, it is reasoned that the fairly similar primary patency rates of above-knee vein and prosthetic grafts plus the much superior results of reoperation if the vein is still available will ultimately lead to a better long-term outcome. That is, the management sequence of initial preferential use of a prosthetic graft for above-knee reconstruction followed by autogenous saphenous vein for patients who do ultimately require secondary repair is preferable.[204]

Michaels extensively reviewed the literature and constructed a mathematical model to test this hypothesis.[205] He concluded that there was a clear overall advantage to using vein for the initial graft, whereas the alternative strategy of prosthetic graft first, vein later if necessary increases the number of additional operations and results in a lower 5-year patency rate when both first and second grafts are considered. Although this is an interesting work, it must be remembered that it is only a model and is limited, as he points out, by a lack of sufficient data from well-controlled trials.

Other studies have shown that the argument sometimes advanced for saving the saphenous vein for possible future use in coronary revascularization is, in fact, rarely necessary.[198, 206] Furthermore, although use of prosthetic grafts is quicker, a corresponding reduction in mortality and morbidity rates has not been conclusively demonstrated by any study. If more second operations are indeed required with initial use of prosthetic grafts, the morbidity rate and the risks of associated complications such as graft infection, which are clearly higher with reoperations, must also be considered.[205] This remains a debated and controversial topic. My own belief is that initial use of prosthetic grafts is indeed an appropriate strategy in certain patients, particularly older patients undergoing operation for noncritical ischemia with fairly good runoff.

As previously noted, an autogenous vein may not be available or may be inadequate for use in infrainguinal bypass in 10% to 40% of patients, depending on the length of the graft and whether it is a primary or secondary operation. In these circumstances, controversy continues about the best substitute conduit. Dacron grafts were initially utilized for lower extremity grafts in the early era of arterial reconstructive surgery, but mediocre long-term results, with 5-year patency rates in the range of 50% to 60%, were generally noted, and even more discouraging results were reported with grafts extending below the knee.[207–210]

Such outcomes and the attractive features of ePTFE grafts, such as the absence of the need for preclotting and the promise of potential lower thrombogenicity, led to a rapid decline in the use of Dacron grafts for femoropopliteal reconstruction. As has been pointed out by Pevec and colleagues, however, this may not be justified.[211, 212] The comparative study by Abbott and colleagues in fact suggested no difference in patency between ePTFE and Dacron above-knee femoropopliteal grafts.[151] Kenney and coworkers reported a 78% 4-year patency rate for externally supported, noncrimped Dacron grafts to the above-knee popliteal artery, which is equivalent to the results of any series of ePTFE grafts.[48]

Nonetheless, ePTFE grafts are clearly the most widely utilized alternative to autogenous vein for lower extremity revascularization procedures. Despite reports of early good experiences,[165, 213–215] the long-term function of ePTFE grafts in below-knee or, particularly, tibial bypasses has been far from ideal.[139, 216–218] However, acceptable results can sometimes be achieved. Veith and colleagues noted a limb salvage rate of 38% at 4 years, similar to that in several other reports.[139] If a patent tibial vessel exists and no autogenous material of any sort is available, bypass to a tibial or peroneal artery is justified in selected patients for attempted limb salvage as opposed to primary amputation.[139, 219]

It is hoped that concepts such as vein cuff interposition and long-term maintenance of warfarin therapy may improve the long-term performance of such grafts. A realistic appraisal of available experience, however, reemphasizes that all efforts to utilize autogenous tissue for infragenicular grafts should be made, serving as a continued stimulus to develop new and improved small-caliber prosthetic grafts.

Extra-anatomic Grafts

Few comparative data exist on the use of Dacron or ePTFE grafts for the variety of remote subcutaneously implanted grafts collectively referred to as *extra-anatomic reconstructions*. Currently, most vascular surgeons regard ePTFE grafts as the graft of choice for axillofemoral, femorofemoral, or axilloaxillary grafts. Although ePTFE patency rates may not be demonstrably higher, the lack of implantation bleeding with ePTFE grafts may be particularly helpful in avoiding hematoma formation in the subcutaneous tunnels compared with knitted Dacron grafts, even when careful preclotting is done. In addition, the relative resistance of ePTFE to compression or kinking and the ease of thrombectomy are valuable features.[103, 220–222]

In these subcutaneous positions, the use of externally supported grafts seems logical, although they are of unproven benefit. A good long-term patency of externally supported Dacron conduits for axillofemoral grafts has also been described.[48, 102] For carotid-subclavian grafts, some authors have documented higher long-term patency rates with ePTFE or Dacron grafts than with vein grafts.[223–225] The relatively small diameter of vein grafts and their potential for kinking and shortening secondary to neck flexion and mobility in contrast to the larger and more rigid prostheses may sometimes preclude their use.

Other Locations

Visceral and renal arterial reconstructions may be performed with prosthetic grafts with good results, and in these reconstructions many surgeons prefer prosthetic grafts. Satisfactory patency is related to their generally short length with high blood flow and to their not being subjected to mechanical stresses around body joints. An exception may be distal renal artery grafts in young patients with fibromuscular disease or visceral or renal procedures that involve bypass to diseased vessels with compromised distal arterial beds. Most experience has been gained with Dacron grafts. Preclotted knitted Dacron seems to be the preferred choice, although currently use of a coated Dacron graft is likely frequent in contemporary practice. Grafts of ePTFE have similar potential benefits and are an equally acceptable choice. However, extensive experience with ePTFE grafts for renal or mesenteric revascularization procedures has not been accumulated.[226]

Grafts of ePTFE may also be used for large-caliber venous replacements in unusual circumstances and for replacement or bypass of the inferior or superior vena cava,[227–229] jugular,[230] and portal[231] veins or for construction of portosystemic shunts for portal hypertension.[232] Stented grafts appear to be advisable for venous grafts.[233] The moderate success of large-caliber supported ePTFE venous grafts may attest to their reduced thrombogenicity and ability to remain patent in lower-flow states. The limited experience with venous reconstructions made with other prosthetic materials has been generally unsuccessful.

When a primary arteriovenous fistula for hemodialysis cannot be performed or has failed, ePTFE grafts are in the opinion of most authorities the prosthetic vessel of choice for angioaccess in contrast to bovine heterografts or other possible alternatives. Its resistance to infection, reasonable long-term patency, ease of revision, satisfactory tissue incorporation, and ability to withstand repeated puncture with less pseudoaneurysm formation have been documented.[234–236]

THE FUTURE

Considerable research is in progress to develop improved vascular substitutes, particularly for small vessel replacement. Such efforts are directed at the creation of new biomaterials with better surface properties and compliance and continued modification of substances already in use in an attempt to lower their flow-surface thrombogenicity.[237] Much emphasis is appropriately focused on a better understanding of the biologic phenomena at the cellular level that occur at the blood-prostheses interface. It is hoped that better knowledge of the cellular, humoral, and enzymatic processes that control the interdependent interactions of platelets, endothelial cells, smooth muscle cells, and other blood and tissue components will permit favorable modification of the graft flow surface, better control of neointimal hyperplasia, and more specific and successful pharmacologic control of the clotting process. Ultimately, a true biologic era of grafts may result; efforts to develop a biologic graft based on cell culture technology are already underway.[238]

Endothelial Cell Seeding

Appreciation of the integral role played by living endothelial cells, with their diverse and dynamic biochemical functions, in maintaining a thrombus-free flow surface in normal vessels or autogenous tissue vascular grafts has quite logically stimulated efforts to produce a similar antithrombogenic lining in prosthetic grafts (Fig. 37–11). It is now clearly established that endothelial regeneration in synthetic vascular grafts, as often demonstrated in various experimental animals, does not occur in the human except within several centimeters of each anastomosis of a graft. Hence, efforts have been directed toward "seeding" prosthetic grafts with mechanically or enzymatically derived autologous endothelial cells at the time of graft implantation in the expectation that subsequent attachment and proliferation of these cells will produce a confluent monolayer of living endothelial cells that will cover the entire graft flow surface and render it less prone to thrombosis (Fig. 37–12).

The concept of endothelial cell seeding was first introduced in 1970 by Mansfield, who employed granulation tissue as a cell source to seed a mixture of endothelial cells, fibroblasts, and macrophages onto Dacron patches implanted into the hearts of dogs.[239] At excision 3 weeks later, the patches seeded with autogenous cells exhibited a surface completely free of thrombus. Since this observation, a voluminous amount of laboratory work has attempted to develop techniques of lining prosthetic grafts with a functional endothelial cell layer, and progress has been made in methods of harvesting, culturing, and seeding techniques.[240, 241]

In the pioneering work of Herring and colleagues, reported in 1978, endothelial cells from veins mechanically scraped with steel wool pledgets were used to seed Dacron grafts in a canine model.[242] The cells were mixed with blood to preclot the grafts, which were immediately implanted in a single-stage technique. When explanted, the seeded grafts showed greater thrombus-free surface over time compared with unseeded controls and also demonstrated significantly thinner inner capsules. Subsequent work confirmed the endothelial nature of the graft lining and showed that seeded ePTFE grafts developed endothelial linings significantly sooner than similar Dacron grafts,[243] suggesting that less porous grafts may be better for seeding or that Dacron is a "less hospitable" material for the endothelial cell.

Because mechanical débridement of cells is relatively cumbersome and inefficient and produces a mixture of smooth muscle as well as endothelial cells, Graham and colleagues developed methods of enzymatic derivation with collagenase.[244] These investigators noted more efficient harvesting using enzymes rather than mechanical scraping. They also cultured the cells before later adding them to blood used to preclot Dacron grafts. Good results in terms of the degrees of endothelialization of both seeded Dacron and ePTFE grafts were noted.[245]

Subsequent work with laboratory animals has suggested that small-caliber endothelial cell–seeded grafts have better early patency, less platelet deposition, greater tolerance to low-flow states, confirmed prostacyclin-generating capacity, and other functional attributes similar to those of the flow surfaces of native vessels.[246–252] Seeded grafts have also been demonstrated to have greater resistance to bacteremic infection due to decreased bacterial adherence to endothelialized graft surfaces as opposed to areas of accumulated surface thrombus.[253] Not all experimental work, however, has confirmed the functional benefits of endothelial seeding.[254, 255]

Although the potential benefits of endothelial cell seeding have been documented, much experimental work has also focused on maximizing the number of cells harvested and improving their adherence to the graft surface. Large numbers of microvascular endothelial cells may be obtained

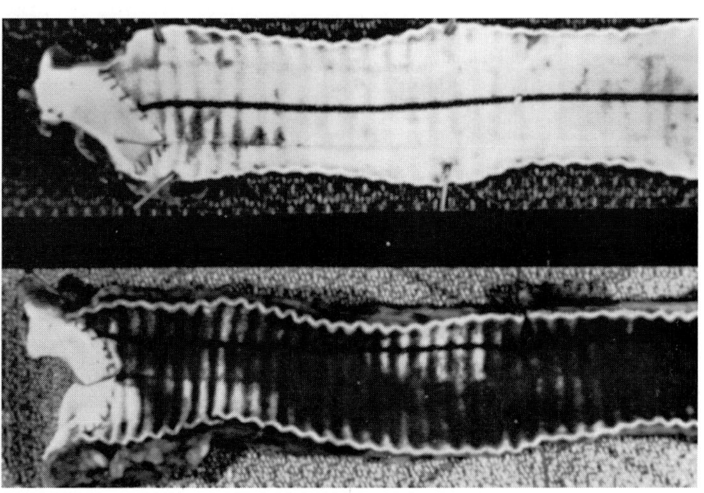

FIGURE 37–11. Endothelial cell-seeded *(upper)* and cell-unseeded *(lower)* Dacron prosthesis 4 weeks after canine thoracoabdominal implantation. Note the thrombus-free surface of the seeded graft compared with typical appearance of the inner surface of the unseeded graft. (Courtesy of J. C. Stanley, M.D.)

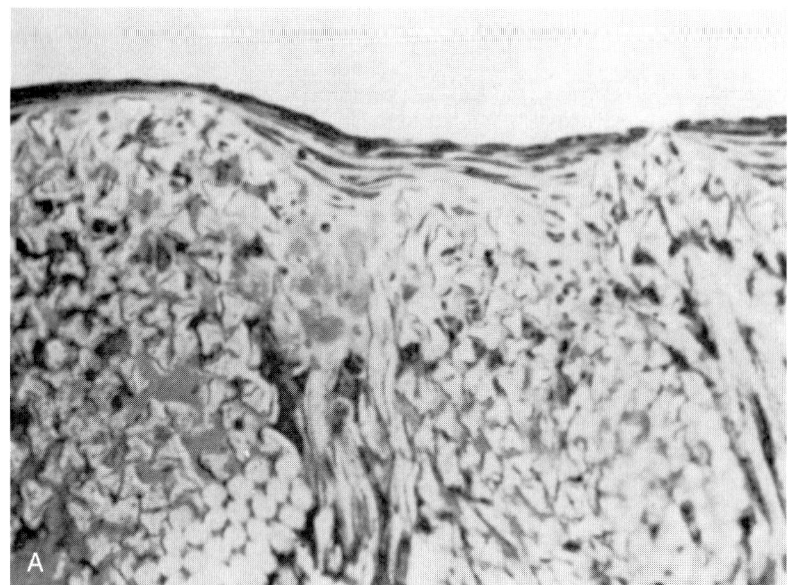

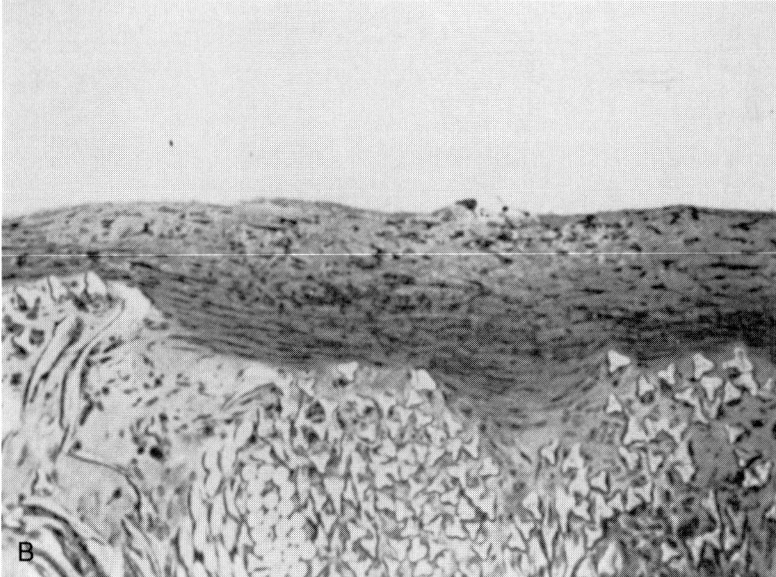

FIGURE 37–12. Photomicrographs of mid-portion of a Dacron prosthesis 4 weeks after canine implantation. *A*, Endothelial cell-seeded graft. Note the thin endothelium-lined flow surface. (×64.) *B*, Thick fibrin-lined surface in unseeded graft. (Methylene blue-basic fuchsin stain, ×40.) (Courtesy of J. C. Stanley, M.D.)

from adipose tissue, but such endothelial cells may not be a pure enough population for successful growth.[256–259] Culture of enzymatically derived cells may provide a larger number of cells for high-density seeding at a later interval, but this process requires considerable time for their growth and increases the risk of bacterial contamination with subsequent inoculation into the host.

Rosenman and associates have characterized the difficulties encountered with satisfactory adherence of seeded endothelial cells to graft surfaces of ePTFE conduits with exposure to blood flow.[260] They noted a 30% detachment of cells within the first 30 minutes, which decreased to 2% per hour over the next 24 hours. However, only about 5% of harvested cells remained attached to the graft 72 hours after seeding. Seeger[261, 262] demonstrated that precoating ePTFE grafts with fibronectin significantly improved endothelial cell adherence, and Ramalanjaona and coworkers[263] confirmed a sixfold increase in cell retention in ePTFE grafts pretreated with fibronectin.

There is limited clinical experience with endothelial cell seeding in humans. In 1984, Herring and coworkers described seeding of Dacron femoropopliteal, axillofemoral, and femorofemoral grafts.[264] No difference in patency was observed between seeded and nonseeded grafts, although early patency of seeded grafts was worse in patients who continued to smoke. Herring and coworkers also documented the first evidence of endothelialization in a human with a seeded ePTFE graft.[265]

Ortenwall and colleagues found significantly less platelet deposition in seeded limbs of Dacron aortic bifurcation grafts than in unseeded opposite limbs, seeming to imply an antiplatelet effect.[266, 267] In a subsequent series of 23 lower extremity grafts, these investigators seeded half of each ePTFE implant with autogenous endothelial cells. Seeded segments accumulated significantly fewer platelets at 1 and 6 months after surgery than unseeded portions, suggesting a reduced surface thrombogenicity in the seeded areas.[268] Short-term results of several small clinical series of seeded femoropopliteal grafts appear to favor seeded versus unseeded grafts, although the results are not statistically significant.[269–271] Another clinical trial failed to show any significant patency differences.[272]

The wealth of promising animal and laboratory results have not yet been duplicated in humans. The ability to harvest cells and seed the graft in the operating room requires simplified methods. The ability of seeded cells to adhere to and grow on a particular graft surface and to resist the sheer surface of flowing blood needs to be improved. It also remains to be established conclusively that seeded cells will maintain their anticoagulant and other favorable biologic functions in ways that will translate into better long-term patency of small vessel grafts. This work remains an exciting and potentially valuable concept for prosthetic grafts, however, and the use of recombinant gene technology to allow genetic modification of the function of seeded endothelial cells is perhaps a revolutionary influence on the horizon.[273–275]

Biodegradable Prostheses

The advantages of autogenous tissue vascular grafts and the potential adverse long-term mechanical and biochemical effects of blood and tissue interaction with prosthetic materials have continually spurred efforts to develop satisfactory biologically derived tissue conduits. A relatively recent example of this is the development of an absorbable prosthetic graft. In theory, subsequent tissue ingrowth and incorporation would eventually result in a conduit whose functional attributes were those of the regenerated host tissues themselves.

The concept of using a totally biodegradable mesh prosthesis with acceptable implant porosity was initially investigated in several laboratories.[276, 277] Animal studies demonstrated the capabilities of many components of an animal artery to regenerate over a scaffold of material such as an absorbable woven polyglactin acid (Vicryl) prosthesis. Microscopic studies showed that the polyglactin prostheses had almost entirely disappeared after several months and were replaced by regenerating endothelialized vessels containing smooth muscle-like myofibroblasts and dense fibroplasia, without thrombosis or infection. A tendency toward dilatation or frank aneurysm was noted, however.

The clinical efficacy of bioresorbable vascular prostheses depends in part on the development of adequate strength of the regenerated tissue before loss of strength of the absorbable prosthesis itself.[278] If this is a problem in potential human implantation, as appears likely, "compound" grafts might be constructed from yarns containing both bioresorbable and more permanent inert materials, or prostheses can be constructed of a mix of different biodegradable components that are resorbed at slower rates, thereby promoting early tissue ingrowth while the more slowly resorbed component remains as a mechanical strut.

Laboratory work along these lines has been reported.[279–281] Although intriguing and potentially clinically useful, at present bioresorbable vascular prostheses remain an experimental example of a "bioprosthetic compound" vascular graft.

Impregnated Grafts

In addition to coating or impregnating grafts with albumin, collagen, or gelatin to reduce implantation porosity and bleeding, investigators have incorporated substances within grafts or on their flow surfaces that might improve some aspect of their performance. Although infection after implantation of vascular prostheses is relatively infrequent in current practice (2% to 6%), infections do occur despite use of prophylactic systemic antibiotics or local irrigation with antibiotic solutions and they remain a challenging complication.

An appealing concept is a process that would render grafts more resistant to infection. Conventional antibiotic usage or soaking a prosthetic graft in an antibiotic solution immediately before implantation is relatively ineffective owing to the brief presence of the drug at the implantation site. In contrast, direct incorporation of antibacterial agents into the graft can theoretically prolong residence of drugs at the immediate graft site. In 1974, Clark and Margraff described experimental treatment of prosthetic grafts with a silver-allantoin-heparin complex that significantly resisted infection in dogs.[282]

Further work on the bonding of antibiotics to Dacron and ePTFE grafts, employing carriers such as a benzalkonium-oxacillin complex, tridodecylmethyl ammonium chloride (TDMAC), and other compounds, has been reported with promising laboratory results.[283–288] Incorporation of silver along with the antibiotic appears to enhance antibacterial activity and prolong retention of the antibiotic in the graft, slowing the washout effect of blood flow and permitting a slower steady diffusion.[289] Moore and associates used collagen as the vehicle for bonding amikacin to knitted Dacron grafts.[290] Such grafts were found to be much more resistant than control implants in the canine aorta to intravenously administer bacterial challenges. Most recent experimental and clinical work has focused on the incorporation of rifampicin onto Dacron grafts.[291–295]

These trials remain experimental. Further efforts are needed to find the best method of affixing antibiotics to grafts and improving their retention and release. Furthermore, translation of results of animal studies to humans may be difficult. Nonetheless, this developmental approach remains promising.

In related work, heparin bonding as a means of reducing the thrombogenicity of prosthetic materials and potentially improving their function as small-diameter vessel substitutes has been investigated. Gott and associates bound heparin directly to prosthetic surfaces using benzalkonium chloride and graphite as absorbed anchoring molecules.[296] Refinement of this concept led to development of the Gott shunt for bypass of the thoracic aorta without systemic heparinization in repair of thoracic aneurysms.

Esquivel and associates described covalent bonding of heparin to ePTFE and polyurethane prostheses, noting a significant reduction of thrombogenicity in a sheep laboratory model.[297] Bonding of antithrombotic pharmacologic agents other than heparin, such as urokinase or the potent antithrombin agent hirudin, and affixation of endothelial cell mitogens such as growth factor to enhance potential endothelialization, have also been studied, but such studies are in their early stages, and results are inconclusive thus far.[16, 52, 298, 299]

Alternative Grafts

Both theoretical concepts and laboratory and clinical experience with prosthetic grafts continue to lead to new graft materials and designs. Most have been investigated only in the laboratory and remain experimental; a few have had limited clinical application.

Alternative polymers for construction of small-caliber synthetic grafts have included various polyurethanes. Despite their promise of low thrombogenicity and relatively high implant compliance, such grafts have not had as good patency rates when tested in vivo.[300, 301] These polyurethanes and other polymers have also exhibited a disturbing tendency toward later degeneration and aneurysm formation.[302]

A unique replamineform graft has been described by White and colleagues.[303, 304] This conduit is formed with the sea urchin spine as a cast of uniform microporosity. The structure is impregnated with polyurethane and polymerized. Finally, the urchin bioskeleton is dissolved with 5% hydrochloric acid, yielding a polyurethane tube with uniform pores measuring 15 to 20 μm. Any advantage of this uniform pore size and geometric arrangement over that of microporous ePTFE grafts remains to be established.

Attempts to modify interactions favorably at the blood-prosthesis interface on the graft flow surface have also been made. The normal intraluminal polarity of the normal blood vessel is negative. Because blood cells are also negatively charged, it is logical that a repulsive negative charge interface normally exists between the vessel wall and the blood components, resulting in decreased thrombogenicity.[301] Sawyer and associates have emphasized such electrochemical forces to produce an "ion cloud" to help make a graft surface "invisible" to blood.[305] Grafts coated with carbon or bioelectrical polyurethane to impart a negative intraluminal charge have also been utilized but with limited success.[306–309] Carbon and other compound coats on grafts can also alter other important physical characteristics of the basic prosthetic material, such as porosity, and need further investigation.

SUMMARY

Nearly five decades of clinical experience with arterial reconstruction have demonstrated the importance of prosthetic grafts in the treatment of patients with vascular disease. A variety of synthetic and biologically derived conduits have been developed, often by innovative vascular surgeons in response to a particular clinical need. When vessel reconstruction with autogenous tissue grafts is not feasible, a number of generally satisfactory alternative prosthetic grafts exist for each specific clinical requirement. Although no consensus on the optimal prosthetic choice for a particular procedure exists, the vascular surgeon can make a reasoned selection based on the particular advantages and disadvantages unique to each type of prosthesis. Considerations include the attributes of each material in a particular location, anatomic requirements, patient status, handling characteristics of the material, cost, and individual preferences of each surgeon.

As some of the biologic mysteries of prosthesis-host interactions become unraveled, a better understanding of the events occurring at these interfaces will lead to new concepts and designs of prosthetic grafts. Whether the ideal prosthetic graft—that is, a vessel substitute with a live intima and a permanently stable and compliant wall that truly parallels the complex dynamic functions of an artery—will ever be developed is uncertain. It is important to remember Szilagyi's admonitions that any clinical introduction of newly modified prostheses should be preceded by careful and extended laboratory studies and that commercial introduction should occur only after a period of controlled clinical use with careful and thorough analysis by critically minded and unbiased investigators.[1]

REFERENCES

1. Szilagyi DE: Vascular substitutes, 1981: Achievements, disappointments, prospects. J Cardiovasc Surg 23:183, 1982.
2. Callow AD: Historical overview of experimental and clinical development of vascular grafts. *In* Stanley JC (ed): Biologic and Synthetic Vascular Prostheses. New York, Grune & Stratton, 1982, pp 11–26.
3. Sauvage LR, Berger KE, Wood SJ, et al: Interspecies healing of porous arterial prostheses. Arch Surg 109:698, 1974.
4. Scales JT: Tissue reactions to synthetic materials. Proc R Soc Med 46:647, 1953.
5. Sauvage LR: Biologic behavior of grafts in arterial system. *In* Haimovici H (ed): Vascular Surgery: Principles and Techniques, 3rd ed. Norwalk, Conn, Appleton & Lange, 1989, pp 136–160.
6. Edwards WS: The effect of porosity in solid plastic grafts. Surg Forum 8:446, 1957.
7. Boyd DP, Midell AI: Woven Teflon aortic grafts: An unsatisfactory prosthesis. Vasc Surg 5:148, 1971.
8. Fry WJ, DeWeese MS, Kraft RO, et al: Importance of porosity in arterial prostheses. Arch Surg 88:836, 1964.
9. Weslowski SA, Fries CC, Karlson KE, et al: Porosity: Primary determinant of ultimate fate of synthetic vascular grafts. Surgery 50:91, 1961.
10. Weslowski SA: The healing of vascular prostheses. Surgery 57:319, 1965.
11. Mathisen SR, Wu H-D, Sauvage LR, et al: The influence of denier and porosity on performance of a warp-knit Dacron arterial prosthesis. Ann Surg 203:382, 1986.
12. Campbell CD, Goldfarb D, Roe A: A small arterial substitute: Expanded microporous PTFE: Patency vs. porosity. Ann Surg 182:38, 1975.
13. White RA: Evaluation of small diameter graft parameters using replamineform vascular prostheses. *In* Wright CB (ed): Vascular Grafting. Littleton, Mass, John Wright PSG, 1983, pp 315–325.
14. Szilagyi DE: Arterial substitutes: Current problems and preferences. *In* Najarian JS, Delaney JP (eds): Advances in Vascular Surgery. Chicago, Year Book Medical Publishers, 1983, pp 81–90.
15. Greisler HP: Vascular graft healing: Interfacial phenomena. *In* Greisler HP (ed): New Biologic and Synthetic Vascular Prostheses. Austin, Texas, RG Landes, 1991, pp 1–19.
16. Esquivel CO, Blaisdell FW: Why small caliber vascular grafts fail: A review of clinical and experimental experience and the significance of the interaction of blood at the interface. J Surg Res 41:1, 1986.
17. Berger K, Sauvage LR, Rao AM, et al: Healing of arterial prostheses in man: Its incompleteness. Ann Surg 175:118, 1972.
18. Sauvage LR, Berger K, Beilin LB, et al: Presence of endothelium in an axillary femoral graft of knitted Dacron with an external velour surface. Ann Surg 186:749, 1975.
19. Kaplan S, Marcoe KF, Sauvage LR, et al: The effect of predetermined thrombotic potential of the recipient on small-caliber graft performance. J Vasc Surg 3:311, 1986.
20. Sauvage LR, Walker MW, Berger K, et al: Current arterial prostheses: Experimental evaluation by implantation in the carotid and circumflex coronary arteries of the dog. Arch Surg 114:687, 1979.
21. Sauvage LR, Smith JC, Davis CC: Dacron arterial grafts: Comparative structures and basis for successful use of current prostheses. *In* Kambic HE, Kantrowitz A, Sung P (eds): Vascular Graft Update: Safety and Performance. Philadelphia, American Society of Testing and Materials, 1986, pp 16–24.

22. Sanders RJ, Kempczinski RF, Hammond W, DiClementi D: The significance of graft diameter. Surgery 88:856, 1980.
23. Abbott WM, Cambria RP: Control of physical characteristics (elasticity and compliance) of vascular grafts. *In* Stanley JC (ed): Biologic and Synthetic Vascular Prostheses. New York, Grune & Stratton, 1982, pp 189–220.
24. Imparato AM, Bracco A, Kim GE, Zeff R: Intimal and neointimal fibrous proliferation causing failure of arterial reconstructions. Surgery 72:1007, 1972.
25. Gaylis H: Pathogenesis of anastomotic aneurysms. Surgery 90:509, 1981.
26. O'Donnell TF, Mackey W, McCullough JL, et al: Correlation of operative findings with angiographic and noninvasive hemodynamic factors associated with failure of polytetrafluoroethylene grafts. J Vasc Surg 1:136, 1984.
27. Kidson IG, Abbott WM: Low compliance and arterial graft occlusion. Circulation 58(Suppl I):1, 1978.
28. Walden R, L'Italien G, Megerman J, et al: Matched elastic properties and successful arterial grafting. Arch Surg 115:1166, 1980.
29. Voorhees AB Jr, Jaretzke AL III, Blakemore AH: The use of tubes constructed from Vinyon-"N" cloth in bridging arterial defects. Ann Surg 135:332, 1952.
30. Blakemore AH, Voorhees AB Jr: The use of tubes constructed from Vinyon-N cloth in bridging arterial defects: Experimental and clinical. Ann Surg 140:324, 1954.
31. Edwards WS, Tapp JS: Chemically treated nylon tubes as arterial grafts. Surgery 38:61, 1955.
32. Edwards WS, Tapp JS: A flexible aortic bifurcation graft of chemically treated nylon. Surgery 41:723, 1957.
33. Edwards WS: Progress in synthetic graft development: An improved crimped graft of Teflon. Surgery 45:298, 1959.
34. Deterling RA, Bhonslay SB: An evaluation of synthetic materials and fabrics suitable for blood vessel replacement. Surgery 38:71, 1955.
35. Harrison JH: Synthetic materials as vascular prostheses: A comparative study in small vessels of nylon, Dacron, Orlon, Ivalon sponge and Teflon (I and II). Am J Surg 95:3, 1958.
36. Creech O Jr, Deterling RA Jr, Edwards WS, et al: Vascular prostheses: Report of Committee for Study of Vascular Prostheses for the Society of Vascular Surgery. Surgery 41:62, 1957.
37. Weslowski SA, Dennis C: Fundamentals of Vascular Grafting. New York, McGraw-Hill, 1963.
38. DeBakey ME, Jordan GL Jr, Abbott JP, et al: The fate of Dacron vascular grafts. Arch Surg 89:757, 1964.
39. Snyder RW, Botzko KM: Woven, knitted, and externally supported Dacron vascular prostheses. *In* Stanley JC (ed): Biologic and Synthetic Vascular Prostheses. New York, Grune & Stratton, 1982, pp 485–508.
40. Lindenauer SM: The fabric vascular prosthesis. *In* Rutherford RB (ed): Vascular Surgery, 3rd ed. Philadelphia, WB Saunders, 1989, pp 450–460.
41. Hall CW, Liotta D, Ghidoni JJ, et al: Velour fabrics applied to medicine. J Biomed Mater Res 1:179, 1967.
42. Lindenauer SM, Lavanway JM, Fry WJ: Development of a velour vascular prosthesis. Curr Top Surg Res 2:491, 1970.
43. Sauvage LR, Berger K, Wood SJ, et al: An external velour surface for porous arterial prostheses. Surgery 70:940, 1971.
44. Sauvage LR, Berger KE, Mansfield PB, et al: Future directions in the development of arterial prostheses for small and medium caliber arteries. Surg Clin North Am 54:213, 1974.
45. Goldman M, McCollum CN, Hawker RJ, et al: Dacron arterial grafts: The influence of porosity, velour, and maturity on thrombogenicity. Surgery 92:947, 1982.
46. Wu H-D, Zammit M, Sauvage LR, Steicher MD: The influence of inner wall filamentousness on the performance of small- and large-caliber arterial grafts. J Vasc Surg 2:255, 1985.
47. Yates SG, Barros D'Sa AAB, Berger K, et al: The preclotting of porous arterial prostheses. Ann Surg 188:611, 1978.
48. Kenney DA, Sauvage LR, Wood SJ, et al: Comparison of noncrimped, externally supported (EXS) and crimped, non-supported Dacron prostheses for axillo-femoral and above-knee femoropopliteal bypass. Surgery 92:931, 1982.
49. Quinones-Baldrich WJ, Moore WS, Ziomek S, Chvapil M: Development of a "leak-proof," knitted Dacron vascular prosthesis. J Vasc Surg 3:895, 1986.
50. Ruhland D, Wigger J, Botleher K, et al: Fate of collagen following implantation of Microvel Hemashield grafts in the dog. Angiol Arch 9:22, 1985.
51. McGee GS, Shuman TA, Atkinson JB, et al: Long-term assessment of a damp-stored, albumin-coated, knitted vascular graft. Ann Surg 55:174, 1989.
52. Greisler HP: Biohybrids—biological coatings in synthetic grafts. *In* Greisler HP (ed): New Biologic and Synthetic Vascular Prostheses. Austin, Tex, RG Landes, 1991, pp 33–46.
53. Siverhus DJ, Schmitt DD, Edmiston CE, et al: Adherence of mucin and non–mucin-producing staphylococci to preclotted and albumin-coated velour knitted grafts. Surgery 104:613–619, 1990.
54. Kottke-Marchant K, Anderson JM, Umemura Y, et al: Effect of albumin coating on the in vitro compatibility of Dacron arterial prostheses. Biomaterials 110:147, 1989.
55. Lyman DJ, Klein KG, Brosh JJ, et al: Platelet interaction with protein coated surfaces. Thromb Diath Haemor 42(Suppl):109, 1970.
56. Canadian Multicenter Hemashield Study Group: Immunological response to collagen-impregnated vascular grafts: A randomized prospective study. J Vasc Surg 12:741, 1990.
57. Norgren L, Holtas S, Persson G, et al: Systemic response to collagen-impregnated versus non-treated Dacron velour grafts for aortic and aortofemoral reconstructions. Eur J Vasc Surg 4:379, 1990.
58. De Mol Van Otterloo JCA, Van Bockel JH, Ponfoort ED, et al: The effects of aortic reconstruction and collagen impregnation of Dacron prostheses on the complement system. J Vasc Surg 16:774, 1992.
59. Rumisek JD, Wade CE, Brooks DE, et al: Heat-denatured albumin coated Dacron vascular grafts: Physical characteristics and in vivo performance. J Vasc Surg 4:136, 1986.
60. Stegmann TH, Haverich A, Borst HG: Clinical experience with a new collagen-coated Dacron double-velour prosthesis. Thorac Cardiovasc Surg 34:54, 1986.
61. Reigel MM, Hollier LH, Pairolero PC, Hallett JW Jr: Early experience with a new collagen-impregnated aortic graft. Am Surg 54:134, 1988.
62. Freischlag JA, Moore WS: Clinical experience with a collagen-impregnated knitted Dacron vascular graft. Ann Vasc Surg 4:449, 1990.
63. Branchereau A, Rudondy P, Gournier J-P, Espinoza H: The albumin-coated knitted Dacron aortic prosthesis: A clinical study. Ann Vasc Surg 4:138, 1990.
64. Kang SS, Petsikas D, Murchan P, et al: Effects of albumin coating of knitted Dacron grafts on transinterstitial blood loss and tissue ingrowth and incorporation. Cardiovasc Surg 5:184–189, 1997.
65. Al-Khaffaf H, Charlesworth D: Albumin-coated vascular prostheses: A five year follow-up. J Vasc Surg 23:686–690, 1996.
66. Chakfe N, Beaufigeau M, Nicolini P, et al: Albumin-impregnated prosthetic graft for infrarenal aortic replacement: Effects on the incidence and volume of perioperative blood transfusion. Ann Vasc Surg 11:588–595, 1997.
67. Reid DB, Pollack JG: A prospective study of 100 gelatin-sealed aortic grafts. Ann Vasc Surg 5:320–324, 1991.
68. Cavallaro A, Sciacca V, Gallo P: Pretreatment of Dacron prosthesis with gelatin: Experimental research and clinical evaluation. J Vasc Surg 17:83–89, 1989.
69. Drury JK, Ashton TR, Cunningham JD, et al: Experimental and clinical experience with a gelatin impregnated Dacron prosthesis. Ann Vasc Surg 1:542, 1987.
70. Balzer K, Werner HH, Adamek L, et al: Results after implantation of gelatin-impregnated bifurcated grafts. Thorac Cardiovasc Surg 36:351–355, 1988.
71. Cooke PA, Nobis PA, Stoney RJ: Dacron aortic graft failure. Arch Surg 108:101, 1974.
72. Perry MO: Early failure of Dacron prosthetic grafts. J Cardiovasc Surg 16:318, 1975.
73. Blumenberg RM, Gelfand ML: Failure of knitted Dacron as an arterial prosthesis. Surgery 81:493, 1977.
74. May J: Multiple aneurysms in Dacron velour graft. Arch Surg 113:320, 1978.
75. Watanabe T, Kusaka A, Kuma H, et al: Failure of Dacron arterial prostheses caused by structural defects. J Cardiovasc Surg 24:95, 1983.
76. Lundqvist B, Almgren B, Bowald S, et al: Deterioration and dilation of Dacron prosthetic grafts. Acta Chir Scand Suppl 29:81, 1985.
77. Wilson SE, Krug R, Mueller G, Wilson L: Late disruption of Dacron aortic grafts. Ann Vasc Surg 11:383–386, 1997.
78. Riepe G, Loos J, Imig H, et al: Long-term in vivo alterations of

polyester vascular grafts in humans. Eur J Vasc Endovasc Surg 13:540–548, 1997.
79. Berger K, Sauvage LR: Late fiber deterioration in Dacron arterial grafts. Ann Surg 193:477, 1981.
80. Nunn DB, Freeman MH, Hudgins PC: Postoperative alterations in size of Dacron aortic grafts. Ann Surg 189:741, 1979.
81. Blumenberg RM, Gelfand ML, Barton EA, et al: Clinical significance of aortic graft dilation. J Vasc Surg 14:175, 1991.
82. King MW, Guidoin R, Blais P, et al: Degeneration of polyester arterial prostheses: A physical or chemical mechanism? *In* Fraker AC, Griffin CD (eds): Corrosion and Degradation of Implant Materials: Second Symposium, ASTM STP 859. Philadelphia, American Society for Testing and Materials, 1985, pp 295–307.
83. Pourdeyhimi B, Wagner D: On the correlation between the failure of vascular grafts and their structural and material properties: A critical analysis. J Biomed Mater Res 20:375, 1987.
84. Nunn DB, Carter MM, Donohue MT, et al: Postoperative dilation of knitted Dacron aortic bifurcation graft. J Vasc Surg 12:291, 1990.
85. Hunter GC, Bull DA: The healing characteristics, durability, and long-term complications of vascular prostheses. *In* Bernhard VM, Towne JB (eds): Complications in Vascular Surgery. St. Louis, Quality Medical Publishing, 1991, pp 65–86.
86. Ottinger LW, Darling RC, Wirthlin LS, Linton RR: Failure of ultralightweight knitted Dacron grafts in arterial reconstruction. Arch Surg 111:146, 1976.
87. Yashar JJ, Richmond MH, Dyckman J, et al: Failure of Dacron prostheses caused by structural defect. Surgery 84:659, 1978.
88. Kim GE, Imparato AM, Nathan I, et al: Dilatation of synthetic grafts and junctional aneurysms. Arch Surg 114:1296, 1979.
89. Claggett GP, Salander JM, Eddleman WL, et al: Dilation of knitted Dacron aortic prostheses and anastomotic false aneurysms: Etiologic considerations. Surgery 93:9, 1983.
90. Boyce B: Physical characteristics of expanded polytetrafluoroethylene grafts. *In* Stanley JC (ed): Biologic and Synthetic Vascular Prostheses. New York, Grune & Stratton, 1982, pp 553–561.
91. Soyer Y, Lempinen M, Cooper P, et al: A new venous prosthesis. Surgery 72:864, 1972.
92. Matusmoto H, Hasegawa T, Fuse K: A new vascular prosthesis for a small caliber artery. Surgery 74:518, 1973.
93. Campbell CD, Brooks DH, Webster MW, et al: The use of expanded microporous polytetrafluoroethylene for limb salvage: A preliminary report. Surgery 79:485, 1976.
94. Campbell DC, Brooks DH, Webster MW, et al: Aneurysm formation in expanded polytetrafluoroethylene prostheses. Surgery 79:491, 1976.
95. Mathisen SR, Wu HD, Sauvage LR, et al: An experimental study of eight current arterial prostheses. J Vasc Surg 4:33, 1986.
96. Kohler TR, Stratton JR, Kirkman TR, et al: Conventional versus high-porosity polytetrafluoroethylene grafts: Clinical evaluation. Surgery 112:901, 1992.
97. Clowes AW, Kirkman TR, Reidy MA: Mechanisms of arterial graft healing. Rapid transmural capillary ingrowth provides a source of intimal endothelium and smooth muscle in porous PTFE prostheses. Am J Pathol 123:220, 1986.
98. Zacharias RK, Kirkman TR, Clowes AW: Mechanisms of healing in synthetic grafts. J Vasc Surg 6:429, 1987.
99. Kempczinski RF: Physical characteristics of implanted polytetrafluoroethylene grafts: A preliminary report. Arch Surg 114:917, 1979.
100. Jarowenko MV, Buchbinder D, Shah DM: Effect of external pressure on axillo-femoral bypass grafts. Arch Surg 193:274, 1981.
101. Cavallaro A, Sciacca V, DiMarzo L, et al: The effect of body weight compression on axillo-femoral bypass patency. J Cardiovasc Surg 29:476, 1988.
102. Schultz GA, Sauvage LR, Mathisen SR, et al: A five- to seven-year experience with externally supported Dacron prostheses in axillofemoral and femoropopliteal bypass. Ann Vasc Surg 1:214, 1986.
103. Harris JE, Taylor LM, McConnell DB, et al: Clinical results of axillofemoral bypass using externally supported polytetrafluoroethylene. J Vasc Surg 12:416, 1990.
104. Burnham SJ, Flanigan DP, Goodreau JJ, et al: Ankle pressure changes in distal bypass grafts during knee flexion. Surgery 87:652, 1980.
105. Taylor RS, McFarland RJ, Cox MI: An investigation into the causes of failure of PTFE grafts. Eur J Vasc Surg 1:335, 1987.
106. Hurwitz RL, Johnson JM, Hufnagel CE: Femoropopliteal bypass using externally supported polytetrafluoroethylene grafts: Early results in a multi-institutional study. Am J Surg 150:574, 1985.
107. Dunn MM, Robinette DR, Peoples JB: Comparison between externally stented and unstented PTFE vascular grafts. Am Surg 54:324, 1988.
108. Gupta SK, Veith FJ, Kram HB, Wengerter KR: Prospective, randomized comparison of ringed and nonringed polytetrafluoroethylene femoropopliteal bypass grafts: A preliminary report. J Vasc Surg 13:162, 1991.
109. Flinn WR, Rohrer MJ, Yao JST, et al: Improved long-term patency of infragenicular polytetrafluoroethylene grafts. J Vasc Surg 7:685, 1988.
110. Miller JH, Foreman RK, Ferguson L, Faris I: Interposition vein cuff for anastomosis of prosthesis to small artery. Aust N Z J Surg 54:283, 1984.
111. Tyrrell MR, Wolfe JHN: New prosthetic venous collar anastomotic technique: Combining the best of other procedures. Br J Surg 78:1016, 1991.
112. Taylor RS, Loh A, McFarland RJ, et al: Improved technique for polytetrafluoroethylene bypass grafting: Long-term results using anastomotic vein patches. Br J Surg 79:348, 1992.
113. Tyrrell MR, Chester JF, Vipond MN, et al: Experimental evidence to support the use of interposition vein collars/patches in distal PTFE anastomoses. Eur J Vasc Surg 4:95, 1990.
114. Wolfe JHN, Tyrrell MR: Justifying arterial reconstruction to crural vessels—even with a prosthetic graft. Br J Surg 78:897, 1991.
115. Stonebridge PA, Howlett R, Prescott R, et al: Randomized trial comparing polytetrafluoroethylene graft patients with or without Miller cuff. Br J Surg 82:555–556, 1995.
116. Harris PL, Bakran A, Enabi L, Nott DM: ePTFE grafts for femorocrural bypass: Improved results with combined adjuvant venous cuff and arteriovenous fistula? Eur J Vasc Surg 7:528–533, 1993.
117. Pappas PJ, Hobson RW, Meyers MG, et al: Patency of infrainguinal polytetrafluoroethylene bypass grafts with distal interposition vein cuffs. Cardiovasc Surg 1998; 6:19–26, 1998.
118. Corson JD, Reinhardt R, von Grondell A, et al: Clinical and experimental evaluation of aortic polytetrafluoroethylene grafts for aneurysm replacement. Arch Surg 123:453, 1988.
119. Corson JD, Baraniewski HM, Shah DM, et al: Large diameter expanded polytetrafluoroethylene grafts for infrarenal aortic aneurysm surgery. J Cardiovasc Surg 31:702, 1990.
120. Cintora I, Pearce DE, Cannon JA: A clinical survey of aortobifemoral bypass using two inherently different graft types. Ann Surg 208:625, 1988.
121. Burke PM Jr, Herrmann JB, Cutler BS: Optimal grafting methods for the small abdominal aorta. J Cardiovasc Surg 28:420, 1987.
122. Mohan CR, Hoballah JJ, Martinasevic M, et al: The aortic polytetrafluoroethylene graft: Further experience. Eur J Vasc Endovasc Surg 11:158–163, 1996.
123. Lord RSA, Nash PA, Raj PT, et al: Prospective randomized trial of polytetrafluoroethylene and Dacron aortic prosthesis: I. Perioperative results. Ann Vasc Surg 3:248, 1988.
124. Friedman SG, Lazzaro RS, Spier LN, et al: A prospective randomized comparison of Dacron and polytetrafluoroethylene aortic bifurcation grafts. Surgery 117:7–10, 1995.
125. Shah DM, Darling RC III, Kreienberg PB, et al: A critical approach for longitudinal clinical trial of stretch PTFE aortic grafts. Cardiovasc Surg 4:414–418, 1997.
126. Polterauer P, Prager M, Holzenbein TH, et al: Dacron versus polytetrafluoroethylene for Y-aortic bifurcation grafts: A six-year prospective randomized trial. Surgery 111:626, 1992.
127. Veith FJ, Gupta S, Daly V: Management of early and late thrombosis of expanded polytetrafluoroethylene (PTFE) femoropopliteal bypass grafts: Favorable prognosis with appropriate reoperation. Surgery 87:581, 1980.
128. Bergamini TM, Bandyk DF, Govostis D, et al: Infection of vascular prostheses caused by bacterial biofilms. J Vasc Surg 7:21, 1988.
129. Bandyk DF, Bergamini TM, Kinney EV, et al: In situ replacement of vascular prostheses infected by bacterial biofilms. J Vasc Surg 13:575, 1991.
130. Shah PM, Ito K, Clauss RH, et al: Expanded microporous polytetrafluoroethylene (PTFE) grafts in contaminated wounds: Experimental and clinical study. J Trauma 23:1030, 1983.
131. Schmitt DD, Bandyk DF, Pequet AJ, Towne JB: Bacterial adherence to vascular prostheses. J Vasc Surg 3:732, 1986.

132. Harris JM, Martin LF: An in vitro study of the properties influencing *Staphylococcus epidermidis* adhesion to prosthetic vascular graft materials. Ann Surg 207:612, 1987.
133. Hamlin GW, Rajah SM, Crow MJ, et al: Evaluation of the thrombogenic potential of three types of arterial grafts studied in an artificial circulation. Br J Surg 65:272, 1978.
134. Goldman M, Hall C, Dykes J, et al: Does 111-indium platelet deposition predict patency in prosthetic arterial grafts? Br J Surg 70:635, 1983.
135. Allen BT, Sicard GA, Welch MJ, et al: Platelet deposition in vascular grafts: The accuracy of in vivo quantification and the significance of in vivo platelet reactivity. Ann Surg 203:318, 1986.
136. Shoenfeld NA, Connolly R, Ramberg K, et al: The systemic activation of platelets by Dacron grafts. Surg Gynecol Obstet 166:454, 1988.
137. Shepard AD, Gelfand JA, Callow AD, O'Donnell TF Jr: Complement activation by synthetic vascular prostheses. J Vasc Surg 1:829, 1984.
138. Quiñones-Baldrich WJ, Ziomek S, Henderson T, Moore WS: Primary anastomotic bonding in polytetrafluoroethylene grafts? J Vasc Surg 5:311, 1987.
139. Veith FJ, Gupta SK, Ascer E, et al: Six-year prospective multicenter randomized comparison of autogenous saphenous vein and expanded polytetrafluoroethylene grafts in infrainguinal arterial reconstruction. J Vasc Surg 3:104, 1986.
140. Mehigan DG, Fitzpatrick B, Browne HI, Boucher-Hayes DJ: Is compliance mismatch the major cause of anastomotic arterial aneurysms? Analysis of 42 cases. J Cardiovasc Surg 26:147, 1985.
141. Echave V, Koornick AR, Haimov M, et al: Intimal hyperplasia as a complication of the use of the polytetrafluoroethylene graft for femoropopliteal bypass. Surgery 86:791, 1979.
142. Sottiurai VS, Yao JS, Flinn WR, et al: Intimal hyperplasia and neointima: An ultrastructural analysis of thrombosed grafts in humans. Surgery 93:809, 1983.
143. Sladen JG, Maxwell TM: Experience with 130 polytetrafluoroethylene grafts. Am J Surg 141:546, 1981.
144. Clowes AW, Gown AM, Hanson SR, Reidy MA: Mechanisms of arterial graft failure: 1. Role of cellular proliferation in early healing of PTFE prostheses. Am J Pathol 118:43, 1985.
145. Kuwano H, Hashizume M, Yang Y, et al: Patterns of pannus growth of the expanded polytetrafluoroethylene vascular graft with special attention to the intimal hyperplasia formation. Am Surg 52:663, 1986.
146. Oblath RW, Buckley FO, Green RM, et al: Prevention of platelet aggregation and adherence to prosthetic grafts by aspirin and dipyridamole. Surgery 84:37, 1978.
147. Hagen PO, Wang ZG, Mikat EM, Hackel DB: Antiplatelet therapy reduces aortic intimal hyperplasia distal to small diameter vascular prostheses (PTFE) in nonhuman primates. Ann Surg 195:328, 1982.
148. Green RM, Roedersheimer R, DeWeese JA: Effects of aspirin and dipyridamole on expanded polytetrafluoroethylene graft patency. Surgery 92:1016, 1982.
149. Barbalinardo RJ, Citrin P, Franco CD, et al: A comparison of isobutyl 2-cyanoacrylate glue, fibrin adhesive, and oxidized regenerated cellulose for control of needle hole bleeding from polytetrafluoroethylene vascular prostheses. J Vasc Surg 4:220, 1986.
150. Miller CM, Sangiolo P, Jacobson JH II: Reduced anastomotic bleeding using new sutures with a needle-suture diameter ratio of one. Surgery 101:156, 1987.
151. Abbott WM, Green RM, Matsumoto T, et al: Prosthetic above-knee femoropopliteal bypass grafting: Results of a multicenter randomized prospective trial. J Vasc Surg 25:19–28, 1997.
152. Brewster DC, LaSalle AJ, Robison JG, et al: Factors affecting patency of femoropopliteal bypass grafts. Surg Gynecol Obstet 157:437, 1983.
153. Dale WA: Alternatives for femoropopliteal reconstruction. *In* Dale WA (ed): Management of Vascular Surgical Problems. New York, McGraw-Hill, 1985, pp 166–189.
154. Veith FJ, Moss CM, Sprayregen S, Montefusco C: Preoperative saphenous venography in arterial reconstructive surgery of the lower extremity. Surgery 85:253, 1979.
155. Brewster DC, LaSalle AJ, Robison JG, et al: Femoropopliteal graft failures: Clinical consequences and success of secondary reconstructions. Arch Surg 118:1043, 1983.
156. Graham JW, Lusby RJ: Infrapopliteal bypass grafting: Use of upper limb vein alone and in autogenous composite grafts. Surgery 91:646, 1982.
157. Harris RW, Andros F, Salles-Cunha SX, et al: Totally autogenous venovenous composite bypass grafts. Arch Surg 121:1128, 1986.
158. Taylor LM Jr, Edwards JM, Brant B, et al: Autogenous reversed vein bypass for lower extremity ischemia in patients with absent or inadequate greater saphenous vein. Am J Surg 153:505, 1987.
159. Edwards WS, Gerety E, Larkin J, et al: Multiple sequential femoral tibial grafting for severe ischemia. Surgery 80:722, 1976.
160. Jarrett F, Berkoff HA, Crummy AB, Belzer FO: Femorotibial bypass grafts with sequential technique. Arch Surg 116:709, 1981.
161. Flinn WR, Ricco JB, Yao JST, et al: Composite sequential grafts in severe ischemia: A comparative study. J Vasc Surg 1:449, 1984.
162. Dale WA, Pridgen WR, Shoulders HH Jr: Failure of composite (Teflon and vein) grafting in small human arteries. Surgery 51:258, 1962.
163. Hobson RW II, O'Donnell JA, Jamil Z, Mehta K: Below-knee bypass for limb salvage: Comparison of autogenous saphenous vein, polytetrafluoroethylene, and composite Dacron-autogenous vein grafts. Arch Surg 115:833, 1980.
164. Baker WH, Hadcock MM, Littooy FN: Management of polytetrafluoroethylene graft occlusions. Arch Surg 115:508, 1980.
165. Burnham SJ, Flanigan DP, Goodreau JJ, et al: Nonvein bypass in below-knee reoperation for lower limb ischemia. Surgery 84:417, 1978.
166. Linton RR, Wirthlin LS: Femoropopliteal composite Dacron and autogenous vein bypass grafts: A preliminary report. Arch Surg 107:748, 1973.
167. Lord JW Jr, Sadranagani B, Bajwa G, Rossi G: New technique for construction of composite Dacron vein grafts for femoro-distal popliteal bypass in the severely ischemic leg. Ann Surg 181:670, 1975.
168. LaSalle AJ, Brewster DC, Corson JD, Darling RC: Femoropopliteal composite bypass grafts: Current status. Surgery 92:36, 1982.
169. Snyder SO Jr, Gregory RT, Wheeler JR, Gayle RG: Composite grafts utilizing polytetrafluoroethylene-autogenous tissue for lower extremity arterial reconstructions. Surgery 90:881, 1981.
170. Wheeler JR, Gregory RT, Snyder SO Jr, Gayle RG: Gore-Tex autogenous vein composite grafts for tibial reconstruction. J Vasc Surg 1:914, 1984.
171. Lundqvist B, Bowald S, Eriksson I: Composite grafts for femorodistal bypass surgery. Acta Chir Scand 529(Suppl):69, 1985.
172. Scribner RG, Beare JP, Harris EJ, et al: Polytetrafluoroethylene vein composite grafts across the knee. Surg Gynecol Obstet 157:237, 1983.
173. Feinberg RL, Winter RP, Wheeler JR, et al: The use of composite grafts in femorocrural bypasses performed for limb salvage: A review of 108 consecutive cases and comparison with 57 in situ saphenous vein bypasses. J Vasc Surg 12:257–263, 1990.
174. Chang JB, Stein TA: The long-term value of composite grafts for limb salvage. J Vasc Surg 22:25–31, 1995.
175. Benedetti-Valentini F, Gossetti B, Irace I, et al: Composite grafts for critical ischemia. Cardiovasc Surg 3:372–376, 1996.
176. Karacagil S, Holmberg A, Narbani A, et al: Composite polytetrafluoroethylene/vein bypass grafts: Conventional distal vein segment or vein cuff? Eur J Vasc Endovasc Surg 12:337–341, 1996.
177. Landrey GL, Ramsey DE, Hodgson KJ, et al: Infrapopliteal bypass for severe ischemia: Comparison of autogenous vein, composite, and prosthetic grafts. J Vasc Surg 13:631–636, 1991.
178. Fichelle JM, Marzelle J, Colacchio G, et al: Infrapopliteal polytetrafluoroethylene and composite bypass: Factors influencing patency. Ann Vasc Surg 9:187–196, 1995.
179. McCarthy WJ, Pearce WH, Flinn WR, et al: Long-term evaluation of composite sequential bypass for limb-threatening ischemia. J Vasc Surg 15:761, 1992.
180. Verta MJ: Composite sequential bypasses to the ankle and beyond for limb salvage. J Vasc Surg 1:381, 1984.
181. Crawford ES: Thoraco-abdominal and abdominal aortic aneurysms involving renal, superior mesenteric, and celiac arteries. Ann Surg 179:763, 1974.
182. Brewster DC, Darling RC: Optimal methods of aortoiliac reconstruction. Surgery 84:739, 1978.
183. Brewster DC, Cooke JC: Longevity of aortofemoral bypass grafts. *In* Yao JST, Pearce WH (eds): Long-Term Results in Vascular Surgery. Norwalk, Conn, Appleton & Lange, 1993, pp 149–161.
184. Crawford ES, Bomberger RA, Glaeser DH, et al: Aortoiliac occlusive disease: Factors influencing survival and function following recon-

structive operation over a twenty five year period. Surgery 90:1055, 1981.
185. Szilagyi DE, Elliott JP Jr, Smith RF, et al: A thirty-year survey of the reconstructive surgical treatment of aortoiliac occlusive disease. J Vasc Surg 3:421, 1986.
186. Cronenwett JL: Factors influencing the long-term results of aortic aneurysm surgery. *In* Yao JST, Pearce WH (eds): Long-Term Results in Vascular Surgery. Norwalk, Conn, Appleton & Lange, 1993, pp 171–179.
187. Meadox Medical, personal communication.
188. Quarmby JW, Burnand KG, Lockhart SJ, et al: Prospective randomized trial of woven versus collagen-impregnated knitted prosthetic Dacron grafts in aortoiliac surgery. Br J Surg 85:775–777, 1998.
189. Veterans Administration Cooperative Study Group 141: Comparative evaluation of prosthetic, reversed, and in situ vein bypass grafts in distal popliteal and tibial-peroneal revascularization. Arch Surg 123:434, 1988.
190. Bennion RS, Williams RA, Stabile BE, et al: Patency of autogenous saphenous vein versus polytetrafluoroethylene grafts in femoropopliteal bypass for advanced ischemia of the extremity. Surg Gynecol Obstet 160:239, 1985.
191. Budd JS, Brennan J, Beard JD, et al: Infrainguinal bypass surgery: Factors determining late graft patency. Br J Surg 77:1382, 1990.
192. Weisel RD, Johnston KW, Baird RJ, et al: Comparison of conduits for leg revascularization. Surgery 89:8, 1981.
193. Bergan JJ, Veith FJ, Bernhard VM, et al: Randomization of autogenous vein and polytetrafluoroethylene grafts in femoro-distal reconstruction. Surgery 92:921, 1982.
194. Quiñones-Baldrich WJ, Martin-Paredero V, Baker JD, et al: Polytetrafluoroethylene grafts as first-choice arterial substitute in femoropopliteal revascularization. Arch Surg 119:1238, 1984.
195. Quiñones-Baldrich WJ, Busuttil RW, Baker JD, et al: Is the preferential use of polytetrafluoroethylene grafts for femoropopliteal bypass justified? J Vasc Surg 8:219, 1988.
196. O'Donnell TF, Farber SP, Richmond DM, et al: Above-knee polytetrafluoroethylene femoropopliteal bypass graft: Is it a reasonable alternative to the below-knee reversed autogenous vein graft? Surgery 94:26, 1983.
197. Rosen RC, Johnson WC, Bush HL, et al: Staged infrainguinal revascularization: Initial prosthetic above-knee bypass followed by a distal vein bypass for recurrent ischemia: A valid concept for extending limb salvage. Am J Surg 152:224, 1986.
198. Sterpetti AV, Schultz RD, Feldhaus RJ, Peetz DJ: Seven-year experience with polytetrafluoroethylene as above-knee femoropopliteal bypass graft: Is it worthwhile to preserve the autologous saphenous vein? J Vasc Surg 2:907, 1985.
199. Patterson RB, Fowl RJ, Kempczinski RF, et al: Preferential use of ePTFE for above-knee femoropopliteal bypass grafts. Ann Vasc Surg 4:338, 1990.
200. Prendiville EJ, Yeager A, O'Donnell TF, et al: Long-term results with above-knee popliteal expanded polytetrafluoroethylene graft. J Vasc Surg 11:517, 1990.
201. Budd JS, Langdon I, Brennan J, Bell PRF: Above-knee prosthetic grafts do not compromise the ipsilateral long saphenous vein. Br J Surg 78:1379, 1991.
202. Whittemore AD, Clowes AW, Couch NP, Mannick JA: Secondary femoropopliteal reconstruction. Ann Surg 193:35, 1982.
203. Edwards JM, Taylor LM, Porter JM: Treatment of failed lower extremity bypass grafts with new autogenous vein bypass grafting. J Vasc Surg 11:136, 1990.
204. Moore WS: The preferential use of PTFE for initial femoropopliteal bypass. *In* Veith FJ (ed): Current Critical Problems in Vascular Surgery. Vol 2. St. Louis, Quality Medical Publishing, 1990, pp 59–61.
205. Michaels JA: Choice of material for above-knee femoropopliteal bypass graft. Br J Surg 76:7, 1989.
206. Houser SL, Hashmi FH, Jaeger VJ, et al: Should the greater saphenous vein be preserved in patients requiring arterial outflow reconstruction in the lower extremity? Surgery 95:467, 1984.
207. Stephen M, Loewenthal J, Little JM, et al: Autogenous veins and velour Dacron in femoropopliteal arterial bypass. Surgery 81:314, 1977.
208. Christenson JT, Eklof B: Sparks mandril, velour Dacron and autogenous saphenous vein grafts in femoropopliteal bypass. Br J Surg 66:514, 1979.
209. Yashar JJ, Thompson R, Burnhard RJ, et al: Dacron vs vein for femoropopliteal arterial bypass. Arch Surg 116:1037, 1981.
210. Rosenthal D, Evans D, McKinsey J, et al: Prosthetic above-knee femoropopliteal bypass for intermittent claudication. J Cardiovasc Surg 31:462, 1990.
211. Pevec WC, Darling RC, L'Italien GJ, Abbott WM: Femoropopliteal reconstruction with knitted, non-velour Dacron versus expanded polytetrafluoroethylene. J Vasc Surg 16:60, 1992.
212. Pevec WC, Abbott WM: Femoropopliteal Dacron graft: Five- to ten-year patency. *In* Yao JST, Pearce WH (eds): Long-Term Results in Vascular Surgery. Norwalk, Conn, Appleton & Lange, 1993, pp 273–277.
213. Campbell CD, Brooks DH, Webster MW, et al: Expanded microporous polytetrafluoroethylene as a vascular substitute: A two-year follow-up. Surgery 85:177, 1979.
214. Veith FJ, Moss CM, Fell SC, et al: Comparison of expanded polytetrafluoroethylene and autologous saphenous vein grafts in high-risk arterial reconstructions for limb salvage. Surg Gynecol Obstet 147:749, 1978.
215. Haimov M, Giron F, Jacobson JH: The expanded polytetrafluoroethylene graft. Arch Surg 114:673, 1979.
216. Hallett JW, Brewster DC, Darling RC: The limitations of polytetrafluoroethylene in reconstruction of femoropopliteal and tibial arteries. Surg Gynecol Obstet 152:189, 1981.
217. Charlesworth PM, Brewster DC, Darling RC, et al: The fate of polytetrafluoroethylene grafts in lower limb bypass surgery: A six-year follow-up. Br J Surg 72:896, 1985.
218. Whittemore AD, Kent KC, Donaldson MC, et al: What is the proper role of polytetrafluoroethylene grafts in infrainguinal reconstruction? J Vasc Surg 10:299, 1989.
219. Davies MG, Feeley TM, O'Malley MK, et al: Infrainguinal polytetrafluoroethylene grafts: Saved limbs or wasted effort? A report on ten years' experience. Ann Vasc Surg 5:519, 1991.
220. Connolly JE, Kwan JHM, Brownell D, et al: Newer developments of extraanatomic bypass. Surg Gynecol Obstet 158:415, 1984.
221. Chang JB: Current status of extraanatomic bypasses. Am J Surg 152:202, 1986.
222. Garcia-Rinaldi R, Revuelta JM, Vaughan GD III, et al: The versatility of Gore-Tex grafts for extra-anatomic bypass. Vasc Surg 18:294, 1984.
223. Craido FJ: Extrathoracic management of aortic arch syndrome. Br J Surg 69(Suppl):45, 1982.
224. Ziomek S, Quiñones-Baldrich WJ, Busuttil RW, et al: The superiority of synthetic arterial grafts over autogenous veins in carotid-subclavian bypass. J Vasc Surg 3:140, 1986.
225. Perler BA, Williams GM: Carotid-subclavian bypass—a decade of experience. J Vasc Surg 12:716, 1990.
226. Langneau P, Michel JB, Charrat JM: Use of polytetrafluoroethylene grafts for renal bypass. J Vasc Surg 5:738, 1987.
227. Dale WA, Harris J, Terry RB: Polytetrafluoroethylene reconstruction of the inferior vena cava. Surgery, 95:625, 1984.
228. Chan EL, Bardin JA, Bernstein EF: Inferior vena cava bypass: Experimental evaluation of externally supported grafts and initial clinical application. J Vasc Surg 1:675, 1984.
229. Fujiwara Y, Cohn LH, Adams D, et al: Use of Gore-Tex grafts for replacement of the superior and inferior venae cavae. J Cardiovasc Surg 67:774, 1974.
230. Comerata AJ, Harwick RD, White JV: Jugular venous reconstruction: A technique to minimize morbidity of bilateral radical neck dissection. J Vasc Surg 3:322, 1986.
231. Norton L, Eiseman B: Replacement of portal vein during pancreatectomy for carcinoma. Surgery 77:280, 1975.
232. Sarfeh IJ, Rypins EB, Mason GR: A systematic appraisal of portacaval H-graft diameters. Clinical and hemodynamic perspectives. Ann Surg 204:356, 1986.
233. Robinson RJ, Peigh PS, Fiore AC, et al: Venous prostheses: Improved patency with external stents. J Surg Res 36:306, 1984.
234. Raju S: PTFE grafts for hemodialysis access: Techniques for insertion and management of complications. Ann Surg 206:666, 1987.
235. Palder SB, Kirkman RL, Whittemore AD, et al: Vascular access for hemodialysis. Patency rates and results of revision. Ann Surg 202:235, 1985.
236. Hurt AV, Batello-Cruz M, Skipper BJ, et al: Bovine carotid artery heterografts versus polytetrafluoroethylene grafts. A prospective randomized study. Am J Surg 146:844, 1983.

237. Taylor DEM: How may vascular grafts be modified to improve patency? *In* Greenhalgh RM, Jamieson W, Nicolaides AN (eds): Vascular Surgery: Issues in Current Practice. London, Grune & Stratton, 1986, pp 175–186.
238. Weinberg CB, Bell E: A blood vessel model constructed from collagen and cultured vascular cells. Science 231:397, 1986.
239. Mansfield PB: Tissue cultured endothelium for vascular prosthetic devices. Rev Surg 27:291, 1970.
240. Welch M, Durrans D, Car HMH, et al: Endothelial cell seeding: A review. Ann Vasc Surg 6:473, 1992.
241. Stansby G, Berwanger C, Shukla N, Hamilton G: Endothelial cell seeding of vascular grafts: Status and prospects. Cardiovasc Surg 5:543, 1994.
242. Herring MB, Gardiner A, Glover JL: A single-staged technique for seeding vascular grafts with autogenous endothelium. Surgery 84:498, 1978.
243. Herring MB, Baughman S, Glover JL, et al: Endothelial seeding of Dacron and polytetrafluoroethylene grafts: The cellular events of healing. Surgery 96:745, 1984.
244. Graham LM, Vinter DW, Ford JW, et al: Endothelial cell seeding of prosthetic vascular grafts—early experimental studies with cultured autologous canine endothelium. Arch Surg 115:929, 1980.
245. Graham LM, Burkel WE, Ford JW, et al: Expanded polytetrafluoroethylene vascular prostheses seeded with enzymatically derived and cultured endothelial cells. Surgery 91:550, 1982.
246. Stanley JC, Burkel WE, Ford JW, et al: Enhanced patency of small-diameter externally supported Dacron iliofemoral grafts seeded with endothelial cells. Surgery 92:994, 1982.
247. Clagett GP, Burkel WE, Sharefkin JB, et al: Platelet reactivity in vivo in dogs with arterial prostheses seeded with endothelial cells. Circulation 69:632, 1984.
248. Sicard GA, Allen BT, Long JA, et al: Prostaglandin production and platelet reactivity of small diameter grafts. J Vasc Surg 1:774, 1984.
249. Sharp WV, Schmidt SP, Donovan DL: Prostaglandin biochemistry of seeded endothelial cells on Dacron prostheses. J Vasc Surg 3:256, 1986.
250. Budd JS, Allen K, Hartley J, et al: Prostacyclin production from seeded prosthetic vascular grafts. Br J Surg 79:1151, 1992.
251. Smyth JV, Welch M, Carr HM, et al: Fibrinolysis profiles and platelet activation after endothelial cell seeding of prosthetic vascular grafts. Ann Vasc Surg 9:542, 1995.
252. Baitella-Eberle G, Groscurth P, Zilla P, et al: Long-term results of tissue development and cell differentiation on Dacron prostheses seeded with microvascular cells in dogs. J Vasc Surg 18:1019, 1993.
253. Birinyi LK, Douville EC, Lewis SA, et al: Increased resistance to bacteremic graft infection after endothelial cell seeding. J Vasc Surg 5:193, 1987.
254. Conte MS, Choudhry RP, Shirakowa M, et al: Endothelial cell seeding fails to attenuate intimal thickening in balloon-injured rabbit arteries. J Vasc Surg 21:413–421, 1995.
255. Jensen N, Lindblad B, Ljungberg J, et al: Early attachment of leukocytes, platelets and fibrinogen in endothelial-cell-seeded Dacron venous conduits. Br J Surg 84:52, 1997.
256. Jarrell BE, Williams SK, Stokes G, et al: Use of freshly isolated capillary endothelial cells for the immediate establishment of a monolayer on a vascular graft. Surgery 100:392, 1986.
257. Sterpetti AV, Hunter WJ, Schultz RD: Seeding with endothelial cells derived from the microvessels of the omentum and from the jugular vein: A comparative study. J Vasc Surg 7:677, 1988.
258. Rupnick MA, Hubbard FA, Pratt K, et al: Endothelialization of vascular prosthetic surfaces after seeding or sodding with human microvascular endothelial cells. J Vasc Surg 9:788, 1989.
259. Williams SK, Jarrell BE, Rose DG, et al: Human microvessel endothelial cell isolation and vascular graft sodding in the operating room. Ann Vasc Surg 3:146, 1989.
260. Rosenman JE, Kempczinski RF, Pearce WH, et al: Kinetics of endothelial cell seeding. J Vasc Surg 2:778, 1985.
261. Seeger JM: Improved endothelial cell seeding density after flow exposure in fibronectin-coated grafts. Surg Forum 36:450, 1985.
262. Seeger JM: Improved endothelial cell seeding efficiency with cultured cells and fibronectin coated grafts. J Surg Res 38:641, 1985.
263. Ramalanjaona G, Kempczinski RF, Rosenman JE, et al: The effect of fibronectin coating on endothelial cell kinetics in PTFE grafts. J Vasc Surg 3:264, 1986.
264. Herring MB, Gardner A, Glover JL: Seeding human arterial prostheses with mechanically derived endothelium: The detrimental effect of smoking. J Vasc Surg 2:279, 1984.
265. Herring MB, Baughman S, Glover JL: Endothelium develops on seeded arterial prosthesis. A brief clinical report. J Vasc Surg 2:727, 1985.
266. Ortenwall P, Wadenvik H, Kutti J, et al: Reduction in deposition of indium 111–labelled platelets after autologous endothelial cell seeding of Dacron aortic bifurcation grafts in humans: A preliminary report. J Vasc Surg 6:17, 1987.
267. Ortenwall P, Wadenvik H, Kutti J, et al: Endothelial cell seeding reduces thrombogenicity of Dacron grafts in humans. J Vasc Surg 11:403, 1990.
268. Ortenwall P, Wadenvik H, Risbert B: Reduced platelet deposition on seeded versus unseeded segments of expanded polytetrafluoroethylene grafts: Clinical observations after a 6 month follow-up. J Vasc Surg 10:374, 1989.
269. Herring MB, Compton RS, Legrand DR, et al: Endothelial seeding of polytetrafluoroethylene popliteal bypasses: A preliminary report. J Vasc Surg 6:114, 1987.
270. Zilla P, Fasol R, Deutsch M, et al: Endothelial cell seeding of polytetrafluoroethylene vascular grafts in humans: A preliminary report. J Vasc Surg 6:535, 1987.
271. Leseche G, Ohan J, Bouttier S, et al: Above-knee femoropopliteal bypass grafting using endothelial cell seeded PTFE grafts: Five-year clinical experience. Ann Vasc Surg 9(Suppl):S15–S23, 1995.
272. Walker MG, Thompson GJL, Shaw JW: Endothelial cell seeded versus non-seeded ePTFE grafts in patients with severe peripheral vascular disease: Preliminary results. *In* Zilla P, Fasol R, Deutsch M (eds): Endothelialization of Vascular Grafts. Basel, S Karger, 1987, pp 245–248.
273. Callow AD: The vascular endothelial cell as a vehicle for gene therapy. J Vasc Surg 11:793, 1990.
274. Stanley JC: Genetic manipulation of seeded endothelial cells in vascular prostheses. J Vasc Surg 13:736, 1991.
275. Kotnis RA, Thompson MM, Eady SL, et al: Attachment, replication and thrombogenicity of genetically modified endothelial cells. Eur J Vasc Endovasc Surg 9:335, 1995.
276. Bowald S, Busch C, Eriksson I: Arterial regeneration following polyglactin 910 suture mesh grafting. Surgery 86:722, 1979.
277. Greisler HP: Arterial regeneration over absorbable prostheses. Arch Surg 177:1425, 1982.
278. Greisler HP: Bioresorbable vascular grafts. *In* Greisler HP (ed): New Biologic and Synthetic Vascular Prostheses. Austin, Tex, RG Landes, 1991, pp 70–86.
279. Greisler HP, Endean ED, Klosak JJ, et al: Polyglactin 910/polydioxanone biocomponent totally resorbable vascular prostheses. J Vasc Surg 7:697, 1988.
280. Van der Lei B, Nieuwenhuis P, Molenaar I, Wildevuur CR: Long-term biologic fate of neoarteries regenerated in microporous, compliant, biodegradable, small-caliber vascular grafts in rats. Surgery 101:459, 1987.
281. Galletti PM, Aebischer P, Sashen HF, et al: Experience with fully bioresorbable aortic grafts in the dog. Surgery 103:231, 1988.
282. Clark RE, Margraff HW: Antibacterial vascular grafts with improved thromboresistance. Arch Surg 109:159, 1974.
283. Harvey RA, Alcid DV, Greco RS: Antibiotic bonding to polytetrafluoroethylene with tridodecylmethylammonium chloride. Surgery 92:504, 1982.
284. Greco RS, Harvey RA: The role of antibiotic bonding in the prevention of vascular prosthetic infection. Ann Surg 195:168, 1982.
285. Greco RS, Harvey RA, Smilow PC, et al: Prevention of vascular prosthetic infection by a benzalkonium-oxacillin–bonded polytetrafluoroethylene graft. Surg Gynecol Obstet 155:28, 1982.
286. White JV, Benvenisty A: Simple methods for direct antibiotic protection of synthetic vascular grafts. J Vasc Surg 1:372, 1984.
287. Webb LX, Myers RT, Cordell AR, et al: Inhibition of bacterial adhesion by antibacterial surface pretreatment of vascular prostheses. J Vasc Surg 4:16, 1986.
288. Shue WB, Worosilo SC, Donetz AP, et al: Prevention of vascular prosthetic infection with an antibiotic-bonded Dacron graft. J Vasc Surg 8:600, 1988.
289. Modak SM, Sampath L, Fox CL Jr, et al: A new method for the direct incorporation of antibiotic in prosthetic vascular grafts. Surg Gynecol Obstet 164:143, 1987.

290. Moore WS, Chvapil M, Seiffert G, Development of an infection resistant vascular prosthesis. Arch Surg 116:1403, 1981.
291. Torsello G, Sandmann W, Ghert A, et al: In situ replacement of infected vascular prosthesis with rifampin-soaked vascular grafts: Early results. J Vasc Surg 17:768, 1993.
292. Naylor AR, Clark S, London NJM, et al: Treatment of major aortic graft infection: Preliminary experience with total graft excision and in situ replacement with a rifampicin bonded prosthesis. Eur J Vasc Endovasc Surg 9:252, 1995.
293. Lachapelle K, Graham AM, Symes JF: Antibacterial activity, antibiotic retention, and infection resistance of a rifampin-impregnated gelatin-sealed Dacron graft. J Vasc Surg 19:675, 1994.
294. Torsello G, Sandmann W: Use of antibiotic-bonded grafts in vascular graft infection. Eur J Vasc Endovasc Surg 14(Suppl A):84, 1997.
295. Gupta AK, Bandyk DF, Johnson BL: In situ repair of mycotic abdominal aortic aneurysms with rifampin-bonded gelatin-impregnated Dacron grafts: A preliminary case report. J Vasc Surg 24:472, 1996.
296. Gott VL, Whiffen JD, Dutton RC: Heparin bonding on colloidin graphite surfaces. Science 142:1927, 1963.
297. Esquivel CO, Bjorck C-G, Bergentz S-E, et al: Reduced thrombogenic characteristics of expanded polytetrafluoroethylene and polyurethane arterial grafts after heparin bonding. Surgery 95:102, 1984.
298. Greisler HP, Klosak JJ, Dennis JW, et al: Biomaterial pretreatment with ECGF to augment endothelial cell proliferation. J Vasc Surg 2:393, 1987.
299. Berceli SA, Phaneuf MD, LoGerfo FW: Evaluation of a novel hirudin-coated polyester graft to physiologic flow conditions: Hirudin bioavailability and thrombin uptake. J Vasc Surg 27:1117, 1998.
300. Geeraert AJ, Callaghan JC: Experimental study of selected small calibre arterial grafts. J Cardiovasc Surg 18:155, 1977.
301. Cronenwett JL, Zelenock GB: Alternative small arterial grafts. *In* Stanley JC (ed): Biologic and Synthetic Vascular Prostheses. New York, Grune & Stratton, 1982, pp 595–620.
302. Yeager A, Callow AD: New graft materials and current approaches to an acceptable small diameter vascular graft. Trans Am Soc Artif Organs 34:88, 1988.
303. White RA, White EW, Hanson EL, et al: Preliminary report: Evaluation of tissue ingrowth into experimental replamineform vascular prostheses. Surgery 79:229, 1976.
304. White RA, Klein SR, Shors EC: Preservation of compliance in a small diameter microporous, silicon rubber vascular prosthesis. J Cardiovasc Surg 28:485, 1987.
305. Sawyer PN, Sophie Z, O'Shaughnessy A: Vascular prostheses: Innovative properties. *In* Kambic HE, Kantrowitz A, Sung P (eds): Vascular Graft Update: Safety and Performance. ASTM Special Technical Publication No. 898. Philadelphia, American Society of Testing and Materials, 1986, pp 290–305.
306. Haubold A: Carbon in prosthetics. Ann N Y Acad Sci 283:383, 1977.
307. Sharp WV, Teague PC, Scott DL: Thromboresistance of pyrolytic carbon grafts. Trans Am Soc Artif Organs 24:223, 1978.
308. Scott SM, Gaddy LR, Parra S: Pyrolytic carbon-coated vascular prostheses. J Surg Res 29:395, 1980.
309. Bacourt F and Associates, Universitaire de Recherche en Chirurgie: Prospective randomized study of carbon-impregnated polytetrafluoroethylene grafts for below-knee popliteal and distal bypass: Results of 2 years. Ann Vasc Surg 11:596, 1997.

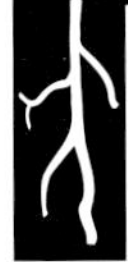

CHAPTER 38

Endovascular Grafts

Geoffrey H. White, M.D.,
and James May, M.D.

Endovascular grafts are transluminally implanted vascular devices that combine a "prosthetic" fabric with a vascular stent and are designed for use as a less invasive treatment of aneurysmal and atherosclerotic vascular diseases. They represent a natural outgrowth of the techniques developed for vascular stents and transluminal endovascular interventions. The principal application, to date, has been in treatment of aortic aneurysms in patients at high risk. The advantages of the technique are related to the absence of surgical exposure of the aorta and avoidance of aortic cross-clamping. Rapid progress has seen endovascular grafts being applied to many other common problems in vascular surgery, including thoracic aneurysms, anastomotic and false aneurysms, aortic dissections, peripheral aneurysms, arterial occlusive disease, and vascular trauma (Table 38–1). These less invasive techniques have the potential to reduce the mortality and morbidity associated with conventional open repair procedures and offer the opportunity to treat patients with severe coexisting diseases or risk factors.

OVERVIEW

Nomenclature

The term *endovascular graft* has come to denote a transluminally placed vascular prosthesis, usually a vascular prosthetic fabric and one or several vascular stents. Essential elements in this new technology have been the introduction of the graft device into the vascular system via a remote, usually easily accessible, site such as the femoral artery, and the implantation of the graft within the vessel lumen (as opposed to the conventional surgical methods of sutured end-to-end or end-to-side anastomosis). Functional specifications for an optimal device vary, depending on the lesion and the anatomic site.

Commonly used terms have included (1) "endovascular graft," (2) "endoluminal graft," (3) "stent-graft," (4) "stented graft," (5) "transluminal graft," (6) "transluminally placed endovascular graft" (TPEG), (7) "covered stent," and (8)

TABLE 38–1. APPLICATIONS OF ENDOVASCULAR GRAFTS

1. Aneurysms
   a. Abdominal aortic aneurysms
   b. Thoracic aortic aneurysms
   c. Iliac aneurysms
   d. Popliteal and other peripheral aneurysms
   e. Anastomotic aneurysms
2. Traumatic arteriovenous fistulae and false aneurysms
3. Peripheral vascular occlusive disease
4. Aortic dissection
5. Venous occlusion and portal hypertension (TIPS)
6. Nonvascular applications

TIPS = transjugular intrahepatic portosystemic shunt.

"coated stent." The terminology is very likely to evolve, reflecting more accurately the nature of various devices as technologic advances continue to be made.

History

The concept of internal repair of blood vessels by transluminal structural reinforcement or splinting is nearly 30 years old and has been credited to Dotter, who experimented with coiled springs and similar devices in benchtop and animal studies.[1] Initial clinical work addressed the internal support of stenosed or occluded arteries by vascular stents used in conjunction with balloon angioplasty techniques. Balloon-expanded and self-expanding variations of vascular stent designs were developed.[2–4]

The use of vascular stents as an intraluminal attachment mechanism for prosthetic vascular grafts was investigated in animal experiments during the 1980s.[5, 6] Parodi recognized the potential for stent-graft combination devices for repair of aneurysms and published the first report of clinical success in 1991.[7] Volodos and coworkers, in Russia, were apparently trialing endovascular devices in the aorta at the same time.[8] Early devices were custom made; a conventional vascular graft was sutured to an arterial stent before it was compressed and placed into the aorta via a catheter introduced through the femoral artery.[9–11] The technology has developed rapidly, and a number of commercial devices have been developed that are currently in various stages of clinical trial or marketing. All current systems of endovascular grafting rely on some form of arterial stent or wireform framework for graft attachment (Fig. 38–1).

Balloon-Expanded Devices

Endoluminal grafts can be divided into two groups according to whether they are deployed by balloon expansion or by a self-expanding stent. Current vascular stents are constructed of stainless steel, elgiloy, tantalum, or nitinol. Grafts based on each form of stent were developed in parallel, but it is instructive to trace the history of each device.

In 1991, Dr. Juan Parodi of Beunos Aires ignited the imagination of many vascular surgeons when he reported the results of the first clinical use of transfemoral endovascular grafting to exclude aortic aneurysms in humans.[7] His innovation was the concept that balloon-deployed vascular stents could be used in place of sutures to secure the proximal and distal ends of a fabric graft within the lumen of the aorta to "exclude" the aneurysm from the circulation. He successfully treated four patients with his device, which was made of a modified, large Palmaz stent sutured to a thin-walled, crimped polyester (Dacron) graft, the entire device then being deployed into the aorta with a 23-mm valvuloplasty balloon via a 22 French (Fr.) sheath (Fig. 38–2). In the first three patients, the graft was anchored only by a proximal stent positioned in the aortic neck below the renal arteries. In one of these patients, Parodi noted a large reflux of blood flow around the distal aspect of the graft, back into the aneurysm sac. This convinced him that a distal stent was also required to fix the graft against the aortic wall near the aortic bifurcation.

Experience in these early cases generated several observations: (1) precise preoperative measurement of the aortic anatomy was important, (2) it was necessary to have adequate lengths of proximal and distal "neck" for attachment and fixation of the tube portion of endoluminal graft, and (3) narrow or tortuous iliac arteries presented difficulties of access. Parodi also raised important questions about the fate of the aneurysm after it was excluded and the natural history of patent lumbar or mesenteric arteries that had been excluded by the graft. In addition, the risk of embolization of thrombotic material as a result of manipulation of guide wires and sheaths was highlighted.[10]

Other balloon-expandable stent-grafts were developed, most utilizing Palmaz stents in conjunction with polyester or polytetrafluoroethylene (PTFE) material.[12–14] These were generally improvised devices constructed in the operating room and often had an aortouni-iliac configuration. One exception was the White-Yu endovascular graft, which fea-

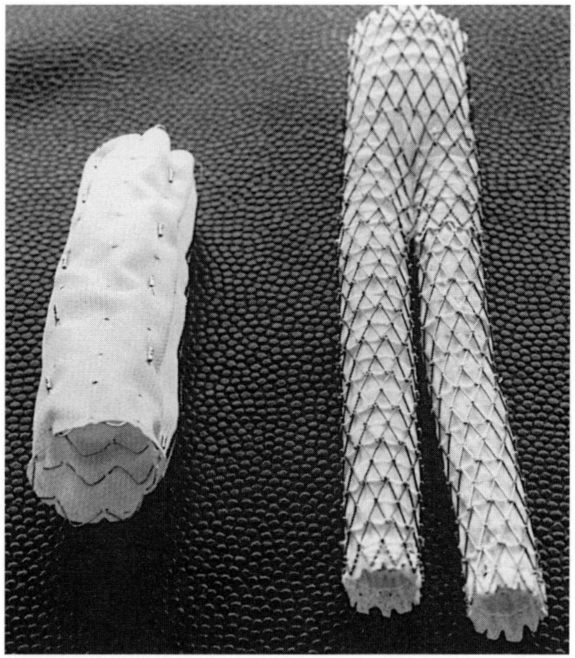

FIGURE 38–1. Two designs of prosthetic graft used for endovascular repair of abdominal aortic aneurysms. The tube graft on the left is deployed by balloon expansion of stent-like wireforms within its wall, whereas the bifurcated graft on the right is deployed and supported by a self-expanding stent framework.

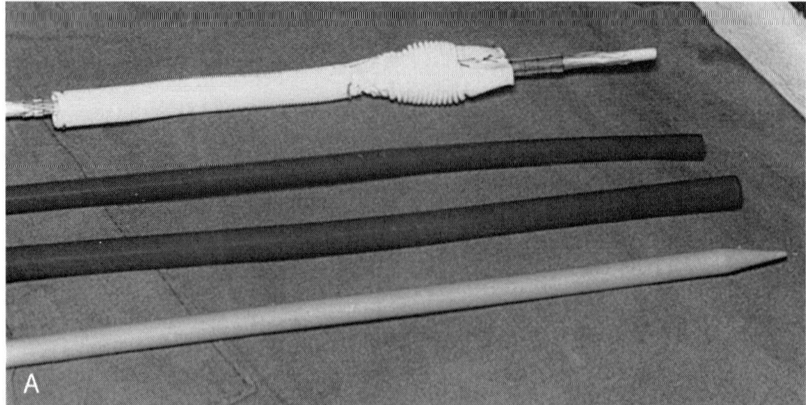

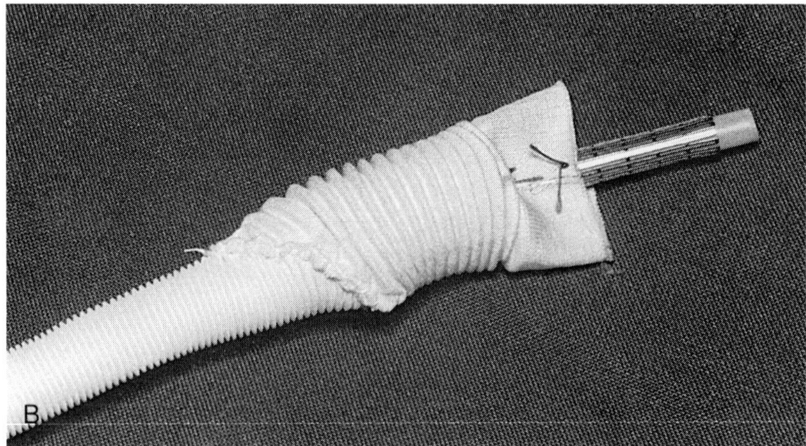

FIGURE 38–2. Modified Parodi endovascular graft technique for endovascular repair of abdominal aortic aneurysm. *A,* The tapered graft used for aorto-iliac configuration with a proximal and distal stent is shown beside the large-diameter sheath and introducing trocar used in early cases. *B,* A close-up view of the top end of the same graft showing the method of attaching the stent to the graft by simple sutures. The first part of the graft is made of a highly compliant material that expands to the size of the stent. Distal to it are segments of conventional crimp graft formed in a tapered configuration.

tured an intermittent stainless steel wireform interwoven with the graft material, in lieu of the vascular stent.[15]

Self-Expanding Devices

Dotter has been credited with developing the first arterial stent designed for insertion through a remote artery. A simple expansile coil, it was plagued by low expansion ratios and episodes of thrombosis.[1] This device was improved somewhat by taking advantage of the special thermal properties of nitinol. The nitinol coil stent was introduced in a cooled system as a straight wire. Once in the bloodstream, and warmed, it expanded to its preformed diameter in the coil shape. In a dog, a tightly wound version of this stent was found to limit extravasation of blood enough to permit healing of an experimental traumatic aneurysm, the first case of endoluminal aneurysm repair from a remote site. Another helical stent developed by Maas was capable of expanding to aortic diameters.[16] Maas successfully implanted helical stents in dogs and calves and proposed that a stent could be combined with a microporous synthetic fabric to serve as a barrier.

Balko and coworkers can probably be credited with the first experimental use of a stent-graft combination for the treatment of artificial aneurysm.[5] In their experiments, a novel form of nitinol, the Z-stent, was combined with a sleeve of polyurethane and tested in a sheep model of aortic aneurysm. The first radiographically guided aortic graft implantations were reported by Lawrence and coworkers, in 1987.[17] They used a chain of stainless steel Gianturco Z-stents within a tube of woven polyester. This stent-graft combination was implanted in the abdominal aortas of six dogs and the thoracic aortas of three others. At follow-up, after 7 to 35 weeks, all but one graft remained patent, although stenosis had developed in two. Graft stenosis and occlusion was thought to be largely due to folding and kinking of the inelastic fabric. Upon explanation, all grafts were found to be lined by a layer of endothelial cells and incorporated into the surrounding arteries by fibrosis of varying degrees.

In an effort to avoid graft stenosis and occlusion, a knitted nylon-Lycra combination fabric was substituted for the woven polyester graft of the earlier experiments. The new prosthesis was implanted transfemorally using percutaneous technique, in both normal canine aortas and a canine model of aortic aneurysm. All but one of the grafts in the latter series were patent at 6 months, but so were the adjacent side branches, owing to the porosity of the knitted fabric. Only one prosthesis carried barbs; the others had an entire stent protruding from the proximal end of the graft to act as an anchor. The single case of migration involved an unbarbed prosthesis. An interesting finding was the proliferation of granulation and connective tissue between the endovascular graft and the aortic wall.

These stent-graft combinations led to the development of several similar devices, notably the endovascular grafts used by Dake and Lawrence-Brown and their respective coworkers.[18–21] In Dake's system, which was used to treat thoracic aortic aneurysms, a self-expanding endoskeleton was fashioned that linked Gianturco Z-stents to one another with loops of suture,[18] whereas Mirich's group had joined their stents with metal struts,[6] and Lawrence-Brown sutured the stents independently to the graft wall, interspersed by a small gap.[20] Another system that relied on self-expanding Z-stents appears to have been developed independently in Russia; although in the majority of cases, the prosthesis was placed directly into the artery after conventional surgical exposure and control.[8] The importance of arterial stents in the development of endovascular grafting is illustrated by the evolution of the Lazarus device from a reliance on staples, which were neither sufficiently secure nor sufficiently hemostatic, to the use of a self-expanding stent, like that in the Guidant/EndoVascular Technologies (EVT, Menlo Park, Calif.) device.[22–24]

TYPES OF ENDOVASCULAR GRAFT DEVICES

There are two general groups of devices (Table 38–2), covered stents and stent-grafts. Covered stents, or coated stents, are single stent devices in which the internal or external walls are covered by a prosthetic graft barrier material. These are typically short, cylindrical tubes that look much like a vascular stent. Stent-graft devices are endovascular or endoluminal devices fixed by a stent at both ends or supported by multiple stents along their length. They may be tubular, tapered, or bifurcated, and many designs are modular, having multiple component pieces (Fig. 38–3).

Covered Stents

The simplest forms of stented grafts can be created by applying a covering of prosthetic graft to a single balloon-expandable or self-expanding stent.[25, 26] These types of covered stents were first made by suturing a segment of thin-walled PTFE graft to a Palmaz stent and were used to treat false aneurysms of peripheral arteries (Fig. 38–4).[26–30] Similar devices based on other stents are useful for treating traumatic lesions of small or medium-sized peripheral vessels.[31, 32] If the covered stent is deployed by balloon, the graft coating alters the expansile behavior of the stent; with this type of device, the balloon used for expansion should actually be slightly shorter than the stent itself.[33] The central portion of the stent is deployed first; then, the ends are fully expanded. If the stent is deployed in the conventional fashion (i.e., with a balloon longer than the stent), the ends flare first, the sutures break, and the graft material is compressed inward toward the central portion of the stent, leaving most of the stent bare.

TABLE 38–2. VARIATIONS OF ENDOVASCULAR GRAFT TECHNOLOGY

Single stent with prosthetic or autogenous barrier layer
Covered stent
Coated stent
Autologous tissue–stent combinations
Multiple stent with prosthetic graft layer
End-fixation stent grafts
Fully supported stent-grafts
Modular, multisegment stent-grafts

Covered stents are sometimes also referred to as *coated stents,* but this term is confusing, since coating the bare struts of metallic stents with various materials such as heparin is now being tried. In these instances, the apertures between the struts are not covered. A further complication arises from the fact that one method of applying thin, prosthetic, expansile coverings to stents now involves dipping the stents into a liquid form of the material, which then coats the struts and fills in the apertures.

Commercial versions of covered stents have been available in Europe and Australia for some time and are undergoing evaluation trials in the United States. Most are self-expanding nitinol devices covered with polyester (Fig. 38–5). This device can be deployed percutaneously through a 12 Fr. sheath into vessels with diameters up to 14 mm, to treat aneurysms of the peripheral circulation without the need for surgical access. Covered stents rely on friction for fixation.

Stent-Grafts

Typical end-supported stent-graft devices use balloon-expandable or self-expanding stents as anchoring mechanisms at the ends of graft material.[34, 35] In this sense, the stents act as a substitute for the surgical anastomosis, leaving unsupported graft material between the various attachment devices (Fig. 38–6). This method was described in initial reports of endovascular therapy for abdominal aortic aneurysms (AAAs) by Parodi and coworkers[7] and has been used for occlusive disease as well.

Problems with rotation, twisting, or kinking of unsupported parts of the endograft[35, 36] have inspired the majority of designs that now feature full-length support along the graft fabric with multiple stents or a continuous pattern of stent wireform. These grafts are available in both tube and bifurcated versions.

Modular Endovascular Grafts

Implanting a bifurcated graft inside the aorta via remote access presents problems of manipulating the two graft limbs into the iliac arteries. To date, two main techniques have been used.

1. Single-piece bifurcated grafts, such as the EVT endograft[24] and the Chuter device,[11] feature a single-piece bifurcated graft, which is initially introduced into the aorta, one limb ("the contralateral limb") being manipulated into position by guide wires and pull wires directed across the aortic bifurcation by conventional interventional techniques.
2. Modular bifurcated grafts are two- or three-piece designs. The various component grafts are overlapped within the aorta or iliac arteries to construct the bifurcated configuration (Fig. 38–7). The second iliac limb is inserted by separate contralateral femoral artery access via antegrade puncture. Modular designs allow some degree of customization of graft component length and diameter to an individual patient's anatomy. Differences between single-piece and modular designs of bifurcated grafts are presented in Table 38–3.

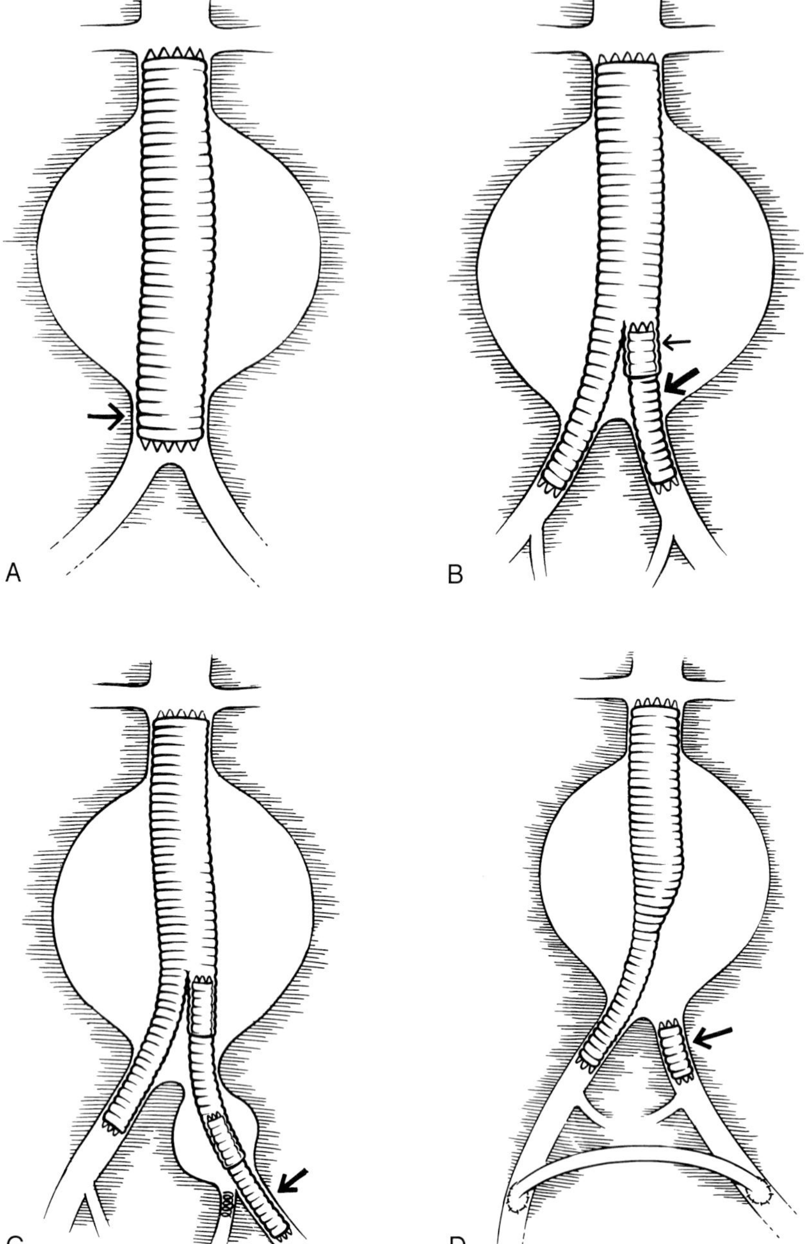

FIGURE 38–3. Four major forms of endovascular graft are used for endovascular repair of abdominal aortic aneurysms: tube grafts, bifurcated grafts, bifurcated grafts with iliac extension limbs, and aortomonoiliac grafts. *A,* The tube, or straight, graft configuration may be used in patients whose aneurysm has a well-formed distal neck, or "cuff" *(arrow)*, above the aortic bifurcation. This configuration is well suited to anastomotic aneurysms and saccular aneurysms. *B,* Configuration of bifurcated endovascular graft. Here, a modular design is shown; the contralateral iliac graft limb *(thick arrow)* is deployed separately by overlap within the stump of the main graft trunk *(thin arrow)*. *C,* Configuration of bifurcated endovascular graft with additional iliac extension graft limb. This configuration is used for an iliac artery aneurysm associated with an abdominal aortic aneurysm. The extension limb *(arrow)* is overlapped within the bifurcated graft components, and retrograde blood flow from the internal iliac artery back into the iliac aneurysm is prevented by implantation of embolization coils. *D,* Configuration of aortomonoiliac graft. In general, a tapered graft is used with distal deployment into the most favorable iliac artery. The contralateral common iliac artery is blocked by an occluder *(arrow)*. Blood flow to the contralateral leg is reestablished by a surgical femorofemoral bypass graft.

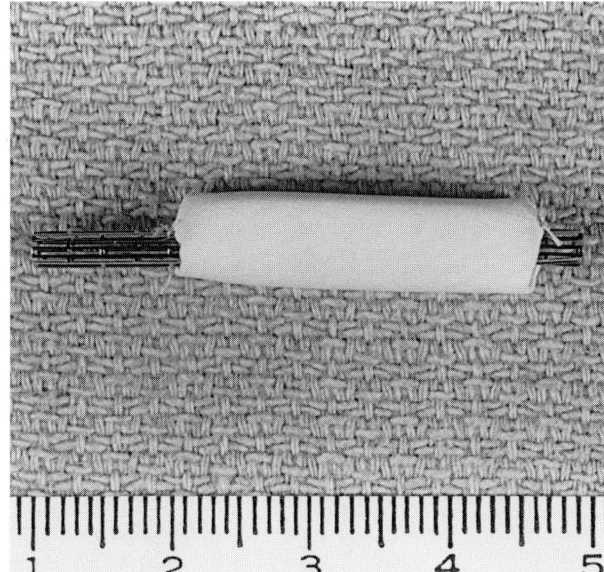

FIGURE 38–4. Basic form of covered stent. A segment of a 6-mm-diameter polytetrafluoroethylene graft has been sutured to the other surface of a Palmaz stent.

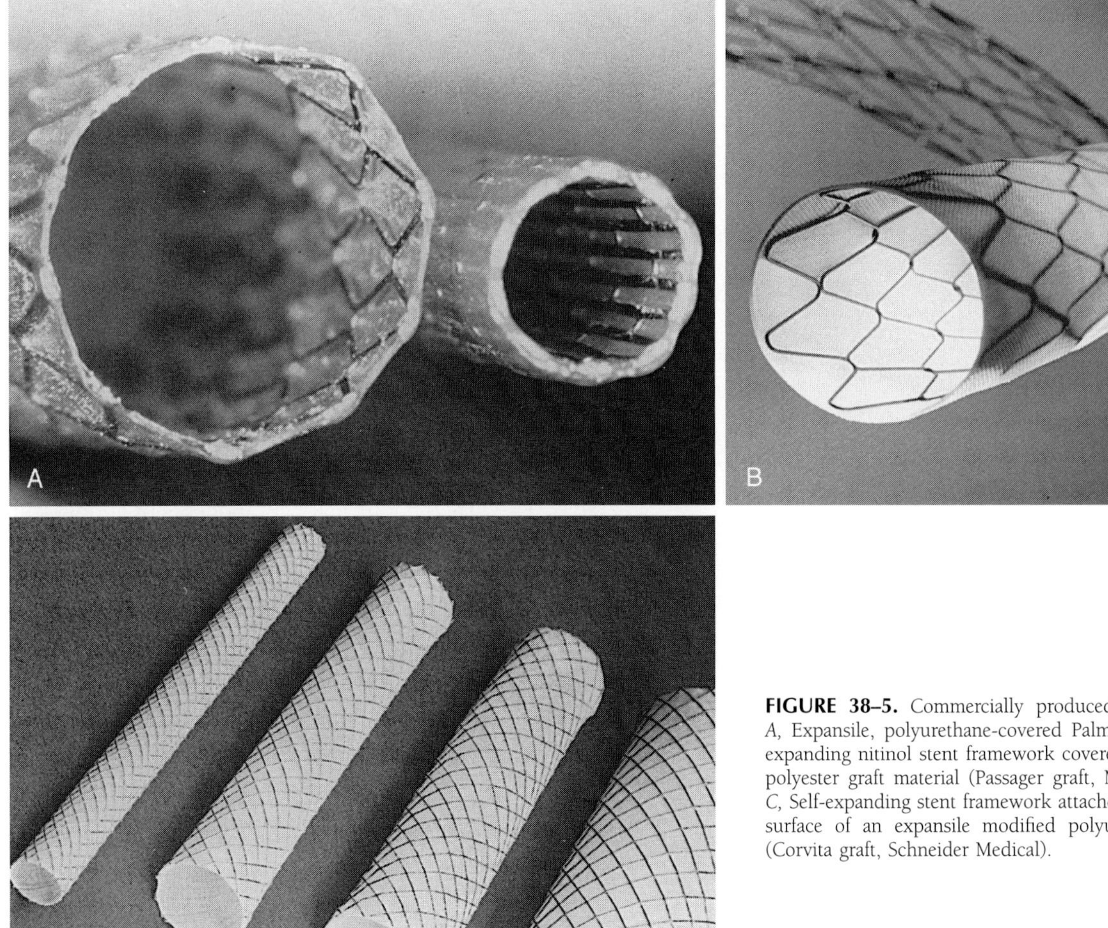

FIGURE 38–5. Commercially produced covered stents. *A*, Expansile, polyurethane-covered Palmaz stent. *B*, Self-expanding nitinol stent framework covered by thin-walled polyester graft material (Passager graft, Meadox Medical). *C*, Self-expanding stent framework attached to the external surface of an expansile modified polyurethane material (Corvita graft, Schneider Medical).

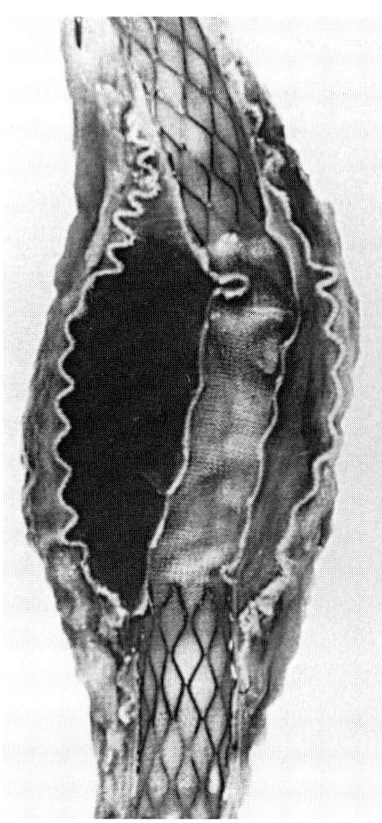
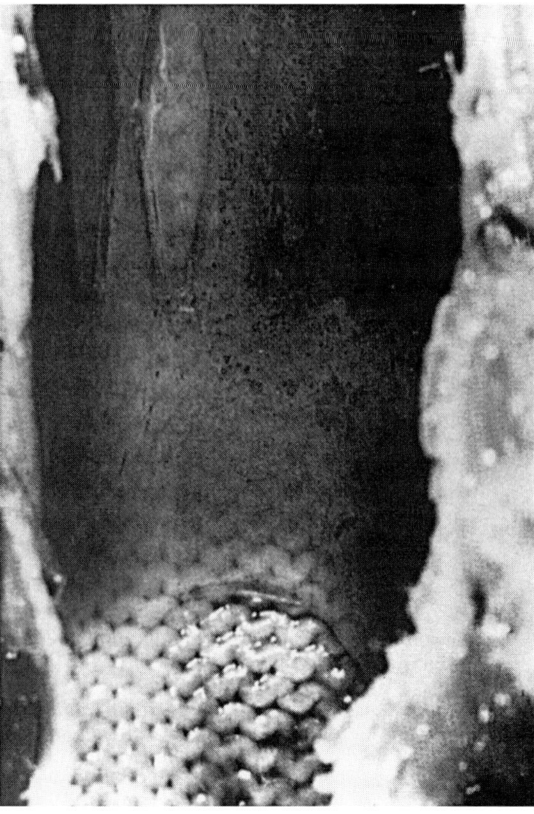

FIGURE 38–6. End-supported stent graft. Shown is the original Parodi stent graft, featuring a polyester graft fabric supported at each end by a Palmaz stent. The view on the *left* illustrates the tendency of nonsupported segments of the graft wall to kink or narrow; the close-up view on the right shows formation of neointima over the prosthetic fabric.

Modular component devices now include the Vanguard[37, 38] (Meadox Medical, Oakland, N.J.), AneuRx[39] (Medtronic, Eden Prairie, Minn.), Baxter[40] (Baxter Healthcare, Irvine, Calif.) and Talent[41] (World Medical Manufacturing, Miami, Fla.) endografts. All these devices are currently in clinical trials in the United States, and their designs involve both modularity and a metallic internal stent support (endoskeleton) or external stent (exoskeleton). The Talent and Vanguard endografts have an uncovered proximal stent, which affords the possibility of implantation over the renal arteries. Although this remains a controversial issue, such an approach may be beneficial when a short proximal neck makes attachment of more conventional endografts potentially less reliable.

TABLE 38–3. COMPARISON OF SINGLE-PIECE AND MODULAR BIFURCATED ENDOVASCULAR GRAFTS

SINGLE-PIECE	MODULAR (MULTIPIECE)
Complex graft construction and delivery system	Simple graft components and delivery system
Graft dimensions determined at time of manufacture	Customized graft component selection may be available at time of procedure
Requires preliminary insertion of iliac crossover catheter	Requires guide wire access to the contralateral graft stump to place iliac limb
Single-piece construction eliminates potential for leak or graft failure	Potential for leakage, disconnection, or stenosis at graft overlap zone
Difficult to deliver fully stented; may require additional stents implanted into graft limbs	Can be delivered as a fully supported stent-graft

Modified from Chuter TAM: Chuter-Gianturco bifurcated stent-grafts for abdominal aortic aneurysm exclusion. *In* Hopkinson B, Yusuf W, Whitaker S, Veith F (eds): Endovascular Surgery for Aortic Aneurysms. London, WB Saunders, 1997, pp 88–104.

COMPONENTS OF ENDOVASCULAR DEVICES

Table 38–4 lists the four main components of endovascular graft device systems:

TABLE 38–4. COMPONENTS OF ENDOVASCULAR GRAFT SYSTEMS

1. Delivery and deployment catheters and sheaths
2. Graft fabric materials
3. Graft attachment systems
   a. Self-expanding stents
   b. Balloon-expanded stents
   c. Integrated wireforms
   d. Hooks, barbs, anchors
   e. Others
4. Accessories
   Guide wires
   Balloons
   Angiocatheters
   Access sheaths
   Snares
   Guiding catheters
   Power injector
   Intravascular ultrasound catheters

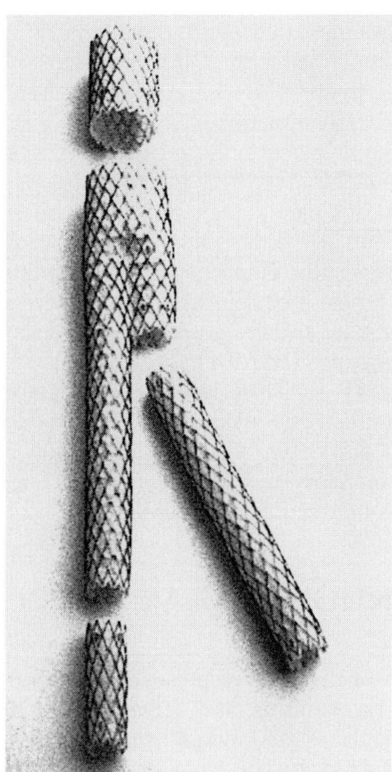

FIGURE 38–7. Modular bifurcated graft concept. The basic graft structure can be modified by proximal graft cuffs or by distal graft extensions to adapt the graft to the individual patient's anatomy.

- Delivery system
- Prosthetic graft fabric
- Stent or anchoring system
- Accessory guide wires, balloons, and special interventional catheters

Delivery Systems

The methods of delivering and deploying an endovascular graft have included simple sheaths and trocars, deployment capsules, and retractable covers. These introducer sheaths and delivery catheters must be narrow enough to pass through the access vessels without causing dissection or perforation, rigid enough to resist kinking, and flexible enough to follow the angulations and twists of diseased iliac arteries and other conduits. A major requirement of the delivery system is that it have a valve system or other extremely efficient hemostatic mechanism.

Fabrics

The graft material must be strong enough to resist late deterioration yet thin enough to compress within the narrow sheath of the delivery system. There is thus strong impetus to develop thin-walled materials whose strength is comparable to that of grafts currently used in open surgery. To date, conventional polyester (Dacron) has been preferred for endovascular grafts used in aneurysm repair, although many designs have already tried thinner polyester variations. PTFE has been tested mainly in grafts used for peripheral vessel trauma or occlusive disease, although some companies are now developing PTFE grafts for endovascular repair of AAAs. Other materials, such as polyurethane, polycarbonate, and other polymers are also under investigation.

Attachment Systems

It seems axiomatic that the attachment of the graft to the vessell wall must be as secure as a sutured anastomosis; however, this may not necessarily be true in all situations, since the graft is implanted in an intact vessel. To date, attachment and fixation systems have, in the main, been variations of self-expanding or balloon-expanded stents, which are designed to form a friction seal inside the arterial wall, in many cases aided by series of hooks or barbs. It has been conjectured that organic glues or mechanical stapling systems may also prove valuable.

It should be noted that the ability of a stent to provide long-term attachment of a prosthetic graft to the aorta remains unproven. Detachment from the aortic neck has been reported in several series, often 1 to 3 years after implantation. Whether stent fixation will be secure against the dynamic stresses and hemodynamic forces of the living human aorta and cyclical blood flow will be determined only by closely monitored prospective studies.

Deployment Accessories

Standard tools of endovascular surgery and interventional radiology are essential accessory devices for successful endovascular graft procedures. Principal amongst these are state-of-the-art guide wires (floppy to "super-stiff"), dilatation balloons, guiding catheters of numerous configurations, angiographic catheters, and snares. A list of the additional equipment and accessories required for endovascular graft procedures is presented in Table 38–5.

BIOLOGICAL RESPONSE TO ENDOVASCULAR GRAFTS

The healing response and other biologic reactions to endoluminal grafts appear to be quite different when compared

TABLE 38–5. ADDITIONAL EQUIPMENT FOR ENDOVASCULAR GRAFT PROCEDURES

1. Fluoroscope with digital angiography capabilities
   a. C-arm or fixed unit
   b. Cine-loop recording and image-recall facility desirable
2. Power injector
   a. Recommended for intraoperative and completion fluoroscopy studies
   b. Radiopaque vascular contrast media
3. Radiopaque (centimeter) ruler or marker board
4. Guide wires
   a. A selection of guide wires of adequate lengths (140–260 cm), including Amplatz Super-Stiff (0.035- or 0.038-inch diameter), Terumo hydrophilic non-kink guide wires, Bentson 0.035-inch wires
5. Angioplasty balloons
6. Angiocatheters, access sheaths, and guiding catheters
   a. Assorted diameters and shapes
7. Snares
8. Intravascular ultrasound catheters and machine
   a. Optional, for selected cases only

to standard vascular bypass grafts. Contradictory findings have been demonstrated in animal studies examining the cellular responses to intraluminal stent-grafts. Weatherford and colleagues have shown that intra-arterial PTFE stent-grafts placed after balloon injury to the vessel exhibited significantly greater endothelialization and less intimal hyperplasia as compared with conventional interposition graft.[42] Ohki and coworkers also found that intraluminal placement enhanced endothelialization of PTFE grafts but resulted in greater anastomotic intimal hyperplasia at the distal stent "anastomosis."[43] In comparison to bare stents, both nitinol stents covered with Dacron[44] and Palmaz stents covered with PTFE[45] showed increased neointimal development in the graft, as compared with the bare stent. The neointimal formation proceeded from the ends toward the center of the covered stents with minimal transgraft tissue penetration, and early thrombus formation at the stent-graft interface appeared to promote neointimal development.[45] In dogs with aortic aneurysms created by vein patch aortoplasty, stent-graft struts were incorporated into an elastin-poor, collagen-rich neointima. Laminated thrombus formed in the aneurysm sac, but microscopic evidence of thrombus recanalization developed.[46] It should be borne in mind that these cellular responses can vary considerably in diseased or aneurysmal human vessels.

Endovascular grafting is associated with greater hemodynamic and metabolic stability than open repair.[47] In a comparative study, patients undergoing open repair showed significant changes in cardiac output, mean arterial pressures, and systemic vascular resistence related to aortic cross-clamping and lower limb reperfusion, whereas the only significant change during endovascular repair was a transient increase in systemic vascular resistance secondary to femoral artery clamping.[47]

On the other hand, early in the experience with the Stentor device, several teams of investigators noted unexpected blood pressure decreases intraoperatively at the time of deployment of the graft. Norgren and associates showed that these were related to release of tumor necrosis factor (TNF).[48] In comparing these reactions to open repair of AAA, they found that release of cytokines occurred and reported indirect evidence of activation of white cells.[49, 50] Granulocyte and monocyte counts decreased significantly. Circulating TNF was detected only in the endoluminal group, whereas interleukin-6 concentrations increased in both groups, but significantly more so in open repair.[49] These investigators also observed that, in aneurysms without extensive device manipulation or a large volume of thrombus, the biological responses were less pronounced or absent.[50] The thrombus within the sac is considered to be an active element, and various inflammatory reactions may be associated with changes in activity, cellular content, and permeability in the thrombus.[51]

The most widely reported late response to successful endovascular exclusion of AAA is shrinkage of the sac diameter,[52–54] sometimes to the extent of total aneurysm regression.[55, 56] Aneurysm sac diameter is related to complete exclusion of luminal and collateral flow from the sac. Expansion of the aneurysm occurs with persistent endoleak.[52–54] Successful endovascular graft implantation produces a marked drop in pressure in the aneurysm; Chuter's group recorded a mean aneurysm pressure of 36.5/33.8, as compared with radial artery pressures of 118.5/50.5 mmHg after implantation of aorto-iliac graft.[57] Other factors, such as downregulation of autoantigens involved in the inflammatory changes that occur in aneurysms, may be involved in the shrinkage. A "post-implantation syndrome" has been recognized that consists of fever, malaise, and back pain that are not associated with elevated white cell count or other parameters of infection.[48, 58, 59] There is evidence that C-reactive protein levels are elevated. The process tends to be self-limiting over several days, and the symptoms are usually alleviated by nonsteroidal anti-inflammatory drugs (NSAIDs).

In the femoral site, early endovascular graft procedures frequently resulted in a syndrome of intense local pain and fever.[60] This may have been due to closure of collateral supply, inflammatory reactions to the graft, or the thrombotic process between the graft and arterial walls.

ENDOVASCULAR DEVICES

This portion of the chapter presents details of the design, deployment mechanisms, and delivery systems for each of the endovascular graft devices* that have been used in clinical series to date. The range of devices used for endovascular repair of AAA is presented in Tables 38–6 and 38–7. The surgical techniques for endovascular graft implantation in general are summarized in the next section, and only the special techniques relevant to each individual graft device are provided. The results, complications, and other clinical details are presented in Chapters 32, 53, 72, and 90.

Parodi Balloon-Expanded Endograft

Initially, the Parodi stent-graft comprised a modified Palmaz stent sutured onto a compliant vascular graft fabric[7] with a second (distal) stent that was deployed independently by a separate balloon. Later versions featured proximal and distal balloons deployed through the same delivery system.

Components

The important components of the Parodi Expanded Endograft[10, 61] and the rationale for their use are listed next. Similar components are found in many of other designs of commercial endovascular grafts used in AAA repair, although most of them use a self-expanding mechanism.

1. A super-stiff guide wire, diameter 0.038 inch, is used to facilitate passage of the sheath and device through tortuous iliac arteries and to hold the axis of the device parallel to that of the aorta. It was also hoped that the stiff guide wire would help to minimize manipulations of the system that could cause embolization.

2. Balloon-expandable stents are modified Palmaz stents made from laser-cut, stainless steel, cylindrical tubes with longitudinal slots that open into a diamond lattice shape

*In the United States, most of these devices are made available for use only in prospective Food and Drug Administration (FDA) Phase I or Phase II trials and Individual Device Exemption (IDE) studies.

TABLE 38–6. ENDOVASCULAR GRAFTS FOR ABDOMINAL AORTIC ANEURYSM

	DEVICE CHARACTERISTICS			DELIVERY SYSTEM		
MANUFACTURER	**Graft Material**	**Stent Material**	**Stent Pattern**	**Size (Outside Diameter)**	**Method of Expansion**	**Method of Fixation**
EndoVascular Technologies	Polyester	Elgiloy	Stent at proximal and distal ends only	27 Fr.	Self-expanding + balloon	Hooks
Boston Scientific	Polyester thin-walled	Nitinol	Continuous mesh (internal)	22 Fr.	Self-expanding + heat	Small hooks + friction
World Medical	Polyester	Nitinol	Intermittent	26 Fr.	Self-expanding	Friction + compression fit
Medtronic	Polyester thin-walled	Nitinol	Continuous mesh (external)	22 Fr.	Self-expanding	Friction + compression fit
Cook	Polyester	Stainless steel (Gianturco type)	Repetitive (total cover)	22 Fr.	Self-expanding	Friction + hooks
Baxter	Polyester	Elgiloy	Intermittent	22 Fr.	Balloon-expandable	Friction + crimps
Gore	Polytetrafluoroethylene	Nitinol	Continuous	22 Fr.	Self-expanding	Friction + small hooks

TABLE 38–7. IMPROVISED, NONCOMMERCIAL ENDOVASCULAR GRAFTS FOR ABDOMINAL AORTIC ANEURYSM

	DELIVERY SYSTEM			DEVICE CHARACTERISTICS		
DEVICE	**Method of Expansion**	**Device Type**	**Method of Fixation**	**Graft Material**	**Stent Material**	**Stent Pattern**
Parodi graft[7]	Balloon	Tube graft	Friction	Polyester (compliant)	Stainless steel (Palmaz)	Proximal and distal
GAD graft (White-Yu[55])	Balloon	Tube, aortoiliac, and bifurcated	Friction + crimps	Polyester	Stainless steel	Intermittent
Parodi variations (May[9], Bray,[14] Adiseshiah[14]	Balloon	Tube or aortoiliac	Friction	Polyester or PTFE	Stainless steel (Palmaz)	Proximal and distal
Montefiore[18]	Balloon	Aortoiliac	Friction	Dilated PTFE	Stainless steel (Palmaz)	Proximal and distal
Leicester[86]						
Dake graft[18]	Self-expanding	Thoracic tube	Friction + small hooks	Polyester	Stainless steel (Gianturco type)	Repetitive (total cover)
Chuter graft[11]	Self-expanding	Bifurcated	Friction + compression fit	Polyester	Stainless steel (Gianturco type)	Proximal and distal
Ivancev-Malmo graft[84]	Self-expanding	Aortouni-iliac	Friction + compression fit	Polyester	Stainless steel	Proximal and distal
Lauterjung[88]	Self-expanding	Bifurcated	Friction	Polyester	Nitinol	Intermittent
Hartley-Lawrence Brown device[21]	Self-expanding	Bifurcated	Friction + small hooks	Polyester	Stainless steel (Gianturco type)	Repetitive (total cover)

PTFE = polytetrafluoroethylene.

when expanded. The stent used for the majority of cases was 35 mm long and expanded from 5 to 30 mm in diameter.

3. Knitted polyester graft fabric 0.2 mm thick, and of 15% compliance for most of the graft length, but 45% in the region of the stent to allow expansion of the stent. The diameter and length of each graft are tailored to the individual patient.

4. A balloon catheter of 9 Fr. with one or two balloons attached to the shaft at positions that correspond to the distal stent (single balloon) or the proximal and distal stents (two balloons).

5. Polytetrafluoroethylene (Teflon) introducing sheath, of 21 Fr. internal diameter with an attachable hemostatic valve at the proximal end.

Early experience with 70 high-risk patients,[61, 62] in addition to animal experiments, led to identification of these important features of endovascular grafting of aneurysms:

1. Adequate fixation of the stent-graft device required at least 10% to 15% balloon expansion of the stent over the aortic diameter, but there was danger of vessel rupture with extreme oversizing.

2. The large size of the introducer sheaths risked spasm and injury of the "access" femoral or iliac artery.

3. Massive embolization due to dislodgment of aneurysm contents was a significant risk that in a number of early cases led to death of the patient from multisystem failure.

4. Folding or kinks in the graft fabric tended to occur in areas where there was no stent support.

5. If there was adequate proximal and distal neck (2 cm), an aortoaortic tube graft could be deployed, whereas if the distal neck was absent, the transfemoral technique was altered to an aortoiliac tapered graft in conjunction with a femorofemoral crossover graft to restore blood flow to the contralateral leg (see Fig. 38–3). Retrograde flow via the contralateral iliac artery was prevented by occluding the lumen with detachable balloons or by ligation.

6. The excluded aneurysm sac thrombosed, with later reduction in aneurysm diameter.

7. Late dilatation of the distal aorta or dislodgment of the distal stent led to problems in some patients who had undergone aortoaortic tube graft, a finding that suggested that a bifurcated or aortoiliac graft configuration would have been preferable in these cases. The first documented attempt at bifurcated endograft using Parodi's device was performed by White and May in July 1992. Unfortunately, the graft could not be deployed correctly by the balloon expansion technique and conversion to open repair was required.[63] Successful bifurcated grafting was achieved in 1993 by Chuter, who used self-expanding stents.[11]

Chuter Bifurcated Endovascular Prosthesis

Chuter's bifurcated endoluminal graft, which featured a thin, uncrimped, woven polyester material attached by three self-expanding modified Gianturco stents, was used in a number of animal studies,[64] and then in a clinical series of bifurcated endoluminal repairs.[11]

The Device

A single-piece bifurcated prosthesis, this stent-graft is passed up into the aorta from a femoral access site, and the two iliac limbs are then manipulated down into the iliac arteries on each side.

Delivery System

The delivery system has a single primary sheath that is inserted with the prosthesis preloaded. The procedure commences with passage of a crossover guide wire over the aortic bifurcation to the contralateral femoral artery to establish access to both iliac arteries. The proximal Gianturco Z-stent has eight points, and the outer 8-mm portion of the stent has no fabric covering. Coils soldered to eight of the limbs provide points of attachment for the graft, and small pairs of barbs are also mounted on four of the proximal stent limbs. One barb of each pair extends proximally to the level of the stent angles, where it bends caudad to form a hook. The other barb extends distally, parallel to the long axis of the stent. The stents at the distal ends of the iliac limbs protrude 2 mm beyond the fabric and are smaller, having a diameter of 17 mm when expanded. These have no barbs. Chuter has reported on the surgical techniques required and the results.[11, 35, 64]

Ancure Endografts

The Guidant/EVT endograft was the first commercial device to undergo clinical trials, which commenced in 1993. Its design is based on concepts developed by Lazarus. Early designs documented in the patient literature featured balloon-driven stapling of the graft to the vessel wall,[22] whereas the current design uses a balloon to augment the implantation of hooks on the self-expanding stent.[23, 24]

The Device

The EVT endograft consists of a polyester vascular graft with proximal and distal attachment stents. The stents are self-expanding, zig-zag elgiloy metal with eight angled hooks attached to the aortic stent and three to the iliac stents (Fig. 38–8). The stents are hand-sewn to the graft fabric, which is woven polyester. The devices are available as tube graft, bifurcated, and aortoiliac configurations (Fig. 38–9). The polyester fabric of the tube graft and the trunk section of the other grafts is "noncrimped," whereas the iliac limbs of the bifurcated and aortoiliac versions are crimped to increase resistance to kinking or angulation caused by tortuosity of the iliac vessels. Thin clusters of polyester fuzz material are sewn to the outside of the graft at the proximal and distal ends (see Fig. 38–9), with the aim of improving the seal around the graft limbs by promoting thrombosis outside the graft. Platinum radiopaque markers are sewn along the length of the grafts 18 mm apart, and they extend along the lateral sides of the iliac limbs.

Delivery System

The Guidant/EVT delivery system consists of an expandable introducer sheath (27 Fr. outer diameter) and a 23 Fr.

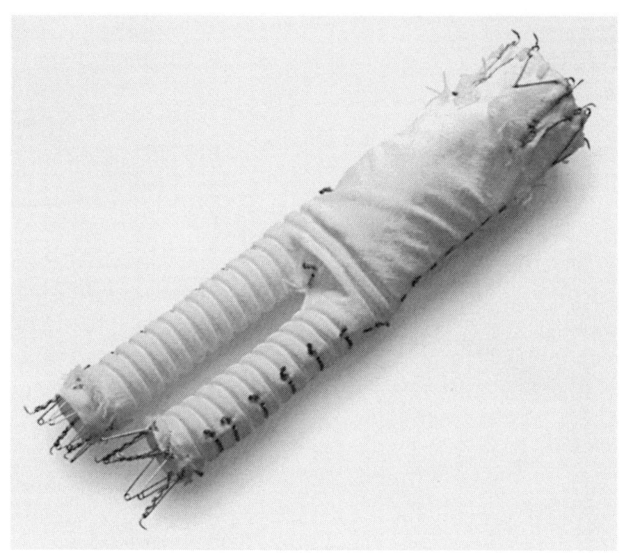

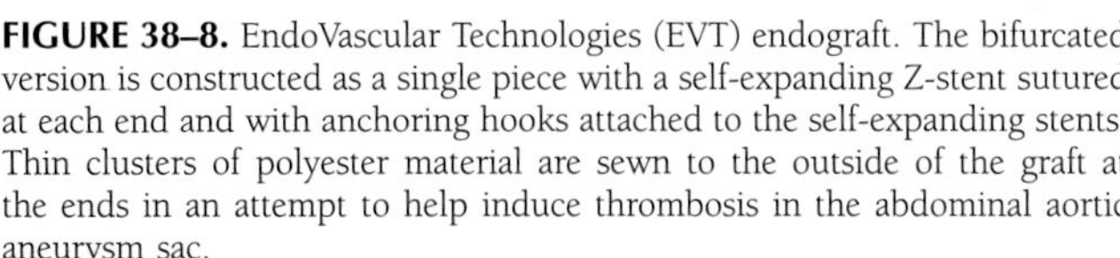

FIGURE 38–8. EndoVascular Technologies (EVT) endograft. The bifurcated version is constructed as a single piece with a self-expanding Z-stent sutured at each end and with anchoring hooks attached to the self-expanding stents. Thin clusters of polyester material are sewn to the outside of the graft at the ends in an attempt to help induce thrombosis in the abdominal aortic aneurysm sac.

coaxial delivery catheter (Fig. 38–10). The expandable sheath facilitates introduction of the delivery system by straightening the common and external iliac access vessels, thus dilating minor areas of narrowing and minimizing vessel tortuosity along the route of introduction. The outer end of the sheath has a hemostatic valve system composed of spring and thumbwheel diaphragm valves, which are a few centimeters apart. Hemostasis is maintained while introducing instruments into the chamber between the valves by opening the spring valve. Access into the sheath is then obtained by opening the thumbwheel valve. The expandable sheath has a tapered dilator to fully expand the sheath. After the dilator is removed, the delivery catheter can be introduced.

The delivery catheter is a coaxial system composed of a single-lumen main catheter, an inner triple-lumen balloon catheter, and an outer jacket. The endograft is preloaded, folded around the balloon catheter. Its attachment systems are housed in compressed form by superior and inferior metal capsules. The capsule of the superior attachment system is fixed to the balloon catheter. The capsule of the inferior or ipsilateral attachment system is fixed to the main catheter.

The system contains two handles. The distal handle is connected to the balloon catheter and controls movement of the superior capsule, and thus release of the superior attachment system. The proximal handle is connected to the main catheter. It enables retraction of the inferior capsule. The capsule for the contralateral attachment system of the bifurcated endograft is connected to a pull wire

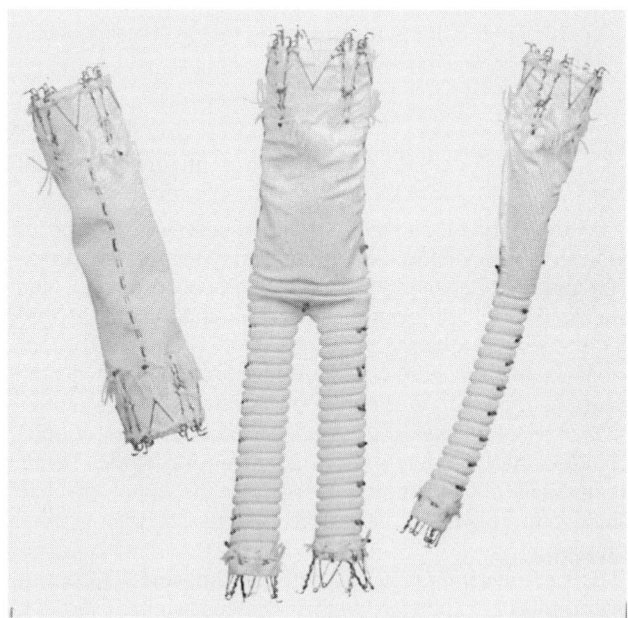

FIGURE 38–9. EndoVascular Technologies endograft. The three configurations are shown: the tube graft *(left)*, the bifurcated graft *(center)*, and the aortoiliac graft *(right)*.

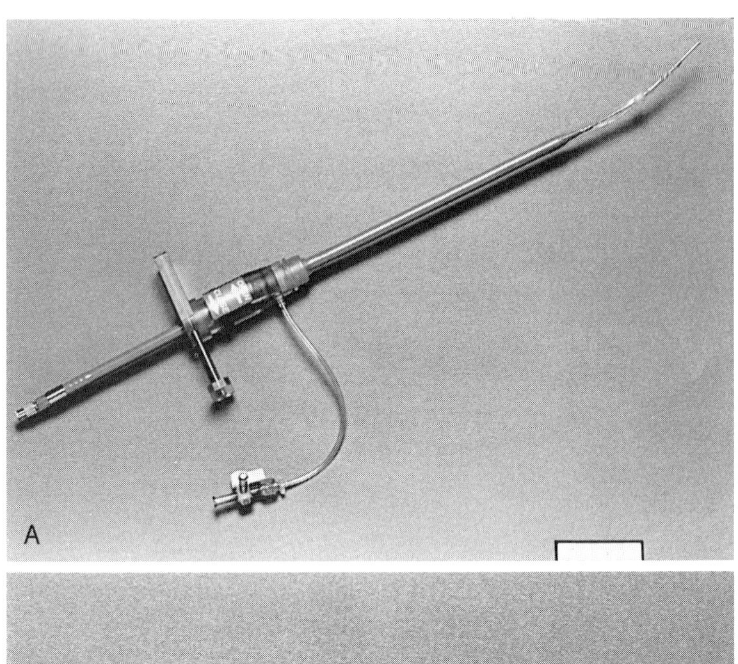

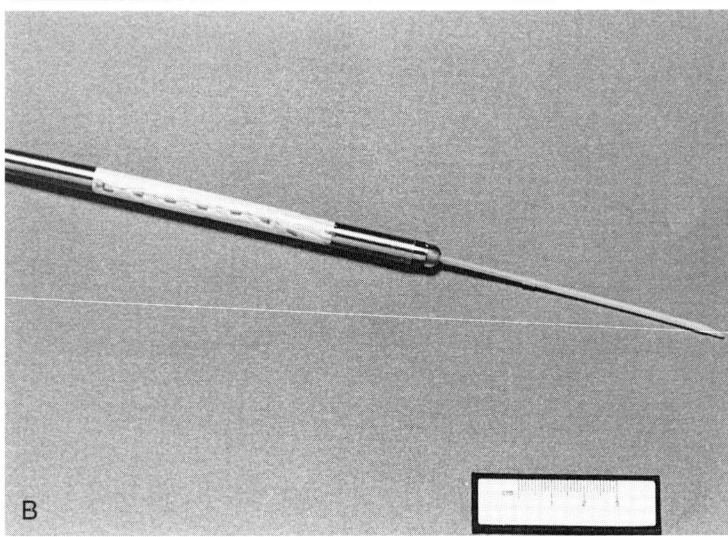

FIGURE 38–10. EndoVascular Technologies (EVT) endograft. *A*, EVT introducer sheath and the tapered dilator. The sheath features a proximal hemostatic valve and an expandable distal segment. *B*, An early version of the EVT tube graft is shown within its delivery capsule on the introducing catheter.

assembly, which is guided in the direction opposite that of the contralateral limb and runs along the prosthesis beyond the tip of the delivery system.

Accessories

The delivery system includes a number of accessories that improve the accuracy and efficacy of graft implantation:

1. *Guidant/EVT marker board.* This accessory is used to indicate the planned position for deployment of the proximal and distal attachment stents. Radiopaque marker bars are cased in a radiolucent, flat box, which is placed behind the patient. The bars can be moved according to the on-table angiogram, and remain visible on the fluoroscopic image as indicators during the procedure.
2. *AngioScale angiography catheter.* This 6 Fr. multihole, pigtail catheter contains 15 to 25 platinum marker bands at intervals of 10 mm and is used for the initial on-table angiogram to verify the correct length for the implant prosthesis.
3. *Contralateral torque catheter.* The Guidant/EVT contralateral torque catheter is a single-lumen, flexible tube that is used only in bifurcated graft procedures. It is inserted over the pull wire assembly through a 12 Fr. introducer sheath and has a locking system at the distal end to hook onto the contralateral capsule. A Luer lock mechanism at the proximal end helps to maintain hemostasis. The contralateral torque catheter corrects for twist in the contralateral limb and is subsequently used to retract the contralateral capsule to release the contralateral limb attachment system.
4. *Iliac balloon catheter.* The hooks of the distal attachment systems of the bifurcated prothesis must be implanted into the arterial wall with a separate balloon catheter. The Guidant/EVT iliac balloon catheter is introduced over the wire through the 12 Fr. introducer sheath on the contralateral side and through the main sheath on the ipsilateral side. The balloon diameters range from 9 to 13 mm, and they can be adjusted to the diameter of the distal attachment systems.

Surgical Technique

Particular aspects of the surgical technique required for the Guidant/EVT graft depend on the methods of access to the artery and of release of the graft from its capsule. For deployment of the tube endograft, in most cases a preferable access site can be selected on the basis of anatomic details of the iliac and common femoral arteries. Deployment of the graft consists of six steps:

1. Positioning of the upper end of the graft attachment system just below the renal arteries, followed by retraction of the outer jacket of the delivery catheter.
2. Advancement of the superior capsule to deploy the proximal attachment stent.
3. Balloon inflation within the proximal stent to embed the hooks into the aortic wall.
4. Retraction of the inferior capsule to release the distal attachment stent.
5. Repositioning of the balloon within the distal stent and inflation to drive the hooks into the wall of the distal neck or cuff of aorta.
6. Retraction of the delivery system into the jacket and removal of the catheter.

Deployment of the bifurcated graft requires bilateral access to the common femoral arteries. After insertion of the sheaths, a crossover wire is passed over the aortic bifurcation to the contralateral side by a snare-loop technique, and this wire is used to retract the contralateral limb of the graft back down into the iliac artery after the main sheath and the graft trunk have been released in the aorta. Any torsion of the device must be corrected before implantation. This correction is achieved by the primary catheter for the graft trunk and by a specific torque catheter, which is introduced on the contralateral side and hooked onto the contralateral graft limb capsule. Self-expanding stents anchor the iliac limbs, and their fixation is aided by balloon inflation to drive the attachment hooks into the arterial wall.

The results achieved with the Guidant/EVT endograft in several prospective multicenter FDA Phase I and Phase II studies have been reported on behalf of the investigators by Moore,[34, 65] Matsumura and coworkers,[53, 66] and others. Other experiences with the Guidant/EVT grafts have been reported by the groups of Balm[67] and May.[68]

Stentor Endovascular Graft

The Miahle Stentor Graft (Mintec, La Ciotat, France) was developed as a modification of the Cragg peripheral stent-graft.[69] The fabric wall for this device was constructed by stitching a polyester sheet into a tubular graft. In clinical use it was plagued by a high rates of material tears and failure, particularly along this suture line.[59, 70] The design was improved after the device was acquired by Boston Scientific/Meadox, particularly the quality of the graft material, and the revised device is now marketed as the Vanguard.

Vanguard Endovascular Aortic Graft

The Vanguard device is currently in Phase II trial in the United States and has been marketed commercially for some time in Europe and Australia. The aortic graft is the Vanguard, and the graft for peripheral or iliac vessels is the Passager.

The Device

The Vanguard endoprosthesis is a flexible, self-expanding tubular prosthesis constructed of a nitinol wire frame covered by a thin-walled woven polyester fabric.[37, 58] It is manufactured in two configurations: straight (tube) graft and bifurcated (Fig. 38–11). The graft fabric is fully supported by the internal metallic framework, which is constructed in segments from "shape-memory wire" bent into a series of zigzag stents. Each segment is of unitary construction, made from a single length of nitinol wire, and held in the predeployment configuration by polypropylene

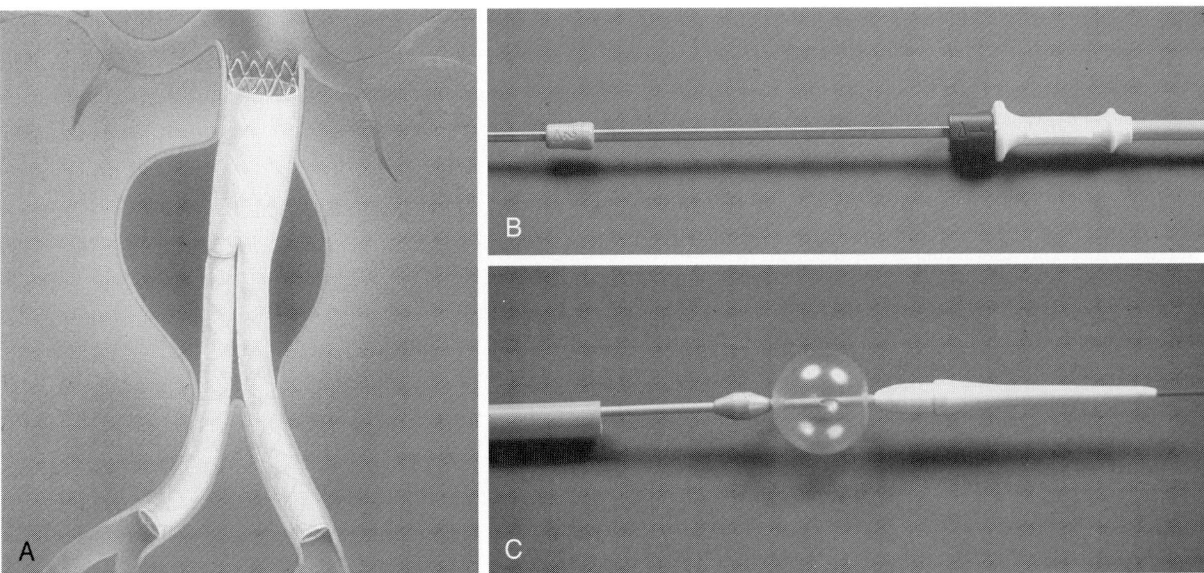

FIGURE 38–11. Boston Scientific/Meadox endovascular grafts. *A,* Bifurcated graft system with modular iliac limb, which interlocks with the stump of the ipsilateral trunk graft. *B,* Close-up view of the proximal end of the deployment catheter for the second iteration (Vanguard II) device. The camlocks on the metal shaft are used to release segments of the deployment sheath to allow expansion of the graft and its ipsilateral limb. *C,* The distal end of the deployment catheter for the Vanguard II device features a tapered nose cone and a compliant latex balloon for stent molding.

ties. The ties are positioned at the apex of the zigs but allow the zigs to move relative to each other, which may afford some changes in geometry of the graft framework after deployment.

The metal frame assemby is attached to the inside wall of the graft material component by polyester sutures. The graft is a seamless, ultrathin, low-porosity woven material similar to the woven grafts made by the same company (Boston Scientific/Meadox) for standard surgical AAA repair. The graft material is attached to the nitinol framework only at the proximal and distal ends of the device. Small barbs on the proximal end of the frame help to anchor the device.

Delivery System

The three-stage delivery system has an outer diameter of 22 Fr. and comprises five components: an introducer sheath, an aortic pusher, an iliac pusher, the stent-graft, and a latex balloon (Fig. 38–11*B* and *C*). There are side ports for irrigation with cold fluid before and during the procedure. The bifurcated endoprosthesis is designed for placement in the abdominal aorta immediately below the renal arteries, and it has a tapered stump that interlocks with the contralateral iliac limb graft, which is introduced via a contralateral femoral approach.

Surgical Technique for Deployment

The technique of implanting the stent-graft has four major steps (Fig. 38–12). Under fluoroscopic control, the delivery system is inserted through a right or left femoral surgical incision, advanced over a stiff 0.035-inch guide wire (Amplatz, Meditech, Watertown, Mass.), and positioned at the level of the renal arteries.

For straight grafts, the aortic pusher is held in a fixed position and the outer sheath of the delivery system is retracted. As the sheath is retracted, the proximal part of the graft is exposed and expands to a tubular shape. The proximal stents are then fully expanded and anchored by inflation of the latex balloon. The outer sheath is then withdrawn completely to fully deploy the implant. For bifurcated stent-grafts, the outer sheath is withdrawn until the radiopaque marker of the contralateral iliac stump (attachment site for the secondary iliac limb component) is seen to jump free. After balloon fixation of the proximal part of the device, the outer sheath is then withdrawn completely while the iliac pusher is held in position to deploy the ipsilateral fixed iliac limb within the iliac artery on the side of access. To complete the bifurcated graft, the second iliac limb section of the implant is inserted percutaneously or by cutdown approach to the contralateral femoral artery using a 10 or 12 Fr. introducer sheath system, and overlapped within the stump of the aortoiliac section previously implanted (Fig. 38–12*A*).

There are various techniques to gain guide wire access to the contralateral stump, to complete the bifurcated graft procedure:

- Direct catherization of the stump of the aortic section using a torquable 6 Fr. or 7 Fr. selective catheter
- Crossover access from the ipsilateral graft limb using a preshaped guiding catheter
- Access from above via the brachial artery,

For the latter two, a snare or loop device is used to grasp the wire within the contralateral iliac artery (Fig. 38–12*C*).[69]

Talent Endoluminal Stent-Graft

The Talent Endoluminal Stent-Graft System (World Medical Manufacturing, Sunrise, Fla.) was specially designed for endovascular treatment of aortic aneurysms, based on a system first used in animals by Balko in 1982. The device can be inserted as a tube or a bifurcated prosthesis.[71]

The Device

The prosthesis is composed of a skeleton of self-expanding nitinol stents (similar in configuration to Z-stents) connected by a stabilizing bar to which polyester graft material is annealed over the aortic segment. In the bifurcated system, the iliac limbs are also covered with polyester, which covers both the inside and the outside of the nitinol stents.

The ends of the stent-graft are made in two configurations (Fig. 38–13). They may be serrated (open-web configuration) or have an open stent segment (bare wire configuration) at one or both ends, which allows the open stent region of the graft to be placed across the orifice of renal, mesenteric, left subclavian, or internal iliac arteries without occluding antegrade blood flow. This may be of benefit when the vessel is tortuous or the neck of the aneurysm is relatively short.

Delivery System

Grafts designed for use in the abdominal aorta typically are delivered through a 24 Fr. sheath. Tube graft segments up to 46 mm in diameter are available for use in the thoracic aorta. For these, a 27 Fr. delivery sheath is required. To date, grafts have been made available from a series of standard catalogue sizes or have been custom-made to measurements acquired by angiography or computed tomography (CT).

Surgical Technique for Deployment

The deployment techniques are similar to that for the Vanguard graft described earlier. The modular bifurcated device trunk with the ipsilateral limb segment is initially deployed, followed by access to the contralateral limb stump by guide wire and deployment of the iliac extension limb.

Medtronic AneuRx Stent-Graft

The Medtronic AneuRx Stent-Graft (Medtronic, Cupertino, Calif.) is a thin-walled polyester graft supported externally by self-expanding stents. The zigzag-shaped nitinol stents are connected by polyester multifilament braided sutures in such a way as to form diamond-shaped apertures, and they cover the whole of the external surface of the graft.

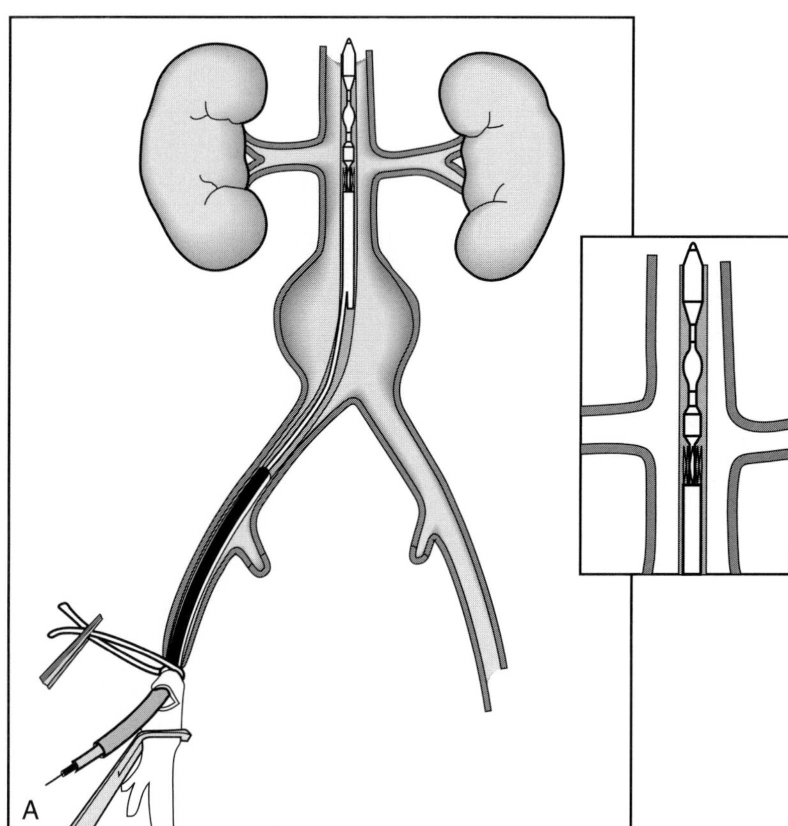

FIGURE 38–12. Deployment of the Boston Scientific/Meadox Vanguard endovascular graft. *A,* The delivery catheter for the bifurcated graft system is initially advanced over a guide wire, to a position several centimeters above the level of the renal arteries. *Inset,* The position of the nose cone and balloon relative to the distal stent within the delivery sheath is shown. *B,* The Vanguard graft device bifurcated trunk is released by retraction of the delivery sheath, and full expansion of the internal nitinol supporting stents is achieved by expanding the balloon. The insets show the recommended positioning of the graft immediately below the renal arteries and the relationship of the graft markers to the stent and graft fabric. Since the graft fabric is mounted below the upper part of the stent framework, the first two wireforms may alternatively be placed above the renal arteries to provide improved attachments in patients with a short or angulated aortic neck.

Illustration continued on following page

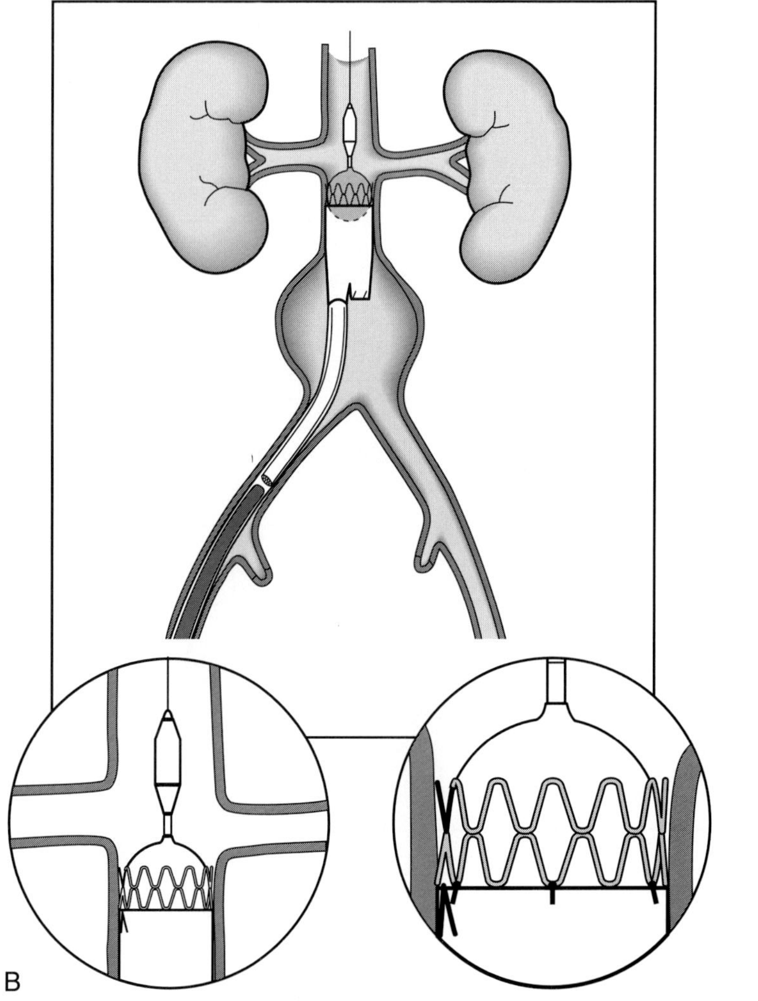

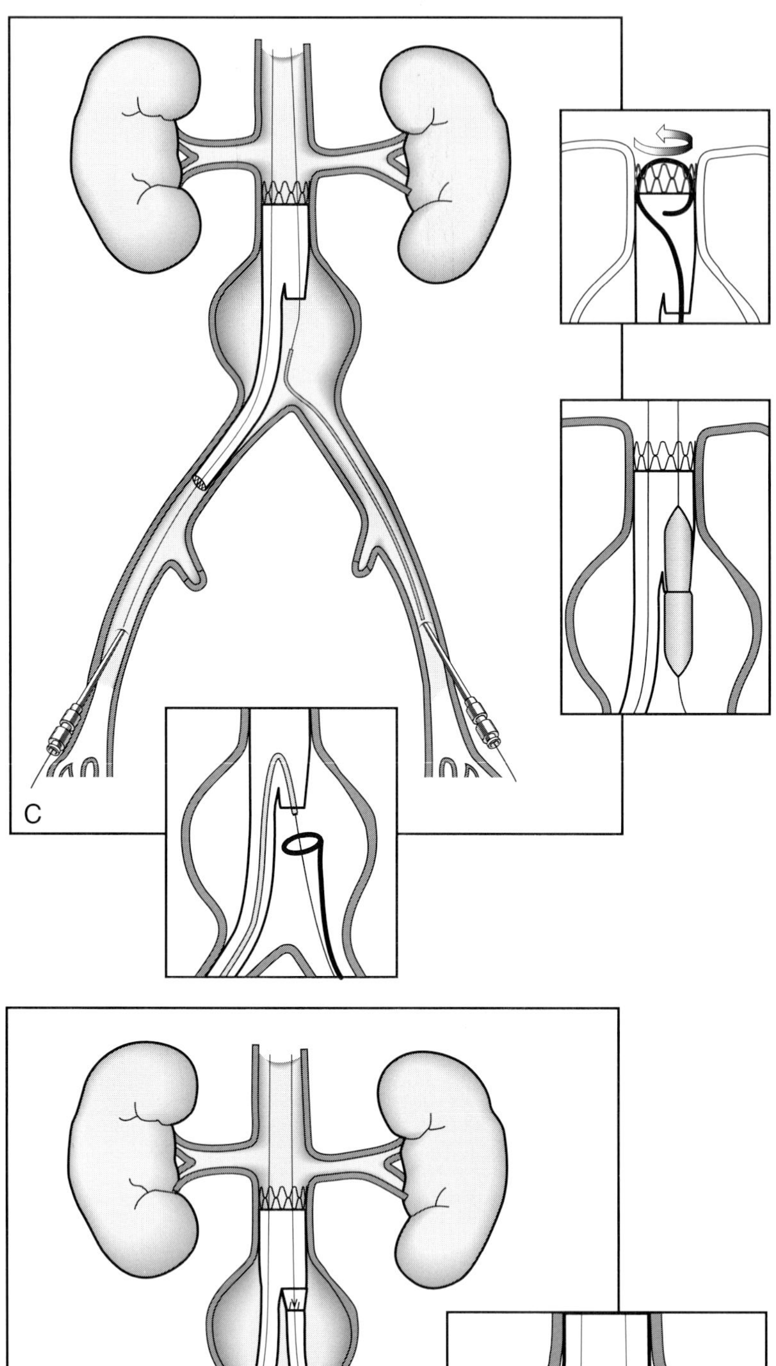

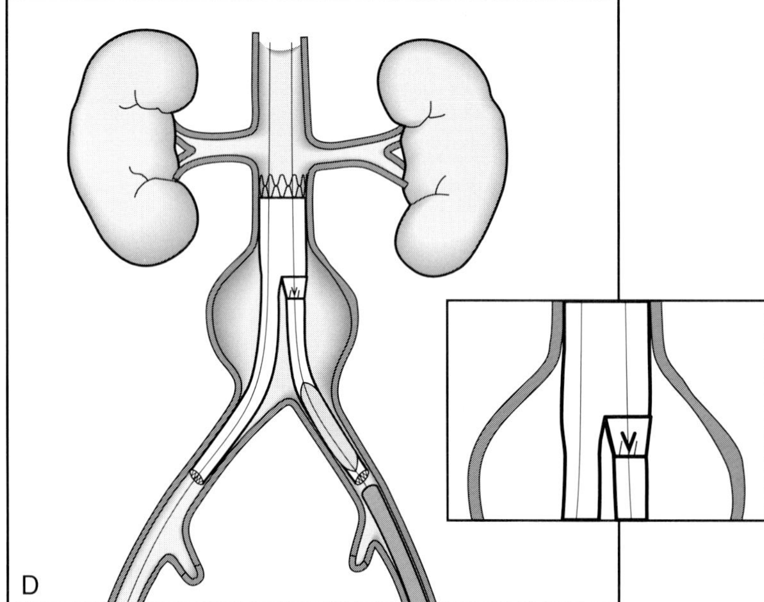

FIGURE 38–12. *Continued C,* The stump of the contralateral limb is cannulated after passage of a guide wire. It may be very difficult to position the guide wire in the limb, and sometimes access must be gained by a crossover catheter technique from within the graft lumen *(lowest inset).* Once the guide wire has been passed, its position within the stump lumen should be confirmed by rotation of a pigtail catheter *(upper right inset)* or by inflation of a balloon within the stump *(lower right inset). D,* The modular graft is completed by deploying the contralateral iliac limb, overlapped within the contralateral stump. The inset shows a close-up view on the overlap zone.

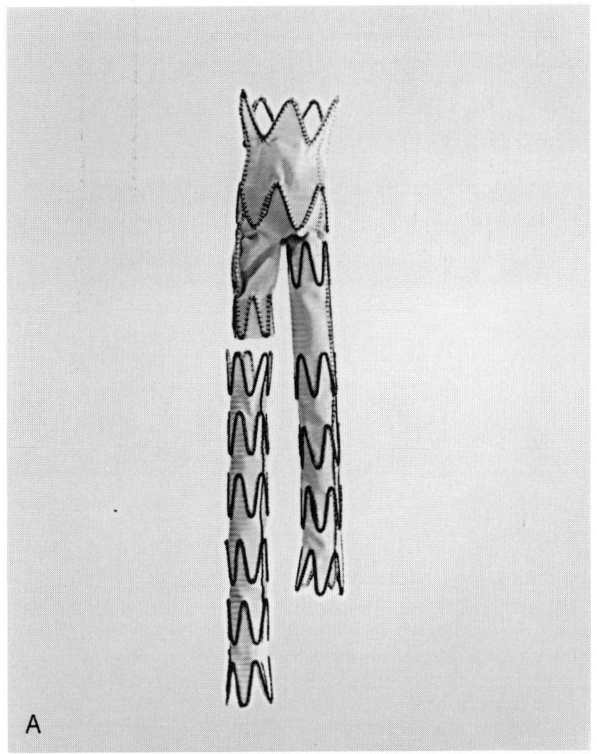

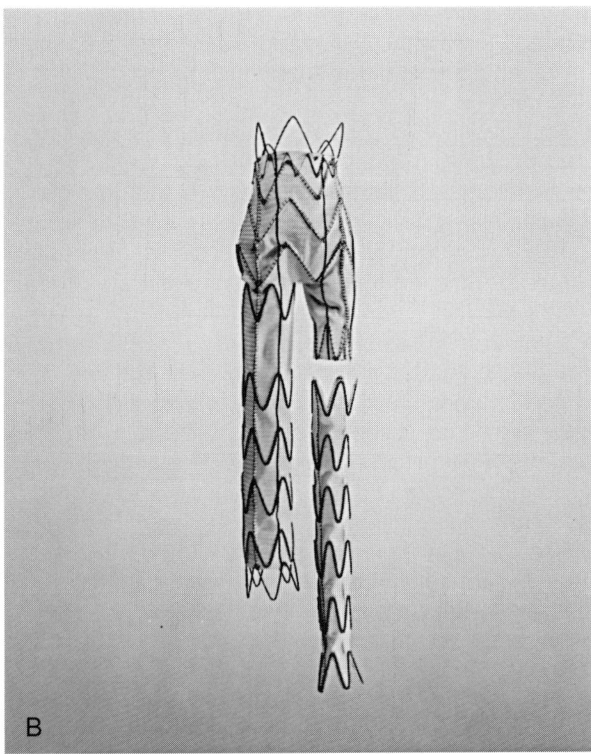

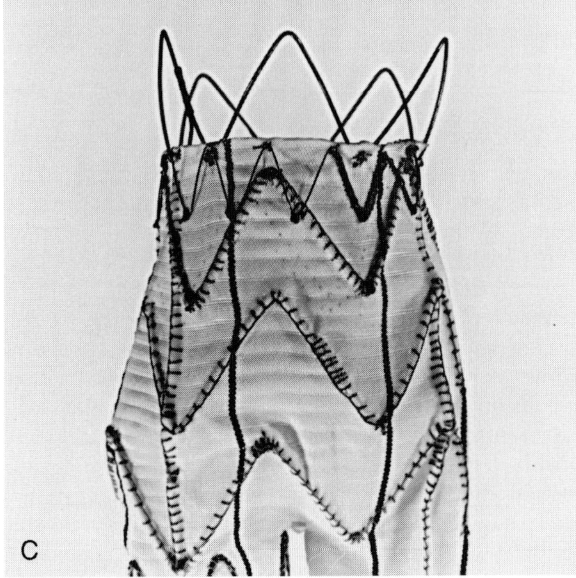

FIGURE 38–13. World Medical Talent endovascular graft. The basic graft design features two variations of the proximal, infrarenal section. *A*, Talent bifurcated graft with modular iliac limb and V-shaped cutout segments of the proximal aspect of the graft wall. *B*, Talent bifurcated graft variation featuring a proximal bare stent that may be placed over the renal artery orifices. *C*, Close-up view of the proximal bare stent.

The Device

The AneuRx stent-graft is a modular system similar to the Vanguard graft in concept, except that the nitinol stent support exoskeleton is sewn to the outer wall of the woven, thin-walled, polyester graft (Fig. 38–14).[39,72,73] The stent is a shape-memory alloy 0.009 to 0.015 inch thick. The polyester graft material has wall thickness of 0.004 to 0.005 inch. The graft material has relatively high porosity of 150 to 400 cc/min/cm^2.

The graft is supplied preloaded in a delivery catheter and is deployed by retracting the outer cover of the delivery catheter to release the stent-supported graft wall into the bloodstream. Two graft lengths are available (135 and 165 mm). The bifurcated trunk graft is available in diameters from 20 to 28 mm, and the iliac limbs in diameters of 12 to 16 mm, the iliac limbs being fixed at half the trunk diameter plus 2 mm (for example, a 26-mm diameter trunk graft has iliac limbs 15 mm in diameter). In addition to the range of devices used to form the bifurcated graft during the procedure, "extension cuffs" are available to help correct errors of placement or of size mismatch at the aortic neck (aortic extension cuff) or in the iliac artery (iliac extension cuff). These may also be used to extend or line segments of the graft that have not formed an adequate seal and are permitting endoleak or as extensions at the proximal or distal ends, respectively, in case of misplacement or inadequate graft length (see Fig. 38–7).

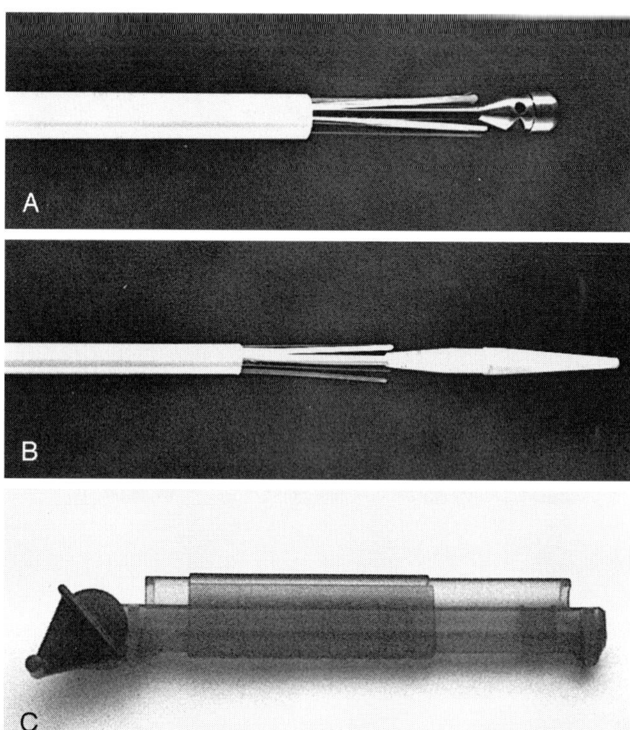

FIGURE 38–15. Delivery system for the Medtronic AneuRx endovascular graft. The distal aspect of the AneuRx delivery catheter, showing the metal nose cone, which is used to orient the graft, and the metallic runners, which reduce friction to allow controlled deployment of the graft by mechanical retraction of the sheath. *B,* Alternative version of the distal tip of the delivery system, showing a tapered nose cone for less traumatic introduction through the access vessels. *C,* AneuRx handle, which is attached to the proximal end of the delivery catheter and contains a central auger used for mechanical retraction of the sheath, to deploy the graft.

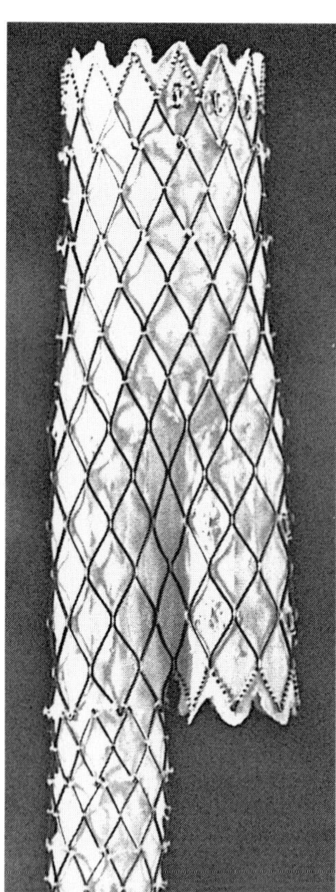

FIGURE 38–14. Medtronic AneuRx endovascular graft. This graft is of thin-walled polyester fabric, supported externally by a nitinol stent framework, or "exoskeleton."

Delivery System

The delivery system has been designed to overcome the outward friction of the nitinol stents against the internal surface of the sheath. To this end, it features a number of thin metallic runners that lie between the stents and the delivery catheter wall. The catheter, which has an outer diameter of 22 Fr., is withdrawn mechanically by manual levered rotation of a central shaft connected to an auger screw within the separate deployment handle, permitting expansion of the preloaded graft unit by the attached self-expanding stents (Fig. 38–15). This action is achieved by turning a crank. This is somewhat similar in concept to the control knob that is turned to retract the jacket of the EVT graft. The central shaft of the delivery catheter is attached to the nose cone and runners. The metallic nose cone has a central hole and a notch to one side to assist in orienting the device before deployment. Oversizing the graft diameter by several millimeters (10% to 20%) with respect to the aortic neck diameter is recommended. The deployment handle is marketed separately and may be resterilized for reuse.

During deployment, the stainless steel runners attached to the delivery catheter facilitate smooth deployment of the graft by reducing frictional forces between the graft wall and the interior of the delivery sheath. In addition to the delivery catheter that houses the device, a separate introducer sheath of larger diameter (Rapid-Trak Introducer Sheath, outside diameter 25 Fr.) is also available. The contralateral iliac limb is deployed in similar fashion from a preloaded 16 Fr. catheter, using the same mechanical deployment handle device.

Surgical Technique for Deployment

The insertion and deployment procedure is essentially the same as for the Vanguard graft (see earlier), with the following exceptions:

1. *Graft markers and orientation.* The metallic nose cone of the delivery catheter and the four radiopaque tantalum graft markers sewn to the fabric of the trunk graft are used to orient the graft before its release (see Figs. 38–14 and 38–15*A*).
2. *Deployment handle.* The mechanical action of this device is used in place of hand-held retraction of the sheath (see Fig. 38–15*C*).
3. *Delivery catheter runners.* These are present only in the AneuRx graft (see Fig. 38–15*B*).

Cook Zenith Endograft

The Zenith endovascular graft (previously known as the Hartley & Lawrence-Brown [HLB] endoluminal stent-graft) is marketed by Cook (Cook, Indianapolis, Ind.). This endoluminal graft for infrarenal aortic aneurysm repair, developed by Hartley and Lawrence-Brown,[20, 21, 74] has been in use in Australia since 1994 and has evolved in parallel with other similar systems used elsewhere. The graft is now available in a bifurcated and an aortouni-iliac form. Each device is custom-made to the patient's requirements, within the limits of designated selection criteria.[21]

Description of The Device

The bifurcated Cook device is a modular, self-expanding endovascular graft constructed of stainless steel and polyester (Fig. 38–16). The prosthetic material is standard, woven, noncrimped polyester, 0.15 mm thick. The main section consists of a bifurcated graft with one long limb and one short one. It is introduced via one femoral artery and positioned in the aorta with the short limb above the bifurcation. The second section is introduced via the contralateral iliac artery and positioned in the appropriately placed short leg. The device is supplied preloaded with each component in its own introduction system.

Each end of the graft is held within a cap; inadvertent release during positioning within the aorta is prevented by a safety catch (Fig. 38–17). This also allows the graft to be rotated to ensure correct orientation. The full length of the graft material is stent-supported to prevent graft torsion or compression. The stents are sutured onto the outside except at the points of proximal and distal attachment or seal. The stents are modified Gianturco Z-stents, with small gaps between each stent to allow some flexibility. The uncovered anchor stents have a hook or barb on each strut.

The graft is also available as an aortoiliac, tapered tube graft. This system is usually used in conjunction with femorofemoral crossover graft and occlusion of the contralateral iliac artery. It is used for the treatment of AAA when access and deployment to the aorta is possible through only one iliac artery.

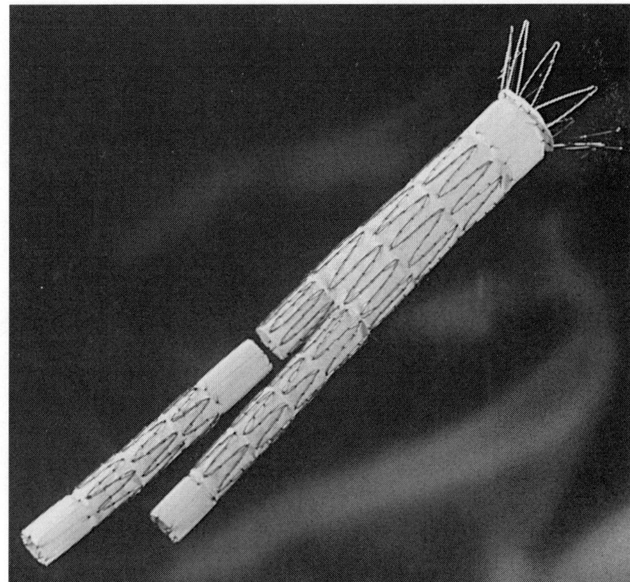

FIGURE 38–16. Cook Zenith bifurcated endovascular graft. This modular bifurcated self-expanding graft has a series of stainless steel stents and polyester graft fabric. The fabric is fully supported along its length by stents of Gianturco type. The proximal anchor stent is uncovered and has a hook or barb on each strut; this portion of the device may be implanted over the origin of the renal and mesenteric vessels.

Delivery System

The graft is delivered through a 20 Fr. Teflon sheath (22 Fr. outer diameter) mounted on a modified Coons dilator, which features a cap to contain the barbed anchor stent and a trigger safety wire mechanism at each end of the graft to control deployment and release.

There are 10 main steps in the deployment sequence:

1. The main system (delivery sheath plus graft body) is inserted via the chosen side to the level of the renal arteries.
2. The system is rotated to bring the "short limb" to an anterolateral position on the contralateral side.
3. The sheath is withdrawn to the level where the short limb is released and expands.
4. The short limb is accessed by guide wire.
5. An angiogram of the top graft position is obtained by injecting contrast medium through the top cap.
6. The top "anchor" stent is released by removing a safety lock and removing a trigger wire.
7. The contralateral "extension leg" is positioned over the guide wire and deployed.
8. The main graft iliac limb is deployed.
9. The distal catheter attachment device is advanced and is docked to the top cap. Then, both are withdrawn as a unit.
10. The graft is inflated with a latex balloon throughout its length, as appropriate, and a final ("completion") angiogram is obtained.

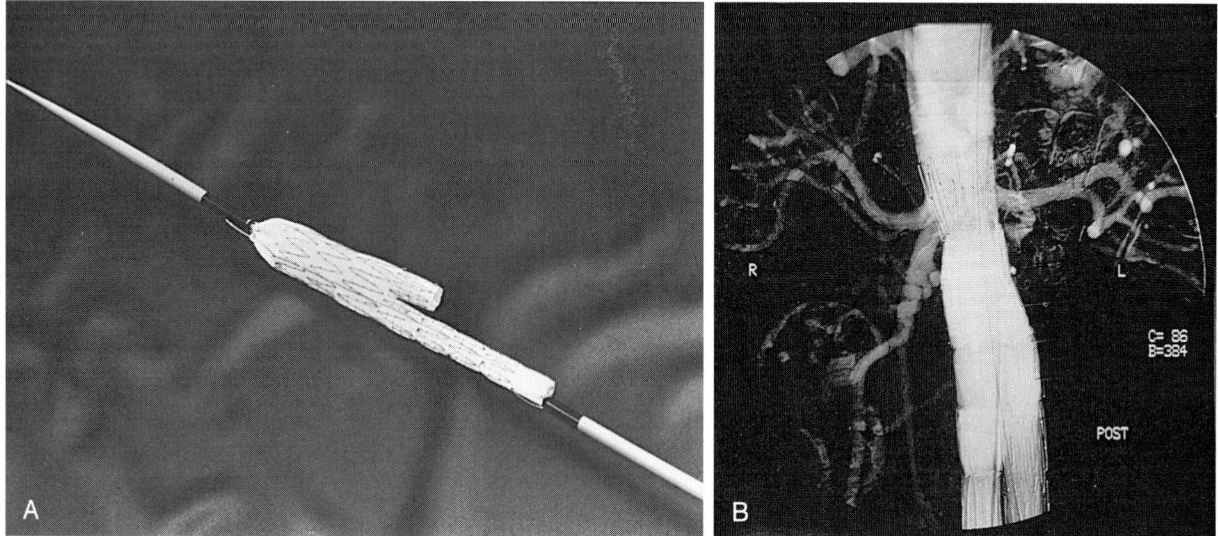

FIGURE 38–17. Cook Zenith bifurcated endovascular graft. *A*, Bifurcated endovascular graft mounted in preparation for delivery sheath. The device is held at both ends by trigger wires, which are used to control graft release. *B*, Angiogram following deployment of the endovascular graft. Note the bare stent across the origin of the renal arteries and also across the origin of the superior mesenteric artery.

Schneider Wallgraft Endoprosthesis

The Wallgraft (Schneider Minneapolis, Minn.) is a development of the self-expanding Wallstent, which already has an established role in treatment of arterial occlusive disease. It is actually a form of spiral stent in which several spirals are braided together to enhance resistance to compression, improve expansion ratios, and reduce shortening. The Wallgraft is currently being tried in applications for complex iliac artery occlusive disease and peripheral arterial aneurysmal disease and trauma.[75–77]

Description of The Device

The Schneider Wallgraft endoprosthesis is a covered stent (Fig. 38–18). It is composed of biomedical superalloy monofilament wire braided in a tubular mesh configuration

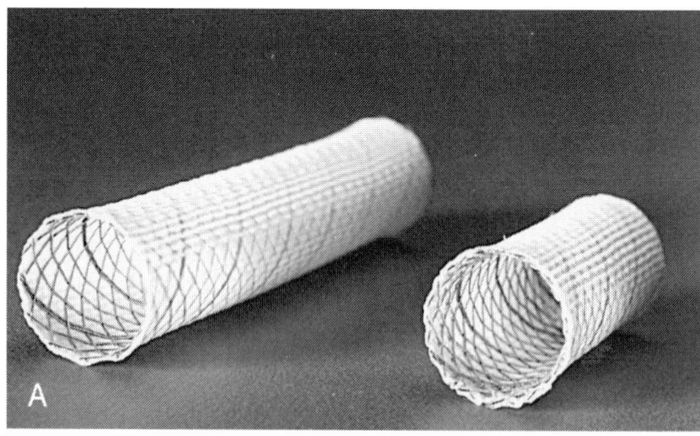

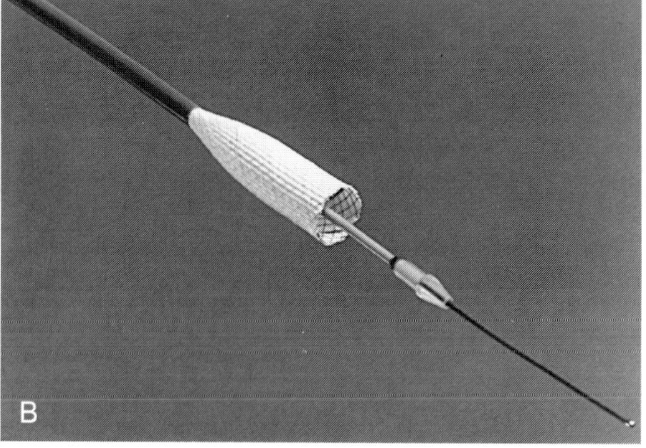

FIGURE 38–18. *A*, The Wallgraft endoprosthesis. This consists of a modified Wallstent with an external covering layer of thin polyester. *B*, Deployment of the Wallgraft by self-expanding mechanism from its delivery sheath.

and covered by polyethyleneterephthalate (PET) graft material. This self-expanding configuration results in an endoluminal graft that is flexible and compliant.

Delivery System

The delivery system (Unistep Plus) consists in part of coaxial tubes. The exterior tube serves to constrain the endoprosthesis until it is retracted during delivery. When desired, the endoprosthesis can be reconstrained before full deployment and repositioned. Radiopaque marker bands reveal the graft's position on fluoroscopic imaging during deployment, and a radiopaque tracer wire indicates the extent of graft material. The delivery system accommodates a 0.035-inch guide wire and can be inserted through a hemostatic introducer sheath.

Corvita Stent-Graft

Corvita vascular grafts are composed of inner meshed polyurethane fibers and an outer layer of meshed polyester reinforcement.[78] In the Corvita stent-graft, a self-expanding stent is integrated with polycarbonate urethane and has the benefits of a high expansion ratio, allowing percutaneous insertion for the smaller-diameter grafts. Larger grafts are used for AAA.[79, 80]

Description of The Device

The Corvita endoluminal graft is a modular system that includes a bifurcated aortic trunk and two iliac leg endoprostheses (Fig. 38–19). The endoprostheses are composed of a biomedical superalloy wire stent lined with a porous polycarbonate elastomer (Corethane). The liner facilitates tissue ingrowth and maintains hemostasis after implantation. The endoprostheses are manually cut to the appropriate length by the user and then compressed and loaded into the delivery systems.

Delivery System

The introducer (Placehit) is similar to the coaxial tube system used for the Wallgraft. The exterior tube constrains the endoprosthesis until it is retracted during delivery. If desired, the endoprosthesis can be reconstrained before full deployment and the device repositioned. Radiopaque markers facilitate imaging during deployment. The delivery systems accommodate an 0.035- or 0.038-inch super-stiff guide wire.

Gore-Tex Hemobahn Endovascular Device

The Hemobahn Endovascular Prosthesis (W. L. Gore, Flagstaff, Ariz.) is a flexible, self-expanding endoluminal prosthesis. This was one of the first commercial endovascular grafts to use expanded ePTFE as the graft material.

The Device

The prosthesis is a flexible, self-expanding endoluminal prosthesis that consists of an PTFE graft with an external nitinol support stent extending along its entire length. The nitinol support is secured to the graft by fluorinated ethylene propylene (FEP) and ePTFE tape (Fig. 38–20*A*). The prosthesis is folded to allow introduction into the vasculature via a percutaneous approach.

A larger-diameter version (Aortic Excluder) is being developed for use in AAA repair.

Delivery System

The folded prosthesis is attached to the leading end of a dual-lumen, over-the-wire, polyethylene delivery catheter (Fig. 38–20 *B* and *C*). Knotted removable loops made of ePTFE fiber are used to maintain the folded prosthesis securely on the delivery catheter. To facilitate accurate prosthesis placement, two radiopaque metallic bands attached to the catheter shaft mark the ends of the folded prosthesis. Two oval beads, or "olives," enclose the radiopaque mark-

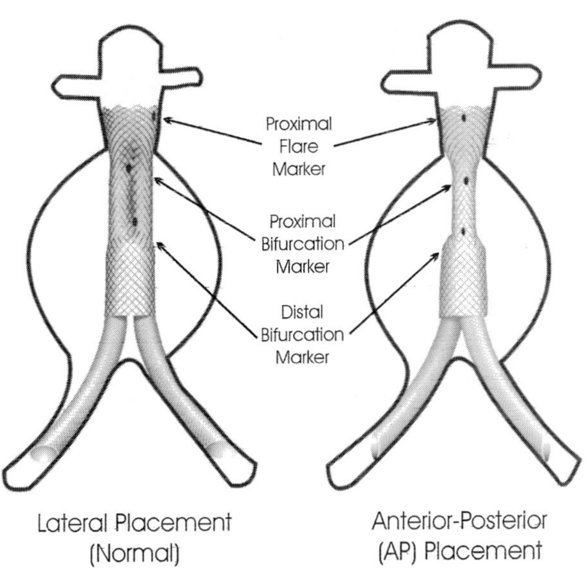

FIGURE 38–19. Corvita bifurcated endoluminal graft system. The two iliac limbs are implanted in the central bifurcation section of the infrarenal trunk graft.

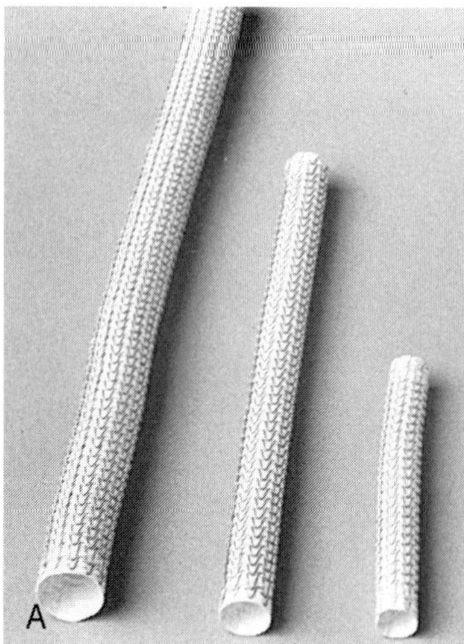

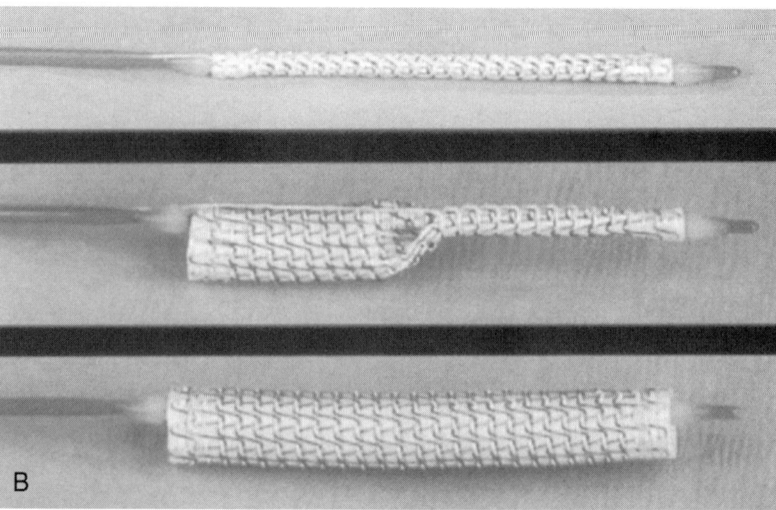

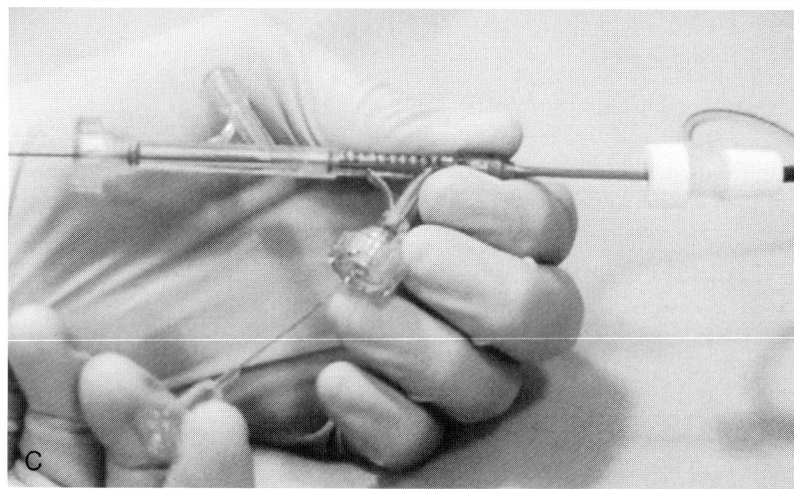

FIGURE 38–20. Hemobahn endovascular prosthesis. *A,* The 12-, 8-, and 6-mm diameter tubular grafts. *B,* Mechanism of deployment of the Hemobahn by pulling on a catch thread, which releases the graft from the proximal aspect to the distal end. *C,* Deployment of the Hemobahn. This illustration shows the pull wire, which is used to initiate release of the graft.

ers. The olives provide a smooth transition from the catheter to the slightly larger profile of the folded prosthesis. The larger lumen of the delivery catheter is used for flushing and guide wire introduction. The smaller lumen contains elements of the deployment mechanism.

The trailing end of the delivery catheter is attached to a three-port, clear plastic adapter, which includes a central port for guide wire introduction, one port for system flushing, and a third port for the deployment system. A final length of ePTFE fiber, called the *deployment line,* extends from the knotted removable loops and is fixed to the deployment knob of the delivery catheter.

Introduction into the vasculature can be accomplished by either percutaneous or surgical cutdown techniques. The prosthesis is properly positioned at the target deployment site under fluoroscopic guidance. To release the prosthesis, the deployment knob is pulled, effectively pulling the deployment line and removing the row of stitches from the prosthesis, which allows it to self-expand. A percutaneous transluminal angioplasty balloon is then used to smooth and seal the prosthesis against the arterial wall. In the vessel segment treated with the prosthesis, blood flows through the prosthesis and is excluded from contact with the vessel wall.

The prosthesis is available in a variety of diameters and lengths. Selection of a prosthesis of appropriate size is based on the diameter and nature of the vessel segment that requires treatment and on the length of the target lesion(s). More than one prosthesis may be used in an overlapping fashion to properly treat the affected vessel segment.

Baxter Endovascular Graft System

The Baxter endovascular graft system (Baxter CVG, Irvine, Calif.) is based on a concept developed in 1993 by White and colleagues.[81] They described a balloon-expandable prosthesis composed of a commercially available woven polyester graft with metallic graft attachment devices incorporated into the fabric of the graft and extending throughout its length (Fig. 38–21). The prosthesis, in tube, aortoiliac, and bifurcated configurations, has been extensively tested in clinical use.[55, 68, 82] In 1996, Baxter Healthcare Corporation commenced the task of turning the "home-made" product, which only its originators had used, into a commercially available device that others could use.

Description

The Baxter endovascular graft is made of woven PET with walls approximately 0.3 mm thick. The graft's strength, durability, and porosity are similar to those of conventional

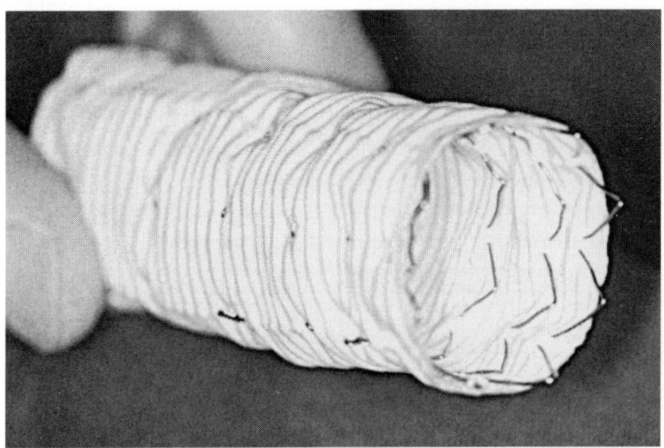

FIGURE 38–21. Balloon-expanded White-Yu tube graft, featuring intermittent wireforms interwoven with the polyester fabric wall. This was the prototype graft for the Baxter endovascular graft.

prostheses. Rather than stents, it features wireform supports composed of annealed elgiloy, a lightweight wire made from a corrosion-resistant alloy that has excellent fatigue resistance. It has an extensive clinical history as a long-term implantable material, including use in Baxter's Carpentier-Edwards bioprostheses (e.g., porcine and pericardial mitral and aortic valves). Annealing the material is necessary to allow balloon expansion of the device. Elgiloy wire segments are formed into curvilinear configurations and are woven into the graft wall so that alternating crests of each wire are outside the graft and the remainder of the wire material is inside it. The free ends of each segment are mechanically connected with a crimped elgiloy splice to complete the wireform. Separate wireforms are woven into the graft material in series, running the length of the graft (Fig. 38–22).

The bifurcated endovascular graft system is made up of three individual units: a bifurcated graft trunk and two iliac extension limbs (see Fig. 38–22*B*). All are balloon deployed, and each is contained in its own delivery system. The top, or proximal, portion of the bifurcated graft trunk contains four independent wireforms of annealed elgiloy interwoven into the polyester graft matrix. The iliac extension graft contains independent wireforms of annealed elgiloy placed throughout the length of each graft to act as attachment devices after deployment via balloon expansion. The proximal portions of the extension grafts are anchored in the limbs of the bifurcated graft trunk (at least 2 cm overlap is required). The distal portions are anchored in their respective iliac arteries.

Delivery System

The delivery system is composed of two primary units, the introducer sheath and the endovascular graft delivery unit, provided as an integral system for transluminal placement of the graft. The introducer-sheath assembly is comprised of a tapered introducer and an introducer sheath. The tapered introducer has a flexible, tapered tip. The introducer sheath has an internal diameter of 18 Fr. and an external diameter of 22 Fr. and a usable length of 21.5 cm. The endovascular graft delivery unit is comprised of a graft loader assembly, a catheter assembly, and a pusher assembly. The catheter assembly consists of an 8 Fr. coaxial nylon (wire-reinforced) catheter body with a noncompliant PET balloon.

The pusher assembly tubing butts up against the com-

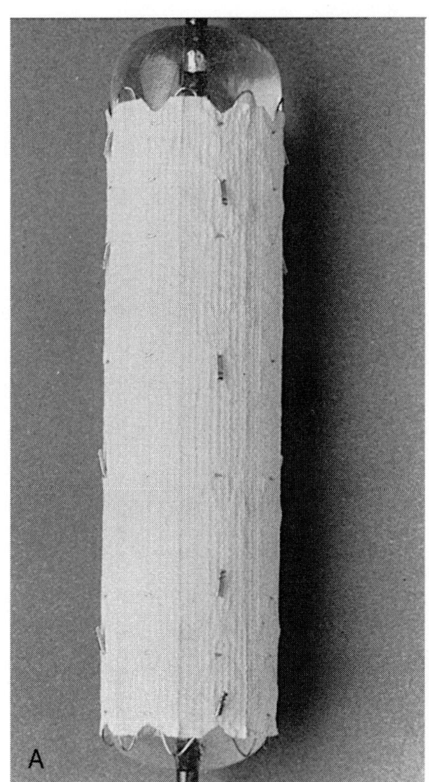

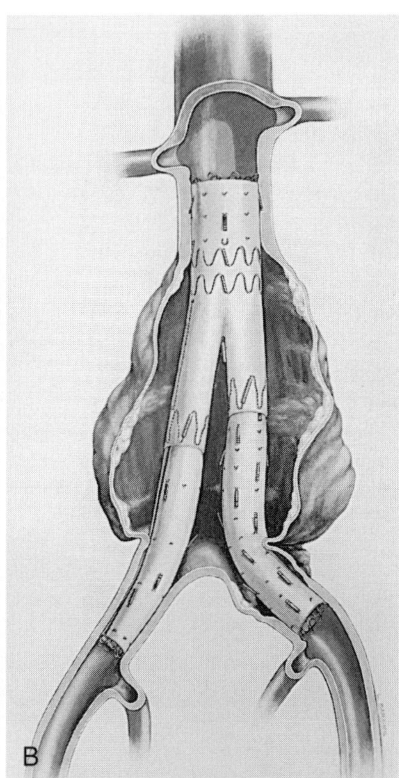

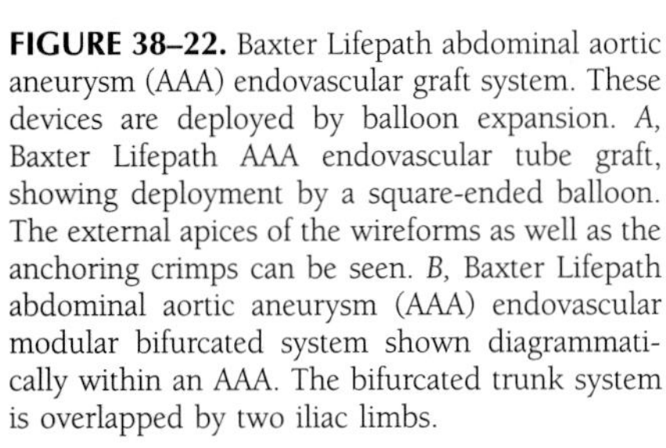

FIGURE 38–22. Baxter Lifepath abdominal aortic aneurysm (AAA) endovascular graft system. These devices are deployed by balloon expansion. *A*, Baxter Lifepath AAA endovascular tube graft, showing deployment by a square-ended balloon. The external apices of the wireforms as well as the anchoring crimps can be seen. *B*, Baxter Lifepath abdominal aortic aneurysm (AAA) endovascular modular bifurcated system shown diagrammatically within an AAA. The bifurcated trunk system is overlapped by two iliac limbs.

pressed endovascular graft to prevent retraction during placement. Oversizing the prosthesis by 10% over the diameter of the proximal neck is recommended. This measure creates sufficient radial force to anchor the device and effect a seal between the aneurysm sac and the general circulation in the aortic lumen. Chaufour and coworkers[83] have confirmed the safety of dilating the aorta with such an oversized balloon and have documented the limits of this maneuver.

Surgical Technique for Deployment

For tube graft procedures, the "trombone technique"[82] is employed with the Baxter system to simplify sizing the length of the prosthesis. With this technique, the first tube prosthesis, 9 cm long, is deployed immediately below the renal arteries. The 6-cm second prosthesis is deployed within and overlapping the first prosthesis, so that it resides immediately above the aortic bifurcation. Provided there is a minimum of 2 cm overlap, the length of the prosthesis can be determined at operation. For bifurcated graft procedures, the bifurcated trunk segment is implanted first, followed by the two iliac limbs. A directional catheter technique is used to achieve cannulation of the contralateral stump (Fig. 38–23).

Other Endovascular Graft Systems

Ivancev-Malmo system

The homemade Ivancev-Malmo device is an aortoiliac tapered, woven, polyester graft based on two barbed Gianturco Z-stents that are situated, respectively, at the proximal (aortic) and distal (iliac) ends.[54, 84] A feature of this system is the central cannula of the delivery system, which carries a suture loop to the cranial end of the prosthesis to pull it through the 23 Fr. introducer sheath. The tapered aortoiliac graft is custom-made according to the patient's vascular dimensions, by suturing together two cylindrical segments of different diameters, and it has been used in conjunction with occlusion of the contralateral iliac artery and femorofemoral bypass.[84, 85] Because it is not supported by stents along its length, insertion of an adjunctive Wallstent has been necessary when graft kinking occurred. A similar endovascular aortoiliac device and technique have been used by the Nottingham group in the United Kingdom.[86]

Stretched Polytetrafluoroethylene Stent Combinations

Devices made from overexpanded PTFE have been described by several groups.[14, 87, 88] In general, these grafts are prepared by stretching an ePTFE prosthesis to a predetermined diameter using a graded series of angioplasty balloons.[87] Usually, the graft is tapered and secured proximally to a large Palmaz stent, mounted over a large-diameter vascular balloon, and back-loaded into a delivery sheath (modified Parodi technique). Applications of this graft design have been reported by the vascular surgery groups at Montefiore Hospital, Bronx, N.Y.[12, 89] and at Leicester, England,[88] both of whom used it in aortomonoiliac configuration in association with femorofemoral crossover graft. The contralateral common iliac artery is occluded by a closed stent-graft.

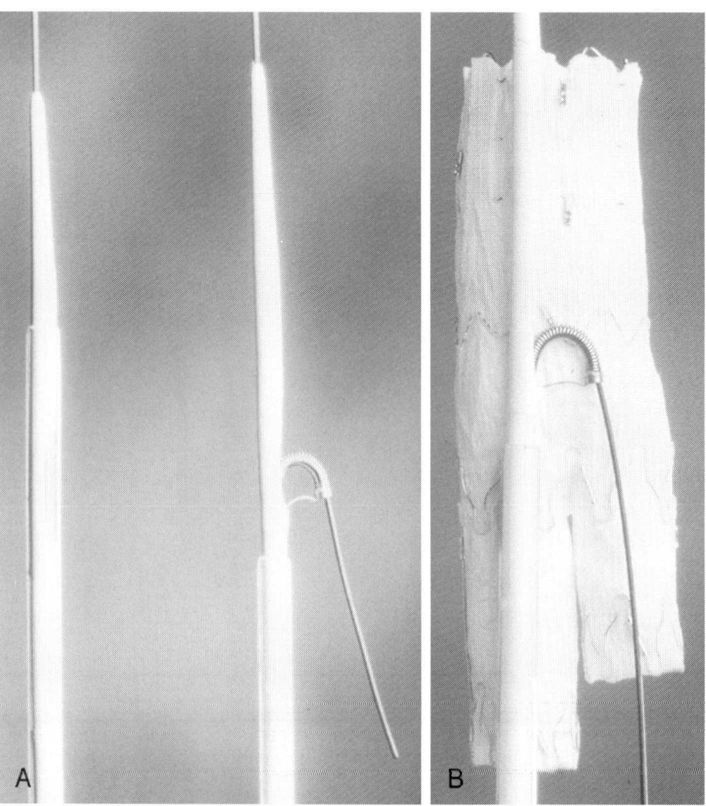

FIGURE 38–23. Baxter Lifepath abdominal aortic aneurysm directional catheter for use in simplifying contralateral stump access with the modular bifurcated system. *A,* The distal end of the directional catheter is shown before deployment of the deflecting tip *(left)* and then after deployment of the tip, *(right)* with a non-kink guide wire from one limb of the graft to the other. *B,* The distal end of the directional catheter is shown against the background of the bifurcated graft body to demonstrate the application of this catheter in passing a guide wire from one limb of the graft to the other.

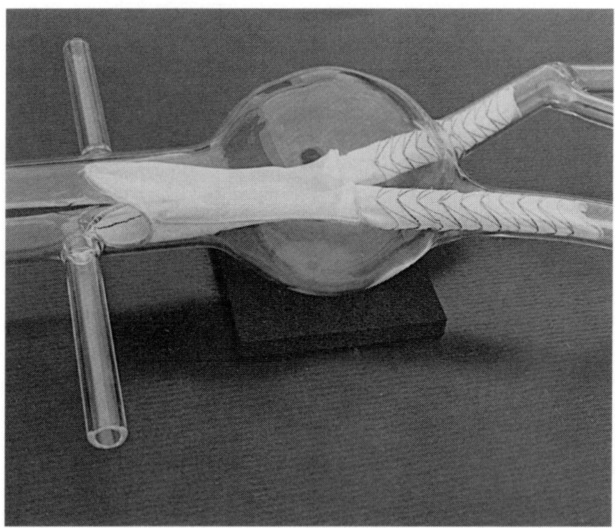

FIGURE 38–24. Vascutek Lauterjung bifurcated graft, featuring a proximal "fish-mouth" shape and two externally supported iliac limbs.

Vascutek/Lauterjung Design

The Vascutek/Lauterjung experimental device is made up of standard polyester graft fabric with a sinusoidal nitinol wire reinforcement at the ends that is used to deploy the graft and attach it to the vessel wall by friction seal (Fig. 38–24).[90]

Other Endovascular Grafts in Development

Many companies involved in vascular surgery, including Cordis, Bard, and Intervascular, are currently developing alternative designs of endovascular grafts.

CLINICAL CONSIDERATIONS

Comparison with Conventional Grafts

Less invasive management of vascular disease involves treatment via remote access to the vascular system. For a vascular graft to be suitable for insertion from such a remote site and internal fixation to the graft wall, some changes in graft characteristics are necessary. The graft material must be compressed into a profile narrow enough to fit a delivery sheath or catheter, yet must maintain enough strength to resist bursting, tearing, and excessive late dilatation. It is not yet known whether endoluminal grafts must have the same porosity characteristics as standard arterial grafts. When the endovascular graft will be contained within an intact aneurysm sac, greater porosity may be acceptable because interstitial bleeding will be contained within the aorta until fibrin or thrombus deposition occludes the pore.[91] On the other hand, if this thrombotic seal still allows transmission of arterial pressure to the contents of the aneurysm sac, the aortic wall may continue to expand. If endovascular grafts are to be used in treatment of ruptured aneurysms, the graft material must be impervious.

Guidelines[91] for the development and use of endovascular prosthetic grafts and reporting standards[92] have been published. Endovascular graft procedures have a range of specific complications, many of which are unique to this technology (Table 38–8).

Tube Versus Bifurcated Grafts for Abdominal Aortic Aneurysm

Although tube graft repair is preferred whenever possible for open repair of AAA, it has become apparent that stent-graft treatment for infrarenal AAA requires a bifurcated graft system in the majority of cases. The anatomy of the proximal neck and the iliac arteries are the major determinants of graft selection. In the large majority of patients assessed for this procedure, the distal neck, or aortic cuff, is unsuitable for successfully implanting a tube graft.[93–95] Even when the distal aortic cuff is 10 to 15 mm long, it is often lined with thrombus and is prone to late expansion, which may result in endoleak.

For a safe and lasting seal, at least 15 to 20 mm of secure attachment and contact with the wall is generally required.[96] Problems with achieving a good seal in the distal aorta are increased by the fact that accurate determination of length for a tube graft may be difficult because of the curved, tortuous path of the vessel[20]; this aspect is not so vital if a bifurcated graft is used, since there is a longer attachment site within the iliac artery. One way of overcoming this problem with tube grafts is by customizing the graft's length at the time of the procedure by overlapping several tube devices.[82]

Several studies have shown that, according to current criteria, as few as 5% of patients may be candidates for tube grafts.[92, 95, 97] In most series, bifurcated grafts are being used for more than 90% of endoluminal graft procedures, and aortoiliac tapered grafts make up the difference. There may be a temptation to overreact and suggest that "non-tube" configurations be used for all endoluminal repairs for AAA. A more moderate approach, however, would be to

TABLE 38–8. COMPLICATIONS PECULIAR TO ENDOVASCULAR GRAFTS

Early

1. Radiation (x-ray) exposure
   - Potential risk to patients and staff
2. Trauma to access arteries
   - Perforation, dissection, thrombosis of femoral or iliac artery
3. Microembolization
   - Due to dislodgment of mural components or thrombus from the abdominal arterial aneurysm sac
4. Graft displacement or misplacement
5. Occlusion of major branch arteries
   - Renal, accessory renal, mesenteric, and so on
6. Endoleak
7. "Post-implantation syndrome"
   - Fever, backache, malaise
8. Graft limb compression, stenosis, occlusion
9. Contrast allergy or renal failure

Late

1. Graft migration
2. Endoleak
3. Late stenosis, kink or thrombosis of graft or graft limb
4. Graft tear or failure, material fatigue, stent breakage
5. Aneurysm rupture

"tighten" the criteria for using tube prostheses, so that the length of the distal neck would be in the range of 2.0 to 2.5 cm.[96] Tube grafts are suitable for many saccular, anastomotic, or false aneurysms. With decreasing mortality and morbidity rates, and with increasing information on the intermediate and long-term outcomes of endoluminal repair, it is likely that there will be a move toward treating smaller AAAs earlier, when they are more suitable for the endoluminal method. Many of these smaller AAAs have proximal and distal necks and are suitable for tube graft implantation.

The implantation procedure for bifurcated grafts is more complex, and the limbs of bifurcated grafts are more prone to thrombotic occlusion, especially when compromised by external compression or kinked by tortuous iliac vessels. Fixed angulation of the proximal segment of the common iliac artery and associated calcification (especially in patients with chronic renal failure) can present an almost impenetrable barrier to safe access to the aorta, and perforation of these segments is common. In such cases, and for some patients with stenosis or aneurysm of the iliac artery on one side, an aortoiliac graft may be preferable, used in conjunction with femoral crossover graft.

Operative Technique for Endoluminal Grafting of Abdominal Aortic Aneurysm

The operative techniques for all devices have many features in common, the principal variations being in the details of deployment. The patient is positioned on the operating table so that a mobile C-arm can image the lower thoracic and abdominal aorta and the iliac arteries.

A radiopaque ruler is placed beneath the patient and positioned immediately to the left of the aorta. The common femoral artery on the side of the least tortuous iliac arteries is usually chosen for primary access. The shape of the AAA and the perceived risk of dislodging mural thrombus are other factors in the choice of the side to be used for primary access. Bilateral femoral access is used for bifurcated grafts. The patient is "heparinized" with 5000 IU administered intravenously. A regular guide wire is passed into the thoracic aorta, and a calibrated pigtail catheter is introduced over it. Aortography is performed after removal of the guide wire and positioning of the pigtail end of the catheter opposite the renal arteries, usually at the level of the upper half of the second lumbar vertebra. The positions of the renal arteries, aortic bifurcation, and internal iliac arteries are noted with reference to the radiopaque ruler.

An extra-stiff or super-stiff guide wire is introduced into the pigtail catheter, and the catheter is then removed. The delivery system catheter is introduced over this guide wire through a transverse femoral arteriotomy to the level of the renal arteries. Conditions that interfere with smooth introduction of the expandable sheet and delivery system are occlusive arterial disease and pronounced tortuosity or angulation of these arteries. When both sides are suitable for access, a right-handed surgeon usually selects the right common femoral artery. The systolic blood pressure is adjusted to 120 mmHg or less, and the deployment process commences.

After implantation of the endovascular graft, a pigtail catheter is passed over the guide wire to enable a completion angiogram to be performed. Contrast-enhanced CT is performed within a week of operation, at 6 and 12 months after operation, and annually thereafter.

Most devices now available effect initial aneurysm exclusion if the patient has relatively straight aortic neck and iliac arteries and a long (>2 cm) implantation zone of healthy arterial wall. Unfortunately, such patients are the minority among those with an AAA or a thoracic aneurysm greater than 5 cm in diameter, and the treating team needs to call on a variety of additional skills and adjunctive techniques to successfully manage the other cases.[98]

Compromising factors include a proximal aortic neck shorter than 15 mm or wider than 26 mm or one that is angulated, conical, lined with thrombus, or irregular in shape. Tortuosity, stenosis, and aneurysm of the iliac arteries each present particular difficulties, especially when the vessels are heavily calcified. In some cases, the solution to these problems requires complex interventional skills and devices; in others, a combination of endovascular and conventional surgical techniques may be applied.[99]

Since endovascular graft devices cannot be resized or modified during the procedure, thorough and precise preprocedural planning is critical. High-quality, quantitative digital angiography and helical CT are used to measure the proximal neck diameter and length and the diameters of the iliac vessels to ensure optimal patient selection.

Endoluminal Repair of Iliac Artery Aneurysms

Repair of iliac artery aneurysms has been reported in several series.[89, 100, 101] Tube grafts of diameters from 10 to 16 mm are usually used, and adjunctive coil embolization of the internal iliac artery is often required to prevent retrograde flow into the aneurysm sac. The smaller-diameter grafts may be implanted by percutaneous technique.[101]

Thoracic Aortic Aneurysms

The most extensive experience of stent-graft repair of thoracic aneurysms has been reported by Dake and coworkers.[18, 19, 102] The devices used are usually larger in diameter than those used in the abdomen (≤40 mm). Special considerations for endovascular grafts suitable for the thoracic aorta include the large-diameter grafts and sheath systems, which may need to be introduced via the common iliac artery or the abdominal aorta.[18] In most cases, this requires a self-expanding stent mechanism, since balloons of this diameter are not readily available. Balloon-expanded grafts have also been successfully deployed, however, to exclude aneurysms or dissections of the thoracic aorta.[55, 103]

Aortic Dissection

Dissections of the thoracic aorta may sometimes be treated by thoracic endovascular grafts, as thoracic aneurysms are.[81, 103] The graft should be positioned to close both the entry and exit points of the dissection, to obliterate the false channel, and to depressurize any aneurysm arising from it. Endovascular graft repair of infrarenal aortic dissections has also been reported.[55, 104]

Anastomotic Aneurysms

Several clinical studies have reported good results for endograft placement for management of anastomotic aneurysms after aortic or aortoiliac graft procedures.[105–107] In many of these cases, a tube graft can be used. These procedures can be done with great success, low morbidity, and short hospital stays.

Applications in Peripheral Vessels

A variety of coated stent and stent-graft devices are being developed for specific applications in the peripheral vessels. Some of the current endovascular grafts for iliac or peripheral arteries are listed in Table 38–9. It is likely that specific variations will be designed for the different applications to management of aneurysms, occlusive disease, and trauma.

Aneurysms in Peripheral Arteries

Peripheral[108] and visceral[109] aneurysms may be treated transluminally by remote access, usually via the femoral artery. This method has been applied particularly to popliteal aneurysms,[110, 111] and initial results have been satisfactory but graft thrombosis has been frequent at mid-term follow-up.

Vascular Trauma, False Aneurysms, and Arteriovenous Fistulae

The use of covered stents or endovascular grafts in trauma cases has great appeal, since there is the potential to transform a quite difficult, hazardous open procedure into a simple, safe transluminal repair via remote access.[30, 31, 106, 111, 112] Endografts can be used in the acute phase to repair the vessel wall and stop hemorrhage, or in the late phase to manage arteriovenous fistula or false aneurysm.[29, 31] The technique may be particularly valuable when injuries occur to vessels in the chest or abdomen, including the subclavian artery or visceral branches, and may be combined with interventional embolization techniques using coils, detachable balloons, or other occluding materials.[26, 27, 113] Endograft implantation for emergency treatment of traumatic aortic rupture has also been reported.[114]

To date, Palmaz stents lined with PTFE or polyester appear to have been used in the majority of trauma cases, although the Corvita endovascular graft is also being tried for this application.[78, 113] A new generation of PTFE-lined nitinol stent-grafts is also entering trials. Autogenous tissue such as veins or fascia should be considered as a covering for the stent in cases of acute trauma with wound contamination.[30] The principal concern about widespread use of endovascular grafts in trauma is the potential for graft infection or loss of patency secondary to stenosis or late occlusion of the prosthesis in young patients.

Arterial Occlusive Disease

Covered stents or endovascular grafts may have valuable applications in treating atherosclerotic peripheral vascular disease, especially when simple stents have produced poor results owing to aggressive restenosis.[115] Stents have been shown to reduce the immediate failure rate after balloon angioplasty of the femoropopliteal segment vessels, but late patency has been adversely affected by a high rate of restenosis. It has been shown that the ingrowth of neointimal hyperplasia through the interstices of stents is reduced by the mechanical barrier of a prosthetic coating, but early thrombosis or mid-term reactions at the ends of stent-grafts used in these situations has led to early failure in some cases.[116] In a trial of endovascular graft lining of recanalized iliac arteries, Marin and colleagues described satisfactory early patency, but frequent demand for reintervention for failing grafts over the longer term.[117]

Cragg and Dake developed a stent-graft "endoluminal bypass" technique for use after percutaneous revascularization of long-segment femoropopliteal occlusions[118] using a 6-mm PTFE, thin-walled graft attached to a self-expanding stent constructed of a nitinol wire. This graft was delivered by compressing it into a tubular loading catheter and pushing it through a 12 Fr. sheath. Deployment was then accomplished by withdrawing the sheath, followed by balloon molding of the lumen of the externally supported, self-expanding stent-graft. Problems were encountered with grafts placed in regions of flexion, and graft thrombosis was common. A polyester-covered version was developed (EndoPro System, Mintec, La Ciotat, France) in which the fabric was bonded with fractionated heparin. Initial experience with this device indicates a high incidence of technical success in femoral lesions, but, again, there were problems with early thrombosis.[119] A unique complication of this endoprosthesis was the development of fever and severe pain at the site of implantation, sometimes associated with perivascular inflammation.[120]

Further trials of similar devices are under way for the treatment of both focal stenotic lesions of the superficial femoral artery and long-segment diffuse disease of the iliac and femoropopliteal sites. Attempts have been made to improve the results by initial debulking or disobliteration of the vessel by atherectomy or closed endarterectomy with ring strippers, followed by endobypass.[121–123] The importance of stent support along the total length of the graft wall has been stressed. Most current designs of stent-grafts for application in peripheral vessels are constructed of nitinol stents covered with polyester (e.g., Passager graft) or PTFE (e.g., Hemobahn graft). The combination of stent-grafts and various coating or pharmacologic materials may prove to be of value, particularly if local genetic manipulation can also be achieved.

Miscellaneous Applications

Stent-grafts have also been proposed for use as conduits in transjugular intrahepatic portosystemic shunts (TIPS),[124] carotid aneurysms,[125–127] gastrointestinal malignancy,[127, 128] aortocoronary saphenous vein grafts,[129] superior vena cava syndrome,[130] and other applications.

UNRESOLVED ISSUES

Thin-Walled Versus Standard Vascular Prosthetic Materials

There is considerable impetus to use thin-walled prosthetic graft materials in the construction of endovascular graft

TABLE 38–9. ENDOVASCULAR GRAFTS FOR ILIAC OR PERIPHERAL VESSELS

DEVICE MANUFACTURER (BRAND NAME)	DEVICE CHARACTERISTICS			DELIVERY SYSTEM			
	Graft Material	**Stent Material**	**Stent Pattern**	**Size (Outside Diameter)**	**Method of Expansion**	**Method of Fixation**	**Main Applications**
Boston Scientific (Passager)	Polyester thin-walled	Nitinol	Continuous mesh (internal)	12 Fr.	Self-expanding + heat	Small hooks + friction	Occlusive disease
World Medical (Talent)	Polyester	Nitinol	Intermittent	16 Fr.	Self-expanding	Friction + compression fit	Iliac limb of bifurcated graft
Medtronic (AneuRx)	Polyester thin-walled	Nitinol	Continuous mesh (external)	16 Fr.	Self-expanding	Friction + compression fit	Iliac limb of bifurcated graft
Schneider (Wallgraft)	PTFE (?)	Titanium (Wallstent)	Continuous mesh (external)	12 Fr.	Self-expanding	Friction	Occlusive disease
Schneider (Corvita)	Polyurethane	Stainless steel	Continuous mesh (external)	12 Fr.	Self-expanding	Friction	Trauma
Baxter	Polyester	Elgiloy	Intermittent	22 Fr.	Balloon-expandable	Friction + crimps	Iliac limb of bifurcated graft
Gore (Hemobahn)	PTFE	Nitinol	Continuous	22 Fr.	Self-expanding	Friction	Occlusive disease

PTFE = polytetrafluoroethylene.

devices, since this allows compression of the graft into narrower delivery systems and deployment sheaths. But thin-walled material may have a greater tendency to dilate, tear, or burst when used to treat aneurysmal conditions, jeopardizing long-term results. Graft material disintegration[60] or tearing[131, 132] with thin-walled polyester has been reported and has led to endoleak or aneurysm rupture. The healing patterns, endurance, and integrity of modified thin PTFE material were investigated by Palmaz and coworkers.[13] PTFE explanted from animals at 3, 6, and 12 months showed no structural deterioration and no changes in internodal distance. Thickness and axial tensile strengths varied by 12% and 17%, respectively, from those in controls.

Conventional polyester grafts used for open surgical repair have proven durability but usually require larger sheath systems when used in an endovascular graft, and these thicker graft materials may also have a tendency to form longitudinal folds or to bunch up when used in endoluminal grafts.[17]

Should the Stent Component Be Placed Over the Renal Arteries?

Implantation of the bare stent component of a stent-graft over or above the renal artery orifices may provide some benefit in fixation of the graft, prevention of endoleak, and reduction of the tendency for late graft displacement or migration (Fig. 38–17*B*). This technique would seem to be particularly so when the aortic neck is short or has unfavorable features such as mural thrombus, irregular shape, or wide diameter. On the other hand, this practice may carry increased risk of renal artery thrombosis or embolization or may result in occlusion of renal artery blood flow by the graft component of the device.[133] Early experimental work with woven Dacron graft material attached to Gianturco Z-stents showed that collateral branches covered by the graft became occluded, whereas those covered by the stent remained open.[17] A thin neointima covered the stents, and a much thicker neointima covered the fabric.

With devices that feature a section of bare stent above the graft material, the full length of the aneurysm neck usually must maintain contact with the graft fabric to prevent proximal endoleak; thus, there is little room for bare metal in the infrarenal region unless the neck is unusually long. Implantation of a close-meshed stent over the renal orifices may lead to ostial occlusion by inducing intimal hyperplasia, whereas more open Z-stent styles would have only one metallic strut across an orifice, which should not provide a "scaffold" for intimal hyperplasia.[17, 21, 134] In clinical studies to date, covering the renal arteries with the open section of Gianturco Z-stents or with nitinol stents does not seem to affect renal function in early follow-up.[134]

Dilatation of the Residual Infrarenal Aorta After Endovascular Exclusion of Abdominal Aortic Aneurysm

The long-term fate of the aortic neck in a patient with aneurysmal disease placed under continuous radial force from a stent is not known. It has been postulated that late dilatation of the neck may occur secondary to continuation of the aneurysmal pathologic process or to stretching and damage from the stent implanted within it, and that this dilatation may lead to endoleak and, eventually, to displacement of the endovascular graft. In this respect, there may be important differences between the effects of a self-expanding and a balloon-expanded stent attachment, since the continued force of an oversized, self-expanding stent against the aortic wall may progressively dilate the neck to the diameter of the device and cause associated weakening of the structure of the wall that could predispose to further late dilatation.

Sonesson and coworkers, using a self-expanding device based on Gianturco Z-stents, showed that there was a significant dilatation of the aneurysm neck at mean follow-up of 25 months that was not associated with concurrent dilatation of the suprarenal aorta.[135] Similar results were reported by May and associates[136] (proximal neck dilatation 1 to 2 mm at 6 months, but no progressive changes). On the other hand, Matsumura and colleagues reported that, 1 year after implantation of EVT tube grafts, there was no change in the diameter of the supraceliac or infrarenal aortic diameter, whereas the diameter of the distal neck enlarged, on average, 1 to 3 mm.[53]

Should Barbs, Hooks, or Anchors Be Used?

Migration of endovascular graft devices was noted even with the earliest experimental work in animals, and subsequently devices were fitted with barbs on the leading stent.[17] The argument for barbs is that they provide more secure attachment to the arterial wall and therefore help prevent migration. However, barbs or hooks may traumatize the vessel or perforate its wall. Perforation of the aorta by an uncovered portion of the stent has been reported.[137] Inclusion of barbs on the stent also usually requires a wider sheath for delivery of the device.

Risk of Infection

Cultures of the aortic wall and mural thrombus associated with aortic aneurysms often grow pathogenic organisms.[138] It is possible, therefore, that implantation of an endovascular graft may place the patient at increased risk for graft infection. A recent study that examined this issue in an experimental model suggested that infection of a stent-graft with *Staphylococcus aureus* would be more severe than infection in a surgically placed conventional graft.[139]

Infection of an aortic endograft (PTFE/Palmaz stent construction) is mentioned briefly in one report.[14] Endovascular graft infection of a nitinol-polyester stent-graft (BSC Vanguard) placed percutaneously into the iliac system for management of aneurysm of the common iliac artery has also been reported,[140] and we have encountered a similar case in our own practice. Infection of metallic stents in the iliac artery has also been encountered, but it remains rare.[141]

To date, there have been no published reports of infection of endovascular grafts placed in the aorta, although development of aortoenteric fistula has been reported.[142] Anecdotal reports of five cases of infected endovascular aortic grafts were elicited in an informal poll of investigators at a recent conference. Since these devices have now been used longer than 5 years, the apparent low incidence of infection at this stage suggests that they may not, in fact, be less resistant to infection than a conventional graft placed by open surgery.

Endoleak

Endoleak, a complication peculiar to endoluminal aneurysm repair, is defined as the persistence of blood flow outside the graft lumen but within the aneurysm sac or adjacent vessels in which the graft is deployed.[143–147] Endoleak that occurs at initial deployment may be due to a number of factors, and it often arises at the proximal or distal site of fixation of the device. In selected cases, further endovascular intervention to repair such primary endoleaks may be successful.[43, 144–149]

Trauma to the device fabric at implantation has also resulted in both early and late endoleaks.[43, 96] Some early postoperative endoleaks appear to seal spontaneously, although the long-term outcome of such sealed endoleaks is not known,[147] and they have been reported to recur.[144, 145] Aneurysm rupture due to untreated or undetected endoleak has been reported.[144, 150] There was also recently a report of AAA rupture after an endoleak was sealed,[65] and experimental studies have demonstrated that "seal" by embolization coils does not necessarily relieve pulsatility or pressure in the aneurysm sac.[151] Endoleak can often be identified with color duplex ultrasonography to identify flow in the sac,[144] but contrast-enhanced CT is the favored method of follow-up[96] and has become the imaging modality of choice. If an endoleak is suspected, further investigation should be carried out with angiography.

Risk of Branch Artery Occlusion

In addition to the risk of occlusion of the renal arteries (or inadvertent occlusion of accessory ones), risks are associated with routine blocking of antegrade flow in the inferior mesenteric artery, lumbar, intercostal, and other branch vessels. In the future, this problem may be addressed by fenestrated stent-grafts[152] or stent-grafts that feature extension sleeves that can be inserted into branch vessels. In the course of treatment of aortoiliac aneurysms or isolated aneurysms of the iliac vessels, the internal iliac arteries must often be occluded by placing an iliac extension graft across their origin or by preprocedural coil embolization of their branches.[87] This can result in gluteal claudication, colonic ischemia, and other severe complications, especially when bilateral internal iliac artery occlusion is performed.

Risk of Microembolization

Microembolization has been reported from several series of endovascular repair procedures, and it has been fatal in some cases.[12, 149] In an experimental study, microembolization during conventional and endovascular aneurysm repairs was quantified by insonating the superficial femoral artery with a 2-MHz Doppler probe.[153] Both particulate and gaseous embolization are more common with endovascular procedures, and the number of particulate emboli corresponds with clinical sequelae. Particulate embolization is most apparent during endoluminal manipulations in the aneurysm sac, the numbers of gaseous, particulate, and total emboli being significantly greater with endovascular repairs than with open repairs.[154] The incidence of this complication seems to decrease with operator experience and with strategies to minimize manipulation of large device components within the AAA sac.

Late Geometric Changes in the Grafts

Recent follow-up data for several types of endovascular grafts have indicated that the devices are prone to distortion and kinking, which may be associated with decreased AAA sac diameter and shortening of the aneurysm (longitudinal shrinkage) after effective treatment.[155] These effects may result in disruption or disconnection of components of a modular graft and detachment of the proximal or distal stents. Paradoxically, effective exclusion of the aneurysm sac itself may lead to changes in graft geometry that eventually lead to complications.[132, 155]

Need for Secondary Interventions

Many series of endoluminal repair of aneurysms have reported a high incidence of secondary interventions, both radiologic and surgical, to correct graft problems such as endoleak, stenosis, kink, and thrombosis.[156] Surgeons who undertake endovascular repair should be prepared for these procedures.

SUMMARY

Today, endovascular aneurysm repair is the most frequent application of endograft technology. It involves transfemoral intravascular implantation of an endograft within the aneurysm, with the aim of completely excluding the sac from the circulation, thus preventing aneurysm expansion or rupture. The endograft is anchored in place by self-expanding or balloon-expandable stents or wireforms, which may support all or part of the graft wall. Structural failure of the stents or attachment hook[34] and the prosthetic fabrics[59, 131, 132] has been documented, and the biological reactions to endografts are ill understood.

Patients who undergo successful endovascular graft procedures require long-term surveillance, including multiple imaging studies, and there is a possibility that late secondary procedures will become necessary to maintain integrity of the endograft. This eventuality would result in further radiation exposure and expense.

Although the technical success and short-term efficacy of endovascular grafts have now been demonstrated for most applications, long-term durability of grafts used in the aorta and patency of smaller endovascular graft conduits used for trauma or occlusive disease remain to be proven. No long-term data are yet available on device durability or patient outcome beyond the initial few years. Recent evidence shows that the ability of endovascular grafts to cause shrinkage and regression of aortic aneurysms may have the paradoxical effect of distorting the endograft itself, thus causing geometric changes in the supporting metallic framework, and, ultimately device failure.

Thus, the desired positive effect of the device may, ironically, lead eventually to its failure. It is clearly essential that endovascular graft technology be subjected to rigorous prospective evaluation for each of its applications. Registries,[157] concurrent comparative studies,[158–160] and randomized trials[161] will all play roles. Of primary importance will be the late and long-term results.

REFERENCES

1. Dotter CT: Transluminally-placed coilspring endarterial tube grafts: Long-term patency in canine popliteal artery. Invest Radiol 4:329–332, 1969.
2. Palmaz JC, Laborde JC, Rivera FJ, et al: Stenting of the iliac arteries with the Palmaz stent: Experience from a multicenter trial. Cardiovasc Interv Radiol 15:291–297, 1992.
3. Strecker EP, Hagen B, Liermann D, et al: Treatment of atherosclerotic occlusive disease of the aortic bifurcation with balloon expandable tantalum stents. Eur Radiol 3:536–540, 1993.
4. Zollikofer CL, Antonucci F, Pfyffer M, et al: Arterial stent placement with use of the Wallstent: Midterm results of clinical experience. Radiology 179:449–456, 1991.
5. Balko A, Piasecki GJ, Shah DM, et al: Transfemoral placement of intraluminal polyurethane prosthesis for abdominal aortic aneurysm. J Surg Res 40:305–309, 1986.
6. Mirich D, Wright KC, Wallace S, et al: Percutaneously placed endovascular grafts for aortic aneurysms: Feasibility study. Radiology 170:1033–1037, 1989.
7. Parodi JC, Palmaz JC, Barone HD: Transfemoral intraluminal graft implantation for abdominal aortic anuerysms. Ann Vasc Surg 5:491–499, 1991.
8. Volodos NL, Karpovich IP, Troyan VI, et al: Clinical experience of the use of a self-fixing synthetic prosthesis for remote endoprosthetics of the thoracic and the abdominal aorta and iliac arteries through the femoral artery and as intraoperative endoprosthesis for aorta reconstruction. Vasa 33(Suppl):93–95, 1991.
9. May J, White GH, Yu W, et al: Endoluminal grafting of abdominal aortic aneurysms: Causes of failure and their prevention. J Endovasc Surg 1:44–52, 1994.
10. Parodi JC: Endovascular repair of abdominal aortic aneurysms. Adv Vasc Surg 1:85–106, 1993.
11. Chuter TAM, Wendt G, Hopkinson BR, et al: Transfemoral insertion of a bifurcated endovascular graft for aortic aneurysm repair: The first 22 patients. Cardiovasc Surg 3:121–128, 1995.
12. Marin ML, Veith FJ, Cynamon J, et al: Initial experience with transluminally placed endovascular grafts for the treatment of complex vascular lesions. Ann Surg 222:449–469, 1995.
13. Palmaz JC, Tio FO, Laborde JC, et al: Use of stents covered with polytetrafluoroethylene in experimental abdominal aortic aneurysm. J Vasc Interv Radiol 6:879–885, 1995.
14. Adiseshiah M, Bray AJ, Bergeron P, Raphael MJ: Endoluminal repair of large abdominal aortic aneurysms using PTFE: A feasibility study. J Endovasc Surg 4:286–289, 1997.
15. White GH, Yu W, May J, et al: A new nonstented balloon-expandable graft for straight or bifurcated endoluminal bypass. J Endovasc Surg 1:16–24, 1994.
16. Maas D, Zollikofer CL, Largiader F, et al: Radiological follow-up of transluminally inserted vascular endoprostheses: An experimental study using expanding spirals. Radiology 152:659–663, 1984.
17. Lawrence DD, Charnsangavej C, Wright KC, et al: Percutaneous endovascular graft: Experimental evaluation. Radiology 163:357–360, 1987.
18. Dake MD, Miller DC, Semba CP, et al: Transluminal placement of endovascular stent-grafts for the treatment of descending thoracic aortic aneurysms. N Engl J Med 331:1729–1734, 1994.
19. Dake MD, Semba CP: Endovascular repair of thoracic aneurysm. *In* Hopkinson B, Yusuf W, Whitaker S, Veith F (eds): Endovascular Surgery for Aortic Aneurysms. London, WB Saunders, 1997, pp 180–193.
20. Lawrence-Brown MMD, Hartley D, MacSweeney STR, et al: The Perth endoluminal bifurcated graft system—development and early experience. Cardiovasc Surg 4:706–712, 1996.
21. Lawrence-Brown M, Sieunarine K, Hartley D, et al: The Perth HLB bifurcated endoluminal graft: A review of the experience and intermediate results. Cardiovasc Surg 6:220–225, 1998.
22. Lazarus HM: Intraluminal graft device: System and method. US Patent No. 4,787,799, 1988.
23. Lazarus HM: Endovascular grafting for the treatment of abdominal aortic aneurysms. Surg Clin North Am 72:959–968, 1992.
24. Lazarus HM: The EVT endoluminal prosthesis: Developmental concepts and design. *In* Chuter TA, Donayre CE, White RA (eds): Endoluminal Vascular Prostheses. Boston, Little, Brown, 1995.
25. White RA, Kopchok G, Zalewski M, et al: Comparison of the deployment and healing of thin-walled expanded PTFE stented grafts and covered stents. Ann Vasc Surg 10:336–346, 1996.
26. Becker GJ, Benenati JF, Zemel G, et al: Percutaneous placement of a balloon-expandable intraluminal graft for life-threatening subclavian arterial hemorrhage. J Vasc Interv Radiol 2:225–228, 1991.
27. May J, White GH, Waugh RC, et al: Transluminal placement of a prosthetic graft-stent device for treatment of subclavian artery aneurysm. J Vasc Surg 18:1056–1059, 1993.
28. Quinn SF, Sheley RC, Semonsen KG, et al: Endovascular stents covered with preexpanded polytetrafluoroethylene for treatment of iliac artery aneurysms and fistulas. J Vasc Interv Radiol 8:1057–1063, 1997.
29. Marin ML, Veith FJ, Panetta TF, et al: Percutaneous transfemoral insertion of a stented graft to repair a traumatic arteriovenous fistula. J Vasc Surg 18:299–302, 1993.
30. Parodi JC, Schonholz C: Endovascular treatment of traumatic arterial lesions with stent-grafts. Endovasc Impact 1:31–34, 1996.
31. Marin ML, Veith FJ, Panetta TF, et al: Transluminally placed endovascular stented graft repair for arterial trauma. J Vasc Surg 20:466–473, 1994.
32. Dorffner R, Winkelbauer F, Kettenbach J, et al: Successful exclusion of a large femoropopliteal aneurysm with a coated nitinol stent. Cardiovasc Interv Radiol 19:117–119, 1996.
33. Katzen BT, Becke GJ, Beneeati JF, Zemel G: Stent grafts for aortic aneurysms: The next interventional challenge. Am J Cardiol 81:33E–43E, 1998.
34. Moore WS, Rutherford RB: Transfemoral endovascular repair of abdominal aortic aneurysms: Results of the North American EVT phase I trial. J Vasc Surg 23:543–553, 1996.
35. Chuter TAM: Chuter-Gianturco bifurcated stent-grafts for abdominal aortic aneurysm exclusion. *In* Hopkinson B, Yusuf W, Whitaker S, Veith F (eds): Endovascular Surgery for Aortic Aneurysms. London, WB Saunders 1997, pp 88–104.
36. Boyle JR, Thompson MM, Clode-Baker EG, et al: Torsion and kinking of unsupported endografts: Treatment by endovascular intervention. J Endovasc Surg 5:216–221, 1998.
37. Blum U, Voshage G: Abdominal aortic aneurysm repair using the Meadox/Vanguard prosthesis: Indications, implantation technique and results. Tech Vasc Interv Radiol 1:19–24, 1998.
38. Blum U, Voshage G, Beyersdorf F, et al: Two-center German experience with aortic endografting. J Endovasc Surg 4:137–146, 1997.
39. White RA, Donayre CE, Walot I, et al: Modular bifurcation endoprosthesis for treatment of abdominal aortic aneurysms. Ann Surgery 226:381–391, 1997.
40. May J, White GH, Yu W: Aorto-aortic Prosthesis: The Baxter Endovascular Graft. *In* Yusuf W, Marin ML, Ivancev K, Hopkinson BR (eds): Operative Atlas of Endoluminal Aneurysm Surgery. Oxford, Isis Medical Media, 1998.
41. Uflacker R, Robinson JG, Brothers TE, et al: Abdominal aortic aneurysm treatment: Preliminary results with the Talent stent-graft system. J Vasc Interv Radiol 9:51–60, 1998.
42. Weatherford DA, Ombrellaro MP, Schaeffer DO, et al: Healing characteristics of intraarterial stent grafts in an injured artery model. Ann Vasc Surg 11:54–61, 1997.
43. Ohki T, Marin ML, Veith FJ, et al: Anastomotic intimal hyperplasia: A comparison between conventional and endovascular stent graft techniques. J Surg Res 69:255–267, 1997.
44. Schurmann K, Vorwerk D, Uppenkamp R, et al: Iliac arteries: Plain and heparin-coated Dacron-covered stent-grafts compared with noncovered metal stents—an experimental study. Radiology 203:55–63, 1997.
45. Dolmatch BL, Tio FO, Li XD, Dong YH: Patency and tissue response to two types of polytetrafluoroethylene-covered stents in the dog. J Vasc Interv Radiol 7:641–649, 1996.

46. Eton D, Warner DL, Owens C, et al: Histological response to stent graft therapy. Circulation 94(Suppl II):182–187, 1996.
47. Baxendale BR, Baker DM, Hutchinson A, et al: Haemodynamic and metabolic response to endovascular repair of infra-renal aneurysms. Br J Anaesth 77:581–585, 1996.
48. Norgren L, Albrechtsson U, Swartbol P: Side effects of endovascular grafting to treat aortic aneurysm. Br J Surg 83:520–521, 1996.
49. Swartbol P, Norgren L, Albrechtsson U, et al: Biological responses differ considerably between endovascular and conventional aortic aneurysm surgery. Eur J Vasc Endovasc Surg 12:18–25, 1996.
50. Norgren L, Swartbol P: Biological responses to endovascular treatment of abdominal aortic aneurysms. J Endovasc Surg 4:169–173, 1997.
51. Adolph R, Vorp DA, Steed DL, et al: Cellular content and permeability of intraluminal thrombus in AAA. J Vasc Surg 25:916–926, 1997.
52. May J, White GH, Yu W, et al: A prospective study of changes in morphology and dimensions of abdominal aortic aneurysms following endoluminal repair: A preliminary report. J Endovasc Surg 2:343–347, 1995.
53. Matsumura JS, Pearce WH, McCarthy WJ, Yao JST: Reduction in aortic aneurysm size: Early results after endovascular graft placement. J Vasc Surg 25:113–123, 1997.
54. Malina M, Ivancev K, Chuter TAM, et al: Changing aneurysm morphology after endovascular grafting: Relation to leakage or persistent perfusion. J Endovasc Surg 4:23–30, 1997.
55. White GH, Yu W, May J, et al: Three-year experience with the White-Yu endovascular GAD graft for transluminal repair of aortic and iliac aneurysms. J Endovasc Surg 4:124–136, 1997.
56. White RA, Donayre CE, Walot I, et al: Regression of an AAA after endograft exclusion. J Vasc Surg 26:133–137, 1997.
57. Chuter T, Ivancev K, Malina M, et al: Aneurysm pressure following endovascular exclusion. Eur J Vasc Endovasc Surg 13:85–87, 1997.
58. Blum U, Voshage G, Lammer J, et al: Endoluminal stent-grafts for infrarenal abdominal aortic aneurysms. N Engl J Med 336:13–20, 1997.
59. Stelter WJ, Umsheid T, Ziegler P: Three-year experience with modular stent-graft devices for endovascular AAA treatment. J Endovasc Surg 4:362–369, 1997.
60. Hayoz D, Do D, Mahler F, et al: Acute inflammatory reaction associated with endoluminal bypass grafts. J Endovasc Surg 4:354–360, 1997.
61. Parodi JC, Schonholz C, La Mura R: The Parodi system. *In* Hopkinson B, Yusuf W, Whitaker S, Veith F (eds): Endovascular Surgery for Aortic Aneurysms. London, WB Saunders, 1997, pp 164–179.
62. Parodi JC: Endovascular repair of abdominal aortic aneurysms and other arterial lesions. J Vasc Surg 21:549–557, 1995.
63. May J, White GH, Yu W, et al: Conversion from endoluminal to open repair of abdominal aortic aneurysms: A hazardous procedure. Eur J Vasc Endovasc Surg 14:4–11, 1997.
64. Chuter TAM, Green RM, Ouriel K, et al: Transfemoral endovascular graft placement. J Vasc Surg 18:185–187, 1993.
65. Moore WS: The role of endovascular grafting technique in the treatment of infrarenal abdominal aortic aneurysm. Cardiovasc Surg 3:109–114, 1995.
66. Matsumura JS, Moore WS, EVT Investigators: Clinical consequences of periprosthetic leak after endovascular repair of abdominal aortic aneurysm. J Vasc Surg 27:606–613, 1998.
67. Balm R, Eickleboom BC, May J, et al: Early experience with transfemoral endovascular aneurysm management (TEAM) in the treatment aortic aneurysms. Eur J Vasc Endovasc Surg 11:214–220, 1996.
68. May J, White GH, Yu W, et al: Early experience with the Sydney and EVT prostheses for endoluminal treatment of abdominal aortic aneurysms. J Endovasc Surg 2:240–247, 1995.
69. Mialhe C, Amicabile C, Becquemin JP: Endovascular treatment of infrarenal abdominal aneurysms by the Stentor system: Preliminary results of 79 cases. J Vasc Surg 26:199–209, 1997.
70. Torsello GB, Klenk E, Kasprzak B, et al: Rupture of abdominal aortic aneurysm previously treated by endovascular stentgraft. J Vasc Surg 28:184–187, 1998.
71. Fry PD, Machan L, Doyle DL, Morris C: The Talent graft for endoluminal aortic aneurysm repair: Initial experience (Abstract). J Endovasc Surg 4(Suppl):I11–112, 1997.
72. Biasi GM, Piglionica MR, Meregaglia D, et al: Infrarenal AAA endoluminal repair using the Medtronic AneuRx stent-graft: A European one-year multicenter experience (Abstract). J Endovasc Surg 5(Suppl):14–15, 1998.
73. Zarins CK, White RA, Schwarten D, et al: AneuRx stent graft vs. open repair of abdominal aortic aneurysms: Multicenter prospective clinical trial. J Vasc Surg 29:292–308, 1999.
74. Gordon MK, Lawrence-Brown MMD, Hartley D, et al: A self-expanding endoluminal graft for treatment of aneurysms: Results through the development phase. Aust N Z J Surg 66:621–625, 1996.
75. Krajcer Z, Diethrich EB: Successful endoluminal repair of arterial aneurysm by Wallstent prosthesis and PTFE graft: Preliminary results with a new technique. J Endovasc Surg 4:80–87, 1997.
76. Krajcer Z, Sioco G, Reynolds T: Comparison of Wallgraft and Wallstent for treatment of complex iliac artery stenosis and occlusion: Preliminary results of a prospective randomized study. Tex Heart Inst J 24:193–199, 1997.
77. Krajcer Z, Khoshnevis R, Leachman DR, Herman H: Endoluminal exclusion of an iliac artery aneurysm by Wallstent endoprosthesis and PTFF vascular graft. Tex Heart Inst J 24:11–14, 1997.
78. Akiyama N, Esato K, Fujioka K, Zempo N: A comparison of Corvita and expanded polytetrafluoroethylene vascular grafts implanted in the abdominal aortas of dogs. Surg Today 27:840–845, 1997.
79. Henry M, Amor M, Henry I, et al: Initial experience with the Corvita endoluminal graft in peripheral arteries (Abstract). J Endovasc Surg 4(Suppl I):I-14–I-15, 1997.
80. Dereume JP, Ferreira J, Dehon P, et al: Treatment of abdominal aortic aneurysm by application of a Corvita endoprosthesis: Medium term results of a feasibility study. Chirurgie 121:428–431, 1996.
81. White GH, Yu W, May J, et al: A new non-stented balloon-expandable graft for straight or bifurcated endoluminal bypass. J Endovasc Surg 1:16–24, 1994.
82. Yu W, White GH, May J, et al: Endoluminal repair of abdominal aortic aneurysms using the Trombone technique. Asian J Surg 19:37–40, 1996.
83. Chaufour X, White GH, Yu W, et al: Evaluation of the risks of using an oversized balloon catheter in the human infrarenal abdominal aorta. Eur J Vasc Endovasc Surg 16:142–147, 1998.
84. Ivancev K, Malina M, Lindblad B, et al: Abdominal aortic aneurysms: Experience with the Ivancev-Malmo endovascular system for aortomonoiliac stent-grafts. J Endovac Surg 4:242–251, 1997.
85. Yusuf SW, Whitaker SC, Chuter TA, et al: Early results of endovascular aortic aneurysm surgery with aortouniiliac graft, contralateral iliac occlusion and femorofemoral bypass. J Vasc Surg 25:165–172, 1997.
86. Yusuf SW, Baker DM, Hind RE, et al: Endoluminal transfemoral abdominal aortic aneurysm repair with aortouni-iliac graft and femorofemoral crossover. Br J Surg 82:916, 1995.
87. Richter GM, Palmaz JC, Allenberg JR, Kauffmann GW: Die transluminale Stentprosthese beim Bauchaortenaneurysma. Radiologie 34:511–518, 1994.
88. Sayers RD, Thompson MM, Nasim A, Bell PRF: Endovascular repair of abdominal aortic aneurysms: Limitations of the proximal stent technique. Br J Surg 81:1107–1110, 1994.
89. Marin M, Veith FJ, Lyon RT, et al: Transfemoral endovascular repair of iliac artery aneurysms. Am J Surg 170:179–182, 1995.
90. Heiss M, Lauterjung L: Endovascular exclusion of thoracic aneurysm with a new stent-graft system (Abstract). J Endovasc Surg 5:172–173, 1998.
91. Veith FJ, Abbott WM, Yao JST, et al: Guidelines for development and use of transluminally placed endovascular prosthetic grafts in the arterial system. J Vasc Surg 21:670–685, 1995; and J Vasc Interv Radiol 6:477–492, 1995.
92. Ahn SS, Rutherford RB, Johnston KW, et al: Reporting standards for infrarenal endovascular abdominal aortic aneurysm repair. J Vasc Surg 25:405–410, 1997.
93. Parodi JC: Endovascular repair of abdominal aortic aneurysms and other arterial lesions. J Vasc Surg 21:549–557, 1995.
94. Chuter TAM, Green RM, Ouriel K, De Weese JA: Infrarenal aortic aneurysm structure: Implications for transfemoral repair. J Vasc Surg 20:44–50, 1994.
95. Andrews SM, Cumig R, MacSweeney STR, et al: Assessment of feasibility for endovascular prosthetic tube correction of aortic aneurysms. Br J Surg 82:917–919, 1995.
96. May J, White GH, May J, et al: Importance of graft configuration in outcome of endoluminal aortic aneurysm repair: A five year analysis by life table method. Eur J Vasc Endovasc Surg 15:406–411, 1998.

97. Schumacher H, Eckstein HH, Kallinowski F, Allenberg JR: Morphometry and classification in abdominal aortic aneurysms: Patient selection for endovascular and open surgery. J Endovasc Surg 4:39–44, 1997.
98. Ivancev K, Chuter TAM: Adjunctive manoeuvres for endovascular exclusion of abdominal aortic aneurysm. *In* Hopkinson B, Yusuf W, Whitaker S, Veith F (eds): Endovascular Surgery for Aortic Aneurysms. London, WB Saunders, 1997, pp 57–71.
99. May J, White GH, Waugh RC: Treatment of complex abdominal aortic aneurysms by a combination of endoluminal and extraluminal aortofemoral grafts. J Vasc Surg 19:924–933, 1994.
100. Cardon JM, Cardon A, Joyeux, Vidal V: Endovascular repair of iliac artery aneurysms with endosystem: 1. A multicentric French study. J Cardiovasc Surg 37(Suppl1):45–50, 1996.
101. Dorros G, Cohn JM, Jaff MR: Percutaneous endovascular stent-graft repair of iliac artery aneurysms. J Endovasc Surg 4:370–375, 1997.
102. Mitchell RS, Miller DC, Dake MD: Stent-graft repair of thoracic aortic aneurysms. Semin Vasc Surg 10:257–271, 1997.
103. White GH, May J, Yu W, et al: Endovascular treatment of thoracic aneurysms and thoracic aortic dissections by balloon-expandable and self-expanding stent-grafts (in press).
104. Ferko A, Krajina A, Jon B, et al: Dissection of the infrarenal aorta treated by stent graft placement. Eur Radiol 8:298–300, 1998.
105. Yuan JG, Marin ML, Veith FJ, et al: Endovascular grafts for non-infected aortoiliac anastomotic aneurysms. J Vasc Surg 26:210–221, 1997.
106. May J, White GH, Yu W, et al: Endoluminal repair: A better option for the treatment of complex false aneurysms. Aust N Z J Surg 68:29–34, 1998.
107. White RA, Donayre CE, Walot I, et al: Endoluminal graft exclusion of a proximal para-anastomotic pseudoaneurysm following aortobifemoral bypass. J Endovasc Surg 4:88–94, 1997.
108. Rousseau H, Gieskes L, Joffre F, et al: Percutaneous treatment of peripheral aneurysms with Cragg Endopro system. J Vasc Interv Radiol 7:35–39, 1996.
109. Bui B, Oliva V, Leclerc G, et al: Renal artery aneurysm: Treatment with percutaneous placement of a stent-graft. Radiology 195:181–182, 1995.
110. Marcade JP: Stent-graft for popliteal aneurysms. Six cases with Cragg Endo-Pro system 1 Mintec. J Cardiovasc Surg 37:41–44, 1996.
111. Criado E, Marston WA, Ligush J, et al: Endovascular repair of peripheral aneurysms, pseudoaneurysms, and arteriovenous fistulas. Ann Vasc Surg 11:256–263, 1997.
112. Parodi JC: Endovascular repair of aortic aneurysms, arteriovenous fistulas, and false aneurysms. World J Surg 20:655–663, 1996.
113. Donayre CE: Intraluminal grafts: Current status and future perspectives. *In* White RA, Fogarty TJ (eds): Peripheral Endovascular Interventions. St. Louis, Mosby–Year Book, 1996, pp 364–408.
114. Scharrer-Pamler R, Gorich J, Orend KH, et al: Emergent endoluminal repair of delayed abdominal aortic rupture after blunt trauma. J Endovasc Surg 5:134–137, 1998.
115. Cragg AH, Dake MD: Treatment of peripheral vascular disease with stent-grafts. Radiology 205:307–314, 1997.
116. Diethrich EB, Papazoglou K: Endoluminal grafting for aneurysmal and occlusive disease in the superficial femoral artery: Early experience. J Endovasc Surg 2:225–239, 1995.
117. Marin ML, Veith FJ, Panetta TF, et al: Transfemoral endovascular stented graft treatment of aortoiliac and femoropopliteal occlusive disease for limb salvage. Am J Surg 168:156–162, 1994.
118. Cragg AH, Dake MD: Percutaneous femoropopliteal graft placement. Radiology 187:643–648, 1993.
119. Henry M, Amor M, Ethevenot G, et al: Initial experience with the Cragg Endopro System 1 for intraluminal treatment of peripheral vascular disease. J Endovasc Surg 1:31–43, 1994.
120. Link J, Muller-Hulsbeck S, Brossmann J, et al: Perivascular inflammatory reaction after percutaneous placement of covered stents. Cardiovasc Interv Radiol 19:345–347, 1996.
121. Moll FL, Ho GH: Closed superficial femoral endarterectomy: A 2-year follow-up. Cardiovascular Surg 5:398–400, 1997.
122. Casselman F, Van Elst F, Spoelstra H: Femoropopliteal endobypass: A feasibility study in 41 patients. Acta Chir Belg 97:23–26, 1997.
123. Bray AE: Superficial femoral endarterectomy with intra-arterial PTFE grafting. J Endovasc Surg 2:297–301, 1995.
124. Haskal ZJ, Davis A, McAllister A, Furth EE: PTFE-encapsulated endovascular stent-graft for transjugular intrahepatic portosystemic shunts: Experimental evaluation. Radiology 205:682–688, 1997.
125. Link J, Feyerabend B, Grabener M, et al: Dacron-covered stent-grafts for the percutaneous treatment of carotid aneurysms: Effectiveness and biocompatibility—experimental study in swine. Radiology 200:397–401, 1996.
126. May J, White GH, Waugh RC, Brennan J: Endoluminal repair of internal carotid artery aneurysm: A feasible but hazardous procedure. J Vasc Surg 26:1055–1060, 1997.
127. Reiter BP, Marin ML, Teodorescu VJ, Mitty HA: Endoluminal repair of an internal carotid artery pseudoaneurysm. J Vasc Interv Radiol 9:245–248, 1998.
128. Severini A, Mantero S, Tanzi MC, et al: Polyurethane-coated, self-expandable biliary stent: An experimental study. Acad Radiol 2:1078–1081, 1995.
129. Heuser RR, Reynolds GT, Papazoglou K, Diethrich EB: Endoluminal grafting for percutaneous aneurysm exclusion in an aortocoronary saphenous vein graft: The first clinical experience. J Endovasc Surg 2:81–88, 1995.
130. Chin DH, Petersen BD, Timmermans H, Rosch J: Stent-graft in the management of superior vena cava syndrome. Cardiovasc Interv Radiol 19:302–304, 1996.
131. Torsello GB, Klenk E, Kasprzak B, Umsheid T: Rupture of abdominal aortic aneurysm previously treated by endovascular stent-graft. J Vasc Surg 28:184–187, 1998.
132. Alimi YS, Chakfe N, Rivoal E, et al: Rupture of an abdominal aortic aneurysm after endovascular graft placement and aneurysm size reduction. J Vasc Surg 28:178–183, 1998.
133. Malina M, Lindh M, Ivancev K, et al: The effect of endovascular aortic stents placed across the renal arteries. Eur J Vasc Endovasc Surg 13:207–213, 1997.
134. Malina M, Brunkwall J, Ivancev K, et al: Renal arteries covered by aortic stents: Clinical experience from endovascular grafting of aortic aneurysms. Eur J Vasc Endovasc Surg 14:109–113, 1997.
135. Sonesson B, Malina M, Ivancev K, et al: Dilatation of the infrarenal aneurysm neck after endovascular exclusion of abdominal aortic aneurysm. J Endovasc Surg 5:195–200, 1998.
136. May J, White GH, Yu W, et al: A prospective study of changes in morphology and dimensions of abdominal aortic aneurysms following endoluminal repair: A preliminary report. J. Endovasc Surg 2:343–347, 1995.
137. Malina M, Brunkwall J, Ivancev K, et al: Late aortic arch perforation by graft-anchoring stent: Complication of endovascular thoracic aneurysm exclusion. J Endovasc Surg 5:274–277, 1998.
138. Ernst CB, Cambell HC, Daugherty ME, et al: Incidence and significance of intraoperative bacterial cultures during abdominal aortic aneurysmectomy. Ann Surg 185:626–632, 1977.
139. Parsons RE, Sanchez LA, Marin ML, et al: Comparison of endovascular and conventional vascular prostheses in an experimental infection model. J Vasc Surg 24:920–926, 1996.
140. Kolvenbach R, El Basha M: Secondary rupture of a common iliac artery aneurysm after endovascular exclusion and stent-graft infection (Letter). J Vasc Surg 26:351–353, 1997.
141. Deiparine MK, Ballard JL, Taylor FC, Chase DR: Endovascular stent infection. J Vasc Surg 23:529–533, 1996.
142. Norgren L, Jernby B, Engellau L: Aortoenteric fistula caused by a ruptured stent-graft: A case report. J Endovasc Surg 5:269–272, 1998.
143. White GH, May J, Yu W: "Endoleak"—a proposed new terminology to describe incomplete aneurysm exclusion by an endoluminal graft. J Endovasc Surg 3:124–125, 1996.
144. White GH, Yu W, May J, et al: Endoleak as a complication of endoluminal grafting of abdominal aortic aneurysms: Classification, incidence, diagnosis and management. J Endovasc Surg 4:152–168, 1997.
145. Wain RA, Marin ML, Ohki T, et al: Endoleaks complicating endovascular graft treatment of aortic aneurysms: Classification, risk factors and outcome. J Vasc Surg 27:69–80, 1998.
146. White GH, May J, Waugh RC, et al: Type III and type IV endoleak: Towards a complete definition of bloodflow in the sac following AAA repair. J Endovasc Surg 5:305–309, 1998.
147. Beebe HB, Bernhard VM, Parodi JC, White GH: Leaks after endovascular therapy for aneurysm: Detection and classification. J Endovasc Surg 3:445–448, 1996.
148. Kato N, Semba CP, Dake MD: Embolization of perigraft leaks after endovascular stent-graft treatment of aortic aneurysms. J Vasc Interv Radiol 7:805–811, 1996.

149. Parodi JC, Barone A, Piraino R, Schonholz C: Endovascular treatment of abdominal aortic aneurysms: Lessons learned. J Endovasc Surg 4:5–12, 1997.
150. Lumsden AB, Allen RC, Chaikof EL, et al: Delayed rupture of aortic aneurysms following endovascular stent grafting. Am J Surg 170:174–178, 1995.
151. Marty B, Sanchez LA, Ohki T, et al: Endoleak after endovascular graft repair of experimental aortic aneurysms: Does coil embolization with angiographic "seal" lower intraaneurysmal pressure? J Vasc Surg 27:454–462, 1998.
152. Park JH, Chung JW, Choo IW, et al: Fenestrated stent-grafts for preserving visceral arterial branches in the treatment of abdominal aortic aneurysms: Preliminary experience. J Vasc Interv Radiol 7:819–823, 1996.
153. Thompson MM, Smith J, Naylor AR, et al: Ultrasound-based quantification of emboli during conventional and endovascular aneurysm repair. J Endovasc Surg 4:33–38, 1997.
154 Thompson MM, Smith J, Naylor AR, et al: Microembolization during endovascular and conventional aneurysm repair. J Vasc Surg 25:179–186, 1997.
155. Harris P, Brennan J, Martin J, et al: Longitudinal aneurysm shrinkage following endovascular aortic aneurysm repair is a source of intermediate and late complications. J Endovasc Surg 6:11–16, 1999.
156. Dorffner R, Thurnher S, Polterauer P, et al: Treatment of abdominal aortic aneurysms with transfemoral placement of stent-grafts: Complications and secondary radiologic intervention. Radiology 204:79–86, 1997.
157. Harris PL, Buth J, Miahle C, et al: The need for clinical trials of endovascular abdominal aortic aneurysm repair: The Eurostar project. J Endovasc Surg 4:72–79, 1997.
158. May J, White GH, Yu W, et al: Concurrent comparison of endoluminal repair versus no treatment for small abdominal aortic aneurysms. Eur J Vasc Endovasc Surg 13:472–476, 1997.
159. White GH, May J, McGahan T, et al: Historical control comparison of outcome for endoluminal versus open repair of abdominal aortic aneurysms. J Vasc Surg 23:201–212, 1996.
160. May J, White GH, Yu W, et al: Concurrent comparison of endoluminal versus open repair in the treatment of abdominal aortic aneurysms: Analysis of 303 patients by life-table method. J Vasc Surg 27:213–227, 1998.
161. Thompson MM, Sayers RD, Bell PRF: Endovascular aneurysm repair: Proof before publicity (Editorial). BMJ 314:1139–1140, 1997.

SECTION VII

Common Complications of Vascular Surgery: Prevention and Management

K. Wayne Johnston, M.D., F.R.C.S.(C.)

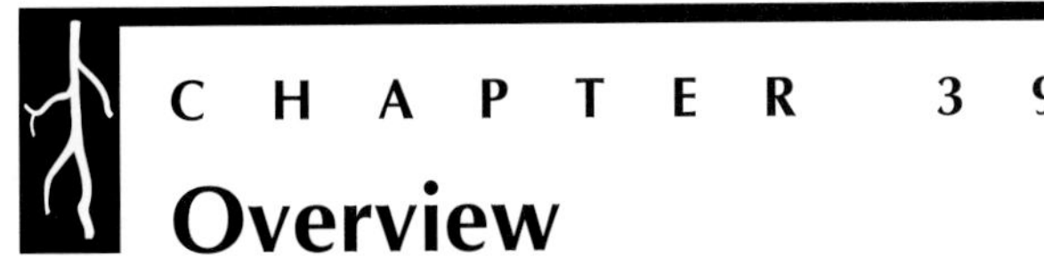

CHAPTER 39

Overview

K. Wayne Johnston, M.D., F.R.C.S.(C.)

The complications associated with vascular surgery can be classified as (1) nonvascular systemic, (2) nonvascular local, (3) vascular local, and (4) remote ischemic vascular (Tables 39–1 to 39–4). Their incidence and severity can be reduced if the vascular surgeon pays attention to preventive measures, early recognition, and specific treatment.

Meticulous attention to detail is the most important aspect of *prevention*. The initial step is to establish an accurate vascular diagnosis by appropriate clinical assessment, noninvasive studies, and angiography. Patient selection should be based on knowledge of the untreated natural history of the underlying disease process and the indications for and limitations of surgery. The preoperative evaluation should include careful assessment of the severity and risks of coexisting medical problems, especially cerebrovascular, cardiac, respiratory, hepatic, renal, and hematologic diseases, and detailed preparation for surgery. The operation and the approach thereto, based on the indications for surgery and the patient's general status, should be considered carefully.

The surgery should be conducted meticulously to avoid errors in technique; in particular, it is important to recognize that congenital anomalies may complicate dissection, diseased vessels can be damaged easily, equipment such as vascular clamps or Fogarty catheters must be used with care, and hemostasis should be complete. Intraoperative objective assessment may be necessary to confirm the success of the procedure. Specific measures to prevent vascular complications, including thrombosis and infection, and general complications (e.g., atelectasis, myocardial infarction, thromboembolism) should be considered. When a complication arises, *early recognition* and *prompt treatment* offer the best opportunity for a good result.

The complications specific to the surgical management of lower extremity arterial disease are described in various chapters. This section includes chapters on the complications that warrant individual consideration either because of their seriousness or because they pose inherent risks in any vascular operation. The following text briefly summarizes the pathogenesis, diagnosis, and management of the complications included in this section.

CARDIAC COMPLICATIONS AND SCREENING (see Chapter 40)

Most persons with occlusive and aneurysmal arterial disease have some degree of coronary artery disease (CAD). Complications of CAD are the most common cause of early and late mortality in this patient group. Preoperative cardiac screening and risk stratification, when appropriate, are intended to identify those patients at increased risk for perioperative events.

An initial assessment using clinical factors and a resting electrocardiogram (ECG) can provide an estimate of low, intermediate, or high perioperative risk. Additional noninvasive screening tests, including exercise electrocardiography, radionuclide ventriculography, continuous electrocardiographic monitoring (Holter), and dipyridamole-thallium scintigraphy, are of greatest benefit for the intermediate-risk group. Although there is continuing controversy regarding the predictive value and cost-effectiveness of such investigations, dipyridamole-thallium scintigraphy in particular has emerged as a widely employed means of further selective evaluation of the intermediate-risk patient. Patients with positive noninvasive findings, in addition to those found to be at high risk in the initial clinical assessment, may be considered for coronary angiography and possible coronary bypass or angioplasty prior to the planned vascular procedure.

A surgeon must weigh the natural history of the vascular disease process against the risks of the proposed operations, including any associated risks of preoperative cardiac investigations and interventions. Preoperative screening and risk stratification provide information that may allow aggressive medical or surgical management of coexisting cardiac disease. This information may lead the surgeon to consider an

TABLE 39–1. NONVASCULAR COMPLICATIONS, SYSTEMIC

0. None
1. Cerebrovascular
2. Cardiac
   2.1. Myocardial infarction
      2.1.1. Enzyme changes only
      2.1.2. ST-T wave changes; positive test for MB isoenzyme of creatinine phosphokinase
      2.1.3. Q waves or loss of R waves
      2.1.4. Death
   2.2. Arrhythmia
      2.2.1. Atrial
      2.2.2. Ventricular
      2.2.3. Heart block
   2.3. Congestive heart failure
3. Pulmonary
4. Renal
   4.0. No change renal function
   4.1. Creatinine increase less than 2 times baseline
   4.2. Creatinine increase more than 2 times baseline
   4.3. Temporary dialysis
   4.4. Permanent dialysis
5. Gastrointestinal, including hepatobiliary and pancreatic
6. Venous thromboembolism
   6.1. Deep vein thrombosis
      6.1.1. Suspected
      6.1.2. Proven
   6.2. Pulmonary embolism
      6.2.1. Suspected
      6.2.2. Proven
7. Coagulation complications
8. Drug and blood reactions
9. Other

Modified from Rutherford RB, Flanigan DP, Gupta SK, et al: Suggested standards for reports dealing with lower extremity ischemia. J Vasc Surg 4:80, 1986.

TABLE 39–2. NONVASCULAR COMPLICATIONS, LOCAL

0. None
1. Fluid accumulation (early or persistent)
   1.1. Sterile
   1.2. Infected
2. Wound
   2.1. Infection (record specific organisms)
      2.1.1. Superficial
      2.1.2. Deep, not involving graft
      2.1.3. Deep, involving graft
   2.2. Separation
   2.3. Evisceration
   2.4. Hematoma
   2.5. Pain
3. Lymphatic disruption
   3.1. Peripheral site
      3.1.1. Lymphocele
      3.1.2. Lymph fistula
   3.2. Central site
      3.2.1. Chylothorax
      3.2.2. Chylous ascites
4. Vascular injury
   4.1. Artery
   4.2. Vein
5. Ureteric injury
6. Pleural, pneumothorax
7. Nerve injury
8. Sexual dysfunction
   8.1. Neurogenic
   8.2. Vasculogenic

Modified from Rutherford RB, Flanigan DP, Gupta SK, et al: Suggested standards for reports dealing with lower extremity ischemia. J Vasc Surg 4:80, 1986.

TABLE 39–3. VASCULAR COMPLICATIONS, LOCAL

0. None
1. Hemorrhage
   1.1. Intraoperative
   1.2. Postoperative, not requiring reoperation; record blood loss and time
   1.3. Postoperative, requiring reoperation
2. Infection of graft (record specific organisms)
   2.1. Suspected
   2.2. Proven
3. Pseudoaneurysm
4. Graft
   4.1. Dilatation
   4.2. Degeneration, aneurysm
   4.3. Stenosis, intimal hyperplasia
   4.4. Stenosis, atherosclerosis
   4.5. Elongation, kinking
5. Thrombosis or unsatisfactory hemodynamic result
6. Fistulization
   6.1. Vein
   6.2. Bowel
   6.3. Biliary tract
   6.4. Ureter
7. Injury to artery or vein

Modified from Rutherford RB, Flanigan DP, Gupta SK, et al: Suggested standards for reports dealing with lower extremity ischemia. J Vasc Surg 4:80, 1986.

alternative surgical technique or to cancel or defer any vascular procedure altogether, and it may influence intraoperative and postoperative management and monitoring.

PULMONARY COMPLICATIONS IN VASCULAR SURGERY (see Chapter 41)

In the older vascular surgery population, who often require major surgery and may have underlying pulmonary disease, it is important to identify which patients are at risk for respiratory insufficiency. Predisposing patient factors include advanced age, chronic obstructive pulmonary disease, a history of heavy tobacco use and poor nutrition, and procedure-related risk factors (e.g., thoracic or upper abdominal incisions, hypoperfusion, massive blood transfu-

TABLE 39–4. ISCHEMIC VASCULAR COMPLICATIONS, REMOTE*

0. None
1. Limb ischemia (see Ref. 1)
2. Bowel ischemia
3. Renal ischemia
4. Spinal cord and cauda equina ischemia
5. Cerebral ischemia (use stroke severity scale)
   5.0. Asymptomatic
   5.1. Transient ischemic attack (<24 hours)
   5.2. Temporary stroke with full recovery (24 hours to 3 weeks)
   5.3. Permanent stroke, minor (>3 weeks)
   5.4. Permanent stroke, major (>3 weeks)
   5.5. Nonspecific dysfunction
6. Nerve ischemia and dysfunction
7. Muscle (compartment syndrome)
8. Other

Modified from Rutherford RB, Flanigan DP, Gupta SK, et al: Suggested standards for reports dealing with lower extremity ischemia. J Vasc Surg 4:80, 1986.

*That is, due to effects of ischemia, thromboembolism, steal, or dissection on limb or end organ.

sion). Screening is by a careful history of chronic cough, sputum production or shortness of breath, physical examination that demonstrates wheezing, hypoinflation or hyperinflation, chest x-ray study, and, when indicated, pulmonary function tests and arterial blood gas measurements.

In some cases, preoperative therapy with vigorous chest physiotherapy, cessation of smoking, a walking program, weight loss, bronchodilators, and antibiotics may be of benefit. For patients with pulmonary disease, the pulmonary risk may be minimized with regional anesthesia, transverse versus midline incision, and appropriate fluid volume replacement. If postoperative ventilation is necessary, standard cardiovascular monitoring provides appropriate surveillance of the multiple factors that influence ventilation and the balance between oxygen delivery and consumption.

Management of respiratory complications depends on recognition of the specific cause. Nonpulmonary parenchymal causes include central nervous system (CNS) depression, mechanical problems of ventilation, and upper airway obstruction. Parenchymal causes include atelectasis, pneumonia, pulmonary edema, adult respiratory distress syndrome (ARDS), and pulmonary embolus. Pulmonary complications can be rapidly fatal; in most cases, however, they are self-limited and, if properly recognized, respond to treatment.

RENAL COMPLICATIONS

(see Chapter 42)

Associated with angiography and arterial reconstructive surgery, renal dysfunction can range from minor abnormalities of function to anuric acute renal failure. Of the prerenal causes (hypovolemia, low cardiac output, septic shock, and renal artery occlusion) in the patient with diffuse atherosclerosis and impaired cardiac function, the distinction between hypovolemia and cardiogenic causes can be problematic even with the use of invasive hemodynamic monitoring. Postrenal causes (obstruction of ureter, bladder, or catheter) of oliguria are the easiest to correct when diagnosed correctly. Parenchymal causes of renal failure may be the result of ischemic injury (suprarenal aortic or renal artery clamping, hypovolemic or cardiogenic shock, or atheroembolism) or toxic injury by angiographic contrast agents, drugs, or myoglobin.

After aortic surgery, the incidence of renal impairment depends on the patient's preoperative renal function, intraoperative technical management (juxtarenal and repetitive cross-clamping) and fluid management, and postoperative complications. Approaches to protect renal function include preoperative fluid hydration, limiting the period of warm renal ischemia, careful aortic clamping to prevent direct renal artery damage and atheromatous embolization, and maintenance of optimum blood volume and cardiac function. The consequences of renal ischemia may be minimized by mannitol or other diuretic administration, regional renal hypothermia, or other investigational methods.

PERIOPERATIVE HEMORRHAGE

(see Chapter 43)

Prevention of hemorrhage begins in the *preoperative* period. Before any vascular surgery, patients should be asked if they have a history of easy bruising, bleeding, or petechiae or a family history of a coagulopathy, and in selected cases coagulation screening tests should be performed. Chapter 43 outlines diagnosis, prevention, and alternatives for correction of preexisting inherited disorders (von Willebrand's disease, hemophilia, and disorders of fibrinogen) and acquired coagulopathies related to liver disease, vitamin K deficiency or administration of oral anticoagulants, uremia, specific and global inhibitors, fibrinolysis, disseminated intravascular coagulopathy (DIC), thrombocytopenia, abnormal platelet function, antiplatelet drugs, and heparin administration.

Intraoperative prevention is directed toward technical details, including:

- The use of blended electrocautery dissection
- Minimal arterial dissection
- Avoidance of excessive heparin and reversal of its effect with protamine at the end of the procedure
- Selection of the appropriate graft
- Suture of the anastomosis with appropriate deep bites and tension
- Evaluation of the proximal anastomosis by declamping
- Caution in applying clamps to the graft to minimize the chances of disrupting the fabric

If large amounts of blood must be transfused, 1 or 2 units of fresh frozen plasma should be administered for every 4 to 6 units of blood transfused, and all the platelets harvested from 6 units of fresh plasma should be administered after 6 to 8 units of blood have been given. When an autotransfusion device is used, platelets and plasma are removed in the washing process; if large volumes of blood are reinfused, platelets and fresh frozen plasma should be administered to prevent coagulopathy.

Intraoperative bleeding is usually related to technical problems and is controlled by local pressure, suture, or both, but in some cases topical hemostatic agents are required (gelatin sponge, oxidized cellulose, microfibrillar collagen, thrombin). Coagulopathies may be caused by dilution of clotting factors, hypothermia, acidosis, or mechanical trauma to cells and proteins in a reperfusion device; a systemic consumptive coagulopathy (DIC) may also occur. Prevention of hypothermia and acidosis and administration of fresh frozen plasma and platelets during a prolonged operation are standard therapy. DIC is associated with tissue hypoperfusion, shock, and multiple transfusions, and if the initial stimulus continues, the reserves of coagulation factors are consumed and hemostasis fails. During the initial phase, anticoagulation may be indicated; during the later phase, replacement therapy is necessary.

BLOOD LOSS AND TRANSFUSION IN VASCULAR SURGERY (see Chapter 44)

When the possibility of blood transfusion is being considered, it is important to balance the risks and benefits of transfusion treatment. The overall incidence of transfusion effects is 5%, including acute and delayed immune hemolytic reactions and fever. Acute hemolytic reaction should be considered if unexplained circulatory collapse occurs in an anesthetized patient receiving a blood transfusion. Similarly, a symptom complex of fever, malaise, hyperbilirubinemia, and falling hematocrit within 10 days after a transfusion suggests a delayed hemolytic reaction. Febrile reactions are usually benign but have been reported to be associated with leukocyte-mediated pulmonary infiltrates, producing an ARDS-type syndrome.

Human blood can transmit various microbes from the donor to the recipient. Cytomegalovirus (CMV) is the most commonly transmitted pathogen in allogeneic blood products; in the immune competent patient, however, it rarely results in clinical disease. Although the transmission of human immunodeficiency virus (HIV) is quoted at 1: 650,000, new highly sensitive screening processes have reduced this risk significantly. Hepatitis C is the most common pathogen to result in significant disease. Bacterial parasitic organisms can be transmitted by blood transfusion, but this is unusual. Although causation has not been established conclusively, some data suggest that allogeneic blood transfusion can result in immune suppression, leading to increased susceptibility to bacterial infection and increased incidence of malignancy.

Stored blood can affect patient physiology in several ways. Elevated potassium levels and decreased diphosphoglycerate (2, 3-DPG) levels result in decreased release of oxygen (O_2) and also can result in changes in hemostasis of the patient. Normal cardiac function can be maintained over a wide range of hemoglobin levels; however, when a patient has CAD, the hemoglobin level appears to have an increasingly important role in oxygen delivery. Experimental trials suggest that a hemoglobin level of 8 mg/dl provides a safe margin for oxygen delivery. Coagulation can also be affected by blood transfusion. Patients who receive large volumes of transfusions should have their platelet International Normalized Ratio (INR) and partial thromboplastin time (PTT) monitored and corrected when necessary.

The awareness and understanding of the potential morbidity associated with allogeneic blood products have modified recent transfusion practices. Transfusions should be based on individual physiologic need and the ability to compensate, not on defined numerical levels. In avoiding transfusion in elective vascular surgery patients, preoperative evaluation of the patient's coagulation status is important. In the resuscitation and treatment of emergency hemorrhage, controversy exists with respect to the degree of resuscitation and the type of fluid to be administered.

Dilution of coagulation factors results in a progressive coagulopathy, and factor replacement should be considered after the administration of a single blood volume. Hypothermia, DIC, and impaired liver function may be contributory factors to coagulopathy and should be considered (i.e., replacement of coagulation factors should not be prophylactic but should be based on laboratory documentation of a factor deficiency).

Heparinization has often been considered to increase the transfusion requirements in the vascular patient; however, some studies suggest that the proper use of heparin does not increase blood loss and in fact may prevent morbidity from CAD. In peripheral vascular surgery, administration of desmopressin (DDAVP) and aprotinin does not reduce blood loss; they should only be administered if there is evidence of a specific factor deficit or platelet dysfunction.

Alternatives to allogeneic blood include predonation of autologous blood, acute normovolemic hemodilution, hypovolemic hemodilution, and autotransfusion. Combinations of these techniques may be the best method to minimize use of allogeneic blood transfusion.

TECHNICAL ADEQUACY AND GRAFT THROMBOSIS (see Chapter 45)

Early graft thrombosis (<30 days postoperatively) results from problems with technique, inflow, outflow, the conduit, and rarely, hypercoagulable states. Although technical errors have been reduced in recent years by advancements in operative technique and routine use of strategies for the intraoperative detection, they remain the most common cause of early failure. Intraoperative angiography, Doppler ultrasonography, duplex scanning, and angioscopy can prevent early thrombosis by identifying anastomotic and graft problems.

If early postoperative thrombosis does occur, reoperation with thrombectomy and intraoperative imaging is indicated in the majority of cases. Reasonable long-term patency may result when it is possible to identify and correct technical errors. In the remaining cases, when no surgically correctable cause is found, the late results are poor. These patients may be screened for hypercoagulable states (e.g., low antithrombin III and protein C or S levels, heparin-induced platelet aggregation, hyperfibrinogenemia, and circulatory lupus anticoagulant). The effectiveness of antithrombotic drugs after early graft failure has been generally disappointing.

Late graft failure is usually due to neointimal hyperplasia and progression of atherosclerosis that impairs inflow and outflow. Vein grafts can be narrowed by atherosclerosis, intimal thickening, and fibrous stenosis. Surveillance can identify threatened grafts and permit appropriate intervention before thrombosis. If late thrombosis occurs, thrombolysis may be useful to restore patency and has the potential to identify any underlying lesion. In most instances, endovascular treatment or surgical intervention is indicated, depending on the site and nature of the lesion.

Reoperation may involve revision of the existing graft with patch angioplasty or replacement of the bypass graft. When the bypass graft is replaced, the choice of conduit is influenced by such factors as availability of autogenous vein, patient age, coexisting cardiac disease and other comorbidity, and the vascular status of the contralateral limb. If no lesion can be found, long-term anticoagulation therapy may be justified.

VASCULAR THROMBOSIS DUE TO HYPERCOAGULABLE STATES

(see Chapter 46)

Patients who have experienced thromboembolic events should be investigated for a possible underlying hypercoagulable state if they are young or have recurrent or multiple thromboses, a family history of thrombosis, thrombosis in an atypical location, or arterial thrombosis in the absence of atherosclerosis. Hereditary or acquired anticoagulant protein deficiencies associated with the highest risk for venous and rarely arterial thrombosis include antithrombin III, protein C, and protein S deficiencies. These patients require life-long anticoagulation.

Patients with antithrombin III deficiency require fresh frozen plasma before anticoagulation therapy with heparin. Warfarin decreases protein C and protein S levels, and therefore patients who already have deficiencies in these proteins should be have systemic anticoagulation with heparin before beginning warfarin therapy. Resistances to activated protein C due to a mutation in factor V, homocystinemia, and prothrombin 20210 polymorphism are the most common, recently discovered, and less severe protein defects associated with a moderately increased risk of thrombosis. Abnormal fibrinogens and defective fibrinolysis are rare causes of hypercoagulability. An increased risk of thrombosis also occurs in a number of clinical syndromes in association with the presence of antiplatelet antibodies (heparin-induced thrombocytopenia and thrombosis) or antiphospholipid antibodies (lupus anticoagulant).

INFECTION OF PROSTHETIC VASCULAR GRAFTS (see Chapter 47)

Early and late graft infections are serious complications of arterial reconstructive surgery because of their associated high rates of morbidity (requiring amputation) and mortality. Microorganisms can infect the prosthesis through direct implantation at the time of surgery, through the wound if there is a complication of healing, or through hematogenous or lymphatic routes from remote sites of infection. The environment around and within the interstices of biomaterials is conducive to the formation of a bacterial biofilm, which tends to protect the bacteria from both host defenses and antibiotics. Although the inflammatory response stimulated by the bacteria may localize the infection, alternatively, the combined inflammatory responses to the infection and to the biomaterial may result in spread along the graft, involvement of adjacent structures, or significant local tissue damage with possible arterial wall or anastomotic disruption and hemorrhage.

The pathologic consequences depend on the virulence of the organism, the host responses, and the site of graft infection. *Early* graft infections are relatively uncommon and are usually associated with virulent pathogens and serious complications (e.g., systemic sepsis, infected false aneurysm, enlargement and erosion into bowel, and external drainage). *Late*-appearing graft infections are commonly the result of less virulent bacteria (e.g., *Staphylococcus epidermidis*), which can grow within a biofilm and can remain indolent.

Preventive measures include administration of prophylactic antibiotics, attention to meticulous sterile technique, careful multilayer wound closure, early recognition and aggressive treatment of wound infection, and education of the patient that late graft colonization is possible at the time of certain procedures (e.g., dental work, cystoscopy) and that prophylactic antibiotics are recommended.

The diagnosis is often difficult and may be delayed but can be made on the basis of the clinical presentation or routine laboratory studies; however, late graft infections may require investigations, including ultrasonography, computed tomography (CT), magnetic resonance imaging (MRI), contrast sinography, aspiration and culture, white blood cell scans, and angiography. Operative exploration may be necessary. Routine culture techniques may not recover organisms of low virulence; mechanical or ultrasonic disruption of the bacteria from the surface of the graft may be necessary.

Depending on the extent of involvement, the infected graft limb or the entire graft is removed, and the arteriotomy is closed with monofilament suture and an autogenous patch if it is necessary to maintain patency of the artery at the site of arteriotomy. The perigraft tissues and arterial wall should be débrided and the area drained. Extra-anatomic bypass grafts and in situ grafts made with superficial femoral vein or cryopreserved homografts are the options.

Culture-specific antibiotics are indicated. In selected cases of infection with low-virulence organisms that are presumably confined to the "slime" layer around the prosthesis, local graft removal and prosthetic graft replacement in situ can be considered.

ANASTOMOTIC AND OTHER PSEUDOANEURYSMS (see Chapter 48)

The surgeon can minimize the risk of a false aneurysm by using synthetic sutures, taking relatively large bites in the artery, preventing hematomas by paying careful attention to hemostasis and obliteration of dead space, avoiding excessive tension on the anastomosis, not performing an excessive endarterectomy, and administering prophylactic antibiotics to prevent graft infection. It may not be possible to protect these pseudoaneurysms against stress from joint movement or atherosclerotic degeneration of the wall.

The clinical presentation depends on the site (intra-abdominal versus extremity) and the presence of complications (expansion and pressure on surrounding nerves and veins, distal emboli from a mural thrombus, thrombosis of the aneurysm with concomitant occlusion of the native artery or bypass graft, or rupture into soft tissues or adjacent hollow viscera). Femoral pseudoaneurysms are the most common. Diagnosis is made by clinical examination, ultrasonography or CT scan. Angiography is rarely required.

Although the natural history of an untreated anastomotic aneurysm has not been documented, most aneurysms continue to enlarge and therefore should probably be repaired surgically. Dissection of the aneurysm is avoided. Proximal and distal control is obtained; often it is safer to obtain distal control with intraluminal balloon catheters. Although it may be possible to simply resuture the anastomosis, most often a short segment of the graft is removed, healthy arterial wall tissue identified, and a new segment of graft reanastomosed. In the presence of suspected infection, autogenous repair is preferred or extra-anatomical bypass is used.

AORTOENTERIC FISTULAE

(see Chapter 49)

An aortoenteric fistula is one of the most serious complications that can occur after aortic surgery. The fistula can develop between the bowel and the suture line, the side of the body, or limb of the prosthetic graft (paraprosthetic). When the suture line is involved, recurrent significant bleeding episodes eventually result in massive hemorrhage, whereas a paraprosthetic fistula is usually associated with minor bleeding through the interstices of the graft or from the edge of the bowel. In either case, there may be evidence of local or systemic infection.

If time permits, investigations include endoscopy to rule out other causes of gastrointestinal bleeding and occasionally to visualize the mucosal abnormality associated with the fistula; arteriography to demonstrate a false aneurysm and rarely the site of bleeding; and multiple cultures along the aortic graft at the time of angiography, CT scan, or gallium scan.

Prevention is directed toward elimination of the common etiologic factors: (1) direct erosion (which is prevented by separation of the prosthesis and bowel by interposing an appropriate retroperitoneal tissue layer), (2) false aneurysm, (3) graft redundancy, and (4) primary graft infection.

Treatment includes (1) high-dose broad-spectrum antibiotics; (2) control of the aorta by cross-clamping, usually at the level of the diaphragm; (3) removal of the aortic graft; (4) suture of the aortic stump and coverage with omentum; (5) closure of the defect in the bowel; and (6) revascularization by extra-anatomic bypass if necessary. If feasible, extra-anatomical repair is carried out before laparotomy to minimize cardiac stress.

ISCHEMIC NEUROPATHY

(see Chapter 50)

"Ischemic neuropathy" is the term used to describe any injury of peripheral nerve caused by reduction in blood supply and may follow acute or chronic ischemia. If acute ischemia is of short duration or is mild, function in peripheral nerve is impaired in a transient manner; however, with prolonged or severe ischemia, damage may be permanent. With chronic arterial insufficiency, nerves show a combination of segmental demyelination and axonal degeneration, and there may be evidence of remyelination and axonal regeneration.

With chronic ischemia, sensory symptoms (burning pain, hyperesthesia, hyperalgesia) occur in a stocking distribution or involve patchy localized areas in the foot and must be distinguished from symptoms caused by persistent ischemia. Small muscles of the foot may be wasted and weak, and there may be slight ankle weakness and depression of the ankle reflex compared with the normal side.

The diagnosis is confirmed by electromyography. Symptoms associated with chronic ischemia are often mild and improve after arterial reconstruction; however, the symptoms may be severe and persist even after adequate revascularization. In this situation, it is important to recognize that the patient's symptoms are neuropathic in origin and that further arterial reconstructive surgery will not be of benefit. The more severe cases call for treatment with analgesics or amitriptyline.

After the acute ischemia is corrected, the symptoms of ischemic neuropathy usually improve spontaneously. However, if flow is not reestablished within several hours, symptoms and signs of neurogenic dysfunction may persist when circulation is restored, and the deficit may be permanent.

Ischemia may cause neuropathy of individual nerves: peroneal, femoral, and lumbosacral plexus. It is important to distinguish lumbosacral plexus involvement from lesions of the lower spinal cord or cauda equina, which have a very poor prognosis for recovery.

LYMPHATIC COMPLICATIONS OF VASCULAR SURGERY (see Chapter 51)

Several factors may contribute to the development of post-bypass leg edema; however, the major causes are increased production of interstitial fluid associated with successful revascularization (increased lymphatic load) and lymphatic interruption or compression. In femoral and popliteal incisions, lymphatic interruption can be minimized by limiting the extent of arterial dissection with a femoral incision that is slightly lateral to the femoral pulse to allow medial retraction of the lymphatics and by opening the popliteal vascular sheath directly over the artery.

The vascular surgeon can prevent lymphatic fistulae and lymphoceles by these methods and, in addition, by cauterizing and ligating any divided lymphatic tissue and by carefully closing the incision in layers. A conservative approach is justified if the lymphatic drainage is of low volume and subsides quickly; otherwise, operative ligation of the divided lymphatics should be considered to shorten the hospital stay and to reduce the possibility of a graft or wound infection. Small lymphoceles can be observed because they may be reabsorbed spontaneously; however, enlarging or symptomatic lymphoceles are considered indications for operation. Special considerations are given to the management of thoracic duct lymph fistulae in the neck, retroperitoneal lymphoceles, chylous ascites, and chylothorax.

SEXUAL DYSFUNCTION AFTER AORTOILIAC REVASCULARIZATION

(see Chapter 52)

Sexual dysfunction can result from any of the following causes: impaired pelvic blood supply, sympathetic or parasympathetic nerve damage, psychogenic causes, drugs, and endocrine disorders. After abdominal aortic surgery, erectile and ejaculatory dysfunction can result if the bypass reduced pelvic blood flow or the parasympathetic or sympathetic nerve plexuses were damaged in the para-aortic plexus, superior hypogastric plexus (inferior mesenteric artery region), or common iliac artery plexus. The surgeon can reduce the incidence of sexual dysfunction by planning the bypass to maintain or to improve the pelvic blood flow and by avoiding damage to the autonomic nerve plexuses by using minimal aortic dissection, which is best achieved through a right lateral aortic approach just below the renal arteries.

ANGIOGRAPHY AND PERCUTANEOUS VASCULAR INTERVENTIONS: COMPLICATIONS AND QUALITY IMPROVEMENT (see Chapter 53)

Angiography and percutaneous techniques, including percutaneous transluminal balloon angioplasty (PTA), stenting, thrombolysis, and atherectomy, are fundamental modalities for the diagnosis and treatment of vascular problems. Chapter 53 describes criteria for evaluating the adequacy of an intervention and the complications of these techniques and suggests standards for performing the procedures based on the suggestions of the Society of Cardiovascular and Interventional Radiology (SCVIR).

Several complications can occur after angiography. Puncture site complications (e.g., thrombosis, hematoma, pseudoaneurysm, arteriovenous fistula) that require surgery or transfusion are rare, less than 0.1%. Catheter-related complications are now rare and include dissections or subintimal injections. They are not usually significant because they are retrograde and thromboembolism from the catheter can be prevented by flushing with heparinized solution. Although cholesterol embolization is commonly noted in autopsy series, blue toe syndrome or other embolic sequelae are rare. Many systemic complications are related to the patient's underlying co-morbidity; however, prevention of contrast reactions and nephrotoxicity requires particular attention. Specific complications can result from neurologic, renal, and other procedures.

PTA is associated with a higher incidence of complications that include puncture site hematoma (because the catheter is larger and there is more manipulation), thrombosis, dissection, and perforation; however, major sequelae are rare. When a stent is placed, the complication rate is further increased slightly because of embolization, vessel rupture, and dissection. Systemic thrombolysis is generally associated with a higher bleeding rate than regional therapy. Urokinase and recombinant tissue plasminogen activator (rt-PA) are preferred over streptokinase because of a lower risk of bleeding and a higher success rate. Reported complications vary but include local or remote bleeding, embolization, reperfusion and compartment syndromes, and mortality.

In aiming to provide optimum quality care, SCVIR has proposed guidelines for training, including the number and nature of cases, practice guidelines, and standards for outcomes (results and complications). The tables in Chapter 53 provide threshold values to serve as a basis for quality improvement.

URETERAL OBSTRUCTION

This discussion is included to cover the problem of ureteral obstruction that may be seen after abdominal aortic reconstructive surgery.

Cause

Ureteral obstruction, hydronephrosis, and consequent urinary sepsis and renal failure can follow an aortobifemoral bypass or abdominal aortic aneurysm surgery. Obstruction may be caused by direct operative trauma to the ureter, ischemic damage to the ureter, kinking of the ureter during tunneling when the periureteric tissue is inadvertently grasped, or formation of dense, fibrotic tissue around the prosthesis that invades the muscular wall of the ureter. Although the ureter may be trapped by a graft placed anterior to it, this mechanism does not appear to be a major factor.

Following early reports of patients with ureteral obstruction after aortic surgery, most vascular surgeons accepted the theory that direct compression of the ureter between the prosthetic graft and the iliac artery is the principal cause of late obstruction. Later reports by Sant and colleagues[2] and Kaufman and coworkers,[3] however, have shown that the ureter is most commonly bound down in localized fibrosis around the graft and that direct compression by an anteriorly placed graft is an important factor in only half of the reported cases.

Clinical Pathology

The consequences of ureteral damage after aortic surgery are of three clinical types. Early transient hydronephrosis occurs in 10% to 15% of these cases owing to edema from the dissection and is of no clinical significance because it usually resolves.[4] Early persistent hydronephrosis is uncommon, occurring in approximately 1% to 2% of aortic cases.[4] Affected patients require continued follow-up, but operation is necessary only for those in whom further complications develop.

Wright and colleagues[5] clarified the pathology associated with delayed-onset hydronephrosis, which occurred in 1.2% of their series. In 50% of the patients, delayed ureteral obstruction was due to a dense local fibrotic reaction, the etiology of which is unknown. To detect this complication, during late follow-up, patients should be studied by ultrasonography, CT scan, or intravenous pyelography (IVP). The other 50% of their cases had associated graft complications, including thrombosis, false aneurysm, graft-enteric fistula, and infection.[5, 6] Thus, patients who present with ureteral complications should be investigated for associated graft complications; conversely, patients who present with aortic graft complications should have a full urologic evaluation because 5% will have an abnormality.

Diagnosis

Sant and colleagues[2] reported that 13% of patients with obstructive uropathy were asymptomatic, 31% had nonurologic symptoms (anorexia, hypertension, nephrotic syndrome), and 56% had urologic symptoms (flank pain, anuria, frequency). Investigations are oriented toward four specific areas:

1. The presence of hydronephrosis may be detected by IVP, ultrasonography, or CT scan.
2. The diagnosis of ureteral obstruction and assessment

of the site of involvement are determined by retrograde pyelography.

3. Renal function is assessed by isotope renography, creatinine clearance measurement by insertion of a percutaneous nephrostomy in the affected kidney, or evaluation of improvement in renal function after temporary decompression.

4. The position of the ureter relative to the graft is determined by a simultaneous retrograde pyelogram and angiogram.

Management

Ureteral dilatation in the early postoperative period is usually the result of edema from operative trauma but in rare instances may be due to ischemia from local interruption of the ureter's blood supply. Conservative treatment is usually successful, but surgery may be indicated if progressive hydronephrosis, renal deterioration, or recurrent pyelonephritis develops.

Chronic ureteral obstruction with symptoms, evidence of impaired renal function, or recurrent infection requires surgery. However, for poor-risk patients, if the cause is fibrosis, the use of a permanent ureteral stent can be considered. Although stents are associated with risk of infection and may be occluded by debris, this approach is relatively noninvasive and can be used on a long-term basis.

If the ureter lies *anterior* to the graft, ureterolysis is performed and subsequent fibrosis is minimized by omental wrapping and possibly steroid administration. A severely scarred and narrowed segment of ureter may have to be excised and continuity reestablished by primary anastomosis, usually over a stent and protected by a proximal diversion and omental wrapping. Other procedures used to reestablish ureteral continuity include ureteroneocystotomy with or without a bladder flap or anastomosis to the contralateral ureter through a retroperitoneal tunnel.

If the ureter lies *posterior* to the graft, the graft can be divided and reanastomosed posteriorly to the ureter, or perfusion can be reestablished by an extra-anatomic bypass, such as a femoral crossover graft. The ureter is freed by ureterolysis. Alternatively, the ureter can be divided and reanastomosed anteriorly to the graft as described above. There are no reports of the long-term results of ureteral repair.

REFERENCES

1. Rutherford RB, Flanigan DP, Gupta SK, et al: Suggested standards for reports dealing with lower extremity ischemia. J Vasc Surg 4:80, 1986.
2. Sant G, Heaney JA, Parkhurst EC, Blaivas JG: Obstructive uropathy—Potentially serious complication of reconstructive vascular surgery. Urology 19:16, 1983.
3. Kaufman JE, Parsons CL, Gosink BB, Schmidt JD: Retrospective study of ureteral obstruction following vascular bypass surgery. Urology 19:278, 1982.
4. Goldenberg SL, Gordon PB, Cooperberg PL, McLoughlin MG: Early hydronephrosis following aortic bifurcation graft surgery: A prospective study. J Urol 140:1367, 1988.
5. Wright OJ, Ernst CB, Evans JR, et al: Ureteral complications and aortoiliac reconstruction. J Vasc Surg 11:29, 1990.
6. Schubart P, Fortner G, Cummings D, et al: The significance of hydronephrosis after aortofemoral reconstruction. Arch Surg 120:377, 1985.

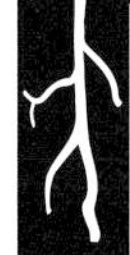

CHAPTER 40

Cardiac Complications and Screening

Mark R. Nehler, M.D., and William C. Krupski, M.D.

There is a great deal to be said for the conservative management of arteriosclerosis and being content to allow patients to grow old gracefully.

A. M. Boyd[17]

Atherosclerosis is a systemic disease that affects one in four adults in Western cultures. The annual mortality rate of cardiovascular disease in the United States exceeds 1 million, higher than all other disease rates combined.[106] Although a patient may present with a "peripheral vascular disorder" (PVD), in reality the patient has a systemic illness that will ultimately determine both the early and the late outcomes. Seventy per cent of early and late morbidity and mortality after peripheral vascular operations is due to coronary artery disease (CAD). The annual morbidity rate exceeds 2.5 million, including 1.5 million myocardial infarctions (MIs), 600,000 strokes, and 400,000 cases of congestive heart failure (CHF).[106] Total morbidity and mortality costs per year surpass $83 billion.[165] As a result, the cornerstone of clinical vascular surgery is the evaluation of risks versus benefits for patients being considered for operative intervention.

Specific indications for various peripheral vascular operations are discussed elsewhere. The purpose of this chapter is to review the current approaches to cardiac screening for the vascular surgery patient and the cardiac complications after vascular surgery. The degree of cardiac disease detected by careful preoperative screening must be weighed carefully against the natural history of the underlying vascular disorder so that the benefits of intervention exceed the risks of surgery. There is great controversy about the positive predictive values of screening tests, the best methods for risk stratification, the likelihood that intervention for CAD will improve early postoperative outcomes, the accuracy of studies promoting cardiac intervention to prolong life in vascular patients, and the socioeconomic and ethical implications of widespread screening for CAD in vascular patients.

BACKGROUND

The systemic nature of atherosclerotic vascular disease is illustrated by the finding that for patients with PVD the risk of amputation due to vascular insufficiency is significantly less than the risk of death during the same time interval.[69] Principal causes of late death in patients with PVD are coronary artery disease (40% to 60%), malignancy (7% to 23%), and cerebrovascular disease (2% to 15%).[7] The systemic complications of atherosclerosis constitute the leading causes of death in patients with PVD.

In 1960, Boyd emphasized the ominous implications of PVD.[17] In a natural history study of patients who had intermittent claudication, he reported that 39% had a nonfatal MI or stroke within 10 years of the onset of extremity symptoms; remarkably, only 22% of patients were alive 15 years after the onset of symptoms.[17] Similarly, Källerö found that patients aged 55 to 69 years with abnormal segmental limb pressure measurements had a 2-fold increased risk of death and a 14-fold increased risk of MI at 10 years.[85]

In a landmark 1985 study, Criqui and colleagues demonstrated that even in asymptomatic patients, decreased ankle-brachial indices (ABIs) strongly correlated with increased mortality from coronary disease compared with individuals with normal ABIs.[27] Criqui and coworkers later showed that for patients with symptomatic or severe PVD the risk of death from CAD is 10 to 15 times greater than those free of PVD.[28]

In a series of 871 patients requiring vascular reconstruction, Hertzer demonstrated that the cumulative cardiac mortality rate (30%) at 10 years was markedly increased for patients with suspected but uncorrected CAD compared with the rates for patients without evidence of synchronous CAD or those who had undergone myocardial revascularization.[69] This uncontrolled study has led some to recommend aggressive coronary revascularization before vascular operations. The merits of this approach are discussed in detail later.

Based on these observations, one can anticipate that half of those patients with severe CAD at the time of diagnosis of PVD will sustain a fatal cardiac complication within the ensuing 5 years. Analysis of pooled data from 50 study series composed of more than 10,000 patients who had operations for abdominal aortic aneurysms, carotid artery

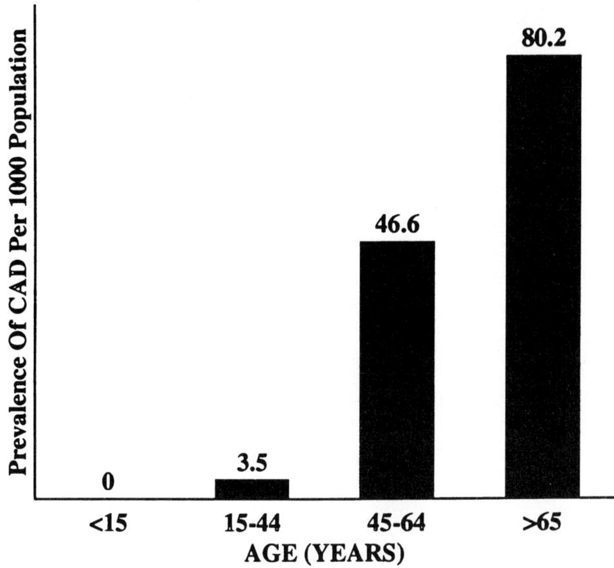

FIGURE 40–1. Prevalence of coronary artery disease (CAD) in four age groups. (From the National Center for Health Statistics, U.S. Public Health Service, Department of Health and Human Services, Washington, DC, 1988.)

disease, or lower extremity ischemia showed that clinical CAD was present in approximately 50% of patients.[103]

PREVALENCE OF CORONARY ARTERY DISEASE

Despite evidence that cardiovascular death rates have decreased by 20% to 30% during the past two decades, atherosclerotic cardiac disease and PVD continue to be major problems.[165] The prevalence of cardiovascular disease increases with age (Fig. 40–1), and the average age of the United States population is rapidly increasing. More than 25 million Americans are older than 65 years, including 2.7 million older than 85.[31] The most rapidly growing group of individuals are those between 80 and 85 years. By the middle of the 21st century, the population older than 65 is expected to reach 66 million. It is projected that nearly 9 million people over age 65 will have symptomatic atherosclerosis by the year 2010 (Table 40–1).

In addition, the incidence of "silent" or asymptomatic CAD, which is prognostically similar to clinically manifest

TABLE 40–1. INCIDENCE AND PREVALENCE OF CORONARY ARTERY DISEASE IN THE UNITED STATES

YEAR	INCIDENCE	PREVALENCE
1980	692,117	5,977,405
1985	729,235	6,700,639
1990	759,583	7,230,904
1995	792,006	7,625,001
2000	834,522	7,973,869
2005	888,438	8,385,046
2010	953,750	8,939,816

From Weinstein MC, Coxson PG, Williams LW, et al: Forecasting coronary heart disease incidence, mortality, and cost. The Coronary Heart Disease Policy Model. Am J Public Health 77:1417, 1987.

CAD, is frequently underappreciated. Cohn estimated that 2 to 5 million individuals have subclinical CAD.[29] He concluded that silent cardiac ischemia (documented by ambulatory electrocardiographic [ECG] monitoring [Holter] or exercise ECG) occurs in 2.5% to 10% of middle-aged men never having signs or symptoms of CAD, 18% of asymptomatic patients after MIs, and 40% of patients with angina pectoris. Thus, current statistics underestimate the true incidence of CAD in the general population. In 1990, Mangano conservatively estimated that more than 25 million patients required noncardiac surgery, 7 to 8 million of whom were considered at risk for cardiac morbidity or mortality by standard criteria[106]; now a substantially higher number of patients are at increased risk.

The true prevalence of CAD in patients with PVD is difficult to determine. Numerous invasive and noninvasive methods have been used to diagnose CAD in vascular patients, including the landmark study by Hertzer and colleagues in which 1000 consecutive patients with aortic aneurysms, carotid artery disease, and leg ischemia underwent routine coronary angiograms regardless of whether they had cardiac symptoms or known abnormalities.[71] Although the studies with coronary angiography do provide useful anatomic information (Table 40–2), results can be biased because patients not considered operative candidates were not studied or because not all patients agreed to coronary angiograms.

The pooled results of angiographic studies suggest that of patients with CAD symptoms, 77% have one significant vessel stenosis and more than 44% have three-vessel disease. Of note, 9% to 20% of asymptomatic patients have stenoses in three vessels.

Some positive noninvasive studies that suggest the presence of significant vascular disease are listed in Table 40–3. A wide disparity can be seen, with positive studies in as few as 16% and in as many as 64% of patients evaluated. This large disparity can in part be explained by differences in patient populations between studies. More importantly, there are great differences in the sensitivities and specificities of various tests (Fig. 40–2). The positive predictive value for cardiac events is quite disappointing.

In most patients with PVD the incidence of severe CAD is independent of the extent of peripheral arterial occlusive disease.[71] However, Källerö and colleagues have shown increased mortality rates, mainly caused by MIs, in patients with arterial occlusive disease in the popliteal trifurcation.[86] Patients with the lowest ABIs have a greater late overall mortality rate than those with higher ABIs, but the incidence of MI was surprisingly equal in all groups.[77]

Moreover, the location of vascular disease is unrelated to the degree of CAD (Table 40–4). The accuracy of clinical detection of CAD is often handicapped by the limitations in activity imposed by PVD.[68] This contributes to the surprisingly high incidence of significant CAD in patients with no clinical indication of CAD as determined by Hertzer (Table 40–5).

FREQUENCY OF ADVERSE CARDIAC EVENTS AFTER VASCULAR SURGERY

Perioperative cardiac morbidity, defined as the occurrence of MI, unstable angina, CHF, serious dysrhythmia, or cardiac death during the intraoperative or in-hospital postoperative period, is the leading cause of death after anesthesia and surgery.[106] Cardiac morbidity is often heralded by the onset of myocardial ischemia. Yet perioperative myocardial ischemia is typically silent, occurs with unexpected frequency, and is often suggested only by persistent tachycardia, making detection difficult.[109–111] Patients are vulnerable throughout the perioperative period, and, because accurate detection is difficult, the reported rates of adverse cardiac outcomes vary markedly.

Comparisons of cardiac morbidity between different studies are often misleading because the frequency of occurrence of cardiac complications depends on the vigor with which the diagnosis is pursued. Retrospective reviews generally report perioperative MI rates of about 3%, whereas more intensive prospective surveillance leads to detection rates as high as 10% to 15%.[168] Unless cardiac enzyme values and ECGs are routinely obtained, postoperative MI rates are substantially underestimated.[25] Moreover, in a series of patients with known CAD undergoing vascular

TABLE 40–2. PREVALENCE OF CORONARY ARTERY DISEASE BASED ON ROUTINE CORONARY ANGIOGRAPHY BEFORE AORTIC RECONSTRUCTION

			ASYMPTOMATIC CORONARY ARTERY DISEASE		SYMPTOMATIC CORONARY ARTERY DISEASE	
AUTHOR	YEAR	NO. OF PATIENTS	≤1 Vessel (%)	3 Vessel (%)	≤1 Vessel (%)	3 Vessel (%)
Tomatis et al[155]*	1972	100	28	16	—	—
Hertzer et al[71]*	1984	1000	37	15	78	44
Young et al[170]*	1986	302	46	20	85	52
Blombery et al[13]†	1986	84	48	9	44	22
Orecchia et al[128]*	1988	59	64	29	84	36
Average		1545 (Total)	40	16	77	44

From Cutler BS: Assessment and importance of coronary artery disease in patients with aortoiliac occlusive and aneurysmal disease. *In* Ernst CB, Stanley JC (eds): Current Therapy in Vascular Surgery, 2nd ed. Philadelphia, BC Decker, 1991, pp 382–388. By permission of Mosby–Year Book.

*Critical stenosis greater than or equal to 70%.

†Critical stenosis greater than or equal to 50%.

TABLE 40–3. RESULTS OF SPECIAL CARDIAC SCREENING TESTS BEFORE VASCULAR SURGERY

AUTHOR	YEAR	SCREENING MODALITY	NO. OF PATIENTS	ABNORMAL TEST (%)	MI OR DEATH (%)	POSITIVE PREDICTIVE VALUE (%)	NEGATIVE PREDICTIVE VALUE (%)
Cutler et al[34]	1981	ETT	130	39	4	16	99
Arous et al[3]	1984	ETT	808	17	NS	21	—
Boucher et al[16]	1985	DTS	48	33	6	19	100
von Knorring and Lepantalo[161]	1986	ETT	105	25	3	8	99
Cutler and Leppo[32]	1987	DTS	116	47	11	20	100
Raby et al[135]	1989	Holter	176	18	7	38	99
Eagle et al[47]	1989	DTS	200	41	8	16	98
Pasternack et al[130]	1989	Holter	200	40	5	NS	NS
Mangano et al[107]	1990	Holter	474	20	18	NS	NS
Mangano et al[110]	1991	DTS	60	37	22	27	82
Lalka et al[98]	1992	D-E	60	50	15	23	93
Hendel et al[66]	1992	DTS	327	51	9	14	99
Lette et al[101]	1992	DTS	355	45	8	17	99
Eichelberger et al[50]	1993	D-E	75	36	3	7	100
Brown and Rowen[19]	1993	DTS	231	33	5	13	100
Kirwin et al[93]	1993	Holter	96	9	11	NS	NS
Davila-Roman et al[37]	1993	D-E	88	23	2	10	100
Poldermans et al[133a]	1993	D-E	131	27	4	14	100
Baron et al[4]	1994	DTS	457	35	5	4	96
Bry et al[20]	1994	DTS	237	46	7	11	100

*Also includes unstable angina and congestive heart failure.

MI = myocardial infarction; ETT = exercise tolerance test; DTS = dipyridamole-thallium scintigraphy; Holter = ambulatory electrocardiographic monitoring; D-E = dobutamine echocardiography; NS = not stated.

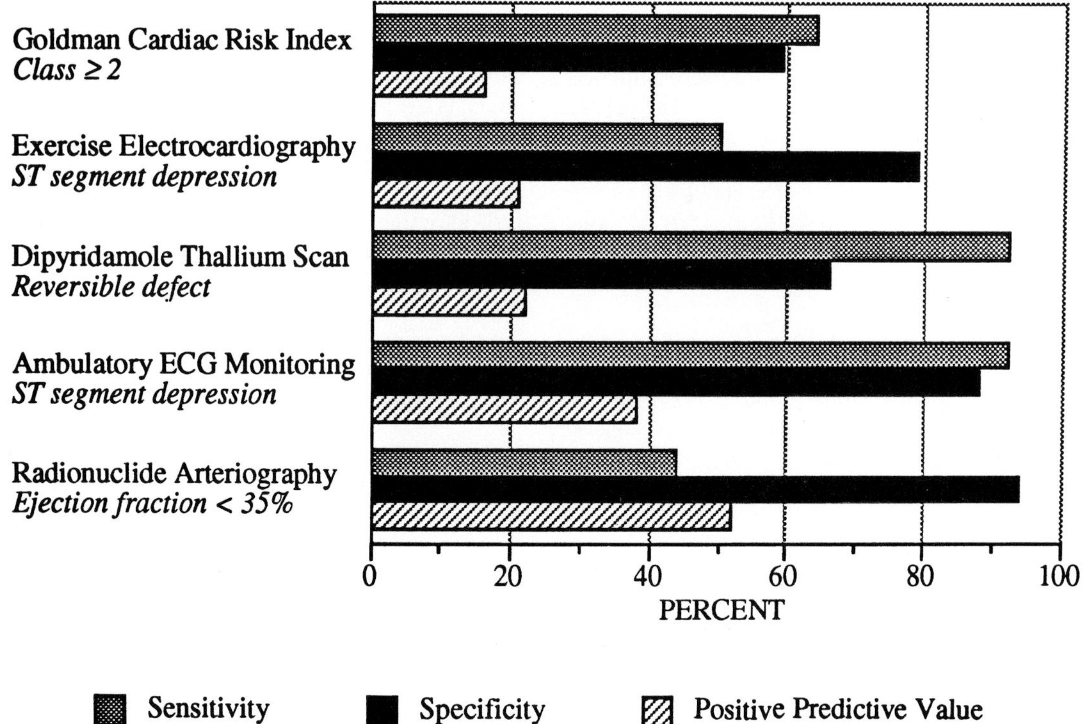

FIGURE 40–2. Comparison of current modalities to predict adverse perioperative cardiac events and cardiac death in patients undergoing vascular reconstruction. ECG = electrocardiogram. (Adapted from Yeager RA: Basic data related to cardiac testing and cardiac risk associated with vascular surgery. Ann Vasc Surg 4[2]:193–197, 1990. Reprinted by permission of Blackwell Scientific Publications, Inc.; and Raby KE, Goldman L, Creager MA, et al: Predictive value of preoperative electrocardiographic monitoring. Figure adapted from data published in The New England Journal of Medicine 322:1296–1300, 1989.)

TABLE 40–4. CLASSIFICATION OF CORONARY ARTERY DISEASE (CAD) AS RELATED TO UNDERLYING VASCULAR DISEASE

CATEGORY OF DISEASES	ABDOMINAL AORTIC ANEURYSM	LOWER EXTREMITY ISCHEMIA	CEREBROVASCULAR DISEASE	OTHER	TOTAL
Normal coronary arteries	16 (6%)	38 (10%)	27 (9%)	4 (7%)	85 (8%)
Mild to moderate CAD	77 (29%)	125 (33%)	94 (32%)	21 (34%)	317 (32%)
Advanced but compensated CAD	77 (29%)	111 (29%)	80 (27%)	21 (34%)	289 (29%)
Severe, correctable CAD	81 (31%)	79 (21%)	77 (26%)	14 (23%)	251 (25%)
Severe, inoperable CAD	12 (5%)	28 (7%)	17 (6%)	1 (2%)	58 (6%)

From Hertzer NR, Beren EG, Young JR, et al: Coronary artery disease in peripheral vascular patients: A classification of 1000 coronary angiograms and results of surgical management. Ann Surg 199:223, 1984.

surgery, 63% were found to have clinically silent postoperative myocardial ischemia by ambulatory ECG monitoring, and more than half of these patients subsequently experienced a clinically significant adverse outcome (MI, CHF, or unstable angina).[129]

The Coronary Artery Surgery Study (CASS) provided additional useful information about the risk of noncardiac surgery in patients with defined coronary disease. The risk of postoperative cardiac death in the general population is 0.5%, but this increases nearly fivefold (to 2.4%) in patients with CAD.[54]

Foster and colleagues reported an 8.7% incidence of postoperative chest pain in patients with CAD undergoing noncardiac surgery, nearly double that of patients without CAD or with a previous coronary artery bypass graft (CABG).[54] Given the silent nature of most postoperative ischemia, this small percentage of patients with postoperative chest pain probably underestimates the true incidence and represents only a fraction of clinical events. The observation that 50% to 90% of postoperative ischemic events detected by ambulatory ECG (Holter) monitoring are silent supports this contention.[109, 118, 129, 130] The incidence of MI after noncardiac surgery ranges from 0% to 0.7%, but the incidence increases substantially to 2% to 6.4% in patients undergoing elective vascular reconstruction, and nearly half of these are fatal.[168]

Although reinfarction rates vary from 5% to 8% in patients with a history of MI, these rates increase to 15% in patients undergoing vascular surgery and to 37% in patients who have had a recent MI.[106] Some studies suggest that implementation of risk stratification, aggressive intraoperative monitoring, and extended stay in the intensive care unit (ICU) can substantially reduce reinfarction rates in patients with a history of MI who are undergoing vascular reconstruction.[8, 137] However, there is a growing number of vascular surgeons who do not agree with this (including some who were originally proponents), citing the low positive predictive value of screening tests and the dearth of studies on the value of intraoperative and ICU monitoring.[154, 168, 169]

In summary, postoperative cardiac morbidity is the primary cause of death after anesthesia and surgery, especially after vascular operations. Approximately 50,000 patients per year sustain a perioperative MI, and 20,000 of these are fatal.[106] The cardiac risk associated with noncardiac surgery is due primarily to clinically silent or apparently stable CAD that is unmasked by the stress of surgery. To minimize adverse outcomes, all patients undergoing vascular reconstruction require careful preoperative evaluation with attention paid to all organ systems, but cardiac morbidity is the overwhelming determinant of both early and late outcome.

The risk of neurologic events associated with noncardiac vascular surgery is surprisingly low (0.4.% to 0.9%),[65, 70] and, although preexisting pulmonary or renal disease can contribute to postoperative morbidity, these conditions, like carotid artery disease, are rarely the primary cause of postoperative death.[22, 64, 140] A thoughtful surgeon must consider the type of surgery, the likelihood of an adverse event, the relative usefulness of confirmatory tests, and the therapeutic options for patients at risk.

TABLE 40–5. CLASSIFICATION OF CORONARY ARTERY DISEASE (CAD) AS RELATED TO CLINICAL PRESENTATION

	CLINICAL CAD	
CATEGORY OF DISEASE	No Indication	Clinically Suspected
Normal coronary arteries	64 (14%)	21 (4%)
Mild to moderate CAD	218 (49%)	99 (18%)
Advanced but compensated CAD	97 (22%)	192 (34%)
Severe, correctable CAD	63 (14%)	188 (34%)
Severe, inoperable CAD	4 (1%)	54 (10%)

From Hertzer NR, Beven EG, Young JR, et al: Coronary artery disease in peripheral vascular patients: A classification of coronary angiograms and results of surgical management. Ann Surg 199:223, 1984.

CLINICAL RISK FACTORS

The likelihood that cardiac morbidity will occur during noncardiac surgery can be predicted partly on the basis of simple clinical information.[40] Age, previous MI, cigarette smoking, CHF, valvular heart disease, angina pectoris, dysrhythmias, diabetes mellitus, and the type of operative procedure for PVD have been implicated as important risk factors for postoperative cardiac morbidity.[106] Since 1980, numerous studies have attempted to identify which clinical risk factors are most predictive of perioperative cardiac risk. Few studies, however, have had more influence on this topic than the seminal work of Goldman and associates.[63]

Goldman and associates were among the first investigators to demonstrate that estimates of perioperative cardiac risk could be derived from information available in a careful history and physical examination.[63] Of the clinical variables examined, recent MI and CHF were the strongest predictors of adverse cardiac outcome. Additional factors identified include (in order of decreasing importance):

1. Abnormal rhythm
2. More than five premature ventricular contractions per minute
3. Intra-abdominal, intrathoracic, or aortic surgery
4. Age more than 70 years
5. Significant aortic valvular stenosis
6. Emergency operation
7. Poor general medical condition

Although no current consensus exists on the best cardiac risk indicators, the following discussion reviews several that are consistently proposed as important.

Age

As many data support the predictive value of age[23, 54, 63] as refute it.[16, 106, 160] Although age does not affect ejection fraction, regional wall motion, or left ventricular volume,[80] it does depress cardiac response to stress and catecholamines.[11] Carliner and coworkers reported a 38% incidence of ischemia, MI, or cardiac death in patients older than 70 years versus 7% in those aged 40 to 49 years.[23] In the series of Goldman and coworkers, the risk of preoperative cardiac death was increased 10-fold for patients older than 70 years.[63]

Baron and associates in Paris prospectively studied 457 consecutive patients undergoing elective aortic surgery and found that an age of more than 65 years, known CAD, and an ejection fraction below 50% were the best predictors of postoperative MI.[4] An age of more than 65 years was the *only* characteristic associated with postoperative mortality in the multivariate analysis. In contrast, Driscoll and coworkers reported that age was a significant predictor only when other factors were present.[44]

Valentine and colleagues have shown that coronary disease is highly prevalent among patients with premature vascular disease.[158] In a group of 59 men whose PVD became symptomatic before age 45 years, significant CAD was present in 71%. Among the 43 patients in the study with CAD, 32 (74%) experienced an MI and 23 (53%) required interventional procedures to control angina. Eight per cent of the study population died of atherosclerotic complications in the 42-month study period.

Previous Myocardial Infarction

In 1964, Topkins and Artusio reported the first comprehensive, large-scale study relating previous MI to the cardiac risk of subsequent noncardiac surgery.[156] They found that the incidence of postoperative MI in patients without previous MI was 0.66% compared with 6.5% in patients with documented prior MI. The mortality rate of postoperative MI in patients without previous MI was 26.5%, but increased to a staggering 72% in patients who had had an antecedent MI! Reinfarction occurred in 54.5% of patients when a previous MI had occurred within 6 months of surgery compared with 4.5% in patients who suffered an MI more than 6 months earlier. Thus, both the history of a prior MI and its temporal relationship to the planned operative procedure determine susceptibility to postoperative adverse cardiac events.

These trends are corroborated in a later series in which reinfarction rates of 36% at 3 months or less, 26% at 3 to 6 months, and 5% at more than 6 months were found.[137] Overall, after vascular surgery, postoperative reinfarction rates average 2% to 6.4%, and more than half of these patients die as a consequence.[168]

Rivers and colleagues have challenged the concept that major vascular surgery must be avoided shortly after an acute MI.[139] They treated 30 patients requiring urgent or emergent vascular procedures in the first 6 weeks after an MI (median, 11 days). There were four postoperative deaths (three cardiac related) and two nonfatal reinfarctions, for an overall cardiac complication rate of 17%. The authors attributed their improved results to the extracavitary nature of the procedure and to advances in anesthetic and perioperative management.

Cigarette Smoking

Cigarette smoke causes numerous adverse endothelial, serologic, and hematologic effects that influence myocardial oxygen supply and demand. Acutely, smoking produces increased coronary vascular resistance (particularly in the presence of preexisting stenosis) and increased carboxyhemoglobin levels; the raised rate-pressure product results in increased myocardial oxygen demand.[125] Chronically, smoking causes endothelial injury, vasoconstriction, increased serum fibrinogen levels (with consequent adverse effects on blood viscosity), increased hematocrit, increased low-density lipoprotein levels, and enhanced platelet aggregation.[95]

Thus, intuitively, cigarette smoking would seem to be a risk factor for perioperative cardiac morbidity. However, in cases from the CASS registry, Foster and associates found that cigarette smoking was neither a univariate nor a multivariate predictor of adverse cardiac outcome after noncardiac operations.[54] Few other data are available.

Congestive Heart Failure

The incidence of CHF doubles in each decade of life after age 45 years, and fewer than half of patients with CHF remain alive 5 years after the time of diagnosis.[106] Nonsurgical patients who retain normal left ventricular (LV) function after MI have a 7% 1-year mortality rate; in contrast, the 1-year mortality rate increases to 44% in those whose ejection fraction deteriorates to less than 30% or who cannot complete an exercise test after MI.[45] Similar data have led some to suggest that it is the degree of myocardial dysfunction, not the time from infarction or the extent of CAD, that determines perioperative mortality.[41, 142] Furthermore, in most cardiac risk indexes, CHF is among the most heavily weighted predictors.[63, 167] Yet CHF is a constellation of clinical symptoms rather than a specific disease.

There is controversy over which marker of heart failure is most predictive of cardiac prognosis. Pathologic heart sounds (S_3, S_4 gallop), jugular venous distention,[62, 167] alveolar pulmonary edema,[54] dyspnea on exertion, LV wall motion abnormalities, and LV ejection fraction of less than

30%[100, 133] have been proposed as predictors of adverse outcome. Arguably, the most objective finding is quantification of LV dysfunction by measurement of ejection fraction.

In patients undergoing either aortic surgery[131] or lower extremity revascularization,[133] Pasternack and colleagues demonstrated that the degree of LV dysfunction as measured by radionuclide angiography correlated with the risk of perioperative MI. In these studies 80% of patients undergoing aortic surgery and 70% of patients undergoing infrainguinal operations sustained an adverse perioperative cardiac event when the ejection fraction was found to be less than 30%. Although these findings have been challenged by some,[55, 119] Bunt[21] has demonstrated that the detection of CHF by physical examination and by the quantification of LV function by ejection fraction helps to stratify the perioperative cardiac risk and further directs the decision to proceed directly to surgery or to obtain additional tests.

Valvular Heart Disease

The prognosis for patients with valvular heart disease depends on which valve is diseased and on the extent of disease. Because of the confounding factors associated with valvular heart disease, such as left ventricular dysfunction, the perioperative risk caused by valvular disease per se is difficult to quantitate. Limited data suggest that aortic stenosis is associated with excessive perioperative mortality.

In their classic study, Goldman and associates reported a 14-fold increased perioperative mortality rate in patients with aortic stenosis who underwent noncardiac surgery.[63] The diagnosis of aortic stenosis was made largely by physical examination, however, without objective measurement of degree of stenosis. Although the incidence of postoperative CHF was increased by the presence of mitral stenosis or insufficiency in that study, only aortic stenosis was associated with increased mortality.

Angina Pectoris

By analyzing the pooled data of angiographically confirmed CAD and autopsy data, Diamond and Forrester estimated that 90% of males older than 40 years and 90% of females older than 60 years with angina have significant CAD.[40] Surprisingly, they suggested that up to 20% of similarly aged *asymptomatic* patients have significant CAD. Goldman and associates determined by univariate and multivariate analyses that angina was conspicuously absent as a significant predictor of perioperative cardiac morbidity.[62, 63]

These results should not be viewed as contradictory if one considers that most perioperative ischemia is clinically silent.[109, 111] In contrast, Eagle and associates concluded that angina was one of five major predictors of perioperative cardiac morbidity.[47]

Arrhythmias

Cardiac arrhythmias are not uncommon, and in patients without significant heart disease they are normally benign. If significant CAD is present or LV function is compromised, however, the development of rhythm disturbances can be lethal.[12] Rhythm disturbances that arise in patients with acute MI or concurrent hypokalemia and ischemia are frequent causes of sudden death.[120, 143] Although few studies have adequately addressed the importance of postoperative arrhythmias, the available data do suggest that frequent premature ventricular contractions or rhythms other than normal sinus rhythm on preoperative ECG are independent predictors of outcome in patients undergoing noncardiac surgery.[54, 62, 63]

Diabetes Mellitus

An unquestionable association exists between diabetes and the development of atherosclerosis. Patients with diabetes appear to be more susceptible to CAD, MI, and premature death than nondiabetics.[11, 163] Although controversial, some studies suggest that people with diabetes are at increased cardiac risk after noncardiac surgery.[54, 68] In our experience, diabetics who require infrainguinal operations have a markedly increased risk of developing myocardial ischemia that is consistent with a more advanced stage of systemic atherosclerosis.[96]

Operative Procedure

The anatomic location of the planned vascular operation has little bearing on postoperative cardiac morbidity. The reported incidences of MI after vascular surgery vary widely, ranging from 0 to 16%, but rates are not uniformly dependent on the type of procedure performed (Tables 40–6, 40–7, and 40–8).[21, 30, 133, 154] The criteria for diagnosing an MI are important in this disparity in reported MI rates, in addition to the vigor with which the diagnosis is pursued (as discussed earlier).

In a comprehensive review of the literature, Yeager estimated that when the diagnosis of MI was made by retrospective review, the incidence of MI after vascular surgery averaged 3%.[168] When the diagnosis of MI was made pro-

TABLE 40–6. INCIDENCE OF PERIOPERATIVE MYOCARDIAL INFARCTION (MI) IN ELECTIVE INFRARENAL AORTIC OPERATIONS

AUTHOR	YEAR	NO. OF PATIENTS	MI (%)	FATAL MI (%)
Ameli et al[2]	1990	105	6.7	4.7
Clark et al[26]	1990	200	1.5	1.5
Mason et al[112]	1990	144	4.2	1.4
Isaacson et al[80]	1990	102	2.0	1.0
Sedwitz et al[144]	1990	109	3.7	0
Golden et al[61]	1990	500	3.0	1.2
Shah et al[148]	1991	280	—	2.5
Bunt[21]	1992	156	0	0
Seeger et al[145]	1994	146	—	0.6
Baron et al[4]	1994	457	4.8	2.2
Lord et al[104]	1994	329	—	1.2
Sicard et al[152]	1995	145	—	1.4
Huber et al[79]	1995	722	—	1.5
Carrel et al[24]	1995	216	4.6	1.9
Henderson and Effeney[67]	1995	538	10	3.7
Erickson et al[52]	1996	209	3.8	1.0
Shueppert et al[151]	1996	144	2.1	0.7
Jarvinen et al[83]	1996	400	4.2	2.3
D'Angelo et al[35]	1997	113	1.8	0.9
Mingoli et al[122]	1997	238	0.9	0.4

TABLE 40–7. INCIDENCE OF PERIOPERATIVE MYOCARDIAL INFARCTION (MI) IN FEMOROPOPLITEAL AND FEMOROTIBIAL OPERATIONS

AUTHOR	YEAR	NO. OF PATIENTS	MI (%)	FATAL MI (%)
Towne et al[157]	1991	361	—	2.2
Taylor et al[153]	1991	498	5.2	2.2
Bunt[21]	1992	249	1.6	0.8
Wagner et al[162]	1992	107	5.6	4
Donaldson et al[42]	1993	585	3.2	1.5
Bergamini et al[6]	1994	252	—	2.7
Kalman et al[87]	1994	275	4.4	—
Hood et al[76]	1996	157	5.0	1.3
Matsura et al[116]	1997	205	3.4	2.9

spectively based on ECG changes *and* cardiac enzyme elevation, the incidence of MI rose to 9.7%. When MIs were diagnosed prospectively based on MB isoenzyme elevation as the only criterion, the average postoperative MI rate was a striking 14.7%.

Most articles on preoperative cardiac screening describe patient cohorts considered for aortic surgery for either occlusive disease or abdominal aortic aneurysms. The frequent occurrence of adverse cardiac events was usually attributed to the stress on myocardium caused by anesthetic induction, aortic clamping, declamping hypotension, washout acidosis, blood loss, large fluid shifts, and metabolic abnormalites.[45] Infrainguinal vascular operations generally do not produce such profound hemodynamic and physiologic alterations, and therefore they might be expected to cause fewer cardiac complications.

To address this question, we prospectively compared cardiac morbidity in 140 patients undergoing aortic (n = 53) and infrainguinal reconstructions (n = 87).[96] Presumably because coronary disease was even higher in patients having "less stressful" infrainguinal procedures, we observed that the number of postoperative cardiac events (cardiac death, MI, unstable angina, CHF, ventricular tachycardia) was similar to patients undergoing major abdominal aortic procedures (Fig. 40–3). In addition, 57% of patients undergoing infrainguinal operations had documented is-

TABLE 40–8. INCIDENCE OF PERIOPERATIVE MYOCARDIAL INFARCTION (MI) IN CAROTID ENDARTERECTOMY

AUTHOR	YEAR	NO. OF PATIENTS	MI (%)	FATAL MI (%)
Salenius et al[141]	1990	331	—	0
Maini et al[105]	1990	246	0.8	—
Bunt[21]	1992	114	0	0
Freischlag et al[56]	1992	141	1.4	0
NASCET[126]	1991	328	1.2	0.3
Hobson et al[75]	1993	211	4.2	1.9
Berman et al[9]	1994	203	2.5	0
Shah et al[149]	1994	654	0.3	0.3
Ombrellaro et al[127]	1995	266	1.5	0
ACAS[53]	1995	724	—	0.1
Mattos et al[115]	1995	2243	—	0.7
Dardik et al[36]	1997	201	2.5	0.5
Hertzer et al[72]	1997	2228	—	0.4

ACAS = Asymptomatic Carotid Atherosclerosis Study.

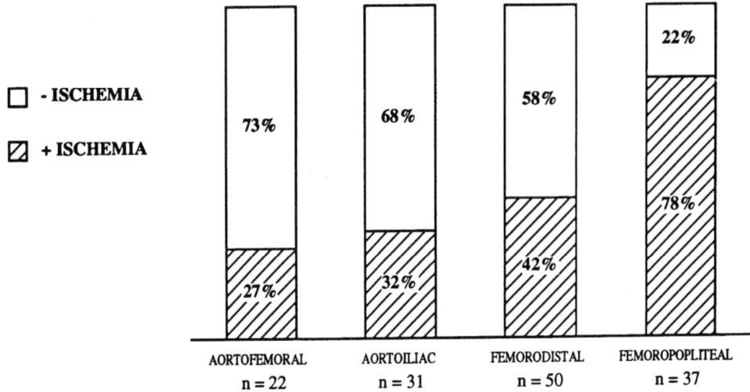

FIGURE 40–3. Incidence of postoperative myocardial ischemia documented by continuous ambulatory electrocardiography in patients undergoing aortic or infrainguinal vascular reconstruction. (Adapted from Krupski WC, Layug EL, Reilly LM, et al: Comparison of cardiac morbidity between aortic and infrainguinal operations. Study of Perioperative Ischemia [SPI] Research Group. J Vasc Surg 15:354, 1992.)

chemia by ambulatory ECG monitoring compared with 31% of patients undergoing aortic reconstruction (p = .005). Interestingly, the ischemia was clinically silent in nearly all (98%) patients, consistent with previous reports that most postoperative ischemia is asymptomatic.[109, 111]

Late cardiac outcomes in patients having operations for infrainguinal occlusive disease are even worse than for patients having aortic operations. A later follow-up of the patient cohort described in the preceding paragraph revealed that at 2 years 25% of all patients had died, about half due to cardiac disease.[97] Twenty of 81 (25%) patients who had infrainguinal procedures compared with 4 of 48 (8%) patients who had aortic operations had adverse cardiac events in late follow-up (p = .04). Multivariate analysis showed that a history of diabetes (p = .001) and preoperative CAD (p = .01) were independently associated with adverse outcomes after both types of PVD operations.

L' Italien and colleagues described a similar analysis of cardiac morbidity in patients undergoing aortic (n = 321), infrainguinal (n = 177), and carotid (n = 49) operations.[103] Perioperative MI occurred in 6% of patients undergoing aortic and carotid artery surgery and in 13% of patients undergoing infrainguinal procedures (p = .019).

Although carotid operations usually have lower cardiac morbidity rates than aortic and infrainguinal operations (see Table 40–8), the study of L' Italien and colleagues shows that surprisingly high rates have occasionally been reported.[103] Ennix and coworkers reported outcomes in 1546 consecutive carotid endarterectomies in 1238 patients over a 10-year period.[51] Although the overall rate of perioperative MI was only 1.6%, MIs occurred in 12.9% of 85 patients with *symptomatic* CAD. More recently, Musser and coworkers reviewed 562 patients who had carotid endarterectomies at a community hospital, and only 10 (1.8%) suffered MIs, 6 (1.1%) being fatal.[123]

RISK STRATIFICATION

Risk stratification has three purposes: (1) to identify patients for whom the cardiac risks outweigh the potential benefits of therapy, (2) to identify patients with clinical problems that might be corrected before surgery, and (3) to identify those who are most likely to benefit from risk-reducing interventions. Methods of risk stratification include clinical risk indexes, resting electrocardiograms (ECGs), exercise treadmill testing, ambulatory ECG (Holter) monitoring, cardiac nuclear imaging (dipyridamole-thallium scintigraphy [DTS], radionuclide ventriculography [RNVG]), dobutamine stress echocardiography, and coronary angiography. These tests attempt to quantify risk in patients who are in danger of perioperative coronary events.

CLINICAL RISK INDEXES

The history alone can detect CAD in a large subset of patients. Physical examination may reveal signs of CHF, cardiac dysrhythmia, or valvular heart disease; it also helps to clarify the patient's general medical status. The physical examination together with a careful history form the basis of all clinical risk indexes. In fact, features elicited by the history and physical examination alone account for 35 of 53 points in the Goldman cardiac risk index (GCRI), with the remaining points derived from simple laboratory tests and an ECG (Fig. 40–4).

As noted previously, Goldman and associates were among the first to attempt to quantify the relative risks of cardiac morbidity and mortality in patients undergoing noncardiac surgical procedures by clinical markers. Multivariate analyses of 39 clinical variables in 1001 surgical patients identified nine features that were predictive of perioperative cardiac morbidity. Points were assigned to each variable to reflect its statistical weight in the analysis, and the GCRI thus was formulated.[63]

The GCRI was subsequently validated in several studies.[25, 38, 150, 171] For example, Shah and coworkers, using stepwise logistic regression, retrospectively analyzed 24 preoperative variables in 688 patients undergoing noncardiac operations who either had cardiac disease (which they defined as previous MI, unstable or stable angina, previous CABG, CHF, valvular heart disease, or ECG abnormality) or were older than 70 years of age.[150] They identified eight variables predictive of perioperative cardiac morbidity (age more than 70 years, emergency operation, chronic stable angina, previous MI, ECG signs of ischemia, type of surgical procedure, hypokalemia). Of these eight variables, only two (chronic stable angina and ECG signs of ischemia) do not have a counterpart on the GCRI.

Unfortunately, no uniform agreement on the utility of a predictive preoperative risk index exists, particularly when

	GOLDMAN CRI	DETSKY CRI	EAGLE CRITERIA
RISK FACTOR	*WEIGHTED RISK FACTOR SCORE*		
AGE >70	5	5	1
MI			1
< 6 months	10	10	
> 6 months		5	
ANGINA			
Class III		10	1
Class IV		20	
Unstable		10	
DIABETES			1
OPERATION			
Emergency	4	10	
Aortic, Abdominal, Thoracic	3		
CHF	11		1
≤ 1 week		10	
> 1 week		5	
ELECTROCARDIOGRAM			
Rhythm other than sinus	7	5	
> 5 PVC / min	7	5	
POOR MEDICAL STATUS	3	5	
CARDIAC RISK	*SUMMED RISK FACTOR SCORES*		
LOW	0-12	0-15	0
INTERMEDIATE	13-25	16-30	1-2
HIGH	> 25	> 30	≥ 3

FIGURE 40–4. Comparison of clinical cardiac risk indexes (CRI) commonly employed in the preoperative risk assessment of patients scheduled for noncardiac surgery. CHF = congestive heart failure; MI = myocardial infarction; PVC = premature ventricular contractions. (Data from Detsky AS, Abrams HB, Forbath N, et al: Cardiac assessment for patients undergoing noncardiac surgery: A multifactorial clinical risk index. Arch Intern Med 146:2131-2134, Copyright 1986, American Medical Association; Eagle KA, Singer DE, Brewster DC, et al: Dipyridamole-thallium scanning in patients undergoing vascular surgery: Optimizing preoperative evaluation of cardiac risk. JAMA 257:2185–2189, Copyright 1987, American Medical Association; and Goldman L, Caldera DL, Nessbaum SR, et al: Multifactorial index of cardiac risk in noncardiac surgical procedures. Reprinted with permission from The New England Journal of Medicine 297: 845, 1977.)

applied to vascular surgery patients. In a study by Lette and colleagues, 125 consecutive patients undergoing vascular reconstruction were evaluated with cardiac risk indexes (CRIs) and DTS.[102] They found that vascular surgery patients classified as Goldman or Detsky class 1 (i.e., lowest risk) still had a 10.4% incidence of perioperative cardiac morbidity. All clinical scoring systems studied (Dripps-ASA [American Society of Anesthesiologists],[43] CRI,[63] Detsky CRI,[39] Eagle criteria,[48] Yeager criteria,[169] and Cooperman probability[30]) failed to predict adverse perioperative outcome (cardiac death or postoperative MI).

Wong and Detsky reexamined the conclusions of Lette and colleagues using Bayesian logic and reached different conclusions.[167] Their analysis suggests that a higher GCRI score (class 3) accurately predicted increased perioperative cardiac risk, but all clinical indexes appear to lack sufficient sensitivity to identify very-low-risk subsets of patients. Thus, their analysis suggests that clinical risk indexes may help to predict perioperative cardiac complications that are of intermediate or high risk.

Despite the lack of a consensus, the studies support the application of risk indexes, like the GCRI, to stratify patients according to estimated perioperative cardiac morbidity. As a result, patients who may potentially benefit from further preoperative evaluation, changes in the planned operative procedure, or modification of the planned perioperative management can be identified. Although a universally accepted risk index does not exist, the evolution of prognostic indexes demonstrates that useful information can be obtained by a thorough history and physical examination.

DIAGNOSTIC TESTING PREDICTORS

Rational recommendations for additional preoperative tests for patients with suspected CAD must be based on several assumptions: (1) perioperative cardiac complications occur sufficiently frequently to justify commitment of significant resources in an attempt to lower their incidences, (2) the proposed tests accurately identify patients at risk, and (3) effective treatment exists to lower the risk of complications significantly in the selected patients.[154] Clinical predictors of cardiac risk are relatively insensitive for patients with vascular disease whose exercise tolerance is limited by either intermittent claudication or previous amputation. The impairment in ambulation imposed by occlusive vascular disease may mask symptoms of exertional angina or CHF.

As a result, attention has been focused on the development of adjunctive preoperative cardiac testing that may enhance the sensitivity and specificity of preoperative risk assessment. Surgical patients who have either symptomatic ischemic heart disease or global LV dysfunction are at greatest risk for perioperative complications and are usually easily identified.[21, 63, 106, 167] Conversely, a significant number of patients appear to be at significant risk due to occult cardiac disease unmasked only by the stress of surgery.[71]

The proliferation of adjunctive tests to help quantify cardiac risk has further complicated the evaluation of intermediate-risk patients. Information from a test alters the estimate of an individual patient's risk for developing a cardiac complication. Patients who have a positive test result are expected to have a higher than average chance of having a cardiac complication, whereas those with a negative test result are expected to have a lower than average risk.[167] However, the procedures are expensive, of uncertain utility, and sometimes risky either as a direct result of the procedure or because of how the information is subsequently used.[82]

In reviewing their own data, Eagle and associates suggested that an adverse cardiac event rate of 10% to 15% may be expected in vascular surgery patients who are determined to be at intermediate or high risk after clinical assessment,[46, 48] whereas less than 5% of vascular patients in the low-risk category may experience an adverse cardiac event. These percentages represent the pretest probability of an adverse cardiac event. Additional testing should be performed only if the post-test probability is increased significantly compared with the pretest probability.[167]

In patients already deemed to be at low or high risk, additional tests (and subsequent clinical management) are unlikely to change the pretest probabilities substantially enough to justify their use (when post-test probability is equal to or less than pretest probability). Conversely, in patients considered to be at intermediate risk, adjunctive tests may provide sufficient information to alter the patients' clinical management enough to justify screening (post-test probability greater than pretest probability).

The most commonly employed screening tests include resting ECG, exercise treadmill testing, ambulatory ECG (Holter) monitoring, DTS, dobutamine stress echocardiography, and coronary angiography. However, a consensus regarding the best test or approach to be used for preoperative risk assessment of vascular surgery patients has *not* been reached. Furthermore, studies of adjunctive tests must be reviewed with caution and analyzed with respect to the following critical limitations:

1. Only selected patients had the recommended diagnostic procedure.
2. The *degree* of ischemia could not be quantified by the diagnostic study.
3. Patients were excluded for poorly defined reasons.
4. Patients enrolled in the study had undergone prior myocardial revascularization.
5. Studies were not blinded, and therefore physicians could employ therapeutic interventions that altered outcome.
6. Data were retrospectively analyzed.
7. Interpretation of the diagnostic test was arbitrary.
8. Length of the postoperative period (typically, $\leq$ 72 hours) precluded identification of adverse cardiac events occurring later in the postoperative course.

Resting Electrocardiogram

Data on the predictive value of preoperative resting ECG are conflicting. However, considering the prevalence of CAD in vascular surgery patients specifically, it is hard to justify the surgeon *not* obtaining a baseline ECG.[159] ECG abnormalities are common. Numerous studies have documented that an abnormal preoperative ECG is a statistically significant predictor of adverse cardiac outcome.[33, 159, 160] An abnormal resting ECG has been associated with up to a threefold increase in perioperative cardiac complications. Hertzer and associates found that 44% of patients with a clinical history of cardiac disease and an abnormal ECG (evidence of previous MI; ST-T segment changes) had *severe* CAD as determined by angiography (more than 70% stenosis of one or more coronary arteries) compared with only 22% of those with normal ECGs.[71]

Of 12,654 patients undergoing major noncardiac surgery, von Knorring prospectively studied 214 patients with ECG patterns suggestive of previous MI, LV hypertrophy or strain, or myocardial ischemia.[160] Of these 214 patients with abnormal preoperative ECGs, 17.7% sustained a postoperative MI with a cardiac mortality rate of 32%. Type of surgery, anesthetic techniques or duration, and patient factors such as history of chest pain, diabetes, age, and sex were not predictive.

Although an abnormal ECG suggests underlying CAD, a normal resting ECG may be misleading. From 25% to 50% of previous MIs are missed on ECG because the test is misread or lacks the pathognomonic findings of an old MI. Using findings from routine coronary arteriograms, Hertzer and colleagues reported that 37% of vascular patients with *normal* resting ECGs had significant stenosis (more than 70%) of one or more coronary arteries.[71] Similarly, Benchimol and associates found angiographic evidence of significant three-vessel CAD in 15% of patients who had completely normal ECGs.[5] These studies illustrate that an abnormal ECG may denote the presence of significant underlying CAD, but a normal ECG should not reassure the physician that significant CAD is absent. Thus, the resting ECG cannot be used as the sole diagnostic test to estimate perioperative cardiac risk.

Special Cardiac Screening Tests

A decision to obtain additional tests should be made only after the operative indications, the patient's general health status, and the cardiac risk profile have been considered. Several investigators have suggested that special preoperative testing should be employed for stratifying cardiac risk only in patients considered to be at intermediate or high clinical risk.[16, 47, 135] In their studies of patients undergoing noncardiac surgical procedures, only 4% of patients clinically identified as low risk suffered nonfatal cardiac events. In contrast, 9% to 21% of patients identified as intermediate or high clinical risk suffered adverse perioperative cardiac events. Patients with previous MI, angina pectoris, or CHF warrant periodic testing regardless of the requirement for noncardiac surgery. In the absence of these criteria, subsets of patients or operative procedures in which the perioperative cardiac event rate exceeds 10% *may* benefit from additional screening tests.

Numerous studies illustrate that patients with high scores on clinical CRIs (GCRI greater than 12 or Detsky index greater than 15) or more than three of the five Eagle criteria (age over 70 years, diabetes mellitus, angina, Q waves on ECG, or ventricular arrhythmias) are at the greatest risk for MI or cardiac death following vascular surgery.[38, 39, 47, 48, 63, 135] Patients identified clinically to be at low cardiac risk and not limited by their PVD or general medical condition are unlikely to benefit from further testing. It is doubtful whether additional tests in this subset of patients would provide additional information sufficient to alter management.

Alternatively, patients considered to be at high risk by clinical criteria are unlikely to benefit from further risk stratification because the clinical evidence of increased perioperative cardiac morbidity is overwhelming.[167] Some authorities recommend that most such patients require intervention for their heart disease in preparation for an elective PVD procedure, although this recommendation is based solely on retrospective, uncontrolled, and nonrandomized studies. The following discussion on special cardiac screening tests focuses on methods of further stratifying patients categorized as *intermediate* risk by clinical scoring.

Exercise Treadmill (Stress) Testing

The enhanced respiratory, metabolic, and cardiovascular work required in the postoperative period increases myocardial stress. In patients with the physical capacity to exercise, ECG stress testing is an inexpensive, noninvasive, and suitable method of predicting postoperative cardiac morbidity. Inability to exercise at low cardiac workloads or the presence of ST-segment abnormalities on ECG during exercise correlates with an increased risk of adverse postoperative cardiac outcomes. Gerson and coworkers found that an inability to exercise was 80% sensitive and 53% specific for postoperative cardiac morbidity.[60]

Exercise-induced ST-segment changes clearly predict cardiac risk. Cutler and colleagues reported the occurrence of perioperative MI in 37% of vascular patients with positive results on stress ECGs compared with an incidence of 1.5% in those with normal studies.[34]

Stress ECG is the most popular method of unmasking myocardial ischemia, but it has less applicability for vascular surgery patients. Patients with vascular disease are often older and deconditioned and are therefore unable to exercise adequately. Submaximal effort leads to an increased frequency of false-negative results.[47] Gage and associates found that patients screened by exercise treadmill testing (ETT) before noncardiac surgery were often unable to complete the examination owing to dyspnea or claudication (24%), and the results were often unreliable because of the increased false-positive (40%) and false-negative (15%) rates.[57] Port and colleagues performed a 12-lead ECG test on 58 patients with intermittent claudication while the patients pedaled a bicycle.[134] Fourteen patients (24%) had positive test results, and 2 of the 14 (14.3%) had fatal postoperative MIs. Arm exercise testing has also been proposed for patients limited by leg claudication, but heart rates are not predictably elevated to sufficient levels with this exercise.

Analysis of the CASS registry data revealed that of 2045 patients with a history of angina pectoris, 65% of men and 33% of women with angiographically documented significant CAD had *normal* ETT results.[164] Subset analysis of men and women matched for age, presence (31%), and extent of CAD demonstrated that the false-positive (44% versus 51%) and false-negative (12% versus 14%) rates were the same regardless of sex.

The accuracy of exercise stress testing is controversial.

False-negative tests are common.[94, 114] Iskandrian and coworkers compared ETT score and thallium perfusion in 617 men and 217 women; all patients subsequently had coronary angiograms.[81] Concordance between the ETT score and thallium occurred in only 273 patients (33%), and neither study correlated well with the degree of angiographic CAD.

The ECG response to exercise when used as an objective finding to confirm or exclude CAD is affected by the prevalence of the disease in the population studied. In a population in whom the prevalence of CAD is high, a positive ETT only slightly increases the likelihood of CAD, whereas a negative stress test correlates poorly with the absence of CAD.[164] Therefore, ECG stress tests have limited application for elderly patients with diffuse atherosclerosis, in those whose claudication or medical condition precludes maximum exercise, and in those who are strongly suspected to have CAD on the basis of the cardiac history or baseline ECG.

Ambulatory Electrocardiographic (Holter) Monitoring

Holter monitoring is commonly used to evaluate cardiac dysrhythmia. During the 1980s it was employed in preoperative risk analyses of patients undergoing noncardiac surgical procedures.[15, 58, 109, 111, 118, 130, 136] Approximately 18% to 40% of surgical patients with or at risk for CAD demonstrate frequent ischemic episodes during the 48-hour interval preceding surgery.

Most (> 75%) ischemic episodes are clinically silent.[96] In a prospective study using multivariate analysis, Raby and colleagues found that preoperative ischemia diagnosed by ambulatory ECG was the most significant predictor of postoperative cardiac events. Ischemia on Holter monitoring remained an independent predictor of adverse cardiac events even after all other preoperative risk factors were controlled. Less than 1% of patients without detectable ischemia had perioperative cardiac morbidity.[135]

Similarly, Pasternack and associates reported that silent ischemia detected by Holter monitoring occurred in more than 60% of patients undergoing vascular surgical procedures.[130] Patients who sustained postoperative MI had longer-duration individual perioperative ischemic episodes, more perioperative ischemic episodes, and longer total perioperative ischemic time (percentage of total monitoring time). Only preoperative silent MI and angina at rest were predictive of perioperative MI. No patient experienced perioperative cardiac morbidity in the absence of preoperative evidence on Holter monitoring of ischemia.

In studies of patients undergoing noncardiac surgery, Mangano and colleagues found that 28% of patients had documented preoperative ischemia on Holter monitoring, and the incidence of ischemia nearly doubled in the postoperative period.[109, 111] Most (94%) ischemic episodes were silent and peaked in severity on the third postoperative day. Ischemia occurred throughout the postoperative weeklong (7-day) monitored period, further emphasizing the underestimated incidence and late time course of perioperative cardiac morbidity. All adverse cardiac outcomes (unstable angina, MI, cardiac death) were heralded by postoperative ischemia detected on Holter monitoring, but, due to the blinded design of the study, no interventions were performed on the basis of these findings.

The advantages of ambulatory ECG monitoring over other noninvasive methods, such as DTS, to determine cardiac risk include its wider availability and lower cost. Disadvantages include the fact that 10% or more of patients have underlying resting ECG abnormalities that limit or preclude the interpretation of ST-segment depression, and ECG patterns such as LV hypertrophy may lead to false-positive evidence of ST-segment depression that is not due to CAD.[47]

Finally, a prospective study by Kirwin and associates questioned the predictive value of silent myocardial ischemia in PVD surgery patients.[93] Ninety-six patients having elective vascular reconstructions underwent preoperative Holter monitoring for a 24-hour period. Patients with and without preoperative silent myocardial ischemia had no statistically significant difference in the incidence of postoperative MIs (11% versus 16%).

Stress-Thallium Imaging (Dipyridamole-Thallium Scintigraphy)

Stress-thallium imaging, performed under conditions of near-maximal coronary blood flow (exercise or injection of dipyridamole), is more sensitive than resting imaging and can detect heterogeneous perfusion due to stenoses as small as 50%.[48] Boucher and coworkers first reported DTS as an accurate, safe, and noninvasive alternative to exercise stress testing for patients in whom claudication precluded exercise.[16] Since that report, hundreds of articles have been published on this technique.

Thallium 201 is taken up by myocardial cells in proportion to blood flow. Intravenous dipyridamole dilates coronary vessels, thus increasing blood flow to parts of the myocardium supplied by nonstenotic vessels. Dipyridamole acts by inhibiting myocardial cellular reuptake and endothelial transport of endogenously produced adenosine, a potent coronary vasodilator. As adenosine accumulates in the interstitium, coronary vasodilation ensues. Administration of dipyridamole, through its adenosine effect, results in an increase in coronary flow by twofold to threefold.[49, 117]

Myocardium supplied by stenotic vessels has poor uptake on early scintigraphic scans, however, resulting in relative absence of thallium uptake in that portion of the heart. In effect, intravenous dipyridamole produces a *steal* phenomenon because nonstenotic arteries enjoy enhanced flow, whereas stenotic arteries cannot vasodilate. Later, this defect resolves if viable myocardium is present, suggesting the presence of an area of myocardium that is potentially at risk during periods of increased stress (late uptake of thallium 201 in areas of myocardium that are initially underperfused is termed *redistribution*). In contrast, a persistent defect on thallium scan suggests an area of prior MI infarction and, therefore, myocardium that is already irreversibly injured (myocardial scarring).[49]

Several studies have suggested that normal DTS findings in a patient scheduled for vascular surgery indicate low risk for cardiac complications.[16, 32, 33, 47, 49, 99] The prognostic implications of a scan that detects either a fixed or reversible defect is less certain. When DTS is used as a guide to selection of patients for preoperative diagnostic angiography, it may be possible to identify subsets of patients at risk for ischemic complications of noncardiac vascular operations.[59]

With DTS Lette and colleagues studied 125 consecutive patients before elective vascular surgery and found that no clinical risk index (GCRI, Dripps-ASA, Detsky CRI, Eagle criteria, Yeager criteria, Cooperman probability) accurately predicted adverse perioperative outcomes, whereas 21% of patients with reversible defects suffered a postoperative cardiac event.[102] If the defects were further quantified by the severity and extent of reversibility of defects (i.e., myocardium at risk), 85% of patients with a substantial amount of myocardium determined to be at risk by DTS suffered cardiac death or MI.

The failure of clinical indexes to be predictive in part reflects the study design (retrospective) and the study endpoints (cardiac death, MI). Furthermore, the low specificity of DTS when interpreted only as positive (reversible defect) or negative ("normal" or fixed defect) illustrates the low yield if it is applied to all patients referred for vascular surgery. Such a conclusion is supported by our findings in a prospective study of 60 patients undergoing elective vascular surgery.[110] DTS was performed preoperatively in all patients, and the treating physicians were blinded to the results. No association could be found between redistribution defects and adverse cardiac outcomes, risk of adverse outcome with redistribution defect, or risk of perioperative ischemia (Holter monitoring, ETT) with redistribution defect. These results led us to conclude that routine use of DTS for preoperative screening is unwarranted.

Similar conclusions were reached by other investigators studying much larger numbers of patients. In France, Baron and coworkers obtained DTS in 457 consecutive patients undergoing elective abdominal aortic surgery.[4] Eighty-six patients (19%) had one or more postoperative cardiac complications: prolonged myocardial ischemia (61 patients), MI (22), CHF (20), and severe ventricular tachycardia (2). DTS did not accurately predict adverse cardiac outcomes, and the authors concluded that the routine use of DTS for screening before abdominal aortic surgery is not justified.

In 1996, Shueppert and colleagues evaluated *routine* DTS in 394 consecutive patients being considered for elective vascular surgery.[151] Routine screening with DTS had no impact on the perioperative MI rate, and the authors no longer use this test on a routine basis. A positive DTS did, however, correlate with late cardiac events in a mean follow-up period of 40 months. Adverse cardiac outcomes were significantly more frequent in patients with reversible defects on DTS. Late MIs occurred in 9% of patients with normal DTS versus 20% of those with reversible defects (late cardiac mortality was 4% versus 19% [$p < .05$]).

Routine stress-thallium cardiac scanning was also evaluated by Seeger and colleagues from the University of Florida.[145] Preoperative stress-thallium scans (DTS, adenosine-thallium scintigraphy, or Bruce protocol exercise-thallium scintigraphy) from 146 patients undergoing aortic reconstruction were evaluated prospectively. Postoperative cardiac complications and long-term survival rates in these patients were compared with results from 172 patients having aortic surgery without previous stress-thallium scanning. Patients with positive studies underwent coronary arteriography and myocardial revascularization "when appropriate." In the thallium cohort, 41% underwent coronary angiography and 11.6% underwent CABG compared with 14.7% and 4.1%, respectively, in the control group. Cardiac mortality, serious cardiac complications, and long-term cardiac mortality rates were not different between groups. Although intraoperative complications and advanced age predicted postoperative cardiac events, a positive stress-thallium test did not. Seeger and colleagues also noted a high incidence of adverse coronary events in patients with normal tests (23%), a finding unique to their study.[145]

Finally, the cost-effectiveness of DTS in vascular surgery patients must be considered. Bry and coworkers determined the positive predictive value (PPV) and cost-effectiveness of DTS screening in 237 patients before aortic or infrainguinal operations.[20] The PPV of DTS was only 19% for all patients with reversible defects. The total cost of screening was $732,697, averaging $3,092 per patient (including costs of subsequent intervention in some patients, such as cardiac catheterization). The authors calculated a cost-effectiveness of $392,253 per life saved and $181,039 per MI averted.

Radionuclide Ventriculography

LV dysfunction is reflected by diminution of ejection fraction (EF). EF can be reliably measured by nuclear cardiologic techniques, which are variously called *multiple uptake gated acquisition* (MUGA) scans, *gated heart pool* scans, *radionuclide angiography*, and *radionuclide ventriculography*. RNVG has been used to assess cardiac function and preoperative risk since the late 1970s. In addition to EF determination, RNVG can show ventricular wall motion abnormalities (akinesis, hypokinesis, dyskinesis) and left ventricular systolic and diastolic dysfunction, which may be present at rest or with exercise.

After several preliminary studies in small groups of patients indicated that RNVG could select patients at high risk for cardiac complications after aortic operations, Pasternack and associates showed that in patients having either aortic or lower extremity operations, the degree of LV dysfunction as measured by radionuclide angiograms identified those patients at greatest risk for postoperative MIs.[132, 133] Although there were no perioperative MIs in patients with EFs above 56%, 80% of patients having aortic and 70% of patients having infrainguinal operations sustained an adverse perioperative cardiac event when the EF was less than 30%. Kazmers and associates at the Seattle Veterans Affairs Medical Center published several reports confirming the utility of RNVG in patients having carotid, aortic, or infrainguinal vascular surgery.[89–92] Of interest, these reports confirmed findings at the Cleveland Clinic and the San Francisco Veterans Affairs Medical Center that the incidence and severity of underlying CAD were unrelated to the underlying PVD diagnosis (see Table 40–4). Although not all studies have substantiated the accuracy of RNVG for predicting postoperative cardiac morbidity,[55] measurement of EF with this technique is one of the strongest predictors of late survival after vascular or cardiac surgery.[146, 147]

Dobutamine Stress Echocardiography

Dobutamine is a beta-receptor agonist that causes myocardial ischemia differently than adenosine or dipyridamole.

Myocardial oxygen demand is increased by the increased heart rate and contractility produced by dobutamine infusion. Two-dimensional echocardiography can detect regional wall abnormalities resulting from myocardial ischemia that may result from dobutamine infusion and can therefore identify CAD.[10]

Lalka and colleagues recently reported 60 patients undergoing elective aortic surgery who had preoperative dobutamine ECG.[98] Eleven adverse cardiac events occurred in 38 patients (29%) who had an abnormal dobutamine stress ECG; conversely, only 1 of 22 patients (4%) with a normal study had a cardiac event. The difference in event rates between patients with positive and negative studies (29% versus 4.6%) was statistically significant ($p < .025$). Sensitivity and specificity of dobutamine stress ECG for diagnosing CAD range from 54% to 96% and from 57% to 95%, respectively, among eight reports comparing it with coronary angiography.[1, 37]

Coronary Angiography

Indications to perform coronary angiography before vascular surgery are unclear. Some investigators recommend it for each vascular surgery patient with clinical or noninvasive evidence of CAD, whereas others believe it is rarely necessary.[69, 71, 74, 154] Again, obtaining coronary angiography presupposes that some intervention will be performed for positive findings. The controversy over prophylactic CABG or percutaneous transluminal coronary angioplasty (PTCA) is discussed later. In addition to enhancing the safety of peripheral vascular surgery, CABG or PTCA may improve late survival in selected patients.

STRATEGIES FOR RISK STRATIFICATION

Routine Comprehensive Screening with Liberal Cardiac Catheterization and Revascularization

Although the policy to perform routine cardiac catheterization before vascular operations is no longer followed in the Cleveland Clinic, surgeons there remain aggressive with respect to surgical correction of significant CAD. In a landmark study, CABG was performed in 70 of 250 (28%) patients with infrarenal abdominal aortic aneurysm (AAAs), 63 of 295 (21%) with cerebrovascular disease, and 70 of 381 (18%) of patients with lower extremity vascular insufficiency before vascular reconstruction.[69] Seventy-two per cent of these 203 patients with surgically correctable CAD who underwent CABG were alive 5 years later. In marked contrast, only 15 of 35 (43%) candidates for CABG who refused the operation and 12 of 54 (22%) patients with severe, uncorrectable CAD remained alive at 5 years (Fig. 40–5).

Subset analyses by the Cleveland Clinic group showed CAD intervention to be beneficial for patients presenting with both aortic aneurysms and lower extremity ischemia.[73, 74] Of 246 patients with aneurysms, 70 (28%) received myocardial revascularization; four fatal complications occurred (5.7%). The 5-year survival rate was 75%. In contrast, the cumulative survival rate in a small subset (n = 16) of patients with severe, uncorrected CAD was

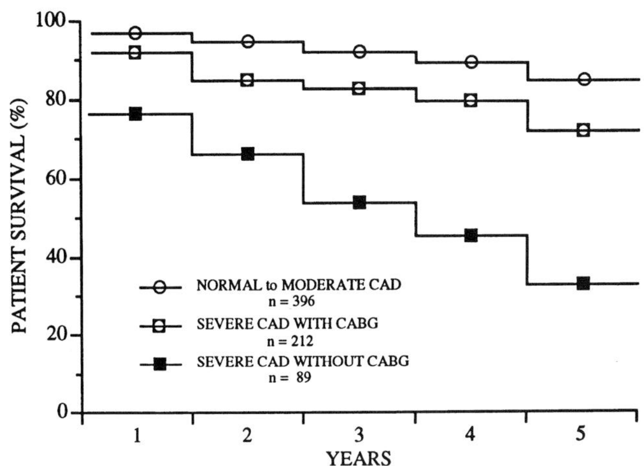

FIGURE 40–5. Cumulative 5-year survival of patients following elective vascular reconstruction stratified according to angiographic severity of coronary artery disease (CAD). CABG = coronary bypass graft prior to elective vascular reconstruction. (Adapted from Hertzer NR: The natural history of peripheral vascular disease: Implications for its management. Circulation 83 [Suppl]:I-12, 1991. Copyright 1991, American Heart Association.)

only 29% ($p = .0001$). Of 286 patients undergoing 407 operations for lower extremity ischemia, 68 (18%) received myocardial revascularization, and three fatal complications occurred (4.4%). In these patients, the 5-year cumulative survival rate was 72% and the cardiac mortality rate was 16%. In comparison, among 36 other patients with severe uncorrected CAD, these rates were 21% and 56%, respectively ($p = .0002$).

Similar results have been reported from the Mayo Clinic.[138] Fifty patients under 70 years of age who underwent preoperative myocardial revascularization had 5-year survival rates comparable with those of 237 patients with no coronary disease (66% versus 83%).

Ennix and coworkers reported outcomes in 1546 consecutive carotid endarterectomies in 1238 patients over a 10-year period that also support the protective effect of CABG before vascular surgery.[51] Although the overall rate of perioperative MI was only 1.6%, MIs occurred in 12.9% of 85 patients with *symptomatic* CAD. In contrast, the MI incidence was reduced to 2.6% in 155 patients with symptomatic CAD who had undergone previous or simultaneous CABG.

Few data are available that address the prophylactic effect of PTCA on the immediate or late outcome of patients with CAD undergoing noncardiac operations. Multiple reports of patients undergoing preoperative coronary arteriography demonstrate that few (6% or less) of all patients have anatomy suitable for PTCA, reflecting the diffuse nature of atherosclerosis in PVD patients.[20, 114, 119]

A 1992 report from the Mayo Clinic described the results of PTCA in 55 patients before noncardiac surgery.[78] Five of 50 patients had unsuccessful angioplasty and were excluded from subsequent analysis (thereby potentially confounding the results according to the "intention to treat" statistical method). All five patients underwent CABG. Fifty-four operations were eventually performed in the 50 patients who had successful preliminary PTCA. The overall frequency of postoperative MI was 5.4% (3 of 54), and operative mortality rate was 1.9%.

Based on data obtained in the aforementioned series that suggest improved outcomes in vascular patients, Bunt recommended extensive cardiac risk assessment for patients with PVD.[21] He prospectively studied 630 patients undergoing vascular surgery to ascertain degree of cardiac risk, which then determined the choice of procedure, type of anesthesia, and level of hemodynamic monitoring. All patients had standard evaluations, including RNVG. Thirty-two per cent of patients had no abnormalities on initial examination and proceeded directly to vascular surgery; 68% (n = 428) had clinical evidence of CAD, and stress-thallium testing was performed. Of the patients undergoing thallium studies, 93% had no perfusion defects and proceeded to surgery, whereas 7% (n = 44) with fixed or reversible defects underwent coronary angiography.

This strict protocol resulted in an enviable 0.7% postoperative MI rate, ranging from 0% in patients undergoing aortic or carotid surgery to 1.6% in those undergoing infrainguinal revascularization. However, several concerns have been raised about Bunt's study: (1) cardiac enzymes were routinely obtained only for the first 48 hours, and many MIs occur on the third postoperative day or even later[1, 4]; (2) the outcomes of the 44 patients with positive thallium studies (41 of whom had coronary angiograms) are not described, and potential morbidity and mortality from CABG could affect the analysis; (3) the high rate of negative thallium studies (93%) is unusual, especially in view of the Cleveland Clinic data; and (4) the many negative studies reduced the cost-effectiveness of this strategy.

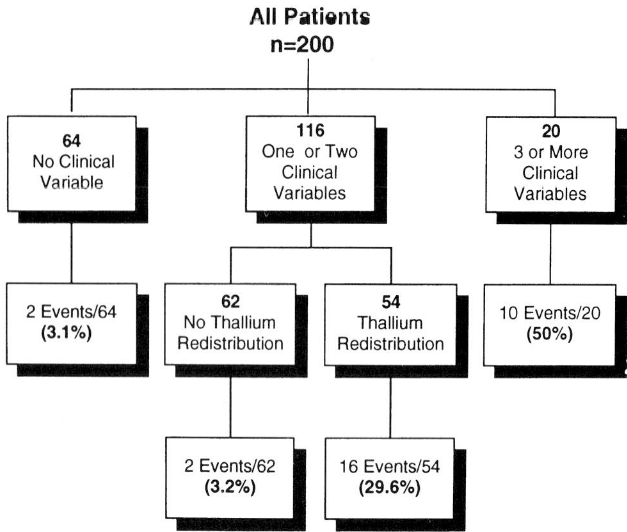

FIGURE 40–6. Results of selective application of dipyridamole scintigraphy in 200 consecutive patients before peripheral vascular operations. Event refers to postoperative cardiac ischemic events, including unstable angina, pulmonary edema, myocardial infarction, and cardiac death. (From Eagle KA, Singer DE, Brewster DC, et al: Dipyridamole-thallium scanning in patients undergoing vascular surgery: Optimizing preoperative evaluation of cardiac risk. JAMA 257:2185, 1987. Copyright 1987, American Medical Association.)

Selective Cardiac Screening

The *selective* use of preoperative DTS in vascular surgery patients has been investigated by Eagle and colleagues.[47, 49] In the initial study, five clinical markers (age over 70 years, Q waves, diabetes mellitus, angina, and arrhythmias requiring treatment) identified in a retrospective analysis of 61 patients scheduled for vascular surgery predicted perioperative cardiac morbidity.[49] These clinical variables were then applied prospectively to 50 consecutive patients undergoing vascular surgery. Only 3% of those who had no clinical indicators sustained an adverse postoperative cardiac event. In this low-risk group, 52 DTSs were performed; nine revealed reversible defects, and only one patient had an adverse ischemic event (angina). In contrast, 29% of patients with one or more clinical markers suffered an adverse cardiac event, and a reversible defect was present in 33 of 59 patients (56%).

In a subsequent study, Eagle and colleagues corroborated their initial findings and were able to identify further an intermediate-risk group in whom DTS was most useful (Fig. 40–6).[47] Again, in the low-risk group (no clinical markers), a 3% postoperative cardiac event rate was noted. Patients considered to be at intermediate risk (one to two clinical predictors) and high risk (three or more clinical predictors) had cardiac event rates of 33% and 50%, respectively. Performance of DTS in the intermediate-risk group demonstrated that in patients with normal thallium scans the cardiac event rate (3.2%) approximated that of the low-risk group, whereas 30% of those with thallium redistribution suffered postoperative cardiac morbidity.

Therefore, DTS appears to add little to the preoperative evaluation of the low-risk and high-risk groups because accurate cardiac risk assessment is possible by clinical criteria alone. The identification of an intermediate-risk group by clinical criteria permits selective application of DTS and additional stratification—that is, the absence of thallium redistribution suggests a 3% probability of an adverse cardiac event, whereas the presence of thallium redistribution increases the probability of an adverse cardiac event to 30%.

The findings of Eagle and colleagues support the contention that *routine* preoperative DTS is not justified. DTS appears to be most useful for patients deemed to be at intermediate risk by clinical analysis, who may benefit from coronary revascularization before elective vascular surgery.[167] This selective strategy has subsequently been adopted at several prominent vascular centers.[18, 33]

Minimal Screening

In 1992, Taylor and associates at the Oregon Health Sciences University (OHSU) reported impressive results using a "minimalist" approach to preoperative cardiac screening.[154] In 491 consecutive patients, 534 vascular procedures (105 aortic, 87 carotid, 207 infrainguinal, 51 extra-anatomic, 84 other) were performed. Basic cardiac evaluation consisted of history, physical examination, and resting ECG. Only 5.8% of patients with severe symptomatic CAD had additional studies, which included cardiology consultation, DTS, evaluation of cardiac EF, and coronary arteriography.

This conservative application of special studies to evaluate cardiac risk resulted in an overall postoperative MI rate of only 3.9%. Predictably, those having emergency operations suffered more MIs than those having elective procedures (8.2% versus 2.8%), respectively. Criticisms of this economical strategy include (1) patients were routinely studied for only the first 72 postoperative hours, (2) nearly one-third of patients did not have cardiac enzyme levels obtained for the full 72 hours, and (3) one-fifth of the patients in the study had previous myocardial revascularization.

Despite these potential flaws, the OHSU results have led to several reexaminations of the more aggressive approaches to CAD in vascular surgery patients. Although the Cleveland Clinic results are impressive, it must be remembered that, although the cardiac catheterizations were performed consecutively and prospectively, the results of prophylactic CABG were retrospectively analyzed. Moreover, comparison of patients eligible for CABG with those having unreconstructable CAD is not equitable.

Recommendation of prophylactic CABG or angioplasty must be tempered by recognition of potential hazards of this strategy. For example, the operative mortality rate of a CABG before elective vascular surgery in one study was 5.2%.[71] Thus, the benefit of risk reduction by prophylactic coronary revascularization is realized only by those who survive bypass surgery *and* subsequent vascular reconstruction.

Cutler and Leppo have also shown the potential downside of prophylactic CABG.[32] They performed DTS in 116 patients scheduled for aortic surgery; 6% of patients were referred for CABG based on DTS results. The operative deaths occurred in the patients undergoing aortic surgery without CABG. However, there was one death in the six patients referred for CABG—a mortality rate of 16% attributable to precautionary CABG. In addition, one patient died of a ruptured aneurysm awaiting CABG.

Mesh and associates have shown that coronary artery bypass in vascular patients is a relatively high-risk procedure.[121] They reviewed a cohort of 680 patients undergoing elective CABG and examined complication-free survival, morbidity, and mortality rates. Fifty-eight patients had significant vascular disease. Overall, CABG mortality was 2.5%, with statistically similar, but relatively higher, rates for PVD patients than for non-PVD patients. In contrast, major morbidity occurred at rates 3.6-fold higher in PVD patients (39.7%) than in disease-free patients (16.7%).

D'Angelo and colleagues reviewed their experience with 113 consecutive patients who underwent elective aortic aneurysm repair.[35] Seventy-four patients had only an ECG before surgery. The remaining patients underwent special testing (DTS, n = 20; echocardiogram, n = 18; MUGA scan, n = 3; cardiac catheterization, n = 8; and some combination, n = 9). There were no differences in postoperative complications between those who had no cardiac workup and those who had special tests. There were three deaths in the entire series (2.7%), and one of these occurred in the group of patients who underwent special cardiac studies. The authors concluded that most patients with AAA can safely undergo repair with no cardiac workup and that cardiac workup before AAA repair contributes little information that affects treatment or final clinical outcome.

In 1997, Massie and coworkers reported an analysis of 70 patients who underwent coronary angiography after abnormal DTS (two or more redistribution defects) and compared their outcomes with those of 227 patients with multiple areas of redistribution on DTS who underwent the same PVD operation without undergoing preliminary cardiac catheterization.[114] Twenty-five of the 70 patients having coronary angiography underwent coronary revascularization. Adverse outcomes affected 46% of the coronary angiography group and 44% of the control group (p = ns). Although patients who underwent coronary angiography had fewer cardiac events with a subsequent vascular operation than did control subjects, any possible benefits from invasive cardiac evaluation was offset by the three deaths and two MIs that complicated the cardiac evaluation. There were no significant differences between the angiography group and the control group in incidences of perioperative non-fatal MI (13% versus 9%), fatal MI (4% versus 3%), late non-fatal MI (16% versus 19%), or late cardiac death (10% versus 13%). The authors concluded that, in the majority of vascular patients with a positive DTS, coronary angiography does not provide additional useful information.

A decision analysis paper from Stanford confirmed the inadvisability of extensive cardiac evaluation.[113] Three strategies were compared. The first strategy was to proceed directly to vascular surgery. The second was to perform coronary angiography followed by selective coronary revascularization before proceeding with vascular surgery and to cancel vascular surgery in patients with severe inoperable coronary artery disease. The third was to perform coronary angiography followed by selective revascularization before proceeding to vascular surgery and to perform vascular surgery in patients with inoperable CAD. Proceeding directly to vascular surgery led to a lower morbidity rate and lower costs in the base case analysis. The coronary angiography strategy led to a higher mortality rate if vascular surgery was performed in patients with inoperable CAD, but led to a slightly lower mortality rate if vascular surgery was cancelled for patients with inoperable CAD. The coronary angiography strategy also led to a lower mortality rate when vascular surgery was particularly dangerous.

The authors concluded that vascular surgery without preoperative coronary angiography usually leads to better outcomes.[113] Preoperative coronary angiography should be reserved for patients whose estimated mortality from vascular surgery is substantially higher than average.

ACC/AHA Task Force Report: Guidelines for Preoperative Cardiovascular Evaluation for Non-Cardiac Surgery

In 1996, the Committee on Perioperative Cardiovascular Evaluation for Non-Cardiac Surgery provided the American College of Cardiology/American Heart Association (ACC/AHA) Task Force report.[1] This extensive document discusses at great length the goals of preoperative studies before vascular surgery. The report describes in detail the positive and negative predictive values of special preoperative tests. A comprehensive review of this article is beyond the scope of this chapter, but the reader is strongly advised to review the report.

The Future

The Department of Veterans Affairs has recently funded a pilot study with the acronym CARP (Coronary Artery

Revascularization Prophylaxis). This pilot study has been designed to assess the merits of intervention for CAD before vascular operations. In brief, after giving informed consent, patients with clinical indicators that suggest CAD undergo preoperative cardiac catheterization. If significant CAD is identified, patients are randomized to either preoperative coronary (CABG or PTCA) intervention or best preoperative medical care.

If this pilot study reveals that recruiting can be successful, the trial will be expanded to include multiple Department of Veteran Affairs Hospitals. The controversy over best strategy for management of CAD before vascular surgery may best be answered by such a prospective randomized study.

SUMMARY

The patient with vascular disease has a systemic disease—*atherosclerosis*. Unequivocally, the greatest perioperative risk to such a patient is intimately related to the extent of involvement of other organ systems, in particular the degree of underlying cardiac disease, which may or may not be obvious. Although the optimal strategy to identify this risk remains controversial, a careful preoperative evaluation is necessary to assist in a rational selection of therapy.

The studies discussed in this chapter suggest that improved results after vascular reconstruction may be achieved through careful preoperative evaluation, risk assessment, and risk reduction. A modification of the algorithm proposed by Wong and Detsky[167] illustrates and incorporates many of the principles of preoperative evaluation that have emerged from studies conducted during the 1980s and 1990s.

Risk assessment begins with a clinical scoring system. An estimate of perioperative risk (low, intermediate, or high) is assigned. Although estimates of low risk do not preclude the presence of perioperative complications, further testing adds little additional information to the estimates obtained with the clinical scoring system. Conversely, patients with high cardiac risk scores are clearly at increased risk of experiencing postoperative complications, but further investigations are needed only if knowledge of the functional severity or degree of myocardial ischemia will alter subsequent management. In these patients, ambulatory ECG, DTS, or coronary arteriography may be useful if the vascular surgery can be delayed until myocardial revascularization is completed. Otherwise, the additional information provided is unlikely to alter the perioperative management.

Patients identified as intermediate risk by clinical scoring benefit most from additional tests. Although a consensus has not yet been reached, DTS is the most popular noninvasive test to evaluate the intermediate-risk patient. Alternatively, we as well as others have demonstrated that ambulatory ECG monitoring is an equally effective noninvasive method of determining cardiac risk. Coronary artery bypass surgery should be recommended only on the basis of the patient's cardiac symptoms and anatomy, not necessarily on the procedure's potential for reducing perioperative risk or the complications associated with the proposed vascular procedure.

The surgeon has many therapeutic options for both intermediate-risk and high-risk patients: proceeding with surgery, instituting aggressive perioperative monitoring and anti-ischemic therapy, performing coronary arteriography and myocardial revascularization before the elective operation, selecting a lower-risk surgical procedure, and canceling the planned procedure. Recent advances in surgical and anesthetic techniques as well as intraoperative and postoperative monitoring have resulted in lower morbidity and mortality rates in elective noncardiac procedures, but none can substitute for sound surgical judgment. In view of the potential combined morbidity and mortality of preoperative cardiac intervention, cardiac screening may ultimately be most useful for patients with the option to abort the vascular procedure (e.g., for claudication, asymptomatic carotid lesions, or modest-sized aortic aneurysms).

REFERENCES

1. ACC/AHA Task Force on Practice Guidelines: ACC/AHA guidelines for perioperative cardiovascular evaluation for non-cardiac surgery. Circulation 93:1280, 1996.
2. Ameli FM, Stein M, Provan JL, et al: Predictors of surgical outcome in patients undergoing aortofemoral bypass reconstruction. J Cardiovasc Surg 31:333–339, 1990.
3. Arous EJ, Baum PL, Cutler BS: The ischemia exercise test in patients with peripheral vascular disease: Implications for management. Arch Surg 119:780, 1984.
4. Baron JF, Mundler O, Bertrand M, et al: Dipyridamole-thallium scintigraphy and gated radionuclide angiography to assess cardiac risk before abdominal aortic surgery. N Engl J Med 330:663, 1994.
5. Benchimol A, Harris CL, Desser KB, et al: Resting electrocardiogram in major coronary artery disease. JAMA 224:1489, 1973.
6. Bergamini TM, George SM Jr, Massey HT, et al: Pedal or peroneal bypass: Which is better when both are patent? J Vasc Surg 20:347–356, 1994.
7. Bergan JJ, Wilson SE, Wolf G, et al: Unexpected, late cardiovascular effects of surgery for peripheral artery disease. Arch Surg 127:1119, 1992.
8. Berlauk JF, Abrams JH, Gilmour IJ, et al: Preoperative optimization of cardiovascular hemodynamics improves outcome in peripheral vascular surgery. A prospective, randomized clinical trial. Ann Surg 214:289, 1991.
9. Berman SS, Bernhard VM, Erly WK, et al: Critical carotid artery stenosis: Diagnosis, timing of surgery, and outcome. J Vasc Surg 19:1015–1020, 1994.
10. Berthe C, Pierad LA, Hiernaux M, et al: Predicting the extent and location of coronary artery disease in acute myocardial infarction by echocardiography during dobutamine infusion. Am J Cardiol 58:1167, 1986.
11. Bertrand YM, Boelens D, Collin L, et al: Preoperative assessment in geriatric patients for elective surgery. Acta Anaesthesiol Belg 35(Suppl):155, 1984.
12. Bigger JTJ, Fleiss JL, Kleiger R, et al: The relationship among ventricular arrhythmias, left ventricular dysfunction, and mortality in the 2 years after myocardial infarction. Circulation 69:250, 1984.
13. Blombery PA, Ferguson IA, Rosengarten DS, et al: The role of coronary artery disease in complications of abdominal aortic aneurysm surgery. Surgery 101:150, 1987.
14. Borer JS, Brensike JF, Redwood DR, et al: Limitations of the electrocardiographic response to exercise in predicting coronary disease. N Engl J Med 293:367, 1975.
15. Boucher CA, Brewster DC, Darling RC, et al: Correlation between preoperative ischemia and major cardiac events after peripheral vascular surgery. N Engl J Med 321:1296, 1989.
16. Boucher CA, Brewster DC, Darling RC, et al: Determination of cardiac risk by dipyridamole-thallium imaging before peripheral vascular surgery. N Engl J Med 312:389, 1985.

17. Boyd AM: The natural course of arteriosclerosis of the lower extremities. Angiology 11:10, 1960.
18. Brewster DC, Okada RD, Strauss W, et al: Selection of patients for preoperative coronary angiography: Use of dipyridamole-stress-thallium myocardial imaging. J Vasc Surg 2:504, 1985.
19. Brown KA, Rowen M: Extent of jeopardized viable myocardium determined by myocardial perfusion imaging best predicts perioperative cardiac events in patients undergoing noncardiac surgery. J Am Coll Cardiol 21:325, 1993.
20. Bry JD, Belkin M, O'Donnell TF, et al: An assessment of the positive predictive value and cost-effectiveness of dipyridamole myocardial scintigraphy in patients undergoing vascular surgery. J Vasc Surg 19:112, 1994.
21. Bunt TJ: The role of a defined protocol for cardiac risk assessment in decreasing perioperative myocardial infarction in vascular surgery. J Vasc Surg 15:626, 1992.
22. Bush HL: Renal failure following abdominal aortic reconstruction. Surgery 93:107, 1983.
23. Carliner NH, Fisher ML, Plotnick GD, et al: Routine pre-operative exercise testing in patients undergoing major non-cardiac surgery. Am J Cardiol 56:51, 1985.
24. Carrel T, Zund G, Jenni R: Prediction of early cardiac morbidity and mortality following aorto-iliac reconstruction: Comparison between clinical scoring systems, echocardiography, and dipyridamole-thallium scanning. Vasa 24:362–367, 1995.
25. Charlson ME, MacKenzie CR, Ales K, et al: Surveillance for postoperative myocardial infarction after noncardiac operations. Surg Gynecol Obstet 167:407, 1988.
26. Clark ET, Gewertz BL, Bassiouny HS, et al: Current results of elective aortic reconstruction for aneurysmal and occlusive disease. J Cardiovasc Surg 31:438–441, 1990.
27. Criqui MH, Coughlin SS, Fronek A: Noninvasively diagnosed peripheral vascular disease as a predictor of mortality: Results from a prospective study. Circulation 72:768, 1985.
28. Criqui M, Langer R, Fronek A, et al: Mortality over a period of 10 years in patients with peripheral arterial disease. N Engl J Med 326:381, 1992.
29. Cohn PF: Silent myocardial ischemia. Ann Intern Med 109:312, 1988.
30. Cooperman M, Pflug B, Martin EW, et al: Cardiovascular risk factors in patients with peripheral vascular disease. Surgery 84:505, 1978.
31. U.S. Department of Commerce: Current population reports. Series 148. Washington, DC: Bureau of the Census, 1995.
32. Cutler BS, Leppo JA: Dipyridamole thallium 201 scintigraphy to detect coronary artery disease before abdominal aortic surgery. J Vasc Surg 5:91, 1987.
33. Cutler BS, Hendel RC, Leppo JA: Dipyridamole-thallium scintigraphy predicts perioperative and long-term survival after major vascular surgery. J Vasc Surg 15:972, 1992.
34. Cutler BS, Wheeler HB, Paraskos JA, et al: Applicability and interpretation of electrocardiographic stress testing in patients with peripheral vascular disease. Am J Surg 141:501, 1981.
35. D'Angelo AJ, Puppalla D, Faber A: Is preoperative cardiac evaluation for abdominal aortic aneurysm repair necessary? J Vasc Surg 25:152, 1997.
36. Dardik A, Williams GM, Minken SL, Perler BA: Impact of a critical pathway on the results of carotid endarterectomy in a tertiary care university hospital: Effect of methods on outcome. J Vasc Surg 1997;26:186–192, 1997.
37. Davila-Roman RG, Waggoner AD, Sicard GA, et al: Dobutamine stress echocardiography predicts surgical outcome in patients with an aortic aneurysm and peripheral vascular disease. J Am Coll Cardiol 21:957, 1993.
38. Detsky AS, Abrams HB, Forbath N, et al: Cardiac assessment for patients undergoing noncardiac surgery: A multifactorial clinical risk index. Arch Intern Med 146:2131, 1986.
39. Detsky AS, Abrams HB, McLaughlin JR, et al: Predicting cardiac complications in patients undergoing non-cardiac surgery. J Gen Intern Med 1:211, 1986.
40. Diamond GA, Forrester JS: Analysis of probability as an aid in the clinical diagnosis of coronary artery disease. N Engl J Med 300:1350, 1979.
41. Dirksen A, Kjoller E: Cardiac predictors of death after non-cardiac surgery evaluated by intention to treat. Br Med J 297:1011, 1988.
42. Donaldson MC, Whittemore AD, Mannick JA: Further experience with an all-autogenous tissue policy for infrainguinal reconstruction. J Vasc Surg 18:41–48, 1993.
43. Dripps RD, Lamont A, Eckenhoff JE: The role of anesthesia in surgical mortality. JAMA 178:261, 1961.
44. Driscoll AC, Hobika JH, Etsten BE, Proger S: Clinically unrecognized myocardial infarction following surgery. N Engl J Med 26:633, 1961.
45. Dwyer EMJ, Greenberg HM, Steinberg G: Clinical characteristics and natural history of survivors of pulmonary congestion during acute myocardial infarction. The Multicenter Postinfarction Research Group. Am J Cardiol 63:1423, 1989.
46. Eagle KA, Boucher CA: Cardiac risk of noncardiac surgery. N Engl J Med 321:1330, 1989.
47. Eagle KA, Coley CM, Newell JB, et al: Combining clinical and thallium data optimizes preoperative assessment of cardiac risk before major vascular surgery. Ann Intern Med 110:859, 1989.
48. Eagle KA, Singer DE, Brewster DC, et al: Dipyridamole-thallium scanning in patients undergoing vascular surgery: Optimizing preoperative evaluation of cardiac risk. JAMA 257:2185, 1987.
49. Eagle KA, Strauss HW, Boucher CA: Dipyridamole myocardial perfusion imaging for coronary heart disease. Am J Cardiac Imaging 2:292, 1988.
50. Eichelberger JP, Schwartz KQ, Blacker, et al: Predictive value of dobutamine echocardiography just before non-cardiac vascular surgery. Am J Cardiol 72:602, 1993.
51. Ennix CL, Lawrie GM, Morris GC, et al: Improved results of carotid endarterectomy in patients with symptomatic coronary disease: An analysis of 1,546 consecutive carotid operations. Stroke 10:122, 1979.
52. Erickson CA, Carballo RE, Freischlag JA, et al: Using dipyridamole thallium imaging to reduce cardiac risk in aortic reconstruction. J Surg Res 60:422–428, 1996.
53. Executive Committee for the Asymptomatic Carotid Atherosclerosis Study: Endarterectomy for asymptomatic carotid artery stenosis. JAMA 273:1421–1428, 1995.
54. Foster ED, Davis KB, Carpenter JA, et al: Risk of noncardiac operation in patients with defined coronary disease: The Coronary Artery Surgery Study (CASS) registry experience. Ann Thorac Surg 41:42, 1986.
55. Franco CD, Goldsmith J, Veith FJ, et al: Resting gated pool ejection fraction: A poor predictor of perioperative myocardial infarction in patients undergoing vascular surgery for infrainguinal bypass grafting. J Vasc Surg 10:656, 1989.
56. Freischlag JA, Hanna D, Moore WS: Improved prognosis for asymptomatic carotid stenosis with prophylactic carotid endarterectomy. Stroke 23:479–482, 1992.
57. Gage AA, Bhayana JN, Balu V, et al: Assessment of cardiac risk in surgical patients. Arch Surg 112:1488, 1977.
58. Gardine RL, McBride K, Greenberg H, et al: The value of cardiac monitoring during peripheral arterial stress testing in the surgical management of peripheral vascular disease. J Cardiovasc Surg (Torino) 26:258, 1985.
59. Gersh BJ, Rihal CS, Rooke TW, et al: Evaluation and management of patients with both peripheral vascular and coronary artery disease. J Am Coll Cardiol 18:203, 1991.
60. Gerson MC, Hurst JM, Hertzberg VS, et al: Cardiac prognosis in noncardiac geriatric surgery. Ann Intern Med 103:832, 1985.
61. Golden MA, Whittemore AD, Donaldson MC, Mannick JA: Selective evaluation and management of coronary artery disease in patients undergoing repair of abdominal aortic reconstruction: Sixteen-year experience. Ann Surg 212:415–420, 1990.
62. Goldman L: Cardiac risks and complications of noncardiac surgery. Ann Intern Med 98:504, 1983.
63. Goldman L, Caldera DL, Nessbaum SR, et al: Multifactorial index of cardiac risk in noncardiac surgical procedures. N Engl J Med 297:845, 1977.
64. Halperin BD, Feeley TW: The effect of anesthesia and surgery on renal function. Int Anesthesiol Clin 22:157, 1984.
65. Harris EJ, Moneta GL, Yeager RA, et al: Neurologic deficits following noncarotid vascular surgery. Am J Surg 163:537, 1992.
66. Hendel RC, Whitfield SS, Villegar BJ, et al: Prediction of late cardiac events by dipyridamole thallium imaging in patients undergoing elective vascular surgery. Am J Cardiol 70:1243, 1992.
67. Henderson A, Effeney D: Morbidity and mortality after abdominal aortic surgery in a population of patients with high cardiovascular risk. Aust NZ J Surg 65:417–420, 1995.

68. Hertzer NR: Myocardial ischemia. Surgery 93:97, 1983.
69. Hertzer NR: The natural history of peripheral vascular disease: Implications for its management. Circulation 83(Suppl I):I-12, 1991.
70. Hertzer NR, Beven EG, Young JR, et al: Incidental asymptomatic carotid bruits in patients scheduled for peripheral vascular reconstruction: Results of cerebral and coronary angiography. Surgery 96:535, 1984.
71. Hertzer NR, Beven EG, Young JR, et al: Coronary artery disease in peripheral vascular patients: A classification of 1000 coronary angiograms and results of surgical management. Ann Surg 199:223, 1984.
72. Hertzer NR, O'Hara PJ, Mascha EJ, et al: Early outcome assessment for 2228 consecutive carotid endarterectomy procedures: The Cleveland Clinic experience from 1989 to 1995. J Vasc Surg 26:1–10, 1997.
73. Hertzer NR, Young JR, Beven EG, et al: Late results of coronary bypass in patients presenting with lower extremity ischemia: The Cleveland Clinic Study. Ann Vasc Surg 1:411, 1986.
74. Hertzer NR, Young JR, Beven EG, et al: Late results of coronary bypass in patients with infrarenal aortic aneurysms. Ann Surg 205:360, 1986.
75. Hobson RW, Weiss DG, Fields WS, et al: Efficacy of carotid endarterectomy for asymptomatic carotid stenosis. N Engl J Med 328:221–227, 1993.
76. Hood DB, Weaver FA, Papanicolau G, et al: Cardiac evaluation of the diabetic patient prior to peripheral vascular surgery. Ann Vasc Surg 10:330–335, 1996.
77. Howell MA, Colgan MP, Seeger RW, et al: Relationship of severity of lower limb peripheral vascular disease to mortality and morbidity: A six-year follow-up study. J Vasc Surg 9:691, 1989.
78. Huber KC, Evans MA, Breshnahan JF, et al: Outcome of noncardiac operations in patients with severe coronary artery disease successfully treated preoperatively with coronary angioplasty. Mayo Clin Proc 67:15, 1992.
79. Huber TS, Harward TR, Flynn TC, et al: Operative mortality rates after elective infrarenal aortic reconstructions. J Vasc Surg 22:287–294, 1995.
80. Isaacson IJ, Lowdon JD, Berry AJ, et al: The value of pulmonary artery and central venous monitoring in patients undergoing abdominal aortic surgery. J Vasc Surg 170:385–389, 1990.
81. Iskandrian AS, Ghads M, Helfeld H, et al: The treadmill exercise score revisited: Coronary arteriographic and thallium perfusion correlates. Am Heart J 124:1581, 1992.
82. Isner JM, Rosenfield K: Reducing the cardiac risk associated with vascular surgical procedures: Balloons as prophylactics. Mayo Clin Proc 67:95, 1992.
83. Jarvinen O, Laurikka J, Sisto T, Tarkka MR: Intestinal ischemia following surgery for aorto-iliac disease. A review of 502 consecutive aortic reconstructions. Vasa 25:148–155, 1996.
84. Kaaja R, Sell H, Erkola O, Harjula A: Predictive value of manual ECG-monitored exercise test before abdominal aortic or peripheral vascular surgery. Angiology 44:11, 1993.
85. Källerö KS: Mortality and morbidity in patients with intermittent claudication as defined by venous occlusion plethysmography: A ten-year follow-up study. J Chronic Dis 34:455, 1981.
86. Källerö KS, Bergquist D, Cederholm C, et al: Late mortality and morbidity after arterial reconstruction: The influence of arteriosclerosis in popliteal artery trifurcation. J Vasc Surg 2:541, 1985.
87. Kalman PG, Johnston KW, Walker PM, Lindsay TF: Preoperative factors that predict hospital length of stay after distal arterial bypass. J Vasc Surg 20:70–75, 1994.
88. Kannel WB, McGee DL: Diabetes and cardiovascular risk factors: The Framingham Study. Circulation 59:8, 1979.
89. Kazmers A, Cerqueira M, Zierler RE: Perioperative and late outcome in patients with left ventricular ejection fraction <35% who require major vascular surgery. J Vasc Surg 8:307, 1988.
90. Kazmers A, Cerqueira M, Zierler RE: The role of preoperative radionuclide left ventricular ejection fraction (EF) for risk assessment in carotid surgery. Arch Surg 123:416, 1998.
91. Kazmers A, Cerqueira M, Zierler RE: The role of preoperative radionuclide ejection fraction in direct abdominal aortic aneurysm repair. J Vasc Surg 8:128, 1988.
92. Kazmers A, Moneta GL, Cerqueira MD, et al: The role of preoperative radionuclide ventriculography in defining outcome after revascularization of the extremity. Surg Gynecol Obstet 171:481, 1990.
93. Kirwin JD, Ascer E, Gennaro M, et al: Silent myocardial ischemia is not predictive of myocardial infarction in peripheral vascular surgery patients. Ann Vasc Surg 7:27, 1993.
94. Kramer N, Susmano A, Shekelle RB: The false negative treadmill exercise test and left ventricular dysfunction. Circulation 57:763, 1978.
95. Krupski WC: The peripheral vascular consequences of smoking. Ann Vasc Surg 5:291, 1991.
96. Krupski WC, Layug EL, Reilly LM, et al: Comparison of cardiac morbidity between aortic and infrainguinal operations. Study of Perioperative Ischemia (SPI) Research Group. J Vasc Surg 15:354, 1992.
97. Krupski WC, Layug EL, Reilly LM, et al: Comparison of cardiac morbidity rates between aortic and infrainguinal operations: Two-year follow-up. Study of Perioperative Ischemia (SPI) Research Group. J Vasc Surg 18:609, 1993.
98. Lalka SG, Sawada SG, Dalsing MC, et al: Dobutamine stress echocardiography as a predictor of cardiac events associated with aortic surgery. J Vasc Surg 15:831, 1992.
99. Lane SE, Lewis SM, Pippin JJ, et al: Predictive value of quantitative dipyridamole-thallium scintigraphy in assessing cardiovascular risk after vascular surgery in diabetes mellitus. Am J Cardiol 64:1275, 1989.
100. Lazor L, Russell JC, DaSilva J, et al: Use of the multiple uptake gated acquisition scan for the preoperative assessment of cardiac risk. Surg Gynecol Obstet 167:234, 1987.
101. Lette J, Waters D, Cevino M, et al: Preoperative coronary artery disease risk stratification based on dipyridamole imaging and a simple three-strop, three segment model for patients undergoing noncardiac vascular surgery or major general surgery. Am J Cardiol 69:1553, 1992.
102. Lette J, Waters D, Lassonde J, et al: Multivariate clinical models and quantitative dipyridamole-thallium imaging to predict cardiac morbidity and death after vascular reconstruction. J Vasc Surg 14:160, 1991.
103. L'Italien GJ, Cambria RP, Cutler BS, et al: Comparative early and late cardiac morbidity among patients requiring different vascular surgery procedures. J Vasc Surg 21:935, 1995.
104. Lord RS, Crozier JA, Snell J, Meek AC: Transverse abdominal incisions compared with midline incisions for elective aortic reconstructions: Predisposition of incisional hernia in patients with increased intraoperative blood loss. J Vasc Surg 20:27–33, 1994.
105. Maini BS, Mullins TF, Catline J, O'Mara P: Carotid endarterectomy: A ten-year analysis of outcome and cost of treatment. J Vasc Surg 12:732–740, 1990.
106. Mangano DT: Perioperative cardiac morbidity. Anesthesiology 72:153, 1990.
107. Mangano DT, Browner WS, Hollenberg M, et al: Association of perioperative myocardial ischemia with cardiac morbidity in men undergoing non-cardiac surgery: The study of Perioperative Ischemia Research Group. N Engl J Med 323:1781, 1990.
108. Mangano DT, Browner WS, Hollenberg M, et al: Long-term cardiac prognosis following noncardiac surgery. JAMA 268:233, 1992.
109. Mangano DT, Hollenberg M, Fegert G, et al: Perioperative myocardial ischemia in patients undergoing noncardiac surgery. I. Incidence and severity during the 4 day perioperative period. The Study of Perioperative Ischemia (SPI) Research Group. J Am Coll Cardiol 17:843, 1991.
110. Mangano DT, London MJ, Tubau JF, et al: Dipyridamole thallium-201 scintigraphy as a preoperative screening test: A reexamination of its predictive potential. Circulation 84:493, 1991.
111. Mangano DT, Wong MG, London MJ, et al: Perioperative myocardial ischemia in patients undergoing noncardiac surgery. II. Incidence and severity during the 1st week after surgery. J Am Coll Cardiol 17:851, 1991.
112. Mason RA, Newton GB, Cassel W, et al: Combined epidural and general anesthesia in aortic surgery. J Cardiovasc Surg 31:442–447, 1990.
113. Mason JJ, Owens DK, Ryan A, et al: The role of coronary angiography and coronary revascularization before noncardiac vascular surgery. JAMA 273:1919, 1995.
114. Massie MT, Rohrer MJ, Leppo JA, Cutler BS: Is coronary angiography necessary for vascular surgery patients who have positive results of dipyridamole thallium scans? J Vasc Surg 25:975, 1997.
115. Mattos MA, Modi JR, Mansour A, et al: Evolution of carotid endarter-

ectomy in two community hospitals: Springfield revisited—seventeen years and 2243 operations later. J Vasc Surg 21:719–728, 1995.
116. Matsura JH, Sobel M, Wong J, et al: The limits of generalized cardiac screening tests for predicting cardiac complications after infrainguinal arterial reconstruction. Ann Vasc Surg 11:620–625, 1997.
117. Mays AE, Cobb FR: Relationship between regional myocardial blood flow and thallium 201 redistribution in the presence of coronary artery stenosis and dipyridamole-induced vasodilation. J Clin Invest 73:1359, 1984.
118. McCann RL, Clements FM: Silent myocardial ischemia in patients undergoing peripheral vascular surgery: Incidence and association with perioperative cardiac morbidity and mortality. J Vasc Surg 9:583, 1989.
119. McEnroe CS, O'Donnell TFJ, Yeager A, et al: Comparison of ejection fraction and Goldman risk factor analysis to dipyridamole-thallium 201 studies in the evaluation of cardiac morbidity after aortic aneurysm surgery. J Vasc Surg 11:497, 1990.
120. McGovern B: Hypokalemia and cardiac arrhythmias. Anesthesiology 63:127, 1985.
121. Mesh CL, Cmolik BL, Van Heekeren DW, et al: Coronary bypass in vascular patients: A relatively high-risk procedure. Ann Vasc Surg 11:612, 1997.
122. Mingoli A, Sapienza P, Feldhaus RJ, et al: Aortoiliofemoral bypass graft in young adults: Long-term results in a series of sixty-eight patients. Surgery 121:646–653, 1997.
123. Musser DJ, Nichoals GG, Reed JF: Death and adverse cardiac events after carotid endarterectomy. J Vasc Surg 19:615, 1994.
124. Myers WO, Gersh BJ, Fisher LD, et al: Medical versus early surgical therapy in patients with triple vessel disease and mild angina pectoris: A CASS registry study of survival. Ann Thorac Surg 44:471, 1987.
125. Nicod P, Rehr R, Winniford MD, et al: Acute systemic and coronary hemodynamic and serologic responses to cigarette smoking in long-term smokers with atherosclerotic coronary artery disease. J Am Coll Cardiol 4:964, 1984.
126. North American Symptomatic Carotid Endarterectomy Trial Collaborators: Beneficial effect of carotid endarterectomy in symptomatic patients with high-grade carotid stenosis. N Engl J Med 325:445–453, 1991.
127. Ombrellaro MP, Dieter RA, Freeman M, et al: Role of dipyridamole myocardial scintigraphy in carotid artery surgery. J Am Coll Surg 181:451–458, 1995.
128. Orecchia PM, Berger PW, White CJ, et al: Coronary artery disease in aortic surgery. Ann Vasc Surg 2:28, 1988.
129. Ouyang P, Gerstenblith G, Furman WR, et al: Frequency and significance of early postoperative silent myocardial ischemia in patients having peripheral vascular surgery. Am J Cardiol 64:1113, 1989.
130. Pasternack PF, Grossi EA, Baumann FG, et al: The value of silent myocardial ischemia monitoring in the prediction of perioperative myocardial infarction in patients undergoing peripheral vascular surgery. J Vasc Surg 10:617, 1989.
131. Pasternack PF, Imparato AM, Bear G, et al: The value of radionuclide angiography as a predictor of perioperative myocardial infarction in patients undergoing abdominal aortic aneurysm resection. J Vasc Surg 1:320, 1984.
132. Pasternack PF, Imparato AM, Bear G, et al: The value of radionuclide angiography as a predictor of postoperative myocardial infarction in patients undergoing abdominal aortic aneurysm resection. J Vasc Surg 1:320, 1994.
133. Pasternack PF, Imparato AM, Riles TS, et al: The value of radionuclide angiogram in the prediction of perioperative myocardial infarction in patients undergoing lower extremity revascularization procedures. Circulation 72(Suppl II):II-13, 1985.
133a. Poldermans D, Fionetti PM, Forster J, et al: Dobutamine stress echocardiography for assessment of perioperative cardiac risk in patients undergoing major vascular surgery. Circulation 87:1506–1512, 1993.
134. Port S, Coff FR, Coleman RE, Jones RH: Effects of age on response of the left ventricle to exercise. N Engl J Med 303:1133, 1980.
135. Raby KE, Goldman L, Creager MA, et al: Correlation between preoperative ischemia and major cardiac events after peripheral vascular surgery. N Engl J Med 321:1296, 1989.
136. Raby KE, Goldman L, Creager MA, et al: Predictive value of preoperative electrocardiographic monitoring. N Engl J Med 322:931, 1990.
137. Rao TL, Jacobs KH, El-Etr AA: Reinfarction following anesthesia in patients with myocardial infarction. Anesthesiology 59:499, 1983.
138. Reigel MM, Hollier LH, Kazmier FJ, et al: Late survival in abdominal aortic aneurysm patients: The role of selective myocardial revascularization on the basis of clinical symptoms. J Vasc Surg 5:222, 1987.
139. Rivers SP, Scher LA, Gupta SK, Veith FJ: Safety of peripheral vascular surgery after recent myocardial infarction. J Vasc Surg 11:70, 1990.
140. Sachs RN, Tellier P, Larmignat P, et al: Risk factors of postoperative pulmonary complications after vascular surgery. Surgery 105:360, 1989.
141. Salenius JP, Harju E, Riekkinnen H: Early cerebral complications in carotid endarterectomy: Risk factors. J Cardiovasc Surg 31:162–166, 1990.
142. Sanz G, Castaner A, Betriu A: Determinants of prognosis in survivors of myocardial infarction. N Engl J Med 306:1065, 1982.
143. Schultz RAJ, Strauss HW, Pitt B: Sudden death in the year following myocardial infarction: Relation to ventricular premature contractions in the late hospital phase and left ventricular ejection fraction. Am J Med 62:192, 1976.
144. Sedwitz, MM, Hye RJ, Freischlag JA, Stabile BE: Zero operative mortality in 109 consecutive elective aortic operations performed by residents. Surg Gynecol Obstet 170:385–389, 1990.
145. Seeger JM, Rosenthal GR, Self SB, et al: Does routine stress-thallium cardiac scanning reduce postoperative cardiac complications? Ann Surg 219:654, 1994.
146. Sergeant P, Flameng W, Lessaffre E, Suy R: The value of ejection fraction as a predictor of early and late survival following aortocoronary bypass surgery in patients with moderate to severe depression of left ventricular function. Thorac Cardiovasc Surg 35:87, 1987.
147. Sergeant P, Wouters L, Dekeyser L, et al: Is the outcome of coronary artery bypass surgery predictable in patients with severe ventricular function impairment? J Cardiovasc Surg (Torino) 27:618, 1986.
148. Shah DM, Chang BB, Paty PS, et al: Treatment of abdominal aortic aneurysm by exclusion and bypass: An analysis of outcome. J Vasc Surg 13:15–21, 1991.
149. Shah DM, Darling RC III, Chang BB, et al: Carotid endarterectomy in awake patients: Its safety, acceptability, and outcome. J Vasc Surg 19:1015–1020, 1994.
150. Shah KB, Kleinman BS, Rao TL, et al: Angina and other risk factors in patients with cardiac diseases undergoing noncardiac operations. Anesth Analg 70:240, 1990.
151. Shueppert MT, Kresowik TF, Corry DC, et al: Selection of patients for cardiac evaluation before peripheral vascular operations. J Vasc Surg 23:802, 1996.
152. Sicard GA, Reilly JM, Rubin BG, Thompson RW, et al: Transabdominal versus retroperitoneal incision for abdominal aortic surgery: Report of a prospective randomized trial. J Vasc Surg 21:174–183, 1991.
153. Taylor LM Jr, Hamre D, Dalman RL, Porter JM: Limb salvage vs amputation for critical ischemia: The role of vascular surgery. Arch Surg 126:1251–1258, 1991.
154. Taylor LJ, Yeager RA, Moneta GL, et al: The incidence of perioperative myocardial infarction in general vascular surgery. J Vasc Surg 15:52, 1992.
155. Tomatis LA, Fierens EE, Verbrugge GP: Evaluation of surgical risk in peripheral vascular disease by coronary arteriography: A series of 100 cases. Surgery 71:429, 1971.
156. Topkins MJ, Artusio JF: Myocardial infarction and surgery: A five-year study. Anesth Analg 43:716, 1964.
157. Towne JB, Bandyk DF, Seabrook GR, Schmitt DO: Experience with in situ saphenous vein bypass during 1981 to 1989: Determinant factors of long-term patency. J Vasc Surg 13:137–149, 1991.
158. Valentine RJ, Grayburn PA, Eichorn EJ, et al: Coronary artery disease is highly prevalent among patients with premature peripheral vascular disease. J Vasc Surg 19:668, 1994.
159. Velanovich V: The value of routine preoperative laboratory testing in predicting postoperative complications: A multivariate analysis. Surgery 109:236, 1991.
160. von Knorring J: Postoperative myocardial infarction: A prospective study in a risk group of surgical patients. Surgery 90:55, 1981.
161. von Knorring J, Lepantalo M: Prediction of perioperative cardiac complications by electrocardiographic monitoring during treadmill exercise before peripheral vascular surgery. Surgery 99:610, 1986.
162. Wagner WH, Levin PM, Treiman RL, et al: Early results of infrainguinal arterial reconstruction with a modified biological conduit. Ann Vasc Surg 6:325–333, 1992.

163. Waller BF, Palumbo PJ, Lie JT, et al: Status of the coronary arteries at necropsy in diabetes mellitus with onset after age 30 years: Analysis of 229 diabetic patients with and without clinical evidence of coronary heart disease and comparison to 183 control subjects. Am J Med 69:498, 1980.
164. Weiner DA, Ryan TJ, McCabe CH, et al: Correlations among history of angina, ST-segment response and prevalence of coronary artery disease in the coronary artery surgery study (CASS). N Engl J Med 301:230, 1979.
165. Weinstein MC, Coxson PC, Williams LW, et al: Forecasting coronary heart disease incidence, mortality, and cost: The Coronary Heart Disease Policy Model. Am J Public Health 77:1417, 1987.
166. Weitz HH: Cardiac risk stratification prior to vascular surgery. Med Clin North Am 77:377, 1993.
167. Wong T, Detsky AS: Preoperative cardiac risk assessment for patients having peripheral vascular surgery. Ann Intern Med 116:743, 1992.
168. Yeager RA: Basic data related to cardiac testing and cardiac risk associated with vascular surgery. Ann Vasc Surg 4:193, 1990.
169. Yeager RA, Weigel RM, Murphy ES, et al: Application of clinically valid cardiac risk factors to aortic aneurysm surgery. Arch Surg 121:278, 1986.
170. Young JR, Hertzer NR, Beven EG, et al: Coronary artery disease in patients with aortic aneurysm: A classification of 302 coronary angiograms and results of surgical management. Ann Vasc Surg 1:36, 1986.
171. Zeldin RA: Assessing cardiac risk in patients who undergo noncardiac surgical procedures. Can J Surg 27:402, 1984.

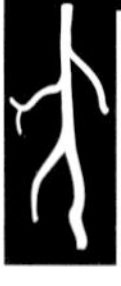

C H A P T E R 4 1

Pulmonary Complications in Vascular Surgery

Charles J. Shanley, M.D., and
Gerald B. Zelenock, M.D.

Postoperative pulmonary insufficiency occurs to some extent in most patients undergoing major vascular surgical procedures. Therefore, pulmonary insufficiency is one of the most frequently encountered complications in vascular surgery. A variety of patient-specific and procedure-specific factors predispose patients undergoing vascular surgical procedures to the development of postoperative pulmonary complications. *Patient-specific risk factors* include advanced age, the presence of chronic obstructive pulmonary disease, a history of heavy tobacco use, poor preoperative nutritional status, and the frequent presence of significant medical co-morbidities. *Procedure-specific risk factors* include the need for urgent or emergent procedures, prolonged general anesthesia, the need for thoracic or upper abdominal incisions, prolonged preoperative or intraoperative hypoperfusion, the requirement for massive transfusion of blood products, and prolonged postoperative ileus or immobility.

The severity of pulmonary insufficiency in postoperative patients ranges from minor atelectasis that is generally benign and self-limited to fulminant acute respiratory failure with an exceedingly high mortality rate. Thus, a clear understanding of the pathophysiology, prevention, and management of postoperative pulmonary insufficiency is essential to the practicing vascular surgeon.

PATHOPHYSIOLOGY

Predictable abnormalities in pulmonary function occur after all major surgical procedures.[3–5] The normal spontaneous breathing pattern includes intermittent deep breaths to maximal lung inflation. This pattern is altered in postoperative patients secondary to general anesthesia, postoperative pain, and narcotic analgesics. Shallow tidal breathing in the postoperative period eventually results in significant alveolar collapse or atelectasis with associated abnormalities in pulmonary mechanics and gas exchange (Fig. 41–1).

It is instructive to review the pathophysiology of alveolar collapse in postoperative patients because it provides an interesting exercise in applied respiratory physiology (Fig. 41–2). Postoperatively, tidal breaths are directed preferentially to the anterior and superior pulmonary segments in the supine patient. Conversely, pulmonary blood flow is directed posteriorly and inferiorly by gravitational forces. In the absence of periodic maximal inflations, the end result is partial or complete collapse of dependent posterior and inferior pulmonary segments. Alveolar collapse leads to predictable changes in pulmonary mechanics, including a reduction in functional residual capacity (FRC), decreased pulmonary compliance, and an increase in the work of breathing (Fig. 41–3).

With respect to postoperative changes in pulmonary gas exchange, an alveolus can contribute to gas exchange only to the extent that it remains inflated. In fact, small amounts of supplemental oxygen will completely saturate pulmonary arterial blood perfusing even partially inflated alveoli. In contrast, completely collapsed alveoli are perfused but not ventilated. Therefore, desaturated pulmonary venous blood from collapsed alveolar units mixes in the left atrium with fully saturated pulmonary venous blood from ventilated

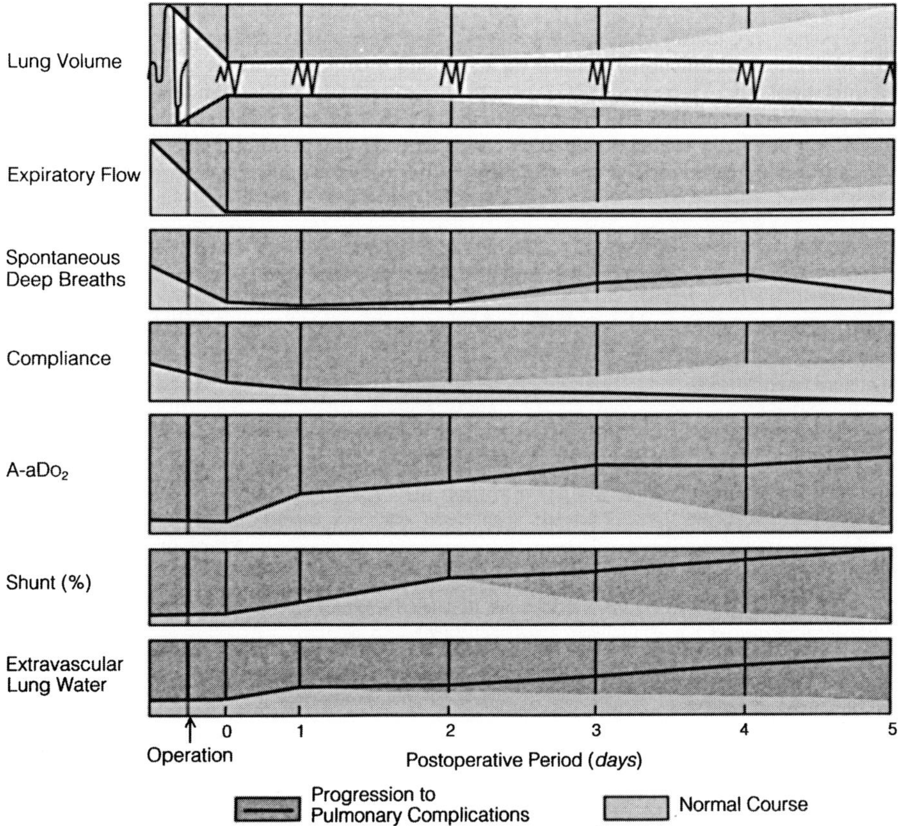

FIGURE 41–1. Normal and pathologic postoperative changes in pulmonary mechanics and gas exchange. (From Bartlett RH: Pulmonary insufficiency. *In* Wilmore DW, Brennan MF, Harken AH, et al [eds]: Care of the Surgical Patient. New York, Scientific American, 1989, p 11.)

lung units. This "admixture" of saturated and desaturated pulmonary venous blood leads to systemic arterial hypoxemia that is refractory to supplemental oxygen in direct proportion to the extent of alveolar collapse. Thus, there is little rationale for the use of high concentrations of supplemental oxygen in postoperative patients with hypoxemia secondary to atelectasis. To the contrary, even low concentrations of supplemental oxygen may be deleterious in those patients with preexistent chronic obstructive pulmonary disease (COPD) who are dependent on a hypoxemic respiratory drive. Furthermore, high concentrations of supplemental oxygen may actually promote collapse by diluting alveolar nitrogen and decreasing surfactant production from type II alveolar epithelial cells.[6]

Thus, if one wishes to improve oxygenation in postoperative patients with hypoxemia secondary to alveolar collapse, the physiologic approach is to minimize supplemental oxygen and to maximize alveolar inflation by encouraging regular deep breaths to total lung capacity.[3, 7, 8] On the other hand, even in the presence of significant atelectasis, relative hyperventilation of the remaining inflated alveoli is generally more than adequate to avoid hypercarbia in patients without preexisting lung disease. This occurs because carbon dioxide diffuses across the alveolar-capillary membrane approximately 20 times more rapidly than oxygen.

Fortunately, this pattern of shallow tidal breathing reverts to normal over the first 2 to 3 days following operation in most patients (see Fig. 41–1). In others, progressive atelectasis is associated with fever and pooling of bronchial secretions in poorly ventilated lung units. This dependent pooling of secretions leads to an increase in sputum production. Inspissation of secretions may lead to plugging of terminal bronchioles and worsening atelectasis. Moreover, stagnation of this protein-rich fluid predisposes patients to development of bacterial pneumonia. Ironically, the administration of poorly humidified supplemental oxygen may inadvertently contribute to alveolar collapse through inspissation of secretions. These tendencies toward alveolar collapse are obviously compounded in elderly and debilitated vascular surgery patients with poor cough and weakened respiratory muscles. Moreover, the development of atelectasis clearly exacerbates pulmonary dysfunction in patients with preexisting parenchymal lung disease.

In addition to alveolar collapse, the development of interstitial and occasionally alveolar pulmonary edema contributes significantly to the mechanical and gas exchange abnormalities noted in postoperative vascular surgery patients (Fig. 41–4). Cardiogenic or hydrostatic pulmonary edema may develop in any patient with left ventricular dysfunction or mitral valve disease. In addition to hydrostatic pulmonary edema, however, a reproducible increase in pulmonary capillary permeability and extravascular lung water occurs after aortic cross-clamping.[9–11] This phenomenon is secondary to the host of ischemic inflammatory mediators that are released into venous blood following lower extremity or visceral reperfusion. The resultant activation of pulmonary endothelial cells, neutrophils, and macrophages results in a reproducible increase in microvascular permeability. This leads to the accumulation of inter-

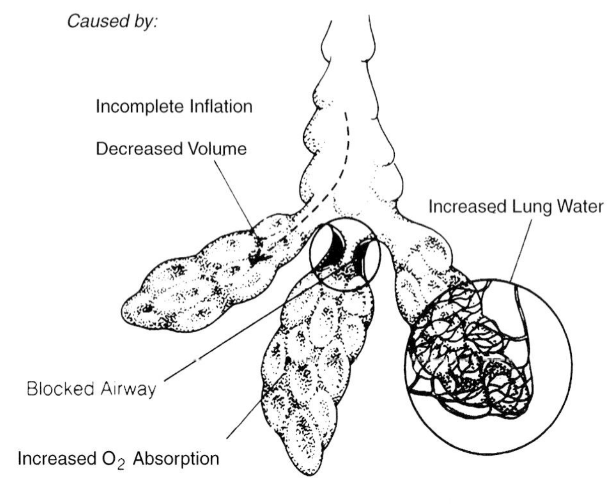

Leads to:	Ventilation-Perfusion Imbalance / Shunt Hypoxemia Decreased Functional Residual Capacity Decreased Compliance Increased Work
Treatment:	Maximize Inflation - Incentive Spirometry, IPPB, CPAP - Mechanical Ventilator (PIP≤ 40 cm H_2O) Maintain Lowest Possible F_IO_2 Decrease Lung Water Treat Infection Optimize Nutrition

FIGURE 41–2. Pathogenesis and pathophysiology of postoperative alveolar collapse. (PIP = peak inspiratory pressure; IPPB = intermittent positive pressure breathing; CPAP = continuous positive airway pressure. (Adapted from Bartlett RH: Pulmonary insufficiency. *In* Wilmore DW, Brennan MF, Harken AH, et al [eds]: Care of the Surgical Patient. New York, Scientific American, 1989, p 6.)

stitial pulmonary edema that is exacerbated by excessive administration of crystalloid fluids during prolonged procedures such as major aortic reconstruction.[12]

The accumulation of interstitial pulmonary edema inhibits alveolar expansion and leads to "cuffing" of the pulmonary arterioles and respiratory bronchioles with further mismatching of ventilation and perfusion. Eventually, fluid accumulation outstrips the capacity for lymphatic clearance, resulting in alveolar flooding (Fig. 41–5). Flooded alveoli are unable to contribute to gas exchange, leading to progressive hypoxemia secondary to transpulmonary shunt. Furthermore, alveolar collapse in dependent lung regions is compounded under the weight of boggy, edematous lung tissue.[13] This further exacerbates the hypoxemia and greatly increases the work of breathing. An increase in the work of breathing may ultimately lead to respiratory muscle fatigue, further reductions in ventilatory volumes, and worsening pulmonary insufficiency.

The extent and duration of these changes in pulmonary function are related to the site of operation, the duration of anesthesia, and preexisting lung disease. Abnormalities are more commonly observed after thoracic and upper abdominal operations and less common after cervical and extremity procedures. Similarly, prolonged general anesthesia can result in significant atelectasis if proper attention is not paid to maximizing alveolar inflation and minimizing excessive fluid administration. Clearly, inadequate removal of tracheobronchial secretions or aspiration of gastric contents exacerbates these abnormalities.

Finally, it should be self-evident that these functional abnormalities are superimposed on preexistent pulmonary dysfunction and are exacerbated in older or malnourished patients with weakened respiratory musculature. Therefore, expected postoperative changes in pulmonary function, if unanticipated and uncorrected, may lead to a vicious circle of alveolar collapse and pulmonary edema, culminating in acute respiratory failure and increased mortality risk. Thus, it is incumbent on the vascular surgeon to maintain strict attention to the details of postoperative ventilatory management in patients undergoing major vascular surgical procedures.

PREVENTION

Preoperative Assessment

As is the case for any patient undergoing a major surgical procedure, prevention of postoperative pulmonary complications begins in the office with a careful history and physical examination. With respect to pulmonary insufficiency, the goal of the history is to identify those patients at high risk for pulmonary complications.[3, 7, 14, 15] It should be self-evident that a history of chronic cough, sputum production, wheezing, and exercise intolerance are harbingers of risk for pulmonary complications; similarly ominous signs on physical examination are auscultation of wheezes, rales, or rhonchi; morphologic evidence of hypoinflation or hyperinflation; and digital evidence of tobacco staining, cyanosis, or clubbing.

As part of routine physical examinations, all patients should be asked to inhale to maximum followed by a vigorous forced expiration (a vital capacity maneuver).[3] Observation of the volume and sound of the forced expiration provides useful information. It is generally possible to estimate the volume of inspiration (at least 1 L/50 kg) and forced expiration (at least 2 L/50 kg) and the expiratory flow rate (most of the exhaled volume within 1 second, and without wheezing). Evidence of reduced volumes and flows suggests the need for formal pulmonary function testing. Alternatively, the forced expiratory volume can be measured directly with a hand-held spirometer. Stair climbing is another inexpensive test of cardiopulmonary reserve.[3, 16] Patients who cannot climb two flights of stairs at a steady pace and without dyspnea may have significant respiratory or cardiac disease, suggesting the need for more sophisticated testing. Finally, the surgeon should obtain routine chest radiography in all patients undergoing major vascular reconstruction who are older than 60 years of age or who have evidence of significant cardiac or pulmonary dysfunction.[3]

On the basis of a careful history and detailed physical examination, the vascular surgeon should feel compelled to

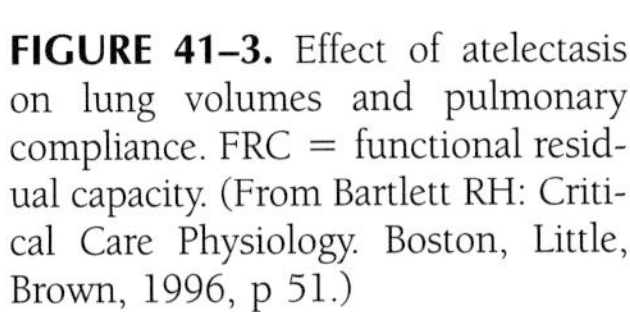

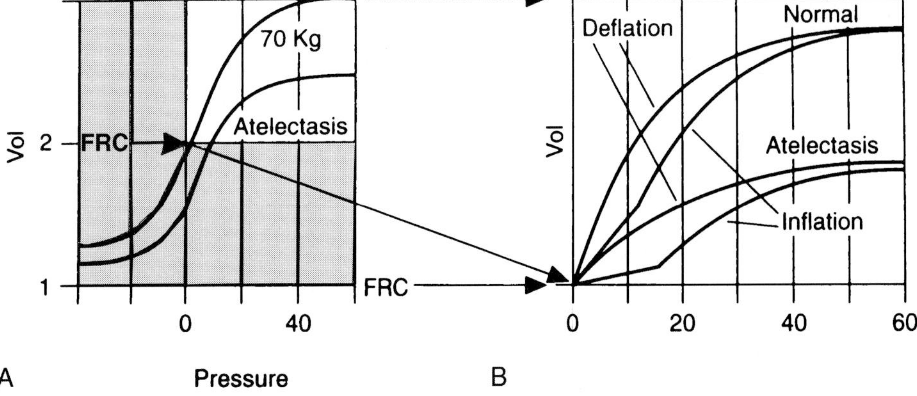

FIGURE 41–3. Effect of atelectasis on lung volumes and pulmonary compliance. FRC = functional residual capacity. (From Bartlett RH: Critical Care Physiology. Boston, Little, Brown, 1996, p 51.)

obtain preoperative pulmonary function testing in any patient deemed to be at significant risk for postoperative complications.[3, 17, 18] Formal pulmonary function testing includes spirometric measurements of tidal volume (V_T), inspiratory capacity (IC), vital capacity (FEV, $FEV_{1.0}$), and maximal voluntary ventilation (MVV). Results are reported as a percentage of the predicted values for age, gender, and size-matched normal patients. Normal values are between 80% and 120% of predicted. Values less than 70% of predicted are abnormal and may be secondary to a variety of factors, including small airway or obstructive lung disease, loss of lung volume, and generalized muscle weakness. An MVV less than 50% of predicted appears to correlate best with the incidence of postoperative pulmonary insufficiency.

Arterial blood gases should be determined as a preoperative baseline in patients with known or suspected pulmonary dysfunction.[19] A room air arterial P_{CO_2} greater than 45 mmHg at rest indicates significant alveolar hypoventilation, which may be secondary to chronic bronchitis, bronchospasm, or respiratory muscle weakness. When feasible, aggressive efforts must be made to correct or optimize these conditions preoperatively. Similarly, a room air arterial P_{O_2} below 70 mmHg suggests a significant abnormality in gas exchange. More detailed testing can differentiate between the various causes of arterial hypoxemia. In order of frequency, these include ventilation-perfusion imbalance, transpulmonary shunt, and diffusion block.

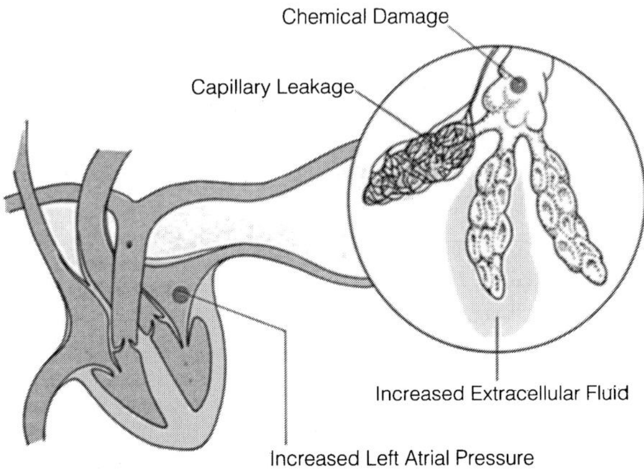

FIGURE 41–4. Pathogenesis and pathophysiology of increased extravascular lung water (pulmonary edema). (From Bartlett RH: Pulmonary insufficiency. *In* Wilmore DW, Brennan MF, Harken AH, et al [eds]: Care of the Surgical Patient. New York, Scientific American, 1989, p 9.)

Preoperative Maneuvers

To prevent postoperative pulmonary complications, the surgeon should make a vigorous effort to address any potentially reversible risk factors. All patients must be encouraged to stop smoking for a minimum of 2 weeks prior

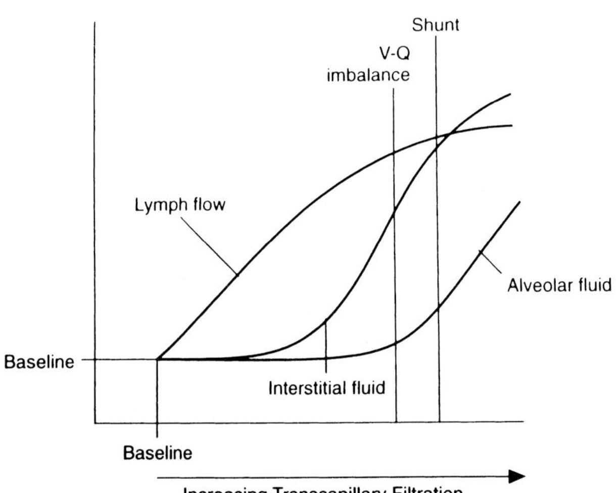

FIGURE 41–5. Effect of increased extravascular lung water on pulmonary lymph flow. V-Q = ventilation-perfusion. (From Bartlett RH: Critical Care Physiology. Boston, Little, Brown, 1996, p 71.)

to any elective procedure. Patients should also be instructed in deep breathing maneuvers and incentive spirometry.[3, 7, 14] If possible, the patient should begin a walking program and weight loss should be encouraged for obese individuals. When feasible, nutritional status should be optimized and any underlying pulmonary edema, bronchospasm, or infection should be treated aggressively prior to operation.

Intraoperative Maneuvers

For patients with known pulmonary risk factors, regional or epidural anesthetic techniques are generally preferred because they appear to cause less central nervous system (CNS) depression and hypoventilation.[20, 21] If general anesthesia is used, especially in prolonged cases, efforts should be made to avoid alveolar collapse by ensuring regular maximal inflations (i.e., 20 ml/kg/min).[3] Excessive administration of crystalloid fluids may exacerbate the development of interstitial pulmonary edema in the postoperative period and should be avoided.[12, 22] Finally, in patients with compromised pulmonary reserve, transverse abdominal incisions appear to be less painful and are preferable to midline incisions in order to encourage deep breathing and expectoration of secretions in the postoperative period.[3]

Postoperative Maneuvers

To prevent the development and progression of postoperative pulmonary insufficiency, the surgeon should maintain and optimize alveolar inflation by encouraging goal-based incentive spirometry and by avoiding fluid overload. Adequate pain control to encourage deep breathing, expectoration of secretions, and early ambulation are obviously of paramount importance.[21] Similarly, optimal nutritional support may help not only to avoid infection but also to maintain strength in the respiratory musculature.[1]

MANAGEMENT

Alveolar Collapse

The most important goal in the management of postoperative pulmonary insufficiency is to optimize alveolar inflation (see Fig. 41–2). Every effort should be made to avoid mechanical impediments to deep inspiration such as severe incisional pain or abdominal distention. Similarly, with respect to diaphragmatic excursion, a seated position is mechanically preferable to the supine position for spontaneously breathing patients (Fig. 41–6).[2, 3] Supplemental oxygen should be used judiciously and carefully titrated to optimize systemic oxygen delivery.

In the spontaneously breathing patient, alveolar inflation is optimized by ensuring regular maximal inflations to total lung capacity through the use of deep breathing exercises. For most patients, volumetric incentive spirometry with any of the commercially available devices is the most convenient and cost-effective means of achieving this goal.[3, 7, 14] It should be evident that appropriate instruction in the proper use of the incentive spirometer is essential to achieve optimal results. Furthermore, the best time for this instruction is *before* the operative procedure in order to minimize the confounding effects of postoperative pain and analgesics. In patients who cannot or will not cooperate with the regular use of an incentive spirometer, properly applied intermittent positive pressure breathing (IPPB), by means of a mechanical ventilator in conjunction with a tight-fitting mask or mouthpiece is also very effective.[3, 23] As with any mechanical ventilatory assist device, it is important to limit inspiratory pressures to less than 30 cm H_2O to avoid deleterious effects of iatrogenic barotrauma.

As discussed previously, pooling of bronchial secretions in dependent lung regions contributes significantly to the pathogenesis of alveolar collapse and pulmonary insufficiency. Optimal pulmonary hygiene is therefore of paramount importance in elderly patients, especially those with preexisting pulmonary parenchymal disease. Avoidance of inspissation of secretions is achieved by ensuring adequate hydration of supplemental oxygen as well as the judicious use of nebulized mist treatments and mucolytic agents. Further, a policy of aggressive chest physiotherapy, including percussion and postural drainage maneuvers, can assist in mobilizing secretions. If management of secretions proves problematic, the careful use of tracheal suctioning may be appropriate; however, tracheal suctioning actually promotes atelectasis by applying negative pressure to the airway.[3] As such, tracheal suctioning should never be used routinely and should be restricted to the removal of tena-

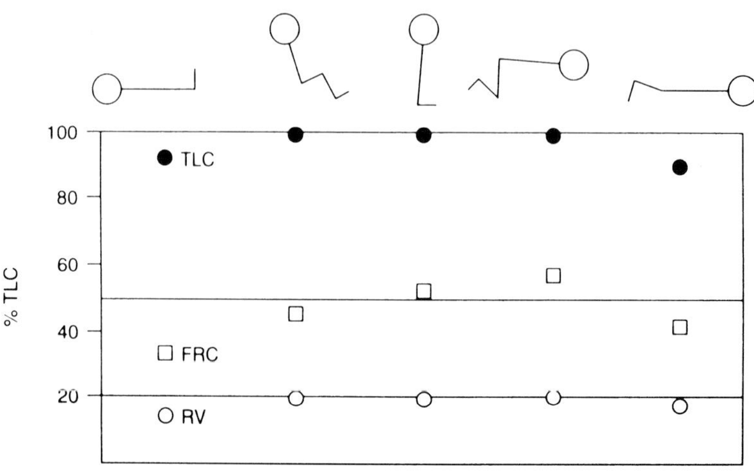

FIGURE 41–6. Effect of positional changes on lung volumes. TLC = total lung capacity. (From Bartlett RH: Critical Care Physiology. Boston, Little, Brown, 1996, p 54.)

cious secretions. Finally, if the aforementioned maneuvers prove to be inadequate, bronchoscopy is a useful adjunct.

Unfortunately, an inordinate emphasis has been placed on the encouragement of coughing as a postoperative technique to prevent pulmonary complications.[3] It should be remembered that coughing is a *forced expiratory maneuver;* at best, it can clear secretions from airways proximal to *inflated* alveoli; at worst, excessive coughing is extremely painful and may contribute to alveolar collapse both mechanically and by discouraging deep breathing.

Pulmonary Edema

Physiologic management of pulmonary edema centers on reduction of extravascular lung water (see Fig. 41–4).[1, 2, 22] For patients with left ventricular dysfunction, hydrostatic edema is best managed by the appropriate use of inotropic drugs and the aggressive use of diuresis to reduce left atrial pressure and improve hemodynamics. For patients with normal left ventricular function, emphasis is placed on avoiding excessive administration of crystalloid fluids, which clearly exacerbates interstitial edema in the presence of increased microvascular permeability. Diuresis is also used to achieve a net negative fluid balance and thereby reduce extracellular lung water while reducing total extracellular fluid volume. In patients with acute respiratory failure in whom diuresis is ineffective or impossible, the judicious use of continuous hemofiltration or dialysis should be considered.

Clearly, reduced plasma colloid oncotic pressure contributes to the formation of interstitial pulmonary edema. As such, an aggressive approach to optimizing nutritional status and correction of anemia is warranted in all vascular surgery patients. However, the use of intravenous albumin is expensive and controversial. Although albumin does theoretically increase plasma colloid oncotic pressure, exogenously administered albumin equilibrates throughout the extracellular space (including the pulmonary interstitium) within 4 to 12 hours following intravenous administration. Thus, any improvement in the plasma oncotic pressure is at best a transient phenomenon.[24, 25] Furthermore, excessive administration of exogenous albumin may theoretically worsen interstitial pulmonary edema by increasing oncotic pressure in the interstitium. Therefore, if exogenous albumin therapy is used at all, it should be used only in combination with aggressive diuresis, and only in patients with documented hypoproteinemia, to take advantage of transient improvements in plasma oncotic pressure.

Acute Respiratory Failure

The optimal approach to the management of acute respiratory failure remains controversial. Conventional management focuses on the intelligent use of controlled positive pressure ventilation.[1–3] Positive pressure ventilation is a mechanical support technique; as such, it is desirable that it not contribute to the ongoing pathophysiology of acute respiratory failure. It is also noteworthy that positive inflation pressure in mechanically ventilated patients is not sufficient to prevent alveolar collapse. Even in mechanically ventilated patients, ventilator settings should be adjusted to achieve periodic maximal inflations. Optimal results are achieved using positive pressure ventilation only when its application is guided by sound physiologic principles and only if it is used with a clear understanding of the potential deleterious effects of positive airway pressure on lung function and recovery.

The primary goal for the physiologic management of critically ill patients with acute hypoxemic respiratory failure is to optimize systemic oxygen delivery (DO_2) relative to oxygen consumption (VO_2).[1, 2] Under normal conditions, DO_2 is approximately four to five times VO_2. Thus, 20% to 25% of the oxygen that is normally delivered to the tissues is extracted from arterial blood and mixed-venous blood is normally 75% to 80% saturated when arterial blood is fully saturated. Acute changes in either DO_2 or VO_2 result in corresponding changes in cardiac output in order to maintain the normal DO_2/VO_2 ratio. If the DO_2/VO_2 ratio is persistently less than 4:1, peripheral oxygen extraction increases to maintain VO_2. An increase in oxygen extraction increases the difference between arterial and mixed-venous blood oxygen content ($a - v\ DO_2$) and correspondingly decreases mixed-venous oxygen saturation (SvO_2). Thus, the overall status of the DO_2/VO_2 relationship is most accurately reflected in the amount of oxygen remaining in mixed-venous blood (Fig. 41–7). Because most of the oxygen in venous blood is bound to hemoglobin, SvO_2 is the best index of systemic oxygen kinetics. Conveniently, SvO_2 can be monitored continuously in the intensive care unit by means of a fiberoptic pulmonary artery catheter.

The primary determinants of systemic DO_2 are the native cardiac output and arterial oxygen content (Table 41–1).

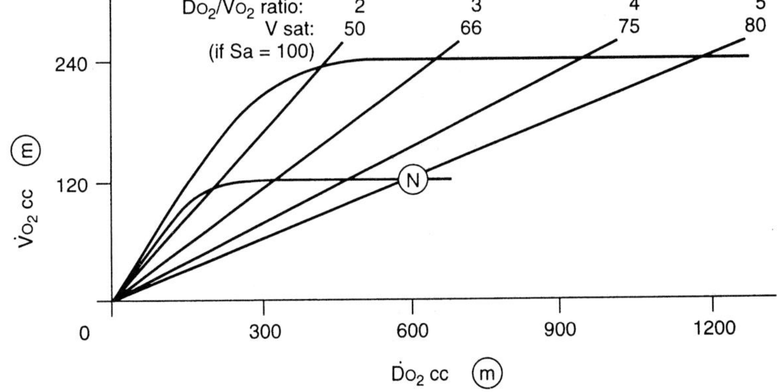

FIGURE 41–7. Theoretical relationship between systemic oxygen consumption (VO_2) and oxygen delivery (DO_2) under conditions of normal metabolism and hypermetabolism. DO_2/VO_2 ratios are represented by isobars corresponding to mixed-venous oxygen saturation (SvO_2). (From Bartlett RH: Critical Care Physiology. Boston, Little, Brown, 1996, p 17.)

TABLE 41–1 OXYGEN KINETICS

$$Cao_2 = (Hb \times Sao_2 \times 1.36) + (0.0031 \times Pao_2)$$
$$Cvo_2 = (Hb \times Svo_2 \times 1.36) + (0.0031 \times Pvo_2)$$
$$a - v\ Do_2 = (Cao_2 - Cvo_2)$$
$$Do_2 = CO \times Cao_2$$
$$Vo_2 = CO\ (a - v\ Do_2)$$

Cao_2 = arterial oxygen content (ml O_2/dl blood); Cvo_2 = mixed-venous oxygen content (ml O_2/dl blood); a − v Do_2 = arteriovenous oxygen difference (ml O_2/dl blood); Do_2 = systemic oxygen delivery (ml O_2/min/m^2); Vo_2 = systemic oxygen consumption (ml O_2/min/m^2); CO = cardiac output (ml/min/m^2); Hb = hemoglobin concentration (mg/dl); Sao_2 = arterial oxygen saturation; Svo_2 = mixed-venous oxygen saturation; Pao_2 = arterial partial pressure of oxygen (mmHg); Pvo_2 = mixed-venous partial pressure of oxygen (mmHg).

Because the hypoxemia of acute respiratory failure is overwhelmingly due to shunting of desaturated pulmonary arterial blood past nonventilated alveoli, efforts to optimize systemic Do_2 should focus on ensuring an adequate cardiac output and arterial hemoglobin concentration in addition to improving alveolar inflation. Furthermore, *optimizing* the Do_2/Vo_2 ratio is quite different from blindly *maximizing* Do_2. For example, a *normal* value for Do_2 may be profoundly *subnormal* if Vo_2 is elevated or *supranormal* if Vo_2 is depressed. Thus, it is best to define *optimal* Do_2 as the level at which the Do_2/Vo_2 ratio is *optimized*, as reflected by continuously measured Svo_2.

Optimizing Svo_2, and hence the Do_2/Vo_2 ratio, can be accomplished by increasing Do_2 or by decreasing Vo_2. Do_2 can be increased by improving oxygenation, correcting anemia, and optimizing cardiac output. Vo_2 can be decreased by modifying those factors that tend to increase metabolic rate; this is accomplished by:

1. Decreasing inflammatory stimuli (e.g., avoiding hypoperfusion, treating infection).
2. Decreasing stimuli for catecholamine release (adequate analgesia, sedation, preventing hypothermia; controlled beta-blockade).
3. Decreasing excessive skeletal muscle activity (sedation, paralysis).
4. Controlling severe hyperthermia (active cooling).

In the modern management of acute respiratory failure, all interventions are carefully and logically titrated to ensure an optimal Do_2/Vo_2 ratio based on continuously measured Svo_2.

It is instructive to review the pathophysiology of acute lung injury in vascular surgery patients because these changes provide the rationale for a physiologic approach to the management of acute respiratory failure. After reperfusion of ischemic tissues, inflammatory mediators are released into venous blood and reach the lung. Neutrophils and platelets adhere to the pulmonary capillary endothelium, activating a variety of inflammatory cascades and leading to diffuse endothelial cell injury and increased capillary permeability. The increase in capillary permeability leads to interstitial pulmonary edema, which gradually progresses to alveolar flooding and collapse. Endothelial cell injury also leads to microvascular hemorrhage and thrombosis, which further reduces the capillary surface area available for gas exchange. Injury to alveolar epithelial cells leads to a loss of surfactant, which increases surface tension and exacerbates postoperative alveolar collapse. A vicious circle is thus established, leading to a profound loss of functional alveolar volume, reduced pulmonary compliance, and an increase in work of breathing and systemic Vo_2. The requirements for minute ventilation in these circumstances often exceed 15 to 20 L/min, necessitating the institution of mechanical ventilation.[1–3] At the same time, systemic Do_2 is obviously compromised secondary to hypoxemia.

It is apparent that in patients with acute hypoxemic respiratory failure, emphasis should be placed on maintaining adequate pulmonary gas exchange and systemic Do_2 without exacerbating lung injury and compromising cardiac output. In cases of severe hypoxemic respiratory failure, high inflation pressures and volumes are often employed in an attempt to compensate for reduced lung efficiency. Unfortunately, these high pressures and volumes are directed toward the remaining inflated lung units, which are more compliant. This leads to regional overdistention of these relatively normal lung units, increasing microvascular permeability and leading to mechanical disruption of the alveolar-capillary membrane.[6] This iatrogenic lung injury has been termed *barotrauma*, or *volutrauma*. Moreover, elevated intrathoracic pressures can significantly retard venous return, reduce cardiac output, and severely compromise systemic Do_2. Thus, although completely safe tidal volumes and peak inspiratory pressures have not been identified, it seems logical in mechanically ventilated patients to manipulate tidal volume, inspiratory time, and inspiratory flow rate to keep the peak inspiratory pressure as low as possible, certainly less than 40 mmHg.[1]

Positive end-expiratory pressure (PEEP) is frequently used to improve oxygenation in acute respiratory failure.[13] PEEP improves oxygenation by preventing alveolar collapse, thereby promoting recruitment of alveoli, increasing functional residual capacity (FRC), and improving pulmonary compliance. Improved alveolar inflation improves oxygenation and reduces transpulmonary shunt. Analogous to the situation with high inflation pressures, the adverse effects of PEEP include an increase in mean intrathoracic pressure, a reduction in venous return, and a reduction in cardiac output. Therefore, the level of PEEP should be physiologically titrated to maximize alveolar inflation and oxygenation while simultaneously avoiding the adverse effects of increased intrathoracic pressure on cardiac output and Do_2.[1–3] Consequently, PEEP is also most logically titrated based on continuously measured Svo_2.

New approaches to mechanical ventilation include the use of pressure-controlled inverse ratio ventilation (PC-IRV) and continuous positive airway pressure (CPAP).[1, 2] During PC-IRV, the inspiratory time is prolonged to more than half the respiratory cycle, allowing more time for recruitment of collapsed alveoli and improving oxygenation at lower airway pressures. CPAP increases lung volumes during spontaneous breathing by maintaining increased airway pressure throughout the respiratory cycle. CPAP also reduces the work of breathing by decreasing airway resistance.

A variety of new ventilatory strategies are currently undergoing prospective clinical trials. The ultimate goal of these new techniques is obviously to improve gas exchange while avoiding iatrogenic lung injury caused by high inflation pressures and lung volumes. At present, it is unclear whether any of these techniques has a clear-cut advantage over conventional mechanical ventilation that is carefully applied and physiologically directed.

In the management of acute respiratory failure, too little emphasis is placed on the profoundly adverse consequences of anemia on arterial oxygen content (Fig. 41–8). For example, a reduction in arterial hemoglobin concentration from 15 to 10 mg/dl in the postoperative patient results in a 33% reduction in arterial oxygen content and therefore systemic Do_2.[1, 2] Although reasonably tolerated in the patient with normal arterial saturation, this degree of anemia can have severe consequences in the patient with acute hypoxemic respiratory failure. This is especially true for older vascular surgery patients with significant coronary or cerebrovascular atherosclerotic occlusive disease and reduced physiologic reserve. Every effort should be made to optimize arterial oxygen content in these patients, and a liberal policy of red blood cell transfusion to avoid anemia appears to be warranted.

With respect to the administration of supplemental oxygen, the shape of the oxyhemoglobin dissociation curve dictates that under steady-state conditions, arterial oxyhemoglobin saturation is adequate as long as the arterial Po_2 is greater than 65 to 70 mmHg.[1–3] Therefore, supplemental oxygen should be titrated based on continuously measured arterial or mixed-venous oxyhemoglobin saturation rather than Po_2. The physiologic goal in these patients, as always, is to optimize the Do_2/Vo_2 ratio based on continuously measured Svo_2.

The role of adequate nutritional support in critically ill patients with acute respiratory failure cannot be overemphasized.[1–3] In a hypermetabolic, catabolic postoperative patient, energy and protein requirements are often markedly increased. During fasting, these requirements are met by endogenous sources. Conversely, these requirements can be met by exogenous sources in the form of enteral or parenteral nutritional support. The consequences of failing to meet these requirements are progressive deterioration of organ function, impaired immunity, infection, and death. Thus, avoidance of malnutrition is fundamental to the physiologic support of patients with acute respiratory failure.

Whenever possible, nutritional support should be administered by an enteral route. Gut mucosal atrophy develops rapidly in the absence of enteral nutrients. Furthermore, early enteral nutrition is considered an effective way to prevent mucosal atrophy. Therefore, if the patient does not tolerate total enteral nutritional support, partial enteral nutrition is recommended to maintain mucosal integrity. If enteral therapy is not feasible, total parenteral nutrition (TPN) should be used as needed to achieve positive caloric and nitrogen balance.

Any intelligent approach to nutritional support requires well-defined physiologic end-points. In a critically ill patient, the most accurate method of determining energy expenditure is the direct measurement of Vo_2 using indirect calorimetry. Because the energy released during oxidation of various nutritional substrates is well known, Vo_2 per minute can be mathematically converted to caloric requirements per day. Unfortunately, overfeeding is also potentially detrimental in the patient with acute respiratory failure. Excessive carbohydrate calories promotes hepatic lipogenesis, leading to increased carbon dioxide production and ventilatory requirements. The ultimate goals of nutritional support are to avoid a caloric deficit and to minimize endogenous protein catabolism. The physiologic approach to nutritional support is to provide sufficient calories and protein to achieve positive caloric and nitrogen balance while avoiding overfeeding. Therefore, caloric support should be based on calorimetry studies. Similarly, protein and amino acid supplementation should be based on daily nitrogen balance studies.

Adjunctive measures for the management of severe respiratory failure include (1) the use of prone positioning and permissive hypercapnia, (2) reducing extravascular lung water, and (3) avoiding high inspired oxygen concentrations. Prone positioning improves ventilative-perfusive matching by diverting pulmonary blood flow from the more collapsed posterior lung segments to the better inflated anterior ones.[13, 26, 27] Permissive hypercapnia employs

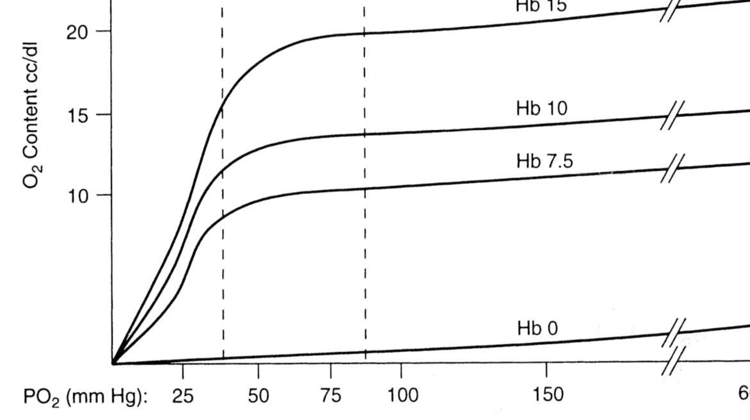

FIGURE 41–8. Effect of anemia on oxygen content. Hb = hemoglobin. (From Bartlett RH: Critical Care Physiology. Boston, Little, Brown, 1996, p 7.)

pressure limited, low tidal volume ventilation to avoid iatrogenic lung injury. Arterial P_{CO_2} is permitted to increase and acidosis is treated pharmacologically. PEEP is adjusted to maintain alveolar inflation and improve oxygenation.

Efforts to reduce extravascular lung water clearly improve gas exchange and pulmonary compliance and appear to reduce mortality from acute respiratory failure. These efforts include aggressive diuresis and fluid restriction. If these maneuvers are unsuccessful, hemofiltration and dialysis are useful adjuncts. Finally, high concentrations of inspired oxygen should be avoided because they tend to promote alveolar collapse not only by washing out alveolar nitrogen but also through toxicity to alveolar epithelial cells, thereby reducing surfactant production.

As discussed previously, mechanical ventilation and positive airway pressure (PAP) are life-saving supportive maneuvers. However, these techniques clearly have the potential to exacerbate the lung injury that necessitated their use in the first place. Unfortunately, patients with the most severe forms of acute respiratory failure are the ones in which the iatrogenic effects of mechanical ventilation may prove the most lethal. It is in this group of patients that extracorporeal gas exchange may represent a superior life support technique. *Extracorporeal life support* (ECLS) refers to the use of prolonged extracorporeal circulation to provide temporary gas exchange or perfusion support for a period of days to weeks. By providing gas exchange, ECLS avoids the damaging effects of positive-pressure ventilation, allowing time for the injured lungs to heal. In the future, continued improvements in the safety and techniques of ECLS may allow increased application of this modality for vascular surgery patients with refractory respiratory failure.

Bacterial Pneumonia

Unfortunately, the development of pneumonia is an all too frequent and potentially lethal complication of vascular surgical procedures. The universal development of alveolar collapse in the postoperative period clearly predisposes patients to this complication. Pooling of contaminated, protein-rich secretions from the upper airway in consolidated, dependent lung regions provides a relatively fertile environment for the development of bacterial pneumonia. This tendency is clearly exacerbated in patients with impaired mucociliary clearance secondary to heavy tobacco use and in patients who are elderly or malnourished.

The development of pneumonia is heralded by worsening hypoxemia, fever, tachypnea, tachycardia, purulent sputum production, and a new or worsening infiltrate on chest radiography. Intelligent therapy requires an accurate diagnosis; therefore, every effort should be undertaken to obtain accurate specimens for culture, including bronchoscopy if necessary. Aggressive, culture-specific antibiotic therapy in conjunction with optimal management of secretions and efforts to optimize alveolar inflation is the cornerstone of physiologic management. Unfortunately, even well-treated pneumonia has a mortality rate of 10% in postoperative patients. This rate increases to 40% in patients with acute respiratory failure and to more than 90% in patients with multiple organ dysfunction syndrome.[28] Thus, every effort must be made to prevent the development of postoperative bacterial pneumonia if optimal results are to be obtained in vascular surgery patients.

SUMMARY

Pulmonary insufficiency is the most frequent and potentially lethal complication for patients undergoing major vascular surgical procedures. The pathophysiology of postoperative pulmonary insufficiency relates to a loss of functional alveolar volume and an increase in pulmonary interstitial fluid. If uncorrected, these changes can progress to acute respiratory failure. The cornerstones of the prevention and management of this problem center on optimizing alveolar inflation and reducing extravascular lung water. One can best meet these objectives by emphasizing physiologic principles to improve systemic D_{O_2} while avoiding the adverse effects of iatrogenic lung injury and bacterial pneumonia.

Acknowledgment: The primary author (C.J.S.) gratefully acknowledges the mentorship and contributions of Robert H. Bartlett, M.D., Professor of Surgery and Director of Surgical Critical Care at the University of Michigan. The principles outlined in this chapter are a humble attempt to summarize his philosophy and approach to the prevention and management of pulmonary insufficiency in surgical patients.

REFERENCES

1. Shanley CJ, Bartlett RH: The management of acute respiratory failure. Curr Opin Gen Surg 1:7–16, 1994.
2. Bartlett RH: Respiratory physiology and pathophysiology. *In* Bartlett RH (ed): Critical Care Physiology. Boston, Little, Brown, 1996.
3. Bartlett RH: Pulmonary insufficiency. *In* Wilmore DW, Brennan MF, Harken AH, et al (eds): Care of the Surgical Patient. New York, Scientific American, 1989.
4. Lee AB, Kinney JM, Turino G, et al: Effects of abdominal operations on ventilation and gas exchange. J Natl Med Assoc 61:164–174, 1969.
5. Okinaka AJ: The pattern of breathing after operation. Surg Gynecol Obstet 125:785, 1967.
6. Parker JC, Hernandez LA, Peevy KJ: Mechanisms of ventilator induced lung injury. Crit Care Med 21:131–143, 1993.
7. Bartlett RH, Gazzaniga AB, Geraghty TR: Respiratory maneuvers to prevent postoperative pulmonary complications: A critical review. JAMA 224:1017–1021, 1973.
8. Bartlett RH, Krop P, Hanson LE, et al: Physiology of yawning and its application to postoperative care. Surg Forum 21:222, 1970.
9. Klausner JM, Paterson IS, Valeri R, et al: Limb ischemia-induced increase in permeability is mediated by leukocytes and leukotrienes. Ann Surg 208:755, 1988.
10. Klausner JM, Anner H, Paterson IS, et al: Lower torso ischemia-induced lung injury is leukocyte dependent. Ann Surg 208:761, 1988.
11. Klausner JM, Paterson IS, Kobzik L, et al: Leukotrienes but not complement mediate limb ischemia-induced lung injury. Ann Surg 209:462, 1989.
12. Simmons RS, Berdine GG, Seidenfeld JJ, et al: Fluid balance and the adult respiratory failure syndrome. Am Rev Respir Dis 135:924, 1987.
13. Gattinoni L, D'Andrea L, Pelosi P, et al: Regional effects and mechanism of positive end-expiratory pressure in early acute respiratory distress syndrome. JAMA 269:2122–2127, 1993.
14. Bartlett RH, Brennan ML, Gazzaniga AB, Hanson EL: Studies on the pathogenesis and prevention of postoperative pulmonary complications. Surg Gynecol Obstet 137:925, 1973.
15. Garibaldi RA, Britt MR, Coleman ML, et al: Risk factors for postoperative pneumonia. Am J Med 70:677, 1981.

16. Bolton JWR, Weimann DS, Haynes JL, et al: Stair climbing as an indicator of pulmonary function. Chest 92:783, 1987.
17. Lawrence VA, Page CP, Harris GD: Preoperative spirometry before abdominal operations: A critical appraisal of its predictive value. Arch Intern Med 149:280, 1989.
18. Kispert JF, Kazmers A, Roitman L: Preoperative spirometry predicts perioperative pulmonary complications after major vascular surgery. Am Surg 58:491–495, 1992.
19. Jayr C, Matthay MA, Goldstone J, et al: Preoperative and interoperative factors associated with prolonged mechanical ventilation: A study in patients following major vascular surgery. Chest 103:1231–1236, 1993.
20. Bendixen HH, Bullwinkle B, Hedley-White J: Atelectasis and shunting during spontaneous ventilation in anesthetized patients. Anesthesiology 25:297, 1964.
21. Cucheri RJ, Morran CG, Howie JC, et al: Postoperative pain and pulmonary complications: Comparison of three analgesic regimens. Br J Surg 72:495, 1985.
22. Mitchell JP, Schuller D, Calandrino FS, et al: Improved outcome based on fluid management in critically ill patients requiring pulmonary artery catheterization. Am Rev Respir Dis 145:990, 1987.
23. Celli BR, Rodriquez KS, Snider GL: A controlled trial of intermittent positive pressure breathing, incentive spirometry, and deep breathing exercises in preventing pulmonary complications after abdominal surgery. Am Rev Respir Dis 130:12, 1984.
24. Demling RH, Manohar M, Will JA, et al: The effect of plasma oncotic pressure on the pulmonary microcirculation after hemorrhagic shock. Surgery 86:323, 1979.
25. Skillman JJ, Parikh BM, Tanenbaum BJ: Pulmonary arteriovenous admixture: Improvement with albumin and diuresis. Am J Surg 119:440, 1970.
26. Albert RK, Leasa D, Sanderson M, et al: Prone positioning improves arterial oxygenation and reduces shunt in oleic acid induced acute lung injury. Am Rev Respir Dis 135:628–633, 1987.
27. Gattinoni L, Pelosi P, Vitale G, et al: Body position changes redistribute lung computed tomographic density in patients with acute respiratory failure. Anesthesiology 74:15–29, 1991.
28. Shanley CJ, Bartlett RH: Multiple organ dysfunction syndrome: Pathogenesis, prevention and management. *In* Nyhus LM, Baker RH, Fischer JE (eds): Mastery of Surgery, 3rd ed. New York, Little, Brown, 1997.

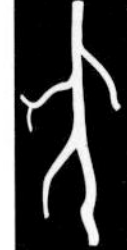

CHAPTER 42
Renal Complications

Kimberley J. Hansen, M.D.,
and Jonathan S. Deitch, M.D.

Fluid shifts and renal function are much better understood now than they were in the 1970s. Consequently, surgeons are better able to perform complex aortic, visceral, and renal vascular reconstructions while still maintaining adequate excretory renal function. Insight into the causes of renal dysfunction complicating vascular surgery, however, remains fragmentary. Despite the increased awareness of the need for fluid resuscitation and the frequent use of invasive monitoring devices, renal dysfunction is not infrequent. The surgeon's limited ability to alter the natural history of acute tubular necrosis (ATN) once it is established and the significant morbidity associated with acute renal failure (ARF) are evidence of the importance of renal dysfunction complicating vascular surgery.

To understand the mechanism and presentation of potential renal insults associated with vascular surgery, one must first consider normal renal physiology. From this reference point, a variety of aberrations in renal function are presented in this chapter.

NORMAL RENAL FUNCTION

A complete discussion of normal renal physiology is beyond the scope of this chapter. A basic understanding of intrarenal and excretory renal function is necessary, however, to appreciate abnormal renal function complicating the evaluation and management of vascular disorders. The following paragraphs provide an overview of normal renal function.

The kidneys are the dominant site for maintenance of normal intravascular volume and composition. Under normovolemic, unstressed conditions, the kidneys receive approximately 25% of the cardiac output. With a 5 L/min cardiac output, the kidneys receive approximately 900 L/day of plasma flow. Because the glomeruli filter 20% of the renal plasma flow and the normal 24-hour urinary output for a 70-kg man is less than 1.8 L, the kidney's tubular system must reabsorb more than 99% of the 180 L/day of filtered plasma to maintain homeostasis. Moreover, the initial composition of the ultrafiltrate is the electrolyte and solute concentration of plasma. Therefore, electrolytes and other solutes such as glucose must also be almost totally reabsorbed.[1]

Reabsorption of electrolytes from the tubular fluid occurs by both active transport and passive back-diffusion. The sodium ion is reabsorbed in the early proximal tubule by its cotransportation with organic solutes, bicarbonate, and divalent cations through an active transport mechanism. Similarly, sodium is actively transported in the late proximal tubule in combination with chloride transport. Because water freely follows this movement of solutes and ions, the tubular fluid is isosmotic to plasma as it enters the loop of Henle.

Depending on their location, the tubular cells of the loop of Henle vary in their permeability. This variable permeability establishes a hypotonic tubular fluid and medullary osmotic gradient. Although the descending loop of Henle is permeable to water but relatively impermeable to sodium and chloride, the ascending loop of Henle is impermeable to water but actively transport the chloride ion, with sodium passively following. The resulting countercurrent mechanism produces a medullary osmotic gradient that regulates urine osmolality from 50 to 1200 mOsm. Distal tubular reabsorption of sodium is also active. In the distal tubule and in the proximal collecting ducts, sodium is actively and almost completely reabsorbed under the control of aldosterone (Fig. 42–1). Of the approximately 25,000 mEq of sodium filtered daily, only 50 to 200 mEq is ultimately excreted (<1%).

Filtered potassium is almost totally reabsorbed in the proximal tubule and in the loop of Henle. Influenced by the electrochemical gradient and the intracellular concentration of potassium, however, potassium is also passively secreted by the distal tubules and early collecting ducts into the tubular lumen. Essentially all of the potassium in the urine is transported there through this process.[1, 2]

NEUROENDOCRINE MODULATORS OF RENAL FUNCTION

Intravascular volume is regulated primarily by a series of stretch or baroreceptors located in the arterial tree and the atria. Because these receptors not only sense pressure or volume changes (atrial receptors) but also monitor the rates of change during the cardiac cycle, they govern the effective circulating volume. Factors that decrease cardiac performance alter the intravascular volume perceived by these receptors and thereby also alter the renal function to retain water and increase the effective circulating volume. Similarly, when the concentration of circulating plasma proteins is reduced, there is a net diffusion of intravascular water

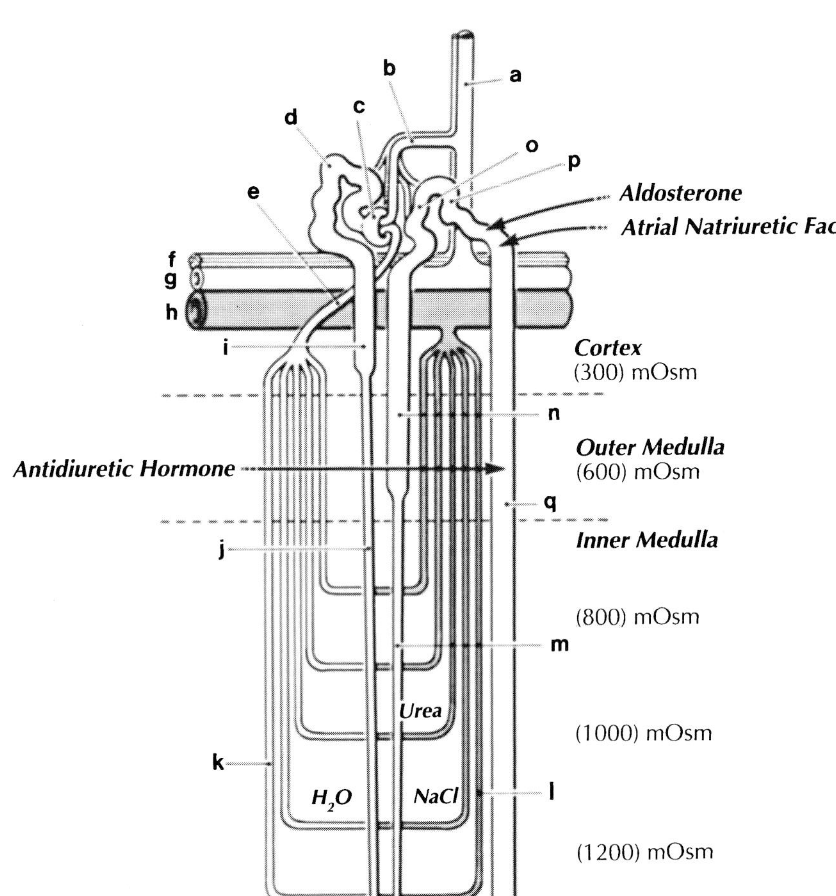

a. Interlobular artery
b. Afferent arteriole
c. Glomerulus
d. Proximal convoluted tubule
e. Efferent arteriole
f. Renal sympathetic nerve
g. Arcuate artery
h. Arcuate vein
i. Thick descending loop of Henle
j. Thin descending loop of Henle
k. Vasa recta
l. Venula recta
m. Thin ascending loop of Henle
n. Thick ascending loop of Henle
o. Macula densa & juxtaglomerular apparatus
p. Distal convoluted tubule
q. Collecting duct

FIGURE 42–1. *a–q*, Anatomic depiction of the nephron and its major hormonal regulators.

into the extravascular space secondary to the decreased intravascular oncotic pressure. This net decrease in circulating volume is sensed by the same receptors, and neuroendocrine regulators of urinary output inhibit excretion of water to correct the volume deficiency.

When the baroreceptors perceive a reduction in circulating volume, their afferent signals are reduced, which decreases their tonic inhibition over the neuroendocrine system. This leads to increased secretion of vasopressin, beta-endorphins, growth hormone, and adrenocorticotropic hormone through the central nervous system (CNS) and to an increase in release of epinephrine from the adrenal medulla. Within the kidneys, at the level of the nephron, baroreceptors within the macula densa cells of the juxtaglomerular apparatus perceive a decrease in intravascular pressure or plasma ion concentration and stimulate juxtaglomerular cells to release renin (Fig. 42–2). Renin, in turn, stimulates the production of angiotensin I from angiotensinogen, which ultimately forms angiotensin II. Angiotensin II raises blood pressure by direct vasoconstriction, and, through its stimulation of aldosterone, it indirectly increases circulating plasma volume.

The primary hormonal regulators of fluid and electrolyte balance are aldosterone, cortisol, vasopressin, and angiotensin. The interactions between insulin, epinephrine, plasma glucose concentration, acid-base balance of the plasma, and other factors, however, play a vital role in modulating the release of these hormones and directly affect the renal tubular management of water and the respective filtered solutes.[1–3] Discussion in this chapter of these interactions and their affect on renal function and fluid shifts is limited to the situation of major vascular surgery.

FLUID SHIFTS ASSOCIATED WITH AORTIC SURGERY

Reconstruction of the abdominal aorta is associated with volume shifts within fluid compartments that normally exist in the unstressed state. These shifts stem from local tissue trauma that occurs with operative dissection, from hemodynamic consequences occurring with aortic clamping and unclamping, and from operative blood loss. The changes are usually mediated through transcapillary and transcellular movement of fluid.

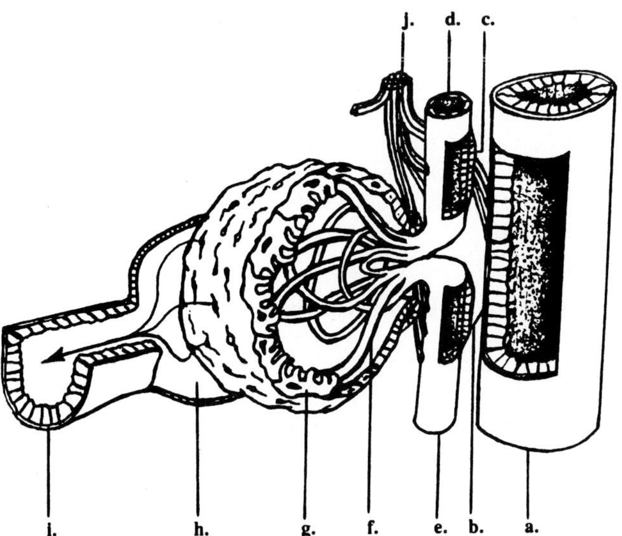

FIGURE 42–2. Juxtaglomerular apparatus (JGA) of the nephron. *a*, Thick ascending loop of Henle. *b*, Macula densa. *c*, Juxtaglomerular cells. *d*, Afferent arteriole. *e*, Efferent arteriole. *f*, Glomerular capillary. *g*, Mesangial cell. *h*, Bowman's space. *i*, Proximal convoluted tubule. *j*, Renal sympathetic nerves.

The net movement of water and solutes from the intravascular, extracellular compartment (plasma) to the interstitium (extracellular or third space) normally occurs at the precapillary level due to increased hydrostatic pressure at that level. The reentry of fluid into the intravascular compartment in the distal capillaries is favored by the presence of intravascular protein, namely albumin, which exerts an oncotic pressure gradient. Normally, 7% of intravascular albumin arriving at the capillary level crosses the capillary membrane into the interstitial space. This extravascular protein eventually enters lymphatics and ultimately returns to the intravascular pool.

After operative dissection that occurs during aortic surgery, disruption of lymphatic channels and the presence of inflammatory mediators causing both local and systemic alterations in tissue perfusion contribute to an increase in permeability of capillary membranes to albumin.[4] The exact mechanisms involved remain obscure, but the resultant effects are those of a flux of albumin into the interstitium and subsequent decrease in water reabsorption into the intravascular space. Indeed, postoperative hypoalbuminemia is a normal finding early after aortic surgery. It is mainly caused by albumin redistribution and not by metabolic changes. The net effects of this, in turn, are decreased intravascular volume and activation of the neuroendocrine mechanisms that decrease renal excretion of sodium and free water. In addition, there is a net movement of sodium and water into the intracellular space from the extracellular compartment. This process is due to a relative deterioration in the normal cellular transmembrane potential after a state of ischemia-reperfusion or shock secondary to blood loss.[5] Why membrane failure occurs is unclear, but it is in part caused by impaired function of the Na^+,K^+-ATPase pump and a loss of active ion transport. This cellular swelling is also governed by a change in intracellular calcium homeostasis and an increase in the intracellular level of calcium.[6] During periods of resuscitation, abnormalities of intracellular sodium concentration and water are reversed.

The normal homeostatic method of contending with a decreased circulating intravascular volume is to mobilize the extracellular (third-space) interstitial fluid. The extravascular fluid space is expanded as a consequence of the aforementioned response to the stress of major intra-abdominal surgery. This excess extravascular third-space fluid might be conceptually described as "entrapped" by its greater oncotic pressure, and the functional reserve of fluid available for return to the plasma for expansion of the contracted intravascular volume is reduced. When one considers the additive impact of temporary ischemia to tissue beds during major vascular surgery, the ensuing shift in acid-base balance in the involved tissue beds, the adverse impact of unreplaced blood loss, the potential reductions in cardiac performance during aortic cross-clamping, and the stimulation of stress response neuroendocrine mechanisms, one can appreciate the vicious circle of events leading to the shift of total body water from the functional circulating blood volume into the third space.[7, 8]

The determination of the intravascular volume and its associated solutes after major surgery has been of dramatic benefit in the intraoperative and early postoperative fluid management of patients undergoing major vascular surgery. The increased obligatory losses of intravascular volume associated with major surgery has led to the current use of balanced salt solutions (5% dextrose Ringer's lactate) for volume replenishment.[9] No theoretical advantages to albumin replacement therapy in the early postoperative period have demonstrated clear benefit. Of equal importance in postoperative management is the appreciation that hourly parenteral fluid replacement requirements during surgery are severalfold those required during a resting state and may vary from 100 to 500 ml/hr. However, even this range of additional replacement fluids is inadequate during and after acute blood loss. These increased fluid replacement requirements continue in the immediate postoperative period owing to continued sequestration of fluid into the areas of the operative dissection.[10]

Mobilization of the sequestered third-space fluid is delayed for several (2 to 5) days depending on the magnitude of operative and postoperative stress, cardiac performance, and intravascular oncotic pressure. Reabsorption of third-space fluid usually begins on the second or third postoperative day. If not managed with appropriate reduction in maintenance parenteral fluid administration or addition of diuretic therapy, reabsorption of third-space fluid can lead to intravascular volume overload and acute congestive heart failure.

RENAL DYSFUNCTION

Sequelae

Renal dysfunction after vascular surgery varies widely in its causes and severity, ranging from a mild natriuresis to fulminant ARF requiring dialysis. For this discussion, events causing renal dysfunction are classified as prerenal, renal, or postrenal in nature (Table 42–1). Although the incidence of renal dysfunction complicating vascular surgery has decreased with the development of appropriate perioperative fluid rescusitation, better surgical techniques, and less nephrotoxic radiocontrast materials, ARF still carries a significant mortality rate, ranging from 10% to 80% depending on the associated presence of multiorgan system failure.[11, 12]

TABLE 42–1. CLASSIFICATION OF EVENTS CAUSING RENAL DYSFUNCTION

PRERENAL	PARENCHYMAL	POSTRENAL
Low cardiac output, cardiogenic shock	Nephrotoxic drugs	Catheter kinking
Increased vascular space	Radiologic contrast	Catheter clot
Septic shock	Myoglobinuria	Bladder clot
Hypovolemia	Acute tubular necrosis	Ureteral obstruction
Blood loss	Other causes	Renal pelvic obstruction
Dehydration		
Third-space sequestration		

Diagnosis

The patient with postoperative renal dysfunction is usually identified by oliguria or increases in serum creatinine level. Consideration of the many possible causes of postoperative renal dysfunction helps the clinician develop an organized plan of diagnosis and treatment. The general evaluation must include a thorough physical examination of the patient. Evidence of intravascular volume depletion, hemodynamic instability, sepsis, or congestive heart failure directs the differential diagnosis toward possible prerenal, renal, and postrenal causes for renal dysfunction. As mentioned, prerenal causes are the most frequent source of acute renal dysfunction in the early postoperative period.

An evaluation of the patient's intravascular volume status and cardiac performance is then carried out. The patient with signs of volume depletion, such as flat neck veins, dry mucous membranes, and reduced filling pressures, requires replenishment of intravascular volume with physiologic saline. Because renal failure is a possibility, potassium-containing solutions and blood products are avoided. If examination reveals that diminished cardiac performance is responsible for the oliguria, as suggested by findings of distended neck veins, S_3 gallop, pulmonary edema, acute electrocardiographic changes, dysrhythmias, decreased cardiac output, and elevated filling pressures, judicious inotropic support is provided and indices of cardiac performance are measured.[13]

If correction of filling pressures or myocardial performance fails to improve urinary output, samples of urine and blood are obtained and diuretic therapy is begun. Serum electrolytes, blood counts, and urine studies permit evaluation of other possible sources of oliguria and renal failure such as ATN and myoglobinuria. Urine studies include urinalysis; urine sodium, urea, and creatinine concentrations; urine osmolality; and estimation of fractional excretion of sodium.

An interpretation of these blood and urinary parameters is provided in Table 42–2. When these prerenal sources of renal dysfunction are excluded, renal artery occlusive disease is evaluated by renal duplex sonography. We proceed with renal duplex, however, only if we are prepared to follow the scan with angiographic confirmation and surgical intervention.

Categories of Dysfunction

Prerenal Dysfunction

Prerenal causes are the most frequent source of acute renal dysfunction in the early postoperative period. Renal failure from a prerenal cause is usually the direct result of a contracted intravascular volume secondary to inadequate fluid replacement during intraoperative and postoperative fluid losses. Less commonly, acute renal dysfunction is secondary to a primary reduction in cardiac performance, which triggers neurohormonal reflexes to increase intravascular volume by increasing tubular reabsorption of sodium and water. In their pure forms, these two causes of reduced

TABLE 42–2. BLOOD AND URINARY PARAMETERS ASSOCIATED WITH RENAL DYSFUNCTION

CHARACTERISTIC	PRERENAL DYSFUNCTION	RENAL PARENCHYMAL DYSFUNCTION	POSTRENAL DYSFUNCTION
Urine specific gravity	>1.020	1.010	1.012
Urine osmolarity (mOsm/L)	>400	300 ± 20	300 ± 40
Urine/plasma (U/P) osmolarity	>1.5	1	1
Urine sodium (Na) (mEq/L)	<20	>30	<30*
Fractional excretion of Na	<1%	>1%	<1%*
UNa/[U/P creatinine (Cr)]	<1	>1	<1
BUN:Cr	20	10	10–20*
U/P Cr	>40	<20	<20

Adapted from Muther RS: Acute renal failure. *In* Civetta JM, et al (eds): Critical Care, 2nd ed. Philadelphia, JB Lippincott, 1992.
*First 24 hours only.
BUN = blood urea nitrogen; UNa = urinary sodium.

renal function are easily discernible. Whereas hypovolemia is associated with flat neck veins, dry mucous membranes, and reduced pulmonary artery wedge pressure, renal dysfunction secondary to poor cardiac performance is associated with distended neck veins, clinical fluid overload, and elevated pulmonary artery wedge pressure. Obviously, the therapy for hypovolemic prerenal azotemia is to increase intravascular volume by administration of balanced salt solution and red blood cells as needed. Conversely, therapy for renal dysfunction of cardiogenic origin is directed at improving myocardial performance by administration of afterload-reducing agents and inotropic agents and instituting diuretic therapy as needed to diminish the preload of the failing left ventricle.

Because the atherosclerotic patient who is undergoing major vascular surgery frequently has associated coronary artery disease and impaired left ventricular function, distinction between these two causes of prerenal dysfunction (hypovolemic versus cardiogenic) can be difficult. In this circumstance, preexisting heart disease may raise the baseline total body volume for an individual to higher central filling pressures, and apparently normal or low-normal cardiac filling pressures may in fact reflect relative hypovolemia. In this clinical situation, we maintain a constant infusion of afterload-reducing agents and inotropic agents (e.g., dobutamine) and cautiously administer small boluses of balanced salt solutions while monitoring cardiac output and pulmonary artery wedge pressure. If no urinary response is noted once filling pressures begin to rise, diuretic therapy is added to treat the cardiac origin of the reduced urinary output. One should have reliable estimates of cardiac function and filling pressures before instituting diuretic or inotropic therapy because exacerbation of compromised renal function can result.[14, 15]

A recently recognized prerenal cause of both acute and chronic renal insufficiency is occlusive disease of the renal arteries. Also termed *ischemic nephropathy,* this diagnosis is made by exclusion of other causes. If other causes have been excluded, renal duplex sonography is used to determine whether there is occlusive disease of the main renal arteries. Because intense interstitial swelling from parenchymal causes of ATN can dramatically increase renal parenchymal resistance, ATN is characterized by a marked decrease in the diastolic velocity from the renal artery spectral analysis. In contrast, hemodynamically significant renal artery stenosis or occlusion is characterized by focal increase in the peak systolic velocity with distal turbulent Doppler waveforms or absence of Doppler flow. In the absence of acute or chronic renal parenchymal disease, the diastolic velocity is increased, reflecting a compensatory decrease in renovascular resistance.[16] When duplex sonography is positive and correction of a renovascular occlusion may be contemplated, we perform contrast angiography to clarify the presence of the occlusion and to plan its correction (see Chapter 123).

Postrenal Dysfunction

Postrenal mechanisms represent the least frequent cause of postoperative oliguria leading to renal dysfunction. The pathophysiology involved in this process is obstructive and is usually at the level of the urethra or urinary catheter and less commonly at the level of the ureters. Hematuria or traumatic catheter insertion can predispose to clots, obstruction of indwelling urinary catheters, and associated obstructive uropathy. For this reason, when rapid cessation of urine flow is detected, initial maneuvers should be directed toward catheter irrigation or replacement, which is usually successful at restoring urinary flow. Problems may be encountered with catheter insertion, such as the presence of clots and urethral strictures. Similarly, catheter kinking should be avoided, as it can occasionally be the cause of obstruction.

Postrenal oliguria can also be caused by ureteral or renal pelvic obstruction, and such obstruction should be sought after other causes of oliguria have been excluded. Causes include iatrogenic injury or compression of the ureters associated with aortic surgery and graft placement and or stone disease. Preliminary diagnosis can be suggested on the basis of renal ultrasound or isotope renography and can be confirmed with retrograde urography. Therapy may require the placement of ureteral stents or percutaneous nephrostomy to relieve the obstruction.[13]

Acute urinary retention leading to obstructive uropathy can on rare occasion accompany urinary catheter removal. Clinical situations in which obstructive uropathy can arise include voiding dysfunction after urinary catheter removal in patients in whom epidural catheters are placed for pain control and urinary retention in patients with prostatic hypertrophy. To avoid urinary retention, we usually wait 6 to 12 hours after epidural analgesia is discontinued before removing urinary catheters. Prostatitis or traumatic urinary catheter insertion in combination with general anesthesia can also precipitate acute urinary retention. Both of these problems, if recognized early, are easily treatable by catheter reinsertion, and they rarely progress to obstructive uropathy.

Renal Parenchymal Dysfunction

Parenchymal causes of acute renal dysfunction are diverse and pose the greatest risk for permanent compromise of excretory renal function. The associated pathophysiologic features depend on the specific cause. For discussion, it is best to categorize the types of renal failure commonly seen as they relate to vascular surgery. In the broadest sense, ATN is used to describe all renal parenchymal causes of ARF. More specifically, the pathophysiologic mechanism of ATN involves a decrease in cellular adenosine triphosphate (ATP), which is associated with a loss in the actin cytoskeleton. Loss of actin causes a loss of renal tubular cell membrane polarity with subsequent loss of intercellular tight junctions.[1, 17]

Shedding of the apical portion of tubule cells into the tubules can cause tubular obstruction and lead to a further reduction or cessation of glomerular filtration in the nephron.[17, 18] This cessation ultimately results in ARF, manifested clinically by an abrupt rise in the serum creatinine level either with or without a change in urinary output (oliguria). It is sometimes possible to detect the presence of tubular cells in the urinary sediment with microscopic urinary evaluation. Although ATN may be transient and self-limited, its causes as it relates to vascular surgery include ischemic injury (shock, acute renal artery occlusion, multiorgan failure, and atheroembolic injury) and toxic injury (myoglobinuria and dye-related injury).[13]

ISCHEMIC INJURY

Acute Ischemic Injury

Acute ischemic injury caused by either temporary periods of interrupted renal perfusion or periods of systemic hypoperfusion associated with major vascular procedures, and its pathophysiologic mechanisms are twofold. First, as a consequence of the magnitude and duration of ischemia, tubular cell swelling occurs following reperfusion. This, in turn, can cause tubular obstruction, leading to further reduction or cessation of glomerular filtration in the nephron. Second, tubular cells can either lose their basement membrane attachment secondary to the interstitial edema that develops after reperfusion or undergo cell death during ischemia, subsequently being sloughed into the tubule. The medullary thick ascending loop of Henle and the pars recta of the proximal tubule appear to be the segments of the tubular epithelium that are most sensitive to ischemia. After loss of the tubular cell, a back-leak of glomerular filtrate into the renal parenchyma then develops.[17–19]

The risk of renal dysfunction after vascular surgical intervention is greatest for aortic surgery. Aortic repair requiring a suprarenal cross-clamp poses a significant risk for ischemic renal insult, and the risk is even greater for repair of thoracoabdominal aneurysm when longer periods of renal ischemia can be anticipated. Rates of ARF approaching 18% have been routinely quoted in larger series of patients undergoing elective repair of thoracoabdominal aneurysms.[20] Ultimate recovery of renal function after suprarenal aortic cross-clamping relates to preexisting renal dysfunction as well as to patient age and the duration of renal ischemia. Periods of hypotension related to blood loss, myocardial dysfunction, or sepsis can also diminish renal blood flow and incite ARF.[20–22] The occurrence of renal failure reported after infrarenal aortic aneurysm repair varies between 1% and 13%.[23–29]

Acute renal artery occlusion can result from emboli from a cardiac event, trauma, or aortic or renal artery dissection. When the occlusion is related to a cardioembolic event, the diagnosis is often delayed; the ultimate recovery of renal function depends on the magnitude of the occlusion as well as the presence of preexisting collaterals to the kidneys. Back, flank, or abdominal pain, new onset of hypertension, hematuria, and elevated serum lactate dehydrogenase (LDH) level may help determine the diagnosis and treatment.[30] Traumatic renal artery occlusion can be suggested by the presence of hematuria and nonvisualization of kidney on intravenous pyelogram. Prompt angiography is necessary to confirm the process, although the success of revascularization largely depends on the ischemic period, which is frequently delayed. Dissection of the renal artery can be caused by catheter-related injury or can arise from preexisting disease (fibromuscular dysplasia). The treatment and opportunity for functional recovery are based on the extent of dissection and, in cases of complete occlusion of the renal artery, the period of ischemia before surgical revascularization.

Vascular procedures complicated by sepsis, myocardial dysfunction, and reperfusion injury can incite transient or permanent degrees of renal dysfunction. In these instances, recovery of excretory renal function depends on elimination of the septic focus and improvement in left ventricular performance to ensure adequate renal perfusion.

Atheroembolism to the renal arteries has been increasingly recognized as a cause of acute renal failure and can cause renal damage culminating in end-stage renal disease. Catheter-based peripheral and coronary angiography and endoluminal interventions such as coronary artery balloon angioplasty are well recognized sources of renal atheroemboli. Moreover, atheromatous disease from proximal diseased aortic segments can complicate suprarenal cross-clamping or manipulation of the aorta. It can also occur spontaneously from these proximal sources or from renal artery atheromatous plaques. The clinical diagnosis is suggested by the presence of deterioration in renal function in a patient who may display other extrarenal manifestations of atheroembolism (i.e., blue toe syndrome) and is highly suggested by the laboratory finding of eosinophilia (71%). The diagnosis is confirmed by renal biopsy, and the treatment is supportive.[31–34]

Chronic Ischemia–Ischemic Nephropathy

Ischemic nephropathy is the term used to describe reduced renal excretory function in combination with renovascular disease. Usually, the renovascular disease is bilateral in distribution or involves a solitary kidney in order to attribute elevated serum creatinine to diminished renal artery perfusion. The significance of ischemic nephropathy is that it tends to be rapidly progressive and may be responsible for as much as 20% of cases of dialysis-dependent renal failure. Uncorrected renovascular disease as a cause of end-stage renal disease is associated with the most rapid rate of death during the follow-up period, with a median survival of only 27 months after the initiation of dialysis and a 5-year survival rate of only 12%. Although dialysis dependence places the patient at increased operative risk, those who survive successful operation have an improved probability of long-term survival.[35]

In patients with risk factors for atherosclerosis, a recent worsening of renal function, and hypertension or worsening of renal function while taking an angiotensin-converting enzyme inhibitor, the presence of ischemic nephropathy should be sought.[36] Unlike renovascular hypertension secondary to unilateral renal artery stenosis, where hypertension is renin dependent, the hypertension in ischemic nephropathy tends to be volume dependent. Thus, patients with this pattern of disease present with severe hypertension, elevated serum creatinine level, and volume overload. Alternatively, the clinical presentation may be that of recurrent episodes of flash pulmonary edema. This entity almost always coexists with some element of intrinsic renal parenchymal disease.[36–39]

Toxic Injury and Angiography

Chemical injury to the kidney can result from many sources. Nephrotoxic agents should be known and prescribed with caution, particularly for the vascular patient with compromised renal clearance. Aminoglycosides are the most common compounds responsible for such injury in the postoperative period, but myoglobin and radiologic contrast media have also been implicated. Aminoglycosides appear to exert their renal toxicity at the tubular cell level and cause mitochondrial damage, cell membrane destruction, phospholipase activation, and lysosomal changes.[40] Because of this relationship and the frequent history of reduced renal function in postoperative vascular surgery patients requiring the administration of aminoglycosides, it is important to identify risk factors that can contribute to nephrotoxicity. These factors include preexisting renal insufficiency, advanced patient age, extracellular volume depletion, and the concomitant use of other nephrotoxins. Furthermore, the routine use of aminoglycoside blood levels to predict or prevent nephrotoxicity is probably not warranted.[13] Although alternative antibiotics with less nephrotoxicity have lessened the use of aminoglycosides by the vascular surgical patient, all agents should be administered with caution and doses adjusted for renal clearance.[40, 41]

Myoglobinuria is an important cause of renal failure in patients submitted to revascularization after prolonged periods of limb ischemia. Circulating as a breakdown product of muscle death, myoglobin is freely filtered by the glomerulus. Myoglobin exerts its toxicity through direct tubular cell injury and through precipitation and obstruction of the tubule.[42] Hematuria after reperfusion of the profoundly ischemic extremity suggests pigment toxicity, and the urine can be tested for myoglobin if a suspicion arises. Alternatively, myoglobinuria is suggested when a urine dipstick test is positive for blood but no red cells are present on microscopic analysis. Once diagnosed, injury to the kidney may be lessened by maximizing the urine flow rate through intravenous crystalloid infusion and diuretics (mannitol) administration and by alkalinizing the urine (sodium bicarbonate).[43]

Of importance as it relates to vascular surgical practice and renal complications is contrast-induced nephrotoxicity. Conventional contrast agents have iodine incorporated into their structures to absorb x-ray photons, thereby achieving visualization of the vasculature. The nephrotoxicity of such iodinated contrast agents has been recognized for many years. The principal site of contrast-induced nephrotoxicity is the renal tubule, and the overall effect on glomerular function appears to be mild.[44] The ionization and high osmolarity of early contrast agents may contribute to their nephrotoxicity. Nonionic contrast agents (e.g., iohexal) are now available that provide comparable absorption of x-ray photons yet are significantly less charged than traditional agents. It was hoped that this would decrease the nephrotoxicity, but the incidence of severe adverse renal events did not differ between ionic and nonionic contrast media in a large randomized clinical trial.[45]

Renal nephrotoxicity after exposure to ionic agents occurs most commonly in patients with preexisting renal insufficiency (3.3 relative risk) alone or in combination with diabetes mellitus, especially when the diabetes is juvenile onset (type 1). Other risk factors such as dehydration, volume of contrast used, multiple myeloma, heavy proteinuria, and simultaneous exposure to other nephrotoxins contribute to the likelihood of acute contrast nephrotoxicity. Overall, the incidence of acute renal dysfunction after contrast angiography varies from 0% to 10%, although these estimates are skewed by several studies that included only type 1 diabetes patients. In one study, hospital-acquired nephropathy occurred in 12% of patients.[46] In patients with normal renal function, however, the incidence of contrast nephropathy is only 1% to 2%.[47] The impact of diabetes on the risk of ARF after angiography appears to be dependent on the type of diabetes and the magnitude of secondary diabetic nephropathy. Patients with type 1 diabetes appear to be more susceptible to contrast-induced ARF than are those with mature-onset (type 2) diabetes.[48, 49] Harkonen and Kjellstrand found that 22 of 26 patients (76%) with a prestudy serum creatinine level of greater than 2 mg/dl who underwent excretory urography developed acute renal failure.[48] Weinrauch and associates reported that ARF after coronary angiography developed in 12 of 13 patients (92%) with type 1 diabetes and severe diabetic nephropathy. In addition, the cause of chronic renal insufficiency appears to affect recovery from contrast-induced acute renal failure. Although both diabetic and nondiabetic patients with renal insufficiency are at increased risk for contrast-induced ARF, those with diabetes appear to recover less often and are at greater risk of permanent dependence on dialysis as a consequence of contrast-induced ARF.[48–50]

Specific measures used to minimize the risk of contrast-induced ARF remain controversial and lack controlled studies to confirm their efficacy. Nevertheless, the basic relationship between the use of contrast material and the risk for any of the currently used agents to cause ARF appears to be related to the amount of time the kidney is exposed to the contrast material. For this reason, the surgeon should consider steps that maximize urine flow rate during and immediately after angiography and limit the quantity of contrast agent used. Maximal urine flow rate should be achieved by preliminary intravenous hydration of the patient. Studies that examined the optimal preparation for patients with renal insufficiency indicate that hydration with 0.45% saline provides better protection against acute decline in renal function associated with radiocontrast agents than does hydration with 0.45% saline plus mannitol or furosemide.[51] We routinely have any patient with the above risk factors admitted to the hospital 12 hours before angiography for intravenous hydration at 1.5 ml/kg/hr. Immediately before angiography the patient usually receives a bolus of intravenous fluid (3 to 5 ml/kg). Finally, intravenous hydration is continued for 4 to 6 hours after completion of the study.

Though attempts to calculate a safe upper limit of contrast material have been somewhat successful, no definitive limit currently exists. Even small doses (30 to 60 ml) may induce renal failure in patients with extreme renal insufficiency (glomerular filtration rate ≤15 ml/min). Conversely, more than 300 ml of contrast material may be safely administered to other patients with no risk factors for ARF.[52] Our practice is to limit the quantity of nonionized contrast agent to less than 50 to 75 ml for patients with a significant reduction in glomerular filtration rate (<20 to 30 ml/min). If additional contrast material is required to complete the vascular evaluation, we postpone further study and approach the total evaluation in a sequential manner. In some instances, the use of digital substraction techniques has been useful in limiting the quantity of contrast material required. Nevertheless, we have found that a single midstream aortic injection, using 30 to 40 ml of nonionic contrast material and conventional cut-film techniques, is just as safe as digital substraction angiography. In this setting, the conventional study provides improved renal artery detail and intrarenal imaging.

Future reduction in renal toxicity will probably result from the development and application of noncontrast studies. The use of carbon dioxide gas as an intraarterial agent is reported to provide accurate and useful arterial imaging with minimal risk.[53, 54] Although influenced by the method of acquisition and post-processing, nuclear magnetic imaging holds great promise for vascular imaging free of nephrotoxicity. Noncontrast methods discussed in detail in Chapter 120.

SPECIAL CONSIDERATIONS

Renal Failure Associated with Aortic Surgery

After aortic surgery, ARF continues to be associated with an extremely high mortality rate. Although it is reported to have an incidence of 1% to 13% in elective aortic surgery,[23–29] ARF depends on the clinical circumstances of the operation, the level of aortic repair undertaken, preoperative renal function, intraoperative and postoperative events, and the overall prior health status of the patient. Data from several series regarding rates of ARF after operations performed for ruptured abdominal aortic aneurysms are summarized in Table 42–3.[27, 29, 55–58] The incidence of ARF complicating rupture of aortic aneurysms and ARF's associated mortality have remained formidable despite a 20-year period of surgical and technologic advancement. Nevertheless, recognition of the clinical syndrome of multiorgan system failure has shed some light on factors that increase this mortality. In patients with postoperative renal failure as an isolated system failure, the associated mortality ranges from 25% for nonoliguric renal failure to 70% for oliguric renal failure. Determinants of outcome include the preexisting disease and precipitating events. In contrast, when renal failure is only one of several system failures, the mortality rate is extremely high, approaching 100% when three or more organs fail simultaneously.[11, 59, 60] It might be surmised that one simply needs to prevent or provide improved treatment for multiorgan system failure to improve the probability of survival in this group with renal failure. To date, however, the prevention of multiorgan system failure has been an illusive goal.

ARF after procedures involving the juxtarenal aorta seldom parallels pure pathophysiologic models but rather results from a combination of underlying causes. In this discussion, however, the respective causes are addressed as independent sources of ARF with the understanding that all of the mechanisms may be active in the production of postoperative renal failure in an individual patient.

A temporary isolated period of renal ischemia because of suprarenal aortic cross-clamping, temporary renal artery occlusion, a single episode of hypovolemic shock, post-clamp hypotension, or cardiogenic shock in the perioperative period is the most common cause of acute renal dysfunction and renal failure associated with aortic surgery. After observations of patients and use of investigative models, Myers and associate have postulated that a pathophysiologic cascade of events following temporary renal ischemia leads to ARF.[61–64] Renal biopsy materials from and autopsy studies in patients with postischemic acute renal failure have demonstrated minimal if any disturbance in glomerular architecture, yet they have demonstrated profound disruption of tubular morphology. These findings led Oliver and colleagues to suggest that this form of ARF is initiated through tubular luminal obstruction caused by sloughed tubular cells, as discussed earlier.[65]

Clinical observation for rates of renal failure after aortic surgery may be subdivided according to the level of aortic repair undertaken. In a large series of patients undergoing thoracoabdominal aneurysm repair, Svensson and colleagues found an 18% incidence of renal failure (serum creatinine level > 3.0 mg/dl) and a 9% rate of dialysis-dependent renal failure.[66] In a recent series in which regional renal hypothermia for renal protection and a clamp and sew technique were used, ARF occurred in 11.5% of patients.[67] Factors identified to predict renal dysfunction included a preoperative creatinine level greater than 1.5 mg/dl and a total cross-clamp time greater than 100 minutes. These results do not appear to differ from those from series in which partial left heart bypass and distal aortic perfusion were utilized.[67] In cases of juxtarenal and suprarenal abdominal aortic aneurysms, preservation of renal function may be enhanced through the use of renal hypo-

TABLE 42–3. INCIDENCE OF ACUTE RENAL FAILURE AFTER REPAIR OF RUPTURED ABDOMINAL AORTIC ANEURYSM

AUTHOR	YEAR	NO. OF PATIENTS	NO. OF PATIENTS WITH ACUTE RENAL FAILURE (%)	MORTALITY RATE (%)
Chawla et al (Chicago)[55]	1975	43	14 (33)	33
Hicks et al (Rochester, NY)[56]	1975	56	10 (18)	70
McCombs and Roberts (Philadelphia)[27]	1979	38	8 (21)	50
Gornick and Kjellstrand (Minneapolis)[29]	1983	30	N/A	64
Fielding et al (UK)[57]	1984	198	4 (24)	66
Gordon et al (UK)[58]	1994	91	18 (20)	44

thermia.[68] For elective infrarenal aortic surgery, a preoperative creatinine clearance rate of less than 45 ml/min has been associated with a significant risk of subsequent renal failure. In the same series, no patient with a preoperative serum creatinine level below 1.5 mg/dl required postoperative dialysis, whereas 8% of patients with a preoperative serum creatinine level above 1.8 mg/dl required postoperative dialysis support.[69]

An alternative cause of ARF in aortic surgery that may be considered a permanent form of ischemic insult is renal atheroembolism. Although this mechanism receives much less attention than the pathophysiologic consequences of temporary ischemia, it may be the dominant cause of ARF in patients without prolonged renal ischemia, excessive blood loss and hypotension, or other recognized nephrotoxic insult to renal function.[70] Obviously, the quantity of microembolization produced during manipulation of the juxtarenal aorta during dissection depends on the embologenic potential of the atheromatous debris and on the operative techniques employed to prevent such an event. Furthermore, the clinical impact of such renal microembolization depends on the quantity of functioning renal parenchyma embolized and on the presence of other causes of ARF. In the absence of other factors that favor ARF and a normal mass of functioning nephron units, relatively large amounts of atheromatous microemboli can occur without immediate impact on renal function.[71] Alternatively, if there is a minimal renal reserve, the added insult of even minor microembolization can lead to decompensation and ARF.

PROTECTION OF RENAL FUNCTION

Measures for protection of renal function during aortic surgery are widely practiced. These include limiting the period of warm renal ischemia, providing adequate circulating blood volume before the operation by preoperative intravenous fluid hydration and adequate blood volume replacement during and immediately after surgery, avoiding repetitive or prolonged renal ischemia, and maintaining maximal parameters of cardiac performance. Additional modalities include the use of mannitol, furosemide, and other diuretics, renal hypothermia, renal vasodilating drugs, and other, more investigational techniques.[72–77] Conceptually, all of these modalities are directed toward reduction of the severity or duration of renal tubular ischemia, reduction of renal tubular metabolic needs during periods of ischemia, and prevention of tubular obstruction by sloughed tubular cells. No single modality or combination of modalities prevents the insult of aortic surgery on renal function, but, by using these preventive measures, one can lessen the severity and duration of renal dysfunction.[78, 79]

Careful attention should be given to limiting the period of warm renal ischemia. For the normally perfused kidney, less than 40 minutes of warm ischemia is well tolerated. For the chronically ischemic kidney, the duration of safe warm ischemic time is extended for an unknown period depending on the amount of collateral flow that has developed. Preoperative evaluation and intraoperative preparation can help to reduce the ischemic time and diminish the chances of time-consuming intraoperative complications.

In addition to routine heparinization and confirmation of systemic anticoagulation by measurement of activated clotting time (ACT), intravenous administration of mannitol, 12.5 to 25 gm, before aortic cross-clamping is a widely practiced measure to prevent ARF. Extensive investigation suggests that mannitol not only acts as an osmotic diuretic to increase urine flow rate but may also attenuate the reduction in cortical blood flow that occurs during and immediately after aortic cross-clamping. Additionally, mannitol acts as a free radical scavenger.[73] Compared with saline administered before aortic cross-clamping in patients undergoing infrarenal aortic aneurysm repair, mannitol causes a reduction in subclinical glomerular and renal tubular damage.[78] It should be noted, however, that these results are not uniformly reproduced; some investigators have found no clinical benefit from using mannitol and dopamine compared with volume expansion alone.[80]

Profound and sustained alterations in renal hemodynamics are observed in patients with impaired renal function or when surgical occlusion of the aorta is prolonged. ARF after aortic surgery requires aggressive therapy, and goals should be aimed at correcting extracellular volume deficits. Once restoration of intravascular volume and cardiac output are ensured, the addition of vasodilatory doses of dopamine (1.5 to 3 μg/kg/min) may then improve urinary volume. The conversion of oliguric renal failure to a nonoliguric state is associated with fewer complications and an improved survival rate.[59]

Induction of regional renal hypothermia has been used sporadically for many years to protect renal function during periods of ischemia. Its use is based on the valid premise that even modest decreases in core temperature significantly reduce metabolic needs. These unmet metabolic needs during ischemia lead to a series of events that produce ARF. The technique usually employs the infusion of 500 ml to 1 L of cold (4 to 5°C) crystalloid solution with or without other additives into the isolated segment of the aorta containing the renal arteries or directly into the renal artery ostia via a handheld cannula or infusion balloon catheters. The protective effect of minimal changes in core temperature has recently been evaluated in rats. Postoperative serum creatinine levels and renal tubular morphology data revealed that a protective effect occurred with a minimal, sustained decrease in core temperature to 35°C.[81]

Finally, we cannot overstate the importance of operative technique in preventing microembolization of atheromatous debris during juxtarenal aortic dissection and control. One should avoid repetitive cross-clamping as this increases the risk of atheroembolization to the renal arteries from proximal atheromatous debris. Because the embologenic potential of the debris cannot be judged definitively until after the aorta is opened, one should assume the worst until it is proven otherwise. For this reason, we temporarily occlude renal artery flow immediately before the application of the aortic clamp whenever the aortogram suggests the presence of complicated perirenal atherosclerosis. This applies to both infrarenal and suprarenal aortic cross-clamping. Although we can provide only anecdotal support for this maneuver, we believe it has been an important adjunct in minimizing the incidence of postoperative ARF among our patients.

REFERENCES

1. Robaczewski DL, Dean RH: Basic science of renovascular hypertension. *In* Sidawy AN, Sumpio BE, Depalma RG (eds): The Basic Science of Vascular Disease. Armonk, NY, Futura Publishing Co, 1997, pp 691–721.
2. Valtin H, Schafer JA: K+ balance: Renal handling of K+. *In* Renal Function, 3rd ed. Boston, Little, Brown, 1995, pp 235–256.
3. Shires GT III: Management of fluids and electrolytes. *In* Sabiston DC Jr, Lyerly HK (eds): Sabiston's Essentials of Surgery, 2nd ed. Philadelphia, WB Saunders, 1994, p 36.
4. Granger H, Dhar J, Chen, HI, et al: Structure and function of the interstitium. Proceedings of the Workshop on Albumin, Bethesda, National Institutes of Health, 1976, pp 114–125.
5. Smeets HJ, Kievit J, Dulfer FT, et al: Analysis of post-operative hypoalbuminemia: A clinical study. Int Surg 79(2):152–157, 1994.
6. Humes HD: Role of calcium in pathogenesis of acute renal failure. Am J Physiol 250:F579–189, 1986.
7. Lucas CE, Ledgerwood AM: The fluid problem in the critically ill. Surg Clin North Am 63(2):439–454, 1983.
8. Dawson CW, Lucas CE, Ledgerwood AM: Altered interstitial fluid space dynamics and post-resuscitation hypertension. Arch Surg 116(5):657–662, 1981.
9. Bomberger RA, McGregor B, Depalma RG. Optimal fluid management after aortic reconstruction. A prospective study of two crystalloid solutions. J Vasc Surg 4(2):164–167, 1986.
10. Nielsen OM, Engell HC: Effects of maintaining normal plasma colloid osmotic pressure on renal function and excretion of sodium and water after major surgery: A randomized study. Dan Med Bull 32(3):182–185, 1985.
11. Brezis M, Rosen S, Epstein FH: Acute renal failure. *In* Brenner BM, Rector FC (eds): The Kidney, 4th ed. Philadelphia, WB Saunders, 1991, pp 993–1061
12. Bullock ML, Umen A, Finkelstein M, Keane WF: The assessment of risk factors in 462 patients with acute renal failure. Am J Kidney Dis 5:97–103, 1985.
13. Muther RS: Acute renal failure: Acute azotemia in the critically ill. *In* Civetta JM, Taylor RW, Kirby RR (eds): Critical Care, 2nd ed. Philadelphia, JB Lippincott, 1992, pp 1583–1598.
14. Bush HC Jr: Renal failure following abdominal aortic reconstruction. Surgery 93:107–109, 1983.
15. Rice CL, Hobelman CF, John DA, et al: Central venous pressure or pulmonary capillary wedge pressure as the determinant of fluid replacement in aortic surgery. Surgery 84(3):437–440, 1978.
16. Hansen KJ, Tribble RW, Reavis SW, et al: Renal duplex sonography: Evaluation of clinical utility. J Vasc Surg 12(3):227–336, 1990.
17. Molitoris BA: New insights into the cell biology of ischemic acute renal failure. J Am Soc Nephrol 1(12):1263–1270, 1991.
18. Mason J, Joeris B, Welsch J, et al: Vascular congestion in ischemic renal failure: The role of cell swelling. Miner Electrolyte Metab 15(3):114–124, 1989.
19. Mohaupt M, Kramer HJ: Acute ischemic renal failure: Review of experimental studies on pathophysiology and potential protective interventions. Renal Failure 11(4):177–185, 1989–1990.
20. Safi HJ, Harlin SA, Miller CC, et al: Predictive factors for acute renal failure in thoracic and thoracoabdominal aortic aneurysm surgery. J Vasc Surg 24(3):338–344, 1996.
21. Schepens MA, Defauw JJ, Hamerlijnck RP, et al: Risk assessment of acute renal failure after thoracoabdominal aortic aneurysm surgery. Ann Surg 219(4):400–407, 1997.
22. Breckwoldt WL, Mackay WC, Belkin M, et al: The effect of suprarenal cross-clamping on abdominal aortic aneurysm repair. Arch Surg 127(5):520–524, 1992.
23. Gardner RJ, Lancaster JR, Tarney TJ, et al: Five year history of surgically treated abdominal aortic aneurysms. Surg Gynecol Obstet 130:981–987, 1970.
24. O'Donnell D, Clarke G, Hurst P: Acute renal failure following surgery for abdominal aortic aneurysm. Aust NZ J Surg 59:405–408, 1989.
25. Thompson JE, Hollier JH, Patman RD, et al: Surgical management of abdominal aortic aneurysms: Factors influencing mortality and morbidity—a 20-year experience. Ann Surg 181:654–661, 1975.
26. Bergqvist D, Olsson P-O, Takolander R, et al: Renal failure as a complication to aortoiliac and iliac reconstructive surgery. Acta Chir Scand 149:37–41, 1983.
27. McCombs PR, Roberts B: Acute renal failure following resection of abdominal aortic aneurysm. Surg Gynecol Obstet 148:175–178, 1979.
28. Diehl JT, Cali RF, Hertzer NR, Beven EG: Complications of abdominal aortic reconstruction: An analysis of perioperative risk factors in 557 patients. Ann Surg 197(1):49–56, 1983.
29. Gornick CC Jr, Kjellstrand CM: Acute renal failure complicating aortic aneurysm surgery. Nephron 35:145–157, 1983.
30. Ouriel K: Renal artery embolism. *In* Ernst CB, Stanley JC (eds): Current Therapy in Vascular Surgery, 3rd ed. St. Louis, Mosby–Year Book, 1995, pp 821–823.
31. Lye WC, Cheah JS, Sinniah R: Renal cholesterol embolic disease: Case report and review of the literature. Am J Nephrol 13(6):489–493, 1993.
32. Blankenship JC: Cholesterol embolisation after thrombolytic therapy. Drug Safety 14(2):78–84, 1996.
33. Thadani RI, Camargo CA Jr, Xavier RJ: Atheroembolic renal failure after invasive procedures. Natural history based on 52 histologically proven cases. Medicine 74(6):350–358, 1995.
34. Sakalayan MG, Gupta S, Suryaprasad A, et al: Incidence of atheroembolic renal failure after coronary angiography: A prospective study. Angiology 48(7):609–613, 1997.
35. Fuller SB, Dean RH: Renovascular disease. *In* Dean RH, Yao JS, Brewster DC (eds): Current Diagnosis and Treatment in Vascular Surgery. Norwalk, Conn, Appleton and Lange, 1995, pp 276–281.
36. Textor SC: Renal failure related to angiotensin converting enzyme inhibitors. Semin Nephrol 17(1):67–76, 1997.
37. Navis G: Ace inhibitors and the kidney: A risk benefit assessment. Drug Safety 15(3):200–211, 1996.
38. Toto RD: Renal insufficiency due to angiotensin-converting enzyme inhibitors. Miner Electrolyte Metab 20(4):193–200, 1994.
39. Kalra PA, Mamtora H, Holmes AM: Renovascular disease and renal complications of angiotensin-converting enzyme inhibitor therapy. Q J Med 77(282):1013–1018, 1990.
40. Moore RD, Smith CR, Lipsky JJ, et al: Risk factors for nephrotoxicity in patients treated with aminoglycosides. Ann Intern Med 100(3):352–357, 1984.
41. Boucher BA, Coffey BC, Kuhl DA, et al: Algorithm for assessing renal

dysfunction risk in critically ill trauma patients receiving aminoglycosides. Am J Surg 160(5):473–480, 1990.
42. Braum SR, Weiss FR, Keller AL, et al: Evaluation of the renal toxicity of hemoproteins and their derivatives: A role in the genesis of acute tubular necrosis. J Exp Med 131:443, 1979.
43. Eneas JF, Schoenfeld BY, Humphreys MH: The effect of infusion of mannitol-sodium bicarbonate on the clinical course of myoglobinuria. Arch Intern Med 139:801–805, 1979.
44. Donadio C, Tramonti G, Lucceshi A, et al: Tubular toxicity is the main renal effect of contrast media. Renal Failure 18(4):647–656, 1996.
45. Rudnick MR, Goldfarb S, Wexler L, et al: Nephrotoxicity of ionic and nonionic contrast media in 1196 patients: A randomized trial. The Iohexol Cooperative Study. Kidney Int 47(1):254–261, 1995.
46. Hou SH, Burchinsky DA, Wish JB, et al: Hospital acquired renal insufficiency: A prospective study. Am J Med 74:243, 1983.
47. Parfrey PS, Griffiths SM, Barrett BJ, et al: Contrast material-induced renal failure in patients with diabetes mellitus, renal insufficiency, or both. N Engl J Med 320:143–149, 1989.
48. Harkonen S, Kjellstrand CM: Exacerbation of diabetic renal failure following intravenous pyelography. Am J Med 63:939, 1977.
49. Shieh SD, Hirsch SR, Boshell BR, et al: Low risk of contrast media induced acute renal failure in nonazotemic type 2 diabetes mellitus. Kidney Int 21:739, 1982.
50. Weinrauch LA, Healy RW, Leland OS, et al: Coronary angiography and acute renal failure in diabetic azotemic nephropathy. Ann Intern Med 86:56–59, 1977.
51. Solomon R, Werner C, Mann D, et al: Effects of saline, mannitol and furosemide to prevent acute decreases in renal function induced by radiocontrast agents. N Engl J Med 331(21):1416–1420, 1994.
52. Cigarroa RG, Lang RA, Williams RH, Hillis LD: Dosing of contrast material to prevent contrast nephropathy in patients with renal disease. Am J Med 86:649–652, 1989.
53. Weaver FA, Pentecost MJ, Yellin AE: Carbon dioxide digital subtraction arteriography: A pilot study. Ann Vasc Surg 4(5):437, 1990.
54. Seeger JM, Self S, Harward TR, et al: Carbon dioxide gas as an arterial contrast agent. Ann Surg 217(6):688–697, 1993.
55. Chawla SK, Najafi H, Ing TS, et al: Acute renal failure complicating ruptured abdominal aortic aneurysm. Arch Surg 110(5):521–526, 1975.
56. Hicks GL, Eastland MW, De Weese JA, et al: Survival improvement following aortic aneurysm resection. Ann Surg 181:863–869, 1975.
57. Fielding JL, Black J, Ashton F, et al: Ruptured aortic aneurysms: Postoperative complications and their aetiology. Br J Surg 71(7):487–491, 1984.
58. Gordon AC, Pryn S, Collin J: Outcome of patients who required renal support after surgery for ruptured abdominal aortic aneurysm. Br J Surg 81(6):836–838, 1994.
59. Anderson RJ, Linas SL, Berns AS, et al: Nonoliguric acute renal failure. N Engl J Med 296(20):1134–1138, 1977.
60. Mann HJ, Fuhs DW, Hemstrom CA: Acute renal failure. Drug Intel Clin Pharm 20(6):421–438, 1986.
61. Myers BD, Moran SM: Hemodynamically mediated acute renal failure. N Engl J Med 314:97–105, 1986.
62. Myers BD, Miller DC, Mehigan JT, et al: Nature of the renal injury following total renal ischemia in man. J Clin Invest 73:329–341, 1984.
63. Moran SM, Myers BD: Course of acute renal failure studied by a model of creatinine kinetics. Kidney Int 27:928–937, 1985.
64. Hilberman M, Myers BD, Carrie G, et al: Acute renal failure following cardiac surgery. J Thorac Cardiovasc Surg 77:880–888, 1979.
65. Oliver J, MacDowell M, Tracy A: Pathogenesis of acute renal failure associated with traumatic and toxic injury. Renal ischemia, nephrotoxic damage, and the ischemuric episode. J Clin Invest 30:1305, 1951.
66. Svensson LG, Crawford ES, Hess KR, et al: Experience with 1509 patients undergoing thoracoabdominal and aortic operations. J Vasc Surg 17(2):357–368, 1993.
67. Kashyap VS, Cambria RP, Davison JF, et al: Renal failure after thoracoabdominal aortic surgery. J Vasc Surg 26(6):949–955, 1997.
68. Allen BT, Anderson CB, Rubin BG, et al: Preservation of renal function in juxtarenal and suprarenal abdominal aortic aneurysm repair. J Vasc Surg 17(5):948–958, 1993.
69. Powell RJ, Roddy SP, Meier GH, et al: Effect of renal insufficiency on outcome following infrarenal aortic surgery. Am J Surg 174(2):126–130, 1997.
70. Iliopoulos JI, Zdon MJ, Crawford BG, et al: Renal microembolization syndrome: A cause for renal dysfunction after abdominal aortic reconstruction. Am J Surg 146(6):779–783, 1983.
71. Smith MC, Ghose MK, Henry AR: The clinical spectrum of renal cholesterol embolization. Am J Med 71(1):174–180, 1981.
72. Miller DC, Myers BD: Pathophysiology and prevention of acute renal failure associated with thoracoabdominal or abdominal aortic surgery. J Vasc Surg 5(3):518–523, 1987.
73. Abbott WM, Abel RM, Beck CH: The reversal of renal cortical ischemia during aortic occlusion by mannitol. J Surg Res 16:482–489, 1974.
74. Hanley MJ, Davidson K: Prior mannitol and furosemide infusion in a model of ischemic acute renal failure. Am J Physiol 241:F556–F564, 1981.
75. Ochsner JL, Mills NL, Gardner PA: A technique for renal preservation during suprarenal abdominal aortic operations. Surg Gynecol Obstet 159:388–390, 1984.
76. Hilberman M, Maseda J, Stinson EB, et al: The diuretic properties of dopamine in patients after open-heart operations. Anesthesiology 61:489–494, 1984.
77. Lindner A, Cutler RE, Bell AJ: Attenuation of nephrotoxic acute renal failure in the dog with angiotensin-converting enzyme inhibitor (SQ-20,881). Circ Res 51:216–224, 1982.
78. Salem MG, Crooke JW, McLoughlin GA, et al: The effect of dopamine on renal function during aortic cross clamping. Ann Coll Surgeons Engl 701(1):9–12, 1988.
79. Nicholson ML, Baker DM, Hopkinson BR, et al: Randomized control trial of the effect of mannitol on renal reperfusion injury during aortic aneurysm surgery. Br J Surg 83(9):1230–1233, 1996.
80. Paul MD, Mazer CD, Byrick RJ, et al: Influence of mannitol and dopamine on renal function during elective infrarenal aortic clamping in man. Am J Nephrol 6(6):427–434, 1986.
81. Pelkey TJ, Frank RS, Stanley JJ, et al: Minimal physiologic temperature variations during renal ischemia alter functional and morphologic outcome. J Vasc Surg 15:619–625, 1992.

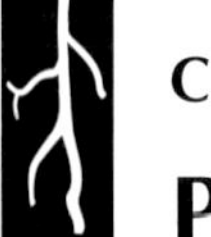

CHAPTER 43

Perioperative Hemorrhage

Cynthia K. Shortell, M.D., Karl A. Illig, M.D.,
and Kenneth Ouriel, M.D.

Hemorrhage in the perioperative period is relatively common and ranges in severity from trivial to life-threatening. The successful treatment of the patient with major perioperative hemorrhage depends on prompt identification of both the nature of the problem and its cause. Causes of perioperative hemorrhage include technical error, vascular pathology, and disorders of hemostasis, and treatment strategies vary significantly, depending on which factors are responsible for the problem. This chapter discusses the mechanisms of hemostasis and provides guidelines for prevention and treatment of perioperative hemorrhage.

OVERVIEW OF NORMAL HEMOSTASIS

General Principles

Inherent in the physiology of hemostasis is a series of checks and balances made by activators and inhibitors and designed to minimize hemorrhage while maximizing perfusion. Almost every step in the clotting cascade triggers a response designed to counteract an earlier one in order to prevent diffuse coagulation, but is itself regulated to avoid diffuse hemorrhage.

The initial response to vascular injury is retraction and spasm of the vessel itself, followed by activation of hemostatic mechanisms inherent in the blood that produce a more complex and definitive response to bleeding. The basic response to bleeding consists of four steps:

1. Response of the vascular endothelium.
2. Platelet activation and aggregation (primary hemostasis).
3. Activation of the coagulation cascade (secondary hemostasis).
4. Lysis of the clot and restraint of coagulation (Fig. 43–1).

Vascular Endothelium

Endothelial cells comprise the lining of the vascular lumen at every level and are critically important in a large variety of physiologic and pathologic processes, including atherosclerosis, hemostasis, thrombolysis, and thrombosis. The endothelium is considered the largest organ in the body, with a surface area of approximately 5000 m^2.[1] Uninjured endothelium does not react with circulating blood elements, whereas injured endothelial cells may set off a variety of acute or chronic responses such as thrombosis and atherosclerosis. The functions of uninjured endothelial cells are to maintain blood fluidity and to regulate vascular integrity and permeability, whereas injured endothelium serves to initiate hemostasis, either directly or through its absence.

A variety of factors contribute to the thromboresistance of endothelium.[2–5] Prostaglandin I_2, a potent inhibitor of platelet aggregation, is synthesized by endothelial cells, as are thrombomodulin and heparan sulfate, both of which inhibit the action of thrombin. Plasminogen activators, such as tissue plasminogen activator (t-PA), are also synthesized by endothelial cells, resulting in the degradation of fibrin. Other receptors on the endothelial cell surface bind thrombin and facilitate its inactivation by circulating antithrombin III (AT III). The negative charge of the endothelial cell can also serve to discourage adherence of platelets, as they are negatively charged as well. Endothelial cells also secrete nitric oxide (NO), a potent vasodilator and anti-inflammatory molecule that inhibits platelet adhesion.[4, 6] When vascular injury occurs, endothelium is denuded and the subendothelial surface becomes exposed to both platelets and coagulation factors within the bloodstream.

Platelets

Under circumstances of normal laminar blood flow, red blood cells form a central column, with a more peripheral layer of plasma and an outermost layer of platelets that marginate to the vessel wall both by convection and by currents of plasma transport.[7–9] Platelets play a crucial role in the initiation of hemostasis through a multistep process. During this sequence of events, platelets undergo adhesion, spreading, secretion of bioactive substances, aggregation, and acceleration of the coagulation process.[3]

Platelet activation, a term that encompasses the processes of adhesion, secretion, and aggregation, is stimulated by a variety of agents (platelet agonists) in vivo and in vitro, including collagen, thrombin, adenosine diphosphate (ADP), epinephrine, and arachidonic acid. Activated platelets are characterized physically by the loss of their discoid shape and the appearance of microtubules and physiologically by conversion of their membrane to a procoagulant surface and the secretion of a number of procoagulant substances (Fig. 43–2). Activation of platelets somehow activates platelet receptors, causing either conformational change or translocation (perhaps from the inside of the phospholipid membrane). These glycoprotein (GP) receptors (Table 43–1) bind subendothelial and plasma proteins and clotting factors such as fibrinogen, von Willebrand's

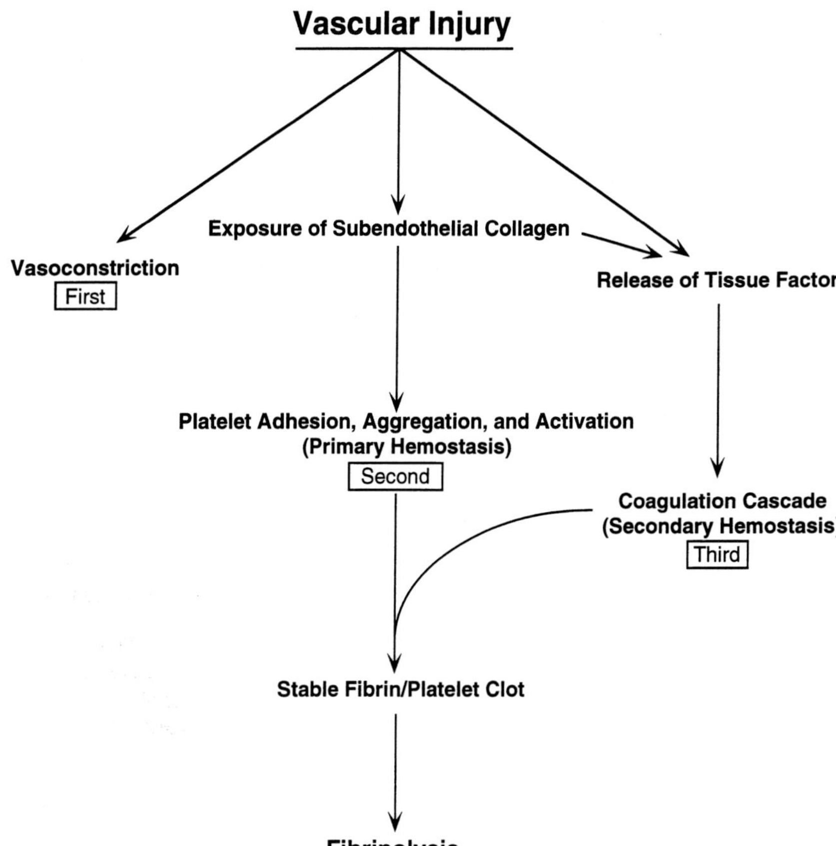

FIGURE 43–1. A simplified schematic of the process of coagulation. All steps interact with each other. Vasoconstriction occurs first, followed by platelet activation and stimulation of the coagulation cascade, primarily via the tissue factor: factor VII complex–mediated activation of factor X (extrinsic pathway). The coagulation cascade requires activated platelets for optimal function and results in cross-linked fibrin, which stabilizes the initial platelet plug. (Modified from Schwartz, SI: Hemostasis, surgical bleeding, and transfusion. *In* Schwartz SI, Shires GT, Spencer FC [eds]: Principles of Surgery, 6th ed. New York, McGraw-Hill, 1994, p 96. Courtesy of the McGraw-Hill Companies.)

factor (vWF), and activated factor V, causing signal transduction across the platelet membrane. Factor V, the essential procoagulant catalytic cofactor for factor Xa, is both secreted by the activated platelet and present in the circulating bloodstream. Factor Va binds factor Xa on the surface of the platelet membrane, forming prothrombinase, the factor responsible for converting prothrombin to thrombin.[10–14]

Platelets do not adhere to intact endothelium but recognize, via their glycoprotein receptors, molecules such as subendothelial collagen (via GPIa/IIa) exposed only after endothelial damage. Subendothelial vWF also mediates

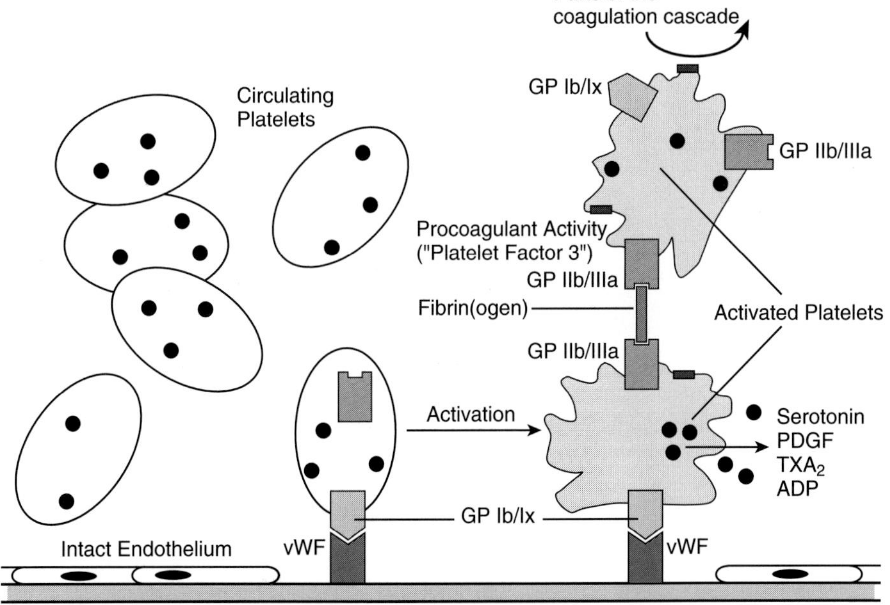

FIGURE 43–2. Schematic representation of platelet activation in response to endothelial injury. In general, von Willebrand factor (vWF) mediates platelet-subendothelial interactions, and fibrinogen mediates platelet-platelet interactions. The fibrinogen receptor, glycoprotein (GP) IIb/IIIa, is not functional until the platelet is activated. PDGF = platelet-derived growth factor; TXA_2 = thromboxane A_2; ADP = adenosine diphosphate. (Modified from Scott-Connor, CEH, Rigdon, EE, Rock WA: Hematology. *In* O'Leary P [ed]: The Physiologic Basis of Surgery. Baltimore, Williams & Wilkins, 1993, p 414.)

TABLE 43–1. PLATELET GLYCOPROTEIN (GP) RECEPTORS

GP RECEPTOR	LIGAND
Ia/IIa	Collagen
Ib	Thrombin
Ib/Ix/V	von Willebrand's factor
Ic/IIa	Fibronectin
IIb/IIIa	Fibrinogen, von Willebrand's factor, and others
IV	Thrombospondin

platelet adherence (via GPIb/Ix), especially at high shear rates. After adhesion, platelets change their shape and spread out on the injured endothelial surface. More platelets then accumulate, adhering to the initial monolayer (platelet aggregation).[15–17]

Platelet degranulation and secretion then occurs, stimulated by a variety of substances, including ADP, platelet-activating factor (PAF), and thromboxane A_2. Elevation of cytoplasmic calcium, which induces fusion of the granule membrane with the outer platelet membrane, is believed to be the common mechanism. There are three types of platelet granules:

- Dense granules (which contain serotonin and ADP)
- α-granules (fibrinogen, vWF, factor V, platelet factor 4, and platelet-derived growth factor)
- Lysosomes (acid hydrolases)

Modulation of platelet activation and degranulation is achieved by endothelial secretion of substances such as thrombomodulin and ADPase and by stimulation of cyclic adenosine monophosphate (cAMP) production within the platelet cytoplasm by arachidonic acid products.[17–19]

To review hemostasis as discussed to this point, the first response to injury is local vasoconstriction. Very quickly, platelets adhere to subendothelial molecules newly exposed by injured, denuded endothelium. Platelets become activated, change shape, and degranulate. The contents of these granules are chemotactic and stimulatory to platelets. More platelets accumulate, forming the initial platelet plug of primary hemostasis and providing a surface on which many of the reactions of the coagulation cascade take place.

Coagulation Cascade

Secondary hemostasis refers to the process of fibrin formation and stabilization of the initial platelet plug and clot, and it is caused by sequential activation of the coagulation cascade. The coagulation cascade (Fig. 43–3) is generally di-

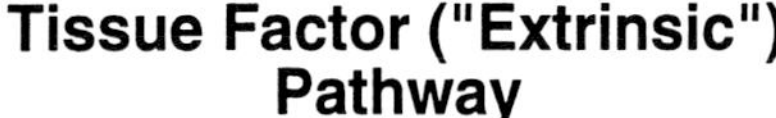

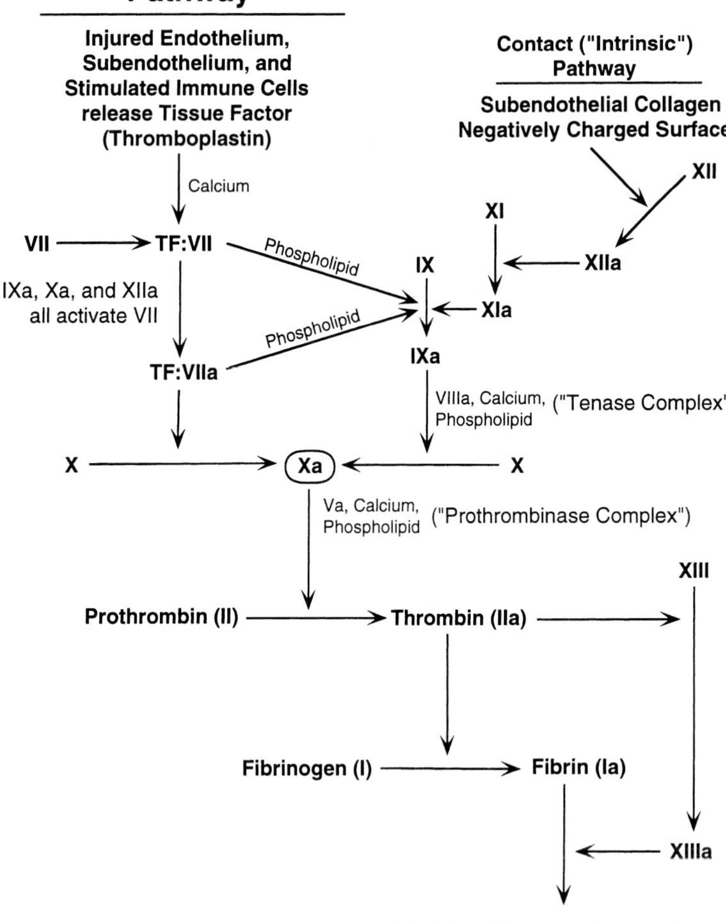

FIGURE 43–3. Schematic representation of the coagulation cascade illustrating the primary role of the tissue factor (TF) (extrinsic) pathway. Note the central role of the TF factor VII and VIIa complexes, which directly activate both factors IX and IX. Thrombin (factor II) activates both fibrinogen (I) and factor XIII, the latter necessary for stabilization of the initial fibrin clot. Factors IXa, Xa, and XIIa all promote activation of factor VII, and it has been suggested that they (along with factor VIIIa) are merely amplification factors for the tissue factor pathway. (From Thijs LG, de Boer JP, de Groot MCM, et al: Coagulation disorders in septic shock. Intensive Care Med 19[Suppl]:58, 1993.)

TABLE 43–2. COAGULATION FACTORS

FACTOR NO.	NAME
I	Fibrinogen
II	Prothrombin
III	Tissue factor (tissue thromboplastin)
IV	Calcium ions
V	Proaccelerin
VII	Proconvertin
VIII	Antihemophiliac factor
IX	Plasma thromboplastin component (Christmas factor)
X	Stuart-Prower factor
XI	Plasma thromboplastin antecedent
XII	Hageman factor
XIII	Fibrin-stabilizing factor

Note: There is no factor VI; it was originally used to denote what was discovered to be factor Va.

vided into two pathways of thrombin generation: the *intrinsic* ("contact") and *extrinsic* ("tissue factor") pathways. These terms actually have little clinical relevance and overlap at multiple points, but they are useful for descriptive purposes.

The intrinsic system is initiated by surface contact. The first protein in this pathway is factor XII, or Hageman factor (Table 43–2), which is activated by contact with negatively charged substances such as collagen, endotoxin, and subendothelium.[3, 20] The substrates of activated factor XII (factor XIIa) are factor XI and kallikrein, and factor XIIa is subject to both positive and negative feedback by kallikrein. Factor XIa converts factor IX, one of the vitamin K–dependent factors, to factor IXa, which then converts factor X to Xa, a process greatly accelerated by the presence of the factor VIII-vWF complex and calcium.[20]

The extrinsic pathway is activated by extravascular substances resulting from injury, classically tissue factor (TF; also called *tissue thromboplastin*). TF and calcium bind to factor VII, a complex that itself can activate factors IX and X or can become activated to factor VIIa (thus, TF and factor VII can both initiate intrinsic and extrinsic pathways). The TF-VIIa complex, however, possesses a 100-fold greater activity than does TF-VII.[21] The activation of factor VII to VIIa in turn undergoes both positive and negative feedback by factor Xa. TF pathway inhibitors, a new class of anticoagulants, block the action of TF-VIIa on both factor IX and factor X (intrinsic and extrinsic pathways, respectively).[22–24]

The two pathways unite permanently when factor X is activated, but this occurs in two slightly different ways. Via the intrinsic, contact pathway, factors IXa and VIIIa and phospholipid, collectively called the *tenase complex,* cleave factor X in the presence of calcium on activated platelet and endothelial membranes.[20, 25, 26] Via the extrinsic, "TF" pathway, the TF-VIIa complex on monocyte or endothelial cell membranes cleaves X, which (as Xa) remains membrane bound.[3, 22]

Factor Xa (produced by both pathways), factor Va, calcium, and phospholipid combine on the platelet membrane to form the prothrombinase complex, which converts prothrombin (factor II) to thrombin (factor IIa). The formation of thrombin by the TF pathway is faster than by the contact pathway, and, in fact, evidence is mounting that the TF pathway is the clinically most significant means of thrombin generation,[23] and it has even been suggested that factors VIII, IX, and XI be considered merely amplification factors for the TF pathway.[27]

The conversion of fibrinogen (factor I) to fibrin (factor Ia) by thrombin is the ultimate outcome of the coagulation cascade and results in a stable clot in which platelets and thrombus are stabilized into a network of cross-linked fibers. Fibrinogen, a large glycoprotein, is found in platelet granules and as a soluble plasma protein. Thrombin binds to the central domain of fibrinogen, liberating fibrinopeptides A and B and generating the formation of fibrin monomers and polymers. Growth of the fibrin strand occurs both longitudinally and laterally, with the lateral growth being of greatest importance in clot strength. Resistance to degradation is conferred by the presence of fibrin cross-links, produced by factor XIIIa (Fig. 43–4). The mature fibrin mesh entraps aggregated platelets and further controls hemorrhage at the site of injury. Fibrin also assists in platelet-endothelium interactions through the action of

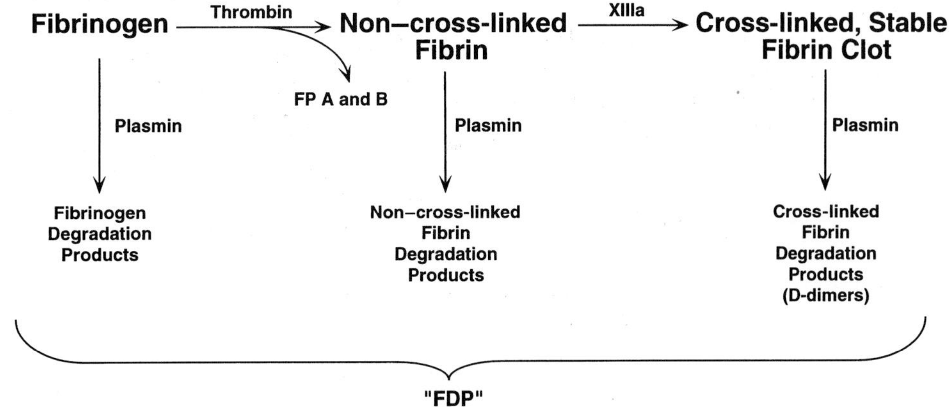

FIGURE 43–4. Fibrinogen activation and degradation. Note that plasmin attacks all forms of fibrin(ogen). Hence overactivation of plasmin (disseminated intravascular coagulation or primary fibrinolysis) will result in fibrinogen depletion and elevation of fibrin degradation products (FDP), the generic name for breakdown products of any form of fibrin. D-dimers, however, imply breakdown of mature, cross-linked clot and are thus (in theory) seen only during primary fibrinolysis. (Modified from Francis CW, Marder VJ: Mechanisms of thrombolysis. *In* Beutler E, Lichtman MA, Coller BS, et al [eds]: Williams' Hematology, 5th ed. New York, McGraw-Hill, 1995, p 1256. Courtesy of the McGraw-Hill Companies. Original source: Colman RW, Hirsh J, Marder VJ, et al: Hemostasis and Thrombosis: Basic Principles and Clinical Practice, 3rd ed. Philadelpha, JB Lippincott, 1994, p 1256.)

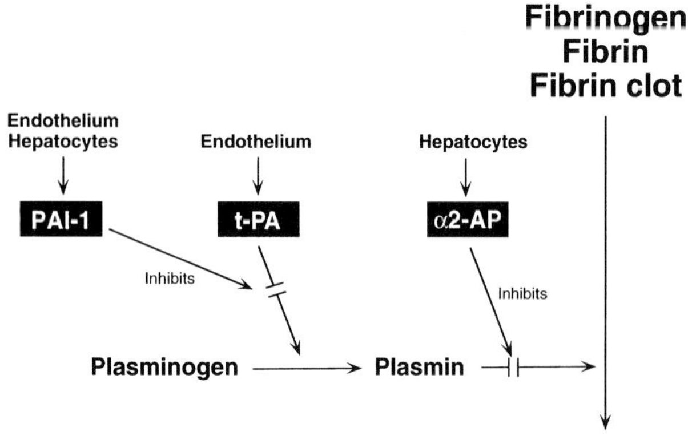

FIGURE 43–5. Fibrinolytic molecules and their inhibitors. Tissue plasminogen activator (t-PA), as well as other physiologic and therapeutic molecules, lyses clot indirectly by cleaving plasminogen to plasmin. Plasminogen activator inhibitors (PAIs), the most common being PAI-1, inhibit t-PA and other plasminogen inhibitors, while α_2-antiplasmin (α_2-AP) directly inhibits plasmin's action on fibrin(ogen). (From Illig, KA, Green, RM, Ouriel, K, et al: Primary fibrinolysis during supraceliac clamping. J Vasc Surg 25:245, 1997.)

proteins such as fibronectin, which has affinity for cross-linked fibrin as well as for collagen present in the injured vessel wall.[28, 29]

Fibrinolysis and Restraints

There are several mechanisms that restrict the coagulation process to the area where it is needed to control local hemorrhage, thus preventing diffuse activation throughout the vascular system. These mechanisms include dilution of factors by flowing blood, inhibition of coagulation factors by negative feedback loops and specific plasma proteins, and fibrinolysis. An example of self-limitation is that thrombin itself inactivates factors Va and VIIIa. Other important components of the restraint system include AT III and protein C; AT III binds and inactivates thrombin, while activated protein C inactivates factors Va and VIIIa.[30–33]

Fibrinolysis, the degradation of cross-linked fibrin, represents an additional pathway limiting thrombosis. The conversion of plasminogen to plasmin by plasminogen activators is the final common pathway for this event, and it is greatly enhanced if plasminogen is bound to fibrin at fibrin's lysine-binding sites. There are a variety of plasminogen activators and inhibitors, including t-PA (released by endothelial cells) and urokinase-type plasminogen activators. Excess plasmin activation (and subsequent fibrin degradation) is prevented by direct plasmin inhibition (α_2-antiplasmin, free floating and bound to fibrin within the clot) and plasminogen activator inhibitors (PAIs) (Fig. 43–5).[34–37]

TESTS OF COAGULATION

To understand, diagnose, and treat hemorrhagic problems, a knowledge of common clinically available tests of coagulation is essential (Table 43–3).

Prothrombin Time

The prothrombin time (PT) is a rough assessment of the extrinsic pathway of coagulation and is measured by subjecting citrated plasma to clotting in response to TF, phospholipid, and calcium. The PT is highly sensitive to the function of the four vitamin K–dependent factors, II, VII, IX, and X, as well as to V.[38–40] Vitamin K–dependent factors are inhibited by warfarin, and the resultant therapeutic anticoagulation is most easily monitored by the PT and its more accurate derived value, the International Normalized Ratio (INR), used to lessen interlaboratory variability.

Elevations in the PT are usually due to iatrogenic warfarin use, vitamin K deficiency (malnutrition or biliary obstruction, most commonly), disseminated intravascular coagulation (DIC), and liver dysfunction and can best be corrected by administration of fresh frozen plasma (FFP) or vitamin K. PT can also be elevated in the setting of high doses of heparin or argatroban because of factor II inhibition.[41]

Activated Partial Thromboplastin Time

The activated partial thromboplastin time (aPTT) roughly measures function of the intrinsic pathway and is sensitive, in varying degrees, to most factors other than VII.[40] Interestingly, mild deficiencies of a single factor may not prolong the aPTT, but the effect of multiple factor deficiencies seems to be exponential. aPTT is measured by subjecting citrated plasma to clotting after exposure to a partial thromboplastin phospholipid alone (PTT) or with a contact factor activator (aPTT).[39, 40] The aPTT is consistently elevated during heparin and argatroban administration due to factor II inhibition, but because low-molecular-weight heparin has relatively little AT III and hence anti-II activity, it will affect the aPTT in a less predictable way.[42, 43]

The aPTT is often elevated as part of a global coagulopathy and often responds to protamine administration even if heparin has not been given or has been adequately reversed. If the aPTT is abnormal, either a factor deficiency or a circulating anticoagulant (e.g., heparin or lupus anticoagulant) is present. If the aPTT normalizes with the addition of normal plasma, the factor deficiency exists; if not, a circulating anticoagulant should be suspected.

The PT and aPTT, as relatively global tests of overlapping factor function (see Fig. 43–3), often co-vary in the setting of coagulopathy, and high doses of any anticoagulant (warfarin, heparin, or other) usually increase both values. If the PT is elevated but the aPTT is normal, a factor VII defi-

TABLE 43–3. TESTS OF COAGULATION*

TEST	MEASURES	COMMON CAUSES OF ABNORMALITIES	CLINICAL USEFULNESS
Prothrombin time (PT)	II, V, VII, IX, and X [proteins C and S]	Warfarin use Liver dysfunction, malnutrition Consumptive coagulopathy	Monitor warfarin effect ID coagulopathy
Activated partial thromboplastin time (aPTT)	Most factors	Heparin use Consumptive coagulopathy Lupus anticoagulant	Monitor heparin, argatroban effect ID coagulopathy
Activated clotting time (ACT) monitoring	Global clotting function	Heparin use	Intraoperative
Thrombin time (TT)	Fibrinogen function	Fibrinolysis or dysfibrinogenemia Heparin Consumptive coagulopathy	Monitor systemic fibrinolysis
Bleeding time (BT)	Platelet number and function	Aspirin use Uremia Thrombocytopenia	Assess platelet dysfunction
Euglobulin clot lysis time (ECLT)	Fibrinolysis	Primary fibrinolysis	ID primary fibrinolysis
Fibrinogen, FDP	Fibrinolysis	Consumptive coagulopathy	ID coagulopathy
Platelet aggregation	Platelet aggregation	Rare platelet disorders [HATT]	Specific disorders
Thromboelastography (TEG)	Clotting kinetics	Multiple	Liver transplantation

*This list is not meant to be all-inclusive.
ID = identification; FDP = fibrin(ogen) degradation products; HATT = heparin-associated thrombosis/thrombocytopenia. Brackets denote related hypercoagulable mediators [proteins C and S] and diseases [HATT].

ciency must exist, usually due to vitamin K deficiency (biliary obstruction or malnutrition) or inhibition (warfarin use). In contrast, if the aPTT is elevated but the PT is normal, this indicates either hemophilia or the presence of a low to moderate dose of heparin.[40]

Activated Clotting Time

Closely related to the aPTT is the activated clotting time (ACT). This is a gross measure of the time needed for whole blood to clot when exposed to a coagulant-accelerating matrix, often diatomaceous earth. The ACT is helpful because it takes only a few minutes, and it is thus most useful in the operating room to assess adequacy of elective heparinization.

Thrombin Time

The thrombin time (TT) measures the thrombin-induced conversion of fibrinogen to fibrin and, as such, is a sensitive method to assess function of the very end of the coagulation pathway (see Fig. 43–3). It can be normal even with severe "upstream" coagulopathy (e.g., hemophilia or liver disease), but is very sensitive to low levels or abnormal forms of fibrinogen as well as to circulating inhibitors such as heparin or fibrin(ogen) degradation products (FDPs) associated with DIC.[40] The TT is abnormal in the setting of inherited dysfibrinogenemias, DIC (due to both hypofibrinogenemia and FDP), and in the presence of heparin, and it has been recommended by some to be the most clinically useful test to monitor therapeutic fibrinolysis (assuming heparin is not being infused).[44]

In our experience, other, more commonly obtained tests (fibrinogen and FDP levels) are as useful in this setting, and the TT is rarely used. Standard fibrinogen assays require the absence of anticoagulant and thus are notoriously inaccurate during therapeutic fibrinolysis as a result of circulating FDPs or concurrent heparin administration.

Bleeding Time

The bleeding time (BT) is the time needed for a superficial wound to clot and assesses primary hemostasis (platelet plug formation). It is sensitive to platelet number, platelet function, and, although not clinically relevant, to vasoconstriction. Because the platelet number can easily be measured, the BT is most valuable as a test of platelet function. It can be elevated whenever platelet function is abnormal (e.g., during aspirin use, uremia, or von Willebrand's disease) or thrombocytopenia exists, and it can be lengthened by decreased fibrinogen and factor V levels. Heparin can also increase the BT, probably because of platelet inhibition and interactions with vWF.[45]

The BT is measured by making a controlled wound with a template in the forearm (Ivy) or earlobe (Duke), and the time needed to clot is then measured with a timer.[46] Values over 5 minutes are typically abnormal. Unfortunately, however, BT is of no use as a preoperative screening test[47] and thus should be reserved for specific indications.

Euglobulin Clot Lysis Time

The euglobulin clot lysis time (ECLT) assesses the time needed for a clot to lyse in a test tube (less than 2 hours is abnormal); however, adequate clot formation is required in the first place. Thus, it is usually not helpful in the setting of DIC in which clot formation and lysis are abnormal. It can be quite helpful, however, when a primary fibrinolytic state is suspected.[33, 48, 49]

Thromboelastography

Thromboelastography (TEG) is a somewhat qualitative means of measuring overall coagulation and fibrinolytic function. Blood is placed in an oscillating chamber, and the changing resistive forces created by the clotting and lysing blood are expressed as a function of time. With values derived from the plot, it is possible to measure or estimate whole blood clotting time, platelet and factor function, fibrinolysis, and hypercoagulability.[50, 51] Although interesting in concept, TEG has not gained widespread acceptance, primarily because it is somewhat cumbersome and technician-dependent and the information it yields can be obtained more simply by judicious use of the tests discussed earlier. It is probably most useful during liver transplantation, when multiple channels can be run simultaneously as the cause of coagulopathy changes with different phases of the operation.[52]

Other Tests

Several other tests are commonly used. Fibrinogen levels are used to assess systemic proteolysis during fibrinolysis, whether therapeutic (e.g., intra-arterial urokinase) or pathologic (DIC); ongoing lysis lowers the fibrinogen level. Equally as useful is measurement of the degradation products of fibrin and fibrinogen, such as FDP and D-dimers. Specific factors can also be measured and are invaluable in the diagnosis of specific factor deficiencies (discussed later). Platelet aggregability is used for diagnosis and characterization of rare platelet disorders.

DISORDERS OF HEMOSTASIS

Disturbances of any of the elements responsible for normal hemostasis can result in excessive bleeding. An excessive bleeding disorder can be temporary or permanent, inherited or acquired, idiopathic or iatrogenic. Recognition of the problem requires an understanding of the disease process involved in each of the disorders. Clinically, disorders of platelet performance result in failure to initiate the hemostatic response, with excessive intraoperative bleeding that is controlled by local pressure and rarely recurs. In contrast, patients with disorders of blood coagulation experience clinical signs of failure to activate and amplify the coagulation cascade, which results in an excessive hemorrhage not responsive to local pressure and usually requiring administration of appropriate blood products to correct the problem.

Inherited Disorders of Hemostasis

Table 43–4 lists some of the most common hereditary causes of abnormal bleeding, tests designed to make the diagnoses, and general treatment strategies.

Platelet Abnormalities

Qualitative (abnormal function) or quantitative (thrombocytopenia) platelet defects can result in failure of hemostasis at the level of initiation—platelets fail to adhere, secrete, or aggregate. Defects in platelet membrane glycoprotein receptors characterize Glanzmann's thrombasthenia and Bernard-Soulier syndrome. In Glanzmann's thrombasthenia, GPIIb/IIIa (which binds fibrinogen and vWF, mediating platelet-platelet interactions) is lacking or defective, and platelet aggregation is impaired. In Bernard-Soulier syndrome, fewer GPIb/Ix/V, which collectively act as the major receptor for vWF, are present, and platelet adhesion is adversely affected. Patients have also been identified who

TABLE 43–4. COMMON HEREDITARY CAUSES OF BLEEDING AND TREATMENT STRATEGIES

DISORDER	CAUSE	DIAGNOSIS	TREATMENT
Glanzmann's thrombasthenia	Abnormal platelet GPIIb/IIIa (defective aggregation)	BT, platelet aggregation studies	Platelet transfusion
Bernard-Soulier syndrome	Reduced platelet GPIb/IX/V (defective adhesion)	BT, platelet aggregation studies	Platelet transfusion, DDAVP
Storage pool and release mechanism diseases	Defective platelet degranulation and secretion	BT, platelet aggregation studies	Platelet transfusion, DDAVP
von Willebrand's disease	Varies, most commonly reduced vWF	BT, platelet aggregation studies	DDAVP, vWF, cryoprecipitate
Hemophilia A	Reduced factor VIII	Factor assay	Factor VIII
Hemophilia B	Reduced factor IX	Factor assay	Factor IX
Fibrinogen disorders	Abnormal fibrinogen	Fibrinogen levels and analysis	Cryoprecipitate
Prothrombin disorders	Abnormal prothrombin and related factors	Specialized assays	Variable replacement
Specific factor deficiencies	Specific deficits	Factor assays	Specific factors

BT = bleeding time; DDAVP = desmopressin acetate (1-deamino-8-D-arginine vasopressin); vWF = von Willebrand's factor.

have deficient GPIa/IIa receptors, the collagen-binding site. Although these disorders are genetically and biochemically different, they are identical clinically. In both, bleeding problems are moderate to severe despite normal platelet counts, and diagnosis is made by platelet aggregation studies.

Abnormalities of platelet secretion include storage pool deficiency (diminished ADP in dense granules) and release deficiency (normal ADP with defective secretory mechanism). These disorders, also diagnosed by specialized platelet aggregation studies, are associated with only moderate bleeding.[53, 54]

von Willebrand's disease (vWD) is characterized by a quantitative or qualitative defect in the adhesive proteins vWF or factor VIII and is the most common inherited bleeding disorder, with an estimated incidence ranging as high as 1%.[55] vWF, via GPIb and GPIIb/IIIa, is required for platelet adhesion to injured endothelium and exists alone or, more commonly, as a complex with factor VIII, depending on whether its location is intravascular, endothelial, or within the platelet granule or megakaryocyte (because factor VIII and vWF are often associated, they were originally thought to be one molecule).

There are at least three primary types (with multiple subgroups) of vWD, most of which are transmitted in an autosomal dominant pattern. The most common type, *type I*, is due to decreased levels of vWF. The clinical picture in patients with vWD is varied. When mild, the condition can remain undetected well into adulthood, often until a surgical challenge occurs. A history of bleeding from mucocutaneous surfaces, easy bruisability, and prolonged bleeding from lacerations is common. The diagnosis is made on the basis of a prolonged BT combined with a reduced ristocetin-induced platelet aggregation response. Therapy is rarely required in the absence of surgery or major trauma.[55–57]

Hemophilias A and B

Hemophilias A and B are less variable and more severe in their clinical manifestations, and they are indistinguishable clinically from each other. Both are X-linked recessive disorders and hence occur almost exclusively in males. Hemophilia A (80% of cases) is the result of a deficiency or absence of factor VIII, whereas hemophilia B (Christmas disease) is the result of a deficiency or absence of factor IX. Patients with hemophilia experience little bleeding from superficial lacerations because of their intact platelet function. Spontaneous hemorrhage into joints and deep muscle spaces after minimal trauma and massive intraoperative hemorrhage, however, are more common.

The severity of bleeding encountered in daily life and in surgical procedures can be predicted by measurement of plasma levels of factors VIII and IX in hemophilias A and B, respectively. Patients with factor levels less than 1% of normal are classified as having severe hemophilia; those with levels greater than 5% of normal, mild; and those with intermediate values, moderately severe.[58–61]

Disorders of Fibrinogen

Disorders of fibrinogen structure and function (hypofibrinogenemia and dysfibrinogenemia) can be hereditary or acquired and are variable in expression. Diagnosis is based on identification (with specialized reagents) of low fibrinogen levels and prolonged clotting times.[62] Disorders involving fibrinogen also affect platelet function. Patients with congenital afibrinogenemia, interestingly, rarely manifest spontaneous bleeding.

Other Inherited Hemostatic Defects

Inherited disorders of prothrombin conversion include abnormalities and deficiencies of factors II (prothrombin), V, VII, and X, all of which are synthesized in the liver, and (with the exception of factor V) they require vitamin K for synthesis. The clinical features of these rare disorders are similar to those of the hemophilias, including variable penetrance and clinical severity. Disorders involving prothrombin itself (hypoprothrombinemia and the dysprothrombinemias) are characterized by variable elevations of the PT and aPTT, with normal TT. Definitive diagnosis involves functional and immunologic prothrombin assays.

Deficiencies of factor V, the essential procoagulant cofactor for factor Xa, are transmitted in an autosomal recessive pattern and are definitively diagnosed by factor V assay. Patients with factor VII deficiency have an unusually variable clinical presentation and characteristically exhibit prolonged PT with normal aPTT and TT; again definitive diagnosis depends on performance of a specific assay for factor VII. Factor X deficiency results in prolongation of the PT and aPTT and is also diagnosed by specific factor assay.[63]

Acquired Disorders of Hemostasis

Table 43–5 lists some of the most common nonhereditary causes of abnormal bleeding, tests designed to make the diagnoses, and general treatment strategies.

Platelet Disorders

Acquired platelet disorders include a wide variety of abnormalities, including functional, anatomic, and quantitative defects. Thrombocytopenia is the most common manifestation. Such disorders are usually part of a larger disease process such as uremia, hypersplenism, hematologic malignancies (and their treatment), immune thrombocytopenic purpura (ITP), and thrombotic thrombocytopenic purpura (TTP).

Acquired vWD can occur in patients with hematologic malignancies and immunologic disorders. It probably results from the development of antibodies against vWF or factor VIII. Severity of bleeding is variable, but the diagnosis should be considered for patients with myeloproliferative and associated disorders who experience excessive bleeding complications.[53, 64]

Uremia

The primary hemostatic abnormality in patients with renal failure involves poor platelet function or other defects of primary hemostasis. Mechanisms are numerous and incompletely understood, but they include abnormalities within the platelets themselves as well as impaired excretion of toxins that impede platelet function—thus some hemor-

TABLE 43–5. COMMON NONHEREDITARY CAUSES OF BLEEDING AND TREATMENT STRATEGIES*

SITUATION	CAUSE	DIAGNOSIS	TREATMENT
Heparin use	Antifactor II (via AT III)	Elevated aPTT (and PT)	Protamine
Argatroban use	Direct anti-II	Elevated aPTT (and PT)	FFP
Warfarin use Hepatic failure Malnutrition Biliary obstruction	Inhibition of II, VII, IX, and X	Elevated PT (with normal aPTT)	FFP, Vitamin K
Dilution	Fewer molecules and cells	Clinical situation, global dysfunction	Replace missing substances
Marrow failure	Thrombocytopenia	Thrombocytopenia, smear, marrow biopsy	Platelet transfusions
Acidosis	Diminished enzyme function	Clinical situation, global dysfunction	Correct cause, bicarbonate
Hypothermia	Diminished enzyme and platelet function	Clinical situation, global dysfunction	Warm
Disseminated intravascular coagulopathy	Global activation of entire clotting system	Clinical situation, elevated FDP, PT, aPTT, reduced fibrinogen, and platelets	Correct the cause, replace as needed
Thrombolytic therapy	Reduced fibrinogen, clot lysis	Clinical situation, elevated FDP, TT, ECLT	Cryoprecipitate
Primary fibrinolysis	Reduced fibrinogen, clot lysis	Clinical situation, elevated FDP, TT, ECLT	Antifibrinolytics
Uremia	Impaired platelet/endothelial binding	Lengthened BT	DDAVP
Aspirin use	Permanent platelet dysfunction	Lengthened BT	Platelet transfusions
Specific inhibitors	Antifactor (usually VIII)	Resistance to factor replacement	High doses, immunosuppression

*Table is not all-inclusive.
AT III = antithrombin III; PT = prothrombin time; aPTT = activated partial thromboplastin time; FFP = fresh frozen plasma; FDP = fibrin(ogen) degradation products; TT = thrombin time; ECLT = euglobulin clot lysis time; BT = bleeding time; DDAVP = desmopressin acetate (1-deamino-8-D-arginine vasopressin).

rhagic tendencies correct with dialysis, while others persist. Possible platelet defects in uremia include abnormal GPIIb/IIIa, functional cyclooxygenase defect due to abnormal prostaglandin synthesis, abnormal platelet serotonin, cAMP, and storage pool ADP levels, and elevated platelet calcium content. Uremic products adversely affecting platelet function include inhibitors of glucose utilization, fibrinolysis, serotonin release, aggregation, and thromboxane production.[53, 65]

Vitamin K–Related Disorders

Factors II, VII, IX, and X, the four vitamin K–dependent clotting factors, must undergo γ-carboxylation to become active, and vitamin K acts as the essential cofactor. Thus, these factors are inactive without it, and when vitamin K availability is reduced, can precipitate coagulopathy.[38, 66–68] Vitamin K is fat-soluble, and thus depends on adequate bile secretion, nutrition, and gut absorptive function to be assimilated into the bloodstream. Hence, biliary obstruction, malnutrition, gut bacterial overgrowth, and other functional disturbances are common causes of bleeding problems in hospitalized patients.

Liver Disease

The liver is the sole or primary site of synthesis for essentially all of the important coagulation factors, proteins C and S, plasminogen, α_2-antiplasmin, plasminogen activator inhibitor-a (PAI-1), and other regulatory proteins such as AT III and C1 inhibitor. In addition, the liver plays a major role in the clearance of activated coagulation factors and plasminogen activators. Reduced synthesis of the four vitamin K–dependent factors contributes substantially to bleeding in patients with liver failure, but abnormal fibrinogen synthesis, thrombocytopenia, functional platelet defects, and low-grade, chronic DIC also contribute significantly.[33, 53, 68–72] In the operating room, of course, the relatively high portal pressure and resultant fragile, extensive collateralization also increase the risk of hemorrhage.

Disseminated Intravascular Coagulation

Although *consumptive coagulopathy* is a more accurate descriptive term for the clinical syndrome usually called *disseminated intravascular coagulopathy* (DIC), the latter name remains in common use. Like the pulmonary system, the coagulation system has a limited ability to respond to injury. The final common pathway for many insults, including bacteremia (endotoxemia), trauma (especially burns with extensive tissue damage), necrotic tissue and severe infection, malignancy with release of tumor necrosis factor (TNF), intravascular prosthetic devices with destruction of circulating blood cells, other metabolic toxins, extremes of temperature and pH, hypoperfusion, and even pain, is uncontrolled systemic activation and consumption of all clotting mediators, including thrombin, platelets, and the fibrinolytic system. This leads to two simultaneous events: (1) uncontrolled, inappropriate systemic coagulation (excess systemic thrombin) and (2) ongoing secondary fibrinolysis (excess systemic plasmin).[27, 39, 68, 73, 74]

DIC seems to be a disorder of the TF (extrinsic) coagulation pathway. All the stimuli above, either directly or via cytokines such as interleukin-1 (IL-1) or TNF, cause release of TF from subendothelium or other cells. Thrombocytopenia usually coincides with or precedes the triggering of the coagulation cascade, as platelets are consumed peripherally at the site of infection or tissue damage or coated with immunoglobulin G (IgG) or specific antibodies. The consequent membrane damage and partial or complete activation causes their membranes either to transform into procoagulant surfaces (generally called *platelet factor 3*) or to express TF. This uncontrolled and ongoing release of TF causes widespread activation of factor VII and the formation of TF-VIIa complex, which in turn leads to generation of factor Xa, which triggers an intense exponential "explosion" of thrombin production.[27, 68, 74]

Although all activated clotting factors are subject to inhibition, they are relatively protected while on procoagulant surfaces. Moreover, the excess thrombin diffuses to create larger and larger zones of activation, upstream and downstream, and further amplifies fibrin production. Plasmin is produced to compensate for the widespread fibrin production. This plasmin originally plays a protective role by lysing microvascular clot. Excessive plasminogen activation, however, can outstrip its restraints and inhibitors to result in attack on the coagulation factors themselves.[75] The progressive consumption of fibrinogen, factor V, and factor VII by unrestricted activation and their destruction by plasmin as part of plasma proteolysis worsen the situation. If the original pathologic stimuli are sustained, the reserves of coagulation factors are exhausted, and the production of fresh coagulation factors is finally outstripped by their consumption (hence the term *consumptive coagulopathy*).

Should thrombin generation and fibrin accumulation continue to be amplified, fibrin microthrombi are produced. These microthrombi lodge in the microcirculation, especially in the vascular beds of the kidney, brain, lung, adrenal glands, and skin, impairing blood flow, nutrient delivery, and organ function. Polymerization of fibrin monomers initiates compensatory plasmin activation and (secondary) fibrinolysis. The degree of organ damage from occlusion of the microcirculation by these fibrin-rich microthrombi depends on the balance between their formation and lysis by plasmin. Thus, the secondary fibrinolysis that occurs as part of DIC is critical and should not be inhibited.[75, 76] Unfortunately, this necessary fibrinolysis further impairs hemostasis because the products of fibrinogen and fibrin degradation (FDP, D-dimers, and various fibrinopeptides) themselves are anticoagulants in large quantities, acting as antithrombins, potentiating thrombolysis, and interfering with fibrin polymerization.[77, 78]

DIC is probably not an "all-or-nothing" event, but exists, to varying degrees, in many conditions and commonly arises from other, inadequately treated problems. For example, in a patient who is cold and underperfused, coagulopathy may initially be simply an enzymatic dysfunction. If the initial insult is not corrected and bleeding persists, however, the worsened hypothermia, acidosis, and toxemia induced by ischemic tissue may push the coagulation system into true DIC. Many patients with abdominal aortic aneurysms (AAA) display asymptomatic laboratory evidence of DIC ("chronic DIC").[79, 80]

DIC can be distinguished from simpler disturbances, in a philosophical but clinically very important sense, by the fact that it tends to be very resistant to correction once it is in full bloom. This is for several reasons:

1. The insult that leads to it is often relatively chronic and is often persistent despite all efforts to the contrary.
2. Activation is usually widespread, ongoing, and massive, exceeding the ability of the body to replace needed factors.
3. Many of the degradation products produced by the syndrome are active anticoagulants (notably FDP), which easily initiate a positive-feedback loop.

Therefore, prevention is critical.

DIC is usually a clinical diagnosis, obvious from the situation, and associated with evidence of consumption of all elements of the coagulation system, especially fibrinogen, thrombin, and platelets. This is manifest by prolonged coagulation tests (PT, aPTT, TT, and ACT), thrombocytopenia, prolonged bleeding times, and hypofibrinogenemia. FDP and D-dimer levels are usually elevated, and the ECLT may show early lysis (if fibrinolysis predominates) or may reveal an inability to form clot at all (if consumption predominates).

Primary Fibrinolysis

Primary fibrinolysis should be distinguished from the secondary fibrinolysis seen as part of DIC. In DIC, fibrinolytic activation occurs as a secondary event, acting to lyse intravascular microthrombi. As such, it is therapeutic, vital to tissue perfusion, and should not be inhibited. In contrast, in primary fibrinolytic states, fibrinolysis occurs de novo as the primary problem, and direct inhibition is often beneficial.[68, 75]

The mechanism by which bleeding occurs differs somewhat from that of DIC. In primary fibrinolysis, direct plasminogen activation is the primary problem rather than being secondary to high thrombin and fibrin clot levels as it is in DIC. Plasmin saturates its inhibitors, especially PAI-1 and α_2-antiplasmin so that free plasmin builds up in the circulation (see Fig. 43–5). "Upstream" substances (factors V and VIII) as well as fibrin and fibrinogen are destroyed. Plasmin generated on the surface of platelets and endothelial cells, as well as within clot, attacks the cell membranes and their receptors and inappropriately lyses hemostatic plugs. Compensatory thrombin generation is quickly amplified, and platelets are recruited in an effort to restore endothelial competence and hemostasis. Platelets are not destroyed, but their function is impaired. Fibrin monomers and FDP are created. In both circumstances, microvascular coagulation occurs when the reticuloendothelial and macrophage-phagocyte systems become overwhelmed. Thus occurs the paradoxical development of microvascular thrombosis and massive hemorrhage observed in both DIC and primary fibrinolysis.[33, 81, 82]

Primary fibrinolysis is caused by high levels of fibrinolytic enzymes in the circulation and occurs in several situations. Best described is the elevation in t-PA seen in cirrhosis and liver failure, possibly due to deficient synthesis of competent PAI-1 and other barriers to plasminogen activation or to inadequate clearance of plasminogen activators[33, 71] and during the anhepatic phase of liver transplantation.[52, 83] Rapid synthesis and release of activators by various neoplasms can also occur, and several venomous snakes secrete antifibrinolytics.[33, 84] More relevant to the vascular surgeon, however, are the iatrogenic administration of fibrinolytic agents for arterial and venous thrombosis and the elevation in t-PA levels seen during supraceliac aortic clamping for paravisceral and thoracoabdominal aneurysm repairs, presumably due to hepatic hypoperfusion.[49, 85] t-PA is extremely rapidly metabolized by the liver[86]; thus, restoring hepatic perfusion and stopping any infused agent are usually adequate, especially if the duration of insult is short.

Drug-Induced Disorders of Hemostasis

In many instances, patients requiring either elective or emergency operation are receiving antithrombotic or thrombolytic agents. Decisions must be made on an individual basis regarding whether the agent should be discontinued prior to the procedure.

Heparin is a naturally occurring glycosaminoglycan, with a molecular weight ranging from 2000 to 40,000 daltons. It binds to and dramatically increases the ability of AT III to inactivate the components of the intrinsic coagulation cascade, factors IXa, Xa, XIa, XIIa, and especially thrombin. Heparin anticoagulation results in prolonged aPTT and ACT, but in moderate doses it does not affect BT or PT. Heparin can be administered only parenterally, either intravenously or subcutaneously. Its half-life is predictable when the intravenous route is utilized (~1.5 hours), but is less so when the subcutaneous route is selected (due to both slower absorption and altered metabolism); the effect of heparin administered by this route may persist up to 8 hours.[87, 88]

Low-molecular-weight (LMW) heparin (4000 to 8000 daltons) is being used instead of unfractionated heparin with increasing frequency. Advantages of LMW heparin include the ability to provide both full anticoagulation and prophylaxis via the subcutaneous route without the need to monitor coagulation parameters. Because its bioavailability, and metabolism are more predictable, LMW heparin acts primarily by inhibition of factor Xa and has a much higher anti-Xa:anti-IIa activity than does conventional heparin. As such, LMW heparin does not affect the aPTT as reliably as conventional heparin does.[42, 43, 89]

Argatroban (Novastan, Texas Biotechnology) is a new direct antithrombin agent currently in clinical trials for the treatment of heparin-induced thrombocytopenia and thrombosis. It has shown much promise with few side effects and may be available for clinical use in the near future.[41] Other novel antithrombotics are also in various stages of development.

Warfarin, an orally administered anticoagulant, interferes with the action of vitamin K on the hepatic synthesis of factors II, VII, IX, and X. Vitamin K is responsible for γ-carboxylation and generation of calcium-binding sites on these factors; without vitamin K, they are synthesized in a nonfunctional form. Anticoagulation with warfarin requires concomitant use of heparin for the first several days, for two reasons:

1. The half-life of prothrombin (factor II), responsible for the anticoagulant effects of warfarin, is longer than that of factor VII, most responsible for elevations in the PT. Therefore, although the PT may be elevated within 24 hours, a therapeutic anticoagulant state may not yet be in effect.
2. Warfarin also inhibits the anticoagulant proteins C and S, which have the shortest half-lives of all. Therefore, early after warfarin administration, a paradoxic hypercoagulable state can occur.[38, 90]

Antiplatelet agents are commonly administered to patients with vascular disease. Aspirin, clopidogrel, and ticlopidine irreversibly inhibit platelet aggregation. Aspirin inactivates platelet cyclooxygenase, inhibiting platelet synthesis of thromboxane A_2, whereas clopidogrel and ticlopidine alter the platelet membrane structure, decreasing expression of GPIIb/IIIa by blocking the ADP receptor. The effects of these agents usually persist for 4 to 7 days after medication is stopped, until enough new, functional platelets have been synthesized.[91]

Specific Inhibitors

Inhibitors to specific procoagulant proteins can be acquired, and catastrophic bleeding can arise if surgery is undertaken in such a patient. These inhibitors arise in 3% to 15% of persons with hemophilia (more commonly hemophilia A and when no native protein activity is present; i.e., the most severely affected patients), and, for this reason, surgery should not be performed in persons with hemophilia or other individuals who lack specific clotting activities until laboratory tests confirm that the substitution or replacement therapy given before operation is adequate to support surgical hemostasis.

Antibodies against factor VIII are by far the most frequently encountered; inhibitors of factor IX activity are much less frequent.[58–60, 92–94] In contrast to a simple deficiency of clotting activity, inhibitors prevent further enzyme activation in the enzyme sequence, and a barrier to activation of subsequent coagulation factors is created at the site of inhibition. The degree of inhibition and the impediment to hemostasis depend on the kinetics of the reaction between the antibody and its target coagulation factor antigen.

Inhibitors can occur in patients with no history of hemostatic problems, such as women early in the postpartum period, in patients with autoimmune or rheumatic connective tissue diseases, as part of systemic hypersensitivity (particularly a reaction to penicillin), in patients with malignancies (especially lymphomas), and in elderly patients without any obvious disease. The pathogenesis of these inhibitors is unclear. A genetic predisposition is suggested by twin studies.[92]

Fortunately, these inhibitors occur rarely and are always accompanied by abnormal coagulation test results. Unfortunately, because there is usually no history of bleeding at previous surgery and no history of bruising, a detailed history directed toward eliciting subtle recent changes in hemostasis may not have been taken, screening tests may not have been performed, and bleeding can be entirely unanticipated.

Global Inhibitors

The specific antibodies described earlier must be differentiated from global, nonspecific inhibitors. Nonspecific inhibitors are immunoglobulins directed against phospholipids and thus are generally called *antiphospholipid antibodies* (APAs). Because they were first seen in patients with systemic lupus erythematosus (SLE) and originally diagnosed by their ability to prolong the aPTT in vitro, they were originally named *lupus anticoagulants.* This name is a double misnomer. APAs are, in fact, procoagulants in vivo, and lupus anticoagulants are merely a special case within the general family of APAs, which include anticardiolipin antibodies as well.[92, 93, 95]

Because APAs are directed against phospholipids, they prolong the aPTT by interfering with multiple steps in the coagulation pathway. Analysis shows a variably decreased activity of factors XII, XI, and occasionally IX. This decrease is rarely (if ever) complete, and usually 30% to 50% of the activity remains and thrombin generation is not impaired. The effect of this interference is to prevent the factors from interacting with one another in vitro, but not to inhibit any specific clotting activity in vivo. Normal hemostasis with its intense procoagulant focus overrides the interference; as a result, these APAs are usually associated with hypercoagulation in vivo. Only antibodies targeted toward a specific clotting factor jeopardize hemostasis. Unfortunately, the mechanism whereby they act as procoagulants in vivo is poorly understood. Hypotheses include platelet activation, endothelial damage or inhibition of PGI_2 secretion, or interference with fibrinolysis.[92, 93]

Therapeutic Thrombolysis

All presently available thrombolytic agents, including streptokinase, urokinase, and t-PA, act indirectly, through conversion of plasminogen to plasmin. As such, the agents are known as *plasminogen activators,* and they lack activity in the absence of plasminogen. When administered systemically, two events occur.

First, both nonpathologic and pathologic thrombi are dissolved. Thus, the useful fibrin-platelet plug sealing a recent trivial defect in an intracerebral vessel is just as susceptible to thrombolytic dissolution as the pathologic thrombus obstructing a coronary artery. Second, systemic thrombolytic therapy produces widespread conversion of plasminogen to plasmin, producing systemic plasminemia, which leads to nonspecific proteolysis, including breakdown of circulating fibrinogen (see Fig. 43–5).

In the ideal situation, therapeutic peripheral arterial fibrinolysis is localized to the site of pathologic clot, usually by catheter-directed infusion, and systemic lysis does not occur. Unfortunately, the doses required to achieve rapid clot dissolution are high enough to produce a systemic proteolytic state similar to that observed with systemic therapy, and it must be assumed that any individual receiving or having recently received peripheral thrombolytic therapy may have a systemic lytic state. The pathophysiology is similar to that of primary fibrinolytic states, with low fibrinogen levels and high degradation products. The PT and aPTT may be normal (if factors have not been attacked by the excess plasmin), but the TT will be prolonged and the ECLT will be abnormally shortened.[96]

REPLACEMENT RESOURCES

To prevent or treat bleeding rationally, it is important to understand what options are available and what specific functions the various replacement resources have (Table 43–6). The reader is referred to several consensus statements and editorials on the use of blood products in the modern era for both medical and surgical indications.[97–103]

Packed Red Blood Cells

Packed red blood cells (PRBCs) are used to restore oxygen-carrying capacity. Their use as a volume expander has all but disappeared because of blood-borne transmissible diseases. Apparently as a result of an article published in 1942, for years the "gold standard" was to transfuse until a hemoglobin level of 10 mg/dl (a hematocrit of roughly 30%) was reached.[104, 105] Given the risk of disease transmission, along with the increasing realization that outcome is acceptable with a lower hematocrit (in part due to the beneficial effects of lowered blood viscosity), current consensus is that lower levels are safe. The National Institutes of Health (NIH) consensus conference recommendations are that otherwise healthy patients should have their hemoglobin levels maintained at 7 mg/dl or more. Obviously, treatment must be individualized, and alternative strategies for blood conservation such as preoperative autologous donation, erythropoietin use, acute normovolemic hemodilution, and intraoperative cell-saver devices should be considered in appropriate circumstances.[97, 100, 103, 106]

Fresh Frozen Plasma

Most coagulation factors, with the exception of factor VIII, are adequately replaced with fresh frozen plasma (FFP). FFP is most useful when an elevated PT is present, often after warfarin administration, or when liver dysfunction or a global coagulopathy is present. Again, because of the risk of blood-borne diseases, FFP should not be used as a volume expander, but rather reserved for situations in which multiple factor deficiencies or ongoing factor destruction exists (e.g., consumptive coagulopathy) or for the acute reversal of warfarin.[107] There is widespread consensus that physicians currently overuse FFP.[100, 102] FFP is immunogenic and should be given in an ABO, Rh-specific manner. It is the agent of choice for treatment of isolated factor deficiencies when a specific factor (e.g., factor V) is not available, but safe, recombinant factors VIII and IX have made FFP obsolete for treatment of the hemophilias.[58, 60, 94, 102]

Platelets

Platelets should be transfused for thrombocytopenia and probably used as the first prophylactic option during massive hemorrhage.[100] They are especially useful in the latter situation both because the resultant thrombocytopenia is usually the most important cause of resultant bleeding and because platelet concentrates contain a substantial amount of FFP and factor V. Although a platelet count of approximately 20/μl is usually adequate for maintenance of normal hemostasis, in the setting of active bleeding a target of 50 to 70/μl (even higher at times, to allow for ongoing loss or destruction) is usually recommended.[101]

TABLE 43–6. REPLACEMENT RESOURCES*

RESOURCE	CONTAINS OR REPLENISHES	COMMON USES	DOSE AND EFFECTS†
Packed red blood cells	Red cells	Replace oxygen-carrying capacity	1 unit (350 ml) increases hematocrit 3%
Platelets	Platelets Substantial clotting factors	Replace deficient or abnormal platelets Treat undefined clotting factor deficiency	1 unit (50 ml) increases platelets 10/μl
Fresh frozen plasma	Most clotting factors except V and VIII	Treat elevated PT	250 ml per unit
Cryoprecipitate	Rich in VIII, vWF, fibrinogen	Treat hypofibrinogenemia	20 ml contains 200 mg fibrinogen, 70 U VIII
DDAVP	Stimulates vWF release	Treat uremic platelet dysfunction	0.3–0.4 μg/kg
Vitamin K	Simulates II, VII, IX, and X	Treat elevated PT, hepatic dysfunction, warfarin overdosage	10–20 mg IM, SC, or IV
Protamine sulfate	Heparin antagonist	Reverse heparin, treat elevated aPTT	10 mg/1000 units of heparin
Amicar	Plasminogen inhibitor	Treat primary fibrinolysis	0.1 gm/kg load, 1 gm/hr
Aprotinin	Plasmin inhibitor	Treat primary fibrinolysis	3.75 mg/kg
Specific factors	Treat specific deficiencies	Many or most are now available in recombinant form with zero risk of disease transmission	

*Table is not all-inclusive.
†Doses, effects, and volumes are approximate and can vary by institution, indication, or formulation.
PT = prothrombin time; DDAVP = desmopressin acetate (1-deamino-8-D-arginine vasopressin); vWF = von Willebrand's factor; IM = intramuscular; SC = subcutaneous; IV = intravenous; aPTT = activated partial thromboplastin time; IU = international unit.

Cryoprecipitate

Cryoprecipitate is rich in factor VIII, vWF, and fibrinogen.[108, 109] It is most commonly used to increase fibrinogen levels during consumptive coagulopathy or when troublesome bleeding occurs during therapeutic thrombolysis. One bag (usually about 20 ml) contains about 200 to 250 mg fibrinogen and 70 units of factor VIII.

Desmopressin

Desmopressin acetate (1-deamino-8-D-arginine vasopressin [DDAVP]) is a synthetic vasopressin analogue. Although it has little vasoconstrictor activity, it has powerful hematologic effects. DDAVP increases factor VIII and vWF levels and thereby improves platelet adhesiveness to injured endothelium.[110, 111] Levels of both factors increase very quickly, and tachyphylaxis occurs, suggesting that DDAVP stimulates release of preformed molecules. DDAVP is especially useful in patients with uremic platelet dysfunction,[112] after cardiopulmonary bypass,[113] and in patients with mild type I vWD (who have low levels of vWF with normal vWF receptors),[55, 66] shortening the BT and reducing bleeding in each. Although prophylactic DDAVP use should be considered when major blood loss is anticipated, its effects have not been consistent.[114–116] DDAVP retains some antinatriuretic properties, and sodium and water balance should be monitored carefully in patients requiring large doses.[109]

Vitamin K

Vitamin K acts to carboxylate already synthesized factors stored in hepatocytes, which are released within about 6 hours after parenteral infusion; the PT usually normalizes within 18 to 24 hours.[66, 67] FFP is best for rapid correction of warfarin effect; the action of vitamin K is slower but more durable, making it harder for the patient to become reanticoagulated.

Protamine Sulfate

Protamine, which is positively charged, reverses the activity of a negatively charged heparin molecule by binding to it and restoring AT III to its native, relatively inactive state.[117] A ratio of approximately 10 mg protamine per 1000 units of heparin is usually used for reversal, but with increasing time after heparin administration, less protamine is needed due to heparin's relatively short half-life. It is our practice to titrate protamine administration to the ACT or observed intraoperative bleeding—if none is present, protamine need not be given. This is an issue both because of protamine's potential side effects (systemic hypotension, pulmonary hypertension, frank anaphylaxis, and death)[118, 119] and because of a report of worsened outcome after carotid endarterectomy when protamine had been given.[120]

Side effects to protamine have been associated with fish allergy (presumably because protamine is derived from salmon semen), prior vasectomy (presumably because of cross-reactive autoantibodies), and previous insulin use (possibly because of sensitization to the protamine contained in neutral protamine Hagedorn [NPH] insulin).[118, 121–124] "Designer" variants have been created to reduce the incidence of these problems, thus far without much success.[87] Protamine itself can have anticoagulant properties because of TF inhibition.[125] Late bleeding can occur after initially adequate reversal, but it is unclear whether this is due to a "heparin rebound" effect or to protamine's anticoagulant effects.[126]

Antifibrinolytic Agents

If primary fibrinolysis is suspected, direct antifibrinolytic agents such as ε-aminocaproic acid (EACA, Amicar), tran-

TABLE 43–7. CHARACTERISTICS OF THE VARIOUS CLOTTING FACTORS REQUIRED FOR SAFE SURGICAL HEMOSTASIS

FACTOR	IN VIVO HALF-LIFE	LEVEL REQUIRED FOR OPERATIVE HEMOSTASIS	STABLE IN PLASMA IF	BEST OPTIONS FOR REPLACEMENT
I (fibrinogen)	3–4 days	100 mg/dl	4°C	FFP, cryoprecipitate
II	2–5 days	20%–40%	4°C	FFP, concentrates
V	15–36 hr	Less than 25%	Frozen	FFP, platelets
VII	4–7 hr	10%–20%	4°C	FFP, concentrates
VIII	9–18 hr	80% or more	Frozen	Concentrates, cryoprecipitate, FFP
IX	20–24 hr	50% or more	4°C	Concentrates, FFP
X	32–48 hr	10%–20%	4°C	FFP, concentrates
XI	40–80 hr	15%–25%	4°C	FFP, concentrates
XII	48–52 hr	None	4°C	Not necessary
XIII	12 days	Less than 5%	4°C	FFP, cryoprecipitate
vWF	A few hours	25%–50%	Frozen	Cryoprecipitate, concentrates, FFP

Adapted from Edmunds LH, Salzman EW: Hemostatic problems, transfusion therapy, and cardiopulmonary bypass in surgical patients. *In* Colman RW, Hirsh J, Marder VJ, et al (eds): Hemostasis and Thrombosis: Basic Principles and Clinical Practice, 3rd ed. Philadelphia, JB Lippincott, 1994, p 958.
FFP = fresh frozen plasma; vWF = von Willebrand's factor.

examic acid (AMCA, Cyklokapron), or aprotinin (Trasylol), all of which block plasminogen directly or block the action of plasmin on fibrin and fibrinogen, can be considered.[127–130] Their use, however, is contraindicated in consumptive coagulopathy. In this setting the fibrinolysis is secondary to widespread microvascular thrombosis, and clot lysis, critical for removing capillary thrombus, should not be inhibited.

Specific Factors

Specific factors, especially VIII and IX, are available for specific deficiencies (Table 43–7). These are most often used electively when surgery must be performed on a patient with a known deficiency and are usually given in collaboration with a hematologist. Pooled factors once carried a high risk of disease transmission, but are now treated to effectively inactivate human immunodeficiency virus (HIV) and hepatitis B virus.[94, 109] Recombinant factors are also becoming available.

PREOPERATIVE SCREENING AND PREVENTION

History, Physical Examination, and Laboratory Testing

The history and physical examination are excellent preoperative screening tools for potential perioperative hemorrhage. A series of carefully directed questions to elicit a personal or family history of bleeding can alert the surgeon in advance of possible bleeding complications and offers an opportunity to correct underlying defects or postpone the proposed procedure. The patient should be specifically questioned regarding prolonged bleeding from skin or mucosal surfaces after injury, excessive gynecologic or obstetric bleeding, bleeding into or swelling of joints, easy bruising, prolonged bleeding during prior surgical or dental procedures, blood transfusion reactions, family history of bleeding diathesis, and ingestion of any medication that might affect hemostasis, such as aspirin, nonsteroidal anti-inflammatory agents, or warfarin. Similarly, the physical examination should be directed toward the identification of any sign of a bleeding tendency, such as the presence of petechiae or bruises, hepatosplenomegaly, joint effusions, or occult blood on rectal examination.

Repeated studies and consensus statements uniformly agree that nondirected, "shotgun" laboratory screening is of no benefit (in terms of clinical efficacy or cost-effectiveness) in otherwise healthy patients without historical factors to suggest bleeding problems.[47, 131–133] From the results of the history and physical examination, however, one can apply the practical guidelines put forth by Rapaport regarding the likelihood of increased bleeding risk.[134]

In *level 1,* the history and physical findings are negative and the proposed procedure is minor; no further testing is required. In *level 2,* the patient has a negative history and physical examination result, but the proposed procedure is major. An aPTT and platelet count are indicated to screen for occult disorders.

Level 3 applies to patients who have a history somewhat suspicious for major bleeding diathesis and whose proposed procedure will result in significant bleeding (e.g., AAA repair), altered hemostatic mechanisms (e.g., cardiopulmonary bypass), large areas of raw surface or critical requirements for hemostasis (e.g., craniotomy). Tests recommended for patients at level 3 include an aPTT, platelet count, PT, and BT.

Level 4 includes patients whose history is strongly suggestive of a major hemostatic defect. Testing in these patients should include BT after aspirin ingestion to rule out vWD, specific factor assays for factors VIII and IX (patients with mild forms of hemophilia A and B may have a normal aPTT), and a TT to rule out dysfibrinogenemia. Consultation with a hematologist is strongly recommended as well.

Once a specific defect has been identified, treatment can

be tailored to the patient, including consideration of the medical necessity of the procedure. For example, the surgeon and patient may decide that the risks outweigh the benefits of a femoropopliteal bypass for claudication in a level 4 situation.

Prevention and Correction of Preexisting Problems

Inherited Disorders

Platelet transfusions may be required because of thrombocytopenia or an acquired or inborn functional abnormality of platelet function. The hemophilias represent a special challenge. In the absence of bleeding, the factor VIII concentration required to maintain hemostatic integrity and to prevent spontaneous hemorrhage is only about 3%. In the presence of bleeding, however, a factor VIII level of approximately 30% is necessary to achieve cessation of minor hemorrhage, and a level of 50% is necessary to control major bleeding. As discussed earlier, although some factor IX formulations can be thrombogenic, modern factors are essentially free of risk of viral disease transmission, whether because of treatment or recombinant etiology, and thus specific factors are now used almost exclusively (see Table 43–7).

For patients undergoing elective surgical procedures, it is desirable to achieve a factor VIII level of 80% to 100% preoperatively and to maintain the level at at least 30% for 2 weeks after the procedure. The dose required is determined by the patient's baseline factor VIII level; each unit of factor VIII infused raises the plasma level by 2%. Half the initial dose should be given every 8 to 12 hours, the half-life of factor VIII.[59, 94, 135, 136] In patients with hemophilia B, the desired plasma levels of factor IX are 20% to 30% for minor bleeding and 50% to 100% for major hemorrhage and surgery, and a level of 20% to 40% should be maintained for 2 weeks postoperatively. The half-life of factor IX is 24 hours, and it can be given half as frequently as factor VIII.[61, 136] Again, because of the risk of specific, antifactor inhibitors, factor activity should be measured before surgery is begun to verify adequate hemostasis.

Patients with vWD require enough functional vWF to obtain improved or normalized primary hemostasis (as reflected by the BT). DDAVP increases vWF levels and clearly shortens the BT in patients with type I vWD, but its actual mechanism, despite the "conventional wisdom" that it releases vWF from endothelial cells, is unknown.[55, 57, 66] DDAVP is probably the first-line treatment for mild type I vWD, but in other situations direct replacement therapy with cryoprecipitate or factors is best. Although factor VIII concentrate is ineffective because it lacks vWF, factor VIII-vWF preparations are available and efficient. Because the different types of vWD vary in molecular mechanism and only type I (fortunately composing 80% of vWD cases) should be treated with DDAVP, early consultation with a hematologist is strongly recommended.

Treatment of inherited and acquired disorders of prothrombin conversion depends on the severity of the disorder. From 10 to 20 ml/kg of FFP is sufficient to restore hemostasis in most cases, unless bleeding is very severe. Isolated factor replacement can be used in these extreme cases. The frequency and volume of replacement with FFP vary based on the factor deficiency.[63]

Liver Disease and Vitamin K Deficiency

In mild hepatic insufficiency, it is possible to replace the coagulation factors by an infusion of FFP. In frank liver failure, however, this is rarely possible, especially if there is ongoing consumption, because 8 L of plasma would be required each day and because, as discussed earlier, the coagulopathy associated with hepatic failure is usually multifactoral. Hepatic insufficiency is often associated with compromised renal function, which limits the volume that can be infused.

For patients with hepatic insufficiency who must undergo operation, an infusion of plasma is begun 2 to 3 hours before the procedure. It is preferable to use FFP rather than stored plasma because FFP contains all the coagulation factors, including higher levels of the labile factors V and VIII, complement, and cold insoluble globulin. Primary fibrinolysis is occasionally caused by liver disease. A 24-hour infusion of ϵ-aminocaproic acid or tranexamic acid, beginning just before surgery and continuing during and after surgery, may be beneficial in this circumstance.

Coagulopathy caused by vitamin K deficiency, whether due to malabsorption or warfarin administration, is usually relatively easy to correct. FFP quickly restores the PT to normal because of direct factor replacement. Parenteral vitamin K also restores factor levels by the carboxylation of presynthesized molecules. This can be quite fast (6 to 24 hours), but it makes reanticoagulation slower.

Uremia

Because the hemostatic defect in renal failure involves both intrinsic platelet abnormalities and inhibitors, treatment is aimed at both factors. In patients with anemia, simple transfusion to a hematocrit of 30% can improve hemostasis through hemodynamic effects by improving platelet margination and enhancing platelet-endothelial contact and interaction. Erythropoietin has a similar, though more delayed, benefit. Dialysis is somewhat effective in removing circulating inhibitors of platelet function, but is seldom successful in restoring hemostasis completely.

Platelet function can also be temporarily boosted by the administration of DDAVP. In addition to its above mentioned effects in vWD, DDAVP promotes elevated concentrations of norepinephrine in the circulating plasma for 1 to 4 hours after infusion. This results in improved platelet-endothelial interactions, probably by sensitizing or activating the α-adrenergic receptors of platelets. Infusion of 10 units of cryoprecipitate results in immediate and nearly complete hemostatic competence that lasts 4 to 12 hours and should be utilized preoperatively in all uremic patients in whom major operative intervention is planned. Cryoprecipitate, rich in factor VIII, vWF, and fibrinogen, is also effective in this situation.[110–112]

Factor-Specific Inhibitors

If the presence of an inactivating inhibitor is not identified preoperatively but suspected intraoperatively (i.e., in the setting of sudden collapse of hemostasis without other cause), cryoprecipitate should be the first therapy. Cryoprecipitate contains factor VIII, which is the target of the specific inhibitors in the majority of cases. Once the specific inhibitor has been identified, overwhelming amounts of the target factor should be administered until hemostasis has been achieved.[61, 93, 94] If only tenuous hemostasis can be achieved, clotting activity can be supplemented by exchange transfusion with normal FFP, usually via plasmapheresis.

Alternatively, preparations of procoagulants isolated and concentrated from pooled donors can be infused. These are designed to bypass the inhibited activity and trigger the sequence of clotting enzyme reactions beyond the inhibited activity, thus generating thrombin. For example, if factor VIII coagulant activity is inhibited, concentrates from the prothrombin complex isolated from plasma (factors II, VII, IX, and X) can be infused in an attempt to bypass the barrier of factor VIII inhibition.

Patients Undergoing Thrombolysis

An increased risk of bleeding may occur from the unavoidable leakage of a thrombolytic agent into the systemic circulation (a cause of primary fibrinolysis) and, as such, will cease quickly as the agents are rapidly metabolized. A longer-lasting effect, however, may occur from circulating anticoagulants (FDP) released as fibrin is degraded. Fibrin is probably the most frequent and troublesome cause of bleeding complications during therapeutic thrombolysis. Hypofibrinogenemia alone is not usually responsible for abnormal bleeding (patients with congenital afibrinogenemia rarely manifest spontaneous bleeding); diminished fibrinogen levels are easily corrected with FFP or cryoprecipitate.

Other Considerations

Although individual response is variable, most authors and clinicians still recommend that elective operation not take place unless the platelet count (assuming normal function) exceeds 50 to 70/μl.[26] Aspirin use is similarly controversial. Although many believe it causes clinically relevant bleeding, study results are inconsistent.[91, 137, 138] Aspirin clearly improves graft patency[139] as well as cerebrovascular and coronary morbidity and mortality in a variety of settings,[140–142] and thus it is our recommendation that patients specifically receive it the night before operation and continue taking aspirin afterward. If cessation is desired, the aspirin should be stopped at least 3 or 4 days preoperatively to allow restoration of platelet function through new platelet production (although the life span of a platelet is 7 to 10 days, after 3 to 4 days enough new platelets are available). Nonsteroidal medications act similarly, but because their effects on platelets are only temporary, they pose even less of a problem intraoperatively.[91]

DIAGNOSIS AND MANAGEMENT OF INTRAOPERATIVE BLEEDING

Despite the most aggressive attempts to identify and correct potential bleeding problems preoperatively, it is inevitable that eventually serious intraoperative bleeding will occasionally arise. When faced with unexpected intraoperative bleeding, the basic strategy is first to identify the cause and then to treat it appropriately. The simplest strategy is to determine whether the bleeding is due to a global coagulopathy or a mechanical problem—obviously, treatments differ considerably (Fig. 43–6).

Diagnosis

The most common cause of intraoperative hemorrhage is mechanical bleeding from surgically correctable sites, which are usually fairly easily handled (see later). Surgically correctable bleeding is usually localized, may be torrential, and is often (if arterial) manifest by a visible jet. Bleeding due to coagulopathy, in contrast, is often diffuse and manifest as a slow ooze that cannot be controlled by local methods.

Management of Coagulopathy

Clotting factors are enzymes, and, like all enzymes, function optimally within a narrow range of temperature and pH, centered around normal values (Fig. 43–7). When these ranges are exceeded, most commonly due to hypothermia or acidosis, function is impaired and clotting progressively becomes abnormal.

Hypothermia

Intraoperative hypothermia is usually encountered with prolonged operative time (due to heat loss to the environment), global hypoperfusion (often due to critical illness or injury), and intraoperative replacement with nonwarmed fluids in large volumes.[143] Because many laboratories measure clotting tests with samples warmed to 37°C, a clinically obvious coagulopathy in a cold patient may be associated with apparently normal test results.[144] Hypothermia can also cause platelet dysfunction[145, 146] and precipitate full-blown DIC.

Like many situational factors causing coagulopathy, the resultant bleeding leads to worsened perfusion, greater fluid requirements, and a longer operation, thus creating a vicious circle. In addition, hypothermia is notoriously difficult to correct, once established. Therefore, prevention is absolutely critical. Operative time is often relatively fixed by the problem at hand. Although speed is not the goal, if quality is preserved then a short operation is better than a long one. If a "high-risk" situation can be identified beforehand (e.g., a ruptured aneurysm or trauma victim with a prolonged extrication time), warming the room before the patient arrives seems prudent. When fluid requirements are expected to be more than minimal, infusion through fluid warmers is required.

Although not all agree whether warming inspired air is helpful, systems that deliver warmed air to exposed parts of the body not in the surgical field (Bair Hugger, Augustine Medical, Inc.) clearly are of value. Finally, although maintaining optimal global perfusion is a critical goal for many reasons, it aids in maintaining temperature as well as reducing the stimulus for elaboration of anticoagulant and fibrinolytic factors.

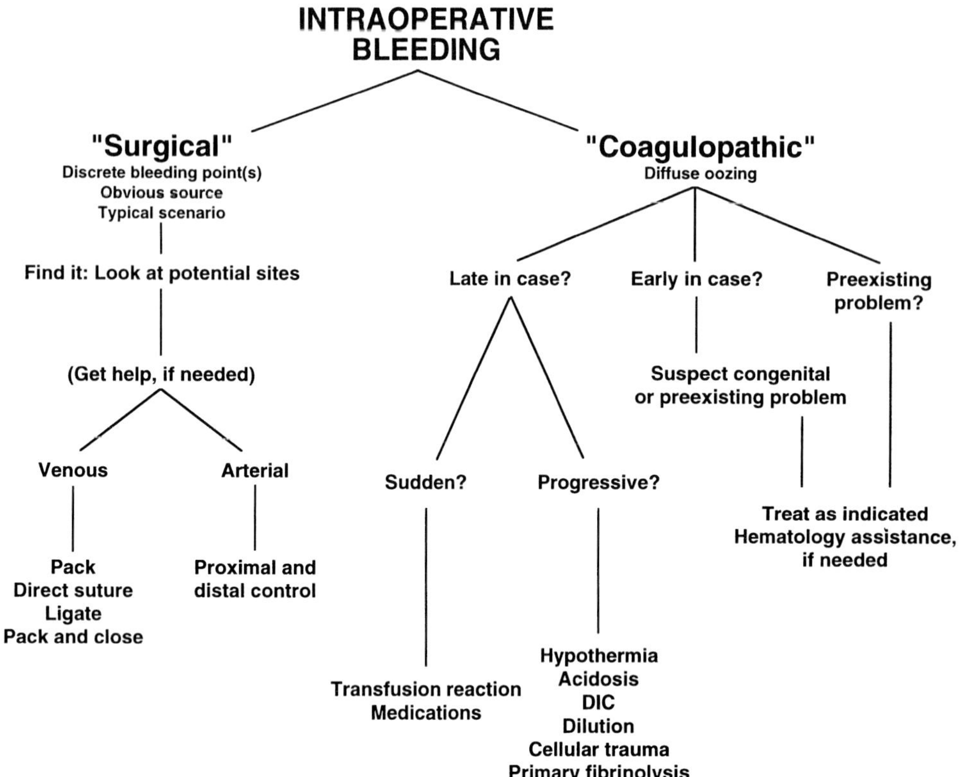

FIGURE 43–6. Algorithm for management of intraoperative bleeding. A nonsurgical coagulopathy that occurs late in a case, especially if slowly progressive, is likely due to a problem that is relatively resistant to treatment, such as disseminated intravascular coagulopathy (DIC), acidosis, hypothermia, or dilution, or injury to proteins and cells. In this situation, terminating the operation to allow resuscitation in an intensive care unit assumes higher priority as time goes on.

Acidosis

Acidosis is a common problem in vascular surgery. It is seen most commonly in the setting of significant bacteremia, global or local hypoperfusion, and after reperfusion of a large ischemic area. The best treatment is prevention by correcting ischemic problems early and maintaining global hemodynamics and by prediction of situations that cannot be prevented and treating them quickly. When a large mass of tissue (e.g., a leg or the small bowel) has been ischemic for more than a short time, acidosis (as well as hyperkalemia, myoglobinemia, and high levels of other anticoagulant toxins) results when perfusion is restored. In this situation, therefore, treatment should ideally coincide with or even precede the event. For example, respiratory and metabolic alkalosis can be established before arterial clamp removal. In addition, unusually close attention should be paid to clinical and laboratory evidence of coagulopathy and the operation not terminated until hemostasis is adequate.

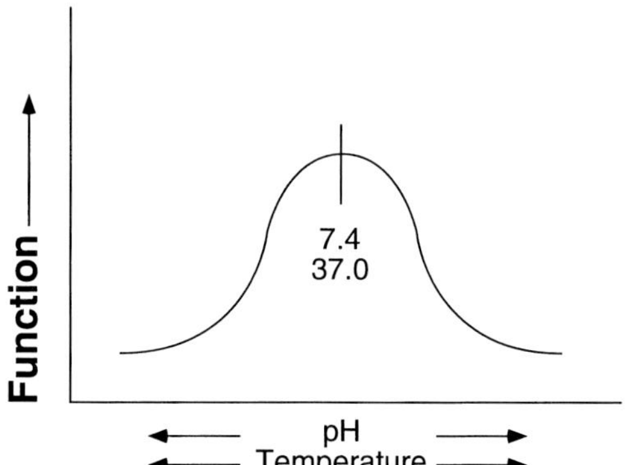

FIGURE 43–7. Schematic curve of enzyme activity (in this case, coagulation factors) versus pH and temperature. Function is maximal at normal physiologic values (7.4 and 37.0, respectively) but falls off as these values change on either side of the norm. Platelet function is also adversely affected, at least by hypothermia, but its relation to pH is less well characterized.

Dilution

Dilution is also a common problem, but one that is often overlooked in the "heat of the battle." With massive transfusion, defined as transfusion of 1 to 2 full blood volumes in a finite time span, platelets and factors are lost and their levels decline as the result of dilution with the crystalloid necessary to maintain cardiac filling and output. Interestingly, there is no consensus as to how clinically significant this loss is. Although thrombocytopenia is usually the major change observed after massive transfusion, there is no specific cutoff that predicts bleeding, and FFP and platelets should probably be transfused only for specific deficiencies. Even in the face of massive blood loss, enough coagulation proteins almost always remain to maintain function.[39, 105] The best strategy, probably, is to be aware of this possibility and to measure platelet count and factor function (by means of PT, aPTT, and ACT) frequently if massive blood loss occurs. Occasionally, loss is so rapid that waiting for laboratory testing before transfusion may not be in the patient's best interest, especially because all blood products become increasingly safe.

Disseminated Intravascular Coagulopathy

DIC usually arises in characteristic clinical settings. The usual scenario is that of a gradual deterioration in previously adequate hemostasis in a critically ill patient (e.g., with sepsis, trauma, or uncontrolled bleeding), with generalized bleeding, particularly from previously hemostatic areas. Primary fibrinolysis usually occurs in patients with cirrhosis or liver failure from other causes in whom PAI synthesis and t-PA clearance are impaired. Relevant to vascular surgery, it also occurs in the setting of hepatic hypoperfusion resulting from supraceliac clamping.[49, 85]

DIC is probably not an "all-or-nothing" event; it commonly arises from previous, inadequately treated problems. For example, in a patient who is cold and underperfused, coagulopathy may initially be simply an enzymatic dysfunction. If the initial insult is not corrected and bleeding persists, however, the worsened hypothermia, acidosis, and toxemia induced by ischemic tissue may push the coagulation system into true DIC.

Because DIC, once established, is often extraordinarily resistant to treatment, prevention is paramount. Early recognition is critical because of DIC's propensity to become autonomous and self-perpetuating. Once DIC is established, general support while the underlying problem is corrected is the best option. In the short term, measures designed to reduce operative time, maintain perfusion, and keep the patient warm and at normal physiologic parameters are important, as discussed earlier. In the longer term, maintenance of adequate nutrition, control of undrained spaces and débridement of ischemic tissues, control of pain, and control of systemic infectious problems are of equal importance. Clotting factors and platelets should be replaced at the rate they are consumed, as determined by frequent laboratory testing and continued administration of FFP, platelets, cryoprecipitate to increase fibrinogen levels, and, as directed, more exotic factors. Antifibrinolytic agents should probably seldom, if ever, be used because the secondary fibrinolysis occurring during DIC is beneficial, cleaning the capillaries of thrombus and restoring perfusion. The mainstay of treatment is correction of the underlying stimulus directly while halting the vicious circle and replacing cells and factors as fast as they are consumed.

Primary Fibrinolysis

Treatment of primary fibrinolysis requires replacement therapy and the use of fibrinolytic inhibitors. Target substrates of plasmin—fibrinogen, factor V, and, to a lesser extent, factor VIII—must be replaced. Platelet infusions may be necessary to supply factor V. Fibrinolytic inhibitors such as EACA, tranexamic acid, and aprotinin, can be beneficial, but antifibrinolytics are contraindicated in DIC because the secondary fibrinolysis that occurs as part of DIC is necessary to clear microvascular thrombi and restore capillary perfusion.

Mechanical Trauma to Clotting Factors and Platelets

Mechanical trauma can occur, usually iatrogenically while the patient is on cardiopulmonary bypass or using the Cell Saver.[106, 147, 148] Autotransfusion devices in which the cells are washed before they are returned to the patient may reduce the risk of DIC, but result in removal of important coagulation factors. In contrast, the non–cell-washing devices return all the blood proteins, but may also return certain triggers of DIC, such as activated complement and damaged cellular elements. The use of extracorporeal circulation results in several abnormalities of hemostasis; both qualitative and quantitative platelet abnormalities and, less commonly, significant reductions in factors V and VIII occur. Rarely, DIC may occur. The most important coagulation abnormalities may result from the massive doses of heparin required to prevent thrombosis within the perfusion system. Treatment of bleeding associated with cardiopulmonary bypass is best addressed by reversal of the two most important factors, thrombocytopenia and hyperheparinemia.

Other Problems

Other less common causes of coagulopathy in the operating room should also be considered. Obviously, an iatrogenic coagulopathy, such as overheparinization or warfarin administration, should be suspected in the appropriate clinical setting; correction is usually easily accomplished by appropriate doses of protamine sulfate, FFP, and vitamin K, as appropriate. If bleeding occurs in a uremic patient, DDAVP should be given as discussed earlier. Low-molecular-weight dextrans interfere with coagulation because of effects on the fibrin clot, hemodilution, and platelet function.[39] Platelet number and function are adversely affected after placement of a large vascular prosthesis.[149, 150] This is not usually a problem in the operating room, however, and in our experience it is solely a laboratory finding. Although increasingly rare, a transfusion reaction should be suspected if abnormal, diffuse bleeding abruptly occurs while the patient is receiving blood products. The transfusion should immediately be stopped and consideration given to aborting the operation, depending on the clinical situation.

Finally, hereditary disorders can occasionally be first detected during an operative procedure. Although relatively rare, such a disorder should be suspected if other causes do not seem to be present. In this setting (e.g., coagulopathic bleeding occurring early in an otherwise uneventful procedure) a full battery of coagulation tests, including thrombin time and factor levels, should be obtained, and intraoperative consultation with a hematologist should be considered.

Technical Problems

The cause of surgically correctable bleeding, by definition, is an open vessel. This can occur for several reasons: spontaneously (a ruptured aneurysm), as the result of prehospital injury, or as the result of iatrogenic, intraoperative injury.

Management, though differing in detail, is conceptually the same in all situations. First, in all but the most minor situations, two things are critical: exposure and assistance. Packing or digital control can often buy time to improve both, and if bleeding can temporarily be controlled, the situation can be thought through, a plan developed, and the problem addressed in an unhurried, logical fashion. Of all parameters, adequate, properly trained help is probably the best resource available—four hands and eyes are better than two.

Arterial and venous bleeding are approached differently.

In all but the most minor arterial injuries, the first priority should be obtaining direct proximal and distal control. Often this is best accomplished by proximal control at a remote site, allowing dissection away from the hematoma or site of temporary control, and distal control with the same technique or a balloon occlusion catheter from within the opened lumen. If bleeding is localized, the patient is stable, and bleeding is expected to be easily handled, heparinization is advisable. However, if the risk of coagulopathy is great, as typified by many ruptured aneurysms, the risks of heparinization may exceed its benefits. Once controlled, the injury can be exposed, explored, and repaired. Simple injuries, including stab wounds, can often be directly sutured. More complex wounds, however, usually require more complex repair, as discussed elsewhere.

Venous bleeding, however, is often approached differently. Because of large size, thin walls, and abundant feeding tributaries, proximal and distal control can often be more problematic and injury can be more diffuse. Because of low venous pressure, spontaneous thrombosis is more likely. For both of these reasons, simple packing, especially when the injury is difficult to expose, is often the best option. Essentially, any vein with the exception of the suprarenal vena cava can be ligated; this is a reasonable option if bleeding is vigorous and the patient's life is at risk.[151, 152]

More commonly encountered in elective surgery is surgical bleeding from less obvious sources. The first step is to conduct a thorough, systematic search. Several sources are common and should be specifically sought out. After aneurysm repair, for example, previously patent but nonbleeding vessels, such as the lumbar or inferior mesenteric arteries or even the cut edge of the aneurysm sac, can bleed as distal perfusion is restored. The splenic bed is a potential source after splenectomy and should be routinely inspected. The spleen itself is often injured (up to 25% of cases) during left medial visceral rotation and should be routinely inspected after this exposure. If the spleen is injured after a complex aortic repair, the surgeon should have a low threshold for splenectomy to reduce the risk of missing or misinterpreting postoperative hemorrhage.

After any vascular anastomosis, whether bleeding or not, all parts of all suture lines should be inspected. If bleeding is found from the suture line itself, repair sutures are placed. Repair sutures should usually be placed in a mattress fashion, over a pledget if any weakness or gap exists, to reduce strain on the surrounding tissues. After the hole has been identified, the inflow artery can be reclamped and the graft decompressed. Caution is required, however, because ill-placed pledgets can obscure visualization of and access to continued bleeding points, if not controlled the first time. Certainly, areas that are relatively inaccessible, such as the back wall of a proximal aortic anastomosis, should be carefully inspected before the distal anastomosis is fashioned and access lost.

If any doubt exists as to the integrity of the tissue, pledgets should be used during initial anastomotic construction. In difficult situations, such as with diffusely friable tissues, a long strip of fabric can be used to reinforce the cuff while the anastomosis is sewn. This has the effect of distributing the force of the suture itself over a wider area, and it can protect friable tissues from the sutures pulling through.

Needle hole bleeding is a different situation. This, almost exclusively, is a problem seen after bypass using polytetrafluoroethylene (PTFE). If needle hole bleeding is seen after a polyester (Dacron) graft has been used, a careful search should be made for gaps, especially related to crimps in the fabric. The surgeon can reduce needle hole bleeding by paying extra attention to following the curve of the needle and by using the best match between suture and needle diameter. True needle hole bleeding almost always stops within 5 or 10 minutes, especially if the hemostatic function is normal (e.g., after protamine administration). Although patience and mechanical control such as packing with oxidized cellulose gauze (Surgicel, Johnson) are usually adequate, rarely a repair suture is required. Obviously, more needle holes are created by a repair suture; maneuvers such as using adjacent bits of tissue as a pledget and not passing through the full thickness of the PTFE are of value. Another cause of bleeding after graft placement, especially if Dacron is used, is inadequate preclotting or abnormal bleeding from the interstices. Again, this almost always stops within a few minutes if coagulation is otherwise normal.

Operative Management

If abnormal bleeding occurs in the operating room, the first step is to identify the cause. If the cause is mechanical, the source should be identified and corrected expeditiously with exposure, local or remote control, and adequate assistance. There are several mechanical resources available. As discussed, packing is an excellent technique, especially for relatively inaccessible venous injuries. Surgicel, although not directly hemostatic, provides an excellent mechanical scaffolding for platelet and fibrin deposition. It is inexpensive and probably the first line of therapy for troublesome but minor bleeding that is expected to stop (such as needle hole bleeding).

More specific pharmacologic therapies are available. Topical bovine thrombin (Gentrac), especially when combined with an absorbable gelatin sponge (Gelfoam) is directly hemostatic and relatively inexpensive. Microfibrillar collagen (Avitene) is a powder that can be sprinkled on diffuse, raw, oozing areas and is quite effective, especially when combined with packing. Topical cryoprecipitate and Amicar are also available, although we have no experience with either.

Occasionally one may encounter bleeding that is uncontrollable despite all possible measures. In this setting, packing, cessation of surgery, and transfer to the intensive care unit (ICU) with a temporary abdominal closure for resuscitation with planned reoperation may be life-saving. Most widely explored by trauma surgeons, this "bail-out" technique assumes that the best resuscitation (warmth, correction of acid-base problems, and coagulopathy) can be carried out in the ICU.[153] This technique is applicable only for coagulopathy and when mechanical bleeding, usually venous, cannot be quickly controlled surgically but can be controlled with packing. It is not applicable when major arterial bleeding is present.

DIAGNOSIS AND MANAGEMENT OF POSTOPERATIVE BLEEDING

Postoperative bleeding can be encountered as a continuation of intraoperative coagulopathy or as a new, unexpected problem. The first step is diagnosis, and an appropriate level of suspicion is required. In a patient who tolerates an otherwise uneventful operation without bleeding (i.e., no intraoperative coagulopathy is present), new postoperative bleeding is almost certainly surgical. In other words, unless a specific cause is present (e.g., consumptive coagulopathy or transfusion), de novo postoperative bleeding should be assumed to be due to an open blood vessel.

There are two questions to answer: (1) is bleeding occurring? and (2) what is the cause? Most bleeding can be easily diagnosed by observation of both the patient's clinical course, including unexplained tachycardia, and basic laboratory parameters, such as the hematocrit, PT and aPTT, and platelet count. If consumptive coagulopathy is suspected, fibrinogen levels, FDP, and TT should be followed as well. ECLT can identify primary fibrinolysis. Monitoring the hematocrit, PT, aPTT, platelet count, and fibrinogen levels every 6 hours is probably optimal to allow time for correction between repeated testing. Bleeding that affects these variables faster than this should be clinically obvious.

The benefit of treating a coagulopathy in an ICU setting is to allow for resuscitation. Warmth is critical, as discussed earlier. An ICU setting allows warming by means of air blankets, radiant heaters, infused fluids, and, probably most important, because the patient's skin has been closed and the patient removed from the usually cold operating room. Acid-base status can be closely monitored and corrected, and global tissue perfusion and hemodynamic status can be optimized, all of which will shift platelet and clotting enzyme function toward normalcy.

Finally, ongoing stimuli for bleeding can be better identified and corrected in the ICU. All dead tissue should be removed, by means of débridement or formal amputation, when benefit exceeds risk. Thus, an irreversibly ischemic foot in a critically ill patient with thrombocytopenia can probably be left alone for the time being, while a cadaveric leg with no other cause of DIC in which DIC is developing should be amputated expeditiously. Abscesses must be drained and pain relieved.

Although the best way to "cure" a coagulopathy is to remove stimuli for its existence and to restore general homeostasis, ongoing replacement therapy is often required (see Table 43–6). Most commonly needed are blood, platelets, and clotting factors. Packed red blood cells (PRBCs) are used for restoring oxygen-carrying capacity. As discussed earlier, although tissue oxygenation is excellent at much lower levels, a hematocrit of 30% is still the target in the setting of ongoing bleeding to allow a margin for error in the setting of ongoing loss. In general, 1 unit of PRBCs increases the hematocrit by 3%. If the increase is less than this, ongoing loss (or dilution) should be suspected. Platelets should be transfused for low platelet counts. Again, although a count of approximately 20 μl is usually adequate for maintenance of normal hemostasis, in the setting of active bleeding a target of 50 to 70 μl (even higher at times to allow for ongoing loss or destruction) is usually recommended. An elevated PT is usually correctable by administration of FFP (to restore new factors) and vitamin K (to counteract liver dysfunction and warfarin effects), whereas an elevated aPTT, often associated with global coagulopathy, can often be corrected with protamine, even if heparin was not given or was apparently adequately reversed.

If bleeding is ongoing, the next step is to look for rarer causes, again to rule out surgical bleeding, or to look for correctly identified but inadequately treated problems. Cryoprecipitate restores factor VIII and fibrinogen levels, and DDAVP improves platelet-endothelial interactions via an increase in vWF. DDAVP is especially useful in uremia and after cardiopulmonary bypass. If primary fibrinolysis is suspected, antifibrinolytic agents can be considered, but their use is contraindicated in DIC.

In general, replacement therapy should be directed by laboratory parameters. Two general exceptions exist:

1. When a defined coagulopathy is known to be present, such as DIC, primary fibrinolysis, or a hereditary disorder. In this setting, initial treatment can be empirical, specifically directed against the presumed problem, while laboratory workup is pending.
2. When coagulopathy is massive and immediately life-threatening. Again, laboratory evaluation should be expeditious, but before the answer is found, treatment should be empirical. In this setting, an old aphorism is "give them everything you can spell." While not very scientific, this "shotgun" approach usually does more good than harm.

In a general sense, treat the most common things first (with PRBCs, platelets, and FFP, often in massive doses) while the laboratory tests are pending.

SUMMARY

Because of the nature of vascular surgery, bleeding complications are common and often serious. All patients for whom a surgical procedure is contemplated should undergo appropriate screening by means of history, physical examination, and, when indicated, laboratory evaluation. Perioperative bleeding can be caused by coagulopathy, either preexisting or acquired, by mechanical, surgically correctable sources, or, frequently, by a combination of each. Many such problems but not all, can be identified and controlled preoperatively.

Many of the stimuli for acquired coagulopathic bleeding are the direct result of blood loss and the systemic problems it creates; thus, all bleeding can cause a vicious circle of ongoing loss, further derangements, and worsened coagulopathy. Because of this possibility, prevention is, by far, the most critical step. Once bleeding occurs, however, a thorough understanding of the coagulation system and replacement strategies is vital to plan and execute rational treatment.

REFERENCES

1. Davies MG, Hagen PO: The vascular endothelium: A new horizon. Ann Surg 218:593, 1993.

2. Jaffe EA: Biochemistry, immunology, and cell biology of endothelium. *In* Colman RW, Hirsh J, Marder VJ, et al (eds): Hemostasis and Thrombosis: Basic Principles and Clinical Practice, 3rd ed. Philadelphia, JB Lippincott, 1994, p 718.
3. Colman RW, Marder VJ, Salzman EW, et al: Overview of normal hemostasis. *In* Colman RW, Hirsh J, Marder VJ, et al (eds): Hemostasis and Thrombosis: Basic Principles and Clinical Practice, 3rd ed. Philadelphia, JB Lippincott, 1994, p 3.
4. Vanhoutte PM: Endothelial dysfunction and atherosclerosis. Eur Heart J 18(Suppl E):E19, 1997.
5. Cain BS, Meldrum DR, Selzman CH, et al: Surgical implications of vascular endothelial physiology. Surgery 122:516, 1997.
6. Robbins RA, Grisham MB: Nitric oxide. Int J Biochem Cell Biol 29:857, 1997.
7. Leonard EF: Rheology of thrombosis. *In* Colman RW, Hirsh J, Marder VJ, et al (eds): Hemostasis and Thrombosis: Basic Principles and Clinical Practice, 3rd ed. Philadelphia, JB Lippincott, 1994, p 1211.
8. Weiss HJ: Flow-related platelet deposition on subendothelium. Thromb Haemost 74:117, 1995.
9. Nemerson Y, Turitto VT: The effect of flow on hemostasis and thrombosis. Thromb Haemost 66:272, 1991.
10. Miletich JP, Jackson CM, Majerus PW: Properties of the factor V binding site on human platelets. J Biol Chem 253:6908, 1978.
11. Bennett JS, Vilaire G: Exposure of the platelet fibrinogen receptors by ADP and epinephrine. J Clin Invest 64:1393, 1979.
12. Colman RW: Platelet receptors. Hematol Oncol Clin North Am 4:27, 1990.
13. Clemetson KJ: Platelet activation: Signal transduction via membrane receptors. Thromb Haemost 74:111, 1995.
14. Celi AC, Lorenzet R, Furie B, et al: Platelet-leukocyte-endothelial cell wall interaction on the blood vessel wall. Semin Hematol 34:327, 1997.
15. Weiss HJ, Turitto VT, Baumgartner HR: Platelet adhesion and thrombus formation on subendothelium in platelets deficient in glycoproteins IIb-IIIa, Ib, and storage granules. Blood 67:322, 1986.
16. Weiss HJ, Hawinger J, Ruggeri ZM, et al: Fibrinogen-independent platelet adhesion and thrombus formation on subendothelium mediated by glycoprotein IIb-IIIa complex at high shear rates. J Clin Invest 83:288, 1989.
17. Colman RW, Cook JJ, Niewiarowski S: Mechanisms of platelet interaction. *In* Colman RW, Hirsh J, Marder VJ, et al (eds): Hemostasis and Thrombosis: Basic Principles and Clinical Practice, 3rd ed. Philadelphia, JB Lippincott, 1994, p 508.
18. Holmsen H: Platelet secretion (release reactions): Mechanism and pharmacology. Adv Pharmacol Ther 4:97, 1978.
19. Holmsen H, Weiss HJ: Secretable storage pools in platelets. Annu Rev Med 30:119, 1979.
20. DeLa Cadena RA, Wachtfogel YT, Colman RW: Contact activation pathway: Inflammation and coagulation. *In* Colman RW, Hirsh J, Marder VJ, et al (eds): Hemostasis and Thrombosis: Basic Principles and Clinical Practice, 3rd ed. Philadelphia, JB Lippincott, 1994, p 219.
21. Zur M, Radcliffe RD, Oberdick J, et al: The dual role of factor VII in blood coagulation: Initiation and inhibition of a proteolytic system by a zymogen. J Biol Chem 257:5623, 1982.
22. Nemerson Y: The tissue factor pathway of coagulation. *In* Colman RW, Hirsh J, Marder VJ, et al eds: Hemostasis and Thrombosis: Basic Principles and Clinical Practice, 3rd ed. Philadelphia, JB Lippincott, 1994, p 81.
23. Semoraro N, Colucci M: Tissue factor in health and disease. Thromb Haemost 78:759, 1997.
24. Broze GJ: Tissue factor pathway inhibitor. Thromb Haemost 74:90, 1995.
25. Ahmad SS, Rawal C, Sheikh RR, et al: Comparative interactions of factor IX and factor IXa with human platelets. J Biol Chem 264:3244, 1989.
26. Limentani SA, Furie BC, Furie B: The biochemistry of factor IX. *In* Colman RW, Hirsh J, Marder VJ, et al (eds): Hemostasis and Thrombosis: Basic Principles and Clinical Practice, 3rd ed. Philadelphia, JB Lippincott, 1994, p 94.
27. Thijs LG, de Boer JP, de Groot MCM, et al: Coagulation disorders in septic shock. Intensive Care Med 19(Suppl):S8, 1993.
28. Blomback B: Fibrinogen and fibrin: Proteins with complex roles in hemostasis and thrombosis. Thromb Res 83:1, 1996.
29. Muszbeck L, Adany R, Mikkola H: Novel aspects of blood coagulation factor XIII. I: Structure, distribution, activation, and function Crit Rev Clin Lab Sci 33:357, 1996.
30. Tans G, Nicholaes GA, Rosig J: Regulation of thrombin formation by activated protein C: Effect of the factor V Leiden mutation. Semin Hematol 34:244, 1997.
31. Aiach M, Borgel D, Gaussem P, et al: Protein C and protein S deficiencies. Semin Hematol 34:205, 1997.
32. van Boven HH, Lane DA: Antithrombin and its inherited deficiency states. Semin Hematol 34:188, 1997.
33. Francis RB: Clinical disorders of fibrinolysis: A critical review. Blut 59:1, 1989.
34. Collen D, Lijnen HR, Todd PA, et al: Tissue-type plasminogen activator: A review of its pharmacology and therapeutic use as a thrombolytic agent. Drugs 38:346, 1989.
35. Erikson LA, Shleef RR, Ny T, et al: The fibrinolytic system of the vascular wall. Clin Haematol 14:513, 1985.
36. Kruithoff EKO: Plasminogen activator inhibitors: A review. Enzyme 40:113, 1988.
37. Sprenger ED, Kluft C: Plasminogen activators and inhibitors. Blood 69:381, 1987.
38. Liem T, Silver D: Coumadin: Principles of use. Semin Vasc Surg 9:364, 1996.
39. Weaver DW: Differential diagnosis and management of unexplained bleeding. Surg Clin North Am 73:353, 1993.
40. White GC, Marder VJ, Colman RW, et al: Approach to the bleeding patient. *In* Colman RW, Hirsh J, Marder VJ, et al (eds): Hemostasis and Thrombosis: Basic Principles and Clinical Practice, 3rd ed. Philadelphia, JB Lippincott, 1994, p 1134.
41. Lewis BE, Walenga JM, Wallis DE: Anticoagulation with Novastan (argatroban) in patients with heparin-induced thrombocytopenia and heparin-induced thrombocytopenia and thrombosis syndrome. Semin Thromb Hemost 23:197, 1997.
42. Rosenberg RD: Biochemistry and pharmacology of low molecular weight heparin. Semin Hematol 34(Suppl 4):2, 1997.
43. Kessler CM: Low molecular weight heparins: Practical considerations. Semin Hematol 34(Suppl 4):35, 1997.
44. Conrad J, Samama M: Theoretic and practical consideration on laboratory monitoring of thrombolytic therapy. Semin Thromb Hemost 13:212, 1987.
45. Heiden D, Mielke CH, Rodvien R: Impairment by heparin of primary haemostasis and platelet [^{14}C] 5-hydroxytryptamine release. Br J Haematol 36:427, 1987.
46. Bowie EJ, Owen CA: The bleeding time. Prog Hemost Thromb 2:249, 1974.
47. Peterson P, Hayes TE, Arkin CF, et al: The preoperative bleeding time test lacks clinical benefit. Arch Surg 133:134, 1998.
48. Blix S: Studies on the fibrinolytic system in the euglobulin fraction of human plasma. Scand J Clin Lab Invest 13(Suppl 58):3, 1961.
49. Illig KA, Green RM, Ouriel K, et al: Primary fibrinolysis during supraceliac clamping. J Vasc Surg 25:244, 1997.
50. Overview of Thrombelastograph Coagulation Analyzer: A Unique Analytical Device. Haemoscope Corporation, Morton Grove, Ill, 1991.
51. DeNicola P, Mazzetti GM: Evaluation of thrombelastography. Am J Clin Pathol 25:447, 1955.
52. Kang YG, Martin DJ, Marquez J, et al: Intraoperative changes in blood coagulation and thrombelastographic monitoring in liver transplantation. Anesth Analg 64:888, 1985.
53. Fuse I: Disorders of platelet function. Crit Rev Oncol Hematol 22:1, 1996.
54. Levy-Toledano S, Caen JP, Breton-Gorius J, et al: Gray platelet syndrome: Alpha granule deficiency: Its influence on platelet function. J Lab Clin Med 98:831, 1981.
55. Nichols WL, Ginsberg WC: von Willebrand disease. Medicine 76:1, 1997.
56. Colman RW: Platelet receptors. Hematol Oncol Clin North Am 4:27, 1990.
57. Mannucci PM: Treatment of von Willebrand's disease. J Int Med 242(Suppl 740):120, 1997.
58. Cahill MR, Colvin BT: Haemophilia. Postgrad Med J 73:201, 1997.
59. Shopnick RI, Brettler DB: Hemostasis: A practical review of conservative and operative care. Clin Orthop Rel Res 328:34, 1996.
60. Berntorp E, Boulyjemnkov V, Brettler D, et al: Modern treatment of haemophilia. Bull WHO 73:691, 1995.
61. Roberts HR, Eberst ME: Current management of hemophilia B. Hematol Oncol Clin North Am 7:1269, 1993.

62. McDonagh J, Carvell N, Lee MH: Dysfibrinogenemia and other disorders of fibrinogen structure and function. *In* Colman RW, Hirsh J, Marder VJ, et al (eds): Hemostasis and Thrombosis: Basic Principles and Clinical Practice, 3rd ed. Philadelphia, JB Lippincott, 1994, p 314.
63. Roberts HR, Lefkowitz JB: Inherited disorders of prothrombin conversion. *In* Colman RW, Hirsch J, Marder VJ, et al (eds): Hemostasis and Thrombosis: Basic Principles and Clinical Practice, 3rd ed. Philadelphia, JB Lippincott, 1994, p 200.
64. Tefferi A, Nichols WL: Acquired von Willebrand disease: Concise review of occurrence, diagnosis, pathogenesis, and treatment. Am J Med 103:536, 1997.
65. Remuzzi G: Bleeding in renal failure. Lancet 1:1205, 1988.
66. Shearer MJ: Vitamin K. Lancet 345:229, 1995.
67. Thorp JA, Gaston L, Caspers DR, et al: Current concepts and controversies in the use of vitamin K. Drugs 49:376, 1995.
68. Baglin T: Disseminated intravascular coagulation: Diagnosis and treatment. BMJ 312:683, 1996.
69. Lechner K, Niessner H, Thaler E: Coagulation abnormalities in liver disease. Semin Thromb Haemost 4:40, 1977.
70. Joist JH: Hemostatic abnormalities in liver disease. *In* Colman RW, Hirsh J, Marder VJ, et al (eds): Hemostasis and Thrombosis: Basic Principles and Clinical Practice, 3rd ed. Philadelphia, JB Lippincott, 1994, p 906.
71. Hersh S, Kunelis T, Francis RB: Pathogenesis of accelerated fibrinolysis in liver cirrhosis: A critical role for tissue plasminogen activator inhibitor. Blood 69:1315, 1987.
72. Rock WA: Laboratory assessment of coagulation disorders in liver disease. Clin Lab Med 4:419, 1984.
73. Feinstein DI: Treatment of disseminated intravascular coagulation. Semin Thromb Hemost 14:351, 1988.
74. Levi M, van der Poll T, ten Cate H, et al: The cytokine-mediated imbalance between coagulant and anticoagulant mechanisms in sepsis and endotoxaemia. Eur J Clin Invest 27:3, 1997.
75. Williams E: Disseminated intravascular coagulation. *In* Loscalzo J, Schafer A (eds): Thrombosis and Hemorrhage. Boston, Blackwell Science, 1994, p 1023.
76. Hesselvik JF, Blomback M, Brodin B, et al: Coagulation, fibrinolysis, and kallikrein systems in sepsis: Relation to outcome. Crit Care Med 17:724, 1989.
77. Atik M: Hemostasis and thrombosis. *In* Peters RM, Peacock EE, Benfield JR (eds): The Scientific Management of the Surgical Patient. Boston, Little, Brown, 1983, p 229.
78. Weitz JI, Leslie B, Ginsberg J: Soluble FDP potentiates tissue plasminogen activator-induced fibrinogen proteolysis. J Clin Invest 87:1082, 1991.
79. Micallef-Eynaud PD, Ludlam CA: Aortic aneurysms and consumptive coagulopathy. Blood Coagul Fibrinol 2:477, 1991.
80. Mulcare RJ, Royster TS, Phillips LL: Intravascular coagulation in surgical procedures on the abdominal aorta. Surg Gynecol Obstet 143:730, 1976.
81. Declerck PJ, Juhan-Vague I, Felez J, et al: Pathophysiology of fibrinolysis. J Int Med 236:425, 1994.
82. Francis CW, Marder VJ: Mechanisms of fibrinolysis. *In* Beutler E, Lichtman MA, Coller BS, et al (eds): Williams' Hematology, 5th ed. New York, McGraw-Hill, 1995, p 1252.
83. Dzik WH, Arkin CF, Jenkins RL, et al: Fibrinolysis during liver transplantation in humans: Role of tissue-type plasminogen activator. Blood 71:1090, 1988.
84. Illig KA, Ouriel K: Ancrod: Understanding the agent. Semin Vasc Surg 9:303, 1996.
85. Eagleton M, Illig KA, Riggs PN, et al: Visceral perfusion ameliorates primary fibrinolysis during supraceliac aortic cross-clamping. Surg Forum 1997, p 419.
86. Collen D, Lijnen HR, Todd PA, et al: Tissue-type plasminogen activator: A review of its pharmacology and therapeutic use as a thrombolytic agent. Drugs 38:346, 1989.
87. Wakefield TW, Stanley JC: Intraoperative heparin anticoagulation and its reversal. Semin Vasc Surg 9:296, 1996.
88. Hirsch J, Raschke R, Warkentin TE, et al: Heparin: Mechanism of action, pharmakokinetics, dosing considerations, monitoring, efficacy, and safety. Chest 108(Suppl):258S, 1995.
89. Donayre CE: Current use of low molecular weight heparins. Semin Vasc Surg 9:362, 1996.
90. Hirsch J, Dalen JE, Deykin D, et al: Oral anticoagulants, mechanism of action, clinical effectiveness, and optimal therapeutic range. Chest 108(Suppl):231S, 1995.
91. Schafer AI: Effects of nonsteroidal antiinflammatory drugs on platelet function and systemic hemostasis. Clin Pharmacol 35:209, 1995.
92. Feinstein DI: Immune coagulation disorders. *In* Colman RW, Hirsch J, Marder VJ, et al (eds): Hemostasis and Thrombosis: Basic Principles and Clinical Practice, 3rd ed. Philadelphia, JB Lippincott, 1994, p 881.
93. Sallah S: Inhibitors to clotting factors. Ann Hematol 75:1, 1997.
94. Seremetis SV, Aledort LM: Congenital bleeding disorders: Rational treatment options. Drugs 45:541, 1993.
95. Khamashta MA, Cuadrado MJ, Mujic F, et al: The management of thrombosis in the antiphospholipid antibody syndrome. N Engl J Med 332:993, 1995.
96. Kandarpa K: Complications of local intraarterial thrombolysis for lower extremity occlusions. *In* Ouriel K (ed): Lower Extremity Vascular Disease. Philadelphia, WB Saunders, 1995, p 359.
97. NIH Consensus Conference: Perioperative red blood cell transfusion. JAMA 260:2700, 1988.
98. American College of Physicians: Practice strategies for elective red blood transfusion. Ann Intern Med 116:403, 1992.
99. Consensus Conference: Blood management and surgical practice guidelines. Am J Surg 170(Suppl 6A):1S, 1995.
100. NIH Consensus Conference: Fesh frozen plasma: Indications and risks. JAMA 253:551, 1985.
101. NIH Consensus Conference: Platelet transfusion therapy. JAMA 257:1777, 1987.
102. Avoiding the misuse of fresh frozen plasma (editorial). BMJ 307:395, 1993.
103. Spence RK: Emerging trends in surgical blood transfusion. Semin Hematol 34(Suppl 2):48, 1997.
104. Adams RC, Lundy JS: Anesthesia in cases of poor surgical risk: Some suggestions for decreasing the risk. Surg Gynecol Obstet 74:1011, 1942.
105. Lipsett PA, Perler B: The use of blood products for surgical bleeding. Semin Vasc Surg 9:347, 1996.
106. Ouriel K, Shortell CK, Green RM, et al: Intraoperative autotransfusion in aortic surgery. J Vasc Surg 18:16, 1993.
107. Triulzi DJ: Plasma Alternatives. Transfusion Medicine Update. Institute for Transfusion Medicine, 1997.
108. Rutledge R, Sheldon GF, Collins ML: Massive transfusion. Crit Care Clin 2:791, 1986.
109. Ratnoff OD: Some therapeutic agents influencing hemostasis. *In* Colman RW, Hirsh J, Marder VJ, et al (eds): Hemostasis and Thrombosis: Basic Principles and Clinical Practice, 3rd ed. Philadelphia, JB Lippincott, 1994, p 1104.
110. Mannucci PM, Ruggeri ZM, Pareti FI, et al: 1-Deamino-8-D-arginine vasopressin: A new pharmacological approach to the management of hemophilia and von Willebrand's disease. Lancet 1:869, 1987.
111. Sakarisen KS, Catteneo M, vd Berg A, et al: DDAVP enhances platelet adherence and platelet aggregate grown on human artery subendothelium. Blood 64:229, 1984.
112. Mannucci PM, Remuzzi G, Pusineri F, et al: Deamino-8-D-arginine vasopressin shortens the bleeding time in uremia. N Engl J Med 308:8, 1983.
113. Salzman EW, Weinstein MJ, Reilly D, et al: Adventures in hemostasis: Desmopressin in cardiac surgery. Arch Surg 128:212, 1993.
114. Clagett GP: Desmopressin, hemostasis, and vascular surgery. Semin Vasc Surg 9:340, 1996.
115. Kobrinsky NL, Letts RM, Patel LR, et al: 1-Deamino-8-D-arginine vasopressin (desmopressin) decreases operative blood loss in patients having Harrington rod spinal fusion surgery. Ann Intern Med 107:446, 1987.
116. Clagett GP, Valentine J, Myers SI, et al: Does desmopressin improve hemostasis and reduce blood loss from aortic surgery? A randomized, double-blind study. J Vasc Surg 22:223, 1995.
117. Okajima Y, Kanayama S, Maeda Y, et al: Studies on the neutralizing mechanism of antithrombin activity of heparin by protamine. Thromb Res 24:21, 1981.
118. Gupta SK, Veith FJ, Ascer E, et al: Anaphylactoid reactions to protamine: An often lethal complication in insulin-dependent patients undergoing vascular surgery. J Vasc Surg 9:342, 1989.
119. Morel DR, Zapol WM, Thomas SJ, et al: C5a and thromboxane generation associated with pulmonary vaso- and bronchoconstriction during protamine reversal of heparin. Anesthesiology 66:597, 1987.

120. Mauney MC, Buchanan SA, Lawrence WA, et al: Stroke rate is markedly reduced after carotid endarterectomy by avoidance of protamine. J Vasc Surg 22:264, 1995.
121. Knape JT, Schuller JL, de Hann P, et al: An anaphylactic reaction to protamine in a patient allergic to fish. Anesthesiology 55:324, 1981.
122. Samuel T: Antibodies reacting with salmon and human protamines in sera from infertile men and from vasectomized men and monkees. Clin Exp Immunol 30:181, 1977.
123. Levy JH, Zaiden JR, Faraj B: Prospective evaluation of risk of protamine reactions in patients with NPH insulin dependent diabetes. Anesth Analg 65:739, 1986.
124. Levy JH, Schweiger IM, Zaiden JR, et al: Evaluation of patients at risk for protamine reactions. J Thorac Cardiovasc Surg 98:200, 1989.
125. Anderson MN, Mendelow M, Alfano GA: Experimental studies of heparin-protamine activity with special reference to protamin inhibition of clotting. Surgery 46:1060, 1959.
126. Teoh KH, Young E, Bradley CA, et al: Heparin binding proteins: Contribution to heparin rebound after cardiopulmonary bypass. Circulation 88(II):420, 1993.
127. Sherry S, Marder VJ: Therapy with antifibrinolytic agents. *In* Colman RW, Hirsh J, Marder VJ, et al (eds): Hemostasis and Thrombosis: Basic Principles and Clinical Practice, 3rd ed. Philadelphia, JB Lippincott, 1994, p 335.
128. Alkjaersig N, Fletcher AP, Sherry S: Epsilon-aminocaproic acid: An inhibitor of plasminogen activation. J Biol Chem 234:832, 1959.
129. de Peppo AP, Pierri MD, Scafuri A, et al: Intraoperative antifibrinolysis and blood-saving techniques in cardiac surgery: Prospective trial of 3 antifibrinolytic drugs. Texas Heart Inst J 22:231, 1995.
130. Robert S, Wagner BKJ, Boulanger M, et al: Aprotinin. Ann Pharmacother 30:372, 1996.
131. Golub R, Cantu R, Sorrento JJ, et al: Efficacy of preadmission testing in ambulatory surgical patients. Am J Surg 163:565, 1992.
132. Narr BJ, Hansen TR, Warner MA: Preoperative laboratory screening in healthy Mayo patients: Cost-effective elimination of tests and unchanged outcomes. Mayo Clin Proc 66:155, 1991.
133. Velanovich V: Preoperative laboratory evaluation. J Am Coll Surg 183:79, 1996.
134. Rapaport SI: Preoperative hemostatic evaluation: Which tests, if any? Blood 61:229, 1983.
135. Post M, Telfer MD: Surgery in hemophiliac patients. J Bone Joint Surg 57A:1136, 1975.
136. Hermens WT: Dose calculation of human factor VIII and factor IX concentrates for infusion therapy. *In* Brinkhous KM, Hemker HC (eds): Handbook for Hemophilia. New York, Elsevier America, 1975, p 569.
137. Tuman KJ, McCarthy RJ, O'Connor CJ, et al: Aspirin does not increase allogenic blood transfusion in reoperative coronary artery surgery. Anesth Analg 83:1178, 1996.
138. Ferraris VA, Ferraris SP: Preoperative aspirin ingestion increases operative blood loss after coronary artery bypass grafting (update). Ann Thorac Surg 59:1036, 1995.
139. Antiplatelet Trialists' Collaboration: Collaborative overview of randomized trials of antiplatelet therapy—II: Maintenance of vascular graft or arterial patency by antiplatelet therapy. BMJ 308:159, 1994.
140. Hobson RW, Krupski WC, Weiss DG: Influence of aspirin in the management of asymptomatic carotid artery stenosis. J Vasc Surg 17:257, 1993.
141. ISIS-2 (Second International Study of Infarct Survival) Collaborative Group: Randomised trial of intravenous streptokinase, oral aspirin, both, or neither among 17,187 cases of suspected acute myocardial infarction: ISIS-s. Lancet 2:349, 1988.
142. Steering Committee of the Physicians' Health Study Research Group: Final report on the aspirin component of the ongoing physicians' health study. N Engl J Med 321:129, 1989.
143. Ferrera A, MacArthur JD, Wright HK, et al: Hypothermia and acidosis worsen coagulopathy in the patient requiring massive transfusion. Am J Surg 160:515, 1990.
144. Reed RL, Johnston TD, Hudson JD, et al: The disparity between hypothermic coagulopathy and clotting studies. J Trauma 33:465, 1992.
145. Yoshihara H, Yamamoto T, Mihara H: Changes in coagulation and fibrinolysis occurring in dogs during hypothermia. Thromb Res 37:503, 1985.
146. Valeri CR, Feingold H, Cassidy G, et al: Hypothermia-induced reversable platelet dysfunction. Ann Surg 205:175, 1987.
147. Edmunds LH: Blood-surface interactions during cardiopulmonary bypass. J Cardiol Surg 8:404, 1993.
148. Woodman RC, Harker LA: Bleeding complications associated with cardiopulmonary bypass. Blood 76:1680, 1990.
149. Clagett GP, Russo M, Hufnagel H: Platelet changes after placement of aortic prostheses in dogs. I: Biochemical and functional alterations. J Lab Clin Med 97:345, 1981.
150. Harker LA, Slichter SJ, Sauvage LR: Platelet consumption by arterial prostheses: The effects of endothelialization and pharmacologic inhibition of platelet function. Ann Surg 186:594, 1977.
151. Mullins RJ, Huckfeldt R, Trunkey DD: Abdominal vascular injuries. Surg Clin North Am 76:813, 1996.
152. Aucar JA, Hirshberg A: Damage control for vascular injuries. Surg Clin North Am 77:853, 1997.
153. Rotondo MF, Zonies DH: The damage control sequence and underlying logic. Surg Clin North Am 77:761, 1997.

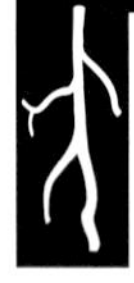

CHAPTER 44

Blood Loss and Transfusion in Vascular Surgery

Richard K. Spence, M.D., F.A.C.S

The specialty of vascular surgery was made possible, in part, by the development of modern transfusion science that made blood and blood products readily available to the surgeon. Successful vascular surgery depended in the past on a capable blood bank. The risks of transfusion were thought to be minimal, and both red blood cells and component products were used by the vascular surgeon with impunity. Renewed recognition of the risks and inherent dangers of *allogeneic*, or banked, volunteer donor, blood has spurred the recent movement toward bloodless surgery and the search for alternatives to allogeneic blood in vascular surgery. This chapter reviews anemia, bleeding, and transfusion in vascular surgery, with guidelines for present practice and an eye toward the future.

RISKS OF ALLOGENEIC BLOOD

The risks of allogeneic blood can be classified broadly into (1) transfusion reactions, (2) disease transmission, and (3) immunomodulation. Transfusion reactions can be divided into three main groups: (1) acute intravascular immune hemolytic from ABO incompatibility, (2) delayed immune hemolytic, and (3) febrile reactions.[117] Reactions occur in approximately 5% of transfusion recipients. The risk of a fatal hemolytic reaction is less than 1:1,000,000; risks of nonfatal hemolytic reactions and febrile reactions are 1:25,000 and 1:100, respectively.[139]

Symptoms of ABO incompatibility reactions include (1) hemoglobinuria, (2) fever, (3) chills, (4) coagulopathy, (5) chest pain, and (6) circulatory collapse. In the unconscious, anesthetized patient, acute reactions present as either sudden hypotension in the euvolemic patient or unexpected bleeding secondary to disseminated intravascular coagulation (DIC).[203] Awareness of this symptom complex is paramount, because such reactions may be misidentified by the vascular surgeon.

Delayed hemolytic reactions are caused by non-ABO antigen-antibody incompatibilities. Symptoms appear within 3 to 10 days after transfusion and include fever, malaise, hyperbilirubinemia, and falling hematocrit. A falling hematocrit during the immediate postoperative period in a recently transfused patient is often attributed to recurrent or continued bleeding. A danger exists in continuing to transfuse such a patient with incompatible blood. In the worst-case scenario, an acute hemolytic reaction can be precipitated if blood has not been cross-matched again since the original transfusion. A delayed hemolytic reaction should be ruled out by appropriate antibody testing in any patient with a falling, postoperative hematocrit and no evidence of ongoing bleeding.[207]

Febrile reactions, the most common type of reaction, are caused by circulating recipient antibodies to donor leukocyte or platelet contaminants. Although these reactions usually produce only minor discomfort in the patient, serious leukocyte-mediated pulmonary infiltrates and insufficiency have been reported.[91] The incidence of febrile reactions can be diminished greatly by the use of a leukodepletion filter.[128] Transfusion-related acute lung injury (TRALI) is clinically indistinguishable from adult respiratory distress syndrome (ARDS), producing pulmonary edema and hypoxia.[187] This reaction may be caused by either recipient alloimmunization (i.e., reaction of the recipient's anti–human leukocyte antigen [anti-HLA] antibodies to donor leukocytes) or direct infusion of high levels of anti-HLA antibody in donor plasma (usually from a multiparous female donor).

Graft-versus-host disease (GVHD) results from the engraftment of immunocompetent T lymphocytes, typically in a reicpient who is immunosuppressed, although the syndrome has been seen after cardiac surgery, cholecystectomy, prostatectomy, and normal delivery.[185] GVHD is characterized by fever, skin rash, and gastrointestinal symptoms and is almost always fatal. GVHD is most common following directed donations from immediate family members who are first-degree relatives or who share an HLA haplotype. Fortunately, the offending lymphocytes are sensitive to γ-irradiation and can be eliminated by pretransfusion treatment with cesium 137 or cobalt 60 at doses that do not damage red blood cells.[138]

Blood can carry and transmit a wide variety of viral, parasitic rickettsial and bacterial diseases. The risks of contracting various diseases are listed in Table 44–1. State-of-the-art human immunodeficiency virus (HIV) testing, which includes screening of high-risk patients, p24 HIV antigen analysis, and antibody testing, has all but eliminated the risk of transmitting this virus by transfusion.[125]

Hepatitis C virus accounts for 98% of the risk to patients in terms of both disease transmission and mortality.[5] Cytomegalovirus (CMV), a member of the herpes family, is present in up to half the units of allogeneic blood transfused.[247] This virus presents a small but troublesome risk, especially to seronegative-status adults who may need multiple transfusions (e.g., those with a ruptured abdominal aortic aneurysm or those who have suffered a blunt trauma). Clinical symptoms vary in severity and may include pulmonary, gastrointestinal, and systemic manifestations. Physicians can avoid exposing patients to CMV by eliminating unnecessary transfusions, screening for antibodies, and filtering leukocytes, which carry the virus.[128]

Many other diseases can be transmitted by transfusion, including malaria, Chagas' disease, Q fever, and Lyme disease. Vascular surgeons should remember that allogeneic blood has the potential to transmit infectious disease despite their best efforts.

A variety of animal and human studies have demonstrated systemic immunomodulation caused by allogeneic transfusion.[21, 118, 228] Both cellular and humoral factors seem to play a role. Macrophage function is altered, resulting in decreased migratory capabilities and decreased eicosanoid and interleukin-2 (IL-2) production. Lymphocyte responses to both antigen and mitogen are suppressed; suppressor cell activity is increased with concomitant declines in helper suppressor cell ratios. Both an increased susceptibility to bacterial infection and an increased cancer-related mortality rate following allogeneic transfusion have been reported.[228, 234]

TABLE 44–1. RISKS OF ALLOGENEIC TRANSFUSION (UNITS OF BLOOD TRANSFUSED)

Noninfectious Risks	
Fatal ABO incompatibility reaction	1:1,000,000
Nonfatal hemolytic reaction	1:25,000
Febrile reaction	1:100
Immunosuppression	? (potentially 1:1)
Graft-versus-host disease (GVHD)	Rare
Infectious Risks	
Human immunodeficiency virus type 1 (HIV-1)	1:650,000
Human T-cell lymphoma virus (HTLV)	Minimal
Viral hepatitis	1:5000
Bacterial infection	Rare
Chagas' disease	Unknown

Data from Lackritz EM, et al: N Engl J Med 333:1721–1725, 1995[125]; Linden JV, Pisciotto PT: Trans Med Rev VI:116–123, 1992[138]; Klein HG: Am J Surg 170(Suppl 6A):21S–26S, 1995[117]; Leiby DA, et al: Transfusion 37:259–263, 1997[135]; Dodd RY: Hematol Oncol Clin North Am 9:137–154, 1995.[56]

Although the clinical impact of transfusion-related immunosuppression has not been established definitively, the surgeon should be aware of the potential risks to patients. Surgeons can help eliminate or reduce this problem by avoiding allogeneic blood transfusion or using leukodepletion filters.[128]

Attention has recently been focused on the damage done to red blood cells and platelets during storage.[114] These so-called storage lesions may produce elevated levels of potassium and decreased levels of 2,3-diphosphoglycerate (2,3-DPG).[66] Infusion of potassium in quantity, as in massive transfusion protocols, can lead to cardiac arrhythmias. Lack of 2,3-DPG results in a higher than desired red blood cell oxygen affinity, causing impaired release of oxygen to tissues. Recovery of sufficient 2,3-DPG levels to correct this problem may take 24 to 48 hours, depending on the length of pretransfusion storage. Platelets develop a progressive storage lesion during their 5-day residence in the blood bank, but the lesion does not usually result in impaired effectiveness.[132, 166] Both allogeneic and *autologous*, or one's own, blood may also be contaminated by overgrowth of bacteria, such as *Yersinia enterocolitica*, during storage.[19] Transfusion of contaminated blood typically produces overwhelming sepsis and death.

THE TRANSFUSION DECISION

Physiologic Responses to Anemia

Maintenance of oxygen delivery and consumption depends on both adequate amounts of hemoglobin and a normally functioning heart. When the hemoglobin level drops, the heart increases cardiac output through either an increase in stroke vloume or an increase in heart rate (Table 44–2).[85, 178] As the hematocrit falls, blood viscosity decreases, leading to an increase in venous return or augmentation of preload. Increases in heart rate are thought to be caused by stimulation of aortic chemoreceptors and the release of catecholamines. The ability of the heart to respond is affected by multiple factors, including (1) underlying disease, (2) the patient's overall condition (e.g., shock and volume status), and (3) the types and amounts of medications given, including anesthetics and beta-blockers.

Because the heart extracts approximately 80% of the oxygen delivered under normal conditions, its ability to increase output is limited by its ability to increase its own oxygen consumption. Cardiac oxygen extraction is improved by coronary artery dilation, which increases coronary flow. In the presence of coronary artery disease, the heart may be unable to provide the work needed to increase total body oxygen delivery without risk to the myocardium.[224] Under these conditions, coronary blood flow is shifted from the endocardium to the epicardium, thereby placing subendocardial tissue at an increased risk of ischemia. Continued demands on the stressed heart to provide oxygen may come at the expense of conversion to an anaerobic metabolic state and eventual subendocardial infarction.[9, 85]

Animal studies of normovolemic hemodilution have shown that the lower limit of cardiac tolerance for anemia lies around 3 to 5 gm/dl in the absence of underlying disease.[70, 252] Clinical trials have shown that in healthy subjects a target hematocrit of 20% to 25% (hemoglobin level of 7.0 to 8.0 gm/dl) is feasible and safe for the patient. Kreimeier and Messmer have demonstrated in humans that intraoperative target hemoglobin levels of 5.0 gm/dl and less have been tolerated by surgical patients without adverse effects.[121] In one study, pediatric patients (1 to 8 years of age) underwent hemodilution with either hydroxyethyl starch or dextran in conjunction with major surgery. A decrease in hematocrit to 17% (equivalent to a hemoglobin level of 5.6 gm/dl) was well tolerated, with no signficant decrease in oxygen delivery and global tissue oxygenation.[6]

Peripheral tissues may also compensate for anemia by increasing oxygen delivery, either by recruiting more capillaries or by increasing blood flow through existing beds.[90] Some tissues, particularly those that are supply-dependent, may compensate by increasing oxygen extraction. In the chronically anemic patient, increases in stroke volume and, therefore, in cardiac output are supplemented by increased levels of 2,3-DPG. These intracellular changes shift the oxyhemoglobin curve to the right, facilitating oxygen offload and increasing oxygen delivery.

Compensatory changes are similar in patients with chronic anemia. Georgieva and Georgieva demonstrated alterations in both the microcirculation and the heart in 299 female patients with severe iron-deficiency anemia.[72] Most patients showed increased diameter and irregularity of the microcirculation. At lower hemoglobin levels, significant enlargement of the left ventricle and increased cardiac output and stroke volume were observed. A slight reduction in myocardial contractility was found only in those patients with severe anemia. Treatment with parenteral iron induced a complete reversibility of both myocardial and microcirculatory changes with moderate and slight degrees of iron-deficiency anemia.

Anemia also affects blood coagulation. This is most apparent in the patient who has suffered extensive blood loss and has undergone massive transfusion. Dilutional

TABLE 44–2. HEMOGLOBIN LEVEL AND OXYGEN TRANSPORT RELATIONSHIPS

PARAMETER	FORMULA	NORMAL RANGE
Cardiac output (CO)	Stroke volume (SV) × heart rate (HR)	4–6 L/min
Arterial oxygen content (Ca_{O_2})	$1.34 \times Hb \times Sa_{O_2} + (0.003 \times Pa_{O_2})$	15–22 ml/dl
Mixed venous oxygen content (Cv_{O_2})	$1.34 \times Hb \times Sv_{O_2} + (0.003 \times Pv_{O_2})$	12–17 ml/dl
Oxygen delivery (D_{O_2})	$CO \times Ca_{O_2} \times 10$	500–750 ml/min/m^2
Oxygen consumption (V_{O_2})	$CO \times (Ca_{O_2} - Cv_{O_2}) \times 10$	100–300 ml/min/m^2
Oxygen extraction ratio (O_2ER)	V_{O_2}/D_{O_2}	0.23–0.30

Hb = hemoglobin.

coagulopathy may occur in the trauma patient, depending on the amount of blood lost and transfused.[48, 217] Standard teaching relates this defect in coagulation to loss or dilution of platelets.

Red blood cells and platelets, however, work in conjunction to promote hemostasis. Red blood cells disperse platelets to the periphery of vessels, where they come into contact with the endothelium more readily.[242] Red blood cells can stimulate platelets to release thromboxane A_2.[243] Red blood cell transfusions correct bleeding times and improve platelet function in patients with chronic renal failure.[141]

The exact hematocrit necessary to cause these changes is unknown. When hematocrit is in the 25% to 35% range, blood viscosity–mediated shear stress induces red blood cells to release adenosine diphosphate (ADP), which affects platelet function.[4] Much more work is needed to clarify the interactions between hematocrit, red blood cells, and platelets as well as their impact on the clinical decision to transfuse.

Transfusion Triggers in Vascular Surgery

Traditionally the degree of anemia has played the most significant role in the transfusion decision in surgery, since most transfusions are based on isolated hemoglobin and hematocrit values[47, 83, 147] The National Institutes of Health (NIH) consensus conference, convened in 1988 to address the topic of perioperative red blood cell transfusion, focused primarily on the risks of transfusion and the need to modify transfusion practices. It also produced recommendations for a new hemoglobin-based transfusion trigger that represented an update over the traditional *10/30 rule* that had existed for years.[1] The target, or trigger, hemoglobin level was lowered to 8 gm/dl, and guidelines for transfusion were given that directed attention toward a global assessment of physiologic status, clinical need, and symptoms rather than numbers alone.

Current policies that focus on global triggers state that, ideally, blood should be transfused only when there is a documented need to increase oxygen delivery in those patients who cannot meet demands through normal cardiopulmonary mechanisms.[6, 225, 239] This criterion is reasonable because the primary function of red blood cells is to transport oxygen to tissues. Therefore, any red cell transfusion should be performed based on the patient's physiology (i.e., to provide the additional oxygen delivery needed to correct or protect against the development of tissue hypoxia).[148]

Optimization of the patient's cardiopulmonary hemodynamics should precede red blood cell transfusion.[85] Improved oxygen delivery and cardiodynamics can be achieved in many patients through a variety of means, including increased inspired oxygen, fluid infusions to increase preload, and the use of inotropes. Such interventions are more likely to be successful in patients under 50 years of age who have good cardiac function.[148]

Robertie and Gravlee recommend that surgeons accept a transfusion trigger of 6 gm/dl for well-compensated patients with no heart disease and no postoperative complications, but raise the trigger to 8 gm/dl for patients with stable cardiac disease and an expected blood loss of 300 ml or more.[195] Older patients and those with postoperative complications who cannot increase cardiac output to compensate for hemodilution should be given a transfusion when the hemoglobin level reaches 10 gm/dl.

In most clinical settings, oxygen consumption is relatively independent of hemoglobin level across a wide range of oxygen delivery values because of compensations made in cardiac output and oxygen extraction (Fig. 44–1). Symptoms of exertional dyspnea do not appear in the otherwise healthy individual until hemoglobin level reaches 7 gm/dl.[30] Even at this and lower levels, symptoms and signs are variable.[165] Because vascular surgical patients typically have coronary artery disease and may not be able to compensate readily for anemia during acute blood loss (i.e., during

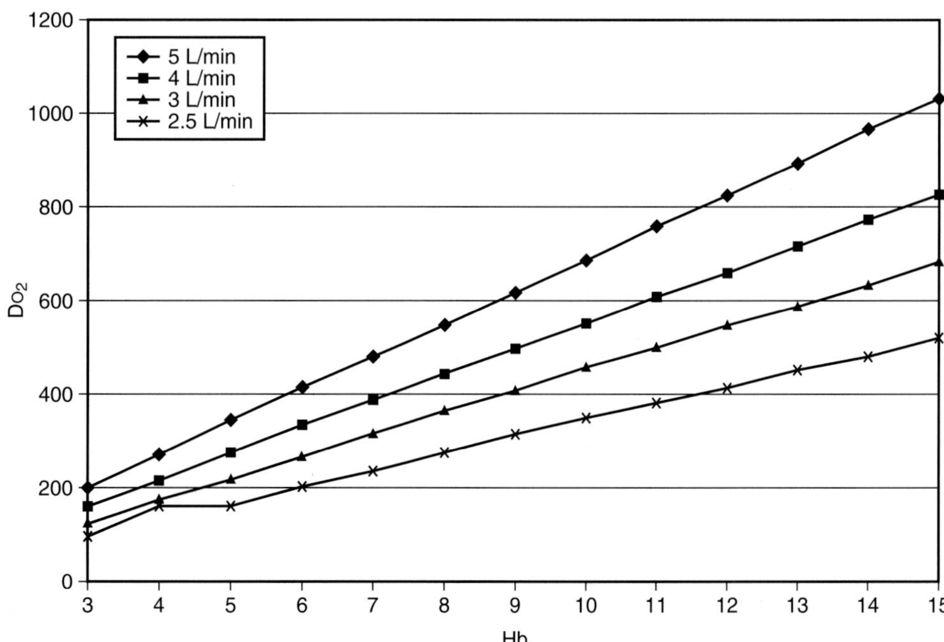

FIGURE 44–1. Influence of hemoglobin (Hb) and cardiac output on oxygen delivery (Do_2).

abdominal aortic surgery), it is appropriate to consider a hemoglobin level higher than 7 to 8 gm/dl.

This position is supported by retrospective analyses of nontransfused, anemic patients and the few clinical trials of transfusion practice that exist. In a study of mortality rate and hemoglobin level in Jehovah's Witnesses by Carson and coworkers, preoperative cardiac disease (as defined by the Multifactorial Cardiac Risk Index) appeared to worsen outcome.[34] An increased incidence of electrocardiographic evidence of myocardial ischemia in postoperative vascular patients with a hematocrit below 29% was found by two separate investigators.[40, 169] These studies suggest that patients with cardiac disease may need hemoglobin levels higher than 8 gm/dl, although no study accounted for the presence or severity of underlying heart disease.

The issue was addressed further in a retrospective, cohort study of 1958 adult Jehovah's Witnesses surgical patients by Carson and associates.[33] This work, which demonstrated that the nontransfused Jehovah's Witnesses patient with cardiopulmonary disease was at increased risk of dying as the hemoglobin level dropped below 10 gm/dl, further supports the decision to maintain a hemoglobin level above 8 gm/dl in the vascular surgical patient.

The appropriate hemoglobin trigger for vascular surgical patients was analyzed by Bush and associates in their prospective, randomized trial of two treatment strategies designed to test the transfusion trigger of 10 gm/dl.[28] Ninety-nine patients undergoing elective aortic and infrainguinal arterial reconstructions were prospectively randomized preoperatively to receive transfusions to maintain a hemoglobin level of either 10 or 9 gm/dl. There were no significant differences in mortality and cardiac morbidity rates, length of hospital stay, or oxygen consumption between the two groups. A multicenter, randomized, controlled pilot study of two transfusion triggers (one restrictive, 7 to 9 gm/dl; one liberal, 10 to 12 gm/dl) in the treatment of critically ill patients showed no difference in intensive care unit (ICU) 30-day and 120-day mortality.[97, 98]

Unfortunately, evidence that red blood cell transfusions are beneficial remains elusive. A meta-analysis of clinical trials designed to maximize oxygen delivery in ICU patients by raising parameters to supranormal levels, which included the use of red blood cell transfusion, was unable to demonstrate any reduction in mortality rate.[102] A recent analysis of almost 10,000 hip fracture patients by Carson and coworkers showed that transfusion had no impact on either 30-day or 90-day mortality rate.[32] Finally, an extensive review of all of the relevant literature on clinical transfusion trials, risks, and benefits found no conclusive evidence of benefit from red blood cell transfusion.[99]

In conclusion, the decision to transfuse should be based on the specific patient's physiologic needs and condition. Transfusion need should be assessed for each patient on a case-by-case basis. This assessment should include (1) a history and physical examination, (2) a review of pertinent laboratory data, (3) consideration of the operation planned and expected amount of blood loss, and (4) analysis of risk factors that may contribute to increased morbidity and mortality.

The history and physical examination should focus on preexisting diseases and conditions that may increase the risk of blood loss or the need for increased oxygen delivery. Cardiac, pulmonary, and other atherosclerotic disease processes should be assessed and quantified when possible. Patients with coronory artery disease and pulmonary hypoxia usually require higher perioperative hemoglobin levels than those with normal hearts and lungs to avoid ischemia and undue cardiac stress. Current evidence, although limited, supports the decision to maintain a perioperative hemoglobin level between 9 and 10 gm/dl in vascular surgical patients.

FACTORS AFFECTING BLOOD LOSS AND TRANSFUSION

Transfusion Practices

Little is known about transfusion practices in vascular surgery. Surveys of blood product use in a variety of surgical procedures consistently have shown extensive interhospital and surgeon-to-surgeon variability in both the types of patients undergoing transfusing and the amount of blood given. The use of alternatives to allogeneic transfusion is also inconsistent.[90, 95, 227, 233] It is safe to conclude that the variabilities found in other surgical procedures can be found in vascular surgical practice. The vascular surgery literature covers both the types of procedures in which blood loss can be expected and the factors than can contribute to blood loss and need for transfusion. These most common factors include (1) trauma,[42, 172, 176] (2) repair of both ruptured and elective abdominal aortic aneurysms,[28, 93, 109, 110, 145, 153, 175] (3) direct venous surgery including thrombectomy and thrombolysis,[46, 171, 246] and (4) thoracoabdominal aneurysm repair.[68, 245] Less common factors include (1) resection of major vessels in conjunction with urologic tumor resections[129] and (2) retroperitoneal hematoma following cardiac catheterization (Fig. 44–2).[116] Factors associated with need for allogeneic transfusion and amount of blood loss include (1) the surgeon's experience, (2) the length of the operation, (3) patient age and preoperative hematocrit, and (4) the use of alternative procedures such as autotransfusion and technical approaches. The role of hematocrit and the use of alternatives are discussed later in this chapter.

Coagulation abnormalities are an important cause of operative bleeding in suprarenal aortic surgery and reflect the need for the vascular surgeon to specifically measure and correct clotting factor deficits and fibrinolysis.[27, 73] In the only specific survey of vascular surgical transfusion practices published to date, Milne and Murphy found that the majority of 31 vascular surgeons practicing in Scotland followed a blood-ordering schedule for both elective and emergency surgeries. Surgeons typically used twice as much blood (8 units) for emergency surgery than for elective surgery.[157]

Several studies have demonstrated that transfusion guidelines, practice policies, and transfusion algorithms can bring some sense to transfusion practices while reducing the risk of exposure to allogeneic blood.[61, 164, 184, 218, 221, 238] The first step in this process is for the vascular surgeon to review his or her transfusion practices to become familiar with which patients need transfusion and how much blood is used. Blood losses should be calculated, not estimated.[23]

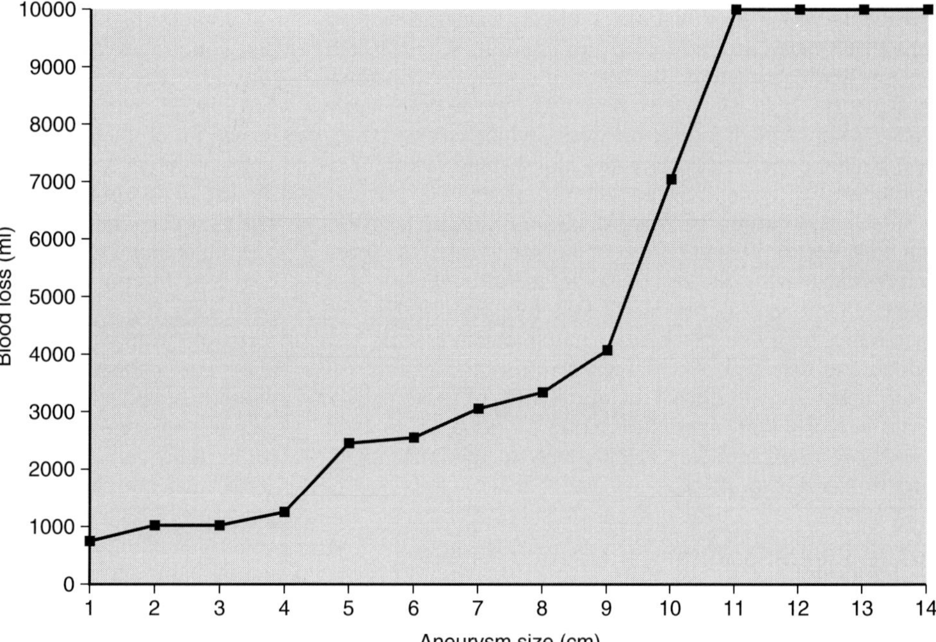

FIGURE 44–2. Influence of aneurysm size on blood loss. (Adapted with permission from Lord RSA, Hardman DTA, Margovsky A: Use of the Cell Saver in aortic aneurysm reconstruction. *In* Tawes RL [ed]: Autotransfusion: Therapeutic Principles and Trends. Detroit, Gregory Appleton, 1997, p 151.)

With this information, the surgeon can establish a blood-ordering schedule to serve as a personal guideline for both allogeneic blood use and institution of appropriate alternatives. The overall impact of such efforts can be determined only after further, randomized trials with appropriate outcomes measures are performed.[201]

Bleeding in Surgical Patients

Although blood is a part of vascular surgery, it does not follow that blood *loss* must or should be a part of vascular surgery. Vascular surgeons routinely clamp, cut, and repair the major blood vessels that other surgeons meticulously avoid while resecting or revising adjacent structures. Because of the nature of the operations vascular surgeons perform, it is essential that they understand how to avoid or minimize bleeding. The next portion of the chapter reviews approaches to this problem for both the elective and emergency vascular surgical patient.

Preoperative Aspects

Careful preoperative evaluation of the patient is essential if blood loss is to be reduced and appropriate plans made for transfusion alternatives. Preoperative measurement of hemoglobin level and hematocrit detects the presence of anemia, which can be analyzed further with red blood cell indices. When time allows, iron-deficiency anemia should be corrected by iron supplementation and attention to nutrition.

Many vascular surgeons measure prothrombin time (PT) and partial thromboplastin time (PTT) in all patients who are to receive heparin anticoagulation; some reserve these tests for those patients who are to undergo major vessel (i.e., aortic) surgery. A preferable approach is to question each patient about any bleeding history because most significant bleeding problems are congenital and have occurred in childhood or they are related to specific medications and disease processes.

All patients should be asked about their use of warfarin-based anticoagulants, aspirin, and nonsteroidal anti-inflammatory drugs (NSAIDs) because they all can lead to increased bleeding. When feasible, patients should stop taking these agents well in advance of any planned surgery.[213] Cephalosporin antibiotics that contain a methylthiotetrazole side chain (e.g., cefamandole, cefotetan, moxalactam, cefoperazone) have been associated with hypoprothrombinemia and bleeding and should be used with caution for prophylaxis.[112]

Coagulation studies should be performed only for patients with clinical indications (e.g., a history of liver disease, malignancy, renal failure, and anticoagulant therapy).[62, 150] Similarly, routine platelet measurements are of little value, because deficiencies caused by abnormal production or increased destruction can be detected primarily by a good history and physical examination and because qualitative defects are not be reflected in abnormally low counts.[155, 190]

The presence of a major coagulation disorder, such as hemophilia A or B, is not an absolute contraindication to surgery. Rudowski and associates have reported that major surgical procedures can be performed with acceptable blood loss and outcomes in such affected patients as long as hemostasis can be corrected to normal or near-normal levels with factor replacement therapy.[200]

The vascular surgeon who operates on a hemophiliac patients, however, should be aware that some hemophiliac patients have circulating antibodies to factors that may counteract replacement therapy.[87] Determination of the presence of such inhibiting antibodies and consultation with a hematologist to devise appropriate therapy should be an essential part of every hemophiliac patient's preoperative care. Bleeding that occurs despite factor replacement usually responds to porcine factor VIIIC or cryoprecipitate.[96]

Patients with von Willebrand's disease can be classified into three types depending on the amount of factor VIII present and on whether the factor is normal or abnormal in structure.[162] Patients may have variants of both factor VIII and von Willebrand factor (vWF), which can be identified by prolonged bleeding time and specific factor measurements.[160]

Intravenous administration of desmopressin (DDAVP) can raise factor VIII–vWF levels in type I patients (those with normal factor but low levels) by recruiting factor from tissue endothelial stores.[162] DDAVP infusions should be tried as a first line of therapy in all patients with von Willebrand disease before surgery to prevent bleeding because it has shown efficacy in up to 85% of these patient regardless of disease type. Restriction of blood component therapy to nonresponders helps greatly to minimize exposure to transfusion risks.

Acute Bleeding in the Emergency Patient

Patients who arrive for treatment through the emergency room with active bleeding present a special challenge to the vascular surgeon. Patients who fit into this category include those with bleeding varices, a ruptured aneurysm, or an injured major vessel. The need for transfusion can be decreased primarily through reduction of blood loss. In the bleeding patient, traditionally the first priority has been to correct volume losses and to reverse hypotension with infusions of colloid and crystalloid solutions. The endpoint is to stabilize the patient and improve oxygen delivery by increasing cardiac output as quickly as possible.

This approach has been questioned because of the perception that fluid resuscitation designed to correct hypovolemia and raise blood pressure may prolong or reinitiate hemorrhage. Several investigators have demonstrated in animal models of uncontrolled hemorrhage that attempts to stabilize the animal with intravenous fluid infusions led to continued blood loss and increased mortality rate.[17, 119] This issue was adressed clinically in a prospective study of the effect of fluid resuscitation in hypotensive patients who had sustained penetrating truncal injuries.[152] No significant difference was noted in mortality between two groups of patients assigned to either initial or delayed resuscitation, although the trend was toward a higher death rate in those undergoing initial resuscitation.

These results can be viewed as supporting the traditional approach to early resuscitation as doing no significant harm; however, they do not show its benefit. Delaying fluid resuscitation until hemorrhage is controlled appears to be as safe as the traditional approach and may have the added benefit of reducing transfusion need. The role of small-volume, hypertonic saline resuscitation, with or without colloid, remains controversial.[120]

Early action to control hemorrhage can affect the ability to reduce allogeneic blood exposure in the patient bleeding from a ruptured aorta, an injured vessel, or varices. Prompt diagnosis and timely surgical intervention directed at controlling hemorrhage are the mainstays to limit allogeneic blood exposures in these situations. Early surgery for a leaking or ruptured abdominal aortic aneurysm (AAA) can lead to a successful outcome for most patients, whereas delay leads to increased mortality.[14, 51]

Diagnosis of bleeding or an injury needing vascular repair is not always obvious (e.g., a leaking AAA, a retroperitoneal hematoma in a victim of multiple trauma, and upper gastrointestinal tract bleeding). *Insistence* on radiologic confirmation of bleeding in a patient with obvious clinical signs of active hemorrhage is to be condemned. Although the use of computed tomography (CT) to identify a leaking aneurysm in clinically stable patients has a definite role, one must not assume that the absence of radiologic evidence of bleeding in those patients with symptoms supports delaying surgery. Most series of patients studied that seem to promote the benefits of CT scanning contain at least one patient whose nonleaking aneurysm ruptured while hospitalized and awaiting surgery.[124, 206] Surgical repair of the symptomatic nonruptured aneurysm within 24 to 36 hours remains the standard.[153]

Vascular injuries of the extremities are usually not exsanguinating. Ongoing bleeding can be controlled via direct compression and exploration to attain proximal control followed by either direct repair or bypass.[244] The use of a stent-graft combination to treat a traumatic femoral arteriovenous fistula has been described by Marin and colleagues.[151]

Exsanguination remains the critical factor that determines outcome in isolated, major vascular injuries.[107, 143] The traditional teaching regarding a retroperitoneal or pelvic hematoma in a blunt trauma patient is to leave it alone lest uncontrollable venous bleeding be unleashed. For the patient with a suspected large vessel injury, this approach may lead to continued hemorrhage and deterioration. Braithwaite and Rodriguez recommend opening all central hematomas in blunt trauma victims after proximal and distal aortic control has been established.[22] This approach, based on sound, vascular surgical principles, allows expeditious repair of major injuries while minimizing blood loss.

Angiography remains the standard not only in identifying pelvic vascular injury but also in controlling bleeding by embolization or coil occlusion. Identification of a bleeding vessel with intraoperative ultrasonography may avoid the delays and dangers inherent in angiography.[253] Occlusion, either by catheter or direct ligation, is appropriate in smaller vessels and in areas where collateral circulation is sufficient to maintain perfusion of the affected distal tissues or in life-threatening situations. Occlusion of a proximal iliac vessel can be disastrous, however, and lead to high amputation rates. A cross-femoral bypass graft performed with iliac artery ligation can help salvage a limb.[202]

Autotransfusion equipment should be ready so that as much shed blood as possible can be saved and returned from the thoracic, abdominal, or thigh compartment. Even though the blood appears to have clotted, such lost blood can be successfully gathered, washed, and returned as red cells to the patient. The total amount of blood lost should be estimated early so that appropriate replacements can be ordered from the blood blank to supplement that replaced by autotransfusion. Emergency vascular surgery cannot be performed routinely without the use of allogeneic, or banked, blood.

In contrast to treatment of the trauma patient, for whom early surgical intervention to stop bleeding is the norm, it is common practice, in the patient with bleeding varices, to determine the need for surgery based on the number of

TABLE 44–3. HEMOSTATIC CAUSES OF INTRAOPERATIVE BLEEDING

Massive transfusion or dilution
Hemolytic transfusion reaction
Fibrinolysis and disseminated intravascular coagulation
Undiagnosed bleeding disorder
Drugs
Hypothermia

units of blood lost or transfused within 12 to 24 hours. By using such guidelines, not only do we magnify the risk of allogeneic blood exposure but we also increase mortality in direct proportion to the number of units transfused.

Lee and coworkers studied 101 patients admitted to the ICU with bleeding from varices.[134] Patients who received more than 10 units in less than 24 hours—30.6% of the cohort—had a significantly higher mortality rate than the others. Multiple blood transfusion was a significant independent predictor of death, and both the degree of blood loss and the failure to stop bleeding contributed to the high mortality rate. *Outcomes*, defined as both survival and a reduction in use of allogeneic blood, can be improved significantly by a more aggressive interventional approach to variceal bleeding.

Most bleeding varices can be controlled initially with a stepwise treatment plan that may include (1) endoscopy, vasopressin, or somatostatin infusion; (2) balloon tamponade; (3) banding; (4) sclerotherapy; and (5) transvenous intrahepatic portosystemic shunting (TIPS) followed by selective decompression with a shunt for persistent or recurrent bleeding.[77] Different types of therapy have different rates of morbidity and mortality, and therapy should be chosen based on careful planning, availability, and experience (see Chapter 114). It is crucial to act without delay if the morbidity and mortality associated with blood loss and transfusion are to be reduced.

Intraoperative Aspects: Bleeding

Bleeding during surgery may also arise from hemostatic defects (Table 44–3). Coagulopathy in the patient with traumatic or massive vascular bleeding is partially dilutional but is also related to both the degree and the length of hypotension and hypoperfusion.[45] Nearly 37% of the original blood elements remain in circulation following the controlled exchange of a single blood volume (10 units in a 70-kg adult). The remaining levels of coagulation factors and platelets (>100,000/mm^3) are usually adequate to maintain hemostasis. With progressive exchanges of two volumes (equivalent to a 20-unit transfusion), blood elements drop to levels of approximately 5%, and coagulopathy follows.[217] These levels serve only as basic estimates in the clinical setting, since both platelet counts and amounts of circulating clotting factors vary, depending on both rate of blood loss and rate of transfusion. Associated injury to the uterus, lung, or prostate, organs rich in plasminogen activators, may result in their release into the circulation and subsequent fibrinolysis.[7] Tissue hypoxia following injury or prolonged cross-clamping of visceral blood supply may also lead to release of plasminogen activators and thromboplastins.

Coagulation factor and platelet depletion are not as common a cause of intraoperative hemorrhage as one might assume. Hypothermia can be a contributing factor.[27, 64] It may be difficult to correlate the clinical observation of bleeding directly with prolongation of the PT and activated partial thromboplastin time (aPTT), which are reagent- and temperature-dependent.[16] Because coagulation testing is routinely performed at 37°C rather than at the patient's actual in vivo temperature, normal coagulation test results can be obtained even when there is clinical evidence of a coagulopathy.[196] Normal test results in this setting suggest that sufficient clotting factors are available for coagulation if normothermia is restored.[174]

Dilutional coagulopathy may be mistaken for or aggravated by the development of DIC.[44, 101, 146] DIC in the setting of massive transfusion occurs in 5% to 30% of trauma patients and is associated with high morbidity and mortality rates of nearly 70%.[48, 105] Tissue injury and hemolysis with release of cytokines and tissue thromboplastin into the circulation may cause immediate activation of both the coagulation and the fibrinolytic systems, resulting in severe DIC.[16]

At present, no single laboratory test can confirm or exclude the diagnosis of DIC; however, the combination of a low platelet count, a low fibrinogen level, an elevated D-dimer, and the presence of soluble fibrin monomers in the context of the patient's underlying condition are the most helpful indicators of DIC. In the patient who has received multiple units of blood, dilutional thrombocytopenia begins to appear after 1.5 blood volumes (or 20 units) have been replaced. Clinical evidence of thrombocytopenia includes diffuse microvascular bleeding and oozing from mucosa, raw wounds, and puncture sites. The exact activity levels of clotting factors needed for hemostasis when multiple-factor deficiencies coexist are not well defined. Hiippala and associates found that critical levels of platelets and clotting factors were not reached with blood loss and replacement until more than two estimated blood volumes (~30 to 40 units) had been replaced. However, fibrinogen deficits appeared much earlier.[103]

Stored allogeneic blood maintains sufficient levels of all coagulation factors except factors V and VIII; however, levels decrease over time.[217] If available, whole blood obtained via acute normovolemic hemodilution can be used to restore coagulation factors and platelets. In a study of 39 patients who received plasma-depleted blood, either from the blood bank or from cell salvage and autotransfusion, Leslie and Toy documented significant platelet decreases in 75% of those who received more than 20 units.[136] PT and PTT were prolonged in 33% of those who received

TABLE 44–4. GUIDELINES FOR COMPONENT THERAPY IN MASSIVE BLOOD LOSS AND TRANSFUSION

COMPONENT	INDICATIONS
Platelets	Platelet count < 80–100 × 10^9/L
Fresh frozen plasma (FFP)	PT or aPTT > 0.5 times normal
Cryoprecpitate and AHP	Fibrinogen < 10 mg/L

PT = prothrombin time; AHP = antihemophilic factor; aPTT = activated partial thromboplastin time.

less than 12 units and in all who received more than 12 units. In a prospective, randomized study of patients needing 12 or more units of blood in 12 hours, Ciavarella and coworkers found no benefit to giving 6 units of platelets or 2 units of fresh frozen plasma (FFP) prophylactically for every 12 units of red blood cells transfused.[40a]

Surgeons can replace coagulation factors and platelets when needed by infusing FFP or platelets. Table 44–4 lists guidelines for specific component therapy during massive transfusion in patients with clinical evidence of microvascular bleeding. *Massive* transfusion is commonly defined as transfusion approximating or exceeding the patient's blood volume within a 24-hour period. In an adult man who weighs 70 kg, this translates to an estimated replacement of 4 to 5 L of blood loss, or transfusion of 16 to 20 units of packed red blood cells. Although specific guidelines can aid one in deciding when to use component therapy, they may also lead to undertransfusion if the decision is based only on laboratory values. Bleeding in vascular patients may be multifactorial and may not correlate directly with laboratory measurements.[240]

The location and extent of injury, the duration of shock, the response to resuscitation, and the risk of complicating factors, such as intracranial bleeding, are important clinical considerations. With prompt management of bleeding and the skilled use of component therapy, the coagulopathy can usually be controlled. In the end, clinical judgment must prevail, even if it results in what appears, based on laboratory measurements, to be overuse of components.

Institutional reviews of the use of FFP and platelets to "correct" undocumented coagulation abnormalities have shown consistently that this practice is both inappropriate and wasteful.[127, 238] In general, "cookbook" formulae for replacement of FFP and platelets according to the number of units transfused should be avoided because they have little value and they increase patient risk by multiple donor exposure. Platelets and FFP should be given to correct *proven* coagulation abnormalities (see Table 44–4).[167]

Intraoperative Aspects: Technique

The most common cause of intraoperative bleeding during vascular surgical procedures is probably surgical misadventure, such as inadvertent venous injury or disruption of a friable, diseased vessel after clamp placement. This type of bleeding can be prevented only through careful surgical technique and experience. Dissection along anatomic, avascular planes is essential and requires a thorough knowledge of anatomy. "Rip and tear" surgical techniques only lead to avulsion of vessels and increased bleeding.

All potentially vascular structures should be clamped and tied before they are cut. Any vessel inadvertently cut or any unexpected bleeding, no matter how minor, must be controlled. Attention to what may seem to be an insignificant detail at the time can lead to diminished blood loss. Blood loss from unattended small vessels during the course of an operation may build up gradually, especially in the hypertensive patient.[53]

A variety of cutting devices, including electrocautery devices, argon beam coagulators, ultrasonic dissectors, and laser, can reduce blood loss in specific settings.[183] In my experience, reduced blood loss is a result more of the surgeon's skill than of the device itself.

Modification of operative approaches can minimize blood loss in vascular surgery. Both the retroperitoneal approach to the abdominal aorta and the exclusion-bypass technique have been reported to be superior to traditional surgical approaches and handling of the aorta in terms of blood loss, although some controversy exists. In their study of a standard, transperitoneal approach, Leather and colleagues estimated that blood loss averaged 1700 ml. By switching to a retroperitoneal approach and excluding the aneursym, the surgeon was able to decrease blood loss to 900 ml, a reduction of almost half.[133] Carrel and coworkers[31] found a decrease from 1300 to 630 ml in 42 retroperitoneal operations compared with 121 transperitoneal cases, and Laohapensang and associates[130] found a similar decrease in 43 consecutive patients. In contrast, neither Cambria and coworkers[29] nor Sieunarine and colleagues[211] found a significant transfusion advantage to using one approach over the other in two series of 69 and 100 patients, respectively, randomized to either a retroperitoneal or transperitoneal operation.

Exclusion of the AAA sac prior to bypass has been used successfully by several groups of vascular surgeons to reduce intraoperative blood loss.[37, 182, 192] Such an approach should be ideal for some religious groups, such as Jehovah's Witnesses. When coupled with a retroperitoneal incision, this procedure appears to result in less postoperative morbidity than a standard aneurysm repair.

The value of a laparoscopy-assisted approach to abdominal aortic surgery in reducing blood loss is not yet known. Chen and associates reported an average blood loss of 1 L in 10 patients when they used this approach.[38] In the lower extremity, Hans and associates noted a greater blood loss with femoral popliteal bypass in situ versus reversed saphenous vein bypass.[94] They attributed this increased blood loss to an increased operative time and to more release of blood when the vein was tested.

Controversy exists about the benefit of using relatively impervious grafts to reduce blood loss. Woven polyester (Dacron) grafts with minimal porosity, albumin, or gelatin-sealed grafts can essentially eliminate direct blood loss caused by extravasation during aortic bypass and replacement, but their effect on reducing the need for transfusion is questionable.[113]

Chakfe and colleagues used albumin-impregnated, polyester, prosthetic grafts for AAA repair in 218 cases (190 elective and 28 emergency) and in another 72 patients with occlusive disease of the aortic bifurcation.[36] The incidence of transfusion overall was 40.4% and 42.6%, respectively, in the two groups, with a mean of 1.4 and 1 units, respectively, of red blood cells transfused. Barral and colleagues found similar results in a randomized trial of high-density, knitted Dacron grafts versus identical grafts that had been impregnated with collagen.[12] Both groups of investigators concluded that impregnated grafts did not significantly reduce perioperative blood loss or transfusion need.

Reid and Pollock reported that gelatin-sealed grafts had "no measurable blood loss at implantation."[191] However, 47 patients still required transfusion for blood losses of greater than 750 ml or on clinical grounds. Fisher and colleagues, in an analysis of double-velour woven Dacron grafts compared with polytetrafluoroethylene (PTFE) grafts with sophisticated blood loss measurement techniques, concluded that neither graft had an advantage over the other in decreasing blood loss or preventing transfusion.[65] Their results may have been skewed by a significantly lower preoperative erythrocyte volume in the Dacron group, which may have accounted for increased transfusion need. It is difficult to know the true benefit of impregnated grafts because none of these studies had a consistent transfusion policy, which affects overall transfusion rates. The amount of blood loss may depend as much on the surgeon as on the graft.

Early studies of endovascular stent grafting of the abdominal aorta reported mixed results with regard to blood loss. It stands to reason that blood loss should be less because the aorta is not directly opened. Eight of the 39 patients (20.5%) who underwent this procedure successfully as part of the North American Endovascular Trial (EVT) Phase 1 trial had to be transfused.[163]

White and coworkers, from Australia, performed a historic control, cohort analysis of 62 patients treated by endovascular techniques for an AAA compared with a selected group of patients treated by open repair.[249] Blood loss was significantly less in the endovascular group: 873 versus 1422 ml. White and colleagues, reported a similar experience with 16 patients who had an average blood loss of 1100 ml.[250] Blood loss decreased as the study progressed, showing the effect of a learning curve. Blood replacement in all but three patients (81%) was accomplished by autotransfusion or banked autologous blood replacement.

Although these early results are encouraging, significant blood can be lost during this procedure because large-diameter devices are introduced into the femoral artery without adequate means to control back-bleeding. This problem should be solved as devices evolve for endovascular approaches. Elimination of the learning curve effect will require both training and experience.

Direct treatment of the aortic wall may facilitate surgical repair while reducing transfusion need. Chen and associates have used direct application of a 25% glutaraldehyde solution to the aortic wall in five cases of aortic dissection.[39] This approach strengthened the fragile aortic wall and helped to prevent catastrophic bleeding caused by further perioperative aortic disruption.

The choice of both anesthetic technique and operation can influence the amount of blood lost during surgery. Regional anesthetic techniques have been associated with decreased blood loss in orthopedic surgery. Bridenbaugh found less blood loss in patients who underwent total hip replacement under continuous epidural anesthesia than in those who received general anesthesia.[24]

Oxygen consumption is reduced 15% to 20% in most patients under general anesthesia.[18] Narcotic anesthesia may add another 5% to 10% reduction, providing a greater margin of safety. Many anesthesiologists favor narcotic anesthesia, usually with fentanyl, for anemic patients. If inhalational anesthetic agents are used, isoflurane is usually chosen because it has less inhibitory effect on the heart's conductivity. These anesthetic agents do not directly minimize blood loss, but they can provide a somewhat safer environment for the stressed, anemic patient who may need increased cardiac reserves.

Postoperative Care

For the ICU patient, the first postoperative 24 to 48 hours are the most critical period. The controlled setting of the operating room, where the patient has undergone ventilation and anesthesia, is replaced by a period of increased stress and pain. Oxygen consumption, which was reduced intraoperatively by both anesthesia and ventilation, increases and may become directly dependent on delivery. Hemoglobin level fluctuates as the intraoperative fluid load shifts. Neither hemoglobin concentration nor oxygen-derived parameters are completely reliable transfusion triggers. Increased cardiac work puts demands on myocardial oxygen delivery such that patients with quiescent coronary artery disease may experience arrhythmias or subendocardial ischemia.

In this setting, the surgeon may choose to maintain the most critically ill patients in an anesthetized, ventilated state to lessen oxygen consumption. Measures should be taken to prevent shivering because it can increase oxygen consumption 35% to 40%. Postoperative blood conservation measures are primarily continuations of those taken both preoperatively and intraoperatively. These measures include attention to nutritional support and iron restoration as well as the use of erythropoietin to stimulate red cell mass replacement. Shed blood may be collected from mediastinal or chest tubes and returned.

Unfortunately, blood loss frequently continues in the postoperative period in the form of phlebotomy for laboratory tests.[214] "Cookbook" order sheets that include standing orders for frequent and often unnecessary laboratory tests should be avoided. Blood samples should be obtained only for essential studies, with the surgeon relying instead on noninvasive monitoring systems to gain information. For example, it is preferable to follow a patient's oxygen status with a transcutaneous oxygen monitor and check blood gases only when acute changes occur rather than measure blood gases every 6 hours. When blood tests are necessary, pediatric collection tubes and microsamples should be used. Flush solutions should be returned to arterial and central lines to avoid wastage.

Pharmacologic Agents Associated with Blood Loss

A variety of drugs that affect either blood loss or transfusion need are available to the vascular surgeon. These drugs can be grouped by their intended actions that (1) limit blood loss, (2) stimulate regeneration of red blood cells, and (3) act as blood substitutes (Table 44–5).

Vitamin K and Vasopressin

Vascular surgeons are familiar with the preoperative use of *vitamin K* to correct a prolonged PT in the patient who has been taking warfarin. Vitamin K, administered by intramuscular injection, restores normal clotting function within a few days by promoting replacement of liver-derived clotting factors. *Vasopressin* can be used intraoperatively during portacaval shunting to reduce blood loss. An infusion of 0.4 U/min of vasopressin started before the skin incision is made produces subcutaneous vasoconstriction and limits bleeding.

TABLE 44–5. PHARMACOLOGIC AGENTS ASSOCIATED WITH SURGICAL BLEEDING AND TRANSFUSION

To limit blood loss
- Vitamin K
- Protamine
- DDAVP
- Tranexamic acid
- EACA
- Aprotinin
- Factors VIII and IX
- Vasopressin
- Topical agents
  - Fibrin glue
  - Surgicel, Hemopad, and so forth

To regenerate red blood cells
- Oral iron
- Intravenous iron
- Erythropoietin
- Steroids
- Intravenous nutrition

Blood substitutes
- Crystalloids
- Colloids
- Hemoglobin derivatives
- Perfluorocarbons

DDAVP = desmopressin; EACA = ϵ-aminocaproic acid.

Heparin

Heparin is used in most vascular surgical procedures to prevent thrombotic complications.[158] The dosage used may vary among surgeons. Concerns over the amount of blood loss and the need for transfusion associated with heparin use were addressed by Thompson and coworkers and the Joint Vascular Research Group in a prospective, multicenter study of 284 patients undergoing AAA surgery.[232] Patients were randomized to receive intravenous heparin or no heparin during surgery. Blood loss was similar in the two groups (median, 1400 versus 1500 ml of blood) as was the amount of blood transfused (4.0 units in both groups). The authors did note a significantly higher incidence of fatal, perioperative myocardial infarction in the nonheparinized group. One can conclude that the risk of bleeding from heparinization is not great, but the risk of avoiding its use is. Cole and colleagues demonstrated that depletion of circulating fibrinogen with preoperative ancrod was as successful as heparin in preventing graft complications and did not increase blood loss.[43]

Protamine

Protamine is used intraoperatively to reverse the effects of heparin during major cardiovascular surgery. The dose administered is calculated initially from the amount of heparin given and is titrated against clotting times. Jobes and coworkers found that titration and administration of protamine based on specific, point-of-service measurement of coagulation factors resulted in less postoperative bleeding and decreased transfusion need (671 versus 1298 ml) and fewer patients received transfusion (9/22 versus 18/24) with fewer donor exposures than with a conventional regimen.[108]

Despotis and colleagues obtained similar results in 244 patients monitored with an on-site, algorithm-driven system.[55] Adding to the controversy, however, is the recent report from Shore-Lesserson and colleagues that there were no differences in blood loss or transfusion requirements in 135 cardiac surgical patients.[209]

Although protamine is given almost universally after procedures that require cardiopulmonary bypass, there is no consistent pattern for protamine in aortic and peripheral vascular procedures when bypass is not employed.[157] In these cases, heparin is usually given in smaller amounts based on body weight and clotting times are rarely followed. Some surgeons routinely use protamine after graft placement; others simply rely on heparin clearance to promote clotting. There is little information available on the role of protamine in preventing bleeding caused by heparin in vascular surgery.

Dorman and coworkers found that the use of protamine in a mix of aortic, infrainguinal, and carotid procedures did not reduce either blood loss or transfusion need.[57] These investigators used systemic heparinization with 90 U/kg of body weight during surgery in 128 patients, randomizing them to reversal with either protamine or saline. No differences were found in either blood loss or transfusion requirements. Of interest is the finding that intraoperative bleeding following drug administration was *greater* with protamine (318 ± 33 versus 195 ± 18 ml; $p < .05$).

Desmopressin

The vasopressin analogue desmopressin (1-desamino-8-D-arginine vasopressin [DDAVP]) has minimal vasopressor activity. Its potential usefulness during vascular surgery derives from its ability to elevate both factors VIII and VIII-vWF twofold to threefold above normal levels. DDAVP can have a significant advantage for the hemophiliac patient with low factor VIII levels.[200]

DDAVP's role in surgical patients, however, is controversial. Clagett and coworkers found no advantage in using DDAVP to reduce blood loss in their randomized study of patients undergoing aortic surgery.[41] Lethagen and coworkers reported a tendency for reduced blood loss with DDAVP in 50 patients undergoing surgery for aortoiliac occlusive disease, but the difference seen was not statistically significant when compared with control values.[137]

DDAVP is not innocuous. It has a variety of side effects, which range from mild facial flushing and headache through tachycardia and hypertension to tachyphylaxis. Based on the studies of Clagget and coworkers[41] and Lethagen and colleagues,[137] and on the extensive review and meta-analysis of the literature of Laupacis and coworkers,[131] which concluded that DDAVP was of no benefit in reducing blood loss during cardiac surgery, the drug's role in vascular surgery is questionable. DDAVP may, however, have a limited usefulness in correcting identifiable platelet defects, such as those caused by aspirin.[53, 67]

Aprotinin

Aprotinin (Trasylol), a serine protease inhibitor, has been used successfully to reduce blood loss during cardiovascular surgery in a number of clinical trials.[52, 199, 216] In their meta-analysis, Laupacis and coworkers concluded that aprotinin use resulted in decreased blood loss during cardiac surgery.[131] Aprotinin is thought to work by inhibiting kallikrein and plasmin or by preserving platelet adhesion membrane receptors during cardiopulmonary bypass.[50]

Like DDAVP, aprotinin may have an important role in treating patients with aspirin-induced platelet abnormalities. Wildevuur and colleagues demonstrated significant reductions in both bleeding time and postoperative blood loss in aprotinin-treated patients who had received aspirin before coronary artery bypass.[251]

Experience with aprotinin in vascular surgical patients is limited but has shown similar results. Ranaboldo and colleagues were unable to find any significant benefit in reducing transfusion requirements in their study of aprotinin use in 136 aortic surgery patients, although they did see reductions in both intraoperative and 24-hour postoperative blood loss.[188] Lord and colleagues have suggested that aprotinin may provide an additional benefit by minimizing neutrophil impairment following aortic procedures.[144] Aprotinin must undergo further study to document both safety and efficacy in vascular surgery before it is ready for general use.

Other Agents

Other pharmacologic agents may be helpful in reducing surgical blood loss. ε-Amino caproic acid (EACA) and tranexamic acid have been shown to help reduce blood loss in cardiac surgery and liver transplantation.[69, 131, 198, 205] Bombesin, pentoxifylline, and prostacyclin are purported to work on the vascular system, bombesin by counteracting opioid-induced vasodilatation and pentoxifylline and prostacyclin by improving microcirculatory flow and tissue oxygen delivery.[222] The clinical role of these drugs remains unproven, although pentoxifylline and prostacyclin may have some benefit for septic or critically ill patients who need maximized peripheral oxygen consumption.

Recombinant human erythropoietin (rHuEPO) is not approved by the Food and Drug Administration (FDA) for use in patients with either cardiac or vascular disease because of concerns over potential drug-induced hypertension, cerebrovascular accidents, and thrombotic complications. Most of this fear is based on early reports of renal dialysis patients.[58, 212] Some of these patients experienced occlusion of shunts, probably from the effect of a rising hematocrit rather than from rHuEPO. Several large-scale studies of rHuEPO in both orthopedic and cardiac surgical patients have proved its value as an alternative to allogeneic transfusion.[11, 81]

There is little reported experience of the use of rHuEPO in vascular patients. I have used rHuEPO successfully in a number of such patients (Jehovah's Witnesses) to restore red cell mass, both preoperatively and postoperatively, with none of the mentioned adverse effects.[219] It is important with erythropoietin to ensure that the patient's iron stores are replenished because existing iron is rapidly depleted by the drug. Iron dextran infusions to replace depleted iron stores can be used to treat acute, critical surgical anemia.[80]

Fibrin glue is made by reaction of a source of fibrinogen, which can be obtained from a variety of sources, including human cryoprecipitate and platelet-rich plasma, with bovine thrombin.[20, 74] Fibrin sealants are generally commercially produced from processed human, animal, or synthetic sources. These materials adhere well to biologic surfaces and have been effective in controlling bleeding in a variety of settings.[74] Glimaker and colleagues used fibrin glue to reinforce the sewn aortic stump in two patients who underwent removal of infected grafts.[78] Other investigators have used fibrin glue in myocardial laceration repairs and as part of septal defect repairs. Milne and coworkers found fibrin sealant to be an effective hemostatic agent when applied to suture lines and arteriotomies in a variety of vascular procedures.[157, 159]

Several authors have reported successful sealing of iatrogenic arteriotomy sites with fibrin products.[10, 63, 106] Agus and associates evaluated a ready-to-use hemostatic agent consisting of a collagen sheet coated with human fibrinogen, bovine thrombin, and bovine aprotinin on one side.[3] Hemostatic control was considered good in 125 surgical operations, which included vascular, hepatic, and urologic procedures.

Unfortunately, fibrin glue derived from multiple allogeneic donors can be a source of disease transmission. Whenever possible, autologous, not allogeneic, plasma should be used if exposure to blood products is to be avoided. Commercially produced, virus-free sealants may solve this problem.

Blood substitutes, whether perfluorocarbon-based or hemoglobin-derived, are undergoing clinical trials and are not available for general use. Initial reports of the utility of these agents as temporary oxygen carriers that provide a "bridge to transfusion" are encouraging.[84, 86, 193, 204] Determination of their usefulness in vascular surgery necessitates further clinical trials.

ALTERNATIVES TO ALLOGENEIC BLOOD

Directed Donor Blood

Although most patients prefer directed donor blood, its use does not reduce transfusion risk because this blood is allogeneic.[210] Directed donor blood carries significant risks, including disease transmission and presence of GVHD. The use of directed donor blood may be an acceptable option in specific settings (e.g., neonatal or pediatric surgery), but in general surgeons should discourage its use and should instruct patients about its potential dangers.

Predonated Autologous Blood

Predonated autologous blood is an alternative source that can reduce dependence on allogeneic blood.[25, 50, 223] Average reductions in allogeneic blood usage range from 30% to 50%, and decreases from 3 to 1 unit of blood transfused per patient are common. Successful autologous predonation depends on:

1. Adequate time for donation.
2. A hemoglobin level greater than 11.0 gm/dl.
3. Absence of significant patient disease (i.e., severe aortic stenosis or active angina).
4. Selection of appropriate patients based on anticipated blood loss and transfusion need.

5. The cooperation of both patient and physician.

The ideal patient for predonation is one who has an anticipated need for blood transfusion with a window of 2 or more weeks before surgery to donate (i.e., a patient scheduled for an elective AAA repair). Both Tedesco and colleagues[231] and Georgiev and coworkers[71] have used a combination of predonation and autotransfusion successfully in more than 150 vascular patients to reduce allogeneic blood exposure. Godet and colleagues combined predonation with the use of platelet-rich plasma and obtained similar results.[79]

Most patients can successfully complete a predonation program without incident. Relative contraindications to predonation include a history of congestive heart failure, valvular heart disease, recent myocardial infarction, angina, arrhythmias, hypertension requiring multiple drug therapy, seizures, and cerebrovascular disease. An increased incidence of reactions is associated with a donor age under 17 years, a weight under 110 pounds, female gender, and a history of previous reactions.[223] Adverse reactions to predonation may occur more often than initially thought in patients with coronary artery disease.

Although some of the reactions can be minimized by saline infusion during phlebotomy and with apheresis collection techniques, these approaches require additional logistics and medical expertise that add to the cost of autologous predonation. Emergency or urgent surgery may eliminate predonation as an option for up to 50% of otherwise eligible patients.

Approximately 10% to 15% of patients do not have the acceptable hemoglobin level of 11 gm/dl for predonation. Male gender and higher initial hematocrit are independent factors associated with successful completion of a 4-unit order. Treatment with rHuEPO can facilitate predonation for mildly anemic patients scheduled for orthopaedic surgery. Although not FDA approved for use in patients with vascular disease in the United States, rHuEPO has been used successfully in Europe in vascular patients to aid predonation.[11, 161, 237]

Unfortunately, predonated blood is rarely used by vascular surgical patients, although the ability of predonation to reduce allogeneic blood exposure has been clearly demonstrated. Only 1 of 31 surgeons surveyed by Milne and Murphy used predonation.[157] Similar results were found in a survey in Germany.[115] Concerns about cost-effectiveness may limit its use, or vascular surgeons simply may not have considered predonation to be a safe alternative for their patients.[122] Predonation may become more useful in the future as vascular surgeons analyze their transfusion needs based on specific procedures and learn more about this alternative.

Acute Normovolemic Hemodilution

There are times when the surgeon wants to use autologous blood but there is not sufficient time before surgery to schedule predonation. In these cases, autologous blood is still available in the form of acute *normovolemic hemodilution*, the process of removing and temporarily storing blood just before or immediately after the induction of anesthesia and replacing with either a crystalloid or colloid solution. The removal of 1 to 4 units is possible when the patient has a normal hematocrit and a postdilutional hematocrit is 20% to 30%.[225]

The amount of blood to be removed can be calculated from measured preoperative hematocrit and estimated blood volume (EBV).[140] The amount of blood to be removed (V) is calculated from the EBV, initial hematocrit (H_i), desired hematocrit (H_f), and the average of the two hematocrits (H_{av}):

$$V = \frac{EBV \times (H_i - H_f)}{H_{av}}$$

For practical purposes, blood volume can be estimated as a percentage of body weight, with 7% for men and 6.5% for women.[88]

Hemodilution can be performed with crystalloid, colloid, or a combination of the two as a diluent. A disadvantage of salt solutions is their short intravascular dwell time and rapid excretion, but they can be removed rapidly with diuretics if needed. A colloid infusion requires less fluid but otherwise offers no significant advantage over less expensive crystalloids.[89] Usable colloids include albumin, dextran, and hydroxyethyl starch.

Kreimeier and Messmer provide an excellent review of state-of-the-art hemodilution, prompted by the renewed interest in this alternative to allogeneic blood.[121] Determination of the usefulness of hemoglobin-based and perfluorocarbon oxygen carriers (i.e., blood substitutes) as facilitators of hemodilution necessitates the results of ongoing trials.[204]

The advantages of acute normovolemic hemodilution include an improvement in tissue perfusion secondary to decreased viscosity and loss of fewer red blood cells from bleeding. A decrease in viscosity produces an increase in cardiac output, primarily in response to an augmented venous return. Increases in cardiac output range from 25% to 35%, depending on the final hematocrit and the patient's tolerance for the procedure. Loss of blood with a hematocrit of 20% is better equated with less red cell mass depletion than is loss of blood with hematocrit of 30% or 40%.

Although some surgeons avoid hemodilution because of a perception that it is time-consuming and requires extensive monitoring, the opposite is true. Acute normovolemic hemodilution can be performed safely and rapidly with a team approach as part of the preinduction routine. Monitoring is dictated primarily by the patient's condition and the type of surgery, not by the use of hemodilution.

At present, a major disadvantage of hemodilution is the need for an experienced anesthesiologist. Although this may seem like a trivial matter, because hemodilution is performed in the operating room on anesthetized patients, most anesthesiologists trained in the United States have little experience with the procedure. Further education can solve this problem.

The factor that limits nadir hemoglobin during hemodilution appears to be ventricular function. Robertie and Gravlee point out in their review of hemodilution in cardiac surgery that patients with normal ventricular function can tolerate hematocrits of 22% without postoperative myocardial problems.[195] Studies of cardiac and vascular patients have suggested that those with left ventricular dysfunction may be at greater risk of ischemia during hemodilution.[189,

[215, 248] Others have shown what may be a protective benefit from hemodilution.

Catoire and colleagues studied the effect of acute normovolemic hemodilution on cardiac function in a series of patients with known coronary artery disease undergoing aortic surgery.[35] The results showed that hemodilution minimized adverse changes in ventricular wall-motion and consequent cardiac hemodynamics seen with aortic cross-clamping.

Although hemodilution studies limited to vascular procedures are few, benefits have been shown in both improved oxygenation and decreased reliance on banked blood.[123, 208] Parris and coworkers reported an improvement in P50 in vascular patients intentionally hemodiluted with autologous blood compared with those who received allogeneic blood.[180] Hemodilution is most often used in combination with other techniques, such as autotransfusion.[115] In his report of an extensive 5-year experience in the treatment of AAAs with a combined approach of hemodilution, autotransfusion, and predonation, Hallett suggested that hemoglobin levels of 8 gm/dl or less are acceptable if no symptoms or signs of myocardial ischemia appear and if hemodynamics remain stable.[92] Others have reported similar successes with hemodilution as part of an overall approach to blood conservation that combines multiple techniques.[149, 184]

The combination of preoperative use of erythropoietin to stimulate the production of red cells with hemodilution may help reduce the lead time and risk associated with autologous predonation of blood.[237] The addition of intraoperative cell salvage and return to these techniques provides a logical and readily accessible approach to blood conservation for the vascular surgeon.

In the United States, hemodilution techniques have been used most frequently during open heart surgery in the form of platelet sequestration. In this process, 1 unit of blood is removed preoperatively before heparin infusion and the institution of bypass. The collected blood is then separated in the Cell Saver (Haemonetics, Braintree, Mass.) into a platelet-rich plasma component and packed red blood cells. Red blood cells are given as needed during the surgery; the plasma component is reinfused as the patient is taken off bypass, and heparin is reversed.

The infusion of autologous clotting factors and platelets that have not been exposed to the pump or to heparin can significantly reduce both bleeding and the need for allogeneic blood transfusion. Tawes and Duvall attained a 45% reduction in allogeneic blood need using plasma sequestration in 41 patients undergoing aortic procedures.[229] Giordano and Jones[75] have recounted the controversy surrounding the use of platelet-rich plasma in Jones and Beall's extensive review of autotransfusion.[111]

Surgeons are perhaps more familiar with hypervolemic hemodilution than with intentional isovolemic hemodilution. Most surgical patients are treated in this fashion when they receive large volumes of crystalloid or colloid intraoperatively. Most anesthesiologists replace blood losses of up to 20% using a formula of 3 ml of crystalloid to every 1 ml of blood lost, which produces a transient hypervolemic hemodilution.

Trouwborst and associates evaluated the effects of this approach on 16 patients who underwent surgery to determine if it could help reduce the need for allogeneic blood transfusion.[235] All patients received hemodilution therapy preoperatively with Ringer's lactate and dextran infusions. Hematocrit dropped from 36.9% to 26.3%. Transesophageal ultrasound monitoring showed increases in the cardiac index of approximately 27.5%. Oxygen consumption, it was noted, decreased slightly. All patients tolerated the surgery without need for allogeneic blood.

Mielke and coworkers found similar results in 49 patients receiving hemodilution therapy with hydroxyethyl starch.[156] Although this procedure appears to be safe, it should be used cautiously because of the dangers of volume overload from intentional hypervolemia.

Autotransfusion

Autotransfusion collection and reinfusion of shed blood is the most common form of autologous blood used in vascular surgery.[255] This alternative does reduce dependence on allogeneic blood by up to 75% of overall transfusion needs during vascular surgical procedures.[2, 76, 158, 186, 220, 229, 254] Autotransfusion may be life-saving in emergency vascular surgery when blood loss is high. Marty-Ane and colleagues found that autotransfusion was the predominant intraoperative factor that correlated with decreased mortality in a series of 61 patients with ruptured AAAs (Table 44–6).[153]

Intraoperative autotransfusion can be performed either with systems that collect blood directly, anticoagulate it, and reinfuse it through filters or with systems that collect the blood, wash it, and reinfuse a packed red blood cells product.[75] Systems without washing capability collect shed blood via a suction wand that simultaneously adds either heparin or citrate-phosphate-dextrose anticoagulant into a collection chamber.[126] The collected blood is returned to the patient through a filter, which is the only means of preparing the blood. Filters are capable of removing large debris (e.g., bone chips) and smaller particulate matter (e.g., cellular fragments). After filtration, the salvaged blood represents red blood cells suspended in plasma, containing platelets, fibrinogen, and clotting factors.

Unwashed blood can contain vasoactive contaminants, activated clotting factors, fibrin degradation products, and free hemoglobin, all of which can be dangerous. Bartels and colleagues compared differences in hemostatic, hemolysis, and hematologic parameters after autotransfusion of washed Cell Saver blood versus unprocessed, shed whole blood during major aortic surgery in 32 patients.[13] Levels of bilirubin, free hemoglobin, lactic dehydrogenase, D-dimers, and fibrin degradation products were significantly higher before transfusion in whole blood than in Cell Saver blood. Moreover, patients who received unprocessed whole blood had significantly higher circulating levels of these products and of D-dimers after autotransfusion.

High postoperative serum levels of cholecystokinin (CK) and lactate dehydrogenase (LDH) enzymes after infusion of autotransfused blood were observed by Nguyen and coworkers in their study of over 300 patients.[173] Shed mediastinal blood contained extremely high levels of these enzymes. The authors caution that presence of these enzymes may be mistaken for evidence of new myocardial infarction.

Transfusion reactions in patients who receive filtered,

TABLE 44–6. AUTOTRANSFUSION IN AND SURVIVAL AFTER RUPTURED ABDOMINAL AORTIC ANEURYSMS

PREDICTIVE FACTOR	PARAMETER (β RISK)	STANDARD ERROR	*p* VALUE	ODDS RATIO
Intraoperative autotransfusion	3.24	0.98	0.0009	25.45
Age	0.18	0.06	0.0039	N/A
Type of revascularization	1.95	0.95	0.0397	7.04
Preoperative blood pressure	0.02	0.01	0.0692	N/A

Adapted from Marty-Ane CH, Alric P, Picot M, et al: Ruptured abdominal aortic aneurysm: Influence of intraoperative management on surgical outcome. J Vasc Surg 22:780–786, 1995.

unwashed blood, characterized by increasing blood pressure, chills, fever, and rigors, may be caused by leukocyte-derived vasoactive contaminants. Washing shed blood reduces, but does not completely eliminate, leukocytes from the infused product.[185]

Shed blood can be collected postoperatively from thoracoabdominal aneurysm patients via mediastinal chest tubes. The ability of systems that wash shed blood to process small volumes (125 ml) coupled with their portability make it possible to process small amounts of blood collected from wound drainage during the postoperative period in the ICU. After a retrospective analysis of 336 patients, de Varennes and coworkers suggested that reinfusion of mediastinal shed blood following cardiac surgery limited the rate of postoperative reexploration for bleeding.[54] Although this study suggests a role for postoperative autotransfusion beyond its impact on allogeneic blood use, this group's findings need to be corroborated, especially because other surgeons have seen no impact on postoperative bleeding from autotransfusion.[100]

Systems that wash blood and concentrate red blood cells have the advantage of providing a cleaner product, free of the contaminants found in unwashed blood. With these systems, blood is collected from the operative field, filtered, anticoagulated, and temporarily stored in a reservoir. The blood is transferred to a centrifuge bowl, which spins at approximately 5000 rpm, thereby separating the red blood cells from plasma. The cells are washed and resuspended in saline to attain a hematocrit of 40% to 60% before they are reinfused.[229]

Disadvantages include the loss of the plasma component, the need for expert help in the form of a perfusionist to run the equipment, the longer set-up time required, and the expense (Table 44–7). Cost has become an increasingly important issue in the age of managed care. Some surgeons have reduced their use of autotransfusion to save money.[8] Others have found that a concerted effort to manage an overall blood conservation program that includes autotransfusion also leads to cost savings.[179, 231] Goodnough and coworkers suggest that washing blood for autotransfusion becomes cost-effective only when blood losses of 1000 ml or greater are encountered.[82]

Unfortunately, such blood loss can be predicted in only some cases (e.g., ruptured AAAs). As suggested earlier, all vascular surgeons would benefit from a systematic review of their own blood loss rates for specific procedures. These rates provide a basis for a rational, cost-effective use of autotransfusion as well as of other alternatives.[197]

Relative contraindications to the use of autotransfused blood, whether washed or not, include the presence of infection or bowel contamination, malignancy, and obstetric procedures contaminated with amniotic fluid.[60] These contraindications rarely present a problem in vascular surgery. When they do (e.g., during further surgery for an infected aortic graft), the surgeon must weigh the potential benefit obtainable from autotransfusion against the risks. Standard cell-washing systems can be modified into closed circuits to make them more acceptable to such groups as Jehovah's Witnesses.[220]

Dzik thoroughly reviewed the literature on the controversy about whether to wash shed blood before autotransfusion and concluded that washing is preferable to not washing.[59] He points out, however, that clinical studies of unwashed blood show that its use is safe under specific circumstances, a finding corroborated by several vascular surgeons.[126, 181, 236, 241] Safety depends on infusion of small quantities and restriction of collection and reinfusion times to 6 hours or less. The surgeon can also reduce toxicities by avoiding skimming, using a second suction wand for blood unsuitable for reinfusion, and avoiding chemical

TABLE 44–7. COMPARISON OF WASHED VERSUS UNWASHED AUTOTRANSFUSION BLOOD

	ADVANTAGES	DISADVANTAGES
Washed	Packed red blood cells	No coagulants
	Eliminates allogeneic risk	More time for set-up
	No cytokine, etc., contamination	Usually requires technical support
	No coagulants added	Requires special equipment
		Less volume
		More expensive
Unwashed	Larger volume	Free hemoglobin, nephrotoxicity
	Faster	Active cytokines, lipids, and enzymes
	No technical support required	Transfusion reactions?
	Less expensive	DIC?
	Disposable; no special equipment	Diluted red cell mass
	Coagulants present, but amount variable	Stroma elements
	Eliminates allogeneic risk	Tissue procoagulants
		Products of fibrinolysis
		Biologic contaminants; urine
		Drug contaminants
		Heparin or anticoagulant citrate dextrose added

DIC = disseminated intravascular coagulation.

TABLE 44–8. ALTERNATIVE STRATEGIES FOR SURGICAL TRANSFUSION

Preoperative
- Stop antiplatelet and anticoagulant drugs
- Optimize cardiopulmonary status
- Autologous predonation
- Erythropoietin
- Iron, oral or intravenous

Intraoperative
- Acute normovolemic hemodilution
- Autotransfusion or cell salvage
- Antifibrinolytics
- Fibrin glue or sealant
- Surgical techniques
- Blood substitutes

Postoperative
- Autotransfusion or cell salvage
- Blood substitutes
- Erythropoietin
- Iron, oral or intravenous

agents (e.g., topical hemostatics) and biologic substances (e.g., urine).[170, 218]

SUMMARY

Successful transfusion strategies in vascular surgery are multifactorial and require an understanding of basic physiology, clinical patient characteristics, the effects of technique and medications on bleeding, and available transfusion alternatives (Tables 44–8 and 44–9). Of primary importance is the vascular surgeon's individual attention to analysis of his or her transfusion practices. Such data collection combined with appropriate knowledge can improve both transfusion practices and overall patient outcomes.

TABLE 44–9. FACTORS TO CONSIDER IN THE SURGICAL TRANSFUSION DECISION

- Clinical history
  - Cardiopulmonary disease
  - Existing coagulopathy, congenital or acquired
  - Anemia
  - Trauma classification
    - Mechanism of injury
    - Injury severity score
- Medications
  - Antiplatelet medications
  - Anticoagulants
- Clinical symptoms
  - Dyspnea on exertion
  - Angina
- Hemoglobin and hematocrit level
- Oxygen delivery and consumption
  - Oxygen extraction ratio
  - Oxygen partial pressure (PvO_2)
  - Oxygen saturation (SvO_2)
  - Serum lactate
  - Base deficit
- Surgical procedure
  - Elective versus emergency
  - Laparoscopic versus open
- Maximum surgical blood-ordering schedule
- Estimated and calculated blood loss
- Religious groups (e.g., Jehovah's Witnesses)

REFERENCES

1. Adams RC, Lundy JS: Anesthesia in cases of poor surgical risk: Some suggestions for decreasing the risk. Surg Gynecol Obstet 74:1011–1019, 1942.
2. Adhoute BG, Nahaboo K, Reymondon L, et al: Autotransfusion applied in elective vascular surgery. J Cardiovasc Surg (Torino) 20:177–184, 1979.
3. Agus GB, Bono AV, Mira E, et al: Hemostatic efficacy and safety of TachoComb in surgery: Ready to use and rapid hemostatic agent. Int Surg 81:316–319, 1996.
4. Alkhamis TM, Beissenger RL, Chediak JR: Artificial surface effect on red blood cells and platelets in laminar shear flow. Blood 75:1568–1575, 1990.
5. Alter HJ: Transfusion transmitted hepatitis C and non-A, non-B, non-C. Vox Sang 67(Suppl 3):19–24, 1994.
6. Aly Hassan A, Lochbuehler H, Frey L, Messmer K: Global tissue oxygenation during normovolaemic haemodilution in young children. Paediatr Anaesth 7:197–204, 1997.
7. Ambrus JL, Mittleman A: Hematologic management of the aged and high risk surgical patient. *In* Siegel JH, Chodoff P (eds): The Aged and High Risk Surgical Patient: Medical, Surgical and Anesthetic Management. New York, Grune & Stratton, 1976, pp 211–229.
8. Ammar AD: Cost-efficient carotid surgery: A comprehensive evaluation. J Vasc Surg 24:1050–1056, 1996.
9. Astiz ME, Rackow EC, Falk JL, et al: Oxygen delivery and consumption in patients with hyperdynamic septic shock. Crit Care Med 15:26–28, 1987.
10. Atkinson JB, Gomperts ED, Kang R, et al: Prospective, randomized evaluation of the efficacy of fibrin sealant as a topical hemostatic agent at the cannulation site in neonates undergoing extracorporeal membrane oxygenation. Am J Surg 173:479–484, 1997.
11. Baron JF: Autologous blood donation with recombinant human erythropoietin in cardiac surgery: The Japanese experience. Semin Hematol 33(Suppl 2):64–67, 1996.
12. Barral X, Gay JL, Favre JP, Gournier JP: Do collagen-impregnated knitted Dacron grafts reduce the need for transfusion in infrarenal aortic reconstruction? Ann Vasc Surg 9:339–343, 1995.
13. Bartels C, Bechtel JV, Winkler C, Horsch S: Intraoperative autotransfusion in aortic surgery: Comparison of whole blood autotransfusion versus cell separation. J Vasc Surg 24:102–108, 1996.
14. Bauer EP, Redaelli C, von Segesserm LK: Ruptured abdominal aortic aneurysms: Predictors for early complications and death. Surgery 114:31–35, 1993.
15. Berard P: Surgical treatment of hemorrhage from ruptured esophageal varices by an orally introduced clip to provoke sclerosis of the lower esophagus and ligation of the peri-esophageal veins through a thoracic approach: Results in 108 cases treated over a period of 5 years. J Chir (Paris) 121:389–393, 1984.
16. Bick RL: Disseminated intravascular coagulation and related syndromes: A clinical review. Semin Thromb Hemost 14:299–305, 1988.
17. Bickell WH, Bruttig SP, Millnamoro GA, et al: The detrimental effects of intravenous crystalloid after experimental aortotomy in swine. Surgery 110:529–534, 1991.
18. Bjoraker DG: Blood transfusion: What is a safe hematocrit? Prob Crit Care 5:386–399, 1991.
19. Bosenberg A, Bosenberg E, Sibrowski W: [Bacterial infection within the scope of hemotherapy.] Infusionsther Transfusionsmed 21(Suppl 1):51–57, 1994.
20. Bouvy BM, Rosin E, Frishmeyer KJ: Evaluation of bovine fibrin sealant in the dog. J Invest Surg 6:241–250, 1993.
21. Bradley JA: The blood transfusion effect: Experimental aspects. Immunol Lett 29:127–132, 1991.
22. Brathwaite CE, Rodriguez A: Injuries of the abdominal aorta from blunt trauma. Am Surg 58:350–352, 1992.
23. Brecher ME, Monk T, Goodnough LT: A standardized method for calculating blood loss. Transfusion 37:1070–1074, 1997.
24. Bridenbaugh LD: Regional anesthesia for outpatient surgery—a summary of 12 years' experience. Can Anaesth Soc J 30:548, 1983.
25. Britton LW, Eastlund DT, Dziuban SW, et al: Predonated autologous blood use in elective cardiac surgery. Ann Thorac Surg 47:529–532, 1989.
26. Burroughs AK, Hamilton G, Phillips A, et al: A comparison of

sclerotherapy with staple transection of the esophagus for the emergency control of bleeding from esophageal varices. N Engl J Med 321:857–862, 1989.
27. Bush HL Jr, Hydo LJ, Fischer E, et al: Hypothermia during elective abdominal aortic aneurysm repair: The high price of avoidable morbidity [see comments]. J Vasc Surg 21:392–400, 1995.
28. Bush RL, Pevec WC, Holcroft JW: A prospective, randomized trial limiting perioperative red blood cell transfusions in vascular patients. Am J Surg 174:143–148, 1997.
29. Cambria RP, Brewster DC, Abbott WM, et al: Transperitoneal versus retroperitoneal approach for aortic reconstruction: A randomized prospective study. J Vasc Surg 11:314–325, 1990.
30. Carmel R, Shulman IA: Blood transfusion in medically treatable chronic anemia: Pernicious anemia as a model for transfusion overuse. Arch Pathol Lab Med 113:995–997, 1989.
31. Carrel T, Pasic M, Turina M, et al: The retroperitoneal approach: An excellent alternative to the transperitoneal route in elective aortic surgery. Int J Angiogr Winter:1–5, 1992.
32. Carson JL, Duff A, Berlin JA, et al: Perioperative blood transfusion and postoperative mortality [see comments]. JAMA 279:199–205, 1998.
33. Carson JL, Duff A, Poses RM, et al: Effect of anaemia and cardiovascular disease on surgical mortality and morbidity. Lancet 348:1055–1060, 1996.
34. Carson JL, Spence RK, Poses RM, Bonavita G: Severity of anemia and operative mortality and morbidity. Lancet 2:727–729, 1988.
35. Catoire P, Saada M, Liu N: Effect of preoperative normovolemic hemodilution on left ventricular segmental wall motion during abdominal aortic surgery. Anesth Analg 75:654–659, 1992.
36. Chakfe N, Kretz G, Petit H, et al: Albumin-impregnated polyester vascular prosthesis for abdominal aortic surgery: An improvement? Eur J Vasc Endovasc Surg 12:346–353, 1996.
37. Chaoui Z, Gutsche J, Kuhnert M, et al: [Posterolateral retroperitoneal approach and exclusion technique in therapy of infrarenal aortic aneurysm: Initial experiences]. Zentralbl Chir 122:752–756, 1997.
38. Chen MH, D'Angelo AJ, Murphy EA, Cohen JR: Laparoscopically assisted abdominal aortic aneurysm repair: A report of 10 cases. Surg Endosc 10:1136–1139, 1996.
39. Chen YF, Chou SH, Chiu CC, et al: Use of glutaraldehyde solution in the treatment of acute aortic dissections. Ann Thorac Surg 58:833–835, discussion 836, 1994.
40. Christopherson R, Frank S, Norris E, et al: Low postoperative hematocrit is associated with cardiac ischemia in high-risk patients (Abstract). Anesthesiology 75:A100, 1991.
40a. Ciavarella D, Reed RL, Counts RB, et al: Clotting factor levels and the risk of diffuse microvascular bleeding in the massively transfused patient. Br J Haematol 67:365, 1987.
41. Clagett GP, Valentine RJ, Myers SI et al: Does desmopressin improve hemostasis and reduce blood loss from aortic surgery? A randomized, double-blind study. J Vasc Surg 22:223–229, 1995.
42. Coimbra R, Hoyt D, Winchell R, Simons R, et al: The ongoing challenge of retroperitoneal vascular injuries. Am J Surg 172:541–544, 1996.
43. Cole CW, Bormanis J, Luna GK, et al: Ancrod versus heparin for anticoagulation during vascular surgical procedures. J Vasc Surg 17:288–292, discussion 293, 1993.
44. Collins JA: Problems associated with the massive transfusion of stored blood. Surgery 75:274–278, 1974.
45. Collins JA: Recent developments in the area of massive transfusion. World J Surg 11:75–81, 1987.
46. Comerota AJ, Aldridge SC, Cohen G, et al: A strategy of aggressive regional therapy for acute iliofemoral venous thrombosis with contemporary venous thrombectomy or catheter-directed thrombolysis [see comments]. J Vasc Surg 20:244–254, 1994.
47. Corwin HL, Parsonnet KC, Gettinger A: RBC transfusion in the ICU: Is there a reason? Chest 108:767–771, 1995.
48. Counts RB, Haisch C, Simon TL, et al: Hemostasis in massively transfused trauma patients. Ann Surg 190:91–96, 1979.
49. D'Ambra MN, Kaplan DK: Alternatives to allogeneic blood use in surgery: Acute normovolemic hemodilution and preoperative autologous donation. Am J Surg 170(Suppl 6A):49S–52S, 1995.
50. D'Ambra MN, Risk SC: Aprotinin, erythropoietin, and blood substitutes. Int Anesth Clin 28:237–240, 1990.
51. D'Angelo F, Vaghi M, Mattassi R: Changing trends in the outcome of urgent aneurysm surgery: A retrospective study on 170 patients treated in the years 1966–1990. J Cardiovasc Surg (Torino) 34:237–239, 1993.
52. Davis R, Whittington R: Aprotinin: A review of its pharmacology and therapeutic efficacy in reducing blood loss associated with cardiac surgery. Drugs 49:954–983, 1995.
53. de Figueiredo LF, Coselli JS: Individual strategies of hemostasis for thoracic aortic surgery. J Cardiovasc Surg 12:222–228, 1997.
54. de Varennes B, Nguyen D, Denis F, et al: Reinfusion of mediastinal blood in CABG patients: Impact on homologous transfusions and rate of re-exploration. J Cardiovasc Surg 11:387–395, 1996.
55. Despotis GJ, Joist JH, Hogue CW Jr, et al: The impact of heparin concentration and activated clotting time monitoring on blood conservation: A prospective, randomized evaluation in patients undergoing cardiac operation [see comments]. J Thorac Cardiovasc Surg 110:46–54, 1995.
56. Dodd RY: Transfusion-transmitted hepatitis virus infection. Hematol Oncol Clin North Am 9:137–154, 1995.
57. Dorman BH, Elliott BM, Spinale FG, et al: Protamine use during peripheral vascular surgery: A prospective randomized trial. J Vasc Surg 22:248–255, 1995.
58. Dunn CJ, Wagstaff AJ: Epoetin alfa: A review of its clinical efficacy in the management of anaemia associated with renal failure and chronic disease and its use in surgical patients. Drugs Aging 7:131–156, 1995.
59. Dzik WH: Blood salvage: Washed versus nonwashed. *In* Tawes RL (ed): Autotransfusion: Therapeutic Principles and Trends. Detroit, Gregory Appleton, 1997, pp 319–328.
60. Dzik WH, Sherburne B: Intraoperative blood salvage: Medical controversies. Trans Med Rev IV:208–235, 1990.
61. Eisenstaedt RS: Modifying physicians' transfusion practice. Transfus Med Rev 11:27–37, 1997.
62. Erban SB, Kinman JL, Schwartz JS: Routine use of the prothrombin and partial thromboplastin times. JAMA 263:2428–2432, 1989.
63. Falstrom JK, Goodman NC, Ates G, et al: Reduction of femoral artery bleeding post catheterization using a collagen enhanced fibrin sealant. Cathet Cardiovasc Diagn 41:79–84, 1997.
64. Ferrara A, MacArthur JD, Wright HK: Hypothermia and acidosis worsen coagulopathy in the patient requiring massive transfusion. Am J Surg 160:515–518, 1990.
65. Fisher JB, Dennis RC, Valeri CR, et al: Effect of graft material on loss of erythrocytes after aortic operations. Surg Gynecol Obstet 173:131–136, 1991.
66. Fitzgerald RD, Martin CM, Dietz GE, et al: Transfusing red blood cells stored in citrate phosphate dextrose adenine-1 for 28 days fails to improve tissue oxygenation in rats [see comments]. Crit Care Med 25:726–732, 1997.
67. Flordal PA: Pharmacological prophylaxis of bleeding in surgical patients treated with aspirin. Eur J Anaesthesiol Suppl 14:38–41, 1997.
68. Frank SM, Parker SD, Rock P, et al: Moderate hypothermia, with partial bypass and segmental sequential repair for thoracoabdominal aortic aneurysm [see comments]. J Vasc Surg 19:687–697, 1994.
69. Fremes SE, Wong BI, Lee E, et al: Metaanalysis of prophylactic drug treatment in the prevention of postoperative bleeding. Ann Thorac Surg 58:1580–1588, 1994.
70. Geha AS, Baue AE: Graded coronary stenosis and coronary flow during acute normovolemic anemia. World J Surg 2:645–652, 1978.
71. Georgiev G, Zakhariev T, Chirkov A: [Blood autotransfusion in vascular surgery (predeposited blood)]. Khirurgiia 48:97–102, 1995.
72. Georgieva Z, Georgieva M: Compensatory and adaptive changes in microcirculation and left ventricular function of patients with chronic iron-deficiency anaemia. Clin Hemorheol Microcirc 17:21–30, 1997.
73. Gertler JP, Cambria RP, Brewster DC, et al: Coagulation changes during thoracoabdominal aneurysm repair. J Vasc Surg 24:936, 1996.
74. Gibble JW, Ness PM: Current perspectives on the use of fibrin glue (sealant) in the United States in the 1990s. *In* Tawes RL (ed): Autotransfusion: Therapeutic Principles and Trends. Detroit, Gregory Appleton, 1997, pp 250–260.
75. Giordano GF, Prust RS, Wallace BA: The use of platelet-rich plasma in cardiac operations. *In* Tawes RL (ed): Autotransfusion: Therapeutic Principles and Trends. Detroit, Gregory Appleton, 1997, pp 217–223.
76. Giordano GF, Giordano DM, Wallace BA et al: An analysis of 9,918

consecutive perioperative autotransfusions. Surg Gynecol Obstet 176:103, 1993.

77. Gliedman ML, Langer B, Rikkers LF, et al: Management of variceal bleeding. Contemp Surg 41:49–62, 1992.
78. Glimaker HC, Bjorck C, Hallstensson S, et al: Avoiding blow-out of the aortic stump by reinforcement with fibrin glue. A report of two cases. Eur J Vasc Surg 7:346–348, 1993.
79. Godet G, Canessa R, Arock M, et al: [Effects of platelet-rich plasma on hemostasis and transfusion requirement in vascular surgery (see comments)]. Ann Fr Anesth Reanim 14:265–270, 1995.
80. Goldberg MA: Erythropoiesis, erythropoietin, and iron metabolism in elective surgery: Preoperative strategies for avoiding allogeneic blood exposure. Am J Surg 170(Suppl 6A):37S–43S, 1995.
81. Goodnough LT, Monk TG, Andriole GL: Erythropoietin therapy. N Engl J Med 336:933–938, 1997.
82. Goodnough LT, Monk TG, Sicard G, et al: Intraoperative salvage in patients undergoing elective abdominal aortic aneurysm repair: An analysis of cost and benefit. J Vasc Surg 24:213–218, 1996.
83. Goodnough LT, Vizmeg K, Riddell J 4th, Soegiarso RW: Discharge haematocrit as clinical indicator for blood transfusion audit in surgery patients. Transfus Med 4:35–44, 1994.
84. Gould SA, Moore EE, Moore FA, et al: Clinical utility of human polymerized hemoglobin as a blood substitute after acute trauma and urgent surgery: A study of desmopressin and blood loss during spinal fusion for neuromuscular scoliosis: A randomized, controlled, double-blinded study. J Trauma 43:325–331, 1997.
85. Greenburg AG: A physiologic basis for red blood cell transfusion decisions. Am J Surg 170(Suppl 6A):44S–48S, 1995.
86. Greenburg AG, Kim HW: Current status of stroma-free hemoglobin. Adv Surg 31:149–165, 1997.
87. Gringeri A, Santagostino E, Mannucci PM: Failure of recombinant activated factor VII during surgery in a hemophiliac with high-titer factor VIII antibody. Haemostasis 21:1–4, 1991.
88. Gross JB: Estimating allowable blood loss: Corrected for dilution. Anesthesiology 58:277–280, 1983.
89. Group, Expert Working: Guidelines for red blood cell and plasma transfusion for adults and children. Can Med Assoc J 156(Suppl 11):S1–S24, 1997.
90. Group, the Sanguis Study: Use of blood products for elective surgery in 43 European hospitals. Trans Med 4:251–268, 1994.
91. Gu YJ, de Vries AJ, Boonstra PW, van Oeveren W: Leukocyte depletion results in improved lung function and reduced inflammatory response after cardiac surgery. J Thorac Cardiovasc Surg 112:494–500, 1996.
92. Hallett JW Jr: Minimizing the use of homologous blood products during repair of abdominal aortic aneurysms. Surg Clin North Am 69:817–826, 1989.
93. Halpern VJ, Kline RG, D'Angelo AJ, Cohen JR: Factors that affect the survival rate of patients with ruptured abdominal aortic aneurysms. J Vasc Surg 26:939–948, 1997.
94. Hans SS, Masi J, Goyal V, et al: Increased blood loss with in situ bypass. Am Surg 56:540–542, 1990.
95. Hasley PB, Lave JR, Hanusa BH, et al: Variation in the use of red blood cell transfusions: A study of four common medical and surgical conditions. Med Care 33:1145–1160, 1995.
96. Hay CRM, Bolton-Maggs P: Porcine factor VIIIC in the management of patients with factor VIII inhibitors. Trans Med Rev V:145–151, 1991.
97. Hebert PC, Wells G, Marshal J, et al: Transfusion requirements in critical care: A pilot study. Canadian Critical Care Trials Group. JAMA 273:1439–1444, 1995.
98. Hebert PC, Wells G, Martin C, et al: A Canadian survey of transfusion practices in critically ill patients: Transfusion requirements in Critical Care Investigators and the Canadian Critical Care Trials Group. Crit Care Med 26:482–487, 1998.
99. Hebert PC, Wells G, Tweeddale M, et al: Does transfusion practice affect mortality in critically ill patients? Transfusion Requirements in Critical Care (TRICC) Investigators and Canadian Critical Care Trials Group. Am J Respir Crit Care Med 155:1618–1623, 1997.
100. Helm RE, Klemperer JD, Rosengart TK, et al: Intraoperative autologous blood donation preserves red cell mass but does not decrease postoperative bleeding. Ann Thorac Surg 62:1431–1441, 1996.
101. Hewson JR, Neame PB, Kumar N, et al: Coagulopathy related to dilution and hypotension during massive transfusion. Crit Care Med 13:387–392, 1985.
102. Heyland DK, Cook DJ, King D, et al: Maximizing oxygen delivery in critically ill patients: A methodologic appraisal of the evidence [see comments]. Crit Care Med 24:517–524, 1996.
103. Hiippala ST, Myllyla GJ, Vahtera EM: Hemostatic factors and replacement of major blood loss with plasma-poor red cell concentrates. Anesth Analg 81:360–365, 1995.
104. Hojlund K, Andersen LI, Huttel MS, et al: [Rational transfusion therapy: A study of transfusion practice and possibilities of optimization in elective coronary bypass surgery]. Ugeskr Laeger 158:7237–7240, 1996.
105. Humphries JE: Transfusion therapy in acquired coagulopathies. Hematol Oncol Clin North Am 8:1181–1201, 1994.
106. Ismail S, Combs MJ, Goodman NC, et al: Reduction of femoral arterial bleeding post catheterization using percutaneous application of fibrin sealant. Cathet Cardiovasc Diagn 34:88–95, 1995.
107. Jackson MR, Olson DW, Beckett WC Jr: Abdominal vascular trauma: A review of 106 injuries. Am Surg 58:622–626, 1992.
108. Jobes DR, Aitken GL, Shaffer GW: Increased accuracy and precision of heparin and protamine dosing reduces blood loss and transfusion in patients undergoing primary cardiac operations. J Thorac Cardiovasc Surg 110:36–45, 1995.
109. Johnston KW: Nonruptured abdominal aortic aneurysm: Six-year follow-up results from the multicenter prospective Canadian aneurysm study. Canadian Society for Vascular Surgery Aneurysm Study Group. J Vasc Surg 20:163–170, 1994.
110. Johnston KW: Ruptured abdominal aortic aneurysm: Six-year follow-up results of a multicenter prospective study. Canadian Society for Vascular Surgery Aneurysm Study Group. J Vasc Surg 19:888–900, 1994.
111. Jones JW, Beall AC Jr: Intraoperative plateletpheresis: Technical tips and critical appraisal. *In* Tawes RL (ed): Autotransfusion: Therapeutic Principles and Trends. Detroit, Gregory Appleton, 1997, pp 234–239.
112. Kaiser WC, McAuliffe JD, Barth RJ: Hypoprothrombinemia and hemorrhage in surgical patient treated with cefotetan. Arch Surg 126:524–525, 1991.
113. Kang SS, Petsikas D, Murchan P, et al: Effects of albumin coating of knitted Dacron grafts on transinterstitial blood loss and tissue ingrowth and incorporation. Cardiovasc Surg 5:184–189, 1997.
114. Karger R, Kretschmer V: [The importance of quality of whole blood and erythrocyte concentrates for autologous transfusion: A literature survey and meta-analysis of in vivo erythrocyte recovery]. Anaesthesist 45:694–707, 1996.
115. Kasper SM, Kiencke P, Lynch J, et al: [Autologous blood transfusion in the Federal Republic of Germany—results of a questionnaire in 1993: 2. The use of autologous transfusion in the old and new federation]. Anaesthesist 45:606–613, 1996.
116. Kent KC, Moscucci M, Mansour KA, et al: Retroperitoneal hematoma after cardiac catheterization: Prevalence, risk factors, and optimal management. J Vasc Surg 20:905–910, 1994.
117. Klein HG: Allogeneic transfusion risks in the surgical patient. Am J Surg 170(Suppl 6A):21S–26S, 1995.
118. Klein HG: Immunologic aspects of blood transfusion. Semin Oncol 21(Suppl 3):16–20, 1994.
119. Krausz MM, Meital BZ, Rabinovici R, et al: "Scoop and run" or "stabilize" hemorrhagic shock by normal saline or small-volume hypertonic saline. J Trauma 33:6–9, 1992.
120. Krausz MM: Controversies in shock research: Hypertonic resuscitation—pros and cons. Shock 3:69–72, 1995.
121. Kreimeier U, Messmer K: Hemodilution in clinical surgery: State of the art 1996. World J Surg 20:1208–1217, 1996.
122. Kruskall MS, Yomtovian R, Dzik WH, et al: On improving the cost-effectiveness of autologous blood transfusion practices. Transfusion 34:259–264, 1994.
123. Kuznetsov NA, Isaev AF, Vasilev VE: Hemodilution in the prevention of complications after surgery of the major arteries. Khirurgiia (Mosk) 3:100–104, 1989.
124. Kvilekval KH, Best IM, Mason RA: The value of computed tomography in the management of symptomatic abdominal aortic aneurysms. J Vasc Surg 12:28–33, 1990.
125. Lackritz EM, Satten GA, Aberle-Grasse J, et al: Estimated risk of transmission of the human immunodeficiency virus by screened blood in the United States [see comments]. N Engl J Med 333:1721–1725, 1995.
126. Lagana S, Cattaneo F, Hackenbruch W: [Autologous blood transfu-

sion: Results with routine use of autologous blood transfusion, normovolemic hemodilution and postoperative retransfusion of drainage blood salvaged with the Solcotrans system]. Swiss Surg 2:244–251, 1996.

127. Lahrmann C, Hojlund K, Kristensen T, Georgsen J: [Use of fresh frozen plasma in patient treatment: Indications illustrated by a literature review and a study of practice at a university hospital]. Ugeskr Laeger 158:3467–3470, 1996.

128. Lane TA: Leukocyte reduction of cellular blood components: Effectiveness, benefits, quality control, and costs. Arch Pathol Lab Med 118:392–404, 1994.

129. Langenburg SE, Blackbourne LH, Sperling JW, et al: Management of renal tumors involving the inferior vena cava. J Vasc Surg 20:385–388, 1994.

130. Laohapensang K, Pongcheowboon A, Rerkasem K: The retroperitoneal approach for abdominal aortic aneurysms. J Med Assoc Thai 80:479–485, 1997.

131. Laupacis A, Fergusson D, Brown RS, et al: Drugs to minimize perioperative blood loss in cardiac surgery: Meta-analyses using perioperative blood transfusion as the outcome. The International Study of Peri-operative Transfusion (ISPOT) Investigators. Tranexamic acid is effective in decreasing postoperative bleeding and transfusions in primary coronary artery bypass operations: A double-blind, randomized, placebo-controlled trial. Anesth Analg 85:963–970, 1997.

132. Leach MF, AuBuchon JP: Effect of storage time on clinical efficacy of single-donor platelet units [published erratum appears in Transfusion 33:887, 1993]. Transfusion 33(8):661–664, 1993.

133. Leather RP, Shah DM, Kaufman JL, et al: Comparative analysis of retroperitoneal and transperitoneal aortic replacement for aneurysm. Surg Gynecol Obstet 168:387–393, 1989.

134. Lee H, Hawker FH, Selby W: Intensive care treatment of patients with bleeding esophageal varices: Results, predictors of mortality, and predictors of the adult respiratory distress syndrome. Crit Care Med 20:1555–1563, 1993.

135. Leiby DA, Kerr KL, Campos JM, Dodd RY: A retrospective analysis of microbial contaminants in outdated random-donor platelets from multiple sites. Transfusion 37:259–263, 1997.

136. Leslie S, Toy P: Laboratory hemostatic abnormalities in massively transfused patients given red blood cells and crystolloid. AJCP 96:770–773, 1991.

137. Lethagen S, Rugarn P, Bergqvist D: Blood loss and safety with desmopressin or placebo during aorto-iliac graft surgery. Eur J Vasc Surg 5:173–178, 1991.

138. Linden JV, Pisciotto PT: Transfusion-associated graft-versus-host disease and blood irradiation. Trans Med Rev VI:116–123, 1992.

139. Linden JV, Kaplan HS: Transfusion errors: Causes and effects. Transfus Med Rev 8:169–183, 1994.

140. Lisander B: Preoperative hemodilution. Acta Anaesthesiol Scand 32(Suppl 89):63–70, 1988.

141. Livio M, Gotti E, Marchesi D, et al: Uremic bleeding: Role of anemia and beneficial effect of red cell transfusions. Lancet 2:1013–1015, 1982.

142. Lohr JW, Schwab SJ: Minimizing hemorrhagic complications in dialysis patients. J Am Soc Nephrol 2:961–975, 1991.

143. Lopez-Viego MA, Snyder WH 3rd, Valentine RJ: Penetrating abdominal aortic trauma: A report of 129 cases. J Vasc Surg 16:332–335, 1992.

144. Lord RA, Roath OS, Thompson JF: Effect of aprotinin on neutrophil function after major vascular surgery. Br J Surg 79:517–521, 1992.

145. Lord RS, Markovsky A: [The use of the Cell-Saver method of blood preservation in reconstructions of aortic aneurysms]. Vestn Khir Im I I Grek 154:99–104, 1995.

146. Lucas CE, Ledgerwood AM: Clinical significance of altered coagulation test after massive transfusions for trauma. Am Surg 47:125–129, 1981.

147. Lum G: Should the transfusion trigger and hemoglobin low critical limit be identical? Ann Clin Lab Sci 27:130–134, 1997.

148. Lundsgaard-Hansen P: Safe hemoglobin or hematocrit levels in surgical patients. World J Surg 20:1182–1188, 1996.

149. Mackay Z, Shugufta Q, Din M, Guru AA: Hemodilution in complicated high velocity vascular injuries of limbs. J Cardiovasc Surg (Torino) 37:217–221, 1996.

150. Macpherson CR, Jacobs P, Dent DM: Abnormal peri-operative haemorrhage in asymptomatic patients is not predicted by laboratory testing. S Afr Med J 83:106–108, 1993.

151. Marin ML, Veith FJ, Panetta TF, et al. Percutaneous transfemoral insertion of a stented graft to repair a traumatic femoral arteriovenous fistula. J Vasc Surg 18:299–302, 1993.

152. Martin RR, Bickell WH, Pepe PE, et al: Prospective evaluation of preoperative fluid resuscitation in hypotensive patients with penetrating truncal injury: A preliminary report. J Trauma 33:354–362, 1992.

153. Marty-Ane CH, Alric P, Picot MC, et al: Ruptured abdominal aortic aneurysm: Influence of intraoperative management of surgical outcome. J Vasc Surg 22:780–786, 1995.

154. McCormick PA, Dick R, Burroughs AK: Review article: The transjugular intrahepatic portosystemic shunt (TIPS) in the treatment of portal hypertension. Aliment Pharmacol Ther 8:273–282, 1994.

155. McIntyre AJ: Blood transfusion and hemostatic management in the perioperative period. Can J Anaesth 39:R108–R114, 1992.

156. Mielke LL, Entholzner EK, Kling M, et al: Preoperative acute hypervolemic hemodilution with hydroxyethylstarch: An alternative to acute normovolemic hemodilution? Anesth Analg 84:26–30, 1997.

157. Milne AA, Murphy WG: Current blood transfusion practice in aortic aneurysm surgery in Scotland: The Scottish Vascular Audit Group. J R Coll Surg Edinb 40:104–108, 1995.

158. Milne AA, Murphy WG, Reading SJ, Ruckley CV: Fibrin sealant reduces suture line bleeding during carotid endarterectomy: A randomised trial. Eur J Vasc Endovasc Surg 10:91–94, 1995.

159. Milne AA, Murphy WG, Reading SJ, Ruckley CV: A randomised trial of fibrin sealant in peripheral vascular surgery. Vox Sang 70:210–212, 1996.

160. Mollison PJ, Engelfriet CP, Contreras M: The transfusion of platelets, leucocytes and plasma components. *In* Mollison PJ, Engelfriet CP, Contreras M (eds): Blood Transfusion in Clinical Medicine. London, Blackwell Scientific, 1993, pp 638–676.

161. Mollmann M, Lubbesmeyer HJ, von Bormann B: [Erythropoietin therapy during frequent autologous blood donations: Dose-finding study]. Anaesthesist 44:624–630, 1995.

162. Montgomery RR, Coller BS: von Willebrand disease. *In* Colman RW, Hirsh J, Marder VJ, Salzman EW (eds): Hemostasis and thrombosis: Basic principles and clinical practice, 3rd ed. Philadelphia, JB Lippincott, 1994, pp 134–168.

163. Moore WS, Rutherford RB: Transfemoral endovascular repair of abdominal aortic aneurysm: Results of the North American EVT phase 1 trial. EVT Investigators. J Vasc Surg 23:543–553, 1996.

164. Morrison JC, Sumrall DD, Chevalier SP, et al: The effect of provider education on blood utilization practices. Am J Obstet Gynecol 169:1240–1245, 1993.

165. Muller G, N'tita I, Nyst M, et al: Application of blood transfusion guidelines in a major hospital of Kinshasa, Zaire [Letter]. AIDS 6:431–432, 1992.

166. Muller-Steinhardt M, Janetzko K, Kirchner H, Kluter H: [Effect of whole blood preparation and leukocyte filtration on storage of erythrocyte concentrates over 42 days]. Beitr Infusionsther Transfusionsmed 34:53–57, 1997.

167. Muntean W: Rational perioperative use of clotting factor concentrates and fresh frozen plasma (FFP). Acta Anaesthesiol Scand 111(suppl):263–264, 1997.

168. Nagasue N, Kohno H, Ogawa Y, et al: Appraisal of distal spinal renal shunt in the treatment of esophageal varices: An analysis of prophylactic emergency and elective shunts. World J Surg 13:92–99, 1989.

169. Nelson AH, Fleisher LH, Rosenbaum SH: The relationship between postoperative anemia and cardiac morbidity in high risk vascular patients in the ICU. Crit Care Med 21:860–866, 1993.

170. Nelson CL, Fontenot HJ: Ten strategies to reduce blood loss in orthopedic surgery. Am J Surg 170(Suppl 6A):64S–68S, 1995.

171. Nevelsteen A, Lacroix H, Suy R: Autogenous reconstruction with the lower extremity deep veins: An alternative treatment of prosthetic infection after reconstructive surgery for aortoiliac disease. J Vasc Surg 22:129–134, 1995.

172. Nezhat C, Childers J, Nezhat F, et al: Major retroperitoneal vascular injury during laparoscopic surgery. Hum Reprod 12:480–483, 1997.

173. Nguyen DM, Gilfix BM, Dennis F, et al: Impact of transfusion of mediastinal shed blood on serum levels of cardiac enzymes. Ann Thorac Surg 62:109–114, 1996.

174. Nicholls MD, Whyte G: Red cell, plasma and albumin transfusion decision triggers. Anaesth Intens Care 21:156–162, 1993.

175. O'Hara PJ, Hertzer NR, Krajewski LP, et al: Ten-year experience with

abdominal aortic aneurysm repair in octogenarians: Early results and late outcome. J Vasc Surg 21:830–837, 1995.

176. Ombrellaro MP, Freeman MB, Stevens SL, et al: Predictors of survival after inferior vena cava injuries. Am Surg 63:178–183, 1997.
177. Orloff MJ, Bell RH Jr, Orloff MS, et al: Prospective randomized trial of emergency portacaval shunt and emergency medical therapy in unselected cirrhotic patients with bleeding varices [see comments]. Hepatology 20:863–872, 1994.
178. Ostgaard G: [Perioperative and postoperative normovolemic anemia. Physiologic compensation, monitoring and risk evaluation]. Tidsskr Nor Laegeforen 116:57–60, 1996.
179. Ovrum E, Holen EA, Tangen G, Oystese R: Cost savings with autotransfusion in connection with coronary surgery. Tidsskr Nor Laegeforen 117:2616–2618, 1997.
180. Parris WCW, Kambam JR, Blanks S: The effect of intentional hemodilution on P50. J Cardiovasc Surg 29:560–562, 1988.
181. Patra PE, Sellier E, Chaillou P: [Blood salvage: Decisive progress in vascular surgery]. J Mal Vasc 21:13–21, 1996.
182. Paty PS, Darling RC 3rd, Chang BB, et al: A prospective randomized study comparing exclusion technique and endoaneurysmorrhaphy for treatment of infrarenal aortic aneurysm. J Vasc Surg 25:442–445, 1997.
183. Pearlman NW, Stiegmann GV, Vance V, et al: A prospective study of incisional time, blood loss, pain, and healing with carbon dioxide laser, scalpel, and electrosurgery [see comments]. Arch Surg 126:1018–1020, 1991.
184. Perttila J, Leino L, Poyhonen M, Salo M: Leucocyte content in blood processed by autotransfusion devices during open-heart surgery. Acta Anaesthesiol Scand 39:445–448, 1995.
185. Petz LD, Calhoun L, Yam P, et al: Transfusion-associated graft-versus-host disease in immunocompetant patients: Report of a fatal case associated with transfusion of blood from a second-degree relative, and a survey of predisposing factors [see comments]. Transfusion 33:742–750, 1993.
186. Pukacki F, Oszkinis G, Piszczek J, et al: [Preoperative autotransfusion and hemodilution and its value in reconstructive vascular surgery]. Wiad Lek 49:26–35, 1996.
187. Ramsey G: The pathophysiology and organ-specific consequences of severe transfusion reactions. New Horiz 2:575–581, 1994.
188. Ranaboldo CJ, Thompson JF, Davies JN, et al: Prospective randomized placebo-controlled trial of aprotinin for elective aortic reconstruction [Study of amount of bleeding in endoscopic sinus surgery]. Br J Surg 84:8–11, 1997.
189. Rao TLK, Montoya A: Cardiovascular, electrocardiographic and respiratory changes following acute anemia with volume replacement in patients with coronary artery disease. Anesth Rev 12:49–54, 1985.
190. Ratnatunga CP, Rees GM, Kovacs IB: Preoperative hemostatic activity and excessive bleeding after cardiopulmonary bypass. Ann Thorac Surg 52:250–257, 1991.
191. Reid DB, Pollock JG: A Prospective study of 100 gelatin-sealed aortic grafts. Ann Vasc Surg 5:320–324, 1991.
192. Resnikoff M, Darling RC 3rd, Chang BB, et al: Fate of the excluded abdominal aortic aneurysm sac: Long-term follow-up of 831 patients. J Vasc Surg 24:851–855, 1996.
193. Riess JG, Krafft MP: Advanced fluorocarbon-based systems for oxygen and drug delivery, and diagnosis. Artif Cells Blood Substit Immobil Biotechnol 25:43–52, 1997.
194. Ring EJ, Lake JR, Roberts JP, et al: Using transjugular intrahepatic portosystemic shunts to control variceal bleeding before liver transplantation [see comments]. Ann Intern Med 116:304–309, 1992.
195. Robertie PG, Gravlee GP: Safe limits of hemodilution and recommendations for erythrocyte transfusion. Int Anesthesiol Clin 28:197–204, 1990.
196. Rohrer MJ, Natale AM: Effect of hypothermia on the coagulation cascade. Crit Care Med 20:1402–1408, 1992.
197. Rosengart TK, Helm RE, DeBois WJ, et al: Open heart operations without transfusion using a multimodality blood conservation strategy in 50 Jehovah's Witness patients: Implications for a "bloodless" surgical technique. J Am Coll Surg 184:618–629, 1997.
198. Rousou JA, Engelman RM, Flack JE 3rd, et al: Tranexamic acid significantly reduces blood loss associated with coronary revascularization [see comments]. Ann Thorac Surg 59:671–675, 1995.
199. Royston D: Blood-sparing drugs: Aprotinin, tranexamic acid, and epsilon-aminocaproic acid. Int Anesthesiol Clin 33:155–179, 1995.
200. Rudowski WJ, Scharf R, Ziemski JM: Is major surgery in hemophiliac patients safe? World J Surg 11:378–386, 1987.
201. Rutherford RB: Vascular surgery—comparing outcomes. J Vasc Surg 23:10–17, 1996.
202. Samuels LE, Gross CF, DiGiovanni RJ: External iliac artery occlusion due to pelvic fracture: Management with a cross-femoral bypass graft. South Med J 86:572–574, 1993.
203. Sazama K: Reports of 355 transfusion-associated deaths: 1976 through 1985. Transfusion 30:583–588, 1990.
204. Scott MG, Kucik DF, Goodnough LT, Monk TG: Blood substitutes: Evolution and future applications. Clin Chem 43:1724–1731, 1997.
205. Scudamore CH, Randall TE, Jewesson PJ: Aprotinin reduces the need for blood products during liver transplantation. Am J Surg 169:546–549, 1995.
206. Seeger JM, Kieffer RW: Preoperative CT in symptomatic abdominal aortic aneurysms: Accuracy and efficacy. Am Surg 52:87–90, 1986.
207. Seyfried H, Walewska I: Immune hemolytic transfusion reactions. World J Surg 11:25–29, 1987.
208. Shcheglov VI, Vasiukov LA, Ukhanov AP: Artificial normovolemic hemodilution with preoperative blood preservation in reconstructive operations in the aortoiliac region. Vestn Khir 144:89–91, 1990.
209. Shore-Lesserson L, Reich DL, DePerio M: Heparin and protamine titration do not improve haemostasis in cardiac surgical patients [see comments]. Can J Anaesth 45:10–18, 1998.
210. Sibrowski W, Schneider C: [Possibilities of family blood donation for children and adults]. Infusionsther Transfusionsmed 21(Suppl 1):69–72, 1994.
211. Sieunarine K, Lawrence-Brown MM, Goodman MA: Comparison of transperitoneal and retroperitoneal approaches for infrarenal aortic surgery: Early and late results. Cardiovasc Surg 5:71–76, 1997.
212. Singbartl G: Adverse events of erythropoietin in long-term and in acute/short-term treatment. Clin Invest 72:S36–S43, 1994.
213. Smith MS, Muir H, Hall R: Perioperative management of drug therapy, clinical considerations. Drugs 51:238–259, 1996.
214. Smoller BR, Kruskall MS: Phlebotomy for diagnostic laboratory tests in adults. Pattern of use and effect on transfusion requirements. N Engl J Med 314:1233–1235, 1986.
215. Spahn DR, Schmid ER, Seifert B, Pasch T: Hemodilution tolerance in patients with coronary artery disease who are receiving chronic beta-adrenergic blocker therapy. Anesth Analg 82:687–694, 1996.
216. Speekenbrink RG, Vonk AB, Wildevuur CR, Eijsman L: Hemostatic efficacy of dipyridamole, tranexamic acid, and aprotinin in coronary bypass grafting. Ann Thorac Surg 59:438–442, 1995.
217. Spence RK, Jeter EK: Transfusion in surgery and trauma. *In* Mintz R (ed): Transfusion Practice. Bethesda, Md, American Association of Blood Banks (AABB), 1998 (in press).
218. Spence RK: Surgical red blood cell transfusion practice policies. Blood Management Practice Guidelines Conference. Am J Surg 170(Suppl 6A):3S–15S, 1995.
219. Spence RK: Emerging trends in surgical blood transfusion. Semin Hematol 34:48, 1997.
220. Spence RK, Alexander JB, DelRossi AJ, et al: Transfusion guidelines for cardiovascular surgery: Lessons learned from operations in Jehovah's Witnesses. J Vasc Surg 16:825–829; discussion, 829–831, 1992.
221. Spence RK, Atabek U, Alexander JB, et al: Preoperatively assessing and planning blood use for elective vascular surgery. Am J Surg 168:192–196, 1994.
222. Spence RK, Cernaianu AC: Pharmacological agents as adjuncts to bloodless vascular surgery. Semin Vasc Surg 7:114–120, 1994.
223. Spiess BD: Pro: Autologous blood should be available for elective cardiac surgery. J Cardiothorac Vasc Anesth 8:231–237, 1994.
224. Stehling L, Simon TL: The red blood cell transfusion trigger: Physiology and clinical studies. Arch Pathol Lab Med 118:429–434, 1994.
225. Stehling L, Zauder HL: Acute normovolemic hemodilution. Transfusion 31:857–868, 1991.
226. Stiegmann GV, Goff JS, Michaletz-Onody PA, et al: Endoscopic sclerotherary as compared with endoscopic ligation for bleeding esophageal varices. N Engl J Med 326:1527–1532, 1992.
227. Stover EP, Siegel LC, Parks R, et al: Variability in transfusion practice for coronary artery bypass surgery persists despite national consensus guidelines: A 24-institution study. Institutions of the Multicenter Study of Perioperative Ischemia Research Group. Anesthesiology 88:327–333, 1998.
228. Tartter PI: Transfusion-induced immunosuppression and perioperative infections. Beitr Infusionther 31:52–63, 1993.

229. Tawes RL, Duvall TB: Autotransfusion in cardiac and vascular surgery: Overview of a 25-year experience with intraoperative autotransfusion. *In* Tawes RL (ed): Autotransfusion: Therapeutic Principles and Trends. Detroit, Gregory Appleton, 1997, pp 147–148.
230. Tawes RL Jr, Sydorak GR, Duvall TB, et al: Avoiding coagulopathy in vascular surgery. Am J Surg 160:212–216, 1990.
231. Tedesco M, Sapienza P, Burchi C, et al: [Preoperative blood storage and intraoperative blood recovery in elective treatment of abdominal aorta aneurysm]. Ann Ital Chir 67:399–403, 1996.
232. Thompson JF, Mullee MA, Bell PR, et al: Intraoperative heparinisation, blood loss and myocardial infarction during aortic aneurysm surgery: A Joint Vascular Research Group study [see comments]. Eur J Vasc Endovasc Surg 12:86–90, 1996.
233. Thomson A, Contreras M, Knowles S: Blood component treatment: A retrospective audit in five major London hospitals. J Clin Pathol 44:734–737, 1991.
234. Triulzi D, Blumberg N, Heal J: Association of transfusion with postoperative bacterial infection. Crit Rev Clin Lab Sci 28:95–107, 1990.
235. Trouwborst A, van Woerkens EC, van Daele M, Tenbrinck R: Acute hypervolaemic haemodilution to avoid blood transfusion during major surgery [see comments]. Lancet 336:1295–1297, 1990.
236. Trubel W, Gunen E, Wuppinger G, et al: Recovery of intraoperatively shed blood in aortoiliac surgery: Comparison of cell washing with simple filtration. Thorac Cardiovasc Surg 43:165–170, 1995.
237. Tryba M: Epoetin alfa plus autologous blood donation and normovolemic hemodilution in patients scheduled for orthopedic or vascular surgery. Semin Hematol 33(Suppl 2):34–36, 1996.
238. Tuckfield A, Haeusler MN, Grigg AP, Metz J: Reduction of inappropriate use of blood products by prospective monitoring of transfusion request forms [see comments]. Med J Aust 167:473–476, 1997.
239. Tuman KJ: Tissue oxygen delivery: The physiology of anemia. Anesthesiol Clin North Am 9:451–469, 1990.
240. Vahl AC, Mackaay AJ, Huijgens PC, et al: Haemostasis during infrarenal aortic aneurysm surgery: Effect of volume loading and cross-clamping. Eur J Vasc Endovasc Surg 13:60–65, 1997.
241. Valbonesi M, Carlier P, Florio G, et al: Intraoperative blood salvage (IOBS) in cardiac and vascular surgery. Int J Artif Organs 18:130–135, 1995.
242. Valeri CR, Crowley JP, Loscalzo J: The red blood cell transfusion trigger: Has a sin of commission now become a sin of omission? Transfusion 38:602–610, 1998.
243. Valeri CR, MacGregor H, Cassidy G, et al: Effects of temperature on bleeding time and clotting time in normal male and female volunteers. Crit Care Med 23:698–704, 1995.
244. van Wijngaarden M, Omert L, Rodriguez A: Management of blunt vascular trauma to the extremities. Surg Gynecol Obstet 177:47–48, 1993.
245. Verdant A, Cossette R, Page A, et al: Aneurysms of the descending thoracic aorta: Three hundred sixty-six consecutive cases resected without paraplegia. J Vasc Surg 21:385–390, 1995.
246. Ward AS, Andaz SK, Bygrave S: Thrombolysis with tissue-plasminogen activator: Results with a high-dose transthrombus technique [see comments]. J Vasc Surg 19:503–508, 1994.
247. Weber B, Doerr HW: Diagnosis and epidemiology of transfusion-associated human cytomegalovirus infection: Recent developments. Infusionsther Transfusionsmed 21(Suppl 1):32–39, 1994.
248. Weisel RD, Charlesworth DC, Mickleborough LL: Limitations of blood conservation. J Thorac Cardiovasc Surg 88:26–38, 1984.
249. White GH, May J, McGahan T, et al: Historic control comparison of outcome for matched groups of patients undergoing endoluminal versus open repair of abdominal aortic aneurysms. J Vasc Surg 23:201–211, 1996.
250. White RA, Donayre CE, Walot I, et al: Modular bifurcation endoprosthesis for treatment of abdominal aortic aneurysms. Ann Surg 226:381–389, 1997.
251. Wildevuur RH, Eijsman L, Gu YJ, et al: Aprotinin reduces bleeding during cardiopulmonary bypass in aspirin treated patients. J Cardiovasc Surg 31:34, 1990.
252. Wilkerson DK, Rosen AL, Sehgal LR, et al: Limits of cardiac compensation in anemic baboons. Surgery 103:665–670, 1988.
253. Williams DM, Dake MD, Bolling SF, et al: The role of intravascular ultrasound in acute traumatic aortic rupture. Semin Ultrasound CT MR 14:85–90, 1993.
254. Williamson KR, Taswell HF: Intraoperative autologous transfusion (IAT): Experience in over 8000 surgical procedures. Transfusion 28:11S, 1988.
255. Williamson KR, Taswell HF: Intraoperative blood salvage: A review. Transfusion. Transfusion 31:662-675, 1991.

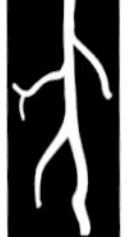

CHAPTER 45

Technical Adequacy and Graft Thrombosis

Daniel B. Walsh, M.D.

Graft thrombosis occurring either early or late after operation is a signal failure for the vascular surgeon. The causes of graft failure are myriad. At present, technical errors are responsible for 4% to 25% of failures early after revascularization.[21, 80, 86, 89] If results of arterial revascularization are to be optimized, technical precision during construction of the revascularization is mandatory. Many techniques exist to accurately assess intraoperatively the adequacy and precision of the revascularization. The subject first addressed in this chapter is the selection and application of these modalities to specific arterial reconstructions.

The remainder of this chapter focuses on the surgeon's response once graft thrombosis has occurred. To achieve the best outcome for patients in this most difficult circumstance, one must make the correct choice among the many available therapeutic options. Understanding the etiology, presentation, and current experience with available treatment options is crucial for achieving the best and most long-lasting results.

TECHNIQUES OF ASSESSMENT

Inspection, Palpation, and Flow Measurement

The most available methods of assessing technical adequacy of a revascularization are inspection and pulse palpation.

This process includes not only inspection of the revascularization for kinks, twists or stenoses but also examination of the target artery and the revascularized tissue if possible. Intuitive in this process are the surgeon's expectations. Does the distal carotid have a new, easily palpable pulse? Is the foot pink? Has capillary refill time been shortened? Is there a pulse now palpable in the foot?

This process is facilitated by having the target organ, as much as possible, prepared into a sterile field and available to the surgeon for intraoperative postrevascularization examination. For example, for aortobifemoral or more distal bypasses, clear plastic bags covering the sterilely prepared feet allow rapid examination after bypass completion. However, inspection and palpation are subjective and thus are susceptible to observer bias. After a complex reconstruction, the surgeon's expectations may cloud the evaluation of capillary refill time in the feet. Arteries calcified by the complications of diabetes may transmit improved pulses poorly. The effects of anesthesia combined with chronic superficial femoral artery occlusions may delay appearance of adequate lower extremity reperfusion. More important, false-negative results can occur when a graft has a strong pulse owing to distal outflow obstruction.

Measurement of arterial inflow and outflow is often severely affected by anesthesia. Furthermore, small hemodynamically insignificant defects in the graft may also result in failure. Low-flow measurements also may accurately predict graft failure, but the finding does not localize a defect once discovered. Studies using an ultrasound flowmeter have confirmed the inability of graft flow alone to predict future graft function.[11] Flow measurement using ultrasonically measured transit times has been reported to be sensitive and specific for graft defects.[73] Again, these studies have appeared cumbersome and have required other adjunctive measures to localize and identify specific graft defects. Because of these problems and the ease and effectiveness of other techniques, these measures of blood flow have been used infrequently.

Arteriography

Since its introduction, intraoperative arteriography has been the gold standard for evaluating anatomically the technical adequacy of arterial reconstructions. Arteriography is uniquely capable of assessing the anatomy of outflow arteries, which is particularly important when preoperative studies have not adequately demonstrated runoff vessels. Although this is an invasive procedure associated with potential complications due to arterial puncture (intimal injury, dissection), injection (air embolism), radiographic contrast (renal failure, anaphylaxis), or radiation exposure, the actual observed complication rate has been negligible in large series.[17, 18, 45] The technique varies according to individual application, but it involves insertion of an 18- to 20-gauge plastic angiocatheter into the arterial graft to allow subsequent injection of 10 to 30 ml of radiographic contrast agent. Temporary occlusion of the arterial inflow maximizes the concentration of the contrast agent without the need for excessively rapid injection. A portable x-ray generator can be used, but use of an overhead x-ray generator at ceiling height above the operating table allows the entire limb to be filmed in a single exposure via one long cassette (Fig. 45–1).

There are several weaknesses inherent in the technique of arteriography. In lower extremity bypass grafts, frequently the proximal anastomosis is not evaluated. Air bubbles or overlying structures may lead to false-positive interpretations. A potential source of false-negative results is the use of a single plane to analyze a multidimensional target. This method can result in underestimation of the stenosis from a small defect, such as an intimal flap or platelet aggregate.[8] Another problem associated with arteriography is the heavy but variable concentration of dye. This variation, on the one hand, can lead to complete coverage of a minor defect which would be better seen with lesser amounts of dye; on the other hand, lesser amounts of dye may suggest defects at valve sites or anastomoses where none exist.

To avoid these problems, intra-arterial digital subtraction arteriography (DSA) using a portable, axially rotatable imaging device can more easily obtain views from different angles.[14] The small amounts of dye and cine nature of modern digital subtraction machines allow visualization of particular areas of the graft with varying concentrations of dye that allow for a more accurate interpretation of images. DSA technology is more expensive but is increasingly available in contemporary operating rooms because of its use in endovascular, orthopedic, and other procedures. DSA also allows use of smaller amounts of contrast agents and real-time video replay. DSA is more applicable to a localized

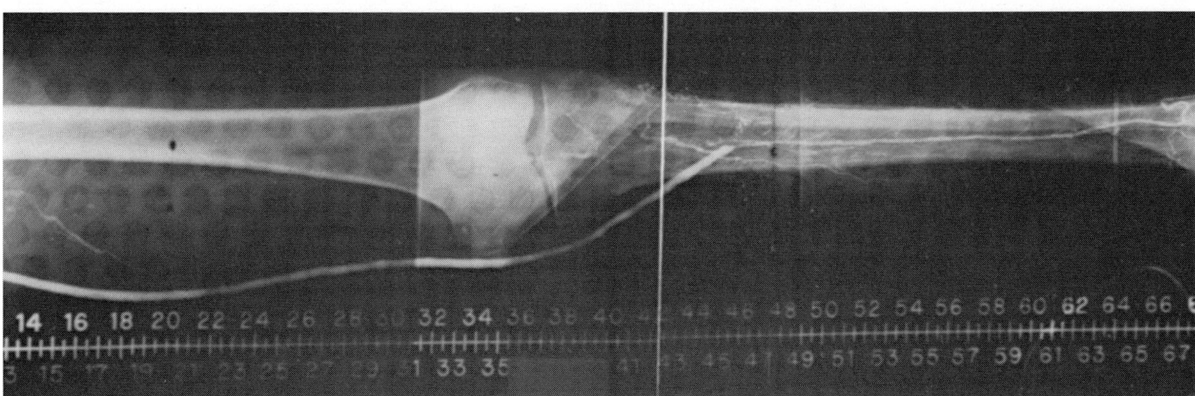

FIGURE 45–1. Normal intraoperative completion arteriogram of a femoral-peroneal in situ saphenous vein graft. A ceiling-mounted x-ray generator allows visualization of nearly the entire leg with a single exposure. A radiopaque ruler facilitates the localization of any graft defects.

area, such as carotid endarterectomy or a distal anastomosis and pedal runoff, than to an entire extremity. An entire extremity can be filmed with this technology using repeated injections of small amounts of contrast to obtain sequential angiographic images (Fig. 45–2).

Ultrasonography

The development of Doppler ultrasound technology has provided multiple noninvasive modalities for the intraoperative assessment of arterial reconstructions. The simplest and least expensive ultrasound device is a continuous wave (CW) Doppler device with an 8- to 10-MHz pencil probe. The major advantage of these probes is that they are easily sterilized by gas and they are readily available for intraoperative use. Their small size allows insonation of arteries in areas less accessible to larger probes. With sterile saline used as an acoustic coupling, the probe can be passed along the graft or endarterectomy site where localized increases in the audible sound frequency or audible turbulence indicate a potential defect. Patent residual vein branches in in situ saphenous vein bypasses can be readily identified by presence of a locally increased frequency, continuous flow, and flow outside the graft boundary. Successively compressing the graft from the proximal distal end while listening for residual proximal flow with a Doppler can also localize these arteriovenous fistulae.

Use of the audible continuous wave Doppler technique is quite subjective and operator-dependent. Considerable experience is required for maximum accuracy. The presence of high-frequency sound waves within the graft or at the distal end of anastomosis is worrisome. However, some authors have shown that the continuous wave Doppler device is not highly sensitive.[52] Most surgeons use this modality as an easy, available, and inexpensive screening device to guide their use of a more precise evaluatory technique.

To increase the objectivity of this technique, one may use a fast Fourier transform spectral analysis computer to quantitate changes in frequency or velocity. A further potential refinement is the use of a high-frequency (20 MHz) pulse Doppler device contained in a small needle probe that allows easy access to all operative sites.[8] Considerable experience with pulsed Doppler probes is required to achieve accurate results, however, and the technique fails to provide anatomic images that are reassuring to most surgeons considering arterial re-exploration.

B-Mode Ultrasonography

B-mode ultrasonography has been used intraoperatively to obtain anatomic imaging noninvasively. Initial experimental studies established its ability to detect small arteriographic defects in subjects comparable with that of arteriography.[16] With arterial defects created in dogs, arteriography and B-mode ultrasonography were both nearly 100% specific in excluding arterial defects. However, ultrasound has significantly greater sensitivity in detecting defects (92% overall) compared with a sensitivity of 70% for serial biplanar arteriography and only 50% for portable arteriography. These techniques had comparable accuracy in detecting stenoses. Clinical experience tends to confirm these findings, since patency after carotid endarterectomy—even with the detection of small defects by B-mode ultrasound—did not lead to any significant increase in stroke rate or restenosis over a 4-year follow-up.[71]

B-mode ultrasonography has also been used in the lower extremity. Kresowik and associates[43] followed up 106 patients. Intraoperative B-mode ultrasonography detected defects in 20% of these patients; half of these defects were deemed important enough to warrant correction. In follow-up, there were no early graft occlusions in the B-mode group, and no residual defects were discovered with duplex follow-up in the postoperative period.[43]

Intraoperative use of B-mode ultrasonography, however, is not without its problems. Because B-mode ultrasonogra-

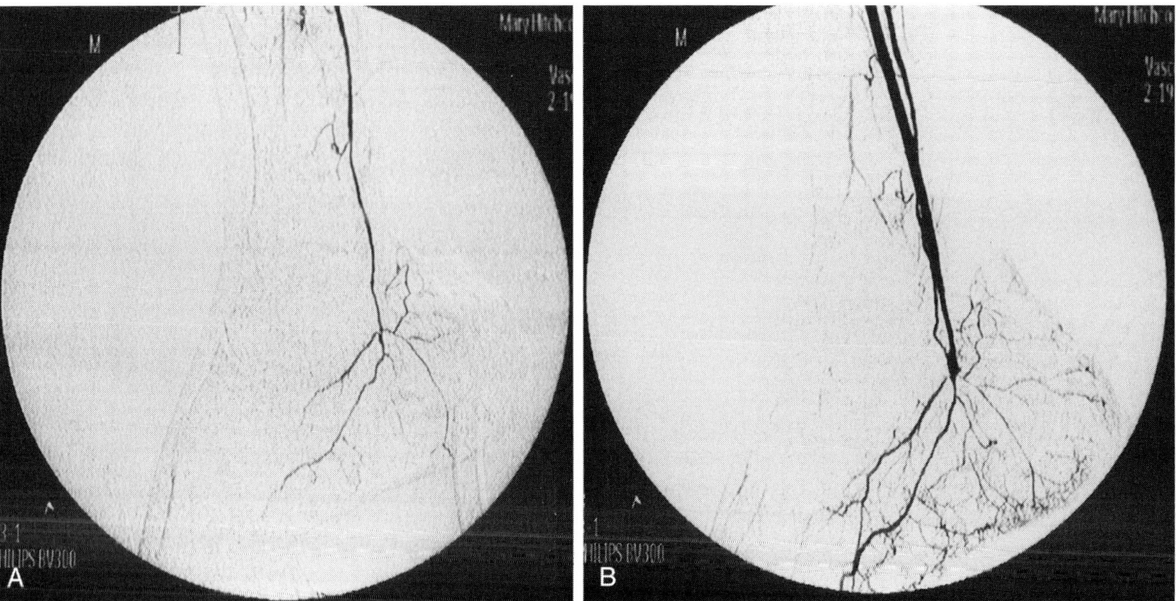

FIGURE 45–2. Intraoperative digital subtraction angiographic images of the plantar circulation performed prior to *(A)* and after *(B)* bypass.

phy does not evaluate blood flow, this technique cannot differentiate fresh thrombus from flowing blood, which has the same echogenicity. In comparison with Doppler pencil probes, B-mode ultrasound probes are larger and cannot be sterilized. Thus, their use is more cumbersome. These probes require a sterile covering containing a gel to maintain an appropriate acoustic interface. Significant operator experience is required to obtain optimal images and to achieve accurate interpretations. In clinical situations, one difficulty with the technique is determining the significance of the many defects identified, because most do not require repair. The lack of accompanying blood flow information makes this decision more difficult. In one study, B-mode ultrasound failed to create images technically adequate for evaluation in nearly 25% of patients. This inadequacy was due to the technical difficulty of imaging the distal internal carotid artery with the large probe. Carotid patch angioplasty prostheses often interfered with the acquisition of acoustic images. Because of these problems, visualization of the endarterectomy end-point at the distal internal carotid artery was often difficult to obtain satisfactorily. This study also pointed out again the problem of the false-positive results associated with defects seen with this technique.[33]

Duplex Ultrasonography

With the addition of flow measuring capability to B-mode ultrasound technology, duplex scanning brings a more powerful, expensive, and complex tool to the operating room. Like B-mode ultrasound probes, duplex probes are larger, cannot be sterilized, and require considerable operator skill not only to obtain accurate images but also to position the probe over the sample target appropriately so that accurate velocity measurements can be made. In this regard, duplex color flow technology provides continuous Doppler signals along the artery at multiple points. Color imaging facilitates identification of areas of increased velocity, albeit at a significant increase in equipment cost (Fig. 45–3).[46] The large probe heads remain difficult to manipulate in small operative fields, creating difficulties in imaging very proximal or distal targets.

Examination of outflow arteries is less precise than with arteriography, although the information provided is physiologic rather than anatomic. Duplex scanning does provide an easier mechanism for identifying defects in proximal arterial anastomoses compared with arteriography, as imaging the proximal anastamosis from a more distally placed catheter is often difficult.[20] Duplex scanning can identify low graft velocities that are undetectable by arteriography. Furthermore, there is an increasing experience with intraoperative duplex in both the carotid and infrainguinal positions.

These experiences, although largely anecdotal, demonstrate a increased sensitivity to technical defects with duplex technology. Early results with intraoperative duplex scanning demonstrate an association between these defects and optimal results in the postoperative period.[41, 42, 57, 85, 90] It is noteworthy that duplex scanning is unable to access polytetrafluoroethylene (PTFE) and polyester (Dacron) grafts because they contain air that prevents ultrasound penetration. This can be a problem with the patient in the carotid artery position when prosthetic patch material is used. A very thin-walled Dacron patch has been introduced that may alleviate this problem.

Angioscopy

Since the introduction of small flexible catheters containing high-resolution optical systems, intraoperative angioscopy has become an attractive technique for evaluation of arterial reconstructions. Angioscopy requires irrigation with saline accompanied by inflow and, sometimes, outflow occlusion to provide a visually clear image. The presence of any red blood cells can completely obscure accurate visualization of the luminal image. The use of a specifically designed infusion pump with high-flow and low-flow rates has greatly facilitated visualization.[50] Experience is required to manipulate both the angioscope and the visual target in order to obtain complete and clear visualization of the item in question.

Angioscopy has been most widely used to inspect in situ saphenous vein grafts to ensure complete valvulysis, to exclude unligated venous branches, and to assess the quality of the venous conduit (Fig. 45–4). Most commonly, our institution employs the 1.4-mm-diameter angioscope in lower extremity vein grafts and inserts the angioscope through an introducer in the most proximal end of the vein or through the most proximal vein branch left unligated for this purpose. Saline irrigation is administered through a sheath. Prior to angioscopy it is useful to identify and ligate as many venous side branches as possible to optimize distal visualization while minimizing irrigation required to clear red blood cells. Angioscopy can be used in other sites if blood flow can be temporarily occluded. This sometimes necessitates the use of balloon occlusion catheters if proximal control is not surgically accessible. Angioscopy appears particularly important in detecting abnormalities within arm veins that may not be apparent at external visual inspection.[47, 67, 81]

Because angioscopy is an invasive intraluminal procedure, related complications are possible. These include endothelial injury leading to late hyperplasia, creation of intimal flaps, and fluid overload due to excess irrigation. Experimental studies have documented that mild intimal injury does occur but only after multiple repeated passages of the larger-diameter scopes.[44] The long-term effects of this mild trauma are not firmly established, but there do not appear to be significant late clinical consequences of angioscopy that uses few passes of a small diameter (~1.4 mm) angioscope in human vein grafts. Several studies have shown that the infusion of irrigation solution can be limited to 500 ml or less in most patients, an amount that has not caused complications, especially when planned as a part of the overall fluid administration during the procedure.[39, 50]

Intravascular Ultrasonography

The newest potential modality for intraoperative evaluation of arterial procedures, the intravascular ultrasound device is based on a flexible catheter-based system and generates two-dimensional cross-sectional images by circumferential rotation of a miniaturized (10 to 30 MHz) ultrasound crystal at the catheter tip. In experimental studies, this

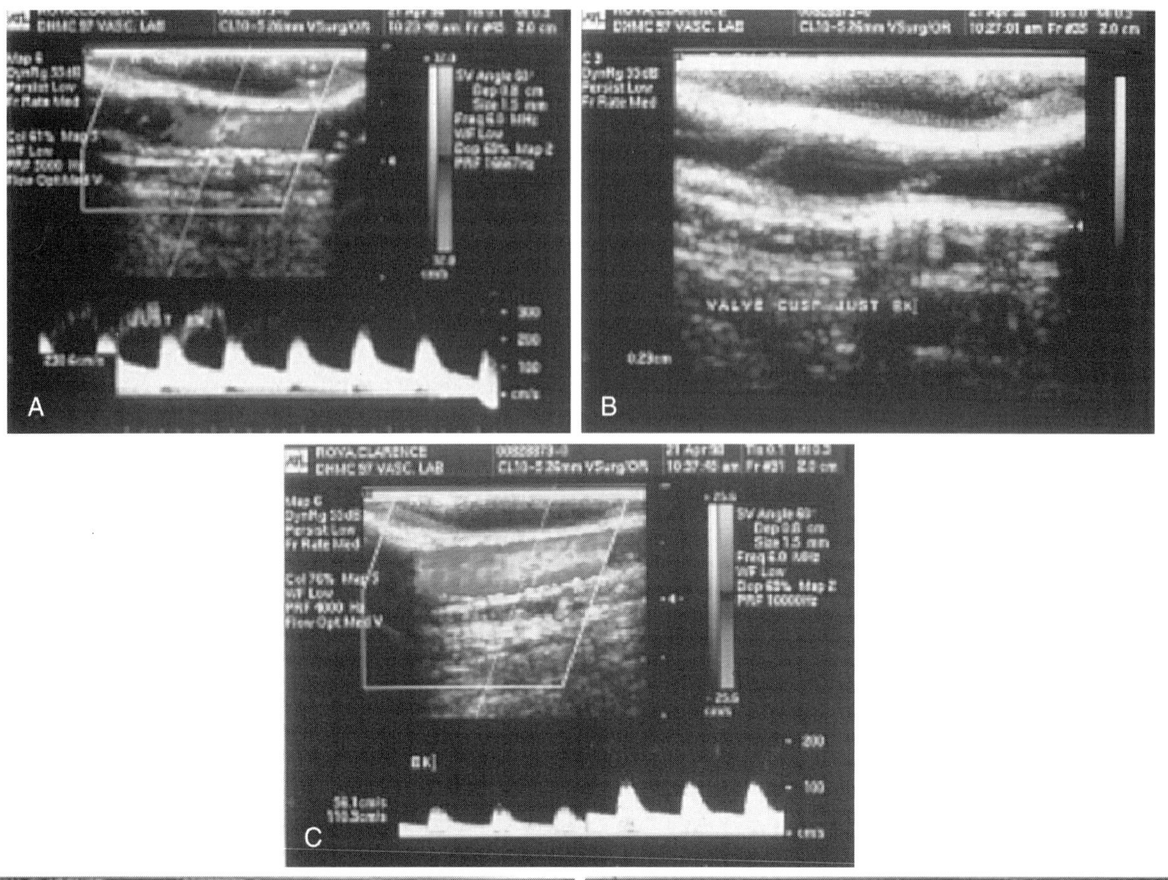

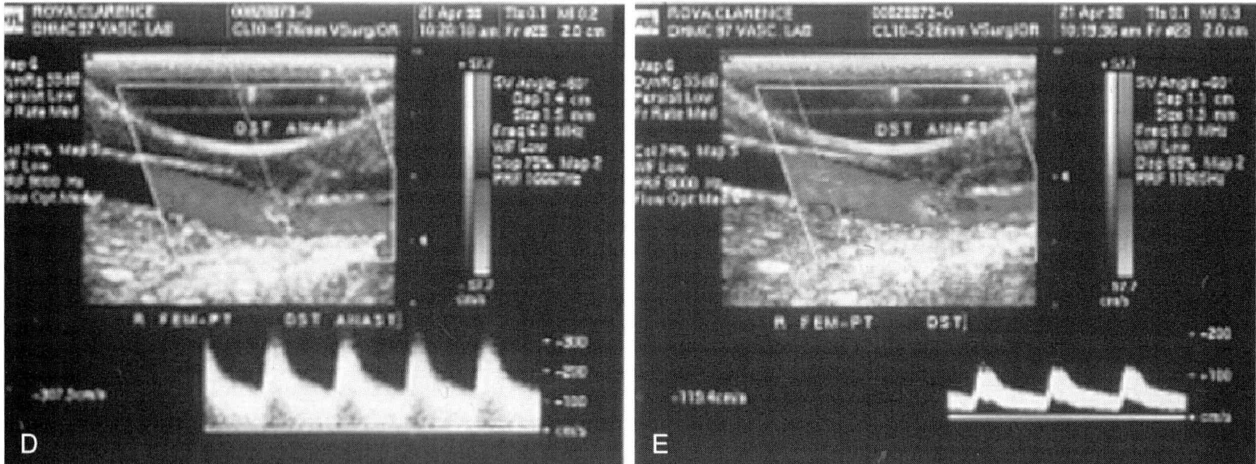

FIGURE 45–3. *A* and *B*, Retained valve cusp in an in situ bypass detected intraoperatively. *C*, Same area after valve lysis; note the decreased velocity after lysis. The distal anastomosis *(D)* of the same graft appears in spasm. The velocity decreases significantly after the injection of papaverine *(E)*.

technique has proved to be quite accurate for measuring luminal diameter and for identifying stenoses caused by atherosclerosis or intimal hyperplasia.[28, 55, 77, 83] As expected, this ultrasound technique is insensitive to detecting thrombus because of the equivalent echogenicity of fresh clot and flowing blood. Both intravascular ultrosonography and angioscopy were found to be 100% accurate in detecting 2-mm intimal flaps in canine femoral arteries compared with only 60% accuracy for single plane arteriography.[54]

Few clinical studies of this device have established its efficacy and potential role. Intravascular ultrasound imaging does appear to provide useful information in evaluation of lesions appropriate for stent graft placement (Fig. 45–5). The technique also appears useful in evaluating the efficacy of the placement of stents and stent grafts.[26] Whether this modality provides information that is different and useful enough to justify its cost, particularly in comparison with the cost of other intraoperative techniques, remains to be proven.

Indirect Methods

In addition to the direct methods of evaluating arterial reconstructions intraoperatively, several indirect methods

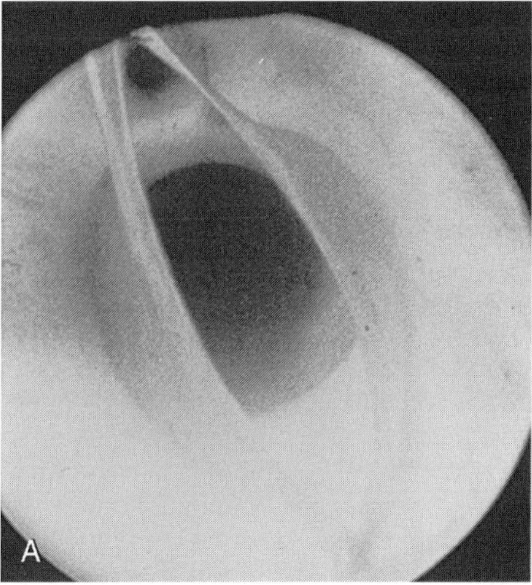

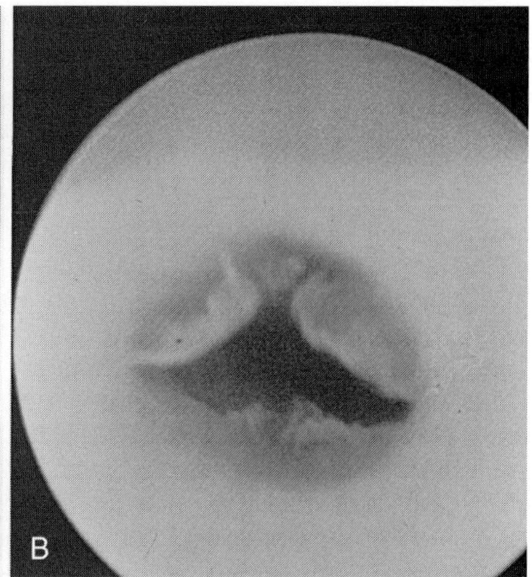

FIGURE 45–4. *A*, Photograph of a valve via an angioscope prior to lysis. *B*, Photograph of an angioscopic image of a valve after lysis. (*B*, from McCaughan JJ Jr, Walsh DB, Edgcomb LP, et al: In vitro observations of greater saphenous vein valves during pulsatile and nonpulsatile flow and following lysis. J Vasc Surg 1:356–361, 1984.)

can measure resistance within the graft or within the outflow bed that may help to evaluate the adequacy of revascularization. This is most easily accomplished intraoperatively with a continuous wave Doppler probe placed over a distal artery, with the examiner listening for audible augmentation in the waveform after release of temporary graft occlusion.

We can obtain a more quantitative assessment by measuring the distal extremity pressure using a sterile blood pressure cuff intraoperatively. In patients with more proximal reconstructions and residual outflow abnormalities, the ankle pressure may not be maximal intraoperatively and may increase only gradually in the postoperative period. Thus, this intraoperative pressure measurement does not have an absolute criterion and must be selectively interpreted on the basis of the preoperative arteriographic anatomy of each patient. Other similar modalities, including pulse volume recording, strain-gauge plethysmography, photoplethysmography, or even transcutaneous oxygen tension, can be used intraoperatively to evaluate the restoration of distal blood flow, with the examiner looking for a significant change in magnitude with and without graft occlusion.

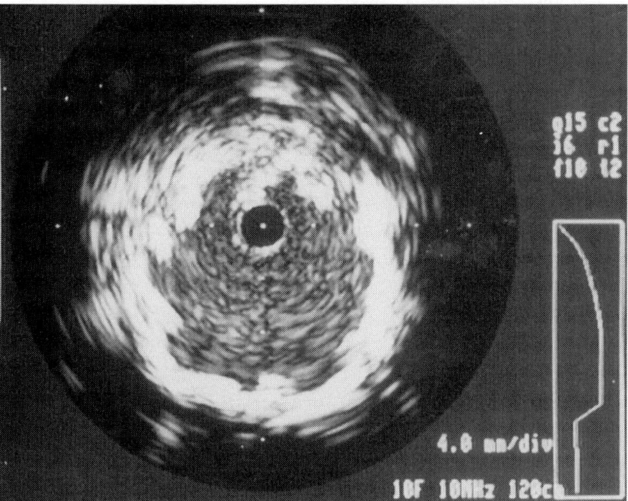

FIGURE 45–5. This is an intravascular ultrasound image of a stent graft. The rippled, uneven appearance of the inner wall represents infolds of the graft between the stent frame.

Although there are more direct methods for assessing the quality of a vein graft, Schwartz and coworkers[73] described a technique that accurately identifies problems within grafts. Unfortunately, this method identifies only increased resistance within a graft. The specific location of the potential problem is not identifiable. Thus, other adjunctive measures are required.

Outflow resistance has been measured intraoperatively to predict subsequent graft failure in extremity bypasses. This technique enables one to calculate outflow resistance based on the pressure measured while saline is injected into the distal end of a bypass graft at a known rate. Ascer and colleagues[4] found that grafts with an outflow resistance of more than 1.2 resistant units (mmHg pressure divided by ml/min flow) all experienced failure within 30 days. Other groups, however, have not confirmed this observation and have reported long-term patency in grafts with high-outflow resistance, especially vein grafts.[59] Like other indirect methods, this technique does not provide anatomic information sufficient to isolate the cause of the high outflow resistance and thus requires adjunctive anatomic study of the graft and its outflow to identify potentially correctable problems. In most instances high-outflow resistance is due to severe distal disease and cannot be improved. In a few cases, this technique may lead to identification of distal anastomotic problems or the need for extension of a proximal graft to a more distal site for improved outflow. In practice, most surgeons have found these techniques complicated and cumbersome.

CLINICAL APPLICATIONS

Cerebrovascular Reconstructions

The efficacy of cerebrovascular surgery for preventing stroke is predicated on a low operative complication rate. The technical requirements for these procedures, including the most frequently performed procedure—carotid endarterectomy—are demanding. Technical performance is best assessed by the operative complication rate, which for carotid endarterectomy is indexed by the rate of postoperative stroke, residual stenosis, and late stenosis or stroke.

Given that most reports describe postoperative stroke rates of less than 5%, one would expect the detection rate for intraoperative technical defects during carotid endarterectomy to be similarly low. Surprisingly, this has not been the case when the technical adequacy of the endarterectomy has been investigated with any of a variety of techniques. In a collected review of more than 2000 endarterectomies evaluated intraoperatively, residual defects were found in an average of 12% of procedures, with a range of 5% to 43%.[9] Although most defects were found in the external carotid artery (because of the blind nature of this portion of the endarterectomy), defects were found in the internal carotid artery in 6.5% of these collected cases, usually at the distal end of the endarterectomy. In a similar review of 1500 carotid endarterectomies, the average frequency of residual defects found by postoperative arteriography or noninvasive testing was 5.7%, with the lowest incidence reported in a series employing some type of intraoperative evaluation.[9]

In contradistinction to lower extremity revascularization, the technical results of carotid endarterectomy do not appear to have changed over time. With various types of techniques used to evaluate technical adequacy, the range of technical defects found requiring at least concern and, in many cases, re-exploration ranged from 4% to 40%.[30, 31, 33, 57]

Because early and late stroke rates in these patients continue to be considerably less than the rate of technical defects detected, it is clear that not all residual defects after carotid endarterectomy cause symptoms. Nonetheless, it is axiomatic that technical defects should be eliminated if possible. This has led most surgeons to use some form of intraoperative assessment after carotid endarterectomy and other vertebral or subclavian artery reconstructions. Although there is usually some hesitation to re-explore a completed carotid endarterectomy because of a *possible* technical defect, there is widespread agreement that this step does not increase morbidity.[27, 32] Reluctance to re-explore an artery is easily overcome when the surgeon has confidence in the method of assessing technical adequacy.

Use of intraoperative arteriography has lead to carotid re-exploration in 2% to 26% of reported cases.[18, 30] After introducing routine intraoperative carotid arteriography, Courbier and colleagues[18] found a reduction in the rate of stroke from 8.2% to 2%, compared with historical controls not undergoing arteriography. Using this approach, these authors found that 5% of the patients' carotid endarterectomies required re-exploration to correct significant technical defects. They further noted that intraoperative arteriograms helped to refine their endarterectomy techniques, progressively reducing the incidence of defects detected.

Donaldson and coauthors,[30] in a series of 410 carotid endarterectomies, found 71 defects that warranted correction in 16% of cases. The operative mortality and morbidity in this series were low, with an ipsilateral stroke rate below 2%. Interestingly, with this aggressive program to achieve technical perfection at the time of initial endarterectomy, over time 7.3% of these patients demonstrated restenosis of greater than 80%. Nearly 4% of these patients required reoperation for recurrent carotid stenosis, a figure comparable to that of other series in which the assessment of technical adequacy was not as comprehensive.

A unique advantage of carotid arteriography, compared with other assessment techniques, is the capability of obtaining intracranial images, if needed, to exclude distal problems such as residual thrombus after acute carotid thrombosis. Using digital subtraction techniques in 50 consecutive patients, Bredenberg and associates found that 12% of their patients required re-exploration after carotid endarterectomy to correct defects in the internal carotid artery (end-point stenosis or nonocclusive platelet thrombi).[14] The usual complaints against arteriography are the cumbersome nature of the technique in the operating room and the great variation in the quality of images seen. The technical inconvenience and imaging variance clearly can be reduced with routine performance of the procedure as the authors previously mentioned have demonstrated.

Continuous wave Doppler ultrasonography alone is the most commonly used assessment of technical adequacy in carotid surgery at present. In experienced hands, Doppler examination of a carotid endarterectomy appears to be quite sensitive. Seifert and Blackshear[76] detected 4.3% residual defects in 229 carotid endarterectomies by continuous wave Doppler inspection, of which 70% were confirmed by re-exploration or arteriography.[76] No false-negative results were reported. Barnes and coworkers[9] reported the detection of internal carotid stenoses in 8% of the 125 carotid endarterectomies, although only 30% of these were found to require exploration as judged by subsequent arteriography, since 70% were related only to spasm at the distal clamp.[9]

Thus, the continuous wave Doppler technique appears to be sensitive but not specific enough to justify re-exploration without a confirmatory additional study. The exception to this occurs when the Doppler findings are so abnormal as to demand re-exploration—a very-high-pitched frequency sound at the distal internal carotid artery or a short, abruptly ending diastolic sound in the internal carotid artery.

Using pulse Doppler spectral analysis, Bandyk and associates[6] found that 20 (8%) of 250 patients undergoing carotid endarterectomy had severe flow defects according to the criterion of the focal velocity increase of more than 150 cm/sec with uniform spectral broadening.[6] Of these, 50% had confirmatory arteriography and re-exploration for end-point stenosis, intimal flaps, or platelet aggregates. The remaining 10 patients had less than 30% stenosis, demonstrated on intraoperative arteriography, and did not undergo re-exploration. Two of these latter patients later had postoperative neurologic deficits and thrombosis caused by platelet aggregates. In an additional three patients not undergoing exploration, residual carotid stenosis of more than 50% developed within 3 months following surgery. This suggested that pulse Doppler spectral analysis detected some important residual lesions (especially platelet aggregates) that had been missed by arteriography. The authors further noted that 10% of the arteriograms were of inadequate quality and concluded that pulse Doppler ultrasonography was more accurate in their hands.

Flanigan and colleagues,[32] using B-mode ultrasonography to evaluate 55 carotid endarterectomies, found that 19% of patients had a common or internal carotid artery defect, of which most (73%) were intimal flaps, with stenosis being next most frequent.[32] In only 7% of these cases was the decision made to re-explore the endarterectomy using the criterion of a stenosis of 30% diameter reduction or more or intimal flap of at least 3 mm long. Although the study emphasizes the sensitivity of B-mode ultrasonography for identifying arterial defects after carotid endarterectomy, a large number of apparently insignificant defects were detected. The same group addressed these issues in a subsequent study, which demonstrated that "lesser defects" did not result in either early or late stroke or residual stenosis after late follow-up using duplex ultrasound.[71] They concluded that "minor" defects detected by B-mode ultrasonography after carotid endarterectomy were benign and did not need re-exploration.

In direct comparison using both arteriography and B-mode ultrasound, Dilly and Bernstein[27] found significant defects requiring re-exploration of 8.3% of 158 patients undergoing carotid endarterectomy. They noted that both techniques had a false-positive rate of 5% to 8% and that combining the techniques improved accuracy. These authors concluded that the use of intraoperative assessment helped to improve their assessment of endarterectomy but, in their hands, no assessment technique was thought to be perfect.

Using gray scale duplex ultrasound intraoperatively, Schwartz and associates[74] found arterial defects requiring re-exploration in 11% of 76 patients undergoing carotid endarterectomy. The authors used Doppler velocity criteria to differentiate significant from trivial intimal flaps observed with B-mode imaging and concluded that this technique represents a major advantage over B-mode ultrasonography alone. In their experience using duplex ultrasound to evaluate 131 carotid endarterectomies, Reilly and coworkers found that 11% of arteries required re-exploration to correct technical defects, of which 5% involved the external carotid artery, 5% the internal carotid artery, and 1% the common carotid artery.[61] They found it difficult to obtain adequate images in 14% of arterial segments but noted a positive correlation between the size of unrepaired intraoperative defects and the severity of artery restenosis. These authors agreed that minor anatomic defects visualized by the B-mode ultrasound but not accompanied by Doppler flow alterations are benign and should not be repaired.

In 1993, Bandyk, Towne, and others reported on an experience in 430 patients who required 461 carotid endarterectomies, all of whom underwent duplex scanning and pulsed Doppler spectral analysis to assess the adequacy of the carotid endarterectomy. This experience included the previously reported 268 patients who underwent ultrasound examination and arteriography and added 142 who underwent duplex scanning and pulse Doppler spectral analysis. All patients were observed in the postoperative period with duplex ultrasonography. Fewer than 6% of patients required intraoperative revision based on intraoperative abnormalities, and 2.6% of patients suffered neurologic deficits, half of which were permanent. Patients with normal intraoperatively flow findings had a significantly lower rate of late ipsilateral stroke. Patients who had an incidence of 50% diameter reducing stenosis or who were not studied had a significantly increased risk of ipsilateral stroke in the late follow-up. This study emphasizes the importance of optimal results at initial carotid endarterectomy so that the perioperative neurologic deficit rate would be reduced and the rate of late ischemic neurologic events would also be minimized.[42]

In a smaller study, Papanicolaou and colleagues[57] confirmed the findings from the Medical College of Wisconsin. Patients who underwent 86 carotid endarterectomies were evaluated with duplex ultrasonography intraoperatively. Of the patients, 11% required re-exploration at the time of initial surgery to correct intimal flaps and platelet thrombi demonstrated on duplex examination. No patients suffered neurologic deficit in the perioperative period, and no carotid restenosis was identified in the follow-up of 43 patients. Although this study was small, it tends to confirm the findings from Kinney and associates,[42] particularly that normal intraoperative duplex findings after carotid endarterectomy appear to decrease the incidence of both perioperative cerebrovascular events and subsequent carotid artery stenosis.

Limited experience using intraoperative angioscopy following carotid endarterectomy has been reported.[33, 49] Gaunt and coworkers[33] evaluated 100 consecutive patients intraoperatively using transcranial Doppler imaging and angioscopy. The arteries were also evaluated with continuous wave Doppler imaging and B-mode ultrasonography. Their findings were interesting, in that continuous wave Doppler ultrasonography was technically inadequate in 9% of patients. B-mode ultrasonography was technically inadequate in 24% of patients. Angioscopy demonstrated significant technical errors in 12% of patients; transcranial Doppler ultrasonography detected shunt malfunction in 13% of patients, emboli that occurred during operative dissection in 23% of the patients, and early postoperative carotid thrombosis in three patients. None of the patients in whom angioscopy detected abnormalities that were subsequently repaired suffered postoperative thrombosis or neurologic deficits in the perioperative period. The authors found angioscopy to be simple in both its application and its interpretation. Another advantage of angioscopy was that these defects were detected and corrected prior to restoration of flow, thus avoiding the need for re-exploration. The authors suggested that angioscopy was likely too sensitive, in that 27% of patients had defects visible at the time of surgery, not all of which required repair or caused perioperative stroke.

When used routinely, these various methods of intraoperative evaluation of carotid endarterectomy have led to re-exploration rates of 4% to 16% in medical centers of recognized excellence and, in the opinion of Gaunt and colleagues, have improved the technical results in most series. The need for intraoperative assessment of technical adequacy clearly depends on each surgeon's complication rate. Given the frequency of this procedure and its high visibility, most surgeons would benefit from use of one or more of these techniques.

Our practice has been to use the continuous wave Doppler probe routinely following carotid endarterectomy and to employ either duplex ultrasound or arteriography intraoperatively if any focally increased frequency or visible defect is detected along the endarterectomy site. Although our perioperative neurologic deficit rate and our restenosis rate are low, the reports described earlier have led us to scrutinize the use of duplex ultrasonography to evaluate in more detail the technical results of our carotid endarterectomies. Once the initial start-up inconveniences were overcome, we have been pleased with the sensitivity provided by the B-mode image combined with the physiologic parameters provided by the Doppler interrogation of the carotid endarterectomy site. We were initially frustrated with the large number of patients who required patch arterioplasty in whom the character of the patch impeded duplex interrogation. The development of thinner prosthetics has obviated much of this difficulty.

Extremity Revascularization

Although intraoperative assessment techniques can be applied equally well after arterial endarterectomy, thrombectomy, embolectomy, or intraoperative balloon angioplasty, most experience has been acquired with lower extremity bypass grafts. Despite improved overall results, the early failure rate in most reported series of infrainguinal vein grafts varies from 5% to 10%, often due to correctable graft or anastomotic defects.[23, 80] Since achievement of long-term patency after graft thrombosis in the early postoperative period is unlikely, efforts to detect and correct any defect in a graft during the initial revascularization attempt are justified.[12, 53, 65]

Early studies using completion arteriography found that the introduction of this technique reduced the early graft thrombosis rate from 18% to 0 due to its ability to detect defects in 27% of the patients undergoing extremity endarterectomy.[62] Using intraoperative arteriography in more than 1800 arterial reconstructions, Courbier and investigators[18] detected significant technical problems in 4.6%. When only bypass grafts were studied, Courbier's group[18] found technical problems in 2.2% of patients. These included emboli, thrombosis, twisted and kinked vein grafts, distal anastomotic stenoses, and intimal flaps. Similarly, Liebman and colleagues[45] found that intraoperative arteriography identified defects in 5.2% of 250 lower extremity bypass grafts with a false-positive rate below 1%.[45] These early reports demonstrate the impact of intraoperative arteriography on the development of better techniques for vascular surgery as well as the evaluation of individual procedures.

In 1992, Mills and coauthors reviewed an experience in 214 consecutive infrainguinal bypass grafts. They found that 8% of grafts were demonstrated at intraoperative arteriography to have technical problems significant enough to require revision. Arteriography missed only two (<1%) defects that caused graft failure within the first 30 days. Those grafts were able to be salvaged. This led the authors to conclude that routine completion arteriography should be considered the standard for intraoperative bypass assessment.[52] Similar experience was reported by Chalmers and investigators[15] in 298 in situ bypasses. Eight per cent required surgical revision of defects detected at intraoperative arteriography.

Two reports of small, highly selected series have suggested that completing arteriography after infrainguinal revascularization is neither sensitive nor cost-effective.[13, 22] Most, however, believe that completion arteriography after infrainguinal revascularization provides valuable information regarding the state of the conduit, the distal anastomosis, and the runoff circulation. Completion arteriography remains a mainstay of confirming technical adequacy of extremity revascularization.

To evaluate pulsed Doppler spectral analysis, Schmitt and coworkers[72] assessed 83 lower extremity in situ saphenous vein grafts intraoperatively.[72] By measuring the peak systolic velocity in the small diameter of the distal vein, they found that 93% of patients had a peak systolic velocity of greater than 40 cm/sec, and there were no postoperative failures in this group. In the remaining 7% of grafts with slower velocities, however, two thirds met with graft failure early or required intraoperative correction of the defect identified with the confirmatory arteriogram. The authors found a slow velocity to be quite specific for graft luminal defect, sclerosed vein segment, or large vein diameter (>5 mm). In previous reports, these authors had also found that a focal decrease in Doppler velocity indicated a potential graft or endarterectomy stenosis.[8] They recorded a 40% incidence of false-positive detection of small significant defects, however, and thus recommend this method as a companion for intraoperative arteriography.

Sigel and associates,[78] using real-time B-mode ultrasound imaging during 165 vascular reconstructions, compared the results with those achieved with intraoperative arteriography. Defects were detected by ultrasound examination in 29% of cases, but only 8% were judged significant enough to warrant re-exploration. In a subset of patients who underwent simultaneous intraoperative arteriography, the authors determined that the accuracy of the ultrasound or arteriography was 96% and 85%, respectively. They concluded that the sensitivity of ultrasound in detecting potential defects is high but that many insignificant abnormalities are also detected not requiring repair. They substantiated this conclusion by noting the lack of subsequent graft failure in patients with small defects that were not corrected. However, B-mode ultrasonography still resulted in unnecessary re-explorations in 14% of patients whose results were false-positive. This illustrates the major difficulty of this technique, namely the selection of defects that are significant enough to warrant re-exploration since many small abnormalities are identified.

In an attempt to define the hemodynamic severity of defects detected by B-mode ultrasound, Cull and colleagues[20] studied 56 lower extremity bypasses using duplex scanning intraoperatively. They considered a lesion hemodynamically significant if the peak systolic velocity focally increased by more than 50% or was lower than 45 cm/sec at any point along the graft, excluding increases in peak systolic velocity immediately beyond the distal anastomosis, where a significant diameter reduction often occurs. Duplex scanning identified technical defects in 39% of these grafts, of which 50% were judged clinically significant enough to warrant re-exploration. Four of these defects were missed by completion arteriography, and one defect identified by arteriography was missed by duplex scanning. Interestingly, 50% of the grafts with uncorrected defects that were detected by duplex scanning became occluded within 1 month of surgery, suggesting that these duplex identified defects were more significant than originally judged on clinical grounds. Unlike B-mode ultrasonography used alone, duplex scanning was not overly sensitive, because it produced only one false-positive study result, which led to an unnecessary graft exploration. These authors concluded that both arteriography and duplex scanning had good sensitivity (88% for both) for identifying graft defects, with the combination of both modalities being even more accurate. They concluded that these techniques were complementary. Despite the combination of both techniques, however, the authors reported a 9% early graft failure rate, similar to that reported by other authors who had not used duplex scanning to evaluate their grafts.

In 1994, Bandyk and colleagues[7] reviewed their experience with intraoperative duplex scanning during arterial reconstructions. They found defects in 18% of 135 infrainguinal vein bypasses that required revision. Intraoperative arteriography was performed in 81% of these procedures and added no additional diagnostic information. Their criteria for defect identification or graft function focused on peak systolic velocity and velocity ratios. For peak systolic velocities less than 125 cm/sec and velocity ratios of 1:1.4, they recommended no further evaluation of this normal flow pattern. Importantly, none of these grafts failed. For peak systolic velocity ratios from 125 cm/sec to 180 cm/sec with velocity ratios of 1:1.5 to 1:2.4, they felt that repeat scanning during the same procedure and intraoperative arteriography would help them decide whether this residual flow abnormality was significant and required exploration. In a later study, peak systolic velocities above 180 cm/sec with spectral broadening and velocity ratios greater than 1:2.5 were thought to be significant abnormalities necessitating exploration and repair. Using these criteria, the authors revised 16% of 275 grafts. Only three bypasses (1%) failed within 30 days of operation; 2.2% (6 bypasses) required revision in the early postoperative period. Critically important was the achievement of normal peak systolic velocity in the repaired vein grafts. Once this lower peak systolic velocity was achieved, no grafts failed. The authors pointed out that most of the defects were related to blind retrograde valvulotomy or to imperfections found in non-reverse translocated grafts. They readily admitted that reversing grafts required significantly fewer revisions.[5]

Considerable experience in the use of angioscopy to evaluate lower extremity reconstructions has been reported. Graft defects that require surgical corrections (including stenoses, webs, and bands resulting from recanalization of intimal flaps, thrombus and anastomotic strictures, and kinks) have been identified in 10% to 20% of these cases.[10, 37, 88] The largest experience with angioscopy has been obtained during evaluation of infrainguinal vein grafts, especially the detection of residual valve cusps and unligated vein branches in in situ saphenous vein grafts.[50] The incidence of angioscopically detected defects has been significantly higher in these grafts, residual cusps being found in 19% to 47% and unligated vein branches in 35% to 75%.[35, 37, 50] Arm vein grafts in particular are prone to recanalization defects (webs or bands), which are detected in 74% of these grafts, perhaps due to trauma of previous venipuncture.[81]

Baxter and colleagues[10] found that arteriography was 95% as specific as angioscopy but only 67% as sensitive. They reported a 20% false-positive rate for arteriography related to small filling defects that could not be substantiated and a 7% false-negative rate for detecting intimal flaps. In a similar comparison of 102 infragenicular area bypasses Woelfle and associates[89] found completion angiography to have a sensitivity of 46% and a specificity of 98% in the detection of significant abnormalities. Stonebridge and associates[81] noted that neither continuous wave Doppler study nor arteriography could identify webs or bands in recanalized arm veins and that introducing angioscopy reduced the early failure rate of these veins from 11% to 0.

Miller and coworkers[50] noted that nearly 50% of the 259 angioscopies performed in lower extremity grafts led to important surgical decisions. They pointed out the utility of angioscopy for monitoring the correction of defects after they were detected intraoperatively. Furthermore, they noted that even after considerable experience with in situ techniques, 10% of the recent in situ saphenous vein grafts had residual valve cusps, which presumably increase the risk of graft failure. This conclusion has not been firmly established, however, since studies using angioscopy detected far more defects than studies using arteriography without obvious changes in the rate of early graft failure. Thus, the remaining key question concerning small defects detected only by angioscopy is the extent to which they effect subsequent graft failure, which would determine the appropriate criteria for repairing them intraoperatively. Although the need for repair of all defects detected by angioscopy has not been firmly proved, it is clear that this is the most sensitive modality for detecting such defects.

Another advantage of using the angioscope is a decrease in residual valve cusps if the valvulotomy is angioscopically directed.[51] If Bandyk's group had employed this technique in their in situ saphenous vein grafts, the number of defects found by B-mode ultrasonography would have been significantly reduced.[5]

In an attempt to resolve questions about determining the optimal method of intraoperative in situ saphenous graft evaluation, my group[35] performed a blinded prospective comparison of arteriography and angioscopy in duplex ultrasound in 20 patients using prospectively defined criteria for defects detected by each modality. Sensitivity in detecting residual unligated vein branches was highest for angioscopy (66%) and arteriography (44%), whereas gray scale duplex scanning detected only 12% of these vein branches. Angioscopy was significantly more sensitive (100%) than either duplex scanning (11%) or arteriography (22%) in detecting residual valve cusps. No anastomotic stenoses were confirmed in our study, although six were suggested, yielding a false-positive rate for erroneous detection of stenosis, 20% for arteriography, 10% for duplex ultrasound, and 0 for angioscopy. The time required to complete these studies was 17 to 20 minutes and did not vary among the three modalities. No stenoses, occlusions, or arteriovenous fistulae have been detected in any of these grafts by postoperative duplex surveillance during a 10-month mean follow-up interval. In this study, arteriography or duplex ultrasound used alone would have missed more than 75% of the actual residual valve cusps that occurred in 30% of these bypass grafts.

Our own practice is to perform angioscopically directed valvulotomy after ligation of all visible vein branches. During that examination, if other patent vein branches are found, they are ligated. Once the distal anastomosis is completed, we perform DSA of the distal anastomosis and runoff bed. Since the late 1980s, we have found very few technical errors in the anastomosis with any technique.

DSA allows evaluation to rule out twists in the graft and any obvious anastomotic problems, and it provides very helpful information about the runoff bed that is not as easily obtained with any other modality. We have used continuous wave Doppler or duplex ultrasound examination of the graft to confirm that all fistulae are ligated. We have been reassured by the experience of Bandyk and associates that a duplex finding of a peak systolic velocity of less than 125 cm/sec or a low velocity ratio is an indicator of excellent long-term graft function, and we are using this modality with increasing frequency.

In addition to bypass grafts or endarterectomy, intraoperative assessment can also yield important information after arterial embolectomy or thrombectomy. Although these procedures are often performed without intraoperative assessment of adequacy, we found that completion arteriography detected 87% of complications occurring after balloon-catheter usage compared with only 23% of complications that were recognized without arteriography.[19] Since many of these complications led to the need for subsequent operations and limb loss, some intraoperative technique is needed to identify distal peudoaneurysms, arteriovenous fistulae, arterial disruption, intimal injury, or inadequate thrombus extraction. Several studies have reported the efficacy of intraoperative angioscopy to confirm the adequacy of graft or arterial thromboembolectomy by direct inspection to identify residual thrombus. This inspection led to complete thrombectomy or alterations in the surgical procedure in more than 80% of these cases, and the authors[75, 87] believe that this contributed substantially to the success of the procedure. They also pointed out the usefulness of angioscopy in directing subsequent attempts at thrombus retrieval, including the ability to guide balloon catheters selectively into tibial branches.

In our own practice, the addition of fluoroscopy and DSA to our operating room has significantly aided the ease of reevaluation after thromboembolectomy. The ability to direct guide wires, to perform intraoperative road mapping, and to pass catheters over directed guide wires with repetitive imaging with small doses of contrast dye have significantly increased the efficiency and accuracy of catheter thromboembolectomy.

Transabdominal Revascularization

As a result of the large size of aortoiliac reconstruction, small technical defects causing flow disturbances that affect graft patency are much less frequent than they are in carotid artery or lower extremity reconstructions. Because iliac intimal flaps occasionally cause immediate or a delayed graft thrombosis, however, intraoperative assessment is required. When aortoiliac bypass or endarterectomy has been uneventful, we rely on the palpation of a normal distal aortoiliac or femoral pulse supplemented with comparable continuous wave Doppler insonation of the anastomoses or endarterectomy end-points, looking for focal increases in frequency or marked turbulence. If a major defect is found, we immediately re-explore the site. In less certain cases, we employ intraoperative duplex ultrasonography. We find that duplex scanning provides more accurate and precise information than arteriography in the abdomen, where the large volume of contrast needed requires a rapid injection to obtain an adequate study. These examinations are often further limited by the inadequate penetration afforded by portable x-ray generators. In practice, it is infrequent that anything more than continuous wave Doppler examination is required in the aortoiliac system, a conclusion supported by the low incidence of postoperative stenoses or thromboses in this region.

For an aortofemoral graft, especially if it is extended into the profunda femoris artery, a more precise determination of technical adequacy is required because the small diameter of the femoral arteries is more easily influenced by minor imperfections. Accordingly, we routinely employ continuous wave Doppler ultrasonography in this area, supplementing it with intraoperative duplex scanning or DSA as required. Good-quality intraoperative arteriography is significantly easier to obtain at this site if we inject a contrast agent into the aortobifemoral graft limb using a temporary proximal graft occlusion to maximize contrast concentration in the femoral graft. We do not advocate this procedure routinely but believe that duplex ultrasound or arteriography should be used liberally if any question is raised about an anastomotic stricture by continuous wave Doppler examination, especially at the profunda femoris anastomosis.

As in the femoral location, renal and mesenteric arterial reconstructions also require careful intraoperative evaluation because small technical defects are likely to lead to graft failure which, when occurring in the early postoperative period, can be catastrophic. The major difficulty associated with evaluation of these endarterectomies or reconstructions is the anatomic location of the arteries, which are often difficult to approach with anything but a small Doppler probe. We have had difficulty in obtaining optimal arteriograms of these arteries because their reconstruction usually requires examination of an aortic anastomosis, making it difficult to achieve sufficient contrast concentration and good x-ray penetration. Furthermore, intraoperative arteriography for the evaluation of renal artery reconstructions has a major theoretical disadvantage, in that the majority of these patients have some degree of renal insufficiency that may be exacerbated by concentrated radiographic contrast injection. Accordingly, we rely initially on continuous wave Doppler inspection followed by intraoperative duplex scanning.

To assess intraoperative duplex ultrasound after renal artery repair, Hansen and colleagues[38] evaluated 57 renal artery reconstructions, including both bypass grafts and thromboendarterectomies. They found defects on B-mode scans in 23% of these repairs, of which half (11%) were confirmed as major defects by increases in peak systolic velocity of 200 cm/sec or greater. This change corresponded to a stenosis with an estimated 60% or greater reduction in diameter. The defects consisted of vein graft anastomotic stenoses and flaps or residual disease in the endarterectomized segment. Postoperatively, duplex and arteriographic evaluation indicated that 98% of the patients without major intraoperative duplex abnormalities had patent arteries that were free of critical stenoses, demonstrating the specificity of duplex assessment. Of the six renal arteries that were revised because of major defects detected on duplex scanning, four remained patent, one became stenotic, and one became occluded. The authors were confident that all the major defects that they explored based on intraoperative duplex evaluation were significant and would have led to the failure of the revascularization, suggesting a low false-positive rate. According to this experience, renal artery procedures that show only minor B-mode ultrasound defects without Doppler spectral changes do not require revision.

In a similar study that used intraoperative duplex ultrasonography after 83 renal and mesenteric reconstructions, Okuhn and coworkers[56] found minor duplex defects in 31% of their repairs and major defects that required re-exploration in 5% based on obviously abnormal duplex signals. They determined that the intraoperative duplex ultrasonography had a sensitivity of 85%, a specificity of 75% in the evaluation of these visceral arterial repairs. These authors also found arteriography to be suboptimal in this location but reported excellent results using duplex ultrasound assessments. Bandyk and colleagues[7] have reported 23 visceral or renal artery reconstructions interrogated by duplex intraoperatively. They found and corrected significant defects in one patient, leading to excellent graft performance.[7]

As experience grows, it appears that duplex ultrasonography has an increasing role in the evaluation of technical defects after revascularization. This is particularly true in the visceral and renal circulations, where angiography or angioscopy is frequently thwarted for technical reasons.

GRAFT THROMBOSIS

Despite the surgeon's best effort at achieving technical perfection, revascularizations may be unsuccessful. Depending on the type of arterial reconstruction, between 0.3% and 10% fail in the early postoperative period.[1, 23, 25] With detailed, long-term follow-up, nearly 50% of vascular reconstructions develop some degree of restenosis or frank failure.[2, 23, 25] When a thrombosed revascularization is evident, therapeutic alternatives range from expectant supportive care through anticoagulation to attempt at an entirely new arterial reconstruction. The best results in these most difficult circumstances require rapid decisions by the surgeon regarding (1) the etiology of the thrombosis, (2) selection of the technique, (3) timing of the multiple possible therapies, and (4) assessment of complex patient risk factors. These circumstances are made more difficult by the fact that few vascular surgeons have current experience with the many situations possible in a failed arterial reconstruction. Since the 1960s, the results of arterial revascularizations have consistently improved, so that any individual surgeon's experience with graft thrombosis is relatively infrequent. This discussion summarizes a reliable set of therapeutic guidelines for the most common among the possible scenarios, when patients present with thrombosis of an arterial reconstruction.

Initial Approach

Regardless of the specific circumstances of the failed revascularization, several factors, which may contribute to any graft failure, should be investigated. If not previously established, the patient's coagulation status should be determined (see Chapters 8 and 36). Graft thrombosis at any time after placement can be the consequence of a previously unrecognized hypercoagulable state.[29] Blood should be sent immediately (prior to anticoagulation) for measurement of standard coagulation parameters, including platelet count, functional activitated protein C resistance, and antithrombin III and protein S determinations. A history of previous exposure to heparin, with consequent heparin associated antibodies causing platelet aggregation, should be investigated. Less likely causes of hypercoagulability leading to thrombosis, such as increased blood viscosity from dehydration or polycythemia or sepsis, can easily be diagnosed with physical examination and routine hematologic screening. Acute or chronic cardiac decompensation is an uncommon but real cause of arterial revascularization failure. Again, these conditions can be rapidly detected at the time of patient presentation with electrocardiography or echocardiography as indicated. A rapid cardiac assessment in these patients is also critical in assessing risk associated with the various possible therapeutic options.

Once the diagnosis of graft thrombosis has been confirmed, the surgeon must give immediate consideration to minimize clot propagation with systemic anticoagulation. A short period of time can be taken to obtain coagulation studies just mentioned. If regional anesthesia is preferred for a surgical attempt at graft salvage, systemic anticoagulation can be delayed until anesthesia is obtained. If immediate operation is not required or regional anesthesia is contraindicated, systemic heparin anticoagulation should be instituted to inhibit further thrombosis.

A primary determinant of the timing required for therapy is the patient's neurologic status at the time of initial presentation. If there is no neurologic compromise, diagnostic or therapeutic maneuvers, which may take considerable time to succeed, can be considered. As the level of neurologic dysfunction increases from dysesthesia to paralysis, the necessity for rapid resolution of the situation increases. Consequently, the time available for lengthy diagnostic or therapeutic measures outside of the operating room decreases correspondingly.

Etiology

The first element fundamental to achieving successful therapy of a failed revascularization is accurate determination of the cause of the thrombosis. Time from the initial revascularization to patient presentation is the single most important characteristic that aids in the determination of the etiology of graft failure (Fig. 45–6). Early (<30 days) thromboses of vascular reconstructions are usually attributed to technical errors. As already mentioned, however, the number of technical causes for early failure has significantly decreased over the past 30 years. Technical errors now cause 20% or less of the arterial reconstruction thromboses in the early postoperative period. Other likely causes include graft thrombogenicity, patient-related hypercoagulable states, and poor selection of the artery targeted for distributing the runoff from the graft. Sauvage and coworkers[70] suggested that there is a critical threshold velocity for sustaining early graft patency. This threshold velocity is a

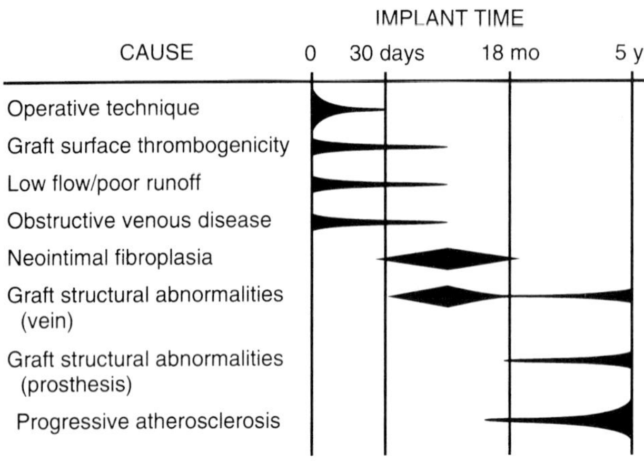

FIGURE 45–6. Factors contributing to graft occlusion with time. (Modified from Rutherford RB: The prevention and management of graft thrombosis. *In* Kempczinski RF [ed]: The Ischemic Leg. Chicago, Year Book Medical Publishers, 1985.)

function of the inflow, the bypass conduit, and the condition of the bypass's runoff bed.

Another method of determining the cause of an unsuccessful arterial revascularization is to examine each of the elements required for effective function of any arterial reconstruction. There are five critical elements for function of any revascularization:

- Inflow
- Outflow
- Conduit
- Technique
- Patient's coagulation function

For any revascularization to function, blood pressure and blood flow at the origin of the reconstruction must be systemic. A gradient between the proximal reconstruction and the central systemic arterial pressure demonstrates the existence of a significant proximal arterial stenosis. No revascularization can long succeed with its inflow compromised.

The quality of outflow for a revascularization can be extremely difficult to characterize. For instance, the carotid artery circulation is a very-low-resistance, high-flow runoff bed. For the lower extremity, however, runoff beds may be composed of only a few small vessels that seem, at arteriography, too sparse to support long-term graft function (Fig. 45–7). No arteriographic criteria have been found to be reliable predictors of graft patency. In the figure, a runoff bed is based on the lateral plantar artery. This graft has been patent for more than 5 years. Measurement of outflow bed resistance also has been predictive of graft failure.[4] However, most surgeons find these methods cumbersome and lacking in the level of accuracy needed for confident recommendation for conversion of a revascularization attempt to a primary amputation.

A pressure gradient measured at the distal end of the arterial reconstruction is evidence of a significant abnormality within the reconstruction that will likely cause early graft thrombosis.[72] When decreased pressure is noted at the distal end of a reconstruction, the cause of the decreased pressure must be identified and rectfied if an enduring revascularization is to be achieved.

When considering timing of occurrence of failed arterial revascularizations, most surgeons use two temporal categories: early (within 30 days of placement) and late (after 30 days). This discussion focuses on infrainguinal revascularizations, since these form the largest single group of revascularizations that fail and confront the surgeon with a multitude of therapeutic options.

Lower Extremity Bypass Failure

Early Graft Failure (0 to 30 days)

Despite maturation of infrainguinal vein graft revascularization techniques, 5% to 10% of grafts fail within 30 days of placement.[23] The response to early graft failure begins in the latter stages of the initial revascularization. As described earlier, technical adequacy of the bypass must be confirmed prior to incision closure. When the techniques described are used to confirm technical adequacy at bypass completion, the likelihood that a technical flaw has caused graft failure is low.

In 1990, a review of our institutional experience demonstrated that technical errors accounted for 25% of our early graft failures.[86] Since that time, the number of graft failures in our series caused by errors in technique have declined sharply, likely a result of our increasing use of angioscopy, duplex scanning, and DSA to confirm the technical adequacy of our revascularizations. This confirmation also allows a prospective, qualitative determination of the likelihood that graft failure will occur and a recognition that should such a failure occur, it is most likely related to the conduit or the quality of the runoff bed. This evaluation greatly simplifies further therapeutic decision making. If a graft fails that has been constructed using the only available autogenous vein conduit and the only possible target runoff vessel and has shown no evidence of anastomosis or a conduit problem at the time of placement, early amputation speeds most patients toward their best available outcome. In such patients, further reoperative attempts at thrombectomy, anastomosis improvement, conduit replacement, or

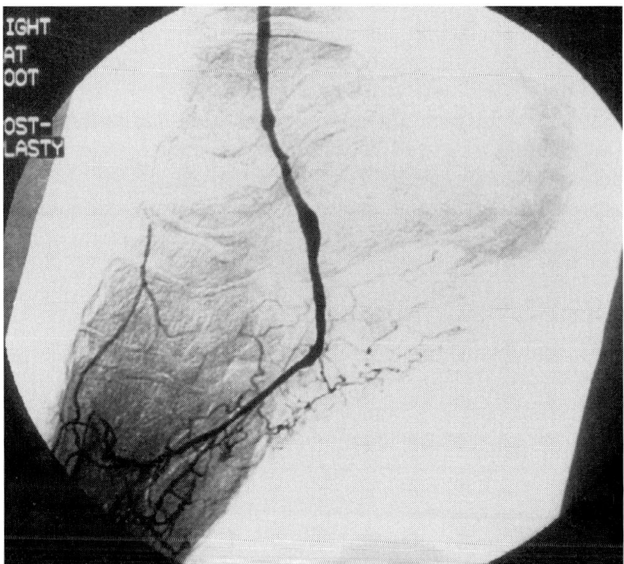

FIGURE 45–7. Intraoperative completion arteriogram demonstrating sparse runoff from a lateral plantar artery.

runoff substitution are only likely to increase morbidity, mortality, and expense, with little improvement in limb salvage.[65]

Thus, when graft thrombosis is initially recognized, the first question is "Can the graft be salvaged?" Because this first bypass probably employed the most appropriate conduit and target vessel, most surgeons would answer, "Yes." Once it has been determined to proceed with attempted salvage of the initial bypass graft, the decision is whether the thrombectomy should be surgical or chemical. The choice of which technique to employ is difficult because the results of either are discouraging in the early postoperative period no matter which type of conduit or procedure is performed.

After thrombolysis is attempted in the early postoperative period, patency of thrombosed vein grafts ranges between 15% and 20% at 1 year.[12, 53] Results with lysis of prosthetic grafts are slightly better, although this is likely related to the better runoff that usually exists when prosthetic graft material is employed as conduit for an initial bypass attempt.[63] Time since initial vein graft placement has been found to be predictive of both short-term and long-term graft patencies after lysis. The more recently placed the graft, the less likely there will be any chance of success with thrombolytic therapy. This is particularly true among patients with diabetes. In our own series, no patient with diabetes and a recently placed graft achieved secondary graft patency with thrombolysis. Of our patients successfully treated with thrombolysis, 44% required early amputation. When thrombolysis failed, the amputation rate rose to 69%.

The results of surgical thrombectomy, even with an adjunctive procedure such as patch angioplasty of the distal anastomosis, are also uniformly poor. Robinson and coauthors[65] reported a cumulative secondary patency rate of 47% at one year. In this series, 26% of the patients required amputation within 1 month of graft thrombectomy. The incidence of patients requiring amputation rose to 41% at 1 year. The results of surgical thrombectomy significantly improved if, at exploration, technical problems (e.g., a twist in the graft or a retained valve cusp in an in situ saphenous vein bypass graft) were identified. In our own experience, long-term graft patency of grafts that thrombosed owing to correctable technical problems approached that of grafts experiencing no complications in the postoperative period. As mentioned, however, the number of technical flaws causing graft failures has decreased dramatically with improved techniques of graft placement.[65] These statements are even more true in regard to bypass grafts performed with prosthetic materials. Our own bias is that surgical thrombectomy of these grafts is technically straightforward and significantly less time-consuming and thus less expensive. At the time of graft thrombectomy, pressure measurements at the inflow and outflow sights as well as proximal and distal arteriography can be performed in order to evaluate the cause of graft failure. Reparative procedures can be undertaken at that time to correct the cause of the graft failure. If not, re-exploration will have caused few confounding problems for other possible therapies.

Our own practice has been to immediately perform re-exploration of any patient whose graft has failed soon after initial revascularization if we expect good graft function, no matter which conduit has been used. We have not found thrombolysis useful because of the time required for lysis, the additional risk of bleeding during thrombolysis, and poor long-term results. In this group of patients, thrombectomy, anticoagulation, and repair of any possible technical problems appear to achieve the best results.[48, 66, 69]

In at least 50% of patients whose grafts undergo exploration for early failure, no cause of the thrombosis is found.[80] In these desperate circumstances, when a correctable problem has not been found and poor conduit or disadvantaged runoff does not appear to be the cause of thrombosis, we have placed a 20-gauge polyethylene catheter in a convenient proximal side-branch of the vein graft after thrombectomy. Through this catheter, nitroglycerin (0.05 μg/min) and heparin (10 units/min) are infused while the patient is held in the postanesthesia recovery unit or the intensive care unit. This measure is an attempt to counteract presumed but undocumented thrombogenicity within the revascularization, whether it is related to runoff spasm or to graft harvest trauma. These catheters are usually removed at the bedside or in the operating room after 24 to 36 hours of infusion. Eight of 10 grafts so treated have remained patent over a mean follow-up of 17 months.[86]

If all measures of diagnosis and salvage of a thrombosed infrainguinal graft fail in the early postoperative period, only two options remain. The first is expectant therapy combined with anticoagulation. This likely leads to amputation even though limb loss is not inevitable.[64, 82] If autogenous vein remains in adequate length, particularly for target vessels with runoff of good quality, as often happens with a failed prosthetic-based revascularization, a repeated bypass using the best available autogenous vein often yields satisfying results.[24]

Late Graft Failure

When a graft has failed more than 1 month after placement, all of the aforementioned general considerations for evaluation and patient therapy continue to apply. The major difference in treatment strategy focuses on the disappearance of technical error from the list of potential causes of graft failure, the improvement of results using thrombolysis, and the increased difficulty of the surgical dissection of previously operated vessels.

Time from graft placement is a strong predictor of success of thrombolysis of thrombosed vein grafts. The longer a graft has been in place, the greater the likelihood the patient and graft patency will benefit from intragraft thrombolysis. Factors critical in predicting success appear to be (1) graft age of approximately 1 year or older since time of placement and (2) the absence of diabetes. In the Dartmouth-Hitchcock Medical Center series, only 1 of 15 failed grafts (7%) among patients with diabetes had a graft patent 1 year after successful thrombolysis. In patients without diabetes whose grafts had been patent for at least 12 months prior to thrombosis, 44% of patients were alive with a patent graft 2 years after thrombolysis.

Once patency has been restored, all series reporting bypass graft salvage demonstrate that the requirement for further endovascular or surgical therapy exceeds 85%. Therapeutic options available include (1) balloon angioplasty of intragraft or juxta-anastomosis stenoses, (2) open vein patch angioplasty, and (3) interposition vein bypass. Although the results of these techniques used to maintain patency of threatened grafts (so-called primary assisted patency) are not comparable to results obtained in failed grafts patent after thrombolysis, experience in the former "threatened" group is much larger and provides a significant body of data from which useful direction can be drawn.

Patency after surgical treatment of vein graft lesions has been achieved in 86% of grafts after 21 months of follow-up. Patency of lesions treated with percutaneous angioplasty was achieved in 42% of patients in the same series.[68] This difference is particularly noteworthy, because the surgical group (in the opinion of the authors) suffered from more extensive disease than the patients treated percutaneously; however, other groups have reported significantly better results for angioplasty of graft stenoses.[40] Excellent results using either technique have been published.

Our personal bias is that percutaneous transluminal angioplasty is best used to maintain graft patency until operative repair can be undertaken, to treat straightforward, short stenoses that are difficult to approach surgically, or to dilate critical stenoses in patients with medical contraindications to anesthesia or surgery. In the patient whose prosthetic bypass graft has failed proximal to atherosclerotic disease that has developed distal to the graft since the graft has been placed, we look to the data related to angioplasty of those specific lesions after graft patency has been reestablished. In the typical patient with new infragenicular popliteal, tibial peroneal trunk, or tibial runoff vessel atherosclerosis, percutaneous treatment with angioplasty of these lesions is justified only when there are no reasonable surgical alternatives.[36, 79]

Selection of patch angioplasty versus interposition graft for repair of a vein graft lesion discovered after lysis should best be made according to (1) lesion location and appearance, (2) availability of usable autogenous vein, and (3) the surgeon's preference as determinants. A detailed review of an experience using both techniques demonstrates that results are similar.[83] Our experience suggests that removal of the hyperplastic intimal lesion vein and replacement with a vein interposition graft should lead to better results. However, the two additional anastomoses within the graft carry their own complication rate. For juxta-anastomotic problems in the distal graft, exposure of the distal target artery beyond the initial anastomosis is technically simpler and results in less morbidity than reoperating at the initial anastomotic site. This option is possible only if suitable lengths of autogenous vein adequate for bypass graft extension are available.

The optimal autogenous vein conduit for replacement of a short segment of vein graft is a segment of remaining ipsilateral saphenous vein or lesser saphenous vein. Interposition of a segment of contralateral greater saphenous or arm vein to provide a short interposition should be avoided to preserve these longer conduits for other uses.

In patients whose older grafts have suffered diffuse deterioration after successful lysis and in patients with diabetes or whose grafts have failed in less than 1 year, we would forego thrombolysis because of the small likelihood of achieving any significant secondary graft patency. For these groups, a repeated bypass has the greatest chance of achieving successful long-term revascularization. Of course, quality distal target vessels and adequate autogenous vein conduit are mandatory if another bypass is to be attempted.

Figure 45–8 compares long-term graft patencies achieved by all techniques of graft salvage from repeated bypass and graft revision to thrombolysis under the best of circumstances. Despite the obvious benefit of repeated bypass in this comparison, it is important to remember that these patient groups are only superficially comparable. In this series conduit availability, condition of runoff, coagulation status, and other important circumstances are either not comparable or not known. For example, in our own patients with failed vein grafts undergoing thrombolysis, a repeated bypass was possible in only 1 of 44 patients. This emphasizes again the complexity of these patients and the importance of understanding the condition of all five elements needed for successful bypass at the time of initial bypass completion and at the time of thrombosis.

Conduit availability and selection constitute another example of the complexity of the decision making involved when a vein graft has failed. Contralateral greater saphenous vein has long been thought to be the optimal conduit for bypass when the ipsilateral greater saphenous vein is not available because of disease or prior use. Concern that the donor leg might require bypass in the future or that the saphenous vein might be required for coronary artery bypass has been outweighed by the immediate need and the belief that the reduced survival of these patients made the need for future bypass elsewhere unlikely. However, examination of the infrainguinal bypass experience at Dartmouth-Hitchcock Medical Center revealed that 20% of our patients required contralateral lower extremity revascularization at a mean of 31 months after initial ipsilateral bypass.[84] The intervention rate in our patients by life-table analysis was relatively linear at 6% per year. Of these interventions, 83% were contralateral infrainguinal vein bypass. Factors that predicted the need for intervention were (1) younger age, (2) presence of diabetes, (3) overt coronary artery disease, and (4) lower contralateral ankle-brachial index at the time of initial ipsilateral revascularization.

In our series, patients with only unilateral lower extremity atherosclerosis severe enough to require operation, the likelihood of future contralateral intervention was less than 10% during the following 5 years. Thus, the contralateral saphenous vein—the optimal bypass conduit—should be used to revascularize the contralateral leg in older patients with atherosclerosis isolated to one limb. In this patient group, the surgeon can proceed, confident that the requirement for the use of this vein elsewhere is very unlikely. Unfortunately, only 8% of patients who typically require infrainguinal revascularization have only isolated unilateral lower extremity atherosclerosis; in actuality, 32% of our infrainguinal bypass patients had both diabetes and coronary artery disease. Of these patients, 31% required intervention for ischemia of the contralateral leg within 5 years of the initial infrainguinal revascularization. Of our patients, 22% had diabetes, coronary artery disease, and low contralateral ankle-brachial index, and half of these patients required later contralateral intervention during follow-up. Therefore, we believe that the selection of a bypass conduit, when ipsilateral greater saphenous vein is not available, is complex.

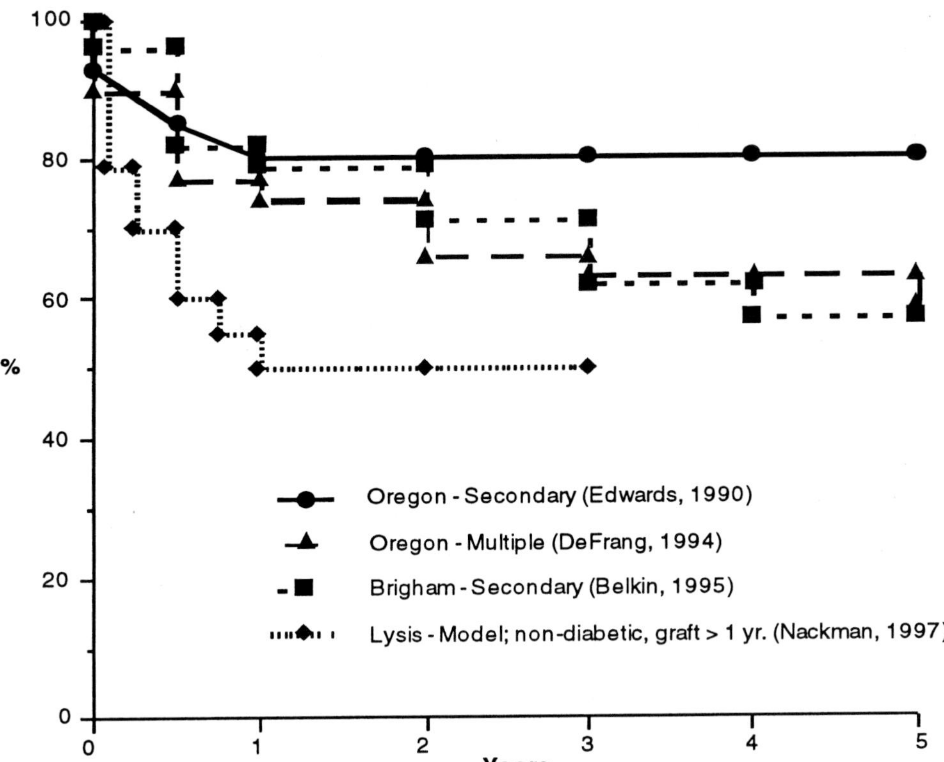

FIGURE 45–8. Comparison of long-term patency of secondary bypass, initial bypass salvage vein surgery, and thrombolysis among the patient groups with the best results. (From Walsh DB: Management of the thrombosed infrainguinal vein graft. Adv Vasc Surg 6:190, 1998.)

The arm vein, deemed acceptable by preoperative duplex evaluation and intraoperative angioscopic examination, is our secondary bypass or rebypass conduit of choice. Although the need for graft revision is greater for bypass grafts using the arm vein as a conduit, the primary assisted patency is 72% over 5 years.[34] We believe that vein grafts spliced together from the lesser saphenous vein and the remaining ipsilateral saphenous vein have a patency equivalent to that of the arm vein but carry with them the added morbidity of distal incisions in a presently ischemic, previously operated limb. Use of the arm vein as a conduit also minimizes the number of venovenostomies. Utilization of the profunda femoris or endarterectomy of the superficial femoral artery to lessen the conduit length required for bypass are also preferred techniques. Others advocate repeated infragenicular bypass using a prosthetic conduit aided by distal vein cuffs or an arteriovenous fistula or with prosthetic conduit alone.[3, 58, 60] We use these techniques rarely and only as a last resort. Despite optimistic reports of others, our results in these patients have not been comparable to repeated bypass with autogenous vein.

As in the circumstance of a failed lower extremity bypass, failure in the early postoperative period after carotid endarterectomy or after revascularization within the abdominal circulation is usually identified by acute ischemia of the profused organ bed and requires immediate return to the operating room for another revascularization in order to avoid catastrophic ischemic damage to the target organ. All of the suggestions mentioned, regarding the confirmation of technical adequacy and the response to graft failure, apply. Only if there is no demonstrable ischemic damage to the organ targeted for revascularization should nonoperative expectant therapy be employed.

When late failure of a cerebrovascular or abdominal revascularization has occurred, the tenets of determining surgical therapy also apply. Optimal methods of surveillance and response to recurrent stenosis or thrombosis of the primary revascularization are also discussed in other chapters. Thus, if the revascularization fails and the organ is ischemic, one should consider a second revascularization; if there is no ischemic injury to the target organ, one can consider expectant therapy.

SUMMARY

The best results in managing failed arterial revascularizations are achieved by instituting protocols that maximize prevention. The first step toward prevention is discovery and correction of any problems at the initial revascularization. This is achieved with (1) rigorous assessment of each revascularization by measuring inflow pressure, (2) direct inspection of the revascularization as well as its inflow and outflow, and (3) performance of intraoperative technical assessments to evaluate the technical function of each revascularization as well as its outflow bed. At the conclusion of each case, one should honestly assess the likely long-term patency of the revascularization. Fruitless re-explorations can be avoided with the recognition that technical errors are unlikely if techniques for confirming the adequacy of the revascularization are used. The lack of another suitable conduit or bypass targets often precludes further reasonable revascularization attempts.

Unexpected early failure of a revascularization warrants screening for hypercoaguable states and immediate surgical re-exploration with thorough evaluation of inflow, outflow, and conduit using repair or a repeated bypass augmented with chronic systemic anticoagulation. Aggressive follow-up of revascularization function can detect patency-threatening lesions prior to thrombosis to ensure maintainance of optimal revascularization function. Patients in whom revascularizations fail in the month after initial operation should be evaluated for the potential benefits of thrombolysis or surgery to reestablish flow in the revascularization. Critical factors in treatment planning include the availability of autogenous vein for conduit and the condition of other distal arterial targets. Patient factors, such as age, diabetes, age of the graft, and presence and severity of coronary artery disease, significantly affect the selection of salvage techniques.

Vascular surgeons should be familiar with the techniques available for maintaining the long-term function of each revascularization they perform and with techniques that can restore perfusion in a severely ischemic target organ. Vascular surgeons are the last hope for preventing permanent ischemic damage in most patients who suffer from severe disseminated atherosclerosis.

REFERENCES

1. AbuRhama AF, Khan JH, Robinson PA, et al: Prospective randomized trial of carotid endarterectomy with primary closure and patch angioplasty with saphenous vein, jugular vein, and polytetrafluoroethylene: Perioperative (30-day) results. J Vasc Surg 24:998, 1996.
2. AbuRhama AF, Robinson PA, Saiedy S, et al: Prospective randomized trial of carotid endarterectomy with primary closure and patch angioplasty with saphenous vein, jugular vein, and polytetrafluoroethylene: Long-term follow-up. J Vasc Surg 27:222, 1998.
3. Ascer E, Gennaro U, Pollina RM, et al: Complementary distal arteriovenous fistula and deep vein interposition: A five-year experience with a new technique to improve infrapopliteal bypass patency. J Vasc Surg 24:134, 1996.
4. Ascer E, Veith FJ, Morin L, et al: Components of outflow resistance and their correlation with graft patency in lower extremity arterial reconstructions. J Vasc Surg 1:817, 1984.
5. Bandyk DF, Johnson BL, Gupta AK, et al: Nature and management of duplex abnormalities encountered during infrainguinal vein bypass grafting. J Vasc Surg 24:438, 1996.
6. Bandyk DF, Kaebnick HW, Adams MB, et al: Turbulence occurring after carotid bifurcation endarterectomy: A harbinger of residual and recurrent carotid stenosis. J Vasc Surg 7:261, 1988.
7. Bandyk DF, Mills JL, Gahtan V, et al: Intraoperative duplex scanning of arterial reconstructions: Fate of repaired and unrepaired defects. J Vasc Surg 20:426, 1994.
8. Bandyk DF, Zierler RE, Thiele BL: Detection of technical error during arterial surgery by pulsed Doppler spectral analysis. Arch Surg 119:421, 1984.
9. Barnes RW, Nix ML, Nichols BT, et al: Recurrent versus residual carotid stenosis. Incidence detected by Doppler ultrasound. Ann Surg 203:652, 1986.
10. Baxter BT, Rizzo RJ, Flinn WR, et al: A comparative study of intraoperative angioscopy and completion arteriography following femorodistal bypass. Arch Surg 125:997, 1990.
11. Beard JD, Scott DJA, Skidmore R, et al: Operative assessment of femorodistal bypass grafts using a new Doppler flowmeter. Br J Surg 76:925, 1989.
12. Berkowitz HD, Kee JC: Occluded infrainguinal grafts: When to choose lytic therapy versus a new bypass graft. Am J Surg 170:136, 1995.
13. Blankensteijn JD, Gertler JP, Brewster DC, et al: Intraoperative determinants of infrainguinal bypass graft patency: A prospective study. Eur J Vasc Endovasc Surg 9:375, 1995.
14. Bredenberg CE, Iannettoni M, Rosenbloom M, et al: Operative angiography by intraarterial digital subtraction angiography: A new technique for quality control of carotid endarterectomy. J Vasc Surg 9:530, 1989.
15. Chalmers RT, Synn AY, Hoballah JJ, et al: Is the use of intraoperative post-reconstruction angiography following in situ saphenous vein bypass redundant? Am J Surg 166:141, 1993.
16. Coelho JCU, Sigel B, Flanigan DP, et al: An experimental evaluation of arteriography and imaging ultrasonography in detecting arterial defects at operation. J Surg Res 32:130, 1982.
17. Courbier R, Jausseran JM, Reggi M: Detecting complications of direct arterial surgery: The role of intraoperative arteriography. Arch Surg 112:1115, 1977.
18. Courbier R, Jausseran JM, Reggi M, et al: Routine intraoperative carotid angiography: Its impact on operative morbidity and carotid restenosis. J Vasc Surg 3:343, 1986.
19. Cronenwett JL, Walsh DB, Garrett HE: Tibial artery pseudoaneurysms: Delayed complication of balloon catheter embolectomy. J Vasc Surg 8:483, 1988.
20. Cull DL, Gregory RT, Wheeler JR, et al: Duplex scanning for the intraoperative assessment of infrainguinal arterial reconstruction: A useful tool? Ann Vasc Surg 6:20, 1992.
21. Cuming R, Blair SD, Powell JT, et al: The use of duplex scanning to diagnose perioperative carotid occlusions. Eur J Vasc Endovasc Surg 8:143, 1994.
22. Dalman RL, Harris EJ, Zarins CK: Is completion arteriography mandatory after reversed-vein bypass grafting? J Vasc Surg 23:637, 1996.
23. Darling RC 3rd, Chang BB, Shah DM, et al: Choice of peroneal or dorsalis pedis artery bypass for limb salvage. Semin Vasc Surg 10:17, 1997.
24. DeFrang RD, Edwards JM, Moneta GL, et al: Repeat leg bypass after multiple prior bypass failures. J Vasc Surg 19:268, 1994.
25. Desiron Q, Detry O, Van Damme H, et al: Comparison of results of carotid artery surgery after either direct closure or use of a vein patch. Cardiovasc Surg 5:295, 1997.
26. Diethrich EB: Endovascular treatment of abdominal aortic occlusive disease: The impact of stents and intravascular ultrasound imaging. Eur J Vasc Surg 7:228, 1993.
27. Dilly RB, Bernstein EF: A comparison of B-mode real-time imaging and arteriography in the intraoperative assessment of carotid endarterectomy. J Vasc Surg 4:457, 1986.
28. DiMario C, The SH, Madretsma S, et al: Detection and characterization of vascular lesions by intravscular ultrasound: An in vitro study correlated with histology. J Am Soc Echocardiogr 5:135, 1992.
29. Donaldson MC, Belkin M, Whittemore AD, et al: Impact of activated protein C resistance on general vascular surgical patients. J Vasc Surg 25:1054, 1997.
30. Donaldson MC, Ivarsson BL, Mannick JA, et al: Impact of completion angiography on operative conduct and results of carotid endarterectomy. Ann Surg 217:682, 1993.
31. Dorffner R, Metz VM, Trattnig S, et al: Intraoperative and early postoperative colour Doppler sonography after carotid artery reconstruction: Follow-up of technical defects. Neuroradiology 39:117, 1997.
32. Flanigan DP, Douglas DJ, Machi J, et al: Intraoperative ultrasonic imaging of the carotid artery during carotid endarterectomy. Surgery 100:893, 1986.
33. Gaunt ME, Smith JL, Ratliff DA, et al: A comparison of quality control methods applied to carotid endarterectomy. Eur J Vasc Endovasc Surg 11:4, 1996.
34. Gentile AT, Lee RW, Moneta GL, et al: Results of bypass to the popliteal and tibial arteries with alternative sources of autogenous vein. J Vasc Surg 23:272, 1996.
35. Gilbertson JJ, Walsh DB, Zwolak RM, et al: A blinded comparison of angiography, angioscopy, and duplex scanning in the intraoperative evaluation of in situ saphenous vein bypass grafts. J Vasc Surg 15:121, 1992.
36. Gray B, Olin J: Limitations of percutaneous transluminal angioplasty with stenting for femoropopliteal arterial disease. Semin Vasc Surg 10:8, 1997.
37. Grundfest WS, Litvack F, Glick D, et al: Intraoperative decisions based on angioscopy in peripheral vascular surgery. Circulation 78:I-13, 1988.
38. Hansen KJ, O'Neil EA, Reavis SW, et al: Intraoperative duplex sonography during renal artery reconstruction. J Vasc Surg 14:364, 1991.
39. Hashizume M, Yang Y, Galt S, et al: Intimal response of saphenous vein to intraluminal trauma by simulated angioscopic insertion. J Vasc Surg 5:862, 1987.

40. Houghton AD, Todd C, Pardy B, et al: Percutaneous angioplasty for infrainguinal graft-related stenoses. Eur J Vasc Endovasc Surg 14:380, 1997.
41. Jackson MR, D'Addio VJ, Gillespie DL, et al: The fate of residual defects following carotid endarterectomy detected by early postoperative duplex ultrasound. Am J Surg 172:184, 1996.
42. Kinney EV, Seabrook GR, Kinney LY, et al: The importance of intraoperative detection of residual flow abnormalities after carotid artery endarterectomy. J Vasc Surg 17:912, 1993.
43. Kresowik TF, Hoballah JJ, Sharp WJ, et al: Intraoperative B-mode ultrasonography is a useful adjunct to peripheral arterial reconstruction. Ann Vasc Surg 7:33, 1993.
44. Lee G, Beerline D, Lee MH, et al: Hazards of angioscopic examination: Documentation of damage to the arterial intima. Am Heart J 116:1530, 1988.
45. Liebman PR, Menzoian JO, Mannick JA, et al: Intraoperative arteriography in femoropopliteal and femorotibial bypass grafts. Arch Surg 116:1019, 1981.
46. Machi J, Sigel B, Roberts A, et al: Operative color Doppler imaging for vascular surgery. J Ultrasound Med 11:65, 1992.
47. Marcaccio EJ, Miller A, Tannebaum GA, et al: Angioscopically directed interventions improve arm vein bypass grafts. J Vasc Surg 17:994–1004, 1993.
48. McMillan WD, McCarthy WJ, Lin SJ, et al: Perioperative low molecular weight heparin for infrageniculate bypass. J Vasc Surg 25:796–802, 1997.
49. Mehigan JT, Olcott C IV: Video angioscopy as an alternative to intraoperative arteriography. Am J Surg 152:139, 1986.
50. Miller A, Stonebridge PA, Jepsen SJ, et al: Continued experience with intraoperative angioscopy for monitoring infrainguinal bypass grafting. Surgery 109:286, 1991.
51. Miller A, Stonebridge PA, Tsoukas AI, et al: Angioscopically directed valvulotomy: A new valvulotome and technique. J Vasc Surg 13:813, 1991.
52. Mills JL, Fujitani RM, Taylor SM: Contribution of routine intraoperative completion arteriography to early infrainguinal bypass patency. Am J Surg 164:506, 1992.
53. Nackman GB, Walsh DB, Fillinger MF, et al: Thrombolysis of occluded infrainguinal vein grafts: Predictors of outcome. J Vasc Surg 25:1023, 1997.
54. Neville RF, Hobson RW, Jamil Z, et al: Intravascular ultrasonography: Validation studies and preliminary intraoperative observations. J Vasc Surg 13:274, 1991.
55. Neville RF Jr, Yasuhara H, Watanabe BI, et al: Endovascular management of arterial intimal defects: An experimental comparison by arteriography, angioscopy, and intravascular ultrasonography. J Vasc Surg 13:496, 1991.
56. Okuhn SP, Reilly LM, Bennett JB III, et al: Intraoperative assessment of renal and visceral artery reconstruction: The role of duplex scanning and spectral analysis. J Vasc Surg 5:137, 1987.
57. Papanicolaou G, Toms C, Yellin A, et al: Relationship between intraoperative color-flow duplex findings and early restenosis after carotid endarterectomy: A preliminary report. J Vasc Surg 24:588, 1996.
58. Parsons RE, Sanchez LA, Marin ML, et al: Comparison of endovascular and conventional vascular prostheses in an experimental infection model. J Vasc Surg 24:920, 1996.
59. Peterkin GA, LaMorte WW, Menzoian JO: Runoff resistance and early graft failure in infrainguinal bypass surgery. Arch Surg 123:1199, 1988.
60. Raptis S, Miller JH: Influence of a vein cuff on polytetrafluoroethylene grafts for primary femoropopliteal bypass. Br J Surg 82:487, 1995.
61. Reilly LM, Okuhn SP, Rapp JH, et al: Recurrent carotid stenosis: A consequence of local or systemic factors? The influence of unrepaired technical defects. J Vasc Surg 11:448, 1990.
62. Renwick S, Royle JP, Martin P: Operative angiography after femoropopliteal arterial reconstruction: Its influence on early failure rate. Br J Surg 55:134, 1968.
63. Rickard MJ, Fisher CM, Soong CV, et al: Limitations of intra-arterial thrombolysis. Cardiovasc Surg 5:634, 1997.
64. Rivers SP, Veith FJ, Ascer E, et al: Successful conservative therapy of severe limb-threatening ischemia: The value of nonsympathectomy. Surgery 99:759, 1986.
65. Robinson KD, Sato DT, Gregory RT, et al: Long-term outcome after early infrainguinal graft failure. J Vasc Surg 26:425, 1997.
66. Rutherford RB, Jones DN, Bergentz SE, et al: The efficacy of dextran 40 in preventing early postoperative thrombosis following difficult lower extremity bypass. J Vasc Surg 1:765, 1984.
67. Sales CM, Marin ML, Veith FJ, et al: Saphenous vein angioscopy: A valuable method to detect unsuspected venous disease. J Vasc Surg 18:198, 1993.
68. Sanchez LA, Suggs WD, Marin ML, et al: Is percutaneous balloon angioplasty appropriate in the treatment of graft and anastomotic lesions responsible for failing vein bypasses? Am J Surg 168:97, 1994.
69. Sarac TP, Huber TS, Back MR, et al: Warfarin improves outcome of infrainguinal vein bypass grafts at high risk failure. J Vasc Surg 28:446, 1998.
70. Sauvage LR, Berger KE, Mansfield PB, et al: Future directions in the development of arterial prostheses for small and medium caliber arteries. Surg Clin North Am 54:213, 1974.
71. Sawchuk AP, Flanigan DP, Machi J, et al: The fate of unrepaired minor technical defects by intraoperative ultrasonography during carotid endarterectomy. J Vasc Surg 9:671, 1989.
72. Schmitt DD, Seabrook GR, Bandyk DF, et al: Early patency of *in situ* saphenous vein bypasses as determined by intraoperative velocity waveform analysis. Ann Vasc Surg 4:270, 1990.
73. Schwartz LB, Belkin M, Donaldson MC, et al: Validation of a new and specific intraoperative measurement of vein graft resistance. J Vasc Surg 25:1033, 1997.
74. Schwartz RA, Peterson GJ, Noland KA, et al: Intraoperative duplex scanning after carotid artery reconstruction: A valuable tool. J Vasc Surg 7:620, 1988.
75. Segalowitz J, Grundfest WS, Treiman RL, et al: Angioscopy for intraoperative management of thromboembolectomy. Arch Surg 125:1357, 1990.
76. Seifert KB, Blackshear WM Jr: Continuous-wave Doppler in the intraoperative assessment of carotid endarterectomy. J Vasc Surg 2:817, 1985.
77. Siegel RJ, Ariani M, Fishbein MC, et al: Histopathologic validation of angioscopy and intravascular ultrasound. Circulation 84:109, 1991.
78. Sigel B, Coelho JCU, Flanigan DP, et al: Detection of vascular defects during operation by imaging ultrasound. Ann Surg 196:473, 1982.
79. Stanley B, Teague B, Raptis S, et al: Efficacy of balloon angioplasty of the superficial femoral artery and popliteal artery in the relief of leg ischemia. J Vasc Surg 23:679, 1996.
80. Stept LL, Flinn WR, McCarthy WJ III, et al: Technical defects as a cause of early graft failure after femorodistal bypass. Arch Surg 122:599, 1987.
81. Stonebridge PA, Miller A, Tsoukas A, et al: Angioscopy of arm vein infrainguinal bypass grafts. Ann Vasc Surg 5:170, 1991.
82. Sullivan TR Jr, Welch HJ, Iafrati MD, et al: Clinical results of common strategies used to revise infrainguinal vein grafts. J Vasc Surg 24:909, 1996.
83. Tabbara MR, Mehringer CM, Cavaye DM, et al: Sequential intraluminal ultrasound evaluation of balloon angioplasty of an iliac artery lesion. Ann Vasc Surg 6:179, 1992.
84. Tarry WC, Walsh DB, Fillinger MF, et al: The fate of the contralateral leg following infrainguinal bypass. J Vasc Surg 27:1039, 1998.
85. Walker RA, Fox AD, Magee TR, et al: Intraoperative duplex scanning as a means of quality control during carotid endarterectomy. Eur J Vasc Endovasc Surg 11:364, 1996.
86. Walsh DB, Zwolak RM, McDaniel MD, et al: Intragraft drug infusion as an adjunct to balloon catheter thrombectomy for salvage of thrombosed infragenicular vein grafts: A preliminary report. J Vasc Surg 11:753, 1990.
87. White GH, White RA, Kopchok GE, et al: Angioscopic thromboembolectomy: Preliminary observations with a recent technique. J Vasc Surg 7:318, 1988.
88. White GH, White RA, Kopchok GE, et al: Intraoperative video angioscopy compared with arteriography during peripheral vascular operations. J Vasc Surg 6:488, 1987.
89. Woelfle KD, Kugelmann U, Bruijnen H, et al: Intraoperative imaging techniques in infrainguinal arterial bypass grafting: Completion angiography versus vascular endoscopy. Eur J Vasc Endovasc Surg 8:556, 1994.
90. Yu A, Gregory D, Morrison L, et al: The role of intra-operative duplex imaging in arterial reconstructions. Am J Surg 171:500, 1996.

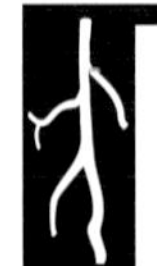

C H A P T E R 4 6

Vascular Thrombosis Due to Hypercoagulable States

Thomas W. Wakefield, M.D., and
Alvin H. Schmaier, M.D.

A number of conditions can lead to a hypercoagulable state and subsequent vascular thrombosis. This area of medicine is a rapidly expanding field, with the three most common causes for thrombosis being recognized within the past few years. Classification of the molecular causes for thrombosis can be made on the basis of their frequency or the severity of thrombosis with which the protein defect is associated (Table 46–1). The first protein defects associated with thrombosis, antithrombin III deficiency and protein C and protein S deficiency, are the most severe. Recent clinical information suggests that patients with these defects who have thrombosis should receive anticoagulation therapy for life. The most common defects associated with thrombosis—resistance to activated protein C (factor V Leiden), hyperhomocystinemia, and prothrombin 20210—are fortunately less severe defects. Much less common causes for thrombosis, abnormal fibrinogens and plasminogens, are usually associated with less severe thrombotic states, although because their frequency is so low, few prognostic studies are available.

In addition to these well-characterized protein defects, a number of clinical syndromes are associated with variable degrees of thrombosis: heparin-induced thrombocytopenia (HIT) and heparin-induced thrombocytopenia and thrombosis syndrome (HITTS), lupus anticoagulant and antiphospholipid syndrome, hyperactive platelets, and other defects in fibrinolysis not yet described. In this chapter, defects associated with thrombosis are classified according to their severity (see Table 46–1).

TABLE 46–1. CAUSES OF THROMBOSIS

FREQUENCY	SEVERITY
Factor V Leiden (20%–40%)	*High Risk for Thrombosis*
Hyperhomocystinemia (10%)	Antithrombin III deficiency
Prothrombin 20210 (4%–5%)	Protein S deficiency
Protein C deficiency (3%–5%)	Protein C deficiency
Protein S deficiency (2%–3%)	*Lower Risk for Thrombosis*
Dysfibrinogenemia (1%–3%)	Factor V Leiden
Antithrombin III deficiency (1%–2%)	Hyperhomocystinemia
Dysplasminogenemia (<1%)	Prothrombin 20210
HIT/HITTS	Dysfibrinogenemia
Lupus anticoagulant	Dysplasminogenemia
Activated platelets	*Variable Risk for Thrombosis*
	HIT/HITTS
	Lupus anticoagulants
	Hyperactive platelets

HIT/HITTS = heparin-induced thrombocytopenia/heparin-induced thrombocytopenia and thrombosis syndrome.

DEFECTS WITH HIGH RISK FOR THROMBOSIS

Antithrombin III Deficiency

Antithrombin III deficiency, either on a congenital or acquired basis, accounts for approximately 1% to 2% of episodes of venous thromboses. Episodes of native arterial and arterial graft thrombosis have also been described in antithrombin III deficiency.[79] Although uncommon, this defect is a significant risk factor for recurrent, life-threatening thrombosis. This syndrome usually manifests early in life, with most cases apparent by 50 years of age. Antithrombin III is a serine protease inhibitor (serpin) of thrombin, kallikrein, and factors Xa, IXa, VIIa, and XIa with a half-life of 2.8 days. The diagnosis should be suspected in a patient who cannot be adequately anticoagulated on heparin or who develops thrombosis on heparin. Heparin is an anticoagulant because of its ability to potentiate the anticoagulant effects of antithrombin III. We can make the diagnosis by measuring antithrombin III antigen and activity levels when patients are not taking anticoagulants. In fact, heparin itself decreases antithrombin III levels 30%, and this effect can be seen up to 10 days after stopping intravenous heparin therapy. Alternatively, warfarin increases antithrombin III levels. During significant thrombotic episodes, antithrombin III levels may also be low due to antithrombin III consumption. The nephrotic syndrome also has been reported to result in antithrombin III (M_r = 59 kD) deficiency because of the loss of intermediate-sized proteins into the urine along with albumin (M_r = 68 kD), with subsequent acute thrombosis of renal veins and arterial bypass grafts.[72]

Additional causes of antithrombin III deficiency include liver disease (site of production), malignancy, disseminated intravascular coagulation (DIC), malnutrition, and decreased protein production.[23] Less frequent causes of antithrombin III deficiency include defective antithrombin III activity with normal quantitative levels (progressive deficiency) and antithrombin III deficiency with an abnormal interaction between antithrombin III and heparin.[17] Homozygous individuals usually die in utero, whereas heterozygous patients usually demonstrate levels less than 70%.

Treatment for a patient with antithrombin III deficiency who needs to be anticoagulated with heparin usually requires the administration of fresh frozen plasma, 2 units every 8 hours decreasing to 1 unit every 12 hours, followed by the administration of oral anticoagulants. Antithrombin III concentrates are also available.[56] Although there is limited experience with their use in vascular reconstructive surgery, they should become the replacement therapy of choice in patients with antithrombin III deficiency for any reason.

Protein C and S Deficiencies

Protein C and its cofactor protein S are both synthesized in the liver. Activated protein C functions as an anticoagulant by inactivating factors Va and VIIIa in the coagulation prothrombinase and Xase complexes, respectively. This effect results in less thrombin formation, the main clotting enzyme, and therefore a cooling down of the clot promoting system. Additionally, activated protein C inhibits the inhibitor to tissue plasminogen activator, thus increasing the fibrinolytic (clot lysis) potential of blood. Protein C is activated to activated protein C (APC) through the interaction of thrombin binding to the endothelial cell receptor, thrombomodulin.[8] Thrombomodulin brings protein C in close proximity to thrombin to be activated. The half-life of protein C and protein S is approximately 4 to 6 hours. Although the majority of cases of protein C or protein S deficiency involve venous thrombosis, cases of arterial thrombosis have been reported, especially in patients younger than 51 years of age.[18] Both protein C and S deficiencies exhibit congenital and acquired forms and when present are significant risk factors for thrombosis. When present as a homozygous state at birth, infants usually die from unrestricted clotting and secondary clot lysis, a condition of extreme DIC that is termed *purpura fulminans*. Patients heterozygous for protein C deficiency usually have antigenic protein C levels less than 60% of normal.[33] Acquired deficiency states for protein C occur with liver failure, DIC, and nephrotic syndrome.

Protein S is a cofactor to activated protein C. Its deficiency results in clinical states like protein C deficiency. Nephrotic syndrome can also lead to a reduction in free protein S (M_r = 42 kD) levels and, subsequently, a hypercoagulable state because of the loss of protein S in the urine.[72] Moreover, inflammatory states such as systemic lupus erythematosus can result in an elevation of C4b binding protein, which complexes with protein S and reduces free protein S. It is free protein S that serves as a cofactor to APC activity. The diagnosis of protein C or S deficiency is made by protein C and S level measurements. For protein C, both antigen and activity levels are measured, whereas for protein S, only antigen levels are measured, because its coagulant assay has a high coefficient of variation. The clinically important value of protein S is to measure its free protein S antigen. A condition also exists in which there is an abnormality in the function of the protein C molecule itself, resulting in a decrease in protein C activity without a decline in antigenic protein C. Thrombosis usually occurs in those between 15 and 30 years of age for deficiency of both of these proteins. When the diagnosis is made with episodes of thrombosis, treatment consists of anticoagulation, initially with heparin, followed by lifelong oral anticoagulation. However, not all patients with low levels of these factors thrombose, and there have been reports that in large populations of asymptomatic blood donors, low protein C levels may be found in asymptomatic patients. Many heterozygous family members of homozygous protein C–deficient infants also are unaffected.[19] Thus, institution of anticoagulation therapy in patients should occur only after they manifest the phenotype of thrombosis.

During the initiation of oral anticoagulation, blood may become transiently hypercoagulable as the vitamin K–dependent factors with short half-lives are inhibited (proteins C and S and factor VII) before the other vitamin K–dependent factors (factors II, IX, and X). In a patient already partially deficient in protein C or S, the levels of these anticoagulant factors will diminish even further with the initiation of warfarin, thus resulting in a temporary hypercoagulable state. This situation can result in thrombosis in the microcirculation and the syndrome of warfarin-induced skin necrosis.[9] The syndrome leads to full-thickness skin loss, especially over fatty areas where blood supply is poor to begin with, such as the breasts, buttocks, and abdomen. To prevent this devastating complication, warfarin therapy should be begun under the protection of systemic heparin anticoagulation (standard heparin or low-molecular-weight heparin) at lower loading doses, especially in patients initiating oral anticoagulation for thromboembolic disease.

DEFECTS WITH LOWER RISK FOR THROMBOSIS

Resistance to Activated Protein C (Factor V Leiden)

This relatively newly described syndrome, resistance to activated protein C, has been reported to be present in 20% to 60% of cases of idiopathic venous thrombosis.[77] It is the most common cause of thrombosis, although it alone is a relatively low risk factor for thrombosis. A common polymorphism of factor V causing activated protein C resistance is present in 1% to 2% of the general population. The syndrome is much more common in whites than in minority Americans.[67] The defect is due to a resistance to inactivation of factor Va by activated protein C as a result of the substitution of a single amino acid, glutamine for arginine, at position 506 in the gene for factor V[37] and is called factor V Leiden. This single amino acid substitution is due to a single base pair mutation in the gene for factor V. Thrombotic manifestations are noted in those individuals either homozygous or heterozygous for this mutation. As opposed to those with other hypercoagulable states, persons homozygous for this mutation usually do not die in infancy. Additionally, the incidence of thrombosis is correlated with the presence of additional risk factors for thrombosis, especially in women using oral contraceptives.[37]

Combined defects with other hypercoagulable states, such as protein C and S deficiency,[40, 41] result in a markedly increased thrombotic risk. The relative risk for thrombosis in patients heterozygous for factor V Leiden is sevenfold, whereas in those homozygous for factor V Leiden, the relative risk for thrombosis is 80-fold.[70] In addition to the large number of cases of venous thrombosis caused by this defect, recurrent venous thrombosis is also more common in patients with this entity, with an increase in recurrent venous thrombosis relative risk of 2.4-fold.[74] Although venous thrombosis predominates in patients with this syndrome, arterial thrombosis, especially involving lower extremity revascularizations, has also been reported.[61] The prevalence of this abnormality has been suggested to be increased in patients with peripheral vascular occlusive disease, measured both by the functional assay[16, 24] and by genetic analysis.[24]

The diagnosis of activated protein C resistance is made by a clot-based assay with the addition of activated protein C. More than 90% of individuals with activated protein C resistance have the factor V Leiden mutation (the arginine to glutamine substitution at position 506). Two patients with activated protein C resistance also were found to have a mutation of the arginine at position 306 of factor Va. Treatment options for activated protein C resistance include anticoagulation, initially heparin, followed by oral anticoagulation. The long-term use of warfarin is controversial. No data exist that suggest that long-term warfarin should be given after a first episode of venous thrombosis in a patient with this syndrome. The fact that activated protein C resistance is a relatively low risk for recurrent thrombosis (2.4-fold) suggests that not all patients after their first episode of thrombosis need long-term anticoagulant treatment and that patients must be evaluated in light of their overall risk factors for thrombosis.

Hyperhomocystinemia

Hyperhomocystinemia has been known to be a risk factor for atherosclerosis and vascular disease for more than 25 years.[65, 81] It also has been found to be a risk factor for venous thrombosis in people younger than 40 years of age[20] and for recurrent venous thrombosis in patients between 20 and 70 years of age.[13] Additionally, high plasma homocysteine levels have been found to be a risk factor for deep venous thrombosis in the general population, with an especially strong association in older women.[14] The combination of homocystinuria with factor V Leiden has been suggested to result in an increased risk of thrombosis, venous, arterial, or both.[54] The mechanism of this hypercoagulable state is multifactorial. Impaired endothelium-dependent vasodilation has been experimentally demonstrated, suggesting that the bioavailability of nitric oxide may be decreased in hyperhomocystinemic patients.[51, 78, 82] Additionally, homocysteine increases lipid peroxidation, which impairs nitric oxide synthetase and directly degrades nitric oxide.[4, 7, 47] Some have suggested that homocysteine has a toxic effect on vascular endothelium[76] and the clotting cascade and that abnormal methionine metabolism affects the methylation of deoxyribonucleic acid (DNA) and cell membranes.[65, 81] Elevated levels of homocysteine reduce protein C activation on thrombomodulin,[34, 69] increase thromboxane B_2 while decreasing prostacyclin levels, and result in reduced tissue plasminogen activation of plasminogen.[27, 38] Although the association between hyperhomocystinemia and venous thrombosis has been established, treatment to lower homocysteine levels using folic acid, vitamin B_6, or vitamin B_{12} and the long-term effects of such treatment on procoagulant activity have yet to be validated.

Prothrombin 20210 Polymorphism

A recently recognized genetic polymorphism in the distal 3′ untranslated region of the prothrombin gene has been described in patients with venous thrombosis. This base pair polymorphism, G20210A, has been found to increase the risk for venous thrombosis by 5.4-fold.[12] Of 219 patients with confirmed venous thrombosis, 12 (5.5%) were found to be heterozygous carriers of the 20210A allele, whereas the incidence in a corresponding group of healthy controls was 1.2%. Additionally, this genotype, although not increased in frequency in patients with arterial disease, has been found to be significantly associated with venous thrombosis in simple heterozygotes with a family history of venous thrombosis, and in double heterozygotes for other procoagulant conditions, and to have synergistic interaction with factor V Leiden.[21] Further, prothrombin 20210 has been shown to be associated with younger women with myocardial infarction.

Defective Fibrinolysis

Another cause of a hypercoagulable state is defective fibrinolytic activity. Abnormal plasminogens (dysplasminogenemias), although quite rare (<1%), have been described in cases of spontaneous arterial or venous thrombosis. Other defects in fibrinolysis that are not well defined may affect up to 10% of the normal population.[80] A report has suggested that the presence of an acquired abnormal fibrinogen capable of aggregating red blood cells with rouleaux formation led to digital ischemia of both hands and feet.[42] This patient was successfully treated by ancrod. Abnormal fibrinogens (dysfibrinogenemia) are other causes of venous thrombosis. Abnormal fibrinogens may account for 1% to 3% of patients with thrombosis.

Other pathways for fibrinolysis could contribute to thrombosis if defective. To date, however, no specific defects have been characterized. Tissue plasminogen activator (t-PA) is released from endothelium in response to thrombin, histamine, and bradykinin. The binding of thrombin to thrombomodulin activates protein C, which inactivates the t-PA inhibitor, thus enhancing fibrinolysis.[68] Although factors of the contact activation system are direct activators of plasminogen, recent evidence indicates that prekallikrein activation on endothelial cells results in kinetically favorable single-chain urokinase activation with subsequent plasmin formation.[57] Corresponding to these fibrinolytic activators, inhibitors include alpha $_2$-antiplasmin and plasminogen activator inhibitor (PAI). Elevated PAI-1 has been associated with deep venous thrombosis and myocardial infarction in epidemiologic studies. Defective fibrinolysis may also occur because of a decreased content or release of plasminogen activators or an increase in their inhibitors.[60] It has been observed that in the postoperative period, there is a fibrinolytic shutdown because of increased inhibitors to t-PA. Although the relationship between venous thrombosis and abnormal fibrinolysis is debated, it is clear that there is a relationship between impaired postoperative fibrinolysis and venous thrombosis.[63] Additionally, secretion of PAI-1 is upregulated by thrombin, endotoxin, and interleukin-1, explaining the elevated circulating levels of PAI-1 during certain infections. Alternatively, tumor necrosis factor (TNF) downregulates protein C and thus decreases the ability of activated protein C to inactivate PAI-1, which is also upregulated during sepsis.[62] Both of these mechanisms result in increased PAI-1 and decreased total fibrinolysis.

DEFECTS ASSOCIATED WITH VARIABLE RISK FOR THROMBOSIS

Heparin-Induced Thrombocytopenia (HIT) and Thrombosis Syndrome (HITTS)

Heparin-induced thrombocytopenia (HIT), also known as *heparin-associated thrombocytopenia* (HAT), occurs in 0.6% to 30% of patients in whom heparin is administered, although severe thrombocytopenia associated with thrombosis (heparin-induced thrombocytopenia and thrombosis syndrome [HITTS]) is seen much less frequently.[3] In an analysis of 11 prospective studies, the incidence was reported to be 3%, with thrombosis in 0.9%.[35] Morbidity and mortality rates as high as 61% and 23%, respectively, have been reported.[73] HIT is caused by a heparin-dependent antibody immunoglobulin G (IgG), which—when conjoined to platelet factor 4 (PF_4)—binds to platelets and induces them to aggregate when exposed to heparin.[38] It has been demonstrated that the antibody is directed against a heparin-PF_4 complex and it activates platelets by platelet Fc receptors. The antibody may not be heparin specific, as the degree of sulfonation of the heparin-like compound has been suggested to be critical for aggregation.[30] Activation of platelets in this setting presents as a spectrum of illness from mild thrombocytopenia to thrombosis, embolic episodes, and death.

A model for the pathophysiology of thrombosis has been summarized[5]:

1. Heparin combines with PF_4.
2. At the platelet and endothelial cell surface, IgG forms to the heparin-PF_4 complex.
3. The IgG then binds by its Fc moiety to a platelet receptor (FcγRIIA).
4. Platelet activation occurs probably through tyrosine phosphorylation.
5. Platelet release and platelet aggregation occur.
6. Platelet-derived microparticles are formed.
7. Mediators such as cytokines and catecholamines enhance platelet aggregation.
8. Immunoglobulins, including IgM, IgA, and complement, are deposited on the surface of endothelial cells, stimulating the production of tissue factor.

The combination of platelet aggregation, microparticle formation, and endothelial cell activation leads to a procoagulant microenvironment, which if extensive enough, results in clinical thrombocytopenia and thrombosis.

Both bovine and porcine standard unfractionated heparins as well as low-molecular-weight heparins have been found to cause the syndrome. HIT usually begins 3 to 14 days after heparin administration. Both arterial and venous thromboses have been reported, and even small exposures to heparin, as with the heparin coating on indwelling catheters or tubing, have been known to cause the syndrome.[26, 43] The diagnosis should be suspected in a patient who experiences a 50% drop in platelet count or when there is a fall in platelet count below 100,000/μl during heparin therapy or in any patient who experiences thrombosis during heparin administration.[25] This entity is a difficult diagnosis to make because many hospitalized patients have multiple reasons for declines in their platelet count, such as sepsis or DIC.

The laboratory diagnosis of HIT/HITTS is made by a number of assays. The serotonin release assay (SRA) is the "gold standard" assay. In this test, donor platelets are radiolabeled with ^{14}C-5-hydroxytryptamine. Patient plasma is mixed with variable concentrations of heparin (or low-molecular-weight heparin if it is the offending agent) and the degree of serotonin release is measured when the heparinized patient's plasma is mixed with donor platelets. A heparin-induced platelet aggregation (HIPA) assay is available to directly detect the ability of heparin to induce aggregation of the patient's platelet-rich plasma. This aggregation test is specific but not very sensitive,[29] whereas the serotonin assay using various doses of heparin has sensitivity and specificity up to 94% and 100%, respectively.[71] A new enzyme-linked immunosorbent assay (ELISA) test detecting the antiheparin antibody in the patient's plasma directed against the heparin-PF_4 complex has been described,[36] as has fluorescence-activated cell sorter (FACS) analysis for the platelet microparticles.[44] Because of its convenience, the ELISA assay may turn out to be the assay of choice.

Treatment consists of stopping heparin and allowing the heparin effect to wear off. Because these patients have circulating platelet microparticles, they have an ongoing prothrombotic state, which when treated with warfarin, potentiates the seriousness of the conduction. Warfarin is contraindicated in this condition until adequate anticoagulation has been established with an alternative anticoagulant. Its presence in the face of circulating platelet microparticles creates a prothrombotic state similar to that seen when warfarin is given in patients with protein C or S deficiency and may lead to venous limb gangrene if an alternate anticoagulant is not given.[86] Aspirin has been used with only limited success. Iloprost, a prostacyclin analogue, has been found useful for this syndrome,[32] but because of its strong vasodilatory and hypotensive effects, it is no longer recommended for use. Low-molecular-weight heparins (enoxaparin and dalteparin) have 92% cross-reactivity with standard heparin antibodies on the serotonin release assay and, therefore, should not be substituted for standard heparin in patients with HIT, although some have suggested that if a low-molecular-weight heparin tests negative in vitro, it may be used clinically.[75]

A number of new anticoagulants are now available. These include danaparoid sodium (Orgaran), a heparinoid prepared from porcine intestinal mucosa with a low number of sulfonations (combination of heparin sulfate, dermatan sulfate, and chondroitin sulfate). This drug has a low level (approximately 24%) of cross-reactivity with heparin in this syndrome.[53] The glycoprotein platelet IIb/IIIa receptor antagonist C7E3 has been used to prevent platelet activation. However, it is not recommended for general use because of potential bleeding risks.[48] The defibrinating agent ancrod has been used, but 12 hours of defibrination is necessary before adequate anticoagulation is achieved.[10]

Last, the direct thrombin inhibitors hirudin[31] and argatroban are the likely treatment of choice.[46] These agents show no cross-reactivity to heparin antibodies. Orgaran can be used for vascular surgery and cardiopulmonary bypass surgery when needed.[26] Lepirudin (Refludan) has recently been approved by the Food and Drug Administration (FDA) for this condition. With early diagnosis and appropriate treatment, morbidity and mortality rates have declined to 6% and 0%, respectively.[2]

Lupus Anticoagulant/Antiphospholipid Syndrome

It is unfortunate that this syndrome is called "anticoagulant" because it is associated with or results in a hypercoagulable state. This syndrome is associated with antiphospholipid antibodies, usually IgG, which through a number of etiologic factors result in thrombosis.[28] The antiphospholipid antibody syndrome consists of the presence of an antiphospholipid antibody in association with episodes of thrombosis, recurrent fetal loss, thrombocytopenia, and livedo reticularis. Strokes, myocardial and visceral infarctions, and extremity gangrene may occur.

The diagnosis is suspected in a patient with a prolonged activated partial thromboplastin time (aPTT) with other standard coagulation tests within normal limits and the presence of a measured antiphospholipid or anticardiolipin antibody. The prolongation in the aPTT is strictly a laboratory artifact. The antiphospholipid antibody interacts with the anionic phospholipids in the aPTT assay, prolonging the assay. The diagnosis may be made on clinical grounds with either an abnormal clot-based functional assay off anticoagulants or by direct ELISA antibody measurement.

There is imperfect agreement between diagnostic tests for this abnormality. Approximately 80% of patients with a positive aPTT test (lupus anticoagulant) have a positive ELISA antiphospholipid antibody, but only 10% to 50% of patients with a positive ELISA antiphospholipid antibody have a positive aPTT test. Patients with both tests positive are reported to have the same thrombotic risk as those with either test alone.[49] The prolonged aPTT appears to be a better predictor for thrombotic events, whereas a high-titer antiphospholipid antibody (especially an IgG anticardiolipin antibody) is more predictive of recurrent fetal loss.[52] In fact, 10% of women with two or more unexplained abortions are found to have a positive antiphospholipid antibody. Although low-titer antibody occurs in 2% of healthy young women (0.2% high-titer antibody), apparent healthy women with high-titer antibody have approximately a 28% chance of fetal loss.[50] The mechanisms responsible for fetal loss are unknown, although new data suggest that levels of annexin V in trophoblasts and endothelial cells are reduced in the presence of antiphospholipid antibodies.[64] Annexin V is a phospholipid-binding protein with potent anticoagulant activity.

Although the lupus anticoagulant has been reported in 5% to 40% of patients with systemic lupus erythematosus (SLE), it can exist in patients without SLE and can be induced in patients by medications, cancer, and certain infectious diseases. A number of possible thrombotic mechanisms have been suggested, including (1) inhibition of prostacyclin synthesis or its release from endothelial cells,[6] (2) inhibition of protein C activation by thrombin/thrombomodulin,[11] (3) raised plasminogen activator inhibitor levels,[85] (4) direct platelet activation,[84] and (5) the coexistence of endothelial cell activation with antiphospholipid antibodies.[22] Increased tissue factor expression on monocytes and low free protein S plasma levels also have been noted in patients with the antiphospholipid syndrome and a history of thrombosis.[66] Although each of these mechanisms has been supported in the literature, no one dominant theme has emerged suggesting that the cause of thrombosis in these patients is multifactorial, characteristic of a syndrome.

Thrombosis can involve both the arterial and venous circulations, especially peripheral vessels of the extremities.[87] At least one third of patients with lupus anticoagulants have a history of one or more thrombotic events, with more than 70% in the venous circulation.[28] One half of a series of 18 arterial vascular bypass grafts thrombosed in patients positive for antiphospholipid antibody.[1] In a second series, the incidence of graft thrombosis was 27% in the presence of either a lupus anticoagulant or heparin-induced thrombocytopenia compared with 1.6% when no hypercoagulable state was identified.[15] In a third series, antibodies to cardiolipin were associated with an increased risk of vein graft failure over a 6-month follow-up.[59]

The incidence of antiphospholipid antibodies was also found to be elevated (26%) in a group of young white men (≤45 years of age) with chronic lower leg ischemia compared with control patients (13%).[83] However, a recent prospective comparison of elective infrainguinal bypass grafting revealed that even though one third of patients were positive for antiphospholipid antibodies, there was minimal difference in primary or assisted patency rates, limb salvage, or survival rates between positive and negative patients.[45]

Treatment of the antiphospholipid antibody syndrome involves anticoagulation in the face of thrombotic events.[50] Higher levels of warfarin (International Normalized Ratio > 3.0) have been recommended for the treatment of the antiphospholipid syndrome.[39] For recurrent fetal loss, heparin or low-molecular-weight heparin use through the pregnancy is recommended. In patients with lupus anticoagulants, heparin therapy can be monitored successfully with a thrombin time or anti–factor Xa level. Warfarin therapy can be monitored by factor X levels.

Abnormal Platelet Aggregation

There are two clinical settings in which abnormal platelet aggregation has been associated with thrombosis, although platelet aggregation testing is not routinely available in most hospital laboratories. These clinical settings are advanced malignancy of the lung and uterus and after carotid endarterectomy. Hyperactive platelets have also been seen during graft thrombosis in peripheral vascular reconstructions.[18] Diabetes mellitus, which is known to be associated with hyperactive platelets, may be a contributor to these conditions. Because of the limited ability to determine quantitative platelet aggregation and because platelet function testing is not a highly developed quantitative assay, the importance of abnormal platelet aggregation to the hypercoagulable condition is really unknown. Antiplatelet agents alone are thus not very likely to eliminate a thrombogenic hypercoagulable potential.[55]

REFERENCES

1. Ahn SS, Kalunian K, Rosove M, et al: Postoperative thrombotic complications in patients with the lupus anticoagulant: Increased risk after vascular procedures. J Vasc Surg 7:749, 1988.
2. Almeida J, Coats R, Liem TK, Silver D: Reduced morbidity and mortality rates of the heparin-induced thrombocytopenia syndrome. J Vasc Surg 27:309, 1998.
3. Ansell JE, Price JM, Shah S, et al: Heparin-induced thrombocytopenia: What is its real frequency? Chest 88:878, 1985.
4. Blom HJ, Kleinveld HA, Boers GH, et al: Lipid peroxidation and susceptibility of low-density lipoprotein to in vitro oxidation in hyperhomocysteinemia. Eur J Clin Invest 25:149, 1995.
5. Cancio LC, Cohen DJ: Heparin-induced thrombocytopenia and thrombosis. J Am Coll Surg 186:76, 1998.
6. Carreras LO, Defreyn G, Machin SJ, et al: Arterial thrombosis, intrauterine death, and "lupus" anticoagulant: Detection of immunoglobulin interfering with prostacyclin formation. Lancet 1:244, 1981.
7. Chin JH, Azhar S, Hoffman BB: Inactivation of endothelium derived relaxing factor by oxidized lipoproteins. J Clin Invest 89:10, 1992.
8. Clouse LH, Comp PC: The regulation of hemostasis: The protein C system. N Engl J Med 314:1298, 1986.
9. Cole MS, Minifee PK, Wolma FJ: Coumadin necrosis: A review of the literature. Surgery 103:271, 1988.
10. Cole CW, Fournier LM, Bormanis J: Heparin-associated thrombocytopenia and thrombosis: Optimal therapy with ancrod. Can J Surg 22:207, 1990.
11. Comp PC, DeBault LE, Esmon NL, Esmon CT: Human thrombomodulin is inhibited by IgG from two patients with non-specific anticoagulants (Abstract). Blood 62(Suppl 1):299a, 1983.
12. Cumming AM, Keeney S, Salden A, et al: The prothrombin gene G20210A variant: Prevalence in a U.K. anticoagulant clinic population. Br J Haematol 98:353, 1997.
13. den Heijer M, Blom HJ, Gerrits WB, et al: Is hyperhomocysteinaemia a risk factor for recurrent venous thrombosis? Lancet 345:882, 1995.
14. den Heijer M, Koster T, Blom HJ, et al: Hyperhomocysteinemia as a risk factor for deep-vein thrombosis. N Engl J Med 334:759, 1996.
15. Donaldson MC, Weinberg DS, Belkin M, et al: Screening for hypercoagulable states in vascular surgical practice: A preliminary study. J Vasc Surg 11:825, 1990.
16. Donaldson MC, Belkin M, Whittemore AD, et al: Impact of activated protein C resistance on general vascular surgical patients. J Vasc Surg 25:1054, 1997.
17. Eby CS: A review of the hypercoagulable state. *In* Penner JA, Hassouna HI (eds): Coagulation disorders: Part II. Hematol Oncol Clin North Am 7:1, 1993.
18. Eldrup-Jorgensen J, Flanigan DP, Brace L, et al: Hypercoagulable states and lower limb ischemia in young adults. J Vasc Surg 9:334, 1989.
19. Esmon CT: The regulation of natural anticoagulant pathways. Science 235:1348, 1987.
20. Falcon CR, Cattaneo M, Panzeri D, et al: High prevalence of hyperhomocyst(e)inemia in patients with juvenile venous thrombosis. Arterioscler Thromb 14:1080, 1994.
21. Ferraresi P, Marchetti G, Legnani C, et al: The heterozygous 20210 G/A prothrombin genotype is associated with early venous thrombosis in inherited thrombophilias and is not increased in frequency in artery disease. Arterioscler Thromb Vasc Biol 17:2418, 1997.
22. Ferro D, Pittoni V, Quintarelli C, et al: Coexistence of anti-phospholipid antibodies and endothelial perturbation in systemic lupus erythematosus patients with ongoing prothrombotic state. Circulation 95:1425, 1997.
23. Flinn WR, McDaniel MD, Yao JS, et al: Antithrombin III deficiency as a reflection of dynamic protein metabolism in patients undergoing vascular reconstruction. J Vasc Surg 1:888, 1984.
24. Foley PW, Irvine CD, Standen GR, et al: Activated protein C resistance, factor V Leiden and peripheral vascular disease. Cardiovasc Surg 5:157, 1997.
25. George JN, Alving B, Ballem P: Platelets. *In* McArthur JR, Benz EJ (eds): Hematology—1994: The Educational Program of the American Society of Hematology. Washington, DC, American Society of Hematology, 1994, p 66.
26. Gitlin SD, Deeb GM, Yann C, Schmaier AH: Intraoperative monitoring of danaparoid sodium anticoagulation during cardiovascular operations. J Vasc Surg 27:568, 1998.
27. Graeber JE, Slott JH, Ulane RE, et al: Effect of homocysteine and homocystine on platelet and vascular arachidonic acid metabolism. Pediatr Res 16:490, 1982.
28. Greenfield LJ: Lupus-like anticoagulants and thrombosis. J Vasc Surg 7:818, 1988.
29. Greinacher A, Michels I, Kiefel V, et al: A rapid and sensitive test for diagnosing heparin-associated thrombocytopenia. Thromb Haemost 66:734, 1991.
30. Greinacher A, Michels I, Mueller-Eckhardt C: Heparin-associated thrombocytopenia: The antibody is not heparin specific. Thromb Haemost 67:545, 1992.
31. Greinacher A, Vopel H, Potzsch B: Recombinant hirudin in the treatment of patients with heparin-induced thrombocytopenia (HIT) (Abstract). Blood 88:281a, 1996.
32. Gruel Y, Lermusiaux P, Lang M, et al: Usefulness of antiplatelet drugs in the management of heparin-associated thrombocytopenia and thrombosis. Ann Vasc Surg 5:552, 1991.
33. Hassouna HI: Laboratory evaluation of hemostatic disorders. *In* Penner JA, Hassouna HI (eds): Coagulation disorders: Part II. Hematol Oncol Clin North Am 7:1161, 1993.
34. Hayashi T, Honda G, Suzucki K: An atherogenic stimulus homocysteine inhibits cofactor activity of thrombomodulin and enhances thrombomodulin expression in human umbilical vein endothelial cells. Blood 79:2930, 1992.
35. Hirsh J, Raschke R, Warkentin TE, et al: Heparin: Mechanism of action, pharmacokinetics, dosing considerations, monitoring, efficacy, and safety. Chest 108:258S, 1995.
36. Jackson MR, Krishnamurti C, Aylesworth CA, et al: Diagnosis of heparin-induced thrombocytopenia in the vascular surgery patient. Surgery 121:419, 1997.
37. Kalafatis M, Mann KG. Factor V Leiden and thrombophilia. Arterioscler Thromb Vasc Biol 17:620, 1997.
38. Kelton JG, Smith JW, Warkentin TE, et al: Immunoglobulin G from patients with heparin-induced thrombocytopenia binds to a complex of heparin and platelet factor 4. Blood 83:3232, 1994.
39. Khamashta MA, Cuadrado MJ, Mujic F, et al: The management of thrombosis in the antiphospholipid-antibody syndrome. N Engl J Med 332:993, 1995.
40. Koeleman BP, Reitsma PH, Allaart CF, et al: Activated protein C resistance as an additional risk factor for thrombosis in protein C-deficient families. Blood 84:1031, 1994.
41. Koeleman BP, van Rumpt D, Hamulyak K, et al: Factor V Leiden: An additional risk factor for thrombosis in protein S deficient families? Thromb Haemost 74:580, 1995.
42. Kwaan HC, Levin M, Sakurai S, et al: Digital ischemia and gangrene due to red blood cell aggregation induced by acquired dysfibrinogenemia. J Vasc Surg 26:1061, 1997.
43. Laster J, Silver D: Heparin-coated catheters and heparin-induced thrombocytopenia. J Vasc Surg 7:667, 1988.
44. Lee DH, Warkentin TE, Hayward CP, et al: The development and evaluation of a novel test for heparin induced thrombocytopenia (Abstract). Blood 84:188a, 1994.
45. Lee RW, Taylor LM Jr, Landry GJ, et al: Prospective comparison of infrainguinal bypass grafting in patients with and without antiphospholipid antibodies. J Vasc Surg 24:524, 1996.
46. Lewis BE, Iaffaldano R, McKiernan TL, et al: Report of successful use of argatroban as an alternative anticoagulant during coronary stent implantation in a patient with heparin-induced thrombocytopenia and thrombosis syndrome. Cathet Cardiovasc Diagn 38:206, 1996.
47. Liao JK, Shin WS, Lee WY, et al: Oxidized low-density lipoprotein decreases the expression of endothelial nitric oxide synthase. J Biol Chem 270:319, 1995.
48. Liem TK, Teel R, Shukla S, et al: The glycoprotein IIb/IIIa antagonist c7E3 inhibits platelet aggregation in the presence of heparin-associated antibodies. J Vasc Surg 25:124, 1997.
49. Lockshin MD: Antiphospholipid antibody syndrome. JAMA 268:1451, 1992.

50. Lockshin MD. Antiphospholipid antibody: Babies, blood clots, biology. JAMA 277:1549, 1997.
51. Loscalzo J: The oxidant stress of hyperhomocyst(e)inemia. J Clin Invest 98:5, 1996.
52. Lynch A, Marlar R, Murphy J, et al: Antiphospholipid antibodies in predicting adverse pregnancy outcome: A prospective study. Ann Intern Med 120:470, 1994.
53. Magnani HN. Heparin-induced thrombocytopenia (HIT): An overview of 230 patients treated with Orgaran (Org 10172). Thromb Haemost 70:554, 1993.
54. Mandel H, Brenner B, Berant M, et al: Coexistence of hereditary homocystinuria and factor V Leiden—effect on thrombosis. N Engl J Med 334:763, 1996.
55. Meade TW, Vickers MV, Thompson SG, et al: Epidemiological characteristics of platelet aggregability. Br Med J 290:428, 1985.
56. Menache D: Antithrombin III concentrates. *In* Penner JA, Hassouna HI (eds): Coagulation disorders: Part I. Hematol Oncol Clin North Am 6:1115, 1992.
57. Motta G, Rojkjaer R, Hasan AA, et al: High molecular weight kininogen regulates prekallikrein assembly and activation on endothelial cells: A novel mechanism for contact activation. Blood 91:516, 1998.
58. Nehler MR, Taylor LM Jr, Porter JM: Homocysteinemia as a risk factor for atherosclerosis: A review. Cardiovasc Surg 5:559, 1997.
59. Nielsen TG, Nordestgaard BG, von Jessen F, et al: Antibodies to cardiolipin may increase the risk of failure of peripheral vein bypasses. Eur J Vasc Endovasc Surg 14:177, 1997.
60. Nilsson IM, Ljungner H, Tengborn L: Two different mechanisms in patients with venous thrombosis and defective fibrinolysis: Low concentrations of plasminogen activator or increased concentration of plasminogen activator inhibitor. Br Med J Clin Res Ed 290:1453, 1985.
61. Ouriel K, Green RM, DeWeese JA, et al: Activated protein C resistance: Prevalence and implications in peripheral vascular disease. J Vasc Surg 23:46, 1996.
62. Paramo JA, Perez JL, Serrano M, et al: Types 1 and 2 plasminogen activator inhibitor and tumor necrosis factor alpha in patients with sepsis. Thromb Haemost 64:3, 1990.
63. Prins MH, Hirsh J: A clinical review of the evidence supporting a relationship between impaired fibrinolytic activity and venous thromboembolism. Arch Intern Med 151:1721, 1991.
64. Rand JH, Wu XX, Andree HA, et al: Pregnancy loss in the antiphospholipid-antibody syndrome—a possible thrombogenic mechanism. N Engl J Med 337:154, 1997.
65. Rees MM, Rodgers GM: Homocysteinemia: Association of a metabolic disorder with vascular disease and thrombosis. Thromb Res 71:337, 1993.
66. Reverter JC, Tassies D, Font J, et al: Hypercoagulable state in patients with antiphospholipid syndrome is related to high induced tissue factor expression on monocytes and to low free protein S. Arterioscler Thromb Vasc Biol 16:1319, 1996.
67. Ridker PM, Miletich JP, Hennekens CH, et al: Ethnic distribution of factor V Leiden in 4047 men and women: Implications for venous thromboembolism screening. JAMA 277:1305, 1997.
68. Rodgers GM: Hemostatic properties of normal and perturbed vascular cells. FASEB J 2:116, 1988.
69. Rodgers GM, Conn MT: Homocysteine, an atherogenic stimulus, reduces protein C activation by arterial and venous endothelial cells. Blood 75:895, 1990.
70. Rosendaal FR, Koster T, Vandenbroucke JP, et al: High risk of thrombosis in patients homozygous for factor V Leiden (activated protein C resistance). Blood 85:1504, 1995.
71. Sheridan D, Carter C, Kelton JG: A diagnostic test for heparin-induced thrombocytopenia. Blood 67:27, 1986.
72. Siddiqi FA, Tepler J, Fantini GA: Acquired protein S and antithrombin III deficiency caused by nephrotic syndrome: An unusual cause of graft thrombosis. J Vasc Surg 25:576, 1997.
73. Silver D, Kapsch DN, Tsoi EK: Heparin-induced thrombocytopenia, thrombosis and hemorrhage. Ann Surg 198:301, 1983.
74. Simioni P, Prandoni P, Lensing AW, et al: The risk of recurrent venous thromboembolism in patients with an $Arg^{506}\rightarrow$Gln mutation in the gene for factor V (factor V Leiden). N Engl J Med 336:399, 1997.
75. Slocum MM, Adams JG Jr, Teel R, et al: Use of enoxaparin in patients with heparin-induced thrombocytopenia syndrome. J Vasc Surg 23:839, 1996.
76. Starkebaum G, Harlan JM: Endothelial cell injury due to copper-catalyzed hydrogen peroxide generation from homocysteine. J Clin Invest 77:1370, 1986.
77. Svensson PJ, Dahlback B: Resistance to activated protein C as a basis for venous thrombosis. N Engl J Med 330:517, 1994.
78. Tawakol A, Omland T, Gerhard M, et al: Hyperhomocyst(e)inemia is associated with impaired endothelium-dependent vasodilation in humans. Circulation 95:1119, 1997.
79. Towne JB, Bernhard VM, Hussey C, et al: Antithrombin deficiency—a cause of unexplained thrombosis in vascular surgery. Surgery 89:735, 1981.
80. Towne JB, Bandyk DF, Hussey CV, et al: Abnormal plasminogen: A genetically determined cause of hypercoagulability. J Vasc Surg 1:896, 1984.
81. Ueland PM, Refsum H, Brattstrom L: Plasma homocysteine and cardiovascular disease. *In* Francis RB Jr (ed): Atherosclerotic Cardiovascular Disease, Hemostasis, and Endothelial Function. New York, Marcel Dekker, 1993, p 183.
82. Upchurch GR, Welch GN, Randev N, et al: The effect of homocysteine on endothelial nitric oxide production (Abstract). FASEB J 9:A876, 1995.
83. Valentine RJ, Kaplan HS, Green R, et al: Lipoprotein (a), homocysteine, and hypercoagulable states in young men with premature peripheral atherosclerosis: A prospective, controlled analysis. J Vasc Surg 23:53, 1996.
84. Vermylen J, Blockmans D, Spitz B, et al: Thrombosis and immune disorders. Clin Haematol 15:393, 1986.
85. Violi F, Ferro D, Valesini G, et al: Tissue plasminogen activator inhibitor in patients with systemic lupus erythematosus and thrombosis. BMJ 300:1099, 1990.
86. Warkentin TE, Elavathil LJ, Hayward CP, et al: The pathogenesis of venous limb gangrene associated with heparin-induced thrombocytopenia. Ann Intern Med 127:804, 1997.
87. Williams FM, Hunt BJ: The antiphospholipid syndrome and vascular surgery. Cardiovasc Surg 6:10, 1998.

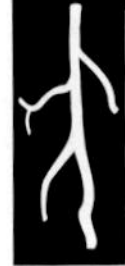

CHAPTER 47

Infection in Prosthetic Vascular Grafts

Dennis F. Bandyk, M.D.

The use of vascular prosthetic devices (grafts, stents, and endovascular stent-grafts) has permitted palliation of vascular conditions that otherwise would have been fatal or disabling. Morbidity rates attributable to fabrication or biomaterial failure (dilatation, rupture, fatigue) or allergic foreign body reaction is low (<5%). Although thrombosis is the most common mode of prosthetic implant failure, infection is the most serious sequela of implantation. Infection dramatically alters patient outcomes and can result in limb loss, organ dysfunction, or death. Surgical therapy is always required, often coupled with prosthesis excision, as antibiotics alone are insufficient to eradicate an established infectious process. Even when treatment is successful, morbidity can be significant, with outcomes often worse than those of the natural history of the vascular disease that led to implantation.

Prosthetic graft infection presents as a *spectrum* of clinical manifestations dependent on anatomic location and virulence of the pathogen. This feature permits surgeons to individualize treatment. The reported incidence of infections involving vascular prostheses varies (from 0.5% to 5% of operations) and is influenced by implant site, indication for intervention, underlying disease, and host defense mechanisms (Table 47–1). The incidence of graft infection after repair of a nonruptured aortic aneurysm in a prospective, multicenter Canadian trial was 0.2%.[50a] The long-term incidence may be higher because many graft infections do not present until years after implantation. Prosthetic graft infection is more common after emergency procedures (e.g., for ruptured abdominal aortic aneurysm, acute arterial ischemia) or when the prosthesis is anastomosed to the femoral artery or placed in a subcutaneous tunnel (e.g., with axillofemoral or femorofemoral bypass). The incidence of infection following percutaneous placement of endovascular grafts or stents is low (<1%), but case reports indicate that endoluminal grafts are susceptible to bacterial colonization.

Multiple surgical options are available. Surgical intervention should be individualized and undertaken after consideration of several important factors, including clinical presentation, anatomic location, extent of infection, type of graft material, virulence of infecting organism, signs of invasive infection, and overall status of the affected individual. Mortality is higher with aortic graft infections, whereas limb loss is highest with lower-limb graft infections. Sepsis and rupture of a mycotic aneurysm associated with graft infection are grave clinical signs, requiring emergent intervention and total graft excision. For less virulent infections, in situ replacement with autologous conduits, allografts, or antibiotic-impregnated grafts can be considered if certain principles are followed. Appropriate patient selection and successful outcomes require accurate diagnostics, administration of culture-specific antibiotics, and sugical intervention to excise or replace the infected biomaterial. For some patients, graft retention combined with biologic or muscle flap coverage of exposed prosthetic graft is appropriate. This chapter reviews the scientific basis and surgical principles in the management of prosthesis-associated vascular infections as well as patient risk factors and techniques for preventing complications.

TABLE 47–1. INCIDENCE OF PROSTHETIC VASCULAR GRAFT INFECTIONS RELATIVE TO IMPLANT SITE

GRAFT IMPLANT SITE	INCIDENCE (%)
Descending thoracic aorta	0.7–3
Aortoiliac	0.4–1.3
Aortofemoral	0.5–3
Femorofemoral	1.3–3.6
Axillofemoral	5–8
Femoropopliteal	0.9–4.6
Femorotibial	2–3.4
Carotid patch	0–0.2
Carotid-subclavian	0.5–1.2
Axillary-axillary	1–4.1
Iliac stent	<1
Aortic stent-graft	<1

PATHOGENESIS

Etiologic Factors

A vascular prosthesis exposed to microorganisms (bacteria or fungi) can result in clinical infection by three major mechanisms:

1. Perioperative contamination.
2. Bacteremia seeding of the biomaterial.
3. Mechanical erosion to skin, bowel, or genitourinary tract tissue.

Perioperative Contamination

Skin is a major reservoir of bacteria. Biomaterial surfaces can contact microorganisms (1) by a *direct route* during implantation, (2) through the surgical wound (in the event of a healing complication), or (3) by *hematogenous* or *lymphatic* spread from remote sites of infection or colonization (e.g., urinary tract infection, tinea pedis, pneumonia, venous or arterial catheter sepsis, endocarditis, ischemic foot ulcers). Important potential sources of direct graft contamination include breaks in aseptic operative technique; contact with the patient's endogenous flora harbored in sweat glands, lymph nodes, diseased artery walls (e.g., atherosclerotic plaque or aneurysm thrombus), disrupted lymphatics, or intestinal bag effluents; and injury to or opening of the gastrointestinal or genitourinary tract. If the surgical wound does not develop a fibrin seal or heal promptly after operation, the underlying vascular prosthesis is susceptible to colonization via initially trivial superficial wound problems (e.g., erythema, dermal necrosis, lymphocele). With persistent wound drainage, a septic focus can develop in ischemic or injured tissue and progress by deep extension to involve the prosthesis.[10]

Diseased artery walls are frequently an unrecognized source of bacteria, especially of coagulase-negative staphylococci, as are "reoperation" wounds. Candidates for graft revision for failed vascular reconstructions commonly harbor bacteria in scar tissue and lymphoceles and on the surfaces of previously implanted prosthetic vascular grafts and suture material. In explanted graft material, microorganisms were cultured from 90% of grafts associated with anastomotic aneurysms and from 69% of thrombosed grafts.[4]

Bacteremia

Bacterial seeding of the prosthesis via a hematogenous route is an uncommon but potentially important mechanism of graft and stent infection. Experimentally, intravenous infusion of 10^7 colony-forming units (CFUs) of *Staphylococcus aureus* produces a clinical graft infection in nearly 100% of animals during the immediate post-implantation period. Bacteremia from sources such as intravascular catheters, an infected urinary tract, or remote tissue infection (e.g., pneumonia or an infected foot ulcer) is common in elderly persons who have vascular disease, particularly during the postoperative period. It is best that such patients at high risk or who are leukopenic or septic do not receive a prosthetic graft when possible. Experimentally, parenteral antibiotic therapy significantly decreased the risk of graft colonization from bacteremia and is the basis for culture-specific antibiotic therapy in patients with known infection at remote sites. The prosthesis becomes less susceptible to colonization as the luminal pseudointimal lining develops and matures over time, but vulnerability to infection from bacteremia has been documented beyond 1 year after implantation.

Transient bacteremia, in combination with altered immune status, may account for graft infections occurring years after the original operation. It is also possible for a low-grade graft infection manifested only as an absence of graft incorporation to become secondarily infected by a remote bacterial challenge. For example, *Escherichia coli* bacteremia from a urinary tract infection might inoculate a susceptible perigraft space formed as a result of central nervous system biofilm infection. Clinicians should consider these mechanisms before they assume that virulent bacteria have remained dormant on graft surfaces since implantation.

Mechanical Erosion

Erosion of a vascular prosthesis through the skin or into the gastrointestinal or genitourinary tract results in perigraft infection. *Graft-enteric erosion* (GEE) can develop as a result of pulsatile pressure transmitted via the graft to the overlying adherent bowel. In a series of 3652 aortic graft implants performed at the Cleveland Clinic, the incidence of aortoenteric fistula or erosion was 0.36%. Theoretically, this complication can be avoided by adequate coverage of the graft with retroperitoneal tissue or omentum at the time of implantation. The pathogenesis of *graft-enteric fistula* (GEF) is more complex, since communication with the suture line is often present and pseudoaneurysm of the aortic anastomosis is present in half of cases. In most patients, the clinical history suggests that infection of the aortic prosthesis occurs first, followed by extension to involve the suture line and subsequent pseudoaneurysm formation. The microflora recovered from an aortic graft with secondary aortoenteric fistula are commonly gram-positive organisms except when bile staining of graft surfaces occurred. From such sites duodenal or intestinal flora are recovered, typically *E. coli*.

Classification and Time of Appearance

Prosthetic graft infections (Table 47–2) can be classified by:

- Appearance time
- Relationship to postoperative wound infections (Szilagyi's classification)
- Extent of graft involvement (Bunt's classification)

The development of early (<4 months after implantation) infection correlates with clinical manifestations, the type of pathogen, and the various surgical options appropriate for treatment. There is evidence that even Szilagyi type I and II wound infections increase the likelihood of a late-appearing graft infection. Bunt proposed using standardized terminology to reflect the spectrum of infections and permit

TABLE 47–2. CLASSIFICATION OF PROSTHETIC GRAFT INFECTIONS

Appearance Time After Implantation or Revision

Early: <4 mo
Late: >4 mo

Szilagyi's Classification (Applicable to Immediate Postoperative Infections)

Grade I: cellulitis involving wound
Grade II: infection involving subcutaneous tissue
Grade III: infection involving the vascular prosthesis

Bunt's Classification (Modified)

Peripheral Graft Infection

P0 graft infection: Infection of cavitary graft. Examples: aortic (abdominal, thoracic) interposition, aortoiliac, aortofemoral.

P1 graft infection: Infection of a graft whose entire anatomic course is noncavitary—not anastomosed to the aorta or its proximal branches within the pleural or peritoneal cavity. Examples include axillofemoral, femorofemoral, femorodistal, carotid-subclavian graft infections.

P2 graft infection: Infection of the extracavitary portion of a graft whose origin is cavitary. Examples include aortofemoral, aortocarotid, and thoracofemoral graft infections.

P3 graft infection: Infection involving a prosthetic patch angioplasty. Examples include carotid and femoral endarterectomies with patch closure.

Graft-Enteric Erosion or Fistula
Aortic Stump Sepsis

comparison of treatment outcomes. Categories include perigraft graft infection, GEE, GEF, and aortic stump sepsis. The majority of early graft infections are apparent within 3 to 4 months after implantation. From extended patient follow-ups, it is evident that more than half of all graft infections present beyond the "perioperative period." Reports of aortic graft infection documented mean appearance times of 25 to 70 months. Extracavitary graft infections appear sooner (within 7 months) than aortic graft infections (40 months) and typically are sequelae of postoperative wound infection.

The most common cause of graft infection is *microorganism contamination* of the graft during implantation or in the perioperative period. The pathogenesis of a vascular device infection involves several fundamental steps:

1. Bacterial adhesion to graft or stent surfaces.
2. Microcolony formation within a bacterial biofilm.
3. Activation of host defenses.
4. An inflammatory response involving perigraft tissues and the graft-artery anastomosis.

Bacterial adherence to the prosthesis depends on cell wall and growth characteristics of the bacterial species and on physical and chemical properties of the biomaterial. Early postoperative infections are most commonly caused by *S. aureus*. The prevalence of staphylococcal biomaterial infections can be explained in part by the relative increased adherence of gram-positive bacteria to biomaterials. Under experimental conditions, *Staphylococcus* species adhere in greater numbers (10 to 1000 times more) to vascular graft materials (e.g., polyester [Dacron], polytetrafluoroethylene [PTFE]) than do gram-negative bacteria.[11] The increased adherence of staphylococci is due to specific capsular adhesins that mediate microorganism attachment and colonization. Antibodies to these specific cell-surface glycoproteins have been developed, and their application to graft surfaces can inhibit adherence of adhesin-producing strains to prosthetic graft surfaces.

The vascular prosthesis and the adherent bacteria act together as a co-inflammatory stimulus to activate the immune system, in particular the inflammatory cytokines. The result is an inflammatory process that attempts to localize the infection but is accompanied by tissue-damaging effects, including the recruitment of polymorphonuclear granulocytes, production of tumor necrosis factor-alpha (TNF-α), and activation of other humoral and cellular defenses (Fig. 47–1). The prosthesis is not an "innocent bystander"; by eliciting an immune foreign body reaction, it produces an acidic ischemic microenvironment conducive to bacterial biofilm formation and proliferation. Unlike autogenous grafts, implanted prosthetic grafts do not develop rich vascular connections with surrounding tissue, and this prevents immune defenses and antibiotics from exerting maximal effects on infecting organisms. The extent of perigraft inflammation and tissue injury depends on the virulence of the infecting organism, but even with indolent infections, tissue autolysis can occur that leads to vessel wall or anastomotic disruption and hemorrhage. Initially, the perigraft infection produces a failure of graft incorporation (healing) and formation of a perigraft cavity or abscess. As the infectious process spreads along the length of the graft, adjacent structures (e.g., adjacent artery, skin, bowel) can be involved. The pathobiology can be manifested clinically as a spectrum of signs, including graft sepsis, localized perigraft abscess, anastomotic pseudoaneurysm, graft cutaneous sinus tract, or GEE or GEF (aortoduodenal fistula).

Early postoperative infections, typically caused by virulent hospital-acquired bacteria, present with sepsis evidenced by fever, leukocytosis, and bacteremia and other signs of wound infection. If the infection is not recognized and treated promptly, anastomotic bleeding can occur. Late infections result from colonization of biomaterials by "low-virulence organisms" such as *Staphylococcus epidermidis* or *Candida* species. The nature of infection is more indolent without signs of sepsis, and because of the low titer of microorganisms, cultures of perigraft fluid or tissue often

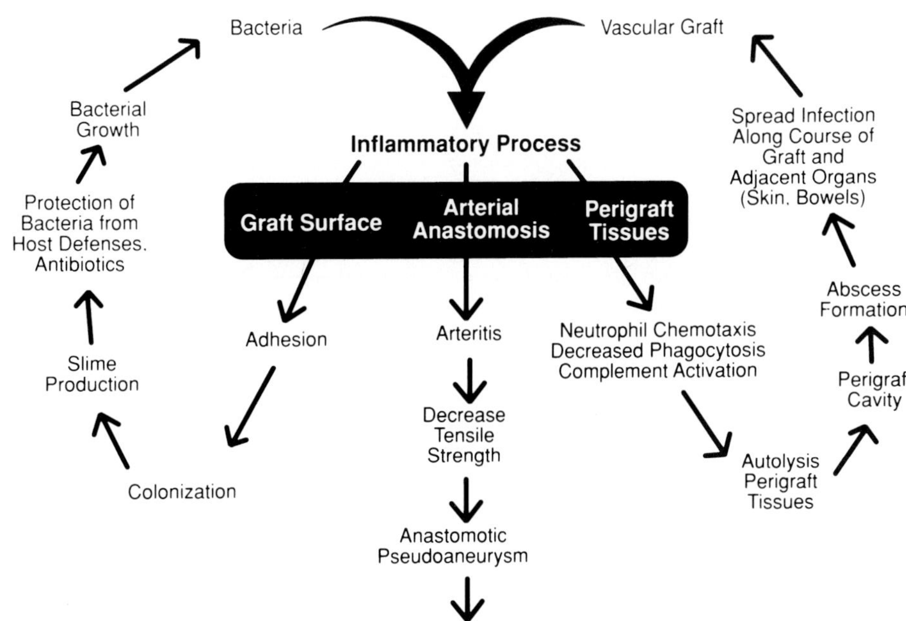

FIGURE 47–1. Pathogenesis of vascular biomaterial–associated infections.

TABLE 47–3. RISK FACTORS FOR GRAFT INFECTION

Bacterial Contamination of the Graft
Faulty sterile technique
Prolonged preoperative hospital stay
Emergency surgery
Extended operating time
Reoperative vascular procedure
Simultaneous gastrointestinal procedure
Remote infection
Postoperative superficial wound infection
Altered Host Defenses
Local factors
Biomaterial involvement
Slime production
Systemic factors
Malnutrition
Leukopenia
Malignancy
Corticosteroid administration
Chemotherapy
Diabetes mellitus
Chronic renal failure
Autoimmune disease

yield no growth. Often the only features that suggest infection are the absence of graft incorporation with surrounding tissue and the presence of perigraft fluid containing large numbers of white blood cells.

Predisposing Factors

Graft infections are commonly associated (1) with operative events that lead to bacterial contamination of the graft or (2) with patient risk factors that predispose to infection (i.e., impaired host defenses) (Table 47–3). The skin is an important reservoir of bacteria. Some graft infections originate from a break in sterile surgical technique that affords graft colonization from the patient's endogenous flora rather than from the operating room environment or the surgical team. A number of factors can promote this mechanism, including prolonged preoperative hospital stay (allowing skin colonization by more resistant organisms), emergency procedures, operative procedures longer than 4 hours, and reoperation for hematoma or graft thrombosis.[57] The increased risk of infection after reoperative vascular procedures reflects the higher frequencies of arterial wall and wound colonization and increased rates of wound complications (e.g., hematoma, lymphocele, dermal necrosis). Concomitant biliary (e.g., cholecystectomy), bowel (e.g., colon resection), and urinary tract (e.g., ureter repair) procedures also increase the risk of graft colonization by bacteria during the procedure. More often, however, colonization results from a postoperative complication such as bile fistula or anastomosis breakdown.

More than 90% of patients have one or more risk factors for graft infection. Early graft infections are usually the result of wound sepsis, reoperation for hematoma, concomitant remote infection, or impaired immunocompetence. Patients with late-appearing graft infections often have a history of multiple operations for graft thrombosis or false aneurysm.

Immune system factors associated with the biomaterial itself (e.g., foreign body reaction) or products of bacterial growth on graft surfaces can impair neutrophil chemotaxis and bactericidal function and result in an indolent, low-grade perigraft infection. The architectural features of the graft material may permit bacteria to grow in the interstices of the biomaterial (e.g., in woven and knitted Dacron prostheses). Products of the bacteria, such as the extracellular glycocalyx called *slime*, protect the bacteria from both host defense mechanisms and antibiotics.[10] Slime production is an indicator of the virulence and pathogenicity of both gram-positive and gram-negative bacteria. Body surface culture results indicate that most patients who undergo prosthetic implant procedures are colonized with pathogenic (i.e., slime-producing) strains of coagulase-negative staphylococci.[57] Coagulase-negative staphylococci are primary opportunists, infecting foreign bodies, injured tissues, and patients with profound leukopenia. The altered immune function associated with malignancy, lymphoproliferative disorders, and some drugs (e.g., steroids, chemotherapy) can predispose patients to graft infection even with low numbers of contaminating bacteria.

PREVENTION

Prevention of graft infection is an important concept, and every surgeon must be cognizant of preoperative, operative, and postoperative prophylactic measures. The preoperative hospital stay should be as short as possible to avoid skin colonization with flora resistant to commonly used antibiotics (i.e., hospital-acquired strains). Prophylactic antibiotic administration is recommended before vascular prosthetic implantation and has been shown to decrease the risk of wound infections that potentially lead to graft infection.[4] Systemic antibiotics should be administered before incision of the skin and at regular intervals during the procedure to maintain tissue drug levels above the minimal bactericidal concentration for expected pathogens (Table 47–4). Additional dosing may be needed during the operation, depending on the rate of elimination and volume of distribution of the antibiotic, larger or more frequent doses being necessary for patients with prolonged procedures (>4 hours) or excessive changes in blood volume, fluid administration, or renal blood flow during the procedure. Culture-specific antibiotics should be prescribed for patients undergoing vascular graft implantation who have coexisting infections of the leg or another remote site. At some vascu-

TABLE 47–4. SURGICAL PROPHYLAXIS IN ADULTS UNDERGOING PROSTHETIC GRAFT OR PATCH IMPLANTATION DURING CLEAN PROCEDURES*

1. Cefazolin, 1 gm IV, at induction of anesthesia and repeated every 8 hr for 24 hr.
2. When methicillin-resistant *Staphylococcus aureus* is cultured on body surfaces or is a known important pathogen in hospitalized patients, add vancomycin, 1 gm IV infused over 1 hr.
3. If patient has a cephalosporin allergy, give aztreonam, 1 gm IV every 8 hr.
4. If patient has a vancomycin allergy give clindamycin, 900 mg IV over 20–30 min.

*There is no evidence to support prophylaxis until central venous or Foley catheters are removed.
IV = intravenous.

lar disease centers, prophylactic antibiotics are given for 3 to 5 days to patients deemed to be at high risk for infection from bacteremia, prolonged pre-procedure hospitalization, or high institutional wound infection rates (>10%).

Attention to meticulous sterile technique is imperative to avoid bacterial contamination of the graft, especially during emergency procedures and prolonged reconstructive procedures. The graft should be protected from contact with any potentially contaminating sources, especially the exposed skin adjacent to the operative field, by the use of iodine-impregnated plastic drapes or antibiotic-soaked towels or cotton pads. Simultaneous gastrointestinal procedures should be avoided during grafting procedures to prevent graft contamination with enteric organisms. If an unplanned enterotomy should occur during celiotomy, graft implantation should be postponed and arterial reconstruction scheduled for a few days later, with planned implantation of an antibiotic-impregnated prosthesis.

A possible exception to the admonition against simultaneous gastrointestinal procedures is cholecystectomy for asymptomatic cholelithiasis, which can safely be performed in patients undergoing aortic graft implantation. An 18% incidence of postoperative acute cholecystitis has been reported in patients with cholelithiasis after elective abdominal aortic aneurysm repair.[18] The risk of aortic graft infection when concomitant cholecystectomy is performed is low, but a large retrospective review of the Mayo Clinic experience documented an increased complication rate. Gallbladder removal should be performed only after the aortic graft has been implanted and covered with retroperitoneum. After prosthetic graft implantation, patients should be informed of the potential risks for graft colonization and infection via bacteremia, especially after interventional procedures such as dental work, colonoscopy, and cystoscopy. Antibiotic prophylaxis is recommended in these instances.

Early recognition and aggressive treatment of postoperative wound infections are absolute necessities to minimize the risk of extension to the underlying graft. Careful handling of the tissues, meticulous hemostasis to prevent hematoma formation, and closure of the groin incisions in multiple layers (to eliminate dead space) are important technical measures that decrease wound healing problems and secondary infections. Wound irrigation with topical antibiotics before closure or incubation of Dacron grafts in rifampin (1 mg/ml) appears to decrease the incidence of groin wound infection after aortofemoral bypass grafting.

BACTERIOLOGY

Although virtually any microorganism can infect a vascular prosthesis, *S. aureus* is the most prevalent pathogen, accounting for one quarter to one half of infections, depending on the implant site (Table 47–5). Since the early 1970s, infections caused by *S. epidermidis* or gram-negative bacteria have increased in frequency. This change in the microbiology of graft infections is the result of reporting both early and late-appearing infections: many late infections are associated with GEE or GEF. Surgeons have also become aware of microbial sampling errors in late-appearing infection when small numbers of bacteria are present. Infections associated with negative culture results, despite clinical and anatomic signs of a perigraft infection, are caused by *S. epidermidis* or other coagulase-negative staphylococci, and on occasion by *Candida* species. Infections due to gram-negative bacteria such as *E. coli* and *Pseudomonas*, *Klebsiella*, *Enterobacter*, and *Proteus* species are particularly virulent. The incidence of anastomotic dehiscence and artery rupture is high and is due to the ability of the organisms to produce destructive endotoxins (e.g., elastase and alkaline protease) that compromise vessel wall structural integrity.[19, 20] Fungal infections of grafts (e.g., with *Candida*, *Mycobacterium*, and *Aspergillus* species) are rare, and most patients with such infections either are severely immunosuppressed or have an established fungal infection elsewhere.

Graft infections that occur within 4 months of implantation are associated with virulent pathogens, with *S. aureus*

TABLE 47–5. BACTERIOLOGY OF PROSTHETIC VASCULAR GRAFT INFECTIONS: INCIDENCE FROM 1258 COLLECTED CASES

	INCIDENCE (%)					
PATHOGEN	**AEF**	**AI**	**AF**	**FD**	**TA**	**ICS**
Staphylococcus aureus	4	3	27	28	22	50
Staphylococcus epidermidis	2	3	26	11	25	20
Streptococcus species	9	3	10	11	2	—
Escherichia coli	18	30	12	7	2	—
Pseudomonas species	3	7	6	16	14	—
Klebsiella species	5	10	5	2	2	10
Enterobacter species	5	13	2	2	—	—
Enterococcus species	8	10	2	7	4	—
Bacteroides species	8	3	3	2	—	—
Proteus species	4	—	4	7	2	—
Candida species	3	—	1	1	4	—
Serratia species	1	—	1	2	—	—
Other species	3	2	4	6	0	—
No growth culture	18	13	2	2	16	20

AEF = aortoenteric fistula or erosion (n = 397); AI = aortoiliac or aortic tube graft (n = 39); AF = aortobifemoral or iliofemoral graft (n = 460); FD = femoropopliteal, femorotibial, axillofemoral, or femorofemoral graft (n = 251); TA = thoracic aorta graft (n = 55); ICS = innominate, carotid, or subclavian bypass graft or carotid patch following endarterectomy (n = 56).

predominating. Coagulase-positive strains produce hemolysis and toxins to leukocytes that provoke intense local and systemic host responses and permit early recognition of the infectious complications. Gram-negative organisms such as *Proteus*, *Pseudomonas*, *Klebsiella*, and *Enterobacter* species can also be involved in early postoperative graft infections; anastomotic hemorrhage is most often associated with a *Pseudomonas aeruginosa* infection. Graft healing complications, such as GEE and GEF, even when they present months to years after implantation, are associated with infections caused by gram-negative enteric bacteria, and thus signs more typical of an early infection are commonplace.

Late-appearing graft infections (i.e., those occurring more than 4 months after implantation) are commonly associated with less virulent bacteria. *S. epidermidis* and other coagulase-negative staphylococci are common pathogens for graft infections that occur months to years after implantation. These organisms are present in normal skin flora but have the ability to adhere to and colonize biomaterials and to grow in a biofilm adherent to the prosthetic surfaces; thus, they can produce an indolent infection. The bacterial biofilm is eventually recognized by host defense mechanisms, causing inflammation of the perigraft tissue and adjacent artery and leading to the subsequent clinical manifestations of a late graft infection.

DIAGNOSIS

Prompt diagnosis and treatment of prosthetic graft infections are essential to avoid complications (e.g., sepsis, hemorrhage) and death. Clinical manifestations are varied and may be subtle, particularly those associated with cavitary graft infections. Operative exploration is the most accurate method for confirming infection of a vascular prosthesis and may be necessary when clinical suspicion of GEE exists. In equivocal cases, the vascular surgeon must prove that a graft infection is not present. Most graft infections are detected more than 4 months after graft implantation,[6, 7, 66, 75] and fewer than 20% are found in the early postoperative period. The urgency of diagnostic evaluation depends on the presentation and the clinical status of the patient. In general, intervention is based on clinical signs, the nature of the abnormalities as demonstrated by vascular imaging, and microbiologic analysis of the graft.

Clinical Manifestations

History

Because graft infections are often subtle in presentation, the vascular surgeon must develop a low threshold for diagnostic testing when any symptom or sign suggests graft infection. Aortic grafts confined to the abdomen can present as unexplained sepsis, prolonged postoperative ileus, or abdominal distention and tenderness as the only clinical signs. If the infection involves an extracavitary graft segment (i.e., in leg, groin, or neck incisions), local signs of graft infection are usually apparent by findings of an inflammatory perigraft mass, cellulitis, a drainage sinus tract, or a palpable anastomotic pseudoaneurysm. Patients with an aortic graft infection and GEF often present with upper or lower gastrointestinal herald bleeding. Any patient with massive gastrointestinal bleeding and an aortic graft should be considered to have graft infection and GEE or GEF until another source of bleeding is conclusively identified or until no graft-bowel communication is verified at operation.[6, 66, 75, 103]

In patients with vague symptoms and ultrasound or computed tomography (CT) evidence of perigraft fluid, careful review of the operative history and surgical notes may furnish clues that further support the diagnosis of graft infection and provide the rationale for more detailed and invasive diagnostic testing. The patient should also be asked about recent medical illnesses that may have resulted in hematogenous or lymphatic seeding of the graft with bacteria. Early graft infections due to *S. aureus* or other gram-negative bacteria appear within weeks of the procedure with the signs of fever, leukocytosis, and obvious perigraft purulence.

Bacteremia, a late sign, is associated with artery wall or mural thrombus infection or with secondary endocarditis. Patients with a graft infection due to *S. epidermidis* present months to years after implantation with healing complications (e.g., anastomotic aneurysm, perigraft cavity with fluid, or graft cutaneous sinus tract), although systemic signs of sepsis (e.g., fever, leukocytosis, and bacteremia) are characteristically absent.

Physical Examination

The clinician performing the physical examination should closely scrutinize the site or sites of graft implantation for signs of inflammation. Surgical incisions should be carefully inspected for healing complications or draining sinuses. Masses near anastomotic sites can represent perigraft abscesses or anastomotic pseudoaneurysms. The extremities should be examined for signs of septic embolization (i.e., a cluster of petechiae downstream from the infected graft). Other sources of infection, such as infected foot lesions, osteomyelitis, and infected urinary calculi, should be sought because these conditions can predispose to hematogenous bacterial seeding and graft colonization.

Laboratory Studies

An elevated white blood cell count (15,000 to 18,000 cells/ml) with leftward-shifted differential and an increased erythrocyte sedimentation rate (>20 mm/min) are common but nonspecific findings in patients with graft infection and fever. Routine laboratory tests should also include urinalysis, blood cultures, and cultures of any other potential sources of infection, such as foot and surgical wound drainage material. A stool guaiac test for blood is indicated for patients with suspected GEF or GEE, but findings are positive in only some two thirds of patients who have documented lesions. All laboratory test results may be normal in patients with late-appearing perigraft infections due to *S. epidermidis*.

Vascular Imaging

A number of vascular imaging modalities are useful for detecting prosthetic graft infections. Anatomic evidence of

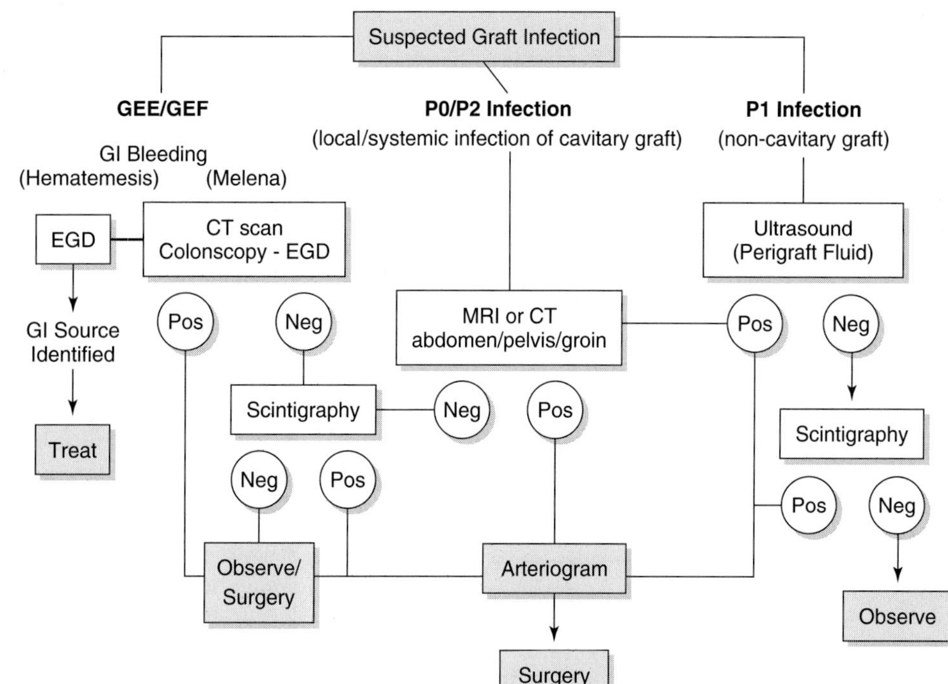

FIGURE 47–2. Algorithm for evaluation of infected prosthetic arterial graft. GEE = graft-enteric infection; GEF = graft-enteric fistula; EGD = esophagogastroduodenoscopy; CT = computed tomography; MRI = magnetic resonance imaging; GI = gastrointestinal; Pos = positive; Neg = Negative.

graft infection, such as perigraft abscess or anastomotic aneurysm, can be identified by ultrasonography, CT, magnetic resonance imaging (MRI), arteriography, and contrast sinography. Functional radionuclide imaging can confirm the presence of a clinically suspected graft infection when anatomic signs of perigraft abscess are equivocal. The combination of anatomic and functional vascular imaging techniques is highly accurate (sensitivity, 80% to 100%; specificity, 50% to 90%) for confirming the presence of infection, planning management, and assessing operative sites for residual or recurrent infection (Fig. 47–2). Arteriography is useful in developing a treatment strategy and should be routine. Anatomic definition of the infectious process identifies safe sites for placing vascular clamps and minimizes the likelihood of vascular injury or organ ischemia secondary to anatomic anomalies or concomitant arterial occlusive disease.

Contrast-Enhanced Computed Tomography

Contrast-enhanced CT is the preferred initial imaging technique for suspected peripheral (P1, P2, P3) graft infections. Findings suggestive of infection include loss of normal tissue planes of the retroperitoneal structures (indicative of inflammation), abnormal collections of fluid or gas around the graft, false aneurysms, hydronephrosis, adjacent vertebral osteomyelitis, and juxta-aortic retroperitoneal abscess (Fig. 47–3). The presence of fluid and air surrounding an aortic prosthesis is normal in the early postoperative period, but it should resolve with time. Any gas in the periprosthetic tissues on CT should be judged as abnormal beyond 6 to 7 weeks after implantation. CT should be performed with intravenous and oral contrast media to better identify the graft lumen, to delineate any periprosthetic abscess, and to define the relationship of the duodenum and small bowel to the aortic prosthesis.

Scanning can be performed quickly enough to be useful in evaluating symptomatic but hemodynamically stable patients with suspected GEE or GEF. CT is 96% sensitive and 88% specific in identifying late-appearing bacterial biofilm graft infections. CT-guided aspiration of perigraft fluid is useful for isolating the infecting pathogen or verifying a process consistent with *S. epidermidis* infection (white blood cells on Gram's stain; no growth on culture).

Ultrasonography

Ultrasonography is a readily available imaging technique that is suited for "portable" examination of patients with suspected extracavitary (P2, P3) graft infections. Color du-

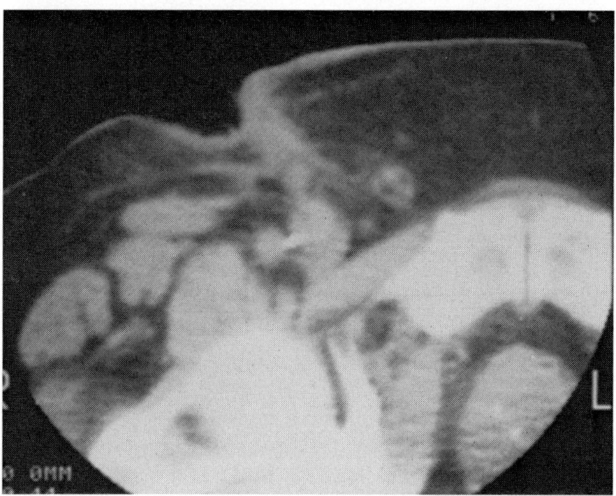

FIGURE 47–3. Computed tomographic scan of an infected aortofemoral graft limb showing perigraft inflammation extending to the skin. The patient presented with groin sinus tract. Graft culture of isolated *Staphylococcus epidermidis*.

plex scanning can reliably differentiate perigraft fluid collections from anastomotic pseudoaneurysms or hematomas and thus is useful in evaluating pulsatile masses. Diagnostic accuracy depends on the skill of the examiner and on the relative "visibility" by imaging of the graft. The area of interest can be obscured by abdominal distention secondary to large amounts of intestinal gas or by body fat. Duplex scanning is the most useful initial imaging technique for verifying vessel or graft patency and for assessing pulsatile masses adjacent to grafts in the groins and limbs.

Magnetic Resonance Imaging

MRI has been used since 1985 for the diagnostic evaluation of graft infections (Fig. 47–4). Its most useful feature is its ability to distinguish between perigraft fluid and perigraft fibrosis, thanks to signal intensity differences between T1- and T2-weighted images. Inflammation is readily demonstrated by inhomogeneously increased signal intensities in tissues adjacent to the vascular prosthesis. In a review by Olofsson and colleagues, MRI clearly identified perigraft fluid collections and inflammation in 11 of 14 patients who proved at operation to have an aortic graft infection.[67] In contrast, CT impressions were correct in only four of 10 patients who had a verified graft infection. MRI and CT share this limitation: They cannot distinguish perigraft abscess fluid from sterile perigraft fluid, and they cannot detect GEE.

Contrast Sinography

Percutaneous localization of perigraft fluid followed by injection of contrast can demonstrate the extent of the perigraft cavity along the graft limb. The contrast sinogram, however, is not routinely recommended because of the risks of contaminating a sterile graft. In addition, the contrast material injected into a perigraft space does not necessarily demonstrate the full extent of the graft infection.

Gram's stain and culture of fluid aspirated from the perigraft space may identify the causative organism. Gram's stain of tissue or perigraft fluid showing no organisms does not reliably rule out infection. It is not uncommon, with a late-appearing graft infection, for only white blood cells to be seen on Gram's stain and for no bacteria to be isolated by a swab culture plated on agar media.[6, 11]

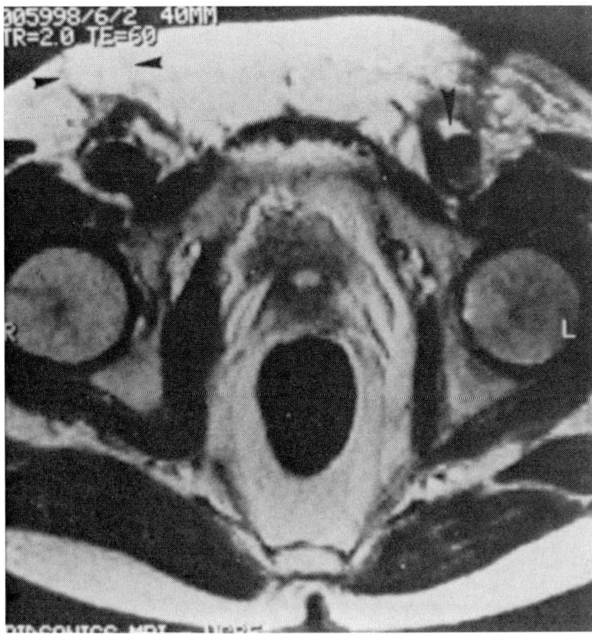

FIGURE 47–4. Magnetic resonance image of prosthetic graft infection. Soft tissue inflammation delineated by *arrowheads*. (From Olofsson PA, Auffermann W, Higgins CB, et al: Diagnosis of prosthetic aortic graft infection by magnetic resonance imaging. J Vasc Surg 8:99, 1988.)

Functional White Blood Cell Scanning

A number of radionuclide scintigraphic techniques (gallium 67 citrate, indium 111–labeled leukocyte, indium 111–labeled immunoglobulin G, technetium 99m hexametazime–labeled leukocyte) are useful for demonstrating sites of leukocyte accumulation that might indicate graft infection. These functional imaging techniques are not useful during the early postoperative course because of nonspecific radionuclide uptake in the perigraft tissues. Although false-negative scan findings are unusual, exclusion of early graft infection is possible; however, normal findings have been reported in late-appearing aortic graft infections complicated by GEE. Three to 4 months after graft implantation, the accuracy of the functional imaging scans in detecting graft infection (especially of indium 111–labeled and technetium 99m hexametazime leukocyte scans) approaches 90%.

Positive findings are associated with a positive predictive value of 80%. At some centers, an immunoglobin G (IgG) scan is preferred over a leukocyte scan because the radionuclide is easy to prepare, does not expose staff to the patient's blood, requires no red blood cell or platelet imaging, and has a long shelf life. Functional imaging studies can be used with MRI and CT to accurately delineate the extent of graft involvement. Patients with nonspecific symptoms and scintigrapic findings of infection should undergo operative exploration of the prosthesis to exclude infection.

Endoscopy

Endoscopy is an important diagnostic modality for suspected secondary aortoenteric fistula or erosion (Fig. 47–5). It is essential that the entire upper gastrointestinal tract be inspected, including the third and fourth portions of the duodenum, which are the most common sites of GEF. Patients with a recent history of massive gastrointestinal hemorrhage should be examined *in the operating room*, where preparations should already have been made should exsanguination from the fistula be induced.[54]

Endoscopy can sometimes visualize the graft eroded through the bowel mucosa or the clot at the bleeding site, but its main purpose is to rule out other sources of bleeding, such as gastritis or ulcer disease. Negative findings *do not* rule out the possibility of an aortoduodenal fistula.

Arteriography

Although arteriography cannot be used to make the diagnosis of graft infection, it can accurately identify infection-

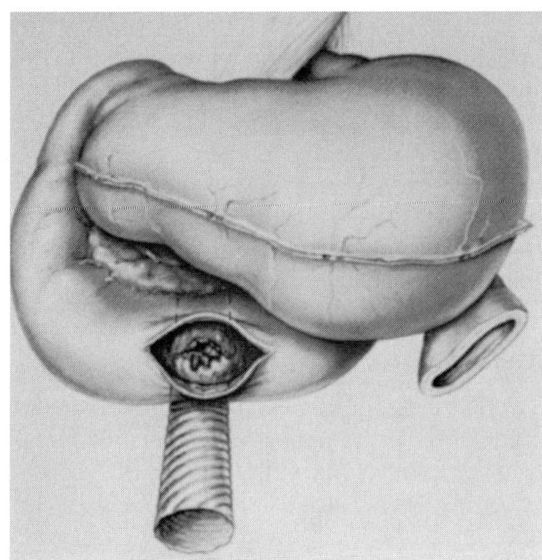

FIGURE 47–5. Graft-enteric fistula.

associated complications such as graft rupture and anastomotic aneurysm. Biplanar angiography should be performed on all patients with confirmed or suspected aortic graft infection to assess the patency of the involved vessels and grafts and to evaluate the status of the proximal and distal vessels as potential sites for extra-anatomic bypass grafts.

Microbiologic Methods

Recovery of microorganisms from sites of suspected prosthetic graft infections is necessary to confirm the diagnosis and to select appropriate antibiotic therapy. Routine culture of graft surfaces and perigraft fluid is usually adequate in patients who have graft infections associated with fever, leukocytosis, or perigraft abscess with cellulitis. Virulent organisms such as *S. aureus*, streptococci, and gram-negative bacteria, which produce systemic signs of graft sepsis by invading the perigraft tissues and blood, are readily identified; however, surface swabs *do not* recover less virulent pathogens that do not produce invasion of the perigraft tissues. Failure of Gram's stain of tissue or perigraft fluid to show organisms is not sufficient to exclude a low-grade infection. Low numbers and virulence of infecting microorganisms, concomitant antibiotic administration, absence of tissue invasion, and activation of host defenses contribute to sampling errors in routine culture techniques.

Use of tryptic soy broth media and mechanical disruption (tissue grinding, ultrasonic tissue disruption of explanted tissue or graft) reliably increases the rate of recovery of bacteria (Fig. 47–6). Culture tubes containing graft specimens should be maintained for 5 to 7 days to exclude growth of coagulase-negative staphylococci. In clinical series of late graft infections, culture of the graft material with mechanical disruption and broth media identified the bacteria (typically *S. epidermidis*) in more than 80%, despite negative findings on Gram's stain and culture of the perigraft tissue and fluid.

Operative Findings

The definitive diagnostic test for suspected graft infection is operative exploration. Operation permits the surgeon to inspect the graft and surrounding tissues for signs of infection, including graft incorporation, perigraft fluid, anastomotic integrity, and GEF. Exploration, graft excision, and culture of the graft material are often the only reliable methods of identifying the pathogens.[6, 11] Operation is also an essential diagnostic test for patients with a history of aortic surgery and gastrointestinal bleeding when all other sources of bleeding have been excluded.

Fewer than half of cases of GEF are conclusively identified by the preoperative testing methods described earlier.[66, 75] Thorough mobilization and exploration of the duodenum, the small bowel, and the aortic graft and proxi-

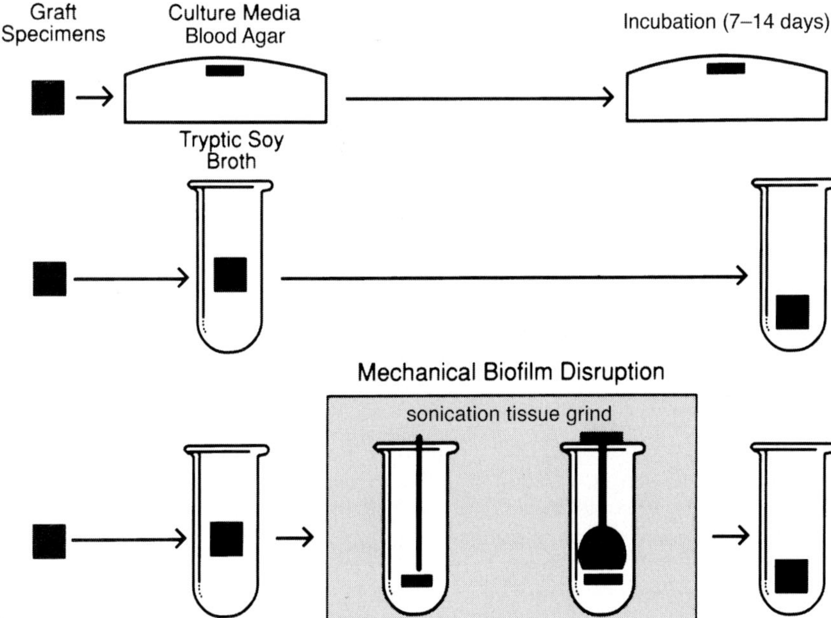

FIGURE 47–6. Culture techniques for recovery of bacteria from prosthetic vascular grafts.

mal anastomoses identify infections in this situation in more than 80% of cases. Successful treatment can be expected if the diagnosis is established before the development of life-threatening complications, such as hypotension and sepsis.

MANAGEMENT STRATEGIES

The clinical spectrum of prosthetic graft infections permits surgeons to individualize treatment. A number of treatment options are available, including graft excision without revascularization, graft excision coupled with ex situ bypass, and graft replacement in situ (see Fig. 47–4). Some reports have emphasized the safety of replacement in situ using a variety of conduits: large-caliber venous autografts, arterial allografts, or antibiotic-bonded prostheses. Observed advantages, compared with the "standard" treatment of graft excision and ex situ bypass, include shorter operative time, less surgical stress, reduced rates of limb loss, and improved graft patency. Judicious patient selection is key, since replacement in situ is most efficacious for low-grade graft infections evident by the absence of sepsis or anastomotic infection, and quantitative cultures of perigraft tissue with fewer than 10^5 CFUs/gm of tissue.

General Principles

Preparing the Patient for Surgery

When a patient presents in septic shock or with hypovolemia secondary to anastomotic bleeding from an infected graft, there is little time for preparation. Adequate resuscitation with restoration of blood and fluid volumes, perioperative cardiopulmonary monitoring, administration of broad-spectrum high-dose antibiotics, and careful planning of the surgical approach are the essential elements of urgent preoperative treatment for these critically ill patients.

Fortunately, most cases of graft infection are discovered in time to allow adequate preoperative preparation, identification of the infecting pathogen, and determination of the extent of graft infection. Patients should be prepared, physiologically and psychologically, for the most extensive operation that might be required. Cardiac function should be determined, and the cardiac index and peripheral vascular resistance should be optimized with administration of nitrates, antiarrhythmia medications, beta-blockers, and alpha-antagonists. The patient's pulmonary status should be evaluated and augmented with bronchodilators and respiratory therapy, as needed. Baseline renal function should be established and renal perfusion improved by hydration or low-dose dopamine (3 to 5 mg/kg/min). Patients who have depleted nutritional reserves or "are anergic" to a battery of standard skin tests should be given enteral or parenteral nutrition when time permits. Glucose levels should be closely monitored and controlled in patients with diabetes. The bowels should be cleansed with mechanical and antibiotic preparations in patients who have an intra-abdominal graft infection. Arterial circulation to the upper and lower extremities should be assessed by Doppler-derived pressure measurements and arteriography to select the appropriate revascularization alternative to maintain perfusion after graft excision.

If autologous replacement in situ is planned, duplex ultrasonography should be used to assess the lower limb deep and superficial veins for caliber and changes indicative of chronic venous disease. Systemic antibiotics should be selected according to isolated or suspected pathogens. Other sites of infection (e.g., urinary tract, lungs, feet) should be appropriately evaluated and treated.

Determining the Extent of Graft Infection

Persistent infection of a nonexcised graft segment or in the arterial graft bed is the major reason for treatment failure and the major cause of morbidity and death.[75] Local control of infection is more successful when there is no gross purulence and when culture results are negative or *S. epidermidis* is recovered. CT, MRI, and leukocyte radionuclide scans are helpful in localizing the infected portion of the graft, but surgical exploration remains the most reliable method of determining the extent of graft infection. Hydronephrosis is a reliable sign of advanced aortic graft infection that denotes diffuse graft involvement.

Removing the Graft

Removal of the entire infected graft is essential to eradicating the infectious process in patients who are septic, present with anastomotic bleeding, or have complete involvement of the graft. Attempts at graft preservation with antibiotic therapy and serial wound débridements have been reported, but infection can persist, particularly if the infected graft is made of Dacron. Patients remain at risk for exsanguination from anastomotic or arterial rupture during the period of treatment. Calligaro and coworkers have recommended specific selection criteria and treatment principles that, when adhered to, led to successful prosthetic preservation in approximately 70% of cases (Table 47–6).[19, 20]

For patients with infections localized to only a portion of an aortofemoral, a single treatment approach is not applicable or appropriate. Excision of the entire graft and extra-anatomic bypass are associated with amputation and mortality rates of 11% to 27% (see Table 47–4). Morbidity continues to be high, owing to persistent infection of the aortic stump (10% incidence), recurrent infection of the extra-anatomic bypass (5% to 10% incidence), and multiple secondary procedures for treatment of the failed extra-

TABLE 47–6. CRITERIA AND TREATMENT ADJUNCTS FOR SELECTIVE GRAFT PRESERVATION FOR EARLY EXTRACAVITARY INFECTIONS

Selection Criteria

1. Graft is patent and not constructed of polyester (Dacron).
2. Anastomoses are intact and not involved with infection.
3. Patient is not systemically septic.

Treatment Adjuncts

1. Repeated and aggressive wound débridements in operating room.
2. Three changes of wound dressing daily utilizing dilute povidone-iodine (1 ml 1% povidone-iodine in 1 L normal saline).
3. Prolonged administration of culture-specific antibiotic.
4. Selective use of rotational muscle flap coverage.

anatomic bypass (25% to 50%). The use of staged procedures lower limb revascularization (axillofemoral bypass) followed in 1 or 2 days by excision of the aortic graft is associated with reduced morbidity.

In special cases, morbidity (death, amputation) may be decreased if the surgeon excises only the infected portion of the graft (partial graft excision), with distal revascularization via remote bypass (obturator, axillofemoral) through tissues not involved with infection. At the site of graft retention, culture specimens should be obtained and topical antibiotics instilled via wound irrigation systems to cleanse perigraft tissues. The quantity and the virulence of the pathogens, the adequacy of local and systemic host defenses, and the extent of the infection are critical factors that influence decision making and treatment outcomes.

Débridement of the Arterial Wall Perigraft Tissues and Drainage

After graft excision, débridement of all inflamed tissues and drainage of the graft bed are important principles for preventing persistence of the infectious process. The artery wall adjacent to the infected graft is a potential reservoir of bacteria, and positive culture specimens of the artery wall increase the risk of aorta stump or artery disruption.[5, 7] The artery wall and perigraft tissues should be débrided to normal-looking tissue, especially in the presence of purulence or false aneurysm. Adequate débridement of the aorta should be confirmed by histologic examination, and if culture results of the arterial wall are positive, patients should be treated with long-term antibiotic therapy.[5]

It is essential to use monofilament permanent sutures to close the artery. Closed suction drainage should be positioned in the infected graft bed when gross purulence is present. Coverage of the arterial closures with viable, noninfected tissue (e.g., omental pedicle or rotational muscle flaps) lessens the risk of stump blowout and separates the arterial closures from adjacent organs, the graft bed, and drains.

Antibiotic Therapy

When the pathogen or pathogens can be identified before operation, bactericidal antibiotics should be administered in large doses preoperatively and perioperatively, and in selected instances an antibiotic is prescribed for the rest of the patient's life (Table 47–7). If the infecting organism has not been identified, broad-spectrum antibiotics, such as an aminoglycoside plus semisynthetic penicillin, a second-generation cephalosporin, or ampicillin plus sulbactam, should be given. If *S. aureus* or *S. epidermidis* is the suspected pathogen, an intravenous first-generation or second-generation cephalosporin and vancomycin would be appropriate. It is essential that antibiotics be administered preoperatively and that adequate tissue levels be maintained throughout the operation.

TABLE 47–7. ANTIBIOTIC THERAPY FOR PROSTHETIC GRAFT INFECTIONS

	ANTIBIOTIC ADMINISTRATION	
MICROORGANISM ISOLATED	**Perioperative (Parenteral)**	**Lifelong (Oral)**
None	Vancomycin, gentamicin	None
Staphylococci/ streptococci	Vancomycin, ampicillin/ sulbactam	None
Gram-negative polymicrobial	Culture-specific antibiotic	Culture-specific
Salmonella spp.	Ciprofloxacin, amoxicillin	Amoxacillin
Candida spp., fungi	Amphotericin B	Fluconazole

Before closure of the incision, topical antibiotics (kanamycin and bacitracin) should be used in combination with a wound pulsed-irrigation system to cleanse tissues and remove debris. Once the graft infection has been treated and the operative cultures have isolated the bacteria, antibiotic coverage should be modified according to antibiotic susceptibility testing of the recovered strains.

The duration of antibiotic administration after graft excision is unclear. Reilly and associates recommended at least 2 weeks of systemic antibiotics.[75] Patients who received long-term antibiotics (parenteral antibiotics for 6 weeks, followed by oral antibiotics for 6 months) had significantly better results than patients treated with short-term therapy (10 to 14 days). The incidence of recurrent infection and aortic stump blowout may be decreased with long-term antibiotic administration, especially in patients with positive arterial wall culture findings[5]; in patients with negative findings, parenteral antibiotics should be administered for 2 to 4 weeks, followed by 3 months of oral therapy specific to the infecting pathogen or pathogens.

Revascularization of Organs and Limbs

Rarely can graft excision alone, without revascularization, be performed for the treatment of a patent, infected prosthetic graft. Occluded grafts and grafts implanted to alleviate symptoms of claudication may be treated by total graft excision without revascularization or in combination with endovascular angioplasty. An end-to-side anastomotic configuration permits reconstruction of the native arteries via autogenous patch angioplasty alone or in combination with endarterectomy. If a phasic Doppler arterial signal is present at the ankle after graft excision or if arterial systolic pressure is greater than 40 mmHg at the ankle or forearm, delayed reconstruction is an option because sufficient collaterals have been preserved. In the presence of critical limb ischemia (i.e., when no distal Doppler signal is audible), arterial revascularization should not be delayed because of the associated risks of increased morbidity and limb loss.

It is preferable to perform limb revascularization before the infected graft is removed; in the presence of anastomotic bleeding and shock, however, control of hemorrhage takes precedence. Autogenous tissue grafts (from the greater saphenous vein, deep femoral vein, or endarterectomized iliac or superficial femoral artery), if available, are the conduits of choice for limb or organ revascularization. If a prosthetic graft is used for an ex situ bypass, PTFE conduits are preferred to Dacron grafts, although eventually antibiotic-impregnated grafts may be the conduits of choice for the treatment of established graft infections by either in situ replacement or extra-anatomic bypass grafting.

Trout and coworkers[99] and Reilly and associates[75] demonstrated decreased morbidity and mortality with staged or

TABLE 47–8. SELECTION CRITERIA AND TREATMENT COMPONENTS OF IN SITU PROSTHETIC GRAFT REPLACEMENT FOR BACTERIAL BIOFILM GRAFT INFECTION

Selection Criteria
- Clinical
  - Presentation months to years after graft implantation
  - No systemic signs of infection: no fever, normal serum white blood cell count, sterile blood culture
- Anatomic
  - Adjacent tissue and artery wall inflammation
  - Perigraft cavity and fluid
  - Absence of graft incorporation
  - Anastomotic dehiscence
- Microbiologic
  - Perigraft fluid Gram stain: white blood cells, no bacteria
  - Perigraft fluid culture: no growth
  - Graft biofilm culture: coagulase-negative staphylococci (*Staphylococcus epidermidis*)

Treatment Components
- Preoperative and perioperative administration of vancomycin
- Gram's stain of perigraft fluid to exclude bacteria
- Wide débridement of inflamed (abnormal) perigraft tissue
- Excision of anastomotic sites
- Cleansing/débridement of tissues with a wound irrigation system
- Use of polytetrafluoroethylene or rifampin-bonded, gelatin-impregnated polyester (Dacron) prosthesis
- Muscle flap coverage of replacement graft if feasible
- Prolonged (6-wk) administration of culture-specific antibiotics

sequential treatment as compared with traditional treatment (i.e., total graft excision followed by immediate extra-anatomic bypass). Preliminary revascularization can be performed without increasing the risk of death, amputation, or new graft infection, and with staged treatment (i.e., revascularization followed 1 to 2 days later by total graft excision), the physiologic stress on the patient may be reduced. Sequential treatment (i.e., preliminary revascularization followed by graft excision) prevents lower limb ischemia and obviates keeping the patient heparinized during total graft excision and closure of the artery or aorta stump.

In situ replacement can be applied in carefully selected cases. When infection involves the thoracic aorta, it may be the only practical approach. The perigraft infectious process should be a low-grade one and not associated with anastomotic hemorrhage, and cultures should be sterile, *or* the anatomic and microbiologic characteristics of the graft infection should suggest infection with *S. epidermidis*. In situ prosthetic replacement has also been used successfully to treat secondary aortoduodenal fistula, but associated operative mortality is 19%. Patients with GEE and minimal retroperitoneal infection fared best.

In situ replacement appears to be a safe option for patients with graft infections secondary to *S. epidermidis*. From 1987 to 1996, this author treated 28 patients with aortoiliofemoral grafts infected by bacterial biofilms with in situ prosthetic replacement. Selection criteria and components of surgical management are outlined in Table 47–8. Presenting signs were localized to the groin, and they included 10 femoral false aneurysms, 10 graft-cutaneous sinus tracts, and eight perigraft abscesses. No deaths or early procedural failures occurred, and during follow-up all replacement grafts remained patent and showed no signs of infection. Two patients required resection of the retained aortic Dacron graft at 1 and 2 years, respectively, after in situ replacement of a distal aortofemoral graft limb.

In situ treatment of bacterial biofilm graft infections is effective for localized graft healing problems, but because of the indolent nature of this type of biomaterial infection, subsequent infection of previously uninvolved graft segments may be expected. When advanced biofilm aortic graft infections are encountered (i.e., a P0 infection), in situ replacement using the neoaortoiliac segment (NAIS) procedure or an arterial allograft is preferred (Table 47–9). In situ graft replacement should be avoided when GEF or GEE is the presenting problem.

Treatment of Infected Graft Sites

Aortoiliac or Aortic Interposition Graft Infections

Aortoiliac or aortic interposition graft infections are best treated by preliminary (right-sided) axillobifemoral bypass grafting through clean, uninfected tissues, followed during the same operation by total graft excision of the infected aortic graft (i.e., sequential treatment). Preliminary remote bypass is safe and is associated with less morbidity than that seen with traditional treatment.[66, 75, 99] In stable patients, extra-anatomic bypass grafting can be performed before contaminated abdomen or retroperitoneum is entered. Because the aortic graft is confined to the abdomen, the distal axillofemoral anastomoses can usually be attached to the common femoral arteries bilaterally.

After completion of the extra-anatomic bypass grafting, all wounds should be closed and covered with sterile,

TABLE 47–9. RESULTS OF "STANDARD" TREATMENT FOR AORTIC GRAFT INFECTIONS

AUTHOR	NO. OF CASES	MORTALITY RATE (%)	EARLY AMPUTATION (%)	STUMP BLOWOUT (%)	SURVIVAL >1 YEAR (%)	INFECTION OF EXTRA-ANATOMIC BYPASS (%)
Bandyk et al, 1984[6]	18	11	11	0	66	17
O'Hara et al, 1986[66]	84	18	27	22	58	25
Reilly et al, 1987[75]	92	14	25	13	73	20
Schmitt et al, 1990[82]	20	15	5	6	75	6
Yeager et al, 1990[106]	38	14	21	4	76	22
Quinones-Baldrich et al, 1991[73]	45	24	11	0	63	20
Watson et al, 1993	45	27	18	0	61	20
Kuestner et al, 1995*	33	27	9	9	75	15

*Treatment of secondary aortoenteric fistula.

TABLE 47–10. RESULTS OF IN SITU REPLACEMENT FOR AORTIC GRAFT INFECTION

AUTHOR	NO. OF CASES	MORTALITY RATE (%)	EARLY AMPUTATION (%)	GRAFT PATENCY AT 1 YR (%)	SURVIVAL > 1 YEAR (%)	RECURRENT INFECTION (%)
Prosthetic						
Bandyk et al, 1984[6]	28	0	0	100	94	9
Neoaortoiliac						
Clagett, 1994	21	10	10	85	85	0
Nevelsteen et al, 1997	35	17	6	76	82	0
Allograft						
Kieffer et al, 1986	103	19	5	70	82	7
GEE/GEF						
Jacobs et al, 1991[50]	27	25	0	—	70	20
Bahnini et al, 1997[4]	32	40	0	—	55	10

GEE = graft-enteric erosion; GEF = graft-enteric fistula.

protective dressings. Celiotomy is then performed to afford excision of the infected aortic graft. Heparinization should be used during the revascularization procedure but should be reversed during excision of the infected graft. In cases with proximal and distal end-to-side anastomoses, in situ autogenous reconstruction should be considered (Table 47–10). This scenario is uncommon, however, because the majority of aortic interpositions and aortoiliac grafts were implanted to treat aneurysmal disease rather than atherosclerotic occlusive disease. Allograft replacement of an infected aortic graft has been advocated as a "bridge," but cadaver aorta retrieval and maintaining a tissue bank are not possible at most institutions.

The entire infected abdominal aortic graft should be excised. Achieving proximal control at the supraceliac aorta before approaching the proximal anastomosis is of value, especially in patients who have a proximal anastomotic aneurysm or a juxtarenal anastomosis. Meticulous care must be exercised to dissect adherent viscera and duodenum from the graft capsule. If GEE or GEF is present, débridement of all necrotic or inflamed bowel wall is imperative, and primary end-to-end anastomosis of the bowel is preferred. The iliac arteries distal to the graft should also be mobilized for distal control before the graft is excised. Culture of explanted graft material should be performed with standard broth and biofilm culture techniques.

The aorta should be débrided back to normal-looking wall and closed with interlocking monofilament sutures. A pedicle of omentum should be passed through the transverse mesocolon and carefully positioned around the aortic stump and into the bed of the excised aorta and graft. When necessary, the aorta can be excised to above the level of the renal arteries, in which case renal revascularization is achieved via bypasses originating from the splenic or hepatic arteries.[63] Fortunately, infection involving the juxtarenal aorta is rare. Closed suction drains should be placed in the infected graft bed and brought out near the flank opposite the axillofemoral graft limb.

The distal aorta or iliac arteries should also be closed with monofilament suture. The ureter should be located and protected from injury throughout the procedure. Preoperative placement of ureteral stents can be helpful; however, they are usually not necessary unless hydronephrosis is present. The site and the method of iliac artery ligation should be chosen to sustain perfusion to the colon, the pelvis, and the buttock muscles. After infrarenal aortic ligation, pelvic circulation can be adequately maintained via retrograde blood flow from the extra-anatomic femoral bypass through the external and internal iliac arteries. With excision of an infected aorta–external iliac graft, salvage of perfusion to one iliac artery via autogenous reconstruction should be considered. Inflow to a single internal iliac artery is usually sufficient to maintain adequate pelvic perfusion because of the abundant collateral flow via the visceral and deep femoral arteries.

Aortobifemoral Graft Infections

Aortobifemoral graft infections are more difficult to treat because involvement of the groin complicates lower limb revascularization and mandates distal anastomoses of the ex situ bypass to the deep femoral, superficial femoral, or popliteal arteries. Preoperative vascular imaging studies can identify localized aortofemoral graft limb infection, thus permitting partial graft excision, typically of the distal groin segment. Patients should have no anatomic evidence of infection involving the proximal aorta and an intact aorta-graft anastomosis. If the graft infection is localized to the femoral region only and the distal anastomosis is not involved, local treatment by drainage of the perigraft abscess without graft excision, radical débridement of the perigraft tissues, and topical povidone-iodine irrigation have been successful.[56] Muscle flap coverage of the exposed graft facilitates graft coverage and enhances wound healing.[73]

Treatment without graft excision is appropriate only in carefully selected patients and is not recommended when patients are septic, the prosthetic graft is occluded, anatomic signs of arterial infection are present, or the infecting organism is a *Pseudomonas* species.[19, 20] Patients treated by graft preservation should be monitored in the intensive care unit, and persistence of perigraft purulence or systemic signs of infection should prompt the surgeon to recommend total graft excision.

If infection is localized to the femoral region of a single aortofemoral graft limb but sepsis or anastomotic involvement (e.g., femoral pseudoaneurysm or bleeding) is present, graft excision is recommended. When vascular imaging studies indicate that the graft infection is limited to the groin, a retroperitoneal approach through an oblique, suprainguinal incision is recommended to confirm that the retroperitoneal aortic graft limb is not involved and to obtain proximal control (Fig. 47–7). If the graft limb is well incorporated and culture results of the excised graft are negative, the graft limb is removed and the remainder of the graft is retained.

After division of the graft limb through the retroperitoneal approach, adjacent tissue should be interposed between the oversewn proximal and distal ends of the graft. The retroperitoneal incision should then be closed, and the infected femoral graft limb should be excised through an inguinal incision. The entire graft-artery anastomosis to the femoral artery should be excised, the adjacent artery wall débrided, and autogenous patch closure attempted. Local endarterectomy may be required to facilitate closure.

Salvage of the common femoral artery is important in maintaining retrograde flow into the pelvis. If the superficial femoral artery is open, an alternative method is to anastomose the superficial femoral artery to the deep femoral artery end to end in order to maintain pelvic flow via collaterals from the deep femoral system (Fig. 47–8).

After graft excision, all arterial ligation sites or anastomoses should be covered with viable tissue. A rotational sartorius muscle flap is particularly useful for groin infections. The groin wound should be left open and treated with topical 0.1% povidone-iodine or antibiotic dressings.

Revascularization of the limb should be performed as necessary to maintain limb viability. Alternatives to revascularization depend on the patency of the distal circulation and can be performed to the deep femoral artery, the superficial femoral artery, or the popliteal artery. Revascularization should be accomplished via noninfected tissue planes using crossover femorofemoral grafts with medial tunneling or tunneling in the retropubic or suprapubic space, obturator bypass via the obturator canal, or lateral tunneling through the psoas tunnel to course diagonally distal to the distal outflow artery. These bypasses are usually performed with PTFE or with saphenous vein if it is large enough (i.e., ≥5 mm in diameter).

Carefully selected cases of femoral graft limb infection that are localized to the groin, that occur late in the postoperative course, and that are secondary to *S. epidermidis* may be treated by graft excision and in situ replacement. Perioperative and postoperative use of antibiotics, both systemic and topical, is imperative in treatment with graft excision and in situ replacement. Wide débridement of all inflamed perigraft tissues, including the inflamed adjacent artery wall, is essential. In situ replacement with a PTFE prosthesis is recommended, because it does have the best early graft healing rate after in situ replacement, both experimentally and clinically.[7, 10] It is recommended that patients continue to take intravenous antibiotics for 2 to 4 weeks after treatment and then oral antibiotics for 3 months.

Results of Treatment

In some series, treatment of aortic graft infections with extra-anatomic bypass and excision of the entire graft has resulted in high operative mortality rates and early amputa-

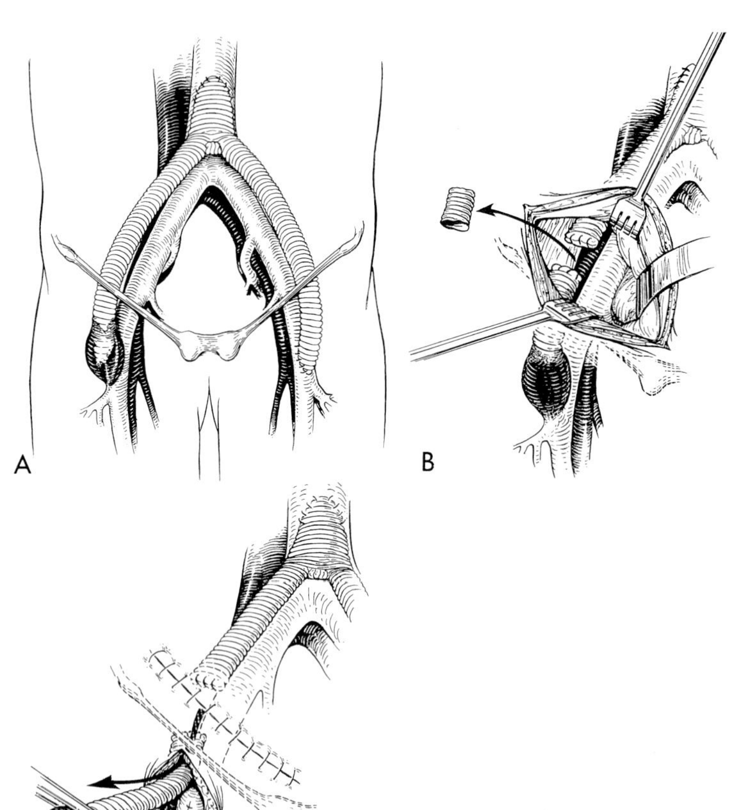

FIGURE 47–7. Excision of an infected femoral graft. *A*, Localized groin infection. *B*, Retroperitoneal exposure of noninfected graft segment. *C*, Excision of infected graft segment. (See text for details.)

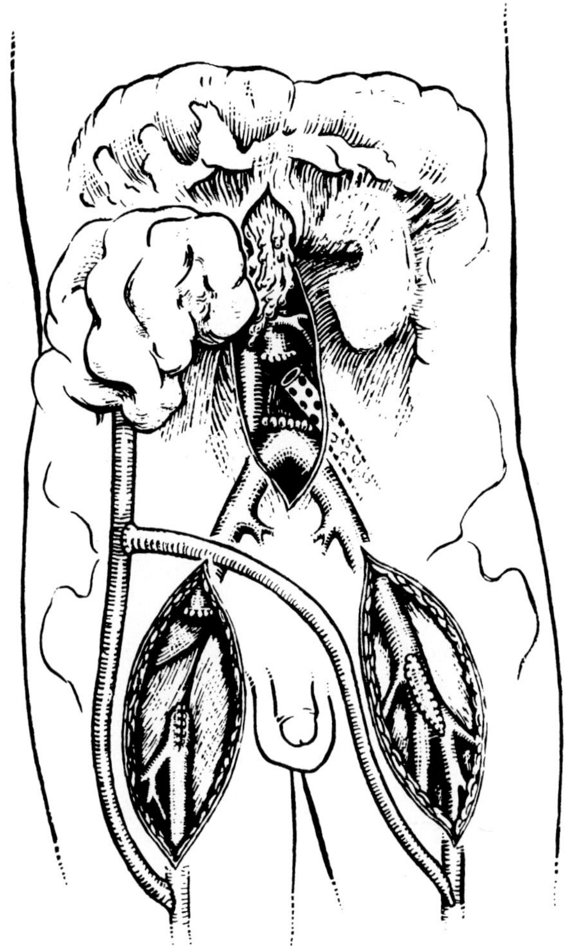

FIGURE 47–8. Excision of an infected aortobifemoral graft with extra-anatomic bypass.

tion rates (see Tables 47–8 and 47–9). Persistent sepsis and aortic stump blowout are the major causes of early and late mortality, but their incidence has decreased. Reilly and associates report a 21% decline in mortality, 19% in aortic disruption, and 27% in limb loss during a contemporary treatment interval (1980 to 1992).[75, 76] Improved outcomes were attributed to wide débridement of infected tissue beds, reduced intervals of lower body ischemia, and advances in perioperative management. Lower extremity amputation and recurrent infections of the extra-anatomic bypass are major causes of late morbidity. The risks of major amputation of the extremity and of failure of extra-anatomic bypass grafts are greater for aortic grafts with *groin* infections than for infected *aortoiliac* grafts.[91] Subsequent infection of an axillofemoral graft is associated with a significantly higher amputation rate than is an infection-free extra-anatomic bypass graft that fails because of thrombosis.[106]

The morbidity and mortality of extra-anatomic bypass grafting and total graft excision, combined with the high rate of late infection or failure of extra-anatomic bypass resulting in late lower extremity amputation, have prompted investigations into alternative methods of treatment in carefully selected patients. Infected aortobifemoral prostheses that are limited to the groin in a patient without sepsis and with an intact distal anastomosis can be treated with local operative débridement, antibiotics, and muscle flap coverage, as reported in several small series with good results.[62, 70]

Calligaro and associates achieved complete graft preservation and wound healing in 16 of 22 cases (73%) of graft infection due to gram-negative bacteria and in 23 of 33 cases (70%) due to gram-positive bacteria.[20] The potential for treatment failure exists nevertheless, and patients must be carefully monitored. All four deaths in this series (10% mortality) were due to graft sepsis; nine patients ultimately required total graft excision, and seven patients' surgical wounds never healed. *Pseudomonas* was a particularly virulent pathogen and was associated with failure of wound healing, anastomotic disruption, and arterial bed hemorrhage. Selective graft preservation carries a small but definite risk of hemorrhage owing to destruction of an anastomosis by the septic process. Findings of one study indicated that preservation of exposed or infected Dacron grafts was less successful than that of PTFE grafts.[19]

In situ replacement after prosthetic graft infections has been reported sporadically. Initial reports describe high (>50%) mortality rates in patients with GEF. More recent reports by Jacobs and coworkers[50] and Robinson and Johansen[78a] indicated mortality rates of less than 20% and long-term survival in 70% of patients when this procedure was applied for low-grade infections. Treatment of bacterial biofilm graft infections by in situ replacement was uniformly successful in one report, but confirmation from additional vascular centers is warranted.[7]

Endovascular Stent and Stent-Graft Infections

Infection of an endovascular device is a rare but grave complication, typically presenting with sepsis, mycotic aneurysm, and septic emboli. *S. aureus* is the most common pathogen. Treatment should consist of removal of the device and the involved arterial segment, followed or preceded by bypass ex situ. For low-grade infections that did not resolve with antibiotic therapy, replacement in situ with autologous vein or arterial allografts may be considered.

Femoral, Popliteal, and Tibial Graft Infections

Once the diagnosis of infrainguinal prosthetic bypass graft infection is made, excision of the entire graft is recommended in the context of anastomotic disruption or graft sepsis. The same principles that apply to aortic graft infection should be followed, including removal of the entire graft; radical débridement of infected perigraft tissues; débridement of the artery wall back to noninfected, uninflamed tissue; closure of the arteriotomies with monofilament suture; and administration of systemic and topical antibiotics. Often, a staged approach is advantageous, beginning with drainage of perigraft abscess and wound débridement, followed after several days by graft excision and vein bypass grafting via adjacent or remote tunneling. The treatment of peripheral graft infections is associated with a low mortality rate but a high amputation rate compared with treatment of aortic graft infections (Table 47–11).

Heparin should be administered intravenously when limb viability is jeopardized by graft excision. Patients

TABLE 47–11. RESULTS OF TREATMENT OF FEMOROPOPLITEAL OR TIBIAL PROSTHETIC GRAFT INFECTIONS

AUTHOR	NO. OF CASES	MORTALITY RATE (%)	AMPUTATION RATE (%)
Szilagyi et al, 1972[90]	10	0	50
Liekweg and Greenfield, 1977[58]	55	9	33
Yashar et al, 1978[105]	3	0	67
Durham et al, 1986[34]	3	0	67

whose prosthetic grafts were inserted because of claudication may be treated with graft excision alone. Patients with limb-threatening ischemia resulting from excision of the infected bypass should undergo revascularization, preferably with autogenous tissue. Frequently, however, autogenous tissue is not available, and reconstruction with prosthetic graft via remote, noninfected planes should be performed in lieu of amputation.

The local treatment of infrainguinal graft infections by aggressive perigraft tissue débridement, antibiotics, and muscle flap coverage, without graft excision, has been successful in patients who did not have graft sepsis or anastomotic disruption. Multiple small series[20, 59, 62] have shown that this alternative treatment can achieve healing in approximately 70% of cases and may not harm the patient as long as early, aggressive management by graft excision is undertaken when sepsis or anastomotic bleeding occurs.[70] When local treatment is successful, it may decrease rates of limb amputation for infrainguinal graft infection; however, there is no conclusive evidence to support this treatment in favor of the more conventional therapy of total graft excision, and remote or in situ vein revascularization as needed.

Thoracic Aortic Graft Infections

Thoracic aortic graft infection is a very grave complication (Table 47–12). The principles of graft excision and extra-anatomic bypass are not applicable to most cases of prosthetic aortic valve or ascending or transverse aortic arch graft infection.[28, 46] The principle of in situ maintenance of circulation must be followed. The operative approach to this severe infection should be wide débridement of the infected tissues, graft excision and replacement if anastomotic areas are involved or disrupted because of the infection, and coverage of the graft with viable, noninfected tissues. Pericardial fat pads, adjacent muscle (including pectoralis major, rectus abdominis, and latissimus dorsi) and the greater omentum pedicle have been used for graft coverage. These principles of treatment were used by Coselli and colleagues in 40 patients.[28] There were five operative deaths: two due to coagulopathy and hemorrhage and three to cardiopulmonary or renal complications. Twenty-eight patients (70%) were alive and showed no evidence of recurrent graft infection 4 months to 6.5 years later.

TABLE 47–12. COLLECTED SERIES RESULTS OF TREATMENT OF THORACIC, INNOMINATE, CAROTID, OR SUBCLAVIAN PROSTHETIC INFECTIONS

GRAFT SITE	NO. OF CASES	OPERATIVE DEATHS	PERIOPERATIVE STROKES*	SURVIVAL > 1 YEAR†
Thoracic	50	6	0	42
Innominate, carotid, or subclavian	33	9	3	14
Carotid patch	11	3	2	5

Data from Kieffer E et al, 1986[52]; Ehrenfeld et al, 1979[35]; and Bergamini et al, 1993.[12]

*All patients with strokes were treated by carotid ligation without reconstruction, which resulted in four operative deaths and one late death.

†Late follow-up was not reported for 13 patients with an innominate, a carotid, or a subclavian bypass graft and for one patient with a carotid patch.

Infections involving prosthetic grafts in the descending thoracic aorta may be amenable to graft excision and revascularization through clean, uninfected planes. A remote bypass graft can be placed through a median sternotomy from the ascending aorta to the abdominal aorta, tunneling through the diaphragm in clean, uninfected tissue. This graft should be placed before excision of the descending thoracic graft. After placement of this graft, the patient should undergo graft excision via left-sided thoracotomy.[46, 46a] The aortic closure should be covered with viable tissue transferred locally.

Innominate, Subclavian, and Carotid Graft Infections

Management of infection of a bypass or patch graft of an innominate, subclavian, or carotid artery should be based on the principles used for lower extremity graft infections. The risks of treatment of prosthetic infections at this site include not only persistent sepsis and death but also stroke (see Table 47–12). The surgical approach to an infected transthoracic bypass graft often requires a median sternotomy and preparation for cardiopulmonary bypass and total circulatory arrest if these are needed for proximal control.[52] Treatment should include total graft excision, parenteral and topical antibiotics, and remote bypass, preferably with autogenous tissue, if needed. There have been reports of successful treatment of infected prostheses with local irrigation, but this is not recommended because graft excision and remote revascularization are usually possible.

An infected transthoracic or extrathoracic bypass graft for upper extremity ischemia can often be removed without the need for immediate revascularization. Ligation of the proximal innominate or subclavian arteries, unlike ligation of the iliac or common femoral arteries, is often tolerated and does not provoke extremity ischemia. A subsequent bypass, if needed, can be performed after the infection clears. Only one case of upper extremity amputation after removal of a subclavian bypass graft for infection has been reported.[52] When upper extremity ischemia results from graft excision, bypass with autogenous tissue through remote planes is preferred. Patients with transthoracic bypass grafts to the innominate and subclavian arteries often have multivessel disease of the aortic arch, necessitating that remote bypasses use the femoral artery, the descending thoracic aorta, or the supraceliac abdominal aorta as the inflow vessel.

Remote bypass after excision of an infected carotid-subclavian bypass can be performed with a carotid-carotid bypass using saphenous vein or an axilloaxillary bypass using vein or PTFE (Fig. 47–9). After excision of an infected axilloaxillary graft, blood flow can be successfully reestablished with a supraclavicular subclavian-subclavian bypass, a carotid-carotid bypass, or a femoroaxillary bypass.

Patients with prosthetic infections of bypasses to the carotid arteries or with prosthetic patch infections of a carotid artery endarterectomy frequently do not tolerate simple ligation. In review of the reported cases of treatment of carotid prosthetic infections, all five perioperative strokes occurred in patients treated by ligation without reconstruction. Simple ligation of the common or internal carotid artery may be safely performed in patients with stump pressures higher than 70 mmHg, but reconstruction of the artery to maintain cerebral blood flow and prevent stroke should be performed when possible.

After graft excision, revascularization is best done with autogenous tissue. The anatomy of the extracranial carotid artery often does not permit remote bypass through noninfected, uninflamed tissues, and it often requires autogenous bypass in infected areas. Coverage of the bypass with muscle can be useful in this situation in preventing recurrence of infection. Autogenous bypasses with saphenous vein or internal iliac artery are successful alternatives.[35]

Treatment of carotid prosthetic patch infections is usually best achieved by excising the patch and reconstructing the vein. Carotid shunts have been successfully and safely used to maintain cerebral perfusion during these difficult, challenging procedures. Stroke, recurrent infection, and carotid pseudoaneurysm formation are late complications in 12% of cases.[12]

FUTURE DIRECTIONS

Dissatisfaction with the morbidity and mortality associated with treating graft infections, regardless of location, by total graft excision and remote bypass has been an impetus to the investigation of selective graft retention or in situ reconstruction. Selection criteria for these less aggressive treatment options have not been clinically verified, but experimental models have shown that treatment outcome depends on the virulence of the infecting organism, the extent of graft-artery infection, and the immune status of the patient. Appropriately designed and executed clinical trials are required to determine which patient group or groups are likely to benefit from these alternative treatments.

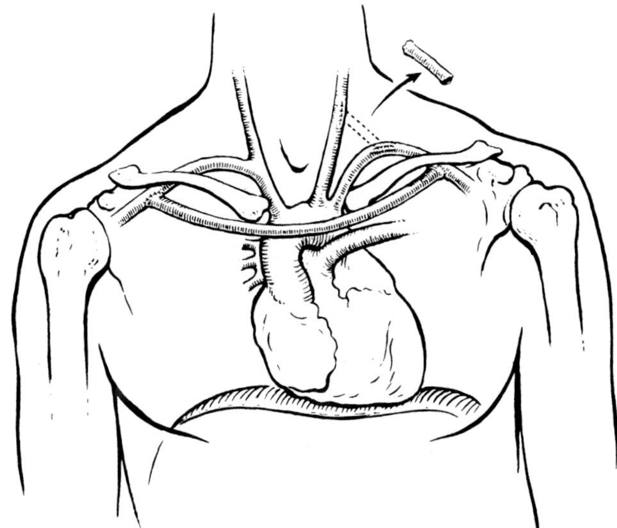

FIGURE 47–9. Excision of an infected carotid-subclavian graft with axilloaxillary bypass.

More studies are also warranted to investigate infection-resistant arterial conduits. The durability of cadaveric venous and aortic allografts is being studied as replacements after excision of an infected prosthetic vascular graft.[40, 51] Antibiotic-impregnated grafts are also on the clinical horizon. Experimentally, antibiotic bonding to vascular biomaterials is now possible, and its efficacy has been demonstrated under a variety of conditions (i.e., bacteremia, direct graft inoculation, and treatment of an established graft infection). Antibiotic-bonded grafts will probably afford the greatest clinical benefit to patients who are at high risk for graft infection or who have established low-grade graft infection and who are candidates for in situ replacement. The roles of omental or muscle coverage of infected or replacement bypass grafts are also under study. Future investigations of the pathogenesis, microbiology, anatomy, clinical presentation, and treatment of graft infection will benefit all surgical specialists who use biomaterials.

REFERENCES

1. Aarnio P, Hannukainen J: Aortic graft-enteric fistula. Ann Chir Gynaecol 78:329, 1989.
2. Abbott WM, Green RM, Matsumoto T, et al: Prosthetic above-knee femoropopliteal grafting: Results of a multicenter trial. J Vasc Surg 25:19, 1997.
3. Arnold PG, Pairolero PC: Intrathoracic muscle flaps in the surgical management of life-threatening hemorrhage from the heart and great vessels. Plast Reconstr Surg 81:831, 1988.
4. Bahnini A, Plissonnier D: Techniques et resultats des allogreffes arterielles dans les infections prothétiques aorto-iliaques. Presente a la 2 Reunion de l'Association pour la Transplantation Vasculaire, Paris, 25 Janvier 1997.

4a. Bakker-deWekker P, Alfieri O, Vermeulin F, et al: Surgical treatment of infected pseudoaneurysms after replacement of the ascending aorta. J Thorac Cardiovasc Surg 88:447, 1984.

5. Bandyk DF: Vascular graft infections: Epidemiology, microbiology, pathogenesis and prevention. *In* Bernhard VM, Towne JB (eds): Complications in Vascular Surgery. St. Louis, Quality Medical Publishing, 1991, pp 223–234.
6. Bandyk DF, Berni GA, Thiele BL, et al: Aortofemoral graft infection due to *Staphylococcus epidermidis*. Arch Surg 119:102, 1984.
7. Bandyk DF, Bergamini TM, Kinney EV, et al: In situ replacement of vascular prostheses infected by bacterial biofilms. J Vasc Surg 13:575, 1991.
8. Becker RM, Blundell PE: Infected aortic bifurcation grafts: Experience with fourteen patients. Surgery 80:544, 1976.
9. Bennion RS, Hiatt JR, Williams RA, et al: Surgical management of unilateral groin infection after aortofemoral bypass. Surg Gynecol Obstet 156:724, 1983.
10. Bergamini TM: Vascular prostheses infection caused by bacterial biofilms. Semin Vasc Surg 3:101, 1990.
11. Bergamini TM, Bandyk DF, Govostis D, et al: Identification of *Staphylococcus epidermidis* vascular graft infections: A comparison of culture techniques. J Vasc Surg 9:665, 1989.
12. Bergamini TM, Seabrook GR, Bandyk DF, et al: Symptomatic recur-

rent carotid stenosis and aneurysmal degeneration following endarterectomy. Surgery 113:580, 1993.
13. Blaisdell FW, DeMattei GA, Gauder PJ: Extraperitoneal thoracic aorta to femoral bypass graft as replacement for an infected aortic bifurcation prosthesis. Am J Surg 102:583, 1961.
14. Branchereau A, Magnan PE: Results of vertebral artery reconstruction. J Cardiovasc Surg 31:320, 1990.
15. Brenner WI, Richman H, Reed GE: Roof patch repair of an aortoduodenal fistula resulting from suture line failure in an aortic prosthesis. Am J Surg 127:762, 1974.
16. Buchbinder D, Leather R, Shah D, et al: Pathologic interactions between prosthetic aortic grafts and the gastrointestinal tract. Am J Surg 140:192, 1980.
17. Busuttil RW, Rees W, Baker JD, et al: Pathogenesis of aortoduodenal fistula: Experimental and clinical correlates. Surgery 85:1, 1979.
18. Calligaro KD, Veith FJ: Surgery of the infected aortic graft. *In* Bergan JJ, Yao JST (eds): Aortic Surgery. Philadelphia, WB Saunders, 1989, pp 485–496.
19. Calligaro KD, Westcott CJ, Buckley RM, et al: Infrainguinal anastomotic arterial graft infections treated by selective graft preservation. Ann Surg 216:74, 1993.
20. Calligaro KD, Veith FJ, Gupta SK, et al: A modified method of management of prosthetic graft infections involving an anastomosis to the common femoral artery. J Vasc Surg 11:485, 1990.
21. Carter SC, Cohen A, Whelan TJ: Clinical experience with management of the infected Dacron graft. Ann Surg 158:249, 1963.
22. Champion MC, Sullivan SN, Coles JC, et al: Aortoenteric fistula: Incidence, presentation, recognition, and management. Ann Surg 3:314, 1982.
23. Cherry KJ, Roland CF, Pairolero PC, et al: Infected femorodistal bypass: Is graft removal mandatory? J Vasc Surg 15:295, 1992.
24. Cohn R, Angell WW: Late complications from plastic replacement of aortic abdominal aneurysms. Arch Surg 87:696, 1968.
25. Conn JH, Hardy JD, Chavez CM: Infected arterial grafts: Experience in 22 cases with emphasis on unusual bacteria and techniques. Ann Surg 171:704, 1970.
26. Connelly JE, Kwaan JHM, McCart PM, et al: Aortoenteric fistula. Ann Surg 4:402, 1981.
27. Conte CC, Ellison LH: Management of extracranial carotid artery aneurysms. Conn Med 50:501, 1986.
28. Coselli JS, Crawford ES, Williams TW, et al: Treatment of postoperative infection of ascending aorta and transverse aortic arch, including use of viable omentum and muscle flaps. Ann Thorac Surg 50:868, 1990.
29. Crawford ES, DeBakey ME, Morris GC Jr, et al: Evaluation of late failures after reconstructive operations for occlusive lesions of the aorta and iliac, femoral, and popliteal arteries. Surgery 17:79, 1960.
30. Criado FJ: Extrathoracic management of aortic arch syndrome. Br J Surg 69(Suppl):S45, 1982.
31. Dean RH, Allen TR, Foster JH, et al: Aortoduodenal fistula: An uncommon but correctable cause of upper gastrointestinal bleeding. Am Surg 44:37, 1978.
32. DeBakey ME, Crawford ES, Morris GC Jr, et al: Patch graft angioplasty in vascular surgery. J Cardiovasc Surg 3:106, 1962.
32a. Deiparine MK, Ballard JL, Taylor FC, Chase DR: Endovascular stent infection. J Vasc Surg 23:529, 1996.
33. Diethrich EB, Noon GP, Liddicoat JE, et al: Treatment of infected aortofemoral arterial prosthesis. Surgery 68:1044, 1970.
34. Durham JR, Rubin JR, Malone JM: Management of infected infrainguinal bypass grafts. *In* Bergan JJ, Yao JST (eds): Reoperative Arterial Surgery. Orlando, Fla, Grune & Stratton, 1986, pp 359–373
35. Ehrenfeld WK, Wilbur BG, Olcott CN, et al: Autogenous tissue reconstruction in the management of infected prosthetic grafts. Surgery 85:82, 1979.
36. Elliott JP, Smith RF, Szilagyi DE: Aortoenteric and paraprosthetic-enteric fistulas. Arch Surg 108:479, 1974.
37. Ferris EJ, Koltay MRS, Koltay OP, et al: Abdominal aortic and iliac graft fistulae—unusual roentgenographic findings. Surgery 94:416, 1965.
38. Flye MW, Thompson WM: Aortic graft-enteric and paraprosthetic-enteric fistulas. Am J Surg 146:183, 1983.
39. Fry WJ, Lindenauer SM: Infection complicating the use of plastic arterial implants. Arch Surg 94:600, 1966.
40. Fujitani RM, Bassiouny HS, Gewertz BL, et al: Cryopreserved saphenous vein allogenic homografts: An alternative conduit in lower extremity arterial reconstruction in infected fields. J Vasc Surg 15:519, 1992.
41. Fulenwider JT, Smith RB, Johnson RW, et al: Reoperative abdominal arterial surgery—a ten-year experience. Surgery 93:20, 1983.
42. Garrett HE, Beall AC, Jordan GL Jr, et al: Surgical considerations of massive gastrointestinal tract hemorrhage caused by aortoduodenal fistula. Am J Surg 105:6, 1963.
43. Geary KJ, Tomkiewicz ZM, Harrison HN, et al: Differential effects of a gram-negative and a gram-positive infection on autogenous and prosthetic grafts. J Vasc Surg 11:339, 1990.
44. Goldstone J, Moore WS: Infection in vascular prostheses: Clinical manifestations and surgical management. Am J Surg 128:225, 1974.
45. Graver JM, Mulcare RJ: Pseudoaneurysm after carotid endarterectomy. J Cardiovasc Surg 27:294, 1986.
46. Hargrove WC III, Edmunds H Jr: Management of infected thoracic aortic prosthetic grafts. Ann Thorac Surg 37:72, 1984.
46a. Hennes N, Sandmann W, Torsello G, et al: Infection of a vascular prosthesis: A retrospective analysis of 99 cases. Chirurg 67:37, 1996.
47. Hoffert PW, Gensler S, Haimovici H: Infection complicating arterial grafts. Arch Surg 90:427, 1965.
48. Humphries AW, Young JR, deWolfe VG, et al: Complications of abdominal aortic surgery. Arch Surg 86:43, 1963.
49. Jamieson GG, DeWeese JA, Rob CG: Infected arterial grafts. Ann Surg 181:850, 1975.
50. Jacobs MJHM, Reul GJ, Gregoric I, et al: In situ replacement and extra-anatomic bypass for the treatment of infected abdominal aortic grafts. Eur J Vasc Surg 5:83, 1991.
50a. Johnston KW: Multicenter prospective study of nonruptured abdominal aortic aneurysm: Part II. Variables predicting morbidity and mortality. J Vasc Surg 9:437, 1989.
51. Kieffer E, Bahnini A, Koskas F, et al: In situ allograft replacement of infected infrarenal aortic prosthetic grafts: Results in 43 patients. J Vasc Surg 17:349, 1993.
52. Kieffer E, Petitjean C, Bahnini A: Surgery for failed brachycephalic reconstruction. *In* Bergan JJ, Yao JST (eds): Reoperative Arterial Surgery. Orlando, Fla, Grune & Stratton, 1986, pp 581–607.
53. Kitka MJ, Goodson SF, Rishara RA, et al: Mortality and limb loss with infected infrainguinal bypass grafts. J Vasc Surg 5:566, 1987.
54. Kleinman LH, Towne JB, Bernhard VM: A diagnostic and therapeutic approach to aortoenteric fistulas: Clinical experience with twenty patients. Surgery 86:868, 1979.
55. Kozol RA, Bredenberg CE: Alternatives in the management of atherosclerotic occlusive disease of aortic arch branches. Arch Surg 116:1457, 1981.
56. Kwaan JHM, Connolly JE: Successful management of prosthetic graft infection with continuous povidone-iodine irrigation. Arch Surg 116:716, 1981.
57. Levy MF, Schmitt DD, Edmiston CE, et al: Sequential analysis of staphylococcal colonization of body surfaces of patients undergoing vascular surgery. J Clin Microbiol 28:664, 1990.
58. Liekweg WG Jr, Greenfield LJ: Vascular prosthetic infections: Collected experience and results of treatment. Surgery 81:335, 1977.
59. Lorentzen JE, Nielsen OM, Arendrup H, et al: Vascular graft infection: An analysis of sixty-two graft infections in 2411 consecutively implanted synthetic vascular grafts. Surgery 98:81, 1985.
60. Martinez NS: Extracranial carotid aneurysm: A complication of carotid endarterectomy. Illinois Med J 150:583, 1976.
61. McCollum CH, Wheeler WG, Noon GP, et al: Aneurysms of the extracranial carotid artery. Am J Surg 137:196, 1979.
62. Mixter RC, Turnipseed WD, Smith DJ Jr, et al: Rotational muscle flaps: A new technique for covering infected vascular grafts. J Vasc Surg 9:472, 1989.
63. Moncure AC, Brewster DC, Darling RC, et al: Use of the splenic and hepatic arteries for renal revascularization. J Vasc Surg 3:196, 1986.
64. Najafi H, Javid H, Dye WS, et al: Management of infected arterial implants. Surgery 65:539, 1969.
65. Ochsner JL, Mills NL: Profound hypothermia and circulatory arrest in control and repair of infected aortic prostheses. J Cardiovasc Surg 20:1, 1979.
66. O'Hara PJ, Hertzer NR, Beven EG, et al: Surgical management of infected abdominal aortic grafts: Review of a 25-year experience. J Vasc Surg 3:725, 1986.
67. Olofsson PA, Auffermann W, Higgins CB, et al: Diagnosis of prosthetic aortic graft infection by magnetic resonance imaging. J Vasc Surg 8:99, 1988.

68. O'Mara CS, Williams GM, Ernst CB: Secondary aortoenteric fistula. Am J Surg 142:203, 1981.
69. Pinkerton JA: Aortoduodenal fistula. JAMA 225:1196, 1973.
70. Piotrowski JJ, Bernhard VM: Management of vascular graft infections. *In* Bernhard VM, Towne JB (eds): Complications in Vascular Surgery. St. Louis, Quality Medical Publishing, 1991, pp 235–258.
71. Popovsky J, Singer S: Infected prosthetic grafts. Arch Surg 115:203, 1980.
72. Proctor CD, Rice KL, Lucas MR: Comparison of ankle-brachial indexes and magnetic resonance flowmetry in predicting outcome in diabetic foot lesions (Abstract). J Vasc Surg 15:242, 1992.
73. Quinones-Baldrich WJ, Hernandez JJ, Moore WS: Long-term results following surgical management of aortic graft infection. Arch Surg 126:507, 1991.
74. Raskind R, Doria A: Wound complications following carotid endarterectomy: Report of two cases. J Vasc Surg 1:127, 1967.
75. Reilly LM, Stoney RJ, Goldstone J, et al: Improved management of aortic graft infection: The influence of operation sequence and staging. J Vasc Surg 5:421, 1987.
76. Reilly LM, Altman H, Lusby RJ, et al: Late results following surgical management of vascular graft infection. J Vasc Surg 1:36, 1984.
77. Reul GJ Jr, Cooley DA: False aneurysms of the carotid artery. *In* Bergan JJ, Yao JST (eds): Reoperative Arterial Surgery. Orlando, Fla, Grune & Stratton, 1986, pp 537–553.
78. Rhodes VJ: Expanded polytetrafluoroethylene patch angioplasty in carotid endarterectomy. J Vasc Surg 22:724, 1995.
78a. Robinson JA, Johansen K: Aortic sepsis: Is there a role for in situ graft reconstruction? J Vasc Surg 13:677, 1991.
79. Rosato FE, Barker C, Roberts B: Aorto-intestinal fistula. J Thorac Cardiovasc Surg 53:511, 1967.
79a. Rosenthal D, Archie JP, Garcia-Rinaldi R, et al: Carotid patch angioplasty: Intermediate and long-term results. J Vasc Surg 12:326, 1990.
80. Samson RH, Veith FJ, Janko GS, et al: A modified classification and approach to the management of infections involving peripheral arterial prosthetic grafts. J Vasc Surg 8:147, 1988.
81. Santschi DR, Frahm CJ, Pascale LR, et al: The subclavian steal syndrome: Clinical and angiographic considerations in 74 cases in adults. J Thorac Cardiovasc Surg 51:103, 1966.
82. Schmitt DD, Seabrook GR, Bandyk DF, et al: Graft excision and extra-anatomic revascularization: The treatment of choice for the septic aortic prosthesis. J Cardiovasc Surg 31:327, 1990.
83. Schroeder T, Hansen HJH: Arterial reconstruction of the brachycephalic trunk and the subclavian arteries. Acta Chir Scand 502:122, 1980.
84. Shaw RS, Baue AE: Management of sepsis complicating arterial reconstructive surgery. Surgery 53:75, 1963.
85. Seeger JM, Wheeler JR, Gregory RT, et al: Autogenous graft replacement of infected prosthetic grafts in the femoral position. Surgery 93:39, 1983.
86. Smith RB III, Lowry K, Perdue GD: Management of the infected arterial prosthesis in the lower extremity. Am Surg 33:711, 1967.
87. Snyder SO, Wheeler JR, Gregory RT, et al: Freshly harvested cadaveric venous homografts as arterial conduits in infected fields. Surgery 101:283, 1987.
88. Spanos PK, Gilsdorf RB, Sako Y, et al: The management of infected abdominal aortic grafts and graft-enteric fistulas. Ann Surg 183:397, 1976.
89. Sproul G: Rupture of an infected aortic graft into jejunum: Resection and survival. JAMA 182:1118, 1962.
90. Szilagyi DE, Smith RF, Elliott JP, et al: Infection in arterial reconstruction with synthetic grafts. Ann Surg 176:321, 1972.
91. Taylor SM, Mills JL, Fujitani RM, et al: The influence of groin sepsis on extra-anatomic bypass patency in patients with prosthetic graft infection. Ann Vasc Surg 6:80, 1992.
92. Thompson JE: Complications of carotid endarterectomy and their prevention. World J Surg 3:155, 1979.
93. Thistlethwaite JR, Hughes RK, Smyth NPD, et al: Spontaneous arteriovenous fistula between the abdominal aorta and vena cava. Arch Surg 81:79, 1960.
94. Thomas WEG, Baird RN: Secondary aorto-enteric fistulae: Towards a more conservative approach. Br J Surg 73:875, 1986.
95. Thompson BW, Read RC, Campbell GS: Operative correction of obstructed subclavian or innominate arteries. South Med J 71:1366, 1978.
96. Thompson BW, Read RC, Campbell GS: Operative correction of proximal blocks of the subclavian or innominate arteries. J Cardiovasc Surg 21:125, 1980.
97. Thompson JE, Kartchner MM, Auston DJ, et al: Carotid endarterectomy for cerebrovascular insufficiency (stroke): Follow-up of 359 cases. Ann Surg 163:751, 1966.
98. Tobias JA, Daicoff GR: Aortogastric and aortoileal fistulas repaired by direct suture. Arch Surg 107:909, 1973.
99. Trout HH, Kozloff L, Giordano JM: Priority of revascularization in patients with graft enteric fistulas, infected arteries, or infected arterial prostheses. Ann Surg 199:669, 1984.
100. Turnipseed WD, Berkoff HA, Detmer DE, et al: Arterial graft infections: Delayed v. immediate vascular reconstruction. Arch Surg 118:410, 1983.
101. Van De Water JM, Gaal PG: Management of patients with infected vascular prostheses. Am Surg 31:651, 1965.
102. Veith FJ, Hartsuck JM, Crane C: Management of aortoiliac reconstruction complicated by sepsis and hemorrhage. N Engl J Med 270:1389, 1964.
103. Walker WE, Cooley DA, Duncan JM, et al: The management of aortoduodenal fistula by in situ replacement of the infected abdominal aortic graft. Ann Surg 205:727, 1987.
104. Welling RE, Cranley JJ, Krause RJ, et al: Obliterative arterial disease of the upper extremity. Arch Surg 116:1593, 1981.
105. Yashar JJ, Weyman AK, Birnard RJ, et al: Survival and limb salvage in patients with infected arterial prostheses. Am J Surg 135:499, 1978.
106. Yeager RA, Moneta GL, Taylor LM, et al: Improving survival and limb salvage in patients with aortic graft infection. Am J Surg 159:466, 1990.

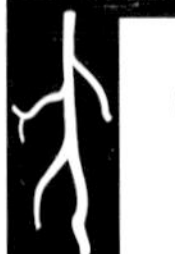

CHAPTER 48

Anastomotic and Other Pseudoaneurysms

Lewis B. Schwartz, M.D., Elizabeth T. Clark, M.D., and
Bruce L. Gewertz, M.D.

Pseudoaneurysms result from a variety of mechanisms, including infection, trauma, and surgical procedures (Fig. 48–1). All have in common the disruption of arterial continuity with extravasation of blood into surrounding tissues. This process ultimately results in the formation of a fibrous tissue capsule that progressively enlarges owing to unrelenting arterial pressure. This chapter focuses on the pathogenesis and natural history of pseudoaneurysms and considers the diverse clinical presentations, diagnostic modalities, and treatment options.

HISTORY

Considerable attention has been given throughout ancient and modern history to the cause and treatment of pseudoaneurysms. Pseudoaneurysm formation was a frequent complication of bloodletting, a practice that was popular for more than 2000 years.[1] In fact, the first successful direct arterial repair, by Lambert in 1759, was performed for a brachial artery pseudoaneurysm after phlebotomy.[2] Subsequent successful reports of traumatic pseudoaneurysm repair by Matas,[3] Lexer,[4] and Pringle[5] at the turn of the twentieth century confirmed the feasibility of arterial suture and led to the development of modern vascular surgery.

Pseudoaneurysms continued to be clinical challenges in recent times. Early prosthetic grafting operations were often complicated by pseudoaneurysm formation due to the frequent degeneration of silk sutures used in the anastomoses.[6–8] Traumatic pseudoaneurysms have become more commonplace as a result of escalation of civilian violence in western society. Finally, the widespread use of percutaneous arterial techniques, beginning in the late 1970s, has ensured that pseudoaneurysms remain a frequent finding in vascular surgical practice.

ANASTOMOTIC PSEUDOANEURYSMS

Etiology

Anastomotic pseudoaneurysms occur as a result of arterial reconstructions or repairs. Their incidence reflects the site of the procedure in that anastomoses under tension or anatomically predisposed to traction are more at risk. The use of prosthetic materials has long been associated with pseudoaneurysm formation because, regardless of the extent of soft tissue "incorporation," mesenchymal tissue ingrowth alone is inadequate to provide the required strength. The integrity of the union between artery and prosthetic graft, therefore, depends forever on the durability and purchase of the suture material. Before 1967, when silk suture material was widely used, up to one fourth of all anastomoses between prosthetic grafts and femoral arteries resulted in pseudoaneurysm formation. There appears to be a decline in the incidence of pseudoaneurysms, owing to improvements in technique, suture strength, and graft design. Nonetheless, graft-arterial disruption remains common, even though few of these disruptions produce clinically important symptoms.

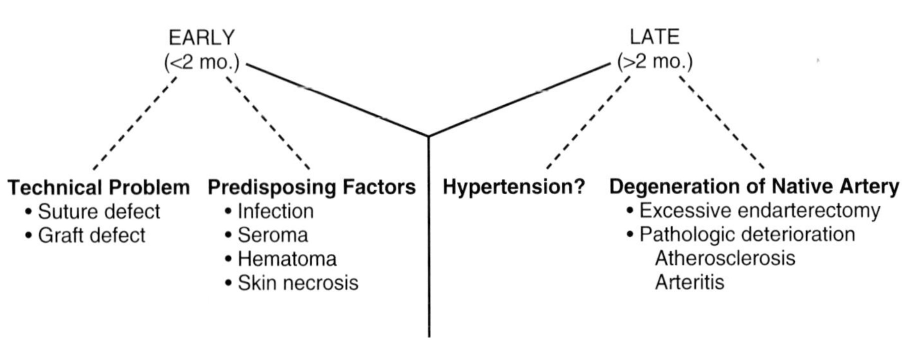

FIGURE 48–1. The etiology and evolution of pseudoaneurysms. A disruption of arterial continuity usually precedes pseudoaneurysmal development, which is propagated by unrelenting arterial pressure.

Other factors implicated in anastomotic aneurysm formation include differences in compliance between native arteries and graft materials, shearing forces along anastomotic lines, vibratory fatigue, graft positioning, and anticoagulation; in all of these situations, blood may escape from the vessel via partial "dehiscence" of the suture line. Theoretically, elongated end-to-side anastomoses may result in localized dilatation and increased tangential tension according to Laplace's law,

$$\text{tension} = \frac{\text{pressure}}{\text{radius}}$$

Because most graft materials are less compliant than native arteries, there is preferential dilatation of the artery, which results in potentially disruptive stresses on the anastomosis.

Loss of structural integrity results not only from suture material fatigue and prosthesis degeneration but also from progressive disease of the host vessel. Fibrous degeneration of the media leads to decreased elasticity, which inhibits arterial adaptability to diverse mechanical stresses. Other causes of host vessel degeneration include the expected progression of atherosclerotic disease, the accumulation of perigraft fluid collections, aggressive endarterectomy, and extensive artery mobilization during the initial procedure.

Graft infection undoubtedly plays a role in the development of pseudoaneurysms. In surgically treated pseudoaneurysms with no clinical evidence of infection, as many as 60% are culture-positive when meticulous bacteriologic recovery techniques are employed.[9] The most common organisms are *Staphylococcus epidermidis* and other coagulase-negative staphylococcal species. Bacteria-borne cytolysins cause disincorporation of the graft from host tissues and increase the propensity for pseudoaneurysm formation.

Diagnosis and Treatment

Most pseudoaneurysms present as asymptomatic pulsatile masses. Some cause local symptoms such as pain, rapid expansion, or venous obstruction. Owing to the mechanisms discussed earlier, the most common site of presentation is the groin. The average patient age at presentation of 62 years, with a range of 20 to 86 years.[10–16] The average graft age is 6.2 years, with a range of 2.5 months to 19 years. Earlier presentation is often correlated with infection or multiple operations.

Diagnosis is aided by ultrasonography and duplex imaging, computed tomography (CT), and angiography. Ultrasonography is useful for defining the size and extent of the pseudoaneurysm and perigraft fluid. Color flow Doppler images have additional utility for detecting blood flow into pseudoaneurysmal cavities and have a diagnostic sensitivity and specificity of 95%.[17] CT scanning is particularly helpful for evaluating pseudoaneurysm morphology and the integrity of surrounding structures such as the retroperitoneum. Angiography is most useful for planning operative strategy.

Femoral Anastomotic Pseudoaneurysms

Femoral pseudoaneurysms are by far the most common type of pseudoaneurysm and account for more than 75% of all clinically important lesions (Fig. 48–2). The most

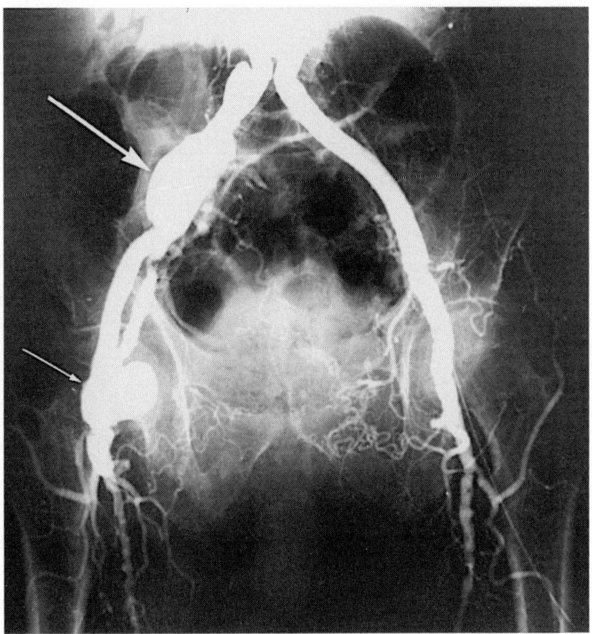

FIGURE 48–2. Femoral and graft-graft pseudoaneurysm formation in a 71-year-old man presenting with a pulsatile right groin mass 6 years after emergent reoperation of iliac-to-femoral interposition grafting. Note the pseudoaneurysms at the graft-graft *(large arrow)* and femoral artery *(small arrow)* anastomoses.

common cause is disruption of a prosthetic arterial anastomosis after either aortofemoral or infrainguinal bypass. With vigorous surveillance, they are detected after 14% to 44% of femoral anastomoses,[18–20] although the cumulative risk of clinically important pseudoaneurysms is probably less than 10%.[13, 21, 22] The appearance of femoral anastomotic aneurysms is clearly a function of time because the risk increases with the age of the patient and graft.

When left untreated, femoral pseudoaneurysms can be complicated by thrombosis, distal embolization, or rupture. It is generally accepted that these sequelae are unusual if the pseudoaneurysm is asymptomatic and less than 2 cm in diameter. Because the morbidity of emergent operation far exceeds that of elective repair, early diagnosis and treatment are the standard of care. Placement of an interposition conduit, composed of either prosthetic material or saphenous vein, is usually the preferred procedure (Fig. 48–3). The operation is generally well tolerated, with less than 4% mortality and more than 90% 2-year patency.[16] In contrast, emergent procedures are associated with excessive rates of amputation and mortality.

The treatment of mycotic (infected) femoral pseudoaneurysms is considerably more problematic. The general principles that guide therapy include drainage and débridement of all infected material and selective revascularization with autologous tissue or extra-anatomic reconstruction. Reddy and associates reviewed the course of 54 patients with intravenous drug abuse (IVDA)–related femoral artery pseudoaneurysms.[23] When the pseudoaneurysm was confined to a single arterial segment (common femoral, superficial femoral, or profunda femoris), that artery could be sacrificed without limb loss. Patients in whom the common femoral or superficial femoral artery was ligated generally

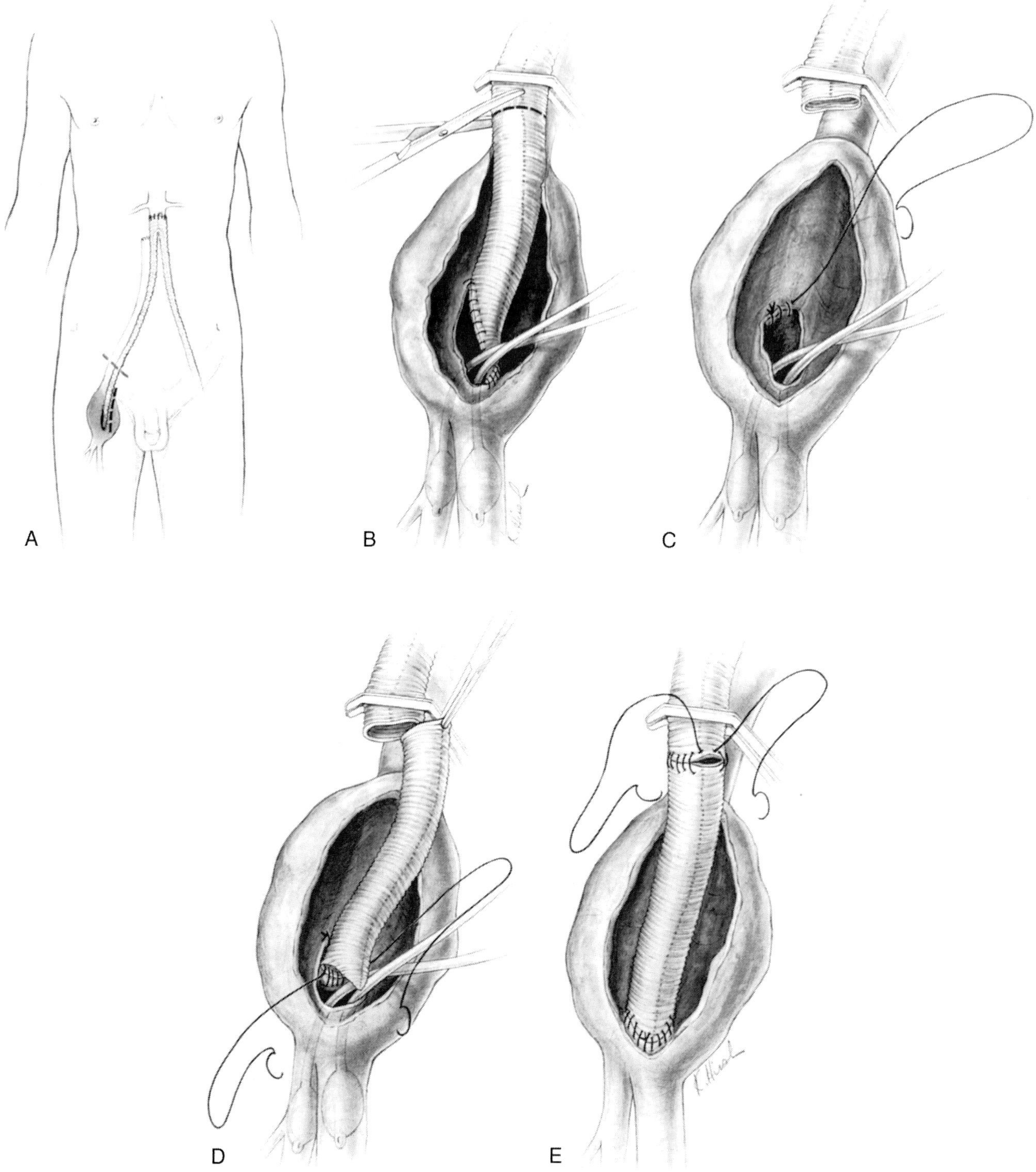

FIGURE 48–3. Surgical repair of femoral anastomotic pseudoaneurysm. *A,* Most femoral pseudoaneurysms can be repaired through the previous groin incision. *B,* The pseudoaneurysm is exposed anteriorly, and control of the limb of the aortofemoral bypass is obtained above the aneurysm. After systemic heparinization, the graft is clamped and the aneurysm is entered. The superficial and deep femoral branches are controlled from within the aneurysm with balloon catheters. The limb of the aortofemoral bypass is transected, the distal anastomosis is excised, and the distal graft segment is removed. *C,* The orifice of the native common femoral artery is oversewn from within the aneurysm. *D,* A new segment of prosthetic Dacron graft, with a diameter matching that of the original graft limb, is sutured to the orifices of the superficial femoral and deep femoral arteries. Large, deep bites are taken to ensure full-thickness passage of each suture. *E,* After completion of the distal anastomosis, the balloon catheters are removed, and a clamp is placed on the Dacron graft for hemostasis. The new graft is then anastomosed end-to-end to the original Dacron graft. (From Zarins CK, Gewertz BL: Atlas of Vascular Surgery. New York, Churchill Livingstone, 1989, pp 195, 197.)

developed claudication, but its treatment could be delayed until after the infection had resolved.

In contrast, attempts at treatment of pseudoaneurysms involving the femoral bifurcation by "triple ligation" (common femoral, superficial femoral, and profunda femoris arteries) are generally unsuccessful, resulting in acute ischemia and amputation in one third of the patients. These patients are best treated by immediate revascularization.[23, 24] If autologous vein is available, the best option for reconstruction is in situ interposition grafting. This avoids potential contamination of remote sites during extra-anatomic bypass. Frequently, however, the saphenous vein is not available. For these patients, the infected skin should be excluded from the surgical field and an obturator, femoral crossover, axillopopliteal, or axilloprofunda bypass performed through noninfected tissue planes.[24] Revascularization of a single outflow vessel is usually adequate for preservation of the extremity. More complete vascularization can be rendered, if necessary, after the infection is resolved.

At the University of Chicago, we have used both in situ repair and extra-anatomic bypass with cryopreserved veins as a temporizing procedure.[25] After the local infection has resolved, more durable reconstructions can be undertaken with autologous tissue or even prosthetic grafts.

Aortic Anastomotic Pseudoaneurysms

Aortic anastomotic pseudoaneurysms are rare, complicating only about 2% to 10% of all aortic operations.[18, 19, 26, 27] They are generally thought to be more common after emergent procedures. In the absence of symptoms, they are difficult to diagnose and are often found during evaluations for other conditions. Patients may occasionally note the presence of a pulsatile abdominal mass, back pain, or weight loss. Unfortunately, many of these lesions present catastrophically, with acute expansion, rupture, infection, or distal embolization (Fig. 48–4).

Patients with aortic anastomotic pseudoaneurysms that are more than 50% the diameter of the graft or are symptomatic should be considered for surgical repair. Direct aortic reconstruction is usually preferred, and the mortality rate of elective operations is less than 10%.[28] In contrast, survival after emergent repair is rare. Because of the difficulty in reoperative aortic surgery, endoluminal exclusion has been advocated for treatment of these lesions.[29, 30]

Carotid Pseudoaneurysms

Carotid endarterectomy is rarely associated with pseudoaneurysm formation; the incidences in various studies range from 0.15% to 0.6%,[31, 32] and only about 400 cases appear in the literature.[33] Other causes include penetrating trauma (Fig. 48–5),[34–36] blunt trauma,[37] and, rarely, fibromuscular dysplasia.[38] Symptoms generally occur 4 to 6 months after operation and may include a painful pulsatile cervical mass, transient ischemic attacks secondary to embolization, and hoarseness due to recurrent laryngeal nerve compression. Differential diagnosis includes chemodectoma of the carotid body, lymphadenopathy, peritonsillar abscess, and kinking of an endarterectomized carotid artery. These causes usually can be distinguished from pseudoaneurysmal disease by duplex imaging. Before 1960, roughly half of all carotid pseudoaneurysms that occurred after endarterectomy were associated with prosthetic patching. Their occurrence may be more rationally attributed to the use of silk suture, however. Various reports from that era confirm an extremely high incidence of pseudoaneurysm formation (as great as 80%) when silk suture material was utilized.[39]

Most patients with pseudoaneurysms after carotid endarterectomy should undergo operative correction to eliminate the risk of embolization. Because simple ligation is associated with at least a 20% incidence of major stroke, revascularization with interposition grafting is preferred. The dissection may be tedious owing to the presence of scar and difficulty in preserving the vagus and hypoglossal nerves.

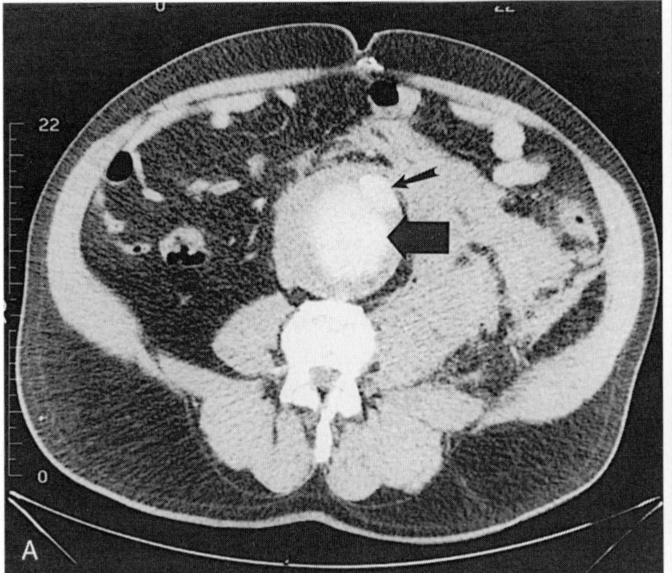

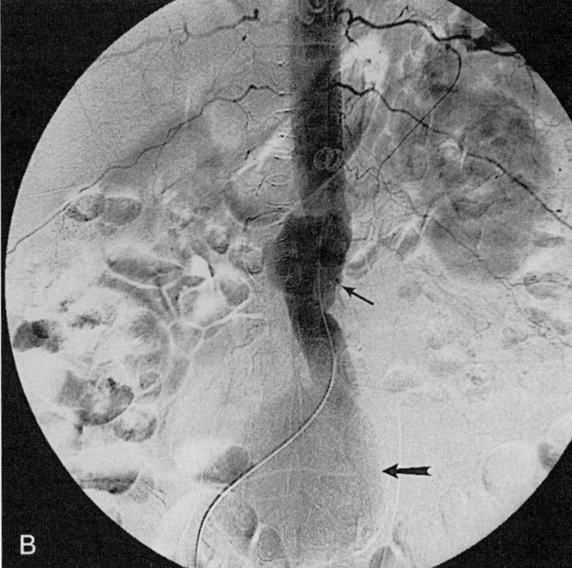

FIGURE 48–4. Massive aortic anastomotic pseudoaneurysm in a 69-year-old man who underwent aortic aneurysm repair 20 years prior to presentation. *A*, contrast-enhanced CT scan showing opacification of graft lumen *(small arrow)* and anastomotic pseudoaneurysm *(large arrow)*. *B*, Anteroposterior aortogram showing massive distal anastomotic pseudoaneurysm *(large arrow)* and smaller proximal anastomotic pseudoaneurysm *(small arrow)*.

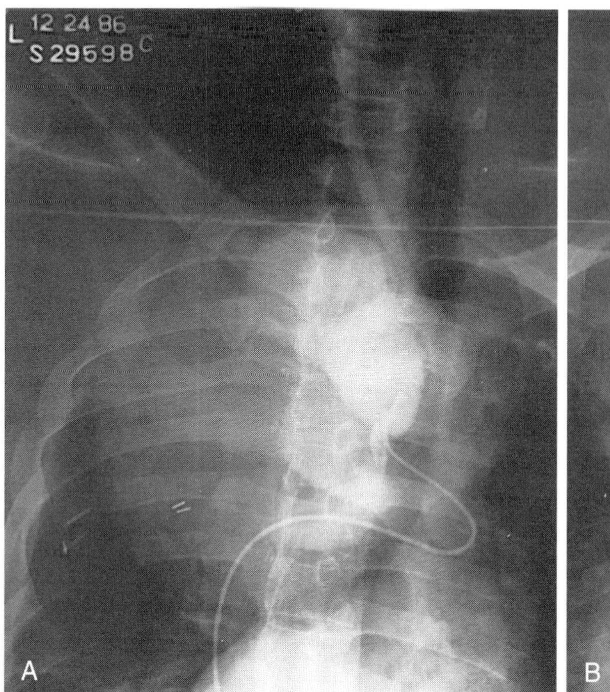

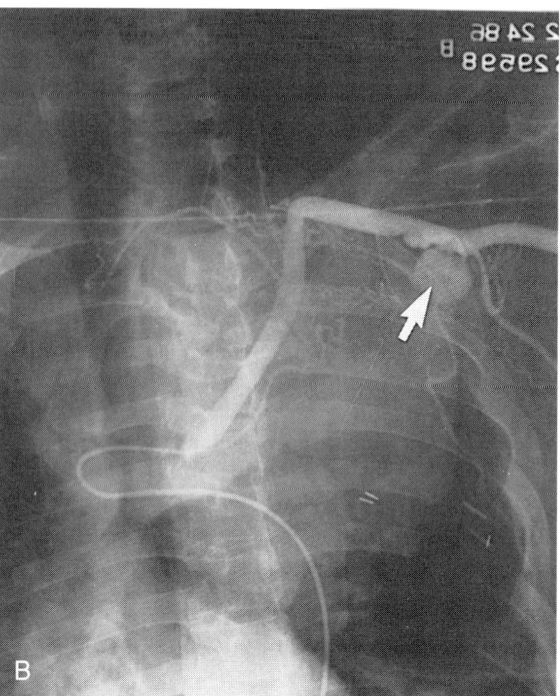

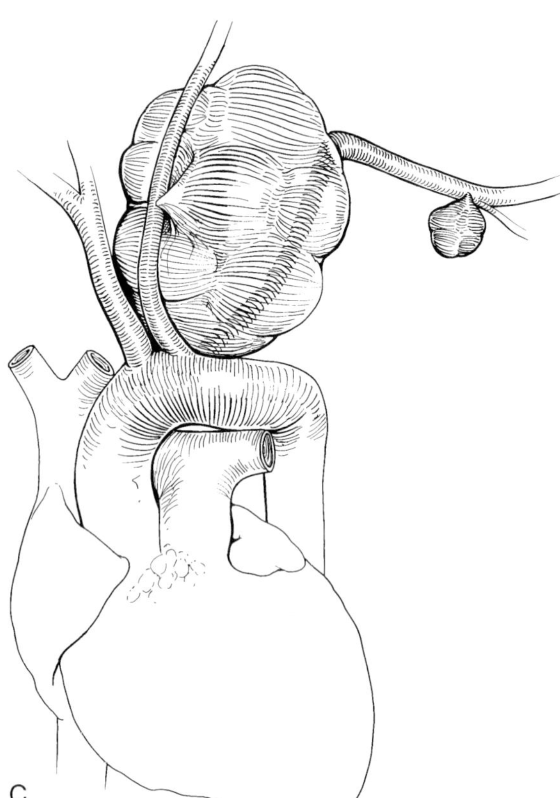

FIGURE 48–5. Traumatic pseudoaneurysm of the left common carotid and subclavian arteries in a 37-year-old man with a remote history of penetrating chest and arm trauma. The suspicion of malignancy prompted a course of chemotherapy before the diagnosis was confirmed. *A,* Direct left common carotid injection demonstrating a massive pseudoaneurysm. *B,* Left subclavian injection demonstrating another pseudoaneurysm. *C,* Drawing of lesions. (From Schwartz LB, McCann RL: Traumatic false aneurysm of the common carotid artery presenting as a mediastinal mass. J Vasc Surg 10:281–284, 1989.)

Manipulation of the aneurysmal sac should be minimized; control of the common, internal, and external carotid arteries should be obtained first. Exposure of the distal internal carotid artery may be facilitated by division of the posterior belly of the digastric muscle with or without mandibular subluxation. Once vascular control is established, the aneurysmal sac is opened and a shunt placed as indicated. Infection must be considered, and cultures of thrombus, prosthetic material, and degenerated arterial wall should be obtained.

Several options for repair are available based on the size of the defect and the virulence of infection. If the defect is small and sterile, primary closure may be undertaken. If the defect is large, patch angioplasty with either prosthetic material or saphenous vein may be required. If the bifurcation has completely degenerated, a saphenous vein bypass from the more proximal common carotid artery to the internal carotid artery may be necessary. Although the mortality rate of repair in early studies was 40%,[40] series in the modern era have reported minimal mortality and neurologic deficit.[38, 41, 42] The feasibility of selected pseudoaneurysm obliteration with endovascular stenting has also been demonstrated.[30, 43]

Primary *mycotic* carotid pseudoaneurysms are rare, but they are associated with lethal complications. An aneurysmal abscess or pseudoaneurysm should be suspected in any drug-abusing patient with a painful neck mass and cellulitis. Although the diagnosis may be confirmed by duplex imaging, angiography is indicated to define the extent of the pseudoaneurysm and to assess the adequacy of collateral flow. Most lesions involve the common carotid rather than the internal carotid artery. Severe cellulitis should be treated with parenteral antibiotics for 7 to 14 days, at which time ligation of the involved artery and evacuation of infected hematoma are performed. Revascularization with autologous bypass grafting is only rarely technically feasible.

IATROGENIC PSEUDOANEURYSM AFTER PERCUTANEOUS ARTERIAL ACCESS

Etiology

Iatrogenic pseudoaneurysm results from failure of hemostasis after arterial puncture. Its frequency can be minimized by the judicious choice of needle size and strict adherence to proper technique. Samples for blood gas analysis can routinely be obtained with a 23-gauge needle, and indwelling arterial pressure monitoring cannulas should only rarely exceed 20-gauge. Femoral artery cannulation for diagnostic arteriography or cardiac catheterization can readily be performed with a 5 French (Fr.) or even a 4 Fr. sheath, and intra-aortic balloon counterpulsation devices have been scaled down to 8 Fr. Very large sheaths (10 to 18 Fr.) may be necessary for advanced interventional procedures such as balloon valvuloplasty and endoluminal grafting, but meticulous attention to technique can prevent pseudoaneurysm formation even in these circumstances.

In short, pseudoaneurysm is a consequence of hemostatic failure after arterial decannulation. As the needle or sheath is withdrawn from the artery, pressure should be applied evenly over the puncture site, allowing time for the smooth muscle to contract and a platelet plug to form. The use of clamps or other compression devices is acceptable, but proper orientation and monitoring are critical. Improper compression, whether manual or mechanical, permits blood to extravasate freely into the loosely packed perivascular tissues, forming a *hematoma*. Although small hematomas are well tolerated and absorbed, large collections can result in morbid local and systemic events, including excessive blood loss, venous compression, and skin necrosis. The incidence of serious hematomas or persistent hemorrhage after femoral puncture is estimated at 0.08% to 0.68%, depending on the series.[44–50]

If the arterial puncture site contributing to the hematoma fails to seal, blood may freely enter and exit its fluid center. A hematoma with a liquid center that communicates freely with the parent artery constitutes a *pseudoaneurysm*.

Incidence and Risk Factors

Iatrogenic pseudoaneurysms occur most commonly in the groin and antecubital fossa, the two most common sites of peripheral arterial access. In a recent review of the literature, including over 180,000 collected femoral arterial access procedures, the incidence of pseudoaneurysm formation was estimated to be about 0.2%.[51] The incidence of pseudoaneurysm complicating brachial artery access is even lower, although the increased risk of thrombosis at this site makes it less attractive to interventionalists. Even though catheter size has been minimized and technical proficiency has matured, the risk of access complications has probably increased as a result of its expanded procedural complexity and liberal application.[52, 53]

Several risk factors for the development of iatrogenic pseudoaneurysm have been identified. Procedural risk factors include:

- Large catheter size[50]
- Therapeutic versus diagnostic procedures[50, 54–59]
- Use of multiple catheters[60] and punctures[61, 62]
- Prolonged procedure time[44, 62, 63]
- Limited operator experience[44, 63]
- Concomitant use of thrombolytic agents[48, 55, 61, 64]

Patient risk factors include (1) female gender,[48, 55, 65, 66] (2) extremes of age[48, 55, 67–69] and body weight,[50, 55, 70] and (3) the presence of systemic hypertension[54, 60, 71] and congestive heart failure.[55]

In the groin, the most important risk factor for the development of pseudoaneurysm is misidentification of the common femoral artery, with resultant cannulation of the external iliac, superficial femoral, or profunda femoris vessels.[47, 49, 50, 72–76] Puncture of the common femoral artery is optimal because the femoral sheath is circumferentially intact at this level and the immediately posterior femoral head provides a firm scaffold for compression. Effective compression of the superficial femoral or profunda femoris artery is difficult to maintain, often resulting in hematoma or pseudoaneurysm formation. Cannulation of the external iliac artery should generally be avoided due to the risk of significant hemorrhage into the potential retroperitoneal space.

Presentation and Diagnosis

Iatrogenic pseudoaneurysms usually become evident shortly after percutaneous arterial access, although the diagnostic interval may be months or years in some cases. The most frequent complaint is pain in the area of puncture. Other symptoms include swelling, discoloration, presence of a pulsatile mass, and paresthesia and sensory loss over the thigh or brachium. Many patients are asymptomatic, and the diagnosis is made during routine physical examination after arterial intervention.

The classic physical finding is a pulsatile groin mass. Although an uncomplicated hematoma may transmit a pulse, a pseudoaneurysm is pulsatile in a radial direction on palpation of the lateral margins of the mass. Physical examination may also reveal discoloration from hematoma formation, generalized or local edema, and skin excoriation. Uncomplicated pseudoaneurysms generally do not cause luminal encroachment, but this should be confirmed by examination of the peripheral pulses and continuous wave Doppler signals. Neurovascular compromise and impending skin necrosis are indications for urgent surgical therapy.

The clinical impression can be readily confirmed by Doppler duplex ultrasound examination (Fig. 48–6*A*) (see Color Plate).[55, 60, 61, 70, 77–79] Duplex is extremely reliable in this setting, with sensitivity and specificity approaching 100%. The examination provides an opportunity for diagnosis as well as therapy (see below). Arteriography is only rarely required.

Natural History and Indications for Intervention

Reports of iatrogenic pseudoaneurysms have emphasized their propensity for enlargement, embolization, rupture, or infection, and routine prophylactic surgical repair was advised. It has become clear, however, that, like iatrogenic arteriovenous fistulas, many pseudoaneurysms spontaneously thrombose, and the projected dangers of expectant management have probably been overstated. A recent report documented spontaneous closure in 90% of selected iatrogenic postcatheterization femoral pseudoaneurysms over 2 months.[80] The results of this study and others[59, 81, 82] have led to a wider acceptance of nonoperative management in selected cases. Surgical therapy is still indicated in many clinical situations, however (Table 48–1), and should be applied liberally to optimize clinical results.

TABLE 48–1. INDICATIONS FOR SURGICAL THERAPY FOR IATROGENIC FEMORAL PSEUDOANEURYSM

Absolute
Active hemorrhage, expansion
Shock
Compartment syndrome
Femoral nerve compression
Infection
Embolization, distal ischemia
Impending skin necrosis
Severe pain
Unsuccessful or severe pain during ultrasound-guided compression
Relative (May Be Candidates for Ultrasound-Guided Compression)
Pseudoaneurysm >3 cm
Pseudoaneurysm with short neck
Pseudoaneurysm <1 cm from skin surface
Coexistent arteriovenous fistula
Requirement for chronic anticoagulation
Patient to undergo major surgery
Patient unable or refusing to return for follow-up
Patient desirous of prompt resolution

Ultrasound-Guided Compression

Patients with relative indications for surgical correction may also be candidates for a trial of ultrasound-guided compression, which was first described in 1991.[83, 84] One performs ultrasound-guided compression by applying direct vertical pressure with the ultrasound scan head with sufficient force to occlude the neck of the pseudoaneurysm

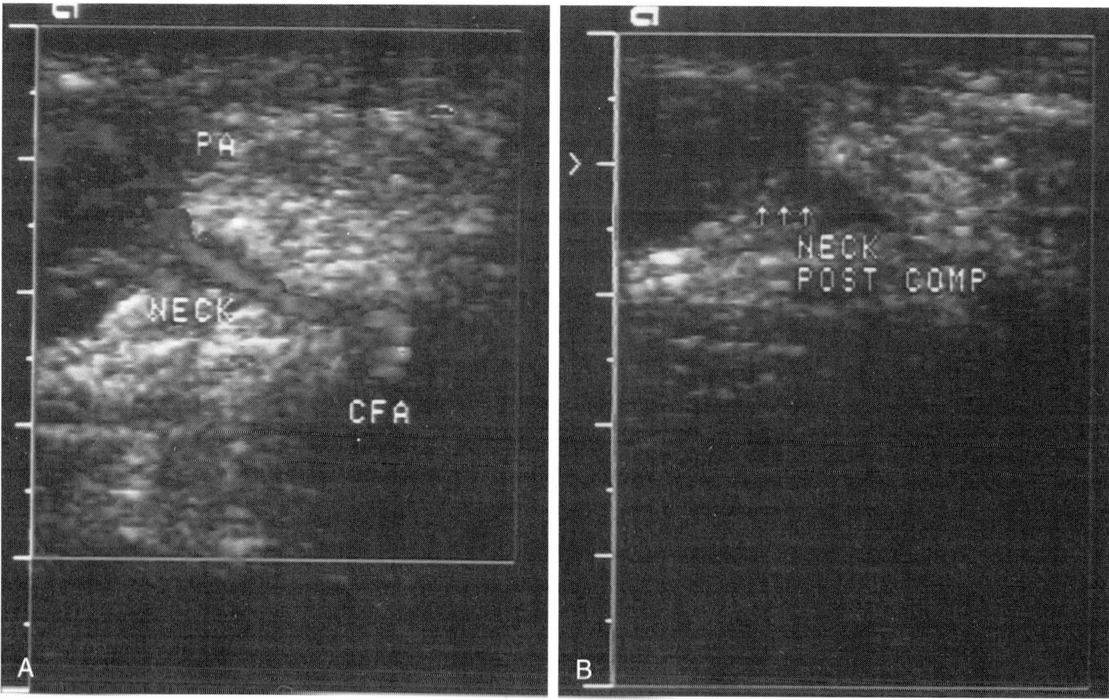

FIGURE 48–6. Common femoral artery (CFA) iatrogenic pseudoaneurysm in a 42-year-old woman 1 day after cardiac catheterization. *A*, Duplex image with color flow mapping showing the CFA, pseudoaneurysm neck (NECK), and pseudoaneurysm cavity (PA). *B*, Duplex image at same location after successful ultrasound-guided compression. Note the obliteration of the neck following compression *(arrows)*. See Color Plate.

while maintaining antegrade arterial flow. Compression is held at 10- to 20-minute intervals and then gently released to evaluate its progress (Fig. 48–6*B*). The examination is often uncomfortable but well tolerated when augmented with intravenous sedation.

Ultrasound-guided compression has enjoyed widespread application, and more than 500 successful cases have been reported in the literature.[85–100] In general, compression is successful in about 90% of patients. Reliable clinical predictors of failure have been elusive because closure has been achieved even with large pseudoaneurysms in anticoagulated patients. Complications are rare, but arterial thrombosis,[83] deep venous thrombosis,[101] distal embolization,[98] rupture,[91, 92, 102] femoral nerve compression,[92] and recurrence[90] have all been reported. The role of adjuncts such as percutaneous coil placement[103–105] and thrombin injection[106] await further definition.

Surgical Repair

The absolute and relative indications for surgical repair are listed in Table 48–1. The operation is usually straightforward and can be performed under local or regional anesthesia. A longitudinal groin incision is made overlying the pulsatile mass. Proximal vascular control of large or inaccessible pseudoaneurysms may be gained with a separate retroperitoneal incision, but this is only rarely necessary. The pseudoaneurysm is entered sharply, and the pinpoint arterial defect is identified and controlled digitally. A single repair suture is usually all that is required. For more complex defects, the arteriotomy may be extended and vascular control maintained intraluminally with balloon catheters. After repair, the residual hematoma should be evacuated and closed-suction drainage established.

The results of over 200 iatrogenic femoral pseudoaneurysm repairs are reported in the literature.[44–50, 54, 55, 57, 58, 60–62, 65, 70, 74, 75, 107, 108] Mortality from the operation is infrequent, although postoperative death from concomitant severe cardiac disease has been reported.[47, 55]

OTHER PSEUDOANEURYSMS

Traumatic (Non-iatrogenic) Pseudoaneurysm

Pseudoaneurysms occurring as a result of immediate or occult trauma have been reported in virtually every artery in humans, including the carotid arteries,[34, 43] vertebral arteries,[109] thyrocervical trunks,[110] innominate artery,[111] subclavian arteries,[34] axillary arteries,[112] digital arteries,[113] aorta,[114, 115] visceral arteries,[116] splenic artery,[117] renal arteries (Fig. 48–7),[118, 119] cystic artery,[120] gluteal arteries (Fig. 48–8*A*),[121, 122] popliteal arteries,[123, 124] and tibial arteries.[125] Their presentations vary with anatomic location. These

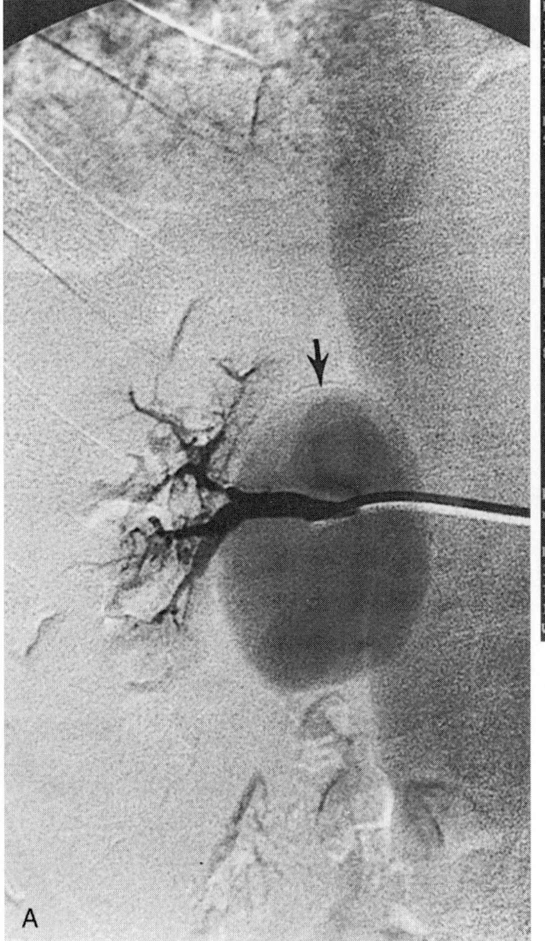

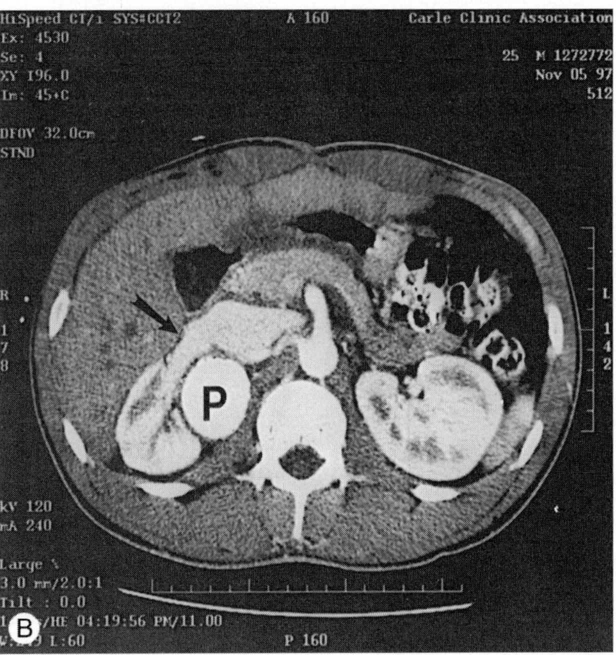

FIGURE 48–7. Traumatic pseudoaneurysm and arteriovenous fistula of an upper pole right renal artery in a 25-year-old man who sustained a gunshot wound to the abdomen 4 years before presenting with malignant hypertension and an abdominal bruit. *A,* Anteroposterior arteriogram with direct injection of the upper pole right renal artery showing large pseudoaneurysm *(arrow)*. *B,* Contrast-enhanced CT scan revealing pseudoaneurysm (P) as well as contrast in the right renal vein *(arrow)*.

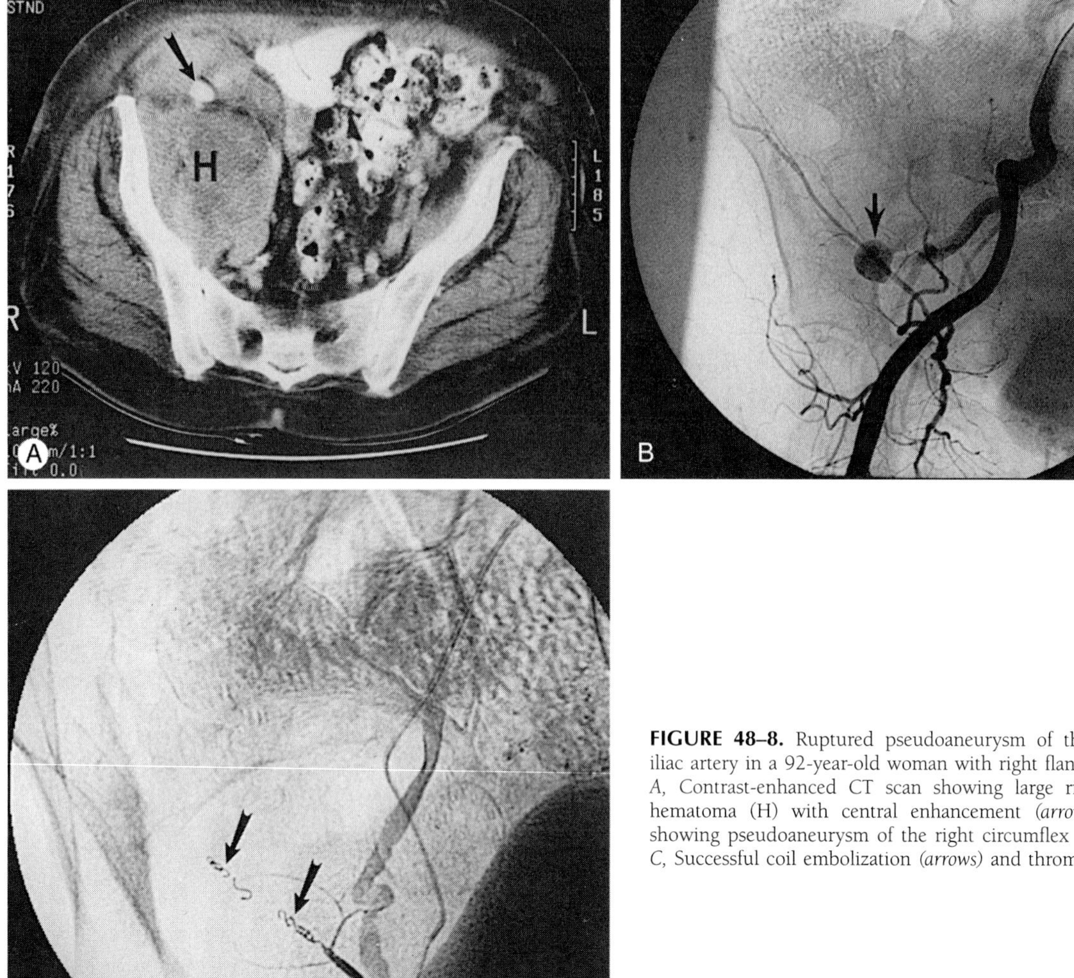

FIGURE 48–8. Ruptured pseudoaneurysm of the right circumflex iliac artery in a 92-year-old woman with right flank pain and anemia. *A,* Contrast-enhanced CT scan showing large right retroperitoneal hematoma (H) with central enhancement *(arrow). B,* Arteriogram showing pseudoaneurysm of the right circumflex iliac artery *(arrow). C,* Successful coil embolization *(arrows)* and thrombosis.

lesions can frequently be treated with endovascular coil embolization with good results (Fig. 48–8*B*). Pseudoaneurysms with short necks or those occurring in vital arteries may require surgical repair and reconstruction.

Other Causes

Other causes of pseudoaneurysm formation include bacterial, mycobacterial,[115] or amebic[126] infection, inflammatory processes such as pancreatitis,[127] arterial degeneration from Marfan's syndrome[128] or fibromuscular dysplasia,[38] malignant erosion,[123] and vasculitis. Treatment usually focuses on controlling the underlying pathologic process as well as reconstruction of the affected artery.

SUMMARY

Pseudoaneurysms result from a variety of processes and occur most commonly after prosthetic bypass or arterial puncture. Avoidance of pseudoaneurysms requires meticulous surgical technique during the initial procedure. The use of a permanent synthetic suture is mandatory, and anastomotic tension must be minimized. Suture depth should be adequate to ensure full-thickness purchase on the arterial wall. An appropriate-sized graft should be attached at an acute angle to dissipate shear and hoop stress. Meticulous hemostasis and sterile technique remain basic but important variables to avoid fluid collections and infection.

Diagnosis and treatment of pseudoaneurysms vary according to etiology and symptoms. In the absence of infection, interposition grafting with prosthetic material is widely accepted as the best form of treatment. When infection is obvious or suspected, autogenous vein remains the optimal conduit. Excellent long-term results may be anticipated for the majority of lesions when the principles of diagnostic suspicion, early recognition, and thoughtful surgical repair are followed.

REFERENCES

1. Hiatt JR, Hiatt N: Bloodletting in ancient and modern times. Contemp Surg 48:164–168, 1996.
2. Lambert R: Giving an account of a new method of treating aneurysm. Med Observ Inq 1761, June 15.
3. Matas R: Traumatic aneurysm of left brachial artery. Med News 53:462, 1888.
4. Lexer E: Die ideale operation des arteriellen und des arteriovenousen aneurysm. Arch Klin Chir 83:1907, 1907.
5. Pringle JH: Two cases of vein grafting for the maintenance of a direct arterial communication. Lancet 1:1795, 1913.
6. Stoney RJ, Albo FJ, Wylie EJ: False aneurysms occurring after arterial grafting operations. Am J Surg 110:153–161, 1965.
7. Gardner TJ, Brawley RK, Gott VL: Anastomotic false aneurysms. Surgery 72:474–478, 1972.
8. Moore WS, Hall AD: Late suture failure in the pathogenesis of anastomotic false aneurysms. Ann Surg 172:1064–1068, 1970.
9. Seabrook GR, Schmitt DD, Bandyk DF, et al: Anastomotic femoral pseudoaneurysm: An investigation of occult infection as an etiologic factor. J Vasc Surg 11:629–634, 1990.
10. Nichols WK, Stanton M, Silver D, Keitzer WF: Anastomotic aneurysms following lower extremity revascularization. Surgery 88:366–374, 1980.
11. Sedwitz MM, Hye RJ, Stabile BE: The changing epidemiology of pseduoaneurysms: Therapeutic implications. Arch Surg 123:473–476, 1988.
12. Knox WG: Peripheral vascular and anastomotic aneurysms: A fifteen-year experience. Ann Surg 183:120–123, 1976.
13. Millili JJ, Lanes JS, Nemir P: A study of anastomotic aneurysms following aortofemoral prosthetic bypass. Ann Surg 192:69–73, 1980.
14. Richardson JV, McDowell HA: Anastomotic aneurysms following arterial grafting: A 10-year experience. Ann Surg 184:179–182, 1976.
15. Sawyers JL, Jacobs JK, Sutton JP: Peripheral anastomotic aneurysms: Development following arterial reconstruction with prosthetic grafts. Arch Surg 95:802–809, 1967.
16. Dennis JW, Littooy FN, Griesler HP, Baker WH: Anastomotic pseudoaneurysms: A continuing late complication of vascular reconstructive procedures. Arch Surg 121:314–317, 1986.
17. Coughlin BF, Paushter DM: Peripheral pseudoaneurysms: Evaluation with duplex ultrasound. Radiology 168:339–342, 1988.
18. Sieswerda C, Skotnicki SH, Barentz JO, Heystraten FMJ: Anastomotic aneurysms—an underdiagnosed complication after aorto-iliac reconstructions. Eur J Vasc Surg 3:233–238, 1989.
19. Edwards JM, Teefey SA, Zierler RE, Kohler TR: Intraabdominal paraanastomotic aneurysms after aortic bypass grafting. J Vasc Surg 15:344–353, 1992.
20. Van den Akker PJ, Brand R, van Schilfgaarde R, et al: False aneurysms after prosthetic reconstructions for aortoiliac obstructive disease. Ann Surg 210:658–666, 1989.
21. Ernst CB, Elliott JP Jr, Ryan CJ, et al: Recurrent femoral anastomotic aneurysms: A 30-year experience. Ann Surg 201:401–409, 1988.
22. Ernst CB: Anastomotic aneurysm. *In* Ernst CB, Stanley JC (eds): Current Therapy in Vascular Surgery. St. Louis, Mosby–Year Book, 1995, pp 415–419.
23. Reddy DJ, Smith RF, Elliott JP Jr, et al: Infected femoral artery false aneurysms in drug addicts: Evolution of selective vascular reconstruction. J Vasc Surg 3:718–724, 1986.
24. Fromm SH, Lucas CE: Obturator bypass for mycotic aneurysm in the drug addict. Arch Surg 100:82–83, 1970.
25. Fujitani RM, Bassiouny HS, Gewertz BL, et al: Cryopreserved saphenous vein allogenic homografts: An alternative conduit in lower extremity arterial reconstruction in infected fields. J Vasc Surg 15:519–526, 1992.
26. McCann RL, Schwartz LB, Georgiade GS: Management of aortic graft complications. Ann Surg 217:729–734, 1993.
27. Bastounis E, Georgopoulos S, Maltezos C, Balas P: The validity of current vascular imaging methods in the evaluation of aortic anastomotic aneurysms developing after abdominal aortic aneurysm repair. Ann Vasc Surg 10:537–545, 1996.
28. Treiman GS, Weaver FA, Cossman DV, et al: Anastomotic false aneurysms of the abdominal aorta and the iliac arteries. J Vasc Surg 8:268–273, 1988.
29. White RA, Donayre CE, Walot I, et al: Endoluminal graft exclusion of a proximal para-anastomotic pseudoaneurysm following aortofemoral bypass. J Endovasc Surg 4:88–94, 1997.
30. Parodi JC: Endovascular repair of abdominal aortic aneurysms and other arterial lesions. J Vasc Surg 21:549–557, 1995.
31. Hertzer NR: Postoperative management and complications following carotid endarterectomy. *In* Rutherford RB (ed): Vascular Surgery, 3rd ed. Philadelphia, WB Saunders, 1989, pp 1451–1471.
32. Thompson JE: Complications of carotid endarertectomy and their prevention. World J Surg 3:155–165, 1979.
33. Schechter DC: Cervical carotid aneurysms: Parts I and II. N Y State Med J 79:892–901, 1042–1048, 1979.
34. Schwartz LB, McCann RL: Traumatic false aneurysm of the common carotid artery presenting as a mediastinal mass. J Vasc Surg 10:281–284, 1989.
35. Deysine M, Adiga R, Wilder JR: Traumatic false aneurysm of the cervical internal carotid artery. Surgery 66:1004–1007, 1969.
36. Arpin EJ, Downs AR: Two false aneurysms of the common carotid artery: A delayed complication of penetrating cervical trauma. J Trauma 15:976–980, 1975.
37. Solheim K: Common carotid artery aneurysm after blunt trauma. J Trauma 19:707–709, 1979.
38. Moreau P, Albat B, Thèvenet A: Surgical treatment of extracranial internal carotid artery aneurysm. Ann Vasc Surg 8:409–416, 1994.
39. Branch CL Jr, Davis CH Jr: False aneurysm complicating carotid endarterectomy. Neurosurgery 19:421–425, 1986.
40. Winslow N: Extracranial aneurysm of the internal carotid artery. Arch Surg 13:689–729, 1926.
41. McCollum CH, Wheeler WG, Noon GP, DeBakey ME: Aneurysms of the extracranial carotid artery. Twenty-one years' experience. Am J Surg 137:196–200, 1979.
42. Faggioli G, Freyrie A, Stella A, et al: Extracranial internal carotid artery aneurysms: Results of a surgical series with long-term follow-up. J Vasc Surg 23:587–595, 1996.
43. Huang A, Baker DM, Al-Kutobi AA, Mansfield AO: Endovascular stenting of internal carotid artery false aneurysm. Eur J Vasc Endovasc Surg 12:375–377, 1996.
44. Adams HL, Adams HL: Complications of coronary arteriography: A follow-up report. Cardiovasc Radiol 2:89–96, 1979.
45. Babu SC, Piccorelli GO, Shah PM, et al: Incidence and results of arterial complications among 16,350 patients undergoing cardiac catheterization. J Vasc Surg 10:113–116, 1989.
46. Kaufman J, Moglia R, Lacy C, et al: Peripheral vascular complications from percutaneous transluminal coronary angioplasty: A comparison with transfemoral cardiac catheterization. Am J Med Sci 297:22–25, 1989.
47. Lilly MP, Reichman W, Sarazen AA, Carney WI: Anatomic and clinical factors associated with complications of transfemoral arteriography. Ann Vasc Surg 4:264–269, 1990.
48. Oweida SW, Roubin GS, Smith RB, Salam AA: Postcatheterization vascular complications associated with percutaneous transluminal angioplasty. J Vasc Surg 12:310–315, 1990.
49. Richardson JD, Shina MA, Miller FB, Bergamini TM: Peripheral vascular complications of coronary angioplasty. Am Surg 55:675–680, 1989.
50. Skillman JJ, Ducksoo K, Baim DS: Vascular complications of percutaneous femoral cardiac interventions: Incidence and operative repair. Arch Surg 123:1207–1212, 1988.
51. Schwartz LB, McCann RL: Vascular complications of cardiac catheterization. *In* Califf RM, Mark DB, Wagner GS (eds): Acute Coronary Care. St. Louis, Mosby–Year Book, 1995, pp 687–695.
52. Schwartz LB, Belkin M: Femorofemoral bypass for limb ischemia during intra-aortic balloon pump therapy. Adv Vasc Surg 3:55–65, 1995.
53. Roberts AC: Ultrasound-guided compression of iatrogenic femoral pseudoaneurysms: Indications and results. *In* Perler BA, Becker GJ (eds): Vascular Intervention: A Clinical Approach. New York, Thieme Medical Publishers, 1998, pp 429–436.
54. Messina LM, Brothers TE, Wakefield TW, et al: Clinical characteristics and surgical management of vascular complications in patients undergoing cardiac catheterization: Interventional versus diagnostic procedures. J Vasc Surg 13:593–600, 1991.
55. McCann RL, Schwartz LB, Pieper KS: Vascular complications of cardiac catheterization. J Vasc Surg 14:375–381, 1991.

56. Burrows PE, Benson LN, Williams WG, et al: Iliofemoral arterial complications of balloon angioplasty for systemic obstructions in infants and children. Circulation 82:1697–1704, 1990.
57. Criber A, Savin T, Berland J, et al: Percutaneous transluminal balloon valvuloplasty of adult aortic stenosis: Report of 92 cases. J Am Coll Cardiol 9:381–386, 1987.
58. Wyman RM, Safian RD, Portway V, et al: Current complications of diagnostic and therapeutic cardiac catheterization. J Am Coll Cardiol 12:1400–1406, 1988.
59. Allen BT, Munn JS, Stevens SL, et al: Selective non-operative management of pseudoaneurysms and arteriovenous fistulae complicating femoral artery catheterization. J Cardiovasc Surg 33:440–447, 1992.
60. Fitzgerald EJ, Bowsher WG, Ruttley MST: False aneurysm of the femoral artery: Computed tomographic and ultrasound appearances. Clin Radiol 37:585–588, 1986.
61. Sheikh KH, Adams DB, McCann RL, et al: Utility of Doppler color flow imaging for identification of femoral arterial complications of cardiac catheterization. Am Heart J 117:623–638, 1989.
62. Brener BJ, Couch NP: Peripheral arterial complications of left heart catheterization and their management. Am J Surg 125:521–526, 1973.
63. Lang EK: A survey of the complications of percutaneous retrograde arteriography. Radiology 81:257–263, 1963.
64. Topol EJ, O'Neil WW, Langburd AB, et al: A randomized, placebo-controlled trial of intravenous recombinant tissue-type plasminogen activator and emergency coronary angioplasty in patients with acute myocardial infarction. Circulation 45:420–428, 1987.
65. Bourassa MG, Noble J: Complication rate of coronary arteriography: A review of 5250 cases studied by a percutaneous femoral technique. Circulation 53:106–114, 1976.
66. Harris JM: Coronary angiography and its complications: The search for risk factors. Arch Intern Med 144:337–341, 1984.
67. Booth P, Redington AN, Shinebourne EA, Rigby ML: Early complications of interventional balloon catheterization in infants and children. Br Heart J 65:109–112, 1991.
68. Ino T, Benson LN, Freedom RM, et al: Thrombolytic therapy for femoral artery thrombosis after pediatric cardiac catheterization. Am Heart J 115:633–639, 1988.
69. Rothman A: Arterial complications of interventional cardiac catheterization in patients with congenital heart disease. Circulation 82:1868–1871, 1990.
70. Cohen GI, Chan KL: Physical examination and echo Doppler study in the assessment of femoral arterial complications following cardiac catheterization. Cathet Cardiovasc Diagn 21:137–143, 1990.
71. Schoonmaker FW, King SB: Coronary arteriography by the single catheter percutaneous femoral technique. Circulation 50:735–740, 1974.
72. Altin RS, Flicker S, Naidech HJ: Pseudoaneurysm and arteriovenous fistula after femoral artery catheterization: Association with low femoral punctures. Am J Radiol 152:629–631, 1989.
73. Chiverton SG, Murie JA: Incidence and management of arterial injuries from left heart catheterization. J R Coll Phys Lond 20:126–128, 1986.
74. McMillan I, Murie JA: Vascular injury following cardiac catheterization. Br J Surg 71:832–835, 1984.
75. Rapoport S, Sniderman KW, Morse SS, et al: Pseudoaneurysm: A complication of faulty technique in femoral arterial puncture. Radiology 154:529–530, 1985.
76. Kim D, Orron DE, Skillman JJ, et al: Role of superficial femoral artery puncture in the development of pseudoaneurysm and arteriovenous fistula complicating percutaneous transfemoral cardiac catheterization. Cathet Cardiovasc Diagn 25:91–97, 1992.
77. Abu-Yousef MM, Wiese JA, Shamma AR: Duplex Doppler evidence of femoral artery pseudoaneurysm. Am J Radiol 150:632–634, 1988.
78. Helvie MA, Rubin JM, Silver TM, Kresowik TF: The distinction between femoral artery pseudoaneurysms and other causes of groin masses: Value of duplex Doppler sonography. Am J Radiol 150:1177–1180, 1988.
79. Mitchell DG, Needleman L, Bezzi M, et al: Femoral artery pseudoaneurysm: Diagnosis with conventional duplex and color Doppler ultrasound. Radiology 165:687–690, 1987
80. Toursarkissian B, Allen BT, Petrinec D, et al: Spontaneous closure of selected iatrogenic pseudoaneurysms and arteriovenous fistulae. J Vasc Surg 25:803–809, 1997.
81. Kent KC, McArdle CR, Kennedy B, et al: A prospective study of the clinical outcome of femoral pseudoaneurysms and arteriovenous fistulas induced by arterial puncture. J Vasc Surg 17:125–133, 1993.
82. Kresowik TF, Khoury MD, Miller BV, et al: A prospective study of the incidence and natural history of femoral vascular complications after percutaneous transluminal coronary angioplasty. J Vasc Surg 13:328–336, 1991.
83. Fellmeth BD, Roberts AC, Bookstein JJ, et al: Nonsurgical repair of post angiographic femoral artery injuries using ultrasound guided compression. Radiology 178:671–675, 1991.
84. Chou YH, Tiu CM, Chiang BN, Chang T: Real-time and image-directed Doppler ultrasonography in deep femoral artery pseudoaneurysm: A new observation with graded compression of the femoral artery. J Clin Ultrasound 19:438–441, 1991.
85. Fellmeth BD, Baron SB, Brown PR, et al: Repair of postcatheterization femoral pseudoaneurysms by color flow ultrasound guided compression. Am Heart J 123:547–551, 1992.
86. Feld R, Patton GM, Carabasi RA, et al: Treatment of iatrogenic femoral artery injuries with ultrasound-guided compression. J Vasc Surg 16:832–840, 1992.
87. Hajarizadeh H, LaRosa CR, Cardullo P, et al: Ultrasound-guided compression of iatrogenic femoral pseudoaneurysm failure, recurrence, and long-term results. J Vasc Surg 22:425–433, 1995.
88. Rocha-Singh KJ, Schwend RB, Otis SM, et al: Frequency and nonsurgical therapy of femoral artery pseudoaneurysm complicating interventional cardiology procedures. Am J Cardiol 73:1012–1014, 1994.
89. Trerotola SO, Savader SJ, Prescott CA, Osterman FA Jr: US-guided pseudoaneurysm repair with a compression device. Radiology 189:285–286, 1993.
90. Cox GS, Young JR, Gray BR, et al: Ultrasound-guided compression repair of postcatheterization pseudoaneurysms: Results of treatment in one hundred cases. J Vasc Surg 19:683–686, 1994.
91. Dol JA, Reekers JA, Kromhout JG: Rupture of pseudoaneurysm during attempted US-guided compression. Radiology 185:284, 1992.
92. Kazmers A, Meeker C, Nofz K, et al: Nonoperative therapy for postcatheterization femoral artery pseudoaneurysms. Am Surg 63:199–204, 1997.
93. Currie P, Turnbull CM, Shaw TRD: Pseudoaneurysm of the femoral artery after cardiac catheterization: Diagnosis and treatment by manual compression guided by Doppler colour flow imaging. Br Heart J 72:80–84, 1994.
94. Schwend RB, Hambsch KP, Kwan KY, et al: Color duplex sonographically guided obliteration of pseudoaneurysm. J Ultrasound Med 12:609–613, 1993.
95. Paulson EK, Kliewer MA, Hertzberg BS, et al: Ultrasonographically guided manual compression of femoral artery injuries. J Ultrasound Med 9:653–659, 1995.
96. Sorrell KA, Feinberg RL, Wheeler JO, et al: Color-flow duplex-directed manual occlusion of femoral false aneurysms. J Vasc Surg 17:571–577, 1993.
97. Moote DJ, Hilborn MD, Harris KA, et al: Postarteriographic femoral pseudoaneurysms: Treatment with ultrasound-guided compression. Ann Vasc Surg 8:325–331, 1994.
98. Coley BD, Roberts AC, Fellmeth BD, et al: Postangiographic femoral artery pseudoaneurysms: Further experience with US-guided compression repair. Radiology 194:307–311, 1995.
99. Schaub F, Theiss W, Heinz M, et al: New aspects in ultrasound-guided compression repair of postcatheterization femoral artery injuries. Circulation 90:1861–1865, 1994.
100. Weatherford DA, Taylor SM, Langan EM, et al: Ultrasound-guided compression for the treatment of iatrogenic femoral pseudoaneurysms. South Med J 90:223–226, 1997.
101. Hilborn M, Downey D: Deep venous thrombosis complicating sonographically guided compression repair of a pseudoaneurysm of the common femoral artery. Am J Roentgenol 161:1334–1335, 1993.
102. Birchall D, Fields JM, Chalmers N, Walker MG: Delayed superficial femoral artery pseudoaneurysm rupture following successful compression therapy. Clin Radiol 52:629–630, 1997.
103. Saito S, Arai H, Kim K, et al: Percutaneous transfemoral spring coil embolization of a pseudoaneurysm of the femoral artery. Cathet Cardiovasc Diagn 26:229–231, 1992.
104. Pan M, Medina A, Suarez de Lezo J, et al: Obliteration of femoral pseudoaneurysm complicating coronary intervention by direct puncture and permanent or removable coil insertion. Am J Cardiol 80:786–788, 1997.

105. Jain SP, Roubin GS, Iyer SS, et al: Closure of an iatrogenic femoral artery pseudoaneurysm by transcutaneous coil embolization. Cathet Cardiovasc Diagn 39:317–319, 1996.
106. Liau C-S, Ho F-M, Chen M-F, Lee Y-T: Treatment of iatrogenic femoral artery pseudoaneurysm with percutaneous thrombin injection. J Vasc Surg 26:18–23, 1997.
107. Dorros G, Cowley MJ, Simpson J, et al: Percutaneous transluminal coronary angioplasty: Report of complications from the National Heart, Lung, and Blood Institute PTCA Registry. Circulation 67:723–730, 1983.
108. Roberts SR, Main D, Pinkerton J: Surgical therapy of femoral artery pseudoaneurysm after angiography. Am J Surg 154:676–680, 1987.
109. Lin T-K, Lin P-J, Chang C-N, Cheng W-C: Direct repair of a giant extracranial vertebral artery pseudoaneurysm through the aneurysmal cavity. J Trauma 42:1140–1143, 1997.
110. Abrokwah J, Shenoy KN, Armour RH: False aneurysm of the thyrocervical trunk: An unconventional surgical approach. Eur J Vasc Endovasc Surg 11:373–374, 1996.
111. Kraus TW, Paetz B, Richter GM, Allenberg JR: The isolated posttraumatic aneurysm of the brachiocephalic artery after blunt thoracic contusion. Ann Vasc Surg 7:275–281, 1993.
112. Szendro G, Golcman L, Klimov A, et al: Successful non-surgical management of traumatic pseudoaneurysm of the axillary artery by duplex guided compression obliteration. Eur J Vasc Endovasc Surg 13:513–514, 1997.
113. Abouzahr MK, Coppa LM, Boxt LM: Aneurysms of the digital arteries: A case report and literature review. J Hand Surg 22A:311–314, 1997.
114. Chase CW, Layman TS, Barker DE, Clements JB: Traumatic abdominal aortic pseudoaneurysm causing biliary obstruction: A case report and review of the literature. J Vasc Surg 25:936–940, 1997.
115. Ohtsuka T, Kotsuka Y, Yagyu K, et al: Tuberculous pseudoaneurysm of the thoracic aorta. Ann Thorac Surg 62:1831–1844, 1996.
116. Stambo GW, Hallisey MJ, Gallagher JJ Jr: Arteriographic embolization of visceral artery pseudoaneurysms. Ann Vasc Surg 10:476–480, 1996.
117. Nagar H, Kessler A, Weiss J: Traumatic intraparenchymal splenic pseudoaneurysms in a child: Nonoperative management. J Trauma 43:552–555, 1997.
118. Chazen MD, Miller KS: Intrarenal pseudoaneurysm presenting 15 years after penetrating renal injury. Urology 49:774–776, 1997.
119. Farrell TM, Sutton JE, Burchard KW: Renal artery pseudoaneurysm: A cause of delayed hematuria in blunt trauma. J Trauma 41:1067–1068, 1996.
120. Maw A, Mander BJ, Nandi SC, et al: Pseudoaneurysm of the cystic artery. Eur J Surg 163:307–309, 1997.
121. Holland AJA, Ibach EG: False aneurysm of the inferior gluteal artery following penetrating buttock trauma: Case report and review of the literature. Cardiovasc Surg 4:841–843, 1996.
122. Stephen DJG: Pseudoaneurysm of the superior gluteal arterial system: An unusual case of pain after a pelvic fracture. J Trauma 43:146–149, 1997.
123. Ballaro A, Fox AD, Collin J: Rupture of a popliteal artery pseudoaneurysm secondary to a fibular osteochondroma. Eur J Vasc Endovasc Surg 14:151–152, 1997.
124. Manns RA, Duffield RGM: Intravascular stenting across a false aneurysm of the popliteal artery. Clin Radiol 52:151–153, 1997.
125. Vasudevan A, Patel D, Brodrick P: Pseudoaneurysm of the dorsalis pedis artery. Anesthesia 52:926–927, 1997.
126. Gopanpallikar A, Rathi P, Sawant P, et al: Hepatic artery pseudoaneurysm associated with amebic liver abscess presenting as upper GI hemorrhage. Am J Gastroenterol 92:1391–1393, 1997.
127. LiPuma JP, Sachs PB, Sands MJ, et al: Splenic artery pseudoaneurysm associated with pancreatitis. Am J Radiol 169:262–263, 1997.
128. Vasseur MA, Doisy VC, Prat AG, Stankowiak C: Coil embolization of a gluteal false aneurysm in a patient with Marfan syndrome. J Vasc Surg 27:177–179, 1998.

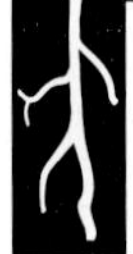

CHAPTER 49

Aortoenteric Fistulae

Sean P. O'Brien, M.D., and
Calvin B. Ernst, M.D.

An *aortoenteric fistula* (AEF) is an uncommon but potentially lethal condition that challenges the surgeon's diagnostic and therapeutic proficiency. This problem can affect either the diseased abdominal aorta (a primary AEF) or the reconstructed aorta (a secondary AEF) and involves a direct communication between the aorta and the enteric tract. The first description of a primary AEF between the infrarenal aorta and the duodenum was published in 1829 by Sir Astley Cooper.[22] The first reported secondary AEF appeared in 1953 by Brock, who described a fistula between the proximal anastomosis of an aortic homograft and the duodenum.[9] Zenker performed the first repair of a primary *aortoduodenal fistula* (ADF) in 1954 with primary closure.[47] MacKenzie and colleagues performed the first successful repair of a homograft secondary to ADF in 1958.[61]

The subtleties of presentation, limitations of definitive diagnostic studies, and complexities of treatment have all contributed to the high morbidity and mortality rates of AEF. A high index of suspicion, along with the application of established surgical principles, offers the patient the best chance for a successful outcome. This chapter reviews the pathophysiology, diagnostic methods, and treatment guidelines for successful management of AEFs.

INCIDENCE AND CLASSIFICATION

AEFs are classified as either (1) primary or (2) secondary. A *primary* AEF is a communication between the aorta, usually aneurysmal, and the enteric tract. The communication most frequently occurs between the diseased infrarenal

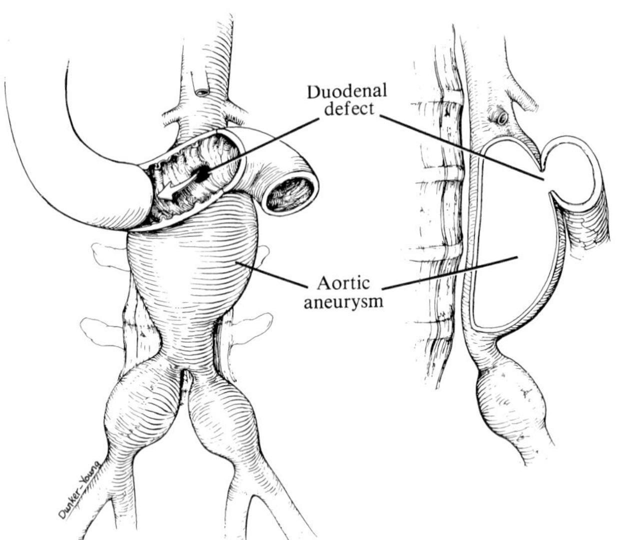

FIGURE 49–1. An abdominal aortic aneurysm with associated aortoenteric fistula. (From Ernst CB: Aortoenteric fistulas. *In* Haimovici H [ed]: Vascular Emergencies. New York, Appleton-Century-Crofts, 1982.)

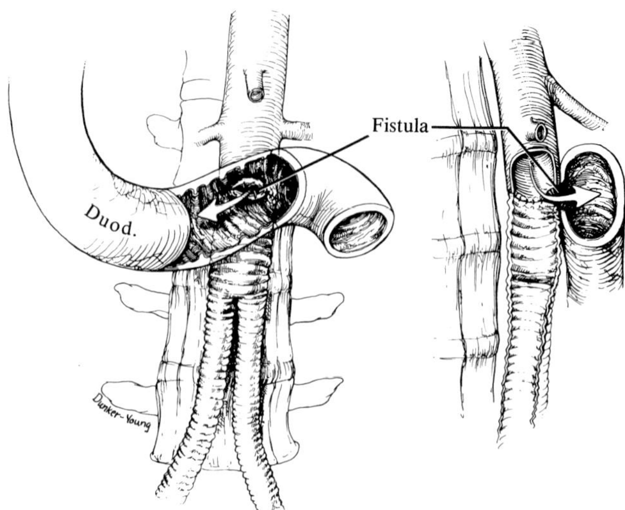

FIGURE 49–2. Secondary aortoduodenal fistula. (From Ernst CB: Aortoenteric fistulas. *In* Haimovici H [ed]: Vascular Emergencies. New York, Appleton-Century-Crofts, 1982.)

aorta and the third or fourth portion of the duodenum (83% of patients), because of the anatomic contiguity of the duodenal-jejunal flexure and the anterior bulge of the aneurysm (Fig. 49–1).[30, 31, 36, 81] Occasionally, other segments of the bowel may be involved, including esophagus, stomach, jejunum, ileum, appendix and colon.[26, 32, 59, 95] Usually the aneurysm is sterile and secondary to arteriosclerotic degeneration of the aorta; however, it is infected in up to 30% of patients, *Staphylococcus aureus* and *Staphylococcus epidermidis* being the most frequent isolates.[100] Other infrequent causes of primary AEF include neoplastic erosion into the bowel and adjacent aorta, peptic ulcer perforation into the aorta, tuberculous mesenteric lymphadenitis, primary aortitis, pancreatic pseudocyst penetration, and irradiation.[17, 32, 39, 44, 67, 72, 91, 94]

Secondary AEFs usually follow aortic reconstructive procedures with prosthetic grafts or homografts, although they may also follow other reconstructive procedures, including endarterectomy and aortorenal bypass.[14, 23, 35, 54, 90] Secondary AEFs occur in two forms: (1) anastomotic communication between aortic lumen and bowel lumen and (2) the less common aortoparaprosthetic-enteric sinus (Figs. 49–2 and 49–3).[8, 36] A paraprosthetic-enteric sinus forms between the outer connective tissue capsule of the prosthesis and the bowel lumen (Fig. 49–4). There is no communication with the aortic lumen except through the interstices of the graft. The eroded edges of bowel mucosa also may be the source of bleeding. A sinus can evolve into a fistula if the paraprosthetic sinus erodes into the aortic lumen or spreads to include the proximal or distal suture lines.[11, 34] Secondary AEFs were more common than the primary type and were reported in as many as 10% of early experiences after aortic reconstructive procedures.[29, 35, 50] With improvements in operative technique, the incidence has declined to 0.4% to 2.4%.[11, 31, 45, 97] The incidence increases up to 40% with primary aortic graft infection, however.[13, 30, 49, 83]

Attempts have been made to classify AEFs uniformly. Vollmar and Kogel designated direct aortoenteric communications as *type I* fistulae.[102] They subclassified type I fistulae according to the absence (*type IA*) or presence (*type IB*) of an associated pseudoaneurysm. *Type II* AEFs are graft-enteric erosions. Buchbinder has classified aortic disruptions as either fistulae or erosions, based on their pathologic appearance.[10] An AEF, whether primary or secondary, represents a direct communication between aorta and bowel, whereas a graft-enteric erosion designates a paraprosthetic sinus.

PATHOPHYSIOLOGY

The pathogenesis of primary and secondary AEFs is thought to involve both mechanical and infectious processes. These processes include erosion into the bowel by an aneurysm or prosthesis, infection, aneurysm rupture, duodenal trauma or ischemia incurred during aortic recon-

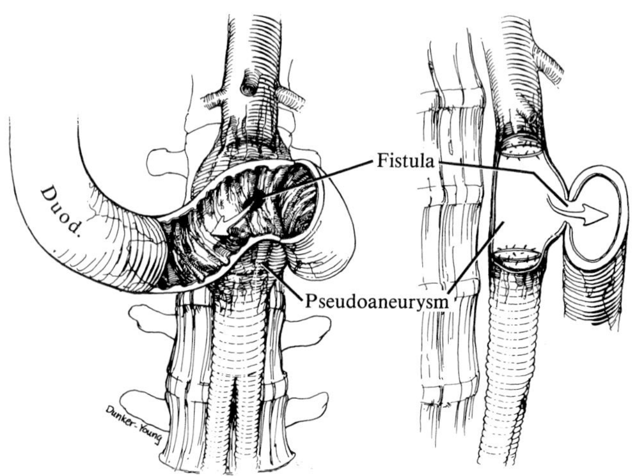

FIGURE 49–3. An aortoduodenal fistula associated with an anastomotic aneurysm. (From Ernst CB: Aortoenteric fistulas. *In* Haimovici H [ed]: Vascular Emergencies. New York, Appleton-Century-Crofts, 1982.)

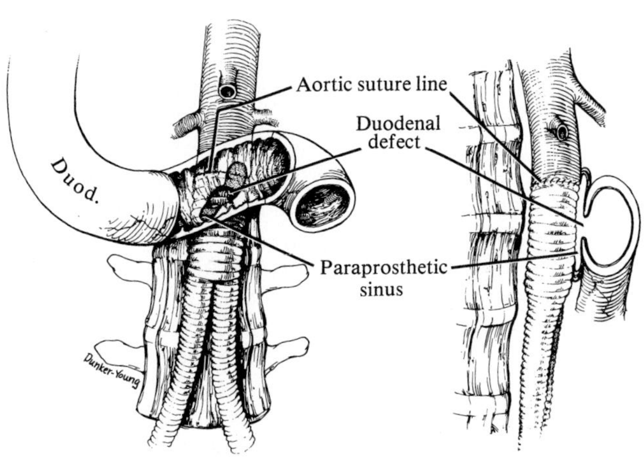

FIGURE 49–4. An aortoparaprosthetic sinus. The prosthesis has eroded into the duodenum. The paraprosthetic sinus tract extends up to the proximal anastomosis *(right)*. (From Ernst CB: Aortoenteric fistulas. *In* Haimovici H [ed]: Vascular Emergencies. New York, Appleton-Century-Crofts, 1982.)

struction, anastomotic degeneration, inadequate prosthetic coverage, and kinking of the graft. Several types of graft materials have been associated with AEF, including polyester (Dacron), polytetrafluoroethylene (Teflon), nylon, and homografts.[9, 20, 28, 34] Duodenal erosion subsequent to the inflammatory foreign body response of the adjacent pulsating noncompliant prosthesis may initiate the process.[28] Operative trauma or ischemia to the duodenum also contributes to the erosion.[34] After bowel perforation, bacteria and digestive enzymes bathe the graft, causing graft infection, retroperitoneal inflammation, and formation of an aortoenteric sinus. With progression of the process and extension of the sinus, the proximal suture line eventually erodes, resulting in a true AEF.[10, 13, 34, 55, 74]

Another proposed mechanism of secondary AEF formation implicates aortic suture line disruption as the primary event. A proximal anastomotic aneurysm forms and eventually erodes into the adjacent bowel. Suture line disruption may be secondary to hypertension, suture fatigue, local infection, or aortic wall degeneration.[21, 50] Events that predispose to infection increase the likelihood of anastomotic disruption.[40, 55, 78] Busuttil and associates reported that repair of ruptured aneurysms was associated with a 1.7% incidence of AEF, as compared with 0.7% after elective aneurysm resection and 0.2% after elective aortic reconstruction for aortoiliac occlusive disease.[13] A flawed proximal anastomosis with inclusion of the proximal flare of the aneurysm when repairing ruptured aortic aneurysms may account for development of such anastomotic aneurysms. The incidence of AEF development was higher in the 1950s and 1960s, when silk suture was used for arterial anastomoses.[69] No reports have implicated end-to-side (more than end-to-end) anastomoses in pseudoaneurysm formation.

The erosive mechanism is supported by the success of contemporary aortic reconstructive techniques as well as by current recommendations for treating primary AEFs. Standard aortic reconstructive procedures may be performed with virtually no delayed infectious complications, supporting a purely erosive and perforating event rather than an infectious process. Another factor supporting the erosive mechanism is the decreased frequency of AEF in reports emphasizing the interposition of viable tissue as a buttress between the prosthesis and the bowel during aortic reconstruction.[7, 27, 34] Large prostheses, especially those larger than 22 mm in diameter, often have inadequate retroperitoneal coverage and are more predisposed to erosion and AEF formation.[55, 78] Current opinion favors a mechanical erosive process, followed by secondary infection in most cases of secondary AEF.

CLINICAL PRESENTATION

The classic triad of symptoms associated with AEF includes gastrointestinal bleeding, sepsis, and abdominal pain. Finding all three symptoms in one patient is uncommon, occurring in fewer than 30%.[11, 26, 95] Classically, gastrointestinal hemorrhage is the initial symptom, occurring in more than 70% of AEFs and manifesting as hematemesis, hematochezia, melena, or chronic anemia.[11, 26, 95] Massive hemorrhage without antecedent bleeding is rare, accounting for fewer than 5% of initial bleeding episodes.[95] Most often, patients present with a "herald bleed," having limited, hemodynamically insignificant bleeding episodes over several hours to days, as the fistulous tract intermittently opens and seals with clot.[11, 95] Voyles noted that 27% of patients with AEF survived less than 6 hours, 14% survived 16 to 24 hours, and 46% were alive after 24 hours.[104] Massive gastrointestinal hemorrhage, uncommon with paraprosthetic sinuses, occurs in fewer than 33% of patients.[11, 83]

The interval from aortic reconstruction to the onset of hemorrhage averages 2 to 6 years after graft placement[7, 15, 24, 41, 55, 87] but it may range from 2 days to 15 years.[87, 107] Massive gastrointestinal hemorrhage inevitably follows the herald bleed, although the interval varies. In 90% of patients, ample time is available to pursue a definitive diagnosis before exsanguinating hemorrhage occurs. Clinically insignificant gastrointestinal bleeding in some form is sometimes encountered after an aortic operation; the cause is rarely AEF. Pabst and coworkers identified 74 episodes of gastrointestinal bleeding in 52 patients after aortic reconstruction.[77] The bleeding occurred over an interval of 46 months postoperatively, but only one episode represented an AEF.

Signs of infection are found most often with paraprosthetic-enteric sinuses, occurring in 60% of patients, in contrast to only 15% of patients with secondary AEFs. Fever of unknown origin, generalized malaise, and unexplained leukocytosis may be manifestations of AEF. Septicemia results from bacterial absorption through venous or lymphatic channels, and blood cultures may be positive for enteric organisms.[86] Bacteria may translocate through the interstices of the graft, onto the prosthetic lining, and occasionally they present as septic emboli to the legs. Clinical signs include purulent, draining groin wounds, petechial leg rashes, and localized leg cellulitis.[5, 43, 64, 93]

Abdominal pain is the least common symptom of AEF but is mostly associated with a primary AEF from aneurysm expansion.[95] Paraprosthetic sinuses present with pain in 20% of patients, whereas only 11% complain of pain with secondary AEFs.[11] Aneurysms are palpable in fewer than

25% of patients who have primary AEFs, whereas aortic anastomotic aneurysms are even less often palpable.[55, 74, 79, 95, 107]

DIAGNOSIS

Multiple diagnostic studies are available, but none is completely reliable. Thus, any patient with an abdominal aortic aneurysm or a history of aortic reconstruction who develops gastrointestinal bleeding should be considered to have an AEF until it is proven otherwise, with the knowledge that AEFs are rare.[11, 34, 42, 55, 77] Although patients with a history of aortic reconstruction who develop gastrointestinal bleeding have only a 2% chance of having an AEF, without prompt diagnosis, death from exsanguinating hemorrhage can rapidly ensue. While preoperative diagnosis is only 15% to 30% accurate, an attempt should be made to identify the source of bleeding if the patient is clinically stable.[11, 55, 86] Upper gastrointestinal endoscopy, aortography, and contrast-enhanced computed tomography (CT) all have clearly defined roles in the preoperative evaluation. The roles of magnetic resonance imaging (MRI), gastrointestinal barium contrast studies, and radiolabeled isotope scans are less clearly defined.

If hemorrhage is massive and the patient is unstable, emergency celiotomy for diagnosis and treatment should be performed promptly if the history suggests an AEF or a paraprosthetic sinus.[75] Usually, the patient remains stable after the initial herald bleed, and this allows time to conduct a deliberate but expeditious evaluation. Unfortunately, only 50% of AEFs can be definitively diagnosed preoperatively, although more may be suspected.[4, 12, 66, 76, 92] Physical examination may reveal a palpable abdominal aortic aneurysm or signs of septic emboli. Downstream blood cultures occasionally identify enteric organisms, suggesting the presence of an AEF. If lower extremity arterial blood cultures yield gram-negative organisms while peripheral culture specimens from arm veins are negative, AEF is very likely the diagnosis.[34] If all available tests are nonconfirmatory, diagnostic celiotomy should be undertaken to confirm or exclude an AEF.

Upper gastrointestinal endoscopy is the initial study of choice in a clinically stable patient.[4, 12, 55, 92] The study should be performed by an experienced endoscopist and includes complete examination of the duodenum through the third and fourth portions.[14, 77] Findings suggestive of an AEF include visualization of an extrinsic mass compressing the duodenum, punctate mucosal ulcerations of the distal duodenum, and bleeding from the duodenal wall. The graft may be seen by the endoscopist in one third of AEFs, the proximal suture line or a bile-stained prosthesis being apparent. Other sources of hemorrhage, such as a gastroesophageal junction tear, bleeding peptic ulcer, or gastric varices, may confound the diagnosis. Patients may bleed from more than one source, and hemorrhage should not be attributed to another cause until an AEF has been definitively excluded. During endoscopy, the tamponading thrombus may become dislodged, precipitating sudden hemorrhage.[78] Consequently, some surgeons recommend performing endoscopy in the operating room with preparations at hand for emergency celiotomy should severe hemorrhage occur.[55, 78, 100]

Contrast-enhanced CT is a good complementary study when endoscopic studies are not definitive. CT cannot consistently differentiate AEF from perigraft infection, but in a retrospective study, CT documented the presence of one or the other of these complications with high sensitivity (94%) and specificity (85%).[60] CT findings consistent with the diagnosis of AEF include perigraft fluid or gas bubbles apparent more than 6 weeks after aortic reconstruction, leakage of oral contrast medium, pseudoaneurysm formation at the proximal anastomosis, and thickening of adjacent bowel wall.[49, 60, 62] Mark and colleagues correctly diagnosed AEF in six of six patients and excluded it in four of four who had no fistula on CT.[63] Culture specimens of perigraft fluid may be obtained with CT-guided needle aspiration to confirm infection, but this does not confirm the presence of a fistula or graft erosion.[25, 51]

Aortography documents findings consistent with AEF in approximately one third of patients, although an actual fistula with contrast extravasation is rarely identified.[71, 89, 98, 99] Aortography may document an anastomotic aneurysm or a kink in a redundant graft, both contributing factors to bowel erosion (Fig. 49–5)[70, 82]; however, aortography cannot document an aortoparaprosthetic sinus. An aortogram does provide valuable anatomic information for aortic reconstruction and important information on visceral vessel patency and the need for lower extremity revascularization. Gastrointestinal contrast studies must be deferred until after the aortographic studies to avoid obscuring radiographic findings.

Barium contrast studies of the upper gastrointestinal tract are seldom helpful. Such contrast studies are infrequently diagnostic and have very low specificity. Radiographic find-

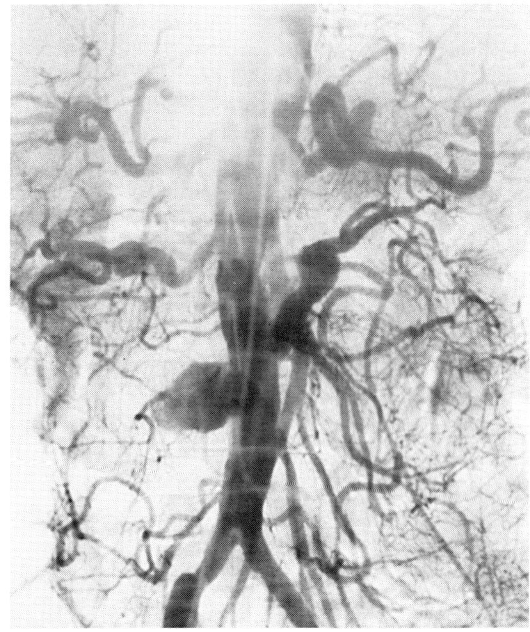

FIGURE 49–5. Aortogram documenting anastomotic aneurysm of right polyester (Dacron) aortorenal bypass. The patient presented with massive upper gastrointestinal hemorrhage. (From Campbell HC Jr, Ernst CB: Aortoenteric fistula following renal revascularization. Am Surg 44:155, 1978.)

ings that may be helpful include duodenal irregularities, such as clot in the duodenum or extrinsic duodenal compression, and the "coiled-spring" configuration from gut contrast extravasation outlining the aortic prosthesis.[106, 108] Actual leakage of contrast medium is very rare, with only 5% of patients having the coiled-spring sign.[11] Furthermore, residual barium makes subsequent CT imaging impossible owing to scanning artefact and obscures possible arteriographic findings.

Other tests that are potentially useful in the evaluation of AEF include MRI, indium 111–labeled leukocyte or red blood cell (RBC) scanning, and indium 111–labeled immunoglobulin G imaging. MRI is accurate in revealing perigraft infection and may be useful with AEF.[3, 73] Nuclear imaging techniques also have high sensitivity for detecting graft infection, but currently their efficacy in the diagnosis of an AEF is unclear.[57, 58] In an anecdotal report, tagged RBC studies documented an aortoappendiceal fistula when findings of all other investigations were negative.[1]

In general, the recommended sequence of diagnostic testing begins with an appropriate history and physical examination to elicit all potential risk factors. For a stable patient with suspected AEF, upper gastrointestinal endoscopy should be the first study, and preparations should be made for immediate celiotomy if necessary (Fig. 49–6). CT should follow a negative or indeterminate endoscopic study. Aortography helps in planning the operative procedure when endoscopy or CT documents an AEF. A "negative CT scan" may be followed by other diagnostic tests, including MRI, indium 111–labeled white blood cell scanning, gastrointestinal contrast studies, and tagged RBC scanning. Diagnostic celiotomy is the most reliable and definitive procedure, when all test findings remain negative. An unstable patient who presents with gastrointestinal hemorrhage should immediately undergo celiotomy.

TREATMENT

Surgical Options

Successful treatment of an AEF requires operative management; otherwise, death from either exsanguinating hemorrhage or sepsis is certain. Diagnostic tests and preparations for definitive treatment must proceed simultaneously. The chance of survival is inversely related to the interval between the onset of bleeding and surgical intervention.[55] Five surgical principles should be followed:

- Confirmation of the diagnosis
- Control of hemorrhage
- Repair of the bowel defect
- Eradication of associated infection
- Restoration of distal circulation

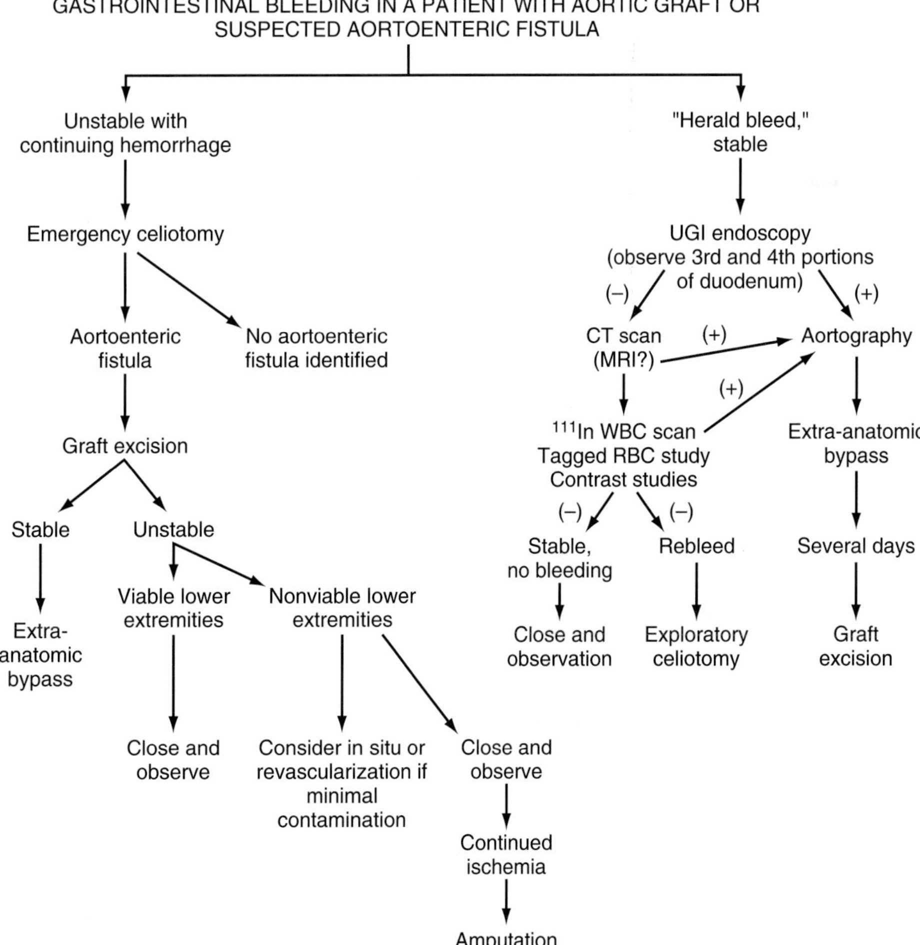

FIGURE 49–6. Algorithm for the management and treatment of secondary aortoenteric fistulae. UGI = upper gastrointestinal tract; RBC = red blood cell; CT = computed tomography. (From Ernst CB: Aortoenteric fistula. *In* Shackelford RT [ed]: Surgery of the Alimentary Tract, 4th ed. Philadelphia, WB Saunders, 1996.)

The patient should be optimally prepared preoperatively with fluid resuscitation, blood typing and cross-matching, and initiation of broad-spectrum antibiotic therapy. Preoperative placement of central monitoring lines should include Swan-Ganz catheterization. The surgeon then has several options, depending on the location of the AEF, the presence of a true communication or a paraprosthetic sinus, and the degree of retroperitoneal infection.

Primary Aortoenteric Fistula

The surgical treatment for primary AEF is less standardized than that for secondary AEF because primary AEF is much less common. Infection usually is of little importance in a primary AEF. Consequently, repair can be successfully accomplished by standard aortic reconstruction with concomitant duodenal repair or segmental bowel resection.[26, 31] The aortic reconstruction may be performed with an in situ prosthetic graft. Daugherty and colleagues, among several other investigators, have advocated this conservative approach and have documented long-term success and almost no infectious sequelae.[26, 95, 96, 103] Bacterial infection is rarely problematic and, when present, is usually confined to the proximate tissues around the fistulous tract. If extensive duodenal spillage is encountered during the dissection, the communication should be treated as a secondary AEF, as described later. With limited infection, however, the recommended treatment of primary AEF consists of aortic aneurysmectomy, duodenorrhaphy, and standard aortic reconstruction.[26, 31]

Secondary Aortoenteric Fistula

Several treatment options are available for managing a secondary AEF, depending on the clinical situation. These options include local repair, graft excision with in situ replacement, graft excision without coincident vascular reconstruction, and graft excision with restoration of arterial flow by selective extra-anatomic revascularization. Successful results can be achieved with each of these procedures in selected patients. Each particular situation must be continuously reassessed and the treatment tailored appropriately. However, the high mortality rates associated with local repair (67%) and graft excision without revascularization (71%) reflect the limited applicability of these options (Table 49–1).[11] Local treatment results in high rates of recurrent fistulization and sepsis, because some degree of retroperitoneal infection is invariably present.[13, 55]

Complete graft excision is required when the graft and retroperitoneum are infected. Extra-anatomic bypass may be indicated, depending on the viability of the lower extremities. Because most secondary AEFs occur after aortic reconstruction for aneurysms (rather than occlusive disease), compensatory collateral vessels are usually minimally developed. Thus, revascularization is necessary to prevent lower extremity limb loss. When the original reconstruction is performed for aortoiliac occlusive disease, preexisting collateral channels may obviate immediate lower extremity revascularization. Although circulation may be marginal and signs of ischemia may be present, collateral blood flow is usually adequate for limb salvage. If the original aortic reconstruction included an end-to-side proximal anastomosis, adequate peripheral blood flow may be maintained through the native aorta after graft excision and aortic repair. If the original reconstruction was renal revascularization, the most appropriate treatment of the secondary AEF usually entails graft excision, lateral aortorrhaphy, and nephrectomy if indicated.[14, 79]

The timing and sequence of graft excision and extra-anatomic reconstruction depend on the mode of presentation. When the diagnosis is uncertain in an unstable patient with ongoing life-threatening hemorrhage, life-saving celiotomy and graft excision must precede extra-anatomic bypass. Several potential risks are inherent with this operative sequence. Prolongation of lower extremity ischemia may lead to critical ischemia and amputation. The increased cardiac afterload following closure of the aortic stump also increases the risk of a myocardial event. Immediate graft excision remains the safest course under such emergent conditions. Selective lower extremity revascularization is then performed when necessary, preferably as a staged, delayed procedure 2 to 3 days later. Immediate extra-anatomic bypass after graft excision taxes the already stressed patient, a fact reflected in the much different mortality rates associated with concomitant (37%) or staged (13%) revascularizations.[84]

When the diagnosis of a secondary AEF has been established preoperatively in a stable patient, a two-stage approach is most appropriate. Preliminary extra-anatomic reconstruction should be performed, followed by graft excision, bowel repair, and aortic stump closure 2 to 3 days later. This approach ensures lower limb viability. Potential problems with this approach include bacterial seeding of the new prosthesis, risk of continuing hemorrhage from the AEF before definitive repair, and thrombosis of the extra-anatomic bypass from decreased blood flow secondary to competing parallel blood flow channels. However, the incidence of secondary infection of the extra-anatomic bypass was only 16% in one report.[84] Additionally, the actual risk of ongoing hemorrhage from the AEF is small, and improved patient survival is associated with the less stressful two-stage approach.[84]

Finally, thrombosis of the extra-anatomic graft from competitive blood flow is not a valid concern.[37] When possible, occlusion of the limbs of the original prosthesis during the initial extra-anatomic revascularization procedure induces graft thrombosis, which simplifies later excision of the infected graft.[35]

The most feared complication of graft excision is aortic stump dehiscence. Aortic stump closure in a potentially infected field can eventuate in this complication. Several variations of stump coverage have been suggested, including omental flaps, muscle flaps, and serosal patches; however, despite these various techniques of closure, aortic stump blowout remains the leading cause of early death after graft excision, occurring in as many as one third of patients.[65, 74]

In situ graft replacement has been suggestesd to obviate aortic stump blowout and to decrease the stress associated with multiple operations.[6, 48, 85, 97, 105] Kieffer and coworkers emphasized in situ replacement of the aortic prosthesis with preserved allografts obtained from cadavers.[52] Their report included 43 patients with an infected graft or secondary AEF, and follow-up averaged almost 14 months.

TABLE 49–1. OPERATIVE MORTALITY OF VARIOUS APPROACHES TO THE REPAIR OF AORTOENTERIC FISTULAS

				OPERATION NO. OF PATIENTS (DEATHS)						
AUTHOR	YEAR	PATIENTS (NO.)	MORTALITY (%)	None	Local	GE/NR	GE/IS	GE/EAB	Celiotomy	Other
Kleinman et al[55]	1979	20	65	5(5)	2(2)	4(2)	2(2)	7(2)	—	—
Puglia and Fry[80]	1980	22	59	5(5)	3(2)	—	4(2)	9(3)	1(1)	—
Buchbinder et al[10]	1980	16	44	—	2(2)	—	—	14(5)	—	—
Perdue et al[78]	1980	16	38	3(3)	—	—	4(1)	7(1)	—	2(1)
Kiernan et al[53]	1980	20	80	—	3(3)	3(3)	5(4)	6(4)	—	3(3)
O'Mara et al[75]	1981	17	88	—	3(2)	1(1)	3(3)	8(7)	2(2)	—
Champion et al[15]	1982	22	77	1(1)	5(5)	4(4)	2(0)	6(3)	3(3)	1(1)
Moulton et al[68]	1986	22	45	—	2(2)	3(2)	2(0)	13(4)	2(2)	—
Thomas and Baird[97]	1986	8	25	—	4(0)	1(1)	2(0)	1(1)	—	—
Walker et al[105]	1987	23	22	—	—	—	23(5)	—	—	—
Harris et al[46]	1987	14	64	2(2)	7(4)	—	5(3)	—	—	—
Vollmar and Kogel[102]	1987	11	45	—	—	2(2)	3(2)	6(1)	—	—
Higgins et al[48]	1990	15	27	—	2(0)	1(0)	4(0)	7(3)	1(1)	—
Kuestner et al[56]	1994	33	18	—	—	—	—	33(6)	—	—
van Baalen et al[101]	1996	27	41	6(6)	—	2(0)	8(0)	6(0)	5(5)	—
TOTAL		286	49	22(22)	33(22)	21(15)	67(22)	123(40)	14(14)	6(5)
MORTALITY (%)				100	67	71	33	33	100	83

GE/NR = graft excision without reconstruction; GE/IS = graft excision with replacement in situ; GE/EAB = graft excision plus extra-anatomic bypass.

They documented 88% initial survival, 81% operative success, and 25% late graft-related complications. This group has suggested such in situ grafting as a bridge to delayed prosthetic aortic reconstruction or maintaining in situ allograft reconstruction as a permanent conduit.[52]

Successful in situ grafting in a minimally infected retroperitoneum has been documented when extra-anatomic bypass was not possible.[2, 16] This has been accomplished with lifelong or long-term antibiotic therapy; however, with a grossly contaminated field, aortic reconstruction in situ is contraindicated. Long-term follow-up is necessary after in situ aortic reconstruction to identify late complications such as recurrent infection, recurrent AEF, and anastomotic aneurysm formation.

Each clinical scenario dictates the method of operative management. Graft excision with selective extra-anatomic bypass remains the recommended approach. If the patient has had a herald bleeding episode and remains hemodynamically stable with a confirmed AEF, a two-stage approach is suggested. The extra-anatomic bypass, preferably an axillobifemoral one, is constructed first. With previous placement of an aortobifemoral graft, the extra-anatomic bypass must be placed through clean tissue planes to distal arterial segments that are free of infection. Consequently, the distal anastomoses may be attached to the distal superficial femoral, deep femoral, or proximal popliteal arteries.

Operative Technique

Celiotomy requires preparing and draping the entire abdomen, thorax, neck and upper arms, groins, and upper thighs. An autotransfusion device should be available. The abdomen is entered through a vertical midline incision. A thorough exploration of the peritoneal cavity to identify any other abnormalities is in order, particularly if a definitive preoperative diagnosis has not been made. The supraceliac aorta should be initially isolated at the diaphragmatic hiatus by dividing the gastrohepatic omentum and the diaphragmatic crura (Fig. 49–7). This measure allows proximal control of the aorta in the event that bleeding is encountered from the fistula during dissection of the infrarenal aorta. Proximal and distal control of the infrarenal aorta is then obtained by placing the vascular clamps above and below the prosthesis or aneurysm. The bowel overlying the aortic aneurysm or aortic prosthesis must be fully mobi-

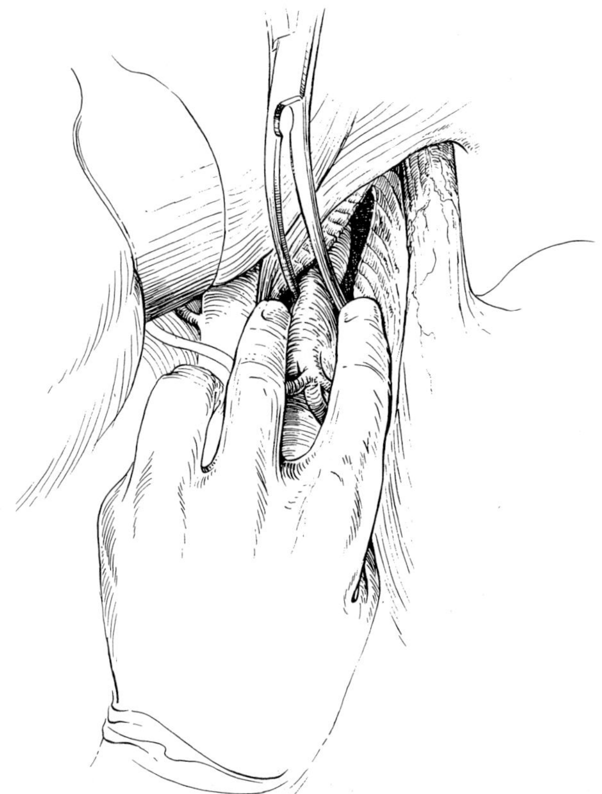

FIGURE 49–7. Method of applying a supraceliac aortic clamp. The diaphragmatic crus has been incised to provide access to the supraceliac aorta. The left lobe of the liver is retracted to the right. (From Ernst CB: Aortoenteric fistula. *In* Shackelford RT [ed]: Surgery of the Alimentary Tract, 4th ed. Philadelphia, WB Saunders, 1996.)

lized so that a fistula or paraprosthetic sinus can be identified. Such mobilization requires sharp dissection to separate all loops of adherent bowel from the aneurysm or graft.

Primary Aortoenteric Fistula

If the diagnosis of primary AEF has been confirmed preoperatively and the patient is not actively bleeding, proximal and distal control of the aorta may be obtained below the renal arteries and below the aneurysm on the aorta or iliac vessels. With massive bleeding, supraceliac aortic occlusion should initially be obtained until adequate infrarenal aortic dissection with clamping has been achieved. After satisfactory infrarenal clamping, the supraceliac clamp is removed. An unstable patient with active bleeding may require rapid division of the fistula before aortic dissection, with immediate tamponade of the hemorrhage. The aortic defect may be adequately controlled by placement of a large balloon-tipped catheter into the defect (Fig. 49–8).[14, 38] If the hole is small, temporary suturing can control the bleeding.

A large defect in the bowel should be temporarily sutured to limit retroperitoneal soiling. The defect is definitively repaired after resection of the aortic aneurysm. A small defect (≤1 cm) may be definitively repaired before the aneurysm resection. Although enterorrhaphy alone usually suffices, segmental resection may be necessary with large, friable, contused, or ischemic bowel defects.

Standard aortic reconstruction is the preferred method of management of a primary AEF. The aneurysm wall must be thoroughly débrided. Culture samples of the aortic wall are obtained, including aerobic, anaerobic, bacterial, and fungal organisms, so that subsequent antibiotic administration can be organism-specific. The proximal anastomosis must be secured to healthy and substantial aortic wall. The site of the distal anastomosis depends on the extent of aneurysmal or occlusive disease. The graft is then covered with débrided aortic wall or wrapped with a viable pedicle of omentum, separating the bowel and the contaminated retroperitoneum from the prosthesis (Figs. 49–9 and 49–10).[26, 31, 95] The retroperitoneum must be thoroughly irrigated before closure to minimize potential graft sepsis.

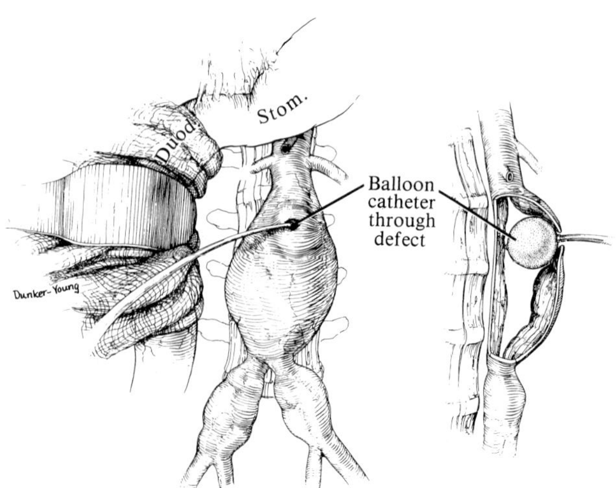

FIGURE 49–8. Inflated balloon-tipped catheter placed into aortic defect of primary aortoduodenal fistula. (From Ernst CB: Aortoenteric fistulas. *In* Haimovici H [ed]: Vascular Emergencies. New York, Appleton-Century-Crofts, 1982.)

Secondary Aortoenteric Fistula or Aortoenteric Paraprosthetic Sinus

Stable patients with secondary AEFs should undergo preliminary axillofemoral reconstruction, particularly when the initial operation was for aneurysmal disease. The axillobifemoral bypass is constructed from the side of the nondominant arm or the arm with the higher blood pressure. The axillary artery is isolated, beginning at the lateral border of the first rib. The common femoral, superficial femoral, and deep femoral arteries are also isolated.

The axillary and groin incisions are connected with a subcutaneous tunnel placed along the mid-axillary line (Fig. 49–11). The graft is tunneled deep to the pectoralis major muscle, then subcutaneously to the groin. Polytetrafluoroethylene with external ring support is the preferred conduit. Axillary and femoral anastomoses are constructed, and the femorofemoral component is completed through a suprapubic tunnel, from the distalmost axillofemoral graft to the opposite common femoral or deep femoral (profunda femoris) artery.

Contamination of groins from a previous aortobifemoral bypass necessitates graft placement through clean tissue fields with distal anastomoses to other sites. Options include the distal deep or distal superficial femoral artery and bilateral axillofemoral bypass. Autogenous vein may be used in contaminated fields when clean, uncontaminated tissue planes are not available.[33]

A recent innovation has been autogenous tissue aortic reconstruction, termed a *neo-aortoiliac system*, using lower extremity venous conduits, principally the superficial femoral vein.[18] Results have been encouraging, and reconstructions have proved durable for at least 36 months without evidence of subsequent infectious complications.[19] Such autogenous tissue reconstructions are technically challenging and arduous and, consequently, are not appropriate under urgent or emergent circumstances.

The patient's condition is assessed after all incisions are closed and after the graft is functioning. If the operative time has been relatively short (≤4 hours) and the patient's condition is satisfactory, the original graft may be excised at the same operation. Otherwise, a 48- to 72-hour delay is recommended before graft excision if the patient remains clinically stable with no evidence of active bleeding.

The abdomen is entered through a vertical midline incision to avoid interference with the axillobifemoral graft. A thorough exploratory celiotomy is performed to assess all potential sources of hemorrhage. Supraceliac control of the aorta is obtained, as described. The infrarenal aorta is then isolated above and below the prosthesis, and the graft is completely excised.

The aortic stump must be securely closed with two rows of nonabsorbable sutures. The closure is performed distal to the renal arteries. All nonviable aortic wall is removed, with only healthy aortic wall used for the closure. Running horizontal mattress sutures construct the proximal row, and the distal row is fashioned with an over-and-over baseball stitch. If the necrotic aorta extends up to the renal ostia and available aorta is insufficient for safe closure, hepatorenal or

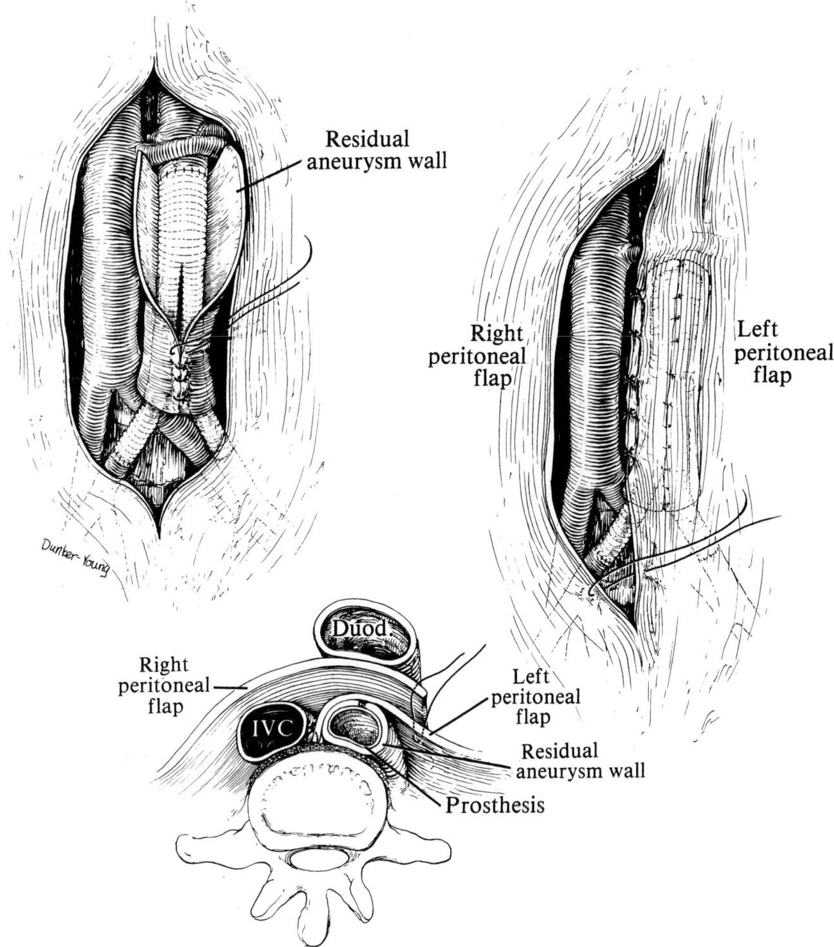

FIGURE 49–9. Method of separating prosthesis from duodenum following aneurysmectomy. Residual débrided aneurysm wall graft *(upper left)*. Left peritoneal flap is sutured to connective tissue between inferior vena cava and graft *(upper right)*. Right peritoneal flap is imbricated over left *(lower)*. (From Ernst CB: Aortoenteric fistulas. *In* Haimovici H [ed]: Vascular Emergencies. New York, Appleton-Century-Crofts, 1982.)

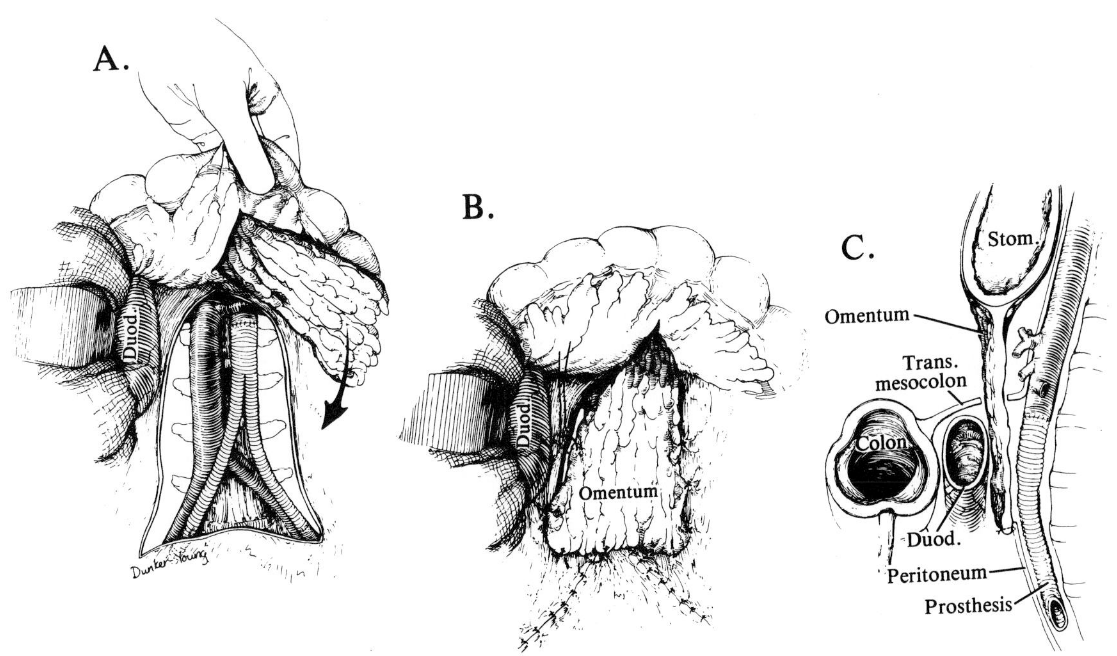

FIGURE 49–10. *A*, Omentum is passed through incision in transverse mesocolon. *B*, The omentum, sutured to retroperitoneal tissues, covers the prosthesis, separating the prosthesis from the duodenum. *C*, Sagittal view showing omentum passed through transverse mesocolon and interposed between prosthesis and duodenum. (From Ernst CB: Aortoenteric fistulas. *In* Haimovici H [ed]: Vascular Emergencies. New York, Appleton-Century-Crofts, 1982.)

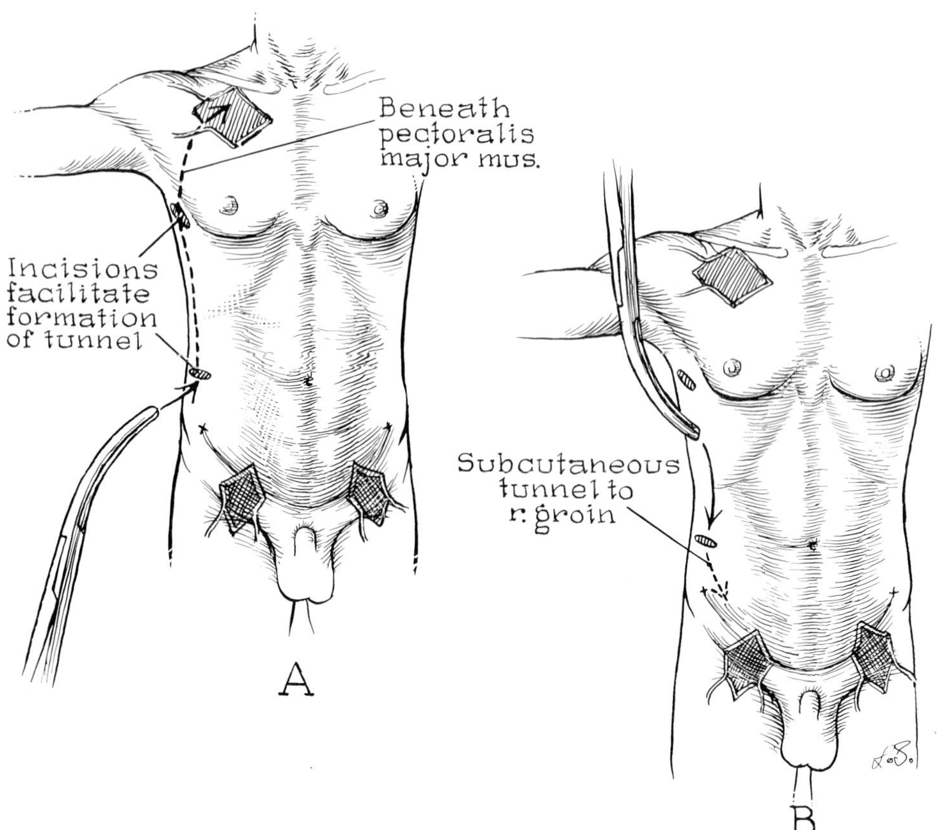

FIGURE 49–11. Axillary femoral tunnel for a right axillofemoral bypass. One or two transverse incisions equidistant between axillary and groin incisions are required for tunnel formation. Tunnel lies in the midaxillary line and passes medial to anterior superior iliac spine. (From Ernst CB: Axillobifemoral bypass. *In* Nyhus LM, Baker RJ [eds]: Mastery of Surgery, 2nd ed. Boston, Little, Brown, 1992.)

splenorenal bypass may be necessary to preserve renal blood flow.[82] The aortic stump is buttressed with a tongue of omentum or healthy surrounding soft tissue (Fig. 49–12).

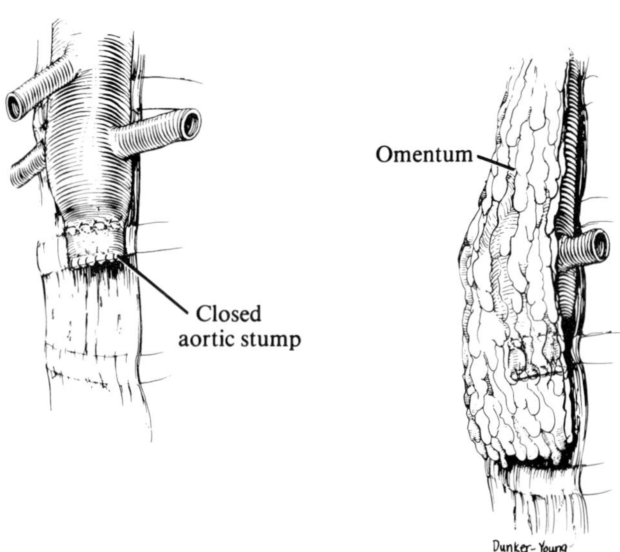

FIGURE 49–12. Method of closing the infrarenal aorta after prosthesis excision. The proximal row of continuous sutures is followed by a distal row of a continuous over-and-over stitch *(left)*. Omental graft passed through transverse mesocolon and sutured over the aortic stump provides additional buttressing and protection *(right)*. (From Ernst CB: Aortoenteric fistula. *In* Brewster D [ed]: Common Problems in Vascular Surgery. Chicago, Year Book Medical Publishers, 1989.)

The distal anastomoses for the original aortic reconstruction may have been to the aorta, iliac vessels, or femoral arteries. When the iliac vessels are involved, they are oversewn with nonabsorbable suture material through the abdominal incision. If the distal anastomoses were made to the femoral vessels, the distal graft limbs are oversewn during the axillobifemoral reconstruction and stuffed cephalad into the retropertitoneum through the groin incision. Later, during the abdominal phase, the graft limbs are delivered into the abdomen and removed with the entire remaining prosthesis.

The bowel defect is closed transversely. If bowel involvement precludes primary closure, the third portion of the duodenum is oversewn and a loop of jejunum is anastomosed to the side of the proximal duodenum, preferably the second portion.[55, 75] When the AEF involves the jejunum, primary closure or segmental resection with end-to-end anastomosis is recommended.

Graft excision must precede extra-anatomic reconstruction for patients with massive bleeding, an equivocal diagnosis, or an AEF encountered unexpectedly during celiotomy for upper gastrointestinal tract bleeding. In these situations, the sequence of procedures is reversed. A patient with well-developed collaterals may tolerate graft excision alone if the original operation was for aortoiliac occlusive disease. Additionally, excision alone may be sufficient if an end-to-side aortic anastomosis was performed originally, when the original graft has thrombosed, or for an amputee.[55] The need for subsequent axillobifemoral bypass grafting depends on the condition of the lower extremities after graft excision. Extra-anatomic reconstruction may be required immediately or within several weeks of the graft excision. When Doppler imaging cannot detect blood flow in the lower extremities or if the extremities appear nonviable, immediate axillobifemoral bypass is necessary. The patient must be stable enough to tolerate the additional procedures. If the patient's condition is so precarious as to preclude extra-anatomic reconstruction, amputation may be the only alternative.

Results

Success of standard aortic reconstruction as the definitive treatment of primary AEF has been documented in several reports, with both short-term and long-term follow-up.[26, 95, 96, 103] Placing a prosthesis in a potentially infected field appears safe. In a collective review of 118 patients with primary AEF, 34 were treated operatively with a mortality rate of 35%.[95] Primary duodenal repair with standard aortic reconstruction was performed in 19 of the 22 survivors. Graft-related complications were found in fewer than 5% of the long-term survivors, an observation that supports the safety of this operative approach.

Without operative treatment, secondary AEFs are uniformly fatal.[11, 34, 55, 75] Survival rates range from 10% to 87% (see Table 49–1).[30] Local aortic anastomotic repair is associated with an average mortality rate of 67%, whereas graft excision without revascularization carries an average mortality of 71%. These poor results render them unacceptable treatments unless aortic graft excision without revascularization is being performed in the presence of occlusive disease with adequate collateralization.

Favorable results have been reported with several other forms of treatment. The average operative mortality for graft excision with extra-anatomic bypass is 33%, and some studies record mortality rates as low as 15%.[10, 15, 30, 53, 55, 75, 78, 88, 97, 102] One report of secondary AEFs treated with extra-anatomic bypass and graft excision mentioned a perioperative mortality rate of only 18% and a 3-year cumulative cure rate of 70%.[56] The incidence of extra-anatomic bypass failure was 18.2%, whereas the incidence of major limb amputation was 9.1%.

The results for graft excision and in situ bypass have been encouraging. Clagett and colleagues reported exceptional results in a few carefully selected patients using autogenous tissue reconstructive techniques employing veins harvested from the legs.[18, 19] Nonetheless, they admittedly limit such reconstructions for these high-risk patients with AEFs and suggest the staged approach, as described. Walker and associates have reported operative mortality for graft excision with in situ prosthetic regrafting to be 22%,[105] whereas Kieffer's group reported operative mortality for in situ cadaver regrafting to be only 12%.[52] Van Baalen and colleagues noted better results with in situ bypass than with extra-anatomic bypass after excision of the infected grafts[101]; however, these results have not been universal.[48, 53, 55, 75] The in situ approach prevents the potential complication of aortic stump blowout, the leading cause of postoperative death, and is an option with minimally infected retroperitoneum. The surgeon must be aware, however, that the tradeoff is reinfection of the in situ graft. Currently, the preferred treatment remains staged operations with extra-anatomic bypass grafting preceding total graft excision by 2 to 3 days for clinically stable patients.

REFERENCES

1. Alfrey EJ, Stanton C, Dunnington G, et al: Graft appendiceal fistulas. J Vasc Surg 7:814, 1988.
2. Atnip RG: Mycotic aneurysms of the suprarenal abdominal aorta: Prolonged survival after in situ aortic and visceral reconstruction. J Vasc Surg 10:635, 1989.
3. Auffermann W, Olofsson PA, Stoney RJ, et al: MR imaging of complications of aortic surgery. J Comput Assist Tomogr 11:982, 1987.
4. Baker BH, Baker MS, vander Reis L, et al: Endoscopy in the diagnosis of aortoduodenal fistula. Gastrointest Endosc 24:35, 1977.
5. Baker MS, Fisher JH, vander Reis L, et al: The endoscopic diagnosis of an aortoduodenal fistula. Arch Surg 111:304, 1976.
6. Bergquist D, Alm A, Claes G, et al: Secondary aortoenteric fistulas—an analysis of 42 cases. Eur J Vasc Surg 1:11, 1987.
7. Bernhard VM: Aortoenteric Fistula. Orlando, Fla, Grune & Stratton, 1985, pp 513–525.
8. Brennaman BH, Shepard AD, Ernst CB: Aortoenteric and caval fistulae. *In* Bergan JJ, Yao JST (eds): Aortic Surgery. Philadelphia, WB Saunders, 1989, pp 497–510.
9. Brock RC: Aortic homografting: A report of six successful cases. Guys Hosp Rep 102:204, 1953.
10. Buchbinder D, Leather R, Shah D, et al: Pathologic interactions between prosthetic aortic grafts and the gastrointestinal tract. Am J Surg 140:192, 1980.
11. Bunt TJ: Synthetic vascular graft infections: II. Graft-enteric erosions and graft-enteric fistulas. Surgery 94:1, 1983.
12. Bunt TJ, Doerhoff CR: Endoscopic visualization of an intraluminal Dacron graft: Definitive diagnosis of aortoduodenal fistula. South Med J 77:86, 1984.
13. Busuttil RN, Reese W, Baker JD, et al: Pathogenesis of aortoduodenal fistula: Experimental and clinical correlates. Surgery 85:1, 1979.
14. Campbell HC Jr, Ernst CB: Aortoenteric fistula following renal revascularization. Am Surg 44:155, 1978.
15. Champion MC, Sullivan SN, Coles JC, et al: Aortoenteric fistula: Incidence, presentation, recognition, and management. Ann Surg 195:314, 1982.
16. Chan FY, Crawford ES, Coselli JS, et al: In situ prosthetic graft replacement for mycotic aneurysm of the aorta. Ann Thorac Surg 47:193, 1989.
17. Chaphery AD, Gupta RL, Currie RD: Carcinoma of head of pancreas with aortoduodenal fistula. Am J Surg 111:580, 1966.
18. Clagett GP, Bowers BL, Lopez-Viego MA, et al: Creation of a neo-aortoiliac system from lower extremity deep and superficial veins. Ann Surg 210:239, 1993.
19. Clagett GP, Valentine RJ, Hagino RT: Autogenous aortoiliac/femoral reconstruction from superficial femoral-popliteal veins: Feasibility and durability. J Vasc Surg 25:255, 1997.
20. Claytor H, Birch L, Cardwell ES, et al: Suture-line rupture of a nylon aortic bifurcation graft into the small bowel. Arch Surg 73:947, 1956.
21. Conn JH, Hardy JD, Chavez CM, et al: Infected arterial grafts. Ann Surg 171:704, 1970.
22. Cooper A: The lectures of Sir Astley Cooper on the Principles and Practice of Surgery with Additional Notes and Cases by F. Tyrell, 5th ed. Philadelphia, Haswell, Barrington, and Haswell, 1939.
23. Cordell AR, Wright RH, Johnston FR: Gastrointestinal hemorrhage after abdominal aortic operations. Surgery 48:997, 1960.
24. Crawford ES, Manning LG, Kelly TF: "Redo" surgery after operations for aneurysm and occlusion of the abdominal aorta. Surgery 81:41, 1977.
25. Cunat JS, Haaga JR, Rhodes R, et al: Periaortic fluid aspiration for recognition of infected graft: Preliminary report. AJR 139:251, 1982.
26. Daugherty M, Shearer GR, Ernst CB: Primary aortoduodenal fistula: Extra-anatomic vascular reconstruction not required for successful management. Surgery 86:399, 1979.
27. DeWeese MS: Discussion. Elliott JP Jr, Smith RF, Szilagyi DE: Aortoenteric and paraprosthetic enteric fistulas. Arch Surg 108:479, 1974.

28. DeWeese MS, Fry WJ: Small bowel erosion following aortic resection. JAMA 179:882, 1962.
29. Donovan TJ, Bucknam CA: Aorto-enteric fistula. Arch Surg 95:810, 1967.
30. Dossa CD, Ernst CB: Aortoenteric fistula. *In* Greenhalgh RM, Hollier LH (eds): Emergency in Vascular Surgery. London, WB Saunders, Ltd, 1992, pp 18.1–18.15.
31. Dossa CD, Pipinos II, Shepard AD, Ernst CB: Primary aortoenteric fistula: Part I. Ann Vasc Surg 8:113, 1994.
32. Dossa CD, Pipinos II, Shepard AD, Ernst CB: Primary aortoenteric fistula: Part II. Primary aortoesophageal fistula. Ann Vasc Surg 8:207, 1994.
33. Ehrenfeld WK, Wilbur BG, Olcott CN, et al: Autogenous tissue reconstruction in the management of infected prosthetic grafts. Surgery 85:82, 1979
34. Elliott JP, Smith RF, Szilagyi DE: Aortoenteric and paraprosthetic-enteric fistulas. Arch Surg 108:479, 1974.
35. Ernst CB: Aortoenteric fistula. *In* Shackelford RT (ed): Surgery of the Alimentary Tract, 4th ed. Philadelphia, WB Saunders, 1996, pp 70–82.
36. Ernst CB: Aortoenteric fistulas. *In* Haimovici H (ed): Vascular Emergencies. New York, Appleton-Century-Crofts, 1982, pp 365–385.
37. Ernst CB: Axillary-femoral bypass graft patency without aortofemoral pressure differential. Ann Surg 181:424, 1975.
38. Foster JH, Morgan CV, Threlkel JB: Proximal control of aorta with balloon catheter. Surg Gynecol Obstet 132:693, 1971.
39. Frosch HL, Horowitz W: Rupture of abdominal aorta into duodenum through sinus tract created by tuberculous mesenteric lymphadenitis. Ann Intern Med 21:481, 1944.
40. Fry WJ, Lindenauer SM: Infection complicating the use of plastic arterial implants. Arch Surg 94:600, 1967.
41. Fulenwider JT, Smith RB, Johnson RW, et al: Reoperative abdominal arterial surgery: A ten-year experience. Surgery 93:20, 1982.
42. Garrett HE, Beall AC Jr, Jordan GL Jr, et al: Surgical considerations of massive gastrointestinal tract hemorrhage caused by aortoduodenal fistula. Am J Surg 105:6, 1963.
43. Gordon SL, Nicholas GG, Carter SL, et al: Aortoenteric fistula presenting as multicentric osteomyelitis. Clin Orthop 131:255, 1978.
44. Gupta RK, Rogers KE: A unique case of aortoduodenal fistula following carcinoma of cervix. Am J Obstet Gynecol 131:110, 1978.
45. Hallett JW Jr, Marshall DM, Petterson TM, et al: Graft-related complications after abdominal aortic aneurysm repair: Reassurance from a 36-year population-based experience. J Vasc Surg 25:277, 1997.
46. Harris JP, Sheil AGR, Stephen MS, et al: Lessons learnt in the management of aortoenteric fistula. J Cardiovasc Surg 28:449, 1987.
47. Heberer A: Diagnosis and treatment of aneursysms of the abdominal aorta. Ger Med Monatchr 2:203, 1957.
48. Higgins RSD, Steed DL, Julian TB, et al: The management of aortoenteric and paraprosthetic fistulae. J Cardiovasc Surg 31:81, 1990.
49. Higgins RSD, Steed DL, Zajko AB, et al: Computed tomographic scan confirmation of paraprosthetic enteric fistula. Am J Surg 162:36, 1991.
50. Humphries AW, Young JR, deWolfe VG, et al: Complications of abdominal aortic surgery. Arch Surg 86:43, 1963.
51. Katz BH, Black RA, Colley DP: CT-guided fine-needle aspiration of a perigraft collection. J Vasc Surg 5:762, 1987.
52. Kieffer E, Bahnini A, Koskas F, et al: In-situ allograft replacement of infected infrarenal aortic prosthetic grafts: Results in forty-three patients. J Vasc Surg 17:349, 1993.
53. Kiernan PD, Pairolero PC, Hubert JP Jr, et al: Aortic graft-enteric fistula. Mayo Clin Proc 55:731, 1980.
54. King RM, Sterioff S, Engen DE: Renal artery graft-to-duodenum fistula: Unusual presentation of a recurrent flank abscess. J Cardiovasc Surg 26:509, 1985.
55. Kleinman LH, Towne JB, Bernhard WM: A diagnostic and therapeutic approach to aorto-enteric fistulas: Clinical experience with twenty patients. Surgery 86:868, 1979.
56. Kuestner LM, Reilly LM, Jicha DL, et al: Secondary aortoenteric fistula: Contemporary outcome with use of extraanatomic bypass and infected graft excision. J Vasc Surg 21:184, 1995.
57. LaMurglia GM, Fischman AJ, Strauss HW, et al: Utility of Indium-111–labeled human immunoglobulin G scan for the detection of focal vascular graft infection. J Vasc Surg 10:20, 1989.
58. Lawrence PF, Dries DJ, Alazraki N, et al: Indium 111–labeled leukocyte scanning for detection of prosthetic graft infection. J Vasc Surg 2:165, 1985.
59. Lorimer JW, Goobie P, Rasuli P, et al: Primary aortogastric fistula: A complication of ruptured aortic aneurysm. J Cardiovasc Surg 37:363, 1996.
60. Low RN, Wall SD, Jeffrey RB, et al: Aortoenteric fistula and perigraft infection: Evaluation with CT. Radiology 175:157, 1990.
61. MacKenzie RJ, Buell AH, Pearson SC: Aneurysm of aortic homograft with rupture into the duodenum. Arch Surg 77:965, 1958.
62. Mark AS, McCarthy SM, Moss AA, et al: Detection of abdominal aortic graft infection: Comparison of CT and In-labeled white blood cell scans. AJR 144:315, 1985.
63. Mark AS, Moss AA, McCarthy SM, et al: CT of aortoenteric fistulas. Invest Radiol 20:272, 1985.
64. Martin A, Copeman PWM: Aorto-jejunal fistula from rupture of Teflon graft with septic emboli in the skin. Br Med J 2:155, 1967.
65. McCann RL, Schwartz LB, Georgiade GS: Management of abdominal aortic graft complications. Ann Surg 217:729, 1993.
66. Mir-Madjlessi SH, Sullivan BH Jr, Farmer RG, et al: Endoscopic diagnosis of aortoduodenal fistula. Gastrointest Endosc 19:187, 1973.
67. Morrow C, Safi H, Beall AC Jr: Primary aortoduodenal fistula caused by *Salmonella* aortitis. J Vasc Surg 6:415, 1987.
68. Moulton S, Adams M, Johansen K: Aortoenteric fistula: A 7 year experience. Am J Surg 151:607, 1986.
69. Nelken N: Aortoenteric fistula. *In* Callow AD, Ernst CB (eds): Vascular Surgery: Theory and Practice. Stamford, Conn, Appleton & Lange, 1995, pp 1311–1323.
70. Ng E, Copperman LR: Erosion of the small intestine with hemorrhage following aortic resection: Roentgen findings. Clin Radiol 21:87, 1970.
71. O'Donnell TF Jr, Scott G, Shepard A, et al: Improvements in the diagnosis and management of aortoenteric fistulas. Am J Surg 149:481, 1985.
72. Odze RD, Begin LR: Peptic ulcer induced aortoenteric fistula: Report of case and review of the literature. J Clin Gastroenterol 113:682, 1991.
73. Olofsson PA, Auffermann W, Higgins CB, et al: Diagnosis of prosthetic graft infection by magnetic resonance imaging (MRI) J Vasc Surg 8:99, 1988.
74. O'Mara CS, Imbembo AL: Paraprosthetic enteric fistula. Surgery 81:556, 1977.
75. O'Mara CS, Williams GM, Ernst CB: Secondary aortoenteric fistula. A 20 year experience. Am J Surg 142:203, 1981.
76. Ott DJ, Kerr RM, Gelfand DW: Aortoduodenal fistula. Gastrointest Endosc 24:296, 1978.
77. Pabst TS III, Bernhard VM, McIntyre KE Sr, et al: Gastrointestinal bleeding following aortic surgery: The place of laparotomy to rule out aortoenteric fistula. J Vasc Surg 8:280, 1988.
78. Perdue GD Jr, Smith RB, Ansley JD, et al: Impending aortoenteric hemorrhage: The effect of early recognition on improved outcome. Ann Surg 192:237, 1980.
79. Perry MO, Melichar R, Heimbach DM: Duodenal erosion by aorto-renal Dacron graft. J Cardiovasc Surg 18:77, 1977.
80. Puglia E, Fry PD: Aortoenteric fistulas: A preventable problem? Can J Surg 23:74, 1980.
81. Reckless JPD, McColl I, Taylor GW: Aortoenteric fistulae: An uncommon complication of abdominal aortic aneurysms. Br J Surg 59:458, 1972.
82. Reilly LM, Altman H, Lusby RJ, et al: Late results following surgical management of vascular graft infection. J Vasc Surg 1:36, 1984.
83. Reilly LM, Ehrenfeld WK, Goldstone J, et al: Gastrointestinal tract involvement by prosthetic graft infection: The significance of gastrointestinal hemorrhage. Ann Surg 202:342, 1985.
84. Reilly LM, Stoney RJ, Goldstone J, et al: Improved management of aortic graft infection: The influence of operative sequence and staging. J Vasc Surg 5:421, 1987.
85. Robinson JA, Johansen K: Aortic sepsis: Is there a role for in situ graft reconstruction? J Vasc Surg 13:677, 1991.
86. Rosenthal D, Deterling RA Jr, O'Donnell TF, et al: Positive blood culture as an aid in the diagnosis of secondary aortoenteric fistula. Arch Surg 114:1041, 1979
87. Salo J, Verkkala K, Ketonen P, et al: Graft enteric fistulas and erosions, complications of synthetic aortic grafting. Vasc Surg March/April: 88, 1986.

88. Schmitt DD, Seabrook GR, Bandyk DF, et al: Graft excision and extra-anatomic revascularization: The treatment of choice for the septic aortic prosthesis. J Cardiovasc Surg 31:327, 1990.
89. Schütte HE: Angiographic signs of aortic graft-enteric fistulae. Clin Radiol 38:503, 1987.
90. Sheil AGR, Reeve TS, Little JM, et al: Aortointestinal fistulas following operations on the abdominal aorta and iliac arteries. Br J Surg 56:840, 1969.
91. Sindelar WF, Mason GR: Aortocystoduodenal fistula: Rare complication of pancreatic pseudocyst. Arch Surg 114:953, 1979.
92. Skibba RM, Greenberger NJ, Hardin CA: Paraprosthetic-enteric fistula: Role of preoperative endoscopy. Dig Dis 20:1081, 1975.
93. Spanos DK, Gilsdorf RB, Sako Y, et al: The management of infected abdominal aortic grafts and graft-enteric fistulas. Ann Surg 183:397, 1976.
94. Sternberg A, Nava HR, Irac AT, et al: Perforation of a benign gastric ulcer into the supradiaphragmatic aorta. Am J Gasteroenterol 82:579, 1987.
95. Sweeney MS, Gadacz TR: Primary aortoduodenal fistula: Manifestations, diagnosis, and treatment. Surgery 96:492, 1984.
96. Taheri SA, Kulaylat MN, Grippi J, et al: Surgical treatment of primary aortoduodenal fistula. Ann Vasc Surg 5:265, 1991.
97. Thomas WEG, Baird RN: Secondary aorto-enteric fistulae: Towards a more conservative approach. Br J Surg 73:875, 1986.
98. Thompson WM, Jackson DC, Johnsrude IS: Aortonteric and paraprosthetic enteric fistulas: Radiologic findings. Am J Roentgenol 127:235, 1976.
99. Thompson WM, Johnsrude IS, Jackson DC, et al: Late complications of abdominal aortic reconstructive surgery: Roentgen evaluation. Ann Surg 185:326, 1976.
100. Trout HH III, Kozloff L, Giordano JM: Priority of revascularization in patients with graft enteric fistulas, infected arteries, or infected arterial prostheses. Ann Surg 199:669, 1984.
101. van Baalen JM, Kluit AB, Maas J, et al: Diagnosis and therapy of aortic prosthetic fistulas: Trends over a 30-year experience. Br J Surg 83:1729, 1996.
102. Vollmar JF, Kogel H: Aorto-enteric fistulas as postoperative complication. J Cardiovasc Surg 28:479, 1987.
103. Voorhoeve R, Moll FL, Bast TJ: The primary aortoenteric fistula in The Netherlands—the unpublished cases. Eur J Vasc Endovasc Surg 11:429, 1996.
104. Voyles WR, Moretz WH: Rupture of aortic aneurysms into gastrointestinal tract. Surgery 43:666, 1958.
105. Walker WE, Cooley DA, Duncan JM, et al: The management of aortoduodenal fistula by in situ replacement of the infected abdominal aortic graft. Ann Surg 205:727, 1987.
106. Wyatt EM, Rauchway MI, Sputz HB: Roentgen findings in aortoenteric fistulae. Am J Roentgenol 126:714, 1976.
107. Yeager RA, Sasaki TM, McConnell DB, et al: Clinical spectrum of patients with infrarenal aortic grafts and gastrointestinal bleeding. Am J Surg 153:459, 1987.
108. Youmans CR, Derrick JR: Gastrointestinal erosion after prosthetic arterial reconstructive surgery. Am J Surg 114:711, 1967.

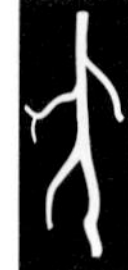

CHAPTER 50
Ischemic Neuropathy

J. Jean E. Turley, M.D., F.R.C.S.(P.), and
K. Wayne Johnston, M.D., F.R.C.S.(C.)

Ischemic neuropathy is a term used to describe any injury of peripheral nerve caused by a reduction in blood supply. These disorders may be associated with diseases of large or small arteries. Large artery lesions may be acute (e.g., those due to arterial embolism, thrombosis, or injury) or chronic (e.g., those due to atherosclerosis). Small endoneurial arteries may be involved in periarteritis nodosa, rheumatoid vasculitis, Churg-Strauss syndrome, and Wegener's granulomatosis. Capillary disease may be significant in diabetic neuropathy. For the surgeon, ischemic disorders of nerve resulting from large artery disease are important.

PERIPHERAL NERVES

Anatomy and Physiology

Peripheral nerves are composed of fascicles of nerve fibers. The fascicles are made up of nerve fibers, Schwann's cells, collagen, small vessels, and endoneurial fluid. Nerve fibers are bathed in endoneurial fluid that is maintained within narrow metabolic limits by blood-nerve and perineurial barriers.

Structural proteins and macromolecules are produced in the nerve cell body and transported in the axon. Axon transport is energy-dependent and requires oxygen and glucose, which are supplied locally to the endoneurial fluid by endoneurial vessels. Transmission of nerve impulses is accomplished by transient depolarization of limited portions of the axonal membrane, during which time sodium and potassium diffuse across the membrane and are then restored to resting levels. This flow uses stored energy that is replenished by glycolysis in the Krebs cycle through aerobic metabolism. Although the nerve continually uses energy to maintain resting ionic gradients, the oxygen requirement of mammalian nerve is small, and even when this requirement is increased by activity, it is less than that of other tissues.[1] As a result, peripheral nerves are relatively resistant to ischemia.

Blood Supply

The metabolic needs of large nerves are met by intraneural blood vessels, the vasa nervorum, whereas those of small nerves are met by diffusion from surrounding tissues. The vasa nervorum arise from nearby major arteries and enter nerve trunks at multiple levels, frequently near joints. The epineural arteries branch, and arteriolar and precapillary branches then penetrate the perineurium to perfuse the endoneurium. There is a complete terminal network of capillaries through the perineurium that supplies blood to nerve at some distance from the nutrient arteries.[1–4] The abundant collateral circulation pattern of peripheral nerve explains why it is difficult to injure a peripheral nerve by occlusion of one or even several nutrient arteries. Regional nutrient arteries have been ligated over considerable lengths of a nerve trunk without disturbing blood supply to nerve or adversely affecting the structure and function of nerve fibers.[5] Extensive studies of the microvasculature of peripheral nerve have demonstrated that the organization of vasa nervorum is such that a total interruption of circulation in nerves is very unlikely unless drastic interference with the blood supply is produced.[6]

The pattern of epineural vessels varies in different nerves, and some nerves may be more susceptible than others to ischemia.[5] In some cases, a single nutrient artery provides the major blood supply to a considerable length of nerve, and this may predispose to ischemic damage to the nerve trunk. At its upper end, the human sciatic nerve receives an arterial branch from the inferior gluteal artery. As the sciatic nerve enters the popliteal fossa, its blood supply is taken over by the popliteal artery and its branches. The tibial nerve is intimately related to the posterior tibial artery, which supplies a large number of direct nutrient arteries.

The peroneal nerve, in contrast, diverges from the main vessels and is supplied in the region of the fibular head by small adjacent arteries. At the neck of the fibula, the major intraneural vessels occupy a superficial position that may expose them to damage from pressure. In the calf, the posterior tibial and peroneal nerves receive branches from the anterior and posterior tibial arteries. The intraneural arterial pattern in the buttock and thigh contains several arterial channels of fairly large caliber, whereas below the knee, one major vessel usually dominates. The peroneal nerve at the knee, and perhaps the more distal portions of the peroneal and posterior tibial nerves, may therefore be more prone to ischemic damage.[5] In an animal model of large vessel ligation, Kelly and colleagues[7] produced an ischemic neuropathy in animals, all of which showed clinical evidence of neuropathy in 1 week confirmed by nerve conduction studies. Examination of corrosion casts showed an area of underfilling of the microcirculation in the region of the proximal tibial nerve with good filling of vessels proximal and distal to this, indicating that in generalized hypoperfusion states (such as large vessel occlusion) the area of poorest perfusion is a watershed zone between two adjacent nutrient vessels to the nerve.

Sympathetic nerve fibers innervate vessels in the epineurium and perineurium. High sympathetic drive may significantly reduce intraneural circulation. Sympathetically mediated vasoconstriction may be important in the pathogenesis of reflex sympathetic dystrophy and chronic pain.[3]

ISCHEMIC NERVES

Pathophysiology

Many studies have been carried out to determine the effect of anoxia on nerve function. A short period of experimental ischemia results in disturbed function of nerve, which can recover if circulation is restored. Severe acute ischemia appears to result in decreased or abolished conduction of impulses. Thus, if ischemia is of short duration or is mild, function in peripheral nerve can be impaired in a transient manner.[8] The slight metabolic needs of nerve and the diffusion of nutrients from surrounding tissues enable it to survive. If ischemia is prolonged or severe, damage may be permanent.[5, 9]

Exactly how these functional changes of nerve occur is unknown. Obviously, ischemia impairs the metabolic processes that maintain the ionic gradient necessary for impulse transmission. Fast axoplasmic transport also depends on an adequate blood supply. The transport of material in the axon is impaired by ischemia at the same time that conduction is impaired, suggesting that both depend on the same sources of energy.[10] The block of fast axoplasmic transport becomes irreversible after 6 to 8 hours of ischemia. The permeability of endoneurial vessels during ischemia is impaired after 8 to 10 hours.[11] Metabolic factors, including anoxia, hypercapnia, hyperkalemia, and acidosis, are probably important. Potassium accumulation in the extracellular space during anoxia may cause irreversible depolarization of cell membrane.[2, 12]

There is controversy about the relative vulnerabilities of nerve and muscle to ischemia. The idea is entrenched in the literature that muscle is more sensitive, and Dyck,[11] in a review of hypoxic neuropathy, still considers skeletal muscle to be more vulnerable to ischemic injury than nerve. Korthals and coworkers[13] ligated the abdominal aorta and femoral artery in cats and found necrotic changes in muscle at 2 to 3 hours, whereas no nerve lesions appeared until 5 hours of ischemia. However, a study by Chervu and associates[14] of the relative sensitivities of skeletal muscle and peripheral nerve function to ischemia and reperfusion suggests that peripheral nerve is more susceptible to ischemia than skeletal muscle.

Pathologic Changes

Pathologic studies have been performed of peripheral nerves in ischemic limbs. Farinon and colleagues,[15] examining muscle and nerve biopsy specimens from patients with chronic arterial insufficiency, found a combination of segmental demyelination and axonal degeneration. They believed that large fibers and small fibers were equally affected and further noted that the severity of the nerve pathology did not correlate well with the severity of vascular disease.

Eames and Lange[16] described the pathologic changes in sural nerve biopsy specimens from eight patients with vascular disease. They found evidence of segmental demyelination and remyelination, axonal degeneration and regeneration, and an increase in endoneurial collagen. The unmyelinated fibers were essentially normal. Rodriguez-Sánchez[17] and associates examined morphologic alterations in the sural nerve from patients with chronic atherosclerotic disease. Both axonal degeneration and regeneration, and demyelination and remyelination were seen. In cases of atherosclerotic disease of large vessels, the lumina of the epineurial and endoneurial vasa nervorum in the sural nerves have been found to be markedly narrowed and the walls thickened.[16]

A later study by Nukada and coauthors[18] examined the

pathology of nerves taken from amputated limbs of seven acutely and nine chronically ischemic legs. In acutely ischemic nerves, axonal degeneration of both myelinated and unmyelinated nerve fibers was prominent if ischemia was present for more than 24 hours. Chronically ischemic limbs showed demyelination, remyelination, endoneurial edema and relative preservation of unmyelinated nerves. All changes except the high rate of demyelination and remyelination have been described in experimental models of acute ischemic and reperfusion injury. The authors concluded that "pathological alterations in chronic ischemic neuropathy may be due to the combined effects of acute ischemia/reperfusion and chronic hypoxia."

Many experimental studies have examined the morphology of animal nerve.[19–23] Sladky and coworkers[24] produced 50% to 75% endoneurial blood flow reduction in rats and found that nerve conduction velocities fell by 25% to 30%; morphologic studies showed structural abnormalities at nodes of Ranvier and mild axonal atrophy. The authors suggested that reduced endoneurial blood flow insufficient to cause infarction may result in measurable functional and morphologic abnormalities in peripheral nerves. In general, large myelinated fibers, particularly in the center of nerves, seem to undergo axonal degeneration.

ISCHEMIC POLYNEUROPATHY

Association with Chronic Arterial Insufficiency

In humans, neither the effects of chronic ischemia on the structure and function of nerves, nor the limit of tolerance of peripheral nerve to ischemia is well defined.

The incidence of neurologic deficits in patients with chronic peripheral vascular disease has not been ascertained. Peripheral nerve involvement in atherosclerosis is probably underestimated because neuropathic symptoms—pain, sensory changes, and even weakness—may be confused with claudication or rest pain. A number of series have reported symptoms such as painful burning and signs varying from sensory impairment to reflex loss, muscle wasting, and weakness in patients with peripheral arterial occlusive disease.

Hutchison and Liversedge found peripheral nerve dysfunction, as manifested by sensory deficits and absent reflexes, in 50% of their patients with peripheral vascular disease.[25] They believed that the presence of neuropathy was related to the severity of the vascular disease. Eames and Lange[16] found impaired sensation in 88% of their 32 atherosclerotic patients, muscle weakness in 50%, and decreased or absent reflexes in 41%. Again, the extent of the deficit was proportional to the degree of ischemia. All patients with claudication after walking less than 100 yards had a neurologic abnormality. Twenty patients had a superficial femoral artery occlusion, and the remainder had proximal vascular disease. Hunter and colleagues[26] found neurologic deficits in 22% of ischemic limbs. Miglietta[27] found decreased ankle jerks and decreased vibration sense in 54% of his patients with atherosclerosis.

When electrophysiologic studies are added to the clinical evaluation, neurologic abnormalities are uncovered in an even greater number of individuals who have no apparent clinical symptoms or signs. Miglietta and Lowenthal[28] found slowing of motor conduction velocity in peroneal nerves in nearly all patients with severe vascular disease and no neurologic signs, but many patients had diabetes. Hunter and colleagues[26] found abnormal peroneal nerve compound muscle action potential amplitudes in 86% and abnormal conduction velocities in the lower extremities in 36% of atherosclerotic patients, whereas only 22% had clinical neurologic abnormalities.

Therefore, it seems that peripheral neuropathy develops in some patients with chronic occlusive vascular disease. The precise location and the severity of the requisite arterial lesion have not been defined, nor has the precise incidence. Nevertheless, there is considerable clinical importance in detecting the presence of neuropathy before surgery. If some of the patient's symptoms are neuropathic in origin, it is to be expected that improvement of vascular supply to the limb may not immediately relieve all of the symptoms, even if adequate revascularization is achieved.

Following Acute Arterial Insufficiency

Incidence

Acute arterial occlusion due to embolism, thrombosis, or arterial injury is often associated with acute neural dysfunction. The motor and sensory deficit usually has a distal limb distribution, but selective peroneal palsy has been described.[29] The frequency of clear neurologic signs in the acutely ischemic limb has seldom been carefully analyzed. Haimovici[30] reported that 22% of his patients presented with sensory symptoms, but no data are presented on physical signs. A number of other reports[1] have documented neurologic deficits with motor signs in about 20% and sensory deficits in 50%. After acute arterial occlusion, if flow is not reestablished within several hours (and this time limit has not been clearly defined), symptoms and signs of neurologic dysfunction may persist when circulation is restored and the neurologic deficit may be permanent.

Clinical Features

The clinical features of ischemic neuropathy following trauma to major blood vessels were summarized by Sunderland.[5] He reported that sensory loss is distal and of a stocking-and-glove type; it is associated with distal muscle wasting and weakness and is sometimes accompanied by late fibrosis and contracture. Wilbourn and coworkers[31] subsequently described 14 cases of ischemic monomelic neuropathy in a single limb, with pain, paresthesia, and paralysis following the restoration of blood flow after acute occlusion of a proximal limb artery.

The precise incidence of ischemic neuropathy and the various factors that predispose to the development of neuropathy in an ischemic limb have not yet been characterized by the publication of a large series or by a prospective study. After an episode of severe ischemia, however, it is not unusual for patients with a satisfactorily revascularized leg to continue to complain of pain that is due to neuropathy. The neuropathic pain is burning and paresthetic in nature, is frequently worse with rest and at night, and is unaffected or relieved by walking, in marked contrast to the pain of claudication. The patient perceives the foot to be cold, although it is in fact warm. The patient may remark on loss of mobility of the toes.

Examination no longer reveals signs of significant ischemia. Instead, the small muscles of the affected foot are wasted compared with those of the normal side, and they are weak. There may be slight ankle weakness, and the ankle reflex may be depressed compared with that of the normal side. There is a unilateral stocking sensory loss, particularly to vibration sense. Unlike the findings in neuropathies caused by diabetes, uremia, drug intoxication, or alcoholism, the findings in ischemic neuropathy are asymmetric, with sensory and motor findings exclusively or prominently in the limb that was afflicted by severe ischemia.

Diagnosis

Vascular Assessment

The severity of ischemia can be assessed clinically or may be determined more objectively by noninvasive methods, including the measurement of ankle and toe pressures and Doppler waveform recordings. If the ankle pressure is greater than 50 to 60 mmHg or the toe pressure is greater than 30 mmHg, ischemic rest pain is unlikely and the diagnosis of ischemic neuropathy should be suspected. Flat or monophasic Doppler waveforms confirm that the arterial disease is severe. If clinical examination and noninvasive assessment confirm that the peripheral circulation is adequate, the pain is probably not due to ischemia. If the perfusion is inadequate, the pain may be due to ischemia, neuropathy, or both, and treatment should be directed first toward improvement of the limb blood flow.

Electrophysiologic Studies

Careful electrophysiologic studies can establish the diagnosis of ischemic neuropathy and define its severity. Typically, a unilateral axonal neuropathy involving distal nerves is present.

Motor nerve conduction studies show a decrease in or an absence of the compound *muscle action potential* amplitude from the extensor digitorum brevis muscle when the peroneal nerve is stimulated and from the flexor hallucis brevis muscle when the posterior tibial nerve is stimulated in the affected foot. Frequently, the distal posterior tibial nerve is more involved than the distal peroneal nerve. The abnormality is always most severe in the distal nerves. The distal latency, if one can be recorded, and the velocity of conduction in the calf portion of the peroneal and posterior tibial nerves are relatively well preserved. These findings are in sharp contrast to those in diabetic and uremic neuropathies, in which distal latencies and conduction velocities tend to be symmetrically reduced well below normal velocities at an early stage in *both* lower limbs.

Sensory nerve conduction studies show decreased or absent sensory potential amplitudes from sural, superficial peroneal, and plantar nerves, whereas sensory conduction velocity, when recordable, is normal.

Needle electrode examination reveals the changes of muscle denervation in the small muscles of the affected foot, particularly in the sole of the foot, with fibrillation potentials at rest and large motor units of long duration in much reduced numbers. Lesser denervation changes are seen in the muscles of the calf if the ischemia has been severe.

Treatment

Once a diagnosis of ischemic neuropathy has been made by clinical and electrophysiologic investigations, what treatment can be offered? If peripheral blood flow is significantly reduced, vascular reconstructive surgery is justified. However, if perfusion is adequate, conservative treatment is indicated. Wilbourn and coworkers[31] suggest that phenytoin, tricyclic antidepressants, and analgesics are ineffective but that carbamazepine produces partial relief. Three of their patients had sympathectomy, and two reported pain relief. Persistent pain that is uncontrolled by such drugs, if dramatically relieved by sympathetic blocks, may well deserve sympathectomy, particularly if the passage of time does not indicate spontaneous regression is taking place. Many clinicians believe that tricyclic antidepressants, sometimes in combination with small amounts of phenothiazine, are effective.

Kihara and colleagues[32, 33] have produced experimental ischemic neuropathy in rat sciatic nerve, treating with hyperbaric oxygen and limb cooling. They found that hyperbaric oxygen 2 hours per day for 7 days beginning within 30 minutes of ischemia was effective in rescuing fibers from ischemic degeneration if ischemia was not extreme. In limbs with the same degree of ischemia, limbs that were hypothermic suffered less ischemic nerve fiber damage. These findings have not yet been applied clinically.

Prognosis

The prognosis is uncertain. After other types of axonal nerve injury, peripheral nerves show a considerable capacity to regenerate, and regeneration has been seen in animal models after ischemia. Therefore, particularly in the absence of any other causes of neuropathy, such as diabetes, uremia, blood dyscrasias, or carcinoma, axon repair might be expected to occur slowly, with relief of symptoms.

ISCHEMIC MONONEUROPATHY ASSOCIATED WITH ATHEROSCLEROTIC DISEASE OF LARGE ARTERIES

Ischemic mononeuropathy is a frequent occurrence in diseases of small vessels associated with vasculitis and diabetes. Ischemic mononeuropathies that seem distinct from compressive neuropathies have occasionally been documented in the literature in association with atherosclerotic disease of large vessels.

Peroneal Neuropathy

Ferguson and Liversedge[29] reported seven cases of peroneal palsy with vascular disease; three resulted from cardiac emboli, and four were associated with atherosclerosis. The precise location of the arterial occlusions was not documented angiographically. As described earlier, the nature of the vascular supply to the peroneal nerve at the fibular head certainly predisposes to ischemic damage, although the nerve is also prone to compression in the same area.

Peroneal neuropathy presents as weakness of dorsiflexion and eversion of the ankle, with preservation of inversion and plantar flexion, which are functions of the posterior calf muscles. The sensory deficit is confined to the dorsum of the foot and perhaps to the lateral calf, and the ankle jerk is preserved. It is possible to confirm the diagnosis with nerve conduction studies, which demonstrate abnormality in peroneal function while all other nerve conduction is intact. It is usually possible to distinguish a compressive peroneal neuropathy, which produces a local area of conduction slowing and block at the fibular head, from an ischemic lesion, which is primarily axonal in nature and produces a uniform conduction velocity throughout the length of the nerve and a reduction in the motor and sensory potential amplitudes.

Femoral Neuropathy

Whether a femoral neuropathy occurs with vascular occlusion in the absence of compression, traction, or hemorrhage is unclear. Chopra and Hurwitz[34] reported slight wasting and weakness of the quadriceps muscle in 1 of 29 patients with atherosclerosis and claudication symptoms, and Archie[35] reported a femoral neuropathy due to common iliac artery occlusion in a nondiabetic. D'Amour and associates[36] reported two cases of femoral neuropathy, one following surgery for abdominal aortic aneurysm with aortobifemoral bypass grafting and one following placement of an intra-aortic balloon pump.

The main trunk of the femoral artery receives nutrient arteries from the iliac branch of the iliolumbar artery, from the deep circumflex iliac artery in the iliac fossa, and from the lateral circumflex femoral artery in the femoral triangle.[5]

A femoral nerve lesion results in flaccid paralysis of the quadriceps muscle, an absent knee jerk, and loss of sensation over the anterior and medial thigh and the inner aspect of the calf down to the level of the medial malleolus. Electrophysiologic studies show decreased or absent motor evoked response from the quadriceps muscle when the femoral nerve is stimulated in the groin and an absent saphenous sensory potential at the ankle, together with fibrillation potentials and motor unit loss, on needle electrode examination of the quadriceps muscle. Other nerves in the limb are normal. Femoral neuropathy is a frequent complication of diabetes and is presumably due to abnormalities of the vasa nervorum. The prognosis for recovery in both traumatic and diabetic femoral neuropathy is excellent. The incidence of and prognosis for ischemic femoral neuropathy await further reports.

Lumbosacral Plexus Lesions

Whether lumbosacral plexus lesions rather than lower cord or cauda equina lesions result from occlusive vascular disease is not well documented.

The lumbosacral plexus really has two parts: (1) a lumbar plexus arising from the second, third, and fourth lumbar roots and forming the femoral and obturator nerves, and (2) a sacral plexus arising from the fourth and fifth lumbar roots and the first three sacral roots and forming the superior and inferior gluteal nerves and the sciatic nerve. Blood supply to the lumbosacral plexus is through five lumbar arteries from each side of the abdominal aorta, the deep circumflex iliac artery, a branch of the external iliac artery, and the iliolumbar and gluteal branches of the internal iliac artery.[5]

Usubiaga and colleagues[37] described a lumbosacral plexus lesion after resection of an abdominal aortic aneurysm and aortobifemoral grafting. At autopsy, the plexus was totally infarcted. Voulters and Bolton[38] reported lumbosacral plexus damage following aortofemoral bypass grafting for repair of an abdominal aortic aneurysm. D'Amour and associates[36] described a number of cases, one following aortofemoral bypass grafting for stenosis of the common and external iliac arteries; one following acute occlusion of an aortobifemoral graft; one following aortofemoral bypass and femoropopliteal thrombectomy for occlusion of the common iliac, internal iliac, and superficial femoral arteries; and one following occlusion of the common iliac and femoral arteries. In these instances, the sciatic nerve seemed to be mainly involved. In two cases, neurologic symptoms appeared following vascular occlusion before surgery. Partial slow recoveries were reported. Gloviczki and coworkers[39] reported on a non–insulin-dependent diabetic patient who had bilateral leg weakness following aorta–profunda femoris bypass grafting for internal iliac disease. The patient experienced slow partial recovery.

Clinical evaluation of the patient with unilateral lower limb dysfunction can often distinguish a lesion of the lumbosacral plexus from one affecting the spinal cord or a major peripheral nerve. When the abnormality resides in the plexus, motor and sensory loss affect more than one peripheral nerve and dermatomal segment. Weakness involves proximal muscles (the iliopsoas, hip adductors and abductors, or glutei) as well as distal muscles. The limb is flaccid and areflexic, with no response to plantar stimulation. This is in contrast to spinal lesions, which produce a spastic, hyperreflexic limb with extensor plantar response and dissociated sensory loss. Electromyography is usually essential to confirm the diagnosis. Localization to the lumbosacral plexus depends on the unilateral absence of sensory potentials (these are preserved in cauda equina and proximal root lesions), the absence of paraspinal denervation, and the presence of denervation changes in muscles innervated by multiple nerves and roots.

It is important to attempt to distinguish the precise level of the lesion when severe unilateral limb dysfunction occurs. Whereas lesions of the lower spinal cord or cauda equina have a very poor prognosis, there is some hope of recovery if the damage has occurred to part of the lumbosacral plexus.

SUMMARY

Nerve injury due to ischemia has been discussed. Although there has been an enormous amount of publication of experimental animal studies, the association of atherosclerotic disease with clinical neuropathic lesions in humans has not been as clearly reported. Occlusive vascular disease, both acute and chronic, seems capable of producing a painful unilateral axonal polyneuropathy, and major vascular occlusion may occasionally cause a mononeuropathy or lumbosacral plexus lesion. In the clinical setting, attempts should be made to detect the location and severity of the neurologic lesion precisely so that clearer therapeutic and prognostic guidelines can be established. In general, if significant ischemia is present, revascularization is indicated; if perfusion is adequate, a conservative approach is justified.

REFERENCES

1. Daube JR, Dyck PJ: Neuropathy due to peripheral vascular diseases. *In* Dyck PJ, Thomas PK, Lambert EH, et al (eds): Diseases of the Peripheral Nervous System. Philadelphia, WB Saunders, 1984, p 1458.
2. Olsson Y: The involvement of vasa nervorum in diseases of peripheral nerves. *In* Vinken PJ, Bruyn GW (eds): Handbook of Clinical Neurology. Vol XII. Amsterdam, North Holland Publishing, 1972, p 644.
3. Lundborg G: Intraneural microcirculation. Orthop Clin North Am 19:1, 1988.
4. Lundborg G: The intrinsic vascularization of human peripheral nerves: Structural and functional aspects. J Hand Surg 4:34, 1979.
5. Sunderland S: Nerve and Nerve Injuries. Edinburgh, Churchill Livingstone, 1978.
6. Lundborg G: Ischemic nerve injury: Experimental studies on intraneural microvascular pathophysiology and nerve function in a limb subjected to temporary circulatory arrest. Scand J Plast Reconstr Surg Suppl 6:3, 1970.
7. Kelly CJ, Augustine C, Rooney BP, et al: An investigation of the pathophysiology of ischaemic neuropathy. Eur J Vasc Surg 5:535, 1991.
8. Parry GJ, Linn DJ: Transient focal conduction block following experimental occlusion of the vasa nervorum muscle and nerve. Muscle Nerve 9:345, 1986.
9. Schmetzer JD, Zochodne E, Low PA: Ischemic and reperfusion injury of rat peripheral nerve. Proc Natl Acad Sci U S A 86:16, 1989.
10. Leone J, Ochs S: Anoxic block and recovery of axoplasmic transport and electrical excitability of nerve. J Neurobiol 9:229, 1978.
11. Dyck PJ: Hypoxic neuropathy: Does hypoxia play a role in diabetic neuropathy? The 1988 Robert Wartenberg Lecture. Neurology 39:111, 1989.
12. Fox JL, Kenmore PI: The effect of ischemia on nerve conduction. Exp Neurol 17:403, 1967.
13. Korthals JK, Maki T, Gieron MA: Nerve and muscle vulnerability to ischemia. J Neurol Sci 71:283, 1985.
14. Chervu A, Moore WS, Homsher E, et al: Differential recovery of skeletal muscle and peripheral nerve function after ischemia and reperfusion. J Surg Res 47:12, 1989.
15. Farinon AM, Marbini A, Gemignani F, et al: Skeletal muscle and peripheral nerve changes caused by chronic arterial insufficiency: Significance and clinical correlations—histological, histochemical and ultrastructural study. Clin Neurol 3:240, 1984.
16. Eames RA, Lange LS: Clinical and pathological study of ischemic neuropathy. J Neurol Neurosurg Psychiatry 30:215, 1967.
17. Rodriguez-Sánchez C, Medina Sánchez M, Malik RA, et al: Morphological abnormalities in the sural nerve from patients with peripheral vascular disease. Histol Histopathol 6:63, 1991.
18. Nukada H, van Rij AM, Packer SG, et al: Pathology of acute and chronic ischaemic neuropathy in atherosclerotic peripheral vascular disease. Brain 119:1449, 1996.
19. Benstead TJ, Dyck PJ, Sangalang V: Inner perineurial cell vulnerability in ischemia. Brain Res 489:177, 1989.
20. Korthals JK, Korthals MA, Wisniewski HM: Peripheral nerve ischemia: 2. Accumulation of organelles. Ann Neurol 4:487, 1978.
21. Parry GJ, Brown MJ: Selective fiber vulnerability in acute ischemic neuropathy. Ann Neurol 11:147, 1981.
22. Nukada H, Dyck PJ: Acute ischemia causes axonal stasis, swelling, attenuation, and secondary demyelination. Ann Neurol 22:311, 1987.
23. McManis PG, Low PA: Factors affecting the relative viability of centrifascicular and subperineurial axons in acute peripheral nerve ischemia. Exp Neurol 99:84, 1988.
24. Sladky JT, Tschoepe RL, Greenberg JH, et al: Peripheral neuropathy after chronic endoneurial ischmia. Ann Neurol 29:272, 1991.
25. Hutchison EC, Liversedge LA: Neuropathy in peripheral vascular disease: Its bearing on diabetic neuropathy. Q J Med 25:267, 1956.
26. Hunter GC, Song GW, Nayak NN, et al: Peripheral nerve conduction abnormalities in lower extremity ischemia: The effects of revascularization. J Surg Res 45:96, 1988.
27. Miglietta O: Electrophysiologic studies in chronic occlusive peripheral vascular disease. Arch Phys Med Rehabil 48:89, 1967.
28. Miglietta O, Lowenthal M: Nerve conduction velocity and refractory period in peripheral vascular disease. J Appl Physiol 17:837, 1962.
29. Ferguson FR, Liversedge LA: Ischemic lateral popliteal nerve palsy. Br Med J 2:333, 1954.
30. Haimovici H: Peripheral arterial embolism. Angiology 1:20, 1950.
31. Wilbourn AJ, Furlan AJ, Hulley W, et al: Ischemic monomelic neuropathy. Neurology 33:447, 1983.
32. Kihara M, McManis PG, Schmelzer JD, et al: Experimental ischemic neuropathy: Salvage with hyperbaric oxygenation. Ann Neurol 37:89, 1995.
33. Kihara M, Schmelzer JD, Kihara Y, et al: Efficacy of limb cooling on the salvage of peripheral nerve from ischemic fiber degeneration. Muscle Nerve 19:203, 1996.
34. Chopra JS, Hurwitz LJ: Femoral nerve conduction in diabetes and chronic occlusive vascular disease. J Neurol Neurosurg Psychiatry 31:28, 1968.
35. Archie JP Jr: Femoral neuropathy due to common iliac artery occlusion. South Med J 76:1073, 1983.
36. D'Amour ML, Lebrun LH, Rabbat A, et al: Peripheral neurological complications of aortoiliac vascular disease. Can J Neurol Sci 14:127, 1987.
37. Usubiaga JE, Kolodny J, Usubiaga LE: Neurologic complications of prevertebral surgery under regional anaesthesia. Surgery 68:304, 1970.
38. Voulters L, Bolton C: Acute lumbosacral plexus neuropathy following vascular surgery. Can J Neurol Sci 10:153, 1983.
39. Gloviczki P, Cross SA, Stanson AW, et al: Ischemic injury to the spinal cord or lumbosacral plexus after aorto-iliac reconstruction. Am J Surg 162:131, 1991.

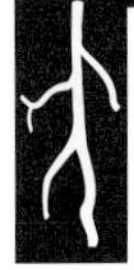

C H A P T E R 51

Lymphatic Complications of Vascular Surgery

Peter Gloviczki, M.D., and
Robert C. Lowell, M.D., F.A.C.S., R.V.T.

Injury to the lymphatic system during vascular reconstructions may be unavoidable. Lymph vessels usually run parallel to corresponding arteries and veins, and major groups of lymph nodes are close to major vessels. However, the ability of transected or ligated lymphatics to regenerate and reestablish normal lymphatic transport is remarkable. Lymphatic injury frequently heals spontaneously and causes minimal or no morbidity. Injury to the lymphatics is, however, a major contributor to the development of edema of a lower extremity after infrainguinal reconstruction.[1–11] Interruption of lymphatic vessels during surgical dissection may also cause a lymphatic fistula[12–17] or lymphocele.[17–27] Rarely, injury to the para-aortic or mesenteric lymphatics may result in chylous ascites,[22, 28–46] and thoracic duct injury during thoracic or thoracoabdominal aortic reconstruction[31, 47–56] or after high translumbar aortography[57] may result in chylothorax. This chapter reviews the pathophysiology, diagnosis, and management of the most frequent lymphatic complications following vascular reconstructions and suggests guidelines for prevention.

POST-BYPASS EDEMA

Lower extremity edema occurs in 50% to 100% of patients who undergo successful infrainguinal arterial reconstruction for chronic ischemia.[2, 7] Leg swelling after femoropopliteal or femorotibial bypass becomes evident with dependency, usually when the patient resumes ambulation. Pitting edema usually subsides within 2 to 3 months after reconstruction. During this period, normal ambulation may be impaired and wound healing delayed. In some patients, the edema may become chronic and cause persistent functional disability despite successful arterial reconstruction.

Etiology and Pathogenesis

Lymphedema develops when the rate of production of protein-rich interstitial fluid exceeds the capacity of the lymphatic system to remove the increased volume of lymph. Insufficiency of lymphatic transport plays the most important role in the development of post-bypass edema.[58] Lymphatic insufficiency has two main causes (Fig. 51–1). First, increased production of interstitial fluid after successful revascularization results in a significant increase in the lymphatic load. Second, the transport capacity of the lymphatic system is reduced because of lymphatic injury and obstruction of deep and superficial lymph channels during dissection in the popliteal space, along the greater saphenous vein and at the groin.

Increased capillary filtration results from elevated arterial pressure after revascularization, alterations in the regulation of the microcirculatory flow, and probable endothelial and smooth muscle injury from chronic ischemia.[1, 7] Decreased arterial and arteriolar smooth muscle tone as a cause of hyperemia following revascularization was first proposed in 1959 by Simeone and Husni.[59] Eickhoff,[8] however, demonstrated that abnormalities in local blood flow regulation normalized within about a week after reconstruction, whereas edema persisted much longer in these patients. Although derangement of the microcirculation contributes to post-bypass edema to some degree, Eickhoff's experiments support the theory that lymphatic obstruction due to surgical injury is the most important cause of post-bypass edema.

If the number of functioning major lymph channels decreases to a critical level, lymphedema develops. In one study, in which patients underwent lymphangiography after infrainguinal bypass, the average number of patent superficial lymph vessels visualized was reduced to 1.7 per patient, as compared with the normal average of 9.5.[1] In a similar series of 37 patients, edema was not significant when more than three intact superficial lymph vessels were visualized on the postoperative lymphangiogram.[4]

AbuRahma and colleagues examined the involvement of the lymphatic system in the pathophysiology of edema formation in patients undergoing femoropopliteal bypass grafting.[9] Edema developed in 29 of the 72 patients (40%). Leg swelling occurred in 85% (17 of 20) of the patients treated by conventional dissection of the femoropopliteal arteries. When careful dissection was performed that preserved the lymphatics, edema developed in only two of 20 patients (10%). Postoperative lymphangiography showed normal anatomy in six of the eight patients without edema, but the anatomy was markedly abnormal in all eight patients with edema who underwent lymphangiography. Persson and coworkers found less edema in those patients who needed less dissection during surgery.[10] Significantly less swelling was observed in patients with prosthetic grafts than in those with vein grafts. Patients with above-knee grafts also had less edema than those with below-knee bypasses.[10]

Studies using albumin clearance in patients with postrevascularization edema also support the idea that edema is mainly lymphatic in origin. A reduction in plasma albumin level with a concomitant increase in the extremity albumin

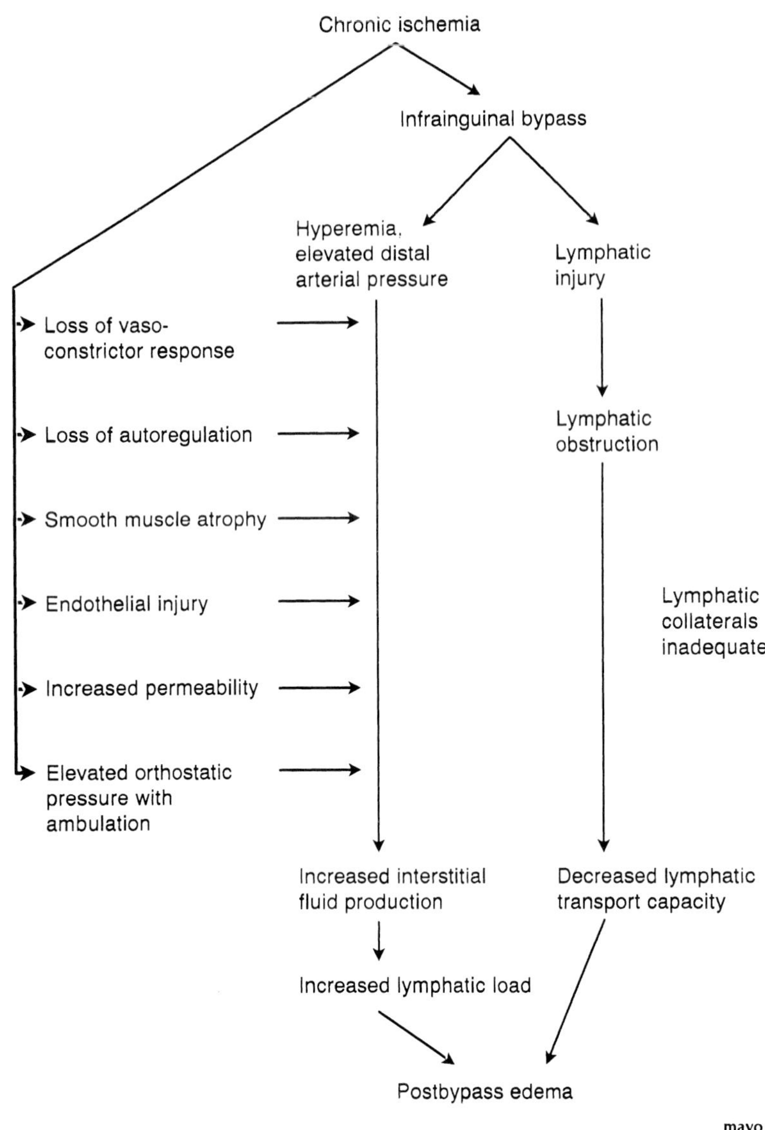

FIGURE 51–1. Mechanism of post-bypass edema. (Adapted from Gloviczki P, Bergman RT: Lymphatic problems and revascularization edema. *In* Bernhard VM, Towne JB [eds]: Complications in Vascular Surgery, 2nd ed. St. Louis, Quality Medical Publishing, 1991, p 366.)

content was noted after femoropopliteal bypass.[60] The increase in albumin content was three times greater in limbs revascularized by femoropopliteal bypass than in those revascularized by aortoiliac grafts. These data correspond to the clinical observation that edema rarely develops after aortofemoral revascularization.

Although venous thrombosis has been proposed as a cause of postoperative leg edema,[61, 62] studies have demonstrated a low incidence of deep venous thrombosis in patients with post-bypass edema.[63, 64] In one series, normal venous hemodynamics and morphology were confirmed in 41 of 45 patients with leg edema after arterial bypass.[65] The incidence of deep venous thrombosis after femoropopliteal bypass was found to be similar in patients who had edema (7%) and in those who did not (10%).[9] Deep venous thrombosis, therefore, seems to play a minor role in post-bypass edema in most patients.[7, 58, 66]

Diagnosis

Mild, partially pitting ankle edema appears on the second or third postoperative day and resolves almost completely with leg elevation and bed rest, Deep venous thrombosis should be excluded as a cause of postoperative edema when there is excessive postoperative swelling, cyanosis, muscle tenderness, or unusual pain. Duplex scanning of the deep veins is the test of choice for excluding deep venous thrombosis. If the cause of the edema is still in question, lymphoscintigraphy confirms lymphedema (Fig. 51–2).

Management

Postoperatively, mild edema of the extremity should be treated with frequent elevation of the limb and some restriction of ambulation. Cardiac failure should be treated promptly to help preserve the normal pressure gradient and to allow venous return and lymph flow toward the heart. Moderate to severe post-bypass edema is treated with compression stockings. In general, the authors prescribe calf-length therapeutic elastic stockings with compression of 30 to 40 mmHg at the ankle level. For patients with a below-knee in situ bypass or any bypass to the distal tibial

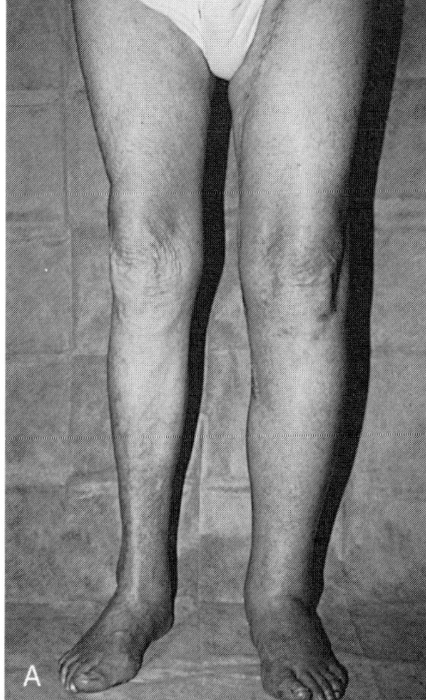

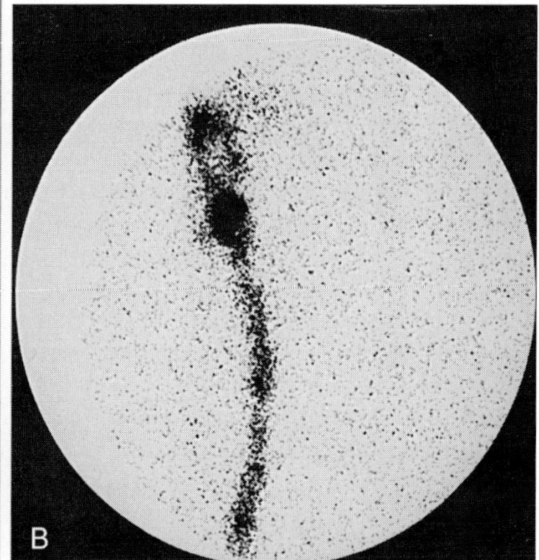

FIGURE 51–2. *A*, Edema of the left lower extremity in an 88-year-old man 4 weeks after left femoropopliteal saphenous vein bypass performed for severe chronic ischemia. *B*, Lymphoscintigraphy confirmed the severe lymphedema of the left leg with no visualization of the lymph vessels or inguinal lymph nodes. Lymphatic transport was normal on the right.

or pedal arteries, management is individualized to avoid direct compression of the subcutaneous vein graft. Attempts to prevent or limit post-bypass edema pharmacologically with steroids, mannitol, terbutaline, or furosemide have not proved effective[10] and are not recommended.

Prevention

Meticulous, lymph-preserving surgical dissection is needed to minimize post-bypass edema.[9, 58] For infrainguinal bypass, a vertical groin incision slightly lateral to the femoral pulse should be made in an attempt to preserve the patency of lymph vessels and the integrity of lymph nodes. The inguinal lymphatics should be retracted medially, and a vertical incision should be made in the femoral sheath to dissect the femoral arteries. Loupe magnification facilitates identification of lymph nodes and lymph vessels. The lymphatics should be carefully preserved; if they must be divided, they should be ligated or cauterized to avoid lymph leakage. Attempts should be made to preserve as much lymphatic tissue as possible between the saphenofemoral junction and the femoral artery. A skin bridge should be left between the groin incision and the incision made in the thigh to dissect the more distal portion of the saphenous vein. Multiple short skin incisions to dissect the saphenous vein disrupt fewer superficial lymphatics.[9]

Dissection around the popliteal artery should be performed with the same care to avoid lymphatic disruption. The vascular sheath should be opened longitudinally without dissection of the popliteal vein or the posterior tibial nerve in the neurovascular bundle. Fibroadipose tissue, which contains the deep lymphatics in the popliteal fossa, should be left intact.

The increasing use of minimally invasive techniques to harvest the greater saphenous vein for lower extremity or coronary bypass should, it is hoped, decrease wound healing problems and associated lymphatic complications. Video-assisted saphenous vein harvest requires fewer and shorter skin incisions in the leg. In a series of 68 lower extremity bypass procedures, only one bleeding complication was related to the video-assisted harvest and two seromas developed at the arterial dissection sites.[67]

LYMPHATIC FISTULA

Because of the rich lymphatic network of the femoral triangle, lymphatic fistulae following vascular reconstructions most often occur at the groin. In 4000 vascular operations, Kalman and associates observed lymphatic fistulae in 45 patients (incidence, 1.1%).[16] In other series, the incidence of this complication was similar, ranging from 0.8% to 6.4%.[13, 68, 69]

Etiology

Important factors that contribute to lymphatic leakage are failure to ligate or to cauterize divided lymphatics and failure to approximate the tissue layers properly at closure. Lymphatic leakage occurs more frequently in older diabetic patients with poor wound healing. Excessive early limb motion, infection of the operated leg or foot, reoperation, and placement of a prosthetic graft to the groin are other possible causes.[16]

Diagnosis

Persistent leakage of clear yellow fluid from a groin incision establishes the diagnosis. Lymphoscintigraphy to confirm that the fluid is of lymphatic origin is seldom necessary when the fistula develops within days or a few weeks after the operation. When lymphatic leakage occurs several months or years after vascular reconstruction, lymphoscintigraphy is helpful; in such cases, however, computed tomography (CT), white blood cell scanning, and sometimes fistulography must be performed to exclude infection of an underlying vascular graft. CT is also valuable for diagnosis of concomitant retroperitoneal lymphatic injury because retroperitoneal lymphocele or chylous ascites can present with lymphatic fistulae at the groin.[58]

Management

Early diagnosis and management of lymphatic fistula are important to prevent prolonged hospitalization and delayed wound healing. Although in one study of 35 patients with lymphatic leakage, infection of an underlying vascular graft was not noted,[14] most studies have reported a small but definite risk of deep wound infection from persistent lymph leakage.[13, 16] In the first few days, conservative management is indicated and should include local wound care, administration of systemic antibiotics, and bed rest with leg elevation to reduce lymph flow.

Like other authors,[13, 16] we favor surgical closure in the operating room when the fistula continues to produce large volumes despite several days of conservative management. First, 5 ml of isosulfan blue (Lymphazurin dye) is injected subcutaneously into the first and third interdigital spaces in the foot (Fig. 51–3).[15, 58] The groin incision is then opened, and the site of the lymphatic injury is readily apparent by the leakage of blue fluid droplets. The area is oversewn, and the wound is closed in multiple layers over a small polyethylene drain. When it is impossible to oversew the damaged tissue, injection of "tissue glue" may be useful.

THORACIC DUCT FISTULA

Injury to the thoracic duct may occur after dissection of the proximal left common carotid artery or after left subclavian or vertebral artery dissection.[22] Neglected cases of thoracic duct cutaneous fistula may lead to malnutrition, lymphocytopenia, anemia, or infection of an underlying prosthetic graft. Early operation with lateral closure using 7-0 or 8-0 nonabsorbable monofilament sutures is the optimal treatment. If lateral closure is not possible, ligation of the thoracic duct at the neck is an accepted alternative because the collateral lymphatic circulation is usually adequate. The incision is closed over a subcutaneous drain, which is left in place for a short time postoperatively.

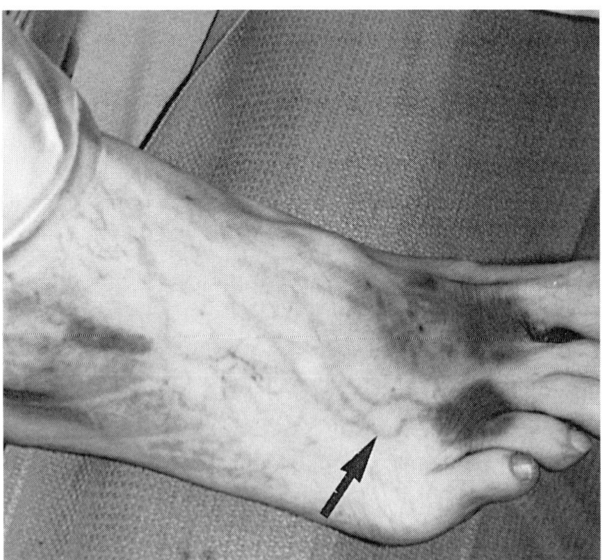

FIGURE 51–3. Injection of isosulfan blue (Lymphazurin) dye into the first and third interdigital spaces of the foot immediately visualizes the foot lymphatics *(arrow)* and during surgery helps to identify the site of lymphatic injury at the groin.

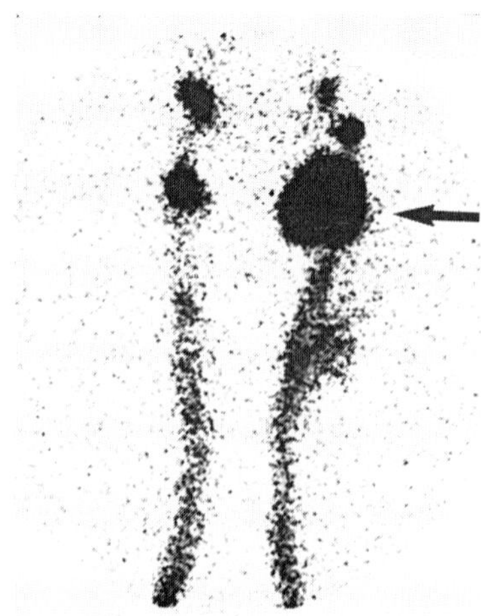

FIGURE 51–4. Bilateral lower extremity lymphoscintigraphy demonstrates a large left groin lymphocele *(arrow)* and extravasation of the colloid in the left thigh.

LYMPHOCELE

A lymphocele is a localized collection of lymph. Early after injury to the lymphatic pathways, the lymph collects between tissue planes. Unless the lymph reabsorbs spontaneously or drains through a cutaneous fistula, a pseudocapsule develops. In contrast to a seroma, a lymphocele usually has a well-localized connection with one or more of the lymphatic channels. For this reason, lymphoscintigraphy can readily demonstrate a lymphocele (Fig. 51–4).

Groin Lymphocele

As with lymphatic fistulae, the most frequent site of lymphoceles after vascular reconstructions is the groin. Most lymphoceles develop in the early postoperative period but may appear later. Large lymphoceles cause local discomfort, pain, and leg swelling. Hematoma, seroma, and wound infection should be considered in the differential diagnosis. The presence of a soft, fluid-filled cyst and intermittent drainage of clear lymph through a fistula confirms the diagnosis of lymphocele. Ultrasonography is helpful in distinguishing a solid, dense hematoma from a cystic lymphocele. CT is performed when a lymphocele develops several weeks to months after the operation. CT is helpful for excluding graft infection or for identifying retroperitoneal lymphocele extending to the groin.

Small lymphoceles can be observed because they may reabsorb spontaneously. For enlarging or symptomatic lymphoceles or lymphoceles that lie close to a prosthetic graft, we advocate early surgery to reduce the risk of graft infection. Injection of isosulfan blue into the foot is helpful for identifying the lymphatic channels supplying the lymphocele. The lymphocele is excised, and the lymphatic pedicle is ligated or oversewn (Fig. 51–5). The wound is closed in multiple layers over a small subcutaneous drain.

Retroperitoneal Lymphocele

Symptomatic retroperitoneal lymphoceles are rare. In a review of more than 4000 aortic reconstructions, an incidence of 0.1% was reported by Garrett and colleagues.[25] In reviewing the literature, we found 11 well-documented cases of this complication following aortic reconstruction.[18, 19, 21–23, 25, 58] The number of unreported and asymptomatic cases is undoubtedly higher. Retroperitoneal lymphoceles have been reported more frequently after renal transplantation (incidence 0.6% to 18%).[26, 70–74] In these patients, however, lymphocele develops not only because of injury to the recipient pelvic lymphatics but also because of increased lymph production and lymph leakage from the donor kidney.[26]

Diagnosis

The most common symptoms of retroperitoneal lymphocele are abdominal distention, nausea, and abdominal pain, and the most frequent finding is an abdominal or a flank mass. Although signs or symptoms may develop early, in almost half of the patients the lymphocele is discovered a year or several years after the operation.[58] Patients who present with signs or symptoms of a retroperitoneal lymphocele should be examined with CT (Fig. 51–6). In five of 11 published cases of retroperitoneal lymphocele, a groin mass was also present.[58] Evaluation of these patients showed a communication between the groin lymphocele and a retroperitoneal lymphocele. This observation illustrates the importance of CT when a groin mass develops after aortofemoral reconstruction. If infection is suspected, white blood cell scanning should also be performed unless CT has already confirmed graft infection. Lymphoscintigraphy can be diagnostic of a retroperitoneal lymphocele and should distinguish it from a perigraft seroma. Nevertheless, lymphoscintigraphic confirmation of a lymphocele does not rule out graft infection.

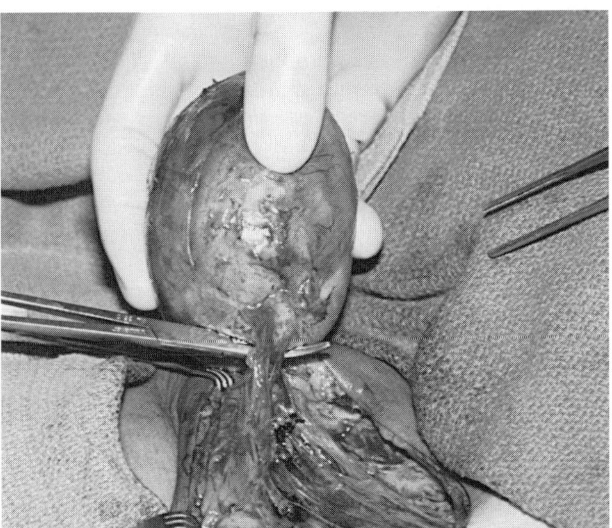

FIGURE 51–5. Intraoperative photograph of a dissected left groin lymphocele with an easily identifiable lymphatic pedicle. The pedicle was ligated, and the lymphocele was removed.

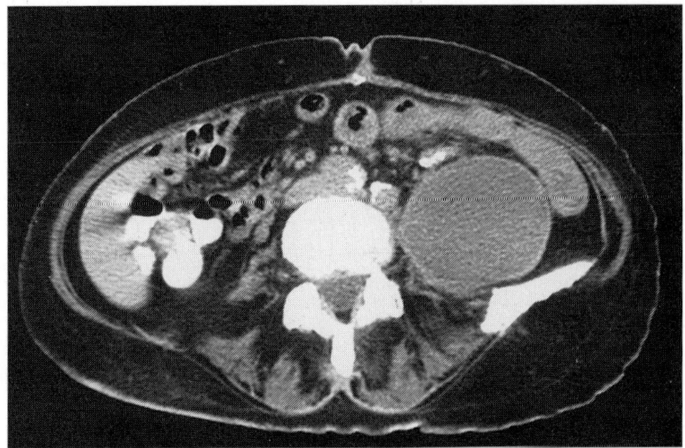

FIGURE 51–6. Computed tomographic scan of a 70-year-old woman reveals a large left retroperitoneal lymphocele 9 months after repair of a thoracoabdominal aortic aneurysm.

Management

For patients with a small asymptomatic retroperitoneal lymphocele, observation with serial ultrasonography or CT is warranted. If the lymphocele increases in size or causes local compression to adjacent structures, needle aspiration under CT or ultrasound guidance is performed. This maneuver is both diagnostic and therapeutic. In four of 11 patients, aspiration alone was used with success.[58] Placement of an indwelling irrigation-drainage system is associated with a risk of infection. Garrett and colleagues discussed two patients whose prosthetic grafts became infected after an irrigation-drainage system was placed for retroperitoneal lymphocele.[25] Therefore, when repeated aspiration is unsuccessful, operative repair should be considered.

Abdominal exploration is performed after injection of 5 ml of isosulfan blue into the ipsilateral foot according to the technique detailed earlier. The lymphocele is unroofed, and the site of the lymphatic injury is oversewn, ligated, or both. If the prosthetic graft is exposed, it is covered by retroperitoneal tissue or omentum. When preoperative aspiration confirms the presence of chyle in the cyst, 24 ounces of cream is given through a nasogastric tube 4 hours before exploration. Absorption of the cream helps to identify the site of lymphatic leakage in the mesenteric lymphatics around the left renal vein or at the cisterna chyli (Fig. 51–7). Whereas the mesenteric lymphatic trunks should be ligated or oversewn, lateral closure of the cisterna should be attempted first with loupe magnification.

For post-transplant lymphocele, peritoneal fenestration has been recommended for treatment.[70, 71] Since the advent of surgical laparoscopy, however, several reports have described aspiration and peritoneal fenestration under laparoscopic visualization.[72, 73] A tongue of omentum is brought down and placed through the peritoneal window to prevent

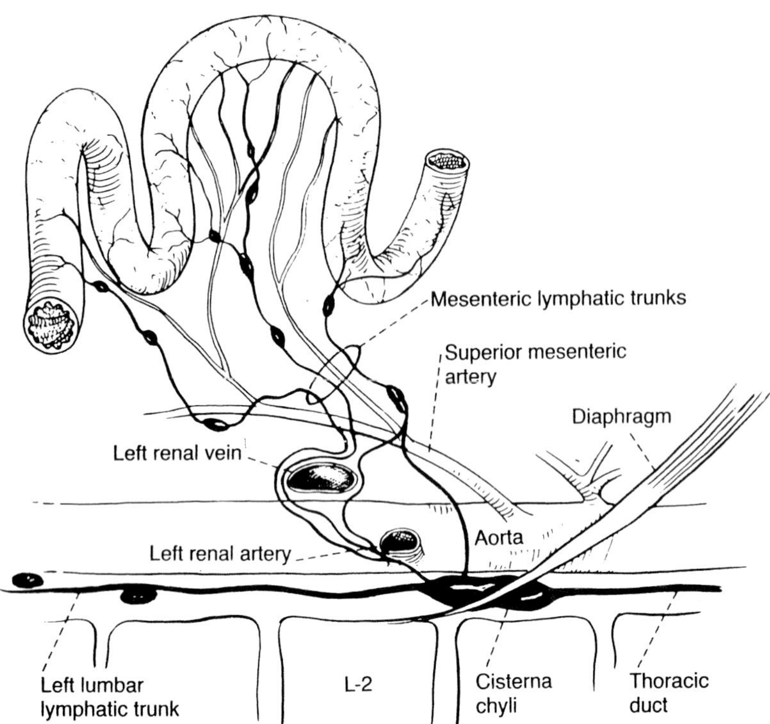

FIGURE 51–7. Anatomy of the mesenteric and ascending lumbar lymphatic trunks and the cisterna chyli. (From Gloviczki P, Bergman RT: Lymphatic problems and revascularization edema. *In* Bernhard VM, Towne JB [eds]: Complications in Vascular Surgery, 2nd ed. St. Louis, Quality Medical Publishing, 1991, p 366.)

premature closure and recurrence of the cyst. One study analyzed results of 12 laparoscopic and 23 open surgical internal marsupializations of pelvic lymphoceles. Laparoscopic lymphocelectomy required a longer operative time, but it resulted in shorter hospital stays, faster convalescences, and fewer recurrences of the lymphocele.[72] Laparoscopic transperitoneal drainage may become a useful addition to the vascular surgeon's armamentarium for the occasional treatment of lymphoceles after vascular reconstruction.

CHYLOUS ASCITES

The development of chylous ascites after abdominal aortic reconstructions is rare, but morbidity and mortality related to this complication can be significant. In reviewing the literature, we found 23 patients who were reported to have chylous ascites after aortic reconstruction.[22, 28–46, 74] Eighteen patients (78%) underwent repair of an abdominal aortic aneurysm, and five (22%) had surgery for occlusive disease. Ascites developed in the first 6 weeks after surgery in all but one patient.

Diagnosis

Symptoms of chylous ascites include progressive abdominal pain, dyspnea, and nausea. Abdominal distention can be significant, and the loss of proteins and fat may result in malnourishment. Lymphopenia and anemia can also develop, frequently resulting in poor immune function. Ascites can usually be detected by physical examination and confirmed by ultrasonography or CT. Paracentesis is necessary to verify the presence of chyle in the ascitic fluid. Chyle is an odorless, sterile, alkaline fluid that is milky in appearance. Its specific gravity is greater than 1012 gm/dl. Its protein content is usually above 3 gm/dl, and its fat content ranges from 0.4 to 4 gm/dl. The fat in the fluid stains with Sudan stain.

Management

Although chylous ascites in patients with abdominal malignancies carries an ominous prognosis, the outcome when chylous ascites develops after aortic surgery is somewhat better. Still, after aortic surgery, four of 23 patients with this complication died (mortality rate, 17%).[22, 31, 47, 74] The causes of death were sepsis in two patients and pulmonary embolus and malnutrition in one patient each.[22, 31, 42, 74]

Most patients with chylous ascites after aortic surgery can be successfully treated without operation. The mainstay of treatment in patients with mild to moderate ascites is a medium-chain triglyceride diet to decrease chyle formation. For severe cases, however, complete bowel rest and total parenteral nutrition must be instituted. Repeated paracentesis results in resolution of the symptoms in most patients. Placement of a peritoneovenous shunt was reported in five patients, but sepsis caused death in one.[74] If repeated paracentesis is unsuccessful, exploration and closure of the site of the lymphatic injury should be performed. Larger mesenteric or para-aortic lymphatic channels should be ligated or oversewn, but lateral closure of the injured cisterna chyli can be attempted with fine monofilament sutures, as mentioned earlier. Of the six patients who underwent exploration and surgical closure of the fistula, all recovered without recurrence.[28, 34, 39, 41, 44, 45]

Prevention

Injury to the retroperitoneal and mesenteric lymphatics during aortic dissection should be carefully avoided. The cisterna chyli is formed by the right and left lumbar and the mesenteric lymphatic trunks; it is usually located at the level of the second lumbar vertebra, between the inferior vena cava and the abdominal aorta.[58] In half of patients, a well-developed cisterna chyli is absent. Several large mesenteric lymph vessels are located on the anteroinferior aspect of the left renal vein (see Fig. 51–7). Injury to these vessels results in leakage of chyle. Failure to close the divided lymphatics may lead to the development of chylous ascites or retroperitoneal lymphocele. All large lumbar, para-aortic, and mesenteric lymph vessels should be ligated or clipped when division is necessary during aortic dissection. Lateral closure of the injured cisterna chyli should be attempted with 7-0 monofilament sutures.

CHYLOTHORAX

Effusion of chyle into the pleural cavity after vascular procedures is uncommon; it occurs in 0.2% to 1% of cases after cardiothoracic surgery.[55] It is more common in neonates and small children operated on for congenital vascular anomalies, most frequently for aortic coarctation.[51–56] Chylothorax after repair of thoracic aortic aneurysm has been reported,[47–50] and in one patient it occurred after repair of an abdominal aortic aneurysm.[31] Chylothorax may develop as a complication of transthoracic dorsal sympathectomy[48] or after high translumbar aortography.[57]

Diagnosis

Pleural effusion is confirmed by chest x-ray studies or CT. Analysis of the fluid obtained through thoracentesis or through the thoracostomy tube confirms the diagnosis. Laboratory analysis of the milky or serous fluid is similar to that described for chylous ascites.

Management

Because respiratory embarrassment is frequent, drainage of the chylous fluid through a thoracostomy tube is usually necessary. The principles of treatment for decreasing chyle formation are the same as those for chylous ascites. Conservative management, consisting of closed drainage through a thoracostomy tube and nutritional support, has been effective in most cases. If a low-fat, high-protein diet with medium-chain triglyceride supplementation is not successful, intravenous hyperalimentation is started. Rarely, surgical closure of the site of the leak by oversewing or ligating the thoracic duct must be performed. Pleurodesis facilitates closure of the pleural space and decreases the potential for recurrence. Of the six patients who had chylothorax after aortic aneurysm repair, only one patient needed thoracotomy to treat a large chylous pseudocyst[47]; however, one patient who was treated conservatively died after a long postoperative course that was complicated by both chylous ascites and chylothorax.[31]

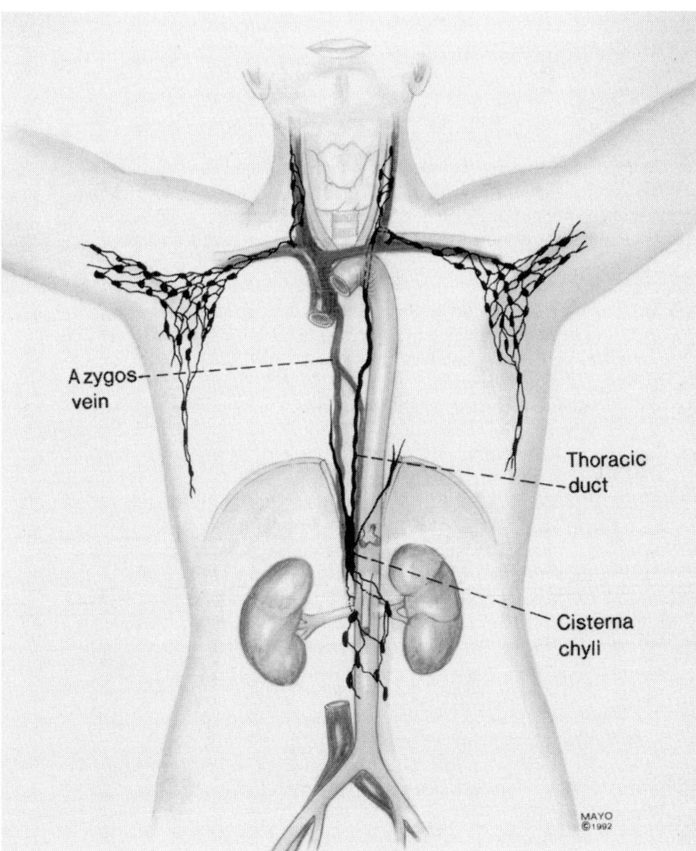

FIGURE 51–8. Anatomy of the thoracic duct. (By permission of Mayo Foundation.)

Prevention

Injury to the thoracic duct during thoracic aortic dissection should be carefully avoided. The thoracic duct extends upward from the cisterna chyli and enters the posterior mediastinum through the aortic hiatus, slightly to the right of the aorta and to the left of the azygos vein (Fig. 51–8). In the posterior mediastinum, it is mostly a right-sided structure. The thoracic duct enters the superior mediastinum behind the aortic arch and subclavian artery, to the left of the esophagus. It is thus exposed to injury during dissection of the proximal thoracic aorta, the aortic arch, or the proximal subclavian artery. Once injury to the thoracic duct is recognized, an attempt at lateral closure should be made using 7-0 monofilament sutures with loupe magnification. When this is not successful, ligation of the thoracic duct should be performed. Adequate collateral lymphatic circulation usually develops.

REFERENCES

1. Vaughan BF, Slavotinek AH, Jepson RP: Edema of the lower limb after vascular operations. Surg Gynecol Obstet 133:282, 1970.
2. Porter JM, Lindell TD, Lakin PC: Leg edema following femoropopliteal autogenous vein bypass. Arch Surg 105:883, 1972.
3. Storen EJ, Myhre HO, Stiris G: Lymphangiographic findings in patients with leg oedema after arterial reconstructions. Acta Chir Scand 140:385, 1974.
4. Schmidt KR, Welter H, Pfeifer KJ, et al: Lymphographic investigations of oedema of the extremities following reconstructive vascular surgery in the femoropopliteal territory. ROEFO 128:194, 1978.
5. Stillman RM, Fitzgerald JF, Varughese G, et al: Edema following femoropopliteal bypass: Etiology and prevention. Vasc Surg 18:354, 1983.
6. Stranden E: Edema in the lower limb following arterial reconstruction for atherosclerosis: A study of pathogenetic mechanisms. J Oslo City Hosp 34:3, 1984.
7. Schubart PJ, Porter JM: Leg edema following femorodistal bypass. *In* Bergan JJ, Yao JST (eds): Reoperative Arterial Surgery. Orlando, Fla, Grune & Stratton, 1986, p 311.
8. Eickhoff JH: Local regulation of subcutaneous blood flow and capillary filtration in limbs with occlusive arterial disease: Studies before and after arterial reconstruction. Dan Med Bull 33:111, 1986.
9. AbuRahma AF, Woodruff BA, Lucente FC: Edema after femoropopliteal bypass surgery: Lymphatic and venous theories of causation. J Vasc Surg 11:461, 1990.
10. Persson NH, Takolander R, Bergqvist D: Edema after lower limb arterial reconstruction: Influence of background factors, surgical technique and potentially prophylactic methods. Vasa 20:57, 1991.
11. Esato K, Ohara M, Seyama A, et al: ^{99m}Tc-HSA lymphoscintigraphy and leg edema following arterial reconstruction. J Cardiovasc Surg 32:741, 1991.
12. Stolzenberg J: Detection of lymphaticocutaneous fistula by radionuclide lymphangiography. Arch Surg 113:306, 1978.
13. Kwaan JHM, Berstein JM, Connolly JE: Management of lymph fistulae in the groin after arterial reconstruction. Arch Surg 114:1416, 1979.
14. Murphy JL, Cole WC, White PM, et al: Lymphatic fistula after vascular reconstruction: A case control study. Can J Surg 34(1):76, 1991.
15. Weaver FA, Yellin AE: Management of postoperative lymphatic leaks by use of isosulphan blue (Letter). J Vasc Surg 14(4):566, 1991.
16. Kalman PG, Walker PM, Johnston KW: Consequences of groin lymphatic fistulae after vascular reconstruction. Vasc Surg 25:210, 1991.
17. Khauli RB, Mosenthal AC, Caushaj PF: Treatment of lymphocele and lymphatic fistula following renal transplantation by laparoscopic peritoneal window. J Urol 147(5):1353, 1992.
18. Dillon ML, Postlethwait RW: The management of an abdominal mass recurring after resection of abdominal aortic aneurysm. Surg Clin North Am 50:1021, 1970.
19. Fitzer PM, Sallade RL, Graham WH: Computed tomography and the diagnosis of giant abdominal lymphocele. Va Med Q 107:448, 1980.
20. Patel BR, Burkhalter JL, Patel TB, et al: Interstitial lymphoscintigraphy for diagnosis of lymphocele. Clin Nucl Med 10:175, 1985.
21. Puyau FA, Adinolfi MF, Kerstein MD: Lymphocele around aortic femoral grafts simulating a false aneurysm. Cardiovasc Intervent Radiol 8:195, 1985.
22. Jensen SR, Voegeli DR, McDermott JC, et al: Lymphatic disruption following abdominal aortic surgery. Cardiovasc Intervent Radiol 9:199, 1986.
23. Pardy BJ, Harris P, Mourad K, et al: Case reports: Upper abdominal lymphocele following urgent aortorenal bypass grafting. J R Soc Med 79:674, 1986.
24. Scott AR: A report on the management of a lymphocyst after vascular surgery. Aust N Z J Surg 57:205, 1987.
25. Garrett HE Jr, Richardson JW, Howard HS, et al: Retroperitoneal lymphocele after abdominal aortic surgery. J Vasc Surg 10:245, 1989.
26. Malovrh M, Kandus A, Buturovic-Ponikvar J, et al: Frequency and clinical influence of lymphoceles after kidney transplantation. Transplant Proc 22:1423, 1990.
27. Velanovich V, Mallory P, Collins PS: Lower extremity lymphocele development after saphenous vein harvesting. Mil Med 156:149, 1991.
28. Bradham RR, Gregorie HB, Wilson R: Chylous ascites following resection of an abdominal aortic aneurysm. Am Surg 36:238, 1970.
29. Klippel AP, Hardy DA: Postoperative chylous ascites. Mo Med 68:253, 1971.
30. DeBartolo TF, Etzkorn JR: Conservative management of chylous ascites after abdominal aortic aneurysm repair: Case report. Mo Med 73:611, 1976.
31. Lopez-Enriquez E, Gonzalez A, Johnson CD, et al: Chylothorax and chyloperitoneum: A case report. Bol Assoc Med P R 71:54, 1979.
32. Meinke AH III, Estes NC, Ernst CB: Chylous ascites following abdominal aortic aneurysmectomy: Management with total parenteral hyperalimentation. Ann Surg 190:631, 1979.
33. Stubbe LTHFL, Terpstra JL: Chylous ascites after resection of an abdominal aortic aneurysm. Arch Chir Neerlandicum 31:111, 1979.
34. McKenna R, Stevick CA: Chylous ascites following aortic reconstruction. Vasc Surg 17:143, 1983.
35. Savrin RA, High JR: Chylous ascites after abdominal aortic surgery. Surgery 98:866, 1985.
36. Sarazin WG, Sauter KE: Chylous ascites following resection of a ruptured abdominal aneurysm. Arch Surg 121:246, 1986.
37. Fleisher HL III, Oren JW, Sumner DS: Chylous ascites after abdominal aortic aneurysmectomy: Successful management with a peritoneovenous shunt. J Vasc Surg 6:403, 1987.
38. Schwein M, Dawes PD, Hatchuel D, et al: Postoperative chylous ascites after resection of an abdominal aortic aneurysm: A case report. S Afr J Surg 25:39, 1987.
39. Williamson C, Provan JL: Chylous ascites following aortic surgery. Br J Surg 74:71, 1987.
40. Boyd WD, McPhail NV, Barber GC: Case report: Chylous ascites following abdominal aortic aneurysmectomy: Surgical management with a peritoneovenous shunt. J Cardiovasc Surg 30:627, 1989.
41. Heyl A, Veen HF: Iatrogenic chylous ascites: Operative or conservative approach. Neth J Surg 41:5, 1989.
42. Ablan CJ, Littooy FN, Freeark RJ: Postoperative chylous ascites: Diagnosis and treatment. Arch Surg 125:270, 1990.
43. Bahner DR Jr, Townsend R: Chylous ascites after ruptured abdominal aortic aneurysm. Contemp Surg 36:37, 1990.
44. Sultan S, Pauwels A, Poupon R, et al: Ascites chyleuses de l'adulte aspects étiologiques, térapeutiques et évolutifs: A propos de 35 cas. Ann Gastroenterol Hepatol (Paris) 26:187, 1990.
45. Williams RA, Vetto J, Quinones-Baldrich W, et al: Chylous ascites following abdominal aortic surgery. Ann Vasc Surg 5:247, 1991.
46. Sanger R, Wilmshurst CC, Clyne CA: Chylous ascites following aneurysm surgery: Case report. Eur J Vasc Surg 5:689, 1991.
47. Mack JW, Heydorn WH, Pauling FW, et al: Postoperative chylous pseudocyst. J Thorac Cardiovasc Surg 77:773, 1979.
48. Kostiainen S, Meurala H, Mattila S, et al: Chylothorax: Clinical experience in nine cases. Scand J Thorac Cardiovasc Surg 17:79, 1983.
49. Okabayashi H, Tamura N, Hirose N, et al: Aortic aneurysm associated with coarctation of the aorta. Kyobu Geka 42(12):1032, 1989.
50. Sachs PB, Zelch MG, Rice TG, et al: Diagnosis and localization of laceration of the thoracic duct: Usefulness of lymphangiography and CT. AJR Am J Roentgenol 157:703, 1991.
51. Hallman GL, Bloodwell RD, Cooley DA: Coarctation of the thoracic aorta. Surg Clin North Am 46(4):893, 1966.

52. Bortolotti U, Faggian G, Livi U, et al: Postoperative chylothorax following repair of coarctation of the aorta: Report of a case with unusual clinical manifestation. Thorac Cardiovasc Surg 30:319, 1982.
53. Fairfax AJ, McNabb WR, Spiro SG: Chylothorax: A review of 18 cases. Thorax 41:880, 1986.
54. Baudet E, Al-Qudah A: Late results of the subclavian flap repair of coarctation in infancy. J Cardiovasc Surg 30:445, 1989.
55. Cooper P, Paes ML: Bilateral chylothorax. Br J Anaesth 66:387, 1991.
56. Chun K, Colombani PM, Dudgeon DL: Diagnosis and management of congenital vascular rings: A 22 year experience. Ann Thorac Surg 53:597; discussion, 602, 1992.
57. Negroni CC, Ortiz VN: Chylothorax following high translumbar aortography: A case report and review of the literature. Bol Assoc Med P R 80:201, 1988.
58. Gloviczki P, Bergman RT: Lymphatic problems and revascularization edema. *In* Bernhard VM, Towne JB (eds): Complications in Vascular Surgery, 2nd ed. St. Louis, Quality Medical Publishing, 1991, p 366.
59. Simeone FA, Husni EA: The hyperemia of reconstructive arterial surgery. Ann Surg 150:575, 1959.
60. Campbell H, Harris PL: Albumin kinetics and oedema following reconstructive arterial surgery of the lower limb. J Cardiovasc Surg 26:110, 1985.
61. Taylor GW: Arterial grafting for gangrene. Ann R Coll Surg Engl 31:168, 1962.
62. Hamer JD: Investigation of oedema of the lower limb following successful femoropopliteal by-pass surgery: The role of phlebography in demonstrating venous thrombosis. Br J Surg 59:979, 1972.
63. Myhre HO, Dedichen H: Haemodynamic factors in the oedema of arterial reconstructions. Scand J Thorac Cardiovasc Surg 6:323, 1972.
64. Myhre HO, Storen EJ, Ongre A: The incidence of deep venous thrombosis in patients with leg oedema after arterial reconstruction. Scand J Thorac Cardiovasc Surg 8:73, 1974.
65. Husni EA: The edema of arterial reconstruction. Circulation 35(Suppl):I169, 1967.
66. Cass AJ, Jennings SA, Greenhalgh RM: Leg swelling after aortic surgery. Int Angiol 5(3):207, 1986.
67. Jordan WD, Voellinger DC, Schroeder PT, McDowell HA: Video-assisted saphenous vein harvest: The evolution of a new technique. J Vasc Surg 26:405, 1997.
68. Skudder PA, Geary J: Lymphatic drainage from the groin following surgery of the femoral artery. J Cardiovasc Surg (Torino) 28:460, 1987.
69. Johnston KW: Multicenter prospective study of nonruptured abdominal aortic aneurysm: II. Variables predicting morbidity and mortality. J Vasc Surg 9:437, 1989.
70. Howard RJ, Simmons RL, Najarian JS: Prevention of lymphoceles following renal transplantation. Ann Surg 18:166, 1976.
71. Clayman RV, So SSK, Jendrisak MD, et al: Laparoscopic drainage of a posttransplant lymphocele. Transplantation 51:725, 1991.
72. Gill IS, Hodge EE, Munch LC, et al: Transperitoneal marsupialization of lymphoceles: A comparison of laparoscopic and open techniques. J Urol 153:706, 1995.
73. Melvin WS, Bumgardner GL, Davies EA, et al: The laparoscopic management of post-transplant lymphocele: A critical review. Surg Endosc 11:245, 1997.
74. Servelle M, Nogues CL, Soulie J, et al: Spontaneous, postoperative and traumatic chylothorax. J Cardiovasc Surg (Torino) 21:475, 1980.

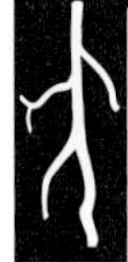

CHAPTER 52

Postoperative Sexual Dysfunction After Aortoiliac Revascularization

D. Preston Flanigan, M.D.

The relationship between altered male sexual function and arterial occlusive disease in the aortoiliac system is now established. Also well known is the complication of postoperative sexual dysfunction in male patients undergoing aortoiliac reconstructive surgery. In 1923, Leriche first pointed out the association between aortic occlusion and impotence.[27] Classic Leriche's syndrome consists of weakness of the thigh muscles, impotence, and terminal aortic occlusion.[28] Historically, surgery on the aortoiliac vessels carries a high risk of iatrogenic sexual dysfunction, but it also has the possible benefit of reversing preoperative impotence. Numerous investigators have demonstrated that approximately 25% of patients with preoperative sexual dysfunction regain normal sexual function after aortoiliac revascularization.[5, 9, 17, 18, 31, 35, 43, 46, 49]

Although sexual improvement after aortoiliac revascularization was presumed to be secondary to an improvement in pelvic circulation, not until the application of Doppler technology to the measurement of penile blood pressure could the actual relationship between sexual function and penile circulation be established. Using Doppler-derived penile blood pressure measurements preoperatively and postoperatively, Queral and coworkers conclusively demonstrated the relationship between improved or worsened sexual function after aortoiliac revascularization and improved or worsened penile perfusion.[41]

The significant interconnections between the sympathetic and the parasympathetic nerves at the levels of the para-aortic and superior hypogastric plexuses have been demonstrated.[38] Both erection and ejaculation may be impaired after injury to these nerve plexuses. When these nerve plexuses have been spared during aortoiliac surgery, the incidence of postoperative sexual dysfunction has decreased.[5, 9, 43] Thus, it is important for vascular surgeons to maintain or improve pelvic circulation *and* to avoid injury to autonomic nerve plexuses during aortoiliac revascularization if the incidence of postoperative sexual dysfunction is to be lessened.

TABLE 52–1. ETIOLOGY OF IMPOTENCE

Psychogenic	Iatrogenic
Neurogenic	Developmental
Vasculogenic	Endocrinologic
Pharmacologic	Traumatic

Women do not seem to be susceptible to iatrogenic sexual dysfunction after aortoiliac surgery, probably because of the lush pelvic collateral circulation to the female sex organs and because female sexual sensation depends locally on intact pudendal somatic nerve fibers.[40] The pudendal nerve is covered by a thick layer of endopelvic fascia and is unlikely to incur surgical injury.

Although the previously mentioned considerations are important, they are not the only factors that may affect sexual function in vascular patients. These patients may have other preoperative and postoperative risk factors for sexual dysfunction, including neurogenic, psychogenic, and pharmacologic causes (Table 52–1). Vascular surgeons must be well versed in the anatomy and physiology of male sexual function, the various causes of sexual dysfunction, the diagnostic methods used in the evaluation of sexual dysfunction, the methods of preventing iatrogenic sexual dysfunction during revascularization, and the treatment of postoperative sexual dysfunction.

ANATOMY

The blood supply to the penis is through the aortoiliac segment. Flow to the penis is via the dorsal artery of the penis, the deep penile artery, and the urethral artery. These arteries are the terminal arteries of the internal pudendal artery, which is a branch of the anterior division of the internal iliac artery (the hypogastric artery). Arterial obstruction anywhere in this arterial axis has been shown to be associated with sexual dysfunction.

At the penile level, there are two paired corpora cavernosa and a single corpus spongiosum. Each corpus cavernosum is surrounded by a thick fibrous sheath that encases multiple interconnected lacunar spaces lined by vascular endothelium. The arterial circulation to the corpora cavernosa is from paired cavernosal arteries. Numerous muscular corkscrew-shaped and helicine arteries lead from the cavernosal arteries directly to the lacunar spaces. Venous drainage from the corpora is through subtunical venules, which coalesce to form larger emissary veins that pierce the tunica albuginea. Drainage proceeds through the deep dorsal vein and the cavernosal and crural veins.

Innervation of the vessels of the penis is by sympathetic nerves arising from the 11th thoracic through the second lumbar segments, whereas parasympathetic innervation and somatic innervation arise from the second through the fourth lumbar segments. Somatic innervation is via the pudendal nerves. Erectile function is thought to be controlled primarily by parasympathetic innervation, whereas ejaculation is primarily a sympathetically mediated function[50]; however, numerous interconnections between the two systems have been demonstrated in the para-aortic plexus and the superior hypogastric plexus.[38] These plexuses are particularly susceptible to injury during infrarenal aortic dissection (Fig. 52–1).

PHYSIOLOGY

Erection occurs as a result of local genital stimulation or through central psychogenic stimuli. Genital stimulation is mediated by a spinal reflex pathway. Several areas of the brain have been implicated in psychogenic erection, including the thalamic nuclei, the rhinencephalon, and the limbic structures. Hypothalamic projections to the spinal cord have been identified; they probably control thoracolumbar sympathetic and sacral parasympathetic outflow to the penis.

Erection is the result of penile arterial smooth muscle relaxation. Cavernosal and helicine artery dilatation leads to filling of the lacunar spaces, which become dilated, thus causing penile engorgement. Increased pressure within the tunica albuginea compresses subtunical venules, resulting in restriction of venous outflow from the lacunar spaces, which maintains tumescence. Loss of erection is the result

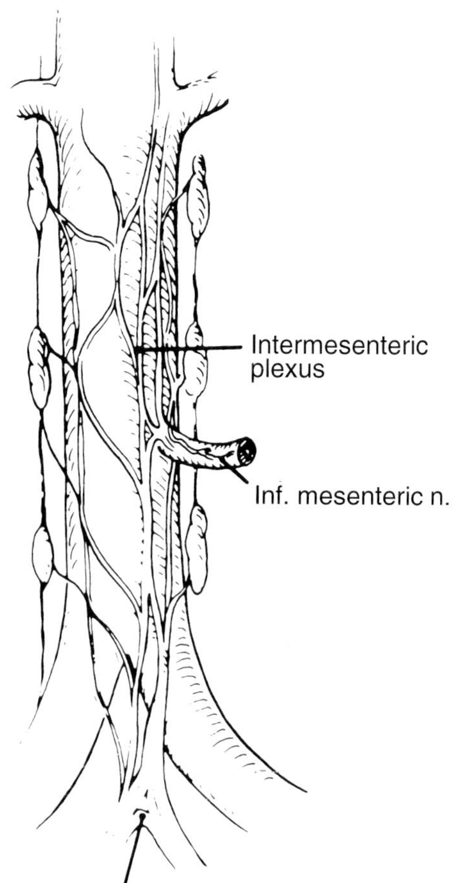

FIGURE 52–1. Anatomy of the autonomic nerve plexuses at the level of the infrarenal aorta and the proximal iliac arteries. The nerves are predominantly on the left side of the aorta and cross the proximal left common iliac artery as they course distally. (From Weinstein MH, Machleder HI: Sexual function after aortoiliac surgery. Ann Surg 181:787, 1975.)

of penile arterial smooth muscle vasoconstriction, which reduces arterial inflow and causes collapse of the lacunar spaces and decreased venous outflow resistance.[25]

Control of penile arterial smooth muscle is through adrenergic nerves, cholinergic nerves, and nerves immunoreactive to vasoactive intestinal peptide. Adrenergic nerves cause smooth muscle constriction through norepinephrine release, whereas smooth muscle relaxation is via cholinergic neurotransmitters. The latter work through effects on other neuroeffector systems. Vascular endothelium can also influence underlying smooth muscle tone, possibly through the release of endothelium-derived relaxing factor, endothelium-derived hyperpolarizing factor, prostaglandins, and the peptide endothelin.[25]

INCIDENCE AND ETIOLOGY

The incidence of male sexual dysfunction has not been accurately assessed. Pertinent to vascular surgery, however, is the incidence of preoperative sexual dysfunction in patients being considered for aortoiliac revascularization. Flanigan and coworkers showed this incidence to be 27% in 110 patients, an incidence similar to that reported in other surgical series.[9] The cause of impotence in vascular patients is not always circulatory. Multiple etiologic factors, such as diabetes mellitus, drug therapy, psychogenic factors, and previous surgery, are often present. Impotence in diabetic patients has been reported to be as high as 50%.[32]

There are numerous causes of impotence that must be considered (see Table 52–1) *Psychogenic* impotence is thought to be the most common form. Although this form is usually not a major postoperative consideration, there may be a perception of change in body image and decreased masculinity that follows major abdominal surgery. *Neurogenic* sexual dysfunction can be secondary to nerve injury or diabetic neuropathy. *Vasculogenic* impotence is usually the result of decreased pelvic blood supply due to either arterial occlusive disease or surgery. Malfunction of the venous occlusive mechanism can also cause vasculogenic impotence.[8]

Pharmacologic sexual dysfunction most commonly results from antihypertensive medications, but numerous other agents have been implicated (Table 52–2). (For an exhaustive list of drugs associated with male sexual dysfunction, see *The Medical Letter*, vol. 29 [issue 744], July 17, 1987.)

TABLE 52–2. DRUGS ASSOCIATED WITH IMPOTENCE

Antihypertensive agents
Thiazide diuretics
Guanadrel
Clonidine
Methyldopa
Propranolol
Angiotensin-converting enzyme inhibitors
Calcium channel blockers
Hydralazine
H_2 receptor antagonists
Cimetidine
Ranitidine
Antipsychotic agents
Tricyclic antidepressants
Central nervous system depressants
Anticancer drugs

Iatrogenic impotence is usually the result of urologic or vascular surgery. Developmental causes, including hypospadias, are rare. Except for diabetes mellitus, *endocrinologic* causes are also unusual; they include such states as eunuchoidism, hypopituitarism, hypothyroidism, Cushing's syndrome, and prolactin disorders. It has been postulated that sexual dysfunction secondary to circulatory impairment might, at least in part, be due to decreased production of testosterone secondary to testicular hypoperfusion.[12] Traumatic sexual dysfunction usually follows spinal or pelvic trauma and is mostly neurogenic in nature.

Although a detailed discussion of the etiology, diagnosis, and management of sexual dysfunction (specifically vasculogenic impotence) is beyond the scope of this chapter, a knowledge of causes other than iatrogenic ones is important for the vascular surgeon in both the preoperative and the postoperative evaluation of men with sexual dysfunction. Documentation of the presence and cause of sexual dysfunction before elective aortoiliac revascularization is obviously important for medicolegal reasons and for informing the patient about the possibilities for postoperative improvement.

DIAGNOSIS OF SEXUAL DYSFUNCTION

The etiology of impotence can often be determined solely by the patient's history and physical examination. Recent psychological trauma or marital problems may be associated with the onset of impotence. A careful medication history may detect the use of agents associated with sexual dysfunction. Developmental and traumatic problems should be easily discovered. Known endocrine pathology may be associated with impotence. A history of the onset of impotence after surgery should be sought.

Of primary importance in the diagnosis of sexual dysfunction is differentiating *psychogenic* from *organic* causes. Organic impotence is nonsituational. Psychogenic impotence may be intermittent, partner-specific, and absent during masturbation. Psychologic impotence can probably best be differentiated from organic impotence through the use of nocturnal penile tumescence studies. All males from 3 to 79 years of age have nocturnal penile tumescence during normal sleep, with the amount being a function of age.[48] Nocturnal penile tumescence monitoring during sleep has been shown to be approximately 80% accurate in differentiating psychogenic from organic impotence.[12]

If organic impotence is suspected based on the history, physical examination findings, and results of nocturnal penile tumescence studies, penile blood pressure measurement and penile duplex ultrasonography with penile papaverine injection are reliable diagnostic tests for detecting the presence of vasculogenic impotence. If this testing indicates that arterial inflow obstruction is probably present, arteriography with selective pelvic catheterization is indicated as a guide to the type of therapy that should be considered.

If the results of vascular studies are normal and if developmental, traumatic, surgical, and pharmacologic causes have been ruled out, neurogenic or endocrinologic causes are most likely. Neurogenic impotence may be associated with an absent bulbocavernosus reflex, abnormal findings on perineal electromyographic studies, and abnormal cystometrographic findings. These abnormal study results are often seen in diabetic patients with sexual dysfunction. The diagnosis of endocrine dysfunction is usually made through the measurement of hormone levels.

PREVENTION

Analysis of the major surgical series addressing sexual function changes associated with aortoiliac revascularization indicates that approximately 25% of patients are impotent preoperatively.[5, 9, 17, 18, 29, 31, 35, 43, 46, 49] Postoperatively, about 25% of such patients regain normal sexual function, and 25% of patients with normal preoperative sexual function experience impotence after surgery.[10] Both erectile dysfunction and ejaculatory dysfunction can follow aortoiliac revascularization, and collected surgical series published before 1975 demonstrated an average 43% incidence of postoperative retrograde ejaculation.[10] The authors of these studies postulated that postoperative sexual dysfunction was secondary to reduced pelvic blood supply, and they demonstrated that injury to the para-aortic and hypogastric nerve plexuses could cause both impotence and retrograde ejaculation. The association between postoperative impotence and postoperative decreases in penile perfusion pressure has now been well documented.[41] Thus, prevention of iatrogenically induced sexual dysfunction after aortoiliac revascularization requires preservation of pelvic circulation and avoidance of injury to the para-aortic and hypogastric autonomic nerve plexuses.

Preservation of pelvic blood flow requires careful evaluation of arteriographic findings and consideration of the type of proximal aortic anastomosis. End-to-side anastomoses do not divert pelvic blood flow but may not be desirable for other reasons. End-to-side aortic anastomoses may carry a greater risk of atheroembolization, may preclude routine retroperitoneal coverage of the graft, and may create a competitive flow situation with the native iliac arteries. It has been suggested that end-to-side anastomoses may have a lower patency rate than end-to-end anastomoses.[39] When end-to-end anastomoses are used, pelvic flow may be diverted if there is not adequate retrograde flow up the external iliac arteries postoperatively. Examples of disease distributions that probably should not be treated with end-to-end anastomoses are shown in Figure 52–2. The requirement for retrograde external iliac artery flow is probably important even if there is occlusion of the hypogastric arteries.

Bilateral hypogastric occlusion or ligation is thought to be associated with a high risk of pelvic ischemia. Although it is commonly believed that hypogastric flow is necessary for normal sexual function, several studies have indicated that this may not always be the case. Kawai showed that branches of the femoral artery may provide significant collateral circulation to the penis in the face of hypogastric artery occlusion.[23] Iliopoulos and associates showed that hypogastric collateral flow in the presence of acute hypogastric artery ligation is more dependent on the ipsilateral external iliac artery than it is on the contralateral hypogastric artery, although in the chronic state lush collateralization between the left and the right internal iliac arteries is common (Fig. 52–3).[19]

Ohshiro and Kosaki suggested that preservation of the hypogastric nerve plexus is more important than preservation of hypogastric blood flow and showed that little correlation exists between postoperative sexual dysfunction and hypogastric circulation.[37] Of 26 patients with bilateral hypogastric atherosclerotic occlusion or bilateral hypogastric artery ligation at the time of surgery who were studied by Flanigan and coworkers, 17 had normal sexual function postoperatively.[9] Although hypogastric artery patency may not be necessary for normal sexual function in all patients, in many patients it is necessary[41] not only for sexual function but also for preventing colon or buttock ischemia.[20]

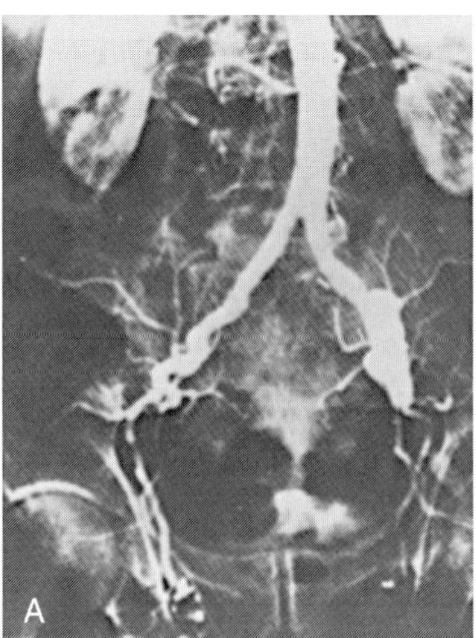

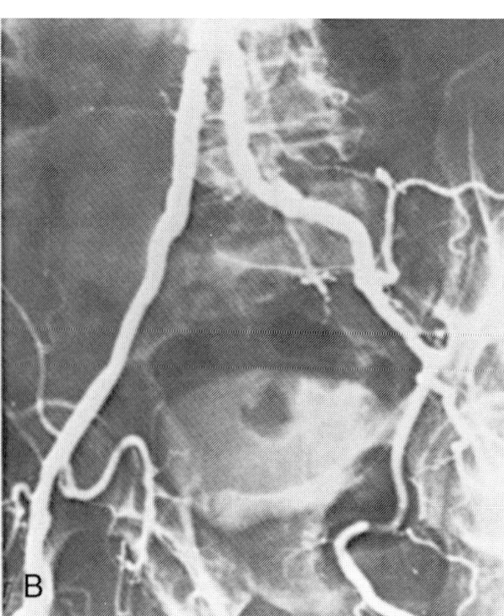

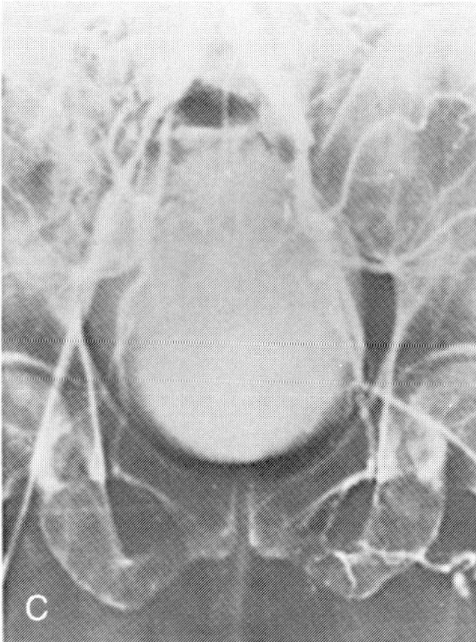

FIGURE 52–2. Examples of disease distribution in which end-to-end aortic anastomoses should be avoided if possible. *A*, Bilateral external iliac artery occlusion. *B*, Unilateral external iliac artery occlusion and contralateral internal iliac artery occlusion. *C*, Unilateral external iliac artery occlusion and contralateral external iliac artery stenosis. (*A–C*, From Flanigan DP, Schuler JJ, Keifer T, et al. Elimination of iatrogenic impotence and improvement of sexual dysfunction after aortoiliac revascularization. Arch Surg 117:544, 1982. Copyright 1982, American Medical Association.)

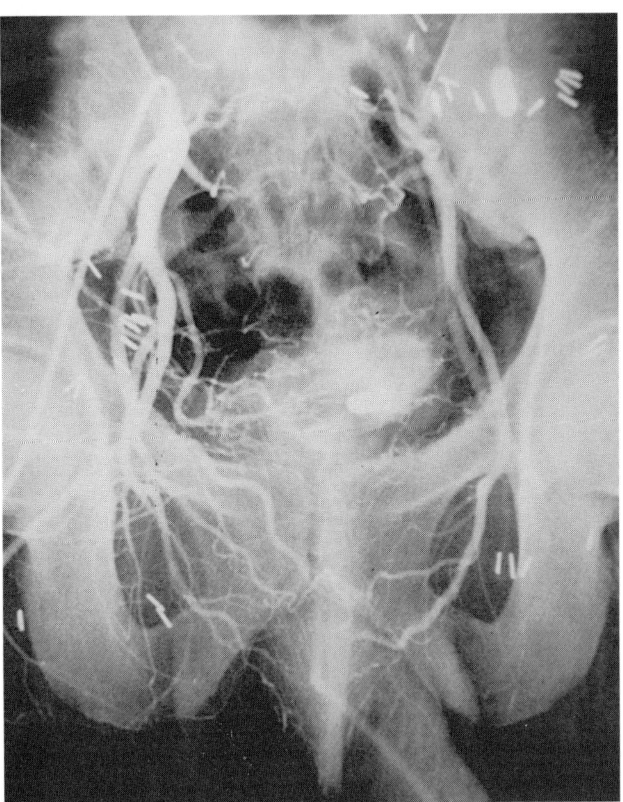

FIGURE 52–3. Selective right internal iliac artery arteriogram demonstrating lush pelvic collaterals filling the contralateral left internal iliac artery circulatory bed. (From Flanigan DP, Schuler JJ: Sexual function and aortic surgery. *In* Bergan JJ, Yao JST [eds]: Aortic Surgery. Philadelphia, WB Saunders, 1989, pp 547–560.)

The important role of the hypogastric circulation in sexual function is further supported by evidence of improved sexual function after internal iliac artery revascularization. Flanigan and associates demonstrated that revascularization of the internal iliac artery at the time of aortoiliac revascularization reversed vasculogenic impotence in five of five men.[11] Subsequently, Gossetti and colleagues studied 148 patients with vasculogenic impotence who were undergoing aortoiliac revascularization and found that 14 of 18 patients (77%) who had had concomitant hypogastric revascularization had normal postoperative sexual function.[15]

Caution dictates that at least unilateral hypogastric flow be maintained whenever possible during aortoiliac revascularization. Nevertheless, bilateral hypogastric artery ligation or exclusion may be unavoidable in some patients. No clear criteria have emerged that indicate the need for direct hypogastric revascularization in such patients. Iwai and coworkers used transanal Doppler monitoring as a guide, but more experience is needed to establish clear guidelines for revascularization.[21] When there is uncertainty regarding the adequacy of pelvic circulation, hypogastric revascularization should probably be performed. This may take the form of internal iliac endarterectomy, side-to-side anastomosis between a bifurcation graft limb and an iliac vessel, or a graft between a bifurcation graft limb and a hypogastric artery.[4, 9, 15]

The incidence of iatrogenic neurogenic sexual dysfunction is lessened through nerve-sparing dissections of the aortoiliac segment. This is best achieved with a right lateral aortic approach just below the renal arteries (Fig. 52–4). Tissues over the anterior aorta are reflected rather than transected. Tunnels are created posterior to the ureters and superior hypogastric plexus. When iliac anastomoses are required, dissection over the iliac arteries is carried out in the longitudinal plane, with the surgeon taking meticulous care not to transect the autonomic nerves. The wall of aortic aneurysms should not be resected, and inferior mesenteric artery control should be achieved from within the aneurysm cavity. When iliac aneurysms are present, graft limbs can often be tunneled through the iliac aneurysm to avoid dissection and incision of the iliac aneurysm, thereby avoiding damage to the overlying autonomic plexus (Fig. 52–5).

Another approach for avoiding iatrogenic impotence is the use of revascularization procedures that do not require dissection of the aortoiliac segment. Endovascular grafts, axillofemoral bypass, femorofemoral bypass, and aortoiliac transluminal balloon angioplasty all achieve this purpose. In addition, as with aortoiliofemoral bypass, these procedures can reverse vasculogenic impotence in selected patients.[1, 3, 7, 9, 34, 42, 44] It is important to inform prospective candidates for aortoiliac revascularization of the risk of iatrogenic sexual dysfunction and of the availability of alternative methods of revascularization that essentially eliminate this risk but may provide a less durable revascularization.

Flanigan and coworkers demonstrated that when careful operative planning is undertaken to avoid diversion of

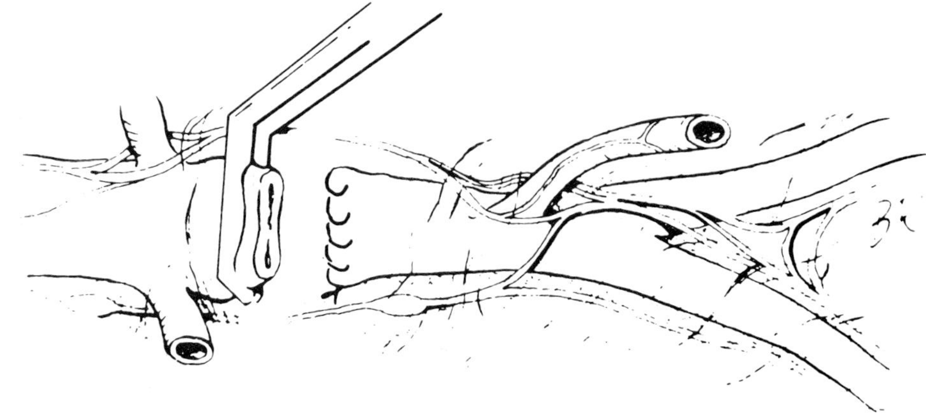

FIGURE 52–4. Suggested approach to aortic dissection and clamping: a right lateral approach to the aorta just below the renal arteries lessens possible injury to the para-aortic and superior hypogastric plexuses. (From DePalma RG, Levine SB, Feldman S: Preservation of erectile function after aorto-iliac reconstruction. Arch Surg 113:958, 1978. Copyright 1978, American Medical Association.)

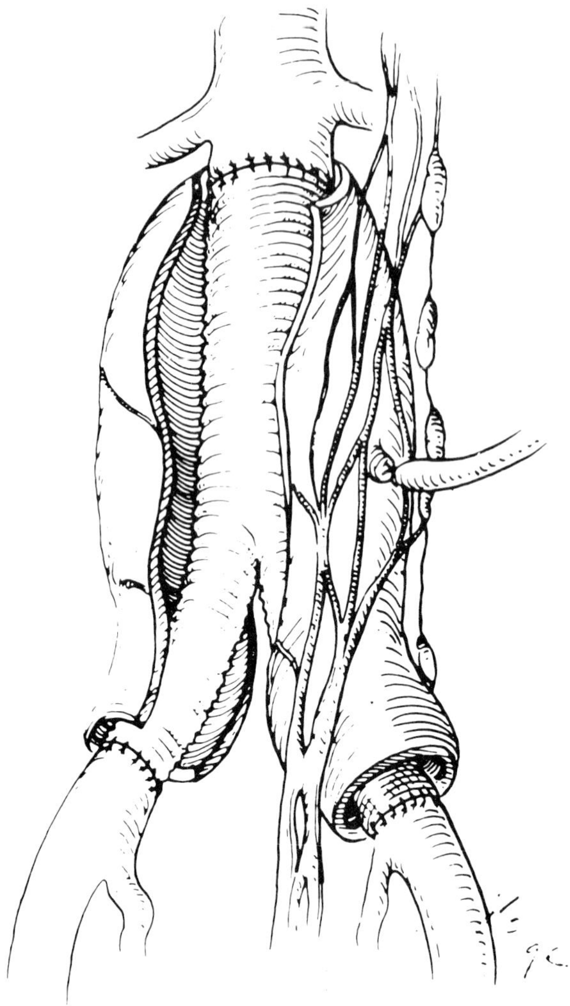

FIGURE 52–5. Bifurcation graft limbs may often be tunneled through iliac aneurysms, thus avoiding transection of the overlying hypogastric nerve plexus. (From Weinstein MH, Machleder HI: Sexual function after aortoiliac surgery. Ann Surg 181:787, 1975.)

pelvic blood flow, nerve-sparing aortoiliac dissections are carried out, and indirect methods of aortoiliac revascularization are selectively employed, iatrogenic impotence can be eliminated and many patients can regain normal sexual function postoperatively.[9] In a series of 110 patients undergoing direct and indirect aortoiliac revascularization, 45% of patients with preoperative vasculogenic impotence regained normal sexual function postoperatively, no patients with normal preoperative sexual function were rendered impotent, and only two patients developed retrograde ejaculation.[9] Despite the use of these techniques, however, patients requiring iliac dissections and those with ruptured aneurysms remain susceptible to iatrogenic sexual dysfunction, especially retrograde ejaculation secondary to nerve injury.

TREATMENT

The treatment of postoperative sexual dysfunction depends on an accurate assessment of the etiologic factors. This fact emphasizes the need for a careful preoperative assessment of the cause of sexual dysfunction in patients being considered for aortoiliac revascularization. Before treatment of postoperative impotence, a complete diagnostic evaluation may be required, as described earlier, especially if no preoperative workup was performed. If sexual dysfunction is determined to be iatrogenic, it is due to either reduced pelvic blood flow and penile ischemia or to nerve injury.

Penile ischemia can sometimes be corrected by penile revascularization. This may take the form of angioplasty, endarterectomy, or bypass to the hypogastric vessels. Direct penile revascularization has also been attempted, with mixed results.[6] Currently, direct revascularization of the penis is accomplished by inferior epigastric artery anastomosis to the dorsal penile[14] or cavernosal[33] arteries. Alternatively, a vein graft can be used.[26] Good results have been reported in 31% to 80% of patients.[6, 14, 45] Older men with diffuse atherosclerosis have poorer results, and vein grafts in some cases may provide excess flow, resulting in priapism.[5]

Treatment of neurogenic impotence requires the placement of a penile prosthesis. This may also be useful in patients with vasculogenic impotence in whom revascularization is not possible or is unsuccessful. Several models of penile prostheses are available.[25] Approximately 90% of patients with a penile prosthesis report satisfactory results.[16, 30] Infection rates vary from 1% to 9% and reoperation because of mechanical failure is necessary in 14% to 44% of patients.[2, 13, 22, 24, 47]

Vacuum constriction devices suck blood into the penis, causing tumescence, and maintain erection through constriction of the venous outflow at the base of the penis.[51] With these devices, patients may have ejaculatory restriction (12%), initial pain (41%),[52] and penile ecchymosis or petechiae (10% to 27%), although satisfactory use is generally achieved.[36]

The best approach to the problem of iatrogenic sexual dysfunction is prevention through the use of appropriate preoperative evaluation, the use of nerve-sparing aortoiliac dissections or indirect methods of aortoiliac revascularization, and intraoperative attention to the maintenance of pelvic blood flow through the use of proper graft configurations and selective hypogastric revascularization.

REFERENCES

1. Blaisdell FW, Hall AD: Axillary-femoral artery bypass for lower extremity ischemia. Surgery 54:563, 1963.
2. Carson CC: Infections in genitourinary prostheses. Urol Clin North Am 16:139, 1989.
3. Castaneda-Zuniga WR, Smith A, Kaye K, et al: Transluminal angioplasty for treatment of vasculogenic impotence. AJR 139:371, 1982.
4. Cronenwett JL, Gooch JB, Garrett HE: Internal iliac artery revascularization during aortofemoral bypass. Arch Surg 117:838, 1982.
5. DePalma RG, Levine SB, Feldman S: Preservation of erectile function after aorto-iliac reconstruction. Arch Surg 113:958, 1978.
6. DePalma RG, Olding M, Yu GW, et al: Vascular interventions for impotence: Lessons learned. J Vasc Surg 21:576, 1995.
7. Dewar ML, Blundell PE, Lidstone, et al: Effects of abdominal aneurysmectomy, aortoiliac bypass grafting and angioplasty on male sexual potency: A prospective study. Can J Surg 28:154, 1985.
8. Ebbehoj J, Wagner G. Abnormal drainage of the corpora cavernosa causing erectile dysfunction. *In* Zorgniotti AW, Rossi G (eds): Vasculogenic Impotence. Springfield, Ill, Charles C Thomas, 1980, p 309.

9. Flanigan DP, Schuler JJ, Keifer T, et al: Elimination of iatrogenic impotence and improvement of sexual dysfunction after aortoiliac revascularization. Arch Surg 117:544, 1982.
10. Flanigan DP, Schuler JJ: Sexual function and aortic surgery. *In* Bergan JJ, Yao JST (eds): Aortic Surgery. Philadelphia, WB Saunders, 1989, pp 547–560.
11. Flanigan DP, Sobinsky KR, Schuler JJ, et al: Internal iliac artery revascularization in the treatment of vasculogenic impotence. Arch Surg 120:271, 1985.
12. Foresta C, Ruzza G, Mioni R, et al: Male hypogonadism in aorto-iliac arteriopathies. Arch Androl 9:297, 1982.
13. Furlow WL, Goldwasser B, Gundian JC: Implantation of model AMS 700 penile prosthesis: Long term results. J Urol 139:741, 1988.
14. Goldstein I: Overview of types and results of vascular surgical procedures for impotence. Cardiovasc Intervent Radiol 11:240, 1988.
15. Gossetti B, Gattuso R, Irace L, et al: Aorto-iliac/femoral reconstructions in patients with vasculogenic impotence. Eur J Vasc Surg 5:425, 1991.
16. Gregory GJ, Purcell MH: Scott's inflatable penile prosthesis: Evaluation of mechanical survival in the series 700 model. J Urol 137:676, 1987.
17. Hallbrook T, Holmquist B: Sexual disturbances following dissection of the aorta and the common iliac arteries. J Cardiovasc Surg 11:255, 1970.
18. Harris JD, Jepson RP: Aorto-iliac stenosis: A comparison of two procedures. Aust J Surg 34:211, 1965.
19. Iliopoulos JI, Hermreck AS, Thomas JH, et al: Hemodynamics of the hypogastric arterial circulation. J Vasc Surg 9:637, 1989.
20. Iliopoulos JI, Horwanitz PE, Pierce GE, et al: The critical hypogastric circulation. Am J Surg 154:671, 1987.
21. Iwai T, Sakurazawa K, Sato S, et al: Intra-operative monitoring of the pelvic circulation using a transanal Doppler probe. Eur J Vasc Surg 5:71, 1991.
22. Kaufman JJ, Linder A, Raz S: Complications of penile prothesis surgery for impotence. J Urol 128:1192, 1982.
23. Kawai M: Pelvic hemodynamics before and after aortoiliac vascular reconstruction: The significance of penile blood pressure. Jpn J Surg 18:514, 1988.
24. Kessler R: Surgical experience with the inflatable penile prosthesis. J Urol 124:611, 1980.
25. Krane RJ, Goldstein I, De Tejada IS: Impotence. N Engl J Med 321:1648, 1989.
26. Krotovsky GS, Turpitko SA, Gerasimov VB, et al: Surgical treatment and prevention of vasculopathic impotence in conjunction with revascularization of the lower extremities in Leriche's syndrome. J Cardiovasc Surg (Torino) 32:340, 1991.
27. Leriche R: Des obliterations arterielles hautes (obliteration de la terminaison de l'aorte) comme causes des insuffisances circulatoires des members inferieurs. Bull Mem Soc Chir 49:1404, 1923.
28. Leriche R, Morel A: The syndrome of thrombotic obliteration of the aortic bifurcation. Ann Surg 127:193, 1948.
29. Magee TR, Scott DJ, Dunkly A, et al: Quality of life following surgery for abdominal aortic aneurysm. Br J Surg 79:1014, 1992.
30. Malloy TR, Wein AJ, Carpeniello VL: Reliability of AMS M700 inflatable penile prosthesis. Urology 28:385, 1986.
31. May AG, DeWeese JA, Rob CG: Changes in sexual function following operation on the abdominal aorta. Surgery 65:41, 1969.
32. McCulloch DK, Campbell IW, Wu FC, et al: The prevalence of diabetic impotence. Diabetologia 18:279, 1980.
33. McDougal WS, Jeffery RF: Microscopic penile revascularization. J Urol 129:517, 1983.
34. Merchant RF, DePalma RG: Effects of femorofemoral grafts on postoperative sexual function: Correlation with penile pulse volume recordings. Surgery 90:962, 1981.
35. Miles JR, Miles DG: Aortoiliac operations and sexual dysfunction. Arch Surg 117:1177, 1982.
36. Nadig PW, Ware JC, Blumoff R: Noninvasive device to produce and maintain an erection-like state. J Urol 27:126, 1986.
37. Ohshiro T, Kosaki G: Sexual function after aorto-iliac vascular reconstruction. Which is more important, the internal iliac artery or hypogastric nerve? J Cardiovasc Surg (Torino) 25:47, 1984.
38. Pick J: Anatomy of the Autonomic Nervous System. Philadelphia, JB Lippincott, 1979, pp 439–441.
39. Pierce GE, Turrentine M, Stringfield S, et al: Evaluation of end-to-side v end-to-end proximal anastomosis in aortobifemoral bypass. Arch Surg 117:1580, 1982.
40. Queral LA, Flinn WR, Bergan JJ, et al: Sexual function and aortic surgery. *In* Bergan JJ, Yao JST (eds): Surgery of the Aorta and Its Body Branches. New York, Grune & Stratton, 1979, pp 263–276.
41. Queral LA, Whitehouse WM, Flinn WR, et al: Pelvic hemodynamics after aortoillac reconstruction. Surgery 86:799, 1979.
42. Ravimandalam K, Rao VR, Kumar S, et al: Obstruction of the infrarenal portion of the abdominal aorta: Results of treatment with balloon angioplasty. AJR Am J Roentgenol 156:1257, 1991.
43. Sabri S, Cotton LT: Sexual function following aortoiliac reconstruction. Lancet 2:1218, 1971.
44. Schuler JJ, Gray B, Flanigan DP, et al: Increased penile perfusion and reversal of vasculogenic impotence following femorofemoral bypass. Br J Surg 69(Suppl):S6, 1982.
45. Sharlip ID: Treatment of iatrogenic impotence by penile revascularization. *In* Proceedings of the Sixth Biennial International Symposium for Corpus Cavernosum Revascularization and Third Biennial World Meeting on Impotence. Boston, October 6, 1988, p 135.
46. Spiro M, Cotton LT: Aorto-iliac thrombo-endarterectomy. Br J Surg 57:161, 1979.
47. Thomalla JV, Thompson ST, Rowland RG, et al: Infectious complications of penile prosthetic implants. J Urol 138:65, 1987.
48. Wasserman MD, Pollak CP, Spielman AJ, et al: The differential diagnosis of impotence. JAMA 243:2038, 1980.
49. Weinstein MH, Machleder HI: Sexual function after aortoiliac surgery. Ann Surg 181:787, 1975.
50. Whitelaw GP, Smithwick RH: Some secondary effects of sympathectomy. N Engl J Med 245:121, 1951.
51. Witherington R: Vacuum constriction device for management of erectile impotence. J Urol 141:320, 1989.
52. Witherington R: Suction device therapy in the management of erectile impotence. Urol Clin North Am 15:123, 1988.

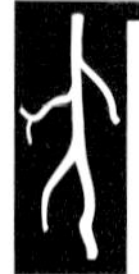

CHAPTER 53

Angiography and Percutaneous Vascular Interventions: Complications and Quality Improvement

David Sacks, M.D.

With choice comes responsibility. There is a wide array of choices in vascular diagnosis and therapy, not only in terms of which modality to use but also who will use it. Vascular diagnoses can be made noninvasively with physical examination segmental pressures, duplex ultrasonography, and magnetic resonance angiography (MRA) or invasively with angiography. Therapy can be "minimally invasive" with percutaneous endovascular techniques of balloon (percutaneous transluminal angioplasty [PTA]) or laser angioplasty, atherectomy, stenting (covered or bare), or thrombolysis or invasive using open surgical techniques of endarterectomy, thrombectomy, patch angioplasty, and bypass.

It is the responsibility of physicians to choose and perform those procedures best suited to the needs of the patients. How one chooses is based on published results and the results achievable locally.[58] It is therefore the responsibility of each institution to maximize successful results and minimize failures and complications regardless of which physician or specialty performs vascular procedures.

This chapter describes definitions and standards for documenting and improving outcomes in endovascular procedures, specifically diagnostic peripheral and neuroangiography, peripheral angioplasty, stents, and thrombolysis. These standards serve as a quality benchmark for the performance of endovascular procedures.

DEFINITIONS OF OUTCOMES

The outcomes of interest in assessing the quality of vascular procedures are success, failure, and complications. These outcomes need to be clearly defined to be useful. Some of the definitions are obvious, such as a successful diagnostic procedure provides sufficient information on which to make a therapeutic decision. Some definitions are more ambiguous, as will be seen with complications.

Success

The definitions of success for therapeutic procedures also depend on a definition of whether a therapeutic procedure has been attempted. For example, if a patient is evaluated for treatment of a femoropopliteal bypass graft occlusion, is it a failure of therapy if the origin of the graft cannot be catheterized? Or if the graft can be catheterized but is found to be sclerotic and thrombosed and one chooses not to start lytic therapy? Or if the graft is found to be sclerotic and thrombosed but is treated anyway with the inability to lyse the clot? When does a lytic procedure start—with attempts to catheterize an occlusion or with the institution of drug infusion?

These questions are not irritating legalisms. If one physician is routinely able to cross an occlusion and another is not, unless one is able to document this result as a success or failure, there is no way to distinguish good and bad outcomes and greater and lesser skilled practitioners.

The Society of Cardiovascular and Interventional Radiology (SCVIR) has a committee assigned to create uniform definitions of success and complications. The committee is creating these standards through the use of examples such as those mentioned. A procedure is defined to have begun with the intention to treat. This includes attempts at passing a wire or catheter across a stenosis or occlusion. Failure to cross the diseased segment is considered a failure of that therapeutic modality (e.g., lysis, PTA, or stent). The "guide wire traversal test" is not considered a diagnostic test; however, if the physician changes therapy based on additional anatomic information (such as deciding not to try lysis when a vein graft is demonstrated to be diffusely sclerotic after being selectively catheterized), this is not considered a failure of the initial therapy. It is understood that there can be different interpretations of these examples. What is important is that definitions be clear and uniformly applied so that outcomes can be equally clearly reported and compared.

Diagnostic Peripheral Angiography

Peripheral angiography should provide a complete and adequate evaluation of the clinical problem, be appropriately and permanently recorded, and be judged diagnostic by others with skill in interpreting angiograms. The angiogram should be followed by a report summarizing the findings, technical aspects, and any immediate complications. The study should be completed in a single sitting.[139] For atherosclerotic occlusive disease, the study should fully characterize the extent of vascular disease that might contribute to the symptomatology.[117] This includes an evaluation of circulation distal to any occlusion, usually requiring imaging to the ankle or foot.

Diagnostic Neuroangiography

Neuroangiography should be sufficient to establish or exclude pathology of the extracranial and intracranial circulation.[26] Unless severe occlusive disease prohibits safe selective catheterization, a selective study is necessary to achieve this goal. The study should be completed in a single sitting. This definition of success states that evaluation of the carotid bifurcation alone is an incomplete diagnostic neuroangiogram. This may strike some as unreasonable if the area of clinical interest is an extracranial carotid stenosis. The rationale for assessing the distal circulation is that it allows detection of significant intracranial vascular pathology that would alter therapy of a carotid bifurcation lesion.[159] This is analogous to evaluating the runoff in the leg distal to an occlusive lesion.

Peripheral Balloon Angioplasty and Stents

This involves a more complex series of definitions dealing with technical, hemodynamic, anatomic, and clinical factors, as well as short-term, intermediate, and long-term results. The need for standardized outcome definitions in these procedures has been eloquently addressed by Porter.[120] Many of the definitions have been borrowed from those used for surgical revascularization procedures,[127] but some have been tailored for endovascular therapy. An attempt has been made to unify and standardize the following definitions for endovascular procedures[128]:

Anatomic success: Less than 30% diameter final residual lumen stenosis measured at the narrowest point of the vascular lumen. In the presence of an angiographically visible dissection at the angioplasty site, the residual lumen is measured from the widest opacified lumen regardless of cracks. This definition is chosen because a residual stenosis of more than 30% has been reported to predispose patients to restenosis,[22] but it is acknowledged that the ability to measure this accurately on postangioplasty angiograms is poor.[155] There are no standards for anatomic success using other imaging modalities such as intravascular ultrasound, MRA, angioscopy, or computed tomographic (CT) angiography. The results with duplex ultrasonography have been controversial.[99, 130]

Hemodynamic success: The ankle-brachial index should be improved by 0.1 or greater above the baseline value and not be deteriorated by more than 0.15 from the maximum early postprocedural level. For patients with noncompressible vessels, the pulse volume recording distal to the treated site should be maintained at 5 mm above the pretreatment tracing. Direct intravascular pressures across the treated site have also been advocated as a measure of success and are widely used clinically to determine the need for a vascular stent following angioplasty. Thresholds of 5 mmHg mean, 10 mmHg mean, 10 mmHg peak, 10% of systemic blood pressure, and others have been proposed,[5, 19, 132, 155] but there is no consensus as to the most appropriate standard to define a successful result.

Clinical success: The Rutherford criteria for acute or chronic limb ischemia must be improved by at least one category immediately after the intervention and be sustained during follow-up by at least one category above the pretreatment clinical level (Tables 53–1 and 53–2).[127] Patients with tissue loss must improve by at least two categories and reach the level of claudication to be considered improved.

Technical success: Meets the criteria for both anatomic and hemodynamic success in the immediate postprocedural period.

Improvement: Meets the combined definitions of hemodynamic and clinical success, as categorized by Rutherford (Table 53–3).[127] Improvement may depend on the results of combined endovascular and surgical procedures. In this case, the standard is to consider the success of either procedure to be determined by the success of the combined revascularization procedures.[127]

Patency: Continued flow through the treated segment. This definition is more useful in the evaluation of bypass grafts rather than angioplasty or stents, where the presence of recurrent stenosis is of greater interest than simply the presence of continued flow.

Thrombolysis

Thrombolysis also involves multiple definitions. At one extreme, a thrombolytic procedure may be successful without restoring antegrade flow if the additional anatomic information provided following clot lysis allows a better or more limited surgical revascularization to be performed. At the other extreme, lysis is successful when there is restoration of antegrade flow with no need for surgery and the limb is returned to its preocclusion clinical status. The following definitions of levels of success are intended to be

TABLE 53–1. CLINICAL CATEGORIES OF ACUTE LIMB ISCHEMIA

CATEGORY	DESCRIPTION/ PROGNOSIS	SENSORY LOSS	MUSCLE WEAKNESS	DOPPLER SIGNALS	
				Arterial	Venous
1. Viable	Not immediately threatened	None	None	Audible	Audible
2. Threatened					
a. Marginally	Salvageable if promptly treated	Minimal (toes) or none	None	Inaudible	Audible
b. Immediately	Salvageable with immediate revascularization	More than toes, associated with rest pain	Mild, moderate	Inaudible	Audible
3. Irreversible	Major tissue loss or permanent nerve damage inevitable	Profound, anesthetic	Profound, paralysis (rigor)	Inaudible	Inaudible

Modified from Rutherford RB, Baker JD, Ernst C, et al: Recommended standards for reports dealing with lower extremity ischemia: Revised version. J Vasc Surg 26:517–538, 1997.

TABLE 53–2. CLINICAL CATEGORIES OF CHRONIC LIMB ISCHEMIA

GRADE	CATEGORY	CLINICAL DESCRIPTION	OBJECTIVE CRITERIA
0	0	Asymptomatic: no hemodynamically significant occlusive disease	Normal treadmill or reactive hyperemia test
I	1	Mild claudication	Completes treadmill exercise (5 min at 2 mph on 12% incline); post-exercise ankle pressure >50 mmHg but at least 20 mmHg < resting value
	2	Moderate claudication	Between categories 1 and 3
	3	Severe claudication	Cannot complete standard treadmill exercise and post-exercise ankle pressure <50 mmHg
II	4	Ischemic rest pain	Resting ankle pressure <40 mmHg; flat or barely pulsatile ankle or metatarsal plethysmogram (PVR); toe pressure <30 mmHg
III	5	Minor tissue loss: nonhealing ulcer; focal gangrene with diffuse pedal ischemia	Resting ankle pressure <60 mmHg; ankle or metatarsal PVR flat or barely pulsatile; toe pressure <40 mmHg
	6	Major tissue loss: extending above transmetatarsal level; functional foot no longer salvageable	Same as category 5

From Rutherford RB, Baker JD, Ernst C, et al: Recommended standards for reports dealing with lower extremity ischemia: Revised version. J Vasc Surg 26:517–538, 1997.
PVR = pulse volume recording.

applicable to both pharmacologic and mechanical methods of clot lysis.[115]

Technical or lytic success: Complete or near complete lysis (95% by volume) of the thrombus.

Clinical success: Improvement or resolution of the presenting symptoms in the immediate postprocedural period. Because the clinical success of lytic therapy often depends on the success of subsequent adjunctive therapy it is important to assess the effect of lysis on the type of subsequent revascularization or level of amputation.[111] Table 53–4 provides definitions of the clinical success of lytic treatment.

TABLE 53–3. RECOMMENDED SCALE FOR GAUGING CHANGES IN CLINICAL STATUS FOR CHRONIC LIMB ISCHEMIA*

GRADE	DESCRIPTION
+3	*Markedly improved:* no ischemic symptoms; any foot lesions completely healed; ABI > 0.9
+2	*Moderately improved:* no open foot lesions; still symptomatic but only with exercise and improved by at least one category; ABI not normalized but increased by >0.10
+1	*Minimally improved:* >0.10 increase in ABI but no categorical improvement or vice versa (i.e., upward categorical shift without an increase in ABI of >0.10)
0	*No change:* no categorical shift and <0.10 change in ABI
−1	*Mildly worse:* no categorical shift but ABI decrease >0.10, or downward categorical shift with ABI decrease <0.10
−2	*Moderately worse:* one category worse or unexpected minor amputation
−3	*Markedly worse:* more than one category worse or unexpected major amputations

From Rutherford RB, Baker JD, Ernst C, et al: Recommended standards for reports dealing with lower extremity ischemia: Revised version. J Vasc Surg 26:517–538, 1997.
*Categories refer to chronic limb ischemia (see Table 53–2).
ABI = ankle-brachial index.

Complications

Complications are even more difficult to define and standardize than success. One possible definition of a complication is an unexpected event related to a procedure that harms a patient. Does harm have to produce symptoms or

TABLE 53–4. CLINICAL SUCCESS OF LYSIS*

−1: Ischemia is worse (by at least one major or minor category from Table 53–1) following lysis (failure, possibly with complication). Subsequent surgical revascularization may be necessary at the same or greater level†

0: No change following lysis (failure). Subsequent surgical revascularization may be necessary at the same level. Endovascular revascularization is not possible.

1: Ischemia is improved
- a. Revascularization with lysis alone
  - 1. Amputation necessary but at a lesser level
- b. Adjunctive surgical revascularization necessary but at a lesser level†
  - 1. Amputation necessary but at a lesser level‡
- c. Adjunctive endovascular revascularization necessary (PTA, stent, atherectomy, mechanical thrombectomy)
  - 1. Amputation necessary but at a lesser level

From Patel N, Technology Assessment Committee of the SCVIR: Reporting standards for thrombolytic therapy for lower extremity arterial and graft occlusions. J Vasc Interv Radiol (in press).
*Lysis includes both pharmacologic and mechanical techniques of treating thrombus. The categories a, b, and c do not imply greater or lesser degrees of success.
†Levels of surgical revascularization:
(1) *major:* insertion of new bypass graft; replacement of an existing bypass graft; excision or repair of an aneurysm.
(2) *moderate:* graft revision, patch angioplasty; endarterectomy; profundaplasty.
(3) *minor:* thrombectomy/embolectomy; fasciotomy.
‡Levels of amputation: (1) above the knee; (2) below the knee; (3) transmetatarsal; (4) toe.
PTA = percutaneous transluminal angioplasty.

signs, such as abdominal pain or decreased walking distance, or is a laboratory abnormality sufficient, such as an elevated creatinine level? If the patient is placed at significant risk of harm by an unexpected event but is not harmed, does this qualify as a complication? If the patient suffers no harm but the cost of the procedure increases as a result of an unexpected event, is this a complication? These questions can be illustrated by the following examples.

EXAMPLE 1:

A common iliac artery stenosis is treated with balloon dilation. Because of an angioplasty-induced dissection there is a residual pressure gradient, which is successfully treated with a stent. Is this a failure of angioplasty or a complication?

EXAMPLE 2:

A common iliac artery stenosis is treated with a stent. An iatrogenic dissection extends beyond the stent and compromises flow. It is successfully treated with a second adjacent stent. The patient has suffered no harm but might be at increased risk for thrombosis or intimal hyperplasia as a result of having a greater length of metal in the vessel. There is an increased cost of the second stent and possibly a second balloon. One series has defined this scenario as a complication,[7, 8] whereas others consider the lack of measurable morbidity to preclude this from being called a complication.[104]

EXAMPLE 3:

A balloon ruptures as a stent is being placed in a renal artery. During attempts to extract the ruptured balloon, the stent migrates back into the aorta and is deployed in the iliac artery. The final stent placement in the renal artery is successful. The patient has suffered no morbidity, but again there is increased expense and a nontarget vessel has been treated with a stent with the theoretical risks of intimal hyperplasia and thrombosis. Is this a complication or merely a challenging case?

EXAMPLE 4:

During an iliac artery angioplasty, a clot embolizes to the ipsilateral common femoral artery. This is successfully treated with a 30-minute infusion of urokinase from the same catheterization. There is the increased cost of the drug plus the increased risk of bleeding either locally or systemically. No bleeding occurred, and there was no morbidity. Is this a complication or a challenging case?

EXAMPLE 5:

During a urokinase infusion into an occluded femorolpopliteal graft, embolization of a clot occurs into the popliteal trifurcation. The patient's symptoms of ischemia worsen. The embolus is successfully treated by placing an infusion wire coaxially into the clot through an infusion catheter. By the time the graft clears, the trifurcation is clear as well. Is this a complication or a frequently expected event from the therapy that required additional treatment?

Similar to the issues faced in the definitions of success, the standards used for defining complications may seem arbitrary and controversial, but they attempt to bring uniformity to reporting for valid comparisons and the ability to improve quality. It is felt that unexpected events that either harm the patient or place the patient at significant risk of being harmed either during the procedure or in the future need to be reported. The easiest way to report these events is as complications, even if the patient has suffered no harm. The severity of the complication determines whether it is considered major or minor. The SCVIR categorizes these as noted in Table 53–5. The purpose of the "X" modifier is to identify minor adverse events that need to be followed for quality purposes.

When these categories are applied to the previous examples, *Example 1* is considered a failure of angioplasty but not a complication unless the patient was made clinically worse by the failure. The additional cost of the stent is not considered sufficient to call this event a complication, particularly since in some series at least 40% of patients treated initially with PTA will require a stent to achieve an optimal result.[155]

TABLE 53–5. CLASSIFICATION OF COMPLICATIONS BY OUTCOME

Minor complications:

A. No therapy, no sequela
B. Minor therapy or minor sequela; includes unplanned overnight hospital admission for observation only (<24 hr)

Major complications

C. Requires major therapy or unplanned hospitalization (24–48 hr)
D. Requires major therapy, unplanned increase in the level of care, prolonged hospitalization (>48 hr)
E. Permanent adverse sequelae
F. Death

An "X" modifier should be used for A and B categories to indicate laboratory values or imaging findings that suggest a significant potential for future harm.

From Citron S, Wallace R, Standards of Practice Committee of the SCVIR: Quality improvement guidelines for neuroangiography. J Vasc Interv Radiol (in press).

Example 2 is a level B complication. The additional stent within the same vessel segment is considered minor therapy. *Example 3* is a B "X" complication because the stent is placed in a non-target vessel. *Example 4* is a C complication. A new type of therapy (lysis) was necessary to treat an adverse event. This therapy has placed other organ systems at risk of hemorrhage, even though the patient ended up suffering no harm.

Example 5 involves an unexpected event, even though it does occur commonly during thrombolysis. The extra manipulation of an infusion wire into a previously nontarget vessel makes this a B complication. If no extra manipulation were necessary, this would be an A complication. If the embolus occluded one of three patent tibial vessels but no therapy was needed for this asymptomatic occlusion, this would be considered an A "X" complication since the loss of a runoff vessel may be of major consequence in the future.

Diagnostic Peripheral Angiography

The complications of peripheral angiography can be divided into three groups: (1) puncture site, (2) catheter-related, and (3) generalized or systemic reactions.

Puncture Site Complications

Puncture site complications that require treatment have been reported in older literature in about 0.5% of femoral punctures and 1.7% of axillary punctures.[59] The recent use of smaller diagnostic catheters has reduced the rate of femoral puncture site complications requiring surgery or transfusion to less than 0.1%.[85, 168] Hematomas occur commonly and rarely need surgical treatment. The rate of hematoma formation depends on the definition of hematoma. If a hematoma includes collections larger than 5 cm in diameter, the incidence is as high as 18%, but the incidence of hematomas larger than 5 cm is only 1.2%.[33]

Although one intuitively expects the risk of hematoma to increase with larger catheters, hypertension, and coagulopathy, the importance of these factors has been variable in several studies. Cragg found no increased risk of large hematomas (>5 cm) when comparing 5 and 7 French (Fr.) catheters, although there was a statistically increased risk of smaller hematomas. There was no increased risk for older age, systolic blood pressure above 150, partial thromboplastin time (PTT) more than 1.5 times the control, or platelet count below 50,000. The greatest risk was patient obesity.[33] Others have found an increased risk of hematomas larger than 4 cm in diameter with platelet counts below 100,000 and catheter size larger than 5 French but no increased risk from an elevated PTT or a prothrombin time (PT) of up to 18 seconds.[34] Similarly, the risk of pelvic, anterior abdominal wall, and retroperitoneal hematomas increases with coagulopathy.[121] The risk of femoral artery pseudoaneurysm is less than 0.05% from diagnostic peripheral procedures using 5 Fr. catheters[168] and 0.2% from diagnostic cardiac procedures using 5 Fr. sheaths.[177] The risk of pseudoaneurysm has been found to increase with a low puncture site, increasing catheter size, hypertension, the use of thrombolytics, and anticoagulation and is therefore higher in therapeutic than in diagnostic procedures.[97, 119, 177]

To avoid puncture site complications, the prudent angiographer uses the smallest catheter that can be easily manipulated. Coagulopathy may be corrected, but this depends on the risks of delaying a study and the possible need for anticoagulation during the procedure. The most effective preventive method is to puncture the femoral artery over the mid-femoral head. High punctures into the external iliac artery increase the risk of intraperitoneal and retroperitoneal hemorrhage.[158] Low punctures increase the risk of pseudoaneurysm.[123, 177] A low puncture with a double-wall puncture technique also increases the risk of arteriovenous fistula, since the femoral vein lies posterior to the bifurcation of the common femoral artery.[11] The puncture site should be checked fluoroscopically to overlie the middle of the femoral head.[1, 11, 123, 126] Punctures guided by surface anatomic landmarks can be misleadingly low in obese patients and high in thin patients. Hemostasis can also be improved by using external compression devices[25, 28, 118, 140] as well as devices that seal the arteriotomy,[20] although these devices may be uncomfortable and expensive and may produce emboli or vessel wall damage. When a pseudoaneurysm or arteriovenous fistula occurs, it may be effectively treated with ultrasound-guided compression[30] or percutaneous thrombin injection,[72a] although almost half will resolve spontaneously.[157]

Catheter-Related Complications

Catheter-related complications include dissections and subintimal injections as well as embolization from the catheter. The incidence of dissection and subintimal injection is under 0.5%.[168] Although most of these complications are not symptomatic because the dissections produced are retrograde and are pushed closed by the direction of blood flow, some can lead to acute occlusions or extensive chronic dissections.[9, 131] Thromboembolism from the catheter occurs in less than 0.5% of patients[143] and is related to operator experience.[72] It can be prevented by using forceful injections of heparinized flush[36] or systemic heparinization.[4, 19a, 38, 167] Cholesterol embolization is a clinically rare complication but has been observed in an autopsy series in as many as 30% of patients following aortography.[122] It can occur from catheter manipulation within a diseased vessel or from the force of contrast or flush injections against the wall of the vessel[48, 56] and may produce blue toe syndrome, gangrene, renal failure, pancreatitis, or death.

Generalized and Systemic Complications

Systemic complications include death, cardiac arrest or dysrhythmia, myocardial infarction, vasovagal syncope, sepsis, persistent nausea or vomiting, contrast reaction, contrast nephrotoxicity, and radiation injury. Because many procedures are performed on ill patients it may be impossible to distinguish a procedure-related complication from progression of the underlying disease. For example, Baum and coworkers[12] found a similar number of systemic complications among those patients who had undergone angiography and those awaiting elective angiography. Complications from contrast can be reduced with adequate hydration and the use of low osmolar contrast in high-risk patients (history of severe allergic reactions, unstable cardiac disease, azotemia particularly associated with diabetes).[10, 41] Although there is a negligible incidence of clinically significant bacteremia,[27, 133, 141] puncture site septic complications have been reported in the cardiology literature in 0.1% to 0.3% of cases,[103, 152] usually in the setting of repeat puncture of the same femoral artery or prolonged sheath placement for interventional procedures.[91]

Radiation injury is unlikely to occur during routine diagnostic angiography but can occur during prolonged procedures and complex interventions. Skin burns can develop after exposure to 2 Gy (200 rad), which is an exposure that can be reached after approximately 1 hour of fluoroscopy over a single site.[166] Higher radiation doses have produced skin necrosis requiring skin grafts.[142] Radiation exposure from filming is additive to the fluoroscopy dose and is significant, particularly if rapid frame cine is used, which has 30 to 60 times the radiation dose as digital subtraction imaging.[79, 109] Radiation exposure is cumulative over time, and repeat procedures over the same area increase the risk of radiation injury.[142] Mild skin injuries may go unnoticed because the injury is usually on the skin of the back if the x-ray tube is located beneath the patient, which is the most common arrangement in angiography rooms. The radiation dose can be minimized by limiting fluoroscopy times, using pulsed fluoroscopy, limiting the use of magnification during fluoroscopy, limiting the duration and frame rate of filming, keeping the image intensifier as low as possible, rotating the x-ray beam slightly to alter the skin entrance site, minimizing oblique imaging, increasing x-ray tube filtration, using a higher energy x-ray beam, and collimation of the x-ray beam as tightly as possible.[89, 166]

In response to reports of radiation injuries, the Food and Drug Administration (FDA) has recommended that institutions establish standard procedures and protocols for each procedure, including consideration of fluoroscopic exposure, determining radiation dose rates for specific fluoroscopy systems, assessing each protocol for the potential for radiation injury to the patient and attempting to minimize absorbed dose to any specific skin area, and recording information in the patient's record that permits estimation of the absorbed dose to the skin from interventional procedures with the potential to exceed a threshold dose of 1 Gy (100 rad).[43–45] Such procedures include radiofrequency cardiac catheter ablation, vascular embolization, transjugular intrahepatic portosystemic shunt placement, and percutaneous endovascular reconstruction. Compliance with these recommendations is considerably easier with the newest generation of angiography rooms, which include radiation dosimeters and calculate cumulative radiation dose during a procedure.

Diagnostic Neuroangiography

The puncture site, catheter-related, and systemic complications are similar to diagnostic peripheral angiography. There are additional complications of neurologic injury when these complications affect the central nervous system. For those patients studied because of symptoms of transient ischemic attack (TIA) or stroke, a subsequent TIA or stroke that occurs within 24 hours of angiography may be catheter-related or due to progression of the underlying disease. To avoid ambiguity, most studies include all neurologic events that occur within 24 hours of a neuroangiogram as procedure-related,[26, 55, 85, 110, 168] although this results in a higher complication rate than may be truly caused by the procedure.

The overall risk of TIA (neurologic deficit < 24 hours' duration) from diagnostic neuroangiography ranges from 0 to 11%, with the largest series reporting rates of about 1% or less.[42, 55, 85, 110, 144, 162, 168] The risk of stroke (neurologic deficit > 24 hours' duration) ranges from 0 to 5%, with the largest series reporting rates of 0.1% to 0.4%.[42, 55, 85, 110, 144, 162, 168] Stroke can also be *reversible* (resolves within 7 days) and *irreversible* (duration > 7 days).[26] The risk of neurologic injury is higher in patients studied for cerebrovascular occlusive disease, as well as subarachnoid hemorrhage, and lowest in patients studied for tumor, seizure, or headache. Complications are more frequent in prolonged procedures and in elderly patients,[55, 84] probably indicating that these procedures are technically more difficult. Most complications are thromboembolic, and their incidence can be reduced by the use of forceful injections of heparinized flush[36] or systemic heparinization,[4, 19a, 38, 167] similar to that used with peripheral angiography.

Peripheral Angioplasty

The complications of peripheral angioplasty include all the risks of a diagnostic study with the added risks of a larger vascular access frequently associated with anticoagulation, injury to the PTA site, and longer procedure times with greater radiation exposure. Whereas diagnostic angiography can be performed through 3 or 4 Fr. catheters, PTA usually requires catheter shaft diameters of 5 Fr. and larger, occasionally with the use of larger vascular sheaths. For this reason, the risk of puncture site hematoma following PTA is double that following diagnostic angiography.[83] The risk of puncture site pseudoaneurysm or arteriovenous fistula ranges from 0 to 3%,[172] but in most series the incidence is under 0.5%.[13, 16, 70] Puncture site thrombosis is even less common.[172]

Complications at the PTA site include thrombosis, dissection, perforation, branch vessel occlusion, and spasm. The incidence of acute thrombosis ranges from 0 to 7%,[172] with most series in the range of 1% to 2%. The risk increases in patients with small vessels, poor flow, or hypercoagulability. Heparin and aspirin can help prevent thrombosis, and lytics can be used to treat the thrombosis if it should occur.

Dissection can be produced by subintimal passage of the guide wire as it crosses a stenosis or occlusion, from subintimal injection of contrast, or from the angioplasty itself. Although the reported incidence of dissection as a complication of PTA ranges from 0 to 6%, dissection is always present at the PTA site whether or not it is angiographically visible.[65] Dissections that produce a significant pressure gradient are less common, but even this definition is ambiguous. As noted earlier, there is no consensus on the size of a pressure gradient that is significant.

The original iliac artery Palmaz stent trial[113] used a definition of 5 mmHg mean gradient after injection of vasodilators as an indication of a failed PTA requiring stent placement. Although this definition is widely quoted, the clinical relevance of this gradient has been questioned in a Dutch stent trial[155] in which a mean gradient of 10 mm across the PTA site following vasodilator injection was considered significant and appropriate for stenting. Use of the 10-mm gradient definition reduced stent placement by 50% compared with the number of stents that would have been placed using the 5 mm gradient definition of a failed PTA[155] and reduced stent placement by 63% compared with primary stenting.[154] Most American practitioners continue to use peak gradients rather than mean, sometimes with flow augmentation with vasodilators or reactive hyperemia and sometimes at rest.[19] Complicating the issue further is the question whether a pressure gradient immediately following PTA predicts a clinical angioplasty failure. Angioplasty-induced dissections remodel over time, and the ankle-brachial index (ABI) can improve over the span of a month, indicating reduction of the post-PTA pressure gradient.[74] This has also been seen with an improvement over time of elevated velocity measurements following PTA using duplex ultrasound at the PTA site.[129] For these reasons, the use of dissection as a measurable complication of angioplasty is of very limited value.

Perforation and vessel rupture are uncommon complications. The incidence ranges from 0 to 10%, but most series have an incidence of about 0.3%.[172] Guide wire perforation alone may be of no clinical consequence, but vessel rupture during balloon dilation may produce life-threatening hemorrhage, particularly in the iliac arteries, where the retroperitoneum can accommodate a large hematoma without producing tamponade. Rupture is usually due to the use of an oversized balloon and is accompanied by sudden pain and hypotension. Hemorrhage is rapidly controlled with reinflation of the balloon across the lesion to stabilize the patient prior to surgical repair.[49] Prolonged balloon inflation may also allow the arterial tear to seal and obviate surgery,[6, 32, 71, 107, 146] although the long-term integrity and risk of pseudoaneurysm development of ruptures treated in this fashion is not known. Alternatively, covered stents may allow definitive endovascular repair of these injuries.[86]

Occlusion of branches following PTA may not be considered a complication if the PTA is otherwise successful and therefore may be underreported. One series has reported this in 1.5% of cases.[22] In locations where a branch may be critical, such as at the origins of tibial vessels, placing a second safety wire or balloon catheter into the branch vessel preserves access and allows simultaneous "kissing balloon" inflation to prevent plaque from being displaced into the branch.[98]

Arterial spasm is more common in the renal and tibial vessels but is rarely reported as a complication.[172] Sublingual nifedipine has been used to prevent spasm,[14] although this route of administration has been criticized, particularly when used to treat hypertension.[53, 160] Spasm can also be treated locally with direct catheter injections of nitroglycerin or papaverine into the affected vessel.[14]

Embolization may occur downstream from the PTA site in 1% to 5% of cases, with most series in the range of 2% to 3%.[172] Most of the occurrences are asymptomatic but when necessary can be treated with percutaneous aspiration thrombectomy or thrombolysis if the embolized material is thrombus. Embolization is more likely to occur when treating occluded vessels.[18, 29, 101] Cholesterol embolization may also occur rarely.

Peripheral Stents

Peripheral stents include the complications of the angioplasty plus complications specific to stent deployment. Overall major complications range from 1% to 19% but in most studies are approximately 10%.[8, 40, 57, 81, 87, 105, 106, 114, 134, 150, 151, 165] Puncture site complications are more common because of the need for a larger delivery sheath of 7 to 10 Fr. inner diameter, compared with the 5 Fr. outer diameter of most angioplasty balloon catheters. Anticoagulation is also frequently used during and following stenting, particularly for femoropopliteal stents, which adds to the incidence of puncture site complications.[87] The lowest incidence of puncture site complications, 2%, was reported by Henry and colleagues[57] and was attributed to the use of smaller Palmaz stents that can be deployed through 6 to 8 Fr. guiding catheters. Open arteriotomy does not necessarily reduce access site complications. In a surgical series in which more than 60% of stents were placed through an open arteriotomy, no hematomas, arteriovenous fistulas, or pseudoaneurysms were reported, but there was an 8% incidence of superficial wound infections.[173] Complications from the routine use of general or regional anesthesia in this series were not reported.

When stents are used to treat occluded vessels, distal embolization may occur. The embolization rate is approximately 5% to 7%.[40, 81, 124, 164] The risk of embolization has been reduced by treating occlusions with intentional underdilation prior to stenting[163] or with primary stent placement without attempting balloon dilation first.[40] Most cases of distal embolization have been successfully treated percutaneously with thrombolysis or suction thrombectomy, but some cases have required surgical thrombectomy.

Vessel rupture has been reported in 1% to 3% of patients,[8, 81, 105, 106, 114, 124] although some large series have reported no ruptures.[87] In most cases, the rupture has been due to balloon dilation prior to stent placement. If primary stenting is performed, however, there is no way to distinguish perforation due to stenting versus perforation that would have occurred from the balloon dilation without the stent being present.

As noted earlier, dissection extending beyond the stented segment has been considered by some authors to be a complication of stent placement. Ballard and colleagues[8] described an overall complication rate of 19% from iliac artery stenting. Dissections occurred in 13% of patients and either were treated with additional stents or required no therapy. Others have not considered such dissections to be complications.[104]

Stent infection has been anecdotally reported and is, fortunately, rare.[8, 21, 24, 51, 62, 80, 93, 102, 156] To prevent this complication, some authors have recommended placing a new delivery sheath if the patient is not treated at a single sitting and the use of prophylactic antibiotics.[51] As noted by Hoffman and Murphy,[62] the incidence of stent infection is so rare that it would be difficult to demonstrate benefit from preventive therapy.

Thrombolysis

Thrombolytic agents may be administered systemically intravenously or regionally through a catheter-directed infusion. Although some studies have reported good results with systemic therapy,[88] such therapy for peripheral arterial thrombosis generally carries a lower success and higher systemic bleeding rate than regional therapy[3, 17] and has been replaced by catheter-directed thrombolysis for treatment of peripheral vascular thrombus. Streptokinase (SK), urokinase (UK), and recombinant tissue plasminogen activator (rt-PA) have all been used for peripheral arterial thrombolysis. Because SK has a success rate one third lower and a bleeding complication rate three to four times higher than either of the other two drugs,[52, 95] SK is rarely used despite its lower price.

Several studies that compared UK and rt-PA found similar success rates. rt-PA was more rapid in effect, but at the cost of increased bleeding.[52, 100, 136a] Meyerovitz and colleagues[100] reported major bleeding in 12.5% of patients treated with UK compared with 31% of patients treated with rt-PA. Minor bleeding occurred in no patients with UK and 12.5% of patients with rt-PA. Graor[52] reported major bleeding complications in 6% of patients treated with UK with no intracranial bleeding compared with 12% treated with rt-PA including a 2% incidence of intracranial bleeding. In a randomized trial of UK, rt-PA, and surgery, the rate of intracranial hemorrhage was 0.9% for UK and 1.5% for rt-PA, but the overall efficacy and bleeding complications from the two drugs were similar.[149] A larger European randomized trial comparing UK and rt-PA similarly found more rapid lysis with rt-PA with no major bleeding complications during lysis in either group, although the incidence of large groin hematomas was 8% for UK and 15% for rt-PA.[136a]

In most of these studies, the sample sizes were small and the differences in bleeding complications did not reach statistical significance. It is possible that the optimal dose of rt-PA for peripheral infusion was not used in these comparisons,[35, 125] but because of the preceding results, UK is the drug most commonly used in the United States for catheter-directed thrombolysis in the peripheral arteries.

Complications of arterial lysis are divided into hemor-

TABLE 53–6. COMPLICATIONS WITH INTRA-ARTERIAL/INTRAGRAFT INFUSIONS OF UROKINASE

	OVERALL (%)	RANGE (%)
A. **Bleeding Complications**	5.9	3–17
1. Major hemorrhage		
a. Local	3.9	2–9
b. Remote	0.8	1–2
c. Intracranial	0.2	0–2
2. Minor hemorrhage	12.8	4–24
a. Local	12.1	4–23
b. Remote	0.7	1–4
B. **Nonbleeding Complications**		
1. Embolization	7.2	2–40
a. Requiring therapy	1.8	1–12
2. Pericatheter thrombosis	1.9	2–10
a. Requiring therapy	0.8	0–6
3. Reperfusion syndrome	0.1	0–1
4. Compartment syndrome	0.9	1–8
5. Renal failure	1.7	1–5
6. Acute myocardial infarction	0.8	0–5
7. Miscellaneous major complications	2.5	0–16
C. **Mortality and Amputation**		
1. Death from procedure	0.9	0–2
2. All deaths at 30 days	5.2	1–18
3. Amputations from procedure	0.8	0–4
4. All amputations at 30 days	11	2–18

Modified from Kumpe DA, Durham JD: Complications of regional fibrinolytic therapy. *In* Ansell G, Bettman MA, Kaufman JA, Wilkins RA (eds): Complications in Diagnostic Imaging and Interventional Radiology, 3rd ed. Cambridge, Blackwell Science, Inc, 1996, p 372.

rhagic and nonhemorrhagic categories and have been summarized by Kumpe and Durham[77] (Table 53–6). Major hemorrhage is defined as requiring transfusion, surgery, or discontinuation of lytic therapy and occurs in approximately 6% of patients. Most major and minor bleeding events occur at the catheter insertion site and can be controlled with local compression or exchanging for a larger catheter or sheath. The use of micropuncture needle sets and small catheters may prevent puncture site bleeding. Systemic heparin is usually administered during regional thrombolysis to prevent pericatheter thrombosis in low flow vessels,[95] although this increases the risk of bleeding complications.[112] In the presence of hemorrhage, the heparin can be reduced, discontinued, or reversed with protamine. Urokinase can be reversed with cryoprecipitate, fresh frozen plasma, tranexamic acid, ε-aminocaproic acid, or aprotinin. Reversal is rarely necessary because UK has a biologic half-life of less than 20 minutes.[15, 37] Pseudoaneurysm at the catheter insertion site has been reported in 0.8% to 3% of cases.[77, 112]

Intracranial hemorrhage can be fatal but is fortunately rare, occurring in 0.1% to 2% of patients.[50, 96, 111, 112, 149] Risk factors that predispose patients to intracranial hemorrhage during arterial infusion are poorly defined. The Thrombolysis or Peripheral Arterial Surgery (TOPAS) trial found that when aspirin and therapeutic heparin were prohibited during lysis, the rate of intracranial hemorrhage decreased from 5% to 0.5%.[112] McNamara and colleagues[96] have recommended controlling hypertension. Laboratory values such as fibrinogen level have been of no value in predicting which patients will have a bleeding complication.[77, 96]

Embolization as the thrombus dissolves during therapy is reported on average in 7% of cases (see Table 53–6) but is probably underreported because it rarely requires therapy other than continued infusion and may be considered part of the expected course of thrombolysis. The randomized TOPAS trial reported a rate of distal embolization during lysis of 14%.[112] Embolization requiring surgery occurs in about 2% of cases but has been reported in as many as 4% to 8% of cases.[39, 145] Embolization from a cardiac thrombus during arterial infusion is rare[82] but has been reported anecdotally.[116] It is not necessary routinely to obtain a cardiac ultrasound to look for a cardiac thrombus before starting lytic therapy for a peripheral embolus.[77, 82, 96, 175]

Both compartment and reperfusion syndromes can occur as a consequence of successful revascularization of ischemic or necrotic tissue and occur in under 1% of patients. The incidence of these complications depends on the severity and duration of ischemia prior to and during treatment.[94]

Shaking chills during UK infusion are of little clinical consequence but can be uncomfortable for the patient and alarming for the physician. Matsumoto and associates[90] found that 28% of their patients experienced rigors during UK therapy beginning in 1990, whereas there were no cases before 1990. Others report an incidence of rigors of less than 1%.[112] No cause has been found for the rigors, but it has been speculated to be due to larger bolus doses of the drug given over short periods of time. Treatment with intravenous meperidine has been rapidly effective.[75, 90, 135]

In an attempt to minimize the complications of lytic therapy, lists of absolute and relative contraindications have been compiled (Table 53–7). These recommendations were first made in 1980[108] regarding systemic therapy and have been widely quoted[88, 169, 175] without formal study. These recommendations should be taken as a list that reasonably indicates which patients are at higher risk of having a complication from lytic therapy rather than a list of abso-

TABLE 53–7. CONTRAINDICATIONS TO THROMBOLYTIC THERAPY

A. **Absolute**
1. Established cerebrovascular event (including TIAs) within past 2 months
2. Active bleeding diathesis
3. Recent gastrointestinal bleeding (<10 days)
4. Neurosurgery (intracranial, spinal) within past 3 months
5. Intracranial trauma within past 3 months

B. **Relative Major**
1. Cardiopulmonary resuscitation within past 10 days
2. Major nonvascular surgery or trauma within past 10 days
3. Uncontrolled hypertension: >180 mmHg systolic or >110 mmHg diastolic
4. Puncture of noncompressible vessel
5. Intracranial tumor
6. Recent eye surgery

C. **Minor**
1. Hepatic failure, particularly those with coagulopathy
2. Bacterial endocarditis
3. Pregnancy
4. Diabetic hemorrhagic retinopathy

From Working Party on Thrombolysis in the Management of Limb Ischemia: Thrombolysis in the management of lower limb peripheral arterial occlusion—a consensus document. Am J Cardiol 81:207–218, 1998. Reprinted with permission of Excerpta Medica, Inc.

TIA = transient ischemic attack.

lute contraindications. As in any medical therapy, the potential risks and benefits of lysis must be weighed against the potential risks and benefits of alternative therapies for the individual patient.

QUALITY IMPROVEMENT

The preceding information on success, failure, and complications needs to be used to maintain and improve quality. In 1986, the Joint Commission on Accreditation of Healthcare Organizations (JCAHO)[66] published its Agenda for Change, which required the creation of quality improvement programs in hospitals. The JCAHO identified 10 steps in monitoring and evaluation:

1. Assign responsibility for the department monitoring and evaluation efforts.
2. Delineate the scope of care or service that the department provides.
3. Identify the important aspects of the services that should be monitored.
4. Identify indicators of quality and appropriateness for the identified important aspects of care.
5. Establish the criteria that will be used to evaluate the indicators. The criteria are thresholds that, if exceeded, will trigger a review to determine the cause of the problem.
6. Collect and analyze the data.
7. If a threshold is exceeded, evaluate care to determine the cause of the problem.
8. Take actions to solve identified problems.
9. Assess the actions and document improvement by continuing to monitor and reevaluate the care.
10. Communicate the relevant information to the organization's quality assurance program.

The JCAHO has modified the 10-step program into a framework using a cycle for improving performance. One method to implement this framework is to use a program such as Plan-Do-Check-Act, in which one plans how to improve a process, implements a change on a small scale, checks the results, and then fully implements the change. Critical to the program is the goal of collecting valid, reliable data to assess how well a process is working and what can be improved. Rather than simply comparing current performance to historical patterns of performance within the institution, it is recommended that the comparison also be made to standards from outside the individual hospital. Such standards can come from health care associations, payers, the government, professional societies, and expert panels.[67]

Quality improvement programs are relevant to peripheral endovascular diagnostic and interventional procedures. There are now multiple specialties with many different training guidelines for performing these procedures.[78, 136, 148, 170, 171] The American Heart Association (AHA) criteria, in addition to specific numbers of cases, state that the outcomes of the training cases must be acceptable.[78] There are no accepted guidelines for the numbers of cases necessary for continued competency in peripheral interventions,

TABLE 53–8. DIAGNOSTIC ANGIOGRAPHY QUALITY IMPROVEMENT STANDARDS

INDICATOR	THRESHOLD
I. **Indications**	95%
1. Evaluation of vascular disease, for diagnosis and staging	
2. Evaluation of malignant disease, for diagnosis and staging	
3. Evaluation of gastrointestinal bleeding	
4. Preoperative planning for portosystemic shunts	
5. Evaluation of benign conditions, for diagnosis and preoperative planning	
II. **Success Rates**	95%
III. **Complications**	
1. Puncture site complications	
a. Hematoma (requiring transfusion, surgery, or delayed discharge)	0.5%
b. Occlusion	0.2%
c. Pseudoaneurysm/arteriovenous fistula	0.2%
2. Catheter-induced complications, other than puncture site	
a. Distal emboli	0.5%
b. Arterial dissection/subintimal passage	0.5%
c. Subintimal injection of contrast	0.5%
3. Contrast-induced renal failure (elevation in baseline serum creatinine or blood urea nitrogen necessitating care that delays discharge, requires unexpected admission or readmission, or results in permanent impairment of renal function)	0.2%
IV. **Overall Procedure Threshold for Major Complications** The overall procedure threshold for major complications is determined by the following formula: $\frac{\text{No. of patients undergoing only diagnostic angiography with complications}}{\text{No. of patients undergoing only diagnostic angiography}} \times 100$	1%

Modified from Society of Cardiovascular and Interventional Radiology: Standard for diagnostic arteriography in adults: Standards of Practice Committee of the Society of Cardiovascular and Interventional Radiology. J Vasc Interv Radiol 4:385–395, 1993.

but it has been amply documented for percutaneous coronary interventions that better outcomes are achieved among physicians and institutions with a greater volume of cases.[54, 76] Each specialty has an interest in starting or continuing to perform these procedures, particularly as endovascular therapies improve to the point of replacing traditional surgical treatment for diseases such as aortic aneurysms and carotid stenosis.[161] There is therefore a need for outcome standards or guidelines to be used as a benchmark for training and as a means of ensuring and improving quality among the many physicians performing peripheral endovascular procedures. Outcome guidelines for diagnostic peripheral and cerebral angiography and peripheral arterial PTA and stenting have been created by the SCVIR.[26, 132, 137, 139] The guidelines for diagnostic angiography are under revision,[143a] and the revised guidelines are used in this chapter. The guidelines for cerebral angiography[26] were created in collaboration with the American Society of Interventional and Therapeutic Neuroradiology (ASITN) and the American Society of Neuroradiology (ASNR) (Tables 53–8 to 53–11). Guidelines for thrombolysis are under development.

For the SCVIR guidelines, indicators of appropriateness are considered along with rates of success, failure, and complications to be measurable aspects of quality of care. These outcome guidelines are distinct from practice guidelines that create algorithms to guide which kind of diagnostic test or treatment is chosen for a particular patient problem or how the procedure is performed. Practice guidelines for performing angiography and PTA have been written,[23, 139] as have guidelines for selecting appropriate patients for PTA.[117, 138] The appropriateness indicators are necessary to determine if physicians are treating an inappropriate number of high-risk lesions or patients.[2] These guidelines will alter as technology improves (i.e., a lesion that is a poor candidate for PTA may be a good candidate for a bare or covered percutaneous stent)[138, 153] and are used as a means of achieving the thresholds described in the outcome guidelines.

The SCVIR practice guidelines have been developed by committee members with scientific and clinical expertise in the field. The initial guidelines were created by roundtable consensus (see Tables 53–8 and 53–10).[137, 139] The more recent outcome guidelines and revisions to prior guidelines (see Tables 53–9 and 53–11)[26, 132, 143a] were created using established rules of evidence,[31, 174] evidence tables, and a modified Delphi technique for reaching consensus.[47] The guidelines were then compared with national registry data from the SCVIR Hi-IQ database for validation. Because of the different methods used for the initial and later guidelines there are differences in some of the complication thresholds, such as for renal failure and puncture site hematoma.

There are problems with using outcome guidelines for quality improvement. For example, published rates for individual types of complications are based on series comprising hundreds of patients, a number larger than most practitioners are likely to treat. If a physician has performed a low number of procedures, such as early in a quality improvement program, a single complication can place the physician over a complication-specific threshold without being statistically valid. It is of little value to identify a single complication when poor quality cannot be distinguished from the sporadic occurrence of the complication.[147] The SCVIR outcome guidelines recognize this and provide both complication-specific thresholds and thresholds for overall complication rates.

The complication and success rates also depend on patient selection and referral patterns. For example, one of the references used to derive the outcome guidelines for

TABLE 53–9. DIAGNOSTIC NEUROANGIOGRAPHY QUALITY IMPROVEMENT STANDARDS

INDICATOR	REPORTED RATES	THRESHOLD
I. **Indications**		99%
1. Define presence/extent of thromboembolic phenomena and atherosclerotic occlusive disease		
2. Define etiology of cranial hemorrhage (subarachnoid, intraventricular, parenchymal, craniofacial)		
3. Define presence, location, and anatomy of intracranial aneurysms and vascular malformations		
4. Evaluation of vasospasm related to subarachnoid hemorrhage		
5. Define presence or extent of trauma to cervicocerebral vessels (e.g., dissection, pseudoaneurysm)		
6. Define vascular supply to tumors		
7. Define presence or extent of vasculitis (infectious, inflammatory, drug-induced)		
8. Diagnose or define congenital or anatomic anomaly (e.g., vein of Galen fistula)		
9. Define presence of veno-occlusive disease (e.g., dural sinus, cortical, deep)		
10. Determine efficacy of therapeutic measures		
II. **Success Rates**	98%	98%
III. **Complications**		
1. Neurologic (within 24 hr of the procedure)		
a. Reversible neurologic deficit	0–2.3%	2.5%
b. Permanent neurologic deficit	0–5%	1%
2. Other major complications		
a. Renal failure	0–0.15%	0.2%
b. Arterial occlusion requiring therapy	0–0.4%	0.2%
c. Arteriovenous fistula or pseudoaneurysm	0.01–0.22%	0.2%
d. Hematoma requiring transfusion, surgery, or delayed discharge	0.26–1.5%	0.5%
IV. **Overall Major Complications**		2%

From Citron S, Wallace R, Standards of Practice Committee of the SCVIR: Quality improvement guidelines for neuroangiography. J Vasc Radiol (in press).

TABLE 53–10. PERIPHERAL ANGIOPLASTY QUALITY IMPROVEMENT STANDARDS

INDICATOR	THRESHOLD
I. **Indications**	95%
A. Presence of one of the following:	
1. Intermittent claudication, which limits lifestyle and is documented by appropriate noninvasive tests	
2. Ischemic rest pain	
3. Ischemic ulceration or tissue loss	
B. And one of the following:	
1. One or more short (<10 cm in length), hemodynamically significant arterial stenoses, with definable continuous runoff below	
2. Short segment (<10 cm in length) occlusion with definable continuous runoff below	
3. More extensive disease than the above in patients who are poor operative risks or who lack suitable bypass material	
4. Stenosis is associated with a bypass graft	
II. **Success Rates**	
A. Iliac	95%
B. Superficial femoral and popliteal	90%
C. Tibial and peroneal	80%
III. **Complications**	
A. Emergency surgery	3%
B. Severe bleeding or hematoma	4%
C. Puncture site occlusion	0.5%
D. Angioplasty site occlusion	3%
E. Distal embolization causing tissue damage	1%
F. Vessel perforation requiring surgery	0.5%

Modified with permission from Society of Cardiovascular and Interventional Radiology (SCVIR): Guidelines for establishing a quality assurance program in vascular and interventional radiology. Fairfax, Va, SCVIR, 1989. Copyright © 1989.

iliac stents excluded patients with poor runoff,[87] which may not be the situation in clinical practice. A tertiary referral center may have a population of patients with more severe peripheral vascular and systemic disease. Severity of disease can be stratified and used to adjust for outcomes,[127, 176] but the adjustment may not be reliable.[64] The thresholds have, in general, been set at a rate higher than the published rates to account for such differences in patient populations but may need to be tailored for an individual institution.

The SCVIR guidelines focus on major complications, described earlier as complications that have real potential for clinically significant sequelae, require prolonged hospitalization (>24 hours) or major therapy, or have permanent adverse sequelae (categories D, E, and F and "X" modifiers from Table 53–5). Minor complications tend to occur more frequently than major complications and can be an earlier and more sensitive indicator of systematic quality problems. For example, it is easier to use minor complication rates to identify quality differences between two physicians who have minor complication rates of 10% and 20%, respectively, but major complication rates of only 1% and 2%.

A greater problem is that a quality improvement system that relies on complication thresholds tends to reward those who hide complications and penalizes those who are honest in their reporting.[147] Given the ambiguity in some of the definitions of complications, as described earlier, there is a possibility of bias in reporting results. For this reason, there must be objective documentation of procedures. Images must be permanently recorded of both diagnostic and interventional procedures. Pre- and post-intervention images must be recorded. Objective measures of success should be obtained using pressure measurements for revascularization interventions.[127] Ideally, measures of functional status should be performed,[60, 92] but this is not easily performed outside of a research environment.

The JCAHO requires that these quality benchmarks be applied uniformly within an institution.[68] If physicians from multiple specialties perform a procedure, there should be an open and joint quality improvement process, which includes indications, success rates, and complication rates. This ensures uniform use of definitions, unbiased reporting, and comparison of quality results between physicians.

LEGAL IMPLICATIONS OF QUALITY IMPROVEMENT STANDARDS

Practice parameters and outcome guidelines and standards have potential legal implications. Practice parameters are more relevant to legal issues, because they are guides on how to practice medicine. Deviation from these guides, in combination with a bad outcome, can be used as evidence of malpractice. Johnson and associates[61, 69] have examined this issue in detail and state that unless the practice parameters are written as standards rather than guidelines, variations from practice parameters are not per se (conclusive) indicators of quality or utilization problems. These variations should merely be a signal for further peer review. As long as the practice parameter recognizes that individual circumstances may require deviation from the guide (as is noted in the SCVIR guidelines), the reasonableness of the deviation will be determined in court. The defendant has the burden to prove why the deviation was appropriate.[73] The credibility of the parameter will be affected by the reliability of the parameter and the group issuing it, the degree to which the parameter provides specific clinical

TABLE 53–11. AORTOILIAC STENT QUALITY IMPROVEMENT STANDARDS

INDICATOR		THRESHOLD
I. **Indications**		95%
A. Presence of one of the following that is likely to be caused by the lesion being treated:		
1. Disabling claudication documented by appropriate noninvasive tests		
2. Critical limb ischemia (rest pain, ulceration, or tissue loss)		
3. Blue toe syndrome		
4. Vasculogenic impotence		
B. And one or more of the following:		
1. Angioplasty result with immediate elastic recoil producing a 30% or greater stenosis and/or a residual trans-stenotic systolic gradient >10 mmHg or >10% ratio drop		
2. Flow limiting dissection or intimal flap		
3. Recanalization of chronic iliac occlusion		
4. Iliac ulceration associated with symptoms		
5. Restenosis after previously performed angioplasty		
6. Complex lesions for which primary stenting may give more satisfactory results*		
II. **Success Rates**		
A. Crossing the stenosis		
1. Short stenosis <3 cm		98%
2. Long stenosis >3 cm		95%
B. Crossing the occlusion		
1. Short occlusion <6 cm		85%
2. Long occlusion >6 cm		Insufficient data
C. Attempted percutaneous stent placement		98%
D. Successful percutaneous vascular access for stent placement		99%
E. Successful stent deployment		98% If lesion is crossed
F. Patency		
1. Short stenosis		90% at 1 year
2. Long stenosis		85% at 1 year
3. Chronic occlusion		70% at 1 year
	REPORTED RATE	**THRESHOLD**
III. **Complications**		
A. Stent-related	2%	3%
1. Thrombosis (periprocedural <30 days)		
2. Dislodgment or malposition		
3. Pseudoaneurysm at stent site		
B. Arterial injury prior to stent deployment	2%	3%
1. Pseudoaneurysm, rupture, perforation after angioplasty at the treatment segment		
C. Puncture site (major)	4%	4%
1. Large hematoma, bleeding, thrombosis, pseudoaneurysm, arteriovenous fistula		
D. Distal embolization associated with:		
1. Stenosis	1%	2%
2. Occlusion	3–6%	7%
E. Post-procedure myocardial infarction	1%	2%
F. Mortality within 30 days	1%	2%
IV. **Overall Major Complications**		
1. Stenosis	4%	6%
2. Occlusion	9%	10%

V. **Appendix**

It is considered a technical failure of percutaneous therapy when an endovascular procedure (arteriogram, angioplasty, atherectomy, vascular stent, or stent/graft) initially intended to be performed percutaneously is converted to an open surgical procedure because of a failure to obtain vascular access. Similarly, the conversion of a percutaneous procedure to an open procedure because of a failure to cross the lesion is considered a failure of the percutaneous procedure. These technical failures require a major unplanned increase in the level of care even if the procedure is subsequently completed through an open access. If the patient has also been injured during the failed attempt to enter the vessel percutaneously or cross the lesion, the procedure is a failure with a complication.

Rarely, endovascular procedures are performed open without an attempt at a percutaneous approach. These are procedures that are intended to be combined with an open bypass operation at the same access site, which involve devices too large to be inserted percutaneously, or involve access sites that are so severely diseased or occluded that percutaneous access is not possible. Routine angioplasty, atherectomy, and stent placement is a percutaneous procedure. For this reason, a threshold of 98% has been set for attempted percutaneous stent placement. It is expected that 99% of percutaneous vascular access attempts will be successful. Therefore, including failures of percutaneous vascular access, fewer than 3% of stents should be placed during an open surgical procedure.

Modified from Sanchez O, Lewis C, Standards of Practice Committee of the SCVIR: Quality improvement guidelines for aorto-iliac arterial stents. J Vasc Interv Radiol (in press).

*The data to support this indication are evolving and unpublished. This indication is therefore reached by consensus of the Standards of Practice Committee of the Society of Cardiovascular and Interventional Radiology.

guidelines applicable to the circumstances of the case, and the nature and purpose of the parameter (i.e., cost containment versus quality of care parameters).

Compliance with a parameter does not establish lack of negligence but may be helpful supportive evidence. In a survey of malpractice cases, Hyams and colleagues[63] found that guidelines were used by both the defense and the plaintiffs but that the guidelines were used three times more frequently as evidence against physicians than supporting physicians. This survey may be biased by cases being dropped if the guidelines support the physician. These authors conclude that compliance with guidelines can reduce the number of claims and lead to claims being dropped, but noncompliance with guidelines can lead to suits and loss of suits.

Malpractice requires that a patient must suffer a significant injury as a result of a breach in the standard of care. Courts have been adopting a national standard of care.[147] These national standards involve the practice of medicine rather than outcome standards. Outcome standards do not indicate that any one bad outcome was or was not a result of negligence. A physician can have outstanding overall outcomes but still have provided negligent care for an individual patient.

Outcome standards are relevant to the liability of the hospital in terms of granting and maintaining credentials to physicians. Under the theory of corporate liability, the hospital may be held responsible for the actions of independent physicians for care provided in the hospital setting. Even though credentials are recommended by the medical staff, the hospital board is responsible for properly selecting, and credentialing, and monitoring its staff physicians and for restricting clinical privileges when a physician provides negligent care.

The hospital board of trustees is expected to meet the standard of care ordinarily exercised by the average hospital in granting staff privileges. The hospital is liable if it knew, or should have known, that the physician whose negligence caused an injury to a patient was providing substandard care to his or her patients.[46] Isolated negligent acts of an otherwise competent independent physician are not generally evidence of hospital negligence. If that physician has a complication and failure rate higher than national quality assurance standards, however, this may be supportive evidence that the physician is not otherwise competent. The evidence may be even stronger if the physician has not met nationally accepted minimum training standards or if other physicians practicing in that community do meet national standards. Under these circumstances, one might argue that if the physician subsequently provides negligent care, the hospital should have known that this was likely to occur. There is no case law holding that individual members of the medical staff may also be liable for these credentialing decisions.

SUMMARY

Quality improvement programs should give patients the assurance that they are being treated by capable physicians and should give physicians the tools to improve outcomes. A successful quality improvement program requires uniform definitions of success, failure, and complications and appropriate outcome standards to which physicians are held accountable. Outcome standards must be applied uniformly within an institution, particularly if there are multiple specialties performing the same procedures. This chapter has provided such definitions and standards and has addressed the ambiguity inherent in some of the definitions.

REFERENCES

1. Altin RS, Flicker S, Naidech HJ: Pseudoaneurysm and arteriovenous fistula after femoral artery catheterization: Association with low femoral punctures. Am J Roentgenol 152:629–631, 1989.
2. American Medical Association (AMA): Using practice parameters in quality assessment, quality assurance and quality improvement programs. Chicago, AMA Office of Quality Assurance 1992, pp 1–9.
3. Amery A, Deloof W, Vermylen J, et al: Outcome of recent thromboembolic occlusions of limb arteries treated with streptokinase. Br Med J 4:639–644, 1970.
4. Anderson JH, Gianturco C, Wallace S, et al: Anticoagulation techniques for angiography: An experimental study. Radiology 111:573–576, 1974.
5. Archie JP Jr: Analysis and comparison of pressure gradients and ratios for predicting iliac stenosis. Ann Vasc Surg 8:271–280, 1994.
6. Ashenburg RJ, Blair RJ, Rivera FJ, et al: Renal arterial rupture complicating transluminal angioplasty: Successful conservative management. Radiology 174:983–985, 1990.
7. Ballard J: Regarding "Complications of iliac artery stent deployment" response to letter to the editor. J Vasc Surg 25:961, 1997.
8. Ballard JL, Sparks SR, Taylor FC, et al: Complications of iliac artery stent deployment. J Vasc Surg 24:545–553, 1996.
9. Bariseel H, Batt M, Rogopoulos A, et al: Iatrogenic dissection of the abdominal aorta. J Vasc Surg 27:366–370, 1998.
10. Barrett BJ: Contrast nephrotoxicity. J Am Soc Nephrol 5:125–137, 1994.
11. Baum PA, Matsumoto AH, Teitelbaum GP, et al: Anatomic relationship between the common femoral artery and vein: CT evaluation and clinical significance. Radiology 173:775–777, 1989.
12. Baum S, Stein GN, Kuroda KK: Complications of "no arteriography." Radiology 86:835–838, 1966.
13. Beck AH, Muhe A, Ostheim W, et al: Long-term results of percutaneous transluminal angioplasty: A study of 4750 dilatations and local lyses. Eur J Vasc Surg 3:245–252, 1989.
14. Becker GJ, Katzen BT, Dake MD: Noncoronary angioplasty. Radiology 170:921–940, 1989.
15. Bell WR, Sasahara AA: Review of Thrombolytic Therapy and Thromboembolic Disease. Glenview, Ill, Physicians & Scientists Publishing Co, 1989, pp 35–37.
16. Belli AM, Cumberland DC, Knox AM, et al: The complication rate of percutaneous peripheral balloon angioplasty. Clin Radiol 41:380–383, 1990.
17. Berridge DC, Gregson RH, Hopkinson BR, et al: Randomized trial of intra-arterial recombinant tissue plasminogen activator, intravenous recombinant tissue plasminogen activator and intra-arterial streptokinase in peripheral arterial thrombolysis. Br J Surg 78:988–995, 1991.
18. Blum U, Gabelmann A, Redecker M, et al: Percutaneous recanalization of iliac artery occlusions: Results of a prospective study. Radiology 189:536–540, 1993.
19. Bonn J: Percutaneous vascular intervention: Value of hemodynamic measurements. Radiology 201:18–20, 1996.

19a. Bookstein JJ, Arun K: Experimental investigation of hypercoagulant conditions associated with angiography. J Vasc Interv Radiol 6:197–204, 1995.

20. Bos J, Hunink M, Mali W: Use of a collagen hemostatic closure device to achieve hemostasis after arterial puncture: A cost-effectiveness analysis. J Vasc Interv Radiol 7:479–486, 1996.
21. Bunt TJ, Gill HK, Smith DC, et al: Infection of a chronically implanted iliac artery stent. Ann Vasc Surg 11:529–532, 1997.
22. Capek P, McLean GK, Berkowitz HD: Femoropopliteal angioplasty: Factors influencing long-term success. Circulation 83:170–180, 1991.

23. Cardella JF, Casarella WJ, DeWeese JA, et al: Optimal resources for the examination and endovascular treatment of the peripheral and visceral vascular systems: AHA Intercouncil report on peripheral and visceral angiographic and interventional laboratories. Circulation 89:1481–1493, 1994.
24. Chalmers N, Eadington DW, Gandanhamo D, et al: Case report: Infected false aneurysm at the site of an iliac stent. Br J Radiol 66:946–948, 1993.
25. Christenson R, Staab EV, Burko H, et al: Pressure dressings and postarteriographic care of the femoral puncture site. Radiology 119:97–99, 1976.
26. Citron S, Wallace R, Standards of Practice Committee of the Society of Cardiovascular and Interventional Radiology: Quality improvement guidelines for neuroangiography. J Vasc Interv Radiol (in press).
27. Clark H: An evaluation of antibiotic prophylaxis in cardiac catheterization. Am Heart J 77:767–771, 1969.
28. Colapinto RF, Harty PW: Femoral artery compression device for outpatient angiography. Radiology 166:890–891, 1988.
29. Colapinto RF, Stronell RD, Johnston WK: Transluminal angioplasty of complete iliac obstructions. Am J Roentgenol 146:859–862, 1986.
30. Coley BD, Roberts AC, Fellmeth BD, et al: Postangiographic femoral artery pseudoaneurysms: Further experience with US-guided compression repair. Radiology 194:307–311, 1995.
31. Cook DJ, Guyatt GH, Laupacis A, et al: Rules of evidence and clinical recommendations on the use of antithrombotic agents. Chest 102:305S–311S, 1992.
32. Cooper SG, Sofocleous CT: Percutaneous management of angioplasty-related iliac artery rupture with preservation of luminal patency by prolonged balloon tamponade. J Vasc Interv Radiol 9:81–83, 1998.
33. Cragg AH, Nakagawa N, Smith TP, et al: Hematoma formation after diagnostic angiography: Effect of catheter size. J Vasc Interv Radiol 2:231–233, 1991.
34. Darcy MD, Kanterman RY, Kleinhoffer MA, et al: Evaluation of coagulation tests as predictors of angiographic bleeding complications. Radiology 198:741–744, 1996.
35. Dawson KJ, Hamilton G: Recombinant tissue-type plasminogen activator versus urokinase in peripheral arterial occlusions (Letter). Radiology 178:283–284, 1991.
36. Dawson P, Strickland NH: Thromboembolic phenomena in clinical angiography: Role of materials and technique. J Vasc Interv Radiol 2:125–132, 1991.
37. de Bono DP, More RS: Prevention and management of bleeding complications after thrombolysis. Int J Cardiol 38:1–6, 1993.
38. Debrun GM, Vinuela FV, Fox AJ: Aspirin and systemic heparinization in diagnostic and interventional neuroradiology. Am J Roentgenol 139:139–142, 1982.
39. DeMaioribus CA, Mills JL, Fujitani RM, et al: A reevaluation of intraarterial thrombolytic therapy for acute lower extremity ischemia. J Vasc Surg 17:888–895, 1993.
40. Dyet JF, Gaines PA, Nicholson AA, et al: Treatment of chronic iliac artery occlusions by means of percutaneous endovascular stent placement. J Vasc Interv Radiol 8:349–353, 1997.
41. Ellis JH, Cohan RH, Sonnad SS, et al: Selective use of radiographic low-osmolality contrast media in the 1990s. Radiology 200:297–311, 1996.
42. Executive Committee for the Asymptomatic Carotid Atherosclerosis Study: Endarterectomy for asymptomatic carotid artery stenosis. JAMA 273:1421–1428, 1995.
43. Food and Drug Administration (FDA): Important information for physicians and other health care professionals: Avoidance of serious x-ray-induced skin injuries to patients during fluoroscopically-guided procedures. Rockville, Md, Center for Devices and Radiologic Health, FDA, September 9, 1994.
44. Food and Drug Administration (FDA): Important information for physicians and other healthcare professionals: Recording information in the patient's medical record that identifies the potential for serious x-ray-induced skin injuries following fluoroscopically guided procedures. Rockville, Md, Center for Devices and Radiologic Health, FDA, September 15, 1995.
45. Food and Drug Administration (FDA): Public health advisory: Avoidance of serious x-ray-induced skin injuries following fluoroscopically guided procedures. Rockville, Md, Center for Devices and Radiologic Health, FDA, September 30, 1994.
46. Feegel JR: Liability of health care entities for negligent care. *In* American College of Legal Medicine (ed): Legal Medicine, 3rd ed. St. Louis, Mosby–Year Book, 1995, p 156.
47. Fink A, Kosecoff J, Chassin M, et al: Consensus methods: Characteristics and guidelines for use. Am J Public Health 74:979–983, 1984.
48. Gaines PA, Cumberland DC, Kennedy A, et al: Cholesterol embolisation: A lethal complication of vascular catheterisation. Lancet 1:168–170, 1988.
49. Gardiner GA Jr, Meyerovitz MF, Stokes KR, et al: Complications of transluminal angioplasty. Radiology 159:201–208, 1986.
50. Gardiner GAJ, Sullivan KL: Complications of regional thrombolytic therapy. *In* Kadir S (ed): Current Practice of Interventional Radiology. Philadelphia, BC Decker, 1991, pp 87–91.
51. Gordon GI, Vogelzang RL, Curry RH, et al: Endovascular infection after renal artery stent placement. J Vasc Interv Radiol 7:669–672, 1996.
52. Graor RA: Efficacy and safety of intraarterial local infusion of streptokinase, urokinase, or tissue plasminogen activator for peripheral arterial occlusion: A retrospective review. J Vasc Med Biol 2:310–315, 1990.
53. Grossman E, Messerli FH, Grodzicki T, et al: Should a moratorium be placed on sublingual nifedipine capsules given for hypertensive emergencies and pseudoemergencies? JAMA 276:1328–1331, 1996.
54. Hannan EL, Racz M, Ryan TJ, et al: Coronary angioplasty volume-outcome relationships for hospitals and cardiologists. JAMA 277:892–898, 1997.
55. Heiserman JE, Dean BL, Hodak JA, et al: Neurologic complications of cerebral angiography. AJNR Am J Neuroradiol 15:1401–1407, 1994.
56. Henderson MJ, Manhire AR: Cholesterol embolization following angiography. Clin Radiol 42:281–282, 1990.
57. Henry M, Amor M, Ethevenot G, et al: Palmaz stent placement in iliac and femoropopliteal arteries: Primary and secondary patency in 310 patients with 2- to 4-year follow-up. Radiology 197:167–174, 1995.
58. Hertzer NR: Outcome assessment in vascular surgery—results mean everything. J Vasc Surg 21:6–15, 1995.
59. Hessel SJ, Adams DF, Abrams HL: Complications of angiography. Radiology 138:273–281, 1981.
60. Hiatt WR, Hirsch AT, Regensteiner JG, et al: Clinical trials for claudication: Assessment of exercise performance, functional status, and clinical end points: Vascular Clinical Trialists. Circulation 92:614–621, 1995.
61. Hirshfeld EB: From the Office of the General Counsel: Practice parameters and the malpractice liability of physicians. JAMA 263:1556, 1559–1562, 1990.
62. Hoffman AI, Murphy TP: Septic arteritis causing iliac artery rupture and aneurysmal transformation of the distal aorta after iliac artery stent placement. J Vasc Interv Radiol 8:215–219, 1997.
63. Hyams AL, Brandenburg JA, Lipsitz SR, et al: Practice guidelines and malpractice litigation: A two-way street. Ann Intern Med 122:450–455, 1995.
64. Iezzoni LI: The risks of risk adjustment. JAMA 278:1600–1607, 1997.
65. Isner JM, Rosenfield K, Losordo DW, et al: Percutaneous intravascular US as adjunct to catheter-based interventions: Preliminary experience in patients with peripheral vascular disease. Radiology 175:61–70, 1990.
66. Joint Committee on Accreditation of Healthcare Organizations (JCAHO): Monitoring and evaluation of the quality and appropriateness of care: A hospital example. Qual Rev Bull 326–330, 1986.
67. Joint Committee on Accreditation of Healthcare Organizations (JCAHO): Performance improvement in health care. *In* Using Performance Improvement Tools in Health Care Settings. Oakbrook Terrace, Ill, JCAHO, 1996, pp 1–14.
68. Joint Committee on Accreditation of Healthcare Organizations (JCAHO): Medical Staff Standard. Oakbrook Terrace, Ill, The Comprehensive Accreditation Manual for Hospitals 1998; Medical Staff Standard 6.8:MS-79.
69. Johnson KB, Kelly JT, Bierig JR, et al: Legal Implications of Practice Parameters. Chicago, American Medical Association, 1990, p 90.
70. Johnston KW, Rae M, Hogg-Johnston SA, et al: 5-year results of a prospective study of percutaneous transluminal angioplasty. Ann Surg 206:403–413, 1987.
71. Joseph N, Levy E, Lipman S: Angioplasty-related iliac artery rupture: Treatment by temporary balloon occlusion. Cardiovasc Intervent Radiol 10:276–279, 1987.

72. Judkins MP, Gander M: Complications of coronary arteriography. Circulation 49:599–602, 1974.
72a. Kang SS, Labropoulos N, Mansour MA, et al: Percutaneous ultrasound guided thrombin injection: A new method for treating post-catheterization femoral pseudoaneurysms. J Vasc Surg 27:1032–1038, 1998.
73. Kapp MB: 'Cookbook' medicine: A legal perspective. Arch Intern Med 150:496–500, 1990.
74. Karanjia ND, Loosemore TM, Ray SA, et al: The differences in early haemodynamic response between surgery and angioplasty after successful re-opening of the superficial femoral artery. Eur J Vasc Surg 7:717–719, 1993.
75. Kerns SR: Rigors with thrombolysis (Letter). J Vasc Interv Radiol 5:787, 1994.
76. Kimmel SE, Berlin JA, Laskey WK: The relationship between coronary angioplasty procedure volume and major complications. JAMA 274:1137–1142, 1995.
77. Kumpe DA, Durham JD: Complications of regional fibrinolytic therapy. *In* Ansell G, Bettman MA, Kaufman JA, Wilkins RA (eds): Complications in Diagnostic Imaging and Interventional Radiology, 3rd ed. Cambridge, Blackwell Science, Inc, 1996, p 372.
78. Levin DC, Becker GJ, Dorros G, et al: Training standards for physicians performing peripheral angioplasty and other percutaneous peripheral vascular interventions: A statement for health professionals from the Special Writing Group of the Councils on Cardiovascular Radiology, Cardio-Thoracic and Vascular Surgery, and Clinical Cardiology, the American Heart Association. Circulation 86:1348–1350, 1992.
79. Lichtenstein DA, Klapholz L, Vardy DA, et al: Chronic radiodermatitis following cardiac catheterization. Arch Dermatol 132:663–667, 1996.
80. Liu P, Dravid V, Freiman D, et al: Persistent iliac endarteritis with pseudoaneurysm formation following balloon-expandable stent placement. Cardiovasc Intervent Radiol 18:39–42, 1995.
81. Long AL, Sapoval MR, Beyssen BM, et al: Strecker stent implantation in iliac arteries: Patency and predictive factors for long-term success. Radiology 194:739–744, 1995.
82. Lonsdale RJ, Berridge DC, Makin GS, et al: Detection of left heart thrombus by echocardiography is not essential before peripheral arterial thrombolysis. J R Coll Surg Edinb 37:19–22, 1992.
83. Lossef S, Barth K: Incidence of hematomas in contemporary practice of vascular and interventional radiology: Results of the SCVIR contrast registry. Society of Cardiovascular and Interventional Radiology, San Diego, California, March 1994. J Vasc Interv Radiol 5:38, 1994.
84. Mani RL, Eisenberg RL: Complications of catheter cerebral arteriography: Analysis of 5,000 procedures: III. Assessment of arteries injected, contrast medium used, duration of procedure, and age of patient. Am J Roentgenol 131:871–874, 1978.
85. Mani RL, Eisenberg RL, McDonald EJ Jr, et al: Complications of catheter cerebral arteriography: Analysis of 5,000 procedures: I. Criteria and incidence. Am J Roentgenol 131:861–865, 1978.
86. Marin ML, Veith FJ, Panetta TF, et al: Percutaneous transfemoral insertion of a stented graft to repair a traumatic femoral arteriovenous fistula. J Vasc Surg 18:299–302, 1993.
87. Martin EC, Katzen BT, Benenati JF, et al: Multicenter trial of the wall stent in the iliac and femoral arteries. J Vasc Interv Radiol 6:843–849, 1995.
88. Martin M, Fiebach BJ: Short-term ultrahigh streptokinase treatment of chronic arterial occlusions and acute deep vein thromboses. Semin Thromb Hemost 17:21–38, 1991.
89. Marx MV: Radiation exposure in interventional radiology. *In* Ansell G, Bettman MA, Kaufman JA, Wilkins RA (eds): Complications in Diagnostic Imaging and Interventions, 3rd ed. Cambridge, Blackwell Science, Inc, 1996, p 133.
90. Matsumoto AH, Selby JB Jr, Tegtmeyer CJ, et al: Recent development of rigors during infusion of urokinase: Is it related to an endotoxin? J Vasc Interv Radiol 5:433–438, 1994.
91. McCready RA, Siderys H, Pittman JN, et al: Septic complications after cardiac catheterization and percutaneous transluminal coronary angioplasty. J Vasc Surg 14:170–174, 1991.
92. McDaniel MD, MacDonald PD, Mangione TW, et al: Interventionalists' guide to the patient's experience of lower extremity arterial occlusive disease. J Vasc Interv Radiol 6:30S–35S, 1995.
93. McIntyre KEJ, Walser E, Hagman J, et al: Mycotic aneurysm of the common iliac artery and distal aorta following stent placement. Vasc Surg 31:551–557, 1997.
94. McNamara TO, Bomberger RA, Merchant RF: Intra-arterial urokinase as the initial therapy for acutely ischemic lower limbs. Circulation 83:I106–I109, 1991.
95. McNamara TO, Fischer JR: Thrombolysis of peripheral arterial and graft occlusions: Improved results using high-dose urokinase. Am J Roentgenol 144:769–775, 1985.
96. McNamara TO, Goodwin SC, Kandarpa K: Complications of thrombolysis. Semin Interv Radiol 11:134–144, 1994.
97. Messina LM, Brothers TE, Wakefield TW, et al: Clinical characteristics and surgical management of vascular complications in patients undergoing cardiac catheterization: Interventional versus diagnostic procedures. J Vasc Surg 13:593–600, 1991.
98. Mewissen MW, Beres RA, Bessette JC, et al: Kissing-balloon technique for angioplasty of the popliteal artery trifurcation. Am J Roentgenol 156:823–824, 1991.
99. Mewissen MW, Kinney EV, Bandyk DF, et al: The role of duplex scanning versus angiography in predicting outcome after balloon angioplasty in the femoropopliteal artery. J Vasc Surg 15:860–865, 1992.
100. Meyerovitz MF, Goldhaber SZ, Reagan K, et al: Recombinant tissue-type plasminogen activator versus urokinase in peripheral arterial and graft occlusions: A randomized trial. Radiology 175:75–78, 1990.
101. Morgenstern BR, Getrajdman GI, Laffey KJ, et al: Total occlusions of the femoropopliteal artery: High technical success rate of conventional balloon angioplasty. Radiology 172:937–940, 1989.
102. Mossad SB, Longworth DL, Olin JW: Infected pseudoaneurysm at the site of an iliac artery Palmaz stent: Case report and review. J Vasc Med Biol 5:277–281, 1994.
103. Muller DW, Shamir KJ, Ellis SG, et al: Peripheral vascular complications after conventional and complex percutaneous coronary interventional procedures. Am J Cardiol 69:63–68, 1992.
104. Murphy TP: Regarding "Complications of iliac artery stent deployment" (Letter). J Vasc Surg 25:960–961, 1997.
105. Murphy TP, Khwaja AA, Webb MS: Aortoiliac stent placement in patients treated for intermittent claudication. J Vasc Interv Radiol 9:421–428, 1998.
106. Murphy TP, Webb MS, Lambiase RE, et al: Percutaneous revascularization of complex iliac artery stenoses and occlusions with use of wall stents: Three-year experience. J Vasc Interv Radiol 7:21–27, 1996.
107. Nichols D, Goff D, Baker R: Iliac artery rupture during percutaneous angioplasty. Clin Radiol 43:142–145, 1991.
108. NIH Consensus Conference: Thrombolytic therapy in treatment: Summary of an NIH Consensus Conference. Br Med J 280:1585–1587, 1980.
109. Norbash AM, Busick D, Marks MP: Techniques for reducing interventional neuroradiologic skin dose: Tube position rotation and supplemental beam filtration. AJNR Am J Neuroradiol 17:41–49, 1996.
110. Olivecrona H: Complications of cerebral angiography. Neuroradiology 14:175–181, 1977.
111. Ouriel K, Veith FJ, Sasahara AA: Thrombolysis or peripheral arterial surgery: Phase I results: TOPAS Investigators. J Vasc Surg 23:64–73, 1996.
112. Ouriel K, Veith FJ, Sasahara AA: A comparison of recombinant urokinase with vascular surgery as initial treatment for acute arterial occlusion of the legs: Thrombolysis or Peripheral Arterial Surgery (TOPAS) Investigators. N Engl J Med 338:1105–1111, 1998.
113. Palmaz JC, Garcia OJ, Schatz RA, et al: Placement of balloon-expandable intraluminal stents in iliac arteries: First 171 procedures. Radiology 174:969–975, 1990.
114. Palmaz JC, Laborde JC, Rivera FJ, et al: Stenting of the iliac arteries with the Palmaz stent: Experience from a multicenter trial. Cardiovasc Intervent Radiol 15:291–297, 1992.
115. Patel N, Technology Assessment Committee of the SCVIR: Reporting standards for thrombolytic therapy for lower extremity arterial and graft occlusions. J Vasc Interv Radiol (in press).
116. Paulson EK, Miller FJ: Embolization of cardiac mural thrombus: Complication of intraarterial fibrinolysis. Radiology 168:95–96, 1988.
117. Pentecost MJ, Criqui MH, Dorros G, et al: Guidelines for peripheral percutaneous transluminal angioplasty of the abdominal aorta and lower extremity vessels: A statement for health professionals from a special writing group of the Councils on Cardiovascular Radiology,

Arteriosclerosis, Cardio-Thoracic and Vascular Surgery, Clinical Cardiology, and Epidemiology and Prevention, the American Heart Association. Circulation 89:511–531, 1994.

118. Petula SM, Hudacek S: The FemoStop compression device: Utilization guidelines for the critical care nurse. Dimens Crit Care Nurs 14:259–264, 1995.
119. Popma JJ, Satler LF, Pichard AD, et al: Vascular complications after balloon and new device angioplasty. Circulation 88:1569–1578, 1993.
120. Porter JM: Endovascular arterial intervention: Expression of concern. J Vasc Surg 21:995–997, 1995.
121. Quint LE, Holland D, Korobkin M, et al: Role of femoral vessel catheterization and altered hemostasis in the development of extraperitoneal hematomas: CT study in 44 patients. Am J Roentgenol 160:855–858, 1993.
122. Ramirez G, O'Neill WM Jr, Lambert R, et al: Cholesterol embolization: A complication of angiography. Arch Intern Med 138:1430–1432, 1978.
123. Rapoport S, Sniderman KW, Morse SS, et al: Pseudoaneurysm: A complication of faulty technique in femoral arterial puncture. Radiology 154:529–530, 1985.
124. Reyes R, Maynar M, Lopera J, et al: Treatment of chronic iliac artery occlusions with guide wire recanalization and primary stent placement. J Vasc Interv Radiol 8:1049–1055, 1997.
125. Risius B, Graor RA, Geisinger MA, et al: Thrombolytic therapy with recombinant human tissue-type plasminogen activator: A comparison of two doses. Radiology 164:465–468, 1987.
126. Rupp SB, Vogelzang RL, Nemcek AA Jr, et al: Relationship of the inguinal ligament to pelvic radiographic landmarks: Anatomic correlation and its role in femoral arteriography. J Vasc Interv Radiol 4:409–413, 1993.
127. Rutherford RB, Baker JD, Ernst C, et al: Recommended standards for reports dealing with lower extremity ischemia: Revised version. J Vasc Surg 26:517–538, 1997.
128. Sacks D, Marinelli DL, Martin LG, et al: Reporting standards for clinical evaluation of new peripheral arterial revascularization devices: Technology Assessment Committee. J Vasc Interv Radiol 8:137–149, 1997; errata, 8:492, 658, 1997.
129. Sacks D, Robinson ML, Marinelli DL, et al: Evaluation of the peripheral arteries with duplex US after angioplasty. Radiology 176:39–44, 1990.
130. Sacks D, Robinson ML, Summers TA, et al: The value of duplex sonography after peripheral artery angioplasty in predicting subacute restenosis. Am J Roentgenol 162:179–183, 1994.
131. Sakamoto I, Hayashi K, Matsunaga N, et al: Aortic dissection caused by angiographic procedures. Radiology 191:467–471, 1994.
132. Sanchez O, Lewis C, Standards of Practice Committee of the Society of Cardiovascular and Interventional Radiology: Quality improvement guidelines for aorto-iliac arterial stents. J Vasc Interv Radiol (in press).
133. Sande MA, Levinson ME, Lukas DS, et al: Bacteremia associated with cardiac catheterization. N Engl J Med 281:1104–1106, 1969.
134. Sapoval MR, Long AL, Raynaud AC, et al: Femoropopliteal stent placement: Long-term results. Radiology 184:833–839, 1992.
135. Sasahara AA: Prophylaxis with urokinase thrombolysis (Letter). J Vasc Interv Radiol 5:787–788, 1994.
136. SCVIR (Society of Cardiovascular and Interventional Radiology): Credentials criteria for peripheral, renal, and visceral percutaneous transluminal angioplasty. Radiology 167:452, 1988.
136a. Schweizer J, Altmann E, Stosslein F, et al: Comparison of tissue plasminogen activator and urokinase in the local infiltration thrombolysis of peripheral arterial occlusions. Eur J Radiol 22:129–132, 1996.
137. Society of Cardiovascular and Interventional Radiology (SCVIR): Guidelines for establishing a quality assurance program in vascular and interventional radiology. Fairfax, Va, 1989.
138. SCVIR: Guidelines for percutaneous transluminal angioplasty: Standards of Practice Committee of the Society of Cardiovascular and Interventional Radiology. J Vasc Interv Radiol 1:5–15, 1990.
139. SCVIR: Standard for diagnostic arteriography in adults: Standards of Practice Committee of the Society of Cardiovascular and Interventional Radiology. J Vasc Interv Radiol 4:385–395, 1993.
140. Semler HJ: Transfemoral catheterization: Mechanical versus manual control of bleeding. Radiology 154:234–235, 1985.
141. Shawker TH, Kluge RM, Ayella RJ: Bacteremia associated with angiography. JAMA 229:1090–1092, 1974.
142. Shope TB: Radiation-induced skin injuries from fluoroscopy. Radiographics 16:1195–1196, 1996.
143. Sigstedt B, Lunderquist A: Complications of angiographic examinations. Am J Roentgenol 130:455–460, 1978.
143a. Singh H: Quality improvement guidelines for diagnostic arteriography. J Vasc Interv Radiol (in press).
144. Skalpe IO: Complications in cerebral angiography with iohexol (Omnipaque) and meglumine metrizoate (Isopaque cerebral). Neuroradiology 30:69–72, 1988.
145. Smith CM, Yellin AE, Weaver FA, et al: Thrombolytic therapy for arterial occlusion: A mixed blessing. Am Surg 60:371–375, 1994.
146. Smith T, Cragg AH: Non-surgical treatment of iliac artery rupture following angioplasty. J Interv Radiol 4:16–18, 1989.
147. Spies JB: Malpractice, risk management, and quality improvement in radiology. *In* Ansell G, Bettman MA, Kaufman JA, Wilkins RA (eds): Complications in Diagnostic Imaging and Interventional Radiology, 3rd ed. Cambridge, Blackwell Science, Inc, 1996, p 631.
148. Spittell JA Jr, Nanda NC, Creager MA, et al: Recommendations for peripheral transluminal angioplasty: Training and facilities: American College of Cardiology Peripheral Vascular Disease Committee. J Am Coll Cardiol 21:546–548, 1993.
149. STILE Investigators: Results of a prospective randomized trial evaluating surgery versus thrombolysis for ischemia of the lower extremity: The STILE trial. Ann Surg 220:251–266, 1994.
150. Strecker EP, Boos IB, Gottmann D: Femoropopliteal artery stent placement: Evaluation of long-term success. Radiology 205:375–383, 1997.
151. Sullivan TM, Childs MB, Bacharach JM, et al: Percutaneous transluminal angioplasty and primary stenting of the iliac arteries in 288 patients. J Vasc Surg 25:829–838, 1997.
152. Swann HK: Cooperative study on cardiac catheterization: Infectious, inflammatory, and allergic complications. Circulation 37:1–101, 1968.
153. TASC (TransAtlantic Inter-Society Consensus) on the Management of PAOD (Peripheral Arterial Occlusive Disease) (in press).
154. Tetteroo E, Haaring C, van der Graaf Y, et al: Intraarterial pressure gradients after randomized angioplasty or stenting of iliac artery lesions: Dutch Iliac Stent Trial Study Group. Cardiovasc Intervent Radiol 19:411–417, 1996.
155. Tetteroo E, van Engelen AD, Spithoven JH, et al: Stent placement after iliac angioplasty: Comparison of hemodynamic and angiographic criteria: Dutch Iliac Stent Trial Study Group. Radiology 201:155–159, 1996.
156. Therasse E, Soulez G, Cartier P, et al: Infection with fatal outcome after endovascular metallic stent placement. Radiology 192:363–365, 1994.
157. Toursarkissian B, Allen BT, Petrinec D, et al: Spontaneous closure of selected iatrogenic pseudoaneurysms and arteriovenous fistulae. J Vasc Surg 25:803–808, 1997.
158. Trerotola SO, Kuhlman JE, Fishman EK: Bleeding complications of femoral catheterization: CT evaluation. Radiology 174:37–40, 1990.
159. Ullrich C, Moore A, Parsons R: The arteriographic diagnosis of extracranial cerebrovascular disease. *In* Robicsek F (ed): Extracranial Cerebrovascular Disease: Diagnosis and Management. New York, Macmillan, Inc, 1986, pp 108–140.
160. van Harten J, Burggraaf K, Danhof M, et al: Negligible sublingual absorption of nifedipine. Lancet 2:1363–1365, 1987.
161. Veith FJ, Marin ML: Endovascular technology and its impact on the relationships among vascular surgeons, interventional radiologists, and other specialists. World J Surg 20:687–691, 1996.
162. Vitek JJ: Femoro-cerebral angiography: Analysis of 2,000 consecutive examinations, special emphasis on carotid arteries catheterization in older patients. Am J Roentgenol Radium Ther Nucl Med 118:633–647, 1973.
163. Vorwerk D, Guenther RW: Mechanical revascularization of occluded iliac arteries with use of self-expandable endoprostheses. Radiology 175:411–415, 1990.
164. Vorwerk D, Guenther RW, Schurmann K, et al: Primary stent placement for chronic iliac artery occlusions: Follow-up results in 103 patients. Radiology 194:745–749, 1995.
165. Vorwerk D, Gunther RW, Schurmann K, et al: Aortic and iliac stenoses: Follow-up results of stent placement after insufficient balloon angioplasty in 118 cases. Radiology 198:45–48, 1996.
166. Wagner LK, Eifel PJ, Geise RA: Potential biological effects following high x-ray dose interventional procedures. J Vasc Interv Radiol 5:71–84, 1994.

167. Wallace S, Medellin H, De Jongh D, et al: Systemic heparinization for angiography. Am J Roentgenol Radium Ther Nucl Med 116:204–209, 1972.
168. Waugh JR, Sacharias N: Arteriographic complications in the DSA era. Radiology 182:243–246, 1992.
169. Weitz JI, Byrne J, Clagett GP, et al: Diagnosis and treatment of chronic arterial insufficiency of the lower extremities: A critical review. Circulation 94:3026–3049, 1996.
170. Wexler L, Dorros G, Levin D, et al: Guidelines for performance of peripheral percutaneous transluminal angioplasty: The Society for Cardiac Angiography and Interventions, Interventional Cardiology Committee, Subcommittee on Peripheral Interventions. Cathet Cardiovasc Diagn 21:128–129, 1990.
171. White RA, Fogarty TJ, Baker WH, et al: Endovascular surgery credentialing and training for vascular surgeons. J Vasc Surg 17:1095–1102, 1993.
172. Wilkinson LS, Wilkins RA: Complications of percutaneous angioplasty. *In* Ansell G, Bettman MA, Kaufman JA, Wilkins RA (eds): Complications in Diagnostic Imaging and Interventional Radiology, 3rd ed. Cambridge, Blackwell Science Inc, 1996, p 346.
173. Williams JB, Watts PW, Nguyen VA, et al: Balloon angioplasty with intraluminal stenting as the initial treatment modality in aorto-iliac occlusive disease. Am J Surg 168:202–204, 1994.
174. Woolf SH: Practice guidelines, a new reality in medicine: II. Methods of developing guidelines. Arch Intern Med 152:946–952, 1992.
175. Working Party on Thrombolysis in the Management of Limb Ischemia: Thrombolysis in the management of lower limb peripheral arterial occlusion—a consensus document. Am J Cardiol 81:207–218, 1998.
176. Wu AW: The measure and mismeasure of hospital quality: Appropriate risk-adjustment methods in comparing hospitals. Ann Intern Med 122:149–150, 1995.
177. Zahn R, Thoma S, Fromm E, et al: Do 5-F catheters reduce the incidence of a pseudoaneurysm? Int Angiol 15:257–260, 1996.

SECTION VIII

ACUTE ISCHEMIA AND ITS SEQUELAE

KENNETH OURIEL, M.D.

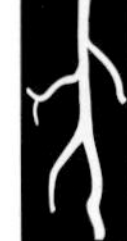

CHAPTER 54

Acute Limb Ischemia

Kenneth Ouriel, M.D.

Acute limb ischemia is one of the most challenging problems encountered by the contemporary vascular practitioner. Its incidence approximates 1.7 cases per 10,000 population per year.[1] Blaisdell and colleagues,[2] in a review of 35 series published after the advent of the balloon thromboembolectomy catheter, documented a mortality rate of 26% and an amputation rate of 37% in more than 3000 cases of acute peripheral arterial thrombosis or embolism. Despite improvements in patient care and operative technique, the morbidity and mortality remain high, with mortality rates in excess of 25% and amputation in 20% of the survivors.[3] Clearly, the morbidity of acute limb ischemia cannot be solely attributable to the ischemia itself; these patients usually present in a severely compromised state as a result of coexistent medical illnesses (Table 54–1). This feature, in part, explains the high rate of morbidity and mortality of acute limb ischemia.

The ischemic process begins with thrombosis of a peripheral artery or bypass graft. The inciting event may be embolism or thrombosis. The process can develop slowly, with gradual progression of an arterial lesion to hemodynamic significance and finally occlusion. In these cases, collateral channels will have had time to develop and patients describe the insidious onset of claudication symptoms. When the process develops rapidly, as in the case of embolization or graft thrombosis, patients present with signs and symptoms of severe ischemia. Pain at rest, mottling or cyanosis of the skin, and sensorimotor changes are common. Patients with such severe symptoms tend to present early, whereas patients with claudication may wait weeks or months before seeking medical advice.

PATHOPHYSIOLOGY

Severe hypoperfusion of a limb, if left untreated, inevitably progresses to tissue infarction and irreversible cell death. Distinct cells have widely varying tolerances to ischemia, tolerances that are dependent on the metabolic rate of the particular cell type. For example, the brain and heart are especially vulnerable to hypoxia because of their high oxygen requirements. Cerebral infarction can occur after just 4 to 6 minutes of total ischemia. Peripheral nerves and muscle, although not as sensitive as the brain and heart, are much more vulnerable than skin and subcutaneous tissue. Histologic changes are observed after only 4 hours of warm ischemia, and irreversible infarction may develop within 6 hours. This critical period, however, is highly dependent on the presence of collateral circulation around

TABLE 54–1. MEDICAL CO-MORBIDITIES IN PATIENTS PRESENTING WITH ACUTE LIMB ISCHEMIA

	TRIAL			
CO-MORBIDITY	Rochester	TOPAS-I	TOPAS-II	Total/Weighted Average
No. of patients	114	213	544	871
Cerebrovascular disease	NR	15.4%	11.5%	11.6%
Congestive heart failure	NR	15.5%	12.5%	13.3%
Coronary artery disease	56.1%	47.1%	42.5%	45.4%
Diabetes mellitus	28.1%	36.7%	29.0%	30.8%
Hypercholesterolemia	31.6%	29.6%	23.5%	26.0%
Hypertension	63.2%	60.9%	59.5%	60.3%
Malignancy	NR	11.9%	11.5%	11.6%
Tobacco history	51.8%	79.3%	77.5%	74.6%

NR = not reported; TOPAS = Thrombolysis Or Peripheral Arterial Surgery.

the occluded vascular segment.[4] Skin and subcutaneous tissue are relatively resistant to hypoxia and will survive periods of ischemia that the underlying muscle and nerve do not, occasionally resulting in a limb with surface viability in the presence of complete functional loss (Fig. 54–1).

The canine gracilis muscle preparation is an excellent experimental model of complete muscle ischemia. The muscle is isolated, leaving only the nutrient artery and draining vein attached. Muscle damage is studied using technetium 99m (^{99m}Tc) pyrophosphate as a marker of cell death. Using this model, Blebea and colleagues[5] studied the effects of the duration of ischemia on muscle viability. After 4 hours of ischemia, the amount of ^{99m}Tc-pyrophosphate accumulation was only slightly greater than control but rose to more than twice the control level at 6 hours and more than four times the control level at 8 hours.[5]

Three pathophysiologic events occur during acute arterial occlusion, each of which worsens the ischemic insult and decreases the chance of reversing the process. First, the arterial thrombus may propagate, occluding the orifices of collateral side branches and, eventually, the collaterals themselves. Second, the ischemic tissues accumulate fluid and swell, leading to compression of the vascular channels within a tight fascial compartment, the so-called compartment syndrome. Third, the cells of the small vessels become edematous, causing significant narrowing of the lumen and obstruction of the arterioles, capillaries, and venules.

Occlusion of the microvasculature after large vessel revascularization is responsible for the "no reflow" phenomenon, a term coined to characterize the clinical paradigm of absent distal perfusion despite an apparently successful revascularization procedure. Urokinase, administered prior to reperfusion in the dog gracilis muscle preparation, resulted in a significant reduction in the percent of muscle infarcted and the amount of muscular edema, presumably (although not demonstrated statistically) as a result of improved postischemic blood flow.[6]

Ischemic injury is not limited to the damage that occurs during the period of hypoperfusion. Additional injury develops during the initial period of reperfusion ("reperfusion injury"), as highly active oxygen metabolites such as the superoxide (O^{-}_{2}) and hydroxyl (OH•) radicals accumulate and compound the cellular insult.[7] Free radical scavengers, such as mannitol and superoxide dismutase, have been shown experimentally to be partially protective against reperfusion injury when administered prior to restoration of arterial flow.[8] A period of controlled, slow reperfusion may diminish tissue damage. In an amputated rat hindlimb model, controlled reperfusion over a protracted period of time was associated with improved postischemic muscle function and a decrease in the amount of edema.[9] Some have suggested that controlled reperfusion is an advantage of thrombolytic therapy, in contrast to the sudden reperfusion associated with surgical revascularization.[10] This contention, although well demonstrated in cardiac tissue, remains unproved in the periphery.

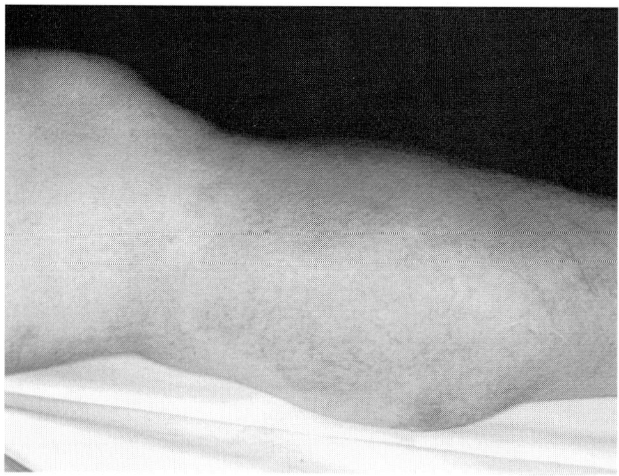

FIGURE 54–1. Calf of a patient after successful reperfusion of an acute superficial femoral artery occlusion. The skin was viable, but the underlying muscle was edematous and partially necrotic. An above-knee amputation was necessary despite the presence of open large vessels.

Reperfusion of an ischemic extremity may be associated with systemic effects in addition to the aforementioned local abnormalities. Acid, potassium, and cardiodepressants such as thromboxane accumulate in the ischemic limb and are discharged systemically on reperfusion.[11] In 1960, Haimovici[12] described the association of acute muscle infarction, myoglobinuria, and renal failure. A decade later, the systemic consequences of reperfusion were more extensively studied by Fisher, Fogarty, and Morrow[13] when they described the biochemical consequences of embolic occlusion of the femoral artery. These investigators sampled the femoral venous effluent following reperfusion, comparing the values with those collected from the systemic venous blood. There was a significantly higher amount of potassium and a lower pH in the venous blood after reperfusion. These observations explain the appearance of sudden cardiac arrhythmias after reperfusion of the legs after removal of a large embolus.[14]

ETIOLOGY OF ACUTE LIMB ISCHEMIA

Acute limb ischemia can be grouped into two distinct etiologic categories: *thrombosis* and *embolism*. Acute *traumatic* occlusions are associated with sudden, profound ischemia caused by the lack of collateral channels. Traumatic injuries are not discussed further in this chapter. *Nontraumatic* thromboses almost always develop in the setting of an underlying lesion in a native artery or bypass graft. In contrast, embolic events generally occur in normal vessels that merely represent the depository for thrombotic material originating from a distant site. These etiologic features of thrombotic versus embolic events hold important implications that determine the rapidity of symptom onset, the severity of the process, and the most appropriate intervention to achieve limb salvage. Although the distinction between thrombotic and embolic etiology is fraught with inaccuracies, recent series suggest that thrombotic occlusions outnumber embolic occlusions by a ratio of almost 6:1.[15] Bypass graft thrombosis appears to present slightly more often than native artery occlusion by a ratio of approximately 5:4.

Native Arterial Thrombosis

Thrombosis of a native arterial segment usually represents the final stage in the progression of an atherothrombotic arterial lesion. Atheromatous plaques develop at predictable locations within the peripheral arterial tree. The distal aorta, iliac system, and popliteal bifurcation are frequent sites of atherosclerotic disease, but the femoral artery at the adductor canal is probably the most common location for the development of a symptomatic peripheral arterial lesion. Zarins and associates[16] observed an equal distribution of atherosclerotic disease along the length of the femoral artery. They suggested that the normal process of arterial dilatation in response to the deposition of atheroma is blunted at the adductor canal, which might explain the preponderance of stenotic lesions at this level.

The progression from a mild atherosclerotic lesion to vessel occlusion begins with the slow deposition of lipids in the intimal layer of the artery. Over time, calcium is deposited within the lesion, and the lipid-calcium concretion represents the "atherosclerotic core." Initially, the atherosclerotic core is isolated from the vessel lumen by a "fibrous cap."[17] The integrity of the fibrous cap may become disrupted, possibly in conjunction with chemotaxis of macrophages and alterations in the levels of metalloproteinase, enzymes with activity directed against the components of the fibrous cap.[18] The atheromatous core is the most thrombogenic component of the atherosclerotic lesion, and exposure of the core can result in rapid progression from stenosis to occlusion.[19] This progression is correlated with the thickness of the cap; coronary arteries have been found to be at greatest risk for thrombosis when the cap is very thin. The risk of occlusion may actually be more dependent on the thickness of the fibrous cap than the arteriographic severity (per cent diameter reduction) of the lesion; these mechanisms explain why sudden occlusion may develop in mildly stenotic lesions of 50% diameter reduction or less.

Occasionally, native artery thrombosis occurs in the absence of a preexisting stenotic lesion (Fig. 54–2). This scenario should prompt a thorough search for a hypercoagulable disorder. Subclinical endothelial disintegrity from minor trauma or early atherosclerosis may underlie the occlusive event even in these patients.

Bypass Graft Thrombosis

With the increasing application of bypass graft procedures for symptomatic peripheral arterial disease, graft thrombosis is becoming the most common cause of acute lower extremity ischemia. Autogenous grafts fail in association with an anastomotic lesion of intimal hyperplasia or a fibrotic valve within the body of the graft itself (Fig. 54–3).[20] By contrast, an underlying lesion may not be detected when a prosthetic graft occludes. Whether this observation relates to the inherent thrombogenicity of the foreign material (Fig. 54–4), kinking of the graft as it crosses a joint, or the inadequacies in present imaging technology remains undetermined.

Embolic Occlusion

Peripheral arterial embolism (see Chapter 55) is responsible for the sudden onset of profound ischemia as a result of a paucity of preexisting collateral vessels. Emboli almost always lodge at arterial bifurcations, obstructing flow into two parallel channels and compounding the problem. The differentiation between emboli and in situ thrombosis is sometimes difficult, but the presence of normal peripheral pulses in the contralateral extremity and a history of cardiac arrhythmia are clues to an embolic event.

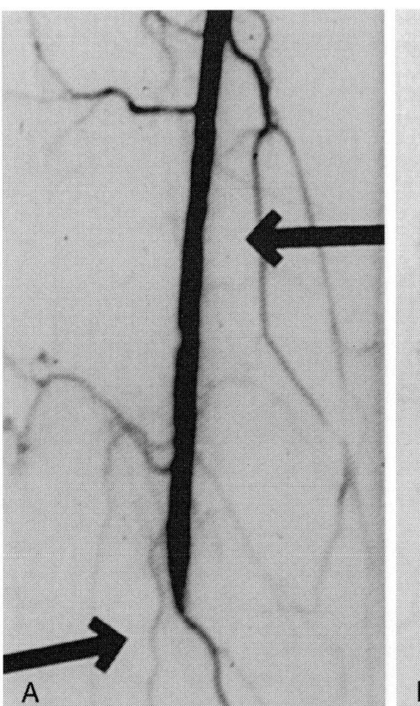

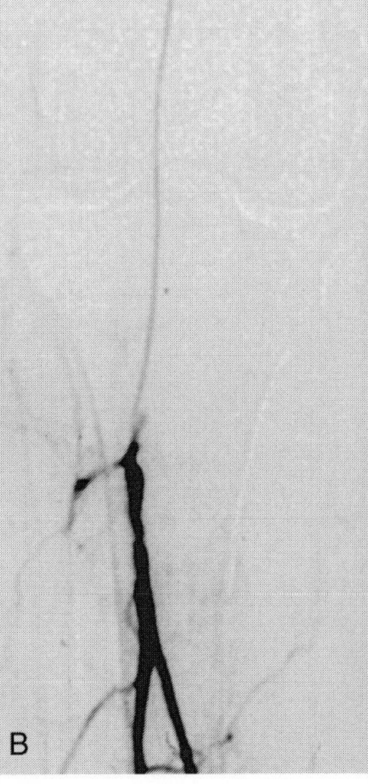

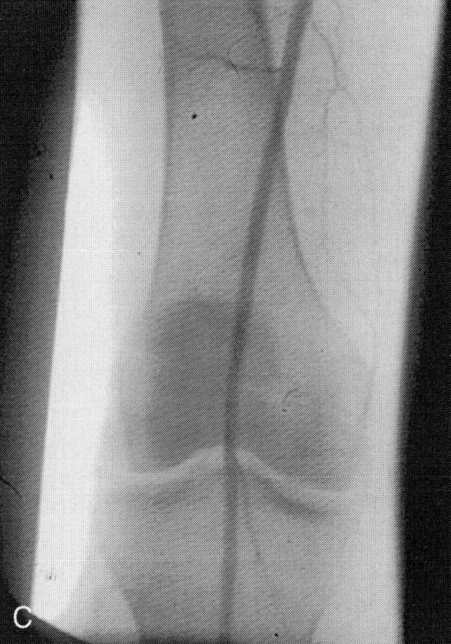

FIGURE 54–2. Acute occlusion of the popliteal artery. *A,* A relatively normal distal superficial femoral and proximal popliteal artery *(top arrow),* terminating abruptly at a medial geniculate artery. *B,* Outflow into an open tibioperoneal trunk vessel with some mural thrombus present. The anterior tibial artery is occluded. *C,* After 20 hours of urokinase thrombolysis, the popliteal artery is completely open, without evidence of an underlying arterial lesion to explain the acute event. The patient had elevated anticardiolipin antibody titers on laboratory evaluation, indicative of the antiphospholipid syndrome.

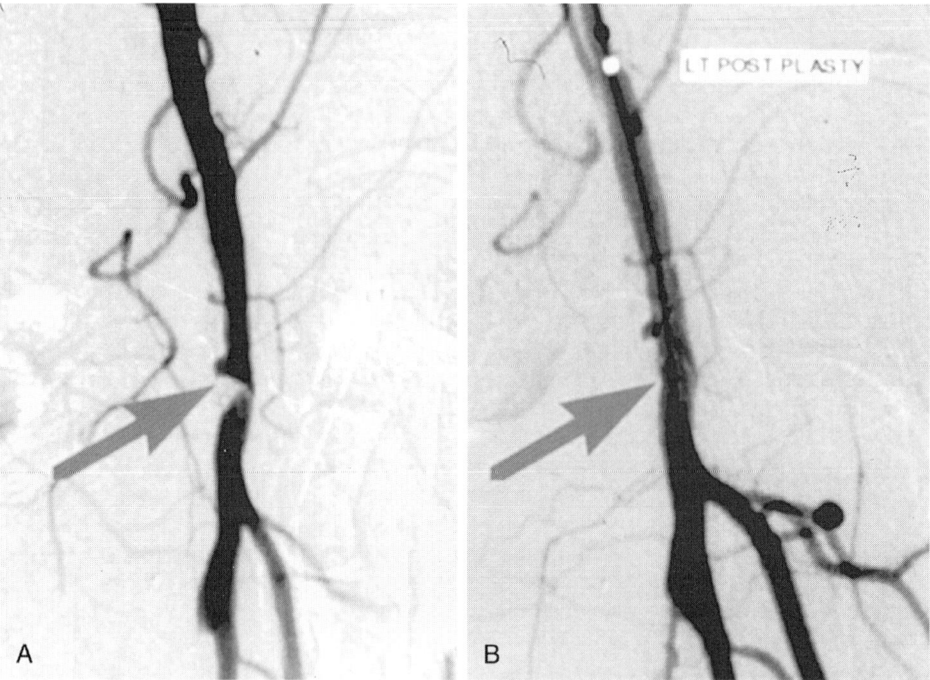

FIGURE 54–3. Occlusion of a recently placed femoropopliteal vein graft. *A*, The diagnostic arteriogram revealed a tight stenosis of the common femoral artery, probably representing a clamp injury that occurred at the time of the procedure. The lesion was thought to be a likely etiologic factor in graft occlusion. *B*, The lesion was treated with a balloon angioplasty prior to thrombolysis of the vein graft.

Other Causes

Patients with severe low-flow states arising from entities such as cardiogenic shock or systemic sepsis often present with acute ischemia of the lower extremities. Drugs such as cocaine or vasopressors may be associated with such intense arterial spasm that the extremity becomes acutely ischemic. The process is almost always bilateral and is usually limited to distalmost aspects of the extremity, beginning with cyanotic discoloration of the toes that may rapidly progress to gangrene of the forefoot. Similar findings in the fingers frequently accompany the lower extremity problems.

Vasculitides represent a rare cause of acute arterial occlusion. Takayasu's arteritis, although most commonly encountered in the aortic branch vessels to the upper extremities, may also occur in the abdominal aorta and lower extremity vessels.[21, 22] Hypercoagulable states associated with malignancy, the antiphospholipid syndrome, activated protein C resistance (either from factor V Leiden mutation or the idiopathic variety), protein C or S deficiency, and antithrombin III deficiency may be associated with acute arterial thrombosis in the absence of demonstrable arterial pathology.

CLINICAL CLASSIFICATION AND DIAGNOSIS

Patients with acute occlusion of a lower extremity artery experience symptoms of a degree that is dependent on the

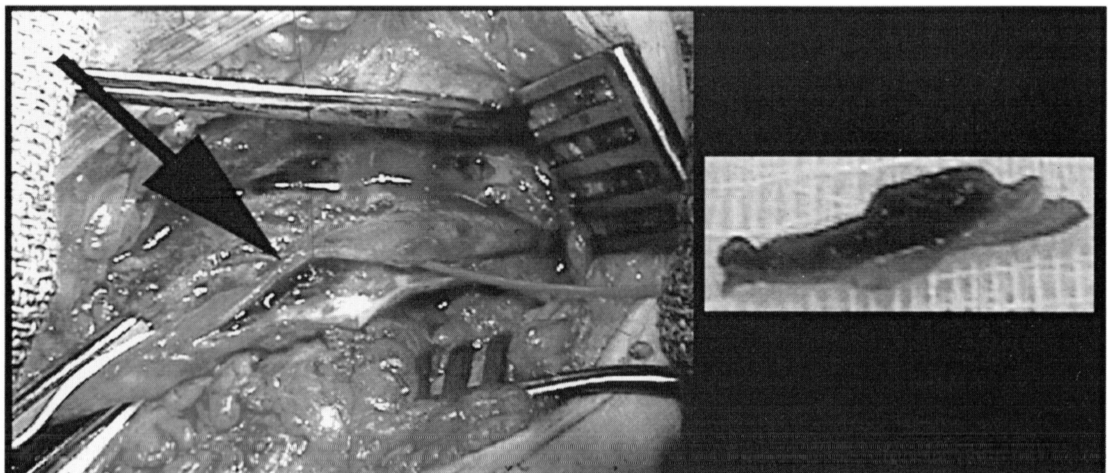

FIGURE 54–4. An occluded expanded polytetrafluoroethylene graft that was successfully recanalized with urokinase thrombolysis. A mural thrombus *(arrow)* was adherent to the wall of the graft. The material was granular in appearance *(inset)*, suggestive of a high platelet content.

TABLE 54–2. CLINICAL CATEGORIES OF ACUTE LIMB ISCHEMIA

CATEGORY	DESCRIPTION	FINDINGS		DOPPLER SIGNALS	
		Sensory Loss	Muscle Weakness	Arterial	Venous
I. Viable	Not immediately threatened	None	None	+	+
II. Threatened					
a. Marginally	Salvageable with prompt treatment	Minimal (toes)	None	–	+
b. Immediately	Salvageable with immediate treatment	More than toes, rest pain	Mild to moderate	–	+
III. Irreversible	Major permanent tissue loss	Anesthetic	Paralysis	–	–

From Rutherford RB, Baker JD, Ernst C, et al: Recommended standards for reports dealing with lower extremity ischemia: Revised version. J Vasc Surg 26:517–538, 1998.

anatomic extent of the process and the ability of parallel, collateral channels to compensate for the reduction in arterial blood flow. Thus, a patient with acute occlusion of the femoral artery with an underlying stenosis at the adductor canal is likely to experience symptoms of claudication alone. As such, the onset may be insidious and a considerable duration may elapse before the patient seeks medical advice. Unlike thrombotic occlusions, emboli to the common femoral bifurcation are almost always associated with the rapid onset of severe ischemia of the entire extremity. The obstruction of blood flow into the deep and superficial femoral systems and the lack of preexisting collateral channels account for this presentation. In these cases, irreversible tissue infarction results if revascularization is not promptly accomplished.

The "six P's" characterize the signs and symptoms of acute ischemia; pulselessness, pallor, pain, coolness (poikilothermia), paresthesia, and paralysis. Whereas patients with mild ischemia experience claudication symptoms alone, patients with severely diminished blood flow experience rapid progression to muscle infarction and rigor. The variability in describing and reporting the signs and symptoms of acute leg ischemia led to the formulation of standards for dealing with lower extremity ischemia. The Joint Council of The Society for Vascular Surgery and the North American Chapter of the International Society for Cardiovascular Surgery developed reporting standards for lower extremity ischemia, the revised version of which was published in 1997.[23] Limb ischemia is stratified into three categories of severity (Table 54–2).

Category I limbs are viable and are not immediately threatened. Examples might include the sudden onset of severe claudication in a patient with an acute femoral artery thrombosis overlying a chronic stenosis and abundant collaterals.

Category II includes those limbs with threatened viability but in which amputation may be averted if revascularization is undertaken in a timely manner. This category has been subdivided into IIa and IIb, differentiated by the requirement for *prompt* treatment in category IIa versus *immediate* treatment in IIb. For instance, a patient with acute occlusion of a femoropopliteal graft associated with mild forefoot numbness falls into category IIa. By contrast, a similar patient who experiences rest pain, diminished sensation of the entire foot, and calf muscle weakness falls within category IIb.

Patients with *category III* ischemia, by definition, suffer profound, permanent neuromuscular damage, irrespective of therapy. Major amputation is the only option.

An examination of the peripheral pulses provides clues to both the etiology and localization of the occlusive process (Table 54–3). Patients with common femoral emboli manifest easily palpable femoral pulses, often with a "water-hammer" character representing the rapid upstroke and downstroke associated with outflow obstruction. The semiliquid consistency of the fresh thrombus preserves a palpable femoral pulse early on; only when the thrombus becomes densely compacted does the pulse disappear. Emboli to the femoral artery may be differentiated from thrombosis by palpation of the vessel itself. A soft, rubbery consistency, occasionally accompanied by tenderness along the course of the vessel, suggests embolism, whereas a rocky, calcific contour is most common when thrombosis overlies chronic atherosclerotic disease.

TABLE 54–3. ARTERIAL OBSTRUCTION THROUGH PALPATION OF PERIPHERAL PULSES

PULSES PALPABLE				
Femoral	Popliteal	Pedal	LOCATION	POSSIBLE CAUSE
–	–	–	Aortoiliac segment	1. Aortoiliac atherosclerosis; 2. embolus to common iliac bifurcation
+	–	–	Femoral segment	1. Thrombosis, femoral atherosclerosis; 2. common femoral embolus
+	+ +	–	Distal popliteal ± tibials	Popliteal aneurysm with embolization
+	+	–	Distal popliteal ± tibials	1. Popliteal embolus; 2. popliteal/tibial atherosclerosis, diabetic

Doppler segmental pressures play a very useful role in objectively documenting the severity of the arterial occlusion. Examination at the ankle level should include a search for audible signals in the veins as well as the arteries, because the most severe ischemia is associated with a loss of flow in both the venous and arterial segments. When Doppler arterial signals are audible, an ankle-brachial pressure index should be measured. Next, segmental pressure measurements should be obtained, with an appropriate-sized pneumatic cuff placed below the knee, above the knee, and at high thigh levels. A pressure drop of 30 mmHg between two adjacent levels accurately identifies the site of the most proximal occlusion.

Duplex ultrasonography can be used to localize the site of occlusion, imaging the common femoral, superficial femoral, and popliteal vessels. The diagnosis of bypass graft occlusion is easily confirmed using the duplex instrument, and emboli at the common femoral or popliteal level are readily imaged. In addition, duplex can be used to guide access to a thrombosed bypass graft when the origin of the graft is poorly visualized at the time of arteriography.

Contrast arteriography remains the "gold standard" for the diagnosis and localization of acute arterial occlusion. Previously, it was common practice to bring these patients directly to operation, without an arteriogram. More recently, preoperative arteriography has been recommended in virtually all patients.[24] An exception to this rule is the patient with a classic presentation for a femoral embolus; in these instances, arteriography is sometimes forgone in favor of immediate operative embolectomy.

The initial diagnostic arteriogram should be performed from a site distant to the arterial occlusion, usually through the contralateral femoral artery. The use of a distant site allows the safe administration of a thrombolytic agent, minimizing the risk of bleeding from dissolution of the fibrin at the site of arterial access, both surrounding the catheter or sheath as well as through inadvertent needle holes created at the time of initial cannulation. A brachial approach is acceptable in cases of bilateral iliac occlusion and absent femoral pulses. The diagnostic film should include the entire abdominal aorta, iliac arteries, and infrainguinal vessels to the level of the feet. Digital subtraction images are used in most centers, minimizing the contrast load. Carbon dioxide has been used as a substitute contrast agent in patients with renal failure or contraindications to the use of standard agents.[25, 26] Although carbon dioxide arteriography provides acceptable images, especially in the infrainguinal vessels, the present technology yields films of inferior quality to those obtained with the use of standard contrast material.

The arteriogram is evaluated for the location of the occlusion and the presence of associated arterial disease. The arteriogram helps to determine the cause of the occlusion. For instance, a popliteal artery occlusion in the presence of medial displacement of a patent contralateral popliteal artery cinches the diagnosis of popliteal artery entrapment as the etiologic problem. Similarly, popliteal artery occlusion with a popliteal aneurysm in the open contralateral vessel suggests that the occlusion is a result of aneurysm thrombosis. Rare causes of ischemia, such as vasculitis, arterial dissection, and low-flow states, may be identified.

It is important to note that the arteriographic differentiation between an embolic or thrombotic cause cannot always be made with certainty. Nevertheless, localized thrombus at an arterial bifurcation, filling defects in multiple arterial beds, and normal adjacent and contralateral vasculature are all consistent with embolic occlusion. In addition to providing clues to the cause of the occlusion, the diagnostic arteriogram can provide useful information about the status of the proximal and distal vessels, information that is of great importance when planning a revascularization procedure. The arteriogram, however, is not the most sensitive test for the identification of lesions responsible for the occlusive event. Intravascular ultrasonography, in our experience, is associated with far greater sensitivity for the detection of otherwise occult bypass graft stenoses.

TREATMENT

Amputation was the only treatment available for ischemia of the lower extremity until just five decades ago. Dos Santos[27] is credited with pioneering lower extremity revascularization when he performed the first femoral endarterectomy to restore adequate arterial perfusion to the leg. Thereafter, saphenous vein bypass attained popularity and became the treatment of choice for long occlusions.[28] With improvements in operative technique, bypass to the tibial and even the inframalleolar arteries of the foot became feasible, with patency rates of more than 70% 5 years following the procedure. The treatment of lower extremity vascular disease was quite simple: embolectomy for localized embolic events and thrombectomy and bypass graft placement or revision for thrombotic occlusions.

Following Blaisdell's series of excess cardiopulmonary mortality with immediate operation, a policy of high-dose heparin therapy and delayed operative revascularization became popular. Delayed operative revascularization was actually recommended by Couch and colleagues[28a] more than a decade prior to the Blaisdell report.[2] After observing a 75% early graft failure rate in patients with recent femoropopliteal occlusions, the authors advocated deferring vascular repair whenever possible. These data, however, are not representative of recent series. Innovations in operative technique and patient care are responsible for improved outcome. Presently, limb salvage is achieved in 70% to 80% of patients, although early operative mortality rates still average 15% or more.[15, 29]

An interesting trend emerged in the surgical treatment of acute bypass graft occlusion. Thrombectomy of the graft, usually with patch angioplasty of the distal anastomosis, was formerly a well-accepted and widely performed method of treating graft occlusion.[30, 31] More recently, replacement of the bypass graft is preferred if an adequate length of appropriate conduit is available.[32] For example, optimal treatment of an occluded prosthetic femoropopliteal graft is insertion of a new saphenous vein graft rather than thrombectomy and revision of the old conduit.

As an alternative to open surgical revascularization, thrombolytic therapy was entertained when, in the mid-1950s, investigators such as Tillet and associates[33] and Clifton[34] separately reported preliminary results using streptokinase in patients with arterial occlusion. Dotter and coworkers[35] popularized the intra-arterial route for thrombolytic infusion, administering the agent directly into the thrombus. McNamara and Fischer[36] used a relatively high dose of thrombolytic agent to dissolve arterial thrombus, popularizing a "graded" infusion of intra-arterial urokinase, administered in a stepwise, decreasing dose. Generally, infusions of 4000 IU/min were continued until antegrade blood flow through the thrombus was achieved. Thereafter, urokinase was continued at 1000 IU/min until complete dissolution was accomplished. Frequent, serial arteriography guided advancement of the catheter to keep the infusion within the substance of the thrombus. Successful thrombolysis was achieved in 77% of 100 infusions, with infusion periods averaging 18 hours.[37]

Today, the technique of thrombolysis has undergone minor, yet important modifications from the original protocols of McNamara. The advent of multiple side-hole catheters allows more efficient infusion of thrombolytic agent into a long length of thrombus. The "infusion guide wire" further increases the length over which thrombolytic infusion may be administered. These guide wires can be placed through the multiple side-hole catheter in a "coaxial" fashion such that even some of the longest bypass grafts can undergo continuous infusion of thrombolytic agent along their entire length. This method of infusion obviates the need for frequent arteriograms and catheter repositioning.

Multicenter thrombolytic trials have confirmed the safety of a dose of 4000 IU/min of urokinase, decreasing to 2000 IU/minute after 4 hours and continuing at that rate until complete dissolution of the thrombus is accomplished.[15, 38] Urokinase, recombinant tissue plasminogen activator (rt-PA), and reteplase are the most commonly employed thrombolytic agents for peripheral vascular indications in the United States, and thrombolysis may be considered a "standard of care" for patients with acute arterial occlusions. Thrombolysis allows one to identify the lesion responsible for the occlusive event (Fig. 54–5), providing the opportunity to directly address this lesion with an operation or endovascular procedure that may be a great deal less invasive than would otherwise have been required.[15]

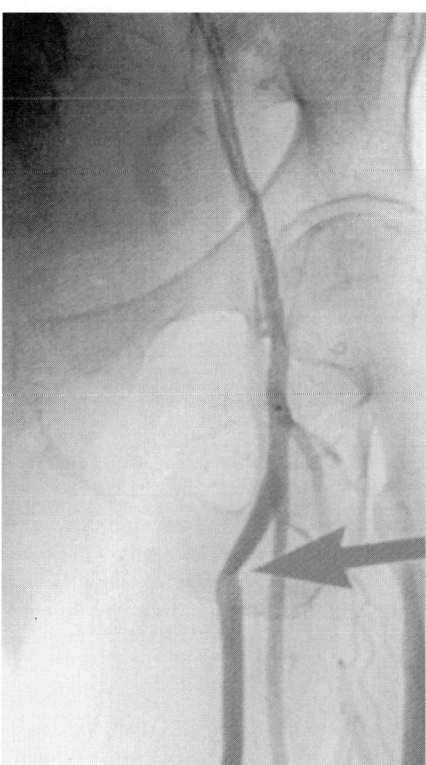

FIGURE 54–5. After successful urokinase thrombolysis, a kink of an expanded polytetrafluoroethylene femoropopliteal graft was uncovered. This technical error was likely responsible for the graft failure.

Patient Subgroups Appropriate for Thrombolysis

Logically, patients with acute limb ischemia represent the most ideal patient subgroup for thrombolysis. Perioperative mortality rates are highest in those patients with the most severe ischemia, and it is within this category that a thrombolytic treatment strategy has been shown to increase survival. In a study of patients presenting within 1 week of symptom onset, the Rochester trial of urokinase versus surgery documented a lower mortality rate in the patients randomized to the thrombolytic group.[39] This benefit appeared to be related to a decreased incidence of cardiopulmonary complications when immediate surgery was avoided. Although adjuvant surgical procedures were necessary to correct unmasked lesions in more than two thirds of the patients randomized to thrombolysis, the procedures that followed successful thrombolysis were often of a lesser magnitude of severity and were performed electively with a well-prepared patient.

Some multicenter trials have generated information on which patient subgroups are best treated with thrombolysis. The study of Surgery or Thrombolysis for the Ischemic Lower Extremity (STILE trial) evaluated two thrombolytic agents, rt-PA and urokinase, comparing them with a group undergoing primary operation for lower extremity ischemic symptoms of less than 6 months' duration. The primary end-point was a composite outcome index that included ongoing or recurrent ischemia, death or major amputation, life-threatening hemorrhage, any perioperative complication (e.g., cardiopulmonary, anesthesia-related), renal failure, vascular complications requiring surgical repair (e.g., dissection, occlusion, false aneurysm), or post-interventional wound complications, such as hematoma formation. Amputation and mortality were not themselves primary end-points.

The goal was to enroll approximately 1000 patients into the trial. At the point of the first interim analysis, after 393 patients had been entered into the study, the safety committee prematurely terminated the trial because of poorer results in the thrombolytic groups. The authors reported no differences in safety or efficacy when patients were given rt-PA or urokinase, and the groups were subsequently pooled for purposes of data analysis. The primary end-point (adverse outcome index) was achieved in a significantly greater proportion of patients treated with thrombolysis, primarily because of an increased rate of ongoing or recurrent ischemia in the thrombolytic treatment group. There were, however, no differences in the rate of major amputation or death between the two groups. A post hoc subgroup analysis was performed to look at patients with recent symptom onset versus those with more chronic symptoms. With a threshold of 14 days, patients with more acute symptoms had a lower amputation rate when given thrombolytic therapy, whereas those with chronic symptoms had fewer amputations when treated with surgery.

Subsequent to the primary STILE publication, two subset analyses appeared. The first provided data on the native artery stratification group and concluded that the results of thrombolytic therapy were poorer than primary operation in this subgroup of patients.[40] Although the mortality rates were equal and the thrombolytic patients had a reduction in their predetermined surgical procedure, the amputation rate was significantly higher when compared with primary operation, 10% versus 0%. The second analysis reported the results of thrombolysis in patients with bypass graft occlusions and concluded that thrombolytic therapy was associated with significant benefits over primary operation in this group of patients.[41] The thrombolytic group manifested a reduction in the predetermined surgical procedure as well as a lower amputation rate at 1 year.

The Thrombolysis Or Peripheral Arterial Surgery (TOPAS) trial evaluated 757 patients randomly allocated to recombinant urokinase or immediate operation, the first 213 in a preliminary dose-ranging study[38] and the subsequent 544 in a head-to-head comparison between the "best" dose of urokinase and primary operation.[15] Although no statistically significant differences between the thrombolytic and operative groups were detected with regard to the primary endpoint of amputation-free survival, thrombolysis was associated with a reduction in the number and magnitude of interventions over 1 year of follow-up. Not unexpectedly, there was a higher incidence of bleeding complications in the thrombolytic group. These complications, however, did not result in an increase in the length of hospitalization or patient mortality. A subsequent multifactor analysis identified the length of the occlusion as a parameter associated with outcome.[42] Patients with longer occlusions (>30 cm in length) fared better with thrombolysis, whereas the reverse was true for patients with shorter occlusions. This observation may relate to the absence of a suitable target vessel for an operative bypass in patients with long thrombotic occlusions.

Treatment Protocol for Patients with Acute Limb Ischemia

The care of patients with acute limb ischemia should proceed in an orderly, systematic fashion, given the multiplicity of therapeutic choices and the frailty of the patients. An accurate history and physical examination should be performed to obtain a diagnosis of arterial occlusion, determine the timing and severity of the problem, and gain insight into the location of the thrombotic process. The limbs should be evaluated with the Doppler ultrasound instrument, and one should listen for signals in the pedal arteries as well as veins. Ankle-brachial pressure indices (ABIs) should be measured.

One must determine whether the ischemia is severe enough to warrant immediate operation without arteriography. This is rarely the case; the performance of a diagnostic imaging study is usually well worth the delay. Similarly, one must determine whether *any* intervention is indicated. For instance, it may not be appropriate to subject a patient with a minimally symptomatic femoropopliteal bypass graft occlusion to the inherent risks of surgical revision or thrombolysis.

If the patient is thought to have a localized embolus to the common femoral artery, arteriography is not always performed and immediate operative exploration is acceptable. Alternatively, preoperative arteriography provides valuable information about the location of propagated thrombus or additional emboli. Occasionally, the arteriogram may suggest that a presumed embolus is more likely a thrombotic process overlying chronic atherosclerotic disease.

After reviewing the diagnostic arteriogram and the clinical presentation, one must determine whether a thrombolytic or operative approach is most appropriate. If the patient has an inflow site and a target vessel appropriate for the conduit available, operative revascularization may be best. For example, a patient with a thrombosed popliteal aneurysm, a patent outflow vessel in the calf, and adequate saphenous vein to bridge the gap from a femoral inflow site should undergo operative bypass without an attempt at thrombolysis. Similarly, a new graft should be placed in a patient with a thrombosed prosthetic femoropopliteal bypass graft, an open popliteal outflow site, and an adequate length of graft material appropriate for the particular revascularization. In contrast, thrombolysis is advantageous in the same patient with a failed saphenous vein graft, providing the possibility of preserving a precious autogenous conduit.

If a thrombolytic strategy is elected, one must ensure that the infusion catheter can be positioned within the substance of the thrombus. Certain tactics can be used to cannulate the graft, including duplex localization of the proximal anastomosis and direct graft puncture techniques. An open operative approach is necessary when access to the thrombus cannot be achieved.

Successful thrombolysis should be followed by endovascular or open surgical revision of any lesions unmasked after dissolution of the thrombus. Endovascular modalities, such as balloon angioplasty with or without stenting, can be performed at the conclusion of thrombolysis, usually through the same access site used for the infusion. When an open surgical approach is more appropriate because of the nature of the lesion, timing of treatment becomes crucial. In the absence of a systemic proteolytic state or therapeutic anticoagulation, infusion catheters can be removed almost immediately following termination of the thrombolytic infusion. Systemic anticoagulation therapy is begun shortly thereafter and is continued until the culprit lesions are surgically repaired. If an offending lesion cannot be identified after successful thrombolysis, even after additional diagnostic interrogations, the patient should receive long-term anticoagulation therapy.

SUMMARY

Patients with acute limb ischemia represent a subpopulation with a variety of serious concurrent medical illnesses. These illnesses predispose the patient to complications after any intervention, be it open surgery, an endovascular procedure, or thrombolytic therapy. Thus, therapy must be well planned and well executed if mortality rates are to be kept to an acceptable level. Adequate arteriographic imaging is crucial in order to determine the most appropriate intervention in a patient. The particular intervention chosen will depend on the clinical severity of ischemia, the anatomy of the occlusion, and the experience of the treating clinician. Long-term results are not equivalent to those achieved in elective procedures because of the medical status of patients, the extent of ischemic tissue damage, and the limited array of options for revascularization.

REFERENCES

1. Davies B, Braithwaite BD, Birch PA, et al: Acute leg ischaemia in Gloucestershire. Br J Surg 84:504–508, 1997.
2. Blaisdell FW, Steele M, Allen RE: Management of acute lower extremity arterial ischemia due to embolism and thrombosis. Surgery 84:822–834, 1978.
3. Jivegård L, Holm J, Shersten T: Acute limb ischemia due to arterial embolism or thrombosis: Influence of limb ischemia versus pre-existing cardiac disease on postoperative mortality rate. J Cardiovasc Surg 29:32–36, 1988.
4. Balas P, Bonatsos G, Xeromeritis N, et al: Early surgical results on acute arterial occlusion of the extremities. J Cardiovasc Surg 26:262–269, 1985.
5. Blebea J, Kerr JC, Franco CD, et al: Technetium 99m pyrophosphate quantitation of skeletal muscle ischemia and reperfusion injury. J Vasc Surg 8:117–124, 1988.
6. Quinones-Baldrich WJ, Chervu A, Hernandez JJ, et al: Skeletal muscle function after ischemia: "No reflow" versus reperfusion injury. J Surg Res 51:5–12, 1991.
7. Ouriel K, Smedira NG, Ricotta JJ: Protection of the kidney after temporary ischemia: Free radical scavengers. J Vasc Surg 2:49–53, 1985.
8. Ricci MA, Graham AM, Corbisiero R, et al: Are free radical scavengers beneficial in the treatment of compartment syndrome after acute arterial ischemia? J Vasc Surg 9:244–250, 1989.
9. Beyersdorf F, Matheis G, Kruger S, et al: Avoiding reperfusion injury after limb revascularization: Experimental observations and recommendations for clinical application (Review). J Vasc Surg 9:757–766, 1989.
10. McNamara TO: Thombolysis as the initial treatment for acute lower limb ischemia. *In* Comerota AJ (ed): Thrombolytic Therapy for Peripheral Vascular Disease. Philadelphia, JB Lippincott, 1995, pp 253–268.
11. Mathieson MA, Dunham BM, Huval WV, et al: Ischemia of the limb stimulates thromboxane production and myocardial depression. Surg Gynecol Obstet 157:500–504, 1983.
12. Haimovici H: Arterial embolism with acute massive ischemic myopathy and myoglobinuria. Surgery 47:739–746, 1960.
13. Fisher RD, Fogarty TJ, Morrow AG: Clinical and biochemical observations of the effect of transient femoral artery occlusion in man. Surgery 68:323–328, 1970.
14. Green R, DeWeese JA, Rob CG: Arterial embolectomy before and after the Fogarty catheter. Surgery 77:24–33, 1975.
15. Ouriel K, Veith FJ, Sasahara AA: A comparison of recombinant urokinase with vascular surgery as initial treatment for acute arterial occlusion of the legs. N Engl J Med 338:1105–1111, 1998.
16. Zarins CK, Weisenberg E, Kolettis G, et al: Differential enlargement of artery segments in response to enlarging atherosclerotic plaques. J Vasc Surg 7:386–394, 1988.
17. Stary HC, Chandler AB, Dinsmore RE, et al: A definition of advanced types of atherosclerotic lesions and a histological classification of atherosclerosis: A report from the Committee on Vascular Lesions of the Council on Arteriosclerosis, American Heart Association. Circulation 92:1355–1374, 1995.
18. Shah PK, Falk E, Badimon JJ, et al: Human monocyte-derived macrophages induce collagen breakdown in fibrous caps of atherosclerotic plaques: Potential role of matrix-degrading metalloproteinases and implications for plaque rupture. Circulation 92:1565–1569, 1995.
19. Fernandez-Ortiz A, Badimon JJ, Falk E, et al: Characterization of the relative thrombogenicity of atherosclerotic plaque components: Implications for consequences of plaque rupture. J Am Coll Cardiol 23:1562–1569, 1994.
20. Ouriel K, Shortell CK, Green RM, DeWeese JA: Differential mechanisms of failure of autogenous and non-autogenous bypass conduits: An assessment following successful graft thrombolysis. Cardiovasc Surg 3:469–473, 1995.
21. Arend WP, Michel BA, Bloch DA, et al: The American College of Rheumatology 1990 criteria for the classification of Takayasu arteritis. Arthritis Rheum 33:1129–1134, 1990.
22. Ishikawa K: Patterns of symptoms and prognosis in occlusive thromboaortopathy (Takayasu's disease). J Am Coll Cardiol 8:1041–1046, 1986.
23. Rutherford RB, Baker JD, Ernst C, et al: Recommended standards for reports dealing with lower extremity ischemia: Revised version. J Vasc Surg 26:517–538, 1997.
24. Parsons RE, Marin ML, Veith FJ, et al: Fluoroscopically assisted thromboembolectomy: An improved method for treating acute arterial occlusions. Ann Vasc Surg 10:201–210, 1996.
25. Kerns SR, Hawkins IFJ, Sabatelli FW: Current status of carbon dioxide angiography. Radiol Clin North Am 33:15–29, 1995.
26. Weaver FA, Pentecost MJ, Yellin AE, et al: Clinical applications of carbon dioxide/digital subtraction arteriography. J Vasc Surg 13:266–272, 1991.
27. Dos Santos JC: Sur la des obstruction des thrombus arterielles anciennes. Mem Acad Chir 73:409–415, 1949.
28. Veith FJ, Gupta SK, Ascer E, et al: Six-year prospective multicenter randomized comparison of autologous saphenous vein and expanded polytetrafluoroethylene grafts in infrainguinal arterial reconstructions. J Vasc Surg 3:104–114, 1986.

28a. Couch NP, Wheeler HB, Hyatt DF, et al: Factors influencing limb survival after femoropopliteal reconstruction. Arch Surg 95:163–169, 1967.

29. Yeager RA, Moneta GL, Taylor LM Jr, et al: Surgical management of severe acute lower extremity ischemia. J Vasc Surg 15:385–393, 1992.
30. Veith FJ, Gupta S, Daly V: Management of early and late thrombosis of expanded polytetrafluoroethylene (PTFE) femoropopliteal bypass grafts: Favorable prognosis with appropriate reoperation. Surgery 87:581–587, 1980.
31. Ascer E, Collier P, Gupta SK, Veith FJ: Reoperation for polytetrafluoroethylene bypass failure: The importance of distal outflow site and operative technique in determining outcome. J Vasc Surg 5:298–310, 1987.
32. Edwards JE, Taylor LM Jr, Porter JM: Treatment of failed lower extremity bypass grafts with new autogenous vein bypass grafting. J Vasc Surg 11:136–145, 1990.
33. Tillet WS, Johnson AJ, McCarty WR: The intravenous infusion of the streptococcal fibrinolytic principle (streptokinase) into patients. J Clin Invest 34:169–185, 1955.
34. Cliffton EE: The use of plasmin in humans. Ann N Y Acad Sci 68:209–229, 1957.
35. Dotter CT, Rösch J, Seaman AJ: Selective clot lysis with low-dose streptokinase. Radiology 111:31–37, 1974.
36. McNamara TO, Fischer JR: Thrombolysis of peripheral arterial and graft occlusions: Improved results using high-dose urokinase. AJR Am J Roentgenol 144:769–775, 1985.
37. McNamara TO, Bomberger RA: Factors affecting initial and 6 month patency rates after intraarterial thrombolysis with high dose urokinase. Am J Surg 152:709–712, 1986.
38. Ouriel K, Veith FJ, Sasahara AA: Thrombolysis or peripheral arterial surgery: Phase I results: TOPAS investigators. J Vasc Surg 23:64–73, 1996.
39. Ouriel K, Shortell CK, DeWeese JA, et al: A comparison of thrombolytic therapy with operative revascularization in the initial treatment of acute peripheral arterial ischemia. J Vasc Surg 19:1021–1030, 1994.
40. Weaver FA, Comerota AJ, Youngblood M, et al: Surgical revascularization versus thrombolysis for nonembolic lower extremity native artery occlusions: Results of a prospective randomized trial. The STILE Investigators: Surgery versus Thrombolysis for Ischemia of the Lower Extremity. J Vasc Surg 24:513–521, 1996.
41. Comerota AJ, Weaver FA, Hosking JD, et al: Results of a prospective, randomized trial of surgery versus thrombolysis for occluded lower extremity bypass grafts. Am J Surg 172:105–112, 1996.
42. Ouriel K, Veith FJ: Acute lower limb ischemia: Determinants of outcome. Surgery 124:336–341, 1998.

CHAPTER 55

Arterial Thromboembolism

Roy K. Greenberg, M.D., and
Kenneth Ouriel, M.D.

Acute ischemia of an extremity may result from in situ thrombosis of a native artery, occlusion of a bypass graft, or embolization. Formerly, thrombotic or embolic occlusion of native arteries accounted for the overwhelming majority of cases of limb ischemia. With the refinement and widespread utilization of peripheral arterial revascularization procedures, occlusion of a bypass graft has replaced native arterial occlusion as the most common underlying etiologic factor in this problem.

HISTORICAL BACKGROUND

The term "embolus" was coined by Virchow in 1854 and is derived from the original Greek term *embolos*, meaning plug. Arterial embolism describes the clinical scenario of sudden obstruction of an artery by material that originated from a distant site. The material may consist of platelet-fibrin thrombus, cholesterol debris, or a foreign body that gained access to the vascular system. Despite significant advances in the management of cardiovascular disease, arterial embolism remains a common cause of limb-threatening ischemia. Although new devices have greatly simplified the surgical approach, the morbidity and mortality associated with embolic events continue to be substantial and remain a challenge to the vascular surgeon.

Less than 100 years ago, the treatment of an arterial thromboembolus was solely observational and the event often terminated in limb loss or death. Following the first successful reports of surgical removal of an embolus in the early 1900s,[1] operative management slowly gained acceptance. Recognition of the necessity for early intervention to avoid irreversible intimal damage and secondary thrombosis distal to the point of embolic occlusion followed.[2–4] The introduction of heparin[5] for use before, during, and after surgical intervention represented the next major advance in the care of the patient with thromboembolic disease.

The complete removal of the thromboembolic material, particularly when it is accompanied by large amounts of propagated thrombus, remains problematic. A variety of methods, including arterial flushing[6, 7] and suction catheters,[8] were attempted, some with relatively good success. The advent of the balloon catheter, introduced by Fogarty and associates in 1963, offered a significant advance for the retrieval of thrombus distal and proximal to the arteriotomy site.[9] For the first time, intravascular thromboembolic material could be removed from a single, strategically placed arteriotomy, with relatively little trauma to the vessel. Despite the ease with which thrombus could be removed, the mortality associated with acute peripheral arterial occlusion remained high, averaging 10% to 25%.[10–19] The risk of mortality was a result not of the limb ischemia per se but, rather, concurrent medical co-morbidities, principally cardiac, that often coexist in these patients.

In the past, patients presenting with acute peripheral arterial occlusion were most often in the fifth decade of life.[20–22] These data were gathered, however, in an era when rheumatic heart disease, associated mitral valvular deformity, and resultant peripheral embolization were the most common causes of ischemia. By contrast, the mean age of patients with acute peripheral arterial occlusion today is 70 years, principally a result of the shift in etiology from rheumatic to atherosclerotic heart disease and the increased frequency of peripheral atherosclerosis as an inciting cause of occlusion.[11, 23] Advanced age and associated medical problems in conjunction with chronic arterial occlusive diseases are factors that appear to have offset the technical advances in surgical treatment and improvements in supportive care factors that would have been expected to decrease morbidity and mortality to a greater extent than has been realized.

PERIPHERAL ARTERIAL EMBOLISM

Etiology

Cardiac Emboli

Arterial embolism can occur spontaneously or iatrogenically. The heart is by far the predominant source of spontaneous arterial emboli, cited as the origin in 80% to 90% of cases. This statistic has remained remarkably constant over the last 50 years in cases of non-iatrogenic emboli, despite a shift underlying heart disease from rheumatic valvular disease to atherosclerotic coronary vascular disease. Presently, atherosclerotic heart disease has been implicated as a causative factor in 60% to 70% of all cases of embolus,[11, 24, 25] with rheumatic mitral valve disease and associated atrial fibrillation in the remaining 30% to 40%. Concomitant atrial fibrillation linked to rheumatic heart disease of the mitral valve is the responsible causative factor in these cases.

The close association of atrial fibrillation with modern-day heart disease may explain the rather constant appearance of arterial emboli despite the markedly diminished incidence of rheumatic disease.[26] Regardless of the cause of atrial fibrillation, this dysrhythmia is currently associated with two thirds to three quarters of peripheral emboli.[11, 15, 25]

As a result of stasis, clot formation in these patients is particularly common in the left atrial appendage. In this location, transthoracic echocardiographic techniques have had only intermediate success in the detection of such emboli.[27, 28] Although transesophageal echocardiography offers a more thorough and accurate evalution of the heart,[29–32] the sensitivity of this modality has also been disappointing. Consequently, the absence of detected thrombus does not rule out the heart as a potential source.

Next to atrial fibrillation, myocardial infarction is the second most frequent entity associated with peripheral arterial embolization. In a series of 400 patients with peripheral emboli, Panetta and coworkers determined that myocardial infarction was the causative factor in 20%.[15] Thrombus within the left ventricle most frequently follows an anterior transmural myocardial infarction.[33, 34] Despite the frequent presence of left ventricular thrombus, the incidence of embolization is less than 5% in this patient population.[35, 36] Darling and associates[20] reported on the timing of embolic complications in relation to the initial cardiac insult. They noted a lag in the development of symptoms, ranging from 3 to 28 days, with a mean of 14 days. Electrocardiographic changes were noted in 64% of all patients presenting with acute extremity ischemia requiring surgical intervention.[37] The presence of electrocardiographic changes predicted a higher morbidity and mortality.

Occasionally, embolic symptoms may be the first clinical manifestation of a "silent myocardial infarct." This adds to the importance of careful evaluation of the electrocardiogram (ECG) and serum cardiac enzymes of patients presenting with acute ischemic syndromes. Delayed presentation of emboli originating from the heart as a result of myocardial infarction is frequently associated with the formation of a left ventricular aneurysm. Thrombus has been found to be present in 50% of cases, with 5% of patients experiencing peripheral embolization.[38] It is the sheer magnitude of the prevalence of coronary artery disease that makes this a common cause of arterial emboli.

Cardiac valvular prostheses are another common source of emboli. Thrombus formation may occur around the sewing ring in a caged-ball or caged-disc valve.[39] Tilting disc valves predispose to thrombus formation at the hinge points, which correspond to sites of low-velocity blood flow. Permanent anticoagulation therapy is required in patients with prosthetic mechanical valves, and embolic complications are particularly common when postimplantation anticoagulation is inadequate or discontinued. Biosynthetic valves, such as the porcine xenograft, are not as thrombogenic as prosthetic valves, and anticoagulation may not be required.[40]

Intracardiac tumors, such as atrial myxomas, are a rare source of peripheral arterial emboli.[20] Similarly, vegetations from mitral or aortic leaflets in patients with bacterial or fungal endocarditis can also be a cause. Despite the improved spectrum of antibiotic regimens, the incidence of endocarditis has increased largely as a result of intravenous drug abuse. This etiologic factor should be suspected in younger patients and in those without a history of atherosclerotic or rheumatic heart disease.[41–43] Histologic examination of the surgical embolic specimen may provide a clue as to the etiology of the insult, especially if leukocytes or bacteria are visualized in the material.

Noncardiac Emboli

Spontaneous emboli originating from noncardiac sources are noted in 5% to 10% of patients.[11] Noncardiac emboli often originate from atherosclerotic disease of more proximal vessels. Downstream embolization of mural thrombus associated with aortoiliac, femoral, or popliteal aneurysms has been reported.[44] Proximal aneurysms in the upper extremity as a result of thoracic outlet syndrome may also contribute to the incidence of this phenomenon.[45–47]

Noncardiac tumors and other foreign bodies may gain access to the arterial circulation and form arterial emboli. This event is more commonly noted in tumors that tend to invade the pulmonary vasculature or heart, such as primary or metastatic lung carcinoma.[48, 49] Bullet emboli have also been reported.[50, 51] "Paradoxical embolization" occurs when a thrombus arising within the venous circulation passes from the right side of the heart to the left side through an intracardiac communication, most often a patent foramen ovale, to become an arterial embolus.[52, 53] This scenario most commonly occurs after the occurrence of a pulmonary embolism, in which acute pulmonary hypertension is associated with the development of a right-to-left shunt.

In addition to venous-derived thrombus, tumor and foreign body paradoxical emboli have been reported.[54] Mixed symptoms of arterial and venous obstruction, a history of deep venous thrombosis (DVT) or pulmonary embolism in a patient presenting with acute arterial occlusion should prompt consideration of this entity. Echocardiography and cardiac catheterization are helpful to identify the right-to-left shunt and to accurately define its location.[29, 55–57]

An additional 5% to 10% of spontaneous emboli originate from a source that remains unidentified, despite an apparently thorough diagnostic interrogation.[20, 58, 59] These have been termed *cryptogenic* emboli. The frequency of this diagnosis has diminished significantly with improvements in imaging techniques. In some instances, confusion arises when one attempts to differentiate in situ thrombosis from peripheral embolism. This is particularly true in the absence of an embolic source. Hypercoagulable states have been suspected particularly in younger patients without evidence of concomitant occlusive disease or in patients with malignancy.[60]

Incidence

Today, the overall incidence of arterial embolism may be shifting yet again. In one study, Sharma and associates[61] noted that 45% of all atheroemboli were iatrogenic in nature. The majority of these (85%) occurred during angiographic manipulation in the abdominal aorta, iliac, or femoropopliteal artery, and the remaining 15% arose during surgery. Although the use of platelet glycoprotein IIb/IIIa receptor antagonists has been controversial, it significantly decreases the incidence of embolic problems associated with angiographic interventions.[62] As the frequency and magnitude of endovascular procedures increase, a larger proportion of arterial emboli are likely to result from intravascular manipulation.

Approximately 20% of emboli involve the cerebrovascular circulation, and 10% involve the visceral vessels.[20] It is likely, however, that embolization to these sites is markedly underdiagnosed. The axial limb vasculature is involved in 70% to 80% of all embolic disease.[15, 20, 63] Emboli lodge within the lower extremities five times as often as in the upper extremity. The abrupt change of vessel diameter at branching sites makes these areas the most common locations of embolic occlusions. The increasing incidence of occlusive disease in our aging population produces multiple areas of stenoses unrelated to bifurcations that can also serve as anchoring sites for emboli. The presence of preexisting collateral vessels may provide enough distal circulation to prevent severe symptoms, adding to the confusion in discriminating between embolization versus thrombosis overlying an atherosclerotic stenosis.

Overall, the femoral bifurcation is the most frequent site of embolic occlusion, noted in 35% to 50% of cases (Fig 55–1).[12, 15, 20, 23–25, 58, 59] The popliteal artery is the second most frequent site and, taken together, the femoral and popliteal arteries are involved more than twice as often as the aorta and iliac vessels. This reflects the simple mechanical fact that only a thrombus of considerable size can lodge at the aortic or iliac bifurcation unless it occurs in the setting of significant aortoiliac occlusive disease.

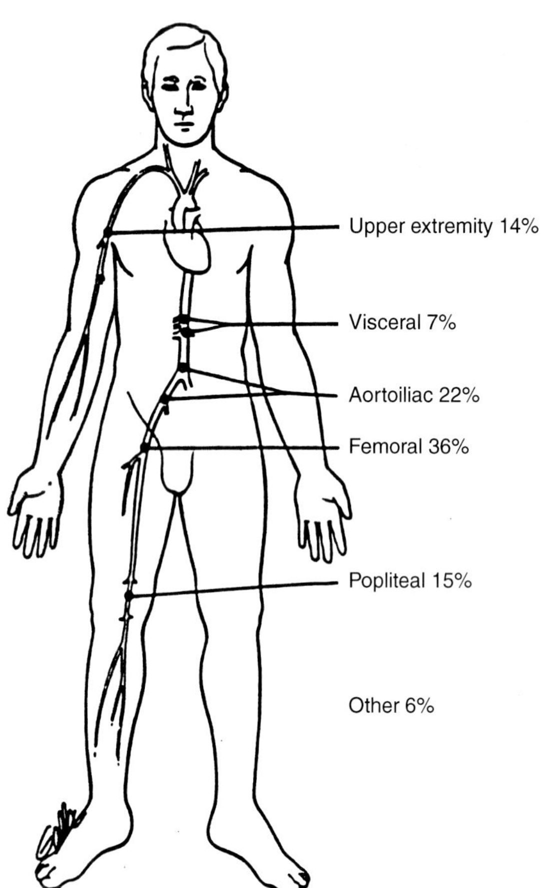

FIGURE 55–1. Incidence of embolic occlusions at different sites. Data compiled from 1303 embolic events at the Massachusetts General Hospital[11] and Stanford University.[25]

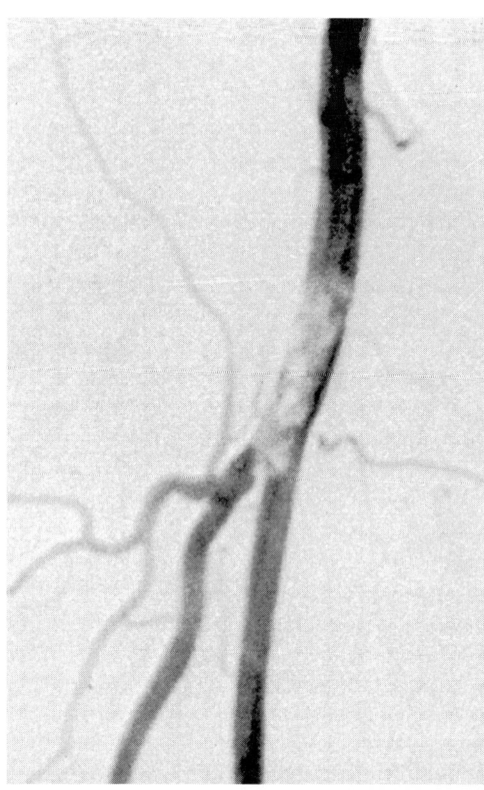

FIGURE 55–2. An embolus is lodged at the bifurcation of the profunda femoris artery and the superficial femoral artery. The diameter of the common femoral artery is large enough to allow the intravascular debris to travel through it, but the individual diameters of the profunda femoris artery and the superficial femoral arteries are too small. This photograph emphasizes the finding that most emboli lodge at branch point.

Prognosis

The clinical outcome of an embolic event depends mainly on the amount of collateral blood flow. Characteristically, emboli lodge at bifurcations and obstruct the main channel of arterial flow. In addition, they can occlude parallel collateral pathways that would ordinarily be adequate to prevent severe ischemia (Fig. 55–2). The common femoral bifurcation is the best example of this phenomenon. Obstruction of the superficial and deep femoral arteries accounts for the greater degree of ischemia with embolic occlusion compared to that observed with atherosclerotic superficial femoral disease alone.

Treatment

Historically, a great deal of emphasis has been placed on intervention within the 4 to 6 hours following onset of symptoms, because this was thought to represent the maximal length of tolerable ischemia. Although this may be true in some instances, it is now well recognized that no arbitrary time limit can be imposed on the timing of interventions. The physiologic state of the limb, determined mainly by a balance between metabolic supply and demand, rather than the elapsed time from the onset of occlusion, is the best predictor of limb salvage.

Aggravating Factors

Following arterial obstruction, three events may aggravate ischemia:

- Propagation of thrombus
- Fragmentation of the embolus
- Venous thrombosis

Proximal and distal thrombus propagation was decribed by Linton in 1941.[64] The extension of thrombus markedly impairs the collateral circulation and thus represents a major secondary factor worsening ischemia. The prevention of the thrombus propagation and the protection of the collateral circulation are the primary reasons for early and aggressive anticoagulation. Secondary thrombus may develop in a noncontinuous fashion.

Fragmentation of an embolus may occur, resulting in migration of debris into the distal circulation. Additionally, associated venous thrombosis may occur in the setting of prolonged arterial ischemia. This is presumably due to a combination of sluggish flow and ischemic injury to the intima of the involved veins. In fact, pulmonary embolism has been historically cited as a significant cause of mortality in patients initially suffering from arterial thromboembolism.[20, 65]

Patients with severe ischemia resulting from embolic occlusions are susceptible to serveral other systemic and metabolic complications. Haimovici[66] estimated that one third of the deaths from peripheral arterial thromboembolism occur as the result of metabolic complications following revascularization. The "reperfusion syndrome" has been the focus of a great deal of attention, characterized by the triad of peripheral muscle infarction, myoglobinemia, and myoglobinuric renal failure. Laboratory evidence of injury is attributed to the participation of heme, heme-oxygenase, and the hydroxyl radical. The site of renal injury is primarily in the proximal renal tubule,[67] and the damage may be mediated by endothelin.[68] Although volume repletion, free radical scavengers, and urinary alkalinization have been the recommended treatments, it now appears that once appropriate volume expansion has been achieved, the addition of free radical scavengers and bicarbonate may be unnecessary.[69]

The content of venous blood in the severely ischemic limb reflects the metabolic consequences of severe hypoxia in a muscular organ. High concentrations of potassium, lactic acid, myoglobin, and cellular enzymes, such as serum glutamic-oxaloacetate transaminase (SGOT), result largely from rhabdomyolysis. In a series of patients with acute limb ischemia the mean venous effluent pH was 7.07, whereas the serum potassium level was elevated to 5.77 mEq/L 5 minutes after surgical embolectomy.[70] After revascularization, the sudden release of these accumulated products into the systemic venous circulation has profound consequences. Hyperkalemia, metabolic acidosis, and myoglobinuria are the key features of the syndrome.

Significant edema may also follow revascularization. The integrity of the capillary wall is compromised to a degree proportional to the duration and severity of ischemia. Capillary disintegrity results from both the ischemic insult itself and the effects of reperfusion.[65] Large quantities of oxygen free radicals are released and tend to overwhelm the intracellular scavenger systems, causing damage to the phospholipid cell membrane and other intracellular organelles. Cell membrane damage results in the transudation of fluid into the interstitial space, producing edema. Substantial edema can further reduce local perfusion and exacerbate tissue injury. This effect is termed the *no-reflow phenomenon*, whereby peripheral tissue hypoperfusion persists despite adequate large vessel revascularization. The no-reflow phenomenon occurs as a result of two processes, massive edema into a fixed space (the compartment syndrome) and capillary endothelial cellular edema with consequent vascular obstruction. The process can rapidly progress to large vessel reocclusion. While fasciotomy may correct the compartment syndrome, small vessel obstruction is more difficult to ameliorate.[71–73]

Clinical Presentation

Cardinal Signs

The sudden onset of arterial ischemia is often manifested by some or all of the five cardinal signs denoted by the "five Ps":

- Pulselessness
- Pain
- Pallor
- Paresthesia
- Paralysis

Temperature changes are often described as "poikilothermic," thus adding a sixth P to the mnemonic. Although the five Ps may be a useful axiom for instruction of house staff, these characteristics represent the nonspecific results of acute arterial occlusion. Considerable diagnostic acumen is required to gauge the severity of ischemia.

The sudden *loss of a previously palpable pulse* may differentiate embolism from other causes of ischemia such as thrombosis over a preexistent atherosclerotic stenosis,[74, 75] but the prior pulse status of the limb is usually unknown or poorly documented. Additionally, a normal or even hyperdynamic pulse may be felt at the actual site of embolic occlusion, representing the transmitted pulse waves through the semi-liquid thrombus.

The site of occlusion can be accurately determined from a careful physical examination of the extremity, with evaluation of the location of pulse disappearance and point of temperature demarcation. Thus, common femoral emboli are associated with a palpable femoral pulse but absence of the popliteal pulse and skin changes will begin at the level of the knee. By contrast, a popliteal embolus is associated with a palpable popliteal pulse, absent pedal pulses, and coolness beginning at the level of the lower leg.

Pain is characteristically severe and steady. Typically, the major muscle groups below the level of obstruction become symptomatic. For instance, symptoms from a common femoral embolus begin with pain and numbness in the toes, rapidly progressing to involve the tissues of the calf and thigh.

Occasionally, sensory disturbances predominate and may mask the primary complaints of pain. In these situations, the patient may complain of *numbness* or *paresthesias*, without a prominent component of pain. The sensory changes occur as a result of ischemia of nerve.

The skin distal to the occlusion initally takes on a pale or waxy appearance, progressing to marbled mottling over time. If left untreated, the skin changes proceed to necrosis and desquamation.

Paralysis is, at first, the result of motor nerve ischemia, but subsequent muscle ischemia compounds the problem. The extent of the motor deficit is a good index of the degree of tissue anoxia and correlates well with ultimate prognosis. Complete motor paralysis is a late symptom signaling impending gangrene, representing a combination of both end-stage muscle and neural ischemia. When paralysis proceeds to rigor and the initial "doughy" consistency of the muscle progresses to "woody" hardness and involuntary muscle contracture (rigor), irreversible ischemia has developed. Although the limb may be salvaged, ultimate function is severely compromised and the systemic metabolic consequences of revascularization may be lethal.

Classification of Limb Findings

Clinical findings and assessment of distal arterial and venous Doppler signals allow limbs to be categorized into clinically relevant groups: (1) viable, (2) threatened, and (3) irreversibly ischemic. These categories were formulated and revised by the Society for Vascular Surgery/International Society for Cardiovascular Surgery (SVS/ISCVS) committee on reporting standards[75] and are fully enumerated in Chapter 54.

PERIPHERAL ARTERIAL THROMBOSIS

Peripheral arterial thrombotic events develop in the setting of an underlying native arterial stenosis or a hypercoagulable state or as the result of occlusion of a bypass graft conduit. Whereas native artery thrombosis may be associated with almost imperceptible changes in the patient's symptomatology due to preexisting collateral channels, symptoms of occlusion secondary to hypercoagulability or bypass graft failure may be sudden and catastrophic. Additional aspects of peripheral arterial thrombotic problems are covered in Chapter 54.

Contemporary series identify *bypass graft failure* as the cause of acute peripheral arterial thrombosis in most occlusions. In the Thrombolysis Or Peripheral Arterial Surgery (TOPAS) trial,[76] 302 of 466 (65%) thrombotic events were related to bypass graft occlusions; the remaining 164 events (35%) were a result of native artery occlusion. Similarly, 63 (70%) of 90 patients with thrombotic events entered into the Rochester trial had bypass graft occlusions, while 27 patients (30%) had native artery thromboses in situ.[77] Hypercoagulability is being increasingly recognized as a cause of acute peripheral arterial occlusion. Although most hypercoagulable states are associated with venous thrombotic events, arterial thrombosis occurs most notably with malignancy, antiphospholipid syndrome, antithrombin III deficiency, and the vasculitides. When patients present with peripheral arterial thrombosis in the absence of underlying atherosclerosis, a search for a hypercoagulable syndrome should be undertaken.

The goal of revascularization in patients with acute thrombosis of a peripheral artery or bypass graft is the rapid restoration of adequate arterial perfusion without the development of morbid local or systemic complications. Herein lies the yet unsolved problem inherent in urgent arterial revascularization. Hypercoagulability, liberation of acid, potassium, myoglobin, and cardiac depressants as well as the frequent presence of systemic atherosclerosis and chronic pulmonary disease compound the ischemic problem and account for a high mortality rate in these patients.

The observation of a mortality rate approaching 30% led Blaisdell and colleagues[78] to advocate a radical change in the management of acute limb ischemia. Reasoning that the risk of death was correlated with the fragile medical state of the patient who had an acutely ischemic limb, they suggested that immediate operation be avoided. Instead, large doses of heparin might lower mortality without increasing the rate of limb loss. Thereafter, an operative procedure, if neccessary, could be performed in the elective setting. These workers demonstrated the feasibility of this concept in a small series of patients.

Despite Blaisdell's personal success with high-dose heparin and delayed revascularization, this treatment paradigm never achieved universal acceptance. In its place, clinicians began to explore options of thrombolytic therapy, which, unlike heparin alone, could produce dissolution of the obstructing thrombus. Lesions responsible for the occlusive event could be identified after successful thrombolysis, and a more limited and directed surgical or endovascular approach might then be performed on an elective basis in a well-prepared patient. Unlike anticoagulation, thrombolysis can open outflow sites previously occluded and unavailable for an operative bypass. In some cases, a popliteal thrombus may be dissolved and a femoropopliteal bypass may be feasible, whereas before a femorotibial reconstruction would have been necessary. This benefit becomes very important in patients without adequate autogenous conduit material.

The theoretical advantages of thrombolytic therapy have translated into clinical benefit in certain patients. For instance, the patients in the Rochester trial, representing a group with very severe ischemia of recent onset, experienced improved survial when thrombolysis with urokinase was employed as initial therapy. A diminished rate of amputation was confirmed in the Surgery or Thrombolysis for the Ischemic Lower Extremity (STILE) trial when patients presenting within 2 weeks of symptoms were treated with thrombolytic modalities.[79] In the largest trial of thrombolysis versus primary operation (TOPAS), a lower rate of mortality was not found in patients treated with a recombinant urokinase. Thrombolytic patients did, however, benefit with respect to a lowered requirement for open surgical procedures, concurrent with equivalent rates of limb-salvage and survival compared with the operative group.

In general, one should consider thrombolytic agents as an option in the therapeutic armamentarium when acute lower extremity ischemia is encountered. The underlying lesion, if identified, can be addressed on an elective basis, with either endovascular or open surgical techniques. Although short stenotic lesions of the iliac system, and occasionally of the infrainguinal arterial segments, may be appropriately treated with balloon angioplasty with or without

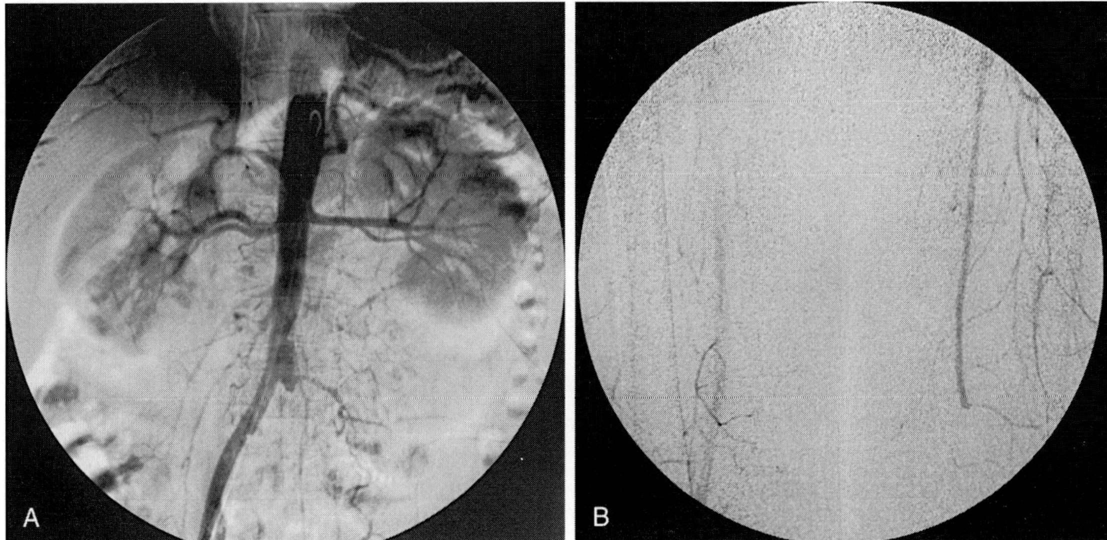

FIGURE 55–3. *A*, Left iliac artery embolus. *B*, Acute occlusion of the superficial femoral artery in the adductor canal. The presence of the proximal embolus, lack of significant disease apparent in the proximal portion of the superficial femoral artery, and lack of a well-developed collateral blood supply suggest that the superficial femoral artery occlusion is also embolic. This hunch proved correct on examination of embolectomized specimens following a surgical procedure.

stenting, longer lesions should be managed with open operative bypass. Chronic occlusions are best treated operatively except in the hands of the most skilled interventionists. With this treatment paradigm, the morbidity and mortality of peripheral arterial occlusion can be expected to fall well below those rates observed several decades ago.

DIFFERENTIAL DIAGNOSIS

Acute arterial occlusion secondary to an embolus is frequently difficult to distinguish clinically from in situ thrombosis of an artery from occlusive or aneurysmal disease. Whereas embolectomy is often successful in a patient after an acute embolic event, attempts at thrombectomy in the setting of thrombotic occlusion usually fail and sometimes exacerbate ischemia.

Several clues to the diagnosis may be obtained from a careful history and physical examination and may assist in the differentiation between embolus and thrombosis. A history of claudication is usually absent in the patient with an embolus, and often no evidence of occlusive disease is present in the contralateral limb on pulse examination or angiography. The level of temperature change is more clearly demarcated in embolic occlusion in contrast to the patient with preexisting occlusive disease with a better-developed collateral system.

A recognizable source of the embolus, most commonly atrial fibrillation or recent myocardial infarction, is another clue. Aortic dissection is an infrequent cause of acute limb ischemia but should be considered, particularly in patients with a history of hypertension and young patients with a marfanoid body habitus. Phlegmasia cerulea dolens can also be confused with acute arterial ischemia. The swelling associated with this condition often makes pulses difficult to palpate; in late stages, secondary arterial insufficiency may in fact develop. However, the cyanotic congestion and rapid onset of massive edema can be contrasted with the typical pallor and collapsed superficial venous system seen with acute arterial insufficiency. Neurologic disorders and low output states can also resemble acute embolic disease, particularly when superimposed on chronic arterial insufficiency.

Angiography can be helpful in differentiating emboli from thrombosis. Emboli typically have a sharp cutoff, sometimes with a convex filling defect, or "reversed meniscus," in an otherwise fairly normal vessel. Scant and poorly developed collateral vessels in the region of the occlusion suggest an acute event. The absence of symmetric disease also dissuades one from the diagnosis of thrombosis in situ.

Multiple filling defects within several arterial beds is probably the most accurate angiographic sign of embolization (Fig. 55–3). The location of the occlusion is more frequently at a bifurcation in embolic disease, whereas acute thrombosis occurs in regions commonly afflicted with atherosclerotic disease, such as Hunter's canal. Unfortunately, many of these findings may become obscured with the propagation of clot (Table 55–1).

TABLE 55–1. DIFFERENTIATION OF EMBOLISM FROM THROMBOSIS

	EMBOLISM	THROMBOSIS
Identifiable Source	Frequently detected	None
Claudication	Rare	Frequent
Physical Findings	Proximal and contralateral pulses normal	Ipsilateral and contralateral evidence of peripheral vascular disease
Angiography	Minimal atherosclerosis, sharp cutoff, few collaterals, multiple occlusions	Diffuse atherosclerotic disease, tapered and irregular cutoff, well-developed collateral circulation

Angiography is extremely useful in the planning of operative procedures and is recommended in all but the most straightforward cases. Only in the most obvious presentation of a femoral embolus, when little doubt in the diagnosis is coupled with an acutely ischemic limb, is there little need for angiography. Alternatively, patients without a clear history, a threatened yet viable limb, emboli distal to the femoral bifurcation, and significant propagation of clot are all best served with preprocedural angiographic evaluation. Furthermore, initial angiographic evaluation may offer an alternative thrombolytic or endovascular means of restoring blood flow, an option that can be determined only from a detailed knowledge of the anatomy of the process, provided by adequate imaging studies.

THERAPY

Knowledge of available surgical options, pharmacologic (primarily thrombolytic) therapies, and mechanical thrombectomy devices can allow one to delineate the most appropriate treatment path for individual patients. Unfortunately, no large prospective randomized trials have compared the various therapeutic options in the treatment of embolic lower extremity ischemia. Nevertheless, much can be learned from the information provided in studies assessing patients with acute limb ischemia if the data are stratified by the etiology of the occlusion.

Surgical, thrombolytic, and percutaneous mechanical thrombectomy techniques are considered individually. Each has advantages and disadvantages, and the therapeutic modality chosen should be based on (1) the clinical status of the leg, (2) the degree of thrombus propagation, and (3) the medical condition of the patient.

Regardless of the intended therapy, rapid systemic anticoagulation is necessary to prevent the proximal and distal propagation of the embolus. Laboratory and electrocardiographic evaluation is required. Preoperative bilateral documentation of pulse examination and ankle-brachial indices (ABIs) is mandatory. The duration and severity of ischemia in conjuction with concomitant medical conditions determine the need for invasive monitoring such as a radial arterial line or pulmonary artery catheter. Cardiac dysrhythmias and dramatic acid-base shifts are likely to occur during revascularization of an acutely ischemic limb if the occluding process is in the proximal vasculature or if therapy has been significantly delayed. In this regard, a patient who does not appear overtly ill can deteriorate rapidly in the operating room, angiography suite, or intensive care unit. Thus, proper and timely preoperative preparation is prudent.

Endovascular Modalities

Thrombolytic Therapy

Catheter-directed thrombolytic treatment strategies were popularized in the 1970s by Dotter,[80] who suggested that fibrinolytic dissolution would occur more rapidly and with fewer system adverse effects if the agent were delivered directly into the thromboembolus through an indwelling catheter. Despite many retrospective reports, the validation of this treatment modality awaited the completion of prospective randomized trials comparing it to open surgical therapy. The Rochester trial[77] demonstrated that thrombolytic therapy in patients with symptoms less than 7 days in duration was associated with a reduction in cardiopulmonary complications. This translated into better survival compared with primary operation. The rate of limb salvage was identical in the thrombolytic and surgical groups.

The data provided by the Rochester trial prompted interest in the development of a pivotal trial of a recombinant form of urokinase (r-UK). The trial was performed in two parts: (1) a 213 patient dose-ranging trial,[81] and (2) a 544 head-to-head comparison of the best dose of r-UK versus primary operation.[76] The multicenter trial included patients with lower extremity arterial occlusion of 14 days or less in duration. The study identified an optimal dose of 4000 IU/min r-UK for 4 hours followed by 2000 IU/min for acute peripheral arterial occlusion. Compared with primary operation, similar rates of limb salvage and patient survival were achieved with r-UK, concurrent with a lower requirement for open surgical procedures at 12 months' follow-up.

A number of interesting facts are brought to light when attempting to apply the data from clinical trials to patients with peripheral arterial embolization. First, acute limb ischemia secondary to embolization affected a minority of patients; native artery or bypass graft in situ thrombosis represented approximately 80% of patients with acute arterial occlusion. Second, the short-term clinical results of thrombolytic treatment for emboli did not differ significantly from those achieved in patients with thrombosis, with successful thrombolytic dissolution of thrombus in approximately 70% of patients over a mean period of 36 to 40 hours.[77] In contrast to the early results, significant differences between patients with emboli and thrombosis in situ were observed at 1 year. Although the numbers of patients in the subgroups were small enough to preclude statistical analysis, patency and survival appeared to be higher in the patients with embolism. Thrombolytic therapy can be used successfully in patients with embolic arterial occlusion, just as it can in patients with in situ thrombosis.

Percutaneous Mechanical Thrombectomy

The ability to perform a percutaneous thrombectomy has appealed to physicians for a number of reasons. The need for angiographic diagnostic evaluation of the arterial anatomy mandates arterial access, which can then be used for therapeutic purposes. Currently available thrombolytic agents are associated with reperfusion over a period measured in hours; some limbs are incapable of tolerating such a delay. Hemorrhagic complications, both local and remote from the site of access, may also be encountered. With these limitations in mind, a variety of percutaneous thrombectomy devices have been evaluated both in vitro and clinically.

Percutaneous mechanical thrombectomy devices can be classified by the mechanism by which they bring about clot removal or dissolution. Greenfield and associates[82] introduced a method of mechanical thrombectomy in 1969, using a 12 French double-lumen, balloon-tipped catheter with a steerable handle. A suction cup was mounted on the tip of the catheter. Once the cup was in apposition with the thrombus, continuous suction was applied to the cup and the thrombus was withdrawn, initially through an incision and later percutaneously through a sheath. Although its size and steerability limit the use of this device, large pulmonary emboli have been successfully removed in this fashion.

Even though a smaller version of Greenfield's device has been used for the retrieval of arterial emboli, the simple combination of a sheath with a removable hemostatic valve and a large, thin-walled angiographic catheter can also be used percutaneously to remove thromboemboli. Following sheath placement and traversal of the thrombus with an angiographic wire and catheter, the wire is withdrawn and suction is applied to the catheter. As the catheter is pulled through the thrombus, it drags the material into the sheath. The hemostatic valve is removed, and the catheter with the attached thromboembolus is withdrawn from the sheath. The valve is then replaced, and the process is repeated until a satisfactory angiographic result is obtained.[83] It is important to place a sheath in close proximity to the thrombus to prevent the need to pull the offending clot through long distances of flowing blood. Despite strict adherence to these technical considerations, clot-fracture with distal embolization remains a significant risk. Consequently, the use of thrombolytic therapy may be required in conjunction with suction-catheter thromboembolectomy.[84]

Technical success has been reported for percutaneous thromboembolectomy, comparing outcome with that of historical controls treated with open surgical intervention. In a series of 85 patients undergoing percutaneous aspiration embolectomy, Wagner and coauthors[85] noted an initial success rate of 86%, with 1- and 4-year limb salvage rates of 88% and 86%, respectively. Many modifications to this method of thrombus extraction have been described. Clot-trapping bags,[86] expanding catheters,[87] and sheaths coupled with Fogarty embolectomy catheters[88, 89] have all been evaluated.

A variety of devices have been designed and implemented to effect thrombus dissolution via pulverization and aspiration (Fig. 55–4). While some of the devices have received Food and Drug Administration (FDA) approval for the treatment of failed arteriovenous hemodialysis fistulas, none have been approved for the treatment of peripheral arterial emboli. Thromboembolic material can be fragmented by the generation of a hydrodynamic vortex using either a high-speed rotational motor or the establishment of a Venturi effect with retrograde-directed fluid jets.[90] Thrombus is then recirculated in the vortex, producing progressive maceration and presumably smaller and fewer emboli. Because a hemolytic effect has also been noted with the use of these devices,[91] however, a balance must be achieved between the degree of recirculation required and the extent of hemolysis occurring.

Sharafuddin and Hicks[90] published a comparative review of mechanical thrombolytic devices. Examples included the Trac-Wright catheter,[92, 93] Amplatz Thrombectomy Device,[94, 95] Impeller-Basket catheter,[96] Thrombolizer,[97] Angiojet,[91] Hydrolyzer,[98] and Shredding Embolectomy Thrombectomy Catheter.[99] Work in vitro demonstrated that one variable predicting the amount of embolic debris was the degree of distal stenosis. In the presence of a severely stenotic lesion, the thrombus is trapped and fewer or smaller emboli are liberated. This can be mimicked to a certain extent by temporary proximal or distal flow obstruction.[100] Consequently, the application of these devices in absence of stenotic lesions must be done in conjunction with a careful scrutiny of the distal circulation before and after embolectomy. Mechanical thromboembolectomy instruments that do not use suction or recirculation rely on high-speed rotational devices designed to break apart thrombus without inducing significant endothelial damage. These instruments are commercially available and include the Cragg Thrombolytic Brush Catheter[101] and the Trerotola Percutaneous Thrombectomy Device.[102] Rotational devices combined with suction provide a mechanism by which thrombus can be fractured into particles more easily removed by aspiration; these devices include the Gunther Thrombectomy Catheter,[103] Transluminal Extraction Catheter,[104] and Amplatz Maceration Aspiration Thrombectomy Catheter.[105]

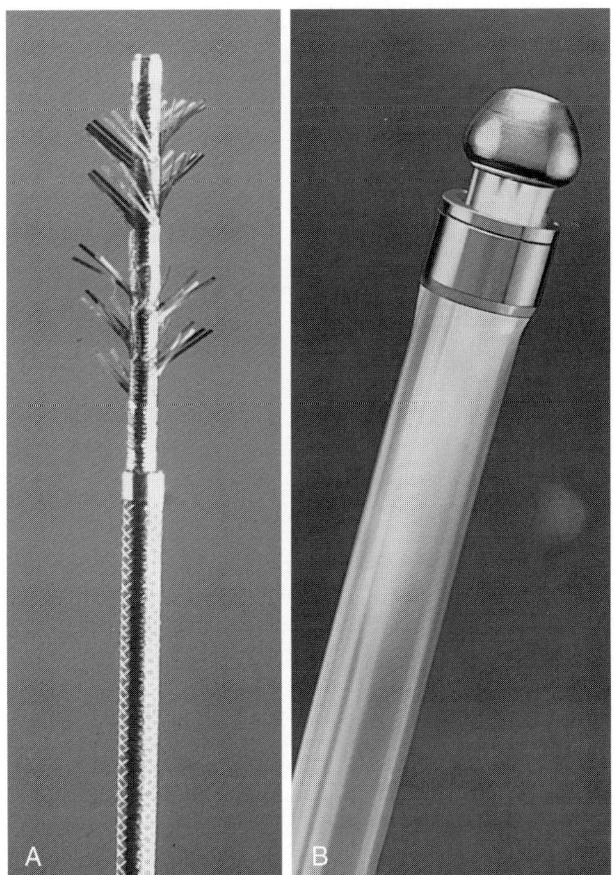

FIGURE 55–4. *A*, The Cragg thrombolytic brush. The brush is placed into the clot using an over-the-wire technique. The clot is then macerated into fine particles. *B*, The AngioJet system relies on the Venturi effect to remove friable thrombus. Both systems represent mechanical thrombectomy devices that are placed percutaneously.

Ultrasound-Accelerated Thrombolysis

Ultrasound energy can be utilized to ablate thrombus by an effect described as acoustic cavitation[106] or to improve the delivery and efficacy of a thrombolytic agent.[107] This has been shown in vitro with both intravascular (catheter-based) and extravascular (transdermal) devices.[108, 109] The effects of ultrasound are dependent on the frequency employed. Low-frequency transducers are associated with a great range of tissue penetration and are suitable for transdermal applications; high-frequency devices are utilized with intravascular devices in catheter-based systems. Although ultrasound improves the rate of thrombolysis, tissue heating is a major concern. Clinical applicability awaits demonstration of safety and efficacy in early feasibility trials presently being organized.

Surgical Modalities

The standard therapy for arterial emboli remains surgical. Ideal treatment consists of expeditious diagnosis of acute arterial ischemia, recognition of the embolic source, rapid systemic anticoagulation, and surgical embolectomy. Historically, embolectomy was popularized with the advent of the Fogarty embolectomy catheters in 1963. Before this, only 23% of arterial emboli were treated with an embolectomy technique, in contrast to 88% of emboli treated with surgical embolectomy between the years 1964 and 1980.[11] With the advent of thrombolytic therapy and percutaneous embolectomy devices, the number of patients undergoing open surgical intervention is likely to diminish once again.

The use of local anesthesia and limited incisions is helpful in decreasing the operative risk in critically ill patients. Adequate communication between the anesthesiologist and the surgeon should eliminate unexpected changes in the hemodynamic state. Additionally, prolonged procedural times are likely detrimental to outcome.

Acute Aortic Occlusion

Patients with acute occlusion of the abdominal aorta are in an extremely compromised state. The patient's status will likely further deteriorate at the instant of reperfusion, and sudden cardiovascular collapse is commonly encountered with the release of accumulated metabolic by-products into the circulation. For this reason, a limited operative approach is often advisable, especially in patients whose occlusion is truly embolic in nature ("aortic saddle embolus").

The transfemoral route is frequently employed as a means of aortic embolectomy, but a bilateral approach is mandatory. The placement of a single ballon catheter is conceptually flawed by the fact that inflation to achieve aortic diameters prevents withdrawal of the catheter and thrombus through a single iliac artery. Furthermore, fracture of the thrombus can occur, resulting in contralateral embolization. Thus, bilateral femoral cutdowns are performed and dual balloon catheters can be placed, simultaneously inflated, and subsequently withdrawn through their respective outflow tracts. If good inflow cannot be restored, often as a result of preexisting occlusive disease, a direct transperitoneal or retroperitoneal approach to the aorta is indicated. A less attractive, but sometimes necessary, alternative is to simply bypass the emboli with an aortobifemoral or axillary bifemoral reconstruction.

A recent report from Albany Medical Center described 48 patients presenting with acute aortic occlusion over 12 years. A mix of acute emboli and thromboses was represented. The investigators noted a 27% mortality rate, and only 10% of the patients had disease amenable to isolated thromboembolectomy; the remainder required either a direct aortic or extra-anatomic bypass procedure.[110]

Iliac and Femoral Thromboemboli

Lower extremity emboli lodging at the iliac or, more frequently, the femoral bifurcation can usually be successfully managed through a groin incision and a femoral arteriotomy. The common, superficial, and deep femoral (profunda femoris) arteries are exposed and controlled with vessel loops or gentle vascular clamps. A transverse arteriotomy is performed unless if the femoral artery is markedly diseased. In this case, a longitudinal arteriotomy is helpful, facilitating closure of the artery with a patch or anastomosis of a bypass graft if necessary.

The technique of catheter embolectomy is familiar to all vascular surgeons. The most common approach involves the insertion of a ballon embolectomy catheter through the arteriotomy with blind passage proximally and distally. Several modifications in catheter design and adjunctive maneuvers have been developed to improve results. "Over-the-wire" embolectomy catheters can be utilized in conjunction with intraoperative fluoroscopy and routine catheter and wire manipulations to accurately direct the catheter into the desired vessel without traumatic injury.

Regardless of technique, the importance of proper sizing cannot be underestimated. Oversized balloons can damage endothelium and cause rupture or dissection, particularly at vessel branch points. Undersized balloons may fragment thrombus, causing embolization to the distal circulation. The iliac vessel is best thrombectomized with a No. 5 catheter; a No. 4 catheter is appropriate for most femoral vessels. Generally, a No. 3 or 4 balloon catheter is used for thromboembolectomy of the profunda femoris artery or the popliteal artery, whereas a No. 2 or 3 catheter is best for the smaller tibial vessels.

Several passes of the catheter are made until no further thrombus is extracted. When performing a thromboembolectomy of inflow vessels, the surgeon's goal should be the restitution of forceful, pulsatile blood flow. Similarly, vigorous back-flow after distal thromboembolectomy is reassuring. Back-flow may not occur in patients without abundant collateral channels, even in the absence of residual thrombus. It is important that the same surgeon inflate and withdraw the catheter to regulate the appropriate amount of traction and inflation pressure to be used, thereby minimizing the risk of iatrogenic vascular injury. Overly forceful attempts to pass the catheter should be avoided. Vessel angulation or tortuosity may hamper distal passage of the catheter. Helpful maneuvers consist of simultaneously inserting multiple catheters, varying the angle of the knee joint, creating a bend at the tip of the catheter followed by rotation of the catheter during induction, and the use of fluoroscopically guided "over-the-wire" catheters.

One should remain cognizant of the length of the catheter passed in order to minimize the risk of vascular perforation. Perforation is most frequent at the terminus of the popliteal artery or at the bifurcation of the tibioperoneal trunk. Extracted thrombus should always be examined. A smooth taper is suggestive of adequate clot removal, while a sharp, fragmented cutoff implies retained thrombus. After satisfactory thromboembolectomy of the proximal and distal vasculature, heparinized saline (1000 units in 50 ml saline) may be infused prior to reocclusion with gentle vascular clamps.

It is essential for the surgeon to assess the adequacy of revascularization after thromboembolectomy. Early studies noted a 35% to 40% incidence of residual thrombus when routine post-thromboembolectomy arteriography was employed.[111] Arteriographic evaluation does not supplant the need for clinical examination of the limb and palpation of distal pulses. These criteria are sometimes difficult to evaluate immediately after revascularization, but Doppler pressure measurements or pulse volume recordings aid in evaluating the success of revascularization.[112] Intravascular ultrasound (IVUS) can readily demonstrate the completeness of thrombus removal. IVUS can detect significant amounts of residual thrombus not apparent arteriographically in up to 60% of patients.[113]

If the intraoperative evaluation suggests incomplete thrombus removal, additional steps must be taken. Standard balloon embolectomy catheters are effective in the removal of soft, fresh thrombus. In contrast, older, more organized, and adherent thrombus and thrombus within areas of atherosclerotic disease may be more difficult to remove. Low-profile graft thrombectomy catheters consisting of latex covered spiral coils or bare wire elements of varying diameters allow the surgeon to exert additional traction on the wall of the lumen, a feature that is particularly useful for removing the mature adherent pseudointima often found in synthetic grafts or arteriovenous fistulae.

Popliteal Thromboemboli

The presence of a palpable, nonaneurysmal popliteal pulse without pedal pulses localizes the process to the distal popliteal artery and, when acute and especially in the absence of diabetes or a hypercoagulable state, is pathognomonic for an embolic etiology. The preferred approach to distal emboli is still debated. Many surgeons utilize a groin incision and pass an embolectomy catheter into the distal circulation through a femoral arteriotomy. Adequate retrieval of thromboembolic material from the tibial vessels, however, may be quite problematic using this approach. Anatomic studies have shown that a catheter blindly passed from above preferentially enters the peroneal artery in nearly 90% of patients.[114] Abbott and colleagues reported a dismal 49% success rate with a transfemoral approach to popliteal emboli.[115]

Thus, the most efficient approach is via direct exposure of the distal popliteal artery and each of its three tibial outflow branches. The latter technique allows precise, selective passage of a small (e.g., No. 2) embolectomy catheter into the runoff vessels. Completion arteriography is an important feature of a successful embolectomy, and retained thrombotic debris mandates additional intervention.

Distal Tibial Thromboemboli

Despite a direct approach to the below-knee popliteal artery, residual thrombus within the tibial circulation is not uncommon. In such circumstances, direct exploration of the distal tibial vessels at the ankle may be required.[25, 116] Small-vessel arteriotomy, however, is met with frequent rethrombosis in the setting of an acutely ischemic limb. Endothelial damage directly attributable to thrombus or balloon manipulation, or indirectly attributable as a result of ischemia, increases the probability of postoperative reocclusion. Furthermore, the frequent need to explore multiple tibial vessels is associated with a significant risk of postoperative bleeding while therapeutic anticoagulation is maintained.

Thus, it is our preference to treat patients with thrombus lodged in the tibial vasculature using catheter-directed thrombolytic techniques. It is extremely difficult to remove thrombi lodged in the inframalleolar vessels by either thrombolytic or open surgical techniques. The lack of any patent arterial segment distal to the occlusive process is a grave finding and the risk of tissue loss is very high irrespective of the nature or rapidity of therapeutic intervention.

Upper Extremity Emboli

Although embolic occlusion of the upper extremity vasculature is the most common source of acute ischemia of the hand, only 17% of all emboli lodge in this region.[117] The origin of these emboli parallels that seen in the lower extremity. Most occur as a result of intracardiac thrombus, with the remainder arising from subclavian aneurysms, occlusive lesions, or iatrogenic causes, including axillary bypass procedures (Fig. 55–5)[118] and arteriovenous hemodialysis fistulae.[119]

The majority of upper extremity emboli lodge at the bifurcation of the brachial artery into the radial and ulnar vessels. Another common site is at the takeoff of the deep brachial artery. In both scenarios, an antecubital exposure of the brachial bifurcation is appropriate, usually performed using local anesthesia. Although more abundant collateral circulation makes limb loss less likely than with lower extremity events, the relative ease, safety, and excellent results of transbrachial embolectomy justify this treatment for most patients.

Intraoperative Thrombolytic Therapy

In view of the fact that recent surgical procedures are traditionally viewed as a strong contraindication to thrombolytic therapy, it is understandable that clinicians have been reluctant to administer thrombolytic agents at the time of incomplete thromboembolectomy. In separate studies, however, Comerota and Quiñones-Baldrich[120–125] have shown that infusion of thrombolytic agents during operative procedures is safe and often beneficial. Experimental work has demonstrated that blood flow is improved and salvage of ischemic muscle is accomplished with less reperfusion edema and ischemic muscle injury.[124, 125] This result, which is presumably due to restoration of perfusion in the small arteriolar branches of larger axial vessels, is not possible with mechanical catheter thromboembolectomy.

The specific agents employed and dosages utilized vary considerably. Urokinase was the thrombolytic agent used most frequently, although recombinant tissue plasminogen activator (rt-PA) and reteplase have also been administered with success. Urokinase (250,000 to 500,000 IU) is infused

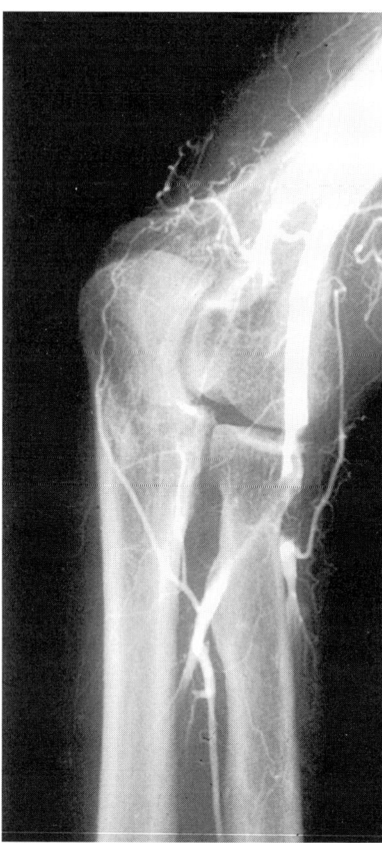

FIGURE 55–5. Embolization to the brachial bifurcation from the stump of a ligated axillofemoral bypass graft.

into the distal vasculature, either as a bolus or, in our preference, as an infusion over approximately 30 minutes. Arteriography is then repeated to assess the results. Gonzalez-Fajardo and associates[126] prospectively evaluated 66 patients undergoing balloon embolectomy, 31 of whom received 250,000 units of urokinase intraoperatively. They noted a statistically significant improvement in the ankle-brachial index (ABI) in these patients, but this hemodynamic improvement did not translate into a reduction in the rate of amputation. Despite these findings, others have noted clinical improvement after regional infusion of thrombolytic agents for acute limb ischemia, and the technique remains promising.[120, 127]

The technique of isolated limb perfusion with oxygenated blood containing a thrombolytic agent has been employed when acutely ischemic limbs without any detectable outflow are judged incapable of withstanding the time required by conventional catheter-directed thrombolytic therapy. In these situations, the lower extremity vessels are exposed just proximal to the level of ischemia and an extracorporeal pump is used to perfuse the limb. Although the technique remains experimental, it has been evaluated in a dog model[128] and successfully employed in a number of patients.[129, 130]

Compartment Syndrome

Following revascularization, significant limb swelling may occur. This situation has the potential to result in a compartment syndrome, most frequently in the anterior compartment. Concomitant venous thrombosis may exacerbate the situation. Such compartmental swelling may lead to neurologic compromise or impairment of distal blood flow. If prolonged severe ischemia has existed prior to embolectomy, the surgeon may elect to perform a fasciotomy empirically in conjunction with the embolectomy.[71–73] Alternatively, because a fasciotomy can be easily performed subsequent to the embolectomy, some surgeons prefer a course of careful observation. The use of compartment pressures may provide some insight into the relative risks of observation versus immediate fasciotomy.[131, 132]

The major risks associated with fasciotomies include both infection and bleeding. It is difficult to weigh the risks and benefits quantitatively; consequently, most decisions regarding fasciotomy in the management of acute embolic ischemia are based on individual preferences, previous clinical experience, and empiricism.

Results of Therapy

The advent of the Fogarty catheter simplified the surgical management and improved the results of operative intervention. These developments have been responsible for a limb salvage rate of between 75% and 90%. Unfortunately, the mortality rate has remained in the range of 10% to 20%. Delays in operative intervention, frequently occurring as a result of late presentation, may be the single most important determinant confounding a successful outcome. In the series by Abbott and coauthors,[11] when treatment began less than 12 hours after onset, the limb salvage rate was 93% and the mortality rate was 19%. In contrast, when there was a delay of more than 12 hours, the limb salvage rate was only 78% and the mortality rate was 31%. Elliott and associates[24] found that within a range of 8 hours to 7 days, the effect of delayed treatment had a linear relationship to severity of ischemic changes and unfavorable results.

Endovascular modalities, including thrombolytic therapy, appear to be promising therapeutic options that must be evaluated in comparison with surgical therapy in well-designed trials. Singh and coworkers[133] stratified 82 patients treated between 1988 and 1993 into three groups. The first group underwent standard surgical treatment; in the second group, intraoperative thrombolytic therapy was combined with balloon embolectomy; and the third group was treated with percutaneous thrombolysis. Although minor differences were noted prior to treatment, an analysis of limb salvage and survival yielded similar results.[133]

In a study comparing thrombolytic versus primary operative intervention in patients with acute limb ischemia, Ouriel and colleagues[77] evaluated outcome in patients with thrombotic or embolic occlusions. Although the number of patients studied was small, the risk of major amputation was the same (~18% at 12 months), regardless of the form of therapy. However, mortality rates were significantly lower in the thrombolytic group (16% versus 42% at 12 months). This observation was explained by a higher frequency of cardiopulmonary complications in the operative group.[77]

It is clear that many factors exert a negative influence on the outcome of patients suffering from acute thromboembolism. These include the underlying source for the embolus, the high incidence of associated atherosclerotic disease, and systemic metabolic complications. As the population ages and patients with emboli make up an older age group, the prevalence of atherosclerotic heart disease increases, as do the risks of both open and percutaneous procedures. It is predictable that the gains from technologic advances may be offset by an increased complexity of medical comorbidities, such that the mortality associated with acute limb ischemia will remain considerable.

SUMMARY

Despite treatment advances, acute peripheral arterial thromboembolism is still associated with substantial morbidity and mortality. Most of these patients are older, have significant co-morbidities and have an underlying cause of the process. Emboli most commonly originate from the heart or as a result of an intra-arterial manipulation. Thrombosis in situ may develop in the setting of an underlying atherosclerotic stenosis or as a result of a hypercoagulable state. Recently, thrombosis of a bypass graft has become a more common cause of acute ischemia of the extremity.

Arterial embolization must be differentiated from acute arterial thrombosis that is due to preexisting occlusive disease. Preoperative arteriography is helpful in all but the most straightforward cases. Prompt treatment is the rule; delays in therapy unquestionably result in less favorable results. Long-term anticoagulation is mandatory in patients with embolic disease and in many cases of thrombotic occlusions of bypass grafts and native arteries.

Despite technologic advances, the morbidity and mortality rates of acute peripheral artery thromboembolism are likely to remain significant owing to an increase in the age and fragility of the population experiencing these events. Appreciable improvements in clinical outcome will be realized only through rapid diagnosis of peripheral thromboembolism, utilization of appropriate surgical or endovascular interventions to restore arterial perfusion, and efficient perioperative care to address the myriad metabolic problems encountered in this group of patients.

REFERENCES

1. Moynihan B: An operation for embolus. Br Med J 2:826, 1907.
2. Key E: Embolectomy in the treatment of circulatory disturbances in the extremities. Surg Gynecol Obstet 36:309, 1923.
3. Key E: Embolectomy on vessels of the extremities. Br J Surg 24:350, 1936.
4. Lerman J, Miller F, Lund C: Arterial embolism and emblectomy. JAMA 94:1128, 1930.
5. Murray D: The use of heparin in thrombosis. Ann Surg 108:163, 1938.
6. Crawford E, DeBakey M: The retrograde flush procedure in embolectomy and thrombectomy. Surgery 40:737, 1956.
7. Keeley J, Rooney J: Retrograde milking: An adjunct in technique of embolectomy. Ann Surg 134:1022, 1951.
8. Dale W: Endovascular suction catheters: For thrombectomy and embolectomy. J Thorac Cardiovas Surg 44:557, 1962.
9. Fogarty T, Cranley J, Krause Rea: A method for extraction of arterial emboli and thrombi. Surg Gynecol Obstet 116:241, 1963.
10. Becquemin J, Kovarsky S: Arterial emboli of the lower limbs: Analysis of risk factors for mortality and amputation. Ann Vasc Surg 9:S32, 1995.
11. Abbott W, Maloney R, McCabe C, et al: Arterial embolism a 44 year perspective. Am J Surg 143:460, 1982.
12. Dale W: Differential management of acute peripheral arterial ischemia. J Vasc Surg 1:269, 1984.
13. Kendrick J, Thompson B, Read R, et al: Arterial embolectomy in the leg: Results in a referral hospital. Am J Surg 142:739, 1981.
14. Santiani B, Gross W, Eans W: Improved limb salvage after arterial embolectomy. Ann Surg 188:153, 1978.
15. Panetta T, Thompson J, Talkington C, et al: Arterial embolectomy: A 34 year experience with 400 cases. Surg Clin North Am 66:339, 1986.
16. Tawes R, Harris E, Brown W, et al: Arterial thromboembolism: A 20-year perspective. Arch Surg 120:595, 1985.
17. Dregelid E, Strangland L, Eide G, et al: Patient survival and limb prognosis after embolectomy. Eur J Vasc Surg 1:263, 1987.
18. Baxter-Smith D, Ashton F, Stanley G, et al: Peripheral arterial embolism: A 20 year review. J Cardiovasc Surg 29:453, 1988.
19. Varty K, St. Johnston J, Beets G, et al: Arterial embolectomy: A long-term perspective. J Cardiovasc Surg 33:79, 1992.
20. Darling R, Austen W, Linton R: Arterial embolism. Surg Gynecol Obstet 124:106, 1967.
21. Warren R, Linton R: The treatment of arterial embolism. N Engl J Med 238:421, 1948.
22. Warren R, Linton R, Scannell J: Arterial embolism: Recent prognosis. Ann Surg 140:311, 1954.
23. Green R, DeWeese J, Rob C: Arterial embolectomy before and after the Fogarty catheter. Surgery 77:24, 1975.
24. Elliott JP Jr, Hageman J, Szilagyi D, et al: Arterial embolization: Problems of source, multiplicity, recurrence and delayed treatment. Surgery 88:833, 1980.
25. Fogarty T, Daily P, Shumway N, et al: Experience with balloon catheter technique for arterial embolectomy. Am J Surg 122:231, 1971.
26. Levine J, Pauker S, Salzman E: Antithrombotic therapy in valvular heart disease. Chest 89:36S, 1986.
27. Shrestha N, Moreno F, Narcisco F, et al: Two-dimensional echocardiographic diagnosis of left-atrial thrombus in rheumatic heart disease: A clinicopathologic study. Circulation 67:341, 1983.
28. Schweizer P, Bardos F, Erbel R: Detection of left atrial thrombi by echocardiography. Br Heart J 45:148, 1981.
29. Daniel W, Mugge A. Transesophageal echocardiography. N Engl J Med 332:1268, 1995.
30. Husain A, Alter M: Transesophageal echocardiography in diagnosing cardioembolic stroke. Clin Cardiol 18:705, 1995.
31. Seward J, Khandheria B, Oh J, et al: Transesophageal echocardiography: Technique, anatomic correlations, implementation, and clinical applications. Mayo Clin Proc 63:649, 1988.
32. Rubin B, Barzilai B, Allen B, et al: Detection of the source of arterial emboli by transesophageal echocardiography: A case report. J Vasc Surg 15:573, 1992.
33. Hellerstein H, Martin J: Incidence of thromboembolic lesions accompanying myocardial infarction. Am Heart J 33:443, 1947.
34. Keeley E, Hillis L: Left ventricular mural thrombus after acute myocardial infarction. Clin Cardiol 19:83, 1996.
35. Asinger R, Mikell F, Elsperger J: Incidence of left ventricular thrombosis after acute transmural myocardial infarction. N Engl J Med 305:297, 1981.
36. Keating E, Gross S, Schlamowitz R: Mural thrombi in myocardial infarction. Am J Med 74:989, 1983.
37. Kuukasjarvi P, Riekkinen H, Salenius J, et al: Prevalence and predictive value of ECG findings in acute extremity ischemia. J Cardiovasc Surg 36:469, 1995.
38. Loop F, Effler D, Navia J, et al: Aneurysms of the left ventricle: Survival and results of a ten-year surgical experience. Ann Surg 178:399, 1973.
39. Perier P, Bessou J, Swanson J, et al: Comparative evaluation of aortic valve replacement with Starr, Bjork, and porcine valve prostheses. Circulation 72:140, 1985.
40. Pipkin R, Buch W, Fogarty T: Evaluation of aortic valve replacement with procine xenograft without long-term anticoagulation. J Thorac Cardiovasc Surg 71:179, 1976.
41. Vo N, Russell J, Becker D: Mycotic emboli of the peripheral vessels: Analysis of forty-four cases. Surgery 90:541, 1981.

42. Kitts D, Bongard F, Klein S. Septic embolism complicating infective endocarditis. J Vasc Surg 14:480, 1991.
43. Freischlag J, Asbun H, Sedwitz M, et al: Septic peripheral embolization from bacterial and fungal endocarditis. Ann Vasc Surg 3:318, 1989.
44. Lord J Jr, Rossi G, Daliana M, et al: Unsuspected abdominal aortic aneurysm as the cause of peripheral arterial occlusive disease. Ann Surg 177:767, 1973.
45. Kempczinski R: Lower-extremity emboli from ulcerating atherosclerotic plaques. JAMA 241:807, 1979.
46. Kwaan J, Vander Molen R, Stemmer E, et al: Peripheral embolism resulting from unsuspected atheromatous plaques. Surgery 78:583, 1975.
47. Machleder H, Takiff H, Lois J, et al: Aortic mural thrombus: An occult source of arterial thromboembolism. J Vasc Surg 4:473, 1986.
48. Harriss R, Andros G, Dulawa L, et al: Malignant melanoma embolus as a cause of acute aortic occlusion: Report of a case. J Vasc Surg 3:550, 1986.
49. Prioleau P, Katzenstein A: Major peripheral artery occlusion due to malignant tumor embolism: Histologic recognition and surgical management. Cancer 42:2009, 1978.
50. Shannon J, Nghia M, Stanton P Jr, et al: Peripheral arterial missile embolization: A case report and 22-year literature review. J Vasc Surg 5:773, 1987.
51. Symbas P, Harlaftis N: Bullet emboli in the pulmonary and systemic arteries. Ann Surg 185:318, 1977.
52. Ward R, Jones D, Haponik E: Paradoxical embolism: An underrecognized problem. Chest 108:549, 1995.
53. Katz S, Andros G, Kohl R, et al: Arterial emboli of venous origin. Surg Gynecol Obstet 174:17, 1992.
54. Schurr M, McCord S, Croce M: Paradoxical bullet embolism: Case report and literature review. J Trauma 40:1034, 1996.
55. Oxorn D, Edelist G, Smith M: An introduction to transesophageal echocardiography: II. Clinical applications. Can J Anaesth 43:278, 1996.
56. Gazzaniga A, Dalen J: Paradoxical embolism: Its pathophysiology and clinical recognition. Ann Surg 171:137, 1970.
57. Laughlin R, Mandel S: Paradoxical embolization: Case report and review of the literature. Arch Surg 112:648, 1977.
58. Hight D, Tilney N, Couch N: Changing clinical trends in patients with peripheral emboli. Surgery 79:172, 1976.
59. Thompson J, Sigler L, Raut P, et al: Arterial embolectomy: A 20 year experience. Surgery 67:212, 1970.
60. Eason J, Mills J, Beckett W. Hypercoagulable states in arterial thromboembolism. Surg Gynecol Obstet 174:211, 1992.
61. Sharma P, Babu S, Shah P, Nassoura Z: Changing patterns of atheroembolism. Cardiovasc Surg 4:573, 1996.
62. EPIC Investigators: Effect of platelet glycoprotein IIb/IIIa receptor inhibition on distal embolization during percutaneous revascularization of aortocoronary saphenous vein grafts. Am J Cardiol 80:985, 1997.
63. Elliott J, Hageman J, Szilagyi D: Arterial embolization: Problems of source, multiplicity, recurrence, and delayed treatment. Surgery 88:833, 1980.
64. Linton R: Peripheral arterial embolism: A discussion of the post-embolic vascular changes and their relation to the restoration of circulation in peripheral embolism. N Engl J Med 224:189, 1941.
65. Walker P: Pathophysiology of acute arterial occlusion. Can J Surg 29:340, 1986.
66. Haimovici H: Muscular, renal and metabolic complications of acute arterial occlusions: Myonephropathic-metabolic syndrome. Surgery 85:461, 1979.
67. Zager R, Burkhard K, Conrad D, Gmur D: Iron, heme oxygenase, and glutathione: Effects on myohemoglobinuric proximal tubular injury. Kidney Int 48:1624, 1995.
68. Karam H, Bruneval P, Clozel J, et al: Role of endothelin in acute renal failure due to rhabdomyolysis in rats. J Pharmacol Exp Ther 274:481, 1995.
69. Homsi E, Barreiro M, Orlando J, Higa E: Prophylaxis of acute renal failure in patients with rhabdomyolysis. Renal Failure 19:283, 1997.
70. Fischer R, Fogarty T, Morrow A: Clinical and biochemical observations of the effect of transient femoral artery occlusion in man. Surgery 68:323, 1970.
71. Padberg F, Hobson RI: Fasciotomy in acute limb ischemia. Sem Vasc Surg 5:52, 1992.
72. Perry M: Compartment syndromes and reperfusion injury. Surg Clin North Am 68:853, 1988.
73. Patman R, Thombosn J: Fasciotomy in peripheral vascular surgery: Report of 164 patients. Arch Surg 101:663, 1970.
74. Rutherford R: Acute limb ischemia: Clinical assessment and standards for reporting. Sem Vasc Surg 5:4, 1992.
75. Rutherford R, Flanigan D, Gupta S, et al: Suggested standards for reports dealing with lower extremity ischemia. J Vasc Surg 64:80, 1986.
76. Ouriel K, Vieth F, Sasahara A: A comparison of recombinant urokinase with vascular surgery as initial treatment for acute arterial occlusion of the legs. N Engl J Med 338:1105, 1998.
77. Ouriel K, Shortell C, DeWeese J, et al: A comparison of thrombolytic therapy with operative revascularization in the initial treatment of acute peripheral arterial ischemia. J Vasc Surg 19:1021, 1994.
78. Blaisdell FW, Steele M, Allen RE: Management of acute lower extremity arterial ischemia due to embolism and thrombosis. Surgery 84:822, 1978.
79. Anonymous: Results of a prospective randomized trial evaluating surgery versus thrombolysis for ischemia of the lower extremity: The STILE trial. Ann Surg 220:251, 1994.
80. Dotter C: Selective clot lysis with low-dose streptokinase. Radiology 111:31, 1974.
81. TOPAS Investigators: Thrombolysis Or Peripheral Arterial Surgery: Phase I results. J Vasc Surg 23:64, 1996.
82. Greenfield L, Proctor M, Williams D, Wakefield T: Long-term experience with transvenous catheter pulmonary embolectomy. J Vasc Surg 18:450, 1993.
83. Sniderman K, Bodner L, Saddekni S, et al: Percutaneous embolectomy by transcatheter aspiration. Radiology 150:357, 1984.
84. Cleveland T, Cumberland D, Gaines P: Percutaneous aspiration thromboembolectomy to manage the embolic complications of angioplasty as an adjunct to thrombolysis. Clin Radiol 49:549, 1994.
85. Wagner H, Starck E, Reuter P: Long-term results of percutaneous aspiration embolectomy. Interv Radiol 17:241, 1994.
86. Ponomar E, Carlson J, Kindlund A, et al: Clot-trapper device for transjugular thrombectomy from the inferior vena cava. Radiology 179:279, 1991.
87. Criado F, Fogarty T, Patten P: New expandable access sheath for endovascular visualization and repair. Cardiovasc Surg 1:61, 1993.
88. Vorweck D, Gunther R, Clerc C: Percutaneous embolectomy: In vitro investigation with a self-expanding tulip sheath. Radiology 182:415, 1992.
89. Vorweck D, Gunther R, Schumann K, et al: Percutaneous balloon embolectomy with a self-expanding tulip: In vivo experiments. Radiology 197:153, 1995.
90. Sharafuddin M, Hicks M: Current status of percutaneous mechanical thrombectomy: Part II. Devices and mechanism of action. J Vasc Interv Radiol 9:15, 1998.
91. Sharafuddin M, Hicks M, Jenson M, et al: Rheolytic thrombectomy with the AngioJet-F105 catheter: Preclinical evaluation of safety. J Vasc Interv Radiol 8:939, 1997.
92. Wholey M, Jarmolowski C: New reperfusion devices: The Kensey catheter, the arthrolytic reperfusion wire, and the transluminal extraction catheter. Radiology 172:947, 1989.
93. Self S, Coe D, Normann S, Seeger J: Rotational atherectomy for treatment of occluded prosthetic grafts. J Surg Res 56:134, 1994.
94. Coleman C, Krenzel C, Dietz C, et al: Mechanical thrombectomy: Results of early experience. Radiology 189:803, 1993.
95. Tadavarthy S, Murray P, Inampudi S, et al: Mechanical thrombectomy with the Amplatz device: Human experience. J Vasc Interv Radiol 5:715, 1994.
96. Schmitz-Rode T, Vorweck D, Gunther R, Biesterfeld S: Percutaneous fragmentation of pulmonary emboli in dogs with the impeller-basket catheter. Cardiovasc Interv Radiol 16:239, 1993.
97. Schmitz-Rode T, Adam G, Kilbinger M, et al: Fragmentation of pulmonary emboli: In vivo experimental evaluation of two high-speed rotating catheters. Cardiovasc Interv Radiol 19:165, 1996.
98. Reekers J, Kromhout J, Spithoven H, et al: Arterial thrombosis below the inguinal ligament: Percutaneous treatment with a thrombosuction catheter. Radiology 198:49, 1996.
99. Vlcol C, Dalichau H, Kohler J, et al: Performance of indirect embolectomy aided by a new developed flush-suction catheter system: Forty-seven experimental embolectomy procedures in test animals. J Cardiovasc Surg 35:193, 1994.

100. van Ommen V, van der Veen F, Dassen W, et al: Distal embolization during thrombectomy with the use of the hydrolyser (hydrodynamic thrombectomy catheter): In vitro testing. J Vasc Interv Radiol 8:933, 1997.
101. Castaneda F, Cragg A, Wyffels P, et al: New thrombolytic brush catheter in thrombosed polytetrafluoroethylene dialysis grafts: Preliminary animal study. Radiology 193:324, 1994.
102. Trerotola S, Davidson D, Filo R, et al: Preclinical in vivo testing of a rotational mechanical thrombectomy device. J Vasc Interv Radiol 7:717, 1996.
103. Gunther R, Vorweck D: Aspiration catheters for percutaneous thrombectomy: Clinical results. Radiology 175:271, 1990.
104. Yedlicka J, Carlson J, Hunter D, et al: Thrombectomy with the transluminal endarterectomy catheter (TEC) system: Experimental study and case report. J Vasc Interv Radiol 2:343, 1991.
105. Pozza C, Gomes M, Qian Z, et al: Evaluation of the newly developed Amplatz maceration and aspiration thrombectomy device using in-vitro and in-vivo models. AJR Am J Roentgenol 162:139, 1994.
106. Rosenschein U, Rassin T: Ultrasound thrombolysis. Sci Med 5:36, 1998.
107. Francis C, Blinc A, Lee S, Cox C: Ultrasound accelerates transport of recombinant tissue plasminogen activator into clots. Ultrasound Med Biol 21:419, 1995.
108. Luo H, Steffen W, Cercek B, et al: Enhancement of thrombolysis by external ultrasound. Am Heart J 125:1564, 1993.
109. Harpaz D, Chen X, Francis C, et al: Ultrasound enhancement of thrombolysis and reperfusion in vitro. J Am Coll Cardiol 21:1507, 1993.
110. Wonatyla S, Darling RI, Lloyd W, et al: Acute and chronic aortic occlusion: Analysis of outcome (Abstract). Proceedings of Eastern Vascular Society 12:82, 1998, Providence, RI.
111. Pleacha F, Pories W: Intraoperative angiography in the immediate assessment of arterial reconstruction. Arch Surg 105:902, 1972.
112. O'Hara P, Brewster D, Darling R, et al: The value of intraoperative monitoring using the pulse volume recorder during peripheralvascular reconstructive operations. Surg Gynecol Obstet 152:275, 1981.
113. Greenberg R, Ouriel K, Waldman D, and Green R: Intravascular ultrasound assessment of the adequacy of thrombolytic therapy. Unpublished data, 1998.
114. Short D, Vaughn GI, Jachimczyk J, et al: The anatomic basis for the occasional failure of transfemoral balloon catheter thromboembolectomy. Ann Surg 190:555, 1979.
115. Abbott W, McCabe C, Maloney R, et al: Embolism of the popliteal artery. Surg Gynecol Obstet 159:533, 1984.
116. Youkey J, Clagett G, Cabellon S, et al: Thromboembolectomy of arteries explored at the ankle. Ann Surg 199:367, 1984.
117. Pentti J, Salenius J, Kuukasjarvi P, Tarkka M: Outcome of surgical treatment in acute upper limb ischemia. Ann Chirurg Gynaecol 84:25, 1995.
118. McLafferty R, Taylor L, Moneta G, et al: Upper extremity thromboembolism after axillary–axillary bypass grafting. Cardiovasc Surg 4:111, 1996.
119. Trerotola S, Johnson M, Shah H, et al: Incidence and management of arterial emboli from hemodialysis graft surgical thrombectomy. J Vasc Interv Radiol 8:557, 1997.
120. Comerota A, White J: Intraoperative intraarterial thrombolytic therapy as an adjunct to revascularization in patients with residual and distal arterial thrombosis. Semin Vasc Surg 5:110, 1992.
121. Parent N, Bernhard V, Pabst T, et al: Fibrinolytic treatment of residual thrombus after catheter embolectomy for severe lower limb ischemia. J Vasc Surg 9:153, 1989.
122. Comerota A, White J, Grosh J: Intraoperative intraarterial thrombolytic therapy for salvage of limbs in patients with distal arterial thrombosis. Surg Gynecol Obstet 169:283, 1989.
123. Quiñones-Baldrich W, Baker J, Busuttil R, et al: Intraoperative infusion of lytic drugs for thrombotic complications of revascularization. J Vasc Surgery 10:408, 1989.
124. Quiñones-Baldrich W, Ziomek J, Henderson T, et al: Intraoperative fibrinolytic therapy: Experimental evaluation. J Vasc Surg 4:229, 1986.
125. Belkin M, Veleri R, Hobson R: Intraoperative urokinase increases skeletal muscle viability after acute ischemia. J Vasc Surg 9:161, 1989.
126. Gonzalez-Fajardo J, Perez-Burkhardt J, Mateo A: Intraoperative fibrinolytic therapy for salvage of limbs with acute arterial ischemia: An adjunct to thromboembolectomy. Ann Vasc Surg 9:179, 1995.
127. Melton S, Croce M, Patton J, et al: Popliteal artery trauma: Systemic anticoagulation and intraoperative thrombolysis improves limb salvage. Ann Surg 225:518, 1997.
128. Quiñones-Baldrich W, Colbum M, Gelabert H, et al: Isolated limb thrombolysis with extracorporeal pump and urokinase. J Surg Res 57:344, 1994.
129. May J, Thompson J, Rickard K, et al: Isolated limb perfusion with urokinase for acute ischemia. J Vasc Surg 17:408, 1993.
130. Greenberg R, Wellander R, Nyman U, et al: Aggressive treatment of acute limb ischemia due to thrombosed popliteal aneurysms. Eur J Radiol 28:211, 1998.
131. Matsen F, Winquist R, Krugmire R: Diagnosis and management of compartment syndromes. J Bone Joint Surg 62:286, 1980.
132. Whitened T, Haney T, Harada H, et al: A simple method of tissue pressure determination. Arch Surg 110:1311, 1975.
133. Singh S, Ackroyd R, Lees, T, et al: Thrombo-embolectomy and thrombolytic therapy in acute lower limb ischemia: A five-year experience. Int Angiol 15:6, 1996.

CHAPTER 56

Atheroembolism and Microthromboembolic Syndromes (Blue Toe Syndrome and Disseminated Atheroembolism)

Jeffrey L. Kaufman, M.D.

BACKGROUND

The observation that some arterial emboli arise from fragmentation of atheromatous plaques or from thrombotic material adherent to these plaques was first documented more than a century ago. Since the mid-1940s,[26] the pathology of plaque degeneration has come to the attention of clinicians as a unifying mechanism for the production of profound cerebrovascular, visceral, cardiac, and limb ischemia. Microembolization of platelet aggregates and cholesterol-laden debris into end-arteries has been documented in every part of the human body.[13, 36, 59, 68] The production of stroke or cerebrovascular insufficiency by this mechanism is discussed in Chapter 127, Section XVIII. Upper extremity microembolic phenomena are discussed in Chapter 78, second part, Section IX, and in Chapter 80. Coronary artery microembolization is a significant factor in the pathogenesis of myocardial ischemia and is discussed elsewhere.[28] This chapter primarily covers embolization to the lower extremities and viscera, but a discussion of the problem of the proximal aorta as a source of systemic microemboli is also included.

Aside from the Hollenhorst plaque in a retinal artery, evidence of atheroembolism is visible to the clinician mainly in the extremities, most often in the feet, uncommonly in the fingers, and in other appendages.[41, 57] Rarely, signs of atheroembolism to the intestine can be discerned by endoscopy.[52] In its classic presentation, the "blue toe syndrome" is marked by a toe that is suddenly cool, painful, and cyanotic in the presence of palpable distal pulses (Fig. 56–1).[37] In its more subtle manifestation, the syndrome may occur in patients without palpable pulses at the ankle. Because patients have seemingly adequate peripheral collateral circulation by vascular laboratory criteria, impending gangrene of a toe is not expected.

The generic term *atheroembolism* refers to cholesterol or atherothrombotic microembolism. Numerous misleading labels have been applied to this condition, including vasospasm, cold injury, localized Raynaud's phenomenon, and idiopathic digital artery thrombosis.[33] Connective tissue and autoimmune disorders, such as vasculitis, polyarteritis, and polymyositis, have also been implicated.[7, 15, 61] The source of this confusion is obvious because these disorders share the pathophysiology of end-arterial occlusion, often with an associated inflammatory response. Despite the long-standing recognition that atheroemboli arise from severely degenerative atherosclerotic plaques in the proximal circulation, many questions remain about the pathophysiology and natural history of this disorder.

Until recently, the general inattention paid to atheroembolism has been likely related, in part, to the lack of understanding and concern about problems of the feet in the medical community at large. The threat to the survival of a single toe may not appear to be of great consequence, but repeated untreated episodes of atheroembolism with continued destruction of the collateral circulation may portend disaster for the leg or life-threatening visceral damage.[13] Diagnostic efforts should be promptly concentrated on the location, stabilization, and, preferably, eradication of the source of such microemboli. Since the 1980s, the increasing importance of proximal aortic plaques as a source of both cerebral and systemic atheroembolism has been recognized. The treatment of these potentially devastating lesions, which often cause symptoms in the context of active coronary artery disease, has become an increasingly common and demanding challenge.

PATHOPHYSIOLOGY

Atheroembolism may originate from a variety of mural lesions, and virtually any artery may degenerate to produce

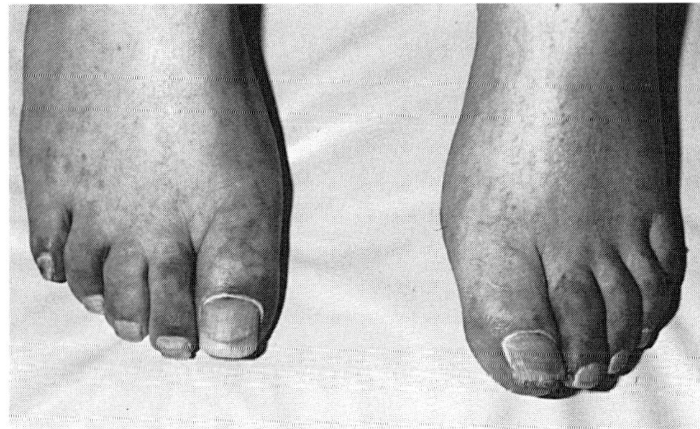

FIGURE 56–1. Typical appearance of the toes after bilateral atheroembolism.

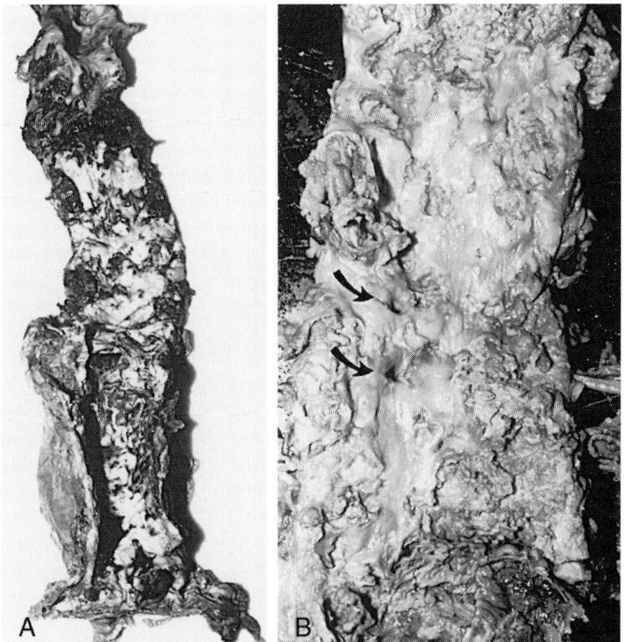

FIGURE 56–2. Surgical specimens from two patients with extensive degenerative atherosclerosis and disseminated atheroembolism. *A*, Total aortic degeneration extending from the ligamentum arteriosum to the iliac arteries. The aorta is diffusely aneurysmal but without the thick laminated thrombus that typically lines infrarenal aneurysms. *B*, View of a visceral aortic segment, showing the friable atheromatous plaques and visceral ostial occlusive disease *(arrows)*.

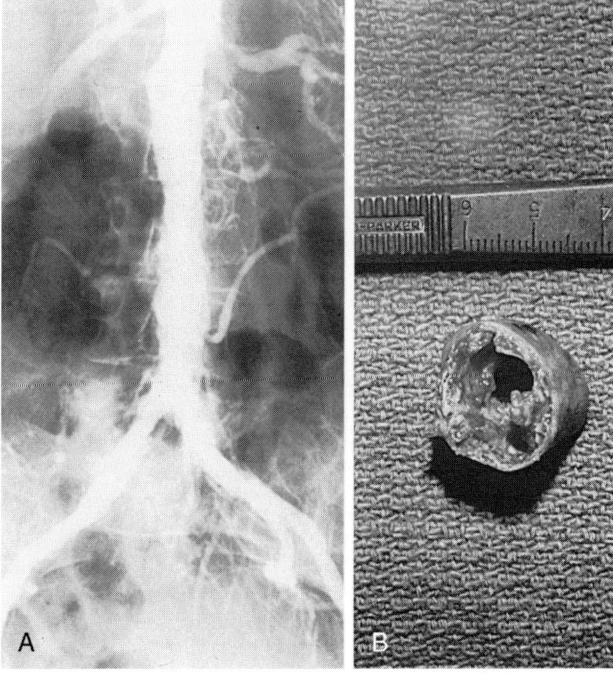

FIGURE 56–3. Same patient as in Figure 56–1. *A*, The angiogram shows severe diffuse irregularity of the aortic wall and stenosis of the inferior mesenteric and left renal arteries. *B*, Cross-sectional appearance of the aorta, a segment removed at the time of aortobifemoral reconstruction. The friability of the "toothpaste"-like atheromatous debris is apparent.

microemboli.[30] Lesions located in the arterial tree from the infrarenal aorta to the distal popliteal arteries account for the majority of emboli to the lower extremities.[48] *Aneurysms* have long been recognized as a source of microemboli, particularly popliteal aneurysms (see Chapter 94). Microembolic "showers" have been noted coincident to occlusion of polytetrafluoroethylene grafts. Nevertheless, the most important sources of emboli are degenerative, stenotic, hemorrhagic, irregular, and ulcerative plaques (Fig. 56–2). Although these lesions have been increasingly documented in the suprarenal aorta, the most common segment responsible for symptomatic embolization is the aortoiliac segment (Table 56–1). Widespread aortic degeneration has been frequently noted, especially in patients who experience symptoms from cardiac catheterization or angiography, and in these cases it is difficult to locate with precision the specific anatomic area responsible for the production of microemboli. In general, *bilateral* atheroembolism signifies a proximal or aortic source, whereas *unilateral* emboli usually arise distal to the aortic bifurcation (Fig. 56–3).[63]

Fragmentation of atheromatous plaques may occur as they undergo central necrosis, with development of virtual liquefaction of cholesterol and calcium debris as well as hemorrhage.[11, 16, 28, 37, 42] With ulceration of the fragile "fibrous cap" overlying this material, debris may be released into the bloodstream, leading to distal embolization. Intact

TABLE 56–1. SOURCES OF RECURRENT MICROEMBOLISM

		EMBOLIC SOURCE			
AUTHOR	**NO. OF CASES**	**Abdominal Aortic Aneurysm**	**Aorta/Iliac**	**Femoral/Popliteal**	**Other**
Baumann et al[6]	62	12	48	10	2
Branowitz and Edwards[11]	4	4			
Carvajal et al[13]	4	4			
Crane[16]	3	2	1		
Jenkins and Newton[35]	15	8	6		
Karmody et al[37]	31	6	2	23	
Keen et al[41]	100	20	47	12	12
Kempczinski[42]	10	8			
Kwaan and Connolly[44]	15	1	5		
McFarland et al[48]	42	14	28		
Mehigan and Stoney[50]	12	5	7		
Schechter[65]	17	3	9	2	
Sharma et al[67]	29	7	16	6	

plaques with stenosis or irregularities may have regions of turbulent blood flow with flow stagnation, analogous to the "coral reef" plaque described in the upper abdominal aorta.[69] Mural thrombi formed in such regions can embolize into distal arteries (Fig. 56–4). Interestingly, the author has observed repeated unilateral distal embolization from aortic sources, which implies that pulsatile flow in the distal aorta is sufficiently laminar to carry microemboli in a repetitive flow pattern.

In the case of aneurysmal sources, emboli may be dislodged from the laminated thrombus that lines the vascular channel. Considerable friability of atheromatous plaques is a common surgical finding, and it is not unusual to find shaggy, frond-like clumps of fibrinoplatelet debris at the site of a high-grade arterial stenosis as a preocclusive phenomenon. These sessile lesions have been well documented during transesophageal echocardiography, which can capture images of the aortic arch and descending aorta. The fact that atheroembolic events occur with arterial catheterization for angiography and with cross-clamping of the ascending aorta has provided additional evidence of the fragility of degenerative plaques.[32, 58, 60] Less often, large fragments of cholesterol debris or crystals may dislodge from severely degenerative plaques.[74] Atheromatous gravel has been observed in the tibial arteries, where it becomes firmly impacted, leading to distal propagation of additional thrombus.[25] It is therefore difficult to determine the exact nature of the atheromatous debris and microthrombotic material that may be involved in the clinical picture of atheroembolism.

Although cholesterol emboli tend to be diffuse and to lodge in arteries 100 to 200 μm in size,[42] small crystals have been observed in capillaries in the end-arterial circulation. The author has observed similar cholesterol crystal

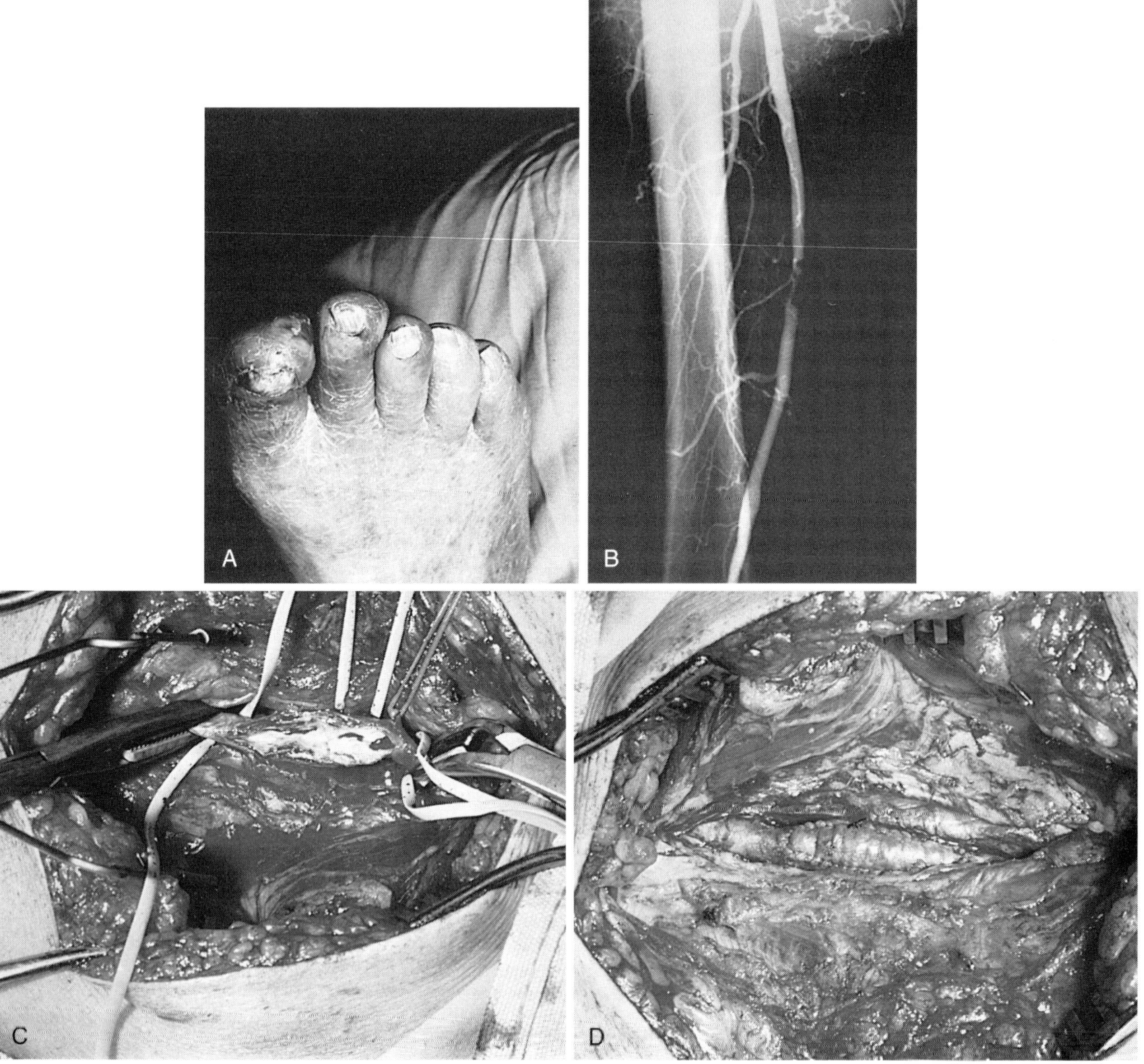

FIGURE 56–4. *A*, Unilateral "blue toe" syndrome. Angiograms demonstrated a high-grade superficial femoral artery stenosis (*B*), on which friable fresh thrombus was found at the time of reconstruction (*C*). A limited endarterectomy and vein patch angioplasty were performed (*D*).

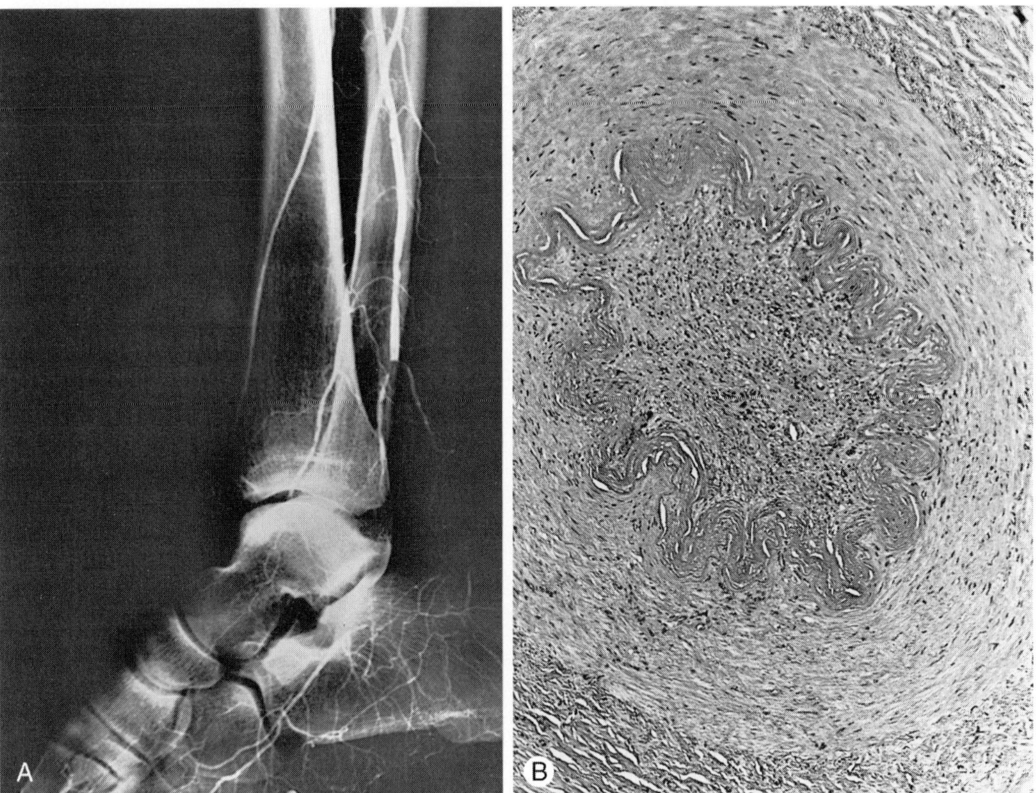

FIGURE 56–5. Atheroembolism from a friable common iliac lesion. Angiography demonstrated a sharp cutoff of the posterior tibial artery (*A*) and multiple intraluminal defects in the peroneal and pedal vessels. After 9 months, a below-knee amputation was performed. The posterior tibial artery contains organized atheromatous debris (*B*).

emboli in the pulmonary capillary circulation. It appears that the smallest elements of this debris may pass through peripheral arteriolar-capillary shunts and thereby return in the venous circulation to lodge in the lung. This phenomenon has been confirmed for the 10- to 20-μm atheromatous debris produced by transcatheter high-speed burr atherectomy.[1] Obviously, digital arteries are most often involved in this embolic phenomenon, but larger emboli have been recovered from the tibial, popliteal, superficial femoral, and brachial arteries (Fig. 56–5). Emboli may occlude the circulation in a cumulative manner, thereby leading to more proximal thromboses. Larger emboli of atheromatous debris appear generally to arise from the aorta and iliac arteries, in which severe atheromatous degeneration may occur.

Pathologists have long noted the autopsy finding of clinically silent extensive degeneration of the whole aorta.[30, 39, 40] Nevertheless, patients with a defined blue toe syndrome remain unusual, and practitioners treating vascular disease exclusively may find patients with atheroembolism a minority within their clinical experience unless they practice in specialties in which microembolic events are more common, such as cardiology and nephrology. In one series, atheroembolism constituted a significant clinical problem in 0.03% of hospitalized patients.[35] As a problem leading to consultation by a nephrologist, atheroembolism has been estimated to cause 5% to 10% of renal failure cases encountered.[47] Fully disseminated atheroembolism carries an autopsy prevalence of 0.79%,[40] and in the Netherlands, this has translated to a prevalence of 6.2 cases per million population per year.[51]

Indeed, it is remarkable that this debris may remain stable and clinically silent in many patients for years. This phenomenon has been confirmed at autopsy.[14, 26] In more recent studies, the presence of such silent degeneration has been documented by intraoperative ultrasonography in the ascending aorta in approximately 20% to 25% of patients undergoing coronary bypass.[60] Why atheroembolism remains a generally silent phenomenon is still unclear.[4] The onset of symptoms does not appear to be directly related to the cumulative burden of debris showering an extremity; some patients with relatively minor plaques have severe symptoms at their first episode, whereas others seemingly tolerate severe arterial degeneration for years. The fact that antiplatelet drugs are useful in treatment (see later) implies a role for platelet-derived humoral factors in the pathogenesis of symptoms and signs.[28, 45]

The type of emboli causing the blue toe syndrome cannot be differentiated on clinical grounds. From aneurysms, the material is usually fragmented laminated clot. Friable granular amorphous thrombus (with the consistency of oatmeal) has been observed to embolize from mural aortic plaques or from isolated iliac or superficial femoral artery stenoses. When cholesterol crystals are found in histologic sections of infarcted tissue, the source is usually the aorta or the common iliac arteries. Atheroembolism is a clinical diagnosis; it is remarkably difficult to find the site of microembolic lodgment or cholesterol debris in peripheral tissues that are infarcted or débrided, even when a pathologist takes care to search for these findings in multiple tissue sections.

Finally, the sequence of clinical events in microembolization of the lower extremity is analogous to that occurring in the carotid circulation, a problem that has achieved far greater clinical recognition. Obviously, this is due to the dramatic nature of stroke and transient ischemic attack symptoms and to the fact that Hollenhorst plaques may be seen in retinal arteries. Many of the issues pertaining to the diagnosis and treatment of peripheral atheroembolism are thus similar to those related to carotid disease.

Physicians must avoid the false sense of security that may occur after patient discomfort subsides from the first embolic episode. Because the symptoms of atheroembolism may be evanescent, a careful history is required to reveal the typical features of the syndrome, in particular the fact that more than one episode has occurred. If the embolic episode is neglected, recurrent microembolization carries the unfortunate consequence of extensive tissue infarction.[11, 65] A significant feature of atheroembolism is the appearance of lesions in crops, as if intermittent showers of debris occur.[50, 65] Collateral circulation in the affected beds is either undeveloped in the presence of this acute shower or destroyed by the emboli, accounting for the progressive nature of the symptoms.

CLINICAL DIAGNOSIS

The typical presentation of microembolism to the lower extremity is the sudden appearance of a painful, small area on the foot, typically a toe, which is mottled blue in color, has sluggish capillary return, and is tender to touch.[22, 37, 55] The discoloration may be patchy, and comparison of both feet shows that the distribution is usually not symmetric. If the presentation is late (1 or more weeks after the onset), early ulceration of the toe tip or eschar formation may be present. There is no history or sign of recent trauma or local infection. Accessory lesions may be present on the lateral and posterior aspects of the heels, which later may develop linear fissures with skin edge gangrene and a dark, necrotic base. Severe atheroembolism from a proximal source may be accompanied by livedo reticularis of the knees, thighs, and buttocks.

The symptoms may last only a few minutes and may cause little noticeable disability. More commonly, the initial insult causes discomfort for several days, long enough to prompt a visit to the patient's local physician or a vascular surgery consultant. If the pain is minor, the lesions generally heal without tissue loss. Occasionally, the presentation of an embolic shower is marked by severe pain, which requires hospitalization and parenteral narcotics for control. The patient often has lesions that progress to gangrene, and, on careful questioning, a history consistent with previous showers is elicited. The outcome is determined by the presence of collateral circulation to the involved skin, and this circulation is dependent on the size of the emboli and the effects of previous or unrecognized embolic episodes. It is important to note that diabetic patients with neuropathy may suffer totally silent atheroembolism resulting in gangrene.

The clinical examination should include assessment of all peripheral arteries, including an examination for aneurysms. In its classic form, microembolism occurs with palpable pedal pulses. A bruit may be present over the affected artery, particularly if the source of microembolism is a highly stenotic common or superficial femoral artery. Duplex ultrasonography may be useful to determine the location of such high-grade stenotic lesions. Ankle blood pressures, ankle-brachial indices, and pulse volume studies should be obtained because they are important in determining the prognosis for healing skin lesions. A Doppler stethoscope can also be used to perform mapping of the digital arteries, which may demonstrate abrupt occlusion sounds (a "tap" or "thunk" without forward systolic or diastolic flow) or absence of flow at the ankle, in the mid-foot, or in affected toes. Since microemboli can traverse relatively large collateral channels, it is possible for a proximal arterial source to lead to the signs and symptoms of atheroembolism even in the presence of chronic occlusive disease.

Patients with stable occlusions, as documented by vascular laboratory studies over time, may heal without a proximal reconstruction if laboratory results are within a range in which healing is expected. The author has found that atheroembolic lesions usually heal if the ankle pressure exceeds 100 mmHg, as measured in compressible arteries, or if metatarsal pulse volume tracings have a standard amplitude above 5 mm (see Chapter 10). In the clinical examination, it is of vital importance to differentiate the chronic disease state that causes most atheroembolism from an acute thrombosis (usually at the adductor canal) that involves concurrent embolization into the distal circulation, a situation that often requires reconstruction for limb salvage.

Patients with evidence of atheroembolism may also require studies with duplex ultrasonography to determine the presence of aneurysms, particularly in the abdominal aorta and femoral popliteal segments. In thin patients, the iliac arteries can be adequately studied with this technique. Not uncommonly, diffuse aneurysmal disease is present throughout the arterial tree, with development of a fusiform dilatation of the aorta extending from the thoracic level to the iliac arteries. Ultrasound studies may define calcified irregular plaques, and the aneurysm may be notable for the absence of laminated thrombus. Computed tomography (CT) may also be helpful, particularly to define iliac aneurysms. With duplex scanning, friable thrombi or fungating plaques in the femoral and popliteal arteries may be documented.

There are no blood or laboratory tests specific to atheroembolism. Eosinophilia has been noted on blood smears and in urine.[75] Renal function is often checked in patients with bilateral lesions. A deterioration in renal function may indicate a suprarenal source of emboli. Insidious ongoing atheroembolism can cause glomerulosclerosis leading to nephrotic syndrome. Proteinuria should therefore not be ignored as a sign of atheroembolism.[31]

Muscle biopsy has received prominent attention in the literature pertaining to atheroembolism, and gastrocnemius muscle biopsies have confirmed atheroembolism in patients with suspicious clinical findings.[2, 5, 13, 66] However, this method has not found widespread use, and the overall accuracy of muscle biopsy has never been determined. It is impressive that the symptoms are usually far more prominent than would be suspected from the degree of vascular occlusion evident in histologic sections of affected tissue.

At present, biplanar angiography is the most accurate diagnostic method for determining the source of emboli. Ideally, this examination should define arteries from the infrarenal aorta to the toes. If the patient has evidence of bilateral embolization, the angiogram should include the lower thoracic aorta. Arterial irregularities may be present in many areas, and a complete examination is therefore necessary to determine the most likely arterial source of emboli. Digital subtraction angiography (DSA) technique is helpful in avoiding excessive contrast loads because often patients are seriously ill. Digital subtraction is also helpful in obtaining good anterior and posterior angiograms of the pedal arches of the foot, where abrupt cutoffs due to impacted atheroemboli may occasionally be visualized. If one is concerned on clinical findings that catheterization for angiography will carry excessive risk of visceral atheroembolism (the "booby-trapped aorta"), CT angiography can be used to define the severity of proximal disease.

It should be stressed that the classic manifestation of atheroembolism is the development of ischemic skin in the presence of a continuous anatomic arterial channel between the source and the foot. Nevertheless, it is still possible for cholesterol debris to move through collateral channels. Therefore, it may be difficult to differentiate lesions resulting from occlusive disease in the foot or caused by local trauma from chronically ischemic or diabetic toes due to atheroembolism. A patient may ultimately need to undergo treatment for both entities in the course of the disease.

DIFFERENTIAL DIAGNOSIS

The manifestations of microemboli are frequently confused with those of other states of abnormal perfusion to the distal lower extremity. While the foot is dangling, a generalized bluish discoloration of the whole forefoot or a discoloration that involves all toe tips equally denotes rubor if it fades into pallor with elevation of the leg. This implies severe proximal occlusive disease, and the pattern of pain may mimic that of atheroembolism if gangrene is impending. Acrocyanosis is associated with abnormal cardiopulmonary function. It usually has a symmetric and constant distribution through all parts of the extremity and may be associated with similar cutaneous discoloration in the hands, nose, helices of the ear, and lips. Confirmation of low cardiac output and abnormal oxygenation may be necessary to make this differentiation.

Patients receiving beta-blocking medications may experience sluggish distal circulation, also symmetric in pattern, but the symptoms occur in the presence of otherwise normal cardiac function. Pain is not a prominent component of the symptom complex, although the sensation of a cool foot may be bothersome. Previous frostbite or exposure injury may leave an extremity sensitive to cold, with early development of bluish discoloration. Connective tissue disorders and microthrombotic episodes due to cryoglobulinemia may also mimic atheroembolism. Signs and symptoms associated with connective tissue disorders are usually more symmetric in nature but may be difficult to differentiate unless specific blood tests are performed. A severe atheroembolic shower may lead to livedo reticularis over the thighs and knees, a finding shared with connective tissue disorders, cold intolerance, and low cardiac output states.

Repeated microthromboembolism or acute thrombosis distal to chronic occlusive disease has been documented in hypercoagulable states, such as protein S or protein C deficiency, antithrombin III deficiency, or occult carcinomatosis.[21] The foot affected by causalgia (reflex sympathetic dystrophy; see Chapter 73) is cool, clammy, and painful and markedly different in appearance from the mottled, patchy, localized lesions of atheroembolism. The purpuric lesions of intravascular coagulopathy may mimic the early lesions of microemboli but are differentiated by the signs and symptoms of systemic sepsis. Nevertheless, a patient may harbor occult endocarditis or a proximal septic arteritis (mycotic aneurysm) as a source of similar lesions in the toes. Localized injury to a diabetic foot may lead to patchy skin discoloration. A careful history and examination of the patient's footwear will assist in substantiating this diagnosis.

Finally, the most important entity to be differentiated from atheroembolism is common impending gangrene of a toe owing to critical lower extremity ischemia. The appearance of the ischemic foot may be identical to that of a repeatedly embolized extremity, and differentiation of these two entities may depend on angiographic or histologic examination of the tissue. Therefore, because early or subsequent episodes of microembolism may be short-lived and may cause few symptoms, the most important aspect of diagnosis is a careful history. Frequently, a family member, rather than the patient, may be able to confirm details of sudden attacks of pain in the calf muscles or previous episodes of skin discoloration.

Obviously, any appearance of the typical symptoms after a catheterization or vascular procedure is most likely to be due to atheroembolization. This includes not only conventional angiography and coronary interventions but also newer endoluminal aortic procedures, as with placement of an aortic graft.[29]

MANAGEMENT

The primary treatment of lower extremity atheroembolism is, first and foremost, removal of the embolic source. Secondarily, if the source is associated with hemodynamically significant proximal occlusive disease, arterial reconstruction may be needed to guarantee healing through improved end-arterial bed perfusion. If the source cannot be eliminated, medical therapy is aimed at suppression of the plaque disruption or clot lamination that is showering the distal circulation.

The long-term therapeutic goals also include palliation of severe pain due to atheroembolism and local care of the damaged skin envelope to minimize the potential for amputation. If an aneurysm is associated with microembolism, conventional operative repair is the best choice. Limited occlusive lesions in the aorta or iliac arteries may be approached by either local endarterectomy or bypass, and conventional anatomic aortofemoral or aortoiliac bypass grafts may be necessary to exclude more extensive diseased segments (see Fig. 56–3).[6, 24, 41, 44, 50, 63] If the source of embolization is a highly stenotic lesion in the femoral or popliteal segments, localized endarterectomy with vein patch angioplasty has proved satisfactory (see Fig. 56–4).[34, 37] If the degree of infrainguinal occlusive disease is extensive, conventional femoropopliteal bypass is indicated, with exclusion of the offending segment from the distal arterial circulation.

Severe plaque degeneration is frequently a generalized phenomenon, and the surgeon should be alert to the possibility of plaque disruption following any manipulation of arteries, particularly with repeated clamping, passage of catheters for angiography,[32, 58] or transluminal balloon angioplasty. Prevention of intraoperative microembolization ("trashing" of the outflow circulation) is particularly important during aortic procedures.[62] It is usually best for the surgeon to clamp the outflow vessels before the aorta is clamped or manipulated in patients undergoing aortic procedures in order to prevent dislodgment of friable material. The graft and proximal arterial cuff should be flushed ("blown out") just before the distal or outflow anastomosis is completed, and initial blood flow for aortofemoral procedures should be directed retrograde into the external iliac arteries before flow is released into the legs. The surgeon must take care in reclamping after testing the proximal aortic suture line for hemostasis; reclamping repeatedly may lead to dislodgment of debris into the renal arteries.

Upon exploring the aorta in a patient with severe degenerative atherosclerosis, the surgeon may encounter severe calcification and rigidity so as to be concerned about the safety of conventional clamping for vascular control (the "lead-pipe aorta"). There are two risks associated with manipulating this type of aorta: (1) atheroembolism and (2) fracture of plaques that then rupture the adventitia, leading to catastrophic hemorrhage when the occluding clamp is released. When this type of arterial injury occurs, it is invariably along the posterior aspect of the aorta, where repair is particularly difficult. In such cases, it is reasonable to abandon attempts at infrarenal repair. In a few case reports, inflow has been achieved at the diaphragm by clamping proximal to the celiac trunk, or retroperitoneal thoracofemoral reconstructions have been performed; however, when the procedure is indicated because of severe atheroembolism, it is reasonable to move to a much less stressful and more easily performed operation—an exclusion-ligation procedure. In this instance, the iliac arteries are ligated, with the surgeon preferably leaving at least one artery patent for retrograde flow from a femoral segment; an axillary-bifemoral bypass is then constructed for inflow to the legs.

Sympathectomy has received attention as a measure for palliation of atheroembolic lesions.[46, 50] It is not only an adjunct to direct surgical treatment of the offending arterial segment but also may be useful to control the pain of severe atheroembolic toe lesions in patients who otherwise cannot undergo direct reconstruction of the embolic source or when correction does not improve distal perfusion. Sympathectomy is easily performed during aortic procedures, or it can be achieved postoperatively through lumbar sympathetic blocks.

In some instances, it may be difficult to identify the exact embologenic area. The author has observed occlusion of infrainguinal bypasses by dislodgment of sizable emboli from the proximal arteries.[25] This is both a frustrating and puzzling phenomenon because the occlusion is associated with a technically adequate reconstruction. When this occurrence is noted, treatment of the proximal circulation with either bypass or endarterectomy may be necessary to remove the offending lesion.

The degree of damage to the lower extremities by atheroemboli may be impressive. After extirpation of the embolic source, extensive healing may ensue. If dry gangrene of the toes is noted after reconstruction, near autoamputation should be allowed before revision or closure. As long as these digits do not become infected, this course preserves the greatest amount of tissue in the foot. Dry dressings are used for protection, and the injured areas are painted twice daily with povidone-iodine liquid. In diabetic patients, the lesions can heal with these measures, but careful home management and frequent office visits are necessary to prevent wet gangrene and disastrous necrotizing infection.

Atheroembolism results in a permanent microvascular insult to the skin, not unlike that occurring with frostbite or exposure injury. Major forefoot injury is treated with conventional transmetatarsal amputation after demarcation has occurred. Amputation through damaged skin may fail to heal properly. Skin flaps must be fashioned and handled with meticulous atraumatic technique and tension-free closure.

Like the controversy associated with the "medical" management of cerebrovascular microembolism leading to a transient ischemic attack or stroke, some disagree about the nonsurgical treatment of lower extremity atheroembolism. Before the initial surgical evaluation, episodes of microembolization are frequently treated by nonsurgical practitioners with a variety of medications, typically aspirin, dipyridamole, warfarin, or steroids.[18] Only one study has examined the efficacy of aspirin for the treatment of atheroembolism, and clinical improvement occurred in more than 50% of patients managed in this way.[53] Because plaque hemorrhage and surface disruption are notable pathologic findings, these medications may actually lead to paradoxical accentuation of atheroembolism by decreasing the stability of the diseased flow surface.[12, 73] After a minor initial embolic event, it is reasonable to give some patients long-term antiplatelet therapy, which appears to carry little morbidity. This decision should be based on the best information about the state of the circulation based on vascular laboratory studies and appropriate angiography. Patients treated in this manner must be observed closely to determine whether treatment failure has occurred.

SPECIAL PROBLEMS: DISSEMINATED ATHEROEMBOLISM FROM PROXIMAL AORTIC DISEASE

The bilateral occurrence of lower extremity atheroembolism is important because it generally indicates a source proximal to the aortic bifurcation.[39, 49, 63] Because the suprarenal aorta or aortic arch may be degenerative (see Fig. 56–2), it is necessary initially to document the patient's renal function and to determine, by history, whether the patient has had symptoms consistent with intestinal atheroembolism (pain, diarrhea, hematochezia, loss of appetite). In the most flagrant form of disseminated atheroembolism, in which the source is in the thoracic aorta and embolization occurs to multiple organ systems, the patient is usually found to have pronounced cardiopulmonary disease, frequently with repeated episodes of congestive heart failure.[13, 17, 39, 56, 68] Renal dysfunction due to multiple episodes of atheroembolism is difficult to treat medically because response to either antiplatelet medication or steroids is poor.

Atheroembolism to the intestinal tract may be confused with diverticular disease, ischemic colitis, pancreatitis, or gastritis.[5, 17, 39] The definitive diagnosis is based on appropriate clinical findings, including weight loss, malaise, bilateral lower extremity lesions, cardiac disease, and recent, rapid deterioration of renal function. Not infrequently, the patient will have undergone visceral endoscopy, with a diagnosis of ulceration, ischemic changes, or nonspecific inflammation.[52] Angiograms demonstrate the severe degenerative atherosclerosis of the suprarenal aorta. Renal, prostatic or rectal biopsy may provide confirmatory evidence of cholesterol embolization to the viscera.[54, 70]

If cardiopulmonary function is good, the theoretical treatment of choice is aortic replacement to remove the offending source, commencing with repair of the aorta proximal to or including the visceral and renal ostia. However, most of these patients are seriously ill at presentation, with marked asthenia, and the prognosis has been early death in 64% to 89% of all cases.[17, 23, 39, 56] In patients with this syndrome, progressive embolization occasionally occurs to the feet, with severe associated pain and impending gangrene. In such cases, an axillary-bifemoral bypass with exclusion ligation of the external iliac arteries may be the only viable alternative.[27, 38] This procedure allows healing of the feet by creation of a new proximal inflow source from an uninvolved subclavian artery and results in gratifying relief of pain. Lumbar sympathetic blocks may be a useful adjunct to this operation.

Short of primary reconstruction of the aorta, there is no satisfactory treatment for documented atheroembolism to the gut or pancreas. Unfortunately, the majority of these cases are diagnosed only after an abdominal catastrophe has occurred or at autopsy. Similarly, little can be done to treat spontaneous atheroembolism to the kidneys if the patient's condition does not permit direct aortic reconstruction. Renal failure in these patients usually develops rapidly during a period when new cutaneous lesions are noted. Because of the friable nature of the involved aorta in these patients, care must be taken during any angiographic studies to prevent further embolization, which may affect adjacent soft tissue structures and the spinal cord. Renal failure after atheroembolism carries a poor prognosis, and early provision of access for hemodialysis or peritoneal dialysis is indicated.[71]

With increasing numbers of people undergoing conventional coronary bypass procedures and catheter-directed coronary interventions, the problem of disseminated atheroembolism from the proximal aorta has become notable. In absolute numbers, although the risk of atheroembolic complications after coronary angiography remains low (on the order of magnitude of 2%), when this event does occur, it can be dramatic and life-threatening.[64] Because of the increase in the number of patients undergoing coronary interventions, however, procedures in the catheterization laboratory have become the cause of more than 40% of clinically significant events seen by vascular surgeons.[67] Through transesophageal ultrasonography of the aortic arch and with intraoperative linear-array studies during coronary revascularization, it is now recognized that many patients have thick plaques (>4 mm) or plaques with fronds of degenerative material waving in the bloodstream.[3, 43] These plaques can be located along any segment of the proximal aorta, and any iatrogenic manipulation, whether clamping or passage of catheters, can lead to disseminated atheroembolism. Plaque disruption has been noted as a complication of intra-aortic balloon assist devices.[72] Paradoxical bursts of atheroembolism may also accompany the use of thrombolytic agents given for treatment of acute myocardial infarction in as many as 14% of cases.[8]

Unfortunately, other than to obtain the history of a previous event of transient or permanent cerebral ischemia, no study or test is available to determine the location and extent of this severe plaque degeneration prior to catheterization of the aorta, and it is therefore no longer rare for a surgeon to be consulted in the management of atheroembolism from a severely diseased aorta. If the patient with symptoms and signs of significant generalized atherosclerosis (claudication, known carotid disease) is undergoing open coronary revascularization, the cardiac surgeon may perform intraoperative ultrasound studies of the ascending aorta and arch.[9] This serves two purposes: it allows (1) placement of the aortic perfusion cannula away from any thick or mobile plaques and (2) safe placement of proximal anastomoses for the coronary grafts.

The presence of dangerous plaques alters the procedure in more than 10% of cases.[19] In a few patients, the plaques may be so extensive that the proximal aorta cannot be manipulated. Methods have been devised to avoid clamping of the aorta in these situations for proximal anastomoses for coronary bypass,[20] and scattered case reports have included use of the subclavian arteries for graft origins. It may be necessary to perform perfusion from the femoral vessels or to reconstruct the ascending aorta as part of the procedure. This adds to the risk of the operation because of the necessity of total hypothermic circulatory arrest. In some cases, the surgeon may determine that the patient cannot tolerate this treatment, and he or she will abandon the operation entirely rather than risk atheroembolism.

As with all cases of manipulation of aortic plaques, the timing of atheroembolism need not coincide with the catheterization or open procedure. The author has observed fragmentation of plaques after coronary surgery with a delay as long as 6 weeks, leading to the typical picture of blue toes, renal failure, and asthenia. In these circumstances, the treatment is no different than noted earlier (primarily supportive), with provision of dialysis if necessary, and appropriate amputation of digits after they demarcate.

For a few patients, plaque degeneration in the ascending aorta has been defined on the basis of continued evidence for low-grade atheroembolism without associated significant coronary disease. One of the key syndromes is the onset of transient cerebral ischemia without high-grade or critical carotid disease, especially if symptoms involve both cerebral hemispheres. In some instances, multi-infarct dementia has been defined from this aortic disease. In a small number of cases, ascending aortic reconstruction without coronary bypass has been accomplished for this indication.[10]

SUMMARY

Atheroembolism and microembolic phenomena are common complications of severe atherosclerosis, most often from limited lesions in the aortoiliac and femoropopliteal segments. The most common clinically apparent manifestation is the blue toe syndrome, but atheroembolism may affect any organ, most significantly the central nervous system as a cause of transient ischemic attacks and stroke. At the occurrence of atheroembolism, diagnostic measures should be aimed at determining the location and character of the source of microemboli and the perfusion state of the involved extremity. Minor single atheroembolic events affecting the feet can be treated with antiplatelet drugs if the source is diffuse degenerative disease, as typically found in the infrarenal aorta. However, patients must have close follow-up because the efficacy of nonsurgical therapy is not well demonstrated and some patients suffer recurrent events, especially after anticoagulant therapy. Because repeated episodes of atheroembolism may result in limb loss, surgical therapy should be focused on removal of the embolic source from the proximal circulation, either by local endarterectomy or bypass procedures.

Disseminated atheroembolism, with associated damage to the viscera and kidneys, has a poor prognosis. If the primary aortic source cannot be replaced in these patients, surgical attention should be focused on providing access for hemodialysis or peritoneal dialysis and on performing exclusion bypass to prevent further embolization to the feet. Patients with thick or sessile plaques in the ascending aorta and arch pose a special problem; they are at risk for disseminated atheroembolism or stroke in the context of coronary artery procedures, both surgical and catheter-directed.

In patients with advanced risk factors for atherosclerosis or with a history of previous stroke, assessment of the aorta may be necessary by transesophageal ultrasonography prior to manipulation or traversing of the aorta.

REFERENCES

1. Ahn SS, Auth D, Marcus DR, Moore WS: Removal of focal atheromatous lesions by angioscopically guided high-speed rotary atherectomy: Preliminary experimental observations. J Vasc Surg 7:292, 1988.
2. Adamson AS, Pittman MR, Karke SG: Atheroembolism presenting as selective muscle embolisation. J Cardiovasc Surg 32:705, 1991.
3. Amarenco P, Cohen A, Tzouria C, et al: Atherosclerotic disease of the aortic arch and the risk of ischemic stroke. N Eng J Med 331:1474, 1994.
4. Amarenco P, Duyckaerts C, Tzourio C, et al: The prevalence of ulcerated plaques in the aortic arch in patients with stroke. N Engl J Med 326:221, 1992.
5. Anderson WR: Necrotizing angiitis associated with embolization of cholesterol: Case report with emphasis on the use of the muscle biopsy as a diagnostic aid. Am J Clin Pathol 43:65, 1965.
6. Baumann DS, McGraw D, Rubin BG, et al: An institutional experience with arterial atheroembolism. An Vasc Surg 8:258, 1994.
7. Berkman M, Berkman N, Favre M, et al: Les embolies de cholesterol: Confrontation clinique, ophthalmoscopique et anatomique, a l'occasion de trois observations. Nouv Presse Med 1:795, 1972.
8. Blankenship JC, Butler M, Garbes A: Prospective assessment of cholesterol embolization in patients with acute myocardial infarction treated with thrombolytic therapy vs conservative therapy. Chest 107:662, 1995.
9. Blauth CI: Macroemboli and microemboli during cardiopulmonary bypass. Ann Thorac Surg 59:1300, 1995.
10. Bojar RM, Payne DD, Murphy RE, et al: Surgical treatment of systemic atheroembolism from the thoracic aorta. Ann Thorac Surg 61:1389, 1996.
11. Branowitz JB, Edwards WS: The management of atheromatous emboli to the lower extremities. Surg Gynecol Obstet 143:941, 1976.
12. Bruns FJ, Segel DP, Adler S: Control of cholesterol embolization by discontinuation of anticoagulant therapy. Am J Med Sci 275:105, 1978.
13. Carvajal JA, Anderson WR, Weiss L, et al: Atheroembolism: An etiologic factor in renal insufficiency, gastrointestinal hemorrhages and peripheral vascular diseases. Arch Intern Med 119:593, 1967.
14. Case records of the Massachusetts General Hospital 50–1977. N Engl J Med 297:1337, 1977.
15. Case records of the Massachusetts General Hospital 30–1986. N Engl J Med 315:308, 1986.
16. Crane C: Atherothrombotic embolism to lower extremities in arteriosclerosis. Arch Surg 94:96, 1967.
17. Dahlberg PJ, Frecentese DF, Cogbill TH: Cholesterol embolism: Experience with 22 histologically proven cases. Surgery 105:737, 1989.
18. Darsee JR: Cholesterol embolism: The great masquerader. South Med J 72:174, 1979.
19. Davila-Roman VG, Barzilai B, Wareing TH, et al: Atherosclerosis of the ascending aorta: Prevalence and role as an independent predictor of cerebrovascular events in cardiac patients. Stroke 25:2010, 1994.
20. Dietl CA Madigan NP, Laubach CA, et al: Myocardial revascularization using the "no-touch" technique, with mild systemic hypothermia, in patients with a calcified ascending aorta. J Cardiovasc Surg 36:39, 1995.
21. Eason JD, Mills JL, Beckett WC: Hypercoagulable states in arterial thromboembolism. Surg Gynecol Obstet 174:211, 1992.
22. Falanga V, Fine MJ, Kapoor WN: The cutaneous manifestations of cholesterol crystal embolization. Arch Dermatol 122:1194, 1986.
23. Fernandez-Samos R, Suarez D, Ortega JM, et al: Multiple cholesterol embolization syndrome: A lethal complication of vascular procedures: Report of two histologically proven cases. J Cardiovasc Surg 36:87, 1995.
24. Fisher DF, Clagett GP, Brigham RA, et al: Dilemmas in dealing with the blue toe syndrome: Aortic versus peripheral source. Am J Surg 148:836, 1984.
25. Flinn WR, Harris JP, Rudo ND, et al: Atheroembolism as a cause of graft failure in femoral distal reconstruction. Surgery 90:698, 1981.
26. Flory CM: Arterial occlusions produced by emboli from eroded aortic atheromatous plaques. Am J Pathol 21:549, 1945.
27. Friedman SG, Krishnasastry KV: External iliac ligation and axillary-bifemoral bypass for blue toe syndrome. Surgery 115:27, 1994.
28. Fuster V, Badimon L, Badimon JJ, Chesebro JH: The pathogenesis of coronary artery disease and the acute coronary syndromes. N Engl J Med 326:310, 1992.
29. Geroulakos G, Homer-Vanniasinkam S, Wilkinson A, et al: Cholesterol embolisation: A lethal complication of instrumentation of an aneurysmal aorta—a case report. Int Angiol 16:69, 1997.
30. Gore L, Collins DP: Spontaneous atheromatous embolization: Review of the literature and a report of 16 additional cases. Am J Clin Pathol 33:416, 1960.
31. Greenberg A, Bastacky SI, Iqbal A, et al: Focal segmental glomerulosclerosis associated with nephrotic syndrome in cholesterol atheroembolism: Clinicopathological correlations. Am J Kidney Dis 29:334, 1997.
32. Harrington JT, Sommers SC, Kassirer JP: Atheromatous emboli with progressive renal failure: Renal arteriography as the probable inciting factor. Ann Intern Med 68:152, 1968.
33. Haygood TA, Fessel WJ, Strange DA: Atheromatous microembolism simulating polymyositis. JAMA 203:423, 1968.
34. Inahara T, Scott CM: Endarterectomy for segmental occlusive disease of the superficial femoral artery. Arch Surg 116:1547, 1981.
35. Jenkins DM, Newton WD: Atheroembolism. Am Surg 57:588, 1991.
36. Karmody AM, Jordan FR, Zaman SM: Left colon gangrene after acute inferior mesenteric artery occlusion. Arch Surg 111:972, 1976.

37. Karmody AM, Powers SR, Monaco VJ, et al: "Blue toe" syndrome: An indication for limb salvage surgery. Arch Surg 111:1263, 1976.
38. Kaufman JL, Saifi J, Chang BB, et al: The role of extra-anatomic exclusion bypass in the treatment of disseminated atheroembolism syndrome. Ann Vasc Surg 4:260, 1990.
39. Kaufman JL, Stark K, Brolin RE: Disseminated atheroembolism from extensive degenerative atherosclerosis of the aorta. Surgery 102:63, 1987.
40. Kealy WF: Atheroembolism. J Clin Pathol 31:984, 1978.
41. Keen RR, McCarthy WJ, Shireman PK, et al: Surgical management of atheroembolism. J Vasc Surg 21:773, 1995.
42. Kempczinski RF: Lower-extremity arterial emboli from ulcerating atherosclerotic plaques. JAMA 241:807, 1979.
43. Khatibzadeh M, Mitusch R, Stierle U, et al: Aortic atherosclerotic plaques as a source of systemic embolism. J Am Coll Cardiol 27:664, 1996.
44. Kwaan JHM, Connolly JE: Peripheral atheroembolism: An enigma. Arch Surg 112:987, 1977.
45. Labs JD, Merillat JC, Williams GM: Analysis of solid phase debris from laser angioplasty: Potential risks of atheroembolism. J Vasc Surg 7:326, 1988.
46. Lee BY, Brancato RF, Thoden WR, et al: Blue digit syndrome: Urgent indication for digital salvage. Am J Surg 147:418, 1984.
47. Mayo RR, Schwartz RD: Redefining the incidence of clinically detectable atheroembolism. Am J Med 100:534, 1996.
48. McFarland RJ, Taylow RS, Woodyer AB, Eastwood JB: The femoropopliteal segment as a source of peripheral atheroembolism. J Cardiovasc Surg 30:597,1989.
49. McLean NR, Irvine BH, Calvert MH: Peripheral embolic phenomena from proximal arterial disease. J R Coll Surg Edinb 29:205, 1984.
50. Mehigan JT, Stoney RJ: Lower extremity atheromatous embolization. Am J Surg 132:163, 1976.
51. Moolenaar W, Lamers CB: Cholesterol crystal embolization in the Netherlands. Arch Intern Med 156:653, 1996.
52. Moolenaar W, Lamers CB: Cholesterol crystal embolization to the alimentary tract. Gut 38:196, 1996.
53. Morris-Jones W, Preston FE, Greaney M, Chatterjee DK: Gangrene of the toes with palpable peripheral pulses: Response to platelet suppressive therapy. Ann Surg 193:462, 1981.
54. O'Brian DS, Jeffers M, Kay EW, et al: Bleeding due to colorectal atheroembolism: Diagnosis by biopsy of adenomatous polyps or of ischemic ulcer. Am J Surg Pathol 15:1078, 1991.
55. Perdue GD, Smith RB: Atheromatous microemboli. Ann Surg 169:954, 1969.
56. Pizzolitto S, Rocco M, Antonucci F, Antoci B: Atheroembolism: A form of systemic vascular disease. Pathologica 83:147, 1991.
57. Quintart C, Treille S, Lefebvre P, et al: Penile necrosis following cholesterol embolism Br J Urol 80:347, 1997.
58. Ramirez G, O'Neill WM, Lambert R, et al: Cholesterol embolization: A complication of angiography. Arch Intern Med 138:1430, 1978.
59. Retan JW, Miller RE: Microembolic complications of atherosclerosis. Arch Intern Med 118:534, 1966.
60. Ribakove GH, Katz ES, Galloway AC, et al: Surgical implications of transesophageal echocardiography to grade the atheromatous aortic arch. Ann Thorac Surg 53:758, 1992.
61. Richards AM, Eliot RS, Kanjuh VI, et al: Cholesterol embolism: A multiple-system disease masquerading as polyarteritis nodosa. Am J Cardiol 15:696, 1965.
62. Robicsek F: Prevention of cholesterol embolism (trash foot) during aorto-iliac reconstruction using a blood filtering device. J Cardiovasc Surg (Torino) 27:63, 1987.
63. Rosenberg MW, Shah DP: Bilateral blue toe syndrome: A case report. JAMA 243:365, 1980.
64. Saklayen MG, Gupta S, Suryaprasad A, et al: Incidence of atheroembolic renal failure after coronary angiography: A prospective study. Angiology 48:609, 1997.
65. Schechter DC: Atheromatous embolization to lower limbs. N Y State Med J 79:1180, 1979.
66. Schipper H, Gordon M, Berris B: Atheromatous embolic disease. Can Med Assoc J 113:640, 1975.
67. Sharma PV, Babu SC, Shah PM, et al: Changing patterns of atheroembolism. Cardiovasc Surg 4:573, 1996.
68. Smith MC, Ghose MK, Henry AR: The clinical spectrum of renal cholesterol embolization. Am J Med 71:174, 1981.
69. Stoney RJ, Skioldebrand CG, Ovarfordt PG, et al: Juxtarenal aortic atherosclerosis: Surgical experience and functional result. Ann Surg 200:345, 1984.
70. Sussman B, Stahl R, Ibrahim IM, et al: Atheroemboli to the lower urinary tract: A marker of atherosclerotic vascular disease—a case report. J Vasc Surg 12:655, 1990.
71. Thadhani RI, Camargo CA Jr, Xavier RJ, et al: Atheroembolic renal failure after invasive procedures: Natural history based on 52 histologically proven cases. Medicine 74:350, 1995.
72. Tierney G, Parissis H, Baker M, et al: An experimental study of intra-aortic balloon pumping with the intact human aorta. Eur J Cardiothorac Surg 12:486, 1997.
73. Willens HJ, Kramer HJ, Kessler KM: Transesophageal echocardiographic findings in blue toe syndrome exacerbated by anticoagulation. J Am Soc Echocardiogr 9:882, 1996.
74. Williams GM, Harrington D, Burdick J, et al: Mural thrombus of the aorta: An important, frequently neglected cause of large peripheral emboli. Ann Surg 194:737, 1981.
75. Wilson DM, Salazer TL, Faroukh ME: Eosinophiluria in atheroembolic renal disease. Am J Med 91:186, 1991.

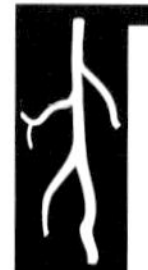

CHAPTER 57

Acute Vascular Insufficiency Due to Drug Injection

R. James Valentine, M.D., and William W. Turner, Jr., M.D.

Substance abuse is a worldwide social concern. Among the many problems associated with drug addiction, acute vascular insufficiency is the most common disorder for which a vascular surgeon is consulted. The modern addict is skilled at achieving intravenous access. The lack of precise anatomic knowledge and inexperience with sterile technique frequently lead to acute complications involving both arterial and venous systems. The more common complications of drug-induced vascular insufficiency are listed in Table 57–1.

ARTERIAL INJURIES

The first report of an accidental intra-arterial drug injection with resulting gangrene appeared more than 55 years ago.[1] Thereafter, several instances of barbiturate-induced vascular insufficiency were described.[2–8] In the earlier years, these problems were due primarily to unintentional intra-arterial injections by physicians or nurses. The complications of intra-arterial injections are now most often associated with illicit drug use. There have been many reports of extremity gangrene following intra-arterial injections of a variety of drugs, and a number of authors have attempted to delineate the mechanisms of the injuries.[2–4, 6, 7, 9–15]

TABLE 57–1. COMPLICATIONS OF DRUG-INDUCED VASCULAR INSUFFICIENCY

Infections	*Vascular complications*
Cellulitis	Compartment syndrome
Abscesses	Rhabdomyolysis
Osteomyelitis	Vasospasm
Septic arthritis	Direct arterial injury
Endocarditis	Intimal disruption
Lymphatic complications	Thrombosis
Puffy hand	Embolism
Neurologic complications	Mycotic aneurysm
Direct nerve injury	Skin ulcers
Polyneuritis	Thrombophlebitis
Ischemic neuritis	Venous aneurysm
Acute transverse myelitis	

Adapted from Ritland D, Butterfield W: Extremity complications of drug abuse. Am J Surg 126:639–648, 1973.

CLINICAL PRESENTATION

There is no way to calculate accurately the incidence of arterial injections associated with drug abuse or to fully describe the variety of resulting vascular insufficiency syndromes. Only the worst complications of intra-arterial drug injections come to medical attention, and it is possible that many inadvertent intra-arterial injections go unnoticed. Several large centers have reported their experiences.[9, 16–25] Complicating the clinical presentation are the multiple and varied manifestations. One report noted hand ischemia secondary to intra-arterial drug injections in five patients who denied any history of substance abuse.[26]

Drug users, depending on "self-taught" skills, may directly inject a superficial artery, or they may enter an artery accidentally while attempting to gain access to any vessel deep in the antecubital fossa or femoral triangle. Only with the production of a "hand trip" does the addict recognize the error of intra-arterial injection.[5] The result has been described as a burning discomfort extending from the point of injection to the tips of the fingers, followed by blanching, severe pain, and subsequent swelling and cyanosis. The exact timing of these events, particularly the development of gangrene, remains unclear. Delay in seeking medical attention is frequent. It is common for digital or even total extremity gangrene to be the presenting complaint (Fig. 57–1).

Before, during, and after the administration of a drug, additional factors can play roles in the development of gangrene. In the quest for vascular access, an individual may use a variety of tourniquets, and the sedative effects of the drug may lead to prolonged tourniquet compression with the induction of venous or arterial thrombosis. The intra-arterially injected drug may remain in sustained contact with the vessel intima prior to release of the tourniquet. Abnormal posturing with arm or thigh flexion or with the extremity compressed under the full weight of the obtunded person may add to circulatory compromise. Experimental studies using catheters placed in normal volunteers have documented marked elevations of intramuscular pressures sufficient to cause muscle and capillary ischemia and local obstruction of the circulation when extremities are placed in postures similar to those assumed by overdosed, sedated, stuporous individuals.[27]

Local injury is a problem associated with arterial access, even when access is performed by skilled clinicians.[28] Arterial injections by the less adept addict may lead to a variety

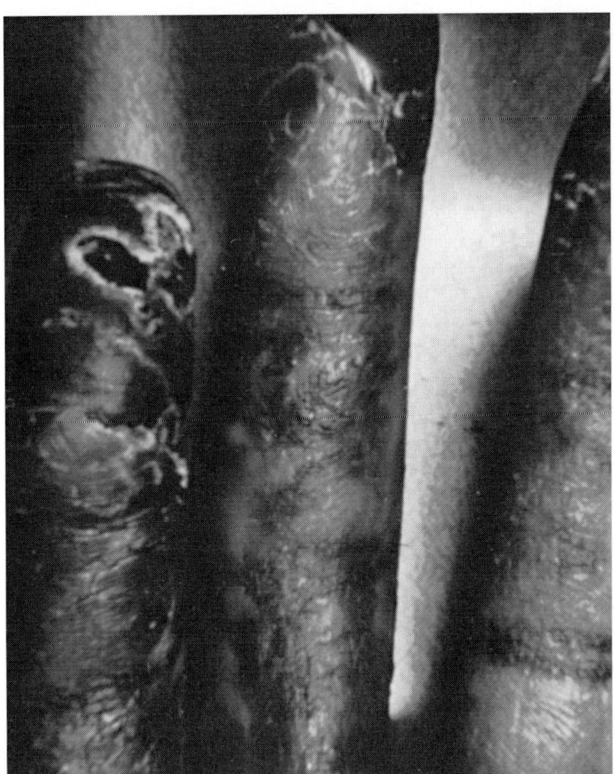

FIGURE 57–1. Distal gangrene following intra-arterial administration of heroin.

of vessel injuries that cause thrombosis at injection sites; these include intimal flaps, perivascular hematomas, and perivascular inflammation. Certain drugs are also more likely to damage the intima directly.[3, 29] Severe damage to arteries at injection sites can cause pseudoaneurysm formation. Pseudoaneurysms may develop at any site as a result of a through-and-through puncture or ineffectual tamponade of a puncture site after removal of a needle. Superimposed infection is common. Mycotic aneurysms are being reported more frequently both at sites of injections and at distant locations, including cerebral, aortic, splenic, coronary, and pulmonary arteries. Other unusual sites for mycotic aneurysms are the inferior mesenteric, carotid, and superior mesenteric arteries.[24, 30–34] The more superficial pseudoaneurysms of the brachial, femoral, and radial arteries are often used by drug addicts for vascular access because they are more easily palpable than peripheral veins (Fig. 57–2).

Upper Extremity

The brachial artery is the most common site of accidental injections in the upper extremity.[35] Pseudoaneurysm is the most common sequela. Patients with pseudoaneurysms frequently present with cellulitis and pain associated with infection or distal ischemia. Severe ischemia accompanies such lesions in approximately 30% of cases. Fortunately, systemic sepsis is usually not a major problem. In a series of 32 patients with upper extremity lesions, only 12% had positive blood cultures.[35]

Mycotic aneurysms associated with intra-arterial injections are treated by ligation and excision, and immediate distal revascularizations are not generally required. This form of treatment has been associated with few complications. For severely involved gangrenous digits, amputation may be necessary.

Lower Extremity

Approximately 75% of all admissions for accidental intra-arterial drug injections involve the lower extremities.[35] Pseudoaneurysm is the most common arterial abnormality, with arteriovenous fistula being second in frequency. The major presenting symptom is a painful, pulsatile mass, often associated with cellulitis. In some cases, the pulsatile mass may be obscured by overlying soft tissue swelling.[36]

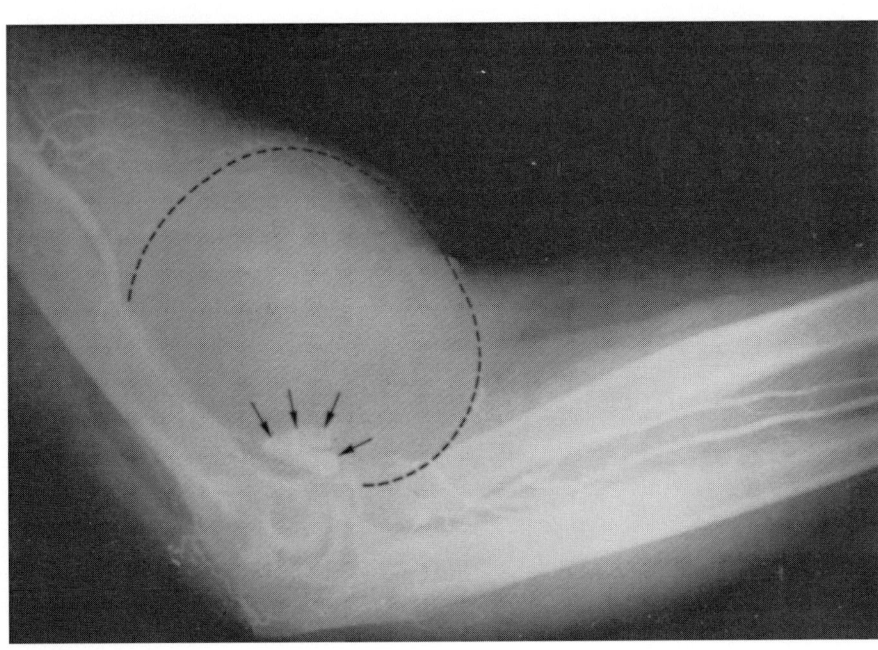

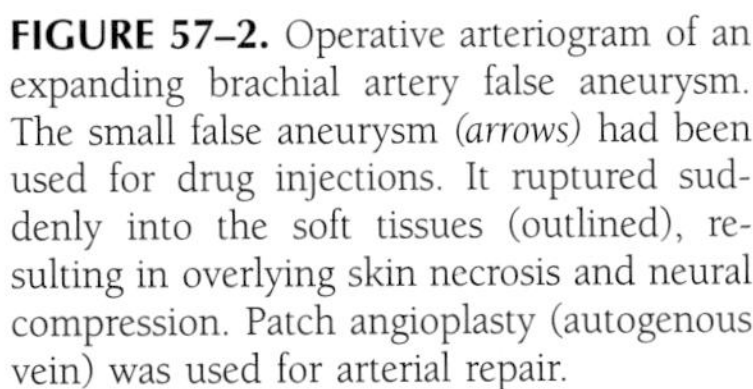

FIGURE 57–2. Operative arteriogram of an expanding brachial artery false aneurysm. The small false aneurysm *(arrows)* had been used for drug injections. It ruptured suddenly into the soft tissues (outlined), resulting in overlying skin necrosis and neural compression. Patch angioplasty (autogenous vein) was used for arterial repair.

Examination often reveals a bruit over the involved area. Local infections are common, and there is a higher incidence of positive blood cultures than with mycotic aneurysms of the upper extremities. The predominant infecting organism is *Staphylococcus aureus*.[36–38]

Optimal treatment of infected femoral artery pseudoaneurysms involves ligation of affected arterial segments to reduce the risk of hemorrhage and débridement of all grossly contaminated tissue to remove the septic focus. The need for subsequent revascularization has been controversial.

In a review of 54 infected femoral artery pseudoaneurysms in drug addicts, 11% of patients required amputations.[40] There was a 33% risk of amputation when the common femoral bifurcation was involved and required excision. Twenty-eight aneurysms were reconstructed by means of either prosthetic grafts or saphenous veins. All synthetic grafts eventually developed septic complications, and graft removal was required. Of 18 patients who were treated by ligations without vascular reconstructions, one third required amputation. This study suggests that if a pseudoaneurysm involves only a single artery, ligation with excision is the treatment of choice. When the common femoral bifurcation is involved, immediate autogenous reconstruction should be considered.

Opponents of revascularization point out that placement of bypass grafts in patients with infected pseudoaneurysms is rarely indicated and is potentially dangerous. Recent experience indicates that ligation and débridement of the common femoral bifurcation without revascularization may be associated with a low risk of amputation.[37, 41] Furthermore, significant complications are frequent after revascularization procedures.

In a study of 18 drug addicts with femoral artery pseudoaneurysms, significant complications developed in all 12 patients who underwent revascularizations.[39] Three patients required amputations, and there were 13 secondary arterial operations in this group. In contrast, no complications occurred in the six patients who underwent primary arterial ligations and débridements. These data suggest that bypass operations may be fraught with risk in drug addicts.

Primary ligation without revascularization may be desirable to prevent serious sequelae, such as life-threatening hemorrhage associated with secondary graft infection.[39, 42] Others have reported amputation rates fewer than 10% in patients who undergo ligation of the common femoral bifurcation without revascularization.[37, 41] All patients have some degree of intermittent claudication, but late amputations are rare. Patients undergoing ligation of all three femoral vessels may be expected to have a higher degree of disability and a lower mean ankle-brachial index (ABI) than patients undergoing ligation of single vessels.[37, 11]

The issue of revascularization in a drug addict is further complicated by poor patient compliance and inadequate autogenous graft material. Post-discharge follow-up of addicts is rare. Repeated use of superficial veins in these patients virtually eliminates autogenous conduits, necessitating the use of prosthetic material in many cases.[36, 38, 39] When, then, should revascularization be considered in these difficult patients?

A rational approach has been suggested by Padberg and associates.[39] Following ligation and removal of the septic focus, limb viability is assessed during surgery by determination of a Doppler signal at the ankle. Revascularization is considered only in patients who have an absent Doppler signal, indicating acute limb ischemia. In these cases, autogenous vein is always the conduit of choice. When superficial veins are not available, the femoral vein may be an excellent alternative.[43] In cases of severe contamination and when prosthetic material is required, obturator bypasses have been utilized successfully for the treatment of mycotic aneurysms in drug addicts.[44] Such extra-anatomic bypass techniques may be excellent alternatives to direct revascularization through contaminated tissues.

Head and Neck

The head and neck are the least common sites of vascular insufficiency secondary to drug abuse. This is perhaps due to the infrequent use of these highly visible areas and to the addict's desire to keep the injection sites hidden. In a review of 172 consecutive patients hospitalized for vascular injuries from drug abuse, only 2% of patients presented with head and neck lesions.[35] The carotid artery was the most commonly involved vessel. There were two carotid pseudoaneurysms, one carotid-jugular arteriovenous fistula, and one arterial wall necrosis. The most common presenting complaint was a pulsatile mass with associated induration and cellulitis. All of the patients were treated with ligations of the common carotid arteries, and no neurologic sequelae resulted from this treatment.

Deep abscesses may be associated with arterial lesions in the neck. Various abused drugs have been implicated, but methylphenidate (Ritalin) has been associated with more than 50% of the deep neck abscesses in some series.[45] Because the majority of these abscesses are acquired outside the hospital, it is not surprising that most cultures reveal staphylococci and streptococci. A less common organism, *Eikenella corrodens,* has been implicated as a synergistic pathogen with streptococci in association with Ritalin-induced abscesses. Oral flora are the most likely source of organisms that contaminate the head and neck.

Needle fragment foreign bodies are a particular problem in addicts who practice self-injection in the neck (Fig. 57–3).[46, 47] Unsuspected neck needles pose significant risk for individuals caring for these patients, especially surgeons. In a report of 50 patients with neck needle foreign bodies related to intravenous drug abuse, only 50% of the patients presented with complaints of retained neck needles and only 10% had complications related to neck needles on presentation.[46] There were no late complications related to the neck needles, suggesting that extraction of asymptomatic fragments is unnecessary. However, seropositivity for human immunodeficiency virus (HIV) was 77%, underscoring the need for strict adherence to universal precautions in intravenous drug abusers who require neck explorations.

Viscera

Gastrointestinal complications in drug addicts are associated most commonly with cocaine use. Acute mesenteric ischemia has been reported following cocaine administration via oral, intravenous, nasal, or respiratory routes.[48, 49]

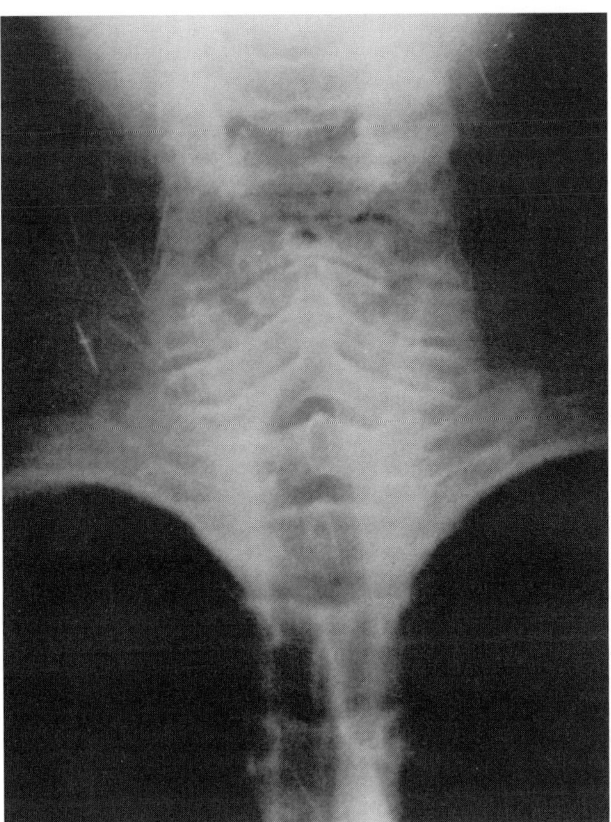

FIGURE 57–3. Multiple needle fragments following self-injections in the neck. (From Williams MF, Eisele DW, Wyatt SH: Neck needle foreign bodies in intravenous drug abusers. Laryngoscope 103:59, 1993. By permission of The Laryngoscope.)

Affected patients usually present with abdominal pain, nausea, and vomiting.[48] Up to half of them have a history of diarrhea.[48]

Angiography usually reveals a "nonocclusive" pattern of mesenteric ischemia, reflecting the intense, cocaine-induced vasospasm associated with this syndrome. Large vessel thrombosis is usually absent.[48–50] Treatment has included resections of infarcted bowel segments, although some patients with less advanced degrees of mesenteric ischemia have recovered after conservative therapy.[48] Pathologic examination of infarcted intestinal segments has disclosed atypical obstructive lesions in small-caliber arterioles within the submucosa.[51]

Other acute visceral ischemia syndromes have been reported following cocaine use, including gastropyloric ulceration,[52] gangrenous cholecystitis,[53] ischemic colitis,[54] and acute hepatocellular necrosis.[55] The underlying pathologic mechanism of these complications has been attributed generally to severe mesenteric vasoconstriction, but recent data suggest that cocaine-induced thrombosis may have contributed to large vessel disease in some patients (Fig. 57–4).[48] We have described two patients with chronic intestinal ischemia caused by intravenous cocaine use who were managed successfully with visceral revascularizations.[48]

Lung

Multiple mycotic pulmonary artery aneurysms have been reported secondary to intravenous drug abuse.[56–58] Patients frequently present with dyspnea, cyanosis, and hemoptysis. Physical examination sometimes reveals a harsh systolic murmur in the left second interspace. Electrocardiographic evidence of right ventricular hypertrophy with right axis deviation is common.[59] These lesions are difficult to manage, as they are frequently multiple and often central in location. Bilaterality occurs, and this precludes surgical treatment by resection and ligation in some cases. To date, fewer than 70 cases have been collected in the world literature. As intravenous drug abuse increases, it is possible that mycotic aneurysms of the pulmonary arteries will be identified more frequently.

Pulmonary hypertension associated with talc granulomas can occur when drugs intended for oral use are injected intravenously. Pulmonary hypertension, and in extreme cases cor pulmonale, result from small vessel occlusions due to excipients.[60, 61]

MECHANISMS OF INJURY

Numerous proposed mechanisms may produce ischemia, for example[7, 18, 19, 23, 62–66]:

- Vessel obstruction by inert particles
- Direct endothelial damage with thrombosis
- Hypersensitivity vasculitis
- Vasospasm
- Venous thrombosis

Inert Particles

Most of these factors lead to thrombosis of the arterial supply to digits as the final common pathway to extremity

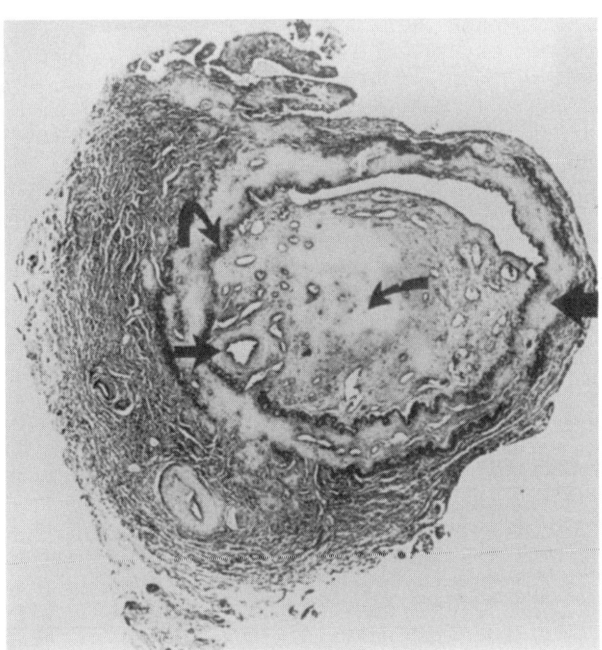

FIGURE 57–4. Photomicrograph of chronic thrombosis in a celiac artery specimen from a cocaine abuser with chronic mesenteric ischemia. *Long arrow* = thrombus; *short arrow* = recanalized channel; *curved arrow* = internal elastic lamina; *broad arrow* = tunica media. (From Myers SI, Clagett GP, Valentine RJ, et al: Chronic mesenteric ischemia caused by intravenous cocaine use: Report of two cases and review of the literature. J Vasc Surg 23:724, 1996. By permission of Journal of Vascular Surgery.)

gangrene. The addict may use pure drugs, but more often the drugs have been "cut" with other materials, either by the producer or by the distributor. Oral preparations are often diluted or suspended and injected along with debris from the tablet (Table 57–2).[24, 67, 68] Each of these additives can compound the vascular injury produced by the specific drug.

Excipients

Excipients may also have systemic effects. Oral suspensions of Ritalin containing talc and cornstarch have been injected intravenously. The excipients have been identified in the retinal fundi and choroid, producing transient blindness and decreased visual acuity as well as neovascularization.[67, 69–74] The microvasculature of the digits may, like the eye, be particularly sensitive to excipient collections. Such effects may result from both intravenous and intra-arterial injections.

Crystals

Crystalline emboli, like excipients, can play a role in producing arterial injury. In one series of experiments, Waters studied in vitro crystallization of thiopental sodium in freshly drawn blood at room and body temperatures.[75] Concentrations of 5%, 2.5%, and 1.25% thiopental were evaluated to show the amount of precipitated thiopental in mixtures with blood. The obstructing capacity of these mixtures was demonstrated by perfusing them through a No. 20 hypodermic needle and, in addition, by postmortem perfusion of a human arm. Crystals formed in 5% and 10% thiopental solutions but occurred less frequently in lower concentration solutions.

Crystal formation does not account for all instances of arterial gangrene. Direct endothelial damage with ensuing thrombosis is another effect associated with injection of some agents. A series of experiments in dogs produced gangrene with dextroamphetamine sulfate (Dexedrine), and promazine hydrochloride (Sparine), ether, and sulfobromophthalein sodium (Bromsulphalein). Temporary occlusion of the femoral artery proximal to the site of injection was necessary in order to produce gangrene. Biopsies and vascular casts of the necrotic tissue demonstrated severe necrosis of the small artery walls with pronounced edema and congestion with thrombi in some of the larger vessels. The vascular casts demonstrated complete occlusion of larger arterioles and small arteries corresponding to the areas of gangrene. It was concluded that these drugs are transported in undiluted forms as boluses of highly irritating solutions that induce gangrene.

TABLE 57–2. COMMON EXCIPIENTS

Caffeine
Lactose
Procaine
Quinine
Starch
Stearic acid
Talcum powder

TABLE 57–3. DRUGS ASSOCIATED WITH HYPERSENSITIVITY VASCULITIS

Allopurinol	Isoniazid
Ampicillin	Levamisole
Bromide	Methylthiouracil
Carbamazepine	Oxyphenbutazone
Chloramphenicol	Phenylbutazone
Chlorpropamide	Phenytoin
Chlortetracycline	Potassium iodide
Chlorthalidone	Procainamide
Cromolyn sodium	Propylthiouracil
Colchicine	Quinidine
Dextran	Spironolactone
Diazepam	Sulfonamides
Diphenhydramine	Tetracycline
Griseofulvin	Trimethadione
Indomethacin	

From McAllister HA Jr, Mullick FG: The cardiovascular system. *In* Riddel RH (ed): Pathology of Drug-Induced and Toxic Disease. New York, Churchill Livingstone, 1982.

Many drugs have been associated with a hypersensitivity vasculitis syndrome. Some of these substances are listed in Table 57–3. Additionally, several drugs have been associated with toxic vasculitis (Table 57–4). A lupus-like syndrome occurring after injection of certain substances has been reported also (Table 57–5).

A study of 10 barbiturate solutions at varying concentrations demonstrated that in addition to crystal formation, hemolysis and platelet aggregation occurred with barbiturates.[62] Since these reports, thiopental has been supplied in the reduced concentration (2.5%), and reports of problems with this drug have become much less frequent.

Vasospasm

Vasospasm secondary to drug acidity, alkalinity, vascular trauma, and norepinephrine or epinephrine release has been studied. The contribution of arterial constriction to the sequelae of intra-arterial drug injection remains controversial. Contraction of aortic strips and ear arteries was produced in rabbits by thiopental.[76] This may have been due to local norepinephrine release or to direct chemical effects.[63] Vasospasm may also result from local trauma or irritation by particulate matter.[77] Most clinical studies that have implicated vasospasm have lacked arteriographic data.[16, 19, 23, 68]

In one experiment, investigators employed micrometer measurements of rabbit femoral arteries before, during, and after injections of 5% thiopental or a buffer of equal pH.[6]

TABLE 57–4. DRUGS ASSOCIATED WITH TOXIC VASCULITIS

Organic arsenicals	Methamphetamine
Gold salts	DDT
Mercurials	Serum
Bismuth	Sulfonamides
Amphetamine	Penicillin

From McAllister HA Jr, Mullick FG: The cardiovascular system. *In* Riddel RH (ed): Pathology of Drug-Induced and Toxic Disease. New York, Churchill Livingstone, 1982.

DDT = dichlorodiphenyl trichloroethane.

TABLE 57–5. DRUGS THAT INDUCE LUPUS-LIKE SYNDROMES

Hydralazine	Tetracycline
Procainamide	Propylthiouracil
Isoniazid	Methylthiouracil
Aminosalicylic acid	Methyldopa
Phenytoin	Barbiturates
Mephenytoin	Griseofulvin
Primidone	Streptomycin
Trimethadione	Quinidine
Ethosuximide	Phenylbutazone
Methsuximide	Chlorpromazine
Reserpine	Methotrimeprazine
Penicillin	Perphenazine
Penicillamine	Promazine
Sulfonamides	

From McAllister HA Jr, Mullick FG: The cardiovascular system. *In* Riddel RH (ed): Pathology of Drug-induced and Toxic Disease. New York, Churchill Livingstone, 1982.

Transient (30-second) vasoconstriction was followed by prompt vasodilatation in response to the thiopental, and no effect was noted from the buffer. In subsequent experiments, tissue necrosis developed after injections of 0.2 ml of 10% thiopental into the central artery of the rabbit ear, followed by application of an intestinal clamp across the base of the ear for 15 minutes. Prolonged observation for 3 to 4 weeks was required before a standard amount of necrosis was seen. In this model, sympathetic denervation by cervical ganglionectomy significantly decreased the area of gangrene, and administration of 2500 units of heparin every 8 hours was also associated with a reduction of the gangrene. When a decreased concentration of thiopental (2.5%) was substituted, the incidence of tissue loss was very low. If procaine or tolazoline was administered following thiopental, no significant reduction in the area of gangrene occurred. The authors concluded that prolonged arterial spasm was not the cause of ischemia after intra-arterial injection of thiopental, since the area of injury could be diminished by lowering the thiopental concentration, by sympathectomy, or by heparinization, but not by vasodilator drugs.

A study in the rabbit ear intra-arterial thiopental model also suggested that vasospasm might have only a limited effect on the clinical events following intra-arterial drug injections. Vasodilators administered after the injection of thiopental had no effect on the course of tissue necrosis.[78] This study did not employ arteriography to assess the degree of vasospasm, and the conclusion that vasospasm played a minor role in the development of gangrene was drawn indirectly from evidence of the ineffectiveness of vasodilators in preventing gangrene. The results of these animal experiments differ from anecdotal cases in humans in which the intra-arterial injection of the vasodilator reserpine produced immediately improved distal perfusion in patients who had injected crushed pentazocine tablets into the brachial arteries.[79]

Although arterial constriction may occupy a debatable position in the etiology of drug-related extremity ischemia, venospasm may play an indirect but significant role. Concentrated drugs can cause venostasis. Repetitive angiography was used to study the effects of 0.4 ml of 10% thiopental on the central arteries and veins of rabbit ears.[12] The study demonstrated dramatic changes in the venous circulation, including marked venospasm along with segmental thrombosis, which probably contributed to the development of ischemia and gangrene. Acute outflow obstruction with transudation into interstitial spaces leading to persistent arterial stasis with thrombosis may have been the mechanism underlying ischemic necrosis.[80] An absence of superficial veins may further contribute to flow reduction and ischemia.[3, 13, 75, 81, 82]

THERAPEUTIC CONSIDERATIONS

Therapy should include immediate measures to relieve pain, to prevent local limb and systemic hypothermia, and to improve venous drainage by patient positioning. Long-term efforts should be directed at discontinuance of drug abuse and cessation of smoking. Arteriography should be performed early, with a catheter positioned proximal to the suspected site of drug injection. An arteriogram can define local arterial injuries, such as an intimal flap, a pseudoaneurysm, an arteriovenous fistula, or thrombosis as well as distal vasospasm or thrombosis. The arteriogram catheter may be left in place for subsequent intraluminal therapy.

Pharmacologic Therapy

Vasodilators

Vasodilating agents can play a role in the treatment of acute arterial ischemia secondary to drugs of abuse.[23, 75, 78, 83–85] Tolazoline (Priscoline) in doses of 25 to 50 mg has been used successfully by injection into the proximal artery.[86] Tolazoline competitively blocks arterial wall alpha-adrenergic receptors, dilates precapillary arterioles, and opens precapillary arteriovenous shunts in the skin. Other vasodilators that have been used in patients following intra-arterial drug injections include verapamil and phentolamine[87, 88]

If vasospasm is not a major component of the process vasodilator, therapy cannot directly alter the response to the drug, although it may serve to maintain collateral circulation.

Anticoagulants

Animal studies have demonstrated a benefit of heparin in reducing gangrene after intra-arterial injections of thiopental.[6, 89] Beneficial reports in humans have included anecdote and a noteworthy description of a patient who reconstituted an occluded palmar arch and also experienced improved digital flow in the hand after the administration of intra-arterial heparin.[9, 18, 23, 86] Evidence suggests that treatment for at least 4 days may be beneficial.[6]

Thrombolytic Agents

Persistent vessel occlusion and poor response to vasodilators may indicate a need for thrombolysis. Low-dose intra-arterial *streptokinase* has been used successfully in patients with palmar arterial thromboses secondary to causes *other* than intra-arterial drug injections.[90, 91] A patient with hand ischemia after forearm arterial drug injection experienced improved hand perfusion within 24 hours of intra-arterial streptokinase.[86] (Fig. 57–5). This patient received an initial intra-arterial dose of 25,000 units of streptokinase followed by 3000 units/hr for 24 hours. Traditionally, the infusion catheter has been placed within the thrombus to produce a high local concentration of the drug and to reduce perfusion of collateral vessels with the drug. This may limit the success of thrombolytic therapy in patients with distal thrombi that are seen frequently after intra-arterial drug injections. Urokinase may have the advantage of fewer allergic reactions, but it is more expensive.

Tissue plasminogen activator (t-PA) is used increasingly in the treatment of intra-arterial thrombosis.[90, 92, 92] Ready availability of recombinant deoxyribonucleic acid (DNA)–produced t-PA has facilitated widespread use. Thrombolysis may be achieved more rapidly with t-PA than with streptokinase, and it is theoretically safer than streptokinase or urokinase because of its affinity for fibrin.[94, 95] A report comparing the success of low-dose streptokinase with that of t-PA demonstrated comparable fibrinolytic effects, shorter duration of therapy required with t-PA, and lower t-PA doses than reported traditionally with the drug.[95] The investigators advocated intra-arterial infusions of t-PA at 0.5 mg/hr, and the median time to achieve reperfusion was 22 hours.

Infusions of thrombolytic agents, even those administered intra-arterially, may cause systemic proteolysis if used for prolonged periods (>48 hours). Although monitoring of plasma fibrinogen levels and other clotting profiles is advocated, evidence supports no reduction in bleeding complications with these measurements.[90]

Steroids

In some studies, chemical endarteritis following intra-arterial drug injections has been ameliorated by intra-arterial dexamethasone sodium phosphate (Decadron).[63, 84, 96] Dexamethasone administered in doses ranging from 40 to 70 mg, followed by 40 mg every 6 hours (orally or intravenously) decreases progressive tissue necrosis.[18, 63] A precautionary note should be made of a case report of digital ischemia resulting from intra-arterial injection of methylprednisolone acetate (Depo-Medrone, Depo-Medrol).[97] This response may have been due to distal small arterial obstruction by the relatively water-insoluble methylprednisolone acetate compared with dexamethasone.

Operative Therapy

Fasciotomy is indicated in selected cases associated with massive edema and compartment syndrome. Clinical findings may be subtle, and compartment pressure measurements may be useful.[3, 65, 98] If drug injections are subfascial, necrotizing fasciitis can develop, necessitating débridement of necrotic tissue and decompression.[19] Local vessel problems may indicate embolectomy, primary repair, resection, or ligation.

Najjar and colleagues observed improvement in a patient with microscopic emboli of the digits who was treated with vasodilator therapy, open arteriotomy, and thorough irrigation of the limb with heparinized saline.[99] Possibly, microscopic debris was irrigated from the vessel. Unfortunately, no follow-up angiogram was obtained to document the effectiveness of the procedure.

VENOUS INJURIES

Habitual use of superficial hand veins as drug injection sites eventually results in venous thrombosis. When combined with lymphatic obstruction secondary to recurrent infection and uptake of injected particulate debris, the result is often the "puffy hand syndrome" (Fig. 57–6).[19, 100] Other than the treatment of acute compartment syndrome, operative management of the puffy hand syndrome is not

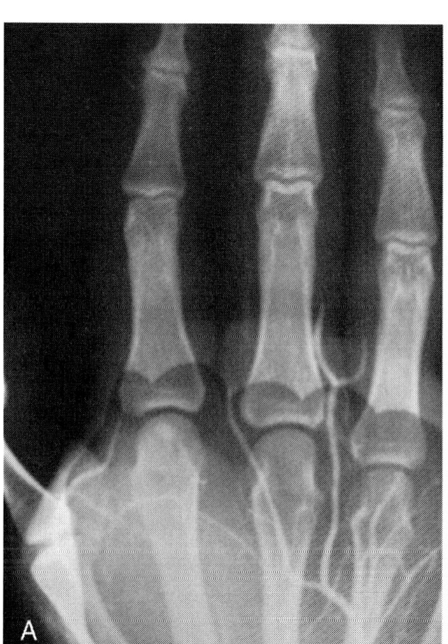

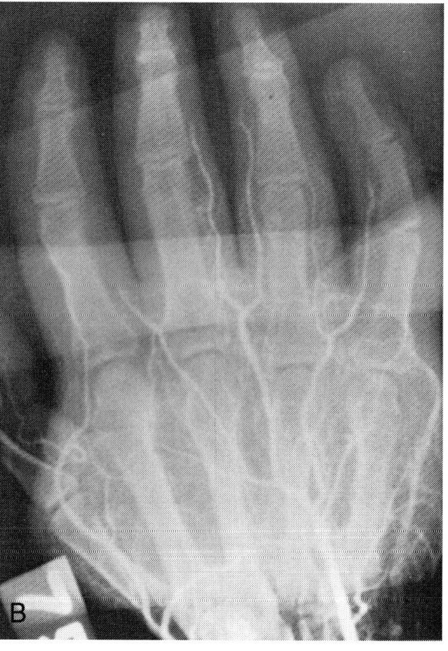

FIGURE 57–5. *A*, Initial arteriogram of the left hand demonstrates absent visualization of the digital arteries. *B*, Arteriogram after intra-arterial streptokinase infusion demonstrates improved flow to all digits of the left hand. (From Silverman SH, Turner WW Jr: Intra-arterial drug abuse: New treatment options. J Vasc Surg 14:111, 1991. By permission of Journal of Vascular Surgery.)

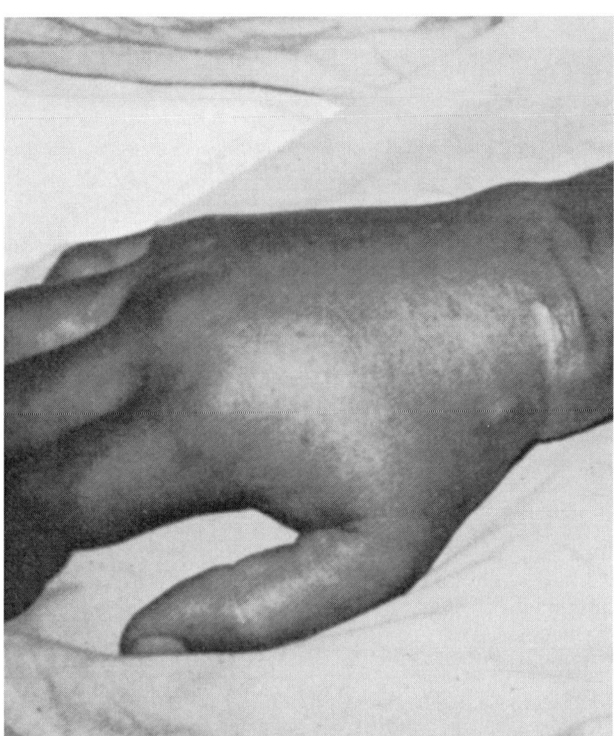

FIGURE 57–6. Puffy hand in an addict secondary to superficial venous and chronic lymphatic obstruction. (From Gellhoed GW, Joseph WL: Surgical sequelae of drug abuse. Surg Gynecol Obstet 139:749, 1974. By permission of Surgery, Gynecology & Obstetrics.)

usually required. Along with elevation, antibiotics and anticoagulation may be indicated. Intractable edema may require management with fitted or pneumatic compression devices.

The appearance of erythema or tenderness over a superficial vein may indicate suppurative thrombophlebitis. The diagnosis is confirmed by needle aspiration, Gram stain, and culture. If suppuration is found, or if elevation and antibiotics do not resolve the infection, operative intervention is indicated. This may include incision or excision of the entire involved superficial vein. Infections by a variety of organisms occur in drug abusers with suppurative thrombophlebitis.[101] Contributing factors are needle sharing, immune system incompetence, and drug injection rituals ("needle licking").[102]

Progressive loss of superficial venous access in chronic drug abusers inevitably leads to deep injections into major venous tributaries. Mechanisms similar to those causing injuries after arterial injections lead to deep venous thrombosis. Absence of venous collateral due to preexisting superficial venous thrombosis may exacerbate the venous hypertension that occurs with deep venous thrombosis. The resulting presentation can be that of catastrophic venous obstruction. Management includes elevation, anticoagulation, and, under conditions of impending gangrene, fasciotomy and venous thrombectomy.

Venous aneurysms may be the consequence of repeated injections into the same area. Because of the close proximity of the femoral vein to the skin, venocutaneous fistula has occurred.[35, 103] Venous pseudoaneurysms have presented also as infected groin masses. Treatment consists of draining the soft tissue abscess, excising the involved venous segment, and ligating the vein proximally and distally.

Poor compliance with prescribed treatment in drug abusers often mandates inpatient treatment with long-term antibiotics and anticoagulants. Long-term central venous catheterization for outpatient antibiotic administration is rarely indicated.

SUMMARY

In summary, acute vascular insufficiency following drug abuse is common in this era of increased use and abuse of a variety of pharmacologic agents. Resultant gangrene and other extremity complications as well as systemic, cerebral, and pulmonary complications are frequent.

Treatment should be aggressive. Success has been greatest when a selective, multimodal approach has been used, including elevation, anticoagulation, vasodilators, thrombolysis, fasciotomy, and operative control of sepsis and gangrene.

REFERENCES

1. van der Post CWH: A case of mistaken injection of pentothal sodium into an aberrant ulnar artery. S Afr Med J 16:182, 1942.
2. Burn JH: Why thiopentone injected into an artery may cause gangrene. Br Med J 2:414, 1960.
3. Cohen SM: Accidental intra-arterial injection of drugs. Lancet 2:361, 1948.
4. Davies DD: Local complications of thiopentone injection. Br J Anaesth 38:530, 1966.
5. Gay GR: Intra-arterial injection of secobarbital sodium into the brachial artery: Sequelae of a "hand trip." Anesth Analg (Cleve) 50:979, 1971.
6. Kinmonth JB, Shepherd RC: Accidental injection of thiopentone into arteries. Br Med J 2:914, 1959.
7. Klatte EC, Brooks AL, Rhamy RK: Toxicity of intra-arterial barbiturates and tranquilizing drugs. Radiology 92:700, 1969.
8. Stone HH, Donnelly CC: Accidental intra-arterial injection of thiopental. Anesthesiology 22:995, 1961.
9. Albo D, Cheung L, Ruth L, et al: Effect of intra-arterial injections of barbiturates. Am J Surg 120:676, 1970.
10. Alix EC, Bogumill GP, Wright CB: Intra-arterial injection of abused drugs. Cardiovasc Res 9:266, 1975.
11. Blackwell SJ, Huang TT, Lewis SR: Intra-arterial drug abuse. Tex Med 74:64, 1978.
12. Ellerston DG, Lazarus HM, Auerbach R: Patterns of acute vascular injury after intra-arterial barbiturate injection. Am J Surg 126:813, 1973.
13. Hewitt JC, Hamilton RC, O'Donnell JF, et al: Clinical studies of induction agents: XIV. A comparative study of venous complications following thiopentone, methohexitone, and propanidid. Br J Anaesth 38:115, 1966.
14. Rumbaugh CL, Fang HCH, Higgins, RE, et al: Cerebral microvascular injury in experimental drug abuse. Invest Radiol 11:282, 1976.
15. Tasker FL, DeBoer B: Vascular changes during oxy- and thiobarbiturate perfusion modified by reserpine and iproniazid. Arch Intern Pharmacodyn 160:223, 1966.
16. Beebe HG, Keats NM: Surgical patients and drug abuse syndrome. Am Surg 38:88, 1973.
17. Daniel DM: The acutely swollen hand in the drug user. Arch Surg 107:548, 1973.
18. Gaspar MR, Hare RR: Gangrene due to intra-arterial injection of drugs by drug addicts. Surgery 72:573, 1972.
19. Geelhoed GW, Joseph WL: Surgical sequelae of drug abuse. Surg Gynecol Obstet 139:749, 1974.

20. Hager DL, Wilson JN: Gangrene of the hand following intra-arterial injection. Arch Surg 94:86, 1967.
21. Hawkins LG, Lisher CG, Sweeney M: The main line accidental intra-arterial drug injection: A review of seven cases. Clin Orthop Relat Res 94:268, 1973.
22. Joseph WL, Fletcher HS, Giordano JM, et al: Pulmonary and cardiovascular implications of drug addiction. Ann Thorac Surg 15:263, 1973.
23. Maxwell TM, Olcott C, Blaisdell FW: Vascular complications of drug abuse. Arch Surg 105:875, 1972.
24. Sternbach G, Moran J, Eliastam M: Heroin addiction: Acute presentation of medical complications. Ann Emerg Med 9:161, 1980.
25. Wilson SE, Van Wagenen P, Passsaro E Jr: Arterial infection. Curr Probl Surg 15:1, 1978.
26. Charney MA, Stern PJ: Digital ischemia in clandestine intravenous drug users. J Hand Surg 16A:308, 1991.
27. Owen CA, Mubarak SJ, Hargens AR, et al: Intramuscular pressures with limb compression: Clarification of the pathogenesis of the drug-induced muscle-compartment syndrome. N Engl J Med 300:1169, 1979.
28. Rich NM, Hobson RW, Fedde CW: Vascular trauma secondary to diagnostic and therapeutic procedures. Am J Surg 126:639, 1973.
29. Citron BP, Halpern M, McCarron M, et al: Necrotizing angiitis associated with drug abuse. N Engl J Med 283:1003, 1970.
30. Espiritu MB, Medina JE: Complications of heroin injections of the neck. Laryngoscope 90:1111, 1980.
31. Ho K, Rassekh ZS: Mycotic aneurysms of the right subclavian artery: A complication of heroin addiction. Chest 74:116, 1978.
32. Lau J, Mattox KL, DeBakey ME: Mycotic aneurysm of the inferior mesenteric artery. Am J Surg 138:443, 1979.
33. Ledgerwood M, Lucas CE: Mycotic aneurysm of the carotid artery. Arch Surg 109:496, 1974.
34. Yellin AE: Ruptured mycotic aneurysm: A complication of parenteral drug abuse. Arch Surg 112:981, 1977.
35. Berguer R, Benitez P: Surgical emergencies from intravascular injection of drugs. *In* JJ Bergan, JST Yao (eds): Vascular Surgical Emergencies. Orlando, Grune & Stratton, 1987, pp 309–318.
36. Levi N, Rordam P, Jensen LP, Schroeder TV: Femoral pseudoaneurysms in drug addicts. Eur J Vasc Endovasc Surg 13:361, 1997.
37. Ting AC, Cheng SW: Femoral pseudoaneurysms in drug addicts. World J Surg 21:783, 1997.
38. Patel KR, Semel L, Clauss RH: Routine revascularization with resection of infected femoral pseudoaneurysms from substance abuse. J Vasc Surg 8:321, 1988.
39. Padberg F Jr, Hobson R II, Lee B, et al: Femoral pseudoaneurysms from drugs of abuse: Ligation or reconstruction? J Vasc Surg 15:642, 1992.
40. Reddy DJ, Smith RD, Elliott JP Jr, et al: Infected femoral artery false aneurysms in drug addicts: Evolution of selective vascular reconstruction. J Vasc Surg 3:718, 1986.
41. Cheng SW, Fok M, Wong J: Infected femoral pseudoaneurysms in intravenous drug abusers. Br J Surg 79:510, 1992.
42. Welch GH, Reid DB, Pollock JG: Infected false aneurysms in the groin of intravenous drug abusers. Br J Surg 77:330, 1990.
43. Clagett GP, Valentine RJ, Hagino RT: Autogenous aorto-iliac/femoral reconstruction from superficial femoral-popliteal veins: Feasibility and durability. J Vasc Surg 25:255, 1997.
44. Fromm SH, Lucas CE: Obturator bypass for mycotic aneurysm in the drug addict. Arch Surg 100:82, 1970.
45. Zemplenyi J, Colman MF: Deep neck abscesses secondary to methylphenidate (Ritalin) abuse. Head Neck Surg 6:858, 1984.
46. Kay DJ, Mirza N: Diagnosis and management of complications of self-injection injuries in the neck. Ear Nose Throat J 75:670, 1996.
47. Williams MF, Eisele DW, Wyatt SH: Neck needle foreign bodies in intravenous drug abusers. Laryngoscope 103:59, 1993.
48. Myers SI, Clagett GP, Valentine RJ, et al: Chronic mesenteric ischemia caused by intravenous cocaine use: Report of two cases and review of the literature. J Vasc Surg 23:724,1996.
49. Gourgoutis G, Das G: Gastrointestinal manifestations of cocaine addiction. Int J Clin Pharmacol Ther 32:136, 1994.
50. Freudenberger RS, Cappell MS, Hutt DA: Intestinal infarction after intravenous cocaine administration. Ann Intern Med 113:715, 1990.
51. Garfia A, Valverde JL, Borondo JC, et al: Vascular lesions in intestinal ischemia induced by cocaine-alcohol abuse: Report of a fatal case due to overdose. J Forensic Sci 35:740, 1990.
52. Lee HS, LaMaute HR, Pizzi WF, et al: Acute gastroduodenal perforations associated with use of crack. Ann Surg 211:15, 1990.
53. Boutros HH, Pautler S, Chakrabarti S: Cocaine-induced ischemic colitis with small-vessel thrombosis of colon and gallbladder. J Clin Gastroenterol 24:49, 1997.
54. Brown DN, Rosenholtz MJ, Marshall JB: Ischemic colitis related to cocaine abuse. Am J Gastroenterol 89:1558, 1994.
55. Perino LE, Warren GH, Levine JS: Cocaine-induced hepatotoxicity in humans. Gastroenterology 93:176, 1987.
56. Morgan JM, Morgan AD, Bradley GW, et al: Fatal hemorrhage from mycotic aneurysms of the pulmonary artery. Thorax 41:70, 1986.
57. Navarro C, Dickinson PCT, Kondlapoodi P, et al: Mycotic aneurysms of the pulmonary arteries in intravenous drug addicts: Report of three cases and review of the literature. Am J Med 76:1124, 1984.
58. SanDretto MA, Scanlon GT: Multiple mycotic pulmonary artery aneurysms secondary to intravenous drug abuse. AJR 142:89, 1984.
59. Boyd LJ, McGavack TH: Aneurysm of the pulmonary artery: Review of the literature and report of two cases. Am Heart J 18:562, 1939.
60. Robertson CH Jr, Reynolds RC, Wilson JE III: Pulmonary hypertension and foreign body granulomas in intravenous drug abusers: Documentation by cardiac catheterization and lung biopsy. Am J Med 61:657, 1976.
61. Waller BF, Brownlee WJ, Roberts WC: Self-induced pulmonary granulomatosis: A consequence of intravenous injection of drugs intended for oral use. Chest 78:90, 1980.
62. Brown SS, Lyons SM, Dundee JW: Intra-arterial barbiturates: Study of some factors leading to intravascular thrombosis. Br J Anaesth 40:13, 1968.
63. Buckspan GS, Franklin JD, Novak GR, et al: Intra-arterial drug injury: Studies of etiology and potential treatment. J Surg Res 24:294, 1978.
64. Goldberg I, Bahar A, Yosipovitch Z: Gangrene of the upper extremity following intra-arterial injection of drugs. Clin Orthop Relat Res 188:223, 1984.
65. Pearlman HS, Wollowick BS, Alvarez EV: Intra-arterial injection of propoxyphene into brachial artery. JAMA 214:2055, 1970.
66. Williams AW, Montgomery GL: Chemical injury of arteries. J Pathol Bacteriol 77:63, 1959.
67. Atlee WE Jr: Talc and cornstarch emboli in eyes of drug abusers. JAMA 219:49, 1972.
68. Lindell TD, Porter JM, Langston JC: Intra-arterial injections of oral medications: A complication of drug addiction. N Engl J Med 287:1132, 1972.
69. Appen RE, Wray SH, Cogan DG: Central retinal artery occlusion. Am J Opthalmol 79:374, 1975.
70. Brucker AJ: Disk and peripheral retinal neovascularization secondary to talc and cornstarch emboli. Am J Ophthalmol 88:864, 1979.
71. Friberg TR, Gragoudas ES, Regan CDJ: Talc emboli and macular ischemia in intravenous drug abuse. Arch Ophthalmol 97:1089, 1979.
72. Kresca LJ, Goldberg MF, Jampol LM: Talc emboli and retinal neovascularization in a drug abuser. Am J Ophthalmol 87:334, 1979.
73. Lee J, Sapira JD: Retinal and cerebral microembolization of talc in a drug abuser. Am J Med Sci 265:75, 1973.
74. Schatz H, Drake M: Self-injected retinal emboli. Ophthalmologica 86:468, 1979.
75. Waters DJ: Intra-arterial thiopentone. Anaesthesia 21:346, 1966.
76. Burn JH, Hobbs R: Mechanism of arterial spasm following intra-arterial injection of thiopentone. Lancet 1:1112, 1959.
77. Begg EJ, McGrath MA, Wade DN: Inadvertent intra-arterial injection: A problem of drug abuse. Med J Aust 2:561, 1980.
78. Crawford CR, Terranova WA: The role of intraarterial vasodilators in the treatment of inadvertent intraarterial injection injuries. Ann Plast Surg 25:279, 1990.
79. Stueber K: The treatment of intra-arterial pentazocine injection injuries with intra-arterial reserpine. Ann Plast Surg 18:41, 1987.
80. Wright CB, Hobson RW, Swan KG, et al: Extremity venous ligation: Clinical and hemodynamic correlation. Am Surg 41:203, 1975.
81. Myers MB, Cherry G: Necrosis due to venous inadequacy: An experimental model in the skin of rabbits. Surg Forum 18:513, 1967.
82. Wright, CB, Swan KG: The hemodynamics of venous occlusion in the canine hindlimb. Surgery 73:141, 1973.
83. Corser G, Masey S, Jacob G, et al: Ischaemia following self administered intra-arterial injection of methylphenidate and diamorphine: A

case report of treatment with intra-arterial urokinase and review. Anaesthesia 40:51, 1985.
84. Enloe G, Sylvester M, Morris LE: Hazards of intra-arterial injection of hydroxyzine. Can Anaesth Soc J 16:425, 1969.
85. Lloyd WK, Porter JM, Lindell TD, et al: Accidental intraarterial injection in drug abuse. Am J Roentgenol Radium Ther Nucl Med 117:892, 1973.
86. Silverman SH, Turner WW Jr: Intraarterial drug abuse: New treatment options. J Vasc Surg 14:111, 1991.
87. Gallacher BP: Intra-arterial verapamil to reverse acute ischemia of the hand after radial artery cannulation. Can J Anaesth 38:138, 1991.
88. Roberts JR, Krisanda TJ: Accidental intra-arterial injection of epinephrine treated with phentolamine. Ann Emerg Med 18:424, 1989.
89. Lazarus HM, Hutto BS, Ellertson DG: Therapeutic prevention of ischemia following intra-arterial barbiturate injection. J Surg Res 22:46, 1977.
90. Earnshaw JJ: Thrombolytic therapy in the management of acute limb ischaemia. Br J Surg 78:261, 1991.
91. Kartchner MM, Wilcox WC: Thrombolysis of palmar and digital arterial thrombosis by intra-arterial thrombolysin. J Hand Surg 1:67, 1976.
92. Buckenham TM, Darby M: Thrombolysis with t-PA. Br J Hosp Med 46:269, 1991.
93. Juhan C, Haupert S, Miltgen G, et al: A new intra-arterial rt-PA dosage regimen in peripheral arterial occlusion: Bolus followed by continuous infusion. Thromb Haemost 65:635, 1991.
94. Dawson KJ, Reddy K, Platts AD, et al: Results of a recently instituted programme of thrombolytic therapy in acute lower limb ischaemia. Br J Surg 78:409, 1991.
95. Earnshaw JJ, Westby JC, Gregson RHS, et al: Local thrombolytic therapy of acute peripheral arterial ischaemia with tissue plasminogen activator: A dose-ranging study. Br J Surg 75:1196, 1988.
96. Treiman GS, Yellin AE, Weaver FA: An effective treatment protocol for intra-arterial drug injection. J Vasc Surg 12:456, 1990.
97. Taweepoke P, Frame JD: Acute ischaemia of the hand following accidental radial artery infusion of Depo-Medrone. J Hand Surg 15:118, 1990.
98. Gall WE, Burr JW, Wright CBV: Noninvasive evaluation and correlation of hemodynamics in "compartment syndrome." Surg Forum 29:222, 1978.
99. Najjar FB, Bridi G, Rizk G: Management of micro-emboli of the digital arteries. J Med Liban 27:467, 1974.
100. Neviaser RJ, Butterfield WC, Wieche DR: The puffy hand of drug addiction: A study of the pathogenesis. J Bone Joint Surg 54-A: 629, 1972.
101. Tuazon CU, Hill R, Sheagren JN: Microbiologic study of street heroin and injection paraphernalia. J Infect Dis 129:327, 1974.
102. Moustoukas NM, Nichols RL, Smith JW, et al: Contaminated street heroin: Relationship to clinical infections. Arch Surg 118:746, 1983.
103. Yeager RA, Hobson RW II, Padberg FT, et al: Vascular complications related to drug abuse. J Trauma 27:305, 1987.

SECTION IX

VASCULAR TRAUMA

KAJ H. JOHANSEN, M.D., Ph.D.

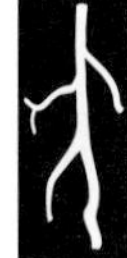

CHAPTER 58

The Epidemiology of Vascular Trauma

Michael T. Caps, M.D., M.P.H.

Epidemiology is the study of the frequency and distribution of diseases or conditions in populations of interest. Such knowledge can facilitate determination of the impact of these disease states or conditions on the population or on selected subgroups. This information can also be used to set priorities for investigation, to determine which segments of the population are candidates for preventive measures and diagnostic screening tests, and to determine the need for treatment facilities.

Because death and disability from trauma are such major public health problems, the epidemiology of trauma has been well characterized. Trauma (both intentional and unintentional injuries) was the leading cause of death among Americans aged 44 years and younger. More importantly, trauma accounted for the largest number of years of life lost, an estimated 3.5 million years in 1995. Measures such as the regionalization of trauma care and the establishment of the National Center for Injury Prevention and Control are examples of the policy changes that have occurred in response to the epidemiologic data on trauma.

Classical epidemiology, which is concerned primarily with questions about disease frequency and etiology *within populations*, is distinct from so-called clinical epidemiology (the study of the *outcome of illness*), which attempts to answer questions about natural history and the most appropriate modes of diagnosis and treatment of *diseased patients*.[41] The study of vascular trauma has necessarily focused on the diagnosis and treatment of patients who have sustained blood vessel injuries. Limiting the analysis of injuries to hospitalized trauma victims, however, results in a skewed picture of the true epidemiology of vascular injury–related morbidity and mortality in the United States population.

In the past, accurate and comprehensive identification of vascular injury cases for epidemiologic study was difficult owing to the complex hospital courses (polytrauma, multiple procedures) of many patients with these injuries. The creation of computerized trauma registries during the past decade has facilitated epidemiologic study of injuries to all major organ systems, including the cardiovascular system.

That stated, the epidemiology of vascular trauma has been incompletely studied and reported. A proper epidemiologic analysis of vascular trauma would include a determination of the incidence of injury to blood vessels, including assessment of temporal trends and identification of population subgroups at particularly high risk. One of the difficulties associated with vascular injury epidemiology has been case definition. In the majority of studies, vascular trauma has been defined on the basis of repair of blood vessel injury. Thus, the *true* epidemiology of vascular injury is poorly characterized because such a definition excludes individuals who die before arriving at a hospital. Furthermore, only irregularly have studies included vascular trauma in persons who die in the hospital before blood vessel repair can be accomplished, or diagnosed blood vessel injuries that are not repaired.

Because most epidemiologic reports on non-iatrogenic vascular injury have not been population-based, direct calculation of incidence rates (number of cases per unit time per person at risk) is not possible. On the other hand, the cumulative incidence (number of cases per person at risk) of iatrogenic vascular injury after invasive diagnostic and therapeutic medical procedures can be directly estimated, because the population at risk is known. This chapter includes an assessment of temporal trends in the incidence of vascular trauma in the United States as well as a description of the characteristics of patients who have sustained blood vessel injuries. For many vascular surgeons, iatrogenic vascular trauma comprises the majority of vascular trauma cases they encounter. Consequently, the epidemiology of this important subgroup of injuries is emphasized.

HISTORICAL AND GEOGRAPHIC SETTINGS

Military Conflicts

Many of the modern principles of treatment of blood vessel injuries were developed during military conflicts of the 20th century. The overwhelming majority of vascular injuries encountered by surgeons during World War II, the

TABLE 58–1. TRENDS IN ANATOMIC DISTRIBUTION OF VASCULAR INJURIES DURING WORLD WAR II, THE KOREAN WAR, AND THE VIETNAM WAR CONTRASTED WITH A LARGE, URBAN CIVILIAN SERIES

ANATOMIC SITE	WORLD WAR II* (NO. = 2471)	KOREAN WAR† (NO. = 304)	VIETNAM WAR‡ (NO. = 1000)	HOUSTON (1958–1988)§ (NO. = 5760)
Neck	1%	4%	5%	12%
Trunk	2%	2%	4%	54%
Extremity	97%	94%	91%	34%

*Data from DeBakey ME, Simeone FA: Ann Surg 123:534, 1946.[12]
†Data from Hughes CW: Ann Surg 147:555, 1958.[17]
‡Data from Rich NM, et al: J Trauma 10:359, 1970.[32]
§Data from Mattox KL, et al: Ann Surg 209:698, 1989.[23]

Korean War, and the Vietnam conflict affected extremity arteries, usually as a result of fragments from exploding devices or bullet injuries.[12, 17, 32] Table 58–1 summarizes the anatomic distributions of vascular injuries in the largest series from each of these three wars, and the largest civilian series of vascular injuries[23] is included for comparison.

Because of reduced prehospital transport times during the Vietnam conflict, a larger proportion of combat casualties (9%) were treated for neck or truncal arterial injuries, which in previous military campaigns had been almost uniformly fatal. The greater proportion of these injuries among cases of civilian vascular trauma probably reflects several factors, including the use of flak jackets in the military, more rapid transport times in urban civilian settings (today, typically less than 20 minutes in most urban United States population centers), and the smaller calibers and lower muzzle velocities of firearms used in civilian settings (which render such injuries more "survivable").

Urban Trauma

In 1989, Mattox and colleagues reported on almost 6000 cardiovascular injuries seen at a single urban trauma center over 30 years.[23] This report provided the most comprehensive epidemiologic survey of urban vascular trauma in the United States published to this time. Perhaps the most startling observation in this study was the increasing incidence of vascular trauma observed in the metropolitan Houston area between 1958 and 1988. Although incidence rates were not calculated in this paper, one can estimate these rates using the Houston population figures provided. This trend in calculated incidence rates, shown in Figure 58–1, demonstrates an epidemic of vascular injuries that evolved over three decades. The patients described in the report were treated at either the Jefferson Davis or Ben Taub Hospitals, the only recognized trauma centers in the greater Houston area until the late 1970s, when a separate trauma service was developed at the University of Texas. Therefore, the incidence rates during the 5-year periods 1979 to 1983 and 1984 to 1988 depicted in Figure 58–1 are *underestimates* of the true rates.

This apparent recent epidemic of vascular trauma in United States cities is further supported by comparative analysis of other large urban trauma series.[5, 6, 13, 16, 35, 40] This trend has been demonstrated for all major mechanisms of vascular injury, penetrating and blunt as well as iatrogenic, and reflects a concomitant increase in assaults, high-speed motor vehicle crashes, falls from heights, and invasive medical procedures. The incidence of blood vessel trauma continued to rise in the late 1980s and the early 1990s, in parallel to the steadily rising incidences of homicide and assault in the United States documented during this period.[11] Although a noteworthy decline in the incidence of homicides and assaults from 1993 to 1996 was noted in nearly all major United States cities, there is no evidence of similar reductions in the incidences of motor vehicle crashes, falls from heights, or invasive medical procedures.

Rural Trauma

Although America's urban trauma centers have provided a rich environment for the clinical study of vascular injury, a significant proportion of blood vessel injuries occur in rural settings, where the epidemiology is markedly different. In 1992, Oller and colleagues presented a review of 978 patients collected over 39 months from North Carolina's statewide trauma registry.[27] Incidence rates could not be directly estimated in this study because the study was not population-based (only persons treated in one of the state's eight trauma centers were included). Since North Carolina is a largely rural state, however, this study provided important information on the characteristics of patients sustaining vascular injuries in rural settings, and the state's sizable urban population allowed direct comparisons of patient characteristics between the two groups. A summary of the pertinent findings from this study is shown in Table

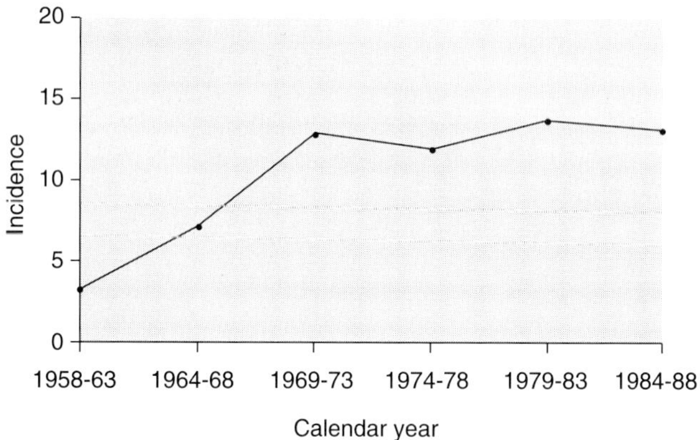

FIGURE 58–1. Estimated incidence of vascular injuries requiring repair in the metropolitan Houston, Texas, area, 1958–1988, per 100,000 person-years. (Redrawn from Mattox KL, Feliciano DV, Burch JM, et al: Five thousand seven hundred sixty cardiovascular injuries in 4459 patients: Epidemiologic evolution 1958 to 1988. Ann Surg 209:698–705, 1989.)

TABLE 58–2. DEMOGRAPHIC AND ETIOLOGIC CHARACTERISTICS OF VASCULAR INJURIES IN RURAL AND URBAN SETTINGS

CHARACTERISTIC	RURAL	URBAN
Demographics		
Age (mean, yr)	51	31
Gender (% male)	79	84
Race (% nonwhite)	38	60
Mechanism		
Blunt trauma (%)	43	27

From Oller DW et al: Vascular injuries in a rural state: A review of 978 patients from a state trauma registry. J Trauma 32(6):740, 1992.

58–2. Among other noteworthy findings, the study demonstrated that patients from rural settings who had vascular injuries were older, more often victims of blunt trauma, more often white, and less often male than were urban patients.

The Oller study[27] was also important because it provided concurrent data on patients with and without vascular injury, allowing comparisons of overall outcomes between these two groups. Table 58–3 highlights the differences between patients with and without blood vessel injuries in this study (data from urban and rural centers were pooled for this comparison). Patients with vascular injuries were more severely injured than trauma patients without vascular injury, as evidenced by their higher injury severity scores and mortality rates, longer hospital stays, and higher hospital charges.

MECHANISMS OF VASCULAR INJURY

Penetrating Trauma

Penetrating trauma remains the dominant cause of non-iatrogenic blood vessel injuries in both urban and rural settings in the United States, accounting for 50% to 90% of all such injuries. The temporal trends in the incidences of homicide and assault (surrogates for the incidence of penetrating vascular trauma) have been noted. Myriad risk factors have been associated with homicide and assault, including age, gender, race, socioeconomic status, education, gun ownership, a criminal record, and alcohol and drug use.[36, 37, 42] In addition to efforts at gun control, community-based interventions have been implemented to reduce the occurrence of violent behavior[18]; the effectiveness of such interventions has been difficult to assess.

The anatomic distribution of penetrating vascular trauma is related to the mechanism of injury. In urban settings, gunshot wounds that cause nonfatal vascular injury are most likely to involve the abdominal vessels, followed by the lower extremities.[23] For vascular injuries secondary to shotgun wounds, this relationship is reversed: truncal shotgun injuries are more frequently fatal. Stab wounds resulting in blood vessel injury are most likely to involve the upper extremities, trunk, or neck.

How such ballistic variables as missile caliber, muzzle velocity, and the use of automatic weapons relate to the incidence of blood vessel injury is not known. It is likely that increasing use of these higher-energy weapons in America's cities has increased the absolute incidence of blood vessel injury; however, a correspondingly larger proportion of these injuries may have resulted in prehospital deaths and thus may have gone unreported, given study designs used in most epidemiologic reports. The increased incidence of penetrating vascular injuries was not attributable to these weapons in the Mattox group's Houston series.[23]

Blunt Trauma

Blunt trauma is an important cause of blood vessel injury. Vascular injury resulting from motor vehicle crashes and, to a much lesser extent, falls from heights and crush injuries, account for as many as 50% of all non-iatrogenic vascular injuries treated in United States hospitals. In a study of geographic variations in mortality rates from motor vehicle crashes, Baker and colleagues[2] found mortality rates ranging from as low as 2.5 per 100,000 population in Manhattan, New York, to as high as 558 per 100,000 population in Esmeralda County, Nevada. Factors associated with the mortality rate from motor vehicle crashes (and with injury severity, for survivors) include population density, travel speeds, road types, vehicle types, alcohol and drug intoxication, use of restraints and inflatable airbags, visual impairment, and sleepiness.[2, 21, 28] Alcohol intake is clearly associated with severity of injury among persons who sustain blunt trauma, but whether this association persists after controlling for other determinants of outcome, such as the severity of impact and the use of restraints, is controversial.[19] While widespread use of seat belts and inflatable automobile air bags is presumed to have a beneficial effect on the incidence and severity of blunt vascular injuries, no direct evidence supports this hypothesis.

Vascular injury secondary to blunt trauma has characteristic anatomic patterns. In motor vehicle crashes, the ab-

TABLE 58–3. INJURY SEVERITY AND OUTCOMES AMONG TRAUMA PATIENTS WITH AND WITHOUT VASCULAR INJURY

CHARACTERISTIC	VASCULAR INJURY	NO VASCULAR INJURY	*p* VALUE
No. of patients	978	25,639	
Injury severity score (mean)	14	10	.0001
Hospital stay (mean days)	13	10	.0001
Intensive care unit (mean days)	5	4	.03
Hospital charges (mean $)	22,500	12,300	.0001
Mortality (%)	13	6	.0001

From Oller DW et al: Vascular injuries in a rural state: A review of 978 patients from a state trauma registry. J Trauma 32(6):740, 1992.

dominal-pelvic, thoracic, and lower extremity vessels are most frequently injured. Arterial injuries to the neck and upper extremities are uncommon after blunt trauma.[7, 23]

Several factors have been associated with increased likelihood of vascular injury after blunt trauma, including the overall severity of the injury and the presence of specific orthopedic injuries. The strong correlation between severity of injury and the presence of vascular injuries in the North Carolina state trauma registry has been mentioned.[27] Several investigators have noted the association between blood vessel injury secondary to blunt trauma and the intensity of the kinetic forces generated in falls from heights and motor vehicle crashes, as evidenced by major injuries to other organ systems. For example, blunt trauma to the carotid, thoracic, and abdominal vessels is frequently associated with severe brain, lung, liver, and pelvic injuries.[8, 10, 16, 22, 29, 35]

Several skeletal injuries are associated with increased risk of vascular injury after blunt trauma. Blunt thoracic vascular injuries are more common among persons who have first rib, scapular, and sternal fractures, all indicators of extreme kinetic forces.[15, 16, 35] Pelvic arterial and venous injuries are unlikely in the absence of pelvic fracture or ligamentous injury.[24] Several patterns of fractures and of dislocations involving the extremities are associated with increased risk of extremity vascular injury[7, 14, 30]; perhaps most noteworthy among them is the association between knee dislocation (with or without bicruciate ligament injury) and popliteal artery disruption. In a study of 115 patients with unilateral knee dislocations who underwent arteriography, Treiman and colleagues documented popliteal artery injury in 23%.[39]

Iatrogenic Trauma

Perhaps the vascular injuries (both arterial and venous) most often evaluated and treated by vascular surgeons are those caused unintentionally by other physicians or by themselves.[25] For example, the number of patients undergoing percutaneous vascular catheterization for diagnostic and therapeutic procedures has increased dramatically over the past few decades. While most iatrogenic blood vessel injuries are related to these procedures, a number of nonvascular operative procedures are associated with sufficient risk of iatrogenic vascular injury to warrant mention.

Vascular injuries due to percutaneous diagnostic or therapeutic arterial procedures usually involve the femoral (and less frequently the brachial) vessels, which serve as access routes. Injuries include, in decreasing order of frequency, hemorrhage and hematoma, pseudoaneurysm, arteriovenous fistula, vessel thrombosis, and embolization. The risk of these local complications is clearly related to the diameter of the device inserted. Rates range from 0.5% for diagnostic procedures to as high as 10% for therapeutic procedures involving stents.[20, 31] Increasing age, female gender, concurrent use of anticoagulation therapy, and the presence of severe atherosclerosis are other important risk factors. Obesity is also a risk factor, in that accurate manual hemostatic pressure frequently cannot be applied in morbidly obese persons. Small children and infants are particularly susceptible to vessel injury secondary to femoral artery catheterization; thrombosis occurs in as many as a third.[38] Increasing interest in endovascular treatment of aneurysms, vascular injuries, and arterial occlusive disease will undoubtedly result in a whole new spectrum of unintended vascular disruptions.

In rare instances, catheter-associated blood vessel injury can occur at remote sites and can take the form of arterial rupture, dissection, occlusion from an initial flap, or embolization. These complications have been reported in the aorta, carotid, renal, and iliac arteries.[33, 43] Vessel rupture occurs in fewer than 1% of patients undergoing balloon angioplasty and has been associated with excessive arterial calcification, the simultaneous presence of both aneurysmal and occlusive arterial disease, and the use of oversized balloons.[4] Dissection is more common, but it is usually treatable with endovascular stenting.[3]

The increased utilization of intra-aortic balloon pumps (IABPs) since the mid-1970s has led to a further increase in the incidence of iatrogenic iliofemoral vascular injuries. Arterial repair is required in as many as 25% of patients treated with IABPs, and morbidity and mortality are significantly higher among those who sustain these injuries than in those who do not.[9]

In 1983, Youkey and colleagues reported the Walter Reed Army Medical Center experience with iatrogenic vascular injuries from 1974 through 1982[43] and contrasted this experience with that of the previous 8 years, 1966 through 1973.[43] The total number of iatrogenic vascular injuries that required surgical intervention (125) increased by 52% during this interval. An increase in the frequency of iliofemoral arterial injuries resulting from percutaneous transluminal dilation procedures was noted, as was a striking increase in major vascular injuries secondary to aggressive surgical attempts at abdominal or retroperitoneal tumor resection.

Several surgical procedures risk blood vessel injury. Hepatic and pancreaticobiliary surgery carries well-known risks of injury to the hepatic arteries and the portomesenteric vessels. Operations involving the lower lumbar spine are occasionally associated with both arterial and venous injuries in the vicinity of the aortic and vena caval bifurcations. As anterior approaches to the lumbar spine have increased in popularity, vascular surgeons have frequently become involved in the establishment of exposure to reduce the risk of serious vascular injury. In a retrospective study of 102 consecutive anterior lumbar spinal procedures, vascular injuries that required surgical repair occurred in 16% of patients.[1] Popliteal artery injury can result from various orthopedic knee procedures, usually as a result of penetrating injury from intra-articular arthroscopic procedures, high tibial osteotomy, or inappropriate screw placement during fracture fixation.[34, 44]

Finally, the dramatic increase in laparoscopic and thoracoscopic procedures during the 1990s has resulted in an increase in associated vascular injuries.[26] Examples include intercostal and epigastric artery injuries during trocar insertion, damage to the aortoiliac or iliocaval vessels during penetration of the peritoneum, and inadvertent damage to the vessels in the hepatoduodenal ligament during laparoscopic cholecystectomy.

PREVENTION

A major goal of trauma epidemiology is the identification of strategies that might reduce the incidence of such injuries in specific populations at risk. A full discussion of the policy implications of trauma epidemiology is beyond the scope of this chapter, but several examples relevant to vascular injury illuminate this point. Means by which the excessive toll of injuries from gunshot wounds might be reduced include restricting access to firearm ownership to licensed persons, tougher sentences for those convicted of firearm-related crimes, taxing weapons or ammunition, and passing enabling legislation to permit lawsuits against firearms manufacturers for injuries sustained by users of their products.

Seat belt and air bag use have clearly had salutary effects on the risks of death and injury from ejection during motor vehicle crashes. Many such vascular injuries occur—from disruption of the heart, thoracic aorta, or great vessels of the thoracic inlet to damage in the extremity vessels.

Similar observations have been made about iatrogenic vascular injuries that are clearly associated with operative or catheter technique. Burgeoning technologic developments will inevitably result in smaller catheters and delivery systems: the potential associated reduction in arterial injuries may be balanced by the ever increasing aggressiveness of interventionalists. Vascular injuries associated with truncal laparoscopic and thoracoscopic procedures will likely continue to occur and will be mitigated only partially by better education of and increased vigilance by surgeons.

SUMMARY

An accurate and detailed understanding of the epidemiology of vascular injury will lead to development of more effective measures aimed at prevention and, in some cases, to improved diagnostic algorithms for patients with suspected vascular injuries. Based on existing data, the incidence of blood vessel injuries appears to have increased significantly during recent decades. Factors responsible for this epidemic include increased incidences of assaults, motor vehicle crashes, and invasive medical procedures. There are significant differences between the epidemiology of vascular trauma in rural and in urban settings, and the anatomic distributions and factors related to increased risk vary with the mechanisms of injury. The importance of this epidemic is highlighted by the increased mortality rates and utilization of medical resources among victims of vascular injury.

REFERENCES

1. Baker JK, Reardon PR, Reardon MJ, et al: Vascular injury in anterior lumbar surgery. Spine 18(15):2227–2230, 1993.
2. Baker SP, Whitfield RA, O'Neill B: Geographic variations in mortality from motor vehicle crashes. N Engl J Med 316(22):1384–1387, 1987.
3. Becker GJ, Palmaz JC, Rees CR, et al: Angioplasty-induced dissections in human iliac arteries: Management with Palmaz balloon-expandable intraluminal stents. Radiology 176(1):31–38, 1990.
4. Belli AM, Cumberland DC, Knox AM, et al: The complication rate of percutaneous peripheral balloon angioplasty. Clin Radiol 41(6):380–383, 1990.
5. Bole PV, Purdy RT, Munda RT, et al: Civilian arterial injuries. Ann Surg 183(1):13–23, 1976.
6. Bongard F, Dubrow T, Klein S: Vascular injuries in the urban battleground: Experience at a metropolitan trauma center. Ann Vasc Surg 4(5):415–418, 1990.
7. Borman KR, Snyder WH III, Weigelt JA: Civilian arterial trauma of the upper extremity: An 11 year experience in 267 patients. Am J Surg 148(6):796–799, 1984.
8. Brown MF, Graham JM, Feliciano DV, et al: Carotid artery injuries. Am J Surg 144(6):748–753, 1982.
9. Busch T, Sirbu H, Zenker D, et al: Vascular complications related to intraaortic balloon conterpulsation: An analysis of ten years experience. Thorac Cardiovasc Surg 45(2):55–59, 1997.
10. Carroll PR, McAninch JW, Klosterman P, et al: Renovascular trauma: Risk assessment, surgical management, and outcome. J Trauma 30(5):547–552, 1990.
11. Cherry D, Annest JL, Mercy JA, et al: Trends in nonfatal and fatal firearm-related injury rates in the United States, 1985–1995. Ann Emerg Med 32(1):51–59, 1998.
12. DeBakey ME, Simeone FA: Battle injuries of the arteries in WWII. Ann Surg 123:534–579, 1946.
13. Drapanas T, Hewitt RL, Weichert RF III, et al: Civilian vascular injuries: A critical appraisal of three decades of management. Ann Surg 172(3):351–360, 1970.
14. Endean ED, Veldenz HC, Schwarcz TH, et al: Recognition of arterial injury in elbow dislocation. J Vasc Surg 16(3):402–406, 1992.
15. Gupta A, Jamshidi M, Rubin JR: Traumatic first rib fracture: Is angiography necessary? A reveiw of 730 cases. Cardiovasc Surg 5(1):48–53, 1997.
16. Hardy JD, Raju S, Neely WA, et al: Aortic and other arterial injuries. Ann Surg 181(5):640–653, 1975.
17. Hughes CW: Arterial repair during the Korean war. Ann Surg 147:555–561, 1958.
18. Kellerman AL, Fuqua Whitley DS, Rivara FP, et al: Preventing youth violence: What works? Annu Rev Public Health 19:271–292, 1998.
19. Li G, Keyl PM, Smith GS, et al: Alcohol and injury severity: Reappraisal of the continuing controversy. J Trauma 42(3):562–569, 1997.
20. Lumsden AB, Miller JM, Kosinski AS, et al: A Prospective evaluation of surgically treated groin complications following percutaneous cardiac procedures. Am Surg 60(2):132–137, 1994.
21. Lyznicki JM, Doege TC, Davis RM, et al: Sleepiness, driving, and motor vehicle crashes: Council on Scientific Affairs, American Medical Association. JAMA 279(23):1908–1913, 1998.
22. Martin RF, Eldrup Jorgensen J, Clark DE, et al: Blunt trauma to the carotid arteries. J Vasc Surg 14(6):789–793, 1991.
23. Mattox KL, Feliciano DV, Burch J, et al: Five thousand seven hundred sixty cardiovascular injuries in 4459 patients: Epidemiologic evolution 1958 to 1988. Ann Surg 209(6):698–705, 1989.
24. Mucha P Jr, Welch TJ: Hemorrhage in major pelvic fractures. Surg Clin North Am 68(4):757–773, 1988.
25. Nehler MR, Taylor LM Jr, Porter JM: Iatrogenic vascular trauma. Semin Vasc Surg 11:283–293, 1998.
26. Nordestgaard AG, Bodily KC, Osborne RW Jr, et al: Major vascular injuries during laparoscopic procedures. Am J Surg 169(5):543–545, 1995.
27. Oller DW, Rutledge R, Clancy T, et al: Vascular injuries in a rural state: A review of 978 patients from a state trauma registry. J Trauma 32(6):740–745, 1992.
28. Owsley C, Ball K, McGwin G Jr, et al: Visual processing impairment and risk of motor vehicle crash among older adults. JAMA 279(14):1083–1088, 1998.
29. Parikh AA, Luchette FA, Valente JF, et al: Blunt carotid artery injuries. J Am Coll Surg 185(1):80–86, 1997.
30. Raskin KB: Acute vascular injuries of the upper extremity. Hand Clin 9(1):115–130, 1993.
31. Ricci MA, Trevisani GT, Pilcher DB: Vascular complications of cardiac catheterization. Am J Surg 167(4):375–378, 1994.
32. Rich NM, Baugh JH, Hughes CW: Acute arterial injuries in Vietnam: 1,000 cases. J Trauma 10(5):359–369, 1970.
33. Rich NM, Hobson RW II, Fedde CW: Vascular trauma secondary to diagnostic and therapeutic procedures. Am J Surg 128(6):715–721, 1974.
34. Rubash HE, Berger RA, Britton CA, et al: Avoiding neurologic and vascular injuries with screw fixation of the tibial component in total knee arthroplasty. Clin Orthop 286:56–63, 1993.
35. Sirinek KR, Gaskill HV III, Root HD, et al: Truncal vascular injury—factors influencing survival. J Trauma 23(5):372–377, 1983.
36. Smith AT Jr, Kuller LH, Perper JA, et al: Epidemiology of homicide in Allegheny County, Pennsylvania, between 1966–1974 and 1984–1993. Prev Med 27(3):452–460, 1998.

37. Spigner C: Race, class, and violence. Research and policy implications Int J Health Serv 28(2):349–372, 1998.
38. Taylor LM Jr, Troutman R, Feliciano P, et al: Late complications after femoral artery catheterization in children less than five years of age. J Vasc Surg 11(2):297–304, 1990.
39. Treiman GS, Yellin AE, Weaver FA, et al: Examination of the patient with a knee dislocation: The case for selective arteriography. Arch Surg 127(9):1056–1062, 1992.
40. Treiman RL, Doty D, Gaspar MR: Acute vascular trauma: A fifteen year study. Am J Surg 111(3):469–473, 1966.
41. Weiss NS: Clinical Epidemiology: The Study of the Outcome of Illness, 2nd ed. New York, Oxford University Press, 1996.
42. Wintemute GJ, Wright MA, Parham CA, et al: Criminal activity and assault-type handguns: A study of young adults [see comments]. Ann Emerg Med 32(1):44–50, 1998.
43. Youkey JR, Clagett GP, Rich NM, et al: Vascular trauma secondary to diagnostic and therapeutic procedures: 1974 through 1982: A comparative review. Am J Surg 146(6):788–791, 1983.
44. Zaidi SH, Cobb AG, Bentley G: Danger to the popliteal artery in high tibial osteotomy. J Bone Joint Surg 77B(3):384–386, 1995.

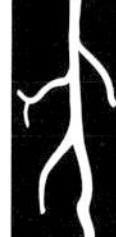

CHAPTER 59

Vascular Injuries of the Extremities

Fred A. Weaver, M.D., Douglas B. Hood, M.D., and Albert E. Yellin, M.D.

Approximately 90% of all peripheral arterial injuries occur in an extremity, lower extremity injuries being more common in the military experience and upper extremity injuries in civilian reports.[42] During World War II, extremity arterial injuries were routinely ligated. For popliteal artery injury, the amputation rate was 73%.[6] The poor results of arterial ligation prompted Hughes and Spencer to perform formal repair of peripheral arterial injuries during the Korean War.[22, 42] Rich and associates reported further refinements of arterial repair during the Vietnam War, decreasing the amputation rate for popliteal artery injuries to 32%.[43] Continuing refinements in arterial surgery over the ensuing three decades have reduced limb loss in most civilian series to less than 10% to 15%[34, 55, 56]; however, long-term disability, predominantly resulting from associated skeletal and nerve injuries, remains a persistent problem for 20% to 50% of patients.[57]

MECHANISM OF INJURY

The initial and ultimate outcome of vascular injury depends in large part on the wounding agent or mechanism of injury. Determining the mechanism of injury is of utmost importance if the surgeon is to utilize available diagnostic and treatment options appropriately. Peripheral vascular injuries in an urban environment most often result from penetrating trauma from knives or bullets. In a recent series of penetrating injuries, arterial injuries were due to gunshot wounds in 64%, knife wounds in 24%, and shotgun blasts in 12%.[40]

With increasing frequency, high-velocity firearms are the causative agent in civilian vascular trauma. In addition to the vascular injury, extensive associated musculoskeletal injury is commonplace. Vascular injuries in this setting result from the dissipation of energy into the surrounding tissues, the blast effect, and fragmentation of the projectile or of bone.[11] Experimental studies have demonstrated a positive correlation between muzzle velocity and the microscopic extent and "length" of damage to the vessel wall.[1] In many ways these wounds mimic lower-velocity shotgun injuries in their devastating combination of penetrating and blunt tissue injury.[31]

Motor vehicle accidents and falls are the most common causes of blunt injury and are becoming more frequent, owing to the ever increasing mobility of modern society.[1, 61] The morbidity of blunt vascular injuries can be magnified by associated fractures, dislocations, and crush injuries to muscles and nerves.

DIAGNOSTIC EVALUATION

Extremity arterial injuries have varied clinical presentations. A minority of patients present with obvious clinical evidence, or "hard signs," of arterial disruption such as pulsatile external bleeding, an enlarging hematoma, absent distal pulses, or an ischemic limb. For patients with overt signs of arterial injury, immediate surgical exploration in the operating room, without further diagnostic testing, is preferred. In most instances, when arteriography is required, an intraoperative arteriogram is sufficient to identify the location and extent of injury and to guide the surgical repair.

A large majority of arterial injuries, however, are clinically occult and pose a diagnostic challenge if they are to be identified. The diagnostic approach has changed substantially since the Korean War. Initially, the severity of soft tissue destruction typical of military wounds prompted the recommendation that all penetrating extremity wounds in proximity to a neurovascular bundle be explored routinely. When applied to civilian injuries, this practice detected normal intact vessels in a large percentage of cases, up to 84% in one series.[19] These patients had undergone expensive, nontherapeutic operations which, occasionally resulted in additional morbidity.

With the appearance of readily available arteriography in most trauma centers, this diagnostic modality supplanted wound exploration, and screening ("exclusion") arteriography became routine and widespread. Like wound exploration, mandatory or routine screening arteriography for proximity wounds, in the absence of other suspicious clinical findings, resulted in a large proportion of normal arteriograms (90%), at significant cost. In addition, arteriograms were found to be less than perfect, having a low, but real, incidence of false-negative and false-positive findings. Because of its invasive nature and the potential nephrotoxicity of contrast media, arteriography also occasionally results in serious complications, thus increasing patient morbidity and further increasing the cost of care.

Increasingly, attention has been directed toward selective, rather than routine, arteriography for patients who might harbor an extremity arterial injury, and the proper role of clinical examination and noninvasive vascular studies has been assessed. For example, in a study designed to determine the diagnostic yield of arteriography when performed for proximity alone or for signs suggestive of an arterial injury,[60] 373 patients with a unilateral penetrating injury to an upper extremity (distal to the deltopectoral groove) or lower extremity (distal to the inguinal ligament) were evaluated during an 18-month period. Arteriograms were obtained when a distal pulse deficit, neurologic deficit, hematoma, history of hemorrhage or hypotension, bruit, fracture, major soft tissue injury, or delayed capillary refill was present *or*, in the absence of these findings, when the path of the penetrating object was judged to run close to a major neurovascular bundle. For 210 of the 373 patients, the posterior tibial/dorsalis pedis or radial/ulnar Doppler pressures in the injured and the uninjured contralateral extremity were obtained and indexed using the brachial Doppler pressure of an uninjured arm as a reference (ankle-arm [brachial] index [ABI]). The minimum ABI (MABI), defined as the lower of the two ABIs at the ankle or wrist, was recorded. All arterial injuries identified by arteriography were categorized as major or minor. Major injuries were defined as injuries to arterial segments that, if interrupted, would likely result in clinically significant limb ischemia (e.g., the superficial femoral artery). All other injuries were termed *minor*.

Of the 373 patients enrolled in this study, 216 presented with one or more abnormal physical findings, and arterial injury was identified arteriographically in 65 (30%). Proximity was the sole indication for arteriography in 157 patients, and an injury was identified in 17 (11%). Stepwise logistic regression analysis revealed that a pulse deficit, neurologic deficit, or shotgun injury each separately correlated ($p < .05$) with arteriographic evidence of either a major or a minor injury. The presence of one or more of these variables identified a high-risk group of 104 patients who had 40 injuries (38%), 15 of which required repair. An intermediate-risk group consisting of patients with an MABI less than 1.00 or with "soft" signs of arterial injury (fracture, hematoma, bruit, decreased capillary refill, history of hemorrhage, hypotension, or soft tissue injury) was identified, 20% (33/165) of whom had an arterial injury. Five of 33 injuries in the intermediate-risk group required intervention. A low-risk group of 104 patients with none of the above findings remained. Nine injuries were identified (9%) in this low-risk group, none of which required therapeutic intervention. These data support the concept that patients with normal clinical findings and ABI rarely have clinically significant arterial injury and, thus, do not require diagnostic arteriography.

To validate this risk stratification scheme and further investigate the ability of Doppler indices to detect occult arterial injuries, a follow-up prospective study was performed in another consecutive cohort of 514 patients with unilateral, isolated penetrating extremity injuries.[44] Arteriography was limited to patients in the high-risk (pulse deficit, neurologic deficit, shotgun injury) or intermediate-risk group (one or more "soft" signs or an MABI less than 1.00). Low-risk patients were observed for 24 hours and did not undergo arteriography. Twenty-two (4%) patients with limb-threatening ischemia or ongoing hemorrhage who required immediate operation and 23 (4%) patients who refused arteriography were excluded from analysis. Of the remaining 469 patients, 213 (45%) were at low risk, 151 (32%) at intermediate risk, and 105 (23%) at high risk for arterial injury. No complication developed in any patient with a low-risk profile during the 24-hour observation period. Arteriography identified injuries in 26% of patients in the intermediate-risk group and 36% in the high-risk group. All patients with a major arterial injury had either a pulse deficit or MABI below 1.00.

For blunt extremity trauma, the indications for arteriography have also been studied. A prospective study analyzed the results of arteriography in 53 patients with unilateral blunt lower extremity trauma.[2] Thirty-one patients had physical findings suggestive of an arterial injury, and an arterial injury was demonstrated in 15. A pulse deficit or decrease capillary refill correlated significantly ($p < .05$) with arteriographic evidence of injury. Of the 15 arterial injuries, 12 were found in patients who had one or both of these findings and four of those injuries required repair. In the remaining 22 patients with neither a pulse deficit nor decreased capillary refill, three minor injuries were found, none of which required repair.

Another series of blunt injuries focused specifically on 115 patients with knee dislocations.[51] Popliteal artery injury was demonstrated arteriographically in 27 of 115 (23%) patients. An abnormal pedal pulse identified popliteal artery injuries with sensitivity of 85% and specificity of 93%. All injuries that required intervention were associated with a diminished pulse. Dennis reported an identical experience in 37 patients with knee dislocations. In all patients who required popliteal repair, pedal pulses were absent.[8] Again, the assertion that the clinical examination can define a subset of high-risk patients who need an arteriogram, and possibly surgical repair, was validated.

Similar evidence for the reliability of the clinical examination combined with noninvasive pressure measurements has been provided by Lynch and Johansen.[27] In a series of

100 patients with blunt or penetrating limb trauma, all patients had ABIs measured and were studied by arteriography. Arterial injuries that required intervention were discovered in 14 cases, and an ABI less than 0.90 predicted the injury with 87% sensitivity and 97% specificity, arteriography being the standard. Because two of the arteriograms were falsely positive, sensitivity and specificity of ABI less than 0.90 were even higher—95% and 97%—when clinical outcome was the standard.

Based on these recently published reports, a patient with a penetrating or blunt injury who has a normal extremity pulse examination and MABI of 1.00 or more does not require arteriography. A period of observation for 12 to 24 hours is all that is necessary. Furthermore, all clinically significant arterial injuries are found in extremities in association with a distal pulse deficit or a MABI less than 1.00. It is in this group of patients that diagnostic arteriography is useful and has its greatest yield.

Finally, although careful physical examination and pressure measurements appropriately select the vast majority of patients (>95%) who have significant arterial injury and require arteriography, occasional injuries are missed. In most cases, however, the missed injuries are clinically unimportant and include occlusive and nonocclusive injuries to minor branch vessels and minimal nonocclusive injuries of major vessels that heal without specific intervention, among others.[7, 15, 49] With these principles in mind, the diagnostic algorithm shown in Figure 59–1 was constructed.[20]

Because of continued improvements in noninvasive vascular imaging, color flow duplex ultrasonography (CFD) has been suggested as a substitute for or complement to arteriography.[33] CFD has several obvious advantages. It is noninvasive and painless. It is portable and can easily be brought to the patient's bedside or the emergency room or operating room. Repeated and follow-up examinations are easily performed without morbidity and are relatively inexpensive.

Bynoe and colleagues reported sensitivity of 95%, specificity of 99%, and accuracy of 98% when CFD was used to evaluate blunt and penetrating injuries of the neck or extremities, and Fry and coworkers[5, 14] documented 100% sensitivity and 97.3% specificity in a similar series. In these two studies, however, a comparison arteriogram was available for only a minority of patients. Bergstein and associates reported on 67 patients who had 75 penetrating extremity injuries, all of whom underwent both CFD and arteriography.[3] Using arteriography as the gold standard, CFD had two false-negative results and one false-positive (sensitivity 50%, specificity 99%). Gagne and coworkers published a series of 37 patients with proximity injuries in 43 extremities.[16] Arteriography identified three injuries to the deep femoral, superficial femoral, and posterior tibial arteries that were not identified by CFD; however, CFD did detect a superficial femoral artery intimal flap that arteriography missed.

Despite some uncertainty about the ability of CFD to detect all arterial injuries, these reports suggest that nearly

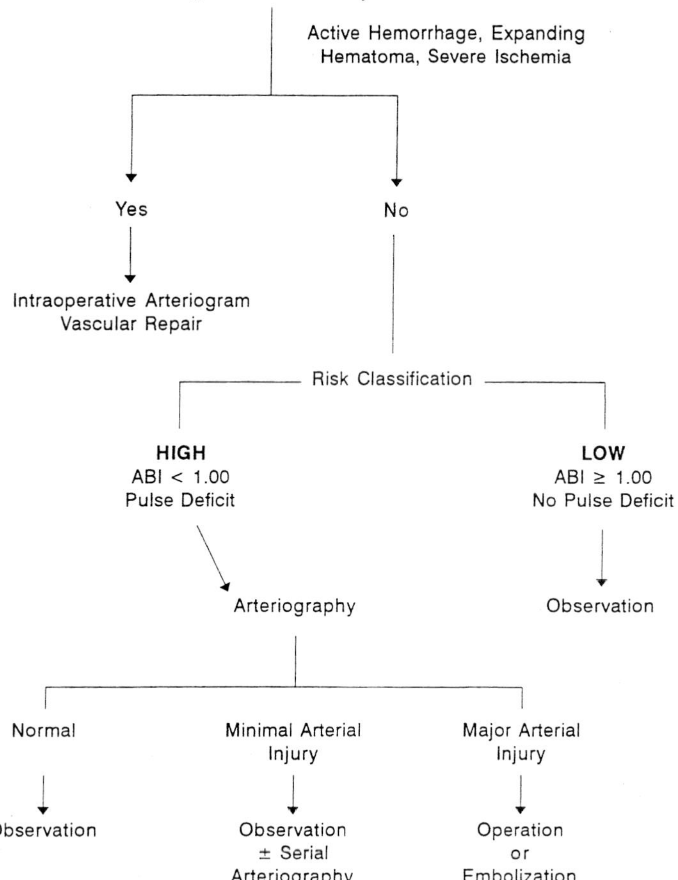

FIGURE 59–1. Diagnostic algorithm for extremity arterial trauma. ABI = ankle-brachial index. (From Hood DB, Yellin AE, Weaver FA: Vascular trauma. *In* Dean R [ed]: Current Vascular Surgical Diagnosis and Treatment. Norwalk, Conn, Appleton & Lange, 1995, p 405.)

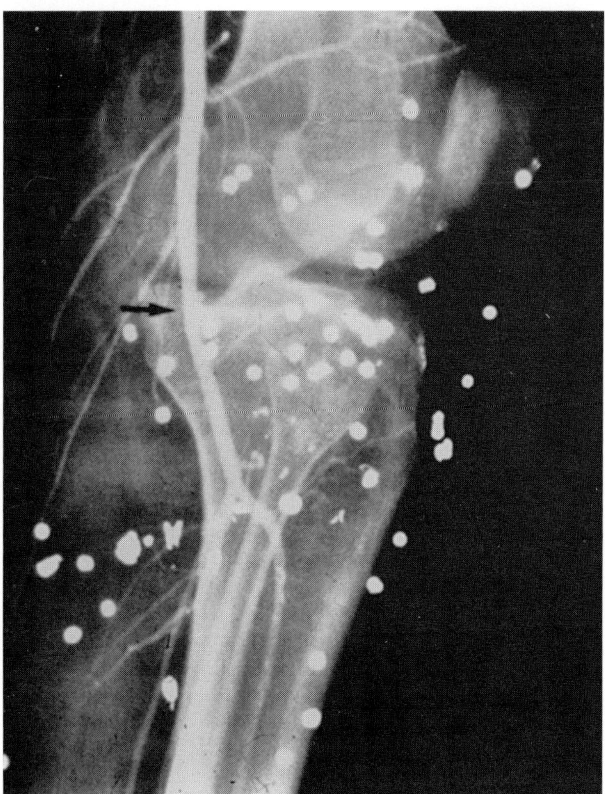

FIGURE 59–2. Popliteal artery shotgun injury with small false aneurysm *(arrow)*, which was managed nonoperatively.

all major injuries that require therapeutic intervention can be identified, potentially at considerable costs savings as compared with arteriography.[33] Ordog has estimated a multimillion dollar cost savings if CFD and outpatient follow-up, rather than arteriography and inpatient observation, were used to exclude extremity arterial injuries.[39]

Our own experience with CFD in the evaluation of extremity trauma has produced an important caveat: CFD is highly operator-dependent and, to be used effectively, requires an institutional investment in experienced vascular technologists and interpreting physicians.[45] This expense could be lessened over the long term if the current effort to train surgeons in the use of diagnostic ultrasound for intracavitary trauma were extended to include extremity vessels.

TREATMENT OF ARTERIAL INJURIES

Nonoperative Management

The management of minimal, nonocclusive, clinically asymptomatic arterial injuries detected by arteriography remains controversial (Fig. 59–2).[59] Some surgeons continue to insist that all detected arterial injuries should be repaired, whereas we[49] and others[7, 15] have proposed using a nonoperative approach when these clinical and radiologic criteria are present:

- Low-velocity injury
- Minimal arterial wall disruption (<5 mm) for intimal defects and pseudoaneurysms
- Adherent or downstream protrusion of intimal flaps
- Intact distal circulation
- No active hemorrhage

When, for a given injury, this approach is selected, follow-up vascular imaging is advisable to document healing or stabilization. Knudson's group has suggested that CFD may be used in lieu of arteriography for serial follow-up.[26]

In a study by Stain and coworkers, 24 nonocclusive minimal arterial injuries were managed nonoperatively and subsequently studied arteriographically at 1 to 12 weeks after injury.[49] Resolution, improvement, or stabilization of the injury occurred in 21 injuries (87%). Progression was noted in three, and only one required repair. There were no cases of acute thrombosis or distal embolization. A similar experience in a group of patients with minimal arterial injuries identified on diagnostic arteriography was reported by Frykberg.[15] Resolution or stability of detected injuries occurred in 89% of the cases during 27 months follow-up. Frykberg's follow-up has now been extended to 10 years with comparable excellent results, further confirming the wisdom of this approach.[7]

Endovascular Management

Transcatheter embolization with coils or balloons can be used to manage selected arterial injuries, such as low-flow arteriovenous fistulae, false aneurysms, and active bleeding from noncritical arteries, particularly in remote anatomic sites. Coils are particularly useful for occluding bleeding vessels and arteriovenous fistulae (Fig. 59–3). Currently available coils are made from stainless steel and are wool or Dacron tufted. Introduced via a 5 or 7 French (Fr.) catheter, they can be extruded at the vessel site that requires

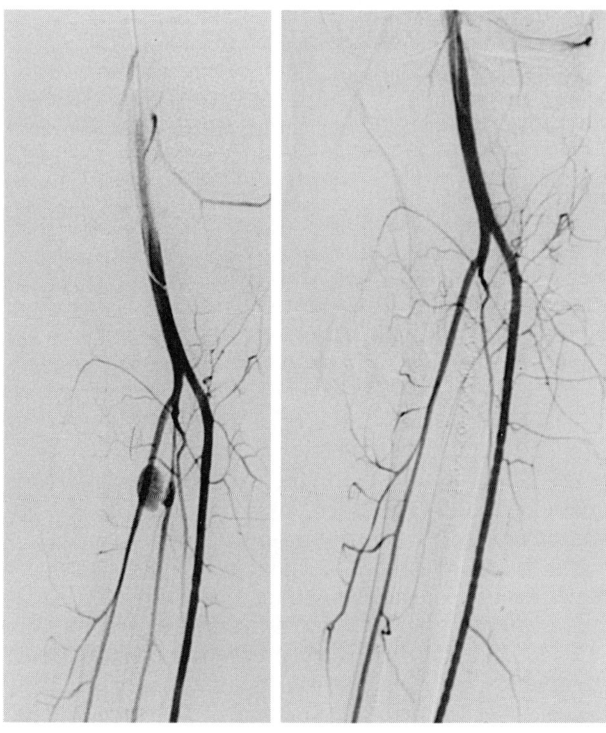

FIGURE 59–3. Large peroneal artery false aneurysm *(left)* was successfully treated by coil embolization *(right)*.

occlusion. Once deployed, the coils expand and lodge at the site of extrusion. The Dacron or wool tuft promotes thrombosis of the vessel. If flow persists 5 minutes after deployment, a second coil is introduced. For arteriovenous fistulae, the coil embolus is placed across the fistula and lodged just on the venous side, so that the fistulous connection is occluded but the supplying artery remains patent. If this is not possible, the next option is to occlude the arterial side of the fistula, preferably by isolating the fistula site with proximal and distal coils. The diameter of the coil must be approximately the same as the diameter of the artery to be embolized; otherwise, it may dislodge and embolize peripherally or centrally.

McNeese reported 11 patients with post-traumatic arteriovenous fistulae, arterial false aneurysms, or uncontrolled bleeding from noncritical vessels that were treated by embolization.[32] Eight patients were treated by wire coil embolization or gelatin clot emboli and one with selective injection of barium-impregnated silicone-like (Silastic) beads sized to the vessel lumen. The last technique was found to be useful in treating arteriovenous fistulae fed by multiple small arteries. Four of the six fistulae were permanently obliterated. Ischemia distal to an obliterated vessel did not occur, and no major complications directly related to the embolization were reported.

Another endovascular approach to extremity injuries uses stent-graft technology. By combining a fixation device such as a stent with a graft, endoluminal repair of false aneurysms or large arteriovenous fistulae is possible. Marin reported the successful treatment of seven vascular injuries by stent-grafts placed endoluminally.[29] As endovascular technology continues to develop, stent-graft repair of peripheral vascular injuries may become commonplace.

Operative Management

The operative management of a peripheral arterial injury requires preparation and draping of the entire injured extremity. In addition, a contralateral uninjured lower or upper extremity should be included in the operative field in the event that repair requires an autogenous vein graft. In most instances, extremity incisions are placed longitudinally, directly over the injured vessel and extended proximally or distally as necessary. Proximal and distal arterial control is obtained prior to exposure of the injury. When proximal control of the traumatized vessel is problematic, as in some axillary and subclavian injuries, endoluminal balloon occlusion of the proximal artery via catheters placed under fluoroscopic guidance from a remote arterial site can provide temporary control. Occasionally, a proximally placed pneumatic tourniquet may help to minimize operative blood loss.

Once control is established, injured vessels are débrided to macroscopically normal arterial wall. Fogarty catheters should be passed gently, both proximal and distal to the arterial injury, to remove any intraluminal thrombus. It is extremely important not to overinflate the balloon, lest the endothelial lining be damaged and arterial spasm or thrombosis result. Both proximal and distal arterial lumens are flushed with heparinized saline solution. Systemic heparinization, particularly for popliteal artery injuries, is a helpful adjunct to prevent thrombosis or thrombus propagation when systemic anticoagulation is not contraindicated.[34, 55] Temporary intraluminal shunting may also be of value for some injuries when the limb is severely ischemic and revascularization will be delayed because of fracture fixation, complex soft-tissue injury, or associated life-threatening injuries.[10, 23, 37] This technique allows early restoration of limb perfusion, which lessens the likelihood of ischemic damage and distal thrombosis. Débridement, fasciotomy, fracture fixation, neurorrhaphy, or vein repair can then be performed in a deliberate and unhurried fashion, before arterial reconstruction.

The type of repair is dictated by the extent of arterial damage. Repair of injured vessels can be accomplished by lateral suture patch angioplasty, end-to-end anastomosis, interposition graft, or, when adjacent soft injury is extensive, a bypass graft. Extra-anatomic bypass grafts are useful in patients with associated extensive soft-tissue injury or sepsis. Stain reported on three axillofemoral, four femorofemoral, one obturator, and one extra-anatomic femoropopliteal graft performed in nine patients who had extensive soft-tissue injuries.[48] Seven patients (78%) had functional extremities salvaged.

Autogenous vein grafts were first used successfully to repair arterial injuries during the Korean War.[22] Later development of prosthetic graft material—expanded polytetrafluoroethylene (ePTFE)—made possible routine use of prosthetic conduits as a substitute for autogenous grafts. Surgical experience suggests that ePTFE is more resistant to infection than other prosthetic grafts and has acceptable patency rates when used in the above-knee position.[53, 54]

In a retrospective civilian series of 188 patients with lower extremity vascular trauma, Martin reported equivalent patencies when ePTFE and vein grafts were used to repair the iliac, femoral, and superficial femoral arteries.[30] There were no infections of ePTFE or vein grafts. A significant difference in immediate patency was apparent, however, when the distal arterial anastomosis was at or below the popliteal artery: failure was more common in patients with ePTFE grafts. Blunt trauma was associated with a higher graft failure rate (35%) than was penetrating trauma (1.2%), and graft failure always resulted in amputation.

Our preference is to use autogenous grafts exclusively for extremity arterial repair, usually the greater saphenous vein harvested from an uninjured leg. An ePTFE graft is used only when autogenous vein is inadequate or unavailable, when the patient is unstable and expeditious repair of the arterial injury is mandatory, or when a large size discrepancy between a vein graft and the native artery would result.

Monofilament 5-0 or 6-0 sutures are suitable for most peripheral vascular repairs, and all completed repairs should be tension free and covered by viable soft tissue. With major soft tissue injury, it may be prudent to enlist the assistance of a plastic or orthopedic reconstructive surgeon to rotate a muscle flap adequate for soft-tissue coverage. We consider intraoperative completion arteriography or duplex scanning to be mandatory to document technical perfection of the vascular reconstruction, visualize arterial runoff, and detect persistent missed distal thrombi. Intra-arterial vasodilators such as papaverine or tolazoline may be helpful, particularly in the pediatric age group, in reversing severe spasm in the distal arterial tree or the repaired arterial segment.

The period immediately following limb reperfusion has been recognized to be an important determinant of ultimate outcome after injury. During reperfusion, toxic oxygen-derived free radicals are generated that overwhelm inherent protective enzyme-scavenging systems such as superoxide dismutase, glutathione peroxidase, and catalase, producing cell injury and death. Viewed clinically, these effects are manifested by the accelerated muscle edema and necrosis seen in compartmental hypertension (see Chapter 62). Experimentally, superoxide dismutase, catalase, mannitol, and allopurinol can interrupt this pathogenetic cascade at various levels and protect against reperfusion injury; decreased muscle necrosis and edema are observed in animals pretreated with these agents.[38]

Wright and colleagues documented similar benefits in animals pretreated with heparin before reperfusion of an ischemic limb.[63] In addition to the experimental evidence that heparin has a mitigating effect on reperfusion injury, its beneficial effects include prevention of thrombosis of distal outflow vessels and collaterals. For all these reasons, the surgeon must be aware of the deleterious effects of reperfusion injury, and systemic mannitol and/or heparin infusion should be considered before an ischemic limb is reperfused. The clinical manifestation of reperfusion injury—compartmental hypertension—must be sought assiduously and treated aggressively.[25]

Specific Arterial Injuries

Subclavian-Axillary Arteries

Injuries to the subclavian-axillary arteries are relatively uncommon because these vessels are protected by the overlying bone and muscle. In most series, penetrating trauma is the most frequent cause. Blunt subclavian-axillary trauma is usually associated with major musculoskeletal and brachial plexus injury.[13] Fracture-dislocation of the first rib, particularly the posterior portion, is associated with an extremely high incidence of subclavian artery injury.

Critical ischemia of the upper extremity is uncommon following subclavian-axillary artery injuries owing to rich collateral circulation around the shoulder. In one report, only 20% of patients had decreased or absent pulses.[18] A high index of suspicion, careful pulse examination, use of Doppler arterial pressure indices, and liberal use of arteriography are thus mandatory for reliable diagnosis of these injuries.

Penetrating injuries of the subclavian-axillary arteries may require median sternotomy for proximal control of right subclavian injuries; left anterolateral or "trapdoor" thoracotomy may be necessary to manage proximal left subclavian injuries, with the more distal subclavian artery exposed through a supraclavicular extension. The axillary artery is approached through a horizontal infraclavicular incision, but proximal supraclavicular control may be necessary for arterial injuries at the thoracic outlet. Resection of the middle third of the clavicle is rarely necessary, but it is an alternative approach for certain injuries at the axillary-subclavian junction.

The primary prognostic factor in blunt arterial injury at this site is the severity of concomitant brachial plexus injury. In patients with a neurologic deficit, the brachial plexus is explored at the time of arterial repair. Complete disruption of the brachial plexus generally results in a permanently paretic, painful, anesthetic limb that ultimately may warrant forequarter amputation. This injury is usually associated with severe vascular disruption and musculoskeletal trauma. A contused but intact brachial plexus may regain all or partial neurologic function in some patients. A recent study by Manord and colleagues demonstrated some degree of neurologic improvement in 87% of such patients.[28] With the exception of patients with spinal root avulsions, significant functional improvement was seen at all levels of brachial plexus injury.

Brachial, Radial, and Ulnar Arteries

Brachial artery injuries are usually due to penetrating trauma and are frequently iatrogenic. Blunt brachial artery injuries are most often associated with supracondylar fractures of the humerus. The location of the brachial artery injury has implications with respect to the associated clinical findings, since injuries below the origin of the profunda brachii may not manifest signs of ischemia owing to the robust collateral networks already present.

Single-vessel injury in the forearm need not be repaired but may be ligated or embolized. Repair is mandatory when one of the vessels, either the radial or the ulnar artery, was previously traumatized or ligated or when the palmar arch is incomplete. When both radial and ulnar arteries are injured, the ulnar artery should be repaired preferentially because it is the dominant vessel.

External Iliac-Femoral Arteries

For proximal control of the external iliac artery, a retroperitoneal approach is ideal. The surgeon extends the femoral incision through the inguinal ligament or makes a separate incision parallel to the lateral border of the rectus sheath and 2 cm above the inguinal ligament (Fig. 59–4). The rectus muscle is retracted mediad, the transversalis fascia is incised, and the retroperitoneal space is entered. The peritoneum and its contents are reflected medially to provide exposure of the distal aorta and the iliac vessels.

Exposure of the common femoral, proximal deep femoral, and superficial femoral arteries is accomplished through a longitudinal thigh incision over the femoral triangle. The common femoral artery lies within the femoral sheath, the common femoral vein lying medial to it and the femoral nerve lateral. Careful dissection is required to avoid iatrogenic injury to the deep femoral artery.

Blunt and penetrating injuries to the superficial femoral artery are very common and are repaired with the techniques described earlier. Injuries of the proximal deep femoral artery should always be repaired in hemodynamically stable patients because of this artery's contribution to the collateral supply of the lower extremity.[17]

Popliteal Artery

Popliteal artery injuries remain among the most challenging of all extremity vascular injuries. Nevertheless, during the

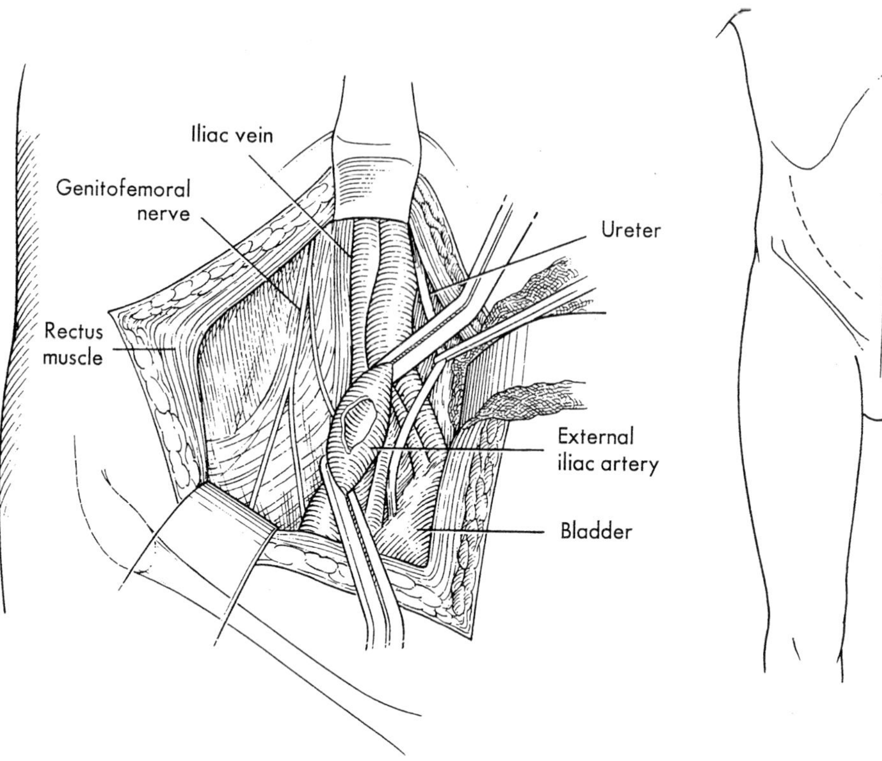

FIGURE 59–4. Retroperitoneal exposure for proximal control of the iliac and proximal common femoral arteries. (From Yellin AE, Weaver FA: Vascular system. *In* Donovan AJ [ed]: Trauma Surgery. St. Louis, Mosby–Year Book, 1994.)

past decade a dramatic reduction has occurred in the rate of amputation after civilian popliteal artery injuries. Amputation rates at our institution have decreased from 23% to 6% for blunt injuries and from 21% to zero for penetrating trauma.[55, 56]

The popliteal vein, infrapopliteal arteries, and tibial nerve are frequently involved in penetrating popliteal injury (20% to 35% of the time). A popliteal artery injury above the knee joint is best repaired through a medial thigh incision; a similar below-knee injury requires a leg incision. An isolated penetrating injury directly behind the knee can be approached from behind (Fig. 59–5). When this approach is used, the contralateral lesser saphenous vein can be harvested if an autogenous graft is required. The outcome of a penetrating popliteal artery injury depends predominantly on the mechanism of injury. The amputation rate for shotgun wounds approaches 20% because of the associated soft-tissue injury and septic sequelae, whereas it is as low as zero for single missile injuries and stab wounds associated with minimal musculoskeletal injury.

In a series of 100 blunt popliteal artery injuries reported from our institution, popliteal artery thrombosis or transection occurred in 97%.[55] Concomitant popliteal vein injury was present in 29%. Repair of the artery was accomplished by end-to-end anastomosis in 49%, vein interposition in 43%, intimal repair and vein patch in 2%, and thrombectomy in 1%. Ten amputations were required because of failure of the arterial repair, and five because of invasive limb sepsis or massive soft tissue injury. Prior to 1980, 12 amputations were necessary; after 1980, only three limbs were amputated. Factors that positively influenced limb salvage included (1) systemic (heparin) anticoagulation, (2) arterial repair accomplished either laterally or end to end, and (3) palpable pedal pulses within the first 24 hours. On the contrary, severe soft tissue injury, deep soft tissue infection, and preoperative ischemia were negative predictors of limb salvage (Table 59–1). Attention to the possibility of compartment syndrome, along with rapid treatment by complete dermotomy/fasciotomy if it is present, is crucial for these patients (see Chapter 62).[25]

In a more recent series, Melton and associates reported a similar experience. In 102 patients with a penetrating or blunt popliteal injury, systemic heparin or local thrombolytic therapy significantly reduced the amputation rate, where all severely traumatized limbs (as characterized by a Mangled Extremity Severity Score [MESS][24] above 8) required amputation.[34]

Tibial Arteries

Isolated occlusive injury to one infrapopliteal artery rarely results in limb ischemia and does not, as a rule, require therapeutic intervention. A single actively bleeding traumatized vessel or arterial pseudoaneurysm can be treated by simple ligation or angiographic embolization; however, when the tibioperoneal trunk or two infrapopliteal arteries are injured, repair is required.[46] The associated nerve, bone, and soft tissue injuries are the essential determinants of limb salvage. In a study by Whitman and colleagues, no amputations occurred in limbs with less than two associated injuries; however, for limbs with all three associated injuries, the amputation rate was 54%.[62]

Pediatric Extremity Arterial Injuries

Management principles for non-iatrogenic arterial injuries in children parallel those for adult trauma, and recent

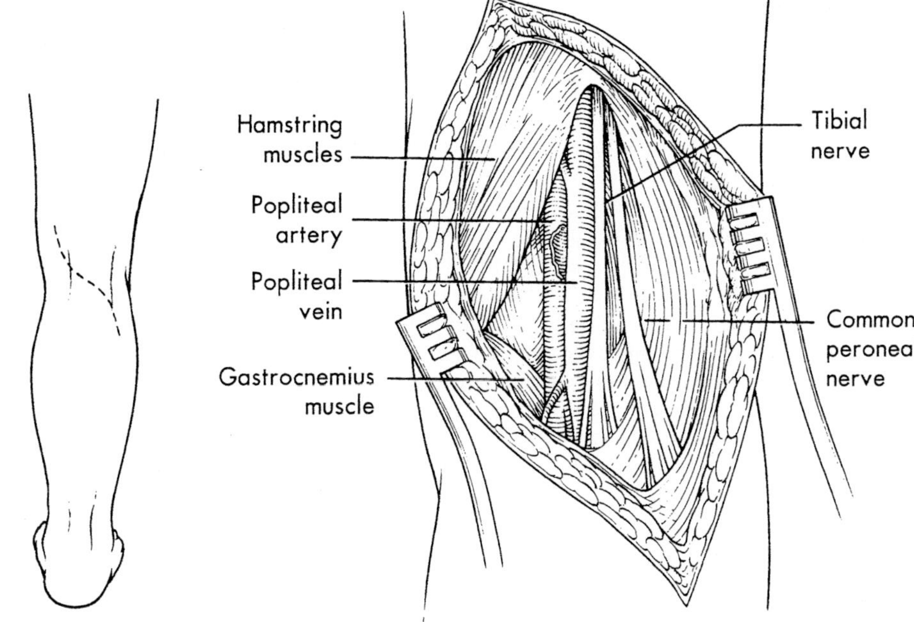

FIGURE 59–5. Posterior approach for a penetrating popliteal injury behind the knee. (From Yellin AE, Weaver FA: Vascular system. *In* Donovan AJ [ed]: Trauma Surgery. St. Louis, Mosby–Year Book, 1994.)

studies suggest that judicious use of arteriography and arterial repair in pediatric vascular injury provides results equivalent to those achieved in adults.[9, 12, 36, 41] Considerations unique to the management of pediatric injuries include the severity of arterial spasm, the unknown long-term consequences of autogenous grafts placed in children, and the long-term effects of diminished blood flow on limb length. The intense arterial spasm associated with pediatric vascular injuries can compromise any arterial repair. Similarly, diagnostic arteriography can exacerbate vasospasm and limb ischemia. Consequently, when diagnostic studies are indicated, a noninvasive modality such as CFD should be considered as an alternative. In a viable limb with an occlusive injury that is neurologically intact, the arterial repair can be deferred, and in a very young child this may be preferable.[47] If repair is not performed, careful follow-up of limb growth is necessary, and arterial repair is indicated if a limb length discrepancy develops.

TABLE 59–1. AMPUTATION RATES IN ASSOCIATION WITH PERIOPERATIVE RISK FACTORS IN BLUNT POPLITEAL ARTERY TRAUMA

RISK FACTOR	PRESENT	ABSENT	*p* VALUE*
Severe soft-tissue injury	13/31 (42%)	2/69 (3%)	<.0001
Deep soft-tissue infection	9/17 (53%)	6/83 (7%)	<.0001
Preoperative ischemia	15/64 (23%)	0/36 (0%)	<.001
Preoperative delay >6 hr	10/40 (25%)	5/24 (21%)	NS
Preoperative delay >12 hr	2/14 (14%)	13/50 (26%)	NS
Systemic anticoagulation	6/71 (8%)	9/29 (31%)	<.01
Primary arterial repair	3/49 (6%)	12/51 (24%)	<.05
Palpable pedal pulse within 24 hr	4/55 (7%)	11/45 (24%)	<.05
Trifurcation arterial injury	6/29 (21%)	9/71 (13%)	NS
Popliteal vein injury	6/29 (21%)	9/71 (13%)	NS
Ligation of venous injury	2/6 (33%)	4/23 (17%)	NS
Fasciotomy (operative or delayed)	11/61 (18%)	4/39 (10%)	NS
Delayed fasciotomy	1/4 (25%)	14/96 (15%)	NS
Preoperative compartment syndrome	2/17 (12%)	13/83 (16%)	NS

Modified from Wagner WH, Caulkins E, Weaver FA, et al: Blunt popliteal artery trauma: 100 consecutive cases. J Vasc Surg 7:736, 1988.

*Two-tailed Fisher's exact test.

NS = not statistically significant.

EXTREMITY VENOUS INJURIES

The most commonly injured major veins of the extremities are the superficial femoral vein (42%), followed by the popliteal vein (23%) and the common femoral vein (14%).[35] When the venous injury is localized and end-to-end or lateral venorrhaphy is possible, repair should be performed unless the patient is hemodynamically unstable. With more extensive venous injuries that require an interposition or panel graft for repair, the advisability and benefit of repair are controversial.[51]

Meyer studied 36 patients with traumatic venous injuries who underwent venous repair.[35] Repairs were studied venographically 7 days after operation. Fourteen (39%) of the venous repairs had thrombosed. Moreover, when an interposition vein graft was used, the thrombosis rate rose to 59%. Limb salvage was 100% successful and was not affected by failure of the venous repair. Timberlake reported a similar outcome, with transient edema in 36% and long-term permanent edema in only 2% of patients with venous injuries.[50] The finding of edema was not related to whether the vein was repaired or ligated. This experience and others suggest that repair of major venous injuries in a stable patient is a reasonable undertaking; however, when venous repair would be complex or the patient is hemodynamically unstable, simple ligation is appropriate. When venous ligation is necessary, postoperative edema can be controlled by extremity elevation and elastic wrapping. For patients undergoing venous repair, patency should be monitored with hand-held Doppler or duplex scan.

ORTHOPEDIC, SOFT TISSUE, AND NERVE INJURIES

The surgical treatment of combined vascular and orthopedic injuries is one of the most difficult problems in the management of trauma patients.[58] Since the duration of ischemia may be critical to the outcome, the arterial repair should usually be performed first to restore circulation to the limb before the orthopedic stabilization is addressed. Sometimes, however, massive musculoskeletal trauma renders a limb so unstable that external fixation must be placed before the vascular procedure. Selective use of intraluminal shunts[10, 23, 37] and rapid installation of an external fixator minimize limb ischemia in this setting. When the vascular repair is performed in advance of orthopedic fixation, it is incumbent on the surgeon to inspect the vascular reconstruction before final wound closure and before the patient leaves the operating room. Patency of the repair must be documented by palpable pulses, arteriography, or CFD.

In patients with major soft tissue injuries, débridement of all clearly nonviable tissue is mandatory. Frequent—and early—returns to the operating room, as often as every 24 to 48 hours, may be required. In these patients, unexplained fever and leukocytosis are assumed to be due to deep tissue infection until proven otherwise. Reexploration of the wound and débridement of necrotic tissue or hematoma is essential for minimizing septic sequelae. Ultimate wound coverage by delayed primary closure, rotational flaps, or free tissue transfer when the soft tissue bed is clean, minimizes the risk of invasive sepsis.

Nerve injuries occur in about 50% of upper extremity and 25% of lower extremity vascular injuries. The nerve injury usually determines the long-term functional status of an injured extremity.[21] If a major nerve has been cleanly transected by a sharp object, primary repair can be performed at the time of vascular repair; however, for most penetrating and all blunt nerve injuries, immediate repair is rarely possible or indicated. Rather, both ends of the injured nerve should be tagged with nonabsorbable suture at the initial operation. This facilitates identification of the nerve at the time of eventual nerve repair or grafting.

Vascular repairs are now performed with such a high rate of success that they exert little influence on ultimate extremity function. Rather, the associated orthopedic, nerve, and soft tissue injuries are the critical factors that determine long-term limb function. A number of scores or indices (e.g., MESS[24]) have been proposed in an attempt to predict early limb salvage and to limit protracted reconstructive efforts aimed at restoring limb function. Unfortunately, application of these indices has often failed to predict functional limb salvage reliably.[4, 34] Currently, for limbs with massive orthopedic, soft tissue, and nerve injuries, primary amputation, rather than complex reconstruction, should be considered, as permanent total functional limb disability—requiring delayed amputation—is common.[58, 62] In hemodynamically unstable patients in whom a complex vascular repair might jeopardize survival, primary amputation should also be considered.

REFERENCES

1. Amato JJ, Billy LJ, Gruber RP, et al: Vascular injuries: An experimental study of high and low velocity missile wounds. Arch Surg 101:167, 1970.
2. Applebaum R, Yellin AE, Weaver FA, et al: The role of routine arteriography in blunt lower extremity trauma. Am J Surg 160:221, 1990.
3. Bergstein JM, Blair JF, Edwards J, et al: Pitfalls in the use of color-flow duplex ultrasound for screening of suspected arterial injuries in penetrated extremities. J Trauma 33:395, 1992.
4. Bonanni F, Rhodes M, Lucke JF: The futility of predictive scoring of mangled lower extremities. J Trauma 34:99, 1993.
5. Bynoe RP, Miles WS, Bell RM, et al: Noninvasive diagnosis of vascular trauma by duplex ultrasonography. J Vasc Surg 14:346, 1991.
6. DeBakey E, Simeone CF: Battle injuries of the arteries in World War II: An analysis of 2,471 cases. Ann Surg 123:534, 1946.
7. Dennis JW, Frykberg ER, Veldenz HC, et al: Validation of nonoperative management of occult vascular injuries and accuracy of physical examination alone in penetrating extremity trauma: 5- to 10-year follow up. J Trauma 44:243, 1998.
8. Dennis JW, Jagger C, Butcher JL, et al: Reassessing the role of arteriograms in the management of posterior knee dislocations. J Trauma 35:692, 1993.
9. deVirgilio C, Mercado PD, Arnell T, et al: Noniatrogenic pediatric vascular trauma: A ten-year experience at a level 1 trauma center. Am Surg 63:781, 1997.
10. Eger M, Golcman L, Goldstein A, et al: The use of a temporary shunt in the management of arterial vascular injuries. Surg Gynecol Obstet 123:67, 1971.
11. Fackler ML: Wound ballistics: A review of common misconceptions. JAMA 259:2730, 1988.
12. Fayiga YJ, Valentine RJ, Myers SI, et al: Blunt pediatric vascular trauma: Analysis of forty-one consecutive patients undergoing operative intervention. J Vasc Surg 20:419, 1994.
13. Fritrige RA, Raptis S, Miller JH, et al: Upper extremity arterial injuries: Experience at the Royal Adelaide Hospital, 1969 to 1991. J Vasc Surg 20:941, 1994.
14. Fry WR, Smith RS, Sayers DV, et al: The success of duplex ultrasonographic scanning in diagnosis of extremity vascular proximity trauma. Arch Surg 128:1368, 1993.
15. Frykberg EP: Advances in the diagnosis and treatment of extremity vascular trauma. Surg Clin North Am 75:207, 1995.
16. Gagne PJ, Cone JB, McFarland D, et al: Proximity penetrating extremity trauma: The role of duplex ultrasound in the detection of occult venous injuries. J Trauma 39:1157, 1995.
17. Gorman JF: Combat arterial trauma analysis of 106 limb-threatening injuries. Arch Surg 98:160, 1969.
18. Graham JM, Feliciano DV, Mattox KL, et al: Management of subclavian vascular injuries. J Trauma 20:537, 1980.
19. Guede JW, Hobson RW, Padberg FT, et al: The role of contrast arteriography in suspected arterial injuries of the extremities. Am Surg 51:89, 1985.
20. Hood DB, Yellin AE, Weaver FA: Vascular trauma. *In* Dean R (ed): Current Vascular Surgical Diagnosis and Treatment. Norwalk, Conn, Appleton & Lange, 1995, p 405.
21. Howe HH, Poole GV, Hansen KJ, et al: Salvage of lower extremities following combined orthopedic and vascular trauma: A predictive salvage index. Ann Surg 53:205, 1987.
22. Hughes CH: Arterial repair during the Korean War. Ann Surg 147:555, 1958.
23. Johansen K, Bandyk D, Thiele B, et al: Temporary intraluminal shunts: Resolution of a management dilemma in complex vascular injuries. J Trauma 22:395, 1982.
24. Johansen K, Daines M, Howey T, et al: Objective criteria accurately predict amputation following lower extremity trauma. J Trauma 30:568, 1990.
25. Johnson SB, Weaver FA, Yellin AE, et al: Clinical results of decompressive dermatomy-fasciotomy. Am J Surg 164:286, 1992.
26. Knudson MM, Lewis FR, Atkinson K, et al: The role of duplex ultrasound arterial imaging in patients with penetrating extremity trauma. Arch Surg 128:1033, 1993.
27. Lynch K, Johansen K: Can Doppler pressure measurement replace

"exclusion" arteriography in the diagnosis of occult extremity arterial trauma? Ann Surg 214:737, 1991.
28. Manord JD, Garrard CL, Kline DG, et al: Management of severe proximal vascular and neural injury of the upper extremity. J Vasc Surg 27:43, 1998.
29. Marin ML, Veith FJ, Panetta TF, et al: Transluminally placed endovascular stented graft repair for arterial trauma. J Vasc Surg 20:466, 1994.
30. Martin LC, McKenney MG, Sossa JL, et al: Management of lower extremity arterial trauma. J Trauma 37:591, 1994.
31. Mayer JP, Lim LT, Schuler JJ, et al: Peripheral vascular trauma from close-range shotgun injuries. Arch Surg 120:1126, 1985.
32. McNeese S, Fink E, Yellin AE: Definitive treatment of selected vascular injuries and post-traumatic arteriovenous fistulas by arteriographic embolization. Am J Surg 140:252, 1980.
33. Meissner M, Paun M, Johansen K: Duplex scanning for arterial trauma. Am J Surg 161:552, 1991.
34. Melton SM, Croce MA, Patton JH, et al: Popliteal artery trauma. Ann Surg 225:518, 1997.
35. Meyer J, Walsh J, Schuler J, et al: The early fate of venous repair after civilian vascular trauma. Ann Surg 206:458, 1987.
36. Myers SI, Reed MK, Black CT, et al: Noniatrogenic pediatric vascular trauma. J Vasc Surg 10:258, 1989.
37. Nichols JG, Svoboda JA, Parks SN: Use of temporary intraluminal shunts in selected peripheral arterial injuries. J Trauma 26:1094, 1986.
38. Odeh M: Mechanisms of disease: The role of reperfusion-induced injury in the pathogenesis of the crush syndrome. N Engl J Med 324:1417, 1991.
39. Ordog GJ, Balasubramanium S, Wasserber J, et al: Extremity gunshot wounds: I. Identification and treatment of patients at high risk of vascular injury. J Trauma 36:358, 1994.
40. Pasch AR, Bishara, Lim LT, et al: Optimal limb salvage in penetrating civilian vascular trauma. J Vasc Surg 3:189, 1986.
41. Reichard KW, Hall JR, Meller JL, et al: Arteriography in the evaluation of penetrating pediatric extremity injuries. J Pediatr Surg 29:19, 1994.
42. Rich NM: Surgeon's response to battlefield vascular trauma. Am J Surg 166:91, 1993.
43. Rich NA, Baugh JH, Hughes CW: Acute arterial injuries in Vietnam: 1,000 cases. J Trauma 10:359, 1970.
44. Schwartz MR, Weaver FA, Yellin AE, et al: Refining the indications for arteriography in penetrating extremity trauma: A prospective analysis. J Vasc Surg 17:166, 1993.
45. Schwartz M, Weaver F, Yellin A, Ralls P: The utility of color flow Doppler examination in penetrating extremity arterial trauma. Am Surg 59:375, 1993.
46. Shah DM, Corson JD, Karmody AM, et al: Optimal management of tibial arterial trauma. J Trauma 28:228, 1988.
47. Smith C, Green RM: Pediatric vascular injuries. Surgery 90:20, 1981.
48. Stain SC, Weaver FA, Yellin AE: Extra-anatomical bypass of failed traumatic arterial repairs. J Trauma 31:575, 1991.
49. Stain SC, Yellin AE, Weaver FA, et al: Selective management of nonocclusive arterial injuries. Arch Surg 124:1136, 1989.
50. Timberlake GA, Kerstein MD: Venous injury: To repair or ligate, the dilemma revisited. Am Surg 61:139, 1995.
51. Timberlake GA, O'Connell R, Kerstein M: Venous injury: To repair or ligate, the dilemma. J Vasc Surg 4:553, 1986.
52. Treiman GS, Yellin AE, Weaver FA, et al: Examination of the patient with knee dislocation: The case for selective arteriography. Arch Surg 127:1056, 1992.
53. Vaughn GD, Mattox KL, Feliciano DV, et al: Surgical experience with expanded polytetrafluoroethylene (PTFE) as a replacement graft for traumatized vessels. J Trauma 19:403, 1979.
54. Veith FJ, Gupta SK, Ascer E, et al: Six-year prospective multicenter randomized comparison of autologous saphenous vein and expanded polytetrafluoroethylene grafts in infrainguinal arterial reconstructions. J Vasc Surg 3:104, 1986.
55. Wagner WH, Caulkins E, Weaver FA, et al: Blunt popliteal artery trauma: 100 consecutive cases. J Vasc Surg 7:736, 1988.
56. Wagner WH, Yellin AE, Weaver FA, et al: Acute treatment of popliteal artery trauma: The importance of soft tissue injury. Ann Vasc Surg 8:557, 1994.
57. Weaver FA, Papanicolaou G, Yellin AE: Difficult peripheral vascular injuries. Surg Clin North Am 76:843, 1996.
58. Weaver FA, Rosenthal RE, Waterhouse G, et al: Combined vascular and skeletal injuries of the lower extremities. Am Surg 50:189, 1984.
59. Weaver FA, Yellin AE: Complications of missed arterial injuries. J Vasc Surg 18:1077, 1993.
60. Weaver FA, Yellin AE, Bauer M, et al: Is arterial proximity a valid indication for arteriography in penetrating extremity trauma? A prospective analysis. Arch Surg 125:1256, 1990.
61. White RA, Scher LA, Samson RH, et al: Peripheral vascular injuries associated with falls from heights. J Trauma 27:411, 1987.
62. Whitman GR, McCroskey BL, Moore EE, et al: Traumatic popliteal and trifurcation vascular injuries: Determinants of functional limb salvage. Am J Surg 154:681, 1987.
63. Wright JG, Kerr JC, Valeri CR, et al: Heparin decreases ischemia-reperfusion injury in isolated canine gracilis model. Arch Surg 123:470, 1988.
64. Yellin AE, Weaver FA: Vascular system. *In* Donovan AJ (ed): Trauma Surgery. St. Louis, Mosby–Year Book, p 207, 1994.

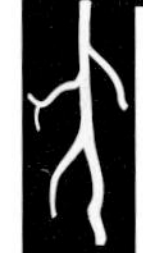

C H A P T E R 6 0

Thoracic and Abdominal Vascular Trauma

Fred Bongard, M.D.

THORACIC VASCULAR TRAUMA

The term *thoracic vascular trauma* typically refers to injuries of the aorta and arch vessels, the pulmonary arteries and veins, the superior and inferior venae cavae, the intercostal vessels, and the internal mammary vessels. These injuries, although life-threatening, constitute only a minority of vascular trauma cases treated at a metropolitan center. In a review of our experience, only 9% of all vascular injuries over a 10-year period were in the chest.[1]

INJURIES OF THE THORACIC AORTA

Interest in the diagnosis and treatment of thoracic aortic injuries stems from the fact that they can be rapidly lethal but often produce minimal, or no, signs and symptoms. Although penetrating mechanisms predominate, the number of patients with aortic disruption due to blunt trauma has continued to increase.[2] It has been estimated that between 7500 and 8000 cases of blunt aortic injury occur each year in the United States.[3, 4] Some 10% to 15% of persons who die from automobile accidents sustain an aortic rupture. Greendyke reported a 27% incidence of rupture for those who were ejected from a vehicle and only 12% for those who were not.[5] The majority of such ruptures occur in patients aged 20 to 30 years, with very few at the extremes of age. Males predominate 9:1. Since the first report of a successful repair in 1958, advances in diagnostic and surgical technique have improved the overall results of management, although morbidity and mortality still remain high.[6] Approximately 10% to 20% of those with acute thoracic aortic disruptions survive the initial trauma. Of these, nearly 30% die within 6 hours, 40% within 24 hours, 72% within the first week, and more than 90% within 10 weeks if no treatment is instituted.[7, 8]

Pathophysiology

The combinations of forces that contribute to traumatic rupture of the thoracic aorta and its branch vessels vary, depending on the location and direction of the force.[9, 10] Theories advanced to explain the predominance of disruption at the aortic isthmus (between the left subclavian artery and the ligamentum arteriosum) are based on the observation that, during a deceleration injury, the heart, the ascending aorta, and the transverse arch continue to move forward, while motion of the isthmus and the descending aorta is limited by their posterior attachments. There is additional evidence that the isthmus is inherently weaker than other parts of the thoracic aorta.[11] Lundevall, using isolated strips of aorta free of adventitia, reported that the isthmus was only two thirds as strong as the ascending aorta. The descending aorta was of intermediate strength.[12] Injuries most commonly become evident as transverse tears beginning at the intima and progressing outward. The adventitia typically remains intact because of its tough collagenous makeup.

Rapid increases in intraluminal pressure can also rupture the aorta.[13] The pressure required may be as low as 580 mmHg or as high as 2500 mmHg.[10, 13] The extent of aortic injury can range from subintimal hemorrhage to complete aortic disruption. In an autopsy study by Parmley, the lesions were classified as (1) intimal hemorrhage, (2) intimal hemorrhage with laceration, (3) medial laceration, (4) complete laceration of the aorta, (5) false aneurysm formation, and (6) periaortic hemorrhage.[14]

The following forces can be responsible for rupture at the isthmus:

1. Vertically directed deceleration after an impact that causes transient stretching of the aorta. Falls that displace the thoracoabdominal aorta caudad are a common example.
2. Compression that follows a frontal impact.
3. Horizontal deceleration, with or without chest compression (e.g., motor vehicle collision).
4. Crush injury.

The mechanical factors thought to contribute to injury at the isthmus include shearing, bending, and torsion stress. Shearing stress is created by different rates of deceleration of the mobile aortic arch and the immobile descending aorta. Shear stress leads to rupture opposite the site of fixation and accounts for the *anterior* location of proximal descending aortic ruptures at the isthmus. Bending stress is created when the heart is displaced caudad and produces flexion of the aortic arch around a fulcrum created by the hilar structures of the left lung. Anteroposterior compression with displacement of the heart to the left produces a pressure wave referred to as *torsion stress*. Torsion stress is also responsible for tears of the *ascending* aorta associated with the vertical deceleration that accompanies falls from heights. The rapid downward displacement of the heart results in acute lengthening of the aorta. The pressure wave thus created produces a water-hammer effect that exerts its greatest effect in the ascending aorta. Aortic valve injury may also occur.

Compression and tension forces sometimes combine to produce tears of the subclavian and innominate arteries. Reporting on the first successful repair of an innominate artery avulsion in 1962, Binet and colleagues theorized that a compressive force would shorten the distance between the sternum and the vertebral column.[15] The decrease in volume would push the heart and the ascending aorta backward and to the left. The curvature of the aortic arch would be accentuated, creating tension on its convex surface at the points of insertion of the brachiocephalic vessels. Binet and colleagues also noted that patients tend to rotate the head to one side to protect against facial injury and, in doing so, place the opposite carotid artery under tension in the longitudinal axis. The tearing force thus created may avulse the carotid artery from the aortic arch. When a first rib is fractured, injuries to the subclavian arteries may also result from being stretched over the rib margin.

An alternative theory advanced by Voigt and Wifert[16] implicates the cranially directed impact of the sternum after contact with a dashboard. When the sternum is fractured, the lower portion is displaced upward and backward. The mediastinum and ascending aorta are forced ("shoveled") superiorly by the sternal fragment. The cranial displacement puts tensile stretch on the proximal descending aorta, which ruptures near its fixed point at the ligamentum arteriosum.[16] Crass and coworkers advanced the theory that aortic isthmus lacerations result from a "pinch" of the aorta between the spine and the anterior bony thorax (manubrium, clavicle, and first ribs) during chest compression caused by abrupt deceleration.[17] The force required to lacerate the aorta in this way is approximately 20,000 newtons (N), far beyond that which can be produced in a motor vehicle accident.[18, 19]

Other thoracic vascular injuries from blunt trauma include *distal* descending aortic tears and disruption of intercostal vessels. The lower descending aorta is most likely ruptured by fracture-dislocations of the lower thoracic spine, whereas intercostal vessel injuries are often associated with rib fractures.

Penetrating injuries include complete and partial transections and arteriovenous fistulae. Because the vessels involved are large, the mechanism of muscular retraction usually fails to control hemorrhage, and rapid blood loss can result.

THE TRAUMA EPIDEMIC

Total Impact Velocity and Injury Risk

IMPACT VELOCITY (miles/hr.)	INJURY RISK (%)		EQUIVALENT FREE FALL	
	morbidity	mortality	MPH	Feet
1–10	2.5	.1	10 →	5
11–20	6	1.0	20 →	13
21–30	25	3.0	30 →	28
≥40	70	40.0	40 →	54
			50 →	84
			60 →	121

FIGURE 60–1. Comparison of automobile deceleration injuries and equivalent free falls.

Diagnostic Findings

A high index of suspicion is the most important factor in initiating a search for thoracic aortic disruption in trauma victims. Because the forces exerted on the aorta are directly related to the energy absorbed, falls from more than three stories or motor vehicle accidents at speeds in excess of 40 mph should arouse suspicion of thoracic vascular injury, even in the absence of physical findings (Fig. 60–1). Circumstances surrounding the incident, such as the death of another automobile occupant or use of harness seat belts (associated with innominate and subclavian injuries) are also suggestive.[20] Abrasions or hematomas across the chest indicate force transmission and should arouse suspicion of thoracic aortic or great vessel injury. Shoulder harnesses leave characteristic marks across the base of the neck and chest (Fig. 60–2). Symptoms on admission are often related to associated injuries. Wilson noted that retrosternal or interscapular pain may result from "stretching" or dissection of the aortic adventitia.[9] A detailed review of the English language literature by Duhaylongsod and colleagues summarized 1188 patients in whom the most frequent presenting symptoms were chest pain (76%) and dyspnea (56%).[21] Loss of consciousness or coma (36.8%) and hypotension (25.9%) were other common presentations.

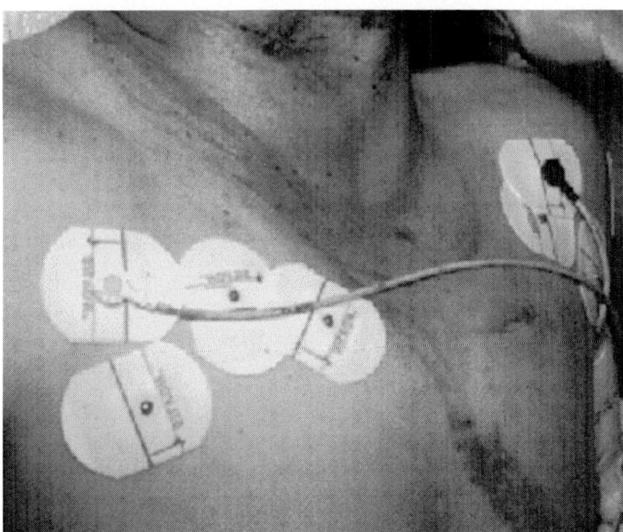

FIGURE 60–2. Classic appearance of a "seat belt" sign. Notice the width and direction of the hematoma. This patient was a passenger, not the driver.

Only a third of those with blunt aortic trauma show physical evidence of thoracic injury on presentation.[10] No single physical finding or combination of findings is diagnostic of acute thoracic aortic rupture. The "acute coarctation syndrome," first reported by Symbas and associates, is characterized by hypertension in the arms and a difference in pulse amplitude between upper and lower extremities.[22] The syndrome may be caused either by intimal dissection and flap or by compression of the aortic lumen by hematoma. Another cause of the hypertension may be stretching or stimulation of receptors in or near the aortic isthmus.[23] A systolic murmur over the precordium or posterior interscapular area that sometimes accompanies the coarctation syndrome is due to the turbulence created as blood flows past the intimal flap. In our experience, the acute coarctation syndrome is uncommon.

Physical findings are summarized in Table 60–1. The frequency of these findings varies considerably among reported series. Clark and coworkers found that a hemothorax of more than 500 ml, pseudocoarctation, or neck hematoma was present in patients at "high risk."[24] Duhaylongsod and colleagues[21] reported that physical findings usually considered "highly suggestive," such as midscapular back pain, differences in pulse amplitude, and generalized hypertension, were not commonly observed; however, preoperative paresis or paraplegia or indeterminate findings on physical examination were present in one third of patients.

Injuries of the ascending aorta are also difficult to diagnose on physical examination. Depending on the distal extent of the disruption, hematomas at the base of the neck or carotid bruits may be present. When a cardiac murmur is noted, a coincident aortic valve injury or fistula at the sinus of Valsalva should be suspected.[18] The two arms may exhibit a blood pressure discrepancy when a distal ascending or aortic arch injury is associated with an innominate artery injury.

Associated injuries are common, and they frequently distract from diagnosis of the underlying thoracic aortic injury. The most commonly reported associated injuries are fractures (both local and remote), pulmonary contusion, closed head injury, intra-abdominal solid organ injury (spleen, kidney, liver), and maxillofacial injuries.[21]

TABLE 60–1. CLINICAL FINDINGS ASSOCIATED WITH TRAUMATIC RUPTURE OF THE THORACIC AORTA

History of high-speed deceleration injury
Multiple rib fractures or flail chest
Fractured first or second rib
Fractured sternum
Pulse deficits
Upper extremity hypertension
Interscapular systolic murmur
Blood in the carotid or subclavian sheaths
Hoarseness or voice change without laryngeal injury
Superior vena cava syndrome

Modified from Wilson RF: Thoracic vascular trauma. *In* Bongard F, Wilson SE, Perry MO (eds): Vascular Injuries in Surgical Practice. Norwalk, Conn, Appleton & Lange, 1991, p 107.

TABLE 60–2. RADIOGRAPHIC FINDINGS ASSOCIATED WITH TRAUMATIC RUPTURE OF THE THORACIC AORTA

Deviation of esophagus to the right at T4 (>1.0 to 2.0 cm)
Superior mediastinal widening
Obscuration of the aortic knob
Obliteration of the outline of descending aorta
Tracheal deviation to the right
Apical cap
Depression of left mainstem bronchus (>40 degrees)
Obliteration of the aortopulmonary window
Obliteration of medial aspect of the left upper lobe
Widened paravertebral stripe
Thickened or deviated paratracheal stripe
Fracture of first or second rib
Fractured sternum

Modified from Wilson RF: Thoracic vascular trauma. *In* Bongard F, Wilson SE, Perry MO (eds): Vascular Injuries in Surgical Practice. Norwalk, Conn, Appleton & Lange, 1991, p 107.

Radiographic imaging remains pivotal in the diagnostic algorithm. The commonly cited findings on plain chest films that suggest rupture of the aorta or brachiocephalic vessels after blunt trauma are summarized in Table 60–2.[25] Recent reports have evaluated the importance of *individual* findings that suggest the diagnosis.[26–28] Of greatest utility are signs with sufficient sensitivity to include all true-positive aortic injuries but adequate specificity to minimize the number of unnecessary angiograms (Fig. 60–3). Supine chest films may falsely enlarge the mediastinal structures because of magnification associated with short focal film distances. Ayella and others suggested "erect" chest radiography to correct for this artifact.[29–31] Mirvis and coworkers found that, although the supine chest radiograph was more sensitive than the erect view for detecting signs of mediastinal hemorrhage, it was the less specific view for demonstrating aortic rupture.[30] However, a subsequent study found that an erect view was normal in 6% of patients who had proven blunt aortic or brachiocephalic arterial ruptures.[32] Therefore, the reduced sensitivity of the erect chest radiograph for signs of mediastinal hemorrhage reduces the number of negative aortograms but does so at the expense of an increased number of missed aortic and brachiocephalic arterial injuries.

In an effort to quantitate mediastinal enlargement, Marsh and Sturm reported that a superior mediastinal transverse width (just above the aortic arch) greater than 8 cm on supine chest films was abnormal.[33] A subsequent report by the same group, however, found that this measurement may exceed 8 cm in as many as 81% of healthy patients.[34] Seltzer and coworkers described the mediastinal width–chest width ratio (M/C), which is calculated by dividing the width of the mediastinum at the aortic arch (M) by the internal diameter of the chest at the same level (C).[31] The initial critical value of 0.25 was later found to produce too many false-positive results, whereas a higher ratio had the potential to overlook true ruptures.[31] Failure of objective measures to predict reliably which patients require aortography has led this author, and others, to rely on the observer's experience and knowledge of mediastinal anatomy to determine the need for aortography.[35] Interobserver variability for mediastinal widening is low, and agreement can usually be reached.[36] It must be noted, however, that the width of the mediastinum in the supine position progressively increases with age, probably owing to atherosclerosis. Thus, mediastinal widening may be a less reliable finding in persons older than 65 years.

Adjunctive findings on chest radiography, such as hemothorax, first rib fracture (unilateral or bilateral), pneumothorax, apical cap, depression of the left mainstem bronchus to more than 40 degrees from the horizontal, deviation of the nasogastric tube to the right, and widening of the right paratracheal stripe, have also been evaluated for their utility in predicting the need for aortography.[30] Extension of a mediastinal hematoma typically displaces

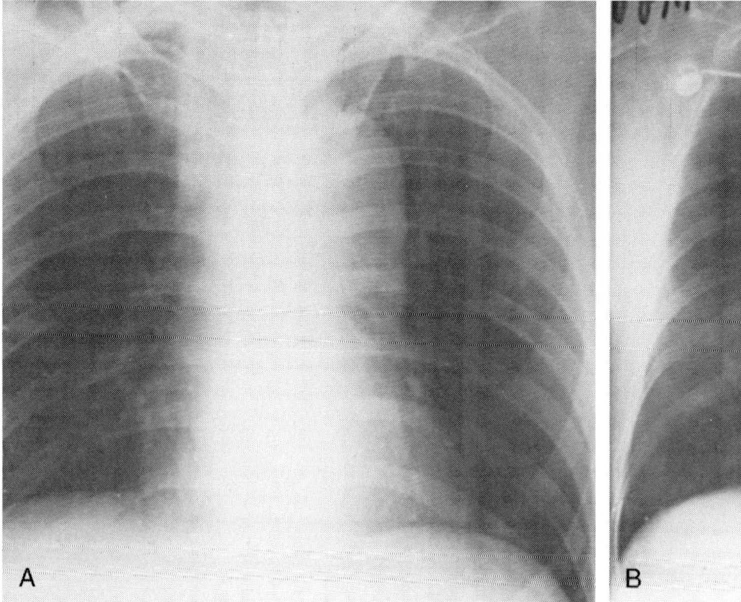

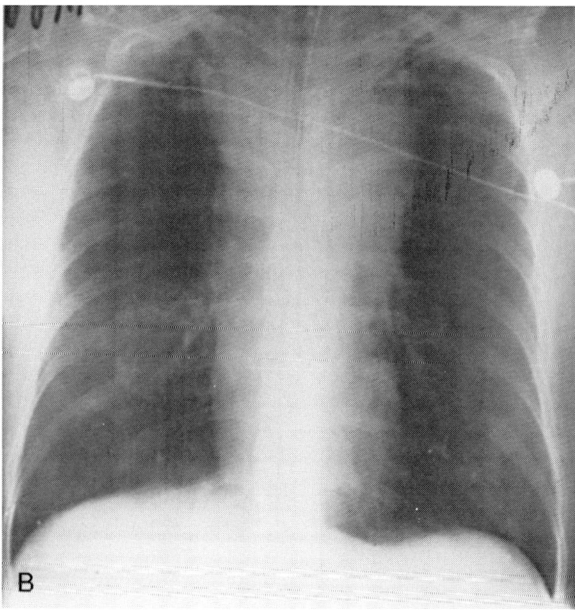

FIGURE 60–3. *A*, Classic appearance of a widened mediastinum on supine chest radiographs. *B*, This abnormal chest film was the result of a malpositioned resuscitation line that infused fluid into a patient's mediastinum. Aortography was normal.

the esophagus to the right. In two series reported by Ayella and Gerlock and associates,[37, 38] no patient with esophageal deviation of less than 1.0 cm from the midline had aortic injury, whereas deviation of more than 2 cm to the right was highly suggestive. When an innominate injury is present, the superior mediastinal hematoma tends to have a pointed shape and often displaces the nasogastric tube to the left. It must be remembered, however, that none of these findings, alone or in combination, is absolutely reliable for the diagnosis of aortic or arch vessel injury. Thoracic skeletal injuries frequently accompany thoracic aortic dissection, and their presence on chest radiography has been used as an indication for arteriography. A recent study by Lee and colleagues found that rib fractures were the only thoracic skeletal injury whose incidence was higher in patients with thoracic aortic disruption.[39] Subjective evaluation of the mediastinum by an experienced observer remains the most valuable tool.

The choice of diagnostic modalities is among the most controversial issues in the management of thoracic aortic injuries. Much debate has attended the question of whether newer modalities can replace the gold standard of contrast aortography. Most authors agree that standard contrast-enhanced dynamic computed tomography (CT) is suboptimal for thoracic aortic injury (Fig. 60–4). A recent multicenter prospective trial by the American Association for the Surgery of Trauma involved 270 patients, 88 of whom underwent CT.[40] In that group, 74% of CT studies were read as positive, 23% were equivocal, and 3% were negative. Thus, the overall diagnostic rate was only 75%. The strength of this study lies in the fact that the diagnosis of blunt aortic injury was made conclusively at autopsy or thoracotomy or by a definitive diagnostic technique. The study used anatomic standards to compare the diagnostic methods. A meta-analysis by Mirvis and associates reviewed 18 series (each having 10 or more patients) that used CT to evaluate the mediastinum after blunt trauma in adults.[41] The authors found the overall sensitivity of CT to be 99.3%, specificity 87.1%, positive predictive value 90.1%, and negative predictive value 99.9%. They concluded that a CT finding of mediastinal hemorrhage alone is sensitive for traumatic aortic injury, but the finding of actual aortic injury is even more diagnostic. False-positive impressions may be caused by thymic tissue, periaortic atelectasis, volume averaging, and pleural effusions.[41]

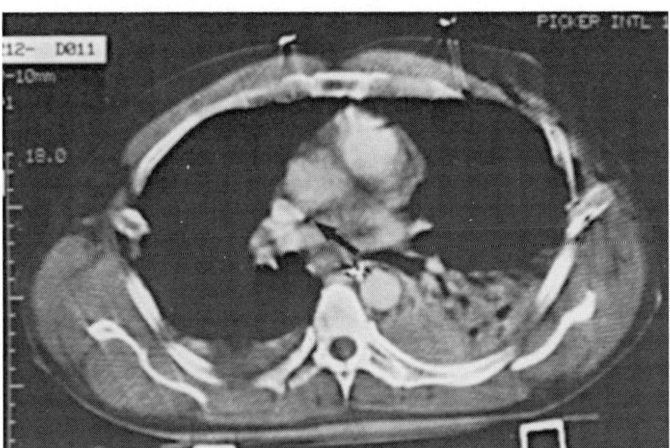

FIGURE 60–4. CT study of a patient after a motor vehicle accident. *Arrow* indicates the widened mediastinum and evidence of hematoma around the proximal aorta.

A recent addition to the CT armamentarium is helical scanning. This is better suited than single-section CT for revealing vascular lesions, because its faster and continuous scanning allows image acquisition to be done consistently during the phase of peak vascular enhancement.[42] One of the obvious shortcomings is that the method requires the appropriate equipment and a skilled operator. Initial reports have been favorable and suggest that helical scanning significantly improves the overall sensitivity of CT. Most surgeons are still reluctant to undertake operative repair solely on the basis of CT findings. Some use CT as a "screening tool" for indications for angiography, proceeding with the latter when CT is positive. Nunez and colleagues correctly state, "Although the CT findings are often diagnostic, the sensitivity and specificity of CT for diagnosing arterial trauma have not yet been established."[42]

Like CT, transesophageal echo (TEE) has continued to evolve as a modality for the detection of thoracic aortic rupture. In a series of 93 patients who underwent TEE, Smith and associates found a sensitivity of 100% and a specificity of 98%. The patients also underwent aortography for confirmation. All injuries detected were in the "classic" area of the descending aorta, near the isthmus.[43] Like helical CT, TEE requires specialized equipment and experienced operators. A significant shortcoming of TEE is that it has a critical "blind spot" between the aorta and the esophagus that is caused by intervening air in the trachea. This obscures the proximal aortic arch. TEE also cannot provide information about the aortic branches or about the distal thoracic aorta.[44] Since up to 20% of thoracic aortic ruptures occur in "nonclassic" areas, vascular injuries may be assessed suboptimally or overlooked when TEE is used as the sole imaging modality.[44] TEE findings can be divided into "direct signs" and "indirect signs."[45] The direct signs include thick stripes within the aortic lumen, false aneurysms, aortic dissection, free-edged intimal flaps, fusiform aneurysms, and complete aortic disruption. Indirect signs include minor increases in aortic diameter, impairment of the aortic Doppler color flow pattern, and increased aorta-probe distance (indicative of hemomediastinum) (Fig. 60–5).

This author's policy for obtaining thoracic aortograms continues to depend on the mechanism of injury and the results of plain chest radiography. With stable patients who are victims of high-speed vehicular accidents or falls from more than three stories, aortograms are usually obtained. Whenever the mediastinum is widened or the severity of associated injuries warrants it, aortography is performed, provided that the patient's condition remains stable.

The author approaches thoracic aortography via the femoral artery, with retrograde introduction of the guide wire and catheter into the ascending arch. When lower extremity pulses are unequal or when pelvic injuries preclude the use of a femoral artery, an axillary or brachial artery may be cannulated. When blunt injury to the innominate artery is suspected owing to the location of the hematoma on plain films, the right axillary artery should not be used.[46] A small amount of oblique angling (15 to 20 degrees left anterior oblique view) aids in evaluating the ascending aorta by

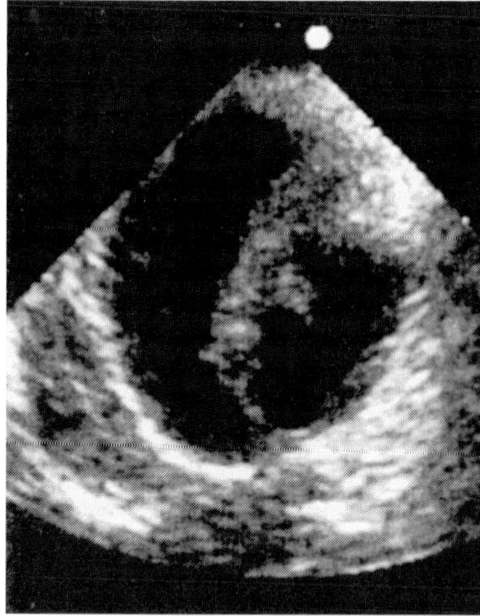
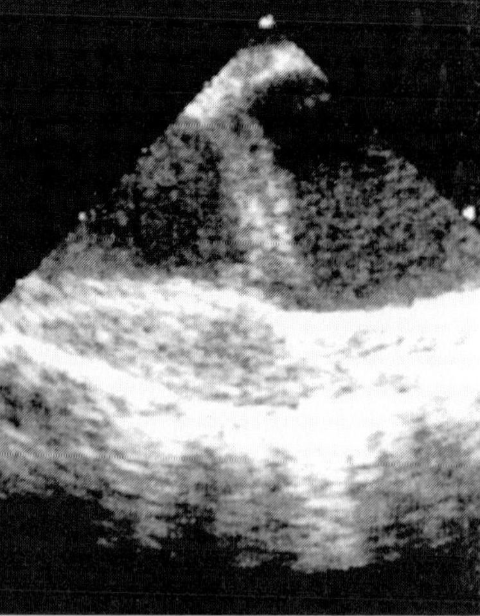

FIGURE 60–5. Two views of a flap seen on transesophageal echocardiography as part of an aortic injury.

rotating it away from the thoracic spine (Fig. 60–6). The most common positive finding is a contained disruption on the anterior surface of the aorta just opposite the ligamentum arteriosum. We have occasionally seen intimal defects and extravasation. When injury to the innominate or subclavian artery has occurred, an oval widening is observed at the orifice of the vessels (Fig. 60–7).[47] In the rare patient with multiple lesions, the need for cardiopulmonary bypass can be appreciated and the appropriate personnel notified. The most common false-positive finding is attributable to the presence of a ductus diverticulum just distal to the origin of the left subclavian artery.[48]

Preoperative Management

Initial management of blunt or penetrating injuries of the thoracic vasculature depends on rapid resuscitation. A secure airway is the first priority. When deceleration is the mechanism, associated cervical spine injuries may be present and hyperextension of the neck must be avoided. In these circumstances, intubation with a fiberoptic bronchoscope or cricothyroidotomy is preferable. After the airway has been secured, adequate gas exchange usually necessitates mechanical ventilation. Patients who have sustained penetrating injuries or blunt trauma with rib fractures are at high risk for development of tension pneumothoraces when positive-pressure ventilation is applied. Bilateral tube thoracostomies may be required, and particular care should be exercised during their placement to avoid disturbing a tamponading periaortic hematoma. The importance of secure and reliable venous access for intravenous fluids and transfusion cannot be overstated. With penetrating injuries of the thoracic inlet, ipsilateral upper extremity access sites are undesirable. In these situations, lower extremity venous

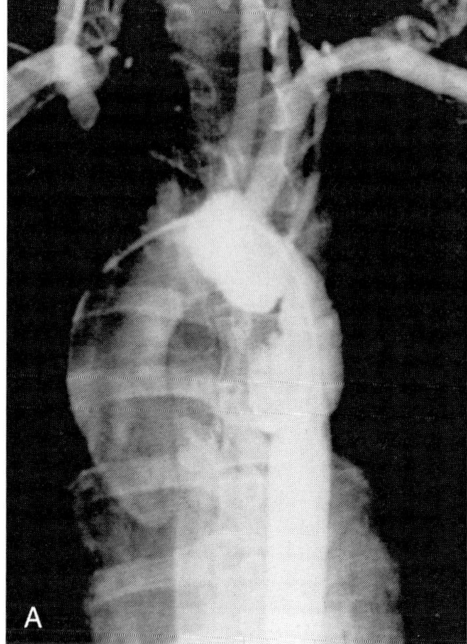

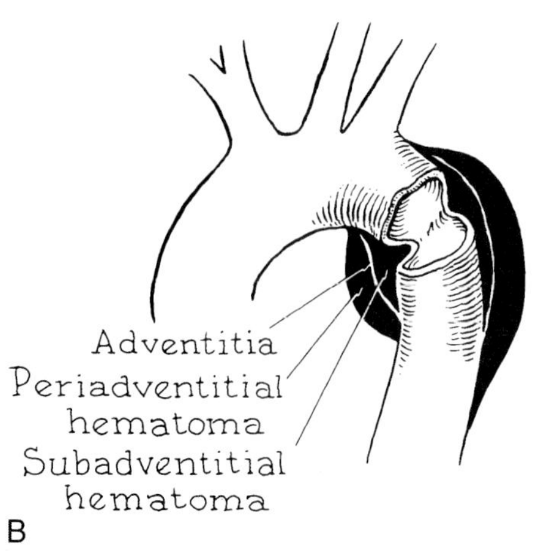

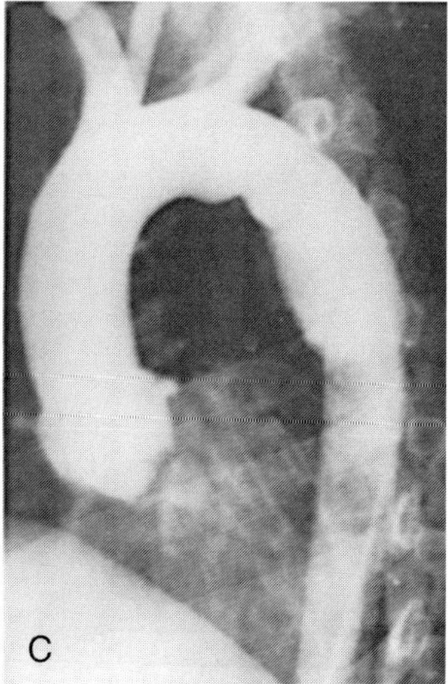

FIGURE 60–6. *A*, Anteroposterior aortogram shows disruption of the aorta at the isthmus with proximal extension. *B*, Schematic representation of injury in *A*. *C*, A similar aortogram shot from an oblique angle "opens" the aortic arch and provides a better view of the injury and great vessels. (*B*, From Wilson RF: Thoracic vascular trauma. *In* Bongard FS, Wilson SE, Perry MO [eds]: Vascular Injuries in Surgical Practice. Norwalk, Conn, Appleton & Lange, 1991, p 119.)

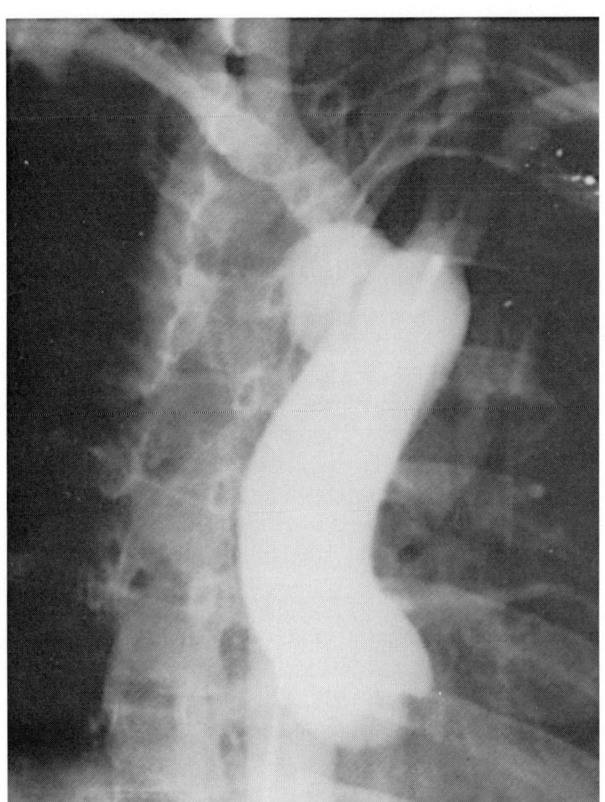

FIGURE 60–7. A gunshot wound to the chest caused a pseudoaneurysm of the innominate artery at its origin from the aorta. Note the oval appearance of the injury.

catheterization is preferred. In patients with associated abdominal trauma, iliac vein or vena cava lacerations may be present, and upper extremity sites should be used. In any case, catheters of sufficient caliber to infuse fluids rapidly are an absolute requirement.

Air emboli can form during resuscitation. Although most common after penetrating injuries, they can also be problematic after blunt trauma associated with rib fractures. Venous air emboli require 100 to 200 ml of air before airlock of the right ventricle occurs.[49] In such cases, the patient should be placed in the left decubitus position with the legs elevated. This displaces air into the apex of the heart and opens the outflow tract. Paradoxical air emboli can form when a patent foramen ovale is present. In contrast to venous air emboli, systemic emboli require less than 1 ml of air to produce devastating effects. Until it is proved otherwise, any dysrhythmia or sudden drop in blood pressure that occurs soon after the application of positive-pressure ventilation should be attributed to systemic air emboli. In this event, the head should be lowered and thoracotomy performed to clamp the lung proximal to the injured area.[9]

Hypotension after penetrating thoracic injury may require *emergency department thoracotomy* to facilitate resuscitation. On the other hand, after blunt injury, resuscitative thoracotomy is seldom successful. Because the thoracic great vessels are located in the superior mediastinum, thoracic inlet, and supraclavicular areas, the approach should be higher than that used for penetrating cardiac injuries. The author prefers to gain access through a third- or fourth-interspace anterolateral thoracotomy. When a penetrating wound is present on the right side, a left-side thoracotomy is still necessary to provide adequate exposure to clamp the descending thoracic aorta.

Once adequate exposure has been achieved, the first priority is localization and identification of the bleeding site. Intercostal vessels are frequently lacerated by rib fractures after blunt injury. The internal mammary artery may be disrupted by a stab wound or during a hastily performed thoracotomy. Pulmonary hilar vessels are also potential bleeding sites.

Wide exposure is the key to success. Frequently, a unilateral thoracotomy must be extended across the sternum to provide bilateral access. A longitudinal incision of the pericardium parallel to the course of the phrenic nerve permits open cardiac massage. Further dissection across the pericardium to the opposite phrenic nerve permits exposure of the intrapericardial portion of the great vessels. When injury of the ascending aorta is present, control can usually be accomplished by placing a partially occluding Satinsky or Wylie-J clamp to isolate the defect. Bleeding from the pulmonary hilum can be secured by applying an aortic vascular clamp across all hilar structures.

Operative Strategy

Operative repair of thoracic injuries requires a preplanned and coordinated approach to optimize outcome. Upon the patient's arrival in the operating room, the following equipment should be available: rib spreaders, saws, aortic cross-clamps, shunts or cardiopulmonary bypass pump tubing (as preferred), and woven grafts of various sizes. The author stores this equipment on the trauma resuscitation "crash cart" kept outside the main trauma surgery suite.

After injury, extrication, transport, and emergency room resuscitation, patients with aortic injuries are frequently profoundly hypothermic. Because of its undesirable effects on myocardial function and the clotting cascade, hypothermia must be aggressively corrected when present. Useful measures in the operating suite include (1) placing a warming pad under the patient, (2) providing a silver-colored thermal blanket (Thermadrape) over the patient to retain body heat, (3) warming all blood products and fluids to be used, and (4) using a heated gas mixture from the anesthesia ventilator.

Patients are positioned on the operating table to facilitate whatever repair is anticipated. In general, exposure and skin preparation should include the anterior neck, thorax, abdomen, and a lower extremity. When a subclavian injury is suspected, the ipsilateral arm should be prepared and draped in a fashion that maintains free mobility of the shoulder, to aid in operative dissection and exposure. The posterolateral thoracotomy provides excellent exposure to virtually all portions of the hemithorax. The contralateral decubitus position brings the affected side into view. The incision extends from behind the medial border of the scapula, below its tip, and then forward to the anterior axillary line. The chest can be entered through the fourth to the seventh intercostal space. Particular care must be exercised when positioning hypotensive patients for this incision, because the decubitus position interferes with venous return and can aggravate the condition. Blood and bronchial contents also may flow to the uninjured dependent lung, causing profound respiratory embarrassment. A split-lumen endotracheal tube allows selective collapse of one lung to facilitate exposure.

When severe shock or hemoptysis precludes using the decubitus position, an anterior thoracotomy may be used instead. This is also the incision of choice for rapid access to the mediastinum for open cardiac massage. The incision should start 2 cm lateral to the sternum to avoid injury to the internal mammary artery. It then follows a gentle curve laterally to the axilla. Overzealous use of rib spreaders usually results in posterior rib fractures, which carry the risk of intercostal vessel disruption. When additional exposure is needed, an anterior thoracotomy may be extended across the sternum in the midline, as a "clamshell" incision. Large shears should be used to transect the sternum, to avoid splintering. Both internal mammary arteries and veins are divided during this rapid approach and must be ligated.

A median sternotomy is preferred for injuries of the ascending aorta and of the innominate and proximal carotid arteries. Extension into the neck along the anterior border of the right sternocleidomastoid muscle affords access to the proximal right subclavian artery and the origin of the right common carotid artery, in addition to the right vertebral artery. Although the author does not prefer leftward extension for exposure of the proximal left subclavian artery, some have noted that, if the shoulders are thrown back by placing a roll vertically between the scapulae, the origin of the left subclavian artery is accessible through this anterior approach.[50]

Controversy continues over what technique is optimal for aortic control and repair, because of concern about spinal cord ischemia and the potential for lower extremity paralysis.[51] Safe time and pressure limits are ill-defined. Several methods for indirect assessment of perfusion are available, and they have received mixed reviews. Intraoperative evaluation of evoked somatosensory potential, monitoring of lumbar spinal fluid pressure, and measurement of distal aortic pressure have all been employed.[52, 53] Because such modalities are awkward in emergency situations, experience in trauma cases is not extensive. The author prefers to perform the operation as expeditiously as possible without these techniques.

Methods of control and repair include partial and complete bypass via an external pump with systemic anticoagulation, external heparin-bonded shunts from the ascending aorta to the descending aorta or femoral artery, and simple clamp and repair. The need for systemic heparin anticoagulation in a patient with multisystem trauma makes widespread hemorrhage a possibility. For this reason, partial or complete cardiopulmonary bypass has largely fallen into disfavor. Patients with thoracic aortic injuries at multiple levels who require extensive repairs are notable exceptions. The torroidal centrifugal pump, which is connected between the left atrium and a femoral artery, can be used with little or no heparin because an oxygenator is not required. It offers the following advantages over complete cardiopulmonary bypass: (1) It does not require systemic anticoagulation. (2) It automatically "deprimes" itself if air enters, effectively reducing the risk of systemic air embolization. (3) It is flow dependent and decreases flow if inflow is obstructed. (4) It is resistance dependent and stops pumping if pressure in the outflow is excessively high.[54–57]

Clamp and repair, without any bypass and by simple suture, prosthetic graft, or sutureless graft, is the most direct method. Its advantages are that it does not require additional equipment, dissection in another area, systemic anticoagulation, or vessel cannulation. Many centers prefer this technique to the more complex bypass or shunt methods.[7, 58–60] There is general agreement that operating times of 30 minutes or less mitigate the risk of paralysis.

The customary operative technique for clamp and repair begins with positioning the patient in the right decubitus position and then creating a left posterolateral thoracotomy in the fourth intercostal space. After retraction of the lung, the area of injury is identified. Vascular tapes are placed sequentially around (1) the aortic arch, between the left common carotid and subclavian arteries, (2) the left subclavian artery just beyond its origin, and (3) the descending aorta just below the injury (Fig. 60–8). Dissection proceeds from distal to proximal, so that the inferior aortic clamp can be moved as close as possible to the site of injury.

Once vascular isolation has been achieved, options for repair include simple repair, graft insertion, and sutureless graft. When a partial laceration is present or the disruption is small, some prefer mobilization, resection of the injured segment, and simple suture repair. Caution is required to ensure adequate mobilization, because tension on the anastomosis increases further after inflow is restored. It is generally believed that only 20% of aortic tears can be repaired by simple suturing.[61] Its advantages include the speed with which it can be performed, the absence of a prosthetic graft, and the decreased risk of prosthetic graft infection.[62]

Prosthetic graft insertion is the customary method of repair, and is obligatory when more than 2 cm of vessel is injured. Although knitted grafts are more flexible and more

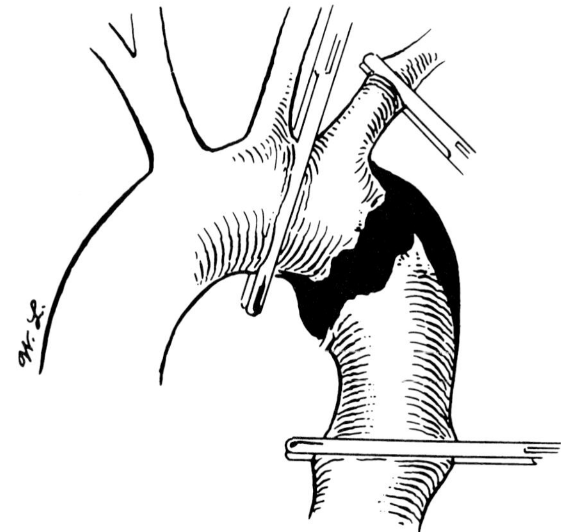

FIGURE 60–8. Control of injuries at the aortic isthmus can be achieved by placing clamps between the left common carotid artery and the left subclavian artery, beyond the origin of the left subclavian and distal to the injury. (From Wilson RF: Thoracic vascular trauma. *In* Bongard FS, Wilson SE, Perry MO [eds]: Vascular Injuries in Surgical Practice. Norwalk, Conn, Appleton & Lange, 1991, p 122.)

easily handled, woven grafts are preferable, because they can be inserted without preclotting. Collagen- or gelatin-impregnated grafts represent a compromise. When the segment of damaged aorta is relatively short, a sleeve patch may be used to bridge the gap. Antunes described the use of a polytetrafluoroethylene (PTFE) graft (18 to 20 mm diameter) that is opened into a sleeve patch.[59] Although two suture lines are still required, the open graft rather than a tubular graft facilitates suturing.

Sutureless grafts are made of woven Dacron and have support rings at each end. The graft is placed through a longitudinal aortotomy with the rings on each side of the defect. The graft is fixed in place with sutures or external rings. Although, theoretically, this graft can reduce cross-clamping time, familiarity with its handling and placement is a prerequisite.

Clamp and repair times depend on a number of variables, including location, associated injuries, and particularly the skill and experience of the surgeon. The decreased distal blood flow during clamp application and the need to control proximal blood pressure with antihypertensives such as sodium nitroprusside compromise spinal cord perfusion. For this reason, many surgeons have opted for extracorporeal shunting with a heparin-bonded shunt. Because of its special surface, clotting is inhibited and the need for systemic anticoagulation is eliminated. After the shunt is filled with heparinized saline, the distal end is clamped. The proximal end is inserted through a pursestring suture into either the ascending aorta or the aortic arch. The distal end can be inserted into the descending thoracic aorta or the femoral artery. Although femoral insertion is preferable to avoid clutter in the field, studies have shown that flow volume is as much as 50% less than that with thoracic aortic insertion.[63] Flow also depends on the size of the shunt; a 7.5-mm cannula can provide 1500 to 2000 ml per minute, whereas a 9.0-mm cannula can provide 3000 to 4000 ml per minute. The presence of a functioning shunt does not, however, provide absolute protection against paraplegia. In a study by Duhaylongsod and colleagues, three of 41 patients (7%) developed paraplegia even after shunting.[21] This result may be related in part to the distal aortic pressure: Cunningham and coworkers observed that a pressure of 60 mmHg or greater beyond the shunt is required to prevent paralysis.[64] Shunt use may be complicated by vessel laceration at the time of placement, by bleeding, or by pseudoaneurysm formation at the insertion site.

In most cases, immediate repair of thoracic aortic injuries is indicated, although delayed repair has been used in selected cases. Soots and coworkers reported on four patients whose repair was delayed (5 to 43 days) because of severe associated injuries.[65] They asserted that major brain injury and pulmonary contusions are indications for delay in hemodynamically stable patients.

In general, unless the patient has multiple and severe associated injuries that are likely to be rapidly fatal, immediate repair is warranted. Studies of minimal vascular injuries in this site are too sparse to support advocating a "wait-and-see" policy.

Several authors have reported on the use of endovascular stents for thoracic aortic injury, although only a few have been placed for classic deceleration-type disruptions. Most patients have had such stents placed for chronic, rather than acute, dissection or for injuries not caused by trauma.[66, 67] The long-term results with these grafts have yet to be determined, as does the rate of complications such as graft migration and endovascular infection. Limitations at this time include the unavailability of grafts longer than 40 cm, the unknown durability of the stent-graft material and the fixation system, and the caliber of the delivery system, which may be excessively large in younger patients.[68] Another potential consideration is that stent-graft placement eliminates the opportunity to reimplant intercostal arteries and may expose the patient to increased risk of paraplegia. Because most thoracic aortic dissections due to blunt trauma occur at the isthmus (which does not include spinal branches), this consideration may be more hypothetical than real.[69]

INJURIES OF THE INTRATHORACIC GREAT VESSELS

Blunt trauma is the cause of the majority of injuries to the great vessels of the chest, the innominate artery being affected most often. A survey of 36 cases of blunt injury to the aortic arch branch vessels identified 22 cases of innominate trauma (61%), seven of the right subclavian artery, and seven of the left subclavian. Eleven patients had associated injuries of the aortic arch proper.[70] Penetrating injuries of the innominate or subclavian arteries typically result from gunshot wounds or inferiorly directed stab wounds.

Like aortic injuries, branch vessel trauma may be associated with stable vital signs or with profound shock. The initial diagnostic impression may be aortic arch injury. The most common findings among victims of blunt trauma are decreased ipsilateral extremity pulses, physical evidence of chest wall trauma, and hypotension.[71] Associated injuries are common, including cranial, tracheal or bronchial, facial, brachial plexus injuries, and abdominal trauma. Penetrating injuries may present with an arteriovenous fistula and palpable distal pulses. Profound shock may be present owing to bleeding into the hemithorax. Occasionally, patients with penetrating thoracic trauma present with a supraclavicular hematoma that expands into the neck. When penetration has extended caudad to the mediastinum, pericardial tamponade may occur.[72]

Subclavian artery injuries are largely due to penetrating mechanisms, although improperly worn shoulder harnesses occasionally cause blunt trauma. The most important sign of a subclavian artery occlusion is absence of the ipsilateral radial pulse. Occasionally, a subclavian steal syndrome may develop when the injury causes stenosis proximal to the origin of the vertebral artery. Associated brachial plexus injuries are common.

Plain chest films typically reveal widening of the superior aspect of the mediastinal silhouette (Fig. 60–9). The mediastinal widening observed with an innominate artery injury is usually in a more superior position than that associated

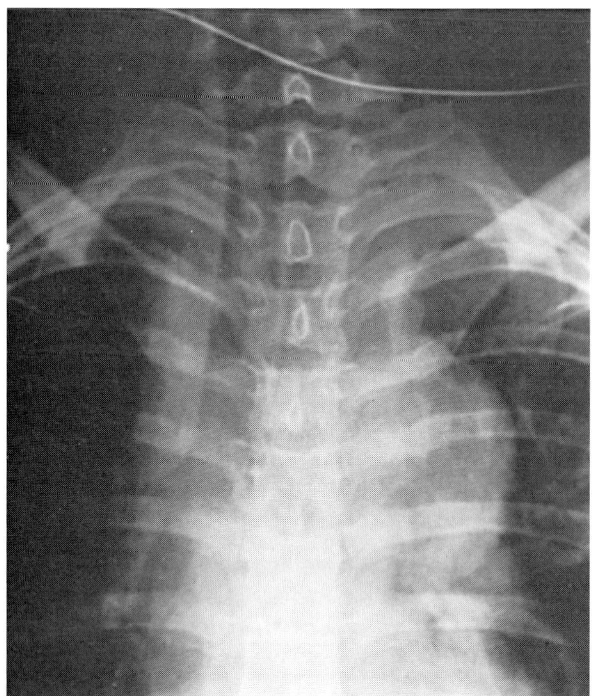

FIGURE 60–9. The mediastinal widening associated with this left subclavian arterial injury is somewhat higher and displaced more laterally than that associated with an injury at the aortic isthmus.

with an aortic injury. With penetrating injuries, a large hemothorax may also be present. When the film is taken with the patient lying supine, only diffuse haziness may be apparent over the involved hemithorax.[9] Arteriography remains the definitive modality for demonstrating branch vessel injuries (Figs. 60–10 to 60–13). A femoral or contralateral axillary approach is preferred. Penetrating injury to the subclavian vessels may be diagnosed by retrograde ipsilateral axillary or brachial arteriography performed in the emergency department.[47] A blood pressure cuff is placed distal to the injury and inflated to 300 mmHg. The action of the blood pressure cuff forces contrast material, injected into either the axillary or brachial artery, backward toward the aortic arch, to demonstrate the injury.

Preoperative Management

Before diagnostic angiography or transport to the operating room, patients must be resuscitated and stabilized using the strategies outlined earlier for injuries of the thoracic aorta. Because of the possibility of concomitant venous trauma, lower extremity venous access sites are preferred.

A penetrating wound of the subclavian artery or vein can result in rapid intrapleural hemorrhage unless it is controlled. When moribund patients have a right-sided injury, emergency high right anterolateral thoracotomy may be performed to allow packing and manual compression of the bleeding site from within the chest.[73] Manual pressure may also be applied to the right supraclavicular fossa to enhance control. When the injury is to the left subclavian artery, an anterolateral thoracotomy is required to gain control of the vessel's proximal intrapleural position. If satisfactory hemostasis is not achieved, digital pressure in the supraclavicular fossa may help.

Operative Strategy for Specific Great Vessel Injuries

Injuries of the Innominate Artery

Access to the innominate artery is best obtained through a median sternotomy. If the proximal right subclavian artery is involved, the incision can be extended into the right side of the neck, as needed. In the absence of profound intraoperative hypotension or an extensive injury that requires simultaneous occlusion of both the innominate and the left common carotid artery, cardiopulmonary bypass or common carotid artery shunting is not necessary. When the repair is likely to be lengthy or when blood pressure is a concern, some have used "stump pressures" to ensure adequate cerebral perfusion.[71] When a carotid shunt is used, it should be placed so that it extends from the proximal ascending aorta to the distal common carotid artery. When injuries involve the aortic arch as well, partial occluding clamps are used to gain control. We have found that cardiopulmonary bypass is seldom required. Vosloo and Reichart reported that inflow occlusion is an alternative to cardiopulmonary bypass.[74] In a patient with partial transection of the innominate artery, they placed clamps on the superior and inferior venae cavae for $1\frac{1}{2}$ minutes, during which time the repair was accomplished.

Blunt injuries typically involve the origin of the innominate artery. Proximal control is obtained with a curved

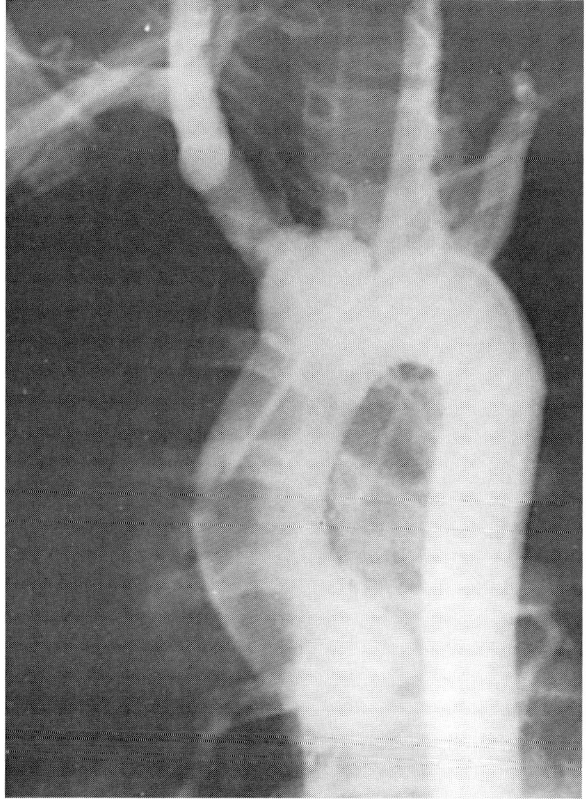

FIGURE 60–10. Blunt injury at the origin of the innominate artery.

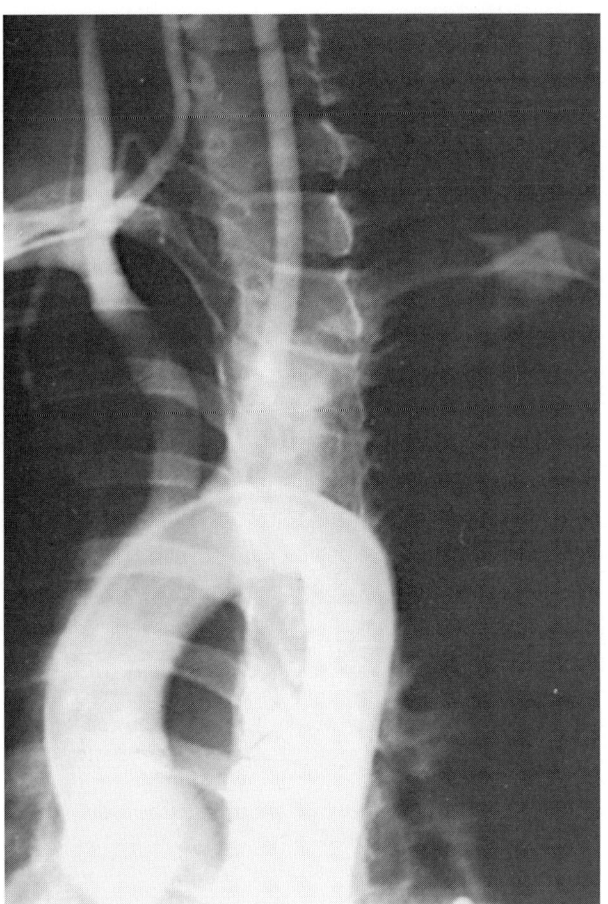

FIGURE 60–11. Occlusion of the proximal left subclavian artery.

instrument such as a Wylie-J clamp. Distal control of the innominate artery is achieved proximal to its bifurcation. When the innominate vein obscures the field, it can be either retracted or divided. An 8- to 12-mm Dacron graft should be placed end-to-side to the proximal ascending aorta, away from the pseudoaneurysm, and then connected to the innominate artery just proximal to its bifurcation. The final step is oversewing of the innominate stump.

Penetrating injuries in the distal portion of the innominate artery are best approached through a median sternotomy extended into the right side of the neck. Removal of the medial portion of the clavicle facilitates exposure and distal control, although this is seldom necessary. The vessel can usually be repaired by lateral arteriorrhaphy, although, occasionally, bypass grafting from the ascending aorta is necessary.

Injuries of the Left Common Carotid Artery

Access to the left common carotid artery is obtained through a median sternotomy extended upward along the anterior border of the left sternocleidomastoid muscle. Proximal control can be achieved at the origin of the vessel from the aortic arch, distal control being obtained cephalad to the injury. The patient's neurologic status dictates what type of repair to perform. Liekweg and Greenfield reported on 233 injuries of the common and internal carotid arteries and found that reconstruction was beneficial for all patients

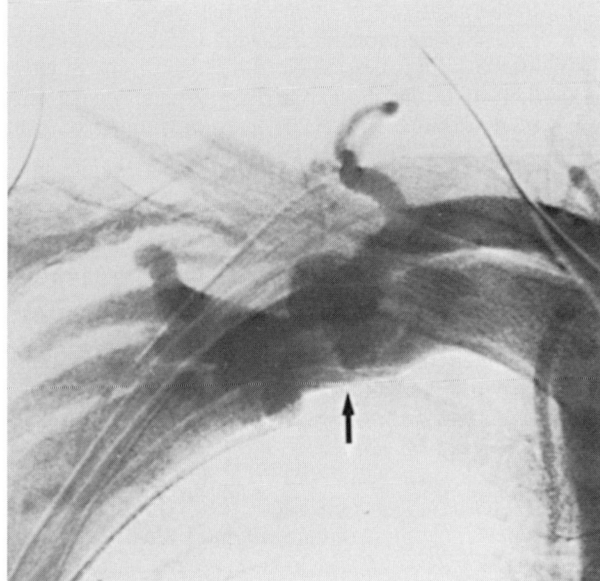

FIGURE 60–12. A digital subtraction angiogram shows a mid-subclavian arteriovenous fistula that occurred after the patient sustained an inferiorly directed knife wound of the supraclavicular fossa.

except those in profound coma.[75] Some surgeons believe that when the patient is seen shortly after injury, repair is warranted because prolonged ischemia may be the more significant threat.[76] Shunts should be used only when intraoperative hypotension is a concern or when both the innominate and the left common carotid artery must be occluded simultaneously.

Injuries of the Subclavian Vessels

Optimal exposure for repair of the proximal right subclavian artery is obtained by a median sternotomy with exten-

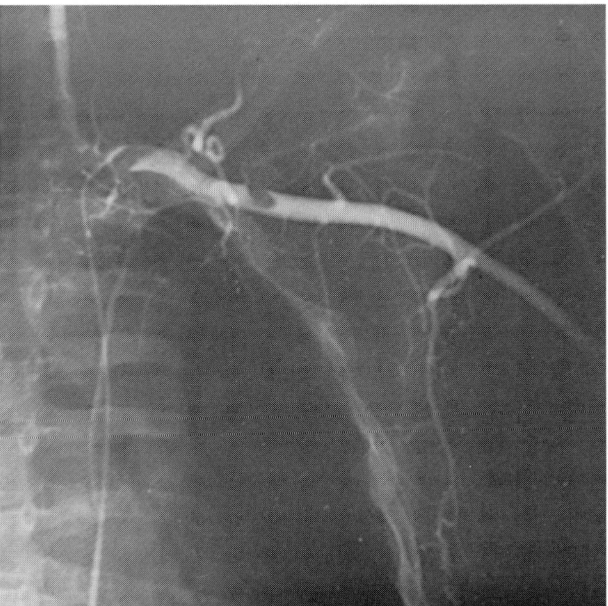

FIGURE 60–13. Traumatic occlusion of the proximal left subclavian artery caused this vertebral steal. The lucency just beyond the vertebral origin is a balloon at the tip of the angiography catheter. Note the second defect in the mid-subclavian artery.

sion into the right side of the neck. Removal of the middle third of the clavicle provides exposure of all three portions of the artery. Injuries to the more distal portions of either subclavian artery can be exposed by supraclavicular incision with removal of the clavicle. Caution must be exercised, because the artery is extremely fragile and can easily be damaged by overzealous dissection.

Because of its intrapleural location, the proximal left subclavian artery is best approached through an anterolateral thoracotomy. Although this incision facilitates proximal control, the more distal extrapleural portions cannot be reached. A supraclavicular incision is added for this purpose. Although many authors speak of the "open book" created when a median sternotomy connects an anterolateral thoracotomy to a supraclavicular incision, the author has found that the approach does not open easily and typically results in multiple posterior rib fractures.

Subclavian artery repairs after penetrating injury can often be performed by débridement and primary anastomosis.[77] For more extensive defects, we have used reversed saphenous grafts successfully. Associated subclavian vein injuries are common and merit repair when possible. For simple lacerations, lateral venorrhaphy is usually adequate. When larger defects are present, a paneled repair may be required to prevent narrowing of the lumen. Although the subclavian artery and vein can be ligated, blunt trauma may disrupt the collateral blood supply around the shoulder and produce effort fatigue of the arm and ischemia of the hand.

Results

The outcome of acute thoracic aortic injury depends not only on the aortic lesion but also on the severity and extent of associated trauma. A study from Duke University examined 108 patients who had sustained blunt trauma.[21] Of the 86% who survived initial resuscitation, 71% survived their injuries. Significantly, only 11 of 42 deaths (26%) were directly attributable to the thoracic aortic injury. Postoperative paraplegia developed in 6.8% of patients.

The survival rate after injuries of the innominate vessels was reported to be 86% in a series by Graham and coworkers.[78] Injuries of the individual common carotid arteries have survival rates near 80%.[79] The mortality rate associated with isolated acute subclavian artery injuries is less than 15%.

ABDOMINAL VASCULAR TRAUMA

The escalation in civilian violence has brought with it increasing numbers of penetrating abdominal vascular injuries in a wide variety of patterns. Tissue destruction depends on the speed, trajectory, and size of the wounding object. If vessel transection occurs, free hemorrhage into the abdominal cavity may result. Occasionally, injury may be partially or completely contained within the retroperitoneum. Rarely, a tangential injury produces thrombosis with ischemia of the respective mesenteric or peripheral bed. Among those undergoing laparotomy for blunt trauma, stab wounds, or gunshots, 3%, 10%, and 25%, respectively, have associated vascular injuries.[80] Arteriovenous fistulae may follow penetrating injuries, although they are somewhat uncommon. The mesenteric, renal, splenic, and iliac vessels can all be affected. Fistulae between the hepatic artery and portal vein, or between the aorta and vena cava have all been reported.[81]

Blunt intra-abdominal vascular injuries are less common than their penetrating counterparts. The usual lesions are avulsions and thromboses. Deceleration or compression produces sufficient shear stress to "avulse" the mobile smaller vessels from their fixed mesenteric origins. This is particularly true of branches that arise from the superior mesenteric artery and from the portal vein. When sufficient energy has been absorbed, affected patients may present in shock secondary to intraperitoneal hemorrhage. In other instances, stretching during deceleration causes intimal tears that lead to vessel thrombosis. Occlusion by an intimal flap is thought to be responsible for the "seat belt aorta" and for occlusions of the proximal renal arteries (Fig. 60–14).

Diagnosis

Patients with intra-abdominal vascular injuries who survive the initial insult typically present with hypotension or frank shock. It has been estimated that only 15% of those who suffer penetrating injuries of the abdominal aorta survive to reach the hospital. Because trauma to the lower thorax may also involve the abdominal aorta, all patients with penetrating injuries between the nipples and the groin should be suspected to harbor an abdominal vascular injury. Retroperitoneal location, a contained hematoma, and hypotension may all be protective, with exsanguination prevented by peritoneal tamponade and decreased pulsatile pressure.[82] As volume resuscitation is instituted, increased

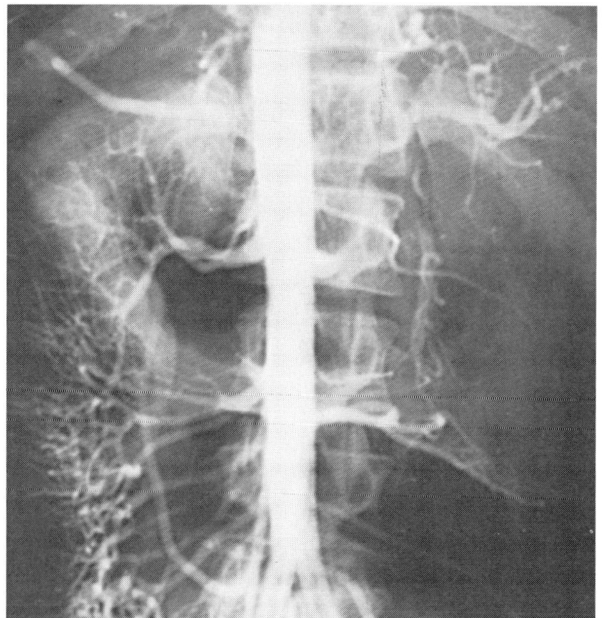

FIGURE 60–14. High-speed motor vehicle accidents may cause arterial intimal stretching and flaps that result in thrombosis. The radiograph shows occlusion of the left renal artery after a motorcycle accident.

cardiac output and blood pressure may expand the hematoma and lead to free hemorrhage.[83] The key to diagnosis is a history of moderate hypotension before arrival and failure to maintain a stable blood pressure after fluid resuscitation.[73]

Rapid and aggressive fluid resuscitation is paramount. Because of the possibility of associated venous injury, the author uses only upper extremity intravenous access sites in these patients. If the patient's condition deteriorates or cardiac arrest ensues, open cardiac massage and cross-clamping of the thoracic aorta is required. These maneuvers decrease intra-abdominal blood loss and may substantially improve the critical coronary and cerebral circulations.[84]

Recently, concern has been expressed about aggressive fluid resuscitation in patients with penetrating truncal injuries who are candidates for immediate operation.[83] Advocates of controlled resuscitation argue that precipitously increasing blood presssure and intravascular volume may actually promote hemorrhage. Until more prospective studies can be completed, this author continues to resuscitate these patients as aggressively as possible. While resuscitation proceeds, physical assessment and radiographic studies are performed. Physical findings of significance include a rapidly expanding abdomen, an audible bruit, and asymmetric lower extremity pulses. An asymmetric femoral arterial pulse is evidence of a common or external iliac artery injury. Normal vascular examination findings do not exclude an arterial injury, however.

Two studies found that 65% of those with iliac injuries had normal findings on vascular examination, although 84% also had "high-risk" clinical findings, which included: entrance wounds below the umbilicus, abdominal tenderness, or hypotension.[84, 85] All patients should have an indwelling urinary bladder catheter in place to monitor resuscitation and provide information about possible renal injury. The author obtains both a chest film and a "one-shot" (single-bolus) intravenous pyelogram (IVP). The chest film helps to exclude associated lesions such as a pneumothorax or a thoracic vascular injury. Additionally, it may reveal missile embolism in patients with venous injuries. The IVP is obtained by infusing 50 ml of Renografin contrast along with the resuscitation fluids. A flat plate view of the abdomen, taken 5 to 10 minutes later, provides information about the kidneys and ureters. Ideally, it demonstrates bilateral renal function and ureteral continuity. This information will be critical for subsequent intraoperative decision making should a perinephric hematoma be found.

Blunt injuries of the abdominal vasculature are more difficult to diagnose. If arterial avulsion is complete, hemorrhage into the peritoneal cavity may produce profound hypotension and signs of peritoneal irritation.[73] When abdominal examination findings are equivocal, diagnostic peritoneal lavage or CT may be helpful.[73]

Diagnostic evaluation of *renal vascular injury* begins with urinalysis. Although 25% to 50% of patients with renal artery injuries have neither gross nor microscopic hematuria, the presence of either should be interpreted with caution.[86–88] A prospective study of 1146 consecutive patients by Mee and colleagues found no significant renal injuries among blunt trauma patients who had microscopic hematuria in the absence of shock.[89] The author has adopted their recommendations that all patients with penetrating trauma to the flank or abdomen and that those with blunt trauma who have either gross or microscopic hematuria and are in shock undergo radiographic evaluation.[89] The IVP seems to be a reasonable tool for patients whose condition is unstable and who require rapid evaluation of renal function. Unfortunately, IVP can have a 30% false-negative rate and can be "uninterpretable" in hypotensive patients.[90] For stable patients who require CT evaluation for intra-abdominal injury, the author routinely includes intravenous contrast injection to examine bilateral renal function. Absence of renal enhancement and excretion, or presence of a "cortical rim" sign, is evidence of thrombosis of the renal artery. When a kidney is not functioning, the author proceeds with arteriography to identify the site and nature of the lesion. Although it has been suggested that CT can substitute for arteriography, this author and others believe that arteriography remains the modality of choice.[91, 92] Once the diagnosis of acute renal artery injury has been made, repair must proceed expeditiously because the chances for functional repair are inversely related to ischemia time. Those whose presentation is significantly delayed cannot anticipate renal salvage.

Operative Management

An operative team familiar with major abdominal surgery is mandatory. Equipment requirements include an aortic compression device or balloon occluders, cardiovascular instruments, and a selection of straight and bifurcated grafts. As a prelude to transporting the hypotensive patient to surgery, emergency department thoracotomy is occasionally necessary. Although this should be avoided whenever possible, thoracic aortic clamp control may be helpful in certain patients who have penetrating abdominal injuries, hypotension, anemia, or abdominal distention. The survival rate for those who require emergency room thoracotomy, however, remains dismal (about 5%).[93]

Conventional teaching has supported the approach of completing repairs during the initial procedure. More recently, however, trauma surgeons have begun to support the concept of "damage control" in selected patients.[94] When injuries are extensive and complex, particularly in the face of hemodynamic instability, a more deliberate approach may be desirable. This is particularly important in patients with a combination of vascular and gastrointestinal injuries in whom definitive repair of all injuries may be ill advised. Application of the principles of damage control dictate addressing the most critical injury and planning reexploration for other problems.

An important sequela of this philosophy applies to abdominal closure. When fluid resuscitation requirements are large and surgery has been lengthy, formal closure may be very difficult. Under these circumstances, temporary closure may be appropriate. Many techniques are available. The author uses an opened 2-L plastic bag of the type commonly used for peritoneal dialysis solutions. A few bags are kept sterile in the operating suite for just such occasions. A corner of the bag is sewn to the skin at the superior or inferior margin of the incision and the bag is then trimmed to fit the defect. This allows rapid closure without placing undue tension on the fascia beneath. A clear adhesive drape is then placed over the closure to make it watertight. An added advantage of this method is that it allows subsequent and frequent inspections of the bowel to ensure that it has not become ischemic. The additional space afforded also helps to prevent development of abdominal compartment syndrome. The temporary closure is removed at a subsequent procedure, when the fascia can be approximated without tension. It is not uncommon to have such a temporary closure in place for a week or more.

Hypothermia should be avoided owing to its adverse effects on the clotting cascade. Equipment for autotransfusion should be available, although this technique should not be used for patients who have bowel injuries and fecal contamination. A significant limitation of devices that wash shed red cells before transfusing them is the removal of plasma proteins, which contributes further to possible coagulopathy when large volumes of autotransfused blood are used.[95]

Abdominal Aortic Injuries

The abdominal aorta is divided into three surgical regions:

1. The diaphragmatic aorta: the aorta at or above the celiac axis.
2. The suprarenal aorta: the portion that extends from the celiac axis to the level of the renal arteries.
3. The infrarenal aorta: the portion that extends from below the renal arteries to the bifurcation into the common iliac arteries (L4).

The patient, having been positioned supine on the operating table, is prepared and draped from the mid-thorax (nipples) to the knees *before induction of anesthesia*. Muscle relaxants used during induction relax the abdominal wall and sometimes relieve tamponade, producing sudden and profound hypotension.

Several incisions have been described for this procedure, including (1) extended midline laparotomy, (2) thoracoabdominal incision, and (3) left thoracotomy with midline laparotomy. The advantage of the added left thoracotomy is that it provides access for immediate control of the descending thoracic aorta when the abdominal injury is so high that subdiaphragmatic control is not possible. The thoracoabdominal approach offers the added advantage of additional exposure in the left upper quadrant.

The author prefers the traditional extended midline laparotomy incision and obtains subdiaphragmatic control just below the aortic hiatus by bluntly dissecting the lesser omentum with the forefinger to gain entry to the lesser sac. This provides access to the posterior peritoneum, which lies over the pancreas and the crura of the diaphragm. The posterior peritoneum is divided, and the muscle fibers of the crura are separated, exposing the periadventitial tissue along the supraceliac aorta.[96] Dissection of the anterior, left, and right walls of the aorta bluntly for about 1 inch enables placement of a slightly curved aortic clamp along the course of the surgeon's fingers. If the aorta is not adequately dissected, the clamp can slip off the dense periaortic tissue. Associated venous injuries, such as aortocaval fistulae, must also be addressed quickly.

Because the veins are fragile, the author prefers to control venous hemorrhage with sponge sticks rather than attempting clamp control. By progressively reducing the length of vein between the sponges, the surgeon can usually control the area of hemorrhage well enough to permit suture repair. When the area of injury contains an avulsion, the proximal and distal ends are controlled with sponges until clamps can be placed accurately around the segments. Blood loss is often considerable during these maneuvers, and it is imperative that, once preliminary hemostasis has been achieved, the surgeon pause long enough to allow the anesthesiologist to replace shed volume, correct metabolic acidosis, and restore platelets as needed.

After hemorrhage has been controlled, a survey should determine whether bowel injuries are present. For small, isolated rents, a few single-layer closures can be performed while the anesthesiologist is correcting metabolic and hematologic derangements. When large segments of intestine have been damaged, noncrushing clamps are used to isolate those segments. Affected bowel should be packed out of the field until the vascular repair has been completed and protected by soft tissue coverage.

Diaphragmatic (Supraceliac) Aortic Injuries

Supraceliac aortic injuries typically have a high mortality rate owing to exsanguination.[97] Upon entering the abdomen, active supramesocolic hemorrhage or an expanding central hematoma signals an aortic injury. Direct pressure controls bleeding until dissection through the lesser omentum allows proximal control. When a large, active hematoma and tissue destruction are present, aortic occluders, transaortic balloon catheters, or transthoracic aortic occlusion may be required. The author has recently employed a balloon catheter inserted through a femoral artery in difficult situations. The drawback to this method is that isolating the femoral artery and introducing the device take the assistant away from the operative field.

Optimal exposure of the supraceliac aorta is obtained via a left lateral retroperitoneal incision with medial rotation of the intestines (Fig. 60–15).[97, 98] The dissection is begun inferiorly along the fusion plane between the left colon and the posterior peritoneum. Further medial mobilization is accomplished by performing blunt dissection of the entire left colon, splenic flexure, spleen, and tail of the pancreas.[96] The left kidney may remain in place or can be rotated medially along with the viscera. Dissection is carried out proximally in the plane of the preaortic fascia to the level of entry of the aorta into the abdomen. In the unlikely event that more proximal exposure is needed, a transthoracic extension can be accomplished by extending the midline incision as a median sternotomy or by making a radial incision in the diaphragm to expose the thoracic aorta. This approach exposes the aorta from T9 to the bifurcation. Potential complications include injury to the spleen, left renal artery, or lumbar arteries.[99]

A right-sided approach may also be used. A wide or extended Kocher maneuver is performed, and the duodenum and head of the pancreas are rotated medially. This produces excellent exposure of the vena cava and aorta below the level of the celiac axis and the superior mesenteric artery. When better exposure of the proximal aorta is needed, the left crus of the diaphragm can be divided at its

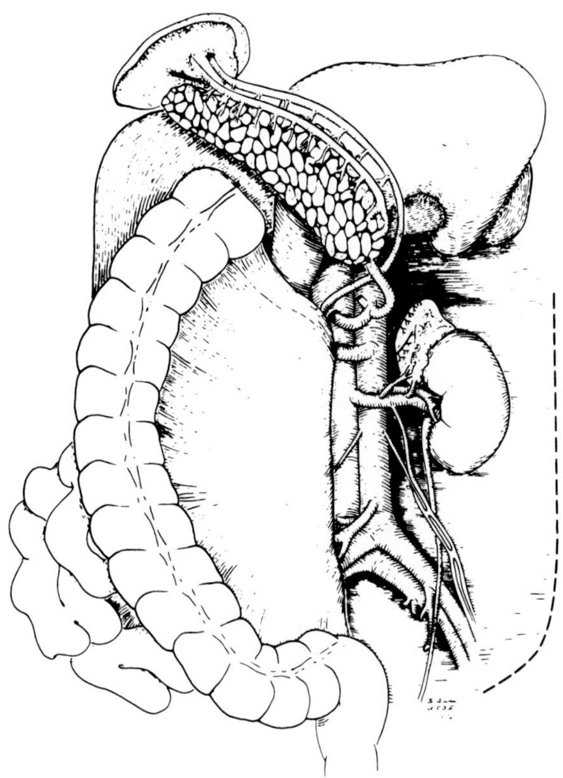

FIGURE 60–15. Incision along the left lateral fusion plane with rotation of the viscera to the midline provides excellent exposure of the aorta and mesenteric vessels. The left kidney may be reflected with the intestines or left in place, as here. (From Shackford SR, Sise MJ: Renal and mesenteric vascular trauma. *In* Bongard FS, Wilson SE, Perry MO [eds]: Vascular Injuries in Surgical Practice. Norwalk, Conn, Appleton & Lange, 1991, p 178.)

insertion with the vertebral body. This provides additional mobility to the esophagus and stomach, allowing exposure of the proximal aorta.[100]

Some authors recommend dividing an injured pancreas to obtain exposure of the superior mesenteric vessels.[101] When this is necessary, a distal pancreatectomy should be performed to avoid a pancreatic anastomosis adjacent to a vascular repair.

The supraceliac aorta typically is repaired with a lateral suture of 3-0 polypropylene. If tissue destruction is extensive near the head of the pancreas along the course of the gastroduodenal arteries, celiac ligation must not be performed, because collateral pathways may have been destroyed. If the aortic defect is sufficiently large to require a patch, we prefer autogenous tissue. Hypogastric artery is usually readily available and can be opened and trimmed to suitable size. This avoids the need to expose, dissect and excise a segment of saphenous vein. Although others have reported routine use of prosthetic materials such as PTFE and Dacron in this site, we avoid them whenever possible, particularly in the presence of gastrointestinal contamination.[102] When a segment of suprarenal aorta must be excised, prosthetic bypass becomes unavoidable. An interesting approach to an intracavitary conduit is to create an end-to-end anastomosis proximally, followed by an end-to-side anastomosis to the distal aorta or to the left common iliac artery, in essence bypassing the aortic injury. The distal stump of the transected aorta should be closed meticulously.

Suprarenal Aortic Injuries

Injuries to the aortic segment between the origin of the renal arteries and the celiac axis carry the highest risk of mortality. Because dense periaortic neural tissue surrounds the celiac axis, the superior mesenteric artery, and the pancreas, this segment is best exposed by medial rotation of the viscera in the same manner described earlier for the supraceliac aorta. When an injury of the inferior vena cava is suspected as well, a right (rather than a left) gutter incision is preferable. With this technique, the right colon, hepatic flexure, and duodenum are mobilized to the left.

Suprarenal aortic injuries are usually repaired with 3-0 monofilament polypropylene via a lateral arteriorrhaphy. When two lacerations closely approximate each other, they can be connected and repaired transversely as a single defect, using a horizontal mattress suture.

Infrarenal Aortic Injuries

Injuries of the infrarenal aorta generally have the best outcome because of their accessibility. Upon entering the abdomen, a large retroperitoneal hematoma extending into the flanks is the first finding. The initial approach requires cephalad traction on the transverse colon mesentery, accompanied by rotation and evisceration of the small bowel to the right. The retroperitoneum is then opened in the midline superiorly, near the transverse colon mesentery. This permits identification of the left renal vein, which serves as a marker for the renal arteries. For most infrarenal injuries, proximal control can be obtained at this level. The left renal vein is usually very mobile and can be retracted superiorly after minimal dissection to expose the renal arteries. When this is not possible, the left renal vein can be ligated medially as it passes over the aorta. If a supraceliac or thoracic aortic cross-clamp has been placed, it can be repositioned below the renal arteries. The author prefers to obtain distal control with a gently curved Crafoord clamp placed tangentially to control the aorta and the lumbar arteries simultaneously. When the injury extends downward toward the bifurcation, the iliac arteries may need to be controlled individually. Particular care must be exercised to prevent injury to the left iliac vein as it passes under the right iliac artery.

When the injury is less than 1 cm long, gentle dissection may provide enough mobility to allow resection and repair. Great care must be exercised to ligate and divide lumbar arteries with clips or suture before mobilization is attempted. Repair is performed with 3-0 monofilament polypropylene suture. Careful closure of the peritoneum over the aorta is imperative.

When a large segment of aorta is damaged, in-line bypass or extra-anatomic bypass with proximal and distal aortic ligation may be performed (see preceding text). Because young trauma victims have relatively small aortas, the maximum size of usable graft is typically 12 to 14 mm. Feliciano and coworkers summarized the results in 33 patients from eight studies and found only one reported graft infection.[103] If the surgeon chooses to use a prosthetic graft, the repair must be meticulously covered with soft tissue and peritoneum before intestinal injuries are repaired. Careful postoperative monitoring is required to detect the earliest evidence of graft infection.

Blunt Aortic Injuries

Blunt trauma to the aorta most often follows motor vehicle accidents or falls. Downward traction produces intimal disruption, particularly in the infrarenal aorta.[104] Bowel injuries are present in 100% of cases when seat belts are the agent of trauma.[104] Typical acute findings include diminished lower extremity pulses in the presence of a normal upper extremity examination. Transaxillary arteriography locates the injury and demonstrates its length. Treatment depends on the extent of the injury and associated findings. Intimal disruption with limited dissection can be repaired by simple suture, whereas lengthy disruptions may require endarterectomy beyond the end-point. Vessel replacement is required when injury is extensive or patient presentation has been delayed.

Iliac Vessel Injuries

Iliac injuries most commonly occur after penetrating trauma and are often accompanied by cecal, sigmoid colon, ureteral, or urinary bladder injuries. Blunt injuries that produce trauma to the common or external iliac vessels are unusual. Hemorrhage is usually due to disruption of branches of the hypogastric artery or vein. A falling hematocrit value after pelvic fracture when there is no other evidence of concomitant injuries is best managed by external fracture stabilization and arteriography for therapeutic embolization.[105] An initial CT scan is helpful in stable patients to demonstrate any retroperitoneal hemorrhage (which would suggest bleeding from a pelvic fracture). Operative ligation of bleeding vessels in this site usually is not necessary.

When laparotomy is performed for penetrating trauma, injuries of the iliac vessels often present as pulsatile and expanding hematomas in the inferior quadrants. Exposure of the right common iliac artery is best obtained by elevating the cecum and terminal ileum toward the left. The left common iliac artery can be exposed by reflecting the sigmoid and left colon toward the right. Exposure of the left iliac vein may require division and reanastomosis of the right common iliac artery.[106] Proximal and distal control must be achieved before the hematoma is entered. Sponge sticks placed on either side of the injury provide rapid hemostasis and permit more careful dissection in a relatively blood-free field. For copious hemorrhage, total pelvic vascular isolation may be necessary for control. This technique requires proximal cross-clamping of both the abdominal aorta and the inferior vena cava above their bifurcations, as well as distal cross-clamping of both the external iliac artery and vein, using one clamp on each side of the pelvis.[107]

Repair of external iliac artery injuries can usually be performed via lateral arteriorrhaphy with 4-0 or 5-0 polypropylene.[108] Resection with mobilization of cut ends provides a tension-free anastomosis for injuries less than 2 cm long. The internal iliac artery makes an excellent autologous graft for short segments. Injuries that extend proximally to include the aortic bifurcation may be repaired by performing an aortoiliac anastomosis on one side, followed by an end-to-side anastomosis of the iliac artery to the contralateral reconstruction. This repositioned "aortic bifurcation" has the advantage of placing the anastomosis out of direct contact with other injured tissue (Figs. 60–16 to

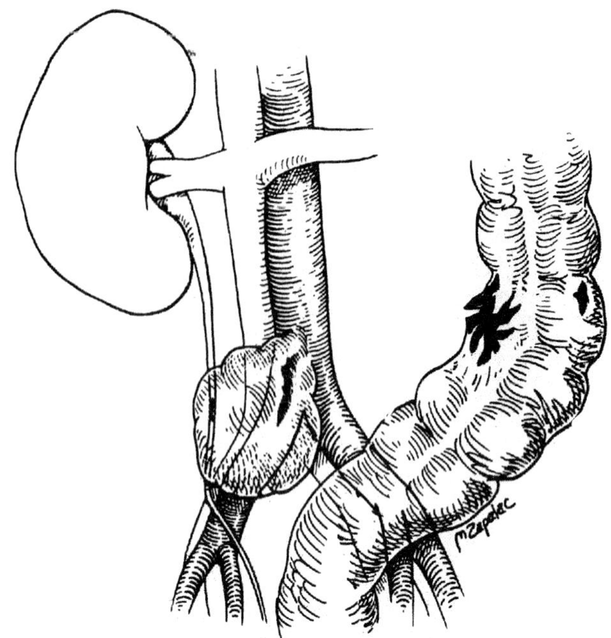

FIGURE 60–16. A typical combined (aorto) iliac and colonic injury.

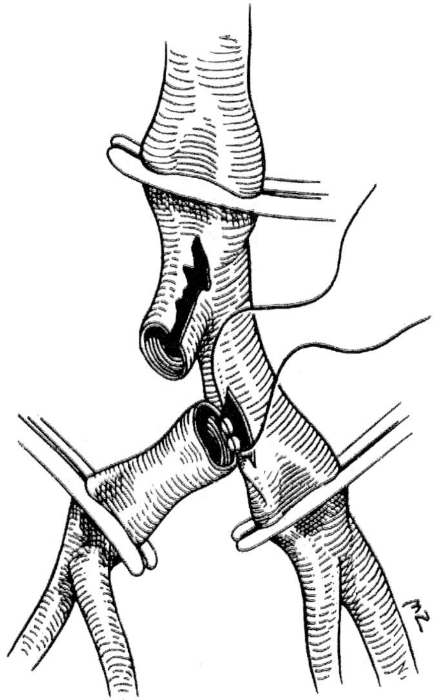

FIGURE 60–17. The proximal right iliac artery has been transposed to the left common iliac artery, thus lowering and "transposing" the aortic bifurcation.

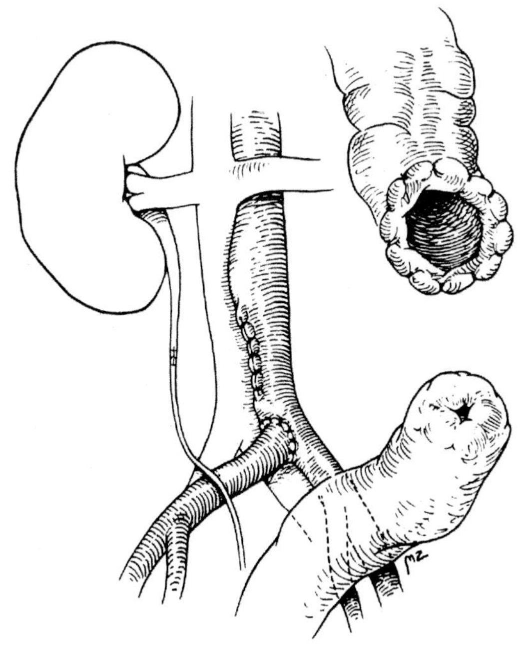

FIGURE 60–18. The proximal right iliac artery has been oversewn, and the distal segment reimplanted. Note that colostomy, rather than a primary repair, has been performed

60–18). Reconstructions should be covered by viable retroperitoneal tissue and replaced in the pelvis.

Iliac venous injuries are exposed by the same methods described earlier for their arterial counterparts. Control is achieved by applying direct pressure or by using sponge sticks. These injuries are usually fairly simple to repair via lateral venorrhaphy, although care must be exercised to prevent narrowing of the vein, which may subsequently lead to thrombosis. When the right iliac artery is divided to repair the left iliac vein, sigmoid mesentery or a pedicle of peritoneum should be placed between the two anastomoses. Although young patients usually tolerate iliac vein ligation well, it should be avoided whenever possible.

A large percentage of patients with iliac vessel injuries have associated gastrointestinal or genitourinary trauma.[109] Contamination of the site risks infection of the vascular repair. Prosthetic grafts must be used with caution in this situation, although good outcomes have been reported by some groups.[109] In general, autogenous tissue should be used whenever possible.[110] In such circumstances, the goal is hemorrhage control rather than vascular repair.[111] If the vessel is oversewn, the suture lines should be bolstered within the retroperitoneum with omentum or psoas muscle, a technique demonstrably useful in preventing disruption of vascular suture lines.[112] If signs of distal ischemia appear after proximal ligation, an extra-anatomic bypass (axillofemoral, femorofemoral, or axillopopliteal) can be performed. When intestinal spillage is modest, the patient is stable, and immediate repair is desirable, the gastrointestinal or genitourinary injury should be addressed immediately after hemorrhage is controlled. Gowns and gloves are changed before the vascular injury is addressed.

Mesenteric and Portal Vessel Injuries

Injuries of the mesenteric and portal vessels are often accompanied by overlying intestinal trauma that renders isolation and repair difficult. Exposure of the origin of the celiac and superior mesenteric arteries is best obtained through lateral mobilization and rightward rotation of the viscera, as outlined for suprarenal aortic injuries. Associated mesenteric venous injuries are common and should be repaired first to prevent venous engorgement of the bowel.[113]

Isolated injuries of the celiac axis are extremely uncommon and can usually be ligated. The common hepatic artery tends to be the largest branch of the celiac artery and can occasionally be repaired with an end-to-end anastomosis or a saphenous vein graft if the patient's overall condition warrants. When necessary, ligation of the common hepatic artery should be done proximal to the origin of the gastroduodenal artery, because this vessel is a large collateral from the superior mesenteric artery (SMA). Several anatomic variants of the celiac axis exist, including a common origin with the superior mesenteric. For this reason, the structures of interest must be clearly identified before any vessels are sacrificed.[82]

The SMA can be divided into four segments, based on their locations and the presence of collateral blood flow: (1) at its origin behind the pancreas proximal to the takeoff of the pancreaticoduodenal artery, (2) in the base of the transverse mesocolon between the pancreaticoduodenal and middle colic branches, (3) beyond the middle colic branch, and (4) at the level of the mesenteric arcades.[114]

At its origin, exposure of the SMA is difficult but can be achieved by rightward rotation of the viscera or by transection of the pancreas. When the proximal SMA is sufficiently damaged to preclude direct repair, splenectomy can be performed and the splenic artery can be turned down with end-to-end anastomosis to the distal stump of the SMA. Alternatively, a graft can be placed from the anterior surface of the aorta to the stump of the superior mesenteric vessel. Care must be exercised, when pancreatic injuries are present, to shield the anastomosis from the potentially disruptive effect of pancreatic enzymes. Ligation of the proximal SMA, if required, is usually tolerated because of collateral flow from the gastroduodenal artery, although associated injuries and vasospasm may threaten midgut viability. Beyond the middle colic branch, SMA repair is obligatory to prevent midgut ischemia.

The superior mesenteric vein lies just to the right of the artery where both vessels cross over the uncinate process of the pancreas and the third portion of the duodenum. Injuries to the artery frequently involve the vein on operative dissection. Repair of the superior mesenteric vein is preferred to ligation, although this may be difficult, especially in the segment that exits from beneath the pancreas. Pancreatic division may be necessary to obtain access and control for repair. Collaterals must be ligated before visualization of posterior venous perforations is possible. Control is obtained with sponge sticks or finger pressure. Repair can be performed with 5-0 or 6-0 polypropylene fashioned to prevent narrowing of the lumen. Methods of repair include saphenous vein interposition, anastomosis to the splenic vein, and ligation. In the author's experience, these injuries are extremely difficult to manage, especially in the face of associated trauma in a marginally compensated hypothermic patient. For these reasons, mesenteric vein injuries that cannot be repaired simply and quickly should be managed by ligation. Ligation of the splenic vein may lead to gastric varices if the spleen is not removed. When the superior mesenteric vein must be ligated, postoperative fluid balance must be monitored carefully, because resultant splanchnic venous congestion leads to peripheral hypovolemia for as long as 72 hours after ligation. "Second-look" laparotomy in 24 to 48 hours is often prudent.

Inferior mesenteric artery injuries are best treated by ligation, as long as SMA and hypogastric collaterals are patent. Assessment of bowel viability is mandatory and is best accomplished by reexploration at 48 to 72 hours, or sooner if indicated.

Repair of portal venous injuries is preferred to ligation when possible. In a hypovolemic and hypotensive patient, portal vein ligation may lead to massive splanchnic congestion and even venous infarction of the gut. Portacaval shunting is difficult to accomplish in this situation and has a high complication rate.[115] Exposure of the portal vein and the confluence of the mesenteric and splenic veins is achieved by mobilizing the hepatic flexure and colon (Fig. 60–19). A Kocher maneuver also facilities exposure. Injuries of the porta hepatis require dissection of the common bile duct and cystic duct, which are then mobilized and displaced. Trauma in this area can also include hepatic artery injuries and may be accompanied by profuse hemorrhage. Placement of a noncrushing clamp across the common bile duct, portal vein, and hepatic artery (Pringle's maneuver) may be necessary. Injuries of the portal vein and hepatic artery to a liver segment result in hepatic ischemia and, if ligated, require segmental hepatectomy. Anterior and left lateral portal vein exposure may require division of the pancreas, which is best accomplished by clamping the head of the pancreas with two straight intestinal clamps and opening between them. Lateral venorrhaphy or end-to-end anastomosis should be performed, although panel grafts may be required when disruption is significant. When the patient's condition is unstable or when a coagulopathy is present, portal venous ligation is required. As in superior mesenteric vein ligation, this produces systemic hypovolemia and requires aggressive fluid resuscitation during the first few days after surgery.

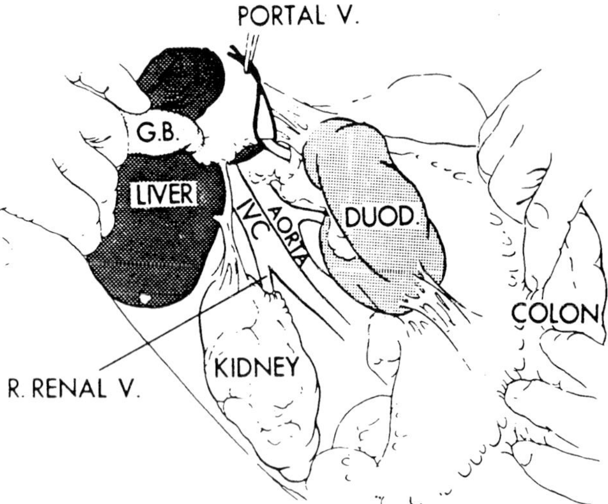

FIGURE 60–19. Exposure of the portal vein is best achieved by incision of viscera along the right fusion line with medial rotation. (From Petersen SR, Sheldon GF, Lim RC: Management of portal vein injuries. J Trauma 19[8]:616–620, 1979. © Williams & Wilkins.)

Renovascular Injuries

At the time of laparotomy, previously unsuspected renovascular injuries are indicated by the presence of a central hematoma or of a pulsatile and expanding lateral perirenal hematoma. Wilson and Zeigler commented that as many as 10% of patients with unexplored perirenal hematomas developed complications that might have been avoided by exploration.[90]

Control of the renal vasculature before exploration of a hematoma is controversial. While classic teaching dictates that the renal pedicle should be secured initially, in practice this is often difficult when a large hematoma extends toward the aorta. In such circumstances, it may be easier to open Gerota's fascia and proceed toward the aorta or inferior vena cava until the renal pedicle can be identified. Investigators recently observed that the need for nephrectomy was influenced more by the severity of renal injury than by the technique used to obtain vascular control.[116] When possible, the proximal renal artery can be exposed either through an incision in the retroperitoneum over the aorta or by mobilizing the viscera from the lateral to the medial aspect. Mobilization of the left renal vein can be achieved by dividing its distal branches, although this maneuver eliminates the possibility of subsequently ligating the vein. Control of the distal left renal artery is achieved by dissecting along the course of the vessel until the hilum is identified. Leftward retraction of the inferior vena cava permits isolation of the right renal pedicle. Care must be taken to ensure that the right renal vein is not avulsed from the inferior vena cava and that posterior lumbar veins are not damaged. Ligation of the right renal vein requires ipsilateral nephrectomy. Very proximal right renal artery injuries may also be controlled by this maneuver, although mobilization of the ascending colon and a Kocher maneuver is usually required to achieve enough exposure to permit repair.

The strategy for repair or ligation of the injured vessel depends on (1) the overall condition of the patient, (2) the extent of injury to the renal artery, (3) the condition of the ipsilateral kidney, and (4) the condition of the contralateral kidney.[82] The duration of renal ischemia is also important. Renal function is severely impaired after 6 hours of warm partial ischemia or after 3 hours of total ischemia.[117] Although successful repairs have been reported after prolonged ischemia, it does not seem prudent to attempt revascularization of a unilateral injury after more than 6 hours. If, however, there is only one kidney or if renal vascular injuries are bilateral, a more aggressive approach is warranted when the patient's condition permits.

After the decision to revascularize has been made, proximal and distal control must be ensured. Lacerations of the distal vessel may be controlled with a sponge stick or with an occluding balloon inserted through the proximal vessel. Simple lacerations should be débrided and repaired end to end, to prevent narrowing of the lumen. If the uninvolved vessel is too short, interposition grafting with saphenous vein is required. Occasionally, the graft must be connected proximally to the aorta. Moving the splenic artery down to replace the left renal artery or the hepatic artery to replace the right renal artery may be possible in a stable patient who has no contralateral renal function. After any type of renal vascular repair, follow-up assessment of renal function by excretion scanning is mandatory. Repairs thought to be successful when first completed may subsequently cause hypertension and require medication or late nephrectomy to correct.[118]

Injuries of the Inferior Vena Cava

Injuries of the inferior vena cava occur in two regions: (1) the infrarenal vena cava, which extends from the junction of the left and right common iliac veins at the level of L5, up to the level of L2, where it receives the left and right renal veins, and (2) the suprarenal and retrohepatic vena cava, which extends cephalad until it enters the right atrium inside the pericardial sac.

Infrarenal Vena Cava Injuries

One third to one half of inferior vena cava injuries occur in this segment. Exposure requires mobilizing the right colon, hepatic flexure, duodenum, and pancreas to the left. Initially, hemostasis is best achieved by placing sponge sticks to isolate the injury. A drop in blood pressure may occur if fluid resuscitation was inadequate. Subdiaphragmatic aortic occlusion may help to restore blood pressure and prevent pooling in the lower extremities. When posterior injuries are present, some hemorrhage may persist from collateral and lumbar veins. The author usually does not completely mobilize the vena cava because such maneuvers can tear the posterior collaterals. For anterior injuries, a side-biting Satinsky clamp controls the injury while permitting some continued venous return. Once controlled, the posterior wall should be inspected carefully for injury. Any small posterior lacerations can be repaired from within the vessel. Suture lines should be kept as short as possible in hope of avoiding later thrombosis.

Most vena caval injuries can be repaired by lateral venorrhaphy, provided the diameter is not narrowed to less than 50%.[119] For large anterior defects, an opened segment of saphenous vein or a panel graft may be required. When an entire segment of vena cava is damaged, replacement or ligation is necessary. Although the creation of spiral vein grafts from a segment of saphenous vein has been described, patients with caval injuries usually are not able to tolerate the long operation required to create such a graft.[115] A number of graft materials and techniques, including creation of distal femorosaphenous arteriovenous fistulae to improve flow through the graft, have been described. The time spent, the potential blood loss, and the likelihood of eventual thrombosis make such efforts inadvisable.[120, 121] For complex injuries the author prefers infrarenal caval ligation to prosthetic repair. Postoperatively, these patients need volume expansion and prevention of lower extremity venous pooling. Venous pumps, elastic wraps, and leg elevation should be maintained for at least 1 week after surgery.

If a small and stable hematoma is discovered on laparotomy, an isolated posterior defect may be responsible. Recently, several authors have proposed management without repair.[122, 123] Experience with this approach is limited, but it may be reasonable under carefully defined and controlled circumstances.[124] Animal studies have confirmed the general absence of sequelae in experimental models.[123]

Suprarenal and Retrohepatic Vena Cava Injuries

Injuries of the suprarenal and retrohepatic vena cava carry a mortality rate of 33% to 67% because of extensive blood loss, difficulty of repair, and associated trauma. When the injury is at the confluence of the renal veins and the inferior vena cava, compression at the site of injury limits hemorrhage until suprarenal and infrarenal sponge sticks or loops can be placed. Once this is done, the left renal vein is looped or ligated medially, and the vena cava is gently mobilized medially until the right renal vein can be visualized and controlled. If the rent is large, a 30-ml Foley catheter can be inserted into the defect and inflated. Particular care is required to prevent too rapid inflation, which results in complete disruption of the injury.

Exposure of suprarenal caval injuries can be achieved with a Kocher maneuver that mobilizes the duodenum and ascending colon toward the midline. Initial hemostasis can be achieved with sponge sticks, finger pressure, or balloon occlusion. Repair is performed in the manner described for infrarenal injuries. Ligation of suprarenal caval injuries carries a high mortality rate.

The retrohepatic portion of the inferior vena cava is the most difficult to expose and control. This segment receives the hepatic veins, which are short and extremely fragile. When initial mobilization of the liver increases hemorrhage, the author packs the area and places downward pressure on the liver to achieve immediate hemostasis. The injury is exposed by dividing the triangular and anterior and posterior coronary ligaments of the overlying hepatic lobe. This limited dissection is occasionally adequate to permit direct repair of the lacerated hepatic veins and vena cava. Pachter and associates have suggested that the hepatic laceration can be extended along the injury tract until the hepatic venous or vena caval injury is exposed.[125] On occasion, extension of the laparotomy to a median sternotomy with radial incision of the diaphragm to the vena caval hiatus is required. Inflow to the area of injury is achieved by aortic occlusion and a clamp applied across the afferent portal and arterial supplies of the liver (Pringle's maneuver).

Vascular isolation of the liver has received much attention but is not much used. Indeed, Nance has commented, "Somewhat like a chicken whose neck has been wrung and still survives, the caval shunt still persists."[126] Multiple techniques and modifications have been described, although most surgeons have had little experience with any of them.[127] The author has found the endotracheal tube technique effective and relatively easy to learn and to apply (Fig. 60–20). A sterile, 7-mm cuffed endotracheal tube is used. A pursestring suture placed widely enough to accept the endotracheal tube is placed in the right atrial appendage. The intrapericardial inferior vena cava is dissected, and a Rumel's tourniquet is placed around it. The proximal end of the endotracheal tube is clamped, and the balloon-tipped end is advanced. A finger palpates for the tip of the tube until it lies just below the renal veins. The tube is withdrawn several centimeters from the atrium, while side holes are cut with rongeurs so that they will lie within the right

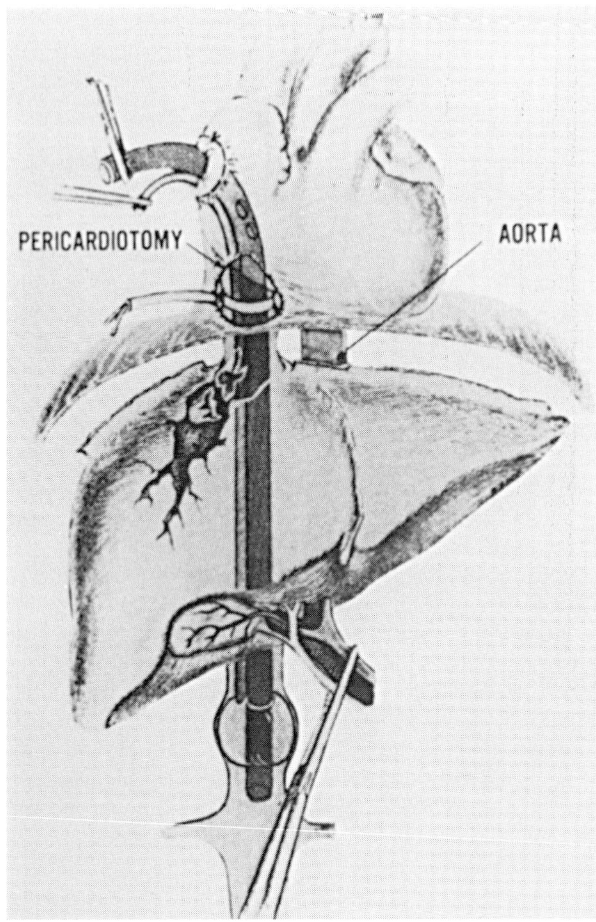

FIGURE 60–20. An endotracheal tube is used to bypass a retrohepatic caval injury. The balloon at the end of the tube eliminates the need for a tourniquet above the renal veins. (From Yellin AE, Chaffee CB, Donovan AJ: Vascular isolation in treatment of juxtahepatic venous injuries. Arch Surg 102:566–573, 1972. Copyright 1971, American Medical Association.)

atrium when the tube is repositioned. The shunt is advanced until the tip lies just *above* the renal veins. The balloon is inflated to secure the shunt in place while the atrial pursestring suture is secured. Care must be taken while the shunt is being advanced, to prevent laceration of tributary veins. Hemostasis in the area is much reduced, although some residual hemorrhage persists because of small tributaries that enter between the renal veins and the hepatic veins.

When the shunt is ready to be removed, the balloon is deflated and the shunt withdrawn through the pursestring. Fluid resuscitation through the exposed portion of the shunt is possible; however, the author prefers not to do this because air embolization would occur were the connectors to become dislodged.[128]

Results

Survival after injury to the abdominal aorta depends largely on the number of associated injuries and on the site of the aortic disruption. Results are best after infrarenal injuries (reported survival 44% to 58%).[98, 129] With suprarenal injuries, the survival rate is slightly lower, from 28% to 46%, although some small studies have reported better results.[98, 129–131] Function is generally good; however, a recent report of follow-up on 11 survivors of abdominal aortic repair found decreased Doppler ankle-brachial pressure indices in five. Pathologic calcifications were noted in the area of repair on CT.[132] Iliac arterial injuries carry a somewhat higher average survival rate, but function of the ipsilateral lower extremity may be suboptimal. Typical survival rates for iliac artery injuries range from 48% to 71%, and for iliac venous injury from 69% to 82%.[133, 134] Ligation of the common or external iliac artery without revascularization is associated with substantial morbidity.[135]

Isolated injuries of the mesenteric vessels are uncommon, so survival rates for patients with these injuries need to be evaluated in the context of associated trauma. Superior mesenteric artery injuries have survival rates of 32% to 67%.[129, 134] Most series are small and their results are not necessarily comparable. Portal vein injuries typically are also found in polytrauma patients; associated mortality is nearly 50%.[103]

Infrarenal vena caval injuries, especially those due to penetrating trauma, typically have good outcomes, survival rates being better than 70%. Suprarenal and retrohepatic caval injuries have lower survival rates, however, and average about 40% to 50%.[135, 136]

REFERENCES

1. Bongard F, Dubrow T, Klein SR: Vascular injuries in the urban battleground: Experience at a metropolitan trauma center. Ann Vasc Surg 4:415, 1990.
2. Feliciano DV, Bitondo CG, Mattox KL, et al: Civilian trauma in the 1980s: A 1-year experience with 456 vascular and cardiac injuries. Ann Surg 199:717, 1984.
3. Jackson DH: Of TRAs and ROCs. Chest 85:585,1984.
4. Mattox KL: Fact and fiction about management of aortic transection. Ann Thorac Surg 48:1, 1989.
5. Greendyke RM: Traumatic rupture of the aorta. Special references to automobile accidents. JAMA 195:527, 1966.
6. Passaro E, Pace WG: Traumatic rupture of the aorta. Surgery 46:787, 1959.
7. DelRossi AJ, Cernaianu AC, Madden LD, et al: Traumatic disruptions of the thoracic aorta: Treatment and outcome. Surgery 108:864, 1990.
8. Avery JE, Hall DP, Adams JE: Traumatic rupture of the thoracic aorta. South Med J 75:653, 1979.
9. Wilson RF: Thoracic vascular trauma. *In* Bongard F, Wilson SE, Perry MO (eds): Vascular Injuries in Surgical Practice. Norwalk, Conn, Appleton & Lange, 1991, p 107.
10. Kirsh MM, Sloan H: Blunt Chest Trauma. Boston, Little, Brown, 1977.
11. Sevitt S: The mechanisms of traumatic rupture of the thoracic aorta. Br J Surg 64:166, 1977.
12. Lundevall J: The mechanism of traumatic rupture of the aorta. Acta Pathol Microbiol Scand 62:34, 1964.
13. Besson A, Saegesser F: Chest Trauma and Associated Injuries. Oradell, NJ, Medical Economics, 1983, p 2.
14. Parmley LF, Mattingly TW, Manion TW, et al: Nonpenetrating traumatic injury of the aorta. Circulation 17:1086, 1958.
15. Binet JP, Langlois J, Cormier JM, et al: A case of recent traumatic avulsion of the innominate artery at its origin from the aortic arch. J Thorac Cardiovasc Surg 43:670, 1962.
16. Voigt GE, Wifert K: Mechanisms of injuries to unrestrained drivers in head-on collisions. *In* Proceedings of the Thirteenth Stapp Car Crash Conference. New York, Society of Automotive Engineers, 1993, pp 295–313.
17. Crass JC, Cohen AM, Motta AO, et al: A proposed new mechanism

of traumatic aortic rupture: The osseous pinch. Radiology 176:645, 1990.
18. Howells GA, Hernandez DA, Olt SL, et al: Blunt injury of the ascending aorta and aortic arch: Repair with hypothermic circulatory arrest. J Trauma 44:716, 1998.
19. Harrington DP, Barth KH, White RI Jr, et al: Traumatic pseudoaneurysm of the thoracic aorta in close proximity to the anterior spinal artery: A therapeutic dilemma. Surgery 87:153, 1980.
20. Wexler L, Silverman J: Traumatic rupture of the innominate artery: A seat-belt injury. N Engl J Med 282:1186, 1970.
21. Duhaylongsod FG, Glower DD, Wolfe WG: Acute traumatic aortic aneurysm: The Duke experience from 1970 to 1990. J Vasc Surg 15:331, 1992.
22. Symbas PN, Tyras DH, Ware RE, et al: Rupture of the aorta: A diagnostic triad. Ann Thorac Surg 15:405, 1973.
23. Fox S, Pierce WS, Waldhausen JA: Acute hypertension: Its significance in traumatic aortic rupture. J Thorac Cardiovasc Surg 75:622, 1973.
24. Clark DE, Zeiger MA, Wallace KL, et al: Blunt aortic trauma: Signs of high risk. J Trauma 30:701, 1990.
25. Fisher RG, Hadlock F, Ben-Menachem Y: Laceration of the thoracic aorta and brachiocephalic arteries by blunt trauma: Report of 54 cases and review of the literature. Radiol Clin North Am 19:91, 1981.
26. Gundry SR, Williams S, Burney RE, et al: Indications for aortography in blunt thoracic trauma: A reassessment. J Trauma 22:664, 1982.
27. Woodring JH: The normal mediastinum in blunt traumatic rupture of the thoracic aorta and brachiocephalic arteries. J Emerg Med 8:467, 1990.
28. Mirvis SE, Bidwell JK, Buddemeyer EU, et al: Value of chest radiography in excluding traumatic aortic rupture. Radiology 163:487, 1987.
29. Ayella RJ, Hankins JR, Turney SZ, et al: Ruptured thoracic aorta due to blunt trauma. J Trauma 17:199, 1977.
30. Mirvis SE, Bidwell JK, Buddemeyer EU: Value of chest radiography in excluding aortic rupture. Radiology 163:487, 1982.
31. Seltzer SE, D'Orsi C, Kirshner R, et al: Traumatic aortic rupture: Plain radiographic findings. AJR 137:1011, 1981.
32. Woodring JH, King JG: The potential effects of radiographic criteria to exclude aortography in patients with blunt chest trauma. J Thorac Cardiovasc Surg 97:456, 1989.
33. Marsh DG, Sturm JT: Traumatic aortic rupture: Roentgenographic indications for angiography. Ann Thorac Surg 21:337, 1976.
34. Sturm JT, Olson FR, Cicero JJ: Chest roentgenographic findings in 26 patients with traumatic rupture of the thoracic aorta. Ann Emerg Med 12:598, 1983.
35. Williams S, Burney RE, MacKenzie J, Cho K: Indications for aortography: Radiography after blunt chest trauma: A reassessment of the radiographic findings associated with traumatic rupture of the aorta. Invest Radiol 18:230, 1983.
36. Burney RE, Gundry SR, Mackenzie JR, et al: Chest roentgenograms in diagnosis of traumatic rupture of the aorta: Observer variation in interpretation. Chest 85:605, 1984.
37. Ayella RJ: Radiologic Management of the Massively Traumatized Patient. Baltimore, Williams & Wilkins, 1978.
38. Gerlock AJ, Muhletaler CA, Coulam CM, et al: Traumatic aortic aneurysm: Validity of esophageal tube displacement sign. Am J Radiol 135:713, 1980.
39. Lee J, Harris JH, Duke JH, et al: Noncorrelation between thoracic skeletal injuries and acute traumatic aortic tear. J Trauma 43:400, 1997.
40. Fabian TC, Richardon JD, Croce MC, et al: Prospective study of blunt aortic injury: Multicenter trial of the American Association for the Surgery of Trauma. J Trauma 42:374, 1997.
41. Mirvis SE, Shanmugaanathan K, Miller BH, et al: Traumatic aortic injury: Diagnosis with contrast-enhanced thoracic CT: Five year experience at a major trauma center. Radiology 200:413, 1996.
42. Nunez D, Rivas L, McKenney K, et al: Helical CT of traumatic arterial injuries. AJR Am J Roentgenol 170:1621, 1998.
43. Smith MD, Cassidy M, Souther S, et al: Transesophageal echocardiography in the diagnosis of traumatic rupture of the aorta. N Engl J Med 332:356, 1995.
44. Ahrar K, Smith DC, Bansal RC, et al: Angiography in blunt thoracic aortic injury. J Trauma 42:665, 1997.
45. Goarin JP, Caoire P, Jacquens Y, et al: Use of transesophageal echocardiography for diagnosis of traumatic aortic injury. Chest 112:71, 1997.
46. Graham JM, Feliciano DV, Mattox KL, et al: Innominate vascular injury. J Trauma 22:647, 1982.
47. O'Gorman RB, Feliciano DV: Arteriography performed in the emergency center. Am J Surg 152:323, 1986.
48. Brasel KJ, Weigelt JA: Blunt thoracic aortic trauma: A cost-utility approach for injury detection. Arch Surg 131:619, 1996.
49. Oppenheimer MJ, Durant TM, Lynch P: Body position in relation to venous air embolism and the associated cardiovascular-respiratory changes. Am J Med Sci 252:362, 1953.
50. Robbs JV, Baker LW, Human RR, et al: Cervicomediastinal injuries. Arch Surg 116:663, 1981.
51. Marvisti MA, Meyer JA, Ford BE, et al: Spinal cord ischemia following operation for aortic transection. Ann Thorac Surg 42:425, 1986.
52. Laschinger JC, Cunningham JN Jr, Nathan IM, et al: Experimental and clinical assessment of the adequacy of partial bypass in maintenance of spinal cord blood flow during operations on the thoracic aorta. Ann Thorac Surg 36:417, 1983.
53. Kewalramani LS, Katta RSR: Atraumatic ischemic myelopathy. Paraplegia 19:352, 1981.
54. Olivier HF, Maher TD, Liebler GA, et al: Use of the BioMedicus centrifugal pump in traumatic tears of the thoracic aorta. Ann Vasc Surg 38:586, 1984.
55. Von Oppell UO, Thierfelder CF, Beningfield SJ, et al: Traumatic rupture of the descending thoracic aorta. S Afr Med J 19:595, 1991.
56. McCroskey BL, Moore EE, Moore FA, et al: A unified approach to the torn thoracic aorta. Am J Surg 162:473, 1991.
57. Hess PJ, Howe HR, Robicsek FR, et al: Traumatic tears of the thoracic aorta: Improved results using the Bio-Medicus pump. Ann Thorac Surg 48:6, 1989.
58. Rich NM, Spencer FC (eds): Injuries of the thoracic aorta. *In* Vascular Trauma. Philadelphia, WB Saunders, 1978, pp 425–440.
59. Antunes MJ: Acute traumatic rupture of the aorta: Repair by simple aortic cross-clamping. Ann Thorac Surg 44:257, 1987.
60. Mattox KL, Holtzman M, Pickard LR, et al: Clamp repair: A safe technique for treatment of blunt injury to the descending thoracic aorta. Ann Thorac Surg 40:456, 1985.
61. Orringer MB, Kirsh MM: Primary repair of acute traumatic aortic disruption. Ann Thorac Surg 35:672, 1982.
62. McBride LR, Tidik S, Stothert JC, et al: Primary repair of traumatic aortic disruption. Ann Thorac Surg 43:65, 1987.
63. Kouchoukos NT, Lell WA: Hemodynamic effects of aortic clamping and decompression with a temporary shunt for resection of the descending thoracic aorta. Surgery 25:58, 1983.
64. Cunningham JN, Lanschinger JC, Merking HA, et al: Measurement of spinal cord ischemia during operations upon the thoracic aorta: Initial clinical experience. Ann Surg 185:196, 1982.
65. Soots G, Warembourg H, Prat A, et al: Acute traumatic rupture of the thoracic aorta: Place of delayed surgical repair. J Cardiovasc Surg 30:173, 1989.
66. Kato N, Dake MD, Milled C, et al: Traumatic thoracic aortic aneurysm: Treatment with endovascular stent grafts. Radiology 205:657, 1997.
67. Semba CP, Kato N, Lee ST, et al: Acute rupture of the descending thoracic aorta: Repair with the use of endovascular stent-grafts. J Vasc Interv Radiol 8:337, 1997.
68. Perreault P, Soula P, Rousseau H, et al: Acute traumatic rupture of the thoracic aorta: Delayed treatment with endoluminal covered stent. A report of two cases. J Vasc Surg 27:538, 1998.
69. Dake M, Miller DC, Semba CP, et al: Transluminal placement of endovascular stent-grafts for the treatment of descending thoracic aortic aneurysms. N Engl J Med 331:1729, 1994.
70. Castagna J, Nelson RJ: Blunt injuries to branches of the aortic arch. J Thorac Cardiovasc Surg 69:521, 1975.
71. Rosenberg JM, Bredenberg CE, Marvast MA, et al: Blunt injuries to the aortic arch vessels. Ann Thorac Surg 48:508, 1989.
72. Knott-Craig CJ, Przybojewski JZ, Barbard PM: Penetrating wounds of the heart and great vessels: A new therapeutic approach. S Afr Med J 62:316, 1982.
73. Feliciano DV, Burch JM, Graham JM: Vascular injuries of the chest and abdomen. *In* Rutherford R (ed): Vascular Surgery, 3rd ed. Philadelphia, WB Saunders, 1989, p 588.
74. Vosloo SM, Reichart BA: Inflow occlusion in the surgical management of a penetrating aortic arch injury: Case report. J Trauma 30:514, 1990.
75. Liekweg WG, Greenfield LJ: Management of penetrating carotid arterial injury. Ann Surg 188:587, 1978.

76. Brown MF, Graham JM, Feliciano DV, et al: Carotid artery injuries. Am J Surg 144:748, 1982.
77. Parmley LF, Mattingly TW, Manion WC: Penetrating wounds of the heart and aorta. Circulation 17:953, 1958.
78. Graham JM, Feliciano DV, Mattox KL, et al: Innominate vascular injury. J Trauma 22:647, 1982.
79. Brown MF, Graham JM, Feliciano DV, et al: Carotid artery injuries. Am J Surg 144:748, 1982.
80. Carillo EH, Bergamini TM, Richardson JD: Abdominal vascular injuries. J Trauma 43:164, 1997.
81. Saunders MS, Riberi A, Massullo EA: Delayed traumatic superior mesenteric arteriovenous fistula after a stab wound: Case report. J Trauma 32:101, 1992.
82. Shackford SR, Sise MJ: Renal and mesenteric vascular trauma. *In* Bongard F, Wilson SE, Perry MO (eds): Vascular Injuries in Surgical Practice. Norwalk, Conn, Appleton & Lange, 1991, p 173.
83. Bickell WH, Wall MJ Jr, Pepe PE, et al: Immediate versus delayed fluid resuscitation for hypotensive patients with penetrating torso injuries. N Engl J Med 331:1105, 1994.
84. Ryan W, Snyder W, Bell T, et al: Penetrating injuries of the iliac vessels and management. Am J Surg 5:144, 1982.
85. Degiannis E, Velmahos GC, Levy RD, et al: Penetrating injuries of the iliac arteries: A South African experience. Surgery 119:146, 1996.
86. Lim RC, Miller SE: Management of acute civilian vascular injuries. Surg Clin North Am 62:113, 1982.
87. Holcroft JW: Abdominal arterial trauma. *In* Blaisdell FW, Trunkey DT (eds): Trauma Management. Vol I. Abdominal Trauma. New York, Thieme-Stratton, 1982, p 253.
88. Cass AS, Bubrick M, Luxenberg M, et al: Renal pedicle injury in patients with multiple injuries. J Trauma 25:892, 1985.
89. Mee SL, McAninch JW, Robinson AL, et al: Radiographic assessment of renal trauma: A 10 year prospective study of patient selection. J Urol 141:1095, 1989.
90. Wilson RF, Zeigler DW: Diagnostic and treatment problems in renal injuries. Am Surg 53:399, 1987.
91. Steinberg DL, Jeffrey RB, Federle MP, et al: The computerized tomography appearance of renal pedicle injury. J Urol 132:1163, 1984.
92. Lang EK, Sullivan J, Frentz G: Renal trauma: Radiologic studies. Radiology 15:1, 1985.
93. Richardson JD, Bergamini TM, Spain DA, et al: Operative strategies for management of abdominal aortic gunshot wounds. Surgery 120:667, 1996.
94. Rotondo MF, Schwab CW, McGonigal MD, et al: "Damage control": An approach for improved survival in penetrating abdominal injury. J Trauma 35:375, 1993.
95. Gentilello LM, Jurkovich GJ: Autotransfusion. *In* Ivatury RR, Cayten CG (eds): The Textbook of Penetrating Trauma. Baltimore, Williams & Wilkins; 1996, p 1007.
96. Talhouk AS, Lim RC, Bongard FS: Abdominal aortic injuries. *In* Bongard F, Wilson SE, Perry MO (eds): Vascular Injuries in Surgical Practice. Norwalk, Conn, Appleton & Lange, 1991, p 165.
97. Accola KD, Feliciano DV, Mattox KL, et al: Management of injuries to the suprarenal aorta. Am J Surg 154:613, 1987.
98. Brinton M, Miller SE, Lim RC, et al: Acute abdominal aortic injuries. J Trauma 22:481, 1982.
99. Mattox KL, McCollum WB, Beall AC, et al: Management of penetrating injuries of the suprarenal aorta. J Trauma 15:808, 1975.
100. Fry WR, Fry RE, Fry WJ: Operative exposure of the abdominal arteries for trauma. Arch Surg 126:289, 1991.
101. Stone HH, Oxford WM, Austin JT: Penetrating wounds of the abdominal aorta. World J Surg 66:1352, 1973.
102. Feliciano DV, Burch JM, Graham JM, et al: Abdominal vascular injury. *In* Mattox KL, Moore EE, Feliciano DV (eds): Trauma. Norwalk, Conn, Appleton-Century-Crofts, 1987, p 519.
103. Feliciano DV, Burch JM, Graham JM: Abdominal vascular injury. *In* Moore EE, Mattox KL, Feliciano DV (eds): Trauma, 2nd ed. Norwalk, Conn, Appleton & Lange, 1991, p 523.
104. Lassonde J, Laurendeau F: Blunt injury of the abdominal aorta. Ann Surg 194:745, 1981.
105. Klein SR, Mehringer CM, Bongard FS: Endovascular occlusive intervention in the management of trauma. Ann Vasc Surg 4:424, 1990.
106. Salam AA, Stewart MT: New approach to wounds of the aortic bifurcation and inferior vena cava. Surgery 98:105, 1985.
107. Feliciano DV, Burch JM, Graham JM. Abdominal vascular injury. *In* Feliciano DV, Moore EE, Mattox KL (eds): Trauma, 3rd ed. Norwalk, Conn, Appleton & Lange, 1996, p 615.
108. Burch JM, Richardson RJ, Martin RR, et al: Penetrating iliac vascular injuries: Recent experience with 233 consecutive patients. J Trauma 30:1450, 1989.
109. Carillo EH, Spain DA, Wilson MA, et al: Alternatives in the management of penetrating injuries to the iliac vessels. J Trauma 44:1024, 1998.
110. Landreneau RJ, Lewis DM, Snyder WH: Complex iliac arterial trauma: Autologous or prosthetic vascular repair? Surgery 114:9, 1993.
111. Pourmoghadam KK, Fogler RJ, Shaftan GW: Ligation: An alternative for control of exsanguination in major vascular injuries. J Trauma 43:126, 1997.
112. Coselli JS, Crawford ES, Williams TW, et al: Treatment of postoperative infection of ascending aorta and transverse aortic arch, including use of viable omentum and muscle flaps. Ann Thorac Surg 50:868, 1990.
113. Courcy PA, Brotman S, Oster-Granite NL, et al: Superior mesenteric vein injuries from blunt abdominal trauma. J Trauma 18:419, 1978.
114. Fullen WD, Hunt J, Altemeier WA: The clinical spectrum of penetrating injury to the superior mesenteric arterial circulation. J Trauma 12:656, 1978.
115. Conti S: Abdominal venous trauma. *In* Blaisdell FW, Trunkey DD (eds): Trauma Management. Vol I. Abdominal Trauma. New York, Thieme-Stratton, 1982, p 253.
116. Atala A, Miller FB, Richardson JD, et al: Preliminary vascular control for renal trauma. Surg Gynecol Obstet 22:223, 1991.
117. Lohse JR, Shore RM, Belzer FO: Acute renal artery occlusion. Arch Surg 117:801, 1982.
118. Maggio AJ, Brosman S: Renal artery trauma. Urology II:125, 1978.
119. State DL, Bongard FS: Abdominal venous injuries. *In* Bongard FS, Wilson SE, Perry MO (eds): Vascular Injuries in Surgical Practice. Norwalk, Conn, Appleton & Lange, 1991, p 185.
120. Lau JM, Mattox KL, Beall AC, et al: Use of substitute conduits in traumatic vascular surgery. J Trauma 23:207, 1983.
121. Johnson V, Eiseman B: Evaluation of arteriovenous shunt to obtain patency of venous autografts. Am J Surg 118:915, 1969.
122. Stewart MT, Stone HH: Injuries of the inferior vena cava. Am Surgeon 52:9, 1988.
123. Posner MC, Moore EE, Greenholz SL, et al: Natural history of untreated inferior vena cava injury and assessment of venous access. J Trauma 26:698, 1986.
124. Burch JM, Feliciano DV, Mattox KL, et al: Injuries of the inferior vena cava. Am J Surg 158:548, 1988.
125. Pachter HL, Spencer FC, Hofstetter S, et al: The management of juxtahepatic venous injuries without an atriocaval shunt: Preliminary clinical observations. Surgery 99:569, 1986.
126. Nance F: Comments. *In* Wieneck RG, Wilson RF (eds): Inferior vena cava injuries: The challenge continues. Am Surg 54:423, 1988.
127. Beall SL, Wards RE: Successful atrial caval shunting in the management of retrohepatic venous injuries. Am J Surg 158:409, 1988.
128. Mattox KL: Abdominal venous injuries. Surgery 91:497, 1982.
129. Kashuk JL, Moore EE, Millikan JS, et al: Major abdominal vascular trauma: A unified approach. J Trauma 18:672, 1978.
130. Millikan JS, Moore EE: Critical factors in determining mortality from abdominal aortic trauma. Surg Gynecol Obstet 160:313, 1985.
131. Buchness MP, LoGerfo FW, Mason GR: Gunshot wounds of the suprarenal abdominal aorta. Ann Surg 42:1, 1976.
132. Soldano SL, Rich NM, Collins GJ, et al: Long-term follow-up of penetrating abdominal aortic injuries after 15 years. J Trauma 28:1358, 1988.
133. Millikan JS, Moore EE, Van Way CW III, et al: Vascular trauma in the groin: Contrast between iliac and femoral injuries. Am J Surg 142:695, 1981.
134. Sirinek KR, Gaskill HV III, Root HD, et al: Truncal vascular injury: Factors influencing survival. J Trauma 23:372, 1983.
135. Cushman JG, Feliciano DV, Renz BM, et al: Iliac vessel injury: Operative physiology related to outcome. J Trauma 42:1033, 1997.
136. Kudsk KA, Bongard F, Lim RC Jr: Determinants of survival after vena caval injury: Analysis of a 14-year experience. Arch Surg 119:1009, 1984.

CHAPTER 61

Cervicothoracic Vascular Injuries

Jeffrey L. Ballard, M.D., and W. Burley McIntyre, M.D.

Arterial and venous trauma to the cervicothoracic region continues to present challenging problems for the surgeon despite advances in vascular diagnostics and surgical technique. Whether these injuries are due to penetrating or blunt mechanisms, the overall incidence is low, whereas morbidity and mortality rates remain high. While the collective experience with cervicothoracic vascular trauma from busy trauma centers has increased, controversies persist about diagnostic evaluation, operative approach, and surgical treatment of these potentially devastating injuries.

Several excellent reviews of this topic have been published.[1–6] Therefore, the primary focus of this chapter is recent advances and controversies surrounding the treatment of cervicothoracic vascular trauma. Pros and cons of duplex ultrasonography (DUS) and angiography in the diagnosis of carotid and vertebral artery injuries are highlighted, and selective (versus mandatory) neck exploration for zone II penetrating injuries is discussed. The importance of increased awareness of blunt carotid artery injury is also emphasized, including management dilemmas frequently associated with it. In addition, this chapter reviews the use of endovascular techniques for management of cervicothoracic vascular injury.

PENETRATING CAROTID ARTERY TRAUMA

Epidemiology

Most penetrating carotid artery trauma results from stab wounds or low-velocity missiles. Victims are generally young, otherwise healthy males who are often under the influence of drugs or alcohol. Carotid artery injuries are coincident to approximately 6% of penetrating neck injuries and account for 22% of all cervical vascular injuries.[5] The common carotid artery is involved more frequently than the internal carotid. Iatrogenic carotid artery injury occurs occasionally during attempts at central venous catheter insertion. Although exact figures are not known, jugular venous injury not infrequently accompanies penetrating carotid artery trauma.

Diagnostic Evaluation

Little controversy exists with regard to the management of the 8% to 25% of patients who present with "hard" signs of vascular injury such as shock, active bleeding, and expanding hematoma. These signs should prompt expeditious transport of the patient to the operating room for stabilization and operative exploration. Penetrating injuries that do not traverse the platysma require no further vascular evaluation; however, controversy surrounds that majority of patients who present with "soft" signs of vascular injury (i.e., history of pulsatile bleeding; small, stable hematoma; cranial nerve injury) or no signs at all but a "proximity" injury.

In 1969, Monson and colleagues proposed the now well-known division of the neck into three anatomic zones.[7] Zone I extends from the sternal notch to 1 cm above the clavicular head; zone II, from 1 cm above the clavicular head to the angle of the mandible; and zone III, from the angle of the mandible to the base of the skull. In the intervening years, it has become generally agreed that stable patients with penetrating zone I and III injuries should be evaluated by arteriography, with selective intervention based on angiographic findings. On the other hand, considerable debate has surrounded the management of penetrating zone II injuries, with strong proponents of either *mandatory* or *selective* operative exploration based on routine angiography. Recent data have demonstrated that DUS may be a substitute for "routine" arteriography of these zone II injuries. Finally, good results have been obtained with diagnostic evaluation of penetrating neck trauma even with physical examination alone.

The largest recent experience that favors mandatory neck exploration was published in 1994 by Apffelstaedt and Muller from South Africa.[8] Over a 20-month period they prospectively explored a remarkable series of 393 consecutive patients whose stab wounds penetrated the platysma in zones I, II, or III. Clinical signs of vascular trauma were absent in 30% of patients whose neck exploration was "positive" and in 58% of those who had "negative" explorations. Overall, the negative exploration rate was 57%. Morbidity and mortality rates for negative explorations were 2.2% and zero, respectively, and length of hospital stay averaged 1½ days. These authors, and others, have cited the unreliability of physical signs for predicting cervical vascular injury.

Those who favor mandatory neck exploration for zone II injuries emphasize that currently available diagnostic studies have variable false-positive and false-negative rates in demonstrating significant cervicothoracic vascular injury. In addition, minimized use of expensive personnel and equipment and overall low morbidity and mortality are cited as advantages of mandatory exploration over a selective approach based on screening diagnostic studies. Detractors point primarily to the high rates (40% to 60%) of negative explorations associated with this approach.[2] In fact, in an extensive review of the literature on this controversy, Asensio and coworkers[9] concluded that neither the mandatory nor the selective approach is clearly superior.

In lieu of mandatory exploration for zone II injuries, routine four-vessel carotid-vertebral arteriography has been proposed. In Demetriades' prospective series of 176 hemodynamically stable patients who underwent arteriography, 19% demonstrated a vascular injury[10]; however, only 8% of these injuries warranted surgical intervention based on the angiographic findings, and all were symptomatic. No nontherapeutic operations were required. These results essentially corroborate those of previous studies, which suggest a low yield for arteriography in asymptomatic patients.[11, 12] Clearly, routine arteriography consumes significant resources; furthermore, some patients are subjected unnecessarily to an invasive procedure and its attendant risks.[13, 14]

The cost and risk of arteriography have fueled the growth of alternative imaging techniques such as DUS, a modality that has proved to be quite accurate in the detection of arterial occlusive disease, particularly in the carotid distribution.[13] Compared with carotid arteriography, it is inexpensive and completely noninvasive.[14] Recent work has focused on the utility of this imaging modality for evaluating cervical vascular trauma.

Fry and colleagues[15] conducted a prospective evaluation of 100 consecutive patients with cervical trauma (89% penetrating, 11% blunt) who had no indication for immediate surgical exploration. The first 15 patients underwent DUS followed by arteriography, and the remaining 85 had arteriography only when ultrasonography suggested an injury. In the first phase of the study, the one arterial injury identified by DUS was confirmed by arteriography. In the second phase, seven arterial injuries were identified by DUS, and all were confirmed by arteriography or operative exploration. Two internal jugular vein injuries were suggested by DUS but were not investigated by venography or operation. The remaining 76 patients without vascular injury shown by DUS remained asymptomatic at 1 week follow-up. The authors noted savings of $1200 per study for DUS over angiography.

Demetriades and associates[16] prospectively evaluated, with both arteriography and DUS, 82 stable trauma patients with penetrating cervical trauma (zones I to III) who had no indication for immediate exploration. Eleven patients (13.4%) had arterial injuries that were identified by arteriography, but only two (2.4%) required operative intervention. DUS correctly identified 10 of 11 injuries, including both of those that required operative repair. Ginzburg and colleagues obtained virtually identical results using a similar protocol.[17] Thus, all three studies concluded that DUS might be a suitable substitute for arteriography as an initial screening test for penetrating cervical trauma that does not warrant immediate surgical exploration. In addition, these authors suggest that, if DUS were the sole diagnostic modality, substantial cost savings—and no decrease in overall accuracy—might result.

Although both arteriography and DUS appear to have excellent diagnostic accuracy, it is apparent that their therapeutic yield is quite low. That is, among patients with soft or absent signs of carotid trauma, the number of vascular injuries that require operative intervention is small. Thus, some propose managing this subgroup only by observation and serial physical examinations.

The primary advocates of this approach have been Frykberg and colleagues in Jacksonville, Florida. In a retrospective review of 110 patients with penetrating zone II injuries (through platysma),[12] 42 whose physical examinations were normal and who had no proximity injuries were observed without further workup. Forty-five other patients with soft signs of a vascular or proximity injury underwent arteriography. Long-term follow-up of 29 (70%) patients who were solely observed demonstrated no missed or late injuries. For the 45 patients studied by arteriography, 27 studies were negative, eight showed injury to noncritical vessels (e.g., branches of external carotid artery), and 10 demonstrated involvement of a major vessel. Only one of those major vascular injuries required surgical intervention, however. The other eight noncritical vessel and nine major vessel injuries were successfully observed without adverse sequelae. The authors concluded that the missed injury rate with physical examination alone was 0.9% (1 of 110).

In a subsequent prospective study of 53 consecutive patients with penetrating zone II injuries, 17 had definite signs of vascular trauma and underwent immediate exploration; two more required operative repair of aerodigestive tract injury, but no vascular disruption was found.[18] Of the remaining 34 patients considered candidates for observation alone, six had arteriograms (all negative). The remainder, who were observed, exhibited no delayed signs of vascular injury at follow-up (mean 1.8 months).[18] A diagnostic approach based on physical examination alone requires extensive experience and the ability to perform careful serial clinical examinations. An obvious concern is the potentially devastating result of missing a significant injury.

It is apparent that good results can be obtained with mandatory exploration, routine arteriography or DUS, or physical examination alone in properly selected patients. Ultimately, the approach adopted should be based on experience, volume, local diagnostic capabilities, and personnel resources. Current opinion supports immediate exploration of all injuries associated with hard signs of vascular trauma (active bleeding, large or expanding hematoma, neurologic deficit, or bruit), while penetrating injuries with soft signs (history of bleeding, small, stable hematoma, or cranial nerve deficit) or a worrisome mechanism (e.g., shotgun blast [Fig. 61–1] or severe direct blunt injury) should be screened by DUS or arteriography, depending on local availability and expertise. Observation for certain penetrating cervical injuries in the context of normal physical findings is appropriate if the patient can be followed closely with serial examinations.

Operative Approach

An oblique incision parallel to the anterior border of the sternocleidomastoid muscle facilitates exposure of the cervical carotid artery. It also affords exploration of nonvascular structures in the neck. It is crucial to prepare and drape the entire chest against the possibility that median sternotomy would be necessary to achieve proximal control of the innominate or either common carotid artery. In fact, for zone I injuries it may be prudent to perform median sternotomy initially or as part of the neck incision. Expo-

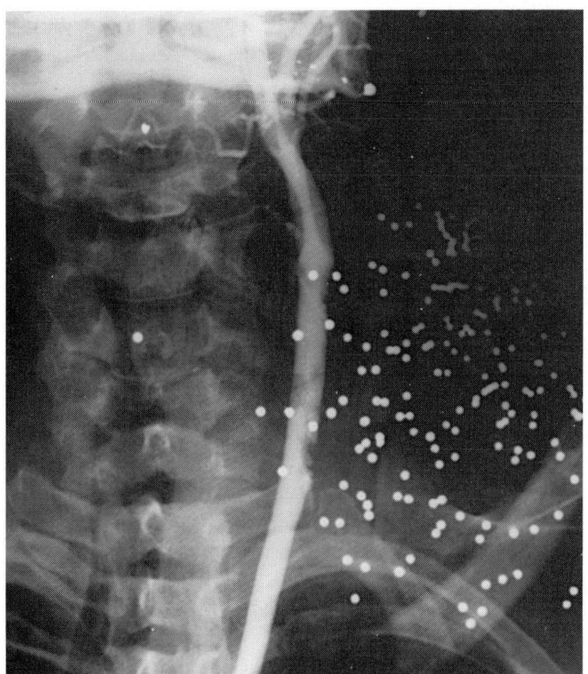

FIGURE 61–1. Shotgun blast injury of left common carotid artery with multiple nonbleeding punctures and mural thrombus.

sure of high zone III injuries can be especially difficult. Maneuvers that have been employed to facilitate this exposure include division of the posterior belly of the digastric muscle, subluxation of the mandible, and mandibular ramus osteotomy.[19] Profuse bleeding near the skull base may be best controlled temporarily with a Fogarty balloon catheter inserted into the injured vessel.[5]

Surgical Management

For significant penetrating carotid artery injuries without concurrent central neurologic deficit, there is fairly universal agreement that all such lesions should be repaired. Available methods include primary repair, patch angioplasty, internal-to-external carotid artery transposition, and interposition grafting with saphenous vein or prosthetic conduit.

Debate persists, however, about treatment of neurologically asymptomatic patients with occlusion of the carotid artery. Concerns about distal embolization during carotid repair are unfounded, although Fry and Fry warn that distal propagation of thrombus might result in delayed neurologic deficit if no repair is made.[20] Recent reports suggest that repair should be performed when it is technically feasible and when retrograde arterial back-flow can be established. This approach has resulted in very little morbidity.[21–23] Restoration of retrograde internal carotid artery (ICA) back-flow by any means other than gentle manual extraction of thrombus (e.g., by passage of an embolectomy catheter) should be performed with great caution to avoid creating a carotid–cavernous sinus fistula. Passing the embolectomy catheter only to the level of the skull base should avoid this serious complication. When potential arterial repair is not technically feasible or ICA back-bleeding cannot easily be established, ligation or subsequent transcatheter balloon occlusion can be performed. The rate of associated subsequent neurologic deficits ranges from zero to 50%.[21, 23] In this difficult situation, some authors have advocated the addition of anticoagulation to prevent thrombus propagation.[21]

Controversy surrounding management of carotid injuries associated with neurologic deficit (including coma) has resulted principally from anecdotal reports of conversion of ischemic infarction to hemorrhagic infarction after revascularization.[2] Despite this concern, all available recent evidence suggests that optimal neurologic outcomes are obtained with operative repair, as most deficits remain unchanged or improve.[2, 5, 6, 21–23] Even patients who are comatose appear to fare best with repair. In collected series, 28 comatose patients treated with carotid ligation had a 61% mortality rate, and only 14% had a normal outcome, whereas 42 comatose patients who had operative repair had a mortality rate of 26%, and 50% were neurologically normal or much improved after arterial reconstruction.[2] Although such results may reflect a certain treatment selection bias based on hemodynamic or other factors, it is crucial to recall that it is not always possible to discern preoperatively which patients have been rendered comatose by shock, alcohol, or drugs as opposed to cerebral ischemia.

Finally, questions about the management of minor carotid artery injury (small intimal defects or small pseudoaneurysms) have arisen. Nonoperative management, at least in neurologically intact patients, appears to be safe[5, 12, 16, 21]; however, long-term follow-up, critical to this approach, is not available and is often difficult to achieve in this patient population.

Most authorities recommend repairing all significant penetrating carotid artery injuries when technically feasible and in almost every circumstance, and reserving ligation or balloon occlusion for critically unstable patients or inaccessible lesions. Anticoagulation, alone or as an adjunct to ligation, should be considered for traumatic distal ICA occlusion in neurologically intact patients. Finally, it may be safe to observe small intimal lesions in neurologically normal patients, but serial carotid DUS examination and close clinical follow-up also seem mandatory.

Outcome

Determining outcome related to penetrating carotid artery injury, as distinct from penetrating cervical trauma, is somewhat difficult, as few studies specifically address the former. Mortality rates of 5% to 20% have been reported.[2] In one retrospective review of identified penetrating carotid artery injuries, there was an overall mortality rate of 17% and a stroke rate of 28%.[23] Mortality rates in this population were significantly higher in the presence of coma or shock (50% and 41%, respectively). Primary determinants of morbidity and survival are severity and duration of shock and neurologic deficit on presentation. Unfortunately, these are factors over which the surgeon has little control.

BLUNT CAROTID ARTERY TRAUMA

Epidemiology

Blunt carotid artery disruption accounts for about 3% to 10% of all carotid injuries.[2, 24–32] Four mechanisms of injury

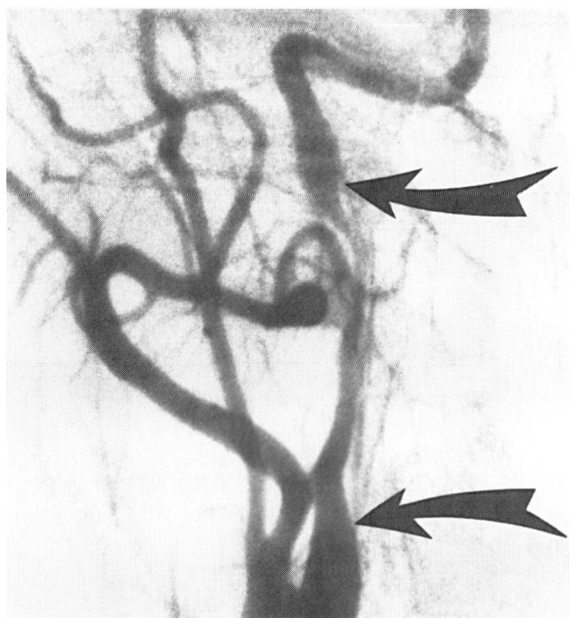

FIGURE 61–2. Left carotid artery dissection *(between arrows)* sustained during a motor vehicle accident.

are recognized: cervical hyperextension/rotation (most common), direct blow to the neck, intraoral trauma, and basilar skull fracture. Injury can result in dissection (Fig. 61–2), thrombosis, pseudoaneurysm formation (Fig. 61–3), carotid–cavernous sinus fistula, or complete arterial disruption.[2] More than 90% of blunt injuries involve the internal carotid artery, often distally, rather than the common carotid artery. Bilateral injury has been reported in 20% to 50% of cases.[24–32] Overall incidence of carotid artery injury in blunt trauma has been variously reported as 0.08% to 0.33%, and as many as half of affected patients show no signs of cervical trauma or neurologic deficit at presentation.[24–32] The low incidence, anatomic site, and variable presentation have made the determination of optimal diagnostic and management strategies difficult. No prospective studies exist.

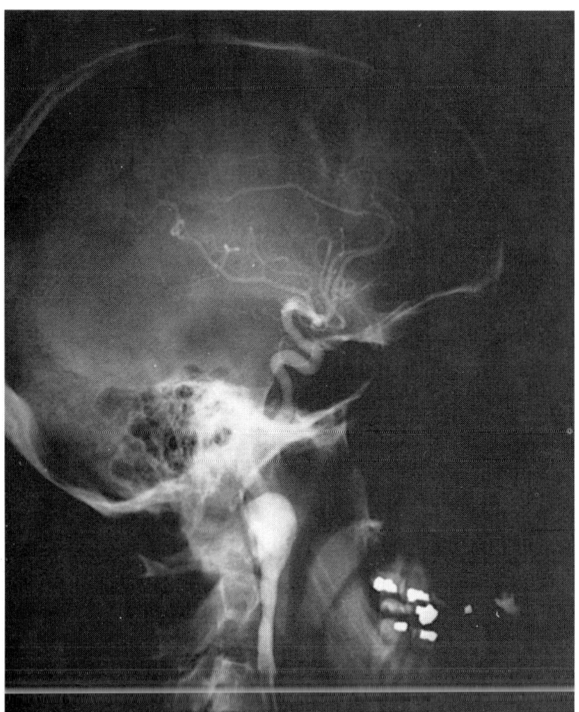

FIGURE 61–3. Large right distal internal carotid artery pseudoaneurysm associated with dissection after direct blunt neck trauma.

Diagnosis

Recognition of these injuries appears to have increased over time, most likely owing to heightened awareness of the problem. Fabian and coworkers[30] noted 96 cases reported up to 1980, 75 cases during the next 10 years, and 309 cases in the subsequent 5 years (1990–1995). This significant increase in diagnosis of injuries probably is not a result of an increase in blunt carotid artery trauma. Nevertheless, even the largest series accumulated fewer than 70 patients over 11 years, and a 6-year multi-institution review involving 11 major trauma centers reported on only 60 blunt carotid artery injuries in 49 patients.[27, 30]

The difficulty in diagnosis is related to the fact that many of these patients present with significant associated intracranial lesions or ethanol or drug intoxication. Others whose neurologic examination is completely normal exhibit delayed (hours to years) development of focal neurologic deficits. In Cogbill's multicenter study of blunt carotid artery trauma, 37% of patients presented with a Glasgow Coma Scale (GCS) score less than 8, whereas 49% had an essentially normal initial neurologic examination (GCS > 12) on admission.[27] More than half of those admitted with a GCS score above 12 developed significant deficits more than 12 hours later.[27] Another recent review of 20 patients found that 47% initially had normal neurologic examination findings and nearly 60% of those who presented without focal deficits subsequently developed them during their admission.[31] Even Fabian and associates,[30] who demonstrated the highest incidence of carotid artery injury in blunt trauma (0.33%), found that 43% of their patients were not diagnosed until a neurologic deficit developed subsequent to the initial presentation. In addition, there was an average delay of 53 hours from injury to definitive diagnosis. Thus, it appears to be the rare patient who presents with specific signs of blunt carotid artery injury or whose problem is diagnosed before neurologic deficits are manifested. This is unfortunate, as early diagnosis is associated with improved outcome.[28–32]

At this time, broad screening does not appear to be practical, particularly given the overall low incidence of significant blunt carotid artery injury, even in high-risk patients with cervicocranial trauma. Routine arteriography clearly is not cost-effective and certainly is not without risk. Although a number of studies demonstrate a role for noninvasive diagnostic studies for penetrating cervical trauma, there is much less experience with DUS in the evaluation of blunt trauma. The most common site of blunt carotid injuries, the distal ICA, is difficult to visualize with DUS.[30] A prospective trial would need to be performed to adequately evaluate the efficacy of DUS expressly for blunt trauma before it could be recommended as a routine screening tool. Similarly, magnetic resonance imaging (MRI) or magnetic resonance angiography (MRA) and transcranial Doppler ultrasonography have not been studied for this application.

Patients presenting with or developing neurologic deficits whose cerebral computed tomographic (CT) scans are normal or do not account for the deficit should undergo further definitive diagnostic evaluation. Additional significant clinical findings include severe cervical soft tissue injury (e.g., contusion, hematoma, bruit), neurologic deficit in a lucid patient, any cranial nerve deficit or Horner's syndrome, and a history of a specific "high-risk" mechanism of injury (e.g., direct cervical blow, significant whiplash). Certain injury patterns (combined head, neck, and chest trauma) also appear to be more frequently associated with blunt carotid injury.[31] Clearly, maintenance of a high index of suspicion is paramount when one is evaluating blunt trauma patients.

Management

Appropriate management of blunt carotid trauma depends on the specific injury and its anatomic site.[2] There is almost universal agreement that carotid–cavernous sinus fistulae should be managed by balloon occlusion techniques, results of which are generally fair to good.[27–31] Conversely, all recently described cases of complete arterial disruption have been fatal.[27, 31] Management of dissection, thrombosis, and pseudoaneurysm, alone or in combination, has been controversial and appears to be evolving.

Older data suggest better outcomes with surgical than with nonsurgical management of dissection and thrombosis.[28] It has become apparent, however, that many of these lesions extend to or beyond the skull base and thus are not amenable to straightforward vascular surgical repair. In addition, it is believed that the majority of neurologic sequelae of these injuries may be related to acute thrombosis, thrombus propagation, or distal embolization. Therefore, surgical reconstruction may be irrelevant. Thus, there is growing support for nonsurgical management of dissections and thromboses—initial systemic heparinization followed by 3 to 6 months of Coumadin therapy.[27–31]

In the largest series to date, Fabian and associates[30] demonstrated significant improvement in clinical outcomes when anticoagulation was instituted for patients who had either minor or major neurologic deficits at the time of diagnosis. In addition, none of the 15 patients who presented with unilateral symptoms but were found to have bilateral injuries developed symptoms referrable to the contralateral injury after heparin therapy was instituted. Parikh and Li and their groups have also suggested improvement of outcomes with anticoagulation alone.[28, 31]

Interestingly, Fabian and coworkers[30] demonstrated that with nonoperative treatment 62% of carotid dissections reverted to normal and 29% progressed to pseudoaneurysms on follow-up angiography. Most thrombosed vessels remained so. Other investigators have documented progression of post-traumatic ICA dissections to severe stenosis over time.[24] Clearly, these injuries should be followed serially with an objective test such as DUS or angiography; MRI/MRA may be useful here. Complications related to anticoagulation range from 13% to 33%, and this mode of treatment may be relatively contraindicated for some trauma patients.[30, 31] Prospective trials comparing surgery with anticoagulation probably are not feasible.

Management of pseudoaneurysms is somewhat less controversial; most authors recommend surgical repair when it is technically feasible.[2, 27, 28, 31] Small or inaccessible pseudoaneurysms have been managed by anticoagulation and proximal ligation with and without extracranial-intracranial bypass. Not only do most ICA pseudoaneurysms fail to resolve spontaneously, but, as noted above, there is evidence that pseudoaneurysms can develop in vessels that initially are found to have only dissection.[30] This observation underscores the need for long-term follow-up of all patients with blunt carotid artery trauma.

In contradistinction to penetrating carotid artery trauma, most authors advocate anticoagulation for the majority of blunt carotid artery dissections or thromboses, operative repair being reserved principally for easily accessible lesions. It is important to follow these patients over the long term for subsequent development of complications, particularly pseudoaneurysms. Pseudoaneurysms should be treated initially with heparin but ultimately should be repaired when technically feasible. Small or inaccessible lesions should be treated with anticoagulation alone. Occasional patients require novel repairs such as extracranial-intracranial bypass or cervical-petrous ICA bypass.[24]

Outcome

In general, the prognosis of blunt carotid artery injury is poor. Recent reports have demonstrated mortality rates of 5% to 43%, with good neurologic outcomes in only 20% to 63% of survivors.[27–31] These authors tend to advocate anticoagulation alone as the primary mode of treatment. Although there is some evidence that anticoagulation therapy improves results, outcome is probably related more closely to diagnostic delay. Emphasis should be placed on maintaining a high index of suspicion for blunt carotid artery injury and on aggressive evaluation of these patients, as a missed or delayed diagnosis can have devastating consequences.

VERTEBRAL ARTERY TRAUMA

Epidemiology

Historically, penetrating or blunt traumatic injury of the vertebral arteries has been exceedingly rare. Several authors have suggested that increased use of diagnostic four-vessel angiography for craniocervical trauma has increased the frequency of diagnosis.[3, 5, 6] That stated, the largest reported series in the literature comprises only 43 patients.[33] Management decisions are complicated both by the anatomic site of the vessel and the relatively few adverse sequelae of its injury.

The clinical presentation and ultimate outcome of vertebral artery trauma are related primarily to associated injuries rather than to the specific arterial lesion itself. Reid and Weigelt found that 32 (72%) of 43 patients with penetrating vertebral artery injuries had no evidence of arterial trauma on physical examination.[33] Furthermore, 38 (88%) of 43 patients had a normal GCS score on presentation, and none presented with or subsequently exhibited vertebrobasilar insufficiency. Similarly, Yee and associates[34] found that 12 (75%) of 16 patients presented with a normal GCS score. In that series, 75% of the 16 neurologic deficits were attributed to associated cervical spinal root or cord injuries or intracranial lesions. Again, no patient showed evidence of vertebrobasilar insufficiency during follow-up.

Although there is substantial anatomic variability in the posterior circulation, Thomas has shown that, with unilateral vertebral artery ligation, the incidence of brain stem ischemia is very low—3.1% for the left artery and 1.8% for the right.[35] Thus, there is general agreement that most injuries to the vertebral artery, including arteriovenous fistulae and pseudoaneurysms, should be managed by proximal and distal artery occlusion.[3, 5, 6, 33, 34] However, controversy surrounds how best to achieve this goal, whether by surgical ligation or by endovascular transcatheter embolization. Arterial repair is reserved for the exceedingly rare circumstance when preoperative arteriography suggests inadequate collateral circulation.[3, 5, 6, 33, 34]

Operative Approach

Surgical exposure of the vertebral artery has been well described.[3, 34, 36] The cervical vertebral artery can be approached anteriorly, as Landreneau's group proposed[37]; however, for proximal injuries the vessel is best approached via a supraclavicular incision centered over the lateral head of the sternocleidomastoid muscle. Extensile exposure can be obtained both proximally and distally by gently curving the medial aspect of this incision upward, along the anterior border of the sternocleidomastoid muscle, or downward, in preparation for median sternotomy. After transverse division of the platysma muscle and the lateral head of the sternocleidomastoid muscle, the omohyoid muscle is divided and the scalene fat pad elevated. The anterior scalene muscle can be divided under direct vision with scissors, care being taken to protect the phrenic nerve, which courses on top of this muscle. This exposure affords excellent access to the subclavian artery and the proximal vertebral artery.

Exposure of the distal vertebral artery is obtained at the level of C1–2 by transection of the sternocleidomastoid muscle at the mastoid to allow palpation of the transverse process of C1. Care must be taken to spare the spinal accessory nerve. The prevertebral fascia, levator scapulae muscle, and tendon of the splenius cervicis muscle are divided to expose the intertransverse space between C1 and C2 where the artery lies. Direct approaches to the interosseous portion of the vertebral artery are available, but they are risky because of the significant dangers of bleeding from surrounding veins and injury to adjacent nerve roots. Persistent bleeding from the vertebral artery in this area has been controlled with hemostatic agents, placement of packs, or balloon catheter occlusion of the distal vessel through a proximal arteriotomy.[3]

Surgical Management

Proponents of surgical ligation of the vertebral arteries cite the findings of Reid and Weigelt in their series of 43 patients with penetrating vertebral artery injury.[33] Although these authors found that arteriography had accuracy of 97% for diagnosing vertebral artery injuries, only 50% of patients' operative findings correlated with the angiographic diagnosis. In particular, a significant number of "angiographic occlusions" were found at operation to be arterial disruptions. In addition, two of 13 patients initially treated with proximal ligation alone required reoperation for distal ligation, whereas none of 28 patients treated initially with proximal and distal ligation required further intervention.

Conversely, the literature describes the use of transcatheter embolization for management of arteriovenous fistulae, pseudoaneurysms, and occlusions.[10, 34, 38, 39] Coil embolization proximal and distal to the injury site has provided satisfactory control of arteriovenous fistulae and pseudoaneurysms (Figs. 61–4 and 61–5). As technology has advanced and experience has increased, successful artery-sparing techniques have been developed for both arteriovenous fistulae and pseudoaneurysms. Beaujeux and coworkers[38] demonstrated occlusion of arteriovenous fistulae with vertebral artery preservation in 32 (91%) of 35 patients. Selected pseudoaneurysms have been managed similarly.[39]

Management of traumatic vertebral artery occlusion is less clear-cut, particularly in light of the older work of Thomas[35] and the intraoperative findings of Reid and Weigelt.[33] Because such lesions frequently are actually arterial disruptions, concerns about rebleeding persist. Although it is possible to perform retrograde embolization via the contralateral vertebral artery, this procedure is technically demanding. Conversely, Yee and Demetriades and

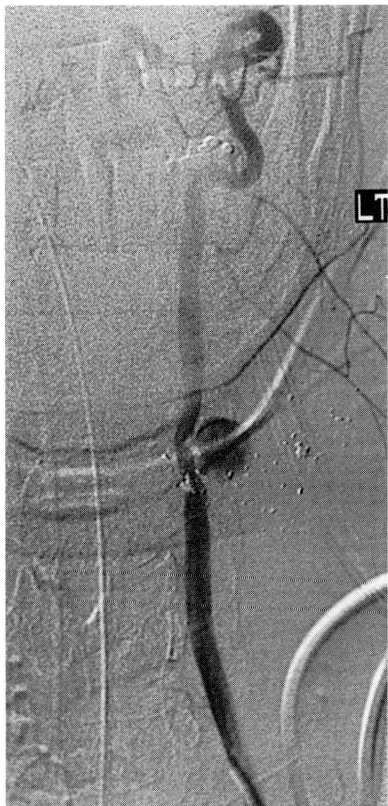

FIGURE 61–4. Gunshot injury of left vertebral artery with pseudoaneurysm. This injury was originally packed during operative exploration and a concomitant internal carotid artery injury was repaired primarily.

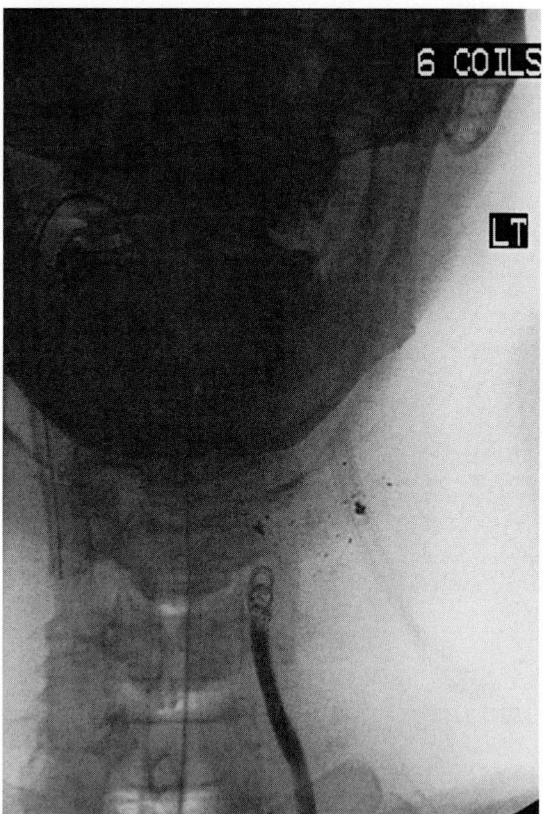

FIGURE 61–5. Successful coil embolization of left vertebral artery injury.

their respective coworkers have successfully observed vertebral artery occlusions without apparent adverse sequelae such as rebleeding or pseudoaneurysm formation, although follow-up is limited.[10, 34]

The current literature thus appears to support operative proximal and distal ligation for hemodynamically unstable patients who require immediate intervention for exsanguinating hemorrhage. "Stable" patients found to have a pseudoaneurysm or arteriovenous fistula should be treated with artery-sparing or occluding transcatheter embolization when available. Patients with vertebral artery occlusion can probably be observed, although proximal and distal transcatheter embolization is not unreasonable, based on the assumption that some arterial occlusions may in fact be complete disruptions. In either case, follow-up with angiography is recommended.

AORTIC ARCH AND GREAT VESSEL TRAUMA

Epidemiology

Arterial trauma to the aortic arch and great vessels is uncommon. Although occasional blunt injuries have been reported (excluding the relatively common proximal descending aortic transection or tear following deceleration trauma), the cause is usually a penetrating injury. These major arterial injuries present particularly challenging problems for surgeons. Management may be complicated by the patient's deteriorating or unstable hemodynamic status, and operative exposure can be difficult. In addition, rates of significant associated injuries to the aerodigestive systems, the lungs and pleura, and the brachial plexus are as high as 80%. Active trauma centers report seemingly low in-hospital mortality rates between 5% and 30%; however, "prehospital" mortality has been estimated to be as high as 48%.[40]

Evaluation

Initial evaluation and management should be based on the Advanced Trauma Life Support (ATLS) protocol. For patients who present in cardiac arrest, one should consider signs of life and vital signs at the scene and in transit when deciding whether to perform resuscitative emergency department (ED) thoracotomy.[41] Johnston and coworkers[42] demonstrated 100% mortality in patients with innominate artery injury who required prehospital cardiopulmonary resuscitation (CPR). Similarly, Wilson and Tyburski[41] found that 32 of 33 (97%) patients who underwent ED thoracotomy died (although they did not specify which of these patients arrived asystolic and which arrested in the ED).

Patients who present in severe shock (systolic blood pressure <50 mmHg) should be transported directly to the operating room for control of hemorrhage. Those in mild to moderate shock (systolic blood pressure between 50 and 90 mmHg) should be rapidly resuscitated concurrent with adjunctive studies such as chest and cervical spine radiography. When shock is persistent or recurrent, resuscitation efforts should continue in the operating room, whereas further diagnostic studies may be pursued if the patient's condition stabilizes appropriately with resuscitation.

Arteriography is currently the gold standard for identification of aortic arch and great vessel trauma. This study should be applied to all stable patients suspected of having possible aortic arch or great vessel injuries. In particular, it should be noted that a normal peripheral pulse is not reliable for ruling out significant injury. Calhoon and colleagues found that 14 of 22 (64%) patients with great vessel injuries had normal distal pulses.[43] At aortography, unsuspected lesions may be identified, and specific localization of the vessel injury will facilitate the appropriate operative approach for achieving proximal arterial control.

Operative Exposure

Interested readers are referred to a recent review of operative exposures of the aortic arch, innominate artery, and proximal subclavian and common carotid arteries.[19] Several important points should be emphasized:

1. Although the standard right or left posterolateral thoracotomy provides excellent exposure of the hemithorax, exposure of the great vessels is limited, and the lateral decubitus position limits access to the abdomen should laparotomy be required.
2. In the setting of resuscitative left anterolateral thoracotomy, extension across the sternum to include right anterolateral thoracotomy (the so-called "clamshell" incision) can provide excellent temporary exposure of arterial structures in the anterior and superior mediastinum for the

purpose of achieving initial, and possibly definitive, control.

3. Attempting repair of zone I injuries to the subclavian or common carotid arteries through a cervical incision alone is generally discouraged, as proximal arterial control may be difficult, if not impossible.

4. Median sternotomy is the most commonly employed and best incision to provide exposure of the aortic arch and innominate artery and the origin of the *right* subclavian artery and both common carotid arteries. Exposure of the superior vena cava and brachiocephalic veins is also facilitated by this incision. This approach will *not* suffice for exposure of the proximal *left* subclavian artery.

5. Extension of the initial median sternotomy above and parallel to the clavicle or along the anterior border of the sternocleidomastoid muscle affords excellent exposure of the more distal *right* subclavian and common carotid arteries. Care should be taken to avoid the phrenic, vagus, and recurrent laryngeal nerves.

6. The origin of the *left* subclavian artery arises from the aortic arch posteriorly and, as noted, cannot be adequately exposed through a median sternotomy incision. Prompt proximal control may be obtained via an anterior left thoracotomy in the third or fourth intercostal space. Subsequent limited sternotomy with left supraclavicular extension (the "trap-door" incision) has been used, with varying success, to provide extended exposure of the left subclavian artery as it courses through the thoracic outlet.

Surgical Management

In general, all identified arterial injuries should be repaired surgically. In the rare case of exsanguinating hemorrhage from a subclavian artery injury, this vessel has been ligated without resulting in significant acute ischemia of the ipsilateral extremity.[44, 45] Depending on the vessel involved and nature of the injury, methods of repair include primary suture, resection with end-to-end anastomosis, interposition grafting, and bypass. Ideally, proximal and distal arterial control should be obtained before an overlying hematoma is entered.[41] After exposure and hemorrhage control, repair of subclavian or common carotid artery injuries is relatively straightforward, with primary suture, resection with end-to-end anastomosis, or interposition grafting, as appropriate.[42–48] Isolated common carotid artery injuries do not require shunting, because the carotid bifurcation remains patent and ipsilateral ICA flow is maintained by collateral flow through the external carotid artery. The use of prosthetic material appears safe.[42–48]

Evolution of management in this area of cervicothoracic vascular trauma has focused principally on aortic arch and innominate artery injuries. Minor aortic lacerations may be repaired with pledgeted sutures using digital control or a side-biting clamp. Intraluminal aortic pressure may be lowered temporarily—for a maximum of 1½ minutes—by inflow occlusion of the vena cava.[41] More extensive injuries requiring aortic cross-clamping demand adjunctive procedures to minimize cardiac stress and distal ischemia, particularly cerebral ischemia. Although full cardiopulmonary bypass can be utilized, it may not be available and requires full heparinization. More practical is a temporary external Y shunt from the proximal ascending aorta to each common carotid artery.[45] This technique has been modified elegantly to allow safe repair of innominate artery injuries.[42, 45] Briefly, a tube or bifurcated graft (as needed) is anastomosed end-to-side to the proximal ascending aorta under side-biting clamp control before the overlying innominate hematoma is entered. Then, with the proximal innominate clamped, end-to-end anastomosis to the distal innominate or both subclavian and common carotid arteries is performed. Subsequently, the innominate stump is oversewn. Johnston and colleagues attribute their significant decrease in mortality from innominate artery injury (from 50% in the 1960s to 11.8% in the 1980s) to the development of this technique.[42]

Outcome

Recently reported mortality rates for injuries to the great vessels have been 7% to 26%.[42–48] Mortality rates have been higher for patients who presented in shock, with central nervous system deficits, with gunshot (versus stab) wounds, or with penetrating (versus blunt) arterial injuries. Except for central nervous system deficits, morbidity is more often related to associated injuries (brachial plexus or aerodigestive systems) than to the specific arterial lesion.[42]

MAJOR VENOUS TRAUMA

Surgical Management

Major cervicothoracic venous injury can significantly complicate management and definitive vascular repair in trauma patients. Operative exposure for venous injuries should follow that of the adjacent artery or arterial lesion. Troublesome venous bleeding can be managed temporarily with digital or sponge-stick pressure until more definitive vascular control has been obtained. In general, severe injuries to brachiocephalic, internal jugular, or subclavian veins can be treated by ligation with relative impunity. This treatment option is recommended for unstable patients or for those who have significant associated injuries. If re-closure of the débrided venous injury would not compromise the lumen by more than 50%, such injuries can be repaired by lateral venorrhaphy.[49, 50] When, however, an entire segment of vein is damaged, ligation (or, rarely, interposition grafting) is necessary. End-to-end anastomosis generally is not feasible once the damaged vessel has been thoroughly débrided. Patch venoplasty or panel or spiral grafting is a time-consuming technique whose use in this setting is imprudent.[49] Repair of the superior vena cava or of one brachiocephalic or internal jugular vein in the presence of bilateral venous injury should be considered to prevent superior vena cava syndrome or acute cerebral edema.[3]

Outcome

Ligation for major cervicothoracic venous trauma is generally well tolerated, although occasional reports have documented long-term disability.[50] Because data suggest more severe venous insufficiency following ligation of large cervicothoracic veins, by inference reestablishment of prograde venous flow in the trauma setting might be reasonable when it does not increase patient risk.[50] Repair of major venous injuries in this area may be appropriate, particularly when there is obvious venous hypertension or when the adjacent major artery has also required concomitant repair.

REFERENCES

1. Perry MO: Vascular injuries in the head and neck. *In* Veith FJ, Hobson RW, Williams RA, Wilson SE (eds): Vascular Surgery: Principles and Practice. New York, McGraw-Hill, 1994, pp 967–964.
2. Byrne MP, Welling RE: Penetrating and blunt extracranial carotid artery injuries. *In* Ernst CB, Stanley JC (eds): Current Therapy in Vascular Surgery. St. Louis, Mosby–Year Book, 1995, pp 598–603.
3. Webb TH, Gewertz BL: Penetrating and blunt vertebral artery trauma. *In* Ernst CB, Stanley JC (eds): Current Therapy in Vascular Surgery. St. Louis, Mosby–Year Book, 1995, pp 604–608.
4. Wilson RF, Tyburski JG: Penetrating trauma to the aortic arch, innominate, and subclavian arteries. *In* Ernst CB, Stanley JC (eds): Current Therapy in Vascular Surgery. St. Louis, Mosby–Year Book, 1995, pp 608–613.
5. Demetriades D, Asensio JA, Velmahos G, Thal E: Complex problems in penetrating neck trauma. Surg Clin North Am 76:661–683, 1996.
6. McConnell DB, Trunkey DD: Management of penetrating trauma to the neck. Adv Surg 27:97–127, 1994.
7. Monson DO, Saletta JD, Freeark RJ: Carotid vertebral trauma. J Trauma 9:987–999, 1969.
8. Apffelstaedt JP, Muller R: Results of mandatory exploration for penetrating neck trauma. World J Surg 18:917–920, 1994.
9. Asensio JA, Valenziano CP, Falcone RE, Grosh JD: Management of penetrating neck injuries: The controversy surrounding zone II injuries. Surg Clin North Am 71:267–296, 1991.
10. Demetriades D, Charalambides D, Lakhoo M: Physical examination and selective conservative management in patients with penetrating injuries of the neck. Br J Surg 80:1534–1536, 1993.
11. North CM, Ahmadi J, Segall HD, et al: Penetrating vascular injuries of the face and neck: Clinical and angiographic correlation. AJR 147:995–999, 1986.
12. Menawat SS, Dennis JW, Laneve LM, et al: Are arteriograms necessary in penetrating zone II neck injuries? J Vasc Surg 16:397–401, 1992.
13. Ballard JL, Fleig K, De Lange M, Killeen JD: The diagnostic accuracy of duplex ultrasound for evaluating the carotid bifurcation. Am J Surg 168:123–126, 1994.
14. Ballard JL, Deiparine MK, Bergan JJ, et al: Cost-effective evaluation of treatment for carotid disease. Arch Surg 132:268–271, 1997.
15. Fry WR, Dort JA, Smith S, et al: Duplex scanning replaces arteriography and operative exploration in the diagnosis of potential cervical vascular injury. Am J Surg 168:693–696, 1994.
16. Demetriades D, Theodorou D, Cornwell E, et al: Penetrating injuries of the neck in patients in stable condition: Physical examination, angiography, or color flow Doppler imaging. Arch Surg 130:971–975, 1995.
17. Ginzburg E, Montalvo B, LeBlang S, et al: The use of duplex ultrasonography in penetrating neck trauma. Arch Surg 131:691–693, 1996.
18. Atteberry LR, Dennis JW, Menawat SS, Frykberg ER: Physical examination alone is safe and accurate for evaluation of vascular injuries in penetrating zone II neck trauma. J Am Coll Surg 179:657–662, 1994.
19. Ballard JL, Killeen JD. Anatomy and surgical exposure of the vascular system. *In* Moore WS (ed): Vascular Surgery: A Comprehensive Review, 5th ed. Philadelphia, WB Saunders, 1997, pp 44–66.
20. Fry WJ, Fry RE: Management of carotid artery injury. *In* Bergan JJ, Yao JS (eds): Vascular Surgical Emergencies. Orlando, Grune & Stratton, 1987, p 587.
21. Kuehne JP, Weaver FA, Papanicolaou G, Yellin AE: Penetrating trauma of the internal carotid artery. Arch Surg 131:942–948, 1996.
22. Rao PM, Ivatury RR, Sharma P, et al: Cervical vascular injuries: A trauma center experience. Surgery 114:527–531, 1993.
23. Ramadan F, Rutledge R, Oller D, et al: Carotid artery trauma: A review of contemporary trauma center experiences. J Vasc Surg 21:46–56, 1995.
24. Ballard JL, Bunt TJ, Fitzpatrick B, Malone JM: Bilateral traumatic internal carotid artery dissections: Case report. J Vasc Surg 15:431–435, 1992.
25. Hellner D, Thie A, Lachenmayer L, et al: Blunt trauma lesions of the extracranial internal carotid artery in patients with head injury. J Craniomaxillofac Surg 21:234–238, 1993.
26. Pretre R, Reverdin A, Kalonji T, Faidutti B: Blunt carotid artery injury: Difficult therapeutic approaches for an under-recognized entity. Surgery 115:375–381, 1994.
27. Cogbill TH, Moore EE, Meissner M, et al: The spectrum of blunt injury to the carotid artery: A multicenter perspective. J Trauma 37:473–479, 1994.
28. Li MS, Smith BM, Espinosa J, et al: Nonpenetrating trauma to the carotid artery: Seven cases and a literature review. J Trauma 36:265–272, 1994.
29. Sanzone AG, Torres H, Soundoulakis SH: Blunt trauma to the carotid arteries. Am J Emerg Med 13:327–330, 1995.
30. Fabian TC, Patton JH, Croce MA, et al: Blunt carotid injury: Importance of early diagnosis and anticoagulant therapy. Ann Surg 223:513–525, 1996.
31. Parikh AA, Luchett FA, Valente JF, et al: Blunt carotid artery injuries. J Am Coll Surg 185:80–86, 1997.
32. Davis J, Holbrook T, Hoyt D, et al: Blunt carotid artery dissection: Incidence, associated injuries, screening, and treatment. J Trauma 30:1514–1517, 1990.
33. Reid JD, Weigelt JA: Forty-three cases of vertebral artery trauma. J Trauma 28:1007–1012, 1988.
34. Yee LF, Olcott CW, Knudson MM, Lim RC: Extraluminal, transluminal, and observational treatment for vertebral artery injuries. J Trauma 39:480–486, 1995.
35. Thomas GI, Andersen KN, Hain RF: The significance of anomalous vertebral-basilar artery communications in operations on the heart and great vessels. Surgery 46:747–757, 1959.
36. Berguer R: Distal vertebral artery bypass: Technique, the "occipital connection," and potential uses. J Vasc Surg 2:621–626, 1985.
37. Landreneau RJ, Weigelt JA, Meier DE, et al: The anterior operative approach to the cervical vertebral artery. J Am Coll Surg 180:475–480, 1995.
38. Beaujeux RL, Reizine DC, Casasco A, et al: Endovascular treatment of vertebral arteriovenous fistula. Radiology 183:361–367, 1992.
39. Halbach VV, Higashida RT, Dowd CF, et al: Endovascular treatment of vertebral artery dissections and pseudoaneurysms. J Neurosurg 79:183–191, 1993.
40. Bladergroen M, Brockman R, Luna G, et al: A twelve-year survey of cervicothoracic vascular injuries. Am J Surg 157:483–486, 1989.
41. Wilson RF, Tyburski JG: Penetrating trauma to the aortic arch, innominate, and subclavian arteries. *In* Ernst CB, Stanley JC (eds): Current Therapy in Vascular Surgery. St. Louis, Mosby–Year Book, 1995, pp 608–613.
42. Johnston RH, Wall MJ, Mattox KL: Innominate artery trauma: A thirty-year experience. J Vasc Surg 17:134–140, 1993.
43. Calhoon JH, Grover FL, Trinkle JT: Chest trauma: Approach and management. Clin Chest Med 13:55–67, 1992.
44. Abouljoud MS, Obeid FN, Horst HM, et al: Arterial injuries of the thoracic outlet: A ten-year experience. Am Surg 59:590–595, 1993.
45. Pate JW, Cole H, Walker WA, et al: Penetrating injuries of the aortic arch and its branches. Ann Thorac Surg 55:586–592, 1993.
46. Hoff SJ, Reilly MK, Merrill WH, et al: Analysis of blunt and penetrating injury of the innominate and subclavian arteries. Am Surg 60:151–154, 1994.
47. Degiannis E, Velmahos G, Krawczykowski D, et al: Penetrating injuries of the subclavian vessels. Br J Surg 81:524–526, 1994.
48. McCoy DW, Weiman DS, Pate JW, et al: Subclavian artery injuries. Am Surg 63:761–764, 1997.
49. Bongard F: Thoracic and abdominal vascular trauma. *In* Rutherford RB (ed): Vascular Surgery, 4th ed. Philadelphia, WB Saunders, 1995, pp 701–702.
50. Perry MO: Injuries of the brachiocephalic vessels. *In* Rutherford RB (ed): Vascular Surgery, 4th ed. Philadelphia, WB Saunders, 1995, pp 705–713.

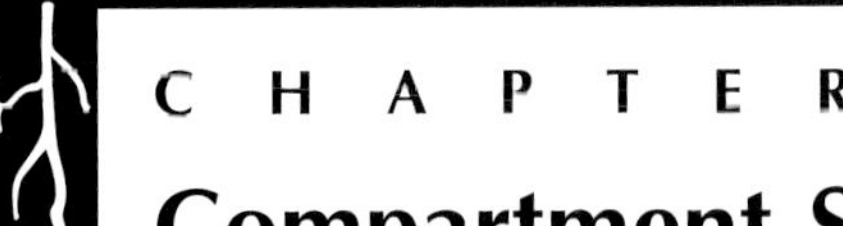

CHAPTER 62

Compartment Syndrome: Pathophysiology, Recognition, and Management

Kaj H. Johansen, M.D., Ph.D., and James C. Watson, Jr., M.S., M.D.

"Compartment syndrome," a constellation of clinical symptoms and signs associated with pathologically elevated tissue pressure, has been observed to complicate a wide spectrum of disorders. Conventionally, however, the term is reserved for post-traumatic or postischemic findings involving skeletal muscle in the extremities.

PATHOPHYSIOLOGY

Compartment syndrome is defined by the development of pathologically elevated tissue pressures within nonexpansile envelopes. Thus, although compartment syndrome is classically identified in osseofascial compartments of the extremities, it shares numerous pathologic similarities with conditions elsewhere in the body that are characterized by sustained elevations in tissue pressure (e.g., closed head injury, testicular torsion, lumbar spinal stenosis, and perhaps even angle-closure glaucoma).

Compartmental pressure rises when either compartmental volume diminishes or compartmental contents expand. The former circumstance is best exemplified by circumstances in which external compression, such as from casts, constrictive dressings, or such devices as the military antishock trousers (MAST suit)[1] exerts pressure on the limb. A circumferential burn wound resulting in a rigid nonexpansile eschar may be another cause for such "extrinsic" compartmental hypertension.

Alternatively, compartmental hypertension can develop in conditions in which compartmental contents increase in volume. Because the bony and fascial bounds of the muscle compartment are inelastic, tissue pressure necessarily rises. Internal compression of the soft tissues within the compartment may result from a space-occupying lesion, such as hematoma, abscess, or synovial fluid (e.g., ruptured Baker's cyst[2]). Iatrogenic causes have been reported for raised intracompartmental pressure (e.g. inadvertent infusion of crystalloid during intraosseous fluid resuscitation[3] or during joint irrigation at the time of arthroscopy[4]).

The most common pathophysiologic cause of compartmental hypertension, however, arises from swelling of the soft tissue contents—primarily skeletal muscle—within the compartment. It has long been understood that post-traumatic soft tissue swelling can result both from an increase in interstitial fluid and from cellular swelling. As long ago as 1910, Rowlands[5] hypothesized that compartment syndrome can occur when ischemia results in a plasma leak and that muscular and neural dysfunction result from elevated compartment pressure. Although we now understand much more about ischemic injury at the cellular and molecular level, Rowlands' "unifying hypothesis" regarding the pathophysiology of compartment syndrome remains relevant today.

Ischemia-Reperfusion

Newer pathophysiologic explanations for compartmental hypertension have arisen out of the development of the *ischemia-reperfusion* theory for cellular injury.[6] According to this theory, ischemia results in the depletion of intracellular energy stores which, after reperfusion and the generation of toxic oxygen radicals, results in a cascade of pathophysiologic consequences. These include (1) activation and adhesion of leukocytes and platelets, (2) calcium influx into cells, (3) disruption of cellular membrane ion pumps, and (4) transudation of fluid; in the aggregate, these consequences produce both cellular swelling and excess interstitial fluid (edema) formation.

The final common pathway for the damage resulting from compartmental hypertension is pathologically raised intracompartmental pressure. Venular pressure, normally 4 to 7 mmHg, rises progressively because of venous outflow obstruction from raised tissue pressure: A vicious circle of steadily increasing capillary pressure exacerbates fluid transudation and cellular swelling, thus further raising intracompartmental pressure. Ultimately, when intracompartmental pressure equals capillary pressure, nutrient blood flow is reduced to zero. Unless compartmental hypertension is relieved, cellular perfusion ceases and tissue infarction commences.

Clinical-Pathologic Correlation

The earliest symptoms of compartment syndrome are neurologic, relating to the fact that the tissues most sensitive to hypoxia are the nonmyelinated type C sensory fibers that carry fine touch and mediate symptoms such as paresthesias. The hypoxic tolerance of tissues increases from nonmyelinated to myelinated nerves, to skeletal muscle, and (most resistant to hypoxia) to skin and bone.

Classically, compartmental pressure greater than 40 to 45 mmHg at any point, or sustained above 30 mmHg for more than 3 to 4 hours, has been considered an indication for compartmental release via fasciotomy.[7,8] However, recent experimental work suggests that such threshold pressure measurements are inadequately sensitive or specific for the diagnosis of compartment syndrome. The physiologic issue of greatest relevance is *arterial perfusion pressure*, the gradient between mean arterial pressure and the interstitial pressure, which of course varies as a function of systemic arterial pressure. Accordingly, intervention is now recommended at a measured compartment pressure 20 mmHg less than systemic diastolic blood pressure or 30 mmHg less than mean blood pressure.[9, 10]

It is not specifically clear, from clinical experience or even from experimental studies, how long pathologically elevated compartmental pressure can be tolerated by skeletal muscle and peripheral nerve before irreversible ischemic changes take place. In acute arterial insufficiency, the likelihood of muscle infarction is overwhelming if revascularization does not take place within 6 to 8 hours. This "grace period" appears relatively constant from both experimental and clinical data, although it may be shortened by the presence of other concurrent problem, such as severe crush injury or compartment syndrome, and may be extended if ischemia is mild because of excellent collateral blood flow. Various data suggest that compartmental hypertension unrelieved for as short a duration as 8 hours also results in irreversible muscle and nerve loss.[11]

Clinical assessment of the success of fasciotomy for the treatment of established compartment syndrome has generally been based on the clinical appearance of the decompressed skeletal muscle and whether it seems to have normal perfusion and contractility. Unfortunately, this assessment may not always be valid; careful histopathologic and nuclear magnetic resonance imaging studies of critically ischemic skeletal muscle demonstrate that nonviable muscle dies "from the inside out."[12, 13] This finding explains the clinical observation that skeletal muscle that appears viable at fasciotomy may proceed over hours to days to progressive muscle necrosis, requiring recurrent débridement and not infrequently resulting ultimately in limb amputation.

Late Pathologic Consequences

Undiagnosed, compartment syndrome progresses inevitably to skeletal muscle infarction. Infection may secondarily supervene, especially in circumstances in which fasciotomy has been performed and wound closure is delayed.[14, 15] Untreated, compartment syndrome may progress to rhabdomyolysis, with release of multiple metabolic toxins—myoglobin, potassium, and organic acids. Haimovici[16] has described the subsequent "myonephropathic-metabolic syndrome" which is characterized by myoglobinuric renal failure, progressive sequential organ failure, and a high mortality rate. This syndrome may warrant emergency amputation as a life-saving procedure.

As previously noted, development of compartmental hypertension is now considered, from a pathophysiologic perspective, to be a manifestation of ischemia-reperfusion. In fact, numerous models of experimental compartment syndrome have been extensively examined as exemplars of ischemia-reperfusion injury. For example, such models have been used to demonstrate that complete ischemia results in more post-reperfusion complications than if partial skeletal muscle perfusion is maintained.[17] Other models have been used to demonstrate that graded reperfusion following an ischemic event, rather than acute restoration of blood flow under systemic pressure, results in fewer and less severe signs of the reperfusion syndrome.[18] Similarly, hypothermia[19] or administration of perfluorocarbons,[20] fibrinolytic agents,[21] heparin,[22] or precursors for adenine nucleotide production[23] during reperfusion appear to mitigate subsequent development of compartment syndrome.

Leukocyte margination, activation, and adhesion to vascular endothelium have been implicated as another pathway for the ischemia-reperfusion injury. Experimental trials have demonstrated that inactivation of white blood cells by anti-adhesion antibodies[24] or depletion of white blood cells by induction of leukopenia with chemotherapeutic agents[25] can mitigate the development of postischemic compartment syndrome. Interference with eicosanoid metabolism,[26] calcium flux,[27] platelet activation,[28] and nitric oxide synthesis[29] appears to diminish the deleterious effects of ischemia-reperfusion.

Finally, in support of the hypothesis that compartment syndrome develops as a consequence of the toxic effects of oxygen radicals generated during ischemia-reperfusion is the demonstration that ischemia-reperfusion injury can be mitigated by pretreatment with mannitol, catalase, or other oxygen radical scavengers prior to the onset of reperfusion.[30–32] Various hyperosmolar volume expanders have also been shown to alleviate compartment syndrome, presumably by reducing interstitial water.[32, 33] These experimental observations have obvious implications relevant to the clinical setting.

CLINICAL PRESENTATION

As with many other disorders, the diagnosis of compartment syndrome is facilitated by the prepared mind. Compartment syndrome occurs primarily in those circumstances, usually post-traumatic or postischemic, in which a substantial expansion in soft tissue volume combines with an intact, inelastic fascial (or other) tissue envelope to produce pathologically elevated compartment pressures. Classically, compartment syndrome has been most commonly seen (1) following major extremity trauma (crush injuries, closed fractures) or (2) as a consequence of reperfusion following severe acute arterial insufficiency, for example, after popliteal thromboembolectomy.

Symptoms include severe pain that is commonly described as being "out of proportion to clinical findings," and that worsens progressively despite appropriate care for the underlying injury (e.g., fracture stabilization). Other important neurologic symptoms are those of distal motor and sensory dysfunction, characteristically weakness and numbness in the distribution of nerves passing through compromised tissue compartments (e.g., the peroneal nerve in the leg and the median nerve in the forearm). This results in weakness of dorsiflexion and numbness in the first dorsal web space in the lower extremity, and numbness in the first web space and weakness in wrist extension in the upper extremity.

Findings on physical examination commonly include tense muscle compartments that are tender to palpation; pain increases with passive motion at the wrist or ankle. The aforementioned motor and sensory deficits are demonstrable. Because compartment syndrome occurs at tissue pressures well below systolic arterial pressure, distal pulses may be intact.

The vascular pathophysiology of compartment syndrome is underscored by the occasional observation of this disorder following massive acute deep venous thrombosis (phlegmasia cerulea dolens)[34] or after successful thromboembolectomy in extremities treated for cardiogenic embolism. However, the fact that the underlying consequences of compartment syndrome are ultimately mediated at the microvascular level is demonstrated by the occasional development of compartment syndrome in circumstances not directly involving large arteries or veins of the extremities. Compartmental syndrome has been reported after electrical injuries, venomous snake bite, or even after massive volume resuscitation for hypovolemic shock.[35] It has also rarely been seen in "medical" conditions such as inherited bleeding disorders,[36] acquired immunodeficiency syndrome (AIDS),[37] hypothyroidism,[38] malignant hyperthermia,[39] and diabetes insipidus.[40]

As previously noted, iatrogenic compartment syndrome has been reported as a consequence of a wide variety of therapeutic interventions, including (1) reaming for tibial nailing,[41] (2) intraosseous fluid administration,[3] (3) irrigation during knee arthroscopic procedures,[4] (4) closure of muscle hernias,[42] (5) prolonged operative positioning, especially in the lithotomy position[43], and (6) successful intra-arterial thrombolysis, either locally or at a remote site.[44, 45]

A substantial diagnostic problem obviously attends evaluation of the patient who is unconscious, intubated, intoxicated, paraplegic or quadriplegic, or who for some other reason cannot sense or communicate sensations of pain in the affected part or cannot participate in the physical examination. For this and other reasons, objective means for measuring compartment pressure have been developed.

OBJECTIVE TESTS

Several of the clinical "hallmarks" of compartmental hypertension are (1) increased tissue tension, (2) dysfunction of the nerves and muscles within the compartments, and (3) occlusion of venous outflow within the compartment. Therefore, objective tests have been developed or modified that may be useful in providing supportive evidence for the effects of compartmental hypertension.

Because diffusely elevated tissue pressure is the sine qua non of compartment syndrome, objective measurement of compartment pressure through the direct percutaneous placement of needles or catheters was proposed.[7, 8] Simple insertion of an intravenous catheter,[46] with pressure transduction using commonly available equipment, is believed by many to be as accurate as more complex catheter systems[47, 48] or self-contained hand-held disposable manometry devices.[49] An automated intravenous infusion device has been cleverly modified to measure compartment pressure.[50]

Determination of the critical compartment pressure required to produce tissue damage requires acceptance of a more dynamic model for the clinical presentation of compartment syndrome, one based not just on absolute tissue pressures but also on the patient's basic cardiovascular status, both regional and systemic. It was initially believed that *any* compartment pressure greater than 40–45 mmHg, or greater than 30 mmHg for more than three hours, warranted fasciotomy.[7, 8] Later physiologic evaluation, however, has suggested that these absolute thresholds for intervention are in practice likely neither sensitive nor specific, because perfusion in muscle compartments is a function of the gradient between diastolic[9] or mean[10] arterial pressure and the tissue pressure in the compartment at risk.

Compartments with increased tissue pressure are tense and turgid to palpation. Steinberg and Gelberman[51] have developed a tissue tonometer for quantifying tissue hardness; in experimental models, their method was found to correlate directly with the results of direct tissue manometry.[51] Because the device is essentially noninvasive, easy to use, and completely portable, it has great logistic appeal for emergency departments and intensive care units.

Above a certain level, increased tissue pressure compromises nerve function, presumably by diminishing perfusion of neural tissues. Distal motor and sensory nerve dysfunction is the result. Present and associates[52] have demonstrated the very high accuracy of somatosensory evoked potential (SSEP) monitoring of nerve dysfunction in the upper and lower extremities with actual or impending compartmental hypertension.[52] Although expensive, invasive, and cumbersome, this technique may be cost-effective and highly accurate in evaluating patients for compartment syndrome, especially those whose clinical status (e.g., intoxication, coma, paralysis) may prevent them from participating fully in a peripheral nerve examination.

If the pathophysiologic mechanisms that result in compartment syndrome are set in motion, one of the first manifestations of raised intracompartmental pressure is venous outflow obstruction. Jones and coworkers[53] pointed out that venous duplex scanning focused on the tibial veins might be an accurate means of indirectly determining the presence of compartmental hypertension because it is not physiologically possible for venous flow dynamics to be normal in the presence of significant compartmental tissue hypertension. Subsequent experimental work by Ombrellaro and colleagues[54] confirmed that abnormal venous hemodynamics, especially loss of normal respiratory venous phasicity, correlate well with elevated tissue pressure. Although duplex scanning of the calf veins cannot by itself *affirm* the presence of pathologically raised tissue pressures, the finding of normally phasic tibial vein flow on duplex scanning of a calf muscle compartment effectively *rules out* elevated tissue pressures in that compartment.

TREATMENT

Fasciotomy

The proper management of established compartment syndrome is decompression by complete dermotomy and fasciotomy. This operation should include all four compartments in the leg or both (some say three[55]) compartments in the forearm. Fasciotomy for other, much less common sites of skeletal muscular hypertension (foot, hand, or thigh) is generally carried out by longitudinal incision over the affected compartment.

Fasciotomy is effective only if performed correctly and in a timely fashion. Although the timing may not always be under the surgeon's control, proper technical performance of the fasciotomy is. The features of a technically successful four-compartment fasciotomy of the lower extremity are:

- Complete incision of the skin overlying the affected compartment or compartments.
- Longitudinal incision of the entire fascia investing each of the compartments.
- Aggressive local wound care followed by timely and complete closure.

In the lower extremity, four-compartment fasciotomy of the calf can be performed through a single lateral incision, started one fingerbreadth anterior to the fibula and carried from near the fibular head to the ankle. As demonstrated in Figure 62–1, access to the anterior, lateral (peroneal), and superficial posterior compartments is straightforward, requiring little more than the raising of relatively narrow skin flaps anteriorly and posteriorly. The deep posterior compartment is more difficult to approach, and the most effective operative strategy is for the surgeon to start distally where the gastrocnemius and soleus muscles become tendinous. The soleus muscle is dissected off the posterior aspect of the fibula, thereby exposing the fascia of the deep posterior compartment. Alternatively, dissecting just anterior to the fibula, beneath the lateral compartment, exposes the interosseous membrane, incision of which releases the posterior compartment.

Perhaps slightly more "user-friendly" for those surgeons not familiar with the details of performing fasciotomy through a single lateral exposure is a two-incision approach (Fig. 62–2). The authors do not consider fibulectomy to be required as a means to decompress the calf muscles. Prior impressions that the tibialis posterior muscle is encompassed in its own fascial compartment and requires separate fasciotomy have been refuted.[56]

In the forearm, a single curvilinear volar incision, starting in the antecubital fossa and ending at the palm of the hand, suffices to decompress both (or all three[55]) of the forearm

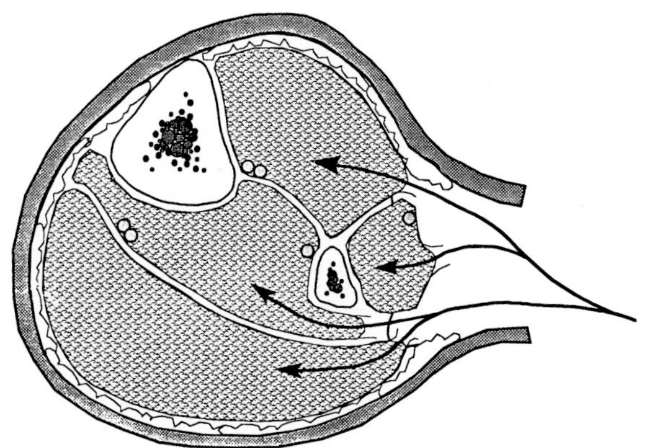

FIGURE 62–1. Lower extremity fasciotomy via a single anterolateral incision. (From Gulli B, Templeman D: Compartment syndrome of the lower extremity. Orthop Clin North Am 25:677–684, 1994.)

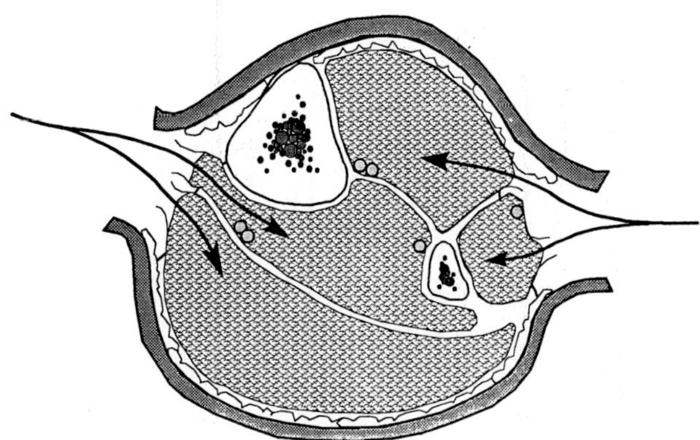

FIGURE 62–2. Lower extremity fasciotomy via anterolateral and medial incisions. (From Gulli B, Templeman D: Compartment syndrome of the lower extremity. Orthop Clin North Am 25:677–684, 1994.)

muscle compartments (Fig. 62–3). The nature of the fascial anatomy in the forearm results in complete compartment release with a single fascial incision. Decompression of the carpal tunnel is obligatory.

Skeletal muscle viability is characterized by color, bleeding, and—most reliable in our view—contraction with galvanic stimulation. This last response should occur independent of whether muscle-relaxant agents have been used during anesthetic induction. Muscle that does not contract should be débrided. Adjunctive measures, such as repair of associated fractures (which now must be treated as open), excision of devitalized tissue, tissue coverage of vascular grafts or orthopedic hardware, and surveillance for further deterioration of skeletal muscle viability, must be carried out. As noted previously, visual evidence of skeletal muscle necrosis may initially be subtle or nonexistent,[12, 13, 50] so frequent repeated examinations are obligatory.

Wound Management and Closure

Timely closure of the fasciotomy wound is crucial. In a comparative study, patients undergoing dermotomy-fasciotomy showed a sharply higher incidence of wound or vascular graft complications when fasciotomy closure was delayed.[14] Methods for wound management and ultimate skin closure include frequent replacement of sterile moist dressings and either skin grafts or delayed primary closure. Immediate skin closure is mentioned only to be condemned: The skin itself can act as a constricting envelope, and consistently unfavorable outcomes after attempts to treat compartment syndrome via minimal skin incisions or with partial or complete wound suture at the time of fasciotomy underscore this fact.

Several methods varying in complexity have been reported to achieve gradual reapposition of skin edges, which tend otherwise to retract, after fasciotomy. Taking advantage of the skin's innate capacity to expand with traction, these methods may be as simple as the use of a plastic vessel-loop threaded between staples placed opposite one another across the wound defect, with serial tightening at the bedside over the next 7 to 10 days,[57] or as complex as commercially available skin traction devices that uniformly distract skin across the fasciotomy wound.[58, 59] Ongoing care must be taken with these techniques, because pathologically ele-

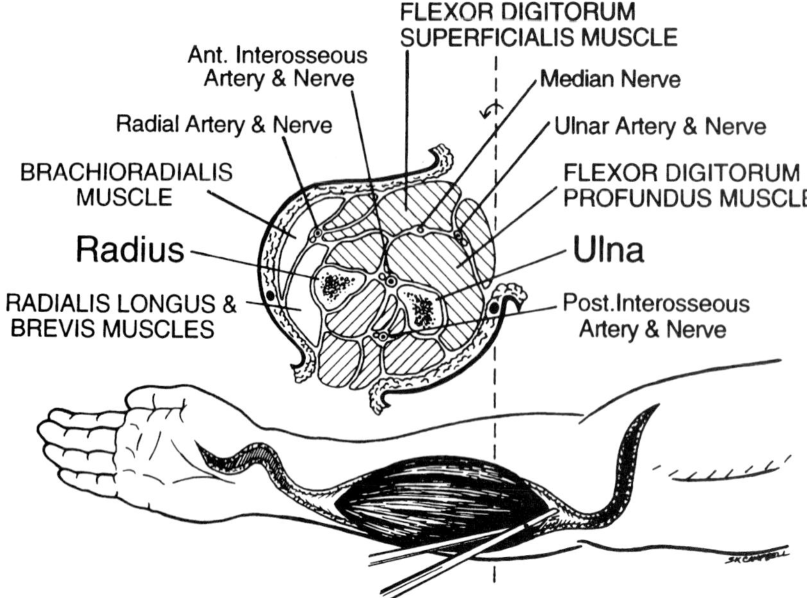

FIGURE 62–3. Upper extremity fasciotomy via a single volar incision. This cross-sectional view demonstrates the location of the ulnar incision, which is rarely required. (From Ombrellaro M, Stevens S: Compartment syndrome: A collective review. Adv Trauma Crit Care 10:85–112, 1995.)

vated tissue pressure has been reported to occur beneath them despite the prior fasciotomy.[60]

Myoglobinuric acute renal failure, especially if recognized and treated late, is a constant concern in patients with compartment syndrome. Proper management consists of aggressive volume expansion, administration of mannitol and loop diuretics, and urine alkalinization by sodium bicarbonate.[61] Hemodialysis may be required, especially if oliguria supervenes; aggressive débridement of devitalized muscle, which may even require amputation, is crucial. The long-term outcome of myoglobulinuric acute renal failure is generally favorable.[61]

Can compartment syndrome be attenuated or even prevented? Experimental data suggesting the important role of oxygen radicals in the pathogenesis of compartment syndrome have revived interest in the utility of mannitol and certain other agents known to scavenge such toxic oxygen species. Indeed, a large clinical series reported by Shah and colleagues[32] at Albany Medical College, where patients with acute arterial insufficiency undergo adjunctive treatment with mannitol, suggests that the severity of compartmental hypertension may be reduced by this treatment, avoiding operation in some cases and appearing to preserve skeletal muscle viability and function in others.[32] Mannitol's effect appears to be based on both its oxygen radical scavenger effect (mitigating ischemia-reperfusion injury) and its hyperosmolar capabilities (reducing tissue edema).[62]

OUTCOMES

The original clinical manifestation of the consequences of neglected compartment syndrome was ischemic contracture of the forearm muscles in children, usually seen following supracondylar humerus fracture and associated brachial artery injury. This so-called Volkmann's contracture[63] has its analogue in equinus deformities of the lower extremity from calf muscle atrophy following compartment syndrome in the lower extremity.

In the lower extremity, loss of one or two muscle compartments can be tolerated, presuming satisfactory wound closure. Ambulation can occur with vigorous retraining, generally with the assistance of splints or ankle-foot orthoses. Loss of more than two muscle compartments in the leg generally warrants amputation and aggressive prosthesis rehabilitation. In the upper extremity, complex microvascular reconstruction with innervated muscle flaps has been successful in restoring hand and arm sensation and motor function.[63]

Unfortunately, because pathologically elevated tissue pressures are transmitted throughout the entire compartment, myonecrosis is global in far-advanced compartment syndrome. Below-knee or even through-knee amputation, both of which require viable calf muscle for wound closure, is rarely feasible to treat compartment syndrome complicated by myonecrosis.

It had previously been thought that the lower extremity calf venous muscle pump depends on an intact fascia to function and that fasciotomy would distort lower extremity venous dynamics. Later studies have demonstrated, however, that the capacitance and function of the lower extremity veins appears to be unaffected by a prior fasciotomy.[64]

When compartment syndrome is managed early, completely, and successfully, affected muscles and nerves appear to function normally. Although a fasciotomy wound can be large and disfiguring at first, the late cosmetic results following either delayed primary closure or even split-thickness skin graft are generally satisfactory.

CHRONIC COMPARTMENT SYNDROME

On occasion, otherwise healthy subjects present with leg pain and foot numbness and weakness in association with vigorous walking or running, and chronic compartment syndrome is diagnosed.[65] This entity, which is confirmed by the development of elevated lower extremity muscle compartment pressures during treadmill exercise, results from the increased leg blood flow associated with exercise and, presumably, the associated expansion of muscle within the leg, most commonly within the anterior compartment.[66] Fasciotomy, with the use of small and cosmetically acceptable skin incisions, is curative.

REFERENCES

1. Templeman D, Lang R, Harris B: Lower extremity compartment syndrome associated with the use of pneumatic anti-shock garments. J Trauma 27:79–81, 1987.
2. Krome J, de Araujo W, Webb LX: Acute compartment syndrome in ruptured Baker's cyst. J South Orthop Assoc 6:110–114, 1997.
3. Galpin RD, Kronick JB, Willis RB, Frewen TC: Bilateral lower extremity compartment syndromes secondary to intraosseous fluid resuscitation. J Pediatr Orthop 11:773–776, 1991.
4. Kaper BP, Carr CF, Shirreffs TG: Compartment syndrome after arthroscopic surgery of knee: A report of two cases managed nonoperatively. Am J Sports Med 25:123–125, 1997.
5. Rowlands RP: Volkmann's contracture. Guy's Hospital Gazette 24:87–92, 1910.
6. Walker PM: Ischemia/reperfusion injury in skeletal muscle. Ann Vasc Surg 5:399–402, 1991.
7. Matsen FA III: Compartmental syndrome: A unified concept. Clin Orthop 113:8–13, 1975.
8. Whitesides TE Jr, Haney TC, Morimoto K, Harada H: Tissue pressure measurements as a determinant for the need of fasciotomy. Clin Orthop 113:43–51, 1975.
9. Matava MJ, Whitesides TE Jr, Seiler JG III, et al: Determination of the compartment pressure threshold of muscle ischemia in a canine model. J Trauma 37:50–58, 1994.
10. Mabee JR, Bostwick TL: Pathophysiology and mechanisms of compartment syndrome. Orthop Rev 22:175–181, 1993.
11. Finkelstein JA, Hunter GA, Hu RW: Lower limb compartment syndrome: Course after delayed fasciotomy. J Trauma 40:342–344, 1996.
12. Labbe R, Lindsay T, Walker PM: The extent and distribution of skeletal muscle necrosis after graded periods of complete ischemia. J Vasc Surg 6:152–157, 1987.
13. Blebea J, Kerr JC, Franco CD, et al: Technetium 99m pyrophosphate quantitation of skeletal muscle ischemia and reperfusion injury. J Vasc Surg 8:117–124, 1988.
14. Johnson SB, Weaver FA, Yellin AE, et al: Clinical results of decompressive dermotomy-fasciotomy. Am J Surg 164:286–290, 1992.
15. Rutgers PH, van der Harst E, Koumans RK: Surgical implications of drug-induced rhabdomyolysis. Br J Surg 78:490–492, 1991.
16. Haimovici H: Muscular, renal, and metabolic complications of acute arterial occlusions: Myonephropathic-metabolic syndrome. Surgery 85:461–468, 1979.
17. Petrasek PF, Walker PM: A clinically relevant small-animal model of skeletal muscle ischemia-reperfusion injury. J Invest Surg 7:27–38, 1994.
18. Anderson RJ, Cambria R, Kerr J, Hobson RW 2d: Sustained benefit of temporary limited reperfusion in skeletal muscle following ischemia. J Surg Res 49:271–275, 1990.
19. Wright JG, Araki CT, Belkin M, Hobson RW 2d: Postischemic hypothermia diminishes skeletal muscle reperfusion edema. J Sura Res 47:389–396, 1989.
20. Mohan C, Gennaro M, Marini C, et al: Reduction of the extent of ischemic skeletal muscle necrosis by perfusion with oxygenated perfluorocarbon. Am J Surg 164:194–198, 1992.
21. Belkin M, Valeri CR, Hobson RW 2d: Intraarterial urokinase increases skeletal muscle viability after acute ischemia. J Vasc Surg 9:161–168, 1989.
22. Hobson RW 2d, Nevill R, Watanabe B, et al: Role of heparin in reducing skeletal muscle infarction in ischemia-reperfusion. Microcirc Endothelium Lymphatics 5:259–276, 1989.
23. Hayes PG, Liauw S, Smith A, et al: Exogenous magnesium chloride–adenosine triphosphate administration during reperfusion reduces the extent of necrosis in previously ischemic skeletal muscle. J Vasc Surg 11:441–447, 1990.
24. Petrasek PF, Liauw S, Romaschin AD, Walker PM: Salvage of postischemic skeletal muscle by monoclonal antibody blockade of neutrophil adhesion molecule CD18. J Surg Res 56:5–12, 1994.
25. Rubin B, Tittley J, Chang G, et al: A clinically applicable method for long-term salvage of postischemic skeletal muscle. J Vasc Surg 13:58–67, 1991.
26. Cambria RA, Anderson RJ, Dikdan G, et al: The influence of arachidonic acid metabolites on leukocyte activation and skeletal muscle injury after ischemia and reperfusion. J Vasc Surg 14:549–556, 1991.
27. Oshiro H, Kobayashi I, Kim D, et al: L-type calcium channel blockers modulate the microvascular hyperpermeability induced by platelet-activating factor in vivo. J Vasc Surg 22:732–739, 1995.
28. Noel AA, Hobson RW 2nd, Duran WN: Platelet-activating factor and nitric oxide mediate microvascular permeability in ischemia-reperfusion injury. Microvasc Res 52:210–220, 1996.
29. Noel AA, Fallek SR, Hobson RW 2d, Duran WN: Inhibition of nitric oxide synthase attenuates primed microvascular permeability in the in vivo microcirculation. J Vasc Surg 22:661–669, 1995.
30. Belkin M, LaMorte WL, Wright JG, Hobson RW 2d: The role of leukocytes in the pathophysiology of skeletal muscle ischemic injury. J Vasc Surg 10:14–18, 1989.
31. Walker PM, Lindsay TF, Labbe R, et al: Salvage of skeletal muscle with free radical scavengers. J Vasc Surg 5:68–75, 1987.
32. Shah DM, Bock DE, Darling RC 3rd, et al: Beneficial effects of hypertonic mannitol in acute ischemia-reperfusion injuries in humans. Cardiovasc Surg 4:97–100, 1996.
33. Hakaim AG, Corsetti R, Cho SI: The pentafraction of hydroxyethyl starch inhibits ischemia-induced compartment syndrome. J Trauma 37:18–21, 1994.
34. Rahm M, Probe R: Extensive deep venous thrombosis resulting in compartment syndrome of the thigh and leg: A case report. J Bone Joint Surg Am 76:18543–18547, 1994.
35. Block EFJ, Dobo S, Kirton OS: Compartment syndrome in the critically injured following massive resuscitation: Case reports. J Trauma 39:787–791, 1995.
36. Naranja RJ Jr, Chan PS, High K, et al: Treatment considerations in patients with compartment syndrome and an inherited bleeding disorder. Orthopedics 20:706–709, 1997.
37. Guidet B, Guerin B, Maury E, et al: Capillary leakage complicated by compartment syndrome necessitating surgery. Intensive Care Med 16:332–333, 1990.
38. Hsu SI, Thadhani RI, Daniels GH: Acute compartment syndrome in a hypothyroid patient. Thyroid 5:305–308, 1995.
39. Steele AP, Inurie MM, Rutherford AM, Bradley WN: Malignant hyperthermia and compartment syndrome. Br J Anaesth 74:343–344, 1995.
40. Geutjens G: Spontaneous compartment syndrome in a patient with diabetes insipidus. Int Orthop 18:53–54, 1994.
41. Tichenko GJ, Goodman SB: Compartment syndromes after IM nailing of the tibia. J Bone Joint Surg 72A:41–44, 1990.
42. Miniaci A, Rorabeck CH: Compartment syndrome as a complication of repair of a hernia of the tibialis anterior: A case report. J Bone Joint Surg Am 68:1444–1445, 1986.
43. Khalil IM: Bilateral compartment syndrome after prolonged surgery in the lithotomy position. J Vasc Surg 5:879–881, 1987
44. Thomas WO, Harris CN, D'Amore TF, Parry SW: Bilateral forearm and hand compartment syndrome following thrombolysis of acute myocardial infarction: A case report. J Emerg Med 12:467–472, 1994.
45. Rudoff J, Ebner S, Canepa C: Limb-compartmental syndrome with thrombolysis (Letter). Am Heart J 128:1267–1268, 1994.
46. Wilson SC, Vrahas MS, Berson L, Paul EM: A simple method to measure compartment pressures using an intravenous catheter. Orthopedics 20:403–406, 1997.
47. Mubarak SJ, Hargens AR, Owen CA: The wick catheter technique for measurement of intramuscular pressure: A new research and clinical tool. J Bone Joint Surg 58A:1016–1020, 1976.
48. Rorabeck CH, Castle GSP, Hardie R: Compartmental pressure measurements: An experimental investigation using the slit catheter. J Trauma 21:446–450, 1981.
49. Styf J: Evaluation of injection techniques in recording of intramuscular pressure. J Orthop Res 7:812–816, 1989.
50. Uppal GS, Smith RC, Sherk HH, Mooar P: Accurate compartment pressure measurement using the Intravenous Alarm Control (IVAC) Pump. J Orthop Trauma 6:87–89, 1992.
51. Steinberg BD, Gelberman RH: Evaluation of limb compartments with suspected increased interstitial pressure: A noninvasive method for determining quantitative hardness. Clin Orthop 300:248–253, 1994.

52. Present DA, Nainzedeh NK, Ben-Yishay A, Mazzara JT: The evaluation of compartmental syndromes using somatosensory evoked potentials in monkeys. Clin Orthop 287:276–285, 1993.
53. Jones WG II, Perry MO, Bush HL Jr: Changes in tibial venous blood flow in the evolving compartment syndrome. Arch Surg 124:801–804, 1989.
54. Ombrellaro MP, Stevens SL, Freeman M, et al: Ultrasound characteristics of lower extremity venous flow for the early diagnosis of compartment syndrome: An experimental study. J Vasc Technol 20:71–75, 1996.
55. Gelberman RH, Zakaib GS, Mubarak SJ: Decompression of forearm compartment syndromes. Clin Orthop 134:225–229, 1978.
56. Ruland RT, April EW, Meinhard BP: Tibialis posterior muscle: The fifth compartment? J Orthop Trauma 6:347–351, 1992.
57. Berman SS, Schilling JD, McIntyre KE, et al: Shoelace technique for delayed primary closure of fasciotomies. Am J Surg 167:435–436, 1994.
58. McKenney MG, Nir J, Fee T, et al: A simple device for closure of fasciotomy wounds. Am J Surg 1771:275–277, 1996.
59. Hirshowitz B, Lindenbaum E, Har-Shai Y: A skin-stretching device for the harnessing of the viscoelastic properties of skin. Plast Reconstr Surg 92:260–270, 1993.
60. Hussmann J, Kucan JO, Zamboni WA: Elevated compartmental pressures after closure of a forearm burn wound with a skin stretching device. Burns 23:154–156, 1997.
61. Zager RA: Rhabdomyolysis and myohemoglobinuric acute renal failure (Editorial). Kidney Int 49:314–326, 1996.
62. Oredsson S, Plate G, Qvarfordt P: The effect of mannitol and reperfusion injury and post-ischaemic compartment pressure in skeletal muscle. Eur J Vasc Surg 8:326–331, 1994.
63. Chuang DC, Carver N, Wei FC: A new strategy to prevent the sequelae of severe Volkmann's contracture. Plast Reconstr Surg 98:1023–1031, 1996.
64. Ris HB, Furrer M, Stronsky S, et al: Four-compartment fasciotomy and venous calf-pump function: Long term results. Surgery 113:55–58, 1993.
65. Detmer D, Sharpe K, Sufit RL, Girdley FM: Chronic compartment syndrome: Diagnosis, management, and outcome. Am J Sports Med 13:162–170, 1985.
66. Turnipseed MD, Hurschler C, Vanderby R: The effects of elevated compartment pressure on tibial arteriovenous flow and relationship of mechanical and biochemical characteristics of fascia to genesis of chronic anterior compartment syndrome. J Vasc Surg 21:810–817, 1995.

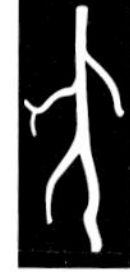

CHAPTER 63

Causalgia and Post-traumatic Pain Syndromes

Ali F. AbuRahma, M.D., and
Robert B. Rutherford, M.D.

BACKGROUND

Post-traumatic pain syndromes, most often called *causalgia* or *reflex sympathetic dystrophy* (RSD), remain some of the most poorly understood and frequently misdiagnosed entities encountered in clinical practice. These painful afflictions can develop after damage to peripheral nerves in a variety of settings. In susceptible patients, the initiating event may be relatively insignificant, even obscure. Although a discussion of the management of all types of post-traumatic pain is beyond the scope of this chapter, the management of causalgia is relevant to the vascular surgeon for several reasons.

First, one form of causalgia is caused by ischemic damage to nerves secondary to delayed revascularization, and, of course, the vascular surgeon may inadvertently injure peripheral nerves during revascularization procedure. Second, the vasomotor phenomena associated with causalgia often cause such patients to be referred to a vascular surgeon. The associated vascular signs often convince the referring physician that he or she is dealing mainly with a painful vascular condition. Such a referral may be fortuitous, because although sympathectomy is now rarely used for vascular disease (see Chapter 73), it is the vascular surgeon who has perfected this procedure and made it safe, and sympathectomy may provide the most dramatic and lasting relief from causalgia.

COMPLEX REGIONAL PAIN SYNDROME

Terminology and New Classification

The term causalgia is derived from the Greek *causos*, meaning heat, and *algos*, meaning pain (i.e., burning pain).[35] Although it was described in detail by Weir Mitchell in 1864,[35] Paré may have reported the first case in the 16th century.[40] These early reports described incomplete peripheral nerve injury secondary to penetrating trauma (e.g., partial rather than complete transection) with subsequent burning pain, autonomic dysfunction, and "limb atrophy." With time, however, symptoms of similar severity were noted to occur subsequent to trauma of a less serious nature, and even in the absence of obvious injury to a peripheral nerve. In 1973, Patman and colleagues consolidated the many terms that had appeared in the literature describing a variety of pain syndromes similar to causalgia, but of different causes, under the name *mimocausalgia*.[41] This term, also derived from the Greek, means "imitating causalgia." Previously, it had been popular to refer to these syndromes as *minor causalgia*, in contrast to the full-blown symptom complex associated with incomplete nerve injuries, referred to as *major causalgia*.

Other commonly used terms are:

- *Minor* and *major traumatic dystrophy*, describing the intensity of the syndrome when it develops after an injury that does not damage a peripheral nerve
- *Shoulder-hand syndrome*, RSD that involves the entire upper extremity
- *Sudeck's atrophy*, a post-traumatic reflex dystrophy with bone involvement demonstrable on radiographs

Table 63–1 includes more than 40 terms from the literature that describe similar symptom complexes that are minor variations from the classic triad of burning pain, sympathetic dysfunction, and limb atrophy.

As a result of the confusion surrounding the various terms used to describe this syndrome, Stanton-Hicks and associates convened a consensus committee on the nomenclature of causalgia and RSD.[50] The committee, which met in Orlando, Florida, in November 1993, determined a need to revise the taxonomic system for RSD. It was agreed that the term RSD had lost all clinical or research utility because of its indiscriminate use without regard to diagnostic or descriptive criteria. The relationship to the sympathetic nervous system was considered to be inconsistent, and the "reflex" implied by the name has never been demonstrated. It was also suggested that the term *dystrophy* was used imprecisely and might not always be present. RSD had also become a "nondiscriminating" diagnosis for patients showing a resistance to therapy for some elements of neuropathic pain.[6]

TABLE 63–1. TERMS USED TO DESCRIBE CAUSALGIA AND POST-TRAUMATIC PAIN SYNDROMES

Acute atrophy of bones	Post-traumatic sympathetic dysfunction
Algodystrophy	Post-traumatic sympathetic dystrophy
Algoneurodystrophy	Post-traumatic vasomotor disorders
Causalgia	Reflex neurovascular dystrophy
Causalgia-like states	Reflex dystrophy
Chronic segmental arterial spasm	Reflex dystrophy of the extremities
Chronic traumatic edema	Reflex nervous dystrophy
Disuse phenomenon	Reflex sympathetic dystrophy
Homans' minor causalgia	Shoulder-hand syndrome
Major causalgia	Steinerocher's shoulder-hand syndrome
Mimocausalgia	Sudeck's atrophy
Minor causalgia	Sudeck's osteodystrophy
Mitchell's causalgia	Sudeck's syndrome
Painful osteoporosis	Sympathalgia
Peripheral trophoneurosis	Sympathetic neurovascular dystrophy
Post-traumatic dystrophy	Traumatic angiospasm
Post-traumatic fibrosis	Traumatic edema
Post-traumatic neurovascular pain syndrome	Traumatic neuralgia
Post-traumatic osteoporosis	Traumatic vasospasm
Post-traumatic pain syndrome	
Post-traumatic painful osteoporosis	
Post-traumatic spreading neuralgia	
Post-traumatic sympathalgia	

Accordingly, the term *complex regional pain syndrome* (CRPS) was developed to replace the terms of "causalgia" and "RSD." CRPS includes a spectrum of conditions that have somewhat similar clinical manifestations that often are grouped together for the sake of clinical utility.[18] Hallmarks of this syndrome include dysfunction and pain of duration or severity out of proportion to what might be expected from the initiating event. The cause of this pain syndrome and the underlying pathophysiology remain obscure; as a consequence, descriptors that implied cause or mechanism (such as the role of the sympathetic nervous system) were excluded from the new nomenclature. The new classification is based on a descriptive method that should allow for future modifications as indicated by new scientific findings.[6, 50]

The following is a summary of the key features of CRPS:

1. *Complex*, denotes the dynamic and varied nature of the clinical presentation, within a single person over time and among persons with seemingly similar disorders. It also includes the autonomic, cutaneous, motor, inflammatory, and dystrophic changes that distinguish this syndrome from other forms of neuropathic pain.

2. *Regional*, describes the wider distribution of the clinical symptoms and findings beyond the area of the original lesion. This is considered a key characteristic of this syndrome. The distal part of a limb is usually affected, but occasionally it occurs in other parts of the body (e.g., the face or torso) and may spread to other body parts.

3. *Pain*, the hallmark of CRPS, is out of proportion to the initiating event. The designation refers to spontaneous burning pain and thermally or mechanically induced allodynia.

Syndrome Types

Two types of CRPS have been recognized. *Type I* corresponds to the former term RSD; *type II*, to the former term causalgia. The definitions of CRPS types I and II contain criteria that exclude (1) pain and other findings that are physiologically, anatomically, and temporally appropriate to some form of injury, and (2) myofascial pain syndrome. The terms *sympathetically maintained pain* (SMP) and *sympathetically independent pain* (SIP) were considered, not as separate entities, but as descriptions of types of pain that can be associated with a variety of pain disorders, including CRPS types I and II.

The diagnostic criteria for CRPS type I (formerly RSD), as adapted from Stanton-Hicks and coworkers[50] and Merskey and Bogduk[33] are these:

1. CRPS type I follows an inciting noxious event.
2. Spontaneous pain or hyperalgesia/allodynia exists beyond the territory of a single peripheral nerve and is disproportionate to the initiating event.
3. Edema, skin blood-flow abnormality, or abnormal sudomotor activity in the region of the pain have developed since the initiating event.
4. The diagnosis is excluded by the presence of conditions that otherwise would account for the degree of dysfunction and pain.

The diagnostic criteria for CRPS type II (formerly causalgia) are as follows:

1. CRPS type II is a syndrome that results specifically from a nerve injury; otherwise, it is similar in all other aspects to CRPS type I. Spontaneous allodynia or pain occurs that is not necessarily limited to the region of the injured nerve.

2. Since the original nerve injury, edema, temperature and skin blood-flow changes, abnormal sudomotor activity, and motor dysfunction in the region of the pain have developed.

3. The diagnosis is excluded by the presence of conditions that would otherwise account for the degree of dysfunction and pain.

Etiology

Three precipitating causes of CRPS have been identified:

- *Traumatic* (fractures, dislocations, sprains, crush injuries, burns, and iatrogenic injuries)
- *Nontraumatic* (prolonged bed rest, neoplasms, metabolic bone disease, thrombophlebitis, myocardial infarction, and cerebral vascular accidents)
- *Idiopathic*

Most cases of CRPS are post-traumatic. The proportion of nerve injuries that result in causalgia (CRPS type II) ranges from 1.8% to 12%.[5] The incidence of CRPS in trauma patients ranges from 0.05% to 5%.[42] CRPS has also been reported in 0.2% to 11% of patients with Colles' fracture[23] and in 12% to 20% of patients with hemiplegia.[13] The incidence of CRPS in myocardial ischemia patients varies between 5% and 20%.[22]

Chronic painful afflictions of the upper extremity subsequent to myocardial infarction have been grouped into a category designated *shoulder-hand syndrome*. This was originally described by Steinbrocker and coworkers, who pointed out that 15% of patients with myocardial infarction developed persistent pain in the shoulder, arm, wrist, or hand sometime during their recovery.[51] The incidence of shoulder-hand syndrome has been reduced significantly, probably because of much more rapid post-infarct mobilization.[22]

Pathogenesis

Many theories have been proposed to explain CRPS, but none have been accepted universally. Most were developed to explain the causalgia associated with nerve injury (CRPS type II). The most popular theory is probably that of "artificial synapses" occurring at the site of a nerve injury, as first proposed by Doupe.[14] According to this theory, a "short circuit" occurs at the point of partial nerve interruption or demyelinization, which allows efferent sympathetic impulses to be relayed back along afferent somatic fibers. Such an artificial synapse has been demonstrated experimentally in crushed nerves,[5] and the interruption of sympathetic efferent impulses may explain the warm, red, and dry extremity seen initially in cases of major causalgia. It has also been demonstrated that stimulation of a sensory nerve along its course makes the nerve more sensitive to the usual types of sensory stimuli.[43] The work of Walker and Nielsen in humans suggests the possibility of an artificial synapse.[57] Stimulation of the postganglionic sympathetics after upper thoracic preganglionic sympathectomy reproduces the causalgia for which the surgery was performed. No such pain was produced, however, in patients whose sympathectomy was performed for a condition other than causalgia. These findings were confirmed by White and Sweet.[58]

One piece of evidence weighing against this theory was the demonstration that, not infrequently, nerve block with local anesthetic beyond the site of the nerve injury (and presumably beyond this artificial synapse) affords relief.[5] Proponents of the artificial synapse theory, however, have countered that the efferent sympathetic impulses that are short-circuited at the site of injury may not always be strong enough by themselves to cause retrograde propagation of impulses, and that summation of these impulses, together with other afferent somatic impulses, may be necessary. Barnes[3] has suggested that impulses at sympathetic–sensory fiber short circuits may travel in both directions. Proximally directed impulses would then cause pain, and those directed distally would release "antidromic" substances, demonstrated by Chapman and coworkers[9] to lower the threshold for sensory stimuli, further increasing the sensory input.

Although these explanations seem plausible in cases of demonstrable nerve injury, obvious difficulties complicate extending them to explain the similar pain experienced without overt nerve injury (CRPS type I). They do not explain the sympathetic overactivity often seen in the later stages of this condition, the pain relief associated with intra-arterial injections of a peripheral adrenergic blocking agent such as tolazoline hydrochloride, or the fact that, in early cases, relief of pain not infrequently lasts beyond the duration of a sympathetic block. A convincing hypothesis for the mechanism of CRPS type I must also explain the modification of pain by emotional and sensory stimuli and the relief of pain by contralateral sympathectomy after failure of an apparently adequate ipsilateral sympathectomy.[44] The hypothesis must also be compatible with the relief of pain by spinal anesthesia below the sympathetic-lumbar outlet and before sympathetic blockade response.[27] Finally, it must explain the failure of sympathectomy in some long-standing cases.

In the late 1930s, Livingston[27] proposed that in causalgia there is a "vicious cycle of reflexes" consisting of three components:

1. Chronic irritation of a peripheral sensory nerve with increasingly frequent afferent impulses.

2. Abnormal heightened activity in the "internuncial pool" in the anterior horn of the spinal cord.

3. Increased efferent sympathetic activity.

This theory was supported experimentally by Toennie's demonstration that individual stimulation of more than one third of the afferent fibers of a cat's saphenous nerve produced not only related impulses cephalad from the spinal center but also in impulses directed back down efferent fibers, including sympathetics.[53] Livingston's theory therefore explains a number of characteristics of CRPS type I that cannot be resolved by the artificial synapse theory of Doupe and colleagues.[14] In particular, it accounts for the high incidence of sympathetic "overactivity" observed in these patients, and for the modifying effect of emotional or sensory stimuli, all of which could act by heightening the background activity in this internuncial pool. It should follow that anything that breaks this vicious cycle, be it interruption of sympathetic efferents by spinal anesthesia or interruption of somatic nerve conduction, could relieve pain.

This latter theory enjoyed only a brief wave of enthusiasm, however, probably because it did not conform to the classic concepts of sensory perception originally proposed by von Frey.[56] According to him, individual receptors exist for pain, touch, warmth, and cold, and these sensations involve simple transmission of a sensory impulse up a modality-specific peripheral nerve fiber, followed by relay from the spinal center to the brain via the spinothalamic tract.[56]

Modern neurophysiology has advanced far from the attractive but simplistic views of von Frey, and, although new knowledge has not supported a return to Livingston's concepts, it has shown that the responsible mechanisms are, indeed, complex. Further understanding has spawned the "gate control" theory of pain mediation.[52] In the substantia gelatinosa of the dorsal horns of the spinal cord, the synapses between the peripheral nerves and those that relay their impulses up the long tracts to the brain are modulated by sympathetic input. Simplified for the sake of explanation, it is as if a gate existed at this point of relay and transmission that controls the relationship between the number or frequency of incoming peripheral impulses and the number or frequency of outgoing pulses reaching the brain. High-frequency stimulation of the latter pathways in awake patients is perceived as burning pain. Thus, when the gate is open—an effect of increased sympathetic activity—sensations of, for example, touch or pressure, which normally would result in lower-frequency impulses being relayed to the brain, might instead be perceived as burning pain because of the higher frequency of the impulses getting through the open gate.

This theory is still under study and will obviously undergo modifications and definition over time, but it does offer an explanation not only for causalgia and the role of sympathetic tone (the susceptible patient, the associated peripheral sympathetic activity, and relief by sympathectomy, which closes the gate), but also for other heretofore unexplained observations (e.g., variations in "pain threshold," relief by transcutaneous nerve stimulators, and the apparent benefit of acupuncture in "receptive" persons).

SYMPATHETICALLY MAINTAINED PAIN AND SYMPATHETICALLY INDEPENDENT PAIN

The terms *sympathetically maintained pain* (SMP) and *sympathetically independent pain* (SIP) describe not separate disorders but, rather, the types of pain that can characterize a variety of pain syndromes, including CRPS types I and II. The role of the sympathetic nervous system in the pain associated with CRPS is unclear. Because of poor understanding of the pathophysiologic mechanisms, it was decided that words that had mechanistic connotations such as those involving the sympathetic nervous system, would not be included in the new nomenclature for CRPS.

SMP was originally described as a pain state maintained by the sympathetic nervous system.[45] Recently, the term SMP has been used to describe the pain maintained by sympathetic efferent innervation, circulating catecholamines, or neurochemical action. SMP denotes pain that can be relieved by pharmacologic blockade or local anesthetic block of the sympathetic ganglia that serve the painful area.[8]

SIP refers to pain states not sustained by the sympathetic nervous system. SMP may vary over time, and a patient may have a pain syndrome in which part of the pain is sympathetically maintained and another part is sympathetically independent (i.e., the patient can have both SIP and SMP at the same time). Alternatively, a patient may have SMP at one time, and SIP later.[18]

Haddox[18] indicated that an important aspect of the role of autonomically mediated pain is that it may be a feature of several types of painful entities and is not a requirement of any one. Both SMP and SIP may include, but are not limited to, CRPS, phantom pain, herpes zoster, neuralgias, and metabolic neuropathies.[50] SMP, accordingly, may or may not be present in a patient with CRPS. CRPS has strict inclusion criteria, but the presence or absence of SMP is not one of them. Thus, SMP is not synonymous with either CRPS type I or II. Provision has been made for some conditions to be present in several variants (e.g., nerve injury plus type II CRPS, or a nerve injury with SMP in which sympathetic block relieves some of the pain), but the presentation does not contain features sufficient for the full CRPS diagnosis.[6]

Clinical Presentation and Diagnosis

Drucker and colleagues[15] have divided the natural history of post-traumatic pain syndromes into three clinical stages:

- *Stage 1, acute.* The clinical course is characterized by warmth, erythema, burning, edema, hyperalgesia, hyperhidrosis, and, after a few months, patchy osteoporosis. At this stage, a good result can be expected with Bier's block or chemical sympathectomy, one that often lasts longer than the normal duration of the block. Spontaneous resolution may occur in this stage, particularly with therapeutic support (see later section on Treatment): the clinical course is reversible.
- *Stage 2, dystrophic.* The clinical course is marked by a good response to sympathetic block; symptoms are present for a fixed interval; and spontaneous resolution is rare. Characteristics include coolness, mottling of the skin, cyanosis, brawny edema, dry, brittle nails, continuous pain, and diffuse osteoporosis. At this stage, not only is a bone scan "positive," but usually changes in bone structure are seen on plain films.
- *Stage 3, atrophic.* Pain always extends beyond the area of injury, and florid trophic changes occur, including atrophy of the skin and its appendages and fixed joint contractures. Radiographs show severe demineralization and ankylosis.

Although these stages oversimplify the condition, they provide a framework for diagnosis, treatment, and prognosis for CRPS. For example, among patients who are in stage 1 or 2, prompt treatment may produce permanent relief of pain, and sympathectomy may not even be required by the former group. For patients in stage 3, however, the likelihood of a poor result is greater, and even sympathectomy may not give lasting relief.

The aforementioned consensus committee that met in Orlando in 1993 were unable to develop a uniform list of symptoms and signs because of the variability of the clinical criteria.[17] The following criteria, which were adapted from Wilson[59] can be used to describe the symptoms and signs of CRPS.

1. Pain is a necessary symptom for the diagnosis of CRPS. This pain is located in the affected extremity and is disproportionate to what would be expected from the initial event. It may be spontaneous or evoked and is usually reported as burning pain or diffuse pain. It is not consistent with the distribution of a peripheral nerve, even if the initial injury involved such a nerve. This important feature distinguishes CRPS from pain of other causes and from more specific neuropathic pain disorders. The pain may be reported as throbbing or aching, intermittent or continuous, and exacerbated by physical or emotional stresses. The patient often adopts a protective posture to protect the affected extremity.

2. Sensory changes are usually reported at some stage, and they include allodynia and hyperesthesia in the region of the pain. Allodynia may occur in response to thermal stimulation (cold or warm), deep pressure, light touch, or joint movement.

3. Sympathetic dysfunction is reported as a sudomotor or vasomotor instability in the affected extremity as compared with the unaffected extremity. This dysfunction may vary in severity from time to time and the patient may report that the extremity is warm and red or cold and blue, purple or mottled. Veldman and associates[55] reported that 92% of patients had altered skin temperature. Sweating, particularly of the palms or soles, may be reported as increased, decreased, or unchanged. Normal sympathetic function may be present at certain times.

4. Swelling may be reported at any stage of the syndrome. This swelling is typically peripheral and may be intermittent or permanent and may be exacerbated by the dependent position of the extremity. There can also be pitting or brawny edema.

5. Trophic changes of the skin may be reported later in the course of the syndrome. The nails may be atrophic or hypertrophic. Hair growth and texture may be decreased or increased, and the skin may become atrophic.

6. Motor dysfunction may include dystonia, tremor, and loss of strength of the affected muscle groups. Joint swelling and stiffness may also be reported, particularly of the digits.

Comprehensive Clinical Evaluation

With the foregoing features in mind, we can enhance the clinical evaluation by focusing on particular aspects or using adjunctive tests:

1. *Sensory examination*. Allodynia may be evaluated by applying non noxious stimuli to the affected extremity (warm, cold, light touch, deep pressure, joint movement) and comparing sensory reports from the affected and a normal extremity. Hyperalgesia can be evaluated by applying noxious stimuli and comparing sensory reports from a normal area and the painful area.

2. *Sudomotor examination*. Resting heat output may be estimated by skin impedance[17] or quinizarin or cobalt blue testing,[16] or as part of the quantitative sudomotor reflex test (QSRT),[29] which measures (1) resting sweat output by hygrometry and (2) changes evoked by iontophoresis of acetylcholine into the skin.[30]

3. *Vasomotor examination*. Simultaneous temperature measurements of both the affected and unaffected extremities are taken at corresponding anatomic sites. The temperature of the digit pads, palms and soles, and forearms and calves can be measured with noncontact thermometry or thermography. Serial measurements should be taken, because peripheral temperatures vary widely under normal circumstances. Skin perfusion can be evaluated visually or by pulse oximetry.

4. *Edema*. Edema is generally judged by clinical impression by comparing one extremity to the other, since most volume displacement methods, which provide quantitative estimates of the extent of the edema and allow objective measurement of the results of treatment, can be cumbersome.

5. *Trophic changes*. The skin, hair, and nails of the two sides are compared.

6. *Motor dysfunction*. The presence of dystonia, tremor, and changes in strength can be measured clinically. Objective measurements should be taken (e.g., apposition and opposition pinch strength, grip, weight bearing on lower extremity).

7. *Psychological changes*. No psychometric instrument has been validated for the treatment of CRPS. The psychiatrist or psychologist generally uses familiar instruments as part of the initial assessment and follow-up.

Radiologic findings of CRPS may take many weeks or months to develop. Osteoporosis and abnormal bone scans (measured by technetium 99) can be found in most cases of CRPS.[12, 24, 25] Asymmetric blood flow is usually seen; flow and uptake are usually increased, but occasionally they are diminished.

The diagnosis of CRPS type II is certain when the clinical presentation includes superficial burning pain in the distribution of a single somatic sensory nerve, hyperesthesia, vasomotor abnormalities, radiographic evidence of osteoporosis, and a good response to sympathetic blockade. In CRPS type I, certain clinical features may be minimal or absent, though the response to sympathetic block may still be a reliable sign. In fact, the ultimate relief obtained by surgical sympathectomy can be predicted by careful documentation of the response to a "one-shot" local anesthetic sympathetic blockade.

The Diagnostic Sympathetic Block

The validity of a clinical diagnosis of CRPS may be greatly strengthened by a positive response to sympathetic blockade. Patients should be encouraged to quantify the degree of pain relief experienced (e.g., 100% relief, 50% relief, and so on). The degree of pain relief a patient enjoys with such a block is an excellent predictor of how much relief can be expected from surgical sympathectomy.[1] Some caution should be exercised here, however, because sympathectomy can afford some degree of nonspecific relief of almost any pain, including ischemic pain.[7, 28] CRPS pain, however is usually dramatically relieved by sympathetic blockade (e.g., almost always 75% to 100% relief), whereas relief of pain of other causes is usually only mild to moderate (25% to 50% at most).

Differential Diagnosis

In the differential diagnosis of post-traumatic pain, one of the most important alternatives is nerve entrapment. Causalgia-like pain may occur if a nerve is caught in a suture, entrapped by scar, or compressed by surrounding structures. Nerve entrapment obviously must be considered when causalgia appears immediately after an operation, but because a nerve can be irritated or injured by any compressing or pinching mechanism, there may be a causalgia component to the pain associated with any nerve compression. This is important, because relieving the compression may only partially relieve the pain and the causalgia component may persist. This is discussed later in relation to residual pain subsequent to operations to relieve herniated disc. If peripheral nerve entrapment is the cause, there is often a "trigger point" where focal application of pressure causes sharp pain. The pain can be relieved by infiltration of a small amount of local anesthetic at that point.

Patients who present with cutaneous signs and symptoms characteristic of Drucker's stage 2 are sometimes thought to have Raynaud's syndrome; however, such a patient's symptoms should be intermittent, related principally to cold exposure, and relieved by warmth. Furthermore, hyperesthesia is rare in Raynaud's syndrome, and its characteristic pain is not usually severe or burning.

The pain of peripheral neuritis is often burning and associated with hyperesthesia and vasomotor phenomena. In fact, the pathogenetic mechanisms for peripheral neuritis and post-traumatic pain can be similar. However, the clinical syndrome associated with peripheral neuritis is more diffuse anatomically and gradual in onset, and the patient has no history of trauma or some other discrete precipitating event.

Treatment

Once a post-traumatic pain syndrome has been temporarily relieved by sympathetic blockade, the question of whether to try to achieve this degree of relief more permanently by sympathectomy typically arises. The answer depends on the clinical stage of development, severity of symptoms, and degree and duration of relief by sympathetic block.

For example, for a patient with pain of recent onset who has enjoyed pain relief from sympathetic blockade that lasted well beyond the known duration of the anesthetic agent used, it is advisable to continue with nonoperative measures (see later). Patients whose condition has persisted for several months, whose pain is disabling, and who receive nearly total relief from sympathetic block but only for the typical "duration" of the anesthetic may be considered candidates for immediate surgical sympathectomy. Patients with symptoms of long duration (many months to years), those who have associated trophic changes, and those whose symptoms are less "classic" and less severe and receive only mild to moderate relief from sympathetic block should be advised that the long-term results are likely to be disappointing. The reader should note that these examples correspond to Drucker's three stages; this is deliberate because sympathectomy is, for the most part, best applied in stage 2, before progression to stage 3, and after stage 1, in patients who are unresponsive to nonoperative therapy.

In the past, when no effective treatment was known, post-traumatic pain syndromes frequently resulted in chronic invalidism, emotional deterioration, and drug addiction. Thus, the basis for proper treatment of CRPS is early recognition and prevention. For patients known to be susceptible to CRPS, such as those who have hemiplegia or myocardial infarction, early mobilization of an injured extremity is critical. When early sympathetic dystrophic changes occur, pain relief and active use of the hand, arm, or leg are indicated. Passive motion by the physical therapist should be avoided, as it may increase the pain and edema. Opiate analgesics, when needed, should be used conservatively. Splinting the hand in a functional position may help.

Other nonoperative therapy, particularly as it applies to stage 1 or early stage 2 disease, consists of drug therapy, intermittent sympathetic blocks, and physiotherapy. Drug therapy may require nonspecific analgesics, but these should be superimposed, and only when necessary, on a "background" of medication designed to attenuate the symptoms by direct effect. Of these, phenytoin, amitriptyline, carbamazepine, and baclofen may be used effectively, usually in that order, because of increasing side effects. Nonsteroidal anti-inflammatory agents may be useful, not only in relieving joint swelling but also in combination with the agents just listed, in allowing dose reduction and producing fewer side effects. Benson[4] recommends amitriptyline hydrochloride (Elavil) in doses of 50 to 75 mg nightly or divided during the day (150 mg maximum). Benson also recommended a phenothiazine such as fluphenazine hydrochloride (Prolixin), which potentiates opiate analgesic effects, possesses an analgesic property of its own, and depresses the response to peripheral stimuli. The recommended dosage is 1 mg three times daily, but doses as large as 10 mg/day can be used.

Treatment of CRPS with either the calcium channel blocker nifedipine or the alpha-sympathetic blocker phenoxybenzamine was assessed in 59 patients by Muizelaar and coworkers[37]; 12 subjects had early CRPS, and 47 had chronic CRPS. In the early CRPS group, three of five patients were cured with nifedipine, and eight of nine (two of whom had earlier received nifedipine) with phenoxybenzamine, for a cure rate of 92% (11 of 12). Among the patients with chronic CRPS, 10 of 30 were cured with nifedipine, and seven of 17 with phenoxybenzamine when it was administered as the first choice; another two of seven patients who had initially received nifedipine were cured, for a total success rate of 40% (19 of 47) for chronic CRPS.

Intensive physical therapy should be initiated, including full range-of-motion exercises and whirlpool exercises. Trudel and associates reported good results in 88% of CRPS patients treated with physical therapy.[54]

Transcutaneous electrical nerve stimulation (TENS) has

been used to treat CRPS.[34] Results have been mixed, but because TENS is easily administered and safe, it may be tried before more aggressive treatment is attempted. In the hands of an experienced practitioner, success or failure of TENS will be apparent by the third to the fifth treatment.[60]

A course of steroids should be tried when the response to physical therapy or TENS is poor. Kozin and collaborators[25] reported a fair to excellent response to steroids in 63 of 67 CRPS patients. The usual daily starting dose of prednisone is 60 mg. The dose is tapered every 3 days by 5 mg, for a total therapy course of about 5 weeks.

Because at least a temporary response to a number of nonoperative treatment modalities is common in early stages of CRPS, a common error in management is to carry attempts at conservative therapy too far, persisting with such treatments too long and shifting repeatedly from one to the other. This not only subjects those who are destined never to respond to such therapy, to wasted time, expense, and suffering; it also may compromise their chances of obtaining complete and lasting relief by surgical sympathectomy. Thus, if the measures described above are not effective in relieving the symptoms promptly, or if symptoms are exacerbated over the course of several days, the physician should proceed directly to sympathetic blocks, which are both diagnostic and therapeutic.

An initial sympathetic block is appropriate early in stage I to confirm the diagnosis and to test its therapeutic potential. The rapid pain relief gained from a sympathetic block can be extremely helpful psychologically. Also, at this stage the condition may be reversible and complete remission can sometimes be achieved, particularly in patients who experience long-lasting relief from serial sympathetic blocks, when it allows aggressive physiotherapy to be applied. When relief is short-lived, however, persisting with repeated blocks is counterproductive and expensive.

Injections of alcohol and phenol have been used instead of surgical sympathectomy in attempts to produce lasting sympathetic denervation but a significant incidence of incomplete or transient sympathetic blocks is associated with this approach. Its risks include painful neuralgia and inflammation with scarring, the latter potentially making subsequent surgery more difficult.[44]

Radiofrequency ablation has been proposed as a more precise method of achieving percutaneous sympathetic denervation.[38] Although it may represent an advance over phenol or alcohol blocks, its effect is not as complete or durable as that of surgical sympathectomy, and the local reaction it produces would seriously interfere with subsequent operation. Furthermore, general anesthesia is necessary.

Such methods have been proposed primarily because of the morbidity of surgical cervical sympathectomy, particularly via the transthoracic route (which may cause significant post-thoracotomy discomfort). However, this latter objection is less compelling now that the procedure can be done safely and precisely thoracoscopically[2, 19, 31] and the patient discharged the next day. Through the modern thoracoscope, with its view enlarged on video screen and using instruments such as those developed for laparoscopic cholecystectomy, removal of the T2 and T3 sympathetic ganglia and division of the rami to the lower part of the stellate ganglion can be performed with precision and safety. The procedure is less predictably successful in the presence of inflammation and scarring.

Others have now reported good results with laparoscopic lumbar sympathectomy[20] (see Chapter 73). In view of this development and the fact that lumbar sympathectomy is tolerated so well, any percutaneous method that does not produce a complete and lasting sympathectomy effect cannot be condoned because it precludes safe sympathectomy later. If surgical sympathectomy is limited to those who obtain excellent relief from sympathetic block with a local anesthetic, nearly 90% of patients enjoy long-term relief.[1, 36]

Cooney[11] summarized a treatment protocol. The first step was to differentiate sympathetic pain from somatic pain (Table 63–2). The RSD score can be helpful. When the pain is somatic, treatment options include (1) isolated nerve block, (2) continuous nerve block, (3) TENS (external), (4) direct electrical nerve stimulation (internal), and (5) nerve ablation. If pain is sympathetic in origin, treatments should include (1) protection of the limb (with a garment or splint) combined with active use, (2) sympathetic blocks (single or continuous), and (3) sympathectomy.

Results of Sympathectomy

The specific techniques of cervicothoracic and lumbar sympathectomy are described in Chapters 73 and 83. The following discussion reviews the results of sympathectomy for CRPS, including our own experience.[1, 36]

The first reports of surgical sympathectomy for causalgia were probably those of Spurling in 1930[49] and of Kwan in 1935.[26] Both described trauma to an extremity that was complicated by causalgia and relieved by sympathectomy. Clinical series from World War II helped to define a role for sympathectomy for causalgia.[21, 32, 48] In 1951, Mayfield[32] reported on 75 patients with causalgia who were treated and followed for 5 years; 73 of them had significant early pain relief, and in 63% of the 73 it was sustained for 5 years. In the other 37%, the pain was significantly relieved but not completely gone at 5 years. In Thompson's 1979 series,[52] 27 patients with causalgia were treated with sympathectomy, and among 120 patients who had minor cau-

TABLE 63–2. DIAGNOSTIC CRITERIA FOR REFLEX SYMPATHETIC DYSTROPHY

Clinical Symptoms and Signs
- Burning pain
- Hyperpathia or allodynia
- Temperature or color changes
- Edema
- Hair or nail growth changes

Laboratory Results
- Thermometry or thermography
- Bone radiography
- Three-phase bone scan
- Quantitative sweat test
- Response to sympathetic block

Interpretation

If total number of positive findings is:
- >6: Reflex sympathetic dystrophy probable
- 3–5: Reflex sympathetic dystrophy possible
- <3: Reflex sympathetic dystrophy unlikely

salgia, 55 were treated with sympathectomy. Among all patients, 82% had excellent pain relief, and 11% good pain relief, and 7% had a poor result. Residual symptoms, largely those secondary to associated injuries, were present in 31%.[52] Olcott and associates also reported 91% good to excellent results in 35 patients.[39]

One of the authors (R.B.R.) has twice published his experience with post-traumatic pain syndromes and sympathectomy. The first series,[61] from Johns Hopkins Hospital, included 27 patients. Immediate pain relief was achieved in 24 patients (all of whom received a successful trial block), and of 15 patients observed for 2 to 17 years, pain relief was sustained in 13. The second series,[36] from the University of Colorado, included 31 patients. All patients in this series were evaluated preoperatively with sympathetic block, and 97% of the patients reported a satisfactory level of immediate pain relief. In extended follow-up, this level of pain relief was sustained in 94%. In a similar, more recent series of 28 patients,[1] the other author (A.F.A.) reported 95% long-term success in patients who had enjoyed an excellent response to a trial block.

An interesting subgroup of patients was identified in two of the aforementioned reports.[1, 36] In the first series,[36] patients with causalgia persisting after disc surgery enjoyed pain relief following sympathectomy equal to that in other patients. These cases constituted more than half of those in which lumbar sympathectomy was performed; this relates both to a high index of suspicion and to indoctrination of local neurosurgeons. In the second series,[1] 10 patients (36% of the total) had had lumbar discectomy and they too reported uniformly excellent results following sympathectomy. Neither the true frequency of persistent postdiscectomy pain nor its nature is known. Once called *arachnoiditis* and thought to be due to inflammation and nerve sheath irritation after disc surgery, it probably reflects residual nerve damage that occurs before nerve root compression is relieved by removal of the herniated nucleus pulposus. Clearly, the recognition of causalgia as a possible component of lumbar disc pain, its persistence after discectomy, and its potential relief by sympathectomy have been inadequately recognized in the medical literature.

Complications

Failure to promptly recognize and to appropriately treat CRPS is unacceptable because the syndrome often results in irreversible changes, including wasting of skin and muscles, fixed joint contractures, and severe demineralization of bone; it also misses the opportunity for permanent pain relief by sympathectomy.

The complications of sympathectomy itself have been described in depth by the authors[1, 46] and are also discussed in Chapter 73. In general, the complications of sympathectomy can be classified as:

- *Preoperative*, in which the anticipated benefit has not been achieved because of improper patient selection
- *Intraoperative*, related to improper technique
- *Postoperative*, encountered after an appropriate and properly executed sympathectomy.

Preoperative complications can be minimized by the use of nerve blocks, sham saline blocks in questionable cases, and, when appropriate, careful psychiatric evaluation. Intraoperative complications can be avoided by meticulous attention to the anatomic relationships and normal variations of anatomy among the structures most frequently injured—the genitofemoral nerve, ureters, lumbar veins, aorta, and inferior vena cava. The most common postoperative complication is postsympathectomy neuralgia, which, though frequent, almost always resolves spontaneously.[3, 36]

When applied selectively for the aforementioned pain syndromes, sympathectomy gives excellent symptomatic relief, far superior to its other indications. Although once associated with significant morbidity and even death when performed on elderly patients with advanced arteriosclerosis, the current technique carries negligible risk and produces very few permanent adverse sequelae in the typically younger and healthier patients who have various forms of sympathetically mediated pain.

REFERENCES

1. AbuRahma AF, Robinson PA, Powell M, et al: Sympathectomy for reflex sympathetic dystrophy: Factors: affecting outcome. Ann Vasc Surg 8:372–379, 1994.
2. Appleby TC, Edwards WH Jr: Thoracoscopic dorsal sympathectomy for hyperhidrosis: Technique of choice. J Vasc Surg 16:121–123, 1992.
3. Barnes R: The role of sympathectomy in the treatment of causalgia. J Bone Joint Surg 35B:172–180, 1953.
4. Benson WF: Discussion of RG Chuinard at Annual Meeting, American Society for Surgery of the Hand, Atlanta, 1980.
5. Bergan JJ, Conn J: Sympathectomy for pain relief. Med Clin North Am 52:147–159, 1968.
6. Boas RA: Complex regional pain syndromes: Symptoms, signs, and differential diagnosis. *In* Janig W, Stanton-Hicks M (eds): Reflex Sympathetic Dystrophy: A Reappraisal. Seattle, IASP Press, 1996, pp 79–91.
7. Bobin A, Anderson WP: Influence of sympathectomy in x-2 adrenoreceptor binding sites in canine blood vessels. Life Sci 33:331, 1983.
8. Campbell JN: Complex regional pain syndrome and the sympathetic nervous system. *In* Pain 1996—An Updated Review. IASP Refresher Courses on Pain Management held in conjunction with the 8th World Congress on Pain. Seattle, IASP Press, 1996, pp 89–96.
9. Chapman LF, Ramos AV, Goodell H, et al: Neurohumoral features of afferent fibers in man. Arch Neurol 4:617–650, 1961.
10. Cheshire NJ, Darzi AW: Retroperitoneoscopic lumbar sympathectomy. Br J Surg 84:1094–1095, 1997.
11. Cooney WP: Somatic versus sympathetic mediated chronic limb pain: Experience and treatment options. Hand Clin 13:355–361, 1997.
12. Davidoff G, Werner R, Cremer S, et al: Predictive value of the three-phase technetium bone scan in diagnosis of reflex sympathetic dystrophy syndrome. Arch Phys Med Rehabil 70:135–137, 1989.
13. Davis SW: Shoulder-hand syndrome in a hemiplegic population: 5-year retrospective study. Arch Phys Med Rehabil 58:353–356, 1977.
14. Doupe J, Cullen CH, Chance GQ: Post-traumatic pain and the causalgic syndrome. J Neurol Psychiatry 7:33–48, 1944.
15. Drucker WR, Hubay CA, Holden WD, et al: Pathogenesis of posttraumatic sympathetic dystrophy. Am J Surg 97:454–465, 1959.
16. Fealey RD: The thermoregulatory sweat test. *In* Low PA (ed): Clinical Autonomic Disorders. Boston, Little, Brown, 1993, pp 217–229.
17. Gibbons JJ, Wilson PR: RSD score: Criteria for the diagnosis of reflex sympathetic dystrophy and causalgia. Clin J Pain 8:260–263, 1992.
18. Haddox JD: A call for clarity. *In* Pain 1996—An Updated Review: IASP Refresher Courses on Pain Management held in conjunction with the 8th World Congress on Pain. Seattle, IASP Press, 1996, pp 97–99.
19. Horgan K, O'Flanagan S, Duignan PJ, et al: Palmar and axillary hyperhidrosis treated by sympathectomy by transthoracic endoscopic electrocoagulation. Br J Surg 71:1002, 1984.
20. Kathouda N, Wattanasirichaigoon S, Tang E, et al: Laparoscopic lumbar sympathectomy. Surg Endosc 11:257–260, 1997.

21. Kirklin JW, Chenoweth AE, Murphy F: Causalgia: A review of its characteristics, diagnosis and treatment. Surgery 21:321, 1947.
22. Kozin F: Reflex sympathetic dystrophy syndrome. Bull Rheum Dis 36:1–8, 1986.
23. Kozin F: The painful shoulder and reflex sympathetic dystrophy syndrome. *In* McCarty DJ (ed): Arthritis and Allied Conditions, 10th ed. Philadelphia, Lea & Febiger, 1985.
24. Kozin F, Genant HK, Bekerman C, et al: The reflex sympathetic dystrophy syndrome: II. Roentgenographic and scintigraphic evidence bilaterally and of periarticular accentuation. Am J Med 60:332–338, 1976.
25. Kozin F, Ryan LM, Carerra GF, et al: The reflex sympathetic dystrophy syndrome: III. Scintigraphic studies, further evidence for the therapeutic efficacy of systemic corticosteroids and proposed diagnostic criteria. Am J Med 70:23–30, 1981.
26. Kwan ST: The treatment of causalgia by thoracic sympathetic ganglionectomy. Ann Surg 101:222, 1935.
27. Livingston WK: Pain Mechanisms: A Physiological Interpretation of Causalgia and Its Related States. New York, Macmillan, 1943, pp 83–113.
28. Loh L, Nathan PW: Painful peripheral states and sympathetic blocks. J Neurol Neurosurg Psychiatry 41:664–671, 1978.
29. Low PA, Pfeifer MD: Standardization of clinical tests for practice and clinical trials. *In* Low PA (ed): Clinical Autonomic Disorders. Boston, Little, Brown, 1993, pp 287–296.
30. Low PA, Wilson PR, Sandroni P, et al: Reflex sympathetic dystrophy: A reappraisal, progress. *In* Janig W, Stanton-Hicks M (eds): Pain Research and Management. Vol. 6, Seattle, IASP Press, 1996, pp 40–43, 212–213.
31. Malone PS, Cameron AE, Rennie JA: Endoscopic thoracoscopic sympathectomy in the treatment of upper limb hyperhidrosis. Ann R Coll Surg Engl 68:93–94, 1986.
32. Mayfield FH: Causalgia. Springfield, Ill, Charles C Thomas, 1951.
33. Merskey H, Bogduk N: Classification of Chronic Pain, 2nd ed. Seattle, IASP Press, 1994.
34. Meyer GA, Fields HL: Causalgia treated by selective large fibre stimulation of peripheral nerve. Brain 95:163–168, 1972.
35. Mitchell SW, Morehouse GR, Keen WW: Gunshot Wounds and Other Injuries of Nerves. Philadelphia, JB Lippincott, 1864, p 164.
36. Mockus MB, Rutherford RB, Rosales C, et al: Sympathectomy for causalgia: Patient selection and long-term results. Arch Surg 122:668–672, 1987.
37. Muizelaar JP, Kleyer M, Hertogs IA, et al: Complex regional pain syndrome (reflex sympathetic dystrophy and causalgia): Management with the calcium channel blocker nifedipine and/or the alpha-sympathetic blocker phenoxybenzamine in 59 patients. Clin Neurol Neurosurg 99:26–30, 1997.
38. Noe CE, Haynsworth RF Jr: Lumbar radiofrequency sympatholysis. J Vasc Surg 17:801–806, 1993.
39. Olcott C, Eltherington LG, Wilcosky BR, et al: Reflex sympathetic dystrophy: The surgeon's role in management. J Vasc Surg 14:488–492, 1991.
40. Paré A: Les Oeuvres d'Ambroise Paré, Paris, Gabriel Bron. Historie de Defunct. Roy Charles 10th book, 1598, p 401.
41. Patman RD, Thompson JE, Persson AV: Management of post-traumatic pain syndromes: Report of 113 cases. Ann Surg 177:780–787, 1973.
42. Plewes LW: Sudeck's atrophy in the hands. J Bone Joint Surg 38:195–203, 1956.
43. Porter EL, Taylor AN: Facilitation of flexion reflex in relation to pain after nerve injuries (causalgia). J Neurophysiol 8:289–294, 1945.
44. Ramos M, Almazan A, Lozano F, et al: Phenol lumbar sympathectomy in severe arterial disease of the lower limb: A hemodynamic study. Int Surg 68:127–130, 1983.
45. Roberts WJ: A hypothesis on the physiological basis for causalgia and related pain. Pain 24:297–311, 1986.
46. Rutherford RB: Complications of sympathectomy. *In* Bernhard VM, Towne JB (eds): Complications in Vascular Surgery. New York, Grune & Stratton, 1980.
47. Schondorf R: The role of the sympathetic skin response in the assessment of autonomic function. *In* Low PA (ed): Clinical Autonomic Disorders. Boston, Little, Brown, 1993, pp 231–241.
48. Shumaker HB Jr, Abramson DI: Post-traumatic vasomotor disorders. Surg Gynecol Obstet 88:417, 1949.
49. Spurling RG: Causalgia of the upper extremity: Treatment by dorsal sympathetic ganglionectomy. Arch Neurol Psychiatry (Chir) 23:704, 1930.
50. Stanton-Hicks M, Janig W, Hassenbusch S, et al: Reflex sympathetic dystrophy: Changing concepts and taxonomy. Pain 63:127–133, 1995.
51. Steinbrocker O, Spitzer N, Friedman HH: The shoulder-hand syndrome in reflex dystrophy of upper extremity. Ann Intern Med 29:22–52, 1948.
52. Thompson JE: The diagnosis and management of post-traumatic pain syndromes (causalgia). Aust NZ J Surg 49:299–304, 1979.
53. Toennie JF: Reflex discharges from the spinal cord over the dorsal roots. J Neurophysiol 1:370, 1938.
54. Trudel J, DeWolfe VG, Young JR, et al: Disuse phenomenon of the lower extremity: Diagnosis and treatment. JAMA 186:1129–1131, 1963.
55. Veldman PHJM, Reynen HM, Arntz IE, et al: Signs and symptoms of reflex sympathetic dystrophy: Prospective study of 829 patients. Lancet 342:1012–1016, 1993.
56. von Frey R: Cited in White JC, Sweet WH: Other varieties of peripheral neuralgia. *In* White JC (ed): Pain and the Neurosurgeon. Springfield, Ill, Charles C Thomas, 1969, pp 87–109.
57. Walker AE, Nielsen S: Electrical stimulation of the upper thoracic portion of the sympathetic chain in man. Arch Neurol Psychiatry 59:599, 1947.
58. White JC, Sweet WH: Other varieties of peripheral neuralgia. *In* White JC (ed): Pain and the Neurosurgeon. Springfield, Ill, Charles C Thomas, 1969, pp 87–109.
59. Wilson PR: Diagnostic algorithm for complex regional pain syndromes. *In* Janig W, Stanton-Hicks M (eds): Reflex Sympathetic Dystrophy: A Reappraisal. Seattle, IASP Press, 1996, pp 93–105.
60. Wilson RL: Management of pain following peripheral nerve injuries. Orthop Clin North Am 12:343–359, 1981.
61. Wirth FP, Rutherford RB: A civilian experience with causalgia. Arch Surg 100:633–638, 1970.

SECTION X

MANAGEMENT OF CHRONIC ISCHEMIA OF THE LOWER EXTREMITIES

RICHARD F. KEMPCZINSKI, M.D.

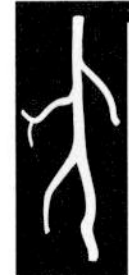

CHAPTER 64

The Chronically Ischemic Leg: An Overview

Richard F. Kempczinski, M.D.

Since the birth of modern vascular surgery in the early 1950s, numerous technical and clinical developments have revolutionized the management of chronic ischemia of the lower extremities. The vascular surgeon is now armed with an amazing array of diagnostic and therapeutic options for the management of arterial occlusive disease. Refinements in traditional angiographic techniques and the introduction of digitized vascular imaging have made detailed visualization of the lower extremity arterial tree routine, and noninvasive methods of hemodynamic testing now provide objective documentation of each patient's physiologic derangement. In addition to a wide variety of traditional bypass and disobliterative (i.e., endarterectomy) techniques, ingenious modifications of the angiographer's catheter have made percutaneous dilatation of arterial stenoses and even the placement of endovascular grafts practical.

Catheter-based management of a wide variety of lesions has evolved from the stage of mere clinical feasibility to the level of reliability and durability required of an integral tool in the treatment of occlusive disease. Percutaneous transluminal angioplasty (PTA) and the use of stents have an established and growing role in the management of lower extremity ischemia. Although using percutaneous methods attempts to extend the role of PTA by laser and atherectomy devices have been disappointing, thrombolytic therapy has allowed some occlusions that in the past would have required open surgery to be treated with endovascular intervention.

An extensive selection of artificial vascular substitutes has been developed and promises to provide durable vascular prostheses for virtually every clinical situation. The resurgence of interest in the use of autogenous saphenous vein in situ for lower extremity bypasses promises to increase the availability of this nearly ideal conduit and to improve long-term patency. Modifications in amputation techniques and prosthetic design have enhanced the rehabilitation of the dysvascular amputee. The indications for lumbar sympathectomy have been defined more clearly. Finally, careful clinical studies and retrospective analyses have clarified the natural history of lower extremity arterial insufficiency and the prognosis for survival and limb loss in patients afflicted with this disease.

This chapter reviews the principles underlying our current understanding of atherosclerosis and the pathophysiology of chronic lower extremity ischemia and covers the following topics:

1. The impact of both gradual arterial occlusion and the development of collateral circulation on lower extremity perfusion.
2. The associated diseases that influence the development and progression of chronic lower extremity ischemia.
3. The general principles that govern vascular reconstruction of the chronically ischemic lower extremity.

Subsequent chapters in Section X cover the nonoperative management of the ischemic limb, describe in detail the indications for and the techniques and results of the various reconstructive procedures, and discuss some of the rarer conditions that may produce lower extremity ischemia.

ETIOLOGY AND PREDISPOSING FACTORS

A thorough understanding of the process and natural history of arterial obliteration is essential for the proper selection of candidates for operation and the appropriate surgical procedures to achieve limb revascularization. The important causes of lower extremity arterial obliteration are:

- Atherosclerosis
- Thromboangiitis obliterans (Buerger's disease)
- Vasculitis
- Arterial trauma

- Popliteal artery entrapment
- Cystic adventitial disease of the popliteal artery

Atherosclerosis is the underlying cause of chronic limb ischemia in the vast majority of patients. Although its etiology remains unclear, its incidence and progression are clearly accelerated by the coexistence of diabetes mellitus, hypertension, lipoprotein abnormalities, and, most important, addiction to the use of tobacco.[11, 19, 20, 25, 31, 47, 55, 58, 60, 63] The already diminished flow through atherosclerotic vessels and the high-resistance collateral channels that have opened to carry blood around them is further compromised by the greater viscosity of the blood in patients with polycythemia and by the reduction in cardiac output from associated heart disease.[32, 47, 73, 75] Alterations in fibrinogen, fibrinolytic activity, and platelet adhesiveness or aggregation may also contribute to the progression of atherosclerosis or may promote thrombosis of already diseased vessels.[23, 46, 47, 50]

Although it is a more common problem in the Middle East and the Far East, *thromboangiitis obliterans* or Buerger's disease is a very infrequent cause of lower limb ischemia in the United States (see Chapter 20).[40] Despite challenges from some investigators as to its very existence, there can no longer be any doubt that Buerger's disease is a distinct pathologic entity.[12, 40, 45, 74] Many cases that in the past would have been classified on clinical grounds as Buerger's disease are now correctly identified, on the basis of more precise angiographic and clinical scrutiny, as peripherally distributed premature atherosclerosis.[12] Occasionally, the two diseases may coexist in the same patient.[45]

Pathologically, thromboangiitis obliterans manifests as a severe, chronic inflammatory process that involves the entire neurovascular bundle of the small vessels of the hands and feet and leads to arterial and venous thrombosis and fibrosis.[12, 40] Its inflammatory nature and distal localization generally preclude direct surgical reconstruction. It typically occurs in individuals during the third and fourth decades of life and is invariably associated with heavy use of tobacco.[40] If the patient can be persuaded to stop using tobacco, the disease process can be halted.

Other types of *vasculitis* may involve the small arteries and arterioles and result in lower extremity ischemia. Proper treatment depends on recognition and management of the underlying disease process and is rarely the direct concern of the vascular surgeon.

Ischemia that is due to *arterial trauma* is usually an acute problem. Nonocclusive arterial trauma occasionally may be overlooked during the initial evaluation of a trauma victim or may be obscured by more pressing or life-threatening injuries. Subsequently, as the patient recovers and resumes ambulation, the arterial injury may become apparent.

Both *entrapment*[34] and *cystic adventitial disease*[21] of the popliteal artery are rare causes of chronic arterial ischemia that generally affect young, otherwise healthy, active individuals. Although these diseases can produce severe disability if they are unrecognized and left untreated, normal circulation can usually be restored in the majority of these patients.

PATHOLOGY OF ATHEROSCLEROSIS

Atherosclerosis is primarily a disease of the arterial intima that extends into the media but usually spares the outer media and adventitia (see Chapter 18).[11] The pathogenesis of its sentinel lesion, the fatty intimal streak, remains the subject of continuing debate.[23, 47, 71] It may begin as a platelet and fibrin thrombus sealing a break in the intima that has exposed subintimal collagen,[46] or increased permeability of the damaged intima to low-density lipoproteins may lead to focal accumulations of this material and cholesterol, particularly in association with proteoglycan, in the vessel wall.[29] Further accumulation of thrombus with the development of fibrosis then leads to plaque formation and progressive luminal encroachment.[11, 23] Continuing lipid accumulation, hemorrhage into the plaque, or deposition of mural thrombus may progressively narrow the lumen until occlusion eventually occurs.[23] Nonocclusive but ulcerated plaques may be the source of peripheral emboli,[27, 51] which can lodge in the smaller, more distal arteries and further aggravate limb ischemia by reducing the runoff bed.

Although atherosclerosis is a generalized disease, it is remarkably segmental in its distribution.[22, 33, 39] It develops at major arterial bifurcations and in areas of posterior fixation or acute angulation.[68] Disruption of laminar flow in these areas creates eddy currents that traumatize the intima and are responsible in part for the increase in atheroma formation at these points.[73] In addition, the marked change in the direction of blood flow at arterial bifurcations and pronounced curves induces a relatively negative force on the intima along the convex inner wall of the curvature (the airfoil effect), which further promotes plaque formation in these areas.[68]

The arterial segment that lies in Hunter's canal and represents the transition between the distal superficial femoral artery and the popliteal artery is the site in the lower extremity most commonly involved with atherosclerosis.[22, 33, 39] It is not only a point of arterial fixation and oblique passage through the adductor magnus tendon but also the site of origin of the large superior genicular branch. Atheromata occur with nearly equal frequency on the posterior wall of the common femoral artery and extend into the proximal superficial femoral and profunda femoris arteries. The infrarenal abdominal aorta commonly has atherosclerotic involvement, which is especially prominent immediately distal to the origin of the inferior mesenteric artery, where it becomes confluent with the plaque arising at the aortic bifurcation. This heavily diseased segment often contains an irregular, ulcerated intima covered by friable, exuberant thrombus that may embolize spontaneously or at the time of surgical manipulation (see Chapter 56).[27]

The true extent of atherosclerotic involvement of the posterior arterial wall may be difficult to appreciate on routine arteriograms taken in a single anteroposterior projection.[42, 61] Careful palpation at the time of surgery, however, usually reveals the magnitude of the problem and permits appropriate modification or extension of the proposed reconstructive procedure.

Other sites for which atherosclerosis exhibits a predilection are[33, 39]:

- Common iliac bifurcation
- Mid-popliteal artery opposite the knee joint
- Popliteal trifurcation, including the proximal portions of the tibial vessels

The experienced clinician who is cognizant of the remarkable propensity of this disorder for segmental localization can usually infer the sites of arterial involvement from a careful history and physical examination, occasionally supplemented by noninvasive hemodynamic measurements, without the need for arteriography.

HEMODYNAMIC CONSIDERATIONS IN THE ISCHEMIC LEG

A complete discussion of hemodynamic principles is presented in Chapter 7. Some of the principles, however, deserve reemphasis to provide the foundation for a rational approach to lower limb revascularization.

Blood Flow

Blood flow is directly proportional to arterial pressure and inversely related to peripheral resistance.[73] *Arterial pressure* is determined by cardiac output, peripheral resistance, and circulating blood volume. *Peripheral resistance* in the normal limb is a function of the precapillary arterioles, blood viscosity, tissue pressure, and venous pressure. A hemodynamically significant obstruction within a major limb artery results in a drop in perfusion pressure distal to the obstruction and an increase in total peripheral resistance that reduces limb blood flow.

Within certain limitations, arterial blood flow is governed by the Poiseuille equation[73]:

$$P_1 - P_2 = \frac{V \cdot 8L\eta}{r^2} = \frac{Q \cdot 8L\eta}{\pi r^4}$$

where Q is flow, $P_1 - P_2$ is pressure differential, η is viscosity, r is radius of the vessel, L is length of the stenosis, and V is mean flow velocity. Therefore, the flow through a stenotic major artery or through narrow collateral vessels is largely governed by the radius of the arterial lumen and by the length of the stenotic segment.

When a main limb artery is occluded, the total resistance to flow that results is the sum of the parallel resistances imposed by the collateral vessels that bypass that segment and is expressed by the formula[73]

$$\frac{1}{r} = \frac{1}{r_1} + \frac{1}{r_2} + \frac{1}{r_n}$$

As the vessels dilate over time, this resistance (r) diminishes and flow improves. If a second segment of the same artery becomes occluded, adding a resistance *in series*, the total resistance is expressed by the formula:

$$r_{total} = r_1 + r_2 + \ldots r_n$$

Thus, the impact of resistance in series is additive and further diminishes the capacity of the arterial tree to meet the functional demands imposed by exercise, infection, or the dissipation of external heat. Finally, even the minimal flow needed to sustain viability is compromised, and tissue necrosis ensues.[67]

Collateral Circulation

Collateral vessels develop from the distributing branches of large and medium-sized arteries.[66] Anatomically as well as functionally, it is convenient to divide the collateral bed into:

- Stem arteries
- Mid-zone collaterals
- Reentry arteries

These vessels, generally preexisting pathways that enlarge when a stenosis or an occlusion develops in a main artery of supply, do not represent neovascularization. Although the precise mechanism that stimulates their development remains unknown, it appears that the pressure differential that develops across the collateral bed as a result of the arterial occlusion causes a reversal of flow in the distal mid-zone collateral channels and increases the velocity of flow through them as they dilate in response to this stimulus (Fig. 64–1). Exercise further enhances this effect by

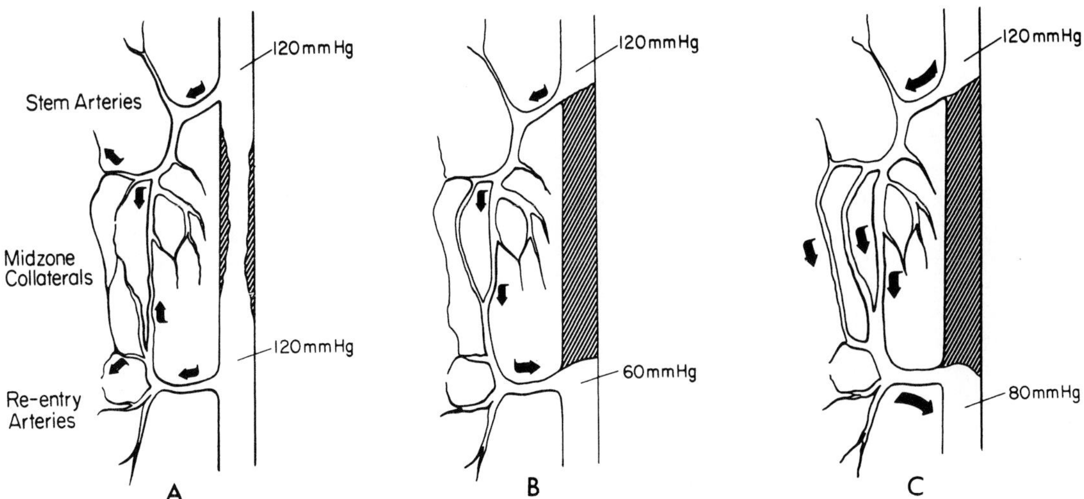

FIGURE 64–1. Hemodynamic theory of collateral formation. *A*, Developing stenosis in main vessel without drop in pressure across it; arrows indicate direction and volume of blood flow in side branches. *B*, Lesion has progressed to acute thrombosis with 60 mmHg pressure drop and reversal of flow in reentry below occlusion. *C*, Over several weeks, collateral flow increases in response to the pressure differential, and the gradient across the lesion decreases.

producing relative tissue hypoxia and acidosis, which reduce peripheral resistance, thus magnifying the pressure gradient across the obstruction.[3]

Collateral channels that form in response to a chronic, unisegmental occlusion can usually provide adequate blood flow to meet the resting needs of the limb and sufficient additional flow to sustain moderate exercise.[39] Sudden occlusion of a previously normal vessel, however, as might occur with an arterial embolus, may not allow sufficient time for the collateral circulation to compensate for the acute ischemia and may result in tissue necrosis or frank gangrene.[66, 67] If the collateral development around an arterial stenosis keeps pace with any progression of the disease, there may be little change in the patient's symptoms or the patient may experience a transient period of severe limb ischemia that gradually relents over the next few weeks as the collateral circulation expands to its ultimate potential (see Fig. 64–1*C*).

Although atherosclerosis usually spares the mid-zone collateral vessels, progressive intimal disease or extension of the main vessel thrombosis may occlude the stem or reentry vessels, thus compromising the effectiveness of the entire collateral network. In the absence of mechanical occlusion, the collateral blood flow may be reduced by decreased cardiac output, increased blood viscosity,[53] hyperfibrinogenemia,[50] or dehydration.

Several well-recognized anatomic patterns of collateral development are illustrated in Figure 64–2. Occlusion of the distal abdominal aorta recruits stem collaterals from the intercostal and lumbar arteries to connect with reentry collaterals of the iliolumbar, gluteal, deep circumflex iliac, and epigastric arteries.[66] A secondary visceral pathway arises from the left colic branch of the superior mesenteric artery, continues through the meandering mesenteric artery, and finally reenters the hypogastric artery via the hemorrhoidal plexus.[18] For external iliac or common femoral artery occlusions, collateral supply develops by way of the hypogastric artery and its gluteal branches with the femoral circumflex branches of the profunda femoris (deep femoral) artery; this important collateral pathway is known as the *cruciate anastomosis.* The relationship between aortoiliac collateral vessels and the visceral circulation explains how occlusive disease involving both systems may predispose the patient to bowel ischemia and necrosis if these channels are disrupted at surgery or if flow through them is altered after aortofemoral bypass.[18, 49, 62, 69]

The interconnection of the perforating branches of the profunda femoris artery and the genicular branches of the popliteal artery readily compensates for occlusion of the superficial femoral artery. This network in the upper leg depends largely on the profunda femoris artery as a critical link between the cruciate and genicular networks and emphasizes the importance of a patent popliteal artery that serves as the reentry vessel for this vital collateral pathway. In similar fashion, the genicular arteries, via their tibial connections, bypass popliteal obstructions.[66] Occlusion of the anterior and posterior tibial arteries is often compensated for by the peroneal artery, which sends large collateral branches to the patent distal segments of the tibial arteries at the ankle.[4] Figure 64–2 graphically illustrates the paucity of collaterals in the lower leg, which helps to explain why even unisegmental occlusion of the distal popliteal and

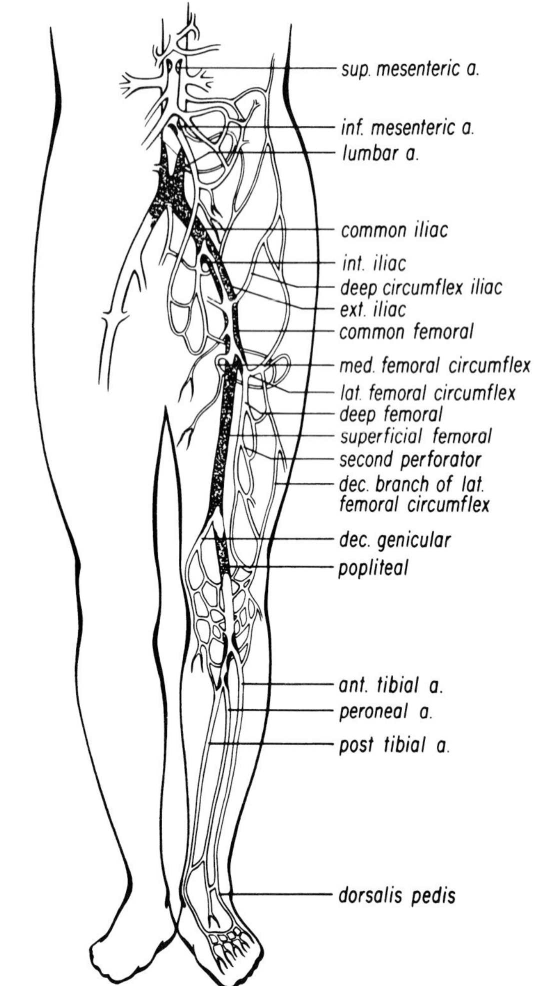

FIGURE 64–2. Diagram of the arterial circulation to the lower extremity, indicating the characteristic segments of obstruction by atherosclerosis *(shaded areas)* and the compensatory collateral network.

proximal tibial arteries may result in such severe ischemia of the distal lower extremity.

CLASSIFICATION

Limb ischemia is classified as (1) "functional" or (2) "critical."

Functional ischemia occurs when blood flow is normal in the resting extremity but cannot be increased in response to exercise; clinically, it manifests as *claudication.* This term, derived from the Latin verb meaning "to limp," indicates one of the best-defined entities in clinical medicine. The single most important symptom of arterial occlusive disease in an extremity, claudication develops whenever blood flow to the exercising muscle mass is unable to meet the requirements of this increased metabolic activity. It consists of three essential features. The pain is:

1. Always experienced in a functional muscle unit.
2. Reproducibly precipitated by a consistent amount of exercise.
3. Promptly relieved by mere stopping of the exercise.

Although a number of syndromes are regularly confused with claudication, careful attention to these features can facilitate accurate diagnosis.[26]

Chronic *critical limb ischemia* (CLI) is defined by either of the following two criteria: (1) recurring ischemic rest pain that persists for more than 2 weeks and requires regular analgesics, with an ankle systolic pressure of 50 mmHg or less, a toe systolic pressure of 30 mmHg or less, or both, or (2) ulceration or gangrene of the foot or toes, with similar hemodynamic parameters.[77]

Unlike claudication, *ischemic rest pain* is experienced not in a muscle group but rather in the foot, specifically the toes and metatarsal heads. It should not be confused with *night cramps*, which are common in patients with atherosclerosis and occur as painful cramps of the calf muscle that usually begin after the patient has fallen asleep and are relieved by massage of the muscle. In its earliest manifestations, rest pain may be experienced as dysesthesias in the foot after it has been elevated for some time. At this stage, the patient can usually relieve the pain by dangling the affected extremity over the side of the bed or, paradoxically, by getting up and walking around. Because this pain typically occurs at night, some clinicians call it *night pain* to distinguish it from the more severe rest pain that is constant and present even with dependency.

Ischemic rest pain implies a reduction of blood flow in the extremity to a level below that required for normal resting tissue metabolism. If left untreated, it almost always results in tissue necrosis. The affected limb is relatively useless or frankly incapacitated by the constant pain, the paresthesias, and the muscle paresis. Because the patient with ischemic rest pain typically keeps the limb dependent, there is often a considerable amount of edema, which further compromises tissue perfusion. Angiography in such extremities invariably demonstrates at least two, and often three or more, serial obstructions of the arterial tree. By contrast, in patients with claudication, usually only one or, at most, two segments are involved.

Although the pathophysiology of CLI is not firmly established, the following hypothesis attempts to incorporate many of the observations on this entity.[77] Arteriolar vasodilatation, probably mediated by local hypotension and the release of vasoactive metabolites, is a microvascular compensation that tends to maintain nutritive flow in the presence of proximal arterial occlusion.[78] Paradoxically, some patients with CLI have increased *total* skin blood flow in the ischemic foot, probably because of maximal vasodilatation in the neighboring ischemic tissue.[79] Therefore, the ultimate cause of CLI is presumably maldistribution of skin microcirculation in addition to reduction in total blood flow. The importance of the microcirculation in CLI is emphasized by the wide overlap found in ankle or toe systolic blood pressures when patients who have CLI are compared with patients who have peripheral arterial disease without CLI.

The ultimate sequence of events leading to decreased capillary perfusion in CLI is not established. However, the potential mechanisms probably include[80]:

1. Collapse of precapillary arterioles because of low transmural pressure.
2. Arteriolar vasospasm.
3. Abnormal vasomotion.
4. Microthrombosis.
5. Capillary occlusion caused by endothelial cell swelling, platelet aggregates, rigid adhesive leukocytes, rigid red blood cells, or blood cell–platelet aggregates.
6. Local activation of the immune system.

Figure 64–3 summarizes the changes that are seen in CLI at different levels of the circulation. Regardless of the precise pathophysiologic mechanisms that are operational, the net result is an inhomogeneous perfusion of the skin microvessels.

Certainly, a clear distinction between the two categories, functional ischemia and CLI, is not always possible. A certain amount of overlap is to be expected because they represent merely two points on the spectrum of the same disease. CLI may develop in a patient with severe claudication without any actual change in limb perfusion who sustains an injury to the ischemic limb or experiences an infection in it. Because there is no functional arterial reserve to meet the increased demands required for healing, the stage is set for progressive necrosis and spreading infection.

The diagnosis of ischemic rest pain may be particularly difficult in the patient with diabetes mellitus. Because atherosclerosis with loss of peripheral pulses is more common in such patients and is often associated with a peripheral neuropathy that can mimic rest pain, the noninvasive vascular laboratory can be very helpful in correctly identifying them.[37] The use of such physiologic testing as well as angiography to define the extent, severity, and operability of the occlusive lesions is discussed in greater detail in Section III.

ASSOCIATED DISEASES

Risk Factor Management

Because the underlying condition (i.e., atherosclerosis) cannot be treated directly, it is important for the clinician to (1) identify any of the associated diseases that are known to influence its course and (2) direct therapeutic efforts against them. This approach, which is described more completely in Chapter 65, should include[11, 19, 55, 63]:

- Abstinence from use of all tobacco products
- Control of hypertension, diabetes mellitus, and hyperlipoproteinemia
- Weight reduction when necessary
- Treatment of congestive heart failure or azotemia

The presence and severity of these problems not only may influence the course of the disease but also may determine whether surgical correction is feasible and which type of reconstruction is most suitable. The importance of meticulous foot care and avoidance of trauma in the ischemic limb cannot be overemphasized.

Diabetes Mellitus

Because of the unique and important role that diabetes mellitus plays in the pathogenesis of atherosclerosis, it is extensively discussed in Chapter 76. This chapter high-

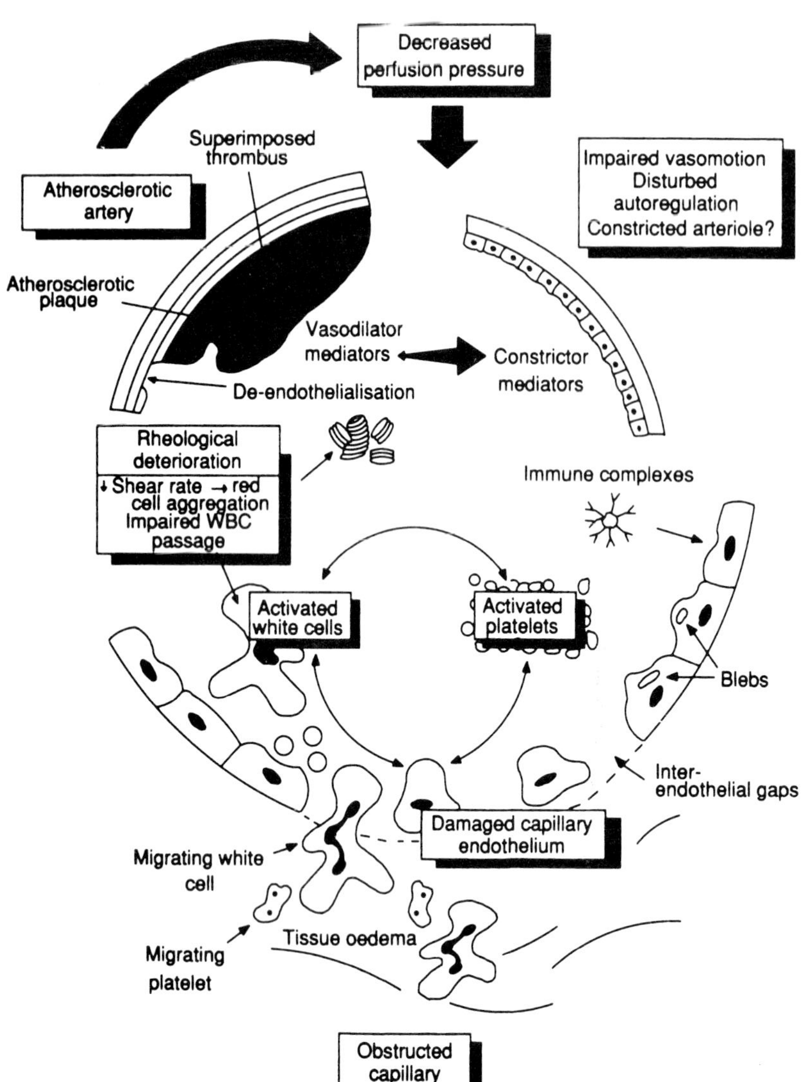

FIGURE 64–3. Summary of suggested pathophysiologic changes in critical leg ischemia at different levels of the circulation. WBC = white blood cell. (From Dormandy J, Verstraete M, Andreani D, et al: Second European Consensus Document on Chronic Critical Leg Ischemia. Circulation 84[Suppl 4]:1, 1991.)

lights some of the more relevant considerations. Although atherosclerosis is not qualitatively different in the patient with diabetes, it appears at an earlier age and progresses more rapidly.[20] Furthermore, its distribution differs significantly.[22, 31, 65] The popliteal, tibial, and profunda femoris arteries are more severely and diffusely involved, whereas the aorta and the iliac arteries may remain largely undiseased.[22, 66]

Although the term "small vessel disease" is commonly used in discussions of diabetes, no anatomically distinct lesion can be identified in the extremity vessels of patients with the disease. The degenerative changes seen in the media of the small arterioles and the basement membrane thickening so often identified in most diabetic patients are, unfortunately, not unique and can be found in nondiabetic patients with advanced atherosclerosis.[76] These lesions are believed to result in impairment of tissue perfusion and nutrition.[2, 5] They may also play a role in the peripheral neuropathy that commonly accompanies diabetes.[31] Because the vascular lesions in patients with and without diabetes are qualitatively similar and differ primarily in frequency of occurrence, severity, and distribution, the pathogenetic mechanisms involved are probably comparable but are accelerated in the diabetic patient.

The combination of neuropathy and peripherally distributed atherosclerosis makes diabetic patients especially vulnerable to foot lesions. It also greatly complicates the evaluation of their frequent complaints of foot pain. In association with the absence of pedal pulses, such pain might be considered ischemic in origin. Attempts to quantitate perfusion noninvasively are frequently confounded by the presence of *calcific medial sclerosis,* which renders the vessels virtually incompressible and makes ankle pressure measurements meaningless. More distal determinations, such as toe pressure measurements, may be needed to help resolve the question.[8]

Even in the absence of demonstrable vascular occlusive disease, diabetic neuropathy and its resulting hypesthesia render the foot insensitive to repeated minor trauma. Such insensitivity may lead to the development of ulcers over pressure points or may provide a portal of entry for bacteria that can spread rapidly and establish extensive, deep-seated infection with remarkably few clinical signs (see Chapter 76).

Finally, diabetic neuropathy may involve the sympathetic nervous system, producing a lower extremity autosympathectomy.[31] This helps to explain the frequent failure of empirically performed surgical sympathectomy to improve skin perfusion in the diabetic patient (see Chapter 73).

Although impaired resistance to infection is commonly invoked to explain the virulence of septic complications in diabetic patients, this concept remains unproven. Nevertheless, such patients appear less able to contain the spread of infection once it becomes established. It is this triumvirate of peripherally distributed atherosclerosis obliterans, neuropathy, and a reduced ability to contain infection that underlies the frequent foot lesions seen in the diabetic person and ultimately results in a significantly higher rate of limb loss.

NATURAL HISTORY

The development of mild to moderate intermittent claudication poses little threat of limb loss to the nondiabetic patient. Approximately three fourths of such patients remain symptomatically stable or actually show some improvement 2 to 5 years after onset of their symptoms, and only 5% to 7% ultimately need amputation of the extremity.[9, 24] This situation is a striking contrast to that in patients who present with ischemic ulceration or rest pain, 19.6% of whom undergo immediate amputation.[25]

The presence and control of coexistent risk factors significantly influence the natural history of atherosclerosis (see Chapter 65). One study showed that 11.4% of those who continued to use tobacco required amputation of a limb, whereas none of those who abstained from smoking did so.[25] Similarly, the presence of diabetes mellitus adversely affects the course of atherosclerosis. Amputations were required in 8% of nondiabetic patients and 34% of diabetic patients.[60] Unfortunately, these risk factors are additive, and the prognosis is worst in diabetics who continue to smoke.

The impact of atherosclerosis on the patient's life expectancy is more important than the risk of amputation. Juergens and colleagues[25] found the overall survival rate for patients with intermittent claudication to be only 72% at 5 years and about 50% at 10 years[25]; the expected 5-year survival rate for age-adjusted control subjects was 90%. Evidence of atherosclerosis in other locations further reduced survival. Thus, in the same study, only 61% of patients with associated cerebrovascular disease and 59% of patients with symptomatic coronary artery disease lived for 5 years. Three quarters of the deaths were due to coronary artery disease. Hypertension had a slightly adverse effect on survival, but hypercholesterolemia had no significant effect on 5-year survival.[25]

Serial angiographic studies indicate that progression of atherosclerosis occurs primarily in the arteries proximal to the initial lesion and suggest that it may exert some type of protective influence on the distal vessels.[15, 33, 44, 72] Following successful bypass of the obstruction, this protection is lost.[72]

In conclusion, most nondiabetic persons with intermittent claudication can expect their symptoms to remain stable, especially if they abstain from tobacco use. Those with ischemic rest pain, ulcers, or gangrene, however, are at high risk for both limb loss and premature death; they deserve an aggressive approach to limb salvage when feasible. Nevertheless, because every patient with symptomatic atherosclerosis is at greater risk for early death, the overall goals of therapy should be to relieve pain and preserve bipedal gait without further jeopardizing the patient's already limited life expectancy.

INDICATIONS FOR INTERVENTION

It is important to decide which patients are candidates for intervention because only these individuals should undergo arteriography. The mere documentation of symptomatic lower extremity atherosclerosis is not an absolute indication for intervention. This decision is facilitated by first assigning patients to one of two categories:

- Patients with functional ischemia
- Patients with CLI

Functional Ischemia

As already discussed, patients with functional ischemia face little risk of limb loss, especially if they are able to abstain from tobacco use, engage in a program of regular exercise, and control associated medical diseases. Often, merely reassuring such patients that they are not facing impending gangrene produces a dramatic improvement in their subjective responses to the disease. If, however, claudication precludes gainful employment or imposes an unacceptable alteration in lifestyle, surgical revascularization or balloon angioplasty should be considered. This decision can be facilitated by physiologic testing of such patients (see Chapter 10).

Stress testing, such as treadmill exercise, can:

- Reproduce patients' symptoms under controlled conditions
- Objectively document the extent of disability
- Exclude more limiting medical conditions, such as coronary artery disease and chronic obstructive pulmonary disease

A further benefit of such testing stems from its ability to localize the arterial lesions with reasonable precision and thus indirectly define the type of arterial repair that would be required to improve the circulation. For example, if a patient with mild to moderate claudication were shown by stress testing to need a revascularization procedure that, if it failed, would entail a significant risk of limb loss, proceeding with arteriography would be foolish. Such risks can be justified only when there is already a serious risk of amputation if the procedure is *not* performed.

Because the determination of disability resulting from functional limb ischemia is relative, it is the patient's prerogative to request revascularization, provided that he or she understands both the risks involved in surgery and the anticipated benefits of the more conservative, nonoperative approach. As the severity of claudication increases, the surgeon is under less constraint to recommend revascularization. It is now incumbent on the surgeon to select the procedure that will improve circulation most effectively, taking into consideration the patient's risk status and the pattern of the vascular disease.

Critical Limb Ischemia

CLI constitutes a definite indication for arterial reconstruction if (1) the patient's disease is sufficiently localized to permit endarterectomy or bypass grafting with a reasonable likelihood of success and (2) the patient can tolerate the proposed procedure.

Even if a patient presents with the recent onset of rest pain or even localized gangrene, amputation or surgical revascularization is not inevitable. If the limb is viable, the condition in approximately 25% to 30% of such patients can be expected to improve, in time, to functional ischemia as collateral circulation develops.

As a result of advances in anesthetic and postoperative management and the development of a variety of percutaneous endovascular techniques for surgical revascularization, currently reported operative mortality rates for most vascular surgical procedures, in the hands of experienced surgeons, are actually lower that those for amputation of an extremity.[17] Furthermore, even temporary graft patency may be sufficient to permit healing of an ischemic ulcer or toe amputation. Subsequent failure of the vascular repair does not inevitably jeopardize survival of the limb. Patients whose grafts become occluded 6 months to 1 year postoperatively frequently maintain a remarkably comfortable foot at rest and enjoy better rehabilitation than would have been possible with amputation and a prosthesis.[4, 48, 67]

Such encouraging exceptions should not, however, delude the vascular surgeon into attempting arterial reconstruction in all patients with CLI on the grounds that "they have little to lose." Although several reports have suggested that a failed vascular reconstruction does not appear to affect the level of subsequent amputation adversely, the mortality and morbidity rates for successive, futile attempts at limb salvage are cumulative, and the emotional and physical toll on the patients, who are often elderly and have a limited life expectancy, is considerable. Furthermore, other experienced vascular surgeons contend that failed distal bypass, especially femoropopliteal bypass, may indeed precipitate an above-knee amputation in the patient for whom a below-knee amputation might have succeeded had the salvage procedure not been attempted.[16, 28, 59] Refinements in amputation techniques that often make it possible to preserve the knee joint, and modern limb prostheses can preserve bipedal gait even in elderly patients, restoring them to a remarkably normal existence. Heroic surgery in hopeless situations does such patients a disservice and is to be condemned.

In the presence of severe multilevel occlusive disease, however, blood flow to the extremities can be so poor that preoperative arteriograms may fail to visualize patent distal vessels that would be suitable for bypass. If Doppler insonation of these vessels reveals audible flow signals and if tissue loss can be confined to the toe or distal metatarsal level, popliteal or tibial artery exploration with intraoperative direct arteriography is a reasonable alternative to empiric major amputation.[57] However, owing to the greater availability of computer-enhanced digital arteriograms to supplement traditional angiograms, this step is rarely necessary.

PRINCIPLES OF VASCULAR RECONSTRUCTION

Like success in so many areas of medicine, success in vascular surgery depends on:

- Judicious patient selection
- Meticulous attention to technical details
- Knowledgeable choice of operative procedure based on certain important principles

Paramount among these principles is the assurance of a relatively unobstructed inflow and a patent distal runoff if both early and long-term patency are to be achieved. For example, if a femoropopliteal bypass is being planned, there must be no significant obstruction in the aorta or the iliac arteries, and a patent segment of popliteal artery with sufficient runoff to sustain a graft must be available.

The auscultation of a femoral bruit or diminution of the femoral pulse, especially after exercise, suggests the presence of significant aortoiliac disease. In some patients, however, this may be difficult to appreciate on the basis of the physical examination alone, and the results of angiography, especially if it is uniplanar, may be confusing.[42, 61] Noninvasive techniques such as duplex scanning of the iliac artery (see Chapter 12) or segmental plethysmography of the thigh may be helpful. If these measures fail to resolve the issue, direct femoral artery pressures can be obtained at the time of angiography or surgery (see Chapter 10).[10] By first recording aortic pressure and then pulling the catheter back into the femoral artery, the clinician can identify the presence of any pressure gradients. A measured pressure differential of 15 mm or more between two adjacent arterial segments in a resting extremity is considered significant. Because some lesions might not produce a 15-mmHg gradient at rest, reactive hyperemia should be produced by using cuff-induced ischemia or the intra-arterial injection of a vasodilator in those patients in whom no initial gradient is seen. The importance of ensuring adequate inflow cannot be overemphasized. In an experimental canine model, graft occlusion regularly occurred when an inflow stenosis was induced, but the graft remained patent despite an equivalent degree of outflow stenosis.[30]

Adequate Runoff

The effectiveness of runoff vessels distal to an obstruction may be difficult to assess. Although a patent common femoral artery with disease-free superficial and profunda femoris arteries or a patent popliteal artery with an intact crural runoff is ideal, the profunda femoris artery can be a perfectly adequate recipient for the entire inflow into the lower extremity.[1, 65] Excellent long-term patency and function can be expected from grafts carried into this vessel despite superficial femoral artery occlusion.[38, 43] Occasionally, an extensive angioplasty of the profunda femoris artery may be necessary before the anastomosis is fashioned (see Chapter 70).

Similarly, extensive disease in the popliteal artery or the tibial vessels does not preclude revascularization in limb-threatening situations. Bypass into a patent popliteal artery without direct runoff into the tibial arteries can be performed, with results comparable to those of conventional femoropopliteal grafting.[36] Distal perfusion relies on the geniculate collateral vessels arising from this so-called isolated popliteal segment to carry blood flow to the more distal vessels of the leg and foot. This approach is particularly suitable for the treatment of rest pain or superficial focal gangrene. When the gangrene is more extensive, higher perfusion pressures are needed to achieve healing, and direct bypass into the tibial arteries is usually required.[4, 48, 52]

Technical Considerations

The technical failure rate for these demanding small vessel anastomoses is higher than that for femoropopliteal bypass, and only 50% to 60% of such anastomoses are still patent 2 years after implantation. Limb salvage rates, however, are higher, averaging 75% over the same period for the reasons already given. Some researchers have suggested that the surgeon can improved these results by performing multiple sequential distal anastomoses to (1) increase the available runoff bed, (2) augment the flow through the graft, and (3) improve long-term patency.[13] Although the sequential bypass technique has great theoretical appeal, sufficient long-term data are not yet available to confirm its effectiveness (see Chapter 69).

Yet another approach for bypass to the infrapopliteal vessels is the use of the autogenous saphenous vein in situ (see Chapter 35). Although a technically more demanding and time-consuming procedure than conventional vein bypass, this technique offers a better size match between the small distal vein and the tibial artery, increased utilization of the vein, and the possibility of improved long-term patency.

Multilevel Occlusions

Most patients selected for vascular reconstruction have arterial obstructions at two or more levels in the same arterial system because chronic unisegmental lesions rarely produce disability serious enough to warrant revascularization. The general principles that govern the choice of operation in these cases are as follows:

1. If all lesions are of equal severity, the most proximal lesion should be corrected first.
2. If the lesions are of greatly differing severity, the more severe occlusion should be corrected first.

If, however, the more proximal lesion is hemodynamically significant, even if it is less severe than the distal lesion, failure to correct it often leads to premature graft occlusion or persistence of the patient's symptoms. The importance of correcting "inflow" disease first is worth reemphasizing.

Collateral Circulation

Restoration of pulsatile arterial flow through or around the proximal obstruction augments circulation through the distal collateral beds sufficiently to ensure limb salvage in most cases and significantly improves exercise tolerance.[5, 35, 43, 67] The simultaneous addition of a distal bypass is rarely required. The most common example of this problem is the patient with significant aortoiliac stenosis and an ipsilateral occlusion of the superficial femoral artery. Aortofemoral bypass into a widely patent profunda femoris artery heals ischemic lesions of the foot, relieves rest pain, and markedly reduces claudication, especially if the distal profunda femoris artery is free of disease and the popliteal artery and its tibial branches are patent.[41] In some instances, even pedal pulses may be restored through these collateral channels (see Chapter 66).[43]

Percutaneous Repairs

Perhaps the most remarkable change in management since the previous edition of this work has been the approach to significant aortoiliac disease. Aggressive, percutaneous dilatation of severely diseased, even occluded, iliac arteries, with or without stents, has made traditional aortoiliofemoral grafting virtually obsolete at some institutions (Chapter 72).

Management of less severe degrees of proximal disease has been a particularly perplexing problem. Surgeons were unwilling to recommend repair of a lesion that was unlikely to improve the patient's arterial hemodynamics, even though they were aware that if left untreated, such lesions would progress with time and jeopardize the distal bypass. The development of PTA has now provided surgeons with an acceptable alternative (see Chapter 72). Before the proposed distal bypass is undertaken, the proximal lesion can be corrected with angioplasty and the hemodynamic improvement of this procedure can be assessed by means of noninvasive tests. If the distal bypass appears to be still necessary, the surgeon can proceed with the assurance that good inflow has now been provided.

Because of the ease and apparent simplicity of PTA, some surgeons have extended its indications to cases in which the symptoms are so mild that surgical revascularization would never have been considered. Unfortunately, failure of the angioplasty may precipitate the need for urgent surgical intervention; PTA should therefore be considered only in those cases in which there are acceptable surgical indications. Conversely, some patients with critical limb ischemia have such severe associated diseases that standard surgical revascularization may be out of the question. PTA in such patients may spell the difference between major amputation and a comfortable, viable extremity.

Another alternative available to the vascular surgeon in the management of such cases is so-called extra-anatomic bypass (see Chapter 68). Although not as durable as more conventional bypass grafts, this procedure can be performed with the use of local anesthesia and can give the patient adequate long-term blood flow to the extremity.

Lumbar Sympathectomy

The role of lumbar sympathectomy in the treatment of chronic lower extremity arterial insufficiency continues to be hotly debated. Although it offers little objective benefit to the patient with functional ischemia, this procedure may relieve mild rest pain or help heal limited areas of superficial gangrene of the pedal skin in some patients who do not have a surgically correctable arterial lesion. The advisability of adding lumbar sympathectomy to an arterial reconstruction remains controversial. Conclusive evidence for either point of view is lacking. Theoretically, the augmented graft flow that undeniably occurs in such circumstances helps to prevent graft occlusion during the early postoperative period, when the pseudointima is forming and thrombosis is most likely. This consideration may be important in situations with poor runoff or in bypasses to small tibial arteries. Lumbar sympathectomy is discussed in greater detail in Chapter 73.

Long-term Follow-up

Because no vascular operation alters or arrests the underlying atherosclerotic process, the patient remains vulnerable to progression of the disease in the vessels contiguous to the bypass or in sites remote from the primary operation. The responsible surgeon thus must accept the obligation to perform continuous long-term follow-up of all patients with symptomatic arterial occlusive disease. The surgeon must:

1. Be vigilant to detect the earliest signs of new occlusive lesions that might threaten the continued patency of the reconstruction.
2. Be alert to possible late deterioration or complications of the bypass graft itself.
3. Remain cognizant of the risk to patient's survival posed by other manifestations of the primary disease and take appropriate steps to control them whenever possible.

SUMMARY

Many ischemic extremities that would certainly have been amputated just a few years ago can now be salvaged by a variety of ingenious techniques available to the trained vascular surgeon. Patients should be carefully selected for elective revascularization, and appropriate reconstructive procedures should be chosen to ensure the maximal improvement in limb perfusion with the least risk to the patient. The surgeon is assisted in making these decisions by a wide range of new tests capable of assessing the physiologic impact of the patient's disease and by significant improvements in angiography that demonstrate the anatomy of the occlusive process with greater clarity. Proper selection of the most appropriate course of management from the bewildering array of alternatives now available requires considerable training and clinical experience. Only through extensive and ongoing involvement in the management of these clinical problems can the vascular surgeon maintain the judgment and technical skill required to achieve optimal results.

REFERENCES

1. Baddeley RM, Ashton F, Slaney G, et al: Late results of autogenous vein bypass grafts in femoropopliteal arterial occlusion. Br Med J 1:653, 1970.
2. Barner HB, Kaiser GC, Willman VL: Blood flow in the diabetic leg. Circulation 43:391, 1971.
3. Barner HB, Kaiser GC, Willman VL, et al: Intermittent claudication with pedal pulses. JAMA 204:100, 1968.
4. Bernhard VM, Ashmore CS, Evans WE, et al: Bypass grafting to distal arteries for limb salvage. Surg Gynecol Obstet 135:219, 1972.
5. Bernhard VM, Militello JM, Geringer AM: Repair of the profunda femoris artery. Am J Surg 127:676, 1974.
6. Bernhard VM, Ashmore CS, Rodgers RE, et al: Operative blood flow in femoral-popliteal and femoral-tibial grafts for lower extremity ischemia. Arch Surg 103:595, 1971.
7. Blaisdell FW, Hall AD: Axillary-femoral artery bypass for lower extremity ischemia. Surgery 54:563, 1963.
8. Bone GE, Pomajzl MJ: Toe blood pressure by photoplethysmography: An index of healing in forefoot amputation. Surgery 89:569, 1981.
9. Boyd AM: Natural course of arteriosclerosis of lower extremities. Proc R Soc Med 53:591, 1962.
10. Brener BJ, Brief DK, Alpert J: The usefulness of intra-arterial pressure measurements in occlusive arterial disease. Vasc Diagn Ther 3:37, 1982.
11. Brown AL, Juergens JL: Arteriosclerosis and atherosclerosis. *In* Fairbairn JF, Juergens JL, Spittell JA (eds): Peripheral Vascular Disease. Philadelphia, WB Saunders, 1972.
12. Brown H, Sellwood RA, Harrison CV, et al: Thromboangiitis obliterans. Br J Surg 56:59, 1969.
13. Burdick JF, O'Mara C, Ricotta J, et al: The multiple sequential distal bypass graft: Improving nature's alternatives. Surgery 89:536, 1981.
14. Burgess EM, Marsden FW: Major lower extremity amputation following arterial reconstruction. Arch Surg 108:655, 1974.
15. Coran AG, Warren R: Arteriographic changes in femoropopliteal arteriosclerosis obliterans. N Engl J Med 274:643, 1966.
16. Dardik H, Kahn M, Dardik I, et al: Influence of failed vascular bypass procedures on conversion of below-knee to above-knee amputation levels. Surgery 91:64, 1982.
17. DeWeese JA, Blaisdell FW, Foster JH: Optimal resources for vascular surgery. Arch Surg 105:948, 1972.
18. Gonzalez LI, Jaffe MS: Mesenteric arterial insufficiency following abdominal aortic resection. Arch Surg 93:10, 1966.
19. Gordon T, Kannel WB: Predisposition to atherosclerosis in the head, heart and legs: The Framingham study. JAMA 221:661, 1972.
20. Guggenheim W, Koch G, Adams AP, et al: Femoral and popliteal occlusive vascular disease: A report on 143 diabetic patients. Diabetes 18:428, 1969.
21. Haid SP, Conn J Jr, Bergan JJ: Cystic adventitial disease of the popliteal artery. Arch Surg 101:765, 1970.
22. Haimovici H: Patterns of arteriosclerotic lesions of the lower extremity. Arch Surg 95:918, 1967.
23. Haust MD, More RH: Development of modern theories on the pathogenesis of atherosclerosis. *In* Wissler RW, Geer JC (eds): The Pathogenesis of Atherosclerosis. Baltimore, Williams & Wilkins, 1972, pp 1–19.
24. Imparato AM, Kim GE, Davidson T, et al: Intermittent claudication: Its natural course. Surgery 78:795, 1975.
25. Juergens JC, Barker NW, Hines EA: Arteriosclerosis obliterans: Review of 520 cases with special reference to pathogenic and prognostic factors. Circulation 21:188, 1960.
26. Kempczinski RF: The differential diagnosis of intermittent claudication. Pract Cardiol 7:53, 1981.
27. Kempczinski RF: Peripheral arterial atheroembolism. *In* Miller DC, Roon AJ (eds): Diagnosis and Management of Peripheral Vascular Disease. Menlo Park, CA, Addison-Wesley Publishing Co, 1982.
28. Kihn RB, Warren R, Beebe GW: The "geriatric" amputee. Ann Surg 176:305, 1972.
29. Kinlough-Rathbone RL, Mustard JF: Atherosclerosis: Current concepts. Am J Surg 141:638, 1981.
30. Kirkpatrick JR, Miller DR: Effects of decreased arterial inflow and runoff on vein graft patency. Surgery 69:870, 1971.
31. Levin ME, O'Neal LW: The Diabetic Foot. St. Louis, CV Mosby, 1973.
32. Levy MN, Share L: The influence of erythrocyte concentration upon the pressure flow relationships in the dog's hind limb. Circ Res 1:247, 1953.
33. Lindbom A: Arteriosclerosis and arterial thrombosis in the lower limb: A roentgenological study. Acta Radiol Suppl 80:1, 1950.
34. Love JW, Whelan TJ: Popliteal artery entrapment syndrome. Am J Surg 109:620, 1965.

35. Malone JM, Moore WS, Goldstone J: The natural history of bilateral aortofemoral bypass-grafts for ischemia of the lower extremities. Arch Surg 110:1300, 1975.
36. Mannick JA, Jackson BT, Coffman JD, et al: Success of bypass vein grafts in patients with isolated popliteal artery segments. Surgery 61:17, 1967.
37. Marinelli MR, Beach KW, Glass MJ, et al: Noninvasive testing vs clinical evaluation of arterial disease: A prospective study. JAMA 241:2031, 1979.
38. Martin P, Frawley JE, Barabas AP, et al: On the surgery of atherosclerosis of the profunda femoris artery. Surgery 71:182, 1972.
39. Mavor GE: The pattern of occlusion in atheroma of the lower limb arteries: The correlation of clinical and arteriographic findings. Br J Surg 43:352, 1956.
40. McKusick VA, Harris WS, Ottesen OE, et al: Buerger's disease: A distinct clinical and pathologic entity. JAMA 181:93, 1962.
41. Mitchell RA, Bone GE, Bridges R, et al: Patient selection for isolated profundaplasty: Arteriographic correlates of operative results. Am J Surg 138:912, 1979.
42. Moore WS, Hall AD: Unrecognized aortoiliac stenosis. Arch Surg 103:633, 1971.
43. Morris GC Jr, Wheeler CG, Crawford ES, et al: Restorative vascular surgery in the presence of impending and overt gangrene of the extremities. Surgery 51:50, 1962.
44. Mozersky DJ, Sumner DS, Strandness DE Jr: Disease progression after femoropopliteal surgical procedures. Surg Gynecol Obstet 135:700, 1972.
45. Mozes M, Cahansky G, Doitsch V, et al: The association of atherosclerosis and Buerger's disease: A clinical and radiological study. J Cardiovasc Surg 11:52, 1970.
46. Mustard JF: Recent advances in molecular pathology: A review: Platelet aggregation, vascular injury and atherosclerosis. Exp Mol Pathol 7:366, 1967.
47. Newman EV, et al: Report by the National Heart and Lung Institute Task Force on Arteriosclerosis, Vol II. Bethesda, Md, National Institutes of Health, 1971. DHEW Publication (NIH) 72–219.
48. Noon GP, Diethrich EB, Richardson WP, et al: Distal tibial artery bypass. Arch Surg 99:770, 1969.
49. Ottinger LW, Darling RC, Nathan MJ, et al: Left colon ischemia complicating aortoiliac reconstruction. Arch Surg 105:841, 1972.
50. Pelgeram LO: Relation of plasma fibrinogen concentration changes to human arteriosclerosis. J Appl Physiol 16:660, 1961.
51. Perdue GD Jr, Smith RB: Atheromatous microemboli. Ann Surg 169:954, 1969.
52. Reichle FA, Tyson RR: Comparison of long-term results of 364 femoropopliteal or femorotibial bypasses for revascularization of severely ischemic lower extremities. Ann Surg 182:449, 1975.
53. Replogle RL, Muselman HJ, Merrell EW: Clinical implication of blood rheology studies. Circulation 36:148, 1967.
54. Roberts B, Gertner MH, Ring EJ: Balloon-catheter dilation as an adjunct to arterial surgery. Arch Surg 116:809, 1981.
55. Rosen AJ, DePalma RG: Risk factors in peripheral atherosclerosis. Arch Surg 107:303, 1973.
56. Samson RH, Gupta SK, Scher LA, et al: Level of amputation after failure of limb salvage procedures. Surg Gynecol Obstet 154:56, 1982.
57. Scarpato R, Gembarowicz R, Farber S, et al: Intraoperative prereconstruction arteriography. Arch Surg 116:1053, 1981.
58. Schadt DC, Hines EA Jr, Juergens JL, et al: Chronic atherosclerotic occlusion of the femoral artery. JAMA 175:937, 1961.
59. Schenker JD, Wolkoff JS: Major amputations after femoropopliteal bypass procedures. Am J Surg 129:495, 1975.
60. Silbert S, Zazeela H: Prognosis in arteriosclerotic peripheral vascular disease. JAMA 166:1816, 1958.
61. Slot HB, Strijbosch L, Greep JM: Interobserver variability in single-plane aortography. Surgery 90:497, 1981.
62. Smith RF, Szilagyi DE: Ischemia of the colon as a complication in the surgery of the abdominal aorta. Arch Surg 80:806, 1960.
63. Stamler J, Berkson DM, Lindberg HA: Risk factors: Their role in the etiology and pathogenesis of the atherosclerotic diseases. *In* Wissler RW, Geer JC (eds): The Pathogenesis of Atherosclerosis. Baltimore, Williams & Wilkins, 1972, pp 41–119.
64. Stary HC: Disease of small blood vessels in diabetes mellitus. Am J Med Sci 252:357, 1966.
65. Stoney RJ, James DR, Wylie EJ: Surgery for femoropopliteal atherosclerosis: A reappraisal. Arch Surg 103:548, 1971.
66. Strandness DF: Collateral Circulation in Clinical Surgery. Philadelphia, WB Saunders, 1969.
67. Taylor GW: Limb salvage arterial surgery for gangrene. Postgrad Med J 47:251, 1971.
68. Texon M, Imparato AM, Helpern M: The role of vascular dynamics in the development of atherosclerosis. JAMA 194:168, 1965.
69. Trippel OH, Jurayj MN, Medell AL: The aorto-iliac steal: A review of this syndrome and a report of one additional case. Ann Surg 175:454, 1972.
70. Vetto RM: The treatment of unilateral iliac artery obstruction with a transabdominal, subcutaneous, femorofemoral graft. Surgery 52:342, 1962.
71. Walton KW: Pathogenetic mechanisms in atherosclerosis. Am J Cardiol 35:542, 1975.
72. Warren R, Gomez RL, Marston JAP, et al: Femoropopliteal arteriosclerosis obliterans—arteriographic patterns and rates of progression. Surgery 55:135, 1964.
73. Weale FE: An Introduction to Surgical Haemodynamics. Chicago, Year Book Medical Publishers, 1967.
74. Wessler S, Ming S, Gurewich V, et al: A critical evaluation of thromboangiitis obliterans: The case against Buerger's disease. N Engl J Med 161:1149, 1960.
75. Whittaker SRF, Winton FR: Apparent viscosity of blood in isolated hind limb of dog and its variation with corpuscular concentration. J Physiol 78:339, 1933.
76. Williamson JR, Kilo C, Crespin SR: Vascular disease. *In* Levin ME, O'Neil LW (eds): The Diabetic Foot. St. Louis, CV Mosby, 1977.
77. Dormandy J, Verstraete M, Andreani D, et al: Second European Consensus Document on Chronic Critical Leg Ischemia. Circulation 84(Suppl 4):1, 1991.
78. Bollinger A, Barras JP, Mahler F: Measurement of foot artery blood pressure by micromanometry in normal subjects and in patients with arterial occlusive disease. Circulation 53:506, 1976.
79. McEwan AJ, Ledingham IM: Blood flow characteristics and tissue nutrition in apparently ischaemic feet. Br Med J 3:220, 1971.
80. Lowe GD: Pathophysiology of critical limb ischaemia. *In* Dormandy J, Stock G (eds): Critical Leg Ischaemia: Its Pathophysiology and Management. Berlin, Springer-Verlag, 1990, pp 17–38.

C H A P T E R 6 5

Natural History and Nonoperative Treatment of Chronic Lower Extremity Ischemia

Lloyd M. Taylor, Jr., M.D., Gregory L. Moneta, M.D., and John M. Porter, M.D.

Vascular surgery in North America occupies an unusual position in the organization of medical specialties. In contrast to the situation of most other surgical disciplines, no widely represented branch of internal medicine is primarily concerned with the diagnosis and treatment of *peripheral arterial disease* (PAD). This means that the vascular surgeon is regularly placed in the roles of diagnostician, primary care provider, and nonoperative therapist for patients with PAD, without the participation of an internal medicine specialist colleague. Thus, vascular surgeons must become as knowledgeable in nonoperative as in operative treatment of vascular disease.

The requirement for such detailed knowledge is nowhere more evident than in the treatment of patients with chronic lower extremity ischemia. PAD affects lower extremities in a continuum of severity ranging from asymptomatic arterial occlusive disease, through symptoms of claudication, to ischemia sufficiently severe that the viability of the limb is threatened. A number of population studies using noninvasive testing have shown that most persons with lower extremity PAD are *asymptomatic*. The examples listed in Table 65–1 include symptomatic:asymptomatic ratios ranging from 1:1.8 to 1:5.3.[24, 31, 46, 109]

The incidence of PAD affecting the lower extremities ranges from 2.2% of a population aged 38 to 82 years to 17% of a population aged 55 to 70 years, emphasizing the rapid rise in prevalence of PAD with increasing age (see Table 65–1). In view of the rapid aging of the population of the United States,[94] it is clear that the absolute number of persons affected by PAD is also increasing rapidly (Fig. 65–1). At present, only about 100,000 operations for treatment of lower extremity ischemia are performed annually in the United States.[105] Clearly, a majority of persons with PAD are currently treated nonoperatively.

A description of the authors' approach to nonoperative treatment of PAD forms the basis for this chapter. The subjects discussed include:

- Natural history of the disease
- Objective diagnostic tests to detect severity and location of occlusive lesions and to evaluate their physiologic significance
- Exercise therapy and cessation of tobacco use
- Foot care
- Interactions with other medical treatments
- Unconventional therapy

NATURAL HISTORY

Operative treatment of lower extremity arterial occlusive disease has been widely performed since the late 1950s. One might think that a large body of data concerning the natural history of unoperated PAD would have been collected before this era, but such is not the case. As has often been true in the history of surgery, acquisition of accurate knowledge about the natural history of a condition unmodified by surgery appears to have been prompted by the evolution of a surgical treatment proposed as a superior alternative to the presumed natural history. Thus, well-documented studies of the natural history of untreated PAD date from the same historical period as the development of surgical treatment methods.

Several aspects of the natural history of PAD are considered here: (1) the available evidence about risk factors for atherosclerotic disease and their relationship to developing PAD; (2) the relationship between PAD and coexisting carotid and coronary artery disease; (3) factors related to progression of existing PAD, especially progression to ische-

TABLE 65–1. INCIDENCE OF PERIPHERAL ARTERIAL DISEASE (PAD) IN VARIOUS POPULATIONS DETERMINED BY OBJECTIVE TESTING

STUDY	COUNTRY	AGE OF POPULATION	PATIENTS WITH PAD (%)	SYMPTOMATIC:ASYMPTOMATIC RATIO
De Backer et al, 1979[31]	Belgium	40–60 yr	4	1:4.4
Schroll and Munck, 1981[109]	Denmark	60 yr	14	1:2.8
Criqui et al, 1985[21]	United States	38–82 yr	2.2	1:5.3
Fowkes et al, 1991[46]	Scotland	55–74 yr	17	1:1.8

TABLE 65–2. EXAMPLES OF INCREASE IN RELATIVE RISK OF PERIPHERAL ARTERIAL DISEASE (PAD) ASSOCIATED WITH VARIOUS RISK FACTORS FOR ATHEROSCLEROSIS

STUDY	COUNTRY	RISK FACTOR	RELATIVE RISK OF PAD (95% CI)
Murabito et al, 1997[86]	United States	Diabetes	2.6 (2.0–3.4)
Fowkes et al, 1992[47]	Scotland	Smoking	3.7 (1.7–8.0)
Bowlin et al, 1994[12]	?	High levels of cholesterol	2.05 (1.44–2.91)
Fowkes et al, 1992[47]	Scotland	High levels of triglycerides	1.7 (1.3–2.1)
Cheng et al, 1997[15]	?	High levels of lipoprotein (a)	2.0
Clarke et al, 1991[17]	United States	High levels of homocysteine	22.3 (1.9–inf.)

CI = confidence interval; inf. = infinity.

mia sufficiently severe to cause limb loss; (4) anticipated survival of persons with PAD; (5) the prognosis associated with the most severe manifestation of PAD, limb-threatening ischemia; and (6) special considerations related to PAD in young persons.

Risk Factors

The familiar risk factors for atherosclerotic coronary heart disease, including diabetes, cigarette smoking, hypertension, lipid abnormalities, elevated plasma fibrinogen levels, and elevated plasma homocysteine values, have all been shown to also be related to the presence of PAD. As seen in Table 65–2, the magnitude of importance of each risk factor is different. Diabetes remains a powerful risk factor. Smoking is related more to PAD than to coronary disease, but elevated cholesterol levels are less important. All known risk factors for coronary disease are also related to PAD, and coexisting risk factors, as often seen in atherosclerotic individuals, vastly increase the risk of PAD just as with coronary disease. For example, in the study reported by Widmer and colleagues,[125] the relative risk of PAD increased from 2.3 for cigarette smoking alone, to 3.3 for the combination of cigarette smoking and diabetes, to 6.3 when hypertension was added to the other two factors.

Associated Coronary and Carotid Artery Disease

The systemic nature of the atherosclerotic disease process that produces PAD is emphasized by the incidence and severity of associated cerebral and coronary vascular disease found in patients with PAD. Multiple studies have contributed important objective and quantitative information about patterns of associated disease.

The first of these is the remarkable patient series accumulated at the Cleveland Clinic under the direction of Hertzer and colleagues,[57] following a policy decision to perform coronary arteriography in 1000 consecutive patients before elective vascular surgery without regard to the presence of symptoms of coronary disease. Angiographically identifiable coronary atherosclerosis was detected in 90% of all patients scheduled for operation to treat claudication (381 of the 1000 patients). The same group of investigators detected only a 47% incidence of coronary disease in similar patients when the clinical history and resting electrocardiographic findings were used for screening,[58] emphasizing the asymptomatic nature of a considerable portion of the coronary disease identified angiographically.

This study demonstrated severe surgically correctable coronary disease in 14% of asymptomatic patients with no historical or electrocardiographic evidence of disease. These important data, shown in Table 65–3, are derived from a population of patients being considered for surgical treatment of lower extremity ischemia who represent the most severe portion of the clinical spectrum of lower extremity occlusive disease. It is reasonable to assume that the coronary artery disease found in these patients is more severe

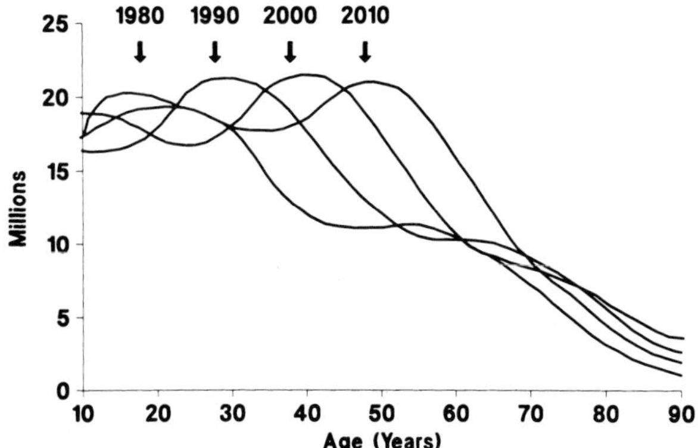

FIGURE 65–1. Age profile of United States population in each decade, 1980 to 2010. Note the rapid increase in mean age of the largest population group. (From Johnson G Jr: The second-generation vascular surgeon. J Vasc Surg 5:213, 1987.)

TABLE 65–3. INCIDENCE OF CORONARY ARTERY DISEASE (CAD) IN 1000 CONSECUTIVE PATIENTS WITH PERIPHERAL DISEASE SCREENED BY CORONARY ANGIOGRAPHY

	CLINICAL ASSESSMENT OF CORONARY DISEASE			
	No Indications of Coronary Disease		Suspected Coronary Disease	
	No. of Patients	*Per Cent*	*No. of Patients*	*Per Cent*
Normal coronary arteries	64	14	21	4
Mild to moderate CAD	218	49	99	18
Advanced but compensated CAD	97	22	192	34
Severe correctable CAD	63	14	188	34
Severe inoperable CAD	4	1	54	10

From Hertzer NR, Beven EG, Young JR, et al: Coronary artery disease in peripheral vascular patients: A classification of 1000 coronary angiograms and results of surgical management. Ann Surg 199:223, 1984.

than in the entire group of patients with PAD, most of whom are insufficiently symptomatic to require surgical intervention.

Completion of the Asymptomatic Carotid Atherosclerosis Study,[43] which demonstrated significant benefit of endarterectomy for patients with greater than 60% internal carotid artery stenosis, makes extremely relevant the number of patients with PAD who have such asymptomatic carotid artery stenoses. Duplex scanning of the carotid bifurcation detects cervical carotid artery disease with accuracy comparable to that achieved with angiography, making it possible to screen large numbers of patients with PAD for carotid artery atherosclerosis. In one study of preoperative patients, 52% were found to have detectable carotid artery disease.[118]

A study by Ahn and coworkers[3] used duplex scanning to examine the carotid arteries of 78 patients with lower extremity vascular disease who had no clinical evidence of carotid artery disease (carotid bruit, abnormal carotid pulses, or neurologic symptoms). They found 16% to 50% stenosis of the internal carotid artery in 33% of the patients, more than 50% stenosis in 14% of the patients, and more than 75% stenosis in 5% of the patients. In the authors' study of patients examined prior to lower extremity bypass surgery for severe limb ischemia, 15.5% of the patients who had no symptoms of carotid artery disease were found to have stenoses greater than 60% in at least one carotid artery.[50]

These studies and others confirm the logical expectation that severe atherosclerosis in lower limb arteries is frequently accompanied by similarly severe disease in the coronary and cerebral beds. As is the case with PAD, a large percentage of cases with coexisting disease are asymptomatic. It is generally true that increasing severity of PAD is accompanied by increasing severity of coronary and cerebral atherosclerosis.

Disease Progression

Intermittent claudication is a clinical condition of lower extremity muscle pain induced by exercise and relieved by short periods of rest. It is caused by fixed arterial obstruction at sites proximal to the affected muscle bed such that the normal exercise-induced increase in muscle blood flow cannot occur to a degree sufficient to meet the metabolic demands of exercising muscle. As mentioned previously, most cases of objectively diagnosed PAD severe enough to produce claudication remain asymptomatic.

In various studies, 50% to 90% of patients with hemodynamic changes sufficient to cause intermittent claudication did not complain of this symptom to their physicians.[61, 98] One explanation is that aging patients appear to accept increasing difficulty in walking as a normal consequence of aging. In one well-documented prospective study, two thirds of patients with arteriographically proven lower extremity arterial occlusions did not complain of having claudication on an initial questionnaire, and one third steadfastly maintained that they were without symptoms even after a detailed interview.[126] These results have an alternative explanation, that claudication is a relative symptom; that is, the patient must both possess a sufficiently significant arterial stenosis and exercise enough to induce relative muscle ischemia.[24] Because the normal lower extremity arterial tree has a vast capacity to increase flow in response to exercise and because most sedentary individuals rarely stress this capacity, it is possible for a tremendous amount of arterial obstruction to result in a great loss of capacity to increase flow without causing symptoms.

This inconstant relationship between severity of PAD and existence of claudication symptoms may explain why different studies have found widely varying ratios of symptomatic to asymptomatic PAD. For example, claudication was more prevalent in a group of farm workers[100] than in a group of office workers,[98] presumably because the more active farm workers required greater physical capacity to perform their occupations.

The most feared consequence of PAD is progression to severe ischemia, with an ultimate need for amputation. Almost all historical studies of large patient groups with claudication have convincingly demonstrated that this progression is an unusual event. Boyd[13] prospectively observed 1440 patients with intermittent claudication and found that after 10 years, only 12.2% required amputation. In the Framingham study, only 1.6% of patients with claudication who were observed for 8.3 years required amputation.[69] The results of multiple historical studies regarding the natural history of claudication are summarized in Table 65–4.

The risk factors associated with greater likelihood of worsening of claudication have been described by many researchers. Continued cigarette smoking has repeatedly been identified as the most consistent adverse risk factor associated with progression of lower extremity ischemia in patients with claudication. Another important risk factor for disease progression is the severity of the initial arterial occlusive disease process, as assessed from symptoms, angiography,[64] or noninvasive segmental pressure measurements.[25, 66] Patients with diabetes have been identified as having a higher likelihood of progression to gangrene and limb loss in some studies,[61, 91] but not in others.[58, 66]

The low long-term likelihood of limb loss in patients with claudication demonstrated by multiple historical studies must be viewed with some skepticism. Clearly, many

TABLE 65–4. HISTORICAL STUDIES OF THE NATURAL HISTORY OF CLAUDICATION PROGRESSION TO SEVERE LIMB ISCHEMIA

STUDY	NO. OF PATIENTS	MEAN FOLLOW-UP (YR)	STABLE OR IMPROVED (%)	WORSE (%)	AMPUTATED (%)
Boyd, 1960[13]	1440	10.0	—	—	12.2
McAllister, 1976[80]	100	6.0	78	22	7
Imparato et al, 1975[64]	104	2.5	79	21	3.8
Peabody et al, 1974[91]	162	8.3	—	—	4.3

TABLE 65–5. NATURAL HISTORY OF CLAUDICATION AS DETERMINED BY OBJECTIVE STUDIES

STUDY	NO. OF PATIENTS	MEAN FOLLOW-UP (YR)	STABLE (%)	WORSE (%)	AMPUTATED (%)
Cronenwett et al, 1984[25]	91	2.5	40	60	—
Rosenbloom et al, 1988[103]	195	8	59	41	—
Jonason and Ringqvist, 1985[66]	224	6	78	22	—
Walsh et al, 1991[123]*	38	3	72	28	—

*Evaluated superficial femoral stenoses only.

patients with leg pain on walking do not have occlusive arterial disease, and this fact may have biased many long-term studies to which patients were admitted on the basis of history alone, without objective documentation of arterial occlusion. An objective method that clearly identifies the patient with claudication and allows quantitation of the severity of the symptoms is readily available. Measurement of the ankle-brachial systolic pressure index (ABI) before and after treadmill walking is a simple noninvasive method that fulfills these requirements.

Interestingly, modern studies for which abnormal findings of a noninvasive lower extremity arterial examination were an entrance requirement have demonstrated a more morbid prognosis than that outlined by historical studies that relied on patient history or on angiographic demonstration of arterial disease without further quantitation of severity. Table 65–5 lists the results of later studies of the natural history of claudication in which objective demonstration of lower extremity arterial occlusive disease was required for inclusion of a patient in the study. Importantly, in each of these studies, the severity of the arterial obstruction as determined objectively at the time of initial patient encounter was the most important factor in predicting the subsequent patient outcome. This objective information is important because it is readily obtained (the ABI is easily measured in any physician's office) and allows classification of patients into high-risk and low-risk groups.

The information in Table 65–5 indicates that by no means all patients with claudication have a benign prognosis and that predicting a benign prognosis on the basis of symptoms alone does not represent the best that medicine has to offer. The published recommended standards for reporting the results of studies of lower extremity ischemia provide a useful format for objective characterization of the severity of ischemia in addition to a description of symptoms.[2]

Survival

All investigations have found that the presence of PAD identifies a patient group with significantly shorter survival than that of age-matched controls. Table 65–6 shows the results of several long-term studies of survival of PAD patients who did not undergo surgery. Table 65–7 gives similar data for patients operated on for claudication. Combining these data permits construction of an approximate life table survival curve, allowing comparison with the anticipated survival of an age-matched control group. As shown in Figure 65–2, this comparison indicates that the predicted mortality rates for patients with claudication at 5, 10, and 15 years of follow-up are approximately 30%, 50%, and 70%, respectively; these mortality rates significantly exceed those observed in control groups.

As is evident from the date in Tables 65–6 and 65–7, the anticipated long-term survival of patients with PAD appears to be related to the severity of ischemia. This stratification of survival risk also applies to patients with more severe ischemia. Thus, the approximate 5-year patient survival rates for various series of patients are:

- 87% in patients with claudication who were treated nonoperatively[100]
- 80% in patients with claudication who were treated by operation[78]
- 48% patients with limb-threatening ischemia who were treated by operation[122]
- 12% in patients requiring reoperative surgery for limb-threatening ischemia[39]

McDermott and colleagues[81] have clearly demonstrated that mortality risk for PAD patients can be classified according to disease severity measured by ABI, just as it can according to severity of symptoms.

The overwhelming cause of death in patients with claudi-

TABLE 65–6. SURVIVAL OF PATIENTS WITH CLAUDICATION OBSERVED WITHOUT OPERATION

STUDY	NO. OF PATIENTS	MEAN FOLLOW-UP (YR)	5-YEAR SURVIVAL (%)	10-YEAR SURVIVAL (%)	15-YEAR SURVIVAL (%)	AGE (YR)
Bloor, 1961[11]	1476	7.0	79.0	54	—	45–54
			72.0	35	—	55–64
			60.0	20	—	65–74
Silbert and Zazeela, 1958[111]	1198	12.0	94.7	71	52	
Kallero, 1981[68]	193	9.7	—	52	—	
Schadt et al, 1961[108]	362	9.0	76.0	59	—	
			54.0	38		
Lefevre et al, 1959[74]	500	5.0	57.0	—	—	

*The top line reflects data for nondiabetics, and the bottom line for diabetics.

TABLE 65–7. SURVIVAL OF PATIENTS WITH CLAUDICATION TREATED BY OPERATION

STUDY	NO. OF PATIENTS	MEAN FOLLOW-UP (YR)	5-YEAR SURVIVAL (%)	10-YEAR SURVIVAL (%)	15-YEAR SURVIVAL (%)
Szilagyi et al, 1979[115]	531	0–15	44	25	6
Hansteen et al, 1975[55]	307	8–16	70	50	37
Crawford et al, 1981[22]	949	0–25	74	50	30
Szilagyi et al, 1986[116]	1648	0–30	70	64	25
Hertzer, 1981[58]	256	6–11	80	60	—
Malone et al, 1977[78]	180	0–15	80	43	26

cation, as predicted from the preceding data, is arteriosclerotic vascular disease and its attendant complications. As seen in Figure 65–3, coronary deaths account for approximately 60% of the deaths in patients with claudication, with cerebrovascular disease causing mortality in another 10% to 15%. Other vascular events, such as visceral infarction and ruptured aneurysm, account for another 10% of the deaths. The remainder have nonvascular causes. Continued cigarette smoking, diabetes, and symptomatic coronary and cerebrovascular disease have been identified as independent risk factors associated with a risk of mortality exceeding that predicted for the entire group of patients with claudication.

Limb-Threatening Ischemia

Limb-threatening ischemia occurs when resting blood flow is insufficient to meet the maintenance metabolic requirements for nonexercising tissue. The clinical manifestations of limb-threatening ischemia are rest pain, ulceration, and gangrene. Ischemic rest pain is typically described as a burning, dysesthetic pain that is usually worse in the forefoot and toes and is frequently worse at night when the patient is recumbent. The pain is typically lessened or relieved if the foot is moved to a dependent position, with the consequent increase in arterial pressure resulting from gravity. Ischemic ulceration occurs when minor traumatic lesions fail to heal because of inadequate blood supply.

Gangrene occurs when arterial perfusion is so inadequate that spontaneous necrosis occurs in the most poorly perfused areas. Progressive gangrene with an ultimate need for amputation is believed by most vascular surgeons to be the inevitable outcome in patients with unrelieved limb-threatening ischemia. An exception to this process is observed in the patient in whom limb-threatening ischemia occurs after an acute thrombotic event, such as closure of a previously stenotic superficial femoral artery. Such a patient may experience a period of days to a few weeks of ischemic rest pain, after which the development of collateral circulation results in stabilization of symptoms at the level of claudication only.

Available data indicate that the true prognosis for limb loss in patients with presumed limb-threatening ischemia is not known with certainty. Progressive gangrenous changes and continuous ischemic rest pain unrelieved by dependency are unstable conditions associated with rapid progression to limb loss. In contrast, a number of patients with advanced ischemia describe occasional episodes of typical nocturnal ischemic rest pain that is easily relieved by limb dependency; in such patients, the symptom complex remains stable for months or even years. Clearly, the clinical symptoms and findings commonly included in the category of limb-threatening ischemia represent a spectrum of severity. In a single patient, the decrease in nutritive blood flow caused by progressive atherosclerosis in primary inflow vessels may be balanced by the development of

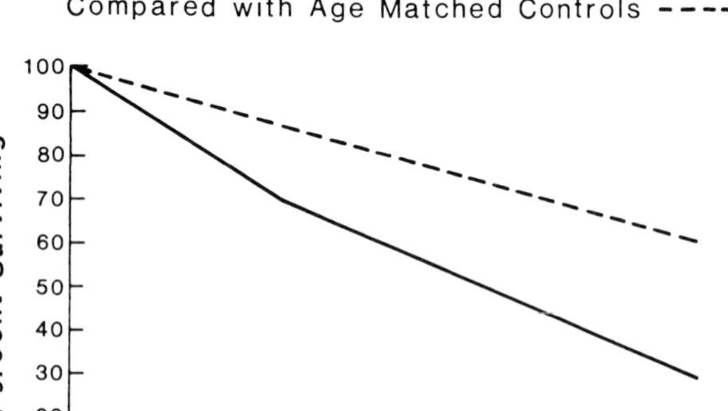

FIGURE 65–2. Survival of patients with claudication compared with controls. (Data from Boyd, 1960[13]; McAllister, 1976[80]; Imparato et al, 1975[64]; Peabody et al, 1974[91]; Cronenwett et al, 1984[25]; Rosenbloom et al, 1988[103]; Jonason and Ringqvist, 1985[66]; and Walsh et al, 1991.[123]).

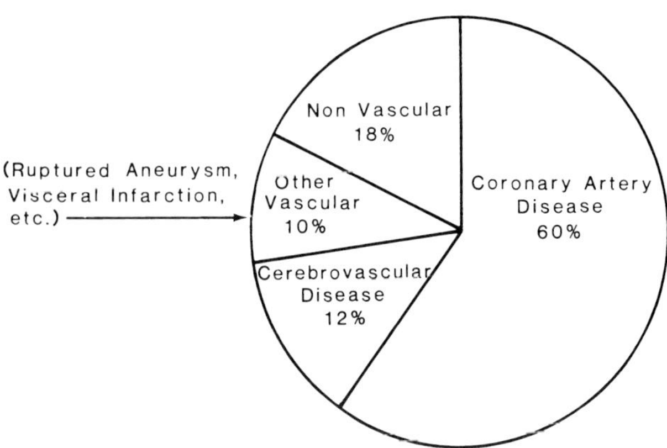

FIGURE 65–3. Causes of death in patients with claudication. (Data from Boyd, 1960[13]; McAllister, 1976[80]; Imparato et al, 1975[64]; Peabody et al, 1974[91]; Cronenwett et al, 1984[25]; Rosenbloom et al, 1988[103]; Jonason and Ringqvist, 1985[66]; and Walsh et al, 1991.[123]).

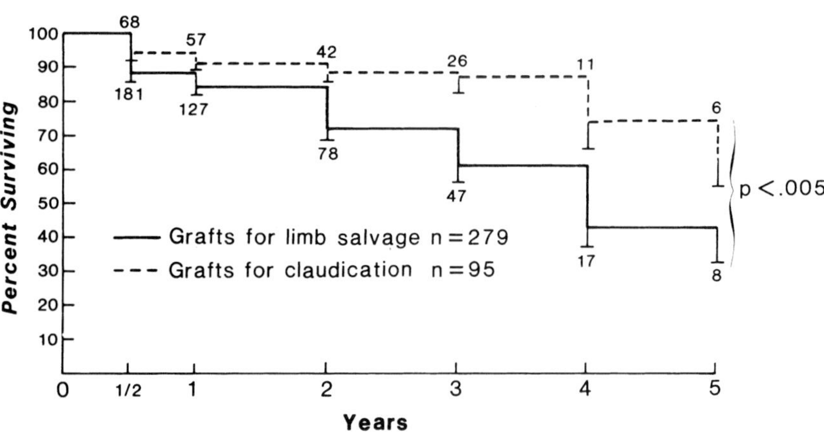

FIGURE 65–4. Survival of patients after surgery for limb salvage compared with patients who underwent surgery for claudication. (From Taylor LM Jr, Porter JM: Current status of the reversed saphenous vein graft. *In* Bergan JJ, Yao J [eds]: Arterial Surgery: New Diagnostic and Operative Techniques. New York, Grune & Stratton, 1987, p 494.)

collaterals so that symptoms remain stable for prolonged periods.

Chronic severe ischemia obviously renders the affected extremity vulnerable, such as when increased blood flow is needed for healing of traumatic lesions or dissipation of external heat. In such cases, minor alterations in capillary flow induced by the improvement in cardiac output resulting from the treatment of congestive heart failure or by specific hemorrheologic drugs may be sufficient to prevent progressive ischemia leading to limb loss.[106] In an important study documenting long-term improvement in a number of limbs with advanced ischemia without specific therapy, Rivers and associates[101] emphasize that the prognosis for patients with severe limb ischemia is not necessarily the early development of gangrene. Their findings clearly point to the critical need for a control population in any study purporting to show a benefit of a specific treatment method in patients with ischemic rest pain.

The results of the few studies including such control groups may be surprising to surgeons accustomed to equating the existence of rest pain or ischemic ulceration with inevitable limb loss. A 1982 Scandinavian trial randomly assigned 22 patients with arterial ischemic ulcers to receive either placebo or prostaglandin treatment and found a 40% rate of ulcer healing in the placebo group.[40] A similar study in the United States of 120 patients reported a 49% incidence of ulcer healing and more than 80% improvement in rest pain in the placebo group.[110] Similar findings have been noted in placebo groups from other studies of patients with ischemic rest pain and gangrenous ulcers, with overall improvement occurring in 25% to more than 50% of the patients.[2, 7] These data obviously indicate that the prognosis for limb loss in patients grouped solely according to *symptoms* of severe lower extremity ischemia is uncertain. Clearly, objective quantitative information to permit better classification of patient groups is essential.

At least some data of this type have been reported, indicating a grim prognosis for the group of patients characterized by the complete absence of pedal arterial flow as assessed by Doppler insonation.[44] The prognosis for survival of patients with severe limb ischemia is more clearly defined than the prospects of limb loss. All researchers agree that patients with ischemic rest pain and gangrene as a group are older and have more advanced coronary and cerebrovascular disease than patients with claudication. The shorter life expectancy for patients operated on for limb-threatening ischemia than for those operated on for claudication is clearly demonstrated in Figure 65–4. In fact, the anticipated survival of patients with limb-threatening ischemia is so short that death is at least as common an outcome as limb loss. Results from several randomized trials of drug therapy for limb-threatening ischemia demonstrate that one half of placebo-treated patients had died or had undergone amputation of the ischemic limb within 6 months of diagnosis.[7, 10, 77, 88] The causes of death in these patients are typically vascular and are quite similar in distribution to those shown in Figure 65–3 for patients with claudication.

Chronic Lower Extremity Ischemia in Young Persons

Arteriosclerosis is generally a disease of later life. Symptomatic peripheral occlusive disease occurring in younger persons is often associated with the presence of identifiable risk factors, such as hyperlipidemia, hypercoagulable states, Buerger's disease, and inborn errors of metabolism. As might be expected from the early age of onset, progression of disease in these patients is especially rapid, with a correspondingly high incidence of amputation reported by most investigators.[32, 89] Most researchers have recommended that arterial reconstruction be avoided, except in cases with clearly threatened limb loss, because of a high anticipated failure rate of the arterial repair in these severely afflicted patients. Several studies have emphasized that a systematic approach to diagnosis should allow assignment of a cause in most patients and that the results of vascular treatment are more favorable when it is combined with vigorous treatment of the associated risk factors.[54, 90]

Physicians must be wary of attributing a vascular cause to all typical leg pain syndromes, especially in young persons. Several unusual syndromes may produce exercise-induced leg pain, which cannot be reliably differentiated from claudication on the basis of the history alone. *Chronic compartment syndrome* is a condition in which muscle exercise results in sudden increases in compartment pressures to a level at which pain and neuromuscular compromise may occur.[119] This syndrome is most often seen in athletes and most frequently involves the anterior and lateral compartments of the calf. Treatment is by fascial incision or limited excision. In *neurogenic claudication,* lower extremity pain induced by walking is caused by stenosis of the spinal canal from any of a number of causes.[85] Both direct compression of the nerve root and compression of the local neural blood supply have been implicated in this syndrome,[4] which may be historically quite similar to claudication caused by large artery obstruction.

The key to diagnosis of these conditions is insistence on objective confirmation of the diagnosis of vascular occlusive disease in suspected claudication with the use of the noninvasive vascular laboratory, as described in the sections that follow and in Chapters 10 and 12. The results of noninvasive testing are abnormal in all patients with arterial vascular claudication, although some patients with mild symptoms may have apparently normal test results at rest. Absence of a vascular abnormality after dynamic testing (treadmill walking or reactive hyperemia) should lead to a search for an alternative explanation for the patient's lower extremity symptoms.

Conclusion

Patients with chronic lower extremity ischemia may present clinically with symptoms ranging from minor claudication to extensive gangrene. The arbitrary division of these patients into two distinct groups, those with claudication and those with threatened limb loss, on the assumption of markedly different natural histories was a serviceable approach in the past but is probably no longer optimal. Great progress has been made in quantitating the extent of ischemia with a variety of noninvasive vascular laboratory methods. Evidence is emerging that the prognosis for patients with chronic lower extremity ischemia is more closely related to these objective findings than to patients' descriptions of symptomatic severity. The missing element in the current method of categorizing patients with chronic lower extremity ischemia is a consistent, objective method of quantitating the rate of progression of the occlusive process. Until this information can be added to the objective description of the current severity of ischemia, the ability of vascular surgeons to prognosticate remains imperfect at best.

Clearly, it is as inappropriate to predict a uniformly satisfactory clinical outcome solely on the basis of a history of claudication as it is to predict the inevitable occurrence of early limb loss in a patient with intermittent ischemic rest pain. Similarly, in the authors' opinion, it is inappropriate to consistently refuse operation in patients with claudication just as it is to always insist on arterial reconstruction in patients with the recent development of an ischemic ulcer that, as noted previously, may heal spontaneously. Careful consideration of the objective findings pertinent to each patient and individualization of therapy on the basis of these findings results in a more favorable clinical outcome than the algorithmic assignment of treatment methods to symptom complexes as if each represented a unique disease process with a predictable clinical outcome.

NONOPERATIVE TREATMENT

Initial Evaluation

The foundation of the initial clinical patient evaluation remains an unhurried and detailed patient history taking and physical examination, the details of which with respect to vascular disease are fully discussed in Chapter 1 and are not repeated here. Lower extremity ischemia is a clinical condition especially suited to objective noninvasive vascular laboratory evaluation, which may be thought of as an extension of the physical examination.

The authors perform complete noninvasive laboratory examination of the lower extremity for all patients with chronic lower extremity ischemia as an integral part of the initial patient evaluation. The testing routinely performed consists of:

1. Palpation of peripheral pulses and recording of Doppler waveforms over the femoral, popliteal, and pedal arteries.
2. Determination of segmental pressure indices at the upper thigh, above-knee, below-knee, ankle, and great toe levels.
3. In patients with incompressible vessels, plethysmographic recordings and toe reactive hyperemia testing.
4. Toe photoplethysmography for detection of significant obstructive disease below the ankle, as is frequently present in diabetic patients.
5. In patients with claudication, treadmill walking followed by measurement of ankle pressure recovery times. The authors' preference is to use a rather slow treadmill speed of 1.5 mph with a 0% grade to duplicate normal ambulation and minimize the cardiopulmonary stress associated with exercise testing.

The clinical and vascular laboratory data obtained at the initial evaluation, an example of which is seen in Figure 65–5, provide the objective information required to form the first impression of the etiology and severity of the patient's symptoms. In addition, the vascular laboratory data serve as a baseline against which to judge progression of disease as well as to evaluate future changes in symptoms or response to therapy objectively.

The initial evaluation should include the identification of risk factors known to influence the natural history of the disease, such as cigarette smoking, diabetes, and hyperlipidemia. Historical details suggesting coronary artery disease should be specifically sought, and objective information relative to coronary disease, such as electrocardiograms, records of previous coronary bypass procedures, and results of dipyridamole–thallium imaging or multiple gated acquisition scanning, should be reviewed if available. In view of the results of the Asymptomatic Carotid Atherosclerosis Study[43] and the documented high prevalence of asymptomatic carotid stenosis in patients with PAD,[50] it is the authors' practice to obtain carotid artery duplex scanning in PAD patients without symptoms of carotid artery

Peripheral Arterial Exam

Common femoral
Popliteal
Posterior Tibial
Dorsal Pedal

Resting Segmental Blood Pressures:

	RIGHT Pressure	RIGHT Leg/Arm Ratio	LEFT Pressure	LEFT Leg/Arm Ratio
Arm	168		168	
Upper thigh	124	.74	127	.76
Above knee	99	.59	115	.68
Below knee	88	.52	100	.59
Ankle D.P.	82	.48	80	.48
P.T.	82	.48	74	.44
Toe .	60	.36	66	.39

Treadmill: 1.5 mph at 0% grade.
Stopped arbitrarily; no discomfort at 5:00 (202 meters)

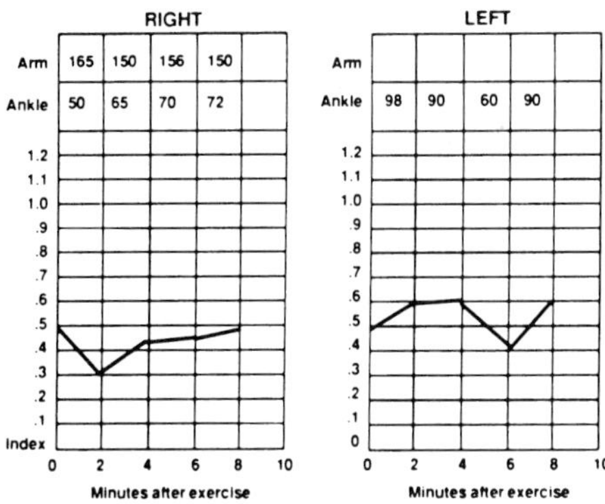

FIGURE 65–5. Information obtained from standard noninvasive peripheral arterial examination provides complete assessment of lower extremity circulation.

disease if they would be candidates for carotid endarterectomy for asymptomatic disease.

Armed with this large body of information, the surgeon can decide whether to recommend operative or nonoperative treatment. Specific nonoperative measures that may be undertaken in the treatment of chronic lower extremity ischemia and the anticipated results of these measures form the basis for the remainder of this chapter.

Cessation of Smoking

It is estimated that 325,000 to 350,000 deaths directly related to cigarette smoking occur yearly in the United States.[93] The direct relationship between tobacco smoking and lower extremity ischemia is well known. Smokers are nine times more likely than nonsmokers to develop claudication.[61] From 98% to 99% of all patients who complain of intermittent claudication smoke cigarettes,[37, 75] as do an equally high percentage of patients undergoing lower extremity amputation for ischemia.[67] Interestingly, the pathophysiologic mechanisms through which smoking exerts its adverse effects on arteries are not known with certainty. This lack of information is in part due to the chemical complexity of cigarette smoke, which has been demonstrated to contain more than 3000 different substances.[126] Multiple individual components of tobacco smoke affect each of the important components of the atherosclerotic process adversely, as outlined in Table 65–8.

Tobacco smoke produces marked alterations in vascular endothelium, prostaglandin metabolism, lipid metabolism, blood viscosity, platelet function, and coagulation function, among other things.[53, 82] Smokers frequently demonstrate chronic vasoconstriction and hypertension, probably as a result of the nicotine in tobacco smoke.

In addition to having adverse influences on atherogenesis, the carbon monoxide component of tobacco smoke has an adverse effect on claudication. Aronow and associates[5] demonstrated an immediate, significant decrease in treadmill walking in patients with claudication who breathed air containing 50 ppm of carbon monoxide. Excellent reviews have more detailed information on the pathophysiologic and epidemiologic association of cigarette smoking with lower extremity ischemia.[21, 45]

TABLE 65–8. ADVERSE EFFECTS OF TOBACCO SMOKING ON COMPONENTS OF ATHEROGENESIS*

1. Endothelial effects
   a. Increased endothelial denudation.[23]
   b. Increased endothelial cell turnover.[23]
   c. Decreased endothelial cell prostacyclin production.[84]
2. Platelet effects
   a. Increased platelet count.[40]
   b. Increased platelet aggregation.[39]
   c. Increased platelet adhesiveness.[7]
   d. Increased thromboxane A_2 production.[42]
3. Lipid effects
   a. Decreased high-density lipoprotein levels.[53]
4. Coagulation effects
   a. Decreased fibrinolytic activity.[54]
   b. Increased blood viscosity.[29]
   c. Increased fibrinogen level.[29]
5. Whole vessel effects
   a. Vasoconstriction.
   b. Hypertension.

*Superscript numbers indicate chapter references.

The overwhelming association between smoking and lower extremity ischemia emphasizes that cessation of all tobacco use is an essential first step in nonoperative treatment of chronic lower extremity ischemia. The initial effort on the part of the vascular surgeon must be to identify clearly the patient's smoking addiction as an important component of the ischemic state. When the surgeon is taking the patient's history, questions such as "Do you still smoke?" or "How much do you smoke?" more effectively convey to the patient the impression that smoking is part of the problem than does the more neutral (and more typically asked) "Do you smoke?" Although almost all smokers are aware of an adverse health influence, most associate tobacco use with pulmonary disease, specifically lung cancer. The increased risks of myocardial infarction and stroke[1, 120] are less well recognized. The strong association with lower extremity ischemia was understood by only 37% of smokers with peripheral vascular disease in the study by Clyne and colleagues.[19]

Surgeons must clearly and unequivocally inform patients that smoking is the most important correctable cause of disease. An unwavering recommendation that a patient with chronic lower extremity ischemia totally cease tobacco use in all forms must be an important part of the initial encounter with the patient and should be repeated at every subsequent encounter. In a study by Kirk and associates,[71] strong and repeated advice by physicians to cease smoking resulted in abstinence by 37% of smokers with arterial disease.

It is important, however, for vascular surgeons to remember that for most smokers, tobacco use represents a powerful chemical addiction, which has been defined by Pollin[93] as the "inability to discontinue smoking despite awareness of the medical consequences." The proportion of the patient population able to cease smoking upon being informed of the importance of this step may be thought of as the population of nonaddicted users. How best to approach the problem of the addicted patient remains unsolved.

In the authors' opinion, it is important that the approach to patients with vascular disease who smoke be positive, nonjudgmental, and oriented toward the future. Poorly chosen statements may imply that the physician is condemning the patient rather than the smoking habit. An admonition to cease smoking accompanied by the threat of refusal to continue treatment if the patient cannot comply is inappropriate, in the authors' opinion, and indicates that the physician does not understand the nature of addiction. It is both appropriate and desirable for the vascular surgeon to indicate carefully and in detail to the patient that cessation of smoking not only removes a strong negative influence but also is associated with tangible positive benefits.

Abundant evidence indicates that abstinence from tobacco use improves the prognosis in patients with chronic lower extremity ischemia. When evaluating studies comparing smokers with nonsmokers or ex-smokers, one must recall the denial and deception common in addicted persons. It is desirable that any study of smoking behavior and its consequences be controlled by objective measurements of smoking markers, such as cotinine or carboxyhemoglobin levels. Studies that rely only on patient history are likely to be skewed by the inclusion of smokers who claim to be abstainers within the group of ex-smokers. It is important to note that this inaccuracy reduces the detected benefit associated with cessation of tobacco use, and studies that demonstrate benefit on the basis of patient history, although probably valid, most likely underestimate the magnitude of the benefit.

Quick and Cotton[96] found that patients with intermittent claudication who stopped smoking (on basis of history) have significant improvement in both ankle systolic pressure and treadmill walking compared with continued smokers.[96] Mean walking distance improved from 214 to 300 m. In the authors' practice, patients with claudication who stop smoking usually experience prompt improvement in walking distance, which averages a doubling of the initial distance.

The prognosis for continued patency of lower extremity arterial repairs has been related to smoking by many studies. Using carboxyhemoglobin blood levels to indicate continued smoking, Greenhalgh and colleagues[52] reported that carboxyhemoglobin levels in patients with failed grafts averaged 2.5 times those found in patients with patent grafts. Provan and associates[95] found significantly improved patency at 5 years in aortofemoral grafts in nonsmokers (71%) and in patients who stopped smoking (77%) compared with continued smokers (42%); this favorable effect could not be confirmed for femoropopliteal grafts in this study, which relied on patient history for smoking information. The study by Myers and coworkers,[87] which also relied on patient history of smoking, demonstrated significantly improved patency of aortofemoral grafts (90% versus 79% at 4 years) and femoropopliteal grafts (80% versus 61%) for patients who smoked fewer than five cigarettes per day. Similar findings were noted by Robicsek and colleagues[102] in patients with aortoiliac disease.

Many studies have documented a better prognosis for prevention of limb loss in patients with chronic lower extremity ischemia who stop smoking. In the study by Jurgens and coworkers,[67] no patients who stopped smoking required amputation, whereas 11.4% of those who continued smoking underwent amputation. Birkenstock and associates[8] found that 85% of persons who stopped smoking experienced improvement in symptoms of lower extremity ischemia, compared with only 20% of those who continued smoking. This difference was maintained even in the subgroup of patients with severe ischemia manifested by ischemic rest pain, gangrene, or both, in which 86% of patients who stopped smoking had improvement and did not require amputation, whereas only 10% of smokers had a similar favorable outcome.

In addition to giving the tobacco-addicted patient the information described, the vascular surgeon should provide a plan of action to achieve the goal of elimination of the addiction. The surgeon must be willing to recognize the limitations of his or her own expertise and to refer addicted patients to colleagues who specialize in substance abuse and addiction. Initial failure or relapse should not be regarded negatively: Multiple attempts are common in the histories of successful abstinence and should be regarded as a necessary part of the process, which for most people who successfully quit requires from 2 to 5 *years* and includes an average of six cycles of abstinence and relapse.[111] Many ex-smokers identify continuing, positively expressed encouragement to stop smoking from physicians, family members, and others as the most important influence leading to success. The prescription of nicotine gum as an aid to ease the transition from tobacco use to abstinence is appropriate. Although the adverse effects of nicotine are well known, studies show that fewer than 5% of successful ex-smokers continue using the gum on a long-term basis.[60]

More than any other factor, current changes in social norms regarding the acceptability of smoking may greatly aid the physician's efforts to influence patients to cease tobacco use. Prohibition of smoking in the workplace and in public places and a growing awareness of the real health risks posed by passive smoking have led to the placement of greater restrictions on smokers. The authors have been impressed with how well their own hospital inpatients, essentially all of whom are smokers, accept the total ban on smoking that exists in all areas of the hospital.

Exercise

Typically, patients with chronic lower extremity ischemia and intermittent claudication greatly reduce their daily walking because of the inevitable discomfort. In addition, many patients with claudication assume that the occurrence of muscle discomfort, which is the hallmark of claudication, indicates tissue damage and should be avoided through voluntary reduction of activity. In fact, the opposite is true. It has long been known that a regular program of walking exercise results in a measurable improvement in walking distance in a large majority of patients with claudication. The improvement produced by exercise programs has ranged from an 80% increase in walking distance in one British study of 21 patients[18] to a 234% increase in a study of 148 patients from Sweden.[41] Exercise programs have ranged from simple recommendations by physicians to increase walking to formal supervised programs using programmed treadmills. All studies have consistently demonstrated benefit, with the greatest benefit coming from supervised programs. A meta-analysis of supervised programs conducted by Gardner and Poehlman[49] found a mean increase of 179% in initial claudication distance and a mean increase of 122% in maximal walking distance.

Despite the frequently confirmed beneficial effects of exercise, not all patients may be able or willing to participate in an exercise training program. Many patients with intermittent claudication have severe coexisting cardiac, pulmonary, arthritic, and other conditions that also limit the safety or applicability of exercise therapy. Others may simply be unwilling. One study from Germany found that 34% of patients with claudication had direct contraindications to exercise treatment and 36% were unwilling to participate, leaving only 30% of a group of 201 patients to whom a planned exercise rehabilitation program could be applied.[33]

The mechanism responsible for improved walking tolerance in patients with claudication following an exercise program is not fully understood. The frequent assumption that exercise results in an improvement in the number of collateral vessels, the size of collateral vessels, or both, with a resulting increase in exercise-induced blood flow, is not supported by available data. Using a variety of techniques, numerous investigators have shown that neither ankle blood pressure nor calf muscle blood flow is better in patients with claudication whose walking tolerance improves after an exercise program.[18, 28, 41, 107, 113] Current opinion indicates that the improved muscle performance caused by exercise training is, at least in part, a result of adaptive changes in muscle enzymes leading to a more efficient extraction of oxygen from the blood.[14] Evidence in support of this mechanism was found when popliteal venous blood from exercising patients with claudication was examined for oxygen content. The extraction of oxygen was significantly increased following regular physical training. In addition, popliteal venous blood lactate levels were not increased, emphasizing that the greater muscle exercise capacity was aerobic in nature.[113]

Although this mechanism of increased exercise tolerance following a regular exercise program seems to be well established, other mechanisms may also be important. At least one study has observed improved hemorrheologic behavior of erythrocytes after regular exercise.[104] Other investigators have speculated that changes in gait to bring nonischemic muscles into greater use, improved mechanical efficiency of muscles, better fatty acid metabolism, and increased muscle fiber:capillary ratios may all play a role.[27, 59] Improvement in claudication after a program of regular walking exercise occurs with sufficient predictability in patients who can or will participate that the surgeon can prescribe such a program with confidence.

In the authors' practice, sedentary patients with claudication have generally experienced at least a doubling of the walking distance by following an exercise program. Interval treadmill examinations in the vascular laboratory may demonstrate incremental increases in walking distance to the skeptical patient before they can be clinically appreciated and thus may increase compliance during early phases of regular exercise. A sedentary lifestyle is a recognized risk factor for the development of atherosclerotic disease, and most patients with claudication have such a lifestyle. It is important for the physician to be aware of the major change in activities represented by the assumption of a regular exercise program and to prescribe a regimen within the range of possibility.

Obviously, exercise programs should be individualized, but for the majority of their patients, the authors have found a recommendation of 1 hour of walking at a comfortable pace each day to be well accepted. The patient should be instructed to (1) walk until claudication occurs, (2) rest until it subsides, and (3) repeat the cycle for 1 hour each day. There is no demonstrated benefit associated with attempting to "walk through the pain," and the level of discomfort produced by this effort is sufficient to discourage even the most dedicated patient. The indoor shopping malls in suburban locations throughout the United States provide a nearly ideal place for walking exercise during inclement weather, free from automobile traffic and often with conveniently spaced benches for periods of rest.

Creasy and coworkers[23] randomly assigned patients with intermittent claudication to treatment with balloon angioplasty or to an exercise therapy program. As expected, the initial improvement in leg circulation, as assessed by ABI, was greater in the angioplasty group. Nevertheless, after 1 year of follow-up, the patients in the exercise group could walk farther, both on the treadmill in the laboratory and as assessed by questionnaire, and there was no longer a significant difference between the ABI values of the two groups. This study demonstrates again the important benefits associated with exercise therapy. In addition, it questions the superiority of invasive therapy presumed by many and indicates that most future studies of claudication treatment should contain a control group that is treated with a regular exercise program rather than not treated at all.

Conclusions About Data on Exercise and Cessation of Smoking

An overwhelming body of data clearly indicates that cessation of smoking and assumption of a regular exercise program favorably influence the natural history of chronic lower extremity ischemia. It is important for physicians to understand that patients' compliance with these recommendations frequently requires profound change of lifelong habits. Physicians recommending basic lifestyle changes must be prepared to deal with a high rate of noncompliance and reversion to noncompliance after initial success. In the past, some investigators recommended that vascular surgeons refuse to treat patients who do not exercise or stop smoking. In the authors' opinion, this is a counterproductive attitude that fails to recognize the difficulty of the recommended tasks and abandons the basic attitude of acceptance of the patient, which is the foundation of a professional physician-patient relationship.

These considerations aside, however, one must be aware that most smokers who successfully quit do so after several initial failures, and most persons who develop the habit of regular exercise do so after a similar series of starts and stops. A disapproving attitude conveyed by the physician may abort this natural process, whereas repeated positive encouragement, based on the very real anticipated benefits outlined previously, may retain in the patient the growing desire for change that ultimately results in success.

In contrast to past times, when physicians may have been the only people encouraging patients to exercise regularly and stop smoking, current societal fashion and public opinion now form strong allies for the medical profession. Family, church, and citizen groups now commonly join in general condemnation of smoking and offer programs to aid those wishing to quit. Health clubs abound, fitness is in vogue, and almost all communities have organized exercise classes and programs specifically intended for the sedentary and infirm wishing to make a change. The vascular surgeon should be aware of such resources in the community and should recommend them as appropriate to patients.

Pharmacologic Therapy

More recent years have witnessed the development of multiple new pharmacologic agents potentially useful in the treatment of chronic lower extremity ischemia, including hemorrheologic agents, prostaglandins, and calcium channel blockers. Use of these agents is described in detail in Chapter 27 and, with the exception of hemorrheologic interventions, is not discussed here.

Hemorrheology

The viscosity of blood has an important influence on blood flow, as is evident from Poiseuille's equation. Active current interest is focused on therapeutic interventions that may improve the flow characteristics of blood in the microcirculation primarily through drug-induced decreases in blood viscosity, an area termed *hemorrheology*. The pharmacologic approaches to this problem are discussed in Chapter 27.

The straightforward approach to a reduction in blood viscosity by simple hemodilution has been evaluated in a blinded, controlled fashion. Ernst and coworkers[42] used hemodilution to treat 24 patients with stable claudication and found significant improvement in resting blood flow and pain-free walking distance, changes that did not occur in control patients. This study obviously indicates further investigation of this relatively simple approach to therapy, especially in patients with abnormally high blood viscosity.

Foot Care

For many patients with stable chronic lower extremity ischemia, the occurrence of minor injuries to the feet may initiate a relentless sequence of unmet demands for increased flow, chronic wounds, infection, further ischemia, gangrene, and ultimate limb loss. An unfortunately common scenario follows the ill-advised application of external heat (e.g., with a "hot pack" or heating pad) to an ischemic foot. It is obvious that the only mechanism by which the extremity can dissipate excess heat is through vasodilatation and increased blood flow. In the setting in which blood flow is fixed by proximal obstructive lesions, the excess heat cannot be dissipated, and full-thickness burns may (and frequently do) result from the application of heating pads set at temperatures that would not injure feet with normal arterial supply. Similarly, surgical operations designed to correct common foot problems may have disastrous consequences if performed in persons with chronic lower extremity ischemia whose blood supply is insufficient to achieve wound healing.

The desirability of preventing these unfortunate events is obvious. Patients with chronic lower extremity ischemia should be specifically instructed in the importance of foot care and the possibility of limb loss resulting from such seemingly inconsequential acts as careless nail or callus trimming. *Any* procedure on the foot should be regarded as a major undertaking and should be preceded by the clear demonstration of palpable pedal pulses; in the absence of pedal pulses, a noninvasive vascular laboratory examination should be performed to assess the potential for healing. The risk inherent in the application of external heat should be described to the patient carefully and in detail. Each patient with chronic lower extremity ischemia should be encouraged to report to the physician immediately the detection of any foot lesion, no matter how apparently minor. Patient instruction sheets are particularly useful in reinforcing the important points of such physician-patient discussions; the instruction sheet that the authors distribute to patients with chronic lower extremity ischemia is shown in Table 65–9.

INFLUENCE OF COEXISTING MEDICAL CONDITIONS AND THEIR TREATMENT

Given the age range, smoking habits, and level of infirmity of most patients with chronic lower extremity ischemia,

TABLE 65–9. GUIDELINES FOR PATIENTS WITH POOR CIRCULATION TO THE FEET

1. It is essential that you not use tobacco in any form.
2. Set aside 1 hour each day for walking exercises. Walk at a comfortable pace until your legs hurt, then stop and rest. When the pain is gone, walk again until they hurt and then rest. Repeat this cycle until an hour has passed.
3. You should take one aspirin tablet every day.
4. Care of your feet is extremely important.
   a. Your feet must be inspected daily for abrasions, ulcerations, or infections.
   b. Clean your feet daily with soap and water, and dry them well.
   c. Dry skin can be treated with any common hand cream.
   d. You should avoid ill-fitting or worn-out shoes.
   e. You should see us before cutting your toenails, trimming any calluses, or performing any other such procedures on your feet.
   f. You should not apply external heat (e.g., heating pad or "hot pack") to your feet, and you should not soak your feet in hot water.
   g. You should avoid trauma to your feet. Do not walk barefoot.
5. Contact us immediately if you develop any problems with your feet.

multisystem disease is the rule rather than the exception. In general, the improvement in cardiac, pulmonary, or renal function and hypertension following careful medical management of each of these conditions beneficially affects patients' chronic lower extremity ischemia as well. A few treatment interactions, however, may produce undesirable results and may not be familiar to internists making primary treatment decisions.

Cardiac function is obviously central to peripheral perfusion, and the adverse influence of lower extremity arterial obstructive lesions may be magnified by significant decreases in cardiac output. All vascular surgeons are familiar with patients with well-compensated chronic lower extremity ischemia in whom rest pain and even ischemic ulcerations develop during periods of decreased cardiac output caused by exacerbation of congestive heart failure. Likewise, patients with mild, previously unrecognized lower extremity occlusive disease may demonstrate impressive signs of peripheral mottling and cyanosis during episodes of decreased cardiac output as, for example, may accompany myocardial infarction. The potential in this situation for mistaken diagnosis of acute arterial occlusion that may lead to the performance of an unnecessary and hazardous operation to revascularize the affected extremity is obvious. In the authors' experience, the true chronic nature of the occlusive process can best be recognized in such patients with the use of objective measurements such as the ABI. The finding of a severely ischemic foot but an ABI of more than 0.4 in a nondiabetic patient with normally compressible arteries should immediately focus attention on decreased cardiac output as the immediate cause of poor distal extremity perfusion.

Treatment of systolic hypertension rarely, in the authors' experience, produces worsening in symptoms of chronic lower ischemia related to blood pressure reduction alone. Beta-adrenergic blocking agents, however, are commonly used to treat hypertension or angina pectoris. Exacerbation of the symptoms of chronic lower extremity ischemia, including claudication, rest pain, gangrene, and symptoms of Raynaud's phenomenon, with the use of these agents has been well described.[51, 79, 97, 121] Although blockade of normal beta-adrenergic peripheral vasodilating influence is part of the involved mechanism, increased sensitivity of peripheral alpha-adrenergic receptors also occurs after beta-blockade.[124] In the study by Marshall and colleagues,[79] symptoms of Raynaud's phenomenon occurred in 50% of patients taking beta-blockers for hypertension but in only 5% of patients achieving similar blood pressure control with the use of methyldopa, emphasizing that the effect is drug specific and is not caused by the decrease in systemic blood pressure. Fortunately, hypertension and angina pectoris can be treated with multiple alternative drug regimens. Beta-adrenergic blockers need not be continued in patients with chronic lower extremity ischemia, and switching to another agent may be associated with sufficient symptomatic improvement to avoid contemplated operative therapy.

NONCONVENTIONAL TREATMENT

Both the considerable expense, risk, and discomfort of surgical treatment and the progressive nature of the underlying disease process provide patients and physicians with strong impetus to seek alternative therapy for chronic lower extremity ischemia. The proven approaches to nonoperative treatment described in the preceding section of this chapter involve primary changes in lifestyle and personal habits that for many patients prove difficult. Thus, new forms of therapy evolve that invariably require less effort by the patient. Unfortunately, appreciation of the variable natural history of chronic lower extremity ischemia is not widespread among patients, physicians, or, sadly, even many investigators. This is particularly true with regard to the natural history of ischemic rest pain and ischemic ulceration, which in the minds of many are symptoms associated with an inevitable progression to gangrene and limb loss. This belief leads to the erroneous attribution of therapeutic benefit to treatment modalities associated with improvement in symptoms of chronic lower extremity ischemia, in the absence of comparison with results in a placebo or control group.

The treatment modalities described in the following section have not been proven to be of benefit in the treatment of chronic lower extremity ischemia. The results reported for these methods are within the range described earlier for the natural history of the conditions being treated.

Epidural Electrical Stimulation

Epidural electrical stimulation was reported to be of benefit in healing skin ulcers, some of which were believed to be ischemic, by Cook and associates[20] in 1976. In 1983, Tallis and coworkers[117] reported improvement in claudication walking distance and exercise tolerance after spinal cord stimulation in six of 10 patients with arterial disease; their study was without controls. A later report by Augustinsson and colleagues[6] described the treatment of 34 patients, 27 of whom had occlusive arterial disease and the remainder of whom had vasospastic disorders. Electrodes were implanted in the epidural space and were connected to a subcutaneous radio receiver. Stimulation was controlled by the patients using a handheld transmitter. Pain relief was described as "adequate" or "complete" in 94% of patients. Ten of the 27 patients with occlusive disease (37%) required amputation at a mean interval of 5.4 months of therapy. This result was believed to be better than that for a historical group of "similar" but otherwise undescribed control patients, who had a 90% amputation rate. A similar study was reported by Jacobs and associates,[65] who found that ischemic ulcers healed in 12 of 20 patients after treatment with epidural stimulation. After 2 years of follow-up, 56% of the limbs in this uncontrolled study had not been lost.

The mechanism of action of spinal cord stimulation is unknown. Pain relief may occur by inhibition of transmission of noxious stimuli, as postulated in the gate control theory of Melzack and Wall,[84] or by stimulation of local endorphin release.[29] Improvement in local blood flow is thought to result from vasodilatation, possibly through an effect on resting sympathetic tone.

The appropriate place for this form of therapy remains to be determined. Although spinal cord stimulation is an established form of pain control, regardless of the cause of the pain, no evidence thus far presented indicates any benefit with regard to limb salvage, ulcer healing, or limitation of localized gangrene when compared with the natural history expected for these symptoms.[76] To date, there have been no controlled studies demonstrating benefit beyond pain relief from electrical epidural stimulation in chronic lower extremity ischemia.

Chelation Therapy

The basis for chelation therapy, an unorthodox and unproven treatment for lower extremity ischemia, lies in the administration of ethylenediaminetetraacetic acid (EDTA) in the hopes that the calcium present in arteriosclerotic plaque will be extracted, solubilized by this chelating agent, and subsequently excreted, with a consequent reduction in the severity of arterial stenoses. Chelation therapy has been recommended by unorthodox practitioners since the 1950s.[16] In its most common form, EDTA is administered intravenously by infusion over several hours, on a near-daily basis for a treatment course of weeks or months. The therapy is most often prescribed as part of an overall approach to the treatment of arteriosclerosis that invariably includes sound recommendations, such as cessation of tobacco use, exercise, and weight reduction.

To date, no evidence has demonstrated effectiveness of chelation therapy for the treatment of arteriosclerosis of any site in a controlled trial setting. The results of numerous clinical reports of effectiveness are within the expected range for the natural history of the conditions being considered.[16, 70, 72, 73] The reasoning behind this approach to therapy is obviously flawed because authorities generally agree that the important events in the generation of atherosclerotic plaques are related to the proliferation of smooth muscle cells and the subsequent deposition by them of collagen, proteoglycans, and elastic fibers, as well as the accumulation of large amounts of lipid. Calcification is a tertiary event, and many significantly occlusive arteriosclerotic plaques contain little or no calcium.

In contrast to many questionably effective therapies that at least involve little or no patient risk, chelation therapy with EDTA carries the potential for significant and even fatal complications. Nephrotoxicity that may produce renal failure is a recognized complication of EDTA therapy.[36] In addition, rapid infusion of EDTA may produce severe hypocalcemia, with resultant tetany and cardiac arrhythmias.[83] A possible role for this drug in the production of serious autoimmune reactions has been suggested.[92]

On the basis of these considerations, statements have been issued by the editors of the *Medical Letter on Drugs and Therapeutics*[38] as well as by the American Medical Association, American Heart Association, American College of Physicians, American Academy of Family Physicians, American Society for Clinical Pharmacology and Therapeutics, American College of Cardiology, and American Osteopathic Association indicating that currently, no basis exists for the use of chelation therapy in the treatment of arteriosclerotic disease.[34] A definitive randomized, controlled trial commissioned by the government of Denmark has conclusively shown no benefit associated with chelation therapy.[112]

Conclusions

Many other nonconventional therapies are proposed for treatment of PAD. A complete listing and discussion of each are considerably beyond the scope of this chapter. Epidural electrical stimulation and chelation therapy are considered because both are invasive and therefore involve risk. Each serves as an example to remind physicians that the benefit of new or unconventional therapies can be evaluated only by controlled trials comparing the new treatment either with currently established treatments or with the untreated natural history of the disease.

SUMMARY

A clear knowledge of the natural history of chronic lower extremity ischemia forms the foundation for all decisions related to therapy for this condition. In the authors' opinion, the classically described benign natural history of claudication and the morbid outcome associated with ischemic rest pain or ulceration are probably too simplistic and are taken from questionable data. More accurate assessment of the prognosis for chronic lower extremity ischemia will be based on objective noninvasive vascular laboratory evaluation of the severity of ischemia.

A marked improvement in symptoms of chronic lower extremity ischemia may follow a regular program of exercise and cessation of tobacco use, both in patients with claudication and in some patients with limb-threatening ischemia. Although not discussed here, the appropriate use of pharmacologic agents as described in Chapter 27 obviously forms an important part of the nonoperative approach to treatment in occasional patients.

The nonconventional therapies described in the final part of this chapter are included because of the need for physicians undertaking the care of patients with chronic lower extremity ischemia to answer frequent patient inquiries regarding such treatment. Familiarity with the natural history of lower extremity ischemia as described in this chapter is critical to the accurate evaluation of treatment results attributed to these therapies.

REFERENCES

1. Abbott RD, Yin Y, Reed DM, et al: Risk of stroke in male cigarette smokers. N Engl J Med 315:717, 1986.
2. Ad Hoc Committee on Reporting Standards, Society for Vascular Surgery, North American Chapter, International Society for Cardiovascular Surgery: Standards for reports dealing with lower extremity ischemia. J Vasc Surg 4:80, 1986.
3. Ahn SS, Baker JD, Walden K, Moore WS: Which asymptomatic patients should undergo routine screening carotid duplex scan? Am J Surg 162:180, 1991.
4. Andersson GBJ, McNeill TW: Definition and classification of lumbar spinal stenosis. *In* Andersson GBJ, McNeill TW (eds): Lumbar Spinal Stenosis. St. Louis, Mosby–Year Book, 1992.
5. Aronow WS, Stemmer EA, Isbell MW: Effect of carbon monoxide exposure on intermittent claudication. Circulation 49:415, 1974.
6. Augustinsson LE, Carlsson CA, Holm J, et al: Epidural electrical stimulation in severe limb ischemia. Ann Surg 202:104, 1985.
7. Belch JJF, McArdle B, Pollack JG, et al: Epoprostenol (prostacyclin) and severe arterial disease: A double-blind trial. Lancet 1:315, 1983.
8. Birkenstock WE, Louw JHY, Terblanche J, et al: Smoking and other factors affecting the conservative management of peripheral vascular disease. S Afr Med J 49:1129, 1975.
9. Birnstingl MA, Brinson K, Chakrabarti BK: The effect of short-term exposure to carbon monoxide on platelet stickiness. Br J Surg 58:837, 1971.
10. Bliss B, Wilkins D, Campbell WB, et al: Treatment of limb-threatening ischaemia with intravenous Iloprost: A randomised double-blind placebo-controlled study. Eur J Vasc Surg 5:511, 1991.
11. Bloor K: Natural history of arteriosclerosis of the lower extremities. Ann R Coll Surg Engl 28:36, 1961.
12. Bowlin SJ, Medalie JH, Flocke SA, et al: Epidemiology of intermittent claudication in middle-aged men. Am J Epidemiol 140:418, 1994.
13. Boyd AM: The natural course of arteriosclerosis of the lower extremities. Angiology 11:10, 1960.
14. Bylund AC, Hammersten J, Holm J, et al: Enzyme activities in skeletal muscles from patients with peripheral arterial insufficiency. Eur J Clin Invest 6:425, 1976.
15. Cheng SWK, Ting ACW, Wong J: Lipoprotein (a) and its relationship to risk factors and severity of atherosclerotic peripheral vascular disease. Eur J Vasc Endovasc Surg 14:17, 1997.
16. Clarke NE, Clarke CN, Mosher RE: The in vivo dissolution of metastatic calcium on approach to atherosclerosis. Am J Med Sci 229:142, 1955.
17. Clark R, Daly L, Robinson K, et al: Hyperhomocysteinemia: An independent risk factor for vascular disease. N Engl J Med 324:1149, 1991.
18. Clifford PC, Davies PW, Hayne JA, et al: Intermittent claudication: Is a supervised exercise class worthwhile? Br Med J 280:1503, 1980.
19. Clyne CA, Arch PJ, Carpenter D, et al: Smoking, ignorance, and peripheral vascular disease. Arch Surg 117:1062, 1982.
20. Cook AW, Oygar A, Baggenstos P, et al: Vascular disease of extremities: Electrical stimulation of spinal cord and posterior roots. N Y State J Med 76:366, 1976.
21. Couch NP: On the arterial consequences of smoking. J Vasc Surg 3:807, 1986.
22. Crawford ES, Bomberger RA, Glaeser DH, et al: Aortoiliac occlusive disease: Factors influencing survival and function following reconstructive operation over a twenty-five year period. Surgery 90:1055, 1981.
23. Creasy TS, McMillan PJ, Fletcher EW, et al: Is percutaneous transluminal angioplasty better than exercise for claudication? Preliminary results from a prospective randomized trial. Eur J Vasc Surg 4:135, 1990.
24. Criqui MH, Fronck A, Klauber MR, et al: The sensitivity, specificity and predictive value of traditional clinical evaluation of peripheral arterial disease: Results from noninvasive testing in a defined population. Circulation 71:516, 1985.
25. Cronenwett JL, Warner KG, Zelenock GB, et al: Intermittent claudication: Current results of nonoperative management. Arch Surg 119:430, 1984.
26. Cronenwett JL, Zelenock GB, Whitehouse WM Jr, et al: Prostacyclin treatment of ischemic ulcers and rest pain in unreconstructible peripheral arterial occlusive disease. Surgery 100:369, 1986.
27. Dahllof A, Bjorntorp P, Holm J, Schersten T: Metabolic activity of skeletal muscle in patients with peripheral arterial insufficiency: Effect of physical training. Eur J Clin Invest 4:9, 1974.
28. Dahllöf AG, Holm J, Sclersten T, et al: Peripheral arterial insufficiency: Effect of physical training on walking tolerance, calf blood flow and blood flow resistance. Scand J Rehabil Med 8:19, 1976.
29. Dahn I, Ekman CA, Lassen NA, et al: On the conservative treatment of severe ischemia of the leg. J Clin Lab Invest 19(Suppl 99):160, 1967.
30. Davis JW, Shelton L, Eigenberg DA, et al: Effects of tobacco and non-tobacco cigarette smoking on endothelium and platelets. Clin Pharmacol Ther 37:527, 1985.
31. De Backer G, Kornitzer M, Sobolski J, Denolin H: Intermittent claudication—epidemiology and natural history. Acta Cardiol 34:115, 1979.
32. DeBakey ME, Crawford ES, Garrett E, et al: Occlusive disease of the lower extremities in patients 16 to 37 years of age. Ann Surg 159:873, 1964.
33. De La Haye R, Diehm C, Blume J, et al: An epidemiological study of the value and limits of physical therapy/exercise therapy in Fontaine stage II arterial occlusive disease. Vasa 38:1, 1992.
34. Diagnostic and Therapeutic Technology Assessment (DATTA): Chelation therapy. JAMA 250:672, 1983.
35. Dintenfass L: Elevation of blood viscosity, aggregation of red cells, hematocrit values and fibrinogen levels in cigarette smokers. Med J Aust 1:617, 1975.
36. Dudley HR, Ritchie AC, Schilling A, et al: Pathologic changes associated with the use of sodium ethylene diamine tetraacetate in the treatment of hypercalcemia. N Engl J Med 255:331, 1955.
37. Eastcott HHG: Arterial Surgery, 2nd ed. London, Pitman Medical Publishers, 1973, p 3.
38. EDTA chelation therapy for arteriosclerotic heart disease. Med Lett Drugs Ther 23:51, 1981.
39. Edwards JM, Taylor LM Jr, Porter JM: Treatment of failed lower extremity bypass grafts with new autogenous vein bypass. J Vasc Surg 11:132, 1990.
40. Eklund AE, Eriksson G, Olsson AG: A controlled study showing significant short term effect of prostaglandin E_1 in healing of ischemic ulcers of the lower limb in man. Prostaglandins Leukot Med 8:265, 1982.
41. Ekroth R, Dahllöf AG, Gundevall B, et al: Physical training of patients with intermittent claudication: Indications, methods and results. Surgery 84:640, 1978.
42. Ernst E, Matrai A, Kollar L: Placebo controlled, double-blind study of hemodilution in peripheral arterial disease. Lancet 1:1449, 1987.
43. Executive Committee for the Asymptomatic Carotid Atherosclerosis Study: Endarterectomy for asymptomatic carotid artery stenosis. JAMA 273:1421, 1995.
44. Felix WR Jr, Sigel B, Gunther L: The significance for morbidity and mortality of Doppler absent pedal pulses. J Vasc Surg 5:849, 1987.
45. Fielding JE: Smoking: Health effects and control. N Engl J Med 313:555, 1985.
46. Fowkes FGR, Housler E, Cawood EHH, et al: Edinburgh Artery Study: Prevalence of asymptomatic and symptomatic peripheral arterial disease in the general population. Int J Epidemiol 20:384, 1991.
47. Fowkes GR, Housley E, Riemersma RA, et al: Smoking, lipids, glucose intolerance and blood pressure as risk factors for peripheral atherosclerosis compared with ischemic heart disease in the Edinburgh Artery Study. Am J Epidemiol 135:331, 1992.
48. Gallasch G, Diehm C, Dorter C, et al: The influence of physical training on blood flow properties in patients with intermittent claudication. Klin Wochenschr 63:554, 1985.
49. Gardner AW, Poelhman ET: Exercise rehabilitation programs for the treatment of claudication pain: A meta-analysis. JAMA 274:975, 1995.
50. Gentile AT, Taylor LM Jr, Moneta GL, Porter JM: Prevalence of asymptomatic carotid stenosis in patients undergoing infrainguinal bypass surgery. Arch Surg 130:900, 1995.
51. Gokal R, Dornan TL, Ledingham JG: Peripheral skin necrosis complicating beta-blockage. Br Med J 1:721, 1979.
52. Greenhalgh RM, Laing SP, Colap V, et al: Progressing atherosclerosis following re-vascularization. *In* Bernhard VM, Towne JB (eds): Complications in Vascular Surgery. New York, Grune & Stratton, 1980, p 39.
53. Hadovic J: Endothelial injury by nicotine and its prevention. Experientia 34:1585, 1978.

54. Hallet JW Jr, Greenwood LH, Robinson JG: Lower extremity arterial disease in young adults. Ann Surg 202:647, 1985.
55. Hansteen V, Lorentsen E, Sivertssen E, et al: Long term follow-up of patients with peripheral arterial obliterations treated with arterial surgery. Acta Clin Scand 141:725, 1975.
56. Henriksen O: Local sympathetic reflex mechanism in regulation of blood flow in human subcutaneous adipose tissue. Acta Physiol Scand 450(Suppl):7, 1977.
57. Hertzer NR, Beven EG, Young JR, et al: Coronary artery disease in peripheral vascular patients: A classification of 1000 coronary angiograms and results of surgical management. Ann Surg 199:223, 1984.
58. Hertzer NR: Fatal myocardial infarction following lower extremity revascularization: Two hundred and seventy-three patients followed six to eleven post-operative years. Ann Surg 193:492, 1981.
59. Hiatt WR, Regensteiner JG, Wolfel EE, et al: Effect of exercise training on skeletal muscle histology and metabolism in peripheral arterial disease. J Appl Phys 81:780, 1996.
60. Hjalmarson AIM: Effect of nicotine chewing gum in smoking cessation. JAMA 252:2835, 1984.
61. Hughson WG, Munn JI, Garrod A: Intermittent claudication: Prevalence and risk factors. Br Med J 1:1379, 1978.
62. Hully SB, Cohen R, Widdowson G: Plasma high-density lipoprotein cholesterol level: Influence of risk factor intervention. JAMA 238:2269, 1977.
63. Hurlow RA, Strachan CJL, George AJ, et al: Thrombosis tests in smokers and non-smokers and patients with peripheral vascular disease. *In* Greenhalgh RM (ed): Smoking and Arterial Disease. London, Pitman Medical Publishers, 1981.
64. Imparato AM, Kim GE, Davidson T, et al: Intermittent claudication: Its natural course. Surgery 78:795, 1975.
65. Jacobs MJHM, Jorning PJG, Beckers RCY, et al: Foot salvage and improvement of microvascular blood flow as a result of epidural spinal cord electrical stimulation. J Vasc Surg 12:354, 1990.
66. Jonason T, Ringqvist I: Factors of prognostic importance for subsequent rest pain in patients with intermittent claudication. Acta Med Scand 218:27, 1985.
67. Jurgens IL, Barker NW, Hines EA: Arteriosclerosis obliterans: A review of 520 cases with special reference to pathogenic and prognostic factors. Circulation 21:188, 1960.
68. Kallero KS: Mortality and morbidity in patients with intermittent claudication as defined by venous occlusion in plethysmography: A ten year follow-up. J Chronic Dis 34:455, 1981.
69. Kannel WB, Skinner JJ, Schwarz MJ, et al: Intermittent claudication: Incidence in the Framingham study. Circulation 41:875, 1970.
70. Kitchell JR, Palmon F, Ayton N, et al: The treatment of coronary artery disease with disodium EDTA: A reappraisal. Am J Cardiol 11:501, 1963.
71. Kirk CJC, Lund VJ, Woolcock NE, et al: The effect of advice to stop smoking on arterial disease patients, assessed by serum thiocyanate levels. J Cardiovasc Surg 21:568, 1970.
72. Lamar CP: Chelation endarterectomy for occlusive atherosclerosis. J Am Geriatr Soc 14:272, 1966.
73. Lamar CP: Chelation therapy of occlusive arteriosclerosis in diabetic patients. Angiology 15:379, 1964.
74. Lefevre FA, Corbacioglu C, Humphries AW, et al: Management of arteriosclerosis obliterans of the extremities. JAMA 170:656, 1959.
75. Lithell H, Hedstrand H, Karlsson R: The smoking habits of men with intermittent claudication. Acta Med Scand 197:473, 1975.
76. LoGerfo FW: Epidural spinal cord electrical stimulation: An unproven methodology for management of lower extremity ischemia. J Vasc Surg 13:518, 1991.
77. Lowe GDO, Dunlop DJ, Lawson DH, et al: Double-blind controlled clinical trial of ancrod for ischaemic rest pain of the leg. Angiology 33:46, 1982.
78. Malone JM, Moore WS, Goldstone J: Life expectancy following aortofemoral arterial grafting. Surgery 81:551, 1977.
79. Marshall AJ, Roberts CJC, Barritt DW: Raynaud's phenomenon as a side effect of beta-blockers in hypertension. Br Med J 1:1498, 1976.
80. McAllister FF: The fate of patients with intermittent claudication managed non-operatively. Am J Surg 132:593, 1976.
81. McDermott MM, Feinglass J, Slavensky R, Pearce WH: The ankle-brachial index as a predictor of survival in patients with peripheral vascular disease. J Gen Intern Med 9:445, 1994.
82. Meade TW, Chakrabarti R, Haines AP, et al: Characteristics affecting fibrinolytic activity and plasma fibrinogen concentrations. Br Med J 1:135, 1979.
83. Meltzer LE, Kitchell JR, Palmon F Jr: The long term use, side effects and toxicity of EDTA. Am J Med Sci 242:51, 1961.
84. Melzack R, Wall PD: Pain mechanism: A new theory. Science 150:971, 1975.
85. Moreland LW, Lopez-Mendez A, Alarcon GS: Spinal stenosis: A comprehensive review of the literature. Semin Arthritis Rheum 19:127, 1989.
86. Murabito JM, D'Agostino RB, Silbershatz H, Wilson PWF: Intermittent claudication: A risk profile from the Framingham Heart Study. Circulation 96:44, 1997.
87. Myers KA, King RB, Scott DF, et al: The effect of smoking on the late patency of arterial reconstructions in the legs. Br J Surg 65:267, 1978.
88. Norgen L, Alwark A, Angqvist KA, et al: A stable prostacyclin analog (Iloprost) in the treatment of ischaemic ulcers of the lower limb: A Scandinavian-Polish placebo-controlled randomised multicentre study. Eur J Vasc Surg 4:463, 1990.
89. Nunn DB: Symptomatic peripheral arteriosclerosis of patients under age 40. Ann Surg 39:224, 1973.
90. Pairolero PC, Joyce JW, Skinner CR, et al: Lower limb ischemia in young adults: Prognostic implications. J Vasc Surg 1:459, 1984.
91. Peabody CN, Kannel WB, McNamara PM: Intermittent claudication: Surgical significance. Arch Surg 109:693, 1974.
92. Peterson GR: Adverse effects of chelation therapy. JAMA 250:2926, 1983.
93. Pollin W: The role of the addictive process as a key step in causation of all tobacco related diseases. JAMA 252:2874, 1984.
94. Projections of the Population of the United States by Age, Sex and Race: 1983–2080. Current Population Reports, Population Estimates and Projections. Washington, DC, U.S. Department of Commerce, 1984. Bureau of the Census, Series P25, No 952.
95. Provan JL, Sojka SG, Murnaghan JJ, et al: The effect of cigarette smoking on the long term success rates of aortofemoral and femoropopliteal reconstructions. Surg Gynecol Obstet 165:49, 1987.
96. Quick CRG, Cotton LT: The measured effect of stopping smoking on intermittent claudication. Br J Surg 69(Suppl):524, 1982.
97. Rees PJ: Peripheral skin necrosis complicating beta-blockade. Br Med J 1:955, 1979.
98. Reid DD, Brett GZ, Hamilton PJ, et al: Cardiorespiratory disease and diabetes among middle aged male civil servants. Lancet 1:469, 1974.
99. Reinders JH, Brinkman HJM, Van Mourik JA, et al: Cigarette smoke impairs endothelial cell prostacyclin production. Arteriosclerosis 6:15, 1986.
100. Renaunen A, Takkunen H, Aromaa A: Prevalence of intermittent claudication and its effect on mortality. Acta Med Scand 537(Suppl):8, 1972.
101. Rivers SP, Veith FJ, Ascer E, et al: Successful conservative therapy of severe limb threatening ischemia: The value of nonsympathectomy. Surgery 99:759, 1986.
102. Robicsek F, Daugherty HK, Mullen DC, et al: The effect of continued cigarette smoking on the patency of synthetic vascular grafts in Leriche syndrome. J Thorac Cardiovasc Surg 70:107, 1975.
103. Rosenbloom MS, Flanigan DP, Schuler JJ, et al: Risk factors affecting the natural history of claudication. Arch Surg 123:867, 1988.
104. Ruell PA, Imperial ES, Bonor FJ, et al: Intermittent claudication: The effect of physical training on walking tolerance and venous lactate concentration. Eur J Appl Physiol 52:420, 1984.
105. Rutkow IM, Ernst CB: An analysis of vascular surgical manpower requirements and vascular surgical rates in the United States. J Vasc Surg 3:74, 1986.
106. Salmasi A-M, Nicolaides A, Al-Katoubi A, et al: Intermittent claudication as a manifestation of silent myocardial ischemia: A pilot study. J Vasc Surg 14:76, 1991.
107. Saltin B: Physical training in patients with intermittent claudication. *In* Cohen LS, Mock MB, Ringqvist I (eds): Physical Conditioning and Cardiovascular Rehabilitation. New York, Wiley, 1981, p 181.
108. Schadt DC, Hines EA, Juergens JHLO, et al: Chronic atherosclerotic occlusion of the femoral artery. JAMA 175:937, 1961.
109. Schroll M, Munck O: Estimation of peripheral arteriosclerotic disease by ankle blood pressure measurements in a population study of 60-year-old men and women. J Chronic Dis 34:261, 1981.
110. Schuler JJ, Flanigan DP, Holcroft JW, et al: Efficacy of prostaglandin E_1 in the treatment of lower extremity ischemic ulcers secondary

to peripheral vascular occlusive disease: Results of a prospective randomized, double-blind, multicenter clinical trial. J Vasc Surg 1:160, 1984.

111. Silbert S, Zazeela H: Prognosis in atherosclerotic peripheral vascular disease. JAMA 166:1816, 1958.
112. Sloth-Nielsen J, Guldager B, Mouritzen C, et al: Arteriographic findings in EDTA chelation therapy on peripheral arteriosclerosis. Am J Surg 162:122, 1991.
113. Sprlie D, Myhre K: Effects of physical training in intermittent claudication. Scand J Clin Lab Invest 38:217, 1978.
114. Stachnik T, Stoffelmayr B: Worksite smoking cessation programs: A potential for national impact. Am J Public Health 73:1395, 1983.
115. Szilagyi DE, Hageman JHY, Smith RF, et al: Autogenous vein grafting in femoropopliteal atherosclerosis: The limits of its effectiveness. Surgery 86:836, 1979.
116. Szilagyi DE, Elliott JP, Smith RF, et al: A thirty-year survey of the reconstructive surgical treatment of aortoiliac occlusive disease. J Vasc Surg 3:421, 1986.
117. Tallis RC, Illip LS, Sedgwich EM, et al: Spinal cord stimulation in peripheral vascular disease. J Neurol Neurosurg Psychiatry 46:478, 1983.
118. Turnipseed WD, Berkoff HA, Belzer FO: Postoperative stroke in cardiac and peripheral vascular disease. Ann Surg 192:365, 1980.
119. Turnipseed W, Detmer DE, Girdley F: Chronic compartment syndrome: An unusual cause for claudication. Ann Surg 210:557, 1989.
120. Ulietstra RE, Kronmal RA, Oberman A, et al: Effect of cigarette smoking on survival of patients with angiographically documented coronary artery disease. JAMA 255:1023, 1986.
121. Vale JA, Jefferys DB: Peripheral gangrene complicating beta-blockade. Lancet 1:1216, 1978.
122. Veith FJ, Gupta SK, Samson RH, et al: Progress in limb salvage by reconstructive arterial surgery combined with new or improved adjunctive procedures. Ann Surg 194:386, 1981.
123. Walsh DB, Gilbertson JJ, Zwolak RM: The natural history of superficial femoral artery stenoses. J Vasc Surg 14:299, 1991.
124. White CB, Udwadia BP: Beta-adrenoreceptors in the human dorsal hand vein and the effects of propranolol and practolol on venous sensitivity to noradrenaline. Br J Clin Pharmacol 2:99, 1975.
125. Widmer LK, Greensher A, Kannel WB: Occlusion of peripheral arteries: A study of 6400 working subjects. Circulation 30:836, 1964.
126. Wynder EL: Tobacco and health: A societal challenge. N Engl J Med 300:894, 1979.

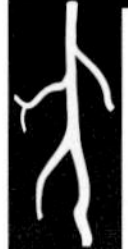

CHAPTER 66

Direct Reconstruction for Aortoiliac Occlusive Disease

David C. Brewster, M.D.

The infrarenal abdominal aorta and the iliac arteries are among the most common sites of chronic obliterative atherosclerosis in patients with symptomatic occlusive disease of the lower extremities.[1] Indeed, atherosclerotic narrowing or occlusion of these vessels, most commonly located at the aortic bifurcation, occurs to various degrees in the majority of patients with symptoms of arterial insufficiency severe enough to require surgical revascularization. Because arteriosclerosis is commonly a generalized process, obliterative disease in the aortoiliac segment frequently coexists with disease below the inguinal ligament. Despite its generalized nature, however, the disease is usually segmental in distribution and is thereby amenable to effective surgical treatment. Even in patients with several levels of disease, successful correction of hemodynamic impairment in the aortoiliac inflow system often provides satisfactory clinical relief of ischemic symptoms. In addition, careful assessment of the adequacy of arterial inflow is important even in patients whose primary difficulty is located in the femoropopliteal or tibial outflow segment if good and durable results of distal arterial revascularization are to be obtained.

Since the introduction of the initial reconstructive methods of thromboendarterectomy and homograft replacement in the late 1940s and early 1950s, great progress has been achieved in the surgical management of aortoiliac occlusive disease. Currently, a variety of methods exist for accurate evaluation of the extent and physiologic severity of the disease process. In addition, improvements in the preoperative assessment of patient risk have helped to clarify the decision about the optimal management in individual patients. Advances in graft materials, surgical techniques, intraoperative management, and postoperative care all have contributed to a steady reduction in perioperative morbidity and mortality and to excellent long-term results. Indications for operation have become fairly well accepted and standardized, and various operative approaches and methods of revascularization are available for use in differing clinical circumstances. With proper patient selection and a carefully performed, appropriate operative procedure, a favorable outcome may be anticipated at low risk to the patient, making surgical management of aortoiliac occlusive disease one of the most rewarding areas of vascular surgical practice today.

CLINICAL MANIFESTATIONS

The symptoms and natural history of the occlusive process are significantly influenced by its distribution and extent

(Fig. 66–1). Truly localized aortoiliac disease (*type I*), with occlusive lesions confined to the distal abdominal aorta and common iliac vessels, is seen infrequently (5% to 10% of patients) and, in the absence of more distally distributed disease, rarely produces limb-threatening symptoms.[2] In such localized aortic obstruction, the potential for collateral blood flow around the aortoiliac arterial segment is great. Collateral pathways include both visceral and parietal routes, such as:

- Internal mammary artery to inferior epigastric artery
- Intercostal and lumbar arteries to circumflex iliac and hypogastric networks
- Hypogastric and gluteal branches to common femoral and profunda femoris (deep femoral) arterial branches
- Superior mesenteric to inferior mesenteric and superior hemorrhoidal pathways via the marginal artery of Drummond (meandering mesenteric artery)

The relatively low incidence of localized aortoiliac disease is based on the angiograms of patients whose symptoms were severe enough for them to be seriously considered for direct surgical intervention. With the increasing use of percutaneous transluminal angioplasty (PTA) and related interventional treatment modalities that may represent "less invasive" forms of management, more liberal application of arteriography earlier in the disease process, when less advanced symptoms are present, may well document a higher incidence of localized occlusive lesions in the aortoiliac segment.[3]

Patients with localized, segmental disease typically present with claudication of varying severity, most often involving the proximal musculature of the thigh, hip, or buttock areas. The symptoms may be equally severe in both limbs, although often, one leg is more severely affected than the other. More advanced ischemic complaints are absent unless distal atheroembolic complications have occurred. In men, impotence is an often associated complaint, present in different degrees in at least 30% to 50% of male patients with aortoiliac disease. Patients with a type I disease pattern are characteristically younger, with a relatively low incidence of hypertension or diabetes but a significant frequency of abnormal blood lipid levels, particularly type IV hyperlipoproteinemia.[4, 5]

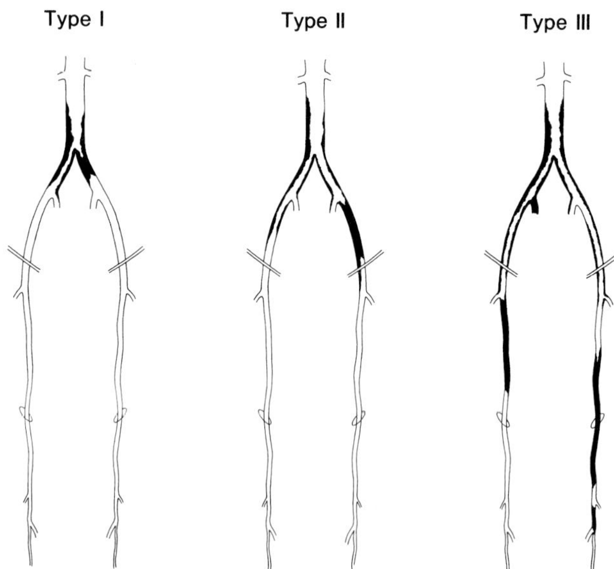

FIGURE 66–1. Patterns of aortoiliac occlusive disease. *Type I*, Localized disease is confined to the distal abdominal aorta and common iliac arteries. *Type II*, More widespread intra-abdominal disease is present. *Type III*, This pattern denotes multilevel disease with associated infrainguinal occlusive lesions.

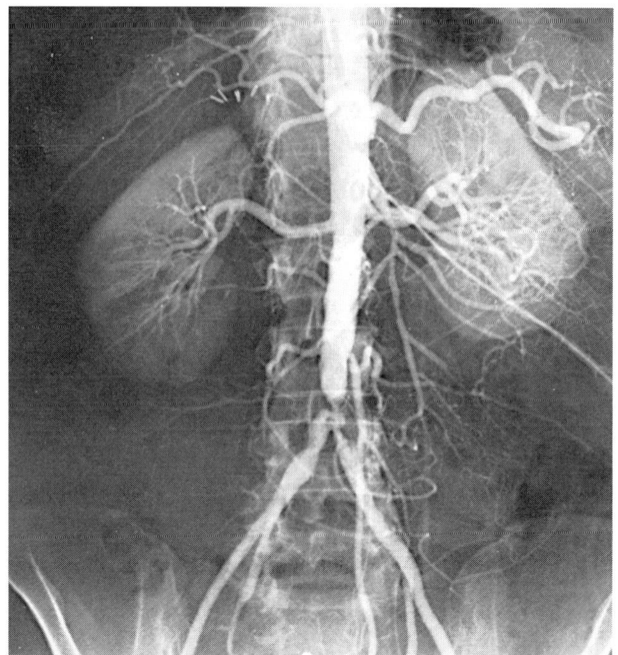
FIGURE 66–2. Translumbar aortogram of a 50-year-old woman with localized type I aortoiliac disease.

In contrast to the usual male predominance in chronic peripheral vascular disease, almost one half of patients with localized aortoiliac lesions are women.[2] Indeed, the frequency of aortoiliac disease in women has been growing substantially, likely reflecting the higher incidence of cigarette smoking in women. Many women with localized aortoiliac disease exhibit a characteristic clinical picture often called the "hypoplastic aorta syndrome" (Fig. 66–2): typically, a woman of about 50 years of age, invariably a heavy smoker, with angiographic findings of small aortic, iliac, and femoral vessels; a high aortic bifurcation; and occlusive disease often strikingly localized to the lower aorta or the aortic bifurcation.[5–8] Commonly, many such patients have experienced an artificial menopause induced by hysterectomy or irradiation.

In more than 90% of symptomatic patients, however, disease is more diffuse. In about 25%, disease is confined to the abdomen (*type II*), and in about 65%, widespread occlusive disease is seen above and below the inguinal ligament (*type III*).[2, 4] Patients in the latter group with such "combined-segment" or "multilevel" disease are typically older, more commonly male (~6:1 male-to-female ratio), and much more likely to have diabetes, hypertension, and associated atherosclerotic disease involving cerebral, coronary, and visceral arteries. Progression of the occlusive process is also more likely in such patients than in patients with more localized aortoiliac disease.[8–10] For these reasons, most patients with a type III pattern manifest symptoms of more advanced ischemia, such as ischemic pain at rest or various degrees of ischemic tissue necrosis, and they require revascularization more often for limb salvage than for relief of claudication alone. In addition, these characteristics not unexpectedly lead to a significant decrease in life expectancy of 10 or more years in patients with diffuse multisegment disease, whereas life expectancy may be nearly normal in patients with localized aortoiliac disease.[11]

DIAGNOSIS

Clinical Evaluation

In most instances, an accurate history and a carefully performed physical examination can unequivocally establish the diagnosis of aortoiliac disease. A reliable description of claudication in one or both legs, possible decreased sexual potency in a man, and diminution or absence of femoral pulses define the characteristic triad often referred to as the *Leriche syndrome*. However, clinical grading of femoral pulses may sometimes be inaccurate, particularly in obese patients or in patients with scarred groins from prior operation.[12, 13] Although proximal claudication symptoms in the distribution of the thigh, hip, and buttock musculature usually constitute a reliable indicator of clinically important inflow disease, a significant number of patients with aortoiliac disease, particularly those with multilevel disease, nonetheless complain only of calf claudication.[14, 15] Audible bruits may commonly be auscultated over the lower abdomen or the femoral vessels, particularly after exercise. Pallor on elevation, rubor on dependency, shiny atrophic skin in the distal limbs and feet, and possible areas of ulceration or of ischemic necrosis or gangrene may be noted, depending on the extent of atherosclerotic impairment.

In some instances, the diagnosis of aortoiliac occlusive disease may not be readily apparent, the pitfalls involving certain complaints that may cause diagnostic confusion. In some patients, pulses and appearance of the feet may be judged to be entirely normal at rest, despite the presence of proximal stenoses that are physiologically significant with exercise. This is often the case in patients presenting with distal microemboli secondary to atheroembolism, the so-called blue toe syndrome.[16, 17] In other instances, complaints of exercise-related pain in the leg, hip, buttock, or even low back may be mistaken for symptoms of degenerative hip or spine disease, nerve root irritation caused by lumbar disc herniation or spinal stenosis, diabetic neuropathy, or other neuromuscular problems. Many such cases may be distinguished from cases of true claudication by the fact that the discomfort from neuromuscular problems is often relieved only by sitting or lying down, as opposed to simply stopping walking. In addition, the typical sciatic distribution of the pain and the fact that the complaints are often brought on simply with standing, as opposed to walking a certain distance, suggest nonvascular causes. In many such circumstances, however, the use of noninvasive vascular laboratory testing modalities, including treadmill exercise, may be extremely valuable.[18, 19]

Objective Assessment

Noninvasive Studies

Use of noninvasive studies not only improves diagnostic accuracy but also allows objective physiologic quantification of the severity of the disease process (see Chapter 10). Such quantification may be of considerable clinical benefit, for instance, in establishing the likelihood of lesion healing without revascularization, or in differentiating neuropathic foot pain from true ischemic rest pain. The results of noninvasive studies may also serve as a reliable and objective baseline by which to follow a patient's disease course.

Finally, they may often help in localization of the disease process. The author and his colleagues have found the use of segmental limb Doppler pressure measurements and pulse volume recordings to be most useful.[20]

Arteriography

If the patient's symptoms and clinical findings indicate sufficient disability or threat to limb survival, angiography is indicated to (1) delineate the extent and distribution of occlusive disease and (2) guide further therapeutic choices. Arteriography is rarely used in a truly diagnostic sense. The presence or absence of occlusive disease as a cause of the patient's symptoms can almost always be reliably established by clinical evaluation supplemented by pre-exercise and post-exercise noninvasive vascular laboratory studies. Instead, angiography is employed to obtain anatomic information for use by the surgeon in selecting and planning the best method of revascularization. On occasion, the angiogram may provide the final bit of data needed for the surgeon to decide whether or not to proceed with operation. In other instances, it may be employed to determine whether occlusive disease is amenable to balloon PTA. Neither of these uses is "diagnostic" in the usual sense of the word but is, rather, part of the therapeutic process.

In addition to noting the actual anatomic distribution of occlusive disease in the aortoiliac segment and distal vessels, the surgeon should examine the angiography films to search for potentially important or critical anatomic variations or associated occlusive lesions in the renal, visceral, or runoff vessels. For example, an enlarged meandering left colic artery (Fig. 66–3) may often be an indicator of associated occlusive disease in the superior mesenteric artery, which can usually be appreciated only on a lateral view. Failure to recognize this fact may lead to catastrophic bowel infarction if the inferior mesenteric artery is ligated at the time of aortic reconstruction.[21]

Approach

The general preference of the author and his colleagues is for a retrograde transfemoral approach, which is feasible from the less involved side in most patients (see Chapter 16). In patients with severe bilateral occlusive disease or total aortic occlusion, a translumbar or transaxillary route may be employed, depending on the preferences of the angiographer or the surgeon. A biplanar study, providing oblique or lateral views, is highly desirable and often greatly enhances the ability to determine the clinical importance of visualized lesions, which often may be underestimated on standard anteroposterior views alone.[12]

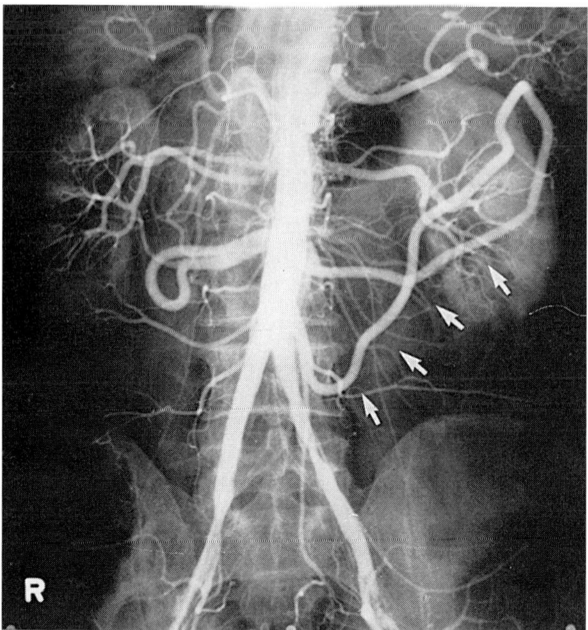

FIGURE 66–3. Aortogram demonstrating enlarged meandering inferior mesenteric and left colic arteries *(arrows)*, indicative of associated occlusive disease in the celiac and/or superior mesenteric arteries.

Extent of Study

For most patients, a complete arteriographic survey of the entire intra-abdominal aortoiliac segment and infrainguinal runoff vessels (runoff views) is advisable. Even if proximal operation alone is planned, knowledge of the status of runoff vessels is important because it (1) helps the surgeon anticipate the probable outcome of proximal operation alone, (2) aids in more effective management of possible technical misadventures, and (3) is needed for future planning. Only such complete studies enable the detection of unusual but highly important variations in the occlusive process that may critically affect the conduct and outcome of operation.

Some investigators believe that aortography is not necessary in patients with complete absence of both femoral pulses. Currently, however, most vascular surgeons hold that even in these cases, angiographic study is important to define the exact anatomic distribution and extent of occlusive disease accurately and to facilitate selection of the appropriate arterial reconstruction.

In general, runoff views are obtained to at least the level of the mid-calf. In selected patients with advanced distal disease and threatened limbs, more distal views may be advisable, including views of the foot itself if the possibility of distal infrapopliteal bypass grafting is considered likely. In such instances, in which the amount of contrast material reaching these distal points may be significantly impaired by multilevel occlusive lesions, supplemental use of digital subtraction angiography (DSA) techniques may enhance visualization and definition of anatomy.

Postangiographic Renal Dysfunction

Despite the relatively nontoxic nature of the contrast agents currently used for diagnostic arteriography, various degrees of deterioration in renal function may be noted following angiographic studies. Such dysfunction may be mild and transient or may lead to severe impairment requiring dialysis. Although the precise risk of acute renal dysfunction after aortic angiography depends on the definition of and criteria for functional impairment, the reported incidence varies between 0 and 10% for patients at low risk for contrast-induced dysfunction and between 30% and 40% for patients at higher risk for this complication.[22] Renal deterioration appears to be related to contrast load and is clearly more likely to occur in patients with preexisting renal insufficiency and azotemia, dehydration, diabetes mellitus, greater age, or other predisposing factors.

Hydration of patients before angiography appears to be beneficial, and it should be liberally employed. The administration of mannitol to patients with preexisting renal disease at the time of angiography has also been recommended. In high-risk patients, DSA appears to be helpful, often providing diagnostic anatomic information with much lower volumes and dosages of contrast media. Whether or not use of non-ionic contrast agents is beneficial in reducing the incidence of contrast-induced renal dysfunction is not clearly established (see Chapter 16).

In general, contrast-induced renal failure usually resolves spontaneously within about 7 days. Because of its possible adverse effects, angiography should precede surgery by an interval sufficient to demonstrate that the serum creatinine concentration has remained stable and that operation is not being carried out at the time of developing renal failure. In current practice, preoperative angiography is usually performed on an outpatient basis prior to admission for surgery, a policy that has therefore alleviated this problem in most instances.[23]

Alternative Imaging Modalities

In recent years, alternative imaging techniques have developed rapidly and in some cases may be used in place of conventional contrast-enhanced angiography. Three-dimensional spiral (helical) computed tomographic angiography (CTA) and magnetic resonance angiography (MRA) are used increasingly to evaluate the carotid artery, the renal artery, aortic aneurysms, and lower extremity occlusive disease.[24–27] At present, however, these modalities cannot match the visual clarity and spatial resolution of conventional arteriograms; thus, their use in evaluation of aortoiliac occlusive disease is currently restricted to special circumstances, such as increased risk of catheter angiography for a variety of reasons (see Chapters 12, 14, and 15).

Femoral Artery Pressure

Although an accurate assessment of occlusive disease is usually possible with traditional clinical evaluation and good-quality arteriography in most patients, difficulty may exist in evaluation of patients with multilevel occlusive disease. Assessment of the hemodynamic significance of occlusive disease at each segmental level is obviously critical in selection of an appropriate reconstructive procedure. It is well recognized that many atherosclerotic lesions visualized on the arteriogram may be of only morphologic significance, with little or no actual hemodynamic importance. In such cases, proximal reconstruction alone often fails to relieve the patient's symptoms adequately. Furthermore, if only moderate proximal disease is present in a patient with advanced distal disease, operative correction of both segmental levels may be required for limb salvage if severe ischemia is present in the foot.

Despite the availability of a wide array of noninvasive vascular laboratory testing methods, none is entirely accurate in establishing the hemodynamic importance of aortoiliac inflow lesions, particularly in the patient with multilevel disease. All the methods appear to be influenced by the presence of infrainguinal occlusive disease, and abnormal results may not always be reliably attributable to the proximal lesions. Deficiencies of segmental limb Doppler pressures or pulse volume recordings are well recognized in this regard.[28–30] Analysis of femoral artery Doppler waveforms or calculation of a pulsatility index is also of questionable accuracy in the presence of multisegment disease because both modalities are affected by distal as well as proximal disease.[12, 31] Other, more complex modifications of Doppler waveform analysis have been devised, but their accuracy and value in combined-segment disease remain uncertain.

Similarly, duplex scanning has been applied to the assessment of lower extremity occlusive disease[32]; however, a threshold criterion for local increase of peak systolic velocity to signify hemodynamically significant iliac disease has not been conclusively established. Duplex scanning examinations also are time-consuming, require very experienced technicians, and may not visualize some arterial segments, all disadvantages that currently limit the applicability of duplex scanning to evaluation of aortoiliac disease.

Reliance on the angiographic appearance of lesions also carries known hazards. Marked interobserver variability is associated with the interpretation of the functional importance of arterial lesions visualized on arteriograms.[33] In addition, although the relationship of a simple arterial stenosis and hemodynamic impairment is well documented, the multiplicity and complexity of lesions occurring in the aortoiliac system make hemodynamic assessment based on morphology alone often inaccurate.[34] In such instances, actual measurement of femoral artery pressure (FAP) may be of considerable value.[12, 35–37]

FAP measurements are usually obtainable in the arteriographic suite at the time of transfemoral catheter aortography. Separate arterial puncture by a relatively small-caliber (19-gauge) needle may occasionally be required if pressure determinations are needed in the femoral artery contralateral to the angiographic catheter insertion site. As illustrated in Figure 66–4, peak systolic pressure in the femoral artery is compared with distal aortic or brachial systolic pressure. Either (1) a resting systolic pressure difference of more than 5 mmHg or (2) a fall in FAP greater than 15% when reactive hyperemia is induced pharmacologically or by inflation of an occluding thigh cuff for 3 to 5 minutes implies hemodynamically significant inflow disease. If revascularization is indicated in patients with such findings, attention should first be directed at correction of the inflow lesions. With negative study findings, the surgeon may more confidently proceed directly with distal revascularization without fear of premature compromise or closure of the distal graft, and without subjecting the patient to an unnecessary inflow operation.[38]

Use of such criteria greatly facilitates selection of patients for an inflow procedure and accurately predicts benefits. In a review by the author's group, 96% of patients with positive results on FAP studies had satisfactory clinical improvement in ischemic symptoms after proximal arterial reconstruction alone, despite uncorrected distal disease in the majority of patients; in contrast, 57% of patients undergoing only proximal operation despite a negative FAP result experienced unsatisfactory relief of symptoms and required

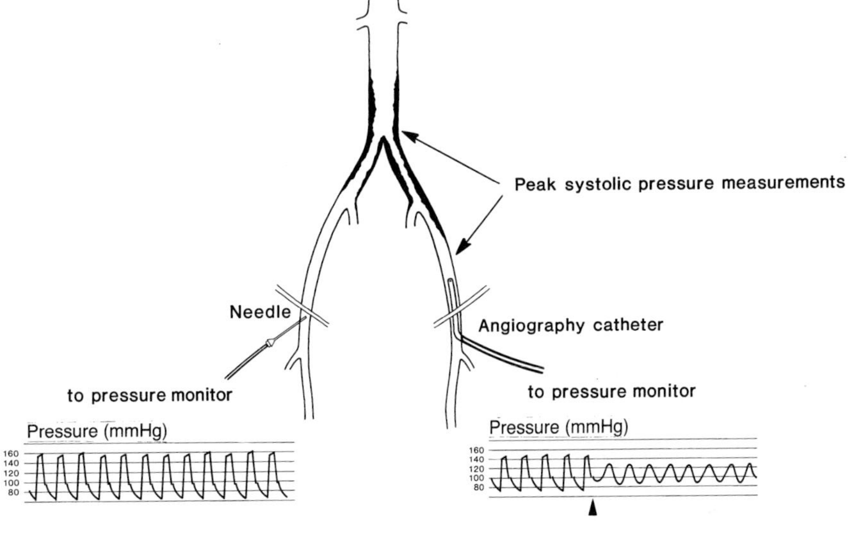

FIGURE 66–4. Femoral artery pressure (FAP) measurement. A significant fall in peak systolic pressure is noted in the tracing on the right *(arrowhead)* as the catheter is withdrawn down the left iliac artery. p̄ = after.

subsequent distal procedures.[14] Similar results have been reported by other investigators using pressure determinations.[37, 39]

TREATMENT

Therapeutic Options

A wide variety of therapeutic options are available for the management of aortoiliac occlusive disease. These may be broadly categorized as:

1. Anatomic or direct reconstructive surgical procedures on the aortoiliac vessels.
2. So-called extra-anatomic or indirect bypasses that avoid normal anatomic pathways.
3. Various nonoperative catheter-based endoluminal therapies that emphasize treatment of the obliterative lesions through a remote, often percutaneous access site to the arterial system.

Although the availability of these numerous alternative therapies is beneficial, enabling the surgeon to select a procedure appropriate to the individual anatomy and risk status of each patient, decision making is often complex and difficult. Substantial differences in reported early and late results of alternative methods have contributed to the confusion. Purported benefits and advantages, particularly of endoluminal techniques, have been accentuated in recent years by the greatly increased emphasis on limiting cost and length of hospitalization. Indeed, the optimal method of management of aortoiliac disease represents one of the most controversial areas of contemporary vascular practice.[40]

Unfortunately, few definitive data exist, and very few prospective randomized studies have been performed with adequate control of the multiple complex variables involved to allow direct comparison of treatment options. Personal bias, previous surgical training, and individual experience remain factors in decision making. In addition, the need to individualize each decision according to specific anatomic distribution of disease and operative risk factors unique to every patient implies that there is no single best method of treatment. The best choice will, and probably should, vary from patient to patient.

Conservative Management

No truly effective medical treatment for aortoiliac occlusive disease is currently available. Nonoperative care is aimed at:

- Limiting disease progression
- Encouraging development of collateral circulation
- Preventing local tissue trauma or infection in the foot

With such care, spontaneous improvement may be noted in a few patients, but in most instances, slow progression of symptoms may be anticipated.

Progression of the atheromatous process may, in some cases, be slowed by altering the patient's risk factors. Complete cessation of cigarette smoking is paramount in this regard and cannot be overemphasized in discussions with the patient. Weight reduction, treatment of hypertension, correction of abnormal serum lipid levels, and regulation of diabetes all seem to be desirable and logical, although the definite benefit of these measures, in terms of stabilization or alleviation of occlusive symptoms, is less well established.

A regular exercise program, often involving nothing more rigorous than regular walking of a specific distance on a daily basis, seems to be the best stimulant to collateral circulation. Good local foot care is extremely important because trauma and digital infection are often the precipitating causes of gangrene and amputation, particularly in the patient with diabetes.

Although numerous vasodilator drugs exist, none is of established benefit in chronic occlusive disease.[41] None of these drugs has been shown to increase the exercising muscle blood flow in the extremity with claudication, the critical requirement for an agent effective in the treatment of claudication. A multi-institution, double-blind, placebo-controlled trial of pentoxifylline (Trental) in the treatment of patients with claudication showed a significant increase in walking distance in patients who received this agent in comparison with those treated with a placebo.[42] In the author's experience, perhaps 25% of patients may find some alleviation of claudication symptoms. It is often difficult to know, however, whether this improvement is attributable to the drug. Pentoxifylline may be used in patients with moderate claudication, but it does not appear to have changed the eventual need for surgical revascularization in patients with severe claudication, resting ischemia, or more advanced symptoms. Newer drugs to alleviate claudication symptoms are being developed and evaluated (see Chapters 19 and 27).

Indications for Intervention

Ischemic pain at rest and actual tissue necrosis, including ischemic ulcerations or frank digital gangrene, are well accepted as indicating advanced ischemia and threatened limb loss. Without treatment, most limbs with these symptoms experience disease progression and require major amputation. Therefore, all surgeons agree that these symptoms represent unequivocal indications for arterial revascularization, if anatomically feasible.

Age per se is rarely an absolute contraindication. Even patients who are elderly or frail or for whom surgery poses high risks because of multiple associated medical problems generally can undergo revascularization with alternative surgical methods, even if direct aortoiliac reconstruction is deemed inadvisable.

Some disagreement remains about the advisability of intervention in patients whose only indication is the presence of claudication. Quite clearly, such decisions must be individualized, with each patient's age, associated medical disease, employment requirements, and lifestyle preferences taken into consideration. However, claudication that jeopardizes the patient's livelihood or significantly impairs the desired lifestyle and daily activities of a patient for whom surgery would be a low risk may be considered to be a reasonable indication for surgical correction if the anatomic situation is favorable for intervention. In such cases, the surgeon should treat the patient conservatively for a time and should thoroughly discuss the merits and possible risks of any invasive therapy. The patient should have demonstrated commitment to the therapeutic program through control of appropriate risk factors, the most important being elimination of cigarette smoking and appropriate weight reduction, when required, and through compliance with a low-fat, low-calorie diet.

In general, most surgeons are more liberal in recommending surgical operation for patients with claudication alone, if symptoms can be attributed to isolated proximal inflow disease, as opposed to patients with additional distal disease in the femoropopliteal arterial segment. This approach seems logical and appropriate because of the generally excellent and long-lasting results currently achieved with aortoiliac reconstruction at low risk to the patient. Similarly, in patients with localized occlusive lesions in the iliac arteries that appear favorable for endovascular treatment by angioplasty or stenting, intervention for relatively modest claudication may be justified (see later).

Another less well-recognized indication for aortoiliac reconstruction is peripheral atheromatous emboli from proximal ulcerated atherosclerotic plaques (see Chapter 56). The aortoiliac system has been recognized as a frequent source of spontaneous atheroembolization to more distal vessels. As already described, clinical evidence of occlusive disease in patients with such emboli may be minimal, with little or no history of claudication and fairly normal pulses at rest. However, if (1) the clinical picture is consistent with a diagnosis of atheroembolization and (2) aortography demonstrates shaggy or ulcerated atherosclerotic plaques in the aortoiliac system, aortofemoral grafting with total exclusion of the host aortoiliac system is commonly indicated to avoid repetitive episodes or even limb loss, even though the occlusive lesions may not be hemodynamically significant.

CATHETER-BASED INTERVENTIONS

Percutaneous Transluminal Angioplasty and Stents

The role of PTA, with or without intravascular stents, and other catheter-based methods of arterial recanalization is discussed more fully in Chapters 32 and 72. PTA may be a valuable treatment modality in some patients with aortoiliac occlusive disease. However, patient selection is paramount.

To be appropriate for PTA, a lesion should be relatively localized and preferably a stenosis rather than a total occlusion. A localized stenosis of the common iliac artery less than 5 cm in length is the most favorable situation for PTA, which achieves good early and late patency rates.[43, 44] Such a situation may exist in perhaps 10% to 15% of patients with aortoiliac disease who undergo arteriographic study.[40] Iliac PTA for focal iliac disease is also a valuable adjunct when combined with distal surgical procedures in appropriate patients with multilevel disease.[45, 46] Although the rate of long-term clinical success even in these favorable subsets of patients appears to be less than that for conventional surgical reconstruction, the likely benefits, in terms of decreased morbidity and probable cost savings, may well justify the use of PTA in these circumstances.

Whether PTA should be employed in patients with milder symptoms who would not normally be considered for standard surgical therapy remains uncertain and controversial. Similarly, whether stents can improve late results of iliac PTA and thereby extend indications for catheter-based interventions to patients with more extensive aortoiliac disease (longer diseased segments, multiple lesions, total occlusions) remains unproven at this time. At present, PTA is generally not recommended for patients with diffuse iliac artery disease, unless they are extraordinarily poor surgical candidates, or for totally occluded iliac arteries, because of the higher incidence of complications or recurrent occlusion. There are almost always alternatives for surgical revascularization in high-risk patients who have conditions that are unfavorable to treatment with PTA.

Stent Grafts

In recent years, some groups have extended endoluminal therapy of aortoiliac occlusive disease to include use of stent grafts for diffuse obliterative disease.[47–49] Such approaches have evolved from initial experience gained with endovascular treatment of abdominal aortic aneurysms.

The basic concept is a combination of conventional prosthetic graft materials with a variety of intraluminal stents designed to secure the prosthetic graft in place while also maintaining a patent vessel lumen. Very aggressive balloon angioplasty recanalizes the aortoiliac system, and the fabric prosthetic portion of the endovascular graft lines the inner wall of the vessel. Unilateral aortoiliac covered stent grafts may be combined with conventional femorofemoral bypass grafts or infrainguinal grafts to treat bilateral or multilevel aortoiliac disease. Although still in its formative stages, this mode of management may prove valuable in some patients as further technologic improvements in endograft design, delivery, and deployment are achieved (see Chapters 38 and 72).

EXTRA-ANATOMIC GRAFTS

Since their introduction in the early 1960s for management of difficult and often desperate technical problems usually related to infection or failure of previous grafts, use of a variety of extra-anatomic bypasses has increased to include wider application in (1) patients judged to be at higher risk with conventional direct aortic surgery and (2) patients with more limited disease not otherwise suitable for PTA or stents. In such patients, the goal is to achieve revascularization by means of grafts that utilize remote, usually subcutaneous pathways and that potentially can be performed with lower morbidity and mortality. Extra-anatomic grafts are discussed more fully in Chapter 68.

There is no question that extra-anatomic grafts are useful alternatives to direct anatomic surgical reconstruction in certain circumstances; much debate continues, however, as to whether their results in current practice have improved sufficiently for the application of such grafts to be expanded. Most controversy in this regard centers on two areas: (1) use of extra-anatomic grafts for treatment of mostly unilateral iliac occlusive disease and (2) possible application of axillofemoral grafts to more patients with bilateral disease.[40, 50, 51] At present, however, extra-anatomic grafts do not appear equivalent in durability or efficacy to aortofemoral grafts. They should therefore be regarded as an occasionally useful and appealing alternative treatment option. In general, the somewhat lower long-term patency rate and less comprehensive revascularization must be accepted as tradeoffs for the lower morbidity and mortality risks of these procedures (see Chapter 68).

DIRECT ANATOMIC SURGICAL RECONSTRUCTION

Since the pioneering development of a fabric arterial graft by Voorhees and colleagues[52] and the initial use of prosthetic aortic grafts in the 1950s,[53, 54] extensive clinical experience has clearly demonstrated that direct aortic grafting is the most durable and efficacious method of revascularization available. Refinements in operative techniques, further improvements in prosthetic graft and suture materials, and striking advances in perioperative anesthetic management and postoperative intensive care have all contributed to steadily improving outcome, lower morbidity and mortality, and generally excellent results in contemporary practice.[2, 55–60] Aortobifemoral grafts continue to be properly regarded as the "gold standard" for the treatment of aortoiliac occlusive disease.[40]

Preoperative Preparation

In addition to angiographic assessment, evaluation of associated cardiac, renal, and pulmonary disease is routinely performed. Any correctable deficiencies are best identified before operation and are appropriately treated. For instance, patients with compromised pulmonary reserve may benefit from a period of preoperative chest physiotherapy, bronchodilator medication, appropriate antibiotic treatment, and so forth. Diminished renal function also requires evaluation, with correction of any prerenal component that is due to dehydration or treatment of other reversible deficiencies. Similarly, cardiac abnormalities demonstrated by clinical evaluation or 12-lead echocardiogram are evaluated and treated appropriately; in many instances, consultation with a cardiologist may be quite helpful.

Without question, the most important and most controversial aspect of the preoperative evaluation is the detection and subsequent management of associated coronary artery disease.[61] Several studies have documented the existence of potentially important coronary artery disease in 40% to 50% or more of patients requiring peripheral vascular reconstructive procedures, 10% to 20% of whom may be relatively asymptomatic largely because of their inability to exercise.[62] Myocardial infarction is quite clearly responsible for the majority of both early and late postoperative deaths. However, most available screening methods suffer from a lack of sensitivity and specificity in predicting postoperative cardiac complications. In addition, many patients with vascular occlusive disease cannot achieve adequate exercise stress as a result of claudication or infirmity. Even with coronary angiography, it is difficult to relate anatomic findings to functional significance and, hence, surgical risk. In addition, coronary angiography is associated with its own inherent risks, and patients undergoing coronary artery bypass grafting or coronary PTA before needed aortoiliac reconstructions are subjected to the risks and complications of both procedures.

In this regard, the author and his colleagues as well as others have found preoperative dipyridamole–thallium 201 imaging to be very valuable in identifying the subset of patients with vascular occlusive disease who may indeed be at high risk for perioperative myocardial ischemic events and perhaps may need more intensive preoperative evaluation.[63–65] This modality has allowed identification of a subset of patients for whom surgery poses a low risk and in whom no further preoperative evaluation or intensive intraoperative monitoring appears to be warranted. Conversely, a subset of patients can be identified for whom surgery poses a high risk and in whom (1) preoperative coronary angiography and, possibly, coronary revascularization should be performed before surgery for vascular occlusive disease or (2) aortic operation may be deferred if more elective indications permit.

Although thallium imaging and, often, preoperative cardiac functional studies may be helpful, the utility of preoperative cardiac evaluation as well as how best to accomplish it remains unsettled. The incidence of major perioperative cardiac events after general vascular procedures is relatively low in contemporary practice,[66] and all screening methods suffer from a poor positive predictive value. Therefore, some surgeons advocate proceeding without extensive cardiac evaluation and managing patients with the assumption that all patients with vascular occlusive disease have coronary disease (see Chapter 40).

Routine testing of coagulation parameters should be part of any preoperative evaluation. Baseline values should be obtained for hematocrit, complete blood count, platelet count, and prothrombin time and partial thromboplastin time measurements. Any abnormalities of such screening studies require further evaluation and correction of specific factor deficiencies. Patients taking aspirin, dipyridamole, or other drugs that may adversely affect platelet function or other aspects of the normal coagulation mechanisms should discontinue such medications about 1 week before operation.

On the day before surgery, the patient is restricted to a liquid diet and a mechanical bowel preparation is ordered. Nonabsorbable oral antibiotics, such as neomycin and erythromycin, may be added if there is reason to believe that gastrointestinal trauma or ischemia may occur, but these agents are generally not used in the author's practice. Prophylactic parenteral antibiotics are routinely given, beginning 1 to 2 hours preoperatively and continuing for about 48 hours after arterial reconstruction. Several randomized studies have clearly established the value of such systemic prophylactic antibiotics in vascular surgery.[67–69]

Aortoiliac Endarterectomy

Aortoiliac endarterectomy may be considered in the group of 5% to 10% of patients with truly localized (type I) disease, and if properly performed in such circumstances, it may give excellent and durable results[2] (see Chapter 67). The principal potential benefit of endarterectomy is avoidance of prosthetic grafts, with their possible complications of dilatation, infection, anastomotic aneurysm, and other graft-related problems. These problems, however, are all relatively unusual with modern-day vascular prostheses.

At present, aortoiliac endarterectomy is rarely used by most vascular surgeons. Most patients have more diffuse disease than is suitable for endarterectomy. Increased use of various catheter-based endoluminal therapies has further reduced the number of patients with relatively localized aortoiliac disease for whom endarterectomy might be appropriate.

Finally, few centers continue to perform an adequate number of endarterectomy procedures for trainees to become skilled in and comfortable with this method of revascularization. For all of these reasons, bypass grafting has become the standard technique.

PRINCIPLES OF AORTIC GRAFT INSERTION

Proximal Anastomosis

The proximal aortic anastomosis may be made either end-to-end or end-to-side. End-to-end anastomosis is clearly indicated in patients with coexisting aneurysmal disease or complete aortic occlusion extending up to the renal arteries. In addition, it is preferred by many vascular surgeons for routine use in most cases for several reasons.

First, it appears to be hemodynamically more sound, with less turbulence, better flow characteristics, and less chance of competitive flow with still patent host iliac vessels. Such considerations have led to better long-term patency and a lower incidence of aortic anastomotic aneurysms in grafts constructed with end-to-end proximal anastomosis in many reported series, although none has been a randomized, prospective trial.[2, 4, 70–72] Other studies, however, have not demonstrated any differences in late patency rates between end-to-end and end-to-side grafts.[73–76]

Second, application of partially occluding tangential clamps for construction of an end-to-side anastomosis may often carry a higher risk of dislodgment of intra-aortic thrombus or debris, which may then be irretrievably carried to the pelvic circulation or lower extremities.

Last, resection of a small segment of host aorta and use of a short body of the prosthetic bifurcation graft for end-to-end anastomosis (Fig. 66–5) allow the prosthesis to be placed in the anatomic aortic bed, greatly facilitating subsequent tissue coverage and reperitonealization and potentially avoiding the late occurrence of aortoenteric fistula formation.[2, 4, 73]

End-to-side anastomosis appears to be potentially advantageous in certain anatomic patterns of disease (Fig. 66–6). First, if a large aberrant renal artery arises from the lower abdominal aorta or iliac artery or if the surgeon wishes to avoid sacrifice of a large patent inferior mesenteric artery (IMA) end-to-side proximal anastomosis is the simplest method to achieve preservation of such vessels. (If end-to-end insertion is preferred, however, these vessels can be preserved and reimplanted into the body of the graft.)

Second, and most important, end-to-side anastomosis appears to be advisable if the occlusive process is located principally in the external iliac vessels. In such instances, interruption of the infrarenal aorta for end-to-end bypass to the femoral level effectively devascularizes the pelvic region because no retrograde flow up the external iliac arteries to supply the hypogastric arterial beds can be anticipated. This problem may potentially increase the incidence of erectile impotence in the sexually potent male.[77, 78] Such hemodynamic consequences may also raise the incidence of postoperative colon ischemia, severe buttock ischemia, or even paraplegia secondary to spinal cord ischemia.[21, 79, 80] Troublesome hip claudication may also continue to plague the patient despite the presence of excellent femoral and distal pulses.

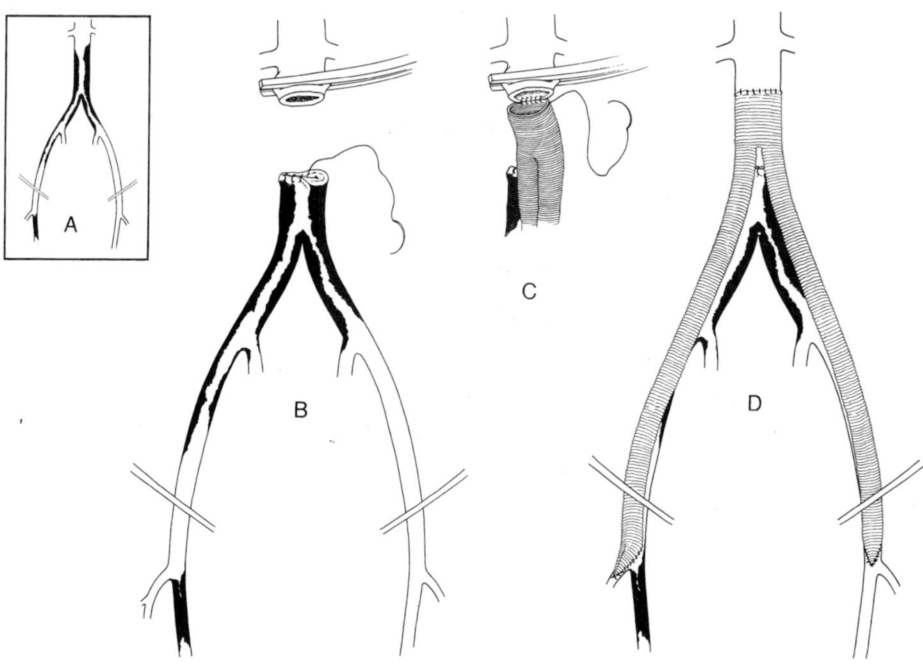

FIGURE 66–5. Aortofemoral graft. *A*, Schematic illustration of a preoperative aortogram. *B*, A segment of diseased aorta is resected, and the distal aortic stump is oversewn. *C*, End-to-end proximal anastomosis. *D*, Completed reconstruction.

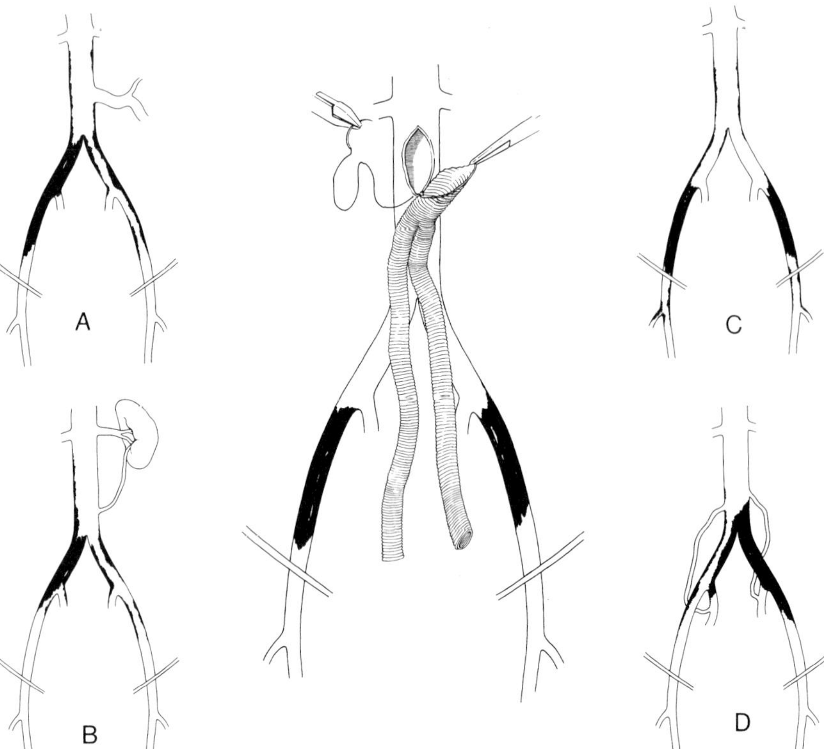

FIGURE 66–6. Anatomic findings or patterns of disease and profunda femoris artery stenosis favoring end-to-side proximal anastomosis of an aortofemoral graft. *A*, Patent and enlarged inferior mesenteric artery. *B*, Low-lying accessory renal artery arising from the distal aorta or proximal iliac vessels. *C*, Occlusive lesions confined largely to the external iliac arteries, with the aorta and common iliac and internal iliac arteries fairly well preserved. In the author's experience, this is the most common indication for end-to-side anastomosis. *D*, Reconstitution of pelvic circulation by collateral sources, which would be interrupted with end-to-end anastomosis. In all of these circumstances, end-to-side aortic anastomosis may be advantageous.

Third, if the limb of the graft becomes occluded in later years, and further revascularization proves to be infeasible, the resulting limb ischemia may be particularly severe and may lead to difficulty with healing after even above-knee amputation. For these reasons, the surgeon may elect to use end-to-side proximal anastomosis in the anatomic circumstances described.

At present, one can only conclude that this area is controversial. Both methods have been advocated by experienced and highly skilled vascular surgeons. Irrespective of the method of proximal anastomosis, the principle of placing the proximal anastomosis high in the infrarenal abdominal aorta, relatively close to the renal arteries in an area almost always less involved by the occlusive process, is of paramount importance to minimize later recurrent difficulties.

Distal Anastomosis

Although the distal anastomosis of the aortic graft may on occasion be constructed at the level of the external iliac artery in the pelvis, it is almost always preferable in patients with occlusive disease to carry the graft to the femoral level, where exposure is generally better and anastomosis is technically easier. With adequate personnel, both femoral anastomoses may often be performed simultaneously. Most important, anastomosis at the femoral level provides the surgeon with an opportunity to ensure adequate outflow into the profunda femoris artery. Experience has clearly demonstrated a higher late failure rate of aorta–external iliac grafts, with a higher incidence of subsequent "downstream" operations as a result of progressive disease at or just beyond the iliac artery anastomosis.[2, 81, 82] With meticulous surgical technique, proper skin preparation and draping, and use of a limited period of prophylactic antibiotic coverage, the higher incidence of infection that was anticipated to occur with extension of grafts to the femoral artery level has not been borne out by extensive experience.[2, 9, 55–60] As a result, aortobifemoral grafting has become the procedure of choice for direct reconstruction in almost all patients with aortoiliac occlusive disease.

Profunda Femoris Artery Runoff

Establishment of adequate graft outflow at the level of the femoral artery anastomosis, via the profunda femoris artery in patients with disease or occlusion of the superficial femoral artery, has been clearly documented to be of paramount importance in early and late graft results.[2, 60, 83, 84] For these reasons, it is imperative that any lesion that might compromise flow in the profunda femoris artery be carefully evaluated and corrected at the time of distal anastomosis.

Preoperative arteriography should visualize the orifice of the profunda femoris artery, particularly when occlusion of the superficial femoral artery is demonstrated. Visualization is usually best accomplished with oblique views of the groin. At operation, the surgeon must look for possible stenosis of the origin of the profunda femoris artery by palpation, gentle passage of vascular probes, or direct inspection. If any stenosis of the profunda femoris origin exists, it should be corrected by endarterectomy or patch angioplasty techniques. The author's preference is for extension of the arteriotomy down the profunda femoris artery beyond the orifice stenosis, with subsequent anastomosis of the beveled tip of the graft as a patch closure (Fig. 66–7).

This maneuver, which achieves hemodynamic correction, is preferable in the author's judgment to true endarterectomy, which may lead to a higher incidence of late pseudoaneurysm formation if the prosthetic graft is sutured to the endarterectomized arterial wall.

Formal endarterectomy of the profunda femoris artery, however, may be required if the vessel is extensively diseased. Subsequent closure can still be achieved with the long, beveled tip of the graft hood. Other surgeons have preferred using autogenous arterial or saphenous vein patches for separate profundaplasty, then anastomosing the prosthesis to the common femoral artery above this site.[84] In any case, it is imperative that the surgeon use precise anastomotic technique at the end-point of the endarterectomy to ensure an adequate profunda femoris artery outflow tract. In the hands of the author and his colleagues, this is usually best achieved by the use of three to five interrupted sutures at the distal end of the anastomosis (see Fig. 66–7*D*), which allows excellent visualization, precise placement, and avoidance of any constricting effect of a running suture line at this critical outflow point.

Although some surgeons have suggested that the mere existence of an occluded superficial femoral artery in itself causes a "functional" stenosis despite the absence of orificial disease of the profunda femoris artery,[85] most evidence suggests that "routine" profundaplasty in all such cases does not improve the hemodynamic result or late patency rate of the graft.[40, 74]

Graft Selection

Although standard fabric prosthetic grafts constructed from polyester (Dacron) or polytetrafluoroethylene (PTFE, Teflon) and used during the initial era of aortofemoral reconstruction have generally performed well, a wide variety of aortic prosthetic grafts have become available to the vascular surgeon in more recent years. Numerous modifications in graft material (e.g., Dacron versus PTFE), methods of fabrication (e.g., knitted versus woven, external velour versus double velour, and porosity differences), and addition of various biologic coatings (e.g., collagen or albumin) to the graft have been devised.

Such alterations have been proposed in the hope of improving the performance and characteristics of the graft, usually:

- Patency
- Durability
- Healing and incorporation within host tissue
- Resistance to infection
- Reduced blood loss through the graft
- Handling qualities

Various claims concerning the benefits of one type over another have been made, although it is often difficult to discern science from salesmanship. Past studies performed to evaluate the differences frequently lacked adequate control to allow an accurate conclusion to be drawn. In one attempt to help clarify this situation, Robicsek and associates[86] used "half-and-half" grafts of woven and knitted Dacron. Implanting a bifurcated Dacron graft constructed with one limb woven and the other knitted allowed them to compare patency of the two limbs directly. Approximately half of their 158 patients underwent replacement procedures for aneurysm; nevertheless, at an average of 5½ years of follow-up, no significant difference was found in patency between the two limbs. In a related study, Robicsek and coworkers[87] also found no difference in platelet deposition between the two varieties of grafts and, hence, presumably no difference in the thrombogenicity.

Many surgeons continue to prefer knitted Dacron grafts

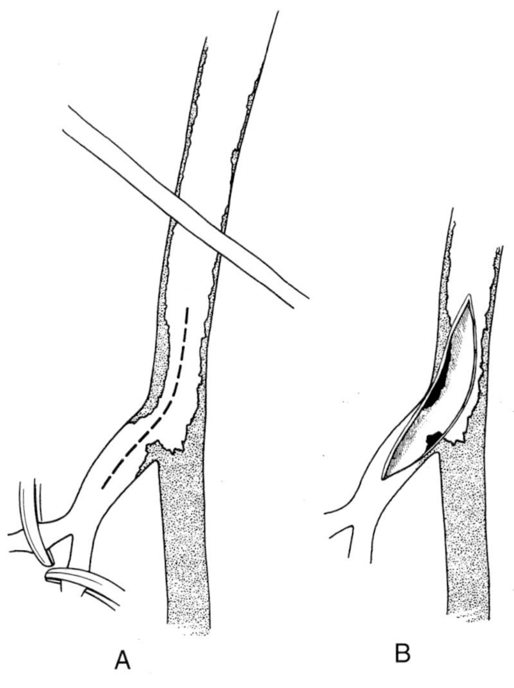

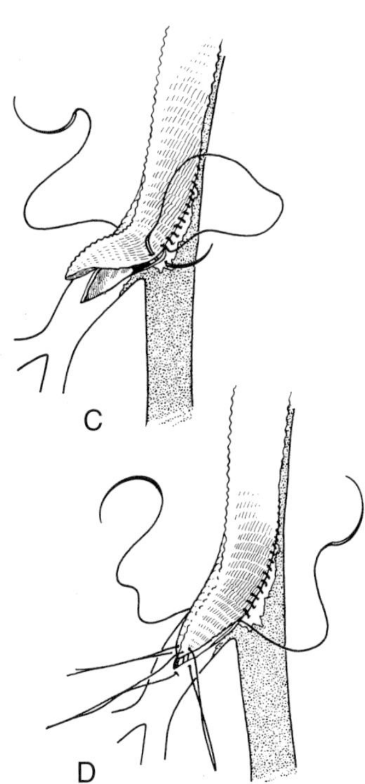

FIGURE 66–7. Femoral anastomosis in a patient with multilevel disease. *A*, With associated femoropopliteal occlusive disease, any disease at the orifice of the profunda femoris artery may limit graft limb runoff and subsequent patency. *B*, Extension of the common femoral arteriotomy into the proximal profunda femoris artery, distal to the orificial stenosis. *C*, The heel of the long, beveled graft hood is anastomosed to the common femoral artery. *D*, The femoral anastomosis is completed with the tip of the graft extended down the profunda femoris artery, thus achieving a patch profundaplasty. Three to five interrupted sutures are first placed at the tip and are not tied down, facilitating visualization and accurate placement without constriction.

for aortofemoral grafting, mainly because of their flexibility and ease of handling and suturing, which is particularly helpful in a difficult profunda femoris artery anastomosis. However, newer manufacturing techniques have begun to blur the former distinct differences in mechanical properties and characteristics between knitted and woven Dacron grafts and to make such considerations less important in current practice. Whether an internal or an external velour surface or a combination of the two is beneficial remains unproven.

Although porosity and incorporation by the host tissue remain desirable theoretical features, the successful use of PTFE grafts in other locations has made these considerations questionable. A study of the use of PTFE grafts in the hypoplastic aorta syndrome by Burke and colleagues[88] suggested better patency results than with Dacron grafts, but the difference was not statistically significant. Similarly, the results of a comparison of PTFE bifurcated grafts and Dacron prostheses by Cintora and associates[89] favored PTFE grafts; although cumulative patency rates at 4 years were not significantly different (97% and 90%, respectively), blood loss was less and late graft-related complications were less frequent with PTFE grafts.

Currently, "zero porosity" biologically coated grafts dominate the market for prosthetic grafts because of their expediency and probably smaller associated blood loss (see Chapter 37). Clearly, both PTFE and biologically coated prosthetics do limit blood loss and facilitate the procedure by obviating preclotting of the graft, but all such grafts are generally more expensive than conventional fabric prostheses, and any improvement in performance is unproven. Their higher cost is often justified by reductions in operative time, need for transfusions, and, perhaps, morbidity because of these factors. One may generally conclude that no single large-caliber graft is clearly superior and that long-term patency is more closely related to proper surgical methods of graft implantation and limitation of disease progression than to the specific graft employed.

Irrespective of the exact type of graft material and fabrication, the use of the proper size graft is important.[90, 91] Previously, many surgeons employed grafts that were too large in comparison with the size of outflow tract vessels, which tended to promote sluggish flow in graft limbs and deposition of excessive laminar pseudointima in the prosthesis. This development often gives rise to a propensity for later fragmentation or dislodgment, leading to occlusion of one or both limbs of the graft. For occlusive disease, a 16 × 8 mm bifurcated graft is most often employed; a 14 × 7 mm or even smaller prosthesis is also used when appropriate, frequently in some female patients. The limb size of such grafts most closely approximates the femoral arteries of patients with occlusive disease or, more particularly, the size of the profunda femoris artery, which often remains as the only outflow tract. In addition, it is now well recognized that many Dacron prosthetic grafts have a tendency to dilate 10% to 20% when subjected to arterial pressure.[92] Selection of a smaller graft helps compensate for this tendency.

Intraoperative Evaluation of Revascularization

At the conclusion of the operative procedure, the surgeon must ensure the technical and hemodynamic integrity of the vascular reconstruction. This is traditionally done by visual inspection of the anastomoses and by palpation of satisfactory pulses at and just beyond the point of graft anastomosis.

If feasible, some means of ensuring adequate distal flow intraoperatively is also advisable. Actual palpation of distal leg and pedal pulses is often cumbersome without contamination of the operative field. In addition, pulses are often difficult to appreciate immediately after reconstruction in the cold and vasoconstricted limb. Some surgeons prefer to prepare and drape the feet in transparent bags so as to allow visualization of their color and appearance, but this method is often rather subjective and uncertain.

It is the practice of the author and his colleagues to obtain pulse volume recordings after restoration of flow to evaluate the hemodynamic adequacy of aortoiliac reconstruction more objectively.[93] Plethysmographic cuffs are placed at the calf or ankle level and are draped out of the operative field. Following graft insertion and release of clamps, postoperative pulse volume recordings are easily obtained by the circulating nurse and can be compared with preoperative tracings to assess the hemodynamic result of proximal revascularization. If more distal sterile draping is necessary, sterile intraoperative cuffs may be used for postreconstructive determinations. Unless extensive uncorrected distal disease is present, such pulse volume recordings should show better amplitude than that in the preoperative tracings.

If extensive distal disease does complicate pulse volume recording monitoring, a sterile cuff may be applied to the distal thigh to ensure adequate revascularization of the profunda femoris artery. Alternatively, some surgeons use postreconstructive determinations of distal ankle Doppler pressures, electromagnetic flow measurements through the open graft limb, or intraoperative duplex scanning with a sterile intraoperative probe. Regardless of the method chosen, the importance of ensuring a satisfactory technical result before the patient leaves the operating room cannot be overemphasized.

SPECIAL CONSIDERATIONS

Retroperitoneal Approach

Although a retroperitoneal approach to the infrarenal abdominal aorta was used by Rob[94] and others during the early era of aortic reconstruction for occlusive or aneurysmal disease, the traditional surgical approach for direct repair of infrarenal aortoiliac occlusive disease has been the transperitoneal route. Several reports have recommended a retroperitoneal approach as an alternative in patients with multiple prior intra-abdominal operations or in patients felt to be at high risk for complications secondary to cardiac or severe pulmonary disease if the standard transperitoneal approach were employed. In this latter group, possible advantages of the retroperitoneal approach are (1) less disturbance of pulmonary function, (2) decreased postoperative ileus, and (3) reduced third-space fluid losses. In other instances of occlusive disease extending close to the renal arteries or in patients with associated occlusive lesions of the visceral or renal arteries, a retroperitoneal approach may permit easier access, control, and repair.[95–97]

The retroperitoneal approach is performed as follows:

1. The patient is placed in a modified left thoracotomy position with the left shoulder and chest elevated to approximately a 45- to 60-degree angle, and the hips and pelvis are rotated posteriorly as far as possible to provide access to the femoral arteries.
2. The mid-point between the left costal margin and the iliac crest is centered over the break in the table, and the table is flexed to widen the left flank. During the operative procedure, the operating table can be rotated either toward or away from the surgeon, who stands on the patient's left side.
3. An oblique flank incision is made beginning at the left lateral border of the rectus muscle several inches below the umbilicus and extended superiorly to the tip of the eleventh rib.
4. Dissection is carried in a retroperitoneal plane, either (a) with dissection anterior to the kidney if standard infrarenal exposure is adequate or (b) with anterior mobilization of the left kidney if access to the supraceliac aorta is necessary.
5. Further medial mobilization of the peritoneal envelope exposes the inferior mesenteric artery, which is divided and ligated close to the aorta, usually facilitating further exposure.

With such an approach, access to the right renal artery is often impossible, and control and repair of the right iliac artery are occasionally difficult. Similarly, tunneling to the right groin and right femoral artery anastomosis may sometimes be difficult, particularly in an obese patient. However, the approach may clearly be helpful in patients with multiple prior intra-abdominal operations, prior aortic surgery, pararenal disease, or similar technical considerations.

Whether or not the retroperitoneal approach is advantageous for standard infrarenal aortic reconstruction in comparison with the conventional transperitoneal approach remains uncertain. A prospective randomized study by Sicard and associates[98] was believed to demonstrate physiologic and cost benefits of a retroperitoneal approach, but the results of a similar original prospective randomized comparison by Cambria and coworkers[99] found no significant differences.

Adjunctive Lumbar Sympathectomy

The use of a concomitant lumbar sympathectomy at the time of aortic reconstruction remains unsettled and controversial (see Chapter 73). Although it is well accepted that sympathectomy increases skin and total limb blood flow, there are few objective data to document more favorable long-term graft patency rates or improved limb salvage results.[100, 101] Available evidence does suggest, however, that decreased pedal vasomotor tone and skin perfusion may be helpful as an adjunct to direct arterial revascularization, particularly in patients with multilevel disease and relatively minor superficial areas of pedal or digital ischemic lesions.[100, 102, 103] Therefore, limited (L2–L3) sympathectomy in conjunction with direct aortic operation may be considered in such cases, particularly when it has been decided to limit operation to inflow reconstruction alone or when distal runoff is considered to be poor. The procedure is easily and quickly accomplished, but it must be acknowledged that the benefit remains unproven.

The Totally Occluded Aorta

Approximately 8% of the author's patients undergoing operation for aortoiliac occlusive disease have chronic totally occluded aorta.[104] In about 50% of these patients, the occlusion has extended retrograde to the level of the renal arteries (Fig. 66–8); in the rest, the occlusion has involved only the distal infrarenal aorta, with the proximal segment remaining open via runoff through a still patent IMA or lumbar vessels.

Surgical management in the latter group is straightforward and is similar to standard aortic graft insertion. With extension of the occluding thrombus to a juxtarenal level, however, the operative approach is more taxing and possible complications are more likely, particularly those complications involving disturbance of renal function.[104–106] Nevertheless, surgery may be advisable in such cases, even if ischemic complaints are relatively mild and stable, because of the potential for more proximal propagation of thrombus with compromise or occlusion of neighboring renal or visceral arteries. The actual threat of proximal propagation of untreated total aortic thrombosis remains controversial, however. Although some series have suggested that the danger is significant,[107, 108] other retrospective reviews have determined that subsequent compromise of renal or mesenteric circulation by further retrograde extension of clot is quite rare unless severe stenosis in renal or visceral arteries is also present.[109, 110]

In almost all patients with juxtarenal occlusion, the bulk of the actual occlusive disease lies in the distal aorta,

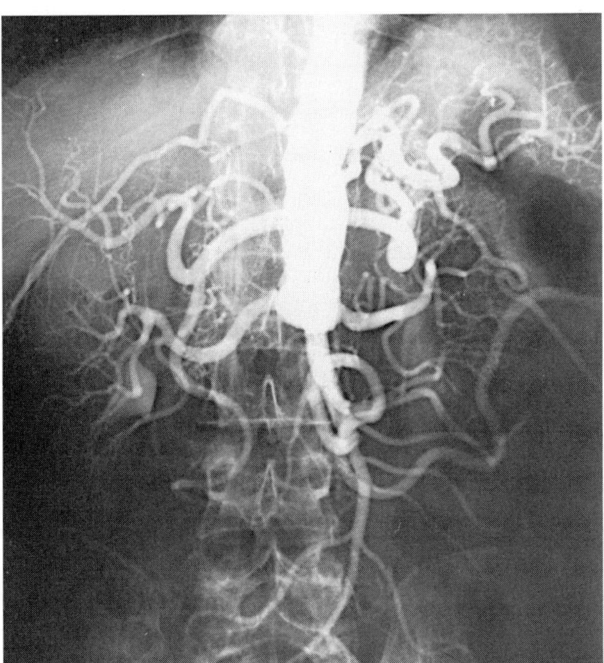

FIGURE 66–8. Transaxillary aortogram demonstrating total juxtarenal aortic occlusion.

with the proximal occlusive material composed largely of secondary thrombus. This proximal plug may almost always be removed with simple thrombectomy followed by routine graft insertion as follows:

1. Adequate dissection is carried out to allow temporary control of the renal arteries by application of gentle bulldog clamps to minimize chances of renal embolization at the time of juxtarenal thrombectomy.
2. Division of the left renal vein may facilitate exposure and is a benign procedure if performed correctly near the insertion of this vein into the vena cava, thereby preserving collateral venous drainage. This division is generally unnecessary, however; the mobilized left renal vein can usually be retracted cephalad or caudad as required for exposure and control of the juxtarenal aorta.[111]
3. The completely occluded aorta is opened through an arteriotomy placed several centimeters below the renal arteries.
4. The infrarenal aorta should *not* be clamped at this juncture, to avoid compression of the apex of the thrombotic material and its possible dislodgment into the renal or mesenteric circulation. Indeed, infrarenal clamping is unnecessary at this stage because the thrombotic plug prevents any bleeding.
5. Thrombectomy of the aortic cuff to the level of the renal arteries is carried out with a blunt clamp. This procedure is usually terminated by the "blowing out" by aortic pressure of a typical organized cap of thrombus representing the apex of the thrombotic occlusion.
6. The suprarenal aorta can now be controlled by manual pressure, or a suprarenal clamp can be temporarily applied.
7. The aorta is flushed, the bulldog clamps are removed from the renal artery, and an appropriate vascular clamp is applied to the now patent infrarenal cuff.
8. The graft is inserted in routine fashion.

Formal endarterectomy is best avoided in most circumstances because this plane may be difficult to terminate without compromise of the renal artery origins. Simple thrombectomy at this level is preferred and is sufficient in almost all cases.

The Calcified Aorta

Occasionally, dense calcification of the infrarenal aorta appears to preclude successful insertion of an aortic graft and leads the surgeon to consider abandoning the procedure. This situation occurs particularly during end-to-side anastomosis with the use of tangential, partially occluding clamps.

Reconstruction can always be accomplished with several possible alterations. First, a high end-to-end proximal anastomosis is preferred. By carrying dissection to or just above the left renal vein after its division or cephalad retraction, the surgeon often finds that the aorta immediately below the renal arteries is less involved and more manageable. Second, endarterectomy of a 1- to 2-cm cuff of totally transected aorta to the level of the infrarenal aortic clamp is usually possible and removes the calcification that always lies in the diseased intima and media. This maneuver greatly facilitates subsequent end-to-end graft anastomosis.

Although the cuff of the endarterectomized aorta, which consists of aortic adventitia and external elastic lamina, always appears fragile, it invariably proves to be adequate for graft anastomosis without later difficulties, such as bleeding, suture line disruption, and pseudoaneurysm formation. The surgeon must employ a tapered (not cutting-tip) needle, and the use of an interrupted mattress suture technique, with each suture backed with a pledget of Teflon felt (Fig. 66–9), is to be particularly recommended.

Clamping of such calcified vessels may also be problematic. It can usually be accomplished just below the renal arteries, where calcification is often less severe. Clamping in an anterior-to-posterior fashion, with the use of an arterial clamp applied from a lateral direction, may also be helpful. In truly difficult situations, the aorta may be clamped above the renal arteries at the level of the diaphragm, or intraluminal methods of vascular control employing balloon catheters may be used.

The Small Aorta

In about 5% to 10% of patients, the infrarenal aorta and the iliac and femoral vessels are small, a feature that makes aortic reconstruction technically difficult. Actual anatomic definition of the small aorta is obviously arbitrary. Cronenwett and associates[5] have defined the syndrome as characterized by an infrarenal aorta measuring (1) less than 13.2 mm just below the renal vessels or (2) less than 10.3 mm

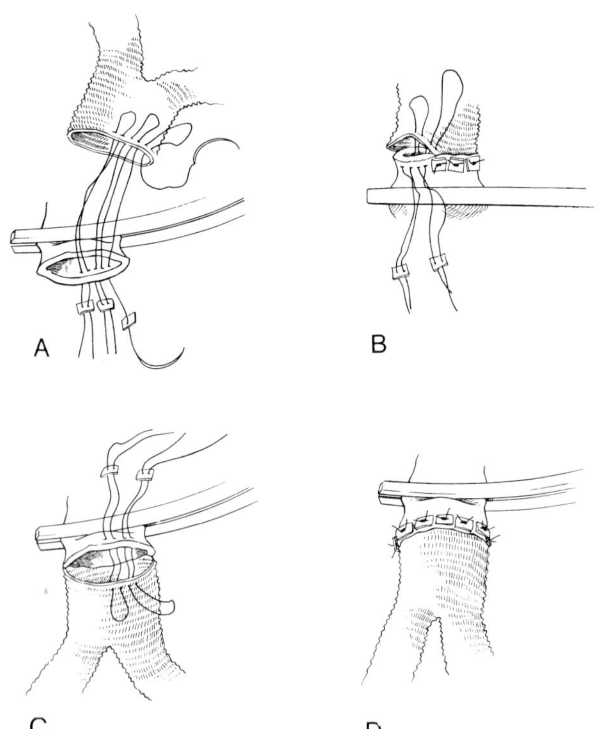

FIGURE 66–9. Interrupted mattress suture technique of aortic anastomosis. *A*, A posterior row of five mattress sutures is placed, with a double-armed suture passed through the posterior graft wall and then through the host aorta. *B*, A posterior row of sutures is tied down over pledgets of polytetrafluoroethylene (Teflon) felt. *C*, The graft is turned inferiorly toward the patient's feet, and a similar anterior row of five mattress sutures is placed with pledgets. *D*, Completed interrupted suture line; this technique is extremely helpful for the small aorta or fragile, diseased vessel.

just above the aortic bifurcation. Iliac and femoral vessels are typically correspondingly small, with the common femoral vessels often measuring only about 5 mm.

These patients appear to form a unique and distinct subgroup and are frequently characterized as having the hypoplastic aorta syndrome.[6–8] Preferred surgical methods for reconstruction in patients with small vessels remain somewhat controversial; some surgeons hold that the small size of the aorta and iliac vessels makes endarterectomy unsuitable, whereas others favoring bypass techniques advocate the use of end-to-side proximal aortic anastomosis to avoid size discrepancies with the usual prosthetic grafts.

Because the occlusive disease in such patients is frequently localized, aortoiliac endarterectomy may be considered. Although the small size of the vessels demands greater care and occasionally requires the use of patch closures, endarterectomy has worked well in the hands of the author and his colleagues.

If occlusive disease is more diffuse, bypass grafting to the femoral vessels is preferred. End-to-side anastomosis, favored by many surgeons to overcome size differences between the graft and the host aorta,[88] is an acceptable technique as long as the infrarenal aorta is not too diseased. A smaller prosthesis should be chosen to avoid the consequences of using inappropriately large grafts. In most cases, a 14 × 7 mm or even a 12 × 6 mm bifurcation graft should be used. The limbs of such grafts, although small, are also much more appropriate for the smaller femoral and outflow vessels of the patient with a small aorta.

Greater technical care must be exercised, but with attention to technical detail, such grafts have not failed as a result of their small size; the author and his colleagues much prefer the insertion of such small grafts to the use of oversized prostheses. A study by Burke and colleagues[88] suggested better patency rates when PTFE aortic bifurcation grafts were used for reconstruction in patients with a small abdominal aorta than when Dacron grafts were used, but statistical significance was not achieved. Adjunctive lumbar sympathectomy may be helpful.

Simultaneous Distal Grafting

A common practical concern in patients with multilevel occlusive disease is whether or not an inflow operation alone will suffice. As already emphasized, such diffuse combined-segment disease (type III) is the most common pattern of occlusive disease, present in between one half and two thirds of the patients coming to surgery.[2, 55–58] Prior reports of patients with multilevel disease, who were treated in a generally accepted fashion with initial aortic reconstruction, have indicated that proximal operation alone may fail to achieve satisfactory relief of ischemic symptoms in up to one third.[10, 14, 56, 70, 74, 112–116] Although symptoms of claudication are lessened in more than 80% of patients with multilevel disease who undergo aortofemoral grafting, only 35% of patients in the author's series experienced total relief of claudication.[14] Many patients with unsatisfactory outcomes must undergo concurrent or subsequent distal bypass grafting. However, identification of patients in whom relief of ischemic symptoms would be insufficient with an inflow procedure alone remains difficult.

In this regard, the author and his colleagues reviewed a 6-year experience comprising 181 patients with multilevel disease who underwent aortofemoral grafting.[14] A well-performed inflow procedure usually suffices if there is unequivocally severe proximal disease in the aortoiliac segment. Such clear-cut proximal disease is best identified from the findings of absence of or clear reduction in the femoral pulse and obvious severe aortic or iliac disease on angiography and is confirmed, if necessary, by the findings of an FAP study.

Several intraoperative criteria may also be used. Restoration of an improved pulse volume recording at the calf or ankle, in comparison with preoperative tracings, can give reassurance of satisfactory improvement in distal circulation. However, improvement in pulse volume recordings or Doppler ankle pressures may not be immediately apparent in the presence of significant distal disease, especially in the cold, vasoconstricted limb. Another useful intraoperative guide in predicting a good clinical response is assessment of the anatomic size of the profunda femoris artery itself. If the proximal profunda femoris artery accepts a 4-mm probe and if a No. 3 Fogarty embolectomy catheter can be passed through it for a distance of 20 cm or more, the profunda femoris artery probably is well developed and will function satisfactorily as an outflow tract and source of collateral circulation.[4, 14, 117]

Possible benefits of simultaneous grafting are (1) a more nearly total correction of extremity ischemia and (2) avoidance of the difficulties and potential complications associated with reoperation in the groin if later distal grafting proves to be necessary. Such advantages are usually outweighed by the greater magnitude of the synchronous two-level grafting and the fact that most properly selected patients are adequately benefited by proximal operation alone (76% in the author's series). Distal bypass may be carried out in the future, if necessary; it was required in 17% of the patients in the author's series who were observed for up to 6 years.[14] Such a figure is in agreement with previously reported experience.[55, 70, 81, 116]

In carefully selected patients with multilevel disease and truly advanced limb-threatening ischemic problems in the foot, synchronous proximal and distal reconstructions seem appropriate.[118] This is particularly pertinent if only modest proximal occlusive disease is present because an inflow procedure is then unlikely to improve blood flow to the foot markedly (Fig. 66–10). The author and his colleagues believe that if the surgeon can reliably predict that a distal graft will almost certainly be necessary in the future for limb salvage, simultaneous grafting is to be preferred because it offers a better chance of limb salvage and avoids a more demanding reoperation in the groin at a later time. Certainly, the use of two surgical teams can minimize the additional operative time required, and it is likely that synchronous grafting will become somewhat more common in the future.[119–124] Although some surgeons have claimed success with preoperative noninvasive hemodynamic studies in selecting such patients,[14, 118, 122, 125] other investigators have found tests of this type to be unreliable indicators of the need for concomitant distal bypass.[74, 81, 113] Good clinical judgment remains most important, with reasoned and pragmatic decisions usually required.

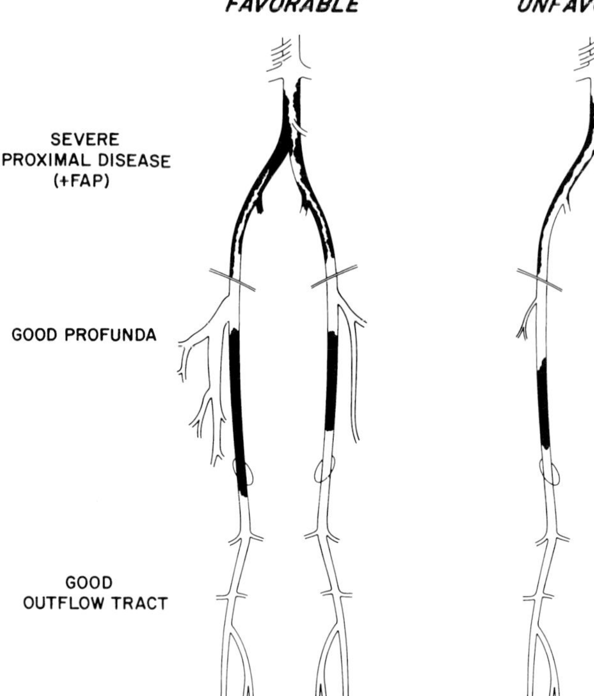
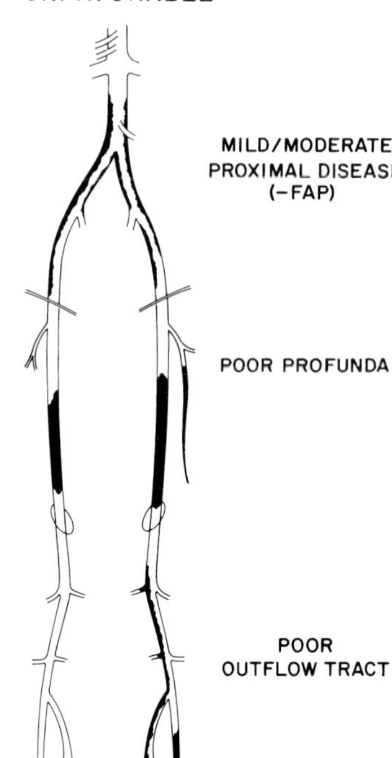

FIGURE 66–10. Clinical circumstances and disease patterns associated with favorable or unsatisfactory outcome of aortofemoral grafts alone in patients with multilevel disease. FAP = femoral artery pressure.

Unilateral Iliac Disease

Not infrequently, proximal occlusive disease may appear unilaterally, with fairly normal pulses and no symptoms in the contralateral extremity. Truly unilateral iliac disease is relatively uncommon because aortoiliac disease is generally a more diffuse and eventually bilateral process. Progression of disease in the aorta or in the untreated contralateral iliac artery may necessitate later reoperation in a significant percentage of patients treated initially with unilateral operations for apparent one-sided disease[82, 126]; estimates of the exact frequency of this occurrence vary considerably, however, and several reports have suggested that it is relatively infrequent.[127–129]

Optimal management of unilateral iliac disease remains controversial, with proponents of both standard aortobifemoral bypass and less extensive extra-anatomic grafts or even endoluminal therapy claiming their approach to be advantageous and preferred.[40, 50] In the patient with a well-preserved aorta and contralateral iliac artery, the use of femorofemoral grafts has become increasingly important, owing to the ease of the procedure and the generally good long-term results.[130–134]

In certain instances, however, the surgeon may wish to avoid the contralateral side and to confine reconstructive efforts to the symptomatic side (e.g., if the contralateral limb is asymptomatic but inflow in the proposed donor limb is of questionable reliability, and the patient is not a good candidate for standard aortobifemoral grafting). In other instances, use of the contralateral groin may be relatively contraindicated because of heavy scarring from prior operative procedures, possible infection, and so forth. In these situations, direct iliofemoral grafting may occasionally be used for disease that is largely unilateral at the time.[135–138] This procedure is used mainly for occlusive disease confined to the external iliac artery, because the ipsilateral common iliac artery must be relatively normal for the proximal graft anastomosis. A retroperitoneal approach through a separate lower quadrant incision (Fig. 66–11) usually provides good exposure and can be carried out with low patient morbidity.

Whether femorofemoral bypass or iliofemoral grafting gives better results is currently debated, although several studies have demonstrated better long-term patency of direct ipsilateral iliofemoral bypass grafts.[139, 140] Nonetheless, femorofemoral grafting is a somewhat simpler procedure, has very low morbidity, and obviates any possibility of interfering with sexual function in men.[141]

In similar situations, retroperitoneal iliac endarterectomy may be employed for relatively localized unilateral inflow lesions via a similar retroperitoneal approach,[128, 142, 143] although with the established success of iliac PTA and possible stenting, this approach has largely been replaced. All methods of unilateral inflow revascularization may be readily combined with concomitant profundaplasty or simultaneous ipsilateral distal bypass and are therefore particularly helpful in patients with mainly unilateral multilevel disease who may require extensive revascularization but in whom the surgeon wishes to limit the extent of the surgical procedure.[45, 118, 127, 142] Similarly, if proximal iliac disease is relatively localized and suitable for PTA, reestablishment of inflow by transluminal angioplasty may be combined with distal surgical procedures, yielding good long term results.[45, 46]

Associated Renal Artery or Visceral Artery Occlusive Lesions

Because of the diffuse nature of atherosclerotic occlusive disease in most patients, it is not surprising that individuals requiring aortic reconstruction for symptomatic lower extremity ischemia may be found to have associated occlusive lesions involving the renal or visceral arteries. Often these lesions are unsuspected and are detected only at the time of preoperative angiography. The dilemma of whether or not to attempt simultaneous correction of both abdominal aortic and visceral lesions is frequently encountered and difficult to resolve.[144, 145]

In these instances, each case must be considered individually and no general recommendations are feasible or appropriate. It is clear that extending aortic reconstruction to include visceral artery revascularization, although theoretically appealing, increases the complexity and magnitude of the operation and hence is associated almost invariably with some increase in morbidity and mortality.[144, 146, 147] For these reasons, truly prophylactic revascularizations should generally be avoided. Serial angiographic studies have demonstrated, however, that renal occlusive disease is progressive in more than 50% of patients and that approximately 10% of high-grade lesions (80% or greater stenosis) proceed to total occlusion, with resultant loss of function in that kidney.[144] Hence, if clinical evaluation suggests that the associated renal lesions are functionally important or preocclusive in severity, simultaneous correction is often appropriate.[144–150]

In the asymptomatic patient with visceral artery disease, careful evaluation of the anatomic pattern of disease on the preoperative arteriogram should indicate whether the patient would be at risk for postoperative intestinal ischemia if the visceral lesions were not treated. As emphasized by Ernst[21] and Connolly and Kwaan,[151] avoidance of this catastrophic postoperative problem requires preservation of an important inferior mesenteric artery in those patients with celiac and superior mesenteric artery occlusive disease or, perhaps, concomitant bypass grafting to the celiac or superior mesenteric artery itself.[21, 151]

It is clear that if associated renal artery disease is present, combined reconstruction may improve associated hypertension or renal function in carefully selected patients.[146–150] Diminished renal function is rarely due to unilateral disease, and significant bilateral disease (either intrarenal or extrarenal) almost always must be present before overall renal function is adversely affected. Adding a unilateral renal bypass without first proving the functional significance of the renal lesion may unnecessarily risk further compromise of excretory function in a patient who may be azotemic predominantly from bilateral arteriolar nephrosclerosis. Therefore, it seems appropriate to assess the functional significance of such a unilateral renal artery lesion preoperatively and to proceed with correction only if study results are positive. If angiographically severe bilateral lesions are present and the patient has significant hypertension or diminished renal function, the addition of renal revascularization of at least one side to the planned aortic reconstruction may well be the best course.

Because the morbidity and mortality of simultaneous aortic operation and bilateral renal artery revascularization are increased,[146, 147] the surgeon may elect to stage the renal artery and aortic procedures, performing an isolated renal artery procedure either before or after the aortic procedure, which is combined with repair of only one renal artery. In

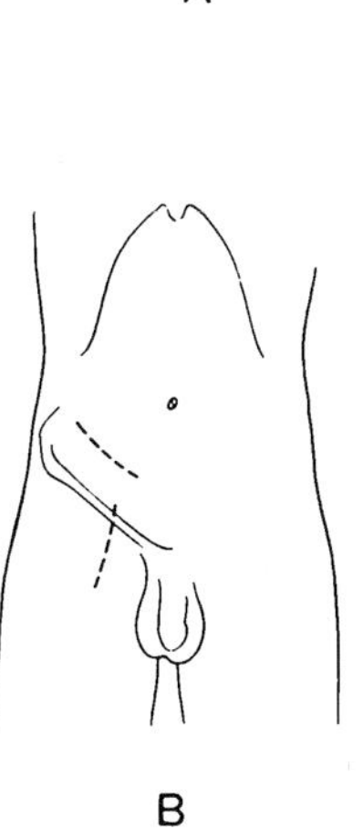

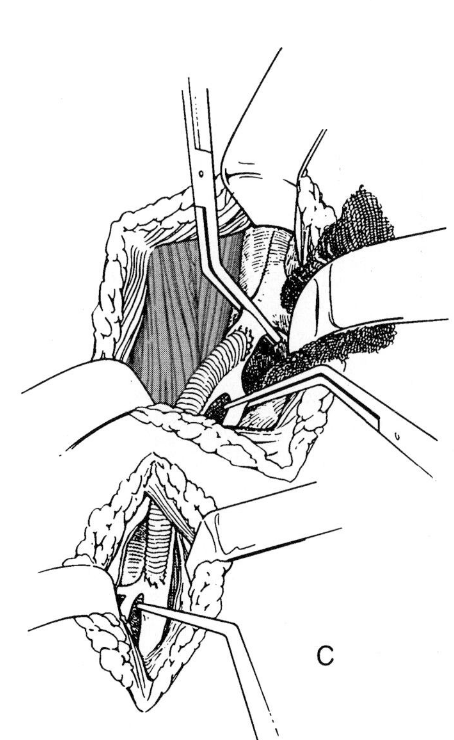

FIGURE 66–11. Unilateral iliofemoral bypass graft. *A*, In this usual situation, such a reconstruction may be considered; occlusive disease is confined largely to one external iliac artery. *B*, Positioning of skin incisions for retroperitoneal exposure of the iliac vessels and standard approach to the femoral arteries. *C*, Iliofemoral graft is inserted.

such situations, the use of extra-anatomic means of renal artery revascularization, such as through the splenic or hepatic arteries, may be particularly helpful in avoiding the necessity of operation in a previously dissected field.[152–154]

Thoracic Aorta to Femoral Artery Bypass

In certain good-risk patients in whom standard abdominal aortic reconstruction is contraindicated or judged to be technically challenging because of hostile abdominal pathology, bypass procedures may be based upon the thoracic aorta. Such procedures may combine the advantages of extra-anatomic grafts, in that they (1) enable the surgeon to avoid operating in a hostile abdomen or potentially unsuitable abdominal aorta but (2) perhaps may be more durable than axillobifemoral bypass. Although used relatively infrequently, grafts based on the thoracic aorta may have appeal for selected clinical circumstances, including:

- Avoidance of the abdominal aorta that has already undergone multiple procedures
- Potential sepsis
- Radiation therapy
- Presence of abdominal stoma
- Technically difficult cases in which the aorta is totally occluded to a juxtarenal level

Most such bypasses originate from the lower descending thoracic aorta and are tunneled through the diaphragm and retroperitoneum to the iliofemoral vessels.[155, 156] Use of the ascending aorta[157] or supraceliac aorta[158] as an alternative inflow site for such grafts has also been described. Usually, a partially occluding clamp can be used for construction of the proximal anastomosis, thereby preserving renal blood flow and minimizing the risks of postoperative renal failure. A bifurcated aortic prosthetic graft may be used, or a unilateral graft may be brought to the left iliac or femoral artery and combined with a standard subcutaneous femorofemoral crossover bypass to the right groin. Good long-term patency rates have generally been reported for all of these reconstructions, which should be kept in mind for possible use in the selected clinical circumstances mentioned.

RESULTS OF DIRECT AORTOILIOFEMORAL RECONSTRUCTION

Currently, generally excellent early and late results of direct aortoiliofemoral reconstructions can be anticipated and are achievable at highly acceptable patient morbidity and mortality rates. A consensus of several large series in the modern era clearly supports this statement, indicating that it is reasonable to expect an 85% to 90% graft patency rate at 5 years and 70% to 75% at 10 years.[2, 55–60, 112] Perioperative mortality rates well under 3% are now commonplace in many centers. The mortality risk for direct reconstructions in patients with relatively localized aortoiliac disease can be expected to be extremely low, whereas those patients with multilevel disease and associated occlusive lesions in coronary, carotid, and visceral vessels quite naturally have a somewhat higher mortality risk. For this latter group of patients, it is hoped that continued improvement of screening methods for associated disease and continued refinements of anesthetic management, intraoperative monitoring, and postoperative intensive care can further reduce the risk of serious morbidity and mortality.

Long-term survival of these patients continues to be compromised, however. The cumulative long-term survival rate for patients undergoing aortoiliac reconstruction remains some 10 to 15 years less than what might be anticipated for a normal age- and sex-matched population. Overall, about 25% to 30% of patients are dead at 5 years, and 50% to 60% at 10 years.[11, 55, 57] Not unexpectedly, most late deaths are attributable to atherosclerotic heart disease. Patients with more localized aortoiliac disease, who have a lower incidence of coronary artery disease, distal occlusive disease, or diabetes, appear to have a much more favorable long-term prognosis, approaching that of a normal population at risk.[11, 112]

COMPLICATIONS AND THEIR PREVENTION

Early Complications

Hemorrhage

With current surgical methods and reliable prosthetic grafts and suture materials, early postoperative hemorrhage is a relatively unusual complication (1% to 2%), most often the consequence of some technical oversight or abnormality of the coagulation mechanism.[159] Gentle surgical technique and proper methods of graft insertion are obviously crucial in avoiding such difficulties. Preoperative routine screening for coagulation abnormalities is essential.

Most currently applied reconstructive techniques emphasize minimal dissection, sufficient only to achieve adequate exposure for securing proper vascular control and graft insertion. Appropriate efforts at hemostasis during dissection are generally easier than localization and securing of bleeding points at the conclusion of the procedure. Normal blood pressure should be restored at the completion of the vascular reconstruction so that an insecure anastomotic suture line or an improperly controlled bleeder is not overlooked.

Leaks from vascular anastomoses, particularly those that are due to tearing of sutures in a fragile arterial wall, may acquire additional sutures, frequently with Teflon pledgets (see Fig. 66–9). Arterial inflow should be clamped briefly while such additional repair sutures are being placed and tied in order to avoid further tears. In many instances, operative bleeding may be due to injury of associated venous structures. Familiarity with the major venous anomalies is important to avoid such injuries.[160] If venous injury is present, bleeding is best controlled by gentle finger tamponade and fine vascular sutures rather than by application of clamps, which may only enlarge the defect in the vein.

Adequate reversal of heparinization after graft insertion is achieved by administration of protamine sulfate; however, considerable variations in individual responses to heparin exist. Monitoring of the activated clotting time before and after heparin administration may be helpful in determination of the proper dose of intraoperative heparin and judgment about the adequacy of its reversal before wound closure.

By far, the most common acquired coagulation deficiency leading to bleeding problems during aortic operations is dilutional coagulopathy. If intraoperative blood loss is excessive and large amounts of avascular fluids and bank blood have been used during surgery, administration of fresh frozen plasma and platelet concentrates is helpful and important and is often guided by serial testing of coagulation parameters.

Finally, prompt recognition of a patient's ongoing volume requirements in the intensive care unit, with early appropriate reoperation as necessary, is essential.

Limb Ischemia

Acute limb ischemia occurring shortly after aortic operation for occlusive disease may be caused either by acute thrombosis of the reconstruction or by more distal thromboembolic complications.[159] Such difficulties are generally recognized from (1) the failure of expected pulses to return after operation, (2) the acute loss of previously present pulses, or (3) ischemic deterioration of the involved extremity. Often this determination may be difficult in patients undergoing operation for multilevel disease, in whom reestablishment of peripheral pulses is not anticipated. In such patients, the use of Doppler signals, limb pressures, and distal pulse volume recordings may be quite helpful. In many patients, the perfusion of distal extremities should continue to improve during the early postoperative period, and a 4- to 6-hour interval of close observation is often justified as long as the femoral pulse remains palpable. Careful clinical judgment, however, is required.

If the diagnosis of acute limb ischemia is established, the patient should be returned promptly to the operating room. If aortoiliac endarterectomy has been performed, the usual causative factors are inadequacies in termination of the endarterectomy at the iliac bifurcation, leading to intimal flaps or constrictive closure of the arteriotomy at this point. In many cases, the basic underlying problem is inappropriate application of the endarterectomy procedure itself in patients with disease extending down the iliac vessels. Generally in such cases, the abdominal incision must be reopened for direct inspection of the endarterectomized segments.

If an aortoiliac bypass graft has been inserted, the surgeon may elect to first explore the groin and pass balloon embolectomy catheters, but often, direct re-exploration is most appropriate. More commonly, an aortofemoral graft will have been extended below the inguinal ligament, and the distal anastomosis can be directly examined by reopening of the groin incision. Acute thrombosis of an aortofemoral graft limb in the early perioperative period occurs in 1% to 3% of patients.[161] Kinking or twisting of the graft limb in the retroperitoneal tunnel may be responsible for acute graft occlusion; most often, however, technical anastomotic problems at the distal femoral artery are responsible. Thrombectomy of the graft limb is easily carried out through a transverse opening in the distal graft hood, which also allows inspection of the interior of the anastomosis and distal passage of embolectomy catheters into the superficial and systems. In the common clinical situation of associated superficial femoral artery occlusion, unobstructed runoff into the profunda femoris artery must be ensured. If the patient has a small or diseased profunda femoris artery and inadequate runoff is believed to be the reason for acute graft limb thrombosis, a distal bypass graft may be required to ensure adequate distal runoff.[161]

Thromboembolic mechanisms of acute limb ischemia may be more common than previously believed.[162, 163] Clot or atheromatous debris may be dislodged from proximal vessels by injudicious application of clamps, or clot that has formed in the graft limb at the time of implantation may be inadequately flushed before flow is restored to the extremity. The surgeon can best prevent thromboembolic occlusion by (1) minimizing manipulation of the aorta, (2) using full systemic heparinization during the procedure, (3) carefully placing gentle vascular clamps on nondiseased portions of the vascular tree, and (4) carefully flushing the reconstruction before restoring flow.

Thromboembolic occlusions of the graft limb or larger outflow vessels may generally be successfully corrected by passage of embolectomy catheters. However, more distal thromboembolic complications may be much more difficult to deal with surgically and are far better prevented, if possible. A truly distal occlusion, involving tibial or digital arteries and colloquially referred to as "trash foot," is a well-recognized and frustrating problem. If pedal pulses are absent, it appears advisable to explore the distal popliteal artery, allowing passage of embolectomy catheters down each of the distal branches of the popliteal artery into the foot and thereby enhancing the possibility of retrieving thrombotic material and improving perfusion. Often, however, if the tibial vessels are patent and the occlusive debris is located in inaccessible foot and digital vessels, little can be done. Systemic heparinization or the use of intravenous low-molecular-weight dextran is often recommended but of no proven benefit. The use of distally injected thrombolytic agents, such as streptokinase or urokinase (see Chapters 28 and 45), also has been suggested but remains of uncertain benefit.[164, 165]

Renal Failure

In the absence of significant preoperative renal functional impairment, postoperative renal failure following elective aortic reconstruction for occlusive disease is currently an unusual event. In their review of the complications of abdominal aortic reconstruction in 557 patients at the Cleveland Clinic, 173 of whom underwent operation for aortoiliac occlusive disease, Diehl and associates[166] found that postoperative acute renal failure (ARF) developed in 4.6% of patients but was not fatal in any. In other reports, the incidence of ARF after elective aortic surgery (both for aneurysm and for occlusive disease) ranges from 1% to 8%, with an overall mortality rate of 40%. Emergency aortic surgery is associated with a higher incidence of ARF, with 50% to 90% mortality.[167]

The most common cause is diminished renal perfusion secondary to a decrease in cardiac output and hypovolemia, which may occur during certain phases of aortic surgery, particularly at the time of declamping. Renal cortical vasospasm secondary to aortic clamping may also contribute by reducing glomerular filtration. Depending on the anatomy of occlusive disease and the required repair, a period of suprarenal clamping may be necessary, or juxtarenal disease may result in intraoperative embolization of the renal circulation. The latter mechanism, producing thrombotic embolization or atheroembolization to the renal circulation, has been recognized as an increasingly important technical point of aortic reconstruction. Hence, in cases of known associated juxtarenal or pararenal atheromatous disease, aortic clamping is more safely accomplished at a supraceliac level, where concomitant occlusive disease is considerably less prevalent. The period of interrupted blood flow is almost certainly safer and better tolerated than causing embolization of atherothrombotic debris into the renal circulation or elevating atherosclerotic perirenal plaques, which may impede renal blood flow.

Other possible mechanisms of acute postoperative renal failure are contrast-induced renal dysfunction following preoperative diagnostic arteriography and the use of potentially nephrotoxic antibiotics or other drugs. Finally, myoglobinuria may result from reperfusion of severely ischemic limbs and the myoglobin may precipitate in renal tubules, resulting in postoperative ARF.[167]

The current low rate of renal failure after elective aortic surgery is attributable to appreciation of the importance of maintaining appropriate intravascular volume through (1) liberal use of intravenous fluids, (2) careful monitoring of pulmonary capillary wedge pressure during operation, and (3) avoidance of declamping hypotension.[167, 168] Administration of intravenous mannitol, furosemide, or both to induce a brisk diuresis before aortic clamping is also used prophylactically by many surgeons, although the benefit of these agents in the prevention of renal failure is uncertain. Similarly, perioperative infusion of low-dose dopamine is believed by some to aid renal blood flow and protect against postoperative dysfunction.

Milder forms of oliguric and nonoliguric renal dysfunction may be observed but rarely require dialysis support. Renal deterioration is much more common in patients with abnormal renal function before operation and in poorly prepared or dehydrated patients requiring emergency reconstruction for acute aortic thrombosis. Most serious and probably irreversible are instances of renal failure secondary to embolization of thrombotic or atheromatous debris into the renal circulation. As noted previously, this complication can be prevented by avoidance of excessive manipulation of the diseased aorta or by protection of the renal arteries with temporary clamping whenever extensive juxtarenal disease makes it advisable.

Intestinal Ischemia

Intestinal ischemia following aortic reconstruction may occur in approximately 2% of cases[21, 169, 170]; it almost always affects the colon, particularly the rectosigmoid region. The incidence of lesser degrees of ischemic colitis, involving only mucosal ischemia and resulting in less devastating consequences than transmural infarction or perforation, is undoubtedly more common, particularly if postoperative colonoscopy is used to identify patients with subclinical ischemic colitis. Small bowel ischemia following aortic operation is distinctly uncommon. Intestinal ischemia is more common after aneurysm repair than after reconstruction for occlusive disease, perhaps owing to a greater incidence of intraoperative hypotension and less well-developed collateral networks.

The etiology of intestinal ischemia is often multifactorial, but it almost always involves a critical loss of blood flow to the involved intestinal segment due to (1) interruption of primary or collateral arterial flow to the bowel wall or (2) operative atheroembolization. Other predisposing causes involve perioperative hypotension and hypoperfusion, manipulative trauma, and prior gastrointestinal tract surgery that has interrupted vital collateral pathways.

Recognition of anatomic situations more likely to result in intestinal ischemia following aortic operation is vital. Hence, the surgeon must examine the preoperative arteriogram for associated occlusive lesions affecting the celiac axis, the superior mesenteric arteries, or both, and for a patent and enlarged IMA, sacrifice of which probably would lead to colon ischemia. Identification of patients with such anatomic patterns of disease allows preservation of the IMA or concomitant revascularization of the superior mesenteric or celiac branches and, it is hoped, prevention of intestinal ischemia.

The status of the hypogastric arteries should be ascertained on the aortogram, and the arterial reconstruction should be designed to maintain flow through at least one of these arteries by direct revascularization or retrograde perfusion from a femoral anastomosis, if possible, especially if a patent IMA must be ligated. If IMA ligation is required, it should be carried out from within the aortic lumen or immediately adjacent to the aortic wall to avoid injury to the ascending and descending branches of the IMA, which then assume greater importance as collateral pathways. Some surgeons have suggested reimplantation of all patent IMAs during aortic reconstruction to minimize the risk of colon ischemia.[171] Although most surgeons do not believe that this procedure is routinely necessary, careful evaluation and assessment are vital whenever a patent IMA is interrupted because such interruption is the most common identifiable factor in the development of clinically significant postoperative colon ischemia, and reimplantation is advisable in selected circumstances.[169] Undue traction on the left colon mesentery must also be avoided.

Intraoperative recognition of intestinal ischemia may be difficult. Although various measures for detecting its presence intraoperatively have been reported, including use of a sterile Doppler probe, measurement of IMA stump pressure, determination of intracolonic pH or transcolonic oxygen saturation, and injection of intravenous fluorescein, none has been found both practical and entirely reliable.[21, 170–172] If colon ischemia is recognized, the surgeon must attempt to increase colonic perfusion through revascularization of the IMA by reimplantation or a short vein graft, superior mesenteric artery bypass, or hypogastric revascularization, depending on the individual circumstances and the anatomic distribution of disease.

Postoperatively, early diagnosis is the key to effective management of intestinal ischemia. Diagnosis often depends on a high level of clinical suspicion and may be facilitated by prompt sigmoidoscopy or colonoscopy. Clinical manifestations immediately after surgery are often masked by incisional discomfort and other problems common to the postoperative period. Findings that suggest the presence of intestinal ischemia include:

- Diarrhea, either liquid-brown or bloody
- Progressive abdominal distention
- Increasing signs of sepsis and peritonitis
- Unexplained metabolic acidosis

Initial supportive care, gastrointestinal tract decompression, and intravenous antibiotic therapy may be used, with careful observation and frequent reexamination, but any evidence of clinical deterioration indicates the need for prompt operative intervention. Resection of nonviable bowel, end-sigmoid colostomy, and formation of a Hartmann pouch are generally necessary. Avoidance of graft exposure during such maneuvers, if feasible, is obviously crucial. Mortality rates for transmural colon infarction remain significant, approximating 50% to 75% in many series.[159, 169]

Spinal Cord Ischemia

Spinal cord ischemia, resulting in paraplegia or paraparesis, is fortunately an unusual complication of aortoiliac surgery for occlusive disease. Szilagyi and associates[173] observed an incidence of 0.25% after 3164 operations involving temporary occlusion of the abdominal aorta, all of which were performed for aneurysmal disease. The incidence of spinal cord ischemia after intervention for ruptured aneurysms is 10 times higher than that after operations for unruptured aneurysmal lesions.[159, 173]

Although the etiology of paraplegia is multifactorial, the usual cause of spinal cord ischemia is interruption of flow through the great radicular artery of Adamkiewicz, the major source of supply to the anterior spinal artery at the lower end of the cord. This vessel normally originates from one of the paired suprarenal intercostal arteries from T8 to T12, but it occasionally has a lower origin. In the latter situation, surgical interruption or thrombosis that is due to prolonged aortic occlusion or intraoperative embolization is believed to cause distal spinal cord ischemia. Because this anatomic variability is unpredictable, the occurrence of spinal cord ischemia is generally considered unavoidable. Preoperative or intraoperative demonstration of the major blood supply to the lower spinal cord is difficult, impractical, and potentially dangerous. Several reports have also emphasized the importance of acute interruption of the pelvic circulation or atheroembolization through the pelvic arteries as another possible mechanism of ischemic neurologic injury.[79, 80, 174]

Currently, it is the consensus of almost all vascular surgeons that this tragic occurrence is essentially unpredictable and therefore not totally preventable in association with infrarenal aortic reconstruction. Monitoring of somatosensory evoked potentials during thoracic aortic surgery has been shown to detect cord ischemia. Practical application of this technique to abdominal aortic reconstruction, however, has not been established. Because of the potential importance of pelvic collateral circulation in a patient with chronic stenosis or occlusion of the artery of Adamkiewicz, preservation of pelvic blood flow through revascularization of at least one hypogastric network or other technical modifications of the operative procedure is advisable; this strategy is similar to the strategies for minimizing the occurrence of postoperative colon ischemia. When ischemic injury to the spinal cord does occur, treatment is confined to supportive care and rehabilitation.

Some investigators recommend the administration of high-dose intravenous steroids to decrease cord edema with the hope of improving perfusion, but the value of this treatment is unproven and controversial.[80] The severity of paraplegia is often directly related to postoperative mortality. In the experience at the Henry Ford Hospital reported by Elliott and coworkers,[175] 76% of patients in whom the initial neurologic deficit was complete died; there were only two complete neurologic recoveries in this group, and one partial recovery. In contrast, of the patients in whom the initial loss was only partial motor or sensory loss or both, 24% died and some degree of recovery was noted in all but one case.

Ureteral Injury

Because the ureter lies immediately adjacent to the operative field and crosses directly anterior to the iliac artery bifurcation, the surgeon must constantly keep in mind the possibility of lacerating, dividing, or ligating the ureter and must avoid injuring it during dissection, graft tunneling, and wound closure. This statement is particularly true of any reoperative surgery. A thorough knowledge of the anatomic relationship of the ureter at the level of the iliac bifurcation is essential. Direct injury to the ureter is best avoided by keeping dissection close to the arterial wall and elevating the ureter from the iliac vessels during retroperitoneal tunneling, particularly during reoperative aortic surgery. Identification of the ureters during closure of the retroperitoneum, particularly the right ureter, is essential to avoid including them in the retroperitoneal closure.

Various degrees of hydronephrosis resulting from ureteral obstruction may also be seen in the late follow-up period, and this complication is probably an underdiagnosed entity. It may occur in up to 10% to 20% of patients but is often asymptomatic and usually is not detected unless intravenous pyelography, ultrasonography, or CT scanning is carried out, often for other purposes.[176, 177] Such ureteral obstruction is most often mild and of no clinical consequence. It is occasionally attributable to placement of the graft limb anterior to the ureter, which entraps the ureter between the graft and the native artery, but is most commonly due to compression by fibrotic changes caused by tissue reaction to the implanted graft. Occasionally, however, hydronephrosis may be a marker of graft complications such as pseudoaneurysm formation or graft infection.[178, 179] Such potential problems need to be carefully considered in patients presenting with severe or symptomatic ureteral obstruction, and the position of the ureters should be assessed before direct reoperative aortic surgery is performed. Occasionally, preoperative placement of ureteral stents is helpful in this regard.

Late Complications

Despite the generally excellent long-term results of aortoiliofemoral reconstruction, late graft-related complications continue to occur throughout the follow-up period and detract from long-term effectiveness of the procedure. In the review of the late outcome of aortoiliac operation for occlusive disease by van der Akker and associates from Leiden,[180] secondary operations for late complications such as reocclusion, pseudoaneurysms, and infection were necessary in 21% of 727 patients observed over a 22-year period and contributed significantly (12.1%) to the causes of late deaths.

Graft Occlusion

The most frequent late complication of aortic operation for occlusive disease is graft thrombosis.[159] Although the exact incidence of late graft occlusions varies from report to report, occlusion may be anticipated in 5% to 10% of patients within the first 5 years after operation and in 15% to 30% of patients observed for 10 years or more postoperatively.[181–183] In the experience of the author and his colleagues, the average interval from original graft insertion to occlusion was 33.8 months.[181]

Most commonly, occlusion affects one limb of an aortofemoral graft, with the contralateral graft limb retaining patency. The resulting lower extremity ischemia is often more severe than that prior to the primary procedure, and not infrequently, urgent reoperation is required for limb salvage. Although thrombosis of an anastomotic aneurysm, compression due to fibrotic scarring, dilatation or degeneration of the graft, hypercoagulable states, or low-output syndromes may occasionally be responsible, the great majority of late graft failures are due to recurrent occlusive disease, usually occurring at or just beyond the distal anastomosis. If aortoiliac endarterectomy or aortoiliac bypass grafting has been performed, progressive occlusive disease in the external iliac artery is commonly responsible.[81, 82] In the most commonly encountered situation, occlusion of an aortofemoral graft limb, occlusive lesions interfering with profunda femoris artery runoff are causative, because the majority of patients undergoing aortofemoral grafting have preexisting chronic occlusion of the superficial femoral artery.[84, 181–184] Recurrent disease compromising the proximal aortic anastomosis generally leads to failure of the entire reconstruction and usually results because the surgeon did not carry the original procedure high enough in the infrarenal aorta.[90] Graft failure, particularly that due to recurrent or progressive inflow or outflow tract occlusive disease, is much more likely to occur in patients with ongoing risk factors for atherosclerosis, especially those who continue cigarette smoking postoperatively.[183, 185–189] This fact deserves repeated emphasis to patients.

Reoperation for occlusion of the entire primary reconstruction almost always requires another aortofemoral grafting if the patient is an appropriate candidate.[82] Axillobifemoral grafting may be considered in the patient for whom a repeated graft procedure poses a high risk. If various technical problems suggest that direct reoperation on the infrarenal abdominal aorta is ill advised or unduly hazardous, the supraceliac aorta, the descending thoracic aorta, or even the ascending thoracic aorta may occasionally be used for the site of proximal anastomosis in reoperative bypass procedures, as previously described.[155–158]

For unilateral limb failure of an aortoiliac procedure, direct reoperation, often employing a retroperitoneal approach, is generally feasible, with extension of the graft to the femoral level. Alternatively, femorofemoral transpubic grafting may be performed if the contralateral iliofemoral system is widely patent.[190]

For unilateral occlusion of one limb of an aortobifemoral graft, inflow can frequently be restored by thrombectomy of the graft limb with the use of a balloon embolectomy catheter.[181, 184] A thromboendarterectomy stripper is often required to complete extraction of the adherent fibrinothrombotic plug.[184, 191] The modification of the standard Fogarty balloon catheter known as the Graft Thrombectomy Catheter also appears to be quite useful for adequate removal of such adherent clots.[192] Once inflow has been reestablished, revascularization of the profunda femoris artery by means of profundaplasty of varying extent or extension of a graft to the more distal profunda femoris artery (Fig. 66–12) is used to restore reliable deep femoral artery outflow.[84, 181, 184, 193–195] In instances in which the profunda femoris artery is small or is extensively diseased, addition of a femoropopliteal or femorotibial bypass may be required to provide adequate outflow and to maintain patency of the reoperated aortofemoral graft limb. Although this decision is often a difficult one, such a bypass was used in one third of such reoperations in the experience of the author and his colleagues[181] and has been advocated by other surgeons as well.[194, 196]

In situations in which graft limb occlusion is more chronic and thrombectomy is not successful, a femorofemoral crossover graft from the patent contralateral graft limb is generally the most useful alternative to reestablish inflow.[130, 132, 134, 190] Direct "redo" aortic surgery for unilateral aortofemoral graft limb occlusion, with replacement of either the entire graft or the involved graft limb, is generally unnecessary because proximal causes are infrequently responsible for unilateral failures and alternative methods of revascularizing the involved extremity are usually successful.[181, 182, 184]

Although such reoperative procedures are often difficult and may tax the skill and ingenuity of even the most experienced vascular surgeon, long-term results suggest that appropriate reoperation is indeed worthwhile, with highly satisfactory extension of graft patency and associated rates of limb salvage.[57, 181]

Anastomotic Pseudoaneurysm

The incidence of anastomotic pseudoaneurysm formation varies between 1% and 5% and is by far most common at the femoral anastomosis of an aortofemoral graft.[57] Although numerous factors may contribute to anastomotic aneurysm formation, degenerative changes within the host arterial wall leading to weakness and dehiscence of the intact suture line appear to be most common.[197] Predisposing factors include:

- Excessive tension on the anastomosis as a result of inadequate graft length
- Poor suture technique using inadequate bites of the arterial wall or excessive spacing between sutures
- A thin-walled artery

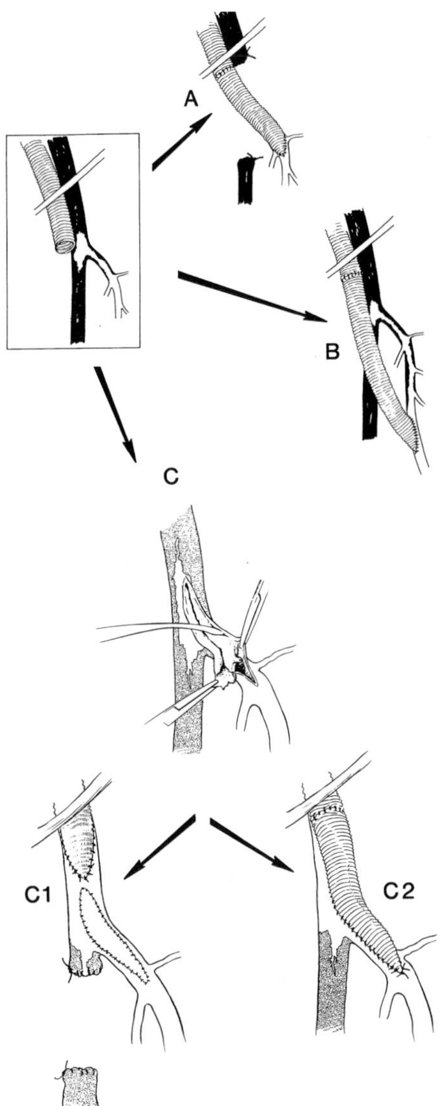

FIGURE 66–12. Options for outflow reconstruction during reoperation for aortofemoral graft limb occlusion. *A*, Addition of a short extension of new prosthetic graft end-to-end to the profunda femoris artery below orificial disease. *B*, If more extensive disease is present, insertion of a longer new graft segment as a bypass to the distal profunda femoris artery is preferred. *C*, Most frequently, endarterectomy of the common femoral artery and profunda femoris artery is performed, with a separate patch closure employing autogenous or prosthetic material and graft reanastomosis above this *(C1)*, or closure with the long beveled tongue of new graft segment *(C2)*. *(A–C2*, From Brewster DC: Surgery of late aortic graft occlusion. *In* Bergan JJ, Yao JST [eds]: Aortic Surgery. Philadelphia, WB Saunders, 1989, p 533.)

Many surgeons also believe that endarterectomy may weaken the arterial wall as a result of a reduction in tensile strength and that the incidence of subsequent pseudoaneurysm formation may be higher if anastomosis is made with such an arterial segment. Rarely, prosthetic suture materials may fracture, or degeneration may occur, leading to late suture line disruption, as was previously seen when silk sutures were used. Infection may be a contributing event and always needs to be considered as a possible etiologic factor when the surgeon is evaluating patients with even bland-appearing anastomotic aneurysms.[198]

Recognition of a femoral anastomotic aneurysm is usually quite simple because a pulsatile mass, which is occasionally tender, is noted by both the patient and the surgeon. Retroperitoneal aortic or iliac anastomotic aneurysm is much less often noted until expansion or rupture produces pain, causes graft occlusion, or erodes into an abdominal hollow viscus. If such an aneurysm is considered to be present, ultrasonography and CT scanning are reliable methods for evaluating intra-abdominal grafts and anastomoses. The true incidence of intra-abdominal anastomotic aneurysms after aortic surgery may be much higher than previously thought; a study by Edwards and coworkers[199] reported a 10% incidence at a mean interval of 12 years following initial operation. This finding suggests that ultrasonography or CT scanning should be a routine part of the late follow-up for patients with aortic grafts.

Diagnosis of a pseudoaneurysm is usually confirmed by angiography. Even if the diagnosis of a femoral anastomotic aneurysm is readily apparent, aortography is generally advisable to evaluate the proximal aortic anastomosis and to help in planning of the operative procedure. Indeed, the presence of a femoral anastomotic aneurysm may be a marker for other graft-related problems. In a report from Emory University of 41 patients who had femoral pseudoaneurysm after aortobifemoral grafting, 70% had bilateral aneurysms and 17% had proximal anastomotic aneurysms.[200]

An anastomotic aneurysm should generally be repaired as soon as it is identified. Even if the aneurysm is asymptomatic, the likelihood of thrombosis or distal embolization warrants elective repair. Such repair is usually easily and successfully carried out at the groin level with the use of a short additional graft segment and reanastomosis to a somewhat more distal arterial segment, often the profunda femoris artery itself. Culture specimens should always be obtained at the time of repair to check for unrecognized infection. Results of repair are generally highly successful, especially if repair is carried out electively rather than as an emergency.[201] Once they have been repaired, anastomotic aneurysms may recur in about 5% to 10% of patients.[202] In such circumstances, occult infection must be seriously considered as a possible contributing cause.[203]

Postoperative Sexual Dysfunction

Although the physiology of penile erection is complex, involving the interaction of psychologic factors, pelvic blood flow, neurologic pathways, and hormonal mechanisms, postoperative disturbance of sexual function in a man should be recognized as a potential consequence of direct aortic operation. A detailed discussion of this topic can be found in Chapters 52 and 77.

Although a high percentage (at least 30% to 50%) of men presenting with aortoiliac occlusive disease significant enough to require surgical correction have various degrees of sexual dysfunction when they are first seen, the incidence of iatrogenic sexual disturbance after aortic reconstruction may approach 25%.[77, 204, 205] As popularized by DePalma and colleagues[206] and others,[204, 205] a nerve-sparing approach to the infrarenal aorta that emphasizes (1) avoidance of autonomic nerve fibers along the left lateral wall of the aorta and (2) minimal dissection in the region of the aortic bifurcation, where such nerves usually cross the proximal common iliac arteries, is helpful. Preservation of hypogastric artery flow by a variety of techniques is also essential.[77, 78, 204, 207, 208]

Whether or not end-to-end proximal aortic anastomosis leads to a higher incidence of erectile dysfunction remains controversial. With appropriate recognition and implementation of such considerations, it is hoped, the surgeon can minimize the incidence of postoperative sexual dysfunction and actually improve sexual function in some patients.[77]

Infection

Infection following aortic reconstruction remains the most feared complication, with formidable morbidity and mortality rates. Fortunately, with current reconstructive methods and the use of prophylactic antibiotics, it remains a rare occurrence, with an incidence of 1% or less.[2, 57, 159, 209–211]

In most series, the highest incidence of infection has been in the inguinal portion of an aortofemoral graft. Important contributing factors are:

- Multiple vascular procedures
- Postoperative wound problems, such as hematoma, seroma, or lymph leakage, particularly in the groin
- Emergency operation

Infectious complications occur almost exclusively after prosthetic graft insertion, being exceedingly rare after autogenous operations such as endarterectomy.

Although graft infection is often not clinically apparent for months to years, it is generally believed that graft contamination occurs most commonly at the time of primary graft implantation. This belief emphasizes the importance of:

1. Meticulous sterile technique at the time of original operation.
2. Avoidance of skin contact with the prosthetic graft by use of adherent plastic drapes.
3. Careful attention to hemostasis and wound closure.
4. General avoidance of concomitant intra-abdominal operations, which may increase the incidence of graft contamination.

Several randomized studies in the literature have documented the efficacy of antibiotic prophylaxis in reducing the incidence of vascular graft infection,[67–69] and its perioperative use in vascular reconstruction is now well accepted. Late graft infection that is due to bacteremic implantation of organisms on the luminal surface of a functioning graft is uncommon but may occur. Because current prostheses are rarely completely healed with a viable endothelial lining, antibiotic prophylaxis should probably be employed in the patient with a previously implanted graft who is exposed to the risk of bacteremia, much as it is in the patient with rheumatic valvular disease or prosthetic heart valves.

Staphylococcus aureus remains the most common responsible organism, but later experience indicates that organisms such as *Staphylococcus albus* and gram-negative bacteria are of increasing importance.[210] In patients presenting with forefoot infection or wet gangrene, it is particularly important to use appropriate specific antibiotic treatment and aggressive débridement before placement of a vascular prosthesis. Several studies have implicated the importance of bacteria in lymph nodes in the groin as the source of subsequent graft infection.[212]

Diagnosis and management of patients with infection following aortoiliofemoral reconstructive procedures are often complex and are discussed more fully in Chapter 47. Graft excision is usually required, and revascularization via remote uncontaminated routes or the use of autogenous methods of anatomic revascularization is often necessary to maintain limb viability.[159, 213–218] If the patient's condition is stable and the diagnosis of graft infection is firmly established, extra-anatomic revascularization preceding graft excision appears to yield a better outcome.[219, 220]

If infection appears localized, as in a single groin, for example, local measures, including antibiotic irrigation, aggressive débridement, and soft tissue coverage with a variety of rotational muscle flaps without graft removal, may sometimes be successful.[221–225] Another approach to treatment of entirely infected aortofemoral grafts consists of graft excision and in situ graft replacement, sometimes with "neo-aortoiliac systems" constructed from autogenous superficial femoral veins[226] (see Chapter 47).

Aortoenteric Fistula

Aortoenteric fistula and associated gastrointestinal hemorrhage are devastating complications, with a continued high incidence of death or limb loss despite efforts at their correction.[159] Communication between the aortic prosthesis and a portion of the gastrointestinal tract invariably leads to massive gastrointestinal bleeding, although initial bleeding episodes may be limited and may allow time for diagnosis and treatment. Such communications involve the third and fourth parts of the duodenum, which overlie the proximal aortic suture line in the majority of cases, but the small bowel or colon may be involved with an iliac anastomotic point in 10% to 20% of cases. Such secondary aortoenteric fistulae must be differentiated from primary fistulae, which occur as a result of the rupture of unoperated aortic or iliac artery aneurysms into adjacent hollow organs.

Secondary aortoenteric fistula formation may occur as a result of several mechanisms. If the adjacent bowel is improperly separated from the prosthesis and suture line, fibrotic adherence and subsequent erosion may occur. In other instances, anastomotic aneurysm formation that is due to mechanical causes or infection may occur first, with subsequent erosion of the pseudoaneurysm into the gastrointestinal tract.

The diagnosis must be suspected whenever an episode of gastrointestinal hemorrhage occurs in a patient who has undergone previous aortic operation. Diagnosis is often elusive. Upper gastrointestinal radiographic evaluation may show distortion or abnormality of the retroperitoneal duodenum, or endoscopy may actually visualize the site of hemorrhage or the prosthesis itself if the distal aspects of the duodenum are examined. Aortography is often nondiagnostic, but it may demonstrate a pseudoaneurysm involving an aortic or iliac artery anastomosis. CT scanning is often helpful, demonstrating anastomotic or perigraft abnormalities.

As with all complications, such difficulties are far more easily prevented than treated. The incidence of aortoenteric fistula formation appears to be higher after end-to-side anastomosis, because it is much more difficult to cover such an anastomotic configuration with viable tissue and avoid contact with the bowel, than after end-to-end proximal anastomosis.[2, 4, 73] In difficult situations, interposition of omentum between the graft and the duodenum is often helpful.

Standard methods of treatment for aortoenteric fistula generally require removal of all prosthetic material, closure of the infrarenal abdominal aorta, repair of the gastrointestinal tract, and revascularization by means of an extra-anatomic graft[227–230] (see Chapter 49). For minimal local sepsis, some reports advocate excision of limited portions of the graft directly in contact with the bowel lumen and in situ repair with a new prosthetic graft, arterial homograft, or an autogenous vein "neo-aorta."[226, 231–236] However, further experience is necessary to determine the safety and wisdom of such an approach in comparison with traditional removal of the graft and remote methods of revascularization. For more discussion, the reader is referred to Chapters 49 and 68.

Despite advances in treatment, death or limb loss continues to occur in 50% or more of patients in whom aortoenteric fistula develops, similar to the results of management of infected aortic grafts, to which aortoenteric fistulae are closely related in terms of mechanism of occurrence and subsequent management. Mortality is often due to continued sepsis, multiorgan system failure, or disruption of the proximal aortic stump closure.

SUMMARY

Arteriosclerotic aortoiliac occlusive disease is a common cause of lower extremity ischemic symptoms. In the majority of patients, occlusive lesions are multifocal, involving the lower abdominal aorta, both iliac arteries, and, frequently, the infrainguinal arterial tree. Before proceeding with aortic reconstructive surgery, the surgeon must document the hemodynamic significance of inflow disease. This may often be accomplished by careful clinical examination supplemented with vascular laboratory hemodynamic data and good arteriographic studies. If any doubt remains, however, direct measurement of femoral artery pressure is helpful.

The key features of aortofemoral grafting are (1) high placement of the proximal anastomosis immediately distal to the renal arteries and (2) careful techniques of distal anastomosis, with or without profundaplasty, to achieve adequate flow into the deep femoral artery. Despite the presence of multilevel disease in the majority of patients, a properly performed inflow operation achieves satisfactory relief of ischemic symptoms in 70% to 80% of cases. Approximately 10% to 15% of patients with advanced distal ischemia may be best managed with simultaneous inflow and outflow reconstruction, but careful patient selection is important.

Clearly, no single option for inflow revascularization is optimal in all instances. In every patient, a decision about which method is best should be made through consideration of several factors; primary factors are the extent and distribution of disease and the anticipated risk of the possible alternatives that might be used. The likely success of various methods in terms of hemodynamic improvement, symptom relief, and sustained patency can usually be predicted with relative accuracy, and such estimates must be judged in the context of patient age, expected length of survival, and specific clinical needs of each patient. Durability must often be balanced against the possible advantages of safety and expediency.

Alternative therapies have a well-established role in the management of occlusive disease of limited extent or lesser severity and in the treatment of patients in whom adverse technical challenges or high operative risk contraindicates conventional direct aortic reconstruction. However, for most patients with diffuse aortoiliac occlusive disease, aortobifemoral grafts remain the most durable and functionally effective means of revascularization and should continue to be rightfully regarded as the gold standard against which other options must be properly compared. As the availability and results of alternative techniques have improved, so too has the safety of standard repair. Indeed, the very definition of a "high-risk" patient is currently much more indistinct than in previous eras. No doubt the future will bring new advances in alternative methods, but it is hoped that properly designed and performed randomized studies, outcome assessment, and cost-benefit analyses will help clarify their role. The need for such information is quite evident; without it, one of the most effective and beneficial procedures that vascular surgeons have to offer may be inappropriately abandoned because of the seductiveness of the axiom "less is best."

Finally, the alternatives for inflow revascularization may not be as competitive with one another as first seems apparent. Each has specific advantages and disadvantages and, when used in appropriate circumstances, can give excellent results. Indeed, it is this very broad spectrum of options that makes treatment of aortoiliac occlusive disease one of the most successful areas of current vascular practice.

REFERENCES

1. DeBakey ME, Lawrie GM, Glaeser DH: Patterns of atherosclerosis and their surgical significance. Ann Surg 201:115, 1985.
2. Brewster DC, Darling RC: Optimal methods of aortoiliac reconstruction. Surgery 84:739, 1978.
3. Brewster DC: Clinical and anatomic considerations for surgery in aortoiliac disease and results of surgical treatment. Circulation 83(Suppl I):142, 1991.
4. Darling RC, Brewster DC, Hallett JW Jr, et al: Aortoiliac reconstruction. Surg Clin North Am 59:565, 1979.
5. Cronenwett JL, Davis JT Jr, Gooch JB, et al: Aortoiliac occlusive disease in women. Surgery 88:775, 1980.
6. DeLaurentis DA, Friedmann P, Wolferth GC Jr, et al: Atherosclerosis and the hypoplastic aortoiliac system. Surgery 83:27, 1978.
7. Greenhalgh RM: Small aorta syndrome. *In* Bergan JJ, Yao JST (eds): Surgery of the Aorta and Its Body Branches. New York, Grune & Stratton, 1979, pp 183–190.
8. Staple TW: The solitary aortoiliac lesion. Surgery 64:569, 1968.
9. Moore WS, Cafferata HT, Hall AD, et al: In defense of grafts across the inguinal ligament. Ann Surg 168:207, 1968.
10. Mozersky DJ, Sumner DS, Strandness DE: Long-term results of reconstructive aortoiliac surgery. Am J Surg 123:503, 1972.
11. Malone JM, Moore WS, Goldstone J: Life expectancy following aortofemoral arterial grafting. Surgery 81:551, 1977.
12. Brewster DC, Waltman AC, O'Hara PJ, et al: Femoral artery pressure

measurement during aortography. Circulation 60(Suppl I):120, 1979.
13. Sobinsky KR, Borozan PG, Gray B, et al: Is femoral pulse palpation accurate in assessing the hemodynamic significance of aortoiliac occlusive disease? Am J Surg 148:214, 1984.
14. Brewster DC, Perler BA, Robison JG, et al: Aortofemoral graft for multilevel occlusive disease: Predictors of success and need for distal bypass. Arch Surg 117:1593, 1982.
15. Johnston KW, Demorais D, Colapinto RI: Difficulty in assessing disease by clinical and arteriographic methods. Angiology 32:609, 1981.
16. Karmody AM, Powers FR, Monaco VJ, et al: "Blue toe" syndrome: An indication for limb salvage surgery. Arch Surg 111:1263, 1976.
17. Kempczinski RF: Lower extremity arterial emboli from ulcerating atherosclerotic plaques. JAMA 241:807, 1979.
18. Goodreau JJ, Creasy JK, Flanigan DP, et al: Rational approach to the differentiation of vascular and neurogenic claudication. Surgery 84:749, 1978.
19. Kempczinski RF: Clinical application of noninvasive testing in extremity arterial insufficiency. *In* Kempczinski RF, Yao JST (eds): Practical Noninvasive Vascular Diagnosis. Chicago, Year Book Medical Publishers, 1982, pp 343–365.
20. Raines JK, Darling RC, Buth J, et al: Vascular laboratory criteria for the management of peripheral vascular disease of the lower extremities. Surgery 79:21, 1976.
21. Ernst CB: Prevention of intestinal ischemia following abdominal aortic reconstruction. Surgery 93:102, 1983.
22. Mason RA, Arbeit LA, Giron F: Renal dysfunction after arteriography. JAMA 253:1001, 1985.
23. Calligaro KD, Dandura R, Dougherty MJ, et al: Same-day admissions and other cost-saving strategies for elective aortoiliac surgery. J Vasc Surg 25:141, 1997.
24. Cambria RP, Kaufman JA, L'Italien GJ, et al: Magnetic resonance angiography in the management of lower extremity arterial occlusive disease: A prospective study. J Vasc Surg 25:380, 1997.
25. Kaufman JA, Yucel EK, Waltman AC, et al: MR angiography in the preoperative evaluation of abdominal aortic aneurysms: A preliminary study. J Vasc Intervasc Radiol 5:489, 1994.
26. Edelman RR: MR angiography: present and future. AJR Am J Roentgenol 161:1, 1993.
27. Raptopoulos V, Rosen MP, Kent KC, et al: Sequential helical CT angiography of aortoiliac disease. AJR Am J Roentgenol 166:1347, 1996.
28. Reidy NC, Walden R, Abbott WA, et al: Anatomic localization of atherosclerotic lesions by hemodynamic tests. Arch Surg 116:1041, 1981.
29. Lynch TG, Hobson RW, Wright CB, et al: Interpretations of Doppler segmental pressures in peripheral vascular occlusive disease. Arch Surg 119:465, 1984.
30. Rutherford RB, Lowenstein DH, Klein MF: Combining segmental systolic pressures and plethysmography to diagnose arterial occlusive disease of the legs. Am J Surg 138:211, 1979.
31. Thiele BL, Bandyk DF, Zierler RE, et al: A systematic approach to the assessment of aortoiliac disease. Arch Surg 118:477, 1983.
32. Kohler TR, Nance DR, Cramer MM, et al: Duplex scanning for diagnosis of aortoiliac and femoropopliteal disease: A prospective study. Circulation 76:1074, 1987.
33. Bruins Slot HB, Strijbosch L, Greep JM: Interobserver variability in single plane aortography. Surgery 90:497, 1981.
34. Flanigan DP, Tullis JP, Streeter VL: Multiple subcritical arterial stenosis: Effect on poststenotic pressure and flow. Ann Surg 186:663, 1977.
35. Brener BJ, Raines JK, Darling RC, et al: Measurement of systolic femoral artery pressure during reactive hyperemia: An estimate of aortoiliac disease. Circulation 49/50(Suppl II):259, 1974.
36. Flanigan DP, Williams LR, Schwartz JA, et al: Hemodynamic evaluation of the aortoiliac system based on pharmacologic vasodilatation. Surgery 93:709, 1983.
37. Moore WS, Hall AD: Unrecognized aortoiliac stenosis: A physiologic approach to the diagnosis. Arch Surg 103:633, 1971.
38. Kikta MJ, Flanigan DP, Bishara RA, et al: Long-term follow-up of patients having infrainguinal bypass performed below stenotic but hemodynamically normal aortoiliac vessels. J Vasc Surg 5:319, 1987.
39. Flanigan DP, Ryan TJ, Williams LR, et al: Aortofemoral or femoropopliteal revascularization? A prospective evaluation of the papaverine test. J Vasc Surg 1:215, 1984.
40. Brewster DC: Current controversies in the management of aortoiliac occlusive disease. J Vasc Surg 25:365, 1997.
41. Coffman JD: Vasodilator drugs in peripheral vascular disease. N Engl J Med 300:713, 1979.
42. Porter JM, Cutler BS, Lee BY, et al: Pentoxifylline efficacy in the treatment of intermittent claudication: Multicenter controlled double-blind trial with objective assessment of chronic occlusive arterial disease patients. Am Heart J 104:66, 1982.
43. Johnston KW, Rae M, Hogg-Johnston SA, et al: Five-year results of a prospective study of percutaneous transluminal angioplasty. Ann Surg 206:403, 1987.
44. Johnston KW: Iliac arteries: Reanalysis of results of balloon angioplasty. Radiology 186:207, 1993.
45. Brewster DC, Cambria RP, Darling RC, et al: Long-term results of combined iliac balloon angioplasty and distal surgical revascularization. Ann Surg 210:324, 1989.
46. Brewster DC: The role of angioplasty to improve inflow for infrainguinal bypasses. Eur J Vasc Surg 9:262, 1995.
47. Marin ML, Veith FJ, Cyanmon J, et al: Initial experience with transluminally placed endovascular grafts for the treatment of complex vascular lesions. Ann Surg 222:449, 1995.
48. Marin ML, Veith FJ, Sanchez LA, et al: Endovascular aortoiliac grafts in combination with standard infrainguinal arterial bypass in the management of limb-threatening ischemia: Preliminary report. J Vasc Surg 22:316, 1995.
49. Sanchez LA, Wain RA, Veith FJ, et al: Endovascular grafting for aortoiliac occlusive disease. Semin Vasc Surg 10:297, 1997.
50. Piotrowski JJ, Pearce WH, Jones DN, et al: Aortobifemoral bypass: The operation of choice for unilateral iliac occlusion? J Vasc Surg 8:211, 1988.
51. Passman MA, Taylor LM Jr, Moneta GL, et al: Comparison of axillofemoral and aortofemoral bypass for aortoiliac disease. J Vasc Surg 23:263, 1996.
52. Voorhees, AB Jr, Jaretzki A III, Blakemore AH: Use of tubes constructed from Vinyon "N" cloth in bridging arterial defects: Preliminary report. Ann Surg 135:332, 1952.
53. Edwards SW, Lyons C: Three years' experience with peripheral arterial grafts of crimped nylon and Teflon. Surg Gynocol Obstet 107:62, 1958.
54. DeBakey ML, Cooley DA: Clinical application of a new flexible knitted Dacron arterial substitute. Am Surg 24:862, 1958.
55. Crawford ES, Bomberger RA, Glaeser DH, et al: Aortoiliac occlusive disease: Factors influencing survival and function following reconstructive operation over a twenty-five year period. Surgery 90:1555, 1981.
56. Malone JM, Moore WS, Goldstone J: The natural history of bilateral aortofemoral bypass grafts for ischemia of the lower extremities. Arch Surg 110:1300, 1975.
57. Szilagyi DE, Hageman JH, Smith RF, et al: A thirty-year survey of the reconstructive surgical treatment of aortoiliac occlusive disease. J Vasc Surg 3:421, 1986.
58. Nevelsteen A, Wouters L, Suy R: Aortofemoral Dacron reconstruction for aorto-iliac occlusive disease: A 25-year survey. Eur J Vasc Surg 5:179, 1991.
59. Poulias GE, Doundoulakis N, Prombonas E, et al: Aorto-femoral bypass and determinants of early success and late favorable outcome: Experience with 1000 consecutive cases. J Cardiovasc Surg 33:664, 1992.
60. Brewster DC, Cooke JC: Longevity of aortofemoral bypass grafts. *In* Yao JST, Pearce WH (eds): Long-term Results in Vascular Surgery. Norwalk, Conn, Appleton & Lange, 1993, pp 149–161.
61. Brewster DC, Edwards JP: Cardiopulmonary complications related to vascular surgery. *In* Bernhard VM, Towne JB (eds): Complications in Vascular Surgery. St. Louis, Quality Medical Publishing, 1991, pp 23–41.
62. Hertzer NR, Beven EG, Young JR, et al: Coronary artery disease in peripheral vascular patients: A classification of 1000 coronary angiograms and results of surgical management. Ann Surg 199:223, 1984.
63. Brewster DC, Boucher CA, Okada RD, et al: Selection of patients for preoperative coronary angiography: Use of dipyridamole-stress thallium myocardial imaging. J Vasc Surg 2:504, 1985.
64. Eagle KA, Coley CM, Newell JB, et al: Combining clinical and thallium data optimizes preoperative assessment of cardiac risk before major vascular surgery. Ann Intern Med 110:859, 1989.

65. Cambria RP, Brewster DC, Abbott WM, et al: The impact of selective use of dipyridamole-thallium scans and surgical factors on the current morbidity of aortic surgery. J Vasc Surg 15:43, 1992.
66. Taylor LM, Yeager RA, Moneta GL, et al: The incidence of perioperative myocardial infarction in general vascular surgery. J Vasc Surg 151:52, 1992.
67. Kaiser AB, Clayson KR, Mulherin JL, et al: Antibiotic prophylaxis in vascular surgery. Ann Surg 188:283, 1978.
68. Pitt HA, Postier RH, MacGowan WL, et al: Prophylactic antibiotics in vascular surgery: Topical, systemic, or both? Ann Surg 192:356, 1980.
69. Hasselgren PO, Ivarsson L, Risberg B, et al: Effects of prophylactic antibiotics in vascular surgery: A prospective, randomized, double-blind study. Ann Surg 200:86, 1984.
70. Mulcare RJ, Royster TS, Lynn RA, et al: Long-term results of operative therapy for aortoiliac disease. Arch Surg 113:601, 1978.
71. Pierce HE, Turrentine M, Stringfield S, et al: Evaluation of end-to-side v. end-to-end proximal anastomosis in aortobifemoral bypass. Arch Surg 117:1580, 1982.
72. Mikati A, Marache P, Watel A, et al: End-to-side aortoprosthetic anastomoses: Long-term computed tomography assessment. Ann Vasc Surg 4:584, 1990.
73. Dunn DA, Downs AR, Lye CR: Aortoiliac reconstruction for occlusive disease: Comparison of end-to-end and end-to-side proximal anastomoses. Can J Surg 25:382, 1982.
74. Rutherford RB, Jones DN, Martin MS, et al: Serial hemodynamic assessment of aortobifemoral bypass. J Vasc Surg 4:428, 1986.
75. Ameli FM, Stein M, Aro L, et al: End-to-end versus end-to-side proximal anastomosis in aortobifemoral bypass surgery: Does it matter? Can Soc Vasc Surg 34:243, 1991.
76. Melliere D, Labastie J, Becquemin JP, et al: Proximal anastomosis in aortobifemoral bypass: End-to-end or end-to-side? J Cardiovasc Surg (Torino) 31:77, 1990.
77. Flanigan DP, Schuler JJ, Keifer T, et al: Elimination of iatrogenic impotence and improvement of sexual function after aortoiliac revascularization. Arch Surg 117:544, 1982.
78. Queral LA, Whitehouse WM Jr, Flinn WR, et al: Pelvic hemodynamics after aortoiliac reconstruction. Surgery 86:799, 1979.
79. Picone AL, Green RM, Ricotta JR, et al: Spinal cord ischemia following operations on the abdominal aorta. J Vasc Surg 3:94, 1986.
80. Gloviczki P, Cross SA, Stanson AW, et al: Ischemic injury to the spinal cord or lumbosacral plexus after aorto-iliac reconstruction. Am J Surg 162:131, 1991.
81. Baird RJ, Feldman P, Miles JT, et al: Subsequent downstream repair after aorta-iliac and aorta-femoral bypass operations. Surgery 82:785, 1977.
82. Crawford ES, Manning LG, Kelly TF: "Redo" surgery after operations for aneurysm and occlusion of the abdominal aorta. Surgery 81:41, 1977.
83. Bernhard VM, Ray LI, Militello JP: The role of angioplasty of the profunda femoris artery in revascularization of the ischemic limb. Surg Gynecol Obstet 142:840, 1976.
84. Malone JM, Goldstone J, Moore WS: Autogenous profundaplasty: The key to long-term patency in secondary repair of aortofemoral graft occlusion. Ann Surg 188:817, 1978.
85. Berguer R, Higgins RF, Colton LT: Geometry, blood flow, and reconstruction of the deep femoral artery. Am J Surg 130:68, 1975.
86. Robicsek F, Duncan GD, Daugherty HK, et al: "Half and half" woven and knitted Dacron grafts in the aortoiliac and aortofemoral positions: Seven and one-half years follow-up. Ann Vasc Surg 5:315, 1991.
87. Robicsek F, Duncan GD, Anderson CE, et al: Indium 111–labeled platelet deposition in woven and knitted Dacron bifurcated aortic grafts with the same patient as a clinical model. J Vasc Surg 5:833, 1987.
88. Burke PM, Herrmann JB, Cutler BS: Optimal grafting methods for the small abdominal aorta. J Cardiovasc Surg 28:420, 1987.
89. Cintora I, Pearce DE, Cannon JA: A clinical survey of aortobifemoral bypass using two inherently different graft types. Ann Surg 208:625, 1988.
90. Robbs JV, Wylie EJ: Factors contributing to recurrent limb ischemia following bypass surgery for aortoiliac occlusive disease, and their management. Arch Surg 193:346, 1981.
91. Sanders RJ, Kempczinski RF, Hammond W, et al: The significance of graft diameter. Surgery 88:856, 1980.
92. Nunn DB, Carter MM, Donohue MT, et al: Postoperative dilation of knitted Dacron aortic bifurcation graft. J Vasc Surg 12:291, 1990.
93. O'Hara PJ, Brewster DC, Darling RC, et al: The value of intraoperative monitoring using the pulse volume recorder during peripheral vascular surgery. Surg Gynecol Obstet 162:275, 1981.
94. Rob C: Extraperitoneal approach to the abdominal aorta. Surgery 53:87, 1963.
95. Sicard GA, Freeman MB, VanderWoude JC, et al: Comparison between the transabdominal and retroperitoneal approach for reconstruction of the infrarenal aorta. J Vasc Surg 5:19, 1987.
96. Williams GM, Ricotta J, Zinner M, et al: The extended retroperitoneal approach for treatment of extensive atherosclerosis of the aorta and renal vessels. Surgery 88:846, 1980.
97. Shepard AD, Tollefson DFJ, Reddy DJ, et al: Left flank retroperitoneal exposure: A technical aid to complex aortic reconstruction. J Vasc Surg 14:283, 1991.
98. Sicard GA, Reilly JM, Rubin BE, et al: Transabdominal versus retroperitoneal incision for abdominal aortic surgery: Report of a prospective randomized trial. J Vasc Surg 21:174, 1995.
99. Cambria RP, Brewster DC, Abbott WM, et al: Transperitoneal versus retroperitoneal approach for aortic reconstruction: A randomized prospective study. J Vasc Surg 11:314, 1990.
100. Barnes RW, Baker WH, Shanik G, et al: Value of concomitant sympathectomy in aortoiliac reconstruction: Results of a prospective randomized study. Arch Surg 112:1325, 1977.
101. Satiani B, Liapis CD, Hayes JP, et al: Prospective randomized study of concomitant lumbar sympathectomy in aortoiliac reconstruction. Am J Surg 143:755, 1982.
102. Imparato AM: Lumbar sympathectomy: Role in the treatment of occlusive arterial disease in the lower extremities. Surg Clin North Am 59:719, 1979.
103. Rutherford RB: The current role of sympathectomy in the management of limb ischemia. Semin Vasc Surg 4:195, 1991.
104. Corson JD, Brewster DC, Darling RC: The surgical management of infrarenal aortic occlusion. Surg Gynecol Obstet 155:369, 1982.
105. Liddicoat JE, Bekassy SM, Dang MH, et al: Complete occlusion of the infrarenal abdominal aorta: Management and results in 64 patients. Surgery 77:467, 1975.
106. Tapper SS, Jenkins JM, Edwards WH, et al: Juxtarenal aortic occlusion. Ann Surg 215:443, 1992.
107. Starrett RW, Stoney RJ: Juxta-renal aortic occlusion. Surgery 76:890, 1974.
108. Deriu GP, Ballotta E: Natural history of ascending thrombosis of the abdominal aorta. Am J Surg 145:652, 1983.
109. McCullough JL, Mackey WC, O'Donnell TF, et al: Infrarenal aortic occlusion: A reassessment of surgical indications. Am J Surg 146:178, 1983.
110. Reilly LM, Sauer L, Weinstein ES, et al: Infrarenal aortic occlusion: Does it threaten renal perfusion or function? J Vasc Surg 11:216, 1990.
111. Gupta SK, Veith FJ: Management of juxtarenal aortic occlusions: Technique for suprarenal clamp placement. Ann Vasc Surg 6:306, 1992.
112. Martinez BD, Hertzer NR, Beven EG: Influence of distal arterial occlusive disease on prognosis following aortobifemoral bypass. Surgery 88:795, 1980.
113. Sumner DS, Strandness DE Jr: Aortoiliac reconstruction in patients with combined iliac and superficial femoral arterial occlusion. Surgery 84:348, 1978.
114. Hill DA, McGrath MA, Lord RSA, et al: The effect of superficial femoral artery occlusion on the outcome of aortofemoral bypass for intermittent claudication. Surgery 87:133, 1980.
115. Galland RB, Hill DA, Gustave R, et al: The functional result of aortoiliac reconstruction. Br J Surg 67:344, 1980.
116. Jones AF, Kempczinski RF: Aortofemoral bypass grafting: A reappraisal. Arch Surg 116:301, 1981.
117. Brewster DC, Darling RC: Aortoiliofemoral bypass grafting. *In* Kempczinski RF (ed): The Ischemic Leg. Chicago, Year Book Medical Publishers, 1985, pp 305–326.
118. Brewster DC, Veith FJ: Combined aortoiliac and femoropopliteal occlusive disease. *In* Veith FJ, Hobson RW, Williams RA, et al (eds): Vascular Surgery: Principles and Practice, 2nd ed. New York, McGraw-Hill, 1994, pp 459–472.
119. Baird RJ: In discussion of Brewster DC, Perler BA, Robison JR, et al: Aorto-femoral graft for multilevel occlusive disease. Arch Surg 117:1593, 1982.

120. Dardik H, Ibrahim IM, Jarrah M, et al: Synchronous aortofemoral or iliofemoral bypass with revascularization of the lower extremity. Surg Gynecol Obstet 149:676, 1979.
121. Harris PL, Cave Bigley DJ, McSweeney L: Aortofemoral bypass and the role of concomitant femorodistal reconstruction. Br J Surg 72:317, 1985.
122. O'Donnell TF Jr, McBride KA, Callow AD, et al: Management of combined segment disease. Am J Surg 141:452, 1981.
123. Eidt J, Charlesworth D: Combined aortobifemoral and femoropopliteal bypass in the management of patients with extensive atherosclerosis. Ann Vasc Surg 1:453, 1986.
124. Dalman RL, Taylor LM Jr, Moneta GL, et al: Simultaneous operative repair of multilevel lower extremity occlusive disease. J Vasc Surg 13:211, 1991.
125. Garrett WV, Slaymaker EE, Heintz SE, et al: Intraoperative prediction of symptomatic result of aortofemoral bypass from changes in ankle pressure index. Surgery 82:504, 1977.
126. Levinson SA, Levinson HJ, Halloran LG, et al: Limited indications for unilateral aortofemoral or iliofemoral vascular grafts. Arch Surg 107:791, 1973.
127. Kram HB, Gupta SK, Veith FJ, et al: Unilateral aortofemoral bypass: A safe and effective option for the treatment of unilateral limb-threatening ischemia. Am J Surg 162:155, 1991.
128. van den Dungen JJAM, Boontje AH, Kropveld A: Unilateral iliofemoral occlusive disease: Long-term results of the semiclosed endarterectomy with the ringstripper. J Vasc Surg 14:673, 1991.
129. Ascer E, Veith FJ, Gupta SK, et al: Comparison of axillounifemoral and axillobifemoral bypass operations. Surgery 97:169, 1985.
130. Brener BJ, Brief DK, Alpert J, et al: Femorofemoral bypass: A twenty-five year experience. *In* Yao JST, Pearce WH (eds): Long-term Results in Vascular Surgery. Norwalk, Conn, Appleton & Lange, 1993, pp 385–393.
131. Brief DK, Brener BJ, Alpert J, et al: Crossover femorofemoral grafts followed up five years or more: An analysis. Arch Surg 110:1294, 1975.
132. Dick LS, Brief DK, Alpert J, et al: A twelve-year experience with femorofemoral crossover grafts. Arch Surg 115:1359, 1980.
133. Eugene J, Goldstone J, Moore WS: Fifteen-year experience with subcutaneous bypass grafts for lower extremity ischemia. Ann Surg 186:177, 1977.
134. Kalman PG, Hosang M, Johnston KW, et al: The current role for femorofemoral bypass. J Vasc Surg 6:71, 1987.
135. Couch NP, Clowes AW, Whittemore AD, et al: The iliac-origin arterial graft: A useful alternative for iliac occlusive disease. Surgery 97:83, 1985.
136. Kalman PG, Hosang M, Johnston KW, et al: Unilateral iliac disease: The role of iliofemoral graft. J Vasc Surg 6:139, 1987.
137. Cham C, Myers KA, Scott DF, et al: Extraperitoneal unilateral iliac artery bypass for chronic limb ischemia. Aust N Z J Surg 58:859, 1988.
138. Darling RC III, Leather RP, Chang BB, et al: Is the iliac artery a suitable inflow conduit for iliofemoral occlusive disease? An analysis of 514 aorto-iliac reconstructions. J Vasc Surg 17:15, 1993.
139. Perler BA, Burdick JF, Williams M: Femoro-femoral or ilio-femoral bypass for unilateral inflow reconstruction? Am J Surg 161:426, 1991.
140. Ricco JB: Unilateral iliac artery occlusive disease: A randomized multicenter trial examining direct revascularization versus crossover bypass. Ann Vasc Surg 6:209, 1992.
141. Brener BJ, Eisenbud DE, Brief DK, et al: Utility of femorofemoral crossover grafts. *In* Bergan JJ, Yao JST (eds): Aortic Surgery. Philadelphia, WB Saunders, 1989, pp 423–438.
142. Taylor LM Jr, Freimanis IE, Edwards JM, et al: Extraperitoneal iliac endarterectomy in the treatment of multilevel lower extremity arterial occlusive disease. Am J Surg 152:34, 1986.
143. Vitale GF, Inahara T: Extraperitoneal endarterectomy for iliofemoral occlusive disease. J Vasc Surg 12:409, 1990.
144. Tollefson DFJ, Ernst CB: Natural history of atherosclerotic renal artery stenosis associated with aortic disease. J Vasc Surg 14:327, 1991.
145. Zierler RE, Bergelin RO, Isaacson JA, Strandress DE Jr: Natural history of atherosclerotic renal artery stenosis: A prospective study with duplex ultrasonography. J Vasc Surg 19:250, 1994.
146. Dean RH, Keyser JE III, Dupont WD, et al: Aortic and renal vascular disease: Factors affecting the value of combined procedures. Ann Surg 200:336, 1984.
147. Tarazi RY, Hertzer NR, Beven EG: Simultaneous aortic reconstruction and renal revascularization: Risk factors and late results in eighty-nine patients. J Vasc Surg 5:707, 1987.
148. Brewster DC, Buth J, Darling RC, et al: Combined aortic and renal artery reconstruction. Am J Surg 131:457, 1976.
149. Cambria RP, Brewster DC, L'Italien G, et al: Simultaneous aortic and renal artery reconstruction: Evaluation of an eighteen-year experience. J Vasc Surg 21:916, 1995.
150. Chaikof, EL, Smith RB III, Salam AA, et al: Empirical reconstruction of the renal artery: Long-term outcome. J Vasc Surg 24:406, 1996.
151. Connolly JE, Kwaan JHM: Prophylactic revascularization of the gut. Ann Surg 190:514, 1979.
152. Brewster DC, Darling RC: Splenorenal arterial anastomosis for renovascular hypertension. Ann Surg 189:353, 1979.
153. Moncure AC, Brewster DC, Darling RC, et al: Use of the splenic and hepatic arteries for renal revascularization. J Vasc Surg 3:196, 1986.
154. Brewster DC, Moncure AC: Hepatic and splenic artery for renal revascularization. *In* Bergan JJ, Yao JST (eds): Arterial Surgery: New Diagnostic and Operative Techniques. Orlando, Fla, Grune & Stratton, 1988, pp 389–405.
155. Criado E, Johnson G Jr, Burnham SJ, et al: Descending thoracic aorta-to-iliofemoral artery bypass as an alternative to aortoiliac reconstruction. J Vasc Surg 15:550, 1992.
156. McCarthy WJ, Mesh CL, McMillan WD, et al: Descending thoracic aorta-to-femoral artery bypass: Ten years' experience with a durable procedure. J Vasc Surg 17:336, 1993.
157. Baird RJ, Ropchan GV, Oates TK, et al: Ascending aorta to bifemoral bypass—a ventral aorta. J Vasc Surg 3:405, 1986.
158. Canepa CS, Schubart PJ, Taylor LM Jr, Porter JM: Supraceliac aortofemoral bypass. Surgery 101:323, 1987.
159. Brewster DC: Complications of aortic and lower extremity procedures. *In* Strandness DE Jr, van Breda A (eds): Vascular Diseases: Surgical and Interventional Therapy. New York, Churchill Livingstone, 1994, pp 1151–1177.
160. Brener BJ, Darling RC, Frederick PL, et al: Major venous anomalies complicating abdominal aortic surgery. Arch Surg 108:159, 1974.
161. Brewster DC: Reoperation for aortofemoral graft limb occlusion. *In* Veith F (ed): Current Critical Problems in Vascular Surgery. St. Louis, Quality Medical Publishing, 1989, pp 341–351.
162. Imparato AM: Abdominal aortic surgery: Prevention of lower limb ischemia. Surgery 93:112, 1983.
163. Starr DS, Lawrie GM, Morris GC Jr: Prevention of distal embolism during arterial reconstruction. Am J Surg 138:764, 1979.
164. Comerota AJ, White JV, Grosh JD: Intraoperative intraarterial thrombolytic therapy for salvage of limbs in patients with distal arterial thrombosis. Surg Gynecol Obstet 169:283, 1989.
165. Parent FN III, Bernhard VM, Pabst TS III, et al: Fibrinolytic treatment of residual thrombus after catheter embolectomy for severe lower limb ischemia. J Vasc Surg 9:153, 1989.
166. Diehl JT, Cali RF, Hertzer NR, et al: Complications of abdominal aortic reconstruction: An analysis of perioperative risk factors in 557 patients. Ann Surg 197:50, 1983.
167. Castronuovo JJ, Flanigan DP: Renal failure complicating vascular surgery. *In* Bernhard VM, Towne JB (eds): Complications in Vascular Surgery. Orlando, Fla, Grune & Stratton, 1985, pp 258–274.
168. Bush HL, Huse JB, Johnson WC, et al: Prevention of renal insufficiency after abdominal aortic aneurysm resection by optimal volume loading. Arch Surg 116:1517, 1981.
169. Brewster DC, Franklin DP, Cambria RP, et al: Intestinal ischemia complicating abdominal aortic surgery. Surgery 109:447, 1991.
170. Bjorck M, Bergqvist D, Troeng T: Incidence and clinical presentation of bowel ischemia after aortoiliac surgery: 2930 operations from a population-based registry in Sweden. Eur J Vasc Endovasc Surg 12:139, 1996.
171. Seeger JM, Doe DA, Kaelin LD, et al: Routine reimplantation of patent inferior mesenteric arteries limits colon infarction after aortic reconstruction. J Vasc Surg 15:635, 1992.
172. Bergman RT, Gloviczki, Welch TJ, et al: The role of intravenous fluorescein in the detection of colon ischemia during aortic reconstruction. Ann Vasc Surg 6:74, 1992.
173. Szilagyi DE, Hageman JH, Smith RF, et al: Spinal cord damage in surgery of the abdominal aorta. Surgery 83:38, 1978.
174. Iliopoulos JI, Howanitz PE, Pierce GE, et al: The critical hypogastric circulation. Am J Surg 154:671, 1987.
175. Elliott JP, Szilagyi DE, Hageman JH, et al: Spinal cord ischemia:

Secondary to surgery of the abdominal aorta. *In* Bernhard VM, Towne JB (eds): Complications in Vascular Surgery. Orlando, Fla, Grune & Stratton, 1985, pp 291–310.

176. McCarthy WJ, Flinn WR, Carter MF, et al: Prevention and management of urologic injuries during aortic surgery. *In* Bergan JJ, Yao JST (eds): Aortic Surgery. Philadelphia, WB Saunders, 1989, pp 539–546.
177. Egeblad K, Brochner-Mortensen J, Krarup T, et al: Incidence of ureteral obstruction after aortic grafting: A prospective analysis. Surgery 103:411, 1988.
178. Schubart P, Fortner G, Cummings D, et al: The significance of hydronephrosis after aortofemoral reconstruction. Arch Surg 120:377, 1985.
179. Wright DJ, Ernst CB, Evans JR, et al: Ureteral complications and aortoiliac reconstruction. J Vasc Surg 11:29, 1990.
180. van der Akker PJ, van Schilfgaarde R, Brand R, et al: Long term success of aortoiliac operation for arteriosclerotic obstructive disease. Surg Gynecol Obstet 174:485, 1992.
181. Brewster DC, Meier GH, Darling RC, et al: Reoperation for aortofemoral graft limb occlusion: Optimal methods and long term results. J Vasc Surg 5:363, 1987.
182. Brewster DC: Surgery of late aortic graft occlusion. *In* Bergan JJ, Yao JST (eds): Aortic Surgery. Philadelphia, WB Saunders, 1989, pp 519–538.
183. Nevelsteen A, Suy R: Graft occlusion following aortofemoral Dacron bypass. Ann Vasc Surg 5:32, 1991.
184. Bernhard VM, Ray LI, Towne JB: The reoperation of choice for aortofemoral graft occlusion. Surgery 82:867, 1977.
185. Wray R, DePalma RG, Hunay CH: Late occlusion of aortofemoral bypass grafts: Influence of cigarette smoking. Surgery 70:969, 1971.
186. Greenhalgh RM, Laing SP, Cole PV, et al: Smoking and arterial reconstruction. Br J Surg 68:605, 1981.
187. Robicsek F, Daugherty HK, Mullen DC, et al: The effect of continued cigarette smoking on the patency of synthetic vascular grafts in Leriche syndrome. J Thorac Cardiovasc Surg 70:107, 1975.
188. Provan JL, Sojka SG, Murnaghan JJ, et al: The effect of cigarette smoking on the long term success rates of aortofemoral and femoropopliteal reconstructions. Surg Gynecol Obstet 165:49, 1987.
189. Myers KA, King BB, Scott DF, et al: Effect of smoking on the late patency of arterial reconstructions in the legs. Br J Surg 65:267, 1978.
190. Nolan KD, Benjamin ME, Murphy TJ, et al: Femorofemoral bypass for aortofemoral graft limb occlusion: A ten-year experience. J Vasc Surg 19:851, 1994.
191. Ernst CB, Daugherty ME: Removal of a thrombotic plug from an occluded limb of an aortofemoral graft. Arch Surg 113:301, 1978.
192. Brewster DC: Aortic graft limb occlusion. *In* Ernst CB, Stanley JC (eds): Current Therapy in Vascular Surgery, 3rd ed. St. Louis, Mosby–Year Book, 1995, pp 419–26.
193. Edwards WH, Jenkins JM, Mulherin JL, et al: Extended profundaplasty to minimize pelvic and distal tissue loss. Ann Surg 211:694, 1990.
194. Sterpetti AV, Feldhaus RJ, Schultz RD: Combined aortofemoral and extended deep femoral artery reconstruction. Arch Surg 123:1269, 1988.
195. Ouriel K, DeWeese JA, Ricotta JJ, et al: Revascularization of the distal profunda femoris artery in the reconstructive treatment of aortoiliac occlusive disease. J Vasc Surg 6:217, 1987.
196. Charlesworth D: The occluded aortic and aortofemoral graft. *In* Bergan JJ, Yao JST (eds): Reoperative Arterial Surgery. Orlando, Fla, Grune & Stratton, 1986, pp 271–278.
197. Szilagyi DE, Smith RF, Elliott JP, et al: Anastomotic aneurysms after vascular reconstruction: Problems of incidence, etiology, and treatment. Surgery 78:800, 1975.
198. Satiani B: False aneurysms following arterial reconstruction: Collective review. Surg Gynecol Obstet 152:357, 1981.
199. Edwards JM, Teefey SA, Zierler RE, et al: Intraabdominal paraanastomotic aneurysms after aortic bypass grafting. J Vasc Surg 15:344, 1991.
200. Schellack J, Salam A, Abouzeid MA, et al: Femoral anastomotic aneurysms: A continuing challenge. J Vasc Surg 6:308, 1987.
201. Goldstone J: Anastomotic aneurysms. *In* Bernhard VM, Towne JB (eds): Complications in Vascular Surgery. St. Louis, Quality Medical Publishing, 1991, pp 87–99.
202. Ernst CB, Elliott JP Jr, Ryan CH, et al: Recurrent femoral anastomotic aneurysms: A 30-year experience. Ann Surg 208:401, 1988.
203. Seabrook GR, Schmitt DD, Bandyk DF, et al: Anastomotic femoral pseudoaneurysm: An investigation of occult infection as an etiologic factor. J Vasc Surg 11:629, 1990.
204. Kempczinski RF: Impotence following aortic surgery. *In* Bernhard VM, Towne JB (eds): Complications in Vascular Surgery. St. Louis, Quality Medical Publishing, 1991, pp 160–171.
205. Weinstein MH, Machleder HI: Sexual function after aorto-iliac surgery. Ann Surg 181:787, 1975.
206. DePalma RG, Levine SB, Feldman S: Preservation of erectile function after aortoiliac reconstruction. Arch Surg 113:958, 1978.
207. Cronenwett JL, Gooch JB, Garrett HE: Internal iliac artery revascularization during aortofemoral bypass. Arch Surg 117:838, 1982.
208. Flanigan DP, Sobinsky KR, Schuler JJ, et al: Internal iliac artery revascularization in the treatment of vasculogenic impotence. Arch Surg 120:271, 1985.
209. Moore WS, Cole CW: Infection in prosthetic vascular grafts. *In* Moore WS (ed): Vascular Surgery: A Comprehensive Review, 3rd ed. Philadelphia, WB Saunders, 1991, pp 598–609.
210. Bandyk DF: Aortic graft infection. Semin Vasc Surg 3:122, 1990.
211. O'Hara PJ, Hertzer NR, Beven EG, et al: Surgical management of infected abdominal aortic grafts: Review of a 25-year experience. J Vasc Surg 3:725, 1986.
212. Rubin JR, Malone JM, Goldstone J: The role of the lymphatic system in acute arterial prosthetic graft infections. J Vasc Surg 2:92, 1985.
213. Piotrowski JJ, Bernhard VM: Management of vascular graft infections. *In* Bernhard VM, Towne JB (eds): Complications in Vascular Surgery. St. Louis, Quality Medical Publishing, 1991, pp 235–258.
214. Reilly LM, Altman H, Lusby RJ, et al: Late results following surgical management of vascular graft infection. J Vasc Surg 1:36, 1984.
215. Quinones-Baldrich WJ, Hernandez JJ, Moore WS: Long-term results following surgical management of aortic graft infection. Arch Surg 126:507, 1991.
216. Yeager RA, Moneta GL, Taylor LM, et al: Improving survival and limb salvage in patients with aortic graft infection. Am J Surg 159:466, 1990.
217. Schmitt DD, Seabrook GR, Bandyk DF, et al: Graft excision and extraanatomic revascularization: The treatment of choice for the septic aortic prosthesis. J Cardiovasc Surg 31:327, 1990.
218. Sharp WJ, Hoballah JJ, Mohan CR, et al. The management of the infected aortic prosthesis: A current decade of experience. J Vasc Surg 19:844, 1994.
219. Reilly LM, Stoney RJ, Goldstone J, et al: Improved management of aortic graft infection: The influence of operation sequence and staging. J Vasc Surg 5:421, 1987.
220. Trout HH III, Kozloff L, Giordano JM: Priority of revascularization in patients with graft enteric fistulas, infected arteries, or infected arterial prostheses. Ann Surg 199:669, 1984.
221. Kwann JWM, Connolly JB: Successful management of prosthetic graft infection with continuous povidone-iodine irrigation. Arch Surg 116:716, 1981.
222. Calligaro KD, Veith FJ, Gupta SK, et al: A modified method for management of prosthetic graft infections involving an anastomosis to the common femoral artery. J Vasc Surg 11:485, 1990.
223. Calligaro KD, DeLaurentis DA, Schwartz, ML, et al: Selective preservation of infected prosthetic arterial grafts: Analysis of a 20 year experience with 120 extracavitary infected grafts. Ann Surg 220:461, 1994.
224. Mixter RC, Turnipseed WD, Smith DJ Jr, et al: Rotational muscle flaps: A new technique for covering infected vascular grafts. J Vasc Surg 9:472, 1989.
225. Perler BA, VanderKolk CA, Manson PM, Williams GM: Rotational muscle flaps to treat prosthetic graft infection: Long-term follow-up. J Vasc Surg 18:358, 1993.
226. Clagett GP, Valentine RJ, Hagino RT: Autogenous aortoiliac/femoral reconstruction from superficial femoral-popliteal veins: Feasibility and durability. J Vasc Surg 25:255, 1997.
227. Bernhard VM: Aortoenteric fistula. *In* Bernhard VM, Towne JB (eds): Complications in Vascular Surgery. Orlando, Fla, Grune & Stratton, 1985, pp 513–525.
228. Connolly JE, Kwaan JHM, McCart PM, et al: Aortoenteric fistula. Ann Surg 194:402, 1981.
229. Perdue GD Jr, Smith RB III, Ansley JD, et al: Impending aortoenteric hemorrhage: The effect of early recognition on improved outcome. Ann Surg 192:237, 1980.

230. Reilly LM, Ehrenfeld WK, Goldstone J, et al: Gastrointestinal tract involvement by prosthetic graft infection: The significance of gastrointestinal hemorrhage. Ann Surg 202:342, 1985.
231. Seeger JM, Wheeler JR, Gregory RT, et al: Autogenous graft replacement of infected prosthetic graft in the femoral position. Surgery 93:39, 1983.
232. Walker WE, Cooley DA, Duncan JM, et al: The management of aortoduodenal fistula by in situ replacement of the infected abdominal aortic graft. Ann Surg 205:727, 1987.
233. Bandyk DF, Bergamini TM, Kinney EV, et al: In situ replacement of vascular prostheses infected by bacterial biofilms. J Vasc Surg 13:575, 1991.
234. Robinson AJ, Johansen K: Aortic sepsis: Is there a role for in situ graft replacement? J Vasc Surg 13:677, 1991.
235. Jacobs MJHM, Reul G, Gregoric I, et al: In-situ replacement and extraanatomic bypass for the treatment of infected abdominal aortic grafts. Eur J Vasc Surg 5:83, 1991.
236. Kieffer E, Bahnini A, Koskas F, et al: In situ allograft replacement of infected infrarenal aortic prosthetic grafts: Results in 43 patients. J Vasc Surg 17:349, 1993.

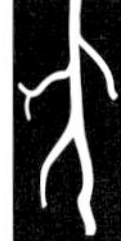

CHAPTER 67

Thromboendarterectomy for Lower Extremity Arterial Occlusive Disease

Eric S. Weinstein, M.D., and
William C. Krupski, M.D.

Since J. C. dos Santos introduced thromboendarterectomy in 1947[1] for the treatment of arteriosclerosis of peripheral arteries and Wylie and coworkers applied it to occlusive disease of the aortoiliac segment in 1951,[2] indications for this technique in the treatment of lower extremity ischemia have changed significantly. Initially, thromboendarterectomy was the procedure of choice for patients with peripheral vascular occlusive disease, but the advent of bypass techniques and the development of prosthetic grafts led to a marked decline in the number of surgeons performing these technically demanding procedures.[3–6] Indeed, the decline in the number of surgeons familiar with these techniques was one of the arguments used to justify the development of vascular surgical training programs in the 1970s.[7]

With the more recent development of endovascular stenting and atherectomy, thromboendarterectomy as a primary procedure in the treatment of lower extremity ischemic disease has been indicated less frequently. However, the advantages of autogenous vascular reconstruction, as well as its utility as an adjunctive technique for patients requiring both aortoiliac and infrainguinal revascularization, continues to make thromboendarterectomy an essential component of the vascular surgeon's armamentarium (Fig. 67–1).

ANATOMIC CONSIDERATIONS

For the surgeon performing endarterectomy, a basic understanding of arterial wall anatomy and the pathology of atherosclerosis is necessary. The normal arterial wall is composed of three layers; from the lumen outward these are (1) the intima, (2) the media, and (3) the adventitia.[8]

The intima extends from the endothelial cells that line the lumen of the vessel to the *internal elastic lamina* (IEL). Extending from the outer surface of the IEL to the inner surface of the *external elastic lamina* (EEL), the media con-

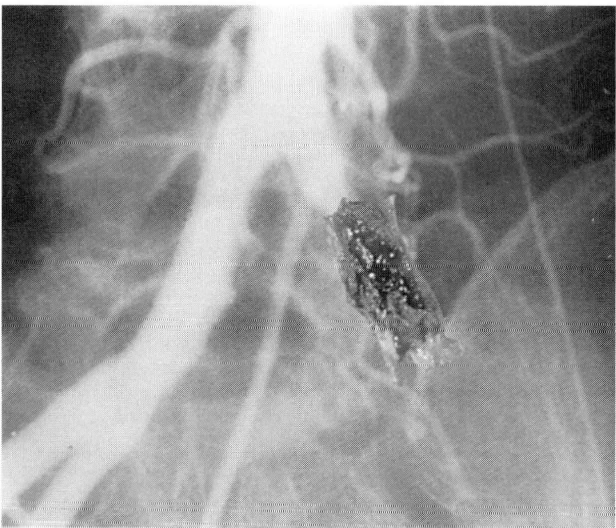

FIGURE 67–1. Aortogram with superimposed left iliac lesion removed by endarterectomy. This short lesion is ideal for thromboendarterectomy; note virtual absence of atherosclerotic occlusive disease on the right. (Courtesy of Anthony Comerata, M.D., Philadelphia, Pa.)

tains two muscular layers consisting of inner circular and outer longitudinally arranged muscle fibers. The EEL marks the beginning of the adventitia, which is composed of connective tissue and the vasa vasorum.

Atherosclerosis initially begins as a disease of the intima, with low-density lipoproteins (LDLs) accumulating within a thin acellular layer, rich in proteoglycans, that lies between the endothelial cells and the IEL. Several theories involving intimal injury, hemodynamic sheer stress, and disorders of lipid metabolism have been advanced to explain this "fatty streak," which some authorities believe is the earliest lesion of atherosclerosis.[8] Tissue macrophages (monocytes) that have migrated from the circulation into the intima esterify and incorporate these lipids, forming foam cells—the characteristic cells of atherosclerotic plaques. As the plaque matures, smooth muscle cells proliferate and collagen deposition occurs, producing the *fibrous plaque*, which also contains extracellular lipid and necrotic debris. As this process advances, calcium accumulates within the plaque, which then extends into the media, disrupting the IEL. Neovascularization of the plaque may occur from the lumen or from the vasa vasorum. Ulceration occurs when the fibrous plaque ruptures.[9]

Three natural cleavage planes exist within muscular arteries: (1) subintimal, (2) transmedial, and (3) subadventitial.[10]

The subintimal cleavage plane is found just outside the internal elastic lamina. The transmedial plane is found between the inner three quarters and outer one quarter of the media, separating the circular and longitudinal muscle fibers. The third cleavage plane separates the adventitia and the media along the inner surface of the external elastic lamina. The nature and extent of the specific atherosclerotic plaque influence the proper cleavage plane for endarterectomy and is determined at the time of operation, but the transmedial plane is optimal. Generally, the subintimal cleavage plane should be avoided because of its association with a higher incidence of postoperative thrombosis, and the subadventitial plane may leave the vessel dangerously attenuated.[10]

The characteristic segmental distribution of atherosclerotic lesions within the aorta and peripheral arteries permits the technique of thromboendarterectomy. Success of the procedure depends on the precise termination of the thromboendarterectomy at the transition zone between normal and diseased intima. This "end-point" needs to be created without disturbing the normal intima in order to prevent the possibility of subintimal dissection by flowing blood, which can produce early postoperative occlusion. Late patency of the endarterectomy is ensured by preservation of adequate inflow and outflow vessels and removal of the entire plaque.[11] Despite the dramatic changes in arterial wall anatomy resulting from endarterectomy, these attenuated vessels can hold sutures and withstand arterial pressure. An increase in arterial wall compliance does occur, but the collagen fibers concentrated in the outer layers of the vessel provide a high degree of elastic stiffness in these arteries[12] and accounts for the low incidence of aneurysmal degeneration seen in large clinical series.[3, 6, 13]

PATTERNS OF ATHEROSCLEROSIS

During the planning of therapeutic interventions for patients with lower extremity arterial insufficiency, it is essential to classify patterns of atherosclerotic involvement as (1) *inflow* arterial disease (aorta, iliac, and femoral arteries) or (2) *outflow* arterial disease (femoral, popliteal, and tibial arteries).

Inflow Disease

Patterns of obstructive atherosclerotic disease affecting the inflow arteries are classically divided into two types. Patients with *type I* disease have atherosclerotic involvement of the infrarenal aorta, the common iliac artery, and the internal iliac artery. Except for the proximal 1 to 2 cm of the external iliac arteries, the remainder of these vessels and the femoral arteries are free of disease. The outflow vessels are also normal unless there has been earlier atheroembolization from the proximal lesions (Fig. 67–2). *Type II* disease includes the type I pattern in addition to involvement of the external iliac arteries and common femoral bifurcations. Often there is diffuse disease of the infrainguinal vessels as well (Fig. 67–3).[11] Type II disease is more common than type I (in a 4:1 ratio) and affects men more often than women (male-to-female ratio for type II, 5:1; male-female ratio for type I, 2:1).

On average, type II patients are 7 years older than type I patients.[14] Because data on the relative incidences of disease patterns have been obtained from symptomatic patients, usually with advanced disease, the true patterns of involvement in the general population may not be known.[15]

Outflow Disease

Like inflow disease, atherosclerotic involvement of the infrainguinal vessels may be *segmental* or *diffuse*. Diffuse atherosclerosis of the outflow vessels with or without inflow disease is more common in patients with strict indications for revascularization. Although segmental occlusive disease is common in the general population, it is often clinically silent or may produce only mild symptoms. However, segmental occlusive disease can produce symptoms severe enough to warrant revascularization if it occurs acutely or in the absence of adequate collateral blood vessels. The superficial femoral artery is the most frequent lower extremity vessel to be involved with segmental occlusive disease, but isolated involvement of the common femoral artery, the profunda femoris artery (deep femoral artery), or the popliteal artery may occur.[16]

CLINICAL PRESENTATION

Claudication is the presenting symptom in most patients with type I disease. The entire leg (buttock, hip, thigh, and calf) or just a portion of it (buttock and thigh alone or calf alone) may be involved. Claudication is also a presenting symptom in patients with type II disease, but usually symptoms are more severe. Manifestations of advanced ischemia (e.g., rest pain, nonhealing ulceration, gangrene) imply concomitant femoral, popliteal, or tibial artery occlusive disease, or *multilevel disease*. Tissue loss is usually absent in patients with type I disease unless atheroembolization has occurred. Impotence may be noted in up to 40% of men with either type I or II disease as a result of hypoperfusion of the internal iliac arteries.[14]

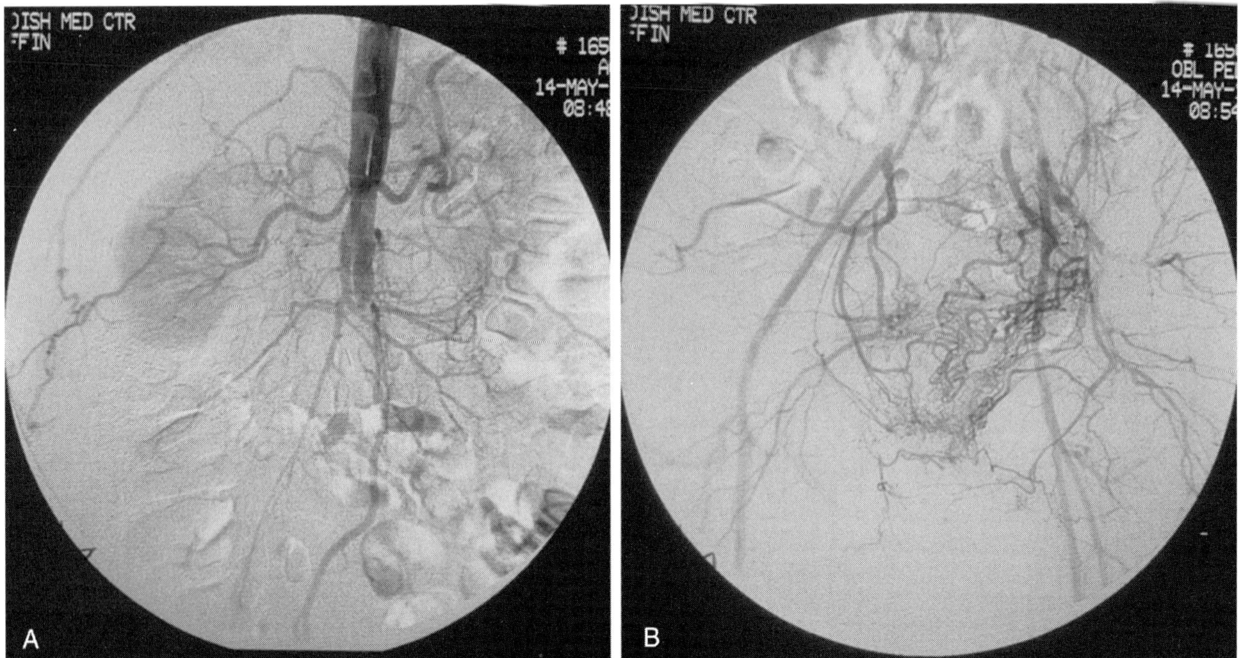

FIGURE 67–2. Digital subtraction aortogram performed via a transaxillary approach in a patient with type I aortoiliac disease. *A*, Occluded aorta just below the inferior mesenteric artery. *B*, Reconstitution of iliac artery bifurcations with external iliac arteries free of disease.

Calf claudication is the predominant symptom in patients with infrainguinal atherosclerosis that is amenable to thromboendarterectomy. Extensive tissue loss and limb-threatening ischemia is often the result of multilevel disease, which is not well treated by this technique alone, because pulsatile blood flow must be restored all the way to the foot in the presence of infrageniculate popliteal or tibial occlusive disease. However, early manifestations of limb-threatening ischemia (e.g., ischemic rest pain, superficial ulceration) may occasionally result from suprageniculate occlusive disease, which may respond to either localized or extensive endarterectomy.

A detailed history and physical examination are mandatory to identify systemic and end-organ manifestations of atherosclerotic disease and to determine the specific risks of therapeutic intervention. Noninvasive vascular assessment is always performed to document the severity of ischemia and to help identify the particular pattern of disease. Segmental pressures, ankle-brachial indices (ABIs), and arterial pulse volume waveform analyses at rest and with exercise or reactive hyperemia are the initial diagnostic studies for identifying and unmasking hemodynamically significant lesions in the aortoiliac and infrainguinal vasculature.

In cases of profunda femoris artery occlusive disease, the functional capacity of the collateral vessels between the profunda and the popliteal-tibial runoff vessels can be determined. Calculation of a *profunda-popliteal collateral index* (PPCI) may be useful in predicting the success of indirect revascularizations of asymptomatic extremity as follows:

$$\text{PPCI} = \frac{\text{above-knee systolic BP} - \text{below knee systolic BP}}{\text{above-knee systolic BP}}$$

where BP = blood pressure.

A low index (<0.25) indicates satisfactory collateral capacity to carry blood beyond a superficial femoral artery occlusion (see Chapter 66).[17]

Advances in duplex ultrasonography have made complete arterial mapping from the juxtarenal aorta to the ankles possible and may eventually replace the need for arteriography.[18, 19] For now, however, biplanar arteriography remains the gold standard for assessing disease patterns and collateral circulation. Coupled with intra-arterial pressure monitoring and provocative testing with intra-arterial vasodilators, these studies can provide both anatomic and hemodynamic assessment of the arterial anatomy. Although the diagnosis and quantification of the severity of occlusive disease can be determined noninvasively, arteriography may be particularly useful in cases of atheroembolization by identifying mildly stenotic nonhemodynamic ulcerative lesions that may be the source of distal emboli.

OPERATIVE INDICATIONS

The threshold for invasive intervention in patients with lower extremity arterial insufficiency caused by aortoiliac disease is somewhat lower than in patients with infrainguinal disease alone. Revascularization in this group of patients is generally undertaken for the treatment of moderate to severe claudication that has not improved with conservative therapy. There are several reasons for this. Because the onset of aortoiliac occlusive disease occurs in the fifth and sixth decades of life before patients have retired from work, claudication may produce significant occupational and lifestyle limitations. In addition, vasculogenic impotence may be an indication for intervention in men in this age group.[11] Patients with aortoiliac atherosclerosis that progresses to aortic occlusion may be at risk for proximal propagation of thrombus with subsequent renal or visceral artery occlusions. Although the true incidence of this event in the natural history of aortic occlusion is unknown, coexistent renal or visceral arterial stenoses may increase the risk of aortic occlusion.[20] As previously noted, patients with aortoiliac occlusive disease may present with digital artery occlusions and limb threat as a result of atheroembolization, or the "blue toe syndrome." Aortoiliac endarterectomy can effectively remove the source of the atheroemboli. Limb-threatening ischemia may also be present in patients with type II disease in whom there is concomitant infrainguinal occlusive disease. In this setting, restoration of inflow alone may be inadequate for limb salvage, and an outflow procedure may be required to restore pulsatile blood flow to the foot.

Patients with atherosclerosis of the femoropopliteal arteries also may present with either claudication or limb-threatening ischemia (e.g., rest pain, nonhealing ulcer, gangrene). Although most authorities agree that revascularization is indicated for such conditions, much debate remains with respect to treatment of patients in this category who have only claudication. Indeed, the controversy has increased with the advent of "less invasive" treatments for atherosclerotic lesions by interventional radiologists. We recommend a conservative approach and treat only patients with this pattern of disease who have limb-threatening or truly *incapacitating* claudication (i.e., the ability to walk less than one block).

Aneurysmal dilatation of the aorta or iliac arteries is the only absolute contraindication to aortoiliac endarterectomy because it is a result of a degenerative process within the media of the vessel and invariably leads to postoperative aneurysm formation.[14] Extensive plaque calcification is a contraindication for the use of closed or semiclosed techniques for either aortoiliac or femoropopliteal endarterectomy because it makes establishing an appropriate cleavage plane for long segment occlusions nearly impossible and leads either to vessel perforation or to inadequate removal of the plaque.[21]

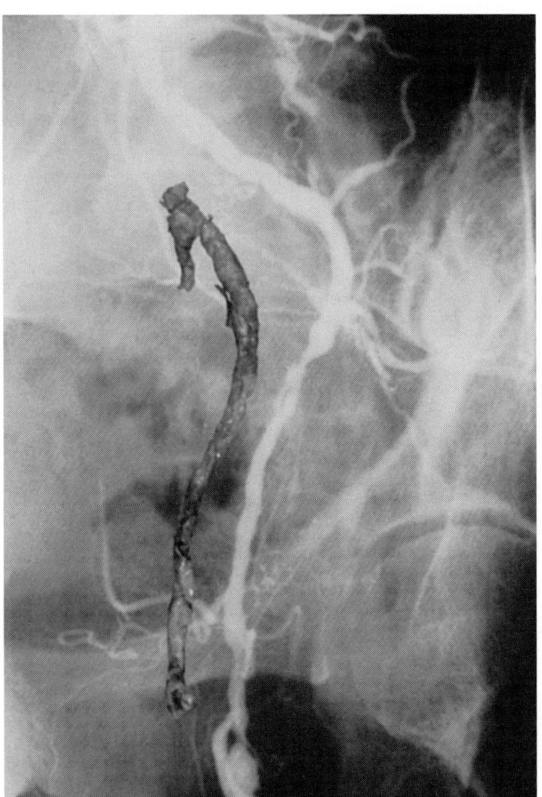

FIGURE 67–3. Aortogram showing type II aortoiliac disease with the endarterectomy specimen superimposed. The atherosclerotic changes in the common femoral bifurcation are often present in type II disease. (Courtesy of Anthony Comerata, M.D., Philadelphia, Pa.)

OPERATIVE TECHNIQUES

Two basic techniques of endarterectomy—*open* and *semi-closed*[10]—may be utilized for aortoiliac or aortoiliofemoral thromboendarterectomy.

Open Technique

The open endarterectomy technique requires that the entire length of the diseased vessel be exposed. A longitudinal arteriotomy is made that extends slightly distal and proximal to the plaque to ensure visualization of the end-points of the endarterectomy. The cleavage plane is directly visualized for the length of the lesion, and with the use of dissectors, the plaque is separated from the arterial wall. A transition zone is usually present at the distal end-point of the plaque, where it tapers to a more superficial cleavage plane. Occasionally, the surgeon must fashion this end-point using a Beaver blade in order to achieve plaque separation. Interrupted tacking mattress sutures may be necessary at the distal end-point to prevent dissection after restoration of blood flow. Autogenous material may be used for patch angioplasty in a longitudinal arteriotomy in a relatively small vessel, in which primary closure would lead to significant vessel narrowing.

Semi-closed Technique

Arteriotomies (longitudinal or transverse) are made at the proximal and distal margins of the plaque. End-points are fashioned through these arteriotomies much as they are in the open technique. Ringed arterial strippers are then placed around the plaque and advanced into the intervening arterial segments. Extensive dissection of the diseased arteries facilitates passage of the ringed strippers by allowing for external circumferential palpation of the vessel along its entire length. This ensures the maintenance of the proper cleavage plane during passage of the stripper and permits confirmation of removal of the entire plaque.

The semi-closed method has been modified by Inahara[7] for patients with type II disease undergoing aortoiliofemoral endarterectomy. In this procedure, the femoral artery is transected just above its bifurcation after the circumflex vessels have been divided. The artery is then mobilized beneath the inguinal ligament and brought into the pelvis, where *eversion thromboendarterectomy* techniques are used to remove the plaque. Once the plaque is removed, the vessel is restored to its proper orientation and is reanastomosed in end-to-end fashion.

Closed Technique

More recently, a third technique for endarterectomy has been described for use in patients with femoropopliteal occlusive disease. In this "closed" endarterectomy technique, the entire plaque is removed via a single incision in the femoral artery. A ring stripper-cutter device is passed down the artery under fluoroscopic guidance until the distal margin of the plaque is reached. The plaque is transected and removed in its entirety, and an intraluminal balloon-expandable stent is used to tack down the distal end-point.[22]

Inflow Disease

Type I Disease: Aortoiliac Endarterectomy

The surgeon dissects the aorta from the level of the renal arteries to the aortic bifurcation along its right anterolateral aspect in order to avoid injury to the autonomic nerve plexus that is adjacent to the left lateral aorta and the origin of the left common iliac artery, thereby preserving sexual function (Fig. 67–4). The inferior mesenteric and lumbar vessels are controlled to prevent back-bleeding during the procedure. Early in the dissection, the external iliac arteries should be palpated to determine whether aortoiliac thromboendarterectomy is feasible. If atherosclerotic plaque extends more than 2 cm beyond the iliac bifurcation, most authorities would abandon the procedure in favor of aortobifemoral bypass.

Distal control of the external iliac artery is obtained at the iliac bifurcation, and control of the internal iliac artery is achieved just beyond its first branch. Again, the surgeon takes care to avoid dissection at the origin of the left common iliac artery so as to prevent injury to the superior hypogastric nerve plexus. After systemic heparinization, atraumatic vascular clamps are placed proximally and distally. Bulldog clamps or vessel loops are placed on the lumbar arteries and the inferior mesenteric artery.

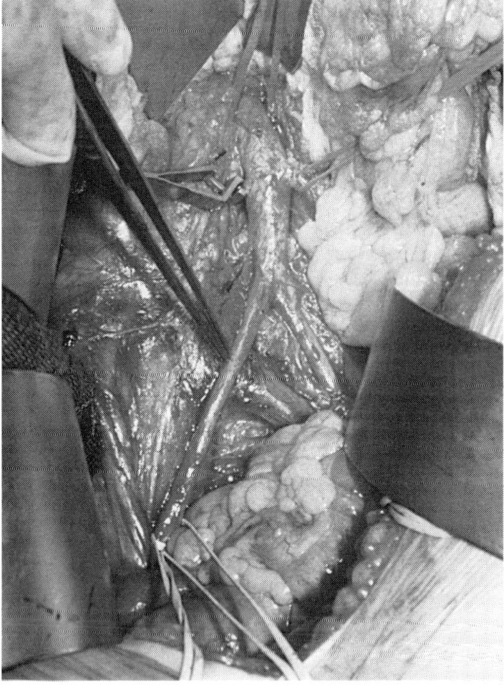

FIGURE 67–4. Operative photograph of patient depicted in Figure 67–1. Forceps point out the lengthy common iliac artery. Vessel loops around right internal and external iliac arteries and inferior mesenteric artery.

A longitudinal aortotomy just to the right of midline is made, extending from the level of the renal arteries to the aortic bifurcation (Fig. 67–5). The surgeon places transverse arteriotomies at each iliac bifurcation and creates end-points at the origins of the external iliac artery using a Beaver blade, carefully beveling the plaque so as to create a smooth transition to normal intima. The plaque is then gently separated from the common iliac vessel and dissected circumferentially. Division of the plaque at the origin of the internal iliac vessel helps to facilitate this maneuver. The remnant of plaque protruding into the internal iliac artery usually extends to its first branch point, and the surgeon may remove it by gently everting the proximal portion of this vessel. A ringed stripper is next advanced over the common iliac plaque and passed retrograde to the aortic bifurcation, where division of the plaque from the aortic component helps to ensure the entire removal of the common iliac plaque (Fig. 67–6). Open endarterectomy techniques are then used to remove the entire plaque from the infrarenal aorta (see Fig. 67–5*B*).

External and internal palpation of the arteries ensures the adequacy of the plaque removal. Any loose debris is removed, and the vessels are irrigated with heparinized saline solution. Tacking of the distal end-point in the external iliac artery is occasionally necessary and can be accomplished with fine, nonabsorbable vertical mattress sutures. The arteriotomies are closed, and flow is restored first into the pelvis and then distally into the lower extremities. In cases of aortic occlusion extending to the level of the renal arteries, individual control of each renal artery must be accomplished to prevent embolization and proximal aortic control is achieved just below the superior mesenteric artery. Removal of the first 5 cm of the aortic atheroma is performed so that the proximal aortotomy can be closed and the clamp lowered to an infrarenal position, thereby minimizing renal ischemia time.

Type II Disease: Aortoiliofemoral Endarterectomy

For some patients with type II inflow disease, application of endarterectomy for the external iliac arteries to the femoral bifurcations is appropriate. The small caliber of the external iliac vessels, their relative inaccessibility beneath the inguinal ligaments, and the adherent nature of the media in this location all make aortoiliofemoral endarterectomy technically demanding. The placement of the distal arteriotomy in these cases is determined by the status of the superficial femoral artery.

If the artery is patent, a transverse arteriotomy is made at the common femoral bifurcation and end-points are fashioned in much the same way as at the iliac artery bifurcation. If the artery is occluded, a longitudinal arteriotomy is made extending onto the profunda femoral artery in order to ensure the completeness of plaque removal and to visualize the distal end-point. (This situation often

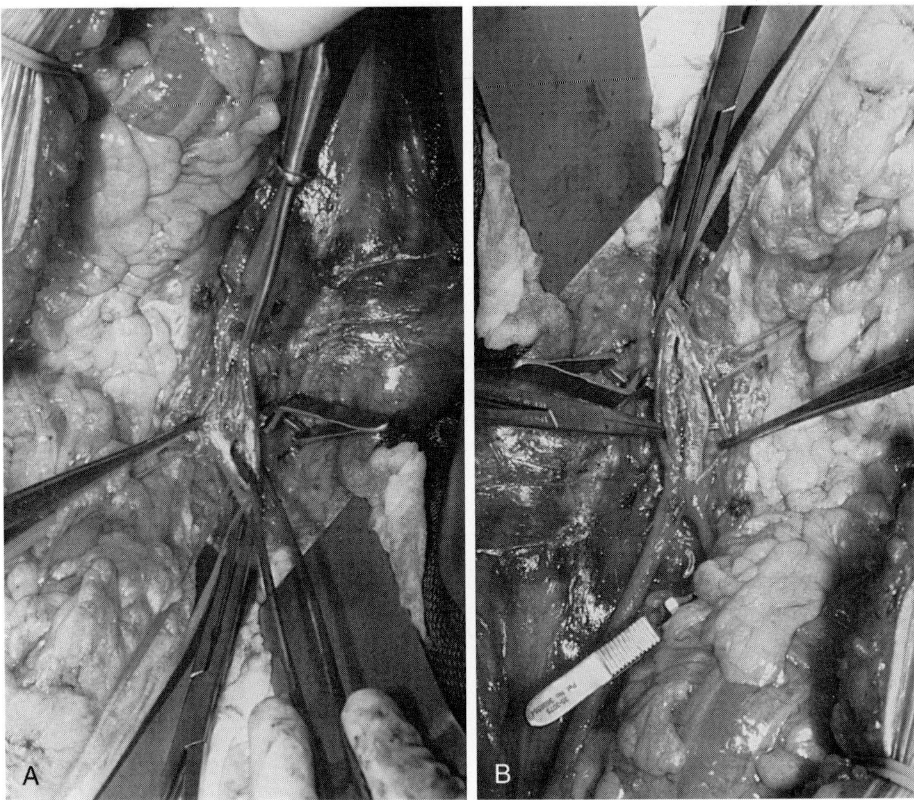

FIGURE 67–5. Open endarterectomy of aorta. *A*, Chronic aortic occlusion beginning at level of inferior mesenteric artery. *B*, Right-angled clamp passed behind plaque in transmedial plane.

calls for patch angioplasty closure using a segment of harvested endarterectomized superficial femoral artery.)

The plaque is dissected circumferentially and passed through the ringed stripper, which is advanced proximally to the common iliac arteriotomy. As described previously, Inhara[7] recommends transection of the artery at the femoral bifurcation, with mobilization of the external iliac artery beneath the inguinal ligament and eversion endarterectomy of this segment under direct vision.

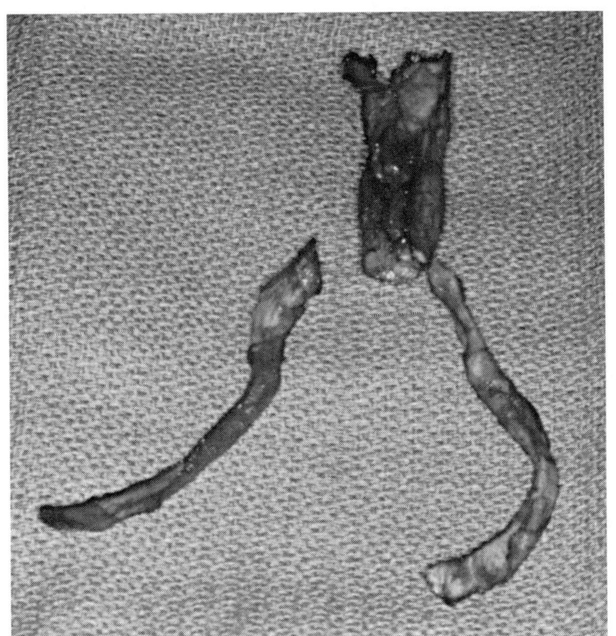

FIGURE 67–6. Operative specimen. Iliac plaques transected at aortic bifurcation to facilitate removal.

Infrainguinal Disease

Segmental Lesions

Localized outflow occlusive disease may affect the common femoral artery, the superficial femoral artery, the profunda femoris artery, or the popliteal arteries (Fig. 67–7). The approach to segmental lesions is similar in all of these vessels. Segmental occlusive disease is best treated with open techniques. The endarterectomy may be performed as the primary method of reconstruction or as a secondary procedure in association with a bypass in order to prepare the vessel as an inflow or recipient site.[23–28] The artery is isolated proximal and distal to the extent of the plaque, and branch vessels are controlled to prevent back-bleeding and allow for blind endarterectomy of their origins. A longitudinal arteriotomy is made long enough to ensure visualization of the distal end-point.

For common femoral artery disease, the patency of the superficial femoral artery and the extent of profunda femoris artery involvement determine the direction of the arteriotomy. If the superficial femoral artery is occluded, the incision on the common femoral artery is brought onto the origin of the profunda to ensure complete visualization of the plaque end-point. To prevent the creation of a blind stump in the origin of the superficial femoral artery and the potential for retrograde propagation of thrombus with the removal of the common femoral artery plaque, transection of the superficial femoral artery origin with suture

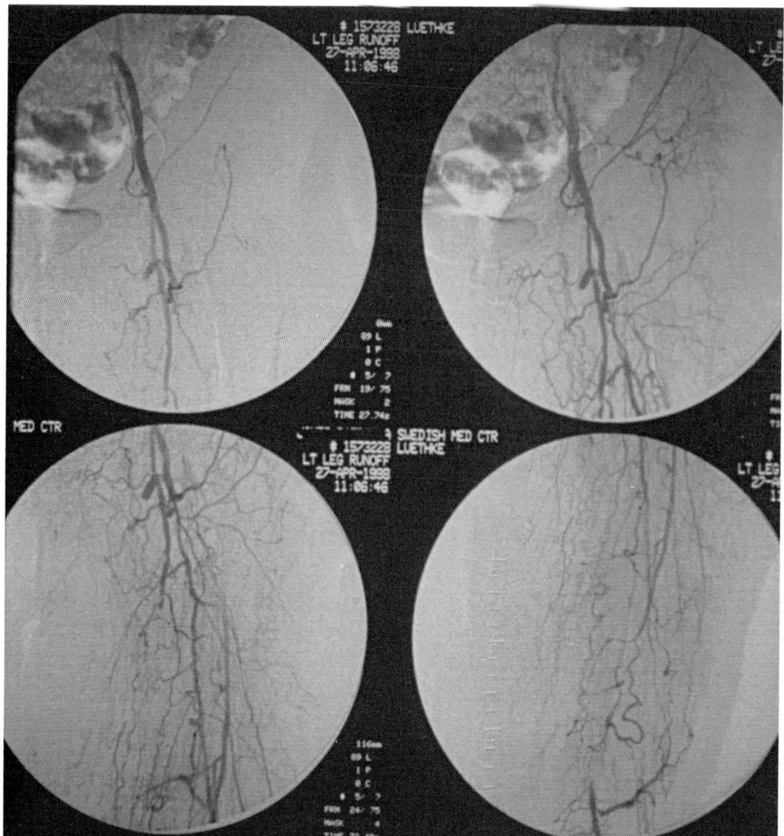

FIGURE 67–7. Digital subtraction arteriogram demonstrating segmental occlusion of the profunda femoris artery.

closure flush with the bifurcation is recommended.[24] The extent of common femoral artery plaque into the profunda femoris artery is often limited to the first profunda femoris artery branch point. When the superficial femoral artery is patent, the common femoral arteriotomy is brought on to the superficial femoral artery origin so that the surgeon might visualize the end-point in this vessel, and the profunda femoris artery origin is cleared by means of blind or eversion endarterectomy techniques.

If the diameter of the vessel is of sufficient size, primary closure may be performed. If the artery is too small to permit primary closure, a patch angioplasty using either a segment of saphenous vein or a segment of endarterectomized, occluded superficial femoral artery is recommended. If the endarterectomy is being performed in association with aortobifemoral bypass and the arteriotomy is short (<3 cm), the anastomosis may be brought onto the arteriotomy for an extended patch angioplasty; otherwise, a patch closure should be completed first and the anastomosis sewn directly to the patch.[27]

Extensive Lesions

Although open endarterectomy, through a series of longitudinal incisions with subsequent vein patch angioplasties, can be employed when atherosclerotic involvement of the femoropopliteal arteries is extensive, semiclosed or closed endarterectomy is the preferred method of treatment of extensive infrainguinal disease.[21–23]

Semi-closed Technique

In the semi-closed technique, the distal arteriotomy is made in the popliteal artery through a medial incision at the knee. The proximal arteriotomy in the common femoral artery permits an open endarterectomy at this level. The surgeon then transects the plaque at the distal end-point using a Beaver blade and directs the plaque through a ringed stripper that is advanced proximally. Passage of the ringed stripper is facilitated by circumferential palpation of the vessel. When the plaque is densely adherent, such as often occurs at the adductor canal, it may be necessary to divide the muscular attachments at this level for the safe completion of this procedure.

Closed Technique

The recently described closed endarterectomy technique is performed through an arteriotomy on the common femoral artery. After threading the core of intima through a conventional ring stripper, the surgeon advances the device prograde down the superficial femoral artery under fluoroscopic guidance through the occluded segment to a predetermined point. The device is removed, and a ring stripper-cutter is then passed along the same cleavage plane until the distal margin of the endarterectomy is reached. The cutter is engaged, and the plaque is transected and removed. A balloon-expandable intraluminal stent is then placed over a previously placed guide wire and inflated so as to secure the distal end point and to prevent dissection. Any loose plaque fragments in the endarterectomized artery are removed with balloon catheters. The surgeon then performs completion angiography to confirm the adequacy of the procedure.

RESULTS

Aortoiliofemoral Disease: Endarterectomy

A number of authors have documented the safety and efficacy of aortoiliac or aortoiliofemoral endarterectomy in the treatment of patients with type I or II atherosclerotic disease patterns.[3, 3a–5, 7, 11, 14] Operative mortality rates have ranged from 1% to 7% for the procedure, with the lower rates reflective of improvements in patient selection and anesthesia techniques.[3–5, 11, 13, 25] Five-year and 10-year patency rates for endarterectomy in patients with type I disease have been impressive and comparable to bypass procedures (Table 67–1). Some authors have claimed similar results for aortoiliofemoral endarterectomy in patients with type II disease patterns,[3, 13, 26] whereas others have reported better patency for prosthetic bypass in this setting.[5]

Proponents of inflow endarterectomy stress the importance of several technical aspects of the procedure that ensure their long-term effectiveness:

1. The endarterectomy of the aorta should begin at the level of the renal arteries. Failure to completely clear the aorta of plaque and maintain adequate inflow will result in restenosis or occlusion of the reconstruction.
2. Endarterectomy should terminate at the iliac artery bifurcation for patients with type I disease and at the common femoral artery bifurcation in patients with type II patterns of atherosclerosis in order to ensure complete disobliteration of the disease process.
3. Unilateral procedures should be avoided because the atherosclerotic process below the bifurcation is essentially always bilateral.
4. The entire medial layer should be removed during the procedure to allow for enlargement of the blood vessel and to create a smooth luminal flow surface.[11, 14] Inahara[14] has noted that the external iliac and common femoral arteries will enlarge by 2 to 5 mm after the procedures and suggests that the change in vessel size contributes the most to the long-term patency of aortoiliofemoral endarterectomy.
5. Unobstructed outflow into the profunda femoris artery must be maintained by extended endarterectomy, if necessary, regardless of the patency of the superficial femoral artery, in order to maintain the patency of aortoiliofemoral endarterectomy for patients with type II disease.

A successful inflow endarterectomy can restore sexual potency in approximately 70% of patients with vasculogenic impotence in addition to improving lower extremity blood flow. With careful operative dissection, ejaculatory function can be retained in 80%.

Infrainguinal Disease: Endarterectomy

Segmental Lesions

Of the three femoral vessels, isolated, segmental occlusive disease least often affects the common femoral artery. However, when such disease is present, these lesions are frequently responsible for symptoms of disabling claudication, more often than isolated lesions in the superficial femoral artery or profunda femoris artery.[29] Limb-threatening ischemia may also be present with isolated femoral artery disease.

In a series by Springhorn and colleagues, 69% of patients undergoing surgery for isolated occlusive disease were classified as having limb-threatening ischemia (rest, pain, ulceration, or gangrene).[30] Of 29 patients in the series by Mukherjee and Inahara,[29] 12 had either rest pain or ulceration. Cumulative patency rates for common femoral endarterectomy at 10 years have been reported as high as 94%.

In regard to the three femoral vessels, isolated occlusion of the superficial femoral artery occurs most commonly. Most patients requiring treatment for anatomic lesion present with claudication—85% in a study by Inahara and Scott[31] and 60% in a study by Ouriel and associates.[32] Five-year cumulative patency rates of 70% were reported by Inahara and Scott. Better results were observed in patients with claudication compared with limb-threatening ischemia, and when the lesions were short (<7.5 cm), Ouriel's group[32] noted an overall cumulative patency rate of 66% at 3 years and 57% at 7 years.

Localized atherosclerotic disease of the profunda femoris artery may also produce disabling claudication or rest pain when it is associated with superficial femoral artery occlusion. The importance of this artery as an alternate blood supply to the lower extremity has been well recognized, and specific circumstances may arise in which revascularization of this vessel is preferable to femoropopliteal reconstruction (see Chapter 70).

TABLE 67–1. CUMULATIVE PATENCY FOR AORTOILIAC AND AORTOILIOFEMORAL THROMBOENDARTERECTOMY

		PATENCY RATE (%)	
SERIES, YEAR	**OPERATION**	**At 5 Yr**	**At 10 Yr**
Butcher and Jaffe, 1971[3a]	AI + AIF TEA	72	—
Inahara, 1972[7]	AIF TEA	96.1	—
Inahara, 1975[13]	AI TEA	—	85
	AIF TEA	—	90
Brewster and Darling, 1978[5]	AI TEA	94	85.2
	AIF TEA	79.6	68.3
Stoney and Reilly, 1987[11]	AI TEA	95	90
	AIF TEA	85	72

AI = aortoiliac; AIF = aortoiliofemoral; TEA = thromboendarterectomy.

As previously noted, direct surgical repair of the profunda femoris artery may be performed as an isolated procedure or in association with a bypass. Taylor and colleagues[33] examined the indications and results of profunda femoris endarterectomy and extended-patch angioplasty in 46 patients. Twenty-one procedures were performed to provide outflow for proximal aortofemoral or femorofemoral bypass:

- Fourteen isolated procedures were performed; four were performed for claudication, and all were successful.
- Three procedures were performed in patients with irreversible gangrene to facilitate healing of a below knee amputation, and all were successful.
- Seven patients were operated on for ischemic rest pain, and two patients subsequently required amputation.

Lawson and colleagues[24] noted an 80% patency rate at 1 year and a limb salvage rate of 87% in a series of 15 limbs revascularized with extended profundaplasty. Tovar-Pardo and Bernhard[27] advocate the use of the profunda-popliteal collateral index to predict which patients might benefit from such procedures, and they stress the importance of having reliable inflow into the profunda femoris artery for success using this indirect method of revascularization.

Diffuse Lesions

The optimal treatment for extensive femoropopliteal atherosclerotic occlusive disease remains a hotly debated topic. Initially, the poor results with extensive open endarterectomy and patch angioplasty techniques performed in the United States led many authors to favor autogenous bypass procedures for patients with severe claudication or limb-threatening ischemia. Darling and Linton[34] identified significant 5-year patency differences for endarterectomy versus bypass (30% versus 74%). Imparato and coauthors[23] reported superiority of vein bypass over open endarterectomy, but patency rates were similar in patients undergoing semiclosed endarterectomy techniques and vein bypass.

The European experience with semi-closed endarterectomy has continued to show promise and has persisted long after most surgeons in the United States abandoned the procedure. The relative ease of the procedure, shorter operative times, and better long-term patency rates for femoropopliteal bypass resulted in only a handful of centers performing extensive femoropopliteal endarterectomy routinely. The development of prosthetic bypass materials had an additional effect on the number of extensive endarterectomies that were being performed because of a lack of autogenous conduit. Recently, refinements that further minimize the "invasiveness" of the revascularization have led to a reevaluation of the usefulness of extended endarterectomy in lower extremity reconstructions.[35–38]

SUMMARY

Thromboendarterectomy remains a viable alternative for aortoiliac and femoropopliteal revascularization in selected patients. Patency and limb salvage results are excellent in reports originating from vascular surgeons with experience and skill using these techniques. Because no prosthetic material is required, thromboendarterectomy carries very little risk of infection, in contrast to conventional bypass grafts. If failure eventually occurs, standard bypasses can still be employed. Thus, thromboendarterectomy should be a part of the armamentarium of all vascular surgeons performing lower extremity revascularizations.

REFERENCES

1. dos Santos JC: Sur la desobstion des thromboses arterielles anciennes. Mem Acad Chir 73:409, 1947.
2. Wylie EJ, Kerr E, Davies O: Experimental and clinical experiences with the use of fascia lata applied as a graft about major arteries after thromboendarterectomy and aneurysmorrhaphy. Surg Gynecol Obstet 93:257, 1951.
3. Gomes MR, Bernatz, PE, Juergens JL: Aortoiliac surgery: Influence of clinical factors on results. Arch Surg 95:387, 1967.

3a. Butcher FR, Jaffe BM: Treatment of aortoiliac disease by endarterectomy. Ann Surg 173:925, 1971.

4. Imparato AM, Sanoudos G, Epstein HY, et al: Results in 96 aortoiliac reconstructive procedures: Preoperative, angiographic and functional classifications used as prognostic guides. Surgery 68:610.1970
5. Brewster DC, Darling RC: Optimal methods of aortoiliac reconstruction. Surgery 84:739, 1978.
6. Crawford ES, Bomberger RA, Glaeser DH, et al: Aortoiliac occlusive disease: Factors influencing survival and function following reconstructive operations over a twenty-five year period. Surgery 90:1055, 1981.
7. Inahara T: Endarterectomy for occlusive disease of the aortoiliac and common femoral arteries. Am J Surg 124:235, 1972.
8. Zarins CK, Glagov S: Artery wall pathology in atherosclerosis. *In* Rutherford R (ed): Vascular Surgery, 3rd ed. Philadelphia, WB Saunders, 1989, p 178.
9. Chisolm GM, DiCorleto PE, Ehrart LA, et al: Pathogenesis of atherosclerosis. *In* Young JR, Graor RA, Olin JW, Bartholomew JR (eds): Peripheral Vascular Diseases. St. Louis, Mosby–Year Book, 1991, p 137.
10. Haimovici H: Endarterectomy. *In* Haimovici H (ed): Vascular Surgery Principles and Techniques. Norwalk, Conn, Appleton and Lange, 1989, p 293.
11. Stoney RJ, Reilly LM: Endarterectomy for aortoiliac occlusive disease. *In* Ernst CB, Stanley JC (eds): Current Therapy in Vascular Surgery. Philadelphia, BC Decker, 1987, p 157.
12. Sumner DS, Hokanson DE, Strandness DE: Arterial walls before and after endarterectomy: Stress-strain characteristics and collagen-elastin content. Arch Surg 99:606, 1969.
13. Inahara T: Evaluation of endarterectomy for aortoiliac and aortoilio-femoral occlusive disease. Arch Surg 110:1458, 1975.
14. Inahara T: Endarterectomy of atherosclerotic aortoiliac and aortofemoral occlusive disease. *In* Ernst CB, Stanley JC (eds): Current Therapy in Vascular Surgery, 2nd ed. Philadelphia, BC Decker, 1991, p 398.
15. Brewster DC: Clinical and anatomical considerations for surgery in aortoiliac disease and results of surgical treatment. Circulation 83(Suppl):42, 1991.
16. Haimovici H: Patterns of atherosclerotic lesions of the lower extremities. Arch Surg 95:918, 1967.
17. Rollins DC, Towne JB, Bernhard VM: Isolated profundaplasty for limb salvage. J Vasc Surg 2:585, 1985.
18. Moneta GL, Yeager RA, Antonovic R, et al: Accuracy of lower extremity arterial duplex mapping. J Vasc Surg 15:275, 1992.
19. Sawchuk AP, Flanigan P, Tober JC, et al: A rapid, accurate, noninvasive technique for diagnosing critical and subcritical stenoses in aortoiliac arteries. J Vasc Surg 12:158, 1990.
20. Reilly LM, Sauer L, Weinstein ES, et al: Infrarenal aortic occlusion: Does it threaten renal perfusion or function? J Vasc Surg 11:216, 1990.
21. van der Heijden FHWM, Eikelboom BC, van Reedt Dortland RWH, et al: Long-term results of semiclosed endarterectomy of the superficial femoral artery and the outcome of failed reconstructions. J Vasc Surg 18:271, 1993.
22. Moll FL, Ho GH: Closed superficial femoral artery endarterectomy: A 2-year follow-up. Cardiovasc Surg 5:398, 1997.

23. Imparato AM, Bracco A, Kim GE: Comparison of three techniques for femoral-popliteal arterial reconstruction. Ann Surg 177:375, 1973.
24. Lawson DW, Gillico GG, Patton AS: Limb salvage by extended profundaplasty of occluded deep femoral arteries. Am J Surg 145:458, 1983.
25. van den Akker PJ, van Schilfgaarde R, Brand R, et al: Long term success of aortoiliac operations for arteriosclerotic obstructive disease. Surg Gynecol Obstet 174:485, 1992.
26. Nash T: Aortoiliac occlusive vascular disease: A prospective study of patients treated by endarterectomy and bypass procedures. Aust N Z J Surg 49:223, 1979.
27. Tovar-Pardo AE, Bernhard VM: Where the profunda femoris artery fits in the spectrum of lower limb revascularization. Semin Vasc Surg 8:225, 1995.
28. Taylor SM, Langan EM, Snyder BA, et al: Superficial femoral artery eversion endarterectomy: A useful adjunct for infrainguinal bypass in the presence of limited autogenous vein. J Vasc Surg 26:439, 1997.
29. Mukherjee D, Inahara T: Endarterectomy as the procedure of choice for atherosclerotic occlusive lesions of the common femoral artery. Am J Surg 157:498, 1989.
30. Springhorn ME, Kinney M, Littooy FN, et al: Inflow atherosclerotic disease localized to the common femoral artery: Treatment and outcome. Ann Vasc Surg 5:234, 1991.
31. Inahara T, Scott CM: Endarterectomy for segmental occlusive disease of the superficial femoral artery. Arch Surg 116:1547, 1981.
32. Ouriel K, Smith CR, De Weese JA: Endarterectomy for localized lesions of the superficial femoral artery at the adductor canal. J Vasc Surg 3:531, 1986.
33. Taylor LM, Baur GM, Eidemiller LR, et al: Extended profundaplasty: Indications and techniques with results of 46 procedures. Am J Surg 141:539, 1981.
34. Darling RC, Linton RR: Durability of femoropopliteal reconstructions: Endarterectomy versus vein bypass grafts. Am J Surg 123:472, 1972.
35. Ahn SS, Reger VA, Kaiura TL: Endovascular femoropopliteal bypass: Early human cadaver and animal studies. Ann Vasc Surg 9:28, 1995.
36. Bray AE: Superficial femoral endarterectomy with intra-arterial PTFE grafting. J Endovasc Surg 2:297, 1995.
37. Vroegindeweij D, Idu M, Buth J, et al: The cost-effectiveness of treatment of short occlusive lesions of the femoropopliteal artery: Balloon angioplasty versus endarterectomy. Eur J Vasc Endovasc Surg 10:40, 1995.
38. Ho GH, Moll FL, Eikelboom BC, et al: Endarterectomy of the superficial femoral artery. Semin Vasc Surg 8:216, 1995.

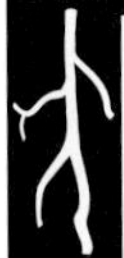

CHAPTER 68

Extra-anatomic Bypass

Robert B. Rutherford, M.D.

The term *extra-anatomic bypass* has been applied to grafts that pass through an anatomic pathway significantly different from that of the natural blood vessels they bypass. Although correctly criticized by purists as a misnomer, the term has gained practically universal acceptance, as opposed to *ex situ bypass*, which has its own problems (e.g., an infrainguinal in situ vein bypass is ex situ with regard to its anatomic pathway). Ordinarily, the use of such a bypass implies deliberate avoidance of the natural location of the vascular supply, either because of a hostile pathologic condition there or because entering the area significantly adds to the risk of the operation (as in entering the abdomen).

The term extra-anatomic bypass commonly applies to an axillofemoral or a femorofemoral bypass or to their combination, the so-called axillobifemoral bypass. Other extra-anatomic arterial bypasses, such as carotid-subclavian, axilloaxillary, splenorenal, and crossover femoropopliteal bypasses, are covered in appropriate chapters elsewhere in this book, as are infrainguinal bypasses, most of which are extra-anatomic to a greater or lesser degree (e.g., the in situ bypass). This chapter focuses on those extra-anatomic routes used to bypass aortoiliac occlusive disease under special circumstances in which (1) the natural inflow has already been or must of necessity be interrupted and (2) direct arterial reconstruction, such as aortobifemoral grafting, is precluded by either "hostile" abdominal disease or the prohibitive operative risk of this approach as a result of impaired function of one or more vital organs. These operations consist primarily of the femorofemoral, axillounifemoral, and axillobifemoral bypasses (Fig. 68–1). In addition, obturator foramen bypass, which is most commonly used to avoid an infected groin, is also discussed in this chapter, partly because it is a proximal extra-anatomic bypass used to avoid hostile pathologic conditions.

HISTORY AND OVERVIEW[1]

Early History

In 1952, Freeman and Leeds[2] described the use of a superficial femoral artery to carry blood directly from one femoral artery to another subcutaneously. In 1958, McCaughan sutured a polyester (Dacron) prosthesis to the left external iliac artery, brought it preperitoneally across to the right groin, and anastomosed it side-to-end to the right profunda femoris (deep femoral) artery and end-to-side to the right popliteal artery, bypassing occlusions of the right iliac, common femoral, and superficial femoral arteries.

In 1959, Lewis resected an abdominal aortic aneurysm but was unable to anastomose the proximal end of a homograft replacement to the abdominal or even the proximal thoracic aorta because of the involvement of both aortic

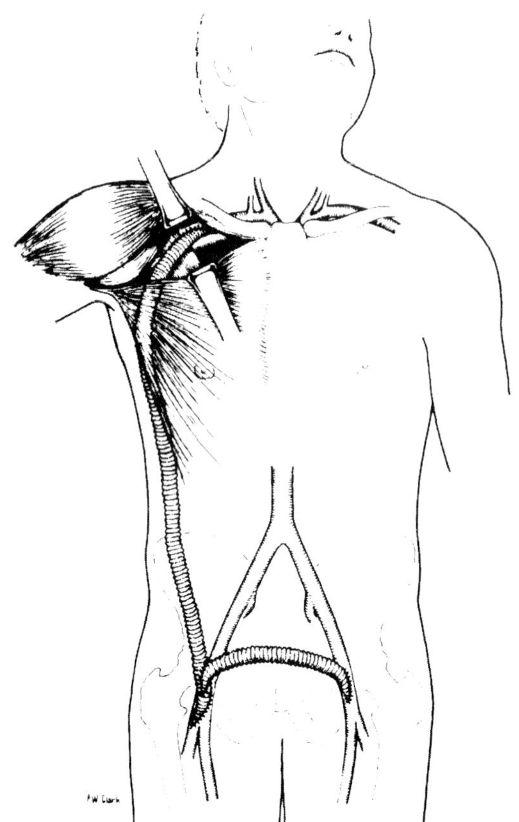

FIGURE 68–1. The axillobifemoral bypass graft represents a combination of axillofemoral and femorofemoral grafts and is employed in preference to bilateral axillofemoral grafts when both lower extremities require revascularization. (From Delaurentis DA, Sala LE, Russell E, McCombs PR: A twelve-year experience with axillofemoral and femorofemoral bypass operations. Surg Gynecol Obstet 147:881–887, 1978. By permission of Surgery, Gynecology & Obstetrics.)

segments with dissecting aneurysm. Therefore, he resected the middle third of the clavicle, sutured a nylon graft end-to-end to the proximal subclavian artery, and brought the graft down the chest wall and into the abdomen at the level of the xiphoid process for anastomosis to the homograft. This somewhat bizarre but ingenious operation showed that arteries in the upper extremity could be used to supply the lower half of the body.

Faced with an infected abdominal aortic prosthesis, Blaisdell and associates[3] anastomosed a Dacron graft to the descending thoracic aorta, brought it out through the chest below the 12th rib and down the lateral abdominal wall, and sutured it to the left common femoral artery. A "side-arm" was then anastomosed to this graft and brought suprapubically across to the right common femoral artery. Warren[4] had earlier reported a bypass between the splenic and iliofemoral arteries. Thus, many surgeons had experimented with ingenious extra-anatomic bypasses before the femorofemoral and axillofemoral grafts were introduced and became the established forms of extra-anatomic bypass in the early 1960s.

In 1962, Vetto[5] reported 10 *transabdominal* subcutaneous femorofemoral graft operations to bypass unilateral iliac occlusive disease in poor-risk patients. The same year, reported almost simultaneously by Blaisdell and Hall[6] and by Louw,[7] Dacron grafts were placed between the axillary and ipsilateral femoral arteries for occlusive disease. Bilateral axillofemoral grafts were placed by Blaisdell and colleagues[8] for revascularization of ischemic extremities after infected aortic prostheses had been removed. Sauvage and Wood[9] are given credit for combining these two procedures, into what they first termed an *axillobifemoral graft procedure*, to avoid the need for bilateral, separate axillofemoral bypasses. The obturator bypass was introduced in 1962 by Shaw and Baue[10] as a means of bypassing graft sepsis localized to the groin.

Changing Perspective

Originally, the use of extra-anatomic bypass grafts was restricted, for the most part, to cases in which there were complications of aortoiliac reconstruction, although even from the outset, extremely ill patients with impending gangrene were treated with both axillofemoral and femorofemoral grafting. Within 5 years of the widespread application of these grafts, however, Alpert and coworkers[11] openly recommended extra-anatomic bypass as the primary reconstructive approach in selected poor-risk patients. By 1970, the same group suggested that the employment of these extra-anatomic bypasses, at least the femorofemoral bypass, had become a matter of "preference rather than compromise."[12] In 1972, they suggested that the femorofemoral bypass actually enhanced the continuing patency of the contralateral or "donor" iliac artery.[13] By 1977, LoGerfo and associates[14] reported that axillobifemoral grafts had almost twice the flow rate and twice the patency rate of unilateral axillofemoral grafts. In August of the previous year, the same group had reported that if one allowed for continuing patency achieved with the aid of thrombectomy, the axillobifemoral graft was comparable to the aortofemoral graft in patency rate but carried only one-fourth the mortality rate.[15]

At the height of this rising enthusiasm for extra-anatomic bypass (in fact, in the same issue of the *Annals of Surgery*), Eugene and coworkers[16] reported a sobering follow-up of the extended experience with extra-anatomic bypass at the San Francisco Veterans' Administration Hospital. Subsequent reports of disappointing long-term results with extra-anatomic bypasses, combined with a steadily decreasing risk with the use of direct transabdominal reconstruction (thanks to improved perioperative monitoring and intensive care), resulted in a more conservative, selective application of these procedures. Later reports of improved long-term results, however, have renewed debate about the more liberal application of axillofemoral and axillobifemoral bypasses[17, 18] versus a preference for aortofemoral bypass in all but the highest-risk patients.[19]

The early reported success of axillofemoral bypass ultimately prompted the use of *extended* extra-anatomic bypass procedures for limb-threatening ischemia when use of the femoral arteries was not feasible. Veith and coworkers[20] reported limited success with axillopopliteal bypass in 1978. Connolly and associates[21] subsequently demonstrated modest success with both axillopopliteal and axillotibial bypass for limb salvage. Two larger series with longer follow-up periods have indicated that axillopopliteal bypass can provide limb salvage for a considerable time in a patient population with relatively limited life expectancy.[22, 23]

Other Applications

Axillobifemoral bypass grafting, in conjunction with ligation of the iliac arteries to induce thrombosis of abdominal aortic aneurysms (AAAs), has been recommended and evaluated as a low-risk alternative to resection in high-risk patients.[24] This combined procedure is discussed in greater detail in Chapter 89. The author mentions it here because it, too, has come under strong criticism on the basis of its poorer patency, difficulty in achieving thrombosis without embolism of patent lumbar arteries, and, most alarming, reports of rupture despite successful aneurysm thrombosis.[25–27] However, this approach may become more popular again because of lower-risk approaches to occlusion of the proximal aorta. Two studies have shown that most of the drawbacks of this approach can be avoided by adding inflow to outflow occlusion of the AAA.[26, 28] Murayama and colleagues[29] have developed a videoscopic retroperitoneal approach to stapling the infrarenal aorta, and cases have been reported in which endovascular occlusion devices, mostly modifications of endograft technology, have been used to occlude the infrarenal aorta proximally and the iliac arteries distally. The extent to which this approach regains popularity, other than simply for anatomically complex, high-risk cases, will probably depend on the long-term results of endograft repair of AAAs.

Nevertheless, there is little argument that axillofemoral bypass is indispensable for treatment of infected aortic grafts and aortoenteric fistulae (see Chapters 47 and 49, respectively). Finally, temporary axillofemoral bypass is occasionally used to supply blood to the lower extremities during difficult operations on the thoracic or abdominal aorta, avoiding the need for pump bypass.

HEMODYNAMIC CONSIDERATIONS

Axillofemoral and femorofemoral bypasses were originally intended only as makeshift or compromise procedures, primarily because it seemed unreasonable to expect one extremity to share its blood supply with another, and particularly when an arm was expected to supply two legs. Furthermore, initially there was concern that if these grafts did provide more than a modest amount of additional flow to "recipient" lower extremities, the increased demand would produce a significant steal phenomenon in the "donor" extremity.

Neither of these fears was justified, however, because they arose from an incomplete appreciation of the hemodynamic principles governing the performance of axillofemoral and femorofemoral grafts. First, the total resistance of parallel circuits, unlike resistances in series, is less than the sum of its parts. Calculated as the reciprocal sum, the resistance to flow through the donor artery is actually significantly reduced by each extremity that the artery supplies, and its flow is increased accordingly. This principle has been confirmed by intraoperative electromagnetic flowmeter measurements.[12] Second, in canine models of a femorofemoral bypass graft, flow through the graft to the recipient extremity could be increased 10-fold without producing a steal in the donor extremity.[30, 31] All of the foregoing studies were performed, however, when no outflow or inflow obstruction was present.

Although resting ankle pressure in the donor limb is often initially decreased after femorofemoral bypass, it soon rises again.[32] In fact, when ankle pressure is related to the brachial or systemic pressure, there is no statistically significant decrease; that is, the ankle-brachial *index* remains unchanged. Moreover, even though the ankle pressure in the donor extremity may drop after exercise, this drop does not constitute a true steal if the donor iliac artery has slight stenosis, because the contralateral ankle pressure drops an equivalent amount. It is possible to produce a steal in the donor extremity after femorofemoral bypass *if* there is outflow occlusive disease (e.g., superficial femoral artery occlusion) on the *donor* side. Even this is not likely to become clinically manifest, however, unless there is greater flow demand (e.g., with exercise), donor iliac artery stenosis, or poor cardiac function.

Although some decrease in ankle pressure in the donor limb has been demonstrated after up to 80% of femorofemoral bypasses, it is rarely clinically significant.[33] Nevertheless, although the fear of significant steal in the donor extremity was proved to be unfounded, the same study showed that when a significant degree of either "inflow" stenosis or "outflow" occlusive disease existed, both the patency rates of these grafts and their likelihood of relieving claudication or salvaging an extremity were reduced despite continued graft patency. In this study, arteriographically documented inflow and outflow occlusive disease was correlated with the success of femorofemoral bypass. In patients without either inflow or recipient outflow occlusive disease, the success rate was 90%. In patients in whom the recipient superficial femoral artery was significantly obstructed, the success rate was more than halved. In all of the patients in whom significant obstruction of the recipient superficial femoral artery was associated with even a moderate degree of obstruction of the donor iliac artery (e.g., 50%), regardless of outflow status, either thrombosis developed in the graft or the graft failed to relieve the symptoms.

Finally, hemodynamic calculations indicate how little flow augmentation in response to exercise could be expected from a femorofemoral graft in the presence of recipient superficial femoral artery occlusion when there was also some stenosis of the donor iliac artery.[32] These hemodynamic considerations are obviously extremely important in the decision to employ extra-anatomic bypasses.

At one time, before the similarity between the peripheral circulation and electrical circuitry (in terms of the effect on flow of resistances in parallel and in series) was appreciated,[34] it was thought that the reasonably good patency rates of these makeshift grafts were attributable to their use for limb salvage in which there was a *continuous* demand for flow rather than the *intermittent* demand in claudication. Although this theory argues against using extra-anatomic bypasses for claudication, the matter is not that simple. In fact, most studies have reported better patencies for patients with claudication, probably because such patients tend to have better runoff.

TABLE 68–1. VARIATION IN REPORTED RESULTS FOR EXTRA-ANATOMIC BYPASS

PROCEDURE	STUDY	OPERATIVE MORTALITY RATE (%)	PATENCY RATE (%) Five-Year Primary	Five-Year Secondary
Femorofemoral	Brief et al, 1975[36]	4	81*	—
	Flanigan et al, 1978[33]	4	74*	—
	Livesay et al, 1979[71]	6	NR	56
	Eugene et al, 1976[16]	15	44	NR
	Kalman et al, 1976[90]	4.1	73.4	NR
	Rutherford et al, 1987[40]	0	74	82
	Chang, 1986[86]	NR	85	NR
	Hepp et al, 1988[87]	4	80	NR
	Ng et al, 1992[43]	1.3	92‡	NR
	Criado et al, 1993[91]	4.5	60	NR
	Farber et al, 1990[92]	4	82	NR
Axillofemoral	Ray et al, 1979[39]	3	NR	67
	LoGerfo et al, 1977[14]	8	NR	37
	Eugene et al, 1976[16]	8	30	NR
	Rutherford et al, 1987[40]	13	19	37
	Ascer et al, 1985[88]	5	44	71
	Chang, 1986[86]	NR	33	NR
	Hepp et al, 1988[87]	5	NR	46
	El-Massry et al, 1993[18]	5	79	NR
	Naylor et al, 1990[93]	11	50	NR
Axillobifemoral	Ray et al, 1979[39]	5	NR	77
	LoGerfo et al, 1977[14]	8	NR	74
	Johnson et al, 1976[15]	2	NR	76
	Eugene et al, 1976[16]	8	33	NR
	Rutherford et al, 1987[40]	11	62	82
	Ascer et al, 1985[88]	5	50	77
	Chang, 1986[86]	NR	75	NR
	Hepp et al, 1988[87]	5	NR	73
	Harris et al, 1990[17]	5	85†	NR
	El-Massry et al, 1993[18]	5	76	NR
	Passman et al, 1996[77]	3.4	74	81
Axillopopliteal	Ascer et al, 1989[22]	8	40	59
	Keller et al, 1992[23]	20	43‡	50‡

*Patency not defined.
†4-year patency.
‡3-year patency.
NR = not reported.

Furthermore, in 1974, Ernst[35] reported the prophylactic use of an axillofemoral bypass graft before repair of a difficult suprarenal aortic aneurysm. Surprisingly, this bypass remained patent despite the absence of a pressure gradient across the native artery it bypassed and, in fact, had to be closed because of disuse atrophy of that vessel, the ipsilateral iliac artery. Brief and associates[36] have claimed that the crossover femorofemoral bypass is preferable to an ipsilateral iliofemoral bypass because the greater flows it produces in the donor iliac artery protect the artery against the atheromatous occlusive process that affected the contralateral vessel. Follow-up angiography of femorofemoral bypasses has shown a tendency toward dilatation of the donor iliac artery, possibly resulting from increased flow.[37] Although other investigators have acknowledged the better-than-expected long-term patency of the donor iliac artery in large series of femorofemoral bypasses, the author has observed donor iliac artery occlusion in 6% of femorofemoral bypasses, a finding that suggests that any protection femorofemoral bypass affords is certainly not absolute.[38]

The final hemodynamic consideration worthy of comment relates to the observation by LoGerfo and coworkers[14] that both flow and patency rates in axillobifemoral grafts were double those in unilateral axillofemoral grafts. Investigators in most reported series have made the same observation, and even in studies in which a significant difference was not found, the mean patency rates have favored the axillobifemoral bypass. This is an important consideration because it forms the basis for (1) the practice of making the anastomosis with the crossover femoral graft as low as possible on the axillofemoral graft to take maximal advantage of this effect[16, 39] and (2) performing an axillobifemoral rather than an axillounifemoral bypass in cases of limb-threatening ischemia on one side only. This issue is discussed later in the section on technique.

INDICATIONS

Femorofemoral Bypass

The femorofemoral bypass has the best overall patency rate of the extra-anatomic bypasses discussed in this chapter (Table 68–1). It is considered by most to be the operation of choice for unilateral iliac artery occlusion in older patients. Before one decides in favor of femorofemoral bypass, several aspects are worth considering:

1. Is the donor iliac artery widely patent?
2. What is the status of the outflow vessels, particularly the superficial femoral artery, and how will this affect patency, likelihood of relief of symptoms, and limb salvage?
3. Is the operation being performed for native iliac artery occlusion or occlusion of one limb of a bifurcation graft?
4. What are the other options, and how do they compare with femorofemoral bypass under the same circumstances?

The status of the donor iliac artery may be determined by biplanar arteriography, but physiologic testing may be more accurate. A normal thigh-brachial index, a thigh plethysmographic tracing with a brisk upslope and good excursion, and a triphasic waveform in an analog Doppler tracing recorded over the femoral artery[33] all indicate a wide-open iliofemoral segment. Direct measurement of femoral artery pressure and its response to a papaverine injection (see Chapter 10) is still the most practical and accurate way of detecting occult iliac artery stenosis, and with a little forethought, it should be obtained at the time of arteriography.

If the superficial femoral artery is occluded, the patency rate of a femorofemoral graft is significantly reduced (from 92% to 52%).[40, 85] Furthermore, in the presence of superficial femoral artery occlusion, the likelihood of symptomatic relief or limb salvage is reduced by more than half (from 90% to 41%).[33] In the author's experience, the patency rate with femorofemoral bypass performed for native iliac artery occlusive disease was 74%, compared with 39% with bypass performed for failure of one limb of a bifurcation graft. As seen in Table 68–2, such factors have a major bearing on outcome and must be taken into consideration in the risk:benefit analysis that determines the indications for surgery in individual cases.

Alternatives to femorofemoral bypass in treating extensive disease or total occlusion of the iliac segments include:

1. Iliofemoral bypass (if the ipsilateral common iliac artery is widely patent).
2. Transluminal angioplasty with or without stenting (if a suitable stenosis or short common iliac artery occlusion is present).
3. Unilateral aortofemoral bypass (if the common iliac is diseased or occluded).
4. Iliofemoral endarterectomy through a retroperitoneal approach (if the disease is confined to the external iliac arteries).
5. Aortobifemoral bypass (in a good-risk patient in whom contralateral iliac artery disease is present but is not hemodynamically significant).

Axillounifemoral bypass is not competitive here because of its significantly lower patency. Transluminal angioplasty is clearly preferred for discrete (<5 cm) stenoses of the common iliac artery, in which the 5-year patency rate approaches 90%.[41] Its use for multiple stenoses or extensive disease of the iliac segment produces much inferior results, and dilatation of external iliac artery lesions fares no better than dilatation of femoropopliteal lesions.[42] Stenting has changed this picture somewhat but has not proved itself yet for the more extensive lesions (see Chapter 72).

Iliofemoral bypass is attractive because in trading an oblique retroperitoneal lower quadrant incision for a groin incision, one avoids a higher risk of graft infection and anastomotic aneurysm, leaves the "normal" femoral artery untouched, and performs a shorter, more direct bypass graft procedure. Comparing patency rates in the literature from individual reports of one or the other operation is not

TABLE 68–2. OVERALL AND SUBGROUP PATENCY RATES FOR EXTRA-ANATOMIC BYPASS

TYPE OF BYPASS	OCCLUSIVE DISEASE		SUPERFICIAL FEMORAL ARTERY		NO.	PATENCY RATE (%)	
	Yes	No	Patent	Occluded		Primary	Secondary
Axillounifemoral	+	+	+	+	15	19	37
	+	+	+	−	7	54	54
	+	+	−	+	8	0	0
Axillobifemoral	+	+	+	+	54	62	81
	−	+	+	+	12	91	100
	+	−	+	+	42	47	69
	+	+	+	−	21	95	100
	+	+	−	+	33	46	60
	+	−	+	−	16	92	92
	+	−	−	+	26	41	58
	Native Artery	**Axillobifemoral Graft Limb**					
Femorofemoral	+	+	+	+	60	67	74
	−	+	+	+	13	39	51
	+	−	+	+	47	74	82
	+	+	+	−	22	79	95
	+	+	−	+	38	53	67
	+	−	+	−	19	92	100
	+	−	−	+	28	52	66

From Rutherford RB, Patt A, Pearce WH: Extraanatomic bypass: A closer view. J Vasc Surg 5:437, 1987.

decisive, and in the four reports in which the two operations have been compared in the same institution, the femorofemoral bypass was superior in two reports[38, 43] and inferior in one,[44] and in the fourth report there was no patency difference between the two procedures.[45] It has also pointed out that one might cause impotence in men in whom the left side is approached in an iliofemoral bypass.[36]

In a comparison of femorofemoral and iliofemoral bypass by Piotrowski and colleagues,[38] it was also observed that aortobifemoral bypass, performed when only one iliac artery had hemodynamically significant narrowing or occlusion, did better than femorofemoral bypass in the patient who also had superficial femoral artery occlusion (72% versus 35% 5-year primary patency rate, respectively). Patencies were equivalent in patients in whom runoff was good.[38] In this experience, femorofemoral bypass was associated with no deaths, compared with 3% mortality for aortobifemoral bypass.

In the presence of unilateral iliac artery occlusion and limited contralateral iliac artery stenosis, percutaneous transluminal angioplasty (PTA) of the stenotic iliac artery can provide adequate donor femoral inflow to permit femorofemoral bypass.[89] Patency with this combined approach is comparable to that with femorofemoral bypass in the absence of donor iliac artery stenosis.[38, 40, 46, 47] Reports of good results with unilateral aortofemoral bypass[48, 49] and iliac artery–based proximal reconstructions[50] have now added to the number of viable alternatives to femorofemoral bypass.

Thus, femorofemoral bypass is a safe operation that results in good patency in a patient with good runoff, and it may be performed even for disabling claudication in such a patient. When superficial femoral artery occlusion is present, this bypass should not be performed for claudication, but it may be performed, with concomitant profundaplasty, for limb salvage in poor-risk patients. Aortofemoral bypass is preferred in good-risk patients whenever the contralateral iliac artery is diseased. When there is forefoot ulceration, gangrene, or infection, concomitant distal bypass is preferable to profundaplasty regardless of the proximal bypass used.[38, 41] Finally, femorofemoral bypass is an acceptable means of handling unilateral occlusion of a bifurcation graft limb that is not amenable to thrombectomy,[51] although it must be realized that the patency rate of the procedure in this setting is definitely inferior to that of a primary bypass.[40]

Axillounifemoral Bypass

Because the axillounifemoral bypass has relatively much poorer 5-year patency rates (see Table 68–1), its application should be limited to use in patients (1) who are clearly in a unilateral limb salvage situation, (2) in whom the abdominal approach is strictly prohibited by either severe anesthetic risk or intra-abdominal disease (e.g., sepsis, irradiation, malignant tumor, stomas), (3) *and* in whom a closer donor artery is not available or cannot be made suitable by PTA.[52] Unfortunately, when this procedure is limited to such patients, the results are poor because of high risk and poor runoff. In the author's experience, the operative mortality rate for this "low-risk alternative" was 11%, and no graft placed proximal to a superficial femoral artery occlusion remained patent for longer than 30 months.[40]

In contrast, when the procedure has been applied with more liberal indications and therefore in patients with better surgical risk and better runoff, surprisingly good results have been obtained (as high as 76% patency[18]), and some surgeons have even claimed that there is no significant difference between axillounifemoral bypass and axillobifemoral bypass. As seen in Table 68–3, however, most of the reports in the literature have shown a significant patency difference in favor of axillobifemoral bypass, and even in the minority of studies that found no statistically significant difference, the mean difference favored axillobifemoral bypass. Therefore, it has been the author's preference to perform the latter procedure even when there is a *critical* degree of ischemia involving only one limb. Axillounifemoral bypass tends to be applied primarily for graft sepsis, as a temporizing measure, when the septic process prohibits femorofemoral crossover grafting.

TABLE 68–3. LONG-TERM PATENCY RATES FOR AXILLOUNIFEMORAL AND AXILLOBIFEMORAL BYPASS

	PATENCY RATE (%)	
STUDY	**Axillounifemoral Bypass**	**Axillobifemoral Bypass**
Significant Difference Observed		
LoGerfo et al, 1977[14]	37	74
Rutherford et al, 1987[40]	19*	62*
Chang, 1986[86]	33*	75*
Hepp et al, 1988[87]	46	73
Illuminati et al, 1996[94]	56	87
Naylor et al, 1990[93]	50*	80*
No Significant Difference Observed		
Ray et al, 1979[39]	67	77
Eugene et al, 1976[16]	30*	33*
Ascer et al, 1985[88]	44*	50*
El-Massry et al, 1993[18]	76*	79*
Harris et al, 1989[95]	53†	68†

*Primary patency; other rates are for secondary patency or not defined.
†3-year patency.

Axillobifemoral Bypass

Axillobifemoral bypass has an overall 5-year patency rate ranging from 33% to 85%. In the author's opinion, it should be performed only rarely for claudication; rather, it should be used in chronic critical ischemia or other situations in which femoral inflow is mandatory and the direct transabdominal reconstructive approach is clearly contraindicated by either prohibitive risk or a hostile intra-abdominal pathologic condition. Such a condition may consist of an infected aortic graft, aortoenteric fistula, mycotic aneurysm, enteric sources of contamination (diverticulitis, ileocolitis, or stoma), failure of a high endarterectomy or bypass with juxtarenal occlusion, irradiation, retroperitoneal fibrosis, metastatic malignant disease, multiple abdominal operations with extensive adhesions, complex ventral hernia, massive obesity, and cirrhosis with ascites.

"Prohibitive anesthetic risk" as an indication for choosing extra-anatomic bypass often requires a decision that is subjective but that should be based as much as possible on objective criteria. The following conditions qualify patients for this indirect form of reconstruction for aortoiliac occlusive disease:

1. Severe cardiac disease (recent myocardial infarction, intractable heart failure, or significant angina pectoris).
2. Chronic renal failure (creatinine clearance rate < 40 mL/hr or the need for hemodialysis).
3. Severe pulmonary insufficiency (dyspnea at rest, oxygen dependency, or a forced expiratory volume < 1 L/sec).
4. Morbid obesity (weight > 45 kg, or at least 100% > ideal body weight).
5. Any uncontrolled malignant or other systemic disease that limits life expectancy to less than 2 years.

The skilled vascular surgeon, working in an optimal environment with good monitoring and intensive care facilities, should adhere to these more limited indications for axillobifemoral bypass, reserving it for very carefully selected patients, and should continue to treat most patients with bilateral aortoiliac occlusive disease with a direct transabdominal reconstruction (see Chapter 66). A lower-morbidity option used by the author with some success employs a limited left lateral retroperitoneal approach to perform the proximal anastomosis and tunnels both graft limbs to the left groin, bringing the right limb across suprapubically, in the manner of a femorofemoral bypass.

Extended extra-anatomic bypass (i.e., to the popliteal artery) should be performed only for limb-threatening ischemia. Indications include the previously enumerated factors that favor axillobifemoral bypass in the presence of concomitant occlusive disease of the common femoral or extensive involvement of both the superficial and the deep femoral branches. Subsequent distal revascularization may be required if a prior axillobifemoral bypass remains patent but fails to achieve clinical improvement.

Finally, when obturator bypass cannot be performed in patients in whom either scarring or sepsis of the ipsilateral groin prohibits a femoral anastomosis, axillopopliteal bypass is indicated.

Obturator Bypass

Although introduced and primarily used as a means of restoring extremity flow when direct vascularization was prohibited by graft sepsis localized to the groin,[10, 53] the ingenious obturator bypass has since been used (1) in the patient with crushing injuries to the groin,[54] (2) for bypassing malignancies involving the inguinal nodes, or (3) when irradiation to that area has resulted in occlusive arteritis.[55–58] More commonly, it has been employed in treatment of infected femoral aneurysms due to nonsterile technique practiced by drug abusers or by physicians performing diagnostic or therapeutic maneuvers through this port of entry (this indication is also discussed in detail in Chapter 97).

Obturator bypass has also been used when the proximal anastomosis of a femorodistal bypass either has become infected or would become infected if suppurative inguinal nodes from a septic foot were ignored. Thus, almost any hostile pathologic condition in the groin can force the surgeon to create a bypass through the obturator foramen. The procedure differs from the other extra-anatomic bypasses discussed previously in that the inflow of another extremity is not being used. Because it is rarely applied electively for occlusive disease, the runoff status of the limb below the point of reentry tends to be normal. As a result, better long-term patency may be achieved than with axillounifemoral bypass. When the superficial femoral and upper popliteal arteries are occluded, the obturator bypass can be terminated in the profunda femoris artery.[59]

TECHNIQUES

Preparation and Positioning

Extra-anatomic bypasses are normally performed with the patient under light general or balanced endotracheal anesthesia because they involve only relatively superficial dissection and subcutaneous tunneling.[31, 60, 61] Obviously, a femorofemoral bypass can be performed satisfactorily with the use of regional anesthesia (e.g., epidural) or even local anesthesia with sedation. Even axillofemoral grafting has been performed in this manner, with heavy narcotics, "amnestic drugs" such as midazolam (Versed), or brief open-mask anesthesia being used during the tunneling process. Ordinarily this is not necessary, and either light general or balanced anesthesia, supplemented with local lidocaine infiltration for skin incisions, is employed in poor-risk patients.

For an *axillofemoral* or *axillobifemoral* bypass, the patient is supine, with the donor arm abducted no more than 90 degrees. Alternatively, the arm may be placed at the side but partly flexed at the elbow. This latter position, which roughly approximates that taken in reaching into a pants pocket, does not pull the axillary artery into the deeper, more tightly stretched position that occurs with abduction, but it still allows access to the axilla and the upper part of the chest (Fig. 68–2).

Ordinarily, for an axillobifemoral graft, the axillary artery on the same side as the more severely ischemic lower extremity is selected as the donor. The accuracy of preoperative noninvasive examination of axillary artery inflow is limited. Calligaro and associates[62] recommend inflow arteriography because they have found both a higher-than-expected incidence of inflow disease (25%) and the failure of

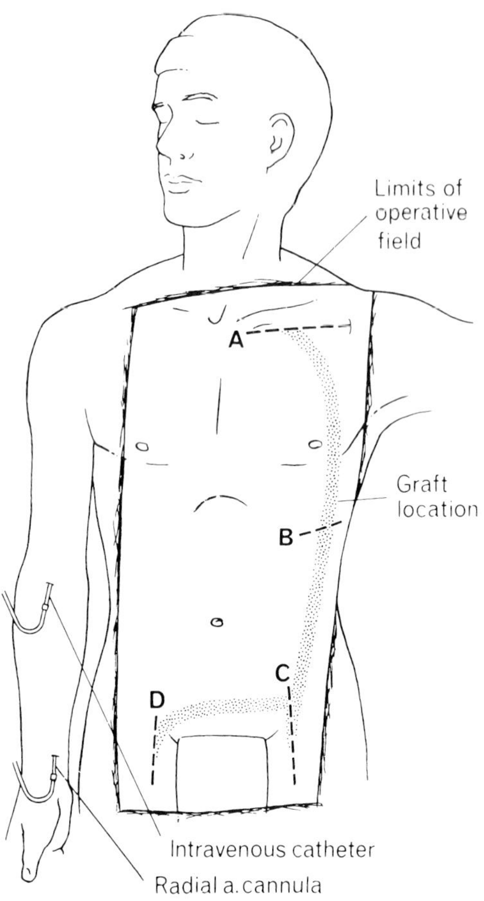

FIGURE 68–2. The position of patient, extent of operative field, location of incisions *(A–D),* and subcutaneous course of grafts for axillobifemoral bypass are represented. (From Rutherford RB: Axillary bifemoral bypass graft. *In* Bergan JJ, Yao JST [eds]: Operative Techniques in Vascular Surgery. New York, Grune & Stratton, 1980.)

noninvasive examination to detect disease in 75% of the patients in whom arteriography revealed significant stenoses. All things being equal, the right subclavian artery is preferred as the donor because it has a much lower risk of currently or eventually having occlusive disease than the left.

If the patient habitually sleeps on a particular side, the surgeon might choose to place the graft on the opposite side because thrombosis seems to develop in a number of axillofemoral grafts during sleep, presumably while they are compressed by the patient's body. This suspicion has not been confirmed by noninvasive studies; however, the two studies with the highest patency rates for axillofemoral bypass used externally supported graft material, which may protect against thrombosis caused by external graft compression.[17, 18] The operative field and the position of the patient for a left axillobifemoral graft are depicted in Figure 68–2.

Axillofemoral Bypass

Axillary exposure is gained through a transverse incision after the fibers of the pectoralis major muscle have been split and the deltopectoral fascia has been opened. The axillary artery, which lies deep and superior to the axillary vein and inferior to the brachial plexus, is identified by dissection toward the palpable pulse or following a branch of the thoracoacromial trunk. Division of the insertion of the pectoralis minor muscle, which appears in the lateral half of the incision, not only aids exposure but also simplifies tunneling of the graft.

Once the axillary artery has been identified, a 5- or 6-cm segment is mobilized. The arteriotomy should be made on the anterior inferior surface of the artery medially, near the chest wall, so that abduction of the upper extremity does not place tension on the anastomosis. Standard advice is that the angle of entry should not be acute, or at least no less than 75 degrees, because disruption of this anastomosis has been reported when the arm has been abducted too much during surgery.[63, 64] Therefore, the previously mentioned precautions are important.

For the same reason, the graft should not be pulled down into the subcutaneous tunnel too tightly. This position not only would threaten the integrity of the anastomosis but might cause the axillary artery to be drawn down into a Y-shaped junction, which would obstruct outflow and contribute to anastomotic stenosis. This complication has been thoroughly reviewed by Taylor and associates.[65] They point out that its incidence is higher than reports in the literature would indicate. It occurred in 11 of 200 patients (5%) in their experience, with 23 cases in the literature, although 67 cases were documented nationwide from 1984 to 1993. These investigators showed techniques for managing the complication according to the type of disruption and suggested another anastomotic configuration to avoid this problem, namely, an acute anastomosis brought laterally with considerable slack before being tunneled toward the ipsilateral groin. Since adopting that technique, they have observed no disruptions.

Occasionally, a single counterincision placed obliquely over the sixth or seventh intercostal space in the *mid-axillary* line is required between the axillary and femoral incisions. In most patients, particularly those who are average or smaller in stature and whose skin and subcutaneous tissue are relatively loose, a long, hollow metal tunneler can be used to connect the axillary and groin incisions, thus avoiding the counterincision. A more anteriorly placed graft (i.e., in front of the mid-axillary line) not only rides over the costal margin and can give rise to aneurysm formation but also is more likely to kink when the patient bends forward.[66, 67]

The femoral vessels are exposed in standard fashion through vertical incisions. If there is occlusive disease of the superficial femoral artery, the profunda femoris artery is exposed at least down to its first major perforator. An end-to-side anastomosis is then constructed into the appropriate outflow vessel in the standard axillounifemoral bypass. This anastomotic configuration may be modified when it is part of an axillobifemoral bypass (see later).

The size of the prosthetic graft used should approximate the diameter of the recipient vessel, usually 8 mm. The author has used both double-velour knitted Dacron and expanded polytetrafluoroethylene (PTFE) prostheses for this operation, with equally good results. The latter graft has the theoretical advantages that it should be less compressible and thrombectomy should be easier if occlusion occurs. Externally supported grafts have produced apparent improvements in patency when compared with historical controls[17, 18]; however, if thrombosis does occur, the supporting rings make surgical thrombectomy more difficult. The author therefore prefers unsupported regular-thickness PTFE to externally supported, thin-walled PTFE for axillofemoral bypasses.

Femorofemoral Bypass

The surgeon performs a femorofemoral bypass by making two vertical incisions over the femoral vessels and anastomosing the graft in the standard fashion on each side after tunneling it in a gentle upward convex curve through the subcutaneous tissue above the pubis and anterior to the rectus sheath. If there are problems with postirradiation changes or subcutaneous infection or if the patient is morbidly obese, it may be preferable to incise the external oblique aponeurosis and pass the graft in a retrofascial plane. The surgeon can even tunnel in the preperitoneal plane behind the rectus muscle and, by exposing the external iliac artery as "donor" through a somewhat more proximal incision, can avoid dissecting the groin on that side completely and obtain a forward-angled end-to-side proximal anastomosis.

Axillobifemoral Bypass

The axillobifemoral bypass essentially combines the two foregoing operations. The manner of combining them in terms of the anastomotic configuration, however, has become the focus of much innovation in an attempt to reduce the risk of thrombosis. Traditionally, after completion of the axillofemoral anastomoses, the first anastomosis of the femorofemoral crossover is usually made into the side of the axillofemoral graft distally. Those surgeons who believe that the extra flow associated with the femoral limb of the graft enhances the patency of the axillofemoral limb usually make this anastomosis quite low so that the graft assumes the configuration of an inverted C[39]; however, it also amounts to a double "piggyback" anastomosis with retrograde flow out through the femorofemoral graft. For this reason, others construct it in a more natural, "lazy S" configuration, with the proximal anastomosis made higher up on the anteromedial surface at the upper edge of the groin incision, which on that side is extended 3 or 4 cm higher than usual. This has the advantage of allowing an acutely angled antegrade takeoff rather than the retrograde flow characteristic of the inverted C anastomosis. In this regard, the results of the European Axillobifemoral Bypass Trial[68] are interesting. Nineteen vascular centers performed a randomized comparison between an axillobifemoral prosthesis with a right-angled (90-degree) side-arm and a newer prosthesis with an acutely angled, antegrade takeoff ("flow splitter"). At 2 years, the latter prosthesis had better than twice the patency rate (84% versus 38%) of the former.

Because both the lazy S and the inverted C configurations of the femorofemoral limb have disadvantages, other alternatives have been advocated (Fig. 68–3). To avoid the double "piggyback" anastomoses of the inverted C configuration yet bring the higher flow all the way to the distal end of the axillofemoral limb, Blaisdell and coworkers[1] recommended mobilizing the common femoral artery and even some of the external iliac artery proximal to this anastomosis, dividing it and oversewing the upper end, and then using the lower end as the site of the proximal anastomosis of the femorofemoral bypass (see Fig. 68–3, *lower right*). Endarterectomy of this segment may be required to make a suitable donor vessel. If this is not feasible, one can construct the proximal stem as a crossover axillofemoral bypass that swings low across the upper end of the ipsilateral groin incision. This allows a very short, antegrade limb to be anastomosed to the undersurface of the main graft. This anastomosis is easier than the lazy S configuration, the "unprotected" segment is short, and all anastomoses have antegrade flow (see Fig. 68–3, *lower left*).

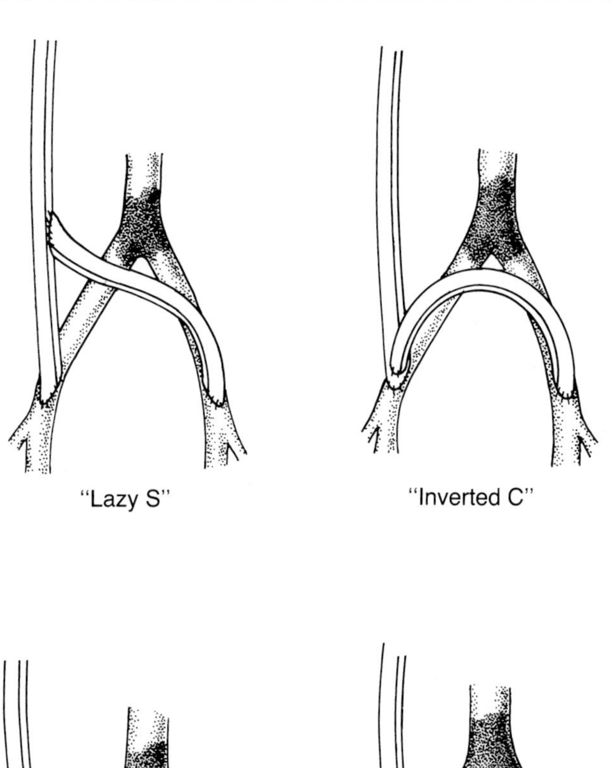

FIGURE 68–3. Some of the more commonly employed configurations for connecting the side limb of an axillobifemoral bypass (see text).

The author has combined these last two techniques, when suitable, into a modification that not only has all antegrade anastomoses *and* brings the higher-flow proximal stem down to the ipsilateral femoral anastomosis but also requires only one graft and three, rather than four, anastomoses. This technique, shown in Figure 68–4, involves mobilization of the upper common femoral artery (after it

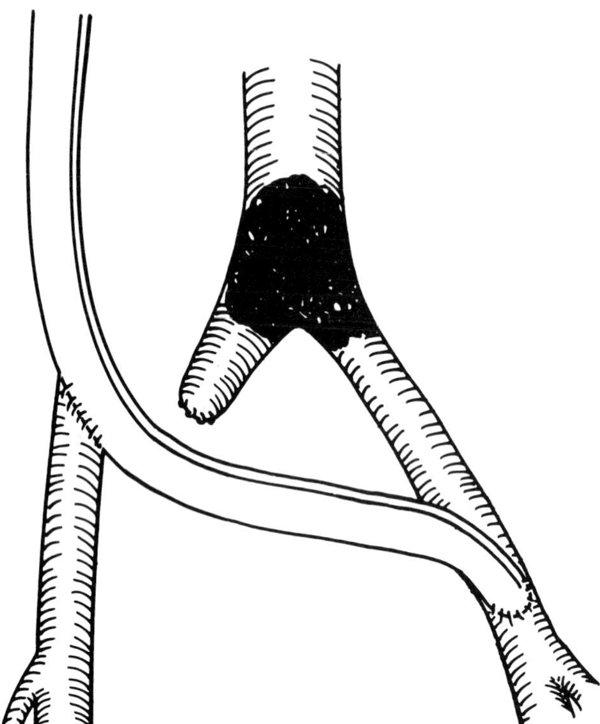

FIGURE 68–4. A modified technique for axillobifemoral bypass in which a single crossover axillofemoral graft is brought down to the contralateral femoral artery and the ipsilateral femoral artery is mobilized, divided, and anastomosed to it. (From Rutherford RB, Rainer WG: A modified technique for axillofemoral bypass [Letter]. J Vasc Surg 10:468, 1989.)

is severed from the external iliac artery and the latter is closed) and anastomosis of it to the underside of an axillary crossover femoral graft as it passes by the upper end of the ipsilateral groin incision.

Finally, some surgeons have simply reversed the order of the anastomoses in the ipsilateral groin, placing the end of the axillofemoral graft into the hood of the proximal femoral bypass, as shown in Figure 68–5. Some may prefer to place this anastomosis a little higher up to minimize retrograde outflow. Clearly, there are many technical modifications to choose from. In the absence of comparative studies, the reader must choose the modification that seems most logical in the given circumstances.

Aftercare for Axillofemoral and Femorofemoral Bypass

These extra-anatomic operations are usually well tolerated because there is minimal blood loss or hemodynamic disturbance. Nasogastric intubation is rarely necessary. In fact, patients usually can resume oral intake the day after surgery. Unless contraindicated, sodium warfarin (Coumadin) is administered on a long-term basis; otherwise, antiplatelet drugs are used. A patency advantage of warfarin therapy in this setting has not been proved at this writing, even though the practice has become popular for these and other long prosthetic grafts (e.g., infrainguinal prosthetic bypasses).

The patient is warned against sleeping on the side of the axillofemoral graft. Compliance can be ensured if a loose wrist gauntlet is attached from the donor wrist to the opposite side of the bed at night until the patient has formed the habit of sleeping on the other side. If the patient needs crutches, it is important that the "Canadian" type, with forearm grips, be used rather than the standard variety. The patient should be taught to feel for the pulses in both limbs of the graft every day to detect graft thrombosis and ensure early attention if this complication develops.

Obturator Bypass

Technique

The patient is placed on the operating table in the supine position, with the entire leg prepared and draped so that it can be rotated laterally and abducted and so that the hip can be flexed to relax the thigh musculature.[69, 70] Any groin wound must be carefully covered with an adherent drape and excluded from the operative field of the abdomen and the thigh. Careful preparation of the skin must be performed because of the likelihood of contamination of the area adjacent to an infection in the groin.

Abdominal exposure may be gained through a right paramedian incision and a transperitoneal approach to the aorta and iliac vessels or the limb of an aortofemoral graft. However, a transverse retroperitoneal approach is preferred if preoperative angiography has confirmed that an iliac artery is suitable as a donor vessel for the graft. This latter approach allows adequate exposure of the obturator membrane for perforation under direct vision.

If the problem for which the procedure is being performed is infection in the groin, it is critical at this point to determine whether infection has extended proximal to the inguinal ligament and up the graft. If the graft is still patent, there is a good possibility that infection may not have extended proximally. If the graft has thrombosis, infection will spread to involve the entire thrombosed segment.

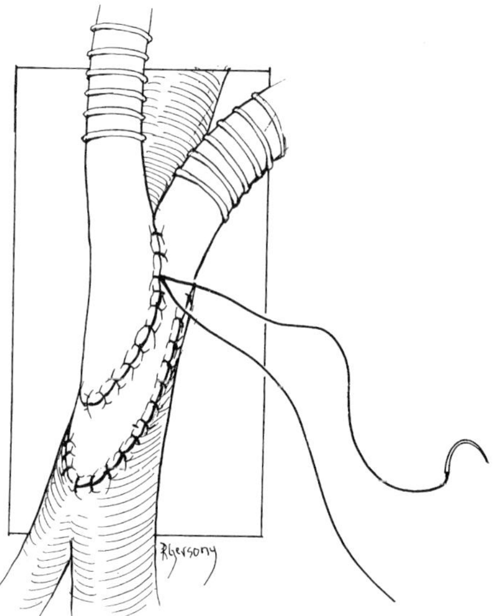

FIGURE 68–5. The axillofemoral graft limb is anastomosed to the hood of the femorofemoral bypass, a reverse of the standard technique intended to improve configuration and reduce flow turbulence. (From Ouriel K, Rutherford RB [eds]: Atlas of Vascular Surgery: Operative Procedures. Philadelphia, WB Saunders, 1998, p 91.)

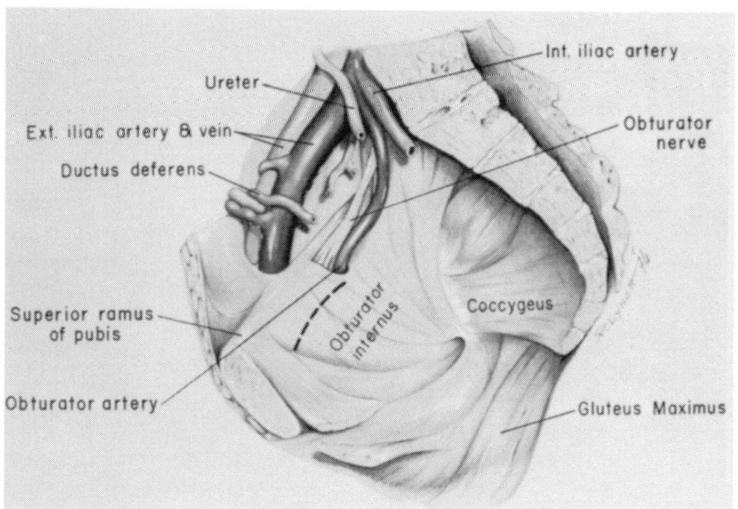

FIGURE 68–6. Anatomy and exposure of the obturator foramen from within the pelvis. Note particularly the avascular area of the foramen and the superior medial portion where the fibers of the obturator internus muscle are separated and the membranous portion is incised.

If the prosthesis shows excellent incorporation by surrounding tissue and overlying peritoneum and if there is no edema, induration, or infected material around it, one can make a reasonable assumption that this portion of the graft is not infected. If time allows, a radioactive indium–labeled leukocyte scan or a computed tomographic scan may help with this determination (see Chapter 47). When this status has been determined, the patent proximal graft can be used as the proximal inflow for an obturator bypass.

If neither the common iliac artery nor the aorta has been previously grafted, either may be selected for the proximal anastomosis. The site selected for anastomosis, of course, depends on the extent of disease present, as determined by palpation and accurate preoperative arteriography. These vessels are then mobilized to afford proximal and distal control. The surgeon must take care at this point in the procedure to identify, mobilize, and preserve the ureter in a safe location.

Next, the obturator foramen is located. As shown in Figure 68–6, it lies just posterior to the superior ramus of the pubis. The surgeon exposes it by reflecting the peritoneum from its surface, beginning at the external iliac artery and proceeding downward over the pubic ramus. Alternatively, the surgeon can locate the obturator foramen by identifying the hypogastric artery and determining the origin of the obturator branch, which usually arises from it and courses downward to and through the foramen. Occasionally, the obturator artery arises from the inferior epigastric artery and travels directly posteriorly over the superior ramus of the pubis to the foramen. The obturator artery, vein, and nerve that serve to identify the exact location of the foramen pass through it at the anterolateral border of the obturator fossa in very close apposition to the edge of bone that forms the lateral superior margin of the canal. In addition, by palpation, the obturator fossa also can be felt behind the superior ramus of the pubis. At the upper edge of the obturator fossa, the vas deferens crosses the pubic ramus and runs posteriorly.

The surgeon now selects an area for making the tunnel through the foramen. This tunnel should be located some distance from where the obturator artery, vein, and nerve pass through to avoid injury to these structures and to traverse the foramen in a relatively avascular location. As shown in Figure 68–6, this point is best located anteriorly and medially, just underneath the superior ramus of the pubis and medial to the vessels. The site for the tunnel should be kept as far anterior as possible to avoid the fleshy, thick obturator internus muscle, which is located more inferiorly. From inside the pelvis, blunt dissection and separation of the fibers of the obturator internus muscle are performed, which will lead to a tough aponeurotic membrane. This is a dense fascial wall lying between the obturator internus and obturator externus muscles, serving as their attachments. This membrane is too tough to break through with blunt finger dissection, and it is better incised sharply. An instrument can then be passed through the tunnel from the pelvis into the thigh.

Attention is then turned to the thigh. The optimal site for the distal anastomosis depends on the individual patient's disease and other considerations. Use of the popliteal artery above the knee has the advantage that a shorter graft is required, but this segment may be atherosclerotic. The popliteal artery below the knee is more likely to be free of disease, but a longer graft is required. A tunneling instrument may be passed from above downward, to lie along the course of the popliteal artery so that one can begin dissection of the thigh above the knee and medially, well below the infected groin wound. This incision is developed with care to avoid injury to the greater saphenous vein, which may be the best graft to use considering the risk of contamination.

The deep fascia is opened, and the sartorius muscle is retracted to expose the proximal popliteal artery in the groove between the sartorius and the vastus medialis muscles. The tendinous margin of the adductor magnus muscle, which may cover the artery, may be divided to facilitate exposure. The fibrous sheath of the popliteal artery is carefully dissected free of its companion veins. The tunnel is then developed with a conventional tunneling instrument. The pectineus, adductor longus, and adductor brevis muscles arise from the anteromedial rim of the obturator foramen. The anterior surfaces of these muscles form the floor and medial boundaries of the femoral triangle. The adductor magnus muscle arises from the posterior rim of the external surface of the foramen, so the tunneler passes through the canal onto the anterior surface of the adductor

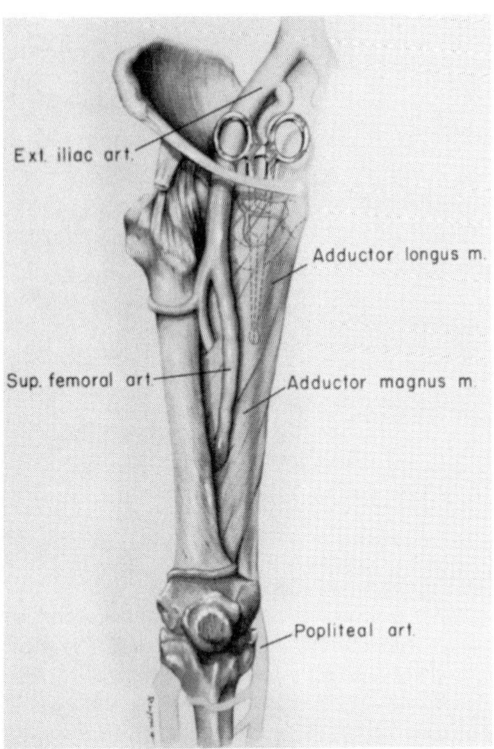

FIGURE 68–7. The tunnel is being created through the obturator foramen, showing the relationships to the pelvis, the major vessels, and the muscles of the thigh. The tunneling instrument lies between the adductor longus and the adductor magnus muscles.

magnus muscle in the thigh (Fig. 68–7). The tunnel is separated from the superficial femoral artery by the anterior mass of the adductor muscles. With gentle pressure and manipulation, the tunneler passes down easily to the vicinity of the adductor hiatus. The hiatus can then be located by palpation in the area where the superficial femoral artery passes through it, and the tunneler is delivered through the hiatus to lie in the popliteal fossa.

If a previous aortofemoral graft is available to be the donor vessel at the iliac level, the prosthesis is divided and sutured end-to-end to the new graft. The distal end of the old graft is then free to be removed later when the groin is débrided. If the iliac artery is the donor vessel, angled vascular clamps are placed on the artery and then rotated laterally so that the arteriotomy is made with the proper orientation for the graft to pass to the obturator foramen. Finally, the external iliac artery is ligated distal to the takeoff of the graft.

The graft is then carefully passed or drawn through the tunnel with the use of the tunneler. After application of the popliteal clamps and reapplication of the iliac artery clamp, the distal suture line is made. The popliteal artery is then usually ligated proximal to the graft to minimize back-bleeding from the superficial femoral artery during the groin dissection.

After restoration of blood flow to the extremity, the peritoneum is closed carefully over the graft. It is best for the new graft to lie along the pelvic wall rather than to run straight across the pelvis. The abdominal and thigh incisions are closed, and dressings are applied. Thereafter, attention is directed to the problem in the groin. If the patient had an infected graft, the distal defunctionalized graft limb can now be removed. The divided proximal end is brought down into the field, and the parent artery is closed. Back-bleeding from the profunda femoris artery is controlled by suture ligature, and infected tissue in the groin is débrided thoroughly. A schematic of the completed operation is shown in Figure 68–8. The groin incision is left open for drainage to allow granulation tissue formation and delayed healing. Appropriate antibiotics are continued during this period.

The preceding description assumes a distal superficial femoral or upper popliteal anastomosis, which is usually feasible. Occasionally, however, anastomosis into the profunda femoris artery in its middle third is necessary. This can be done by using the medial approach to that segment.[59] This exposure is depicted in Figure 68–9. The final appearance and position of the obturator bypass graft with this particular location of distal anastomosis are shown in Figure 68–10.

RESULTS AND COMPLICATIONS

The extra-anatomic bypasses can be associated with all the complications encountered after any arterial prosthetic reconstruction: perigraft hemorrhage, thrombosis, infection, and the like. The very nature of these grafts, the extensive subcutaneous tunneling, the need for groin dissections, and the fact that they are often employed *because* of graft sepsis or other inflammatory intra-abdominal conditions all account for a higher-than-average incidence of each of these complications.[71] Conversely, the incidence of

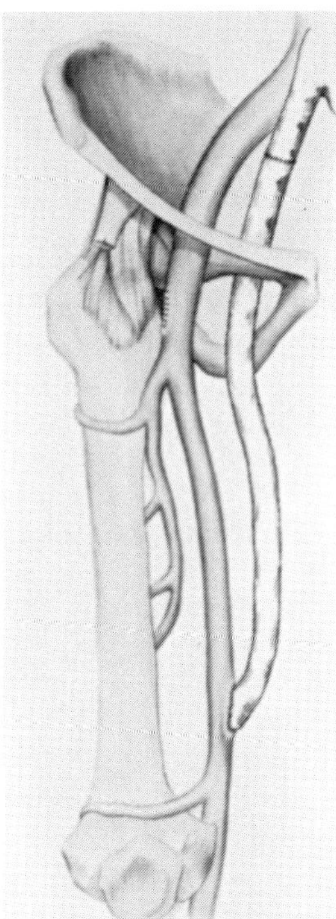

FIGURE 68–8. A graft has been placed from a previous prosthesis and has been continued down to the proximal popliteal artery. The common femoral artery in the septic area has been closed.

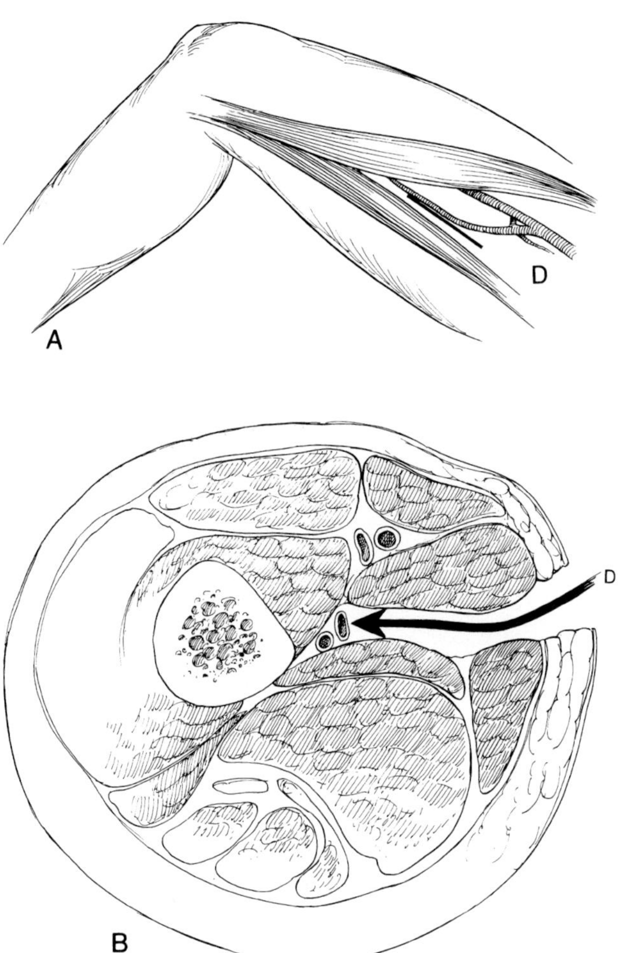

FIGURE 68–9. *A,* When the distal anastomosis of an obturator bypass is made to the profunda femoris artery, the incision is higher on the medial thigh, about the second fifth of a line between the pubic tubercle and the femoral condyle. *B,* This approach, indicated in this cross section by the arrow, enters the thigh just under the adductor longus muscle and follows in beneath it to its inner (lateral) margin, where the sheath around the profunda femoris is encountered. (From Rutherford RB [ed]: Atlas of Vascular Surgery: Basic Techniques and Exposures. Philadelphia, WB Saunders, 1993, p 130.)

general or systemic complications (e.g., pneumonia, ileus, pulmonary embolism, myocardial infarction, renal failure), although probably higher than that generally reported for aortobifemoral bypass grafting, is nevertheless lower than if aortobifemoral bypass had been performed on the same group of patients. This statement also applies to mortality rates, as pointed out later.

In addition, some complications are more or less specific to these procedures, some primarily involving the upper extremity.[72] The likelihood of a steal has already been discussed. Brachial plexus injury, usually because of hyperabduction, has been reported. Occlusion of the subclavian and axillary arteries may result if the graft is inserted under too much tension or becomes tighter as a result of the desmoplastic reaction around it. Occasionally, unrecognized stenoses proximal to the anastomosis result in donor artery thrombosis. The femoral complications are essentially the same as those encountered in aortofemoral bypass grafting.

The results of femorofemoral, axillofemoral, axillobifemoral, and axillopopliteal bypass grafting, as reported in the literature, are summarized in Table 68–1. Roughly fourfold differences in operative mortality and twofold differences in long-term patency are documented. Depending on which of these results one accepts, one might take an enthusiastic or a pessimistic position about applying extra-anatomic bypass. Careful reading of the literature indicates that although some of these differences may be due to technical considerations, most can be explained on the basis of case selection (i.e., liberal versus conservative indications and related patient risk factors) and the criteria for success or failure (i.e., reporting practices).[40, 73–75] The latter relate mainly to the use of secondary as opposed to primary patency rates, because few grafts present a greater opportunity to test the utility of thrombectomy or thrombolysis (i.e., a high thrombosis rate in an accessible graft). For example, one reported comparison of axillobifemoral and aortobifemoral procedures showed a 76% secondary patency rate for the former, but this included a 43% rate of thrombectomy or revision.[15] This cause has been corrected in more recent reports by adherence to accepted reporting standards.

Liberal application of extra-anatomic bypass results in better mortality and patency rates. At the time of this report, Johnson and associates[15] offered axillobifemoral bypass "to anyone over the age of 65, regardless of risk." Most axillobifemoral bypasses reported by Ray and colleagues[39] were performed for claudication. Conversely, conservative application of axillobifemoral bypass results in a paradoxically higher mortality rate for this "low-risk option" than for aortobifemoral bypass (which has benefited by having these high-risk cases removed). By restricting the use of axillofemoral bypass to limb salvage indications, one also can obtain lower patency rates because of poorer cardiac function and the fact that concomitant superficial femoral artery occlusion is almost uniformly present. Clearly, "lumped" or "bottom line" figures can be deceiving. For this reason, the author has published the results for extra-anatomic bypasses broken down according to indications for operation and runoff status and with both primary and secondary patency rates presented.[40] These are summarized in Table 68–2.

The use of externally supported conduits for axillobifemoral bypass has been associated with markedly improved long-term primary patency rates (76% to 85%). However, these reports are also subject to the influence of patient selection. Of the patients reported on by El-Massry and coworkers,[18] 36% had claudication, and although Harris and associates[17] did not report the incidence of claudication in their series, data from a subsequent publication by this group[76] indicated a steadily increasing application of this bypass, as well as the inclusion of cases performed for other indications than occlusive disease and the growing use of concomitant femoropopliteal bypass to mitigate the effects of poor runoff. Whether one credits the externally supported prostheses for the improved patency, or other concomitant changes in technique (e.g., changing the anastomotic configuration in the ipsilateral groin, as described earlier, or performing simultaneous distal bypass) is not as important as whether these improvements justify the more

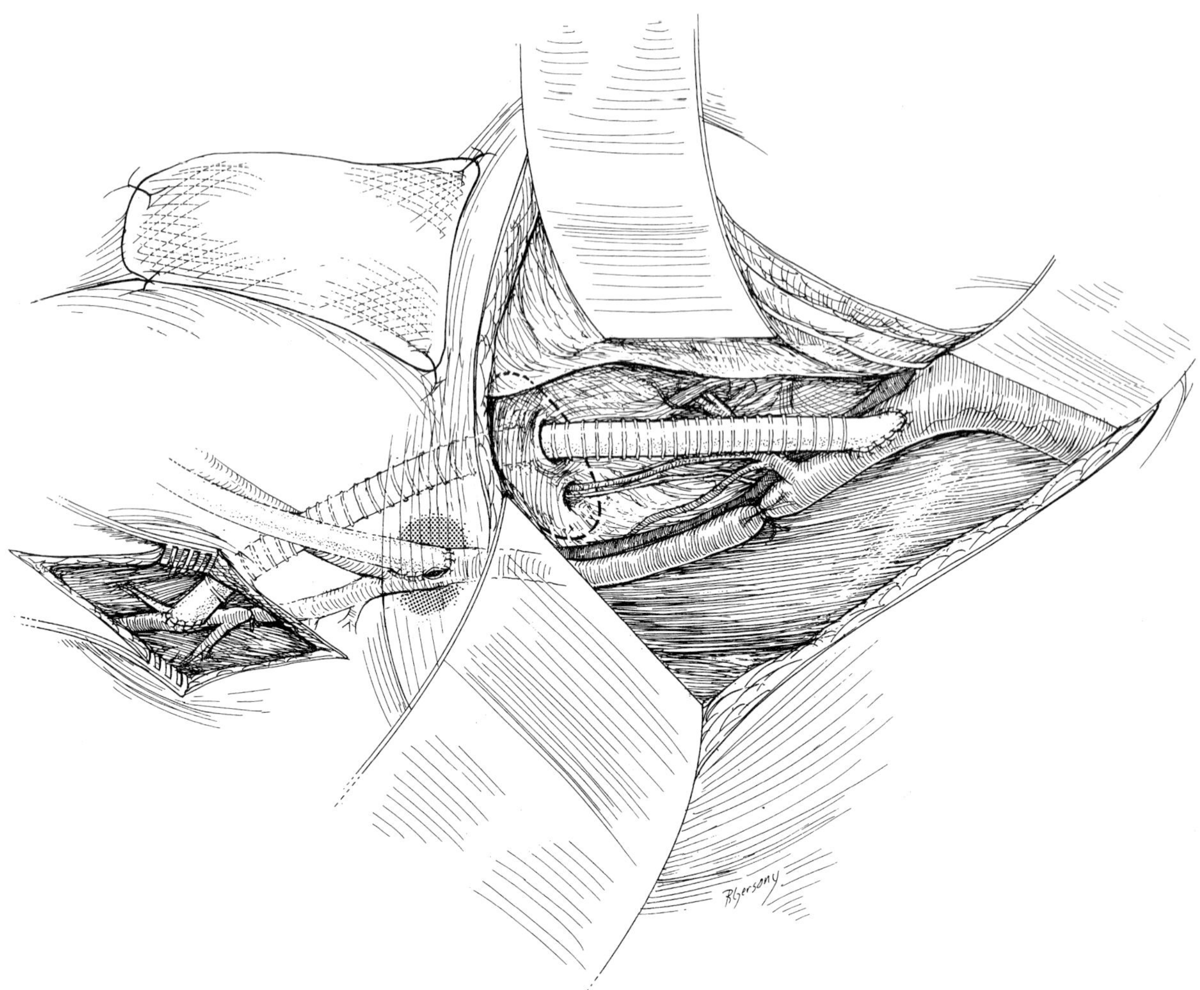

FIGURE 68–10. Final appearance and position of an obturator bypass to the profunda femoris artery before wound closure and removal of the old graft. (From Ouriel K, Rutherford RB [eds]: Atlas of Vascular Surgery: Operative Procedures. Philadelphia, WB Saunders, 1998, p 821.)

liberal application of axillobifemoral bypass in comparison with aortobifemoral bypass.

To this end, Passman and colleagues[77] have published a comparison of the two bypasses as performed at the University of Oregon. As one would expect, the patients undergoing axillobifemoral bypass were a higher-risk group in terms of age, associated heart disease, and "limb salvage" indications, and these attributes were ultimately reflected in a lower patient survival. These investigators, while pointing to a greater complication rate with aortobifemoral bypass, admit to higher 5-year secondary patency rate for the aortobifemoral graft; because there were no other (statistically) significant differences in outcome, however, they conclude that when this procedure is reserved for high-risk patients, the patency and limb salvage rates of axillofemoral bypass are *equivalent* to those of aortofemoral bypass. However, mean data favor the aortobifemoral bypass in both 5-year primary patency (80% versus 74%) and mortality (<1% versus 3.4%).

It is difficult to make valid comparisons between patient groups who differ significantly in known factors affecting outcome, and nowhere else do liberal versus conservative indications magnify these differences more. Neither extreme (liberal or conservative application) is right, however, and as usual, the correct position lies somewhere in between and needs to be based on careful patient selection. In deciding between aortobifemoral and axillobifemoral bypass, one is basically facing, in a given case, a tradeoff between mortality and morbidity and long-term patency. The traditional "life before limb" priority must be honored in patients with prohibitive operative risk and those with hostile abdominal pathologic conditions. The author believes, however, that because of greatly improved perioperative care, the indications for axillobifemoral bypass should not ordinarily be extended beyond these two accepted indications and should not be applied in patients with claudication. It also should be remembered that there are other options to direct transabdominal aortobifemoral bypass, namely, a retroperitoneal aortobifemoral bypass, a thoracic aorta to femoral bypass,[78, 79] and extension of the use of percutaneous balloon dilatation by stenting or thrombolysis. Although the last approach ordinarily cannot be justified in extensive aortoiliac occlusive disease, patients with prohibitive operative risk or "hostile" abdominal pathologic condition and who have limb-threatening ischemia may be justifiable exceptions.

Obturator Bypass Results

Patency rates for obturator bypass range from 66% to 89%.[80] Tilson and Baue[81] and van Det and Brands[82] reported personal series of 10 cases and 13 cases with 89% and 80% patency rates, respectively. Van Det and Brands[82] collected an additional 66 cases from the literature with an overall patency rate of 68%. A later review by Sautner and colleagues[83] reported a 5-year patency rate of close to 60%, which they calculated by combining their 34 cases with 125 cases reported in the literature since 1982. There were no occlusions in their personal series in patients without atherosclerotic occlusive disease during a mean follow-up period of 34 months. Although prosthetic material is often employed, this graft is not subject to acute flexion, and in comparison with femoropopliteal bypasses, it enjoys the advantage of receiving better proximal inflow. Thus, the overall 5-year patency rate of about 60% is not surprising. Except for the expected higher risk of graft sepsis, complications for obturator bypass have been, for the most part, similar to those experienced with any distal bypass.[84]

SUMMARY

Because extra-anatomic bypasses are usually longer grafts and their extra-anatomic position is more subject to external compression, their patency rates generally do not approach those reported with direct arterial reconstruction if runoff and other factors are considered.[15, 39] Mortality will be lower in the same group of high-risk patients, but advances in perioperative monitoring and intensive care have made this a moot consideration in all but patients with the most prohibitive risk factors. Finally, although extra-anatomic bypasses are physiologically much less challenging to the patient, they are usually not technically easier and do not result in significantly reduced operating time.

Unlike obturator bypass, which is used when there is little other choice, axillounifemoral, axillobifemoral, and femorofemoral bypasses often compete in applicability with other procedures. They rarely compete with one another. The correct choice depends on a number of factors in addition to patient risk and hostile abdominal pathologic conditions. The morphology of the occlusive disease may be important, as in the choice between iliac PTA and femorofemoral bypass, and the status of the runoff vessels or the opposite iliac artery may determine the choice between aortobifemoral bypass and femorofemoral bypass (with or without PTA).

On the basis of the foregoing discussions, these decisions may be approached in a logical way and individualized to the particular patient's benefit. An algorithm of this decision-making process is offered in Figure 68–11. Although this algorithm does not, for simplicity's sake, reflect optional reconstructions of the femorofemoral bypass (aortofemoral bypass, iliofemoral bypass, and endarterectomy, as discussed in the text) and other subtler aspects, it should provide a framework for personal decision making.

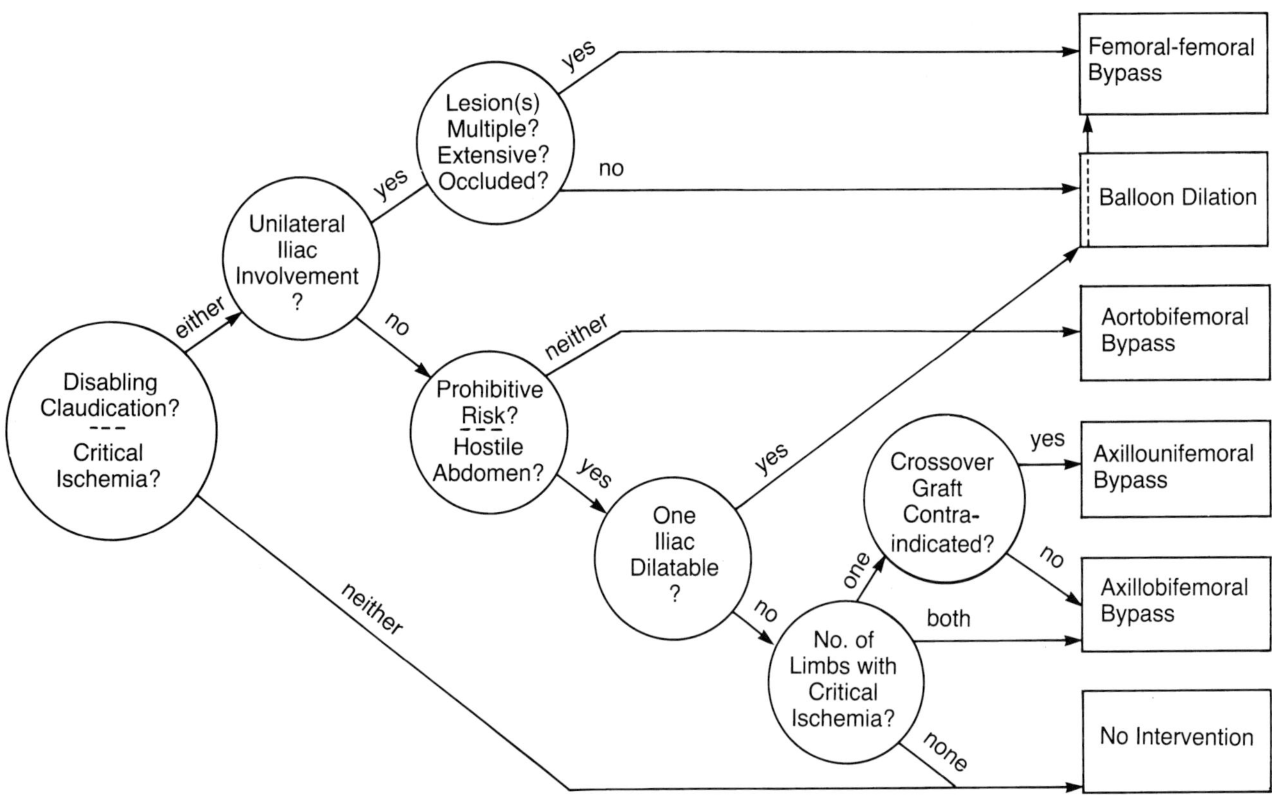

FIGURE 68–11. Algorithm for initial management of aortoiliac occlusive disease.

REFERENCES

1. Blaisdell FW, Holcroft JW, Ward RE: Axillofemoral and femorofemoral bypass: History and evolution of technique. *In* Greenhalgh RM (ed): Extra-anatomic and Secondary Arterial Reconstruction. London, Pitman Medical Publishing, 1982.
2. Freeman NE, Leeds FH: Operations on large arteries: Application of recent advances. Calif Med 77:229, 1952.
3. Blaisdell FW, DeMattei GA, Gauder PJ: Extraperitoneal thoracic aorta to femoral bypass graft as replacement for an infected aortic bifurcation prosthesis. Am J Surg 102:583, 1961.
4. Warren R: Bypass arterial graft between splenic and iliofemoral arteries. Arch Surg 72:57, 1956.
5. Vetto RM: The treatment of unilateral iliac artery obstruction with a transabdominal subcutaneous femorofemoral graft. Surgery 52:342, 1962.
6. Blaisdell FW, Hall AD: Axillary femoral artery bypass for lower extremity ischemia. Surgery 54:563, 1963.
7. Louw JH: The treatment of combined aortoiliac and femoral popliteal occlusive disease by splenofemoral and axillofemoral bypass grafts. Surgery 55:387, 1963.
8. Blaisdell FW, Hall AD, Lim RC Jr, et al: Aortoiliac arterial substitution utilizing subcutaneous grafts. Ann Surg 172:775, 1970.
9. Sauvage LR, Wood SJ: Unilateral axillary bilateral femoral bifurcation graft: A procedure for the poor risk patient with aortoiliac disease. Surgery 60:573, 1966.
10. Shaw RS, Baue AE: Management of sepsis complicating arterial reconstructive surgery. Surgery 53:75, 1962.
11. Alpert J, Brief DK, Parsonnet V: Vascular restoration for aortoiliac occlusion and an alternative approach to the poor risk patient. J Newark Beth Israel Hosp 18:4, 1967.
12. Parsonnet V, Alpert J, Brief DK: Femorofemoral and axillofemoral grafts: Compromise or preference. Surgery 67:26, 1970.
13. Brief DK, Alpert J, Parsonnet V: Crossover femorofemoral grafts: Compromise or preference: A reappraisal. Arch Surg 105:889, 1972.
14. LoGerfo FW, Johnson WC, Corson JD, et al: A comparison of the late patency rates of axillobilateral femoral and axillounilateral femoral grafts. Surgery 81:33, 1977.
15. Johnson WC, LoGerfo FW, Vollman RW: Is axillobilateral femoral graft an effective substitute for aortobilateral iliac femoral graft? Ann Surg 186:123, 1976.
16. Eugene J, Goldstone J, Moore WS: Fifteen-year experience with subcutaneous bypass grafts for lower extremity ischemia. Ann Surg 186:177, 1976.
17. Harris EJ, Taylor LM, McConnell DB, et al: Clinical results of axillobifemoral bypass using externally supported polytetrafluoroethylene. J Vasc Surg 12:416, 1990.
18. El-Massry S, Saad E, Sauvage LR, et al: Axillofemoral bypass using externally-supported, knitted Dacron grafts: A follow-up through twelve years. J Vasc Surg 17:107, 1993.
19. Schneider JR, McDaniel MD, Walsh DB, et al: Axillofemoral bypass: Outcome and hemodynamic results in high-risk patients. J Vasc Surg 15:952, 1992.
20. Veith FJ, Moss CM, Daly V, et al: New approaches to limb salvage by extended extra-anatomic bypasses and prosthetic reconstructions to foot arteries. Surgery 84:764, 1978.
21. Connolly JE, Kwaan JHM, Brownell D, et al: Newer developments of extraanatomic bypass. Surg Gynecol Obstet 158:415, 1984.
22. Ascer E, Veith FJ, Gupta S: Axillopopliteal bypass grafting: Indications, late results, and determinants of long-term patency. J Vasc Surg 10:285, 1989.
23. Keller MP, Hoch JR, Harding AD, et al: Axillopopliteal bypass for limb salvage. J Vasc Surg 15:817, 1992.
24. Karmody AM, Leather RP, Goldman M, et al: The current position of nonresective treatment for abdominal aortic aneurysm. Surgery 94:591, 1983.
25. Inahara T, Geary GL, Mukherjee D, et al: The contrary position to the non-resective treatment of abdominal aortic aneurysm. J Vasc Surg 4:42, 1985.
26. Kim L, Kohler T, Johansen K: Non-resective therapy for aortic aneurysm: Results of a survey. J Vasc Surg 4:469, 1986.
27. Schwartz RA, Nichols WK, Silver D: Is thrombosis of the infrarenal abdominal aortic aneurysm an acceptable alternative? J Vasc Surg 3:448, 1986.
28. Pevec WC, Holcroft JW, Blaisdell FW: Ligation and extraanatomic arterial reconstruction for the treatment of aneurysms of the abdominal aorta. J Vasc Surg 29:629, 1994.
29. Murayama KM, Grune MT, Matamoros A Jr, et al: Staple occlusion of the infrarenal aorta: A videoscopic retroperitoneal approach. J Vasc Surg 25:786, 1997.
30. Ehrenfeld WK, Harris JD, Wylie EJ: Vascular "steal" phenomenon: An experimental study. Am J Surg 116:192, 1968.
31. Shin CS, Chaudhry AG: The hemodynamics of extra-anatomic bypass grafts. Surg Gynecol Obstet 148:567, 1979.
32. Sumner DS, Strandness DE: The hemodynamics of the femorofemoral shunt. Surg Gynecol Obstet 134:629, 1972.
33. Flanigan P, Pratt DG, Goodreau JJ, et al: Hemodynamic and angiographic guidelines in selection of patients for femorofemoral bypass. Arch Surg 113:1257, 1978.
34. Weale FE: The values of series and parallel resistances in steady blood flow. Br J Surg 51:623, 1964.
35. Ernst CB: Axillary femoral bypass graft without aortofemoral pressure differential. Ann Surg 181:424, 1974.
36. Brief DK, Brener B, Alpert J, et al: Crossover femorofemoral grafts followed up five years or more: An analysis. Arch Surg 110:1294, 1975.
37. de Gama AD: The fate of the donor artery in extraanatomic revascularization. J Vasc Surg 8:106, 1988.
38. Piotrowski J, Rutherford RB, Jones DN, et al: Aortobifemoral bypass: The operation of choice for unilateral iliac occlusion. J Vasc Surg 8:211, 1988.
39. Ray LI, O'Connor JB, Davis CC, et al: Axillofemoral bypass: A critical reappraisal of its role in the management of aortoiliac occlusive disease. Am J Surg 138:117, 1979.
40. Rutherford RB, Patt A, Pearce WH: Extra-anatomic bypass: A closer view. J Vasc Surg 5:437, 1987.
41. Rutherford RB, Patt A, Kumpe DA: The current role of percutaneous transluminal angioplasty. *In* Greenhalgh RM, Jamieson CW, Nicolaides AN (eds): Vascular Surgery: Issues in Current Practice. London, Grune & Stratton, 1986.
42. Johnston KW, Rae M, Hogg-Johnston SA, et al: Five-year results of a prospective study of percutaneous transluminal angioplasty. Ann Surg 206:403, 1987.
43. Ng RL, Gillies TE, Baird RN, Horrocks M: Iliofemoral versus femorofemoral bypass: A 6 year audit. Br J Surg 79:1011, 1992.
44. Harrington ME, Harrington EB, Haimov M, et al: Iliofemoral versus femorofemoral bypass: The case for an individualized approach. J Vasc Surg 16:841, 1992.
45. Hanafy M, McLoughlin GA: Comparison of iliofemoral and femorofemoral crossover bypass in the treatment of unilateral iliac artery occlusive disease. Br J Surg 78:1001, 1991.
46. Perler BA, Williams GM: Does donor iliac artery percutaneous transluminal angioplasty or stent placement influence the results of femorofemoral bypass? Analysis of 70 consecutive cases with long term follow up. J Vasc Surg 24:363, 1996.
47. Shah RM, Peer RM, Upson JF, Ricotta JJ: Donor iliac artery angioplasty and crossover femorofemoral bypass. Am J Surg 164:295, 1992.
48. Cham C, Myers KA, Scott DF, et al: Extraperitoneal unilateral iliac artery bypass for chronic lower limb ischemia. Aust N Z J Surg 58:859, 1988.
49. Kram HB, Gupta SK, Veith FJ, Wengerter KR: Unilateral aortofemoral bypass: A safe and effective option for the treatment of unilateral limb-threatening ischemia. Am J Surg 162:155, 1991.
50. Darling RC, Leather RP, Chang BB, et al: Is the iliac artery a suitable inflow conduit for iliofemoral occlusive disease? An analysis of aorto-iliac reconstructions. J Vasc Surg 17:15–19, 1993.
51. Cohn LH, Moore WS, Hall AD: Extra-abdominal management of late aortofemoral graft thrombosis. Surgery 67:775, 1970.
52. Porter JM, Eidemiller LR, Dotter CT, et al: Combined arterial dilatation and femorofemoral bypass for limb salvage. Surg Gynecol Obstet 137:409, 1973.
53. Rudich M, Gutierrez IZ, Gage AA: Obturator foramen bypass in the management of infected vascular prosthesis. Am J Surg 137:657, 1979.
54. Mahoney WD, Whelan TJ: Use of the obturator foramen in iliofemoral artery grafting. Ann Surg 163:215, 1966.
55. DePalma RG, Hubay CA: Arterial bypass via the obturator foramen. Am J Surg 115:323, 1968.
56. Donahoe PK, Froio RA, Nabseth DC: Obturator bypass graft in radical excision of inguinal neoplasm. Ann Surg 166:147, 1967.

57. Hegarty JC, Linton PC, McSweeney ED: Revascularization of the lower extremity through the obturator canal. Arch Surg 98:35, 1969.
58. Mentha C, Launois B, DeLaere J: Les pontages artériels iliofémoraux par le trou obturator. J Chir (Paris) 90:131, 1965.
59. Millis JM, Ahn SS: Transobturator aorto–profunda femoral artery bypass using the direct medial thigh approach. Ann Vasc Surg 7:384, 1993.
60. Delaurentis DA, Sala LE, Russell E, et al: A twelve-year experience with axillofemoral and femorofemoral bypass operations. Surg Gynecol Obstet 147:881, 1978.
61. Rutherford RB: Axillary bifemoral bypass graft. *In* Bergan JJ, Yao JST (eds): Operative Techniques in Vascular Surgery. New York, Grune & Stratton, 1980.
62. Calligaro KD, Ascer E, Veith FJ, et al: Unsuspected inflow disease in candidates for axillofemoral bypass operations: A prospective study. J Vasc Surg 11:832, 1990.
63. White GH, Donayre CE, Williams RA, et al: Exertional disruption of axillofemoral graft anastomosis. Arch Surg 125:625, 1990.
64. Sullivan LP, Davidson PG, D'Anna JA, Sithian N: Disruption of the proximal anastomosis of axillobifemoral grafts: Two case reports. J Vasc Surg 10:190, 1989.
65. Taylor LM, Park TC, Edwards JM, et al: Acute disruption of polytetrafluorethylene grafts adjacent to axillary anastomoses: A complication of axillofemoral grafting. J Vasc Surg 20:520, 1994.
66. Mannick JA, Williams LE, Nabseth DC: The late results of axillofemoral grafts. Surgery 68:1038, 1970.
67. Orringer MB, Rutherford RB, Skinner DB: An unusual complication of axillary femoral artery bypass. Surgery 72:769, 1972.
68. Wittens CHA, van Houtte HJKP, van Urk H: European Axillobifemoral (ABF) Bypass Trial: A prospective randomized multicenter study. Presented at the 5th Annual Meeting of the European Society for Vascular Surgery, Warsaw, September 25–27, 1991.
69. Baue AE, Shaw RS: Bypass grafts using the obturator foramen. *In* Haimovici H (ed): Vascular Surgery, Principles and Techniques. New York, McGraw-Hill, 1976.
70. Guida PM, Moore SW: Obturator bypass technique. Surg Gynecol Obstet 128:1307, 1969.
71. Livesay JJ, Atkinson JB, Baker JD, et al: Late results of extraanatomic bypass. Arch Surg 114:1402, 1979.
72. Kempczinski RF, Penn I: Upper extremity complications of axillofemoral grafts. Am J Surg 136:209, 1978.
73. Schneider JR, Golan JF: The role of extraanatomic bypass in the management of bilateral aortoiliac occlusive disease. Semin Vasc Surg 7:35, 1994.
74. Schneider JR, McDaniel MD, Walsh DB, et al: Axillofemoral pass: outcome and hemodynamic results in high risk patients. J Vasc Surg 15:952, 1992.
75. Rutherford RB: Axillobifemoral bypass: Curent indications, techniques and results. In Veith FJ (ed): Critical Problems in Vascular Surgery, Vol 7. St. Louis, Quality Medical Publishers, 1996.
76. Taylor LM, Moneta GL, McDonnell D, et al: Axillofemoral grafting with externally supported polytetrafluoroethylene. Arch Surg 129:588, 1994.
77. Passman MA, Taylor LM, Moneta GL, et al: Comparison of axillofemoral and aortofemoral bypass for aortoiliac occlusive disease. J Vasc Surg 23:263, 1996.
78. Kalman PG, Johnston KW, Walker PM: Descending thoracic aortofemoral bypass as an alternative for aortoiliac revascularization. J Cardiovasc Surg (Torino) 32:443, 1991.
79. Criado E, Johnson G Jr, Burnham SJ, et al: Descending thoracic aorta to iliofemoral bypass as an alternative to aortoiliac reconstruction. J Vasc Surg 15:550, 1992.
80. Tilson MD, Sweeney T, Gusberg RJ, et al: Obturator canal bypass grafts for septic lesions of the femoral artery. Arch Surg 114:1031, 1979.
81. Tilson MD, Baue AE: Obturator canal bypass graft for infection of the femoral artery. Surg Rounds 2:14, 1981.
82. van Det RJ, Brands LC: The obturator foramen bypass: An alternative procedure in iliofemoral artery revascularization. Surgery 89:543, 1981.
83. Sautner T, Niederle B, Herbst F, et al: The value of obturator canal bypass: A review. Arch Surg 129:718, 1994.
84. Sheiner NM, Sigman H, Stilman A: An unusual complication of obturator foramen arterial bypass. J Cardiovasc Surg 10:324, 1969.
85. Dick LS, Brief DK, Alpert J, et al: A 12 year experience with femorofemoral crossover grafts. Arch Surg 115:1359, 1980.
86. Chang JB: Current state of extraanatomic bypasses. Am J Surg 152:202, 1986.
87. Hepp W, de Jonge K, Pallua N: Late results following extra-anatomic bypass procedures for chronic aortoiliac occlusive disease. J Cardiovasc Surg 29:181, 1988.
88. Ascer E, Veith FJ, Gupta SK, et al: Comparison of axillounifemoral and axillobifemoral bypass operations. Surgery 97:169, 1985.
89. Walker PJ, Harris JP, May J: Combined percutaneous transluminal angioplasty and extraanatomic bypass for symptomatic unilateral iliac artery occlusion with contralateral iliac artery stenosis. Ann Vasc Surg 5:209, 1991.
90. Kalman PG, Hosang M, Johnston KW, Walker PM: The current role of femorofemoral bypass. J Vasc Surg 6:71, 1987.
91. Criado E, Burnham SJ, Tinsley EA Jr, et al: Femorofemoral bypass graft: Analysis of patency and factors influencing long term outcome. J Vasc Surg 18:495, 1993.
92. Farber MA, Hollier LH, Eubanks R, et al: Femorofemoral bypass: A profile of graft failure. South Med J 83:1437, 1990.
93. Naylor AR, Ah-See AK, Engeset J: Axillofemoral bypass as a limb salvage procedure in high risk patients with aortoiliac disease. Br J Surg 77:659, 1990.
94. Illuminati G, Calio FG, Mangialardi N, et al: Results of axillofemoral by-passes for aorto-iliac occlusive disease. Langenbecks Arch Surg 381:212, 1996.
95. Harris KA, Niesobska V, Carrol SE, et al: Extra-anatomic bypass grafting: A rational approach. Can J Surg 32:113, 1989.

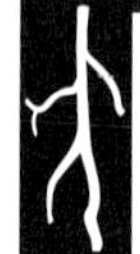

C H A P T E R 69

Infrainguinal Bypass

Anthony D. Whittemore, M.D.,
and Michael Belkin, M.D.

Arterial reconstruction for infrainguinal peripheral vascular occlusive disease has become increasingly successful with regard to long-term palliation of intermittent claudication and salvage of limbs threatened with critical ischemia. Although primary amputation may represent the most humane solution to irrevocable ischemia when extensive infection or tissue necrosis precludes expeditious limb salvage, an initial attempt at reconstruction is usually indicated in all but the most extenuating circumstances. As numerous improvements in perioperative management and surgical technique have evolved, progressively more distal reconstruction has met the challenge imposed by the more extensive disease characteristic of our aging population. The vast majority of patients with claudication achieve long-term palliation, as do those with critical ischemia, for whom an 80% to 90% limb salvage rate may be anticipated.

INDICATIONS

The two major indications for intervention during the natural history of peripheral vascular disease are (1) *claudication* and (2) *limb-threatening critical ischemia*. Claudication is a relative indication because the conditions in the majority of such patients remain stable throughout their lifetime, with ultimate limb loss limited to 1% per year.[28, 75, 96, 153] The conditions of approximately 20% of claudicants deteriorate to the extent that truly incapacitating symptoms require arterial reconstruction. Whether or not claudication constitutes a significant disability depends on the subjective judgment of both patient and surgeon.

Two-block claudication in a younger patient whose livelihood depends on walking tolerance constitutes a more significant disability than the same degree of claudication in an older, retired individual able to attend to his or her daily affairs without significant consequence. Furthermore, the degree of disability cannot be entirely isolated from causative pathologic anatomy. Intervention for relatively moderate symptoms may be justified if excellent results are achieved at low risk. More distal reconstruction associated with less favorable results, higher operative mortality, and increased risk of limb loss may preclude surgery for the same degree of functional impairment. Thus, proximal above-knee reconstruction in a patient with disabling claudication and a patent popliteal artery with excellent runoff may be justified in view of its minimal operative mortality, excellent long-term palliation, and absence of added risk of limb loss beyond that expected from the natural history of the disease process. In contrast, claudicants with diffuse superficial femoropopliteal and tibioperoneal disease are usually not suitable candidates for revascularization because long distal reconstruction does not necessarily provide symptomatic relief and failure of a graft may result in distal arterial thrombosis and a jeopardized limb.

Because most claudicants remain stable for years, it is important to allow sufficient time for a collateral blood supply to develop, since some patients may improve to such an extent that intervention proves unnecessary. For this reason, a structured exercise program is usually initiated for 6 months after the onset of symptoms before a firm decision regarding revascularization is reached.

In contrast, *critical ischemia*, as evidenced by chronic ishemic rest pain or tissue necrosis, is associated with inevitable amputation for most patients unless surgical correction is undertaken. As is true with claudication, ischemic rest pain must be carefully distinguished from other sources of pain in the elderly population, most commonly arthralgia and neuropathy. Although tissue necrosis and gangrene are usually self-evident when the cause is critical ischemia, similar lesions associated with venous stasis, severe anemia, decubitus ulcers, and diabetic neuropathy must be excluded. Patients with the acute onset of critical ischemia deserve special mention. In the absence of progressive neuromotor or sensory deficit, such patients may be maintained on a systemic heparin regimen during preoperative evaluation, which is carried out as it would be for any other patient. The presence of neurologic dysfunction of a progressive nature, however, requires more urgent arteriography and expeditious intervention for limb salvage before irrevocable ischemic nerve damage occurs.

Attempts at revascularization are absolutely contraindicated in the presence of life-threatening sepsis, a situation in which adequate drainage may necessitate major amputation.[98] In contrast, extensive foot infection, as commonly seen in the diabetic population, may be amenable to an initial minor drainage procedure and subsequent revascularization after sepsis is resolved.[57] Well-established flexion contracture and paralysis are additional contraindications, and heroic efforts to salvage a jeopardized limb in a patient with markedly reduced life expectancy are usually not justified.[108, 136] In such individuals, more temporizing procedures, such as percutaneous transluminal angioplasty (PTA) for appropriate localized lesions, might be employed.[73] Reconstruction should be delayed in most individuals with significant acute comorbidity, such as a recent myocardial infarction, unless the limb is imminently threatened and higher perioperative morbidity is acceptable.[119]

PREOPERATIVE EVALUATION

Successful infrainguinal reconstruction for ischemic limbs requires the initial recognition and subsequent management of both the underlying systemic atherosclerotic cardiovascular disease and the associated specific manifestation. Significant comorbidity from the various complications of atherosclerosis in vascular surgery patients has been well documented. The Framingham study unequivocally demonstrated that claudicants harbor a significantly higher incidence of coronary artery insufficiency as well as cerebrovascular and hypertensive disease compared with nonclaudicants.[80] Clinically overt cardiac disease is readily apparent in approximately 50% of the vascular surgery population, and an additional 20% have clinically silent but significant coronary artery disease.[70] The use of ambulatory Holter monitoring has confirmed the high prevalence of clinically silent myocardial ischemia in these patients.[107, 114]

Because myocardial dysfunction is the overwhelming cause of perioperative morbidity and mortality associated with infrainguinal reconstruction, a thorough understanding of the individual patient's cardiac status is required (see Chapter 40). Our approach to preoperative management limits extensive cardiac evaluation to those individuals with clinically overt coronary disease manifested by positive findings on electrocardiography, a history suggestive of coronary insufficiency, or both. Patients with no clinically apparent coronary disease and relatively normal electrocardiographic (ECG) findings can undergo revascularization without significant cardiac morbidity or mortality.[60] At the other extreme, myocardial revascularization of the patient with unstable angina takes precedence over any attempt at infrainguinal reconstruction.

The remaining group of individuals, those with chronic stable angina, sustain the highest incidence of perioperative cardiac morbidity and deserve more exhaustive preoperative evaluation. In this group of patients, we routinely obtain cardiologic consultation for risk assessment and preoperative cardiac optimization. Echocardiography and dipyridamole-sestamibi imaging are employed selectively, but cardiac catheterization is seldom indicated, as preoperative beta blockade and other advances have reduced cardiac morbidity and mortality significantly.

Despite the high prevalence of cigarette smoking in the population undergoing vascular surgery, postoperative pulmonary complications are relatively infrequent with routine postoperative pulmonary care. The increased use of regional anesthesia for infrainguinal procedures may contribute to the overall reduction in pulmonary morbidity. It would be ideal for patients to abstain from smoking long before surgery is planned, but until recently this had been an unrealistic goal for most. With the availability of transcutaneous nicotine patches and other pharmacologic adjuncts, however, preoperative smoking cessation may become a more reasonable expectation.

Routine antihypertensive and cardiac medications are administered as usual until surgery. Patients with chronic renal insufficiency constitute an important group because significant impairment increases operative mortality.[39, 158] Renal function should be optimal before intervention, and patients with end-stage renal disease require dialysis on the day following arteriography and immediately preceding surgery, with reinstitution of dialysis on the first postoperative day. Patients with prosthetic valves or atrial dysrhythmia requiring long-term anticoagulation are advised to discontinue oral anticoagulant use 2 or 3 days before angiography; they continue intravenous dextran and antiplatelet agents perioperatively until oral anticoagulation can sefely be resumed. Finally, it has been our practice to provide aspirin to our patients during the 2 days immediately preceding surgery to ensure adequate tissue levels of antiplatelet activity at the time of intervention.

Local care of ischemic lesions is primarily directed toward minimizing the impact of associated infection. The use of appropriate drainage procedures and preoperative intravenous antibiotics may be advisable before formal revascularization in an effort to reduce the incidence of postoperative wound and graft infection. Adequate drainage may call for minor open amputation with staged revascularization and ultimate revision with primary closure.

Noninvasive evaluation of the lower extremity is often helpful for establishing baseline parameters and for differential diagnosis in the presence of significant comorbidity (see Chapter 9). Segmental Doppler arterial pressure determinations are readily available, as are pulse volume recordings, to interpret spuriously high pressures frequently observed in diabetic patients and in patients in renal failure who have widespread circumferential calcification. For differentiating patients with significant vascular insufficiency from those with primary arthritic or neurogenic comorbidity, exercise testing may prove helpful in equivocal cases. At present, duplex scanning reliably demonstrates the level of critical lesions but does not provide anatomic resolution to the degree necessary for accurate preoperative planning.[69] Duplex mapping of saphenous or alternative veins, however, may be desirable to establish the presence of adequate vein and to plan incisions more accurately. Information obtained with noninvasive duplex scanning regarding the caliber and quality of vein has not been firmly correlated with actual intraoperative findings or outcome. Thus, this modality appears most useful for establishing the presence or absence of vein, with adequacy best determined intraoperatively.

Comprehensive preoperative *arteriography* remains the standard procedure for optimal delineation of the patient's anatomy. Reconstruction should not be abandoned, however, in the absence of angiographic visualization of the distal tibioperoneal vasculature, because direct exploration may reveal patency sufficient for distal outflow. Patency may be determined either by preliminary intraoperative angiography of the proposed isolated outflow vessel or by cannulation of the vessel with a 25-gauge needle to ascertain the presence of blood flow.[53, 69]

Magnetic resonance arteriography (MRA) has been increasingly employed for preoperative arteriographic assessment.[17, 32, 72] Optimal results with this technique depend greatly on the experience of the imager and the quality of the hardware and software. Although most studies have found this technique sufficient for preoperative planning, detail and image quality are generally inferior to those obtained with conventional arteriography. The application of MRA will undoubtedly increase as techniques are simplified and image quality improves.

In patients with borderline ischemia in whom the necessity for intervention is in doubt, transcutaneous oxygen determinations may prove helpful.[118] A limb with a transcutaneous partial pressure of oxygen of less than 22 mmHg almost invariably requires revascularization for healing of an ischemic ulcer or a digital amputation site.[84] Reliable measurements, however, require routine use with well-maintained calibrated equipment.

The preoperative administration of intra-arterial thrombolytic therapy remains controversial, and its role is necessarily individualized.[134, 106] Patients with recent onset of acute ischemia and evidence of distal tibioperoneal thrombus may benefit from preoperative lytic therapy to improve outflow from the distal anastomosis. Lysis following thrombosis superimposed on antecedent localized superficial femoral artery stenosis may allow balloon angioplasty in appropriate patients, thereby avoiding the necessity for a surgical procedure. Although this approach does not provide the durability achieved with conventional revascularization, it may prove to be appropriate for selected patients under extraordinary circumstances.

OPERATIVE MANAGEMENT

Exposure

After the appropriate monitoring lines are inserted, intravenous antibiotics are given, and anasthesia is satisfactorily induced, the appropriate vessels are exposed, an effort greatly facilitated by a two-team approach when available. The site proposed for the distal anastomosis is initially explored. The *above-knee popliteal vessel* is easily exposed through a medial thigh incision, with subsequent posterolateral retraction of the sartorius muscle. The underlying deep muscular fascia is incised over the distal adductor canal for exposure of the above-knee popliteal space. The proximal popliteal artery is dissected free of the accompanying structures just posterior to the femur. The artery should be mobilized as far distally as necessary to ensure an optimal anastomotic site determined by external palpation of plaque distribution.

The *below-knee popliteal artery* is usually exposed through a medial calf incision posterior to the medial femoral condyle and extending distally just medial to the tibial crest (Fig. 69–1). The incision should be located directly over the saphenous vein, if possible, to minimize undermining thin cutaneous flaps. With care taken to minimize trauma to the vein during the exposure and division of appropriate tributaries, the deep muscular fascia is incised and the medial head of the gastrocnemius is reflected posterolaterally to expose the popliteal fossa. The *distal popliteal artery* is mobilized from the posterior tibial nerve posteriorly and the popliteal vein medially. The surgeon can then expose the tibioperoneal trunk, if necessary, by extending the dissection along the anteromedial surface of the distal popliteal artery and transecting the overlying musculotendinous origin of the soleus muscle.

The origin of the *anterior tibial artery* can also be encircled with a loop for control. The proximal halves of both the posterior tibial and the peroneal vessels are most easily exposed by continued distal dissection beyond the bifurcation of the tibioperoneal trunk. (Fig. 69–2) The posterior tibial artery lies more medially on the surface of the reflected soleus muscle or along the posterior tibial muscle. The peroneal artery follows a deeper and more lateral course deep to the flexor hallucis longus. The peroneal artery at this location is frequently invested with multiple surrounding veins that require tedious mobilization for exposure of the desired peroneal segment.

The popliteal artery may also be exposed through a lateral incision, a useful approach for patients with prior reconstruction or sepsis.[144] The popliteal space above the knee is entered by incision of the distal fascia lata and posterior retraction of the biceps femoris tendon. The lat-

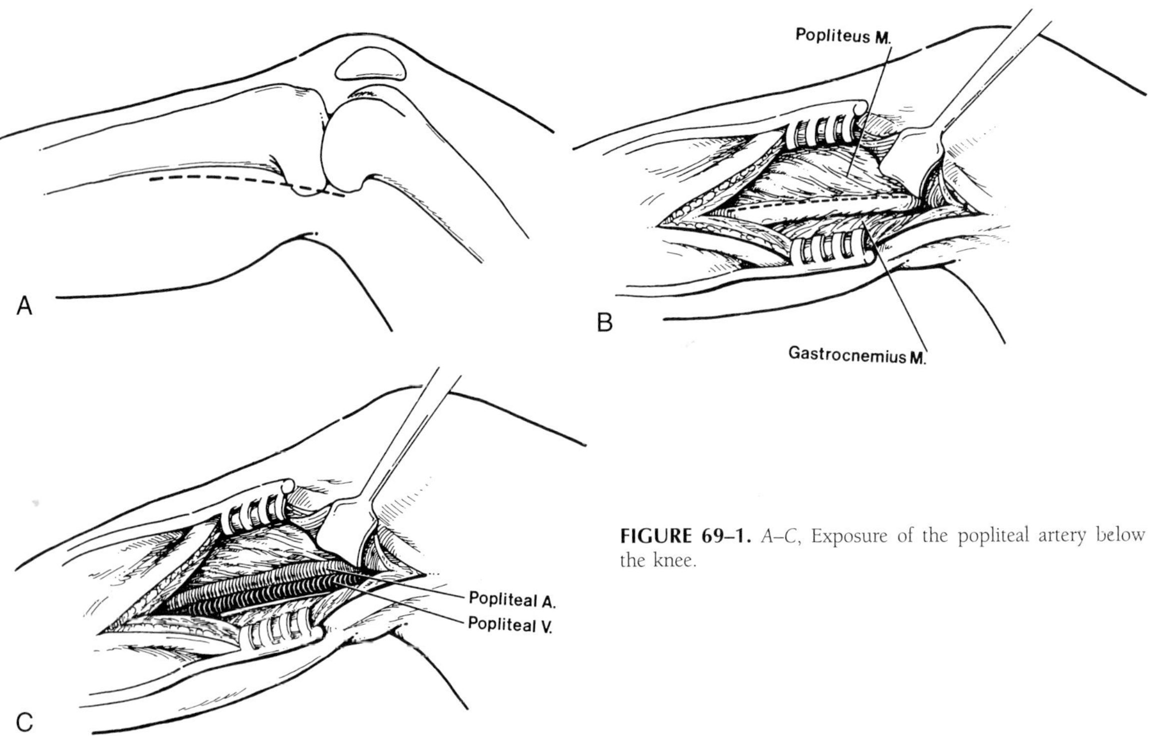

FIGURE 69–1. *A–C*, Exposure of the popliteal artery below the knee.

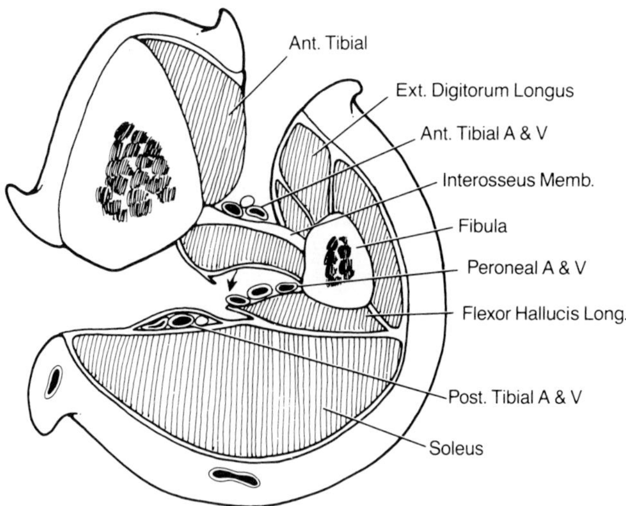

FIGURE 69–2. Anatomic approach to the posterior tibial artery, the anterior tibial artery, and the peroneal artery in the mid-portion of the leg. A = artery; V = vein.

eral approach to the infragenicular popliteal artery requires division of the biceps femoris tendon and excision of the proximal fibula, with care taken to avoid injury to the peroneal nerve.

More distal exposure of the tibial and peroneal vessels is best obtained through individualized incisions (Fig. 69–3). The *distal posterior tibial artery* is easily isolated through an incision just posterior to the medial malleolus, and its medial and lateral plantar branches are exposed by extension of the incision onto the medial surface of the foot.[10] The *anterior tibial artery* is usually approached through a longitudinal incision over the anterior compartment in the distal third of the leg and is exposed by reflection of the anterior tibial muscle anteromedially and the digital extensor muscles laterally.

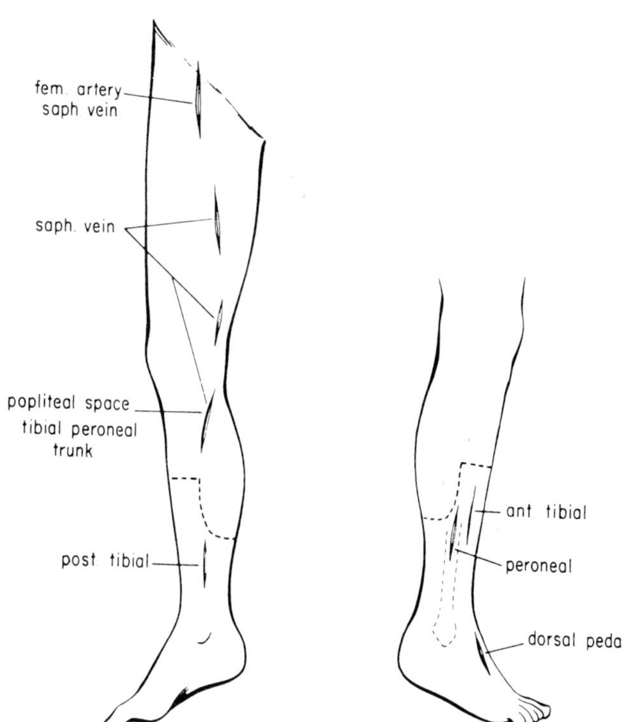

FIGURE 69–3. Placement of incisions for femoropopliteal and femorotibial bypass and for saphenous vein harvest. These should avoid the incision lines for a below-knee amputation.

The distal third of the *peroneal artery* is best exposed through a longitudinal incision over the distal fibula (Fig. 69–4). The long peroneal muscle is mobilized from the bone and reflected posteriorly along with flexor hallucis longus. The periosteum of the fibula is circumferentially scored and elevated, and a 5- to 10-cm length of fibula is resected. The peroneal artery and its accompanying veins lie just deep to the thin layer of fascia directly on the surface of the posterior tibial muscle (see Fig. 69–2).

The *dorsal pedal artery* is easily exposed through an axial incision on the dorsum of the foot just lateral to the extensor hallucis longus tendon (Fig. 69–5). As wide a skin bridge as possible should be provided between the arterial incision and that required for exposure and subsequent mobilization of the distal saphenous vein.[111]

After the surgeon selects and exposes the most appropriate site for distal anastomosis, the proximal incision is made, most frequently in the groin overlying the medial aspect of the common femoral artery (Fig. 69–6). Care must be taken to direct the inferior aspect of this incision posteriorly to avoid undermining a medial flap prone to subsequent necrosis. The native *common femoral artery* is exposed from the level of the inguinal ligament at the origin of the epigastric and circumflex iliac artery branches to its terminal bifurcation. The proximal *superficial femoral artery* is mobilized sufficiently to allow temporary occlusion, or more distally, in the event that it is selected as the site for proximal anastomosis. The profunda femoris artery (*deep femoral artery*) is similarly exposed for a distance appropriate for occlusion, or more distally to the level of its first muscular perforating branches in the event that profundaplasty or extensive endarterectomy is required. Although the lateral femoral circumflex branch of the profunda femoris artery usually orginates from the lateral aspect of the proximal profunda femoris artery, the medial femoral circumflex branch often arises posteriorly from the distal common femoral artery as a separate entity necessitating individual control.

Before anticoagulation and construction of the anastomoses, appropriate tunnels are prepared. For prosthetic conduits, a subsartorial tunnel is usually created between the groin incision and the above-knee popliteal space, either superficial or deep to the deep muscular fascia. Tunnels may be constructed with a variety of instruments, the gentlest of which remain the surgeon's fingers. For below-knee bypass, the tunnel is extended between the heads of the gastrocnemius muscle into the popliteal fossa. No further tunneling is necessary for anastomoses to the exposed posterior tibial or proximal peroneal vessels, but the distal peroneal and anterior tibial vessels require a tunnel from the popliteal space through the interosseous membrane into the mid-anterior compartment. This tunnel is best created by exposing the interosseous membrane directly through the anterolateral calf incision and excising a "postage stamp"–sized segment of the fibrous membrane. A blunt clamp and the surgeon's finger are then serially passed

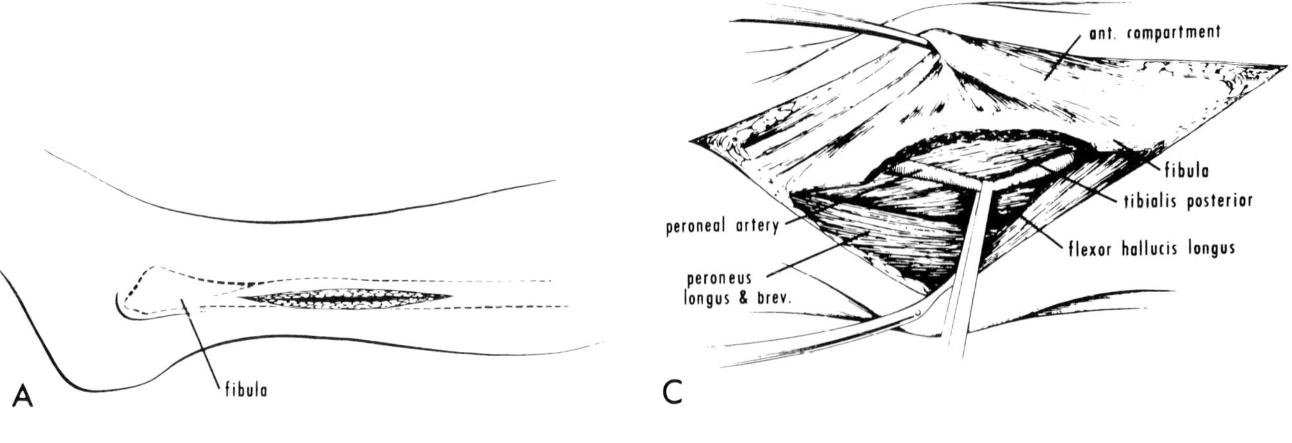

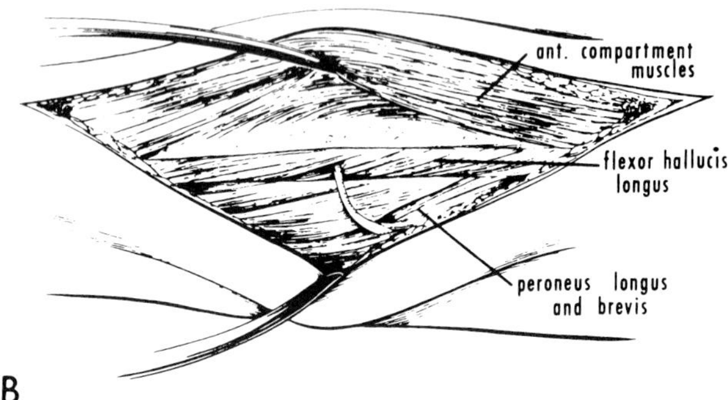

FIGURE 69–4. Lateral approach to the leg for exposure of the distal peroneal artery.

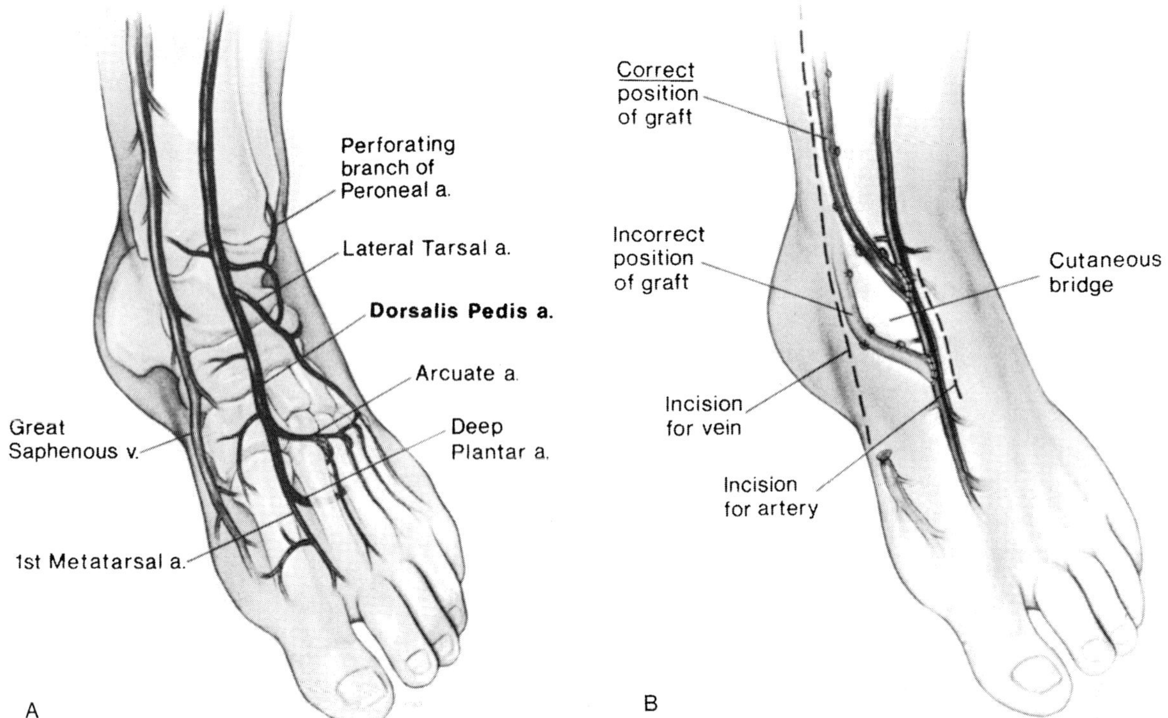

FIGURE 69–5. *A*, The anterior tibial artery continues onto the dorsum of the foot as the dorsal pedal artery, coursing lateral and parallel to the extensor hallucis longus tendon. *B*, Incisions for exposure of both the dorsal pedal artery and the distal greater saphenous vein are illustrated along with the correct and incorrect tunnels under the skin bridge.

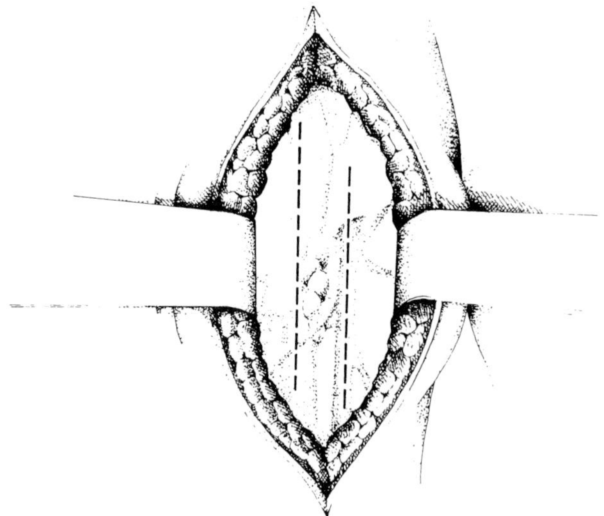

FIGURE 69–6. Separate fascial incisions for exposure of the saphenous vein and common femoral artery in an effort to preserve the lymphatic network.

through the defect to atraumatically create a wide tunnel that will not compress or scar around the graft. Alternatively, subcutaneous tunnels may be constructed from the groin incision, coursing anteriorly over the thigh and the lateral aspect of the knee joint to the anterior compartment.[52] This lateral tunnel is preferable in reoperative situations to avoid a scarred popliteal fossa or residual infection near one of the standard medial incisions.

The in situ technique requires no extensive tunneling except when the below-knee popliteal artery is chosen for the site of the distal anastomosis. In this case, the angle of entry of the vein graft into the distal anastomosis may approach 90 degrees if the vein is brought directly from its below-knee subcutaneous position. The vein is best mobilized to the above-knee level and subsequently tunneled distally between the heads of the gastrocnemius muscle to provide a more optimal angle of anastomosis (Fig. 69–7). Special precautions must also be taken when the in situ graft is being tunneled to the dorsal pedal artery to avoid necrosis of the overlying skin bridge (see Fig. 69–5*B*).[111] After the creation of the required tunnels, the patient customarily receives anticoagulation therapy with heparin at a dose of 5000 to 10,000 units. The sequence of anastomoses varies according to the procedure and the conduit used.

Autogenous Vein Bypass

Reversed Greater Saphenous Vein

Femoropopliteal bypass using autogenous saphenous vein in the reversed position was initially reported by Kunlin in 1949.[83] The vein may be harvested through relatively short longitudinal skin incisions with intervening cutaneous bridges (see Fig. 69–3). Tributaries are divided and ligated, and the vein is removed and prepared with care to minimize mechanical trauma and desiccation. Optimal endothelial preservation may be achieved with external application or perivenous infiltration of a solution containing papaver-

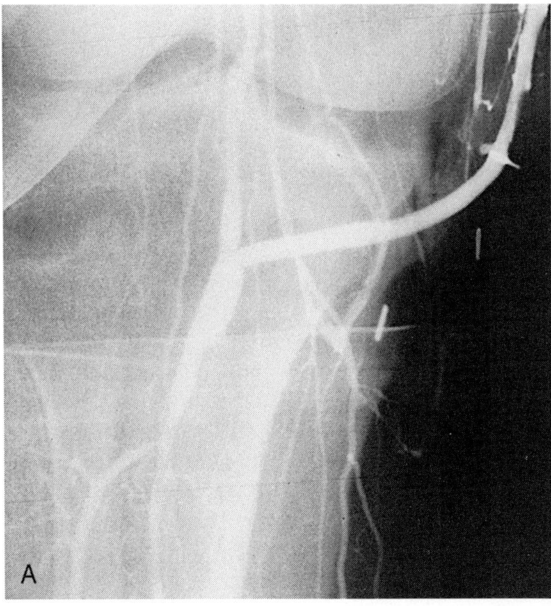

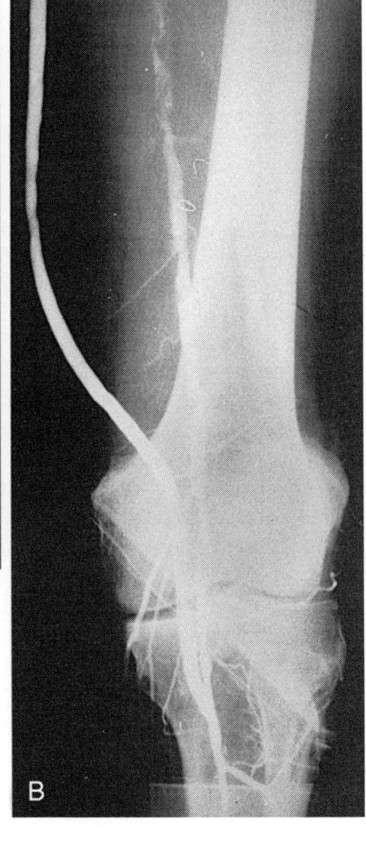

FIGURE 69–7. *A*, Intraoperative completion arteriograms illustrating a kinked vein graft at the distal popliteal anastomosis created by a hyperacute angle of entry when the vein graft is anastomosed directly from its subcutaneous position. *B*, This may be avoided by mobilization of the vein and delivery through a popliteal tunnel from the above-knee position.

ine.[92] After excision, the reversed vein is gently flushed and subsequently stored in chilled autologous blood, Ringer's lactate, or a combined electrolyte solution (Plasma-Lyte) containing both heparin and papaverine to minimize spasm.

The *distal anastomosis* is usually carried out first by means of one of several standard techniques (see Chapter 29), and the graft is delivered through the appropriate tunnel to the groin incision. The graft is gently flushed from the proximal end with the vein preservation solution to ensure against mechanical twist or kink and to establish adequate length and appropriate tension with the leg in the extended position.

Finally, the *proximal anastomosis* is constructed, usually to the common femoral artery, with fine 5-0 or 6-0 monofilament suture. This procedure is completed after careful sequential flushing to minimize embolic events.

In Situ Saphenous Vein

The in situ bypass, initially advocated by Hall,[62] was further modified and popularized by Leather and associates in 1979.[87, 88] The greater saphenous vein is usually exposed throughout the entire length required. A small-caliber vein may be ligated in the distal aspect of the distal incision and partially transected to allow cannulation and gentle flushing with chilled blood, Ringer's lactate, or a combined electrolyte solution containing both heparin and papaverine. This practice minimizes intraoperative venous spasm and lessens the likelihood of injury during subsequent valvulotomy or angioscopy. Partial transection preserves the rotational alignment and orientation of valve cusps to be subsequently lysed. The exposed vein is covered first with sponges or laparotomy pads soaked in vein-preservation solution and then with a barrier to prevent evaporation and desiccation. Alternatively, the skin may be loosely reapproximated over the exposed vein with a stapler during construction of the proximal anastomosis.

Preliminary angioscopy for direct visualization of valve lysis and localization of arteriovenous fistulae has been helpful for some patients by reducing the number of incisions required.[99] Whether this practice favorably influences operating time, length of hospital stay, or incidence of wound complications, however, is debatable. The primary advantage of routine angioscopy may reside in its ability to demonstrate unsuspected endoluminal pathologic features such as phlebitic strictures, webs, and fibrotic valve cusps.[105] This technique may prove most useful with arm veins, in which endoluminal pathology is frequently present and is responsible in part for suboptimal results.[93]

In contrast to reversed vein bypass, the in situ method requires that the proximal anastomosis be initially constructed after transection of the saphenofemoral junction and closure of the common femoral venotomy (Fig. 69–8*A*). Ideally, the proximal anastomosis is located in the distal common femoral artery, but the actual site is frequently dictated by the position of the saphenofemoral junction relative to the bifurcation of the common femoral artery (Fig. 69–8*B*). A portion of the proximal saphenous vein may be mobilized to provide more length and less tension for a distal common femoral anastomosis. To avoid excessive tension, however, the anastomosis must occasionally straddle the common femoral bifurcation. Alternatively, the proximal anastomosis may be located entirely in the proximal superficial femoral artery, which in turn may require preliminary endarterectomy. The cusps of the first venous valve are excised under direct vision in the proximal saphenous vein.

After occlusion of the native arteries with atraumatic vascular clamps, an arteriotomy is usually made in the distal common femoral artery and extended either proximally or distally across the origin of the superficial femoral artery, as indicated by the length of available vein. Preliminary endarterectomy is performed, if necessary, and the proximal anastomosis is then constructed with standard techniques. Before completion of the anastomosis, all vessels should be flushed copiously to avoid distal embolization. After all occluding clamps have been removed, arterial flow is established through the vein graft to the level of the first competent valve.

Although various valvulotomes are available for lysis of valve cusps, our preference has been the modified Mills valvulotome, with the entire vein exposed (Fig. 69–8*C*).[89] Other investigators prefer valvulotomy under direct vision with angioscopic control, but there is little evidence to favor one technique over another. After complete valve lysis and on ensurance of satisfactory inflow from the graft, appropriate control of the distal vessel is secured. Methods of control include (1) application of standard atraumatic external clamps, (2) use of internal balloon catheters, and (3) use of a proximal pneumatic tourniquet.[25] An arteriotomy in the distal vessel is initiated, and the distal vein is appropriately trimmed with the leg extended to ensure adequate length without tension. The transected end is spatulated and sutured to the arteriotomy with fine monofilament suture (Fig. 69–8*D*). Proponents of both the *interrupted* and the *continuous* suture technique have yet to provide convincing data that one method is preferable.

Interest has lately focused on in situ bypasses through more limited incisions. Although angioscopically assisted valve lysis has been employed since the late 1980s, until recently the ligation of patent side branches has required multiple additional incisions. Early experience has suggested that a long retrograde valve cutter may be combined with antegrade passage of a modifed angioscope to cut the valves. Angioscopic identification of patent side branches then allows endoscopic occlusion with small platinum coils.[122] There is a significant learning curve to this technique, and operative times (at least initially) are significantly prolonged. It is hoped that increased experience will lead to fewer wound complications, reduced hospital stays, and shorter recuperation periods.

Nonreversed Saphenous Vein

The relatively high incidence of reoperative infrainguinal bypass surgery, prior coronary artery bypass, or even prior stripping of the greater saphenous vein results in the frequent need for revascularization in the absence of ipsilateral saphenous vein. The practical advantages of the in situ greater saphenous vein, including a better size match between the artery and vein at the proximal and distal anastomoses and an increased vein utilization rate, may be preserved in these situations, however, if the contralateral

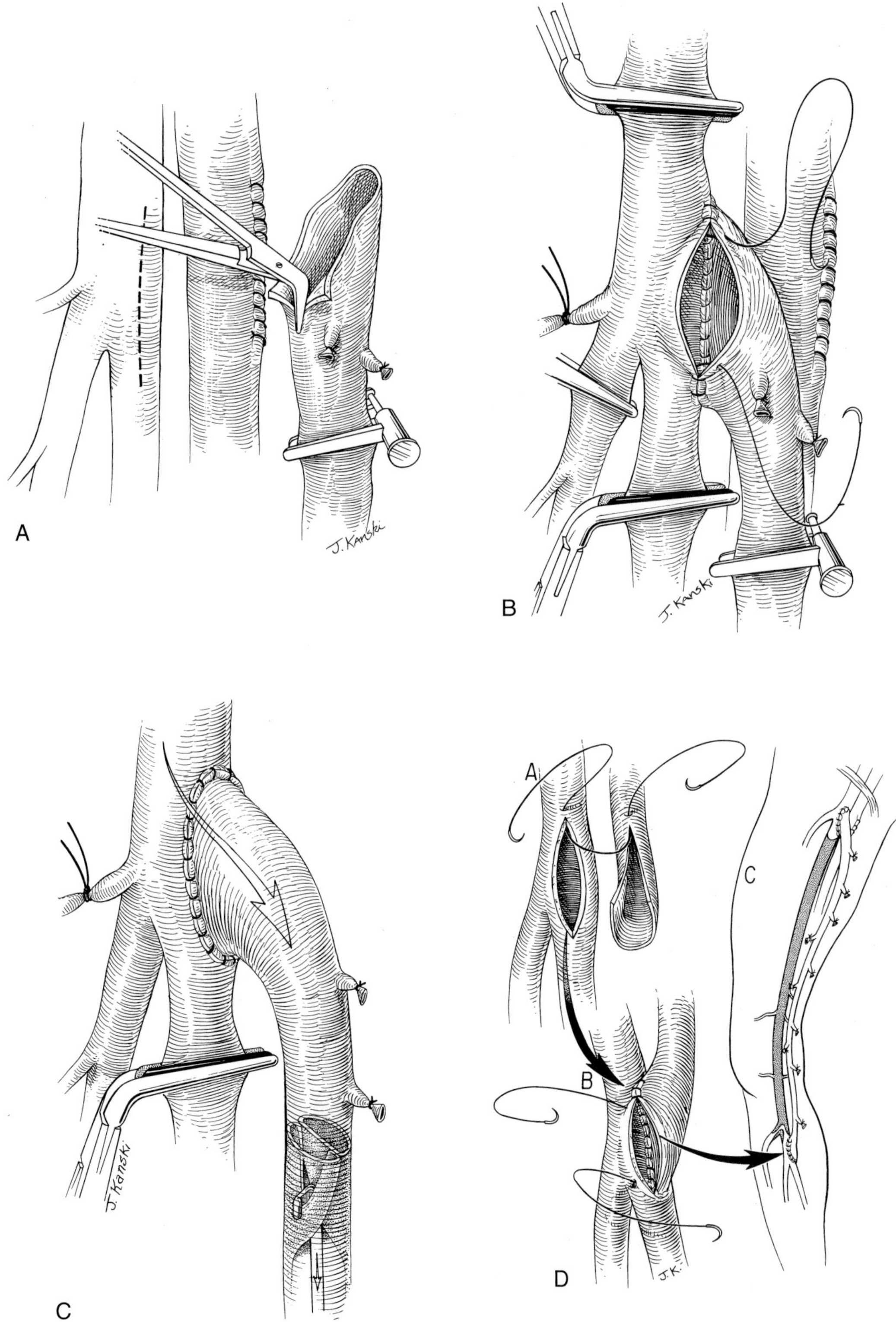

FIGURE 69–8. *A*, In the in situ method of infrainguinal reconstruction, the saphenofemoral junction is transected in the groin, the venotomy in the femoral vein oversewn, and the proximal end of the saphenous vein prepared for anastomosis. *B*, After the first venous valve is excised under direct vision, the graft is anastomosed end-to-side to the femoral artery. *C*, Flow is then restored through the vein graft and the valvulotome inserted through side branches at appropriate intervals to lyse residual valve cusps. *D*, The distal anastomosis is then completed by tying down the heel of the anastomosis (A) and running around to the anterior wall (B). The completed anastomosis, in this case, is to the tibioperoneal trunk (C).

greater saphenous vein is used in a translocated, nonreversed fashion with lysed valves.[19] This technique may also be preferable when extra-anatomic tunneling of the vein graft (e.g., along the anterolateral thigh and calf to the anterior tibial artery), or translocation of the vein graft (e.g., to a more distal inflow artery) is desirable.

The vein is gently harvested from its bed and dilated, as in the reversed vein graft technique. The proximal valve is then excised under direct vision. The proximal anastomosis is completed with standard technique, and the valves are lysed in the same fashion as in the in situ bypass operation. The authors prefer the modified Mill's valvulotome introduced through side branches or the end of the vein graft. Alternatively, before graft implantation, the valves may be lysed while gentle antegrade distention is maintained with electrolyte solution containing heparin.

Sequential Vein

Prominent among the many reasons for failure of long distal reconstructions is the high peripheral resistance in

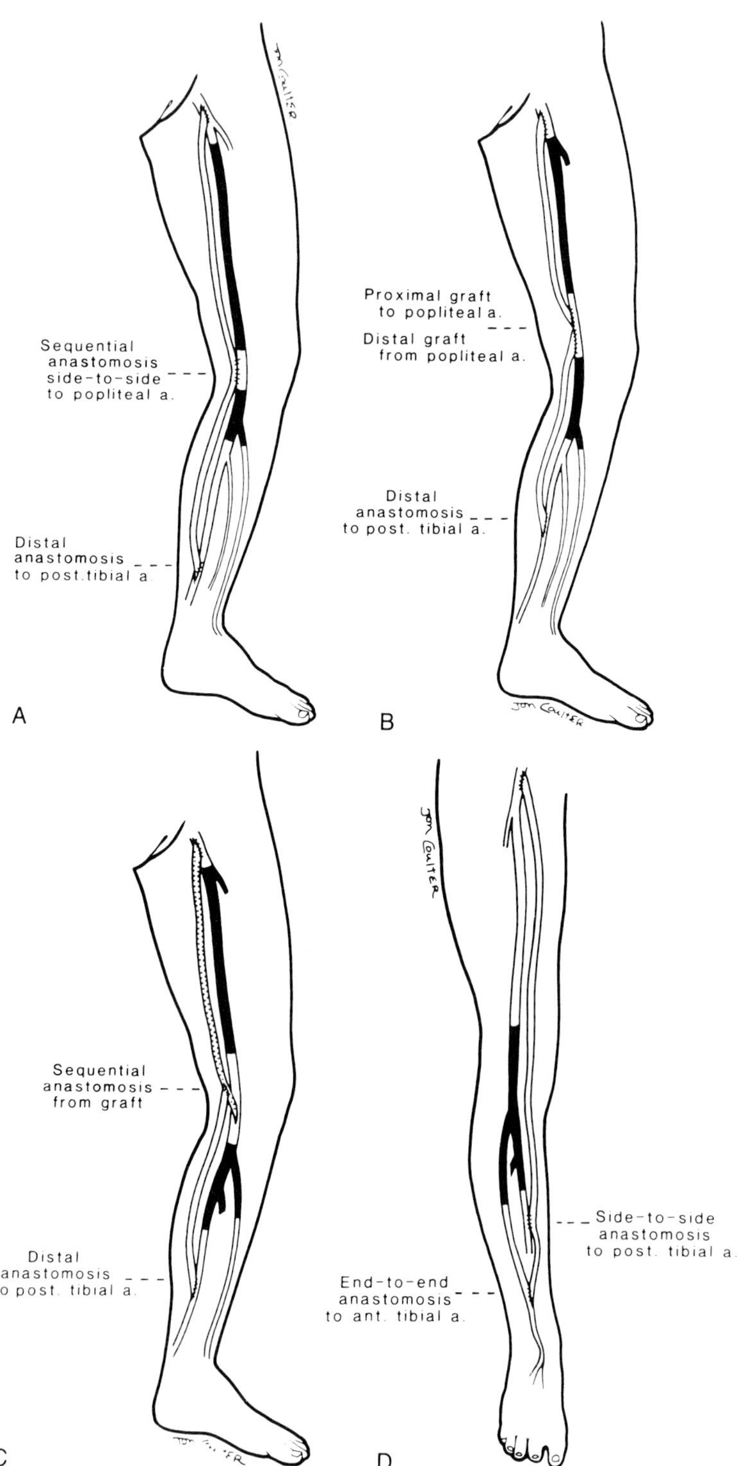

FIGURE 69–9. Four configurations for sequential bypass are possible. In type I (*A*), a single vein or prosthesis is used and a sequential side-to-side anastomosis is constructed to the popliteal artery. In type II (*B*), the proximal portion of the graft is anastomosed end-to-side to the popliteal artery and the distal portion (usually autogenous vein) is sewn to the artery just below, and the distal anastomosis sewn end-to-side to a crural vessel. Type III (*C*) is similar, but the distal portion of the graft takes its origin from the prosthesis rather than from the host artery. Type IV (*D*) is usually employed when the popliteal artery is totally occluded. A side-to-side anastomosis is constructed to one crural vessel proximally, and an end-to-side is made to another more distally in the leg.

the distal outflow bed provided by severely diseased runoff. As initially advocated by DeLaurentis and Friedmann[46] in 1972, sequential bypass is designed to enhance flow through the long arterial limb of the graft by providing two or more distal anastomoses, thereby reducing peripheral resistance. That graft flow is significantly augmented has been established in both laboratory and clinical settings, and the technique is believed by some[76, 77] to improve the long-term patency rates of grafts to restricted-outflow tracts.

Of the several configurations possible, four are illustrated in Figure 69–9. With an adequate length of autogenous vein available, a side-to-side anastomosis may be interposed between the proximal femoral and distal tibial anastomosis. This interposed anastomosis may be constructed to an isolated segment of the popliteal vessel proximally (Fig. 69–9*A*) or to a posterior tibial or peroneal vessel distally (Fig. 69–9*B*). The latter graft may be constructed using an in situ technique. Similar approaches (Fig. 69–9*C* and *D*) are appropriate when shorter segments of vein are available, and the anastomosis may be constructed with either the proximal or distal segment in the in situ configuration. In either case, the interposed sequential anastomosis may be constructed with two separate end-to-side anastomoses or a single side-to-side anastomosis. Alternatively, the distal graft may originate end-to-side from the distal aspect of the proximal graft. These complex reconstructions should clearly be reserved for patients requiring limb salvage and should not be used for palliation of claudication.

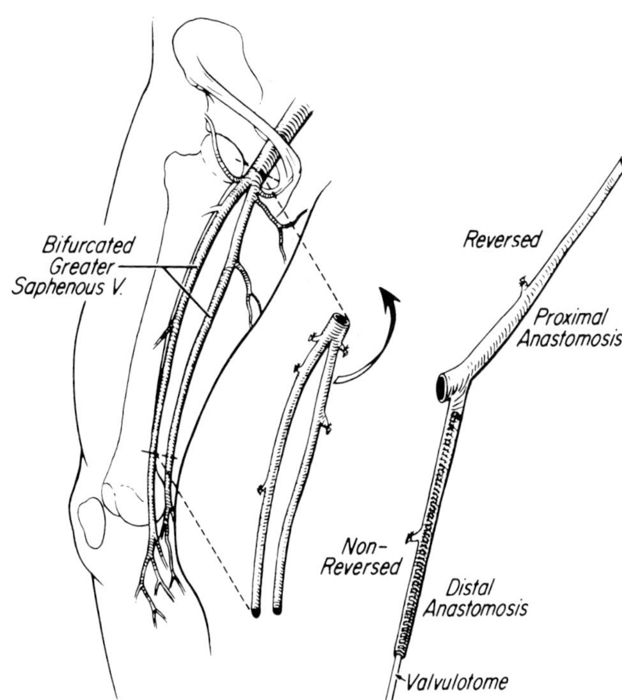

FIGURE 69–10. A short, bifurcated greater superficial saphenous vein may be removed intact and prepared to create a longer vein graft by reversing one limb, lysing the valves in the other nonreversed limb, and oversewing the intervening saphenofemoral junction.

Alternative Autogenous Vein

The use of an autogenous conduit may require some creativity, in view of the frequency of anatomic variants, endoluminal pathology, and prior use for peripheral or coronary procedure. Whereas a single saphenous vein trunk is present in approximately two thirds of patients, a complete double system is present in approximately 10% and an incomplete double system is found in an additional 15%.[132] Double systems may be converted to longer lengths after harvesting of the intact saphenofemoral junction, which is subsequently oversewn (Fig. 69–10).[140] One limb of the duplicated system is then reversed, and the other remains nonreversed after lysis of valve cusps with the valvulotome. Similarly, an inadequate length of autogenous vein may ultimately prove to be sufficient if a more distal site for proximal anastomosis is selected.[11, 145] Generally, a minimum caliber of 3.5 mm is required for optimal results with reversed vein, whereas entirely satisfactory results have been obtained with smaller-caliber grafts with the in situ technique.[154]

In the absence of the suitable greater saphenous vein, either arm vein or lesser saphenous vein may be adequate (see Chapter 35). If the greater saphenous vein is known to be unavailable preoperatively, the lesser saphenous vein is most easily harvested with the patient initially in the prone position. After closure of the posterior calf incision, the patient is turned, reprepared, and draped. Alternatively, the lesser saphenous vein may be harvested through a medial approach, with the patient in the usual supine position following exposure of arterial anastomotic sites.[35] Both arm and lesser saphenous vein may be used in either the reversed or the nonreversed configuration. Our preference is the *nonreversed position*, which usually provides better size matching at the anastomoses but requires preliminary valve lysis with an appropriate valvulotome. There is no evidence, however, that this practice influences ultimate results.

Prosthetic Bypass

Since the mid-1950s, prosthetic grafts have been used in several locations for arterial reconstruction. The earliest types were knitted and woven textile grafts, primarily of polyester (Dacron), which provide consistently favorable results in high-flow, large-caliber settings but perform poorly in the more challenging small-caliber, low-flow conditions characteristic of distal infrainguinal reconstruction. As a result, both human umbilical vein and expanded polytetrafluoroethylene (PTFE) were introduced in the 1970s for clinical use as small-caliber arterial substitutes.[33, 42] Because human umbilical vein proved to be cumbersome, PTFE has been more often used as the conduit of choice in the absence of adequate autogenous saphenous vein. Preliminary reports documented impressive early results comparable to those obtained with saphenous vein, but these results proved to be overoptimistic as patency data matured.[24, 146, 147, 159]

Vein Patch/Collar

Because results achieved with distal PTFE reconstructions proved to be suboptimal, several modifications of the standard approach to prosthetic infrainguinal bypass have been suggested. Common among several mechanisms of failure

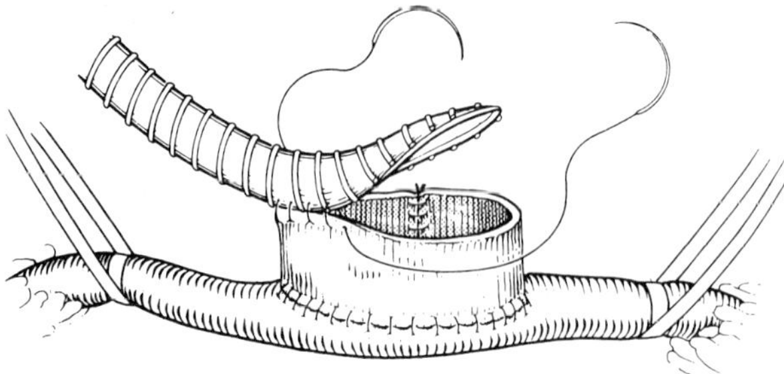

FIGURE 69–11. To minimize the impact of anastomotic intimal hyperplasia, a collar of vein may be interposed between the distal end of the prosthetic graft and the recipient native vessel. (From Miller JH, Foreman RK, Ferguson L, Faris I: Interposition vein cuff for anastomosis of a prosthesis to small artery. Aust N Z J Surg 54:283, 1984.)

associated with PTFE is a particularly vigorous smooth muscle proliferative response at the distal anastomosis, which results in stenosis. A "collar" of vein may be interposed between the distal arteriotomy and the distal PTFE graft (Fig. 69–11).[101] It is theorized that when this is done, the kinetic energy stored in the pulse pressure within the noncompliant graft is more effectively dissipated by the relatively elastic properties of autogenous material. As turbulence is reduced, trauma to the arterial endothelium is diminished, thereby minimizing the proliferative response. A similar approach incorporates an autogenous venous "patch" across the distal anastomosis (Fig. 69–12).[139] For some authors, this practice has improved results and provides a reasonable alternative for limb salvage in patients who would otherwise have to undergo amputation.[142, 143]

Adjunctive Arterial Venous Fistula

A second modification uses an arteriovenous fistula constructed in conjunction with the distal anastomosis (Fig. 69–13) or at a site more remote from the distal anastomosis (Fig. 69–14) in an effort to augment flow through the prosthetic graft and to enhance patency.[74, 109] Preliminary results have been encouraging, but more trials and longer-term data are needed.

The use of a composite prosthetic vein conduit is a third adjunctive method for enhancing prosthetic performance in patients requiring a long reconstruction when the available length of vein is limited (Fig. 69–15). The distal anastomosis of the proximal prosthetic component is constructed end-to-side to a patent popliteal segment and above the knee, whenever possible, to allow the distal venous component to cross the knee joint through an anatomic tunnel.[54] The proximal vein is anastomosed end-to-side to an ellip-

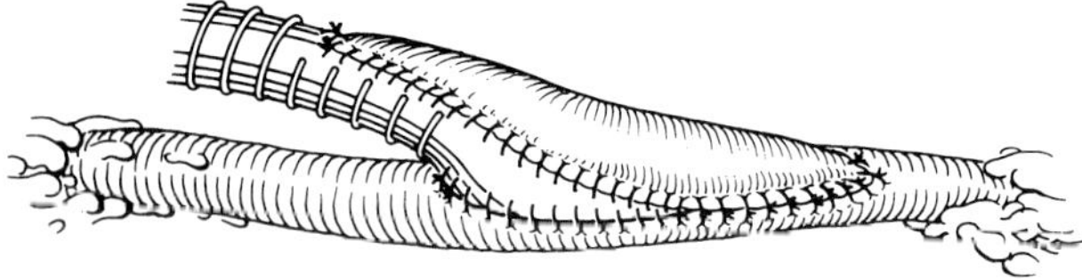

FIGURE 69–12. An alternative method for compensating for inevitable anastomotic intimal hyperplasia consists of a vein patch. (From Taylor RS, McFarland RJ, Cox MI: An investigation into the causes of failure of PTFE grafts. Eur J Vasc Surg 1:335, 1987.)

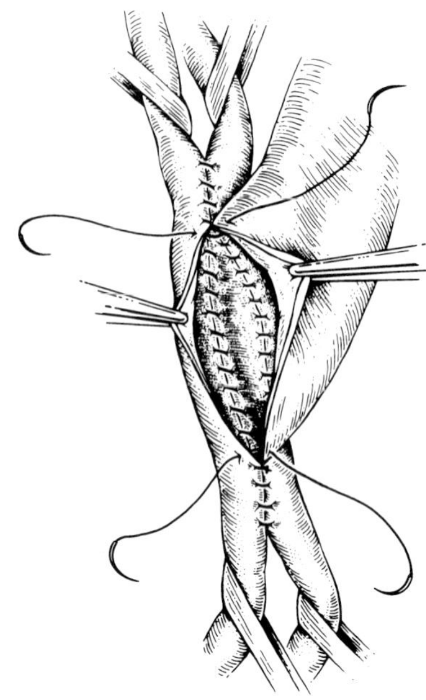

FIGURE 69–13. To increase flow through a prosthetic bypass to limited arterial outflow, the surgeon sometimes creates an anastomotic arteriovenous fistula to enhance graft flow with diversion into the high-capacitance venous system.

tical incision excised from the hood of the distal prosthetic anastomosis. Long-term anticoagulation therapy has also been routinely employed to improve long-term patency in the demanding setting of infrapopliteal prosthetic bypass. Preliminary results in an uncontrolled series suggest that anticoagulation may improve patency rates twofold or threefold.[55]

Biologic Grafts

A third prosthetic material with which considerable experience has been gained is *human umbilical vein* tanned with glutaraldehyde. This prosthesis was introduced in the mid-1970s, at the same time PTFE became popular, and initially provided similar short-term results.[42] This prosthesis has never gained the popularity associated with PTFE for two major reasons. First, it is technically more demanding because an initial irrigation protocol is necessary to remove residual alcohol and aldehyde and meticulous anastomotic technique is required to incorporate the outer reinforcing mesh (Fig. 69–16).[43] Second, a propensity for dilatation and aneurysm formation has gradually become evident.[44, 67] As longer-term results obtained with PTFE have usually proved to be inferior to those achieved with autogenous vein, however, several studies have favorably compared umbilical vein to PTFE, particularly at the above-knee level.[1, 79, 99]

Cryopreserved Vein

Historically, aneurysmal degeneration and dismal patency rates have been problematic in venous and arterial allografting. These poor results have generally been attributed to immune destruction of the graft. Recent advances in the techniques of cryopreservation, including improved cryo-

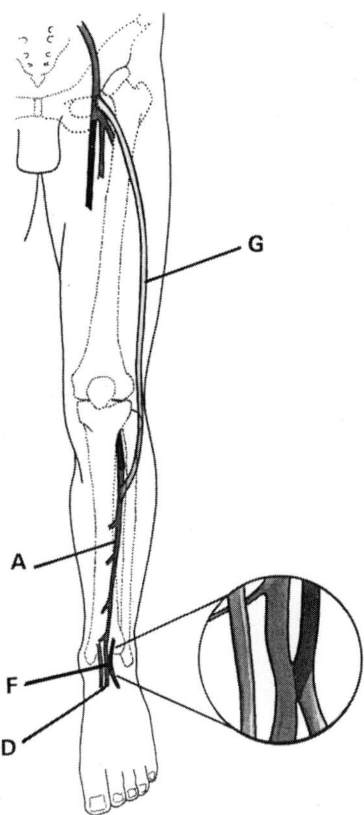

FIGURE 69–14. An alternative approach to enhance flow through a prosthetic graft (G) is the creation of an arteriovenous fistula (F) at a site remote (D) from the distal anastomosis. In theory, flow is also augmented in the intervening arterial segment (A) and its collaterals.

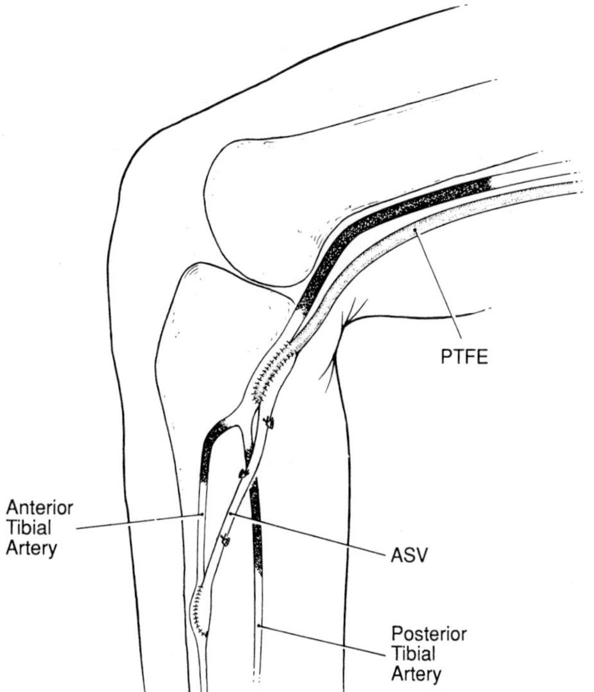

FIGURE 69–15. Composite prosthetic grafting to the popliteal artery is an option in the absence of suitable vein. When possible, the composite anastomosis should be located above the knee, but in some cases a distal popliteal site is required. The distal prosthetic anastomosis is initially an end-to-side construction, and the proximal venous composite anastomosis is constructed to an elliptical incision excised from the hood of the distal prosthetic anastomosis. PTFE = polytetrafluoroethylene; ASV = autogenous saphenous vein.

preservatives and rate-controlled freezing, have held out the hope that improved patency rates may be achieved.[95, 152] These grafts have the advantages of (1) ready availability, (2) a theoretical lower risk of infection, and (3) the initial technical feature of working with a high-quality autogenous vein. Unfortunately, some series continue to demonstrate unacceptably low patency rates and continued problems with aneurysm formation. These problems, coupled with the high expense of the grafts, limit their current applicability to short-term limb salvage applications when infection is a major consideration.

Completion Evaluation

After the bypass procedure is completed, an objective assessment of technical adequacy is mandatory. Completion arteriography is easily performed with a variety of methods (Fig. 69–17). Hand injection of 20 to 25 ml of diluted (50%) diatrizoate (Renografin) antegrafin into the proximal vein graft with the anastomosis occluded provides excellent visualization. Contrast solution may also be injected retrograde to allow opacification in the presence of normal antegrade blood flow. A single injection is sufficient for an above-knee reconstruction, but two injections are required for assessment of the entire length of longer below-knee or infrapopliteal grafts. Although angiography provides excellent opacification of the distal anastomosis and the outflow vessels, as well as of residual arteriovenous fistulae in the case of in situ grafts, endoluminal pathology may be obscured.[18, 59, 100, 160] Completion angioscopy more reliably identifies retained valve cusps and endoluminal pathology. The incidence of retained valve cusps, however, is quite low (4% to 12%), and the most important contribution of angioscopy is the demonstration of unsuspected endoluminal pathology.

Intraoperative completion evaluation with the duplex scan has been increasing in popularity.[13] A 10-MHz color Doppler probe is used to interrogate the entire length of the graft as well as the proximal and distal anastomoses. Areas of flow disturbance are characterized by measuring the peak systolic flow velocity within the lesion as well as within the adjacent normal vein graft. Defects with a peak systolic flow velocity above 180 cm/sec generally merit immediate revision. Similarly, lesions with a peak systolic flow velocity ratio (peak velocity within lesion/peak velocity

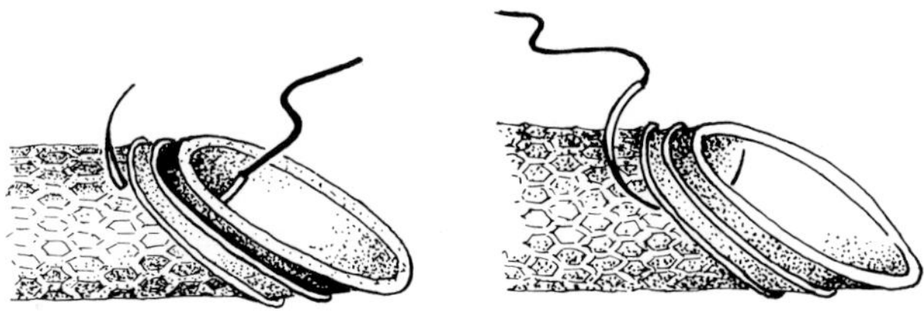

FIGURE 69–16. Proper suture technique for constructing anastomoses with human umbilical vein includes the incorporation of the outer mesh as well as the actual intimal component of the graft in the suture line.

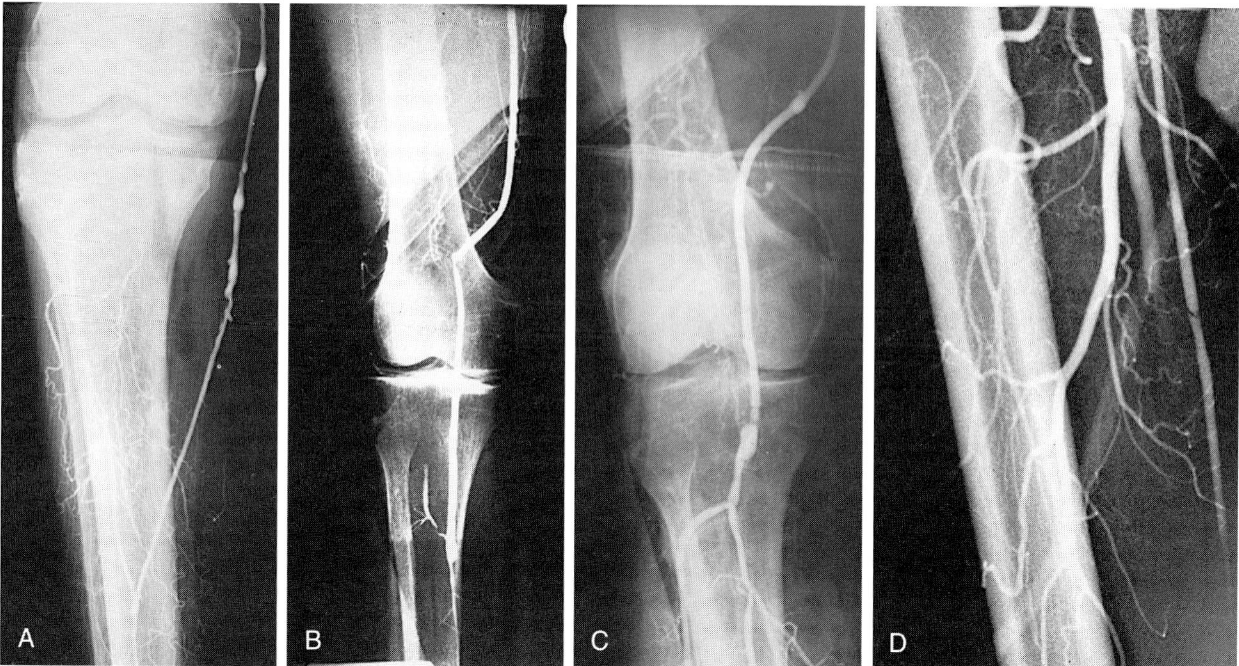

FIGURE 69–17. Intraoperative completion arteriograms demonstrate an endoluminal lesion in the distal aspect of a femoroperoneal vein graft (*A*), a kink in a femoroposterior tibial vein graft as the graft enters the popliteal tunnel above the knee (*B*), a residual platelet plug just proximal to the distal anastomosis in a femoropopliteal vein graft (*C*), and a retained valve cusp in an in situ femoropopliteal graft with a residual arteriovenous fistula (*D*).

within normal adjacent vein) above 2.4 mandate investigation and repair. This protocol has proved useful in identifying all significant intraluminal pathology and technical defects and has reduced early graft failure (to <1%) and has decreased the need for subsequent graft revision (to 2%).[13]

Once the completion study has been performed and is deemed satisfactory, attention is turned to closure. If adequate hemostasis is achieved, anticoagulation therapy is not routinely reversed, and the incisions are closed with continuous absorbable subcutaneous suture and skin staples. For excessively thin skin in the distal third of the leg and foot, subcutaneous closure is not necessary and may prove to be detrimental. Closure of the incisions on the dorsum of the foot required for dorsal pedal in situ bypass is best achieved with interrupted nylon vertical mattress sutures. We believe that this technique offers the most precise approximation of the wound edges and minimizes the tension on the wound.

POSTOPERATIVE MANAGEMENT

If initial recovery is uneventful, most patients do not require routine admission to an intensive care unit. Pulses should be frequently assessed, either by palpation or by monitoring with a Doppler velocity meter during the first 12 hours and several times daily thereafter to ensure sustained patency. If no significant systemic complications have ensued, early graft thrombosis should prompt immediate return to the operating room for thrombectomy, angiography, and revision as necessary.

Patients without significant tissue necrosis routinely begin ambulation on the first postoperative day; patients with healing lesions begin later as indicated. Patients undergoing bypass to the pedal level generally require an additional day of bed rest to allow sufficient wound healing prior to ambulation. Claudicants who have had uncomplicated procedures are usually discharged by the fifth postoperative day, whereas those with systemic complications or cutaneous distal lesions may require longer hospitalization.

After discharge and the initial postoperative outpatient visit, periodic surveillance of all grafts is necessary to identify hemodynamically significant lesions before thrombosis. It has been repeatedly demonstrated that revision of such stenotic lesions results in sustained graft patency, whereas revision of similar lesions following graft thrombosis yields poor results (see Chapter 71).[14, 15, 149, 160]

At present, little clinical evidence is available to support the routine long-term use of oral anticoagulation agents to maintain graft patency.[82] Preliminary evidence suggests that routine anticoagulation therapy may improve the results with infrapopliteal prosthetic bypass.[54] A multicenter Veterans Affairs study assessing the efficacy of warfarin anticoagulation in routine autogenous reconstructions failed to show any significant patency benefits.[78] Patients with unexplained graft thrombosis after thrombectomy and patients with an identifiable hypercoagulopathy, however, are frequently maintained on an oral anticoagulation regimen.

Complications

Perioperative mortality within 30 days of surgery ranges from 2% to 5% and most commonly results from coronary artery disease.[23, 48, 90, 112, 113, 115, 138] Overall morbidity rates vary widely, depending on inclusion criteria, but major systemic complications, the predominant cause of which is again cardiac, develop in 5% to 10% of patients. Local complications include hemorrhage, graft thrombosis, wound infection, and leg edema. Hemorrhage during the first 48 hours is unusual; the incidence in most series is less than 2%.[48, 138] A significant or an expanding hematoma must be evacuated, and a diligent search for its cause must be undertaken. Of identifiable causes, suture line hemorrhage and insecure ligation of an arterial branch or arterialized venous tributary are frequent culprits. Hemorrhage occurring beyond the immediate postoperative period suggests underlying infection of an anastomotic suture line and usually calls for ligation or excision of the graft.

Graft thrombosis within the first 30 days of surgery complicates 2% to 7% of procedures and most often results from technical defects, hypercoagulopathy, inadequate distal runoff, and (rarely) postoperative hypotension.[49] Technical defects are more common with autogenous reconstructions and are responsible for most early failures. Such errors include graft kinks, valvulotome injury, retained leaflets, intimal flaps, significant residual arteriovenous fistulae, and small-caliber vein. Various hypercoagulopathies occur in at least 10% to 14% of the population with vascular problems and are responsible for 20% of early graft thromboses, most commonly resulting from antiphospholipid syndrome and heparin-induced platelet aggregation. Systemic hypotension, which is usually cardiogenic in origin, may also contribute to earlier graft failure.

Although most wound complications are relatively minor and are limited to superficial skin necrosis along the edges of incisions or an erythematous reaction to sutures or staples, significant wound infection occurs with a reported incidence of 8% to 19%.[48, 112, 116] Infection is usually associated with persistent hematoma, lymphocele or lymphorrhea, and significant superficial necrosis. Lymphocele with or without lymphorrhea from the inguinal incision may result from the transection of unrecognized lymphatics during the initial groin exploration. Although immobility with elevation and local care usually results in spontaneous resolution, copious and persistent lymphorrhea should prompt re-exploration of the groin and ligation of lymph channels to minimize the incidence of secondary infection.[129] An infected incision usually responds to appropriate antibiotics and local drainage with acute débridement, but if the suture line of an underlying graft becomes involved, especially if complicated with hemorrhage, excision of the graft is required.[157]

Wound healing may be significantly delayed by the inevitable appearance of edema in the leg after successful revascularization. The edema results from increased interstitial fluid accumulation, lymphatic obstruction, and, to some degree, venous interruption. Of all three potential components, venous interruption seems to be the least important because of the plethora of deep veins available to compensate for ligation during the exposure of distal arteries. In all probability, chronic ischemia attenuates autoregulatory vasomotor responses, which normalize to some extent after reperfusion. Disruption of lymphatic channels, however, is probably the most important factor contributing to lower extremity edema.[4] Patients should be discharged with elastic compression stockings of moderate pressure, with instructions to elevate the legs periodically during early recovery. The edema gradually subsides in most patients over the course of a few weeks, but it may occasionally linger for several months. Delayed wound complications have been reported to occur in as many as 50% of these patients.

RESULTS

Interpretation

Comprehensive assessment of the efficacy of infrainguinal reconstruction, as reported in the literature, is confounded by a frustrating multitude of variables that preclude statistically valid comparisons. Unfortunately, even standardized methods of reporting, as suggested by the Ad Hoc Committee of the International Society for Cardiovascular Surgery/Society for Vascular Surgery (ISCVS/SVS), have not been uniformly adopted.[124, 126] Most authors use life-table methods for reporting graft patency, limb salvage, and patient survival, which in turn allows the reader to assess the actuarial probability of the specific end-point after a given interval of time.

Graft patency rates are customarily reported as primary or secondary. *Primary patency* usually refers to only grafts that either require no further intervention after initial bypass or that need revision or extension while they are still patent. Some authors consider grafts to be primarily patent even though an acute thrombectomy and revision may have been required for acute thrombosis within 48 hours of the original procedure. Still others consider separately grafts that have required some form of revision, while still patent, to have "primary assisted" or "primary revised" patency. *Secondary patency* refers to all grafts that remain primarily patent as well as to thrombosed grafts requiring lysis or thrombectomy with revision; these rates should not be confused with primary patency rates derived from secondary or reoperative procedures.

Successful limb salvage rates customarily include those limbs requiring minor amputation to the transmetatarsal level. Unfortunately, limb salvage rates may be speciously enhanced by inclusion of patients initially operated on for claudication as well as those operated on for critical ischemia. Another common problem in assessing life-table analyses are results reported prematurely, with an insufficient number of grafts at risk at longer-term intervals. For instance, the validity of an 80% mean graft patency rate reported for only one to two limbs at risk may be compromised by a large standard error.

Indications for a particular procedure undergoing analysis may demonstrate extraordinary variation. Claudication is a relatively subjective symptom, and although limb viability is clearly threatened by ischemic tissue necrosis, rest pain also remains a subjective complaint that defies quantitation. Patients in the affected age group often have pain from various sources other than ischemia, including arthritis and neuropathy. Broad interpretation of criteria for determining claudication as disabling and rest pain as truly limb-threatening contributes to considerable variation in reported results.

The site chosen for the distal anastomosis is also important, less so with more tolerant autogenous vein grafts and more so with relatively thrombogenic prosthetic grafts, and it cannot be considered independent from the quality of outflow. Thus, a bypass to a popliteal artery with single-vessel runoff does not fare as well as a similar graft to a popliteal vessel with three unobstructed infrapopliteal vessels for outflow. Although the site of the distal anastomosis is frequently included in analyses of results, the status of the outflow often is not, and it may in fact prove to be the more important variable.[124]

The choice of conduit is a very important determinant of graft patency. In most circumstances, autogenous vein provides a more durable reconstruction than any prosthetic graft, yet several series combine both types of conduit in reporting results.[147] In similar fashion, some reports of all autogenous reconstructions use greater superficial saphenous vein in both reversed and in situ configurations and may include arm, lesser saphenous, and composite vein grafts. Although an appreciable difference between reversed and in situ saphenous vein grafts has not been consistently demonstrated, both usually demonstrate better patency rates than either arm or lesser saphenous vein.[16, 56, 65, 103, 151, 155] In addition, the quality and caliber of vein used are important but not easily documented variables.[23, 154]

Technical considerations also confound accurate comparison of concurrent reports. Methods of vein preparation, magnification, experience of the surgical team, and intraoperative assessment on completion of the bypass are not necessarily uniform. Although completion arteriography has undoubtedly reduced the number of technical complications resulting in early graft failure, both intraoperative duplex scanning and angioscopy are being used with increasing frequency and may favorably or unfavorably influence the ultimate result.

The extent of significant comorbidity also influences the ultimate outcome. Significant susceptibility to myocardial ischemia increases the risk of perioperative cardiac morbidity and mortality and reduces longer-term survival.[27, 31, 60, 107, 114] The presence of diabetes has not significantly altered the results when compared with those observed in nondiabetic patients; in fact, many series have demonstrated better results in patients with diabetes.[23, 48, 125, 138] Patients with mild renal insufficiency and threatened limbs achieve graft patency rates comparable to those in patients with normal renal function, but they sustain higher operative mortality and diminished survival.[36, 50, 63, 127, 158] Patients with end-stage renal disease, however, especially those with diabetes, demonstrate lower patency rates. The relatively recent recognition that a significant number of vascular surgery patients harbor a variety of hypercoagulopathies, most commonly antiphospholipid syndrome and heparin-induced platelet aggregation, represents yet another example of significant comorbidity affecting the outcome of bypass results.[47]

Postoperative management of these patients is of critical importance to sustained graft patency. Patients who persist in using tobacco have significantly lower graft patency and limb salvage rates than do patients who abstain from smoking after reconstruction.[6, 112, 125] There are no clear guidelines for the use of postoperative anticoagulation therapy, and its application has not been consistent. Warfarin enhances the primary patency of long prosthetic grafts and is commonly used after secondary intervention for a failed graft.[82] Although routine use of anticoagulation therapy for autogenous vein grafts has not proved useful, its selective application in high-risk grafts may be. It has been repeatedly shown that repair of an isolated vein graft or perianastomotic stenosis before graft thrombosis provides satisfactory sustained patency rates of approximately 80% after 5 years.[29, 38, 103, 160] In contrast, similar intervention for recently thrombosed grafts, necessitating initial catheter thrombectomy or thrombolysis, yields much lower patency rates (20% to 30%).[20] This observation has spawned various postoperative graft surveillance protocols, which have demonstrated that neither recurrent ischemic symptoms nor reduced ankle-brachial index (ABI) values are as reliable in identifying these stenotic lesions, and therefore incipient graft failure, as is routine serial duplex evaluation.[14, 61, 102, 161] Variations in postoperative surveillance protocols, then, significantly alter secondary patency results and overall limb salvage rates.

Autogenous Vein Bypass

Four representative series of autogenous infrainguinal bypasses (Table 69–1) report operative mortality rates of 1% to 3%.[23, 49, 86, 138] Primary 5-year patency rates ranged from 63% to 75%, and secondary patency rates ranged from 80% to 83%. Limb salvage rates ranged from 84% to 92%, and overall patient survival rates of 28% to 66% were observed at the end of 5 years. In an attempt to arrive at working figures that enable the practicing clinician to make reasonable decisions and discuss potential outcome with patients, we can average results from several series by dividing the sum of the product of the number of limbs and the patency rate (per cent) by the sum of the limbs. This formula represents an effort to correct for variations in the number of patients in each series:

$$\% = \frac{\Sigma(N \times \%)}{\Sigma(N)}$$

TABLE 69–1. INFRAINGUINAL RECONSTRUCTION WITH AUTOGENOUS VEIN

			FIVE-YEAR CUMULATIVE RATES (%)			
			Graft Patency			
STUDY	NO. OF LIMBS	OPERATIVE MORTALITY (%)	*Primary*	*Secondary*	Limb Salvage	Patient Survival
Taylor et al, 1990[138]	516	1	75	80	90	28
Bergamini et al, 1991[23]	361	3	63	81	86	57
Donaldson et al, 1991[48]	440	2	72	83	84	66
Leather et al, 1992[86]	1688	3	70	81	92	58
Total/weighted average	3005	2	70	81	90	54

TABLE 69–2. WEIGHTED-AVERAGE PRIMARY GRAFT PATENCY RATES ASSOCIATED WITH INFRAINGUINAL RECONSTRUCTION USING AUTOGENOUS VEIN

SITE OF DISTAL ANASTOMOSIS	STUDY	TOTAL NO. OF LIMBS	FIVE-YEAR CUMULATIVE PATENCY RATES (%)	
			Primary	Secondary
Popliteal				
Above-knee	Donaldson et al, 1991[48] Taylor et al, 1990[138]	155	75	83
Below-knee	Donaldson et al, 1991[48] Taylor et al, 1990[138] Bergamini et al, 1991[23] Leather et al, 1992[86]	952	74	83
Infrapopliteal	Donaldson et al, 1991[48] Taylor et al, 1990[138] Bergamini et al, 1991[23] Leather et al, 1992[86]	1843	67	78

Although these four series are relatively comparable, three reports are restricted to experience with in situ greater saphenous vein,[23, 48, 86] and Taylor and coworkers[138] reported experience with reversed autogenous vein including arm and lesser saphenous sources. Claudicants constituted fewer than 10% of patients in the series reported by Leather and associates[86] and Bergamini and colleagues,[79] and approximately 70% of their bypasses were carried to the tibial level. In contrast, 20% to 30% of procedures reported by Taylor and coworkers[77] and Donaldson and associates[48] were indicated for claudication, and fewer than 50% were infrapopliteal. Table 69–2 illustrates the weighted average of results from these same four series for autogenous reconstructions to above-knee, below-knee, and infrapopliteal levels.

As techniques have improved, allowing the use of smaller-caliber vein, progressively more distal bypasses have been carried out in patients with more extensive disease who would not have been considered appropriate candidates for reconstruction in the early 1980s. This is evidenced by the increasing number of *femorotibial bypasses*, ranging from 45% to 68% of the series listed in Table 69–1. Bypasses to the peroneal artery, frequently the only suitable alternative in diabetic patients, have provided results as durable as those of bypasses to the anterior or posterior tibial vessels.[23, 48, 90] Increasing use of the in situ technique has enabled the use of smaller-caliber veins of 2.5 mm in diameter,[23, 90, 154] and improved methods of exposure and surgical technique allow anastomoses to be constructed as far distally as the plantar branches.[110] Femorotibial bypasses provided primary patency rates ranging from 63% to 69% and secondary patency rates of 72% to 85% after 5 years (see Table 69–2), and acceptable results have also been reported for various subgroups using these distal vessels. For instance, vein grafts beyond the ankle level provide average patency rates of 50% after 4 to 5 years (Table 69–3). In the absence of sufficient length of saphenous vein for conventional femorotibial bypass, a shorter length of residual vein originating from a patent below-knee popliteal artery provides similar 5-year patency rates of 40% to 55%.[8, 34, 64, 81, 94, 117, 120, 133, 156]

Distal grafts originating from a proximal tibial vessel have also proved satisfactory,[150] as have bypass vein grafts to the plantar vessels, which provide significant salvage of limbs jeopardized by overt distal gangrene.[40, 137] Finally, when outflow is extremely limited, autogenous vein bypass to isolated tibial artery segments may be performed with the expectation of good patency rates, improved foot perfusion, and distal ischemic wound healing.[21]

More recently, series of in situ saphenous vein bypasses that have followed up patients for more than a decade have been reported.[22, 131] These studies have testified to the durability of this procedure with 10-year primary and secondary patency rates of 55% to 60% and 70% to 76%, respectively. Similarly, 10-year limb salvage rates of 84% to 90% were attained.

In the absence of suitable greater saphenous vein, alternative sources include arm vein and the lesser saphenous vein. Primary patency rates associated with arm vein have ranged from 40% at 3 years to 50% after 5 years, with

TABLE 69–3. PARAMALLEOLAR INFRAPOPLITEAL RECONSTRUCTION WITH AUTOGENOUS VEIN

STUDY	NO. OF LIMBS	PRIMARY PATENCY RATES (%)		FOUR- TO FIVE-YEAR LIMB SALVAGE RATE (%)
		Two- to Three-Year	Four- to Five-Year	
Andros et al, 1988[8]	224	62	40	71
Klamer et al, 1990[81]	68	81	81	95
Pomposelli et al, 1990[111]	97	80	—	—
Shah et al, 1992[133]	270	74	61	89
Harrington et al, 1992[64]	73	59	50	74
Total/weighted average	732	70	55	82

secondary patency rates approaching 60% after 5 years and limb salvage rates as high as 82%.[9, 12, 66] A vein is a less reliable conduit than the greater saphenous vein but provides acceptable results, particularly in the setting of severely compromised outflow, in which prosthetic material has proved unsatisfactory.[130] It has been suggested that preliminary intraoperative angioscopy may enable correction of unsuspected endoluminal defects more frequently encountered in arm vein than in other venous conduits and, thereby, may improve overall durability.[93] The lesser saphenous vein, yet another autogenous conduit, has been associated with primary patency rates of 77% at 2 years and 55% after 3 years.

Finally, because of the limited number of patients for whom sequential bypass proves to be appropriate, collective experience has been limited. Reported patency rates, however, have exceeded 80% after 1 year and have ranged from 42% to 64% after 4 years.[30, 31, 85, 121]

The deeper femoral vein and the popliteal vein, additional sources of autogenous material, have been used for femoropopliteal reconstruction despite the risk of significant lower extremity edema and the longer operating time required. Harvesting of the shortest possible length of femoral vein with preservation of the deep femoral vein is desirable. In a series of 100 such reconstructions, Shulman and associates[128] reported a 64% 5-year patency rate and a 70% limb salvage rate. These results also reflect adjunctive profundaplasty and secondary interventions. The incidence of early lower extremity edema is significant, but the magnitude of subsequent chronic disability remains unclear.

Prosthetic Bypass

Results achieved with infrainguinal bypass using PTFE (Table 69–4) have been less satisfactory than those obtained with autogenous vein. The discrepancy has been most pronounced in the challenging low-flow conditions of the femorotibial bypass.[1, 45, 37, 71, 108, 112, 113, 123, 135, 141, 147, 159] On the basis of these studies, infrapopliteal reconstruction with PTFE provides an average patency rate of 14%, rendering autogenous vein from nearly any source the preferred conduit. In contrast, PTFE in the femoropopliteal position provides 5-year patency rates averaging 40%, which differ less from those obtained with autogenous vein. As is true with vein, however, better results are achieved with reconstructions indicated for claudication than with those performed in the more challenging setting required for limb salvage. This finding is most pronounced for above-knee reconstructions, for which overall primary patency rates achieved in claudicants ranged from 42% to 68% at the 5-year interval and averaged 63%.

Because surgical technique and graft material are reasonably standardized, and provided that reporting methods are comparable, the significant variation in the results illustrated in Table 69–4 primarily reflects the different patient selection criteria with regard to indication and the quality of the popliteal vessel and its distal runoff. A prosthetic bypass to a compromised popliteal artery with single-vessel runoff cannot be expected to provide the durability of a similar bypass to a relatively disease-free popliteal artery with two-vessel or three-vessel runoff. Most published series represent the summation of some combination of these extremes, but a preponderance of one or the other shifts overall patency rates to the higher or lower end of the range accordingly.

The claim that prosthetic reconstruction with PTFE in the above-knee location is superior to vein with regard to durability has not yet been substantiated in prospectively randomized patients treated by the same group of surgeons using standardized patient selection criteria.

Initially disappointing results with infrainguinal reconstruction using prosthetic Dacron grafts led to increasing enthusiasm for PTFE shortly after its introductioin in the mid-1970s, when preliminary results obtained with PTFE initially appeared comparable to those achieved with saphenous vein. Now that long-term results with PTFE are well documented, it does not appear to any advantage over the textile Dacron material. In a randomized, prospective

TABLE 69–4. PATENCY RATES FOR INFRAINGUINAL RECONSTRUCTION USING POLYTETRAFLUOROETHYLENE

	FIVE-YEAR PRIMARY PATENCY RATES							
	Femoropopliteal Above-Knee and Below-Knee		Femoropopliteal Above-Knee		Femoropopliteal Above-Knee-Claudication		Infrapopliteal	
STUDY	No.	*Patency (%)*	No.	*Patency (%)*	No.	*Patency (%)*	No.	*Patency (%)*
Hobson et al, 1985[71]	80	22					41	12
Charlesworth et al, 1985[37]	134	24	53	39				
Tilanus et al, 1985[141]	24	37						
Sterpetti et al, 1985[135]			90	58	41	76		
Veith et al, 1986[147]	171	38	91	38			98	12
Whittemore et al, 1989[159]	279	37	182	42	64	62	21	12
Patterson et al, 1990[108]			138	54				
Prendiville et al, 1990[112]			114	42	44	57		
Rosenthal et al, 1990[123]					100	65		
Davies et al, 1991[45]			48	63				
Aalders and van Vroonhoven, 1992[1]			49	39	41	42		
Quiñones-Baldrich et al, 1992[113]	294	59	219	61	110	68	28	22
Pevec et al, 1992[110]	85	27						
Total/weighted average	1067	40	984	50	400	63	202	14

experience with above-knee infrainguinal reconstruction for claudicants, Rosenthal and coworkers[123] reported a 5-year cumulative primary patency rate of 65% for PTFE grafts and 67% for Dacron, a difference that proved to be statistically insignificant. Similarly, in a later randomized prospective comparison, an insignificant difference of 62% 5-year patency for Dacron, compared with 57% 5-year patency for PTFE, was found for above-knee popliteal bypass grafts.[2] More dramatic are results reported by Pevec and associates[110] from a nonrandomized but concurrent experience in which the 48% 5-year cumulative patency rate achieved with Dacron proved statistically superior to the 27% rate associated with PTFE for femoropopliteal reconstruction, both above and below the knee and for all indications.

Experience with human umbilical vein documents 5-year primary patency rates approximating 60% for femoropopliteal grafts and ranging as high as 81% in the above-knee location.[1, 26, 41, 51, 97] In the three randomized series reported, umbilical vein demonstrated results that were statistically either comparable or superior to those achieved with PTFE.[1, 45, 97] Because all three series have reported at 3-year intervals, the overall effect of aneurysmal dilatation of vein grafts cannot be factored into the equation. On the basis of past experience, however, aneurysmal degeneration may be anticipated in as many as 57% of patent grafts after 2 years.[68] Dardik and colleagues[41] reported aneurysmal degeneration in 36% after 5 years and noted dilatation in an additional 21%.

Functional Outcome

Vascular surgeons have historically judged the results of infrainguinal arterial reconstruction on the basis of (1) patency rates, (2) limb salvage rates, and (3) in some cases, maintenance of hemodynamic improvement. More recently, we have begun to focus on the objective measurement of functional patient outcomes after infrainguinal surgery, with greater emphasis placed on physical function and comfort, role function, and general health perception.

An early, small study employed Spitzer's QL-Index to assess quality of life in a series of patients 3, 6, and 12 months after treatment for ischemic lesions of the foot. This index is based on occupational status, activities of daily living, perception of own health, support structure, and outlook on life. Not surprisingly, patients who underwent limb salvage through either conservative management or revascularization had a better outcome than those undergoing immediate or delayed amputation.[5]

A later study demonstrated that preoperative independence and ambulation were the best predictors of postoperative function.[3] Postoperative living and ambulatory independence were maintained in 99% and 97% of patients with preoperative independence. Unfortunately, only 4% of patients not living independently became independent after surgery and 21% of nonambulatory patients became ambulatory postoperatively.

A larger study was reported by Gibbons and colleagues,[58] who assessed 156 patients undergoing infrainguinal reconstruction for limb-threatening ischemia. Questionnaires were administered before treatment and after 6 months of follow-up. Questions focused on general health status, activities of daily living, social activity, mental well-being, and a vitality scale adopted from the SF-36 Health Survey. At 6 months' follow-up, improved mental well-being, vitality, and ability to perform activities of daily living were documented. Patients with better functional status and general well-being at baseline status showed more improvement than patients with poorer baseline status. Despite the documented improvements in well-being and function, only 45% of patients reported that they were "back to normal" at 6 months. This was attributed to the poor general health status of many of the patients and the significant comorbidity (84% with diabetes mellitus, 83% with cardiac problems).

The early results of these studies assessing quality of life thus confirm the salutary effects of successful limb salvage operations in maintaining the quality of life in patients with lower extremity ischemia. Nonetheless, the significant comorbidities affecting these patients may significantly limit the benefits of our interventions.

SUMMARY

Judicious selection of the appropriate method of infrainguinal reconstruction for a given patient requires an appreciation of the results obtained with all available approaches. Although PTA may be appropriate for some patients with short-segment lesions and profundaplasty may be effective in others, most patients with an ischemic limb require conventional surgical bypass. Most claudicants achieve sustained relief, and 80% to 90% of limbs threatened with critical ischemia are salvaged. Of variables influencing the ultimate outcome, choice of conduit is most important, and every effort must be made to use autogenous vein for optimal results. Additional factors influencing outcome include indications, site of distal anastomosis and associated outflow, and extent of significant comorbidity.

Sustained graft patency requires vigilant graft surveillance with secondary intervention before graft thrombosis occurs. A diligent multidisciplinary approach to the patient with atherosclerosis must coordinate management of individual manifestations of the underlying systemic disease process and must reduce predisposing risk factors to further improve results from infrainguinal reconstruction and overall life expectancy.

REFERENCES

1. Aalders GJ, van Vroonhoven TJM: Polytetrafluoroethylene versus human umbilical vein in above-knee femoropopliteal bypass: Six-year results of a randomized clinical trial. J Vasc Surg 16:816, 1992.
2. Abbott W, Green R, Matsumato T, et al: Prosthetic above-knee femoropopliteal bypass grafting: Results of a multicenter randomized trial. J Vasc Surg 25:19, 1997.
3. Abou-Zamzam A, Lee R, Moneta G, et al: Functional outcome after infrainguinal bypass surgery for limb salvage. J Vasc Surg 25:287, 1997.
4. AbuRahma AF, Woodruff BA, Lucente FC: Edema after femoropopliteal bypass surgery: Lymphatic and venous theories of causation. J Vasc Surg 11:461, 1990.
5. Albers M, Fratezi AC, De Luccia N: Assessment of quality of life of patients with severe ischemia as a result of infrainguinal arterial occlusive disease. J Vasc Surg 16:54, 1992.

6. Ameli FM, Stein M, Prosser RJ, et al: Effects of cigarette smoking on outcome of femoral popliteal bypass for limb salvage. J Cardiovasc Surg 30:591, 1989.
7. Andros G, Harris RW, Salles-Cunha SX, et al: Lateral plantar artery bypass grafting: Defining the limits of foot revascularization. J Vasc Surg 10:511, 1989.
8. Andros G, Harris RW, Salles-Cunha SX, et al: Bypass grafts to the ankle and foot, J Vasc Surg 7:785, 1988.
9. Andros G, Harris RW, Salles-Cunha SX, et al: Arm veins for arterial revascularization of the leg: Arteriographic and clinical observations. J Vasc Surg 4:416, 1986.
10. Ascer E, Veith FJ, Gupta SK: Bypasses to plantar arteries and other tibial branches: An extended approach to limb salvage. J Vasc Surg 8:434, 1988.
11. Ascer E, Veith FJ, Gupta SK, et al: Short vein grafts: A superior option for arterial reconstruction to poor or compromised outflow tracts? J Vasc Surg 7:370, 1988.
12. Balshi JD, Cantelmo NL, Menzoian JO, LoGerfo FW: The use of arm veins for infrainguinal bypass in end-stage peripheral vascular disease. Arch Surg 124:1078, 1989.
13. Bandyk D, Johnson B, Gupta A, et al: Nature and management of duplex abnormalities encountered during infrainguinal vein bypass grafting. J Vasc Surg 24:430, 1996.
14. Bandyk DF, Schmitt DD, Seabrook GR, et al: Monitoring functional patency of in situ saphenous vein bypasses: The impact of a surveillance protocol and elective revision. J Vasc Surg 9:286, 1989.
15. Bandyk DF, Bergamini TM, Towne JB: Durability of vein graft revision: The outcome of secondary procedures. J Vasc Surg 113:200, 1991.
16. Batson RC, Sottiurai VS: Nonreversed and in situ vein grafts: Clinical and experimental observations. Ann Surg 201:771, 1985.
17. Baum R, Rutter C, Sunshine J, et al: Multicenter trial to evaluate vascular magnetic resonance arteriography of the lower extremity. JAMA 274:875, 1995.
18. Baxter BT, Rizzo RJ, Flinn WR, et al: A comparative study of intraoperative angioscopy and completion arteriography following femorodistal bypass. Arch Surg 125:997, 1990.
19. Belkin M, Knox J, Donaldson M, et al: Infrainguinal arterial reconstruction with nonreversed greater saphenous vein. J Vasc Surg 24:957, 1996.
20. Belkin M, Donaldson M, Whittemore A, et al: Observations on the use of thrombolytic agents for thrombotic occlusion of vein grafts. J Vasc Surg 11:289, 1990.
21. Belkin M, Welch H, Mackey W, et al: Clinical and hemodynamic results of bypass to isolated tibial artery segments for ischemic ulceration of the foot. Am J Surg 64:281, 1992.
22. Belkin M, Conte M, Donaldson M, et al: The impact of gender on the results of arterial bypass with in situ greater saphenous vein. Am J Surg 170:97, 1995.
23. Bergamini TM, Towne JB, Bandyk DF, et al: Experience with in situ saphenous vein bypasses during 1981 to 1989: Determinant factors of long-term patency. J Vasc Surg 13:137, 1991.
24. Bergan JJ, Veith FJ, Bernhard VM, et al: Randomization of autogenous vein and polytetrafluoroethylene grafts in femoral-distal reconstruction. Surgery 92:921, 1982.
25. Bernhard VM, Boren CH, Towne JB: Pneumatic tourniquet as a substitute for vascular clamps in distal bypass surgery. Surgery 87:709, 1980.
26. Boontje AH: Aneurysm formation in human umbilical vein grafts used as arterial substitutes. J Vasc Surg 2:524, 1985.
27. Boucher CA, Brewster DC, Darling RC, et al: Determination of cardiac risk by dipyridamole-thallium imaging before peripheral vascular surgery. N Engl J Med 312:389, 1985.
28. Boyd AM: The natural course of arteriosclerosis of lower extremities. Proc R Soc Med 55:591, 1962.
29. Brewster DC, LaSalle AJ, Robinson JG, et al: Femoropopliteal graft failures: Clinical consequences and success of secondary reconstructions. Arch Surg 118:1043, 1983.
30. Burdick JF, O'Mara C, Ricotta J, et al: The multiple sequential distal bypass graft: Improving nature's alternatives. Surgery 89:536, 1981.
31. Calhoun TR, Wright RM, Wright RM Jr, et al: Sequential bypass grafting for salvage of lower extremities. South Med J 78:41, 1985.
32. Cambria R, Kaufman J, L'Italien G, et al: Magnetic resonance arteriography in the management of lower extremity occlusive disease: A prospective study. J Vasc Surg 25:380, 1997.
33. Campbell CC, Goldfarb B, Roe R: A small arterial substitute: Expanded microporous polytetrafluoroethylene. Patency versus porosity. Ann Surg 182:138, 1975.
34. Cantelmo NL, Snow JR, Menzoian JO, LoGerfo FW: Successful vein bypass in patients with an ischemic limb and a palpable popliteal pulse. Arch Surg 121:217, 1986.
35. Chang BB, Paty PSK, Shah DM, Leather RP: The lesser saphenous vein: An under-appreciated source of autogenous vein. J Vasc Surg 15:152, 1992.
36. Chang BB, Paty PS, Shah DM, et al: Results of infrainguinal bypass for limb salvage in patients with end-stage renal disease. Surgery 108:742, 1990.
37. Charlesworth PM, Brewster DC, Darling RC, et al: The fate of polytetrafluoroethylene grafts in lower limb bypass surgery: A six-year follow-up. Br J Surg 72:896, 1985.
38. Cohen JR, Mannick JA, Couch NP, Whittemore AD: Recognition and management of impending vein-graft failure. Arch Surg 121:758, 1986.
39. Cohen JR, Mannick JA, Couch NP, Whittemore AD: Abdominal aortic aneurysm repair in patients with pre-operative renal failure. J Vasc Surg 3:867, 1986.
40. Dalsing MC, White JV, Yao JST, et al: Infrapopliteal bypass for established gangrene of the forefoot or toes. J Vasc Surg 2:669, 1985.
41. Dardik H, Miller N, Dardik A, et al: A decade of experience with the glutaraldehyde-tanned human umbilical cord vein graft for revascularization of the lower limb. J Vasc Surg 7:336, 1988.
42. Dardik H, Ibrahim IM, Dardik I: Evaluation of glutaraldehyde-tanned human umbilical cord vein as a vascular prosthesis for bypass to the popliteal, tibial and peroneal arteries. Surgery 83: 577, 1978.
43. Dardik H: The use of glutaraldehyde-stabilized umbilical vein for lower extremity reconstruction. *In* Greenhalgh RM (ed): Vascular Surgical Techniques: An Atlas. London, WB Saunders, 1989.
44. Dardik H, Miller N, Dardik A, et al: A decade of experience with the glutaraldehyde-tanned human umbilical cord vein graft for revascularization of the lower limb. J Vasc Surg 7:336, 1988.
45. Davies MG, Feeley TM, O'Malley MK, et al: Infrainguinal polytetrafluoroethylene grafts: Saved limbs or wasted effort? A report on ten years' experience. Ann Vasc Surg 5:519, 1991.
46. DeLaurentis DA, Friedmann P: Sequential femoropopliteal bypasses: Another approach to the inadequate saphenous vein problem. Surgery 71:400, 1972.
47. Donaldson MC, Weinberg DS, Belkin M, et al. Screening for hypercoagulable states in vascular practice: A preliminary study. J Vasc Surg 11:825, 1990.
48. Donaldson MC, Mannick JA, Whittemore AD: Femoral-distal bypass with in situ greater saphenous vein: Long-term results using the Mills valvulotome. Ann Surg 213:457, 1991.
49. Donaldson MC, Mannick JA, Whittemore AD: Causes of primary graft failure after in situ saphenous vein bypass grafting. J Vasc Surg 15:113, 1992.
50. Edwards JM, Taylor LM, Porter JM: Limb salvage in end-stage renal disease (ESRD): Comparison of modern results in patients with and without ESRD. Arch Surg 123:1164, 1988.
51. Eickoff JH, Broome A, Ericsson BF, et al: Four years' results of a prospective randomized clinical trial comparing polytetrafluoroethylene and modified human umbilical vein for below-knee femoropopliteal bypass. J Vasc Surg 6:506, 1987.
52. Eslami M, Belkin M, Mannick J, et al: Optimal methods for autogenous bypass to the anterior tibial artery. Am J Surg 174:198, 1997.
53. Flanagan DP, Williams, LR, Keifer T, et al: Prebypass operative arteriography. Surgery 92:627, 1982.
54. Flinn WR, Ricco JB, Yao JST, et al: Composite sequential grafts in severe ischemia: A comparative study. J Vasc Surg 1:449, 1984.
55. Flinn WR, Rohrer MJ, Yao JST, et al: Improved long-term patency of infragenicular polytetrafluoroethylene grafts. J Vasc Surg 7:685, 1988.
56. Fogle MA, Whittemore AD, Couch NP, Mannick JA: A comparison of in situ and reversed saphenous vein grafts for infrainguinal reconstruction. J Vasc Surg 5:46, 1987.
57. Gibbons GW: The diabetic foot: Amputations and drainage of infection. J Vasc Surg 5:791, 1987.
58. Gibbons GW, Burgess AM, Guadagnoli E, et al: Return to well-being after infrainguinal revascularization. J Vasc Surg 21:35, 1995.
59. Gilbertson JJ, Walsh DB, Zwolak RM, et al: A blinded comparison of angiography, angioscopy, and duplex scanning in the intraoperative

evaluation of in situ saphenous vein bypass grafts. J Vasc Surg 15:121, 1992.

60. Golden MA, Whittemore AD, Donaldson MC, Mannick JA: Selective evaluation and management of coronary artery disease in patients undergoing repair of abdominal aortic aneurysms: A 16-year experience. Ann Surg 212:415, 1990.
61. Green RM, McNamara J, Ouriel K, DeWeese JA: Comparison of infrainguinal graft surveillance techniques. J Vasc Surg 11:207, 1990.
62. Hall KV: The great saphenous vein used "in situ" as an arterial shunt after extirpation of vein valves. Surgery 51:492, 1962.
63. Harrington EB, Harrington ME, Schanzer H, Haimov M: End-stage renal disease: Is infrainguinal limb revascularization justified? J Vasc Surg 12:691, 1990.
64. Harrington EB, Harrington ME, Schanzer H, et al: The dorsalis pedis bypass: Moderate success in difficult situations. J Vasc Surg 15:409, 1992.
65. Harris PL, How TV, Jones DR: Prospectively randomized clinical trial to compare in situ and reversed saphenous vein grafts for femoropopliteal bypass. Br J Surg 74:252, 1987.
66. Harward TRS, Coe D, Flynn TC, Seeger JM: The use of arm vein conduits during infrageniculate arterial bypass. J Vasc Surg 16:420, 1992.
67. Hasson JE, Newton WD, Waltman AC, et al: Mural degeneration in the glutaraldehyde-tanned umbilical vein graft: Incidence and implications J Vasc Surg 4:243, 1986.
68. Hasson JE, Newton WD, Waltman AC, Fallon JT: Mural degeneration in the glutaraldehyde-tanned umbilical vein graft: Incidence and implications. J Vasc Surg 4:243, 1986.
69. Haysukami TS, Primozich JF, Zierler RE, et al: Color Doppler imaging of infrainguinal arterial occlusive disease. J Vasc Surg 16:527, 1992.
70. Hertzer NR, Beven EG, Young JR, et al: Coronary artery disease in peripheral vascular patients: A classification of 1000 coronary angiograms and results of surgical management. Ann Surg 199:223, 1984.
71. Hobson RW II, Lynch TG, Zafar J, et al: Results of revascularization and amputation in severe lower extremity ischemia: A five-year clinical experience. J Vasc Surg 2:174, 1985.
72. Hoch J, Millis M, Kennell T, et al: Use of magnetic resonance arteriography for the preoperative evaluation of patients with infrainguinal arterial occlusive disease. J Vasc Surg 23:792, 1996.
73. Hunink MGM, Donaldson MC, Meyerovitz MF, et al: Risks and benefits of femoral-popliteal percutaneous balloon angioplasty. J Vasc Surg 17:183, 1993.
74. Ibrahim IM, Sussman B, Dardik H, et al: Adjunctive arteriovenous fistula with tibial and peroneal reconstruction for limb salvage. Am J Surg 140:246, 1980.
75. Imparato AM, Kim G, Davidson T, et al: Intermittent claudication: Its natural course. Surgery 78:795, 1975.
76. Jarrett F, Berkoff HA, Crummy AB, et al: Femoro-tibial bypass grafts with sequential technique. Arch Surg 116:709, 1981.
77. Jarrett F, Perea A, Begelman K, et al: Hemodynamics of sequential bypass grafts in peripheral arterial occlusion. Surg Gynecol Obstet 150:377, 1980.
78. Johnson W, Blebea J, Cantelmo N, et al: Does oral anticoagulation improve patency of vein bypasses? A prospective randomized study. Presented at 51st annual meeting of the Society for Vascular Surgery, June 1, 1997, Boston.
79. Johnson WC, Lee KK, Bartle E, et al: Comparative evaluation of PTFE, HUV and saphenous vein bypasses in fem-pop AK vascular reconstruction. J Vasc Surg (in press).
80. Kannel WB, Skinner JJ, Schwartz MJ, et al: Intermittent claudication: Incidence in the Framingham study. Circulation 41:857, 1970.
81. Klamer TW, Lambert GE, Richardson JD, et al: Utility of inframalleolar arterial bypass grafting. J Vasc Surg 11:165, 1990.
82. Kretschmer G, Wenzl E. Piza F, et al: The influence of anticoagulant treatment on the probability of function in femoropopliteal vein bypass surgery: Analysis of a clinical series (1970 to 1985) and interim evaluation of a controlled clinical trial. Surgery 102:453, 1987.
83. Kunlin J: Le traitment de l'arterite obliterante par la greffe veineuse. Arch Mal Coeur Vaiss 42:371, 1949.
84. Lalka SA, Anderson G, Bernhard VM, et al: Transcutaneous Po_2 and Pco_2 monitoring to determine severity of limb ischemia and predict surgical outcome. J Vasc Surg 7:507, 1988.
85. Lamberth WC Jr, Karkow WS: Sequential femoropopliteal-tibial bypass grafting: Operative technique and results. Ann Thorac Surg 42:531, 1986.
86. Leather RP, Fitzgerald K: Personal communication from Vascular Data Registry, Department of Surgery, Albany Medical College, October 19, 1992.
87. Leather RP, Powers SR, Karmody AM: A reappraisal of the in situ saphenous vein arterial bypass: Its use in limb salvage. Surgery 86:453, 1979.
88. Leather RP, Shah DM, Chang BB, et al: Resurrection of the in situ saphenous vein bypass: 1000 cases later. Ann Surg 208:435, 1988.
89. Leather RP, Shah DM, Corson JD, Karmody AM: Instrumental evolution of the valve incision method of in situ saphenous vein bypass. J Vasc Surg 1:113, 1984.
90. Leather RP, Shah DM, Chang BB, Kaufman JL: Resurrection of the in situ saphenous vein bypass. 1000 cases later. Ann Surg 208:435, 1988.
91. Lette J, Waters D, Lassonde J, et al: Multivariate clinical models and quantitative dipyridamole-thallium imaging to predict cardiac morbidity and death after vascular reconstruction. J Vasc Surg 14:160, 1991.
92. LoGerfo FW, Quist WC, Crawshaw HW: An improved technique of preservation of endothelial morphology in vein grafts. Surgery 90:1015, 1981.
93. Marcaccio EJ, Miller A, Tannenbaum GA, et al: Angioscopically directed interventions improve arm vein bypass grafts. J Vasc Surg 17:994, 1993.
94. Marks J, King TA, Baele H, et al: Popliteal-to-distal bypass for limp threatening ischemia. J Vasc Surg 15:755, 1992.
95. Martin R, Edwards W, Mulherin J, et al: Cryopreserved vein allografts for below-knee extremity revascularization. Ann Surg 219:664, 1994.
96. McAllister FF: The fate of patients with intermittent claudication managed non-operatively. Am J Surg 132:593, 1976.
97. McCollum C, Kenchington G, Alexander C, et al: PTFE or HUV for femoro-popliteal bypass: A multi-center trial. Eur J Vasc Surg 5:435, 1991.
98. McIntyre KE, Bailey SA, Malone JM, Goldstone J: Guillotine amputation in the treatment of nonsalvageable lower extremity infections. Arch Surg 119:450, 1984.
99. Miller A, Stonebridge PA, Tsoukas AI, et al: Angioscopically directed valvulotomy: A new valvulotome and technique. J Vasc Surg 13:813, 1991.
100. Miller A, Marcaccio E, Tannenbaum GA, et al: Comparison of angioscopy and angiography for monitoring infrainguinal bypass vein grafts: Results of a prospective randomized trial. J Vasc Surg 15:1078, 1992.
101. Miller JH, Foreman RK, Ferguson L, Faris I: Interposition vein cuff for anastomosis of prosthesis to small artery. Aust N Z J Surg 54:283, 1984.
102. Mills JL, Harris EJ, Taylor LM, et al: The importance of routine surveillance of distal bypass graft with duplex scanning: A study of 379 reversed vein grafts. J Vasc 12:379, 1990.
103. Moody AP, Edwards PR, Harris PL: In situ versus reversed femoropopliteal vein grafts: Long-term follow-up of a prospective, randomized trial. Br J Surg 79:750, 1992.
104. O'Mara CS, Flinn WR, Johnson ND, et al: Recognition and surgical management of patent but hemodynamically failed arterial grafts. Ann Surg 193:467, 1981.
105. Panetta TF, Marin ML, Veith FJ, et al: Unsuspected pre-existing saphenous vein pathology: An unrecognized cause of vein bypass failure. J Vasc Surg 15:102, 1992.
106. Parent FN, Piotrowski JJ, Bernhard VM, et al: Outcome of intra-arterial urokinase for acute vascular occlusion. J Cardiovasc Surg 32:680, 1991.
107. Pasternak PF, Grossi EA, Baumann FG, et al: The value of silent myocardial ischemia monitoring in the prediction of perioperative myocardial infarction in patients undergoing peripheral vascular surgery. J Vasc Surg 10:617, 1989.
108. Patterson RB, Fowl RJ, Kempczinski RF, et al: Preferential use of ePTFE for above-knee femoropopliteal bypass grafts. Ann Vasc Surg 4:338, 1990.
109. Paty PSK, Shah DM, Saifi J, et al: Remote distal arteriovenous fistula to improve infrapopliteal bypass patency. J Vasc Surg 11:171, 1990.
110. Pevec WC, Darling RC, L'Italien GJ, Abbott WM: Femoropopliteal

reconstruction with knitted, nonvelour Dacron versus expanded polytetrafluoroethylene. J Vasc Surg 16:60, 1992.

111. Pomposelli FB, Jespen SJ, Gibbons GW, et al: Efficacy of the dorsal pedal bypass for limb salvage in diabetic patients: Short term observations. J Vasc Surg 11:745, 1990.
112. Prendiville EJ, Yeager A, O'Donnell TF, et al: Long-term results with the above-knee popliteal expanded polytetrafluoroethylene graft. J Vasc Surg 11:517, 1990.
113. Quiñones-Baldrich WJ, Prego AA, Ucelay-Gomez R, et al: Long-term results of infrainguinal revascularization with polytetrafluoroethylene: A ten-year experience. J Vasc Surg 16:209, 1992.
114. Raby KE, Goldman L, Creager MA, et al: Correlation between preoperative ischemia and major cardiac events after peripheral vascular surgery. N Engl J Med 321:1296, 1989.
115. Rafferty TD, Avellone JC, Farrell CJ, et al: A metropolitan experience with infrainguinal revascularization: Operative risk and later results in northeastern Ohio. J Vasc Surg 6:365, 1987.
116. Reifsnyder T, Bandyk D, Seabrook G, et al: Wound complications of the in situ saphenous vein bypass technique. J Vasc Surg 15:843, 1992.
117. Rhodes GR, Rollins D, Sidaway A, et al: Popliteal-to-tibial in situ saphenous vein bypass for limb salvage in diabetic patients. Am J Surg 154:245, 1987.
118. Ricco JB, Pearce WH, Yao JST, et al: The use of operative prebypass arteriography and Doppler ultrasound recordings to select patients for extended femorodistal bypass. Ann Surg 198:646, 1983.
119. River SP, Scher LA, Gupta SK, Veith FJ: Safety of peripheral vascular surgery after recent acute myocardial infarction. J Vasc Surg 11:70, 1990.
120. Rosenbloom MS, Walsh JJ, Schuler JJ, et al: Long-term results of infragenicular bypasses with autogenous vein originating from the distal superficial femoral and popliteal arteries. J Vasc Surg 7:691, 1988.
121. Rosenfeld JC, Savarese RP, Friedman P, et al: Sequential femoropopliteal and femorotibial bypasses: A ten year follow-up study. Arch Surg 116:1538, 1981.
122. Rosenthal D, Dickson C, Rodriguez F, et al: Infrainguinal endovascular in situ saphenous vein bypass: Ongoing results. J Vasc Surg 20:389, 1994.
123. Rosenthal D, Evans D, McKinsey J, et al: Prosthetic above-knee femoropopliteal bypass for intermittent claudication. J Cardiovasc Surg 31:462, 1990.
124. Rutherford RB, Flanigan DP, Gupta SK, et al: Suggested standards for reports dealing with lower extremity ischemia. J Vasc Surg 4:80, 1986.
125. Rutherford RB, Jones DN, Bergentz SE, et al: Factors affecting the patency of infrainguinal bypass. J Vasc Surg 8:236, 1988.
126. Rutherford RB, Baker JD, Ernst C, et al: Recommended standards for reports dealing with lower extremity ischemia: Revised version. J Vasc Surg 26:517, 1997.
127. Sanchez LA, Goldsmith J, Rivers SP, et al: Limb salvage surgery in end-stage renal disease: Is it worthwhile? J Cardiovasc Surg 33:344, 1992.
128. Schulman ML, Badhey MR, Yatco R, Pillari G: A saphenous alternative: Preferential use of superficial femoral and popliteal veins as femoropopliteal bypass grafts. Am J Surg 152:231, 1986.
129. Schwartz ME, Harrington EB, Schanzer H: Wound complications after in situ bypass. J Vasc Surg 7:802, 1988.
130. Sesto ME, Sullivan TM, Hertzer NR, et al: Cephalic vein grafts for lower extremity revascularization. J Vasc Surg 15:543, 1992.
131. Shah D, Darling R, Chang B, et al: Long-term results of in situ saphenous vein bypass: Analysis of 2058 cases. Ann Surg 222:438, 1995.
132. Shah DM, Chang BB, Leopold PW, et al: The anatomy of the greater saphenous venous system. J Vasc Surg 3:273, 1986.
133. Shah DM, Darling RC, Chang BB, et al: Is long vein bypass from groin to ankle a durable procedure? An analysis of a ten-year experience. J Vasc Surg 15:402, 1992.
134. Sicard GA, Schier JJ, Totty WG, et al: Thrombolytic therapy for acute arterial occlusion. J Vasc Surg 2:65, 1985.
135. Sterpetti AV, Schultz RD, Feldhaus RJ, Peetz DJ Jr: Seven-year experience with polytetrafluoroethylene as above-knee femoropopliteal bypass graft: Is it worthwhile to preserve the autologous saphenous vein? J Vasc Surg 2:907, 1985.
136. Szilagyi DE, Hageman JH, Smith RF, et al: Autogenous vein grafting in femoropopliteal atherosclerosis: The limits of its effectiveness. Surgery 86:836, 1979.
137. Tannenbaum GA, Pomposelli FB, Marcaccio EJ et al: Safety of vein bypass grafting to the dorsal pedal artery in diabetic patients with foot infections. J Vasc Surg 15:982, 1992.
138. Taylor LM, Edwards JM, Porter JM: Present status of reversed vein bypass grafting: Five-year results of a modern series. J Vasc Surg 11:193, 1990.
139. Taylor RS, McFarland RJ, Cox MI: An investigation into the causes of failure of PTFE grafts. Eur J Vasc Surg 1:335, 1987.
140. Thompson RW, Mannick JA, Whittemore AD: Arterial reconstruction at diverse sites using nonreversed autogenous vein: An application of venous valvulotomy. Ann Surg 205:747, 1987.
141. Tilanus HW, Obertop H, Van Urk H: Saphenous vein or PTFE for femoropopliteal bypass: A prospective randomized trial. Ann Surg 202:780, 1985.
142. Tyrrell MR, Chester JF, Vipond MN, et al: Experimental evidence to support the use of interposition vein collars/patches in distal PTFE anastomoses. Eur J Vasc Surg 4:95, 1990.
143. Tyrrell MR, Grigg MJ, Wolfe JHN: Is arterial reconstruction to the ankle worthwhile in the absence of autologous vein? Eur J Vasc Surg 3:429, 1989.
144. Veith FJ, Ascer E, Gupta SK, et al: Lateral approach to the popliteal artery. J Vasc Surg 6:119, 1987.
145. Veith FJ, Gupta SK, Samson RH, et al: Superficial femoral and popliteal arteries as inflow sites for distal bypasses. Surgery 90:980, 1981.
146. Veith FJ, Moss CM, Fell SC, et al: Expanded polytetrafluoroethylene grafts in reconstructive arterial surgery: Preliminary report of the first 100 consecutive cases for limb salvage. JAMA 240:1867, 1978.
147. Veith FJ, Gupta SK, Ascer E, et al: Six-year prospective multicenter randomized comparison of autologous saphenous vein and expanded polytetrafluoroethylene graft in infrainguinal arterial reconstruction. J Vasc Surg 3:104, 1986.
148. Veith FJ, Gupta SK, Samson RH, et al: Progress in limb salvage by reconstructive arterial surgery combined with new or improved adjunctive procedures. Ann Surg 194:386, 1981.
149. Veith FJ, Weiser RK, Gupta SK, et al: Diagnosis and management of failing lower extremity arterial reconstructions prior to graft occlusion. J Cardiovasc Surg 25:381, 1984.
150. Veith FJ, Ascer E, Gupta SK, et al: Tibiotibial vein bypass graft: A new operation for limb salvage. J Vasc Surg 2:552, 1985.
151. Veterans Administration Cooperative Study Group 141: Comparative evaluation of prosthetic, reversed, and in situ bypass grafts in distal popliteal and tibial-peroneal revascularization. Arch Surg 123:434, 1988.
152. Walker P, Mitchell R, McFadden P, et al: Early experience with cryopreserved saphenous vein grafts as a conduit for complex limb salvage procedures. J Vasc Surg 18:561, 1993.
153. Walsh DB, Gilbertson JJ, Zwolak RM, et al: The natural history of superficial femoral artery stenoses. J Vasc Surg 14:299, 1991.
154. Wengerter KR, Veith FJ, Gupta SK, et al: Influence of vein size (diameter) on infrapopliteal reversed vein graft patency. J Vasc Surg 11:525, 1990.
155. Wengerter KR, Veith FJ, Gupta SK, et al: Prospective randomized multicenter comparison of in situ and reversed vein infrapopliteal bypasses. J Vasc Surg 13:189, 1991.
156. Wengerter KR, Yang PM, Veith FJ, et al: A twelve-year experience with the popliteal-to-distal artery bypass. The significance and management of proximal disease. J Vasc Surg 15:143, 1992.
157. Wengrovitz M, Atnip RG, Gifford RRM, et al: Wound complications of autogenous subcutaneous infrainguinal arterial bypass surgery: Predisposing factors and management. J Vasc Surg 11:156, 1990.
158. Whittemore AD, Donaldson MC, Mannick JA: Infrainguinal reconstruction for patients with chronic renal insufficiency. J Vasc Surg 17:32, 1993.
159. Whittemore AD, Kent KC, Donaldson MC, et al: What is the proper role of polytetrafluoroethylene grafts in infrainguinal reconstruction? J Vasc Surg 10:299, 1989.
160. Whittemore AD, Clowes AW, Couch NP, Mannick JA: Secondary femoropopliteal reconstruction. Ann Surg 193:35, 1981.
161. Wolfe JHN, Thomas ML, Jamieson CW, et al: Early diagnosis of femorodistal graft stenoses. Br J Surg 74:268, 1987.

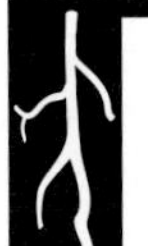

CHAPTER 70

Profundaplasty

Jonathan B. Towne, M.D.,
and Victor M. Bernhard, M.D.

The use of profundaplasty for lower leg revascularization has evolved over the last several decades. Early on, it was a primary means of increasing blood flow to the lower extremities utilizing the very rich collateral vessels between the deep arterial system and the popliteal and intrapopliteal vessels. Since autogenous vein femoral distal bypasses for lower extremity revascularization have become increasingly successful, profundaplasty is used less often.

Currently, profundaplasty is used mainly in patients with lower limb ischemic disease who do not have an adequate saphenous vein or who have infected prosthetic grafts originating or terminating in the groin that require removal and when the procedure is used as a means of revascularizing legs after the failure of prior autogenous lower leg reconstructions. Profundaplasty remains an important tool in the care of patients with lower limb occlusive disease, and all vascular surgeons should understand the anatomy and physiology of the deep femoral system to allow proper selection of patients who might benefit from this procedure.

ANATOMY OF THE DEEP FEMORAL ARTERY

The profunda femoris (deep femoral) artery is the major artery in an extensive chain of longitudinal anastomosing vessels of the lower extremity and provides a collateral network (the cruciate anastomosis) that extends from the internal iliac artery to the tibial vessels. It usually arises 2 to 4 cm below the inguinal ligament, passing posterolaterally to the superficial femoral artery (Figs. 70–1 and 70–2). The medial and lateral circumflex femoral arteries diverge from the proximal profunda femoris artery to form major collateral channels to the internal iliac artery. Variations in the origin of profunda femoris artery and the circumflex arteries may occur frequently.

In 10% of cases, the profunda femoris artery runs medial to the superficial femoral artery,[1, 2] and in 2%, large branches of the profunda femoris artery are found both medial and lateral to the superficial femoral artery. The branching pattern is also variable. That is, in 58% of cases, a common trunk gives rise to both medial and lateral circumflex vessels; in 18%, the medial femoral circumflex artery is a direct branch of the common femoral artery; and in 15%, the lateral femoral circumflex is a direct branch of the common femoral artery.

When the lateral femoral circumflex artery arises directly from the common femoral artery, the main trunk of the profunda femoris artery takes a medial or posteromedial course to the superficial femoral artery. The main trunk of the profunda femoris artery passes inferiorly just medial to the femur and gives off three perforating branches. The terminal portion of the profunda femoris artery (sometimes referred to as the "fourth" perforating branch) anastomoses with the highest genicular branch of the popliteal artery at the adductor hiatus. The lateral femoral circumflex passes transversely and divides into an ascending, transverse, and descending branches. The ascending branch passes upward to the lateral aspect of the hip, thereby making connections with the branches of the inferior gluteal artery. The descending branch passes inferiorly lateral to the femur to the level of the knee, anastomosing with the lateral superior genicular branch of the popliteal artery. The medial femoral circumflex artery passes posteromedially to the area of

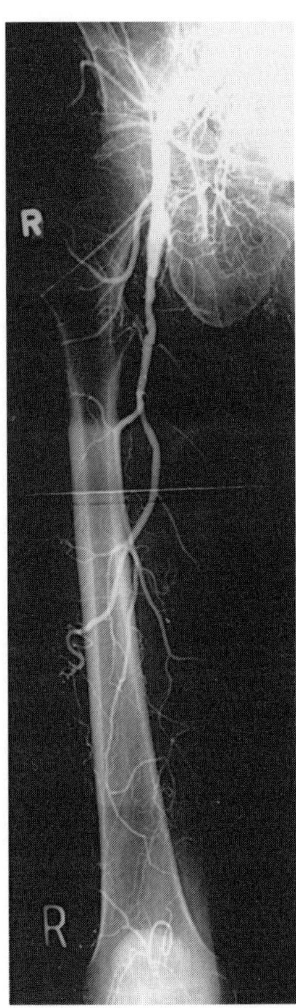

FIGURE 70–1. Angiogram demonstrates the normal branching pattern of the profunda femoris artery. A profundaplasty had previously been constructed. The superficial femoral artery is occluded at its origin.

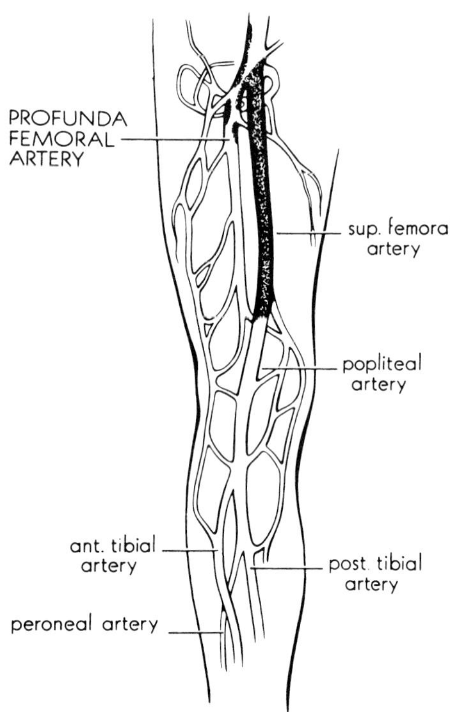

FIGURE 70–2. The profunda femoris provides the major collateral channel to the leg when the superficial femoral artery is obstructed. Atherosclerosis and thrombosis are usually limited to the origin and proximal third of this vessel. (From Bernhard VM, Militello JM, Geringer AM: Repair of the profunda femoris artery. Am J Surg 127:676, 1974.)

the obturator foramen, where it makes connections with branches of the obturator artery.

The profunda femoris artery and its collateral connections are the major source of blood supply to the lower leg in patients who have superficial femoral artery occlusive disease. When both the superficial femoral artery and the popliteal artery are occluded, the profunda femoris artery anastomoses to the tibial vessels via the highest genicular artery with the musculoarticular and saphenous branches, the fourth perforating branch, the descending branch of the lateral femoral circumflex, the genicular collateral network around the knee, and the recurrent tibial arteries.

DISTRIBUTION OF ARTERIAL DISEASE

Arteriosclerotic involvement of the profunda femoris artery is most commonly at its origin. Since the profunda femoris artery often arises from the posterior lateral aspect of the common femoral artery, stenosis of the profunda orifice may not be apparent on anterior posterior views obtained during arteriography; the profunda femoris artery may appear foreshortened, obscuring stenotic arterial lesions. Beales and associates demonstrated stenosis of the profunda femoris artery in 38.8% of patients.[1] In 67.9% of patients with occlusive disease of this artery, the stenotic segment was recognized only on oblique or lateral views, thus demonstrating the necessity of oblique views for adequate roentgenographic assessment.

Patients with atherosclerotic occlusive disease in the lower extremity often have a relatively disease-free profunda femoris artery. Haimovici and colleagues reported an incidence of atherosclerotic involvement in the profunda femoris artery in 9.5% of patients without diabetes and 30.5% in diabetic patients.[3] Margulis and coworkers, in a study of 168 limbs, noted significant atherosclerotic involvement of the profunda femoris artery in only 18%.[4] These two studies demonstrate that in patients with widespread atherosclerotic involvement of the lower extremities, the profunda femoris artery can be a valuable source of inflow into the lower extremity if it is relatively free of disease.

INDICATIONS

The purpose of profundaplasty is to relieve a significant stenosis or an occlusion of the proximal portion of the deep femoral artery in order to restore its function. The procedure is employed most frequently as an adjunct to an inflow procedure, such as treatment of a combined aorto-iliac and femoral popliteal occlusive disease. In addition, when patients have presented with an occluded limb of the aortobifemoral bypass, the profunda femoris artery is often the only major outflow vessel in the groin. A profundaplasty in these patients ensures continued patency of the aortofemoral limb. If a distal bypass fails, profundaplasty occasionally can result in limb salvage. In addition, effective perfusion of the knee joint is the critical factor for healing a below-knee amputation. If extensive pedal gangrene precludes limb salvage in patients with profunda femoris artery stenosis as well as distal femoropopliteal tibial occlusive disease, profundaplasty can be performed in order to lower the amputation site to the more functional below-knee level. It is unusual to obtain healing of a below-knee amputation without unobstructed arterial flow in the deep femoral system.

Profundaplasty is also of value for patients with groin sepsis. The profunda femoris artery can be used as an outflow vessel to the lower extremity, thereby avoiding the septic groin area. This is particularly important when the superficial femoral and popliteal arteries are occluded or when an obturator bypass is not feasible. An axillary/mid–profunda femoris arterial bypass via a lateral approach avoids the groin and can result in limb salvage. Profundaplasty is less frequently performed as an isolated procedure to serve as an alternative to femoropopliteal or femorotibial bypasses. If distal bypass is not feasible, a deep femoral repair may be the only procedure available to improve profusion of an ischemic leg. Although limb salvage may not be achieved in this circumstance, the level of anticipated amputation may be lowered from above to below the knee.

The success of profundaplasty in improving lower leg profusion depends on the adequacy of the collateral vessels at the termination of the profunda femoris artery. These collateral channels can be evaluated both angiographically and noninvasively by a measurement of segmental pressure. Angiographic criteria that reliably predict successful outcome include minimal occlusive disease of the distal profunda femoris artery, well-developed distal profunda femoris artery collaterals, patent popliteal artery, and minimal tibial occlusive disease.[5, 6]

Hemodynamic criteria obtained from segmental Doppler pressure measurements can also reliably determine the extent of occlusive disease in each limb segment by providing an estimate of the resistance in each collateral bed. We have shown that resistance across the knee joint is the most important determinant of the success of profundaplasty. It can be evaluated by the measurement of the profunda popliteal collateral index (PPCI), which is calculated by the formula

$$PPCI = \frac{AKSP - BKSP}{AKSP}$$

where AKSP is the above-knee segmental pressure and BKSP is the below-knee segmental pressure.

An index greater than 0.5 implies high resistance across the knee joint as the result of poor collateral circulation and predicts profundaplasty failure, whereas a PPCI less than 0.19 usually results in limb salvage.[7] McCoy and coworkers found that measurements of the low thigh to ankle pressure gradient correlated with success of profundaplasty.[8] This gradient evaluates the obstruction of flow across the knee as well as obstruction due to tibial artery occlusive disease. We can calculate the low thigh to ankle gradient (TAGI) pressure index by subtracting the ankle pressure from the low thigh pressure and dividing the result by the low thigh pressure. Like the PPCI, the lower the index, the less resistance there is to blood flow. In patients with successful outcomes, the TAGI was 0.39; in patients with an unsuccessful outcome, the TAGI was 0.79.

Roentgenographic criteria also augur well for success of profundaplasty. Sladen and Burgess[6] identified four roentgenographic signs that were associated with poor results:

- No obstruction at the origin of the profunda femoris artery
- A patent superficial femoral artery
- Inadequate development of distal profunda femoris collateral vessels
- Poor visualization of the tibial arteries

All of these authors[5–8] are using different techniques to evaluate the status of the profunda femoris artery collateral bed. For a patient to have a good result, a well-developed collateral channel from the distal profunda femoris artery to either a patent popliteal or tibial vessel with a relative absence of tibial occlusive disease is required.

OPERATIVE TECHNIQUE

In most cases, profunda femoris artery angioplasty is performed as an auxiliary procedure to ensure satisfactory runoff for aortofemoral, axillofemoral, or femorofemoral bypass. In approximately 30% of limbs requiring profunda femoris arterial repair, however, aortoiliac inflow is not obstructed and profundaplasty is performed as the primary procedure. Occasionally, repair is carried out in conjunction with bypass to the popliteal or tibial arteries when it appears that removal of a modest stenosis of the profunda femoris artery itself cannot adequately resolve the ischemic problem.

General anesthesia with full monitoring is mandatory when profundaplasty is performed in conjunction with aortofemoral bypass. For an isolated procedure accomplished through a single groin incision, either caudal anesthesia or local lidocaine infiltration, with anesthetist standby, may be satisfactory and is ideal in the presence of severe cardiopulmonary disease that permits only a limited operation.

A vertical groin incision is made directly over the common femoral artery and is carried 5 cm cephalad of the inguinal crease and 8 cm or more caudally (Fig. 70–3). The distal extension of the incision depends on the length of the profunda femoris artery that must be exposed. The inguinal ligament is partially or completely divided to facilitate dissection of the distal external iliac artery and its deep epigastric and circumflex iliac branches. The common femoral artery is freed throughout its length and circumference so that anatomic variations can be carefully searched for and all significant branches preserved. The superficial femoral artery is exposed for a variable distance both to facilitate dissection of the profunda femoris artery and to make the outer wall of this occluded vessel available as an autogenous patch.

The point of origin of the profunda femoris artery, from the posterior aspect of the common femoral artery, is identified. The surgeon achieves progressive distal exposure by incising the enveloping fatty areolar tissue and dividing the large overlying lateral circumflex femoral vein, which lies deep to the superficial femoral artery and passes over the anterior surface of the profunda femoris artery 1 to 3 cm

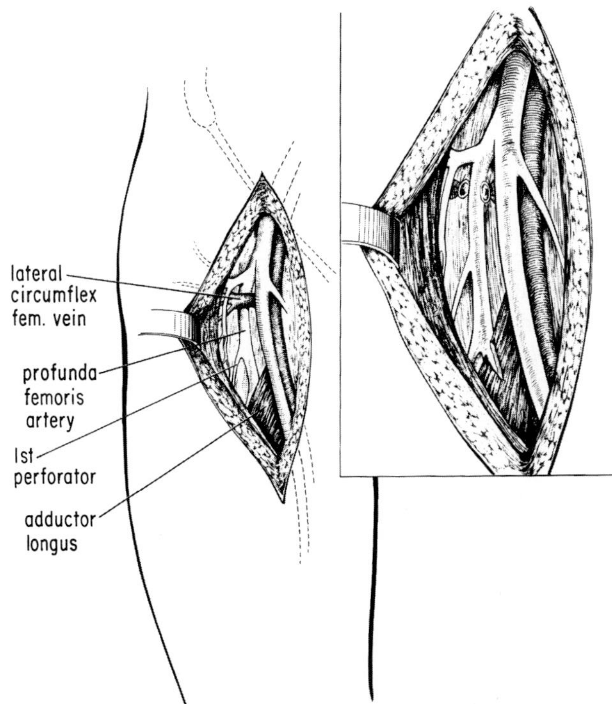

FIGURE 70–3. Identification of the proximal portion of the profunda femoris artery requires division of the large circumflex femoral vein that lies anterior to it. The distal portion of the profunda at and beyond the level of the second perforator is exposed by incising the adductor longus muscle. (From Bernhard VM: The role of profundaplasty in revascularization of the lower extremities. Surg Clin North Am 59:681, 1979.)

distal to its origin. The length of profunda femoris artery that must be dissected free depends on the distal extent of significant atheromatous obstruction. This is readily ascertained by reference to the preoperative arteriogram and direct inspection and palpation of the vessel.

The dissection should be carried at least distal to the lateral circumflex femoral and often beyond the first perforating branch. More distal exposure can be facilitated by lateral rotation of the thigh with modest flexion of the knee and hip. Partial or complete division of the adductor longus muscle may be necessary to expose the artery beyond its second perforator branch.

This direct approach to the profunda femoris artery may be difficult or impossible to achieve in patients with infection or severe inguinal scar formation due to multiple precious vascular repairs. A simple alternative to this dilemma is to approach the mid-portion of the deep femoral artery through an anterior thigh incision that can be readily located distal to the previous groin incision. The sartorius is retracted laterally to expose the superficial femoral vessels, which are retracted medially. Branches of the femoral nerve in this area should be identified and preserved. The fascia deep to the superficial femoral artery is incised to expose the deep femoral vessels between the first and second perforator branches. When infection is present, the incision should be placed lateral to the sartorius muscle, which is retracted medially to more effectively separate the operative field from the area of sepsis. The exposed segment of profunda femoris artery lies distal to the arterial obstruction and can be readily anastomosed to a new or revised inflow graft.

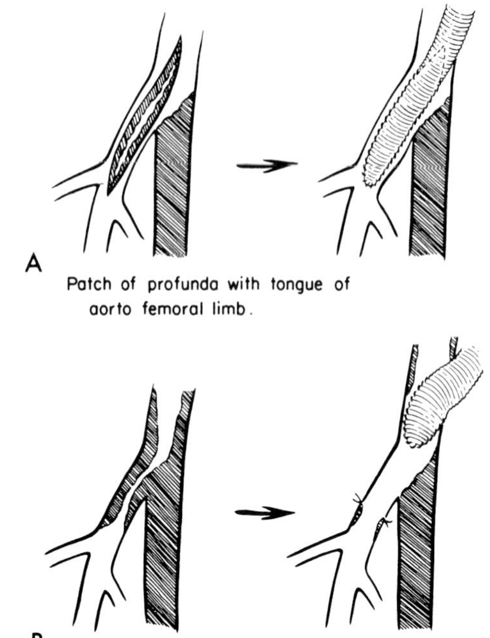

FIGURE 70–4. Operative technique of profundaplasty in association with aortofemoral graft or other procedure for inflow obstruction. *A*, The Dacron limb may be used as an extended tongue to widen a stenotic area in the proximal profunda. *B*, A limited common and deep femoral endarterectomy with suture stabilization of the distal intima can be carried out when the plaque involves only the orifice and not more than 1 cm of the profunda femoris. (*A* and *B*, From Bernhard VM, Militello JM, Geringer AM: Repair of the profunda femoris artery. Am J Surg 127:676, 1974.)

Heparin, 5000 to 7000 units, is given systemically. Thereafter, the branches are controlled with microsurgical clips or latex loop slings, and clamps are applied to the common femoral artery and the distal profunda femoris artery. A vertical incision is made on the anterior aspect of the common femoral artery, and any loose debris and thrombus are removed. Occasionally, the major obstruction is due to a large plaque on the posterior wall of the common femoral artery that obscures the profunda femoris arterial orifice and extends only a few millimeters down the profunda femoris lumen. This plaque can be removed entirely through the common femoral arterial incision, and the intima of the distal profunda femoris artery can be controlled with a few tacking stitches placed from inside the arterial orifice to prevent subsequent dissection (Fig. 70–4). The arteriotomy is then closed with a simple running suture or by end-to-side anastomosis to an inflow graft.

In the majority of cases, however, the obstructing atheroma extends a substantial distance down into the profunda femoris artery. The common femoral arteriotomy is extended through the profunda femoris artery orifice and then distally on to the anterior surface of the deep femoral artery. The arteriotomy must be carefully placed to avoid incision into the crotch between the superficial femoral artery and the deep femoral artery and also to skirt the orifices of major branches. The incision should extend 1 cm or more beyond the usually abrupt point of transition between significant atheromatous encroachment and the relatively normal distal intima. This usually occurs just beyond one of the major profunda femoris arterial branches, and at this level the lumen generally is 4 to 5 mm.

Thromboendarterectomy is carried down to this transition point, which should be at least a few millimeters proximal to the caudal end of the arteriotomy. This facilitates placement of tacking sutures, as needed, to prevent further dissection if a clean break from the distal intima cannot be achieved. Extensions of the plaque into branch orifices should be meticulously avulsed so that these branches will remain open and contribute to the collateral function of the profunda femoris artery.

The arteriotomy is then closed with a patch to ensure an adequate lumen without stenosis into the runoff vessel. When profundaplasty is combined with a procedure designed to restore inflow, the polyester (Dacron) inflow limb can be tailored and sutured over the profunda femoris arteriotomy as an extended tongue for a distance of 2 to 3 cm. Longer arteriotomies are more reliably closed with a patch of autogenous tissue. A segment of adjacent occluded superficial femoral artery can be filleted and prepared by endarterectomy to make a patch of desired length and width (Fig. 70–5). Although a major branch of the saphenous also can be used for the patch, the main saphenous trunk should usually be saved in anticipation of its possible future use for distal bypass or coronary revascularization.[9, 10] Regardless of the material employed, the patch should be tailored and sutured in such a way that it produces a gradually tapering lumen, with the caudal end bluntly rounded to produce a funnel into the distal artery.

COMPLICATIONS

Operative complications are similar to those associated with any other vascular reconstructive procedure. Hemorrhage or hematoma formation requires immediate wound exploration to repair a suture line leak and control other bleeding vessels. If early thrombosis occurs, the groin wound should be promptly explored to remove intraluminal clot and correct technical errors.

Lymphorrhea and lymphocele formations are more common following the extended groin incision associated with profundaplasty than with the routine vascular groin incision. The incidence of this complication can be reduced by (1) avoiding the transection of lymph nodes during groin dissection, (2) ligating all observed open lymph ducts, and (3) ensuring meticulous multilayer closure of the groin wound.

Treatment calls for bed rest, with moderate leg elevation until drainage ceases and groin swelling recedes. Samples of draining fluid should be obtained for culture and appropriate antibiotics given if infection is present. Skin sutures should not be removed until the problem has been resolved unless the wound is septic. If any skin edge necrosis is suspected, the surgeon should perform prompt groin exploration to débride all necrotic tissue and to ligate leaking lymphatic channels.

Superficial wound infections should be drained promptly and treated with local care and antibiotics. Deep infections involving repaired vascular structures or grafts should be managed as described elsewhere. To reduce the incidence of wound infection, prophylactic antibiotics are routinely administered, and all wounds are copiously irrigated with antibiotic saline solution before closure.

Late thrombosis after profunda femoris arterial repair is usually due to progression of the underlying atherosclerotic process in the profunda femoris or in the aortoiliac inflow vessels. Angiography should be carried out promptly to estimate the feasibility of reoperation on the artery and to determine the need for revision or addition of a procedure for inflow obstruction. If the vessel distal to the occlusive process is still patent, revision and extension of the previous profundaplasty, although tedious, is usually successful. Bypass to the mid profunda femoris artery is a reliable alternative when scarring or infection is present. Thrombosis of the associated femoral limb of an aortic bifurcation graft can usually be relieved by Fogarty catheter thrombectomy, and only occasionally is insertion of a new bypass required.

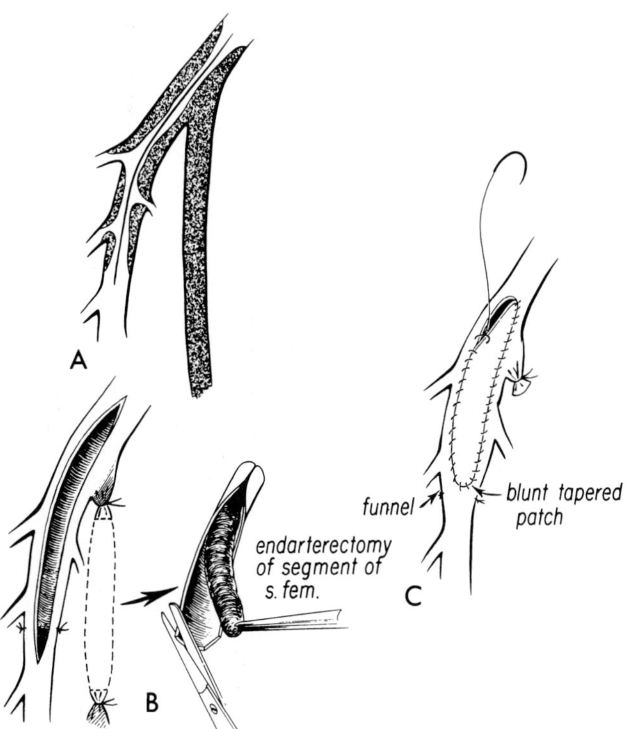

FIGURE 70–5. *A–C,* Technique for long profunda femoris endarterectomy and patch angioplasty utilizing the outer layers of the occluded segment of the superficial femoral artery when a vein is not available for patch.

RESULTS

The operative mortality rate for this procedure is low, and deaths occur almost invariably in those patients who are in desperate need of revascularization to prevent major amputation. In the author's experience with 237 profunda femoris arterial repairs in a series of 209 patients, there were no deaths among those who underwent operation for claudication and five deaths (3%) occurred in the limb salvage group.[11] This difference reflects a more aggressive approach to patients at greater risk in whom the alternative is loss of the limb. Others have reported similar results.[12, 13]

The improvement in limb perfusion after profundaplasty, performed as an adjunct to an inflow procedure, is much greater than that after profundaplasty alone, because the most important level of obstruction is proximal and the popliteal-tibial runoff is usually relatively good. In comparison, patients with a similar degree of ischemia who have unimpaired aortoiliac inflow and require profunda femoris arterial repair to restore its collateral function generally have more severe disease in the leg and foot.

When claudication was the indication for operation in the authors' patients, early patency of the profunda femoris arterial repair was achieved in all patients and was maintained in 77% at 5 years; no significant difference was noted between patients requiring bypass and profundaplasty and those requiring profundaplasty alone (Fig. 70–6). In the authors' experience, marked subjective improvement or complete relief of claudication was achieved in 99% of the 82 limbs managed by inflow and profundaplasty or isolated profundaplasty. Similar results have been reported by Martin and coworkers,[14] Welsh and Repetto,[15] and others. However, a measurable increase in the ankle-brachial pressure index (ABI) of more than 0.1 was noted in only 69% of cases in the authors' series. Only four of seven patients subjected to isolated profundaplasty had a significant increase in treadmill exercise tolerance in the study reported by Strandness,[16] although Fernandes and associates[17] demonstrated a higher incidence of hemodynamic improvement.

Initial patency in limbs operated on for salvage was obtained in 88%; at 5 years, however, there was a progres-

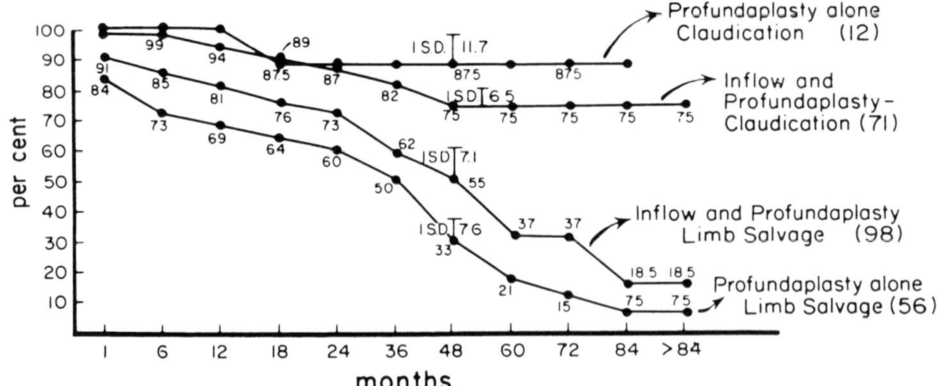

FIGURE 70–6. Cumulative profundaplasty patency of individual groups. (From Towne JB, Bernhard VM, Rollins DL, et al: Profundaplasty in perspective: Limitations in long-term management of limb ischemia. Surgery 90:1037, 1981.)

sive attrition in patency of the repair to 37% in patients managed by an inflow procedure and profundaplasty and to 21% in those receiving profundaplasty alone. Nevertheless, limb salvage was achieved initially in 93% and was retained in 80% of the limbs with the combined procedures, but in only 36% of those with profundaplasty alone after 5 years (Fig. 70–7).

There is considerable debate regarding the value of isolated profundaplasty for limb salvage. Criteria for patient selection for this procedure versus a bypass to the popliteal or tibial vessels have not been consistently applied. Relief of rest pain and healing of necrotic lesions or minor amputations are most likely to be achieved in patients who have severe (>50%) stenosis of the profunda femoris artery, with a patent popliteal segment in continuity with at least one vessel runoff to the pedal arch and a low PPCI. It is noteworthy that immediate success was achieved in 91% of limbs with a PPCI of less than 0.19. Similar results were achieved by McCoy and associates in patients with a TAGI of less than 0.55.[8]

Isolated profundaplasty should be preferred to infrapopliteal bypass as the initial procedure whenever a satisfactory autogenous vein is not available. Furthermore, patients with severe proximal profunda femoris arterial stenosis in whom infrainguinal bypass is not technically feasible should also undergo revascularization of the profunda femoris artery. Although limb salvage is infrequently achieved under these circumstances, amputation at the below-knee level is much more likely to heal if the profunda femoris artery is patent and well perfused.

Profundaplasty is an important adjunct to aortobifemoral bypass and other inflow procedures when any degree of obstruction in the proximal portion of this artery is identified by arteriography, duplex scanning, or intraoperative assessment. If adequate saphenous vein is unavailable in patients with severe multisegmental disease and limb salvage indications for surgery, restoring adequate inflow to the profunda femoris artery usually provides adequate outflow to sustain long-term patency of the inflow procedure and salvage the extremity, especially if the popliteal artery is patent. In fact, even when the profunda femoris artery itself is severely diseased, extended endarterectomy and patch angioplasty of this vessel using endarterectomized superficial femoral artery has yielded surprisingly good results. Pearce and Kempczinski reported limb salvage in 72% of such patients with 5-year patency of the inflow procedure and profunda femoris arterial reconstruction in 86% of patients, although they also reported a 38% incidence of groin wound complications resulting from these long, tedious procedures.[18]

As an isolated procedure, profundaplasty improves claudication distance, relieves rest pain, and permits healing of minor ischemic lesions in some patients if selection criteria are routinely employed. Kalman and coworkers, in a more recent study of isolated profundaplasty, reported excellent results, with a cumulative clinical success rate, considered

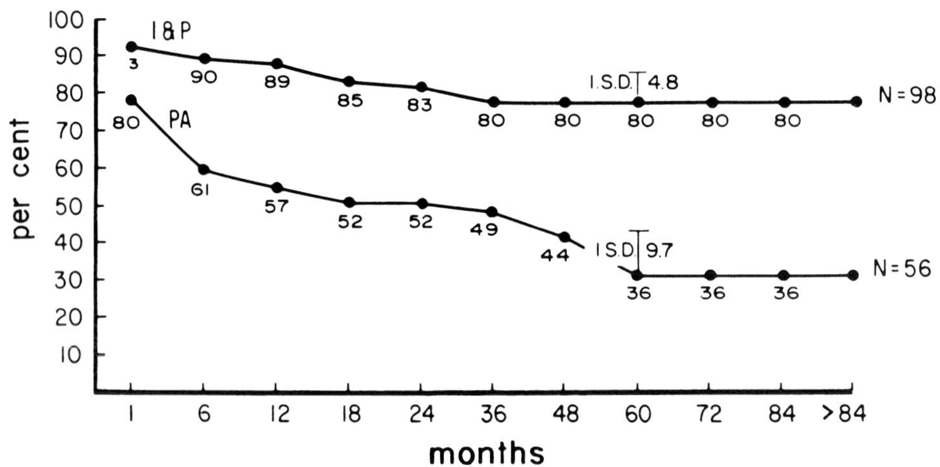

FIGURE 70–7. Cumulative limb salvage of inflow procedure and profundaplasty and profundaplasty alone groups. (From Towne JB, Bernhard VM, Rollins DL et al: Profundaplasty in perspective: Limitations in long-term management of limb ischemia. Surgery 90:1037, 1981.)

as both a patent repair and clinical improvement, of 83% at 30 days, 67% at 1 year, 57% at 2 years, and 49% at 3 years.[19] The cumulative limb salvage rate in this group of patients at 3 years was 76%. The most significant determinant of limb salvage in this series was good tibial outflow; greater success was correlated with good tibial outflow than with poor tibial outflow. "Good" tibial outflow was defined as two or three patent tibial arteries; "poor" outflow was considered as no or one patent artery. Ouriel and coworkers reported 2- and 4-year patency rates of 83% and 76% when the middle and distal profunda femoris arteries were used for the distal anastomosis of an inflow procedure.[20]

SUMMARY

Profundaplasty is a valuable technique with which all vascular surgeons should be familiar. Although not a primary procedure for treating lower limb arterial insufficiency, it often can be used in difficult or extreme cases when all else has failed to salvage an extremity.

REFERENCES

1. Beales JSM, Adcock FA, Frawley JS, et al: The radiological assessment of disease of the profunda femoris artery. Br J Radiol 44:854–859, 1971.
2. Bernhard VM, Ray LI, Militello JM: The role of angioplasty of the profunda femoris artery in revascularization of the ischemic limb. Surg Gynecol Obstet 142:840, 1976.
3. Haimovici H, Shapiro JH, Jacobson HG: Serial femoral arteriography in occlusive disease: Clinical-roentgenologic considerations with a new classification of occlusive patterns. Am J Roentgenol 83:1042, 1960.
4. Margulis AR, Nice CM Jr, Murphy TO: Arteriographic manifestations of peripheral occlusive vascular disease: With the report of two new signs. Am J Roentgenol Rad Ther Nucl Med 78:273–282, 1957.
5. Mitchell RA, Bone GE, Bridges R, et al: Patient selection for isolated profundaplasty: Arteriographic correlates of operative results. Am J Surg 1979;138:912–919.
6. Sladen J, Burgess JJ: Profundaplasty: Expectations and ominous signs. Am J Surg 140:242–245, 1980.
7. Boren CH, Towne JB, Bernhard VM, et al: Profundapopliteal collateral index: A guide to successful profundaplasty. Arch Surg 115:1366–1372, 1980.
8. McCoy DM, Sanchek AP, Schuler JJ, et al: The role of isolated profundaplasty for the treatment of rest pain. Arch Surg 124:441–444,1989.
9. Malone JM, Goldstone J, Moore WS: Autogenous profundaplasty: The key to long-term patency in secondary repair of aortofemoral graft occlusion. Ann Surg 1988:817–823, 1978.
10. Morris-Jones W, Jones CDP: Profundaplasty in the treatment of femoropopliteal occlusion. Am J Surg 127:680–686, 1974.
11. Towne JB, Bernhard VM, Rollins DL, et al: Profundaplasty in perspective: Limitations in the long-term management of limb ischemia. Surgery 90:1037–1046, 1981.
12. Jacobs DL, Seabrook GR, Freischlag JA, Towne JB: The current role of profundaplasty in complex arterial reconstruction. Vasc Surg 29:457–463, 1995.
13. Erdoes LS, Bernhard VM, Berman SS: Aortofemoral graft occlusion: Strategy and timing of reoperation. Cardiovasc Surg 3:277–283, 1995.
14. Martin P, Frawley JE, Barabas AP, et al: On the surgery of atherosclerosis of the profunda femoris artery. Surgery 71:182–189, 1972.
15. Welsh P, Repetto R: Revascularization of the profunda femoris artery in aortoiliac occlusive disease. Surgery 78:389, 1975.
16. Strandness DE Jr: Functional results after revascularization of the profunda femoris artery. Am J Surg 119:240, 1970.
17. Fernandes JF, Nicolaides AN, Angelides NA, et al: An objective assessment of common femoral endarterectomy and profundaplasty in patients with superficial femoral occlusion. Surgery 83:313, 1978.
18. Pearce WH, Kempczinski RF: Extended autogenous profundaplasty and aortofemoral grafting: An alternative to synchronous distal bypass. J Vasc Surg 1:455–458, 1984.
19. Kalman PG, Johnston KW, Walker PM: The current role of isolated profundaplasty. J Cardiovasc Surg 13:107–111, 1990.
20. Ouriel K, DeWeese JA, Ricotta JJ, Green RM: Revascularization of the distal profunda femoris artery in the reconstructive treatment of aortoiliac occlusive disease. J Vasc Surg 6:217–220, 1987.

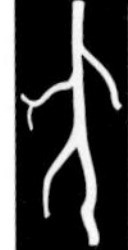

C H A P T E R 7 1

Secondary Arterial Reconstructions in the Lower Extremity

Frank J. Veith, M.D., Ricardo T. Quintos II, M.D., Enrico Ascher, M.D., and Luis A. Sanchez, M.D.

Arterial reconstructions for lower extremity ischemia comprise aortoiliac, aortofemoral, and femorofemoral procedures and bypasses to the popliteal and infrapopliteal arteries. As indicated by the life-table patency rates shown in other chapters, all of these operations have an intrinsic tendency to fail or to become ineffective as time elapses. The proportion of such operations undergoing this fate increases with time and is greater at all times for reconstructions terminating more distally in the arterial tree. Because a sizable minority of patients undergoing these operations have circulatory deterioration at some point in their lives and because this deterioration often is associated with disabling or limb-threatening manifestations, appropriate management of this condition has become an extremely important aspect of vascular surgery to which the competent vascular surgeon must be committed in order to serve the interest of the patient.

This chapter describes the general principles and strategies of this management with a specific focus on the aspects of reoperative vascular surgery that distinguish it from a primary approach to lower extremity ischemia.

INDICATIONS

In general, we believe that arterial reconstructions should rarely be performed for intermittent claudication.[1] Our reasons for this attitude are (1) the relatively high inevitable failure rate of such operations and (2) the fact that failure may be associated with ischemia worse than that prompting the original operation. These factors and the greater difficulty and higher complication rate associated with most secondary operations, particularly if the involved arteries have been dissected, seem to justify our conservative attitude toward *primary* operations for intermittent claudication. This attitude, however, is by no means universal, and present practice accepts "truly disabling" claudication as an indication for primary arterial reconstruction to at least the popliteal level.

In contrast, almost all present-day vascular surgeons tend to avoid secondary arterial operations for intermittent claudication. Thus, gangrene, a nonhealing ischemic ulcer, or severe ischemic rest pain should be the indication for most *secondary* arterial reconstructions, especially those below the inguinal ligament. Interestingly, occasional patients with these classic limb-threatening manifestations and poor noninvasive test results can be effectively managed with conservative measures for protracted periods.[2] Such treatment, if possible, is particularly appropriate in patients who are faced with the need for a difficult distal reoperation. Thus, except for the special circumstances occurring with a "failing graft" (see later), in most patients undergoing secondary arterial reconstruction, the indication for operation is the unquestionable need for immediate limb salvage.

ETIOLOGY OF UNSUCCESSFUL PROCEDURES

Early Reoperations (Within 30 Days)

The need to reintervene soon after a primary arterial reconstruction may be generated by several situations.[3] First, the original repair may undergo thrombosis or may fail in the early postoperative period (i.e., within 30 days). Generally, this occurrence is due to a technical flaw in the operation, poor choice of inflow or outflow sites, insufficient runoff, or progression of soft tissue infection.[4] In addition, thrombosis may occur for no apparent reason, presumably owing to the inherent thrombogenicity of the graft in a low-flow setting. Usually, idiopathic thrombosis occurs only with polytetrafluoroethylene (PTFE) and other prosthetic grafts, but in rare instances it can occur with a vein graft. A transient fall in cardiac output or hypotension can contribute to such unexplained thrombosis.

Second, the original operation, although technically satisfactory and associated with a patent bypass graft, may fail to provide hemodynamic improvement sufficient to relieve the patient's symptoms. This in turn may be due to the choice of the wrong operation (e.g., the performance of an aortofemoral bypass in a patient whose femoral artery pressure was normal and who actually needed a femoropopliteal bypass). Such hemodynamic failure may also occur in the presence of multisegment disease and extensive foot gangrene or infection. In this setting, uninterrupted arterial circulation to the foot may be required, and a primary or secondary sequential bypass may be indicated.[1, 5, 6]

Late Reoperations (After 30 Days)

Failure with graft thrombosis can occur at any time after the first postoperative month. It may be due to some of the factors already mentioned but is usually due to the development of some flow-reducing lesion within the bypass graft or its inflow or outflow tract.

Intimal hyperplasia is a prominent cause of failure and graft thrombosis. It may occur with all kinds of grafts in all positions. The etiology of this process is poorly understood and, fortunately, does not affect most arterial reconstructions. When intimal hyperplasia does occur, it usually produces infrainguinal graft failure between 2 and 18 months after operation.[3, 7, 8] It can involve any portion of a vein graft in a focal or diffuse manner and either anastomosis of vein or prosthetic grafts. Because the lumen of the distal artery is smaller, this site is most vulnerable to flow reduction by this process.

After 18 months, progression of the atherosclerotic disease process involving the inflow or outflow tract of the arterial reconstruction becomes the predominant cause of failure and graft thrombosis. After 3 to 4 years, a variety of other degenerative lesions may also afflict autogenous vein grafts and umbilical vein grafts.[7, 9, 10] These processes, which are rare in autogenous vein grafts but extremely common in umbilical vein grafts, may lead to wall changes and aneurysm formation with thrombosis or embolization.

CONCEPT OF THE FAILING GRAFT

Intimal hyperplasia, progression of proximal or distal disease, or lesions within the graft itself can produce signs and symptoms of hemodynamic deterioration in patients with a prior arterial reconstruction without producing concomitant thrombosis of the bypass graft.[11–14] The authors refer to this condition as a *failing graft* because if the lesion is not corrected, graft thrombosis is almost certain to occur. This concept is important because many difficult lower extremity revascularizations can be salvaged for protracted periods by relatively simple interventions if the lesion responsible for the circulatory deterioration and diminished graft blood flow can be detected before graft thrombosis occurs.

The authors have now been able to detect more than 350 failing grafts and to correct the lesions before graft thrombosis occurred.[12, 20, 21] The majority of these grafts were vein grafts, but approximately one third were PTFE or polyester (Dacron) grafts (Figs. 71–1 and 71–2). Invariably, the corrective procedure was simpler than the secondary operation that would be required if the bypass went on to thrombosis. Many lesions responsible for the failing state were remedied by percutaneous transluminal angioplasty (PTA), although some required a vein patch angioplasty, a short bypass of a graft lesion, or a proximal or distal graft extension.[12, 20–22] Some of the angioplasties of these lesions have failed and required a second reintervention; others have remained effective in correcting the responsible lesion, as documented by arteriography more than 2 to 5 years later (see Fig. 71–1).

Nevertheless, the role of PTA for vein graft lesions remains controversial. Although the authors and some other groups[14, 15] have had many excellent results with PTA of vein graft stenoses, others have not.[16] Moreover, in the authors' experience there were some failures with limb loss.[17] The authors, therefore, currently restrict the use of PTA to lesions shorter than 1.5 cm if they are located in an inaccessible part of the vein. PTA has also been useful in the treatment of some inflow and outflow lesions.[21] Most important, the results of reinterventions for failing grafts, in terms of both continued cumulative patency and limb salvage rates, have been far superior to the results of reinterventions for grafts that have undergone thrombosis and have failed (Fig. 71–3).[8, 11, 13, 20–22]

This difference in results, together with the ease of reintervention for failing grafts, mandates that surgeons performing infrainguinal bypass operations observer their patients closely in the postoperative period and indefinitely thereafter. In the authors' practice, the surgeon examines the peripheral pulses of patients at 6- to 8-week intervals for the first 6 months and every 2 to 4 months thereafter. Ideally, noninvasive laboratory tests, including duplex ultrasonography scanning of vein grafts, should be performed with similar frequency,[14, 18, 19] but the authors have found such tests to be expensive and sometimes impractical to perform in all patients.

If the patient has any recurrence of symptoms or the surgeon detects either any change in peripheral pulse examination or other manifestations of ischemia, the circulatory deterioration is confirmed by noninvasive tests and the patient is admitted for urgent anticoagulation therapy and arteriography. If a lesion is detected as a cause of the failing state, it is corrected urgently by PTA or operation. The authors' aggressive prophylactic intervention for these lesions, even if they are asymptomatic, is based on their dire prognosis if left untreated and the greater difficulty and worse outcome that result if the lesion is untreated and the graft goes on to thrombosis, as it almost certainly will.[11, 20]

Moreover, if the failing graft is a vein bypass, detection of the failing state permits accurate localization and definition of the responsible lesion with arteriography followed by salvage of any undiseased vein. In contrast, allowing the

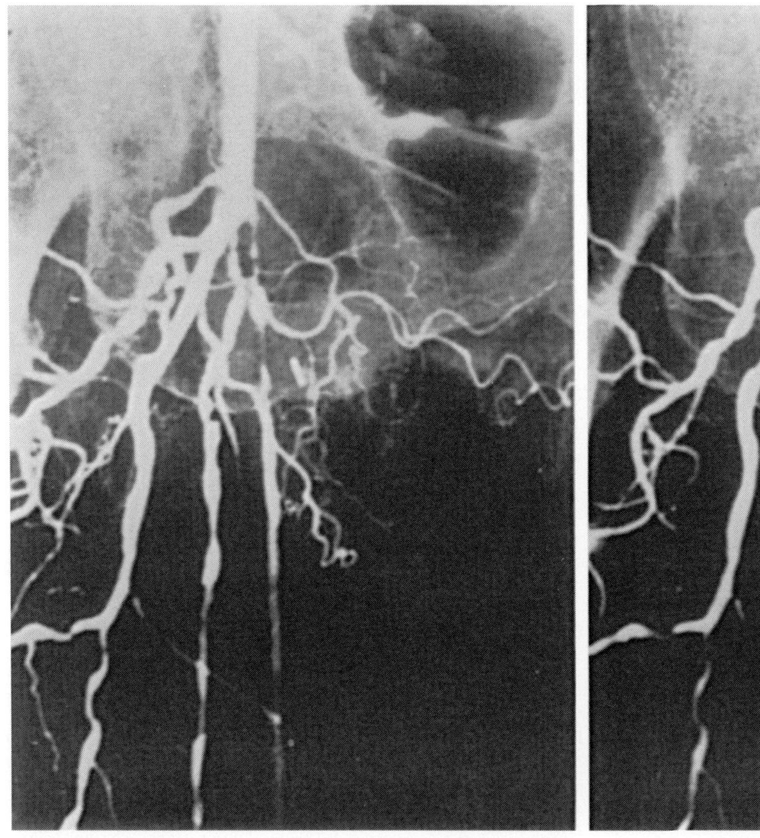
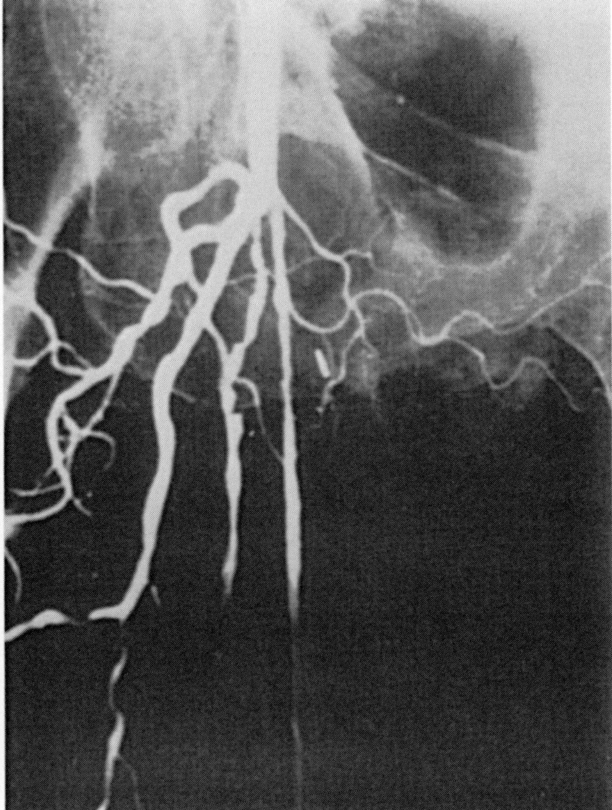

FIGURE 71–1. *Left,* Arteriogram 18 months after a common femoral–anterior tibial bypass. A proximal stenosis produced the "failing state." *Right,* An arteriogram 2 years after the stenosis was corrected by percutaneous transluminal angioplasty. The graft remained patent 5 years later.

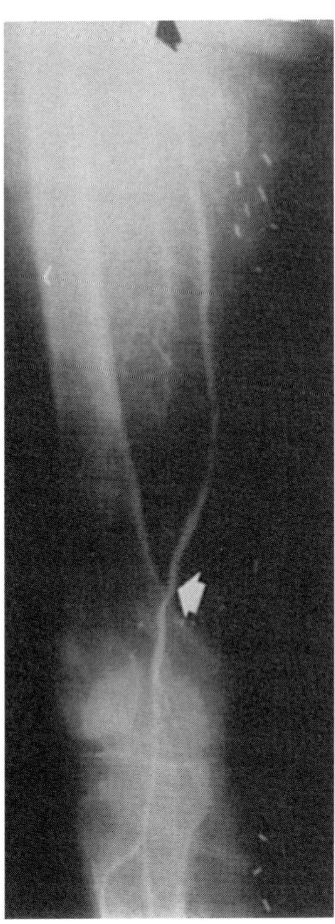

FIGURE 71–2. Arteriogram of a patient with a failing polytetrafluoroethylene femoropopliteal graft 2 years after the initial operation. The arteriogram was performed because of a return of rest pain and the loss of distal pulses. The graft (between *arrows*) was patent despite a proximal occlusion of the common femoral artery and an inflow pressure of only 40 mmHg. A bypass from the external iliac artery to the original graft was performed, and the original graft remained patent until the patient's death 6 years later.

graft to undergo thrombosis has the following consequences:

1. The responsible lesion may be difficult to identify.
2. It may be difficult or impossible to clear the vein with thrombectomy.
3. The results of lytic therapy are imperfect.
4. The patient's best graft—the ipsilateral greater saphenous vein—may have to be sacrificed, rendering the secondary operation even more difficult and more likely to fail, with associated limb loss.

MANAGEMENT STRATEGIES

Patients with circulatory deterioration after an infrainguinal arterial reconstruction present with recurrent symptoms, a decrease in pulses in the involved limb, other changes detected on physical examination, or a decrease in noninvasive vascular laboratory values. These manifestations may occur at any time after operation and are presumptive evidence that the arterial reconstruction has undergone thrombosis, although they may also occur in the absence of graft thrombosis if some lesion is present in, proximal to, or distal to the bypass graft (i.e., with a failing graft).

Presumed Early Graft Failure (Within 30 Days)

If the primary operation was originally justified, a secondary procedure is also mandated. If the primary operation was performed for limb salvage, early (within 30 days) graft failure or thrombosis is always associated with a renewed threat or even a worse threat to the limb. If the original preoperative arteriogram was satisfactory, another arteriography is not necessary.

The patient is given intravenous heparin and returned to the operating room as expeditiously as possible. Because vein grafts can be injured by the ischemia associated with intraluminal clot and because it may be more difficult to remove solid thrombotic material from vein grafts, it is more urgent to reoperate for a failed autogenous vein graft than for a failed PTFE graft. In any event, reoperation should be undertaken less than 12 hours after failure is detected. Even greater urgency is required if calf muscle tenderness or neurologic changes are associated with graft failure.

Vein Grafts

The distal incision over the arterial reconstruction is reopened. The graft thrombosis is confirmed by palpation. Control of the artery proximal and distal to the distal anastomosis is obtained, and a full anticoagulating dose of intravenous heparin (7500 IU) is given. A linear incision is made in the hood of the graft (Fig. 71–4) to visualize the interior of the distal anastomosis.[3] Balloon catheters are gently passed retrograde in the graft to remove the clot (Fig. 71–5). If necessary, any clot is similarly removed from the proximal and distal adjacent host artery, and any visualized anastomotic defect is repaired. The surgeon may

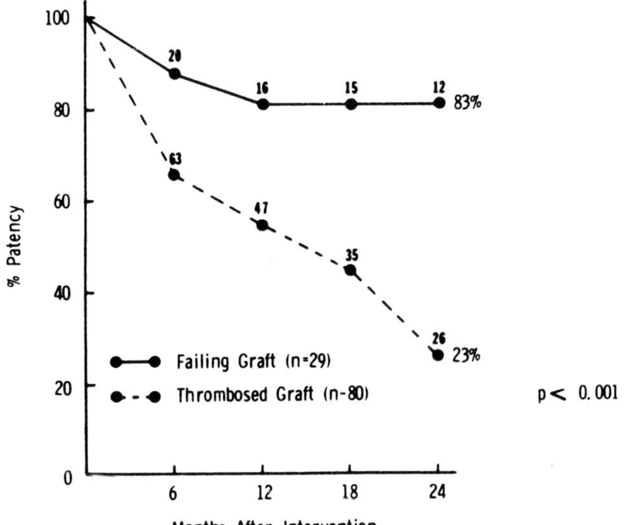

FIGURE 71–3. Comparison of patency rates after reintervention or reoperation for failing and failed (thrombosed) below-knee femoropopliteal and femorodistal polytetrafluoroethylene grafts. Numbers of grafts at risk are shown at 6-month intervals. Standard error for all points is less than 10%. (From Ascer E, Collier PE, Gupta SK, Veith FJ: Reoperation for PTFE bypass failure: The importance of distal outflow site and operative technique in determining outcome. J Vasc Surg 5:298, 1987.)

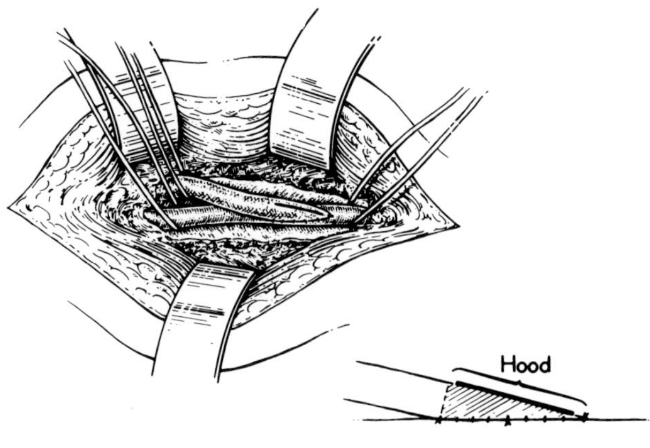

FIGURE 71–4. Operative exposure of the distal anastomosis. The incision in the blood of the graft is made to within 1 mm of the distal end of the graft. This provides optimal exposure of the distal anastomosis and facilitates thrombectomy. (From Ascer E, Collier PE, Gupta SK, Veith FJ: Reoperation for PTFE bypass failure: The importance of distal outflow site and operative technique in determining outcome. J Vasc Surg 5:298, 1987.)

find that valves in the vein graft prevent retrograde passage of the catheter or that it is impossible to restore adequate, normal prograde arterial flow through the graft. In either event, the proximal incision is opened, and the same procedures are performed at the proximal anastomosis.

With flow restored and all openings in the graft closed with fine running monofilament sutures, intraoperative fluoroscopy or arteriography is performed to visualize the graft and the outflow tract. If no defect is seen, adequacy of the reconstruction and the inflow tract is demonstrated by direct arterial pressure measurements, which should reveal no gradient in excess of 15 to 20 mmHg between the distal end of the graft and the brachial or radial artery. Any gradient in excess of 30 mmHg should be localized to the inflow tract or the graft by appropriate needle placement.

If there is a gradient in the vein graft, it should be eliminated by revision. If revision is impossible, the graft should be replaced by a prosthetic (PTFE) graft.[21, 22, 42] Often such unexplained gradients are due to recanalized, thrombophlebitic segments of vein.[23] Unless removed, such segments cause recurrent failure. If an inflow gradient is present, it should be eliminated with a suitable inflow bypass (aortofemoral, femorofemoral, or axillofemoral) or with an intraoperative or postoperative balloon angioplasty with or without a stent.

If disease in the outflow tract is detected and is the presumed cause of graft failure, it generally is best treated with an extension to a more distal, less diseased segment of the same or another outflow artery (Fig. 71–6).

If no defect is detected with arteriography or pressure measurements, the procedure is terminated. Despite older evidence to the contrary,[24] an occasional vein graft undergoes early failure for no apparent reason and remains patent indefinitely after simple thrombectomy. Perhaps the unexplained thrombosis is due to an undetected reduction in cardiac output with hypotension and decreased arterial flow.

With the growing ability to perform distal bypasses to disadvantaged outflow tracts,[1, 21, 25, 26, 42] the authors have encountered some patients whose distal grafts failed early for no apparent reason other than high-outflow resistance. In some of these instances, thrombectomy and extension of the graft to another outflow vessel as a sequential graft have resulted in long-term graft patency and limb salvage.[27]

Polytetrafluoroethylene and Other Prosthetic Grafts

Early thrombosis of PTFE grafts is managed in essentially the same fashion as already described for early failure of vein grafts.[3, 20] Differences include the almost complete freedom from graft defects as a cause of failure, although occasionally a PTFE graft is compressed, kinked, or twisted because of poor tunneling technique and malposition around or through some of the tendinous structures in the region of the knee.

In addition, graft thrombosis for no apparent reason is more common with PTFE grafts than vein grafts, occurring in 56% of the authors' 61 early failures in a series of 882 PTFE infrainguinal grafts (Table 71–1).[28] Simple thrombectomy of the graft with the techniques already described results in patency rates in excess of 50% after 3 years, if no other defect is found and if the distal end of the graft is above the knee joint.[3, 20] The secondary operative treatment in all of the authors' 61 cases was based on the cause of early failure, as shown in Table 71–1. Management techniques were similar to those described for vein grafts, except that in one case, disease just beyond the distal

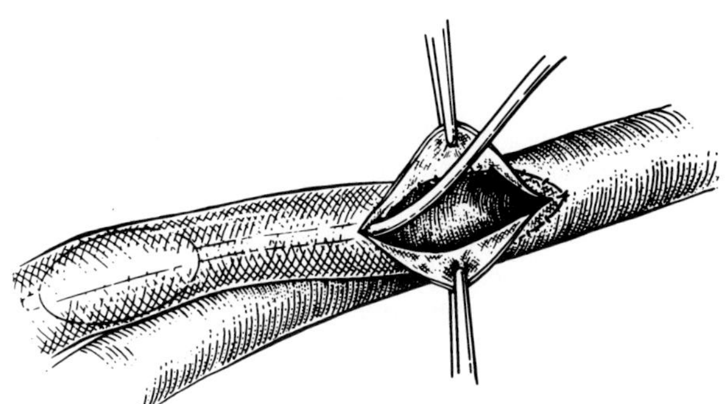

FIGURE 71–5. Thrombectomy alone is performed through the distal graft incision when no cause for graft failure is identified. Clot is removed from the graft and, if needed, from the artery both proximally and distally. (From Ascer E, Collier PE, Gupta SK, Veith FJ: Reoperation for PTFE bypass failure: The importance of distal outflow site and operative technique in determining outcome. J Vasc Surg 5:298, 1987.)

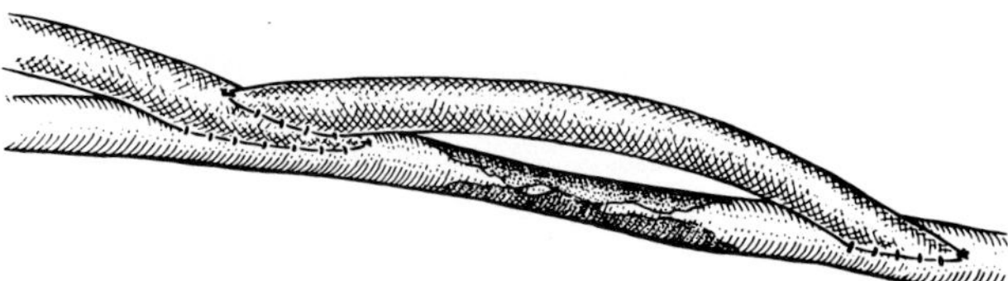

FIGURE 71–6. If disease in the outflow tract is detected, particularly a distal arteriosclerotic lesion, a graft extension is performed. (From Ascer E, Collier PE, Gupta SK, Veith FJ: Reoperation for PTFE bypass failure: The importance of distal outflow site and operative technique in determining outcome. J Vasc Surg 5:298, 1987.)

TABLE 71–1. EARLY (<1 MONTH) OCCLUSION OF POLYTETRAFLUOROETHYLENE BYPASS GRAFT IN 61 FAILED GRAFTS

CAUSE	TREATMENT	NUMBER	INCIDENCE (%)
None found	Thrombectomy alone	34	56
Hypotension	Thrombectomy alone	2	3
Embolus	Thrombectomy alone	2	3
Technical*	Patch graft	1	2
Inflow stenosis	Proximal extension	3	5
Distal disease	Distal extension	19	31

*Unrecognized stenotic lesion just beyond distal anastomosis.

anastomosis was treated with a patch graft angioplasty (Fig. 71–7) rather than a distal graft extension.

Presumed Late Graft Failure (After 30 Days)

Every patient with presumed late (>30 days) graft failure should undergo a standard transfemoral or translumbar arteriogram with visualization of all arteries from the renal arteries to the forefoot.[1] If a failing graft is found, it is urgently treated by a reintervention, as already discussed. If a failed or thrombosed graft is present, the patient is not subjected to reintervention unless the limb is unequivocally threatened.

Surprisingly, even if the original operation was performed for salvage of a limb with critical ischemia,[29] the limb may not be threatened again when the original arterial reconstruction becomes occluded.[3] Ten per cent to 25% of patients are able to tolerate occlusion of a limb salvage bypass and to function effectively indefinitely. This proportion seems to grow as the interval between the primary operation and its failure increases. Presumably, this phenomenon occurs because the original limb-threatening lesion has healed by virtue of the bypass and does not recur with the renewed ischemia. Alternatively, improved collateral vessels maintain the limb better after some graft failures than before the operation for reasons that remain obscure.

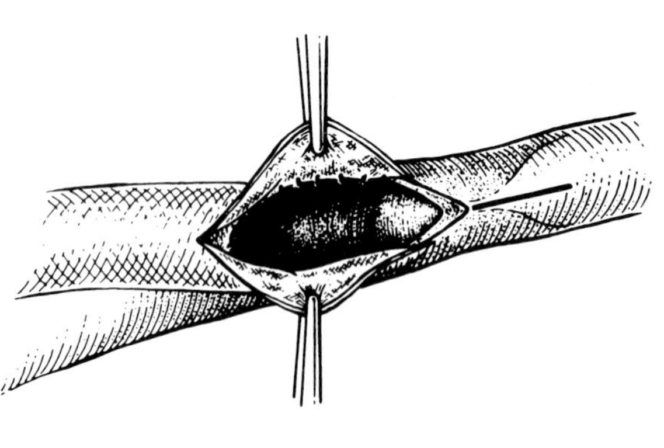

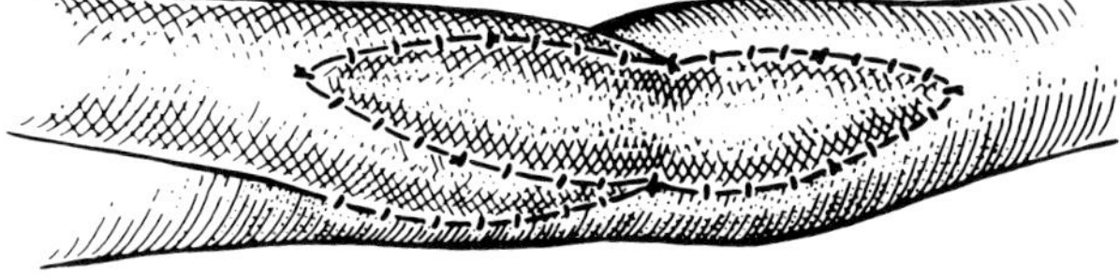

FIGURE 71–7. Stenosis just distal to the anastomosis can be caused by an unrecognized atherosclerotic lesion. This can be corrected by extending the graft incision distally across its apex and down the recipient artery until its lumen is no longer narrowed. A patch of polytetrafluoroethylene or vein is then inserted across the stenosis to widen the lumen. Similar treatment is appropriate for intimal hyperplasia that causes late graft occlusion. (From Ascer E, Collier PE, Gupta SK, Veith FJ: Reoperation for PTFE bypass failure: The importance of distal outflow site and operative technique in determining outcome. J Vasc Surg 5:298, 1987.)

When graft thrombosis *is* associated with renewed critical ischemia and an imminently endangered lower extremity, aggressive reintervention is indicated and is very important to achievement of optimal limb salvage results.[1, 30] Management strategies differ, depending on the type of graft and its location. In all instances, complete arteriography should precede any reintervention.

Axillofemoral and Femorofemoral Grafts

In the patient with failure of an axillofemoral or femorofemoral graft, the inflow tract of the graft should be examined angiographically. With axillofemoral grafts, it is possible to perform an arch arteriogram via the transfemoral or translumbar route.[31] Similar examination should be used to evaluate the inflow or donor iliac system with failed femorofemoral grafts. If significant inflow disease is found, it can be corrected by PTA with or without a stent, or a new bypass from an alternative site must be performed. If, for example, inflow iliac disease has caused failure of a femorofemoral graft, (1) it can be corrected by PTA with or without a stent, (2) an aortobifemoral bypass can be performed, or (3) an aortic limb can be brought to the thrombectomized femorofemoral graft.

The arteriogram should also be used to seek evidence of progression of outflow disease and to identify patent distal segments that can be used to bypass such outflow disease if necessary. An example is progression of deep femoral artery disease in a patient for whom that vessel is providing outflow for an axillofemoral or femorofemoral bypass. In this circumstance, the popliteal artery should be evaluated angiographically, and thrombectomy of the graft should be followed by a profundaplasty or graft extension to the undiseased deep femoral or popliteal artery.

After suitable arteriographic examination, the patient is subjected to a secondary operation. The graft is opened over the hood or hoods of the distal anastomoses so that the interior of the distal anastomosis can be inspected (Fig. 71–8). With axillofemoral grafts, inspection is facilitated if the original femorofemoral limb is placed over the distal end of the axillary limb (Fig. 71–9). In this way, a single opening in the graft permits thrombectomy of all prosthetic grafts, thrombectomy of arteries in one groin, and diagnosis and correction of anastomotic problems at one distal anastomosis (see Fig. 71–8).

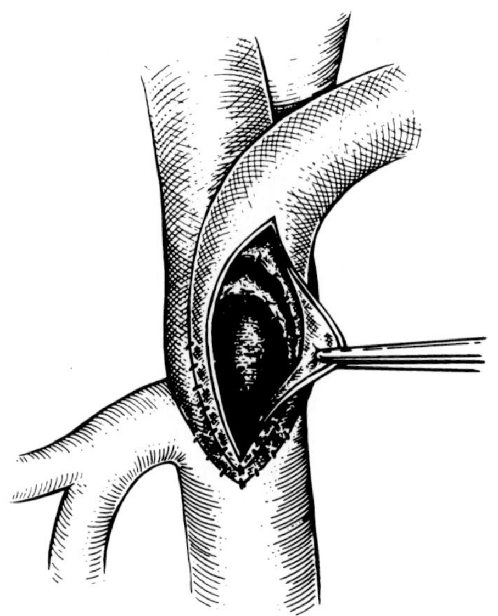

FIGURE 71–8. Approach to an unsuccessful axillobifemoral bypass. The distal anastomosis and adjacent vessels are dissected free and are controlled. An opening is made in the hood of the graft to permit proximal thrombectomy and visualization of the interior of this anastomosis.

Although blind balloon catheter thrombectomy of any distal anastomosis via an opening in the graft remote from the anastomosis is occasionally successful, the authors object strongly to the practice. The chance of damage to the anastomosis, injury of the intima, or disruption of plaque in the adjacent artery is too great. It is true that the anastomosis and adjacent arteries must be dissected free and controlled and that this procedure may be difficult because of scarring, but it is clearly worth the effort. If distal anastomotic intimal hyperplasia is detected as the cause of graft failure, it is treated by a graft extension or by incision across the hyperplastic lesion and insertion of a patch graft (see Fig. 71–7). In the latter circumstance, the incision and patch are usually placed across the origin of the deep femoral artery.

If no cause of failure is found on preoperative arteriography or intraoperative inspection, intraoperative arteriography or fluoroscopy is performed. If no defects or partially obstructing lesions are found, as is often the case with failed axillofemoral grafts, the reoperative procedure is terminated, and good results can be expected.

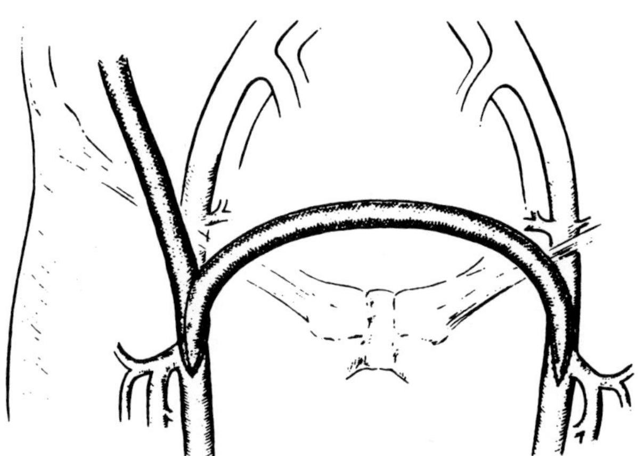

FIGURE 71–9. Crossover portion of axillobifemoral procedure is placed directly over the first femoral anastomosis. (From Ascer E, Collier PE, Gupta SK, Veith FJ: Reoperation for PTFE bypass failure: The importance of distal outflow site and operative technique in determining outcome. J Vasc Surg 5:298, 1987.)

The value of these reoperations for failed extra-anatomic bypasses consists of substantially improved late patency rates[32] with a 3-year *additional* patency rate, calculated from the time of reoperation, of 75%.[20]

Reoperations or Secondary Operations After Failed Femoropopliteal or Infrapopliteal Bypasses

If a failed femoropopliteal or infrapopliteal bypass graft is confirmed by arteriography to have thrombosis, reintervention is undertaken only if the limb is in immediate jeopardy. If this is the case, complete contrast-enhanced arteriography must precede any secondary operation to provide some information (albeit perhaps incomplete) as to why the graft failed and to define possible therapeutic options by demonstrating remaining patent distal arterial segments and the quality of undissected proximal arteries that may be used for bypass origin, such as the mid-portion or distal portion of the deep femoral artery.[33, 34]

Bilateral contrast-enhanced venography should also precede reoperation to define the length and quality of the remaining superficial veins.[35] This step can be helpful in patients with failed vein grafts because it reveals unused accessory greater saphenous veins, unused short saphenous veins, and, occasionally, a main saphenous trunk. The authors have also found that duplex ultrasonography can be useful in predicting the length and diameter of residual venous segments. However, neither technique of preoperative evaluation is totally accurate, and surgical exploration may be the only way to assess vein suitability with certainty. Preoperative venography or duplex ultrasonography is also indicated in the patient who has previously received a prosthetic bypass. The authors have been surprised by how often the greater saphenous vein in such cases has been damaged during the first operation or by scarring.

The usual standard surgical approaches to arteries in patients who have failed bypasses are often rendered more difficult, or even impossible to use, by surgical scarring or infection. For that reason, the authors have developed a variety of new or unusual approaches to all the infrainguinal arteries, which allow these vessels to be reached through virginal tissue planes.[31] These approaches can be helpful in avoiding the scarred standard access routes and can be essential if a previous operation was complicated by infection. The approaches obviate the need to use a scarred or infected groin to trace the deep femoral artery down from its origin.[34] They also permit the distal portions of the artery to be used to provide inflow for a distal shorter vein graft. The authors have now used these direct distal routes to the deep femoral artery in more than 80 secondary procedures.[34]

Another set of unusual approaches are for the above-knee or below-knee popliteal artery.[36] These approaches are particularly useful in the presence of medial incision sepsis and permit use of the popliteal artery for bypass inflow or outflow even in the presence of groin and medial thigh infection.[36] In addition, all three leg arteries can be reached medially or laterally, and adequate exposure can be obtained to perform an anastomosis. The lateral approach involves fibula resection, through which all parts of the tibial and peroneal arteries can be reached.[1, 37–39]

The authors have also devised a method for exposing the lower third of the peroneal artery from a medial approach. This technique involves division of the long flexor muscles and tendons to the toes and foot and is particularly suitable if an in situ bypass to the distal third of the peroneal artery is to be performed.

Finally, the authors have developed surgical approaches to the terminal branches of the posterior tibial artery and the dorsalis pedis artery.[25, 33, 39] Any of these branches, which include the medial and lateral plantar branches of the posterior tibial artery and the lateral tarsal and deep metatarsal arch branches of the dorsalis pedis artery, can be used for secondary bypass operations.[25, 36] The deep metatarsal arch is accessed via a dorsal incision with removal of portions of the shaft of the second and perhaps third metatarsal bones.

Another principle that is particularly useful to the vascular surgeon planning a secondary procedure is the short vein graft or distal origin bypass. Every bypass to the popliteal or infrapopliteal vessels need not originate from the common femoral artery.[40] Grafts to these distal arteries may originate from the superficial femoral, popliteal, or even tibial arteries without compromising late patency results (Fig. 71–10).[25, 40] Such short vein grafts are particularly useful in secondary bypass operations because they allow the surgeon to avoid previously scarred or infected areas and facilitate the use of the limited remaining superficial veins as bypass conduits.[25, 40] Certainly, they are better than prosthetic grafts.[41] Moreover, the authors have shown that short vein grafts probably have better patency rates than long vein grafts, particularly when they are used as bypasses to disadvantaged outflow tracts.[25, 26]

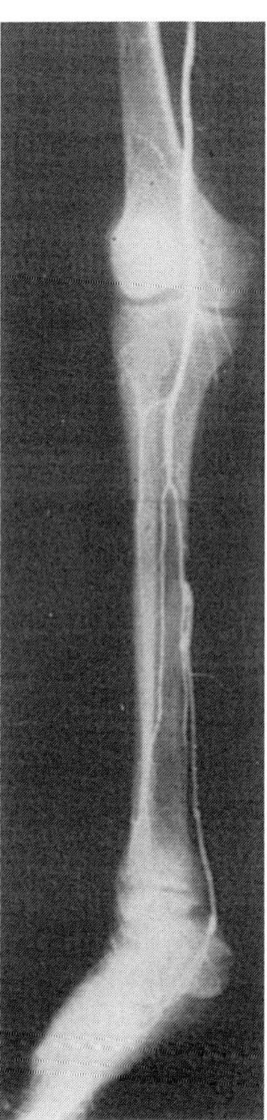

FIGURE 71–10. Arteriogram showing a posterior tibial to posterior tibial bypass, which has now remained patent for more than 8 years. (From Veith FJ, Ascer E, Gupta SK, et al: Tibiotibial vein bypass grafts: A new operation for limb salvage. J Vasc Surg 2:552, 1985.)

Two types of secondary arterial reconstruction are available to the vascular surgeon who is planning a reintervention for a failed infrainguinal bypass. The first, termed by the authors a "reoperation," employs some form of graft thrombectomy and revision or extension in an effort to save all or as much of the original graft as possible. Newer methods for thromboembolectomy using digital cinefluoroscopy and catheter–guide wire endovascular techniques are discussed in detail in Chapter 72. The other type of secondary operation involves placement of a totally new secondary bypass graft, preferably but not necessarily using previously undissected patent arteries for the origin and insertion of the bypass.

The choice of which type of secondary bypass to employ depends on a number of variables, including:

- Type of primary bypass (PTFE or autogenous vein)
- Nature and location of the lesion responsible for the failure of the primary operation
- The surgeon's training and experience
- Residual arterial and superficial venous anatomy
- Most important, the location of the primary bypass

Because of the importance of the last factor, treatments for the different kinds of failed primary operations that require reintervention are considered separately.

Failed Vein Grafts

With failed femoropopliteal or infrapopliteal bypass, thrombectomy of an occluded vein graft is not attempted. If a patent albeit isolated popliteal segment is present, a bypass to that segment is attempted. An effort to perform bypass with a vein graft from the ipsilateral extremity is made with the use of a remnant of the greater saphenous or the lesser saphenous vein. This effort is facilitated by using the distal deep femoral or superficial femoral artery for inflow, if possible, and by keeping the vein graft short.

If no ipsilateral lower extremity vein of adequate length is available, a PTFE graft has good prospects of remaining patent and providing long-term limb salvage, particularly if it is inserted above the knee,[41] and the authors use it in preference to vein from the other leg or the arms. If foot necrosis or infection is extensive in this setting, a sequential femoral-popliteal-tibial bypass should be performed with the use of a short distal vein graft obtained from any extremity of the patient. If no patent popliteal segment is present, as short a vein graft as possible is performed, extending from the distalmost artery with unobstructed proximal flow (i.e., deep or superficial femoral, popliteal, or tibial artery) to the most proximal patent infrapopliteal artery that courses without significant obstruction to its terminal end. For such procedures, autogenous vein from any extremity is used, even if it is only 2.5 to 3 mm in diameter when distended.[25, 42, 43] PTFE grafts should be used for bypasses to infrapopliteal arteries only if absolutely no autogenous vein is available. However, a secondary arterial reconstruction with such a prosthetic graft has a chance of remaining patent for several years and has a moderate chance of saving the involved limb.[41, 42] Accordingly, use of such a graft, though not ideal, is a better option than an amputation.

Failed Polytetrafluoroethylene Bypass

Femoral–Above-Knee Popliteal Artery Bypass

For failure of a femoral–above-knee bypass that threatens the limb and necessitates a secondary intervention, it is the authors' present belief that a reoperation with an attempt at graft salvage is justified and indicated (Table 71–2).[3, 20] If the preoperative arteriogram indicates an inflow problem, the problem is treated appropriately by PTA or a proximal extension. The distal end of the graft is redissected along with its adjacent arteries (see Fig. 71–4), and after administration of 7500 IU of heparin, a vertical incision is made in the distal hood of the graft to permit balloon catheter thrombectomy of the graft and the popliteal artery proximally and distally (see Figs. 71–4 and 71–5). Great care is exercised, and minimal balloon inflation is used when the catheter is passed in arteries to avoid intimal injury. Only if necessary is a proximal incision made. If the presence of a distal lesion is detected on inspection of the anastomosis or by preoperative arteriography, it is treated.

The authors still believe that an incision across the lesion and patch angioplasty are best for intimal hyperplasia (see Fig. 71–7), and a graft extension to a distal patent artery with a PTFE or vein graft (see Fig. 71–6) is best for distal progression of disease. Although this approach requires a difficult redissection of the distal anastomosis (which may be more technically demanding than performance of a totally new bypass), the authors believe it is justified and indicated in view of (1) the acceptable 3-year patency results (Fig. 71–11) and (2) the fact that such an approach preserves the maximal amount of undissected patent distal arterial tree for use if further problems develop.

Femoral–Below-Knee Popliteal or Infrapopliteal Artery Bypass

When failure of a femoral–below-knee popliteal or infrapopliteal artery bypass results in the need for a secondary arterial reconstruction, the authors perform an entirely new secondary bypass, preferably employing an autogenous vein graft and some of the strategies already discussed that minimize graft length and permit use of previously unused segments of arteries or segments approached through virginal tissue planes.[33, 34, 36] The authors' primary reason for departing from the previous strategy of performing a reoperation with an attempt at graft salvage[3] is the poorer additional patency that is obtained with reoperations on these below-knee grafts (see Fig. 71–11) in comparison with the better results of a totally new secondary bypass (>a 40% 2-year patency rate).[20] A second reason for not using the reoperation strategy is the 6% infection rate with such procedures, compared with a rate of less than 1% with a new secondary bypass.[20]

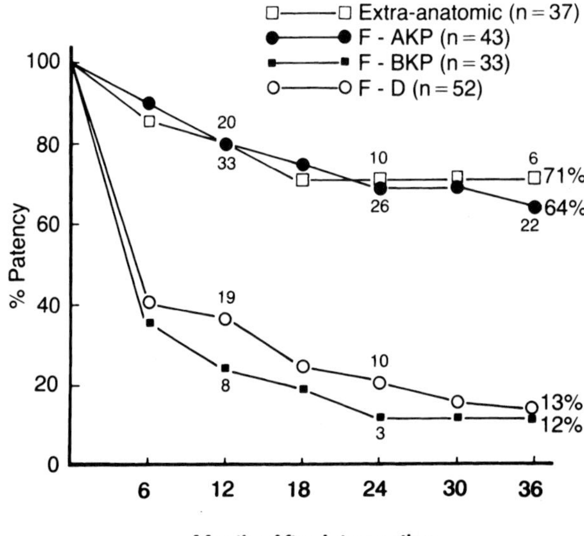

FIGURE 71–11. Cumulative life table patency rates for various types of polytetrafluoroethylene bypasses subjected to one or more reoperations with salvage of the original graft. Numbers of grafts at risk are shown at yearly intervals. Extra-anatomic procedures include axillofemoral and femorofemoral grafts. F-AKP = femoral–above-knee popliteal grafts; F-BKP = femoral–below-knee popliteal grafts; F-D = femoral-infrapopliteal artery grafts. (From Ascer E, Collier PE, Gupta SK, Veith FJ: Reoperation for PTFE bypass failure: The importance of distal outflow site and operative technique in determining outcome. J Vasc Surg 5:298, 1987.)

Failed Secondary Arterial Reconstruction

Although some vascular surgeons are reluctant to undertake multiple attempts at arterial reconstruction to salvage a threatened limb, in the belief that the risks of infection and knee loss outweigh the potential benefits, the authors and others disagree.[1, 3, 8, 20, 30, 44] The results show that many patients can benefit from multiple limb salvage operations and that the benefits outweigh the risks and disadvantages if the principles and strategies already advocated are employed.[1, 3, 8, 20, 30, 42, 44, 45]

TABLE 71–2. CAUSE, INCIDENCE, AND MANAGEMENT OF LATE OCCLUSION IN 104 POLYTETRAFLUOROETHYLENE BYPASS GRAFTS

CAUSE OF FAILURE	NUMBER OF CASES	PERCENTAGE OF TOTAL	TREATMENT
Progression of distal disease	39	37	Thrombectomy and distal graft extension (30) or new bypass to more distal artery (9)
None found	29	28	Thrombectomy alone
Intimal hyperplasia	22	21	Thrombectomy and patch angioplasty
Progression of proximal disease	12	12	Thrombectomy and proximal graft extension
Hypotension/technical	2	2	Thrombectomy alone

Thrombolysis

In the last several years, there has been renewed interest in the use of fibrinolytic agents for lysis of intravascular clots (see Chapters 35, 57, 60, 150, and 154). The administration of low-dose streptokinase or high-dose urokinase by direct intra-arterial injection into thrombosed bypass grafts has been found to be effective in restoring patency.[46–60] With restored bypass patency, some perfusion can be reestablished and the underlying cause for the graft thrombosis may be identified. Additionally, the patencies of occluded but undiseased inflow source and outflow tracts may be regained, thereby facilitating planning for reintervention and possibly converting a major operation into a minor procedure.

Occasionally, intraoperative local lysis may be helpful or necessary when the distal outflow tract is occluded by clots that cannot be retrieved by mechanical means.[55–58] Although early reports did not initially show that these advantages resulted in prolonged graft patency, later accumulated experiences of different groups indicated that adequate results can be achieved in some groups of patients.[50–54, 59, 60] Generally, patients in whom proximal occlusions of short duration can be traversed with a guide wire and whose distal vessels can be visualized on angiogram have good outcomes after lytic therapy and revision for the occluded grafts.[53] The authors and several other groups continue to use urokinase for some graft thromboses with promising results, and this agent as well as the newer human tissue plasminogen activator should continue to be regarded with interest. Nevertheless, more experience is needed before a conclusion can be reached about the exact place of thrombolytic agents in the management of failed infrainguinal arterial reconstruction. Almost certainly they will play an important role.

SUMMARY

Secondary arterial reconstructions play an important part in achieving the ultimate goal of limb salvage after primary infrainguinal interventions fail. By employing the strategies and principles outlined in this chapter, the surgeon can obtain good results, in terms of patency, of the reoperated primary reconstruction or the secondary reconstruction with significantly augmented limb salvage at low cost, that is, in operative morbidity and mortality.[28, 42] These results mandate that vascular surgeons maintain an aggressive attitude toward the use of these secondary operations when (1) a primary procedure fails to achieve or maintain its intended function and (2) a patient is faced with the imminent loss of a lower limb because of distal ischemia.

REFERENCES

1. Veith FJ, Gupta SK, Samson RH, et al: Progress in limb salvage by reconstructive arterial surgery combined with new or improved adjunctive procedures. Ann Surg 194:386, 1981.
2. Rivers SP, Veith FJ, Ascer E, et al: Successful conservative therapy of severe limb-threatening ischemia: The value of nonsympathectomy. Surgery 99:759, 1986.
3. Veith FJ, Gupta SK, Daly V: Management of early and late thrombosis of expanded polytetrafluoroethylene (PTFE) femoropopliteal bypass grafts: Favorable prognosis with appropriate reoperation. Surgery 87:581, 1980.
4. Carsten CG, Taylor SM, Langan EM, Crane MM: Factors associated with limb loss despite a patent infrainguinal bypass graft. Am Surg 64:33, 1998.
5. Veith FJ, Gupta SK, Daly V: Femoropopliteal bypass to the isolated popliteal segment: Is polytetrafluoroethylene graft acceptable? Surgery 89:296, 1981.
6. Flinn WR, Flanigan DP, Verta MJ et al: Sequential femoral-tibial bypass for severe limb ischemia. Surgery 88:357, 1980.
7. Szilagyi DE, Smith RF, Elliot JP, et al: The biologic fate of autogenous vein implants as arterial substitutes: Clinical, angiographic and histopathologic observations in femoropopliteal operations for atherosclerosis. Ann Surg 178:232, 1973.
8. Whittemore AD, Clowes AW, Couch NP, et al: Secondary femoropopliteal reconstruction. Ann Surg 193:35, 1981.
9. Karkow WS, Cranley JJ, Cranley RD, et al: Extended study of aneurysm formation in umbilical grafts. J Vasc Surg 4:486, 1986.
10. Hasson JE, Newton WD, Waltman AC, et al: Mural degeneration in the glutaraldehyde tanned umbilical vein graft: Incidence and implications. J Vasc Surg 4:243, 1986.
11. Veith FJ, Weiser RK, Gupta SK, et al: Diagnosis and management of failing lower extremity arterial reconstruction. J Cardiovasc Surg 23:381, 1984.
12. O'Mara CS, Flinn WR, Johnson ND, et al: Recognition and surgical management of patent but hemodynamically failed arterial grafts. Ann Surg 193:467, 1981.
13. Smith CR, Green RM DeWeese JA: Pseudo-occlusion of femoropopliteal bypass grafts. Circulation 68(Suppl II):88, 1983.
14. Berkowitz HD, Kee JC: Occluded infrainguinal grafts: When to choose lytic therapy versus a new bypass graft. Am J Surg 170:136, 1995.
15. Tonnesen KH, Holstein P, Rordam L, et al: Early results of percutaneous transluminal angioplasty (PTA) of failing below-knee bypass grafts. Eur J Vasc Endovasc Surg 15:51, 1998.
16. Whittemore AD, Donaldson MC, Polak JF, et al: Limitations of balloon angioplasty for vein graft stenosis. J Vasc Surg 14:340, 1991.
17. Sanchez LA, Suggs WD, Marin ML, Veith FJ: Is percutaneous balloon angioplasty appropriate in the treatment of graft and anastomotic lesions responsible for failing vein bypasses? Am J Surg 168:97, 1994.
18. Bergamini TM, George SM, Massey HT, et al: Intensive surveillance of femoropopliteal-tibial autogenous vein bypasses improves long-term graft patency and limb salvage. Ann Surg 221:507, 1995.
19. Wilson YG, Davies AH, Currie IC, et al: Vein graft stenosis: Incidence and intervention. Eur J Vasc Endovasc Surg 11:164, 1996.
20. Ascer E, Collier P, Gupta SK, Veith FJ: Reoperation for PTFE bypass failure: The importance of distal outflow site and operative technique in determining outcome. J Vasc Surg 5:298, 1987.
21. Sanchez L, Gupta SK, Veith FJ, et al: A ten-year experience with one hundred fifty failing or threatened vein and polytetrafluoroethylene arterial bypass grafts. J Vasc Surg 14:729, 1991.
22. Sanchez LA, Suggs WD, Veith FJ, et al: The merit of polytetrafluoroethylene extensions and interposition grafts to salvage failing infrainguinal vein bypasses. J Vasc Surg 23:329, 1996.
23. Panetta TF, Marin ML, Veith FJ, et al: Unsuspected pre-existing saphenous vein disease: An unrecognized cause of vein bypass failure. J Vasc Surg 15:102, 1991.
24. Craver JM, Ottinger LW, Darling C, et al: Hemorrhage and thrombosis as early complications of femoropopliteal bypass grafts: Causes, treatment, and prognostic implications. Surgery 74:839, 1973.
25. Veith FJ, Ascer E, Gupta SK, et al: Tibio-tibial vein bypass grafts: A new operation for limb salvage. J Vasc Surg 2:552, 1985.
26. Ascer E, Veith FJ, Gupta SK, et al: Short vein grafts: A superior option for arterial reconstructions to poor or compromised outflow tracts? J Vasc Surg 7:370, 1988.
27. Ascer E, Veith FJ, Morin L, et al: Components of outflow resistance and their correlation with graft patency in lower extremity arterial reconstructions. J Vasc Surg 1:817, 1984.
28. Collier P, Ascer E, Veith FJ, et al: Acute thrombosis of arterial grafts. *In* Bergan JJ, Yao JST (eds): Vascular Surgical Emergencies. New York, Grune & Stratton, 1987, pp 517–528.
29. Working Party of the International Vascular Symposium: The definition of critical ischemia of a limb. Br J Surg 69(Suppl):S2, 1982.
30. Veith FJ, Gupta SK, Wengerter KR, et al: Changing arteriosclerotic disease patterns and management strategies in lower limb-threatening ischemia. Ann Surg 212:402, 1990.
31. Calligaro KD, Ascer E, Veith FJ, et al: Unsuspected inflow disease in

candidates for axillofemoral bypass operations: A prospective study. J Vasc Surg 11:832, 1990.
32. Ascer E, Veith FJ, Gupta SK, et al: Comparison of axillounifemoral and axillobifemoral bypass operations. Surgery 97:169, 1985.
33. Veith FJ, Ascer E, Nunez A, et al: Unusual approaches to infrainguinal arteries. J Cardiovasc Surg 28:58, 1987.
34. Nunez A, Veith FJ, Collier P, et al: Direct approaches to the distal portions of the deep femoral artery for limb salvage bypasses. J Vasc Surg 8:576, 1988.
35. Veith FJ, Moss CM, Sprayregen S, et al: Preoperative saphenous venography in arterial reconstructive surgery of the lower extremity. Surgery 85:253, 1979.
36. Veith FJ, Ascer E, Gupta SK, et al: Lateral approach to the popliteal artery. J Vasc Surg 6:119, 1987.
37. Veith FJ, Gupta SK: Femoral-distal artery bypasses. *In* Bergan JJ, Yao JST (eds): Operative Techniques in Vascular Surgery. New York, Grune & Stratton, 1980, pp 141–150.
38. Dardik H, Dardik I, Veith FJ: Exposure of the tibial-peroneal arteries by a single lateral approach. Surgery 75:337, 1974.
39. Ascer E, Veith FJ, Gupta SK: Bypasses to plantar arteries and other tibial branches: An extended approach to limb salvage. J Vasc Surg 8:434, 1988.
40. Veith FJ, Gupta SK, Samson RH, et al: Superficial femoral and popliteal arteries as inflow sites for distal bypasses. Surgery 90:980, 1981.
41. Veith FJ, Gupta SK, Ascer E, et al: Six-year prospective multicenter randomized comparison of autologous saphenous vein and expanded polytetrafluoroethylene grafts in infrainguinal arterial reconstructions. J Vasc Surg 3:104, 1986.
42. Parsons RE, Suggs WD, Veith FJ, et al: Polytetrafluoroethylene bypasses to infrapopliteal arteries without cuffs or patches: A better option than amputation in patients without autologous vein. J Vasc Surg 23:347, 1996.
43. Wengerter KR, Veith FJ, Gupta SK: Influence of vein size (diameter) on infrapopliteal reversed vein graft patency. J Vasc Surg 11:525, 1990.
44. Bartlett ST, Olinde AJ, Flinn WR, et al: The reoperative potential of infrainguinal bypass: Long-term limb and patient survival. J Vasc Surg 5:170, 1987.
45. Belkin M, Conte MS, Whittemore AD: Preferred strategies for secondary infrainguinal bypass: Lessons learned from 300 consecutive reoperations. J Vasc Surg 21:282, 1995.
46. Hargrove WC III, Barker CF, Berkowitz HD, et al: Treatment of acute peripheral arterial and graft thromboses with low dose streptokinase. Surgery 92:981, 1982.
47. van Breda A, Robison JC, Feldman L, et al: Local thrombolysis in the treatment of arterial graft occlusions. J Vasc Surg 1:103, 1984.
48. McNamara TO, Fisher JR: Thrombolysis of peripheral arterial and graft occlusions: Improved results using high-dose urokinase. Am J Roentgenol 144:769, 1985.
49. Veith FJ, Gupta SK, Ascer E, et al: Reoperations and other reinterventions for thrombosed and failing polytetrafluoroethylene grafts. *In* Yao JST, Bergan JJ (eds): Reoperative Arterial Surgery. New York, Grune & Stratton, 1986, pp 337–392.
50. Chalmers RT, Hoballah JJ, Kresowik TF, et al: Late results of a prospective study of direct intraarterial urokinase infusion for peripheral arterial and bypass graft occlusions. Cardiovasc Surg 3:293, 1995.
51. Ouriel K, Shortell CK, Green RM, DeWeese JA: Differential mechanisms of failure of autogenous and non-autogenous bypass conduits: An assessment following successful graft thrombolysis. Cardiovasc Surg 3:469, 1995.
52. Bhatnagar PK, Ierardi RP, Ikeda Y, et al: The impact of thrombolytic therapy on arterial and graft occlusions: A critical analysis. J Cardiovasc Surg 37:105, 1996.
53. Comerota AJ, Weaver FA, Hosking JD, et al: Results of a prospective randomized trial of surgery versus thrombolysis for occluded lower extremity bypass grafts. Am J Surg 172:105, 1996.
54. Van Damme H, Trotteur G, Dongelinger RF, Limet R: Thrombolysis of occluded infrainguinal bypass grafts. Acta Chir Belg 97:177, 1997.
55. Quinones-Baldrich WJ, Zierler RE, Hiatt JC: Intraoperative fibrinolytic therapy: An adjunct to catheter thromboembolectomy. J Vasc Surg 2:319, 1985.
56. Beard JD, Nyanekye I, Earnshaw JJ, et al: Intraoperative streptokinase: A useful adjunct to balloon-catheter embolectomy. Br J Surg 80:21, 1993.
57. Comerota AJ, Rao AR, Throm RC, et al: A prospective, randomized, blinded and placebo-controlled trial of intraoperative intra-arterial urokinase infusion during lower extremity revascularization: Regional and systemic effects. Ann Surg 218:534, 1993.
58. Braithwaite BD, Quinones-Baldrich WJ: Lower limb intra-arterial thrombolysis as an adjunct to the management of arterial and graft occlusions. World J Surg 20:649, 1996.
59. Ouriel K, Veith FJ, Sasahara AA: Thrombolysis or peripheral arterial surgery: Phase I results. J Vasc Surg 23:64, 1996.
60. Ouriel K, Veith FJ, Sasahara AA: A comparison of recombinant urokinase with vascular surgery as initial treatment for acute arterial occlusion of the legs. N Engl J Med 338:1105, 1998.

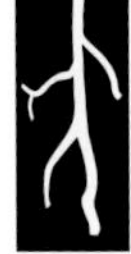

C H A P T E R 72

Endovascular Interventions in the Management of Chronic Lower Extremity Ischemia

Peter A. Schneider, M.D., and
Robert B. Rutherford, M.D.

This chapter describes the role of endovascular intervention in revascularization of the chronically ischemic lower extremity. The most widely accepted and clinically relevant technique for an endovascular approach to occlusive disease is balloon angioplasty. Percutaneous transluminal angioplasty (PTA) provides in-line, autologous reconstruction for a reasonable price and at relatively low morbidity in selected clinical settings. Stents function by holding open an obstructed arterial segment and may be used to supplement balloon angioplasty when necessary. The relative roles of other techniques are also noted. Chapter 32 reviews the principles and fundamental considerations associated with endovascular intervention. The complications of endovascular techniques are detailed in Chapter 53. Thrombolytic therapy and its uses are discussed in Chapter 28.

APPLYING ENDOVASCULAR CONCEPTS TO CLINICAL PRACTICE

Specialists among all disciplines are enthusiastic about the concept of effective, low morbidity therapy for vascular disease introduced through a remote access site. The application of this concept to clinical practice requires a thorough understanding of both the clinical situations and the skills of endovascular intervention. Catheters form the avenue for endovascular surgery; they are disposable, and relatively inexpensive, and most are not complex in design or application. Catheter-based therapy has had a more significant impact on the treatment of lower extremity ischemia than elsewhere in the noncoronary circulation. Occlusive disease is more common and the vasculature more forgiving in the lower extremity than in other locations.[1–3]

Despite advances, there are several reasons why a precise role for endovascular intervention in the lower extremity is still difficult to define:

1. Rapid changes in technology have made it difficult to obtain long-term results with any approach before "improvements" are made in equipment or technique. In this environment, the learning curve for new procedures and modified techniques is continually renewed.
2. Vast differences in lesion and patient mix have made reported results difficult to compare, and relatively few randomized trials have been conducted.
3. Developing technology and maturing endovascular skills have fostered the treatment of increasingly more complex lesions, especially in the iliac and superficial femoral arteries. Often, these procedures are replacing open surgery, even though their results are not comparable to results accumulated for the treatment of focal lesions.
4. Part of the promise of endovascular intervention is less expensive treatment. It is difficult to assess actual costs, however, especially when the cost of maintaining patency may be high and should be included.
5. An "arteriographic schism," an arbitrary division of clinical and technical expertise distributed among various specialties, results in crusades for the exclusivity of one approach or another.
6. Varying local levels of interest and expertise lead to wide variations in the aggressiveness and manner in which endovascular techniques are applied to clinical practice.

Spectrum of Endovascular Practice

Although the precise role in management is difficult to define, it is generally accepted that endovascular approaches play an integral role in the management of chronic infrarenal atherosclerotic occlusive disease. Balloon catheters for PTA have been widely available for more than 20 years, and long-term follow-up data are available for the aortoiliac and infrainguinal arteries.

In the interim, multiple techniques have been developed that are shaping endovascular practice; they include:

- Digital subtraction arteriography
- Refinement and miniaturization of guide wires, catheters, and access sheaths
- Improved balloon technology
- Thrombolytic therapy
- Stents

Higher-resolution imaging permits shorter procedures with smaller loads of contrast agent. Improved guide wires allow more lesions to be traversed safely. Better catheters result in fewer aborted procedures and intraprocedural complications. Thrombolytic therapy facilitates more aggressive treatment of occlusions. Stents have made the management of more complex lesions possible.

These techniques have expanded the spectrum of peripheral arterial occlusive disease that is appropriate for mechanical treatment. Continued advances will likely be supported by enthusiasm among endovascular specialists, the medical device industry, and patients themselves.

Role of Stents

Stents have permitted an endovascular approach to complex infrarenal occlusive lesions that previously would have been manageable only with open operation. Stents provide a "bailout" method of treatment for acute postangioplasty dissections and residual stenoses, thus avoiding emergency operation or acute limb-threatening ischemia (Fig. 72–1).[4–8] Endovascular specialists are tackling lesions that they would not previously have considered for fear of causing catastrophic complications.[9–16] The availability of stents has also supported the development of stent-grafts, which are intended to furnish a completely new endoluminal lining via catheter-based delivery (see Chapter 38).

Stents vary in design, size, length, material, rigidity, method of expansion, and cost. The Palmaz stent* is rigid and balloon-expandable; the Wallstent† is flexible and self-expandable. Both the Palmaz stent and the Wallstent have been approved for limited clinical use in the United States. Both of these stents have been extensively deployed in the iliac arteries and have had a significant effect on endovascular practice. Multiple other stents are in various stages of development or clinical use outside the United States.[6, 17–20]

PATIENT EVALUATION

The decision as to whether a patient with lower extremity ischemia should undergo any procedure is based on the history and physical examination, supplemented as needed with noninvasive vascular testing and evaluation of the severity of disease in other organ systems. Clinical evaluation usually establishes (1) the extent of disability, (2) the threat to limb viability, (3) the general location and severity of the occlusive lesions, (4) the anesthetic risk, and (5) the patient's prospects for long-term survival. Almost any patient who is a candidate for open surgery should also be considered a potential candidate for endovascular intervention. In addition, some patients who are candidates for an endovascular approach would not be considered candidates for open surgery because of co-morbidities that predict excessive surgical risk.

*A product of Cordis, A Johnson & Johnson Company, Miami, Fla.
†A product of Schneider USA, Plymouth, Minn.

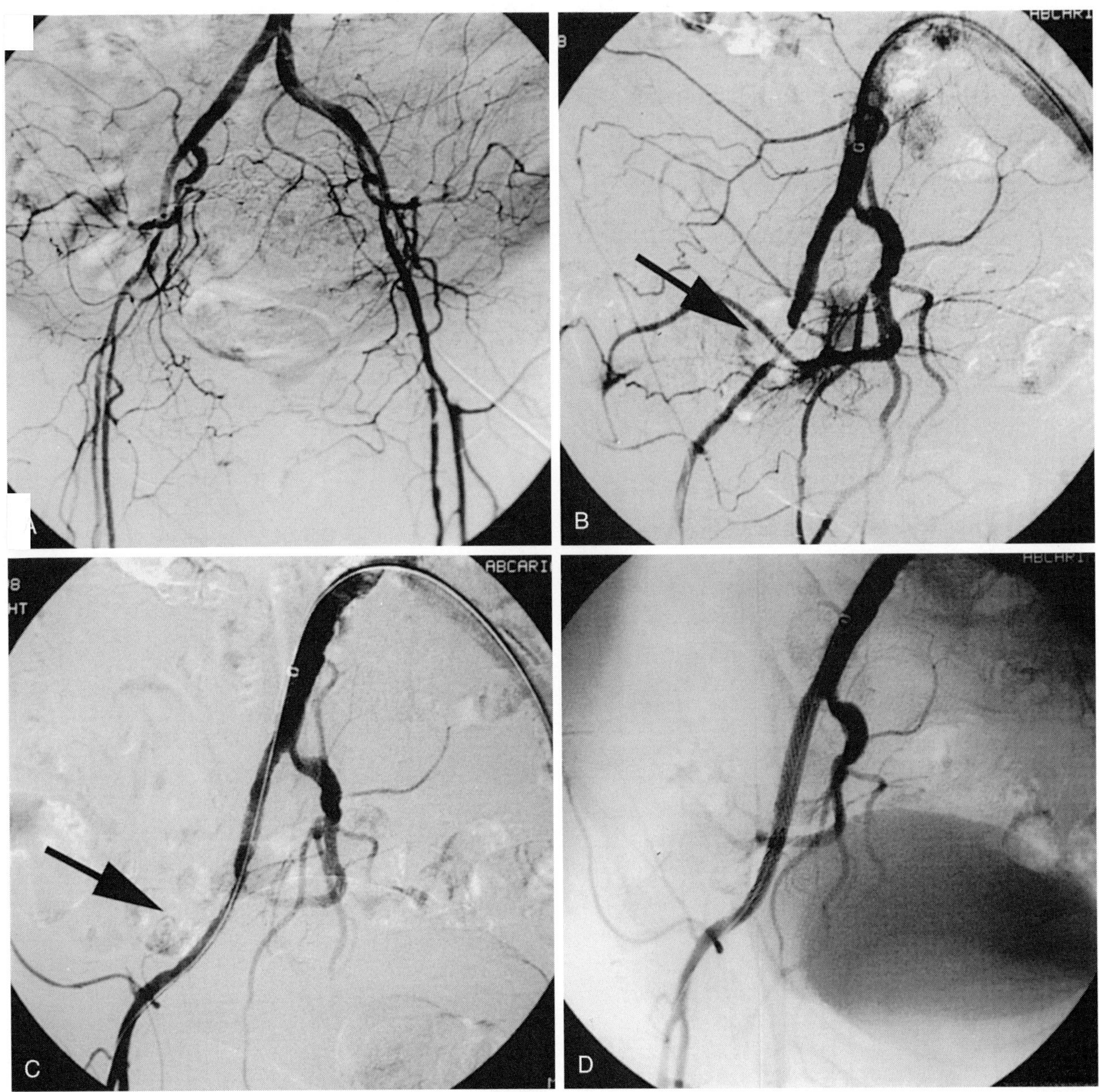

FIGURE 72–1. Stent placement provides a method of treatment for inadequate results after percutaneous transluminal balloon angioplasty (PTA). *A*, Aortogram of a 65-year-old woman with very-short-distance right leg claudication and clinical evidence of iliac artery disease. *B*, Left anterior oblique projection of the right external iliac artery revealed a long, critical stenosis *(arrow)*. *C*, After PTA to 7 mm, there was a residual stenosis and a systolic pressure gradient of 30 mmHg *(arrow)*. *D*, A Wallstent was placed, and another angioplasty was performed. Completion arteriography showed no residual stenosis, and there was no pressure gradient.

The greater cost and risk of surgery must be balanced against the lower durability and more limited applicability of PTA. From evaluation of various factors associated with the lesion and the clinical situation, the likely outcome of PTA can be predicted and can be compared with the anticipated results of arterial reconstruction (see later discussion). Understanding these factors is essential to appropriate evaluation of patients and assessment of their candidacy for endovascular intervention.

Noninvasive Evaluation

Mapping of the aortoiliac and femoropopliteal segments with duplex scanning (duplex mapping) is useful in identifying lesions that are likely to be amenable to PTA.[21–27] A combination of indirect noninvasive tests and aortoiliac duplex mapping may be used to identify inflow stenosis with a high degree of accuracy.[23, 28, 29] Duplex mapping has even better accuracy and greater reproducibility in evaluating the femoropopliteal segment.[21, 23, 24] Stenoses and occlusions may be distinguished and points of reconstitution may be identified. In patients who are candidates for endovascular intervention, noninvasive vascular evaluation serves several purposes; it:

1. Identifies disease that may be treated by PTA.
2. Provides objective baseline evidence of the extent of lower extremity ischemia.

3. Gauges the relative contributions of multiple occlusive lesions to the overall level of ischemia.

Arteriography Is Strategic, Not Diagnostic

Arteriography is invasive and expensive and has associated complications; it should not be used to screen patients for lesions amenable to endovascular intervention.[30–32] Diagnosis can almost always be made on the basis of clinical evaluation and noninvasive testing. As such, the contemporary role of arteriography consists of the strategic planning of revascularization and periprocedural guidance of endovascular interventions.[33] Arteriography is justified when the decision has been made to proceed with revascularization. When possible, arteriography should be performed in a manner that facilitates the performance of PTA during the same procedure, if this option is considered most appropriate.

FACTORS AFFECTING OUTCOME

Factors that influence the results of endovascular intervention for the ischemic lower extremity are (Table 72–1)

- Characteristics of lesion
- Pattern of arterial occlusive disease
- Patient demographics
- The clinical situation
- Intraprocedural factors

Patient demographics and the clinical situation are determined by clinical evaluation. Duplex mapping reveals preliminary information about lesion characteristics and the overall pattern of disease, and the arteriogram provides additional anatomic data. Intraprocedural factors may arise during PTA. In general, larger arteries are more easily and successfully treated than smaller ones, and patients with mild ischemia caused by focal disease with good runoff fare better.

TABLE 72–1. FACTORS AFFECTING OUTCOME OF ENDOVASCULAR INTERVENTIONS FOR CHRONIC LOWER EXTREMITY ISCHEMIA

Lesion characteristics
Location of lesion
Stenosis versus occlusion
Lesion length
Multiple stenoses in same segment
Other morphologic factors
Pattern of vascular disease
Multilevel occlusive disease
Runoff status
Patient demographics
Gender
Diabetes
Clinical situation
Indication for intervention
Recurrent stenosis
Intraprocedural factors
Dissection or residual stenosis after percutaneous balloon angioplasty
Initial hemodynamic response

Characteristics of Lesions

Because the aim of endovascular techniques is to achieve in-line repair of the artery rather than its replacement as with bypass surgery, characteristics of the lesion significantly influence the difficulty of the procedure and its expected outcome.

Location

The long-term patency following PTA depends on the dilatation site. Proximal, larger-caliber arteries offer the best initial and long-term results, with progressively decreasing long-term patency rates for more distal dilatation sites.

The mean patency rate for PTA of infrarenal aortic lesions was 80% at 5 years, compared with 69% for iliac arteries according to pooled data from the literature.[34] Dilatation sites in the common iliac artery have better patency rates than those in the external iliac artery (65% versus 48%, respectively, at 4 years).[35] Many studies have established the superiority of the results of iliac PTA over that of femoropopliteal PTA.[36–40] Among patients in the University of Toronto series, 5-year patency rates were 60% for iliac PTA and 38% for femoropopliteal PTA (Fig. 72–2).[37, 38] PTA of above-knee popliteal lesions was associated with better results than PTA of below-knee popliteal lesions.[38] PTA of the femoropopliteal arteries had twice the initial failure rate of PTA of the iliac arteries (16% versus 8%) and twice the early failure rate at 1 year (20% versus 10%).[39]

Stenosis versus Occlusion

The initial and long-term results of endovascular reconstruction are better for stenoses than for occlusions of the iliac arteries. Technical failure occurs in 10% to 20% of iliac occlusions but only 1% to 5% of iliac stenoses.[34, 35, 41, 42] The University of Toronto data demonstrated 3-year patency rates of 48% for iliac occlusions and 61% for iliac stenoses.[35] More recently, stents have been placed in an attempt to improve results in treating occlusions.[6, 42–47]

Compared with stenoses, occlusions in the femoral and popliteal arteries are associated with a higher rate of technical failures (18% versus 7%) and complications (22% versus 7%).[48] After successful dilatation, however, the long-term results may be similar for the two types of lesions. Some series have shown a 10% to 20% advantage in late outcome favoring stenoses over occlusions,[38, 49, 50] whereas others have found no difference.[48, 51, 52]

Length

The longer the stenosis, the lower the patency rate after PTA.[48, 50, 53, 54] Longer iliac artery stenoses have lower patency rates than shorter lesions after PTA alone or PTA with stent placement.[9, 53, 55–58] Some investigators have suggested that lesion length should be a relative indication for stent placement in the iliac artery, although the results of this approach are not yet conclusive.[10, 58]

Longer lesions have a significantly negative effect on the results of femoropopliteal PTA.[36, 48, 50] A detailed breakdown of femoropopliteal lesion length reveals steadily decreasing 5-year success rates for longer occlusions: 40% for occlusions measuring 0 to 9 cm, 29% for those 9 to 14 cm, and 17% for those longer than 14 cm.[36]

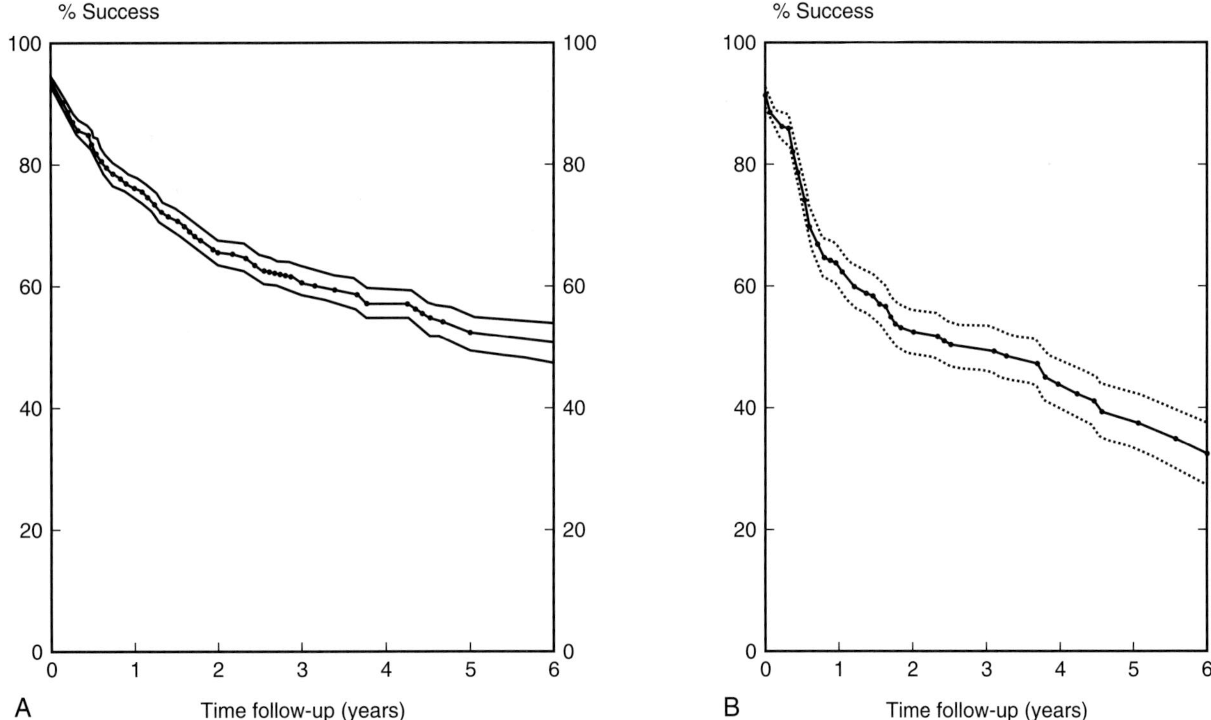

FIGURE 72–2. Results of iliac and femoropopliteal percutaneous transluminal balloon angioplasty (PTA). *A*, This curve represents a Kaplan-Meier life-table analysis of the results of 662 iliac PTAs in the University of Toronto series. The cumulative percentage success (mean ± SE) is plotted against time of follow-up. (From Johnston KW: Iliac arteries: Reanalysis of results of balloon angioplasty. Radiology 186:207–212, 1993.) *B*, This curve represents a Kaplan-Meier life-table analysis of the results of 254 femoropopliteal PTAs in the University of Toronto series. The cumulative percentage success (mean ± SE) is plotted against time of follow-up. (From Johnston KW: Femoral and popliteal arteries: Reanalysis of results of balloon angioplasty. Radiology 183:767–771, 1992.)

Multiple Stenoses in the Same Segment

Lesions composed of multiple stenoses present more potential sites for dissection, residual stenosis, or recurrent stenosis. The outlook after PTA for these lesions is inferior to that for focal stenosis over the long term in both iliac and femoropopliteal segments.[37, 38, 59] The initial success rate for iliac artery occlusions was 80% after dilatation of one site but was 46% when multiple sites required PTA.[35]

Other Morphologic Features

Calcification of a stenotic lesion may affect long-term patency after PTA, but there is no reasonable way to classify lesions according to the extent of calcification. Heavily calcified lesions are more likely to rupture, dissect, or cause a residual stenosis after PTA.

Eccentricity of the lesion is probably not important provided that a good hemodynamic correction has been achieved.[51] Eccentricity has been correlated with inferior results in some studies. Some investigators consider lesion eccentricity in the iliac segment an indication for stent placement. In the femoropopliteal arteries, lesion eccentricity is associated with a higher rate of early failure due to dissection.[48] Intravascular ultrasound may be used in the future to evaluate these lesion characteristics and determine their potential clinical significance.

Pattern of Vascular Disease

The pattern of vascular disease indicates the extent of involvement with atherosclerosis and the presence or absence of runoff lesions that may negatively affect the success at a PTA site.

Multilevel Occlusive Disease

Stenosis or occlusion of more than one arterial segment in an ischemic extremity may still be treated with PTA. Each dilated site has its own failure rate, however, and failure at any site could negatively affect the entire reconstruction. When both common and external iliac arteries require dilatation, the 4-year patency rate is 52%, versus 65% for a common iliac artery PTA alone.[35] In addition, the 3-year clinical benefit of iliac artery stent placement is 92% for focal disease and 61% for multilevel occlusive lesions.[59]

Runoff Status

Although runoff status is not simple to quantify, multiple studies have identified it as a significant prognostic factor in the outcome of endovascular intervention.[38, 48, 53] Good runoff was a strong predictor of success after iliac PTA (73% at 3 years versus 30% for poor runoff).[37] This difference is accentuated in diabetic patients, who often have severe distal disease compromising runoff. In a study of PTA in diabetic patients, there was a 19% difference between groups with good runoff and poor runoff at 1 year (95% versus 76%, respectively), but at 5 years, there was an almost fourfold difference in patency (77% versus 20%).[56]

Most studies of femoropopliteal PTA have found that runoff status influenced the outcome.[50, 51, 60, 61] Krepel and colleagues[51] reported 5-year success rates of 77% and 59% for patients with good runoff and poor runoff, respectively. Gallino and associates[60] reported better early (2-day) and late (2-year) success rates among patients with two or three patent tibial arteries (86% and 71%, respectively) than those who had one or no patent tibial artery (43% and 36%). In the series reported by Johnston and coworkers,[62] the 5-year primary patency rate was 50% for stenoses with good runoff, 38% for stenoses with poor runoff, 34% for occlusions with good runoff, and 20% for occlusions with poor runoff; the length of lesion treated was not taken into account. Another study documented 2-year patency rates after femoropopliteal PTA as 55% in limbs with good runoff and 23% in limbs with poor runoff.[50]

Patient Demographics

Multiple demographic factors may influence the results of endovascular intervention, but these variables are difficult to isolate, and the relative importance of each cannot be independently verified.

Gender

Women have a lower patency rate after external iliac PTA than men (57% versus 34%, respectively, at 3 years).[35] Gender differences for all types of vascular reconstructions have attracted interest recently and will be a subject of scrutiny in years to come.[59]

Diabetes

The presence of diabetes correlates with poorer results in some series.[48, 53, 60, 62, 63] However, diabetes characteristically produces a different distribution of occlusive lesion disease, with proportionally fewer favorable proximal iliac lesions and a high incidence of infrapopliteal occlusive lesions, which result in poor runoff. For the same combination of occlusive lesions, there was no significant difference between diabetic and nondiabetic patients in outcome following angioplasty.[56, 64]

Clinical Situation

The clinical presentation influences the outcome: The worse the ischemia, the less likely is a successful long-term outcome for endovascular intervention.

Indication for Intervention

One of the strongest predictors of outcome is the indication for the procedure; patients with claudication have better long-term success rates and require fewer amputations than patients with limb-threatening ischemia. Limb-threatening ischemia is usually associated with a more diffuse, multilevel pattern of atherosclerosis and poor runoff. Patients who require PTA for limb salvage are also more likely to have other co-morbidities and a more limited life span.[65, 66] The long-term patency rate for both iliac and femoropopliteal PTA procedures is significantly better among patients with claudication than among those with limb-threatening ischemia.[35–38, 40] This is also the case for iliac artery stent placement.[58, 67]

Recurrent Stenosis

Reports on the long-term results of repeat dilatation following failed iliac angioplasties show reasonable results.[53, 60, 62, 68] Several studies found similar initial and long-term success rates following first and second dilatations, although with relatively smaller numbers of patients and shorter follow-up intervals.[60, 62, 69]

The initial success of PTA for recurrent femoropopliteal lesions associated with claudication was 63%; for patients with gangrene and recurrent disease, it was 47%.[69] In another study, second femoropopliteal PTA procedures resulted in a 2-year patency rate of 20%.[70] Stenosis recurring after femoropopliteal PTA has a high chance of recurring after a second procedure; surgical reconstruction should be considered instead. Some surgeons have included second PTA procedures in reporting long-term results so are actually reporting secondary patency rates.[41, 52, 71–73]

Intraprocedural Factors

The previously described factors are determined prior to the endovascular procedure. Additional events may occur during the periprocedural period and subsequently influence long-term results. Prior to the development of stents, intraprocedural complications at the PTA site, such as post-angioplasty dissection, a significant residual stenosis, or a poor hemodynamic result, often caused sudden early failure and occasionally resulted in urgent surgical reconstruction. These events may be corrected with stent placement, the long-term results of which are being evaluated.

Post-PTA Dissection or Residual Stenosis

Flow-limiting dissection or residual stenosis (>30%) occurs after PTA in up to 10% of patients.[5, 6, 40, 74] Stents may be placed to correct inadequate PTA in either the iliac or femoropopliteal artery. The 3-year patency rate for iliac stent placement for post-PTA dissection or residual stenosis ranges from 54% to 86%.[4, 58, 75] It is not clear how the results of stenting these "complicated" cases compare with simple dilatation over the long term. The results of stent placement so far reflect a decrease in early failure rates.[42]

Initial Hemodynamic Response

After angioplasty, the extent of improvement in the ankle-brachial index (ABI) serves as a gauge of the immediate hemodynamic improvement and also as a prognostic indicator. Improvement in the ABI after iliac PTA has been shown to be strongly predictive of sustained patency.[37, 49]

INDICATIONS FOR ENDOVASCULAR INTERVENTION: EMPHASIS ON GUIDELINES

Once the determination has been made that the ischemia is significant enough to warrant mechanical intervention, the role played by endovascular intervention depends on an understanding of its benefits and risks and how they compare with other treatment options. Guidelines were proposed in 1994 by an American Heart Association (AHA) Task Force for PTA in each infrarenal vascular segment.[40] These guidelines were derived from accumulated clinical experience with PTA at the time and from analyses of influential factors and their effect on outcome. The arteriographic extent of disease was divided into four categories, and the appropriateness of endovascular intervention compared with open surgery was indicated in each category. Table 72–2 contains (1) a general description of categories of occlusive disease, (2) an index of the clinical usefulness of endovascular intervention and open surgery in each disease category, (3) recommendations for management of disease in each category with either endovascular intervention or open surgery, and (4) the previously published recommendations of the AHA.

Much has changed since the original AHA guidelines were proposed. More rigorous reporting standards have been instituted, leading to a more accurate assessment of results. Longer post-intervention follow-up is available for PTA in all types of infrarenal occlusive lesions. Intravascular stents are now commonly utilized and must be taken into account by the surgeon considering which lesions to treat with endovascular intervention. Practitioners in multiple specialties have become interested in comparing various endovascular and open surgical treatment options. Therefore, the authors have developed updated guidelines that take these factors into account. Table 72–3 summarizes

TABLE 72–2. INDICATIONS FOR LOWER EXTREMITY ENDOVASCULAR INTERVENTION BASED ON LESION ARTERIOGRAPHIC CATEGORIES OF DISEASE

	GENERAL DESCRIPTION OF DISEASE	CLINICAL USEFULNESS BASED UPON RISKS/BENEFITS		AUTHORS' RECOMMENDATION	AMERICAN HEART ASSOCIATION CATEGORIES OF DISEASE
		PTA	Surgery		
Category 1	Short, focal, stenotic disease at the site of intervention. Mild or no disease in the proximal or distal arterial segments.	+ + +	0	Surgery not indicated as initial treatment.	Lesions for which PTA alone is the procedure of choice. Treatment of these lesions will result in a high technical success rate and will generally result in complete relief of symptoms or normalization of pressure gradients.
Category 2	Moderate-length, focal, stenotic disease at the site of intervention. Mild disease in the proximal or distal arterial segments.	+ +	+	PTA is appropriate initial therapy. Surgery is initial therapy in selected cases, such as young, good risk patients.	Lesions that are well suited for PTA. Treatment of these lesions will result in complete relief or significant improvement in symptoms, pulses, or pressure gradients. This category includes lesions that will be treated by procedures to be followed by surgical bypass to treat multilevel vascular disease.
Category 3	Long stenotic disease or short occlusion at site of intervention. Moderate disease in the proximal or distal arterial segments.	+	+ +	Surgery is initial therapy except in selected cases, such as prohibitive surgical risk.	Lesions that may be treated with PTA, but because of disease extent, location, or severity have a significantly lower chance of initial technical success or long term benefit than if treated with surgery. However, PTA may be performed, generally because of patient risk factors or because of lack of suitable bypass material.
Category 4	Diffuse or extensive stenotic disease or long occlusion at site of intervention. Severe disease in the proximal or distal arterial segments.	0	+ + +	Surgery preferable; PTA not indicated.	Extensive vascular disease, for which PTA has a very limited role because of low technical success rate or poor long-term benefit. In very-high-risk patients or in those for whom no surgical procedure is applicable, PTA may have some place.

Modified from Pentecost MJ, Criqui MH, Dorros G, et al: Guidelines for peripheral percutaneous transluminal angioplasty of the abdominal aorta and lower extremity vessels. Circulation 89:511–531, 1994.

Key: + with minimal disease elsewhere in that segment; + + with mild/moderate occlusive disease elsewhere in that segment; + + + with moderate to severe occlusive disease elsewhere in that segment. PTA = percutaneous transluminal angioplasty.

TABLE 72–3. SUITABILITY OF LESIONS FOR ENDOVASCULAR INTERVENTION OR SURGERY BASED ON EXTENT OF DISEASE

	AORTA	ILIAC ARTERY	FEMOROPOPLITEAL ARTERIES	INFRAPOPLITEAL ARTERIES (USED FOR LIMB SALVAGE ONLY)
Category 1	Short (<2 cm) concentric noncalcified stenosis of the intrarenal aorta (+)	Short (<2 cm) concentric noncalcified stenosis of the common or external iliac artery (+)	Short (<2 cm) stenosis not involving the proximal superficial femoral artery or distal popliteal artery (+)	Short (<1 cm) stenosis of an infrapopliteal artery (+)
Category 2	1. Medium-length (2–5 cm) noncomplex stenosis, or 2. Short (<2 cm) complex (calcified, eccentric) stenosis (+)	1. Medium-length (2–5 cm) noncomplex stenosis of the common or external iliac artery, or 2. Short (<2 cm) complex (eccentric, calcified) stenosis (+)	1. Medium-length (2–5 cm) stenosis, or 2. Short (<2 cm) occlusion (+)	Two or three short (<1 cm) stenoses of an infrapopliteal artery (+)
Category 3	1. Long (>5 cm) simple stenosis, or 2. Medium-length (2–5 cm) complex (calcified, eccentric) stenosis (+ +)	1. Long (5–10 cm) simple stenosis of the common iliac artery, or 2. Medium-length (2–5 cm) complex stenosis of the common or external iliac artery (+ +)	1. Long (5–10 cm) stenosis 2. 2 or 3 short (<2 cm) stenoses 3. Heavily calcified stenosis up to 5 cm 4. Occlusion (2–5 cm) in length) 5. Lesion of the proximal superficial femoral artery or the distal popliteal artery (+ +)	1. Moderate length (1–2 cm) stenosis 2. Tibial trifurcation stenosis 3. Multiple short (<1 cm) stenoses (+ +)
Category 4	1. Long (>5 cm) complex stenosis 2. Aortic occlusion 3. Aortic lesion with abdominal aortic aneurysm or another lesion requiring aortoiliac surgery (+ + +)	1. Any iliac stenosis > 10 cm 2. Occlusion > 2 cm 3. Another lesion requiring aortoiliac surgery 4. External iliac stenosis which extends to the common femoral artery 5. Long (>5 cm) stenosis of the external iliac artery 6. Any complex stenosis > 5 cm (+ + +)	1. Multiple lesions 2. Any stenosis > 10 cm 3. Any occlusion > 5 cm 4. Any heavily calcified lesion > 8 cm 5. Coexisting common femoral artery occlusion 6. Distal popliteal occlusion (+ + +)	1. Tibial occlusion 2. Long (>2 cm) stenosis (+ + +)

Key: + with minimal disease elsewhere in that segment; + + with mild/moderate occlusive disease elsewhere in that segment; + + + with moderate to severe occlusive disease elsewhere in that segment.

the suitability of lesions for treatment with endovascular intervention and open surgery based on arteriographic categories of disease. Categories of disease (1 through 4) were applied to lesions of the aorta, iliac, femoropopliteal, and infrapopliteal arteries through the use of the format previously proposed by the AHA.[40]

Best results are achieved with the use of endovascular intervention for category 1 lesions, which represent the least severe manifestation of occlusive disease and for which PTA is usually the treatment of choice. Endovascular intervention is progressively less useful for the more severe forms of disease in categories 2 and 3. PTA is reasonable as initial therapy for patients with category 2 disease; however, many patients so treated later require surgery for endovascular failures. Most category 3 diseases require open surgery, but it may occasionally be reasonable to attempt PTA in patients with prohibitive surgical risks. Category 4 disease is not amenable to endovascular intervention and is almost always treated surgically.

A number of clinically significant issues essential to patient care cannot be adequately expressed in terms of guidelines; they are:

- Expertise of the treating physician
- Impact of the ischemic symptoms on the patient's life
- Projected life span of the patient (during which time, it is hoped, the properly chosen intervention will continue to relieve ischemia)
- Consequences of failure
- Long-term cost of care

In addition, insufficient data are available to determine the ultimate role of stents and exactly how the indications for endovascular intervention should be modified to include stents, especially in the infrarenal aorta and iliac arteries.

Indications for Endovascular Aortoiliac Intervention

PTA is best for short, focal stenoses of the aorta or iliac arteries that cause significant symptoms (category 1 lesions). The justification for an endovascular approach to a wide variety of other types of lesions in other locations has been based on extrapolation from the excellent results achieved with focal aortoiliac stenosis.

Isolated, focal stenosis of the infrarenal aorta is an uncommon manifestation of vascular disease because aortic disease is usually diffuse, or accompanied by significant iliac occlusive disease, or both. Therefore, the number of cases and length of follow-up are much less for aortic PTA than for iliac PTA. Nevertheless, aortic PTA is appropriate for many lesions in category 1 and some in category 2 (see Table 72–3). Experience with aortic stents is limited but suggests that dissections and residual stenoses after PTA of category 1 or 2 lesions are adequately treated with stent placement. The availability of stents may extend indications for PTA to some patients with category 3 lesions, although the results of this approach are not yet known.

PTA alone is usually all that is required to achieve good results for most patients with iliac lesions in category 1. Stents have had a major impact on endovascular treatment of the diseased iliac segment. The option of stent placement for post-PTA complications provides encouragement for the treatment of many lesions in category 2 and some in category 3 that previously would have qualified only for open operations. The risk and cost of treating long lesions or occlusions with endovascular intervention are higher, however, and the long-term results are inferior to those obtained in the treatment of focal lesions.

Routine, primary stent placement cannot be justified by currently available data, but selective stent placement should be considered for lesions that are recurrent or occluded and for postangioplasty dissection or residual stenosis.

Multilevel lower extremity occlusive disease may be amenable to endovascular intervention for an iliac lesion and distal operative reconstruction. When a discrete iliac stenosis is located opposite a diffusely diseased or occluded contralateral iliac artery or proximal to an ipsilateral infrainguinal occlusion, dilatation of the iliac stenosis may be performed with a femorofemoral or distal bypass, respectively.

Diffuse or excessively lengthy lesions, multiple stenoses in the same segment, severe bilateral iliac disease, long occlusions, and combined aortic and iliac disease are all best treated with arterial reconstruction, provided that the balance between operative risk and the threat of limb loss justifies such intervention. Other types of reconstructive techniques, such as atherectomy, laser, and endovascular grafts, have not matched the results of PTA with selective stent placement in terms of morbidity, cost, or results; these techniques should be considered only as last resorts or experimental alternatives.

Indications for Infrainguinal Endovascular Intervention

PTA is appropriate for short (<2 cm), focal stenoses in the superficial femoral or popliteal arteries (category 1 lesions). AHA guidelines advocate PTA for stenoses and occlusions up to 10 cm in length.[40] This level of aggressiveness with endovascular techniques is probably not justified in patients who are otherwise reasonable surgical candidates.

Long lesions (>5 cm), multiple short stenoses in the same segment, a single critical stenosis in a diffusely involved irregular segment, and most occlusions are all best treated with surgical arterial reconstruction if co-morbidities permit (category 3 and category 4 lesions). Femoropopliteal stent placement has not appreciably extended long-term patency rates and has increased complications and cost. Therefore, it should be considered only for extensive or flow-limiting postangioplasty dissection that is in imminent danger of causing acute occlusion.

Infrapopliteal angioplasty should be considered only for the rare patient with (1) a short, focal tibial artery stenosis that prevents in-line flow to the foot, (2) limb-threatening ischemia, and (3) significant contraindications to operation (see Table 72–3). Improvements in guide wire and catheter technology have contributed significantly to the feasibility of tibial PTA. Stents have not been adapted to the tibial arteries, however, so complications of PTA can usually be treated only with open operation. Results are not reliable or durable enough to justify the use of infrapopliteal PTA for purposes other than limb salvage.

PATIENT SELECTION: BEST-CASE AND WORST-CASE SCENARIOS

Although the lower periprocedural morbidity of an endovascular intervention is usually accompanied by a lower long-term patency rate than standard operative reconstruction, endovascular intervention is often the best choice for well-selected patients. In applying endovascular intervention, the surgeon assumes that PTA is a safe procedure and that it rarely makes matters worse.[76] It allows a wider spectrum of patients to be treated by expanding the array of options available in the treatment armamentarium. Endovascular techniques have the greatest clinical utility in two groups of patients at opposite ends of the spectrum of illness severity, which can be characterized as best-case and worst-case scenarios.

1. Patients with focal disease (category 1 lesions) causing claudication have the most favorable lesions for endovascular intervention. Although this clinical situation carries the most marginal indication for mechanical intervention, it is followed by the best results. Lifestyle-limiting discomfort with ambulation is a relative indication for intervention. Limb threat is not a major concern in this group, unless it occurs as the result of an endovascular procedural complication, such as embolization. If mechanical intervention is not undertaken, the usual alternative is exercise training.
2. A second, smaller group comprises patients with limb-threatening ischemia, usually due to diffuse or multilevel disease (category 3 or 4 lesions), for whom standard surgery poses a high risk. If PTA is used only when surgery is too risky despite absolute indications for intervention, the high proportion of cases with diffuse disease and poor runoff gives poor overall PTA results. Nevertheless, in patients facing certain limb loss and without other options, endovascular reconstruction can occasionally offer limb salvage, even after treatment of lesions that are unfavorable for an endovascular approach (Fig. 72–3).[77, 78]

Endovascular intervention is the best option in a substantial proportion of patients in these two groups. However, there is a less well-developed clinical sense of patient selection for endovascular intervention in the majority of

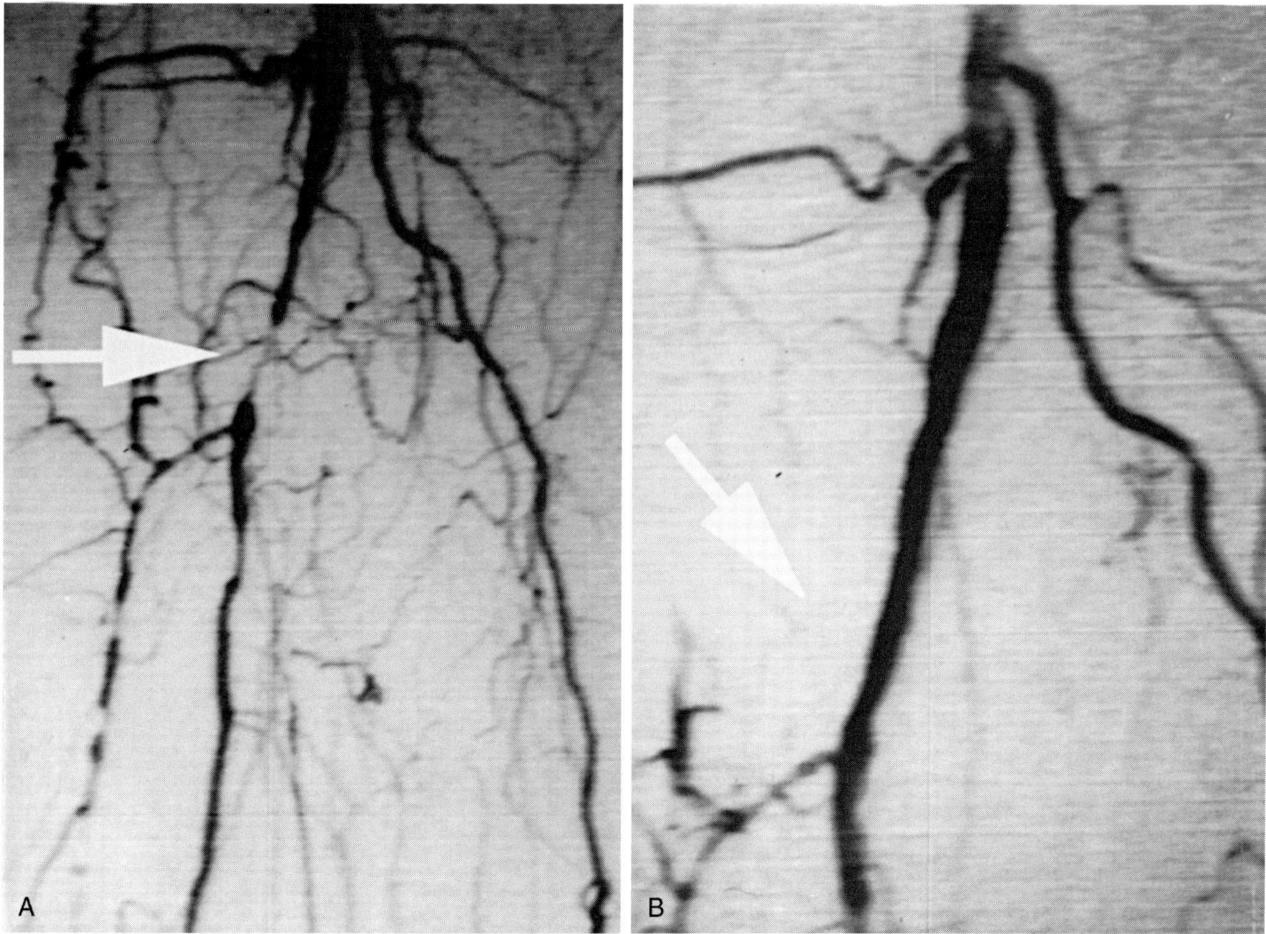

FIGURE 72–3. Distal popliteal percutaneous transluminal balloon angioplasty (PTA) for limb salvage. *A*, Gangrene of the tip of the fifth toe in a 69-year-old woman. Surgical risk was increased by cardiomyopathy, renal insufficiency, and chronic obstructive pulmonary disease. Physical examination suggested, and duplex mapping confirmed, adequate inflow to the popliteal level. A limited lower extremity arteriogram, obtained through an ipsilateral antegrade approach, demonstrated a long, critical stenosis of the distal below-knee popliteal artery *(arrow)*. *B*, The lesion was dilated to 4 mm. The arterial lumen was improved significantly on completion arteriography *(arrow)*. The wound was healed within 2 weeks, and the foot remained intact 2 years after PTA.

patients between these two extremes, for whom endovascular intervention and open surgery may both be options. The opportunity to replace an open operation and its associated risks with a percutaneous procedure and rapid return to activity is enticing. When endovascular techniques are employed indiscriminately, however, the usual results are expensive but short-lived reconstructions. Ischemia may be worsened or limbs lost before eventual definitive therapy can be delivered. The concept of always attempting PTA first, with surgery reserved for endovascular failures, becomes less cost-effective with the treatment of progressively more unfavorable (category 3 and category 4) lesions. There is also an inclination among many endovascular enthusiasts to treat lesions because they are able to do so rather than because they should, to develop a lesion-oriented approach rather than a patient-oriented approach. Patient selection for endovascular intervention is best guided by solid clinical indications in patients with favorable (category 1 or 2) lesions.

TECHNICAL CONSIDERATIONS

Improved overall care of lower extremity ischemia results from a better understanding by clinicians of the technical aspects of endovascular intervention. To the extent that the special procedures suite is a "black box" to many clinicians, the development of a balanced view of the benefits, risks, and clinical role of percutaneous endovascular intervention is a major challenge. Arteriography is detailed in Chapter 16, and general techniques of endovascular intervention are covered in Chapter 32. This discussion briefly describes some selected aspects specific to the endovascular skills required for lower extremity revascularization using balloon angioplasty and stents. Other references are available for additional detail.[79–82]

Conversion of an Arteriographic Procedure to a Therapeutic Procedure

The initial approach in arteriography should be chosen with the target lesion in mind so that PTA may be performed at the time of the arteriogram, if indicated. In general, the best approach for PTA and stent placement is the one that provides the shortest and most direct access to the lesion. Arteriography is usually performed through the femoral artery on the less symptomatic side so that the femoral artery on the more symptomatic side is available for either antegrade or retrograde puncture for PTA.

The simplest approach for most iliac lesions is an ipsilateral retrograde puncture and catheter placement. Lesions at the aortic bifurcation require the simultaneous passage and inflation of balloons in each iliac artery ("kissing balloon" technique). Distal external iliac artery lesions and proximal superficial femoral artery lesions are best approached from the contralateral side through passage of the catheter over the aortic bifurcation. Most infrainguinal lesions can be treated with an antegrade ipsilateral approach, which permits the maximum degree of control.

Crossing the Lesion

A floppy-tip guide wire is passed through the lesion under fluoroscopic guidance. If the guide wire passage fails, secondary choices are:

- Hydrophilic or steerable guide wires
- "Road mapping"
- Passage of the guide wire through a bent-tip, steerable catheter
- Approaching the lesion from another direction

The guide wire should not be forced or passed blindly. After it crosses the lesion, intraluminal position of the guide wire should be confirmed before one proceeds to PTA. Passing a catheter through a preocclusive lesion may stop flow through the lesion. This situation should be anticipated; the operator should consider heparin administration and should be prepared to dilate the lesion quickly. The location of the lesion is indicated on the skin with the use of external markers or bony landmarks. The utility of heparin administration varies for different angioplasty sites. In general, the more distal the site and the more complex the reconstruction, the more likely that heparin is necessary.

Choosing the Best Balloon

The diameter of the "normal" proximal or distal artery as measured on the cut film is used to choose balloon size, providing a slight overdilatation of the artery. If only digital subtraction arteriography is available, the balloon chosen is slightly undersized, and after the "waist" of atherosclerosis is dilated, a larger balloon diameter can be used if necessary. A significant initial overestimation of balloon diameter may result in rupture of the artery. The diameter of the common iliac artery is usually 7 to 10 mm; of the external iliac artery, 6 to 8 mm; of the superficial femoral artery, 5 to 7 mm; and of the popliteal artery, 4 to 6 mm. The balloon should be just long enough to extend slightly beyond the lesion.

Dilating the Lesion

The balloon catheter is passed over the guide wire and into correct position across the lesion, with the use of fluoroscopic guidance and the radiopaque markers on the catheter (Fig. 72–4). The balloon is inflated under fluoroscopic visualization with a 50% solution of contrast agent. As the balloon expands, the waist of atherosclerosis resolves when enough intraluminal pressure has been applied (Fig. 72–5). Inflation is maintained for 30 to 60 seconds, and is usually repeated.

Completion Arteriography

The balloon catheter is withdrawn after complete deflation has been ensured, but the guide wire position is maintained. After iliac PTA, completion arteriography may be obtained either through a catheter placed through the lesion over the same guide wire or through the contralateral iliac artery if a previous contralateral puncture was performed for arteriography. After infrainguinal PTA, completion arteriography is usually obtained through the antegrade sheath that was used to secure access.

Iliac Percutaneous Transluminal Angioplasty and Stent Placement

Single-balloon PTA may be performed in iliac lesions that begin a centimeter or more from the aortic bifurcation. Iliac PTA usually causes flank discomfort. Stent placement should be considered for recurrent stenosis or occluded segments. If completion arteriography reveals residual stenosis or significant dissection, stent placement is warranted (Figs. 72–6 and 72–7).

The choice of the stent is tailored to the lesion to be treated. The Palmaz stent has excellent hoop strength and is best for focal lesions or orifice lesions. Wallstents are more flexible and are useful for long or tortuous lesions.

Infrainguinal Percutaneous Transluminal Angioplasty

Most infrainguinal lesions are treated with an ipsilateral antegrade approach. Heparin is usually administered. The balloon catheter is advanced into the lesion under fluoroscopic guidance, and dilatation is performed (Fig. 72–8). The balloon catheter is removed to allow for completion arteriography. Intermittent fluoroscopic visualization must be obtained during catheter exchanges to ensure that guide wire position is maintained across the lesion. Stent placement should be considered only for post-PTA complications that threaten imminent occlusion at the PTA site.

Intraoperative Techniques

The most clinically useful combination of endovascular and open surgical techniques is iliac angioplasty for inflow followed by an infrainguinal surgical reconstruction. It is reasonable to perform concomitant intraoperative PTA and distal surgery when the iliac lesion is anatomically favorable (category 1 or 2) so that success is virtually assured (with supplementary stent placement if needed).

The patient is positioned on the operating table so that the iliac segment can be visualized with fluoroscopy. The arteries are exposed, the conduit is prepared, tunnels are made, and heparin is administered. The femoral artery is punctured, and a sheath is placed (Fig. 72–9). A guide wire is advanced through the lesion, a balloon catheter is placed, and dilatation is performed. Following completion arteriography, the femoral artery is cross-clamped, and the same arteriotomy is lengthened and used for the proximal anastomosis.

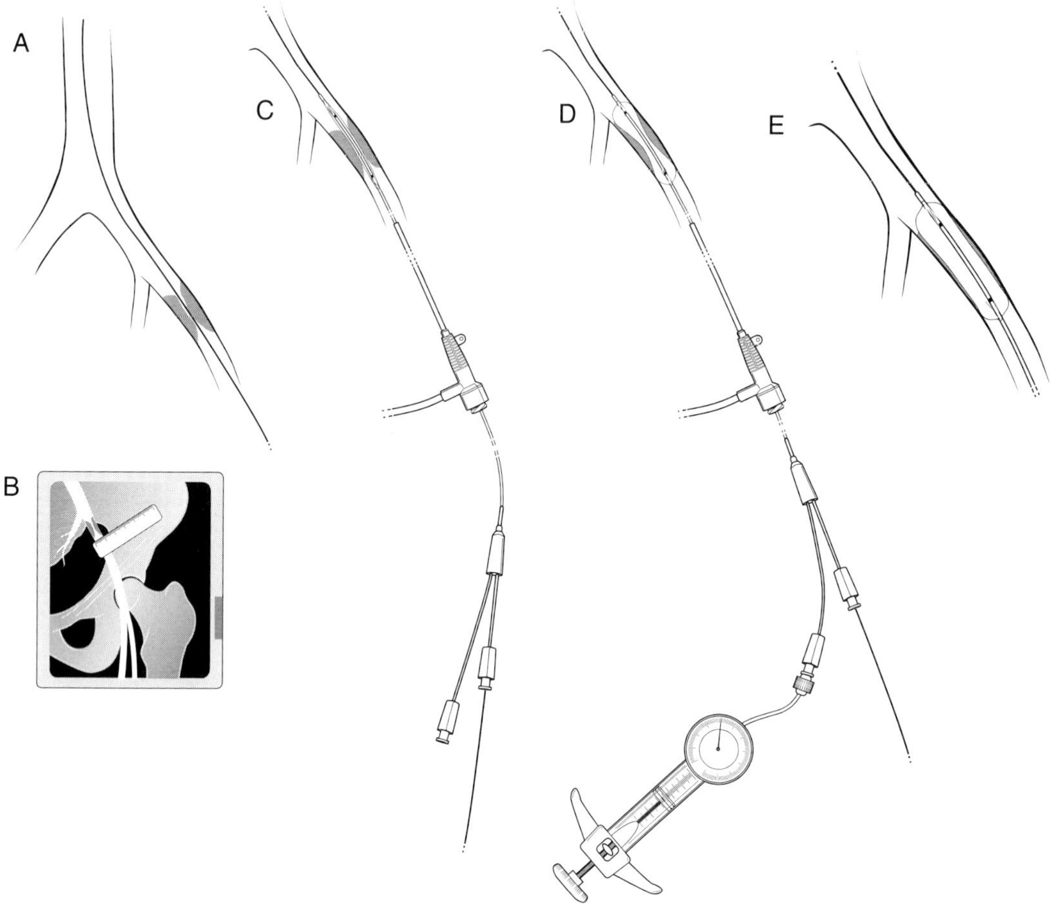

FIGURE 72–4. Technique of iliac artery balloon angioplasty. *A*, The guide wire is placed retrograde across an iliac artery stenosis. *B*, The diameter of the balloon is selected by measuring the diameter of the uninvolved, juxtaposed iliac artery on the cut-film arteriogram. *C*, The balloon catheter is passed over the guide wire, through the hemostatic access sheath, and positioned across the lesion by fluoroscopic guidance. *D*, The balloon is inflated with an inflation device that monitors pressure within the lumen. *E*, The lesion is dilated until the impression of the lesion on the balloon resolves and the balloon assumes a cylindrical shape, as determined on fluoroscopy. (From Schneider PA: Balloon angioplasty: Minimally invasive autologous revascularization. *In* Endovascular Skills. St. Louis, Quality Medical Publishing, 1998, pp 107–117.)

REPORTING RESULTS: EMPHASIS ON STANDARDIZED CRITERIA

The published results of endovascular interventions vary significantly, often because of differences in assessing and reporting results, as discussed in Chapter 3. The need to observe the same reporting standards used for bypass surgery has become more widely recognized.[83, 84] Problematic factors that pertain specifically to reporting results in the field of endovascular intervention for lower extremity ischemia are listed in Table 72–4. These problems have delayed progress in the field and have prompted the development of standards.[40, 85–88]

These standards should facilitate a better understanding of procedural outcomes. The Society of Vascular Surgeons/International Society for Cardiovascular Surgery (SVS/ISCVS) Ad Hoc Subcommittee on Reporting Standards for Endovascular Procedures and the AHA Task Force on PTA Guidelines both advised that the degree of chronic lower extremity ischemia be separated into categories 1 through 6, in the same manner as for surgical revascularization.[83] Arterial lesions should be described by location, type, and length of lesion and status of runoff (Table 72–5).[40, 87] Criteria for improvement after intervention consist of both clinical and hemodynamic assessments (Table 72–6).[83] Anatomic success is defined as a residual stenosis of less than 30%. Long-term results should be assessed in terms of the clinical and hemodynamic status and expressed in life-table format. These criteria are described further in Chapter 3.

The results of endovascular procedures are determined by many different factors, some of which cannot be stratified. Nevertheless, the uniform assessment and reporting of results at least facilitate comparisons between procedures and patient populations, which are essential in supporting advancement in endovascular intervention.

RESULTS OF AORTOILIAC ENDOVASCULAR INTERVENTION

Infrarenal Aorta

Numerous small series have demonstrated that reasonable patency rates may be achieved with PTA for focal stenosis of the infrarenal aorta.[89–94] In the largest series in the literature (38 patients), technical success was achieved in

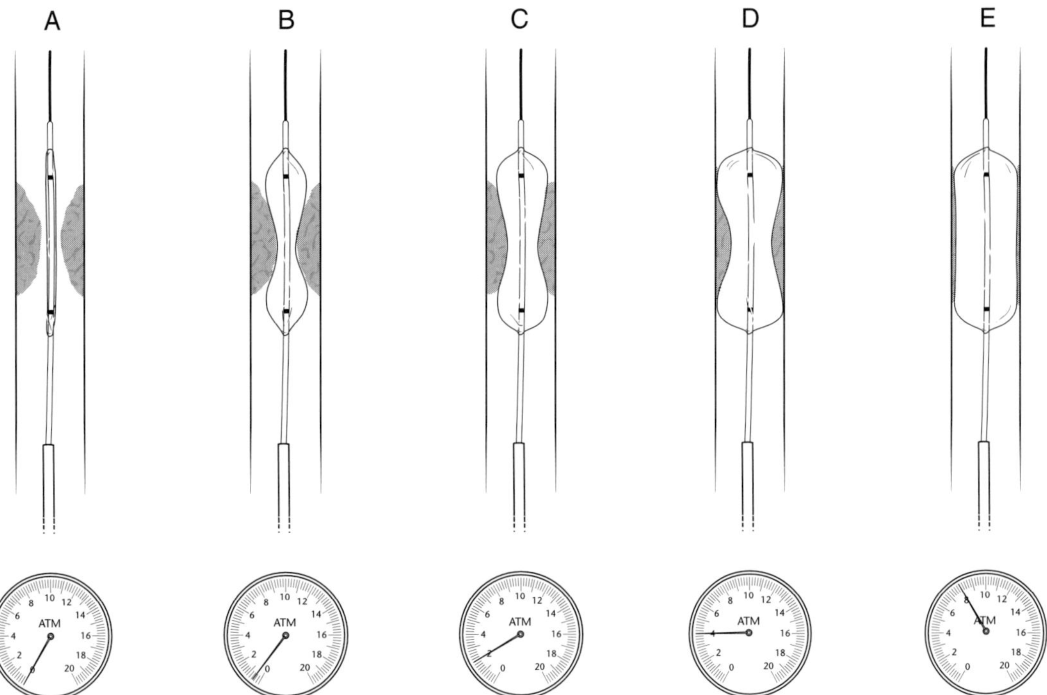

FIGURE 72–5. Dilatation of the atherosclerotic "waist." *A*, The balloon catheter is placed within the lesion. The radiopaque markers straddle the lesion. *B*, The balloon begins to take shape at low pressure. *C*, At 2 atmospheres (at) of pressure, the waist of atherosclerosis is evident. This represents the area of heaviest plaque formation and is usually the last area to be fully dilated. *D*, At 4 at, a substantial residual stenosis is present. *E*, When the pressure is doubled to 8 at, the waist is completely dilated. (From Schneider PA: Balloon angioplasty: Minimally invasive autologous revascularization. *In* Endovascular Skills. St. Louis, Quality Medical Publishing, 1998, pp 107–117.)

94% of cases.[94] All patients underwent follow-up aortography at a mean of 34 months, and 19% had recurrent stenosis. Among the 684 aortoiliac PTA procedures reported from the University of Toronto, only 17 were for focal aortic lesions, and the 5-year patency rate was 70%.[95] Rholl[34] summarized 17 series reported between 1980 and 1993, which ranged in size from 1 to 32 patients, and determined a technical success rate of 95% and patency rates of 98% at 1 year, 87% at 3 years, and 80% at 5 years.

Several reports of stented infrarenal aortic lesions are available.[4, 11–13, 93, 96–98] Stents have been successfully placed for residual stenosis or dissection after PTA[4, 96, 97] and for treatment of embolizing aortic lesions.[93] Thrombolysis has been used in a small number of patients to recanalize chronic aortic occlusions prior to stent placement.[11, 12] In one series, two of seven patients sustained distal embolization during aortic recanalization.[12] The role of aortic stents is not yet defined, and there is no reliable data on their patency.

TABLE 72–4. FACTORS PROMPTING DEVELOPMENT OF STANDARDS FOR ASSESSING AND REPORTING RESULTS OF LOWER EXTREMITY ENDOVASCULAR INTERVENTION

1. Initial failures should be reported so overall patency can be determined.
2. Primary, secondary, and primary assisted patency must be correctly categorized.
3. Objective criteria for determining procedural success must be included, both clinical and hemodynamic.
4. Documentation of the severity of underlying ischemia permits assessment of subsequent improvement and limb salvage rate.
5. Documentation of the severity and morphology of the underlying lesion permits lesion classification so that results may be compared.

Aortic Bifurcation

Occlusive lesions of the aortic bifurcation were initially not considered amenable to angioplasty because of the risk of dislodging aortic plaque. This technical problem was solved by introduction of the "kissing balloon" technique.[4, 41, 99–102] In this technique, a balloon catheter is placed retrograde into each iliac artery, and the balloons, which are of equal size, are inflated simultaneously to dilate the entire aortic bifurcation. Unfortunately, the results of PTA are difficult to interpret because these bifurcation lesions are usually included as part of larger series of iliac artery or aortic lesions. Because these lesions are orifice lesions that involve both iliac arteries, the results of treatment and the need for adjunctive measures, such as stents, may differ from those for isolated iliac stenoses.

A 1992 review of the literature identified 72 cases.[80] Patency rates ranged from 76% to 92% at 3 years. Later studies have demonstrated similar patency rates.[99, 100] The largest series reported to date comprised 79 patients with aortic bifurcation lesions. The cumulative clinical success rate at a mean of 4 years was 80%.[103]

Thrombolysis for aortic bifurcation occlusions has not been widely reported. In one series of note, recanalization was achieved with thrombolysis and PTA in 13 of 25 patients, thus avoiding aortofemoral bypass.[104]

More recently, stents have been used to reconstruct the

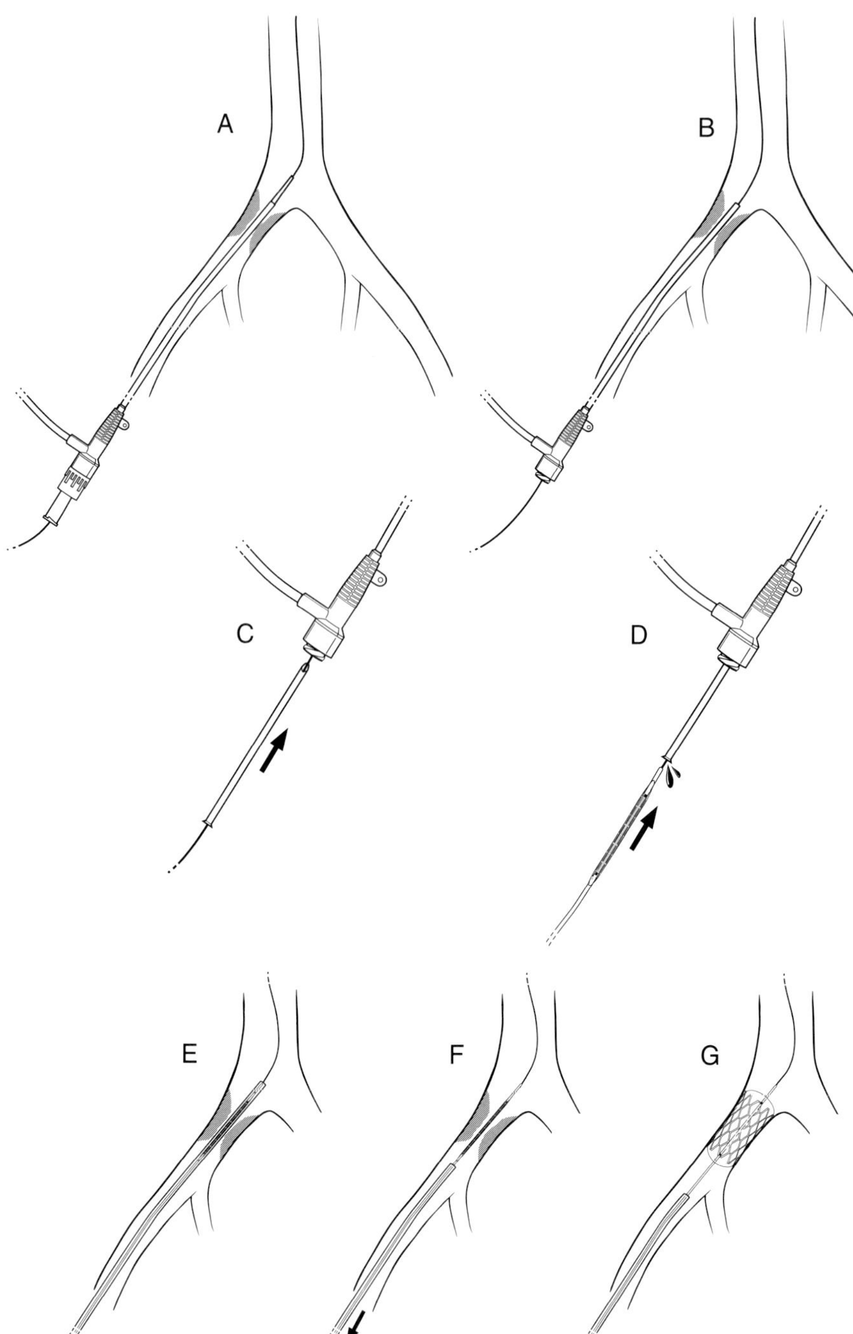

FIGURE 72–6. Technique of Palmaz stent placement. *A*, A long dilator and sheath are advanced across the iliac lesion. B, The dilator is removed, leaving the sheath across the stenosis. *C*, A metal introducer with a beveled end opens the hemostatic valve on the head of the sheath. *D*, The stent, which has been mounted on a balloon of appropriate length and diameter and crimped into place, is advanced into the sheath. *E*, The stent is placed at the desired location within the lesion using fluoroscopic guidance. *F*, The sheath is withdrawn to expose the mounted stent. *G*, The balloon is inflated to deploy the stent. (From Schneider PA: A stent is an intravascular graft. *In* Endovascular Skills. St. Louis, Quality Medical Publishing, 1998, pp 133–164.)

aortic bifurcation.[14, 82, 105] The "kissing stent" technique offers an option for bifurcation PTA that is complicated or inadequate, and it usually produces a strikingly appealing cosmetic result. Most reported patients have fared well, but the overall patency rate is not known and there is very little information on follow-up beyond 1 year.

PTA for Iliac Artery Stenosis

Balloon angioplasty is safe, effective, and durable in selected patients (Fig. 72–10). The results of iliac artery PTA for stenotic lesions are summarized in Table 72–7. The six contemporary studies listed in the table report long-term results using life-table analysis or the Kaplan-Meier product-limit method.[36, 37, 41, 56, 106, 107] Initial success rates range from 88% to 97%. Five-year patency ranges from 34% to 85%.

The largest body of single-institution data available is from the University of Toronto, in which 580 patients undergoing iliac PTA were followed prospectively.[35, 37] Among the variables that significantly influenced results were (1) the indication for revascularization (claudication versus limb salvage), (2) site of the PTA (common versus external iliac artery), and (3) runoff status. Among 313 common iliac artery stenoses treated, the success rate was 97% initially, 81% at 1 year, 71% at 2 years, 68% at 3 years, 65% at 4 years, and 60% at 5 years. The success rate for PTA in 209 external iliac arteries was 95% initially,

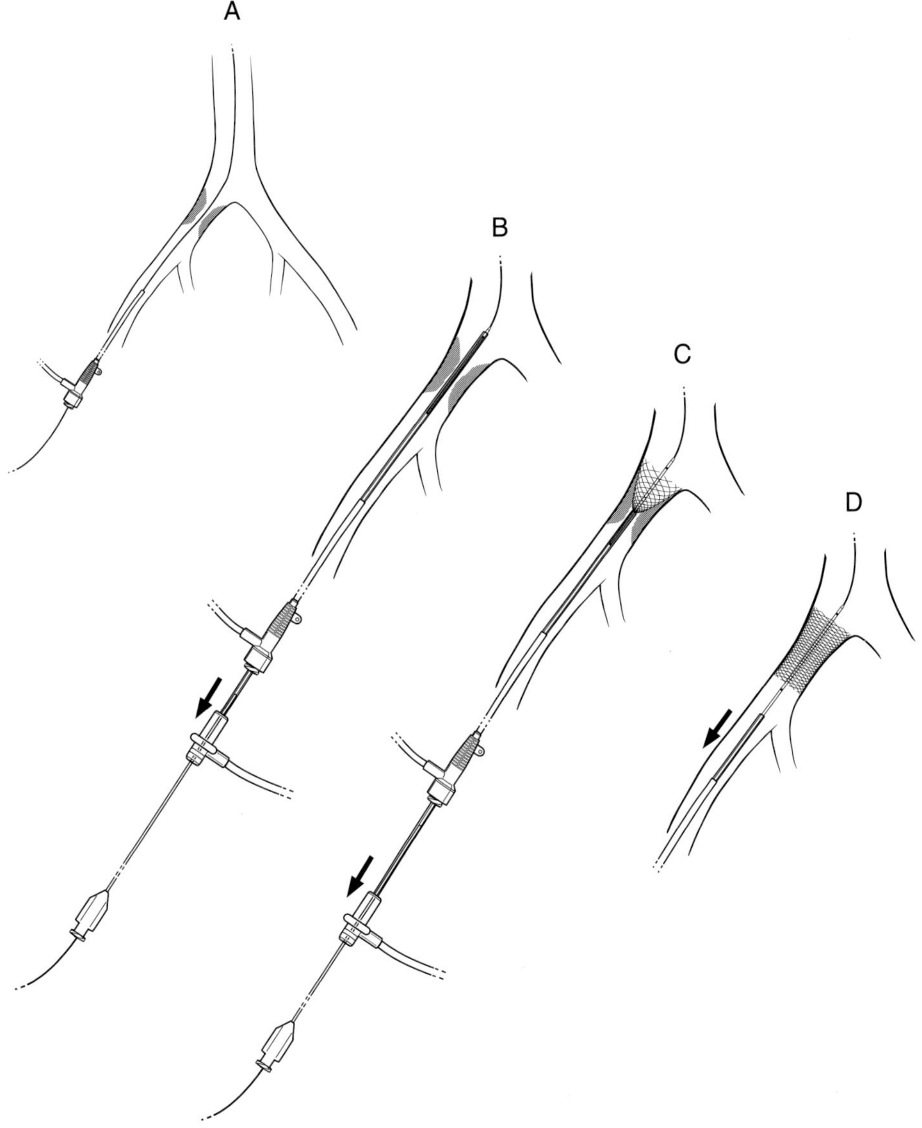

FIGURE 72–7. Technique of Wallstent placement. *A*, The guide wire is placed across the iliac lesion. *B*, The Wallstent delivery catheter is advanced over the guide wire. The proximal radiopaque marker on the delivery catheter is placed proximal to the lesion. The metal pushing rod is held stationary while the valve body is slowly withdrawn *(arrow)*. *C*, The position of the stent is continuously monitored using fluoroscopy. As the stent opens, its position is reassessed. The stent can be "dragged" distally but not advanced. (Some delivery systems permit the stent to be reconstrained if only a short length of the stent has expanded.) As the valve body is withdrawn along the length of the pushing rod *(arrow)* the covering sheath that constrains the stent is removed and the stent expands. *D*, After stent deployment, the stent delivery catheter is removed. Further balloon angioplasty of the stent is usually performed. (From Schneider PA: A stent is an intravascular graft. *In* Endovascular Skills. St. Louis, Quality Medical Publishing, 1998, pp 133–164.)

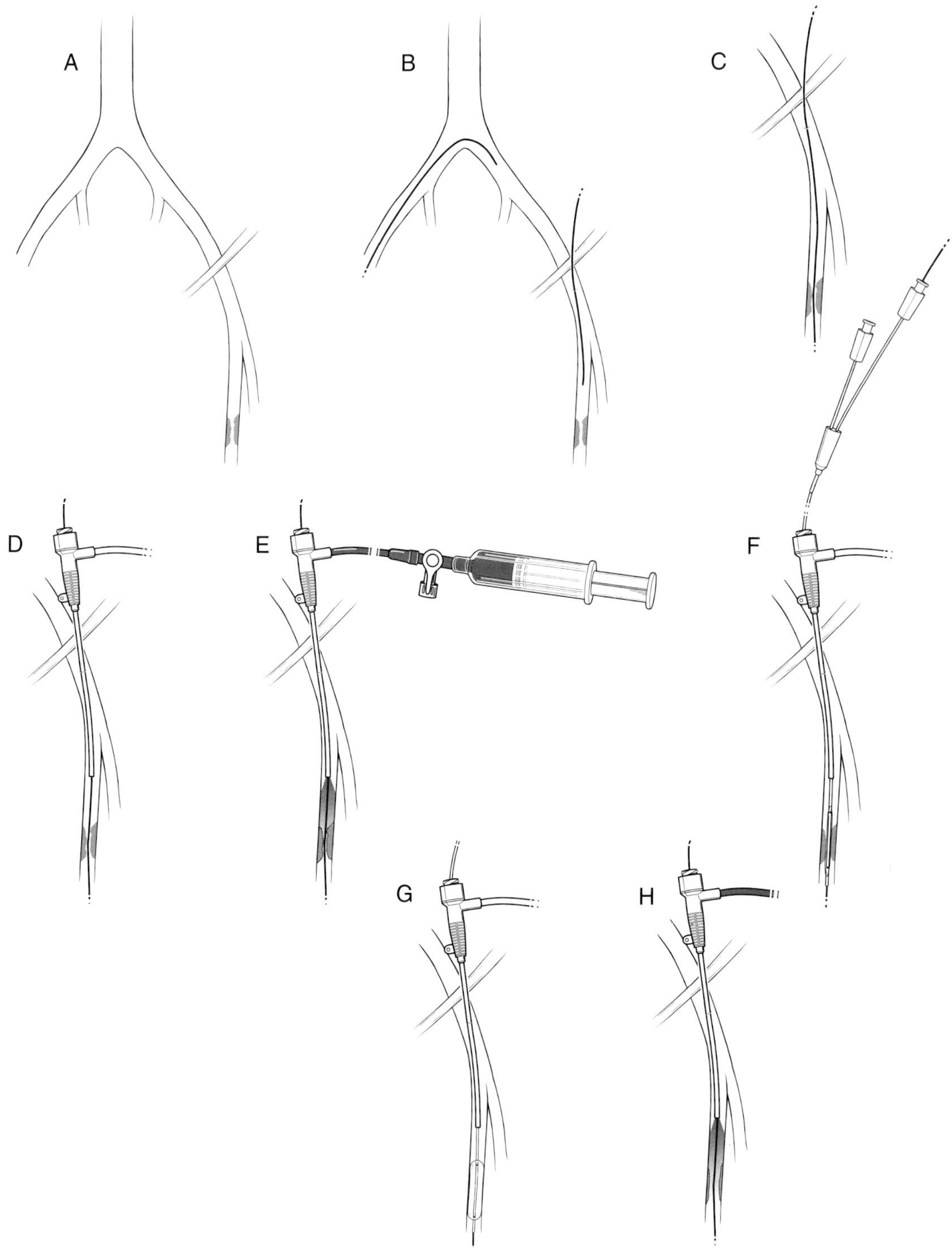

FIGURE 72–8. Technique of superficial femoral artery balloon angioplasty. *A*, Arteriography reveals a superficial femoral artery stenosis which is suitable for percutaneous transluminal balloon angioplasty (PTA). *B*, An antegrade approach to the lesion may be achieved either across the aortic bifurcation from the contralateral femoral artery or through an ipsilateral antegrade common femoral artery puncture. *C*, The guide wire is advanced across the lesion. *D*, A hemostatic access sheath is placed over the guide wire and advanced into the proximal superficial femoral artery. *E*, Femoral arteriography is performed through the side arm of the sheath to evaluate the lesion and confirm intraluminal position of the guide wire. *F*, The appropriate balloon catheter is advanced over the guide wire, through the sheath, and across the lesion. *G*, The lesion is dilated with fluoroscopic guidance. *H*, The balloon catheter is withdrawn, but the guide wire position is maintained across the lesion. Completion arteriography is performed through the side arm of the sheath. (From Schneider PA: Advice about angioplasty and stent placement at specific sites. *In* Endovascular Skills. St. Louis, Quality Medical Publishing, 1998, pp 167–197.)

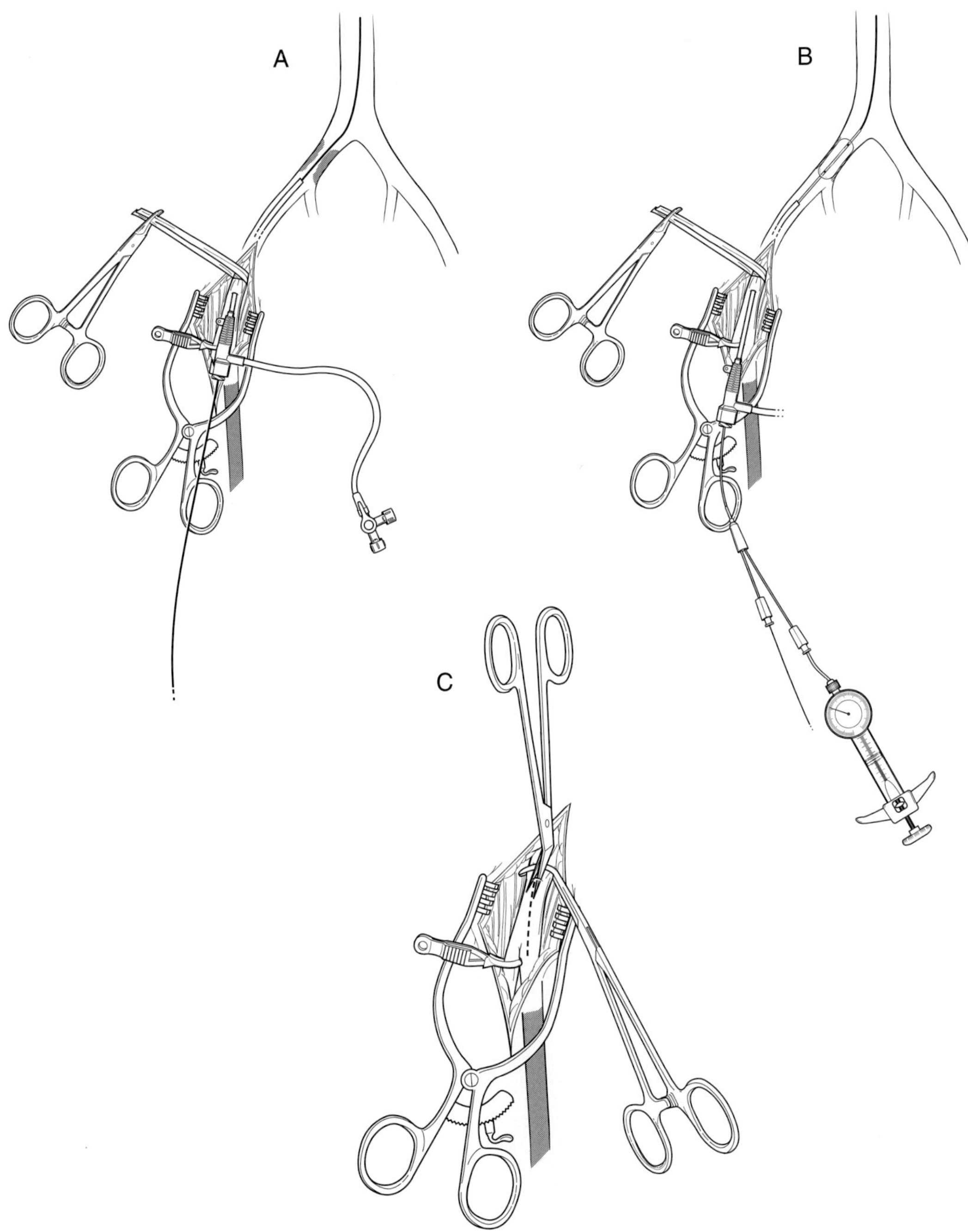

FIGURE 72–9. Technique of combined inflow balloon angioplasty and infrainguinal surgical reconstruction. *A*, After arterial exposure, conduit preparation, tunneling, and heparin administration, the guide wire and hemostatic sheath are placed in the exposed common femoral artery. *B*, Balloon angioplasty of the inflow artery is performed. After completion arteriography confirms the adequate inflow, the guide wire and sheath are removed. *C*, The common femoral artery is clamped, and the arteriotomy is lengthened and prepared for the proximal anastomosis. (From Schneider PA: Endovascular techniques in the operating room. *In* Endovascular Skills. St. Louis, Quality Medical Publishing, 1998, pp 205–212.)

TABLE 72–5. STANDARDS FOR DESCRIPTION OF THE LESION TO BE TREATED WITH ENDOVASCULAR TECHNIQUES

Location
Aorta, common iliac, external iliac, superficial femoral, popliteal, tibioperoneal trunk, tibial

Type
Occlusion vs. stenosis, diffuse vs. focal, eccentric vs. concentric, ulcerated vs. smooth, calcified vs. noncalcified

Length
<2 cm, 2–5 cm, >5–10 cm, >10 cm

Runoff
Aortoiliac procedures
Good = SFA <50% stenosis, poor = SFA > 50% stenosis or occluded
Infrainguinal procedures
Good = 2–3 patent tibial arteries, poor = 0–1 patent tibial arteries

From Ahn SS, Rutherford RB, Becker GJ, et al: Reporting standards for lower extremity arterial endovascular procedures. J Vasc Surg 17:1103–1107, 1993.
SFA = superficial femoral artery.

74% at 1 year, 62% at 2 years, 51% at 3 years, and 48% at 4 years.

More complex lesions, composed of longer stenoses and multiple stenoses, carry lower long-term primary patency rates. Spence and colleagues[73] reported a lower patency rate at 2 years for lesions 2 to 5 cm long than for lesions 1 cm long (75% versus 86%, respectively). Single discrete iliac stenoses had a 3-year patency rate of 91%, compared with 56% for two or more ipsilateral iliac lesions requiring dilatation.[108]

In general, one can expect an overall initial failure rate of 5% to 10%. Further failure rates are 19% to 26% during the first year, 10% to 12% the second year, and 3% to 5% per year in subsequent years. Overall, results of iliac PTA have shown reasonable 5-year patency rates, but consideration of certain characteristics that affect outcome helps in decision making.[39] Long-term patency rates range between 85% and 45%, with an increment of roughly 10% being accounted for by each of the following features: (1) location (common versus external iliac artery), (2) runoff status (superficial femoral patency or occlusion), (3) discreteness of lesion (short versus multiple or long lesions), and (4) clinical stage (claudication versus limb salvage). Excellent

TABLE 72–6. CLINICAL IMPROVEMENT AFTER PERCUTANEOUS INTERVENTIONS FOR LOWER EXTREMITY ISCHEMIA

+3	*Markedly improved:* No ischemic symptoms, and any foot lesions completely healed; ABI essentially "normalized" (increased to more than 0.90)
+2	*Moderately improved:* No open foot lesions, still symptomatic but only with exercise *and* improved by at least one category*; ABI not normalized but increased by more than 0.10
+1	*Minimally improved:* Greater than 0.10 increase in ABI† but no categorical improvement *or* vice versa (i.e., upward categorical shift without an increase in ABI of more than 0.10)
0	*No change:* No categorical shift and less than 0.10 change in ABI
−1	*Mildly worse:* No categorical shift but ABI decreased more than 0.10, or downward categorical shift with ABI decrease less than 0.10
−2	*Moderately worse:* One category worse or unexpected minor amputation
−3	*Markedly worse:* More than one category worse or unexpected major amputation

From Rutherford RB, Baker JD, Ernst C, et al: Recommended standards for reports dealing with lower extremity ischemia: Revised version. J Vasc Surg 26:517–538, 1997.
*Categories refer to clinical classification.
†In cases where the ABI cannot be accurately measured, an index based on the toe pressure, or any measurable pressure distal to the site of revascularization, may be substituted.
ABI = ankle-brachial index.

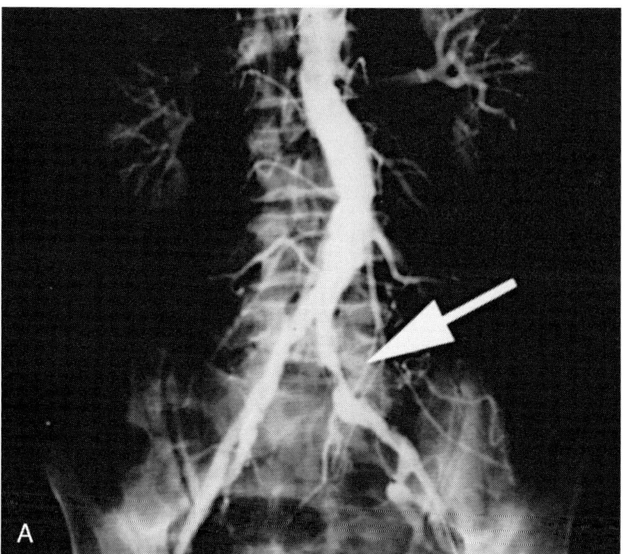

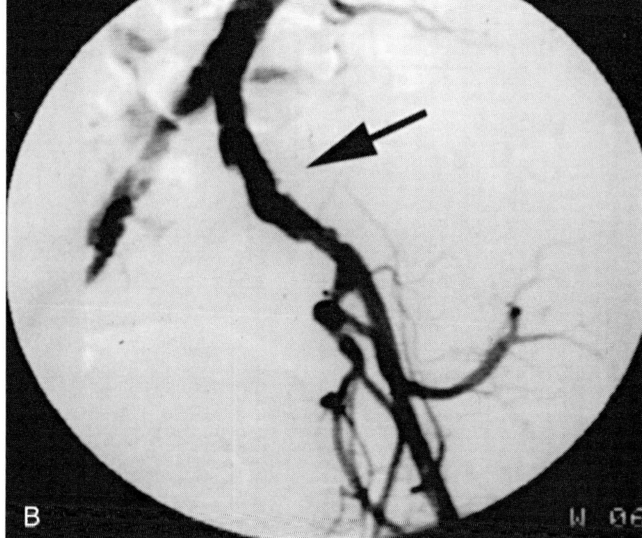

FIGURE 72–10. Iliac artery percutaneous transluminal balloon angioplasty (PTA). *A*, Arteriogram of severe left thigh and buttock claudication in a 75-year-old man. There was a significant, focal left common iliac artery stenosis *(arrow)*. *B*, After PTA, the left iliac artery stenosis resolved and there was no pressure gradient *(arrow)*. Symptoms of claudication resolved after PTA.

TABLE 72–7. RESULTS OF BALLOON ANGIOPLASTY FOR ILIAC ARTERY STENOSIS

STUDY		NO. OF PATIENTS	PATENCY (%)			
Author	Year		Initial	1 Year	3 Years	5 Years
Johnston[37]	1993	580	96	77	61	54
Tegtmeyer et al[41]	1991	200	93	96	89	85
Stokes et al[56]*	1990	53	94	85	67	34
Jeans et al[36]†	1990	180	88	67	60	57
In der Maur et al[106]	1990	157	97	96	92	84
Jorgensen et al[107]	1993	150	93	79	68	63

*Includes 1.8% occlusions.
†Includes 6.0% occlusions.

long-term results may be achieved with iliac PTA through the use of judicious selection of patients with favorable lesions. The unsolved problem of iliac PTA is the achievement of better results in less favorable lesions.

Stent Placement for Iliac Artery Stenosis

Stents have influenced the endovascular management of iliac artery stenosis in several ways:

1. They provide a method of treatment for acute postangioplasty dissection and residual stenosis, thus decreasing the rate of initial failure.
2. They have expanded the variety of lesions that may be treated to include more patients with category 2 lesions and some with category 3 lesions. Better hemodynamic and cosmetic results can be achieved with stents than with PTA alone for longer and more complex lesions and for occlusions. Some of these are lesions that would not have been dilated previously because of concern about the high likelihood of acute failure with PTA alone.
3. Stent placement has also been performed extensively with the hope that it would increase the long-term patency of iliac PTA for all types of lesions.

Some investigators have advocated primary stent deployment as routine at the time of iliac PTA, but the overall effectiveness of this approach has not been proven.[67, 109–114] Others have deployed stents selectively, for specific indications, such as post-PTA dissection or residual stenosis, occlusion, and recurrent stenosis.[4, 5, 16, 75] Other relative indications for stent placement are long or complex lesions (category 3 or 4) and embolizing lesions (category 3).[10] There is also evidence to suggest that stent placement in the external iliac artery improves patency to levels that are similar to those achieved in the common iliac artery.[58]

The results of stent placement lack clarity at present owing to several factors:

1. Indications for stent placement (primary versus selective) are often ambiguous and frequently mixed within the same study.
2. Both stenoses and occlusions have been included in many studies, and the results of each are often not possible to extract.
3. Lesions in categories 1 through 4, for which different results of endovascular intervention are expected, have often been included in the same treatment groups.
4. Most studies have evaluated one of several different stents (e.g., Palmaz, Wallstent, or Strecker), and the results of the different types may not be comparable.

The results of selective stent placement for iliac artery stenosis are presented in Table 72–8. Initial success rates were 97% to 99%, and the 3-year patency rates range from 74% to 86%.[4, 58, 115, 116] The results of primary stent placement for iliac artery stenosis are presented in Table 72–9.[59, 67, 117, 118] The initial success rates varied from 90% to 99%. Patency rates have been reported as 69% at 43 months and 86% at 4 years.[117, 118] The results of primary stent placement and selective stent placement are striking in their similarity. Reported patency rates at 2 years range from 73% to 98% for primary stent placement and from 71% to 91% for selective iliac artery stent placement.

Therefore, the indications for stent placement are not clear, and their effect on long-term patency cannot be predicted. No prospective, randomized trial has been published that compares the long-term results for iliac arteries

TABLE 72–8. RESULTS OF SELECTIVE STENT PLACEMENT AFTER PERCUTANEOUS TRANSLUMINAL ANGIOPLASTY FOR ILIAC ARTERY STENOSIS*

STUDY		NO. OF PATIENTS	STENT	PATENCY (%)					
Author	Year			Initial	1 Year	2 Years	3 Years	4 Years	5 Years
Henry et al[58]	1995	184	Palmaz	99	94	91	86	86	NA
Vorwerk et al[4]	1996	109	Wallstent	97	95	88	86	82	72
Martin et al[116]	1995	140	Wallstent	97	81	71	NA	NA	NA
Cikrit et al[115]	1995	38	Palmaz	NA	87	NA	74	NA	63

*Studies selected had more than 90% of lesions being stenoses and more than 90% of stents placed selectively.
NA = not available.

TABLE 72–9. RESULTS OF PRIMARY STENT PLACEMENT FOR ILIAC ARTERY STENOSIS

STUDY		NO. OF PATIENTS	STENT	PATENCY (%)				
Author	Year			Initial	1 Year	2 Years	3 Years	After 3 Years
Sullivan et al[67]†	1997	288	Wallstent Palmaz	90	89	76	NA	NA
Palmaz et al[117]	1992	486	Palmaz	99	91	84	69	69 at 43 mo
Murphy et al[118]	1995	83	Palmaz	99	89	NA	NA	86 at 4 yr
Laborde et al[59]	1995	455 Type*	Palmaz	NA	92	92	92	
		I 180		NA	100	98	98	
		II 58		NA	86	73	61	
		III 217						

*Type I aortic and common iliac stenosis; type II includes external iliac stenosis; type III includes infrainguinal occlusive disease.
†10% of lesions were occlusions.
NA = not available.

treated with stents and with PTA alone or the results for primary and selective stent placements at iliac PTA sites. In addition, selective stent placement is, by definition, performed for PTA with inadequate results or complications, and one might expect lower patency rates as a result of their use in compromised situations. Conversely, many of the patients undergoing routine, primary stent placement probably had favorable lesions (category 1) that were treatable with PTA alone and may not have required stents at all. These factors suggest that if iliac artery stent placement improves long-term patency, primary stent placement should yield significantly better results than selective stent placement. There is no evidence so far that this is true.

Several studies of note contribute to a partial resolution of the issue. A meta-analysis was performed to compare the results of iliac stent placement (816 patients from eight studies) and of PTA alone (1300 patients from six studies) from studies published in the 1990s (Fig. 72–11).[42] The immediate technical success rate was significantly higher

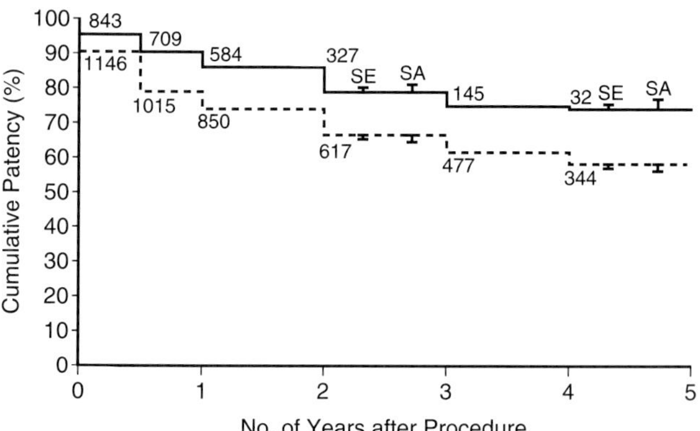

FIGURE 72–11. Iliac percutaneous transluminal balloon angioplasty (PTA) versus iliac stent placement: results of a meta-analysis. Cumulative primary patency after iliac PTA (n = 1,146, *dashed line*) and iliac PTA with stent placement (n = 843, *solid line*), unadjusted for covariates and including technical failures. The cumulative percentage success is plotted against time of follow-up. The number of patients entering each follow-up interval is indicated. The standard error (SE) and the range found in the sensitivity analysis (SA) are given (From Bosch JL, Hunink MGM: Meta-analysis of the results of percutaneous transluminal angioplasty and stent placement for aortoiliac occlusive disease. Radiology 204:87–96, 1997.)

after stent placement (96%) than after PTA alone (91%). Primary patency rates at 4 years were higher after stent placement (77%) than after PTA alone (65%) for the treatment of iliac artery stenosis that was causing claudication. For patients in whom iliac stenosis was treated because of limb-threatening ischemia, the 4-year patency rate was 67% for stent placement and 53% for PTA alone. Unfortunately, this comparison does not accurately represent clinical practice, for several reasons:

1. Most of the published PTA results for comparison were derived from procedures performed in the "pre-stent" era. Patient selection for endovascular intervention emphasized inclusion of more favorable lesions, and there were no reliable endovascular options for treating acute failures.
2. An operator faced with an acute PTA site complication, at present, would selectively place a stent, rather than be forced to accept the sequela of "PTA alone."
3. This meta-analysis could not answer the pertinent clinical question, whether to use primary or selective stenting, because these two approaches were not compared. There is a reasonable possibility that if the correct lesions could be properly chosen for selective stent placement, a benefit may be derived similar to the benefit that would be achieved by placing stents for all iliac PTA procedures.
4. If the early failures in the PTA group in the meta-analysis were converted to successes through placement of stents at the beginning, the advantage for stents would be only 7% to 9% at 4 years.

There are two randomized trials in progress. The Dutch Iliac Stent Trial has randomly assigned 213 patients with claudication to receive primary or selective iliac artery stent placement.[119, 120] Early results show that pressure gradients across iliac lesions could be resolved but that only 37% of the selective group required stent placement to accomplish this resolution. No long-term patency data are yet available. A widely quoted, multicenter, German trial comparing primary and selective iliac stent placement has randomly assigned several hundred patients to either PTA alone or PTA with stents since 1987, but long-term results have been published only in abstract form.[111–114] Preliminary results show that further intervention was required by 36 months in 28% of those treated with PTA compared with 2% of those treated with stents.

In conclusion, the use of stents with PTA for iliac artery stenosis is justified for acute dissection or significant residual post-PTA stenosis, to reduce the technical and hemodynamic failure rates, respectively. Although there is no proof, the use of stents in second dilatations to prevent restenosis has also been generally accepted. Whether primary stent placement to improve long-term patency following PTA is justified will depend on its cost-effectiveness as well as on the results of the trials mentioned previously.

The use of stents to extend the application of endovascular intervention to lesions unfavorable for PTA alone (e.g., categories 3 and 4) is clearly feasible, but the long-term results are not known. Stents are costly ($750 to $1200 per stent), and multiple stents are commonly deployed for a complex reconstruction. Unless significant short-term and long-term advantages over simple unilateral bypass (femorofemoral or iliofemoral) can be shown, iliac artery placement stent for these more complex lesions can be justified only for patients with prohibitive surgical risks.

Multilevel Occlusive Disease with Proximal Iliac Artery Stenosis

Endovascular intervention has been combined with open surgery to treat lower extremity ischemia caused by multilevel occlusive disease (Fig. 72–12).[121–132] This usually involves balloon angioplasty (alone or with stent placement) for iliac inflow and a distal, open operation. This combination of procedures may be performed in a staged fashion, with PTA followed at some interval by a separate, open operation.[121, 126, 129] Staging permits the hemodynamic effect of the PTA to be assessed prior to distal surgery but also results in delay and the cost of a second procedure to complete the revascularization.

An alternative is the simultaneous combination of intraoperative balloon angioplasty with operation at a more distal level, such as infrainguinal bypass, femoral endarterectomy, or femorofemoral bypass.[122, 131] This approach requires an inventory of endovascular supplies and quality fluoroscopic imaging to be available in the operating room but obviates the need for a separate operation. Acute failure of an intraoperative angioplasty site is unlikely because stents may be used to manage inadequate post-PTA results.[132] The advantage of this latter approach is that the scope of surgery may be extended with minimal additional time and operative morbidity to achieve the desired reconstruction immediately.

Both the staged and simultaneous approaches appear to be safe and effective, and excellent results have been published for each. The 5-year primary patency rate for combined reconstructions ranges from 61% to 80%.[121, 125, 129] Three studies have compared the staged and simultaneous approaches, and patency rates were similar.[122–124] Length of hospital stay and rate of complications were lower with the simultaneous approach.[122]

Iliac Artery Occlusion

Many iliac artery occlusions can be recanalized with a combination of thrombolytic therapy and balloon angioplasty. Initial success and long-term patency may be enhanced with stent placement.

The results of PTA alone and PTA with stent placement for iliac artery occlusion are summarized in Table 72–10.[37, 43, 44, 47, 133] Initial success rates appear to be better when stents are placed than when PTA alone is used. Longer-term results are less clear. The only 4-year data available in studies evaluating occlusions alone show no difference between the two approaches (78% versus 76%).[43, 133] In the previously cited meta-analysis, the patency rate at 4 years for iliac occlusions in patients with claudication was 54% for PTA alone and 61% when stents were also placed.[42] The rates for PTA alone and PTA with stents were 44% and 53% at 4 years, respectively, when critical ischemia was the indication for treatment of the iliac artery occlusion.

Thrombolytic therapy can play an important role in treating occlusions. In a study that evaluated the results of balloon angioplasty alone, early success was 100% when thrombolysis was complete, but only 88% when residual thrombus was present at the treatment site.[134] Thrombolytic therapy prior to PTA of an occlusion also enhanced 1-year patency rates.[135]

Alternative approaches also deserve consideration. In one study, thrombolysis and PTA were performed in 46 iliac artery occlusions and stents were placed whenever the results of this approach were inadequate (39% of cases).[16] The initial overall success rate was 98%, and the patency rate at 2 years was 93%. These results compare favorably with those reported for stent placement in all patients with occlusions. Another approach is initial stent placement at the occlusion site without prior thrombolysis.[136, 137] This approach was found to be efficacious in two small studies, but there was no follow-up.

Distal embolization remains a significant problem and may occur in 3% to 10% of patients.[37, 43, 44, 47, 133] This complication is one of the ways that claudication may be converted to limb-threatening ischemia as the result of an endovascular procedure. In addition, if the surgical alternative is a femorofemoral bypass, it can usually be performed with low morbidity.

Summary

Stents have improved the initial success rate of endovascular treatment for iliac artery occlusions. They may also enhance the long-term results of treatment, although this issue is not yet clear. Unless there is a prohibitive risk, bypass surgery is usually the best choice.

RESULTS OF INFRAINGUINAL ENDOVASCULAR INTERVENTION

Angioplasty of the Superficial Femoral and Popliteal Arteries

Neither the initial success rate nor the long-term patency is as high for femoropopliteal angioplasty as it is for iliac procedures.[37–39] Optimal lesions for femoropopliteal PTA are short (<2 cm) stenoses (category 1 lesions) in patients who have claudication and good runoff. Longer lesions and occlusions can be treated by angioplasty, but the initial success and long-term primary patency rates are lower. Extensive post-PTA dissection or significant residual steno-

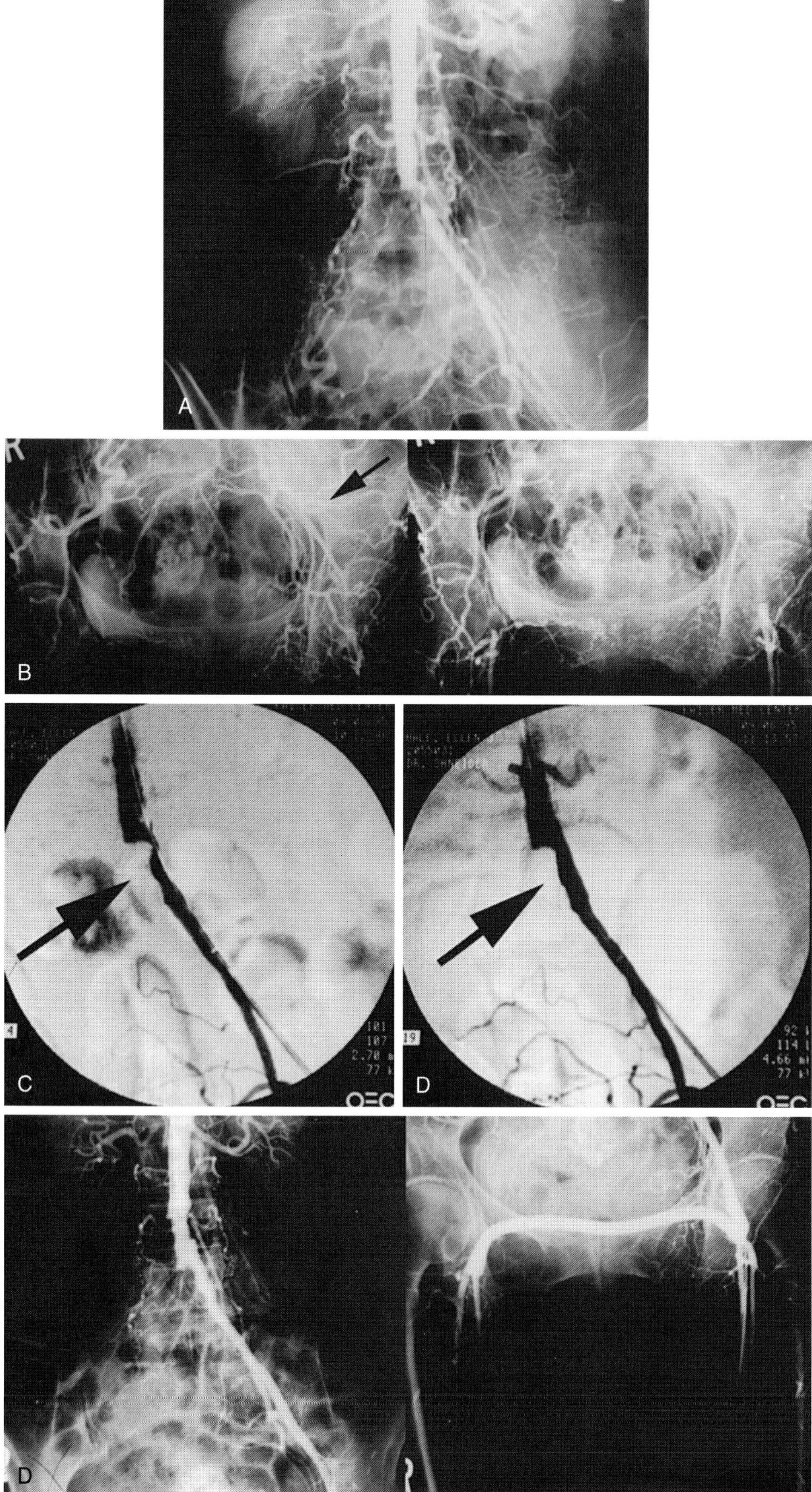

FIGURE 72–12 *See legend on opposite page*

TABLE 72–10. RESULTS OF ENDOVASCULAR INTERVENTION FOR ILIAC ARTERY OCCLUSION

STUDY		NO. OF PATIENTS	PATENCY (%)					
Author	Year		Initial	1 Year	2 Years	3 Years	4 Years	5 Years
PTA alone								
Johnston[37]	1993	82	76	60	53	48	NA	NA
Gupta et al[133]	1993	50	79	79	76	76	76	76
PTA + stent								
Reyes et al[47]	1997	59	92	78	73	72	NA	NA
Dyet et al[44]	1997	72	93	88	NA	NA	NA	NA
Vorwerk et al[43]	1995	103	96	87	83	81	78	NA

PTA = percutaneous transluminal angioplasty; NA = not available.

sis may be treated with stent placement to avoid acute occlusion and its attendant morbidity. However, the long-term results of infrainguinal PTA are not improved by stent placement.

Major contemporary studies with long-term, life-table analysis of patency are summarized in Table 72–11.[38, 48, 50, 138, 139] Initial patency rates for all lesions ranged from 86% to 93%. Patency rate at 1 year ranged from 47% to 71%, and at 5 years from 26% to 60%.

The type of lesion (stenosis versus occlusion) and the runoff status were the best predictors of long-term outcome in the University of Toronto series.[38] Unfortunately, the length of the lesion was not taken into account in this study. The 5-year success rate was 53% for stenoses with good runoff, 36% for occlusions with good runoff, 31% for stenoses with poor runoff, and 16% for occlusions with poor runoff. Patients treated for claudication had a significantly better long-term patency than patients requiring treatment for limb salvage. Thrombolytic infusions have been shown to improve the results of endovascular intervention for chronic infrainguinal arterial occlusion, but at costs of higher complication rates and the need for adjunctive procedures.[135, 140–143]

Adar and associates[139] subjected seven femoropopliteal PTA studies (1461 procedures) to confidence profile analysis. The absolute value they found for the patency of PTA may not be reliable because many of the studies they analyzed did not include initial failures. A separate comparison of claudication versus limb-threatening ischemia, however, demonstrated a significant difference between these two indications (Table 72–12).[139]

Lesion length also correlated with outcome. Femoropopliteal lesions that were shorter than 2 cm (category 1) had significantly better patency than longer lesions (categories 2 and 3).[48, 50] In another study, the 3-year patency rates were 68% for single, short stenoses and 20% for long, multifocal stenoses.[144] Dilatation of long (>5 cm) occlusions (category 4) had dismal results; 22 of 23 initially successful PTA procedures had failed within 6 months.[145]

Although angioplasty of more extensively diseased femoropopliteal segments, either occluded or diffusely stenotic, is less durable, it may be reasonable to dilate such lesions for limb salvage indications in patients with prohibitive surgical risks, especially if they have persistent rest pain or superficial ulceration (Fig. 72–13).[146, 147] The improved arterial circulation is often short-lived (several months), but it may save the extremity without surgical intervention. Rush and associates[63] treated 97 limbs in 86 patients with end-stage arterial occlusive disease in whom vascular reconstruction was not considered either appropriate or possible. Limb salvage was 76% at post-PTA intervals ranging from 1 to 45 months. The 1-year restenosis rate was 57%, and second PTA procedures successfully maintained patency in only 10 limbs. In another study of 50 similar patients, Currie and associates[145] reported the 2-year rate of survival as only 60% and the limb salvage rate as 42%.

Thus, femoropopliteal PTA carries an initial failure rate of 7% to 14%. An additional 20% to 40% of PTA sites fail in the first year. Thereafter, the failure rate continues at 4% to 8% per year. Best-case and worst-case scenarios at 5 years range from 70% to 20%, with increments accounted for by clinical stage (20%, claudication versus limb salvage), type of lesion (10%, occlusion versus stenosis), runoff (20%, 2 to 3 vessels patent versus 0 to 1 vessel patent), and length of lesion (20%, <10 cm or >10 cm).

Stent Placement in the Superficial Femoral and Popliteal Arteries

Early enthusiasm that stents might be able to enhance the marginal long-term results of PTA in the superficial femoral and popliteal arteries has not been supported by subsequent studies. Primary patency rates in nonrandomized

FIGURE 72–12. Intraoperative iliac angioplasty and stent placement and combined femorofemoral bypass. *A*, The patient is a 76-year-old woman who presented with bilateral rest pain and right first toe gangrene. Aortography demonstrated a long-segment right iliac artery occlusion and a significant stenosis at the orifice of the left common iliac artery. *B*, Iliofemoral arteriographic runoff showed bilateral common femoral artery occlusions with reconstitution of the femoral bifurcations. The left external iliac artery was patent but underperfused *(arrow)*. *C*, Intraoperative left common iliac artery balloon angioplasty caused a mild dissection but made minimal improvement in the degree of stenosis *(arrow)*. *D*, A Palmaz stent was placed and a subsequent angioplasty resolved the stenosis *(arrow)*. A left femoral endarterectomy and a femorofemoral bypass were performed. *E*, Follow-up arteriography at 1 year demonstrated a patent iliac stent site and distal reconstruction.

TABLE 72–11. RESULTS OF BALLOON ANGIOPLASTY FOR FEMOROPOPLITEAL ARTERY OCCLUSIVE DISEASE

STUDY		NO. OF PATIENTS	PATENCY (%)			
Author	Year		Initial	1 Year	3 Years	5 Years
Johnston[38]	1992	236	89	63	51	38
Adar et al[139]	1989	1461	86	66	58	60
Stanley et al[50]	1996	176	93	58	38	26
Capek et al[48]	1991	217	90	71	51	48
Matsi et al[138]	1994	106	89	47	NA	NA

NA = Not available.

cohort studies have ranged from 49% to 81% at 12 months.[58, 148–152]

One large study with long-term follow-up employed the Palmaz stent in 126 patients and found a 65% 4-year patency rate in superficial femoral artery lesions.[58] Stents placed for stenosis had a better 4-year patency rate (80%) than did those placed for occlusion (39%). Longer lesions yielded inferior patency rates, 69% at 3 years for lesions longer than 3 cm compared with 82% for lesions shorter than 3 cm. Lesions of the popliteal artery fared worse than those in the superficial femoral artery (50% and 81% patency rates at 1 year, respectively). Another study achieved a 2-year patency rate of 77% and found that the type of lesion (occlusion versus stenosis) affected results.[152]

Early stent thrombosis has been a problem in 5% to 15% of patients.[148, 153] Many studies have employed periprocedural anticoagulation and extended it for several months afterward. White and colleagues[151] used femoropopliteal stents to treat the acute complications of PTA without long-term anticoagulation and achieved an 18-month patency rate of 83%.[151]

In one randomized trial comparing PTA alone and PTA with stent placement, there was no difference; patency rates at 1 year were 85% after PTA and 74% after stent placement.[45] Subsequent occlusion occurred in 21% of patients with stents and 7% of patients undergoing PTA. Another study of note compared PTA with stents and PTA alone for the treatment of long (>3 cm) occlusions.[148] The 1-year patency rates were 42% for PTA with stents and 65% for PTA alone. Stent failures were due to either early thrombosis (one third) or intimal hyperplasia (two thirds).

In conclusion, stent placement does not extend the patency of femoropopliteal PTA. The factors that limit the results of PTA (i.e., occlusion, long lesion) also limit those of stent placement. Stents may be used to treat post-PTA dissection to avoid imminent occlusion, and long-term anticoagulation may not be necessary.

TABLE 72–12. PERCUTANEOUS TRANSLUMINAL ANGIOPLASTY OF THE FEMOROPOPLITEAL ARTERY: COMPARISON OF PATENCY RATES FOR CLAUDICATION AND LIMB THREAT*

LENGTH OF FOLLOW-UP	SUCCESS RATE (%)	
	Claudication	Limb Threat
30 days	89.1 ± 2.5	76.8 ± 4.0
6 mo	81.1 ± 2.7	60.7 ± 4.4
1 yr	69.8 ± 4.2	50.3 ± 6.4
2 yr	63.7 ± 8.1	46.6 ± 6.5
3 yr	62.4 ± 9.1	43.1 ± 7.2

Modified from Adar R, Critchfield GC, Eddy DM, et al: A confidence profile analysis of the results of femoropopliteal percutaneous transluminal angioplasty in the treatment of lower extremity ischemia. J Vasc Surg 10:57–67, 1989.

*The distribution statistics include mean ± SD in per cent.

Angioplasty of Infrapopliteal Arteries

Smaller-diameter guide wires and soft, low-profile catheters have been developed for tibial PTA. The clinical situation in which one might consider infrapopliteal PTA is quite common: limb-threatening ischemia without a good surgical option because of the presence of medical co-morbidities, the lack of a conduit, or other reasons. The anatomic features required for this procedure, however, are very uncommon. The patient must have in-line flow to an ischemic foot that is interrupted by a single, short, focal tibial artery stenosis. Because tibial artery disease tends to be diffuse, especially in diabetic patients, candidates for this procedure must be selected judiciously if the procedure is to be clinically successful. Only patients with limb-threatening ischemia should be considered. If plaque disruption results in occlusion of the PTA site, there may be little recourse because stents have not been adapted to use in the infrapopliteal vasculature.

Numerous series demonstrate that infrapopliteal PTA is feasible and that it contributes to limb salvage in some cases.[154–169] The rate of early clinical success ranges from 71% to 93%, with 1-year limb salvage rates ranging from 60% to 88% and 2-year limb salvage rates from 50% to 83%.[154, 156, 157, 166–169]

Unfortunately, the results of available series are not directly comparable, for the following reasons:

1. Many infrapopliteal PTA procedures were performed distal to iliac or femoropopliteal dilatations in patients with multilevel disease. These proximal dilatations may have been responsible for clinical success in some cases.
2. Many series included patients with one or more of the following confounding variables: acute ischemia, occluded or failing bypass grafts, claudication, need for thrombolysis, and inclusion of PTA of the below-knee popliteal artery.
3. Dilatations were usually performed at several sites in multiple tibial arteries, compounding the difficulty of assessing the individual patency of each PTA site.

Horvath and associates[168] reported on dilatation of 103 tibial lesions in 71 patients, noting a 96% technical success rate and limb salvage rates of 80% at 1 year, 75% at 2 years, and 65% at 3 years. Schwarten[156] reported a 97% technical success rate as well as limb salvage rates at 1 and

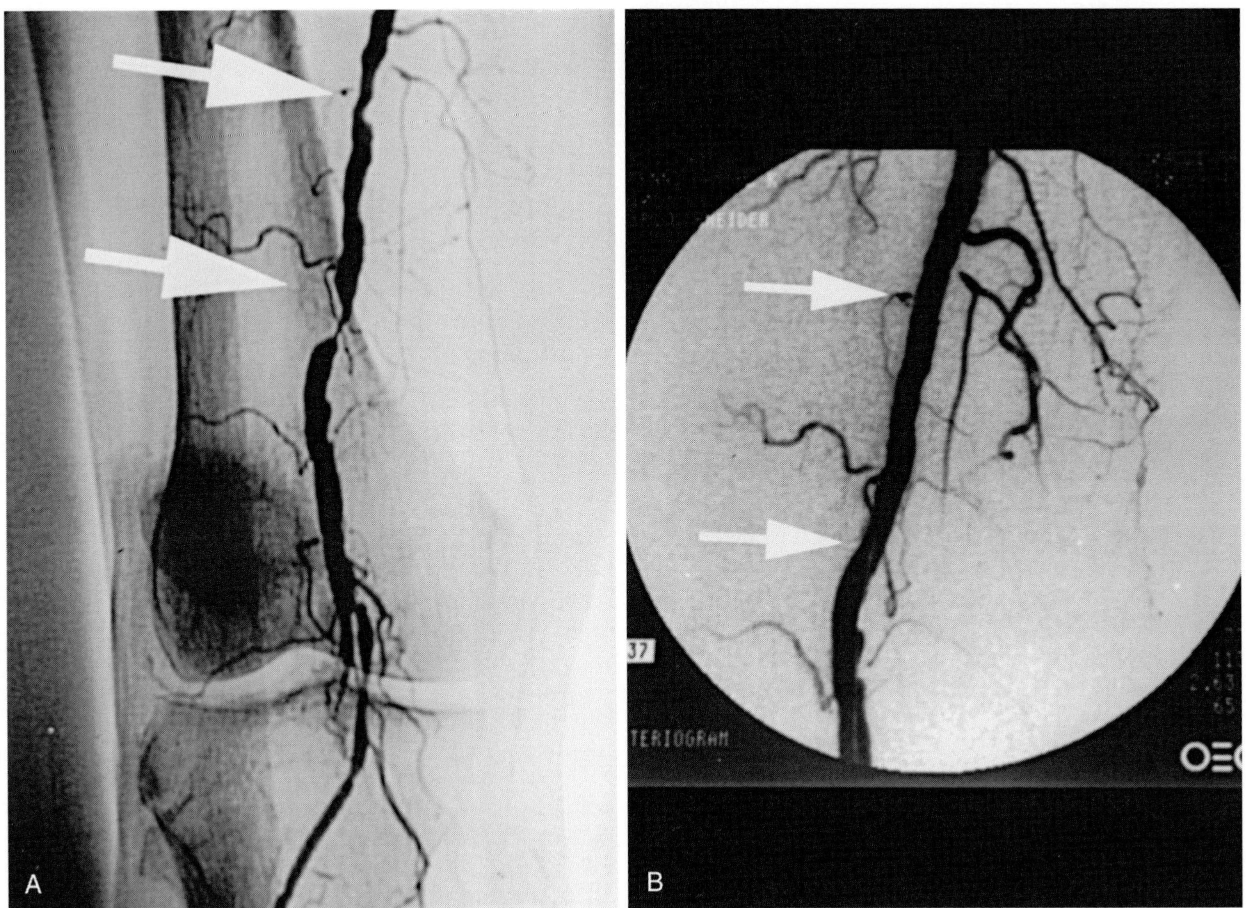

FIGURE 72–13. Superficial femoral artery balloon angioplasty for limb salvage in a patient with prohibitive surgical risk. *A*, Right great toe gangrene in an 85-year-old dialysis-dependent man with cardiomyopathy. The patient was not a candidate for distal bypass. Arteriography identified diffuse infrainguinal occlusive disease, poor runoff, and tandem stenoses in the adductor canal *(arrows)*. *B*, Balloon angioplasty improved the stenotic segments significantly *(arrows)* and ankle-brachial indices increased from 0.22 to 0.58. The wound was healed 1 month later.

2 years of 88% and 83%, respectively, after 146 dilatations in 96 patients. In studies in which patients were observed and evaluated with hemodynamic monitoring, however, the success rates were lower; they were reported as 51% to 59% at 1 year, 32% to 46% at 2 years, and 20% to 36% at 3 years.[163–165]

Difficulty in assessing results makes it impossible to accurately define the role of infrapopliteal PTA in clinical practice; however, several interpretations can be made:

1. PTA of the infrapopliteal arteries has improved significantly in the past 15 years.[170, 171]
2. If in-line flow is restored to the foot, the results are significantly better.[167, 172]
3. Success is much higher when PTA is performed for a single stenosis than for occlusion or multiple stenoses.[154, 157]
4. Infrapopliteal PTA is applicable only to a small minority of patients requiring limb salvage.[156, 159, 160]

Angioplasty of Lesions in Other Locations

Some lower extremity arteries have a less favorable outlook with PTA, such as the common femoral artery and the profunda femoris (deep femoral) artery. Balloon angioplasty can be performed in these vessels under special circumstances, but they are not a common part of endovascular practice.

Common Femoral Artery

Plaque in the common femoral artery is bulky and eccentric, often involves the femoral bifurcation, and is poorly suited to PTA. It is commonly associated with disease of the iliac or superficial femoral arteries. Because the common femoral artery is in an area of high mobility, it would not be expected to fare well following stent placement. Patency rates among 18 cases treated with PTA were 59% at 1 year and 37% at 3 years.[62] Surgical repair of this artery, however, is simple, has relatively low morbidity and high patency, and can be combined with any other endovascular procedure that is required either proximally or distally.[122, 173]

Profunda Femoris Artery

Clinical situations in which a temporary improvement in profunda femoris artery perfusion would salvage a limb certainly occur. The disease in this artery is not generally favorable for PTA, however, because it is usually either an orifice lesion, involving the femoral bifurcation, or diffuse disease along the length of the artery. Also, the profunda femoris artery tends to dissect in response to PTA. Older series suggest a reasonable technical success rate, but no long-term follow-up information is available.[174, 175] As with the common femoral artery, if repair is required in the profunda femoris artery, surgery produces excellent results.

COMPLICATIONS

The complications of endovascular procedures are presented in detail in Chapter 53. The usual motivation for performing an endovascular procedure to treat lower extremity occlusive disease, even though the surgical alternative may offer a better chance of long-term success, is that the morbidity of an endovascular approach should be less. Therefore, the expected rate of complications influences the decision about which procedure to advise.

The AHA Task Force on PTA Guidelines reviewed published complications among 3784 patients in 12 series of balloon angioplasty procedures in various lower extremity arteries (Table 72–13).[40] Complications of the puncture site, PTA site, or distal vessel occurred in approximately 10% of patients, and serious systemic complications or death occurred in 1%. Because these results are derived from retrospectively analyzed series, they may not reflect the true incidence of complications.

Caution in the placement of iliac artery stents is indicated because the incidence of complications with this procedure may be higher than with PTA alone. In the University of Toronto series on iliac PTA, 3.6% of patients had major complications that required treatment.[37] A survey of large iliac stent series reveals a rate of major complications ranging from 4% to 11%.[4, 9, 43, 116, 118, 173] Overall complication rates of 12% to 19% have routinely been reported after stent placement.[43, 59, 67, 110, 116, 176] The incidence of complications in one large study was not altered by operator experience.[117] In addition, unusual but devastating complications of stent placement have been reported, including stent infection, pseudoaneurysm, thromboembolization from stents, retrograde aortic dissection, and stent fracture.[177–190]

TABLE 72–13. COMPLICATIONS OF PERCUTANEOUS TRANSLUMINAL ANGIOPLASTY FOR LOWER EXTREMITY ISCHEMIA

	INCIDENCE (%)
Location	
Puncture site (total)	4.0
Bleeding	3.4
False aneurysm	0.5
Arteriovenous fistula	0.1
Angioplasty site (total)	3.5
Thrombosis	3.2
Rupture	0.3
Distal vessel (total)	2.7
Dissection	0.4
Embolization	2.3
Systemic (total)	0.4
Renal failure	0.2
Myocardial infarction (fatal)	0.2
Cerebrovascular accident (fatal)	0.55
Consequence	
Surgical repair	2.0
Limb loss	0.2
Mortality	0.2

Modified from Pentecost MJ, Criqui MH, Dorros G, et al: Guidelines for peripheral percutaneous transluminal angioplasty of the abdominal aorta and lower extremity vessels. Circulation 89:511–531, 1994.

WHAT ARE THE CONSEQUENCES OF FAILURE?

Acute Failure of Endovascular Reconstruction (<30 days)

The rate of acute failure of endovascular interventions for focal iliac and femoropopliteal lesions has decreased with the improvements in equipment and technique. Acute failures still occur, however, because endovascular intervention is being attempted on an expanding array of morphologically unfavorable lesions.

In a series of 318 iliac artery and femoropopliteal artery PTA procedures, early technical failures occurred in 17%, and none of the affected patients was worse than before the procedure.[191] Technical failures are more common after PTA of occlusions than after PTA of stenoses.[37, 38] After treating 83 iliac artery occlusions, Kalman and associates[35] reported 15 early failures; in only one (6.7%) case, however, did worse ischemia occur. There were eight technical failures of PTA for iliac stenosis among 584 patients; one patient required emergency surgery for ischemia, one patient died of iliac artery rupture, and one patient experienced contrast extravasation. The remaining patients were treated electively.

Vascular stents present an opportunity with risk: They permit treatment of post-PTA dissection and residual stenosis and avoid many acute failures that would have occurred because of these problems. They also, however, have encouraged attempts to treat lesions that never should have been approached with endovascular technique, and acute failures have resulted. Iliac stents have a lower early failure rate than iliac PTA, but the course of patients with acute failure at a stent site has not been well documented.[42, 192, 193]

Later Failure of Endovascular Reconstruction (>30 days)

Endovascular reconstructions of the iliac and femoropopliteal arteries that fail after a month usually do so as a result of recurrent stenosis. The affected patient most often presents with recurrent ischemic symptoms, usually claudication.

Kalman and Johnston[194] have documented that (1) the implications of a failed angioplasty are less ominous than those of a failed graft and (2) recurrent stenosis at the dilatation site or new stenosis in the same arterial segment usually returns the patient to the predilatation clinical condition. They studied 223 eventual failures among 631 angioplasties. Eighty-five per cent of the patients with PTA failure returned to their original level of symptoms, 5.5% remained better off than they were originally, and only 9.5% were clinically worse than before PTA. The 12 amputations in this series were due to advanced atheromatous disease and in no instance were attributed to failure of the PTA. Recurrent lesions can usually be redilated, and many investigators advise also placing stents.[58, 115, 116] Among patients undergoing subsequent reconstructive surgery, a failed PTA had little effect on the type and outcome of the operation.

It is not yet clear how to treat recurrent lesions within stents. Options include a second dilatation, a second stent placement, atherectomy, and surgery.[75, 193, 195] The secondary procedures are usually performed electively because acute ischemia is rarely the first symptom of recurrence.

INCORPORATING ENDOVASCULAR TECHNIQUES INTO THE OPERATIVE ARMAMENTARIUM

Lower extremity revascularization provides a venue for the incorporation of endovascular techniques into the operating room environment.[82, 132] Balloon angioplasty, stent placement, and thrombolytic therapy have all shown the reliability and durability required for their inclusion in the operative armamentarium. The simultaneous combination of endovascular intervention and open surgery is a reasonable option to achieve multilevel revascularization of a chronically ischemic limb. This combination approach requires imaging, equipment inventory, and endovascular expertise to be brought into the operating room. Facility with this approach permits the operator to use these techniques (1) in conjunction with intraoperative arteriography, (2) in the treatment of failed dialysis access grafts or lower extremity bypass grafts, (3) for the management of acute limb ischemia, (4) subclavian occlusive disease, and (5) in stent-graft placement for aneurysm disease. Several series of lower extremity PTA procedures have been published in which the procedures were performed by vascular surgeons, and there was no difference between these results and those available in the literature.[196–199]

COMPARISON OF BALLOON ANGIOPLASTY WITH NONOPERATIVE TREATMENT AND OPEN SURGERY

Comparison of balloon angioplasty, bypass, and nonoperative medical management must take many factors into account:

- Initial and long-term success rates
- Risk (mortality and morbidity)
- Cost-effectiveness
- Consequences of failure

These three modes of therapy constitute a spectrum of options that may be utilized to treat a patient with an ischemic limb, depending on (1) the needs of the patient, (2) the severity of the disease, and (3) the relative risk of intervention. There is some overlap of the treatment options that may be best for an individual. In general, however, PTA stands between surgery and nonoperative management on the basis of these factors.

Percutaneous Transluminal Angioplasty versus Medical Management

The additional cost of PTA (and stents) compared with exercise training in patients with claudication could be justified if functional improvement after endovascular reconstruction were significantly greater and reasonably durable. This is probably the case for PTA in iliac artery disease if favorable lesions are selected. However, PTA for femoropopliteal artery disease may not confer the same benefits.

Two small trials randomly assigned patients with claudication to receive PTA or medical management. In the Oxford Study,[200] 36 patients with claudication who had discrete femoropopliteal disease were prospectively randomly divided into two well-matched groups (by according to ankle-brachial index and walking distance) to receive either exercise training or PTA. The initial (3-month) advantage of PTA was lost by 12 months. By that point, the exercise-trained group was walking significantly further before claudication occurred, almost three times their pretreatment distance. In a similar study of 62 patients from the University of Edinburgh, patients undergoing PTA had fewer occluded arteries after 2 years but they did not have better walking ability.[201] Nevertheless, in many patients with claudication, exercise training fails despite best efforts. Endovascular intervention should be considered on an individual basis.

Percutaneous Transluminal Angioplasty versus Surgery

Since the introduction of PTA, the rate of open surgery for lower extremity ischemia has also increased.[202–204] In at least one major study from the Mayo Clinic, the rate of lower extremity amputation simultaneously decreased.[203]

The optimal use of PTA is among patients with less severe disease. Large series of lower extremity revascularizations have shown that patients selected for PTA more often have claudication, have better long-term survival, are younger, have fewer occlusions, and are less likely to have multilevel disease.[205, 206] When these patients, who are well suited for PTA, are randomly assigned to receive either PTA or surgery, there is no significant difference in outcome. The durability of surgery is better, but the higher morbidity obscures this benefit.[207–209]

In a Veterans Administration Cooperative Study, more than 1300 patients were screened to find 263 who could be treated with either PTA or surgery for lower extremity ischemia.[207] Patients were randomly assigned and treated between 1983 and 1987. Primary success favored bypass. At 2 years, primary patency rates for the treatment of iliac disease were 81% for surgery and 71% for PTA; for the treatment of femoropopliteal disease, the rates were 70% for surgery and 59% for PTA. If the higher cost and morbidity of operation are considered, however, patients with lesser forms of disease should probably be treated with lesser interventions when possible.

PTA is less expensive per procedure than bypass for patients with claudication, length of hospital stay being mainly responsible for the difference.[210–212] If stents are required, the cost of endovascular revascularization may approach that of bypass on a per-limb basis.[213] Endovascular reconstruction, especially of the iliac arteries, may decrease the overall cost of care, to the extent that it prevents the need for open surgery (assuming careful patient selection to minimize failure and the likelihood of either redilatation or eventual bypass). This developing technology may increase the overall cost of care, however, by extending the indications for intervention to patients who previously would have been treated nonoperatively.

The advantages of operative arterial reconstruction are primarily its greater durability and better hemodynamic response and also the fact that it can be applied to a much wider spectrum of patients, regardless of the degree and extent of occlusive disease. However, durability is not the only standard by which to judge a vascular reconstructive procedure. Patients with peripheral vascular disease have a high mortality rate in follow-up, ranging from 25% to 50% at 5 years and from 60% to 90% at 10 years.[3, 66, 214, 215] In view of such high late death rates, the initial advantages of PTA become more significant and may well counterbalance its lesser degree and duration of benefit.

Furthermore, there appears to be a difference in the pattern of failure of surgery and angioplasty. Thrombosis of some bypass grafts is associated with propagation of thrombus or progression of disease into the adjacent native artery, leaving the patient with a worse clinical status than before the bypass. The management of a failed graft with some combination of thrombolysis, balloon angioplasty, surgical thrombectomy, and surgical revision or secondary reconstruction is often more complex and expensive than the original operation. In thrombosed infrainguinal vein grafts, the saphenous vein may be lost.[71] This is not the case with angioplasty, in which redilatation of recurrent stenosis or a new stenosis in the same arterial segment is usually possible. Most patients with failed endovascular reconstruction return to their pretreatment status.

In patients with chronic critical ischemia, bypass is more effective than PTA because the occlusive disease is characteristically much more extensive and the degree of hemodynamic improvement required is greater.[216] Nevertheless, some lesions are amenable to an endovascular approach. In high-risk patients, PTA is often a reasonable option, even when longer lesions are involved and predicted durability is limited.[217] In these cases, even a few months of improved flow are often enough for limb salvage to be achieved.

Although comparisons among these three modalities for claudicants and for those with chronic critical ischemia are valuable, they are unlikely to produce absolute answers or to establish exclusive superiority of one treatment over another. Knowledge of their relative merits in these settings permits appropriate choices to be made in individual patients. These three forms of therapy each contain obvious strengths and weaknesses, and often the choice in *individual* patients is apparent when all factors are considered.

IS THERE A ROLE FOR ADJUNCTIVE DEVICES?

Endovascular reconstruction of the aortoiliac and femoropopliteal segments using PTA (and stents when necessary) has a valuable role in clinical practice. Many other techniques of endovascular surgery are going or have gone through a "boom or bust" cycle. Laser therapy is a "bust" in terms of its application to the management of peripheral arterial occlusive disease. The results of atherectomy have also been generally disappointing. Results with PTA and selective stenting are excellent in some clinical settings. New devices are introduced ostensibly to extend the scope of endovascular intervention to the treatment of more extensive occlusive lesions in a wider array of locations. Any newly introduced endovascular device must surpass the results of PTA in at least some aspect in order to be considered clinically useful.

Unfortunately, the universal response to endovascular trauma is neointimal hyperplasia. This response has been largely responsible for restenosis rates in the range of 30% to 50% within 6 to 12 months for most devices. The long-term outlook for any new endovascular device depends on control of neointimal hyperplasia, an endeavor in which some progress is being made (see Chapter 24).

Stent-Grafts and Covered Stents

Stents and vascular graft material may be combined to create an intraluminal bypass (see Chapter 38). Although this concept has been aggressively applied to the clinical problem of aneurysm disease over the past few years, occlusive disease is also being evaluated as a potential application of this technique. If the entire luminal surface of a severely diseased vessel segment could be relined by a transluminally placed graft, the scope of occlusive disease that could be treated with endovascular intervention would be dramatically increased. Unfortunately, the technology and the science is lagging behind the concept and its potential clinical applications. There have been experimental and clinical reports of periprosthetic thickening and thrombosis in response to covered stents.[218–220]

Several small, cohort series of intraluminal iliofemoral bypasses have been published.[221–232] Early technical success generally exceeds 90%. An operative mortality of 9% in one series led the authors to question whether the procedure was truly less invasive.[22] Patency ranges from 80% to 89% at 6 to 18 months.[221, 222, 232] Intraluminal iliofemoral bypasses have also been combined with infrainguinal bypass, femoral endarterectomy, or femorofemoral bypass to treat multilevel occlusive disease.[227–229]

Intraluminal femoropopliteal bypasses have also been reported.[231, 232] Primary patency was 72% at 8 months in one series and 73% at 12 months in another. Graft thrombosis was a significant problem, occurring in 11 of 55 grafts within 1 month.[232]

Laser and Atherectomy Devices

Laser

Laser energy has been used to penetrate an occluded infrainguinal arterial segment and to produce a channel adequate for introducing a balloon catheter. Laser-assisted balloon angioplasty (LABA) was claimed to produce better results than PTA alone, an 82% 1-year patency; however, when initial failures were included, a 63% patency rate was achieved.[233] This result is similar to published femoropopliteal PTA results achieved at 1 year.[48, 50, 139] Nevertheless, within 2 years, 20,000 LABAs were performed and more than 300 "laser centers" appeared in the United States alone. The pendulum swung back as negative reports emerged, documenting high technical failure rates (16% to 33%), high initial hemodynamic failure rates (13% to 36%), low overall patency rates (22% to 50% at 6 to 12 months), and a higher complication rate than achieved with PTA alone (e.g., 4% to 9% perforation, 5% to 11% hemorrhage, 5% to 17% dissection, and 1.5% to 8.7% amputation).[54, 234–237]

Subsequently, some trials with larger hot-tip probes, eximer (cool) laser, and the computer-guided "smart" laser have proved disappointing despite theoretical advantages.[238–240] None of the laser devices has improved on the results of PTA alone, and lasers carry a significantly higher expense in terms of equipment and procedural costs in addition to their complication rate.

Atherectomy Devices

Many devices have been developed and tested for their ability to remove, rather than displace, plaque in hopes of reducing the likelihood of restenosis. Several devices have been released by the Food and Drug Administration (FDA) for clinical use, but none has an established role in patient care.

The *Simpson Atherocath* has a circular cutter that spins at 2000 revolutions/min (rpm) inside a metal housing with a longitudinal window on one side that can be pressed against the plaque by inflating a balloon located on its opposite side, thereby slicing off strips of plaque and depositing them inside the chamber. Because multiple passes are required and the chamber must be evacuated periodically, the process is time-consuming and labor-intensive and in practice can be used only for short (and, ideally, eccentric) occlusive lesions. Nevertheless, complication rates are lower and patency rates higher than those reported with other devices (possibly because its use is limited to more discrete favorable lesions).

In the initial trial by Simpson and associates,[241] only 69% of patients obtained continued relief of claudication by 6 months. Patients with follow-up angiograms showed a restenosis rate of 36%. Polnitz and colleagues[242] reported an 82% initial success rate and a 72% 1-year patency rate (~60% overall patency). However, Dorros and coworkers reported an angiographic and clinical follow-up of 126 patients in whom restenosis or occlusion occurred in more than 50% of those followed up for more than 5 months.[243]

The *Auth Rotablator* atherectomy device is introduced over a guide wire and comes with variably sized, olive-shaped tips (1.25 to 5.0 mm in diameter). The tip is rotated at 100,000 to 200,000 rpm as it traverses the lesion. It preferentially pulverizes calcified plaque while deflecting the softer and more elastic underlying arterial wall. Its use has been marked by transient hemoglobinuria, perforations, equipment breakage, and thrombosis. Early (6-month) follow-up of 42 procedures showed a 24% incidence of *major* complications (with a 5% amputation rate), 24% hemodynamic failures, and 5% technical failures with only 29% of procedures patent at 6 months.[244]

The *transluminal extraction catheter* (TEC) system is passed over a guide wire. The conical tip contains cutting blades that rotate at 700 rpm. Suction carries the plaque cuttings through the housing while a heparin solution is introduced for irrigation. Because of its size relative to the arterial lumen, "adjunctive" PTA is often required. In a multicenter trial that involved treatment of 126 lesions in 95 patients, 47% required PTA.[245] Only 16 patients had follow-up angiography at 6 months, with a 25% rate of reocclusion. Problems with excessive blood loss or embolization are unique to this device.

Conclusion

The laser and various atherectomy devices have not succeeded in extending the application of PTA to longer or more complex lesions than can be managed by PTA alone because of unacceptable restenosis rates or greater morbidity. Whether other, newer devices can succeed where these have failed remains doubtful, in view of the almost universal myointimal proliferative response to endovascular trauma. Only a means of preventing or minimizing neointimal hyperplasia can be expected to change this picture.

Intravascular Ultrasound

The impact of intravascular ultrasound (IVUS) in general endovascular practice has yet to be felt. IVUS offers adjunctive guidance of therapeutic endovascular procedures and provides information that is not often obtainable with periprocedural arteriography. This technique permits endoluminal imaging, which provides a unique cross-sectional view of the treated segment. IVUS has a role in the deployment of endoluminal grafts for aneurysmal disease and complex stenting procedures.[246–251] Preliminary data suggest that the free lumen area, as measured by IVUS following PTA, may be a strong predictor of outcome.[252] The advantage of IVUS in the evaluation of stent placement appears to be enhanced with smaller stents (<5 mm), in which conventional arteriography is not as accurate.[253] At present it is too expensive and time-consuming for use in routine PTA procedures.

FUTURE OF ENDOVASCULAR INTERVENTION FOR CHRONIC LIMB ISCHEMIA

Endovascular intervention for chronic lower extremity ischemia has matured significantly over the past 20 years. Catheter-based management of a wide variety of lesions has evolved from the stage of mere clinical feasibility to the level of reliability and durability required to become an integral tool in the treatment of occlusive disease. PTA and stents have an established and growing role in the management of lower extremity ischemia. Percutaneous attempts to extend the role of PTA by laser and atherectomy devices have been disappointing, but thrombolytic therapy has allowed some occlusions to be treated with endovascular intervention that would have required open surgery in the past.

Continued efforts to extend the scope of endovascular intervention will likely be successful in the future as they have been in the past. The future of endovascular intervention is likely to be shaped by two relatively unpredictable factors: (1) advances in technology and (2) the political and economic forces of medicine.

Advances in Endovascular Technology

The concept of endovascular intervention has been well supported by the continuous advance of technology, which has regularly had a profound effect on the field. Continued miniaturization of guide wires, catheters, and other devices should increase accessibility of some lesions and decrease overall complication rates. If endoluminal grafts can be made safe enough to place, small enough to be percutaneous, and durable enough to compete with other types of reconstructions, there will be a major role for this type of device. If restenosis could be controlled with radiation, gene therapy, or covered stents, endovascular intervention could be extended to a wider variety of clinical scenarios. These are primarily questions of technology.

Opposing Forces in Endovascular Intervention

Opposing "market" forces will have a major influence on the future development of endovascular intervention. Pressure from patients and insurers to perform a "lesser" procedure may favor more endovascular intervention. Interest in decreasing the overall care costs may stimulate the elimination of procedures for indications other than a threatened life or limb, thus favoring less endovascular intervention. This will be particularly true in capitated managed care programs. It is hoped that competition among the manufacturers of similar medical devices, such as stents, will decrease the astronomical prices being commanded on a per-item basis.

Finally, "opposing forces" are no more apparent than among the different medical disciplines that have a strong interest in endovascular intervention. Some traditional open surgical procedures will most likely be replaced by endovascular approaches. A wider variety of options will increase the spectrum of patients to whom some form of mechanical intervention may be offered. More sophisticated endovascular procedures will be safest if a collaborative approach is used. Although these are just a few of the many dynamic issues to consider, the one reliable constant is that the field of endovascular intervention will likely flourish if the best interests of the patient are kept in mind.

REFERENCES

1. Fowkes FG, Housley E, Cawood EH, et al: Edinburgh artery study: Prevalence of asymptomatic and symptomatic peripheral arterial disease in the general poplulation. Int J Epidemiol 20:384–392, 1991.
2. Criqui MH, Fronek A, Barrett-Connor E, et al: The prevalence of peripheral arterial disease in a defined population. Circulation 71:510–515, 1985.
3. Criqui MH: Peripheral arterial disease and subsequent cardiovascular mortality: A strong and consistent association. Circulation 82:2246–2247, 1990.
4. Vorwerk D, Gunther RW, Schurmann K, et al: Aortic and iliac stenoses: Follow-up results of stent placement after insufficient balloon angioplasty in 118 cases. Radiology 198:45–48, 1996.
5. Gunther RW, Vorwerk D, Antonucci F, et al: Iliac artery stenosis or obstruction after unsuccessful balloon angioplasty: Treatment with a self-expandable stent. AJR Am J Roentgenol 156:389–393, 1991.
6. Hallisey MJ, Parker CB, van Breda A: Current status and extended applications of intravascular stents. Curr Opin Radiol 4:7–12, 1992.
7. Becker GJ, Palmaz JC, Rees CR, et al: Angioplasty-induced dissections in human iliac arteries: Management with Palmaz balloon expandable intraluminal stents. Radiology 176:31–38, 1990.
8. Katzen BT, Becker GJ: Intravascular stents: Status and development of clinical applications. Surg Clin North Am 72:941–957, 1992.
9. Sapoval MR, Chatellier G, Long AR, et al: Self-expandable stents for the treatment of iliac artery obstructive lesions: Long-term success and prognostic factors. AJR Am J Roentgenol 166:1173–1179, 1996.
10. Murphy TP, Webb MS, Lambiase RE, et al: Percutaneous revascularization of complex iliac artery stenoses and occlusions with use of Wallstents: Three year experience. J Vasc Interv Radiol 7:21–27, 1996.
11. Long AR, Gaux JC, Raynaud AC, et al: Infrarenal aortic stents: Initial clinical experience and angiographic follow-up. Cardiovasc Intervent Radiol 16:203–208, 1993.
12. Dietrich EB: Endovascular techniques for abdominal aortic occlusions. Int Angiol 12:270–280, 1993.
13. Martinez R, Rodriguez-Lopez J, Dietrich EB: Stenting of abdominal aortic occlusive disease: Long-term results. Tex Heart Inst J 24:15–22, 1997.
14. Palmaz JC, Encarnacion CE, Garcia OJ, et al: Aortic bifurcation stenosis: Treatment with intravascular stents. J Vasc Interv Radiol 2:319–323, 1991.
15. Long AR, Page PE, Raynaud AC, et al: Percutaneous iliac artery stent: Angiographic long-term follow-up. Radiology 180:771–778, 1991.
16. Blum U, Gabelmann A, Redecker M, et al: Percutaneous recanalization of iliac artery occlusions: Results of a prospective study. Radiology 189:536–540, 1993.
17. Dalsing MC, Ehrman KO, Cikrit DF, et al: Iliac artery angioplasty and stents: A current experience. *In* Yao JST, Pearce WH (eds): Technology in Vascular Surgery. Philadelphia, WB Saunders, 1992, pp 373–386.
18. Busquet J: The current role of vascular stents. Int Angiol 12:206–213, 1993.
19. Palmaz JC, Rivera FJ, Encarnacion CE: Intravascular stents. Adv Vasc Surg 1:107–135, 1993.
20. Ahn SS, Concepcion B: Indications and results of arterial stents for occlusive disease. World J Surg 20:644–648, 1996.
21. Legemate DA, Teeuwen C, Hoeneveld H, et al: The potential of duplex scanning to replace aortoiliac and femoropopliteal angiography. Eur J Vasc Surg 3:49–54, 1989.
22. Kohler TR, Nance DR, Cramer MM, et al: Duplex scanning for diagnosis of aortoiliac and femoropopliteal disease: A prospective study. Circulation 76:1074–1080, 1987.
23. Moneta GL, Yeager RA, Antonovic R, et al: Accuracy of lower extremity arterial duplex mapping. J Vasc Surg 15:275–284, 1992.
24. Cossman DV, Ellison JE, Wagner WH, et al: Comparison of contrast arteriography to color-flow duplex imaging in the lower extremities. J Vasc Surg 10:522–529, 1989.
25. Edwards JM, Coldwell DM, Goldman ML, et al: The role of duplex scanning in the selection of patients for transluminal angioplasty. J Vasc Surg 13:69–74, 1991.
26. Elsman BHP, Legemate DA, van der Heyden FWHM, et al: The use of color-coded duplex scanning in the selection of patients with lower extremity arterial disease for percutaneous transluminal angioplasty: A prospective study. Cardiovasc Intervent Radiol 19:313–316, 1996.
27. Elsman BHP, Legemate DA, van der Heyden FWHM, et al: Impact of ultrasonographic duplex scanning scanning on therapeutic decision making in lower limb arterial disease. Br J Surg 82:630–633, 1995.
28. Langsfeld M, Nepute J, Hershey FB, et al: The use of deep duplex scanning to predict hemodynamically significant aortoiliac stenoses. J Vasc Surg 7:395–399, 1988.
29. Burnham SJ, Jaques P, Burnham CB: Noninvasive detection of iliac artery stenosis in the presence of superficial femoral artery obstruction. J Vasc Surg 16:445–452, 1992.
30. Waugh JR, Sacharias N: Arteriographic complications in the DSA era. Radiology 182:243–246, 1992.
31. Gomes AN, Baker JD, Martin-Paredero V: Acute renal dysfunction after major arteriography. AJR 145:1249–1253, 1985.

32. Dawson P, Trewhella M: Intravascular contrast agents and renal failure. Clin Radiol 41:373–375, 1990.
33. Schneider PA: Strategic arteriography: Surgical approach and analysis of technique. Ann Vasc Surg 5:493–505, 1996.
34. Rholl KS: Percutaneous aortoiliac intervention in vascular disease. *In* Baum S, Pentecost MJ (eds.): Abram's Angiography: Interventional Radiology. Boston, Little, Brown & Co, 1997, pp 225–261.
35. Kalman PG, Sniderman KW, Johnston KW: Technique and six-year follow-up on percutaneous transluminal angioplasty to treat iliac arterial occlusive disease. *In* Yao JST, Pierce WH (eds): Long-Term Results in Vascular Surgery. Norwalk, Conn., Appleton & Lange, 1993, pp 201–212.
36. Jeans WD, Armstrong S, Cole SE, et al: Fate of patients undergoing transluminal angioplasty for lower limb ischemia. Radiology 177:559–564, 1990.
37. Johnston KW: Iliac arteries: Reanalysis of results of balloon angioplasty. Radiology 186:207–212, 1993.
38. Johnston KW: Femoral and popliteal arteries: Reanalysis of results of balloon angioplasty. Radiology 183:767–771, 1992.
39. Rutherford RB, Durham J: Percutaneous balloon angioplasty for arteriosclerosis obliterans: Long-term results. *In* Yao JST, Pearce WH (eds): Technologies in Vascular Surgery. Philadelphia, WB Saunders, 1992, pp 329–345.
40. Pentecost MJ, Criqui MH, Dorros G, et al: Guidelines for peripheral percutaneous transluminal angioplasty of the abdominal aorta and lower extremity vessels. Circulation 89:511–531, 1994.
41. Tegtmeyer CJ, Hartwell GD, Shelby JB, et al: Results and complications of angioplasty in aortoiliac disease. Circulation 83(Suppl I):I53–I60, 1991.
42. Bosch JL, Hunink MGM: Meta-analysis of the results of percutaneous transluminal angioplasty and stent placement for aortoiliac occlusive disease. Radiology 204:87–96, 1997.
43. Vorwerk D, Guenther RW, Schurmann K, et al: Primary stent placement for chronic iliac artery occlusions: Follow-up results in 103 patients. Radiology 194:745–749, 1995.
44. Dyet JF, Gaines PA, Nicholson AA, et al: Treatment of chronic iliac artery occlusions by means of percutaneous endovascular stent placement. J Vasc Interv Radiol 8:349–353, 1997.
45. Vroegindeweij D, Vos LD, Tielbeek AV, et al: Balloon angioplasty combined with primary stenting versus balloon angioplasty alone in femoropopliteal obstructions: A comparative randomized study. Cardiovasc Intervent Radiol 20:420–425, 1997.
46. Gunther RW, Vorwerk D, Bohndorf K, et al: Iliac and femoral artery stenoses and occlusions: Treatment with intravascular stents. Radiology 172:725–730, 1989.
47. Reyes R, Maynar M, Lopera J, et al: Treatment of chronic iliac artery occlusions with guidewire recanalization and primary stent placement. J Vasc Interv Radiol 8:1049–1055, 1997.
48. Capek P, McLean GK, Berkowitz HD: Femoropopliteal angioplasty: Factors influencing long-term success. Circulation 83:(Suppl I): I70–I80, 1991.
49. Kumpe DA, Jones DN: Percutaneous transluminal angioplasty: Radiological viewpoint. Vasc Diagn Ther 3:19, 1982.
50. Stanley B, Teague B, Spero R, et al: Efficacy of balloon angioplasty of the superficial femoral artery and the popliteal artery in the relief of leg ischemia. J Vasc Surg 23:679–685, 1996.
51. Krepel VM, van Andel GJ, van Erp WFM, et al: Percutaneous transluminal angioplasty of the femoropopliteal artery: Initial and long-term results. Radiology 156:325, 1985.
52. Murray RR, Hewes RC, White RI, et al: Long-segment femoropopliteal stenoses: Is angioplasty a boon or a bust? Radiology 162:473, 1987.
53. van Andel GJ, van Erp WFM, Krepel VM, et al: Percutaneous transluminal dilatation of the iliac artery: Long-term results. Radiology 156:321, 1985.
54. Wright JG, Belkin M, Greenfield AJ, et al: Laser angioplasty for limb salvage: Observations on early results. J Vasc Surg 10:29, 1989.
55. Zeitler E, Richter EI, Roth FJ, et al: Results of percutaneous transluminal angioplasty. Radiology 146:57–60, 1983.
56. Stokes KR, Strunk HM, Campbell DR, et al: Five-year results of iliac and femoropopliteal angioplasty in diabetic patients. Radiology 174:977, 1990.
57. Damaraju S, Cuasay L, Le D, et al: Predictors of primary patency failure in Wallstent self-expanding endovascular prostheses for iliofemoral occlusive disease. Tex Heart Inst J 24:173–178, 1997.
58. Henry M, Amor M, Ethevenot G, et al: Palmaz stent placement in the iliac and femoropopliteal arteries: Primary and secondary patency in 310 patients with 2- to 4-year follow-up. Radiology 197:167–174, 1995.
59. Laborde JC, Palmaz JC, Rivera FJ, et al: Influence of anatomic distribution of atherosclerosis on the outcome of revascularization with iliac stent placement. J Vasc Interv Radiol 6:513–521, 1995.
60. Gallino A, Mahler F, Probst P, et al: Percutaneous transluminal angioplasty of the arteries of the lower limbs: A 5-year follow-up. Circulation 70:619, 1984.
61. Graor RA, Young JR, McCandless M, et al: Percutaneous transluminal angioplasty: Review of iliac and femoral dilatations at Cleveland Clinic. Cleve Clin Q 51:149, 1984.
62. Johnston KW, Rae M, Hogg-Johnston SA, et al: Five year results of a prospective study of percutaneous transluminal angioplasty. Ann Surg 206:403, 1987.
63. Rush DS, Gewertz BL, Lu CT, et al: Limb salvage in poor risk patients using transluminal angioplasty. Arch Surg 118:1209, 1983.
64. Davies AH, Cole SE, Magee TR, et al: The effect of diabetes mellitus on the outcome of angioplasty for lower limb ischemia. Diabet Med 9:480–481, 1992.
65. Criqui MH, Coughlin SS, Fronek A: Noninvasively diagnosed peripheral arterial disease as a predictor of mortality: Results from a prospective study. Circulation 72:768–773, 1985.
66. Criqui MH, Langer RD, Fronek A, et al: Mortality over a ten year period in patients with peripheral arterial disease. N Engl J Med 325:556–562, 1992.
67. Sullivan TM, Childs MB, Bacharach JM, et al: Percutaneous transluminal angioplasty and primary stenting of the iliac arteries in 288 patients. J Vasc Surg 25:829–839, 1997.
68. Morin JF, Johnston KW, Wasserman L, et al: Factors that determine the long-term results of percutaneous transluminal dilatation for peripheral arterial occlusive disease. J Vasc Surg 4:68, 1986.
69. Schmidtke I, Roth F-J: Relapse treatment by percutaneous transluminal dilatation. *In* Dotter CT, Grüntzig AR, Schoop W, et al (eds): Percutaneous Transluminal Angioplasty: Technique, Early and Late Results. Berlin, Springer-Verlag, 1983, pp 131–139.
70. Treiman GS, Ichikawa L, Treiman RL, et al: Treatment of recurrent femoral or popliteal artery stenosis after percutaneous transluminal angioplasty. J Vasc Surg 20:577–585, 1994.
71. Berkowitz HO, Spence RK, Freiman DB, et al: Long-term results of transluminal angioplasty of the femoral arteries. *In* Dotter CT, Gruntzig AR, Schoop W, et al (eds): Percutaneous Transluminal Angioplasty: Technique, Early and Late Results. Berlin, Springer-Verlag, 1983, pp 207–214.
72. Neiman HL, Bergan JJ, Yao JST, et al: Hemodynamic assessment of transluminal angioplasty for lower extremity ischemia. Radiology 143:639, 1982.
73. Spence RK, Freeman DB, Gatenby R, et al: Long term results of transluminal angioplasty of the iliac and femoral arteries. Arch Surg 116:1377, 1981.
74. Sniderman KW: Noncoronary vascular stenting. Prog Cardiovasc Dis 39:141–164, 1996.
75. Treiman GS, Schneider PA, Lawrence PT, et al: Does stent placement improve the results of ineffective or complicated iliac artery angioplasty? J Vasc Surg 28:104–112, 1998.
76. Johnston KW, Kalman PG: Percutaneous transluminal angioplasty. *In* Kempczinski RF (ed): The Ischemic Leg. Chicago, Year Book Medical Publishers, 1985, pp 269–278.
77. Auster M, Kadir S, Mitchell SE, et al: Iliac artery occlusion: Management with intrathrombus streptokinase infusion and angioplasty. Radiology 153:385, 1984.
78. Martin EC: Femoropopliteal revascularization. *In* Baum S, Pentecos MJ: Abram's Angiography: Interventional Radiology. Boston, Little Brown & Co, 1997, pp 262–283.
79. Schneider PA, Andros G, Harris RW: Percutaneous balloon angioplasty for lower extremity arterial occlusive disease. *In* Carter DC, Russell RCG: Rob & Smith's Operative Surgery. London, Butterworth-Heinemann, 1994, pp 636–646.
80. Orron DE, Kim D: Percutaneous transluminal angioplasty. *In* Kim D, Orron DE (eds): Peripheral Vascular Imaging and Intervention. St. Louis, Mosby–Year Book, 1992, pp 379–420.
81. Dalsing MC, Harris VJ: Intravasculat stents. *In* White RA, Fogarty TJ (eds): Peripheral Endovascular Interventions. St. Louis, Mosby–Year Book, 1996, pp 315–339.

82. Schneider PA: Endovascular Skills. St Louis, Quality Medical Publishing, 1998.
83. Rutherford RB, Baker JD, Ernst C, et al: Recommended standards for reports dealing with lower extremity ischemia: Revised version. J Vasc Surg 26:517–538, 1997.
84. Rutherford RB: Reporting standards for endovascular surgery: Should existing standards be modified for newer procedures? Semin Vasc Surg 10:197–205, 1997.
85. Spies JB, Bakal CW, Burke DR, et al: Guidelines for percutaneous transluminal angioplasty. Radiology 177:619–626, 1990.
86. Rutherford RB: Standards for evaluating results of interventional therapy for peripheral vascular disease. Circulation 83:(Suppl I): I6–I11, 1991.
87. Ahn SS, Rutherford RB, Becker GJ, et al: Reporting standards for lower extremity arterial endovascular procedures. J Vasc Surg 17:1103–1107, 1993.
88. Myers KA: Reporting standards and statistics for evaluating intervention: Cardiovasc Surg 3:455–461, 1995.
89. Steinmetz OK, McPhail NV, Hajjar GE, et al: Endarterectomy versus angioplasty in the treatment of localized stenosis of the abdominal aorta. Can J Surg 37:385–390, 1994.
90. Ravimandalam K, Rao VR, Kumar S, et al: Obstruction of the infrarenal portion of the abdominal aorta: Results of treatment with balloon angioplasty. AJR Am J Roentgenol 156:1257–1260, 1991.
91. Tadavarthy AK, Sullivan WA, Nicoloff D, et al: Aorta balloon angioplasty: 9-year follow-up. Radiology 170:1039–1041, 1989.
92. Hedeman Joosten PPA, Ho GH, Breuking FA, et al: Percutaneous transluminal angioplasty of the infrarenal aorta: Initial outcome and long term clinical and angiographic results. Eur J Vasc Endovasc Surg 12:201–206, 1996.
93. el Ashmaoui A, Do DD, Triller J, et al: Angioplasty of the terminal aorta: Follow-up of twenty patients treated by PTA or PTA with stents. Eur J Radiol 13:113–117, 1991.
94. Hallisey MJ, Meranze SG, Parker BC, et al: Percutaneous transluminal angioplasty of the abdominal aorta. J Vasc Interv Radiol 5:679–687, 1994.
95. Kalman PG, Johnston KW, Sniderman KW: Indications and results of balloon angioplasty for arterial occlusive lesions. World J Surg 20:630–634, 1996.
96. Vorwerk D, Gunther RW, Bohndorf K, et al: Stent placement for failed angioplasty of aortic stenoses: Report of two cases. Cardiovasc Intervent Radiol 14:316–319, 1991.
97. Sheeran SR, Hallisey MJ, Ferguson D: Percutaneous transluminal stent placement in the abdominal aorta. J Vasc Interv Radiol 8:55–60, 1997.
98. Dietrich EB, Santiago O, Gustafson G, et al: Preliminary observations on the use of the Palmaz stent in the distal portion of the abdominal aorta. Am Heart J 125:490–501, 1993.
99. Sagic D, Grujicic S, Peric M, et al: "Kissing balloon" technique for abdominal aortic angioplasty: Initial results and long term outcome. Int Angiol 14:364–367, 1995.
100. Morag B, Garniek A, Bass A, et al: Percutaneous transluminal aortic angioplasty: Early and late results. Cardiovasc Intervent Radiol 16:37–42, 1993.
101. Yakes WF, Kumpe DA, Brown SB, et al: Percutaneous transluminal aortic angioplasty: Techniques and results. Radiology 172:965–970, 1989.
102. Morag B, Rubinstein Z, Kessler A, et al: Percutaneous transluminal angioplasty of the distal abdominal aorta and its bifurcation. Cardiovasc Intervent Radiol 10:129–133, 1987.
103. Insall RL, Loose HW, Chamberlain J: Long-term results of double-balloon percutaneous transluminal angioplasty of the aorta and iliac arteries. Eur J Vasc Surg 7:31–36, 1993.
104. Pilger E, Decrinis M, Stark G, et al: Thrombolytic treatment and balloon angioplasty in chronic occlusion of the aortic bifurcation. Ann Intern Med 120:40–44, 1994.
105. Kuffer G, Spengel F, Steckmeier B: Percutaneous reconstruction of the aortic bifurcation with Palmaz stents: Case reports. Cardiovasc Intervent Radiol 14:170–172, 1991.
106. In der Maur GTD, Boeve J, Kerdel MC, et al: Angioplasty of the iliac and femoral arteries: Initial and long-term results in short stenotic lesions. Eur J Radiol 11:163, 1990.
107. Jorgensen B, Skovgaard N, Norgard J, et al: Percutaneous transluminal angioplasty in 226 iliac artery stenoses: Role of the superficial femoral artery for clinical success. Vasa 21:382–386, 1993.
108. Rutherford RB, Patt A, Kumpe DA: The current role of percutaneous transluminal angioplasty. *In* Greenlagh KM (ed): Vascular Surgery: Issues in Current Practice. New York, Grune & Stratton, 1986, pp 229–244.
109. Palmaz JC, Richter GM, Noeldge G, et al: Intraluminal stents in atherosclerotic iliac artery stenosis: Preliminary report of a multicenter study. Radiology 168:727, 1988.
110. Palmaz JC, Garcia OJ, Schatz RA, et al: Placement of balloon-expandable intraluminal stents in iliac arteries: First 171 procedures. Radiology 174:969, 1990.
111. Richter G: Balloon-expandable Palmaz stent placement versus PTA in iliac artery stenoses and occlusions: Long term results of a randomized trial. Presented at the Society of Cardiovascular and Interventional Radiologists' Annual Meeting in Washington, DC, 1992.
112. Richter GM, Roeren T, Noeldge G, et al: Prospective randomized trial: Iliac stenting versus PTA (Abstract). Angiology 43:268, 1992.
113. Richter GM, Noeldge G, Roeren T, et al: First long-term results of a randomized multicenter trial: Iliac balloon-expandable stent placement versus regular percutaneous transluminal angioplasty (Abstract). Radiology 177:152, 1990.
114. Richter GM, Roeren T, Brado M, et al: Long-term results: Palmaz's stent. Presented to the Radiological Society of North America, Chicago, 1993.
115. Cikrit DF, Gustafson PA, Dalsing MC, et al: Long-term follow-up of the Palmaz stent for iliac occlusive disease. Surgery 118:608–613, 1995.
116. Martin EC, Katzen BT, Benenati JP, et al: Multicenter trial of Wallstent in the iliac and femoral arteries. J Vasc Interv Radiol 6:843–849, 1995.
117. Palmaz JC, Laborde JC, Rivera FJ, et al: Stenting of the iliac arteries with the Palmaz stent: Experience from a multicenter trial. Cardiovasc Intervent Radiol 15:291–297, 1992.
118. Murphy KD, Encarnacion CE, Le VA, et al: Iliac artery stent placement with the Palmaz stent: Follow-up study. J Vasc Interv Radiol 6:321–329, 1995.
119. Tetteroo E, Haaring C, van der Graaf Y, et al: Intra-arterial pressure gradients after randomized angioplasty or stenting of iliac artery lesions. Cardiovasc Intervent Radiol 19:411–417, 1996.
120. Tetteroo E, Haaring C, van Engelen AD, et al: Therapeutic consequences of variation in intraarterial pressure measurements after iliac angioplasty. Cardiovasc Intervent Radiol 20:426–430, 1997.
121. Brewster DC, Cambria RP, Darling RC, et al: Long-term results of combined iliac balloon angioplasty and distal surgical revascularization. Ann Surg 210:324, 1989.
122. Schneider PA, Abcarian PW, Ogawa DY, et al: Should balloon angioplasty and stents have a role in operative intervention for lower extremity ischemia? Ann Vasc Surg 11:574–580, 1997.
123. Hsiang YN, al-Salman M, Doyle DL, et al: Comparison of percutaneous with intraoperative balloon angioplasty for arteriosclerotic occlusive disease. Aust N Z J Surg 63:864–869, 1993.
124. Alimi Y, Di Mauro P, Barthelemy P, et al: Iliac transluminal angioplasty and distal surgical revascularization can be performed in a one-step technique. Int Angiol 16:83–87, 1997.
125. Bull PG, Schegl A, Mendel H: Combined iliac transluminal angioplasty and femoropopliteal reconstruction for multilevel arterial occlusive disease. Int Surg 78:332–337, 1993.
126. Walker PJ, Harris JP, May J: Combined percutaneous transluminal angioplasty and extraanatomic bypass for symptomatic unilateral iliac artery occlusion with contralateral iliac artery stenosis. Ann Vasc Surg 5:209–216, 1991.
127. Wilkinson JM, Beard JD, Gaines PA: Aortoiliac occlusion treated by a combination of aortoiliac stent and femorofemoral crossover grafting. Eur J Vasc Endovasc Surg 12:372–374, 1996.
128. Wilson SE, White GH, Wolf G, et al: Proximal percutaneous balloon angioplasty and distal bypass for multilevel arterial occlusion: Veterans Administration Cooperative Study No. 199. Ann Vasc Surg 4:351–355, 1990.
129. Peterkin GA, Belkin M, Cantelmo NL, et al: Combined transluminal angioplasty and infrainguinal reconstruction in multilevel atherosclerotic disease. Am J Surg 160:277–279, 1990.
130. van der Vliet JA, Mulling FJ, Heijstraten FM, et al: Femoropopliteal arterial reconstruction with intraoperative iliac transluminal angioplasty for disabling claudication: Results of a combined approach. Eur J Vasc Surg 6:607–609, 1992.
131. Demasi RJ, Snyder SO, Wheeler JR, et al: Intraoperative iliac artery stents: Combination with infrainguinal revascularization procedures. Am Surg 60:854–859, 1994.
132. Schneider PA: Balloon angioplasty and stent placement during opera-

tive vascular reconstruction for lower extremity ischemia. Ann Vasc Surg 10:589–598, 1996.

133. Gupta AK, Ravimandalam K, Rao VRK, et al: Total occlusion of the iliac arteries: Results of balloon angioplasty. Cardiovasc Intervent Radiol 16:165–177, 1993.
134. Motarjeme A, Gordon GI, Bodenhagen K: Thrombolysis and angioplasty of chronic iliac artery occlusions. J Vasc Intervent Radiol 6(Suppl):66S–72S, 1995.
135. Meyerovitz MF, Didier D, Vogel JJ, et al: Thrombolytic therapy compared with mechanical recanalization in non-acute peripheral arterial occlusions: A randomized trial. J Vasc Interv Radiol 6:775–781, 1995.
136. Yedlicka JW, Ferral H, Bjarnson H, et al: Chronic iliac artery occlusions: Primary recanalization with endovascular stents. J Vasc Interv Radiol 5:843–847, 1994.
137. Ballard JL, Taylor FC, Sparks SR, et al: Stenting without thrombolysis for aortoiliac occlusive disease: Experience in 14 high-risk patients. Ann Vasc Surg 9:453–458, 1995.
138. Matsi PJ, Manninen HI, Vanninen RL, et al: Femoropopliteal angioplasty in patients with claudication: Primary and secondary patency in 140 limbs with 1–3 year follow-up. Radiology 191:727–733, 1994.
139. Adar R, Critchfield GC, Eddy DM, et al: A confidence profile analysis of the results of femoropopliteal percutaneous transluminal angioplasty in the treatment of lower extremity ischemia. J Vasc Surg 10:57–67, 1989.
140. Smith CM, Yellin AE, Weaver FA, et al: Thrombolytic therapy for arterial occlusion: A mixed blessing. Am Surg 60:371–375, 1994.
141. Matas Docampo M, Gomez Palones F, Fernandez Valenzuela V, et al: Intraarterial urokinase for acute native arterial occlusion of the limbs. Ann Vasc Surg 11:565–572, 1997.
142. Bhatnagar PK, Ierardi RP, Ikeda I, et al: The impact of thrombolytic therapy on arterial and graft occlusions. J Cardiovasc Surg 37:105–112, 1996.
143. Chalmer RT, Hoballah JJ, Kresowick TF, et al: Late results of a prospective study of direct intra-arterial urokinase infusion for peripheral arterial and bypass graft occlusions. Cardiovasc Surg 3:293–297, 1995.
144. Jorgensen B, Tonnesen KH, Holstein P: Late hemodynamic failure following percutaneous transluminal angioplasty for long and multifocal femoropopliteal stenoses. Cardiovasc Intervent Radiol 14:290–292, 1991.
145. Currie IC, Wakeley CJ, Cole SE, et al: Femoropopliteal angioplasty for severe limb ischemia. Br J Surg 81:191–193, 1994.
146. Lu CT, Zarins CF, Yang CF, et al: Percutaneous transluminal angioplasty for limb salvage. Radiology 142:337, 1982.
147. Ray SA, Minty I, Buckenham TM, et al: Clinical outcome and restenosis following percutaneous transluminal angioplasty for ischemic rest pain or ulceration. Br J Surg 82:1217–1221, 1995.
148. Do-dai-Do, Triller J, Walpoth BH, et al: A comparison study of self-expandable stents versus balloon angioplasty alone in femoropopliteal artery occlusions. Cardiovasc Intervent Radiol 15:306–312, 1992.
149. Rousseau HP, Raillat CR, Joffre FG, et al: Treatment of femoropopliteal stenoses by means of self-expandable endoprostheses: Midterm results. Radiology 172:961–964, 1989.
150. Sapoval MR, Long AL, Raynaud AC, et al: Femoropopliteal stent placement: Long term results. Radiology 184:833–839, 1992.
151. White GH, Liew SCC, Waugh RC, et al: Early outcome and intermediate follow-up of vascular stents in the femoral and popliteal arteries without long-term anticoagulation. J Vasc Surg 21:270–281, 1995.
152. Bergeron P, Pinot JJ, Poyen V, et al: Long-term results with the Palmaz stent in the superficial femoral artery. J Endovasc Surg 2:161–167, 1995.
153. Chatelard P, Guibourt C: Long-term results with a Palmaz stent in the femoropopliteal arteries. J Cardiovasc Surg 37(Suppl 1):67–72, 1996.
154. Bull PG, Mendel H, Hold M, et al: Distal popliteal and tibioperoneal transluminal angioplasty: Long-term follow-up. J Vasc Interv Radiol 3:45–53, 1992.
155. Dorros G, Lewin RF, Jamnadas P, et al: Below-the-knee angioplasty: Tibioperoneal vessels, the acute outcome. Cathet Cardiovasc Diagn 19:170–178, 1990.
156. Schwarten DE: Clinical and anatomical considerations for nonoperative therapy in tibial disease and the results of angioplasty. Circulation 83 (Suppl I):86, 1991.
157. Saab MH, Smith DC, Aka PK, et al: Percutaneous transluminal angioplasty of the tibial arteries for limb salvage. Cardiovasc Intervent Radiol 15:211–216, 1992.
158. Buckenham TM, Loh A, Dormandy JA, et al: Infrapopliteal angioplasty for limb salvage. Eur J Vasc Surg 7:21–25, 1993.
159. Hanna GP, Fujise K, Kjellgren O, et al: Infrapopliteal transcatheter interventions for limb salvage in diabetic patients: Importance of aggressive interventional approach and role of transcutaneous oximetry. J Am Coll Cardiol 30:664–669, 1997.
160. Durham JR, Horowitz JD, Wright JG, et al: Percutaneous transluminal angioplasty of the tibial arteries for limb salvage in the high-risk diabetic patient. Ann Vasc Surg 8:48–53, 1994.
161. Varty K, Bolia A, Naylor AR, et al: Infrapopliteal percutaneous transluminal angioplasty: A safe and successful procedure. Eur J Vasc Endovasc Surg 9:341–345, 1995.
162. Nydahl S, Hartshorne T, Bell PR, et al: Subintimal angioplasty of infrapopliteal occlusions in critically ischemic limbs. Eur J Vasc Endovasc Surg 14:212–216, 1997.
163. Treiman GS, Treiman RL, Ichikawa L, et al: Should percutaneous transluminal angioplasty be recommended for treatment of infrageniculate popliteal artery or tibioperoneal trunk stenosis? J Vasc Surg 22:457–463, 1995.
164. Lofberg AM, Lorelius LE, Karacagil S, et al: The use of below-knee percutaneous transluminal angioplasty in arterial occlusive disease causing chronic critical limb ischemia. Cardiovasc Intervent Radiol 19:317–322, 1996.
165. Favre JP, Do Carmo G, Adham M, et al: Results of transluminal angioplasty of infra-popliteal arteries. J Cardiovasc Surg 37(Suppl 1):33–37, 1996.
166. Bakal CW, Sprayregen S, Scheinbaum K, et al: Percutaneous transluminal angioplasty of the infrapopliteal arteries: Results in 53 patients. AJR Am J Roentgenol 154:171–174, 1990.
167. Brown KT, Schoenberg NY, Moore ED, et al: Percutaneous transluminal angioplasty of the infrapopliteal vessels: Preliminary results and technical considerations. Radiology 169:75–78, 1988.
168. Horvath W, Oertl M, Haidinger D: Percutaneous transluminal angioplasty of crural arteries. Radiology 177:565–569, 1990.
169. Brown KT, Moore ED, Getrajdman GI, et al: Infrapopliteal angioplasty: Long-term follow-up. J Vasc Interv Radiol 4:139–144, 1993.
170. Sprayregen S, Sniderman KW, Sos TA, et al: Popliteal artery branches: Percutaneous transluminal angioplasty. AJR 135:945–950, 1980.
171. Tamura S, Sniderman KW, Beinart C, et al: Percutaneous transluminal angioplasty of the popliteal artery and its branches. Radiology 143:645–648, 1982.
172. Jagust MB, Sos TA: Infrapopliteal revascularization. *In* Baum S, Pentecost MJ (eds): Abram's Angiography: Interventional Radiology. Boston, Little, Brown & Co, 1997, pp 284–293.
173. Wolf YG, Schatz RA, Knowles HJ, et al: Initial experience with the Palmaz stent for aortoiliac stenoses. Ann Vasc Surg 7:254–261, 1993.
174. Motarjeme A, Keifer JW, Zuska AJ: Percutaneous transluminal angioplasty of the deep femoral artery. Radiology 135:613, 1980.
175. Waltman AC: Percutaneous transluminal angioplasty: Iliac and deep femoral arteries. AJR 135:921,1980.
176. Ballard JL Sparks SR, Taylor FC, et al: Complications of iliac artery stent deployment. J Vasc Surg 24:545–553, 1996.
177. Bunt TJ, Gill HK, Smith DC, et al: Infection of a chronically implanted iliac artery stent. Ann Vasc Surg 11:529–532, 1997.
178. Ray CE, Kaufman JA, Waltman AC, et al: Inadvertent compression of intraarterial Palmaz stents during vascular surgery. AJR Am J Roentgenol 166:996–997, 1996.
179. Cisek PL, McKittrick JE: Retrograde aortic dissection after bilateral iliac artery stenting: A case report. Ann Vasc Surg 9:280–284, 1995.
180. Weinberg DJ, Cronin DW, Baker AG: Infected iliac pseudoaneurysm after uncomplicated percutaneous balloon angioplasty and (Palmaz) stent insertion: A case report and literature review. J Vasc Surg 23:162–166, 1996.
181. Vorwerk D, Gunther RW, Keulers P, et al: Surgical and percutaneous management of contralateral thrombus dislodgement following stent placement and dilatation of iliac artery occlusions: Technical note. Cardiovasc Intervent Radiol 14:134–136, 1991.
182. Chalmers N, Eadington DW, Gandanhamo D, et al: Case report: Infected false aneurysm at the site of an iliac stent. Br J Radiol 66:946–948, 1993.
183. Therasse E, Soulez G, Cartier P, et al: Infection with fatal outcome after endovascular metallic stent placement. Radiology 192:363–365, 1994.
184. Hoffman AI, Murphy TP: Septic arteritis causing iliac artery rupture

and aneurysmal transformation of the distal aorta after iliac artery stent placement. J Vasc Interv Radiol 8:215–219, 1997.
185. Cutry AF, Whitley D, Patterson RB: Midaortic pseudoaneurysm complicating extensive endovascular stenting of aortic disease. J Vasc Surg 26:958–962, 1997.
186. Liu P, Dravid P, Freiman D, et al: Persistent iliac endarteritis with pseudoaneurysm formation following balloon-expandable stent placement. Cardiovasc Intervent Radiol 18:39–42, 1995.
187. van Lankeren W, Gussenhoven EJ, van Kints MJ, et al: Stent remodeling contributes to femoropopliteal artery restenosis: An intravascular ultrasound study. J Vasc Surg 25:753–756, 1997.
188. Deiparine MK, Ballard JL, Taylor FC, et al: Endovascular stent infection. J Vasc Surg 23:529–533, 1996.
189. Stoeckelhuber BM, Szeimies U, Spengel FA, et al: Late thromboembolic complication from a Palmaz stent in the common iliac artery. Cardiovasc Intervent Radiol 19:190–192, 1996.
190. Sacks BA, Miller A, Gottlieb M: Fracture of an iliac artery Palmaz stent. J Vasc Interv Radiol 7:53–55, 1996.
191. Armstrong MWJ, Torrie EPH, Galland RB: Consequences of immediate failure of percutaneous transluminal angioplasty. Ann R Coll Surg Engl 74:265–268, 1992.
192. Becker GJ: Intravascular stents: General principles and status of lower extremity arterial applications. Circulation 83(Suppl I):I122–I136, 1991.
193. Sapoval MR, Long AL, Pagny JY, et al: Outcome of percutaneous intervention in iliac artery stents. Radiology 198:481–486, 1996.
194. Kalman PG, Johnston KW: Outcome of a failed percutaneous transluminal dilation. Surg Gynecol Obstet 161:43, 1985.
195. Vorwerk D, Guenther RW, Schurmann K, et al: Late reobstruction in iliac artery stents: Percutaneous treatment. Radiology 197:479–483, 1995.
196. Harris RW, Dulawa LB, Andros G, et al: Percutaneous transluminal angioplasty of the lower extremities by the vascular surgeon. Ann Vasc Surg 5:345–353, 1991.
197. Gross GM, Johnson RC, Roberts RM: Results of peripheral endovascular procedures in the operating room. J Vasc Surg 24:353–361, 1996.
198. Silva MB, Hobson RW, Jamil Z, et al: A program of operative angioplasty: Endovascular intervention and the vascular surgeon. J Vasc Surg 24:963–971, 1996.
199. Clement C, Costa-Foru B, Vernon P, et al: Transluminal angioplasty performed by the surgeon in lower limb arterial disease: One hundred fifty cases. Ann Vasc Surg 4:519–527, 1990.
200. Creasy TS, McMillan PJ, Fletcher EWL, et al: Is percutaneous transluminal angioplasty better than exercise for claudication? Preliminary results from a prospective randomized trial. Eur J Vasc Surg 4:135, 1990.
201. Whyman MR, Fowkes FG, Kerracher EM, et al: Is intermittent claudication improved by percutaneous transluminal angioplasty? A randomized controlled trial. J Vasc Surg 26:551–557, 1997.
202. Davies AH, Ramarakha P, Collin J, et al: Recent changes in the treatment of aortoiliac occlusive disease by the Oxford Regional Vascular Service. Br J Surg 77:1129–1131, 1990.
203. Hallet JW, Byrne J, Gayari MM, et al: Impact of arterial surgery and balloon angioplasty on amputation: A population-based study of 1155 procedures between 1973 and 1992. J Vasc Surg 25:29–38, 1997.
204. Tunis SR, Bass EB, Steinberg EP: The use of angioplasty, bypass surgery, and amputation in the management of peripheral vascular disease. N Engl J Med 22:556–562, 1991.
205. Becquemin JP, Cavillon A, Allaire E, et al: Iliac and femoropopliteal lesions: Evaluation of balloon angioplasty and classical surgery. J Endovasc Surg 2:42–50, 1995.
206. Lorenzi G, Domanin M, Costantini A, et al: Role of bypass, endarterectomy, extra-anatomic bypass and endovascular surgery in unilateral iliac occlusive disease: A review of 1257 cases. Cardiovasc Surg 2: 370–373, 1994.
207. Wilson SE, Wolf GL, Cross AP, et al: Percutaneous transluminal angioplasty versus operation for peripheral arteriosclerosis: Report of a prospective randomized trial in a selected group of patients. J Vasc Surg 9:1–9, 1989.
208. Wolf GL, Wilson SE, Cross AP, et al: Surgery or balloon angioplasty for peripheral vascular disease: A randomized clinical trial: Veterans' Administration Cooperative Study No. 199. J Vasc Interv Radiol 4:639–648,1993.
209. Holm J, Arfvidsson B, Jivegard L, et al: Chronic lower limb ischemia: A prospective randomized controlled study comparing 1 year results of vascular surgery and percutaneous transluminal angioplasty. Eur J Vasc Surg 5:517–522, 1991.
210. Freiman DB, Freiman MP, Spence RK, et al: Economic impact of transluminal angioplasty. Angiology 36:772, 1985.
211. Jeans WD, Danton RM, Baird RN, et al: A comparison of the costs of vascular surgery and balloon dilatation in lower limb ischaemic disease. Br J Radiol 59:453, 1986.
212. Kinnison ML, White RI, Bowers WP, et al: Cost incentives for peripheral angioplasty. AJR 145:1241, 1985.
213. Ballard JL, Bergan JJ, Singh P, et al: Aortoiliac stent deployment versus surgical reconstruction: Analysis of outcome and cost. Presented at the Western Vascular Society, Lanai, Hawaii, 1997.
214. Boyd AM: The natural course of arteriosclerosis of the lower extremities. Angiology 11:10, 1960.
215. DeWeese JA, Rob CG: Autogenous venous grafts ten years later. Surgery 82:775, 1977.
216. Cooper JC, Welsh CL: The role of percutaneous transluminal angioplasty in the treatment of critical ischemia. Eur J Vasc Surg 5:261–264, 1991.
217. Gutteridge W, Torrie EP, Galland RB: Cumulative risk of bypass, amputation or death following percutaneous transluminal angioplasty. Eur J Vasc Endovasc Surg 14:134–139, 1997.
218. Sapoval MR, Gaux JC, Long AL, et al: Transient periprosthetic thickening after covered-stent implantation in the iliac artery. AJR Am J Roentgenol 164:1271–1273, 1995.
219. Tepe G, Duda SH, Hanke H, et al: Covered stents for prevention of restenosis: Experimental and clinical results with different stent designs. Invest Radiol 31:223–229, 1996.
220. Link J, Muller-Hulsbeck S, Brossman J, et al: Perivascular inflammatory reaction after percutaneous placement of covered stents. Cardiovasc Intervent Radiol 19:345–347, 1996.
221. Nevelsteen A, Lacroix H, Stockx L, et al: Stent grafts for iliofemoral occlusive disease. Cardiovasc Surg 5:393–397, 1997.
222. Pernes JM, Auguste MA, Hovasse D, et al: Long iliac stenosis: Initial clinical experience with the Cragg endoluminal graft. Radiology 196:67–71, 1995.
223. Marin ML, Veith FJ, Sanchez LA, et al: Endovascular repair of aortoiliac occlusive disease. World J Surg 20:679–686, 1996.
224. Lacroix H, Stockx L, Wilms G, et al: Transfemoral treatment for iliac occlusive disease with endoluminal stent-grafts. Eur J Vasc Endovasc Surg 14:204–207, 1997.
225. Henry M, Amor M, Ethevnot G, et al: Initial experience with the Cragg Endopro System 1 for intraluminal treatment of peripheral vascular disease. J Endovasc Surg 1:31–43, 1994.
226. Sanchez LA, Marin ML, Veith FJ, et al: Placement of endovascular stented grafts via remote access sites: A new approach to the treatment of failed aortoiliofemoral reconstructions. Ann Vasc Surg 9:1–8, 1995.
227. Cynamon J, Marin ML, Veith FJ, et al: Stent-graft repair of aorto-iliac occlusive disease coexisting with common femoral artery disease. J Vasc Interv Radiol 8:19–26, 1997.
228. Ohki T, Marin ML, Veith FJ, et al: Endovascular aortounifemoral grafts and femorofemoral bypass for bilateral limb-threatening ischemia. J Vasc Surg 24:984–996, 1996.
229. Marin ML, Veith FJ, Sanchez LA, et al: Endovascular aortoiliac grafts in combination with standard infrainguinal arterial bypasses in the management of limb-threatening ischemia: Preliminary report. J Vasc Surg 22:316–324, 1995.
230. Marin ML, Veith FJ: Clinical application of endovascular grafts in aortoiliac occlusive disease and vascular trauma. Cardiovasc Surg 3:115–120, 1995.
231. Spoelstra H, Casselman F, Lesceu O: Balloon-expandable endobypass for femoropopliteal atherosclerotic occlusive disease: A preliminary evaluation of fifty-five patients. J Vasc Surg 24:647–654, 1996.
232. Dietrich EB, Papazoglou K: Endoluminal grafting for aneurysmal and occlusive disease in the superficial femoral artery: Early experience. J Endovasc Surg 2:225–239, 1995.
233. Sanborn TA, Cumberland DC, Greenfield AJ, et al: Percutaneous laser thermal angioplasty: Initial results and 1-year follow-up in 129 femoropopliteal lesions. Radiology 168:121, 1988.
234. Blebea J, Ouriel K, Green RM, et al: Laser angioplasty in peripheral vascular disease: Symptomatic versus hemodynamic results. J Vasc Surg 13:222, 1991.
235. Harrington ME, Schwartz ME, Sanborn TA, et al: Expanded indica-

tions for laser-assisted balloon angioplasty in peripheral arterial disease. J Vasc Surg 11:146, 1990.
236. Perler BA, Osterman FA, White RI, et al: Percutaneous laser probe femoropopliteal angioplasty: A preliminary experience. J Vasc Surg 10:351, 1989.
237. AbuRahma AF, Robinson PA, Kennard W, Boland JP: Intra-operative peripheral Nd:YAG laser-assisted thermal balloon angioplasty: Short-term and intermediate-term follow-up. J Vasc Surg 12:566, 1990.
238. Rosenthal D, Wheeler WG, Seagraves A, et al: Nd:YAG iliac and femoropopliteal laser angioplasty: Results with large probes as "sole therapy." J Cardiovasc Surg 32:186, 1991.
239. Geschwind HJ, Dubois-Rande J, Shafton E, et al: Percutaneous pulsed laser-assisted balloon angioplasty guided by spectroscopy. Am Heart J 117:1147, 1989.
240. Leon MB, Almagor Y, Bartorelli AL, et al: Fluorescence-guided laser-assisted balloon angioplasty in patients with femoropopliteal occlusions. Circulation 81:143, 1990.
241. Simpson JB, Selman MR, Roberson GC, et al: Transluminal atherectomy for occlusive peripheral vascular disease. J Am Coll Cardiol 61:96, 1988.
242. Polnitz A, Nerlich A, Berger H, et al: Percutaneous peripheral atherectomy. J Am Coll Cardiol 15:682, 1990.
243. Dorros G, Iyer S, Lewin R, et al: Angiographic follow-up and clinical outcome of 126 patients after percutaneous directional atherectomy (Simpson AtheroCath) for occlusive peripheral vascular disease. Cathet Cardiovasc Diagn 22:79, 1991.
244. Jennings LJ, Mehigan JT, Ginsberg R, et al: Rotablator atherectomy: Early experience and six-month follow-up. Presented at the Western Vascular Society, Rancho Mirage, Calif, January 1991.
245. Wholey MH, Jarmolowski CR: New reperfusion devices: The Kensey catheter, the atherolytic reperfusion wire device, and the transluminal extraction catheter. Radiology 172:947, 1989.
246. Tabbara MR, White RA, Cavaye DM, et al: In-vivo human comparison of intravascular ultrasound and angiography. J Vasc Surg 14:496–504, 1991.
247. Scoccianti M, Verbin CS, Kopchok GE, et al: Intravascular ultrasound guidance for peripheral vascular interventions. J Endovasc Surg 1:71–80, 1994.
248. Losordo DW, Rosenfield K, Piezcek A, et al: How does angioplasty work? Serial analysis of human iliac arteries using intravascular ultrasound. Circulation 86:1845–1858, 1992.
249. Dietrich EB: Endovascular treatment of abdominal aortic occlusive disease: The impact of stents and intravascular ultrasound imaging. Eur J Vasc Surg 7:228–236, 1993.
250. Cavaye DM, Dietrich EB, Santiago OJ, et al: Intravascular ultrasound imaging: An essential component of angioplasty assessment and vascular stent deployment. Int Angiol 12:212–220, 1993.
251. White RA, Verbin C, Kopchok G, et al: Role of cinefluoroscopy and intravascular ultrasound in evaluating the deployment of experimental endovascular prostheses. J Vasc Surg 21:365–371, 1995.
252. van Lankeren W, Gussenhoven EJ, van der Lugt A, et al: Intravascular sonographic evaluation of iliac artery angioplasty: What is the mechanism of angioplasty and can intravascular sonography predict clinical outcome? AJR Am J Roentgenol 166:1355–1360, 1996.
253. Bolz KD, Hatlinghus R, Wiseth R, et al: Angiographic and intravascular ultrasonographic findings after endovascular stent implantation. Acta Radiol 35:590–596, 1994.

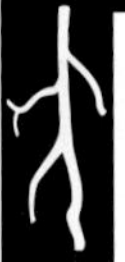

CHAPTER 73

Lumbar Sympathectomy: Indications and Technique

Robert B. Rutherford, M.D.

HISTORICAL BACKGROUND

The concept of sympathetic denervation as a mode of therapy for arterial occlusive disease was first elaborated and tested by Leriche and Jaboulay in 1913.[20] Their experience with periarterial sympathectomy was disappointing because of reinnervation and vasospasm recurring within weeks of operation. Adopting the lumbar sympathetic ganglionectomy technique of Royle and Hunter, Adson and Brown in the United States and Diez in South America secured more lasting relief among patients with symptomatic vasospasm in the 1920s.[1a, 17] These reports marked the beginning of an era in which sympathetic denervation ultimately became widely used for occlusive arterial disease, often as the only surgical alternative to amputation.

During the next 30 years, variable results were reported, but the use of the procedure was not seriously challenged because alternative methods of improving limb perfusion were unavailable. With the development of arterial reconstructive techniques, direct vascularization supplanted sympathectomy as optimal surgical therapy by the 1960s. The transition was aided by experimental studies of the effects of sympathetic denervation that confirmed the growing clinical impression that significant hemodynamic improvement could *not* be achieved with this approach alone. With further improvement in reconstructive techniques, vascular indications for lumbar sympathectomy have become very limited. During this transition, many surgeons persisted in using sympathectomy, admitting its lesser degree of benefit but preferring its lower risk.

Currently, noninvasive vascular testing, performed before and after sympathetic blockade, is being increasingly used preoperatively to provide objective evidence for a potential benefit of sympathectomy rather than being applied empirically in the hope that it might help. In this chapter, the physiologic consequences and the results of lumbar sympathectomy in different clinical settings are presented as the basis for recommended indications and techniques.

PHYSIOLOGIC CONSEQUENCES

Critical understanding of the effects of lumbar sympathectomy requires synthesis of both clinical and experimental data. Although sympathetic denervation clearly increases blood flow to a normal limb, its impact on an extremity afflicted with arterial occlusive disease is less clear. Elucidation of its role in improving microcirculatory hemodynamics and relieving ischemic symptoms can be considered in regard to several aspects:

1. Magnitude, distribution, and duration of the blood flow increase.
2. Effect of the procedure on collateral perfusion in acute and chronic ischemia.
3. Nutritive value of the observed flow increases.
4. Alteration of pain impulse transmission.

The effect of sympathectomy on each of these factors is examined within the context of more recent studies that attempt to define better the potential benefit of sympathectomy in limb ischemia.

Increase in Blood Flow

Lumbar sympathectomy increases total blood flow to an extremity by abolishing both basal and reflex constriction of arterioles and precapillary sphincters. Flow increases ranging from 10% to 200% have been observed and vary with the degree of arterial occlusive disease involving the limb.[2, 11, 41, 68] Indeed, patients with severe, multilevel occlusions may receive no benefit from sympathectomy because their muscular and cutaneous arteries are already maximally dilated at rest. In both normal and diseased limbs, most of the observed flow increase is shunted through cutaneous arteriovenous anastomoses (AVAs) with only small increases in tissue perfusion.[13] This alteration in blood flow distribution is due to elimination of the primary sympathetic function of modulating the musculocutaneous distribution in response to thermal regulatory requirements. After sympathectomy, the positive distributional effects are maximal for the distal cutaneous circulation and characteristically produce the warm, pink foot or hand that, for many years, was thought to reflect the overall improvement in limb perfusion.

This phenomenon of extremity blood flow redistribution is important because improved muscular perfusion was once presumed to parallel increased cutaneous blood flow and justify the application of sympathectomy for claudication. Radioactively labeled microsphere studies by Rutherford and Valenta in a canine arterial occlusion model showed that neither resting nor exertional muscle perfusion are improved by sympathectomy.[56] Using a similar technique in a canine hindlimb study, Cronenwett and Lindenauer[12] corroborated this finding in subjects with both patent and acutely obstructed femoral arteries. These observations are explained by the relative sensitivities of precapillary sphincters in muscle and skin to adrenergic tone; cutaneous sphincters have low resting myogenic tone and are exclusively controlled by sympathetic impulses. Precapillary sphincters in muscle, however, have high resting myogenic tone and respond almost exclusively to local, primarily metabolic, humoral factors.[62] In patients in whom proximal occlusive disease places relatively fixed limitations on arterial inflow, sympathectomy can actually adversely affect the natural redistribution of blood flow to exercising muscle by lowering cutaneous vascular resistance.[56, 62]

Regardless of the patency of the arterial tree, maximum vasodilation is noted immediately after sympathectomy but begins to taper off within 5 to 7 days of denervation. This "fifth day phenomenon" is more noticeable after dorsal sympathectomy, but it occurs in the lower extremities as well. Although at a much lesser level than initially observed, peripheral cutaneous vasodilation and blood flow remain elevated over basal levels for months, persisting in the face of stimuli that provoke vasoconstriction through centrally mediated reflexes (e.g., the vasoconstrictor cold response test).[70] Resting vasomotor tone usually returns to normal levels from 2 weeks to 6 months after sympathectomy. Previous explanations for this return of sympathetic vasomotor tone have included anatomically incomplete denervation, crossover reinnervation, and vascular hyperreactivity to circulating catecholamines. Isolated rabbit ear sympathectomy studies have shown that arteriolar smooth muscle cells are 1.5 times more sensitive to exogenous norepinephrine but are unable to constrict maximally owing to viscoelastic changes in the vessel wall.[3] However, this does not appear to involve endothelium-derived relaxing factor (EDRF).[24] In addition, study of canine adrenergic receptors demonstrates no change in the concentration of extrasynaptic, alpha$_2$-receptors that initiate vasoconstriction in response to blood-borne catecholamines.[6] Although attenuated, the capacity for vasoconstriction and its mediators is *not* obliterated by sympathectomy. The degree of recovery of vasomotor tone after sympathectomy depends on circulating norepinephrine levels and the degree of vascular adaptation to loss of physiologic constriction.

Effect on Collateral Circulation

The effect of lumbar sympathectomy on resting collateral blood flow in response to both acute and chronic arterial occlusion has been studied in human as well as canine models. Using a canine model of acute popliteal arterial occlusion, Dalessandri and associates[15] have shown that lumbar sympathectomy produces a temporary but significant increase in paw blood flow as measured by plethysmographic tracings. This effect was noted after sufficient time had elapsed to allow maximal vasodilation of collateral vessles around the knee. Among patients with chronic foot ischemia as a result of multilevel arterial occlusions, Ludbrook observed submaximal collateral blood flow at rest in 30%. Sympathectomy produced an average 11% increase in distal perfusion among this subgroup of patients with inappropriate resting vasoconstriction.[40] Van der Stricht reported a similar phenomenon and postulates that sympathectomy increases collateral flow by increasing the pressure gradient across fixed obstructions at the femoral and popliteal levels.[67]

Although this improvement is often relatively small and transient, sympathectomy does seem to increase distal perfusion, circumventing proximal obstructions in patients with inappropriate resting vasoconstriction. However, in *most* patients with ischemia at rest, locally released humoral factors maximize flow through existing and newly formed collateral channels.

Nutritive Value of Blood Flow Increase

Central to the debate concerning the utility of sympathectomy is determination of the nutritive value of whatever blood flow increase is observed after denervation. Presuming that cutaneous AVA flow is non-nutritive because capillary perfusion is bypassed, Cronenwett and colleagues[12] maintain that sympathectomy does not increase blood flow to ischemic skin and therefore should have no effect on rest pain or ischemic ulcers. This contention is supported by Welch and Leiberman's studies of cutaneous capillary perfusion using iodine 125-iodoantipyrine clearance in patients with peripheral vascular disease following lumbar sympathectomy or arterial reconstruction; no improved clearance was found in denervated limbs, in contrast to accelerated clearance seen after arterial reconstruction.[72]

Perry and Horton also found no difference in spectrophotometric measurements of transcutaneous oxygen tensions in patients before and after lumbar sympathectomy.[47] Using intradermal xenon 133 clearance, however, Moore and Hall showed improved skin capillary perfusion and observed ischemic ulcer healing after lumbar sympathectomy in patients with severe vascular disease.[43] Uncontrolled clinical series appeared to support Moore and Hall's observations by reporting ischemic ulcer healing in 40% to 67% of patients after sympathectomy.[5, 10, 34, 48]

In spite of conflicting data, it seems fair to concede that in *some* patients sympathectomy produces a small but sufficient increase in nutritive perfusion to facilitate healing of small ulcers or relieve ischemic rest pain. As discussed later, the key to its use is to select appropriate patients.

Alteration of Pain Impulse Transmission

An alternative mechanism to explain the relief of ischemic rest pain (rather than increased perfusion) is both central and peripheral attenuation of painful stimulus transmission by sensory nerves. Although objective assessment of pain threshold changes is difficult, aversive stimuli studies in cats have shown that lumbar sympathectomy enhances tolerance of hindlimb noxious stimuli.[49] Theories concerning a relationship between sympathetic innervation and pain threshold suggest that sympathectomy decreases noxious stimulus perception by both decreasing tissue norepinephrine levels and reducing spinal augmentation of painful stimulus transmission to cerebral centers.[39] This may also explain clinical series, including one randomized trial,[14] reporting a significant portion of patients afflicted with either disabling claudication or rest pain who were subjectively relieved without hemodynamic evidence of improved perfusion.[14] Among the subset with rest pain, Owens suggests that clear differentiation of neuropathic from ischemic pain in patients with absent ankle pulses is not made.[45] Including patients with causalgia (burning pain) in the clinical group with ischemic rest pain would spuriously increase the sympathectomy response rate. Despite this possible flaw in inclusion criteria, both clinical and experimental evidence suggests that lumbar sympathectomy can be efficacious in attenuating pain perception in patients with ischemic rest pain.

Summary of Physiologic Effects

Sympathectomy increases peripheral blood flow by the vasodilation of arterioles primarily in cutaneous vascular beds. Much of this increased flow passes through naturally occurring AVAs. Thus, although overall extremity blood flow may be increased, significant increases in nutritive flow occur only in distal cutaneous beds. Limitations in arterial inflow imposed by proximal occlusive lesions may mitigate this increase, and the return of vasomotor tone toward normal with time may further diminish it. Nevertheless, some patients *may* receive sufficient increases to help heal superficial ischemic ulcers and relieve ischemic rest pain. In addition, although increases in blood perfusion are relatively small in the long run in patients with organic occlusive disease, protection against an exaggerated vasoconstrictor response to cold, amelioration of sympathetic pain, and suppression of sweating are long lasting. These observations determine the appropriate indications for sympathectomy.

INDICATIONS AND RESULTS

It has been said that indications determine results and results determine indications. Nowhere is this more true than for sympathectomy, which has been performed for such diverse indications and with such markedly differing outcomes that quoting overall results is meaningless. Results in specific clinical situations have gradually defined its indications. With the passage of time, performance of sympathectomy for some indications has gradually become more limited and selective with the increasing use of trial blocks, noninvasive testing, and improvement in competitive forms of therapy. For example, better pharmacologic management of the initial stage causalgia and pure vasospastic disorders has significantly reduced the number of patients now being referred for sympathectomy.[25, 37, 51] Furthermore, increasing success with infrapopliteal bypass has further reduced the number of patients in whom sympathectomy is considered in lieu of direct revascularization. Even in these cases, selection criteria have been tightened by noninvasive testing before and after trial blocks.

Alternatives to Ganglionectomy

Attempts at sympathetic denervation for previously inoperable occlusive disease by injections of phenol or alcohol have become increasingly popular, especially outside of North America.[53] More recently, radiofrequency ablation has been tried with some success.[44] At present, however, the high rate of incomplete or transient sympathetic denervation with these methods is still a major drawback. Furthermore, the injection of phenol and alcohol can result in painful complications, and all such attempts, even multiple blocks using local anesthetic agents, ultimately can create enough inflammation and scarring to make subsequent surgical sympathectomy difficult, if not dangerous.

Although further progress may change this perspective, surgical sympathectomy today can be carried out with minimal risk, which may be reduced even further with the increasing use of laparoscopic methods. Thus, it is appropriate to generally condemn *any* percutaneous (injection or coagulation) technique that cannot regularly achieve a complete and durable sympathectomy in patients who might otherwise be considered potential candidates for surgical sympathectomy.

Intermittent Claudication

As previously discussed, there is no objective evidence that sympathectomy improves muscular blood flow in patients with ischemic muscle pain induced by exercise.[63] Muscular perfusion is increased primarily by vasodilation mediated by the acidic products of anaerobic metabolism. Despite this dictum, improvement in walking time among claudicants who show neither hemodynamic improvement after sympathectomy nor enhanced muscular perfusion has been reported.[50] These results, and others from nonrandomized studies, may simply reflect the natural history of claudication or the known pain-modulating effects of sympathectomy. However, there is *no* physiologic or clinical rationale for performing lumbar sympathectomy for claudication.

Causalgia

The central role of the sympathetic nervous system in perpetuating causalgia makes sympathetic denervation particularly suitable for this entity. Uniform success is obtained when the diagnosis and therapeutic potential of sympathectomy are confirmed by trial block. In the authors' more recent experience, early postoperative pain relief was obtained in 96% of patients by trial block, with 84% remaining asymptomatic after a median follow-up interval of 28 months.[42] Similar results have been obtained by other investigators and are superior to those of repeated transcutaneous sympathetic blocks alone.[32] In a report by AbuRahma and colleagues,[1] initial and late satisfactory results of 100% and 95%, respectively, were achieved in patients who showed an excellent response to a trial sympathetic block.

Peripheral Vasospasm

Most patients with Raynaud's phenomenon secondary to vasospasm complain more of upper extremity than of lower extremity discomfort; therefore, this indication is detailed along with contrasting perspectives in Chapters 82 and 86. Occasionally, however, the reverse is true, particularly for patients in colder climates, possibly because it is easier to warm the hands periodically than the feet. Thus, although the procedure is uncommonly needed, lower extremity vasospasm and cold intolerance respond remarkably well to lumbar sympathectomy, possibly even more so than with upper extremity involvement.

Janoff and colleagues reported their experience with 10 patients suffering from episodic distal vasospasm that was refractory to maximal medical management.[31] *Pernio*, or chilblain, a localized itching and painful erythema on the fingers and toes, produced by cold damp weather, was noted in each patient and did not recur after lumbar sympathectomy. Hypothermic toe plethysmographic testing normalized, and all patients remained asymptomatic after 4 years' mean follow-up. Both Felder and Gifford and their associates[22, 26] reported similarly good and lasting symptom relief among a larger group of patients. Despite loss of resting cutaneous vasodilation, reflex digital vasoconstriction in response to regional or remote cold stimuli did not recur in any of the more recently studied patients.

Ischemic Rest Pain

Critical assessment of clinical reports on the efficacy of lumbar sympathectomy for ischemic rest pain is limited by (1) variations in the severity and anatomic distribution of occlusive disease, (2) failure to differentiate this from other forms of lower extremity pain, and (3) differing criteria for determining "inoperability" for distal bypass. With this in mind, the more recent reports cited, it is hoped, better reflect progress in infrapopliteal revascularization, pharmacologic manipulation, and noninvasive testing. Nevertheless, most share the same flaw; that is, they were not prospectively randomized against conservatively treated controls.

Of the two manifestations of critical lower limb ischemia that may be considered categorical indications for lumbar sympathectomy, *rest pain* has a higher response rate than ischemic ulceration, for two reasons:

1. The blood flow increase needed to satisfy oxygen demands at rest is less than the inflammatory response required for tissue healing.
2. Pain impulse attenuation may enhance tolerance of ischemic pain even if perfusion is not very significantly increased.

Selection of patients for lumbar sympathectomy for both of these indications should be based on three simple assessment criteria[48, 69]:

1. An ankle-brachial index (ABI) of greater than 0.3.
2. Absent neuropathy on physical examination.
3. Limited forefoot tissue loss.

To this may be added relief of pain associated with plethysmographic or other objective evidence of improved flow in response to sympathetic blockade.[64]

Critical to the success of lumbar sympathectomy is adequate arterial inflow, as indirectly measured by Doppler segmental limb pressures. Designation of a threshold ABI of 0.3 is based on Yao and Bergan's original observation that arterial inflow below this level was insufficient to allow perfusion augmentation or symptom relief with sympathectomy in 90% of patients.[74] Subsequent studies have defined a range of ABIs centered around 0.3 when patients with spuriously high ankle pressures as a result of incompressible vessels are excluded. In the minds of some investigators, this ABI threshold cast doubt on the efficacy of sympathectomy because the natural history of rest pain alone in a patient with an ABI greater than 0.3 might not be significantly different from the response to sympathectomy.

This question was addressed and partially answered in a prospective, randomized clinical trial conducted by Cross and Cotton in which transcutaneous phenol lumbar sympatholysis was compared with saline sham lumbar injections.[14] Forty-one limbs in 37 patients were objectively and subjectively analyzed at regular intervals up to 6 months after treatment. Among the control group, only 24% of patients reported symptomatic relief, as shown by a decrease in narcotic requirements, in comparison with 84% in the treatment group. This highly significant subjective difference was *not* associated with objective signs of improved perfusion as measured by segmental limb pressures or blood flow and galvanic skin response monitored on the dorsum of the foot. This study reflects both the natural history of ischemic rest pain in "inoperable" patients (25% of whom were spontaneously improved) and the pain impulse modulation effect of sympathetic denervation. Other clinical series report similar symptomatic response rates ranging from 47% to 78%, with early "limb salvage" rates of 60% to 94%.[5, 10, 34] Persson and colleagues[48] report the best results for sympathectomy for this indication.

In patients followed up to 82 months after lumbar sympathectomy, 30 of 35 limbs with an ABI greater than 0.3 (86%) experienced early and sustained elimination or improvement of rest pain, compared with five patients who received no relief and required early amputation. Again, no significant overall improvement in limb perfusion was noted and, reflective of the severity of their systemic atherosclerosis, nearly 50% of the patients suffered myocardial infarction from 6 months to 4 years after operation. These results support a limited role for sympathectomy as a pain control procedure for patients with ischemic rest pain whose occlusive arterial disease is truly not amenable to direct revascularization or transluminal angioplasty and is refractory to maximal medical management (see Chapters 27 and 63).

An unfortunate subgroup of patients are those with diabetes who have not only end-stage extremity arterial disease but also an "autosympathectomy" that is due to progressive diabetic neuropathy. Rest pain in this group is rarely, if ever, responsive to sympathectomy. Not only can increased distal perfusion not be expected, but also the prospect of enhanced pain tolerance is negligible. Imparato and colleagues first noted the relationship between diabetic neuropathy and lack of responsiveness to surgical sympathectomy. He demonstrated the histologic equivalence of diabetic autosympathectomy and surgical lumbar sympathetic ganglionectomy by finding no difference in the number of periarterial sympathetic fibers in lower extremity amputation specimens from both groups.[27, 30] Other clinical series have confirmed that the high frequency of a sensory and sympathetic neuropathy in diabetic patients with limb-threatening ischemia is associated with autosympathectomy and an unresponsiveness to lumbar sympathetic ganglionectomy in the majority of patients.[16]

Finally, the results of sympathectomy in patients with Buerger's disease, and patient selection, are discussed in Chapter 20.

Ischemic Ulceration or Tissue Loss

Assessment of the results of lumbar sympathectomy for distal ischemic ulceration or focal gangrene is subject to the same limitations as were described for rest pain. The additional flow above basal requirements, needed to heal wounds and combat infection, create even greater demands of sympathectomy than combating ischemic rest pain. Radionuclide perfusion studies show that close to a twofold increase in blood flow around the ulcer (hyperemic response) is necessary for healing.[61] Infected or deeper ulcers require even greater increases in regional perfusion. As expected, both clinical and experimental studies indicate that sympathectomy *rarely, if ever,* provides sufficiently increased nutritive perfusion to allow healing of deep ulcers or large areas of skin necrosis, even when secondary infection is not prominent.

Clinical studies, noting partial or complete healing in 35% to 62% of patients with forefoot tissue loss, corroborate the intrinsic limitations of sympathectomy.[5, 10, 34] Again, the best results are reported by Persson and coworkers, who performed sympathectomy on 22 limbs with adequate inflow but, importantly, with no evidence of neuropathy or subcutaneous infection; 77% demonstrated complete ulcer healing, whereas only 22% required amputation.[48]

Lee and colleagues reported somewhat lower healing rates for patients with superficial toe gangrene, with 56% of the involved digits "salvaged" by sympathectomy and a 40% toe salvage rate among those with three or more digits involved.[36] Among "nonresponders" in such reports, the immediate amputation rate ranged from 27% to 38%, suggesting that not all of these cases were doomed without therapeutic intervention and that the level of amputation required was not improved by sympathectomy.

Precise characterization of the ischemic forefoot lesion that is most likely to respond to sympathectomy is difficult to glean from this literature. From a conceptual and practical point of view, however, use of sympathectomy should be confined to small, shallow, uninfected forefoot ulcers or single-digit superficial gangrene in patients with an ABI greater than 0.3 and absent neuropathy. One might expect successful healing in at least 35% of such patients, but no change in amputation level can be anticipated should amputation ultimately be required.

Sympathectomy as an Adjunct to Arterial Reconstruction

Experimental evidence indicates that sympathectomy improves patency of small vessel anastomoses and the repair of traumatized arteries.[7, 58] Some authors have even reported better patency rates for both proximal and distal arterial reconstructions when concomitant sympathectomy is performed.[21, 57] It is difficult, however, to predict which reconstructions would be protected by sympathectomy. Its application in proximal reconstructions that have been performed in the face of distal thromboembolism, poor runoff, or small "hypoplastic" vessels is less problematic because the sympathetic chain can often be exposed through the same incision. With distal reconstruction, however, sympathectomy would constitute an entirely separate surgical procedure and therefore is harder to justify.

Preferably, intraoperative electromagnetic flowmeter studies, documenting low graft blood flow that significantly increases in response to intra-arterial papaverine or tolazoline (Priscoline), should be used to justify the addition of lumbar sympathectomy. However, a multicenter trial has shown that dextran 40 infusions can produce a threefold decrease in early postoperative thrombosis of difficult distal bypass operations.[55] This results from both an increase in flow and a decrease in coagulability and would seem to provide a better alternative to sympathectomy. Prostanoids and hemorrheologic agents may offer future promise in this situation, and it is anticipated that the application of sympathectomy for this indication will be negligible in the future.

Sympathectomy to Speed Up Development of Collateral Circulation

Sympathectomy is a commonly mentioned indication for which there is little scientific proof. Ludbrook has shown that collateral arteries contributed 23% of the resistance at rest and 73% at peak flows in patients with claudication, and 52% of the resistance at rest and 89% at peak flows in patients with rest pain.[40] Decreasing the resistance of the peripheral vascular bed distal to the obstruction by sympathectomy would not greatly decrease overall resistance or increase flow, particularly if the occlusive process was a severe one. In the same situation, however, an equal decrease in the collateral artery resistance would have a very significant effect on overall blood flow.

Therefore, the critical question is, to what extent are the collateral arteries under sympathetic control? Shepherd, using indirect methods of evaluating the collateral circulation, concluded that collateral vessels are indeed under the control of the sympathetic nervous system.[59] However, Dornhorst and Sharpey-Schafer studied the effect of lumbar sympathectomy in 10 patients and found that although the collateral resistance dropped in seven cases, the decreases were quite transient.[18] Similar findings were reported by Barcroft and Swan.[2] Thus, there probably is some improvement in the speed but not in the magnitude of development of collateral circulation after sympathectomy *if* it is performed early enough (i.e., the first few weeks after occlusion). This benefit may result from either vasodilation of the collateral channels themselves or the increased pressure gradient produced across the block by the decrease in distal resistance that results from sympathectomy.

Despite these studies, reduction of collateral resistance is not an accepted indication for sympathectomy. There is rarely a pressing enough need for this to warrant an operative intervention; besides, some pharmacologic agents can produce similar effects.

Summary of Recommended Indications

Within the context of its physiologic consequences and the clinical results just presented, it is evident that lumbar sympathectomy should be applied rarely and very selectively to the following patients: (1) those with lower extremity pain or ischemia, (2) those whose condition is refractory to medical management, and (3) those who are not candidates for more effective revascularization techniques. Regardless of the indication, both subjective and objective preoperative assessment of response to sympathetic blockade greatly enhances the probability of therapeutic success. With these considerations in mind, lumbar sympathectomy may be indicated for the following conditions according to the recommended selection criteria:

1. Causalgia.
2. Inoperable arterial occlusive disease with limb-threatening ischemia causing rest pain, limited ulceration, or superficial digital gangrene.
3. Symptomatic vasospastic disorders.

Causalgia

When detected and treated early (*stage I*), post-traumatic pain syndromes respond to intensive medical therapy in 40% to 60% of cases.[66] Such nonoperative treatment consists of mild analgesics, physiotherapy, tricyclic antidepressants, anticonvulsants, and alpha$_2$-adrenergic blockers administered in a stepwise manner according to symptom responsiveness.[25] Consideration of surgical sympathectomy is usually withheld until conscientious participation in medical therapy has continued for 3 months. Multiple translumbar sympathetic blocks with local anesthetic agents are used to obtain and observe symptom relief, particularly in regard to degree and duration.[60]

Among patients with chronic pain or atypical pain and a "learned helplessness" personality profile, saline placebo injections may help to confirm or to rule out a true cause-and-effect relationship for the reported symptomatic relief.[8] If reproducible pain relief is achieved, lumbar sympathectomy yields a uniformly gratifying and sustained response rate.[1, 42, 76] It should be applied as soon as the patient's relief from sympathetic blockade, which lasts only as long as the effect of the local anesthetic used (*stage II*), wears off. Patients allowed to progress to *stage III* do not respond to sympathectomy (Chapter 63 further describes this indication).

Inoperable Arterial Occlusive Disease

Before specific selection criteria are discussed, the term *inoperable* needs to be defined. In general, the application of direct revascularization techniques for ischemic limbs with severe infrapopliteal occlusive disease is limited by the level and characteristics of the recipient artery, the adequacy of distal runoff, the conduit available for arterial bypass, and the technical expertise of the surgeon. Inadequate runoff (i.e., no distal arteries to bypass) is becoming an infrequent indication, thanks to intra-arterial digital subtraction, color Doppler scanning, and, more recently, magnetic resonance arteriography. Improved application of in situ, translocated, or reversed saphenous vein grafting techniques permits bypass to suitable arteries in the lower calf, ankle, and foot with very acceptable limb salvage rates.[35] With available autogenous vein and patent distal arteries, "inoperability" is determined by the technical proficiency of the surgeon (see Chapter 69).

Rest Pain. Assuming that a critical degree of forefoot ischemia has been demonstrated by objective criteria to confirm the clinical diagnosis of ischemic rest pain, lumbar sympathectomy is preferable to amputation if the following criteria are met:

1. Ankle-brachial index (ABI) greater than 0.3.
2. Absent neuropathy.
3. Symptomatic relief obtained by trial block.

Relief of rest pain from lumbar sympathectomy can be expected in 50% to 85% of patients meeting these criteria.

Limited Tissue Loss. Initial evaluation includes definition of the extent and depth of tissue loss, treatment of secondary infection with limited débridement, topical care, and culture-specific antibiotic therapy. In addition to noninvasive testing, perfusion scans with injections of intravenous thallium or intra-arterial technetium 99m-labeled albumen microspheres permit determination of the hyperemic ratio surrounding the lesion and prediction of healing potential (see Chapter 10).[61] For example, if a perfusion ratio after a thallium 201 intravenous injection was 1.5:1 (<1.75:1 predicts a nonhealing ulcer), but a repeated scan during the time of effect of a sympathetic block rose to 2.5:1, a sympathectomy may be recommended with confidence. Studies predicting nonhealing or the absence of signs of healing after 6 weeks of intensive wound management warrant obtaining arteriograms using special timing or digital subtraction methods to demonstrate "operability."

Other selection criteria for sympathectomy are similar to those used for determining rest pain and include:

1. An ABI greater than 0.3.
2. Absent neuropathy.
3. Limited ulceration or superficial single-digit gangrene.
4. Absence of major deep infection.

Strict adherence to these criteria can be expected to result in healing in 35% to 65% of patients after lumbar sympathectomy.[48, 69]

Lower Extremity Vasospasm

Symptomatic vasospasm of the lower extremity primarily affects patients with Raynaud's phenomenon or victims of frostbite. Discomfort and typical color changes in response to mild environmental cold with painful rewarming hyperemia or even a mild superficial dermatitis (pernio) are noted. Severe vasospasm may produce digital ulcerations in the presence of readily palpable pedal pulses. Digital photoplethysmography discloses either artifactually peaked pulse volume recordings or sustained loss of pulsatile flow in response to a local or distant hypothermic challenge.[31] One can predict a good response to sympathectomy by demonstrating at least a 50% increase in amplitude of the digital pulse volume recording with cold exposure following chemical sympathetic blockade.[64]

Before lumbar sympathectomy is considered, maximal medical therapy with calcium channel blockers, cold avoidance, and cessation of smoking must be earnestly pursued. Vasospasm refractory to these measures warrants lumbar sympathectomy; immediate and lasting symptom resolution has been noted in nearly 90% of patients managed in this stepwise fashion.[22, 26, 31]

Will Minimally Invasive Sympathectomy Change the Indications?

In recent years, there have been increasing reports of early experiences with lumbar sympathectomy carried out by laparoscopic or endoscopic methods. Most of these reports mention a small number of cases, with general enthusiasm and surprisingly few complications or other drawbacks mentioned. Specifically, major vascular injuries, especially the inferior vena cava on the left, do not seem to have been encountered. Only one report suggests that incomplete sympathectomy may be a problem (i.e., only 50% relief of pain at 4 months[29]).

Initially, some of these procedures were carried out transabdominally, with reflection of the colon,[33] but most surgeons now use an extraperitoneal technique with balloon inflation to dissect the extraperitoneal plane.[9, 19, 29, 33] If one presumes that this technique can produce a complete and lasting lumbar sympathectomy with safety and reduced morbidity, it may reduce the reticence to perform the procedure for some indications (e.g., frostbite injury, symptomatic vasospasm, or hyperhidrosis) where the gain is relatively insignificant for an open surgical operation. However, for patients with causalgia or chronic critical ischemia and inoperable arterial occlusive disease facing amputation, the gain is potentially great. Such a procedure would probably speed up the application of sympathectomy for causalgia if it did not increase its use, and it might allow it to compete more favorably with other less effective non-revascularization alternatives (e.g., epidural spinal stimulation, hyperbaric oxygen) and pharmacotherapy in those with inoperable arterial disease and limb threat. However, identifying proper candidates, by objective evaluation of a trial block, will remain the cornerstone of patient selection.

PERFORMING THE PROCEDURE

Anatomic Considerations

Proper performance of lumbar sympathectomy requires appreciation of the anatomic characteristics of the lumbar sympathetic chain. Preganglionic neurons are located in the anteromedial aspect of the thoracolumbar spinal cord. At segmental levels, efferent fibers from preganglionic neurons synapse with postganglionic neurons in paravertebral ganglia via white rami communicantes. A small percentage of preganglionic efferent fibers either bypass the paravertebral ganglia to synapse in more peripherally located intermediate ganglia or cross over to innervate contralateral regions via conventional pathways. Characteristically, preganglionic fibers that supply a specific somatic region either synapse with multiple postganglionic fibers in paravertebral ganglia or proceed more peripherally to synapse in intermediate ganglia that are at a distance from their segmental source. Therefore, complete sympathetic denervation of an extremity requires division of preganglionic fibers along their segmental origin as well as resection of their corresponding relay ganglia and intercommunicating fibers.

Sympathetic outflow to the lower extremities originates in spinal cord segments from T10 to L3. Preganglionic fibers from these segments form extensive synaptic connections in paravertebral ganglia from L1 to S3 for innervation of the entire lower extremity and pelvic region. Sympathetic innervation of the foot and lower leg is primarily conveyed through the L2 and L3 ganglia; the proximal leg region is primarily innervated from the L1 to the L4 ganglia. Variations in the number and location of sympathetic ganglia are most common in the lumbar region, with the majority occurring at the L1, L4, and L5 levels.

Overall, three lumbar ganglia are most commonly found, with the fusion of the L1 and L2 ganglia most commonly accounting for the reduced number.[75] Crossover fibers occur in 15% of patients, with most leaving via the fourth and fifth lumbar ganglia.[71] For most clinical indications, L2 and L3 ganglionectomy is sufficient, but also removing L4 is advised to reduce the possibility of collateral reinnervation. Imparato advocates removal of all encountered lumbar ganglia to ensure that complete lower extremity sympathectomy is accomplished.[30] However, such extensive ganglionectomy is not usually warranted and may result in ejaculatory disturbances in preclimacteric males when bilateral high ganglionectomies (i.e., including L1) are performed. Impotence is also claimed to occur under these circumstances but has no known physiologic basis at this level. It is more likely to be produced by extensive dissection of the distal aorta, particularly around the origin of the left common iliac artery.

Technique

Lumbar sympathectomy begins with proper positioning of the patient so that the interval between the costal margin and iliac crest is "opened." The surgeon can accomplish this objective by raising the flank region approximately 30 degrees by placing padded rolls beneath the hip and thorax. With the mid-flank region centered over the kidney rest, the table is flexed approximately 10 to 15 degrees to widen the distance between the costal margin and the iliac crest. Tension on the ipsilateral psoas muscle is relieved by flexing the patient's upper (ipsilateral) thigh with appropriate padding beneath and between each leg.

An oblique incision is begun at the lateral edge of the rectus muscle, extending toward the middle of the space between the ribs and iliac crest, and ending at the anterior axillary line. The musculofascial layers of the internal and external oblique as well as the transversalis are split in the direction of their fibers or divided in line with the incision. The transversalis fascia should be divided laterally where the peritoneum is stronger, less adherent, and more easily separated from the fascial undersurface. The lateral plane between the transversalis fascia and the peritoneum is easily developed by blunt finger dissection directed toward the vertebral column. Continued separation of the peritoneum is gently performed in medial, caudal, and cephalad directions to maximize retroperitoneal exposure through the relatively small anterior flank incision.

With continued dissection toward the posterior midline, the surgeon should take care to remain close to the peritoneum and anterior to the psoas muscle rather than dissect into the retroperitoneal fat or posterolateral flank muscles, where bleeding may be encountered. The ureter and gonadal vessels are left attached to overlying peritoneum and are lifted off the psoas muscle as the dissection proceeds medially. The ureter should always be clearly visualized to avoid inadvertent injury.

The lumbar sympathetic chain is located medial to the psoas muscle and lies over the transverse processes of the lumbar spine. The lumbar chain should not be confused with the genitofemoral nerve, which lies more laterally over the medial third of the psoas muscle itself. On the left, the lumbar ganglia lie adjacent and lateral to the abdominal aorta; on the right, the chain lies just beneath the edge of the inferior vena cava.

Tactile identification of the lumbar chain by plucking discloses a characteristic "snap" as a result of tethering of the nodular chain by rami communicantes. Other vertical, band-like structures in this region (genitofemoral nerve, paravertebral lymph nodes, or ureter) do not recoil as briskly. Once identified, the mid-portion of the sympathetic chain is dissected free of surrounding tissues and retracted with a right angle clamp or a nerve hook to draw it up under tension from the surrounding tissue. The ganglia are mobilized by division of tethering rami with prior metal clip application. The surgeon facilitates orientation and ganglion numbering by identifying the sacral promontory and an adjacent lumbar vein that usually crosses the sympathetic chain in front of or behind the third lumbar ganglion. A large space between the first and second lumbar ganglia is often found with the first ganglion partially obscured by the lumbocostal arch. Metal clip application to all elements of the sympathetic chain prior to division prevents unexpected bleeding from vessels mistaken for rami or injury to non-neural structures during attempts to control the latter. Once the chain, with at least two lumbar ganglia, is removed, hemostasis is secured, and the incision is closed in layers after the table is flexed.

This anterolateral approach of Flowthow is most popular because the incision is well tolerated, dissection remains retroperitoneal, and exposure is adequate.[23] The posterior approach of Royle is not favored because of significant postoperative paraspinal muscle spasms.[54] The anterior approach of Adson is applicable only for sympathectomy combined with an abdominal aortic or other intraperitoneal procedure.[1] Using this anterior, transperitoneal approach, the surgeon identifies the right lumbar chain by dissecting along the right lateral aspect of the inferior vena cava. Exposure of the left lumbar chain is best accomplished by mobilization and medial reflection of the left colon along the white line of Toldt. This approach avoids dissection through lymphatic and vascular tissue immediately lateral to the aorta.

The technique of laparoscopic lumbar sympathectomy is not described fully here, but by the time this text is published, there should be numerous articles on technique in addition to those already mentioned.[9, 19, 33] The same instruments and dissection maneuvers, along with videoscopic magnification, that have proved so effective in thoracoscopic dorsal sympathectomy are employed. However, although the access will be different, the anatomy is the same, and the exposure must be adequate because the same segments of sympathetic chain must be removed and in a safe, controlled manner, for the risk and consequences of injury to adjacent vessels is greater than with dorsal sympathectomy.

Complications

Major complications result from failure to appreciate normal anatomic relationships, with resultant injury to the genitofemoral nerve, ureter, lumbar veins, aorta, and inferior vena cava. Although reported, such injuries are avoidable by attention to anatomic detail and prevention of hemorrhage from vessels lying outside the proper plane of dissection.

The most common complication after lumbar sympathectomy is postsympathectomy *neuralgia*. This sequela appears in up to 50% of patients from 5 to 20 days after sympathectomy.[38, 42] The pain is characterized as an annoying "ache" in the anterolateral thigh region that is worse at night and is unaffected by activity or level of cutaneous stimulation. The discomfort responds to moderate analgesics and spontaneously remits within 8 to 12 weeks after onset. Counseling patients about this annoying complication before surgery is essential and often attenuates overreactions. The cause is still speculative, and various technical maneuvers have not reduced its overall incidence.

In men, sexual derangement consists of retrograde ejaculation, which affects 25% to 50% of patients undergoing bilateral L1 sympathetic ganglionectomy.[52, 73] This complication rarely occurs after unilateral ganglionectomy, especially when the surgeon takes care to preserve the first lumbar ganglion. Although potency should not be affected, many experienced surgeons insist that such derangements in sexual function do occur in men. Careful preoperative questioning about sexual function is important to evaluate any changes reported after lumbar sympathectomy.

Systemic arterial *steal syndromes* resulting from lumbar sympathectomy have been reported but are largely unsubstantiated by careful analysis. Nonetheless, paradoxical gangrene of the contralateral extremity has been reported but has been due to intrinsic arterial occlusion of the affected leg rather than to selective hypoperfusion at the aortoiliac level.[4] Similarly, mesenteric arterial insufficiency with bowel infarction has been attributed to intrinsic mesenteric occlusive disease rather than to aortoiliac steal.

Apart from postsympathectomy neuralgia, the second most common "complication" is *failure to achieve the desired objectives of pain relief or tissue healing*. Additionally, attenuation of initially favorable results has been previously considered to be secondary to technical errors or inadequate sympathectomy. Further elucidation of the consequences, as well as its intrinsic limitations, of lumbar sympathectomy has shown that these sequelae are unavoidable. Within the context of the criteria and indications outlined in this chapter, however, complications of this nature should be infrequent.

Proper patient selection for operation, and evaluation, in terms of standard anesthetic risk factors, as well as improvement in perioperative management protocols, have markedly reduced the mortality of this procedure. Although Haimovici and associates,[28] Palumbro and Lulu,[46] and Taylor[65] have reported mortality rates ranging from 2.9% to 6.0% in older series, the authors and others have noted no operative deaths among a large series of high-risk patients.[10, 34, 42, 48] Modern surgical care, therefore, permits performance of lumbar sympathectomy with an almost negligible risk of perioperative death.

SUMMARY

The role of lumbar sympathectomy in the modern management of lower extremity vascular disease is relatively minor; in carefully selected patients with no other surgical options, however, sympathetic denervation may sufficiently increase distal perfusion and cutaneous capillary nutritive flow to allow healing in situations of limited ischemic tissue loss as well as decrease ischemic pain perception. Causalgia remains its best indication, and though the procedure is also effective in cold-induced vasospasm, the level of disability caused is so low and the success of nonoperative management is so high that sympathectomy is rarely warranted here. Although the procedure is very effective in controlling hyperhidrosis, this is uncommonly a consideration in the lower extremities (in contrast to the upper extremities), where desiccating foot powders can be helpful. Further elucidation of the influence of lumbar sympathectomy on microcirculatory hemodynamics in patients with end-stage arterial occlusive disease may refine criteria and indications for future use. Unless the potential of laparoscopic lumbar sympathectomy is realized, it is likely that improved pharmacologic agents (e.g., prostacyclin analogues), rather than an increased application of sympathectomy, will fill this void.

REFERENCES

1. AbuRahma AF, Robinson PA, Powell M, et al: Sympathectomy for reflex sympathetic dystrophy: Factors affecting outcome. Ann Vasc Surg 8:372, 1994.

1a. Adson AW, Brown CE: Treatment of Raynaud's disease by lumbar ramisection and ganglionectomy and perivascular sympathectomy neurectomy of the common iliac arteries. JAMA 84:1908, 1925.

2. Barcroft H, Swan HJC: Sympathetic Control of Human Blood Vessels. London, Arnold and Co, 1953.
3. Beran RD, Tsuru H: Functional and structural changes in the rabbit ear artery after sympathetic denervation. Circ Res 49:478, 1981.
4. Bergan JJ, Trippell OH: Arteriograms in ischemic limbs worsened after lumbar sympathectomy. Arch Surg 85:135, 1962.
5. Blumenberg RM, Gelfand L: Lumbar sympathectomy for limb salvage: A goal-line stand. Am J Surg 138:241, 1979.
6. Bobik A, Anderson WP: Influence of sympathectomy on alpha-2 adrenoreceptor binding sites in canine blood vessels. Life Sci 33:331, 1983.
7. Casten DF, Sadler AH, Furman D: An experimental study of the effect of sympathectomy on patency of small blood vessel anastomoses. Surg Gynecol Obstet 115:462, 1962.
8. Chapman SL, Brena SF: Learned helplessness and responses to nerve blocks in chronic low back pain patients. Pain 14:355, 1982.
9. Cheshire NJ, Darzi AW: Retroperitoneoscopic lumbar sympathectomy. Br J Surg 84:1094, 1997.
10. Collins GI, Rich NM, Claggett GP, et al: Clinical results of lumbar sympathectomy. Am Surg 47:31, 1981.
11. Cronenwett JL, Lindenauer SM: Direct measurement of arteriovenous anastomotic blood flow after lumbar sympathectomy. Surgery 82:82, 1977.
12. Cronenwett JL, Lindenauer SM: Hemodynamic effects of sympathectomy in ischemic canine hind limbs. Surgery 87:417, 1980.
13. Cronenwett JL, Zelenock GB, Whitehouse W Jr, et al: The effect of sympathetic innervation of canine muscle and skin blood flow. Arch Surg 118:420, 1983.
14. Cross FW, Cotton LT: Chemical lumbar sympathectomy for ischemic rest pain. A randomized, prospective controlled clinical trial. Am J Surg 150:341, 1985.
15. Dalessandri KM, Carson SM, Tillman P, et al: Effect of lumbar sympathectomy in distal arterial obstruction. Arch Surg 118:1157, 1983.
16. DaValle MJ, Bauman FG, Mintzer R, et al: Limited success of lumbar sympathectomy in the prevention of ischemic limb loss in diabetic patients. Surg Gynecol Obstet 152:784, 1981.
17. Diez J: Un nuevo metodo de simpatectomia periferica para el tratamiento de affecionas trofilas y gangrenosas de los miembros. Bol Soc Cir Buenos Aires 8:10, 1924.
18. Dornhorst AC, Sharpey-Schafer EP: Collateral resistance in limbs with

arterial obstruction: Spontaneous changes and effects of sympathectomy. Clin Sci 10:371, 1951.
19. Elliot TB, Royle JP: Lararoscopic extraperitoneal lumbar sympathectomy: Technique and early results. Aust N Z Surg 66:400, 1996.
20. Ewing M: The history of lumbar sympathectomy. Surgery 70:791, 1971.
21. Faenza A, Splare R, Lapilli A, et al: Clinical results of lumbar sympathectomy alone or as a complement to direct arterial surgery. Acta Chir Belg 76:101, 1977.
22. Felder DA, Simeone FA, Linton RR, et al: Evaluation of sympathetic neurectomy in Raynaud's disease. Surgery 26:1014, 1949.
23. Flowthow PG: Anterior extraperitoneal approach to the lumbar sympathetic nerves. Am J Surg 127:953, 1948.
24. Funahashi S, Komori K, Itoh H, et al: Effects of lumbar sympathectomy on the properties of both endothelium and smooth muscle of the canine femoral artery and autogenous vein grafts under poor runoff conditions. J Surg Res 64:184, 1996.
25. Ghostine SY, Gomair YG, Turner DM, et al: Phenoxybenzamine in the treatment of causalgia: Report of 40 cases. J Neurosurg 60:1263, 1984.
26. Gifford RS Jr, Hines EA Jr, Craig WM: Sympathectomy for Raynaud's phenomenon: Follow-up study of 70 women with Raynaud's disease and 54 women with secondary Raynaud's phenomenon. Circulation 17:5, 1958.
27. Groch JM, Bauman FG, Riles TS, et al: Effect of surgical lumbar sympathectomy on innervation of arterioles in the lower limb of patients with diabetes. Surg Gynecol Obstet 153:39, 1981.
28. Haimovici H, Steenman C, Karson IH: Evaluation of lumbar sympathectomy. Arch Surg 89:1089, 1964.
29. Hourlay P, Vangertruyden G, Verdyckt F, Trimpeneers F, Hendrickx J: Endoscopic extraperitoneal lumbar sympathectomy. Surg Endosc 9:530, 1995.
30. Imparato AM: Lumbar sympathectomy. Role in the treatment of occlusive arterial disease in the lower extremities. Surg Clin North Am 59:719, 1979.
31. Janoff KA, Phinney ES, Porter JM: Lumbar sympathectomy for lower extremity vasospasm. Am J Surg 150:147, 1985.
32. Je'bara VA, Saade B: Causalgia: A wartime experience: Report of twenty treated cases. J Trauma 27:519, 1987.
33. Kathouda N, Wattanasirichaigoon S, Tang E, et al: Laparoscopic lumbar sympathectomy. Surg Endosc 11:257, 1997.
34. Kim GE, Ibrahim IM, Imparato AM: Lumbar sympathectomy in end-stage arterial occlusive disease. Am Surg 183:157, 1976.
35. Leather RP, Karmody AM: In situ saphenous vein arterial bypass for the treatment of limb ischemia. Adv Surg 19:175, 1986.
36. Lee BY, Madden JL, Tuoden WR, et al: Lumbar sympathectomy for toe gangrene. Long-term follow-up. Am J Surg 145:398, 1983.
37. Lindenauer SM, Cronenwett JL: What is the place of lumbar sympathectomy? Br J Surg Suppl 69:532, 1982.
38. Litwin MS: Post-sympathectomy neuralgia. Arch Surg 84:591, 1962.
39. Loh L, Nathan PW: Painful peripheral states and sympathetic blocks. J Neurol Neurosurg Psychiatry 41:664, 1978.
40. Ludbrook J: Collateral arterial resistance in human lower limbs. J Surg Res 6:423, 1966.
41. May AG, DeWeese JA, Rob CG: Effect of sympathectomy on blood flow in arterial stenosis. Ann Surg 158:182, 1968.
42. Mockus MB, Rutherford RB, Rosales C, et al: Sympathectomy for causalgia. Arch Surg 122:668, 1987.
43. Moore WS, Hall AD: Effects of lumbar sympathectomy on skin capillary blood flow in arterial occlusive disease. J Surg Res 14:151, 1973.
44. Noe CE, Haynsworth RF Jr: Lumbar radiofrequency sympatholysis. J Vasc Surg 17:801, 1993.
45. Owens JC: Causalgia. Am Surg 23:636, 1957.
46. Palumbro LT, Lulu DJ: Lumbar sympathectomy in peripheral vascular disease. Arch Surg 86:182, 1963.
47. Perry MO, Horton J: Muscle and subcutaneous oxygen tension. Measurements by mass spectrometry after sympathectomy. Arch Surg 113:176, 1973.
48. Persson AV, Anderson LA, Padberg FT Jr: Selection of patients for lumbar sympathectomy. Surg Clin North Am 65:393, 1985.
49. Petten CV, Roberts WJ, Rhodes DL: Behavioral test of tolerance for aversive mechanical stimuli in sympathectomized cats. Pain 15:177, 1983.
50. Pistolese GR, Speziale F, Taurino M, et al: Criteria for prognostic evaluation of the results of lumbar sympathectomy: Clinical, hemodynamic and angiographic findings. J Cardiovasc Surg 23:411, 1982.
51. Porter JM, Rivers SP: Management of Raynaud's syndrome. *In* Bergan JJ, Yao JST (eds): Evaluation and Treatment of Upper and Lower Extremity Circulatory Disorders. New York, Grune & Stratton, 1983, pp 181–202.
52. Quale JB: Sexual function after bilateral lumbar sympathectomy and aortoiliac bypass surgery. J Cardiovasc Surg 21:215, 1980.
53. Ramos M, Almazán A, Lozano F, et al: Phenol lumbar sympathectomy in severe arterial disease of the lower limb: A hemodynamic study. Int Surg 68:127, 1983.
54. Royle ND: A new operative procedure in the treatment of spastic paralysis and its experimental basis. Med J Aust 1:77, 1924.
55. Rutherford RB, Jones DH, Bergentz SE, et al: The efficacy of dextran-40 in preventing early postoperative thrombosis following difficult lower extremity bypass. J Vasc Surg 1:776, 1984.
56. Rutherford RB, Valenta J: Extremity blood flow and distribution: The effects of arterial occlusion, sympathectomy and exercise. Surgery 69:332, 1971.
57. Satiani B, Liapsis CD, Hayes JP, et al: Prospective randomized study of concomitant lumbar sympathectomy with aortoiliac reconstruction. Am J Surg 143:755, 1982.
58. Sandmann W, Kremer K, Wust H, et al: Postoperative control of blood flow in arterial surgery: Results of electromagnetic blood flow measurement. Thoraxchir Vask Chir 25:427, 1977.
59. Shepherd JT: The effects of acute occlusion of the femoral artery on the blood supply to the calf of the leg before and after release of sympathetic vasomotor tone. Chir Sci 9:355, 1950.
60. Shumacker HB Jr: A personal overview of causalgia and other reflex dystrophies. Ann Surg 201:278, 1985.
61. Siegel ME, William GM, Giargiano FA Jr, et al: A useful objective criterion for determining the healing potential of an ischemic ulcer. J Nucl Med 21:993, 1975.
62. Smith RB, Dratz AF, Coberly JC, et al: Effect of lumbar sympathectomy on muscle blood flow in advanced occlusive vascular disease. Ann Surg 37:247, 1971.
63. Strandness DE, Bell JW: Critical evaluation of the results of lumbar sympathectomy. Ann Surg 160:1021, 1964.
64. Sumner DS, Strandness DE Jr: An abnormal finger pulse associated with cold sensitivity. Ann Surg 175:294, 1972.
65. Taylor I: Lumbar sympathectomy for intermittent claudication. Br J Clin Pract 27:39, 1973.
66. Thompson JE: The diagnosis and management of post-traumatic pain syndromes (causalgia). Aust N Z J Surg 49:299, 1979.
67. van der Stricht J: Lumbar sympathectomy in occlusive diseases. Int Angiol 4:345, 1985.
68. Vautinnen E, Luberg MV, Sotaranta M: The immediate effect of lumbar sympathectomy on arterial blood flow measured by electromagnetic flowmetry. Scand J Thorac Cardiovasc Surg 12:101, 1978.
69. Walker PM, Johnston KW: Predicting the success of a sympathectomy: A retrospective study using discriminant function and multiple regression analysis. Surgery 87:216, 1980.
70. Walsh JA, Glynn CJ, Cousins MJ, et al: Blood flow, sympathetic activity and pain relief following lumbar sympathetic blockade or surgical sympathectomy. Anaesth Intensive Care 13:18, 1985.
71. Webber RH: An analysis of the cross communications between the sympathetic trunks in the lumbar region in man. Ann Surg 145:365, 1957.
72. Welch GH, Leiberman DP: Cutaneous blood flow in the foot following lumbar sympathectomy. Scand J Clin Lab Invest 45:621, 1985.
73. Whitelaw GP, Smithwick RH: Some secondary effects of sympathectomy, with particular reference to disturbance of sexual dysfunction. N Engl J Med 245:121, 1951.
74. Yao JST, Bergan JJ: Predictability of vascular reactivity relative to sympathetic ablation. Arch Surg 107:676, 1973.
75. Yeager GH, Cowley RA: Anatomical observations on the lumbar sympathetics with evaluation of sympathectomies in organic peripheral vascular disease. Ann Surg 127:953, 1948.

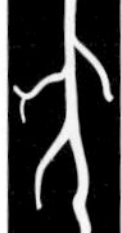

CHAPTER 74

Adventitial Cystic Disease of the Popliteal Artery

Lewis J. Levien, M.B., B.Ch., Ph.D., F.C.S.(S.A.),
and John J. Bergan, M.D.

Adventitial cystic disease of the popliteal artery is a very unusual cause of lower limb ischemic symptoms. Nevertheless, it is an important consideration in the differential diagnosis in young individuals complaining of leg claudication. Even though the etiology and pathogenesis of the condition are poorly understood, a correct diagnosis of this condition frequently enables the treating physician to restore limb blood supply to normal.

HISTORICAL PERSPECTIVE

Adventitial cystic disease was first described more than 50 years ago by Atkins and Key[5] in 1947. Their first description of this condition was, except for the anatomic site of the cyst, typical of the usual presentation of adventitial cystic disease. Their patient was a 40-year-old man with a 4-month history of progressive severe thigh and calf claudication. Surgical exploration of a mass that subsequently appeared above the inguinal ligament in the region of the external iliac artery revealed the features seen normally during operation on a conventional ganglion. Myxomatous tissue was found to be arising from the posterior aspect of the middle third of the external iliac artery.

Eight years later, Ejrup and Hiertonn[47] described a similar condition in what has subsequently been found to be the most common location for adventitial cystic disease, the popliteal artery.[52, 74] Ten years after the condition was first described, only four cases of popliteal adventitial cystic disease had been described in the literature.[66] Characteristically, the patients were all young men presenting with intermittent claudication subsequently demonstrated at operation to be due to a popliteal cyst filled with a mucoid material. Microscopic examination revealed a cystic lesion lined by a simple cellular lining closely resembling a ganglion in appearance and lying in the adventitial layer of the artery (Fig. 74–1). The intramural mucinous degeneration was clearly different from Erdheim's cystic medial necrosis. Investigators reporting cases of adventitial cystic disease have frequently commented on the absence of associated atherosclerotic changes in patients with adventitial cystic disease.[46, 89]

Although many case reports followed,[69, 117, 124, 143, 156, 159] the cause of adventitial cystic disease remained unexplained. Subsequent reviews by Flanigan and colleagues[52] in 1979 and Jasinski and colleagues[76] in 1987 have established that adventitial cystic disease occurs in a number of sites where large arteries lie in close proximity to adjacent joint spaces. Although the popliteal artery remains the most commonly affected location (Fig. 74–2), other sites of occurrence are the femoral and external iliac arteries, the radial or ulnar arteries in proximity to the wrist joint, and the brachial artery adjacent to the elbow. Adventitial cystic disease has also been reported in the veins of the leg,[3, 55, 57, 74] in the femoral vein adjacent to the hip joint,[118] and in the saphenous vein near the ankle joint.[91] Similar types of ganglion-like cysts have been reported in the lateral popliteal nerve.[27, 114] To date, a total of 321 cases of adventitial cystic disease have been documented in the literature,[89] although many cases probably remain unreported.

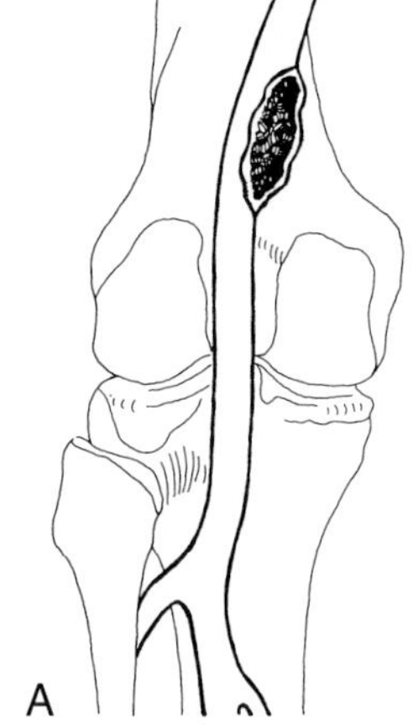

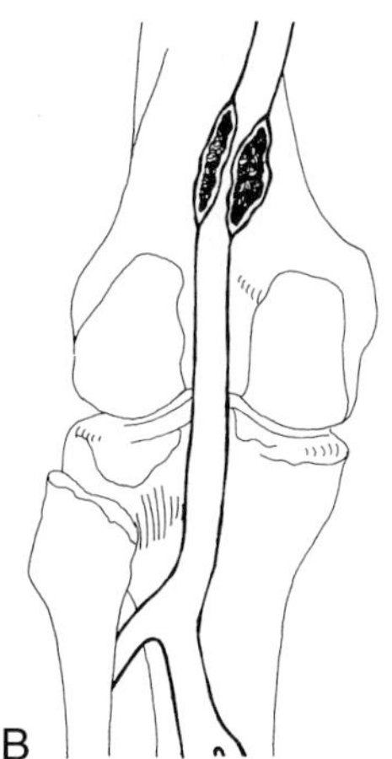

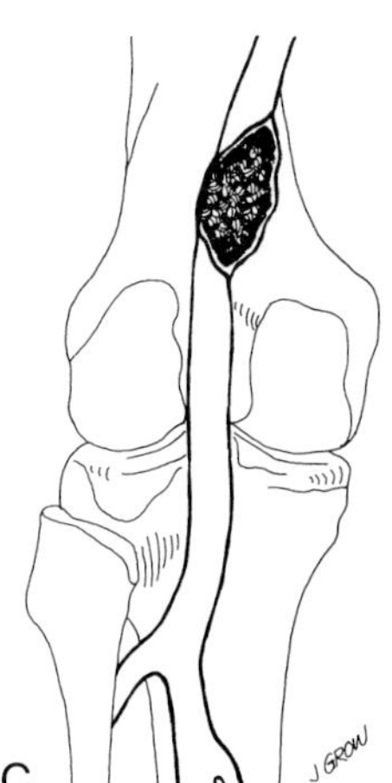

FIGURE 74–1. Adventitial cysts may appear in variable locations on the popliteal artery. The expanding cyst may indent the artery *(A)*, the scimitar sign; encircle the artery *(B)*, the hourglass sign; or completely occlude the vessel *(C)*.

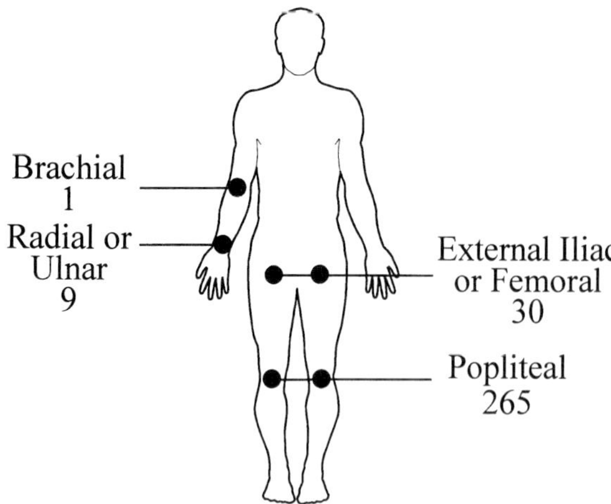

FIGURE 74–2. Anatomic location and sex in 321 published cases of adventitial cystic disease.

The presence of a communication with the adjacent joint demonstrated both in many arterial cases of adventitial cystic disease and in cysts of the lateral popliteal nerve strongly favors some form of developmental anomaly. In 1963, Bliss and colleagues[13, 14] acknowledged that the cause of the condition was unknown but stated that the clinical picture, pathologic features, and treatment were well defined. Various investigators have advanced several theories in an attempt to explain the diverse manifestations of adventitial cystic disease, but convincing evidence in support of any one theory remains elusive.

Bergan[52] in 1979 surveyed the authors of previous reports to obtain long-term follow-up on patients who had been treated for popliteal adventitial cystic disease. He reported 27 patients with follow-up of more than 2 years, with the longest follow-up being 30 years. In no instance was amputation required, and no serious disability was recorded. No patient experienced adventitial cystic disease of the contralateral popliteal artery or, indeed, of any other artery, and in no instance did joint disease or evidence of any systemic connective tissue disorder develop.

DEMOGRAPHICS AND PATHOPHYSIOLOGY

The condition of adventitial cystic disease of the popliteal artery chiefly affects males in the ratio of approximately 15:1 and appears in the fourth and fifth decades. The youngest reported patient was 10 years old, and the oldest a man of 77 years. In women, the condition appears in the sixth decade.[52]

The prevalence of popliteal adventitial cystic disease as a cause of claudication was found to be 1 in 1200 cases, with the condition being found in 1 in 1000 angiograms, suggesting an incidence in claudication of about 0.01%.[90]

Although the onset of symptoms is usually sudden, it is probable that the cyst arises over a long period, producing progressive stenosis of the artery with preservation of patency. The cyst appears to enlarge slowly and progressively within the arterial wall, producing a localized stenosis in the affected vessel. Initially, as in other causes of vascular stenosis, velocity of blood through the diseased segment increases. With progressive compromise of the vascular lumen, it is possible that flow occurs only with peak systole,[75] giving rise to the important clinical sign of a bruit in the popliteal fossa first described by Eastcott.[45] Ishikawa and colleagues[73] contributed an important diagnostic sign when they noted that normal distal pulses may be obliterated when the knee is sharply flexed in patients whose cystic disease has resulted in stenosis without total occlusion. In time, the popliteal artery may undergo total occlusion owing to the mass lesion produced by progressive enlargement of the cyst and its contents. However, possibly because of the healthy proximal and distal arteries and the slowly progressive nature of the occlusion, no case of acute limb threat due to adventitial cystic disease has been reported. Once the intracystic pressure exceeds that of the adjacent artery, or possibly as the physical size of the cyst increases, occlusion of the affected vessel results. Importantly, thrombosis may not be superimposed immediately, as evidenced by the fact that simple cyst evacuation may result in full arterial patency, even in cases of arteriographically proven occlusion.

The pathophysiologic consequences of the occlusion subsequent to localized arterial occlusion is no different from that produced by other causes of arterial constriction. Claudication without critical ischemia is a regular finding in these cases. Noninvasive tests demonstrate features of single-segment occlusive disease.

ETIOLOGY

The exact cause of adventitial cystic disease of the popliteal artery and other blood vessels affected by this condition is unknown. Schramek and Hashmonai[133] in 1973 and subsequently Flanigan's group[52] in 1979 reviewed the following four theories of possible etiology and pathogenesis of adventitial cystic disease:

- Systemic disorder theory
- Repetitive trauma theory
- Ganglion theory
- Developmental theory

Some concepts of formation of adventitial cystic disease involve a combination of more than one of these theories of causation.

The first theory, of a "mucinous" or myxomatous *systemic* degenerative condition associated with a generalized disorder,[62] was initially proposed by Linquette and coworkers,[92] who based their hypothesis on an abnormal skin biopsy. This theory has failed to gain substantial support because long-term follow-up has not demonstrated systemic manifestation of disease in any patient, nor has a contralateral or other adventitial cyst in a second site been reported in any patient presenting initially with adventitial cystic disease.[52] This theory also does not explain the preponderance of adventitial cysts in the popliteal artery. The name "myxomatous cystic degeneration" seems to be a misnomer.[90]

The single theory that has enjoyed the widest support is that of *repetitive trauma*.[14] Proximity of the popliteal artery to the knee joint is proposed to render the artery unduly prone to stretch and distortion. This repetitive trauma of the popliteal artery has been postulated to cause possible destruction and cystic degeneration of the adventitia of the adjacent vessel.[8, 66–68, 74, 125] It is thought that small detachments of the adventitia from the media cause intramural bleeds,[2, 98] resulting in cystic formation by chemical enzymatic activity within the adventitia.[84]

A further modification of the trauma theory suggests that joint-related structures may undergo repeated trauma,[59] with joint capsule degeneration leading to connective tissue changes in which cells secrete a material derived from ground substance or collagen that contains hydroxyproline.[61] These cells then form cysts, which may invade the adventitia.[52] It is suggested that such cysts enlarge, coalesce to form multilocular cysts, and grow rapidly to encroach on the arterial lumen, or possibly cause medial damage by direct compression of the arterial wall and subsequent arterial thrombosis.[84] In addition, a shearing stimulus has been suggested to arise mechanically from an element of entrapment of the vessels by fascia and tendons of the gastrocnemius muscle.[59, 60, 147]

Despite the attraction of these proposals, there is a lack of compelling evidence in support of the traumatic theory[128] because (1) a history of recurrent trauma is lacking in most cases of adventitial cystic disease and (2) the condition has been reported to occur in school-aged children. This theory also fails to explain the occurrence of adventitial cystic disease in the radial, ulnar, and external iliac arteries as well as the low frequency of the condition in laborers and athletes, who presumably sustain far greater mechanical stresses to their popliteal vessels than the normal population.

Adventitial cysts have been reported to be biochemically and histologically similar to ganglia,[39, 83, 138, 140] leading to the *ganglion theory*, whereby adventitial cysts arise as capsular synovial structures that then enlarge and track, either during development or later in life, along vascular branches to involve the adventitia of the adjacent major vessel.[140] The ganglion theory of origin is supported by a rich content of hyaluronic acid and a positive alcian blue stain response of the adventitial cystic contents.[41]

Further support for the theory of ganglion involvement of adjacent structures is provided by case reports in which such cystic lesions have involved adjacent vascular structures. These cases include adventitial cystic disease involving the lesser saphenous vein,[91] lesions connected to Baker's cyst,[134] and further reports of adventitial cystic disease involving the radial artery.[43, 89] Attempts by various researchers[22, 48, 86] to confirm the ganglion hypothesis through study of the histochemistry of the cyst lining and chemical analysis of the fluid contents, however, have failed to provide convincing evidence in support of the theory.

The fourth proposal, the *developmental theory*, is that adventitial cystic disease is a developmental manifestation of mucin-secreting cells derived from the mesenchyme of the adjacent joint.[52, 100, 110] This theory implies that such cells are included in the adventitia of the artery or vein during development.[51, 59, 120, 140] This idea, also called the "cellular inclusion theory," is supported by the reported demonstration of a communication between the cyst and the neighboring joint in a substantial number of case reports in which this phenomenon has been actively sought at surgery.[21, 52, 70, 86, 110, 114, 121, 140]

A refinement of the developmental theory is the possibility that a joint-related ganglion-like structure is incorporated into the vessel during embryologic development and that this synovial rest or ganglion secretes and enlarges over the years.[15, 66] It develops within the adventitial wall at a later stage in life, invoking both ganglion and developmental theories.[124] This idea provides a concept of development consistent with surgical experience. When the cyst is entirely adventitial, it is readily removed, leaving the intact artery. Otherwise, when sequestered cells are the cause of cystic formation within the deeper layers of the artery, enucleation is impossible, and the affected arterial segment must be resected.

In support of the developmental theory, Levien and Benn[89] have drawn attention to the embryologic derivation of those arteries that are affected by adventitial cystic disease and have concluded that all such blood vessels are nonaxial arteries. Their study suggests that during limb bud development, cell rests derived from condensations of mesenchymal tissue destined to form the knee, hip, wrist, or ankle joints are incorporated into the nearby and adjacent nonaxial vessels during development of these vessels at 15 to 22 weeks. These newly forming nonaxial vessels develop from vascular plexuses during the same stage of development and in close proximity to the adjacent condensing joint structures. These cell rests are then responsible for the formation of adventitial cystic disease later in life, when the mucoid material secreted results in a mass lesion within the arterial or venous wall.

Ulex europaeus 1 (UEA1) histochemical markers are present in vascularly derived endothelium. The absence of UEA1 reactivity of the endothelium-like cells of the lining of adventitial cysts[41] tends to exclude a vascular origin for this lesion and is advanced in support of a synovial or joint-related origin. Adventitial cyst fluid has a much higher concentration of hyaluronic acid than synovial fluid. These findings, described by Jay and colleagues,[77] support the hypothesis that inclusion of mesenchymal mucin-secreting cells has occurred as a result of embryologic aberration and contradict the concept that adventitial arterial cysts are formed and maintained by communication with a synovial space. The suggestion that synovial rests are sources of the cyst is unlikely because (1) synovial cavity forms through liquefaction of the limb bud mesenchyme rather than from specialized cell types[10, 12, 59] and (2) histochemical markers for synovium are absent in adventitial cysts.[39, 41, 83, 128] These findings, however, do not exclude the possibility that mesenchymal cell rests secreting a mucin-like substance may be incorporated into the vessel wall during development and that these cell rests give rise to the adventitial cystic manifestation with anatomic and chemical characteristics different from those of normal synovial tissues.

CYST CONTENT

Chemical analysis of cyst fluid by Hiertonn and Lindberg[67] showed that the viscous mucinous substance, when incubated with hyaluronidase, turned into a thin, cloudy fluid. Paper chromatography revealed amino acids but no carbohydrates. Cholesterin and calcium could not be detected. Other investigators reported that mucoproteins or mucopolysaccharides were the most common findings.[26, 37, 48, 77] Hyaluronic acid and hydroxyproline were also found, and these substances, of course, indicated a connective tissue origin for the fluid.[36, 61] Table 74–1 summarizes the result of chemical studies reported by Leaf[86] from Case 2 collected by Lewis and coworkers.[90] Although it has been suggested that the material originates from collagen tissue because of the significant amounts of hydroxyproline present, this hypothesis remains unconfirmed.

The chemical and histologic analyses indicate that ganglia and adventitial cysts are quite similar.[86, 90] After sophisticated investigation, Endo and coworkers[48] described the degree of confusion regarding the origin of the cyst and its contents:

> *The results of the chemical, enzymatic, and electrophoretic studies together with infrared spectrum indicated that the major component (0.5 M Fr) in the cyst of mucoid degeneration was proteohyaluronic acid. Although the substance separated from the cyst of cystic mucoid degeneration is shown to be identical to the proteohyaluronic acid obtained from normal human umbilical cord, the mechanism of the accumulation of proteohyaluronic acid in the cyst of this disease remains to be solved.*

The presence of proteohyaluronic acid identical to that found in normal human umbilical cord, however, does lend some support to the hypothesis that the cells from which adventitial cystic disease is derived originate from primitive mesenchyme.

TABLE 74–1. AMINO ACID COMPOSITION OF PROTEIN FROM POPLITEAL CYST COMPARED WITH COLLAGEN AND ELASTIN*

	CYST PROTEIN	COLLAGEN	ELASTIN
Aspartic acid	38.4	50.5	15.6
Threonine	24.4	19.3	13.4
Serine	23.2	38.5	10.5
Glutamic acid	52.9	75.5	23.1
Proline	23.6	127.2	117.3
Hydroxyproline	0	96.2	11.4
Glycine	87.0	338.0	318.7
Alanine	41.0	115.6	223.6
Cystine	19.0	0	0
Valine	29.0	26.5	136.7
Methionine	4.3	6.0	2.0
Isoleucine	6.4	9.5	30.5
Leucine	32.3	27.2	67.2
Tyrosine	11.2	3.8	12.7
Phenylalanine	18.8	14.8	36.4
Lysine	42.3	22.5	8.2
Histidine	9.5	5.6	1.9
Arginine	19.9	51.2	9.8
Glucosamine	29.2	—	—
Hydroxylysine	0	9.3	—

From Leaf G: Amino acid analysis of protein present in a popliteal artery cyst. Br Med J 3:416, 1967.

*Values are expressed as μmoles amino acid per 10^5/gm dry matter for the unknown protein, and μmoles per 10^5 gm protein for collagen (human tendon) and elastin (bovine aorta).

CLINICAL FINDINGS

The typical patient with symptoms due to adventitial cystic disease of the popliteal artery is a male in his mid-40s with a sudden onset of claudication, often with ischemic neuropathy. Usually, the history of symptoms is short, often measured in days to weeks rather than months to years. The claudication is usually severe, limiting walking distance to 50 meters or less. Occasionally, ischemic neuropathy may cause paresthesias, burning pain, or coldness.

Reduction or absence of popliteal and foot pulses is characteristic of popliteal adventitial cystic disease. If the lesion is producing only stenosis, however, a bruit may be heard in the popliteal fossa, and evidence of total occlusion appears only during acute knee flexion, when distal pulses disappear. Stenosis rather than occlusion is present in approximately two thirds of cases. Lewis and associates[90] have reported that a bruit could be heard over the popliteal artery of one of their patients in whom the symptoms had recurred after the cyst had been incompletely excised.

The phenomenon of disappearing distal arterial pulses was noted by Barnett and colleagues[7] in their 61-year-old patient who had normal limb pulses and oscillometric readings. Ankle pulses disappeared on exercise, and a loud murmur appeared over the popliteal artery at that time. Other investigators have reported hemodynamic alterations produced by exercise.[147]

Imaging of the cyst and its relationship to the parent artery is easily achieved by ultrasonography. B-mode scans allow determination of the shape, dimensions, and number of cysts present. The boundary between the cyst contents and vessel lumen is seen as a fine bright line that pulsates in real time. The absence of both atherosclerotic plaques and flow signals within the cyst in the presence of a distinctive sign of aneurysmal enlargement of the artery can be considered signs pathognomonic for adventitial cystic disease.[149]

Computed tomography (CT) can show circumferential involvement of the artery and even cyst recurrence after supposedly successful primary resection.[123] CT guidance lends itself to percutaneous cyst aspiration.[50] This approach should be viewed cautiously, however, because complete decompression may be difficult to achieve and ultimate recurrence is possible.[142]

Magnetic resonance imaging (MRI) and magnetic resonance angiography have been used both to image the cyst and to determine the extent of the arterial involvement. There appears little evidence that MRI is superior to other forms of imaging and conventional angiography for the diagnosis and planning of therapy of adventitial cystic disease.

ARTERIOGRAPHIC FINDINGS

Early in the course of popliteal adventitial cystic disease, arteriography demonstrates stenosis of the artery.[2] The lesion is usually in the mid-portion of the vessel, extending from 1 to 8 cm. There is no medial deviation of the artery, as is seen in cases of types I to III of the popliteal artery entrapment syndrome. The vessel above and below the lesion is surprisingly free of atheromatous degeneration. There are a few marginal irregularities.[46] When the smooth tapering is concentric, the lesion is described as having an "hourglass" appearance (Fig. 74–3). If the cyst is eccentrically located, the artery tapers smoothly above and below it; this shape has been described as a "scimitar sign." The artery may be displaced medially or, more commonly, laterally.

The stenosis may be missed on conventional anteroposterior films, appearing only on lateral projections.[7] The arteriographic findings are sufficiently characteristic to be diagnostic. The condition is easily differentiated from atherosclerosis and from the more commonly encountered popliteal artery entrapment syndromes. Adventitial cystic disease should not be confused with an extrinsic mass lesion, such as that seen with a hematoma or occlusion of the artery from true joint cyst.[132, 133]

TREATMENT

Because of the rarity of this condition, experience in any one center is limited and anecdotal. No randomized studies are available to indicate the best therapy. At present, optimal treatment of this condition would appear to be surgical. More conservative approaches such as aspiration have been successful in eradicating the arterial occlusion but have been characterized by early recurrence of the mass lesion. Percutaneous transluminal angioplasty (PTA) has proved manifestly unsatisfactory simply because, unlike in atherosclerosis, the intima in cystic disease is normal, and it is the arterial wall that is affected.[54] Furthermore, if the secretory lining of the cyst remains functional, the cyst contents are likely to reaccumulate with time.

The operative findings are relatively uniform. On exposure, the artery is found to be enlarged and sausage-shaped, just as in the first case described by Hiertonn and coworkers.[66, 67] Adhesions may be present, binding the adventitial cystic structure to adjacent vein or to the posterior aspect of the joint capsule. The cyst itself is usually unilocular but may be multilocular with septa. The fluid is usually crystal clear but may be faintly yellow or even the color of currant jelly, depending on the amount of recent or old hemorrhage.

Incision into the cyst and evacuation of its contents are usually sufficient to restore arterial patency, unless the artery has undergone thrombosis as a consequence of protracted occlusion. Because the condition is rare and preoperative diagnosis was rarely made in the past, a number of cases were treated by excision of the cyst with its adjacent artery and insertion of various grafts, with good results. Cyst evacuation, however, is currently the preferred treatment if the artery has not become occluded. Now that the condition is becoming better known, this method is being used with growing frequency. If the process has progressed to total arterial occlusion with thrombosis, however, graft replacement or bypass is preferred, with the adjacent long or short saphenous vein used as the arterial substitute.

The tendency has been to perform minimally invasive correction of the underlying arterial stenosis or occlusion.

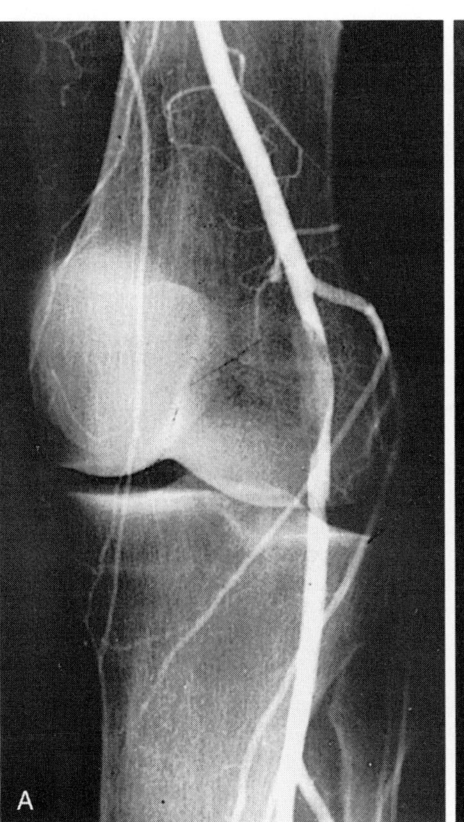

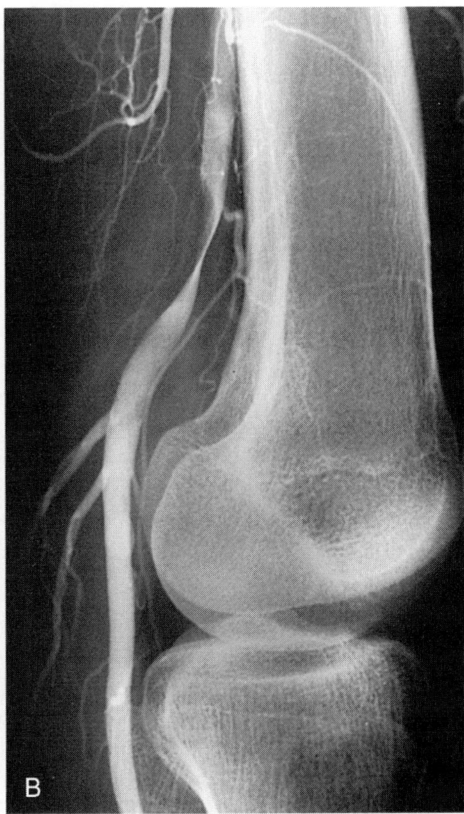

FIGURE 74–3. *A*, Femoral angiogram showing compression of right popliteal artery by adventitial cyst. *B*, Lateral view of same patient showing anterior compression of the popliteal artery above the knee.

Aspiration of the cyst under ultrasound or CT guidance has resulted in improved luminal caliber. Although this method permits restoration of a flow channel, the medium-term patency rate of this approach has been low,[142] presumably because of ongoing secretion by the cyst lining and progressive occlusion of the artery. Thrombolytic therapy has been employed to clear recent thrombus in an occluded arterial segment, followed by PTA.[127] With this approach, too, early failure has occurred, presumably owing to ongoing secretion by the cyst lining. After total occlusion of the artery, operative intervention has proved to be the most successful method of restoring arterial flow permanently. Continuing reports suggest that both short-term and long-term outcomes are better after complete removal of the cyst. Although some surgeons have treated this condition without arterial reconstruction, majority opinion holds that autogenous arterial repair remains the treatment of choice.[101]

A review of 115 case reports has been completed to allow an evaluation of treatment procedures.[52] Simple cyst evacuation has restored arterial blood flow in 56 instances. Prosthetic grafts, homografts, and autogenous vein grafts were used to restore flow in 42 patients. Patches were used to perform angioplasty in some cases, and in a patient who refused other surgery, rest pain was relieved with a sympathectomy. Curiously, the popliteal fossa in this instance was punctured, and a quantity of jelly was aspirated from the cyst.[102] Cyst aspiration under CT guidance has also been accomplished,[38] but most surgeons report disappointing results and rapid reaccumulation of cyst fluid.

Recurrent occlusions due to the cysts have been treated by needle aspiration, with recovery of varying amounts of gelatinous material and subsequent restoration of arterial flow.[90] Because simple cyst evacuation is effective treatment, it should be employed in situations in which the afflicted artery has not become occluded.[52] If simple cyst evacuation cannot be done, local angioplasty should be avoided. None of these procedures has been as effective as replacement of the vessel by grafting. When total occlusion of the popliteal artery by the cyst is encountered, replacement of the artery or bypass should be performed with the use of the best surgical technique available.

SUMMARY

Adventitial cystic disease of arteries remains a rare and interesting cause of stenosis and occlusion. Naturally, the cause of such an anomaly remains a fascination. It is an unforgettable experience to apply clamps to a pulsating blood vessel, incise its adventitia, and be treated to the vision of crystal-clear fluid instead of blood pouring under pressure from the arteriotomy. In such a circumstance, the relation of this disorder to simple ganglia seems irrefutable. Whereas ganglia of nonpopliteal locations are common, cystic arterial disease itself is rare and, in volar or dorsal carpal locations, rare indeed (nine cases). The location of cystic arterial disease in the popliteal fossa and along the external iliac artery is remote from the usual locations of ganglia. Logical as these facts are, however, the fluid remains clear and colorless, tantalizing in its similarity to the familiar content of a simple ganglion. The cause, therefore, remains obscure, even though meticulously performed dissections have shown connection of cyst wall to the knee joint.[139]

Treatment of this condition remains as illogical as the lesion is curious. What could be less likely to cure an arterial occlusion than evacuation of the cyst? To a vascular surgeon trained in performing bypass or vein graft procedures to restore arterial patency, simple cystotomy seems too easy. Yet there is no doubt now that this, rather than resection, is the treatment of choice if the artery is not occluded.[32] If total evacuation can be accomplished without violating the integrity of the arterial intima, cystotomy suffices. Otherwise, if the artery is completely blocked, arterial bypass must be performed. Although spontaneous resolution of adventitial cystic disease has been reported, such an outcome is not to be expected regularly.[113]

REFERENCES

1. Anderson RH, Ashley GT: Growth and development of the cardiovascular system–anatomical development. *In* Davies JA, Dobbing J (eds): Scientific Foundations of Pediatrics. Philadelphia, WB Saunders, 1974, p 165.
2. Andersson T, Gothman B, Lindberg K: Mucinous cystic dissecting intramural degeneration of the popliteal artery. Acta Radiol 52:455, 1959.
3. Annetts DL, Graham AR: Cystic degeneration of the femoral vein. Br J Surg 67:287, 1980.
4. Arey LB: Developmental Anatomy, 7th ed. Philadelphia, WB Saunders, 1995.
5. Atkins HJB, Key JA: A case of myxomatous tumor arising in the adventitia of the left external iliac artery. Br J Surg 34:426, 1947.
6. Backstrom CG, Linell F, Ostberg G: Cystic myxomatous adventitial degeneration of the radial artery with development in the connective tissue. Acta Chir Scand 129:447, 1965.
7. Barnett AJ, Dugdale L, Ferguson I: Disappearing pulse syndrome due to myxomatous degeneration of the popliteal artery. Med J Aust 2:355, 1966.
8. Barnett AJ, Morris KN: Cystic myxomatous degeneration of the popliteal artery. Med J Aust 2:793, 1964.
9. Bartos J, Kalus M, Possner J: Cystische adventitielle Degeneration der Arteria poplitea. Langenbecks Arch Klin Chir 314:177, 1966.
10. Baumann G, Schmidt FC, Becker HM, et al: Cystische Wanddegeneration der Arteria iliaca externa und Arteria femoralis communis. Chirurg 38:520, 1967.
11. Begg MW, Scott JE: Hyaluronic acid and protein in simple ganglia and Heberden's nodes. Ann Rheum Dis 25:145, 1966.
12. Berger MF, Weber EE: MR imaging of recurrent cystic adventitial disease of the popliteal artery. J Vasc Interv Radiol 4:695, 1993.
13. Bliss BP, Rhodes J, Harding Rains AJ: Cystic myxomatous degeneration of the popliteal artery. Br Med J 2:847, 1963.
14. Bliss BP: Cystic myxomatous degeneration of the popliteal artery. Am Heart J 68:838, 1964.
15. Blum L, Giron F: Adventitial cyst of the popliteal artery with secondary inflammatory entrapment. Mt Sinai J Med 43:471, 1976.
16. Borrelli M, Bracco E, Scarrone A, et al: Cystic adventitial degeneration of the common femoral artery: A case report. Radiol Med (Torino) 89:350, 1995.
17. Bounameaux H, Schneider PA, Faidutti B: Cystic adventitial degeneration of the popliteal artery: An unusual cause of intermittent claudication. Schweiz Med Wochenschr 118:692, 1988.
18. Boyd AM, Ratcliffe AH, Jepson RP, James GWH: Intermittent claudication. J Bone Joint Surg 318:325, 1949.
19. Brunner U, Soyka P: Gesichtspunkte der arteriellen Adventitiazysten. Vasa 6:105, 1977.
20. Campbell RT, McCluskey BC, Andrews MIJ: A case of polycystic adventitial disease of the left external iliac and femoral artery. Br J Surg 57:865, 1970.

21. Campbell WB, Millar AW: Cystic adventitial disease of the common femoral artery communicating with the hip joint. Br J Surg 72:537, 1985.
22. Cavallaro A, diMarzo L, Sciacca V: Cystic adventitial degeneration of the popliteal artery: A case report. Vasa 19:443, 1985.
23. Chandler JJ: Popliteal artery occlusion by subadventitial pseudocyst. Surgery 69:474, 1971.
24. Chevrier JL: Un cas de degénérescence colloide de l'adventice de l'artère poplitée. Mem Acad Chir 88:261, 1962.
25. Chiche L, Baranger B, Cordoliani YS, et al: Two cases of cystic adventitial disease of the popliteal artery: Current diagnostic approach. J Mal Vasc 19:57, 1994.
26. Cholet M, Rousseau H, Ferro P, et al: Adventitial cyst of the popliteal artery: Imaging and percutaneous treatment. J Radiol 77:201, 1996.
27. Clark K: Ganglion of the lateral popliteal nerve. J Bone Joint Surg 43:778, 1961.
28. Clarke JM, McCann BG, Colin JF: Artery occlusion by a popliteal (Bakers) cyst. Eur J Vasc Surg 2:61, 1988.
29. Colburn GL, Lumsden AB, Taylor BS, Skandalakis JE: The surgical anatomy of the popliteal artery. Am Surg 60:238, 1994.
30. Costa M, Colaianni N, Badessi S: Stenosis of the popliteal artery due to adventitial cysts. Minerva Chir 45:1411, 1990.
31. Crolla RM, Steyling JF, Hennipman A, et al: A case of cystic adventitial disease of the popliteal artery demonstrated by magnetic resonance imaging. J Vasc Surg 21:706, 1995.
32. Cystic degeneration of the popliteal artery (Leading Article). Br Med J 4:699, 1970.
33. Darling RC, Buckley CJ, Abbott WM, et al: Intermittent claudication in young athletes: Popliteal artery entrapment. J Trauma 14:543, 1974.
34. De Majo A, Pricolo R, D'Alessandro A: Cystic adventitial disease of the popliteal artery: Report of 2 cases and review of the literature. Minerva Chir 44:1315, 1989.
35. Delannoy E, Martinot M: Dégénérescence colloide de l'adventice de l'artère poplitée. Mem Acad Chir 86:824, 1962.
36. DeLaurentis DA, Wolferth CC Jr, Wolf FM, et al: Mucinous adventitial cysts of the popliteal artery in an 11 year old girl. Surgery 74:456, 1973.
37. Descotes J, Grobert J, Chavent J, et al: Dégénérescence colloide de l'adventice de l'artère poplitée. Lyon Chir 62:898, 1966.
38. Deutsch AL, Hyde J, Miller SM, et al: Cystic adventitial degeneration of the popliteal artery: CT demonstration and directed percutaneous therapy. Am J Roentgenol 145:117, 1985.
39. Devereux D, Forrest H, McLeod T, et al: The non-arterial origin of cystic adventitial disease of the popliteal artery in two patients. Surgery 88:723, 1980.
40. di Marzo L, Peetz DJ Jr, Bewtra C, et al: Cystic adventitial degeneration of the femoral artery: Is evacuation and total cyst excision worthwhile as a definitive therapy? Surgery 101:587, 1987.
41. diMarzo L, Rocca CD, d'Amati G, et al: Cystic adventitial degeneration of the popliteal artery: Lectin-histochemical study. Eur J Vasc Surg 8:16, 1994.
42. Dunant JH, Eugenidis N: Cystic degeneration of the popliteal artery. Vasa 2:156, 1973.
43. Durham JR, McIntyre KE Jr: Adventitial cystic disease of the radial artery. J Cardiovasc Surg 30:517, 1989.
44. Eastcott HHG: Cystic degeneration of the popliteal artery. Br Med J 1:111, 1971.
45. Eastcott HHG: Cystic myxomatous degeneration of popliteal artery. Br Med J 2:1270, 1963.
46. Ehringer VH, Denck H: Zystische Adventitiadegeneration. Wien Med Wochenschr 120:49, 1970.
47. Ejrup B, Hiertonn T: Intermittent claudication: Three cases treated by free vein graft. Acta Chir Scand 108:217, 1954.
48. Endo M, Tamura S, Minakuchi S, et al: Isolation and identification of proteohyaluronic acid from a cyst of cystic mucoid degeneration. Clin Chim Acta 47:417, 1973.
49. Evans HM: On the development of the aortae, cardinal and umbilical veins and other blood vessels of vertebrate embryos from capillaries. Anat Rec 3:498, 1909.
50. Fitzjohn TP, White FE, Loose HW, et al: Computed tomography and sonography of cystic adventitial disease. Br J Radiol 59:933, 1986.
51. Flanc C: Cystic degeneration of the popliteal artery. Aust N Z J Surg 36:243, 1967.
52. Flanigan DP, Burnham SJ, Goodreau JJ, Bergan JJ: Summary of cases of adventitial cystic disease of the popliteal artery. Ann Surg 189:165, 1979.
53. Flueckiger F, Steiner H, Rabl H, Waltner F: Cystic adventitia degeneration of the popliteal artery: Sonographic confirmation of the diagnosis. Ultraschall Med 12:84, 1991.
54. Fox RL, Kahn M, Alder J: Adventitial cystic disease of the popliteal artery: Failure of percutaneous transluminal angioplasty. J Vasc Surg 2:464, 1985.
55. Fyfe NCM, Silcocks PB, Browse NC: Cystic mucoid degeneration in the wall of the femoral vein. J Cardiovasc Surg 21:703, 1980.
56. Gertsch P, Stamm B, Burri B, et al: Die arterielle Adventitiazyste der Arteria poplitea. Angio 3:191, 1980.
57. Gomez-Ferrer F: Cystic degeneration of the wall of the femoral vein. J Cardiovasc Surg 7:162, 1966.
58. Gripe K: Intramural cystisk arterial mukoiddegeneration. Nord Med 70:1381, 1963.
59. Haid SP, Conn J Jr, Bergan JJ: Cystic adventitial disease of the popliteal artery. Arch Surg 101:765, 1970.
60. Hamming JJ, Vink M: Obstruction of the popliteal artery at an early age. J Cardiovasc Surg 6:516, 1965.
61. Harris JD, Jepson RP: Cystic degeneration of the popliteal artery. Aust N Z J Surg 34:265, 1965.
62. Hart Hansen JP: Cystic mucoid degeneration of the popliteal artery. Acta Chir Scand 131:171, 1966.
63. Hayashi S, Hamanaka Y, Sueda T, et al: A case of adventitial cystic disease of the popliteal artery preoperatively diagnosed by magnetic resonance imaging. Nippon Geka Gakkai Zasshi 94:314, 1993.
64. Hiertonn T, Karacagil S, Bergqvist D: Long term follow-up of autologous vein grafts: 40 years after reconstruction for cystic adventitial disease. Vasa 24:250, 1995.
65. Hiertonn T, Hemmingsson A: The autogenous vein graft as a popliteal artery substitute. Acta Chir Scand 150:377, 1984.
66. Hiertonn T, Lindberg K, Rob C: Cystic degeneration of the popliteal artery. Br J Surg 44:348, 1957.
67. Hiertonn T, Lindberg K: Cystic adventitial degeneration of the popliteal artery. Acta Chir Scand 113:72, 1957.
68. Hofmann KT, Consiglio L, Hofmeier G, et al: Die zystische Gefassdegeneration. Brun's Beitr Klin Chir 217:284, 1969.
69. Holmes JG: Cystic adventitial degeneration of the popliteal artery. JAMA 173:654, 1960.
70. Hunt BP, Harrington MG, Goodle JJ, Galloway JMD: Cystic adventitial disease of the popliteal artery. Br J Surg 67:811, 1980.
71. Inoue Y, Iwai T, Ohashi K, et al: A case of popliteal cystic degeneration with pathological considerations. Ann Vasc Surg 6:525, 1992.
72. Ishibashi S, Namiki K, Abe M, et al: Cystic adventitial disease of the popliteal artery—a case of young boy. Tohoku J Exp Med 176:173, 1995.
73. Ishikawa K, Mishima Y, Kobayashi S: Cystic adventitial disease of the popliteal artery. Angiology 12:357, 1961.
74. Ishikawa K: Cystic adventitial disease of the popliteal artery and of other stem vessels in the extremities. Jpn Surg 17:221, 1987.
75. Jacquet GH, Meyer Burgdorff G: Arterielle Durchblutungsstörung infolge cysticher Degeneration der Adventitia. Chirurg 31:481, 1960.
76. Jasinski RW, Masselink BA, Partridge RW, et al: Adventitial cystic disease of the popliteal artery. Radiology 163:153, 1987.
77. Jay GD, Ross FL, Mason RA, Giron F: Clinical and chemical characterisation of an adventitial popliteal cyst. J Vasc Surg 3:448, 1989.
78. Koppensteiner R, Katzenschlager R, Ahmadi A, et al: Demonstration of cystic adventitial disease by intravascular ultrasound imaging. J Vasc Surg 23:534, 1996.
79. Kuijpers PJ, Mol PCM, Hoefsloot FAM: Idiopathic cystic degeneration of the left common femoral artery. Arch Chir Neerl 21:77, 1969.
80. Lambley DG: Intermittent claudication due to cystic degeneration of popliteal artery. Br Med J 2:849, 1963.
81. Larsen WJ: Development of the limbs. *In* Larsen WJ (ed): Human Embryology. New York, Churchill Livingstone, 1993, pp 281–307.
82. Larsen WJ: Development of the vasculature. *In* Larsen WJ (ed): Human Embryology. New York, Churchill Livingstone, 1993, pp 181–184.
83. Lassonde J, Laurendeau F: Cystic adventitial disease of the popliteal artery. Am Surg 48:341, 1982.
84. Lau J, Kim HS, Carcia-Rinaldi R: Cystic adventitial disease of the popliteal artery. Vasc Surg 11:299, 1977.
85. Lazic V, Stierli P: Adventitia resection in cystic degeneration of the popliteal artery. Helv Chir Acta 60:883, 1994.

86. Leal G: Amino-acid analysis of protein present in a popliteal artery cyst. Br Med J 3:415, 1967.
87. Leu HJ, Ruttner JR: Pathologie, Klinik, Radiologie und Chirurgie der zystichen Adventitia degeneration peripherer Blutfegasse. Vasa 6:94, 1977.
88. Leu HJ: Pathogenese und Histologie der zystischen Adventitia degeneration peripherer Blutgefasse. Vasa 6:94, 1977.
89. Levien LJ, Benn CA: Adventitial cystic disease: A unifying hypothesis. J Vasc Surg 28:193, 1998.
90. Lewis GJT, Douglas DM, Reid W, et al: Cystic adventitial disease of the popliteal artery. Br Med J 3:41, 1967.
91. Lie JT, Jensen PL, Smith RW: Adventitial cystic disease of the lesser saphenous vein. Arch Pathol Lab Med 115:946, 1991.
92. Linquette M, Mesmacque R, Beghin B, et al: Dégénérescence colloide de l'adventice de l'artère poplitée. Semaine Hôp (Paris) 43:3005, 1967.
93. Little JM, Goodman AH: Cystic adventitial disease of the popliteal artery. Br J Surg 57:708, 1970.
94. Lord JW: *In* Haid SP, Conn J Jr, Bergan JJ: Cystic adventitial disease of the popliteal artery. Arch Surg 101:765, 1970.
95. Lossef SV, Rajan S, Calcagno D, et al: Spontaneous rupture of an adventitial cyst of the popliteal artery: Confirmation with MR imaging. J Vasc Interv Radiol 3:95, 1992.
96. Lowe DK, Winegarner FG, Jesseph JE: Cystic adventitial degeneration of the common femoral artery. Surgery 76:511, 1974.
97. Malleux P, Mairy Y, Coulier B, et al: Adventitial cyst of the common femoral artery: Computerized tomography demonstration of the articular origin of this disorder. J Belge Radiol 75:1, 1992.
98. Marzoli GP, Meyer Burgdorff G, Jacquet GH: Sulle pseudocisti dell parete arteriosa. Chirurgia Italiana 14:290, 1962.
99. McAnespey D, Rosen RC, Cohen JM, et al: Adventitial cystic disease. J Foot Surg (United States) 30:160, 1991.
100. McEvedy BV: Simple ganglia. Br J Surg 49:585, 1962.
101. Melliere D, Ecollan P, Kassab M, Becqemin JP: Adventitial cystic disease of the popliteal artery: Treatment by cyst removal. J Vasc Surg 8:638, 1988.
102. Mentha C: Dégénérescence kystique adventitielle ou bursite de l'artère poplitée. J Chir 89:173, 1965.
103. Mentha C: La dégénérescence mucoide des veines. Presse Med 71:2205, 1963.
104. Meuche C, Heidrich H, Langholz JP, et al: Mucoid cystic adventitial degeneration of the popliteal artery with simultaneous arteriosclerosis. Vasa 19:167, 1990.
105. Meyer JN, Lyndrup P, Schroeder TV: Cystic adventitial degeneration: A rare cause of intermittent claudication. Ugeskr Laeger (Denmark) 156:2096, 1994.
106. Milliken JC: Cystic degeneration of the popliteal artery in a female. Br Med J 2:769, 1971.
107. Nemec P, Joukai M, Fikulka J, Cerny J: Cystic degeneration of the adventitia of the popliteal artery. Rozhl Chir (Czechoslovakia) 67:51, 1988.
108. Nicolau H, Calen S, Gourul JC, et al: Adventitial cysts of the popliteal artery. Ann Vasc Surg 2:196, 1988.
109. O'Neill JS, Drury RAB, Bliss BP: Cystic myxomatous degeneration of the femoral vein. Eur J Vasc Surg 1:359, 1987.
110. O'Rahilly R, Gardener E: The embryology of movable joints. *In* Sokoloff L (ed): The Joints and the Synovial Fluid. New York, Academic Press, 1978, pp 49–103.
111. Ohta T, Kato R, Sugimoto I, et al: Recurrence of cystic adventitial disease in an interposed vein graft. Surgery 116:587, 1994.
112. Olcott C 4th, Mehigan JT: Popliteal artery stenosis caused by a Baker's cyst. J Vasc Surg 4:403, 1986.
113. Owen ERTC, Speechly Dick EM, Kour NE, et al: Cystic adventitial disease of the popliteal artery—a case of spontaneous resolution. Eur J Vasc Surg 4:319, 1990.
114. Parkes A: Intraneural ganglion of the lateral popliteal nerve. J Bone Joint Surg 43B:784, 1961.
115. Parks RW, Barros D'Sa AAB: Critical ischemia complicating cystic adventitial disease of the popliteal artery. Eur J Vasc Surg 8:508, 1994.
116. Patel J, Cormier JM: La dégénérescence kystique ou colloide de l'adventice artériel. Presse Med 71:244, 1963.
117. Patel J, Facquet J, Piwnica A: Dégénérescence kystique ou colloide de l'adventice. Presse Med 66:1164, 1958.
118. Paty PSK, Kaufman JL, Koslow AR, et al: Adventitial cystic disease of the femoral vein: A case report and review of the literature. J Vasc Surg 15:214, 1992.
119. Pierangeli A, De Rubertis C: Degenerazione cistica avientiziale dell'arteria poplitea. Arch Ital Chir 92.108, 1966.
120. Powis SJA, Morrissey DM, Jones EL: Cystic degeneration of the popliteal artery. Surgery 67:891, 1970.
121. Richards RL: Cystic degeneration. Br Med J 3:997, 1963.
122. Riviere J, Soury P, Poli P, et al: Importance of complementary peroperative examinations in the treatment of adventitial cystic degeneration of the popliteal artery. J Mal Vasc 19:251, 1994.
123. Rizzo RJ, Flinn WR, Yao JST, et al: Computed tomography for evaluation of arterial disease in the popliteal fossa. J Vasc Surg 11:112, 1990.
124. Robb D: Obstruction of popliteal artery by synovial cyst. Br J Surg 48:221, 1960.
125. Ruppel V, Sperling M, Schott H, Kern E: Pathological anatomical observations in cystic adventitial degeneration of the blood vessels. Beitr Path Bd 144:101, 1971.
126. Saeed M, Wolf YG, Dilley RB: Adventitial cystic disease of the popliteal artery mistaken for an endoluminal lesion. J Vasc Interv Radiol 4:815, 1993.
127. Samson RH, Willis PD: Popliteal artery occlusion caused by cystic adventitial disease: Successful treatment by urokinase followed by nonresectional cystotomy. J Vasc Surg 12:591, 1990.
128. Savage PEA: Arterial cystic degeneration. Postgrad Med J 48:603, 1972.
129. Savage PEA: Cystic disease of the popliteal artery. Br J Surg 56:77, 1969.
130. Schaberle W, Eisele R: Ultrasound diagnosis, follow-up and therapy of cystic degeneration of the adventitia: 2 case reports and review of the literature. Ultraschall Med 17:131, 1996.
131. Schafer K, Sell G, Schafer B, Rumpelt HJ: Degeneration of the adventitia of the popliteal artery as a possible sequela of entrapment syndrome. Chirurg 66:154, 1995.
132. Schlenker JD, Johnston K, Wolkoff JS: Occlusion of popliteal artery caused by popliteal cysts. Surgery 76:833, 1974.
133. Schramek A, Hashmonai M: Subadventitial haematoma of the popliteal artery. J Cardiovasc Surg 14:447, 1973.
134. Schroe H, Van Opstal C, De Leersnijder J, et al: Baker's cyst connected to popliteal artery cyst. Ann Vasc Surg 2:385, 1988.
135. Senior HD: The development of the human femoral artery, a correction. Am J Anat 17:271, 1920.
136. Senior HD: Abnormal branching of the human popliteal artery. Am J Anat 44:111, 1929.
137. Senior HD: The development of the arteries of the human lower extremity. Am J Anat 25:55, 1919.
138. Shabbo FP: Cystic disease of the popliteal artery. Proc R Soc Med 69:362, 1976.
139. Shannon R: Cystic degeneration of the popliteal artery. Aust N Z J Surg 40:290, 1971.
140. Shute K, Rothnie NG: The aetiology of cystic arterial disease. Br J Surg 60:397, 1973.
141. Sietz Castello J: Adventitial cystic disease of the popliteal artery: A clinical case. Angiologia 43:126, 1991.
142. Sieunarine K, Lawrence-Brown M, Kelsey P: Adventitial cystic disease of the popliteal artery: Early recurrence after CT-guided percutaneous aspiration. J Cardiovasc Surg 32:702, 1991.
143. Simon R: Dégénérescence colloide de l'adventice de l'artère poplitée traitée par prosthèse en Dacron. Mem Acad Chir 89:849, 1963.
144. Simpson CJ, Gillespie G: Cystic degeneration of the popliteal artery in a female patient—case report. Scott Med J 31:187, 1986.
145. Sipponen J, Lepantalo M, Kyosola K, et al: Popliteal artery entrapment. Ann Chir Gynaecol (Finland) 78:103, 1989.
146. Sperling M, Schott H, Rüppell V: Die cystische Adventitiadegeneration der Blutgefässe. Chirurg 43:37, 1972.
147. Stallworth JM, Brown AG, Burges GE, et al: Cystic adventitial disease of the popliteal artery. Am Surg 5:455, 1985.
148. Stapff M, Steckmeier B, Kuffer GV, Spengel FA: A patient with cystic adventitia degeneration and entrapment syndrome of the popliteal artery. Bildgebung 56:77, 1987–1989.
149. Stapff M, Zoller WG, Spengel FA: Image-directed Doppler ultrasound findings in adventitial cystic disease of the popliteal artery. J Clin Ultrasound 17:689, 1989.
150. Steffen CM, Ruddle A, Shaw JF: Cystic disease: Multiple cysts causing femoral artery occlusion. Eur J Vasc Endovasc Surg 9:118, 1995.
151. Stirling GR, Aarons BJ: Cystic myxomatous degeneration of the popliteal artery. Alfred Hosp Clin Rep 14:91, 1967.

152. Suy R, Van Osselaer G, Pakdaman A, et al: The pseudocyst of the adventitia of the popliteal artery. J Cardiovasc Surg 11:103, 1970.
153. Tabata D, Arikawa K, Umebayashi Y, et al: A case report of cystic adventitial degeneration communicating with the hip joint in the external iliac artery. Nippon Geka Gakkai Zasshi 92:611, 1991.
154. Taylor H, Taylor RS, Ramsay CA: Cyst of popliteal artery. Br Med J 4:109, 1967.
155. Tracy GD, Ludbrook J, Rundle FF: Cystic adventitial disease of the popliteal artery. Vasc Surg 3:10, 1969.
156. Tytgat H, Derom F, Galinsky A: Dégénérescence kystique de l'artère poplitée traitée par greffe en nylon. Acta Chir Belg 57:188, 1958.
157. Van Berge Henegouwen DP, Salzmann P, Lindner F: Entrapment and cystic degeneration of the adventitia as a cause of occlusion of the popliteal artery. Chirurg 57:797, 1986.
158. Velasques G, Zollikofer C, Nath HP, et al: Cystic adventitial arterial degeneration. Radiology 134:19, 1980.
159. Vollmar J: Die zystische Adventitiadegeneration der Schlagadern. Z Kreislaufforsch 52:1028, 1963.
160. Ward AS, Reidy JF: Adventitial cystic disease of the popliteal artery. Clin Radiol 38:649, 1987.
161. Wehmann TW: Computed tomography in the diagnosis and management of popliteal artery entrapment syndrome. J Am Osteopath Assoc 93:1039, 1993.
162. Wilbur AC, Spigos DG: Adventitial cyst of the popliteal artery: CT-guided percutaneous aspiration. J Comput Assist Tomogr 10:161, 1986.
163. Zinicola N, Ferrero S, Odero A: Adventitial cyst of the popliteal artery: Case report. Minerva Cardioangiol 21:474, 1973.

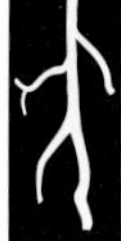

CHAPTER 75

Popliteal Artery Entrapment

Richard J. Fowl, M.D., and
Richard F. Kempczinski, M.D.

In 1879, T. P. Anderson Stuart,[21] a medical student at the University of Edinburgh, writing a "Note on a Variation of the Popliteal Artery," described the anomaly of popliteal artery entrapment concisely: "The popliteal artery, after passing through the opening in the adductor magnus, instead of, as it usually does, coursing downwards and outward towards the middle of the popliteal space, so as to lie between the two heads of the gastrocnemius muscle, passes almost vertically downward internally to the inner head of the gastrocnemius. It reaches the bottom of the space by turning round the inner border of that head, and then passes downwards beneath it—between it and the lower end of the shaft of the femur." It was not until almost a century later, in 1959, that the recognition of this anomaly was resurrected and its management was described by Hamming and Vink[13] of the Netherlands. Additional cases were reported by Servello in Italy in 1962,[20a] Carter and Eban[4] in England in 1964, and Love and Whelan[16] in the United States in 1965. A 1991 review of the English literature on popliteal artery entrapment disclosed 249 reported cases of this anomaly.[17]

This chapter summarizes the clinical features of this uncommon disorder.

ANATOMIC FEATURES AND CLASSIFICATION

Popliteal artery entrapment results from a developmental defect in which the popliteal artery passes medial to and beneath the medial head of the gastrocnemius muscle or a slip of that muscle, with consequent compression of the artery. Rarely, an anomalous fibrous band or the popliteal muscle deep to the medial head of the gastrocnemius muscle is the compressing structure.[12] Concomitant entrapment of the popliteal vein with the artery has been reported in only 7.6% of cases.[17]

The most widely accepted classification recognizes five types of popliteal artery entrapment,[18] with one addition:

Type I: The medial head of the gastrocnemius muscle arises normally, and the artery is displaced in an exaggerated loop that passes medially around and beneath the muscle origin (Fig. 75–1).

Type II: The medial head of the gastrocnemius muscle arises from a point more lateral than its normal origin. The popliteal artery descends in a relatively straight course but still passes medial to and beneath the muscular origin (Fig. 75–2).

Type III: The popliteal artery is compressed by an accessory slip of muscle from the medial head of the gastrocnemius muscle that arises more laterally than the medial head. The artery descends in a relatively straight course, as in type II (Fig. 75–3).

Type IV: The entrapment of the popliteal artery is by the deeper popliteal muscle or from a fibrous band in the same location.[8] The artery may or may not pass medially around the medial head of the gastrocnemius muscle (Fig. 75–4).

Type V: This type consists of any of the preceding types with the addition that the *popliteal vein* is entrapped along with the popliteal artery.

"Type VI": In 1997, Levien[15] described a "functional" type

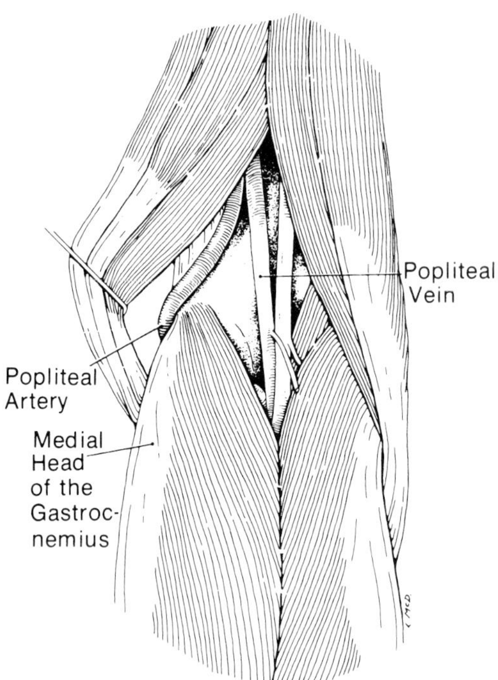

FIGURE 75–1. Type I popliteal entrapment. Exaggerated medial looping of the popliteal artery around and under normally arising head of the gastrocnemius muscle. Medial hamstring muscles have been retracted. (From Haimovici H: Vascular Surgery: Principles and Techniques, 2nd ed. New York, McGraw-Hill, 1984.)

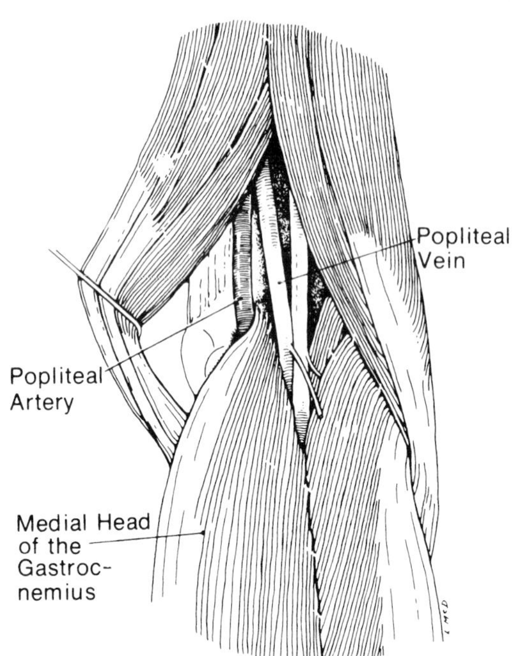

FIGURE 75–2. Type II popliteal entrapment. The course of the popliteal artery is straighter but still medial to and beneath the medial head of the gastrocnemius, which arises more laterally than normal. (From Haimovici H: Vascular Surgery: Principles and Techniques, 2nd ed. New York McGraw-Hill, 1984.)

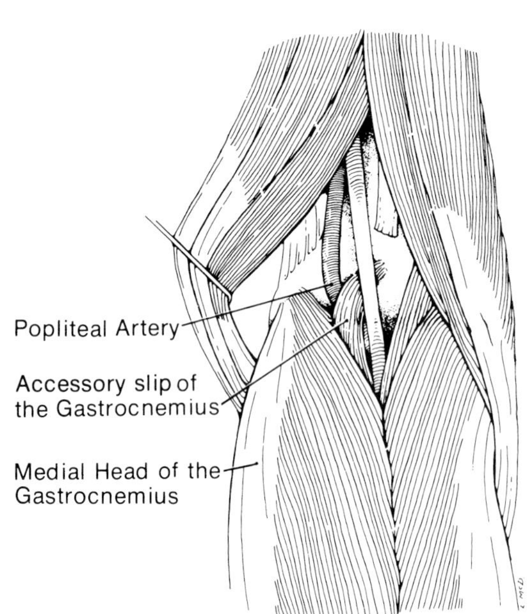

FIGURE 75–3. Type III popliteal entrapment. The structure compressing the popliteal artery is an accessory muscle or fascial slip arising more laterally than the medial head of the gastrocnemius muscle. (From Haimovici H: Vascular Surgery: Principles and Techniques, 2nd ed. New York, McGraw-Hill, 1984.)

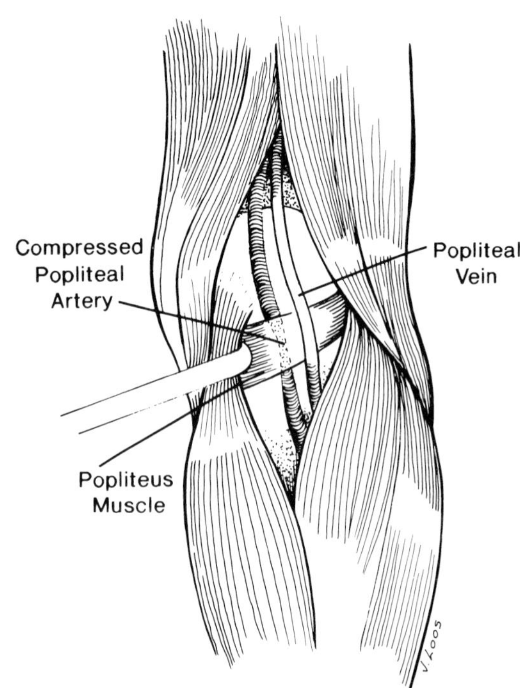

FIGURE 75–4. Type IV popliteal entrapment. The popliteal artery is entrapped by the popliteal muscle or a fibrous band in this location. The artery may or may not pass medial to the medial head of the gastrocnemius muscle.

of popliteal artery entrapment in which the popliteal artery becomes occluded with plantar flexion but no anatomic abnormality exists. He has postulated that it may be due to acquired hypertrophy of a somewhat laterally inserted muscular belly of the medial head of the gastrocnemius muscle. In a series of 73 cases of popliteal artery entrapment, 25 (34%) were of this type and three of the patients presented with an occluded popliteal artery. Levien[15] has labeled this variant type VI.

Other variations are rare and consist of hypertrophied gastrocnemius, plantaris, or semimembranosus muscles in highly trained and athletic individuals.[2, 19] Soleus and plantaris muscle entrapment of the popliteal artery in well-conditioned athletes has also been reported.[23]

According to a 1995 review, type I accounts for 19% of cases of popliteal artery entrapment; type II for 25%; type III for 30%; and type IV for 8%; the remaining 18% consist of the other types.[20]

PATHOLOGY

There are three stages of pathologic findings in the popliteal artery entrapment syndrome[15]:

Stage I: There is adventitial thickening and fibrosis with neovascularization of the adventitia.

Stage II: With disease progression, fragmentation of the external elastic lamina occurs. The medial smooth muscle is replaced by collagen, and invasion of the media by new vessels and fibrosis predisposes the artery to aneurysm formation.

Stage III: The degenerative process results in near-total destruction of the media with fibrous tissue replacement. Later, the internal elastic lamina is destroyed and is replaced by fibrous tissue, making the artery susceptible to thrombosis. Therefore, a popliteal artery that has undergone thrombosis owing to entrapment should no longer be considered salvageable. It must be replaced by a vein graft, not subjected to thrombectomy or endarterectomy.

INCIDENCE

Hamming and Vink,[13] who described the first surgical case of popliteal artery entrapment, reported four additional cases and claimed that the incidence of popliteal artery entrapment was 40% in patients younger than 30 years with calf and foot claudication. In their overall population of 1200 patients with claudication, 12 were younger than 30 years; of these, 5 patients had popliteal artery entrapment. The condition, although described infrequently in the literature, is more common than originally thought.[2, 10, 14] Gibson and associates,[10] in a study of 86 autopsy specimens, demonstrated the anomaly in four cases (3.5% incidence). In a review of 20,000 Greek soldiers, Bouhoutsos and Daskalakis[2] found 45 instances of the anomaly in 33 subjects (0.17%).

CLINICAL FINDINGS

Claudication in the calf and foot of a young man should suggest popliteal artery entrapment syndrome. Table 75–1 summarizes the pertinent clinical data from a review of the literature. This entity occurs nine times more frequently in men. The onset of the symptoms is often sudden, occurring during an episode of intense lower extremity activity, such as during the running of an obstacle course.[3, 6, 16] Although claudication is the only symptom in 69% of cases, paresthesias occur in 14%, and rest pain or ulcer is present in 11%.[17] The symptoms usually are correlated with the development of segmental occlusion of the mid-popliteal artery. This correlation was noted in 53% of reported cases.[17] In the remainder, the patients had symptoms even though

TABLE 75–1. CHARACTERISTICS OF POPLITEAL ARTERY ENTRAPMENT

CHARACTERISTIC	NO. OR PERCENTAGE OF PATIENTS*
Demographics	189 patients
Sex distribution	
Male	90%
Female	10%
Age (yr)	
>30	67%
<30	33%
Age Range (yr)	
Male	12–63
Female	14–53
Distribution	
Unilateral:	66%
Right	50%
Left	50%
Bilateral	34%
Symptoms	159 patients
Claudication	69%
Paresthesias	14%
Rest pain or ulcer	11%
Other	6%
Pedal pulse findings	88 patients
Absent	63%
Decreased	10%
Palpable	16%
Absent with plantar flexion	11%
Popliteal artery angiogram findings	199 patients
Occlusion	53%
Stenosis	34%
Normal	13%
Occlusion or stenosis with plantar flexion	24%
Operative approach	122 patients
Posterior	79%
Medial	21%
Operative procedure	196 patients
Myectomy only	32%
Myectomy and arterial repair	37%
Vein graft arterial repair only	20%
Thromboendarterectomy ± patch	5%
Other	6%

Data from Persky JM, Kempzinski RF, Fowl RJ: Entrapment of the popliteal artery. Surg Gynecol Obstet 173:84, 1991.

*Number of patients is given for each characteristic, because information on each characteristic was not available for all patients.

their arteries were patent, albeit compressed or stenotic (see Table 75–1).

The symptoms described by these patients include cramping in the calf and foot and coldness, blanching, paresthesias, and numbness in the foot associated with walking and relieved by rest. Symptoms are generally unilateral despite the subsequent demonstration of bilateral involvement.[8] In a few of the patients with arterial compression only and without occluding thrombus, the claudication has had unusual characteristics; for example, the claudication occurs with walking but not with running or it begins immediately with the first steps rather than after the patient has walked a finite distance.[4, 6] Some patients have presented with frank popliteal artery aneurysms beyond the site of arterial compression.[6]

In most cases, the anomaly is suspected from the patient's history. Certain physical findings, however, may reinforce the suspicion. Pedal pulses are absent in 63% of cases, diminished in 10%, and palpable in 16%; in 11%, pulses palpable at rest disappear with passive dorsiflexion or active plantar flexion (see Table 75–1). In addition, there may be evidence of increased collateral circulation around the knee. Geniculate arteries may be palpable over the anteromedial and anterolateral aspects of the knee, which is warm.

In patients who have characteristic symptoms but palpable popliteal and pedal pulses, the pathophysiologic finding is a compressed but nonoccluded popliteal artery. In this situation, two maneuvers must be added during palpation of the pedal pulses: passive dorsiflexion of the foot and active plantar flexion against resistance. With these maneuvers, the gastrocnemius muscle is tensed across the compressed artery, thus obliterating the pedal pulses. This portion of the physical examination may be quantitated using an ankle pulse volume recording (PVR) and documenting a decrease in PVR amplitude as evidence of arterial compression with the stress maneuvers (Fig. 75–5). Auscultation of the popliteal artery may demonstrate a systolic bruit if the artery is sufficiently compressed. The maneuvers just described should also be performed on the opposite, asymptomatic limb, because the predisposing anatomic abnormality may be bilateral.

Palpation of a popliteal artery aneurysm in a young man should suggest the presence of the anomaly. Evaluation of the venous system for evidence of obstruction at the popliteal level, namely, distended superficial veins, edema, and dependent cyanosis, completes the evaluation of the lower extremities.

The remainder of the evaluation consists of efforts to exclude diffuse arterial disease, that is, arteriosclerosis, arteritis, collagen vascular disease, or a proximal source for arterial embolus. If the more probable diagnoses have been eliminated by careful general examination, a localized anomaly in the popliteal artery is likely.

DIAGNOSTIC EVALUATION

The critical examination is bilateral femoral arteriography. The diagnosis of popliteal artery entrapment is unequivocally established when two or more of the following findings are noted on neutral, nonstressed views:

- Medial deviation of the proximal popliteal artery
- Segmental occlusion of the mid-popliteal artery
- Post-stenotic dilatation

In addition, "stress arteriograms" should be performed with the leg actively plantarflexed against resistance or passively dorsiflexed in order to show compression that may not be seen in the neutral position (see Fig. 75–5).[11]

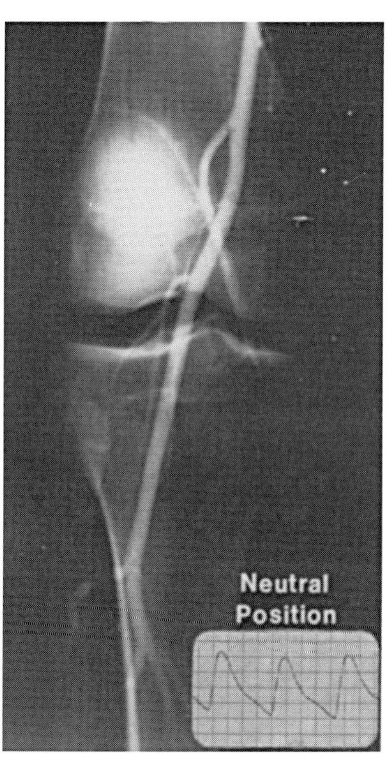

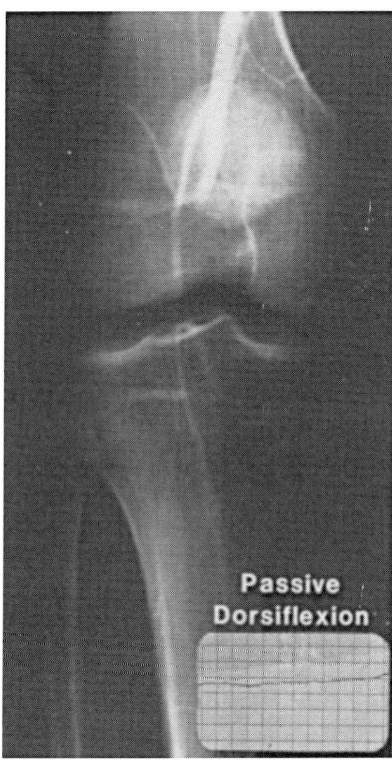

FIGURE 75–5. *Left,* Angiogram reveals a normal course of the popliteal artery with a normal ankle pulse volume recording (PVR) *(inset)* when the foot is in the neutral position. *Right,* With passive dorsiflexion of the foot, the popliteal artery becomes occluded and the ankle PVR becomes flat *(inset).*

The most characteristic radiologic feature of the anomaly is the medial deviation. Segmental occlusion of the mid-popliteal artery is confused with only one other entity, adventitial cystic degeneration (popliteal artery cyst) with *thrombosis* (see Chapter 74). The same segment of the artery is involved in both entities, whereas degenerative disease or inflammatory diseases of arteries is almost never so focal and located in the mid-popliteal artery. Prior to thrombosis, a popliteal artery cyst presents the arteriographic picture of a smooth curvilinear filling defect encroaching upon the arterial lumen. Another important finding is post-stenotic dilatation, which is present in 12% of patients with this anomaly.[17]

Duplex scanning of the popliteal artery may be used to identify popliteal compression. A baseline scan is first obtained of the popliteal artery. Decrease or disappearance of popliteal artery flow with active plantar flexion suggests popliteal artery entrapment.[5] One must interpret the duplex scan in relation to the patient's clinical symptoms and other diagnostic studies, however, because popliteal occlusion with active plantar flexion can be seen on duplex scanning in more than 50% of normal people.[1, 7]

Computed tomography (CT) and, more recently, helical CT have been utilized to determine relationships in the popliteal fossa when the artery has thrombosis because arterial anatomy in the crucial area cannot be delineated by arteriography in this instance.[22] A popliteal artery cyst as well as anomalous insertion of muscle can be delineated by CT scan.[24] Magnetic resonance imaging (MRI) has also been able to define the anatomy preoperatively.[9]

If (1) the remaining patent distal arteries and proximal femoral arteries are normal, (2) the characteristic radiologic findings are present, and (3) the physical findings are not suggestive of generalized arterial disease, preparation can be made for operative correction of the arterial occlusion, if present, and resection of the anomalous anatomy.

If there is any question of more generalized arterial disease, additional arteriography and appropriate tests to rule out metabolic or immunologic aberrations may be required. These procedures are seldom necessary in popliteal artery entrapment syndrome. The localized symptoms of calf and foot claudication on one side, if due to this entity, usually are seen in a young person who is otherwise healthy.

OPERATIVE INTERVENTION

All cases of popliteal artery entrapment should be surgically corrected whether the artery is occluded or not. This philosophy applies not only for symptomatic limbs but also for asymptomatic limbs in which the anomaly is incidentally identified on routine bilateral arteriography or other imaging modalities. It would be unacceptable to risk progression of the anomaly to popliteal occlusion and potential lower extremity ischemic injury in such young, healthy patients. Table 75–1 lists the various procedures that have been reported from the literature in 196 patients with this anomaly.

The posterior approach to the popliteal artery has been most commonly used because it most clearly delineates all variations of this anomaly. Although the medial calf approach (Szilagyi incision) has been utilized and is satisfactory for type I, it may be cumbersome and may pose problems in the management of types II, III, and IV. When the occlusion extends to the popliteal bifurcation, a medial incision may be more appropriate. Table 75–2 emphasizes the advantages and disadvantages of each approach.

Epidural or endotracheal general anesthesia is applicable. The patient lies prone on the table with the leg slightly flexed, 10 to 15 degrees. The incision is S-shaped, with the cephalad vertical portion of the S placed over the posteromedial thigh, the caudad vertical portion on the posterolateral aspect of the calf, and the horizontal limb in the popliteal crease (Fig. 75–6*A* and *B*).

Wide flaps are raised in the subcutaneous tissue, exposing the deep fascia. The surgeon then incises the deep fascia longitudinally, avoiding injury to the median cutaneous sural nerve, which lies immediately subfascial at this level. The accompanying lesser saphenous vein may be sacrificed in order to afford better exposure.

The first of the deep structures to be identified is the tibial nerve, which is mobilized as the vessels are approached. The vein, unless it participates in the anomaly, is found in the deep popliteal fossa, passing between the heads of the gastrocnemius muscle. The artery is not present in the normal location but is identified high in the popliteal space as it exits from the adductor canal. With distal dissection along the arterial adventitia, the surgeon verifies the anomalous course medial to the medial head of the gastrocnemius muscle.

Transection of the compressing muscle or fascial band is begun at the point where the artery passes deep to it. The tight compression of the artery between the muscle and the posterior femur and knee joint capsule is remarkable. The transection must be complete, and the entire artery must be mobilized. If the artery is compressed but not occluded, and secondary fibrotic changes have not taken place in the arterial wall, nothing further is necessary. The medial head of the gastrocnemius may be resected without disturbing function, or if desired, the transected head may be attached to the femur medial to the corrected course of the artery.[6]

For patients with "functional" entrapment (type VI), myotomy of the medial head of the gastrocnemius muscle through a medial incision has resulted in complete relief of symptoms.[15] Turnipseed and Pozniak[23] described an unusual variant of popliteal artery entrapment in which the popliteal artery was compressed by hypertrophied soleus and plantaris muscles in well-conditioned athletes. Symp-

TABLE 75–2. OPERATIVE APPROACHES TO THE POPLITEAL ARTERY

POSTERIOR APPROACH	MEDIAL APPROACH
Better identification of the anomaly; surgeon does not miss it	May miss the anomaly; recurrences more likely
Adequate exposure for most cases	Better exposure for infrapopliteal vessel involvement
Limited access to saphenous vein	Better access to saphenous vein

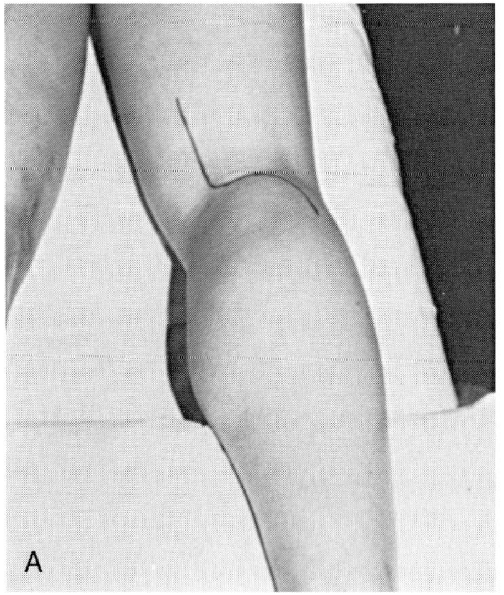

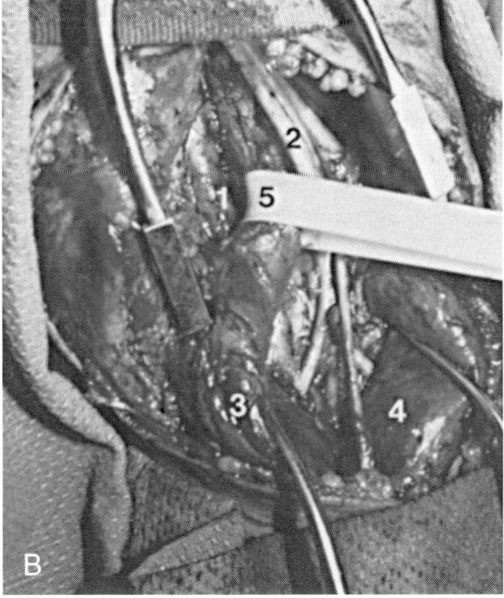

FIGURE 75–6. *A,* The S-shaped incision in the popliteal fossa is used for the posterior approach. *B,* Anatomic structures identified through the posterior incision are (1) the popliteal artery, (2) the tibial nerve, (3) the medial head of the gastrocnemius muscle, (4) the lateral head of the gastrocnemius muscle, and (5) a Penrose drain wrapped around the accessory slip of the gastrocnemius muscle, causing arterial compression.

toms were relieved by surgical release of the soleus muscle from the tibia and resection of the plantaris muscle.

Intra-arterial thrombolytic agents have been utilized to disobliterate a recently clotted artery.[11] However, arterial bypass or replacement is usually necessary for a patent artery in which lysis of the thrombus has been successful, because of arterial wall injury and subsequent fibrosis and thickening from the long-standing entrapment. If organized thrombus with a poor line of cleavage between thrombus and vessel wall is present, or if the vessel is narrowed owing to fibrosis, resection and vein graft interposition are indicated.[14] The graft can be obtained from the greater saphenous vein in the medial flap in the lower thigh. Alternatively, a short bypass vein graft can be utilized without resection of the thrombosed segment.

If a popliteal aneurysm has developed as an extension of the process of post-stenotic dilatation, resection and replacement vein graft with ligation or resection of the aneurysmal segment should be performed.[4] It should be emphasized that in all operations for this condition, the surgeon must first relieve the entrapment by transection of the offending muscle. The wound is closed without drainage. Patients should perform quadriceps-setting exercises hourly until the second to third postoperative day, when they are allowed to ambulate.

RESULTS

Table 75–1 summarizes the frequency with which the various operative procedures have been used. For patients requiring arterial reconstructions, the most successful procedure is vein graft bypass. Of 40 such procedures reported, only two bypasses (5%) became occluded in the immediate postoperative period. Thromboendarterectomy, with or without a patch, has had the poorest results, with acute postoperative thrombosis developing in five of nine patients (55%); therefore, this operation is not recommended for popliteal artery entrapment. Of 119 patients for whom results of surgical treatment were available, results in 103 (87%) were described as "good." Eight patients required early reoperation, and in another eight, problems developed more than 1 month postoperatively.[17]

Several complications may follow operation for popliteal artery entrapment:

- Thrombosis of the graft
- Bleeding
- Infection
- Deep venous thrombosis (DVT)

Graft thrombosis is indicated by loss of pedal pulses and is confirmed by arteriography. Reoperation should be carried out promptly to rectify the technical error and restore circulation. Although bleeding is seldom a problem, hematoma developing shortly after operation should be evacuated in the operating room under sterile conditions, with control of all bleeding points and thorough irrigation of the wound.

DVT is the only indication for anticoagulation in the immediate postoperative period. Because adequate heparinization in the early postoperative period predisposes the patient to bleeding and hematoma formation, anticoagulation should be instituted only when DVT is confirmed by venography or duplex scanning. As for most vascular surgical procedures, prophylactic antibiotics should be used preoperatively, and two to three doses should be administered postoperatively.

SUMMARY

Although popliteal artery entrapment is uncommon, it is an important cause of arterial insufficiency in younger patients. Accurate diagnosis depends on a high index of suspicion combined with dynamic noninvasive testing and "stress arteriography." Although arteriographic demonstration of medial deviation of the artery is diagnostic, absence of this finding does not exclude the diagnosis. Positional arteriography may be necessary in such cases.

Surgical exploration should be performed through a posterior approach because it both facilitates identification of the precise anatomic variant and allows easy arterial repair if necessary. The condition of the popliteal artery must dictate the extent of the surgical procedure. If the artery is normal, relief of the constricting lesion alone suffices. If the artery appears to have disease or thrombosis, myotomy and arterial reconstruction must be undertaken. Reconstruction is best accomplished by bypass grafting with the use of autogenous vein. Thromboendarterectomy of an occluded popliteal artery is contraindicated.

REFERENCES

1. Akkersdijk WL, de Ruyter JW, Lapham R, et al: Colour duplex ultrasonographic imaging and provocation of popliteal artery compression. Eur J Vasc Endovasc Surg 10:342, 1995.
2. Bouhoutsos J, Daskalakis E: Muscular abnormalities affecting the popliteal vessels. Br J Surg 68:501, 1981.
3. Brightmore TGJ, Smellie WAB: Popliteal artery entrapment. Br J Surg 58:481, 1971.
4. Carter AE, Eban R: A case of bilateral developmental abnormality of the popliteal arteries and gastrocnemius muscles. Br J Surg 51:518, 1964.
5. di Marzo L, Cavallaro A, Sciacca V, et al: Diagnosis of popliteal artery entrapment syndrome: The role of duplex scanning. J Vasc Surg 13:434, 1991.
6. Darling RC, Buckley CJ, Abbott WM, et al: Intermittent claudication in young athletes: Popliteal artery entrapment syndrome. J Trauma 14:543, 1974.
7. Erdoes LS, Devine JJ, Bernhard VM, et al: Popliteal vascular compression in a normal population. J Vasc Surg 20:978, 1994.
8. Ezzet F, Yettra M: Bilateral popliteal artery entrapment: Case report and observations. J Cardiovasc Surg 2:71, 1971.
9. Fujiwara H, Sugano T, Fujii N: Popliteal artery syndrome: Accurate morphological diagnosis utilizing MRI. J Cardiovasc Surg 33:160, 1992.
10. Gibson MHL, Mills JG, Johnson GE, et al: Popliteal artery entrapment syndrome. Ann Surg 185:34, 1977.
11. Greenwood LH, Yiezarry JM, Hallett JW: Popliteal artery entrapment: Importance of the stress run-off for diagnosis. Cardiovasc Intervent Radiol 9:93, 1986.
12. Haimovici H, Sprayregen S, Johnson F: Popliteal artery entrapment by fibrous band. Surgery 72:789, 1972.
13. Hamming JJ, Vink M: Obstruction of the popliteal artery at early age. J Cardiovasc Surg 6:516, 1965.
14. Insua JA, Young JR, Humphries AW: Popliteal artery entrapment syndrome. Arch Surg 101:771, 1970.
15. Levien LJ: Popliteal artery thrombosis caused by popliteal entrapment syndrome. *In* Greenhalgh RH, Powell JT (eds): Inflammatory and Thrombotic Problems in Vascular Surgery. London, WB Saunders Co, Ltd, 1997, p 158.
16. Love JW, Whelan TJ: Popliteal artery entrapment syndrome. Am J Surg 109:620, 1965.
17. Persky JM, Kempczinski RF, Fowl RJ: Entrapment of the popliteal artery. Surg Gynecol Obstet 173:84, 1991.
18. Rich NM, Collins GJ Jr, McDonald PT, et al: Popliteal vascular entrapment. Arch Surg 114:1377, 1979.
19. Rignault DP, Pailler JL, Lunely F: The "functional" popliteal artery syndrome. Int Angiol 4:341, 1985.
20. Rosset E, Hartung O, Brunet C, et al: Popliteal artery entrapment syndrome: Anatomic and embryologic bases, diagnostic and therapeutic considerations following a series of 15 cases with a review of the literature. Surg Radiol Anat 17:161, 1995.

20a. Servello M: Clinical syndrome of anomalous position of the popliteal artery. Circulation 26:885, 1962.

21. Stuart TPA: Note on a variation in the course of the popliteal artery. J Anat Physiol 13:162, 1879.
22. Takase K, Imakita S, Kuribayashi S, et al: Popliteal artery entrapment syndrome: Aberrant origin of gastrocnemius muscle shown by 3D CT. J Comput Assist Tomogr 21:523, 1997.
23. Turnipseed WD, Pozniak M: Popliteal entrapment as a result of neurovascular compression by the soleus and plantaris muscles. J Vasc Surg 15:285, 1992.
24. Williams LR, Flinn WR, McCarthy WJ, et al: Popliteal artery entrapment: Diagnosis by computed tomography. J Vasc Surg 3:360, 1986.

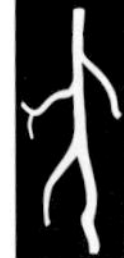

C H A P T E R 7 6

Management of Foot Lesions in the Diabetic Patient

Gary R. Seabrook, M.D., and
Jonathan B. Towne, M.D.

Patients with diabetes mellitus are afflicted with a combination of vascular occlusive disease and peripheral neuropathy that places them at significant risk for injury to the integument, invasive soft tissue infection, osteomyelitis, chronic ulceration, derangement of the skeletal architecture, and gangrene. Foot ulcers and soft tissue infections in diabetic patients are referred for care to vascular surgeons because of their expertise in dealing with the atherosclerotic complications of the disease. Chronic ischemia and sensory and motor neuropathy place the skin and soft tissue of the feet at risk for destructive insults, which often result from only trivial injury. It may be difficult to predict the degree of peripheral neuropathy or arterial ischemia based on the clinical severity of a patient's diabetes. Some patients who have diabetes of many years' duration and who require significant doses of insulin are spared foot complications, while other patients with disease of relatively recent onset are confronted with devastating complications.

The magnitude of this problem is illustrated by the observation that gangrene occurred 53 times as frequently in diabetic men and 71 times as frequently in diabetic women as in their nondiabetic counterparts.[1] The incidence of atherosclerotic gangrene was also increased in diabetic women, and the usual male predominance of gangrene associated with atherosclerosis was absent in diabetic patients. Knowledge of the pathophysiologic changes caused by diabetes mellitus is essential for proper understanding and treatment of foot problems in these patients.

ARTERIAL OCCLUSIVE DISEASE

Vascular occlusive disease in diabetic patients afflicts arteries in a different distribution and effects changes in the blood vessels themselves in ways that are different from those of atherosclerosis as manifested in patients with cardiovascular risk factors such as hypertension, hypercholesterolemia, and cigarette smoking. In the diabetic population, the aortoiliac segments are frequently free of disease. Although arterial wall calcification develops in the femoral-popliteal system, arterial lumina remain patent. The ravages of atherosclerosis most severely affect the distal popliteal segment, the tibial and metatarsal vessels. The tibial-peroneal trunk and the origin of the anterior tibial artery may be completely obliterated. In some patients segments of the distal tibial vessels are reconstituted, but these conduits often feed diseased runoff arteries in the foot, where the collateral system is likely to be occluded. The peroneal artery may be spared for a significant portion of its course and, via collaterals at the ankle to the anterior tibial and posterior tibial arteries, may provide an excellent supply of reconstituted blood flow.

The pathophysiologic changes are associated with increased calcification adjacent to the internal elastic lamina of the tributaries of the tibial system, including the pedal arch and the metatarsal vessels. At the arteriolar level, microangiopathy results in thickening of the intima at the basement membrane. Electron microscopic examination demonstrates thickening of the basement membrane. Banson and Lacy identified the process in 88% of diabetic specimens but in only 23% from nondiabetic patients.[2] The distribution was patchy: normal capillaries were often interspersed with diseased ones. That basement membrane width increased from biopsy samples taken from the distal extremity, suggested an effect of venous hydrostatic pressure in its formation.[3]

Siperstein and colleagues, in a study of human muscle capillary basement membranes by electron microscopy, noted that the average width in diabetic patients was twice that in nondiabetic persons. Increased basement membrane thickness was common in diabetic patients: 98% demonstrated this lesion. Of interest, this thickening was seen in 50% of patients who were genetically "prediabetic" but had not manifested clinical diabetes. This work suggests that basement membrane thickening is an early lesion of diabetic microangiopathy rather than a disturbance of carbohydrate metabolism.[4] This thickening usually did not occlude the lumen, however, and its role in selective capillary permeability and its effect on endothelial metabolism remain hypothetical. Although arterial patency may be preserved, hypertrophy of the endothelial layer impairs oxygen delivery. Unfortunately, the severity of this destructive process at the arteriolar and capillary levels cannot predictably be ameliorated by rigorous blood glucose control.

PERIPHERAL NEUROPATHY

More insidious than the vascular occlusive process for patients with diabetes mellitus is the development of peripheral neuropathy. Both sensory and motor nerves are subjected to segmental demyelination resulting from a defect in the metabolism of Schwann cells. The clinical manifestation of the process is delayed nerve conduction velocity. Microscopically, the basement membrane surrounding the Schwann cell becomes thickened. In advanced disease there is a breakdown of the medullary sheath into separate, concentric conglomerates. Nerves of the distal part of the leg were more often affected, and both medullated and nonmedullated fibers were involved. There is diminution of anterior horn cells in the spinal cords of some diabetic patients.[5, 6] Degeneration of the dorsal columns, most marked in the lower segments, results in scattered destruction and gliosis.[7]

The cause of this nerve destruction may be an occlusive process of the vasa vasorum enveloping the nerve bundles. This process appears to compromise both motor and sensory nerves. When peripheral nerves are examined, the more distal portions show more extensive demyelination than the proximal portions.[5] Neuropathy generally develops slowly. Initially it consists of night cramps and paresthesias; it progresses to loss of vibratory sense and perception of light touch and pain; and finally deep tendon reflexes are lost. The sensory deficit allows abnormal pressure and minor trauma to go unrecognized, so that the protective function of the nervous system is lost.

When an insult results in an inflammatory process, erythema, swelling, and pain are not appropriately recognized. Deficits in the motor nerves result in malfunction of the intrinsic muscles of the foot that distorts foot architecture. This chronic motor denervation results in extensor subluxation of the toes, the plantar prominences of the metatarsal heads, proximal migration of the metatarsal fat pad, and an imbalance in the action of the toe flexors and extensors. With dislocation of the metatarsophalangeal joints, the metatarsal heads become the strike points during ambulation and multiple abnormal bony prominences develop that are not protected by conventional footwear (Fig. 76–1).[8]

Further progression of this neuropathy leads to failure of the joints between the metatarsal and tarsal bones and to eventual collapse of the entire ankle mechanism. This process leads to Charcot's foot. This manifests initially as collapse of the plantar arch, and, in its most extreme form, without benefit of any neurogenic protection, the disorganized tarsal bones erode through the plantar surface.

SOFT TISSUE INFECTION

Infections in patients with diabetes mellitus become serious and even limb-threatening because of risk factors that impede prompt detection and defects in the patient's defense

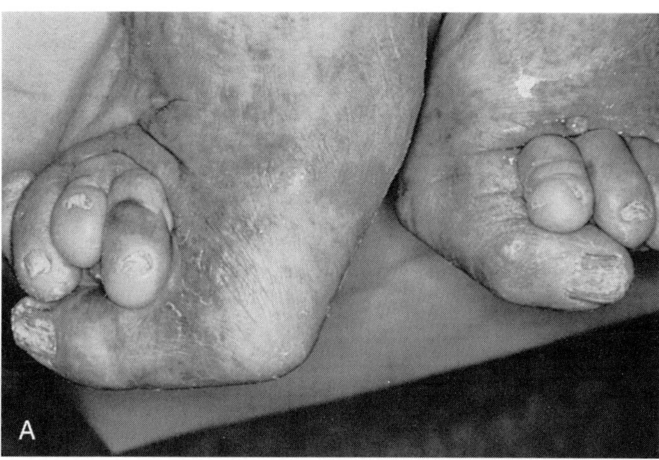

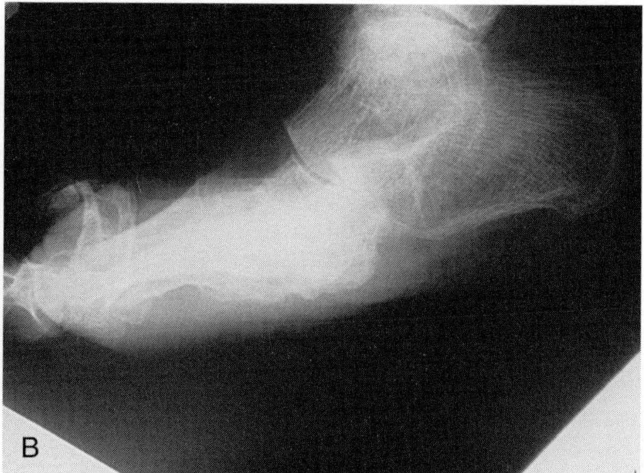

FIGURE 76–1. *A*, Abnormal foot architecture in a diabetic patient with severe peripheral neuropathy. Subluxation and migration of the toes result in many abnormal bony prominences. *B*, Lateral radiograph of Charcot's foot in a diabetic patient. The metatarsal arch has collapsed with chronic dislocation of the tarsal mechanism. The proximal metatarsal elements compose the strike point of the walking surface.

system. Lesions that progress to infection are directly related to the diabetic neuropathy. The diabetic patient cannot sense minor traumatic injuries that progress to soft tissue lesions that become infected secondarily. Once a tissue defect occurs, an infection can rapidly progress without the patient's appreciating even that a lesion is present. When infections do occur, they are likely to progress rapidly and to result in more significant tissue destruction. The arterial occlusive disease is a co-morbid condition that further hinders repair of minor lesions.

The hyperglycemic state enhances conditions that promote infection in diabetic patients. The normal intracellular bactericidal activity of leukocytes is diminished by hyperglycemia. When glucose levels exceed 200 mg/dl, tissue glycosylation occurs, which impairs wound healing by increasing the collagenase activity that reduces the collagen content at the site of tissue injury. The presence of dysfunctional phagocytic cells, coupled with poor wound healing conditions, provides a fertile environment for development of a synergistic microbial infection. Good blood glucose control (≤200 mg/dl) reduces the risk of infection in diabetic surgical patients and should be viewed as an important component in the management of diabetic foot infections.

Polymicrobial infections with aerobic and anaerobic species have the ability to compound the destructive potential of the organisms to a combined virulence that exceeds the individual destructive forces of any of them alone. This "synergistic virulence" accounts for the rapid progression of foot infections and for the fact that broad-spectrum antimicrobial therapy may be required to treat them effectively.

Unlike infected gangrene in a nondiabetic foot, sepsis in a diabetic patient is usually due to infection with multiple organisms, both gram-negative and gram-positive, aerobic and anaerobic.[9] In a classic study, Louie and coworkers identified an average of 5.8 bacterial species per specimen from a diabetic patient's infected foot, among them, on average, 2.3 aerobic organisms and 2.6 anaerobic organisms.[10] When the subgroup with cellulitis was studied, these investigators found an average of 7.3 isolated organisms per specimen, as compared with 4.9 for patients with chronic ulcers. In a more recent series of 26 patients with diabetic foot infections, the author identified 172 bacterial isolates, including 95 aerobes and 77 anaerobes (mean, 6.6 isolates per patient).[11] The incidences and distributions of bacterial species recovered from diabetic foot infections and isolated in our microbiology research laboratory are recorded in Table 76–1.

Peptostreptococci are second only to *Bacteroides* species in anaerobic isolates recovered, and *Peptostreptococcus magnus* is the single most common clinical isolate of the peptostreptococci in diabetes-related infections. This organism produces a potent collagenase capable of disrupting the skin and subcutaneous tissues. This destructive enzyme activity appears to account for the rapid tissue necrosis associated with diabetic foot infections. The microorganism may selectively survive and proliferate because of its ability to break down tissue barriers and invade deeper anatomic spaces.[12]

OSTEOMYELITIS

Diabetic patients are at risk for osteomyelitis, and a destructive bone infection may be present in the absence of severe clinical signs of sepsis. The bone may become colonized via a sinus tract that develops from progression of a small skin injury, ulcer, or fissure. Avascular cartilaginous joint surfaces and sesamoid bones provide a nidus for microbial invasion. In diabetic patients, osteomyelitis is almost always the consequence of an associated contiguous soft tissue infection where the skin envelope has been disrupted. Anatomic defects lead to maldistribution of weight on the foot, and injury results at focal points of pressure and high shear stress. The infection follows an indolent course, and impaired host defenses cannot rid the poorly vascularized bone of the infecting organisms. The disorganized foot architecture of Charcot's foot may mimic osteomyelitis having signs of a chronic inflammatory state, including erythema and edema. If the patient's integument is intact, the erosive or hypertrophic bone changes may not represent infection.

TABLE 76–1. PREDOMINANT MICROBIAL POPULATIONS RECOVERED IN CULTURE FROM DIABETIC FOOT INFECTIONS AND THEIR PREVALENCES

Gram-Negative Aerobes
Proteus spp., 55%
Escherichia coli, 35%
Klebsiella spp., 25%
Pseudomonas aeruginosa, 20%
Other *Pseudomonas* spp., 15%
Morganella morganii, 10%
Enterobacter spp., 25%
Acinetobacter spp., <5%
Citrobacter spp., <5%
Gram-Positive Aerobes
Enterococcus faecalis, 40%
Enterococcus faecium, 5%
Staphylococcus aureus, 30%
Staphylococcus epidermidis, 50%
Streptococcus milleri group, 35%
Streptococcus agalactiae, 10%
Micrococcus spp., 15%
Corynebacterium spp., 15%
Miscellaneous coagulase-negative staphylococci, 25%
Gram-Negative Anaerobes
Bacteroides fragilis group, 65%
Bacteroides fragilis, 45%
Porphyromonas spp., 5%
Fusobacterium spp., 20%
Prevotella spp., 15%
Veillonella parvula, <5%
Bifidobacterium species, <5%
Gram-Positive Anaerobes
Peptostreptococcus magnus, 55%
Peptostreptococcus anaerobes, 15%
Other *Peptostreptococcus* spp., 35%
Actinomyces spp., 5%
Propionibacterium spp., <10%
Clostridium perfringens, <10%
Clostridium spp., <5%

Data from Bacterial Isolate Reference Bank, Surgical Microbiology Research Laboratory, Department of Surgery, Medical College of Wisconsin, Milwaukee, 1998.

CLINICAL EVALUATION

Diabetic foot infections present with a wide spectrum of clinical signs. The most minor finding is cellulitis, a manifestation of inflammation of the skin. It presents as warmth and redness without a defect in the skin structure. Infection that invades the dermis is manifested as skin bullae or fluid-filled blisters. Frequently it is the result of a process by which the interlinking collagen bridges become disrupted and fluid leaks from cell junctions, resulting in increased capillary permeability. The fluid may be sterile, in which case it is protective of the underlying injured tissue. The fluid can also serve as an excellent culture medium, however, and, if it becomes infected, pathogenic organisms may be spread over an underlying injured and compromised surface. Another destructive process at the capillary level may allow bleeding into a skin blister that results in a subcutaneous hematoma. This, too, serves as an excellent culture medium that allows virulent pathogens to penetrate into the deeper tissues of the foot (Fig. 76–2).

A diabetic foot infection may present in a more cryptic fashion when a deeper form of sepsis, often subclinical osteomyelitis, emerges to a superficial level through a sinus tract. The underlying infection produces inflammatory fluid, which travels along fascial planes to the surface. In this process, a chronic condition develops, because fluid is continually removed from the infected site along the sinus tract. Frequently, the sinus tract itself becomes epithelialized, and this further stabilizes and perpetuates a chronic lesion. With this process, underlying bone destruction is not uncommon but, owing to the patient's neuropathy, the skeletal defect goes unrecognized. When such a sinus tract becomes mechanically obstructed, the active infection becomes enclosed and an abscess cavity may quickly develop. This often presents as a paradoxical phenomenon: an obvious, chronic osteomyelitis presents with a very acute soft tissue infection, although often the patient reports having had the clinical signs for only a few hours.

More overt and advanced infections present as epidermal ulceration with exposure and contamination of the underlying subcutaneous tissue (Fig. 76–3). A more aggressive form of this process that destroys the muscle and fascia presents as myonecrosis. This severe tissue destruction leads to interruption of nutrient blood supply, and the lesion progresses to gangrene. Compromised blood supply in the absence of virulent infection may lead to the development of an area of dry gangrene. That devitalized tissue then becomes secondarily involved in an active and destructive soft tissue infection.

One clinical sign of arterial compromise in the foot of a diabetic patient is muscle atrophy, the result of chronic malnourishment, which precludes maintenance of normal muscle mass. Furthermore, motor denervation may render a muscle nonfunctional leading to atrophy. Loss of intrinsic muscle structures results in dysfunctional alignment of the foot bones. This leads to migration of the toes away from the metatarsal heads, collapse of the plantar arch, and even destruction of the ankle joint.

Ischemia results in thickened nails (the result of cornification from extraordinarily slow growth at the nailbed) and predisposes to chronic fungal infections. Chronic ischemia leads to loss of hair growth over the foot and lower leg, another sign of chronic arterial insufficiency. In conducting a physical examination of a patient with chronic ischemia, the examiner will note decreased capillary refill, dependent rubor secondary to chronic vasodilatation, and loss of normal sympathetic control and elevation pallor secondary to decreased arterial perfusion pressures. The examiner must distinguish between cellulitis from an acute infection and the chronic inflammatory process that sometimes accompanies a Charcot's joint.

NONINVASIVE ARTERIAL TESTING

Ulcers and surgical wounds must be assessed for healing potential. A diabetic patient poses unique problems for the application of noninvasive techniques to quantitate lower extremity arterial flow. Because of increased vessel wall calcification in medium-sized and small arteries, it is difficult to compress the vessels when arterial segmental limb pressures are measured. This is most marked with long-standing insulin-dependent diabetes, and it produces erron-

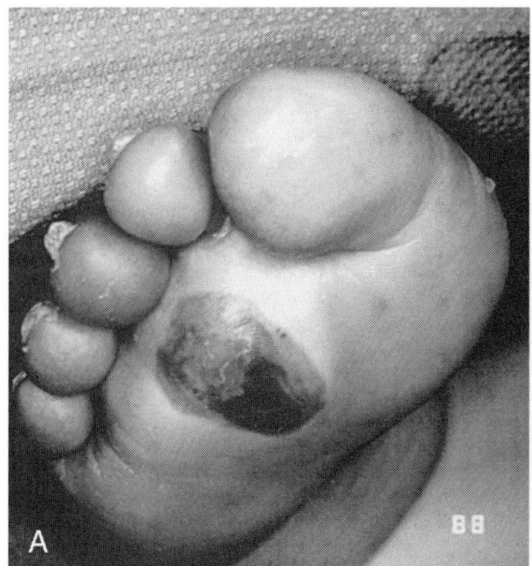

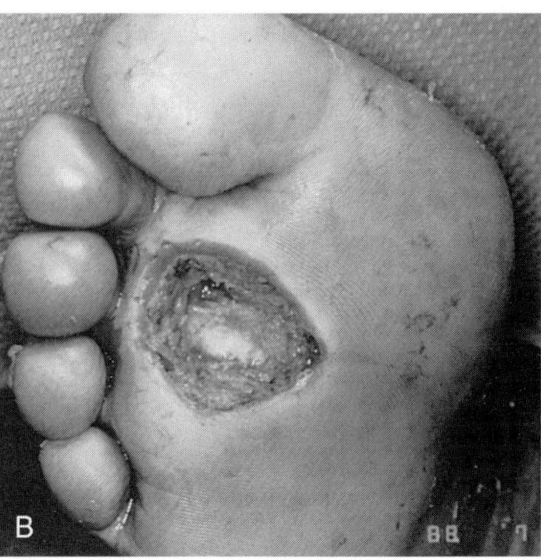

FIGURE 76–2. *A*, Hematoma on the plantar surface over the third metatarsal head in a diabetic patient. The lesion was not associated with symptoms. *B*, Operative débridement of the hematoma revealed extensive soft tissue necrosis extending to the metatarsal head, which is exposed in the base of the wound. A wood sliver was removed from the cavity.

eously high pressure readings. Because calcification of the digital vessels is less pronounced than in proximal metatarsal, plantar, and tibial vessels, toe pressures can be measured accurately.[13] A photoplethysmograph attached with double-sided adhesive tape to the toe distal to a small digital pneumatic pressure cuff provides accurate, reproducible pressures that correlate well with ankle pressures in patients with compressible vessels. These noninvasive tests are of greatest value in assessing the vascular supply of the foot and in evaluating the healing potential of local amputations or ulcerations.[14, 15] Holstein and Lassen reported successful healing of local amputations when toe pressures were greater than 30 mmHg.[16] Only 9% of toe amputation wounds healed when the digital pressure was 20 mmHg or less, whereas those of all 33 patients with pressures greater than 30 mmHg healed. Barnes reported successful healing in patients whose digital pressures were greater than 25 mmHg.[17]

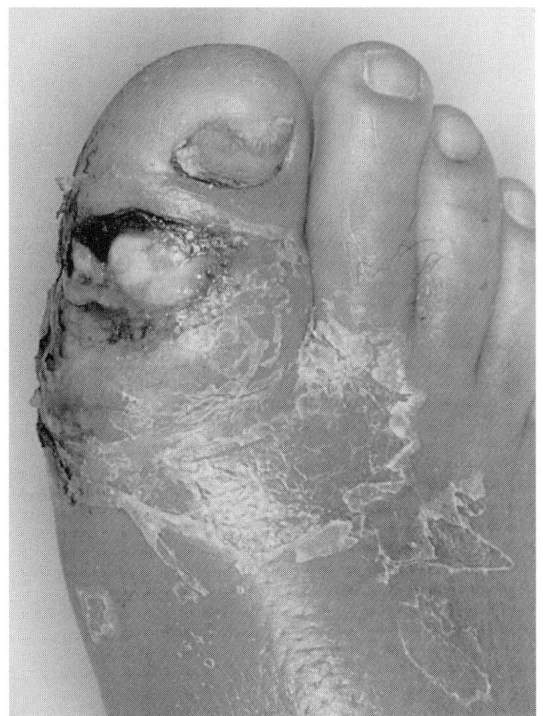

FIGURE 76–3. Diabetic foot infection with ulceration and myonecrosis in a patient with peripheral neuropathy. Although the involved toe was not painful, erythema, edema, and purulent drainage were present.

All other factors being equal, the arterial blood pressure necessary for healing in diabetic patients is higher than that needed by nondiabetics. This is due in part to the aggregate effect of occlusive disease of both large and small vessels, which results in greater resistance and lower arterial flow at any given pressure.[18] Toe pressures have also been helpful in evaluating patients who have combined popliteal and tibial occlusive disease and occlusive disease of the small vessels of the foot. By quantitating the digital blood pressure, we can determine who will require bypass surgery sooner and avoid time-consuming attempts at more conservative therapy that ultimately would prove unsuccessful.

Toe pressures also give an objective measurement of the extent of occlusive disease between the ankle and the toe; however, ankle pressures that are falsely elevated because of calcified, incompressible vessels can skew these results. A normal toe-brachial index is 0.75, and an index of less than 0.25 represents severe occlusive disease. By calculating the toe-brachial index and measuring segmental pressures, the surgeon can evaluate the various segments of the vascular tree, from the femoral artery to the digital artery, and can quantitate the relative contribution of arterial obstruction at each level.

IMAGING STUDIES

Patients who present with an acute diabetic infection should have standard radiographs to examine the skeletal system for osteomyelitis, which is seen as bone destruction in advanced forms of the disease and as cortical irregularities in early forms. Films also identify gas in the soft tissue, which indicates a gas-producing anaerobic infection. Although this is a destructive process that urgently requires surgery, air in the soft tissue of a diabetic foot infection usually is *not* clostridial gangrene associated with necrotizing fasciitis.

Osteomyelitis becomes evident on plain radiographs, owing to inflammatory hyperemia and subsequent deossification. Findings include focal osteopenia and disturbances in the cortex and medullary bone. The process is not evident until significant amounts of bone have been resorbed, which usually takes 2 to 3 weeks from onset of infection.[19, 20]

Technetium phosphate bone scintigraphy can detect infection within days of onset, long before changes can be observed on conventional radiographs. Scintigraphic findings are associated with focal hyperemia. Gallium scanning localizes osseous infection because granulocytes or bacteria take up the tracer. Indium-labeled white blood cell studies are specific for infection, because radiolabeled leukocytes are not incorporated into areas of active bone metabolism.[21] Scans normalize when the infection resolves.

Magnetic resonance imaging (MRI), which demonstrates high tissue contrast, is very sensitive for soft tissue infection. Early changes are detected with low signal intensity on T1-weighted images and high signal intensity on T2-weighted ones. In addition to study of bone structure, MRI allows precise visualization of soft tissue and localization of infection.[22]

CULTURE TECHNIQUES

Although the treatment of polymicrobial diabetic foot infections relies on empirical selection of antibiotics, microbiologic studies should be performed to identify (1) organisms resistant to standard regimens and (2) unusual virulent organisms that may require specific antimicrobial therapy.

The immunocompromised diabetic patient is chronically colonized with a variety of microorganisms, some of which actually have virulent characteristics when associated with a clinical infection. In the treatment of foot infections, it is important to distinguish between constituents of this chronic host flora and organisms that may be responsible for a more destructive process. Thus, culture samples for diagnosis of a foot infection should be collected from the site of most active infection. Surface swabs of material from an ulcer "chronic wound" contain normal colonizing flora and may not recover the predominant microflora responsible for the infection. Swabs are prone to drying and actually carry a relatively small volume of material for culture. Microbial recovery is much enhanced when the volume of the sample is increased.

The ideal specimen for culture is collected by aspiration of purulent material or performing tissue biopsy after careful débridement of the necrotic lesion. Bone tissue is notoriously difficult to "culture," as the organisms may be harbored deep in cancellous bone and may never be exposed to the culture medium. The merits of injecting and then aspirating saline solution from the subcutaneous tissue in an attempt to recover organisms poses a significant risk of contaminating uninfected compartments, and the likelihood of gaining useful clinical information is minimal. This technique should not be used.

Because diabetic foot infections are polymicrobial, the product of both aerobic and anaerobic pathogens, culture techniques should always employ anaerobic collection methods. The specimen should be transported to the laboratory in a gassed-out anaerobic collector. Some transport vessels provide a hydrogen generator that is activated by crushing a sealed capsule. Other systems simply involve use of a closed, serum-capped vial purged of oxygen that contains a charge of hydrogen.

Specimens transported for anaerobic culture should never be refrigerated because oxygen contamination occurs more readily at lower temperatures. Recovery of the anaerobic microbial populations typically associated with diabetic foot infections requires these specialized collection systems. Failure to employ these techniques significantly reduces the yield of the anaerobes that are most frequently associated with these serious infections.[23]

SURGICAL TREATMENT

Surgical débridement is the primary therapy for serious soft tissue infections involving the foot. Because these polymicrobial infections tend to produce significant tissue destruction, it is essential that all devitalized tissue be débrided and all infected material removed, to arrest the infectious process. The anaerobic component of the infection can lead to gas gangrene; therefore, all fascial compartments of the foot that are infected must be opened. Because infection travels readily along the fascia and tendinous planes of the foot, these spaces must be adequately inspected and exposed to make sure no infected tissue is left in the wound.

Some localized wounds can be treated by incision and drainage of an abscess. Care must be taken to unroof the entire infected site. Frequently, the abscess develops under a neurotrophic ulcer. Devitalized tissue and callus should be removed. Strategic placement of incisions in these débridements may allow preservation of parts of the walking surface of the foot.

When the infection begins in a toe, amputation is recommended. If a portion of a toe is destroyed by an infection, seldom can the digit be preserved. The amputation should be performed to remove the proximal phalanx and the opposing metatarsal head. After a toe has been excised, the base of the wound should be débrided of devitalized tissue. A curette easily distinguishes living tissue from dead and is effective in removing residual infected debris. The cartilaginous surface of the metatarsal head, which is avascular, should be removed using a bone rongeur. Because the cartilage covers the entire metatarsal head, care should be taken to resect enough of the bone so that all of the cartilage is removed. When the great toe is amputated, lateral and medial sesamoid bones should also be removed, since they also have limited blood supply and may harbor residual organisms (Fig. 76–4).

Individual digits may be successfully amputated while leaving adjacent structures intact. If the skin in the web space is preserved, surgical incisions should be placed to preserve the adjacent digital arteries. Incisions should be closed with simple sutures or skin staples to prevent ischemia of wound edges. Surgeons should resist the temptation to use mattress sutures or an intradermal closure in an effort to appose skin margins precisely (Fig. 76–5).

When the infection involves all of the digits, transmetatarsal amputation can be performed by removing all of the metatarsal heads and fashioning a flap from the plantar

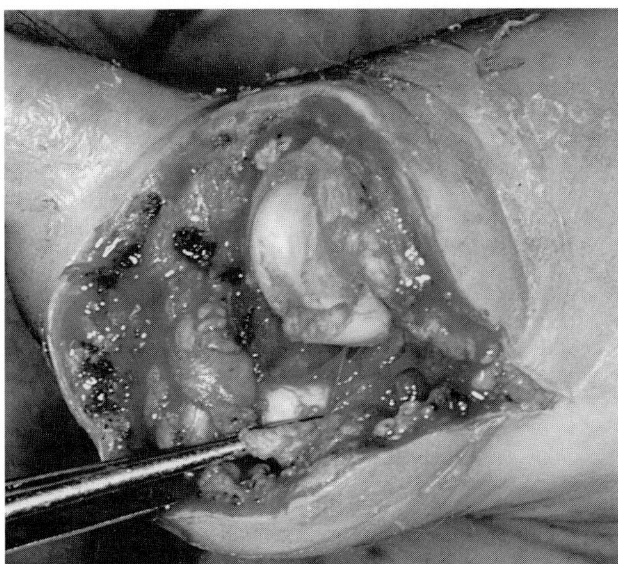

FIGURE 76–4. Amputation of the great toe pictured in Figure 76–3. All necrotic tissue has been débrided. Resection is required for the exposed metatarsal head and sesamoid bone.

surface that can be closed secondarily. The initial surgery should always be directed at removing infection, and no attempt should be made to close any of the underlying soft tissue. Tissue flaps that might appear to be adequate for primary closure of the wound will likely contract. The surgeon should not be discouraged by having to employ a secondary wound closure if the infectious process will be eradicated.

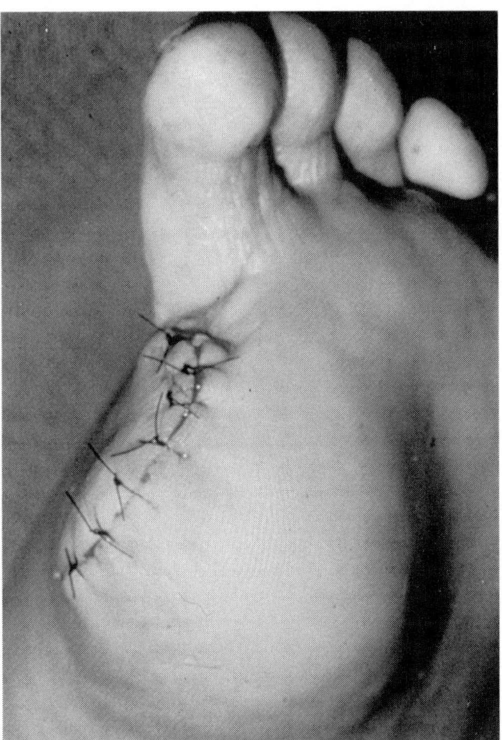

FIGURE 76–5. Wound closure after amputation of the great toe because of chronic osteomyelitis of the phalanx in a diabetic patient. Skin flaps are fashioned and closed with simple sutures to avoid ischemia of the wound margins.

Serious invasive infection can travel along the tendinous planes in the plantar surface, and every diabetic foot infection has the potential to invade the plantar space. At surgery, care should be taken to ensure that no active infection has invaded these deeper fascial compartments. If pus can be expressed from the plantar space, the compartment must be opened. Although preserving the walking surface of the foot is an appropriate goal, a longitudinal incision along the midline of the foot is necessary if infection extends into the plantar space. Such a radical incision can heal, and the foot can return to functional status.

When infection has engulfed the mid-foot, and particularly when necrotic debris is identified at the medial or lateral malleolus, salvage of the foot is seldom possible. Ankle disarticulation is an efficient method of removing the septic focus in an operation that can be performed expeditiously. If the incision is placed just distal to the malleolar heads, the tibiotalar joint can be entered and the foot can be removed by dividing a few soft tissue planes. Fewer lymphatic channels are entered, and tissue compartments remain uncontaminated. Ankle disarticulation must be revised to a formal below-knee amputation.

When an ascending infection spreads from the foot, above the level of the ankle, a "guillotine" amputation is recommended to control the septic process. A circumferential incision is made that is carried directly down to the tibia and fibula, both of which can be divided with a bone saw. The site of amputation should be advanced to a more proximal level if there is evidence of purulent drainage or residual necrotic debris in the wound of the guillotine incision. Formal below-knee amputation is the preferred method of secondary closure, but the surgeon must not leave infected tissue in the wound in an attempt to preserve gastrocnemius or soleus muscle for possible future construction of a posterior flap.

ANTIBIOTICS

Although surgical intervention is the primary treatment for invasive diabetic foot infections, antibiotic therapy is an important adjunct. Antibiotics are not intended to kill microorganisms in soft tissue that has been destroyed by infection; their role is to control invasive microorganisms in adjacent viable tissue. Likewise, bacteria that have been collected by the ascending lymphatic system can be effectively eradicated by proper antibiotic therapy.

Initial therapy should be empirical, and drugs that cover the wide spectrum of microorganisms involving these soft tissue infections should be employed. A semisynthetic penicillin with a beta-lactamase inhibitor covers the majority of aerobic and anaerobic organisms.[24] The quinolones are ideal compounds for the treatment of diabetic foot infections[25–27]; however, the antimicrobial spectra of these agents vary greatly, depending on the "generation." Second-generation quinolones exhibit excellent gram-negative facultative activity but should never be used alone in treating an acute diabetic foot infection because they demonstrate little activity against gram-negative anaerobic populations. Clindamycin or metronidazole should be added to provide effective anaerobic coverage for the microbial flora encountered in a diabetic foot infection.

Historically, empirical therapy for polymicrobial infections always included an aminoglycoside. There is no role for aminoglycosides in serious foot infections of diabetic patients. The nephrotoxicity of aminoglycosides poses too great a risk to these patients, many of whom already suffer from diabetic nephropathy.

The fourth-generation quinolones are agents with excellent aerobic and anaerobic coverage against both gram-positive and gram-negative pathogens encountered in serious foot infections. For the first time, quinolones are available that may be used as single agents for treatment of serious soft tissue infections. These compounds are available in both oral and parenteral compounds, and their pharmacokinetic profiles allow for once daily dosing. Patients may be treated initially in the hospital with the intravenous formulation and then discharged home with oral medication. The quinolones demonstrate concentration-dependent killing, so that as the concentration of the drug increases at the site of infection, enhanced bactericidal activity is noted. The quinolones demonstrate excellent tissue penetration into a wide variety of cells including phagocytic cells, and are equally effective against cells in growth phase or a passive metabolic state.[28, 29] The quinolones exhibit a post-antibiotic effect against both gram-positive and gram-negative bacteria, inhibiting bacterial growth for periods as long as 2 hours, allowing the host immune system to deal with the microbial invader.[30, 31]

WOUND CARE

After surgical treatment and appropriate empirical antibiotic therapy, most diabetic foot infections resolve quickly once the infection is controlled. When blood supply is adequate to support wound healing, granulation tissue begins to develop. Because diabetic patients frequently suffer from arterial insufficiency, early evaluation of the blood supply is important to determine whether vascular reconstruction may be necessary to allow wound healing. A marginal blood supply, which might have been capable of preserving an intact skin envelope, may be inadequate to allow repair of a significant surgical wound.

Wounds involving drainage of a superficial abscess or amputation of an infected digit close secondarily. Granulation tissue should be kept clean, and a moist wound-healing environment should be maintained. Hydrocolloid gel applied to the wound and covered by a semi-occlusive dressing can provide such an environment.[32] Materials composed of calcium alginate allow absorption of wound exudate fluids while keeping the wound surface moist. Commercial adhesive wound dressings provide the additional features of absorbing exudate while protecting adjacent skin surfaces from the toxicity of wound drainage. Although normal in the reparative process, fibrin deposition impairs wound healing and impedes physiologic closure of the wound. Enzymatic agents are effective in removing tenacious build-up of fibrin debris and should be employed to optimize the surface conditions of the wound.[33, 34] Once the depth of the wound has been filled with granulation tissue, epithelialization across the regenerated surface occurs.

Platelet-derived growth factor (PDGF) has proved effective in accelerating the rate of healing of diabetic neurotrophic ulcers that extend into, or deeper than, the subcutaneous layer of the skin. Recombinant agents function much as endogenous PDGF does, by promoting chemotactic recruitment, activation of inflammatory cells, and proliferation of cellular elements in a granulating wound. The growth factors accelerate the wound healing cascade by increasing the activity of fibroblasts, smooth muscle cells, and capillary endothelial cells. Cell mitogenesis and migration are promoted to synthesize protein and the components of the extracellular matrix.[35–39]

Large wounds that constitute significant anatomic defects may close faster if a powered vacuum device is applied. Vacuum-assisted closure is effective in providing mechanical apposition of wound margins and by removing serous drainage and fibrinous exudate. Granulation tissue develops more rapidly in this environment.[40]

Wounds that have developed a granulated surface but are slow to epithelialize may be closed with split-thickness skin grafts. Quantitative cultures should be obtained before grafting to ensure that skin is not transferred onto a colonized field. Although all open wounds harbor some bacteria, bacterial counts greater than 10^5 colony-forming units (CFUs) per gram of tissue are associated with higher incidences of infectious wound-healing complications.[41] Many pathogens of diabetic foot infections are particularly destructive to split-thickness skin grafts.

When a graft is applied, a dressing should be employed to ensure excellent apposition of the grafted skin against the granulation bed. The use of foam dressings or a sealed dressing under which a vacuum device has been inserted can enhance contact. The desire to maintain a dressing over the skin graft to allow invasion of skin buds must be tempered with the need to remove any contaminated exudate that could subsequently contribute to destruction of the graft.

A total contact cast is an effective option for treating diabetic foot ulcers that are not associated with infection. This technique has been championed at the Gillis W. Long Hansen's Disease Center, and often it results in healing of chronic ulcers.[42] Contraindications to cast treatment include acute infection, ischemia, deep ulcers, and draining wounds. When patients have multiple plantar ulcers and peripheral neuropathy limited to the forefoot, consideration should be given to transmetatarsal amputation, which accomplishes two objectives: (1) it removes the area of ulceration, and (2) it places the insensate skin on the non–weight-bearing surface of the foot, as stressed by McKittrick and associates.[43] When blood supply is adequate, these amputations usually heal without difficulty.

After successful healing of these ulcers, patients with severe neuropathy and orthopedic deformation of the feet should wear extra-depth shoes with total-contact inserts to distribute their weight as evenly as possible on the plantar surface and to avoid overloading the protruding metatarsal heads.

Clinical follow-up of diabetic ulcers can be frustrating because the absence of pain in the ulcer makes patient compliance less likely. Poor foot hygiene is also common, in part because of the patient's poor vision secondary to retinopathy. Congestive heart failure, with its resultant leg edema, also complicates ulcer healing. Careful surveillance is necessary to monitor chronic ulcers and to detect changes in foot architecture that might promote development of a plantar space infection. Conservative therapy poses significant risks for patients whose digital pressure is less than 30 mmHg.

A diabetic foot infection does not imply that the blood supply to the soft tissues of the foot is compromised or that the foot cannot be salvaged; however, angiography should be performed when the patient's healing potential is poor. Vascular reconstruction, when technically feasible, is recommended for patients with chronic neurotrophic ulcers associated with critical ischemia. Distal vein bypasses in diabetic patients have excellent patency rates (i.e., equal to those performed in nondiabetic patients).[44]

These data emphasize the need for long-term follow-up of diabetic patients with peripheral neuropathy, foot ulcers, or a history of soft tissue infection. Education for the patient and primary care physician is necessary to identify risks and to detect foot lesions promptly. Aggressive surgical care offers the best chance of avoiding major amputation.[45]

REFERENCES

1. Bell ET: Atherosclerotic gangrene of the lower extremities in diabetic and nondiabetic persons. Am J Clin Pathol 28:27, 1957.
2. Banson BB, Lacy PE: Diabetic microangiopathy in human toes. Am J Pathol 45:41, 1964.
3. Lippman HI: Prevention of amputation in diabetics. Angiology 30:649, 1979.
4. Siperstein MD, Unger RH, Madison LL: Studies of muscle capillary basement membranes in normal subjects, diabetics and prediabetic patients. J Clin Invest 47:1973, 1968.
5. Dolman CL: The morbid anatomy of diabetic neuropathy. Neurology (Minneap) 13:135, 1963.
6. Greenbaum D, Richardson PC, Salmon MJ, et al: Pathological observation on six cases of diabetic neuropathy. Brain 87:201, 1964.
7. Olsson Y, Save-Soderbergh J, Sourander P, et al: A pathoanatomical study of the central and peripheral nervous system in diabetics of early onset and long duration. Pathol Eur 3:62, 1968.
8. Ctercteko GC, Dhanondran M, Hutton WC, et al: Vertical forces acting on the feet of diabetic patients with neuropathic ulceration. Br J Surg 68:608, 1981.
9. Pratt TC: Gangrene and infection in the diabetic. Med Clin North Am 49:987, 1965.
10. Louie TJ, Bartlett JG, Tally FP, et al: Aerobic and anaerobic bacteria in diabetic foot ulcers. Ann Intern Med 85:461, 1976.
11. Seabrook GR, Edmiston CE, Schmitt DD, et al: Comparison of serum and tissue antibiotic levels in diabetes-related foot infections. Surgery 110:671, 1991.
12. Krepel CJ, Gohr CM, Edmiston CE: Anaerobic pathogenesis: Collagenase production by *Peptostreptococcus magnus* and its relationship to site of infection. J Infect Dis 163:1148,1991.
13. Ferrier TM: Comparative study of arterial disease in amputated lower limbs from diabetics and nondiabetics. Med J Aust 1:5, 1967.
14. Bone GE, Pomajzl MJ: Toe blood pressure by photoplethysmography: An index of healing in forefoot amputation. Surgery 89:569, 1981.
15. Gibbons GW, Wheelock FC Jr, Siembieda C, et al: Noninvasive prediction of amputation levels in diabetics. Arch Surg 114:1253, 1979.
16. Holstein P, Lassen NA: Healing of ulcers on the feet correlated with distal blood pressure measurements in occlusive arterial disease. Acta Orthop Scand 51:995, 1980.
17. Barnes RW: Discussion of Gibbons GW, Wheelock FC Jr, Siembieda C, et al: Noninvasive prediction of amputation levels in diabetics. Arch Surg 114:1253, 1979.
18. Tenembaum MM, Rayfield E, Junior J, et al: Altered pressure flow relationship in the diabetic foot. J Surg Res 31:307, 1981.
19. Crim JR, Seeger LL: Imaging evaluation of osteomyelitis. Crit Rev Diagn Imaging 35:201–256, 1994.
20. Longmaid HE III, Kruskal JB: Imaging infections in diabetic patients. Infect Dis Clin North Am 9:163–181, 1995.
21. Newman GL, Waler J, Palestro CJ, et al: Unsuspected osteomyelitis in diabetic foot ulcers. JAMA 266:1246–1251, 1991.
22. Erdman WA, Tamburro F, Jayson HT, et al: Osteomyelitis: Characteristics and pitfalls of diagnosis with MR imaging. Radiology 180:533, 1991.
23. Jousimies-Somers HR, Summanen PH, Finegold S: *Bacteroides*, *Porphyromonas*, *Prevotella*, *Fusobacterium* and other anaerobic gram-negative bacteria. *In* Murray PR, Baron EJ, Pfaller MA, et al. (eds): Manual of Clinical Microbiology, 6th ed. Washington, DC, American Society for Microbiology Press, 1995, pp 603–620.
24. Grayson ML, Gibbons GW, Habershaw DV, et al: Use of ampicillin/sulbactam versus imipenem/cilastatin in the treatment of limb-threatening foot infections in diabetic patients. Clin Infect Dis 18:683–693, 1994.
25. Peterson LR, Lissack LM, Canter K, et al: Therapy of lower extremity infections with ciprofloxacin in patients with diabetes mellitis, peripheral vascular disease, or both. Am J Med 86:801–808, 1989.
26. Gentry LO: Therapy with newer oral beta-lactam and quinolone agents for infections of skin and skin structures: A review. Clin Infect Dis 14:285–297, 1992.
27. Rissing JP: Antimicrobial therapy for chronic osteomyelitis in adults: Role of the quinolones. Clin Infect Dis 25:1327–1333, 1997.
28. DiPiro JT, Edmiston CE, Bohnen JMA: Pharmacodynamics of antimicrobial therapy in surgery. Am J Surg 171:615–622, 1996.
29. Craig W, Dalhoff A: Pharmacodynamics of fluoroquinolones in experimental animals. *In* Kuhlmann J, Dalhoff A, Zeiler HJ (eds): Quinolone Antibacterial. Berlin, Springer-Verlag, 1998, pp 207–232.
30. Edmiston CE, Goheen MP: Impact of subinhibitory concentrations of quinolones on adherence of Enterobacteriaceae to cells of the small bowel. Rev Infect Dis 11(Suppl 5):948–949, 1989.
31. Schmitt DD, Bandyk DF, Edmiston CE, et al: The in-vitro effect of subinhibitory concentrations of quinolones and vancomycin on adherence of slime-producing *Staphylococcus epidermidis* to vascular prostheses. Rev Infect Dis 11 (Suppl 5):947–948, 1989.
32. Varghese MC, Balin AK, Carter DM, et al: Local environment of chronic wounds under synthetic dressings. Arch Dermatol 122:52–57, 1986.
33. Steed DL, Donohoe D, Webster MW: Effect of extensive debridement and treatment of the healing of diabetic foot ulcers. J Am Coll Surg 183:61–64, 1996.
34. Sinclair RD, Ryan TJ: Proteolytic enzymes in wound healing: The role of enzymatic debridement. Australas J Dermatol 35:35–41, 1994.
35. Steed DL: Clinical evaluation of recombinant human platelet-derived growth factor for the treatment of lower extremity diabetic ulcers: Diabetic Ulcer Study Group. J Vasc Surg 21:71–81, 1995.
36. Robson MC, Phillips LG, Thomason A, et al: Platelet-derived growth factor BB for the treatment of chronic pressure ulcers. Lancet 339:23–25, 1992.
37. Musto TA, Curier NR, Allman RM, et al: A phase II study to evaluate recombinant platelet-derived growth factor-BB in the treatment of stage 3 and 4 pressure ulcers. Arch Surg 129:213–219, 1994.
38. Brown GL, Curtsinger I, Jurkiewicz MJ, et al: Stimulation of healing of chronic wounds by epidermal growth factor. Plast Reconstr Surg 88:189–196, 1991.
39. Falanga V, Eaglstein WH, Bucalo B, et al: Topical use of recombinant epidermal growth factor (h-EGF) in venous ulcers. J Dermatol Surg Oncol 18:604–606, 1992.
40. Argenta LC, Morykwas MJ: Vacuum-assisted closure: A new method for wound control and treatment: Clinical experience. Ann Plast Surg 38:563–577, 1997.
41. Robson MC, Sternberg BD, Heggers JP: Wound healing alterations caused by infection. Clin Plast Surg 17:485–492, 1990.
42. Duffy JC, Patout CA Jr: Management of the insensitive foot in diabetes: Lessons learned from Hansen's disease. Mil Med 155:575, 1990.
43. McKittrick LS, McKittrick JB, Risley TS: Transmetatarsal amputation for infection or gangrene in patients with diabetes mellitus. Ann Surg 130:826, 1948.
44. Bergamini TM, Towne JB, Bandyk DF, et al: Experience with in situ saphenous vein bypasses during 1988 to 1989: Determinant factors of long term patency. J Vasc Surg 13:37–49, 1991.
45. Klamer TW, Towne JB, Bandyk DF, et al: The influence of sepsis and ischemia on the natural history of the diabetic foot. Am Surg 53:490, 1987.

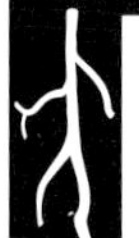

CHAPTER 77

Vasculogenic Impotence

Ralph G. DePalma, M.D., F.A.C.S., and
Richard F. Kempczinski, M.D.

Progress in the diagnosis and treatment of impotence has accelerated dramatically during the past three decades. Beginning with Leriche's[37] 1923 observation that aortoiliac occlusion caused impotence due to inadequate perfusion of the corpora cavernosa, surgeons became interested in the relationship between potency and cavernosal perfusion.[36] Aortic surgical interventions often produced impotence,[32, 43] and beginning in the 1970s, techniques were developed to minimize this complication.[10, 58] It was also postulated that vascular surgical procedures could be applied for revascularization of the corpus cavernosum.[14, 45]

Consequently, corpus cavernosum revascularization was emphasized in the late 1970s and early 1980s. In 1982, however, it was found that erection could be stimulated by injection of the vasoactive agents papaverine[55] and phentolamine[6] into the corpora cavernosa. This discovery helped to illuminate the processes of cavernosal smooth muscle function. Intracorporeal administration of these agents led to effective methods for testing and quantifying various aspects of erectile dysfunction and provided important tools for diagnosis and treatment. Emphasis shifted from simple mechanistic efforts to increase arterial inflow toward sophisticated investigations of corporal smooth muscle function. Import recent contributions are (1) elaboration of the roles of nitric oxide (NO) and oxygen tension in normal erection and (2) delineation of mediators of corporal muscle contraction and relaxation.[3, 52]

Impotence is "inability to achieve or maintain an erection adequate for intromission." Impotence should be distinguished from *retrograde ejaculation*, a neurogenic dysfunction in which bladder neck closure does not occur, so that semen is ejaculated into the bladder. In the latter disorder, the patient is still able to complete coitus and achieve orgasm. Although impotence, by definition, is a disorder limited to men, women with aortoiliac artery obstructive disease might experience insufficient vaginal lubrication and loss of orgasm.[13] This disorder is uncommon clinically, however, because female genital sensation depends more on the integrity of the somatic pudendal nerves and their sensory fibers. Collateral arterial blood supply to the female sexual organs is also extensive, and men present with aortoiliac occlusive disease more frequently in vascular practice than do women.

This chapter reviews current concepts of the physiology of erection as well as the diagnostic and treatment approaches and techniques used in vascular surgery to prevent erectile failure or restore function.

PHYSIOLOGY OF PENILE ERECTION

Penile erection results from a neurally mediated increase of arterial inflow into the corporal bodies along with a reduction or cessation of venous outflow. Findings reported by Rajfer and colleagues[52] support the idea that endothelium-derived relaxant factor (EDRF) is involved in nonadrenergic, noncholinergic neural transmission, which leads to the cavernosal smooth muscle relaxation required for normal erection. Histochemically, nerve fibers positive for the reduced form of nicotinamide adenine dinucleotide phosphate (NADP) and diaphorase are found in human penile tissue, indicating NO synthase activity.[31] Other neurotransmitters, such as vasoactive intestinal polypeptide (VIP) and fibers positive for acetylcholinesterase, are also present.[2] When the penis is flaccid, the corporal smooth muscle is contracted; contraction is due to a normally present overriding adrenergic tone. With erection, smooth muscle relaxation occurs. Various other receptors are present in penile smooth muscle, including those responsive to VIP, dopamine, histamine, prostaglandin (PG), and probably several other substances.

The initiating event of penile erection is vasodilation. With increased intracavernosal flow, a greater amount of oxygen is thought to stimulate NO synthesis by cavernosal nerves and endothelium. Cavernosal oxygenation promotes penile erection, whereas hypoxemia is inhibitory. Testosterone, in addition to its central effects, has been shown experimentally to stimulate NO synthase activity in corporal tissues,[8] enhancing sensitivity to cavernosal nerve stimulation in animals. NO, in turn, activates conversion of guanosine triphosphate to cyclic guanosine monophosphate (GMP). The latter provides the message leading to relaxation of the smooth muscle within the corpora cavernosa.[9] Agents that inhibit hydrolysis of cyclic GMP may increase messenger cyclic GMP, enhancing smooth muscle relaxation and thus promoting penile erection.[4] Cyclic nucleotide phosphodiesterase (PDE) isoenzymes increase hydrolysis of cyclic GMP; among these, PDE_5 and PDE_6 are specific for the substrate in human cavernosal tissue.[28] Inhibitors of PDE constitute a new class of oral agents for treatment of impotence.

HEMODYNAMICS AND DIAGNOSIS

Figure 77–1 illustrates the hemodynamics of the erectile process. In flaccidity, the corporal smooth muscle and cav-

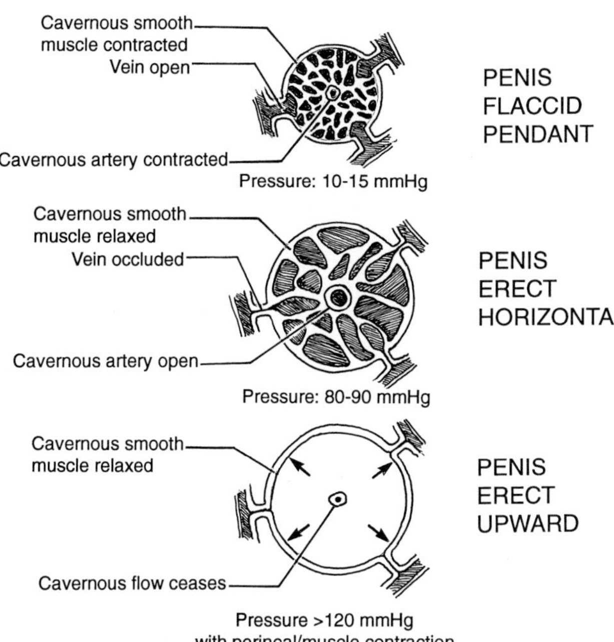

FIGURE 77–1. Current theory of penile erection showing three stages of erection as smooth muscle relaxation occurs. Pressure measurements are those obtained before and after intracavernosal injection of vasoactive agents. Note onset of venous occlusion in the second stage. (From De-Palma RG: New developments in the diagnosis and treatment of impotence. West J Med 164:54, 1996.)

ernosal arteries are contracted, and the emissary and pudendal veins are open. The intracavernosal pressure is equivalent to venous pressure; the blood in the intracavernosal spaces is desaturated. It is important to understand this physiologic process, which has now been reviewed elsewhere.[17]

Current diagnostic methods, such as dynamic infusion cavernosometry and cavernosography (DICC), are used to measure penile blood pressure and flow changes and to detect sites of leakage. The authors usually employ these methods in cooperation with urologic and radiologic colleagues. At low intracavernosal pressure in the flaccid state, a cavernosal or venous leak is always detected radiographically; in other words, every flaccid penis exhibits a venous leak. This fact is key to the understanding of penile physiology and cavernosographic findings.

In the next stage of erection, intracavernosal pressure increases to 80 to 90 mmHg synchronously with progressive smooth muscle relaxation, facilitating an increase in arterial inflow. With full relaxation, the penile veins become obstructed as a result of the occluding action of the subalbugineal smooth muscle. A fully turgid erection, in terms of vascularity, occurs with intracavernosal pressures of about 100 mmHg. With full erection, the cavernosal artery occlusion pressure (CAOP) tends to be equivalent to the intracavernosal pressure, but flow is markedly reduced.

In the final stage, pelvic muscular contraction, suprasystolic pressures are generated, maximum rigidity occurs, and cavernosal artery flow ceases transiently. For diagnostic purposes, flow in the cavernosal artery can be measured by duplex scanning[39] at specific intervals after the intracavernosal injections of vasoactive agents.

During DICC, the pressure at which cavernosal artery flow ceases can be detected by a Doppler probe placed at the penile base. This method uses "artificial erection" generated by a roller pump infusion of warm normal saline solution. The pressure at which the signal returns on pump flow reduction is taken as the CAOP. This value normally ranges from 80 to 90 mmHg, with a gradient of less than 30 mmHg in comparison with a simultaneously obtained brachial pressure.[21, 30] The CAOP is an indirect assessment of the adequacy of arterial flow.

Both large vessel aortoiliac disease and abnormalities of the pudendal arterial supply (Fig. 77–2) cause arteriogenic impotence. The flow to maintain erection is a measure of venous efflux provided that complete smooth muscle relaxation has been obtained. The flow to maintain erection considered to be normal has been taken as less than 40 ml/min, with pressure drops of less than 1 mmHg/sec on flow cessation.

Standardization of DICC depends on maximum muscular relaxation through the intracavernosal administration of vasoactive agents. With a previously described method,[21] 60 mg of papaverine hydrochloride and 2.5 mg of phentolamine were used. Readministration of these agents during DICC has been recommended to achieve maximal muscular relaxation and linear pressure-flow relationships.[54] An understanding of this process is also important for demon-

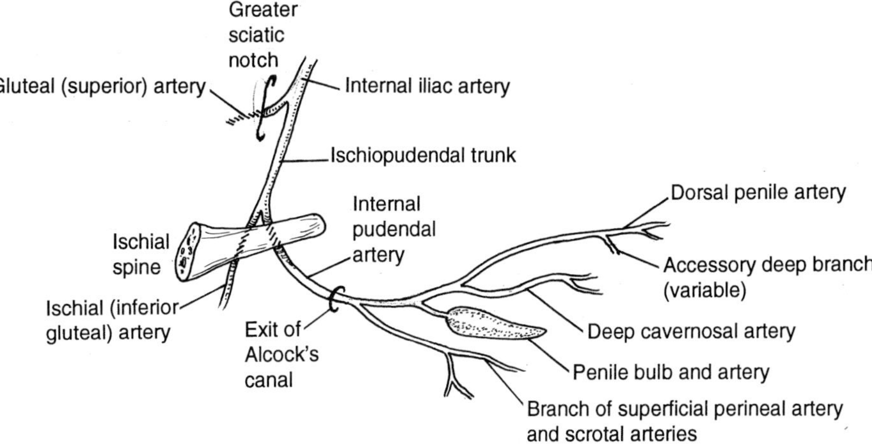

FIGURE 77–2. A right oblique schematic showing the internal iliac artery and the pudendal artery and its branches to the penis. This view can be seen on highly selective pudendal arteriography. Note bony landmarks. (Modified from DePalma, RG: New developments in the diagnosis and treatment of impotence. West J Med 164:54, 1996.)

strating penile arterial anatomy. When the intracavernosal administration of vasoactive agents produces full erection, arteriography causes radiographic artifacts due to cessation of cavernosal artery flow. For visualization of the penile artery, the goal of injection is tumescence, not full erection; therefore, smaller doses of vasoactive agents are used.

GENERAL CAUSES OF IMPOTENCE

As one may infer from a consideration of physiology, erectile failure is a vascular dysfunction. Impotence can also be caused, however, by endocrine, metabolic, neurogenic, and psychologic factors. Some form of arterial inflow abnormality is associated with this complaint in about 50% of patients screened noninvasively.[16] As will be seen, however, this finding is not always caused by inflow compromise. Arteriogenic impotence can also be related to intrinsic abnormalities of the penile arteries or smooth muscle. Endocrine causes of impotence are uncommon[17, 35]; only 3% to 4% of patients screened show lowered testosterone levels. Prolactinomas are also rare, being found in about 0.2% of patients screened. Similarly, restoration of a euthyroid state has not notably improved erectile function in patients with hypothyroidism.

The most common association in arteriogenic impotence is with a variety of antihypertensive drugs; angiotensin-converting enzyme inhibitors are thought to spare erectile function. Antidepressants such as selective serotonin uptake inhibitors reduce libido and thus affect potency. Bupropion, a member of another class of antidepressants, exhibits prosexual effects, including effects on libido, arousal, and the duration and intensity of orgasm.[47] Oral medications for erectile dysfunction include phentolamine, yohimbine, trazodone, pentoxifylline, apomorphine, and sildenafil.[34] Isoxsuprine, an $alpha_1$ blocker, has also been found useful.[22] Sildenafil is an inhibitor of type V phosphodiesterase (PDE_5), the main isoenzyme involved in the metabolism of cyclic GMP in the corpus cavernosum[5]; this agent has been approved for use in the United States.

Psychogenic problems, often observed in impotent men, can produce sufficient anxiety and enhanced adrenergic tone to override even intracavernosal injections (ICIs) of vasoactive agents. Interestingly, heavy cigarette smoking just before injection of 80 mg of papaverine in normal young volunteers has been shown to inhibit erection.[29] In spite of limitations, intracavernosal injection using prostaglandin E_1 (PGE_1) (up to 30 μg) is an important diagnostic and therapeutic tool.[56] An adequate erectile response, while not ruling out proximal arterial disease, suggests that the arterial system is capable of delivering adequate inflow and that corporal relaxation and venous closure are relatively functional. An adequate erection also means that, in addition to ICIs, intraurethral prostadil can be used for treatment.[50]

As can be seen from the consideration of erectile physiology, arterial inflow compromise, in turn, causes venous leakage. DICC alone, even with CAOP measurement, cannot with certainty establish or rule out the diagnosis of venous leakage. When both DICC and pudendal arteriography were used in one study, 23% of men with normal noninvasive parameters and suspected venous leakage were found to have associated arterial obstructive lesions.[11] These relatively young men (average age, 48.8 years) had lesions involving the pudendal and penile arteries. Therefore, before microvascular operations for impotence, both DICC and pudendal arteriography are needed. In the patient with marginal arterial inflow, a venous interruption procedure is unlikely to yield satisfactory results.

Neurologic dysfunction is also important. Diabetic neuropathy can be the dominant factor contributing to impotence when the vascular system appears normal. It is difficult to sort out the exact importance of each factor in these cases, inasmuch as cavernosal smooth muscle dysfunction also contributes to impotence in diabetic patients. Impotence due to nerve damage as well as arterial compromise can follow prostatic, rectal, or aortic operations. Refined surgical techniques are available to avoid such effects in a significant proportion of cases. As further discussed, this complication is particularly relevant in aortic dissection.

Figure 77–3 shows the neural pathways involved in penile erection. Overall, 28% of impotent men screened neurologically exhibited one or more abnormalities in pudendal or tibial evoked potentials or bulbocavernosal reflex times.[24] Normally, mean bulbocavernosal reflex times range from 28.3 to 37.5 ms. The contribution of these abnormalities to erectile failure is difficult to assess, as many men exhibit coexisting vascular abnormalities. However, neurologic testing using pudendal evoked potentials and bulbocavernosal reflex times does yield reproducible values that can be used to assess nerve damage.[25, 49] These techniques measure somatic nerve reflexes. Abnormalities, when present, point to neurogenic deficits involving the genitourinary tract, rectum, and aortoiliac nerve plexuses and the central nervous system itself. Men with these abnormalities are

TABLE 77–1. FACTORS IN VASCULOGENIC IMPOTENCE

FACTOR	PROBABLE CAUSE
Cavernosal	
Arteriolar	Functional or anatomic; helicine vessel abnormalities; blood pressure medication
Fibrosis	Postpriapic; drug administration
Peyronie's disease	Deformity invading cavernosal smooth muscle; venous leakage through tunica albuginea
Refractory smooth muscle	Hormonal: prolactinemia, low testosterone level; blood pressure medication
	Metabolic: diabetes mellitus, uremia
Venous Leakage	
Acquired	Abnormal tunica albuginea; traumatic lesions
Congenital	Isolated leakage from corpus cavernosum into the spongiosum
Arterial	
Aortoiliac atherosclerosis	
Steal due to external iliac disease	
Occlusive disease of pudendal arteries	Atherosclerotic
Occlusive disease of penile arteries	Atherosclerotic; idiopathic proliferative
Atheroembolization	

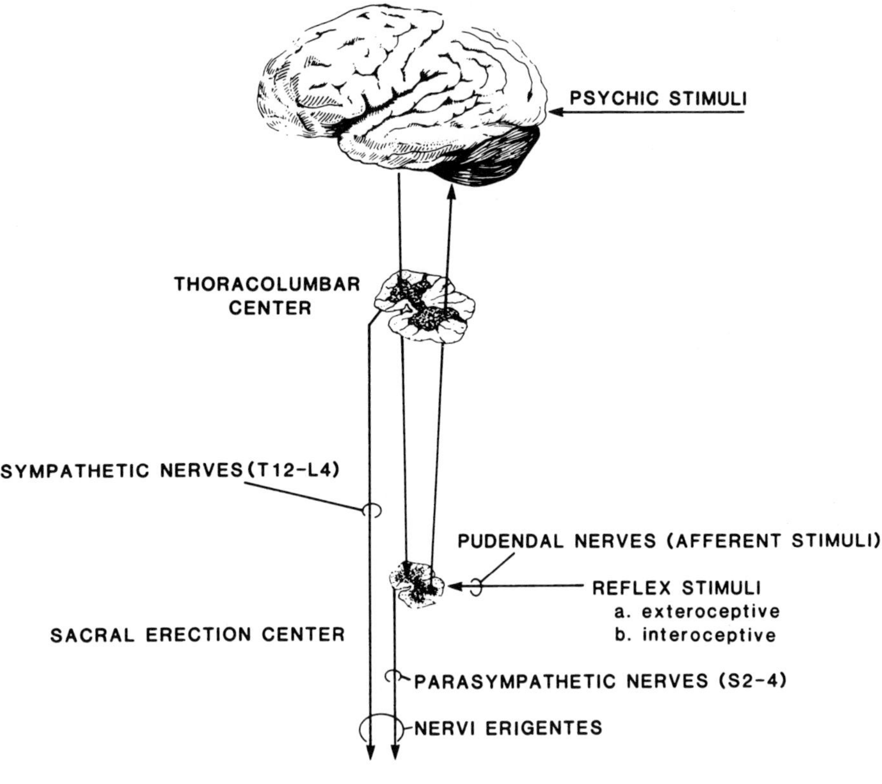

FIGURE 77–3. Diagrammatic representation of neural pathways involved in penile erection.

often exquisitely sensitive to the intracavernosal administration of vasoactive drugs. The detection of nerve conduction deficits is a warning to avoid initially high doses of these agents, which could cause priapism.

The reader can appreciate, from the discussion thus far, that multiple factors contribute to vasculogenic impotence. These factors, summarized in Table 77–1, determine the approaches to diagnosis and treatment.

APPROACH TO DIAGNOSIS

Various noninvasive and invasive alternatives are available to investigate cases of erectile dysfunction. There is as yet no universally accepted approach. One approach is limited and patient goal–directed, depending on the response of the condition to initial therapy.[41] If simple measures such as oral medications fail, more elaborate investigations are advised.[12, 18] Should the intracavernosal administration of vasoactive agents fail or vacuum constrictor devices prove ineffective, evaluation would then progress to invasive tests for delineation of abnormal physiology.

A diagnostic sequence based on noninvasive neurovascular screening can also be used before the office visit for a detailed history and physical examination.[12] Then, at the time of the office visit, depending on the initial findings and the patient's desires, erectile function can be assessed directly by intracavernosal administration of PGE. At the same time, blood specimens are obtained for measurements of prolactin, testosterone, glucose, and prostate-specific antigen. As noted, initial noninvasive neurovascular testing can help determine the diagnostic category of the impotence, that is, vasculogenic or neurogenic. Noninvasive vascular methods of testing are described later in this chapter, and the advantages and limitations of each are considered.[15]

Contributions in this area have been made by vascular surgeons as well as by urologists and radiologists; these are of practical and historical interest and can be adopted by most vascular laboratories. Canning and colleagues[10] noted in 1963 that vascular insufficiency of the pelvic vessels, even in the presence of normal femoral pulses, could cause impotence. They attempted to identify affected patients by palpating penile pulses and performing impedance plethysmography. Subsequently, other investigators assessed penile blood flow using mercury strain-gauge plethysmography, spectrographic or ultrasonic measurement of penile systolic pressure, and pulse volume recordings.[1, 6, 27, 34]

One of the authors (R.F.K.) studied 234 patients using the Doppler velocimeter to measure penile systolic pressure.[34] This value, in turn, was divided by brachial systolic pressure to obtain a penile-brachial index (PBI). Pulse volume waveforms (PVWs) of penile volume change with each systolic ejection were also recorded. The influence of both sexual function and patient age on each of these parameters was then determined. Age exerted a deleterious influence on all variables of penile blood flow independent of the status of sexual potency. Patients younger than 40 years had a mean PBI of 0.99, compared with a PBI of 0.74 for older patients with equal potency; this difference was

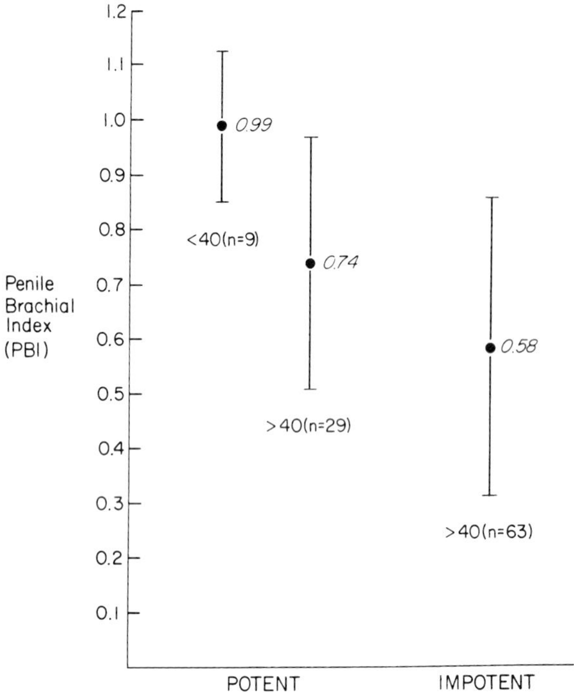

FIGURE 77–4. Distribution of penile-brachial index values (mean ± SD) in patients by age and sexual potency. (Data from Kempczinski RF: Role of the vascular diagnostic laboratory in the evaluation of male impotence. Am J Surg 138:278, 1979.)

statistically significant. In contrast, impotent patients older than 40 years of age had a mean PBI of 0.58, which was also a statistically significant difference (Fig. 77–4). The PVWs of patients younger than 40 years of age were of good to fair quality, and no poor-quality waveforms were observed. With increasing age and sexual dysfunction, a greater percentage of patients had poor-quality waveforms, but this difference was not statistically significant. Similar findings have been confirmed by other investigators, who have emphasized the utility of this type of testing in the initial evaluation of patients with erectile dysfunction.[44, 51]

DePalma and associates[12, 15] employ noninvasive vascular testing in the flaccid penile state by calculating the PBI; the penile pressure is detected with a Doppler probe placed distal to an inflated 2.5-cm cuff. The reappearance of Doppler signals in the dorsal artery branches just proximal to the glans signals reflow. This pressure is normally systemic. A PBI of 0.75 suggests that no major occlusion exists between the aorta and the distal measurement point. A PBI of less than 0.6 relates to major aortoiliac occlusion and almost always to erectile dysfunction. Penile pulse waves are then recorded at mean arterial pressure with the use of a pneumoplethysmographic cuff with a contained transducer. This procedure measures total pulsations of all penile arteries as the cuff compresses the penile tissue. Variables recorded are crest time, waveform, and the presence or absence of a dicrotic notch on a polygraph with a chart speed of 25 mm/sec and a sensitivity setting of 1. In normal men, the upstroke of the waveform is completed by 0.2 second (i.e., a 5-mm space at a chart speed of 25 mm/sec), and normal waveforms range from 5 to 30 mm in height.

Although these noninvasive vascular laboratory tests help define arteriogenic impotence, they do not detect impotence due to venous leak or other causes. In later studies, the sensitivity of these tests was shown to predict an abnormal arteriogram in 85% of cases.[21] Specificity—the percentage of true-negative test results—was 70%. The advantage of plethysmographic testing lies in the ability to define arteriogenic inflow problems before the office visit. These tests can be simply and inexpensively performed by a vascular technologist. One of the authors (R.G.D.) uses this convenient form of screening preoperatively and postoperatively and before progressing to treatment with drugs, intracavernosal injection, or intraurethral prostadil. In the patient with clear arterial compromise, higher initial dosages of vasoactive agents can be used, whereas in patients with normal noninvasive studies and probable neurogenic dysfunction, lower dosages are advisable.

The noninvasive data facilitate a focused history and goal-directed physical examination. A history of gradual onset of erectile failure in the absence of traumatic life events implies an organic cause. The complaint of claudication or the physical findings of aneurysmal or occlusive aortoiliac disease suggest a diagnosis of arteriogenic impotence, which is supported by abnormalities detected by noninvasive arterial testing.[12] A novel observation is that small aneurysms sometimes relate to an abrupt onset of impotence.[20] This event, due to atheroembolism, might be suspected from results of noninvasive studies, as illustrated in Figure 77–5.

The presence of risk factors for atherosclerosis, mainly smoking, hyperlipidemia, hypertension, and diabetes, suggests a diagnosis of arteriogenic impotence, as does a his-

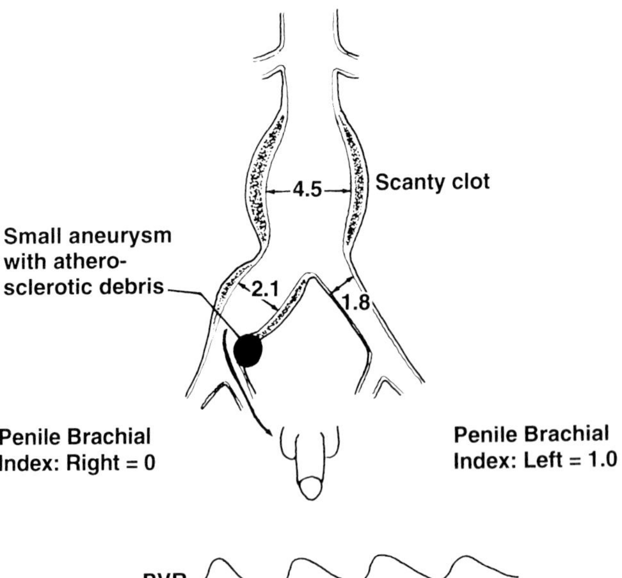

FIGURE 77–5. Aortoiliac aneurysm and associated penile pulse volume recordings and penile-brachial index values in a 60-year-old man with abrupt onset of impotence. Note penile-brachial index of "0" over right dorsal penile artery branches. Embolism is suggested from a small friable aneurysm at bifurcation of common iliac artery found at operation. Pulse volume recording (PVR) exhibited delayed upstroke and sine waves preoperatively and postoperatively. The patient was responsive to intracavernous injection postoperatively. (Modified from DePalma RG, Olding M, Yu GW, et al: Vascular interventions for impotence: Lessons learned. J Vasc Surg 21:76, 1995.)

tory of pelvic or perineal trauma. The onset of impotence immediately after pelvic or arterial surgical therapy is critical. Finally, the patient must be assessed for presence of diabetes and the use of any drugs or alcohol.

Physical examination is often unrevealing when small vessel arterial disease causes impotence. Leg pulse deficits or femoral bruits suggest macroarterial disease. Sensory testing of extremities, perineum, and the glans occasionally detects neuropathy, but neurologic laboratory testing is much more sensitive. After examination of the prostate and rectum, palpation of the corporal bodies for Peyronie's plaques and of the testes completes the examination. At this time, 10 to 30 μg of PGE is administered intracavernosally to observe the quality of erection achieved and to assess the response to therapy. The patient should remain in the office for at least an hour following this procedure to ensure subsidence of the erection.

Duplex scanning can be used at this point to scan the penile vessels after administration of the vasoactive agent.[38, 40] Control values for normal men have been estimated for this procedure. For example, in middle-aged men after the administration of PGE and visual sexual stimulation, a 70% increase in deep cavernosal arterial diameter and a systolic peak blood flow velocity in the range of 30 cm/sec have been described as normal. Duplex scanning is also believed to detect venous leakage with high diastolic flows, although for this issue, the data are less secure. Considerable interest exists in using duplex scanning as a preliminary to invasive procedures such as arteriography and DICC.

The approach used by one of the authors (R.G.D.) is to observe the quality of erection after increasing intracavernosal doses of the vasoactive agent; when erectile failure occurs or a Peyronie's plaque is found, duplex scanning is used to determine the extent of the plaque. Ultrasonography should also be used to scan for previously undetected abdominal aneurysms. Duplex scanning after the intracavernosal administration of a vasoactive agent, however, is more time-consuming than noninvasive vascular studies and requires a physician's presence before and after administration of the agent.

A study reported by Mansour[42] demonstrates the pitfalls in evaluating the veno-occlusive mechanism. Duplex scanning with the evaluation of end-diastolic flow showed 22% false-positive results. When abnormalities of veno-occlusions were detected with the use of end-diastolic flow, subsequent nocturnal penile tumescence (NPT) monitoring studies proved to be normal in eight of 37 men. The findings suggested anxiety in the clinical setting where duplex scanning was done.

NPT monitoring is not used routinely by the authors but is employed when psychogenic impotence is likely or, in cases of injury, with continuing medicolegal issues. It is performed optimally in a formal sleep laboratory with 3 nights of monitoring and the measurement of penile rigidity when erection occurs.[57] Normal penile rigidity or pressure is defined as 400 to 500 gm of axial buckling pressure. This test is both time-consuming and expensive, but it is important because the presence of a normal sleep erection virtually rules out organic erectile dysfunction. For screening purposes, a RigiScan home NPT monitor can also be employed; use of this device may help to establish the diagnosis by minimizing both the expense and the anxiety involved with measurements taken in the clinical setting.

TREATMENT CONSIDERATIONS

Figure 77–6 provides an algorithm for an approach to diagnosis and treatment. Initial treatment is medical. Most relevant for vascular surgeons are aortoiliac dissection techniques that perfuse the internal iliac arteries and spare autonomic nerves to minimize sexual dysfunction when aortic procedures are required.

Not only can iatrogenic impotence be avoided but potency can be restored in 58% of men with aortoiliac involvement. In a 1996 report on 10 years of experience with vascular interventions for impotence, men with the sole complaint of impotence underwent interventions for aortoiliac aneurysms or occlusive disease.[48] Of these patients, 58% experienced resumption of spontaneous penile function during follow-up periods ranging from 33 to 48 months; an additional 15% achieved functional erections with intracavernosally administered agents or with vacuum constrictor devices. These men with aortoiliac disease averaged 61 years of age. In contrast, during the same period, men selected for microvascular procedures for penile artery bypass, deep dorsal vein arterialization, and venous ligation had an average age of 42 to 47.3 years. This age difference was statistically significantly at a *P* value of .001 by analysis of variance. A significant difference between observed and expected frequencies of spontaneous erection was shown between the patients who underwent aortoiliac interventions and those who had penile arterial or venous procedures. At 33 to 48 months after operation, only 27% to 33% of these men undergoing penile arterial or venous procedures reported spontaneous erections. When intracavernosal administration of PGE or vacuum constrictor devices were added to the postoperative treatment, however, 72% to 77% reported functional erections that they previously had been unable to attain.

It is critical that the vascular surgeon understand and avoid causing iatrogenic impotence. Prior to aortoiliac surgery in each patient, careful inquiries should be made as to the importance and frequency of sexual function. Although modern techniques offer greatly improved function, some patients become dysfunctional postoperatively. Such patients in particular are those who experienced atheroembolization, emergency procedures, and internal iliac aneurysms.

DePalma and colleagues[19, 22] have used a nerve-sparing procedure for exposure of the infrarenal aorta that emphasizes the following:

- Approach to the abdominal aorta along its right lateral aspect
- Minimal division of longitudinal periaortic tissues to the left of the infrarenal aorta
- Avoidance of dissection at the base of the inferior mesenteric artery
- Sparing of the nerve plexuses that cross the left common iliac artery

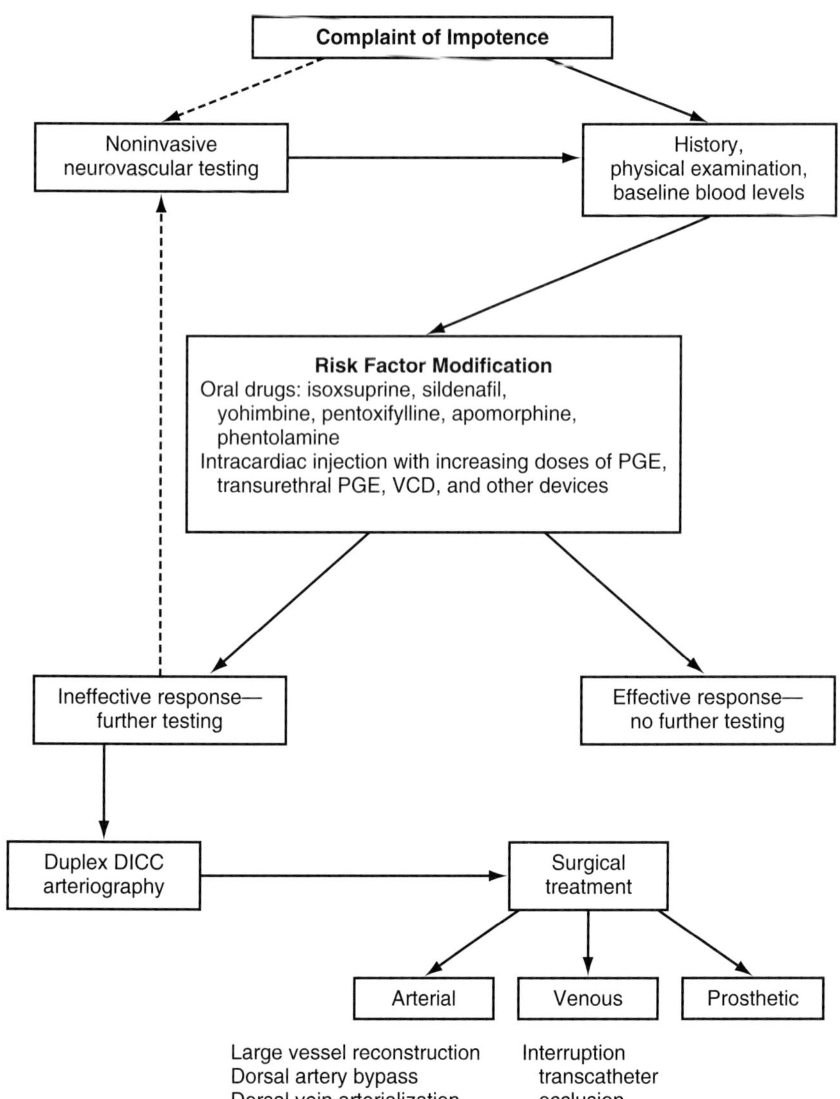

FIGURE 77–6. Algorithm showing sequences of testing and treatment for the complaint of impotence. *Dashed* lines indicate optional steps. Surgical treatment *(bottom right)* is used for only a minority of patients. DICC = dynamic infusion cavernosometry and cavernosography; PGE = prostaglandin E; VCD = vacuum constrictor device. (From DePalma RG: Vascular surgery for impotence: A review. Int J Impot Res 9:61, 1997.)

Using this approach, several other groups have achieved a notable reduction in postoperative impotence in their patients.[26, 46, 53, 58]

Although the findings on conventional angiograms correlate poorly with erectile function, preservation of adequate perfusion into at least one hypogastric artery is a vital component of operations successful in minimizing iatrogenic erectile dysfunction. When possible, direct antegrade perfusion of at least one internal iliac artery should be ensured. This may require thromboendarterectomy of the hypogastric artery orifice, when possible. If both external iliac arteries are occluded or stenotic, and bypass into the common femoral arteries is anticipated, proximal aortic anastomoses should be performed in an end-to-side fashion because retrograde perfusion of the internal iliac artery is compromised in such circumstances and significant reduction of pelvic blood flow occurs.

When proximal disease is so extensive that thromboendarterectomy is impractical and preoperative noninvasive testing has confirmed decreased penile perfusion, aortofemoral grafting might not restore pelvic collateral blood flow enough to relieve vasculogenic impotence. Age and duration of erectile dysfunction also appear to be factors in relief of preoperative impotence. Older patients are less likely to experience resumed function. Preoperative recognition of such cases is not easy, but when preservation of function seems likely, the surgeon can consider reimplanting the hypogastric artery into one limb of the aortofemoral graft or adding a jump graft into the distal hypogastric artery.

In men with unilateral iliac artery occlusive disease, the objectives of nerve sparing, extremity revascularization, and increased hypogastric artery perfusion can also be accomplished with the use of femorofemoral bypass. Several investigators have confirmed the success of this procedure in improving penile blood flow and restoring erectile capability.[44, 53] Femorofemoral bypass is especially useful for young, sexually active males with unilateral disease because it avoids aortic dissection. The use of angioplasty, stents, or both is effective in unilateral disease of the common iliac artery; such procedures are not effective in the internal iliac artery, however, owing to the branched nature of this vessel.[20] Angioplasty, placement of stents, or both in the external iliac artery can also improve function by relieving steal from the internal pudendal–internal iliac artery axis via the superior gluteal artery.

During reconstruction, the surgeon must avoid flushing atheromatous debris into the internal iliac artery. Operative technique should be modified to allow adequate back-bleeding in the internal iliac arteries prior to completion of anastomoses. Unfortunately, emergent aortic surgery, such as the resection of a ruptured abdominal aortic aneurysm, rarely allows time for the careful dissection necessary to avoid nerve damage, and the incidence of iatrogenic impotence is accordingly higher in this situation.

In assessing vascular intervention for treatment of impotence, it is important to define subsets of anatomic patterns of vascular involvement.[23] Hatzichristou and Goldstein[33] have described angiographic patterns for use in procedure selection; their report focuses on planning of microvascular procedures for penile revascularization on the basis of localized disease. The following broader subsets of anatomic patterns can be considered:

- Aortoiliac macrovascular disease
- Pudendal and penile artery segmental obstruction
- Diffuse obliterative penile artery disease
- Cavernosal leakage, congenital or acquired

On the basis of data obtained by meta-analysis, Montague and associates[48] concluded that the results of venous and arterial surgery, predominantly microvascular, did not appear to justify its routine use for treatment of erectile failure. DePalma[23] has reviewed the controversies surrounding vascular and microvascular interventions for impotence. No life-table data on potency have been published in the urologic literature, as are usually shown in reports of graft patency and limb salvage in the vascular literature.

Although most patients show a satisfactory response to medical therapy,[20, 28, 31, 32] a subset of men, approximately 6% to 7% of those complaining of impotence, show no response to medical treatment, intracavernosal injection, or vacuum devices.[48] These men become candidates for either revascularization or prosthetic implantation. Inasmuch as prosthetic implantation precludes a physiologic erection, some might choose revascularization as a first step. The future applicability of microvascular procedures such as dorsal penile artery bypass, deep dorsal vein arterialization, and venous interruption requires scrutiny and long-term follow-up; evaluation based on selected patient cohorts with comparable anatomic and physiologic bases for vasculogenic impotence is needed. Younger patients with pelvic trauma are probably the best candidates for these procedures, but they are not the only candidates. An important exception resides in the challenging group of men with aortoiliac disease, particularly those with aneurysms and localized pelvic artery occlusive disease.

REFERENCES

1. Abelson D: Diagnostic value of the penile pulse and blood pressure: A Doppler study of impotence in diabetics. J Urol 113:636, 1975.
2. Adaikan PG: Physiopharmacological basis of treatment for erectile dysfunction (Abstract). Int J Impot Res 6(Suppl I):PL1, 1994.
3. Azadzoi KM, Nehra A, Siroky MB: Effects of cavernosal hypoxia and oxygenation on penile erection (Abstract). Int J Impot Res (Suppl I):D4, 1994.
4. Beavo, JA: Cyclic nucleotide phosphodiesterases: Functional implication of multiple isoforms. Physiol Rev 75:725, 1995.
5. Boolell M, Allen MS, Ballard SA, et al: Sildenafil: An orally active type 5 cyclic GMP-specific phosphodiesterase inhibitor for the treatment of penile erectile dysfunction. Int J Impot Res 8:47, 1996.
6. Brindley GS: Pilot experiments on the actions of drugs injected into the human corpus cavernosum penis. Br J Pharmacol 87:495, 1986.
7. Britt DB, Kemmerer WT, Robison JR: Penile blood flow determination by mercury strain gauge plethysmography. Invest Urol 8:673, 1971.
8. Brock GB, Zvara P, Sioufi R, et al: Nitric oxide synthase is testosterone dependent (Abstract). Int J Impot Res 6(Suppl I):D42, 1994.
9. Burnett AL: Role of nitric oxide in the physiology of erection. Biol Reprod 52:485, 1995.
10. Canning JR, Bowers LM, Lloyd FA, et al: Genital vascular insufficiency and impotence. Surg Forum 14:298, 1963.
11. DePalma RG, Dalton CM, Gomez CA, et al: Predictive value of a screening sequence for vasculogenic impotence. Int J Impot Res 4:143, 1992.
12. DePalma RG, Emsellem HA, Edwards CM, et al: A screening sequence for vasculogenic impotence. J Vasc Surg 5:228, 1987.
13. DePalma RG, Kedia K, Persky L: Vascular operations for preservation of sexual function. *In* Bergan JJ, Yao JST (eds): Surgery of the Aorta and Its Body Branches. New York, Grune & Stratton, 1979, pp 227–236.
14. DePalma RG, Kedia K, Persky L: Surgical operations in the correction of vasculogenic impotence. Vasc Surg 14:992, 1980.
15. DePalma RG, Michal V: Point of view: Déjà vu—again: Advantages and limitations of methods for assessing penile arterial flow. Urology 36:199, 1990.
16. DePalma RG: Anatomy and physiology of normal erection: Pathogenesis of impotence. *In* Sidawy AN, Sumpio RE, DePalma RG (eds): The Basic Science of Vascular Disease. Armonk, NY, Futura Publishing, 1997, pp 761–773.
17. DePalma RG: New developments in the diagnosis and treatment of impotence. West J Med 164:54, 1996.
18. DePalma RG: What constitutes an adequate impotence workup? World J Urol 10:157, 1992.
19. DePalma RG, Levine SB, Feldman S: Preservation of erectile function after aortoiliac reconstruction. Arch Surg 113:958, 1978.
20. DePalma RG, Olding M, Yu GW, et al: Vascular interventions for impotence: Lessons learned. J Vasc Surg 21:76, 1995.
21. DePalma RG, Schwab FJ, Emsellem HA, et al: Noninvasive assessment of impotence. Surg Clin North Am 70:119, 1990.
22. DePalma RG: Impotence in vascular disease: Relationship to vascular surgery. Br J Surg 69:514, 1982.
23. DePalma RG: Vascular surgery for impotence: A review. Int J Impot Res 9:61, 1997.
24. Emsellem HA, Bergsrund DW, DePalma RG, Edwards CM: Pudendal evoked potentials in the evaluation of impotence. J Clin Neurophysiol 5:359, 1998.
25. Fisher-Santos BL, DeDues Viera AL, dos Santos ES: Bulbocavernosus reflex and evoked potentials in evidently normal males. Int J Impot Res 4:A12, 1994.
26. Flanigan DP, Schuler JJ, Keifer T, et al: Elimination of iatrogenic impotence and improvement of sexual function after aortoiliac revascularization. Arch Surg 117:544, 1982.
27. Gaskell P: The importance of penile blood pressure in cases of impotence. Can Med Assoc J 105:1047, 1971.
28. Gingell C, Ballard SA, Tang K, et al: Cyclic nucleotide phosphodiesterase and erectile function. Int J Impot Res 9(Suppl I):510, 1997.
29. Glina S, Reichelt AS, Leao PP, Dos Reis JM: Impact of cigarette smoking on papaverine-induced erection. J Urol 140:523, 1988.
30. Goldstein I: Vasculogenic impotence: Its diagnosis and treatment. *In* de Vere White J (ed): Problems in Urology: Sexual Dysfunction. Philadelphia, JB Lippincott, 1987, pp 547–563.
31. Gopalakrishnakone P, Adaikan PG, Ponraj G, Ratnam SS: NADPH-diaphorase and VIP positive nerve fibres in human penile erectile tissue (Abstract). Int J Impot Res 6(Suppl I):A26, 1994.
32. Harris, JD, Jepson RP: Aorto-iliac stenosis: A comparison of two procedures. Aust N Z J Surg 34:211, 1965.
33. Hatzichristou D, Goldstein I: Penile microvascular arterial bypass. Surg Annu 2:208, 1993.
34. Kempczinski RF: Role of the vascular diagnostic laboratory in the evaluation of male impotence. Am J Surg 138:278, 1979.
35. Keogh ET, Earle CM, Chew KK, et al: Medical management of impotence (Abstract). Int J Impot Res 6(Supp I):S13, 1994.

36. Leriche R, Morel A: The syndrome of thrombotic obliteration of the aortic bifurcation. Ann Surg 127:193, 1948.
37. Leriche R: Des oblitérations artériele hautes (oblitération de la términation de l'aorte) comme cause de insuffisances circulatoires des membres inférieurs (Abstract). Bull Mem Soc Chir 49:1404, 1923.
38. Lewis RW, King BF: Dynamic color Doppler sonography in the evaluation of penile erectile disorders. Int J Impot Res 7(Suppl I):A30, 1994.
39. Lue TF: Oral medication for erectile dysfunction. Int J Impot Res 9:511, 1997.
40. Lue TF, Hricak H, Marich RW, Tanago EA: Vasculogenic impotence evaluated by high resolution ultrasonography and published Doppler spectrum analysis. Radiology 155:777, 1985.
41. Lue TF: Impotence: A patient's goal-directed approach to treatment. World J Urol 8:67,1990.
42. Mansour MOA: Anxiety mediated impotence mis-diagnosis as venogenic impotence by color duplex scanning: A comparison with nocturnal tumescence monitoring. Int J Impot Res 6(Suppl I):A30, 1994.
43. May AG, DeWeese JA, Rob CG: Changes in sexual function following operation on the abdominal aorta. Surgery 65:41, 1969.
44. Merchant RF Jr, DePalma RG: Effects of femorofemoral grafts on postoperative sexual function: Correlation with penile pulse volume recordings. Surgery 90:962, 1981.
45. Michal V, Kramar L, Pospichal F, Hejel L: Gefasschirurgia erektiver Impotenz. Sex Med Sondertr 5:15, 1976.
46. Miles JR, Miles DG, Johnson G: Aortoiliac operations and sexual dysfunction. Arch Surg 117:1177, 1982.
47. Modell JG, Katholi CR, Modell JD, DePalma RL: Comparative sexual side effects of bupropion, fluoxetine, paroxetine and sertraline. Clin Pharmacol Ther 61:476, 1997.
48. Montague DK, Barada FH, Belker AM, et al: Clinical Guidelines Panel on Erectile Dysfunction: Summary report on the treatment of organic erectile dysfunction. J Urol 156:2007, 1996.
49. Opsomer RJ, Guerit JM, Wese FX, Van Congh DJ: Pudendal cortical somatosensory evoked potentials. J Urol 135:1216, 1986.
50. Padma-Nathan H, Hellstrom-Wayne JG, Kaiser FE, et al: Treatment of men with erectile dysfunction with transurethral alprostadil. N Engl J Med 336:1, 1997.
51. Queral LA, Whitehouse WM, Flinn WR, et al: Pelvic hemodynamics after aortoiliac reconstruction. Surgery 86:799, 1979.
52. Rajfer J, Aronson WJ, Bush PA, et al: Nitric oxide as a mediator of relaxation of the corpus cavernosum in response to nonadrenergic neurotransmission. N Engl J Med 326:90, 1992.
53. Schuler JJ, Gray B, Flanigan DP, et al: Increased penile perfusion and reversal of vasculogenic impotence following femorofemoral bypass. Br J Surg 69:S7, 1982.
54. Udelson, D, Hatzichristou DG, Saenz de Tejada I, et al: A new methodology of pharmacocavernosometry which enables hemodynamic analysis under conditions of known corporal smooth muscle relaxation (Abstract). Int J Impot Res 6(Suppl I):A17, 1994.
55. Virag R: Intracavernous injection of papaverine for erectile failure (Letter). Lancet 2:938, 1982.
56. Waldhauser M, Schramek P: Efficiency and side effects of prostaglandin E_1 in the treatment of erectile dysfunction. J Urol 140:525, 1988.
57. Ware JC, Kryger MH, Roth T, Dement WC (eds): Principles and Practice of Sleep Medicine. Philadelphia, WB Saunders, 1989, pp 689–695.
58. Weinstein MH, Machleder HI: Sexual function after aorto-iliac surgery. Ann Surg 181:787, 1975.

INDEX

Note: Page numbers in *italics* refer to illustrations; page numbers followed by t refer to tables.

E

G

H

J

K

L

M

N

O

Q

R

S

T

W

Y

Z